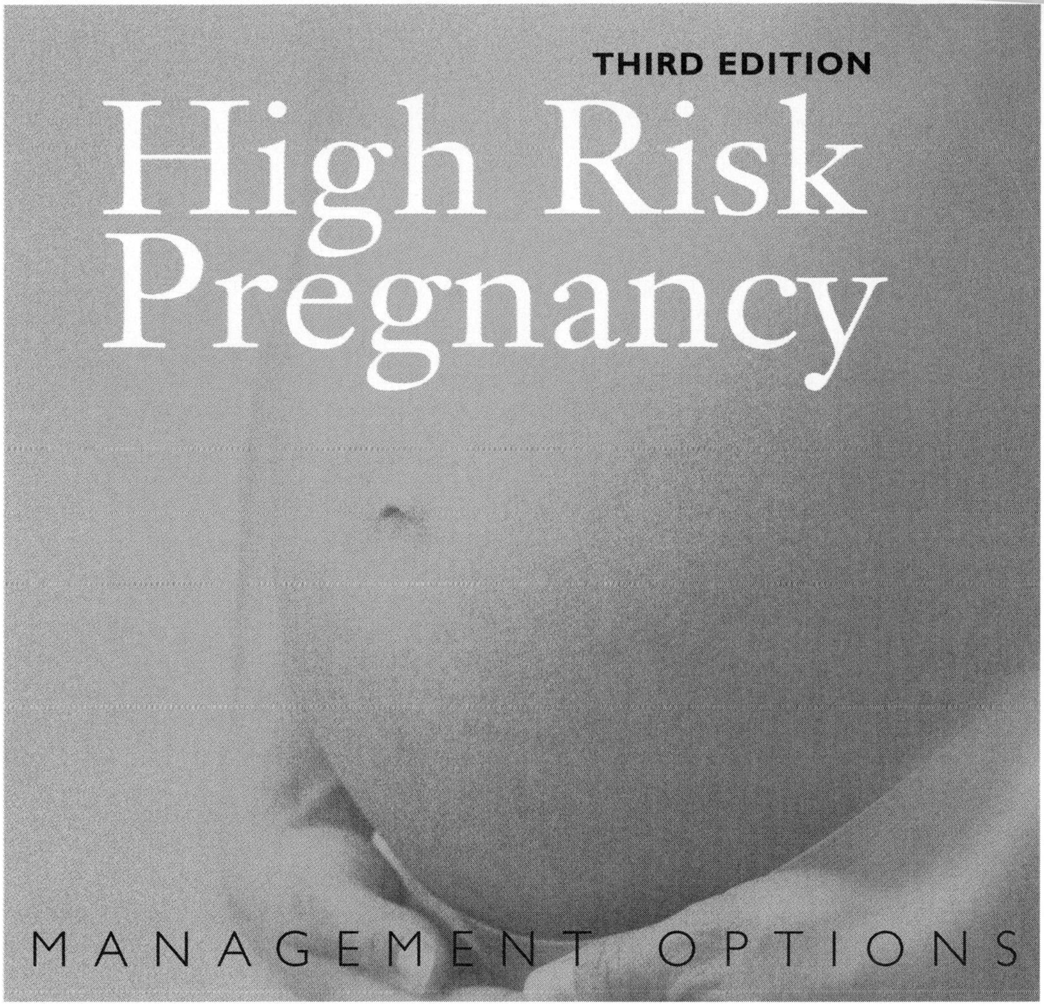

David K. James
MA, MD, FRCOG, DCH
Professor of Fetomaternal Medicine
Director of Medical Education
Queen's Medical Centre
Nottingham
UK

Carl P. Weiner
MD, MBA, FACOG
Professor
Department of Obstetrics, Gynecology,
and Reproductive Sciences
Professor
Department of Physiology
University of Maryland School of Medicine
Baltimore, Maryland

Philip J. Steer
BSc, MD, FRCOG, FCOGSA (hon)
Professor
Faculty of Medicine
Imperial College London
Chelsea and Westminster Hospital
London
UK

Bernard Gonik
MD, FACOG
Professor and Fann Srere
Chair of Perinatal Medicine
Department of Obstetrics and Gynecology
Wayne State University
School of Medicine
Detroit, Michigan

SAUNDERS
ELSEVIER

ELSEVIER
SAUNDERS

1600 John F. Kennedy Blvd.
Ste. 1800
Philadelphia, Pennsylvania 19103-2899

HIGH RISK PREGNANCY: MANAGEMENT OPTIONS, 3/E ISBN 0-7216-0132-4

NOTICE

Knowledge and best practice in this field are constantly changing. As new research and experience broaden our knowledge, changes in practice, treatment and drug therapy may become necessary or appropriate. Readers are advised to check the most current information provided (i) on procedures featured or (ii) by the manufacturer of each product to be administered, to verify the recommended dose or formula, the method and duration of administration, and contraindications. It is the responsibility of the practitioner, relying on their own experience and knowledge of the patient, to make diagnoses, to determine dosages and the best treatment for each individual patient, and to take all appropriate safety precautions. To the fullest extent of the law, neither the Publisher nor the Editors assumes any liability for any injury and/or damage to persons or property arising out of or related to any use of the material contained in this book.

Previous editions copyrighted 1999, 1994

Library of Congress Cataloging-in-Publication Data

High risk pregnancy : management options / David K. James ... [et al.]–3rd ed.
p. cm.
ISBN 0-7216-0132-4
1. Pregnancy–Complications. I. James, D. K. (David K.)

RG571.H46 2005
681.3–dc22

2005046458

Printed in the United States of America

Last digit is the print number: 9 8 7 6 5 4 3 2 1

CONTRIBUTORS

Oqba A. Al-Kuran, MD
Consultant
Maternal Fetal Medicine
Queen's Medical Centre
Nottingham
UK

Anthony Ambrose, MD
Associate Professor
Pennsylvania State University College of Medicine
Hershey, PA
USA

Christine Ang, MBChB, DFFP, ALSO, MD, MRCOG
University of Leicester
Leicester
UK

Marie-Cécile Aubry, MD
Associate
Université Paris V;
Consultant
Hôpital Necker Enfants Malades
Paris
France

John Anthony, MB, ChB, FCOG (SA)
Professor
Obstetrics and Gynaecology
University of Cape Town;
Groote Schuur Hospital
Capetown
South Africa

Vincent T. Armenti, MD, PhD
Professor of Surgery
Abdominal Organ Transplant Program
Temple University School of Medicine
Philadelphia, PA
USA

Robert D. Auerbach, MD
Yale University School of Medicine
New Haven, CT
USA

Loraine Bacchus, BSc, MA, PhD
Research Associate
Kings College London
School of Nursing and Midwifery
London
UK

May Backos, MBChB, MRCOG
Obstetrics and Gynaecology
West Middlesex University Hospital
Isleworth, Middlesex
UK

Philip Baker, BMedSci, BM, BS, MRCOG, DM
Professor
Academic Unit Obstetrics & Gynecology
and Reproductive Health Care
St. Mary's Hospital
Manchester
UK

Ahmet Alexander Baschat, MB, BCh, MD
Assistant Professor
University of Maryland Medical School;
Attending Physician
University of Maryland Medical Center
Baltimore, MD
USA

Susan Bewley, MBBS, MA, FRCOG
Consultant Obstetrician
Maternal-Fetal Medicine
Guy's and St. Thomas' NHS Foundation Trust;
London
UK

Joseph R. Biggio, Jr., MD
Assistant Professor
Department of Obstetrics and Gynecology and Department of Genetics
University of Alabama at Birmingham
Birmingham, AL
USA

Ralph B. Blasier, MD
Professor and Associate Chairman for Orthopedic Research and Education
Orthopedic Surgery
Wayne State University;
Orthopedic Surgery
Sinai-Grace Hospital
Detroit, Michigan
USA

Renee A. Bobrowski, MD
Assistant Professor
Department of Obstetrics and Gynecology
University of Connecticut
Farmington, CT;
Attending Physician
Hartford Hospital
Hartford, CT
USA

D. Ware Branch, MD
Professor
Department of Obstetrics-Gynecology
University of Utah School of Medicine
Salt Lake City, UT
USA

Anneke Brand
Immunohematology and Blood Transfusion Service
Leiden University Medical Center
Leiden
The Netherlands

David Cahill, MD, MRCPI, FRCOG
Consultant Senior Lecturer in Reproductive Medicine
University of Bristol;
Consultant Gynecologist
St. Michael's Hospital
Bristol
UK

Alessandra Capponi
Department of Obstetrics and Gynecology
Università Roma Tor Vergata Ospedale Fatebenefreatelli Isola Tiberina
Rome
Italy

J. Ricardo Carhuapoma, MD
Assistant Professor
Departments of Neurology, Neurological Surgery, and Anesthesiology/Critical Care Medicine
Johns Hopkins University School of Medicine
Baltimore, MD
USA

Tinnakorn Chaiworaponga, MD
Department of Obstetrics and Gynecology
Wayne State University
Detroit, MI
USA

Allan Chang, BS, PhD, FRCOG
Professor
University of Queensland;
Director
Mater Research Support Centre
Mater Health Services
South Brisbane
Australia

Frank A. Chervenak, MD
Professor and Chairman
Department of Obstetrics and Gynecology
Weill Medical College of Cornell University;
Obstetrician and Gynecologist-in-Chief
Weill Cornell Medical Center
New York, NY
USA

Lisa M. Cohen, MD
Clinical Assistant Professor
Department of Dermatology
Tufts University School of Medicine
Boston, MA;
Director
Cohen Dermatopathology
Newton, MA
USA

Joshua A. Copel, MD
Professor and Vice Chair
Obstetrics, Gynecology, and Reproductive Sciences
Yale University School of Medicine;
Attending
Obstetrics and Gynecology
Yale-New Haven Hospital
New Haven, CT
USA

Marc Coppens, MD
Consultant Gynaecologist–Obstetrician
Department of Obstetrics, Gynaecology, and Fertility
AZ Middelheim Hospital
Antwerpen
Belgium

Caroline A. Crowther, MBChB, MD, RCOG, Cert. MFM, FRANZCOG
Department of Obstetrics and Gynaecology
The University of Adelaide
Adelaide, South Australia
Australia

Peter Danielian, MA, MD, FRCOG
Honorary Senior Lecturer
Department of Obstetrics & Gynecology
Aberdeen University Medical School;
Consultant Obstetrician
Department of Obstetrics, Neonatology, and Gynecology
Aberdeen Maternity Hospital
Aberdeen, Scotland
UK

John M. Davies, MA, MD, FRCP, FRCPath
Honorary Senior Lecturer
University of Edinburgh;
Consultant Haematologist
Western General Hospital
Edinburgh, Scotland
UK

John M. Davison, MD
Professor of Obstetrics and Gynaecology
School of Surgical and Reproductive Sciences
University of Newcastle
Newcastle upon Tyne
UK

Isaac Delke, MD
Associate Professor
Obstetrics and Gynecology
University of Florida Health Science Center
Jacksonville, FL
USA

Philip Dennen, MD
Assistant Clinical Professor
Department of Obstetrics and Gynecology
Yale University School of Medicine
New Haven, CT
USA

Jan Deprest, MD, PhD
Consultant
Obstetrics and Gynecology
University Hospitals Leuven
Leuven
Belgium

Jodie M. Dodd, MBBS, FRANZCOG, Cert. MFM
Department of Obstetrics and Gynaecology
The University of Adelaide
Adelaide, South Australia
Australia

Jan E. Dickinson, MD
Associate Professor
Maternal-Fetal Medicine
School of Women's and Infants' Health
The University of Western Australia;
Maternal-Fetal Medicine Specialist
King Edward Memorial Hospital for Women
Perth, Western Australia
Australia

Marc Dommergues, MD
Professor
Service de Gynécologie Obstétrique
Groupe Hospitalier Pitié Salpétiêre
Paris
France

J. M. Ernest, MD
Professor
Department of Obstetrics and Gynecology
Wake Forest University School of Medicine
Winston-Salem, NC
USA

Peter A. Farndon, MSc, MD, FRCP, DCH
Professor of Clinical Genetics
University of Birmingham;
Consultant Clinical Geneticist
West Midlands Regional Clinical Genetics Service
Birmingham Women's Hospital
Birmingham
UK

Roy G. Farquharson, MD, FRCOG
Clinical Director
Obstetrics and Gynecology
Liverpool Women's Hospital
Liverpool
UK

Nicholas M. Fisk, PhD, FRCOG
Professor
Institute of Reproductive and Developmental Biology
Imperial College London;
Consultant
Centre for Fetal Care
Queen Charlotte's Hospital
London
UK

Breton C. Freitag, BS, MD
Clinical Instructor;
Fellow in Neonatal-Perinatal Medicine
Oregon Health and Science University
Portland, OR
USA

Harry Gee, MD
Medical Director
Birmingham Women's Health Care NHS Trust
Birmingham Maternity Hospital
Birmingham
UK

Reynir Tómas Geirsson, MD, PhD, FRCOG
Professor of Faculty of Medicine
Obstetrics and Gynecology
University of Iceland;
Chairman
Department of Obstetrics and Gynecology
Women's Clinic
Landspitali University Hospital
Reykjavík
Iceland

Robert Gherman, MD
Chairman
Department of Obstetrics and Gynecology
Washington Adventist Hospital
Takoma Park, MD
USA

Joanna Girling, MA, MBBS, MRCP, MRCOG
Honorary Senior Lecturer
Imperial College School of Medicine
London;
Consultant Obstetrician and Gynaecologist
West Middlesex University Hospital
Isleworth
UK

Luis F. Gonçalves, MD
Department of Obstetrics and Gynaecology
Wayne State University
Detroit, MI
USA

John M. Grant, MBChB, MRCP, MRCOG, FRCS (Glas)
Consultant Obstetrician and Gynaecologist
Wishaw General Hospital
Wishaw, Lanarkshire
Scotland

Michael G. Gravett, MD
Professor
Department of Obstetrics and Gynecology;
Chief
Division of Maternal–Fetal Medicine
Oregon Health and Science University
Portland, OR;
Senior Scientist
Division of Reproductive Sciences
Oregon National Primate Research Center
Beaverton, OR
USA

Michael Greaves, MBChB, MD, FRCPath, FRCP (Lon), (Edin), (Glas)
Head of School of Medicine
University of Aberdeen;
Honorary Consultant
Haematology
Aberdeen Royal Infirmary
Aberdeen, Scotland
UK

Clare Gribbin, BMedSci, BMBS, MRCOG, MI Psych Med
Specialist Registrar
Obstetrics and Gynaecology
Queen's Medical Centre
Nottingham
UK

David Griffin, MD, FRCOG
Consultant Obstetrician and Gynaecologist
West Herts Hospital HMS Trust
Waterford, Hertferdshire
UK

Mordechai Hallak, MD, MPA
Professor
Ben Gurion University,
Head of Feto-Maternal Medicine Unit
Soroka Medical Center
Beer Sheva
Israel

Roger F. Haskett, MD
Professor of Psychiatry
Department of Psychiatry
University of Pittsburgh;
Medical Director, Adult Services
Western Psychiatric Institute and Clinic
UPMC Presbyterian Shadyside;
Chief
Department of Psychiatry
Magee-Women's Hospital
Pittsburgh, PA
USA

Robert H. Hayashi, MD
J. Robert Willson Professor of Obstetrics
Director of Maternal-Fetal Medicine Fellowship
University of Michigan School of Medicine
Ann Arbor, MI
USA

Elizabeth Helen Horn, MD, FRCP, MRCPath
Consultant Haematologist
Department of Haematology
Royal Infirmary of Edinburgh
Edinburgh, Scotland
UK

David Howe, MD, MRCOG
University of Glasgow
Glasgow
Scotland

Alyson Hunter MD, MRCOG
Senior Lecturer
Department of Obstetrics and Gynaecology
Queen's University of Belfast;
Consultant in Fetal and Maternal Medicine
Royal Jubilee Maternity Hospital
Belfast
Northern Ireland

Jonathon Hyett, MD, MBBS, MRCOG
Harris Birthright Research Centre for Fetal Medicine
King's College Hospital
London
UK

David K. James, MA, MD, FRCOG, DCH
Professor of Fetomaternal Medicine
Director of Medical Education
Queen's Medical Centre
Nottingham
UK

Robin B. Kalish, MD
Assistant Professor
Weill Medical College of Cornell University;
Assistant Professor
New York Presbyterian Hospital
New York, NY
USA

Humphrey H. H. Kanhai, MD, PhD
Professor, Obstetrics
University Medical Center;
Head of Department of Obstetrics in Fetal Medicine and Leiden University Medical Center
Leiden
The Netherlands

Lucy H. Kean, MA, DM, MRCOG
Consultant in Fetal and Maternal Medicine
Department of Obstetrics
City Hospital
Nottingham
UK

Rohna Kearney, MB, MRCPI, MRCOG
National Maternity Hospital
Dublin
Ireland

Anna P. Kenyon, MBChB, MD
Department of Obstetrics
Maternal and Fetal Research Unit
Guys King's and St. Thomas' School of Medicine
London
UK

Lauren Kerzin-Storrar, BA, MS
Lecturer (honorary) MSC Programme Director
University of Manchester;
Consultant Genetic Counsellor
Regional Genetic Service and Academic Unit of Medical Genetics
Manchester
UK

Mark D. Kilby, MBBS (Lond.), MD, MRCOG
Professor of Fetal Medicine
Department of Obstetrics and Gynaecology
Birmingham Women's Hospital
Birmingham
UK

Justin C. Konje, MBBS, FMCOG, MRCOG
Professor
University of Leicester;
Consultant Obstetrician and Gynaecologist
Leicester Royal Infirmary
Leicester
UK

George Kroumpouzos, MD, PhD
Associate Faculty
Department of Internal Medicine
South Shore Hospital
South Weymouth, MA;
Courtesy Faculty
Division of Dermatology
Department of Medical Specialties
St. Vincent Hospital at Worcester Medical Center
Worcester, MA;
Staff Dermatologist
South Shore Medical Center
Norwell, MA
USA

Mark B. Landon, MD
Professor and Vice Chair
Director
Division of Maternal-Fetal Medicine, Obstetrics, and Gynecology
Ohio State University
College of Medicine and Public Health
Columbus, OH
USA

Steven R. Levine, MD
Professor of Neurology
Neurology and Stroke Program
The Mount Sinai School of Medicine;
Director, Cerebrovascular Education
Neurology and Stroke Program
The Mount Sinai Hospital
New York, NY
USA

Liesbeth Lewi, MD
Consultant
Obstetrics and Gynecology
University Hospitals Leuven
Leuven
Belgium

Bertis B. Little, PhD
Tarleton State University
Stephenville, TX
USA

Charles J. Lockwood, MD
The Anita O'Keefe Young Professor
Department of Obstetrics, Gynecology and Reproductive Sciences
Yale University School of Medicine;
Chief
Obstetrics and Gynecology
Yale-New Haven Hospital
New Haven, CT
USA

Mary Ann Lumsden, MB, MD, FRCOG, MRCOG
Department of Obstetrics and Gynaecology
University of Glasgow
Glasgow Royal Infirmary
Glasgow
Scotland

I. Z. MacKenzie, MA, MD, FRCOG, DSc
Reader in Obstetrics and Gynaecology
Nuffield Department of Obstetrics and Gynaecology
University of Oxford;
Honorary Consultant in Obstetrics and Gynaecology
John Radcliffe Hospital
Oxford
UK

Kassam Mahomed, MBChB, MD, FRCOG, FRANZCOG
Associate Professor
Department of Obstetrics–Gynecology
University of Queensland;
Director
Department of Obstetrics and Gynecology
Toowoomba Hospital
Toowoomba
Australia

Michael Maresh, BSc, MD, FRCOG
Honorary Senior Lecturer
Department of Obstetrics and Gynaecology
University of Manchester;
Consultant Obstetrician
St. Mary's Hospital for Women and Children
Manchester
UK

Neil Marlow, DM, FRCPCH
Professor of Neonatal Medicine
University of Nottingham
Queen's Medical Centre
Nottingham
UK

Michael J. Mendelow, MD
Assistant Professor
Orthopedic Surgery
Wayne State University;
Orthopedic Surgery (Pediatric Orthopedic and Scoliosis Surgery)
Children's Hospital of Michigan
Detroit, Michigan
USA

Michael J. Moritz, MD
Professor of Surgery
Director of Abdominal Transplantation
Drexel University College of Medicine
Philadelphia, PA
USA

Robert T. Morris, MD
Associate Professor
Obstetrics and Gynecology
Wayne State University School of Medicine;
Gynecologic Oncology
Barbara Ann Karmanos Cancer Institute;
Director
Gynecologic Oncology
St. John Medical Center
Detroit, MI
USA

Adnan R. Munkarah, MD
Associate Professor
Obstetrics and Gynecology
Wayne State University;
Director
Obstetrics and Gynecologic Oncology
Karmanos Cancer Institute/Detroit Medical Center
Detroit, MI;
Director
Gynecologic Oncology
Oakwood Hospital Medical Center
Dearborn, MI;
USA

Catherine Nelson-Piercy, MA, FRCP
Consultant Obstetric Physician
Guy's and St. Thomas' Hospitals Trust
London
UK

Robert Ogle, MBBS, FRANZCOG, FHGSA (Clinical Genetics)
Senior Staff Specialist
Physician in Molecular and Clinical Genetics
Department of Obstetrics and Fetal Medicine
Royal Prince Alfred Hospital for Women and Babies
Sydney, New South Wales
Australia

Colm O'Herlihy, MD, FRCOG, FRCPI
Professor and Head
Department of Obstetrics and Gynaecology
University College Dublin;
Consultant Obstetrician and Gynaecologist
National Maternity Hospital
Mater Misericordiae Hospital
Dublin
Ireland

Zoë Penn, MD, FRCOG
Honorary Senior Lecturer in Obstetrics
Faculty of Medicine
Imperial College London;
Consultant in Obstetrics
Chelsea and Westminster Hospital NHS Healthcare Trust
London
UK

T. Flint Porter, MD, MPH
Assistant Professor
Obstetrics and Gynecology
University of Utah Health Sciences;
Medical Director
Maternal-Fetal Medicine
LDS Hospital, Urban Central Region of Intermountain Healthcare
Salt Lake City, UT
USA

Raymond Powrie, MD, FRCPEC
Associate Professor of Medicine and Obstetrics and Gynecology
Brown University;
Academic Director Division of Obstetric and Consultative Medicine
Women and Infants Hospital of Rhode Island
Providence, RI
USA

Margaret Mary Ramsay, MA, MD, FRCOG, MRCP
Senior Lecturer in Fetomaternal Medicine
School of Human Development
Nottingham University;
Honorary Consultant in Fetomaternal Medicine
Queen's Medical Centre
Nottingham
UK

Lesley Regan, MD, FRCOG
Head of Department of Obstetrics and Gynaecology
Imperial College London;
Professor and Head Department of Obstetrics and Gynaecology
Director of Early Pregnancy and Recurrent Miscarriage Services
St. Mary's Hospital;
Honorary Consultant in Obstetrics and Gynaecology, Service Director for Gynaecology
Women and Children's Directorate
St. Mary's NHS Hospital Trust
London
UK

John T. Repke, MD, FACOG
Professor and Chairman
Department of Obstetrics and Gynecology
Pennsylvania State University College of Medicine;
Obstetrician–Gynecologist-in-Chief
The Milton S. Hershey Medical Center
Hershey, PA
USA

Laura E. Riley, MD
Assistant Professor Obstetrics and Gynecology and Reproductive Biology
Harvard Medical School
Cambridge, MA;
Medical Director of Labor and Delivery
Massachusetts General Hospital
Boston, MA
USA

Giuseppe Rizzo, MD
Professor
Department of Obstetrics and Gynecology
Università Roma Tor Vergata;
Ospedale Fatebenefreatelli Isola Tiberina
Rome
Italy

Jeffrey S. Robinson, MB, BCh, BAO, FRCOG, FRANZCOG
Professor of Obstetrics and Gynaecology
University of Adelaide
Adelaide, South Australia
Australia

Stephen Robson, MD, MRCOG, MBBS
Professor of Fetal Medicine
School of Surgical and Reproductive Sciences
University of Newcastle upon Tyne
Newcastle upon Tyne
UK

Michael S. Rogers, MBChB, FRCOG, FRCS, MD
Professor
Chinese University of Hong Kong;
Professor and Division Head
Department of Obstetrics and Gynaecology
Chinese University of Hong Kong
Shatin, Hong Kong
China

Roberto Romero, MD
Chief Perinatology Research Branch
Intramural Division, NICHD
Professor
Department of Obstetrics and Gynecology
Wayne State University/Hutzel Hospital, Department of Obstetrics and Gynecology
Detroit, MI
USA

Thomas Roos, MD
Assistant Professor
Department of Obstetrics and Gynecology
University of Regensburg
Attending
Department of Obstetrics
Sahlgrenska University Hospital—East
Gothenburg
Sweden

Jane M. Rutherford, DM, MRCOG
Consultant in Fetomaternal Medicine
Obstetrics and Gynaecology
Queen's Medical Centre
Nottingham
UK

Rodrigo Ruano, MD
Research Fellow
Université Paris V;
Consultant
Hôpital Necker Enfants Molades
Paris
France

Luis Sanchez-Ramos, MD
Professor
Obstetrics and Gynecology
University of Florida Health Science Center
Jacksonville, FL
USA

Veronica L. Schimp, DO
Wayne State University School of Medicine;
Assistant Professor
Wayne State University Karmanos Cancer Institute
Detroit, MI
USA

Neil S. Silverman, MD
Clinical Professor
Department of Obstetrics and Gynecology
Geffen School of Medicine at UCLA;
Medical Director
Inpatient Obstetric Services
Cedars-Sinai Medical Center
Los Angeles, CA
USA

Gordon C. S. Smith, MD, PhD, MRCOG
Professor and Head of Department
Obstetrics and Gynaecology
Cambridge University;
Consultant in Maternal-Fetal Medicine
Addenbrooke's NHS Trust
Cambridge
UK

John Stafan Smoleniec, BSc (Mech. Eng.,) MBBCh, MRCOG, FRACOG, FMFF (UK), DDU, MFMC (Aust.)
Conjoint Appointee
University of New South Wales
Sydney;
Director
Feto Maternal Unit
Liverpool Hospital
Liverpool
Australia

Christopher S. Snyder, MD
Head of Pediatric Electrophysiology
Ochsner Clinic Foundation
New Orleans, LA
USA

Peter William Soothill, BSc, MBBS, MD, FRCOG
Professor of Maternal and Fetal Medicine
Obstetrics and Gynaecology, Clinical Sciences South Bristol
University of Bristol;
Professor of Maternal and Fetal Medicine
Obstetrics and Gynaecology
St Michael's Hospital, UBHT
Bristol
UK

Philip J. Steer, BSc, MBBS, MD, FRCOG
Professor
Academic Department of Obstetrics and Gynaecology
Faculty of Medicine
Imperial College London;
Chelsea and Westminster Hospital
London
UK

Peter Stone, BSc, MBChB MD (Bristol), FRCOG, FRANZCOG, DDU, CMFM
Professor of Maternal Fetal Medicine
Department of Obstetrics and Gynecology
University of Auckland;
Professor of Maternal Fetal Medicine
National Women's Hospital
Auckland Hospital
Auckland
New Zealand

Jane Streltzoff, BS, RDMS
Division of Maternal—Fetal Medicine
Department of Obstetrics and Gynecology
Weill Medical College of Cornell University
New York, NY
USA

Jane Strong, MBChB, MRCP(UK), MRCPath
Consultant Haematologist
Leicester Royal Infirmary
Leicester
UK

John M. Svigos, MBBS, DRCOG, FRCOG, FRANZCOG
Senior Clinical Lecturer
Department of Obstetrics and Gynaecology
University of Adelaide;
Senior Visiting Medical Officer and Obstetric Unit Head
Women's and Children's Hospital
North Adelaide, South Australia
Australia

Myles J. O. Taylor, BA, MRCGP, MRCOG, PhD
Honorary Clinical Senior Lecturer
Peninsula Medical School
Universities of Exeter and Plymouth;
Consultant Obstetrician and Gynaecologist
Subspecialist in Fetal and Maternal Medicine
Royal Devon and Exeter NHS Foundation Trust
Devon
UK

Jim Thornton, MD, FRCOG
Professor in Obstetrics and Gynaecology
School of Human Development
University of Nottingham;
Honorary Consultant Obstetrician and Gynaecologist
Nottingham City Hospital NHS Trust
Nottingham
UK

Mark W. Tomlinson, MD
Clinical Assistant Professor
Obstetrics and Gynecology
Oregon Health and Sciences University;
Obstetrics and Gynecology
Providence St. Vincent's Hospital;
Women's Healthcare Associates
Portland, OR
USA

Lawrence C. Tsen, MD
Associate Professor in Anesthesia
Harvard Medical School;
Director of Anesthesia, Center for Reproductive Medicine
Department of Anesthesiology, Perioperative, and Pain Medicine
Brigham and Women's Hospital
Boston, MA
USA

Sarah Vause, MD, MRCOG
Consultant in Fetomaternal Medicine
St. Mary's Hospital
Manchester
UK

Rasniah Vigneswaran, MD*
Formerly Senior Staff Neonatologist
University of Adelaide
Adelaide Women's and Children's Hospital
Adelaide, South Australia
Australia

Yves Ville, MD, PhD
Professor
Department de Gynecologie Obstetrique et Medecine de la Reproduction
Centre Hôspitalier Intercommunal
Poissy, Cedex
France

Anthony Vintzileos, MD
Professor and Chair
Department of Obstetrics, Gynecology, and Reproductive Sciences
UMDNJ-Robert Wood Johnson Medical School;
Chairman
Department of Obstetrics Gynecology, and Reproductive Sciences
Robert Wood Johnson University Hospital
New Brunswick, NJ
USA

Asnat Walfisch, MD
Instructor
Ben Gurion University;
Department of Obstetrics and Gynecology
Soroka Medical Center
Beer Sheva
Israel

Ann Walker, MBChB
Lead Clinician for Pregnancy
University of Leeds
Leeds
UK

James Walker, MD, FRCOG, FRCP
Professor of Obstetrics and Gynecology
University of Leeds;
Professor of Obstetrics and Gynaecology
St. James University Teaching Hospital
Leeds
UK

Peter Wardle, MD, FRCS (Lond.), FRCOG
Consultant Obstetrician and Gynaecologist
Southmead Hospital
Bristol
UK

D. Heather Watts, MD
Medical Officer
Pediatric, Adolescent, and Maternal AIDS Branch
National Institute of Child Health and Human Development
National Institutes of Health
Bethesda, MD
USA

Carl P. Weiner, MD, MBA, FACOG
Professor
Department of Obstetrics, Gynecology, and Reproductive Sciences;
Professor
Department of Physiology
University of Maryland School of Medicine
Baltimore, MD
USA

Katharine, D. Wenstrom, BA, MA, MD
Professor
Obstetrics and Gynecology
University of Alabama School of Medicine;
Director
Division of Maternal–Fetal Medicine and Reproductive Genetics
University of Alabama Hospital and Clinics
Birmingham, AL
USA

Hajo I. J. Wildschut, MD, PhD
Associate Professor of Obstetrics and Gynecology
Erasmus University Medical Center;
Consultant in Obstetrics and Gynecology
Erasmus University Medical Center
Rotterdam
The Netherlands

David Williams, MBBS, PhD
Senior Lecturer, Maternal Medicine
Imperial College London;
Consultant Obstetric Physician
Department of Obstetrics and Gynaecology
Chelsea and Westminster Hospital
London
UK

*(deceased)

Catherine Williamson, BSc, MBChB, MRCP
Senior Lecturer in Obstetric Medicine
Imperial College London;
Honorary Consultant Obstetric Physician
Queen Charlotte's Hospital
London
UK

Lami Yeo, MD
Associate Professor
Department of Obstetrics, Gynecology, and Reproductive Sciences
UMDNJ—Robert Wood Johnson Medical School;
Director of Perintal ultrasound
Director of Fetal Cardiovascular Unit
Robert Wood Johnson University Hospital
New Brunswick, NJ
USA

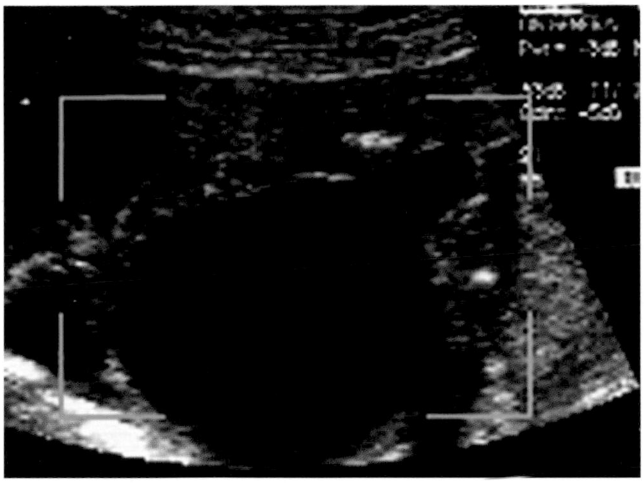

COLOR PLATE 1
A transverse view of lower fetal abdomen on ultrasound at 16 weeks, showing a dilated bladder with a keyhole sign (see Fig. 13–3).

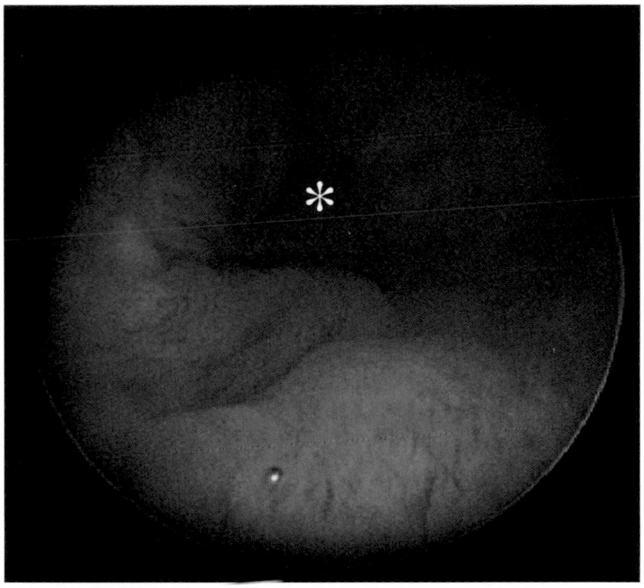

COLOR PLATE 3
Fetal cystoscopic view of a fetal bladder and the proximal urethra (*) (see Fig. 13–6).

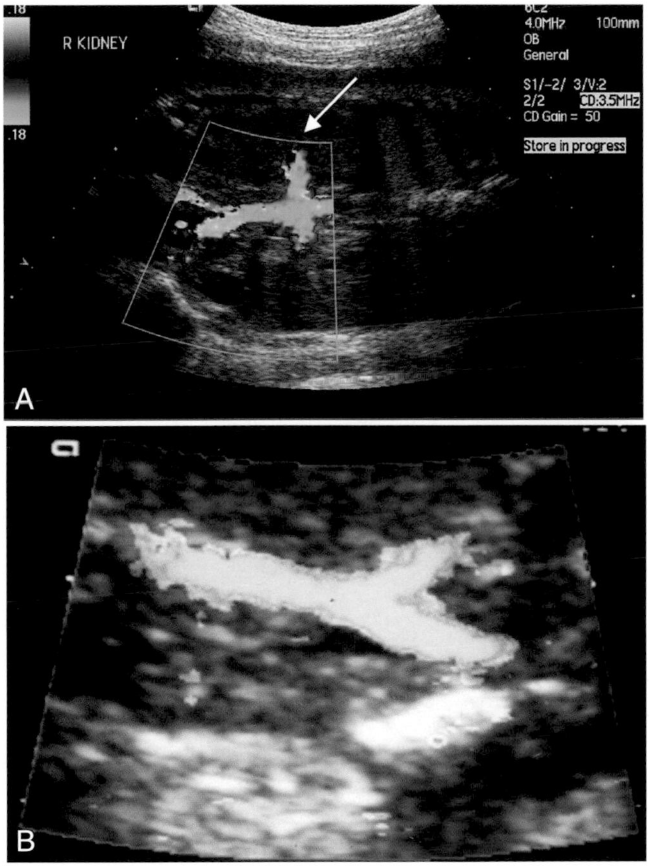

COLOR PLATE 2
Color Doppler/power Doppler showing renal arteries in a normal fetus (*A*) but absent from a fetus with renal agenesis (*B*) (see Fig. 13–5).

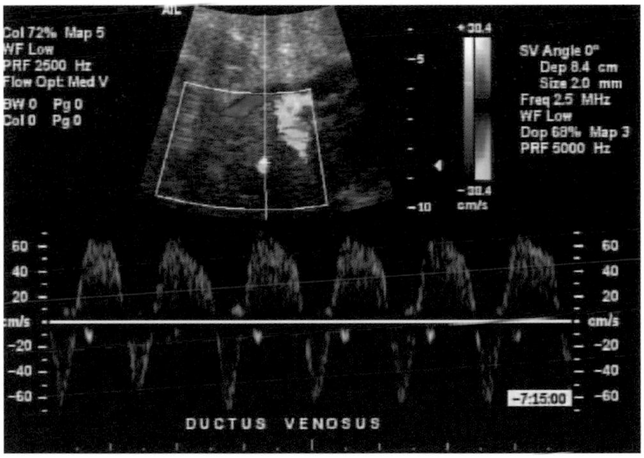

COLOR PLATE 4
Flow in ductus venosus of a fetus with reentrant supraventricular tachycardia. Normal flow is unidirectional in contrast with bidirectional flow shown here (see Fig. 16–3).

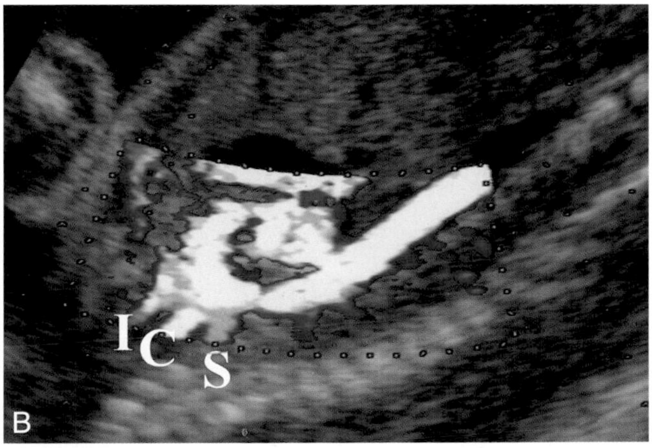

COLOR PLATE 5
B, Same section with power Doppler superimposed showing the arch with its three branches: innominate artery (I), left carotid artery (C) and subclavian artery (S) (see Fig. 17–5).

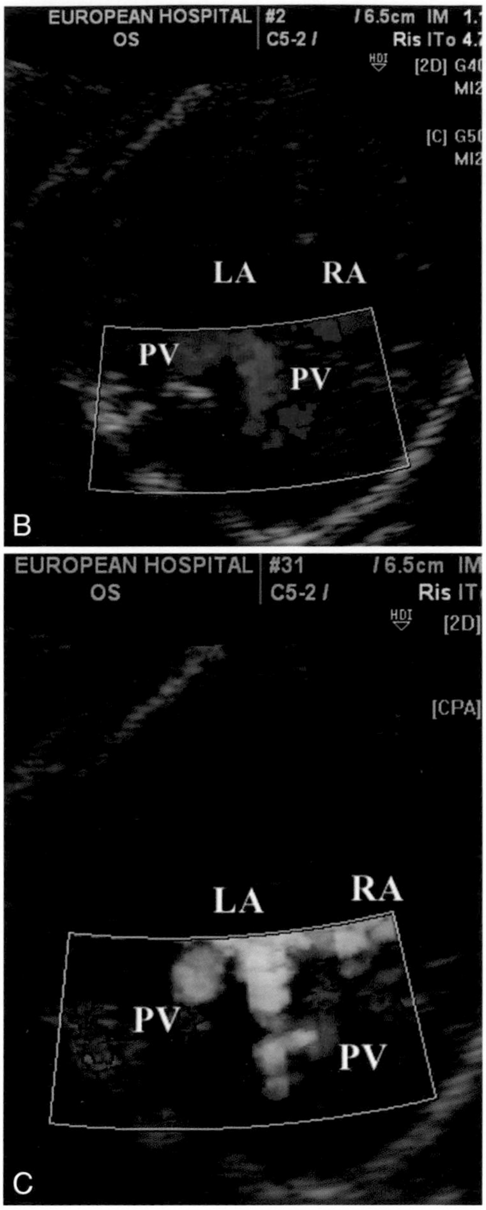

COLOR PLATE 6
Apical four-chamber view of the fetal heart showing the inlet of the pulmonary veins (PV) in the left atrium in real time (*A*) and with the help of color (*B*) and power (*C*) Doppler (see Fig. 17–11).

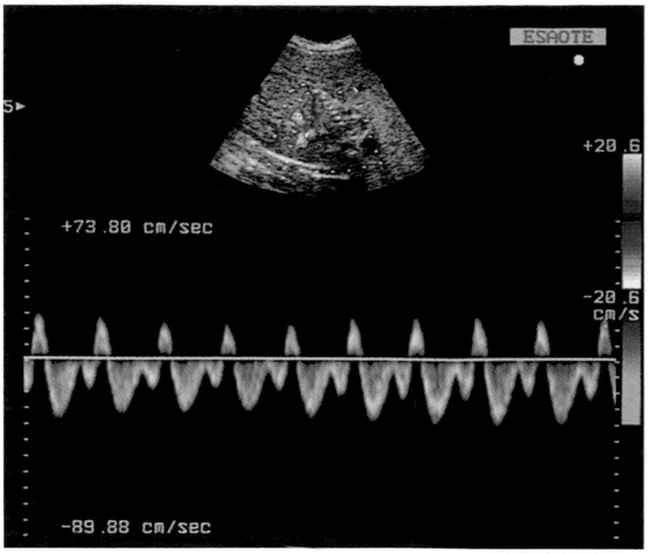

COLOR PLATE 7
Parasagittal view of the fetal trunk with the sample volume placed on the inferior vena cava. Note the typical triphasic morphology with the reverse flow (upper channel) during atrial contraction (A wave) (see Fig. 17–12).

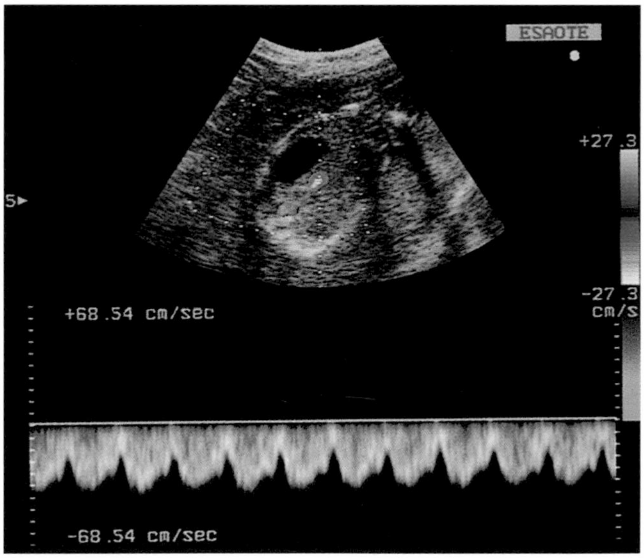

COLOR PLATE 8
Transverse section of the upper fetal abdomen with the sample volume placed on the ductus venosus. Note the typical biphasic morphology (see Fig. 17–13).

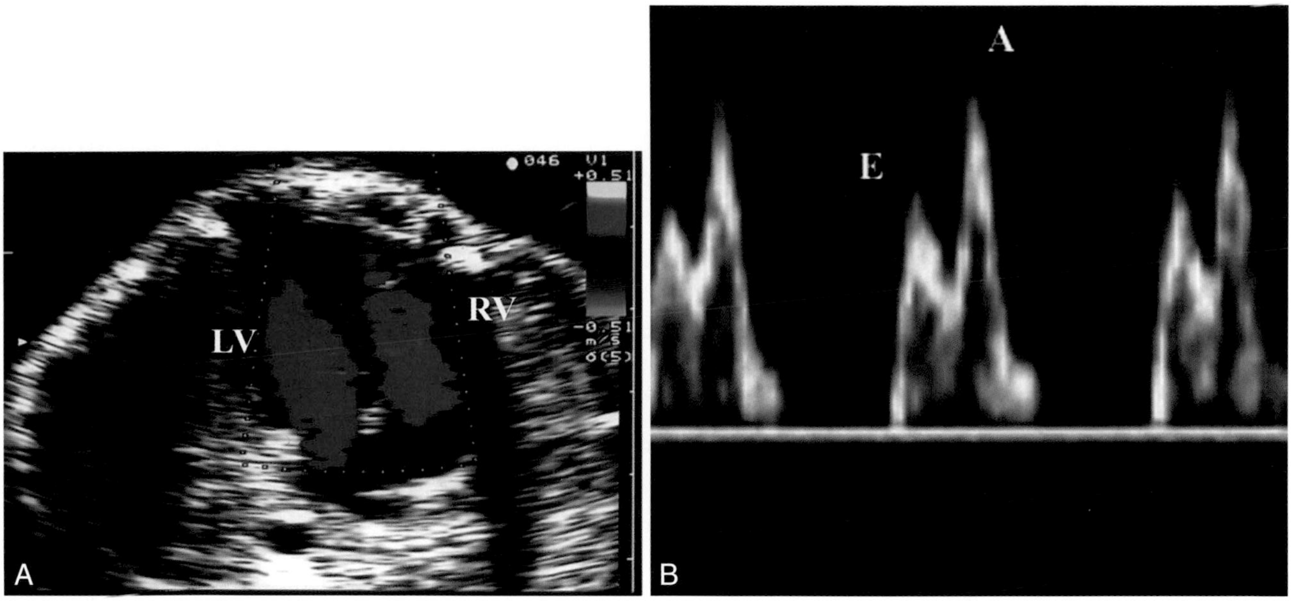

COLOR PLATE 9

A, Apical flow chamber view of the fetal heart showing the normal filling of the two ventricles (*red color*). *B*, Pulsed Doppler tracing from tricuspid valve. Note the typical morphology (E and A waves) and the absence of flow during systole (see Fig. 17–15).

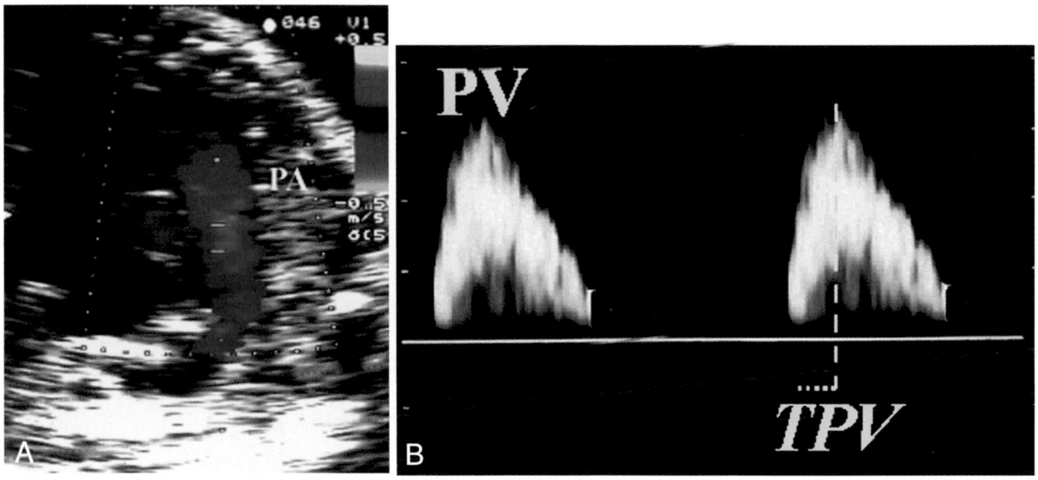

COLOR PLATE 10

A, Short-axis view of the fetal heart with the color Doppler superimposed showing the outflow of the right ventricle (*blue*). *B*, Pulsed Doppler tracing at the level of the pulmonary valve and the typical velocity waveform recorded. PV, peak velocity; TPV, time to peak velocity (see Fig. 17–16).

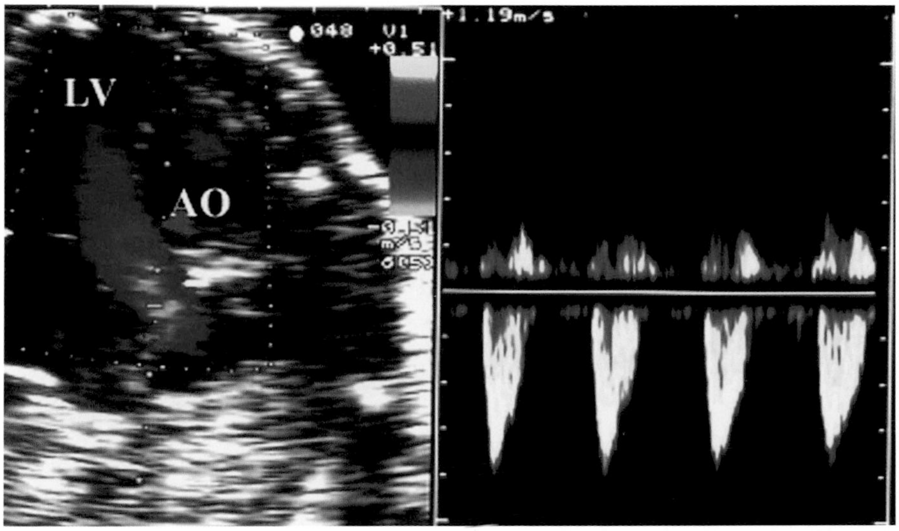

COLOR PLATE 11

Long-axis view of the fetal heart with the color Doppler superimposed showing the outflow of the left ventricle (*blue*). The sample volume is placed at the level of the aorta and the typical velocity waveform recorded (see Fig. 17–17).

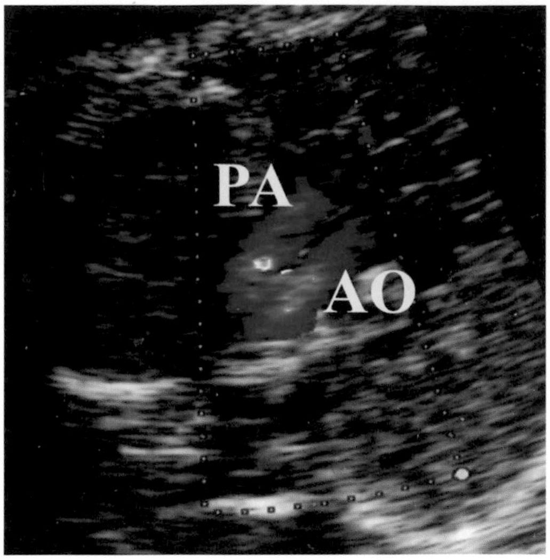

COLOR PLATE 12
Three-vessel view with the color Doppler superimposed showing pulmonary artery (PA) and ascending aorta (AO) with the same flow direction (see Fig. 17–18).

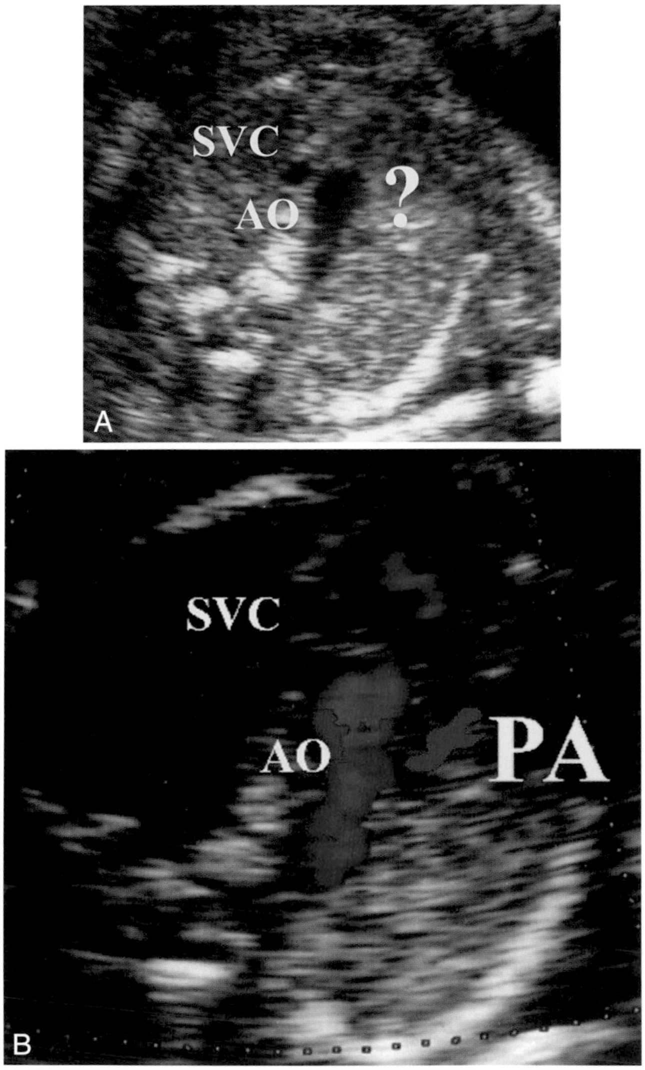

COLOR PLATE 13
Three-vessel view in a fetus with pulmonary atresia. *A*, The pulmonary artery is not evidenced (?) in real-time image. *B*, With the color Doppler superimposed, a small caliber pulmonary artery is identified with reversal flow (*red*) indicating retrograde perfusion from the systemic circulation to pulmonary circulation (see Fig. 17–19).

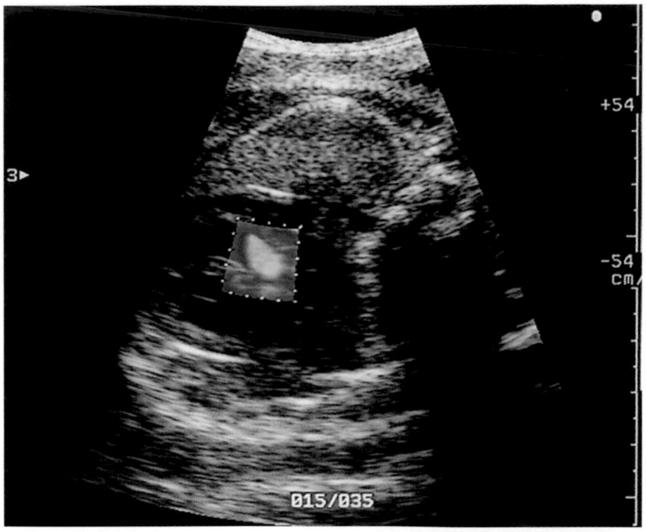

COLOR PLATE 14
This small perimembranous septal defect is visualized with the help of color Doppler. High-velocity jet from the left to the right ventricle is due to the association of aortic stenosis (see Fig. 17–21).

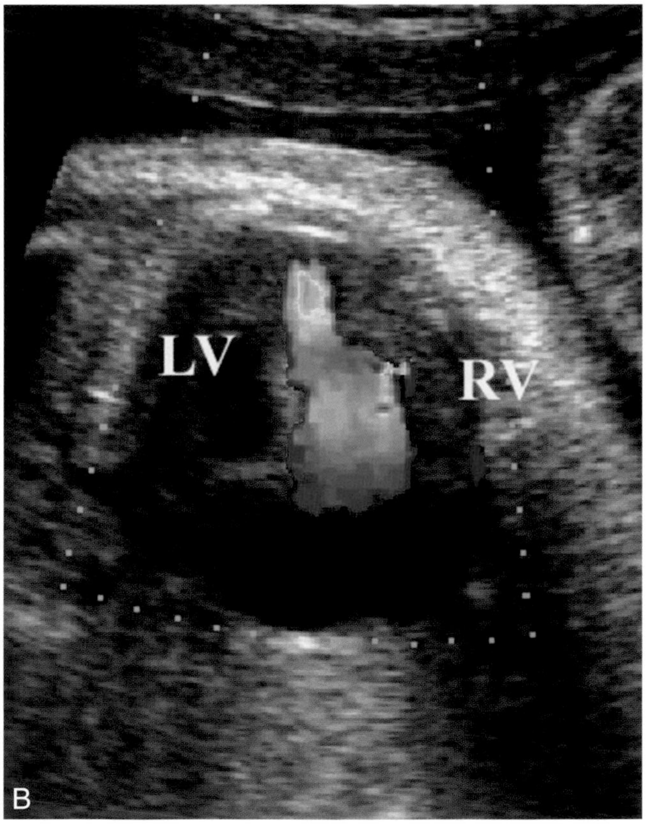

COLOR PLATE 15
The color Doppler shows the normal filling of the right ventricle (*red*) and the absent filling of the left ventricle (mitral atresia). LV, left ventricle; RV, right ventricle (see Fig. 17–25*B*).

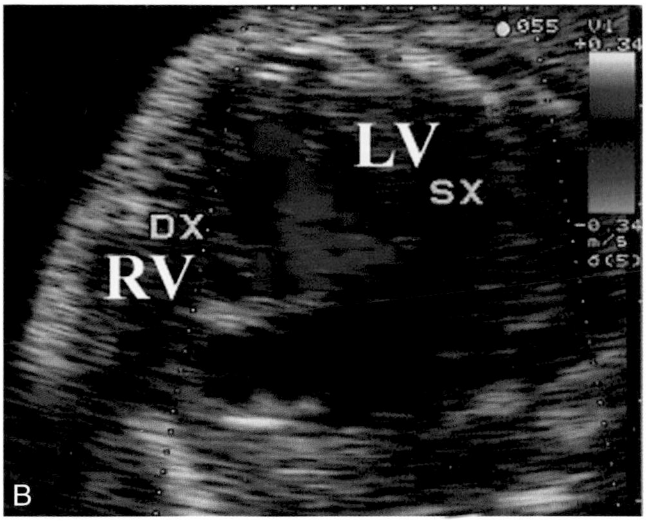

COLOR PLATE 16
Color Doppler shows the absent filling of the right ventricle (tricuspid atresia). LV, left ventricle; RV, right ventricle (see Fig. 17–26*B*).

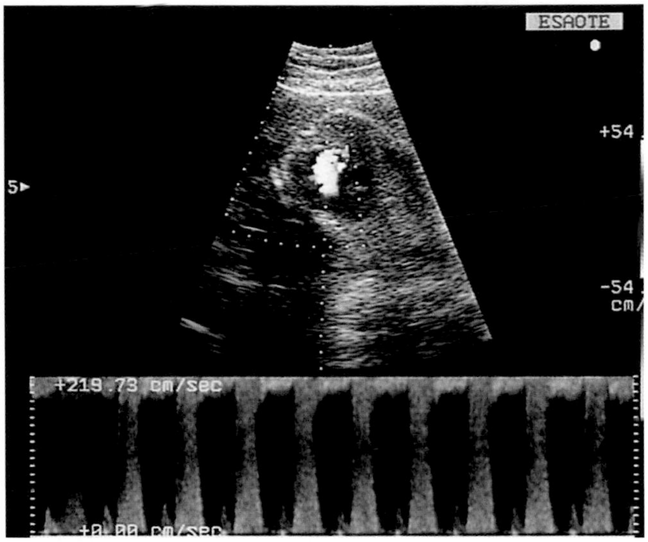

COLOR PLATE 18
Color Doppler image with the pulsed Doppler sample placed on the aortic valve showing high velocities (PV > 220 cm/sec) suggestive of aortic stenosis (see Fig. 17–28).

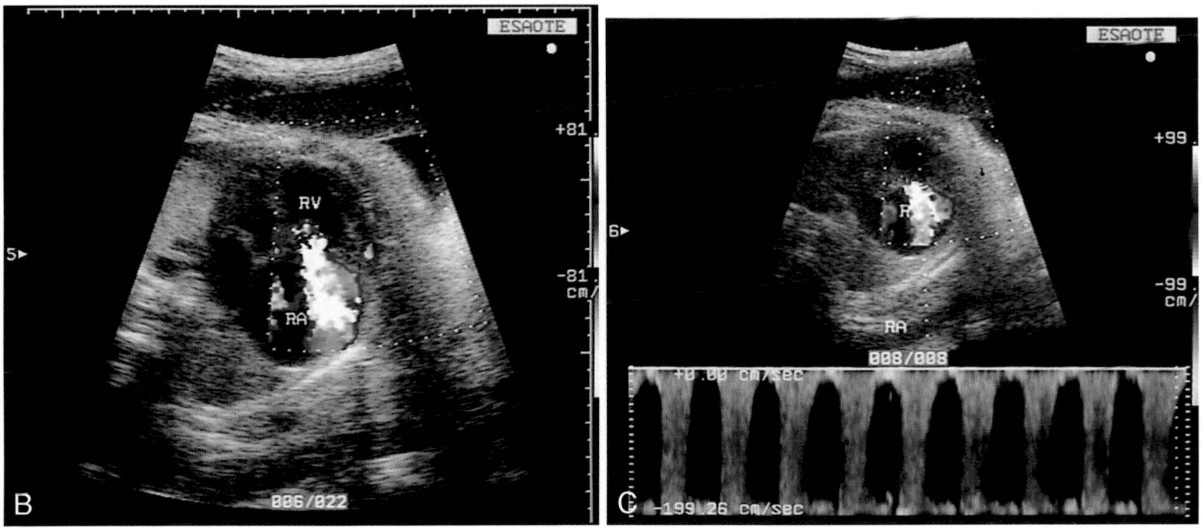

COLOR PLATE 17
Apical four-chamber view in the presence of a pulmonary atresia and intact septum. When the color Doppler is superimposed a high-velocity retrograde jet is seen (*blue*) (*B*) and a holosystolic high velocity (>2 m/sec) tricuspid regurgitation is measured by pulsed Doppler (*C*). LA, left atrium; RA, right atrium; LV, left ventricle; RV, right ventricle (see Fig. 17–27*B*,*C*).

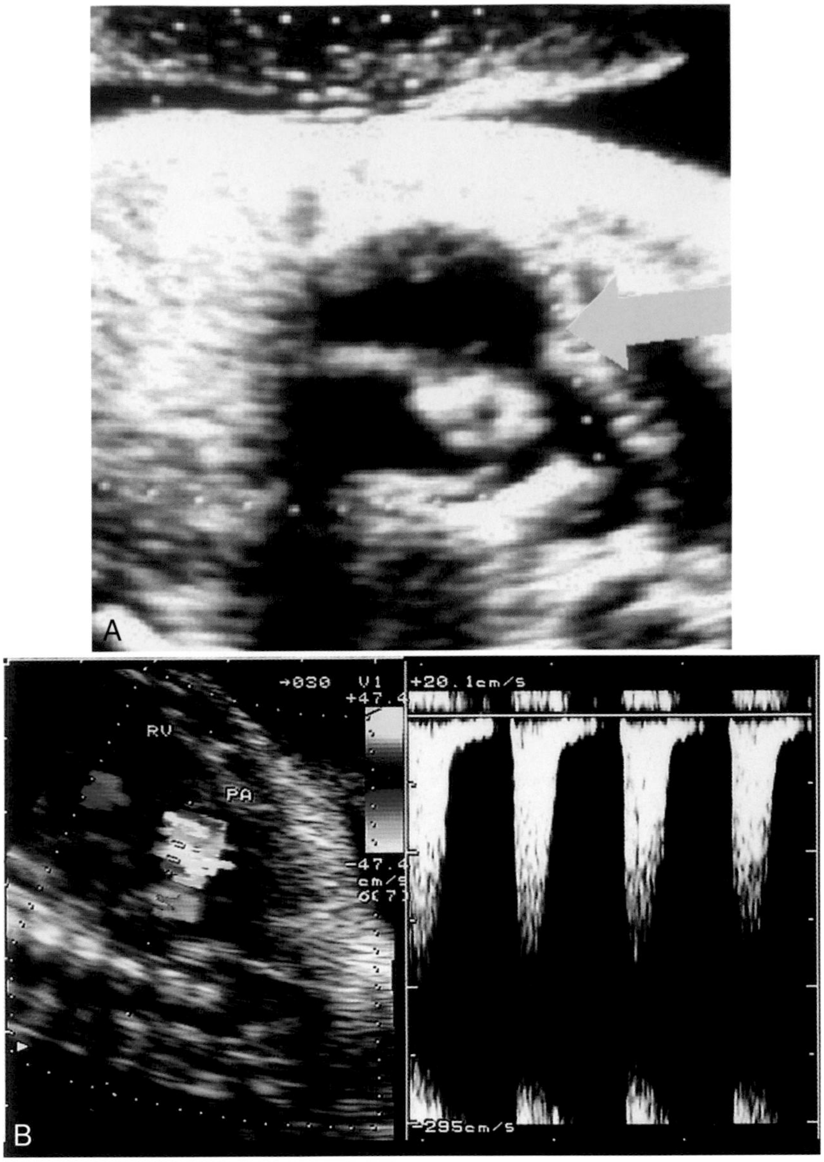

COLOR PLATE 19
Short-axis view of the fetal heart in a fetus with pulmonary stenosis. *A*, Narrowing of the valve. *B*, Color Doppler superimposed showing high velocities in pulmonary artery (PA). Pulsed Doppler demonstrates high-velocity waveforms (180 cm/sec) consistent with pulmonary stenosis (see Fig. 17–30).

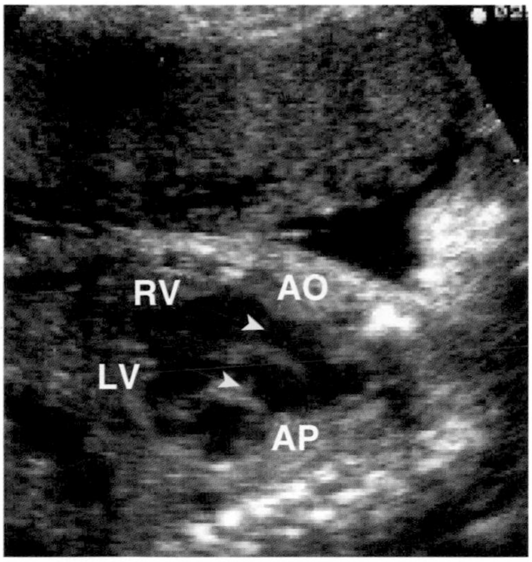

COLOR PLATE 20
Example of correct transposition of great artery with intact septum. The heart is seen in long axis, and in contrast to normal, both great arteries are seen in this projection. They arise in parallel orientation with the aorta (AO) from the anterior right ventricle (RV) and the pulmonary artery (PA) from the posterior left ventricle (LV) (see Fig. 17–31).

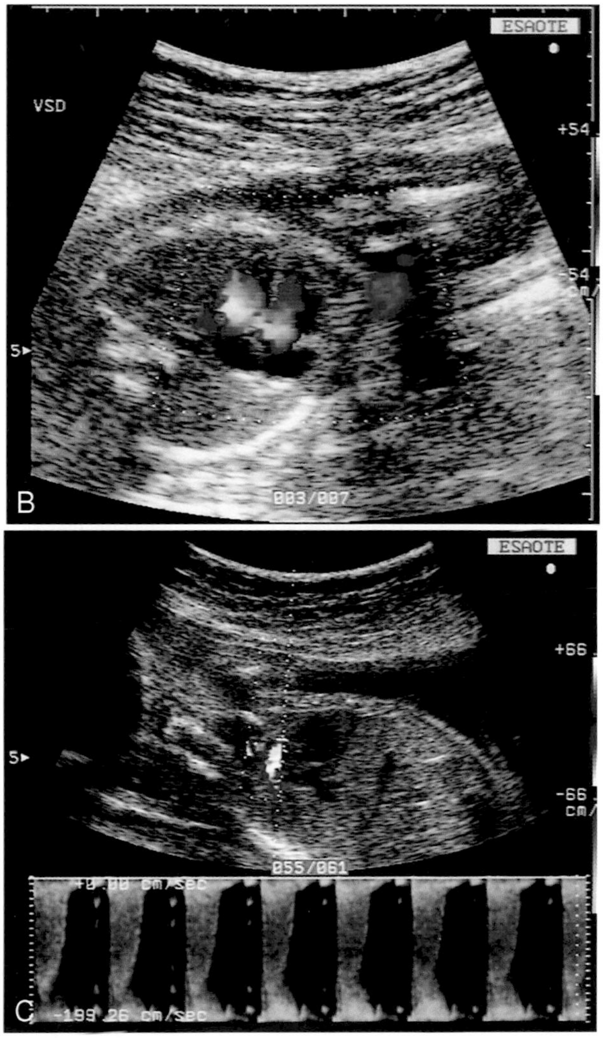

COLOR PLATE 22
Tetralogy of Fallot. Color Doppler demonstrates the presence of the ventricular septal defect (*B*) and pulsed Doppler placed at the level of pulmonary valve demonstrates the presence of high velocities (>2 m/sec) consistent with pulmonary stenosis (*C*) (see Fig. 17–35*B*,*C*).

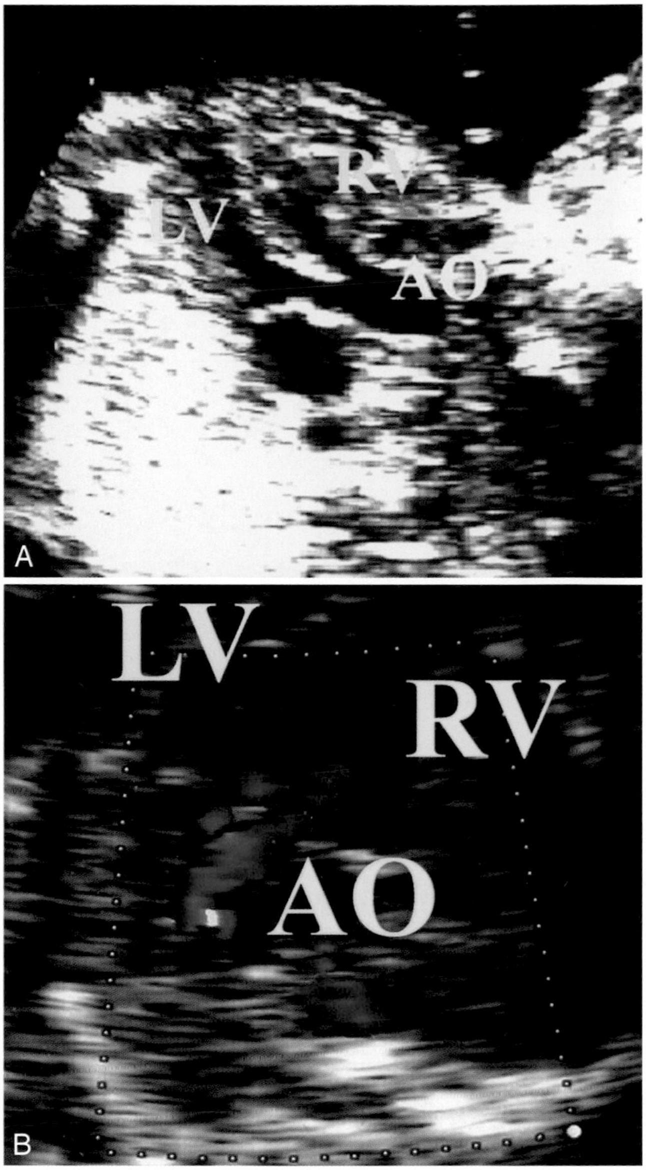

COLOR PLATE 21
Long-axis view of the fetal heart in a fetus with tetralogy of Fallot. *A*, The aorta (AO) is overriding the left (LV) and right ventricles (RV) in real time. *B*, The color Doppler shows the perfusion during systole from the left (LV) and right (RV) ventricles into the overriding aorta (AO) (Y sign) (see Fig. 17–34).

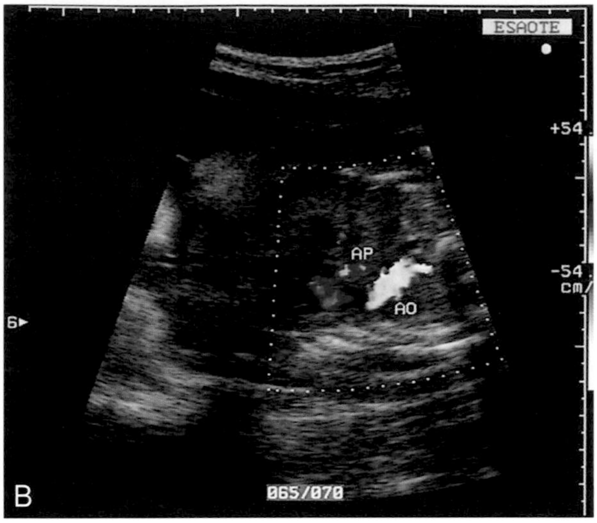

COLOR PLATE 23
Double outlet right ventricle. Both great vessels originate from the right ventricle (RV). Furthermore the PA is atretic and a retrograde flow (*blue*) is evident, suggesting that the pulmonary circulation depends on the aorta (*B*) (see Fig. 17–36*B*).

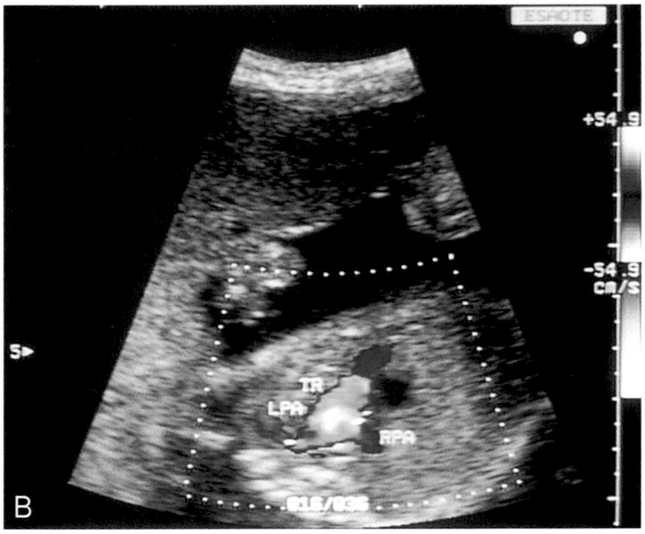

COLOR PLATE 24
Truncus arteriosus. Color Doppler allows the visualization of the origin of the right (RPA) and left (LPA) pulmonary arteries from the truncus (TR) (see Fig. 17–37*B*).

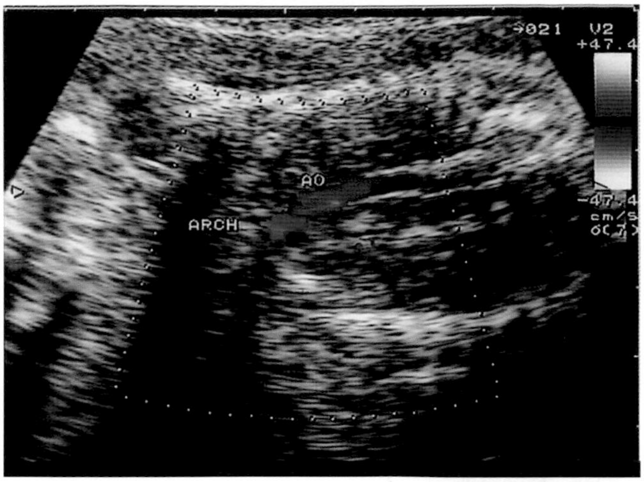

COLOR PLATE 25
Arch view in presence of a hypoplastic left ventricle. The arch is perfused in the reverse direction (blue color is seen instead of red) suggesting that the brain and coronary circulation depend on the right ventricle. AO, aorta (see Fig. 17–39).

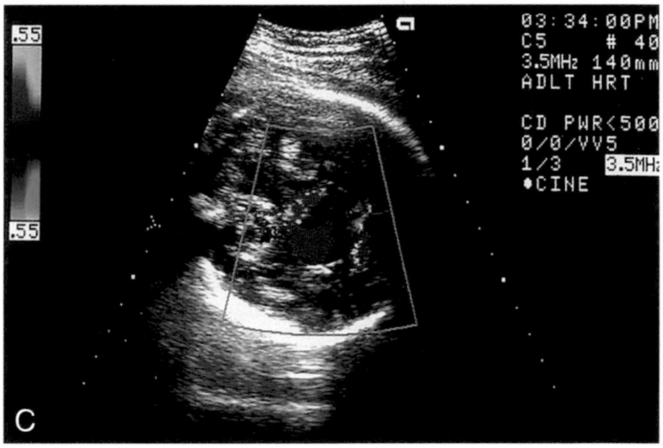

COLOR PLATE 26
Transverse section through fetal head using color Doppler demonstrating blood flow in cystic structure, vein of Galen (see Fig. 18–15*C*).

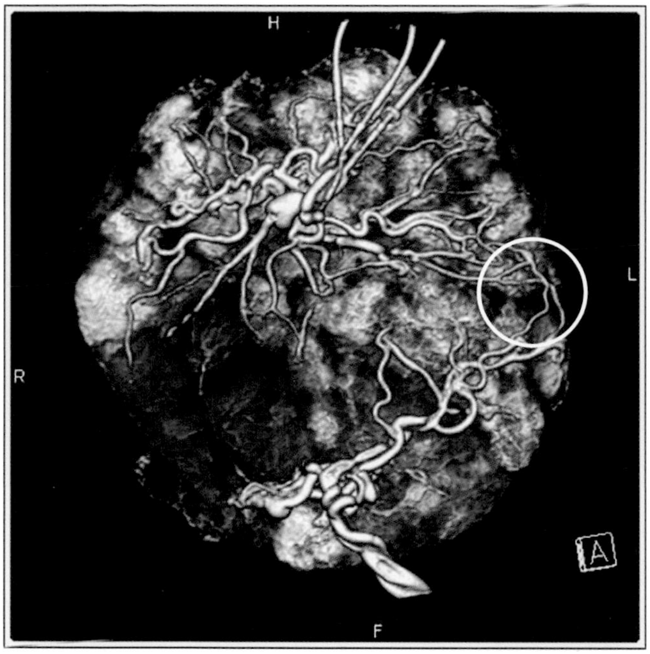

COLOR PLATE 27
Three-dimensional reconstruction of a CT-angiogram of a monochorionic placenta at term, showing an equal distribution of the placental mass and a large arterioarterial and venovenous superficial anastomosis (*arrows*). (see Fig. 24–2). (In collaboration with M. Cannie, UZ Leuven, Belgium.)

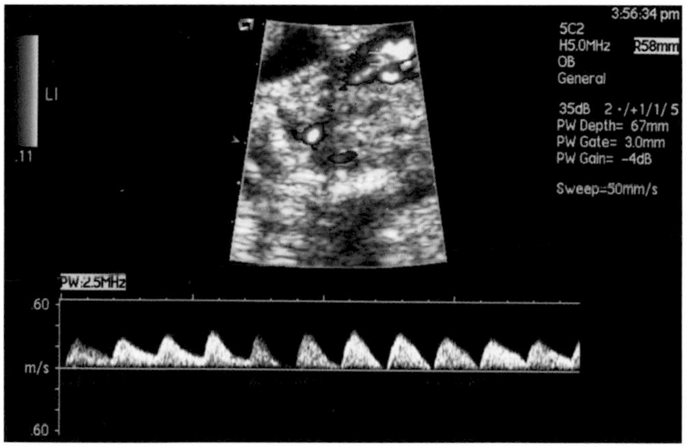

COLOR PLATE 28
Doppler pattern of intermittent absent end-diastolic flow as typically seen in the smaller twin of a monochorionic pair with discordant growth (see Fig. 24–7).

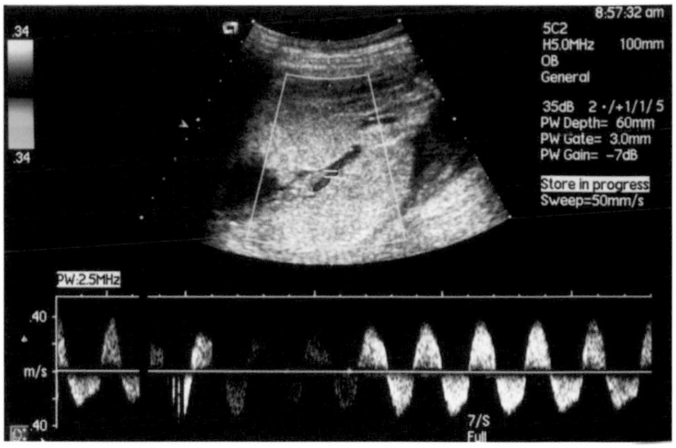

COLOR PLATE 29
Characteristic bidirectional Doppler pattern in an arterioarterial anastomosis, which confirms monochorionicity (see Fig. 24–8).

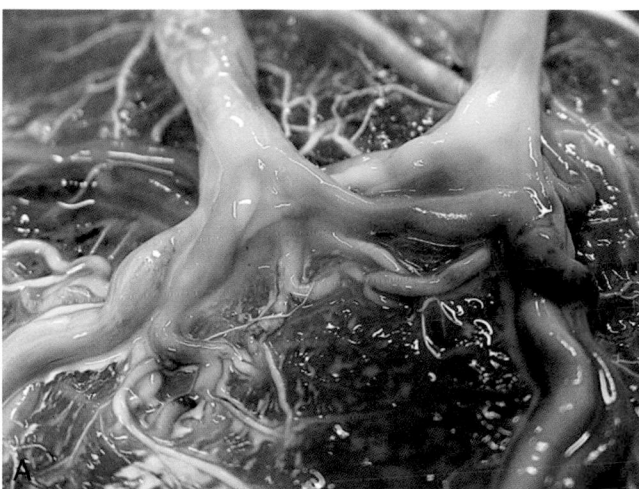

COLOR PLATE 30
Macroscopic image of large-diameter anastomoses and side-to-side insertion of the umbilical cords as typically seen in a monoamniotic twin pregnancy (see Fig. 24–9*A*).

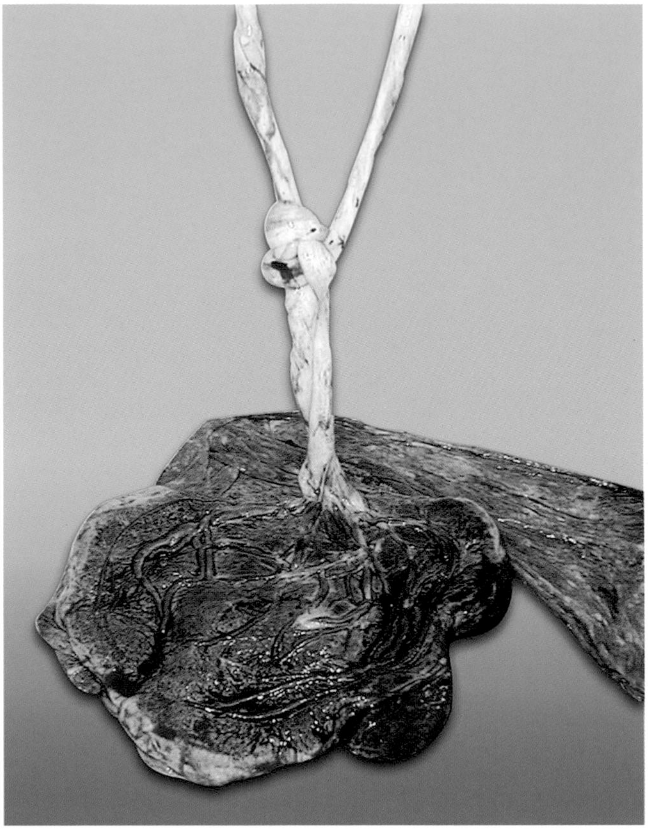

COLOR PLATE 31
Cord entanglement and knotting at birth in a monoamniotic twin pregnancy (see Fig. 24–12). (Courtesy of S. Dobbelaere, H. Hart Hospital, Lier, Belgium.)

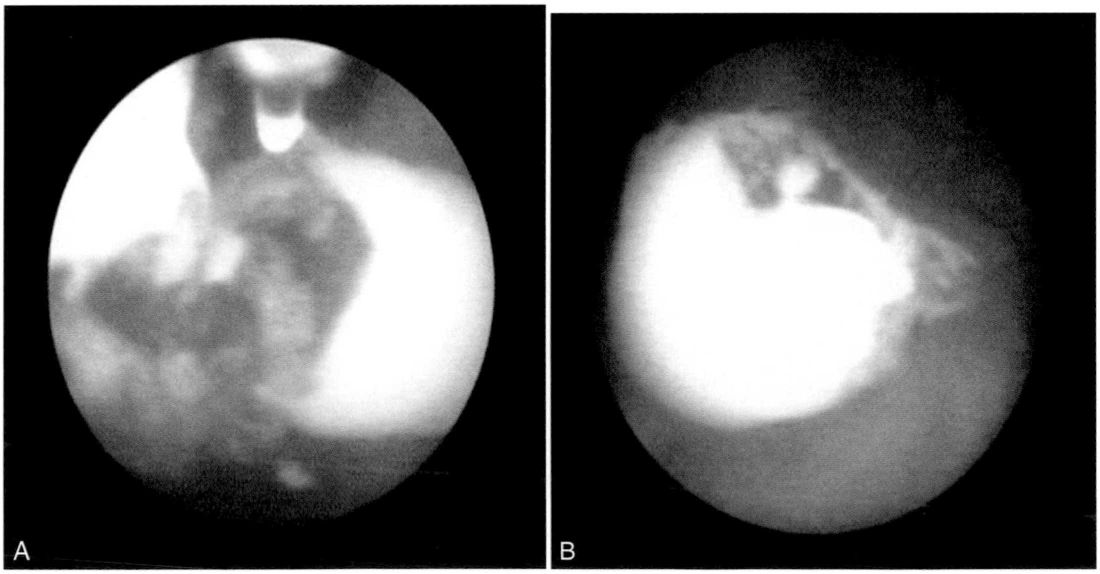

COLOR PLATE 32
Fetoscopic image during (*A*) and after (*B*) umbilical cord transsection by laser in a monoamniotic twin pregnancy with a severe discordant anomaly (see Fig. 24–13).

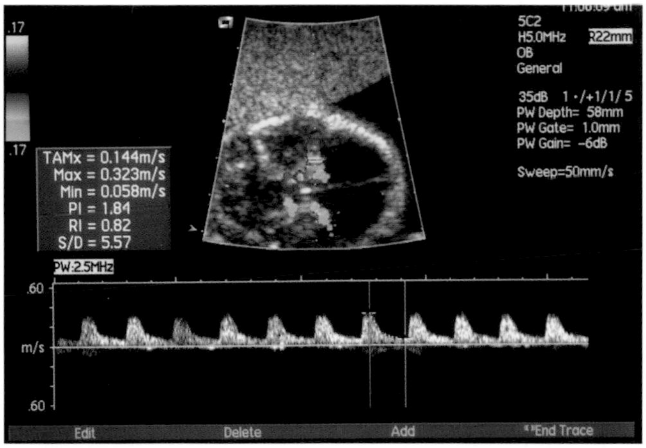

COLOR PLATE 33
Doppler examination of the middle cerebral artery of the surviving twin of a monochorionic pair at 20 weeks' gestation, within 4 days after sIUFD of the growth-retarded co-twin (see Fig. 24–15).

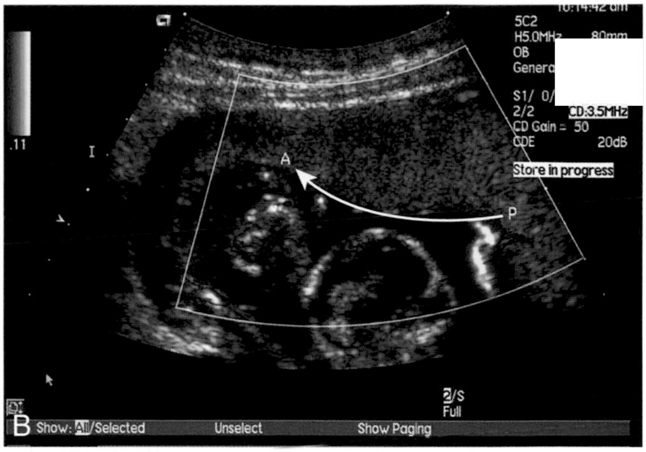

COLOR PLATE 36
Doppler examination at 15 weeks' gestation, demonstrating the typical, retrograde flow from the pump twin toward the acardiac twin over an arterioarterial anastomosis (*arrow*) (see Fig. 24–18*B*).

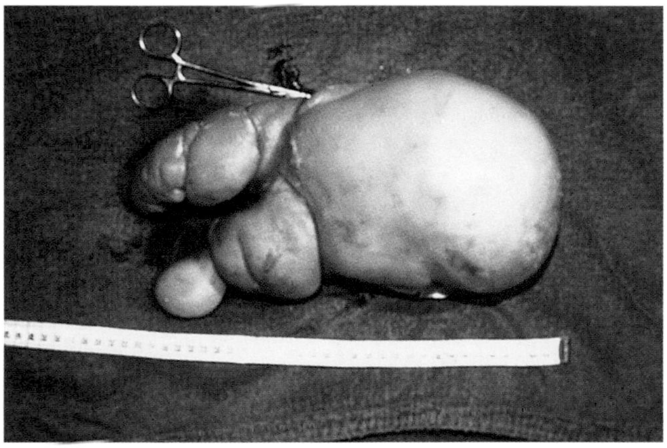

COLOR PLATE 34
Macroscopic image of an acardiac twin with absent head and partial development of lower limbs and abdomen. This acardiac mass weighed about 4 kg and was not diagnosed until the third trimester. The patient delivered at 37 weeks, and the pump twin survived (see Fig. 24–16).

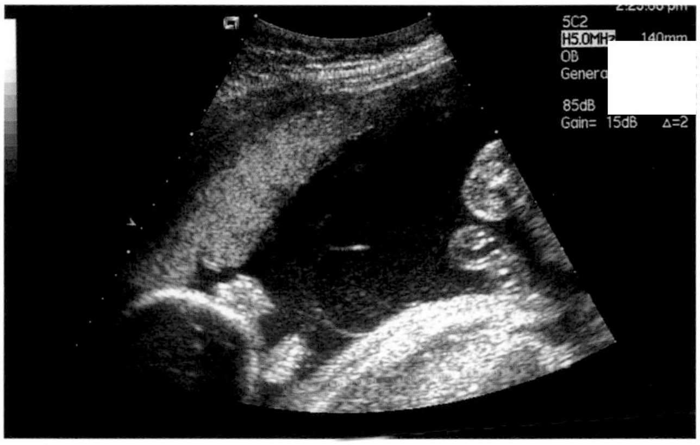

COLOR PLATE 37
Ultrasound image of membrane folding in a monochorionic twin pregnancy, which reflects discordant amniotic fluid in a monochorionic twin pregnancy (see Fig. 24–23).

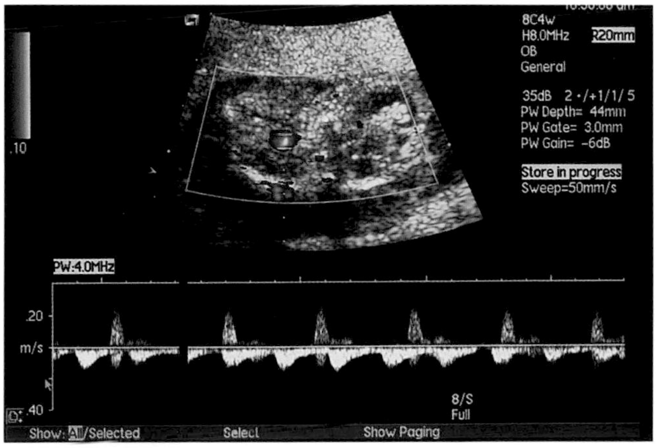

COLOR PLATE 35
Doppler examination demonstrating cardiac activity in the rudimentary heart (70 bpm) of the acardiac twin, with flow in the opposite direction in the aorta (140 bpm) (see Fig.24–17).

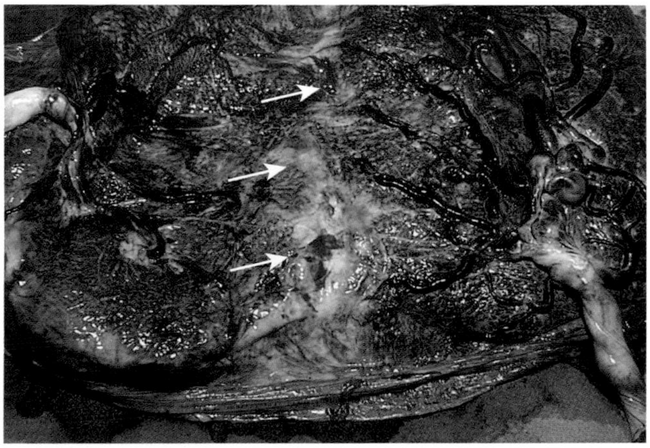

COLOR PLATE 38
Macroscopic image of a placenta at birth demonstrating "bichorionization" and laser impact (*arrows*) on the monochorionic placenta after laser coagulation for twin-to-twin transfusion syndrome (see Fig. 24–24).

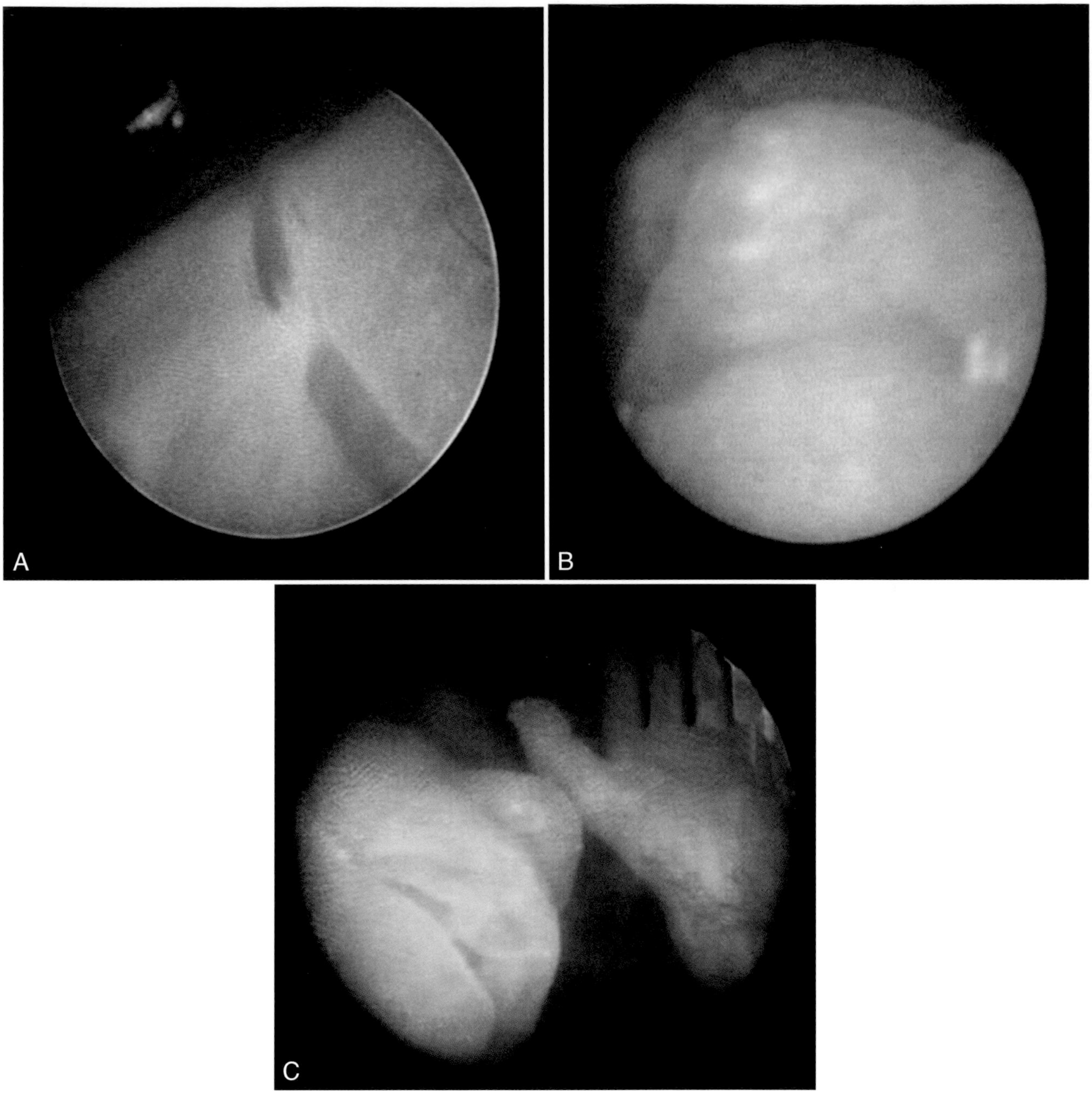

COLOR PLATE 39
A, Fetoscopic image of laser coagulation of an arteriovenous anastomosis for twin-to-twin transfusion syndrome. *B*, Fetoscopic image of the hands of the donor twin, who is stuck behind the intertwin septum. *C*, Fetoscopic image of the face of the recipient, who moves freely in the hydramniotic sac (see Fig. 24–26).

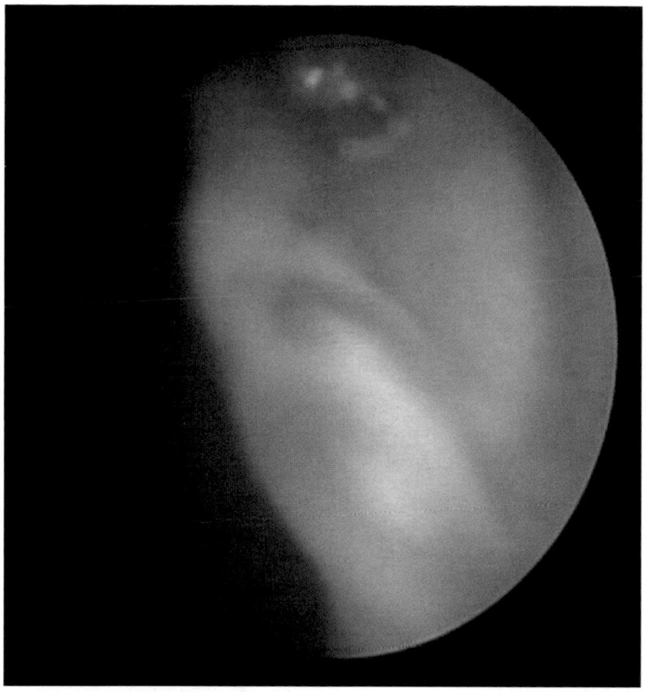

COLOR PLATE 40
Fetoscopic image of laser cord coagulation (see Fig. 24–28).

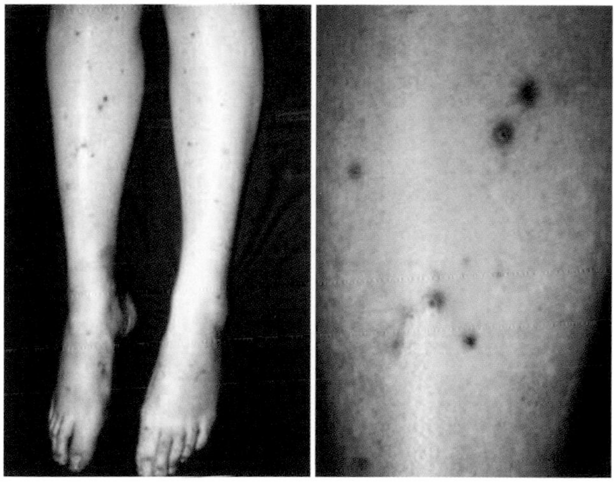

COLOR PLATE 41
Dermatologic features observed in obstetric cholestasis cases: Dermatitis artefacta (see Fig. 48–1).

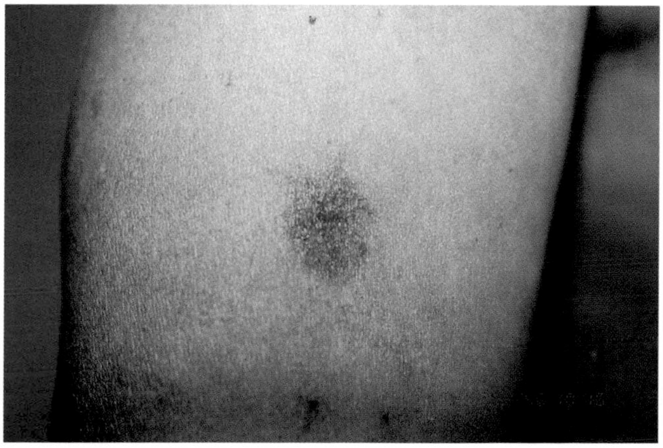

COLOR PLATE 42
Spider angioma (telangiectasia) on the arm (see Fig. 52–1).

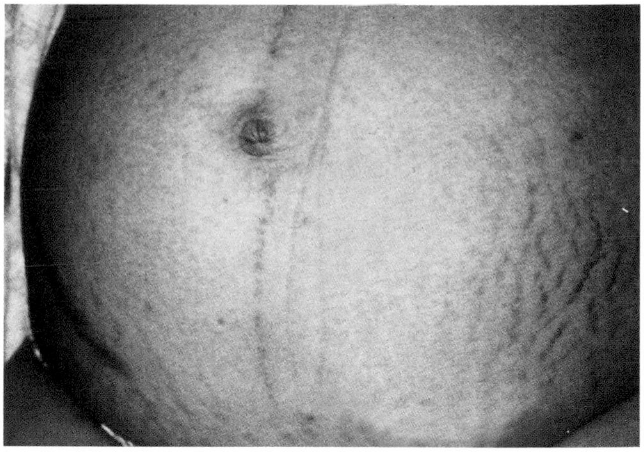

COLOR PLATE 43
Stretchmarks (striae gravidarum) on the lateral aspects of the abdomen and hyperpigmentation of the linea alba, causing development of the *linea nigra* (see Fig. 52–2).

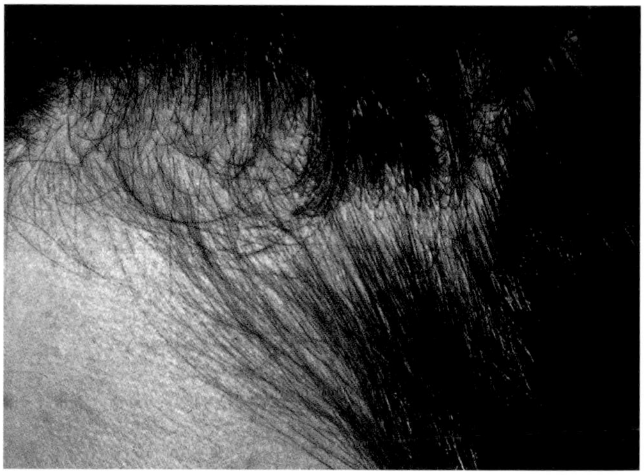

COLOR PLATE 44
Telogen effluvium, which developed in the immediate postpartum period, with typical temporal recession and thinning (see Fig. 52–3).

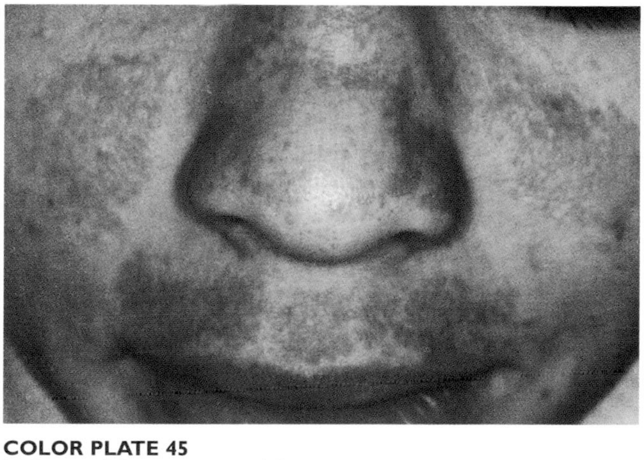

COLOR PLATE 45
Melasma of the entire central face (see Fig. 52–4).

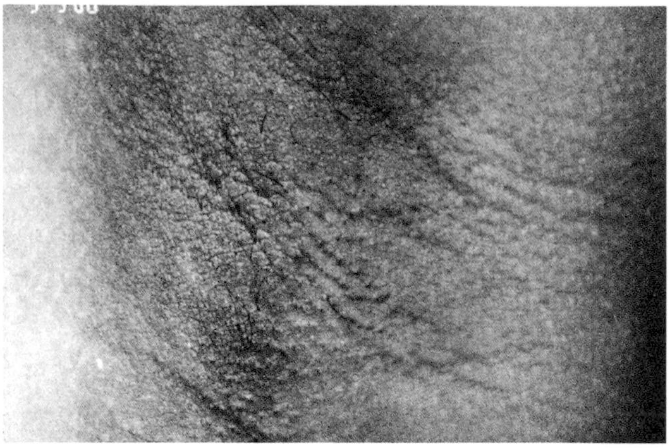

COLOR PLATE 46
Pseudoacanthosis nigricans may develop in skin of color during pregnancy and manifests itself as hyperpigmented velvety plaques on the axillae (as shown) and neck (see Fig. 52–5).

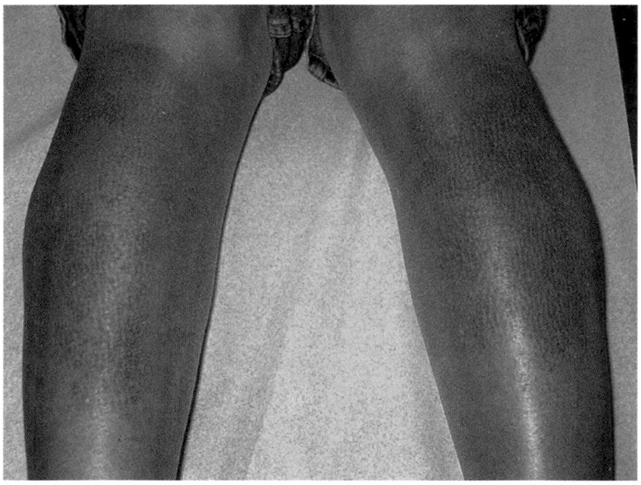

COLOR PLATE 47
Grayish-brown ill-defined patches of dermal melanocytosis may develop in pregnancy and persist in the postpartum period (see Fig. 52–6).

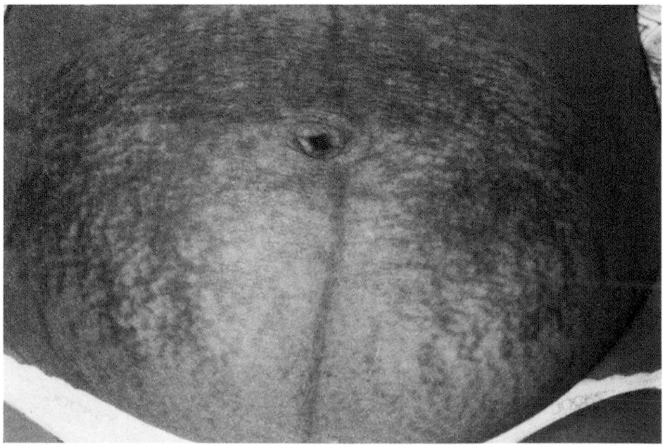

COLOR PLATE 48
Extensive postinflammatory hyperpigmentation secondary to pruritic urticarial papules and plaques of pregnancy in an Asian female (see Fig. 52–7).

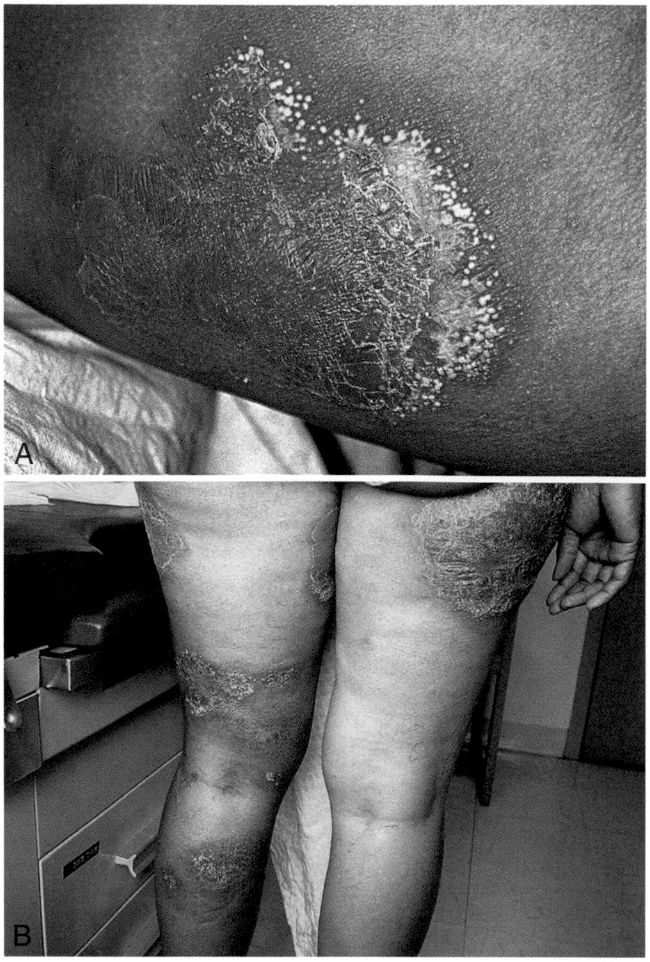

COLOR PLATE 49
A, Early impetigo herpetiformis: discrete group sterile papules at the periphery of erythematous patch. *B*, Generalized advanced lesions of impetigo herpetiformis show crusting or vegetations (see Fig. 52–8). (Photographs courtesy of Aleksandr Itkin, MD.)

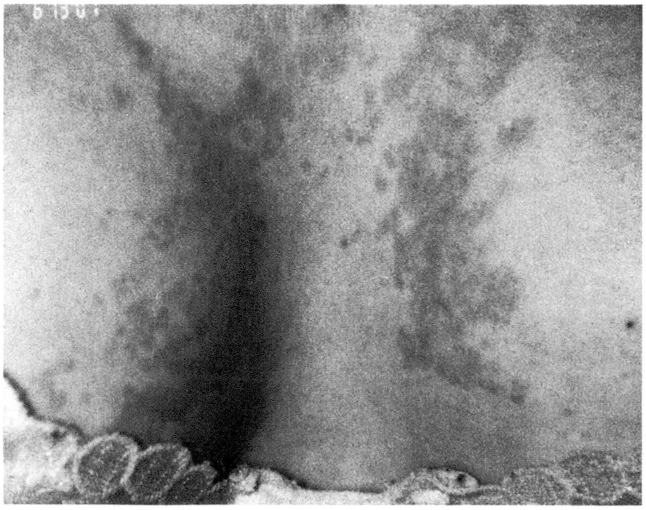

COLOR PLATE 50
Hyperpigmented minimally scaly patches on the chest in a pregnant female with tinea versicolor (see Fig. 52–9).

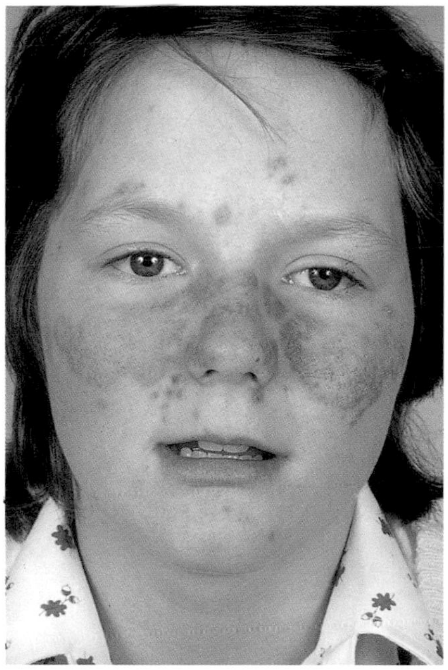

COLOR PLATE 51
Malar erythema in a butterfly distribution in a pregnant woman with systemic lupus erythematosus (see Fig. 52–10). (Photograph courtesy of Cameron Thomas, Campbell Kennedy, and Phillipa Kyle from second edition.)

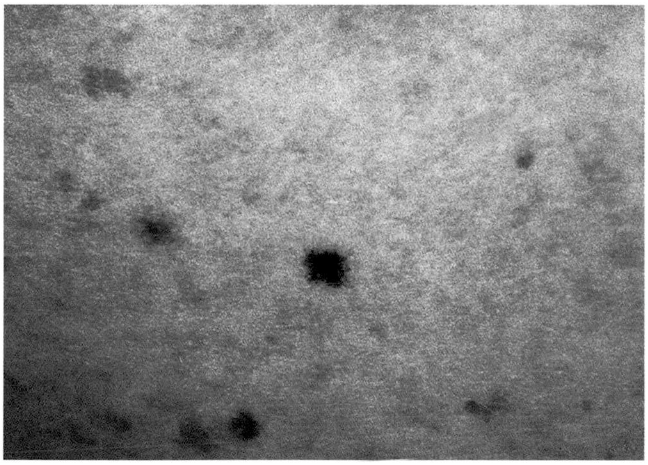

COLOR PLATE 52
Melanocytic nevus that became darker and developed a mild border irregularity during gestation (see Fig. 52–11).

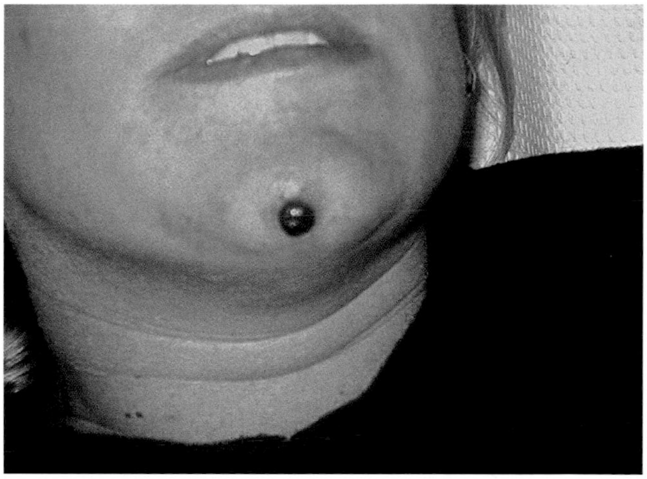

COLOR PLATE 53
Pyogenic granuloma of pregnancy (*granuloma gravidarum*), typically seen on the gingivae, can also develop on extramucosal sites (see Fig. 52–12).

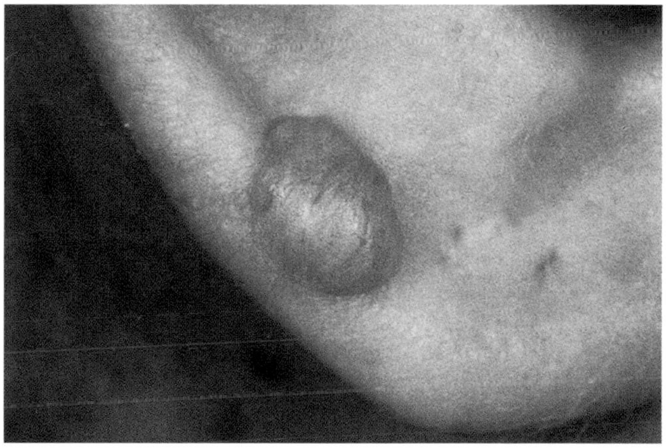

COLOR PLATE 54
Keloid that developed during pregnancy without previous trauma (see Fig. 52–13).

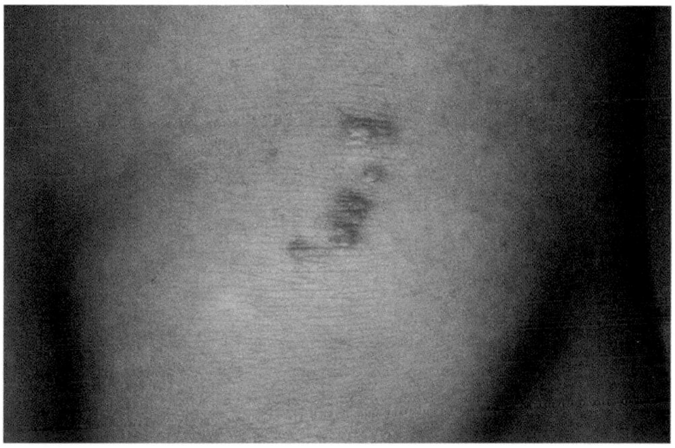

COLOR PLATE 55
Minimal residual skin lesions of sarcoidosis on the knee in a pregnant female who showed severe generalized skin sarcoidosis before gestation (see Fig. 52–14).

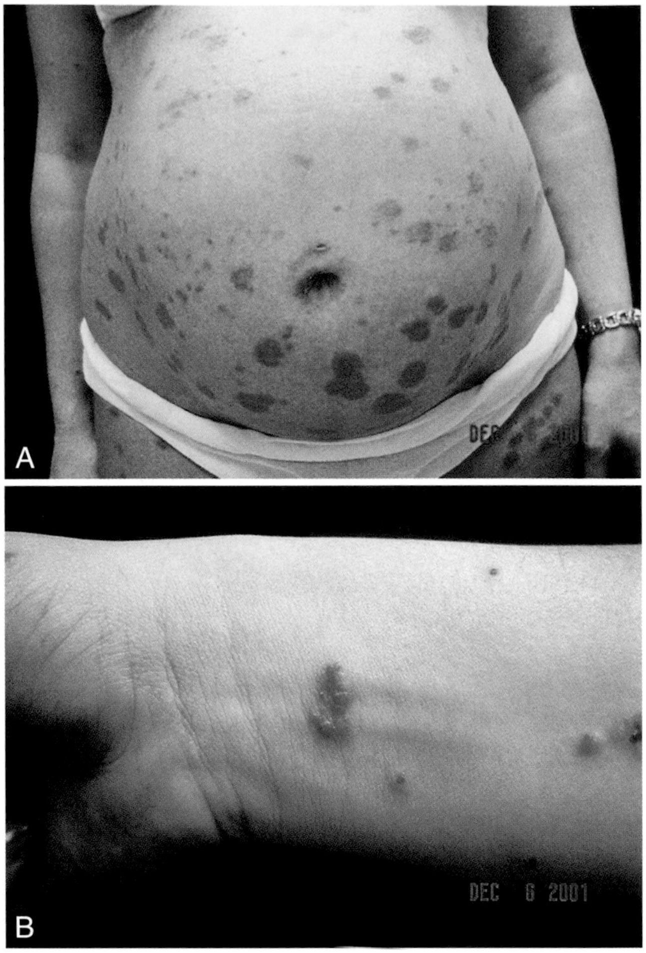

COLOR PLATE 56
A, Pruritic abdominal urticarial lesions usually develop in the early phase of herpes gestationis. *B*, Characteristic tense vesicles on an erythematous base on the forearm in a patient with herpes gestationis. (see Fig. 52–15). (Photographs courtesy of Jeffrey Callen, MD.)

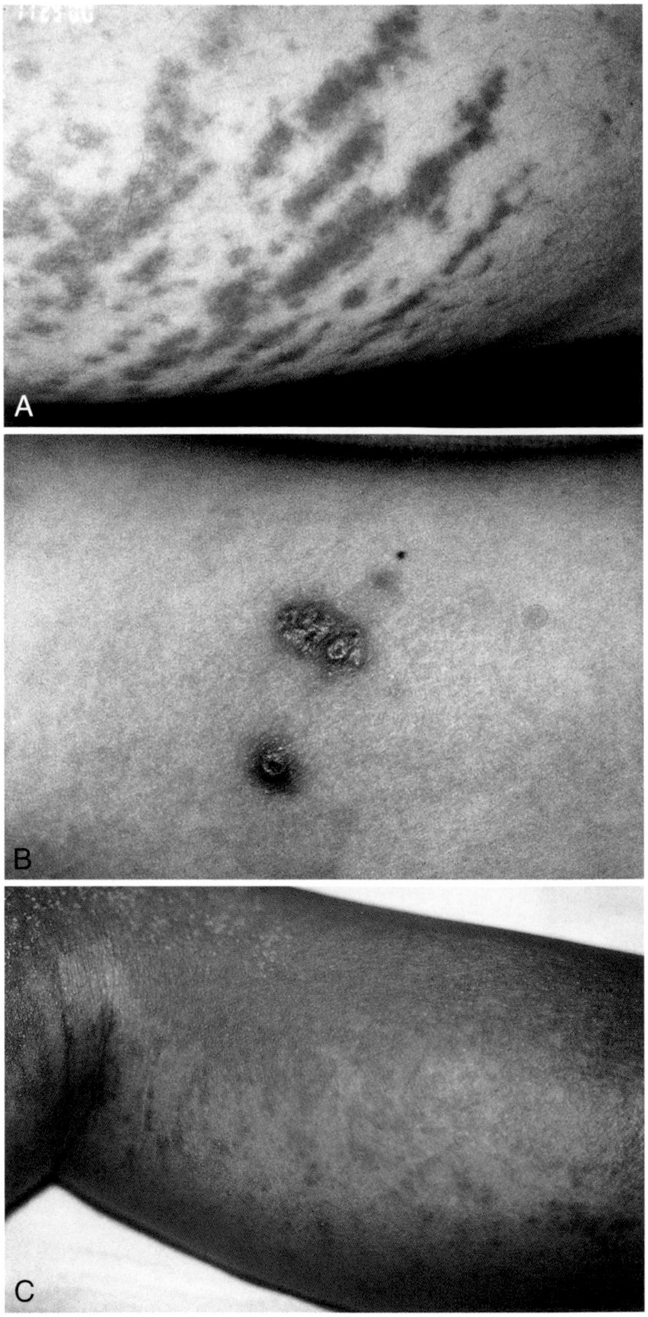

COLOR PLATE 57
A, Early PUPPP showing typical urticarial lesions in the abdominal striae. *B*, Lesions with microvesiculated appearance on the forearm in PUPPP. *C*, Widespread PUPPP may resemble a toxic erythema (see Fig. 52–16). (Photograph courtesy of Helen Raynham, MD.)

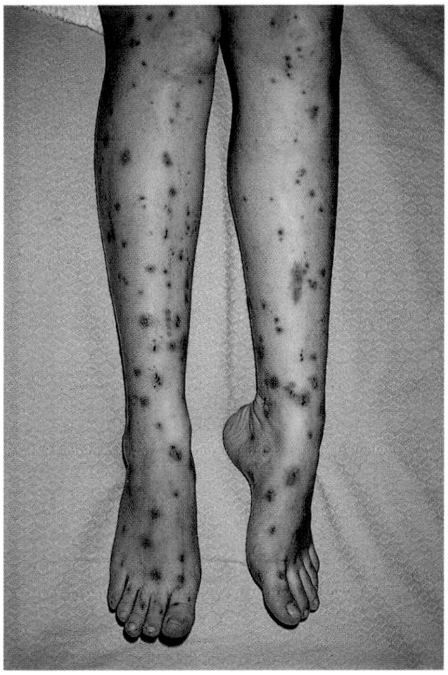

COLOR PLATE 58
Prurigo gestationis: excoriated papules and nodules on the extensor surfaces of the extremities (see Fig. 52–17). (Photograph courtesy of Cameron Thomas, Campbell Kennedy, and Phillipa Kyle from second edition.)

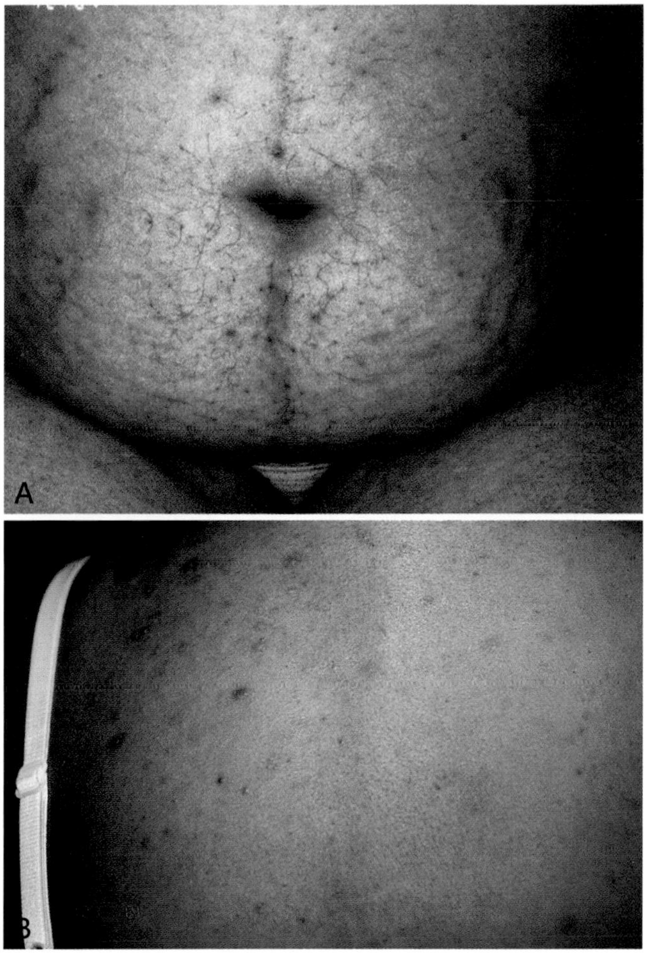

COLOR PLATE 59
A, Pruritic folliculitis of pregnancy: typical follicular erythematous or pigmented papules on the abdomen. *B*, Follicular acneform pustules and papules on the upper back in pruritic folliculitis of pregnancy (see Fig. 52–18).

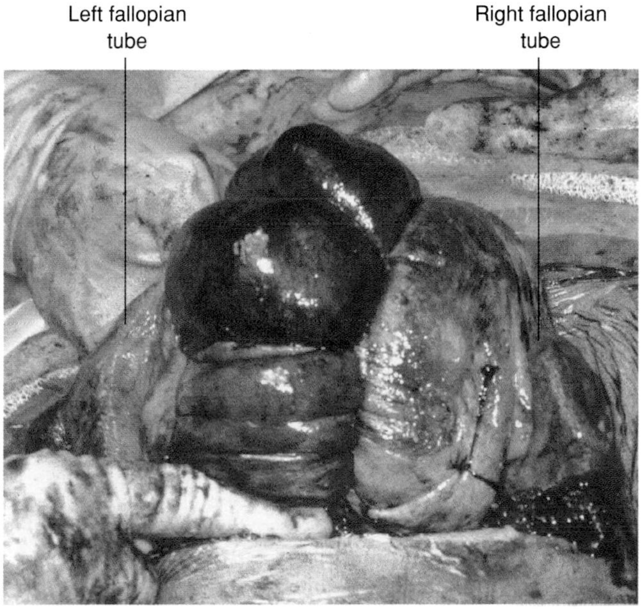

COLOR PLATE 60
Posterior view of compression sutures (see Fig. 77–9). From Hayman RG, Arulkumaran S, Steer PJ: Uterine compression sutures: Surgical management of postpartum hemorrhage. Obstet Gynecol 2002;99:502–506.

EVIDENCE-BASED SUMMARY OF MANGEMENT OPTIONS BOXES

One of the most popular features of the first two editions of High Risk Pregnancy: Management Options was the "Summary of Management Options" (SOMO) Box. The SOMO Box was placed at the end of each chapter or section within a chapter and presented the reader with an *aide memoire* of the main points regarding the management options for a specific condition discussed in detail in the chapter.

In 2003, the SOMO Boxes were compiled into a separate publication: Evidence Based Obstetrics. For that book, however, the SOMO Boxes were expanded to include an evidence-based scoring system. Each management option was scored on the basis of the quality of evidence that underpinned that strategy. The strength of recommendation for a given management option would inevitably result from the quality of evidence, with the highest recommendation being linked with the best quality of evidence.

For the third edition of *High Risk Pregnancy: Management Options* the editors have agreed to include the same evidence-based approach in the SOMO Boxes.

The following is the evidence based scoring system that is used in this book for the SOMO Boxes.

Scoring System for Summary of Management Options Boxes

Quality (Level) of Evidence

Ia Evidence obtained from meta-analysis of randomized controlled trials

Ib Evidence obtained from at least one randomized controlled trial

IIa Evidence obtained from at least one well-designed controlled study without randomization

IIb Evidence obtained from at least one other type of well-designed quasi-experimental study

III Evidence obtained from well-designed non-experimental descriptive studies, such as comparative studies, correlation studies, and case studies

IV Evidence obtained from expert committee reports or opinions and/or clinical experience of respected authorities

Strength (Grade) of Recommendation

A At least one randomized controlled trial as part of a body of literature of overall good quality and consistency addressing the specific recommendation (Evidence Levels Ia or Ib)

B Well-controlled clinical studies available but no randomized clinical trials on the topic of the recommendations (Evidence Levels IIa, IIb, or III)

C Evidence obtained from expert committee reports or opinions and/or clinical experiences of respected authorities. Indicates an absence of directly applicable clinical studies of good quality (Evidence Level IV)

GPP Good Practice Point: recommended best practice based on the clinical experience of the chapter authors and editors

PREFACE TO THE FIRST EDITION

This new international textbook in obstetrics will, we believe, be of major value to all practicing clinicians, be they trainees or established in practice.

It aims to assist with the questions: How do I manage this patient? or How do I perform this procedure?

It presents a wide range of reputable management options. Unlike many traditional texts, based on a single individual's experience and view, all the contributors to each section were asked to give their preferred management in all areas of their section. Each resulting chapter reflects that wide range of acceptable practice. This means you will have a *choice* about which option or combination of options suits you and your patient.

This book is designated to be practical. It addresses those difficult questions which arise in practice, which often stem not only from the medical facts, but from the constraints of time, facilities, finance, and patient acceptability. Moreover, we have standardized the presentation of each topic as far as possible (while still allowing the personality of the original authors to shine through!) to enable the reader to become familiar with the format.

We have deliberately chosen a panel of contributors who are both leaders in their field and who can represent practice in the USA, Europe, and Australasia and this we feel gives the text a unique universality.

Finally it is our intention that the book is comprehensive. We hope that we will have something to say on all the important problems you come across. If you find any exceptions, please let us know, with your comments, in time for the next edition.

PREFACE TO THE THIRD EDITION

Welcome to the third edition of *High Risk Pregnancy: Management Options*. We hope this edition will build on the success of the first two. In particular, we seek its continued growth in reputation as a true International Postgraduate Textbook. Although the majority of contributors come from the United States, the author list includes representatives from all over the world (UK, Ireland, Netherlands, France, Italy, Germany, Belgium, Israel, Iceland, South Africa, Hong Kong, Australia, and New Zealand).

We have made the following significant improvements to the third edition whilst maintaining the key characteristic features of previous editions:

- a major overhaul and revision of the book's appearance to further enhance readability
- a clearer presentation of the text while keeping to the original layout style of
  - "Introduction"
  - "Risks (Maternal and Fetal)"
  - "Management Options (Prepregnancy, Prenatal, Labor and Delivery, Postnatal)"
  - "Summary of Management Options" Box
- The Summary of Management Options Box includes evidence-based scoring for each management strategy proposed. It illustrates how strong the evidence is for your actions
- The majority of the 82 chapters are essentially new contributions designed to address changes in the field:
  - The 14 new chapters are (Prepregnancy antecedents [1], Midpregnancy problems [6], Screening for fetal abnormality [7 and 8], Management of the abnormal screening test [9], Invasive procedures for prenatal diagnosis [10], Critical evaluation of prenatal fetal assessment methods [11], Intrauterine infection, preterm parturition, and the fetal inflammatory response syndrome [27], Pregnancy following transplantation [54], Psychiatric illness [56], Screening for prelabor membrane rupture and preterm labor [61], Shoulder dystocia [70], Perineal repair and pelvic floor injury [73], and Domestic violence [81]]
  - 29 chapters were rewritten by new authors to bring a fresh view [4, 5, 12, 15, 16, 19, 28, 29, 30, 31, 33, 38, 39, 42, 43, 45, 46, 48, 50, 52, 58, 66, 68, 69, 75, 77, 78, 79, 80]
  - The 39 remaining chapters were all extensively updated

As in prior editions, we have appreciated the comments of readers and reviewers and sought to respond to them wherever possible.

We hope you find the third edition of *High Risk Pregnancy: Management Options* an even more valuable but always practical reference manual for the management of problem pregnancies.

David K. James
Philip J. Steer
Carl P. Weiner
Bernie Gonik

CONTENTS

SECTION ONE

Pregnancy

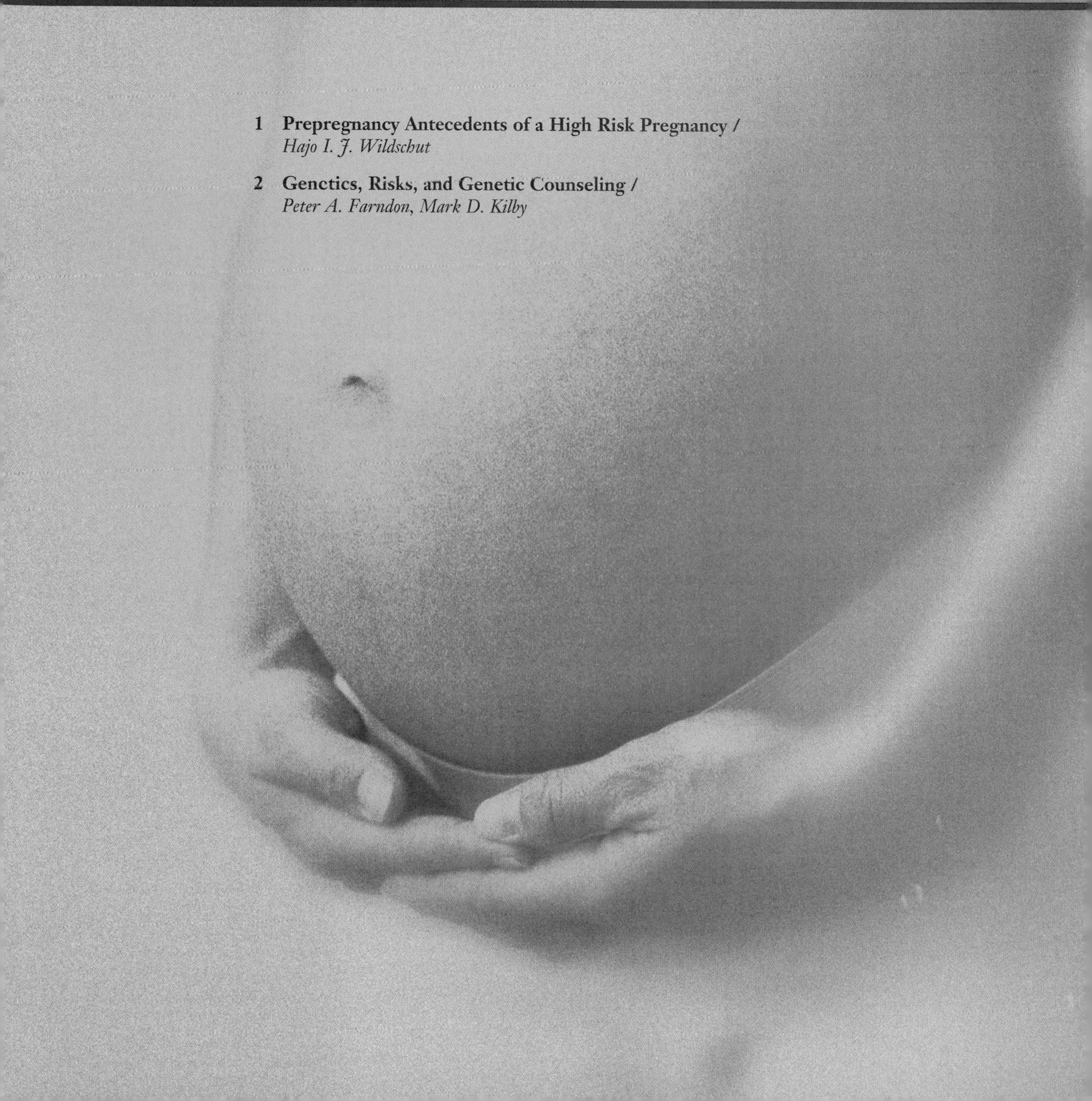

CHAPTER 1

Prepregnancy Antecedents of a High Risk Pregnancy

Hajo I.J. Wildschut

WHAT IS A HIGH RISK PREGNANCY?

Definition

In general, pregnancy should be considered a unique, physiologically normal episode in a woman's life. However, preexisting disease or unexpected illness of the mother or fetus can complicate the pregnancy. *Risk* is defined as the probability of an adverse outcome or a factor that increases this probability. A pregnancy is defined as *high risk* when the probability of an adverse outcome for the mother or child is increased over and above the baseline risk of that outcome among the general pregnant population (or reference population) by the presence of one or more ascertainable risk factors, or indicators. This classification does not take into consideration the magnitude of risk or the importance of the risk to the health outcome of the pregnant population at large.

The Concept of Risk

Risk is a reflection of the incidence of an adverse health outcome arising in a defined population during a given period. The magnitude of risk is usually expressed as a point estimate of probability (ranging from 0 to 1) or odds (ranging from 0 to + ∞ [infinity]) [Table 1–1].

Thus, for example, a risk of 20% of the occurrence of the target condition (e.g., incidence of a disease) equates to a probability (P) of 0.20 (1 of 5) or odds of 0.25 (the likelihood of one individual having an adverse outcome to four not having this outcome). Probability can be computed from odds by the following formula:

$$P \text{ (of the disease)} = \frac{\text{Odds (of the disease)}}{1 + \text{odds (of the disease)}}$$

Conversely, odds can be computed from probability by the following formula:

$$\text{Odds} = \frac{P}{1-P}$$

With lower values (<0.20), risk estimates based on probabilities approximate those based on odds (see Table 1–1).

The terms *relative risk* (or *risk ratio* [RR]) and *odds ratio* (OR) are alternative ways of expressing risk. RR is the likelihood of the target condition occurring in people exposed to a particular risk, compared with people who are not exposed.[1] It indicates how many more times likely exposed people are to have the target condition than nonexposed people. RRs are usually derived from prospective longitudinal studies. Case–control studies allow an estimate of risk as a result of exposure by assessing exposure among those who have been identified with the target condition and their controls. The OR is given by the ratio of the odds of exposure among those with the target condition (cases) and the odds of exposure among those without the target condition (controls). Thus, case–control studies measure the *prevalence*, not the *incidence*, of exposure among those with and without the outcome of interest. RR is not synonymous with OR, although for rare outcomes, these estimates approximate one another.[1] An RR or OR of 1 indicates no difference in the occurrence of the condition of interest between the two comparison groups (exposed and unexposed). An RR or OR of greater than 1 suggests that exposure is associated with increased risk of the target condition

TABLE 1–1

The Relation between Probability and Odds

PROBABILITY	ODDS
0.001	0.001
0.01	0.01
0.02	0.02
0.05	0.05
0.1	0.11
0.2	0.25
0.3	0.43
0.4	0.67
0.5	1
0.6	1.5
0.7	2.3
0.8	4
0.9	9
0.95	19
0.98	49
0.99	99
0.999	999

compared with nonexposure. Conversely, an RR or OR of less than 1 suggests that exposure is associated with decreased risk compared with nonexposure. In these contexts, however, the actual point estimation of risk should be considered together with the 95% confidence intervals. In epidemiology, a statistically significant difference between two groups can be shown only if the 95% confidence intervals do not include 1 (do not cross unity).

The importance of a specific risk factor for the incidence of the outcome of interest in a population is usually expressed as the *population-attributable risk* (i.e., the proportion of disease in a population that results from a specific risk to health). It also gives an indication of the proportion of incidence of disease that could be prevented by total elimination of that risk factor in the population (Fig. 1–1).[2]

Risk as a Proxy for Care

Focusing on risks to health is the key to preventing disease and injury. Over recent decades, the ability to predict and avert adverse reproductive health events has improved greatly. Women with high risk pregnancies can potentially benefit from increased care. The initial assessment of a woman's reproductive health risks may start well before pregnancy occurs (i.e., the preconception period). Ongoing assessment of a woman's health and that of her unborn child is the foundation of modern maternal and fetal care.

Preconception Health Care Model

Preconception care involves risk assessment, health promotion, and intervention.[3] Risk assessment includes questions about the woman's medical, obstetric, family, and genetic history; nutritional habits; drug use; environmental exposures; lifestyle; and social issues. Similar information is obtained about her partner.[4] The Appendix shows an example of a preconception questionnaire.

Primary care health professionals may be involved in providing preconception care, as may be obstetricians, midwives, nurses, clinical geneticists, and genetic counselors. The most common reasons for referral for preconception counseling include previous spontaneous abortion, chronic maternal disease, and previous fetal abnormality.[3,4]

Some women do not seek or receive preconception care. These include women with unplanned pregnancies and those without health insurance. Physicians are not always equipped to address the many time-intensive medical and social problems encountered in couples seeking preconception care.

Finally, few controlled trials show the effectiveness of preconception care (e.g., folic acid to prevent neural tube defects, normalization of blood glucose values in patients with diabetes). More research is needed in this area.

GENETIC AND CONSTITUTIONAL FACTORS

Genetic Factors

The enormous technologic progress in medical genetics in recent decades has enabled implementation of a novel form of prevention based on reproductive choice. The goal is to maximize the chances that individuals at increased risk for having affected offspring will have children free of the disorder. The prepregnancy management options for individuals who are at risk for genetic conditions are discussed in Chapter 2.

Ethnicity

Race and ethnicity are complex, controversial sociologic issues that are difficult to measure accurately. Race and ethnicity are often considered surrogate measures for standard of living and lifestyle.[5] However, both between and within ethnic populations, marked variations occur in cultural beliefs and practices, language, household structure, sexual behavior, contraceptive patterns, general health, perception of illness and disease, childbirth and child-rearing practices, postnatal customs, dietary habits, housing, education, employment, economic status, level of assimilation, stress, and access to health care services.[6–9] Some of these attributes have little to do with health or disease, whereas others may be important factors. In clinical research, the terms *race* and *ethnicity* are often defined inadequately, if at all. Therefore, epidemiologic associations with health problems should be interpreted cautiously. For example, for public health considerations, information about race or ethnicity could be relevant for the identification of specific health problems and medical needs.

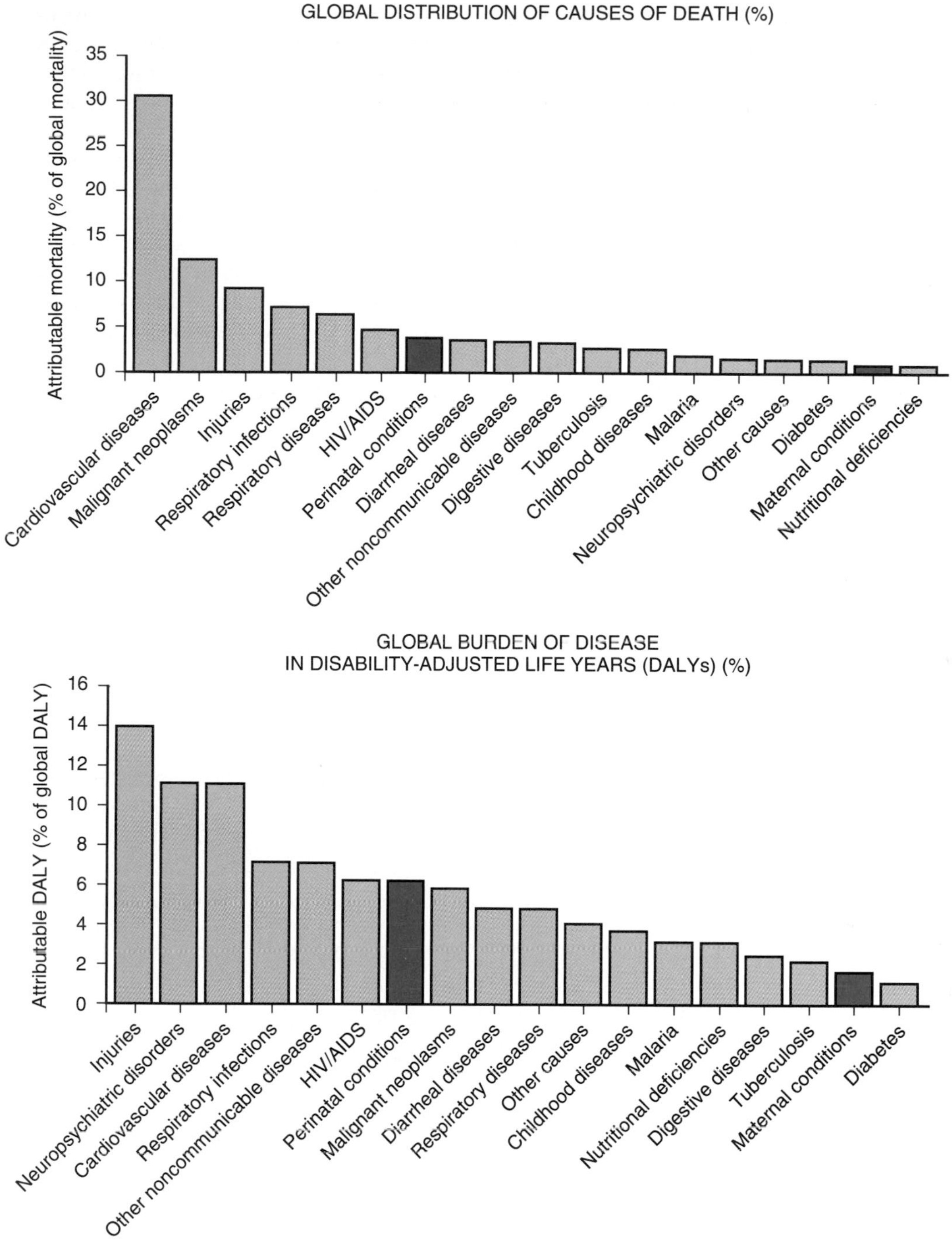

FIGURE 1–1
Attributable mortality (*A*) and burden of disease (*B*) as a result of leading global risk factors. The estimated relative mortality and disease burden are shown in terms of disability-adjusted life years (DALY) for each risk factor considered individually. These risks act in part through other risks as well as jointly with other risks. Consequently, the burden caused by groups of risk factors is usually less than the sum of individual risks. (Reproduced with permission.)

Risks

Ethnicity is one of the factors that is most strongly associated with low birth weight.[8–12] Low birth weight is closely related to infant mortality and childhood morbidity rates.[13] In the United States, preterm birth rather than growth restriction is implicated as the most important cause of low birth weight in black women.[12,14] Given the high rates of preterm delivery, crude survival rates for black infants are less favorable than those for white infants.[12,15,16] The biologic explanation for the high preterm delivery rate among black women is unclear.

Apart from preterm delivery, newborns designated as white and black may show different patterns of intrauterine growth.[17,18] For example, at term, black infants are on average smaller than white infants.[18,19] Moreover, the average duration of gestation in black women is slightly shorter than in white women.[18] It has been argued that birth weight distribution is an intrinsic genetic feature of ethnicity, just like the sex of the infant. Hence, for each ethnic group, different norms for gestational age and birth weight distributions should be applied.[20] Others, however, refute this assumption by claiming that ethnic disparities in birth weight distribution are most likely the result of disparities in maternal health, socioeconomic status, and prenatal care.[10,15,17,21]

It has been suggested that birth weight–specific mortality in preterm black infants is lower than that in preterm white infants. Wilcox and Russell[19,20] postulated that this finding is based on an artifact. They stated that over the whole spectrum of adjusted birth weight, black infants are less likely to survive the perinatal period than white infants. The excess birth weight–specific mortality in black infants may be compounded by a failure to seek or receive optimal medical care.[21]

Many diseases and problems that occur during pregnancy have both ethnic and geographic distributions. The risks are summarized in Table 1–2.

Female circumcision is still practiced in some parts of Africa, in particular the Horn of Africa, and may affect childbirth.[22]

Uterine fibroids occur more often in black women than in white women.[23] Nonengagement of the fetal head late in pregnancy is not uncommon in black primigravidae.[24] The available data on ethnic differences in the frequency of dysfunctional labor are inconclusive. Differences in duration of labor may be attributed to a wide range of confounding variables, including maternal age, stature, birth weight of the infant, poor communication, and unfavorable sociocultural circumstances.[23,25,26]

Management Options

Information, screening, and appropriate counseling services should be made available for communities that are considered at risk for specific diseases (see Table 1–2 and other relevant chapters).

PRENATAL

Communication is often a problem because of language barriers. Video displays and informative pamphlets or

TABLE 1–2

Risks in Pregnancy Associated with Certain Ethnic Groups

ETHNIC GROUP	RISKS
Mediterranean islands, parts of middle East, Southeast Asia, and parts of the Indian subcontinent	Beta-thalassemias: Minor: Anemia in pregnancy, treated with oral iron and folate, but not parental iron Major: Rare to survive to reproductive age, but those who do often have pelvic bony deformities and problems with labor and delivery; also iron overload with subsequent hepatic, endocrinologic, and myocardial damage Major/minor: Possible risk of inheriting the disease, a requiring prenatal counseling and diagnosis Alpha-thalassemias: Minor: Usually asymptomatic Major: Rare, but a spectrum of presentation: in adults, usually manifests as a hemolytic anemia of variable severity Major/minor: Possible risk of inheriting the disease, requiring prenatal counseling and diagnosis; homozygous alpha-thalassemias in the fetus can manifest as hydrops fetalis and associated severe preeclampsia in the mother
Afro-Caribbean, Mediterranean, Middle East, India	Sickling disorders (especially HbSS, HbSC): Maternal: Infection, sickling crises, preeclampsia, renal compromise, jaundice; although HbSC tends to be a milder disease (Hb levels usually within normal limits), it can cause massive sickling crises if the diagnosis has not been made; HbAS (carrier state) mothers are rarely at risk for sickling crises with, for example, anoxia, dehydration, or acidosis Fetus: Possible risk of inheriting the disease, requiring prenatal counseling and diagnosis; growth restriction is a risk with HbSS and HbSC
Mediterranean, American Blacks	Glucose-6-phosphate dehydrogenase deficiency: Mother: Hemolytic anemia Fetus: Risk of inheriting the disease, requiring prenatal counseling and diagnosis; fetal hydrops
Far East	Hepatitis B (chronic carriers): Risk of transmission to the fetus or neonate and health care workers
Africa, Caribbean, Hawaii	HIV infection: Risk to the mother of symptomatic infection; risk to the fetus and health care workers of acquiring the infection
Africa (especially Horn of Africa)	Female circumcision: Problems with vaginal delivery (dystocia, trauma, hemorrhage)
Developing countries	Varied effects of endemic infection on the mother or fetus

HbSC, hemoglobin SC; HbSS, hemoglobin SS.

brochures written in several languages should be made available.[27] Standard information should include guidelines for lifestyle and nutrition as well as preparation for parturition and parenthood, preferably in keeping with sociocultural features of the relevant ethnic communities.[27] The use of interpreters, either in person or by telephone, is advisable for dealing with specific problems.[27]

Once prenatal care has been initiated, women at risk for specific diseases, such as hemoglobinopathies, may be selected for further testing or treatment.[28,29] In parous women, it is important to obtain all necessary information about the course and outcome of previous pregnancies. Immunization status should be checked, and[30] fetal growth should be monitored.[8,10–12]

LABOR AND DELIVERY

The continuous presence of a supportive female companion during labor and delivery benefits maternal well-being by improving her emotional status, shortening labor, and decreasing the need for medical intervention.[31] Psychosocial support may also improve mother–infant bonding. It is unlikely that ethnicity in itself affects the duration of labor and delivery.

POSTNATAL

Breastfeeding should be encouraged.[32] Contraceptive advice should take into account individual sociocultural norms and values.[33,34]

CONCLUSIONS

- Large variations occur in health care coverage and reproductive outcome among different racial and ethnic groups.[5]
- The reasons for differences in pregnancy outcome between ethnic groups are not clear, although social environment, age, parity, and genetic and constitutional factors may play a role.[34]
- Several diseases show clear ethnic differences among pregnant women. These include genetic defects, such as the hereditary hemoglobinopathies; medical disorders, such as chronic hypertension; and specific conditions acquired in endemic areas, such as malaria, AIDS, and tuberculosis.[28,29]
- Each disease or condition requires a separate approach in pregnant women (see Table 1–2 and the Summary of Management Options).

SUMMARY OF MANAGEMENT OPTIONS
Pregnancy in Women from Different Ethnic Backgrounds

Management Options	Quality of Evidence	Strength of Recommendation	References
Prepregnancy			
Provide education, screening, and counseling for communities at specific risk.	III	B	28
Prenatal			
Overcome language and cultural barriers.	IV	C	27
Offer screening and counseling where specific risk exists.	III	B	29
Offer prenatal diagnosis if appropriate.	III	B	28
Provide maternal and fetal surveillance for any specific risk.	IIa	B	8,10–12
Labor and Delivery			
Offer the continuous presence of a supportive companion during labor and delivery.	Ia	A	31
Postnatal			
Encourage breast-feeding.	IV	C	32
Offer contraceptive advice, taking account of individual sociocultural norms and values.	III	B	33,34

ENVIRONMENTAL FACTORS

Prescribed Drugs

The risks and management options for women who take prescribed drugs before pregnancy are discussed in Chapter 35.

Drug Abuse, Cigarette Smoking, and Alcohol

The risks and management options for women who abuse drugs, cigarettes, and alcohol before pregnancy are discussed in Chapter 34.

Vaccines

The risks and management options for individuals who receive vaccines are discussed later in this chapter (see "Air Travel during Pregnancy").

Ionizing Radiation (See also Chapter 53)

Definition

Ionizing radiation is any radiation capable of displacing electrons from atoms or molecules, thereby producing ions. Examples are α-, β-, γ-, and x-rays. Sources of radiation are given in Figure 1–2.[35]

Risks

Two categories of biologic effects of ionizing radiation are described, deterministic and stochastic.[36,37] Deterministic effects pertain to a decrease in or loss of organ function as a result of cell damage or cell killing (apoptosis).[37] Loss of organ function could lead to fetal malformation, mental retardation, or death. For these effects to occur, threshold doses exist. Fetal exposures of less than 100 mGy (historically termed "10 rad") do not increase the incidence of fetal malformation at birth. Doses of more than 100 mGy should be evaluated in the context of the type of radiation and the time of exposure relative to fetal development and may be associated with impaired cognitive development (IQ).[36] The risks of fetal growth restriction and major structural malformation seem small.[36] The 1986 nuclear reactor accident at Chernobyl did not result in a detectable change in the prevalence of major congenital anomalies in neighboring European countries, despite exposure to relatively high radiation doses (200–700 mSv) in the first year after the disaster.[38] Radiation doses greater than 500 mGy result in a significant risk of central nervous system damage, with severe mental retardation, especially when the fetus is exposed 8 to 15 weeks after conception.

Stochastic effects are those that result from radiation changes in cells that retain their ability to divide.[36,37] These modified cells sometimes initiate malignant transformation of a cell that eventually leads to clinically overt cancer. The period between initiation and manifestation of the disease may extend from a few years (e.g., leukemia) to several decades (e.g., colon and liver cancer). In addition, genetic effects may be initiated as a result of irradiation of germ cells. For stochastic effects, no threshold doses are assumed. The probability of their occurrence is believed to be proportional to the dose. Therefore, the probability of tumor induction should be reduced by keeping the dose as low as possible. The estimated mortality risk from radiation-induced cancer in childhood (0–15 years) is 0.06% per 10 mGy.[39]

Because of the low level of radiation exposure, prenatal exposure to ionizing radiation from diagnostic procedures is not associated with an increased risk of adverse pregnancy outcome in terms of perinatal death, congenital abnormalities, or mental retardation (see Table 1–3).[40]

The stochastic effects of radiodiagnostic examinations are typically very limited. For this reason, termination of pregnancy is not warranted when the mother is exposed to diagnostic procedures involving ionizing radiation.[40] Special attention should be given to nuclear examination

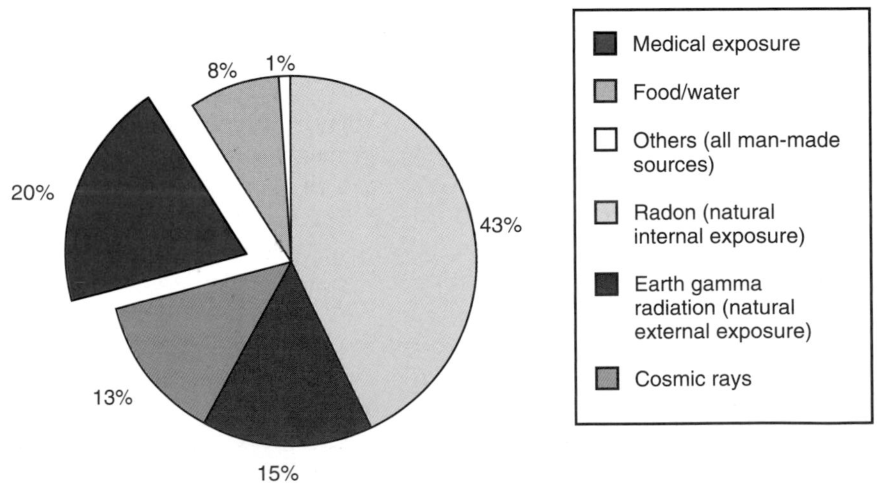

FIGURE 1–2
Sources and distribution of average radiation exposure in the world population. (From http://www.who.int/ionizing_radiation/en, with permission.)

TABLE 1–3
Fetal Radiation Exposure after Diagnostic Procedures

EXAMINATION	FETAL EQUIVALENT DOSE (mSv)*	
	MEAN DOSE	MAXIMUM DOSE
Conventional X-rays		
Abdomen	1.4	4.2
Thorax	<0.01	<0.01
Intravenous urography	1.7	10
Lumbar spine	1.7	10
Pelvis	1.1	4
Skull	<0.01	<0.01
Thoracic spine	<0.01	<0.01
Barium meal	1.1	5.8
Barium enema	6.8	24
Computed Tomography		
Abdomen	8.0	49
Thorax	0.06	0.96
Head	<0.005	<0.005
Lumbar spine	2.4	8.6
Pelvis	25	79
Nuclear Medicine		
^{99m}Tc bone scan	3.3	4.6
^{99m}Tc lung perfusion	0.2	0.4
^{99m}Tc kidney scan	1.5	4.0
^{99m}Tc thyroid scan	0.7	1.6
^{99m}Tc brain scan	4.3	6.5

*The estimated exposure to background radiation in the general population is on average 2 millisieverts (mSv) per year. The sievert is the unit for equivalent dose, which is the average absorbed dose in an organ or tissue multiplied by a radiation weighting factor. The unit for absorbed dose is the gray (Gy) [100 rad]. For almost all radiation used in medicine, the radiation weighting factor equals unity, making Sv and Gy numerically equal. ^{99m}Tc, radiopharmaceutical labeled technetium-99m.
(From www.europa.eu.int/comm/environment/radprot)

with radiopharmaceuticals and radionuclides. In nuclear medicine, unlike x-ray procedures, the woman may be a source of radiation for some time after the examination. For this reason, in certain circumstances, the woman should be advised to avoid pregnancy for an appropriate period after radionuclide administration.[41] Prenatal radiation exposure should be recorded to facilitate estimation of the fetal dose.

In a therapeutic setting, however, high doses of radiation during pregnancy (>100–200 mGy) are associated with an increased risk of impaired cognitive development (IQ).[36] The fetus is particularly vulnerable to the stochastic effects of high doses of ionizing radiation when exposed 8 to 15 weeks after conception. During this period, exposure to ionizing radiation at a dose of 1000 mGy (1 Gy) is associated with a 30-point decrease in IQ.[40]

In young women who have been exposed to radiation therapy below the diaphragm, reproductive problems include the risk of ovarian failure and significantly impaired development of the uterus. The magnitude of risk is related to the radiation field, total dose, and fractionation schedule.[42] Irradiation of either parental gonad in the preconception period is not associated with an increased risk of genetic defects, congenital malformations, or childhood or adulthood cancer.[43]

Management Options

RADIODIAGNOSTIC EXAMINATIONS

- Every woman of childbearing potential who is undergoing a radiodiagnostic examination should be explicitly asked, orally or in writing, whether she might be pregnant or have missed a period. If there is any uncertainty about pregnancy, the planned examination should be postponed or the woman should be treated as if she were pregnant.[36,40]
- There is no need to apply the 10-day rule (i.e., exposure during the first 10 days after the onset of the last menstrual period), unless the radiodiagnostic examination involves radionuclides or radiopharmaceuticals.[40]
- If the woman is pregnant, special attention should be given to the justification and urgency of the radiodiagnostic examination.[36,41,44]
- In pregnant women, alternative diagnostic methods, such as ultrasound or magnetic resonance imaging (MRI), should be considered.[36,40]
- Reduction of the radiation dose to the fetus may be achieved by lead-shielding the abdomen, where

feasible.[36,40] Moreover, reduction of radiation to the fetus can be achieved by adapting radiodiagnostic techniques and taking fewer images.[36,40,44]

- Every woman who is undergoing a nuclear medicine examination should be asked, orally or in writing, whether she is breastfeeding.[40]
- When a pregnant woman is undergoing a nuclear medicine examination, the dose of radionuclide is kept as low as possible without sacrificing radiographic information. The commonly administered radiopharmaceuticals used for lung, gallbladder, kidney, bone, and bleeding scans are labeled with technetium-99m. All deliver whole fetal doses of less than 5 mGy (see Table 1–3).[44]

RADIATION THERAPY

- The presence of pregnancy should be evaluated when radiation therapy is considered in women of reproductive age.[40]
- Appropriate lead shields should be used to protect the gonads of patients undergoing radiation therapy.[36,40]
- If the patient is pregnant, she must be involved in the discussion and decision about radiation therapy.[40]
- Termination of pregnancy should be considered if the radiation dose would lead to severe deterministic effects or a high probability of stochastic effects.[40]
- Patients who have had radiation therapy should not be discouraged from having children.[40]

SUMMARY OF MANAGEMENT OPTIONS

Radiodiagnostic Examinations

Management Options	Quality of Evidence	Strength of Recommendation	References
Prepregnancy			
Postpone planned examination if pregnancy is unconfirmed.	IV	C	40
Prenatal			
If the patient is pregnant, explain the justification for and urgency of radiodiagnostic examination.	III	B	36,41
In a pregnant patient, keep the dose of radionuclide as low as possible without compromising the radiographic examination.	IV	C	40,44
Postnatal			
Ask every woman of reproductive age who is scheduled for nuclear medicine examination whether she is breastfeeding.	IV	C	40

Magnetic Resonance Imaging

Risks

MRI is a powerful imaging tool that does not expose patients to ionizing radiation. MRI requires powerful magnetic fields and a radiofrequency pulse to produce a diagnostic image. Under most circumstances, these fields do not appear to pose a health or safety risk.[45] Although generally considered safe, MRI has some maternal safety issues, including the effects of high magnetic fields on metallic biomedical implants or other metallic foreign bodies.[46] Foreign metallic materials embedded within patients can have ferromagnetic properties that present a potential hazard in the strong fields associated with MRI, precluding MRI examination in these patients. Other hazards of MRI include the potential side effects of contrast agents, anxiety, claustrophobia, and temporary hearing loss as a result of acoustic noise generated by MRI.

SUMMARY OF MANAGEMENT OPTIONS

Magnetic Resonance Imaging

Management Options	Quality of Evidence	Strength of Recommendation	References
Prepregnancy			
Postpone a planned examination if pregnancy is unconfirmed.	IV	C	47

SUMMARY OF MANAGEMENT OPTIONS

Magnetic Resonance Imaging *(Continued)*

Management Options	Quality of Evidence	Strength of Recommendation	References
Prepregnancy			
Evaluate each patient with a written questionnaire followed by oral questioning before imaging to identify those with ferromagnetic foreign bodies or implants anywhere in the body that are electrically, magnetically, or mechanically activated.	IV	C	46
Maintain a high state of vigilance to prevent iatrogenic burns and injuries from ferromagnetic missiles.	IV	C	46
Prenatal			
Magnetic resonance imaging (MRI) is not recommended during the first trimester.	IV	C	48
The use of contrast material for MRI is not recommended in pregnancy.	IV	C	48
Ultrasonography is the initial imaging modality of choice for the evaluation of obstetric patients. In limited cases, however, when the results of ultrasonography are indistinct, MRI may be a clinically useful adjuvant for diagnostic evaluation. Indications for the complementary use of diagnostic MRI in pregnancy include the evaluation of adnexal masses, hydroureteronephrosis, placenta accreta, and fetal abnormalities, in particular those involving the central nervous system.	III	B	47–50

Ultrasound

Risks

Ultrasound has become a widely accepted and valuable diagnostic tool in standard clinical practice. Most ultrasound machines in obstetrics use phased-array real-time technology with a brightness-mode (B-mode) display. Although the potential biophysical effects of ultrasound, such as tissue warming and cavitation, are well established, diagnostic ultrasound in medicine is considered safe.[51,52] As to diagnostic ultrasound in pregnancy, there have been no reports of potential harmful effects in the offspring, other than a few studies showing a statistically significant association of ultrasound and left-handedness in male offspring.[53,54] It is unlikely that this association is the result of brain damage because there is no association between ultrasound exposure in pregnancy and other indicators of brain damage (i.e., impaired motor or speech development, impaired school performance, visual disturbances, or hearing loss).[55] In recent years, there has been a trend to use new diagnostic ultrasound techniques, such as color flow imaging, power Doppler, and pulsed Doppler. These techniques require higher acoustic exposures than those used in B- and M-modes, with pulsed Doppler associated with the highest levels. In pulsed Doppler ultrasound, the beam is focused onto a small volume and kept stationary so that the same tissues are insonated throughout the examination, thereby maximizing the heating effects. Data from animal studies show that pulsed Doppler ultrasound can produce significant thermal effects, particularly near bone.[52] To ensure the continued safe use of diagnostic ultrasound in medicine, modern obstetric ultrasound machines are subject to output regulation only in the United States.[56,57] Ultrasound machines with on-screen displays of "thermal index" and "mechanical index" encourage the ultrasonographer to protect the fetus or embryo from potential harmful levels of acoustic exposure. The thermal and mechanical output indicators, however, do not take account extraneous factors, such as dwell time, examination time, and patient temperature. Hence, thermal index and mechanical index are not perfect indicators of the risks of bioeffects to the fetus, but should be accepted as the most practical and understandable methods of estimating the potential for such risks.[51]

Management Options

For the safe use of diagnostic ultrasound in medicine, the following international recommendations and guidelines are advocated.[52–58]

B- AND M-MODES

Based on scientific evidence of ultrasonically induced biologic effects, there is no reason to withhold B- or M-mode scanning for any clinical application, including the routine clinical scanning of every woman during pregnancy.

DOPPLER FOR FETAL HEART MONITORING

Because low power levels are used for fetal heart rate monitoring (cardiotocograph, CTG), the use of this modality, even for extended periods, is not contraindicated on safety grounds.

DOPPLER MODES (COLOR FLOW IMAGING, POWER DOPPLER, AND PULSED DOPPLER)

Exposures used for Doppler modes are higher than those used for B- and M-modes. There is considerable overlap in the ranges of exposure that may be used for color flow imaging, power Doppler, and pulsed Doppler techniques. The clinical user should be aware that pulsed Doppler at maximum machine outputs and color flow imaging with small color boxes have the greatest potential for biologic effects.

USE OF DOPPLER STUDIES IN THE FIRST TRIMESTER

The embryonic period is particularly sensitive to external influences. Until further data are available, studies using pulsed or color Doppler ultrasound should be carried out with careful control of output levels and exposure times. With increasing mineralization of the fetal bone as the fetus develops, the possibility of heating fetal bone increases. The user should prudently limit exposure of critical structures, such as the fetal skull and spine, during Doppler studies.[52–59]

In general, the informed use of Doppler ultrasound is not contraindicated. However, at the maximum machine output settings, significant thermal effects at bone surfaces cannot be excluded. The user is advised to use the exposure information provided by the manufacturer (e.g., displayed safety indices) to determine the highest output conditions and to act prudently to limit exposure of critical structures, including bone, and regions, including gas. If an online display is not available, care should be taken to minimize exposure times.[52–59]

Caution should be exercised in febrile patients. Doppler ultrasound might present an additional embryonic and fetal risk.

Care should be taken to use the minimum output that will obtain the required diagnostic information and to minimize the duration of pulsed Doppler examinations in pregnancy.[57]

TRANSVAGINAL ULTRASONOGRAPHY

In the absence of long-term, large-scale, follow-up studies after first-trimester transvaginal ultrasound exposure, care is required in the application of transvaginal ultrasonography in early pregnancy. It should be performed only for valid medical reasons that benefit the mother or the embryo.[58]

NONMEDICAL USE IN PREGNANCY

The use of two-dimensional or three-dimensional ultrasound only to view the fetus, obtain a picture, or determine fetal sex, without a medical indication, is inappropriate and contrary to responsible medical practice. Although there are no confirmed biologic effects on patients caused by exposures from current diagnostic ultrasound instruments, such biologic effects may be identified in the future. Thus, ultrasound should be used prudently to provide medical benefit to the patient.[59]

NEW DEVELOPMENTS

Echo-contrast agents can be useful in diagnostic ultrasound, may decrease the threshold for cavitation. As a consequence, the use of echo-contrast agents may change the risk-to-benefit ratio substantially in various clinical applications. Given the increased use of ultrasound, the introduction of new techniques, and a broadening of the medical indications for ultrasound examinations, continuous vigilance is essential to ensure its continued safe use.[58]

SUMMARY OF MANAGEMENT OPTIONS
Ultrasonography

Management Options	Quality of Evidence	Strength of Recommendation	References
Prepregnancy			
The use of echo-contrast agents may change the risk-to-benefit ratio substantially in various clinical applications. Given the introduction of new techniques and a broadening of the medical indications for ultrasound examinations, continuous vigilance is essential to ensure its continued safe use.	IV	C	52–58
Prenatal			
There is no reason to withhold B- or M-mode scanning for any clinical application, including routine clinical scanning of every woman during pregnancy.	Ia	A	52–58

SUMMARY OF MANAGEMENT OPTIONS
Ultrasonography *(Continued)*

Management Options	Quality of Evidence	Strength of Recommendation	References
Prenatal			
Use ultrasound prudently to provide medical benefit to the patient.	IV	C	59
Transvaginal ultrasonography in early pregnancy should be performed only for medical reasons to benefit the mother or embryo.	IV	C	52–58
Limit Doppler ultrasound exposure of critical structures, such as the fetal skull or spine.	IV	C	52–58
Use cautiously in febrile patients. Doppler ultrasound may present an additional embryonic or fetal risk.	IV	C	52–58
Use the minimum output to obtain the required diagnostic information to minimize the duration of pulsed Doppler examinations in pregnancy.	IV	C	52–58
Fetal heart monitoring (cardiotocography, CTG) is not contraindicated, on safety grounds, even when it is to be used for extended periods.	III	B	52–58

Video Display Terminals

Several studies show that exposure to the magnetic fields emitted by video display terminals does not constitute an appreciable risk to the reproductive health of women or a risk to their children.[60,61]

Environmental Health Hazards

From the public health point of view, environmental health hazards can be categorized into five distinct groups: chemical, physical, biologic, mechanical, and psychosocial. Their effects on pregnancy are discussed in other chapters (e.g., infection, prescribed drugs, drugs of abuse).

It is difficult to ascertain the clinical importance of each of these environmental influences on reproductive health. The adverse effect on pregnancy outcome is dependent on the prevalence of exposure and the dose and timing during pregnancy. Information of this kind is often lacking. Furthermore, confounding factors and the interaction of more than one factor hamper the interpretation of potentially adverse effects of a particular environmental agent on reproductive health. For example, increased genetic susceptibility of the individual and the use of medication could mediate the adverse effects of these agents. Moreover, the assessment of a cause-and-effect relationship is hampered because of a considerable time gap between exposure to the environmental risk factor and outcome in terms of disease, disability, or death.

Chemicals

Polychlorinated Biphenyls

Polychlorinated biphenyls (PCBs) have been produced commercially since the late 1920s. They have been used in pesticides, surface coatings, inks, adhesives, flame retardants, and paints.[62] Because PCBs resist both acids and alkali and are relatively heat-stable, they have been used in dielectric fluids in transformers and capacitors. Further environmental contamination may occur from disposal of old electrical equipment containing PCBs. Many countries have severely restricted or banned the production of PCBs.

Highly chlorinated PCB congeners are generally persistent in the environment. The general population is exposed to PCBs in the air, drinking water, and food, particularly meat, fish, and poultry. They are rapidly absorbed from the intestinal tract and distribute to and accumulate in the liver. They also cross the placenta and are excreted in breast milk. Detectable concentrations of PCBs have been found in amniotic fluid, placenta, and fetal tissue samples. Breast-fed infants can have blood levels greater than those of their mothers. Formula is free of PCBs. Much concern exists that PCBs transferred to the fetus across the placenta may induce long-lasting neurologic damage. Recent data from a Dutch cohort study among 418 infants showed that prenatal exposure to PCBs has subtle negative effects on the neurologic and cognitive development of the child up to 6 years of age. Half of the infants were fully breast-fed for at least 6 weeks. Despite higher PCB exposures from breast milk, breast-feeding had a beneficial effect on cognitive development in this cohort of infants.[63] Hence, the beneficial effects of breast-feeding outweigh the potentially adverse effects of PCB exposure from breast milk. Epidemiologic studies suggest that exposure to PCBs is associated with an increased risk of cancers of the digestive system, notably the liver, and malignant melanoma.[62] However, in many studies, the limitation of exposure data, the inconsistency of results, and the presence of confounding factors preclude the identification of a true causal relationship.

Dioxins

Dioxins are a heterogeneous mixture of chlorinated dibenzo-*p*-dioxin and dibenzofuran congeners. The main sources of dioxins are emissions of industrial and municipal incineration processes. Dioxins accumulate in the food chain, and human exposure occurs mainly through contaminated food.[64] Few data are available on the effects of dioxins on female reproductive health. In animal models, dioxin has an antiestrogenic effect. Environmental chemicals have been implicated in the temporal decline in the age of onset of puberty, the development of polycystic ovarian syndrome, and shortened lactation. The prevalence of male reproductive disorders, such as cryptorchisms and hypospadias, need more careful study, particularly because they are linked to testicular cancer and show temporal changes in many countries. The effects of environmental chemicals on sperm quality are inconsistent. Because of methodologic shortcomings in epidemiologic studies, it is unknown whether dioxins affect spontaneous abortion rates or fetal growth restriction.

Pesticides

Pesticides, including fungicides, herbicides, insecticides, and rodenticides, are a reproductive health concern in many countries. They are often found in commercially available food products. However, the almost universal exposure to low concentrations of these compounds makes it very difficult to determine the effect of pesticides on the incidence of fetal abnormalities. Occupational exposure to pesticides has been implicated in increased birth defects rates.[65,66] Birth defects, however, are mostly multifactorial, meaning that other risk factors may also play an important role.

SOCIOECONOMIC STATUS

The importance of maternal social factors on the health and well-being of the offspring has been recognized for a long time. For example, infant mortality is closely associated with social inequality. Large differences in social conditions still exist. Caution should be exercised in interpreting studies of the effect of social conditions on pregnancy outcome. These include variations in definitions and practices associated with time and geographic area, availability of reliable data, and interpretation of the findings.[67–69]

The concept of *social index* is not simple. Various measures of social status are used, some of which tend to be crude and meaningless. In England and Wales, for example, the maternal social class index is traditionally derived from the Registrar General's Classification, which is based on the occupation of the father of the child (Table 1–4).

TABLE 1–4

Social Class by Occupation of the Father

CATEGORY	OCCUPATION
I	Higher professionals
II	Other professionals, including those in managerial positions
IIIa	Skilled workers, nonmanual
IIIb	Skilled workers, manual
IV	Semiskilled workers
V	Unskilled workers

Although there is a strong association between social class, thus defined, and infant mortality, this observation does not explain why some infants die and others do not. Other methods of categorization of socioeconomic status include those based on ranking of educational attainment, income, type of health care coverage, employment profile, legitimacy, family affluence, and household characteristics.[69] Accurate information of this kind is usually not readily available.

Social risk factors, however defined, are descriptive rather than explanatory. Social disadvantage in itself is unlikely to have a direct causal effect on the outcome of pregnancy.[70] Socioeconomic status should be considered merely a risk indicator, identifying high risk groups within the population.[71] Social adversity probably represents a wide range of behavioral, environmental, medical, and psychological factors that are causally related to pregnancy outcome, some of which are more amenable to intervention than others.[10,72–74] In this context, it is assumed that women of higher socioeconomic status have better financial, educational, and medical resources than women of lower socioeconomic status. Many social risk factors are interrelated. In the absence of logically structured multivariate analyses, the independence of their effects cannot be established.[17] In scientific research, correlations with socioeconomic status should be the impetus for further investigation, rather than the endpoint of an analysis.[75]

Risks

Lower socioeconomic status is associated with an increased risk of various adverse pregnancy outcomes, including perinatal mortality, preterm birth, and low birth weight. Smoking has been suggested as the key factor underlying socioeconomic differences in low birth weight and infant mortality.[69,76–78] Differences in care along the social strata may also account for some of the extra risks. The contribution of poor nutrition is discussed in the next section.

Management Options

Prenatal

Socially disadvantaged women are less likely to seek prenatal care and also have more pregnancy complications.

Some claim that apart from recognizing the increased risk associated with socioeconomic disadvantage, there is little to do in terms of prevention. Social support, however, benefits women psychologically, although the effect of social intervention on mean birth weight, low birth weight, and preterm delivery is limited.[31] From a public health point of view, the greatest reduction in adverse pregnancy outcome may be anticipated from prenatal services directed at socially disadvantaged women.[79,80] In this respect, widespread health education and serious antismoking measures are needed.[81]

Labor and Delivery

Intrapartum management need not be substantially modified if no other risk factors are present.

Postnatal

Women of higher socioeconomic status tend to breastfeed more often and longer than women of lower socioeconomic status. Breastfeeding should be encouraged and social support provided, when indicated.[82] Contraception must be discussed when needed.[34]

CONCLUSIONS

- The maternal environment has a pronounced effect on birth weight and pregnancy outcome.
- Knowledge of a pregnant woman's socioeconomic status does not provide direct information about the circumstances in which she lives. Differences in socioeconomic status may reflect differences in material conditions in life and differences in behavior (e.g., smoking habits). Caution must be exercised in the extrapolation of associations between socioeconomic status, however defined, and pregnancy outcome, because the mechanisms underlying these associations are often unclear.
- Clinically, it is difficult to alleviate the effects of social deprivation. Social support may improve the patient's emotional well-being, but there is no evidence that it has any effect on any other outcome variable.[31]

SUMMARY OF MANAGEMENT OPTIONS
Pregnancy in Women of Low Socioeconomic Background

Stage of Pregnancy	Management Options	Quality of Evidence	Strength of Recommendation	References
Prepregnancy				
	Recommend health education measures specifically directed at smoking cessation and family planning.	Ib	A	81
Prenatal				
	Encourage patients to seek early antenatal care.	III	B	39
	Provide specific and directed social support.	Ia	A	31
	Look for clinical evidence of poor fetal growth.	III	B	76
Labor and Delivery				
	No additional measures are needed on the basis of adverse socioeconomic factors alone.	–	–	–
Postnatal				
	Encourage breastfeeding.	Ib	A	82
	Provide specific and directed social support.	Ib	A	80
	Discuss contraception.	III	B	34

NUTRITIONAL FACTORS

Risks

General

Nutritional conditions during key periods in early pregnancy are believed to be of major importance in determining health in later life.[83,84] The long-term effects on adult health, such as type 2 diabetes, hypertension, and coronary heart disease, are considered consequences of fetal programming. This describes the phenomenon whereby a stimulus or an injury at a critical period in early fetal life can produce lasting changes in physiology and metabolism.[83,85] The central concept is that despite current levels of nutrition in western countries, intrauterine nutrition is suboptimal because the nutrients available are unbalanced or their delivery is constrained by changes in the structure and function of the placenta.[83] Evidence suggests that after an intrauterine lesion, regulatory mechanisms may maintain homeostasis for many years, until further damage, caused by age, obesity, or other effects, initiates a self-perpetuating cycle of progressive functional loss.[83] Follow-up studies of the war-induced Dutch famine of 1944–1945 showed a relative increase in placental weight in infants whose mothers' nutrition was compromised around conception or in the first trimester of pregnancy.[86] The increase in the placenta weight-to-birth weight ratio is interpreted as a compensatory mechanism after reduced caloric intake in early pregnancy.[87,88] An increased ratio is also seen with maternal anemia, tobacco use in pregnancy, and births at high altitude.[87] Fetal cardiovascular adaptations are a recognized feature of intrauterine growth restriction and divert nutrient-rich, highly oxygenated blood to spare the growth of the brain and other critical organs. Furthermore, reduced availability of micronutrients may affect fetal body composition. The relative amounts of fetal bone and lean and fat mass influence the risk of adult obesity and type 2 diabetes.[83] Placental size also has an important effect on fetal endocrinology and metabolism, with lasting effects on health in later life. When undernutrition during early development is followed by improved nutrition, many animals and plants have accelerated, or compensatory, growth.[83] Compensatory growth has costs, however; in animals, these risks may include reduced life span.[84] It has been reported in humans that undernutrition and small size at birth followed by rapid childhood growth may lead to cardiovascular disease and type 2 diabetes in later life.[83]

Caffeine

Caffeine has been a controversial topic in pregnancy nutrition for more than a decade. A 1980 study by the U.S. Food and Drug Administration (FDA) found that caffeine, when fed to pregnant rats, caused birth defects and delayed skeletal development in their offspring. At that time, although the human implications were unknown, the FDA advised pregnant women to eliminate caffeine from their diets.[89] Subsequent epidemiologic studies showed inconsistent results. Some studies found significant effects of caffeine on pregnancy outcomes, whereas others did not. Risks associated with maternal caffeine consumption during pregnancy and perinatal outcomes have proved difficult to estimate. Caffeine consumption is difficult to measure, and substantial misclassification occurs when consumption does not account for the actual cup size used. Moreover, cigarette smoking may confound the association of caffeine consumption with pregnancy outcomes.[89]

Vitamins

The current reference daily intakes (RDI) for vitamins are summarized in Table 1–5.[90] Pregnancy may increase vitamin requirements. Mechanisms underlying vitamin deficiency include inadequate dietary intake and abnormal metabolism.

FOLATE

Most evidence of the relation between maternal nutritional status and pregnancy outcome is derived from studies of the association between folate and neural tube defects. Folate is a water-soluble vitamin and is found mainly in polyglutamated form. Folic acid (folacin) is the synthetic form present as a monoglutamate in vitamin tablets and fortified foods. Folate is important for the biosynthesis of DNA and RNA. It also plays an important role in the conversion of homocysteine to methionine, an essential amino acid. An adequate level of folate should be established before conception and maintained during the first trimester to reduce the risk of neural tube defects. Fruits, green vegetables, beans, nuts, and bread are the primary sources of folate. Cooking may destroy some forms of dietary folate. The RDI is 400 μg/L.[90] In pregnancy, folate requirements are usually increased.

TABLE 1–5

Current Reference Daily Intakes for Vitamins

VITAMIN	DAILY VALUE
Vitamin A	1500 μg (5000 IU)
Vitamin C	60 mg
Vitamin D	10 μ (400 IU)
Vitamin E	20 mg (30 IU)
Vitamin K	80 μg
Vitamin B_6	2 mg
Vitamin B_{12}	6 μg
Folate	400 μg
Thiamin	1.5 mg
Riboflavin	1.7 mg
Niacin	20 mg

(From Fairfield KM, Fletcher RH: Vitamins for chronic disease prevention in adults: Scientific review. JAMA 2002;287:3116–3126.)

A low folate plasma concentration could be caused by inadequate dietary intake or the use of anticonvulsant drugs, such as phenytoin, phenobarbital, and carbamazepine, which are known folate antagonists. Moreover, folate deficiency could be the result of inherited metabolic disorders, associated, for instance, with methylenetetrahydrofolate reductase (MTHFR) gene polymorphism. MTHFR is a key enzyme in homocysteine metabolism.[91] The homocysteine plasma concentration is considered a sensitive biomarker of the levels of folate and vitamins B_6 and B_{12}. In pregnancies complicated by a fetal neural tube defect, maternal plasma homocysteine levels are elevated and plasma folate concentration is decreased, suggesting a defect in the folate-dependent homocysteine metabolism. Hyperhomocystinemia is also associated with various conditions characterized by placental vasculopathy, such as preeclampsia and abruption, and with recurrent pregnancy loss.[92]

OTHER VITAMINS

Vitamin A is the family of fat-soluble compounds called *retinoids* that have vitamin A activity.[90] The current RDI is 1500 µg/L (5000 IU).[90] Isotretinoin, a derivative of vitamin A, is a powerful prescription drug for the treatment of severe recalcitrant nodular acne. High doses of vitamin A can cause birth defects (e.g., heart defects, craniofacial anomalies), beginning at doses of only three times the daily allowance. Since its approval, isotretinoin has been labeled as pregnancy category X, meaning that it should not be used during pregnancy. Another derivative of vitamin A, etretinate, is a prescription drug for the treatment of psoriasis. This drug is also contraindicated in pregnant women and those who are likely to become pregnant while taking it. In adults, vitamin A toxicity results in hepatotoxicity and visual changes.[90] Xerophthalmia, night blindness, and increased susceptibility to disease characterize vitamin A deficiency.

Vitamin B_6 (pyridoxine, pyridoxal, and pyridoxamine) is water-soluble and is found in various plant and animal products. The current RDI for vitamin B_6 is 2 mg.[90] Vitamin B_6 is involved in many enzymatic reactions. Deficiency is uncommon.

Vitamin B_{12} (cyanocobalamin) is water-soluble and found in animal products only. The current RDI for vitamin B_{12} is 6 µg.[90] Cyanocobalamin has no known physiologic role, but must be converted to a biologically active form (i.e., methylcobalamin of adenosylcobalamin). Methylcobalamin is an essential cofactor in the conversion of homocysteine to methionine.[91] When this reaction is impaired, hyperhomocysteinemia occurs and folate metabolism is deranged. The cobalamins are involved in fat and carbohydrate metabolism, protein synthesis, and hematopoiesis. Deficiency can result from poor intake, including strict veganism, malabsorption from the absence of intrinsic factor, and rare enzyme deficiencies. Vitamin B_{12} deficiency results in macrocytic anemia and neurologic abnormalities. There are no consistent adverse effects of high intake.[90]

Vitamin C (ascorbic acid) is water-soluble and acts as a cofactor in hydroxylation reactions, which are required for collagen synthesis. It is also a strong antioxidant. The current RDI for vitamin C is 60 mg.[90] Vitamin C deficiency leads to bruising and easy bleeding (scurvy). Large doses (≤2000 mg) of vitamin C are generally well tolerated.

Vitamin D (calciferol) is not a true vitamin because humans can synthesize it with adequate sunlight exposure. The current RDI for vitamin D (1,25-dihydroxyvitamin D_3) is 0.01 mg (400 IU).[90] Vitamin D deficiency is associated with rickets in children. In adults, vitamin D deficiency leads to secondary hyperparathyroidism, with subsequent bone loss and increased fracture risk. There is evidence that genetic polymorphisms strongly affect fracture risk.[90] Inadequate vitamin D intake is more common than previously believed, particularly among housebound women of specific ethnic minority groups.[90] There is no documented evidence of vitamin D deficiency and adverse pregnancy outcome, apart from neonatal hypocalcemia. Given the relatively high prevalence of vitamin D deficiency in certain communities, vitamin D supplementation at a dosage of 0.01 mg (400 IU) is advocated. High intake of vitamin D (>0.05 mg or 2000 IU) results in hypercalcemia and soft tissue calcification.[90]

Vitamin E is a family of eight related compounds, the tocopherols and the tocotrienols. With the possible exception of hemolytic anemia and retinopathy in preterm infants, vitamin E deficiency as a result of dietary limitations has not been seen in humans. However, genetic deficiencies in apolipoprotein B or α-tocopherol transfer protein lead to severe vitamin E deficiency syndromes, with symptoms including hemolytic anemia, muscle weakness, and brain dysfunction.[90] The current RDI for vitamin E is 20 mg (30 IU).[90] With doses of 800 to 1200 mg/day, antiplatelet effects and bleeding may occur.[90] Because of its antioxidative properties, vitamin E is believed to prevent diseases associated with oxidative stress, such as cardiovascular diseases, cancer, chronic inflammation, and neurologic disorders. It is assumed, but not proven, that vitamin E requirements increase during pregnancy. Supplementation with vitamins C and E may help to prevent preeclampsia in women at risk for the disease. There is, however, insufficient evidence to recommend this strategy (see also Chapter 36).[93]

Vitamin K is fat-soluble and essential for normal clotting, especially for the production of prothrombin and factors VII, IX, and X, and protein C and S. Vitamin K has two subtypes, vitamin K_1 and K_2. Vitamin K_1, or phylloquinone, is found in most vegetables and dairy products. Vitamin K_2, or menaquinone, is synthesized by the intestinal flora and absorbed only in small amounts.[94] The current RDI for vitamin K is 80 µ/L.[90] Vitamin K deficiency occurs when dietary intake is inadequate or intestinal bacteria, which synthesize vitamin K, are altered. Newborn infants are at risk for vitamin K deficiency because of poor placental transfer, lack of intestinal bacteria, and low content in breast milk.[94] The risk of vitamin K deficiency is higher in the breast-fed infant because breast milk contains lower amounts of vitamin K than modern formula or cow's milk.[94] A single dose of either oral or intramuscular vitamin K, 1 mg, to all infants is advocated to prevent hemorrhagic disease of the newborn in the first week after birth.[94] Women using antiepileptic drugs, including phenytoin, carbamazepine, and phenobarbital, are particularly at risk for vitamin K deficiency in their offspring. They are advised to use an oral dose of vitamin K, 10 mg daily, from the 36th week of gestation to prevent neonatal hemorrhagic disease.[95]

IODINE AND ZINC

Trace minerals, such as iodine, are needed in greater quantities during pregnancy. Deficiencies of trace minerals, such as iodine and zinc, are also implicated in low birth weight, perinatal mortality, mental retardation, childhood hearing and speech disorders, and birth defects.[96]

IRON

In Europe, iron deficiency is an important nutritional disorder, affecting large fractions of the population, particularly children, menstruating women, and pregnant women. Factors that affect iron deficiency include the type of contraception in women, blood donation, and minor pathologic blood loss (e.g., hemorrhoids, gynecologic bleeding). Moreover, women, especially vegetarians, vegans, and patients with malabsorption, are at increased risk for iron deficiency. A reduction in body iron is associated with a decrease in the level of functional compounds, such as hemoglobin (see also Chapter 39).

Management Options

General

From a recent overview of randomized controlled trials, no firm conclusions could be drawn about the implications of nutritional advice to prevent or treat impaired fetal growth.[88] Most physicians agree that RDIs, except those for iron and folic acid, can be obtained through a proper diet. Pregnant teenagers, smokers, drug users, alcohol drinkers, and strict vegetarians tend to be deficient in various vitamins.[97–99] Multivitamin supplements can be of value.

To reduce the incidence of neural tube defects, most countries advocate folic acid supplementation in a dosage of 0.4 mg/day to all women from at least 4 weeks before until 8 weeks after conception.[89]

Large quantities of caffeine consumption (>600 mg daily) should be avoided. Caffeine is associated with reductions in birth weight equivalent to those associated with smoking 1 to 10 cigarettes.[89]

SUMMARY OF MANAGEMENT OPTIONS

Nutritional Preparation for Pregnancy

Stage of Pregnancy	Management Options	Quality of Evidence	Strength of Recommendation	References
Prepregnancy				
	Offer counseling to women at risk for nutritional deficiency.	III	B	100, 103
	Recommend folate supplements (0.4 mg/day) for all women contemplating pregnancy.	Ia	A	101
	Offer continuing folate supplementation (0.4 mg/day) to all women at increased risk for neural tube defects in pregnancy.	Ia	A	101
Prenatal				
	The decision to recommend supplements is based on individual requirements.	Ia	A	102
	Routine iron supplementation is warranted in populations in which iron deficiency is common.	Ia	A	104

SUMMARY OF MANAGEMENT OPTIONS

Nutritional Preparation for Pregnancy *(Continued)*

Stage of Pregnancy	Management Options	Quality of Evidence	Strength of Recommendation	References
Prenatal				
	Avoid excess vitamin A (i.e., more than the daily allowance).	III	B	90
	Advise supplemental vitamin K (10 mg/day from 36 weeks gestation) to women who take antiepileptic drugs to prevent neonatal hemorrhagic disease.	IIa	A	95
	Advise women to avoid large amounts of caffeine (>600 mg daily, which is equivalent to six 10-ounce cups of coffee).	III	B	84
Labor and Delivery				
Postnatal				
	Give a single dose (1 mg) of either intramuscular or oral vitamin K to the newborn to prevent classic hemorrhagic disease. Vitamin K prophylaxis improves biochemical indices of coagulation status at 1 to 7 days.	Ib	A	94

MATERNAL WEIGHT AND WEIGHT GAIN

Although routine weighing of pregnant women has become an important feature of prenatal care, surprisingly little is known about the effectiveness of weighing as a screening procedure for predicting fetal demise or about the clinical and practical implications of "abnormal" weight changes in pregnancy. Epidemiologically, prepregnancy weight may be considered a risk indicator, identifying women who are at increased risk for pregnancy complications and poor reproductive outcome. Prepregnancy weight is a crude reflection of nutritional status, which is largely determined by maternal genotype and environmental factors, including a woman's lifelong health status, beginning at her own conception. Weight gain is arguably directly related to birth weight and the subsequent health of the child.

Underweight Women

Definitions

Perhaps the best way to assess abnormalities of nutritional status, namely undernutrition and obesity, is to refer to standard height and weight tables, using information on maternal height and prepregnancy weight. Body mass index (BMI), also known as Quetelet's index (weight [kg]/height[m]^2), is commonly used. Naeye[105] classified pregnant women into four categories according to arbitrary BMI values: "thin," less than 20; "normal," 20 to 24; "overweight," 25 to 30; and "obese," greater than 30. In clinical practice, however, these standard definitions of BMI are difficult to apply because information on prepregnancy weight is usually unavailable at the first prenatal visit. Therefore, many investigators have limited the definitions for abnormal nutritional status to information on body weight. In this regard, subjective criteria for "initial" body weight have been proposed. Values of 45 kg (99 lb) or less are used to describe "underweight" women and values of 85 kg (187 lb) or greater are used to describe "overweight" women.[106] Alternatively, skinfold thickness measurements are used to define maternal constitution in terms of body fat content. Estimates of skinfold measurements, however, are affected by alterations in maternal body composition during pregnancy.[107,108] Because it is impossible to rely fully on the accuracy of these measurements during pregnancy, the results should be interpreted carefully. Also, from a practical viewpoint, most institutions do not routinely record this measurement.

Nutritional deprivation may arise as a result of starvation, dieting, or chronic eating disorders, such as anorexia nervosa and bulimia. Eating disorders are a public health concern in affluent societies.[97]

Anorexia nervosa is a syndrome characterized by severe weight loss, a distorted body image, and an intense fear of becoming obese.[97,109] Anorexia nervosa is not synonymous with bulimia, although bulimic symptoms may occur in women with anorexia nervosa.

Bulimia is characterized by recurrent episodes of secretive binge eating followed by self-induced vomiting, fasting, or the use of laxatives or diuretics.[97] Depression and alcohol and drug abuse are also prominent features of this disorder.[110] Patients show frequent weight fluctuations, but are not likely to have significant weight loss, as seen in women with anorexia nervosa. Both syndromes, which primarily affect adolescents and young adults from middle-class and upper middle-class families, are often associated with oligomenorrhea and amenorrhea.[97] Despite menstrual irregularities, women with chronic eating disorders may become pregnant. Stewart and colleagues reviewed the outcome of pregnancies in women with anorexia and bulimia.[100]

Risks

Nutritional deprivation has a negative effect on birth weight.[86,111] Underweight women are more likely than women of normal weight to give birth to infants who are small for gestational age.[105,112,113] Poor fetal growth may result in birth asphyxia and complications, such as neonatal hypoglycemia and hypothermia.[114] Underweight women my be more susceptible to anemia.[76] In "thin" women (Quetelet's index <20), the perinatal mortality rate is increased.[105]

The outcome of pregnancy in women with anorexia and bulimia varies. If the eating disorder is in remission, then an uneventful pregnancy and a favorable pregnancy outcome can be anticipated. However, expectant women with active anorexia nervosa or bulimia at the time of conception may have a number of severe health problems, including electrolyte imbalances, dehydration, depression, social problems, and poor fetal growth. Appropriate psychiatric treatment is warranted.[100,109]

Management Options

PREPREGNANCY

Women who have anorexia or bulimia and wish to become pregnant are advised to wait until the eating disorder is in remission.[100] The treatment of underweight women with anovulatory infertility should be focused on restoration of weight by an integrated multidisciplinary approach rather than on ovulation induction.[97]

PRENATAL

In view of the increased risk of low birth weight, prenatal care should focus on early detection of impaired fetal growth.[109] Careful dating of gestation is important. Adequate weight gain should be ensured. However, the beneficial effects of dietary advice, with or without specific food supplements, are controversial.[88,97,115]

LABOR AND DELIVERY

If fetal growth restriction is suspected, the patient should be admitted to a specialist unit. Continuous electronic fetal heart rate monitoring is advised.[113] Emergency neonatal services should be readily available for resuscitation.

POSTNATAL

Approximately 40% of women with eating disorders have a history of affective disorders, which also puts them at risk for postpartum depression.[109] No additional specific management strategies need to be considered. Treatment with antidepressant drugs may be warranted.

Overweight Women

Definitions

According to the recommendations of the World Health Organization, overweight is defined as a BMI of more than 25.0 kg/m^2 and obesity is defined as a BMI of greater than 30 kg/m^2.[116] The degree of obesity is classified into three categories: grade I (BMI 30.0–34.9 kg/m^2), grade II (BMI 35.0–39.9 kg/m^2), and grade III (BMI > 40 kg/m^2).

Risks

Hypertensive disorders, including preexisting hypertension and pregnancy-induced hypertension, are more common in women with excess weight, although prevalence rates in different reports vary widely (7%–46%).[117] Gestational diabetes is also more frequent, affecting 7% to 17% of obese women.[117] Other problems associated with obesity include gallstones, urinary tract infections, postnatal hemorrhage, and possibly thrombophlebitis.[118,119] Obese women are more likely to give birth to large-for-gestational-age infants. Poor fetal growth is not usually seen in obese women.[118] Despite the higher mean birth weight of the infant, there is no clear evidence that obese women without prenatal complications are at increased risk for labor and delivery complications, such as dysfunctional labor, shoulder dystocia, and birth asphyxia.[118,120] Moreover, obese women without prenatal complications do not appear to be more prone to either augmentation with oxytocin for poorly progressing labor or cesarean section for dystocia when compared with matched nonobese control subjects.[118,119]

There is conflicting evidence about the effect of obesity on perinatal mortality. Based on the findings of the Collaborative Perinatal Study in the United States, Naeye[105] concluded that perinatal mortality rates are directly related to Quetelet index values, even when the effects of demographic factors, smoking, and prenatal complications were considered. He showed that nearly half the increase in perinatal mortality among obese women could be ascribed to preterm birth. The increased rate of twin births may also partially explain the relatively high rates of preterm birth and subsequent increased perinatal mortality rates among obese women.[105] Other investigators could not confirm this association between perinatal mortality and obesity. Such a lack of association could be the effect of prenatal care, through early recognition and appropriate management of prenatal complications in the obese woman.[117] Various studies suggested that the cesarean section rate for obese women is slightly higher than that for women of normal weight.[119] In fact, the increased need for abdominal delivery in obese women can be attributed mainly to the relatively high rate of prenatal complications and to factors such as advanced age and high parity. When surgical delivery is required, obese women are more prone to wound infection compared with nonobese women.[117,121]

Management Options

PREPREGNANCY

If an obese woman wishes to reduce her weight, she should be encouraged to lose weight before or after pregnancy. There are several potentially effective programs for weight loss.[122] It has been suggested that weight loss programs should aim initially at a reduction of body weight by 10% from baseline, at a rate of 1 or 2 pounds (approximately 0.5–1 kg) per week, for 6 months.[122] Diets with a deficit of 500 to 1000 kcal/day produce weight loss of 300 to 1000 g/wk, depending on the patient's weight.[123] Starvation diets, with energy intake of less than 200 kcal/day, are no longer used. Dietary manipulation should not be advocated during pregnancy. It is difficult to achieve, offers no benefit to the mother, and may have ill effects on fetal weight and the subsequent health of the child.[111,124] Apart from a balanced diet, daily exercise programs should be promoted[116,122] (see "Physical Activity"). If a woman insists on severe caloric restriction for weight reduction, the problem of maintaining reduced weight for prolonged periods should be addressed. The recurrence rate of obesity after weight reduction is high.[125] Massively obese women who cannot achieve dietary control sometimes opt for surgical treatment of obesity. Pregnancies that occur after intestinal bypass surgery are often complicated by fetal growth restriction.[125] In contrast, most pregnancies that occur after gastric bypass surgery appear to have a generally benign course; this procedure is seldom associated with nutritional and metabolic abnormalities.[126] Pregnancy should be avoided if electrolyte imbalance is present.

PRENATAL

Prepregnancy weight and maternal height should be documented routinely in the prenatal health records or medical records. Weight is usually recorded at each prenatal visit, using calibrated scales. Blood pressure should also be monitored with an appropriately sized cuff. Obese women may show artificially high readings when a standard cuff is used.[127]

In grossly obese women, it can be difficult to assess fetal growth and well-being. Ultrasonic measurements of fetal size may be untrustworthy if adipose tissue limits proper visualization of the fetus. Ascertainment of fundal height in overweight women by either palpation or measurement could also present problems in terms of accurate estimation of fetal size. There is no simple solution. Moreover, in massively obese women, it may be difficult to determine fetal presentation. Ultrasonography is particularly important in resolving problems of presentation. Before delivery, anesthesia consultation is needed if medical problems arise, such as hypertension, diabetes mellitus, or pulmonary dysfunction.

Obese women should be evaluated for gestational diabetes at the first prenatal visit. Testing should be repeated in the second or third trimester if the previous findings were normal.[119] Women should be screened for asymptomatic bacteriuria by culture and colony count of clean-catch voided urine.[128] Screening for asymptomatic bacteriuria, with subsequent treatment, reduces the risk of pyelonephritis and its consequences.[128]

LABOR AND DELIVERY

Fetal macrosomia is strongly associated with problems in labor, including poor progress as a result of cephalopelvic disproportion, shoulder dystocia, and birth asphyxia.[120] Attempts to derive a prediction score to identify large-for-gestational-age infants have been unsuccessful because of unacceptably high false-positive rates.[129]

PROCEDURE

CESAREAN SECTION IN THE OBESE PATIENT

Preoperative Considerations

Anesthesia

In view of technologic advances, there should no longer be a hesitancy to perform a cesarean section in morbidly obese women. In nonemergent deliveries, epidural anesthesia warrants serious consideration. Even in the massively obese woman, epidural anesthesia is technically possible and is preferred over general anesthesia, at least in experienced hands.[118,130]

Prophylactic Measures

The use of prophylactic antibiotics during both elective and emergency cesarean section significantly reduces the risks of maternal wound infection and febrile morbidity.[131] Additionally, prophylactic administration of low-molecular-weight heparin is recommended, beginning preoperatively and continuing until the patient is fully ambulatory.[132]

Type of Incision

In obese women, the type of incision for abdominal delivery, midline vertical versus low-transverse (Pfannenstiel), is often subject to debate. Gross[133] reviewed the benefits and risks of the two operative approaches in obese women. He concluded that the favorable aspects of the Pfannenstiel incision are: (1) less postoperative pain and early ambulation, thus avoiding atelectasis and embolism; (2) a more secure closure; and (3) less adipose tissue to incise. Moreover, the Pfannenstiel incision gives a better cosmetic result than the midline incision. The potential adverse effects of the Pfannenstiel incision are: (1) greater likelihood of infection because the incision is located in a warm, moist area; (2) potentially restricted access to the infant; and (3) more difficult exposure of the upper abdomen.

In theory, prolongation of surgery increases the risk of wound infection. The extent to which the type of incision affects the duration of surgery in overweight women is unknown. The total duration of the operation in obese women appears to be only marginally affected by the type of incision used. The interval from incision to delivery with the Pfannenstiel technique may be somewhat longer because extraction of the infant may be more difficult, particularly when the infant is large. Incision closure may be more difficult when a midline incision is used. Exteriorization of the uterus to facilitate repair of the uterine incision is commonly practiced when exposure is particularly difficult. The value of this technique, however, remains to be established.[134] Use of a "full-thickness" or "one-layer" closure technique (incorporating peritoneum together with rectus sheath) with nonabsorbable suture material could avoid the problem of wound dehiscence. Placing surgical drains at the time of closure of the abdomen in obese women is a matter of debate. There is no conclusive evidence about how the skin should be closed after cesarean section.[135]

POSTNATAL

Specific complications after abdominal delivery in obese women include wound infection, wound dehiscence, atelectasis, and pulmonary emboli. Prophylactic administration of anticoagulants should be continued until the patient is fully mobilized. Early mobilization appears to improve maternal outcome.

In newborn infants born to grossly obese women, especially those that are large for gestational age, the postnatal blood sugar level should be monitored during the first hours of life.

CONCLUSIONS

- Obese women are more likely to have prenatal complications, including hypertensive disorders, gestational diabetes, urinary tract infection, cesarean section, large-for-gestational-age infants, and intrapartum and postpartum complications.
- Maintaining awareness of the specific medical and obstetric problems associated with obesity will enable the clinician to maximize efforts to improve maternal health and fetal outcome.

Weight Gain in Pregnancy

The total weight gain of a healthy nulliparous woman eating without restriction is approximately 12.5 kg (27.5 lb).[108] However, large variations in weight gain are seen in women with normal outcomes.[108,136] In western societies, average total weight gain ranges from 10 to 16 kg (22–35 lb).[137] This variation is a function of prepregnancy weight, age, parity, and dietary habits during pregnancy. In healthy, well-nourished women with uncomplicated pregnancies, the proportional weight gain (i.e., total weight gain at term expressed as a proportion of the weight before pregnancy) is 17% to 20%.[107] The increase is mostly accounted for by an increase in total body water (averaging approximately 7.5 kg [16.4 lb] when no edema is present) and body fat mass (approximately 2.2–3.5 kg [5.0–7.7 lb]).[108,137,138] The rest, approximating 0.9 kg (2 lb), is caused by an increase in protein content, half of which is fetal. Mean weight gain in pregnancy, from conception to birth, does not show a linear trend. The normal, lean nulliparous woman, who eats to appetite, gains only a little weight during the first trimester (0.65–1.1 kg [1.4–2.4 lb] by 10 weeks).[108,137] In the second trimester, average weekly weight gain is approximately 0.45 kg (1 lb); thereafter, it is approximately 0.36 kg (0.8 lb).[118] Weight loss or failure to gain weight over a 2-week interval in the third trimester is not uncommon in both nulliparous and parous women. The average weight gain in parous women may be slightly less than in nulliparous women. The maximum rate of weight gain occurs between 17 and 24 weeks of pregnancy.[136] Subcutaneous fat is laid down over the abdomen, back, and upper thighs, mainly in the first and second trimesters.[117]

A study from the Netherlands showed that in a highly selective group of healthy women, postpartum weight was 2.9 kg (6.4 lb) greater than weight before pregnancy.[138] After delivery, the most rapid weight loss occurs between 4 and 10 days postpartum, mainly from loss of fluid. In the following weeks, weight loss is much more gradual, approximately 0.25 kg (0.55 lb) per week, consistent with a gradual mobilization of fat stores.[139] Eventually, the average woman loses most of the weight she gains during pregnancy, taking into account the effects of age and weight gain over time.[108,140] Pregnancy does not have a lasting effect on body fat mass. Breast-feeding for longer than 60 days has a favorable effect on the rate of postpartum weight loss because it is assumed that maternal caloric consumption is generally insufficient to meet the increased needs of lactation.[141]

Risks

There is a positive correlation between maternal weight gain and birth weight, regardless of maternal age and parity.[136,141] Women who gain little weight in pregnancy are at increased risk for having low–birth weight infants. The magnitude of the association between inadequate maternal weight gain and low birth weight depends on prepregnancy weight: women of low prepregnancy weight who have little weight gain during pregnancy are more likely to give birth to a low–birth weight infant than overweight women who have a similar net weight gain during pregnancy. Net weight gain in underweight women is strongly related to birth weight. In overweight women, net weight gain is only marginally related to birth weight.[142] The optimum weight gain in terms of minimum perinatal mortality is 7.3 kg (16 lb) for overweight women, 9.1 kg (20 lb) for women of normal weight, and 13.6 kg (30 lb) for underweight women.[108] The possibility of an eating disorder should be considered in women who do not gain appropriate weight or who have intractable vomiting.[100]

Management options

PRENATAL

Dietary policies vary markedly from hospital to hospital, but the rationale for dietary management of pregnant women with "inappropriate" weight gain is unclear. Over the last several decades, significant changes have been made in the recommendations made to women about weight gain during pregnancy. Until the 1970s, it was common practice to advise women to restrict food intake. These recommendations were aimed at curtailing weight gain to approximately 6.8 kg (15 lb) or 11.3 kg (25 lb) at most.[142] The main objectives for dietary restriction were threefold: (1) reduction of the incidence of preeclampsia, (2) promotion of easier labor, and (3) preservation of the woman's figure after birth.[142] Later, when the association between low birth weight and inadequate weight gain was recognized to be less strong than originally thought, and in view of the fact that dietary restriction could not avert preeclampsia, medical attitudes toward weight gain in pregnancy were relaxed.[124]

Caloric restriction in women cannot be recommended because there is no scientific evidence that such policy has a beneficial effect on maternal and fetal health, in terms of preventing preeclampsia, perinatal mortality, preterm birth, or impaired fetal growth.[88,102,124,143] By increasing energy intake, however, the pregnant woman can promote excessive fat accretion.[137] A modest reduction in nutrient intake may reduce the likelihood of retaining undesirable amounts of fat postpartum.[137] If a woman wishes to pursue this approach, a dietitian should advise her about a healthy, well-balanced diet, taking into account her background, assets, and lifestyle.

LABOR AND DELIVERY

Important considerations were discussed in the previous section.

CONCLUSIONS

- Mean infant birth weight is a function of maternal weight before pregnancy and weight gain during pregnancy.
- Weight gain during pregnancy seems to have a far greater effect on the birth weight of infants born to underweight women than on those born to overweight women.

SUMMARY OF MANAGEMENT OPTIONS
Underweight Women

Management Options	Quality of Evidence	Strength of Recommendation	References
Prepregnancy			
Advise women with eating disorders who wish to become pregnant to wait until the eating disorder is in remission.	III	B	100
Use a multidisciplinary approach for eating disorders.	III	B	97

Continued

SUMMARY OF MANAGEMENT OPTIONS
Underweight Women *(Continued)*

Management Options	Quality of Evidence	Strength of Recommendation	References
Prenatal			
Check for fetal growth restriction.	III	B	100,113
Provide multidisciplinary treatment for women with eating disorders not yet in remission.	III	B	109,113
Labor and Delivery			
Provide continuous electronic fetal heart rate monitoring if the fetus is small.	IIa	B	114
Postnatal			
Monitor signs of maternal depression, and provide treatment if indicated.	III	B	109

SUMMARY OF MANAGEMENT OPTIONS
Overweight Women

Management Options	Quality of Evidence	Strength of Recommendation	References
Prepregnancy			
Provide advice on intervention for weight reduction.	Ia	A	130
Explain the risks of hypertension, diabetes, urinary infections, large fetal size, and postpartum hemorrhage.	III	B	118,119
Prenatal			
Avoid attempts to manipulate the diet during pregnancy.	Ib	A	123
Screen for hypertension, diabetes, and bacteriuria.	III	B	118
Monitor the blood pressure of women with large arms with an appropriately sized cuff.	III	B	127
Monitor for fetal growth with ultrasound.	III	B	120,129
Labor and Delivery			
Look for cephalopelvic disproportion and shoulder dystocia.	III	B	120
Cesarean section:			
Use regional rather than general anaesthesia.	IIa	B	118
Give prophylactic antibiotics.	Ia	A	130
Give prophylactic low-dose subcutaneous heparin.	IV	C	128
There is no agreement over which incision is best.	Ia	A	132
Wound drains may be of value.	IIa	B	135,144
Postnatal			
Give subcutaneous heparin until the patient is fully ambulatory.	IV	C	132
Recommend early mobilization.	IV	C	132
Continue with measures to lose weight.	IV	C	116

SUMMARY OF MANAGEMENT OPTIONS

Abnormal Weight Gain

Management Options	Quality of Evidence	Strength of Recommendation	References
Prenatal			
Check for abnormal fetal growth.	Ib	A	124
Consider physical and organic causes.	IIb	B	143
Offer advice on improving diet.	Ia	A	139,124,143
Advice on reducing weight is not useful.			
Labor and Delivery			
See the recommendations for Overweight Women.	–	–	–

PHYSICAL ACTIVITY

Definition

Physical activity is of two types: (1) daily activities, including household, occupational, and commuting-related activities; and (2) leisure activities, such as sports and exercise, including aerobics. Physical activity accounts for 15% to 40% of total energy expenditure. The magnitude of the physiologic response to physical activity is determined by age, fitness, body weight, body position, concurrent physical adaptations to pregnancy, and psychological factors.[145] Because physical activity has many interrelated dimensions, its quantification is complex. Indirect assessment of physical activity by questionnaire is the most practical and widely accepted approach in epidemiologic studies.[146]

Risks

General Health

There are clear associations between physical activity and health and between diet and health. These relationships are often linked through obesity.[116] Although obesity, an unhealthy diet, and physical inactivity are independent risk factors, they are often found together and are a common risk factor for type 2 diabetes, hypertension, cardiovascular disease, and stroke.[116]

Pregnancy

Research focused on physical activity in the workplace shows that physically and emotionally demanding work during pregnancy is associated with an increased risk of hypertension, low birth weight, and preterm birth[147] (see "Occupational Factors"). Research focused on leisure time physical activity during pregnancy has not identified similar associations.[147] Research findings indicate that the overall effect of regular recreational exercise on pregnancy outcome is positive for both mother and fetus, in terms of maternal cardiovascular reserve, placental growth, and functional capacity.[147–149] This also holds true for vigorous exercise, including aerobics and competitive sports.[150,151] Activities with a high risk of abdominal trauma should be avoided.[148] Scuba diving should be discouraged throughout pregnancy, because the fetus is not protected from decompression problems and is at risk for malformation and gas embolism after decompression disease.[148,152]

Management Options

A woman's overall health, including obstetric and medical risks, should be evaluated before an exercise program is prescribed.[148] The American College of Obstetricians and Gynecologists (ACOG) recommends healthy pregnant women to engage in 30 minutes or more of moderate exercise daily, provided there are neither medical nor obstetric complications.[148] Healthy pregnant women are allowed to exercise vigorously or take part in competitive sports, provided that there are no noticeable health hazards to themselves or their infants.[145,148,150,151]

SUMMARY OF MANAGEMENT OPTIONS

Exercise in Pregnancy

Management Options	Quality of Evidence	Strength of Recommendation	References
Advise healthy pregnant women to engage in daily exercise if there are no medical or obstetric complications.	III	B	145,148,150,151
Warn patients to avoid activities with a high risk of abdominal trauma.	IV	C	148
Discourage scuba diving in pregnancy.	IIb	B	152
Exercise is associated with higher self-esteem and confidence.	Ia	A	151
Regular exercise carries no demonstrable harm to the mother or fetus.	Ia	A	151

OCCUPATIONAL FACTORS

Risks

The number of women in paid employment has increased over the last decades in both developing and developed countries.[153] With increasing participation in the workforce, many women have become vulnerable to unsafe and unhealthy conditions, such as exposure to toxic chemicals, radiation, and physically or mentally demanding work.

Women's occupations are multidimensional. They may undertake paid work at home or may combine part-time or full-time work with household activities and the care of children. They are likely to move in and out of the paid labor force during different life stages. For these reasons, a simple occupational category is seldom sufficient as a guide for establishing specific health risks.[69,154]

Determining both exposure and outcome may be problematic. Data on meaningful indicators of reproductive health hazards in the workplace are usually scarce, and occupational morbidity is frequently unquantified and largely invisible. The same is true for occupational hazards associated with household work, for instance, exposure to toxic chemicals, such as cleaning fluids, bleach, detergents, insecticides, and pesticides. Furthermore, little information is available on the physical effort and emotional strain associated with the daily care of young children, which may be demanding, especially when there is little support from the woman's partner, friends, or family. Despite considerable progress in integrating women into the labor force, many women are still found in jobs where employment conditions are relatively unfavorable. Many jobs often held by women (e.g., salesperson, hairdresser, teller, cashier) require static work, monotonous tasks, and repetitive movements that may result in physical and mental health problems. Migrant workers are of special concern because they are often underpaid and work in exploitative conditions. The adverse effects of poor working environment can be magnified by problems of isolation, stress, tiredness, and depression.

Physical violence is a major contributor to women's health risks, either in the home or in the formal workplace. Unemployment and poverty have led many women to work in the sex industry. Although the occupational health risks of sex workers vary with the setting and context, these workers are at increased risk for violence and sexually transmitted diseases (see Chapter 81).

The list of occupational exposures suspected to be harmful to the fetus is long. For instance, occupational exposures to anesthetic agents, laboratory chemicals, organic solvents, and pesticides have been linked to adverse pregnancy outcomes.[155,156] However, interpretation of the findings of studies in occupational settings is often hampered by methodologic shortcomings. A recent meta-analysis of working conditions and adverse pregnancy outcomes concluded that physically demanding work is significantly associated with preterm birth (OR, 1.22; 95% CI, 1.16, 1.29), fetal growth restriction (OR, 1.37; 95% CI, 1.30, 1.44), and hypertension or preeclampsia (OR, 1.60; 95% CI, 1.30, 1.96). Other occupational exposures significantly associated with preterm birth include prolonged standing (OR, 1.26; 95% CI, 1.13, 1.40) and shift and night work (OR, 1.24; 95% CI, 1.06, 1.46).[157] No adverse outcomes are seen in women with less strenuous jobs or in those who can modify their work activity.[158] These data suggest that interventions to reduce physical exertion among pregnant women could improve birth outcomes. French investigators developed a useful scale for identifying strenuous working conditions. This "fatigue index" comprises five sources of potential occupational hazards:

posture, type of work, physical exertion, mental stress, and situational factors (e.g., exposure to noise and heat). They showed a strong relationship between preterm delivery and adverse working conditions, as reflected by the fatigue index.[159] Several studies noted an association between stress and fatigue related to the work or home environment and increased risk of adverse pregnancy outcome (pooled OR, 1.63; 95% CI, 1.33, 1.98).[157] The underlying mechanism of these adverse effects on pregnancy outcomes is unclear.

Legislation to protect women in the workplace has been enacted in most countries. Such legislation is frequently used to exclude women from specific industries, either because the work is too physically demanding or because it poses unwarranted risks to the outcome of pregnancy. Implementation of these protective health and safety measures is often problematic. For instance, informal sector employment is generally excluded from protective legislation, leaving women vulnerable to workplace hazards.

Management Options

A careful workplace history should be taken, including level of activity, hazardous exposures, and ease of workplace modification.[158] Precautions should be taken to protect women from specific occupational health risks, such as exposure to toxic chemicals or radiation.[153] Women whose work is physically or emotionally demanding should be monitored carefully throughout pregnancy for evidence of hypertension, intrauterine growth restriction, and symptoms of preterm labor.[157] It is important for health care professionals, family members, and employers to recognize the potential negative effect of adverse working conditions on pregnancy outcome.

The ultimate decision on continuation of employment during pregnancy should be made by the pregnant woman after careful counseling by her physician, involving the company medical officer and the employer, when indicated.

SUMMARY OF MANAGEMENT OPTIONS

Work and Pregnancy

Management Options	Quality of Evidence	Strength of Recommendation	References
Precautions should be taken to protect women against specific occupational health risks, such as exposure to toxic chemicals or radiation.	IV	C	153
Warn patients to avoid long hours of standing and walking.	Ia	B	157
Tell patients to avoid excess lifting and exercise.	Ia	B	157
Recommend that patients continue to work if they wish to work and are not unduly tired.	Ia	B	157,159
There is no evidence that video display units (VDUs) are associated with adverse pregnancy outcome.	III	B	60,61

ADOLESCENT PREGNANCY

Definitions

The term *adolescent* is often used synonymously with *teenager*. In this sense, *adolescent pregnancy* is pregnancy in a girl or woman aged 10 to 19 years.[160] Epidemiologically, a distinction is often made between pregnancy (or birth) rates among adolescents aged 15 to 19 years and those among adolescents aged 10 to 14 years. Some investigators advocate the use of the terms *reproductive age* and *gynecologic age* as measures of physiologic maturity.[161–164] *Reproductive age* is the interval from the age of menarche (i.e., onset of first menses) to the chronologic age at conception, whereas *gynecologic age* is the time span from the age of menarche to the chronologic age at delivery. Conception or delivery within 2 years after the onset of menarche represents the lower extreme of the distribution of reproductive or gynecologic ages, respectively.

With the improvement of socioeconomic conditions, the median age of menarche has shown a downward trend. Currently, the median age of menarche among girls in developed countries is approximately 12.5 years.[160]

Incidence

The incidence of teenage pregnancy shows marked variation between developed countries. The lowest teenage pregnancy rates are found in the Netherlands (14/1000 among 15- to 19-year-olds), whereas in Sweden and England and Wales combined, they are considerably higher. According to recent figures for England and Wales, the teenage pregnancy rate (15–19 years) is 45/1000, the abortion rate is 19/1000, and the birth rate is 26/1000.[160] The highest pregnancy rates in developed countries are found in the United States. In the mid-1990s, among teenagers 15 to 19 years old, the pregnancy rate was 83.6, the abortion rate was 29.2, and the birth rate was 54.4.[165] In the United States, approximately 1 in every 11 girls aged 15 to 19 years becomes pregnant each year.

Risks

Teenage pregnancy is associated with both social and medical problems, in particular, preterm birth.[160,162,166] Many teenage mothers originate from working-class families and ethnic minorities. Many are themselves the children of teenage or very young parents.[167] Most teenage pregnancies are unplanned and unwanted. Consequently, in western societies, abortion rates among adolescents are quite high, ranging from 30% to 60% of all confirmed pregnancies in this age group.[168]

Reports on complications of pregnancy in adolescents are contradictory and difficult to interpret because of the confounding effects of adverse social circumstances and poor attendance for prenatal care. Typically, cigarette smoking and illicit drug use are common among pregnant adolescents.[160] Medical complications associated with adolescent pregnancy include preterm birth and low birth weight, perinatal mortality, short interval to next pregnancy, and sudden infant death syndrome. Moreover, adolescents who become pregnant are at particular risk for nutritional deficiencies, anemia, HIV infection, and other sexually transmitted diseases.[160] The increased incidence of pregnancy-induced hypertension among pregnant adolescents is largely explained by nulliparity.[160] It has been suggested that competition for nutrients between the fetus and the mother could affect pregnancy outcome in adolescents by interrupting the normal growth process.[169] However, contrary to common belief, biologic "immaturity" does not affect appreciably the reproductive performance of teenagers in terms of length of labor and route of delivery.[160,162,169] In facts, the likelihood of operative delivery is not increased.[160]

Management Options

Prevention and Prepregnancy Management

Primary prevention focuses on preventing pregnancy through sexual education in schools, with an emphasis on the importance of family planning and related issues.[168,170–172] Teenagers should be encouraged to discuss openly with their friends and classmates the realities of pregnancy and parenthood.[173] The media could play an important role in this area. Education should also include information about values, responsibilities, and the right to say "no." Secondary prevention is directed at sexually active women through a flexible approach to the use and provision of contraceptives for both males and females.[171] Some family planning clinics require parental notification if a teenager attends the clinic for birth control. Such policy may have a positive effect of including motivated parents in guiding their children's sexual behavior and contraceptive decision-making. However, such policy may also discourage teenagers from attending family planning clinics for fear of discovery and potential repercussions, in particular when they are raised with the idea that premarital sex is wrong. Motivation to use birth control is rarely hampered by negative attitudes toward contraception. In fact, positive ideas about "getting pregnant" and indifference toward "having a baby" are justifications that are frequently mentioned by childbearing teenagers for not having used contraceptives before conception.[172] Tertiary prevention involves adolescents who become pregnant. They are encouraged to seek early adequate prenatal care and to discuss options for the resolution of pregnancy.[174–176]

Prenatal

Compliance with prenatal care tends to be poor, especially among teenagers in their second pregnancy. Obviously, the provision and use of health care services is beneficial to both mother and child, although it is not clear to what extent prenatal care per se exerts a positive effect on pregnancy outcome. Routine ultrasonography during early pregnancy is advisable to confirm gestational age. Furthermore, timely identification of risk factors is important. Strategies for intervention should be focused on individual medical and social risk factors, in particular, poor nutritional status, adverse health habits, and perceived isolation. It is often difficult to determine the real needs of the pregnant teenager, her partner, and her family. Nevertheless, pregnant adolescents should be offered social support when feasible, preferably in close cooperation with the family physician, an empathetic midwife, or a social worker.[31] Also, information on pregnancy, delivery, and child-rearing should be made available.

Labor and Delivery

There are usually no specific programs for the intrapartum management of teenage pregnancies. The well-being of both the mother and the child must be monitored effectively. If possible, continuous emotional support during labor should be provided by a professional (e.g., nurse, midwife) or nonprofessional caregiver (e.g., spouse, friend, relative).[31] The patient may be hospitalized in a regular maternity unit if she has no risk factors other than age. In exceptionally young adolescents, specialized care is advisable because of the increased likelihood of obstructive labor in patients with a small, immature pelvis.[177]

Postnatal

Infant feeding practices, infant growth, and infant safety should be reviewed. Symptoms of medical problems in the infant must be considered. Social and financial concerns should be discussed.[176] Teenage girls should be encouraged to continue secondary education.[173] Effective contraception should be implemented. A large percentage of teenagers who give birth before the age of 17 years have a repeat pregnancy before they are 19 years old.[178,179] Home visitation programs by public health nurses can have a positive effect on the health of the adolescent mother and her child.[178,179]

CONCLUSIONS

- Pregnancy has a tremendous effect on the adolescent and her family.
- Detrimental effects of age can be explained largely by poor social circumstances.
- Data indicate that most pregnant adolescents are biologically mature when they conceive.
- Teenagers tend to delay seeking prenatal care and typically do not use prenatal care facilities appropriately.
- Attention should be focused on individual risk factors.

SUMMARY OF MANAGEMENT OPTIONS
Pregnancy in Adolescence

Management Options	Quality of Evidence	Strength of Recommendation	References
Prepregnancy			
Education and advertising directed toward sexual behavior and family planning.	IIa	B	160,170,171
Emphasize self-referral for care when pregnant.	III	B	174–176
Prenatal			
Encourage early referral for routine prenatal care and regular attendance.	III	B	174,175
Confirm gestation with early ultrasonography.	III	B	174
Provide advice about diet and adverse habits (e.g., smoking).	III	B	178
Mobilize social support.	III	B	176
Labor and Delivery			
Ensure adequate psychological support.	Ia	A	31
Schedule delivery in a special unit if dystocia is anticipated.	III	B	177
Postnatal			
Provide advice and support for maternal and child care.	III	B	179
Discuss contraception.	III	B	171,172

ADVANCED MATERNAL AGE

Incidence

In the late 1960s and early 1970s, there was a decrease in the number of live births generally and a decrease in the proportion of mothers aged 35 years and older.[180,181] In the last three decades, there has been a trend toward deferred childbearing, especially among healthy, well-educated women with career opportunities.[182–184] The proportion of pregnant women aged 35 years and older varies from country to country. Both socioeconomic circumstances and the nature of the population of elderly women have changed with time. Formerly, pregnant women aged 35 years and older tended to have several unplanned children, whereas today, the proportion of first births to "elderly" pregnant woman is growing.

Risks

Advanced maternal age is a risk indicator for several pregnancy complications, including spontaneous miscarriage; ectopic pregnancy; stillbirth; chromosomal abnormalities; twins; uterine fibroids; hypertensive disorders; gestational diabetes; prolonged labor; cephalopelvic disproportion necessitating operative delivery; bleeding disorders, including placenta previa; low birth weight; antepartum and intrapartum fetal loss; and neonatal mortality.[183–186] However, most reports of pregnancy outcome in elderly primiparous women have not taken into account effects other than age, such as details of general health, smoking habits, and reproductive history (including a history of miscarriage or infertility and its treatment).[182] Information about whether the first pregnancy was postponed deliberately is often lacking. In the early 1990s, Berkowitz and colleagues[184] reported that although pregnancy complications are more common in primiparous women aged 35 years and older, the risk of poor neonatal outcome is not appreciably increased. The women in their study represented a highly selected group of private patients who were predominantly white, married, college-educated, and nonsmoking, and who were delivered of a single infant in a tertiary care center. Hence, their study population was not representative of the population at large. The findings of this study should be interpreted with caution because they may not be applicable to other populations.

Maternal age at conception is highly correlated with the risk of spontaneous miscarriage, regardless of parity or the number of previous miscarriages (Fig. 1–3).[186]

It is assumed that the increased risk of spontaneous miscarriage among older women is a function of the age-related risk of chromosomal abnormalities. Approximately 40% to 60% of conceptions that abort are chromosomally abnormal.[182] The relative frequency of chromosomally normal miscarriages also increases with age, possibly resulting in a decline in uterine function with age.[182] Maternal age has no effect on the incidence of birth defects of unknown etiology.[187]

The topic of maternal age and chromosomal abnormalities is addressed in Chapter 2.

Advanced paternal age has little or no independent effect on the risk of autosomal trisomies when the effect of maternal age is taken into account.[188]

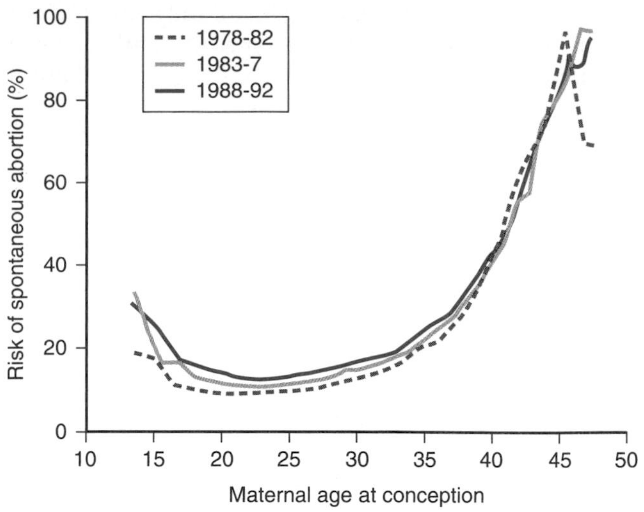

FIGURE 1–3
Risk of spontaneous abortion according to maternal age at conception, stratified according to calendar period, based on Danish civil registry data from 1978–1992. During this period, a total of 634,272 women had 1,221,546 pregnancies, of which 126,673 ended in fetal loss, 285,022 in an induced abortion, and 809,762 in a live birth. (From Andersen A-MN, Wohlfahrt J, Christens P, et al: Maternal age and fetal loss: Population-based register linkage study. BMJ 2000;320:1708–1712, with permission.)

Management Options

Preconception and Prenatal

In clinical practice, maternal age normally refers to the age of the pregnant woman at the time she consults the physician or midwife for the first prenatal visit. This information is particularly important for genetic counseling about the maternal age–specific risks of chromosomal abnormalities because these are typically based on maternal age at the time of delivery. Moreover, counseling should carefully distinguish the risk of a chromosomal abnormality in a live birth from the risk of a fetal chromosomal abnormality that is detectable in early pregnancy or midpregnancy.[189–191] This notion is also important for the proper interpretation of the risk estimates derived from first- and second-trimester screening tests for fetal abnormalities (see Chapters 7, 8, and 9). Fetal chromosomal abnormalities can be diagnosed with chorionic villus sampling or amniotic fluid sampling (amniocentesis) [see Chapter 10].The timing of chorionic villus sampling should take into account the higher baseline rate of spontaneous first-trimester miscarriages in women of advanced maternal age.[186,192]

Although medical and obstetric complications tend to be more common in women aged 35 years and older (discussed earlier), in practice, normal prenatal care usually is not modified unless another risk factor or complication is identified.

Labor and Delivery

Elderly women are usually advised to be delivered in a specialized unit because of the risk of dystocia during labor. However, the impression is often gained that the woman's age in itself contributes strongly to the decision to intervene.[184] Close monitoring of fetal condition (intermittent monoaural auscultation or cardiotocography) and progress in the second stage of labor are warranted. However, intrapartum care is not modified substantially because of the extremes of maternal age.

Postnatal

Discussion of long-term contraception is recommended.[193,194]

CONCLUSION

- It is widely held clinically that advanced maternal age is associated with poor reproductive outcome. Only the increased risks of chromosomal abnormalities and spontaneous abortion are proven.

SUMMARY OF MANAGEMENT OPTIONS
Advanced Maternal Age

Management Options	Quality of Evidence	Strength of Recommendation	References
Prepregnancy			
Discuss risks with the goal of putting the risks into perspective.	III	B	183,184
The risk of spontaneous miscarriage increases with maternal age.	III	B	186
Management is not altered in the woman of advanced age, other than discussion about prenatal diagnosis of chromosomal abnormalities. The other risks are considered relatively unimportant.	III	B	188,191
Advanced paternal age has little or no independent effect on the risk of autosomal trisomies when the effect of maternal age is taken into account.	III	B	188
The probability of multiple pregnancy increases with maternal age.	III	B	185
Prenatal			
Discuss prenatal diagnosis of chromosomal abnormalities and serum marker screening of chorionic villus sampling or amniocentesis if requested.	III	B	192
Labor and Delivery			
Delivery in a unit that can manage dystocia and other complications.	III	B	183
Postnatal			
Discuss long-term contraception.	III	B	193,194

MATERNAL PARITY

Incidence

In western societies, nulliparous women constitute approximately half of all pregnant women.

Definitions

Definitions of parity differ from country to country. *Parity* is the number of times a woman has given birth to an infant, dead or alive. However, the gestational threshold may vary (e.g., 23 completed weeks' gestation vs. 27 completed weeks' gestation).

Risks

Differences in mortality risk between the offspring of primiparous and multiparous women are accounted for by birth weight.[17] Parity is closely correlated with maternal age and with socioeconomic status to a certain extent. It is often difficult to establish precisely how these factors are implicated in the etiology of adverse pregnancy outcome. On the whole, the risk of adverse outcome with parity does not show a consistent pattern. Mean birth weight for infants born to nulliparous women is consistently lower than that for infants born to multiparous women.[166] Some investigators suggested that differences in the mean birth weight of infants born to women of different parity could be explained by differences in maternal weight. It is well known that nulliparity is associated with an increased risk of pregnancy-induced hypertension, which in itself is strongly related to low birth weight. Further, in nulliparous women, there is an increased risk of perineal trauma as a result of either episiotomy or spontaneous tear, compared with multiparous women.

Women of high parity tend to receive inadequate obstetric care. They often delay seeking care and show poor attendance for prenatal care. Moreover, it is assumed that women with a history of rapid or precipitated childbirth have an increased risk of unattended out-of-hospital delivery. High parity is associated with an increased likelihood of abnormal fetal presentation and obstetric hemorrhage.[195] Parity, however, does not have a significant effect on the incidence of Down syndrome when the effect of maternal age is taken into account.[196]

Management Options

Prenatal

Nulliparity is a nonspecific risk factor. In this respect, no specific precautions need to be taken, provided the course of pregnancy is uneventful. There is no need for specialist care on the grounds of nulliparity alone.

In parous women, it is of fundamental importance to obtain all clinically relevant details of previous pregnancies. Reproductive history is a very informative predictor of pregnancy outcome. Consequently, this information has implications for the management of subsequent pregnancies. To facilitate the provision of prenatal care to parous women, it is useful to provide space and staff to accommodate the patients' children, who may accompany her.

Labor and Delivery

Empirically, there is a difference in the normal labor patterns of nulliparous and multiparous women. The median duration of the second stage of labor (i.e., from full dilation of the cervix to delivery) is approximately 45 minutes in nulliparous women versus approximately 20 minutes in multiparous women who have experienced a vaginal delivery previously. Clinically, however, the duration of the second stage of labor is highly variable. In both nulliparous and multiparous women, policies for imposing limits on the length of the second stage of labor tend to be subjective and are usually based on uncontrolled observational data. If the maternal and fetal condition is satisfactory and progress is occurring, with descent of the presenting part, obstetric intervention is not warranted. Cephalopelvic disproportion, however, must be considered when progress in labor is slow. To assure proper maternal and fetal surveillance during labor and prevent unattended out-of-hospital delivery, all women should be instructed to make the necessary arrangements for reaching the hospital in time. For women with a history of rapid or precipitated delivery, timely admission to the hospital and elective induction of labor may be considered, although there is no evidence that this approach is beneficial.

Postnatal

Discussion of long-term contraception is recommended.[193,194]

CONCLUSIONS

- First births have a statistically increased risk over second births, although the pattern of risk varies with age and in itself should not affect pregnancy care.
- Parity, age, and socioeconomic status are interrelated, and they all have an effect on birth weight and pregnancy outcome.
- Overall, the relative importance of parity is limited where fetal outcome is concerned.
- Nulliparity is associated with an increased risk of pregnancy-induced hypertension.
- High parity (traditionally five or more) is associated with abnormal fetal presentation and obstetric hemorrhage.
- Empirically, the duration of "normal" labor in multiparous women is shorter than that in nulliparous women.

SUMMARY OF MANAGEMENT OPTIONS
Women at the Extremes of Parity

Management Options	Quality of Evidence	Strength of Recommendation	References
Prepregnancy			
Discuss the risks, with emphasis on the effects of parity alone and nulliparity or high multiparity (≥5).	III	B	195,196
Prenatal			
Encourage regular attendance for care in those of high parity.	III	B	196
Look for pregnancy-induced hypertension in those of nulliparity.	III	B	196
Look for abnormal presentation from 36 weeks' gestation in those of high parity.	III	B	195
Labor and Delivery			
No specific recommendations are needed on the grounds of parity alone.	III	B	195,196
Postpartum hemorrhage is more likely with increasing parity.	III	B	195
Postnatal			
Discuss long-term contraception.	III	B	193,194

AIR TRAVEL DURING PREGNANCY

General Considerations

With commercial air travel becoming more global, health care providers are increasingly confronted with questions from travelers and airline crew members about the safety of long-distance flights. In this context, pregnant women and those contemplating pregnancy need special consideration because of the specific nature of the potential health risks of long-distance flights. These include exposure to cosmic radiation (see Fig. 1–2), reduced arterial oxygen pressure, immobilization, and unforeseen medical and obstetric emergencies encountered during the flight.[197] Little information has been published on this topic, and the recommendations made to airline crew members and travelers are typically based on common sense rather than scientific evidence.[197]

Risks

Radiation Exposure

The annual exposure dose limit for a member of the general public is 1 millisievert (mSv). The occupational limit is 5 mSv.[198] The exposure dose from cosmic radiation at flight altitudes is usually not higher than 0.005 mSv/hr (see also Fig. 1–2).[35] Rough estimates show that it takes a minimum of 200 flight hours to approach the annual dose limit for the general public. More radiation shielding is provided by atmospheric air at lower altitudes. The dose received from cosmic radiation is usually lower during short-haul flights than during long-haul flights because longer flights are usually flown at higher altitudes. The latitude of the flight route also makes a difference in the level of cosmic radiation exposure, with maximum exposures occurring near the equator. Airlines usually restrict commercial airline crew members from long-haul flights once pregnancy is diagnosed.

Fetal and Maternal Hypoxia

On long-distance commercial flights at an altitude of 32,000 feet, cabin pressure is set at the equivalent to an altitude of 6000 feet.[197] Acute ascent to 6000 feet produces transient cardiovascular and pulmonary adaptations, including decreased heart rate, increased blood pressure, and a significant decrease in aerobic capacity.[199,200] These changes are associated with a decrease in partial oxygen pressure that should not affect women with uneventful pregnancies. However, this decrease may affect those with compromised pregnancies. Therefore, pregnant women should be discouraged from air travel if they have a medical or obstetric problem that is exacerbated by a hypoxic environment.[197] If they must travel, supplemental oxygen should be prescribed during air travel.[201]

Venous Thrombosis

There is probably a link between long-distance air travel and deep venous thrombosis. The increased risk of venous thrombosis is ascribed to prolonged immobilization from cramped seats ("economy class syndrome"). The risk, however, appears very small and is largely confined to those with recognized risk factors, such as a history of thrombosis, recent major surgery, hormone treatment, and malignancy.[202–206] However, the risk does not appear to be confined to those traveling in economy class. There are insufficient scientific data on which to base specific recommendations for prevention, other than leg exercise and the use of elastic compression stockings.[203,206,207]

Preterm Labor

There is no evidence that air travel itself increases the risk of preterm labor. However, 5% to 8% of pregnancies are complicated by preterm labor. Women with a history of preterm birth and those with multiple pregnancies are at increased risk for preterm birth. Recent recommendations from the ACOG suggest that pregnant women who have evidence of preterm labor or are at increased risk for preterm birth should avoid long-distance air travel.[201] Pregnant women who plan to travel should be aware that appropriate medical facilities may not be available in the country of destination.

Obstetric Emergencies

Obstetric emergencies, such as antepartum hemorrhage, cord prolapse, and placental abruption, are rare. However, the consequences are potentially fatal for the mother and child. Pregnant women should be aware that there is no guarantee that qualified medical personnel will be on board the flight and that medical equipment is limited.[197]

Seat Belts

Advice for airline seat belt use is the same as that for cars. A recent study showed that the likelihood of adverse pregnancy outcome among belted pregnant women who were involved in a passenger car accident is comparable to that of those who were not pregnant.[208] Because air turbulence cannot be predicted and this risk of trauma is not trivial, pregnant women are advised to use their seat belts continuously while seated.[201]

Vaccines

A woman who is contemplating pregnancy should receive vaccines that are safe and will protect her health and that of her child when she becomes pregnant. However, care must be taken to avoid inappropriate administration of certain vaccines that can be hazardous to an unborn child. This is particularly true for live vaccines. According to the recommendations of the World Health Organization, active vaccination with live attenuated measles, mumps, rubella, bacillus Calmette-Guérin, and yellow fever virus vaccines should be avoided in pregnancy (Table 1–6).[209,210]

The risks and benefits of vaccination should be examined in each case. For instance, women who are more than 13 weeks' pregnant are advised to be vaccinated against influenza virus because they are at increased risk for complications of influenza, including hospitalization for cardiorespiratory conditions, compared with nonpregnant women.[211]

TABLE 1–6

Vaccination in Pregnancy

VACCINE	USE IN PREGNANCY	COMMENTS
Bacille Calmette-Guérin	No	
Cholera	Yes, administer if indicated	Avoid unless high risk
Hepatitis A	Yes, administer if indicated	Safety not determined
Hepatitis B	Yes, administer if indicated	Safety not determined
Influenza	Yes, administer if indicated	Consult a physician
Japanese encephalitis	Yes, administer if indicated	Avoid unless high risk
Measles	No	
Meningococcal disease	Yes, administer if indicated	
Mumps	No	
Poliomyelitis	Yes, administer if indicated	Normally avoided
Rubella	No	
Tetanus and diphtheria	Yes, administer if indicated	
Rabies	Yes, administer if indicated	
Typhoid	Yes, administer if indicated	Avoid unless high risk
Varicella	No	
Yellow fever	Yes, administer if indicated	Avoid unless high risk

(From World Health Organization: International travel and health. Vaccine-preventable diseases. www.who.int/ith/chapter 06_16.html; Thomas RE: Preparing patients to travel abroad safely: Part 2. Updating vaccinations. Can Fam Physician 2000; 46: 646–652, 655–656.)

Malaria Prophylaxis

Four parasitic protozoa of the genus *Plasmodium* (*Plasmodium ovale*, *Plasmodium vivax*, *Plasmodium malariae*, and *Plasmodium falciparum*) cause human malaria. Of the four species, *P. falciparum* causes the most severe morbidity and mortality. All four species are transmitted through the bite of an infected female *Anopheles* species mosquito. At risk for contraction of malaria are nonimmune persons living in or traveling to areas of Central and South America, Hispaniola, sub-Saharan Africa, the Indian subcontinent, Southeast Asia, the Middle East, and Oceania. Resistance of *P. falciparum* to chloroquine is now common in nearly all malaria-endemic countries of Africa, especially in east Africa, thus posing increasing problems for the provision of suitable treatment. The clinical features of malaria in pregnancy depend to a large extent on the immune status of the woman, which in turn is determined by her previous exposure to malaria. In pregnant women with little or no preexisting immunity, such as those from nonendemic areas or travelers to endemic areas, infection is associated with a high risk of severe maternal anemia and low birth weight. These complications are more common in primigravidae than in multigravidae.[212] Preventive strategies include chemoprophylaxis, intermittent preventative treatment with antimalarials, and insecticide-treated bed nets.[212–215] These strategies reduce the risk of severe maternal anemia and low birth weight, in particular among women of low parity.[212–215] Recommendations for the most appropriate strategy depend on the country of destination, the length of stay, and individual preferences.[216] In the absence of medical attention, travelers to endemic areas are increasingly advised to carry emergency medication for self-treatment.[217]

Chemoprophylaxis should be started at least 1 week before the woman enters the endemic area, preferably 2 to 3 weeks before, so that side effects can be detected before travel occurs. If necessary, prophylaxis can be changed to an alternative drug. Chemoprophylaxis should be continued with unfailing regularity throughout the stay in the endemic area and for 4 weeks after the woman leaves the endemic area. Chloroquine, sulfadoxine–pyrimethamine, and mefloquine are considered safe for use in pregnancy. Normal precautions and contraindications should be observed.

Chemoprophylaxis is increasingly hampered by parasite drug resistance and poor patient compliance.[215] Moreover, chemoprophylaxis does not offer 100% protection, and health care professionals should be alert to the clinical symptoms of malaria.[218] Malaria, which can be fatal, must be suspected if fever, with or without other symptoms, develops at any time between 1 week after the first possible exposure and 2 months (or even later in rare cases) after the last possible exposure.[218]

Other Precautions

The risk of travelers' diarrhea is approximately 7% in developed countries and 20% to 50% in the developing world.[219] Routine prophylaxis of travelers' diarrhea, especially with antibiotics, should be discouraged. Oral rehydration is generally important in the treatment of diarrhea, but travelers' diarrhea is not usually dehydrating in adults.[219] Less severe disease can be treated with a variety of nonantibiotic agents, including bismuth subsalicylate-containing compounds and loperamide.[219,220] These drugs are considered safe for use in pregnancy.

MEDICAL FACTORS

The risks of specific medical conditions in pregnancy and the prepregnancy management options are discussed in the relevant chapters.

SUMMARY OF MANAGEMENT OPTIONS

Air Travel in Pregnancy

Management Options	Quality of Evidence	Strength of Recommendation	References
In the absence of predictable obstetric or medical problems, long-distance air travel is safe in pregnancy.	IV	C	197,201
Long-distance flights are not recommended for women up to 36 weeks' gestation with singleton pregnancies and 32 weeks' with multiple pregnancies.	IV	C	201
Air travel is not recommended for infants younger than 7 days old.	IV	C	197
Update travelers on routine immunizations, including tetanus, diphtheria, polio, measles, mumps, rubella, hepatitis A and B, and influenza vaccines. Other immunizations are based on geographic risk.	IV	C	210

Continued

SUMMARY OF MANAGEMENT OPTIONS
Air Travel in Pregnancy *(Continued)*

Management Options	Quality of Evidence	Strength of Recommendation	References
Travel is not recommended at any time during pregnancy for women who have either medical or obstetric problems that could result in emergencies.	IV	C	201
Preventive measures (e.g., supportive stockings, periodic movement of lower extremities) can be used during long hours of air travel to minimize thromboembolic risk. Additional prophylaxis is advised in those with increased thromboembolic risk (see Chapter 43).	Ib	A	201,207
Travelers should be informed about how to protect themselves against mosquito bites in malarial endemic areas.	Ia	A	214
Drugs given to prevent malaria in pregnancy significantly reduce the likelihood of severe maternal anemia and low birth weight, in particular among women of low parity.	Ia	A	215
Malaria should be suspected in all patients who have symptoms after traveling to an area where malaria is endemic. These patients should undergo blood microscopy.	III	B	218

CONCLUSIONS

- The couple's health status, lifestyle, and reproductive and family history before conception may have a major effect on the likelihood of a successful pregnancy.
- The initial assessment of a woman's reproductive health risks may start well before pregnancy occurs (see Appendix).
- The developing fetus is most vulnerable to maternal conditions and environmental exposures in the first trimester of pregnancy.[83,84]
- Preconception health care may improve reproductive outcome.[4,221]
- The key elements of preconception services include the following:
- Identification of women at increased risk for adverse pregnancy outcome, with subsequent counseling about the necessary preventive measures to ensure an optimal outcome
- Provision of health education to all women, regardless of their risk status, to increase the likelihood of optimal reproductive outcome
- Preconception health care services should include a discussion of contraception and timing of pregnancy, nutritional information, and the patient's infection and immunization history.[4]
- A recent systematic review found evidence of the effectiveness of preconception care in the following three areas[221]:
- Screening women who are seeking family planning for high risk conditions
- Folate supplementation in sexually active women of reproductive age
- Women affected with certain metabolic conditions (e.g., diabetes and hyperphenylalaninemia)
- When couples are systematically provided with information and skills to reduce health risks, they are more likely to reduce substance use, stop using tobacco products, practice safe sex, eat healthy foods, and engage in physical activity.[222]
- Physicians who provide primary care to women should include prepregnancy care in their routine encounters with women of reproductive age.[221]

REFERENCES

1. Altman DG: Comparing groups: Categorical data. In Altman, DG (ed): Practical Statistics for Medical Research. London, Chapman and Hall, 199, pp 229–276.
2. Murray CJL, Lopez AD, Mathers CD, Stein C: The Global Burden of Disease 2000 project: aims, methods and data sources. Geneva, World Health Organization, 2001. Available at: www.who.int/evidence/bod
3. Allaire AD, Cefalo RC: Preconceptional health care model. Eur J Obstet Gynaecol Reprod Biol 1998;78:163–168.
4. de Weerd S, van der Bij AK, Cikot RJ, et al: Preconception care: A screening tool for health assessment and risk detection. Prev Med 2002;34:505–511.
5. Terry PB, Condie RG, Settatree RS: Analysis of ethnic differences in perinatal statistics. BMJ 1980;281:1307–1308.
6. Houdek Jimenez M, Newton N: Activity and work during pregnancy and the postpartum period: A cross-cultural study of 202 societies. Am J Obstet Gynecol 1979;135:171–176.
7. Barron SL: Birthweight and ethnicity. Br J Obstet Gynaecol 1983;90:289–290.
8. Helman C: Culture factors in epidemiology. In Helman C (ed): Culture, Health and Illness. Bristol, UK, John Wright, 1986, pp 181–193.
9. Cruickshank JK, Beevers DG: Migration, ethnicity, health and disease. In Cruickshank JK, Beevers DG (eds): Ethnic Factors in Health and Disease. London, Butterworth, 1989, pp 3–6.
10. Kleinman JC, Kessel SS: Racial differences in low birth weight: Trends and risk factors. N Engl J Med 1987;317:749–753.
11. Shiono PH, Klebanoff MA, Graubard BI, et al: Birth weight among women of different ethnic groups. JAMA 1986;255:48–52.
12. Lieberman E, Ryan KJ, Monson RR, Schoenbaum SC: Risk factors accounting for racial differences in the rate of premature birth. N Engl J Med 1987;317:743–748.
13. McCormick MC: The contribution of low birth weight to infant mortality and childhood morbidity. N Engl J Med 1985;312:82–90.
14. Shiono PH, Klebanoff MA: Ethnic differences in preterm and very preterm delivery. Am J Public Health 1986;76:1317–1321.
15. Paneth N, Wallenstein S, Kiely JL, Susser M: Social class indicators and mortality in low birth weight infants. Am J Epidemiol 1982;116:364–375.
16. Behrman RE: Premature births among black women. N Engl J Med 1987;317:763–765.
17. Kline J, Stein Z, Susser M: Preterm delivery: II. Risk factors; Fetal growth and birthweight: I. Indices, patterns and risk factors. In Kline J, Stein Z, Susser M (eds): Conception to Birth: Epidemiology of Prenatal Development. New York, Oxford University Press, 1989, pp 191–230.
18. Alexander GR, Tompkins ME, Altekruse JM, Hornung CA: Racial differences in the relation of birth weight and gestational age to neonatal mortality. Public Health Rep 1985;100:539–547.
19. Wilcox AJ, Russell IT: Birthweight and perinatal mortality: III. Towards a new method of analysis. Int J Epidemiol 1986;15:188–196.
20. Wilcox A, Russell I: Why shall small black infants have a lower mortality rate than small white infants: The case for population specific standard of birthweight. J Pediatr 1990;116:7–10.
21. Rahbar F, Momeni J, Fomufod A, Westney L: Prenatal care and perinatal mortality in a black population. Obstet Gynecol 1985;65:327–329.
22. De Silva S: Obstetric sequelae of female circumcision. Eur J Obstet Gynecol Reprod Biol 1989;32:233–240.
23. Tuck SM, Cadozo LD, Studd JWW, Gibb DMF: Obstetric characteristics in different racial groups. Br J Obstet Gynaecol 1983;90:892–897.
24. Briggs ND: Engagement of the fetal head in the Negro primigravida. Br J Obstet Gynaecol 1981;88:1086–1089.
25. Thom MH, Chan KK, Studd JWW: Outcome of normal and dysfunctional labour in different racial groups. Am J Obstet Gynecol 1979;135:495–498.
26. Doornbos JPR, Nordbeck HJ: Perinatal mortality: Obstetric risk factors in a community of mixed ethnic origin in Amsterdam. PhD thesis. University of Amsterdam, 1985.
27. Shaw-Taylor Y: Culturally and linguistically appropriate health care for racial or ethnic minorities: Analysis of the US Office of Minority Health's recommended standards. Health Policy 2002;62:211–221.
28. Cao A, Rosatelli MC, Galanello R: Control of beta-thalassaemia by carrier screening, genetic counselling and prenatal diagnosis: The Sardinian experience. Ciba Found Symp 1996;197:137–151.
29. Kadkhodaei Elyaderani M, Cinkotai KI, Hyde K, et al: Ethnicity study and non-selective screening for haemoglobinopathies in the antenatal population of central Manchester. Clin Lab Haematol 1998;20:207–211.
30. Zuniga de Nuncio ML, Nader PR, Sawyer MH, et al: A prenatal intervention study to improve timeliness of immunization initiation in Latino infants. J Community Health 2003;28:151–165.
31. Hodnett ED. Support during pregnancy for women at increased risk: Cochrane review. In Cochrane Library, issue 1, 2003. Oxford, UK, Update Software.
32. American Academy of Pediatrics Work Group on Breastfeeding: Breastfeeding and the use of human milk. Pediatrics 1997;100:1035–1039.
33. Garg M: Uptake of family planning services among an ethnically mixed population in a general practice setting. Br J Fam Planning 1998;24:82–83.
34. Baranowski T, Bee DE, Rassin DK, et al: Social support, social influence, ethnicity and the breastfeeding decision. Soc Sci Med 1983;1599–1611.
35. http://www.who.int/ionizing_radiation/en
36. Radiation and your patient: A guide for medical practitioners. Ann Int Commission Radiol Protection 2001;31:5–31.
37. Fry RJ: Deterministic effects. Health Phys 2001;80:338–343.
38. Dolk H, Nichols R, EUROCAT Working Group: Evaluation of the impact of Chernobyl on the prevalence of congenital anomalies in 166 regions of Europe. Int J Epidemiol 1999;28:941–948.
39. Doll R, Wakeford R: Risk of childhood cancer from fetal irradiation. Br J Radiol 1997;70:130–139.
40. Directorate General Environment, Nuclear Safety and Civil Protection of the European Committee: Guidance for protection of unborn children an infants irradiated due to parental medical exposures (http://europa.eu.int/comm/environment/radprot/100/rp-100-en.pdf)
41. Tham TCK, Vandervoort J, Wong RKC, et al: Safety of ERCP during pregnancy. Am J Gastroenterol 2003;98:308–311.
42. Critchley HO, Bath LE, Wallace WH: Radiation damage to the uterus: Review of the effects of treatment of childhood cancer. Hum Fertil (Camb) 2002;5:61–66.
43. Arnon J, Meirow D, Lewis-Roness H, Ornoy A: Genetic and teratogenic effects of cancer treatments on gametes and embryos. Hum Reprod Update 2001;7:394–403.
44. Adelstein SJ: Administered radionuclides in pregnancy. Teratology 1999;59:236–239.
45. Takahashi M, Uematsu H, Hatabu HMR: Imaging at high magnetic fields. Eur J Radiol 2003;46:45–52.
46. Boutin RD, Briggs JE, Williamson MR: Injuries associated with MR imaging: Survey of safety records and methods used to screen patients for metallic foreign bodies before imaging. AJR Am J Roentgenol 1994;162:189–194.

47. Wagenvoort AM, Bekker MN, Go AT, et al: Ultrafast scan magnetic resonance in prenatal diagnosis. Fetal Diagn Ther 2000;15:364–372.
48. Nagayama M, Watanabe Y, Okumura A, et al: Fast MR imaging in obstetrics. Radiographics 2002;22:563–580.
49. Levine D, Barnes PD, Madsen JR, et al: Fetal central nervous system anomalies: MR imaging augments sonographic diagnosis. Radiology 1997;204:635–642.
50. Levine D, Barnes PD, Edelman RR: Obstetric MR imaging. Radiology 1999;211:609–672.
51. ISUOG Bio-effects and Safety Committee: Safety statement, 2000 (reconfirmed 2003). International Society of Ultrasound in Obstetrics and Gynecology (ISUOG). Ultrasound Obstet Gynecol 2003;21:100.
52. Barnett SB, Maulik D: International Perinatal Doppler Society guidelines and recommendations for safe use of Doppler ultrasound in perinatal applications. J Matern Fetal Med 2001;10:75–84.
53. Salvesen KA: EFSUMB: Safety tutorial. Epidemiology of diagnostic ultrasound exposure during pregnancy: European Committee for Medical Ultrasound Safety (ECMUS). Eur J Ultrasound 2002;15:165–171.
54. Neilson JP: Ultrasound for fetal assessment in early pregnancy: Cochrane review. In Cochrane Library, issue 2, 2003. Oxford, UK, Update Software.
55. Abramowicz JS, Kossoff G, Marsál K, Ter Haar G: Literature review by the ISUOG Bioeffects and Safety Committee. Ultrasound J Obstet Gynecol 2002;19:318–319.
56. Barnett SB, Ter Haar GR, Zistin MC, et al: International recommendations and safety guidelines for the safe use of diagnostic ultrasound in medicine. Ultrasound Med Biol 2000;26:355–366.
57. Meltzer RS: Food and Drug Administration ultrasound device regulation: The output display standard, the 'mechanical index' and ultrasound safety. J Am Soc Echocardiogr 1996;9:216–220.
58. European Federation of Societies for Ultrasound in Medicine and Biology: Guidelines for the safe use of Doppler ultrasound for clinical applications. Report from the European Committee for Ultrasound Radiation Safety. http://www.efsumb.org/statement2001.htm
59. American Institute of Ultrasound in Medicine: Official Statements and Reports of the American Institute of Ultrasound in Medicine, 1999. http://www.aium.org/stmts.htm
60. McDonald AD, McDonald JC, Armstrong B, et al: Work with visual display units in pregnancy. Br J Indust Med 1988;45:509–515.
61. Lindbohm ML, Hietanen M: Magnetic fields of video display terminals and pregnancy outcome. J Occup Environ Med 1995;37:952–956.
62. Faroon OM, Keith LS, Smith-Simon C, De Rosa CT: Polychlorinated biphenyls: Human health aspects. International Chemical assessment document No. 55. Geneva, World Health Organization, 2003. http://www.who.int/pcs/cicad/full_text/cicad55.pdf
63. Boersma ER, Lanting CI: Consequences for long-term neurological and cognitive development of the child lactation. Adv Exp Med Biol 2000;478:271–287.
64. Parzefall W: Risk assessment of dioxin contamination in human food. Food Chem Toxicol 2002;40:1185–1189.
65. Garry VF, Schreinemachers D, Harkins ME, Griffith J: Pesticide appliers, biocides, and birth defects in rural Minnesota. Environ Health Perspect 1996;104:394–399.
66. Schreinemachers DM: Birth malformations and other adverse perinatal outcomes in four U.S. wheat-producing states. Environ Health Perspect 2003;111:1259–1264.
67. Jones IG, Cameron D: Social class analysis: An embarrassment to epidemiology. Community Med 1984;6:37–46.
68. Oakley A, Rajan L, Robertson P: A comparison of different sources of information about pregnancy and childbirth. J Biosocial Sci 1990;22:477–487.
69. Krieger N: Women and social class: A methodological study comparing individual, household, and census measures as predictors of black/white differences in reproductive history. J Epidemiol Community Health 1991;45:35–42.
70. Antonovsky A, Bernstein J: Social class and infant mortality. Soc Sci Med 1977;11:453–470.
71. Gunning-Schepers L: The health benefits of prevention: A simulation approach. In Blanpain J, Davis K, Gunji A (eds): Health Policy, vol. 12. Amsterdam, Elsevier, 1989.
72. Chalmers I: Short, Black, Himsworth and social class differences in fetal and neonatal mortality rates. BMJ 1985;2:231–233.
73. Chalmers B: Psychological aspects of pregnancy: Some thoughts for the eighties. Soc Sci Med 1986;16:323–331.
74. Elbourne D, Pritchard C, Dauncey M: Perinatal outcomes and related factors: Social class differences within and between geographical areas. J Epidemiol Community Health 1986;40:301–308.
75. Golding J, Tejeiro A, Rojas Ochoa F: The uses and abuses of national statistics. In Golding J (ed): Social and Biological Effects on Perinatal Mortality, vol. III. Perinatal Analyses: Report on an International Comparative Study Sponsored by the World Health Organization. Bristol, UK, Bristol University, 1990, pp 355–384.
76. Kramer MS, Seguin L, Lydon J, Goulet L: Socio-economic disparities in pregnancy outcome: Why do the poor fare so poorly? Paediatr Perinat Epidemiol 2000;14:194–210.
77. Brooke OG, Anderson HR, Bland JM, et al: Effects on birth weight of smoking, alcohol, caffeine, socioeconomic factors and psychosocial stress. BMJ 1989;289:795–801.
78. Leon DA: Influence of birthweight on differences in infant mortality by social class and legitimacy. BMJ 1991;303:964–967.
79. Greenberg RS: The impact of prenatal care in different social groups. Am J Obstet Gynecol 1983;145:797–801.
80. Langer A, Campero L, Garcia C, Reynoso S: Effects of psychosocial support during labour and childbirth on breastfeeding, medical interventions, and mothers' wellbeing in a Mexican public hospital: A randomised clinical trial. Br J Obstet Gynaecol 1998;105:1056–1063.
81. Lancaster T, Stead LF: Individual behavioural counselling for smoking cessation: Cochrane review. In Cochrane Library, issue 1, 2002. Oxford, UK, Update Software.
82. Donath S, Amir L: Rates of breastfeeding in Australia by state and socio-economic status: Evidence from the 1995 National Health Survey. J Paediatr Child Health 2000;36:164–168.
83. Barker DJP, Eriksson JG, Forsén T, Osmonda C: Fetal origins of adult disease: Strength of effects and biological basis. Int J Epidemiol 2002;31:1235–1239.
84. Metcalfe NB, Monaghan P: Compensation for a bad start: Grow now, pay later. Trends Ecol Evol 2001;16:254–260.
85. Godfrey KM: The role of the placenta in fetal programming: A review. Placenta 2002;23(suppl A):S20–S27.
86. Lumey LH: Compensatory placental growth after restricted maternal nutrition in early pregnancy. Placenta 1998;19: 105–111.
87. Godfrey K, Robinson S, Barjker DJP, et al: Maternal nutrition in early and late pregnancy in relation to placenta and fetal growth. BMJ 1996;312:410–414.
88. Merialdi M, Carroli G, Villar J, et al: Nutritional interventions during pregnancy for the prevention or treatment of impaired fetal growth: An overview of randomized controlled trials. J Nutr 2003;133:1626S–1631S.
89. Bracken MB, Triche EW, Belanger K, et al: Association of maternal caffeine consumption with decrements in fetal growth. Am J Epidemiol 2003;157:456–466.
90. Fairfield KM, Fletcher RH: Vitamins for chronic disease prevention in adults: Scientific review. JAMA 2002;287:3116–3126.

91. Scott JM: Folate and vitamin B12. Proc Nutr Soc 1999;58(2):441–448.
92. Hague WM: Homocysteine and pregnancy. Best Pract Res Clin Obstet Gynaecol 2003;17:459–469.
93. Chappell LC, Seed PT, Briley AL, et al: Effect of antioxidants on the occurrence of pre-eclampsia in women at increased risk: A randomised trial. Lancet 1999;354:810–816.
94. Puckett RM, Offringa M: Prophylactic vitamin K for vitamin K deficiency bleeding in neonates: Cochrane review. In Cochrane Library, issue 1, 2003. Oxford, UK, Update Software.
95. Cornelissen M, Steegers-Theunissen R, Kollee L, et al: Supplementation of vitamin K in pregnant women receiving anticonvulsant therapy prevents neonatal vitamin K deficiency. Am J Obstet Gynecol 1993;168:884–888.
96. Steegers-Theunissen RPM: Maternal nutrition and obstetric outcome. Baillieres Clin Obstet Gynaecol 1995;9:431–443.
97. Herzog DB, Copeland PM: Eating disorders. N Engl J Med 1985;313:295–302.
98. Cohen-Kerem R, Koren G: Antioxidants and fetal protection against ethanol teratogenicity: I. Review of the experimental data and implications to humans. Neurotoxicol Teratol 2003;25:1–9.
99. Dreosti IE: Nutritional factors underlying the expression of the fetal alcohol syndrome. Ann N Y Acad Sci 1993;678:193–204.
100. Stewart DE, Raskin J, Garfinkel PE, et al: Anorexia nervosa, bulimia, and pregnancy. Am J Obstet Gynecol 1987;157: 1194–1198.
101. Lumley J, Watson L, Watson M, Bower C: Periconceptional supplementation with folate and/or multivitamins for preventing neural tube defects: Cochrane review. In Cochrane Library, issue 1, 2003. Oxford, UK, Update Software.
102. Villar J, Merialdi M, Gulmezoglu AM, et al: Nutritional interventions during pregnancy for the prevention or treatment of maternal morbidity and preterm delivery: An overview of randomized controlled trials. J Nutr 2003;133:1606S–1625S.
103. Hytten F: Nutritional requirements in pregnancy: What should the pregnant woman be eating? Midwifery 1990;6:93–98.
104. Mahomed K: Iron supplementation in pregnancy: Cochrane review. In Cochrane Library, issue 2, 2003. Oxford, UK, Update Software.
105. Naeye RL: Maternal body weight and pregnancy outcome. Am J Clinical Nutr 1990;52:273–279.
106. Dawes MG, Grudzinskas JG: Repeated measurement of maternal weight during pregnancy: Is this a useful practice? Br J Obstet Gynaecol 1991;98:189–194.
107. Durnin JVGA: Energy requirements of pregnancy: An integration of the longitudinal data from the five-country study. Lancet 1987;ii:1131–1133.
108. Hytten FE: Weight gain in pregnancy. In Hytten FE, Chamberlain G (eds): Clinical Physiology in Obstetrics, 2nd ed. Oxford, UK, Blackwell, 1991, pp 173–203.
109. Franko DL, Blais MA, Becker AE, et al: Pregnancy complications and neonotal outcomes in women with eating disorders. Am J Psychiatry 2001;158: 1461–1466.
110. Feingold M, Kaminer Y, Lyons K, et al: Bulimia nervosa in pregnancy. Obstet Gynecol 1988;71:1025–1027.
111. Lind T: Nutrition: The changing scene. Would more calories per day keep low birthweight at bay? Lancet 1984;i:501–502.
112. Spuy ZM van der, Steer PJ, McCusker M, et al: Outcome of pregnancy in underweight women after spontaneous and induced ovulation. BMJ 1988;296:962–965.
113. Sollid CP, Wisborg K, Hjort J, Secher NJ: Eating disorder that was diagnosed before pregnancy and pregnancy outcome. Am J Obstet Gynecol 2004;190:206–210.
114. Lin CC, Moawad AH, Rosenow PJ, River P: Acid-base characteristics of fetuses with intrauterine growth retardation during labor and delivery. Am J Obstet Gynecol 1980;137: 553–559.
115. Kramer MS: Balanced protein/energy supplementation in pregnancy: Cochrane review. In Cochrane Library, issue 1, 2003. Oxford, UK, Update Software.
116. Obesity preventing and managing the global epidemic: Report of a WHO consultation on obesity. Geneva, World Health Organization, 1997. World Health Organization Tech Rep Ser 2000;894:i–xii:1–253.
117. Drife JO: Weight gain in pregnancy: Eating for two or just getting fat? BMJ 1986;293:903–904.
118. Kliegman RM, Gross T: Perinatal problems of the obese mother and her infant. Obstet Gynecol 1985;66:299–305.
119. Garbaciak JA, Richter M, Miller S, Barton JJ: Maternal weight and pregnancy complications. Am J Obstet Gynecol 1985;152: 238–245.
120. Robinson H, Tkatch S, Mayes DC, et al: Is maternal obesity a predictor of shoulder dystocia? Obstet Gynecol 2003;101:24–27.
121. Dindo D, Muller MK, Weber M, Clavein PA: Obesity in general elective surgery. Lancet 2003;361:2032–2035.
122. Harvey EL, Glenny A-M, Kirk SFL, Summerbell CD: Improving health professionals' management and the organisation of care for overweight and obese people: Cochrane review. In Cochrane Library, issue 2, 2003. Oxford, UK, Update Software.
123. Astrup A: Dietary approaches to reducing body weight. Baillieres Best Pract Res Clin Endocrinol Metab 1999:109–120.
124. Kramer MS: Energy/protein restriction for high weight-for-height or weight gain during pregnancy: Cochrane review. In Cochrane Library, issue 2, 2003. Oxford, UK, Update Software.
125. Friedman CI, Kim MH: Obesity and its effect on reproductive function. Clin Obstet Gynecol 1985;28:645–663.
126. Richards DS, Miller DK, Goodman GN: Pregnancy after gastric bypass for morbid obesity. J Reprod Med 1987;32:172–176.
127. O'Brien E, Coats A, Owens P, et al: Use and interpretation of ambulatory blood pressure monitoring: Recommendations of the British hypertension society. Br Med J 2000;320:1128–1134.
128. Smaill F: Antibiotics for asymptomatic bacteriuria in pregnancy: Cochrane review. In Cochrane Library, issue 1, 2003. Oxford, UK, Update Software.
129. Scott A, Moar V, Ounsted M: The relative contribution of different maternal factors in large-for-gestational-age pregnancies. Eur J Obstet Gynecol Reprod Biol 1982;13:269–277.
130. Hood DD, Dewan DM: Anesthetic and obstetric outcome in morbidly obese parturients. Anesthesiology 1993;79:1210–1218.
131. Smaill F, Hofmeyr GJ: Antibiotic prophylaxis for cesarean section: Cochrane review. In Cochrane Library, issue 1, 2003. Oxford, UK, Update Software.
132. Greer IA, Gross TL: Prevention of venous thromboembolism in pregnancy. Best Pract Res Clin Haematol 2003;16:261–278.
133. Gross TL: Operative considerations in the obese pregnant patient. Clinics Perinatol 1983;10:411–421.
134. Wilkinson C, Enkin MW: Uterine exteriorization versus intraperitoneal repair at caesarean section: Cochrane review. In Cochrane Library, issue 2, 2003. Oxford, UK, Update Software.
135. Alderdice F, McKenna D, Dornan J: Techniques and materials for skin closure in caesarean section: Cochrane review. In Cochrane Library, issue 2, 2003. Oxford, UK, Update Software.
136. Dawes MG, Grudzinskas JG: Patterns of maternal weight gain in pregnancy. Br J Obstet Gynaecol 1991;98:195–201.
137. Maternal weight gain in pregnancy. Lancet 1991;338:415.
138. Raaij JMA van, Vermaat-Miedema SH, Schonk CM, et al: Energy requirements of pregnancy in the Netherlands. Lancet 1987;ii:953–955.
139. Lawrence M, McKillop FM, Durnin JVGA: Women who gain more fat during pregnancy may not have bigger babies: Implications for recommended weight gain during pregnancy. Br J Obstet Gynaecol 1991;98:254–259.
140. Greene GW, Smiciklas-Wright H, Scholl TO, Karp RJ: Post partum weight change: How much of the weight gained will be lost after delivery? Obstet Gynecol 1988;71:701–707.

141. McAnarney ER: Young maternal age and adverse neonatal outcome. Am J Dis Child 1987;141:1053–1059.
142. Abrams BF, Laros RK: Prepregnancy weight, weight gain, and birth weight. Am J Obstet Gynecol 1986;15:503–509.
143. Theron GB, Thompson ML: The usefulness of a weight gain spurt to identify women who will develop preeclampsia. Eur J Obstet Gynecol Reprod Biol 1998;78:47–51.
144. Allaire AD, Fisch J, McMahon MJ: Subcutaneous drain vs. suture in obese women undergoing cesarean delivery: A prospective, randomized trial. J Reprod Med 2000;45:327–331.
145. Lotgering FK, Gilbet RD Longo LD: Maternal and fetal response to exercise during pregnancy. Physiol Rev 1985;65;1–35.
146. Wildschut HIJ, Harker LM, Riddoch CJ: The potential value of a short self-completion questionnaire for the assessment of habitual physical activity in pregnancy. J Psychsom Obstet Gynaecol 1993;14:17–29.
147. Clapp JF III: Pregnancy outcome: Physical activities inside versus outside the workplace. Semin Perinatol 1996;20: 70–76.
148. ACOG Committee on Obstetric Practice: ACOG committee opinion: Exercise during pregnancy and the postpartum period. No. 267, January 2002. American College of Obstetricians and Gynecologists. Int J Gynaecol Obstet 2002;77:79–81.
149. Clapp JF III, Kim H, Burciu B, Lopez B: Beginning regular exercise in early pregnancy: Effect on fetoplacental growth. Am J Obstet Gynecol 2000;183:1484–1488.
150. Clapp JF III: Exercise during pregnancy: A clinical update. Clin Sports Med 2000;19:273–286.
151. Kramer MS: Aerobic exercise for women during pregnancy: Cochrane review. In Cochrane Library, issue 1, 2003. Oxford, UK, Update Software.
152. Camporesi EM: Diving and pregnancy. Semin Perinatol 1996;20:292–302.
153. Figà-Talamanca I: Reproductive health and occupational hazards among women workers. In Kane P (ed): Women and Occupational Health: Issues and Policy Paper for the Global Commission of Women's Health, 2003, pp 65–73. http://www.who.int/oeh/OCHweb/OCHweb/OSHpages/OSH Documents/Women/WomenOccupHealth.pdf.
154. Dennerstein L: Paid work, Gender and Health. In Kane P (ed): Women and Occupational Health: Issues and Policy Paper for the Global Commission of Women's Health, 2003, pp 50–54. http://www.who.int/oeh/OCHweb/OCHweb/OSHpages/OSH Documents/Women/WomenOccpHealth.pdf
155. McMartin KI, Chu M, Kopecky E, et al: Pregnancy outcome following maternal organic solvent exposure: A meta-analysis of epidemiologic studies. Am J Ind Med 1998;34:288–292.
156. Lindbohm ML: Effects of parental exposure to solvents on pregnancy outcome. J Occup Environ Med 1995;37:908–914.
157. Mozurkewich EL, Luke B, Avni M, Wolf FM: Working conditions and adverse pregnancy outcome: A meta-analysis. Obstet Gynecol 2000;95:623–635.
158. Gabbe SG, Turner LP: Reproductive hazards of the American lifestyle: Work during pregnancy. Am J Obstet Gynecol 1997;176:826–832.
159. Mamelle N, Laumon B, Lazar P: Prematurity and occupational activity during pregnancy. Am J Epidemiol 1984;119:309–322.
160. Treffers PE: Teenage pregnancy, a worldwide problem [Dutch]. Ned Tijdschr Geneeskd 2003;147:2320–2325.
161. Sandler DP, Wilcox AJ, Horney LF: Age at menarche and subsequent reproductive events. Am J Epidemiol 1984;119: 765–774.
162. McAnarney ER: Young maternal age and adverse neonatal outcome. Am J Dis Child 1987;141:1053–1059.
163. Scholl TO, Hediger ML, Salmon RW, et al: Association between low gynaecological age and preterm birth. Paediatr Perinatal Epidemiol 1989;3:361–370.
164. Mitchell LE, Bracken MB: Reproductive and chronologic age as a predictor of low birth weight, preterm delivery and intrauterine growth retardation in primiparous women. Ann Hum Biol 1990;17:377–386.
165. Singh S, Darroch JE: Adolescent pregnancy and childbearing: Levels and trends in developed countries. Fam Planning Perspect 2000;32:14–23.
166. Golding J: Maternal age and parity. In Golding J (ed): Social and Biological Effects on Perinatal Mortality, vol. III. Perinatal Analyses: Report on an International Comparative Study Sponsored by the World Health Organization. Bristol, UK, University of Bristol, 1990; pp 183–218.
167. Adolescent pregnancy. Lancet 1989;2:1308–1309.
168. Fielding JE, Williams CA: Adolescent pregnancy in the United States: A review and recommendations for clinicians and research needs. Am J Prev Med 1991;7:47–52.
169. Sukanich AC, Rogers KD, McDonald NM: Physical maturity and outcome of pregnancy in primiparous women younger than 16 years of age. Pediatrics 1986;78:31–36.
170. Mitchell-DiCenso A, Thomas BH, Devlin MC, et al: Evaluation of an educational program to prevent adolescent pregnancy. Health Educ Behav 1997;24:300–312.
171. Jaccard J, Dittus PJ: Adolescent perceptions of maternal approval of birth control and sexual risk behavior. Am J Public Health 2000;90:1426–1430.
172. Stevens-Simon C, Kelly L, Kulick R: A village would be nice but...it takes a long-acting contraceptive to prevent repeat adolescent pregnancies. Am J Prev Med 2001;21(1):60–65.
173. Hollingsworth DR, Felice M: Teenage pregnancy: A multiracial sociologic problem. Am J Obstet Gynecol 1986;155:741–746.
174. Fraser AM, Brockert JE, Ward RH: Association of young maternal age with adverse reproductive outcomes. N Engl J Med 1995;332:1113–1117.
175. Orvos H, Nyirati I, Hajdu J, et al: Is adolescent pregnancy associated with adverse perinatal outcome? J Perinatal Med 1999;27: 199–203.
176. Quinlivan JA, Petersen RW, Gurrin LC: Adolescent pregnancy: Psychopathology missed. Aust N Z J Psychiatry 1999;33:864–868.
177. Moerman ML: Growth of the birth canal in adolescent girls. Am J Obstet Gynecol 1982;143:528–532.
178. Blankson ML, Cliver SP, Goldenberg RL, et al: Health behavior and outcomes in sequential pregnancies of black and white adolescents. JAMA 1993;269:1401–1403.
179. Koniak-Griffin D, Anderson NL, Brecht ML, et al: Public health nursing care for adolescent mothers: Impact on infant health and selected maternal outcomes at 1 year postbirth. J Adolesc Health 2002;30:44–54.
180. Jones DC, Lowry RB: Falling maternal age and incidence of Down syndrome. Lancet 1975;1:753–754.
181. Holloway S, Brock DJH: Changes in maternal age distribution and their possible impact on the demand for prenatal diagnostic services. BMJ 1988;296:978–981.
182. Stein ZA: A woman's age: Childbearing and child rearing. Am J Epidemiol 1985;121:327–342.
183. Tuck SM, Yudkin PL, Turnbull AC: Pregnancy outcome in elderly primigravida with and without a history of infertility. Br J Obstet Gynaecol 1988;95:230–237.
184. Berkowitz GS, Skovron ML, Lapinski RH, Berkowitz RL: Delayed childbearing and the outcome of pregnancy. N Engl J Med 1990;322:659–664.
185. MacGillivray I, Samphier M, Little J: Factors affecting twinning. In MacGillivray I, Campbell DM, Thompson B (eds): Twinning and Twins. Chichester, John Wiley, 1988, pp 67–97.
186. Andersen A-MN, Wohlfahrt J, Christens P, et al: Maternal age and fetal loss: Population-based register linkage study. Br Med J 2000;320:1708–1712.
187. Baird PA, Sadovnick AD, Yee IML: Maternal age and birth defects. Lancet 1991;337:527–530.
188. Hook EB: Issues in analysis of data on paternal age and 47, +21: Implications for genetic counselling for Down syndrome. Hum Genet 1987;77:303–306.

189. Snijders RJM, Sundberg K, Holzgreve W, et al: Maternal age- and gestation-specific risk for trisomy 21. Ultrasound Obstet Gynecol 1999;13:167–170.
190. Stein Z, Stein W, Susser M: Attrition of trisomies as a maternal screening device: An explanation of the association of trisomy 21 with maternal age. Lancet 1986;1:944–947.
191. Morris JK, Wald NJ, Mutton DE, Alberman E: Comparison of models of maternal age-specific risk for Down syndrome live births. Prenatal Diagn 2003;23:252–258.
192. Alfirevic Z, Gosden CM, Neilson JP: Chorion villus sampling versus amniocentesis for prenatal diagnosis: Cochrane review. In Cochrane Library, issue 2, 2003. Oxford, UK, Update Software.
193. Moos MK, Bartholomew NE, Lohr KN: Counseling in the clinical setting to prevent unintended pregnancy: An evidence-based research agenda. Contraception 2003;67:115–132.
194. Truitt ST, Fraser AB, Grimes DA, et al: Combined hormonal versus nonhormonal versus progestin-only contraception in lactation: Cochrane review. In Cochrane Library, issue 2, 2003. Oxford, UK, Update Software.
195. Babinszki A, Kerenyi T, Torok O, et al: Perinatal outcome in grand and great-grand multiparity: Effects of parity on obstetric risk factors. Am J Obstet Gynecol 1999;181:669–674.
196. Smith GF, Berg JM: Down's Anomaly, 2nd ed. Edinburgh, Churchill Livingstone, 1976.
197. Kingman CEC, Economides DL: Air travel in pregnancy. Obstet Gynaecol 2002;4:188–192.
198. www.who.int
199. Huch R, Baumann H, Fallenstein F, et al: Physiologic changes in pregnant women and their fetuses during jet air travel. Am J Obstet Gynecol 1986;154:996–1000.
200. Artal R, Fortunato V, Welton A, et al: A comparison of cardiopulmonary adaptations to exercise in pregnancy at sea level and altitude. Am J Obstet Gynecol 1995;172:1170–1178.
201. ACOG Committee Opinion No. 264 ACOG Publications 2001.
202. Jacobson BF, Munster M, Smith A, et al: The BEST study: A prospective study to compare business class versus economy class air travel as a cause of thrombosis. S Afr Med J 2003;93:522–528.
203. Mendis S, Yach D, Alwan A: Air travel and venous thromboembolism. Bull WHO 2002;80:403–406.
204. Kesteven P, Robinson B: Incidence of symptomatic thrombosis in a stable population of 650,000: Travel and other risk factors. Aviat Space Environ Med 2002;73:593–596.
205. Giangrande: Air travel and thrombosis. Br J Haematol 2002;117:509–512.
206. Geroulakos G: The risk of venous thromboembolism from air travel. Br Med J 2001;322:188.
207. Scurr JH, Machin SJ, Bailey-King S, et al: Frequency and prevention of symptomless deep-vein thrombosis in long-haul flights: A randomised trial. Lancet 2001;357:1485–1489.
208. Hyde LK, Cook LJ, Olson LM, et al: Effect of motor vehicle crashes on adverse fetal outcomes. Obstet Gynecol 2003;102:279–286.
209. Health Organization: International travel and health: Vaccine-preventable diseases. www.who.int/ith/chapter 06_16.html
210. Thomas RE: Preparing patients to travel abroad safely: Part 2. Updating vaccinations. Can Fam Physician 2000;46:646–652, 655–656.
211. Ahmed F, Singleton JA, Franks A: Influenza vaccination for healthy young adults. N Engl J Med 2001;345:1543–1547.
212. Shulman CE, Dorman EK: Importance and prevention of malaria in pregnancy. Trans R Soc Trop Med Hyg 2003;97:30–35.
213. Shulman CE, Dorman EK, Cutts F, et al: Intermittent sulphadoxine-pyrimethamine to prevent severe anaemia secondary to malaria in pregnancy: A randomised placebo-controlled trial. Lancet 1999;353:632–636.
214. Choi HW, Breman JG, Teutsch SM, et al: The effectiveness of insecticide-impregnated bed nets in reducing cases of malaria infection: A meta-analysis of published results. Am J Trop Med Hyg 1995;52:377–382.
215. Garner P, Gülmezoglu AM: Drugs for preventing malaria-related illness in pregnant women en death in the newborn: Cochrane review. In Cochrane Library, issue 2, 2003. Oxford, UK, Update Software.
216. Thomas RE: Preparing your patients to travel abroad safely: Part 3. Reducing the risk of malaria and dengue fever. Can Fam Physician 2000;46:1126–1131.
217. Nothdurft HD, Jelinek T, Pechel SM, et al: Stand-by treatment of suspected malaria in travellers. Trop Med Parasitol 1995;46:161–163.
218. Casalino E, Le Bras J, Chaussin F, et al: Predictive factors of malaria in travelers to areas where malaria is endemic. Arch Intern Med 2002;162:1625–1630.
219. Ericsson CD: Travellers' diarrhoea. Int J Antimicrob Agents 2003;21:116–124.
220. Thomas RE: Preparing patients to travel abroad safely: Part 4. Reducing risk of accidents, diarrhea, and sexually transmitted diseases. Can Fam Physician 2000;46:1634–1638.
221. Korenbrot CC, Steinberg A, Bender C, Newberry S: Preconception care: A systematic review. Matern Child Health J 2002;6:75–88.
222. World Health Organization: Care in normal birth: A practical guide, 1996 (WHO/FRH/MSM/96.24).

APPENDIX

March of Dimes
Saving babies, together

PRECONCEPTION SCREENING AND COUNSELING CHECKLIST

Upper Hudson Prenatal Services Network

NAME	BIRTHPLACE	AGE

DATE: / / ARE YOU PLANNING TO GET PREGNANT IN THE NEXT SIX MONTHS? __ Y __N

IF YOUR ANSWER TO A QUESTION IS YES, PUT A CHECK MARK ON THE LINE IN FRONT OF THE QUESTION. FILL IN OTHER INFORMATION THAT AI LIES TO YOU

DIET & EXERCISE

What do you consider a healthy weight for you? __________
___Do you eat three meals a day?
___Do you follow a special diet (vegetarian, diabetic, other)?
___Which do you drink (__coffee __tea __cola __milk __water __other soda/pop other ____________________________)?
___Do you eat raw or undercooked food (meat, other)?
___Do you take folic acid?
___Do you take other vitamins daily (__multivitamin __vitamin A __other)?
___Do you take dietary supplements (__black cohosh __ pennyroyal __other)?
___Do you have current/past problems with eating disorders?
___Do you exercise? Type/frequency:________________
Notes:

MEDICATION/DRUGS

___ Are you taking prescribed drugs (Accutane, valproic acid, blood thinners)? List them______________________________________
___ Are you taking non-prescribed drugs?
List them:____
___Are you using birth control pills?
___Do you get injectable contraceptives or shots for birth control?
___Do you use any herbal remedies or alternative medicine?
List:____
NOTES:

WOMEN'S HEALTH

___Do you have any problems with your menstrual cycle?
___ How many times have you been pregnant?
What was/were the outcomes(s)? ______________________________
___Did you have difficulty getting pregnant last time?
___Have you been treated for infertility?
___Have you had surgery on your uterus, cervix, ovaries or tubes?
___Did you mother take the hormone DES during pregnancy?
___Have you ever had HPV, genital warts or chlamydia?
___Have you ever been treated for a sexually transmitted infection (genital herpes, gonorrhea, syphilis, HIV/AIDS, other)? List:___________________
NOTES:

HOME ENVIRONMENT

___Do you feel emotionally supported at home?
___Do you have help from relatives or friends if needed?
___Do you feel you have serious money/financial worries?
___ Are you in a stable relationship?
___Do you feel safe at home?
___Does anyone threaten or physically hurt you?
___Do you have pets (cats, rodents, exotic animals)? List:____________
___Do you have any contact with soil, cat litter or sandboxes?
Baby preparation (if planning pregnancy):
___Do you have a place for a baby to sleep?
___Do you need any baby items?
NOTES:

LIFESTYLE

___Do you smoke cigarettes or use other tobacco products?
How many cigarettes/packs a day? _____________
___Are you exposed to second-hand smoke?
___Do you drink alcohol?
What kind?_________ How often? _________ How much?________
___Do you use recreational drugs (cocaine, heroin, ecstasy, meth/ice, other)?
List:____
___Do you see a dentist regularly?
What kind of work do you do?________________________________
___Do you work or live near possible hazards (chemicals, x-ray or other radiation, lead)? List:______________________________
___Do you use saunas or hot tubs?
NOTES:

MEDICAL/FAMILY HISTORY

Do you have or have you ever had:
___Epilepsy?
___Diabetes?
___Asthma?
___High blood pressure?
___Heart disease?
___Anemia?
___Kidney or bladder disorders?
___Thyroid disease?
___Chickenpox?
___Hepatitis C?
___Digestive problems?
___Depression or other mental health problem?
___Surgeries?
___Lupus?
___Scleroderma?
___Other conditions?
Have you ever been vaccinated for:
___Measles, mumps, rubella?
___Hepatitis B?
___Chickenpox?
NOTES:

GENETICS

Does your family have a history of	or	your partner's family
___Hemophilia?		___
___Other bleeding disorders?		___
___Tay-Sachs disease?		___
___Blood diseases (sickle cell, thalassemia, other)?		___
___Muscular dystrophy?		___
___Down syndrome/Mental retardation?		___
___Cystic fibrosis?		___
___Birth defects (spine/heart/kidney)?		___

Your ethnic background is: ________________________________
Your partner's ethnic background is:__________________________
NOTES:

OTHER

IS THERE ANYTHING ELSE YOU'D LIKE ME TO KNOW?

ARE THERE ANY QUESTIONS YOU'D LIKE TO ASK ME?

Source: http://www.marchofdimes.com/files/preconception_tool_ed.pdf

CHAPTER 2

Genetics, Risks, and Genetic Counseling

Peter A. Farndon / Mark D. Kilby

INTRODUCTION

An abnormal fetal phenotype can be caused by environmental factors, chromosomal abnormalities, specific genes, or more complex genetic mechanisms. For most couples, the finding of fetal anomalies is unexpected, but some have identifiable factors that suggest a high risk of fetal anomaly. These include the following:

- A previous child affected with a single-gene disorder
- A family history of a single-gene disorder
- A parent with a chromosomal anomaly
- Structural anomalies found on ultrasound examination

Because families with single-gene disorders or parental chromosomal anomalies are at increased risk, it is important to identify couples from such families before they undertake pregnancy. An assessment of an individual's risk can often be made by a combination of pedigree analysis, precise clinical diagnosis, and genetic testing, which is available for an increasing number of conditions.

Although the main effect of genetics on current obstetric practice may be aiding the prediction and understanding of fetal anomaly, in the future, it is likely that screening for maternal genetic susceptibility to conditions such as eclampsia will be feasible.

DETERMINING THE GENETIC BASIS OF A CONDITION

To give a family accurate genetic information, it is recommended that the following steps (which are discussed in greater detail later) are undertaken:

- Examine the family tree to detect a pattern of inheritance.
- Refine and confirm the diagnosis by clinical examination and testing.
- Perform karyotype analysis or DNA testing, as appropriate.
- Assess the genetic risks to family members.
- Explain the genetic information to the family ("genetic counseling").
- Discuss the available options.
- Support the family while they make decisions appropriate to their situation.

IDENTIFICATION OF FAMILIES AT INCREASED GENETIC RISK

The couple may have realized that the family tree suggests a genetic disorder and volunteer this information. In other cases, the high risk is appreciated only when a formal history is taken.

The best and easiest way to record genetic information is to draw a pedigree. The standard notation is shown in Figure 2–1. Guidelines include the following:

- Create the tree from the "bottom," starting with the affected child and siblings: "Please give me the names of your children and their dates of birth, in order of age, starting with the oldest."
- Choose one parent (usually the mother) and ask about her siblings and their children, and then her parents, moving from generation to generation.
- Add information about the paternal side of the family.
- Use clear symbols (e.g., circles for females, squares for males). Fill in the symbol if the person is affected.
- Put a sloping line through the symbol (from the bottom left to the top right corner) if the person has died.
- Record all names, dates of birth, and maiden names.
- Ask about miscarriages, stillbirths, or deaths in each partnership: "How many children have you had? Have you lost any children? Have you had any previous partners?"

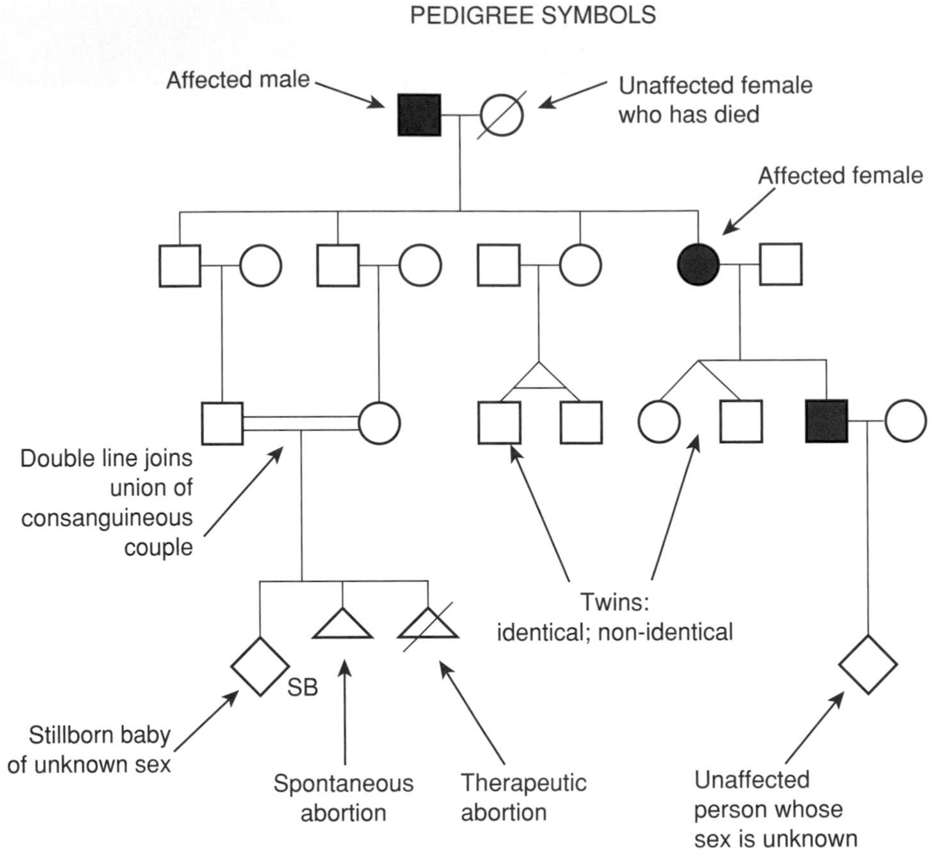

FIGURE 2–1
Symbols used in drawing a pedigree.

- Note parental occupations, medical and drug history, and pregnancy and birth history, especially when a child has a dysmorphic syndrome.
- Record at least basic details for both sides of the family, even when it appears that a disorder is segregating on one side.
- Ask about consanguinity: "Are you and your partner related? Are there any surnames in common in the family?"
- Date and sign the pedigree.

When the mode of inheritance is certain from the diagnosis (e.g., a known autosomal recessive condition), it may not be necessary to record personal details about all family members in as much detail as would be required for an unknown disease.

It is recommended to seek the couple's consent to share their medical information and test results with other family members.

Interpretation of the Pedigree

The precise pattern of affected members may suggest dominant, recessive, or X-linked inheritance, as discussed later. Inherited chromosomal anomalies may show a pattern of unaffected members having children with multiple anomalies and/or several pregnancy losses (Table 2–1).

Consanguinity does not prove autosomal recessive inheritance, but makes it more likely. An isolated case can still have a genetic cause. Illegitimacy may explain discrepancies.

Confirmation of the Diagnosis

Accurate genetic information requires a precise diagnosis. The diagnosis may need to be confirmed by referral to a specialist, who may be able to identify clinical subtypes that have different modes of inheritance. Confirmatory documents, such as specialists' letters and laboratory or necropsy results, may also be required. Apparently unaffected individuals may need to be assessed to exclude mild or early disease, especially in autosomal dominant disorders, such as neurofibromatosis, tuberous sclerosis, myotonic dystrophy, retinitis pigmentosa, and adult polycystic kidney disease.

Genetic Counseling

Genetic counseling is not solely giving a risk figure. Harper[1] defined it as "the process by which patients or relatives at risk of a disorder that may be hereditary are given information about the consequences of the disorder, the probability of developing and transmitting it and the ways in which it may be prevented or ameliorated."

Providing Genetic Counseling

The provision of clinical genetic services varies between countries. In the United Kingdom, trained clinical

TABLE 2–1

Establishing the Mode of Inheritance

Autosomal Dominant Inheritance

Males and females affected in equal proportions
Transmitted from one generation to next ("vertical transmission")
All forms of transmission are observed (i.e., male to male, female to female, male to female, and female to male)

Autosomal Recessive Inheritance

Males and females affected in equal proportions
Individuals affected in a single sibship in one generation
Consanguinity in the parents provides further support

X-Linked Recessive Inheritance

Males affected almost exclusively
Transmitted through carrier females to their sons ("knight's move" pattern)
Affected males cannot transmit the disorder to their sons

X-Linked Dominant Inheritance

Males and females are affected but affected females occur more frequently than affected males
Females are usually less severely affected than males
Affected females can transmit the disorder to male and female children, but affected males transmit the disorder only to their daughters, all of whom are affected

Inherited Chromosomal Anomalies

May give a pattern of unaffected family members having children with multiple abnormalities with growth and developmental retardation
The hallmarks of chromosome anomalies are multiple organ systems affected at different stages in embryogenesis
May give a pattern of multiple pregnancy losses

Mitochondrial Inheritance

If all the children of affected mothers are affected, but no children of affected fathers, consider the possibility of mitochondrial inheritance.

An Apparently Isolated Case

Could be caused by a:

- Phenocopy (caused solely by environmental factors)
- New dominant mutation
- More severe expression in a child of a dominant disorder in a parent
- Recessive condition
- X-linked condition (if a male)
- Chromosome anomaly (either inherited or spontaneous)
- A combination of environmental influences on a genetic predisposition

geneticists, usually supported by a team of genetic counselors, are usually based in tertiary referral centers, but most have clinics in district hospitals.

As part of clinical care, most obstetricians give genetic information about common chromosomal trisomies found at prenatal diagnosis, for instance, but seek advice from a clinical geneticist for DNA diagnosis, familial chromosomal disorders, single-gene disorders, and malformation syndromes.

Giving Genetic Information

Genetic information should be given in a nondirective manner, presenting facts, discussing options, and helping couples and families to reach their own decisions. It may not be easy to be completely nondirective because the professional's views can affect the tone and manner of presentation of the information. There is no "right" or "wrong" decision; a couple must make a decision that they believe is right for them. Whenever possible, the partners should be seen together when discussing genetic information or abnormalities found at prenatal diagnosis.

Timing

Couples who consider themselves to be at potentially high risk for a genetic disorder and who have sought genetic information before embarking on a pregnancy have time to decide which option is the most appropriate.

The diagnosis of a serious genetic disorder or malformation syndrome during pregnancy may require difficult management decisions to be made relatively quickly. The family may have little time to understand the severity and consequences of the disorder, identify the options (including available treatments), and discuss the genetic implications. Families want to know whether the condition is lethal or severely disabling, whether there is a high risk that a future pregnancy will be affected, and whether specific prenatal diagnosis would be available.

Genetic information may play an important role in the consideration of options for future pregnancies and clinical management of the current pregnancy. Options include the following:

- Having no (more) children
- Accepting the risk
- Undertaking prenatal diagnosis, if available
- Seeking adoption
- Having gamete donation
- Seeking preimplantation diagnosis

A couple's choice will depend on social, economic, moral, and practical factors, among others.

DETERMINING RISKS

The mathematical "risk of recurrence" can usually be derived with certainty for a single-gene (mendelian) disorder. For other conditions, empirical figures must be used (discussed later).

Explaining Risks (See also Chapter 1)

Although some people perceive risks only as "high" or "low," most wish to understand how a figure has been reached, when a discussion about modes of inheritance and mechanisms of genetic disease may be helpful. Expressing a risk figure as a fraction (e.g., 1 in 2, 1/2), as odds (50:50), or as a percentage (50%) is less likely to lead to confusion. The perception of what constitutes "high" or "low" risk varies with the individual. Some families find it easier to understand risk figures presented as odds, whereas others prefer to discuss these figures as percentages. Most clinical geneticists use both odds and percentages during a consultation, concentrating on the one that the patients find easiest to understand.

The decision as to what constitutes an "acceptable" risk varies with the disorder and the individual. However, providing some reference points (Table 2–2) may be helpful.

Genetic Risk: Burden and Probability

A "risk" figure has two components: the probability that the condition will occur and the burden of the disease. Families may view the same mathematical figure entirely differently. For example, for autosomal dominant conditions with a "1 in 2" risk, the family may view the effect of the disease as mild (e.g., brachydactyly) or very severe (e.g., Huntington disease). Their view may also be affected by whether screening and treatment are available (e.g., bilateral retinoblastoma, adenomatous polyposis coli). Such issues may need to be discussed during the genetic consultation.

TABLE 2–2

Examples of Approximate Reproductive Risks in Developed Countries

REPRODUCTIVE OUTCOME	RISK ODDS	RISK %
Infertility	1 in 10	10.0
Pregnancy ending in a spontaneous miscarriage	1 in 8	12.5
Perinatal death	1 in 30 to 1 in 100	1.0
Birth of a baby with a congenital abnormality (major and minor)	1 in 30	3.3
Birth of a baby with a serious physical or mental handicap	1 in 50	2.0
Death of a child in the first year after the first week	1 in 150	0.7

SUMMARY OF MANAGEMENT OPTIONS

Genetics, Risks, and Genetic Counseling

Management Options	Quality of Evidence	Grade of Recommendation	References
Population Genetic Screening			
Policies vary on the basis of: • Financial constraints • Prevalence and health burden of the conditions • Political issues	IV	C	2, 3
If screening is implemented, patients should be given the following information: • Nature of the medical condition • Mode of inheritance • Reliability of the screening test • Procedures for giving results • Implications for their future, their existing children, and their family members if the screening test result is positive • Possibility that genetic screening may result in unexpected information being revealed	IV	C	2,3
General (Prepregnancy, Prenatal, and Postnatal)			
Families with single-gene disorders and parental chromosomal anomalies have the highest risks and may be detected by taking a family pedigree.	IV	C	1
Adequate time should be made available in a quiet setting that is free from interruptions.	IIa	B	40
Both partners should be seen together whenever possible.	IIb	B	41
Obtain accurate and comprehensive information to make a secure diagnosis, including taking a family pedigree.	IIa	B	40
Provide nondirective and supportive counseling.	III	B	42, 43
Ensure that stated risks are accurate and up-to-date.	IIa	B	40
What constitutes an "acceptable" risk to an individual varies with the disorder because a risk figure has two components: The probability of occurrence and the burden of disease.	III	B	43
Consider referring complex cases to a clinical geneticist.	III	B	42

TYPES OF GENETIC DISORDERS: MECHANISMS AND RISKS

Humans have approximately 23,000 genes arranged on 23 pairs of chromosomes that allow their physical transmission from cell to cell and generation to generation. Generally, gain or loss of gene function is the underlying mechanism for single-gene and chromosomal disorders. However, isolated congenital anomalies are often the result of multifactorial inheritance. In multifactorial disorders, the condition develops in individuals with a liability above a particular threshold. The liability is composed of "environmental" components that act with a genetic predisposition caused by the summation of the effects of several genes.

CONDITIONS WITH MENDELIAN INHERITANCE: SINGLE-GENE DISORDERS

General

Single-gene (mendelian) disorders behave as though they are under the control of only one pair of genes. They have high risks of recurrence. This mode of inheritance is usually recognized by a combination of clinical diagnosis and pedigree pattern.

Risks can usually be determined from knowledge of the mode of inheritance of a particular condition. However, some conditions, such as retinitis pigmentosa, have dominant, recessive, and X-linked forms, so care is needed.

For many mendelian conditions, DNA tests are available for presymptomatic diagnosis, carrier detection, and prenatal diagnosis (Table 2–3). Up-to-date information should be sought from a clinical genetics department because advances are too rapid for published literature to remain current. In addition, access to online databases is helpful (Appendix). Prenatal diagnostic possibilities may have changed by the time a couple is considering having another child.

TABLE 2–3

Examples of Common Single-Gene Disorders* Detected by DNA Diagnosis

Dominantly Inherited Disorders
Achondroplasia
Adult polycystic kidney disease
Breast cancer (some families)
Familial adenomatous polyposis coli
Familial hypercholesterolemia
Hereditary motor and sensory neuropathy
von Hippel-Lindau disease
Huntington's disease
Marfan syndrome
Multiple endocrine neoplasia
Myotonic dystrophy
Neurofibromatosis
Tuberous sclerosis
Recessively Inherited Disorders
α-1 Antitrypsin
Congenital adrenal hyperplasia
Cystic fibrosis
Friedreich's ataxia
Sickle cell disease
Spinal muscular atrophy
Tay-Sachs disease
Thalassaemia
X-Linked Disorders
Alport syndrome
Becker muscular dystrophy
Duchenne muscular dystrophy
Fragile X syndrome
Hemophilia A and B

*For gene tracking, DNA from the affected person and family studies are required. Consult the Regional Clinical Genetics Service for the availability of DNA diagnosis in other diseases; it is potentially possible for all diseases in which the gene has been localized. Online databases that list DNA tests provided by genetic laboratories are increasingly available. To ensure clinical reliability and validity, it is important to confirm that laboratories that offer testing are part of recognized quality control programs and to ask about the experience of the laboratory with the particular test.

Autosomal Dominant Inheritance (Fig. 2–2)

A dominant trait manifests in a heterozygote (a person with both the abnormal and the normal alleles) and is usually transmitted from one generation to the next ("vertical transmission") [see Fig. 2–2]. Each offspring of a parent with an autosomal dominant trait has a 1 in 2 chance of inheriting the disease gene. Autosomal dominant traits can exhibit variable expressivity, reduced penetrance, and sex limitation. The effects on a fetus from a dominant disorder may be more difficult to predict than suggested by the straightforward simple probability of 1 in 2 of inheriting the disease gene.

Some dominant conditions are so variable in their expression that careful physical examination is needed to detect the minute signs that a parent has the gene. For instance, freckles in the axilla may be the only sign of neurofibromatosis. For some disorders, a fetus may be considerably more affected than the affected parent. For example, the increase in size during maternal transmission of a trinucleotide repeat associated with the gene causing myotonic dystrophy can result in the congenital form of myotonic dystrophy: The parent has minor signs of the disease but the child is severely affected. However, the phenotypes of other dominant conditions never vary (e.g., achondroplasia).

Very rarely, a person who carries the gene for an autosomal dominant condition (with an affected parent and an affected child) has no physical signs of the condition. The gene is said to be "nonpenetrant" in the person who has no signs of the disease.

Some autosomal dominant conditions appear to occur sporadically. If there is no family history and both parents are found to be unaffected after appropriate examinations and investigations, then the child's disease is likely to be caused by a new mutation. The recurrence risk for parents is low, but the child has a 50% risk of passing on the

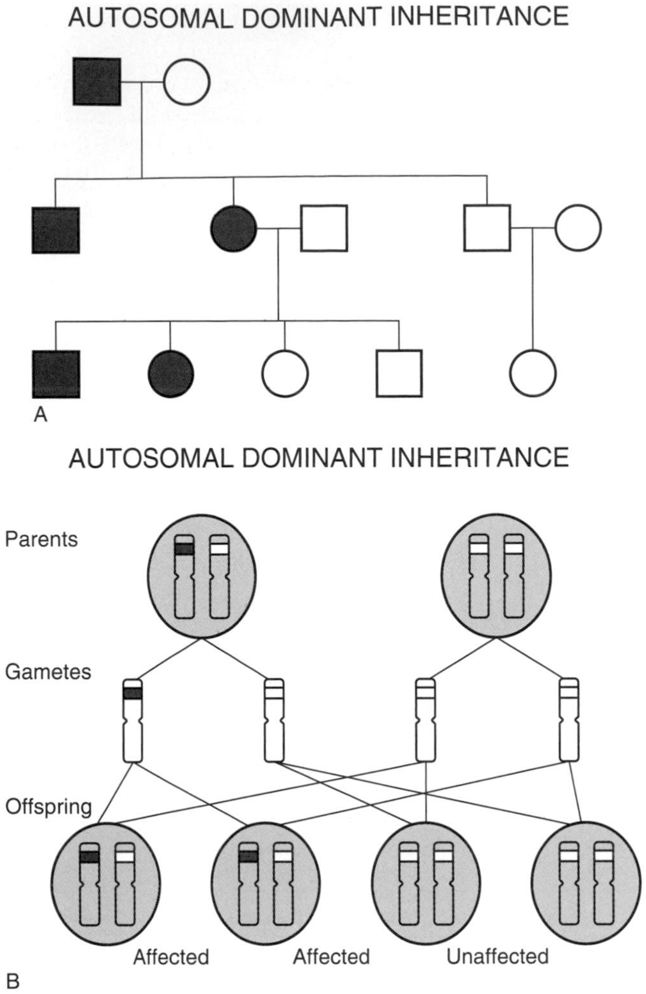

FIGURE 2–2
Single-gene disorders: examples of pedigrees and modes of inheritance. *A*, Autosomal dominant inheritance. Three generations are affected, and male-to-male transmission is shown. *B*, Autosomal dominant inheritance. If one parent is affected by a dominant condition, each offspring has a 50% (1 in 2) risk of inheriting the gene.

disease to offspring. There is a slight chance that a parent of a child with an apparently new dominant mutation has gonadal mosaicism. In this case, the germ line contains two populations of cells: one with the mutation and one with the normal gene. This situation explains the rare cases in which unaffected parents have two children with the same autosomal dominant condition.

Autosomal Recessive Conditions (Fig. 2–3)

Autosomal recessive disorders are manifest only in the homozygous state: the affected person has two copies of the abnormal gene. Heterozygotes (carriers) are normal. When parents are heterozygous for the same autosomal recessive condition, each offspring has a 1 in 4 chance of being affected. An unaffected sibling of an affected person has a 2 in 3 chance of being a carrier (see Fig. 2–3). If an affected person reproduces, the children will be at risk only if the partner is a carrier for the same autosomal recessive condition.

Carriers for some inborn errors of metabolism can be identified by biochemical tests. Unfortunately, for many disorders, the range of results for carriers overlaps with the range of results for noncarriers, with test results generating a probability of being a carrier rather than giving a definitive answer. DNA techniques allow diagnosis of the carrier state for some autosomal recessive conditions in some families. This "genetic testing" is offered when other evidence (usually being closely related to an affected person or a known carrier) suggests increased risk.

For some conditions, DNA diagnosis can be offered to members of a general population with a high proportion of carriers for a specific mutation. In this case, carrier risks can be altered for couples who have no family history. This "genetic screening" is discussed in more detail later.

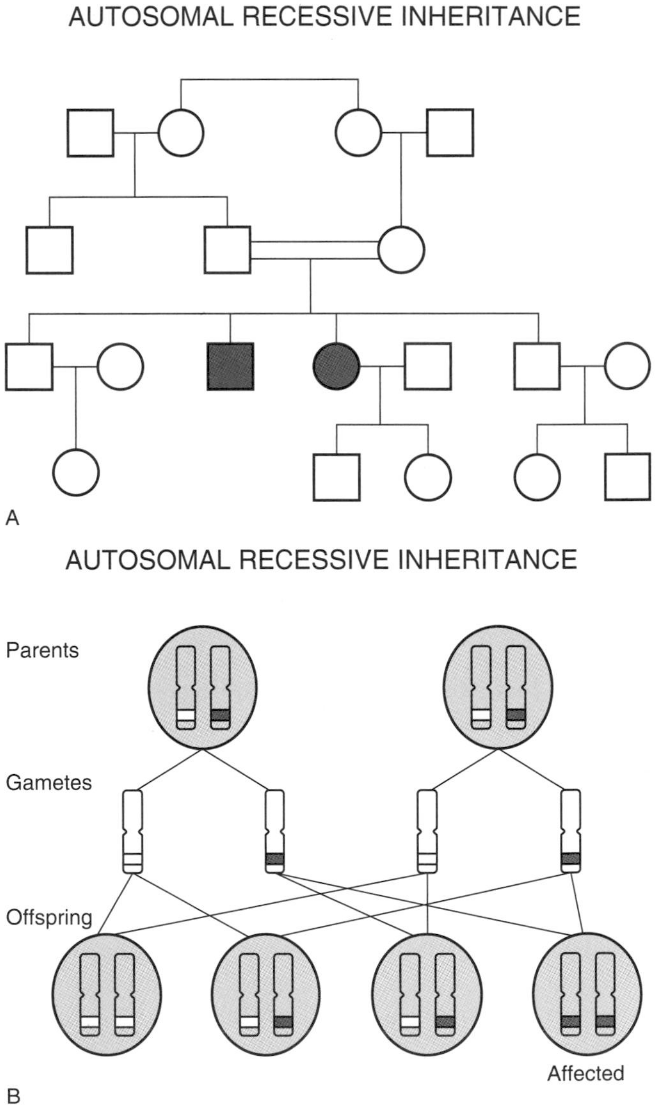

FIGURE 2–3
Single-gene disorders: examples of pedigrees and modes of inheritance. *A*, Autosomal recessive inheritance. Siblings in only one generation are affected. In this family, the parents are first cousins. *B*, Autosomal recessive inheritance. If both parents carry the same abnormal gene for a recessive condition, their offspring have a 25% (1 in 4) risk of inheriting the abnormal gene from both parents and therefore being affected.

Unless the disorder is very common or unless consanguinity is present, the risks for half-siblings, children of affected individuals, and especially children of unaffected siblings are minimally increased over the risks in the general population. The precise risk depends on the frequency of heterozygotes in the population and can be calculated using mendelian principles.

Some couples request sterilization after the birth of a child with an autosomal recessive condition. Very sensitive handling of this request is needed. If the parents separate, either parent may form a new relationship with an unrelated partner; in this case, it is likely that the risk of recurrence would be low.

X-Linked Recessive Inheritance (Fig. 2–4)

Although males and females have similar sets of the 22 pairs of autosomes, the sex chromosome pair is different. Females have two X chromosomes, whereas males have one X chromosome and a Y chromosome. Because sex-linked recessive traits are determined by genes on the X chromosome, they usually manifest only in males because males have a single copy of the genes on the X chromosome. Although females have two copies of the X chromosome, one is inactivated at random early in gestation. In an individual female cell, the genes from either the paternal or the maternal X chromosome are active and most of the genes on the other X chromosome are silenced. Therefore, a female who is heterozygous for an X-linked condition will be a mosaic of normal and affected cells. The proportions of each type in a given tissue are related to the chance pattern of X inactivation. For this reason, carrier detection in X-linked recessive disorders may be difficult. For example, approximately 30% of known carriers of Duchenne muscular dystrophy have biochemical carrier test results within the normal range,

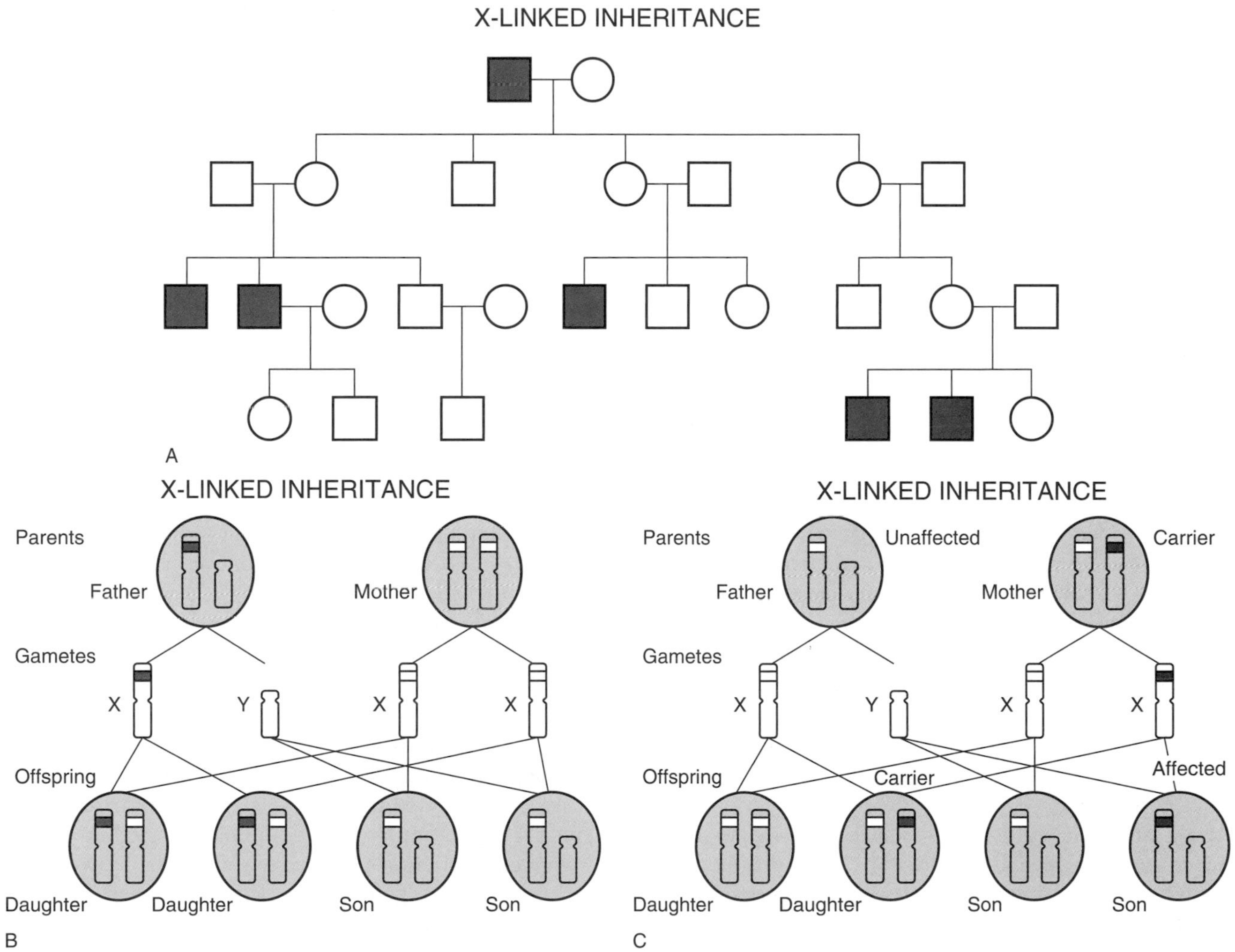

FIGURE 2–4
Single-gene disorders: examples of pedigrees and modes of inheritance. *A*, X-linked inheritance. In this family, the grandfather has a nonlethal X-linked disorder (e.g., hemophilia). Males affected in several generations are linked through unaffected females. Daughters of affected men are obligatory carriers. *B*, X-linked recessive inheritance in which a father is affected. If a father has an X-linked condition, all of his daughters will be carriers, but none of his sons will be affected. (Sons inherit his Y chromosome; that is why they are male!) *C*, X-linked recessive inheritance in which a mother is a carrier. If a woman carries a gene for a recessive condition on one of her X chromosomes, each of her sons has a 1 in 2 risk of being affected and each of her daughters has a 1 in 2 risk of being a carrier.

presumably because, by chance, relatively few muscle cells express the abnormal gene in these women. Many cases of the more serious X-linked diseases are caused by new mutations, which makes counseling difficult unless reliable techniques for carrier detection are available. However, DNA techniques may be able to answer these questions with high precision, either by direct detection of a mutation or by gene tracking (discussed later).

A son of a woman who is heterozygous for an X-linked recessive disorder has a 1 in 2 chance of inheriting the disease allele from his mother and of being affected (see Fig. 2–4*C*). A daughter also has a 1 in 2 chance of inheriting the disease allele, but would be expected to be an unaffected carrier. (Women who are carriers for the fragile X mental retardation syndrome can have daughters who are mentally handicapped; because of the complexities involved, patients should be referred for genetic counseling.)

Daughters of affected males are obligate heterozygotes (see Fig. 2–4*B*).

Rarely, females show signs of an X-linked recessive trait or disease because they are homozygous for the allele (e.g., color blindness), have a single X chromosome (Turner syndrome), have a structural rearrangement of an X chromosome, or are heterozygous with skewed or nonrandom X inactivation.

If male-to-male transmission is shown, then X linkage is excluded.

Unusual Patterns of Inheritance

Unusual inheritance patterns can be explained by phenomena such as genetic heterogeneity, mosaicism, anticipation, imprinting, UPD, and mitochondrial mutations.

GENETIC SCREENING

In genetic screening, members of a particular population are offered a test for a condition or defect when there is no prior evidence of its presence in an individual.

The potential benefits of genetic screening include identifying treatable genetic disorders at an early stage and allowing couples to make informed choices about parenthood. Potential disadvantages of being discovered to be at high risk through genetic screening include whether or not to communicate the information to the family, and when screening is performed in pregnancy, the urgency of deciding about prenatal diagnosis and considering the options available. In the future, it may be possible to identify people with genetic susceptibility to common serious diseases. However, the advantages of early identification will need to be weighed against possible adverse effects on employment prospects and the ability to obtain insurance.

Guidelines for genetic screening programs have been recommended by several organizations.[2–5] These are helpful in determining the aims, limitations, scope, and ethical aspects of a genetic screening program as well as considerations for the storage and registration of data or material, the need for follow-up (including social consequences), and the risk of side effects.

People undergoing genetic investigations are entitled to receive sufficient information about what is proposed and about substantial risks in a way they can understand. They should be given time to decide whether or not to agree to what is proposed. They must be free to withdraw at any time.

Specifically, they should receive information about the following:

- Nature of the medical condition
- Mode of inheritance
- Reliability of the screening test
- Procedures for giving results
- Implications for their future, their existing children, and family members if the result is positive
- Possibility that genetic screening may result in unexpected information being revealed (e.g., non-paternity)

The debate in the United Kingdom over population screening for carriers for the autosomal recessive condition cystic fibrosis illustrates many of these points. The disease is common, with 1 in 25 of the white population in the United Kingdom being a carrier. Routine DNA tests can identify approximately 85% of carriers; these people have the common mutations. A "negative" result for commonly tested mutations does not exclude a member of the population from being a carrier, but greatly reduces the risk. In contrast, DNA testing for sickle cell disease would be expected to detect virtually all carriers.

The current program for screening newborns for cystic fibrosis covers approximately 18% of the population of England and focuses on identifying affected individuals. The incorporation of direct gene analysis into screening based on serum immunoreactive trypsinogen measurement is highly effective.[6] "Cascade testing" can then be offered to the relatives of affected individuals. Compared with other methods, offering testing to relatives of an affected person produces a high ratio of positive test results. This method is up to ten times more powerful than unfocused screening in detecting carriers.[7] Although this method effectively detects carriers in the relatives of affected people, the majority of carriers in the general population are not found by this method.

Indeed, making a CF carrier test available to anyone interested in the general population has been shown to result in a low uptake. In contrast, a high uptake (>70%) followed an invitation during pregnancy to be screened by an interested health professional. However, screening during pregnancy may not allow people to be fully informed or high-risk couples to have the choice of all options.[8] A "two-step" approach in pregnancy has been studied,[9] in which the woman was tested first and testing was offered to men whose partner was found to be a carrier. However, considerable anxiety may occur when the woman is determined to be a carrier and the man is not. An alternative procedure is to regard the couple as the screened unit and to provide information on carrier status only when both partners are carriers.[10]

When the mutations that cause cystic fibrosis in an affected person have been identified, definitive carrier testing is available for family members.

The term "genetic testing" is used when an individual is tested for a condition or defect that other evidence suggests may be present. This may be to confirm a diagnosis or to test for carrier status within a family. Although the same laboratory procedure may be used for both genetic screening and genetic testing, there are important clinical conceptual differences. Those undergoing genetic testing are likely to have more knowledge about the genetic implications because they were identified as being at high risk because of their family history. This is unlikely to be the case in a genetic screening program, where education and information have been shown to be key factors in successful programs (e.g., a carrier screening program for thalassemia in Cyprus, screening for Tay-Sachs disease in Montreal).

The optimal timing of the testing procedure changes as a community becomes more informed. For example, a screening program that is designed to detect newborns affected with a recessive disorder so that treatment may be instituted may encourage relatives to undergo carrier testing. This can increase awareness of the benefits of antenatal screening and may lead to an offer of testing to couples or individuals in the general population[4] before pregnancy. Some communities encourage individuals leaving school to be tested.[5]

It is widely accepted that predictive genetic testing of children should be offered when the condition occurs in childhood or when treatment can be offered, but children should not be tested for adult-onset genetic disease (unless specific preventive measures are available) nor for carrier status until they are old enough to decide whether to undergo testing.[11] However, the U.K. national neonatal screening program to identify people with sickle cell disease will also detect carriers; clinical practice in the United Kingdom for the carrier testing of children in families with genetic disorders may need to be reviewed.

DNA TECHNIQUES IN PRESYMPTOMATIC DIAGNOSIS, CARRIER DETECTION, AND PRENATAL DIAGNOSIS

DNA techniques can be used in single-gene disorders to allow the following:

- Confirmation of the diagnosis, especially when the clinical features can be equivocal
- Confirmation that a family member has not inherited the disease
- Carrier testing, especially when biochemical testing is not available or the results are equivocal
- Presymptomatic diagnosis so that surveillance can be instituted (e.g., familial adenomatous polyposis coli, some types of breast cancer)
- Prenatal diagnosis, especially for conditions for which biochemical or hematologic testing or ultrasound detection of associated structural anomalies were formerly the only possibilities

Identification of Families for DNA Diagnosis

Families are often identified from the pattern of affected members or when a precise diagnosis is made. Each family must be assessed individually because some techniques rely on the family structure and availability of the necessary DNA samples. Therefore, DNA diagnosis may require considerable time. Families are best referred to a clinical genetics unit before pregnancy for completion of the steps outlined in Table 2–4.

TABLE 2–4

Practice Points for Prenatal Diagnosis by DNA Techniques for Single-Gene Disorders*

Identify families through:

- Previously affected child
- Carrier screening programs for autosomal recessive disease
- Family history

Do they wish to proceed to further testing?

Consider the techniques available for prenatal diagnosis:

- Biochemical assays
- Ultrasound
- DNA diagnosis

Is DNA diagnosis possible? Consult the regional Genetics Services. Check before each pregnancy because of the rate of advances.

- Is the clinical diagnosis secure?
- Has the gene been localized or cloned?
- Is the family structure suitable, and are samples available for testing?
- Is sufficient time available for testing?

Explain procedures and the accuracy of results to family.
Collect appropriate samples.
Order laboratory testing:

- Gene tracking
- Direct mutation detection

Explain the results and options.
Proceed with diagnostic testing:

- Presymptomatic
- Prenatal

*A clinical genetics unit can advise and arrange for much of the above. The genetics of some single-gene disorders may be complicated (e.g., retinitis pigmentosa can be inherited as autosomal dominant and autosomal and X-linked recessive).

The Principles of Diagnosis: Gene Tracking and Mutation Detection

Gene Tracking: The Use of Linked DNA Markers

Gene tracking can be used when the chromosomal localization of the disease is known, but the gene has not been isolated. The goal is to identify a DNA marker that is inherited with the disease gene in a family.

The chromosomal region that contains the gene has usually been identified through a linkage study in which many DNA markers spread throughout the genome have been analyzed in families with the disease. After statistical analyses of results from all the families are completed, the chromosomal region that is most likely to contain the gene is identified. This information can be used prospectively for diagnosis in individual families by identifying a familial DNA pattern that is inherited with the disease gene. DNA sequences that vary in length naturally in the population ("polymorphisms") and are next to or within the disease gene are used to generate these "markers" in a family. A class of highly variable CA repeat markers is usually used (Fig. 2–5). The markers are detected by their different positions on a gel after electrophoresis. Figure 2–6 shows an example of an autosomal recessive disease. The fragment "tracking" with the disease gene can be identified by observing which fragment pattern is common to affected family members. An error is associated with the use of linked markers because recombination may occur between the DNA marker and the disease gene. To minimize the risk of misdiagnosis, markers that show no more than 1% recombination with the disease gene are used whenever possible.

Diagnosis by Direct Detection of a Mutation

The definitive diagnostic test is to show a change in DNA that is predicted to disrupt gene function, and this cause disease. When a mutation is predicted to cause truncation of the protein product (usually through a frameshift mutation

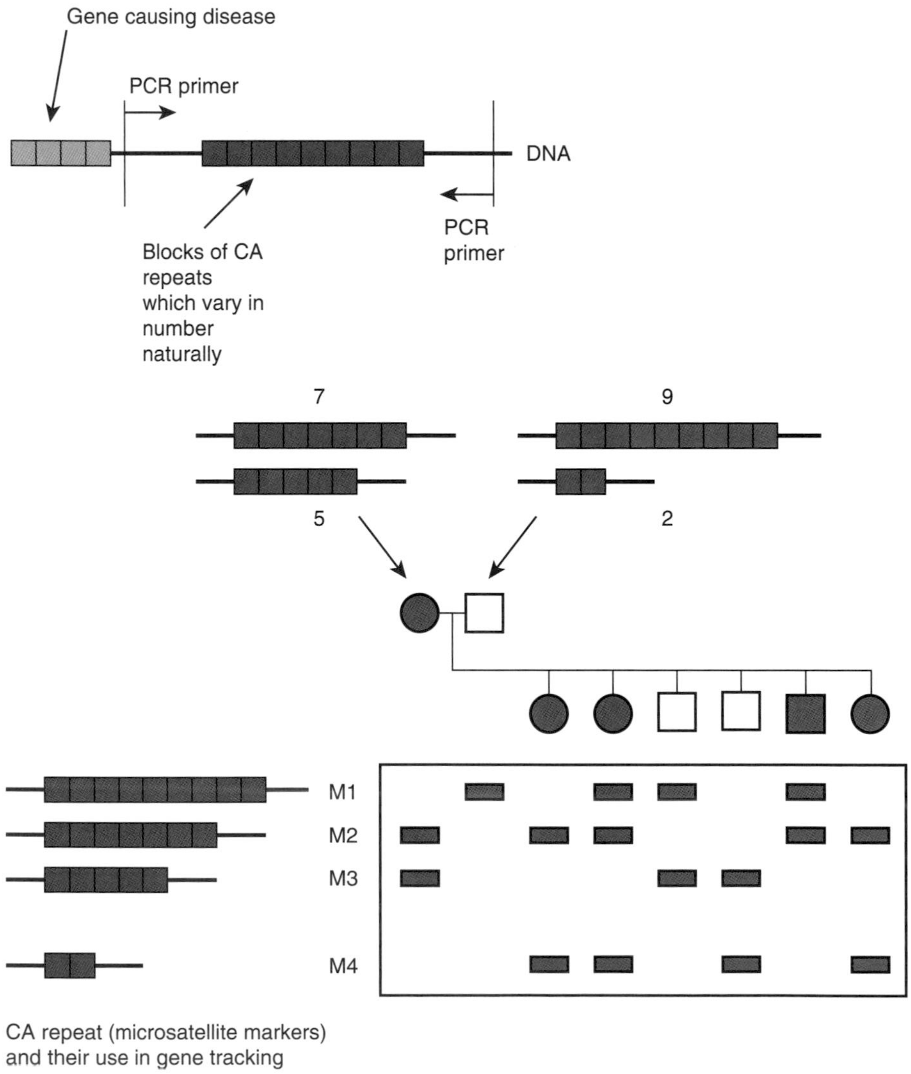

FIGURE 2–5
Principles of gene tracking with CA repeat markers. A variable DNA sequence (consisting of two DNA bases, CA, repeated several times) is fortuitously situated immediately in front of a gene that is known to cause a particular disorder. The length of the $CA_{(n)}$ sequence varies from individual to individual and is usually of no significance. Variation in its length is used as a marker tracking the gene of interest in a family. Members of this family whose symbols are blocked in are affected with an autosomal dominant disorder. DNA is extracted from lymphocytes, and the DNA segment containing the CA repeat is amplified by polymerase chain reaction (PCR) so that there are sufficient copies to be visualized. The different $CA_{(n)}$ lengths are separated by electrophoresis. In this family, the father has CA repeats of lengths 9 and 2, and the mother affected by the dominant disorder has repeats of lengths 7 and 5. Because the CA repeat sequence is acting as a marker of the parental disease gene alleles, all affected children have inherited the same maternal $CA_{(n)}$ allele. This marker allele could be used for diagnosis in other family members. In other families with the same condition, however, the disease will be associated with this CA marker system, but the mutated allele that causes the disease could be tracking with a different length of CA repeat. When using gene tracking, a study of each family is needed to determine which allele is associated with the disease gene.

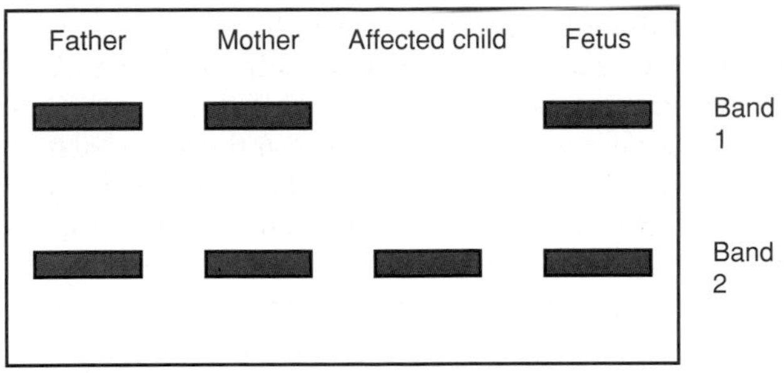

FIGURE 2–6
DNA diagnosis of an autosomal recessive condition by gene tracking. In this family, both parents have two detectable fragments (*1* and *2*) but their son, who is affected with spinal muscular atrophy (SMA), shows only one (*2*). Therefore, the SMA gene must be located on the parental chromosomes that give the fragment labeled *2*. In the next pregnancy, the fetus had two fragments, *1* and *2*, and therefore is predicted to be a carrier, but is not affected with SMA.

or the introduction of a stop codon), this is strong evidence that a pathogenic mutation has been identified. Other sequence changes may be more difficult to interpret, especially missense mutations that result in replacement of one amino acid by another. Additional studies may be needed to determine the likelihood of pathogenicity. These may include testing members of the population to determine if this is a polymorphism or performing a family study to determine whether the DNA change is being inherited with the disease in the case of a dominant disorder, for instance.

For some diseases, common mutations are known (e.g., δ-F508 mutation in cystic fibrosis, G380R mutation in achondroplasia). For most diseases, however, the precise mutation causing the disease in the family must first be identified. Identification may take months, depending on the structure of the gene and the laboratory techniques used. Many laboratories use an initial screening test, but techniques such as single-strand conformation polymorphism (SSCP) appear to detect only approximately 80% of mutations, depending on the gene. It has been argued that direct DNA sequencing of a gene is the "gold standard," but although this method should detect coding sequence variants, it does not detect deletions or large rearrangements. After the mutation is identified, other family members can be offered definitive diagnosis. Even when the genetic code of a gene is known, gene tracking may have to be used if technical constraints make direct mutation testing impractical.

CHROMOSOMAL ABNORMALITIES

The Karyotype Report: Nomenclature

Karyotyping is labor-intensive because high-resolution (extended) chromosome preparations reveal more than 850 bands. These bands are usually analyzed by light microscopy, although computer imaging is beginning to have a major effect. Occasionally, only limited analysis may be possible because of poor elongation of the chromosomes.

The human chromosome composition is reported in an internationally agreed format that gives a precise description of an abnormality. The format has three parts that are separated by a comma: the total number of chromosomes seen, the sex chromosome constitution, and the abnormalities or variants.

- The first figure gives the total number of chromosomes (e.g., 46, 45, 47).
- The second part gives the sex chromosome complement (e.g., XX, XY, X, XXY).
- The third part describes abnormalities or variants affecting the following:
    - Whole chromosomes
    - Arms of chromosomes

The short arm of a chromosome is designated "p" (for *petit*), and the long arm is designated "q" (the next letter in the alphabet). Each arm is further subdivided into bands and subbands.

Breakpoints involved in structural rearrangements are described according to the arm involved, the region of the arm, and then by band and subbands within that region. For example, band Xq27.3 is found on the long arm of the X chromosome, in region 2, band 7, and subband 3. Further examples are given in Table 2–5.

Molecular Cytogenetic Techniques

Some syndromes are caused by submicroscopic deletions of chromosomal material. Molecular techniques (usually fluorescence in situ hybridization, FISH) can be used for diagnosis when the loss or gain of material is beyond the limit of light microscopy. This technique is also helpful for determining the origin of chromosomal material.

This method can also be applied to interphase nuclei to determine the numbers of copies of specific chromosomes, particularly as a rapid screening test for common trisomies.

A Parent with a Chromosome Anomaly

Chromosomal Translocations

A translocation is formed when there has been transfer of material between chromosomes, requiring breakage of both chromosomes, with repair in an abnormal arrangement. If the exchange results in no loss or gain of DNA, the individual is clinically normal and is said to have a "balanced translocation." Such a translocation carrier is, however, at risk of producing chromosomally unbalanced gametes, which may result in a chromosomally abnormal baby, miscarriages, still birth, or infertility depending on the origin and amount of chromosome material involved.

When a translocation is found, other family members should be offered testing for carrier status because of the potentially high risks of having offspring with unbalanced forms of the translocation. Clinical genetics services are used in contacting and dealing with such families.

TABLE 2-5

Examples of Cytogenetic Nomenclature

Normal	
46,XX	Normal female
Sex Chromosome Aneuploidies	
45,X	Monosomy X (Turner syndrome)
47,XXY	Klinefelter syndrome
45,X/46,XX	Mosaic Turner syndrome
Autosomal Aneuploidies	
47,XY, +21	Male with trisomy 21 (Down syndrome)
47,XX, +13	Female with trisomy 13 (Patau syndrome)
Polyploidy	
69,XXY	Triploidy
Deletions	
46,XX,del(18)(q21)	Deletion of part of the long arm of one chromosome 18 from band q21 to the end of the long arm (qter)
46,XX,del(17)(p13)	Female karyotype with a deletion of part of the short arm of chromosome 17, from band p13 to the end of the short arm (pter)
Translocations	
46,XY,t(2;12)(p14;p13)	Male with a balanced reciprocal translocation between chromosomes 2 and 12, with breakpoints on the short arms, at p14 on chromosome 2 and at p13 on chromosome 12
46,XX,der(2)t(2;12)(p14;p13)mat	Female with an unbalanced complement, having received the derivative chromosome 2 from her mother, who carries a translocation between chromosomes 2 and 12; this child would have too little material from chromosome 2 (from p14 to pter) and an additional copy of material from chromosome 12 (from p13 to pter), making her effectively monosomic for 2p and trisomic for 12p
45,XY,rob(14;21)(q10q10)	Carrier of a Robertsonian translocation between one chromosome 14 and one chromosome 21
Other	
46,XY,inv(5)(p14;q15)	Pericentric inversion of one chromosome 5
46,XX,r(15)	Female with one normal and one ring chromosome 15
46,XY,fra(X)(q27.3)	Male with a fragile site in subband 27.3 on the X long arm
46,XX,add(20)(p13)	Additional material of unknown origin attached to band p13 on one chromosome 20

Generally, the smaller the segment involved, the greater the chance of viable offspring. The cytogenetic literature may show whether the birth of a viable child with the potential unbalanced products of the particular translocation has been reported. It may be possible to calculate a theoretical risk figure, so the clinical genetics or cytogenetics services should be consulted. For most couples, the precise risk figure is not the vital consideration because fetal karyotyping in future pregnancies can determine whether the fetus has inherited an abnormal arrangement of chromosomal material.

There are two types of translocations:

RECIPROCAL TRANSLOCATION

In reciprocal translocations, chromosomal material distal to (i.e., beyond) the breaks in two chromosomes is exchanged. The long or short arms of any pair of chromosomes may be involved. Approximately 1 in 500 people is a reciprocal translocation carrier.

When a fetus has inherited an apparently balanced reciprocal translocation from a clinically normal parent, there appears to be no increased incidence of phenotypic abnormality in the child, especially if the translocation is present without effect in several family members.

It appears that the risk of a child with the "balanced" parental karyotype having phenotypic abnormalities due to theoretical possibilities (such as the translocation having a cryptic unbalanced component beyond the resolution of conventional cytogenetics, or uniparental disomy) is remote in practice. A cryptic unbalanced complement is more likely if the parental translocation is de novo.

ROBERTSONIAN TRANSLOCATION (CENTRIC FUSION)

A Robertsonian translocation is one in which effectively all of one chromosome is joined end-to-end to another. Robertsonian translocations involve the acrocentric chromosomes (13, 14, 15, 21, and 22) and are among the most common balanced structural rearrangements in the general population, with a frequency in newborn surveys of approximately 1 in 1000.

Centric fusion may arise from breaks at or near the centromere in two acrocentric chromosomes, with the two products fusing together. This usually results in the production of a single chromosome and most frequently involves chromosomes 13 and 14. Next in frequency are chromosomes 14 and 21. Clinically, the most important fusions are those involving chromosome 21, which give rise to familial Down syndrome.

For female carriers of a Robertsonian 14;21 translocation, the risk of having a liveborn infant with Down syndrome is approximately 10%. The risk is approximately 1% for a male carrier.

A Robertsonian translocation involving both copies of chromosome 21 is rare, but all children of a carrier will have Down syndrome.

Where a Robertsonian translocation involves chromosome 15 and a balanced translocation karyotype is detected at prenatal diagnosis, it is appropriate to offer testing for uniparental disomy (UPD). This is to exclude Angelman syndrome or Prader-Willi syndrome in the fetus caused by UPD for chromosome 15. This can occur by postzygotic "correction" of trisomy 15 when one parental chromosome 15 that is not involved in the Robertsonian translocation is lost during mitosis.

Deletions and Duplications of Chromosomal Material

When a patient with partial autosomal monosomy or trisomy is sufficiently unaffected to have children, the risk that the child will inherit the parental chromosomal abnormality is theoretically 50%, as the child can inherit either the normal homologue or the chromosome with the deletion or duplication.

Inversions

An inversion (inv) affects just one chromosome, with a segment between two breaks inverted and reinserted. Inversions are found in fewer than 1 in 100 individuals. A pericentric inversion has one break in the short arm and one in the long arm. A paracentric inversion has both breaks in the same chromosome arm.

An inversion carrier is usually phenotypically normal, but the inversion may cause chromosomally unbalanced gametes. For the normal and inverted chromosomes to pair at meiosis, they have to adopt an unusual physical configuration. If a crossover occurs between the inverted and the normal chromosomes, in the inverted segment unbalanced products will result. In theory, the larger the inverted segment, the greater the risk of recombination and the greater the risk of having abnormal liveborn children. In contrast, a viable recombinant product is unlikely to come from a chromosome with an inverted segment that is less than one third the length of the chromosome.

The overall risk of having an abnormal child is approximately 1% when there is no family history of the recombinant form, but the individual risk depends on the precise inversion. If the family is identified through the birth of an individual with a recombinant chromosome, then the risk of having an abnormal liveborn child is 5% to 10%.

An otherwise normal carrier of an inversion that involves one chromosome arm and not the centromere (paracentric inversion) has virtually no increased risk of having a chromosomally abnormal child. There are common inversion variants of chromosomes 1, 9, 16, and Y that do not imply an increased risk.

Parents with Trisomies

Few data are available on the risks associated with the rare occurrence of an individual with trisomy 21 having a child. Affected individuals rarely reproduce. From a literature review of approximately 30 pregnancies, an approximate empiric risk of 1 in 3 of having a child with trisomy 21 has been quoted for females, but the risk of a chromosomally normal fetus having a birth defect or being mentally handicapped could be as high as 30%.[12]

Fetal Chromosomal Anomaly Found on Karyotyping during Pregnancy

Aneuploidies

Most structural chromosomal abnormalities are aneuploidy, numerical abnormalities that involve the loss or gain of one, two, or even whole chromosome sets. These anomalies are most commonly caused by nondisjunction, a process that is more common with increased maternal age. Fraser and Mitchell[13] noted a lack of hereditary factors but an association with advanced maternal age in cases of Down syndrome. Subsequently, in a study of 350 cases, Shuttleworth[14] reported a considerable proportion of affected infants born to women approaching the climacteric. Bleyer[15] proposed an association with degeneration of the ovum. Antonarakis and associates[16] examined DNA polymorphisms in infants with Down syndrome and showed that 95% of nondisjunction trisomy 21 is maternal in origin.

In the late 1970s and early 1980s, when prenatal diagnosis was in its infancy, eight large studies were carried out to assess the age-specific prevalence of trisomy 21 in live births.[17–24] Some of these studies had incomplete ascertainment and little information about the distribution of maternal age and the effect of selective abortion after prenatal diagnosis.

However, two studies[19,22] had nearly complete ascertainment. Cuckle and colleagues[25] combined the data from these eight surveys on a total of 3,289,114 births to determine the prevalence of trisomy 21 at each maternal age. Regression analysis was applied to smooth out fluctuations in the observed data.

In the 1970s and 1980s, genetic amniocentesis at 16 to 20 weeks was offered to women 35 years of age or older. This group was considered to be at increased risk for aneuploidy. Similarly, these groups were targeted for chorionic villus sampling between 9 and 14 weeks.

Data from these prenatal studies confirmed that the prevalence of trisomy 21 increased with maternal age and that the prevalence was higher during pregnancy than at birth.

Combined data from two multicenter studies of amniocentesis (one in the United States and one in Europe) showed that the prevalence of trisomies 13, 18, and 21 was approximately 30% higher at 16 to 20 weeks than at birth.[26,27] Similarly, data from fetal karyotyping by chorionic villus sampling showed that the prevalence of these aneuploidies was approximately 50% higher between 9 and 14 weeks than at birth (Fig. 2–7).[28]

Ultrasound studies have demonstrated that major chromosomal defects are often associated with multiple fetal abnormalities. Conversely, in a fetus with multiple abnormalities, the frequency of chromosomal defects is high and the relative risk increases with the number of anomalies identified. However, prenatal karyotyping is often performed because the prognosis for the baby may be dictated not only by the combination of structural anomalies identified but also by marked neurodevelopmental morbidity associated with aneuploidy. The frequency of chromosomal defects, such as aneuploidy, increases with maternal age. Traditionally, counseling of patients about the risk of fetal chromosomal defects depends on the provision of live birth indices of trisomy 21. However, with ultrasound screening, the prevalence must be established for all chromosomal defects that are associated with structural and biometric anomalies.

Chromosome anomalies differ in the rate of intrauterine attrition, and it is important to establish maternal and

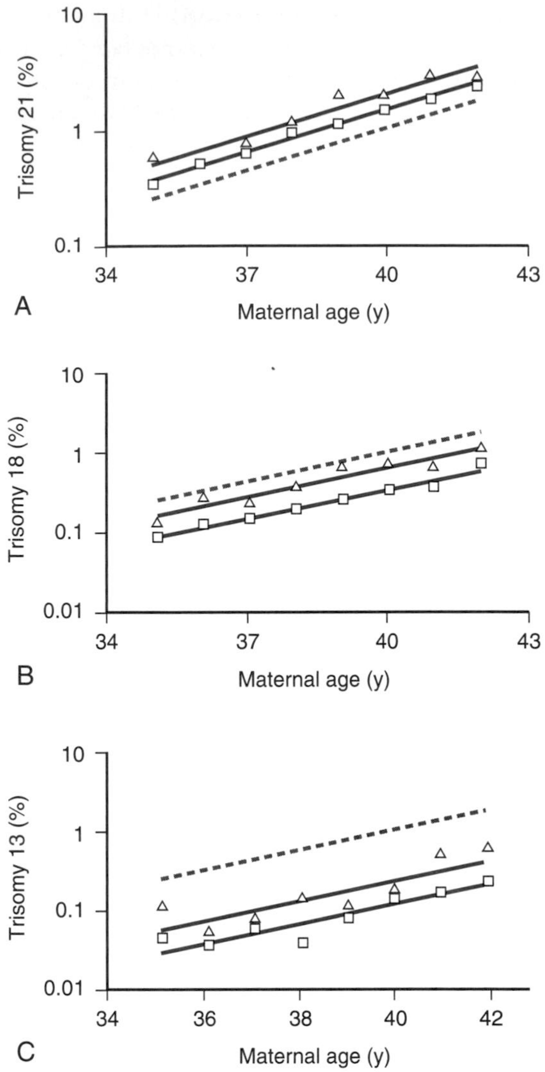

FIGURE 2–7
The prevalence of trisomy 21 (A), trisomy 18 (B), and trisomy 13 (C) at 9 to 14 weeks' gestation (△) and the prevalence of these trisomies at 16 to 20 weeks (□) compared with the prevalence of live births affected with trisomy 21 (–) in women 35 to 42 years old. (From Snijders RJM, Nicolaides KH: Assessment of risk in ultrasound markers for fetal chromosome defects. In Nicolaides KH (ed): Frontiers in Fetal Medicine. London, Parthenon, 1996.)

gestational age-specific risks for each of the common aneuploidies. Data from a subgroup of women 35 to 42 years old have been used to examine the radiance of regression lines that describe the relationship between maternal age and the prevalence of aneuploidy. For trisomy 21 (see Fig. 2–7*A*), trisomy 18 (see Fig. 2–7*B*), and trisomy 13 (see Fig. 2–7*C*), the increase in frequency is nearly parallel, suggesting that there are no maternal age-related differences in the rate of intrauterine loss. If the prevalence of each of the common trisomies in live births is considered to be 1, then the relative prevalence of other gestational ages can be calculated and relative prevalence curves calculated.

The identification of fetal structural abnormalities leads to a stepwise increase in prevalence risk with each additional abnormality. A detailed discussion is beyond the scope of this chapter, but may be found elsewhere (See Snijders and Nicolaides, listed in Further Reading). In the last 10 years, the use of first-trimester scanning to measure nuchal translucency (as related to fetal crown–rump length), combined with maternal serum free βHCG and pregnancy-associated plasma protein A, has been used to screen for aneuploidy (see Chapter 7).

Triploidy

Survival to term of fetuses with triploidy is rare, and those born alive die shortly after birth. Most have partial hydatidiform mole, and the rest are nonmolar, with a normal or hypoplastic trophoblast. It is reasonable to offer prenatal karyotyping in future pregnancies. The phenotypes of the fetus and placenta depend on whether the additional set of chromosomes is paternally or maternally derived. The overall recurrence risk is usually low, but diandric triploidy associated with partial hydatidiform mole has a 1% to 1.5% risk of recurrence, and some women appear to have a predisposition for digynic triploidy.

Structurally Abnormal Chromosomes

When an unexpected structural chromosomal abnormality is found, the first step should be to examine the parental chromosomes. If neither parent has the chromosomal abnormality, gain or loss of chromosomal material may have occurred during gamete formation, with consequent severe clinical effects. If the structural anomaly is present in one parent who is otherwise normal, it is unlikely that a similar anomaly in the child will cause severe problems. Exceptions may occur when chromosomes known to be imprinted are involved, principally chromosome 15. Further cytogenetic advice should be sought.

Structurally Abnormal Additional Chromosomes ("Marker Chromosomes")

If a structurally abnormal extra chromosome (marker, supernumerary, accessory chromosome) or a ring chromosome is discovered, parental karyotyping should be performed urgently. Further advice should be sought in counseling these patients because specialized cytogenetic tests (e.g., painting with chromosome-specific fluorescent probes) may be able to determine whether the fetus is at high or low risk by showing the chromosomal origin and nature. These chromosomes are often found in mosaic form with a normal cell line. The ratio of cell lines in tissue used for prenatal diagnosis cannot be used prognostically. There is no accurate information relating to the residual risk of mental retardation when ultrasound examination shows no fetal anomalies.

Mosaicism

Mosaicism occurs when an individual's tissues or organs contain more than one genetic line of cells. The mutant line of cells may contain a chromosomal anomaly or sometimes a mutant single gene. This is a difficult situation because the phenotype lies somewhere between that of a full disorder and that of a normal individual, and further testing is needed. Even so, the proportion of abnormal cells in one tissue may not be the same as the proportion elsewhere. Similarly, exact figures cannot be given for the risk to offspring of individuals with chromosome or single-gene mosaicism because of the very nature of mosaicism. The risk depends on the numbers and disposition of mutant cells in the gonads.

Placental mosaicism with a chromosomally normal fetus is a well-recognized phenomenon (see Chapter 10). Mosaicism for chromosomes 13, 18, and 21 often predicts fetal abnormality. A high incidence of fetal abnormality is associated with mosaic trisomy 9 and mosaic trisomy 22. Mosaicism for a structurally abnormal additional chromosome appears to carry a greater risk than autosomal trisomy mosaicism. However, another concern when autosomal trisomy mosaicism is found at prenatal diagnosis is that a trisomic fetus may have "lost" one of the three copies of the chromosome in some cells to "correct" the imbalance. If both remaining copies of the chromosome originated from the same parent (UPD), this too could give an abnormal phenotype (discussed later).

De Novo Apparently Balanced Structural Rearrangements

The concern is that there may be a submicroscopic abnormality, either deletion, duplication, or gene disruption, involving the breakpoints. Molecular techniques, such as comparative genomic hybridization, may help to determine whether there is cryptic gain or loss of material in apparently de novo rearrangements found at prenatal diagnosis.

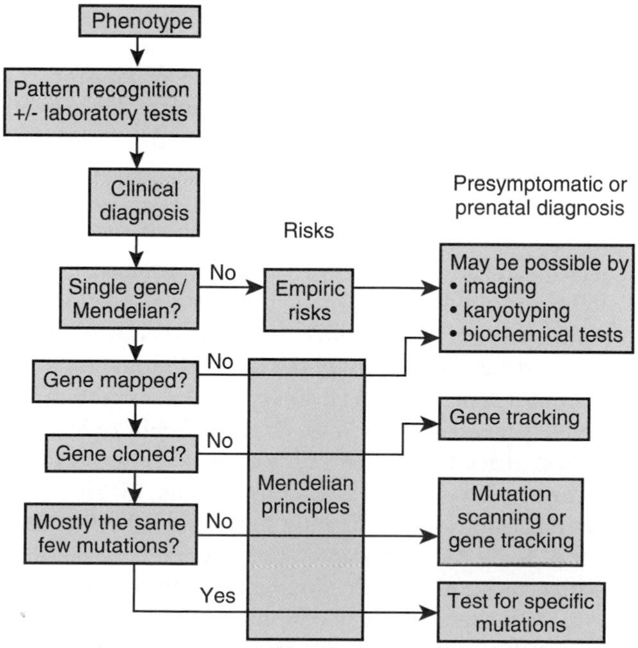

FIGURE 2–8
A flow chart to assist in determining risks and the appropriate type of presymptomatic or prenatal diagnosis.

De Novo Apparently Balanced Reciprocal Translocation

In a very large study, Warburton[29] found that serious malformations were detected in 6.1% of pregnancies at elective termination or in liveborn infants, which is approximately 3% greater than the background risk of malformation that applies to all pregnancies. No prospective data on the risks of cognitive impairment or mental retardation are available. A figure of 5% to 10% is often used to include malformations and neurologic and developmental deficiencies. Negative scan findings may reduce the risks, but cannot predict cognitive outcome. Congenital malformations found on ultrasound indicate likely chromosomal imbalance.

De Novo Robertsonian Translocation

Because the formation of Robertsonian translocations does not disrupt coding sequences, the risk of phenotypic abnormalities is low. When a Robertsonian translocation involves chromosome 14 or 15, fetal UPD studies may be indicated to exclude the small chance that the fetus inherited both copies of chromosome 14 or 15 from the same parent, resulting in dysmorphic and developmental features because of imprinting effects (discussed later).

De Novo Apparently Balanced Inversions

The risk of phenotypic abnormality is increased if the inversion is de novo. Empirically, the risk appears to be approximately 9%. Figures for cognitive impairment are not available.

Other Chromosomal Abnormalities

Duplication is the presence of two copies of a segment of a chromosome. It may originate from unequal crossing-over during meiosis, with the other product of that cell division being a deletion. Duplications are more common than deletions and are generally less harmful. Specific syndromes are associated with certain deletions, but few phenotypes associated with duplications have been given names.

Loss or duplication of part of a chromosome can result in congenital malformations and mental retardation. The precise features depend on the amount of chromosomal material involved and the chromosome from which it was derived.

The clinical effects of the likely chromosomal imbalance may be found from similar cases in the literature. The recurrence risk for a de novo deletion is very low, but not zero. Rare recurrences are likely to be caused by parental mosaicism, which is not usually detected by routine karyotyping. Although recurrence is extremely rare, many couples request prenatal diagnosis for reassurance. When the deletion is caused by an unbalanced product from a familial translocation, the risk of recurrence can be high.

Hereditary fragile sites can occur on several chromosomes, giving the appearance of breakage at a specific point. On autosomes, they appear to be harmless. However, a fragile site near the end of the long arm of the X chromosome at Xq27.3 is a marker for fragile X syndrome, an X-linked mental retardation syndrome. Because of the high risks and complex genetics of this single-gene disorder, families should be referred to the clinical genetics department.

OTHER MECHANISMS OF GENETIC ABNORMALITY: UNIPARENTAL DISOMY AND GENOMIC IMPRINTING

Uniparental Disomy (UPD)

The genomic stimulus for fetal growth is affected by the constant constraints of maternal size, placental function, and nutritional sufficiency. However, the expression of certain genes in both the fetus and the placenta is probably crucial to growth potential. It is probable that the placenta can control not only its own size, but through a variety of mechanisms, that of the fetus. Few studies of the genetic control of fetal and placental growth have been done. However, UPD may be a cause of abnormal fetal growth, especially when it occurs without classic risk factors.

Abnormal growth in utero predisposes the fetus to increased perinatal and neonatal morbidity and mortality. In mammals, reproduction requires the fusion of two haploid chromosome sets, one paternal and the other maternal. The fertilized egg then contains two copies of each chromosome. It is usual, and previously has been assumed invariable, for one member of each chromosome pair to be derived from each parent. However, in UPD, one homologous chromosome pair comes from the same parent (in isodisomy, the chromosomes are identical, but in heterodisomy, the two different maternal or paternal chromosomes are inherited). Catanach and Kirk in 1985 showed UPD in mice that resulted in specific abnormal phenotypes associated with growth disturbance.[30] The progeny of mice with maternal disomy of chromosome 11 were smaller than their normal litter mates. Those with paternal disomy 11 were considerably larger than their litter mates.

Recently, cases have been described in human pregnancies where UPD for specific chromosomes have caused a clinical disorder. The first example was an individual with maternal isodisomy 7 and homozygosity for the cystic fibrosis gene.[31] A similar case was subsequently described by Vosse et al, the progeny showing phenotypically short stature.[32]

Other conditions may be associated with UPD and show the following characteristics:

- Occurrence that is usually sporadic
- No consistent cytogenetic abnormalities
- Abnormal growth patterns and rates of growth

Three separate mechanisms have been postulated for UPD:

- Chromosomal duplication in a monosomic somatic cell after postzygotic loss of a homologous chromosome
- Fertilization of a nullisomic gamete by a disomic gamete
- Loss of a supernumerary chromosome from a trisomic cell, leaving two homologues from the same gamete (trisomic rescue)[33]

Supporting the evidence for this has been provided in recent publications.[34,35] The paper by Purves-Smith reported a confined placental mosaicism for trisomy 15, but an apparently normal karyotype on amniotic fluid cytogenetic and postnatal blood analysis.[34] However, at the age of 2 years, Prader-Willi syndrome was diagnosed clinically and maternal disomy 15 confirmed on molecular studies. The second study reported confined placental mosaicism for trisomy 16 in 4 fetuses with severe intrauterine growth restriction.[35] Subsequent skin karyotyping and molecular studies showed a normal karyotype with maternal disomy of chromosome 16.

Alternatively, postzygotic mitotic recombination could result in "mosaic" UPD. This phenomenon was recently identified in four patients with Beckwith-Wiedemann syndrome.

Further mechanisms for UPD include gamete complementation or monosomic zygote correction; the latter has supporting evidence from some isodisomy cases of Angelman syndrome when no evidence of recombination between chromosome 15 was found.[36] Whatever the mechanism, UPD may play an important role in unresolved genetic syndromes that affect growth.

Similarly, we carried out pilot chromosomal studies of 11 babies born with idiopathic growth restriction. The fetuses had prenatal diagnosis performed before 26 weeks' gestation. In the 11 cases, we showed 5 instances of placental chromosomal mosaicism. The chromosomal abnormalities identified varied from trisomies for chromosomes 7 and 8 to structural abnormalities and deletions. In a further six pregnancies in which chromosomal mosaicism was detected prenatally after first-trimester chorionic villus sampling, three cases occurred involving chromosome 7, one chromosome 8, and two chromosome 15 for utero-placental disomy. In one of these six cases, UPD was found and this was for chromosome 15. Maternal heterodisomy was detected and would have resulted in Prader-Willi syndrome if the pregnancy continued.[37]

Fewer than 100 well-documented pregnancies are reported as having intrauterine growth restriction or fetal death associated with confined placental mosaicism. To date, only 12 chromosomes have been involved: 2, 3, 7, 8,

9, 13, 14, 15, 16, 18, 22, and X.[35] Trisomy 16 is the most common trisomy associated with pregnancy loss and confined placental mosaicism in intrauterine growth restriction. A prospective study investigated the incidence of UPD associated with growth restriction in 35 infants born between 25 and 40 weeks.[38] However, only two fetuses were born before 28 weeks, and both had chromosomal UPD of chromosome 16 plus confirmed placental mosaicism. No other UPD was found for the 12 chromosomes tested. It was concluded that UPD for the chromosomes tested did not explain the etiology of most cases of intrauterine growth restriction. However, many of these cases occurred after 32 weeks, and a higher detection rate is likely in fetuses with severe intrauterine growth restriction before 28 weeks.

Genomic Imprinting

The concept that male and female genomes do not contribute equally to mammalian development derives from observations made in mice two decades ago.[39] In these experiments, the development of uniparental diploid embryos was severely disrupted. Pathogenetic conceptuses developed embryos up to the 25-cell stage but showed only very rudimentary extraembryonic tissues. Androgenic conceptuses were characterized by relatively well-developed extraembryonic membranes and severely perturbed embryos. These reciprocal uniparental phenotypes probably resulted from disruption of the normal parental-specific expression patterns of a subset of imprinted genes. A detailed discussion is outside the scope of this chapter (See Further Reading, Georgiades et al, 2001).

MALFORMATION SYNDROMES

General

The term "dysmorphology" has been applied to the study of birth defects occurring in recognizable syndromic combinations. The causes of these syndromes include chromosomal abnormalities, genetic defects, and teratogens (e.g., drugs, infections, metabolic causes). The cellular pathways involved in the pathogenesis of some malformation syndromes are being delineated, often by analyzing genes identified in other species as vital for normal development. Confirming that mutations in these genes cause specific human syndromes offers the possibility of DNA diagnosis.

Structural Malformations Found at Ultrasound Examination

A detailed screening fetal ultrasound examination may show a pattern of major anomalies that suggests a specific diagnosis (see Chapters 7 and 8). Recognizable patterns are most likely to be caused by chromosomal anomalies, but rare single-gene or dysmorphic syndromes may be diagnosed in utero in the absence of a history of the syndrome. In addition to major structural abnormalities, careful evaluation of the fetus may show other dysmorphic features that are not commonly sought in a routine "screening" ultrasound examination. These abnormalities include micrognathia, hypotelorism, and hypertelorism as well as subtle abnormalities of the hands (e.g., clinodactyly) or feet (e.g., sandal gap of the toe). Careful evaluation of the fetal posture or attitude when the fetus is stationary and moving may also give important diagnostic information.

Evaluation of the features with a clinical geneticist or perinatologist who has a special interest in fetal dysmorphology may aid in the prospective diagnosis of a dysmorphic syndrome. The use of computer databases (see Further Reading) may be helpful in obtaining a diagnosis. It is important to look at photographs in original reports because a description may sound identical but the reported case may look entirely different from the patient.

As with all aspects of genetic counseling, accuracy of the diagnosis is paramount. Information obtained prenatally should be supplemented by information from postnatal examination, or from a detailed examination by a perinatal pathologist if the couple opts for termination or if the fetus is stillborn. Photographs of the main features are helpful when seeking the diagnostic advice of a clinical geneticist.

Syndromes

For many common disorders, empirical risk tables are available (see Further Reading and Harper, P, 1998). If the diagnosis is not clear or no accurate data on which to base a recurrence risk are available, it is advisable to refer the case to a clinical geneticist.

ISOLATED ORGAN AND SYSTEM ANOMALIES

Many disorders that affect specific organ systems appear to have a genetic or inherited component but show no clear pattern of mendelian inheritance or identifiable chromosomal abnormality. The term "multifactorial" has been used to describe this group. In some cases (e.g., Hirschsprung disease, congenital heart disease), the disorder is not a single entity but a heterogeneous group of indistinguishable disorders. Some of these may be inherited in a mendelian fashion, others may result from interplay of an inherited component and environmental factors, and others may be "acquired" in the sense that environmental factors are largely influential. Empiric risk data, obtained from observing recurrences in population studies, are available for many of these conditions (see Further Reading), but a clinical geneticist should be consulted.

SUMMARY OF MANAGEMENT OPTIONS

Counseling Points for Common Conditions

Management Options	Quality of Evidence	Grade of Recommendation	References
Mendelian Inheritance			
High recurrence risks	IV	C	1
Establish an accurate diagnosis and the mode of inheritance before counseling.	IV	C	1
Seek the latest information about carrier detection tests.	IV	C	1
Plan invasive procedures requiring DNA methods in consultation with a laboratory.	IV	C	1
Autosomal Dominant Conditions			
50% risk to offspring of the affected parent	IV	C	1
Potential pitfalls in conditions with variable expression	IV	C	1
Autosomal Recessive Conditions			
25% risk of an affected child when both parents are carriers	IV	C	1
Prenatal diagnosis is possible for some	IV	C	1
Donor gametes may be an acceptable therapeutic option for some; much discussion is required.	IV	C	1
X-Linked Recessive Conditions			
Male-to-male transmission never occurs.	IV	C	1
Daughters of an affected male are carriers.	IV	C	1
Unaffected males never transmit the disease.	IV	C	1
For female carriers, each son has a 1 in 2 risk of being affected and each daughter has a 1 in 2 risk of being a carrier; affected homozygous females are rare.	IV	C	1
Chromosome Abnormalities			
Refer families with translocations to a clinical geneticist so that family studies can be performed to identify the risk of an unbalanced karyotype (which may lead to miscarriage or a child with abnormalities).	IV	C	1
With an unexpected structural chromosome abnormality, examine the parents' chromosomes.	IV	C	1
Duplication or deletion of chromosomal material can result in congenital malformation or mental retardation.	IV	C	1
Predicting the clinical effects of mosaicism is difficult; it may require karyotyping other cell lines.	IV	C	1
De novo chromosomal disorders have a low risk of recurrence; offer fetal karyotyping for reassurance.	IV	C	1
Check karyotype reports with a laboratory if the meaning is in doubt.	IV	C	1
Clarify whether risks relate to "at amniocentesis" or "at delivery".	IV	C	1
Specific Syndromes			
Ensure the accuracy of diagnosis and risks.	IV	C	1
Empiric risk figures are available for some conditions (see "Further Reading").	IV	C	1
Prenatal diagnosis is available for some with a biochemical basis, where a gene has been found, or where a microdeletion or duplication is the cause.	IV	C	1

SUMMARY OF MANAGEMENT OPTIONS
Counseling Points for Common Conditions *(Continued)*

Management Options	Quality of Evidence	Grade of Recommendation	References
Specific Syndromes *(Continued)*			
If the diagnosis or risks are in doubt, refer the patient to a clinical geneticist.	IV	C	I
Organ and System Abnormalities			
For many conditions, information should be obtained from a clinical geneticist.	IV	C	I
Empiric risk figures for siblings and children are available for some conditions (see "Further Reading").	IV	C	I

CONCLUSIONS

- Fetal abnormality is not uncommon, affecting 1% to 2% of newborns.
- Not all abnormalities have a genetic basis or a risk of recurrence in a future pregnancy.
- Families with single-gene disorders and parental chromosomal anomalies have the highest risks and may be detected by taking a family pedigree.
- The more distant the pregnant woman's relationship from a blood relative with a gentic disorder, the lower the risk of the condition.
- For women who have had trisomies, the risk of recurrence applies only to further siblings.
- Accurate and comprehensive information is needed to make a secure diagnosis, including taking a family pedigree before undertaking counseling.
- Close liaison with clinical geneticists is advisable.

FURTHER READING

Baraitser M, Winter RM: Multiple Congenital Anomalies: A Diagnostic Compendium. London, Chapman and Hall, 1996.

Cassidy SB, Allanson JE: Management of Genetic Syndromes. New York, John Wiley and Sons, 2001.

Donnai D, Winter RM: Congenital Malformation Syndromes. London, Chapman and Hall, 1995.

Gardner RJM, Sutherland GR: Chromosome Abnormalities and Genetic Counseling, 3rd ed. Oxford, Oxford University Press, 2004.

Georgiades P, Watkins M, Baxton GJ, Fergusson-Smith AC: Roles of genomic imprinting and the zygotic genome in placental development. Proc Natl Acad Sci, USA, 2001;98:4522–4527.

Harper PS: Practical Genetic Counselling, 5th ed. Oxford, Butterworth-Heinemann, 1998.

Jones KL: Smith's Recognisable Patterns of Human Malformation, 5th ed. Philadelphia, Saunders, 1997.

Scriver CR, Beaudet AL, Sly WS, Valle D: The Metabolic and Molecular Basis of Inherited Disease, 8th ed. New York, McGraw-Hill, 2002.

Shashidhar Pai G, Lewandowski RC, Borgaonkar DS: Handbook of Chromosomal Syndromes. New York, Wiley-Liss, 2002.

Snijders RJM, Nicolaides KH: Assessment of risk in ultrasound markers for fetal chromosome defects. In Nicolaides KH (ed): Frontiers in Fetal Medicine. London, Parthenon, 1996.

Rimoin DL, Connor JM, Pyeritz RE, et al: Emery and Rimoin's Principles and Practice of Medical Genetics, 4th ed. London, Churchill Livingstone, 2001.

Farndon P: Fetal anomalies—the geneticist's approach. In Twinning P, Meltugo JM, Pilling DW (eds.) Textbook of Fetal Abnormalities. Churchill Livingstone, 2000.

Dysmorphology Databases:

The Winter-Baraitser Dysmorphology Database (www.lmdatabases.com)

POSSUM (Pictures of Standard Syndromes and Undiagnosed Malformations)(www.possum.net.au)

REFERENCES

1. Harper PS: Practical Genetic Counselling, 5th ed. Oxford, Butterworth-Heinemann, 1998.
2. Godard B, Ten Kate L, Evers-Kiebooms G, Ayme S: Population genetic screening programmes: Principles, techniques, practices, and policies. Eur J Hum Gen 2003;11(suppl 2): S49–S87.
3. Hoedemaekers R, ten Have H, Chadwick R: Genetic screening: A comparative analysis of three recent reports. J Med Ethics 1997;23:135–411.
4. Kaplan F: Tay-Sachs disease carrier screening: A model for prevention of genetic disease. Genet Test 1998;2:271–292.
5. Mitchell JJ, Capua A, Clow C, Scriver CR: Twenty-year outcome analysis of genetic screening programs for Tay-Sachs and beta-thalassaemia disease carriers in high schools. Am J Hum Genet 1996;59:793–798.
6. Ranieri E, Lewis BD, Gerace RL, et al: Neonatal screening for cystic fibrosis using immunoreactive trypsinogen indirect gene analysis: Four years' experience. BMJ 1994;308:1469–1472.
7. Super M, Schwarz MJ, Malone G, et al: Active cascade testing for carriers of cystic fibrosis gene. BMJ 1994;308:1462–1457.
8. Raeburn JA: Screening for carriers of cystic fibrosis. BMJ 1994;308:1451–1452.
9. Mennie ME, Gilfillan A, Compton M, et al: Prenatal screening for cystic fibrosis. Lancet 1992;340:214–216.
10. Livingstone J, Axton RA, Gilfillan A, et al: Antenatal screening for cystic fibrosis: A trial of the couple method. BMJ 1994;308:1459–1462.
11. Clarke A, Fielding D, Kerzin-Storrar L, et al: The Genetic Testing of Children: Report of the Working Party of the Clinical Genetics Society (UK). J Med Genet 1994;31:785–797.
12. Rani AS, Jyothi A, Reddy PP, Reddy OS: Reproduction in Down's syndrome. Int J Gynaecol Obstet 1990;31:81–86.
13. Fraser J, Mitchell A: Kalmuk idiocy: Report of a case with autopsy. J Mental Sci 1876;98:169–179.
14. Shuttleworth GE: Mongoloid imbecility. BMJ 1909;2: 661–665.
15. Bleyer A: Indication that mongoloid imbecility is a gametogenic mutation of disintegrating type. Am J Dis Child 1934; 47:342.
16. Antonarakis SE, Lewi JG, Adelsberger PA, et al: Parental origin of the extra chromosome in trisomy 21 as indicated by analysis of DNA polymorphisms. N Engl J Med 1991;324:872–876.
17. Hook EB, Chambers GM: Estimates of rates of Down's syndrome in live births by one year maternal age intervals for mothers aged 20–49 in a New York state study. In Bergsma D, Lowry RB, Trimble BK, Feingold M (eds): Numerical Taxonomy of Birth Defects and Polygenic Disorders: Birth Defects. New York, Allan R Liss, 1977.
18. Hook EB, Fabia JJ: Frequency of Down's syndrome in live births by single year maternal age interval: Rresults of the Massachusetts study. Teratology 1978;17:223–228.
19. Hook EB, Lindsjo A: Down's syndrome in live births by single year maternal age intervals in a Swedish study: Comparison with the results of the New York state study. Am J Hum Genet 1978;30:19–27.
20. Trimble BK, Baird PA: Maternal age and Down's syndrome: Age specific incidence rates by single year intervals. Am J Genet 1978;2:1–5.
21. Sunderland GR, Clisby SR, Bloor G: Down's syndrome in South Australia. Med J Aust 1979;2:58–61.
22. Koulisher L, Gillerot Y: Down's syndrome in Wallonia (south Belgium), 1971 to 1978: Cytogenetic in incidence. Hum Gene 1980;54:243–250.
23. Young D, Williams EM, Newcombe RG: Down's syndrome and maternal age in South Glamorgan. J Med Genet 1980;17: 433–436.
24. Huether CA, Gummere GR, Hook EB: Down's syndrome: Percentage reporting of birth certificates and single year maternal age risks for Ohio 1970–1979. Comparisons with up-state New York data. Am J Public Health 1981;71:1367–1372.
25. Cuckle HS, Ward NJ, Thompson SG: Estimating a woman's risk of having a pregnancy associated with Down's syndrome using her age and serum alphafetoprotein level. Br J Obstet Gynaecol 1987;94:387–402.
26. Ferguson-Smith MA, Yates JRW: Maternal age specific rates for chromosome aberrations and factors influencing them: Report of a collaborative European study on 52,965 amniocenteses. Prenat Diagn 1984;4:5–44.
27. Hook EB, Cross PK, Regal RR: The frequency of trisomies 21, 18 and 13 at the upper most extremities of maternal age: Results on 56,094 fetuses studied prenatally and comparisons with data on live births. Hum Genet 1984;68:211–220.
28. Snijders RJM, Sebre N, Nicolaides KH: Maternal age and gestational age-specific risk for chromosome defects. Fetal Diagn Ther 1995;10:215–219.
29. Warburton D: De novo balanced chromosome rearrangements and extra marker chromosomes identified at prenatal diagnosis: Clinical significance and distribution of breakpoints. Am J Hum Genet 1991;49:995–1013.
30. Cattanach B, Kirk M: Differential activity of maternal and paternally derived chromosome regions in mice. Nature 1985;315: 496–498.
31. Spence JE: Uniparental disomy as a mechanism for human genetic disease. Am J Hum Genet 1988;42:217–226.
32. Vosse R: Isodisomy of chromosome 7 in a patient with cystic fibrosis: Could uniparental disomy be common in humans? Am J Hum Genet 1989;45:373–380.
33. Clark AC: Genetic imprinting in clinical genetics. Development 1990;23:131–139.
34. Suani MAH, Barten SC, Norris ML: Development of reconstituted mouse eggs suggest imprinting during gametogenesis. Nature 1984;308:548–550.
35. Purves-Smith SG: Uniparental disomy 15 resulting from correction of an initial trisomy 15. Am J Hum Genet 1992;50: 1348–1350.
36. Kalousek DK: Uniparental disomy of chromosome 16 in humans. Am J Hum Genet 1993;52:8–16.
37. Mutirangura A: Greenbeg F, Butter MG, et al Multiplex PCR of 3 dinucleotide repeats in Prader-Willi/Angelman critical region (15q11-q13): Molecular diagnosis and mechanisms of uniparental disomy. Human Molecular Genetics 1993;2:143–151.
38. Moore GE, Ali Z, Khan RU, et al: The incidence of uniparental disomy associated with intrauterine growth restriction in a cohort of 35 severely affected babies. Am J Obstet Gynecol 1997;176:294–299.
39. Barton S, Surani M, Norris M: Role of paternal and maternal genomes in mouse development. Nature 1984;311;374–376.
40. Marteau TM, Kidd J, Michie S, et al: Anxiety, knowledge and satisfaction in women receiving false positive results on routine prenatal screening: A randomized controlled trial. J Psychosom Obstet Gynecol 1993;14:185–196.
41. Hall S, Bobrow M, Marteau TM: Psychological consequences for parents of false negative results on prenatal screening for Down's syndrome: Retrospective interview study. BMJ 2000;320:407–412.
42. Michie S, Bron F, Bobrow M, Marteau TM: Nondirectiveness in genetic counseling: An empirical study. Am J Hum Genet 1997;60:40–47.
43. Marteau T, Drake H, Bobrow M: Counselling following diagnosis of a fetal abnormality: The differing approaches of obstetricians, clinical geneticists, and genetic nurses. J Med Genet 1994;31:864–867.

APPENDIX

Useful Genetics Web Links

Genetics knowledge, both clinical and scientific, is expanding so rapidly that it is necessary to rely on international databases to ensure that patients have the most up-to-date information. This section lists a selection of useful websites, and many more can be found on the websites of the European and American Societies of Human Genetics. *(www.eshg.org; www.ashg.org)*

OMIM (On-line Mendelian Inheritance in Man)

OMIM is a catalog of mendelian disorders in humans. It was initiated by Victor McKusick at Johns Hopkins Hospital. *(http://www.ncbi.nlm.nih.gov/Omim/searchomim.html)*

GeneClinics

GeneClinics is a clinical information resource that relates genetic testing to the diagnosis, management, and genetic counseling of individuals and families with specific inherited disorders. There is also a listing of laboratories and the tests that they provide. *(http://www.geneclinics.org/)*

EDDNAL (European Directory of DNA Diagnostic Laboratories)

EDDNAL, which is supported mainly by funding from the European Commission, provides standardized information on molecular diagnostic services for heritable syndromes and disorders offered by laboratories in 17 European countries. *(http://www.eddnal.com/)*

UK GTN (United Kingdom Genetic Testing Network)

The UK GTN website lists the diseases and available molecular tests in UK GTN laboratories. (http://www.ukgtn.org).

Public Health Genetics Unit

This site provides news and information about advances in genetics and their effect on public health and the prevention of disease. Its information database has reports, summaries, literature references, and other information about the genetic basis of disease, genetic testing and screening, policy development for genetic services, and ethical issues. *(http://www.phgu.org.uk/index.php)*

AIDS TO LEARNING GENETICS AND GENETICS INFORMATION

The Genetics Education Center at the University of Kansas Medical Center has an excellent listing of resources and is highly recommended. *(http://www.kumc.edu/gec/)*

DNA from the Beginning

DNA from the Beginning is an online learning text that is organized around key concepts of classical genetics, molecules of genetics, and genetic organization and control. The science behind each concept is explained by animation, images, video interviews, problems, biographies, and external links. *(http://vector.cshl.org/dnaftb/)*

Clinical Genetics: A Self-Study for Health Care Providers

This self-study guide from the United States has two sections. The first consists of four lessons designed to increase knowledge about genetics and assist in identifying families for genetic referral. The second section includes reasons for referral, a glossary, a list of resources, and educational tools to use when working with patients and families. *(http://www.vh.org/Providers/Textbooks/ClinicalGenetics/Contents.*

ETHICAL ISSUES

Nuffield Council on Bioethics

The Nuffield Council on Bioethics offers published reports on the ethics of research into genetics, genetics and human behavior, and ethical issues associated with genetic screening. *(http://www.nuffield.org/bioethics/index.html)*

International: Centre for Public Law Research at the University of Montreal

The HumGen site provides information on a wide range of legislation, policy, guidelines, and recommendations of government and nongovernment organizations worldwide. *(http://www.humgen.umontreal.ca/intro.htm)*

INFORMATION FOR PATIENTS

Contact-a-Family

Contact-a-Family is an umbrella group that lists many patient support groups in the United Kingdom. *(http://www. cafamily.org.uk/)*

NORD (National Organization for Rare Disorders)

NORD is a federation of voluntary health organizations that is dedicated to helping people with rare "orphan" diseases and assisting the organizations that serve them. NORD is committed to the identification, treatment, and cure of rare disorders through programs of education, advocacy, research, and service. NORD has an index and a database of rare diseases and information about support groups and other sources of help. *(http://www.rarediseases. org/)*

GIG (Genetics Interest Group)

GIG is an organization in the United Kingdom that represents more than 120 charities that support children, families, and individuals affected by genetic disorders. Its primary goal is to promote awareness and understanding of genetic disorders. The website has video clips of patients discussing their diagnoses, discrimination and stigma, understanding and public awareness, and the prospects for research. *(http://www.gig. org.uk/)*

SECTION TWO

Early Prenatal Care

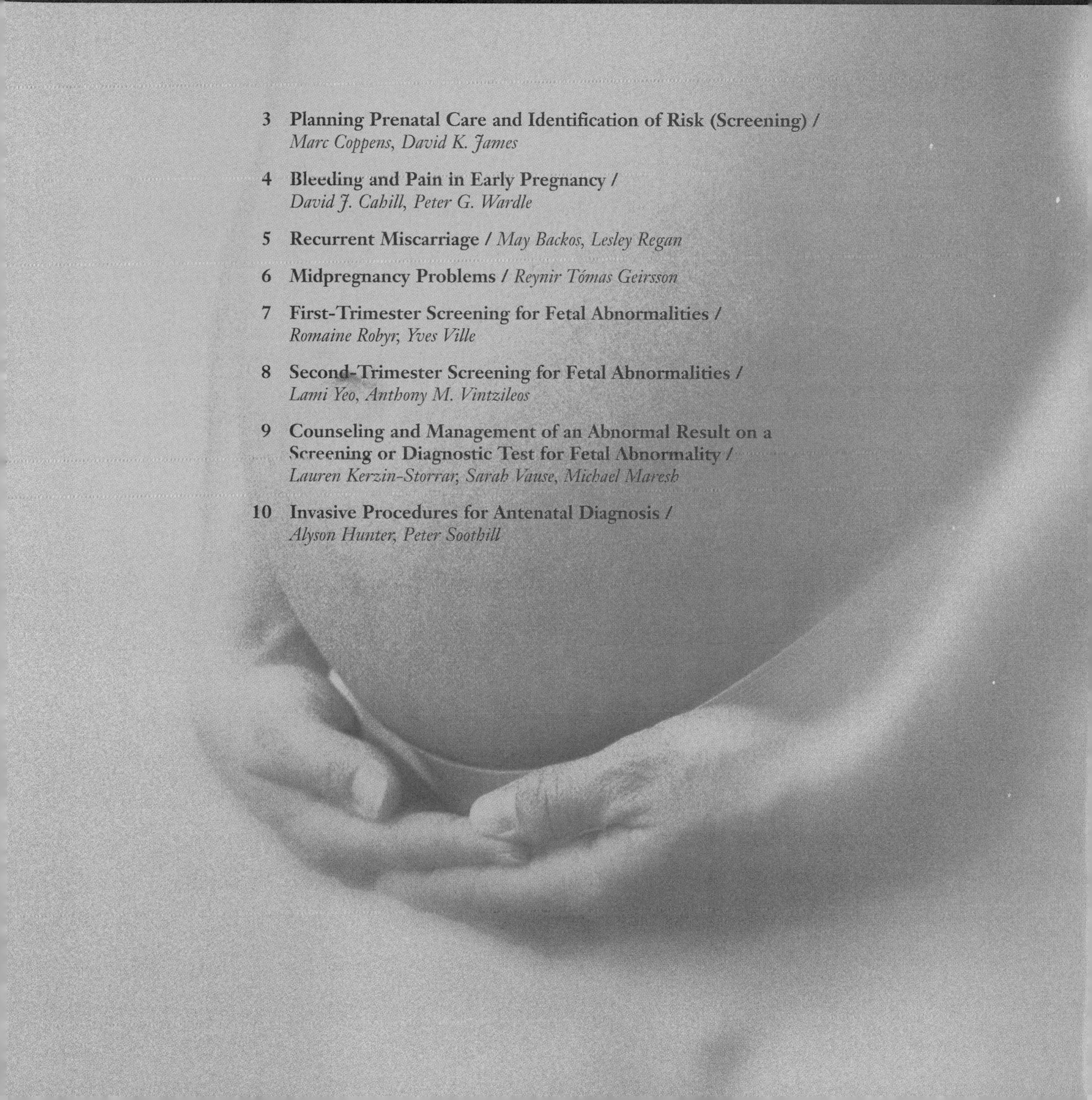

CHAPTER 3

Planning Prenatal Care and Identification of Risk (Screening)

Marc Coppens / David K. James

INTRODUCTION

Definition of Risk

A pregnancy is defined as "high risk" when the likelihood of an adverse outcome for the woman or infant is greater than the incidence of that outcome in the general population.[1]

Aims of Prenatal Care

According to this definition, most pregnancies are not high risk. The aims of care for women with normal "low-risk" pregnancies are as follows[2]:

- To provide advice, reassurance, education, and support for the woman and her family
- To treat minor symptoms associated with pregnancy
- To provide an on-going screening program (clinical and laboratory-based) to confirm that the pregnancy continues to be low risk

For the minority of women who are identified as high risk before, during, or after pregnancy, these aims of prenatal care still apply. However, in addition, there is a fourth aim[2]:

- To prevent, detect, and manage problems and factors that adversely affect the health of the mother or infant

Is Prenatal Care Worthwhile?

Over the last 50 years, many studies of prenatal care, including major national surveys, showed worse pregnancy outcome in women who receive no prenatal care.[3–6] The association between prenatal care and improved pregnancy outcome has been suggested in several European epidemiologic studies.[7,8] Studies in developing countries have also indicated a causal relationship between enhanced prenatal care and a decrease in perinatal and maternal mortality rates.[6,9,10]

In light of these associations, some argue erroneously that prenatal care must be beneficial. However, this argument is flawed.[11,12] Further, what constitutes "prenatal care" varies considerably in practice (discussed later). The controversy over the real effect of prenatal care on pregnancy outcome was reinforced by recent studies. A critical review of studies conducted between 1966 and 1994 showed no conclusive proof of improved pregnancy outcome as a result of prenatal care programs.[13] More recent data have not resolved this controversy.[14] A recent regional audit of perinatal deaths in the Netherlands showed that many deaths were unrelated to women's use of prenatal care.[15]

A much stronger case for prenatal care can be made by examining whether individual components of care have proven benefit in achieving the four aims of prenatal care.[2,16–19] Each suggested strategy for prenatal care can be critically examined and categorized as follows[20]:

- Measures of proven benefit
- Measures for which further evidence is needed
- Measures for which the available evidence shows no benefit or even harm; it is reasonable to argue that this group of strategies should no longer be used in prenatal care

Space does not allow a detailed discussion of the evidence for classifying management strategies into these three groups; this information is available elsewhere.[21] Tables 3–1 through 3–4 show summaries of the evidence of the value of certain management strategies for prenatal care. Evidence for and against specific management options is discussed in greater detail in other chapters.

TABLE 3–1

Evidence That Advice, Reassurance, Education, and Support in Preparation for Childbirth is Effective (Aim No. 1 of Prenatal Care)

Proven Strategy	Level of Evidence	Grade of Recommendation	Benefit
Improved social and psychological support from caregivers	Ia	A	Better communication, satisfaction with care; less anxiety, less postnatal illness, and fewer feeding problems
Antismoking interventions	Ib	A	Reduced smoking and higher mean birthweight
Antenatal classes	III	B	Fewer intrapartum analgesia requirements
Routine ultrasonography with positive feedback	IIb	B	Positive feeling toward baby; lower post-term induction rate
Strategy Needing More Study			
Modifications of work patterns			Possible improvements in maternal and perinatal morbidity
Carbohydrate supplements for malnourished women			Possible higher mean birthweight
Antenatal classes			Possible increase in self-esteem and satisfaction with pregnancy; less pelvic floor trauma after delivery
Iron, folate, multivitamin, and nutritional supplementation for all women			Possible improvements in maternal and perinatal morbidity; higher birthweight, fewer neural tube defects, less preeclampsia
Strategy of No Proven Benefit or Proven Harm			
Failure to involve women in decision-making			
Failure to provide continuity of care			
Physicians involved in the care of all pregnant patients			
Prescribing high-density protein supplements			
Advising restriction of weight gain			
Advising restriction of salt intake			
Prescribing high doses of vitamin A (>4000 IE/day) or vitamin E			

(From Cochrane Pregnancy and Childbirth Group: Abstracts of Cochrane Reviews. The Cochrane Library, issue 2. Oxford, UK, Update Software, 2003.)

CRITICAL REVIEW OF THE EVIDENCE TO JUSTIFY THE OPTIONS AND VARIATIONS IN THE PROVISION AND USE OF PRENATAL CARE

Different measures are used to quantify the use of prenatal care (e.g., percentage of women receiving care, timing of the first visit, percentage of women receiving late or no care, frequency of visits, and indices of adequacy of prenatal care).[20] Data on the use of prenatal care show distinct socioeconomic, ethnic, and geographic differences.[20,22] These differences, also present within western countries, such as the United Kingdom, have led to important differences in perinatal and maternal mortality. For example, it is estimated that the perinatal mortality rate in Pakistani-born mothers in the United Kingdom is twice the national average.[23] In both developed and developing countries, there is great variation in the provision and content of prenatal care. However, there is little evidence to justify the different methods of providing prenatal care.

The Changing Childbirth report[24] explicitly stated that women should be the focus of maternity care. The main goal is to enable women to make informed decisions, based on their needs, after discussing the options fully with the professionals involved.

Reviews of women's views on antenatal care suggest that the aspects of care that women value most are respect, competence, communication, support, and convenience.[25]

Providers

The respective roles of obstetricians, family physicians (general practitioners), and midwives in the delivery of prenatal care vary from one country to another.[20] There is no evidence that physicians need to be involved in the prenatal care of every patient.[26–28] For specific problems, especially social concerns, midwives, family physicians, or other professionals may actually offer more benefit than specialists.[27,29] Midwives and general practitioners are primarily oriented to the care of women with normal pregnancies and, arguably, are more responsive to their needs than specialist obstetricians, whose care is concentrated on problems.[30] Incorporating different medical professionals into one shared antenatal care program can be effective in providing appropriate care for women with low-risk pregnancies.[31,32] Recent studies in Australia showed that continuity of midwifery care can realistically be achieved in a tertiary obstetric referral center without an increase in perinatal mortality and morbidity rates and with increased patient satisfaction.[28] The World Health Organization (WHO) Antenatal Care Trial Research Group evaluated

TABLE 3–2

Evidence That Minor Symptoms Can Be Relieved (Aim No. 2 of Prenatal Care)

Proven Strategy	Level of Evidence	Grade of Recommendation	Benefit
Antiemetics (e.g., antihistamines)	Ia	A	Reduced nausea and vomiting
Antacids	Ib	A	Reduced heartburn
Increased dietary fiber intake	IIb	B	Reduced constipation
Bulking agents and stool softeners	III	B	Reduced constipation
Strategy Needing More Study			
Magnesium supplements			Possible reduced leg cramps
Dilute hydrochloric acid			Possible reduced heartburn
Prostigmine			Possible reduced heartburn
Sodium chloride			Possible reduced leg cramps
Calcium			Possible reduced leg cramps
Quinine			Possible reduced leg cramps
Vitamin D			Possible reduced leg cramps
Strategy of No Proven Benefit or Proven Harm			
Saline cathartics or lubricant oils for constipation			

(From Cochrane Pregnancy and Childbirth Group: Abstracts of Cochrane Reviews. The Cochrane Library, issue 2. Oxford, UK, Update Software, 2003.)

the effectiveness of different antenatal care programs for women with low-risk pregnancies (reduced frequency of prenatal visits, different prenatal care providers).[32] The data showed no differences in selected perinatal outcomes for low-risk pregnant women, regardless of the different prenatal care programs. However, there were differences in satisfaction with the prenatal care provider. When care provided by a midwife and a general practitioner was compared with care provided by an obstetrician and a gynecologist, women's response regarding the continuity of care favored midwife-led shared care.[33] Financial constraints on national medical budgets have reopened the discussion of optimizing the cost-effectiveness of health care delivery. A physician-based prenatal care model for low-risk pregnancies appears to be more expensive without actually improving pregnancy outcome.[27,28,34,35] From a health

TABLE 3–3

Evidence That Antenatal Screening Identifies Women at Risk (Aim No. 3 of Prenatal Care)

Proven Strategy	Level of Evidence	Grade of Recommendation	Risk Identified
Selective fetal ultrasonography or invasive procedure	Ia	A	Fetal abnormality
Maternal serum α-fetoprotein testing or biochemical screening (first or second trimester)	III	B	Neural tube defects, Down syndrome
Fundal height in high-risk pregnancies	Ib	B	Pathologic fetal growth
Regular ultrasound measurements of fetal size	Ia	A	Pathologic fetal growth
Maternal kick charts	Ib	A	Fetal death
Biophysical tests of fetal well-being	III	B	Fetal death
Doppler ultrasound of fetal circulation in high-risk pregnancy	Ia	A	Fetal compromise
Rhesus antibody screening	III	B	Rhesus hemolytic disease
Selective use of ultrasonography	IIa–IIb	B	Fetal viability, gestational age, placental site, fetal presentation
Regular blood pressure measurements and urinalysis	III	B	Preeclampsia
Screening for impaired glucose tolerance	IV	C	Gestational diabetes
Screening for bacteriuria	Ia	A	Asymptomatic bacteriuria and sequelae
Screening for infectious diseases (syphilis, HIV, gonorrhea)	III	B	Maternal, fetal, or neonatal infection
Screening for group B streptococcus carrier status near term	IV	C	Neonatal sepsis
Strategy Needing More Study			
Fundal height in low-risk pregnancies			Pathologic fetal growth
Doppler ultrasound of uteroplacental circulation			Fetal compromise, preeclampsia
Routine screening for toxoplasmosis, cytomegalovirus, chlamydia			Fetal or neonatal infection
Regular herpes swabs in women with a history of herpes			Neonatal infection
Risk scoring, monitoring of uterine activity, screening for vaginal sepsis, cervical assessment (digital, ultrasound)			Spontaneous preterm labor
Maternal and fetal screening			Risk of placental abruption
Maternal and fetal assessment in postdates pregnancy			Maternal and fetal risk

(From Cochrane Pregnancy and Childbirth Group: Abstracts of Cochrane Reviews. The Cochrane Library, issue 2. Oxford, UK, Update Software, 2003.)

TABLE 3–4

Evidence That When a Specific Risk Is Identified, the Subsequent Intervention and Management Improves the Outcome (Aim No. 4 of Prenatal Care)

Proven Strategy	Level of Evidence	Grade of Recommendation	Benefit
Multivitamins and folate supplements in patients with a previous fetus with a neural tube defect	Ia	A	Reduced incidence of neural tube defects in subsequent pregnancy
Amniocentesis vs chorionic villus sampling	Ia	A	Lower miscarriage rate with amniocentesis in the second trimester vs chorionic villus sampling in the first trimester
Anti-D for Rhesus-negative women after delivery of a Rhesus-positive child	Ia	A	Reduced subsequent isoimmunization
Intravascular fetal blood therapy for Rhesus hydrops	IIa	B	Improved perinatal outcome
Routine ultrasound	IIb	B	Reduced postdates induction
Doppler ultrasound of fetal circulation	Ia	A	Reduced perinatal morbidity and mortality
Antihypertensive therapy in women with hypertension	Ia	A	Reduced severe hypertensive pregnancy
Tight control of diabetes (rather than moderate)	Ia	A	Reduced urinary infection, preterm delivery, cesarean section, macrosomia, respiratory distress, congenital anomaly, perinatal mortality
Various antifungals	Ia	A	Reduced persistent candidiasis
Metronidazole after the first trimester	Ib	A	Reduced *Trichomonas* infestation
Intrapartum antibiotics for patients with maternal group B streptococcal vaginal infection	Ia	A	Reduced neonatal colonization and sepsis
Rubella vaccination postpartum	IV	C	Reduced rubella embryopathy subsequently
Cervical cerclage with previous second-trimester miscarriage	III	B	Reduced delivery before 33 weeks, miscarriage, or perinatal death
Intravenous tocolytics (β-mimetics or oxytocin antagonists) in patients with preterm labor	Ia	A	Reduced delivery within 24 hr or 48 hr, and before 37 weeks
Steroids before preterm delivery	Ia	A	Reduced respiratory distress syndrome, periventricular hemorrhage, necrotizing enterocolitis, early neonatal death
Use of antibiotics with steroids after preterm premature rupture of the membranes	Ia	A	Reduced infectious morbidity (maternal and fetal); delay delivery >7 days after initiating antibiotic therapy
Cesarean section for breech presentation at term	Ia	A	Reduced neonatal morbidity and mortality
Antiviral therapy and cesarean section when mother is HIV-positive	Ia	A	Reduced fetal and neonatal infection
Strategy Needing More Study			
Diagnosis of fetal abnormality by ultrasound, biochemical methods, and invasive procedures			Possible reduced incidence of fetal abnormality at birth and reduced maternal morbidity
Identification of pathologic fetal growth			Possible reduced perinatal morbidity and mortality
Maternal kick charts			Possible reduced perinatal morbidity and mortality
Biophysical tests of fetal well-being			Possible reduced perinatal morbidity and mortality
Plasmapheresis in severe Rhesus disease			Possible reduced perinatal morbidity and mortality
Antiplatelet agents in women at risk for preeclampsia and fetal growth deficiency			Possible reduced recurrence risk
Plasma expansion for severe preeclampsia			Possible reduced severe hypertension and renal failure
Hospital admission for nonproteinuric hypertension			Possible reduced development of proteinuria or severe hypertension, and maternal and perinatal morbidity and mortality
Strict bed rest for proteinuric hypertension			Possible reduced fulminating preeclampsia, and maternal and perinatal morbidity and mortality
Treatment of mycoplasma colonization			Possible reduced maternal and perinatal morbidity
Antiviral agents for patients with active genital herpes			Possible reduced persistent infection, and neonatal infection
Cesarean section for patients with herpes with no active disease			Possible reduced neonatal infection
Cervical cerclage for patients with a history other than previous second-trimester miscarriage			Possible reduced preterm delivery and perinatal mortality

TABLE 3-4—(cont'd)

Evidence That When a Specific Risk Is Identified, the Subsequent Intervention and Management Improves the Outcome (Aim No. 4 of Prenatal Care)

Proven Strategy	Level of Evidence	Grade of Recommendation	Benefit
Strategy Needing More Study—cont'd			
Tocolytics (β-mimetics or oxytocin antagonists) after preterm premature membrane rupture			Possible reduced maternal and perinatal morbidity
Use of fibronectin swabs			Possible reduced recurrence of preterm labor in subsequent pregnancy
Use of antibiotics in patients with toxoplasmosis seroconversion			Possible reduced severity of toxoplasmosis-induced congenital abnormality
Oral β-mimetics after inhibition of preterm labor			Possible reduced recurrence of preterm labor
Strategy of No Proven Benefit or Proven Harm			
Prescribing ethanol for inhibition of preterm labor			
Inducing labor routinely at less than 42 weeks			
Biochemical tests of fetal well-being			

(From Cochrane Pregnancy and Childbirth Group: Abstracts of Cochrane Reviews. The Cochrane Library, issue 2. Oxford, UK, Update Software, 2003.)

economics perspective, there is evidence of cost reduction if antenatal care is provided by staff other than obstetrician-gynecologists, without an increase in perinatal and maternal risks.[33,35] However, in many countries, the conceptual framework for prenatal care today is not based on good economics or evidence-based practice. Local and professional habits and traditions, political motives, and cultural and ethical beliefs all contribute.

Within the European community, Denmark and the Netherlands give a pivotal responsibility to midwives, with family physicians playing a supportive role and obstetricians being involved only in problem pregnancies and labor and delivery. In contrast, most of the care is provided by obstetricians in Belgium, Luxemburg, and Germany. In France and the United Kingdom, the sources of care are more diversified; however, in general, family physicians and midwives share the responsibility for prenatal care, with obstetricians involved marginally, if at all, in normal pregnancies. This pattern of care is also seen in Australia and New Zealand. In North America, midwives are uncommon, although there are several pilot studies examining an increasing role for these professionals. Most prenatal care in the United States and Canada is provided by family physicians or obstetricians, and some care is provided by nurse practitioners. Traditional birth attendants (TBAs) do not contribute significantly to prenatal care in developed countries. Involvement of TBAs in more than 5% of pregnancies has been reported in Guatemala, Honduras, and Mexico only.[20] In contrast, in some developing countries, up to 70% of all pregnancy care, including delivery, is provided by TBAs. Properly trained TBAs can serve as an inexpensive additional, yet effective, provider of prenatal care in developing countries without profound economic constraints.[22,36] Apart from the economic advantages of training TBAs, surveys in developing countries show that, during pregnancy and childbirth, many women prefer to receive care from a TBA rather than from other medical professionals.[36]

Education and Use of Prenatal Care

There is great variation in the form, content, and amount of education and advice that women receive during pregnancy, both between and within countries. Women receive much information about pregnancy not from medical professionals but from relatives and friends. One determinant of the quantity and quality of such information may be the professional's qualifications and experience.[37] Communication skills training for midwives and physicians appears to improve their ability to inform patients about pregnancy.[38] Trials in which women were given extra information prenatally in a variety of formats suggest that this information is valued and may reduce anxiety.[39] Providing knowledge (both oral and written) to health care providers can improve preventive measures in common practice (e.g., educating women about preterm labor and delivery).[40] Women tend to absorb information that is provided verbally by health care professionals better than information provided by standard evidence-based leaflets.[40]

On the other hand, in developed countries, specific barriers to free access to prenatal care persist and the number of women who do not seek or receive antenatal care is increasing.[41] The relationship between socioeconomic factors and poor use of prenatal care is well documented.[20,42–45] Providing financial incentives alone does not overcome these barriers to receiving prenatal care.[20,46,47] Additional efforts are needed to facilitate enrollment and enhanced social support services for these specific categories of women.[20,29,48] Home visits by prenatal care providers can be beneficial for women of low socioeconomic status, improving their medical knowledge, health habits, support level, and satisfaction.[48,49] Further research is needed to substantiate its value on a large scale.

In developing countries, these barriers play an even greater role in the low use of prenatal care. The major barriers identified are economic, cultural, and those related to women's perception of their condition.[50–52] Reduction of poverty and economic empowerment of rural women are prerequisites for tangible improvement in the use of antenatal and obstetric delivery services in developing countries.[52] There may be an even greater need to create awareness about obstetric complications through targeted community-based health education interventions to promote early recognition of obstetric emergencies.[52] There is no sound evidence that removing user fees alone increases the use of prenatal care in developing countries.[53] Another major constraint experienced by women seeking health services is lack of satisfaction with the quality of care (e.g., long waiting lists in health centers, no combined maternal–child care, inappropriate communication, lack of transportation).[54]

Frequency of Visits

There is no agreement about the ideal number of prenatal visits. For example, the American College of Obstetricians and Gynecologists recommends a visit every 4 weeks until 28 weeks, every 2 weeks until 36 weeks, and then weekly until delivery.[55] This amounts to 13 visits if the first visit is at 8 weeks and the last is at 40 weeks. In contrast, a recent expert committee suggested a reduction to eight visits for women with normal pregnancies.[56] This is also the proposed number of antenatal visits for women with uncomplicated pregnancies in the United Kingdom.[25] In European countries, the recommended number of prenatal visits varies from 5 to 15.[57] It is likely that the number of prenatal visits can be reduced considerably in normal pregnancies.[58–61] The large WHO Antenatal Care Randomised Trial and a critical review of recent randomized controlled trials of reduced-visit programs in developed and developing countries clearly show that a reduction in the use of resources is possible without adversely affecting prenatal care process variables, pregnancy outcome, or patient satisfaction.[60,62,63] A reduction in the number of antenatal visits, with or without an increased emphasis on the content of the visits, could be implemented without an increase in adverse biologic maternal and perinatal outcomes. Some dissatisfaction with care, especially among women in western countries, has been reported when women receive fewer visits. Women who had fewer visits reported that their expectations were not fulfilled.[33] However, an opposite trend was reflected when these women were asked their preference for the type of care for future pregnancies.

Clinical and Laboratory Screening Programs

Despite much variation in other aspects of prenatal care, the clinical and laboratory-based screening that occurs during pregnancy is similar in most developed countries. Variations are often determined by the prevalence of local problems. Factors that are commonly checked during pregnancy are summarized in Table 3–5. Worldwide, large and unjustified variations in prenatal clinical and laboratory screening services have been observed.[64] This variation is due in part to the unavailability of certain services in some prenatal care units. More important is the observation that in clinics in which screening tests are available, few women are receiving these services. The variation and heterogeneity of antenatal services cast doubts on the rationale for routine antenatal care.[63]

CRITICAL REVIEW OF THE EVIDENCE SUPPORTING DIFFERENT APPROACHES TO RISK MANAGEMENT IN PREGNANCY

The third aim of prenatal care (discussed earlier) is to provide an ongoing screeening program to confirm that the pregnancy remains at low risk (and also to identify women at risk). This identification is based on the woman's history and findings on examination or tests performed before pregnancy, at the first prenatal visit, or during subsequent visits. The fourth aim of prenatal care is effective and appropriate management of women at risk. The goal of management is prevention, amelioration, or treatment of the adverse outcome.

In practice, risk in pregnancy can be identified in two ways:

- General risk scoring
- Specific risk scoring

General Risk Scoring

The main aim of a formal risk scoring system in pregnancy is to permit the classification of women into different categories for which different and appropriate management strategies can be implemented. Other benefits of general risk scoring include aiding teaching and audit, defining populations for epidemiologic purposes, and allocating resources. The main adverse outcome measures for which risk scores have been developed and evaluated to aid management care are as follows[64,65]:

- Perinatal death
- Small-for-gestational age or low-birth-weight fetus
- Preterm labor and delivery
- Perinatal asphyxia
- A combination of these

TABLE 3–5

Risk Factors Commonly Documented in Prenatal Screening

Demographic General Factors
Maternal age
Ethnicity
Socioeconomic status
Marital status
Paternal influences (age, habits, drugs, alcohol, ethnicity)
Nutritional history (vegetarian, anorexia, diet, vitamins)
Occupational and possible exposure dangers
Poor grasp of the English language
Obstetric History
Parity
Ectopic pregnancy or miscarriage
Mode of delivery
Baby pregnancy outcome, gestation, size, normality
Other complications of pregnancy
Postpartum depression
Medical History
Cigarette smoking
Alcohol abuse
Other drug abuse
Maternal medical disorders
Maternal prescribed medication
Previous surgery
Previous anesthetic problems
Previous blood transfusions
Gynecologic History
Subfertility
Contraception
Menstrual regularity
Specific problems
Infections (HIV, syphilis, human papilloma virus, gonorrhea, hepatitis B and C, chlamydia)
Family History
Congenital anomalies
Diabetes
Hypertension
Renal disease
Thromboembolic disease
Physical Examination
Maternal weight
Maternal height
General examination
Pelvic examination (not performed by all obstetricians, especially if there is no indication and routine pelvic ultrasound is offered)
Pregnancy Factors
Multiple pregnancy
Vaginal bleeding
Reduced or abnormal fetal movements
Abnormal uterine size or amniotic fluid volume
Other problems (weight gain in pregnancy is not universally recorded)
Tests
Urinalysis (glucose, protein, blood, ketones)
Complete blood count, blood typing, and antibody screen
Serologic screening for rubella, syphilis, and other infections, depending on local prevalence (e.g., hepatis B and C, HIV, toxoplasmosis, cytomegalovirus)
Biochemical screening for congenital anomalies (Down syndrome, neural tube defects)
Screening for thyroid function
Routine ultrasonography
Cervical smear (depending on local screening policy)
Blood pressure
Group B streptoccocal carrier status

The risk can be calculated in the following three ways[65,66]:

- According to the number of risk factors present
- According to the sum of the mathematically weighted risk for each individual factor
- By correcting the weighted risk by a further mathematical process, such as Bayes' theorem[66]

In primigravidae, the use of weighted risk factors, with or without Bayes' theorem, was superior to the use of unweighted factors. In multigravid women, the difference between the three approaches was marginal.[67]

Theoretically, formal risk scoring may be unsatisfactory in practice. Applying Bayes' theorem to risk assessment in prenatal care has the following limitations[68]:

- Geographic variations and the treatment paradox reduce the reliability of any assessment.
- Most obstetric variables are interdependent.

Formal risk scoring also leads to a simplistic and inflexible view of pregnancy management. "Risking systems" often include risk factors that have little predictive usefulness. The changing risk status during the prenatal period, in labor, and at delivery poses problems for the clinician who relies on risking systems to characterize the likelihood of adverse events. Risk scoring systems are not sufficiently robust for this task.[69] Formal risk scoring carries the inherent danger of ignoring low-risk women. It also requires computerized calculation of scores. These factors contribute to the limited use of risk scoring systems. However, another explanation for their limited use is that, although many formal scoring systems predict the likelihood of an adverse outcome, there is little evidence that their use is associated with a reduction in adverse pregnancy outcome.[64] Further, when risk scoring is applied in practice, there is a real danger that a potential, yet imprecise, risk of an adverse outcome will be replaced by increased surveillance and possible intervention and treatments, many of which may be of unproven value and carry their own risks. Examples include fetal monitoring and measures reported to reduce the risk of preterm labor and delivery.[64,70,71] However, the West Los Angeles Preterm Birth Prevention Project showed a significant reduction in preterm birth among women with high-risk pregnancies who were enrolled in a formal risk scoring program.[72] Since the late 1960s, a formal risk scoring program to evaluate the risk of preterm delivery has been conducted in France, with promising results.[73] However, outside France, these results have not been repeated.[74,75] The conflicting evidence of the efficacy of primary preterm birth prevention programs emphasizes the long-recognized difficulties in implementing and assessing effective primary prevention strategies. Finally, risk scores vary with different populations and for reasons other than prevalence or specific adverse outcomes.[75] The limitations of performance and potential disadvantages mean that formal risk scoring lacks many characteristics of effective screening tests. Recent attempts to use risk scoring models at clinics in Africa did not identify women at risk for pregnancy complications.[76] Despite promising results from Australia,[77,78] formal risk scoring should not be introduced into routine pregnancy care until results from a well-designed randomized trial are available.

Recognition of Specific Risks

In practice, the most common way in which risk in pregnancy is identified is by the recognition of specific risk factors. After a woman is identified as having a risk factor for a specific adverse outcome, she receives specific additional management that may prevent, ameliorate, or treat the specific outcome. This management is in addition to the routine prenatal care received by all women. For example, a woman who weighs more than 85 kg is at increased risk for hypertension and gestational diabetes and, accordingly, the clinical and laboratory-based prenatal screening program must be amended to look specifically for these complications. In practice, the main problem with this approach is that although there may be agreement about what constitutes a risk factor and what the adverse outcome may be, there is less consensus about the appropriate management strategy. For many interventions, scientific proof of benefit is lacking, as discussed earlier (see Tables 3–1 through 3–4). The way in which additional care is provided on the basis of identification of risk factors may be empirical or schematic.

Empirical

After a specific risk factor is identified, the obstetrician chooses additional management strategies. Thus, if the patient weighs more than 85 kg, given the known risk of hypertension and gestational diabetes, the obstetrician may screen for hypertension in several ways, including the following:

- No measures other than paying strict attention to routine blood pressure recordings at routine prenatal visits and using a large sphygmomanometer cuff to obtain the measurements
- Increased frequency of clinic attendance for blood pressure readings
- Giving the woman a self-assessing sphygmomanometer and guidelines for self-referral

Similarly, the obstetrician may screen for gestational diabetes in the following ways:

- Performing random blood glucose testing on one or more occasions
- Performing a fasting glucose test on one or more occasions
- Performing a modified 50-g glucose tolerance test on one or more occasions
- Performing a formal 75-g glucose tolerance test on one or more occasions

Schematic

Every time a given risk factor is identified, the obstetrician implements a specific preagreed management strategy (Tables 3–6 through 3–11).[2] No studies have compared the outcomes of the schematic approach with those of the empirical approach. However, the schematic approach has several advantages, including the following:

- It provides consistent management of specific risk factors.
- It allows comparison of the effectiveness of one management strategy with another.

An implicit requirement of the schematic approach is that the underlying basic prenatal care program for all pregnant women should be documented (Table 3–12).[2]

Decision Analysis

In the future, some form of decision analysis may be applied to the provision of prenatal care.[71,79] This is likely to occur in the following two ways:

- Providing counseling about management options
- Determining the benefits of alternative management strategies on the basis of the literature, but without a randomized trial

Providing Counseling About Management Strategies

A simple example is a 40-year-old woman who seeks advice at 11 weeks about prenatal diagnosis of Down syndrome. In this patient, the likelihood of delivering a baby with the diagnosis is 1:100; the risk of miscarriage is approximately 1:100 for amniocentesis at 16 weeks and 1:50 for chorionic villus sampling at 11 weeks. She is asked to place a relative score, or weighting, on her view of Down syndrome versus miscarriage.

- If she fears Down syndrome three times more than she fears a miscarriage, then she can have either invasive procedure.
- If she fears Down syndrome two times more than she fears a miscarriage, than she should opt for amniocentesis.
- If she fears a miscarriage more than she does Down syndrome, then she should not have an invasive procedure.

TABLE 3–6

Schematic Management of Risk Factors: General Factors

RISK FACTOR	TYPE OF RISK	MANAGEMENT
Vegetarian	Poor nutritional intake	Multivitamins, folate, iron, and other nutritional supplements
Age <18 yr	Poor antenatal attendance, education, and screening	Social worker involvement, home visits
	Hypertensive disease, IUGR	Vigilance for increased blood pressure, grade I fetal check
Age >35 yr	Chromosomal abnormalities	Early consideration for prenatal diagnosis
	Hypertensive disease, IUGR	Vigilance for increased blood pressure, grade I fetal check
Parity >4	IUGR	Grade I fetal check
	Anemia	Iron and folate supplementation
	Further pregnancies	Discuss contraception
	Malpresentation	Check presentation at 36 wk
	Postpartum hemorrhage	Vigilance for uterine atony and hemorrhage
Non-white	Hemoglobinopathy	Hb electrophoresis
	HB-Ag carrier (Far East) or HIV carrier (Africa)	If positive, then clear labeling of notes and implementation of policy guidelines
	Poor English, education, and screening	Interpreter
Single parent, financial and social	Poor antenatal attendance, education, and screening	Home visits if necessary, discussion of plans for labor and delivery, social worker
	IUGR	Grade I fetal check

Grade I fetal check, careful check of fetal growth by fundal height measurements and questioning about fetal activity; Hb, hemoglobin; HB-Ag, hepatitis B antigen; IUGR, intrauterine growth restriction.
(From James DK, Smoleniec J: Identification and management of the at-risk obstetric patient. Hosp Update 1992; 18:885–890.)

Many argue that these decisions are being made intuitively by women and their partners when given the relevant information in a nondirective way and without the need to complicate the issue with mathematical models. For more difficult decisions, there are good reasons to believe that decision analysis rather than intuitive methods will result in decisions that match patient preferences.[71] Changing the age of the woman in this example from 40 years to 37 years and incorporating the results of recent developments in noninvasive antenatal testing into the discussion (first-trimester ultrasound, measurement of nasal bone length or nuchal translucency, first-trimester or second-trimester biochemical testing) will lead to a far more complex decision analy-

TABLE 3–7

Schematic Management of Risk Factors: Obstetric History

RISK FACTOR	TYPE OF RISK	MANAGEMENT
Previous ectopic pregnancy	Recurrence, maternal anxiety	Early ultrasound to confirm intrauterine pregnancy
Previous still birth or neonatal death	Risk depends on cause (not all are recurrent)	Try to establish cause; early review and specific management
Baby weight < 2 SD	Intrauterine growth restriction	Grade II fetal check
Baby weight > 2 SD	Gestational diabetes	Random glucose testing at 28 and 32 wk
	Further large fetus	Grade II fetal check, vigilance in labor
Congenital anomaly	Possible recurrence	Obtain details and diagnosis; possible prenatal diagnosis
Antibodies	Hemolytic disease	Specific protocol
Proteinuric preeclampsia	Recurrence	Assess renal function, grade II fetal check, carefully check blood pressure
Preterm delivery	Recurrence	Specific plan depending on cause
Uterine scar	Uterine rupture, cesarean section	Review of mode of delivery at 36 wk
Short labor	Recurrence and neonatal problems (trauma, asphyxia, hypothermia)	Specific management plan at 36 weeks
Postpartum hemorrhage	Recurrence	Specific plan at 36 wk
Other labor or delivery problems	Recurrence	Specific plan at 36 wk
Problems with baby	Recurrence, maternal anxiety	Obtain details and make a specific plan

< 2SD, less than 2 standard deviations below mean for gestation; > 2 SD, more than 2 standard deviations above mean for gestation; grade II fetal check, careful check of fetal growth by ultrasound every 2–4 wk and use of a fetal movement chart.
(From James DK, Smoleniec J: Identification and management of the at-risk obstetric patient. Hosp Update 1992; 18:885–890.)

TABLE 3–8

Schematic Management of Risk Factors: Medical, Surgical, Gynecologic, and Family History

RISK FACTOR	TYPE OF RISK	MANAGEMENT
Smoking	IUGR, placental problems (placenta previa, solutio placentae)	Advice to reduce or stop smoking, grade I fetal check, ultrasound check of placenta
Excess alcohol	IUGR, fetal alcohol syndrome	Offer specific help, grade II fetal check, alert pediatricians
Chronic disease and prescribed drugs	Possible adverse effects of disease on pregnancy and pregnancy on disease	Obstetric and physician joint care with preagreed specific protocols
Drug abuse	HB-Ag, HC-Ag, HIV, IUGR, neonatal withdrawal	Counseling and serologic testing, grade II fetal check, alert pediatrician
Hemoglobinopathy	Sickle or thalassemia trait: risk of affected fetus Sickle disease: crisis or IUGR	Test partner, offer prenatal diagnosis, encourage hydration, check renal function, regular midstream urine, grade II fetal check
Anesthetic problems	Recurrence	Consultant anesthesist
Family history of diabetes	Gestational diabetes	Random glucose testing at 28 and 32 wk
Family history of congenital anomaly	Possible recurrence, maternal anxiety	Obtain details and diagnosis, consult obstetrician for possible prenatal diagnosis
Subfertility	Anxiety, multiple pregnancy, hypertension, or gestational diabetes with polycystic ovaries	Reassure, vigilance for hypertension, random glucose testing at 28 and 32 wk if polycystic ovaries
IVF/ICSI pregnancy	Congenital anomalies, chromosomal abnormality, IUGR	Consult obstetrician for possible prenatal diagnosis, grade II fetal check
Intrauterine contraceptive device in situ	Miscarriage, preterm labor	Remove if threads visible; if not, check at delivery

Grade I fetal check, careful check of fetal growth by fundal height measurements and questioning about fetal activity; grade II fetal check, careful check of fetal growth by ultrasound every 2–4 wk and fetal movement chart; HB-Ag, hepatitis B antigen; HC-Ag, hepatitis C antigen; IUGR, intrauterine growth restriction; IVF/ICSI, in vitro fertilization/intracytoplasmic sperm injection.

sis for the woman and her partner. The decision will be based on weighing the specificity and sensitivity of different noninvasive tests for Down syndrome and balancing these against procedure-related and age-specific risks.

DECIDING BETWEEN ALTERNATIVE MANAGEMENT STRATEGIES WITHOUT A RANDOMIZED TRIAL

No management strategy should be implemented without the benefit of a randomized trial. An example of how a randomized trial can affect clinical practice is provided by the study of Hannah and colleagues[80] on the mode of delivery of infants with breech presentation at term. Before this study, clinicians had to rely on circumstantial evidence in the literature.[81] The study by Hannah and coworkers shows that the optimal mode of delivery is planned cesarean section after the woman has been offered external cephalic version.[82] A survey of obstetricians showed that most now choose cesarean section as a result of the study.[83] However, attempts to resolve other management options have not been successful. An example is the management of compromised preterm fetuses. It is unlikely that a sufficiently large study could be con-

TABLE 3–9

Schematic Management of Risk Factors: Factors from Examination

RISK FACTOR	TYPE OF RISK	MANAGEMENT
Weight >85 kg	Hypertension, gestational diabetes	Dietary advice, vigilance for increased blood pressure, random glucose testing at 28 and 32 wk
Weight <45 kg	Intrauterine growth restriction	Grade I fetal check
Primigravida and height <1.52 m	Cephalopelvic disproportion, asymptomatic heart disease	Plan for labor if fetal head is unengaged at 40 wk
Cardiac murmur	Maternal clinically significant heart disease, fetal congenital heart disease	Consider cardiologic opinion

Grade I fetal check, careful check of fetal growth by fundal height measurement and questioning about fetal activity.

TABLE 3–10

Schematic Management of Risk Factors: Factors Arising in Pregnancy

RISK FACTOR	TYPE OF RISK	MANAGEMENT
Vaginal bleeding	<20 wk: miscarriage >19 wk: placenta previa, placental abruption	Acute referral to hospital, no long-term additional action Acute referral to hospital, long-term grade II fetal check
Blood pressure >140/90	Preeclampsia, IUGR	• If blood pressure >160/100 or proteinuria, refer for hospital admission and care with preagreed protocol • If blood pressure <160/100 and no proteinuria, refer for day care with preagreed protocol
Multiple pregnancy	Anemia, hypertension, IUGR, preterm delivery, congenital anomalies	Iron and folate supplement, vigilance for increased blood pressure, preterm uterine activity, grade II fetal check, more frequent visits
Fetus small for dates	IUGR	Fetal assessment with preagreed protocol
Fetus large for dates	Big baby and complications, gestational diabetes, hydramnios, multiple pregnancy	Fetal assessment with preagreed protocol, random glucose testing
Polyhydramnios	Big baby and complications, abnormal fetus, diabetes	Fetal assessment with preagreed protocol, random glucose testing
Malpresentation after 35 wk	Delivery problems	Look for cause, make plan for labor
Reduced fetal movement	Poor maternal perception, fetal disease	Immediate nonstress tests, fetal assessment
Preterm rupture of membranes	Preterm labor, amnionitis	Hospital admission, manage with preagreed protocol
Urinary tract infection	Pyelonephritis, preterm labor	Treat (5 days), monthly midstream urine
Group B streptococcus–positive vaginal culture	Neonatal sepsis	Intrapartum intravenous antibiotics

Grade II fetal check, fetal growth by ultrasound every 2–4 wk and fetal movement chart; IUGR, intrauterine growth restriction.

TABLE 3–11

Schematic Management of Risk Factors: Factors from Studies

RISK FACTOR	TYPE OF RISK	MANAGEMENT
Proteinuria	Infection, renal disease, preeclampsia	Midstream urine, blood pressures studies if proteinuria persists
Glycosuria	Decreased renal threshold, gestational diabetes	Random glucose testing at 28 and 32 wk
Hematuria	Infection, renal disease	Midstream urine, renal hematuria studies if persists
No rubella antibodies	Susceptible to rubella	Warn mother, offer puerperal vaccination
Rhesus-negative status	Potential for sensitization	Check antibodies at first visit, 28, and 34 wk; give anti-D at potential sensitization
Antibodies	Fetal hemolytic disease	Specific protocol of management
Increased α-fetoprotein level	Fetal abnormality If normal, intrauterine growth restriction, placental bleeding, preeclampsia	Careful ultrasound scan at 18 wk Grade II fetal check, vigilance for increased blood pressure
Low Hb (<10 g/dL)	Pathologic anemia	Investigate; treat cause with oral therapy; refer to hematologist if uncertain cause, intolerance of therapy, no response to therapy
Increased random glucose level (>7 mM)	Gestational diabetes	Formal 75 g oral glucose tolerance test
Abnormal cervical smear	Possible invasive carcinoma	Refer for colposcopy
Group B streptococcus-positive vaginal swab	Neonatal infection	Intrapartum intravenous antibiotics

TABLE 3–12

Schematic Approach to Prenatal Care: Basic Care (Suggested Minimum Program)

GESTATION (WK)	AIMS AND ACTION TAKEN
8–14 (wk)	Confirm pregnancy Check medical, family, social, and obstetric histories General physical examination Pelvic examination if indicated Tests: • Urinalysis (glucose/protein/blood) • Midstream urine specimen • Complete blood count • ABO/Rhesus grouping and antibody screen • Serologic tests (rubella, syphilis, toxoplasmosis, cytamegalovirus, HIV) • Ultrasound: nuchal translucency; confirm or correct estimated date of delivery Discuss pregnancy, including the offer of screening for neural tube defect or Down syndrome (first trimester or second trimester) and ultrasound scan at 18 wk General advice on diet and hygienic measures if toxoplasmosis or cytomegalovirus-negative (if performed), exercise, breast care, infant feeding, parentcraft classes, smoking, alcohol, family planning, and maternity benefits Complete case notes
16	Serum screening for neural tube defects or Down syndrome (if not performed in first trimester) Check all test results
18	Detailed ultrasound scan Check results from 16-wk ultrasound serum screening Confirm or amend estimated date of delivery (if not performed in first trimester)
22–24	Routine check (history of symptoms, especially vaginal bleeding, reduced or absent fetal movements), measurement of blood pressure, urinalysis, fundal height with tape measure (charted)
28	Routine check (as before, but including fetal heart rate and liquor volume), especially blood pressure and fundal height Complete blood count, Rhesus antibody screen if Rhesus-negative
32	Routine check (as before), especially of blood pressure, fundal height, and the of the 28-wk test Discuss labor and parentcraft
35–37	Routine check (as before), especially of blood pressure, growth, and possible malpresentation Check group B streptococcus-carrier status Complete blood count, Rhesus antibody screen if Rhesus-negative
38–39	Routine check (as before), especially of blood pressure, growth, and possible malpresentation
40	Routine check (as before), especially of blood pressure, growth, and possible malpresentation Discuss labor
41	Review and discuss induction of labor Routine check (as before)

ducted in the near future to determine the optimum mode and timing of delivery. An attempt to answer these questions was started in 1996 (Growth Restriction Intervention Trial).[84] A 2003 update of the results did not provide conclusive answers.[85] Nevertheless, it has been argued from decision analysis of the available literature that cesarean section without a trial of labor is indicated when there is evidence of acidemia before delivery. Otherwise, a careful trial of labor (including maternal oxygen supply, use of the left lateral decubitus position, and cervical ripening before the use of oxytocin) should be considered.[85]

CONCLUSIONS

- There is great variation in the provision and use of prenatal care both between and within countries in terms of who sees pregnant women, when they are seen, and what testing is done. There seems to be more consistency in terms of screening programs empolyed.
- Of the four aims of prenatal care, arguably the most important is the prevention, detection, and management of problems and factors that adversely affect the health of the mother, infant, or both.
- In managing these problems, the obstetrician should know which strategies have proven benefit and which are unproven.

SUMMARY OF MANAGEMENT OPTIONS

Planning Prenatal Care

Management Options	Quality of Evidence	Strength of Recommendation	References
Aims of Prenatal Care			
For the Majority of Pregnancies (Normal to Low Risk)			
Provide advice, reassurance, education, and support (see Table 3–1)			
Improved social and psychological support from caregivers	Ia	A	86
Antismoking interventions	Ib	A	87
Antenatal classes	III	B	29
Routine ultrasound with positive feedback	IIb	B	88
Treat minor symptoms (see Table 3–2)			
Antiemetics (e.g., antihistamines)	–	GPP	–
Antacids	Ib	A	89
Increased dietary fiber intake	IIb	B	90
Bulking agents and stool softeners	III	B	91
Implement an ongoing screening program (clinical and laboratory) to ensure continuing low-risk status (see Table 3–3)	–	GPP	–
Using risk scoring systems in pregnancy predicts the likelihood of adverse outcomes, with little evidence of a reduction in these outcomes	IV	C	64,65
A schematic approach is arguably more scientific than an empirical approach (see Tables 3–6 to 3–11 for examples)	–	GPP	–
For the Minority of Pregnancies (High Risk)			
Implement the above three aims in addition; prevent, detect, and manage risk factors (arguably the most important aim)			
There is no proof that prenatal care per se improves neonatal outcome	III	B	13
Specific interventions that are effective for specific risks can reduce mortality and morbidity (see Table 3–4)	III	B	95
Routine or Normal Prenatal Care			
What constitutes routine or normal prenatal care for a given population varies with the available resources: • Personnel • Buildings and accommodations ("plant") • Laboratory Considerations (see Table 3–12 for example): • Who will see the pregnant women • When they will be seen • What will be done when they are seen	–	GPP	–
The relative role of obstetricians, family physicians (general practitioners), and individuals in the delivery of prenatal care varies between countries.	III	B	20,63
There is no evidence that doctors need to be the medical professionals involved in the prenatal care of every pregnant patient.	Ib	A	27,35,38,48

Continued

SUMMARY OF MANAGEMENT OPTIONS

Planning Prenatal Care *(Continued)*

Management Options	Quality of Evidence	Strength of Recommendation	References
For specific problems, especially social ones, midwives or general practitioners may offer more benefit than specialist obstetric care.	Ia	A	27–29
Incorporating different medical professionals into one shared antenatal care program can be effective in providing appropriate care.	Ia	A	31,32
A physicians based prenatal care model appears to be more expensive without improving pregnancy outcome.	Ia	A	34,35
The frequency of prenatal visits can safely be reduced in low-risk pregnancies.	Ia	A	58,59
Socioeconomic factors and poor use of prenatal care are correlated.	III	B	20,42
Women report that midwife-led care provides better continuity of care.	Ia	A	27,32
In developing countries, well-trained traditional birth attendants can serve as an additional effective, yet inexpensive provider of prenatal care.	IV	C	36
There is great variation in the form, content, and amount of education and advice that women receive during pregnancy.	IV	C	37
Better communication skills by health care providers improve their ability to inform patients.	IV	C	38,39
Western women report dissatisfaction when they receive fewer prenatal visits.	Ia	A	33
Clinical and laboratory-based prenatal screening is similar in European countries.	–	GPP	56
Unjustified variation in clinical and laboratory-based prenatal screening exists worldwide.	III	B	63
The main aim of a formal risk scoring system in pregnancy is to permit the classification of women into different categories for which different and appropriate management options can be implemented.	IV	C	64
Overall risk can be calculated by: • Number of risk factors present • Sum of weighted risk factors • Correcting this weighted risk by mathematical processes, such as Bayes' theorem	IV	C	65
Formal risk scoring leads to a simplistic and inflexible view of pregnancy management.	IV	C	64
When risk scoring is used in practice, there is a real danger that a potential, yet imprecise risk of an adverse outcome is replaced by the introduction of increased surveillance and treatments of unproven value.	IV	C	69
Formal risk scoring should not be introduced into routine pregnancy care.	IV	C	64
The most common way in which risk in pregnancy is identified is by specific risk recognition; this can be done on an empirical basis or on a schematic basis.	–	GPP	–
The schematic approach has advantages over the empirical approach:	–	GPP	–

Continued

SUMMARY OF MANAGEMENT OPTIONS
Planning Prenatal Care *(Continued)*

Management Options	Quality of Evidence	Strength of Recommendation	References
• It allows consistency of management for given risk factors. • It allows comparison of the effectiveness of one management strategy with another.			
Decision analysis will be applicable in the future and is likely to occur in two ways: • Providing counseling about management options • Determining the benefits of alternative management strategies on the basis of published literature, but without the benefits of a randomized trial	IV	C	71,79

REFERENCES

1. James DK: Risk at booking visit. In James DK, Stirrat GM (eds): Pregnancy and Risk. Chichester, UK, John Wiley, 1988, pp 45–80.
2. James DK, Smoleniec J: Identification and management of the at-risk obstetric patient. Hosp Update 1992;18:885–890.
3. Butler NR, Bonham DG: Perinatal Mortality: The First Report of the British Perinatal Survey. Edinburgh, Churchill Livingstone, 1963.
4. Butler NR, Alberman ED: Perinatal Problems: The Second Report of the British Perinatal Mortality Survey. Edinburgh, Churchill Livingstone, 1969.
5. Chamberlain G: A re-examination of antenatal care. J R Soc Med 1978;71:662–668.
6. Swyer PR: Organisation of perinatal/neonatal care. Acta Paediatr Suppl 1993;385:1–18.
7. Gomez-Olmedo M, Delgado-Rodriguez M, Bueno-Cavanillas A, et al: Prenatal care and prevention of preterm birth: A case-control study in southern Spain. Eur J Epidemiol 1996;12:37–44.
8. Barros H, Tavares M, Rodrigues T: Role of prenatal care in preterm birth and low birthweight in Portugal. J Public Health Med 1996;18:321–328.
9. Drazancic A: Antenatal care in developing countries. What should be done? J Perinat Med 2001;29:188–198.
10. Naidu J, Moodley M, Adhikari R, et al: Clinico-pathological study of causes of perinatal mortality in a developing country. J Obstet Gynaecol 2001;5:443–447.
11. Hall MH: Critique of antenatal care. In Turnbull A, Chamberlain G (eds): Obstetrics Edinburgh, Churchill Livingstone, 1989, pp 225–233.
12. Hall MH: What are the benefits of prenatal care in uncomplicated pregnancy? Birth 1991;18:151–152.
13. Fiscella K: Does prenatal care improve birth outcomes? A critical review. Obstet Gynecol 1995;85:468–479.
14. Alexander GR, Kotelchuck M: Assessing the role and effectiveness of prenatal care: History, challenges and directions for further research. Public Health Rep 2001;116:306–316.
15. Wolleswinkel-van den Bosch JH, Vredesvoogd CB, Borkent-Polet M, et al: Substandard factors in perinatal care in The Netherlands: A regional audit of perinatal deaths. Acta Obstet Gynecol Scand 2002;81:17–24.
16. Parboosing J, Kerr M: Innovations in the role of obstetric hospitals in antenatal care. In Enkin M, Chalmers I (eds): Effectiveness and Satisfaction in Antenatal Care. London, Spastics International, 1982, pp 254–256.
17. Stirrat GM: Late antenatal care. In Turnbull A, Chamberlain G (eds): Obstetrics. Edinburgh, Churchill Livingstone, 1989, pp 247–256.
18. Hall MH: The antenatal programme. In Marsh GN (ed): Modern Obstetrics in General Practice. Oxford, Oxford University Press, 1985, pp 85–98.
19. Chamberlain G: Organisation of antenatal care. BMJ 1991;302:647–650.
20. Buekens P: Variations in provision and uptake of prenatal care. Clin Obstet Gynaecol 1990;4:187–205.
21. Cochrane Pregnancy and Childbirth Group: Abstracts of Cochrane Reviews. The Cochrane Library, issue 2. Oxford, UK, Update Software, 2003.
22. Nylander PPS, Adekunle AO: Antenatal care in developing countries. Clin Obstet Gynaecol 1990;4:169–186.
23. Lord Hunt P: The future of public health. World Hosp Health Serv 2002;38:34–40,42,44.
24. Department of Health: Changing Childbirth: Part 1. Report of the Expert Maternity Group. London, HMSO, 1995.
25. http://www.rcog.org.uk/guidelines.asp?PageID=108&GuidelineID=53
26. Hall ML: Identification of high risk and low risk. Clin Obstet Gynaecol 1990;4:65–76.
27. Biro MA, Waldenstrom U, Brown S, Pannifex JH: Satisfaction with team midwifery care for low- and high-risk women: A randomized controlled trial. Birth 2003;30:1–10.
28. Hepburn M: Social problems. Clin Obstet Gynaecol 1990;4:149–168.
29. Support for pregnant women. In Enken M, Keirse MJNC, Neilson J, et al (eds): A Guide to Effective Care in Pregnancy and Childbirth. Oxford, UK, Oxford University Press, 2000, pp 16–23.
30. Lombardo M, Golding G: Shared antenatal care: A regional perspective. Aust Fam Physician 2003;32:133–139.
31. Chan FY, Pun TC, Tse LY, et al: Shared antenatal care between family health services and hospital (consultant) services for low-risk women. Asia Oceania J Obstet Gynaecol 1993; 19:291–298.
32. Khan-Neelofur D, Gulmezoglu M, Villar J: Who should provide routine antenatal care for low-risk women and how often? A systematic review of randomised controlled trials. WHO Antenatal Care Trial Research Group. Paediatr Perinat Epidemiol 1998;1212:7–26.

33. Gravely EA, Littlefield JH: A cost-effectiveness analysis of three staffing models for the delivery of low-risk prenatal care. Am J Public Health 1992;82:180–184.
34. Carroli G, Villar J, Piaggio G, et al: WHO systematic review of randomised controlled trials of routine antenatal care. Lancet 2001;357:1565–1570.
35. Villar J, Ba'aqueel H, Piaggio G, et al: WHO antenatal care randomised trial for the evaluation of a model of routine antenatal care. Lancet 2001;357:1551–1564.
36. Brennan M: Training traditional birth attendants reduces maternal mortality and morbidity. Trop J Obstet Gynaecol 1988;1:44–47.
37. Haas JS, Orav EJ, Goldman L: The relationship between physician's qualifications and experience and the adequacy of prenatal care and low birthweight. Am J Obstet Gynecol 1995;85:1087–1091.
38. Rowe RE, Garcia J, Macfarlane AJ, Davidson LL: Improving communication between health professionals and women in maternity care: A structured review. Health Expect 2002;5:63–83.
39. Sprague A, Stewart P, Niday P, et al: Community education on preterm birth: Does it change practice? Can Fam Physician 2002;48:727–734.
40. O'Cathain A, Walters SJ, Nicholl JP, et al: Use of evidence based leaflets to promote informed choice in maternity care: Randomised controlled trial in everyday practice. BMJ 2002;324:643.
41. Elam-Evans LD, Adams MM, Gargiullo PM, et al: Trends in the percentage of women who received no prenatal care in the United States, 1980–1994: Contributions of the demographic and risk effects. Obstet Gynecol 1996;87:575–580.
42. Meikle SF, Orleans M, Leff M, et al: Women's reasons for not seeking prenatal care: Racial and ethnic factors. Birth 1995;22:81–86.
43. Lewis CT, Mathews TJ, Heuser RL: Prenatal care in the United States, 1980–1994. Vital Health Statistics 1996;21:1–17.
44. Rogers C, Schiff M: Early versus late prenatal care in New Mexico: Barriers and motivators. Birth 1996;23:26–30.
45. Laken MP, Ager J: Using incentives to increase participation in prenatal care. Obstet Gynaecol 1995;85:326–329.
46. York R, Grant C, Gibeau A, et al: A review of problems of universal access to prenatal care. Nurs Clin North Am 1996;31:279–292.
47. Krieger JW, Connell FA, LoGerfo JP: Medicaid prenatal care: A comparison of use and outcome in fee-for-service and managed care. Am J Obstet Gynecol 1992;82:185–190.
48. Blondel B, Breart G: Home visits pregnancy: Consequence on pregnancy outcome, use of health services and women's situations. Semin Perinatol 1995;19:263–271.
49. Gerein N, Mayhew S, Lubben M: A framework for a new approach to antenatal care. Int J Gynaecol Obstet 2003;80:175–182.
50. Fatmi Z, Avan BI: Demographic, socio-economic and environmental determinants of utilisation of antenatal care in a rural setting of Sindh, Pakistan. J Pak Med Assoc 2002;52:138–142.
51. Adamu YM, Salihu HM: Barriers to the use of antenatal and obstetric care services in Kano, Nigeria. J Obstet Gynaecol 2002;22:600–603.
52. Hasan IJ, Nisar N: Women's perceptions regarding obstetric complications and care in a poor fishing community in Karachi. J Pak Med Assoc 2002;52:148–152.
53. Wilkinson D, Gouws E, Sach M, Karim SS: Effect of removing user fees on attendance for curative and preventive primary health care services in rural South Africa. Bull World Health Organ 2001;79:665–671.
54. Mwaniki PK, Kabiru EW, Mbugua GG: Utilisation of antenatal and maternity services by mothers seen in child welfare services in Mbeere District, Eastern Province, Kenya. East Afr Med J 2002;79:184–187.
55. American College of Obstetricians and Gynecologists: Guidelines for Perinatal Care. Washington, DC, American Academy of Pediatrics and American College of Obstetricians and Gynecologists, 1988, pp 54–55.
56. Demographic and Health Surveys: Selected statistics from DHS surveys. Demographic Health Surveys Newsletter 1989;2:10.
57. Hall MH, Chong PK, McGillivray I: Is routine antenatal care worthwhile? Lancet 1980;ii:78–80.
58. Binstock MA, Wolde-Tsadik G: Alternative prenatal care: Impact of reduced visit frequency, focused visits and continuity of care. J Reprod Med 1995;40:507–512.
59. Villar J, Carroli G, Khan-Neelofur D, et al: Patterns of routine antenatal care for low-risk pregnancy. Cochrane Database Syst Rev 2001;4:CD000934.
60. Berglund A, Lindmark G: The impact of obstetric risk factors and socioeconomic characteristics on utilization of antenatal care. J Public Health Med 1998;20:455–462.
61. McDuffie RS Jr, Beck A, Bischoff K, et al: Effect of frequency of prenatal care visits on perinatal outcome among low-risk women: A randomized controlled trial. JAMA 1996;275:847–851.
62. Munjanja SP, Lindmark G, Nyström L: Randomized controlled trial of a reduced-visits programme of antenatal care in Harare, Zimbabwe. Lancet 1996;348:364–369.
63. Piaggio G, Ba'aqueel H, Bergsjo P, et al: The practice of antenatal care: Comparing four study sites in different parts of the world participating in the WHO Antenatal Care Trial Randomised Controlled Trial. Paediatr Perinatol Epidemiol 1998;12:116–141.
64. Alexander S, Keirse MJNC: Formal risk scoring during pregnancy. In Chalmers I, Enkin M, Keirse MJNC (eds): Effective Care in Pregnancy and Childbirth. Oxford, Oxford University Press, 1990, pp 345–365.
65. Chard T: Obstetric risk scores. Fetal Med Rev 1991;3:1–10.
66. Chard T, Chard DT, MacIntosh M: Prediction of future outcome using Bayesian logic. Clin Obstet Gynaecol 1994;8:607–624.
67. Chard T, Harding S, Carroll S, et al: A comparison of different methods for calculating overall risk scores from risk factors ascertained in a computerized obstetric information system. J Perinatol Med 1990;18:23–29.
68. Lilford RJ, Chard T: Problems and pitfalls of risk assessment in antenatal care. Br J Obstet Gynaecol 1983;90:507–510.
69. Orleans M, Haverkamp AD: Are there health risks in using risking systems? The case of perinatal risk assessment. Health Policy 1987;73:297–307.
70. Owen P, Patel N: Prevention of preterm birth. Clin Obstet Gynaecol 1995;9:465–479.
71. Thornton JG: Decision analysis. Clin Obstet Gynaecol 1996;10:677–695.
72. Collaborative Group on Preterm Birth Prevention: Multicenter randomized, controlled trial of a preterm birth prevention program. Am J Obstet Gynecol 1993;169:352–366.
73. Papiernik E, Grange G: Prenatal screening with evaluated high risk scores. J Perinatol Med 1999;27:21–25.
74. Alexander GR, Korenbrot CC: The role of prenatal care in preventing low birth weight. Future Child 1995;5:103–120.
75. Shiono PH, Klebanoff MA: A review of risk scoring for preterm birth. Clin Perinatol 1993;20:107–125.
76. Majoko F, Nyström L, Munjanja S, Lindmark G: Usefulness of risk scoring at booking for antenatal care in predicting adverse pregnancy outcome in a rural African setting. J Obstet Gynaecol 2002;22:604–609.
77. Humphrey MD: The beneficial use of risk scoring in a remote and high-risk pregnant population. Aust N Z J Obstet Gynaecol 1995;35:139–143.
78. Mohamed H, Martin C, Haloob R: Can the New Zealand antenatal scoring system be applied in the United Kingdom? J Obstet Gynaecol 2002;22:389–391.

79. Thornton J, van Lith J: Decision analysis. Eur J Obstet Gynaecol Reprod Biol 2002;94:171–173.
80. Hannah ME, Hannah WJ, Hewson SA, et al: Planned caesarean section versus planned vaginal birth for breech presentation at term: A ransomised multicentre trial. Term Breech Trial Collaborative Group. Lancet 2000;356(9239):1375–1385.
81. Gifford DS, Morton SC, Fiske M, Kahn K: A meta-analysis of infant outcomes after breech delivery. Obstet Gynecol 1995;85:1047–1054.
82. Hannah ME, Hannah WJ, Hodnett ED, et al: Outcomes at 3 months after planned cesarean section vs planned vaginal delivery for breech presentation at term: The international randomized Term Breech Trial. JAMA 2002;287:1822–1831.
83. Hogle KL, Kilburn L, Hewson S, et al: Impact of the international Term Breech Trial on clinical practice and concerns: A survey of centre collaborators. J Obstet Gynaecol Can 2003;25:14–16.
84. When do obstetricians recommend delivery for a high-risk preterm growth-retarded fetus? The GRIT Study Group. Growth Restriction Intervention Trial. Eur J Obst Gynaecol Reprod Biol 1996;67:121–126.
85. GRIT Study Group: A randomised trial of timed delivery for the compromised preterm fetus. Short term outcomes and Bayesian interpretation. Br J Obstet Gynaecol 2003;110:27–32.
86. Hodnett ED: Support during pregnancy for women at increased risk of low birthweight babies: Cochrane review. In Cochrane Library, issue 4. Oxford, Update Software, 2000.
87. Ershoff DH, Quinn VP, Muller PD: Pregnancy and medical cost outcomes of a self-help prenatal smoking cessation program in a HMO. Public Health Rep 1990;105:304–347.
88. Campbell S, Warsof SL, Little D, et al: Routine ultrasound screening for the prediction of gestational age. Obstet Gynecol 1985;65:613–620.
89. Atlay RD, Weekes AR, Entwistle GD, Parkinson DJ: Treating heartburn in pregnancy: Comparison of acid and alkali mixtures. BMJ 1978;2:919–920.
90. Anderson AS, Wichelow MJ: Constipation during pregnancy: Dietary fiber intake and the effect of fiber supplementation. Hum Nutr Appl Nutr 1985;39:202–207.
91. Muller M, Jaquenoud E: Treatment of constipation in pregnant women: A multicenter study in a gynaecological practice. Schweiz Med Wochenschr 1995;125:1689–1693.
92. Keirse MJNC: Interaction between primary and secondary care during pregnancy and childbirth. In Chalmers I, Enkin M, Keirse MJNC (eds): Effective Care in Pregnancy and Childbirth. Oxford, Oxford University Press, 1990, pp 197–201.
93. Blondel B, Pusch D, Schmidt E: Some characteristics of antenatal care in 13 European countries. Br J Obstet Gynaecol 1985;92:565–568.
94. Cheng M, Hannah M: Breech delivery at term: A critical review of the literature. Obstet Gynecol 1993;82:605–618.
95. Weiner CP, Baschat AA: Fetal growth restriction: Evaluation and management. In James DK, Steer PJ, Weiner CP, Gonik B (eds): High Risk Pregnancy: Management Options. London, WB Saunders, 1999, pp 291–308.

CHAPTER 4

Bleeding and Pain in Early Pregnancy

David J. Cahill / Peter G. Wardle

INTRODUCTION

Complications arise more frequently during the first trimester than at any other stage of pregnancy. Most patients have bleeding, pain, or both. Vaginal bleeding occurs in approximately 20% of clinically diagnosed pregnancies.[1] It causes considerable anxiety for the woman and her partner. In most cases, no intervention will alter the outcome. The main aim of clinical management is a prompt, accurate diagnosis, with reassurance if the pregnancy is appropriately developed and viable, or appropriate intervention if not. The differential diagnosis is shown in Table 4–1.

Most studies estimate that 15% to 20% of clinically recognized pregnancies end in miscarriage.[2] When bleeding occurs in the first trimester, approximately 30% of patients have a miscarriage, 10% to 15% have an ectopic pregnancy, approximately 0.2% have a hydatidiform mole, and approximately 5% have termination of the pregnancy. The remaining 50% of pregnancies continue beyond 20 weeks.[3]

Ectopic pregnancy is the most important cause of maternal mortality in the first trimester of pregnancy in the United Kingdom[4] and other western countries[5] and is the single largest cause of death in pregnancy among black American women. The most recent United Kingdom Confidential Enquiry into Maternal Mortality reported 13 deaths as a result of ectopic pregnancy (in contrast to 7 women who died after spontaneous miscarriage and 5 who died of sepsis).

When family size was larger, the loss of a pregnancy, particularly in the first trimester, was often accorded less importance by society and the medical profession. Now, with most couples having fewer children, the loss of an individual pregnancy or child has assumed greater significance. The understanding and appreciation of the psychological effects of early pregnancy loss have lagged behind that of perinatal bereavement.[6] However, there is now greater recognition of the psychological and psychiatric sequelae and the consequent need for support.[7] These considerations should be taken into account in the management of couples who experience early pregnancy loss.

INITIAL MANAGEMENT

Resuscitation and Triage

Heavy bleeding in early pregnancy should never be ignored and should be assessed urgently. The rate and amount of blood loss should be assessed as accurately as possible, including a speculum examination to estimate additional concealed loss from intravaginal blood and clotting. Most women with first-trimester bleeding are young and fit and can maintain their blood pressure, even after substantial blood loss. When the woman's initial blood pressure is low, it is important to visualize the cervix carefully and remove any products of pregnancy, which may be lying within the cervical canal. It is important to differentiate between cervical shock (which responds rapidly to this removal of retained products of conception) and vascular decompensation, which is more likely to be the result of catastrophic hemorrhage requiring rapid resuscitation.

If the patient is in shock and there are no products of conception in the cervical canal, she should be managed as if a major blood loss has occurred, regardless of the amount of bleeding seen.

When severe blood loss is evident or suspected, adequate staff should be available for resuscitation. Pulse and

TABLE 4–1

Differential Diagnosis of First-Trimester Pain or Bleeding

Pregnancy-Related
Miscarriage (threatened, inevitable, incomplete, complete, missed, or septic)
Ectopic pregnancy
Hydatidiform mole
Coincidental to Pregnancy: Gynecologic
Ruptured corpus luteum of pregnancy
Ovarian cyst accident
Torsion or degeneration of a pedunculated fibroid
Coincidental to Pregnancy: Nongynecologic
Appendicitis
Renal colic
Intestinal obstruction
Cholecystitis
Not Related to Pregnancy, but Gynecologic
Pelvic inflammatory disease
Dysfunctional uterine bleeding
Endometriosis

blood pressure should be recorded frequently, and large-bore intravenous access should be established. Blood should be obtained for a complete blood count, clotting screen, and type and crossmatch. A minimum of 4 units of blood would be required for a patient who is in shock. The woman should be assessed rapidly based on her clinical history and examination while resuscitation is proceeding. If this assessment suggests a catastrophic intraperitoneal hemorrhage from a ruptured ectopic pregnancy, it is unlikely that resuscitation will make her clinically stable. Under these circumstances, an emergency laparotomy should be undertaken.

If the woman responds promptly to appropriate resuscitation, or if she is not in shock (most patients), a careful history and examination should be undertaken and investigations arranged.

Diagnosis (See Table 4–1)

History

The date of the woman's last menstrual period, the usual length of her usual menstrual cycle and any variations, and the date of her first positive urinary pregnancy test should define the likely gestational age. The severity of early pregnancy symptoms, particularly nausea and breast discomfort, may be of diagnostic value. Nausea and vomiting in the first trimester are more frequently associated with a positive pregnancy outcome,[8] even among women with a threatened miscarriage.[9] The loss of early pregnancy symptoms around the time of vaginal bleeding is a bad prognostic sign. Increased early pregnancy symptoms also may be associated with molar pregnancies and multiple pregnancies.

The outcome of previous pregnancies should be noted and is an important indicator of the risk of miscarriage, ectopic pregnancy, or gestational trophoblastic disease (GTD). Primigravidae and women with previous live births have a lower risk of miscarriage. The risk of miscarriage increases cumulatively according to the number of previous miscarriages.[10,11] Similarly, women with a previous ectopic pregnancy are at substantially increased risk of another ectopic pregnancy.[12] There is approximately a tenfold increased risk of another hydatidiform mole in women with a history of an affected pregnancy.[13]

The nature and distribution of associated pain can be helpful. Unilateral pelvic pain is not necessarily related to an ectopic pregnancy; it may simply be caused by ovarian capsule distention from a corpus luteum of pregnancy, particularly if the pain radiates to the anterior thigh from irritation of the adjacent cutaneous nerves. Shoulder tip pain suggests diaphragmatic irritation as a result of intra-abdominal bleeding. Although it is more likely with an ectopic pregnancy, it can also occur with retrograde bleeding from a miscarriage. The extent of first-trimester vaginal bleeding provides a useful prognostic guide. Pregnancy is rarely successful if the loss is equivalent to or greater than a woman's normal menstrual blood loss.[14] A common exception is the loss of one of a twin pregnancy, although spontaneous reduction to a single pregnancy often is not accompanied by bleeding (the "vanishing twin" phenomenon).[15]

Examination

The aims of examination should be to differentiate between an early pregnancy complication and a coincidental abdominal pathology and to identify women who need prompt surgical intervention. Pulse and blood pressure should be monitored frequently to identify developing clinical shock early. The abdomen may be distended because of intraperitoneal bleeding or bowel dilation. Rarely, Cullen's sign (bluish tinge of the periumbilical skin or an umbilical "black eye") may be present in cases of ruptured ectopic pregnancy. Generalized lower abdominal guarding or rebound tenderness on abdominal palpation suggest intraperitoneal bleeding. Localized unilateral iliac fossa tenderness may be present with an unruptured ectopic pregnancy but can also be caused by a physiologic corpus luteum cyst of pregnancy.

Vaginal examination with a Cusco speculum should identify any local cause of bleeding due to trauma or cervical bleeding as a result of a polyp or physiologic ectropion (where bleeding can frequently be related to coitus). An open cervical os suggests either incomplete or inevitable miscarriage. Blood loss through the cervical os should be noted, including whether it is fresh or "old." If products of conception are extruding through the cervix, these can be removed with sponge forceps, which may relieve pain and correct reflex shock as a result of cervical distention. If indicated, removed products of conception should be sent for histologic assessment.

Bimanual examination should be done to assess cervical dilation and identify cervical excitation tenderness as a clinical sign of an ectopic pregnancy. The size and shape of the uterus should be assessed. If it is larger than expected based on menstrual dates, the patient may have a multiple pregnancy, a hydatidiform mole, or coincidental uterine pathology, most frequently fibroids. Adnexal palpation may identify a tender mass that may be either an ectopic pregnancy or a normal corpus luteum cyst.

Special Investigations

A urinary βhCG pregnancy test should always be done if not checked previously. Commercial tests are now very sensitive and specific and can be expected to yield a positive result even 2 or 3 days before a missed period. If the result is positive, the critical and complementary diagnostic tests are a transvaginal pelvic ultrasound scan (TV USS) and quantitative serum βhCG measurements.

Ultrasound and βhCG Level

TV USS usually gives more immediate information, but is generally unhelpful in women who are less than 7 days past their missed period (a missed period is conventionally taken to be 4 weeks after the last period). Rapid changes in appearance occur between 4 and 7 weeks of amenorrhea (Table 4–2). Five weeks after the woman's last menstrual period (assuming a regular 28-day cycle), a gestation sac 2 to 5 mm in diameter should be visible (see Table 4–2). However, this sac can be difficult to differentiate from a pseudogestational sac associated with an ectopic pregnancy (where there is simply a small collection of fluid secretions within the uterine cavity) or a decidual cast (when the pregnancy has failed and decidual separation from the basal endometrium has occurred). A genuine intrauterine gestation sac has two recognizable concentric decidual rings surrounding it, whereas a decidual cast or pseudogestation sac has only one ring. Even in practitioners with considerable ultrasound scanning experience, these subtle differences are easily missed.

Confirmation of an intrauterine sac can be made when the yolk sac or fetus becomes visible. The yolk sac is the first structure that becomes identifiable within the gestation sac, usually by 5½ weeks (Fig. 4–1). It usually measures 2 to 5 mm in diameter. Initially, up to about 6 weeks, it is larger than the fetus. However, an excessively large yolk sac (>5.6 mm in diameter) is often an early sign of impending miscarriage.[16] Other early indicators of almost certain miscarriage are a gestational sac whose diameter exceeds 20 mm without a visible yolk sac and a sac that exceeds 25 mm without a visible fetus.

When an intrauterine pregnancy is clearly visible, a useful formula to calculate approximate gestational age (in days from the last menstrual period) is as follows:

[Gestational age (days) = Mean sac diameter (mm) + 30].[17]

This formula is valid up to 9 weeks' gestation. A second, more accurate, but more complex, formula that is valid to at least 12 weeks gestation is as follows:

[Mean sac diameter (mm) = 0.986 (days after ovulation/conception) – 17.1].[18]

The presence of an ongoing intrauterine pregnancy with a live fetus is a good prognostic finding. When a live embryo or fetus is seen on ultrasound, the overwhelming evidence is that the pregnancy is likely to continue (>95% of cases).[19,20] In addition to ultrasound structures, fetal circulation becomes evident at 5½ weeks and is visible in all viable pregnancies by 6 weeks.[18] Initially, the fetal heart rate is slower than normal, but it increases over time, from 85 to 90 beats/min at 6 weeks to up to 180 beats/min at

TABLE 4–2

Ultrasound Findings and βhCG Concentrations for a Singleton Intrauterine Pregnancy at Particular Gestational

	TRANSVAGINAL ULTRASOUND FINDINGS		
WEEKS (DAYS) FROM THE LAST MENSTRUAL PERIOD (ASSUMING A 28–30 DAY CYCLE)	ENDOMETRIAL THICKNESS	GESTATIONAL SAC (AFTER HOLLANDER, 1972[26] AND MILLS, 1992[18])	YOLK SAC (AFTER MILLS, 1992[18])
4 weeks (28 days)	10–15 mm	–	–
5 weeks (35 days)	15–20 mm	3 mm	2 mm
5 1/2 weeks (38-39 days)	20 mm	7–8 mm	3 mm
6 weeks (42 days)	20 mm	10–12 mm	4 mm
6 1/2 weeks (45-46 days)	–	14–15 mm	4.5 mm
7 weeks (49 days)	–	17–18 mm	5 mm

For optimal interpretation, data are presented for half weeks where possible and from more than one source, leading to a range of values in some cells and no data in other cells.

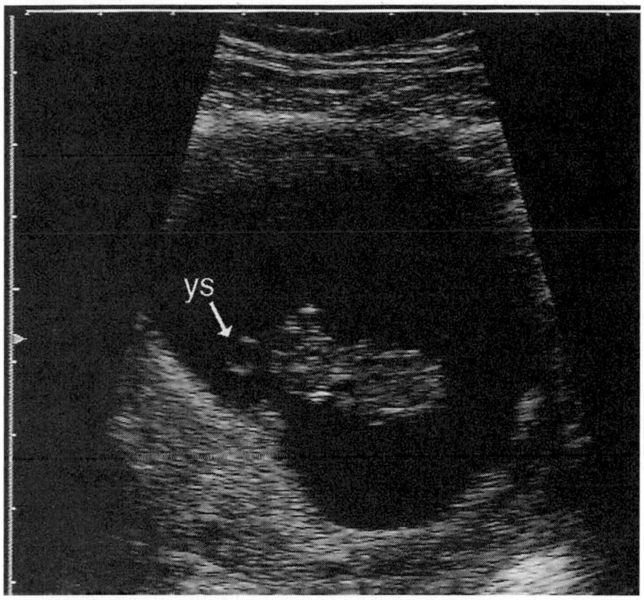

FIGURE 4–1
Pregnancy with a yolk sac (*ys*) at 8 weeks' gestation.

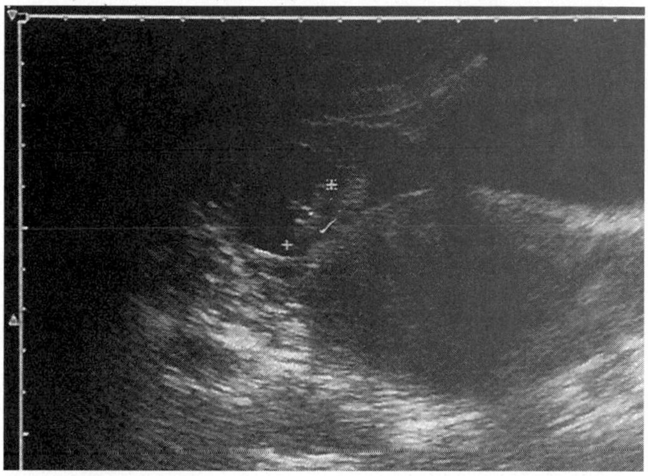

FIGURE 4–2
Uterus with an ectopic pregnancy (crown–rump length, 19 mm) showing fetal heart activity at 9 weeks' gestation.

9 weeks.[21] Rates persistently slower than 100 beats/min are more likely to be associated with a poorer outcome.[21]

Serum βhCG concentrations complement the information available from TV USS in assessing early pregnancy problems. In this chapter, all references to values and ranges of βhCG levels relate to the Third International Standard Preparation (WHO Preparation 75/735). Absolute levels may be helpful in recognizing when a woman with a normal intrauterine pregnancy should be evaluated with TV USS. Levels of βhCG greater than 1500 to 2000 IU/L (depending on local laboratory variations) are almost always associated with the finding of a gestation sac in the uterus if the pregnancy is intrauterine.[22] If it cannot be seen in the uterus, then it should be assumed that there is a pregnancy elsewhere (Fig. 4–2).

This maxim is not universally accepted and is the subject of debate. Caution should be exercised when women have had assisted conception treatment (by in vitro fertilization or ovulation induction). In these situations, more than one embryo might be present; therefore, an intrauterine and an extrauterine pregnancy might coexist (i.e., heterotopic pregnancy) or two intrauterine pregnancies might exist, giving rise to higher βhCG levels without a visible pregnancy on TV USS. Excessively high serum βhCG levels are also found with GTD (≥20 times normal values), and levels up to twice the normal values can be found in pregnancies affected by Down syndrome. Generally, βhCG levels are lower at any given gestational age with ectopic pregnancies than with normal intrauterine pregnancies. However, the overlap in values between the two clinical conditions is too great for this difference to be a diagnostic criterion.

Changes in βhCG levels are more useful clinically. Usually βhCG values are best tested at intervals of 48 hours or longer. A decreasing βhCG concentration in the first few weeks identifies a pregnancy as abnormal. If the

Age Points in Early Fetal Life

CROWN RUMP LENGTH (AFTER HOLLANDER, 1972[26] AND MILLS, 1992[18])	FETAL HEART (RATE) (AFTER MERCHIERS, 1991[21] AND ROBINSON, 1973[27])	SERUM βhCG (IU/L) (MEDIAN VALUES FOR βhCG ASSAY) (FROM THE THIRD INTERNATIONAL STANDARD PREPARATION)
–	–	<100
–	–	600
3–4 mm	–	–
4 mm	85–100	5200
7 mm	–	–
10 mm	125	26,700

βhCG level decreases by more than one half within 48 hours, it suggests that residual trophoblastic activity has ceased and that the pregnancy is likely to resolve without intervention. With a viable intrauterine pregnancy, βhCG values should increase by at least 66% in 48 hours.[23] If the rate of increase is less than 66% or if the βhCG doubling time is more than 2.7 days, there should be a strong suspicion of an ectopic pregnancy. A βhCG doubling time of more than 7 days is never found in a normal pregnancy.[23]

SUMMARY OF MANAGEMENT OPTIONS

Bleeding in Early Pregnancy—Initial and General Management

Management Options	Quality of Evidence	Strength of Recommendation	References
Identify the cause of bleeding by a combination of history, examination, βhCG assay, and transvaginal ultrasound.	III	B	9,11–14,18–21,23–27
Assess the amount and rate of blood loss.	III	B	14
Obtain regular recordings of pulse and blood pressure.	–	GPP	–
Provide intravenous access if there is actual or risk of hemodynamic instability.	–	GPP	–
FBC for all. Perform a clotting screening if coagulopathy is suspected or excess blood loss occurs. Crossmatch blood if excessive blood loss occurs.	–	GPP	–

FBC, full blood count.

SPONTANEOUS ABORTION OR MISCARRIAGE

Definition

Now used synonymously, the terms *spontaneous abortion* and *miscarriage* imply the natural loss of a pregnancy before viability. Until recently, the term *abortion* was generally used in professional communication and *miscarriage* was used in discussion with patients. However, because the term *abortion* (which many patients find offensive) has pejorative connotations of "elective termination of pregnancy," there has been an overall shift away from using *abortion* to describe the spontaneous loss of a pregnancy.[28] Viability implies the ability of the fetus to survive extrauterine life. This is generally considered to occur at approximately 24 weeks' gestation. Rarely, fetuses born before that gestation survive for a short time or at least show some signs of life. The cutoff point for the use of the term *miscarriage* might lie at 22 weeks' gestation (154 days), as recommended by the World Health Organization (WHO).[29] The WHO also includes in this definition the fetus's weight (<500 g). In the United Kingdom, the legal definition changed in 1992 to 24 weeks' gestation (168 days), whereas in North America, the gestational age limit for a miscarriage is 20 weeks.[30]

In addition to these changes in terminology, there has been a marked alteration in the way in which early-pregnancy bleeding and pain are managed. Many of these changes are attributable to the following:

- Availability of rapid access to serum βhCG measurements
- High-resolution TV USS
- Introduction of fast-track referrals to early pregnancy assessment units or clinics (EPU/EPC)

In EPCs, access to integrated evaluation by ultrasonography, serum sampling for βhCG, and the presence of experienced medical and nursing staff has permitted women to be managed as outpatients or in the office, providing a more streamlined service.

Table 4–3 provides a summary of requirements for an EPC service. EPCs have improved the quality of care and produced considerable savings in financial and staff resources. However, as a tool in patient management, EPC services have not been fully evaluated.[31] Management of women through an EPC service is not without its drawbacks. Inappropriate delays in diagnosis of true ectopic pregnancies and overmanagement by laparoscopy of suspected ectopic pregnancies both occur, despite rigid adherence to protocols.

A pregnancy loss may be clinically evident after a patient has bleeding or pain or may be clinically silent and identified on a routine ultrasound scan. The introduction of nearly routine scanning to confirm gestational dates has had a dramatic effect on the

TABLE 4–3

Requirements for an Early Pregnancy Assessment Clinic

Appropriate resources for rostering of ultrasonographic, medical, and nursing staff (Exact calculation of time required is not evidence-based; experience suggests that for a hospital with 5000 deliveries/yr, 3 hours of patient contact time daily for all disciplines and 1 hour of telephone contact time later in the day is reasonable.)
Dedicated clinic space, with rooms for ultrasonography, clinical assessment and investigation, counseling, and a waiting area
Good-quality ultrasound machines with transvaginal capability
Availability of same-day βhCG estimation
A senior member of the clinical staff who is responsible for the development of guidelines and the resolution of diagnostic conflicts and problems

management of early pregnancy loss. Bleeding occurs in one fifth of recognized pregnancies before the 20th week of gestation. However, it is likely that far more pregnancies are lost before they are suspected, recognized, or confirmed (giving rise to the term *pregnancy loss iceberg*[32,33]; Fig. 4–3).

In one study, 12% of pregnancies in which bleeding occurred ended in miscarriage.[34] Other studies reported higher rates (≥16%),[34] but these studies did not include women who did not know they were pregnant (≥22%)[35] or those who did not seek medical advice about their bleeding, knowing that they were pregnant (approximately 12%).[34]

Risks

The maternal risks are blood loss, infection, and the psychological effects of pregnancy loss.

Presentation and Diagnosis

Most women seek care at a hospital, family physician's office, or EPC with one of the following concerns:

- Bleeding without pain
- Bleeding with pain, with possible passage of pregnancy tissue vaginally
- Bleeding with pain, with symptoms and signs of blood loss
- Absence of bleeding, with decreased symptoms of pregnancy

The amount of bleeding can vary from very slight to significant and has some prognostic value. Bleeding without pain is more likely to be associated with a threatened miscarriage. Patients seen at an EPC service often have painless bleeding. Once ongoing pregnancy is confirmed by ultrasound, the practitioner can provide reassurance. In most of these cases, bleeding has a local cause, such as physiologic changes in the cervix. The additional presence of pain is often associated with cervical opening or distention as a result of the passage of tissue or a blood clot, which may

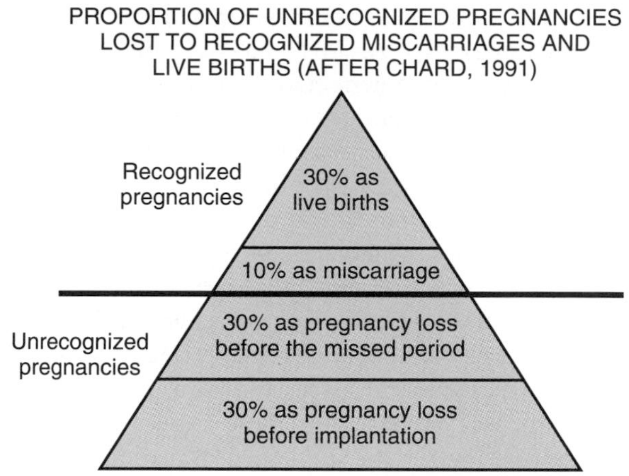

FIGURE 4–3
Proportion of unrecognized pregnancies lost to recognized miscarriages and live births. (From Chard T: Frequency of implantation and early pregnancy loss in natural cycles. Baillieres Clin Obstet Gynaecol 1991;5:179–189.)

be painful. Blood loss can give rise to symptoms in itself, and the passage of tissue through the cervical os can promote a vagal response that causes shock, which is rapidly relieved if the products are removed from the os.

Management Options

Threatened miscarriages are managed expectantly. If bleeding is slight and is not associated with pain, then the woman can be reassured that the pregnancy is likely to continue. Of all pregnancies in which bleeding occurs, more than 50% continue.[3] If bleeding occurs at 10 weeks' gestation, more than 90% continue; at 13 weeks, 99% continue.[36] If the menstrual or gestational age is greater than 6 weeks, then ultrasound may show a healthy, ongoing pregnancy. In such cases, the likelihood of pregnancy loss is less than 3%.[20] Ultrasonography before 6 weeks is less likely to be helpful. If a patient needs the reassurance of an ongoing pregnancy by ultrasound scan, then this evaluation should be undertaken after 6 weeks.

The management options for the loss of an early intrauterine pregnancy are

- Expectant
- Medical
- Surgical

Spontaneous complete miscarriage can be managed expectantly. Most difficulty in the management of bleeding in early pregnancy involves missed or incomplete miscarriage.

In most western countries, the surgical approach (evacuation of retained products of conception [ERPC]) historically has been the most common emergency gynecologic procedure. The procedure was traditionally carried out with ovum forceps and curettage and evolved to vacuum aspiration. Vacuum aspiration is associated with less blood loss and pain and is a shorter procedure than surgical curettage.[37]

Expectant management avoids a surgical procedure and allows the woman to continue her normal daily routine. It is more acceptable to women and causes fewer effects on the quality of life.[38] Primary care physicians in the Netherlands and elsewhere strongly favor the use of expectant management, and it is likely that many miscarriages are managed expectantly in primary care.[39] However, expectant management is associated with more prolonged bleeding than either surgical[40] or medical management.[41] Reports from secondary care settings are less encouraging about expectant management; in one report, the incidence of prolonged bleeding and the success rate of expectant management were so low that its use was considered unjustified in clinical practice.[41]

Medical management has been advocated as an intermediate approach. The treatment regimens used have included misoprostol (often in combination with mifepristone),[42,43] sulprostone,[44] and gemeprost.[45] Women who have medical treatment have greater analgesic needs and more vaginal bleeding compared with those who have surgical management.[45,46] The treatment did not achieve success (ERPC was still required) in 50% to 80% of women in most studies,[45,47,48] although in one uncontrolled study, a success rate of 100% was reported.[44] The authors concluded that although medical treatment reduced the need for surgical evacuation, a significant proportion of patients who underwent medical treatment still needed ERPC. This approach hardly seems an effective treatment or an appropriate use of resources. When medical management is compared with expectant management, no differences are found in the number of days of bleeding, pain scores, blood loss, or complications. Women having medical treatment had a longer convalescence than those treated by expectant management.[42] Medical treatment is not innocuous; 45% of women in one study had gastrointestinal upset.[49]

In the absence of an adequately powered randomized controlled trial evaluating surgical, medical, and expectant management, how should incomplete miscarriages be managed? Can we rationalize the evidence from the assorted studies already undertaken? Gradation of the quality of evidence supporting the choices is provided in the Summary of Management Options. Expectant management should be used for women in the first instance, providing that they are stable. Given a choice, most women favor this approach.[50] It appears difficult to predict for which women expectant management will be effective.[51] Patients must understand that they may bleed for slightly longer,[52] and they must have ready access to hospital services should they require them. Women who choose medical management appear to have better mental health scores subsequently.[38] Perhaps if there is no clear option on clinical grounds, then medical management should be the treatment of choice. Future fertility does not appear to be compromised by adopting this route.[53]

For those who do not want medical or expectant management, surgical management remains an option. Vacuum aspiration is preferred over surgical curettage; it is quicker, safer, and less painful.[37] Whether any women should electively have surgical treatment rather than any other is not clear, although in terminations, women of high parity (more than para 3) are more likely to have a complete abortion after surgical management.[54] Should tissue be sent from all miscarriages for histologic examination? Obvious practical problems arise with medical and expectant management, but it certainly should be requested for patients who undergo surgical curettage. Suspicious findings on ultrasound should direct management to surgery.

Some have suggested that the management option can be determined on the basis of ultrasound and biochemical evaluation. The volume of tissue remaining in the uterine cavity on ultrasound may be a useful guide in management. No intervention is required if there is no tissue or if the products of conception have a mean diameter of less than 15 mm. Medical or expectant management may be considered if the tissue mass is between 15 and 50 mm, and ERPC is probably required if the tissue diameter exceeds 50 mm.[42] More complications (37% vs. 3%) occurred when women with significant intrauterine tissue (intrauterine sac >10 mm in diameter) were managed expectantly compared with surgically.[55] Evidence to recommend the routine use of serum βhCG levels[55,56] or progesterone[56] to determine the need for surgical intervention is insufficient. When color Doppler imaging of uterine blood flow and the intervillous space was examined in missed miscarriages,[57] uterine blood flow could not differentiate between women whose miscarriage resolved spontaneously and those who required ERPC. Intervillous space blood flow was associated with an 80% chance of spontaneous resolution compared with 23% in those for whom flow was absent.[57] Although this technique shows promise, it requires validation. These adjuvant techniques are of little value in determining which women should be managed expectantly or otherwise. Should women undergoing surgical evacuation of the uterus have *Chlamydia* screening in line with other invasive interventions in the uterine cavity? One inadequately powered randomized trial showed no benefit, but because *Chlamydia* screening and selective antibiotic treatment reduces infection in induced abortion, this practice is worth continuing until evidence suggests otherwise.[58]

Thus, much of the management of bleeding in early pregnancy may be in the hands of general practitioners[39] or midwives,[1] but accurate diagnosis of ectopic pregnancies[55] and molar pregnancies[51] remains of particular concern. Rapid access to ultrasound and βhCG assays should remain a fundamental part of the management of bleeding in early pregnancy.

SUMMARY OF MANAGEMENT OPTIONS

Spontaneous Miscarriage

Management Options	Quality of Evidence	Strength of Recommendation	References
Expectant management	Ia	A	42,59
Medical evacuation	Ib	A	42,47,59–61
Surgical evacuation	Ia	A	47,59
An adequately resourced early pregnancy clinic is key to the management of early pregnancy problems.	III	B	31
Many cases do not need hospital admission.	Ia	A	39
Expectant management is the first choice.	Ia	A	42,59
Expectant management does not affect future fertility.	Ib	A	62
Medical management should be undertaken before surgical management.	Ib	A	47,63
Vacuum aspiration is provided to surgical evacuation.	Ia	A	37
Couples require equal psychological support after medical or surgical management of miscarriage.	Ib	A	64

ECTOPIC PREGNANCY

The management of ectopic pregnancy has changed over the last 20 years. The changes that have led to these improvements in management are summarized in Table 4–4.

In line with this shift in practice, there has been a fourfold decrease in the mortality rate associated with ectopic pregnancy over the last 25 years, although the incidence of ectopic pregnancies has increased twofold.[4] The current rate of ectopic pregnancy (ectopic pregnancies per 1000 pregnancies) in the United Kingdom is 11.1 (approximately 1%), and in the United States, it is 20.[65] The mortality rate as a result of ectopic pregnancies in the United Kingdom is 4 per 10,000 (estimated) ectopic pregnancies.[4] In the United States, the rate is 3.4 per 10,000.[65] Complacency would be inappropriate, however, because ectopic pregnancy remains the leading cause of maternal death in early pregnancy.[4] Factors that predispose to ectopic pregnancy are listed in Table 4–5.

TABLE 4–4

Changes Leading to Improved Management of Ectopic Pregnancy

Recognition of high-risk individuals (see Table 4-5)
Increased sensitivity of home pregnancy tests
Early referral to dedicated (early pregnancy) clinics in hospitals
Development and refinement of high-resolution transvaginal ultrasound
Accurate and rapid estimation of serum βhCG)
Laboratory techniques allowing 24-hour access to automated sample processing

Definition

An ectopic pregnancy is one that occurs outside the uterine cavity, usually at an adjacent site, generally, the fallopian tube. In more than 98% of ectopic pregnancies, the primary site is in the fallopian tube. The rest occur in the abdominal cavity, on the ovary, or in the cervix. In the fallopian tube, approximately 80% of pregnancies occur in the ampullary region.

Risks

Risks are blood loss and its consequences, implications for future reproductive performance, and the psychological effects of the loss of the pregnancy.

Diagnosis

Symptoms

Diagnosis of an ectopic pregnancy can be difficult. Some, all, or none of the following symptoms may be elicited in a woman with an ectopic pregnancy:

TABLE 4–5

Specific Risk Factors Predisposing to Ectopic Pregnancy

Peak age-specific incidence 25–34 years
Infertility (fourfold increased risk)
Sexually transmitted disease, especially chlamydia
Increased *Chlamydia* antibody titer
Tubal sterilization and reconstruction
Intrauterine contraceptive device
Endometriosis

- Amenorrhea
- Abdominal pain
- Vaginal bleeding
- Fainting
- Shoulder tip pain

Signs

At presentation to an EPC, many women with an ectopic pregnancy have few or no signs on examination. Unilateral iliac fossa pain is in keeping with ectopic pregnancy, but bilateral pain is not uncommon. Guarding, rigidity, and signs of peritonism may be elicited on abdominal palpation. Guarding may be reduced if the knees are drawn up to relax the abdominal muscles.

On vaginal examination, it may be possible to elicit pain on the affected adnexal side by manipulating the cervix laterally. Because the uterus moves in the opposite direction as a result of rotation around the fulcrum of the transverse cervical ligaments, there is increased tension on the side of the ectopic pregnancy. This is described as the pain of cervical excitation.

The uterus may be softer and even enlarged slightly in the presence of an ectopic pregnancy as a result of the softening effect of increased levels of progesterone on the endometrium and myometrium.

It is now rare in the United Kingdom for women to be admitted with an ectopic pregnancy presenting with hypovolemic shock or severe pain.

Investigations

Ectopic pregnancy must be differentiated from other causes of lower abdominal pain in a woman of reproductive age (see Table 4–1).

Critical to the diagnosis of ectopic pregnancy are TV USS and serum βhCG and, to a lesser extent, serum progesterone. Confirmation of the diagnosis by laparoscopy is not always necessary. Laparoscopy is not even the absolute answer because it has a false-negative rate of 3% to 4% (if done too early) and a false-positive rate of 5% (because of retrograde uterine bleeding).[66]

The complementary roles of TV USS and βhCG measurements were discussed earlier. Serum progesterone is also considered to have a role in the differentiation of an ectopic pregnancy. Its use is not as widespread as βhCG and TV USS. Serum progesterone concentrations well into the normal range for early pregnancy (>80 nmol/L) are associated with a high probability of the pregnancy being normal and intrauterine in site.[25] Conversely, values less than 15 nmol/L are highly likely (98%) to be associated with a nonviable pregnancy.[67] Most ectopic pregnancies have progesterone concentrations between these values that make the test of little value for routine clinical practice. Algorithms have been devised with and without the use of serum progesterone and can be referred to and integrated into local practice guidelines if considered appropriate.[22,68] Figure 4–4 shows an example of a practical algorithm.

The patient who has obvious intra-abdominal bleeding can be diagnosed without difficulty. The less acute clinical scenario, in which a woman has little or no pain, vague symptoms, slowly increasing βhCG levels, and nonspecific findings on ultrasound, is more challenging.

Management Options

Management of the acutely ill woman differs from the more common presentation of a woman who is clinically stable.

The acute presentation that includes hypotension, tachycardia, pain, and other signs of shock, usually, but not always, associated with amenorrhea, is generally treated with laparotomy. The acute symptoms are usually caused by fallopian tube rupture or significant intraperitoneal bleeding. Surgical treatment usually requires partial or total salpingectomy, securing hemostasis, and removing blood and products of conception from the abdominal cavity.

In the less acute situation, there are several treatment options, which include surgical (conservative and radical), medical, and expectant management. The gradation of the quality of evidence is shown in the Summary of Management Options. The algorithm in Figure 4–4 shows the critical criteria that affect management; the trend in serum βhCG and the findings on TV USS. A serum βhCG level that increases above a critical threshold in the absence of an intrauterine gestation sac is usually an indication for surgical intervention. The choice of laparoscopy or laparotomy depends on the patient's surgical history, the findings on TV USS, and the absolute level of βhCG and its rate of increase.

Expectant Management

As shown in Figure 4–4, this management is most appropriate when the woman is hemodynamically stable, with no symptoms of pain. Some authors have suggested exclusion criteria, such as gestation sac size (>4 cm) or the presence of a fetal heartbeat on TV USS.[69] Expectant management is more likely to be effective if the initial serum βhCG concentration is less than 1000 IU/L and decreases thereafter and if a gestation sac is not seen on TV USS.[69] The serum βhCG level (both the initial level and the trend) is generally the most important predictor of successful expectant management.[69] Recent publications suggest that of vaginal bleeding, endometrial thickness, serum βhCG, and serum progesterone, the most useful modality to predict spontaneous resolution was serum progesterone, with a cutoff level of less than 20 nmol/L.[70]

Practically, expectant management involves establishing a reliable diagnosis of early extrauterine pregnancy

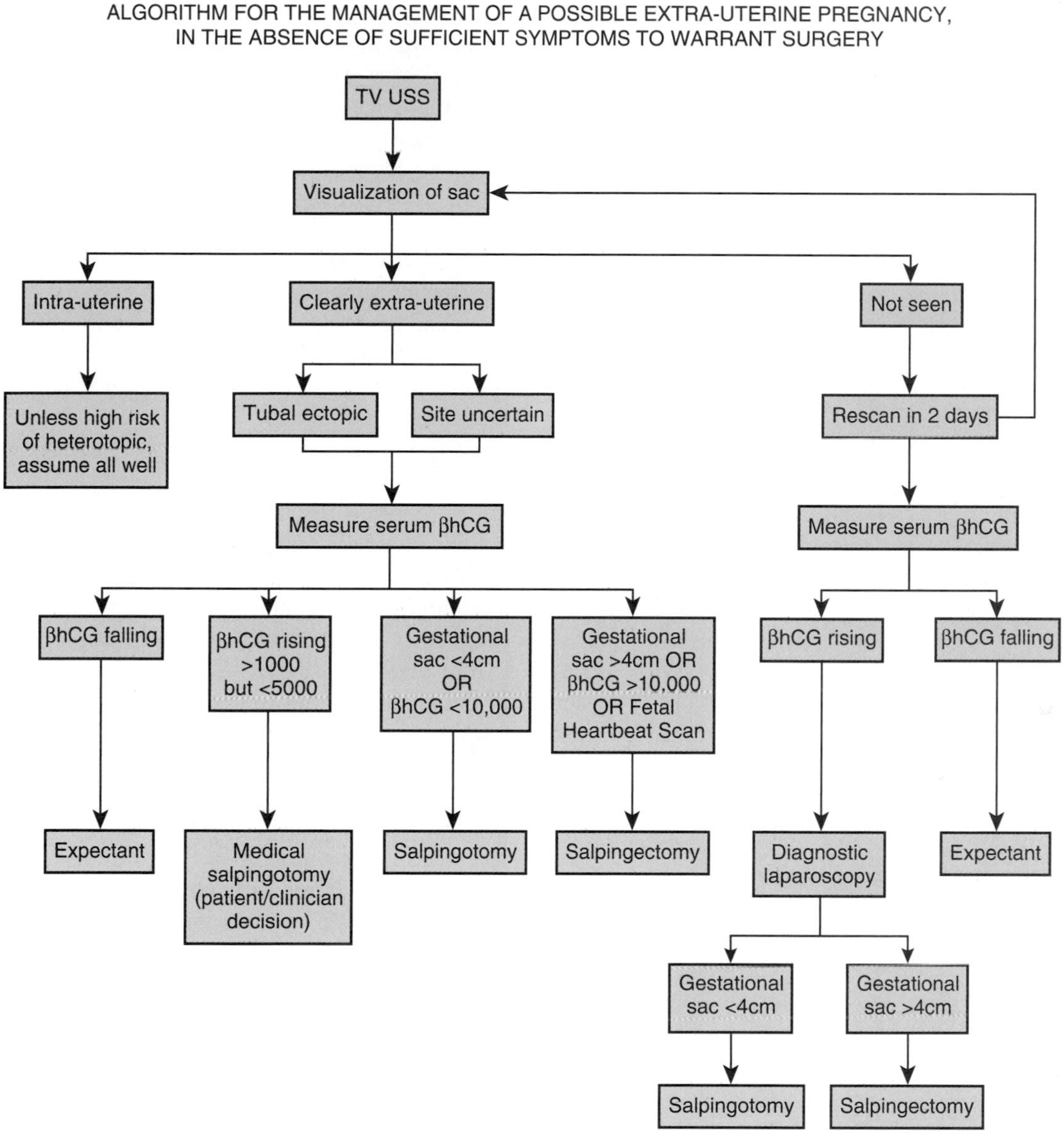

FIGURE 4–4
Algorithm for the management of a possible extrauterine pregnancy in the absence of sufficient symptoms to warrant surgery. FH, fetal heart beat; TV USS, transvaginal pelvic ultrasound scan.

failure, informing the patient of other treatment options, and obtaining consent that this method of management is acceptable. Serum βhCG levels should be monitored every 3 to 4 days until they decrease to less than 10 to 15 IU/L.[67]

Success rates for this approach range from 70% to 75% for βhCG levels of less than 1000 IU/L,[69,70] decreasing to 25% if levels are greater than 2000 IU/L.[71]

Medical Treatment

Current methods of medical management focus on the use of methotrexate, generally as a single dose. Multiple-dose regimens are less commonly used. Methotrexate is a folic acid antagonist. As a chemotherapeutic agent, it is active against rapidly dividing tissues, such as those in the placental trophoblast. Methotrexate can produce side effects through its actions on other tissues, such as the gastrointestinal tract and the hematologic system. Adverse symptoms include stomatitis, gastritis, diarrhea, transient liver enzyme disorders, and rarely, bone marrow suppressive disorders. Single-dose use rarely gives rise to symptoms; daily or alternate-day multiple doses do so more commonly. Folinic acid is given to counteract this effect. Folinic acid is not required when doses are given at greater than weekly intervals.[72] Medical management is particularly appropriate when surgical intervention would be difficult (e.g., cervical and interstitial pregnancies).

Medical treatment has been available for more than 20 years,[73] but has not been adopted extensively. This is lamentable because studies involving large series of women show success rates of approximately 90%.[74] Predictors of success of medical treatment include sac size, fetal cardiac activity, and serum βhCG concentration; βhCG concentration is the most important of these.[74] For values of 2000 to 5000 IU/L, the likelihood of success is 92% (86%–97%; 95% confidence interval [CI]) and higher when values are less than 1000 IU/L (98%, 96–100%; 95% CI).[74] Compared with conservative laparoscopic surgery, methotrexate is associated with a shorter hospital stay but a longer return to normal βhCG levels.[75] In the United Kingdom, most women might be expected to attend an outpatient EPC for diagnosis, so this is not a particular advantage. However, future reproductive expectations are better with methotrexate, with higher intrauterine pregnancy rates and lower ectopic rates subsequently.

The dose of methotrexate used in clinical practice varies. Given systemically, and usually intramuscularly, the dose is either 1 mg/kg or 50 mg/m^2. These doses seem to be equally effective, and most favor the easier dose calculation of the former, with a minimum total dose of 50 mg.[76]

Surgical Treatment

Salpingectomy has long been considered the gold standard treatment for ectopic pregnancy. In emergency treatment of rupture of the fallopian tube, this may still be unavoidable. However, recently, considerable emphasis has been placed on conservation of the fallopian tubes when possible, and debate now hinges on the following questions:

- When is it appropriate to conserve a fallopian tube?
- Does fallopian tube conservation significantly affect subsequent fertility rates?

CONSERVATION OF THE FALLOPIAN TUBE

The Royal College of Obstetricians and Gynaecologists recommends that surgical treatment by laparoscopic salpingectomy is the preferred method of treatment for an ectopic pregnancy when the fallopian tube on the other side is normal.[77] However, until recently, most women in the United Kingdom were having open surgery, not laparoscopy, for the management of ectopic pregnancy.[78] Laparotomy may be the more appropriate route. A meta-analysis, based on the combined results of three studies involving women with unruptured tubal pregnancies, suggests that laparoscopic conservative surgery had more failures than an open surgical approach, when failure was defined as persistence of trophoblastic tissue and increased βhCG levels (relative risk [RR], 0.90; 95% CI, 0.83–0.97).[79]

There is not sufficient evidence from randomized controlled trials to answer the questions raised in the salpingectomy–salpingotomy debate. Opinions vary on this matter. In the management of an ectopic pregnancy, removal of the fallopian tube (salpingectomy) is considered the safest,[80] most clinically effective,[81] and most cost-effective technique.[82] A meta-analysis of nine well-designed comparative studies showed similar intrauterine pregnancy rates whether salpingectomy (49%) or salpingotomy (53%) was used.[76] That report and a separate meta-analysis showed higher subsequent ectopic pregnancy rates after salpingotomy (15% vs. 10%).[76,83] There is general agreement that salpingectomy would be appropriate if a women desired no further children, if a second ectopic pregnancy occurred in the same fallopian tube, if bleeding could not be controlled, or if the tube was severely damaged by the ectopic pregnancy. If salpingotomy is undertaken, further quantitative βhCG monitoring is required to confirm successful treatment because ectopic pregnancy persists in 8% to 19% of cases.[76,84]

In women who had one fallopian tube and underwent a salpingostomy, 54% achieved a subsequent intrauterine pregnancy, but 21% had a further ectopic pregnancy.[76]

The details of surgical techniques are beyond the scope of this chapter. Salpingectomy may be undertaken laparoscopically or by open surgery. Open surgery is more likely to be undertaken if the woman is in shock or is otherwise showing signs of hemodynamically instability. Laparoscopic salpingectomy techniques include resection with diathermy and scissors, loop ligatures, or single-use proprietary stapling instruments. Conservative surgery generally involves a linear incision along the antimesenteric border of the fallopian tube, over the site of the ectopic pregnancy. The pregnancy is removed by flushing with high-pressure hydrodissection, and hemostasis is achieved by (bipolar) diathermy. In two small studies, prophylactic local infiltration of dilute vasopressin was used in 40 hemodynamically stable women with a small unruptured ectopic pregnancy,[85] and diluted oxytocin was used in 25 similar women.[86] These interventions reduced the need for electrocoagulation for hemostasis (RR, 0.36; 95% CI, 0.14–0.95) without side effects, resulting in a significantly shorter operation time, reduced intraoperative and postoperative blood loss, and easier removal of the tubal pregnancy without side effects. However, neither study showed any benefit in reducing the likelihood of persistent trophoblastic disease.

FERTILITY AFTER SURGERY

After salpingectomy, in a woman who has a normal fallopian tube on the contralateral side, the likelihood of any pregnancy being intrauterine is still greater than 50%.[87] After salpingotomy, the likelihood of an intrauterine pregnancy is approximately 65%.[76,88]

Any study of fertility after radical or conservative treatment must consider the fact that there is a higher chance of salpingectomy if the initial ectopic pregnancy ruptured. In studies that considered this important factor, no appreciable difference was found in the subsequent intrauterine pregnancy rates.[89] The factors that altered the likelihood of conception included the woman's age, previous tubal damage, and infertility.[89] This holds true even if the previous ectopic pregnancy ruptured.[90] The reported likelihood of a future ectopic pregnancy after 3 years of follow-up varies. It is 18% to 23% after conservative treatment and 28% after radical treatment.[89,91]

On economic and fertility outcome grounds, there are no clear indicators as to whether salpingectomy or salpingostomy is more appropriate for women who have both fallopian tubes.

Future Advice and Appropriate Treatment

After an ectopic pregnancy, many women are concerned about their future and the likelihood of recurrence. Regardless of the initial form of treatment, the likelihood of a further ectopic pregnancy varies little. Previous tubal rupture does not appear to have a detrimental effect on future fertility. Smoking is an independent risk factor for fertility, and the likelihood of a future intrauterine pregnancy appears to be increased by stopping smoking.[89] Future fertility also decreases if the woman is older (>35 years)[90] or has had previous tubal damage or infertility.[89] For these women, assisted conception may offer a better chance of an intrauterine pregnancy. The risk of a further ectopic pregnancy is strongly increased (three to four times) if the woman was previously nulliparous, if this was not her first ectopic pregnancy, if she has had previous tubal surgery,[91] or if there are adhesions around either fallopian tube.[89]

If a woman has had a previous ectopic pregnancy, any subsequent pregnancy is more likely to be ectopic. Under these circumstances, early review by high-resolution TV USS in a special EPC is advisable so that evaluation can be made of the site and viability of the pregnancy as soon as possible. This will either provide reassurance or allow timely intervention.

SUMMARY OF MANAGEMENT OPTIONS
Ectopic Pregnancy

Management Options	Quality of Evidence	Strength of Recommendation	References
Diagnosis			
Accurate and rapid βhCG level estimation and high-resolution transvaginal ultrasound are key to the management.	III	B	22
Expectant			
Suitable for some ectopic pregnancies if βhCG levels are low and falling (<1000 IU/L)	Ib	A	79,92,93
Medical			
Valid option with no fetal heartbeat and βhCG <5000 IU/L, if patient is asymptomatic and willing to have serial βhCG estimations	III	B	74
Methotrexate local	Ib	A	79
Methotrexate systemic	Ib	A	79,94
Hyperosmolar glucose	Ib	A	79
Prostaglandins and methotrexate	Ib	A	79
Surgery: General			
Laparotomy has higher success rates.	Ib	A	79
Salpingectomy is marginally better than salpingotomy; subsequent fertility rates are no different.	III	B	76,91
Use agents intraoperatively to reduce bleeding.	Ib	A	85,86
Surgery: Laparoscopy/Laparotomy			
Salpingotomy or salpingectomy	Ib	A	79

GESTATIONAL TROPHOBLASTIC DISEASE

GTD is an uncommon cause of vaginal bleeding in the first half of pregnancy. The disease encompasses a wide range of conditions that vary in their clinical presentation, their propensity for spontaneous resolution, local invasion and metastasis, and their overall prognosis. These conditions include complete or partial hydatidiform mole, invasive mole, choriocarcinoma, and placental site trophoblastic tumors.[95–97] The worldwide incidence of GTD is approximately 0.6 to 2.3 per 1000 pregnancies. Most cases are complete or partial hydatidiform moles.[98–100] The most invasive form of GTD, choriocarcinoma, has an incidence of 0.2 to 2.0 per 10,000 pregnancies.

The incidence of all types of GTD is reported to be up to twice as high in the Far East, particularly in Korea and Japan.[99,101] The woman's age is a consistently demonstrated risk factor for hydatidiform mole. Compared with women aged 25 to 30 years, there is approximately a 6-fold excess risk in women who become pregnant before 15 years of age and approximately a 300-fold excess risk in women who become pregnant after 45 years of age.[98,102] This age association is much greater for complete, rather than partial, hydatidiform mole. However, because women at these extremes of reproductive age represent such a small proportion of all pregnancies, more than 90% of molar pregnancies still occur in women aged 18 to 40 years. A history of a previous molar pregnancy is also a risk factor. Women with a history of one hydatidiform mole have at least a 10-fold greater risk of a repeat molar pregnancy, usually the same type of mole as in the preceding pregnancy, which equates to an incidence of approximately 18 per 1000 pregnancies.[103,104]

A complete hydatidiform mole is usually diploid and entirely androgenetic in origin. Most have a 46,XX karyotype; a few have a 46,XY karyotype. A complete molar pregnancy consists of diffuse hydropic chorionic villi with trophoblastic hyperplasia, forming a mass of multiple vesicles. There is usually no evidence of a fetus and minimal embryonal development.

A partial hydatidiform mole is usually triploid, with one maternal and two paternal haploid sets, either from dispermic fertilization or from fertilization with an unreduced diploid sperm. There is usually a fetus and a large placenta. The hydropic villi show a less florid appearance than is seen with a complete hydatidiform mole and are interspersed with normal chorionic villi. The fetus usually dies within a few weeks of conception, and a recent review did not identify any case in which a fetus of paternal (diandric) origin survived to term.[105] Very rarely, a partial molar pregnancy develops with two maternal and one paternal haploid set (digynic). In these cases, the placenta is small, the villi show minimal hydropic changes, and the fetus is growth-restricted. Some of these pregnancies have been reported to result in live births, with subsequent early neonatal death.[106] One study suggested that diandric partial molar pregnancies have a greater malignant potential than digynic partial molar pregnancies. Of 3000 women with partial hydatidiform moles, 0.1% had a choriocarcinoma. All were genetically diandric.[107]

Persistent trophoblastic disease or malignant complications are much more common with a complete molar pregnancy than with a partial hydatidiform mole. The incidence of these complications is approximately 8% and 0.5%, respectively, compared with a risk of approximately 1:50,000 after a full-term pregnancy.

Diagnosis

Presentation and Clinical Features

Abnormal vaginal bleeding in early pregnancy, usually between 8 and 16 weeks' gestation, is the most common presentation. The diagnosis of a molar pregnancy might be suspected based on a number of clinical features (Table 4–6). These features are usually more prominent and develop at an earlier gestational age in women with a complete hydatidiform mole. The mean gestational age at diagnosis 40 years ago was 16 weeks, and this is still the case in many developing countries. In developed countries, most molar pregnancies are now diagnosed before 12 weeks, probably because of the increased use of high-resolution TV USS. With a complete mole, previously, ultrasound scan findings were reported characteristically as a "snowstorm" appearance of mixed echogenicity, representing hydropic villi and intrauterine hemorrhage (Fig. 4–5). This appearance is apparent only in later ultrasound scans when there has been some intrauterine hemorrhage. With increasing resolution and earlier use of ultrasound, a mole often shows a fine vesicular or honeycomb appearance rather than the classic description. The ovaries often contain multiple large theca-lutein cysts as a result of increased ovarian stimulation by excessive βhCG. Ultrasound diagnosis of a partial mole is more difficult. The fetus may still be viable, but may show signs consistent with triploidy, such as unusually

TABLE 4–6

Symptoms and Signs Suggestive of Gestational Trophoblastic Disease and Their Approximate Frequency

Irregular first-trimester vaginal bleeding (>90%)
Uterus large for dates (25%)
Pain from large benign theca-lutein cysts (20%)
Vaginal passage of grapelike vesicles (10%)
Exaggerated pregnancy symptoms:
Hyperemesis (10%)
Hyperthyroidism (5%)
Early preeclampsia (5%)

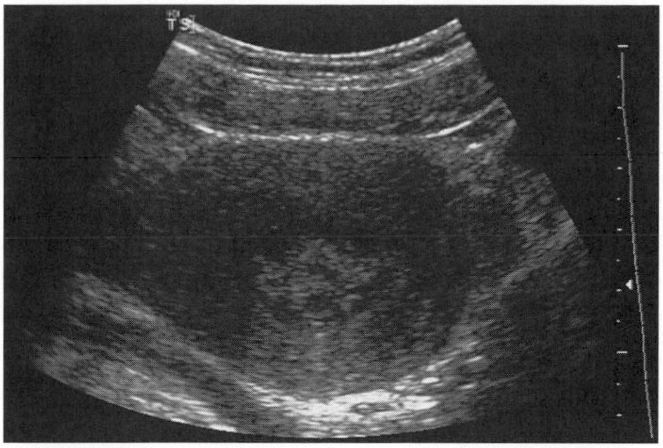

FIGURE 4–5
Ultrasound image of a hydatidiform mole in the first trimester showing a mixed echogenic appearance in the uterine cavity that is characteristically reported as a "snowstorm" appearance of mixed echogenicity, representing hydropic villi and intrauterine hemorrhage.

early growth restriction or developmental abnormalities. There may be only scattered cystic spaces within the placenta, and ovarian cystic changes are usually much less pronounced. When there is diagnostic doubt, the scan should be repeated in 1 to 2 weeks.

The quantitative serum βhCG level is higher than expected in women with a complete mole, often exceeding 100,000 IU/L. This is much less likely in women with a partial mole; in these women, the level is often within the wide range associated with normal pregnancy. Partly as a result of the less elevated βhCG levels, the symptoms and signs of a partial mole are often delayed and mild enough to be missed. These women more often have a missed miscarriage or a spontaneous miscarriage, with the passage of a recognized fetus. The diagnosis of a partial mole is often missed clinically and is frequently made from subsequent histologic assessment of the products of conception. The clinical and pathologic differences between complete and partial hydatidiform moles are summarized in Table 4–7.

Investigations

Investigations directed at disease assessment include a complete blood count, measurement of creatinine and electrolytes, liver function tests, thyroid function tests, and a baseline quantitative βhCG measurement. A careful pelvic and abdominal ultrasound scan should be done to look for evidence of an invasive mole, exclude a coexisting pregnancy, and look for possible metastatic disease. Computed tomography or magnetic resonance imaging of the abdomen and pelvis may provide supplementary information. Chest radiography or computed tomography should be considered if there are symptoms that suggest pulmonary metastases. Computed tomography or magnetic resonance imaging of the brain should also be considered. If cerebrospinal metastases are suspected despite normal findings on imaging, a lumbar puncture may be done to measure βhCG levels in the cerebrospinal fluid. A plasma-to-cerebrospinal fluid ratio for βhCG of greater than 1:60 is strongly suggestive of occult cerebral metastases.[108,109]

Studies that relate to the prognosis include the ABO and Rhesus blood type of the woman and her partner, the ethnic origin of both partners, and a careful history of previous pregnancies and the duration of sex-steroid use by the woman.

TABLE 4–7

Clinical and Pathologic Differences between Complete and Partial Hydatidiform Moles

	COMPLETE MOLE	PARTIAL MOLE
Clinical		
Symptoms	Often severe and early	Often mild, similar to miscarriage
Diagnosis	Usually suspected from clinical and ultrasound features	Often missed clinically and diagnosed histologically from conception products
Persistent trophoblastic disease or tumor	8% of cases	0.5% of cases
Pathologic		
Macroscopic appearance	Grapelike vesicles often recognized; no fetal tissues	Often normal or suspected hydropic miscarriage; fetal tissue may be seen
Microscopic appearance	Diffuse hydropic villi; trophoblastic proliferation	Focal hydropic villi; variable mild trophoblastic proliferation; often focal; microscopic diagnosis sometimes difficult
Karyotype	Usually diploid; paternal chromosomes only	Usually triploid; diploid paternal and haploid maternal contribution

Risks

Risks include hemorrhage, persistent trophoblastic disease, malignant changes, psychological problems related to the loss of pregnancy, and the risks and need for follow-up of persistent or malignant disease.

Management Options

An algorithm for the management of GTD is shown in Figure 4–6.

Evacuation of Molar Pregnancy

Complete and partial molar pregnancies are managed differently.

Suction curettage is the method of choice for uterine evacuation of complete molar pregnancies. A suction catheter of up to 12 mm in diameter is usually sufficient because of the absence of fetal parts. It is best to avoid prior cervical preparation, the routine use of patient oxytocic drugs and sharp curettage, or medical evacuation with a complete mole, to minimize the risk of

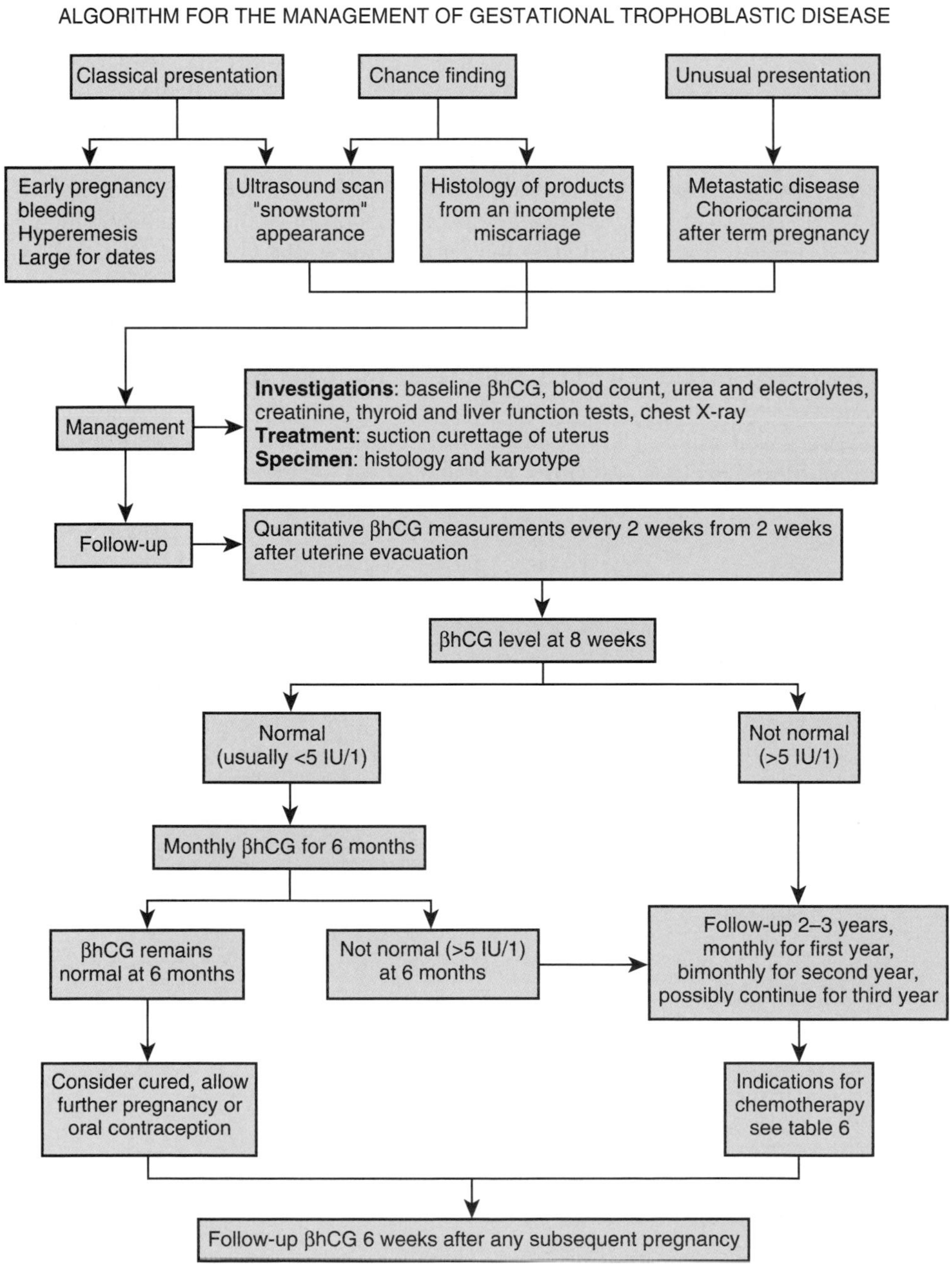

FIGURE 4–6
Algorithm for the management of gestational trophoblastic disease.

dissemination of tissue leading to metastatic disease.[110,111] Oxytocic agents and prostaglandin analogues are best used only after uterine evacuation when there is significant hemorrhage.

In partial molar pregnancies that are recognized before uterine evacuation, suction curettage is the method of choice. However, when pregnancy is more advanced and the size of any fetal parts may reduce the chance of complete suction evacuation, medical termination can be used.

Total abdominal hysterectomy, with the molar pregnancy in situ, can be considered for older women whose families are complete. This approach reduces the risk of persistent trophoblastic disease by up to 50%.[112]

Follow-up After Uterine Evacuation

The aims of follow-up are to confirm successful treatment and to identify women with persistent or malignant GTD who may require adjuvant chemotherapy or surgery at an early stage. Persistent clinical symptoms, particularly vaginal bleeding, and continuing elevation of serum βhCG levels are the main indicators of residual disease. The approach to follow-up and the criteria for initiating chemotherapy vary around the world. The most effective systems are based on regional or national registries that involve experienced specialist oncologists.

Clinical follow-up and βhCG surveillance after uterine evacuation of a molar pregnancy vary in different countries and according to the different prognosis for persistent or malignant GTD between complete and partial hydatidiform moles. The clinical course for women who have had a partial hydatidiform mole is almost always benign after uterine evacuation. Persistent disease occurs in 1.2% to 4% of cases. Metastatic disease occurs in only 0.1% of cases.[113,114] In complete moles, these risks are approximately five times greater after treatment with uterine evacuation and two to three times greater after treatment with hysterectomy.[112,115] The risk of persistent or recurrent GTD is greatest in the first 12 months after evacuation, with most cases evident within 6 months.

In North America, current recommendations for surveillance after uterine evacuation of a molar pregnancy are for βhCG monitoring 48 hours after surgery and then weekly until three normal levels (<5 IU/L) have been obtained. Levels of βhCG are monitored at 2-week intervals for 3 months and monthly for 6 to 12 months for partial and complete molar pregnancies, respectively.

In the United Kingdom, there is a central registry for patients with molar pregnancies. Monitoring is supervised by a small number of screening centers. Monitoring of βhCG levels usually begins 2 weeks after uterine evacuation. The frequency and duration of monitoring is dependent on serum or urinary βhCG levels. With successful treatment by uterine evacuation alone, the serum βhCG level decreases to normal (<5 IU/L) after 8 weeks. Subsequent follow-up is usually by monthly serum or urinary βhCG monitoring for 6 months (for partial hydatidiform mole) or 12 months (for complete hydatidiform mole). If βhCG levels remain normal for 6 months, the risk of malignant GTD is very small, approximately 1:300, and the woman can consider a further pregnancy from that stage.[116]

Use of a combined oral contraceptive is best avoided until after the βhCG levels have returned to normal. Limited data suggest that this slows the rate of decrease of the βhCG level and may increase the risk of persistent GTD. However, the risk associated with an unplanned early pregnancy is greater, and the use of oral contraception is considered acceptable by some North American clinicians.[114,115]

Adjuvant chemotherapy may be required in approximately 10% of women after uterine evacuation. The indications for chemotherapy are shown in Table 4–8. The WHO scoring system uses a point score for different prognostic indicators, such as the woman's age, the hCG level, the ABO blood group of both partners, and the number and site of metastases. This allows the differentiation of women with low risk disease (who are usually treated with single-agent methotrexate and folinic acid rescue) from women with high risk disease (who require multiagent chemotherapy with etoposide, methotrexate, and actinomycin D [EMA], alternating with cyclophosphamide and vincristine [CO]).

After the completion of chemotherapy, serial βhCG measurements are usually assessed monthly for 1 year and then every 2 months for a second year. Cure rates are high, sometimes with additional salvage surgery, and more than 80% of women who wish to conceive are successful in achieving a pregnancy.[117] Monitoring of βhCG is advisable after any subsequent pregnancy, regardless of gestational age or outcome, to exclude recurrent GTD.

Women who have had a previous molar pregnancy should expect to have a normal chance of conception subsequently, even after chemotherapy. There is no evidence of an increase in the risk of fetal abnormalities, miscarriage, ectopic pregnancy, premature delivery, or stillbirth, compared with the normal population.[118–120]

In a subsequent pregnancy after chemotherapy for GTD, an ultrasound scan should be performed at 8 weeks' and 14 weeks' gestation. The risk of further GTD is 1.4% to 2.4%.[120] Monitoring of βhCG levels should be performed 6 weeks and 3 months after delivery.

TABLE 4–8

Indications for Adjuvant Chemotherapy in Gestational Trophoblastic Disease

Serum βhCG levels >20,000 IU/L more than 4 weeks after uterine evacuation
Static or rising βhCG levels at any time after uterine evacuation
Increased βhCG level 6 months after uterine evacuation
Metastases in liver, lung, brain, or gastrointestinal tract
Histologic diagnosis of choriocarcinoma

SUMMARY OF MANAGEMENT OPTIONS

Gestational Trophoblastic Disease

Management Options	Quality of Evidence	Strength of Recommendation	References
Presentation			
Complete moles cause more exaggerated symptoms and signs than partial moles.	III	B	121,122
Partial moles are often missed clinically and by ultrasound scan and are often diagnosed histologically after uterine evacuation of an incomplete miscarriage.			
Surgical Evacuation			
Primary treatment of choice for all moles	III	B	123
Suction curettage for uterine evacuation is safer than sharp curettage, particularly for evacuation of complete moles.	IIb	B	124
Oxytocics, cervical preparation, and medical termination are better avoided, particularly for evacuation of complete moles.	IV	C	116
Medical (for partial moles)			
Methotrexate	III	B	125
Actinomycin-D	III	B	125
Combination therapy	III	B	126,127
Follow-up			
If βhCG levels remain normal 8 weeks to 6 months after evacuation, a woman can be considered cured and further pregnancy allowed.	–	GPP	–
βhCG should be measured 6 weeks after any subsequent pregnancy because of the risk of further trophoblastic disease.	–	GPP	–

RHESUS PROPHYLAXIS

Guidelines from the Royal College of Obstetricians and Gynaecologists and the British Blood Transfusion Society[128] recommend that women who have a miscarriage after 12 weeks' gestation should be given anti-D. Between 12 and 20 weeks' gestation, a Kleihauer test to quantify fetomaternal hemorrhage is not required; treatment with 250 IU anti-D immunoglobulin is adequate.

For miscarriages and ectopic pregnancies earlier than 12 weeks' gestation, the evidence for decision-making is poor. There is general consensus that complete spontaneous miscarriages without surgical intervention do not require anti-D prophylaxis.[128] When surgical evacuation of the uterus is required, even before 12 weeks' gestation, it is associated with a higher chance of transfer of fetal cells to the maternal circulation.[129] Under these circumstances, 250 IU anti-D immunoglobulin should be given to all Rhesus-negative women.[130]

With a threatened miscarriage before 12 weeks' gestation, anti-D is generally not required. However, Rhesus prophylaxis may be prudent if the patient has very heavy bleeding or considerable abdominal pain. If a threatened miscarriage occurs later than 12 weeks, anti-D (≥ 250 IU) should be given. If bleeding is persistent, this may be repeated at intervals of no more than 6 weeks. The half-life of anti-D is 2 weeks. Prophylaxis may be needed at 2-week intervals if bleeding is heavy or if it is indicated by the results of a Kleihauer test.[128]

Most religious groups who have concerns about the use of blood products do not object to the use of anti-D prophylaxis.

If it is indicated, anti-D prophylaxis should be given within 72 hours of the sensitizing episode.[131] A 250-IU dose is sufficient for fetomaternal hemorrhage before 12 weeks' gestation. The use of anti-D immunoglobulin in Rhesus-negative women in later pregnancy is addressed in Chapter 14.

SUMMARY OF MANAGEMENT OPTIONS
Rhesus Prophylaxis

Management Options	Quality of Evidence	Strength of Recommendation	References
Bleeding associated with threatened miscarriage before 12 weeks gestation does not require anti-D.	IV	C	128
Anti-D is required for an incomplete miscarriage only when surgical evacuation is required.	III	B	130

CONCLUSIONS

- Complications, usually vaginal bleeding and pain, are more common in the first trimester than at any other stage of pregnancy.
- These symptoms may be dramatic, and quick assessment, accurate diagnosis, and prompt management are necessary to minimize maternal morbidity and mortality.
- When the symptoms are less acute, careful assessment with high-resolution ultrasound and serum βhCG measurements is critical.
- TV USS and βhCG together usually allow the differentiation of a normal, viable intrauterine pregnancy from the complications of miscarriage, ectopic pregnancy, and hydatidiform mole.
- Management considers the woman's future reproductive expectations. In the case of hydatidiform mole, other specialists may need to be involved and longer-term follow-up may be required.

REFERENCES

1. Krause SA, Graves BW: Midwifery triage of first trimester bleeding. J Nurse Midwifery 1999;44:537–548.
2. Zinaman MJ, Clegg DE, Brown CC, et al: Estimates of human fertility and pregnancy loss. Fertil Steril 1996;65:503–509.
3. Stabile I, Campbell S, Grudinskas JG: Ultrasonic assessment of complications during the first trimester of pregnancy. Lancet 1987;ii:1237–1240.
4. Department of Health: Why mothers die: Confidential enquiry into maternal deaths in the United Kingdom. In Drife J, Lewis G (eds): Norwich, UK: HMSO, 2001, pp 282.
5. Grimes DA: The morbidity and mortality of pregnancy: Still a risky business. Am J Obstet Gynecol 1994;170:1489–1494.
6. Stirtzinger R, Robinson GE: The psychological effects of spontaneous abortion. Can Med Assoc J 1989;140:799–806.
7. Frost M, Condon JT: The psychological sequelae of miscarriage: A critical review of the literature. Aust N Z J Psychiatry 1996;30:54–62.
8. Furneaux EC, Langley-Evans AJ, Langley-Evans SC: Nausea and vomiting of pregnancy: Endocrine basis and contribution to pregnancy outcome. Obstet Gynecol Surv 2001;56:775–782.
9. Weigel MM, Weigel RM: Nausea and vomiting of pregnancy and pregnancy outcome: An epidemiological study. Br J Obstet Gynaecol 1989;96:1304–1311.
10. Regan L, Braude PB, Trembath PL: Influence of past reproductive performance on risk of spontaneous abortion. BMJ 1989;299:541–545.
11. Knudsen UB, Hansen V, Juul S, Secher NJ: Prognosis of a new pregnancy following previous spontaneous abortions. Eur J Obstet Gynecol Reprod Biol 1991;39:31–36.
12. Canis M, Wattiez A, Bruhat M: Multifunctional analysis or fertility after conservative laparoscopic treatment of ectopic pregnancy in a series of 223 patients. Fertil Steril 1991;56:453–460.
13. Semer DA, Macfee MS: Gestational trophoblastic disease: Epidemiology. Semin Oncol 1995;22:109–112.
14. Peckham CH: Uterine bleeding during pregnancy. Obstet Gynecol 1970;78:14–18.
15. Grobman WA, Peaceman AM: What are the rates and mechanisms of first and second trimester pregnancy loss in twins? Clin Obstet Gynecol 1998;41:37–45.
16. Lindsay DJ, Lovett IS, Lyons EA, et al: Yolk sac diameter and shape at endovaginal ultrasound: Predictors of pregnancy. Radiology 1992;183:115–118.
17. Nyberg DA, Filly RA, Mahony BS, et al: Early gestation: Correlation of HCG levels and sonographic identification. Am J Roentgenol 1985;144:951–954.
18. Mills MS: Ultrasonography of Early Embryonic Growth and Fetal Development [thesis]. University of Bristol, UK, 1992, p 358.
19. Jouppila P, Huhtaniemi I, Tapanainen J: Early pregnancy failure: Study by ultrasonic and hormonal methods. Obstet Gynaecol 1980;55:42–47.
20. Wilson RD, Kendrick V, Wittman BK, McGillivary B: Spontaneous abortion and pregnancy outcome after normal first trimester ultrasound examination. Obstet Gynecol 1986;67:352–355.
21. Merchiers EH, Dhont M, De Sutter PA, et al: Predictive value of early embryonic cardiac activity for pregnancy outcome. Am J Obstet Gynecol 1991;165:11–14.

22. Ankum WM, Van der Veen F, Hamerlynck JV, Lammes FB: Laparoscopy: A dispensable tool in the diagnosis of ectopic pregnancy? Hum Reprod 1993;8:1301–1306.
23. Kadar N, DeVore G, Romero R: Discriminatory hCG zone: Its use in the sonographic evaluation for ectopic pregnancy. Obstet Gynecol 1981;58:156–161.
24. Regan L, Rai R: Epidemiology and the medical causes of miscarriage. Best Pract Res Clin Obstet Gynaecol 2000;14:839–854.
25. Stovall TG, Ling FW, Carson SA, Buster JE: Serum progesterone and uterine curettage in differential diagnosis of ectopic pregnancy. Fertil Steril 1992;57:456–458.
26. Hollander HJ: Estimation of gestational age by mean gestational sac diameter. Ultraschalldiagnostik Schwangerschaft 1972:47–53.
27. Robinson HP, Shaw-Dunn J: Fetal heart rates as determined by sonar in early pregnancy. J Obstet Gynaecol Br Commonw 1973;80:805–809.
28. Hutchon DJR, Cooper S: Terminology for early pregnancy loss must be changed. BMJ 1998;317:1081.
29. WHO: Spontaneous and Induced Abortions. Geneva, World Health Organization, 1970.
30. Norwitz ER, Schorge JO: Ectopic pregnancy. In Norwitz ER, Schorge JD: Obstetrics and Gynecology at a Glance. Oxford, Blackwell, 2001, pp 14–15.
31. Bigrigg MA, Read MD: Management of women referred to early pregnancy assessment unit: Care and cost effectiveness. BMJ 1991;302:577–579.
32. Chard T: Frequency of implantation and early pregnancy loss in natural cycles. Baillieres Clin Obstet Gynaecol 1991;5:179–189.
33. Macklon NS, Geraedts JP, Fauser BC: Conception to ongoing pregnancy: The 'black box' of early pregnancy loss. Hum Reprod Update 2002;8:333–343.
34. Everett C: Incidence and outcome of bleeding before the 20th week of pregnancy: Prospective study from general practice. BMJ 1997;315:32–34.
35. Wilcox AJ, Weinberg CR, O'Connor JF, et al: Incidence of early loss of pregnancy. N Engl J Med 1988;319:189–194.
36. Pandya PP, Snijders RJ, Psara N, et al: The prevalence of non-viable pregnancy at 10-13 weeks of gestation. Ultrasound Obstet Gynecol 1996;7:170–173.
37. Forna F, Gulmezoglu AM: Surgical procedures to evacuate incomplete abortion: Cochrane Review. Cochrane Library, issue 1, 2003. Oxford, Update Software.
38. Wieringa-de Waard M, Hartman EE, Ankum WM, et al: Expectant management versus surgical evacuation in first trimester miscarriage: Health-related quality of life in randomized and non-randomized patients. Hum Reprod 2002;17:1638–1642.
39. Ankum WM, Wieringa-de Waard M, Bindels PJE: Management of spontaneous miscarriage in the first trimester: An example of putting informed shared decision making into practice. BMJ 2001;322:1343–1346.
40. Chipchase J, James D: Randomised trial of expectant versus surgical management of spontaneous miscarriage. Br J Obstet Gynaecol 1997;104:840–841.
41. Jurkovic D: Modern management of miscarriage: Is there a place for non-surgical treatment? Ultrasound Obstet Gynecol 1998;11:161–163.
42. Nielsen S, Hahlin M, Platz-Christensen J: Randomised trial comparing expectant with medical management for first trimester miscarriages. Br J Obstet Gynaecol 1999;106:804–807.
43. Wagaarachchi PT, Ashok PW, Narvekar N, et al: Medical management of early fetal demise using a combination of mifepristone and misoprostol. Hum Reprod 2001;16:1849–1853.
44. Henshaw RC, Cooper K, El-Rafaey H, et al: Medical management of miscarriage: Non-surgical uterine evacuation of incomplete and inevitable spontaneous abortion. BMJ 1993;306:894–895.
45. Johnson N, Priestnall M, Marsay T, et al: A randomised trial evaluating pain and bleeding after a first trimester miscarriage treated surgically or medically. Eur J Obstet Gynecol Reprod Biol 1997;72:213–215.
46. Chung T, Leung P, Cheung LP, et al: A medical approach to management of spontaneous abortion using misoprostol: Extending misoprostol treatment to a maximum of 48 hours can further improve evacuation of retained products of conception in spontaenous abortion. Acta Obstet Gynecol Scand 1997;76:248–251.
47. Chung TK, Lee DT, Cheung LP, et al: Spontaneous abortion: a randomized, controlled trial comparing surgical evacuation with conservative management using misoprostol. Fertil Steril 1999;71:1054–1059.
48. Ngai SW, Chan YM, Tang OS, Chung Ho P: Vaginal misoprostol as medical treatment for first trimester spontaneous miscarriage. Hum Reprod 2001;16:1493–1496.
49. Chung TK, Cheung LP, Sahota DS, et al: Spontaneous abortion: Short-term complications following either conservative or surgical management. Aust N Z J Obstet Gynaecol 1998;38:61–64.
50. Luise CL, Jermy K, May C, et al: Outcome of expectant management of spontaneous first trimester miscarriage: Observational study. BMJ 2002;324:873–875.
51. Luise C, Jermy K, Collins WP, Bourne TH: Expectant management of incomplete, spontaneous first-trimester miscarriage: Outcome according to initial ultrasound criteria and value of follow-up visits. Ultrasound Obstet Gynecol 2002;19:580–582.
52. Gronlund L, Gronlund A-L, Clevin L, et al: Spontaneous abortion: Expectant management, medical treatment or surgical evacuation. Acta Obstet Gynecol Scand 2002;81:781–782.
53. Kaplan B, Pardo J, Rabinerson D, et al: Future fertility following conservative management of complete abortion. Hum Reprod 1996;11:92–94.
54. Child TJ, Thomas J, Rees M, MacKenzie IZ: A comparative study of surgical and medical procedures: 932 pregnancy terminations up to 63 days gestation. Hum Reprod 2001;16:67–71.
55. Hurd WW, Whitfield RR, Randolph JF, Kercher ML: Expectant management versus elective curettage for the treatment of spontaneous abortion. Fertil Steril 1997;68:601–606.
56. RCOG: Recommendations from the study group on problems in early pregnancy: Advances in diagnosis and management. London, RCOG, 1997, p 8.
57. Schwarzler P, Holden D, Nielson S, et al: The conservative management of first trimester miscarriages and the use of colour Doppler sonography for patient selection. Hum Reprod 1999;14:1341–1345.
58. Prieto JA, Eriksen NL, Blanco JD: A randomised trial of prophylactic doxycycline for curettage in incomplete abortion. Obstet Gynecol 1995;85:692–696.
59. Geyman JP, Oliver LM, Sullivan SD: Expectant, medical, or surgical treatment of spontaneous abortion in first trimester of pregnancy? A pooled quantitative literature evaluation. J Am Board Fam Pract 1999;12:55–64.
60. Creinin MD, Schwartz JL, Pymar HC, Fink W: Efficacy of mifepristone followed on the same day by misoprostol for early termination of pregnancy: A report of a randomised trial. Br J Obstet Gynaecol 2001;108:469–473.
61. Autry A, Jacobson G, Sandhu R, Isbill K: Medical management of non-viable early first trimester pregnancy. Int J Gynaecol Obstet 1999;67:9–13.
62. Blohm F, Nielsen S, Hahlin M, Milsom I: Fertility after a randomised trial of spontaneous abortion managed by surgical evacuation or expectant treatment. Lancet 1997;349:995.
63. Herabutya Y, Prasertawat O: Misoprostol in the management of missed abortion. Int J Gynaecol Obstet 1997;56:263–266.
64. Lee DTS, Cheung LP, Haines CJ, et al: A comparison of the psychological impact and client satisfaction of surgical treatment with medical treatment of spontaneous abortion: A randomized controlled trial. Am J Obstet Gynaecol 2001;185:953–958.
65. Speroff L, Glass RH, Kase NG: Ectopic pregnancy. In Speroff L, Glass RH, Kase NG (eds): Clinical Gynecological Endocrinology

and Infertility, 6th ed. Baltimore, Williams & Wilkins, 1999, pp 1149–1168.
66. Ling FW, Stovall TG: Update on the diagnosis and management of ectopic pregnancy. In Rock J (ed): Advances in Obstetrics and Gynecology. Chicago, Mosby, 1994, pp 55–83.
67. Lipscomb GH, Stovall TG, Ling FW: Nonsurgical treatment of ectopic pregnancy. N Engl J Med 2000;343:1325–1329.
68. Sau A, Hamilton-Fairley D: Nonsurgical diagnosis and management of ectopic pregnancy. Obstet Gynaecol 2003;5:29–33.
69. Trio D, Strobelt N, Picciolo C, et al: Prognostic factors for successful expectant management of ectopic pregnancy. Fertil Steril 1995;63:469–472.
70. Banerjee S, Aslam N, Woelfer B, et al: Expectant management of early pregnancies of unknown location: A prospective evaluation of methods to predict spontaneous resolution of pregnancy. Br J Obstet Gynaecol 2001;108:158–163.
71. Korhonen J, Stenman UH, Ylostalo P: Serum human chorionic gonadotropin dynamics during spontaneous resolution of ectopic pregnancy. Fertil Steril 1994;61:632–636.
72. Fernandez H, Bourget P, Ville Y, et al: Treatment of unruptured tubal pregnancy with methotrexate: Pharmacokinetic analysis of local versus intramuscular administration. Fertil Steril 1994;62:943–947.
73. Tanaka T, Hayashi H, Kutsuzawa T, et al: Treatment of interstitial ectopic pregnancy with methotrexate: Report of a successful case. Fertil Steril 1982;37:851–852.
74. Lipscomb GH, McCord ML, Stovall TG, et al: Predictors of success of methotrexate treatment in women with tubal ectopic pregnancies. N Engl J Med 1999;341:1974–1978.
75. Fernandez H, Capella-Allouc Yves Vincent S, Pauthier S, et al: Randomized trial of conservative laparoscopic treatment and methotrexate administration in ectopic pregnancy and subsequent fertility. Hum Reprod 1998;13:3239–3243.
76. Yao M, Tulandi T: Current status of surgical and nonsurgical management of ectopic pregnancy. Fertil Steril 1997;67: 421–433.
77. RCOG: The management of tubal pregnancies. London, RCOG, 1999, p 8.
78. Sau AK, Sau M: Can we offer completely non-surgical management for ectopic pregnancy? BMJ 2000;322:793–794.
79. Hajenius PJ, Mol BWJ, Bossuyt PMM, et al: Interventions for tubal ectopic pregnancy: Cochrane Review. Cochrane Library, issue 2, 2003. Oxford, Update Software.
80. Carson SA, Buster JE: Ectopic pregnancy. N Engl J Med 1993;329:1174–1181.
81. Dubuisson JB, Morice P, Chapron C, et al: Salpingectomy: The laparoscopic surgical choice for ectopic pregnancy. Hum Reprod 1996;11:1199–1203.
82. Mol BW, Hajenius PJ, Engelsbel S, et al: Is conservative surgery for tubal pregnancy preferable to salpingectomy? An economic analysis. Br J Obstet Gynaecol 1997;104:834–839.
83. Clausen I: Conservative versus radical surgery for tubal pregnancy: A review. Acta Obstet Gynecol Scand 1996;75:8–12.
84. Gray DT, Thorburn J, Lundorff P, Lindblom B: Laparoscopic treatment of ectopic pregnancy. Lancet 1995;346:706–707.
85. Ugur M, Yesilyurt H, Soysal S, Gokmen O: Prophylactic vasopressin during laparoscopic salpingotomy for ectopic pregnancy. J Am Assoc Gynecol Laparosc 1996;3:365–368.
86. Fedele L, Bianchi S, Tozzi L, et al: Intramesosalpingeal injection of oxytocin in conservative laparoscopic treatment for tubal pregnancy: Preliminary results. Hum Reprod 1998;13:3042–3044.
87. Pouly JL, Chapron C, Manhes H: Multifactorial analysis of fertility after conservative laparoscopic treatment of ectopic pregnancy in a series of 223 patients. Fertil Steril 1991;56:453–460.
88. de la Cruz A, Cumming DC: Factors determining fertility after conservative or radical surgical treatment for ectopic pregnancy. Fertil Steril 1997;68:871–874.
89. Ego A, Subtil D, Cosson M, et al: Survival analysis of fertility after ectopic pregnancy. Fertil Steril 2001;75:560–566.
90. Job-Spira N, Fernandez H, Bouyer J, et al: Ruptured tubal ectopic pregnancy: Risk factors and reproductive outcome. Results of a population-based study in France. Am J Obstet Gynecol 1999;180:938–944.
91. Mol BW, Matthijsse HC, Tinga DJ, et al: Fertility after conservative and radical surgery for tubal pregnancy. Hum Reprod 1998;13:1804–1809.
92. Korhonen J, Stenman UH, Ylostalo P: Low-dose oral methotrexate with expectant management of ectopic pregnancy. Obstet Gynecol 1996;88:775–778.
93. Lang PF, Makinen JI, Irjala KM, et al: Laparoscopic instillation of hyperosmolar glucose vs. expectant management of tubal pregnancies with serum hCG ≤ 2500 mIU/mL. Acta Obstet Gynecol Scand 1997;76:797–800.
94. Laatikainen T, Tuomivaara L, Kaar K: Comparison of a local injection of hyperosmolar glucose solution with salpingotomy for the conservative treatment of tubal pregnancy. Fertil Steril 1993;60:80–84.
95. Rose PG: Hydatidiform mole: Diagnosis and management. Semin Oncol 1995;22:149–156.
96. Bower M, Brock C, Fisher RA, et al: Gestational choriocarcinoma. Ann Oncol 1995;6:503–508.
97. Lage JM, Bagg A, Berchem GJ: Gestational trophoblastic diseases. Curr Opin Obstet Gynecol 1996;8:79–82.
98. Bagshawe KD, Dent J, Webb J: Hydatidiform mole in England and Wales 1973-1983. Lancet 1986;ii:673–677.
99. Palmer JR: Advances in the epidemiology of gestational trophoblastic disease. J Reprod Med 1994;39:155–162.
100. Kohorn EI: The new FIGO 2000 staging and risk factor scoring system for gestational trophoblastic disease: Description and critical assessment. Int J Gynecol Cancer 2001;II:73–77.
101. Kim SJ: Gestational trophoblastic disease. In Hancock BW, Newlands ES, Berkowitz RS (eds): London, Chapman and Hall, 1997, pp 27–42.
102. Sebire NJ, Foskett M, Fisher RA, et al: Risk of partial and complete hydatidiform molar pregnancy in relation to maternal age. Br J Obstet Gynecol 2002;109:99–102.
103. Bracken MB: Incidence and aetiology of hydatidiform mole: An epidemiological review. Br J Obstet Gynecol 1987;94: 1123–1135.
104. Sebire NJ, Fisher RA, Fockett M, et al: Risk of recurrent hydatidiform mole and subsequent pregnancy outcome following complete or partial hydatidiform molar pregnancy. Br J Obstet Gynecol 2003;110:22–26.
105. Petignat P, Billieux MH, Blouin JL, et al: Is genetic analysis useful in the routine management of hydatidiform mole? Hum Reprod 2003;18:243–249.
106. Fryns JP, Van de Kerckhove A, Goddeeris P, Van den Berghe H: Unusually long survival in a case of full triploidy of maternal origin. Hum Genet 1977;38:147–155.
107. Seckl MJ, Fisher RA, Salerno G, et al: Choriocarcinoma and partial hydatidiform moles. Lancet 2000;356:36–39.
108. Bagshawe KD, Harland S: Immunodiagnosis and monitoring of gonadotrophin-producing metastases in the central nervous system. Cancer 1976;38:112–118.
109. Shapter AP, McLellan R: Gestational trophoblastic disease. Obstet Gynecol Clin North Am 2001;28:805–817.
110. Stone M, Bagshawe KD: An analysis of the influence of maternal age, gestational age, contraceptive method and mode of primary treatment of patients with hydatidiform moles on the incidence of subsequent chemotherapy. Br J Obstet Gynaecol 1979;86:782–792.
111. Gillespie AM, Tidy J, Bright N, et al: Primary gynaecological management of gestational trophoblastic tumours and the subsequent development of persistent trophoblastic disease. Br J Obstet Gynecol 1998;107 (suppl 17): 95.
112. Bahar AM, el-Ashnehi MS, Senthilselvan A: Hydatidiform mole in the elderly: Hysterectomy or evacuation? Int J Gynaecol Obstet 1989;29:233–238.

113. Tidy JA, Gillespie AM, Bright N, et al: Gestational trophoblastic disease: A study of mode of evacuation and subsequent need for treatment with chemotherapy. Gynecologic Oncol 2000;78: 309–312.
114. Hancock BW, Tidy JA: Current management of molar pregnancy. J Reprod Med 2002;47:347–354.
115. Curry SL, Hammond CB, Tyrey L, et al: Hydatidiform mole: Diagnosis, management, and long-term follow up of 347 patients. Obstet Gynaecol 1975;45:1–8.
116. RCOG: The management of gestational trophoblastic disease. London, RCOG (Guideline 18), 1999.
117. Berkowitz RS, Goldstein DP: Chorionic tumours. N Engl J Med 1996;335:1740–1748.
118. Lurain JR, Sand PK, Carson SA, Brewer JI: Pregnancy outcome subsequent to consecutive hydatidiform moles. Am J Obstet Gynecol 1982;142:1060–1061.
119. Berkowitz RS, Goldstein DP, Bernstein MR, Sablinska B: Subsequent pregnancy outcomes in patients with molar pregnancies and gestational trophoblastic tumours. J Reprod Med 1987;32:680–684.
120. Garner EIO, Lipson E, Bernstein MR, et al: Subsequent pregnancy experience in patients with molar pregnancy and gestational trophoblastic tumor. J Reprod Med 2002;47:380–386.
121. Szulman AE: Trophoblastic disease: Clinical pathology of hydatidiform moles. Obstet Gynaecol Clin N Am 1988;15: 433–456.
122. Jauniaux E, Kadri R, Hustin J: Partial mole and triploidy: Screening patients with first trimester spontaneous abortion. Obstet Gynaecol 1996;88:616–619.
123. Horn LC, Bilek K: Clinicopathologic analysis of gestational trophoblastic disease: Report of 158 cases. Gen Diagn Pathol 1997;143:173–178.
124. Schlaerth AB, Morrow CP, Rodriguez M: Diagnostic and therapeutic curettage in gestational trophoblastic disease. Am J Obstet Gynecol 1990;162:1465–1471.
125. Matsui H, Iitsuka Y, Seki K, Sekiya S: Comparison of chemotherapies with methotrexate, VP-16 and actinomycin-D in low-risk gestational trophoblastic disease: Remission rates and drug toxicities. Gynecol Obstet Invest 1998;46:5–8.
126. Newlands ES, Bower M, Holden L, et al: Management of resistant gestational trophoblastic tumors. J Reprod Med 1998;43: 111–118.
127. Dobson LS, Lorigan PC, Coleman RE, Hancock BW: Persistent gestational trophoblastic disease: Results of MEA (methotrexate, etoposide and dactinomycin) as first-line chemotherapy in high risk disease and EA (etoposide and dactinomycin) as second-line therapy for low risk disease. Br J Cancer 2000;82:1547–1552.
128. Robson SC, Lee D, Urbaniak S: Anti-D immunoglobulin in RhD prophylaxis. Br J Obstet Gynaecol 1998;105:1091–1094.
129. Matthews CD, Matthews AE: Transplacental haemorrhages in spontaneous and induced abortion. Lancet 1969;1:694–695.
130. RCOG: The management of early pregnancy loss. London, RCOG, 2000, p 8.
131. Murphy KW, Whitfield CR: Rhesus disease in this decade. Contemp Rev Obstet Gynaecol 1994;6:61–67.

CHAPTER 5

Recurrent Miscarriage

May Backos / Lesley Regan

INTRODUCTION

Miscarriage is the most common complication of pregnancy. Approximately 50% of all conceptions[1] and 15% of all recognized pregnancies[2] result in miscarriage. The World Health Organization[3] defined miscarriage as the "expulsion or extraction from its mother of an embryo or fetus weighing 500 g or less." The more accepted definition of miscarriage is "spontaneous expulsion of the conceptus before viability has been achieved."

Recurrent miscarriage, which is defined as the loss of three or more consecutive pregnancies, affects 1% of couples who are trying to achieve a successful pregnancy.[4] Because the incidence of recurrent miscarriage is higher than that expected by chance alone (0.34%),[5,6] a proportion of couples with recurrent miscarriage have a persistent underlying cause for their pregnancy losses. Careful studies are needed to identify potentially treatable factors. Most clinicians agree that there is sufficient justification to initiate diagnostic evaluation of couples after three miscarriages. However, some argue that even two miscarriages warrant investigation because the possibility of finding an underlying causal factor is similar after two or three miscarriages (approximately 50%).[7] A further argument is that couples with two miscarriages should not be subjected to the trauma of another miscarriage before undergoing testing. The contrary argument is that most (80%) of these couples achieve a successful pregnancy outcome without undergoing stressful and expensive investigations.

RISK FACTORS FOR RECURRENT MISCARRIAGE

Recurrent miscarriage is a heterogeneous condition, and more than one factor may underlie recurrent pregnancy loss.

Epidemiologic Factors

Maternal Age

The risk of miscarriage increases with advancing maternal age, regardless of reproductive history, as a result of an age-related increase in chromosomally abnormal conceptions or a decline in uterine and ovarian function. A large prospective register linkage study[8] reported the following age-related risks of miscarriage in recognized pregnancies:

- 13.3% at 12 to 19 years
- 11.1% at 20 to 24 years
- 11.9% at 25 to 29 years
- 15% at 30 to 34 years
- 24.6% at 35 to 39 years
- 51% at 40 to 44 years
- 93.4% at 45 years or older

More recently, advanced paternal age was identified as a risk factor for miscarriage. A large multicenter European study[9] reported that the risk of miscarriage is highest for couples in which the woman is 35 years or older and the man is 40 years of age or older.

Reproductive History

Reproductive history is an independent predictor of future pregnancy outcome. The risk of a further miscarriage increases after each successive pregnancy loss, reaching approximately 40% after three consecutive pregnancy losses. A prospective study[2] concluded that a woman's risk of miscarriage can be quantified by her obstetric history. The single most important predictor is a previous miscarriage. For example, primigravidae and women with a history of live births have a 5% chance of miscarriage in their next pregnancy, a significantly lower risk than that in women whose last pregnancy ended in miscarriage (19%). Similarly, a large Danish study[10] in an unselected population reported a 10% risk of miscarriage in primigravidae. The risk increased to 15%, 24%, 43%, and 54% after one to four previous consecutive miscarriages, respectively. These observations may be partly explained by reproductive compensation. Women whose pregnancy ends in miscarriage tend to embark on more pregnancies at progressively later ages, until they achieve the desired family size. Data from populations with recurrent miscarriage suggest that a previous live birth does not preclude subsequent recurrent miscarriage.[11,12]

Genetic Factors

Chromosomal abnormalities of the embryo account for at least 50% of first-trimester sporadic miscarriages[13] and 29% to 57% of further miscarriages in couples with recurrent miscarriage.[14,15] However, most published studies used conventional cytogenetic analysis, which identifies only gross chromosomal aberrations. Conventional cytogenetic analysis depends on tissue culture before karyotyping and is limited by external contamination, culture failure, and selective growth of maternal cells.[16] More recently, analysis of miscarriage tissue by comparative genomic hybridization (a technique that detects chromosomal abnormalities without the need for culture) showed that conventional cytogenetic analysis underestimates the incidence of chromosomal anomalies and that the contribution of chromosomal abnormalities to first-trimester miscarriage is nearly 70%.[17]

Parental Chromosomal Rearrangement

In approximately 3% to 5% of couples with recurrent miscarriage, one partner carries a balanced structural chromosomal abnormality.[18,19] Women are more likely than men to carry most types of chromosomal rearrangements.[18] The most common types of parental chromosomal abnormalities are balanced translocations, either reciprocal or Robertsonian (Fig. 5–1). In reciprocal translocations, segments distal to breaks in two chromosomes are exchanged. In Robertsonian translocations, two acrocentric chromosomes fuse at the centromeric region, with loss of the short arms. Although carriers of a balanced translocation are usually phenotypically normal, their pregnancies are at increased risk for miscarriage and may result in a live birth of a child with multiple congenital malformations or mental handicaps because of an unbalanced chromosomal arrangement. The risk of miscarriage is affected by the size and genetic content of the rearranged chromosomal segments.

A less common chromosomal abnormality that may cause recurrent miscarriage is a chromosome inversion. This has been reported in 0.2% of couples with recurrent miscarriage.[18]

Embryonic Aneuploidy and Polyploidy

Aneuploidy is caused by nondisjunction during meiosis that leads to the production of an extra chromosome (trisomy) or the deletion of a chromosome (monosomy). Triploidy occurs when there is a complete set of extra chromosomes. This usually arises from fertilization of the oocyte by two spermatozoa or from failure of one of the maturation divisions of either the oocyte or the spermatozoon. Tetraploidy (four times the haploid number) is usually caused by failure to complete the first zygotic division. In couples with recurrent miscarriage, conventional cytogenetic analysis reports the incidence of trisomy, polyploidy, and monosomy X in miscarriage tissue as 30%, 9%, and 4%, respectively.[15] Most trisomies are the result of meiotic error as a result of advanced maternal age[20]; however, gonadal mosaicism and sperm aneuploidies also increase the risk of trisomic conceptions. The risk of sex chromosome monosomy and polyploidy conceptions do not increase with maternal age.[21]

Some couples with a history of recurrent miscarriage are at risk for recurrent aneuploidy. The embryonic karyotype in a previous pregnancy may help to predict the future miscarriage rate. Women with a previous normal

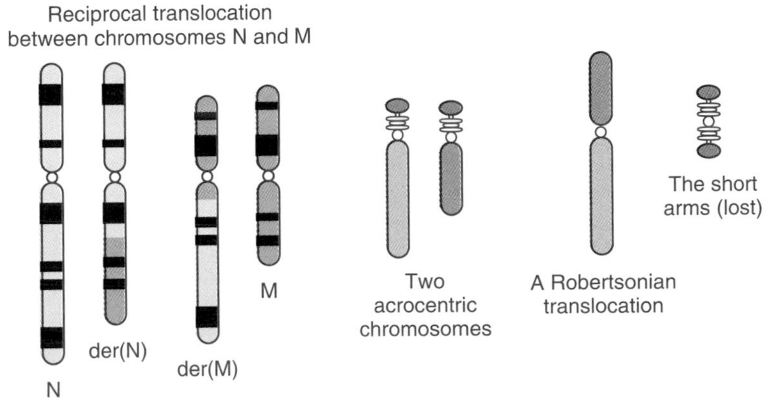

FIGURE 5–1
Parental chromosomal reciprocal and Robertsonian translocations. (Courtesy of Dr. Jonathan Wolfe, Department of Biology, Galton Laboratory, University College, London, UK.)

embryonic karyotype miscarry more frequently than those with an abnormal embryonic karyotype,[14,22] suggesting that mechanisms other than fetal chromosomal abnormalities may account for some cases of recurrent miscarriage.

Molecular Mechanisms

Recent advances in molecular genetic technology highlighted the importance of certain mechanisms, such as single-gene mutations and skewed X chromosome inactivation, in the etiology of pregnancy loss. The role of single-gene mutations, which cause abnormalities in embryonic, placental, or cardiac development, is the subject of current research.[23]

Skewed X chromosome inactivation (preferential expression of either the maternal or paternal X chromosome in most maternal cells) is significantly more common in women with recurrent miscarriage compared with control subjects.[24] These findings suggest that women with skewed X chromosome inactivation may carry an X-linked recessive fetal-lethal trait that makes them susceptible to recurrent miscarriage. Future research may identify the specific X-linked and autosomal genes that are linked to pregnancy loss.

Anatomic Disorders

Congenital Uterine Malformations

Congenital uterine malformations (Fig. 5–2) are the result of disturbances in müllerian duct development, fusion, canalization, and septal reabsorption. The contribution of congenital uterine anomalies to recurrent pregnancy loss is unclear because the true prevalence and reproductive implications of uterine anomalies in the general population are unknown. In patients with recurrent miscarriage, the reported frequency of uterine anomalies varies widely, from 1.8% to 37.6%.[25] This variability may reflect differences in the criteria and techniques used for diagnosis and the fact that available studies included women with two, three, or more miscarriages at both early and late stages of pregnancy. The prevalence of uterine anomalies is highest in women with a history of late miscarriages, which probably reflects the greater prevalence of cervical incompetence in women with uterine malformation.[26]

Using three-dimensional ultrasound as a diagnostic tool, a recent large prospective study[27] reported that the frequency of uterine anomalies was 23.8% in women with recurrent first-trimester miscarriage (three or more consecutive pregnancy losses) compared with a frequency of 5.3% in low-risk women who were referred

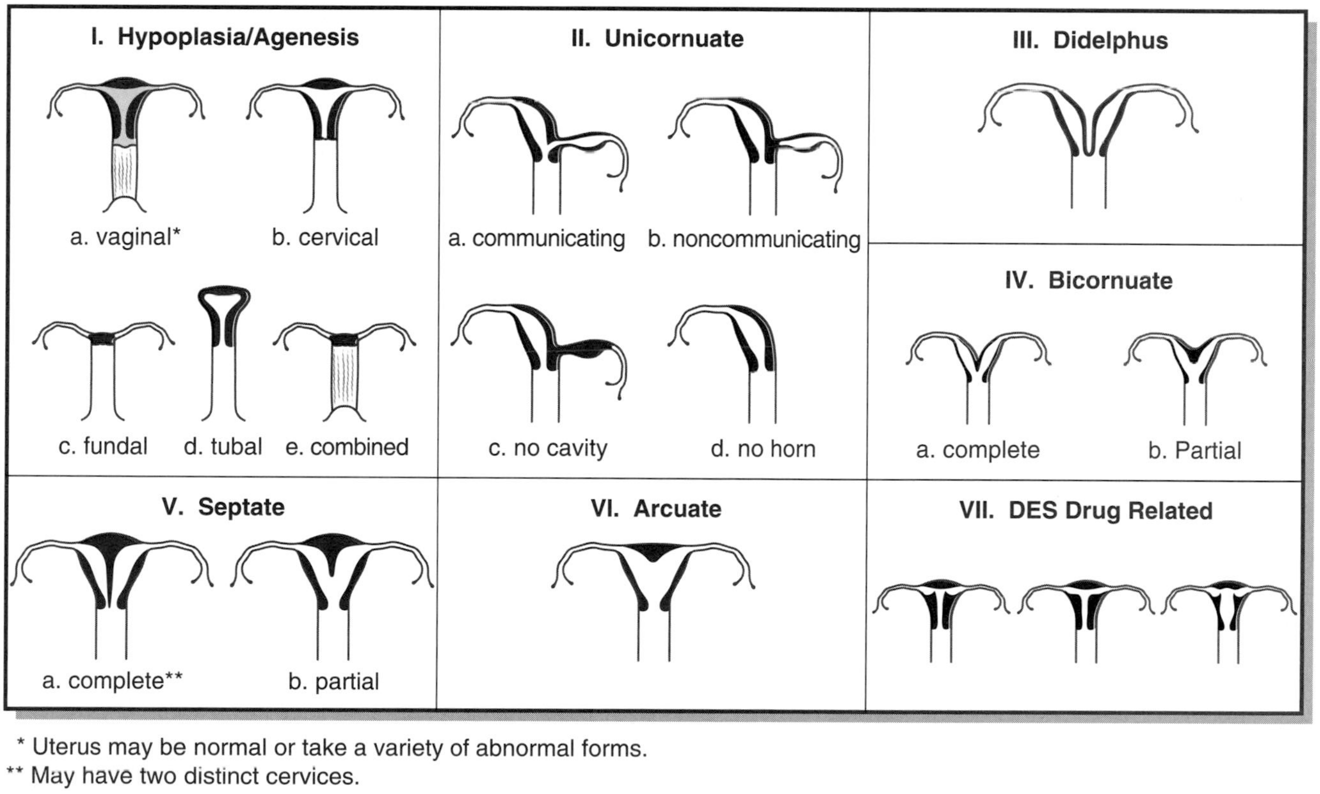

FIGURE 5–2
The American Society for Reproductive Medicine classification of müllerian anomalies. (From The American Fertility Society: The American Fertility Society Classification of adrenal adhesions, distal tubal occlusion, tubal occlusion secondary to tubal ligation, tubal pregnancies, müllerian anomalies and intauterine adhesions. Fertil Steril 1988;49:944–955. Reprinted by permission of the American Society for Reproductive Medicine.)

for ultrasound for a variety of reasons unrelated to reproductive outcome. Further, distortion of uterine anatomy was more severe in women with recurrent miscarriage. These findings suggest that congenital uterine anomalies may contribute to pregnancy loss in a small proportion of women with recurrent miscarriage.

A retrospective review[25] of reproductive performance in patients with untreated uterine anomalies suggested that these women have high rates of miscarriage and preterm delivery and a term delivery rate of only 50%. However, retrospective studies are biased by patient selection. Until well-controlled prospective data become available, the role of uterine anomalies in recurrent miscarriage will be debatable.

Cervical Incompetence

Cervical incompetence is a well-recognized cause of recurrent midtrimester miscarriage. It is defined as the inability to support a term pregnancy because of a functional or structural defect of the cervix. Cervical incompetence occurs along a spectrum of severity. Severe incompetence leads to midtrimester miscarriage, and lesser degrees underlie some cases of preterm delivery.[28] The true incidence of cervical incompetence is unknown, because the diagnosis is essentially clinical and there are no agreed objective criteria for the diagnosis. Crude estimates from epidemiologic studies suggest an approximate incidence of 0.5% in the general obstetric population[29] and 8% in women with previous midtrimester miscarriages.[30]

Although some cases involve mechanical incompetence, such as congenital hypoplastic cervix, previous cervical surgery, and extensive trauma, most women with a clinical diagnosis of cervical incompetence have normal cervical anatomy. When considered as a continuum, premature cervical ripening may represent a final common pathway of a variety of pathophysiologic processes, such as infection, colonization, inflammation, and hormonal or genetic predisposition.[31] The cervix is the main mechanical barrier separating the pregnancy from the vaginal bacterial flora. Many patients who have asymptomatic midtrimester cervical dilation have evidence of subclinical intrauterine infection.[32] It is unclear whether this high rate of microbial invasion is the result or the cause of premature cervical dilation. When premature cervical ripening occurs, the mechanical barrier is disrupted, which may further stimulate processes (e.g., colonization of the upper genital tract) that culminate in spontaneous preterm birth. When cervical incompetence is associated with mechanical weakness, supportive measures such as cerclage may prevent ascending infection and hence may prolong pregnancy. In contrast, if cervical changes result from nonmechanical processes, then cerclage would be less effective, and even harmful in some cases, because of possible inflammatory and infectious complications.

Fibroids

Uterine fibroids have long been associated with a variety of reproductive problems, including pregnancy loss. The extent of the association is affected by the size and location of the fibroids. Although the exact mechanisms are unclear, the presumed theories of pathophysiology include mechanical distortion of the uterine cavity, abnormal vascularization, abnormal endometrial development, endometrial inflammation, abnormal endocrine milieu, and structural and contractile myometrial abnormalities.[33] Evidence of the association between uterine fibroids and recurrent miscarriage is retrospective[34] and insufficient to determine differences in pregnancy outcome or assess the effect of the size and location of the fibroids. Recent data from patients with infertility suggest that only fibroids with a submucosal or an intracavitary component are associated with a reduced implantation rate and an increased rate of miscarriage.[35] Subserous fibroids have no deleterious effect, and the role of intramural fibroids that do not distort the cavity is controversial.[35–37]

Intrauterine Adhesions

Intrauterine adhesions (Asherman's syndrome, an acquired uterine defect of varying severity) result from intrauterine trauma after vigorous endometrial curettage or evacuation of retained products of conception. Intrauterine adhesions are associated with recurrent miscarriage. The presumed mechanisms are decreased uterine cavity volume and fibrosis and inflammation of the endometrium that predispose the patient to abnormal placentation and pregnancy loss. However, evidence of the association is mostly retrospective[38,39] and conflicting,[40] and no robust prospective evidence confirms a causal relationship.

Endocrine Factors

Luteal Phase Defect and Progesterone Deficiency

Luteal phase defect is an entity in which the corpus luteum is defective, with insufficient progesterone production resulting in retarded endometrial development. Because progesterone is necessary for successful implantation and the maintenance of early pregnancy, progesterone deficiency during the luteal phase is associated with recurrent miscarriage. However, standard diagnostic criteria required to assess the true incidence and effect of luteal phase defect as a cause of recurrent miscarriage are lacking. Diurnal variations and pulsatile secretion make serum progesterone measurements unreliable, and the interpretation of the results of endometrial biopsy is susceptible to sampling and interobserver variation.[41] Additionally, serum progesterone levels are not predictive of pregnancy outcome; low progesterone levels in early pregnancy appear to reflect a pregnancy that has already failed.

Moreover, no convincing studies show that treatment of luteal phase defect improves pregnancy outcome in women with recurrent miscarriage.[42,43]

Polycystic Ovary Syndrome, Hypersecretion of Luteinizing Hormone, and Hyperandrogenemia

Polycystic ovary syndrome (PCOS) is linked to infertility and miscarriage. Polycystic ovaries, a high luteinizing hormone (LH) level, and hyperandrogenemia are classic features of PCOS and have been reported as risk factors for recurrent miscarriage. Although polycystic ovaries are found significantly more often among women with recurrent miscarriage than among parous control subjects, polycystic ovaries themselves do not appear to predict future pregnancy outcome in ovulatory women with recurrent miscarriage.[44] A high level of LH or testosterone does not correlate with pregnancy outcome in ovulatory women with recurrent miscarriage.[45] Further, a prospective randomized placebo-controlled trial[46] reported that prepregnancy suppression of high LH does not improve the live birth rate, and the outcome of pregnancy in women in the placebo group was similar to that in women with a normal LH level.

More recently, the association between PCOS and insulin resistance leading to compensatory hyperinsulinemia has come under scrutiny as a risk factor for recurrent miscarriage. Insulin resistance is associated with a higher rate of miscarriage among women with PCOS undergoing ovulation induction compared with those who are not insulin resistant.[47] Preliminary reports[48,49] suggest that metformin treatment (which increases sensitivity to insulin) in women with PCOS during induction of ovulation and early pregnancy may improve endometrial receptivity and implantation and reduce the risk of future miscarriage. However, the role of insulin resistance and the effectiveness and safety of metformin in women with polycystic ovaries and recurrent miscarriage remain to be established in prospective controlled trials.

Systemic Endocrine Factors

Diabetes mellitus and thyroid disease are associated with miscarriage, but there is no direct evidence that they contribute to recurrent miscarriage. Women with diabetes who have high hemoglobin A_{1c} levels in the first trimester are at risk for miscarriage and fetal malformation.[50] In contrast, well-controlled diabetes mellitus is not a risk factor for recurrent miscarriage, nor is treated thyroid dysfunction.[51,52] The prevalence of diabetes mellitus and thyroid dysfunction in women with recurrent miscarriage is similar to that expected in the general population.[19,53,54]

Thyroid autoantibodies are not associated with recurrent miscarriage. Women with recurrent miscarriage are no more likely than fertile control subjects to have circulating thyroid antibodies.[55] The presence of thyroid antibodies in euthyroid women with a history of recurrent miscarriage does not affect future pregnancy outcome.[56]

Coagulation and Immunologic Factors

Thrombophilia

The hemostatic system plays an important role in the establishment and maintenance of pregnancy. A thrombophilic defect is an abnormality in the coagulation system that predisposes an individual to thrombosis. During the last few years, the role of antiphospholipid syndrome (APS), an acquired thrombophilic defect, has become an established and treatable cause of recurrent miscarriage and the potential role of other thrombophilic defects (acquired or inherited) has been explored. The presumed hypothesis is that some cases of recurrent miscarriage and later pregnancy complications are caused by an exaggerated hemostatic response during pregnancy, leading to thrombosis of the uteroplacental vasculature and subsequent fetal demise.

Antiphospholipid Antibodies

Antiphospholipid antibodies (aPLs) are a family of heterogeneous autoantibodies that react with epitopes on proteins that are complexed with negatively charged phospholipids. In the etiology of recurrent pregnancy loss, the two most clinically important aPLs are lupus anticoagulant and anticardiolipin antibodies.

APS is the association between aPLs and pregnancy morbidity or vascular thrombosis.[57] Pregnancy morbidity includes recurrent first-trimester miscarriage, one or more morphologically normal fetal deaths after the 10th week of gestation, and one or more preterm births before the 34th week of gestation as a result of severe preeclampsia, eclampsia, or placental insufficiency. APS in patients with chronic inflammatory diseases, such as systemic lupus erythematosus, is referred to as "secondary APS." In contrast, "primary APS" affects patients with no identifiable underlying systemic connective tissue disease.

A major characteristic of APS is recurrent miscarriage. In 15% of women with recurrent miscarriage, aPLs (lupus anticoagulant and anticardiolipin IgG or IgM antibodies) are present.[58] In comparison, the prevalence of aPLs in women with a low-risk obstetric history is less than 2%.[59] In untreated pregnancies, the chance of successful pregnancy outcome in women with aPLs is exceedingly poor and the live birth rate may be as low as 10%.[60] The mechanisms by which aPLs cause adverse pregnancy outcome are varied, reflecting in part their heterogeneity. Historically, the pathogenesis of aPL-related pregnancy loss focused on placental thrombosis.[61,62] However, thrombosis is neither specific nor universal, and recent research provides new insights into the mechanisms of aPL-related pregnancy failure. Defective decidualization of the endometrium and abnormal early trophoblastic function and differentiation may be the primary pathologic mechanisms.[63–66]

Inherited Thrombophilic Defects

Inherited thrombophilic defects are established causes of systemic thrombosis. These defects include activated protein C resistance (most commonly caused by the factor V Leiden [FVL] gene mutation); protein C, protein S, and antithrombin III deficiencies; hyperhomocysteinemia; and prothrombin gene mutation. Recently, these defects were reported to be associated with fetal loss and late pregnancy complications. Evidence of this association is largely retrospective, and prospective data are inadequate to prove a causal relationship. A recent meta-analysis[67] of pooled data from 31 retrospective studies suggested that the magnitude of the association between inherited thrombophilia and fetal loss varies according to the type of fetal loss and the type of thrombophilic disorder. In that meta-analysis, FVL mutation, an inherited activated protein C resistance, was associated with a history of both early and late recurrent fetal loss and late nonrecurrent fetal loss. Acquired activated protein C resistance was associated with early recurrent fetal loss, and the prothrombin gene mutation was associated with early recurrent and late nonrecurrent fetal loss. Protein S deficiency was associated with late nonrecurrent fetal loss. Methylenetetrahydrofolate mutation, protein C, and antithrombin III deficiencies were not significantly associated with fetal loss. However, because protein C and antithrombin III deficiencies are rare, the number of women available for study was too small to show a difference in pregnancy outcome.

Only one small prospective study[68] showed that women with recurrent miscarriage who carry the FVL mutation are at significantly increased risk for miscarriage compared with those with a normal factor V genotype. However, carrying the FVL mutation did not preclude an uncomplicated pregnancy delivered at term. No test can reliably discriminate between women with recurrent miscarriage and FVL mutation who are destined to miscarry and those who are destined to have a successful pregnancy.

Disorders of Maternofetal Alloimmune Relationships

The hypothesis that successful pregnancy depends on maternal immunologic tolerance of the fetus and that some cases of recurrent miscarriage result from failure of maternal alloimmune recognition of the pregnancy has not been substantiated. No alloimmune mechanisms have been shown unequivocally to cause recurrent miscarriage in humans. No clear evidence supports the hypothesis that HLA incompatibility between couples, the absence of maternal leukocytotoxic antibodies, or the absence of maternal blocking antibodies is related to recurrent miscarriage. These tests should no longer be offered routinely to women with recurrent miscarriage. The role of endometrial immunity in recurrent early pregnancy loss is under investigation. Immune effector cell dysfunction and defects in immunosuppressive factors, cytokines, and growth factors at the local maternofetal interface may be implicated in the pathogenesis of implantation failure and recurrent early pregnancy loss.[69,70] However, further studies are needed.

A Cochrane systematic review[71] found that various forms of immunotherapy, including paternal cell immunization, third-party donor leukocytes, trophoblast membranes, and intravenous immune globulin (IVIG), are of no benefit in women with unexplained recurrent miscarriage. Further, immunotherapy is expensive and has potentially serious side effects, including transfusion reaction, anaphylactic shock, and hepatitis, and it should no longer be offered to women with unexplained recurrent miscarriage outside the context of approved clinical research projects.[72]

Other Factors

Infections

The role of infection in recurrent miscarriage is weak. Any severe infection that leads to bacteremia or viremia can cause sporadic miscarriage. However, for an infective agent to be implicated in the etiology of repeated pregnancy loss, it must persist in the genital tract and avoid detection or cause insufficient symptoms to disturb the woman. Toxoplasmosis, rubella, cytomegalovirus, herpes, and *Listeria* infections do not fulfill these criteria.[73] Although bacterial vaginosis in the first trimester has been reported as a risk factor for second-trimester miscarriage and preterm delivery,[74] evidence of an association with first-trimester miscarriage is inconsistent.[75,76] In women with a history of midtrimester miscarriage or preterm birth, detection and treatment of bacterial vaginosis early in pregnancy may reduce the risk of preterm, prelabor rupture of the membranes and low birth weight, but it did not reduce the risk of preterm birth.[77] Whether this treatment improves neonatal outcome is unclear.

Environmental Factors

Most data on environmental risk factors concentrated on sporadic rather than recurrent miscarriage. The results have been conflicting and undoubtedly biased by difficulties in controlling for confounding factors, the inaccuracy of exposure data, and the measurement of toxin dose. Most studies[78] agree that maternal cigarette smoking is associated with a dose-dependent increased risk of spontaneous miscarriage. Interestingly, however, a recent study challenged these findings.[79] Heavy alcohol consumption is toxic to the embryo and the fetus. Even moderate consumption of five or more units* per week may increase the risk of sporadic miscarriage.[80] Caffeine consumption is associated with a dose-dependent increased risk of miscar-

*1 unit of alcohol is equal to approximately 8g of absolute alcohol, or one small glass of wine.

riage. The risk becomes significant when caffeine intake exceeds 300 mg (3 cups of coffee) daily.[79,81,82] Working with or using video display terminals does not increase the risk of miscarriage.[83] Evidence on the effect of anesthetic gases among theater workers is contradictory. Earlier studies suggested an increase in the risk of spontaneous miscarriage, but more recent studies have reported that exposure to waste anesthetic gases did not increase the risk of miscarriage among theater workers.[84,85]

Psychological Factors

Miscarriage is a stressful life event, and recurrent miscarriage may affect the patient's mental health. A recent study[86] indicated that 33% of women with recurrent miscarriage were clinically depressed, and 21% had levels of anxiety that were equal to or higher than those in typical psychiatric outpatient populations. Animal data[87] indicate that stress may induce miscarriage. A recent small prospective study[88] indicated that among 14 psychological parameters studied, only a high depression scale affected the miscarriage rate in women with a history of two previous miscarriages. Larger prospective studies are needed to address the scope of psychological disorders and their contribution to recurrent miscarriage.

MANAGEMENT OPTIONS

"Prepregnancy" When the Third Miscarriage Occurs

A detailed history of the previous miscarriages is important to identify the underlying etiology. When the third miscarriage occurs, it is important to consider the following factors:

- The underlying causes of first-trimester miscarriage are different from those responsible for midtrimester loss. Therefore, it is important to determine the accurate gestational age, confirmed by ultrasound wherever possible, when the miscarriage occurred.
- If a first-trimester miscarriage occurred, determine whether the loss was biochemical, anembryonic (blighted ovum), embryonic (6–8 weeks), or fetal (>8 weeks). Different pathologic factors affect the various stages of early pregnancy. For example, biochemical and anembryonic losses are more likely to be associated with chromosomally abnormal embryos.
- Note whether fetal heart activity was detected before the miscarriage. Most first-trimester miscarriages associated with APS occur after the establishment of fetal heart activity.
- When surgical evacuation of the products of conception is performed, it is important to document suspected uterine abnormalities, such as a bicornuate or subseptate uterus or fibroids. Tissue should be collected and sent for both histologic examination (to confirm the diagnosis and exclude trophoblastic disease) and fetal karyotype (Table 5–1).
- If a second-trimester miscarriage occurred, note whether the pregnancy loss was preceded by intrauterine fetal death, spontaneous rupture of the membranes, vaginal bleeding, painful uterine contractions, or painless cervical dilation. This information is particularly useful in identifying or excluding a presumed diagnosis of cervical incompetence. The couple should be encouraged to consent to a full fetal postmortem examination, fetal karyotyping, and placental histologic examination.
- Ensure that a follow-up appointment is scheduled for the couple.

TABLE 5–1

Chromosome Analysis of the Products of Conception: Tissue Collection

General	It is a good practice, and in some countries a legal requirement, to obtain patient consent before tissue collection for diagnostic testing. Ensure aseptic technique in tissue handling.
Collection: first-trimester miscarriage	Collect all fetal tissue and placental villi.
Collection: second-trimester miscarriage	Obtain a small sample of full-thickness fetal skin with subepidermal layers. It is important, particularly in cases of intrauterine fetal death and macerated fetus, that in addition to a fetal sample, a placental biopsy is also sent, because culturing of the fetal sample is often unsuccessful. The placental biopsy specimen should be a wedge from the cord insertion site and should include membranes.
Container	Use a sterile universal container containing sterile saline or transport media provided by the cytogenetic laboratory. Do not add formalin. The transport media should be regularly renewed.
Labeling	Record patient details, including name, date of birth, and hospital number on the sample container label. Include a completed referral form. The laboratory should be informed that the sample will be sent.
Transport and storage	Send samples to the laboratory immediately after collection. Transport them at room temperature. Sample can be refrigerated at 4°C if they are not sent until the next day. Do not freeze samples.
Causes for rejection	Samples may be rejected because of gross contamination, necrotic tissue, or the use of fixative.
Limitations	Some products of conception may contain only maternal tissue. Trophoblasts may contain mosaicisms or aneuploidy not present in the fetus.

Prepregnancy Assessment and Counseling after the Third Miscarriage

The loss of a pregnancy at any stage is a tragic event, and sensitivity is required in assessing and counseling couples with recurrent miscarriage. A dedicated recurrent miscarriage clinic is often a better environment in which to provide this care rather than a busy postnatal or general gynecologic clinic. Ideally, the couple should be seen together and given accurate information to facilitate decision-making about future pregnancies (see "Risk Factors for Recurrent Miscarriage"). When possible, the couple should be given written information to take home.

History

A comprehensive history should be obtained from both partners, noting their age and obstetric, gynecologic, medical, surgical, social, psychological, and family histories. Seeking the cooperation of the patient's family physician and other physicians may be necessary to obtain relevant information.

Physical Examination

The physical examination should include height, weight, blood pressure, and a general assessment of signs of endocrine disease. Pelvic examination should assess signs of previous cervical trauma or surgery, genital tract anomalies, and uterine size.

Investigation of Recurrent Miscarriage (Table 5–2)

Testing should include the following:

- Parental karyotyping of both partners is performed to determine abnormal chromosome rearrangements, translocations, or inversions.
- Two-dimensional pelvic ultrasound is performed to identify polycystic ovaries and assess the uterine anatomy. Suspected uterine anomalies may require further studies with hysterosalpingography, hysteroscopy, laparoscopy, or three-dimensional pelvic ultrasound.
- Early follicular phase (days 2–4 of cycle) LH, follicle-stimulating hormone, and testosterone levels are measured for evidence of LH hypersecretion, hyperandrogenemia, and possible high levels of follicle-stimulating hormone.
- All women with recurrent miscarriage should be screened for aPLs before pregnancy. The diagnosis of APS requires at least two positive test results 6 weeks apart of either lupus anticoagulant or anticardiolipin IgG or IgM antibodies in medium or high titers. Women with one positive test result and a second negative test result should have a third aPL test to confirm or refute the APS diagnosis. The detection of aPLs is subject to considerable interlaboratory variation because of temporal fluctuation of aPL titers in individual patients, transient positivity as a result of infection, suboptimal methods of sample collection and preparation, and lack of standardization of laboratory tests for their detection.[89] Therefore, laboratory assays should be performed according to international guidelines.[57] Because maternal aPLs may be down-regulated during pregnancy,[90] tests are best performed preconceptually. Testing for aPLs other than lupus anticoagulant or anticardiolipin antibodies is uninformative.[57] Although no single test detects all lupus anticoagulant, the dilute Russell viper venom time test, together with platelet neutralization, is more sensitive and specific than either the activated partial thromboplastin time or the kaolin clotting time test.[58] Anticardiolipin antibodies are detected with a standardized enzyme-linked immunosorbent assay.
- Screening for APC resistance should include coagulation tests for both unmodified and modified APC resistance and factor V genotyping with polymerase chain reaction.

TABLE 5–2

Investigation of Recurrent Miscarriage

All patients	Karyotype Parental Miscarried tissues (see Table 5–1) Pelvic ultrasound Early follicular phase luteinizing hormone, follicle-stimulating hormone, and testosterone Antiphospholipid antibodies Lupus anticoagulant and IgG and IgM anticardiolipin antibodies Activated protein C resistance Factor V Leiden gene mutation Serology for rubella Blood group and Rhesus type
Selected patients	HSG, hysteroscopy, and laparoscopy Three-dimensional pelvic ultrasound Full thrombophilia screening (in addition to tests performed on all patients): protein C, protein S, antithrombin III, activated protein C resistance, prothrombin gene mutation, MTHFR Glucose tolerance test Thyroid function tests Cervical screening in pregnancy Vaginal swab culture for bacterial vaginosis

HSG, hysterosalpingography; MTHFR, methyleretetrahydrofolate reductase.

Other studies are determined by positive findings on history, examination, and laboratory tests. Table 5–2 shows a complete list of possible tests. It is unlikely that a cause will be found in more than half of the cases of recurrent miscarriage.[7]

Prepregnancy Treatment Options

General Approach

Couples should be treated sensitively and sympathetically. It is important to avoid recommending unproven treatments.

Epidemiologic Factors

Advanced maternal age and the number of previous miscarriages are two important independent risk factors for further miscarriage that should be considered.

Genetic Factors

When a parent carries a balanced chromosome rearrangement, the risk of producing chromosomally unbalanced offspring depends on the specific chromosomes involved, the size of the segments involved in the rearrangement, and the sex of the transmitting parent. The risk of miscarriage in couples with reciprocal translocation is approximately 50%. With robertsonian translocation, the risk is approximately 25%.[91,92] Most couples with balanced chromosome rearrangements have healthy children; however, homologous robertsonian translocations always result in fetal aneuploidy.

The finding of an abnormal parental karyotype warrants genetic counseling. Genetic counseling offers the couple a prognosis for future pregnancies, prenatal diagnostic options, and the opportunity to perform familial chromosomal studies, if desired. If a subsequent miscarriage occurs, karyotyping of the products of conception is essential, regardless of the parental karyotype. Table 5–1 summarizes the procedure for collecting the products of conception for chromosome analysis.

Traditionally, reproductive options in couples with chromosomal abnormality have included proceeding to a further natural pregnancy, with or without prenatal diagnostic tests, chorionic villus sampling, or amniocentesis; gamete donation[93]; and adoption. More recently, preimplantation genetic diagnosis has been explored as a treatment option for translocation carriers[94,95] and couples with unexplained recurrent miscarriage.[96] Preimplantation genetic diagnosis is a technically demanding procedure, and clinical experience is limited. The technique requires the couple to undergo in vitro fertilization to produce embryos. Therefore, couples with proven fertility must be made aware of the high financial cost and low implantation and live birth rates per cycle after in vitro fertilization. Further, the couple should be informed that they have a 40% to 50% chance of a healthy live birth in future untreated pregnancies after natural conception.[92]

Anatomic Factors

As a screening test for uterine anomalies, noninvasive two-dimensional pelvic ultrasound assessment of the uterine cavity, with or without sonohysterography,[19,97] when performed by skilled and experienced staff, is as informative as invasive hysterosalpingography. Because three-dimensional ultrasound offers diagnosis and classification of uterine malformations,[98,99] its use may obviate the need for hysteroscopy and laparoscopy.

A minor defect does not warrant surgical correction. In the past, abdominal metroplasty was advocated for a uterine septum; however, open uterine surgery has not been assessed in prospective trials, is associated with postoperative infertility, and carries a significant risk of scar rupture during pregnancy.[100] These complications are less likely to occur after transcervical hysteroscopic resection of uterine septa, and experience from case series appears promising.[101] However, before a clear judgment can be made, the procedure must be evaluated in a prospective controlled trial. These procedures must be performed by clinicians with appropriate training and experience in hysteroscopic surgery. Metroplasty has been traditionally advocated for bicornuate uterus and uterus didelphys, even though it is of unproven benefit and carries a significant risk of morbidity. Unicornuate uterus is rare and has limited treatment options. Cervical cerclage has been proposed, but is of uncertain value.[102] Uterine anomalies resulting from in utero diethylstilbestrol exposure are rarely amenable to surgical correction, but prophylactic cervical cerclage has been advocated.[103]

Intrauterine adhesions can be corrected by hysteroscopic lysis, placement of an intrauterine device, and administration of estrogen after surgery.

Occasionally, abdominal or hysteroscopic myomectomy is warranted for recurrent miscarriage associated with significant submucous fibroids that distort the uterine cavity or occupy a large subendometrial area. A 3-month course of a gonadotropin-releasing hormone analog preoperatively facilitates surgery by reducing the size and vascularity of the fibroids. More recently, percutaneous thermal ablation of uterine fibroids under real-time magnetic resonance control was studied and appears to be a promising alternative treatment.[104]

Traditionally, the diagnosis of cervical incompetence has been clinical because it relies on a history of late miscarriage preceded by spontaneous rupture of the membranes or painless cervical dilation. The clinical diagnosis has not been evaluated in terms of it its ability to predict future pregnancy outcome. Although hysterosalpingography (HSG) and painless passage of an 8 Hegar dilator have been used to confirm the diagnosis before pregnancy, neither procedure has been studied prospectively. There is no satisfactory objective test to identify nonpregnant women with cervical incompetence. Prepregnancy cervical cerclage is advocated in some cases of assumed cervical incompetence, although its benefit is unproven.

Endocrine Factors

There is no value in performing glucose tolerance tests in women with recurrent miscarriage who have no history suggestive of diabetes mellitus. In women with established diabetes, poor glycemic control increases the risk of pregnancy loss. Consequently, these women require prepregnancy counseling with the aim of obtaining optimal periconceptual glycemic control.[105]

The contribution of luteal phase defect to recurrent miscarriage is controversial, and a review of pregnancy rates after hormonal treatments for luteal phase deficiency concluded that the benefits are uncertain.[43] One meta-analysis[42] reported that progesterone support for pregnancy in women with recurrent miscarriage may have a beneficial effect, but this meta-analysis was based on three small studies. A multicenter placebo-controlled study of hCG supplementation in early pregnancy showed no benefit in pregnancy outcome.[106] Subsequently, a small placebo-controlled study cited that the benefit of hCG is confined to a small subgroup of patients with recurrent miscarriage and oligomenorrhea.[107] Prepregnancy suppression of high LH levels with an LH-releasing hormone analog followed by low-dose ovulation induction in ovulatory women with recurrent miscarriage does not improve pregnancy outcome. Further, the live birth rate without pituitary suppression is excellent.

The role of insulin resistance and the safety and effectiveness of metformin treatment in women with recurrent miscarriage and polycystic ovaries require further study. Metformin should be used only in the context of prospective controlled trials.

Infections

All women with recurrent miscarriage should be screened routinely for rubella antibody status to determine and afford immunization before the next pregnancy. The empirical use of antimicrobial drugs in the treatment of women with recurrent pregnancy loss cannot be justified.

Antiphospholipid Antibodies

Antiphospholipid antibodies are associated with a wide spectrum of pregnancy complications, including recurrent miscarriage, late fetal loss, fetal growth restriction, preeclampsia, placental abruption, preterm birth, and maternal thromboembolic disease.[108–110] Several treatment modalities have been used to improve the pregnancy outcome of these women. The use of steroids during pregnancy leads to significant rates of maternal and fetal morbidity and does not improve pregnancy outcome compared with other treatment modalities.[111,112] The combination of low-dose aspirin and low-dose heparin significantly reduces pregnancy loss by 54% compared with aspirin alone.[113] Further, a recent randomized trial found that aspirin plus heparin is superior to IVIG[114] in the treatment of women with aPL-related pregnancy loss.

The use of low-dose aspirin during pregnancy is considered safe.[115] Because heparin does not cross the placental barrier, it is not teratogenic and does not cause fetal hemorrhage. However, heparin can be associated with maternal complications, including bleeding, hypersensitivity reactions, heparin-induced thrombocytopenia, and when used long term, osteopenia and vertebral bone fractures. However, two prospective studies[116,117] showed that the loss in bone mineral density at the lumbar spine associated with long-term, low-dose heparin therapy is similar to the loss that occurs physiologically during normal pregnancy. Risk–benefit assessment of aspirin plus heparin treatment appears to support its use in women with APS.

After the diagnosis of APS is made, women should be advised to start aspirin and heparin treatment after confirmation of their next pregnancy (at 4–5 weeks). No evidence suggests that preconceptual treatment of APS improves pregnancy outcome.

Hereditary Thrombophilia

The pregnancy outcome for women with a history of recurrent miscarriage associated with FVL mutation is poor when no pharmacological treatment is offered during pregnancy. The efficacy of thromboprophylaxis during pregnancy in women with recurrent miscarriage and inherited thrombophilic defects, who are otherwise asymptomatic, has not been assessed in prospective randomized controlled trials. Uncontrolled studies[118,119] suggest that heparin therapy may improve the live birth rate in these women. Until further evidence becomes available, the poor pregnancy outcome associated with FVL mutation, coupled with the maternal risks during pregnancy, probably justifies routine screening for FVL and antenatal thromboprophylaxis for those with the FVL mutation or evidence of placental thrombosis. Full anticoagulation may be required throughout pregnancy and puerperium in some patients with a personal or family history of thromboembolism (see Chapter 43).

Disorders of Maternofetal Alloimmune Relationships

No alloimmune theory has been substantiated, and no immunologic tests have been identified to predict pregnancy outcome. Further, immunotherapy is of no proven benefit and may actually cause harm. Immunotherapy should only be offered to women with recurrent miscarriage in the context of prospective controlled trials.

Unexplained Recurrent Miscarriage

Despite extensive testing, in approximately 50% of couples with recurrent miscarriage, no cause is identified.[7] Although the mechanism is unclear, several nonrandomized studies[11,12] suggest the benefit of supportive care and attendance at a dedicated early pregnancy clinic. The prognosis for a successful future pregnancy in women with unexplained recurrent miscarriage who receive supportive care alone is approximately 75%; it is worse with increasing maternal age and increasing number of previous miscarriages. These data suggest that empirical treatment in women with unexplained recurrent miscarriage is unnecessary and should be avoided.

General advice about stopping smoking, avoiding excessive alcohol and caffeine intake, losing weight (in obese women), and dietary balance is important. Folic acid (400 μg/day) for at least 2 months before attempting conception is indicated to prevent neural tube defects.

Management during Subsequent Pregnancy, Delivery, and Puerperium

Strategies for management during subsequent pregnancy differ according to the underlying cause of miscarriage. The risk of repeated miscarriage increases with each successive pregnancy loss and with advanced maternal age. Even when the pregnancy progresses beyond 24 weeks' gestation, evidence suggests that women with recurrent miscarriage are at risk for late pregnancy complications (e.g., preeclampsia, intrauterine fetal growth restriction, preterm delivery, perinatal loss, and operative delivery[108,110,120]). Close antenatal surveillance and planned delivery in a unit with specialized obstetric and neonatal intensive care facilities are indicated.

First Trimester

Couples with recurrent miscarriage are understandably anxious and need support and reassurance throughout the first trimester. Ultrasound is important in the management of early pregnancy by confirming or predicting viability and, when fetal heart activity is detected, providing maternal reassurance. Transvaginal ultrasound shows a gestation sac at 5 weeks, a yolk sac at approximately 5.5 weeks, and fetal heart activity in embryos less than 4 to 5 mm at 6 weeks. Thereafter, a scan to show fetal heart activity may be obtained every week or every 2 weeks, until the end of the first trimester. These scans, together with the finding of normal fetal growth and activity, may be reassuring to some couples.

Women with APS should be offered aspirin and heparin treatment. Low-dose aspirin (75 mg/day) should be initiated as soon as the patient has a positive urinary pregnancy test result. Subcutaneous low-dose heparin therapy in the form of low-molecular-weight heparin (enoxaparin [Clexane] [Lovenox] 20 mg/day or dalteparin [Fragmin] [Fragmin] 2500 units/day) or unfractionated heparin ([Calciparine] 5000 IU twice daily) should be initiated when intrauterine pregnancy is confirmed by ultrasound scan (the finding of a gestational sac and a yolk sac within the uterine cavity). Although unfractionated heparin and low-molecular-weight heparin preparations are equally beneficial, low-molecular-weight heparin can be administered once daily because of its longer half-life and increased bioavailability. Women should have a weekly platelet count during the first 3 weeks of heparin treatment to detect heparin-induced thrombocytopenia, which is rare.

Despite significant improvement in live birth rates, pregnant women who have aPLs and are treated with aspirin plus heparin until 34 completed weeks of gestation are at risk for late complications. These complications include pre-eclampsia, intrauterine growth restriction, placental abruption, and preterm delivery.[110] Whether continuation of treatment until delivery effectively reduces the risk of these late pregnancy complications is the subject of current research.

Second Trimester

When cervical incompetence is suspected in pregnancy, transvaginal ultrasonic assessment of the cervix is a noninvasive and objective means of assessing cervical length and shape and predicted preterm birth in high-risk populations.[121–123] The three ultrasound signs that suggest cervical incompetence are shortening of the endocervical canal, funneling of the internal os, and sacculation or prolapse of the membranes into the cervix, either spontaneously or as a result of fundal pressure (Fig. 5–3). A short cervix (<25 mm) is the best independent predictor of spontaneous preterm birth before 34 weeks' gestation.

Cervical cerclage is a recognized treatment for cervical incompetence. However, a meta-analysis[124] of four randomized controlled trials found no conclusive evidence that prophylactic cervical cerclage reduces the risk of pregnancy loss and preterm delivery in women at risk for preterm birth or midtrimester loss because of

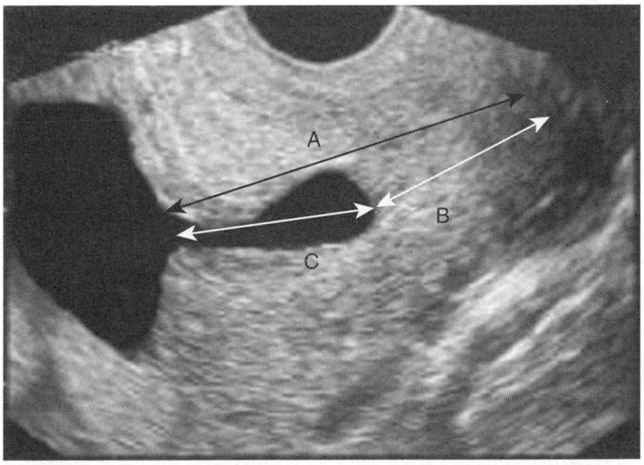

FIGURE 5–3
Transvaginal ultrasound scan of a cervix showing cervical shortening and funneling. A, Total cervical length; B, length of the distal cervical segment; C, depth of the cervical funnel.

cervical factors. Further, the procedure was associated with an increased risk of minor morbidity, but no serious morbidity. A small decrease in the number of deliveries before 33 weeks' gestation was noted in the largest trial.[125] The benefit was greatest in women with three or more second-trimester miscarriages or preterm births. There was no significant improvement in neonatal survival.

The same meta-analysis[124] assessed the role of therapeutic cerclage in women with a short cervix seen on ultrasound. The pooled results from two small randomized controlled trials[126,127] showed no reduction in midtrimester pregnancy loss and preterm delivery before 28 and 34 weeks in women assigned to undergo ultrasound-indicated cerclage. However, the numbers of women randomized were too small to allow firm conclusions to be drawn.

Based on the available evidence, it would seem reasonable to divide women with a history of midtrimester miscarriage that suggests cervical incompetence into two groups, with the therapeutic approach tailored accordingly. The first group includes women at increased risk for second-trimester miscarriage, including those with two or more second-trimester miscarriages without bleeding or clear signs of labor preceding the miscarriage. These women may benefit from prophylactic cervical cerclage at 13 to 16 weeks, with removal at 37 to 38 weeks. Several adjuvant short-term measures may be considered to minimize the risk of infection or other complications. These measures may include a short course of antibiotics and bed rest for 48 hours. Before prophylactic cerclage, these women should be offered ultrasound examination to assess fetal viability and exclude apparent fetal anomalies.

The second group, considered at medium risk, includes women with a history of one second-trimester miscarriage and those with evidence of other causes of preterm delivery (e.g., infection). These women can be offered serial transvaginal cervical ultrasound scanning beginning at 12 weeks and performed weekly or every 2 weeks until 23 weeks to measure cervical length and exclude funneling of the upper cervical canal. Therapeutic cervical cerclage may be offered to women with ultrasound signs of cervical shortening (<25 mm) or with progressive funneling in the absence of uterine activity or evidence of chorioamnionitis. Techniques for cervical cerclage are described in Chapter 6.

Uterine artery Doppler ultrasonography at 22 to 24 weeks may be useful in predicting preeclampsia and intrauterine growth restriction in women with APS and circulating lupus anticoagulant who are at increased risk for these complications.[128]

A glucose tolerance test at 28 weeks may be prudent for women with PCOS because of the increased risk of gestational diabetes. However, no evidence shows that the current management of gestational diabetes leads to improved outcomes for the mother and fetus.[129]

Third Trimester

During the third trimester, serial fetal growth scans and umbilical artery Doppler recordings are advisable. The risk of intrauterine growth restriction is increased in women with a history of recurrent miscarriage, particularly those with APS or inherited thrombophilia (see Chapters 42, 43, and 44).

Delivery and Puerperium

If pregnancy is progressing well, a history of recurrent miscarriage is not an indication for increased intervention. However, many women with a history of recurrent miscarriage request delivery by elective cesarean section. The obstetrician may consider that this approach or elective induction of labor at term is appropriate for psychological reasons.

In women receiving heparin, it is important to plan regional anesthesia to minimize the risk of epidural hematoma, and coordination with the anesthetist is required. Current guidelines[130,131] recommend that regional techniques should not be used until at least 12 hours after the previous prophylactic dose of low-molecular-weight heparin and 6 hours after a dose of unfractionated heparin. Heparin should not be given for at least 4 hours after the epidural catheter is removed.

There are no prospective data on the risk of systemic thrombosis to determine the optimal management of asymptomatic women with inherited thrombophilia. Current guidelines based on expert opinion recommend that postnatal thromboprophylaxis may be indicated in some women with known inherited thrombophilias, depending on the specific type of thrombophilia and the presence of other thrombotic risk factors.[130] Similarly, in women with APS and no symptoms other than recurrent miscarriage, there is no evidence to justify routine postnatal thromboprophylaxis. In women with APS without additional thrombotic risk factors, postnatal thromboprophylaxis is not recommended.

SUMMARY

The management of recurrent miscarriage requires a combination of sensitivity and a systematic approach to care. The goal is to identify a cause and implement appropriate treatment whenever possible. Of the many risk factors, parental karyotype abnormalities, APS, activated protein C resistance, and cervical incompetence are the only established causes of recurrent miscarriage. Of the many treatment options for couples with recurrent miscarriage, only aspirin plus heparin treatment in women with APS has proven benefit. Despite detailed studies, in approximately 50% of couples with recurrent miscarriage, no cause is found. However, even without pharmacologic treatment, the prognosis is good and supportive care appears to play an important role. Empirical treatments for women with recurrent miscarriage should be avoided, and new treatments should be introduced only after their benefit has been assured through properly designed prospective controlled trials.

CONCLUSIONS

- Recurrent miscarriage, defined as the loss of three or more consecutive pregnancies, is a distressing problem that affects 1% of couples.
- Systematic screening of couples with three consecutive miscarriages identifies a probable cause in 50% of cases. The remaining 50% of cases may result from recurrent, but sporadic, chromosomal abnormalities that occur by chance.
- The chance of successful pregnancy outcome after three consecutive miscarriages is high, depending on maternal age, reproductive history, and the underlying cause of miscarriage.
- Parental karyotype abnormalities, cervical incompetence, antiphospholipid syndrome, and activated protein C resistance are established causes of recurrent miscarriage.
- In couples with chromosomal translocations, options include natural conception with or without prenatal diagnosis tests, gamete donation, and preimplantation genetic diagnosis with in vitro fertilization.
- Elective cervical cerclage may confer benefits in women with two or more midtrimester losses as a result of cervical incompetence. Cervical ultrasound screening during pregnancy may be useful in reducing the rate of cervical cerclage when the history is equivocal.
- Low-dose aspirin and heparin treatment is the first-line therapy in women with antiphospholipid syndrome because it results in a live birth rate of 70%.
- Low-dose heparin may confer benefits in women with recurrent miscarriage associated with activated protein C resistance and evidence of placental thrombosis.
- Supportive care in couples with unexplained recurrent miscarriage is associated with an excellent prognosis; empirical treatments should be avoided.

SUMMARY OF MANAGEMENT OPTIONS
Recurrent Miscarriage—Prepregnancy Assessment

Management Options	Quality of Evidence	Strength of Recommendation	References
AT THE TIME OF THE THIRD MISCARRIAGE			
Document the pattern and trimester of the pregnancy loss and whether a live embryo or fetus was present.	–	GPP	–
Carefully document a suspected uterine abnormality at surgical evacuation.	–	GPP	–
Send the products of conception for histologic testing or autopsy and karyotype with consent of the patient, as appropriate (see Table 5–1).	–	GPP	–
A general approach is important (e.g., see the couple together, express sympathy, show sensitivity).	–	GPP	–
Offer follow-up assessment and counseling.	IV	C	6

Continued

SUMMARY OF MANAGEMENT OPTIONS

Recurrent Miscarriage—Prepregnancy Assessment *(Continued)*

Management Options	Quality of Evidence	Strength of Recommendation	References
PREPREGNANCY ASSESSMENT AND COUNSELING AFTER THE THIRD MISCARRIAGE			
History and Examination for Causative and Associated Factors			
Obtain an obstetric history to confirm the diagnosis of "recurrent miscarriage" (e.g., pattern of losses, gestations of former losses, previous confirmation of pregnancy: biochemical, ultrasonographic or histologic).	–	GPP	–
Obtain a general medical history	–	GPP	–
• Features associated with autoimmune disease (e.g., joint pain, rash)			
• Features related to antiphospholipid syndrome (e.g., migraine, epilepsy, vascular thrombosis)			
• Thrombophilia-related features (e.g., personal or family history of vascular thrombosis)			
• Exposure to environmental toxins or drugs			
Obtain a surgical history (cervix, uterus, ovary).	–	GPP	–
Obtain a family history (recurrent miscarriage, polycystic ovarian syndrome, genetic disease, hereditary thrombophilia)	–	GPP	–
Perform a physical examination: to identify signs of endocrine or gynecologic disease, including opportunistic screening (blood pressure, cervical cytology, breast palpation) and checking special risk factors identified by the history.	–	GPP	–
Routine Tests in All Patients (see Table 5–2)			
Karyotype			
• Both partners	III	B	18,19
• Miscarried tissue (with consent, as appropriate)	III	B	14,15,17
Pelvic ultrasound	III	B	97–99
Anticardiolipin antibodies (IgG and IgM)	III	B	58
Lupus anticoagulant	III	B	58
Early follicular phase luteinizing hormone, follicle-stimulating hormone, and testosterone	III	B	53,54
Thrombophilia screening:	IIa	B	68
• Activated protein C resistance and Factor V Leiden mutation testing is indicated in all cases. (Antithrombin III, factor XII, protein C, protein S, prothrombin gene mutation and MTHFR are reserved for patients with a high risk of thrombophilia.)	III	B	67
Prepregnancy opportunistic screening:	–	GPP	–
• Serology for rubella status			
• Blood group and Rhesus type			
Other tests are determined by positive findings on the history or examination (see Table 5–2).	–	GPP	–

SUMMARY OF MANAGEMENT OPTIONS

Recurrent Miscarriage—Prepregnancy Assessment *(Continued)*

Management Options	Quality of Evidence	Strength of Recommendation	References
Counseling with the Following Key Principles and Guidelines			
See the couple together, preferably at a dedicated miscarriage clinic. Take a sympathetic approach.	–	GPP	–
The true rate of recurrent miscarriage is affected by a reproductive compensation effect.	IV	C	6
After three consecutive losses, intensive testing identifies a probable cause in approximately 50% of couples.	III	B	19
The remaining 50% probably result from repeated, but sporadic chromosome abnormalities that occur consecutively by chance.	III	B	14,15
Advanced maternal and paternal age and previous reproductive history are important risk factors for a further miscarriage.	III	B	2,8–10
Anatomic defects of the uterine fundus and cervix, parental chromosomal rearrangements, gene mutations, phospholipid antibodies, and activated protein C resistance also play a role.	III	B	18,19,25,26, 58,60,67,68, 121,122,123
Progesterone deficiency, hypersecretion of luteinizing hormone, infective agents, and immune rejection are not considered causes of recurrent miscarriage. Empirical treatment with progesterone, high luteinizing hormone suppression, or immunotherapy is of no proven benefit.	Ia	A	42–46,71,73
Subclinical thyroid disorders and diabetes mellitus are rare.	III	B	19,53,54
Psychological stress is probably not relevant.	IV	C	6
Even after three miscarriages, the chance of a successful pregnancy without treatment is approximately 60%, apart from women with antiphospholipid syndrome and those with activated protein C resistance. In these women, success rates are lower.	III IIa	B B	2,10 60,68

MTHFR, methylene tetrahydrofolate reductase.

SUMMARY OF MANAGEMENT OPTIONS

Recurrent Miscarriage—Prepregnancy Treatment

Management Options	Quality of Evidence	Strength of Recommendation	References
Do not advocate unproven treatments.	–	GPP	–
Parental translocations			
• Genetic counseling for the couple and relatives	IV	C	18
• Proceeding to a further pregnancy, with or without prenatal diagnosis (amniocentesis or chorionic villus biopsy)	III	B	91–95
• Gamete donation	–	GPP	–
• Artificial insemination with donor sperm	–	GPP	–
• In vitro fertilization with a donor egg	–	GPP	–
• Preimplantation genetic diagnosis with in vitro fertilization	–	GPP	–
• Adoption	–	GPP	–

Continued

SUMMARY OF MANAGEMENT OPTIONS
Recurrent Miscarriage—Prepregnancy Treatment *(Continued)*

Management Options	Quality of Evidence	Strength of Recommendation	References
Uterine abnormalities			
• Uterine septum	III	B	25,100,101
GnRH analog Hysteroscopic septal incision Temporary intrauterine device			
• Intrauterine adhesions	III	B	39
Hysteroscopic division and temporary intrauterine device Postoperative temporary cyclic estrogen and progesterone therapy			
• Fibroids (Significant submucous fibroid or intramural with a significant intracavity component)	III	B	34
Gonadotropin-releasing hormone analog Myomectomy			

SUMMARY OF MANAGEMENT OPTIONS
Management during Subsequent Pregnancy, Delivery, and Puerperium

Management Options	Quality of Evidence	Strength of Recommendation	References
Provide psychological support and reassurance.	III	B	11,12
Do not advocate unproven treatments.	–	GPP	–
There is no evidence that any immunologic therapy is of benefit.	Ia	A	71
Offer low-dose aspirin and heparin to women with antiphospholipid syndrome	Ib	A	3,11,109,114
Offer low-dose heparin to women with activated protein C resistance or other thrombophilia.	IIb	B	9,11,118
Maintain good metabolic control in patients with diabetes mellitus.	IIb	B	105
First trimester			
• Transvaginal ultrasound scan to confirm fetal viability	–	GPP	–
• Serial scans for reassurance	–	GPP	–
Second trimester			
• Suspected cervical incompetence options: Serial cervical ultrasonography with insertion of a cervical suture if there is evidence of shortening/funneling or	Ib	A	126
primary cervical cerclage	Ib	A	125
• Serial vaginal swabs for pathogens	–	GPP	–
• Uterine artery Doppler studies in selected patients	III	B	128
• Prophylactic maternal steroids at 28 weeks in selected patients	–	GPP	–
• Formal GTT at 28 weeks in selected patients	–	GPP	–

SUMMARY OF MANAGEMENT OPTIONS
Management during Subsequent Pregnancy, Delivery, and Puerperium *(Continued)*

Third trimester: Vigilance for fetal growth restriction, preeclampsia, and preterm labor in selected patients	III	B	102,108,110
Labor and delivery: Consider elective LSCS/IOL at term in some patients	III	B	110
Puerperium: Consider postnatal thromboprophylaxis in selected patients	–	GPP	–

GTT, glucose tolerance test; IOL, induction of labor; LSCS, lower segment cesarean section.

REFERENCES

1. Kline J, Stein Z, Susser M (eds): Conception to Birth: Epidemiology of Prenatal Development. In Monographs in Epidemiology and Biostatistics. Oxford, Oxford University Press, 1989.
2. Regan L, Braude PR, Trembath PL: Influence of past reproductive performance on risk of spontaneous abortion. BMJ 1989;299:541–545.
3. WHO recommended definitions, terminology and format for statistical tables related to the perinatal period. Acta Obstet Gynaecol Scand 1977;56:247–253.
4. Stirrat GM: Recurrent miscarriage. Lancet 1990;336:673–675.
5. Alberman E: The epidemiology of repeated abortion. In Beard RW, Sharp F (eds): Early Pregnancy Loss: Mechanisms and Treatment. London, RCOG Press, 1988, pp 9–17.
6. Stirrat GM: Recurrent miscarriage: II. Clinical associations, causes, and management. Lancet 1990;336:728–733.
7. Coulam CB: Epidemiology of recurrent spontaneous abortion. Am J Reprod Immunol 1991;26:23–27.
8. Nybo Anderson AM, Wohlfahrt J, Christens P, et al: Maternal age and fetal loss: Population based register linkage study. BMJ 2000;320:1708–1712.
9. De la Rochebrochard E, Thonneau P: Paternal age and maternal age are risk factors for miscarriage: Results of a multicentre European study. Hum Reprod 2002;17:1649–1656.
10. Knudsen UB, Hansen V, Juul S, Secher NJ: Prognosis of a new pregnancy following previous spontaneous abortions. Eur J Obstet Gynaecol Reprod Biol 1991;39:31–36.
11. Clifford K, Rai R, Regan L: Future pregnancy outcome in unexplained recurrent first trimester miscarriage. Hum Reprod 1997;12:387–389.
12. Brigham SA, Conlon C, Farquharson RG: A longitudinal study of pregnancy outcome following idiopathic recurrent miscarriage. Hum Reprod 1999;14:2868–2871.
13. Boue J, Bou A, Lazar P: Retrospective and prospective epidemiological studies of 1500 karyotyped spontaneous human abortions. Teratology 1975;12:11–26.
14. Carp H, Toder V, Aviram A, et al: Karyotype of the abortus in recurrent miscarriage. Fertil Steril 2001;75:678–682.
15. Stephenson MD, Awartani KA, Robinson WP: Cytogenetic analysis of miscarriages from couples with recurrent miscarriage: A case-control study. Hum Reprod 2002;17:446–451.
16. Goddijn M, Leschot NJ: Genetic aspects of miscarriage. Baillieres Best Pract Res Clin Obstet Gynaecol 2000;14: 855–865.
17. Fritz B, Hallermann C, Olert J, et al: Cytogenetic analyses of culture failures by comparative genomic hybridisation (CGH): Re-evaluation of chromosome aberration rates in early spontaneous abortions. Eur J Hum Genet 2001;9:539–547.
18. de Braekeleer M, Dao TN: Cytogenetic studies in couples experiencing repeated pregnancy losses. Hum Reprod 1990;5:519–528.
19. Clifford K, Rai R, Watson H, Regan L: An informative protocol for the investigation of recurrent miscarriage: Preliminary experience of 500 consecutive cases. Hum Reprod 1994;9:1328–1332.
20. Robinson WP, McFadden DE, Stephenson MD: The origin of abnormalities in recurrent aneuploidy/polyploidy. Am J Hum Genet 2001;69:1245–1254.
21. Hassold T, Chiu D: Maternal age-specific rates of numerical chromosomal abnormalities with special reference to trisomy. Hum Genet 1985;70:11–17.
22. Ogasawara M, Aoki K, Okada S, Suzumori K: Embryonic karyotype of abortuses in relation to the number of previous miscarriages. Fertil Steril 2000;73:300–304.
23. Ward KJ: Genetic factors in recurrent pregnancy loss. Semin Reprod Med 2000;18:425–432.
24. Lanasa MC, Hogge A, Kubik CJ, et al: A novel X chromosome-linked genetic cause of recurrent spontaneous miscarriage. Am J Obstet Gynecol 2001;185:563–568.
25. Grimbizis GF, Camus M, Tarlatzis BC, et al: Clinical implications of uterine malformations and hysteroscopic treatment results. Hum Reprod Update 2001;7:161–174.
26. Acien P: Incidence of Müllerian defects in fertile and infertile women. Hum Reprod 1997;12:1372–1376.
27. Salim R, Regan L, Woelfer B, et al: A comparative study of the morphology of congenital uterine anomalies in women with and without a history of recurrent first trimester miscarriage. Hum Reprod 2003;18:162–166.
28. Althuisius SM, Dekker GA, van Geijn HP: Cervical incompetence: A reappraisal of an obstetric controversy. Obstet Gynecol Surv 2002;57:377–387.
29. Lidegaard O: Cervical incompetence and cerclage in Denmark 1980–1990: A register based epidemiological survey. Acta Obstet Gynecol Scand 1994;73:35–38.
30. Drakeley AJ, Quenby S, Farquharson RG: Mid-trimester loss: Appraisal of screening protocol. Hum Reprod 1998;13:1975–1980.
31. Iams JD, Johnson FF, Sonek J, et al: Cervical competence as a continuum: A study of ultrasonographic cervical length and obstetric performance. Am J Obstet Gynecol 1995;172(4 Pt 1):1097–1103; discussion 1104–1106.
32. Romero R, Gonzalez R, Sepulveda W, et al: Infection and labor: VIII. Microbial invasion of the amniotic cavity in patients with suspected cervical incompetence: Prevalence and clinical significance. Am J Obstet Gynecol 1992;167(4 Pt 1):1086–1091.
33. Richards PA, Richards PD, Tiltman AJ: The ultrastructure of fibromyomatous myometrium and its relationship to infertility. Hum Reprod Update 1998;4:520–525.

34. Li TC, Mortimer R, Cooke ID: Myomectomy: A retrospective study to examine reproductive performance before and after surgery. Hum Reprod 1999;14:1735–1740.
35. Pritts EA: Fibroids and infertility: A systematic review of the evidence. Obstet Gynecol Surv 2001;56:483–491.
36. Hart R, Khalaf Y, Yeong CT, et al: A prospective controlled study of the effect of intramural uterine fibroids on the outcome of assisted conception. Hum Reprod 2001;16:2411–2417.
37. Check JH, Choe JK, Lee G, Dietterich C: The effect on IVF outcome of small intramural fibroids not compressing the uterine cavity as determined by a prospective matched control study. Hum Reprod 2002;17:1244–1248.
38. Schenker JG, Margalioth EJ: Intrauterine adhesions: An updated appraisal. Fertil Steril 1982;37:593–610.
39. Katz Z, Ben-Arie A, Lurie S, et al: Reproductive outcome following hysteroscopic adhesiolysis in Asherman's syndrome. Int J Fertil Menopausal Stud 1996;41:462–465.
40. Valli E, Zupi E, Marconi D, et al: Hysteroscopic findings in 344 women with recurrent spontaneous abortion. J Am Assoc Gynecol Laparosc 2001;8:398–401.
41. Jordan J, Craig K, Clifton DK, et al: Luteal phase defect: The sensitivity and specificity of diagnostic methods in common clinical use. Fertil Steril 1994;62:54–62.
42. Daya S: Efficacy of progesterone support for pregnancy in women with recurrent miscarriage: A meta-analysis of controlled trials. Br J Obstet Gynaecol 1989;96:275–280.
43. Karamardian LM, Grimes DA: Luteal phase deficiency: Effect of treatment on pregnancy rates. Am J Obstet Gynecol 1992;167:1391–1398.
44. Rai R, Backos M, Rushworth F, Regan L: Polycystic ovaries and recurrent miscarriage: A reappraisal. Hum Reprod 2000; 15:612–615.
45. Nardo LG, Rai R, Backos M, et al: High serum luteinizing hormone and testosterone concentrations do not predict pregnancy outcome in women with recurrent miscarriage. Fertil Steril 2002;77:348–352.
46. Clifford K, Rai R, Watson H, et al: Does suppressing luteinising hormone secretion reduce the miscarriage rate? Results of a randomised controlled trial. BMJ 1996;312:1508–1511.
47. Dale PO, Tanbo T, Haug E, Abyholm T: The impact of insulin resistance on the outcome of ovulation induction with low-dose follicle stimulating hormone in women with polycystic ovary syndrome. Hum Reprod 1998;13:567–570.
48. Glueck CJ, Phillips H, Cameron D, et al: Continuing metformin throughout pregnancy in women with polycystic ovary syndrome appears to safely reduce first-trimester spontaneous abortion: A pilot study. Fertil Steril 2001;75:46–52.
49. Jakubowicz DJ, Iuorno MJ, Jakubowicz S, et al: Effects of metformin on early pregnancy loss in the polycystic ovary syndrome. J Clin Endocrinol Metab 2002;87:524–529.
50. Hanson U, Persson B, Thunell S: Relationship between haemoglobin A1C in early type 1 (insulin-dependent) diabetic pregnancy and the occurrence of spontaneous abortion and fetal malformation in Sweden. Diabetologia 1990; 33:100–104.
51. Mills JL, Simpson JL, Driscoll SG, et al: Incidence of spontaneous abortion among normal women and insulin-dependent diabetic women whose pregnancies were identified within 21 days of conception. N Engl J Med 1988;319:1617–1623.
52. Abalovich M, Gutierrez S, Alcaraz G, et al: Overt and subclinical hypothyroidism complicating pregnancy. Thyroid 2002; 12:63–68.
53. Bussen S, Sutterlin M, Steck T: Endocrine abnormalities during the follicular phase in women with recurrent spontaneous abortion. Hum Reprod 1999;14:18–20.
54. Li TC, Spuijbroek MD, Tuckerman E, et al: Endocrinological and endometrial factors in recurrent miscarriage. Br J Obstet Gynaecol 2000;107:1471–1479.
55. Esplin MS, Branch DW, Silver R, Stagnaro-Green A: Thyroid autoantibodies are not associated with recurrent pregnancy loss. Am J Obstet Gynecol 1998;179:1583–1586.
56. Rushworth FH, Backos M, Rai R, et al: Prospective pregnancy outcome in untreated recurrent miscarriers with thyroid autoantibodies. Hum Reprod 2000;15:1637–1639.
57. Wilson WA, Gharavi AE, Koike T, et al: International consensus statement on preliminary classification criteria for definite antiphospholipid syndrome: Report of an international workshop. Arthritis Rheum 1999;42:1309–1311.
58. Rai RS, Regan L, Clifford K, et al: Antiphospholipid antibodies and beta 2-glycoprotein-I in 500 women with recurrent miscarriage: Results of a comprehensive screening approach. Hum Reprod 1995;10:2001–2005.
59. Lockwood CJ, Romero R, Feinberg RF, et al: The prevalence and biologic significance of lupus anticoagulant and anticardiolipin antibodies in a general obstetric population. Am J Obstet Gynecol 1989;161:369–373.
60. Rai RS, Clifford K, Cohen H, Regan L: High prospective fetal loss rate in untreated pregnancies of women with recurrent miscarriage and antiphospholipid antibodies. Hum Reprod 1995;10: 3301–3304.
61. Out HJ, Kooijman CD, Bruinse HW, Derksen RH: Histopathological findings in placentae from patients with intrauterine fetal death and anti-phospholipid antibodies. Eur J Obstet Gynecol Reprod Biol 1991;41:179–186.
62. Peaceman AM, Rehnberg KA: The effect of immunoglobulin G fractions from patients with lupus anticoagulant on placental prostacyclin and thromboxane production. Am J Obstet Gynecol 1993;169:1403–1406.
63. Mak IY, Brosens JJ, Christian M, et al: Regulated expression of signal transducer and activator of transcription, Stat5, and its enhancement of PRL expression in human endometrial stromal cells in vitro. J Clin Endocrinol Metab 2002;87: 2581–2588.
64. Katsuragawa H, Kanzaki H, Inoue T, et al: Monoclonal antibody against phosphatidylserine inhibits in vitro human trophoblastic hormone production and invasion. Biol Reprod 1997;56:50–58.
65. Di Simone N, Castellani R, Caliandro D, Caruso A: Antiphospholid antibodies regulate the expression of trophoblast cell adhesion molecules. Fertil Steril 2002;77:805–811.
66. Sebire NJ, Fox H, Backos M, et al: Defective endovascular trophoblast invasion in primary antiphospholipid antibody syndrome-associated early pregnancy failure. Hum Reprod 2002; 17:1067–1071.
67. Rey E, Kahn SR, David M, Shrier I: Thrombophilic disorders and fetal loss: A meta-analysis. Lancet. 2003;361(9361): 901–908.
68. Rai R, Backos M, Elgaddal S, et al: Factor V Leiden and recurrent miscarriage: Prospective outcome of untreated pregnancy. Hum Reprod 2002;17:442–445.
69. Johnson PM, Christmas SE, Vince GS: Immunological aspects of implantation and implantation failure. Hum Reprod 1999; 14:26–36.
70. King A: Uterine leukocytes and decidualization. Hum Reprod Update 2000;6:28–36.
71. Scott JR: Immunotherapy for recurrent miscarriage. Cochrane Database Syst Rev 2003; 1:CD000112.
72. CBER Letter: Lymphocyte Immune Therapy (LIT). http://www.fda.gov/cber/ltr/lit013002.
73. Regan L, Jivraj S: Infection and pregnancy loss. In MacLean A, Regan L, Carrington D (eds): Infection and Pregnancy. London, RCOG Press, 2001, pp 291–304.
74. Hay PE, Lamont RF, Taylor-Robinson D, et al: Abnormal bacterial colonisation of the genital tract and subsequent preterm delivery and late miscarriage. BMJ 1994;308:295–298.
75. Llahi-Camp JM, Rai R, Ison C, et al: Association of bacterial vaginosis with a history of second trimester miscarriage. Hum Reprod 1996;11:1575–1578.

76. Ralph SG, Rutherford AJ, Wilson JD: Influence of bacterial vaginosis on conception and miscarriage in the first trimester: Cohort study. BMJ 1999;319:220–223.
77. McDonald H, Brocklehurst P, Parsons J, Vigneswaran R: Antibiotics for treating bacterial vaginosis in pregnancy. Cochrane Database Syst Rev 2003; 1:CD000262.
78. Lindbohm ML, Sallmen M, Taskinen H: Effects of exposure to environmental tobacco smoke on reproductive health. Scand J Work Environ Health 2002;28(Suppl 2):84–96.
79. Rasch V: Cigarette, alcohol, and caffeine consumption: Risk factors for spontaneous abortion. Acta Obstet Gynecol Scand 2003;82:182–188.
80. Kesmodel U, Wisborg K, Olsen SF, et al: Moderate alcohol intake in pregnancy and the risk of spontaneous abortion. Alcohol Alcoholism 2002;37:87–92.
81. Fernandes O, Sabharwal M, Smiley T, et al: Moderate to heavy caffeine consumption during pregnancy and relationship to spontaneous abortion and abnormal fetal growth: A meta-analysis. Reprod Toxicol 1998;12:435–444.
82. Leviton A, Cowan L: A review of the literature relating caffeine consumption by women to their risk of reproductive hazards. Food Chem Toxicol 2002;40:1271–1310.
83. Marcus M, McChesney R, Golden A, Landrigan P: Video display terminals and miscarriage. J Am Med Womens Assoc 2000; 55:84–88, 105.
84. Shuhaiber S, Koren G: Occupational exposure to inhaled anesthetic: Is it a concern for pregnant women? Can Fam Physician 2000;46:2391–2392.
85. McGregor DG: Occupational exposure to trace concentrations of waste anesthetic gases. Mayo Clin Proc 2000;75:273–277.
86. Craig M, Tata P, Regan L: Psychiatric morbidity among patients with recurrent miscarriage. J Psychosom Obstet Gynaecol 2002;23:157–164.
87. Arck PC, Merali FS, Stanisz AM, et al: Stress-induced murine abortion associated with substance P-dependent alteration in cytokines in maternal uterine decidua. Biol Reprod 1995;53: 814–819.
88. Sugiura-Ogasawara M, Furukawa TA, Nakano Y, et al: Depression as a potential causal factor in subsequent miscarriage in recurrent spontaneous aborters. Hum Reprod 2002;17:2580–2584.
89. Robert JM, Macara LM, Chalmers EA, Smith GC: Inter-assay variation in antiphospholipid antibody testing. Br J Obstet Gynaecol 2002;109:348–349.
90. Kwak JY, Barini R, Gilman-Sachs A, et al: Down-regulation of maternal antiphospholipid antibodies during early pregnancy and pregnancy outcome. Am J Obstet Gynecol 1994;171:239–246.
91. Neri G, Serra A, Campana M, Tedeschi B: Reproductive risks for translocation carriers: Cytogenetic study and analysis of pregnancy outcome in 58 families. Am J Med Genet 1983;16:535–561.
92. Regan L, Rai R, Backos M, El Gaddal S: Recurrent miscarriage and parental karyotype abnormalities: Prevalence and future pregnancy outcome (abstract). Hum Reprod 2001; 16:177–178.
93. Remohi J, Gallardo G, Levy M, et al. Oocyte donation in women with recurrent pregnancy loss. Hum Reprod 1996;11:2048–2051.
94. Ogilvie CM, Braude P, Scriven PN: Successful pregnancy outcomes after preimplantation genetic diagnosis (PGD) for carriers of chromosome translocations. Hum Fertil (Camb) 2001; 4:168–171.
95. Scriven PN, Flinter FA, Braude PR, Ogilvie CM: Robertsonian translocations: Reproductive risks and indications for preimplantation genetic diagnosis. Hum Reprod 2001;16:2267–2273.
96. Vidal F, Rubio C, Simon C, et al: Is there a place for preimplantation genetic screening in recurrent miscarriage patients? J Reprod Fertil Suppl 2000;55:143–146.
97. Soares SR, Barbosa dos Reis MM, Camargos AF: Diagnostic accuracy of sonohysterography, transvaginal sonography, and hysterosalpingography in patients with uterine cavity diseases. Fertil Steril 2000;73:406–411.
98. Jurkovic D, Geipel A, Gruboeck K, et al: Three-dimensional ultrasound for the assessment of uterine anatomy and detection of congenital anomalies: A comparison with hysterosalpingography and two-dimensional sonography. Ultrasound Obstet Gynecol 1995;5:233–237.
99. Raga F, Bonilla-Musoles F, Blanes J, Osborne NG: Congenital Müllerian anomalies: Diagnostic accuracy of three-dimensional ultrasound. Fertil Steril 1996;65:523–528.
100. Jacobsen LJ, DeCherney A: Results of conventional and hysteroscopic surgery. Hum Reprod 1997;12:1376–1381.
101. Homer HA, Li TC, Cooke ID: The septate uterus: A review of management and reproductive outcome. Fertil Steril 2000;73:1–14.
102. Golan A, Langer R, Wexler S, et al: Cervical cerclage: Its role in the pregnant anomalous uterus. Int J Fertil 1990;35:164–170.
103. Goldberg JM, Falcone T: Effect of diethylstilbestrol on reproductive function. Fertil Steril 1999;72:1–7.
104. Hindley JT, Law PA, Hickey M, et al: Clinical outcomes following percutaneous magnetic resonance image guided laser ablation of symptomatic uterine fibroids. Hum Reprod 2002; 17:2737–2741.
105. Rosenn B, Modovnik M, Combs CA, et al: Pre-conception management of insulin-dependent diabetes: Improvement of pregnancy outcome. Obstet Gynecol 1991;77:846–849.
106. Harrison RF: Human chorionic gonadotrophin (hCG) in the management of recurrent abortion: Results of a multi-centre placebo-controlled study. Eur J Obstet Gynecol Reprod Biol 1992;47:175–179.
107. Quenby S, Farquharson RG: Human chorionic gonadotropin supplementation in recurring pregnancy loss: A controlled trial. Fertil Steril 1994;62:708–710.
108. Branch DW, Silver RM, Blackwell JL, et al: Outcome of treated pregnancies in women with antiphospholipid syndrome: An update of the Utah experience. Obstet Gynecol 1992;80:614–620.
109. Rai R, Cohen H, Dave M, Regan L: Randomised controlled trial of aspirin and aspirin plus heparin in pregnant women with recurrent miscarriage associated with phospholipid antibodies (or antiphospholipid antibodies). BMJ 1997;314:253–257.
110. Backos M, Rai R, Baxter N, et al: Pregnancy complications in women with recurrent miscarriage associated with antiphospholipid antibodies treated with low-dose aspirin and heparin. Br J Obstet Gynaecol 1999;106:102–107.
111. Cowchock FS, Reece EA, Balaban D, et al: Repeated fetal losses associated with antiphospholipid antibodies: A collaborative randomized trial comparing prednisone with low-dose heparin treatment. Am J Obstet Gynecol 1992;166:1318–1323.
112. Silver RK, MacGregor SN, Sholl JS, et al: Comparative trial of prednisone plus aspirin versus aspirin alone in the treatment of anticardiolipin antibody–positive obstetric patients. Am J Obstet Gynecol 1993;169:1411–1417.
113. Empson M, Lassere M, Craig JC, Scott JR: Recurrent pregnancy loss with antiphospholipid antibody: A systematic review of therapeutic trials. Obstet Gynecol 2002;99:135–144.
114. Triolo G, Ferrante A, Ciccia F, et al: Randomized study of subcutaneous low molecular weight heparin plus aspirin versus intravenous immunoglobulin in the treatment of recurrent fetal loss associated with antiphospholipid antibodies. Arthritis Rheum 2003;48:728–731.
115. Duley L, Henderson-Smart D, Knight M, King J: Antiplatelet drugs for prevention of pre-eclampsia and its consequences: Systematic review. BMJ 2001;322(7282):329–333.
116. Shefras J, Farquharson RG. Bone density studies in pregnant women receiving heparin. Eur J Obstet Gynecol Reprod Biol 1996;65:171–174.
117. Backos M, Rai R, Thomas E, et al: Bone density changes in pregnant women treated with heparin: A prospective, longitudinal study. Hum Reprod 1999;14:2876–2880.

118. Brenner B, Hoffman R, Blumfield Z, et al: Gestational outcome in thrombophilic women with recurrent pregnancy loss treated by enoxaparin. Thromb Haemost 2000;83:693–697.
119. Younis JS, Ohel G, Brenner B, et al: The effect of thrombophylaxis on pregnancy outcome in patients with recurrent pregnancy loss associated with factor V Leiden mutation. Br J Obstet Gynaecol 2000;107:415–419.
120. Jivraj S, Anstie B, Cheong YC, et al: Obstetric and neonatal outcome in women with a history of recurrent miscarriage: A cohort study. Hum Reprod 2001;16:102–106.
121. Andrews WW, Copper R, Hauth JC, et al: Second-trimester cervical ultrasound: Associations with increased risk for recurrent early spontaneous delivery. Obstet Gynecol 2000;95: 222–226.
122. Owen J, Yost N, Berghella V, et al: National Institute of Child Health and Human Development, Maternal-Fetal Medicine Units Network: Mid-trimester endovaginal sonography in women at high risk for spontaneous preterm birth. JAMA 2001;19:1340–1348.
123. Guzman ER, Walters C, Ananth CV, et al: A comparison of sonographic cervical parameters in predicting spontaneous preterm birth in high-risk singleton gestations. Ultrasound Obstet Gynecol 2001;18:204–210.
124. Drakeley AJ, Roberts D, Alfirevic Z: Cervical stitch (cerclage) for preventing pregnancy loss in women: Cochrane review. In Cochrane Library, issue 1, 2003.
125. MRC/RCOG Working Party on Cervical Cerclage: Final report of the Medical Research Council/Royal College of Obstetricians and Gynaecologists multicentre randomised trial of cervical cerclage. Br J Obstet Gynaecol 1993;100:516–523.
126. Althuisius SM, Dekker GA, Hummel P, et al: Final results of the Cervical Incompetence Prevention Randomized Cerclage Trial (CIPRACT): Therapeutic cerclage with bed rest versus bed rest alone. Am J Obstet Gynecol 2001;185:1106–1112.
127. Rust OA, Atlas RO, Reed J, et al: Revisiting the short cervix detected by transvaginal ultrasound in the second trimester: Why cerclage therapy may not help. Am J Obstet Gynecol 2001;185:1098–1105.
128. Venkat-Raman N, Backos M, Teoh TG, et al: Uterine artery Doppler in predicting pregnancy outcome in women with antiphospholipid syndrome. Obstet Gynecol 2001;98:235–242.
129. National Institute for Clinical Excellence: Antenatal care. Routine care for the healthy pregnant women. Clinical Guidline 6. October 2003. www.nice.org.uk
130. Royal College of Obstetricians and Gynaecologists: Thromboprophylaxis during pregnancy, labour, and after vaginal delivery. Guideline No. 37. London, RCOG Press, 2004.
131. Bullingham A, Strunin L: Prevention of postoperative venous thromboembolism. Br J Anaesth 1995;75:622–630.

CHAPTER 6

Midpregnancy Problems

Reynir Tómas Geirsson

INTRODUCTION

"Midpregnancy" is most accurately defined in theoretical terms as corresponding to the second trimester, from 12 to 28 weeks after the first day of the last menstrual period. However, in practical terms, it is usually considered to be the time between 15 to 16 weeks and 26 to 28 weeks, a period that encompasses the second phase of trophoblast invasion[1] and the most rapid phase of placental growth.[2] For most women, it is the easiest part of pregnancy, a time when the mother has passed the initial adaptive changes to the pregnant state and feels generally well. She experiences a slow increase in the physiologic and psychological changes associated with pregnancy, the growth and reactivity of the uterus as a living muscle compartment, and the awakening of new life within her. During this time, the development of the fetus is focused on organ maturation rather than physical growth.

Midpregnancy has an "air of healthiness" about it, and it is sometimes referred to as the "quiet stage" of pregnancy. Most mothers need little maternity care in midpregnancy, and antenatal care systems do not emphasize frequent visits during this time. Most problems and questions that arise are minor and require only understanding and adequate explanation based on physiologic knowledge. When a disorder or disease develops, in most cases, the mother becomes symptomatic. This should alert the physician or midwife, allowing diagnosis as well as appropriate and timely treatment.

In some cases, problems in midpregnancy are a considerable threat to the pregnancy, and sometimes a premature end to pregnancy cannot be averted. However, the experience may be used to prevent recurrence of the problem in a subsequent pregnancy. Some women belong to well-defined risk groups for problems in midpregnancy. In this case, advance planning and risk management is needed in asymptomatic women. In the absence of symptoms, both women and caregivers should not look for trouble where it is not expected. Testing is not needed if there are no symptoms. Within a modern screening environment, early data-gathering on maternal health, physical examination, and ultrasound and biochemical screening provide a basis for the completed planning of antenatal care by the early second trimester. Midpregnancy is typically quiet. In the third trimester, more adverse events may be anticipated and routine surveillance is increased.

PHYSIOLOGIC CHANGES OF MIDPREGNANCY

Knowledge of the maternal physiologic adaptations of midpregnancy is essential for the recognition of pathology during midpregnancy (Table 6–1). Fetal development comprises organ growth and maturation in a maternal environment dominated by physiologic adaptation favoring the needs of the fetus. Developments in the mother's body occur in advance of the main fetal growth spurt, reaching their maximum either early or late in midpregnancy. At this time, the maternal–placental supply line far exceeds immediate fetal needs. Changes in cardiac output and plasma volume approach their maximum velocity at approximately 20 weeks, and the red blood cell mass grows at a slower, steadier pace throughout midpregnancy. The result is a decrease in diastolic and systolic blood pressure and hemodilution. Increasing vascular permeability contributes to this as well as the developing low-resistance placental bed. Gastrointestinal motility and absorption, renal perfusion, and excretory changes in the mother begin even before the start of midpregnancy. Pelvic girdle distention and lumbar ligament softening gradually become more evident. Metabolic, hormonal, immunologic, and mental changes in the mother are less evident, but occur and are part of the adaptive process.

Uterine volume grows linearly during pregnancy, but the rate of placental growth is greatest between 20 and 30

TABLE 6–1

The Main Physiologic Adaptations in Normal Midpregnancy

General Changes
Increased cardiac stroke volume or output (inotropic, chronotropic)
Increased peripheral blood flow, decreased vascular resistance, venous dilation
Decreased midpregnancy blood pressure
Extracellular fluid accumulation, sodium retention
Blood and plasma volume expansion, hypervolemia, hemodilution
Increased erythrocyte production, count, increased plasma globulins and fibrinogen
Increased neutrophil count, reactivity, lymphocyte production
Increased platelet count, increased platelet adhesion, coagulation activation
Increased serum lipid level, metabolic and hormonal changes
Decreased pulmonary vascular resistance, increased tidal volume
Increased oxygen consumption, hyperventilation
Decreased gastrointestional motility, increased absorption
Increased renal blood flow, increased renal plasma filtration
Increased renin-angiotensin-aldosterone levels, angiotensin II resistance
Immunosuppression, altered B- and T-cell and complement function
Changes in connective and elastic tissue, change in thermoregulation
Uteroplacental Changes
Placental hormone production
Increased uterine size, contour and position changes
Increased uterine volume, amniotic fluid volume expansion
Increased intrauterine pressure
Increased myometrial mass and contractility
Increased energy production, action potential change, change in ion flow
Increased uterine blood flow
Second-phase invasion of spiral artery
Development of subplacental low-resistance flow compartment
Fastest placental growth rate
Cytotrophoblast shedding, aponecrotic change

weeks' gestation. Placental growth reaches its main velocity and bulk before fetal weight gain begins.[2] This basic physiologic adaptation ensures an adequate nutrition supply for the fetus and allows for third-trimester fetal volume growth. By the end of midpregnancy, the placenta can be thought of as "middle-aged" and well matured, whereas at term, it is reaching "old age." The physiologic adaptation process protects the mother from adverse events in pregnancy and contributes to fetal and maternal well-being.

MISCELLANEOUS SYMPTOMS AND PROBLEMS

Many problems in later pregnancy, including intrauterine growth disturbance, preeclampsia, and gestational diabetes may become evident in midpregnancy, but are discussed in the relevant chapters, as are the problems of multiple pregnancy, Rhesus isoimmunization, and other specific maternal and fetal diseases.

In midpregnancy, the signs and symptoms that indicate a risk of fetal death, late miscarriage, or early preterm delivery are abdominal pain and inappropriate uterine contractility (labor pains), vaginal bleeding and discharge, inappropriate uterine size, and infection. In addition, a vague feeling of "unwellness" should not be ignored.

Abdominal Pain (See Chapters 57 and 58)

Abdominal pain may originate from the pregnancy itself, the uterine muscle, or the ovaries. It may also stem from other intra-abdominal organs. Some pain is related to definite disease states, whereas other pain is functional. Most sources of pain do not pose a significant risk to the pregnancy, such as fibromyoma in the uterine muscle, ovarian cysts, urinary tract infections, pelvic girdle pain, irritable bowel syndrome, and pain caused by spontaneous uterine muscle contractility and tension from the round ligaments. Other sources of pain may have serious consequences because of the associated risk of reflex uterine contractility, intrauterine infection, and preterm labor. Potentially serious causes of abdominal pain include appendicitis, cholecystitis, severe pyelonephritis and urolithiasis, and twisted or ruptured hemorrhagic ovarian cysts. Any intra-abdominal organ may be responsible, and all must be considered in the differential diagnosis.

Appendicitis occurs in approximately 1 in 800 pregnancies.[3] By midpregnancy, the upward and lateral displacement of the ascending part of the large bowel by the growing uterus or the position of a pelvic appendix behind the uterus may mask the diagnosis. A moderate fever, an increased white blood cell count, and an increased C-reactive protein level occur with diffuse and uncharacteristic pain accompanied by nausea and sometimes vomiting. A low threshold of clinical suspicion must be maintained. When appendicitis occurs in midpregnancy, approximately 1 in 7 women deliver prematurely.[3] Early surgery with appendectomy is preferable, but with a ruptured appendix and appendiceal abscess, conservative treatment with appropriate antibiotics may be the first option. Some obstetricians prefer to treat appendicitis themselves, whereas others seek surgical assistance. The primary responsibility for care remains with the obstetric team, because maintenance of the pregnancy with tocolysis and prophylactic administration of steroids is an important goal of management (see Chapter 57).

The management of cholecystitis is conservative, and cholecystectomy is rarely needed. Complications of ovarian cysts are best treated with surgical removal, and pyelonephritis, renal calculi, and related problems are managed by appropriate measures to detect underlying pathology in consultation with a urology team (see Chapters 57 and 58).

Inappropriate Uterine Activity (See also Chapter 62)

Differentiating between normal uterine activity and the start of preterm labor in women with very different thresholds of pain is difficult in midpregnancy. Discomfort as a result of tension and muscle activity in the round ligaments and an increased perception of uterine contractility are common in midpregnancy, but usually harmless. Preterm labor entails both uterine contractions and cervical dilation. Not all women who have contractions are laboring; equally, women may approach delivery without a perception of uterine contractions.[4] Vague abdominal discomfort that is easily ascribed to another abdominal condition (e.g., gastroenteritis, irritable bowel syndrome) may be the only symptom of impending late miscarriage or very preterm delivery. Conversely, in a woman with a noncompliant, collagenous cervix, uterine contractions do not necessarily indicate labor or a risk of preterm delivery.

A thorough history and examination, patience, and careful observation are required. Emphasis must be placed on reaching a diagnosis by cervical assessment with a speculum (occasionally with careful digital palpation) and supplementing this examination with transvaginal ultrasound. Direct inspection of the cervix should be performed to detect dilation, fluid leakage, and cervical insufficiency as well as mucopurulent discharge indicative of intrauterine infection and chorioamnionitis. Endocervical bacterial culture is necessary unless the cervical mucus is clear. Tests for fibronectin, which indicates preterm premature rupture of the membranes, may be required.[5] Ultrasound is done to determine cervical length, identify cervical funneling, and assess amniotic fluid volume, fetal size, and viability in the early stages of midpregnancy. Before 24 weeks, external tocography has limited use, both for practical reasons and because viability is unlikely. To assess pain, the use of palpation and observation is better than attempting to record uterine contractility with an external monitor. Chorioamnionitis is not reflected in uterine tenderness or pain until it reaches an advanced stage, but uterine tenderness can be an early sign of placental abruption.

Treatment must be cause-oriented, but most options are not based on clear evidence. If delivery seems likely or inevitable, the viability of the infant and likelihood of survival without major disability must be considered. In a large study of infants delivered between 24 and 28 weeks' gestation, after adjustment for various confounding factors, no difference was seen between those delivered abdominally and those delivered vaginally.[6] The chance of survival improves with increasing gestational age, absence of maternal hypertension, singleton pregnancy, and antenatal steroid therapy. The rate of cerebral palsy in this study was 11.1%, but 63.1% of the infants were healthy at 2 years of age, regardless of the mode of delivery in these infants of borderline viability. Shennan and associates[7] found that of 383 liveborn infants between 26 and 30 weeks' gestation, before the advent of high-frequency ventilation techniques, 39, or approximately 1 in 10, did not survive. Further, 34, or another 1 in 10, had a significant disability at 1-year follow-up. When infants who died or were disabled were paired with gestational-age-matched infants from the total group, no difference was seen between the groups in the rates of prenatal complications, including prolonged rupture of the membranes and antepartum hemorrhage. However, their condition during labor or at birth was worse among infants who died or were disabled. Therefore, prelabor characteristics do not appear to have major prognostic significance for the pregnancy and are not a useful guide to management. Newer techniques for neonatal support have increased survival rates for infants born between 24 and 28 weeks' gestation, whereas disability rates remains the same, at approximately 14% to 17%.[8–11] However, the outlook for infants born before 25 to 26 weeks is still poor.

Vaginal Discharge (See Chapter 32)

Vaginal discharge can be physiologic or may be a sign of bacterial vaginosis, vaginitis caused by *Trichomonas* or *Candida albicans* infection, a foreign body reaction, or chlamydial or gonorrheal infection of the cervix. In midpregnancy, the risk associated with vaginal discharge is ascending intrauterine infection and chorioamnionitis, with resulting preterm labor and delivery.

Changes in Uterine Size (See Chapters 12 and 13)

Early growth restriction affects not only fetal growth but also placental and amniotic fluid volume. This possibility should be borne in mind when the fundal height is less than expected in midpregnancy. Measuring fundal height is not a sensitive way to detect growth restriction, but it is an inexpensive routine measure that detects approximately 30% of cases. A symphysis–fundus chart must be appropriately constructed and relevant to the population. The fundal height should be approximately equal in centimeters to the gestational age in weeks. After maternal size is considered, a difference of more than 3 cm is a reason for further ultrasound assessment.[12] Growth restriction in midpregnancy is usually caused by an underlying medical disease affecting the peripheral or renal blood vessels. It tends to be serious and affects the fetus and placenta in a symmetrical way. If poor growth is confirmed by ultrasound measurement, Doppler studies of flow in the uterine arteries and fetal umbilical artery, aorta, and cerebral arteries are indicated. Cytogenetic studies and a thorough repeat evaluation of the fetal anatomy may be necessary.

Uterine expansion caused by polyhydramnios may occur as a result of fetal infection (*Parvovirus* infection or toxoplasmosis), congenital anomalies that affect the fetal gut, twin–twin transfusion syndrome, or poorly controlled diabetes.

General Malaise, Tiredness, and Fainting

Although these symptoms are common in normal pregnancy, they can be a clue to a new infectious or medical condition or the exacerbation of a preexisting problem. Many medical disorders are associated with an increased risk of loss in midpregnancy (e.g., cardiac or renal disease, ulcerative colitis, Crohn's disease, sarcoidosis, occult malignancy). Anemia caused by deficiency of iron, folic acid, and B_{12} as well as sickle cell anemia and thalassemia must be considered, along with toxoplasmosis and other zoonotic, bacterial, or viral infections.

SUMMARY OF MANAGEMENT OPTIONS

Miscellaneous Symptoms and Problems in Midpregnancy

Condition	Management Options
Abdominal pain	See Chapters 57 and 58
Inappropriate uterine activity	See Chapter 62
Vaginal discharge	See Chapter 32
Uterine size changes or discrepancies	See Chapters 12 and 13
General malaise, tiredness, and fainting	See relevant chapters
Consider:	
• Pregnancy	
• Medical disorders (especially cardiac, renal, inflammatory bowel)	
• Anemia	
• Infection	

PREVIOUS MIDPREGNANCY LOSS (See also Chapter 62)

Definition

Previous midpregnancy loss is any previous loss of a pregnancy between 12 and 28 weeks' gestation. A diagnosis of failed pregnancy, such as missed miscarriage or fetal death between 12 and 16 weeks, can be considered a prolongation of events originating in the first trimester. These occurrences are handled in a similar manner, usually by evacuation with suction or treatment with prostaglandins and mifepristone, when this drug is available. Problems that occur in the second trimester (e.g., fetal loss or very preterm delivery as a result of cervical insufficiency, intrauterine death as a result of fetal anomaly, ascending or systemic infection, or idiopathic or secondary placental insufficiency) have another cause and require different management.

Risks

Few women miscarry or deliver during midpregnancy. When this occurs, the cause may be fetal or maternal. Fetal causes are related to congenital and chromosomal anomalies as well as intrauterine growth restriction, and the usual outcome is intrauterine fetal death. Maternal causes may be related to uterocervical anomalies, vascular disorders, or infection, and the fetus is usually born alive.[13] The incidence of preterm labor varies from 4% in developed countries with high living standards to 12% to 20% in developing countries, depending on risk factors, such as maternal age, race, poverty, smoking, alcohol and drug use, low prepregnancy weight, poor maternal education, strenuous work, short interpregnancy interval, abnormal bacterial colonization in the vagina, multifetal pregnancy, and uterine malformations. The miscarriage rate of live fetuses between 14 to 22 weeks is approximately 1.3% of all deliveries,[13] but the rate of preterm delivery between 22 and 28 weeks is less than 0.5% of all deliveries and approximately 7% of preterm deliveries before 37 weeks[13–15] The same risk factors apply as a continuum for the period from 14 to 28 weeks.[13] A greater risk is seen with advanced maternal age, lower socioeconomic status, an adverse obstetric history, previous therapeutic termination of pregnancy, and heavy smoking. The spontaneous loss rate in twin pregnancies (3%–7% in the second trimester) is caused by the same factors, but at a higher rate than for singletons. In monozygotic twins, velamentous cord insertion and twin–twin transfusion are additional causes.[16] Although the World Health Organization recommends that birth be recorded from

22 weeks onward, viability is generally accepted from approximately 23 to 24 weeks' gestation.[17,18] The major risk factors for midpregnancy loss are previous loss in the second or early third trimester (up to five times more likely[13]), multiple pregnancy, and bleeding from the uterine cavity in the first trimester and early second trimester. Idiopathic preterm delivery and multiple pregnancy are discussed in Chapters 62 and 60, respectively. Pregnancy-specific conditions and preexisting medical conditions that are exacerbated by pregnancy are rarer causes that are not discussed here. The one remaining cause is increased and premature cervical compliance occurring with normal or increased myometrial activity, leading to early cervical opening (i.e., cervical insufficiency).

Cervical Insufficiency

Premature dilation of the uterine cervix is a major reason for loss or delivery in midpregnancy. Traditionally, the diagnosis of cervical insufficiency has been retrospective, based on a history of midpregnancy or early third-trimester loss associated with cervical dilation that occurs without a maternal sensation of uterine contractions.[19,20] The typical situation is "silent" or "painless" dilation in a patient with the finding of bulging fetal membranes extruding onto or through the external opening of the cervix. Slight vaginal bleeding and discharge, with perineal pressure and a varying sensation of pain, indicative of concomitant chorioamnionitis, often indicates early cervical dilation. This makes diagnosis and treatment difficult. Knowledge of the risks, pathophysiology, and treatment of cervical insufficiency is incomplete and is based on case reports, small observational or case–control studies of limited value, and inconclusive evidence from a few randomized studies.[21] However, transvaginal ultrasound is improving the understanding of the antecedent pathophysiology of the condition and has increased the management possibilities.[22]

The varying incidence of preterm labor affects estimates of how often preterm delivery is caused by cervical insufficiency, particularly in midpregnancy. Older data suggest that, on average, clinicians performed cervical cerclage in 0.5% of women,[21,23] suggesting the approximate frequency of the condition and its diagnosis. If 10% of preterm deliveries occur before 28 weeks' gestation, approximately one in three deliveries between 22 and 28 weeks is because of cervical insufficiency. Among twins, the rate of cervical insufficiency is higher.[16]

Pathophyisology

The pathophysiology of cervical insufficiency is not well understood. Deficiency of collagen, elastin, or the interconnective glycosaminoglycan structures of collagen fibrils may affect the ability of the cervical sphincter mechanism to resist the steady expansion of the uterine cavity and gravitational pressure on the internal os.[14] The higher incidence in multiple pregnancies points to the importance of uterine cavity distention. Recent ultrasound studies showed that the cervix opens by funneling and herniation of the membranes into the cervical canal as it shortens and effaces (Fig. 6–1). The cervix is not a static organ, but living tissue that is constantly adapting to different pressures.[24] Compliance and molding may vary among women, possibly on a genetic basis and is in addition affected by events such as subclinical infection ascending through the cervix and bleeding from the decidua or placental edge.[21,24] Several factors are probably required to initiate the process of cervical softening and effacement. For this reason, it is difficult to treat developing cervical insufficiency. Optimal therapy is by

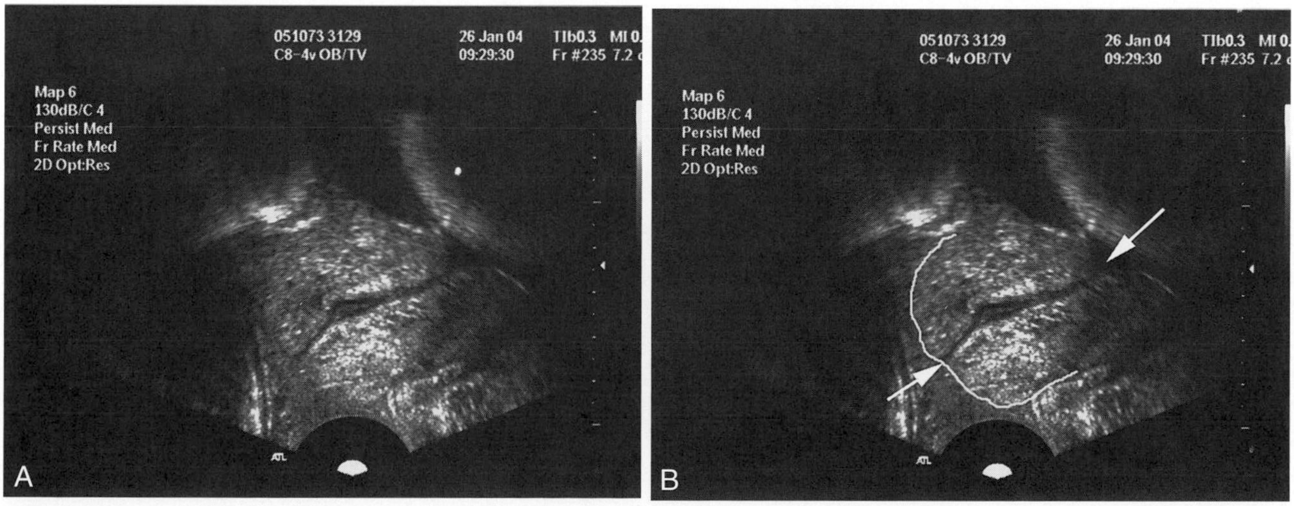

FIGURE 6–1
A, The transvaginal sagittal ultrasound appearance of a normal, undilated midpregnancy cervix. *B*, The cervix marked out; arrows point to the interal and external os.

preventive measures, either prophylactic, based on previous midpregnancy loss, or after a diagnosis is reached in an affected pregnancy. Several measures may be initiated, including cervical cerclage suture, antibacterial prophylaxis, tocolytic drugs, rest, and cessation of smoking, although none is adequately researched or proven.

Diagnosis

Diagnosis of cervical insufficiency is challenging. Typically, there is a history of midpregnancy painless dilation and effacement to 2 to 4 cm, accompanied by a feeling of pressure down onto the perineum and mucoid discharge. To this can be added a history of cervical lacerations from previous deliveries (although these often remain undiagnosed), cone biopsies, and excessive dilation (>9–12 mm) during earlier termination. After conization, only 2% to 3% of women deliver before 28 weeks' gestation, although the overall preterm delivery rate is increased two to five times.[25] However, the risk of early delivery varies with the type and extent of conization and may be higher than 3% after extensive or repeated procedures.

Routine digital examination of the cervix does not help and may be counterproductive. Digital examination increases prostaglandin production and may introduce infection. In a population at low risk for preterm delivery, repeated digital examination doubles the incidence of preterm delivery.[26] Attempts to produce risk scores lacked the necessary predictive value.[26,27] It is now necessary to add ultrasound evidence of funneling and prolapse of the membranes to a measured shortening of the cervical canal. The accepted median length of the normal cervical canal is 3.5 to 3.8 cm. The 10th percentile value is 2.5 cm.[24,28] With effacement, the internal os and cervical canal gradually change from a T to a Y shape and finally assume a V-shaped appearance (Fig. 6–2). This change is accompanied by progressive shortening of the cervical canal below the 2.5-cm mark. The predictive value of these changes for preterm delivery is high, and in the absence of major uterine myometrial activity, a diagnosis of cervical insufficiency is likely if the cervix is less than 2.5 cm long.[24,29–31] There is debate as to whether a lowest critical value exists, but a cervical length of 1.5 cm has been suggested.[32] This value may be realistic in view of a recent randomized trial that showed no benefit of cerclage at 2.5 cm.[33]

Although the risk of delivery increases with a shorter cervical length, there is no known value at which the prediction is absolute. Manual transfundal pressure may make the diagnosis clearer.[30,31] In a large prospective study assessing cervical length between 24 and 28 weeks in 2800 asymptomatic women, decreasing cervical length was positively associated with a risk of earlier delivery.[29] Incorporation of cervical assessment into the 18- to 20-week routine ultrasound examination may be useful because this is also the average time for an ultrasound diagnosis of cervical insufficiency, but this would need follow-up for at-risk women at approximately 24 weeks and awaits confirmation from randomized studies.[22,29,30] This approach may be acceptable to most women, even if it involves additional or repeated vaginal ultrasound.[28] Serial examinations of the cervix by transvaginal ultrasound do not appear to increase the risk of preterm delivery.[34] At an earlier gestational age (<14 weeks), however, there appears to be no appreciable difference in cervical length between women who deliver preterm and those who deliver at term.[22] This suggests that screening at 14 weeks or earlier has little value. This is to be expected because pressure on the internal cervical os does not increase until well into midpregnancy.

Management Options

PREPREGNANCY

For women with a history of previous midpregnancy loss, management of suspected cervical insufficiency first

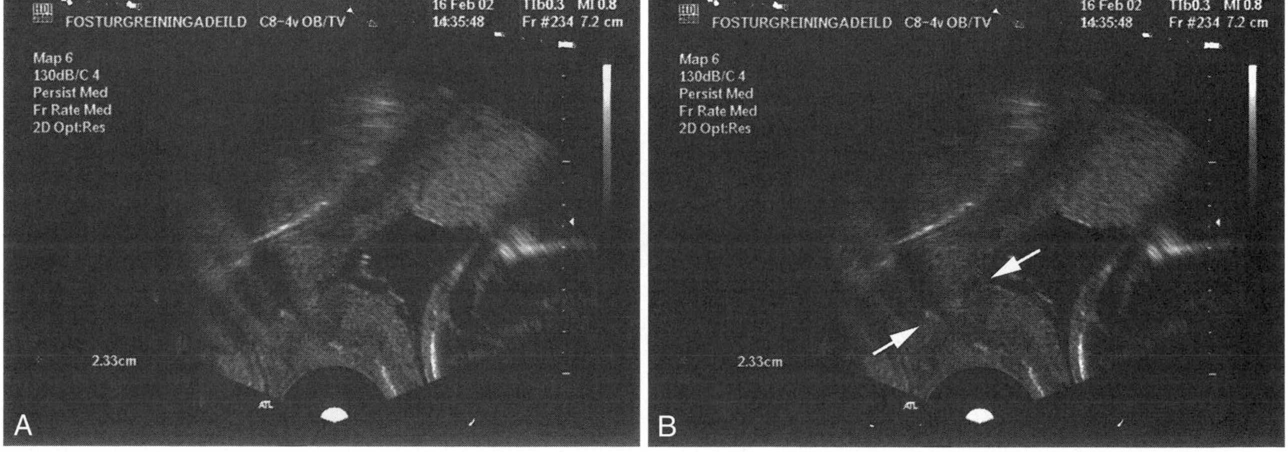

FIGURE 6–2
A, Funnelling of the cervical canal and widening of the interanl os with beginning chorioamnionic membrane herniation into the internal os of the cervical canal. *B*, The arrows mark out the shortened cervix (length 2.3 cm).

involves the repair of cervical lacerations that extend along the vaginal portion of the cervix and possibly above the cervical fornices. This repair should be done before pregnancy, with adequate time allowed for inflammation to resolve before the woman becomes pregnant again.

PRENATAL

Before or shortly after the woman becomes pregnant again, a decision must be made whether to insert a cervical purse-string (cerclage) suture. This procedure is usually done at 12 to 15 weeks' gestation, after fetal viability is established. Before cerclage is performed, screening at 11 to 13 weeks to ensure that the fetal anatomy is normal and that there is a low likelihood of chromosomal anomaly may be appropriate for most prospective parents. Although only one randomized trial has shown a benefit from prophylactic cerclage, and then only after at least two previous midpregnancy losses,[43] clinicians are under considerable pressure to take action.

Three options are currently available:

- Perform observation only, with or without clinical tests to detect and treat abnormal bacterial colonization in the vagina or inside the uterine cavity.
- Perform observation, with regular transvaginal ultrasound to detect cervical shortening and funneling. If necessary, perform a "rescue" cerclage suture procedure.
- Perform a prophylactic cerclage suture operation, either transvaginally or transabdominally. The transabdominal approach is indicated when the vaginal portion of the cervix (portio vaginalis) is very scarred, defective, short, or nonexistent, as may be the case after one or more conizations followed by one or more midpregnancy losses, or after an unsuccessful transvaginal cerclage procedure.

The technique for the abdominal approach was described by Mahran.[35] Series of these procedures have been reviewed, and the results in terms of a successful pregnancy outcome appear good.[36–38] These sutures have the advantage of being placed high on the cervix, near the internal os, in a bacteria-free environment. With a conventional or modified Shirodkar[39,40] or McDonald procedure,[41] the suture is placed transvaginally. Despite the potential for operative morbidity, the abdominal operative method is not difficult, but it requires laparotomy and subsequent cesarean section. Recently, laparoscopic suture insertion before pregnancy (interval suture) was described.[42] The suture may be left in place for a future pregnancy. Successful removal of the suture by culdotomy has been described with subsequent vaginal delivery but may not prove easy near term.

The transvaginal approach is a short, relatively simple procedure in which the suture is placed as high as possible on the vaginal portion of the cervix. Bladder dissection and upward displacement is no longer widely practiced, although the original Shirodkar procedure has a better success rate than a repeat McDonald suture when a previous suture did not prevent midtrimester loss. If the cervix is very deficient, bladder dissection and upward displacement may be unavoidable. Suture removal is usually performed at approximately 35 to 37 weeks or when labor starts and vaginal delivery is the goal. In addition to the mechanical compression effect of the suture, there may be more effective formation of a mucous barrier to bacterial invasion in the cervical canal.[26] Most clinicians prefer either Mersilene tape (two to three stitches required) or a braided double silk suture (five to seven stitches), inserted in a similar manner, with a knot in the anterior fornix.

There is still no consensus as to whether transvaginal cerlage suturing prolongs pregnancy and enhances neonatal survival.[21] Evidence seems to point to an overall benefit in prolonging pregnancy past 34 weeks' gestation for women with a cervix less than 2.5 cm long and for other high-risk groups.[31] The largest trial done for prophylactic historical reasons, before the advent of transvaginal ultrasound assessment,[43] showed a benefit with transvaginal cerclage after two preterm losses and no benefit after cervical conization. Although the complication rate after elective preventive cerclage suture is low (chorioamnionitis develops in 1%–7% of patients), an increased risk of infection after the procedure must be considered and discussed with the patient before a decision is made.

If the option of observing the cervix by transvaginal ultrasound is chosen, it is important for the clinician and the patient to understand that by the time funneling and effacement of the cervix are detected sonographically, a complicated pathophysiologic process may have begun and may be impossible to stop. Evidence is conflicting as to whether screening and placement of a rescue suture is effective. In a recent study of 2702 women evaluated at 23 weeks by transvaginal ultrasound, 43 (1.6%) had a cervical length of less than 1.5 cm. Half of the women were treated expectantly by their clinicians, and of those, 11 of 22 delivered before 32 weeks. The other half had a transvaginal cervical rescue suture inserted; only 1 of 21 delivered before 32 weeks. Although the two groups were comparable and a benefit of suturing was indicated, the study was not randomized.[44] Two small randomized studies and some observational studies suggested a benefit from serial transvaginal ultrasound and suture insertion when the cervical length is less than 2.5 cm,[30,31,45] although one randomized study showed no clear effect of cerclage suture.[33] Moreover, considerable morbidity occurred in the entire group studied and was attributed to prexisting subclinical infection, placental abruption, and preterm labor. The value of this approach and consequent late or emergency (rescue) cerclage is uncertain. Each case requires thorough evaluation of the options because there are no objective guidelines from well-constructed prospective studies.[21,31] When dilation and delivery in a previous pregnancy was accompanied by bleeding and pain indicative of concomitant chorioamniotic infection, transvaginal ultrasound surveillance may be a better option than prophylactic transvaginal cerclage.

In twin or other multiple pregnancy, routine prophylactic cervical cerclage offers no benefit. Serial ultrasound cervical assessments with timely selective cerclage in women with evidence of cervical shortening and funneling may improve outcome, although this hypothesis is unproven.[16,21,31]

When very preterm delivery may be imminent because of advancing cervical shortening or dilation, rescue cerclage suture insertion can be considered. For this to meet with any degree of success, cervical dilation must not be more than approximately 2 cm and the membranes must not protrude out of the external cervical os. When the membranes are visible, the prognosis worsens appreciably.[32] It is then necessary to exclude infection by speculum examination and bacterial culture from the cervix and to evaluate cervical length and appearance by transvaginal ultrasound. If the woman has no fever and a normal white blood cell count and serum C-reactive protein level, chorioamnionitis is less likely. A negative finding on cervicovaginal fibronectin assay (a marker of choriodecidual disruption) may also be useful.[5] Harger[21] suggested a management protocol to exclude infection and identify women who may benefit from late or emergency cervical cerclage suturing. Despite the risk associated with rescue suture, additional time is sometimes gained. Extra time is particularly useful from 24 to 26 weeks' gestation. Complication rates with rupture of the membranes and chorioamnionitis are high, between 20% and 50%. The value of prophylactic measures to maintain a normal vaginal bacterial environment (i.e., low pH, no bacterial vaginosis) is controversial,[46,47] although treatment of established bacterial vaginosis is likely to reduce the risk of preterm birth and is recommended.[47,48]

SUMMARY OF MANAGEMENT OPTIONS

Suspected Cervical Insufficiency

Management Options	Quality of Evidence	Strength of Recommendation	References
Prepregnancy			
Repair cervical lacerations and allow time for inflammation to resolve.	–	GPP	–
Provide counseling about the recurrence risks and options for pregnancy management.	–	GPP	–
Prenatal			
Confirm fetal normality at the end of the first trimester (NT and transvaginal ultrasound).	–	GPP	–
Cervical cerclage:			
Option 1: Elective cerclage at 12–15 wks:	Ib	A	43
• McDonald or Shirodkar	III	B	31
• Transabdominal (especially with previous failed transvaginal approach)	Ia	A	38
Option 2: Serial cervical ultrasound and "rescue" cerclage with evidence of change (shortening or funneling)	IIa III	B B	44 30,31,45
Prophylactic use of antibiotics is controversial.	Ib	A	46
Labor and Delivery			
Vaginal sutures are usually removed at ~36 wk.	III	B	21
Abdominal sutures require cesarean section; removal at the same time depends on the patient's intentions for future pregnancies.	III	B	35,37

NT, nuchal translucency.

MIDTRIMESTER BLEEDING (See also Chapter 59)

Definition

Midtrimester bleeding is any bleeding that occurs during midpregnancy. It has the same causes as bleeding that occurs during the third trimester. It may originate from the vulva, the vagina and the vaginal portion of the cervix, from a low-lying placenta or placenta previa, and from marginal and (rarely) total placental separation.

Risks

Most midtrimester bleeding is not serious,[49] but is associated with a considerably increased risk of repeated bleeding and preterm delivery.[49,50] Repeated first-trimester bleeding, with or without evidence of hematoma on ultrasound, is common and is not associated with a poor prognosis if it resolves before 14 weeks. However, bleeding in the second trimester is likely to be related to abnormality of the placental site, and the risk of an adverse pregnancy outcome is increased twofold to fivefold.[51–53] Among women with painless bleeding in the second and early third trimesters, one third deliver preterm. In women with uterine contractility, two thirds deliver preterm and half of these do so within 1 week.[49] After bleeding in the second trimester, the relative risk of placental abruption increases between 5-fold and 30-fold.[51,53] This bleeding is related to intrauterine growth restriction and fetal distress.[53] Abruption is not common in midpregnancy, probably because of the normal decrease in blood pressure that occurs at this time, but if it occurs, the risk of fetal demise is doubled.[50] Placenta previa also leads to a considerable risk of bleeding in the second trimester.[54] An increased risk of bleeding is also associated with severe early-onset hypertensive disorder, rare cases of women who are carriers of a bleeding diathesis, and medication with anticoagulant drugs.

Management Options

Any bleeding, however slight, with or without pain or uterine contractions, must be investigated. The same considerations for diagnosis and treatment apply as in the third trimester. Cervical or postcoital bleeding may be related to vaginal or cervical infection, a frail ectropion or cervical polyps, the early stages of cervical insufficiency, or rarely, cancerous lesions. Domestic abuse must be kept in mind as well. Blood streaks in the cervical mucus indicate that the origin of the bleeding is the uterine cavity. The most likely source is a decidual blood vessel at the placental edge or a dilating cervix. Bleeding from a low-lying placenta (<2 cm from the internal os) or placenta previa or minor placental abruption (bleeding into the decidua and subplacental space) must be considered.

In 30% of pregnancies, ultrasound screening at approximately 18 to 20 weeks will show a low-lying placenta. A more definitive diagnosis may be made with color Doppler studies. Vaginal ultrasound shows whether funneling of the internal os and shortening of the cervical canal is taking place. A diagnosis at this time makes it possible to warn the mother and to take appropriate precautions.

Cervical polyps originate in the lower part of the cervical external os and arise in response to cervical infection, leading to a tissue reaction in the endocervical glandular tissue. This can produce a 0.5- to 3-cm inflamed protrusion from the cervix that bleeds easily, typically after exertion or intercourse. Diagnosis is made by speculum examination. Management consists of grasping the polyp with a sponge forceps and twisting it loose (taking care not to tear it away) to stop the blood supply and reduce bleeding. The woman should be reassured about the benign nature of the condition and its nonrecurrence, although histopathologic examination should be performed in all cases. Use of an appropriate self-administered antibacterial vaginal cream may be recommended for a few days.

After initial examination by speculum, the first rule is to await developments and not to examine the woman digitally by pushing a finger into or through the cervix. A new scan should not be necessary, unless the bleeding occurred before the 18- to 20-week scan, when it is more likely to be associated with fetal intrauterine death. Fetal viability can be shown easily with a portable handheld Doppler ultrasound fetal heart detector. Intrauterine hematoma can be recognized by an echolucent "stringy" area just above the internal os. The hematoma often lifts the membranes off the decidua or causes a separation of the placental edge. An older hematoma may be more echodense and difficult to detect.

Conservative management with bed rest is usually advised, although no studies show a benefit from this or from oral or parenteral tocolytic drugs or sedatives. It is important to allay the woman's anxiety as much as possible. Advising the woman to avoid strenuous work and to rest periodically throughout the day can be helpful because tiredness provokes uterine contractions that may lead to resumed bleeding. For the same reason and to prevent ascending infection, eradication of bacterial vaginosis or infection and abstaining from sexual intercourse may be helpful.[48] Occasionally, repeated bleeding may lead to anemia. Rarely, blood transfusion is necessary. The value of antifibrinolytic drugs, such as tranexamic acid, is debated.

SUMMARY OF MANAGEMENT OPTIONS
Midtrimester Bleeding

Condition	Management Options
Antepartum hemorrhage	See Chapter 59
Preterm labor	See Chapter 62
Gynecologic conditions	See Chapters 32, 53, and 58
Domestic violence	See Chapter 81

MIDPREGNANCY MEMBRANE RUPTURE (See Chapters 61 and 63)

Definition

Midpregnancy membrane rupture is leakage of amniotic fluid between 12 and 28 weeks. It is particularly significant after 20 weeks (very preterm prelabor rupture of membranes [PPROM]). The condition is serious because of the high likelihood of infection, placental abruption, fetal compromise, and early preterm birth, with its associated neonatal morbidity and mortality and the risks of maternal operative morbidity, infection, and thrombosis.

Risks

The antecedent risk factors are the same as for previous midpregnancy loss (i.e., previous midpregnancy loss or delivery, bacterial vaginosis, ascending bacterial infection with ensuing chorioamnionitis, cervical insufficiency and repeated bleeding from early in pregnancy, cervical conization). Other risk factors include low body mass, lung disease and smoking, strenuous working conditions, and perhaps genetic factors related to genes that regulate tissue breakdown and remodeling (matrix metalloproteinases).[25,48,51,53,55,56] These factors may predict which patients will have the condition, although none is easily recognized in an individual patient, except for cervical insufficiency seen developing on transvaginal ultrasound.

The fetal prognosis is affected by the gestational age at which the membranes rupture, the interval until delivery, the degree of oligohydramnios (which is not always complete), and the degree to which subclinical and overt infection develop. The sequence of events is likely to be initiated when proteolytic bacteria enter the cervical canal (made easier when bleeding from the placental site tracks down behind the membranes and through the cervix) and reach the chorionic membrane, where enzymatic breakdown is accelerated rapidly by proinflammatory mediators.[55,56] Infection affects both membranes and the amniotic fluid compartment, eventually reaching the fetus through the umbilical cord and lungs. Approximately 50% of infants are delivered by 1 week, 70% to 75% are delivered by 2 weeks, and 80% to 85% are delivered by 4 weeks.[56] Earlier rupture usually means a longer latent time until delivery. When very PPROM occurs before 24 to 26 weeks, serious complications related to arrest of lung development, (e.g., intrauterine pneumonia, bronchopulmonary hypoplasia [in approximately 16% of cases], pulmonary hypertension [if the neonate survives]) are major factors that affect survival.[55–57] Another risk factor is skeletal deformity caused by oligohydramnios and severe fetal distress, including that caused by cord entanglement or prolapse. If the membranes have been ruptured for more than 1 week, the risk of pulmonary hypoplasia and limb deformity increases, particularly before 26 weeks' gestation and if the duration of rupture is longer than 5 weeks.[58] With PPROM before 20 weeks, at least half of fetuses have bronchopulmonary hypoplasia, but this rate decreases as gestation advances and the latent time to birth becomes shorter. PPROM occurs in 5% to 7% of all pregnancies, but the interval to delivery is longer than 1 week in only 10% of these pregnancies. Diagnosis is made by clinical observation, ultrasound,[58] and positive signs of infection. The use of proinflammatory factors (interleukins) in amniotic fluid or cervical secretions to identify patients with PPROM is experimental.

Management Options

Treatment is conservative from early in the midtrimester until 28 weeks' gestation. If leakage occurs early in midpregnancy (i.e., before 18–20 weeks), the prognosis for fetal survival is so grave that termination must be discussed with the parents. Most women (but not all) miscarry spontaneously before 20 weeks. If pockets of amniotic fluid remain, the chance of a successful outcome improves. If fetomaternal infection occurs before viability is achieved at 20 weeks, it may be necessary to stimulate uterine activity with vaginal or oral prostaglandins or oxytocin infusion, depending on the degree of cervical dilation. Infection parameters, primarily maternal temperature, white blood cell count, and C-reactive protein level, must be monitored. Antibiotics that cover anaerobic bacteria (clindamycin or metronidazole) should be administered before and during evacuation of the uterus.

An elevated or increasing white cell blood count may be helpful in determining the onset of chorioamnionitic infection necessitating delivery, but its specificity and positive predictive value are low. Measurement of the C-reactive protein level may be more reliable, but only if the value is clearly greater than the upper normal distribution level (two standard deviations). The C-reactive protein level does not increase to a diagnostic level until approximately 12 hours before the infection becomes clinically obvious.[59]

If the pregnancy is continued, the main option after 20 to 22 weeks' gestation, depending on local legislation, is expectant management, usually with initial hospitalization. After initial assessment, discharge home with monitoring for fetal viability and infection is feasible and does not worsen the prognosis.[56] A meta-analysis of the studies of prophylactic antibiotic treatment, dominated by one randomized study (the ORACLE trial), showed improved outcome after 24 weeks, defined as delaying preterm birth for 1 week (relative risk, 0.88; 95% confidence interval, 0.84–0.92), reducing the incidence of chorioamnionitis (relative risk, 0.62; 95% confidence interval, 0.51–0.72), and reducing the incidence of maternal infection (relative risk, 0.85; 95% confidence interval, 0.76–0.96).[56,60] The incidence of neonatal infectious disease, the requirement for oxygen, and the number of abnormal cerebral ultrasound findings were also significantly reduced. The antibiotics of choice are metronidazole and erythromycin. Corticosteroid administration is safe. The need for booster courses is questionable, but tocolysis can be used as indicated (particularly to allow in utero transfer to a tertiary neonatal unit). Amnioinfusion and sealing of the leak site are currently experimental approaches.[56] If PPROM occurs in a patient who has a transvaginal cerclage suture, the suture is usually removed if signs of infection occur. After 24 weeks, it may be possible to maintain the suture with antibiotic treatment.

INCARCERATED UTERUS

Definition

When the pregnant uterus is in a retroverted and retroflexed position and cannot rise out of the pelvic cavity, it is incarcerated. The fixed retroverted position pulls the cervix and vagina forward and cephalad, stretching and pressing on the urethra. Acute urinary retention, the usual symptom, is often preceded for a few days by frequency as a sign of overflow incontinence. Forward bulging may be noted behind the posterior vaginal wall.

Risks

A previously retroverted and retroflexed uterus is the usual antecedent. This uterine position is found in 1 in 5 to 1 in 10 women,[61–63] although the uterus rises out of the pelvis spontaneously after 12 to 15 weeks' gestation in almost all cases. The incidence of incarceration is reported to be only 1 in 3000 pregnancies. Predisposing factors are not known. Uterine wall fibroids or posterior wall adhesions may be implicated in some cases. Potential complications include neuromuscular damage to the bladder, ureteric obstruction and hydronephrosis with renal infection and damage, pressure necrosis of adjoining organs, and uterine rupture. In rare cases, sacculation persists into the third trimester, resulting in abnormal fetal presentation.[62,63]

Management Options

The bladder must be emptied by catheter. The catheter is left on free drainage for 24 to 48 hours. Subsequent ultrasound monitoring of bladder emptying to ensure a residual of no more than 150 to 200 mL is advisable. If the residual is greater, an indwelling catheter is inserted. Recurrent episodes of retention are common until the condition gradually resolves. Ultrasound examination is a necessary adjunct to diagnosis to exclude the alternative diagnosis of ovarian cyst incarceration in the pelvis.[63] Manual repositioning of the uterus may be considered and may need to be done under general anesthesia. Occasionally, ureteric stents or catheters are required to alleviate hydroureter and hydronephrosis.[64] Antibiotic treatment is not required unless there is evidence of infection.

SUMMARY OF MANAGEMENT OPTIONS

Incarcerated Uterus

Management Options	Quality of Evidence	Strength of Recommendation	References
Prenatal			
Encourage bed rest in the prone position.	IV	C	62,63
Encourage regular emptying of the bladder, with ultrasound confirmation that it remains empty (<200 mL).	IV	C	62,63
Consider catheterization for 48 hr if the patient cannot keep the bladder empty by voiding.	IV	C	62,63

CONCLUSIONS

- Midpregnancy is a time of intense physiologic evolution that is relatively undisturbed by intercurrent problems.
- Vague symptoms consistent with maternal adaptation to the growing fetus and ongoing pregnancy must not be confused with developing disease.
- Most serious problems that occur during midpregnancy involve a risk of very early delivery or fetal loss, particularly in patients with repeated previous midpregnancy loss, cervical insufficiency and repeated early bleeding from the placenta implantation site, or very preterm prelabor rupture of the membranes.
- Some potential remedies are designed to delay delivery and counteract infectious morbidity, including cervical cerclage, with or without transvaginal ultrasound follow-up, and antibiotic, tocolytic, and corticosteroid treatment, when indicated.
- Most of these measures have been inconclusively researched, and their value is debated.
- More evidence-based guidelines are needed. Meanwhile, clinicians should be prepared to make therapeutic recommendations based on individual needs and the best available evidence.

REFERENCES

1. Kaufmann P, Black S, Huppertz B: Endovascular trophoblast invasion: Implications for the pathogenesis of intrauterine growth retardation and preeclampsia. Biol Reprod 2003;69:1–7.
2. Geirsson RT: Intrauterine volume in pregnancy. Acta Obstet Gynecol Scand Suppl 1986;136:41–43.
3. Andersen B, Nielsen TF: Appendicitis in pregnancy: Diagnosis, management and complications. Acta Obstet Gynecol Scand 1999;78:758–762.
4. Oláh KS, Gee H: The prevention of preterm delivery: Can we afford to continue to ignore the cervix? Br J Obstet Gynaecol 1992;99:278–280.
5. Honest H, Bachmann LM, Gupta JK, et al: Accuracy of cervicovaginal fetal fibronectin test in predicting spontaneous preterm birth: Systematic review. Br Med J 2002;325:301–304.
6. Kitchen W, Ford GW, Doyle LW, et al: Cesarean section or vaginal delivery at 24 to 28 weeks gestation: Comparison of survival and neonatal and two-year morbidity. Obstet Gynecol 1985;66:149–157.
7. Shennan AT, Milligan JE, Hoskins EM: Perinatal factors associated with death or handicap in very preterm infants. Am J Obstet Gynecol 1985;151:231–238.
8. Sutton L, Bajuk B: Population based study of infants born at less than 28 weeks gestation in New South Wales, Australia in 1992–93. New South Wales Neonatal Intensive Care Unit Study Group. Paediatr Perinat Epidemiol 1999;13:288–301.
9. Finnström O, Olaugsson PO, Sedin G, et al: The Swedish national prospective study on extremely low birthweight (ELBW) infants: Incidence, mortality, morbidity and survival in relation to level of care. Acta Paediatr 1997;86:503–511.
10. Doyle LW for the Victorian Infant Collaborative Study Group: Outcome at 5 years age of children 23–27 weeks gestation: Refining the prognosis. Pediatrics 2001;108:134–141.
11. Ahner R, Bikas D, Rabl M, et al: Ethical implications of aggressive obstetric management at less than 28 weeks gestation. Acta Obstet Gynecol Scand 2001;80:120–125.
12. Steingrimsdottir T, Cnattingius S, Lindmark G: Symfysis-fundus height: Construction of a new Swedish reference curve, based on ultrasonically dated pregnancies. Acta Obstet Gynecol Scand 1995;74:346–351.
13. Ancel PY, Saurel-Cubizolles MJ, Di Renzo GC, et al: Risk factors for 14–21 week abortions: A case-control study in Europe. The Europop Group. Hum Reprod 2000;15:2426–2432.
14. NOMESCO: Health statistics in the Nordic countries 2001. Copenhagen, NOMESCO, 2003.
15. Holmgren PÅ, Högberg U: The very preterm infant: A population-based study. Acta Obstet Gynecol Scand 2001;80:525–531.
16. Grobman W, Peaceman AM: What are the rates and mechanisms of first and second trimester pregnancy loss in twins? Clin Obstet Gynecol 1998;41:37–45.
17. World Health Organization: International Statistical Classification of Diseases and Related Health Problems, 10th revision. Geneva, World Health Organization, 1993.
18. Hack M, Fanaroff AA: Outcomes of children of extremely low birthweight and gestational age in the 1990's. Early Hum Dev 1999;53:193–218.
19. American College of Obstetricians and Gynecologists: Preterm labor: The College Technical Bulletin No. 206. Washington DC, American College of Obstetricians and Gynecologists, 1995.
20. Berghella V, Haas S, Chervoneva I, Hyslop T: Patients with prior second-trimester loss: Prohylactic cerclage or serial transvaginal sonograms? Am J Obstet Gynecol 2002;187:747–751.
21. Harger JH: Cerclage and cervical insufficiency: An evidence-based analysis. Obstet Gynecol 2002;100:313–327.
22. Berghella V, Talucci M, Desai A: Does transvaginal sonographic measurement of cervical length before 14 weeks predict preterm delivery in high-risk pregnancies? Ultrasound Obstet Gynecol 2003;21:140–144.
23. Lidegaard: Cervical incompetence and cerclage in Denmark 1980–90: A register-based epidemiological survey. Acta Obstet Gynecol Scand 1994;73:35–38.
24. Iams JD, Goldenberg RL, Meis PJ, et al: The length of the cervix and the risk of spontaneous premature delivery. N Engl J Med 1996;334:567–572.
25. Kristensen J, Langhoff-Roos J, Wittrup M, Bock JE: Cervical conization and preterm delivery/low birth weight: A systematic review of the literature. Acta Obstet Gynecol Scand 1993;72: 640–644.
26. Mortensen OA, Franklin J, Löfstrand T, Svanberg B: Prediction of preterm delivery. Acta Obstet Gynecol Scand 1987;66: 507–512.
27. Mercer BM, Goldenberg RL, Das A, et al: The preterm prediction study: A clinical risk assessment system. Am J Obstet Gynecol 1996;174:1885–1895.
28. Heath VC, Southall TR, Souka AP, et al: Cervical length at 23 weeks gestation: Relation to demographic characteristics and previous obstetric history. Ultrasound Obstet Gyneco 1998;12:304–311.
29. Rizzo G: Use of ultrasound to predict preterm delivery: Do not lose the opportunity. Ultrasound Obstet Gynecol 1996;8: 289–292.

30. Guzman ER, Mellon C, Vintzileos AM, et al: Longitudinal assessment of endocervical canal length between 15 and 24 weeks gestation in women at risk for pregnancy loss or preterm birth. Obstet Gynecol 1998;92:31–37.
31. Althuisius SM, Dekker GA, van Geijn HP: Cervical incompetence: A reappraisal of an obstetric controversy. Obstet Gynecol Surv 2002;57:377–387.
32. Groom KM, Shennan AH, Bennett PR: Ultrasound-indicated cervical cerclage: Outcome depends on preoperative cervical length and presence of visible membranes at time of cerclage. Am J Obstet Gynecol 2002;187:445–449.
33. Rust OA, Atlas RO, Reed J, et al: Revisiting the short cervix detected by transvaginal ultrasound in the second trimester: Why cerclage therapy may not help. Am J Obstet Gynecol 2001;185:1098–1105.
34. Fox R, James M, Tuohy J, Wardle: Transvaginal ultrasound in the management of women with suspected cervical incompetence. Br J Obstet Gynaecol 1996;103:921–924.
35. Mahran M: Transabdominal cervical cerclage during pregnancy. Obstet Gynecol 1978;52:502–506.
36. Gibb DMF, Salaria DA: Transabdominal cervicoisthmic cerclage in the management of recurrent second trimester miscarriage and preterm delivery. Br J Obstet Gynaecol 1995; 102:802–806.
37. Anthony GS, Walker RG, Cameron, et al: Transabdominal cervico-isthmic cerclage in the management of cervical incompetence. Eur J Obstet Gynecol Reprod Biol 1997;72;127–130.
38. Zaveri V, Aghajafari F, Amankawah K, Hannah M: Abdominal versus vaginal cerclage after a failed transvaginal cerclage: A systematic review. Am J Obstet Gynecol 2002;187: 868–872.
39. Shirodkar VN: A new method of operative treatment for habitual abortion in the second trimester of pregnancy. Antiseptic 1955;52:299–300.
40. Cunningham FG, MacDonald PC, Gant NF, et al: Williams Obstetrics, 20th ed. Stamford Conn, Appleton & Lange, 1997, pp 588–590.
41. McDonald IA: Suture of the cervix for inevitable miscarriage. J Obstet Gynaecol Br Empire 1957;64:346–350.
42. Gallot D, Savary D, Laurichesse H, et al: Experience with three cases of laparoscopic transabdominal cervico-isthmic cerclage and two subsequent pregnancies. Br J Obstet Gynaecol 2003;110:696–700.
43. MRC/RCOG Working Party on Cervical Cerclage: Final report of the Medical Research Council/Royal College of Obstetricians and Gynaecologists multicentre randomised trial of cervical cerclage. Br J Obstet Gynaecol 1993;100:516–523.
44. Heath VC, Souka AP, Erasmus I, et al: Cervical length at 23 weeks gestation: The value of Shirodkar suture for the short cervix. Ultrasound Obstet Gynecol 1998;12:318–322.
45. Berghella V, Daly SF, Tolosa JE, et al: Prediction of preterm delivery with transvaginal ultrasonography of the cervix in patients with high risk pregnancies: Does cerclage prevent prematurity? Am J Obstet Gynecol 1999;181:809–815.
46. Vermeulen GM, Bruinse HW: Prophylactic administration of clindamycin 2% vaginal cream to reduce the incidence of spontaneous preterm birth in women with an increased recurrrence risk: A randomised placebo-controlled double-blind trial. Br J Obstet Gynaecol 1999;106:652–657.
47. Lamont RF, Duncan SL, Mandal D, Bassett P: Intravaginal clindamycin to reduce preterm birth in women with abnormal genital tract flora. Obstet Gynecol 2003;101:516–522.
48. McGregor JA, French JI: Bacterial vaginosis in pregnancy. Obstet Gynecol Surv 2000;55:1–19.
49. Leung TY, Chan LW, Tan WH, et al: Risk and prediction of preterm delivery in pregnancies complicated by antepartum hemorrhage of unknown origin before 34 weeks. Gynecol Obstet Invest 2001;52:227–231.
50. Wolf EJ, Vintizileos AM, Rosenkrantz TS, et al: Do survival and morbidity of very-low-birth-weight infants vary according to the primary pregnancy complication that results in preterm delivery? Am J Obstet Gynecol 1993;169:1233–1239.
51. Toivonen S, Heinonen S, Anttila M, et al: Reproductive risk factors, Doppler findings and outcome of affected births in placental abruption: A population-based analysis. Am J Perinatol 2002;19:451–460.
52. Johns J, Hyett J, Jauniaux E: Obstetric outcome after threatened miscarriage with and without hematoma on ultrasound. Obstet Gynecol 2003;102:483–487.
53. Nagy S, Bush M, Lipinski RH, Gardo S: Clinical significance of subchorionic and retroplacental hematomas detected in the first trimester of pregnancy. Obstet Gynecol 2003;102:94–100.
54. Sheiner E, Shoham Vardi I, Hallak M, et al: Placenta previa: Obstetric risk factors and pregnancy outcome. J Fetal Matern Med 2001;10:414–419.
55. Mercer BM: Preterm premature rupture of membranes. Obstet Gynecol 2003;101:178–193.
56. Lamont RF: Recent evidence associated with the condition of preterm prelabour rupture of membranes. Curr Opin Obstet Gynecol 2003;15:91–99.
57. Nimrod C, Varela-Gittings F, Machin G, et al: The effect of very prolonged membrane rupture on fetal development. Am J Obstet Gynecol 1984;148:540–543.
58. Odibo AO, Talucci M. Berghella V: Prediction of preterm premature rupture of membranes by transvaginal ultrasound features and risk factors in a high-risk population. Ultrasound Obstet Gynecol 2002;20:245–251.
59. Fisk NM, Fysh J, Child AG, et al: Is C-reactive protein really useful in preterm premature rupture of membranes? Br J Obstet Gynaecol 1987;94:1159–1164.
60. Kenyon S, Boulvain M, Neilson J: Antibiotics for preterm premature rupture of membranes. Cochrane Database of Systematic Reviews CD001058, 2001.
61. Donald I: Local abnormalities. In Practical Obstetric Problems, 4th ed. London, Lloyd-Luke, 1969, pp 212–238.
62. O'Connell MP, Ivory CM, Hunter RW: Incarcerated retroverted uterus: A nonrecurring complication of pregnancy. J Obstet Gynaecol 1999;19:84–85.
63. Hamod H, Chamberlain PE, Moore NR, Mackenzie IZ: Conservative treatment of an incarcerated gravid uterus. Br J Obstet Gynaecol 2002;109:1074–1075.

CHAPTER 7

First-Trimester Screening for Fetal Abnormalities

Romaine Robyr / Yves Ville

INTRODUCTION

The first-trimester diagnosis of fetal abnormalities is characterized by the confidentiality surrounding parental decisions. Early termination of pregnancy has considerable medical and psychological benefits for women compared with the effects of late termination. The early first-trimester ultrasound examination is also an opportunity to identify a family history of genetic syndromes or anomalies that warrant more frequent or detailed ultrasound assessments during the pregnancy (see also Chapter 8).

The most common indications for routine ultrasound examination at 11 to 14 weeks are the following:

- Assessment of viability
- Determination of gestational age
- Identification and typing of multiple pregnancies
- Screening for fetal aneuploidy based on the measurement of nuchal translucency (NT) thickness. A combination of ultrasonography and laboratory testing at 11 to 14 weeks' gestation is the best available method for screening for fetal aneuploidy.[1,2]
- Assessment of gross fetal anatomy. Technologic improvements, in particular, high-frequency transvaginal ultrasound probes, allow detection of the most severe fetal structural abnormalities before 14 weeks' gestation.[3,4]

Screening requires standardization and quality control. An ultrasound examination at 11 to 14 weeks includes at least the following three core views of the fetus:

- A strict midsagittal plane is used to allow measurement of the crown–rump length (CRL) and examination of the abdominal wall as well as both cranial and caudal fetal extremities. NT measurement is also performed in this plane.
- An axial view of the skull is used to identify the cranial contour, the midline of the brain, and the posterior fossa.
- A cross-section of the abdomen is used to identify the cord insertion site on the abdomen and the intra-abdominal position of the stomach. The presence of four limbs with three segments is also verified.

The 11- to 14-week window of gestational age is the best compromise to assess gestational age, measure NT thickness, and obtain a potentially detailed anatomic survey (Table 7–1). A more thorough examination of the fetal anatomy is performed when mandated by the patient's history or abnormal findings on a screening examination.

TABLE 7–1

Ultrasound Examination of the Fetal Anatomy at 11 to 14 Weeks' Gestation

Sagittal View to Assess
Crown–rump length
Integrity of the cranial vault
Insertion of the umbilical cord on the abdominal wall
Thickness of the nuchal translucency
Cross-Section Planes Showing
Normal position of the heart in the thorax
Four limbs with three segments, with normal mobility and alignment
Stomach bubble in the abdomen
Bladder
Axial View of the Brain Showing
Midline and falx cerebri
Lateral ventricles filled with choroids plexi
No cystic images

ULTRASOUND EXAMINATION AT 11 TO 14 WEEKS

Identifying a Viable Pregnancy

Ultrasound examination at 11 to 14 weeks is often the first opportunity to diagnose early pregnancy failure (Fig. 7–1). The prevalence of early pregnancy failure in one screening study of 17,870 women at 10 to 13 weeks was 2.8% (501 cases), including 313 (62.5%) missed abortions and 188 (37.5%) anembryonic pregnancies.[5] The diagnosis of a nonviable pregnancy is important because elective evacuation of the retained products of conception is likely more cost-effective and potentially safer than emergency surgery for miscarriage.[5]

The likelihood of pregnancy loss after the successful development of embryonic anatomic landmarks identified on endovaginal ultrasound has been evaluated.[6] Two hundred thirty-two women with positive urinary pregnancy test results and no history of vaginal bleeding underwent endovaginal sonography at their initial visit and then at subsequent visits, as clinically indicated. The presence of anatomic and embryonic structures (gestation sac, yolk sac, embryo) as well as cardiac activity was recorded. Twenty-seven losses were documented in the embryonic period, with 4 losses in the fetal period and 201 live births reported. When a gestation sac was seen, the total subsequent loss rate was 11.5% during the embryonic period; the rate was 8.5% with a yolk sac only, 7.2% with an embryo up to 5 mm, 3.3% with an embryo 6 to 10 mm, and 0.5% with an embryo larger than 10 mm. No pregnancies were lost between 8.5 and 14 weeks. The fetal loss rate after 14 weeks was 2.0%.[6]

Dating the Pregnancy

Dating a pregnancy by menstrual history is often unreliable. Up to 40% of women are uncertain of their menstrual dates, and even when they are certain, gestational

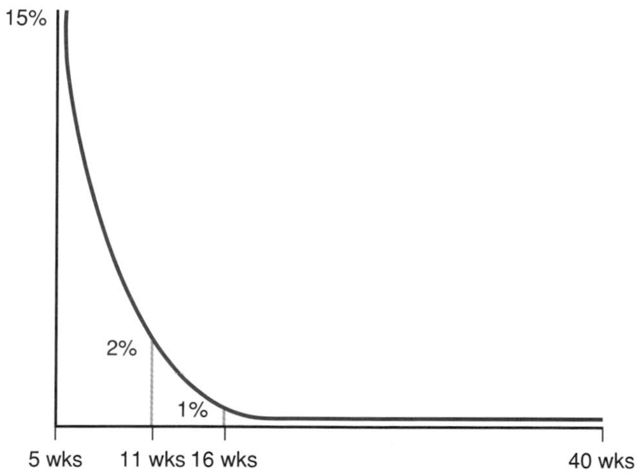

FIGURE 7–1
Risk of spontaneous miscarriage.

age is often overestimated compared with ultrasound findings.[7] Overestimation of true gestational age by menstrual history increases the prevalence of postdated pregnancies.[8] Estimates of the duration of gestation based on the last menstrual period are subject to both random error and a systematic tendency to overstate the duration of gestation, most likely because of delayed ovulation.[9] In a recent study, the prevalence of post-term births was 12.1% based on menstrual history, but only 3.4% based on ultrasound findings. The effect on the cost of delivering obstetric health care is real, considering that more than 8% of pregnant women have unnecessary antenatal surveillance.

Before 6 weeks, dating is done by description and measurement of the gestation sac.[10] The size of the sac can be correlated to gestational age.[11] The gestation sac is always visible by 4 weeks. In 95% of cases, the yolk sac is present by 5 weeks, and in all cases, it is present by 6 weeks. The fetal heart is seen beating in 86% of cases by 6 weeks, and always by 7 weeks.

Of all of the available measurements, the maximum embryo length between 6 and 10 weeks and the CRL up to 14 weeks are the most accurate for determining gestational age. The random error is 4 to 8 days at the 95th percentile.[12–15] The largest study that used a strict method is that of Wisser and Dirscheld,[15] who highlighted potential pitfalls of earlier studies and reported a predictive interval of 4.7 days (standard deviation) in 160 patients who underwent in vitro fertilization, including 21 with multiple pregnancies.[15]

The maximum embryo or fetal length is usually measured excluding the inferior limbs and without correction of the body's flexion. All charts are concordant before 60 mm (predictive interval, 3 days [standard deviation]), but differ significantly thereafter.

The gestational age should not be altered if the discrepancy between the last menstrual period and the CRL measurement is less than 7 days. A discrepancy of more than 1 week suggests inaccurate menstrual dates. However, there is no advantage in considering the last menstrual period when an ultrasound has been performed, even when the date is described as "certain," because the outcome of pregnancy is more closely related to gestational age as determined by ultrasound.[16]

When the CRL is greater than 60 mm, other biometric parameters are more useful for dating the pregnancy up to 20 weeks.[17] These parameters include biparietal diameter, head circumference, femur length, and abdominal circumference. Some authors indicate that long bone measurements can aid in the detection of skeletal dysplasia, although the low prevalence of these abnormalities, together with technical difficulties involved in measurement, leads to a poor positive predictive value when applied to the general population.[18]

First-trimester fetal biometry is underused to diagnose or characterize abnormal fetal development. Fetal growth during the first trimester was previously considered relatively uniform, but increasing evidence shows that anthropometric differences and other growth abnormalities may be expressed in the first trimester. In one series of transvaginal measurements, Kustermann and colleagues[19] observed that fetal biparietal diameter, head circumference, and abdominal circumference correlated better with the CRL than they did with gestational age. Further, direct assessment of early fetal measurements once established on the basis of the CRL may provide more relevant information than the two-step process using biometry based on gestational age. Salomon and associates[16] also found that fetal biometry is better estimated in relation to the CRL than to gestational age. Finally, reliable charts of biparietal diameter, head circumference, and abdominal circumference provide an opportunity to assess the quality of transverse views of the fetal head and abdomen at 11 to 14 weeks' gestation.

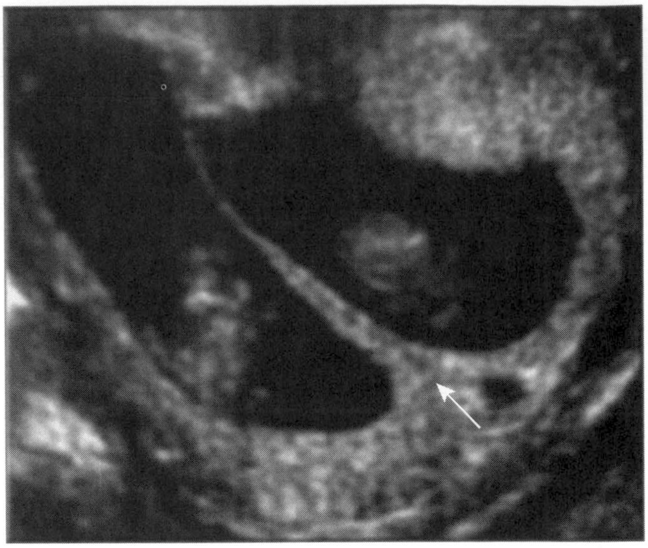

FIGURE 7–2
Dichorionic diamniotic twin pregnancy and the lambda sign.

Detecting Multiple Pregnancies and Determining Chorionicity (See Chapters 24 and 60)

Two percent of all pregnancies are twin pregnancies (Table 7–2). Two-thirds of these are dizygotic (genetically different, or nonidentical), and one-third are monozygotic (genetically identical). An important task of the first-trimester scan is to diagnose twin pregnancy and determine chorionicity. For obstetricians, chorionicity is far more important than zygosity because the management of multiple pregnancies relies mainly on chorionicity. Zygosity is relevant only to specific genetic issues. The relationship between chorionicity and zygosity can be kept simple. Two-thirds of dichorionic pregnancies (two placentas) are dizygotic, but one-third of them are monozygotic. The only way to determine zygosity is through invasive testing, with chorionic villus sampling, amniocentesis, or cordocentesis to analyze the fetal DNA. In 2% of cases, monozygotic twins share organs (Siamese, or conjoined, twins).

The first trimester is the best time to determine chorionicity. Dichorionic twins have two placentas, but in most cases, the placentas are adjacent, making the diagnosis of chorionicity difficult. An ultrasound clue to chorionicity in the first trimester is the lambda sign (Fig. 7–2).[20] This sign is a triangular tissue projection at the base of the intertwin membrane. It is an extension of the two chorion layers within the intertwin membrane that is present only in dichorionic pregnancy. In monochorionic pregnancies, there is no layer of chorion between the two layers of amnion, and the lambda sign is absent. This sign can be seen from 9 weeks onward, and its identification at any stage of pregnancy is proof of dichorionicity. However, the chorion disappears with advancing gestation, and the lambda sign becomes progressively more difficult to identify. At 16 weeks and 20 weeks, respectively, the lambda sign, or twin peak sign, is present in only 98% and 87% of cases.[21]

Identifying Normal Sonographic Features in the First Trimester

Ultrasound examination of the fetal anatomy in the first trimester focuses on embryologic development. Most fetal structures can be visualized at approximately 12 to 13 weeks with either vaginal or abdominal ultrasound (Table 7–3).[3,22–24]

Some sonographic features are similar to those described in the second and third trimesters (see also Chapter 8). Others are characteristic of the first trimester. Normal

TABLE 7–2

Types of Monozygotic Twins and Time of Division after Fertilization

CHORION	AMNION	TIME OF DIVISION (DAY)	FREQUENCY
Dichorionic	Diamniotic	0–3	33%
Monochorionic	Diamniotic	4–8	65%
Monochorionic	Monoamniotic	>8	2%
Monochorionic	Monoamniotic (Siamese)	>13	Rare

(From Wigglesworth JS, Singer DB: Textbook of Fetal and Perinatal Pathology. London, Blackwell, 1991, pp 131)

TABLE 7-3

Gestational Age at Visualization of Anatomic Landmarks

LANDMARK	GESTATIONAL AGE (WK)*	
	TRANSABDOMINAL ULTRASOUND	TRANSVAGINAL ULTRASOUND
Cranium	11,12–13	11–12
Spine	12–13	11
Long bones	12–13	10–11
Feet	12–13	13
Four-chamber view	12–13	12
Kidneys	12–13	11–12
Bladder	12–13	13
Anterior abdominal wall	12–13	12
Face	12–13	12
Stomach	13	11–12

*Gestational age at which organs may be visualized in >70% of fetuses. (From Chitty L, Pandya P: Ultrasound screening for fetal abnormalities in the first trimester. Prenat Diagn 1997; 17: 1269–1281.)

sonographic characteristics at 11 to 14 weeks include the following features.

External Features

Ossification begins at approximately 11 weeks with the occipital bone. The skull appears regular and hyperechogenic compared with the underlying tissues.[25]

Central Nervous System

From 9 weeks onward, the outline of the lateral ventricles, the echogenic choroid plexus, and the midline echo are visible. At 10 to 11 weeks, the third and fourth ventricles become visible, and from 14 weeks onward, the cerebellum and thalami are seen. The ventricles occupy most of the cerebral hemispheres. The diagnosis of hydrocephaly is difficult to establish in the first trimester. The choroids plexus should fill the lateral ventricles completely. Choroid plexus cysts are more common in the first trimester than in the second (incidence, 5.7% vs. 1.4%)[26,27] and are not known to be associated with fetal abnormalities at this early gestation.

Heart

The position, axis, four-chamber view, and symmetry of the heart can be seen in the first trimester. Huggon and associates[28] examined the fetal heart before 14 weeks' gestation. A highly trained cardiologist performed the examinations, and informative images were obtained transabdominally in 84% of cases. With less specialized operators, the four-chamber view was imaged successfully in 76% and 95% of cases transabdominally and transvaginally, respectively at 12 to 13 weeks' gestation.[3] Whitlow and Economides[29] reported that the four-chamber cardiac view was seen in 83% at 11 weeks and in 98% from 13 weeks onward. Women with an increased NT measurement are at risk for cardiac abnormalities (discussed later).[30]

Stomach

The stomach bubble is seen by 8 weeks in 31% of fetuses,[31] and in all cases by 12 to 13 weeks, as a small, sonolucent cystic structure in the upper left quadrant of the abdomen, below the heart. The relationship of this structure to the diaphragm should be noted. Fetal swallowing movements can be seen from 11 weeks onward[31]; fluid production from the intestinal epithelium is the most likely explanation for visualization of a stomach earlier.[32]

Abdominal Wall

The physiologic hernia of the midgut into the umbilical cord is a normal feature of embryonic intestinal development.[31] It is a large, hyperechogenic mass that retracts into the abdominal cavity between 10 weeks and 4 days and 11 weeks and 5 days. Fetuses older than 11 weeks and 5 days should not show herniation.[31] At that point, a differential diagnosis of omphalocele and gastroschisis should be considered.

Bladder and Kidneys

The fetal kidneys are seen in most cases at 12 to 13 weeks and appear more echogenic than the rest of the intra-abdominal contents. Renal echogenicity decreases as excretory function develops.[29] As a result, the fetal bladder is visualized in 80% of fetuses[33] by 11 weeks and in more than 90% by 13 weeks. The sagittal long axis of the bladder is less than 6 mm in the first trimester. In a study of 300 pregnancies at 10 to 14 weeks' gestation, the fetal bladder was always visualized when the CRL was greater than 67 mm. The fetal bladder was visualized in 90% of fetuses with a CRL of 38 to 67 mm.[34]

Skeleton

All three parts of the long bones are consistently seen from 11 weeks onward, although measurement of the long bones before 14 weeks seems clinically irrelevant. Body and limb movements are seen from 9 and 11 weeks onward, respectively. All long bones are similar in size at 11 to 14 weeks, ranging from approximately 6 mm at 11 weeks to 13 mm at 14 weeks.[35]

Nuchal Translucency

Definition

NT is the ultrasound definition of the physiologic collection of fluid under the skin behind the fetal neck at 11 to 14 weeks. NT thickness normally increases with

CRL.[36–38] It is important, therefore, to consider gestational age when deciding whether NT thickness is increased. The 50th percentile value for NT thickness is 1.2 mm and 1.9 mm for a CRL of 45 mm (11 weeks) and 85 mm (13 weeks and 6 days), respectively, and the 95th percentile value is 2 mm and 2.8 mm, respectively. Gestational age can therefore influence the risk calculation significantly (Fig. 7–3).

Because of the need to standardize measurement of the NT, initial attempts to differentiate the NT from cystic hygroma have been abandoned. However, cystic hygroma can be clearly differentiated from an increased simple NT, and further attempts to assess the prognosis of these fetuses are needed. When NT thickness is greater than 3.5 mm, thin septations are seen. The typical ultrasonographic appearance of cystic hygroma is two dilated jugular lymphatic sacs seen on a transverse scan at the level of the neck and separated from the NT (Fig. 7–4).

Measurement

Standardization and quality control in NT measurement is best served by the Fetal Medicine Foundation (FMF) initiative. This initiative established a process for certification in the 11- to 14-week scan to ensure that those performing the examination are adequately trained and maintain an appropriate level of performance through continuing education and audit (*www.fetalmedicine.com*).

To obtain a reliable measurement of fetal NT, the following steps are needed (Fig. 7–5):

- All sonographers who perform fetal scans must be appropriately trained. The ability to measure NT reproducibly improves with training; good results are typically achieved after approximately 100 scans. Intraobserver and interobserver differences in measurements are less than 0.5 mm in 95% of examinations.[39–40]
- The ultrasound equipment must be of good quality, with a video-loop function. The calipers should be able to provide measurements to a tenth of a millimeter.
- NT can be measured successfully by transabdominal ultrasound in approximately 95% of cases; in the rest, transvaginal sonography is required.
- Because the optimal gestational age for the measurement of NT is 11 weeks to 13 weeks and 6 days, the minimum fetal CRL should be 45 mm and the maximum, 84 mm.
- Because fetal NT thickness increases with CRL, gestation must be taken into account when determining whether a given NT increases risk.
- To measure the CRL, a good sagittal section, with the fetus in the neutral position, is needed for accurate measurement of NT.
- The magnification should be such that each increment in distance between calipers is 0.1 mm.
- Care must be taken to distinguish between fetal skin and the amnion. Both structures appear as thin membranes at this gestation. This distinction is made by waiting for spontaneous fetal movement away from the amniotic membrane or by "bouncing" the fetus off of the amnion by having the mother cough or by tapping the maternal abdomen.
- During the scan, more than one measurement is taken, and the maximum technically acceptable measurement is recorded.
- The nuchal umbilical cord is present in approximately 8% of scans, and this finding may falsely increase the NT measurement.[41] In these cases, the measurements of NT above and below the umbilical cord are different. In the calculation of risk, it is more appropriate to use first- or second-trimester laboratory screening results (Fig. 7–6).

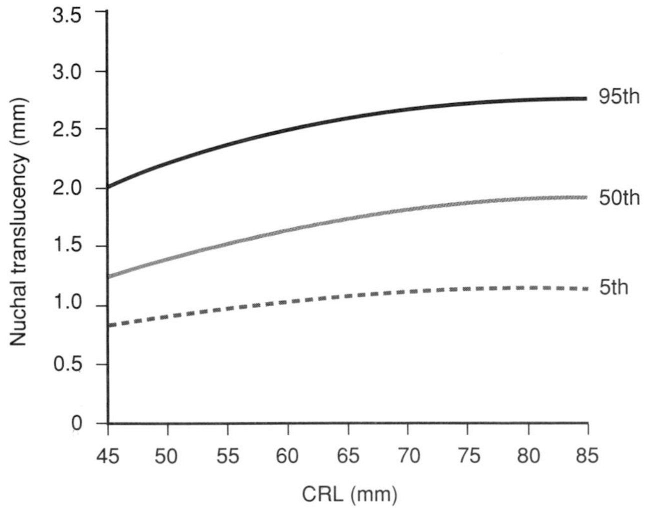

FIGURE 7–3
Changes in nuchal translucency with gestational age, as expressed by crown–rump length (CRL). (Adapted from Pandya PP, Snijders RJM, Johnson SJ, et al: Screening for fetal trisomies by maternal age and fetal nuchal translucency thickness at 10 to 14 weeks of gestation. BJOG 1995;102:957–962.)

Screening for Fetal Aneuploidies

FETAL NUCHAL TRANSLUCENCY AND TRISOMY 21

Down syndrome is the most common chromosomal abnormality, and every woman is at risk for having an affected fetus. This pervasive risk justifies the screening programs that have been established worldwide. A woman's risk of having a fetus with Down syndrome depends on her age, the gestational age, and the woman's history of chromosomal defects. These factors establish the background risk. A 33-year-old woman at 10 weeks' gestation has a 1 in 352 risk of having a fetus with trisomy 21. Because the risk decreases with gestation as a result of the spontaneous death of fetuses with chromosomal abnormalities, the risk is 1 in 547 at 40 weeks.

NT measurement at 11 to 14 weeks, combined with maternal age, provides an effective method of screening

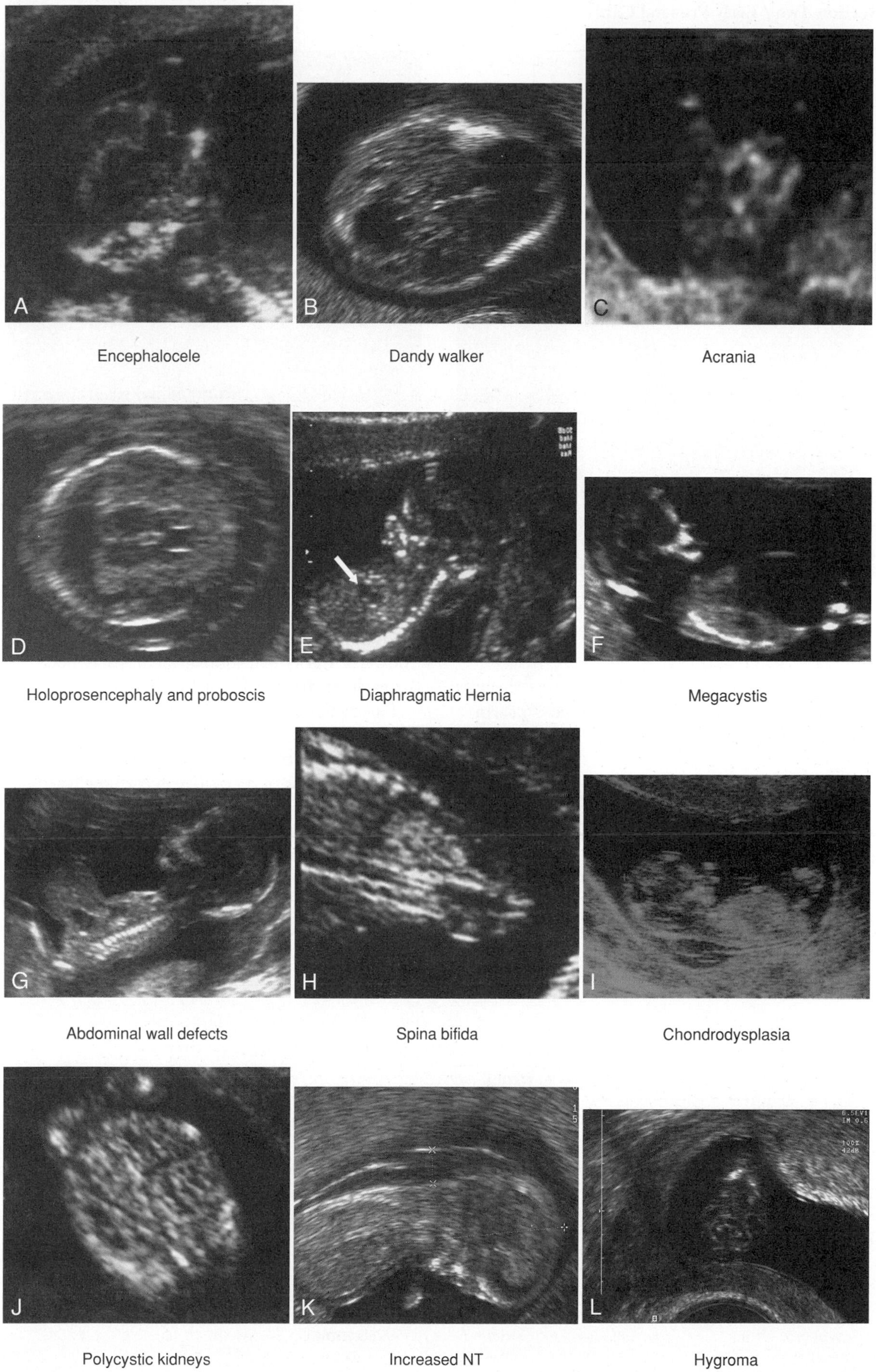

FIGURE 7–4
The most common structural defects diagnosed during screening at 11 to 14 weeks. *A*, encephalocele; *B*, Dandy-Walker syndrome; *C*, acrania; *D*, holoprosencephaly and proboscis; *E*, diaphragmatic hernia; *F*, megacystis; *G*, abdominal wall defects; *H*, spina bifida; *I*, chondrodysplasia; *J*, polycystic kidneys; *K*, increased nuchal translucency; *L*, hygroma.

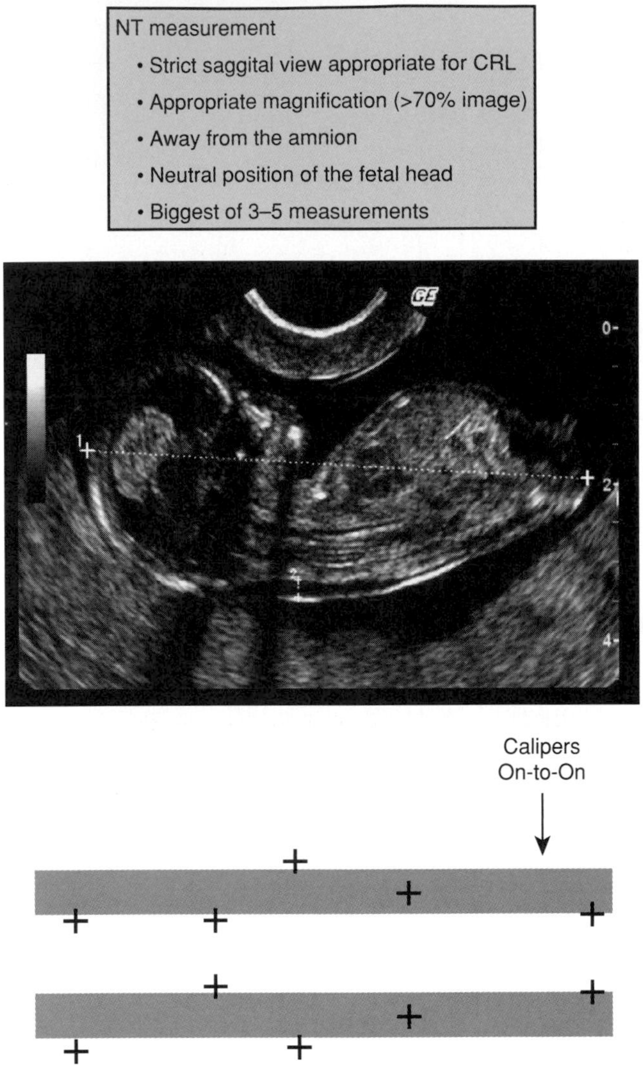

NT measurement
• Strict saggital view appropriate for CRL
• Appropriate magnification (>70% image)
• Away from the amnion
• Neutral position of the fetal head
• Biggest of 3–5 measurements
Calipers
On-to-On

FIGURE 7–5
Measurement of nuchal translucency. A strict sagittal view is appropriate for measuring crown–rump length. Appropriate magnification is greater than 70%. The view should be obtained away from the amnion. The fetal head should be in a neutral position. The largest of three to five measurements is recorded.

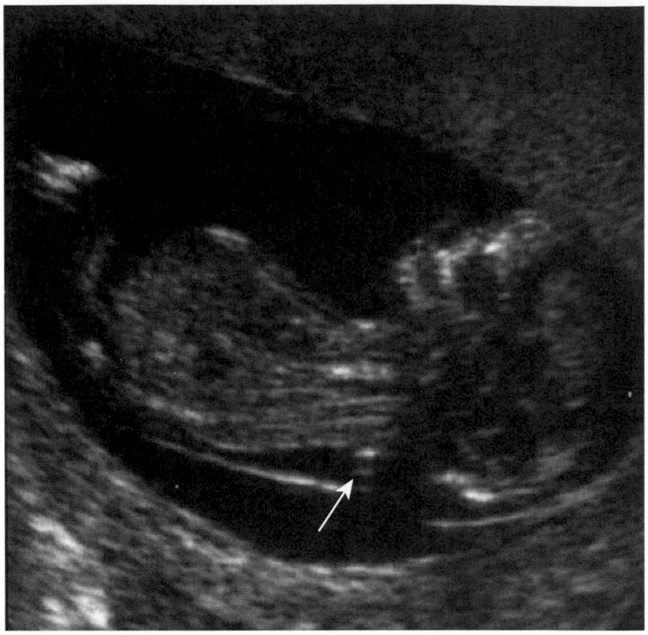

FIGURE 7–6
Umbilical cord around the neck (*arrow*).

for trisomy 21. An association between increased NT thickness and chromosomal defects has been seen since the early 1990s.[36,42–54]

The average detection rate with NT measurement is 77%, for a false-positive rate of 4.7%. The false-positive rate is the percentage of karyotypes potentially performed because of a positive screening test result. This detection rate represents the combined results of 14 prospective studies on NT measurement for chromosomal abnormalities involving 174,473 patients, including 728 with trisomy 21 (Table 7–4).[36,42–54] For comparison, screening by maternal age only, with a cutoff age of 37 years, has a detection rate of 30%, for a false-positive rate of 5%. With second-trimester maternal

TABLE 7–4

Studies Examining the Implementation of Fetal Nuchal Translucency Screening for Trisomy 21

STUDY	*N*	GESTATION (WK)	CUTOFF	FALSE-POSITIVE RATE	DETECTION RATE
Pandya et al., 1995[39]	1 763	10–14	≥2.5 mm	3.6%	3/4 (75%)
Szabo et al., 1995[43]	3 380	9–12	≥3.0 mm	1.6%	28/31 (90%)
Taipale et al., 1997[44]	6 939	10–14	≥3.0 mm	0.8%	4/6 (67%)
Hafner et al., 1998[45]	4 371	10–14	≥2.5 mm	1.7%	4/7 (57%)
Pajkrt et al., 1998[46]	1 547	10–14	≥3.0 mm	2.2%	6/9 (67%)
Snijders et al., 1998[36]	96 127	10–14	≥95th percentile	4.4%	234/327 (72%)
Economides et al., 1998[47]	2 281	11–14	≥99th percentile	0.4%	6/8 (75%)
Schwarzler et al., 1999[48]	4 523	10–14	NT >2.5 mm	2.7%	8/12 (67%)
Theodoropoulos et al., 1998[49]	3 550	10–14	≥95th percentile	2.3%	10/11 (91%)
Zoppi et al., 2000, 2001[50]	12 311	10–14	≥95th percentile	5.0%	52/64 (81%)
Gasiorek-Wiens et al., 2001[51]	23 805	10–14	≥95th percentile	8.0%	174/210 (83%)
Brizot et al., 2001[52]	2 996	10–14	≥95th percentile	5.3%	7/10 (70%)
Audibert et al., 2001[53]	4 130	10–14	≥95th percentile	4.3%	9/12 (75%)
Wayda et al., 2001[54]	6 750	10–12	≥2.5 mm	4.3%	17/17 (100%)
Total	174 473			4.7%	562/728 (77%)

Adapted from Nicolaides KH: Screening for chromosomal defects. Ultrasound Obstet Gynecol 2003;21:313–321.

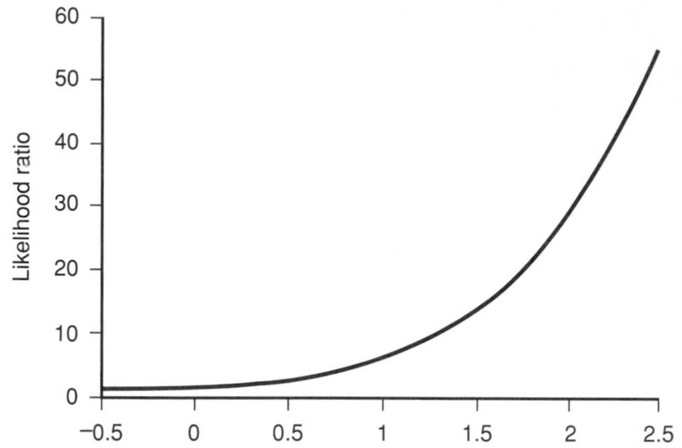

FIGURE 7–7
Likelihood ratios for trisomy 21 in relation to the deviation in fetal nuchal translucency thickness from the expected normal median for crown–rump length. (From Snijders RJM, Nicolaides KH: Assessment of risks. In Ultrasound Markers for Fetal Chromosomal Defects. Carnforth, UK, Parthenon, 1996, pp 63–120.)

serum markers, the detection rate is approximately 60%, for the same false-positive rate.[55]

Whenever a screening test is performed, the background risk is multiplied by the test factor to calculate a new risk. Therefore, in a fetus with a given CRL, each NT measurement is a likelihood ratio that is multiplied by the background risk to provide a new risk (Fig. 7–7).[36,56] A woman's risk of having a fetus with trisomy 21 is higher if the NT measurement is large and lower if it is small (Figs. 7–8 and 7–9).[36,56]

The median NT thickness is approximately 2.0 mm in fetuses with trisomy 21. However, because NT thickness increases with gestation, the use of a cutoff value rather than a continuous assessment with CRL and maternal age leads to a 5% loss in sensitivity.[57]

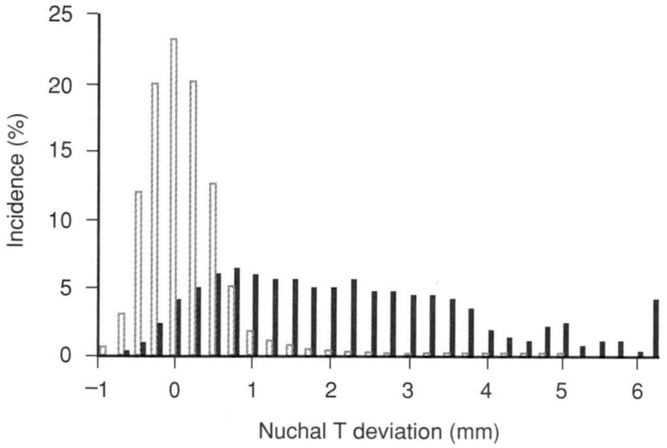

FIGURE 7–8
Distribution of fetal nuchal translucency thickness expressed as deviation from the expected normal value for crown–rump length in chromosomally normal fetuses (*open bars*) and 326 fetuses with trisomy 21 (*solid bars*) (From Snijders RJM, Noble P, Sebire N, et al: UK multicentre project on assessment of risk of trisomy 21 by maternal age and fetal nuchal translucency thickness at 10–14 weeks of gestation. Lancet 1998;351:343–346.)

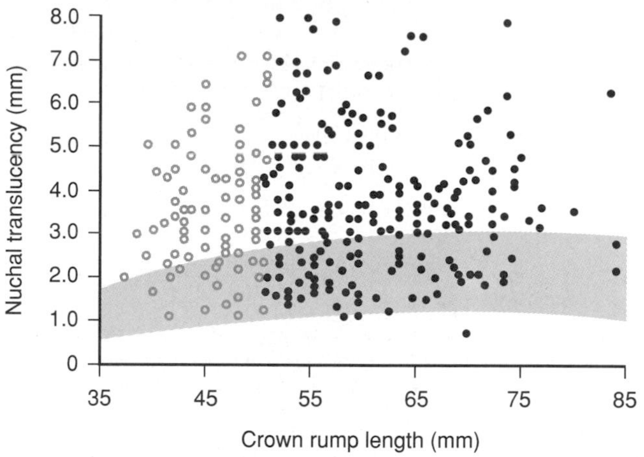

FIGURE 7–9
Nuchal translucency measurements in 326 fetuses with trisomy 21 plotted against the normal range for crown–rump length (95th and 5th percentiles) (From Snijders RJM, Noble P, Sebire N, et al: UK multicentre project on assessment of risk of trisomy 21 by maternal age and fetal nuchal translucency thickness at 10–14 weeks of gestation. Lancet 1998;351:343–346.)

NUCHAL TRANSLUCENCY AND CHROMOSOMAL DEFECTS OTHER THAN TRISOMY 21

Chromosomal abnormalities that are much less prevalent than trisomy 21 are associated with increased NT thickness. In these fetuses, other characteristic sonographic findings are associated with increased NT measurements.

In trisomy 18, early-onset intrauterine growth restriction (IUGR) often occurs and may cause an error in dating the pregnancy. In approximately 30% of these cases, other anomalies, such as exomphalos, are seen after 11 weeks.[58]

Trisomy 13 may also cause early-onset IUGR and severe brain anomalies, mainly holoprosencephaly, in up to 30% of cases at 11 to 14 weeks.[59]

Turner syndrome is characterized by fetal tachycardia in approximately 50% of cases. These fetuses often have large cystic hygromas.[60]

In triploidy, there is early-onset, but asymmetrical IUGR, with an almost normal-sized head. Other severe anomalies are present in approximately 40% of cases, and molar changes in the placenta are seen in approximately one third of cases.[61]

INCREASED NUCHAL TRANSLUCENCY AND NORMAL KARYOTYPE

By definition, 5% of fetuses screened at 11 to 14 weeks have an NT measurement greater than the 95th percentile. Most of these fetuses are chromosomally and anatomically normal antenatally and at birth.[36,62] Fetuses with increased NT thickness but a normal karyotype are at increased risk for major cardiac defects as well as other structural anomalies, rare genetic syndromes, and other unfavorable outcomes (Table 7–5).[63–67]

Souka and colleagues[63] looked at pregnancy outcome in 1320 chromosomally normal fetuses with NT thick-

TABLE 7–5

Anomalies Associated with Increased Nuchal Translucency

Chromosomal abnormalities	Hydroletahlus syndrome
Cardiac defects	Jarcho-Levin syndrome
Diaphragmatic hernia	Joubert syndrome
Exomphalos	Meckel-Gruber syndrome
Achondrogenesis type II	Nance-Sweeney syndrome
Asphyxiating thoracic dystrophy	Noonan syndrome
Beckwith-Wiedemann syndrome	Osteogenesis imperfecta type II
Blomstrand osteochondrodysplasia	Perlman syndrome
Body stalk anomaly	Roberts' syndrome
Campomelic dysplasia	Short-rib polydactyly syndrome
Ectrodactyly-ectodermal dysplasia-cleft palate syndrome	Smith-Lemli-Opitz syndrome
Fetal akinesia deformation sequence	Spinal muscular atrophy type 1
Fryns syndrome	Thanatophoric dysplasia
GM_1 gangliosidosis	Trigonocephaly C syndrome
Sotos syndrome	VACTERL association
	Zellweger syndrome

Adapted from Souka AP, Snidjers RJM, Novakov A, et al: Defects and syndromes in chromosomally normal fetuses with increased nuchal translucency thickness at 10–14 weeks of gestation. Ultrasound Obstet Gynecol 1988;11: 391–400.

ness greater than 3.5 mm in the first trimester. In chromosomally normal fetuses, the chance of a live birth and no structural defects was 86% when the NT thickness was 3.5 to 4.4 mm, 77% when the NT thickness was 4.5 to 5.4 mm, 67% when the NT thickness was 5.5 to 6.4 mm, and 31% when the NT thickness was greater than 6.5 mm. Thus, parents should be counseled that even if the NT thickness exceeds 6.5 mm, there is a one in three chance that the pregnancy will end with the live birth of an infant with no major defects.[63]

CARDIAC DEFECTS

An abnormal NT measurement in a fetus with a normal karyotype is also associated with major abnormalities of the heart and great arteries. The prevalence of major cardiac defects increases with increasing NT thickness.[64] Fetal echocardiography can be performed at 16 weeks, and if the results are normal, the parents can be reassured.[30] However, many recommend a second echocardiogram at 18 to 22 weeks if the first results were normal. One explanation for the association of congenital heart defects and increased NT thickness is aortic arch abnormalities or heart failure. However, this finding is rarely confirmed either later in pregnancy or in the neonatal period.

DIAPHRAGMATIC HERNIA

In a study of 19 fetuses with diaphragmatic hernia, NT thickness was increased in 37%, including 83% of those who died in the neonatal period as a result of pulmonary hypoplasia. Only 22% of the survivors had an increased NT measurement. Increased NT thickness may reflect venous congestion in the head and neck as a result of mediastinal shift or compression and impaired venous return.[68]

EXOMPHALOS

The prevalence of exomphalos is approximately 10 times higher in fetuses with a normal karyotype and an increased NT measurement compared with the general population.[69,70] Other structural defects are associated with increased NT thickness and a normal karyotype.[70]

Increased Nuchal Translucency Measurement and Twin–Twin Transfusion Syndrome

In a study of 132 monochorionic twin pregnancies, an increased NT measurement (above the 95th percentile for CRL) at 11 to 14 weeks was associated with a fourfold increase in the risk of severe twin–twin transfusion syndrome.[71] Although the positive predictive value of this screening test is low, it is important to follow these pregnancies closely for the early diagnosis of twin–twin transfusion syndrome (see also Chapters 24 and 60).

Miscellaneous Associations

The association between increased NT thickness and a wide range of structural abnormalities and genetic syndromes is an indication of the need for long-term follow-up of these children, even when they appear normal at birth. Hiippala and colleagues[72] followed 50 chromosomally normal children 2.4 to 7.1 years of age who had NT thickness greater than 3 mm at 13 to 15 weeks' gestation. Their growth was within normal limits, but 1 in 12 had a previously unrecognized cardiac defect. One child had Noonan syndrome, one had cleidocranial dysplasia, and a third had developmental delays and an undefined syndrome. Webbing was seen in the neck region of two children who were otherwise free of associated pathology.

An increased NT measurement (>3.5 mm) with a normal karyotype is an indication for detailed follow-up ultrasound examinations. An anomaly scan should be performed at 14 to 16 weeks to determine the evolution of the NT to nuchal edema and to diagnose or exclude most fetal defects.[63] Nuchal edema is diagnosed when subcutaneous edema is noted in the midaxial plane of the neck and tremors occur if the uterine wall is tapped, or if the edema measures more than 6 mm.[73] If no obvious abnormalities are seen during the 14- to 16-week scan, echocardiogram should be performed at 20 to 22 weeks, when further genetic testing may be indicated (Fig. 7–10).[63]

An adverse outcome occurred in 18% of fetuses with persistent, unexplained nuchal edema at 20 to 22 weeks,[63] including progression to hydrops, genetic syndromes detected at birth, and cardiac defects (one third) that could have been detected, but were missed antenatally. The prevalence of neurodevelopmental delays in the group with normal findings on follow-up scans was 0.4%, but it was 1.2% in those with persistent nuchal edema. Other studies reported a 3.2% to 5.6% prevalence of residual neurodevelopmental delays in fetuses with increased NT thickness.[74,75] Methodologic issues make it difficult to compare the prevalence of mental retardation in infants with increased NT measurements with the prevalence in the general population, which ranges from 0.5% to 2%.[76] Etiologies include chromosomal abnormalities in 25% of cases and genetic syndromes in 7% to 10% of cases. Mental retardation is unexplained in 30% to 50% of cases,[76] or less than 1% of the population. Children with an isolated NT measurement in utero of greater than 3.5 mm should be followed jointly by pediatricians and geneticists to allow enhanced prenatal counseling (Table 7–6).[62,63,74,75,77,78] Elucidation and integration of these data are essential if the counseling is to be balanced. Otherwise, counseling may resemble this confusing statement: "The good news is that the karyotype is normal, and the bad news is the karyotype is normal."[77,78] This type of uncertainty is potentially lethal, particularly when announced in the first trimester, especially in countries where social termination is an option at 14 weeks, but is challenged or forbidden at a later gestational age.

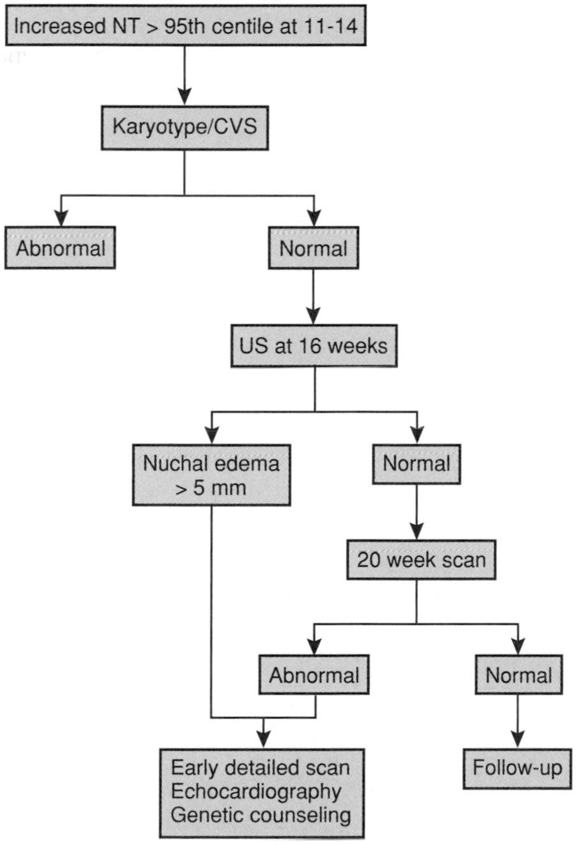

FIGURE 7–10
Follow-up of fetuses with increased nuchal translucency and normal karyotype. CVS, chorionic villus sampling. (From Senat MV, De Keersmaecker B, Audibert F, et al: Pregnancy outcome in fetuses with increased nuchal translucency and normal karyotype. Prenat Diagn 2002;22:345–349.)

Fetal Nasal Bones

Recent studies indicate that the nasal bones are not visible on ultrasound between 11 and 14 weeks in more than 3% of chromosomally normal fetuses and in 60% of fetuses with trisomy 21.[79–82] This finding was first shown in high risk pregnancies and more recently was confirmed in unselected pregnancies. The actual value of screening for absent nasal bones on ultrasound at 11 to 14 weeks in the general population remains to be established. Methodologic problems surrounding that part of the first-trimester scan can generate a high false-positive rate, together with significant interoperator and intraoperator variability.[83]

Ultrasound Diagnosis of Fetal Abnormalities at 11 to 14 Weeks

Reports of detection rates of fetal structural defects in the first trimester other than those associated with increased NT thickness are mostly confined to high-risk groups or selected populations (Table 7–7).[84–87] However, increasing evidence shows that early detailed ultrasonography is technically feasible as a screening test for fetal structural defects in lowrisk pregnancies.[87] Most fetal structures can be visualized at 12 to 13 weeks, and this gestational age offers the earliest opportunity for screening for fetal abnormalities.

In 2853 pregnant women who underwent a routine ultrasound scan at 11 to 14 weeks by operators with different levels of experience,[88] 22.3% of fetal anomalies were detected in the first trimester (n = 130). Operator experience is important. More than half of major fetal abnormalities (1.5%) were identified during first-trimester screening in 20,465 unselected pregnant women who were screened at 13 to 14 weeks.[87] Sensitivity was lowest in the first year (22%) and highest (79%) in the

TABLE 7–6

Outcome of Fetuses with Nuchal Translucency Greater than the 95th Percentile, Normal Karyotype, and Normal Findings on Examination at Birth

STUDY	NO. OF FETUSES	MEAN NT AT 11–14 WK	MEAN POSTNATAL FOLLOW-UP (RANGE)	LOST TO FOLLOW-UP	ADVERSE OUTCOME (*n*)
Cha'ban et al., 1996[78]	19	4.6 mm	18 mo (4–32 mo)	0%	0
Van Vugt et al., 1998[74]	50	3.6 mm	33.5 mo (7–75 mo)	32%	Various minor health problems, 5 (5/50; 10%)
Adekunle et al., 1999[75]	31	NA	23 mo (12–38 mo)	26%	Developmental delay, 2 Noonan syndrome, 1 (3/23; 13%)
Souka et al., 2001[63]	980	4.5 mm	NA	0%	22 adverse outcomes including, 4 with developmental delay (22/980; 2%)
Hippala et al., 2001[72]	59	4.0 mm	56 mo (29–85 mo)	15%	Noonan syndrome, 1 Cleidocranial dysplasia, 1 Unknown syndrome, 1 Delayed speech and visuomotor disturbances, 2 (5/50; 10%)
Senat et al., 2002[62]	58	4.6 mm	39 mo (12–72 mo)	7%	Developmental delay, 2 Delay in walking, 1 Stuttering, 1 Torticolis, 1 (6/54; 11%)

NA, not applicable; NT, nuchal translucency.
Adapted from Senat MV, De Keers Maecker B, Audibert F, et al: Pregnancy outcome in fetuses with increased nuchal translucency and normal karyotype. Prenat Diagn 2002; 22: 345–349.)

last (sixth) year. Adequate sensitivity in screening for major malformations during first-trimester ultrasonography can be achieved after 3 to 4 years of experience.[87]

The most frequently detected anomalies reported are central nervous system defects, such as anencephaly, encephalocele, and holoprosencephaly. The diagnosis of spina bifida is a challenge because the indirect sonographic signs that are characteristic later in gestation are usually missing before 14 weeks.[89] Exomphalos, gastroschisis, and megacystis are also commonly diagnosed in the first trimester. There are also several case reports of first-trimester diagnosis of a wide range of severe skeletal defects (see Fig. 7–4).

Acrania, Exencephaly, and Anencephaly

Anencephaly can be diagnosed reliably on routine 11- to 14-week ultrasound examination. Acrania is the main feature of anencephaly in the first trimester. Fetuses with acrania may have a normal brain or one that shows varying degrees of disruption.[90,91] In a large, multicenter study, screening for fetal abnormalities was performed in 53,435 singleton and 901 twin pregnancies. In this study, 8 of the 47 fetuses with anencephaly were missed during the early scan.[91] The sonographers were then instructed to look specifically for the cranial vault and at brain organization. All subsequent cases of anencephaly were identified at the 11- to 14-week scan.

TABLE 7–7

Most Common Structural Defects Diagnosed Prenatally during Screening at 11 to 14 Weeks

Atrioventricular septal defects and hypoplastic left heart syndrome
Acrania and alobar holoprosencephaly
Omphalocele and gastroschisis
Megacystis
Lethal skeletal defects

Encephalocele

Encephalocele appears as a bony defect in the skull, with brain tissue protruding. It is associated with Meckel-Gruber syndrome.[92,93] In most cases, the lesion arises midline in the occipital area. The main alternative diagnosis is cystic hygroma. Once the diagnosis is suspected, the prognosis usually cannot be ascertained before the late second trimester.

Holoprosencephaly

Holoprosencephaly results from incomplete cleavage of the forebrain. The most severe forms, alobar and semilobar, are amenable to first-trimester ultrasound diagnosis. They are characterized by a monoventricular cavity and fusion of the thalami. These forms are often associated with facial abnormalities.[94,95] The most common related chromosome abnormality is trisomy 13.

Spina Bifida

Sonographic diagnosis of spina bifida aperta is difficult before 14 weeks. At this early gestation, the lemon (frontal bone scalloping) and banana signs (abnormal curvature of the cerebellar hemispheres) are usually absent.[89,96] Other signs, such as a flattened occiput, parallel peduncles, a straight metencephalon, and the acorn sign (frontal bone narrowing) are not consistently present.[89,96] Blaas and colleagues[97] studied high risk pregnancies prospectively and identified three first-trimester fetuses with lumbosacral myelomeningocele characterized by an irregularity in the caudal part of the spine before 10 weeks. Three-dimensional ultrasound examination may be helpful, but is not necessary to make the diagnosis.

Heart Defects

Heart defects were largely covered in the earlier discussion of NT thickness of greater than 3.5 mm. The prevalence of major cardiac defects increases with NT thickness, from 5.4 per 1000 with an NT measurement of 2.5 to 3.4 mm to 233 per 1000 with an NT measurement of greater than 5.5 mm. The sensitivity of NT is 15% to 56% for the diagnosis of major cardiac defects.[57,64–66] Early fetal echocardiography is recommended and can be performed reliably by trained operators from 14 weeks onward.[28–30] Care should be taken in extrapolating the results of these studies to a population in which the initial index of suspicion is not high.

Exomphalos

Reduction of the physiologic midgut hernia ends by 11 weeks and 5 days.[98] An abdominal defect, especially exomphalos, should be suspected if herniation continues after 12 weeks. This defect is sporadic, with a prevalence at birth of approximately 1 in 4000. There are many reports of first-trimester ultrasound diagnosis of omphalocele.[99,100]

Megacystis

Fetal megacystis is defined as a bladder with a longitudinal diameter of 7 mm or more at 10 to 14 weeks' gestation. It is found in approximately 1 in 1500 pregnancies.[34] In a recent study of 145 fetuses with megacystis of 7 to 15 mm, 25% had a chromosomal abnormality, mainly trisomies 13 and 18.[101] In 75% of fetuses with chromosomal abnormalities, NT thickness was also increased, possibly as a result of thoracic compression. Ninety percent of chromosomally normal fetuses had spontaneous resolution, with no obvious adverse effects on the development of the urinary system. The risk of a chromosomal abnormality is lower, approximately 10%, when the longitudinal diameter is more than 15 mm. However, in these fetuses, a strong association with progressive obstructive uropathy is seen.[101] Favre and colleagues[102] also reported a high incidence of chromosomal abnormalities in fetuses with megacystis with a longitudinal diameter of 9 to 15 mm. Parents usually can be reassured when the fetus has megacystis of 7 to 15 mm with a normal karyotype because 90% of cases resolve and renal function is normal. Moreover, vesicoamniotic shunting in midgestation was ineffective treating these fetuses. There is no experience with first-trimester decompression.[103]

Renal Anomalies

Bilateral renal agenesis, hydronephrosis, and multicystic dysplastic kidney have been diagnosed with ultrasound in early pregnancy.[104–106]

Skeletal Defects

Skeletal dysplasias complicate approximately 1 in 4000 births. Twenty-five percent of affected fetuses are stillborn, and 30% die in the neonatal period. Growth impairment is not apparent until later in gestation in some skeletal dysplasias. However, first-trimester diagnosis of isolated cases is reported, mainly because severe skeletal defects in the first trimester are typically associated with increased NT thickness.[107–108]

Three-Dimensional Ultrasound

Three-dimensional ultrasound is used increasingly in obstetric practice. The method seems to offer several advantages in the first trimester because it allows visualization of planes that are otherwise difficult to obtain with two-dimensional scanning. It could potentially minimize actual scanning time and provides an excellent way to store scanned data for later study. However, no randomized controlled trials of three-dimensional versus two-dimensional ultrasound have been published, and the benefits of three-dimensional scanning are speculative. If the two-dimensional images are of poor quality, the resulting three-dimensional images are of little clinical use. As shown by Michailidis and associates,[109] two-dimensional ultrasound seems to be the best way to examine the fetal anatomy in the first trimester. In 93.7% of cases, a complete anatomic survey was achieved with two-dimensional ultrasound. However, it was achieved in only 80.5% of cases with three-dimensional volume acquisition (P <0.001).

There are several reports of the feasibility of obtaining an NT measurement with three-dimensional ultrasound.[110–113] Theoretically, NT measurement could be performed, regardless of the fetal position, significantly shortening examination time. Moreover, tomographic examination of the three-orthogonal sectional images would make it easy to distinguish fetal skin from the amnion. Paul and colleagues[110] studied the feasibility and repeatability of three-dimensional ultrasound for NT measurement. They concluded that reslicing of stored three-dimensional volumes could be used to replicate NT measurements only if the nuchal skin was also clearly seen on two-dimensional ultrasound. When the fetus was lying in a position that precluded clear visualization of the nuchal fold, three-dimensional ultrasound was unlikely to help.[110]

MATERNAL SERUM MARKERS AT 11 TO 14 WEEKS

Median serum concentrations of (α–fetoprotein, estriol, and βhCG (total and free) are independent of maternal age and can be combined in the second trimester to refine the risk of trisomy 21. This testing allows identification of approximately 60% of fetuses with trisomy 21 (compared with 30% based on maternal age alone) with a 5% invasive testing rate.[55,114]

Free βhCG is more discriminant in the first trimester (11–14 weeks), and when combined with pregnancy-associated plasma protein A (PAPP-A) and maternal age, it provides an estimated detection rate of 60%, with a 5% invasive testing rate.[1]

Free β-hCG

The maternal serum concentration of free βhCG is higher in fetuses with trisomy 21 than in chromosomally normal fetuses. The median multiple of the median (MoM) in pregnacies affected with trisomy 21 is approximately 2. First-trimester measurement of free βhCG alone allows for the detection of 35% of fetuses with trisomy 21, with a 5% invasive testing rate. The detection rate is increased to 45% if the findings are integrated with maternal age.[1] The maternal serum free βhCG level is decreased in trisomies 13 and 18.[115,116] It is usually normal in women whose fetus has a sex chromosomal abnormality.[117]

In a recent study, a free βhCG level at or above the 95th percentile (3.85 MoM) was associated with fetal loss only beyond 24 weeks. Levels lower than the 5th percentile (0.36 MoM) were not significantly associated with obstetric complications.[118,138]

PAPP-A

The PAPP-A level normally increases with gestation and is lower in pregnancies in which the fetus is affected with trisomy 21 than in those in which the fetus is chromosomally normal. The median value in trisomy 21 is approximately 0.5 MoM. When used alone in the first trimester, PAPP-A allows for the detection of 40% of fetuses with trisomy 21, with a 5% invasive testing rate. The detection rate increases to 50% when the findings are integrated with maternal age.[1] The maternal serum PAPP-A level is also decreased when the fetus has trisomies 13 and 18 or sex chromosomal abnormalities.[115–117]

In a recent study that excluded fetuses with chromosomal abnormalities, low levels of PAPP-A were associated with pregnancy complications in 11.3% (184 of 1622).[118] Patients with PAPP-A levels of 0.25 MoM or less had higher rates of IUGR (relative risk [RR] = 3.12), preeclampsia (RR = 6.09), and spontaneous abortion (RR = 8.76). Women with PAPP-A levels of 0.50 MoM or less also had higher rates of IUGR (RR = 3.30) and spontaneous abortion (RR = 3.78). A multicenter study was done to determine the frequency and clinical consequences of an extremely high maternal serum PAPP-A level. Among 46,776 tested pregnancies, in 79 pregnancies, PAPP-A levels were greater than 5.0 MoM (0.2%).[119] The authors concluded that the outcome of pregnancies with a high PAPP-A level is similar to the outcome of those with normal marker levels. The issue is controversial, and a recent study confirmed previous reports of increased PAPP-A levels in women who subsequently have preeclampsia.[120]

Free βhCG and PAPP-A

When maternal age is combined with first-trimester maternal serum PAPP-A levels and free βhCG levels, the estimated detection rate for trisomy 21 approximates 60%, with a 5% invasive testing rate.[1,121,122] These rates are similar to those obtained in the second trimester. Screening with a combination of fetal NT measurement and maternal levels of serum PAPP-A and free βhCG allows the detection of approximately 90% of these chromosomal abnormalities, with a 5% invasive testing rate (Table 7–8).[1,123–131]

Logistic and Organizational Issues

There is no significant association between fetal NT measurement and maternal serum free βhCG or PAPP-A

TABLE 7–8

Detection and False-Positive Rates of Screening Tests for Trisomy 21

SCREENING TEST	DETECTION RATE	FALSE-POSITIVE RATE
Maternal age (MA)	30% (or 50%)	5% (or 15%)
MA + serum βhCG + PAPP-A at 11–14 wk	60%	5%
MA + fetal nuchal translucency (NT) at 11–14 wk	75% (or 70%)	5% (or 2%)
MA + fetal NT + nasal bone (NB) at 11–14 wk	90%	5%
MA + fetal NT + serum βhCG + PAPP-A at 11–14 wk	90% (or 80%)	5% (or 2%)
MA + fetal NT + NB + serum βhCG + PAPP-A at 11–14 wk	97% (or 95%)	5% (or 2%)
MA + serum biochemistry at 15–18 wk	60%–70%	5%
Ultrasound for fetal defects and markers at 16–23 wk	75%	10%–15%

PAPP-A, pregnancy-associated plasma protein A.

levels in pregnancies affected by trisomy 21 or chromosomally normal pregnancies. Therefore, ultrasonographic and biochemical markers can be combined in the first trimester to provide more effective screening than either method individually. The same is true for NT measurement and second-trimester biochemical markers.[132] Many European countries have adopted first-trimester screening for chromosomal abnormalities with a combination of ultrasound NT measurement and maternal serum testing.[135–136] In 1997, the 32nd Study Group of the Royal College of Obstetricians and Gynaecologists concluded that the evidence in favor of first-trimester screening for trisomy 21 by NT measurement or biochemical testing was sufficiently well developed to justify moving out of the research phase and into routine practice. They also concluded that ultrasound in early pregnancy would be superior to biochemical screening in the second trimester. Several large studies support these conclusions.[133–140] Spencer and colleagues[2] studied 12,339 women with singleton pregnancies at 10 to 14 weeks' gestation who were screened by measurement of NT and maternal serum markers at 11 to 14 weeks in a one-stop clinic for assessment of risk (OSCAR).[2] The results of a prospective trial in the United States reached a similar conclusion.[139] It is time to shift screening for trisomy 21 from the second to the first trimester.[2]

Fetal Nuchal Translucency Measurement and Maternal Serum Free βhCG and PAPP-A (Combined Screening Test)

Spencer and associates[131] reviewed the findings in 12,339 pregnancies in which first-trimester screening was performed with measurement of NT, serum free βhCG, and PAPP-A. The detection rate for trisomy 21 was 92% (23 of 25). The invasive testing rate was 5.2%. The detection rate was far better than that achieved with second-trimester serum screening. This combined method also identified 94% of all other major chromosomal defects, such as trisomies 13 and 18, triploidy, and Turner syndrome, and 60% of other chromosomal defects, such as deletions, partial trisomies, unbalanced translocations, and sex chromosomal aneuploidy other than Turner syndrome.[133] Wapner and associates[137] found similar results in a prospective study of 8514 patients. With a false-positive rate of 5%, the detection rate was 78.7% (Table 7–9).

Fetal Nuchal Translucency Measurement and Maternal Serum Markers at 14 to 17 Weeks

Sonographic and biochemical screening methods evolved independently. As a result, many women undergo sequential two-stage screening, even when the NT screen result is negative. Each method is designed to generate a 5% invasive testing rate, and a two-stage screening paradigm has a cumulative rate. Thus, the proportion of patients undergoing invasive prenatal diagnostic testing can be as high as 10%, or even higher in countries that offer invasive prenatal diagnosis to women older than 35 years of age, regardless of the screening result. This approach increases both the iatrogenic loss rate of normal pregnancies and all related costs. The rate of invasive testing for fetal karyotyping is an important public health issue that must be controlled. When the combined first-trimester test is not available, one approach is to combine NT measurement and second-trimester maternal serum screening results into a single risk assessment and not to consider the results independently (integrated screening) (Table 7–10).[132]

In women undergoing second-trimester biochemical testing after first-trimester NT screening (with or without maternal serum testing), the background risk must be adjusted to take into account the first-trimester screening results. For example, in a 41-year-old woman whose age-related background risk of having a fetus with trisomy 21 is 1 in 50, the risk decreases if the NT is thin on the first-trimester scan (e.g., 1 in 200). If the risk after second-trimester screening with serum markers is 1 in 100, this woman has an integrated risk of 1 in 400 because the NT measurement allowed a fourfold reduction of the background risk and maternal serum testing has done so by

TABLE 7–9

Major Prospective and Retrospective Studies that Used a Combination of Maternal Age, Fetal Nuchal Translucency, Maternal Serum Pregnancy-Associated Plasma Protein A, and Free βhCG to Detect Down Syndrome

STUDY	*N*	PREVALENCE OF T21	GESTATION (WK)	FALSE-POSITIVE RATE	DETECTION RATE FOR TRISOMY 21
Orlandi et al., 1997[123]	744	0.9%	9–13.4	5%	87%
De Biasio et al., 1999[127]	1467	0.9%	10–13+6	3.3%	85%
Spencer et al., 1999[1]	1156	18%	10–14	5%	89%
Krantz, 2000[124]	5809	0.8%	9–13+6	5%	91%
Hafner et al., 2001[128]	3316	0.3%	10–13	4.1%	90%
Niemimaa et al., 2001[126]	1602	0.3%		5%	80%
Bindra et al., 2003[130]	15,030	0.5%	11–14	5%	90.2%
Von Kaisenberg et al., 2002[125]	3864	0.5%	11–14	6.6%	84.2%
Crossley et al., 2002[129]	12,560	0.2%	10–14	5%	82%
Spencer et al., 2003[131]	12,339	0.2%	10–14	5.2%	92%

TABLE 7–10

Definitions

TERM	DEFINITION
Combined screening	Nuchal translucency measurement + first-trimester serum markers
Fully integrated screening	Nuchal translucency measurement + first-trimester serum markers + second-trimester serum markers
Serum integrated screening	Pregnancy-Associated Plasma Protein A + second-trimester serum markers
Sequential screening	Successive independent risk assessments, leading to cumulative false-positive rates

twofold. Both tests have therefore divided the background risk by 8. Because first-trimester combined screening can identify almost 90% of pregnancies affected by trisomy 21, second-trimester serum testing identifies, at best, 6% of affected pregnancies (60% of the residual 10%), although it doubles the overall invasive testing rate from 5% to 10%. It is theoretically possible to use various statistical techniques to combine NT measurement with different components of first- and second-trimester serum testing.[133] One hypothetical model combined first-trimester NT measurement and PAPP-A testing with second-trimester free βhCG, estriol, and inhibin A testing (fully integrated test), claiming a potential sensitivity of 90%, for a 5% false-positive rate.[138]

In one multicenter interventional study,[132] NT was measured at 12 to 14 weeks' gestation in 9444 women. Maternal serum markers were measured between 14 weeks and 1 day and 17 weeks' gestation. Karyotyping was delayed until after maternal blood was obtained. A combined risk for NT measurement and maternal serum markers was estimated retrospectively. The invasive testing rate generated by sequential two-stage screening was 8.6%, which means that 8.6% of patients underwent amniocentesis because of an increased risk generated by any of these tests. Twenty-one fetuses (0.22%) had trisomy 21. Adjusting for a 5% invasive testing rate, the detection rates would have been 55% and 80% for NT measurement alone and NT measurement combined with second-trimester serum marker testing, respectively. The results of the study suggest a 25% increase in the detection rate with a combination of NT measurement at 12 to 14 weeks and serum marker studies between 14 weeks and 1 day and 17 weeks, with a 5% invasive testing rate and a modest increase in cost. Four other studies reported screening with a combination of fetal NT measurement in the first trimester and maternal serum marker testing in the second trimester, with similar results.[132,134–136]

Sequential (but not integrated) screening programs also increase the invasive procedure-related pregnancy loss rate. This increased rate is an important issue in populations in which the prevalence of Down syndrome is less than 1 in 1000 births. In these populations, an invasive testing rate of 8.6% might be considered unacceptably high in women who are at relatively low risk,[132] compared with the 5% rate generated by a single-test screening program. A single risk assessment that integrates the results of NT measurement, free βhCG levels, and α-fetoprotein levels with maternal age is possible. With such an algorithm, it would be possible to keep the sensitivity as high as that obtained with combined screening while maintaining an invasive testing rate of as low as 5%. However, the cost is also significant because the 25% increase in the detection rate would delay risk calculation and invasive testing by 2 to 4 weeks. Such information should be included in genetic counseling, especially when termination for fetal abnormality is an issue. Further, screening strategies in the first trimester are cost-effective compared with the use of second-trimester biochemical markers.[132]

CONCLUSIONS

- The emphasis in screening for fetal abnormalities has moved to the first trimester.
- This is particularly true for fetal aneuploidies, using a combination of maternal age, gestational age, nuchal translucency, and maternal serum markers.
- The optimal gestational age range is 11 to 14 weeks.
- At this time, testing for viability, gestational age assessment, fetal number, and a fetal anatomic survey can be performed.
- If most pregnant women should be offered an ultrasound examination within this gestational window, there will be important implications for health care planners in terms of resources and teaching programs.
- All sonographers who perform fetal scans must be trained appropriately. The reproducibility of nuchal translucency measurements improves with training, and good results are typically achieved after approximately 100 scans.
- Combined first-trimester screening can be performed at multiple clinical sites.
- Adequate sensitivity in screening for major malformations during first-trimester ultrasonography seems to be achieved after a few years of experience.
- Nuchal translucency measurement combined with serum integrated screening for trisomy 21 has the highest detection rates.
- Chorionic villus sampling is the adjunctive diagnostic test; thus, screening at 11 to 14 weeks may lead to an increase in the demand for this testing.

SUMMARY OF MANAGEMENT OPTIONS

First-Trimester Screening for Fetal Abnormalities

Management Options	Quality of Evidence	Strength of Recommendation	References
General Approach			
Prerequisites: • Details of the history, examination, and routine tests completed and known relevant risk factors identified • Prescan interview, discussions, and counseling	See Chapter 9		
Screening is performed ideally between 11 and 14 weeks	III	B	2
Ultrasound is considered safe in both the short and long terms.	Ib	A	141
First-Trimester Screening—Benefits			
Confirm viability.	III	B	5,6
Dating the pregnancy by crown–rump length before 14 weeks is the most accurate method and decreases the risk of post-term pregnancy.	III	B	8–16
Screening for fetal aneuploidy:			
• Nuchal translucency (NT) measurement, combined with maternal age and maternal serum markers for trisomy 21, has a detection rate of 80% to 90%, for a 5% false-positive rate.	IIa	B	131,132
• Other chromosomal abnormalities are also more likely with increased NT thickness.	III	B	58–61
Detection of structural abnormalities:			
• Some major structural anomalies are detectable as early as 12 weeks. These include anencephaly, holoprosencephaly, abdominal wall defects, and major limb defects.	IIb	B	22–24,63,67
• Detection rates are dependent on sonographer experience.	III	B	87
Multiple pregnancy:			
• Chorionicity is optimally determined by either visualization or absence of the lambda sign.	III	B	20,21
• Twin–twin transfusion syndrome is more likely in monochorionic pregnancies with increased NT thickness.	III	B	71
Examine the uterus and adnexal structures.	IV	C	18

REFERENCES

1. Spencer K, Souter V, Tul N, et al: A screening program for trisomy 21 at 10–14 weeks using fetal nuchal translucency, maternal serum free β-human chorionic gonadotropin and pregnancy-associated plasma protein-A. Ultrasound Obstet Gynecol 1999;13:231–237.
2. Spencer K, Spencer CE, Power M, et al: Screening for chromosomal abnormalities in the first trimester using ultrasound and maternal serum biochemistry in a one stop clinic: A review of three years prospective experience. BJOG 2003;110:281–286.
3. Braithwaite JM, Armstrong MA, Economides: Assessment of fetal anomaly at 12 to 13 weeks of gestation by transabdominal and transvaginal sonography. BJOG 1996;103: 82–85.
4. Timor-Trisch IE, Farine D, Rosen M: A close look at early embryonic development with the high-frequency transvaginal transducer. Am J Obstet Gynecol 1988;159:676–681.
5. Pandya PP, Snijders RJ, Psara N, et al: The prevalence of non-viable pregnancy at 10 13 weeks of gestation. Ultrasound Obstet Gynecol 1996;7:170–173.
6. Goldstein SR: Embryonic death in early pregnancy: A new look at the first trimester. Obstet Gynecol 1994;83:738–740.
7. Campbell S, Warsof SL, Little D, et al: Routine ultrasound screening for the prediction of gestational age. Obstet Gynecol 1985;65:613–620.
8. Gardosi J, Vanner T, Francis A: Gestational age and induction of labour for prolonged pregnancy. BJOG 1997;104:792–797.
9. Savitz DA, Terry JW Jr, Dole N, et al: Comparison of pregnancy dating by last menstrual period, ultrasound scanning, and their combination. Am J Obstet Gynecol 2002;187:1660–1666.
10. Warren WB, Peisner DB, Raju S, et al: Dating the early pregnancy by sequential appearance of embryonic structures. Am J Obstet Gynecol 1989;161:747.
11. Daya S: Accuracy of gestational age estimation by means of fetal crown-rump length measurement. Am J Obstet Gynecol 1987;168:903–908.
12. Robinson HP, Fleming JE: A critical evaluation of sonar 'crown-rump length' measurements. BJOG 1975;82: 702–710.

13. Daya S, Woods S, Ward S, et al: Early pregnancy assessment with transvaginal ultrasound scanning. CMAJ 1991;144:441–446.
14. Lasser DM, Peisner DB, Vollebergh J, Timor-Tritsch I: First-trimester fetal biometry using transvaginal sonography. Ultrasound Obstet Gynecol 1993;3:104–108.
15. Wisser J, Dirscheld P: Estimation of gestational age by transvaginal sonographic measurement of greatest embryonic length in dated human embryos. Ultrasound Obstet Gynecol 1994;4: 457–462.
16. Salomon LJ, Bernard JP, Duyme M, et al: Revisiting first-trimester fetal biometry. Ultrasound Obstet Gynecol 2003;22: 63–66.
17. Hadlock FP: Sonographic estimation of fetal age and weight. Radiol Clin North Am 1990;28:39–50.
18. De Biasio P, Prefumo F, Lantieri PB, Venturini PL: Reference values for fetal limb biometry at 10–14 weeks of gestation. Ultrasound Obstet Gynecol 2002;19:588–591.
19. Kustermann A, Zorzoli A, Spagnolo D, Nicolini U: Transvaginal sonography for fetal measurement in early pregnancy. BJOG 1992;99:38–42.
20. Sepulveda W, Sebire NJ, Hughes K, et al: The lambda sign at 10–14 weeks of gestation as a predictor of chorionicity in twin pregnancies. Ultrasound Obstet Gynecol 1996;7:421–423.
21. Sepulveda W, Sebire NJ, Hughes K, et al: Evolution of the lambda or twin/chorionic peak sign in dichorionic twin pregnancies. Obstet Gynecol 1997;89:439–441.
22. Whitlow BJ, Chatzipapas IK, Lazanakis ML, et al: The value of sonography in early pregnancy for the detection of fetal abnormalities in an unselected population. BJOG 1999;106: 929–936.
23. Economides DL, Whitlow BJ, Braithwaite JM: Ultrasonography in the detection of fetal anomalies in early pregnancy. BJOG 1999;106:516–523.
24. Chitty L, Pandya P: Ultrasound screening for fetal abnormalities in the first trimester. Prenat Diagn 1997;17:1269–1281.
25. Green JJ, Hobbins JC: Abdominal ultrasound examination of the first trimester fetus. Am J Obstet Gynecol 1988;159:165–175.
26. Lazanakis M, Whitlow BJ, Economides DL: The significance of choroids plexus cysts, 'golf ball' sign and pyelectasis in the first trimester of pregnancy. J Obstet Gynecol 1997;17:S32.
27. Bromley B, Lieberman R, Benacerraf BR: Choroid plexus cysts: Not associated with Down syndrome. Ultrasound Obstet Gynecol 1996;8:232–235.
28. Huggon IC, Ghi T, Cook AC, et al: Fetal cardiac abnormalities identified prior to 14 weeks' gestation. Ultrasound Obstet Gynecol 2002;20:22–29.
29. Whitlow BJ, Economides DL: The optimal gestational age to examine fetal anatomy and measure nuchal translucency in the first trimester. Ultrasound Obstet Gynecol 1998;11:258–261.
30. Carvalho JS, Senat MV, Schwarzler P, Ville Y: Increased nuchal translucency and ventricular septal defect in the fetus. Circulation 1999;99:E10.
31. Blaas HG, Eik-Nes SH, Kiserud T, Hellevik LR: Early development of the abdominal wall, stomach and heart from 7 to 12 weeks of gestation: A longitudinal ultrasound study. Ultrasound Obstet Gynecol 1995;6:240–249.
32. Diamant NE: Development of esophageal function. Am Rev Respir Dis 1985;131:S29–S32.
33. Rosati P, Guariglia L: Transvaginal sonographic assessment of the fetal urinary tract in early pregnancy. Ultrasound Obstet Gynecol 1996;7:95–100.
34. Sebire NJ, Von Kaisenberg C, Rubio C, et al: Fetal megacystis at 10–14 weeks of gestation. Ultrasound Obstet Gynecol 1996;8:387–390.
35. Zorzoli A, Kusterman E, Carvelli E, et al: Measurements of fetal limb bones in early pregnancy. Ultrasound Obstet Gynecol 1994;4:29–33.
36. Snijders RJM, Noble P, Sebire N, et al: UK multicentre project on assessment of risk of trisomy 21 by maternal age and fetal nuchal translucency thickness at 10–14 weeks of gestation. Lancet 1998;351:343–346.
37. Pandya PP, Snijders RJM, Johnson SJ, et al: Screening for fetal trisomies by maternal age and fetal nuchal translucency thickness at 10 to 14 weeks of gestation. BJOG 1995;102: 957–962.
38. Braithwaite JM, Morris RW, Economides DL: Nuchal translucency measurements: Frequency distribution and changes with gestation in a general population. BJOG 1996;103:1201–1204.
39. Pandya PP, Altman DG, Brizot ML, et al: Repeatability of measurement of fetal nuchal translucency thickness. Ultrasound Obstet Gynecol 1995;5:334–337.
40. Pajkrt E, Mol BW, Boer K, et al: Intra- and interoperator repeatability of the nuchal translucency measurement. Ultrasound Obstet Gynecol 2000;15:297–301.
41. Schaefer M, Laurichesse-Delmas H, Ville Y: The effect of nuchal cord on nuchal translucency measurement at 10–14 weeks. Ultrasound Obstet Gynecol 1998;11:271–273.
42. Pandya PP, Goldberg H, Walton B, et al: The implementation of first-trimester scanning at 10–13 weeks' gestation and the measurement of fetal nuchal translucency thickness in two maternity units. Ultrasound Obstet Gynecol 1995;5:20–25.
43. Szabo J, Gellen J, Szemere G: First-trimester ultrasound screening for fetal aneuploidies in women over 35 and under 35 years of age. Ultrasound Obstet Gynecol 1995;5:161–163.
44. Taipale P, Hiilesmaa V, Salonen R, Ylostalo P: Increased nuchal translucency as a marker for fetal chromosomal defects. N Engl J Med 1997;337:1654–1658.
45. Hafner E, Schuchter K, Liebhart E, Philipp K: Results of routine fetal nuchal translucency measurement at 10–13 weeks in 4,233 unselected pregnant women. Prenat Diagn 1998;18:29–34.
46. Pajkrt E, van Lith JMM, Mol BWJ, et al: Screening for Down's syndrome by fetal nuchal translucency measurement in a general obstetric population. Ultrasound Obstet Gynecol 1998;12: 163–169.
47. Economides DL, Whitlow BJ, Kadir R, et al: First trimester sonographic detection of chromosomal abnormalities in an unselected population. BJOG 1998;105:58–62.
48. Schwarzler P, Carvalho JS, Senat MV, et al: Screening for fetal aneuploidies and fetal cardiac abnormalities by nuchal translucency thickness measurement at 10-14 weeks of gestation as part of routine antenatal care in an unselected population. BJOG 1999;106:1029–1034.
49. Theodoropoulos P, Lolis D, Papageorgiou C, et al: Evaluation of first-trimester screening by fetal nuchal translucency and maternal age. Prenat Diagn 1998;18:133–137.
50. Zoppi MA, Ibba RM, Floris M, Monni G: Fetal nuchal translucency screening in 12,495 pregnancies in Sardinia. Ultrasound Obstet Gynecol 2001;18:649–651.
51. Gasiorek-Wiens A, Tercanli S, Kozlowski P, et al: Screening for trisomy 21 by fetal nuchal translucency and maternal age: A multicenter project in Germany, Austria and Switzerland. Ultrasound Obstet Gynecol 2001;18:645–648.
52. Brizot ML, Carvalho MHB, Liao AW, et al: First-trimester screening for chromosomal abnormalities by fetal nuchal translucency in a Brazilian population. Ultrasound Obstet Gynecol 2001;18:652–655.
53. Audibert F, Dommergues M, Benattar C, et al: Screening for Down syndrome using first-trimester ultrasound and second-trimester maternal serum markers in a low-risk population: A prospective longitudinal study. Ultrasound Obstet Gynecol 2001;18:26–31.
54. Wayda K, Kereszturi A, Orvos H, et al: Four years experience of first-trimester nuchal translucency screening for fetal aneuploidies with increasing regional availability. Acta Obstet Gynecol Scand 2001;80:1104–1109.
55. Cuckle H: Integrating Down's syndrome screening. Curr Opin Obstet Gynaecol 2001;13:175–181.
56. Snijders RJM, Nicolaides KH: Assessment of risks. In Ultrasound Markers for Fetal Chromosomal Defects. Carnforth, UK, Parthenon, 1996, pp 63–120.
57. Schwarzler P, Carvalho JS, Senat MV, et al: Screening for fetal aneuploidies and fetal cardiac abnormalities by nuchal translucency thickness measurement at 10–14 weeks of gestation as part

of routine antenatal care in an unselected population. BJOG 1999;106:1029–1034.
58. Sherrod C, Sebire NJ, Soares W, et al: Prenatal diagnosis of trisomy 18 at the 10–14-week ultrasound scan. Ultrasound Obstet Gynecol 1997;10:387–390.
59. Snijders RJM, Sebire NJ, Nayar R, et al: Increased nuchal translucency in trisomy 13 fetuses at 10–14 weeks of gestation. Am J Med Genet 1999;86:205–207.
60. Sebire NJ, Snijders RJ, Brown R, et al: Detection of sex chromosome abnormalities by nuchal translucency screening at 10–14 weeks. Prenat Diagn 1998;18:581–584.
61. Jauniaux E, Brown R, Snijders RJ, et al: Early prenatal diagnosis of triploidy. Am J Obstet Gynecol 1997;176:550–554.
62. Senat MV, De Keersmaecker B, Audibert F, et al: Pregnancy outcome in fetuses with increased nuchal translucency and normal karyotype. Prenat Diagn 2002;22:345–349.
63. Souka AP, Krampl E, Bakalis S, et al: Outcome of pregnancy in chromosomally normal fetuses with increased nuchal translucency in the first trimester. Ultrasound Obstet Gynecol 2001;18:9–17.
64. Hyett JA, Perdu M, Sharland GK, et al: Increased nuchal translucency at 10–14 weeks of gestation as a marker for major cardiac defects. Ultrasound Obstet Gynecol 1997;10:242–246.
65. Hyett JA, Perdu M, Sharland GK, et al: Using fetal nuchal translucency to screen for major congenital cardiac defects at 10–14 weeks of gestation: Population based cohort study. BMJ 1999;318:81–85.
66. Mavrides E, Cobian-Sanchez F, Tekay A, et al: Limitations of using first-trimester nuchal translucency measurement in routine screening for major congenital heart defects. Ultrasound Obstet Gynecol 2001;17:106–110.
67. Michailidis GD, Economides DL: Nuchal translucency measurement and pregnancy outcome in karyotypically normal fetuses. Ultrasound Obstet Gynecol 2001;17:102–105.
68. Sebire NJ, Snijders RJ, Davenport M, et al: Fetal nuchal translucency thickness at 10–14 weeks' gestation and congenital diaphragmatic hernia. Obstet Gynecol 1997;90:943–946.
69. Ville Y, Lalondrell C, Doumerc S, et al: First trimester diagnosis of nuchal anomalies: Significance and fetal outcome. Ultrasound Obstet Gynecol 1992;2:314–316.
70. Souka AP, Snidjers RJM, Novakov A, et al: Defects and syndromes in chromosomally normal fetuses with increased nuchal translucency thickness at 10–14 weeks of gestation. Ultrasound Obstet Gynecol 1998;11:391–400.
71. Sebire NJ, Hughes K, D'Ercole C, et al: Increased fetal nuchal translucency at 10–14 weeks as a predictor of severe twin-to-twin transfusion syndrome. Ultrasound Obstet Gynecol 1997; 10:86–89.
72. Hippala A, Eronen M, Taipale P, et al: Fetal nuchal translucency and normal chromosomes: A long-term follow-up study. Ultrasound Obstet Gynecol 2001;18:18–22.
73. Benacerraf BR, Frigoletto FD Jr: Soft tissue nuchal fold in the second-trimester fetus: Standards for normal measurements compared with those in Down syndrome. Am J Obstet Gynecol 1987;157:1146–1149.
74. Van Vugt JM, Tinnemans BW, Van Zalen-Sprock RM: Outcome and early childhood follow-up of chromosomally normal fetuses with increased nuchal translucency at 10–14 weeks' gestation. Ultrasound Obstet Gynecol 1998;11:407–409.
75. Adekunle O, Gopee A, el-Sayed M, Thilaganathan B: Increased first trimester nuchal translucency: Pregnancy and infant outcomes after routine screening for Down's syndrome in an unselected antenatal population. Br J Radiol 1999;72:457–460.
76. Curry CJ, Stevenson RE, Aughton D, et al: Evaluation of mental retardation: Recommendations of a consensus conference: American College of Medical Genetics. Am J Med Genet 1997;72:468–477.
77. Ville Y: Nuchal translucency in the first trimester of pregnancy: Ten years on and still a pain in the neck? Ultrasound Obstet Gynecol 2001;18:5–8.
78. Cha'ban FK, Van Splunder P, Los FJ, Wladimiroff JW: Fetal outcome in nuchal translucency with emphasis on normal fetal karyotype. Prenat Diagn 1996;16:537–541.
79. Cicero S, Curcio P, Papageorghiou A, et al: Absence of nasal bone in fetuses with trisomy 21 at 11–14 weeks of gestation: An observational study. Lancet 2001;358:1665–1667.
80. Otano L, Aiello H, Igarzabal L, et al: Association between first trimester absence of fetal nasal bone on ultrasound and Down's syndrome. Prenat Diagn 2002;22:930–932.
81. Orlandi F, Bilardo CM, Campogrande M, et al: Measurement of nasal bone length at 11–14 weeks of pregnancy and its potential role in Down's syndrome risk assessment. Ultrasound Obstet Gynecol 2003;22:36–39.
82. Zoppi MA, Ibba RM, Axinan C, et al: Absence of fetal nasal bone and aneuploidies at first trimester nuchal translucency screening in unselected pregnancies. Prenat Diagn 2003;23:496–500.
83. Senat MV, Bernard JP, Boulvain M, Ville Y: Intra- and interoperator variability in fetal nasal bone assessment at 11–14 weeks of gestation. Ultrasound Obstet Gynecol 2003;22:138–141.
84. Yagel S, Achiron R, Ron M, et al: Transvaginal ultrasonography at early pregnancy cannot be used alone for targeted organ ultrasonographic examination in a high-risk population. Am J Obstet Gynecol 1995;172:971–975.
85. Rottem S, Bronshtein M: Transvaginal sonographic diagnosis of congenital anomalies between 9 weeks and 16 weeks, menstrual age. J Clin Ultrasound 1990;18:307–314.
86. Rottem S: Early detection of structural anomalies and markers of chromosomal aberrations by transvaginal ultrasonography. Curr Opin Obstet Gynecol 1995;7:122–125.
87. Taipale P, Ammala M, Salonen R, Hiilesmaa V: Learning curve in ultrasonographic screening for selected fetal structural anomalies in early pregnancy. Obstet Gynecol 2003;101:273–278.
88. Carvalho MH, Brizot ML, Lopes LM, et al: Detection of fetal structural abnormalities at the 11–14 week ultrasound scan. Prenat Diagn 2002;22:1–4.
89. Bernard JP, Suarez B, Rambaud C, et al: Prenatal diagnosis of neural tube defect before 12 weeks' gestation: Direct and indirect ultrasonographic semeiology. Ultrasound Obstet Gynecol 1997;10:406–409.
90. Chatzipapas IK, Whitlow BJ, Economides DL: The 'Mickey Mouse' sign and the diagnosis of anencephaly in early pregnancy. Ultrasound Obstet Gynecol 1998;13:196–199.
91. Johnson SP, Sebire NJ, Snijders RJM, et al: Ultrasound screening for anencephaly at 10–14 weeks of gestation. Ultrasound Obstet Gynecol 1997;9:14–16.
92. Bronshtein M, Zimmer EZ: Transvaginal sonographic follow-up on the formation of fetal cephalocele at 13–19 weeks' gestation. Obstet Gynecol 1991;78:528–530.
93. van Zalen-Sprock M, van Vugt JMG, van der Harten HJ, van Geijn HP: Cephalocele and cystic hygroma: Diagnosis and differentiation in the first trimester of pregnancy with transvaginal sonography. Report of two cases. Ultrasound Obstet Gynecol 1992;2:289–292.
94. Turner CD, Silva S, Jeanty P: Prenatal diagnosis of alobar holoprosencephaly at 10 weeks of gestation. Ultrasound Obstet Gynecol 1999;13:360–362.
95. Wong HS, Lam YH, Tang MHY, et al: First-trimester ultrasound diagnosis of holoprosencephaly: Three case reports. Ultrasound Obstet Gynecol 1999;13:356–359.
96. Buisson O, De Keersmaecker B, Sénat MV, et al: Sonographic diagnosis of spina bifida at 12 weeks: Heading towards indirect signs. Ultrasound Obstet Gynecol 2002;19:290–292.
97. Blaas HGK, Eik-Nes SH, Isaksen C: The detection of spina bifida before 10 gestational weeks using two- and three dimensional ultrasound. Ultrasound Obstet Gynecol 2000;16:25–29.
98. Timor-Tritsch IE, Warren W, Peisner DB, Pirrone E: First-trimester midgut herniation: A high frequency transvaginal sonographic study. Am J Obstet Gynecol 1989;161:831–833.
99. van Zalen-Sprock RM, van Vugt JMG, van Geijn HP: First-trimester sonography of physiological midgut herniation

and early diagnosis of omphalocele. Prenat Diagn 1997;17: 511–518.
100. Pagliano M, Mossetti M, Ragno P: Echographic diagnosis of omphalocele in the first trimester of pregnancy. J Clin Ultrasound 1990;18:658–660.
101. Liao AW, Sebire NJ, Geerts L, et al: Megacystis at 10–14 weeks of gestation: Chromosomal defects and outcome according to bladder length. Ultrasound Obstet Gynecol 2003;21:338–341.
102. Favre R, Kohler M, Gasser B, et al: Early fetal megacystis between 11 and 15 weeks of gestation. Ultrasound Obstet Gynecol 1999;14:402–406.
103. Carroll SG, Soothill PW, Tizard J, Kyle PM: Vesicocentesis at 10–14 weeks of gestation for treatment of fetal megacystis. Ultrasound Obstet Gynecol 2001;18:366–370.
104. Bronshtein M, Amit A, Achiron R, et al: The early prenatal sonographic diagnosis of renal agenesis: Techniques and possible pitfalls. Prenat Diagn 1994;14:291–297.
105. Bronshtein M, Bar-Hava I, Blumenfeld Z: Clues and pitfalls in the early prenatal diagnosis of 'late onset' infantile polycystic kidney. Prenat Diagn 1992;12:293–298.
106. Hernadi L, Torocsik M: Screening for fetal anomalies in the 12th week of pregnancy by transvaginal sonography in an unselected population. Prenat Diagn 1997;17:753–759.
107. Fisk NM, Vaughan J, Smidt M, Wigglesworth J: Transvaginal ultrasound recognition of nuchal edema in the first-trimester diagnosis of achondrogenesis. J Clin Ultrasound 1991;19: 586–590.
108. Soothill PW, Vuthiwong C, Rees H: Achondrogenesis type 2 diagnosed by transvaginal ultrasound at 12 weeks' gestation. Prenat Diagn 1993;13:523–528.
109. Michailidis GD, Papageorgiou P, Economides DL: Assessment of fetal anatomy in the first trimester using two- and three-dimensional ultrasound. Br J Radiol 2002;75:215–219.
110. Paul C, Krampl E, Skentou C, et al: Measurement of fetal nuchal translucency thickness by three-dimensional ultrasound. Ultrasound Obstet Gynecol 2001;18:481–484.
111. Clementschitsch G, Hasenohrl G, Schaffer H, Steiner H: Comparison between two- and three-dimensional ultrasound measurements of nuchal translucency. Ultrasound Obstet Gynecol 2001;18:475–480.
112. Kurjak A, Kupesic S, Ivancic-Kosuta M: Three-dimensional transvaginal ultrasound improves measurement of nuchal translucency. J Perinat Med 1999;27:97–102.
113. Chung BL, Kim HJ, Lee KH: The application of three-dimensional ultrasound to nuchal translucency measurement in early pregnancy (10–14 weeks): A preliminary study. Ultrasound Obstet Gynecol 2000;15:122–125.
114. Cuckle H: Biochemical screening for Down syndrome. Eur J Obstet Gynecol Reprod Biol 2000;92:97–101.
115. Tul N, Spencer K, Noble P, et al: Screening for trisomy 18 by fetal nuchal translucency and maternal serum free beta hCG and PAPP-A at 10–14 weeks of gestation. Prenat Diagn 1999;19: 1035–1042.
116. Spencer K, Ong C, Skentou H, et al: Screening for trisomy 13 by fetal nuchal translucency and maternal serum free beta hCG and PAPP-A at 10–14 weeks of gestation. Prenat Diagn 2000;20: 411–416.
117. Spencer K, Tul N, Nicolaides KH: Maternal serum free beta hCG and PAPP-A in fetal sex chromosome defects in the first trimester. Prenat Diagn 2000;20:390–394.
118. Yaron Y, Heifetz S, Ochshorn Y, et al: Decreased first trimester PAPP-A is a predictor of adverse pregnancy outcome. Prenat Diagn 2002;22:778–782.
119. Cuckle H, Arbuzova S, Spencer K, et al: Frequency and clinical consequences of extremely high maternal serum PAPP-A levels. Prenat Diagn 2003;23:385–388.
120. Bersinger NA, Smarason AK, Muttukrishna S, et al: Women with preeclampsia have increased serum levels of pregnancy-associated plasma protein A (PAPP-A), inhibin A, activin A and soluble E-selectin. Hypertens Pregnancy 2003;22:45–55.
121. Krantz DA, Larsen JW, Buchanan PD, Macri JN: First-trimester Down syndrome screening: Free beta-human chorionic gonadotropin and pregnancy-associated plasma protein A. Am J Obstet Gynecol 1996;174:612–616.
122. Haddow JE, Palomaki GE, Knight GJ, et al: Screening of maternal serum for fetal Down's syndrome in the first trimester. N Engl J Med 1998;338:955–961.
123. Orlandi F, Damiani G, Hallahan TW, et al: First-trimester screening for fetal aneuploidy: Biochemistry and nuchal translucency. Ultrasound Obstet Gynecol 1997;10:381–386.
124. Krantz DA, Hallahan TW, Orlandi F, et al: First-trimester Down syndrome screening using dried blood biochemistry and nuchal translucency. Obstet Gynecol 2000;96:207–213.
125. von Kaisenberg CS, Gasiorek-Wiens A, Bielicki M, et al: Screening for trisomy 21 by maternal age, fetal nuchal translucency and maternal serum biochemistry at 11–14 weeks: A German multicenter study. J Matern Fetal Neonatal Med 2002;12:89–94.
126. Niemimaa M, Suonpaa M, Perheentupa A, et al: Evaluation of first trimester maternal serum and ultrasound screening for Down's syndrome in Eastern and Northern Finland. Eur J Hum Genet 2001;9:404–408.
127. De Biasio P, Siccardi M, Volpe G, et al: First-trimester screening for Down syndrome using nuchal translucency measurement with free beta-hCG and PAPP-A between 10 and 13 weeks of pregnancy: The combined test. Prenat Diagn 1999; 19:360–363.
128. Hafner E, Schuchter K, Metzenbauer M, et al: [Combined test in the first trimester of pregnancy in 3,316 unselected pregnant patients for diagnosing Down syndrome] Z Geburtshilfe Neonatol 2001;205:99–103 (German).
129. Crossley JA, Aitken DA, Cameron AD, et al: Combined ultrasound and biochemical screening for Down's syndrome in the first trimester: a Scottish multicentre study. BJOG 2002;109: 667–676.
130. Bindra R, Heath V, Liao A, et al: One-stop clinic for assessment of risk for trisomy 21 at 11–14 weeks: A prospective study of 15,030 pregnancies. Ultrasound Obstet Gynecol 2002;20: 219–225.
131. Spencer K, Spencer CE, Power M, et al: Screening for chromosomal abnormalities in the first trimester using ultrasound and maternal serum biochemistry in a one-stop clinic: A review of three years prospective experience. BJOG 2003;110:281–286.
132. Rozenberg P, Malagrida L, Cuckle H, et al: Down's syndrome screening with nuchal translucency at 12(+0)–14(+0) weeks and maternal serum markers at 14(+1)–17(+0) weeks: A prospective study. Hum Reprod 2002;17:1093–1098.
133. Nicolaides KH: Screening for chromosomal defects. Ultrasound Obstet Gynecol 2003;21:313–321.
134. Thilaganathan B, Slack A, Wathen NC: Effect of first-trimester nuchal translucency on second-trimester maternal serum biochemical screening for Down's syndrome. Ultrasound Obstet Gynecol 1997;10:261–264.
135. Schuchter K, Hafner E, Stangl G, et al: Sequential screening for trisomy 21 by nuchal translucency measurement in the first trimester and maternal serum biochemistry in the second trimester in a low-risk population. Ultrasound Obstet Gynecol 2001;18: 23–25.
136. Audibert F, Dommergues M, Benattar C, et al: Screening for Down syndrome using first-trimester ultrasound and second-trimester maternal serum markers in a low-risk population: A prospective longitudinal study. Ultrasound Obstet Gynecol 2001;18:26–31.
137. Wapner R, Thom E, Simpson JL, et al: First-trimester screening for trisomies 21 and 18. N Engl J Med 2003;349:1405–1413.
138. Malone F, Wald N, Canick J, et al: First and second trimester evaluation of risk (FASTER) trial: Principal results of the NICHD multicenter Down syndrome screening study. Am J Obstet Gynecol 2004;189:abstract 1.

CHAPTER 8

Second-Trimester Screening for Fetal Abnormalities

Lami Yeo / Anthony M. Vintzileos

INTRODUCTION

Every pregnant woman desires a healthy child who is free of anomalies. In the general population, the overall risk of having a child with a major malformation is 3% to 5%. The ability conferred by the increasing sophistication of ultrasonography and biochemical testing to screen for fetal abnormalities is of growing importance to obstetricians and their patients as a greater proportion of women delay childbirth. The shortened reproductive window has increased the pressure on all for a successful outcome. We found that genetic sonography is a patient-driven service. This chapter focuses on noninvasive modalities of screening for fetal abnormalities in the second trimester and reviews the likely continued shift to the use of screening earlier in gestation (see Chapter 7).

In the early 1970s, the only method available to screen for fetal Down syndrome was based on maternal age; amniocentesis was offered to all women 35 years or older. However, maternal age proved a very inefficient screening tool; fewer than one third of fetuses with trisomy 21 were identified. In the 1980s, a new screening method incorporated second-trimester maternal serum biochemical markers in addition to maternal age. In the 1990s, screening for Down syndrome by combining maternal age and fetal nuchal translucency (NT) thickness in the first trimester was introduced. Subsequently, maternal serum biochemical markers of value in the first trimester were identified. Most recently, three-dimensional sonography entered the arena of screening.

Invasive tests, such as amniocentesis, chorionic villus sampling, and cordocentesis, are diagnostic tools and not screening tests. They allow for essentially 100% accuracy in the diagnosis of fetal aneuploidy but carry a real risk of pregnancy loss. Thus, many women choose biochemical and ultrasound screening modalities for aneuploidy detection because the test efficiency (percentage of abnormal fetuses identified) is so much higher than that based on maternal age alone, even though they have a relatively high invasive testing rate (false-positive rate), typically set at 5%. Then, based on the result of the selected screening test, a decision is made as to whether an invasive test for diagnosis is necessary. The combination of screening and diagnostic tests allows the maximum number of patients to gain accurate information about their individual risk status.

FIRST-TRIMESTER SERUM SCREENING (See also Chapter 7)

Maternal serum testing in the second trimester is the standard of care in many countries, including the United States, for screening women at low risk for fetal aneuploidy, neural tube defects, and other fetal anomalies. However, first-trimester screening offers several advantages, including shortening of the diagnostic paradigm by several weeks, which provides either earlier reassurance or the option for termination of an affected fetus.

Many serum analytes have been investigated as first-trimester markers for trisomy 21. The two markers with the greatest discriminatory values are βhCG (human chorionic gonadotropin) and pregnancy-associated plasma protein A (PAPP-A).[1,2] In affected pregnancies, the median free βhCG level is approximately 1.8 multiples of the median (MoM), and the median PAPP-A level is approximately 0.4 MoM. The combination of the two, in addition to maternal age, yields trisomy 21 detection and screen-positive rates similar to those of second-trimester serum screening (63% and 5.5%, respectively).[3] Several caveats are noteworthy. First, free βhCG may not be increased in pregnancies affected by trisomy 21 until 12 weeks. Second, PAPP-A loses its discriminatory value after 13 weeks. Careful timing of the test is essential, and accurate assignment of gestational age is an absolute requirement for the test to be useful.

There is no significant relationship between fetal NT and maternal serum free βhCG or PAPP-A levels in either trisomy 21 or nonaneuploid pregnancies. Thus, sonographic and biochemical markers may be combined and detection rates enhanced. A body of research shows that the combination of maternal age, first-trimester maternal serum screening, and NT allows for 85% to 90% sensitivity, with a 5% screen-positive rate for the detection of trisomy 21 (Table 8–1) [see also Chapter 7].[4] Even a modest increase in NT may be clinically significant when combined with biochemistry findings and maternal age.

Other types of aneuploidy affect first-trimester maternal biochemical markers. For example, PAPP-A and free βhCG levels are lower in women with a trisomy 18 fetus, and it is estimated that 77% of trisomy 18 fetuses could be detected with a 0.5% screen-positive rate.[4] Trisomy 13, too, is associated with lower multiples of the median of free βhCG and PAPP-A. In contrast, PAPP-A levels are lower, but free βhCG is unchanged in pregnancies with fetal Turner syndrome.[4] Combining NT and biochemical screening also increases the sensitivity for other types of aneuploidy. Low levels of free βhCG (0.28 MoM) and PAPP-A (0.18 MoM) plus an increased NT (3.3 MoM) increase the detection rate for trisomy 18 to 89%, with a 1% screen-positive rate.[4]

NORMAL FIRST-TRIMESTER ULTRASOUND

First-trimester scanning requires familiarity with the normal development of the embryo or fetus. The presence or absence of certain sonographic structures may be normal or abnormal, depending on gestational age. Transvaginal sonography improves first-trimester embryo imaging. Embryologists use the term "embryo" to describe the conceptus during the first 9 weeks of pregnancy. The gestational sac is visible at 4.5 weeks menstrual age. The yolk sac is visible at 5 weeks in 95% of cases and in nearly all cases by 6 weeks. A fetal pole should be seen next to the yolk sac by 6 weeks.[5] Fetal heart motion is seen in 86% of cases by 6 weeks, and always by 7 weeks. The fetal heart rate increases steadily from 110 beats/min to 171 to 178 beats/min, with crown–rump lengths of 3 to 4 mm and 15 to 32 cm, respectively. Heart rates outside these ranges are associated with pregnancy failure, and these patients should be monitored closely.[5]

Between 6 and 7 weeks, the first anatomic structure that is sonographically apparent is the primitive neural tube that runs throughout the embryonal length. By week 7, the head is discernible from the rest of the fetal body (Fig. 8–1), and the primitive ventricular system is visible, appearing as a single round sonolucent cavity that almost completely fills the head.[5] At 8 weeks, the primitive brain contains sonolucencies, and the hindbrain, or rhombencephalon, is visualized. With transvaginal imaging, the limbs can be imaged by 8 weeks. The cerebral falx, choroid plexus, thalami, long bones, and fingers appear at 9 weeks' gestation. After 9 weeks, previously developed organs and structures become easier to visualize as a result of rapid fetal growth (Fig. 8–2).[5] The cerebellum is seen by 10 to 11 weeks, when the face, palate, feet, and toes can also be seen. Ossification of the fetal cranium begins and accelerates after 9 weeks (important for ruling out acrania). Active fetal movements can be observed from 10 weeks onward. Midgut herniation into the umbilical cord is an important physiologic phenome-

TABLE 8–1

Various Sensitivities for Fetal Down Syndrome (False-Positive Rate of 5%) with Various Screening Tests in Combination

SCREENING TEST	SENSITIVITY FOR FETAL DOWN SYNDROME
Age	30%
Age, first-trimester biochemistry results	63%
Age, NT	75%
Age, first-trimester biochemistry results, NT	85%–90%
NT, nasal bone	90%
Age, first-trimester biochemistry results, NT, nasal bone	97%
Age, second-trimester triple-screen results	60%–70%
Age, second-trimester quadruple-screen results	67%–75%

NT, nuchal translucency.

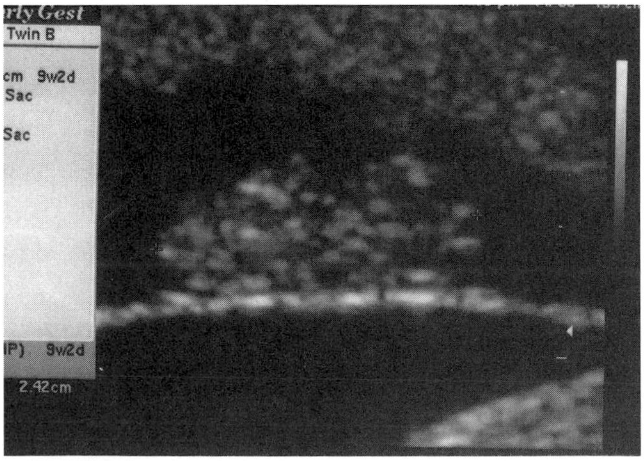

FIGURE 8–1
Enlarged crown–rump length (24.2 mm) of a 9-week fetus of a twin gestation. The fetus is lying on the thick, dividing membrane.

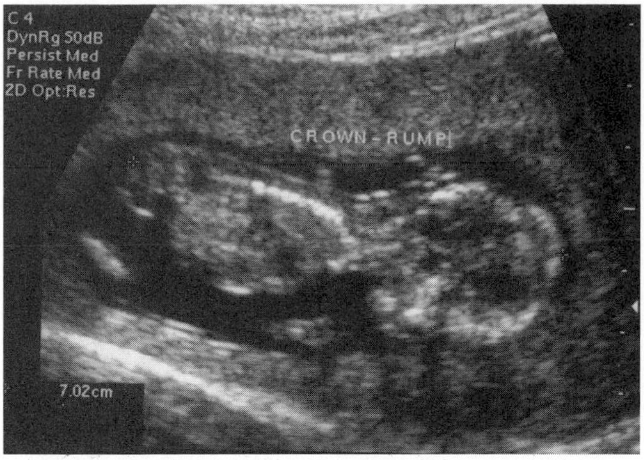

FIGURE 8–2
Crown-rump length of a 12- to 13-week fetus. Anatomic structures are easier to see than in Figure 8–1.

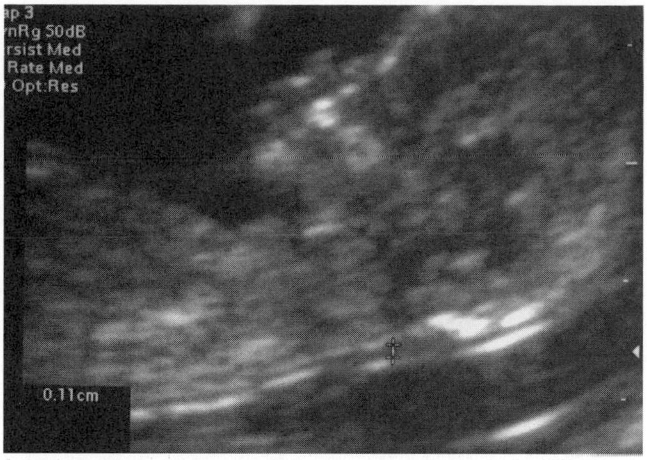

FIGURE 8–3
Normal nuchal translucency (0.11 cm) in a longitudinal section of the fetus, showing the fetal head, neck, and upper thorax.

non that occurs normally between 8 and 10 weeks; the gut returns to the abdomen by 12 weeks.[6] Failure to recognize this normal process may lead to an erroneous diagnosis of omphalocele.

Although the four-chamber view of the heart is seen as early as 11 weeks, it is not readily imaged until 14 weeks, when the four-chamber view and the great vessels should be visible. Although the fetal kidneys can be imaged consistently from 12 to 13 weeks with transvaginal sonography, the bladder is visible in only 50% of cases at 12 weeks, and it is not imaged consistently until 13 weeks. Fetal urine enters the amniotic cavity beginning at approximately 8 to 11 weeks; however, urine does not contribute significantly to the amniotic fluid volume before 15 weeks. Most (but not all) fetal structures can be seen well by 15 weeks with a high-frequency transvaginal probe.[5]

NUCHAL TRANSLUCENCY SCREENING (See also Chapter 7)

In 1866, Langdon Down observed that the skin of individuals with trisomy 21 appeared to be too large for their body. It was observed initially in the 1980s that cystic hygromas in the first trimester appear different (nonseptated vs. septated) from those seen in the second trimester, and they also differed in their association with aneuploidy.[7] Further, cystic hygromas visualized in the first trimester could evolve into increased nuchal thickening or become normal in nuchal thickness but still be associated with aneuploidy. Simultaneously, second-trimester nuchal fold thickening was associated with an increased risk of fetal trisomy 21.[8]

In 1992, Nicolaides and associates[9] coined the term "nuchal translucency" to describe the sonographic anechoic area under the skin at the back of the fetal neck during the first trimester (Fig. 8–3). The concept of measuring NT in all fetuses became the basis for first-trimester ultrasound screening. By 1995, several large studies of NT were published.[10] Increased NT was clearly associated with an increased incidence of trisomy 21. In addition, increased NT was associated with other types of aneuploidy (trisomy 13, trisomy 18, Turner syndrome), congenital heart disease, and a wide range of miscellaneous congenital anomalies. The prevalence of aneuploidy varied from 30% to 86% in fetuses with increased NT.[11] The etiology of increased NT is unclear. Suggested causes include accumulation of lymphatic fluid as a result of delayed or abnormal lymphatic duct development. However, the specific pathophysiologic etiology of increased NT may vary with the underlying condition. For example, the increased "fluid" may be the result of decreased circulation and cardiac function because increased NT is associated with major fetal cardiac abnormalities.[12] Further, differences in skin composition, such as increased collagen and hyaluronan, are associated with increased NT.[13,14] Collagen composition may vary in the various trisomies because of a gene dosage effect that reflects the extra chromosome 13 or 21.[14] Increased amounts of hyaluronan would also lead to excessive hydration of the extracellular matrix.[13] In some cases, these abnormalities of collagen and hyaluronan may explain the known association between increased NT and skeletal dysplasias.

There is wide variation in the reported sensitivities for Down syndrome when NT screening is used (29%–100%), with screen-positive rates of 0.4% to 8.0% (Table 8–2).[15–32] This variation is attributed to differences in the techniques used to measure NT, along with differing criteria and cutoffs for abnormality. Other factors that no doubt contributed to the variable detection rates include inconsistencies in the study populations and variability in training quality, mean values, success in measuring NT, and follow-up (both pregnancy and neonatal). Many initial studies used a specific cutoff value (2.5 or 3 mm). Subsequent studies used gestational age-specific

TABLE 8–2

Reported Sensitivities and False-Positive Rates of Fetal Down Syndrome with Nuchal Translucency Screening

AUTHOR AND YEAR	*N*	GESTATIONAL AGE (WK)	CUTOFF	SENSITIVITY FOR TRISOMY 21	FALSE-POSITIVE RATE
Bewley et al., 1995[15]	1127	8–13	3 mm	33% (1/3)	6%
Hafner et al., 1995[16]	1972	10–13	2.5 mm	50% (2/4)	1.3%
Pandya et al., 1995[17]	1763	10–14	2.5 mm	75% (3/4)	3.6%
Szabo et al., 1995[18]	3380	9–12	3 mm	90% (28/31)	1.6%
Kornman et al., 1996[19]	923	<13	3 mm	29% (2/7)	3.7%
Zimmerman et al., 1996[20]	1151	10–13	3 mm	50% (2/4)	1.9%
Taipale et al., 1997[21]	10,010	10–15.9	3 mm	54% (7/13)	0.8%
Biagiotti et al., 1997[22]	3241	9–13	*Calculated	59% (19/32)	5%
Thilaganathan et al., 1997[23]	2920	10–14	1:200	71% (5/7)	5%
Theodoropoulos et al., 1998[24]	3550	10–14	1:300	91% (10/11)	4.9%
Hafner et al., 1998[25]	4233	10–13	2.5 mm	43% (3/7)	1.7%
Snijders et al., 1998[26]	96,127	10–14	1:300	82% (268/326)	8.3%
Pajkrt et al., 1998[27]	1473	10–14	3 mm	67% (6/9)	2.2%
Economides et al., 1998[28]	2281	11–14	≥ 99th percentile	63% (5/8)	0.4%
Schwarzler et al., 1999[29]	4523	10–14	1:270	83% (10/12)	4.7%
Gasiorek-Wiens et al., 2001[30]	23,805	10–14	1:300	88% (184/210)	13%
Brizot et al., 2001[31]	2996	10–14	≥ 95th percentile	70% (7/10)	5.3%
Wayda et al., 2001[32]	6841	10–12	2.5 mm	100% (17/17)	4.3%

*The risk of Down syndrome was calculated with maternal age and gestational-dependent multiples of the median or delta value.

thresholds combined with maternal age to generate an individual risk estimate, or used a cutoff of greater than the 95th percentile. Further, there is no universal consensus as to what constitutes an increased measurement. The original studies included high-risk women (35 years or older) undergoing first-trimester prenatal diagnosis in referral centers for indications such as advanced maternal age or family history of aneuploidy. Subsequent studies of low-risk women in routine clinical practice settings produced conflicting results.[19,33,34] This variability may be attributable to interobserver and intraobserver variations in NT measurements. More recent reports show sensitivities for the detection of fetal trisomy 21 approaching 70% to 80%, with a 5% screen-positive rate.[4] In 1998, an impressive study from the Fetal Medicine Foundation prospectively screened more than 100,000 women at 22 centers in the United Kingdom (see Table 8–2).[26] Clinicians at all centers were trained in a standardized approach, and quality control measures were in place. The study found 82% sensitivity for trisomy 21, for an 8.3% screen-positive rate. Further, 80% of fetuses with trisomy 13 and trisomy 18 were detected.

The Fetal Medicine Foundation, based in London, England, developed strict criteria and auditing practices to certify practitioners to perform NT screening. The system ensures that the screening test is performed uniformly to maximize efficiency. Consistent, accurate measurements of NT require high-quality sonography, experienced and well-trained sonographers, and continuous quality assessment.

Current criteria for measuring NT include the following[35]: the use of high-quality sonographic equipment with video-loop function and the capability to magnify the image sufficiently to measure to 0.1 mm; screening between 11.3 and 13.6 weeks' gestation (crown–rump length, 45 to 84 mm); placement of the fetus in a sagittal plane in the midline filling more than 50% of the frame; placement of the fetal head in a neutral (straight) position, with the head in line with the spine; care taken to distinguish fetal skin from amnion (both appear as thin membranes); and correct placement of the calipers on the skin and underlying tissue interfaces (Figs. 8–3 and 8–4). The examiner may either wait for spontaneous movement away from the amniotic membrane or bounce the fetus off the amnion by asking the mother to cough or by tapping the maternal abdomen. It is important to measure the maximum thickness of the subcutaneous translucency between the skin and the soft tissue overlying the cervical spine. More than one measurement should be taken during the scan, and the largest measurement that is technically correct is recorded. Only the fetal head, neck, and upper thorax are required to be in the image (see Fig. 8–3). Although NT is usually measured transabdominally, a transvaginal approach may be required in 5% of cases.[36] In one study that compared transabdom-

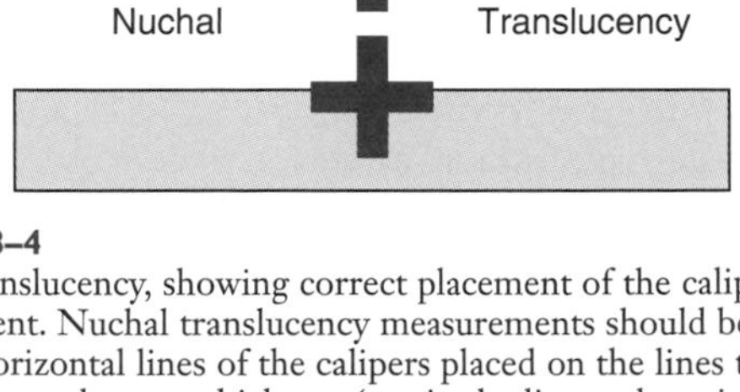

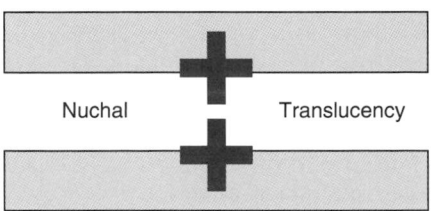

FIGURE 8–4
Nuchal translucency, showing correct placement of the calipers for measurement. Nuchal translucency measurements should be taken with the horizontal lines of the calipers placed on the lines that define the nuchal translucency thickness (not in the line and not in the nuchal fluid).

inal and transvaginal approaches, the authors found that NT could be measured in 92% of pregnancies by transabdominal scanning, in 90% by transvaginal scanning, and in 100% if both approaches were used when necessary.[37] Transabdominal measurements are slightly but significantly larger than those obtained with transvaginal scanning.

The accuracy of NT measurement is highly dependent on technical factors. For example, the position of the fetal neck affects the measurements. Extension of the fetal neck is associated with a mean NT increase of 0.6 mm, whereas neck flexion reduces the measurement by 0.4 mm (compared with the neutral position).[38] NT measurement is most reproducible in the neutral position, where 95% of measurements are within 0.48 mm of each other.

The ability to measure NT reproducibly improves with training. Good results are achieved after 80 and 100 scans for the transabdominal and transvaginal approaches, respectively.[36] Pandya and colleagues[39] reported that intraobserver and interobserver variabilities were 0.54 mm and 0.62 mm, respectively, in 95% of cases. NT can also be used in twins and higher-order multiple gestations. Increased and discordant NT in a monochorionic gestation may indicate an increased risk of subsequent twin–twin transfusion syndrome.[40]

The normal NT measurement is dependent on the crown–rump length, and gestational age must be considered when determining whether NT is increased.[36] Pandya and associates[41] found that median NT increased from 1.3 mm (crown–rump length, 38 mm) to 1.9 mm (crown–rump length, 84 mm). They also observed that the 95th percentile increased from 2.2 mm (crown–rump length, 38 mm) to 2.8 mm (crown–rump length, 84 mm).

The definition of abnormal NT has evolved since the initial descriptions. Initially, a categorical cutoff of 2.5 or 3 mm was used. However, because NT increases with gestational age and the risk varies with the measurement,[28] NT measurements are now expressed relative to either gestational age or crown–rump length as a delta value or multiple of the median.[26] A patient-specific risk is calculated from either the multiple of the median or derived likelihood ratios. This approach also permits the integration of risks based on NT, biochemical markers, and maternal age to generate a combined risk.

Fetuses with increased NT but a normal karyotype are at increased risk for other adverse pregnancy outcomes, such as major cardiac defects, a wide range of structural defects, and rare genetic conditions. Hyett and associates[42] observed that the prevalence of major cardiac abnormalities rose in chromosomally normal fetuses in direct relation to the magnitude of the increase in NT. The prevalence of major cardiac defects rose from 0.8 in 1000 when NT was below the 95th percentile for gestational age to 63.5 in 1000 when NT was greater than the 99th percentile.[12] For fetuses with NT greater than 5.5 mm, the prevalence of major cardiac defects was nearly 20% (195.1 in 1000), more than 100 times the overall prevalence (1.7 in 1000). In total, 55% of nonaneuploid fetuses with a major cardiac defect had NT greater than the 95th percentile. In contrast, Schwarzler and colleagues[29] prospectively studied 4523 women at low risk and found that only 1 of 9 (11%) major cardiac defects were associated with NT of greater than 2.5 mm. Thus, the sensitivity of increased NT as a screening test for major cardiac defects remains uncertain.

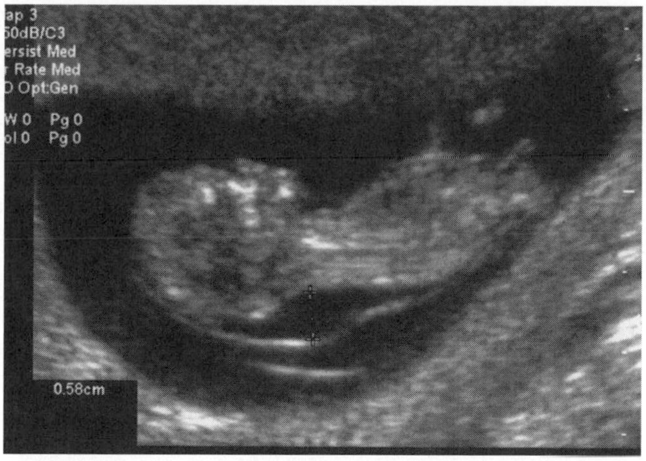

FIGURE 8–5
First-trimester scan showing increased nuchal translucency thickness of 5.8 mm. The karyotype proved to be trisomy 21.

Increased NT (Fig. 8–5) is associated with other anomalies, including diaphragmatic hernia, omphalocele, neural tube defects, and body stalk anomalies. NT is reportedly increased in a number of rare genetic syndromes and skeletal dysplasias, such as Smith-Lemli-Opitz syndrome, Noonan syndrome, arthrogryposis, Pena-Shokeir syndrome, multiple pterygium syndrome, spinal muscular atrophy, Jarcho-Levin syndrome, thanatophoric dysplasia, and thalassemia.[4] Superior mediastinal compression, as might occur with diaphragmatic hernia or with the narrow thorax seen in some skeletal dysplasias, may cause venous congestion in the head and neck. Another possible mechanism for increased NT is failure of lymphatic drainage as a result of impaired fetal movements with fetal neuromuscular disorders, such as the fetal akinesia deformation sequence. In summary, the finding of increased NT during the first trimester mandates a detailed investigation in a fetal ultrasound laboratory to complement the indicated karyotype. This detailed examination may be performed by vaginal sonography at 14 to 16 weeks or by abdominal sonography at 18 to 20 weeks.

FIRST-TRIMESTER DUCTUS VENOSUS DOPPLER VELOCIMETRY

Ductus venosus Doppler sonography may further discriminate between chromosomally normal and abnormal fetuses in the first trimester.[43] In one study, the authors examined 486 fetuses between 10 and 14 weeks' gestation.[43] Of these fetuses, 68 had aneuploidy; in 90.5% of the aneuploid fetuses, flow was either reversed or absent during atrial contraction. Abnormal ductal flow was present in only 3.1% of nonaneuploid fetuses. Interestingly, ductus venosus Doppler imaging may also help to determine which nonaneuploid fetuses with increased NT are at increased risk for cardiac defects. Matias and colleagues[44] studied 142 first-trimester chromosomally normal fetuses with increased NT measurement. Eleven fetuses had reversed or absent flow during atrial contraction; of these, 7 (64%) had major cardiac defects seen on fetal echocardiography. No major cardiac defects were identified in the remaining 131 fetuses with increased NT and normal findings on ductus venosus Doppler studies.

SONGRAPHIC ABNORMALITIES UP TO 15 WEEKS' GESTATION

The progressive improvement in sonographic resolution, coupled with growing expertise, has made the detection of many structural abnormalities during the first trimester a reality.[45] Transvaginal scanning has had a tremendous effect on the ability to detail fetal structures, and targeted ultrasound for fetal anomalies can be performed as early as 14 to 15 weeks.[5] However, not all anomalies are apparent by this time, and expertise in early transvaginal sonography is not widespread. Thus, in most cases, a targeted scan later in gestation is warranted.

Whitlow and colleagues[46] used transabdominal or transvaginal scanning, as necessary, from 11 to 14 weeks. They detected 59% of fetuses with structural abnormalities. Structural abnormalities were seen in 35% of aneuploid fetuses, excluding three fetuses with XXY. However, structural anomalies during the first 14 weeks are more likely to be associated with trisomy 13 and trisomy 18 than with trisomy 21. Only 9% of fetuses with trisomy 21 (2 of 23) had visible structural abnormalities. In another first-trimester study of trisomy 21, the detectable structural abnormality rate was 12.5%.[28] In contrast, holoprosencephaly was diagnosed in 24% and omphalocele in 10% of 46 fetuses with trisomy 13.[47]

Malformations of the fetal head, neck, and spine that are detectable by transvaginal sonography before 15 weeks include acrania (absence of the entire cranium or a major portion of the cranium in the presence of a brain), anencephaly (absence of the cranium above the orbits, with variable amounts of remnant brain tissue), cephaloceles (cranial defects, with herniation of the brain or meninges), holoprosencephaly (failure of the forebrain to differentiate into cerebral hemispheres and lateral ventricles), ventriculomegaly or hydrocephalus, Dandy-Walker malformation (cystic dilation of the fourth ventricle), neural tube defects, and iniencephaly (see Chapter 18). Iniencephaly is a lethal anomaly that includes an occipital defect, retroflexion of the spine, and open spinal defects. The diagnosis of ventriculomegaly in the first trimester or early second trimester may be especially difficult because the lateral ventricles are normally prominent at this stage (Fig. 8–6). In the first trimester, cranial findings associated with neural tube defects (NTDs), such as the lemon or banana signs and hydrocephalus, may be very subtle or absent. Therefore, a follow-up scan in the second trimester is warranted for at-risk fetuses.

Cystic hygromas may also be seen in the first trimester. It is important to differentiate a cystic hygroma from increased NT. Cystic hygromas appear as bilateral, posterior cystic structures that contain characteristic thick septations. They are often associated with hydrops, effusions, or ascites and adverse outcomes. Bronshtein and colleagues[48] reported 125 fetuses with cystic hygroma in the early second trimester and observed that, compared with "nonseptated" cystic spaces (NT), septated cystic hygromas were more likely to persist (56% vs. 2%) and to be associated with aneuploidy (72% vs. 5.6%), hydrops (40% vs. 1.7%), other anomalies (52% vs. 15%), and pregnancy loss (88% vs. 6%). In another series of 56 fetuses with hygromas diagnosed between 9 and 14 weeks, chromosomal abnormalities were found in 29%: 38% had trisomy 18, 31% had trisomy 21, 25% had Turner syndrome, and 6% had 47 XXX. The prevalence of an adverse outcome in fetuses with cystic hygromas and normal chromosomes was 30%.[49]

Facial anomalies that are diagnosable in the first trimester include cleft lip or palate, ocular anomalies (hypertelorism or hypotelorism, anophthalmia, microphthalmia), and fetal cataracts. Cardiac malformations are also diagnosable before 15 weeks. Bronshtein and associates[50] identified 47 fetuses with congenital heart disease among 12,793 fetuses scanned transvaginally at 12 to 16 weeks. Ectopia cordis is reported as early as 12 to 14

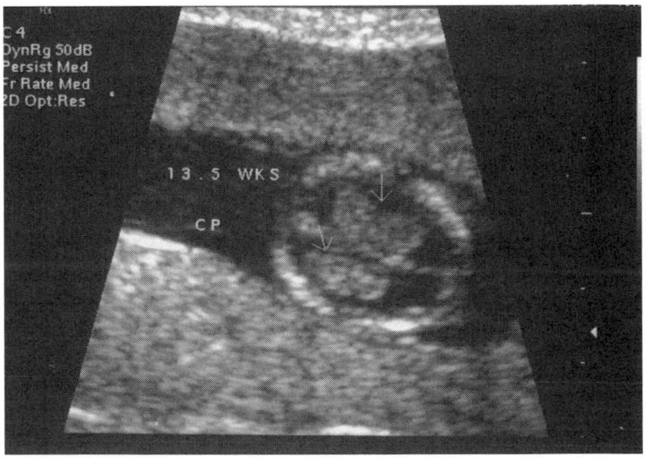

FIGURE 8–6
Axial view of a fetal head at 13.5 weeks, showing prominent lateral ventricles filled with the choroid plexus (*arrows*).

weeks, and pentalogy of Cantrell is noted as early as 11 weeks.[5] Body stalk anomalies are also reported in the first trimester. Umbilical cord cysts and the presence of a single umbilical artery are reported within the first 14 weeks. Although transient umbilical cord cysts do not appear to be associated with either aneuploidy or structural anomalies, persistent cysts detected after the first trimester may be associated with other fetal malformations.

The normal protrusion of the midgut into the umbilical cord between 8 and 10 weeks can easily be confused with omphalocele, which is associated with aneuploidy, especially for trisomy 13 or trisomy 18. The bowel normally returns to the abdominal cavity by 12 weeks.[6] Persistence of this normal gut migration can produce small, bowel-containing omphaloceles. Omphaloceles that include liver have a lower association with aneuploidy, especially if no other fetal anomalies are present. Snijders and associates[51] reported that of omphaloceles detected in the first trimester, aneuploidy (trisomy 13, trisomy 18, or triploidy) was present in 61%. The risk is significantly higher than that observed when omphalocele is first diagnosed in the second or third trimester. Omphalocele is found during the first trimester in 9% of fetuses with trisomy 13, 23% with trisomy 18, and 13% with triploidy.[51] Gastroschisis also can be diagnosed before 15 weeks, although there is no association between gastroschisis and fetal aneuploidy.

Several malformations of the urinary system are visible before 15 weeks, including hydronephrosis, bilateral renal agenesis, multicystic dysplastic and infantile polycystic kidneys, and obstructive uropathy. Before 15 weeks, fetuses with bilateral renal agenesis may have normal fluid volume and a visible bladder. The same is true for severe multicystic or polycystic kidney disease.[5] Osteogenesis imperfecta, sirenomelia (complete or nearly complete fusion of the lower extremities), and various skeletal abnormalities have been diagnosed sonographically before 15 weeks.

Nonstructural sonographic markers of fetal aneuploidy are also sought in the first trimester. Whitlow and colleagues[52] reported the prevalence of three such markers (choroid plexus cyst, renal pyelectasis, and echogenic intracardiac foci) in 5383 women who underwent scanning between 10 and 14 weeks. The prevalence of these markers was 2.2%, 0.9%, and 0.6%, respectively, in normal fetuses. Pyelectasis (likelihood ratio, 8.0) and echogenic intracardiac foci (likelihood ratio, 10.3) were significantly associated with fetal aneuploidy, but choroid plexus cysts were not.[52]

COST-EFFECTIVENESS OF FIRST-TRIMESTER SCREENING

Although routine first-trimester ultrasound offers certain benefits, such as accurate dating, NT measurement, the potential to detect structural abnormalities, and determination of chorionicity in multiple gestations, it has not replaced the second-trimester anatomic survey and creates additional costs. We addressed this issue in a cost–benefit analysis comparing two approaches: the "British" approach of first-trimester NT screening followed by chorionic villus sampling in screen-positive patients and the "American" approach of second-trimester maternal serum screening followed by amniocentesis in screen-positive patients.[53] The costs of first-trimester screening are comparable to those of second-trimester screening if the screening has a sensitivity of at least 80% and a screen-positive rate of no more than 5% for detecting fetal trisomy 21.[53]

SUMMARY OF FIRST-TRIMESTER SCREENING (See also Chapter 7)

Screening for aneuploidy in the first trimester rather than second trimester has the obvious advantage of providing earlier prenatal diagnosis and the ability to terminate the pregnancy with less morbidity. NT screening requires only one measurement but must be preceded by basic training. It also requires ongoing quality control. The risks of fetal aneuploidy and adverse outcome increase progressively with increasing NT. NT is a marker for aneuploidies other than trisomy 21 as well as for other anomalies. The combination of maternal age, first-trimester serum screening, and NT allows 90% sensitivity for the detection of trisomy 21, with a 5% screen-positive rate. Sonographers who perform NT screening must be familiar with normal and abnormal first-trimester fetal anatomy so that they can detect anomalies accurately.

SECOND-TRIMESTER BIOCHEMICAL SERUM MARKER SCREENING

Screening for trisomy 21 in low-risk patients (women younger than 35 years) was initiated in the mid-1980s with the observation that the mean maternal serum concentration of α-fetoprotein was 0.7 MoM in affected pregnancies.[54–56] Subsequently, it was recognized that hCG levels were higher (2.04 MoM) and unconjugated estriol levels were lower (0.79 MoM) in pregnancies with trisomy 21.[57–60] By using the relative risks derived from maternal serum levels, the maternal age-related risk can be modified and a "triple-screen" risk derived for each woman.

Triple-marker screening is used extensively and is the preferred screening modality in some locales for the detection of fetal trisomy 21 in women younger than 35 years.[60–63] In this group, the triple-marker screen identifies approximately 60% of pregnancies affected by trisomy 21 as being at risk, with a 5% screen-positive rate (see Table 8–1). In the population of women 35 years and older, the triple-marker screen identifies 75% or more of pregnancies affected by trisomy 21 and some other aneuploidies.[64] Because the maternal age-related risk of trisomy 21 is the basis of the serum screening protocol, both the trisomy 21 detection rate and the screen-positive rate increase with maternal age.[65] Different laboratories use different screen-positive cutoffs. For example, some use the midtrimester risk of trisomy 21 in a 35-year-old woman (1 in 270). Others apply a screen-positive cutoff that provides an acceptable balance between the detection rate and the screen-positive rate (usually 1 in 190 or 1 in 200).

Maternal serum screening is performed between 15 and 20 weeks but is most accurate between 16 and 18 weeks. Like first-trimester screening, the pregnancy must be dated accurately because errors will affect the assigned risk, causing false-negative and false-positive results. It is important to recalculate the results if the dates are found to be in error, or to have a new sample drawn if the original sample was obtained before 15 weeks.

Serum screening is used primarily to detect trisomy 21, and it does not efficiently detect other fetal aneuploidies, except possibly trisomy 18. Thus, serum screening will miss both lethal (e.g., trisomy 13) and sex chromosomal abnormalities that are not associated with severe physical or developmental limitations or profound mental retardation.

Some investigators believe that, as a marker, the free beta subunit of hCG (βhCG) is superior to the intact hCG molecule, but this has not been proven in the second trimester. Recently, several new analytes of interest have emerged. Dimeric inhibin A is the most promising and is used by many commercial laboratories in combination with the three traditional analytes. This four-analyte combination ("quad screen") detects 67% to 76% cases of fetal trisomy 21 in women younger than 35 years, with a screen-positive rate of 5% or less.[66,67]

Diagnostic options are limited for screening multiple gestations. With twins, the risk of trisomy 21 is calculated by considering the maternal age-related risk and the probability that one or both fetuses will be affected. In a twin gestation in a 33-year-old woman, the midtrimester risk of trisomy 21 in at least one fetus approximates the risk in a singleton pregnancy in a 35-year-old woman, justifying an offer of invasive testing.[68]

FETAL ANATOMIC SURVEY ON SECOND-TRIMESTER SONOGRAPHY

The introduction of two-dimensional static scanning in the early 1970s allowed physicians to view the fetus for the first time. In the late 1970s and early 1980s, real-time B-mode imaging emerged as a widespread clinical tool. Because sonography images with sound waves and not ionizing radiation, it quickly became the most commonly used method during pregnancy. The major advantage of ultrasound is its lack of a demonstrable adverse fetal effect.[69] Despite the apparent safety of this method, some believe that fetal sonography should be used only when there is a clear indication. However, most complicated pregnancies are unexpected, and ultrasound examinations are routinely performed throughout pregnancy in many European countries. Ultrasound resolution has improved dramatically, and a detailed examination of the fetus for both structural anomalies and markers of aneuploidy is possible. The diagnosis and management of specific congenital fetal abnormalities are discussed in other chapters. We focus here on the elements of a complete sonographic fetal anatomic survey.

We believe that all pregnant women should have access to expert obstetric sonography. The examination should be systematic and thorough. Normal findings provide reassurance to patients, and the examination should detect most fetal malformations, along with abnormalities in fetal growth, the placenta, amniotic fluid, and the cervix. We examined the value, from a patient's perspective, of a targeted ultrasound examination performed after an abnormal karyotype was discovered.[70] All women valued the scan because it helped them to visualize the anomalies and accept the diagnosis of aneuploidy, and this in turn affected their plans for pregnancy management. All patients considered the effect of the ultrasound greater than that of the chromosomal diagnosis alone, and all believed that ultrasound should be used for patients in similar clinical situations.

The American Institute of Ultrasound in Medicine first published standards for the performance of obstetric ultrasound in 1994.[71] Minimum requirements in the first trimester include evaluation of the uterus, adnexa, cul-de-sac, gestational sac, crown–rump length, fetal number, and presence of cardiac activity. Minimum requirements in the second and third trimesters include verifying fetal life, number, presentation, and activity (multiple gestations require additional documentation); measuring amniotic fluid volume; determining the placental location, appearance, and relationship to the internal os; visualizing the umbilical cord; measuring the fetal biparietal diameter or head circumference; measuring the limbs; estimating fetal weight (requires the abdominal diameter or circumference); evaluating the cerebral ventricles; evaluating the posterior fossa; obtaining a four-chamber view of the heart and determining its position; and evaluating the spine, stomach, kidneys, bladder, abdominal cord insertion site, uterus, cervix, and adnexa.

The current state of the art requires a more detailed examination than that described by the American Institute of Ultrasound in Medicine for optimal diagnostic accuracy of fetal abnormalities (Table 8–3). Further, sonographer training must be targeted to ensure that these detailed examinations are done appropriately. The sonographer must be familiar with normal fetal anatomy,

TABLE 8–3

Content of Fetal Anatomic Survey on Second-Trimester Sonography at Robert Wood Johnson Medical School

ORGAN STRUCTURES
Head
Cranial shape, mineralization
Cerebral hemispheres, thalami, cerebral peduncles, lateral ventricles and choroid plexus, third and fourth ventricles, cerebellum and vermis, cisterna magna, cavum septum pellucidum
Face and Neck
Profile, orbits, lips and palate, nasal bone, nuchal fold, ear
Thoracic Cavity
Lungs
Configuration of the bony thorax
Heart
Four-chamber views (apical and subcostal), outflow tracts, longitudinal parasternal arches, inferior and superior vena cava, valves, atria and ventricular septa
Abdomen
Situs
Stomach
Liver, gallbladder, spleen
Bowel
Wall and cord insertion site
Genitourinary System
Kidneys
Bladder
Genitalia
Spine
Extremities
Upper, including both hands
Lower, including both feet
Cord
Number of vessels
Biometric Measurements
Biparietal diameter
Head circumference
Atria of lateral ventricles, cisterna magna, nuchal fold (when applicable)
Cerebellum
Thoracic circumference (when applicable)
Abdominal circumference
Femur length, humerus length, radius and ulna lengths, tibia and fibula lengths
Foot length
Nasal bone length
Orbital diameters
Other
Number of fetuses, position
Placenta
Amniotic fluid
Cervix and lower uterine segment

sonographic landmarks, and normal variants. An adequate examination requires proper equipment. The highest-frequency transducer should be used to maximize the resolution of the fetal anatomy.

The entire uterus is scanned both transversely and longitudinally to determine the fetal position, amniotic fluid volume, and placental location. Accurate determination of the right and left sides of the fetus is crucial. Factors that may limit visualization (Table 8–4) include equipment quality, fluid abnormalities, maternal body habitus or tissue density, and other scanning characteristics. Techniques to improve visualization include changing the maternal position (to effectively change the fetal position) and using different scanning probes (including transvaginal). The timing of the second-trimester ultrasound varies with the center and physician preference. Repeating the examination later may aid the resolution of anatomic detail of some structures (e.g., heart) but hinder visualization of others (e.g., extremities). This is not to infer that scanning, even late in pregnancy, cannot provide important information and be highly sensitive for fetal anomalies whose diagnosis will alter pregnancy management. We recommend that the fetal anatomy survey be performed at 18 to 20 weeks to optimize the assessment of anatomy while leaving an adequate window for invasive testing, if necessary. Scans performed at 18 to 20 weeks are less likely than earlier scans to end incompletely and trigger the need for a repeat examination. In addition to evaluating the fetal anatomy, the number and position of fetuses should be determined. The placental appearance, thickness, echogenicity, and location are important to document, along with amniotic fluid volume. Amniotic fluid abnormalities may indicate an anomalous (e.g., anhydramnios is associated with renal agenesis and polyhydramnios with esophageal atresia) or infected fetus. The fetal echocardiogram is best performed between 22 and 24 weeks, when the cardiac structures are larger.

Content of the Fetal Anatomic Survey

The examination begins with the fetal head and proceeds caudally. Imaging the fetal intracranial anatomy is extremely important because central nervous system anomalies can have a devastating effect on perinatal morbidity and mortality. The calvarium can be identified from the late first trimester onward. It should be well

TABLE 8–4

Factors That May Limit Sonographic Examination of the Fetal Anatomy

FACTORS
Equipment quality
Sonographer expertise
Length of time spent scanning
Maternal habitus, tissue density, and scanning characteristics
Incomplete filling or overfilling of the bladder
Fetal positioning
Fluid abnormalities (increased or decreased)
Gestational age (early or late)
Ossification of fetal bony structures (later in gestation)
Fetal movement

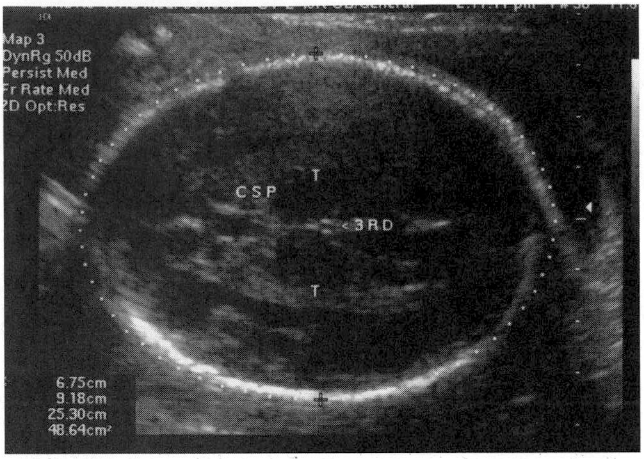

FIGURE 8–7
Axial view through the fetal head showing the thalami (T), falx, third ventricle (3rd) between the thalami, and cavum septum pellucidum (CSP). The calipers also show measurement of the head circumference.

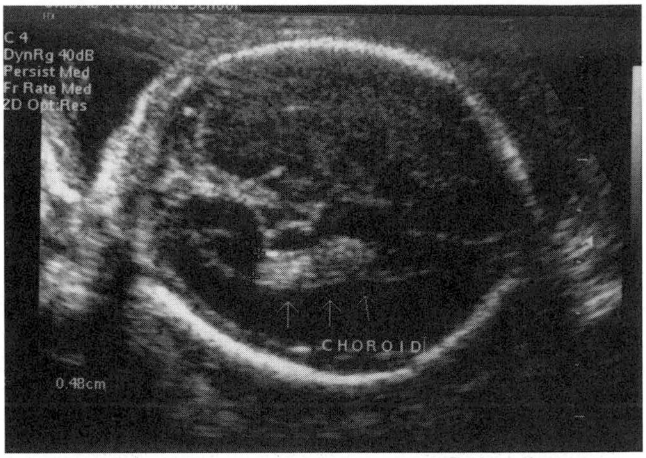

FIGURE 8–8
Transventricular view of the fetal head, showing measurement of the atria of the lateral ventricle (0.48 cm) and the echogenic choroid plexus (*arrows*).

mineralized (hypomineralization may indicate skeletal dysplasia) and elliptical. Brachycephaly (anteroposterior shortening) suggests fetal trisomy 21 or 18 ("strawberry" head). A lemon-shaped head suggests a neural tube defect. Tangential imaging shows cranial sutures (hypoechoic spaces between bones) that are best visualized early in gestation. Premature closure of the sutures occurs in many syndromes (e.g., craniosynostosis) and with several skeletal dysplasias.

The transthalamic view is an axial view through the brain at the level of the thalami (Fig. 8–7). It is here that the biparietal diameter and head circumference are obtained. Biparietal diameter is measured from the outer margin of the near calvarium to the inner margin of the far calvarium (with cranial bones perpendicular to the ultrasound beam). The head circumference is measured circumferentially at the outer margin of the calvarium (see Fig. 8–7). Other structures that are visualized in the transthalamic view include the cavum septum pellucidum (a fluid-filled midline structure anterior to the thalami), midline falx, third ventricle (between the thalami), and frontal horns of the lateral ventricles. A normal cavum suggests proper midline brain formation; its absence may signal abnormalities, such as holoprosencephaly or agenesis of the corpus callosum. The transventricular view is just superior to the transthalamic view and includes the lateral ventricles that contain sonolucent cerebrospinal fluid. Within lies the echogenic choroid plexus that normally fills the atrium and may contain cysts (a potential marker for trisomy 18) [Figs. 8–8 and 8–9]. The cerebral ventricle is measured through the atrium in an axial plane and is normally less than 10 mm. The transcerebellar view contains the cerebellum and vermis, cisterna magna (between the dorsum of the cerebellar hemispheres and inner calvarium), and nuchal fold (Fig. 8–10). Visualization of this area is important to exclude spina

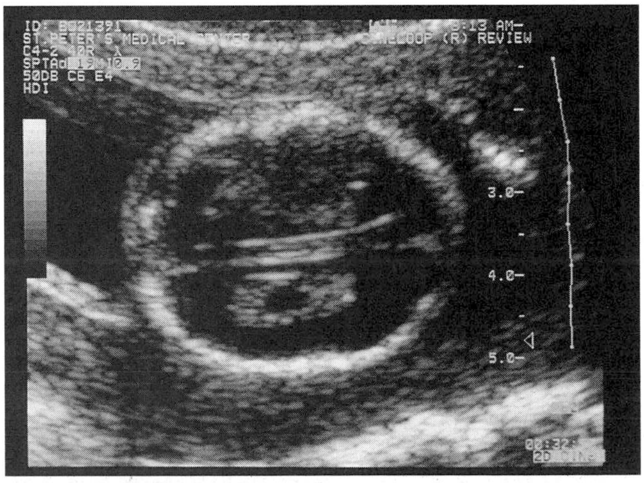

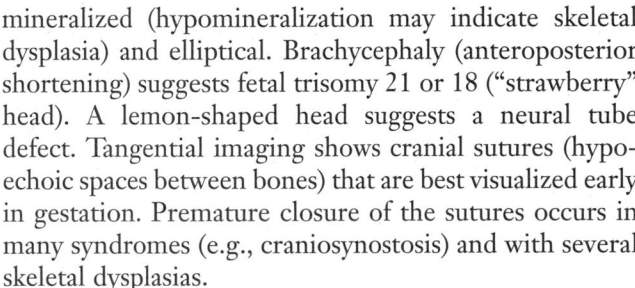

FIGURE 8–9
A single sonolucent choroid plexus cyst in the far lateral ventricle.

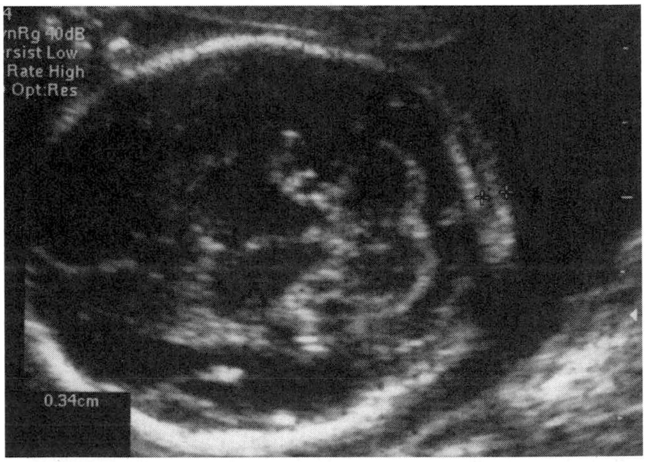

FIGURE 8–10
Transcerebellar view, showing the cerebellar hemispheres and cisterna magna and a normal nuchal fold measurement (0.34 cm).

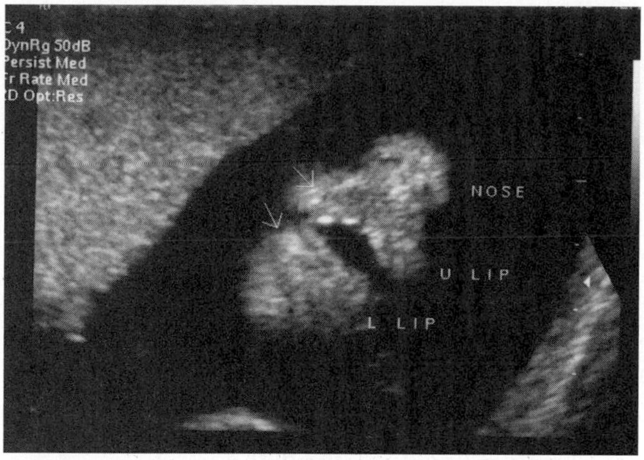

FIGURE 8–11
Coronal view of the fetal face, showing the nose and upper and lower lips (*arrows*).

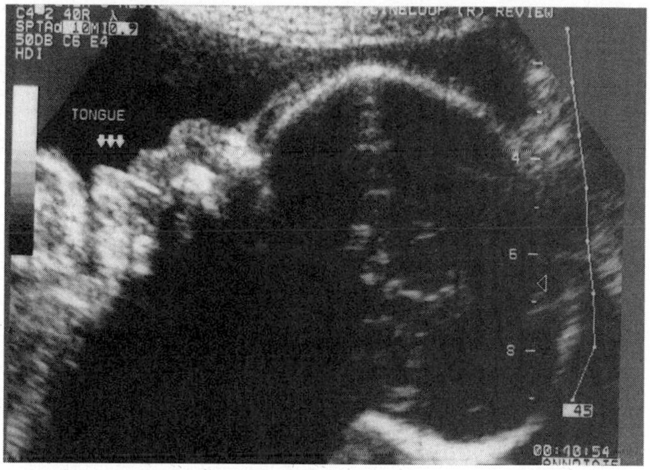

FIGURE 8–12
Sagittal profile of a third-trimester fetus with Down syndrome, showing the tongue protruding between the upper and lower lips.

bifida; obliteration of the cisterna magna and a banana-shaped cerebellum typically occur with this disorder. This view is also used to exclude Dandy-Walker malformation or variant, occipital encephalocele, and cerebellar agenesis or hypoplasia. The nuchal fold should be less than 6 mm, although breech presentations may create false-positive thickening. The transcerebellar diameter provides a useful estimate of gestational age because it is relatively spared by growth restriction. Sometimes the head is low in the pelvis, blocking access to the intracranial structures; in this case, transvaginal scanning may be useful.

The facial structures are especially important for the diagnosis of genetic disorders or syndromes, and they should be examined routinely. This is accomplished with coronal (Fig. 8–11), sagittal (profile) [Fig. 8–12], and axial views. Often, a combination of these planes is optimal. Structures important to image include the chin (for micrognathia), nasal bone (absent or shortened) [Fig. 8–13], nose, lips, anterior palate (to exclude cleft lip or palate), orbits (and diameters, if necessary, to exclude hypertelorism or hypotelorism), and ear (which may be short in aneuploid and nonaneuploid fetuses) [Fig. 8–14].

Next, the fetal spine is imaged in sagittal (Fig. 8–15), transverse, and coronal views, when possible. The overlying skin should be intact to exclude open spina bifida and masses or tumors. Each normal vertebral segment consists of three echogenic ossification centers (two located posteriorly, and one located anteriorly that is the vertebral body) lying in a symmetrical, triangular configuration. In the transverse plane, the posterior processes appear angled in the same way as the roof of a house; if they are splayed, a neural tube defect should be sought (Fig. 8–16). Sagittal and coronal views are useful to observe how well the ossification centers align to exclude hemivertebrae that cause disorganization or absence of ossification centers. The sacrum should curve gently upward.

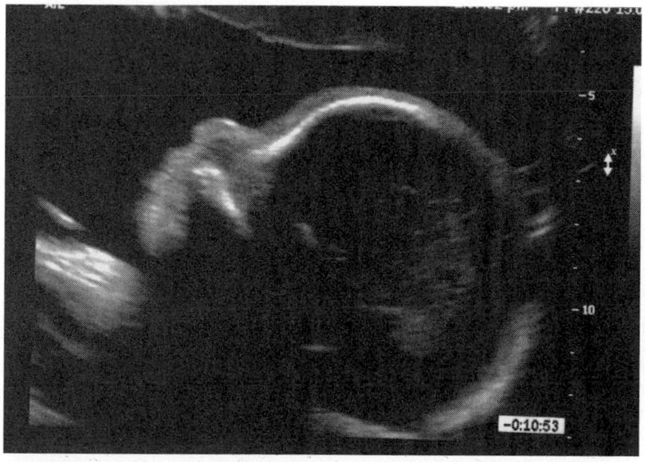

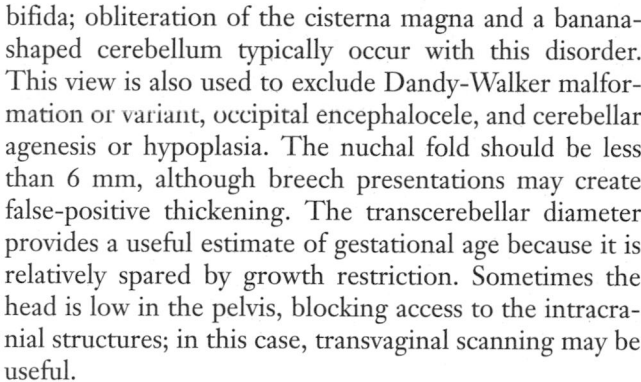

FIGURE 8–13
Profile of a fetus with Down syndrome, showing frontal bone, but no nasal bone.

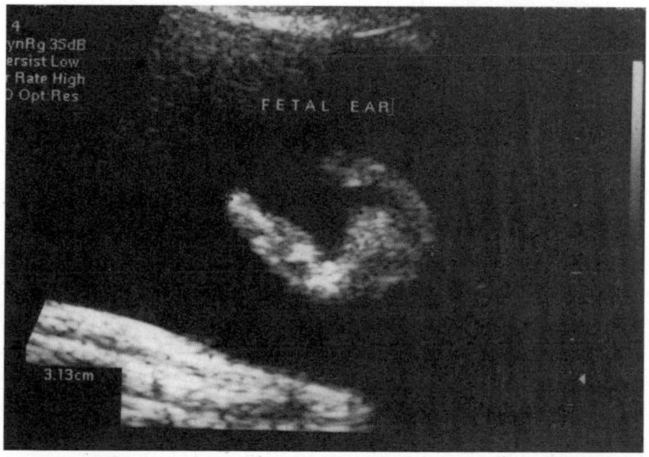

FIGURE 8–14
Frontal view of the fetal ear, showing caliper placement.

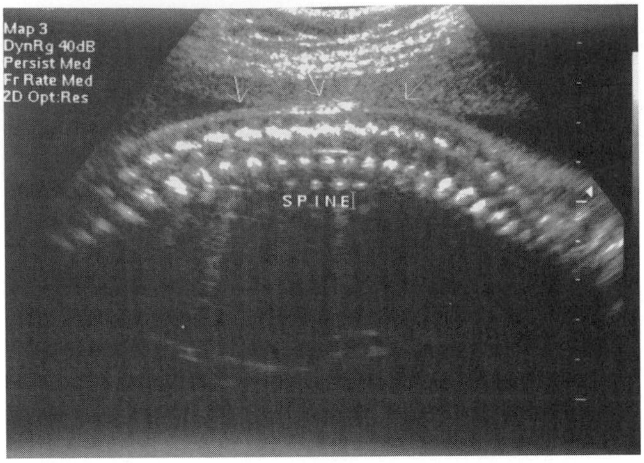

FIGURE 8–15
Normal sagittal view of the fetal spine. The overlying skin (*arrows*) is intact, and the features of the spinal centers are parallel.

The ribs, clavicles, and scapulae are examined next. A normal appearance excludes some types of skeletal dysplasia. Abnormal lung tissue or echogenicity (e.g., cystic adenomatoid malformation) or pleural effusions may be seen. The thoracic circumference is measured to exclude pulmonary hypoplasia, and the diaphragm is examined for evidence of a hernia.

A detailed fetal cardiac examination is perhaps the most challenging task performed by a sonographer. The cardiac rate and rhythm (normally 120–160 beats/min and regular), size (one-third of the fetal thorax), axis and position (apex points to the left at an angle of 45 ± 20 degrees relative to the midline), and situs should be established (liver on the right, stomach on the left). Alterations in position, axis, or both suggest malposition or an intrathoracic mass deviating the mediastinum. Multiple planes and views are used in real time to exclude cardiac defects. Routine imaging of the outflow tracts increases detection sensitivity and should be part of the standard fetal cardiac examination. When screening for cardiac defects, the examination should include, minimally, the four-chamber apical (Fig. 8–17) and subcostal views, outflow tracts, longitudinal parasternal arches (aortic and ductal), inferior and superior vena cava, valves, and atria and ventricular septa. The chambers are roughly equal in size. The pulmonary veins should enter the left atrium; the two atrioventricular valves and septa should be visualized in their entirety and the rate and rhythm documented as well as the axis, position, and size of the heart. The great vessels should cross each other, and there should be no dependent pericardial fluid. Some recommend routine color, M-mode, or pulsed Doppler sonography to assist in the visualization of the heart and great vessels and to exclude significant valvular stenosis or regurgitation (see Chapter 17 for a discussion of specific cardiac abnormalities). An echogenic focus is commonly seen, typically in the left ventricle. It is caused by specular reflection from the papillary muscles and chordae tendineae (Fig. 8–18).[72]

Intra-abdominal organs that are identifiable on ultrasound include the liver (occupying most of the upper abdomen), spleen (solid organ posterior to the stomach), gallbladder (teardrop-shaped organ in the right upper quadrant, at the inferior edge of the liver), stomach, bowel, umbilical vein, and umbilical cord insertion site. Abdominal circumference is the most sensitive fetal growth parameter. It is measured at the transverse level, where the umbilical vein joins the right portal venous system (Fig. 8–19), which should "curve" away from the stomach. If the curve is toward the stomach, persistence of the right umbilical vein is suspected. The stomach and spine should be imaged in this axial plane; the stomach should always be located below the diaphragm. An absent or small stomach despite prolonged scanning to allow for filling suggests esophageal atresia, with or without tracheoesophageal fistula, or a diaphragmatic hernia (stomach located within the chest). Most of the abdomen is

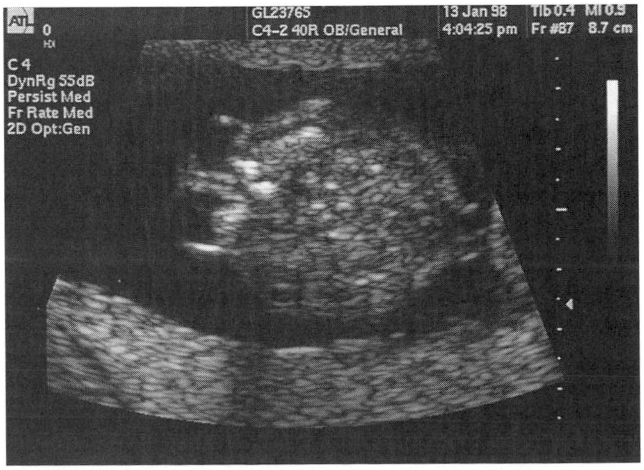

FIGURE 8–16
Transverse plane of the fetal spine, showing a large neural tube defect with splaying of the posterior processes.

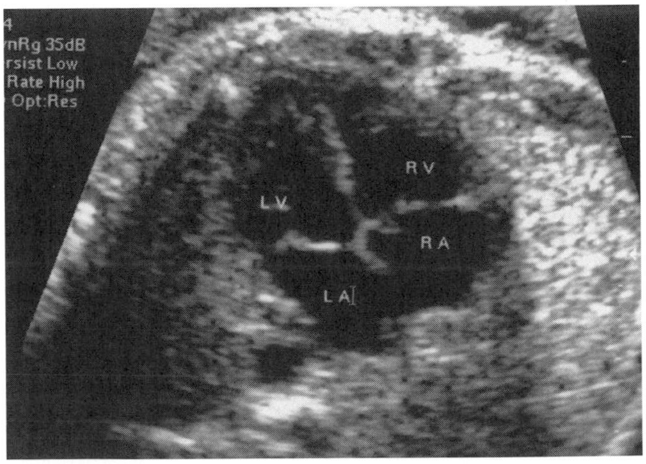

FIGURE 8–17
Apical four-chamber view of the fetal heart, showing the left atrium and ventricle (LA, LV) and right atrium and ventricle (RA, RV).

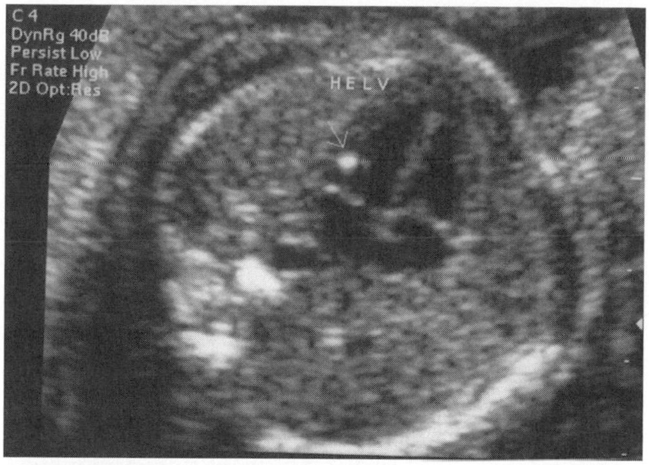

FIGURE 8–18
Apical four-chamber view of the fetal heart, showing a bright, echogenic focus in the left ventricle (HELV).

bowel-filled, and the appearance varies with gestational age. In the second trimester, the bowel appears as midlevel to increased echogenicity filling the abdomen. Hyperechoic bowel is associated with aneuploidy, infection, and bowel abnormalities. In the third trimester, prominent hypoechoic loops of colon may be seen. More dilated loops of bowel may reflect atresia or another cause of obstruction. The umbilical cord insertion and the adjacent ventral abdominal wall should be visualized to exclude ventral wall defects (e.g., omphalocele, gastroschisis). There should be no fetal ascites.

Next visualized is the genitourinary tract, which is a common site for fetal anomalies. The kidneys are bilateral, hypoechoic, paraspinal structures that include the urine-containing renal pelvis. Abnormal findings include dilation of the renal pelvis, calix, or ureter; renal masses; cysts within the parenchyma; hyperechogenicity; and enlargement or absence of the kidneys. Color or power Doppler imaging is useful to identify the renal arteries, especially when the kidneys cannot be seen in their usual location. It is important to distinguish between pyelectasis (dilated renal pelvis) and hydronephrosis (pyelectasis plus upper tract dilation). The bladder is a urine-filled structure located midline, anterior, and low in the fetal pelvis. Absence of the fetal bladder (bladder exstrophy) or a very enlarged bladder (lower obstructive uropathy) should be excluded. The sonographer should confirm that the two umbilical arteries course around the fetal bladder. This image all but excludes a two-vessel cord. Gender is assigned by imaging the genitalia, and not by the lack of an image. Ambiguous genitalia should be excluded. The fetus is male if both the penis and scrotum are seen. The testicles are echogenic and usually descend into the scrotum during month seven. The labia appear as several parallel linear echoes.

Documentation of all fetal extremities is not included in the guidelines for routine obstetric ultrasound examination. However, a survey of all extremities (including hands and feet) may provide important diagnostic information. The five fingers should extend fully (Fig. 8–20). Movement and tone should be normal, and the middle phalanx of the fifth digit should be visualized. Persistently clenched hands with overlapping digits are a highly sensitive (95%) sonographic feature for trisomy 18.[73] The long bones (femur, humerus, radius and ulna, tibia and fibula) should be well mineralized and of normal length. Absence, fractures, contractures, or bowing of these bones is abnormal. The ulna extends farther into the elbow than the radius, and the tibia extends farther into the patella than the fibula. The length of each long bone is measured. Images are obtained with the diaphysis located horizontally in the image (Fig. 8–21) because vertical measurements can falsely "shorten" the length. Multiple images are measured, and the longest technically adequate image is the optimal measurement. The

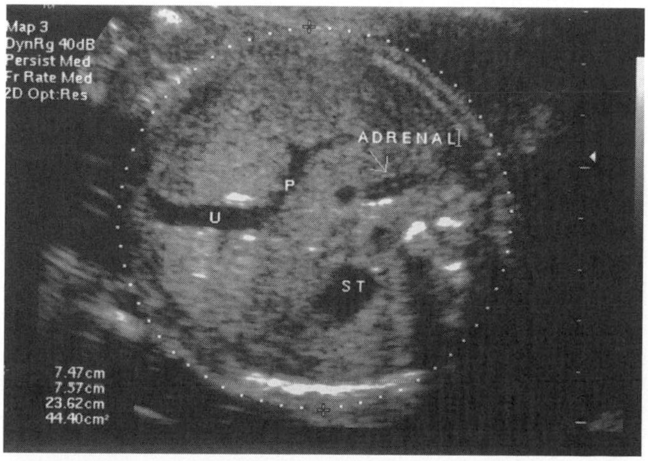

FIGURE 8–19
Correct method for measuring the abdominal circumference. P, portal vein; ST, stomach; U, umbilical vein.

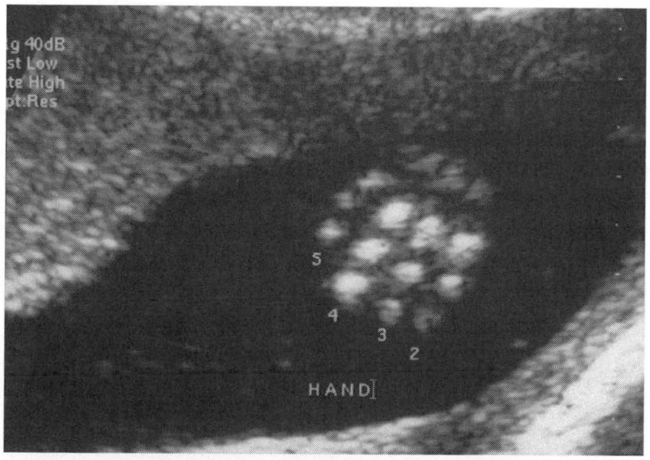

FIGURE 8–20
Fetal hand, showing echogenic phalanges of four fingers, including the fifth digit.

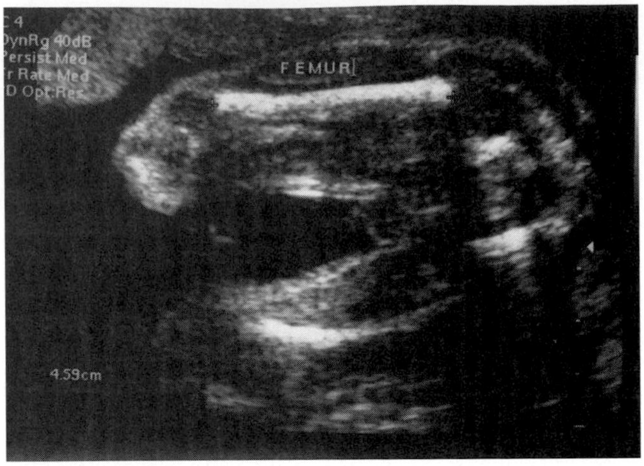

FIGURE 8–21
Femur length measured from the proximal end to the distal metaphysis.

lower extremities should not be clubbed, nor should the plantar surface appear "rocker-bottom." There should be five toes (Fig. 8–22), and they should not appear dysplastic. The foot length can also be measured.

Finally, the umbilical cord is examined. There should be two arteries and one vein. Once the umbilical vein enters the fetal abdomen, it should turn superiorly, enter the liver, and communicate with the portal vein. The umbilical vein continues into the ductus venosus and then into the inferior vena cava and right atrium.

Second-Trimester Ultrasound Screening for Structural Abnormalities

There are many accepted indications for ultrasound examination during pregnancy, and 60% to 70% of all pregnant women in the United States undergo an examination at some stage during pregnancy.[74] The rate is much higher in other industrialized countries. One of the first studies to quantify the diagnostic accuracy of ultrasound in high risk pregnancies was performed in the United Kingdom in the late 1970s and early 1980s; 95% of malformations were correctly diagnosed.[75] Subsequently, many studies examined the efficacy of routine screening ultrasound. Published sensitivities range from 13.3% to 82.4%,[76] with the collaborative world experience approximating 50%.[77] We believe that much of the variation in results reflects differences in the quality of training. In light of these wide variations in detection rates, it is understandable why the reliability and utility of sonographic screening for fetal malformations have been challenged. Even among those who recommend routine ultrasound screening, the number and timing of scans are debated. Because 75% of patients with abnormal fetuses are considered low risk, it is important to review the literature to assess the effect of routine sonography.[76]

The antenatal diagnosis of a fetal abnormality has many advantages. It may trigger additional testing to refine the diagnosis or prognosis, alter pregnancy management (e.g., termination, intrauterine therapy, early delivery, delivery in a tertiary care center), prepare the parents for an adverse pregnancy outcome, and alert the clinician to the possibility of other malformations. For many patients, the benefits of sparing social and psychological costs are also very important. However, there is one fact that no one contests. Sonographic screening performed by inexperienced individuals increases the costs of health care and generates high false-negative and false-positive rates, with serious consequences, such as termination of an actually normal fetus.

Many biases and problems may explain much of the variation in sensitivity.[76] Reasons for the variation include technical issues (e.g., fetal positioning, obesity), lesions that resolve over time, and the undetectability of certain anomalies by ultrasound. However, these factors are unlikely explanations for differences in large studies. Selection bias may play an important role, depending on whether the patient source is a hospital or an office practice. The most important bias is the variation in sonographic skills, capability, and experience of individuals performing the ultrasound examination. In the Helsinki study, which incorporated patient populations from two hospitals, the sonographic sensitivity for detecting anomalies was twofold higher in the university hospital than in the city hospital (77% vs. 36%).[78] A systematic and almost compulsive approach to each examination is necessary, with attention paid to all structures. Each center has different criteria as to what constitutes a detailed ultrasound examination. The less detailed the examination, the lower the sensitivity. The selection of pregnant women is also important. Screening high risk women is likely to be more effective because sonographers become more focused because they expect to find an anomaly. One group noted an average sensitivity of 55% in a low risk population and 92% in a high risk population.[76]

Gestational age at screening also affects sensitivity because various anomalies may appear at different gesta-

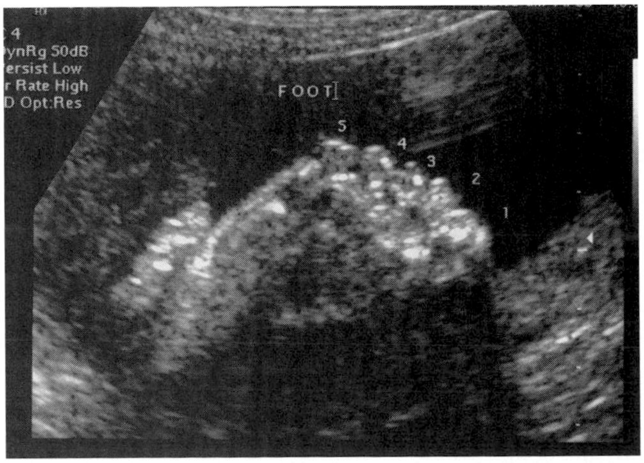

FIGURE 8–22
Third-trimester fetal foot, showing five toes.

tional weeks. Some are seen only later in gestation (e.g., duodenal atresia). The more scans a patient undergoes, the greater the anomaly detection rate. Levi[76] reported that the average sensitivity of studies that included only scans performed once before 20 weeks was 45%. The sensitivity increased to 60% if the scanning was performed several times during the pregnancy.

The prevalence of specific malformations within a population can significantly affect the sensitivity of ultrasound screening. Studies that exclude certain anomalies because they are considered either minor or undetectable can dramatically alter the sensitivity compared with a calculation that includes all anomalies. A 1996 study found that the sensitivity of ultrasound for diagnosing both minor and major anomalies was only 8.7%; however, if only major anomalies detectable by ultrasound were included, the sensitivity rose to 75%.[77]

Finally, other factors may affect the reported fetal anomaly detection rates, such as a lack of autopsies (the "gold standard"), suboptimal neonatal evaluation at birth, and inadequate length of neonatal follow-up (some anomalies may not express themselves immediately after birth).[76]

The Routine Antenatal Diagnostic Imaging with Ultrasound (RADIUS) trial was the first randomized clinical trial of second-trimester ultrasound in the United States.[79] It compared pregnant patients who underwent routine scanning with those who had ultrasound when indicated. An additional scan was performed in the study group early in the third trimester. The goal of the trial was to determine the benefits, if any, of routine ultrasound among pregnant women at low risk. Although the identification rate of anomalies in this study was three times better with routine vs. indicated ultrasound (35% vs. 11%, respectively), the sensitivity of 17% for anomalies detected between 15 and 22 weeks was extremely low.

The findings of the trial underwent intense scrutiny. One potential source of bias was that practice-based patients were used, which may have created an inadvertent selection bias (vs. a community- or hospital-based population). Others criticized the relative simplicity of the scans performed. The investigators reported a relative detection rate of 2.7 (95% confidence interval, 1.3–5.8) for tertiary compared with nontertiary ultrasound units.[79] The detection rate of anomalous fetuses was 35% versus 13% in nontertiary centers. Sonographic screening did not significantly affect the management or outcome of pregnancies complicated by congenital malformations. This was to be expected because there was no standardized response to the sonographic findings. Diagnostic ultrasound is not a therapeutic instrument.

In 1998, Van Dorsten and associates[80] reported that the sensitivity of ultrasound for anomaly detection at a tertiary care center (in women at risk for anomalies) was 89.7%. Although the sensitivity was decreased (47.6%) in the lower-risk population (screening group), it was sufficient to ensure cost-effectiveness for the patients.[80] In 1999, the Eurofetus group reported the results of a study designed to evaluate the sensitivity of routine ultrasound screening for fetal malformations.[81] Nearly 200,000 pregnant women (the largest group among screening studies) were enrolled and evaluated in 60 hospital laboratories in 14 countries. The sensitivity rate was 64% (2363 of 3685), a rate much higher than that in the RADIUS study. However, the two trials may not be comparable. Women in the RADIUS trial were at very low risk because strict exclusion criteria were applied before patient recruitment occurred. Further, the criteria used to designate major fetal anomalies (gold standard) were very liberal. Both of these factors could have lowered sensitivity. In contrast, all women in the Eurofetus trial were studied, regardless of risk status, and only "truly" major abnormalities were considered as endpoints; this classification may have artificially raised the sensitivity of the ultrasound screening.

Women in the Helsinki trial underwent one screening examination in the second trimester; 40% of major fetal anomalies were detected, including most anomalies of the central nervous system or genitourinary system and cases with multiple anomalies. In this trial, screening was less effective in detecting cardiac and gastrointestinal tract anomalies.[82] This finding is logical because many bowel abnormalities are sonographically "silent." In addition, cardiac morphology changes in response to malformations and may not be seen when first imaged unless flow abnormalities are sought. In the 1991 Belgian Multicentric Study,[83] 154 of 381 structurally abnormal fetuses were correctly detected by ultrasound (sensitivity, 40%). The specificity, positive, and negative predictive values were 99.9%, 95%, and 98.6%, respectively.

We examined the efficacy of a complete sonographic survey (as described in this chapter) for the detection of fetal abnormalities and correlated the findings with perinatal autopsy results.[84] Of 88 abnormal autopsy findings, 85 fetuses had one or more abnormal structural sonographic findings, giving a sensitivity of 97% for anomalous fetuses. The low sensitivities reported in the past may be in great part the result of failure to look for specific abnormalities. There were 372 separate abnormalities found on autopsy. Antenatal sonography detected 75% and 18%, respectively, of the 299 major and 73 minor abnormalities. Thus, the sensitivity for minor abnormalities is poor, even when a complete sonographic survey is performed. In 65% of cases, there was either complete agreement or only minor differences between sonographic and autopsy findings.[84]

Because sensitivity for the antenatal sonographic detection of fetal anomalies is highly dependent on the clinical setting and the expertise of the sonographer, there is insufficient evidence to list a single estimate of the sensitivity of routine ultrasound as a screening tool for fetal anomalies. However, the specificity of a fetal anatomic survey exceeds 99% in many studies.[79,85–87] Therefore, in low-risk patients, ultrasound is helpful in excluding anomalies and detecting normal features, but may not be equally reliable in detecting anomalies. The sensitivity of screening programs may continue to improve because of technologic advances (e.g., three-dimensional sonography) and uniform and detailed training of practitioners.[76]

Antenatal detection of an anomalous fetus, especially one with a life-threatening defect, allows the delivery of these infants in a tertiary care center that can provide immediate and appropriate care, maximizing survival. Is this statement supported by evidence in the literature? In the 1994 RADIUS study,[79] screening did not affect the detection, management, or outcome of fetuses with anomalies. However, of the infants with life-threatening anomalies, 75% (21 of 28) survived in the routinely screened group compared with 52% (11 of 21) in the non-screened group.[79] The study may have been inadequately powered to address this specific question, and although many fetal medicine practitioners are convinced, additional studies are required.

Another important question is whether routine ultrasound improves overall perinatal morbidity and mortality rates. For example, routine sonography increases the accurate detection of multiple gestations, gestational age, and placental abnormalities. Table 8–5 summarizes three trials[74,78,88] that investigated the perinatal morbidity and mortality rates of pregnancies in which routine ultrasonography was performed. The perinatal mortality rates were similar in the routine sonography and control groups in both the RADIUS and Stockholm trials.[74,88] However, the perinatal mortality rate in the Helsinki trial was significantly lower in the routine ultrasound group (4.6 of 1000 vs. 9.0 of 1000). This difference was attributable mainly to improved early detection of major malformations, leading to pregnancy termination.[78] There were no differences in perinatal morbidity rates between the study and control groups in these three trials (see Table 8–5).[74,78,88] Although two trials had a similar distribution of birth weights between study groups,[74,78] the third trial had fewer births less than 2500 g in the routine ultrasound group.[88] The mean birth weight was also higher in the routine ultrasound group in women who smoked, and the authors speculate that this difference may be attributable to healthier maternal behaviors after these women saw their fetuses on ultrasound.[88] Although the authors of the RADIUS trial concluded that the adoption of sonographic screening in the United States would increase health care costs without improving perinatal outcome or providing measurable benefit from early detection of fetal anomalies, another study concluded that routine screening for anomalies improves perinatal outcome by leading to termination of pregnancy for certain anomalies and delivery at tertiary care centers for life-threatening malformations.[80] The prospective trials also showed that twin gestations are diagnosed earlier with routine sonography. In the Helsinki trial, 100% of twins were detected before 21 weeks in the routine ultrasound group, compared with 76% in the control group.[78] Further, the perinatal mortality rate was reduced (27.8 of 1000 vs. 65.8 of 1000).

A subgroup analysis was also performed in the RADIUS study for infants who were small for gestational age and neonates born at 42 weeks or later.[74] There was no improvement in overall outcome for these conditions when routine ultrasound was performed. The available evidence indicates that routine sonography will, at a minimum, reduce perinatal outcome in low-risk pregnancies by decreasing perinatal mortality rates because of induced abortions after the detection of fetal abnormalities.

Sonographic screening for anomalies may also provide value to both patients and physicians that is not quantifiable in terms of psychological reassurance, antepartum management, referral, genetic counseling, or preparation of families and health care providers. The benefits discussed earlier may outweigh the "risks" of ultrasound (e.g., false-positive diagnosis). Most patients will choose

TABLE 8–5

Three Trials Comparing Perinatal Morbidity and Mortality Rates in Patients Undergoing Routine Ultrasonography (vs. Control Groups)

TRIAL	PERINATAL MORBIDITY	PERINATAL MORTALITY	*P*	MEAN BIRTH WEIGHT AND NO. OF INFANTS WITH LOW BIRTH WEIGHT (<2500 G)	*P*
Ewigman et al., 1993[74] (RADIUS)	*Similar	Similar	NS	Similar birth weight	NS
Saari-Kemppainen et al., 1990[78] (Helsinki)	†Similar	‡Improved (4.6/1000 vs. 9.0/1000)	<0.05	Similar birth weight	NS
Waldenstrom et al., 1988[88] (Stockholm)	†Similar	Similar	NS	Fewer low-birth-weight infants (2.5% vs. 4%)	0.005
				Smokers: higher mean birth weight (3413 vs. 3354 g)	0.047
				Nonsmokers: higher mean birth weight	NS

*Moderate morbidity defined as neonatal sepsis, grade I or II intraventricular hemorrhage, or stay of >5 days in neonatal unit; severe morbidity defined as ventilation >48 hours or stay of >30 days in neonatal unit.
†Defined as admission to neonatal unit.
‡Attributable to early detection of malformations, leading to termination of anomalous fetuses.
NS, not significant.

anomaly screening if given a choice and counseled on the current diagnostic capability of sonography. Pregnant women usually do not perceive ultrasound as a "test," but rather as a tool to evaluate the fetus as a patient. We agree with this philosophy and argue that examination of the fetus as a patient should be a routine practice, as it is in all aspects of adult medicine.

The last issue to address is the cost–benefit analysis of routine second-trimester sonography. We performed a cost–benefit analysis based on the RADIUS trial, comparing routine second-trimester sonography in low-risk pregnant women with a policy of not offering screening. Routine second-trimester sonographic screening is associated with net benefits only if the sonogram is performed at a tertiary care center.[89] Another study showed that a one-stage second-trimester screening ultrasound was both cost-effective and associated with fewer perinatal deaths.[90] Finally, Van Dorsten[80] and colleagues assessed the cost-effectiveness of anomaly screening in their patient population and concluded that routine screening was cost-effective. There seems to be little doubt that the cost-effectiveness of routine sonographic screening for fetal anomalies rests not on the tool but on the caliber of the sonographer.

Sonographic Aneuploidy Markers and Genetic Sonography

The most common autosomal trisomy in liveborn infants is Down syndrome, or trisomy 21, which was first described by John Langdon Down in 1866. Autosomal trisomies are primarily the result of meiotic nondisjunction, the risk of which increases with maternal age. The first screening method for fetal trisomy 21 was introduced in the early 1970s and was based on maternal age. Amniocentesis was offered to women 35 years or older, based on the findings of an early study that stated that the risk of a procedure-related loss approximated the likelihood that a midtrimester fetus of a 35-year-old woman would have trisomy 21 (1 in 270). There has been a fundamental shift in birth trends over the last three decades, with more births occurring to women older than 35 years.[91] In 1974, women 35 to 49 years old accounted for 4.7% of live births compared with 12.6% in 1997.[91] As a result, the prevalence of fetal trisomy 21 during the second trimester has increased from 1 in 740 in 1974 to 1 in 504 in 1997. However, the fact remains that most infants with trisomy 21 are born to women younger than 35 years. Fetuses with aneuploidy account for 6% to 11% of stillbirths and neonatal deaths,[92] whereas chromosomal defects that are compatible with life, but associated with significant morbidity, occur in 0.65% of newborns.[93]

A large body of literature attests to the specific use of second-trimester genetic ultrasonography for antenatal detection of trisomy 21 by seeking aneuploidy markers. We offer genetic sonography as an option to all (and only) high risk patients (i.e., advanced maternal age at the time of delivery, abnormal serum marker screen results, or both). The information derived from this sonogram is used to generate an adjusted risk of Down syndrome to guide a woman's decision about genetic amniocentesis. When the findings on genetic sonogram are normal in high risk patients, the amniocentesis rate is only 3%.[94] The amniocentesis rate increases in direct proportion to the number of abnormal sonographic markers identified, with almost 100% of women selecting invasive testing when four or more markers are seen. Since the initiation of our genetic sonography service 10 years ago, 4951 women have avoided amniocentesis based on normal findings on genetic sonogram. If the fetal loss rate related directly to amniocentesis is between 1 in 100 and 1 in 300, then between 17 and 50 fetal lives were saved, attesting to the power of genetic sonography.

Screening based on maternal age identifies at most 47% of fetuses with trisomy 21, with a false-positive rate of 13% to 14% (a rate that has increased in recent years).[91] Based on advanced maternal age, 140 amniocentesis procedures are required to detect one fetus with trisomy 21,[95] implying that one healthy fetus will be lost for every two affected fetuses identified. Although the combination of maternal age and triple-screen results increases the detection rate to 60% to 65%,[65] 60 to 70 amniocentesis procedures are required to detect one fetus with trisomy 21.[95] Thus, one healthy fetus will be lost for every three to four fetuses in which trisomy 21 is detected. As a result, some challenged the practice of offering invasive testing to all high risk pregnant women (based on age or triple-screen results).[65] Reducing the screen-positive rate is beneficial, regardless of an individual's personal opinion on testing. Genetic sonography reduces the invasive testing rate by refining the selection of candidates for invasive testing without significantly decreasing detection rates.

Ideally, genetic sonography is performed between 18 and 20 weeks. It is a targeted examination for fetal aneuploidy (predominantly, trisomy 21) during which the sonographer searches for abnormal fetal biometry, fetal structural anomalies, and other markers of aneuploidy.[94] Because only 25% of fetuses with trisomy 21 have a sonographically detectable major anomaly in the second trimester,[95] the examination must include other markers to increase sensitivity (Table 8–6). Markers of aneuploidy that are detectable on ultrasound include shortened long bones, increased nuchal fold thickness (Fig. 8–23), pyelectasis (Fig. 8–24), choroid plexus cysts (see Fig. 8–9), short ear length, wide iliac wing angle, hyperechoic bowel, echogenic intracardiac focus (see Fig. 8–18), sandal gap toes (Fig. 8–25), hypoplastic midphalanx of the fifth digit, clinodactyly, and absent nasal bone (see Fig. 8–13). The risk of fetal trisomy 21 increases with the number of markers present. Each marker alone has low to moderate sensitivity for trisomy 21 and does not necessarily increase the risk of

TABLE 8–6

Aneuploidy Markers of the Genetic Sonogram at Robert Wood Johnson Medical School

ANEUPLOIDY MARKER
Structural anomalies, including cardiac (four-chamber and outflow tracts)
Short femur (observed to expected <10th percentile)
Short humerus (observed to expected <10th percentile)
Pyelectasis (anteroposterior diameter of renal pelvis ≥ 4 mm)
Nuchal fold thickening (≥ 6 mm)
Echogenic bowel (similar to echogenicity of iliac bones)
Choroid plexus cysts (>10 mm)
Hypoplastic middle phalanx of the fifth digit
Wide space between the first and second toes (sandal gap)
Two-vessel umbilical cord
Echogenic intracardiac focus, short tibia, short fibula, short ear (since October 1997)
Absent nasal bone (since 2003)

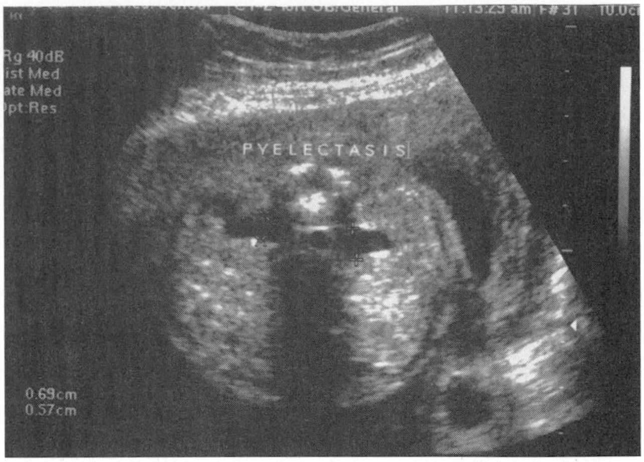

FIGURE 8–24
Bilateral pyelectasis in a second-trimester fetus.

aneuploidy when found in isolation in low risk patients. However, the risk of fetal aneuploidy may increase when multiple sonographic abnormalities or markers are detected in low-risk patients or when isolated markers are seen in high-risk patients.

A thickened nuchal fold (sensitivity, 40%; false-positive rate, 0.1%)[96] is the single most sensitive and specific marker for Down syndrome, although absent nasal bone has also been shown to have 41% sensitivity and 100% specificity for fetal trisomy 21.[97] A short femur length (measurement-to-expected length ≤ 0.91) is found in 24%,[98] and a short humerus (measurement-to-expected length < 0.90) in 50% of affected fetuses, with a false-positive rate of 6.25%.[99] There is a large overlap in bone measurements between affected and normal fetuses. The sensitivity of pyelectasis (anteroposterior diameter of the renal pelvis ≥ 4 mm in the second trimester) for trisomy 21 is 25%.[99] Echogenic bowel has a reported sensitivity of 7% to 12.5%, whereas an echogenic intracardiac focus (see Fig. 8–18) has a reported sensitivity of 18%.[99] We examined the sensitivity of a short sonographic ear length for trisomy 21.[100] Forty-one percent (21 of 51) had an ear length at or below the 10th percentile. However, a short ear length was not as sensitive a marker for trisomy 21 as it was for trisomy 13 (100%) or trisomy 18 (96%). The association between trisomy 21 and choroid plexus cyst is controversial.

Several studies reported the accuracy of genetic sonography in detecting trisomy 21 in high risk populations.[94] When "abnormal" is defined as the finding of at least one marker on ultrasound, the overall sensitivity was 77% (range, 50%–93%) and the false-postive rate was 13% (range, 7%–17%).[94] In 1998, an 11-center collaborative study examined the sensitivity of sonography for the detection of trisomy 21.[101] Eighty-five percent of fetuses with trisomy 21 (n = 241) had at least one abnormal finding on ultrasound. In 2003, an eight-center study evaluated the utility of second-trimester genetic sonography in

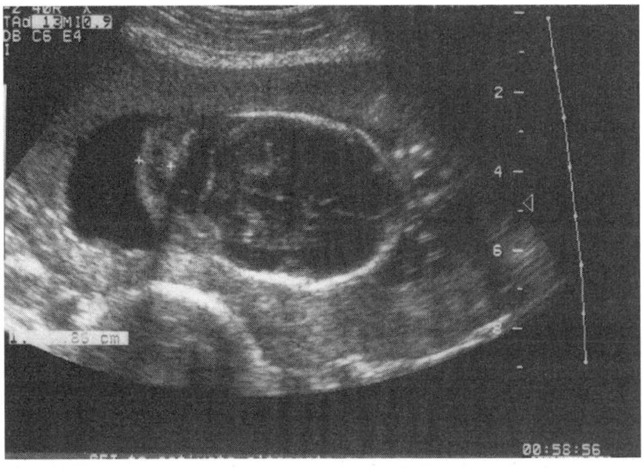

FIGURE 8–23
Thickened nuchal fold (0.86 cm) in a fetus with Down syndrome.

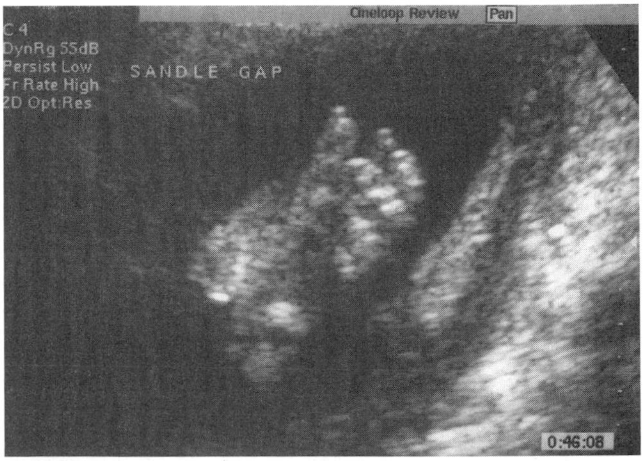

FIGURE 8–25
Sandal gap (wide space between the first and second toes) in a fetus with Down syndrome.

high risk women, including 176 fetuses with trisomy 21.[102] The sensitivity for the detection of trisomy 21 was 72% (center range, 64%–80%). Approximately half (47%) of the fetuses with trisomy 21 had a thickened nuchal fold of 5 mm or more.

In 1996, we published findings on the use of second-trimester genetic sonography to guide clinical management in women at high risk for pregnancy affected by trisomy 21.[103] After analyzing the data through 1999, we began to counsel women that the likelihood of trisomy 21 in the absence of abnormalities or markers was reduced by at least 80% from the a priori risk (triple-screen results or, if unavailable, maternal age).[94] Our experience was reassuring. Since November 1992, we evaluated 5299 fetuses with genetic sonography. The findings were normal in 85% (no markers seen); 12% had one marker, and 3% had two or more markers. When at least one marker was present, the sensitivity, specificity, and positive and negative predictive values for trisomy 21 were 87% (52 of 60), 91% (4395 of 4831), 11% (52 of 488), and 99.8% (4395 of 4403), respectively. Approximately two thirds of fetuses with trisomy 21 had two or more abnormal sonographic markers.

Over the years, we found that more and more high-risk women prefer genetic sonography as their first option rather than amniocentesis (Table 8–7). Since 1998, more than 70% of women chose to begin with genetic sonography. Accordingly, the number of amniocenteses performed has decreased. The total amniocentesis rate (the sum of amniocentesis procedures as the first option plus amniocentesis procedures performed after genetic sonography) decreased from 99.6% in 1993 to 32% in 2002. Recently, we examined the accuracy of genetic sonography for the detection of fetal trisomy 21 according to the indication for testing (advanced maternal age, abnormal triple-screen results, abnormal triple-screen results in women younger than 35 years, and abnormal triple-screen results in women 35 years and older). We also examined the risk of trisomy 21 after normal findings on genetic sonography.[104] The magnitude of the risk adjustment after normal findings on genetic scan is independent of the testing indication, and there are no significant indication-specific variations in the accuracy of genetic sonography.

Although some advocate second-trimester genetic sonography for screening of the general population, we believe that it should be reserved for the high-risk population. First, a high degree of expertise is required to exclude sonographic fetal malformations (especially subtle cardiac defects), and this expertise is not widely available in many countries. Second, the application of genetic sonography to low risk women may be inappropriate and perhaps dangerous, in light of the high screen false-positive rate (12%–15% in the high risk population), which is likely even higher in a low risk population. In low risk women, the a priori risk of trisomy 21 may be so low that the presence of one aneuploidy marker (e.g., pyelectasis) would not elevate the risk enough to justify amniocentesis. Therefore, with this approach, the positive predictive value and perhaps even the sensitivity of genetic ultrasound for fetal trisomy 21 are likely to be decreased in low risk patients. Third, the accuracy of second-trimester aneuploidy markers has been studied mainly in high risk populations. Extrapolation of such accuracy to low risk women may not be appropriate. Some concluded that an isolated marker (other than increased nuchal fold thickness or structural anomalies) should not be used as an indication for amniocentesis testing in the low risk population.[94] Others argue that if it is applied to the low risk population, any risk adjustment must reflect both the a priori risk of trisomy 21 and the sensitivity of the specific marker identified.

Figure 8–26 shows the algorithm we apply to both high and low risk patients. Clinicians should not recommend amniocentesis to low risk patients who have an isolated marker identified because the sensitivity is low (with the possible exception of increased nuchal fold thickness).[105] The incidental finding of an organ or structural anomaly (with few exceptions), nuchal thickening, or two or more aneuploidy markers in a low risk patient should trigger counseling and informed consent with the patient. The patient should be informed that if the accuracy of genetic ultrasound is extrapolated from high risk to low risk women, then the risk of trisomy 21 is likely high enough to justify offering genetic amniocentesis. In these patients, the risk of trisomy 21 is higher than the risk of amniocentesis-related fetal loss, regardless of maternal age or triple-screen results (unless the a priori risk is less than 1 in 10,000). Certain isolated sonographic fetal abnormalities (e.g., gastroschisis) are

TABLE 8–7

Annual Utilization Rates of Genetic Sonography for Detection of Fetal Trisomy 21 at Robert Wood Johnson Medical School

YEAR	CANDIDATES FOR PRENATAL DIAGNOSIS*	GENETIC ULTRASOUND *N* (%)	TOTAL NO. OF AMNIOCENTESES† *N* (%)
1993‡	477	2 (0.4%)	475 (99.6%)
1994	495	82 (17%)	423 (85%)
1995	523	251 (48%)	292 (56%)
1996	594	328 (55%)	279 (47%)
1997	793	510 (64%)	315 (40%)
1998	856	662 (77%)	215 (25%)
1999	1285	956 (74%)	405 (31%)
2000	1537	1114 (73%)	468 (30%)
2001	1497	1062 (71%)	488 (32%)
2002	1526	1110 (73%)	493 (32%)

*Includes advanced maternal age (≥35 years) with or without abnormal serum biochemistry results, abnormal serum biochemistry results in women younger than 35 years, or family history of chromosome abnormality.
†Includes women who underwent genetic amniocentesis only as their first option and women who underwent amniocentesis after genetic sonography.
‡The genetic sonogram service was available for only 2 months in 1993 (November and December).

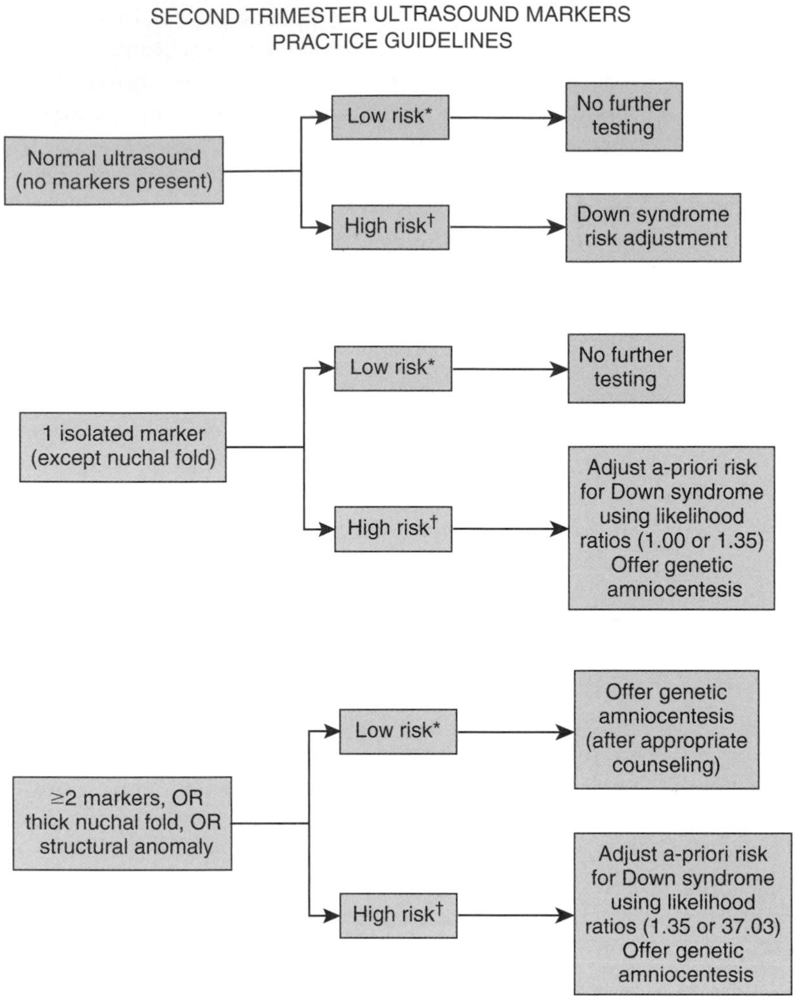

FIGURE 8–26
Algorithm for clinical management based on the results of second-trimester ultrasound (presence or absence of ultrasound markers). *Maternal age younger than 35 years, serum screen result less than 1:274, or both. †Maternal age 35 years and older, serum screen result 1:274 and greater, or both. (Modified from Yeo L, Vintzileos AM: The use of genetic sonography to reduce the need for amniocentesis in women at high-risk for Down syndrome. Semin Perinatol 2003;27:158.)

not usually associated with aneuploidy and do not require further invasive testing.

In high risk patients, we use genetic sonography as an adjunct to maternal age and serum screening (triple or quadruple, whichever is available) to adjust the risk of fetal trisomy 21 for each patient, based on our accuracy (see Table 8–8). The a priori risk is based on serum screening results. If serum screening results are not available or if testing was not performed, the risk is based on maternal age. We then multiply the a priori risk with var-

TABLE 8–8

Ultrasound-adjusted Risk for Fetal Down Syndrome (Maximum Risk 1:2) in Genetic Sonography and Clinical Examples

ULTRASOUND FINDINGS	LIKELIHOOD RATIO	CLINICAL EXAMPLES
Normal scan	0.20	35-year-old woman with no serum screen done 2VC seen 1:274 ÷ 1.00 = 1:274
One marker structural anomalies, including cardiac, short femur length, short humerus length, pyelectasis, nuchal fold thickening, echogenic bowel, HELV, short tibia length, short fibula, short ear length, absent nasal bone	1.35	44-year-old woman with triple-screen risk 1:798 Only pyelectasis seen 1:798 ÷ 1.35 = 1:591 22-year-old woman with quadruple-screen risk 1:200 Increased nuchal fold seen 1:200 ÷ 1.35 = 1:148
One marker choroid plexus cyst >10 mm, hypoplastic middle phalanx of the fifth digit, sandal gap, 2VC	1.00	38-year-old woman with triple-screen risk 1:5000 No markers seen 1:5000 ÷ 0.20 = 1:25,000 16-year-old girl with quadruple-screen risk 1:240 Sandal gap and HELV seen 1:240 ÷ 37.03 = 1:6
Any two or more markers	37.03	

HELV, hyperechoic focus in the left ventricle; 2VC, two-vessel cord.

ious likelihood ratios (LR), depending on the presence or absence of aneuploidy markers. For example, if the a priori risk of fetal trisomy 21 is 1 in 274 and the results of genetic scanning are normal, the adjusted risk of fetal trisomy 21 is (1 in 274 × 0.20), or 1 in 1370, a reduction of at least 80%. The revised risk is discussed with the patient. The patient should be told that the genetic scan can never reduce her risk to 0%. In our experience, the presence of only one of the following markers increases the risk of trisomy 21 by 1.35-fold: structural anomalies, including cardiac; short femur length; short humerus length; pyelectasis; nuchal fold thickening; echogenic bowel; hyperechoic focus in the left ventricle; short tibia length; short fibula length; short ear length; and absent nasal bone. Thus, the adjusted risk of fetal trisomy 21 is (1 in 274 ÷ 1.35), or 1 in 203, which is "abnormal." In our experience, this group of markers in isolation (choroid plexus cyst greater than 10 mm, a hypoplastic middle phalanx of the fifth digit, a sandal gap toe, or a two-vessel cord) is not associated with an increased risk of trisomy 21. Thus, the risk of fetal trisomy 21 remains the same (1 in 274). Once two or more markers are visualized, the a priori risk (in this case, 1 in 274) is modified by an LR of 37.03, and the adjusted risk becomes 1 in 7 (1 in 274 ÷ 37.03). The maximum adjusted risk for Down syndrome reaches 1:2. Other clinical examples are shown in Table 8–9. An adjusted risk of trisomy 21, based on the genetic sonogram, is given, even for high risk patients. For example, based on age alone, a 44-year-old patient is at high risk for fetal trisomy 21. However, if triple-screen results are 1 in 798 (a priori risk) and the findings on genetic sonogram are normal, the adjusted risk for trisomy 21 is 1 in 3990. If the same patient has one marker, the adjusted risk for Down syndrome is 1 in 591 (LR, 1.35) or remains the same at 1 in 798 (LR, 1.00), depending on the marker found.

Although it would intuitively seem that certain markers (e.g., nuchal fold thickening, cardiac defects) in isolation are very "strong" and would increase the risk for trisomy 21 (above an LR of 1.35), we have found these markers most frequently in combination with other markers. Therefore, for any marker in isolation (except the four described above, where the LR is 1.00), we use an LR of 1.35. Either a triple or a quadruple screen risk is acceptable as an a priori risk because most of our findings are based on high risk patients who underwent serum testing.

We and other investigators believe that risk adjustment for trisomy 21 is institution-specific and that the published experience from one center does not necessarily apply to another.[106] Each center performing genetic sonography must monitor their sensitivity for the detection of trisomy 21 to provide patients accurate, detailed, and updated counseling about their degree of risk reduction when scan findings are normal. Considering the range of expertise available in many countries, it is reasonable to suggest limiting genetic sonography to specialized centers.[64]

We analyzed the cost of universal amniocentesis and genetic sonography and concluded that genetic sonography was cost-effective when the sensitivity for the detection of trisomy 21 was greater than 74%.[107] We observed that genetic sonography saved the health care system 9% and reduced the loss rate of normal fetuses as a result of amniocentesis by 87%.[107] Genetic sonography is also cost-effective in women younger than 35 years who are at moderate risk for Down syndrome based on their triple-screen results as well as in patients with advanced maternal age who decline amniocentesis after second-trimester genetic counseling.[108] Offering genetic sonography to these patients is associated with cost savings for most acceptable genetic ultrasound accuracies. Finally, a recent study indicated that the combination of second-trimester genetic sonography with traditional serum markers may further improve diagnostic accuracy.[109] Various integrated algorithms combining serum analytes and sonographic markers have been reported (e.g., nuchal thickness, humerus length, serum α-fetoprotein, hCG) but have not been validated prospectively.

Nasal Bone

Nasal hypoplasia is part of the trisomy 21 phenotype. Cicero and associates[110] reported in 2001 that the nasal bone was sonographically absent in 73% of first-trimester fetuses with trisomy 21, with a false-positive rate of 0.5%. Shortly after that, Sonek and Nicolaides[111] reported a small series of second-trimester scans and noted that two of the three fetuses with trisomy 21 had a sonographically absent nasal bone; the third had a nasal bone length of less than 2.5% for gestational age.

Several studies (Table 8–9) examined the sensitivities and screen false-positive rates for trisomy 21 of a sonographically absent or short fetal nasal bone during the first or second trimester.[97,110–118] First-trimester sensitivity ranged from 60% to 73% (false-positive rate, 0.25%–0.6%), whereas second-trimester sensitivity ranged from 37% to 66% (false-positive rate, 0%–20%).

A recent study suggested that obtaining a fetal profile in the first trimester for the presence or absence of the nasal bone can improve the sensitivity for fetal trisomy 21 to greater than 95% (with a 5% false-positive rate) when combined with maternal age, NT, and the results of first-trimester biochemical serum screening (see Table 8–1).[114] We studied the usefulness of the finding of a sonographically absent nasal bone in a matched case–control study of 40 second-trimester fetuses with trisomy 21.[97] The facial profile was adequate in 29 (72.5%). Of these, 12 had an absent nasal bone, yielding a sensitivity of 41% and a specificity of 100%. Importantly, when absent nasal bone was added to the other sonographic markers of aneuploidy, the sensitivity of genetic sonography increased from 83% (24 of 29) to 90% (26 of 29).[97] Absence of the nasal bone was noted in two fetuses with trisomy 21 with no other ultrasound

TABLE 8–9

Summary of Sensitivity and False-Positive Rates for Absent Fetal Nasal Bone on Sonogram in Detecting Down Syndrome in the First- and Second-Trimesters

AUTHOR AND YEAR	DOWN SYNDROME (*N*)	FIRST-TRIMESTER SENSITIVITY	FALSE-POSITIVE RATE (%)	SECOND-TRIMESTER SENSITIVITY	FALSE-POSITIVE RATE (%)
Cicero et al., 2001[110]	59	73%	0.5%		
Cicero et al., 2002[112]	79	68%	0.5%		
Otano et al., 2002[113]	5	60%	0.6%		
Cicero et al., 2003[114]	100	69%	0.25%		
Sonek and Nicolaides, 2002[111]	3			66%*	NA
Cicero et al., 2003[115]	34			62%†	1.2%
Lee et al., 2003[116]	20			40%–45%	10%–20%
Bromley et al., 2003[117]	16			37%	0.5%
Bunduki et al., 2003[118]	22			59%‡	5%
Vintzileos et al., 2003[97]	40			41%	0

*The third fetus had nasal bone length <2.5% for gestational age.
†Defined as absent nasal bone or nasal bone <2.5 mm.
‡Defined as less than the fifth percentile.
NA, not available.

markers for aneuploidy. Thus, we added this marker to the list of aneuploidy markers evaluated in a genetic scan.

Ossification of the nasal bone in fetuses affected with a trisomy may increase with advancing gestational age, explaining the lower sensitivity in the second trimester compared with the first trimester. Additional studies show absent nasal bone in first-trimester fetuses with trisomy 18 (50%–55%).[110,112] Lee and colleagues[116] reported at least 58 genetic syndromes that may be associated with a sonographically absent nasal bone.

THREE-DIMENSIONAL SONOGRAPHY

Three-dimensional ultrasound was first introduced in the late 1980s. Two-dimensional ultrasound acquires a single plane of image information with traditional transducers. Three-dimensional ultrasound acquires volume data with one of several techniques. The resulting data can be viewed as single or multiple planes, or in combination with a rendered image that conveys the information from the entire volume (the "classic" three-dimensional appearance).[119] The initial machines were somewhat slow, but display times decreased dramatically with the evolution of computer processors. The image quality is directly related to the image quality of the two-dimensional scan used to acquire volumes. In some cases, multiplanar imaging in a standard orientation allows the sonographer to be more confident of a finding compared with conventional two-dimensional imaging.

This technology has the potential to provide both the physician and the patient with more accurate and additional information about the fetus (e.g., extent or size of anomalies) than is possible with traditional two-dimensional sonography. Other advantages of three-dimensional sonography include rapid acquisition of volume data, use of new orientations and planes (not obtainable with two-dimensional scanning), maternal–fetal bonding, and improved comprehension of the fetal anatomy by the patient and family.[119] The study of fetal behavior is facilitated by the rapid acquisition of data, which can be up to 16 frames/sec.[119] Technical problems occur with three-dimensional ultrasound because these scans are at least semimanual (the operator must remain still) and thus are in part limited by the operator's skill. Three-dimensional images are easier to generate with computed tomography because the scanning system is automatic and provides sequential slices.

Three-dimensional imaging can be more useful than conventional two-dimensional scanning for the evaluation of fetal malformations. Merz and colleagues[120] studied 204 anomalous fetuses and found that compared with two-dimensional ultrasound, three-dimensional ultrasound was advantageous in 62%, equivalent in 36%, and disadvantageous in 2%. In a similar study of 63 fetuses with 103 anomalies, three-dimensional sonography was advantageous in 51%, equivalent in 45%, and disadvantageous in 4%.[121] Several anomalies, such as cleft lip and abnormal facies, were seen only with three-dimensional ultrasound. Most anomalies were better visualized with three-dimensional than with two-dimensional imaging.[120,121] Although patient management was altered in only 5% of patients, the improved visualization derived from multiplanar and rendered images can help the physician and family to understand the anomalies.

First Trimester (See also Chapter 7)

Three-dimensional sonography is an excellent tool in the first trimester, allowing extensive and detailed evaluation of the embryo or fetus. Volume data are acquired with transvaginal transducers, and the resulting image is manipulated to identify the desired structures. One group reported that more anatomic structures were identifiable with three-dimensional compared with two-dimensional imaging.[122] As a result, the anatomic survey was more complete, and the detection of anomalies was improved. Obtainable images include the stomach, bladder, umbilical cord insertion, NT, and limbs. Some investigators believe that three-dimensional ultrasonography will allow even greater accuracy and reproducibility of NT compared with two-dimensional sonography.[123] One advantage of three-dimensional imaging is that the embryo can be rotated into a sagittal plane, regardless of the acquisition plane, theoretically allowing NT to be measured in all cases. Hull and associates[122] observed that the actual scanning time for the patient was significantly less with three-dimensional ultrasound (2.7 minutes vs. 14.7 minutes).

Blaas and colleagues[124] studied the brain cavities of human embryos with three-dimensional ultrasound. Visualization was possible as early as 7 weeks. The brain cavities grow and develop with time, and their volumes can be measured accurately with three-dimensional ultrasound. Because the planes examined from transvaginal acquisitions cannot be acquired with two-dimensional ultrasound, the detection of congenital abnormalities should be improved. The detection of conjoined twins and ectopia cordis is reported with three-dimensional sonography.[119] In addition, the volume of the gestational sac can be measured in the first trimester; this measurement is more predictive of a successful pregnancy outcome than maternal hormone levels.[125]

Second- and Third-Trimesters

Three-dimensional imaging is useful in the second and third trimesters to image anomalies of the skull, brain, face, heart, spine, limbs, urinary tract, umbilical cord, and placenta.[119] Other applications being studied include evaluations of the placenta, umbilical cord, cervix, fetal weight, and uterine anomalies (e.g., bicornuate, septate).

One of the most valuable features of three-dimensional sonography is the ability to rotate the face so that it can be viewed directly and in an upright position. Surface-rendered displays are obtained successfully in 70% of patients.[119] Several studies noted that three-dimensional imaging is beneficial for the detection of facial anomalies, such as cleft lip or palate, midface hypoplasia, asymmetric facies, micrognathia, facial masses, hypotelorism or hypertelorism, facial dysmorphia (sloping forehead, flat facies, flat nose), holoprosencephaly, and deformed ears.[119] Three-dimensional imaging is particularly valuable in examining the face for cleft lip or palate, especially the primary, or hard, palate. Some anomalies that were detected on three-dimensional ultrasound were missed on two-dimensional ultrasound. These include cleft lip or palate, micrognathia, flat facies, unilateral orbital hypoplasia, and cranial ossification defect.[119] In one series, two-dimensional ultrasound identified only 45% of fetuses with cleft palate, whereas three-dimensional imaging identified 86%.[126] Artifacts produced from three-dimensional volumes can imitate "clefting" of lips that are actually normal. These artifacts include shadowing from the umbilical cord adjacent to the face, motion during image acquisition, nasal bone shadowing, and identifying a nostril as a cleft.[119]

It is almost always possible to obtain a fetal profile. In addition, rotation of the volume allows consistent and accurate depiction of the midsagittal plane. Three-dimensional imaging of the face may be difficult early in gestation, if there is oligohydramnios, if limbs obscure the face, and when the face is very close to the uterine wall or placenta.[119]

Three-dimensional imaging is valuable in examining fetal skull defects, intracranial pathology and symmetry, and abnormal sutures or fontanelles of the skull. A new view has been suggested ("three-horn view") to examine the lateral ventricles, in which the anterior, inferior, and posterior horns are visualized together.[127] Fluid in the inferior horn is abnormal and is an early sign of ventriculomegaly. By placing the "marker dot" in the volume, the sonographer can "navigate" through ventricles, parenchyma, and cystic structures, and along vascular structures.[119] This knowledge can be important for consulting pediatric neurologists and neurosurgeons. The fetal spine is often imaged more clearly with three-dimensional sonography. Image quality is improved with rendering techniques that optimize the appearance of bone for the diagnosis of scoliosis, hemivertebrae, and neural tube defects. Studies suggest that three-dimensional evaluation of neural tube defects allows more accurate identification of the level, because the transverse and coronal images are viewed simultaneously with the rendered image.[128]

Three-dimensional sonography of the heart is difficult because of its rapid motion. Most current three-dimensional machines acquire only static, nongated volume images.[119] Cardiac abnormalities have been missed or misidentified with nongated acquisitions.[120] However, the great vessels can often be seen well. Cardiac gating is usually necessary to obtain an adequate cardiac image.[119] With gated volume data, the reviewer can slow the heart and evaluate its anatomy from various orientations in multiple planes throughout the cardiac cycle.[119] Sklansky and colleagues[129] found that fetal cardiac anatomy was more consistently shown and less dependent on the orientation (compared with two-dimensional ultrasound) of the volume acquisition when using gated data. Volume-rendered images of the ventricles, atria, great vessels, and valves were useful to assess the anatomy. In the future, volume measurements of the chambers may be helpful to evaluate cardiac function.

Abnormalities of the fetal abdomen and pelvis (and in some cases, their volume) can be imaged with three-dimensional ultrasonography (e.g., gastroschisis, omphalocele, bowel obstruction, hydronephrosis, multicystic dysplastic kidney). However, it is not clear whether additional information is obtained compared with two-dimensional sonography. Abnormalities of the genitalia may also be assessed with three-dimensional imaging.

The fetal extremities can usually be imaged with three-dimensional sonography because of the rapid acquisition. If the limb moves during an acquisition, the volume should be discarded and another one acquired. With conventional two-dimensional ultrasound, motion often obscures limb anatomy or makes assessment difficult. However, once a three-dimensional volume is obtained, the structure can be studied carefully without motion, and the limb can be "rotated" to various orientations for full evaluation. Rendered images can be used to evaluate surface and bony features and the number and position of digits. In evaluating the lower extremities for clubfeet, it is often difficult to determine whether this is a "transient" (false-positive) or "fixed" (true-positive) event. Three-dimensional imaging may help in some cases.

Three-dimensional ultrasound offers several advantages over conventional two-dimensional imaging in fetuses with skeletal dysplasia. Abnormal bone shapes, shortened ribs, and abnormal facies are more accurately identified with volume acquisition.[119] One author reported that three-dimensional ultrasound allowed identification of abnormalities that were not seen on two-dimensional ultrasound in 43% of fetuses (3 of 7) with skeletal dysplasias.[130] Specific bones may be imaged with three-dimensional sonography to narrow the normally wide differential diagnosis of skeletal dysplasias (see Chapter 21).

Three-dimensional sonography has been used to estimate fetal weight. Fetal weight has been estimated with volume data of the abdomen and extremities because it is impossible to obtain an entire fetal volume.[119] Preliminary studies suggest that three-dimensional ultrasound may be more accurate than two-dimensional ultrasound.[131] Fetal liver and lung volumes are also reported.[132,133] Chang and associates[132] found that two-dimensional ultrasound underestimated fetal liver volume.

Another area under investigation is the maternal cervix. Cervical funneling can be imaged with three-dimensional sonography, along with the entire cerclage, if present. Vascular structures and their distribution and extent (e.g., umbilical cord, vasa previa, placenta accreta, velamentous insertions, aneurysm of the vein of Galen) can be evaluated with three-dimensional ultrasound.[119] However, image acquisition may be difficult and time-consuming because of motion, flash artifacts, and the longer time needed to acquire volume with color and power Doppler techniques. Interventional procedures are also being performed with three-dimensional imaging, including oocyte aspiration, embryo transfer, treatment of ectopic pregnancy, and laser surgery.[119]

Perhaps one of the greatest advantages of three-dimensional sonography is improved bonding with the fetus. Among patients who undergo three-dimensional sonography for reassurance, women with a history of fetal or neonatal demise, those with a history of a fetus with congenital anomalies, those carrying fetuses with lethal anomalies, those treated for infertility, and couples who have a surrogate carry their pregnancy seemed to derive the most benefit.[119]

In summary, the world is three-dimensional, and three-dimensional ultrasonography provides anatomic images that are more easily understood by both physicians and patients. It offers women and their care team an improved understanding of the anomalies found on two-dimensional ultrasound, clarifies the extent of the anomaly, and provides visual confirmation of the reality of the abnormality. It also facilitates bonding with the fetus.

SCREENING FOR TRISOMY 18 AND OTHER ANEUPLOIDIES

Trisomy 18 is the second most common autosomal trisomy and has a uniformly poor prognosis. In the multicenter NT trial conducted by the Fetal Medicine Foundation, 325 first-trimester pregnancies were complicated by chromosomal abnormalities other than trisomy 21.[26] Fetal NT was greater than the 95th percentile for crown–rump length in 71%. In addition to increased NT, sonographic findings showed abnormality in many of these fetuses. Trisomy 18 was associated with early-onset intrauterine growth restriction, relative bradycardia, and in 30%, exomphalos.[36] Trisomy 13 was characterized by fetal tachycardia in 66% and by holoprosencephaly or exomphalos in 30%.[36] Approximately 40% of triploid fetuses show early-onset, asymmetrical intrauterine growth restriction, relative bradycardia, holoprosencephaly, exomphalos, or a posterior fossa cyst. Molar placental changes are seen in approximately one third.[36]

First-trimester serum biochemistry results may be abnormal in fetuses with aneuploidies other than trisomy 21.[36] In trisomies 13 and 18, serum free βhCG and PAPP-A levels are decreased. In sex chromosomal abnormalities, the maternal serum free βhCG level is normal, but the PAPP-A level is low. These analytes may also be abnormal in fetal triploidies, depending on the source of the third chromosome set. With paternal origin (diandric triploidy), a partial molar placenta is usually seen. The free βhCG level is greatly increased, and the PAPP-A level is mildly decreased. If the extra set is of maternal origin (digynic triploidy), the normal-appearing placenta is small; the fetus is severely, asymmetrically growth-restricted; and the free βhCG and PAPP-A levels are markedly decreased. Screening with a combination of fetal NT and serum free βhCG and PAPP-A allows identification of approximately 90% of these chromosomal abnormalities, with a screen-positive rate of 1%.[36]

Second-trimester serum triple-marker screening can identify 60% to 75% of fetuses with trisomy 18 when a separate analysis is performed that seeks low levels of all three analytes, with or without consideration of maternal age.[134,135]

Sonography has variable but high sensitivity for detecting trisomy 18 (64%–100%), particularly when the examination is part of a thorough anatomic survey.[73] In a recent study, we found that all fetuses with trisomy 18 had four or more sonographic anomalies (one fetus had 19 separate detectable anomalies). Short ear length was present in 96%, bilateral clenched or closed hands or overlapping digits in 95%, and central nervous abnormalities in 87%. In another study, we observed shortened ear length (at or below the 10th percentile) in 100% of fetuses with trisomy 13, 96% of fetuses with trisomy 18, 75% of those with Turner syndrome, and 91% of those with other various aneuploidies.[100] Many investigators confirmed that abnormal hands are seen in most fetuses with trisomy 18.[73] Other sonographic abnormalities that are common in trisomy 18 include growth restriction, abnormal feet, choroid plexus cysts, and structural cardiac defects. We found intrauterine growth restriction in 63% of fetuses with trisomy 18.[73] Early-onset growth restriction is common in trisomy 13 and triploidy. In particular, triploidy is associated with a characteristic small body relative to the head.

Choroid plexus cysts are visualized in 1% (range, 0.3%–3.6%) of normal fetuses in the second trimester (see Fig. 8–9). These cysts may be associated with trisomy 18,[136] and in the past, genetic amniocentesis was considered even if they were isolated. However, a cyst can be considered "isolated" only after a detailed fetal survey shows no other structural abnormalities or markers. In our study, half of the fetuses with trisomy 18 had a choroid plexus cyst, but they were always associated with multiple other sonographic abnormalities (i.e., never isolated).[73] In another study, none of 98 fetuses with an isolated choroid plexus cyst had aneuploidy, whereas 100% of the 13 fetuses with a choroid plexus cyst and major anatomic abnormalities had trisomy 18.[137] In our experience, the risk of aneuploidy is very low and does not justify amniocentesis if no other anomalies are found (especially if the hands are open and the ear length is normal). Many investigators concur that if the choroid plexus cyst is isolated and the patient is at low risk for fetal aneuploidy, the presence of these cysts should not affect management. Like genetic sonography for screening for fetal trisomy 21, normal findings on a complete anatomic survey in experienced hands should "decrease" a patient's risk of trisomy 18 (regardless of the presence of choroid plexus cysts or abnormal triple-screen results) to a low level sufficient to avoid genetic amniocentesis after appropriate patient counseling.[73]

CRITICAL REVIEW OF THE EVIDENCE ON FIRST- AND SECOND-TRIMESTER SCREENING FOR FETAL ABNORMALITY

Both physicians and patients often ask whether first-trimester screening is more effective than second-trimester screening. Studies show that 85% to 90% of cases of trisomy 21 can be detected (with a 5% screen false-positive rate) in the first trimester (11–14 weeks) with a combination of maternal age, NT thickness, and serum biochemical screening (PAPP-A and free βhCG). This level of sensitivity seems significantly higher than that of second-trimester biochemical screening plus maternal age, which has a 60% detection rate (with a 5% screen false-positive rate). However, it does not account for the increased in utero lethality of trisomy 21 between the first and second trimesters. More than 10% of fetuses with trisomy 21 that are alive at 11 to 13 weeks are lost spontaneously by 16 to 18 weeks.[4] In addition, fetuses with trisomy 21 and increased NT thickness are more likely to be lost spontaneously.[4] These facts raise an important issue. Although first-trimester screening has the definite advantage of early diagnosis, we believe that the intrauterine lethality requires higher sensitivity rates compared with second-trimester screening for equivalent efficiency.

There is no uniform population-based screening for trisomy 21 in the United States. There are even variations in the specific second-trimester serum markers used, depending on the laboratory. Although some centers use integrated first-trimester screening, others use second-trimester serum marker screening, and some couple serum screening with an ultrasound for sonographic markers to derive individual risks for fetal trisomy 21. Although new developments in both first- and second-trimester screening offer women a variety of options for trisomy 21 screening, they increase the complexity of choices. The addition of more screening tests (especially when additive or sequential) can increase false-positive rates, patient anxiety, invasive testing rates, and procedure-related pregnancy loss. However, if sequential tests are interpreted in light of the results of earlier tests, it may be possible to decrease the invasive testing rates while maintaining high sensitivity.[4] Another variable to consider is that if 80% to 90% of fetuses with trisomy 21 are detected by first-trimester screening, the predictive values of second-trimester screening (ultrasonography and biochemical screening) are dramatically reduced.[4] In theory, second-trimester biochemistry will probably identify at best only 6% (60% of the residual 10%) of affected pregnancies while doubling the overall invasive testing rate (from 5% to 10%).

There is also no uniformity in screening for fetal malformations. Table 8–10 lists several approaches that may be used clinically. Examples of approaches are: A and D or E, B and D or E, C only, D only, E only, and F only. We prefer A and B and then D or E. We follow the protocol shown in Figure 8–27 and use the Fetal Medicine Foundation software to calculate a first-trimester risk (using NT and maternal age) for all patients, while noting the absence or presence of nasal bone. We anticipate incorporating first-trimester biochemical testing into the calculated risks once we validate first-trimester risk adjustments clinically. Although very good data support the efficacy of NT screening, we do not use the first-trimester calculated risk as an a priori risk for genetic sonography for several reasons. First, not all examiners or centers performing NT screening do so accurately and with high quality. Second, there are no data on the accuracy of second-trimester genetic sonography when a priori risks are established by NT screening. Third, there are no data to suggest how to combine the findings of second-trimester sonographic markers and NT. Until there is clear evidence, we believe that it is premature to incorporate NT-generated risks as a priori risks in second-trimester genetic sonography.

How to use information obtained from first-trimester calculated risks when performing level II scans is also not clear. There is also a lack of data on the relationship between first- and second-trimester biochemistry results.[36] Therefore, regardless of the first-trimester risk adjustment (whether abnormal or normal), we recommend second-trimester serum screening because it offers additional benefits. For example, elevation of maternal serum α-fetoprotein and hCG can suggest placental disease, future development of intrauterine growth restriction, hypertension, or other abnormalities. A fetal anatomy survey or genetic sonogram is also performed, depending on maternal age and serum screening results (Table 8–10 and Fig. 8–28). Some patients may elect invasive testing (chorionic villus sampling or amniocentesis) as a first choice if they have advanced maternal age or abnormal serum screening results. In summary, although we recommend first-trimester risk calculation for all patients (and counsel accordingly at that time), we do not use these results to alter risk adjustment in the second trimester because of a lack of data.

The best method for patients is unclear. A reasonable approach might be to integrate all available markers into a single reported risk, with the goals of optimizing sensitivity and minimizing screen false-positive results. One group proposed an "integrated test," combining first-trimester NT and PAPP-A levels with the second-trimester quadruple serum screen.[138] Mathematical calculations were performed but not validated clinically. It was estimated that an 85% sensitivity rate for trisomy 21, with a very low 1% invasive testing rate, could be achieved with this approach.[138] For women 35 years and older, the predicted detection rate is 92%, with a screen false-positive rate of 3.3%. However, even if an integrated type of screening gains physician acceptance, its ultimate success will depend on patients' willingness to wait until 16 weeks to receive the combined results. Whether a patient chooses first-trimester screening or waits for an "integrated screen" will most likely vary, and the choice will depend on personal preferences, the types of invasive tests that are available, the risks that are present, the patient's plans for termination, and the patient's previous experiences. This concept may be more complex than it seems. A prospective multicenter trial funded by the National Institute of Health is being performed to address both first- and second-trimester screening (FASTER trial). The findings of this trial should shed important light on these questions and may affect the implementation of screening in the United States.

Two studies specifically examined the effect of first-trimester NT screening on second-trimester biochemical testing.[23,139] In the first study, the positive predictive value of second-trimester screening was initially 1 in 40. However, after the introduction of NT screening, when 83% of fetuses with trisomy 21 were identified in the first trimester, the positive predictive value of biochemical screening decreased to 1 in 200.[139] In the second study, first-trimester NT screening identified 71% of fetuses with trisomy 21, for a screen-positive rate of 2%. The

TABLE 8–10

Various Approaches Used Clinically in Screening for Fetal Malformations

APPROACH	DESCRIPTION	NOTES
A	First-trimester risk adjustment (nuchal translucency, biochemistry results, age), with or without nasal bone	Use FMF software (follow protocol in Fig. 8–27)
B	Second-trimester serum screening (triple or quadruple)	Quadruple screening has higher sensitivity
C	Invasive testing (chorionic villus sampling amnio) offered automatically to patients with advanced maternal age or abnormal serum screen results	Discuss risks and benefits of invasive testing Genetic sonogram not performed
D	Level II anatomy scan; offer amnio, depending on results	Not advanced maternal age or has normal serum screen results No calculated adjusted risk for aneuploidy given
E	Genetic sonogram (only high-risk patients); offer amnio if risk adjustment is abnormal	A priori risk: second-trimester serum screening (first) or maternal age Based on absence or presence of aneuploidy markers or structural anomalies on ultrasound, adjusted risk for Down syndrome given
F	No testing performed	
Ours	Both A and B, then D or E (based on age or results of second-trimester serum screening)	Although we incorporate both schemes (A and B), we do not use first-trimester risk as an a priori risk for genetic sonography If patients want only invasive testing, this is done

Amnio, amniocentesis; FMF, Fetal Medicine Foundation.

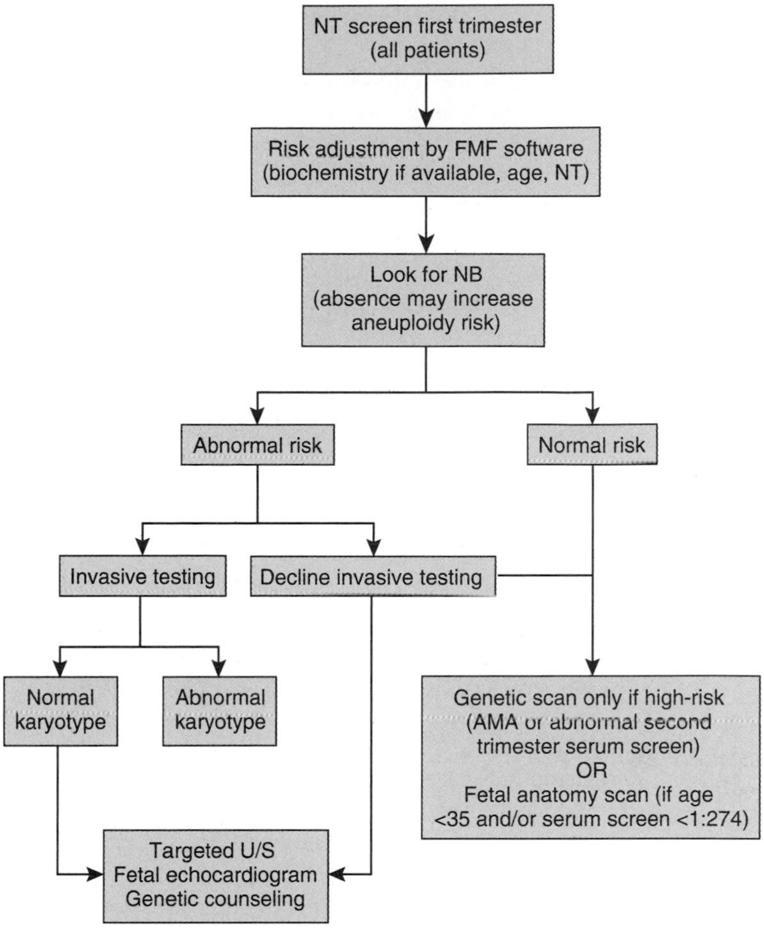

FIGURE 8–27
Algorithm for first-trimester screening used at our institution. AMA, advanced maternal age; FMF, Fetal Medicine Foundation; NB, nasal bone; NT, nuchal translucency; U/S ultrasound.

positive predictive value of second-trimester screening (via quadruple test) was only 1 in 150.[23] These studies suggest that the gain of an integrated approach may not offset the delay in results.

Several studies examined screening with a combination of fetal NT and serum biochemistry in the second trimester. Schuchter and colleagues[140] examined 9342 pregnancies and classified as screen-positive those with NT of 2.5 mm or greater as well as those with an estimated risk from biochemical testing of 1 in 250 or greater. The screen-positive rate was 7.2%, and the sensitivity for trisomy 21 was 95% (18 of 19 cases). Audibert and colleagues[141] examined 4130 pregnancies and classified as screen-positive those with NT of 3 mm or greater those with an estimated risk from biochemical testing of 1 in 250 or greater. The screen-positive rate was 5%, and the sensitivity for trisomy 21 was 90% (9 of 10 cases).

As previously discussed, there are no data on the interrelationship between second-trimester sonographic markers and NT or first- and second-trimester biochemistry findings.[36] It may be reasonable to assume that these factors are independent.[36] However, there may also be exceptions because the concept of sequential screening assumes independence between the findings of different screening results. For instance, the finding of nuchal edema or a cardiac defect during the second-trimester

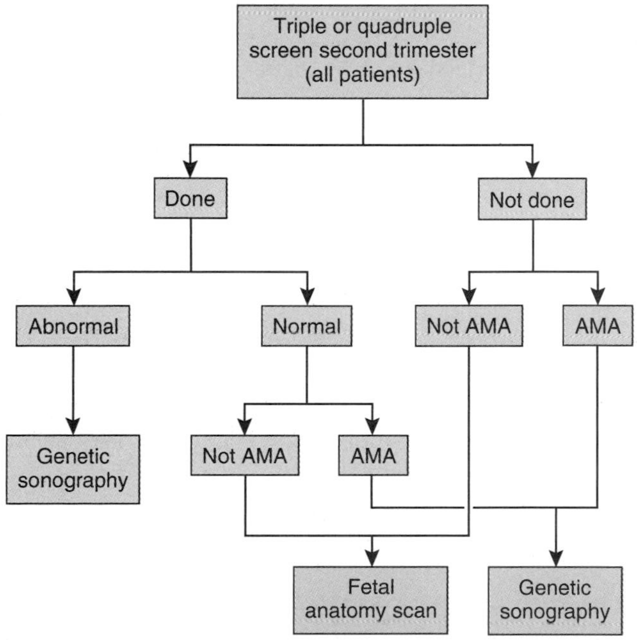

FIGURE 8–28
Algorithm for second-trimester screening used at our institution. AMA, advanced maternal age. Genetic sonography is used only in high-risk patients (advanced maternal age at the time of delivery, abnormal serum screen, or both). For genetic sonography, we use serum screening (first) or maternal age (if the results of serum screening are not available or if the test is not performed) as the basis for the a priori risk.

examination cannot be considered independent of NT measurement in the first trimester.[36]

Potential changes will likely involve using both first- and second-trimester screening in some form. As future studies are published, first-trimester risk assessment (age, biochemistry findings, NT, nasal bone) will likely gain increasing and prominent importance, and may even become the standard of care, because this screening is noninvasive and offers the clear advantages of high sensitivity (97%) and early detection of fetal Down syndrome. Thus, second-trimester serum screening may fall out of clinical favor, with first-trimester calculated risks becoming the a priori risk. However, this screening will never be abandoned because many patients seek prenatal care after the first trimester.

We anticipate that first-trimester calculated risks will eventually be incorporated into second-trimester ultrasonography. Ultrasonography in some form will probably never fall out of favor because it offers many distinct benefits, both clinically and psychologically, for patients and physicians alike. We anticipate that, with growing expertise, more genetic sonograms will be offered as a first choice to high risk patients and will become the standard of care in this group, with targeted fetal scans reserved for the low risk patient. Some patients may prefer first- or second-trimester screening, just as some may prefer chorionic villus sampling to second-trimester amniocentesis. High sensitivity is important for high risk women, whereas low false-positive rates are most desirable among low risk women.

CONCLUSIONS

GENERAL

- Prenatal Diagnosis and Screening for Fetal Abnormalities Performed for Various Reasons
  - To provide reassurance to patients (and obstetricians)
  - To provide information and knowledge to patients
  - To provide opportunities for prenatal invasive testing
  - To provide counseling about the prognosis and modify management
- Some patients specifically request screening for the purposes of pregnancy termination. Other patients may not choose this as an option but wish to be prepared ahead of time, with the ability to have counseling with pediatric surgeons, geneticists, and other specialists well before the actual delivery date.
- Information about specific abnormalities or aneuploidies can optimize management of the pregnancy as well as labor and delivery, including resuscitative measures.
- Knowledge of abnormalities or aneuploidy can affect future pregnancies and alter counseling about prognosis and genetics.
- In practice, patients have many screening options available to them in both the first and second trimesters.
- Each test has advantages and disadvantages as well as varied sensitivities in detecting fetal Down syndrome or other forms of aneuploidy.

FIRST-TRIMESTER BIOCHEMICAL SERUM SCREENING

- Combined with maternal age, the sensitivity and false-positive rates for trisomy 21 are 63% and 5.5%, respectively.
- The two most discriminatory analytes are βhCG and pregnancy-associated plasma protein A.
- The results may also be altered in other types of aneuploidy.

FIRST-TRIMESTER SONOGRAPHY

- Transvaginal scanning should be performed to improve and optimize image quality when transabdominal scanning is suboptimal.
- The sonographer must be familiar with normal anatomic structures to recognize abnormalities.
- Ductus venosus Doppler velocimetry can discriminate between chromosomally normal and abnormal fetuses.

NUCHAL TRANSLUCENCY SCREENING

- Testing is performed only between 11 weeks, 3 days and 13 weeks, 6 days
- Testing is associated with aneuploidy, congenital heart disease, congenital anomalies, and genetic syndromes.
- Sensitivity varies from 29% to 100%, with screen-positive rates of 0.4% to 8%.
- Strict criteria for performance must be followed, and sonographers should be trained appropriately.
- Normal nuchal translucency values depend on the crown–rump length.

SECOND-TRIMESTER SERUM SCREENING

- Accurate dating of the pregnancy is essential.
- Triple-screen sensitivity for Down syndrome in women younger than 35 years is 60%, with a 5% false-positive rate.
- Quadruple-screen sensitivity for Down syndrome in women younger than 35 years is 67% to 76%, with a 5% false-positive rate.

SECOND-TRIMESTER SONOGRAPHY

- The RADIUS trial had low sensitivity for the detection of fetal anomalies; routine ultrasound did not affect the detection, management, or outcome of fetuses with anomalies and did not improve perinatal outcome.
- Much has changed since the RADIUS trial.
- A complete, targeted, and thorough examination should be performed,
- Sensitivity for fetal abnormalities varies widely, depending on the center and other issues.
- Testing is cost-effective in centers with reasonable accuracy for detecting fetal abnormalities.
- Genetic sonography should be offered only to high-risk patients and has sensitivities ranging from 50% to 93% (overall, 77%), with a screen false-positive rate of 13%.
- More patients prefer genetic sonography as their first option compared with invasive testing.
- Absence or shortening of the nasal bone is a sensitive sonographic marker for trisomy 21 in the first and second trimesters.
- Three-dimensional sonography has many advantages in the first and second trimesters.

SUMMARY OF MANAGEMENT OPTIONS
First- and Second-Trimester Screening for Fetal Abnormality

Management Options	Quality of Evidence	Strength of Recommendation	References
General			
Prerequisites: • Details of the history, examination, and routine studies completed; known relevant risk factors identified • Prescan interview, discussions, and counseling	See Chapter 9	–	–
Discuss the screening options in the first and second trimesters and decide on an individual pregnancy management plan (e.g., serum testing, ultrasound, invasive testing)	–	GPP	–
First-Trimester Serum Screening			
Use analytes βhCG and pregnancy-associated plasma protein A	IIa	B	1,2
	IIb	B	
May combine with maternal age, nuchal translucency, nasal bone	IIa	B	114
Use for other types of aneuploidy	IIa	B	4
First-Trimester Sonography			
Improved by the transvaginal method	IV	C	5
Screen all patients with this test	–	GPP	–
Nuchal Translucency Screening			
Screen all patients with this test	–	GPP	–
Express measurements relative to gestational age or crown–rump length as a delta value or multiple of the median. Use multiple of the median and derived likelihood ratios to generate patient-specific risks	IIa	B	26

Continued

SUMMARY OF MANAGEMENT OPTIONS

First- and Second-Trimester Screening for Fetal Abnormality *(Continued)*

Management Options	Quality of Evidence	Strength of Recommendation	References
Nuchal Translucency Screening			
Offer karyotype testing if the results are abnormal; if the karyotype is normal, examine for structural defects (especially cardiac) and various syndromes	IIa IV	B C	4 11
Combine with nasal bone imaging	IIa	B	114
Use ductus venosus Doppler velocimetry to determine which nonaneuploid fetuses with increased nuchal translucency thickness are at risk for cardiac defects	III	B	44
Second-Trimester Serum Screening			
Use quadruple screen testing for greater sensitivity	IIa	B	66, 67
Combine with detailed sonography to screen for aneuploidy	III IIa	B B	94 104
Second-Trimester Sonography			
Perform a detailed survey to increase sensitivity, and screen all patients with this test	–	GPP	–
Genetic sonography should be offered only to high risk patients and performed by experienced laboratories	III	B	94
Use three-dimensional ultrasound to add more information to two-dimensional scanning, if available	IV III	C B	119 120,121
Authors' Practice			
For all patients, perform first-trimester screening (nuchal translucency, age) and look for nasal bone (biochemical screening in the future)	IIa	B	114
For all patients, perform second-trimester serum screening (quadruple preferred)	IIa	B	66,67
For all patients, perform level II or genetic sonography (both detailed examinations for aneuploidy markers and structural anomalies), depending on maternal age or serum screening results.	III IIa	B B	94 104
Invasive testing also discussed as an option, when applicable	–	GPP	–
Perform three-dimensional ultrasound, if necessary	IV III	C B	119 120,121

REFERENCES

1. Wald NJ, George L, Smith D, et al: Serum screening for Down's syndrome between 8 and 14 weeks of pregnancy: International Prenatal Screening Research Group. Br J Obstet Gynaecol 1996;103:407–412.
2. Haddow JE, Palomaki GE, Knight GJ, et al: Screening of maternal serum for fetal Down's syndrome in the first trimester. N Engl J Med 1998;338:955–961.
3. Canick JA, Kellner LH, Saller DN Jr, et al: Second-trimester levels of maternal urinary gonadotropin peptide in Down syndrome pregnancy. Prenat Diagn 1995;15:739–744.
4. Souter VL, Nyberg DA: Sonographic screening for fetal aneuploidy: First trimester. J Ultrasound Med 2001;20:775–790.
5. Monteagudo A, Timor-Tritsch IE: Malformation in the first fifteen weeks. In Nyberg DA, McGahan JP (eds): Diagnostic

Imaging of Fetal Anomalies. Philadelphia, Lippincott Williams & Wilkins, 2003, pp 815–844.
6. Timor-Tritsch IE, Warren WB, Peisner DB, Pirrone E: First-trimester midgut herniation: A high frequency sonographic study. Am J Obstet Gynecol 1989;161:831–833.
7. Bronshtein M, Rottem S, Yoffe N, Blumenfeld Z: First-trimester and early second-trimester diagnosis of nuchal cystic hygroma by transvaginal sonography: Diverse prognosis of the septated from the nonseptated lesion. Am J Obstet Gynecol 1988;161:78–82.
8. Benacerraf BR, Gelman R, Frigoletto FD: Sonographic identification of second trimester fetuses with Down's syndrome. N Engl J Med 1987;317:1371–1376.
9. Nicolaides KH, Azar G, Byrne D, et al: Fetal nuchal translucency: Ultrasound screening for chromosomal defects in first trimester of pregnancy. BMJ 1992;304:867–869.
10. Pandya PP, Kondylios A, Hilbert L, et al: Chromosomal defects and outcome in 1015 fetuses with increased nuchal translucency. Ultrasound Obstet Gynecol 1995;5:15–19.
11. American College of Obstetricians and Gynecologists: First-trimester screening for fetal anomalies with nuchal translucency. Genet Obstet Gynecol 2002:23–24.
12. Hyett J, Perdu M, Sharland G, et al: Using nuchal translucency to screen for major cardiac defects at 10–14 weeks of gestation: Population based cohort study. BMJ 1999;318:81–85.
13. Bohlandt S, von Kaisenberg CS, Wewetzer K, et al: Hyaluronan in the nuchal skin of chromosomally abnormal fetuses. Hum Reprod 2000;15:1155–1158.
14. Von Kaisenberg CS, Krenn V, Ludwig M, et al: Morphological classification of nuchal skin in human fetuses with trisomy 21, 18, and 13 at 12–18 weeks and in a trisomy 16 mouse. Anat Embryol (Berl) 1998;197:105–124.
15. Bewley S, Roberts LJ, MacKinson AM, Rodeck CH: First trimester fetal nuchal translucency: Problems with screening the general population. 2. Br J Obstet Gynaecol 1995;102:386–388.
16. Hafner E, Schuchter K, Philipp K: Screening for chromosomal abnormalities in an unselected population by nuchal translucency. Ultrasound Obstet Gynecol 1995;6:330–333.
17. Pandya PP, Goldberg H, Walton B, et al: The implementation of first-trimester scanning at 10–13 weeks gestation and the measurement of fetal nuchal translucency thickness in two maternity units. Ultrasound Obstet Gynecol 1995;5:20–25.
18. Szabo J, Gellen J, Szemere G: First-trimester ultrasound screening for fetal aneuploidies in women over 35 and under 35 years of age. Ultrasound Obstet Gynecol 1995;5:161–163.
19. Kornman LH, Morssink LP, Beekhuis JR, et al: Nuchal translucency cannot be used as a screening test for chromosomal abnormalities in the first trimester of pregnancy in a routine ultrasound practice. Prenat Diagn 1996;16:797–805.
20. Zimmermann R, Hucha A, Savoldelli G, et al: Serum parameters and nuchal translucency in first trimester screening for fetal chromosomal abnormalities. Br J Obstet Gynaecol 1996;103:1009–1014.
21. Taipale P, Hiilesmaa V, Salonen R, Ylostalo P: Increased nuchal translucency as a marker for fetal chromosomal defects. N Engl J Med 1997;337:1654–1658.
22. Biagiotti R, Periti E, Brizzi L, et al: Comparison between two methods of standardization for gestational age differences in fetal nuchal translucency measurement in first trimester screening for trisomy 21. Ultrasound Obstet Gynecol 1997;9:248–252.
23. Thilaganathan B, Slack A, Wathen NC: Effect of first-trimester nuchal translucency on second-trimester maternal serum biochemical screening for Down's syndrome. Ultrasound Obstet Gynecol 1997;10:261–264.
24. Theodoropoulos P, Lolis C, Papgeorgiou C, et al: Evaluation of first-trimester screening by fetal nuchal translucency and maternal age. Prenat Diagn 1998;18:133–137.
25. Hafner E, Schuchter K, Leibhart E, Philipp K: Results of routine fetal nuchal translucency measurement at weeks 10–13 in 4233 unselected pregnant women. Prenat Diagn 1998;18:29–34.
26. Snijders RJ, Noble P, Sebire N, et al: UK multicentre project on assessment of risk of trisomy 21 by maternal age and fetal nuchal translucency thickness at 10–14 weeks of gestation. Lancet 1998;352:343–346.
27. Pajkrt E, van Lith JM, Mol BW, et al: Screening for Down's syndrome by fetal nuchal translucency measurement in a general obstetric population. Ultrasound Obstet Gynecol 1998;12:163–169.
28. Economides DL, Whitlow BJ, Kadir R, et al: First trimester sonographic detection of chromosomal abnormalities in an unselected population. Br J Obstet Gynaecol 1998;105:58–62.
29. Schwarzler P, Carvalho JS, Senat MV, et al: Screening for fetal aneuploidy and fetal cardiac abnormalities by nuchal translucency thickness measurement at 10–14 weeks gestation as part of routine antenatal care in an unselected population. Br J Obstet Gynaecol 1999;106:1029–1034.
30. Gasiorek-Wiens A, Tercanli S, Kozlowski P, et al: Screening for trisomy 21 by fetal nuchal translucency and maternal age: A multicenter project in Germany, Austria and Switzerland. Ultrasound Obstet Gynecol 2001;18:645–648.
31. Brizot ML, Carvalho MHB, Liao AW, et al: First-trimester screening for chromosomal abnormalities by fetal nuchal translucency in a Brazilian population. Ultrasound Obstet Gynecol 2001;18:652–655.
32. Wayda K, Kereszturi A, Orvos H, et al: Four years experience of first-trimester nuchal translucency screening for fetal aneuploidies with increasing regional availability. Acta Obstet Gynecol Scand 2001;80:1104–1109.
33. Pajkrt E, de Graaf IM, Mol BW, et al: Weekly nuchal translucency measurements in normal fetuses. Obstet Gynecol 1998;91:208–211.
34. Hafner E, Schuchter K, Liebhart E, Philipp K: Results of routine fetal nuchal translucency measurement at 10–13 weeks in 4,233 unselected pregnant women. Prenat Diagn 1998;18:29–34.
35. Pandya P: Nuchal translucency thickness. In Nicolaides KH, Sebire NJ, Snijders RJM (eds): The 11–14 Week Scan: The Diagnosis of Fetal Abnormalities. Diploma in Fetal Medicine Series. Carnforth, England: Parthenon, 1999, p 15.
36. Bindra R, Heath V, Nicolaides KH: Screening for chromosomal defects by fetal nuchal translucency at 11 to 14 weeks. Clin Obstet Gynecol 2002;45:661–670.
37. Braithwaite JM, Economides DL: The measurement of nuchal translucency with transabdominal and transvaginal sonography: Success rates, repeatability and levels of agreement. Br J Radiol 1995;68:720–723.
38. Whitlow BJ, Chatzipapas IK, Economides DL: The effect of fetal neck position on nuchal translucency measurement. Br J Obstet Gynaecol 1998;105:872–876.
39. Pandya PP, Altman DH, Brizot ML, et al: Repeatability of measurement of fetal nuchal translucency thickness. Ultrasound Obstet Gynecol 1995;5:334–337.
40. Sebire NJ, Souka A, Skentou H, et al: Early prediction of severe twin-to-twin transfusion syndrome. Hum Reprod 2000;15:2008–2010.
41. Pandya PP, Snijders RJM, Johnson SP, et al: Screening for fetal trisomies by maternal age and fetal nuchal translucency thickness at 10 to 14 weeks of gestation. Br J Obstet Gynaecol 1995;102:957–962.
42. Hyett JA, Perdu M, Sharland GK, et al: Increased nuchal translucency at 10–14 weeks of gestation as a marker for major cardiac defects. Ultrasound Obstet Gynecol 1997;10:242–246.
43. Matias A, Gomes C, Flack N, et al: Screening for chromosomal abnormalities at 10–14 weeks: The role of ductus venosus blood flow. Ultrasound Obstet Gynecol 1998;12:380–384.
44. Matias A, Huggon I, Areias JC, et al: Cardiac defects in chromosomally normal fetuses with abnormal ductus venosus blood flow at 10–14 weeks. Ultrasound Obstet Gynecol 1999;14;307–310.

45. Souka AP, Nicolaides KH: Diagnosis of fetal abnormalities at the 10–14 week scan. Ultrasound Obstet Gynecol 1997;10:429–442.
46. Whitlow BJ, Chatzipapas IK, Lazanakis ML, et al: The value of sonography in early pregnancy for the detection of fetal abnormalities in an unselected population. Br J Obstet Gynaecol 1999;106:929–936.
47. Snijders RJM, Sebire NJ, Nayar R, et al: Increased nuchal translucency in trisomy 13 fetuses at 10–14 weeks of gestation. Am J Med Genet 1999;86:205–207.
48. Bronshtein M, Bar-Hava I, Blumenfeld I, et al: The difference between septated and nonseptated nuchal cystic hygroma in the early second trimester. Obstet Gynecol 1993;81:683–687.
49. Ville Y, Lalondrelle C, Doumerc S, et al: First-trimester diagnosis of nuchal anomalies: Significance and outcome. Ultrasound Obstet Gynecol 1992;2:314–316.
50. Bronshtein M, Zimmer EZ, Gerlis LM, et al: Early ultrasound diagnosis of fetal congenital heart defects in high-risk and low-risk pregnancies. Obstet Gynecol 1993;82:225–229.
51. Snijders RJ, Sebire NJ, Souka A, et al: Fetal exomphalos and chromosomal defects: Relationship to maternal age and gestation. Ultrasound Obstet Gynecol 1995;6:250–255.
52. Whitlow BJ, Lazanakis ML, Kadir RA, et al: The significance of choroid plexus cysts, echogenic foci and renal pyelectasis in the first trimester. Ultrasound Obstet Gynecol 1998;12:385–390.
53. Vintzileos AM, Ananth C, Smulian JC, et al: Cost benefit analysis of prenatal diagnosis for Down syndrome using the British or American approach. Obstet Gynecol 2000;95:577–583.
54. Cuckle HS, Wald NJ, Lindenbaum RH: Maternal serum alpha-fetoprotein measurement: A screening test for Down syndrome. Lancet 1984;1:926–929.
55. Cuckle HS, Wald NJ, Thompson SG: Estimating a woman's risk of having a pregnancy associated with Down's syndrome using her age and serum alpha-fetoprotein level. Br J Obstet Gynaecol 1987;94:387–402.
56. New England Regional Genetics Group Prenatal Collaborative Study of Down Syndrome Screening: Combining maternal serum α-fetoprotein measurements and age to screen for Down syndrome in pregnant women under age 35. Am J Obstet Gynecol 1989;160:575–581.
57. Bogart MH, Pandian MR, Jones OW: Abnormal maternal serum chorionic gonadotropin levels in pregnancies with fetal chromosome abnormalities. Prenat Diagn 1987;7:623–630.
58. Wald NJ, Cuckle HS, Densem JW, et al: Maternal serum unconjugated oestriol as an antenatal screening test for Down's syndrome. Br J Obstet Gynaecol 1988;95:334–341.
59. Wald NJ, Cuckle HS, Densem JW, et al: Maternal serum screening for Down's syndrome in early pregnancy. BMJ 1988;297: 883–887.
60. Haddow JE, Palomaki GE, Knight GJ, et al: Prenatal screening for Down's syndrome with use of maternal serum markers. N Engl J Med 1992;327:588–593.
61. Cheng EY, Luthy DA, Zebelman AM, et al: A prospective evaluation of a second-trimester screening test for fetal Down syndrome using maternal serum alpha-fetoprotein, hCG, and unconjugated estriol. Obstet Gynecol 1993;81:72–77.
62. Burton BK, Prins GS, Verp MS: A prospective trial of prenatal screening for Down syndrome by means of maternal serum α-fetoprotein, human chorionic gonadotropin, and unconjugated estriol. Am J Obstet Gynecol 1993;169:526–530.
63. Wenstrom KD, Williamson RA, Grant SS, et al: Evaluation of multiple-marker screening for Down syndrome in a statewide population. Am J Obstet Gynecol 1993;169:793–797.
64. American College of Obstetricians and Gynecologists: Prenatal diagnosis of fetal chromosomal abnormalities: 2003 Compendium of Selected Publications. Washington, The American College of Obstetricians and Gynecologists, 2003, pp 547–557
65. Haddow JE, Palomaki GE, Knight GJ, et al: Reducing the need for amniocentesis in women 35 years of age or older with serum markers for screening. N Engl J Med 1994;330:114–118.
66. Wald NJ, Densem JW, George L, et al: Prenatal screening for Down's syndrome using inhibin-A as a serum marker. Prenat Diagn 1996;16:143–153.
67. Wenstrom KD, Owen J, Chu DC, Boots L: Prospective evaluation of free beta-subunit of human chorionic gonadotropin and dimeric inhibin A for aneuploidy detection. Am J Obstet Gynecol 1999;181:887–892.
68. Rodis JF, Egan JF, Craffey A, et al: Calculated risk of chromosomal abnormalities in twin gestations. Obstet Gynecol 1990;76: 1037–1041.
69. American College of Obstetricians and Gynecologists: New ultrasound output display standard. 2003 Compendium of Selected Publications. of Selected Publications. Washington, The American College of Obstetricians and Gynecologists, 2003, pp 69–70.
70. Yeo L, Vintzileos AM, Guzman ER, et al: Targeted ultrasound after an abnormal karyotype: The patient's perspective. Am J Obstet Gynecol 2001;185:S233.
71. American Institute of Ultrasound in Medicine: Standards for Performance of the Antepartum Obstetrical Ultrasound Examination. Laurel, MD, American Institute of Ultrasound in Medicine, 1994.
72. Bowerman RA, Nyberg DA: Normal fetal anatomic survey. In Nyberg DA, McGahan JP (eds): Diagnostic Imaging of Fetal Anomalies. Philadelphia, Lippincott Williams & Wilkins, 2003, pp 1–30.
73. Yeo L, Guzman ER, Day-Salvatore D, et al: Prenatal detection of fetal trisomy 18 through abnormal sonographic features. J Ultrasound Med 2003;22:581–590.
74. Ewigman BG, Crane JP, Frigoletto FD, et al: Effect of prenatal ultrasound screening on perinatal outcome: RADIUS Study Group. N Engl J Med 1993;329:821–827.
75. Campbell S, Pearce JM: The prenatal diagnosis of fetal structural anomalies by ultrasound. Clin Obstet Gynecol 1983;10:475–506.
76. Levi S: Ultrasound in prenatal diagnosis: Polemics around routine ultrasound screening for second trimester fetal malformations. Prenat Diagn 2002;22:285–295.
77. Skupuski DW, Newman S, Edersheim T, et al: Fetus-placenta-newborn: The impact of routine obstetric ultrasonographic screening in a low-risk population. Am J Obstet Gynecol 1996:175:1142–1145.
78. Saari-Kemppainen A, Karjalainen O, Ylostalo P, Heinonen OP: Ultrasound screening and perinatal mortality: Controlled trial systematic one-stage screening in pregnancy. The Helsinki Ultrasound Trial. Lancet 1990;336:387–391.
79. Crane JP, LeFevre ML, Winborn RC, et al: A randomized trial of prenatal ultrasonographic screening: Impact on the detection, management, and outcome of anomalous fetuses. The RADIUS Study Group. Am J Obstet Gynecol 1994;171:392–399.
80. Van Dorsten JP, Hulsey TC, Newman RB, Menard MK: Fetal anomaly detection by second-trimester ultrasonography in a tertiary center. Am J Obstet Gynecol 1998;178:742–749.
81. Grandjean H, Larroque D, Levi S, Eurofetus team: The performance of routine ultrasonographic screening of pregnancies in the Eurofetus study. Am J Obstet Gynecol 1999;181:446–454.
82. Saari-Kemppainen A, Karjalainen O, Ylostalo P, Heinonen OP: Fetal anomalies in a controlled one-stage ultrasound screening trial: A report from the Helsinki Ultrasound Trial. J Perinat Med 1994;22:279–289.
83. Levi S, Hyjazi Y, Schaapst JP: Sensitivity and specificity of routine antenatal screening for congenital anomalies by ultrasound: The Belgian Multicentric Study. Ultrasound Obstet Gynecol 1991;1:102–110.
84. Yeo L, Guzman ER, Shen-Schwarz S, et al: Value of a complete sonographic survey in detecting fetal abnormalities: Correlation with perinatal autopsy. J Ultrasound Med 2002;21:501–510.
85. Chitty LS, Hunt GH, Moore J, Lobb MO: Effectiveness of routine ultrasonography in detecting fetal structural abnormalities in a low risk population. BMJ 1991;303:1165–1169.

86. Levi S, Schaaps JP, De Havay P, et al: End-result of routine ultrasound screening for congenital anomalies: The Belgium Multicentric Study 1984–92. Ultrasound Obstet Gynecol 1995; 5:366–371.
87. Shirley IM, Bottomley F, Robinson VP: Routine radiographer screening for fetal abnormalities by ultrasound in an unselected low risk population. Br J Radiol 1992;65:564–569.
88. Waldenstrom U, Axelsson O, Nilsson S, et al: Effects of routine one-stage ultrasound screening in pregnancy: A randomized controlled trial. Lancet 1988;2:585–588.
89. Vintzileos AM, Ananth CV, Smulian JC, et al: Routine second-trimester ultrasonography in the United States: A cost benefit analysis. Am J Obstet Gynecol 2000;182:655–660.
90. Leivo T, Tuominen R, Saari-Kemppainen A, et al: Cost-effetiveness of one-stage ultrasound screening in pregnancy: A report from the Helsinki ultrasound trial. Ultrasound Obstet Gynecol 1996;7:309–314.
91. Egan JF, Benn P, Borgida AF, et al: Efficacy of screening for fetal Down syndrome in the United States from 1974 to 1997. Obstet Gynecol 2000;96:979–985.
92. Alberman ED, Creasy MR: Frequency of chromosomal abnormalities in miscarriages and perinatal deaths. J Med Genet 1977; 14:313–315.
93. Milunsky A, Milunsky J: Genetic counseling: Preconception, prenatal, and perinatal. In Milunsky A (ed): Genetic Disorders and the Fetus: Diagnosis, Prevention, and Treatment, 4th ed. Baltimore, Johns Hopkins University Press, 1998, pp 1–52.
94. Yeo L, Vintzileos AM: The use of genetic sonography to reduce the need for amniocentesis in women at high-risk for Down syndrome. Semin Perinatol 2003;27:152–159.
95. Vintzileos AM, Egan JF: Adjusting the risk for trisomy 21 on the basis of second trimester ultrasonography. Am J Obstet Gynecol 1995;172:837–844.
96. Benacerraf BR, Barss BA, Laboda LA: A sonographic sign for the detection in the second trimester of the fetus with Down's syndrome. Am J Obstet Gynecol 1985;151:1078–1079.
97. Vintzileos A, Walters C, Yeo L: Absent nasal bone in the prenatal detection of fetuses with trisomy 21 in a high-risk population. Obstet Gynecol 2003;101:905–908.
98. Nyberg DA, Resta RG, Hickok DE, et al: Femur length shortening in the detection of Down syndrome: Is prenatal screening feasible? Am J Obstet Gynecol 1990;162:1247–1252.
99. Bromley B, Benacerraf BR: The genetic sonogram scoring index. Semin Perinatol 2003;27:124–129.
100. Yeo L, Guzman ER, Ananth CV, et al: Prenatal detection of fetal aneuploidy by sonographic ear length. J Ultrasound Med 2003; 22:565–576.
101. Persutte WH, Hobbins JC, Nyberg DA, et al: Trisomy 21 multicenter collaborative project (abstract). Am J Obstet Gynecol 1998;178:S22.
102. Hobbins JC, Lezotte DC, Persutte WH, et al: An eight center study to evaluate the utility of mid-term genetic ultrasounds among high-risk pregnancies. J Ultrasound Med 2003;22:33–38.
103. Vintzileos AM, Campbell WA, Rodis JF, et al: The use of second-trimester genetic sonogram in guiding clinical management of patients at increased risk for fetal trisomy 21. Obstet Gynecol 1996;87:948–952.
104. Vintzileos AM, Guzman ER, Smulian JC, et al: Down syndrome risk estimation after normal genetic sonography. Am J Obstet Gynecol 2002;187:1226–1229.
105. Hobbins JC, Bahado-Singh RO, Lezotte DC: The genetic sonogram in screening for Down syndrome: Response to the JAMA study. J Ultrasound Med 2001;20:269–272.
106. Landwehr JB Jr, Johnson MP, Hume RF, et al: Abnormal nuchal findings on screening ultrasonography: Aneuploidy stratification on the basis of ultrasonographic anomaly and gestational age at detection. Am J Obstet Gynecol 1996;175:995–999.
107. Vintzileos AM, Ananth CV, Fisher AJ, et al: An economic evaluation of second-trimester genetic ultrasonography for prenatal detection of Down syndrome. Am J Obstet Gynecol 1998;179:1214–1219.
108. DeVore GR: Is genetic ultrasound cost-effective? Semin Perinatol 2003;27:173–182.
109. Bahado-Singh R, Cheng CC, Matta P, et al: Combined serum and ultrasound screening for detection of fetal aneuploidy. Semin Perinatol 2003;27:145–151.
110. Cicero S, Curcio P, Papageorghiou A, et al: Absence of nasal bone in fetuses with trisomy 21 at 11–14 weeks of gestation: An observational study. Lancet 2001;358:1665–1667.
111. Sonek JD, Nicolaides KH: Prenatal ultrasonographic diagnosis of nasal bone abnormalities in three fetuses with Down syndrome. Am J Obstet Gynecol 2002;186:139–141.
112. Cicero S, Bindra R, Rembouskos G, et al: Fetal nasal bone length in chromosomally normal and abnormal fetuses at 11–14 weeks of gestation. J Matern Fetal Neonatal Med 2002;11:400–402.
113. Otano L, Aiello H, Igarzabal L, et al: Association between first trimester absence of fetal nasal bone on ultrasound and Down syndrome. Prenat Diagn 2002;22:930–932.
114. Cicero S, Bindra R, Rembouskos G, et al: Integrated ultrasound and biochemical screening for trisomy 21 using fetal nuchal translucency, absent fetal nasal bone, free β-hCG and PAPP-A at 11 to 14 weeks. Prenat Diagn 2003;23:306–310.
115. Cicero S, Sonek JD, McKenna DS, et al: Nasal bone hypoplasia in trisomy 21 at 15–22 weeks' gestation. Ultrasound Obstet Gynecol 2003;21:15–18.
116. Lee W, DeVore GR, Comstock CH, et al: Nasal bone evaluation in fetuses with Down syndrome during the second and third trimesters of pregnancy. J Ultrasound Med 2003;22:55–60.
117. Bromley B, Liberman E, Shipp TD, Benacerraf BR: Fetal nose bone length: A marker for Down syndrome in the second trimester. J Ultrasound Med 2002;21:1387–1394.
118. Bunduki V, Ruano R, Miguelez J, et al: Fetal nasal bone length: Reference range and clinical application in ultrasound screening for trisomy 21. Ultrasound Obstet Gynecol 2003;21: 156–160.
119. Pretorius DH, Nelson TR, James G: Three-dimensional ultrasound in obstetrics. In Nyberg DA, McGahan JP (eds): Diagnostic Imaging of Fetal Anomalies. Philadelphia, Lippincott Williams & Wilkins, 2003, pp 969–988.
120. Merz E, Bahlmann F, Weber G: Volume scanning in the evaluation of fetal malformations: A new dimension in prenatal diagnosis. Ultrasound Obstet Gynecol 1995;5:222–227.
121. Dyson RL, Pretorius DH, Budorick NE, et al: Three-dimensional ultrasound in the evaluation of fetal anomalies. Ultrasound Obstet Gynecol 2000;16:321–328.
122. Hull AD, James G, Salerno C, et al: Three-dimensional ultrasound and the assessment of the first trimester fetus. J Ultrasound Med 2001;20:287–293.
123. Kurjak A, Kupesic S, Ivancic-Kosuta MJ: Three-dimensional transvaginal ultrasound improves measurement of nuchal translucency. J Perinat Med 1999;27:97–102.
124. Blaas HG, Eik-Nes SH, Kiserud T, et al: Three-dimensional imaging of the brain cavities in human embryos. Ultrasound Obstet Gynecol 1995;5:228–232.
125. Steiner H, Gregg AR, Bogner G, et al: First trimester three-dimensional ultrasound volumetry of the gestational sac. Arch Gynecol Obstet 1994;255:165–170.
126. Johnson DD, Pretorius DH, Budorick NE, et al: Fetal lip and primary palate: Three-dimensional versus two-dimensional US. Radiology 2000;217:236–239.
127. Timor-Tritsch I, Monteagudo A, Mayberry P: Three-dimensional ultrasound evaluation of the fetal brain: The three horn view. Ultrasound Obstet Gynecol 2000;16:302–306.
128. Mueller GM, Weiner CP, Yankowitz J: Three-dimensional ultrasound in the evaluation of fetal head and spine anomalies. Ultrasound Obstet Gynecol 1996;88:372.
129. Sklansky MS, Nelson TR, Pretorius DH: Usefulness of gated three-dimensional fetal echocardiography to reconstruct and

display structures not visualized with two-dimensional imaging. Am J Cardiol 1997;80:665–668.
130. Garjan KV, Pretorius DH, Budorick NE, et al: Fetal skeletal dysplasia: Three-dimensional US. Initial experience. Radiology 2000;214:717–723.
131. Lee W, Comstock CH, Kirk JS, et al: Birthweight predictions by three-dimensional ultrasonographic volumes of the fetal thighs and abdomen. J Ultrasound Med 1997;161:799–805.
132. Chang FM, Hsu KF, Ko HC, et al: Three-dimensional ultrasound assessment of fetal liver volume in normal pregnancy: A comparison of reproducibility with two-dimensional ultrasound and a search for a volume constant. Ultrasound Med Biol 1997;23:381.
133. Lee A, Kratochwil A, Stumpflen I, et al: Fetal lung volume determination by three-dimensional ultrasonography. Am J Obstet Gynecol 1996;175:588–592.
134. Canick JA, Palomaki GE, Osathanondh R: Prenatal screening for trisomy 18 in the second trimester. Prenat Diagn 1990;10: 546–548.
135. Palomaki GE, Haddow JE, Knight GJ, et al: Risk-based prenatal screening for trisomy 18 using alpha-fetoprotein, unconjugated oestriol and human chorionic gonadotropin. Prenat Diagn 1995;15:713–723.
136. Gross SJ, Shulman LP, Tolley EA, et al: Isolated fetal choroid plexus cysts and trisomy 18: A review and meta-analysis. Am J Obstet Gynecol 1995;172:83–87.
137. Yeo L, Guzman ER, Vintzileos AM, et al: Isolated vs. non-isolated choroid plexus cysts: Their relationship to aneuploidy and other congenital anomalies. Am J Obstet Gynecol 1999;180 (Part 2):S58
138. Wald NJ, Watt HC, Hackshaw AK: Integrated screening for Down's syndrome on the basis of tests performed during the first and second trimesters. N Engl J Med 1999;341:461–467.
139. Kadir RA, Economides DL: The effect of nuchal translucency measurement on second-trimester biochemical screening for Down's syndrome. Ultrasound Obstet Gynecol 1997;9:244–247.
140. Schuchter K, Hafner E, Stangl G, et al: Sequential screening for trisomy 21 by nuchal translucency measurement in the first trimester and maternal serum biochemistry in the second trimester in a low-risk population. Ultrasound Obstet Gynecol 2001;18:23–25.
141. Audibert F, Dommergues M, Benattar C, et al: Screening for Down syndrome using first-trimester ultrasound and second-trimester maternal serum markers in a low-risk population: A prospective longitudinal study. Ultrasound Obstet Gynecol 2001;18:26–31.

CHAPTER 9

Counseling and Management of an Abnormal Result on a Screening or Diagnostic Test for Fetal Abnormality

Lauren Kerzin-Storrar / Sarah Vause / Michael Maresh

INTRODUCTION

Although medicine benefits from many technologic advances, too often the communication of information about these advances to our patients lags behind. The individuality of patients and their feelings and values must be considered when imparting information.

The goal of current medical practice is to provide a quality service, and we must ensure that our patients are as satisfied as possible. Thus, there is little benefit in providing a scientifically excellent antenatal screening program if our patients are unhappy with the way that the information is presented. Too often, communication issues are considered unexciting and are the subject of very little research in contrast to the vast sums spent developing and evaluating new screening methods. No new screening test should be introduced into routine practice without comprehensive education for those who are in contact with patients, backed up by information leaflets that have been developed in conjunction with patients' groups.

Concept and Perception of Risk

One area that both health professionals and the public have difficulty with is the concept of risk. What is the real meaning to an individual of being told that her unborn baby has a risk of 1% of having a certain condition? To a woman who has a 1 in 4 (25%) risk of having the condition, 1% may seem very low, whereas to another who has a lower background risk (e.g., 1 in 1000), it may seem very high. In addition, the interpretation of the terms "low" and "high" may vary between professionals and parents. In pregnancy, for historic reasons, a cutoff of 1 in 200 or 250 has developed as differentiating between high and low risk (possibly from the perceived risk of miscarriage from amniocentesis). In other areas of medicine and life, other cutoffs may be used. Yet, can a woman compare the risks encountered in other walks of life, such as the risk of having an accident on a certain stretch of road, with the risk of her baby having a major abnormality?

Attributes of a Screening Test

Before the introduction of a screening test, ideally, the test has been shown to have the following attributes:

- **Relevance.** The condition must be a relevant and important medical condition. For example, prenatal screening for a major cardiac abnormality is clearly relevant, but screening for cleft palate is more debatable.
- **Effect on management.** Alternative management options must be available. For example, with a suspected diaphragmatic hernia, management options include planning for delivery in a tertiary care center.
- **Sensitivity.** The screening test must detect the vast majority of cases. For example, serum screening for Down syndrome using only two serum markers is not considered sufficiently sensitive (approximately 60% sensitive for a 5% false-positive rate).
- **Specificity.** The screening test must exclude the vast majority of patients who do not have the condition.
- **Predictive value.** More relevant than specificity and sensitivity in practical counseling is the predictive value of a test. If a woman has a positive result on a screening test for Down syndrome, she wants to know

the likelihood that her baby will have this condition so that she can balance this knowledge with the risks of an invasive diagnostic test, such as amniocentesis.

- **Reproducibility.** When repeated, the test must produce the same results in the same patient. Laboratories that perform serum screening for Down syndrome participate in quality control programs. Routine use of nuchal translucency screening requires appropriate and regularly checked equipment. In addition, the operator must be appropriately trained and involved in the evaluation of data quality.
- **Affordability and availability of resources.** Before the introduction of a test, the resources must be identified for both equipment and personnel. Too often, a suboptimal service is introduced because no time is allowed for counseling.
- **Equity of availability.** If a screening service is being introduced within the context of a national program, then it must be available in all areas (rural and urban) and to all relevant populations, including minority groups.

Ethical Issues

The following ethical issues must be considered as well:

- The ability of caregivers to separate their own moral and ethical viewpoints from the decision-making process.
- Societal and cultural attitudes about disability, not only in general terms, but also regarding the degree of disability. These attitudes may vary enormously in multiethnic environments, such as may be found in parts of Europe or North America. In addition, in some societies, screening is equated with eugenics, whereas in others, it is regarded as a natural right.
- The validity of assessing the costs and benefits of screening by comparing the costs of screening with the costs incurred in life by a person with a disability. Is it possible to put a value on life in this way?

Legal Issues

Some relevant legal issues are discussed briefly here and more fully later. There have been recent reviews of the law in the United Kingdom and the United States.[1,2]

- **Provision of a comprehensive service.** In the United Kingdom, the National Health Service has a statutory responsibility to provide a comprehensive service. Recent recommendations have been made with regard to screening for Down syndrome.[3] If the service is not available as described by a certain date, the hospital or local authority may be liable.
- **Informed consent.** Before a management decision is made, the patient must be counseled and provided with the necessary information to allow her to make an informed decision. For example, if a clinician does not make it clear and document that termination of pregnancy is an option, the clinician may be liable after childbirth if the woman decides in retrospect that she would have preferred to have the pregnancy terminated.
- **Operator skill.** All clinicians must be competent in the areas in which they work. Those involved in invasive procedures must demonstrate that they are performing sufficient numbers of procedures to remain skilled. If a woman miscarries after an amniocentesis and it is clear that the clinician is performing significantly fewer procedures than published guidelines recommend,[4] the court might find the clinician liable.
- **Termination of pregnancy.** English law is complex and involves several separate acts; however, clear summaries are available.[1] There is no gestational age limit for termination of pregnancy for fetal handicap. What is required is that two physicians believe in good faith that there is a substantial risk that the child would suffer from such physical or mental abnormalities as to be seriously handicapped. The imprecise terms "substantial" and "seriously" tend to allow consensus medical opinion to determine the working of the law[5]. In the United States, although laws on the availability of abortion vary from state to state, the judgment in specific cases of fetal abnormality is usually left to health care rather than legal professionals.[2]

Thus, the management of an abnormal screening test result involves many challenges and pitfalls for the health professional. In addition, it puts the staff involved under frequent pressure, and the welfare of the staff involved in this difficult work should not be forgotten. This chapter describes strategies to help women who have an abnormal result on a screening test. The evidence base is regrettably limited, and this is a challenge for the future.

PRETEST COUNSELING

Before a prenatal screening test is performed, counseling is essential to ensure that the woman (and her partner, when relevant) can make an informed choice about whether to have the test and also to prepare her for the possible outcome of an abnormal screening or diagnostic result.[6] Biochemical and ultrasound screening for abnormality is now available to all pregnant women in many centers, regardless of previous risk, and providing quality counseling to large numbers of women has become a challenge in contemporary maternity care. Some express the view that because most screening tests provide reassurance, it is wrong to raise unnecessary anxiety through detailed discussion before a screening test is performed, and that from a resource perspective, more time should be spent counseling women with positive screening or diagnostic test results. However, if the aim of informed consent is to be fulfilled, full and accurate information must be available before a woman decides whether to opt for screening.

Informed Consent: Opting in or Opting Out?

Because screening tests have been incorporated into standard prenatal care, the issue of consent has focused on women who choose to opt out of a process seen as routine, rather than on ensuring that women who do consent have made a positive decision to opt in to a genuinely optional screening program.[7] One approach to promoting choice is to provide pretest information and counseling on a separate day from the screening procedure, so that women who want testing make the positive choice to return to the clinic on another day.[8] Although this approach may inconvenience women who find an additional prenatal visit impractical for socioeconomic reasons, it is important to avoid the presumption that most women want screening tests and that those who do want them must justify their decision.

Needs of Different Patient Groups

Although basic general principles for providing information and counseling apply to all women offered tests in pregnancy, the needs of women may vary according to their previous obstetric and family history as well as their cultural background. Most women who undergo screening tests have a low previous risk of abnormality, and many perceive screening as an opportunity to gain reassurance about the normality of their baby. It has been argued that this perception presents a greater challenge for professionals to ensure informed consent.[9,10] In contrast, some women at high genetic risk may approach testing with a heightened expectation that the baby will be affected. Their needs are therefore focused on receiving access to up-to-date, relevant testing as early as possible. Awareness of these potential differences can improve communication and understanding between clinicians and patients.

Women at High Genetic Risk

Women at increased genetic risk are likely to have the following characteristics:

- History of poor pregnancy outcome
- Anxiety
- Well-informed
- Tentative attitude toward the pregnancy
- Desire to delay routine prenatal care until after testing is complete
- Need for prenatal diagnosis in future pregnancies

Women who Perceive they Are at Increased Risk

Women may believe that they are at increased risk because they have one or more of the following characteristics:

- A previous affected child (although the risk of recurrence may be low)
- A positive screening result in one or more previous pregnancies
- Advanced age

With changes in society, increasing numbers of women are having children in their later reproductive years. These women are at increased risk of having a baby with Down syndrome. Some of these women and also those who have had a previous baby with an abnormality may believe that the uncertainty associated with screening methods is unacceptable and may wish to move straight to a diagnostic test, with its small but definite risk of miscarriage.

A particularly difficult scenario that is becoming increasingly common is that of a woman in her late 30s who, after years of trying to conceive, has done so with the aid of assisted reproduction techniques and has a multiple pregnancy. This is likely to be her only pregnancy, she is at increased risk of having a child with Down syndrome and other congenital anomalies, amniocentesis carries a risk to both pregnancies, and feticide has a significant risk of losing both pregnancies. In addition, there may be the added problem of triplets. This situation raises the further difficult issue of selective reduction. It is incumbent on the assisted reproduction service to ensure that all of these issues have been discussed in advance. In the future, the use of embryo aneuploidy screening may reduce the complexity of the management, although it has its own potential problems. Often it appears to those providing pregnancy care that with the enormous desire of the woman to achieve a pregnancy and the goal of the assisted reproduction service to obtain good results, these issues have not been discussed in depth. As a result, the early part of pregnancy is a time of anxiety while the patient undergoes multiple counseling sessions to determine the best way to proceed.

Women at Population Risk

Women with increased population risk are likely to have the following characteristics:

- Less likely to be well informed
- Unlikely to have personal experience with the conditions that testing may detect
- Usually expect a normal finding

Cultural Issues

Within a multicultural society, specific issues that need to be addressed may include the following:

- Religious beliefs, particularly in relation to pregnancy termination
- Attitudes of the community toward a congenital abnormality or disability
- Role of the partner and extended family in pregnancy decisions
- Language barriers (where English is not the first language)

Assumptions are often made about the views of members of certain racial, cultural, or religious groups on the acceptability of termination of pregnancy. These assumptions may affect the discussion of test results, follow-up diagnostic tests, and the option of termination of the pregnancy.

Clinicians may also, consciously or unconsciously, alter or delay clinic appointments if they do not believe that women from certain ethnic or cultural backgrounds will consent to antenatal tests. Physicians and midwives should be aware of this possibility and take steps to ensure equity and avoid discrimination. Although some evidence shows that women from specific ethnic minority groups, including Pakistani and Bangladeshi Muslims (in the United Kingdom) and Mexican Americans (in the United States), are less likely to accept prenatal screening tests, attitudes among women within the same ethnic group may vary considerably.[9,11–13] Therefore, it is important to avoid generalizations while recognizing potential culturally sensitive issues.

Information Content

There are clear recommendations (Table 9–1) about what information should be made available to women before screening tests are performed.[14,15]

Providing an accurate description of the condition being tested for is essential, and obstetricians and midwives must stay up-to-date on the long-term outlook for affected individuals.[16,17] Although serum screening programs for Down syndrome are often emphasized, opinion varies as to whether information should be provided on other, less common chromosomal conditions that may be identified through screening. Women should be informed that less common conditions can be identified, but detailed descriptions of these conditions are not needed at this point.

In the case of ultrasound screening for abnormality, providing such detailed information would be impossible. Many potential abnormalities could be identified, and much of the information may not be available. In 1997, the Royal College of Obstetricians and Gynaecologists suggested a practical approach to providing information before ultrasound screening (Table 9–2).[14]

Women must be made aware from the outset that an offer of termination of pregnancy is a potential outcome of screening. Some women may decline screening on this basis alone. However, they should also be made aware that screening may detect conditions that can benefit from prompt treatment in the neonatal period and that testing may allow the care of their baby to be optimized.

Providing Information

The provision of information is a process that ideally begins preconception, particularly for those at genetic risk, and continues until after delivery when an abnormality is identified. This emphasis on process is important, and the amount and nature of information needed at each stage vary. The information provided at each stage should address the key decisions currently facing the woman and her partner. These are summarized in Table 9–3.

Many approaches to information provision are used, including written leaflets, touch screens, videos, group discussion, and one-to-one counseling. There is no evidence that a particular method improves understanding or affects participation in screening,[18,19] but several studies reported that the quality (measured in terms of comprehensiveness, accuracy, presentation, and accessibility of language) of both written and spoken information varies considerably.[15,20,21] Peer-reviewed written information leaflets are now available, and these may also be used as a template for individual institutions to produce

TABLE 9–1

Prescreening Information Content[14,15]

Description of the condition
Prognosis
Available management (e.g., medical, social)
Variability
Chance that the baby with have the condition
Procedures and risks to the pregnancy
Accuracy of the test, including the meaning of a screen-positive (increased risk) result and a screen-negative (decreased risk) result
Potential problematic outcomes of the screening process:
Affected pregnancy and offer of termination
Positive screening test result in an unaffected pregnancy
Possibility of identifying an unexpected condition

Adapted from RCOG: Ultrasound screening for fetal abnormalities: Report of the RCOG Working Party. London, Royal College of Obstetricians and Gynaecologists, 1997, and Murray J, Cuckle H, Sehmi I, et al: Quality of written information used in Down syndrome screening. Prenat Diagn 2001;21:138-142.

TABLE 9–2

Prescreening Information Content: Ultrasound Screening for Abnormality[14]

The scan may:
confirm normality
identify a fatal condition
identify significant conditions that are untreatable, but compatible with survival
identify treatable conditions
detect abnormalities with uncertain significance
detect "minor" features or abnormalities
The scan findings may lead to:
the offer of invasive tests, such as amniocentesis
the offer of termination of pregnancy

Adapted from RCOG: Ultrasound screening for fetal abnormalities: Report of the RCOG Working Party. London, Royal College of Obstetricians and Gynaecologists, 1997.

TABLE 9–3

Key Decisions at Different Stages of the Counseling Process

STAGE	DECISIONS
Preconception (particularly for those at increased genetic risk)	Should I have a child? Which reproductive options available are acceptable to me (e.g., prenatal diagnosis, assisted conception)
At the offer of a screening test	Do I want this test? What would I do with a screen-positive result?
After a screen-positive result	Do I want to have further invasive tests? What will I do when I receive the result?
After an abnormal diagnostic result	Should I continue with the pregnancy?
After delivery or termination of a baby with an abnormality	Did I make the right decision? (Was the prenatal diagnosis correct?) Should I have another child?

locally appropriate patient literature, including translated versions for non-English-speaking patients.[22,23]

Who Should Provide Counseling?

A multidisciplinary approach to maternity care means that a wide range of health professionals will be involved in the delivery of screening and diagnostic tests. Primary care physicians, obstetricians, midwives, and nurses may play a role in presenting screening tests and facilitating informed choice; however, this is likely to represent a small proportion of their overall workload. On the other hand, specialists such as those working in fetal medicine units and genetic services may be involved in disclosing abnormal prenatal diagnostic test results and managing the sequelae on a daily basis. Both the "generalists" and the "specialists" play an important role in prenatal screening, and both groups require training in counseling issues.

Important points to consider include the following:

- Knowledge of the test and condition
- Personal attitudes toward screening, termination, and the patient's choices
- Communication skills, including explaining risk and facilitating decision-making

In the United Kingdom, the National Screening Committee commissioned the establishment of a national network of training workshops for midwives, ultrasonographers, obstetricians, and general practitioners, and the Royal College of Obstetricians and Gynaecologists and the Royal College of Radiologists jointly offer courses that include counseling issues.

Communicating Results

An important issue for women is knowing how, when, and by whom they will be informed about the results of screening tests. When possible, women should be given the choice of how they want the results to be given. Some women prefer a face-to-face discussion, whereas others might wish to hear the news by telephone or letter in the privacy of their own home, before coming in for a discussion of a positive result. For women who are at high risk for abnormality, it may be helpful to have a prearranged appointment to discuss the results, given the increased level of anxiety and the expectation of an abnormal result. This also allows the woman's partner to be present when the results are communicated and allows the woman and her partner to prepare emotionally and practically. For all women, the agreed arrangements should be written in the case notes, for reference when the results are available. Arrangements for giving results are also relevant to the vast majority of women who receive screen-negative results. The importance of communicating screen-negative results promptly should not be underestimated.

Communicating results is a more complicated issue in the context of ultrasound screening for abnormality because "results" may emerge during the procedure. This can be stressful for the person performing the scan as well as for the woman and her partner, if present. Although different units have different protocols, the important principle, again, is clarity. Sonographers are governed not only by their own professional body's guidelines, but also by the protocols in their own departments.[24] The sonographer should explain at the start of the scan how concerns will be discussed, whether during the scan, at the end of the scan, after consultation with colleagues within the scan unit, after a report is issued to the obstetrician, or after a further ultrasound scan.

As with other professional groups, appropriate training in communication skills, an awareness of personal limitations, and clear guidelines for working in multidisciplinary teams enable sonographers to provide appropriate care in a difficult situation.[25,26]

COUNSELING FOR SCREEN-POSITIVE RESULTS

General Issues

Every hospital or unit should have a policy for communicating abnormal screening results. These issues should be decided, in conjunction with the woman, before testing. Midwives and sonographers, as front-line professionals, often must break the news of a screen-positive result.

Presenting screen-positive results in a way that allows the woman and her partner to interpret the findings and make a decision about invasive testing is a challenge. Helpful guidelines include the following:

- Use the word "chance" or "likelihood" because "risk" implies an assumption that an affected child would be viewed negatively.
- Give the numeric risk in two forms, such as a percentage and a ratio.
  "There is a 1 in 100, or 1%, chance that the baby will have Down syndrome."
- Reverse the risk to explain the chance that the baby will be unaffected.
  "In other words, there is a 99 in 100, or 99%, chance that the baby will not have Down syndrome."
- Compare the screen-positive figure with the risk before testing or the population risk.
  "Before your screening test, your chance of having a baby with Down syndrome at this age was 1 in 300. Now, with this test result, the risk has increased to 1 in 100."
- Use descriptive analogies if the woman has difficulty understanding the concept of probability.
  "If we had 100 women in the clinic, all of whom had the same screening result as you, we know that one of the women would be carrying a baby with Down syndrome, but the other 99 would be unaffected."
- Avoid the use of descriptive terms that are subjective, such as "low" or "high," other than in response to the woman's interpretation.
  "I understand that you are concerned and that you feel that this is a high risk. It is certainly considered high enough to offer you an amniocentesis, but it is important to remember that there is a 99% chance that the baby does not have Down syndrome."

Although the risk of an invasive test, such as amniocentesis, should also be presented, it should not be considered a direct comparison with the risk of having an affected child. For some women, a miscarriage may be the worst possible outcome, whereas for others, the highest priority is to avoid the birth of an affected child.

Decision to Have Invasive Test

One aim of informed consent before screening is to encourage women to think about what they might do if they receive a screen-positive result or if a possible abnormality is identified on a scan. However, many women do not consider their options until they are faced with the decision of whether to proceed to an invasive test, such as amniocentesis.

There have been few published studies of the number of women who consent to amniocentesis after a screen-positive result for Down syndrome, and this is likely to vary from center to center because of cultural and socioeconomic differences. However, from our own experience and from the limited evidence available, a substantial proportion of women who consent to screening choose not to proceed to invasive testing, given a screen-positive result.[27]

Of women who choose to proceed, not all do so with the intention to terminate. They may choose an invasive test for any of the following reasons:

- To allow them to prepare psychologically and practically in advance of the birth of an affected child
- To influence obstetric management. For example, if ultrasound found severe early-onset growth retardation, a woman might choose to have amniocentesis even though she would not consider termination. If she knew the fetus had trisomy 13, trisomy 18, or triploidy, she might choose not to have further scans, not to be monitored in labor, or not to have a cesarean section.
- To make the decision to terminate an affected child

Specific Screening Problems

Even if women have had adequate pretest counseling, most are poorly prepared for a positive result from a screening test.[28] Although women may be well informed about the practical aspects of the test, they are less well informed about aspects of the test that could inform their decisions about whether to undergo diagnostic testing and prepare themselves for an adverse outcome.[29]

The following specific problems may be encountered in patients who have positive screening test results:

- Ongoing anxiety after false-positive results
- Soft markers
- Inability to provide a specific diagnosis antenatally
- Variations in options for diagnostic testing based on gestation
- Lack of specificity
- Issues associated with multiple pregnancy

False-Positive Results

All screening tests give false-positive and false-negative results, and handling these results presents a significant challenge. Although recently introduced screening tests for Down syndrome have lower false-positive rates than older tests, it is inevitable that they will occur.

False-positive screening test results may lead to ongoing anxiety. Women who receive negative results from a diagnostic test after a false-positive screening test result may have enormous relief initially, but worries often re-emerge later.[30] If the baby doesn't have Down syndrome, what does it have? Women frequently search for explanations of false-positive results. Even after the birth of an unaffected child, these worries can persist.[31]

Younger women with false-positive results often have very high levels of anxiety, even after normal karyotype results. Research shows that women who are classified as high risk on the basis of a blood test have higher levels of anxiety than those with the identical numeric risk based on age alone.[32] Professionals should be aware of these issues and address them in their counseling.

Soft Markers

The concept of soft markers is difficult to explain and can lead to ongoing anxiety about the function of the respective organ. For example, the detection of an echogenic focus in the heart may lead a woman to be concerned about congenital heart abnormalities or cardiac function. Choroid plexus cysts are poorly understood by obstetricians who provide a range of counseling, often advocating unnecessary follow-up. This may lead to ongoing anxiety in women or their partners regarding the "cysts in the brain" and requests for follow-up scans that are at times agreed to.[33] Visual imagery is powerful, and anomalies detected on ultrasound may exaggerate the psychological costs (e.g., nuchal thickening, choroid plexus cysts).[34] Clinicians may alleviate this by taking care to choose appropriate language and to avoid reinforcing the ongoing anxiety by arranging further testing that may or may not show resolution of the marker.

Inability to Provide a Specific Diagnosis or Prognosis

Discussing isolated structural abnormalities is often relatively straightforward. It is far more difficult to counsel a patient when multiple abnormalities are detected or when there is an inability to provide a specific diagnosis. When multiple abnormalities are detected, it is important to convey the concept that each abnormality cannot be taken in isolation and that a combination of abnormalities may indicate an underlying syndrome or genetic disorder. The inability to provide a specific diagnosis or cases in which there may be a variable prognosis may result in ongoing uncertainty for both the woman and staff. For example, isolated ascites with negative test results for viruses, antibodies, and a normal karyotype have an extremely variable prognosis, ranging from a normal baby to a one with a lethal genetic condition. Isolated ventriculomegaly is another such finding in which the neurodevelopmental outcome can vary from normal to significant disability. Such uncertainties in the prognosis should be acknowledged and explained, and referral to a clinical geneticist may be helpful.

Gestation

The point in gestation at which the result of a screening test is available can affect which diagnostic test is offered. A woman who obtains a high risk result after first-trimester screening has the option of undergoing chorionic villus biopsy or waiting until the second trimester for an amniocentesis with a lower risk of miscarriage.

A two-stage integrated test for Down syndrome screening has been proposed. This includes first-trimester screening, with the second part of the test performed in the second trimester. Women must choose whether they wish the results to be revealed in a staged way, and if high risk, after the first stage of testing; whether to have diagnostic testing in the first trimester; or whether to wait until the results of the second-trimester test are integrated. Waiting until after the second-trimester component is obtained reduces the false-positive rate. Counseling, both before and during the testing process, would be extremely difficult.

Lack of Specificity

In addition to being a marker for Down syndrome, an increased nuchal translucency measurement is associated with cardiac abnormalities,[35] other structural abnormalities, and poor pregnancy outcome.[36] If a thickened nuchal translucency is detected but the karyotype is normal, a detailed second-trimester scan and fetal echocardiogram should be considered. Ongoing testing engenders ongoing anxiety. Even if no anomalies are detected on ultrasound, it is difficult to provide complete reassurance because some anomalies may be undetected or are undetectable on ultrasound.[37]

A further example is an increased level of α-fetoprotein, which is associated with structural abnormalities and later growth retardation, preeclampsia, preterm delivery, abruption, and fetal death. Ongoing follow-up should be offered and complete reassurance cannot be given, even if abnormality is excluded.

Multiple Pregnancy (See also Chapters 24 and 60)

In a multiple pregnancy, determination of chorionicity is important and is best done in the first trimester. The incidence of abnormality is higher in multiple pregnancy. Before screening tests are performed, it is important to discuss the options available for diagnostic testing and subsequent termination, if necessary.

If diagnostic testing, such as amniocentesis, is performed in a multiple pregnancy, it is extremely important to document precisely and rigorously which sample comes from which fetus. Features such as the position of the fetus in the uterus, placental site, and fetal sex can be used to identify each fetus. The importance of this documentation becomes apparent when there is one normal result and one abnormal result.

A woman with a twin pregnancy should be made aware of the option of selective reduction. This discussion should include the risk of miscarriage of the healthy twin. The woman should be informed that the terminated fetus remains within the uterus until delivery and that it must be registered as a stillbirth if delivery (not termination) occurs after 24 weeks' gestation. Selective feticide with potassium chloride injection cannot be performed if the twins are monochorionic because the potassium may cross through the placenta into the normal twin. Selective reduction by cord occlusion is possible in monochorionic twins. Potassium chloride feticide can be used for selective reduction in dichorionic twins.

Although structural abnormalities may be diagnosed in a twin around the time of the "20-week" anomaly scan, it may be more appropriate to wait for viability of the other fetus in the early third trimester before performing the selective termination. The advantages of delaying the termination should be explained, and the woman's views on the timing of the termination should be taken into account.

Problems with Diagnostic Tests

Diagnostic tests may produce any of the following:

- Unexpected results (e.g., sex chromosome trisomies, structural rearrangements, mosaicism)
- False reassurance
- Findings that show nonpaternity
- The need for an unexpected and sometimes ethically challenging decision

Unexpected Results

Although prenatal diagnostic testing is often performed because of concerns about trisomy 21, other chromosomal abnormalities may also be detected. In some cases, such as when trisomy 18 or trisomy 13 is detected, the outcome for the infant if the pregnancy continued is predictable. For these conditions, clear information can be given to a couple to enable them to make an informed choice as to whether to continue with the pregnancy or terminate.

In other situations, for example, when a sex chromosome abnormality, a balanced structural rearrangement of the chromosomes, or mosaicism is detected, then predicting the likely outcome for the infant is much more difficult. Involvement of a clinical geneticist is frequently required.

SEX CHROMOSOME ABNORMALITIES (TURNER SYNDROME XO, KLINEFELTER SYNDROME XXY, TRIPLE X SYNDROME XXX, EXTRA Y XYY)

When a sex chromosome abnormality is diagnosed antenatally, the parents should be offered expert counseling by clinical genetics professionals.[38] The obstetrician or other professional who initially discloses the diagnosis must avoid giving inaccurate or out-of-date information on the implications of the chromosomal abnormality. A recent study emphasized the effect of this first information on parents' decisions and on their perception of the more expert information given to them later in the genetics clinic.[19] As more information about the long-term outcome becomes available from prospective studies, more parents opt to continue the pregnancy.[4,39–41] The main issues for parents faced with the decision of whether to continue with a pregnancy in which the fetus has been found to have a sex chromosome abnormality appear to be worries about congenital abnormalities, the risk of mental retardation, behavioral problems, and the prospects for establishing sexual identity, future sexual relationships, and a successful family life.[42]

STRUCTURAL REARRANGEMENTS

If the rearrangement appears balanced, there should be no harmful effects. However, if it occurs de novo and is not found in either parent, it could cause congenital abnormalities or mental retardation. Because the phenotypic effects of a de novo translocation are unpredictable, it is difficult to provide parents with information to use when making decisions about whether to continue with a pregnancy or terminate. Input from clinical geneticists may be useful. Detailed tertiary-level scanning may have a role. If an abnormality is seen on a scan, it would support the assertion that the rearrangement is exerting a phenotypic effect. However, a normal ultrasound provides limited reassurance because it may detect only approximately one third of abnormalities.

MOSAICISM

Chromosomal mosaicism is the mixture of two or more cell lines with different chromosome constitutions. Mosaicism causes difficulty in interpretation and adds uncertainty to counseling. The difficult is in determining whether this represents the pattern in the fetus, reflects confined placental or membrane mosaicism, or is an in vitro artefact. Chromosomal mosaicism confined to placental tissue, with a normal fetal karyotype, is relatively common (1%). This possibility should be mentioned during counseling, before chorionic villus biopsy is performed. Sampling other tissues, such as amniotic fluid or fetal blood, may provide more information, but does not remove the original abnormal result.

False Reassurance

False reassurance may be provided by a rapid fluorescent in situ hybridization (FISH) test for aneuploidy, when karyotype on cultured cells subsequently show a problem. For example, a FISH test may miss a balanced translocation and therefore give false reassurance initially. Women should be made aware of the limitations of the diagnostic test being offered.

Nonpaternity

Nonpaternity may be discovered when investigating Rhesus disease and finding that the fetus is Rhesus-negative and the putative father is homozygous for the Rhesus-positive gene. Such cases should be handled with tact and respect for confidentiality.[43]

Unexpected Decisions

At times, women make unexpected decisions when the results of tests are available. This can create ethical dilemmas for the team of professionals caring for the woman. For example, amniocentesis may be requested and performed because of maternal age, but on learning the sex of the baby, the woman may then request a termination. This creates a difficult situation for the clinicians. If the pregnancy is clearly of less than 24 weeks' duration (in practice, usually no more than 22 weeks), then in England, it would be feasible and legal to perform a termination if two physicians considered that continuation of the pregnancy would cause more risk to the physical or mental health of the woman (or her existing children) than termination. Most physicians are uncomfortable with termination under these circumstances. However, if they decline the request for termination, it is expected that they would at least try to find other physicians who would be prepared to consider the request or to offer other forms of psychosocial support.

Timing of Diagnostic Procedures

Sometimes a scan performed as part of ongoing obstetric management may show an unexpected abnormality that may be associated with karyotypic abnormality. Diagnostic tests must be discussed in relation to the gestation of the pregnancy. For example, if a "double bubble" suggestive of duodenal atresia is noted on a 32-week scan, amniocentesis may be offered. However, the woman should be aware that although she has the option of termination of pregnancy if trisomy 21 is detected, potassium chloride feticide is necessary before the induction of labor. Many women find it extremely difficult to contemplate a termination in the third trimester, find the need for feticide extremely distressing, and are upset at the prospect of induction, labor, and vaginal delivery. Some women therefore decide not to have karyotyping performed later in pregnancy.

When formulating departmental policies on the appropriate gestation for routine scanning, it is important to bear in mind that in the United Kingdom potassium chloride feticide is advised for most terminations from 22 weeks' gestation. The only exceptions are cases in which the abnormality would be lethal in the early neonatal period. In some hospitals, there is a tendency to perform routine scanning after 20 weeks' gestation to maximize visualization of the heart, but if an abnormality is detected and subsequent testing is needed, then it is easy to exceed the 22-week limit before a definitive diagnosis is made and a termination decided on.

COUNSELING AFTER THE DIAGNOSIS

Emotional Effect

The diagnosis of abnormality has a profound emotional effect on the woman and her partner. These parents now face the following prospects:

- Loss of the anticipated normal pregnancy and child
- Possible end to a wanted pregnancy
- Responsibility for deciding whether to continue or terminate the pregnancy
- Guilt over either decision

After the diagnosis of abnormality in a fetus or child, parents experience a bereavement reaction, as they mourn the "perfect" wished-for baby while incorporating the diagnosis into an altered relationship with the affected baby.[44,45] Responses associated with bereavement reactions, including shock, anger, sadness, and helplessness, are common. When the diagnosis is made prenatally, the parents have the additional burden of deciding whether to continue with the pregnancy within a limited time.

Breaking Bad News

The emotional response to hearing that their baby has an abnormality is so strong that the parents are likely to remember the circumstances of being told for the rest of their lives. For this reason, the importance of the way in which bad news is given cannot be overstated. Basic principles include the following:

- Results should be given in the way discussed before testing, according to the woman's wishes.

  "You asked us to arrange an appointment for you and your partner when the results of your amniocentesis were available. We expect these tomorrow, so can you come in tomorrow afternoon?"
- Arrange to give the results in a room that affords adequate privacy and is located away from women who are receiving routine antenatal care.

  "I will see you in my office, which is down the corridor from the clinic."
- When giving the result, lead in with a short "warning shot."

  "I know that you are anxious to hear the result of your amniocentesis. I do have the result here. I'm afraid it's not what we were hoping for."
- Give the result clearly.

  "The baby's chromosome pattern is abnormal. The baby has a serious condition called *Edwards syndrome*, or *trisomy 18*."
- Acknowledge the effect of the news. Show empathy.

  "I am so sorry to have to give you this news. This must be a terrible shock for both of you."

  "Women in this situation often blame themselves; it is important for you to know that there was nothing you did, or didn't do, that caused this to happen."

- Offer further information about the diagnosis.
  "I can give you more information about Edwards syndrome today, but you may find it difficult to concentrate now, so I have this leaflet that you can take with you."
- State the options clearly.
  "You may decide to terminate the pregnancy or to continue. I will be able to make the arrangements if you decide to terminate. If you decide to continue, I will continue to look after your care through the pregnancy."
- Offer counseling to facilitate decision-making.
  "You may find it helpful to see a genetic counselor while you are deciding whether you want to continue with the pregnancy."
  "There is a support group run by other parents who have been in a similar position. Here are the details."
- Emphasize that there is time to decide (within the constraints of the stage of pregnancy).
  "You don't need to decide today. You have time to consider this carefully over the next few days."
- Make clear what happens next.
  "I will ask the genetic counselor to telephone you tomorrow. I will see you again on Monday."

Decision-Making

For most women and their partners, deciding whether to continue with the pregnancy is the most difficult decision they have had to face in their lives. Although analytic decision models do not appear to account for the way in which women arrive at these decisions, broadly, the process involves the following features:

- An objective assessment of the facts
- A subjective interpretation based on personal values, beliefs, experiences, and circumstances

It is not surprising that women with the same diagnostic result will make different decisions. This individuality has been borne out in a number of large quantitative studies that attempted to identify primary factors in the decision-making process; these studies have yielded varied findings.[46–48] It is important to be aware of factors that may affect the decision-making process for a specific patient, including the following:

- Severity of the condition
- Perceived "burden" of the condition (its likely effect on the child, parents, and other family members)
- Gestational age
- Beliefs and values (religious, cultural, or moral)
- Family size
- Experience with the condition, whether personal or indirect
- Practical and social considerations

Most women are able to come to a decision once they have been given full information, opportunity for discussion, and time. In the longer term, few women regret their decisions, although most experience periods of doubt.[49] However, the burden of responsibility weighs heavily, and women may still seek reassurance that they have made the "right" decision. It is possible to offer this reassurance while upholding the ethos of noncoercion, which is sacrosanct:

> "I can tell you have thought carefully about this before coming to your decision. There is no such thing as a 'right' decision, but the important thing is that when you look back, you will be able to say that you made the best decision you could at the time."

Some parents may seek more than reassurance and may ask directly for advice about what to do. The need to maintain neutrality does not eliminate the responsibility for facilitating decision-making. Some parents reported feeling abandoned by their clinicians and felt that they were left to make a decision without support.[50] If the patient asks an awkward question, such as "What would you do in our situation?" a supportive response might be as follows:

> "It sounds as if you are unsure about what to do. Some ("most" or "a few") of my patients in your situation have decided to terminate the pregnancy, whereas others ("many" or "a few") have continued. What can I do to help you with your decision?"

For women who are struggling to make a decision, it is important to offer help in facilitating this process. To help them gain a sense of control and the confidence to make a decision, it may be helpful to encourage them to reflect on how they have coped with previous difficult decisions. A useful counseling strategy is to explore the various potential outcomes that may result from the diagnosis by imagining them as scenarios. This approach enables the woman and her partner to imagine which outcome would be least difficult for them personally.

A smaller group of women have sustained difficulty in reaching a decision. This is more likely to occur if any of the following factors is present:

- Disagreement between the woman and her partner
- Uncertainty about the diagnosis or prognosis
- Religious, cultural, or moral conflict
- Vulnerability because of age or cognitive impairment

For these women, other sources of counseling and support should be considered, including genetic counselors, specialists (e.g., neonatologists, surgeons), lay support groups, trusted professionals (e.g., general practitioner), and religious advisors.

POST-DECISION CARE

Whatever decision women make, they experience feelings of guilt. Many report an expectation that they will be judged by health professionals as well as by family and friends. It is crucial that they receive understanding and nonjudgmental support at this vulnerable time.

Continuing Pregnancy

In the early years of prenatal diagnosis and screening, the presumption was that these services were only for women who intended to terminate an affected pregnancy.[51] In more recent years, there has been an increase in the number of women choosing to continue with their pregnancy after a diagnosis of abnormality, although maternity staff are less familiar with how to care for these women.[52] This group includes women who make an informed choice at the outset that although they would not terminate an affected pregnancy, they would prefer to be warned about a problem in the baby before delivery; others who have tests with the intention of terminating, but who change their mind when faced directly with the decision; and others who entered screening programs unaware that a possible outcome would be the offer of termination.

The choice to continue the pregnancy has been made for a range of abnormalities, including known lethal conditions in which parents would prefer to "allow nature to take its course," structural abnormalities with a reasonable prospect for surgical intervention, and chromosomal conditions with and without an asso ciated mental handicap (e.g., Down syndrome, Turner syndrome).

A different approach to ongoing prenatal care is required for women continuing with a pregnancy affected with a serious abnormality.[52,53] These women understandably feel different from other pregnant women, and these feelings fluctuate through the rest of the pregnancy. Anxiety is usually greatest around the time of diagnosis and again near the expected date of delivery. Many aspects of care for these women should be addressed, including the following:

- The importance of a nonjudgmental approach by health professionals
- The realization that the woman may change her mind and request termination later
- The need for access to detailed information on the likely outcome for the baby at delivery and beyond, which may include input from lay support groups, pediatricians, and pediatric surgeons
- The option to attend prenatal appointments outside routine prenatal clinic sessions, if desired
- Continuity of care with senior staff and careful communication with primary care practitioners
- Avoidance of further ultrasound scans unless strictly indicated or desired by the woman
- The choice of a private room in the hospital, with the recognition that the woman may prefer to be with other women
- Preparation of both parents and staff for delivery of a baby who may die in the neonatal period or require immediate intervention
- Confirmation of the abnormality after delivery and the offer of genetic counseling, when appropriate

Termination of pregnancy (See also Chapter 68)

Before Viability

After the decision to terminate is made, the woman and her partner need to know what will happen next. If the decision to terminate the pregnancy is made before 14 weeks' gestation, either medical or surgical termination may be performed. After 14 weeks' gestation, there may not be a local gynecologist experienced in late surgical termination, so the only option may be medical termination. A thorough explanation of the processes is required. Some obstetricians and midwives find it difficult to discuss these matters frankly, but women who have had terminations have emphasized the importance of this information at the time. Patient support group literature may also be helpful.[54,55]

When there is a choice of methods, the surgical method may appear attractive initially because the woman is spared the pain of contractions and the often lengthy induction process. Instead, the woman wakes from her anesthetic and the termination is complete. However, disadvantages include the following:

- The experience of giving birth may help in the grieving process.[56]
- There is no opportunity to see the fetus.
- Confirmation of a structural anomaly is unlikely, although chromosomal abnormalities can be confirmed.
- If the surgical procedure is incomplete, the woman may pass recognizable fetal parts.

In contrast, the major disadvantages associated with medical methods are the following:

- A delay of approximately 48 hours between the administration of mifepristone and prostaglandin induction is advised.
- The induction process is often long.
- The woman needs adequate pain relief.
- There is a slight risk of an incomplete procedure, and a subsequent surgical procedure may be needed.

Before undergoing a termination, the woman and her partner must also be informed of a number of decisions that they must make shortly after the procedure is complete.

- Whether to see or hold their baby after a medical induction and delivery
- Whether to have photographs taken
- Whether to agree to have a postmortem examination, either full or limited
- Whether they wish to arrange a funeral, cremation, or other type of remembrance

All of these decisions may be very difficult. Good practice emphasizes the importance of offering parents the opportunity to see their baby. Whether they accept this offer is an intensely personal choice for them and should be respected. Seeing the baby can help the parents to acknowledge the reality of their loss and can also provide precious memories. Even externally severe abnormalities can appear less frightening than imagined. For babies without obvious external abnormalities, parents must be prepared that this does not imply that the diagnosis was incorrect. If parents decide not to see their baby, photographs can be taken for access at a later date if they choose.

The issue of postmortem examinations is important in the United Kingdom because of the retention of material for subsequent research.[57] This practice appears to be resulting in a further decrease in the number of postmortem examinations. Attempting to confirm an abnormality that is not externally apparent, but has been diagnosed on ultrasound scan, is important for the woman as well as for quality control for the prenatal diagnostic service. In addition, the necropsy may change the diagnosis from that presumed before delivery. For those who dislike the idea of such an examination, the concept of limited examinations, biopsies, and detailed imaging (possibly including magnetic resonance imaging) must be explored. In addition, a detailed external examination by a clinical geneticist may show subtle external signs of the underlying problem. Such investigations may lead to a specific diagnosis and a more accurate recurrence risk.

Usually, these patients are cared for in the gynecology department when the pregnancy has not advanced beyond fetal viability. However, the nursing staff may not be accustomed to caring for a woman who has terminated a wanted pregnancy and may have difficulty providing optimum care. Midwives may also have difficulty caring for these women in a delivery unit. Each hospital must recognize the important aspects of care and must provide care in the best possible setting, where the woman is most likely to receive the following[58]:

- Care by staff with experience with terminations for abnormality
- Access to adequate pain relief
- Privacy, including privacy from women delivering healthy babies

In addition, staff should avoid making clinical comments about the fetus because often mistakes are made, such as comments that the baby appears normal or mistaking female fetuses for male fetuses.

After Viability (See also Chapters 24 and 68)

Decisions to terminate a pregnancy are sometimes made around the time of fetal viability for a variety of reasons, including the following:

- Most hospitals perform routine anomaly scans around 20 weeks' gestation. However, some hospitals perform these scans at 21 or 22 weeks' gestation. It is likely that if an abnormality is detected and a termination requested, it would be performed around the time of viability.
- At times, further confirmatory scans are needed or other tests, such as amniocentesis, are indicated. The pregnancy may proceed to 22 weeks' gestation before the woman is in a position to make a decision about termination. Similar delays may occur when thalassemia trait in pregnancy is diagnosed.
- At times, women seek care late in pregnancy and anomalies are detected at this point.
- Sometimes the disease occurs late in the pregnancy (e.g., intraventricular hemorrhage).
- Sometimes an anomaly progresses during the pregnancy, with a worsening prognosis. For example, a couple may choose to continue a pregnancy with isolated mild ventriculomegaly, but if this condition progresses during the pregnancy to severe ventriculomegaly, they may reconsider their decision and request late termination.

Although in some countries, including the United Kingdom, terminations can be performed after viability if it is likely that the child will be seriously handicapped, either physically or mentally, induction of labor may result in the baby being born alive. In this case, unless the attending pediatrician believes that the external appearance of the baby is such that it is incompatible with life, resuscitation of the baby must be undertaken, regardless of parental wishes. In the United Kingdom, feticide is necessary from 22 weeks' gestation unless the baby would die in the immediate neonatal period as a result of its abnormality.[5] The woman and her partner need to have been counseled about this possibility. Injecting potassium chloride into the fetus under ultrasound guidance is clearly very traumatic for the woman and her partner. The woman may feel considerable fetal activity just before fetal demise. She must actively cooperate in the feticide procedure by lying still on the ultrasound table and allowing the operator to inject the potassium chloride. She knows exactly when and where her baby died.

In addition, it is very traumatic for all of the staff present, particularly the person giving the lethal injection and watching fetal demise on the ultrasound screen; the staff will need the support of the entire team and sometimes independent counselors.

Occasionally, a woman feels unable to have a feticide procedure. In this case, she must be fully counseled about the steps that the team must take; unless the baby appears to have a condition that is incompatible with life, at least initially, they must provide full resuscitation and neonatal care.

As in early pregnancy, women may request surgical rather than medical termination, so in later pregnancy, women may ask for a cesarean delivery. Although this procedure offers some benefits, such as a speedier process, cesarean section has several disadvantages, including the following:

- The opportunity to deliver normally may help in the grieving process.
- The maternal morbidity rate is greater.
- The hospital stay is longer.
- Subsequent deliveries may be affected.
- The abdominal scar may act as a constant reminder of the baby.

Postdelivery care

How long a woman wishes to stay in the hospital varies depending on many factors, including family support, cultural concerns, and the type of facility. It is often assumed that women want to go home immediately, but some women who stay in the hospital for medical reasons find the continued support from staff helpful. Women must be warned that they may produce milk; if they do, they should be offered suppression of lactation. They also must be advised how long they may bleed. Most units have detailed checklists to be completed before discharge. These include routine postdelivery issues, such as checking Rhesus status, direct notification of primary care practitioners, and arrangements for follow-up.

At follow-up visits, the following issues should be addressed:

- Emotional adjustment
- Test results
- Appointments with other experts (e.g., geneticists)
- Future pregnancies

The woman may not be able to cope with all of these issues in one session, and further appointments may be advised. Unless the woman specifically requests it, these appointments should not take place in prenatal clinics.

Psychological Sequelae

Parents experience grief after termination for abnormality akin to that after the death of a child, as reported by many authors.[45,48,49,59–61] While still in the hospital, many parents describe relief that the termination procedure is behind them. However, this relief is quickly followed by emotions associated with bereavement, including sadness, emptiness, anger, isolation, and guilt. Almost all women experience grief in the first 2 months after the termination. The intensity of psychological distress decreases over time, with most women reaching a sense of resolution within 6 to 24 months. Studies of factors that may predict which women will have a complicated or prolonged grief response are not conclusive, but those who are very young, are not well supported by their partners, have a psychiatric history, or have had other recent stressful life events may be at greater risk. There is no objective evidence that women grieve less after a first-trimester rather than a second-trimester termination.

In addition to coping with their loss, women almost universally experience guilt and shame that can affect their self-esteem. They may feel that they were in some way responsible for the occurrence of the abnormality (even in the presence of a medical explanation to the contrary), and they feel responsible for deciding to end the pregnancy. Even parents who believe that they made the right decision experience periods of doubt. Some women have nightmares in which the baby or other family members chastise them, or where the diagnosis turned out to be wrong. The sense of shame over having a termination may be particularly acute in women with conflicting religious or cultural values, and most women are concerned about how other people would react to their decision to terminate.

After the initial acute grieving period of 4 to 8 weeks, looking ahead to another pregnancy can play an important part in moving forward, and it may be helpful to initiate discussions about a further pregnancy, including options for prenatal diagnosis. One study in the United Kingdom found that 75% of women became pregnant again 14 months after termination for abnormality.[48]

It is important not to overgeneralize the psychological effects of termination for abnormality, and professionals must avoid prescriptive advice and support. Parents must find their own way to grieve, which may include rituals, such as spending time with the baby and having a funeral. Parents must be offered choices, and relevant patient support group literature should be made available.[54,55] Anticipatory guidance about possible psychological sequelae can help to prepare parents for the following reactions:

- They may experience initial feelings of relief after the termination.
- They are likely to experience grief for a period of months.
- The emotions associated with grief become less intense with time.
- The woman and her partner may grieve in different ways. Understanding and supporting each other is very important.
- It may be helpful to prepare what they will tell other people about the loss. The explanation may be different for their other children, extended family, friends, or colleagues.
- The woman may find it difficult to be around other women who are pregnant, particularly family members or close friends. Making a plan for how to deal with this possibility can be helpful.
- Parents may experience guilt and doubt over their decision. Many parents who say that they know they made the right decision still have doubt at some point. Some women experience nightmares in the first few months after the termination.
- Many women feel psychologically ready to consider a further pregnancy within a year after the termination.

Fathers

The psychological needs of fathers are often overlooked, and the partners of women undergoing termination may feel marginalized. The limited data from studies of fathers' experience of termination for abnormality confirm that fathers also experience profound psychological sequelae, although they may manifest in different ways.[62,63] Fathers often take a supportive role toward their partners, and although both they and their partners can benefit from this approach, it may interfere with or delay their own grief response. However, men and women may not express grief in the same way. If the man shows less overt distress, this may be misinterpreted by others as a lack of grief or failure to grieve. Health professionals can respond more effectively to fathers by following these guidelines:

- Acknowledge that he, like his partner, has lost a wanted child.
- Recognize his role as the supportive partner.
- Recognize that he may feel marginalized because he cannot share the physical burden with his partner.
- Reassure him that men may not express emotion openly and that this does not reflect a lack of feeling.
- Show empathy to a father who cries.
- Suggest opportunities for follow-up support, including lay groups and access to published accounts by fathers.[63]

STAFF SUPPORT

It is stressful for any staff members who are involved in the care of a woman with a suspected major fetal abnormality.[64] For some, this is an unusual event (e.g., a midwife working on a delivery unit who is caring for the first time for a woman who is having a very late termination for a fetal abnormality). For others (e.g., fetal medicine specialists in regional centers), counseling women about these decisions and following through with them is almost an everyday occurrence. However, both groups face common issues, such as the following:

- Moral conflicts
- The need to maintain neutrality
- Reaction to patient choices

These can take an emotional toll on the staff, and further training and support may be needed.

Support for Those Involved in General Maternity Care

A midwife working on the delivery unit usually can decide whether to become involved in the care of such women after they leave the hospital. Her colleagues and the unit manager should discuss the issues in a nonjudgmental way, allow her to make her own decision, and allow her to discuss her final decision with them so that if she does not want to become involved in the future she does not feel alienated. The United Kingdom has a statutory midwifery supervision process, and this process must support the decisions of midwives. Midwives in tertiary care units, many of whom work with women who undergo termination for abnormality, should have the opportunity to attend a fetal anomaly ultrasound scanning session. There, they can begin to understand what women and their partners experience, and they can also see the type of work that their clinical colleagues perform every day. This experience is likely to make the decision-making process easier; ideally, midwives should be able to do this before they are faced with an actual patient. Midwives in smaller units (in which termination for abnormality is much less common) should have the opportunity to join a tertiary care fetal medicine unit for a day to see how they work. This experience can supplement their training in related areas, such as care of the bereaved, to allow them to provide good care. These cases must be discussed at routine general clinical meetings, such as perinatal mortality and morbidity meetings, or at adverse event meetings or clinical case presentation sessions, and not just brushed aside as another case of abnormality. This type of discussion allows those who are not involved to begin to understand some of the moral and ethical dilemmas that can face the staff who are directly involved.

Support for Staff Working in Specialized Fetal Medicine Units

For staff working in a fetal medicine unit, caring for women where a major fetal anomaly being diagnosed is almost a daily occurrence, and for those performing feticide with potassium chloride injections, this is also a fairly regular event. Those deciding to enter this field, whether physicians, midwives, or sonographers, must realize that this aspect of care will become part of their routine work. Several strategies are needed to support the members of the team.

- Sharing the workload. The members of the team must try to share the workload as equally as is feasible. In addition, they should be trained to recognize a colleague who appears to be going through a difficult period and should try to lighten this person's workload.
- Weekly clinical meetings. Meeting frequently to discuss recent cases allows the other members of the team to show support for their colleagues who have had difficult cases.
- Support for the patient's decision. It is important to focus on the fact that the woman made a positive informed choice to terminate a pregnancy based on the belief that she was preventing her unborn child from suffering and that this was the best option for her and her family.
- Away days. Scheduling time away from the clinic allows more relaxed discussions about policy, workload, and future developments. This time should make it easier for team members to discuss work-related anxiety.

- Social events. Occasional social gatherings may increase support for the team and allow team members to discuss work-related problems.
- External support. Sometimes additional counseling is needed, and these services must be made available. Some team members may feel shame if they need this support. To minimize negative feelings, team members should be told about these counseling services when they join the team, and the team should be reminded about their availability from time to time.

CONCLUSIONS

- Almost every woman who has antenatal care undergoes some form of screening; therefore, all health care professionals involved must be equipped to counsel and manage patients who have abnormal results.
- Health care professionals should focus on the principle that the aim of offering a screening test is to allow women and their partners to make informed choices about their pregnancy. This choice may include termination, but that is not a prerequisite for testing.
- Health care professionals should provide clinical, psychological, and social support to women throughout pregnancy, especially with respect to screening for fetal abnormality.
- Screening should be offered within a professional ethos of supporting the choices and decisions made by the woman and her family.
- Reflective practice should include consideration of the counseling process.

SUMMARY OF MANAGEMENT OPTIONS

Counseling and Management of an Abnormal Finding on a Screening or Diagnostic Test for Fetal Abnormality

Management Options	Quality of Evidence	Strength of Recommendation	References
Pretest Counseling			
Informed Consent			
Although a prenatal test can be presented as an opt-in or opt-out test, obtaining true informed consent fosters an ethos of opting in to testing.	IIb	B	8
Needs of Different Groups			
Counseling and diagnostic options should be offered according to the patient's clinical history, and access to services should not be restricted because of professional assumptions about the patient's cultural or ethnic background.	IIb	B	9,13
Content of Information			
Recommendations about information content should be followed (see Table 9–1).	IV	C	3,14
Affected individuals should be given access to information abut the long-term outlook.	IIb	B	16,17
Communication of Information			
Quality, peer-reviewed information, available in locally appropriate languages, should be used.	Ib IV	A C	15 24,25
Responsibility for Providing Patient Counseling			
Information may be given by a range of professionals, but a nondirective approach should be used.	III IV	B C	18 3

Continued

SUMMARY OF MANAGEMENT OPTIONS

Counseling and Management of an Abnormal Finding on a Screening or Diagnostic Test for Fetal Abnormality *(Continued)*

Management Options	Quality of Evidence	Strength of Recommendation	References
Communication of Test Results			
Arrangements for communication of results should be discussed with the woman and clearly documented in the records.	IV	C	3
Counseling for Screen-Positive Results			
General Issues			
To promote the patient's understanding of the meaning of a screen-positive result, risk figures should be presented in different formats and in the context of the background risk.	III	B	20
Decision to Have an Invasive Test			
Not all women with a screen-positive result will choose to proceed with an invasive diagnostic test.	III	B	27
Specific Screening Problems			
Women should be made aware of the limitations of screening, including false-positive and inconclusive results.	III	B	10,20
Problems with Diagnostic Tests			
When an unexpected or ambiguous result, such as a sex chromosome abnormality, is identified, referral for expert genetic counseling should be offered.	IIb	B	17,39,40,41
Timing of Diagnostic Procedures			
The options that would be available should a diagnosis be confirmed must be considered before a procedure is performed later than the second trimester.	IV	C	1,2
Counseling after Diagnosis			
Emotional Effect			
Acknowledgement of the profound emotional effect of a diagnosis of abnormality contributes to psychological adjustment.	III	B	45,49,52,56
Breaking Bad News			
Results should be given clearly and empathetically.	IIb	B	17,49
Decision Making			
Women should be supported in making a decision that is consistent with their personal values and circumstances, free of coercion.	IIb III	B B	46,47 48,52
Postdecision Care			
Continuing Pregnancy			
Continuing with an affected pregnancy should be presented as a valid choice.	III	B	54,55
Specialized postdelivery care should be provided.			

SUMMARY OF MANAGEMENT OPTIONS

Counseling and Management of an Abnormal Finding on a Screening or Diagnostic Test for Fetal Abnormality *(Continued)*

Management Options	Quality of Evidence	Strength of Recommendation	References
Termination			
Individualized care plans should consider the most appropriate method and setting for the termination.	IIb	B	48,56,60
Anticipatory guidance about bereavement and common feelings of guilt and responsibility should be offered.	III IIb	B B	48,56,60 49
Fathers			
Acknowledging the father's loss can reduce potential feelings of marginalization.	III	B	63,64
Staff Support			
The emotional toll on staff involved in prenatal diagnosis should be acknowledged. Support should be made available.	–	GPP	–

REFERENCES

1. Montgomery J: Legal issues in prenatal diagnosis in England. In Abramsky L, Chapple J (eds): Prenatal Diagnosis: The Human Side, 2nd ed. Cheltenham, UK, Nelson Thornes, 2003, pp 17–28.
2. Haddow JB: Legal issues in prenatal diagnosis in the USA. In Abramsky L, Chapple J (eds): Prenatal Diagnosis: The Human Side, 2nd ed. Cheltenham, UK, Nelson Thornes, 2003, pp 29–39.
3. Muir Gray JA, Worthington DJ: Antenatal screening for Down's syndrome: National Guidance on Policy and Quality Management. UK National Screening Committee, London, 2003.
4. Whittle MJ: Amniocentesis (8): Clinical Green Top Guidelines. London, Royal College of Obstetricians and Gynaecologists, 2000.
5. Report of the RCOG Ethics Committee: A consideration of the law and ethics in relation to late termination of pregnancy for fetal abnormality. London, Royal College of Obstetricians and Gynaecologists, 1998.
6. Midwives Information and Resource Service: www.midirs.org
7. Press N, Browner CH: Characteristics of women who refuse an offer of prenatal diagnosis. Am J Med Genet 1998;78:433–445.
8. Dormandy E, Michie S, Weinman J, Marteau TM: Variation in uptake of serum screening: The role of service delivery. Prenat Diagn 2002;22:67–69.
9. Press N, Browner C: Why women say yes to prenatal diagnosis. Soc Sci Med 1997;45:979–989.
10. Marteau TM, Dormandy E: Facilitating informed choice in prenatal testing: How well are we doing? Am J Med Genet 2001;106:185–189.
11. Gilbert L, Nichol J, Alex S, et al: Ethnic differences in the outcome of serum screening for Down's syndrome. BMJ 1996;312:94–95.
12. Saridogan E, Djahanbakhch O, Naftalin AA: Screening for Down's syndrome: Experience in an inner city health district. Br J Obstet Gynaecol 1996;108:1025–1211.
13. Sandall J, Grellier R, Ahmed S: Prenatal screening and diagnosis in a multicultural, multiethnic society. In Abramsky L, Chapple J (eds): Prenatal Diagnosis: The Human Side, 2nd ed. Cheltenham, UK, Nelson Thornes, 2003, pp 83–97.
14. RCOG: Ultrasound screening for fetal abnormalities: Report of the RCOG Working Party. London, Royal College of Obstetricians and Gynaecologists, 1997.
15. Murray J, Cuckle H, Sehmi I, et al: Quality of written information used in Down syndrome screening. Prenat Diagn 2001;21:138–142.
16. Williams C, Alderson P, Farsides B: What constitutes "balanced information" in the practitioners' portrayals of Down's syndrome? Midwifery 2002;18:230–237.
17. Abramsky L, Hall S, Levitan J, Marteau TM: What parents are told after prenatal diagnosis of a sex chromosome abnormality: Interview and questionnaire study. BMJ 2001;322: 463–466.
18. O'Cathlain A, Walters SJ, Nicholl JP, et al: Use of evidence based leaflets to promote informed choice in maternity care: Randomised controlled trial in everyday practice. BMJ 2002;324:643.
19. Thornton JG, Hewison J, Lilford RJ, Vail A: A randomized trial of three methods of giving information about prenatal testing. BMJ 1995;311(7013):1127–1130.
20. Marteau TM, Dormandy E: Facilitating informed choice in prenatal testing: How well are we doing? Am J Med Genet 2001;106:185–190.
21. Carroll JC, Brown JB, Reid AJ, Pugh P: Women's experience of maternal serum screening. Can Fam Physician 2000;46:614–620.
22. www.infochoice.org
23. www.marchofdimes.com
24. United Kingdom Association of Sonographers: Guidelines for professional working standards: Ultrasound practice. London, United Kingdom Association of Sonographers, 2001.
25. SATFA: Support after Termination for Abnormality: Guidelines for *ultrasonographers*. Rugby, England, Support after Termination for Abnormality, 1992.
26. Hollingsworth J, Daly-Jones E: The sonographer's dilemma. In Abramsky L, Chapple J (eds): Prenatal Diagnosis: The Human Side, 2nd ed. Cheltenham, UK, Nelson Thornes, 2003, pp 98–106.
27. Priest JH, FitzGerald JM, Haag MM, et al: Acceptance of amniocentesis by women in the state of Montana (USA) who are

screen positive for Down's syndrome. J Med Screen 1998;5:178–182.
28. Statham H, Green J: Serum screening for Down's syndrome: Some women's experiences. BMJ 1993;307:174–176.
29. Smith DK, Shaw RW, Marteau TM: Informed consent to undergo serum screening for Down's syndrome: The gap between policy and practice BMJ 1994;309:776.
30. Tymstra T: False positive results in screening tests: Experience of parents of children screened for congenital hypothyroidism Fam Pract 1986;3:92–96.
31. Marteau TM, Cook R, Kidd J, et al: Psychological effects of false positive results in prenatal screening for fetal abnormality: A prospective study. Prenat Diagn 1992;12:205–214.
32. Abuelo DN, Hopmann MR, Barsel-Bowers G, et al: Anxiety in women with low maternal serum alpha-fetoprotein screening results. Prenat Diagn 1991;11:381–385.
33. Mason GC, Baillie C: Counselling should be provided before parents are told of presence of ultrasonographic 'soft markers' of fetal abnormality. BMJ 1997;315:189–190.
34. Marteau TM: Screening in practice: Reducing the psychological costs. BMJ 1990;301:26–28.
35. Hyett J, Perdu M, Sharland G, et al: Using fetal nuchal translucency to screen for major congenital cardiac defects at 10–14 weeks of gestation: Population based cohort study. BMJ 1999;318(7176):81–85.
36. Souka AP, Snijders RJ, Novakov A, et al: Defects and syndromes in chromosomally normal fetuses with increased nuchal translucency thickness at 10–14 weeks of gestation. Ultrasound Obstet Gynecol 1998;11:391–400.
37. Saari-Kemppainen A, Karjalainen O, Ylostalo P, Heinonen OP: Fetal anomalies in a controlled one-stage ultrasound screening trial: A report from the Helsinki Ultrasound Trial. J Perinat Med 1994;22:279–289.
38. Biesecker B: Prenatal diagnoses of sex chromosome conditions. BMJ 2001;322:463–466.
39. Clayton-Smith J, Andrews T, Donnai D: Genetic counselling and parental decisions following antenatal diagnosis of sex chromosome aneuploidies. J Obstet Gynaecol 1989;10:5–7.
40. Meschede D, Louwen F, Nippert I, et al: Low rates of pregnancy termination for prenatally diagnosed Klinefelter syndrome and other sex chromosome polysomies. Am J Med Genet 1998;80:330–334.
41. Christian SM, Koehn D, Pillay R, et al: Parental decisions following prenatal diagnosis of sex chromosome aneuploidy: A trend over time. Prenat Diagn 2000;20:37–40.
42. Garrett C, Margerison L: Difficult decisions in prenatal diagnosis. In Abramsky L, Chapple J (eds): Prenatal Diagnosis: The Human Side, 2nd ed. Cheltenham, UK, Nelson Thornes, 2003, pp 146–163.
43. Lucassen A, Parker M: Revealing false paternity: Some ethical considerations. Lancet 2001;57:1033–1035.
44. Kennell JH, Slyter H, Klaus MH: The mourning response of parents to the death of a newborn infant. N Engl J Med 1970;283:344–349.
45. Seller M, Barnes C, Ross S, et al: Grief and mid-trimester fetal loss. Prenat Diagn 1993;13:341–348.
46. Schechtman KB, Gray DL, Baty JD, Rothman SM: Decision-making for termination of pregnancies with fetal anomalies: Analysis of 53,000 pregnancies. Obstet Gynecol 2002;99: 216–222.
47. Kramer RL, Jarve RK, Yaron Y, et al: Determinants of parental decisions after the prenatal diagnosis of Down syndrome. Am J Med Genet 1998;79:172–174.
48. Statham H: Prenatal diagnosis of fetal abnormality: The decision to terminate the pregnancy and the psychological consequences. Fetal Matern Med Rev 2002;13:213–247.
49. White-van Mourik MCA, Connor JM, Ferguson-Smith MA: The psychosocial sequelae of a second-trimester termination of pregnancy for fetal abnormality. Prenat Diagn 1992;12:189–204.
50. Dimavicius J: Antenatal screening for Down's syndrome. Lancet 1998;352:1862.
51. Green J: Obstetricians' views on prenatal diagnosis and termination of pregnancy: 1980 compared with 1993. Br J Obstet Gynaecol 1995;102:228–232.
52. Chitty L, Barnes CA, Berry C: For debate: Continuing with pregnancy after a diagnosis of lethal abnormality. Experience of five couples and recommendations for management. BMJ 1996;313:478–480.
53. Fonda Allen JS, Mulhauser LC: Genetic counseling after abnormal prenatal diagnosis: Facilitating coping in families who continue their pregnancies. J Genet Counsel 1995;4:251–266.
54. ARC: Antenatal Results and Choices. London, ARC, 1999.
55. A Heartbreaking Choice: www.aheartbreakingchoice.com, 2003.
56. Suslak L, Scherer A, Rodriguez G: A support group for couples who have terminated a pregnancy after prenatal diagnosis: Recurrent themes and observations. J Genet Counsel 1995;4:169–178.
57. Maternal and Child Health Research Consortium: Confidential enquiry into stillbirths and deaths in infancy: 8th annual report. London, Maternal and Child Health Research Consortium, 2001.
58. Fox R, Pillai M, Porter H, Gill G: The management of late fetal death: A guide to comprehensive care. Br J Obstet Gynaecol 1997;107:4–10.
59. Blumberg B: The emotional implications of prenatal diagnosis. In Emery EH, Pullen IM (eds): Psychological Aspects of Genetic Counselling. London, Academic Press, 1984, pp 201–217.
60. Donnai P, Charles N, Harris R: Attitudes of patients after genetic termination of pregnancy. BMJ 1981;282:621–622.
61. Black RB: A 1 and 6 month follow-up of prenatal diagnosis patients who lost pregnancies. Prenat Diagn 1989;9:795–804.
62. Hall RD: Parents' reactions to termination of pregnancy for fetal abnormality: From a father's point of view. In Abramsky L, Chapple J (eds): Prenatal Diagnosis: The Human Side, 2nd ed. Cheltenham, UK, Nelson Thornes, 2003, pp 199–204.
63. Robson FM: Yes! A chance to tell my side of the story. A case study of a male partner of a woman undergoing termination of pregnancy for foetal abnormality. J Health Psychol 2002;7:183–193.
64. Wiggins J: The human side of carers. In Abramsky L, Chapple J (eds): Prenatal Diagnosis: The Human Side, 2nd ed. Cheltenham, UK, Nelson Thornes, 2003, pp 224–236.

CHAPTER 10

Invasive Procedures for Antenatal Diagnosis

Alyson Hunter / Peter Soothill

INTRODUCTION

Ultrasound in pregnancy fostered the development of invasive techniques to assist in antenatal diagnosis. Methods such as chorionic villus sampling (CVS), amniocentesis, fetal blood sampling (FBS), and fetal tissue biopsy allow testing of fetal materials for chromosomal, genetic, and biochemical abnormalities. The type of procedure selected depends on many factors, including the indication, the gestational age, and how soon the result is needed. Possible applications are increasing rapidly with advances in human genetics and the evolution of molecular tools. All invasive in utero diagnostic techniques carry a risk of fetal injury or death. These risks must be properly explained to the parents so that informed consent can be obtained. Noninvasive approaches, such as measuring free fetal DNA in the mother's blood, show great promise, but are clinically used only in specific areas, such as fetal blood grouping.[1] This chapter summarizes the indications, methods, and complications of the most common invasive diagnostic methods.

ISSUES COMMON TO ALL INVASIVE DIAGNOSTIC TECHNIQUES

All of the techniques described in this chapter share certain features.

Guidelines for Training

The Royal College of Obstetricians and Gynaecologists published guidelines for training in antenatal invasive diagnostic methods, and these guidelines can serve as a global model.[2] Trainees in obstetrics and gynecology should perform at least 30 amniocenteses under supervision before they act independently. After they complete training, physicians who perform amniocentesis should perform at least 30 per year. The College also recommends that amniocentesis for multiple gestation be performed in a tertiary fetal medicine unit. Training in CVS and FBS is not part of general obstetric training and is usually limited to trainees who specialize in fetal and maternal medicine. Units that perform more complex fetal procedures should perform enough procedures each year to maintain skills. They should periodically audit the results and make these available to patients and colleagues. A reasonable minimum number of complex procedures is 12 per year.

Consent

The procedure, its goals, and likely or significant complications must be explained in language that is understandable to the patient so that written informed consent can be given. The specific considerations for each procedure are discussed later.

Sampling Site

Ultrasound is used to determine the best site to obtain the sample, considering the target size, needle length, needle path, and potential injury to structures in the path. The skin site for needle insertion is planned, but the position chosen reflects the ultrasound-guided technique used.

Ultrasound-Guided Needling Technique

Two approaches to ultrasound-guided needling are used: needle guide and freehand.

Needle Guide

The needle guide technique uses a sector or curvilinear ultrasound transducer with a guide that has an attached needle channel. Lines on the ultrasound screen indicate the path of the needle when inserted down the guide. The transducer is moved until these lines cross the intended target. This approach allows the use of thinner needles (i.e., 22–26 gauge) than those needed for a freehand procedure (i.e., 20–22 gauge). Despite the use of a thinner needle and the fact that the entire length of the needle is not usually seen, the tip is visible as a bright dot (Fig. 10–1). Some suggest that because the needle is thin and its movement confined to a single plane, the complication rate may be lower than with the freehand technique.[3] The guide does not seem to increase the need to remove and reinsert the needle, nor is there a relationship between the complication rate and the number of insertions.

Freehand

The freehand technique uses a curvilinear or linear ultrasound transducer. The ultrasound transducer is moved until the intended sampling site is identified and appears on one side of the ultrasound screen, with the skin insertion point on the other. The intended needle path is nearly perpendicular to the ultrasound beam, allowing the entire length of the needle to be imaged (Fig. 10–2). The freehand technique allows the operator to image the entire length of the needle and compensate for a suboptimal insertion or adjust to changes during the procedure (e.g., contractions, interfering fetal movements). It also may facilitate rare procedures in which multiple sites are sampled.

Some operators prefer to have an assistant control the scanning transducer, but then the operator forfeits control of the intended needle path. Others prefer a single operator. With this approach, one hand holds the needle and the other holds the ultrasound transducer. An assistant is required to withdraw the needle stylet, fix a syringe, aspirate at the right time, and place the sample in appropriate containers without spillage, contamination, or mislabeling.

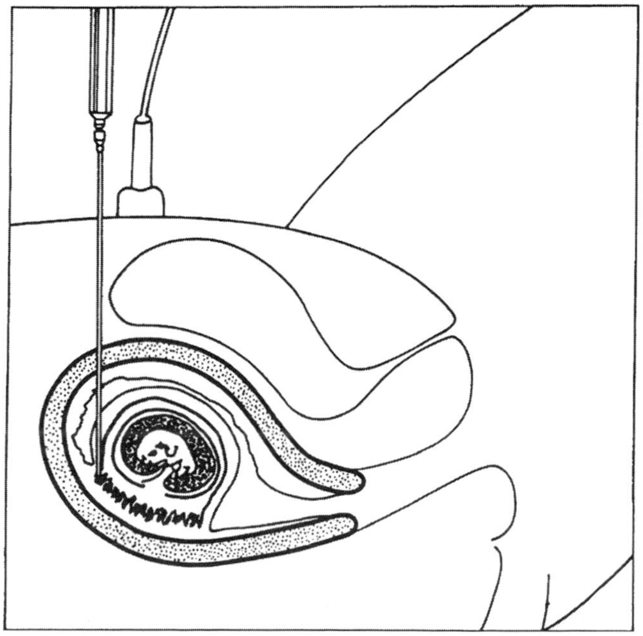

FIGURE 10–1
Line drawing of chorionic villus sampling via the transabdominal route showing the needle.

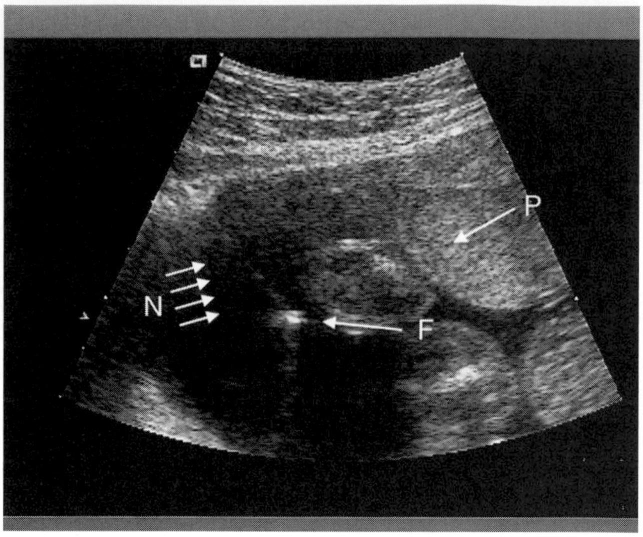

FIGURE 10–2
Ultrasound view of an amniocentesis needle (N) entering a pool of amniotic fluid. F, fluid; P, placenta.

Preparation

The atmosphere should be informal, and any additional staff required should be present for the procedure and introduced to the patient. Anything that gives the patient an image of an "operation" (e.g., surgical masks, hats, drapes) should be minimized or replaced by a scrupulous "no-touch" technique. The length of the needle required depends on abdominal wall thickness, amniotic fluid volume, and fetal and placental positions. An 8- to 12-cm needle is usually sufficient, but if in doubt, the distance should be measured on the screen before the procedure. Detailed ultrasound examination of the fetus is performed before the procedure because the discovery of structural defects, impaired growth, or other problems may alter the physician's and patients' choice. New ultrasound findings may make the procedure unnecessary, or help subsequently, when there is an unusual chromosomal finding such as mosaicism.

Needle Path Selection

The target is visualized on screen, and the transducer is rotated through 180° until a path that avoids fetal parts and maternal vessels is identified. With the freehand technique, the best skin insertion point is determined by observing sonographically the effect of digital pressure on the maternal abdomen. The transducer is adjusted until the sampling site and the skin insertion point are on opposite sides of the screen.

Antiseptic and Anesthetic

The skin insertion site is scrupulously cleaned with antiseptic solution (e.g., chlorhexidine). Procedures that require larger than a 22-gauge needle may be helped by local anesthetic, which is injected first into the skin and then into the abdominal and uterine peritoneum. Anesthetic injection can help to confirm the needle angle required to follow the intended path and may decrease the need to change the direction of the sampling needle during the procedure. Patients who underwent amniocentesis with a 22-gauge needle with and without anesthesia reported that the anesthetic injection is more painful than the procedure.

Postprocedure Considerations

The patient should be shown both the fetus and the motion of the fetal heart on the ultrasound monitor after the procedure. The sample is carefully labeled, and the details are confirmed by the woman before the sample is taken to the laboratory. The information submitted to the laboratory must be sufficient for testing to be done and diagnosis to be made. It should include information about consent, including permission to store DNA and maintain cells lines, if applicable.

Alloimmunization

An invasive procedure associated with placental bleeding doubles the risk of Rhesus sensitivity.[4–6] After an invasive intrauterine procedure, 500 IU rather than 250 IU anti-D immunoglobulin can be given intramuscularly to an at-risk Rhesus-negative woman.

Multiple Pregnancies

In women with multiple pregnancies, invasive procedures should be performed in a fetal medicine unit.[2] The chorionicity should be determined and the placental implantation site mapped in the first trimester.[7] In monochorionic pregnancies, a single amniotic fluid sample may be sufficient unless ultrasound shows discordant abnormalities. In dichorionic pregnancies, both sacs should be sampled separately, either with a single needle through the intertwin septum or with two separate maternal abdominal punctures.[8,9] The operator should be able and willing to perform a selective feticide if an abnormal result is discordant. In skilled hands, ultrasound guidance eliminates the need for indigo carmine. Potentially harmful dyes, such as methylene blue, should not be used.[10] Fetal zygosity can be determined from DNA when there is doubt or when the fetuses are at risk for inheritable syndromes.[11]

Complications

The loss rate after a diagnostic invasive procedure is a combination of the procedure-related loss rate and the background loss rate. The background loss rate is much higher if the fetus has an anomaly (e.g., chromosomal abnormality, intrauterine growth restriction, fetal hydrops).[12] The procedure-related loss rate is the product of many factors, including maternal age, operator experience, type of procedure, and difficulties experienced during the procedure.[3,13] The gestational age at the time of the procedure is also relevant. In one study, the rate of fetal loss in older women after transabdominal and transcervical CVS was 5.8% and 6.2%, respectively, if done before 12 weeks, but 2.4% thereafter.[14] Some portion of the excess loss early in gestation reflects losses destined to occur. Early CVS and diagnosis of aneuploidy may result in termination, with all of the physical and psychological implications for the parents, whereas delayed CVS or amniocentesis may, by virtue of the later gestation, allow time for spontaneous loss to precede the planned procedure. Several multicenter studies did not show consistent procedure-related differences with regard to the safety of CVS compared with other methods.[15,16]

The procedure-related loss rate for CVS, amniocentesis, and FBS is reported in many studies, including those listed in Table 10–1.[3,4,15,17–30] No standard criteria are used to determine background loss rates. Postprocedural loss rates were included up to 28 weeks and up to term in some studies.[4,28] Others suggest that most procedure-related losses occur within 2 weeks of the procedure (Table 10–2).[12] These procedures should be confined to centers with volumes large enough to calculate their own loss rates rather than to quote the rates of other units.

SPECIFIC PROCEDURES

Chorionic Villus Sampling

Introduction

CVS, or placental biopsy, is performed from 11 weeks onward and is used to diagnose many chromosomal and genetic conditions. CVS is usually performed by transabdominal needle aspiration, although some practitioners use a transcervical technique, with catheter aspiration or biopsy. Some suggest that the highest success rates are achieved when the clinician is comfortable using either approach.

Indications

Fetal trophoblast cells, especially the mesenchymal core of the villi, divide rapidly. The advantage of first-trimester CVS is rapid diagnosis in early gestation. If an abnormality is detected, surgical termination, rather than medical induction of labor, can be offered.

TABLE 10–1

Reported Outcomes after Invasive Prenatal Diagnostic Procedures[3,4,17–30]

SERIES	PROCEDURE	STUDY TYPE	REPORTING OF OUTCOMES
MRC, 1978	Amnio	Controlled	Reported outcome until the end of the neonatal period
Tabor et al., 1986	Amnio	RCT	Reported outcome as SA (<16 wk and >16 wk), induced abortion, SB (<36 wk >36 wk)
Canadian trial, 1989	Amnio, CVS	RCT	Reported outcome as induced abortion, loss ≤140 days, between 141–196 days postprocedure
Smidt-Jensen et al., 1992	Amnio, CVS	RCT	Reported outcome until the neonatal period; classified as spontaneous loss before the procedure, elective abortion, postprocedure, and unintentional loss
Johnson et al., 1996	Amnio	RCT	Reported outcome as postprocedure total fetal loss rate until term
Nicolaides et al., 1996	Amnio, CVS	Observational	Outcomes classified as total loss (spontaneous and induced) and spontaneous loss (IUD/NND)
Sundberg et al., 1997	Amnio, CVS	Observational	Reported outcome as total fetal loss rate and neonatal morbidity
Hanson et al., 1987	Amnio, CVS	Observational	Reported outcomes <2 wk, >2 wk, and 28 wk postprocedure
CEMAT, 1998	Amnio	RT	Reported loss as preprocedure abortion, postprocedure abortion (20 weeks), SB, LB, and NND
Rhoads et al., 1989	CVS	Observational	Reported outcome until the end of the neonatal period
MRC European Trial, 1991	CVS	RCT	Reported outcome as spontaneous fetal death <28 wk, termination, SB, and NND
Wapner et al., 1997	CVS	Observational	Reported outcomes until 28 wk
Maxwell et al., 1991	FBS	Observational	Reported losses in pregnancies with normal fetal anatomy, fetal abnormalities, fetal physiologic assessment, nonimmune hydrops; 2-wk cutoff for procedure-related loss
Anandkumar et al., 1993	FBS	Observational	Reported loss when FBS was done for fetal abnormality on scan, normal fetuses, nonimmune hydrops, advanced maternal age; 2-wk cutoff for procedure-related loss
Ghidini et al., 1993	FBS	Observational	Reported outcomes in low-risk groups as total fetal losses <28 wk and >28 wk
Wilson et al., 1994	FBS	Observational	Reported procedure-related loss in cases with normal fetal growth and anatomy, fetal abnormality, or IUGR; 1-wk cutoff for procedure-related loss
Weiner and Okumura, 1996	FBS	Observational	Reported outcomes until term; 2-wk cutoff for procedure-related loss

Amnio, amniocentesis; CVS, chorionic villus sampling; FBS, fetal blood sample; IUD, intrauterine death; IUGR, intrauterine growth restriction; NND, neonatal death; RCT, randomized controlled trial; RT, randomized trial; SA, spontaneous abortion; SB, stillbirth.

Early detection of chromosomal disorders is the most common indication. The introduction and growing availability of first-trimester screening for Down syndrome (e.g., nuchal translucency measurement) has increased the importance of this technique. Noninvasive approaches, such as measuring maternal plasma free fetal DNA, may make invasive testing for sexing unnecessary.[31] Because of the increasing number of diagnosable monogenic disorders, couples with a family history of a genetic disorder should be offered genetic counseling, either before conception or early in pregnancy. Many laboratories provide a rapid direct preparation of the fetal karyotype within 2 to 5 days or fluorescent in situ hybridization (FISH) of chromosomes 13, 18, 21, and Y, if requested. Fetal cells are also cultured for more detailed analysis.

CVS can be used at any time in gestation, and it is a very successful way to obtain a karyotype after delivery when the fetus has died. Although CVS is possible throughout gestation, the cytotrophoblast divides more slowly with advancing gestation, and other procedures, such as amniocentesis and FBS, may be more appropriate.

TABLE 10–2

Overview of Pregnancy Losses after Amniocentesis, Chorionic Villus Sampling, and Fetal Blood Sampling as Classified

TEST	TOTAL	MINUS	KNOWN LETHAL CONDITION	MINUS	> 2/52	= PROCEDURE-RELATED
Amniocentesis	10 (1.8%)		3		3	4 (0.7%)
Chorionic villus sampling	18 (4.1%)		14		3	1 (0.23%)
Fetal blood sampling	18 (10.7%)		16		0	2 (1.19%)

From Nanal RKP, Soothill PW: A classification of pregnancy loss after invasive prenatal diagnostic procedures: An approach to allow comparison of units with a different case mix. Prenat Diagn 2003; 23:488–492.

PROCEDURE

CHORIONIC VILLUS SAMPLING

Consent

The procedure should be described to the patient. Counseling must include the aims of the CVS (i.e., karyotype, DNA analysis) and the risk of a serious complication (often described as 1%), including abortion, either procedure-related or background, should be quoted. The risk of limb defects should also be mentioned. The risk is minimal after 10 weeks. The limitations of a karyotype and the risks of unrelated abnormalities that are not detected by a karyotype should be explained. Patients should also be informed of the small chance that testing will show confined placental mosaicism or sex chromosome abnormality and the possiblility of a further invasive technique to confirm a diagnosis such as amniocentesis or fetal blood sampling. Alternative diagnostic techniques may be discussed. Only after the counseling process is complete is the patient asked to provide written consent.

Sampling Site

The ideal target is a thick part of the placenta that can be sampled at an angle that allows a long needle path through the placenta and avoids a perpendicular path to the chorionic plate (see Fig. 10–1). Rarely, at approximately 11 weeks, transabdominal CVS is difficult if the uterus is retroverted, the placenta is posterior, and a lateral approach is not possible. Some operators switch to a transcervical approach, but we ask the patient to return in a week, when sampling may be easier.

Target Puncture

Transabdominal CVS can be done either freehand or with a needle guide. With the "double-needle" technique, after a local anesthetic has been administered, the first needle is advanced through the maternal skin, through the uterine wall, and into the placenta. The introducing stylet is removed, and a second needle is passed into the placenta and attached to a syringe that contains normal saline. The placental villi are then aspirated.[32,33] By drawing the finer needle into the outer needle during aspiration, the sharp bevel of the first needle seems to cut the villi, reducing the need for needle movement and presumably reducing placental trauma. A placental biopsy forceps may also be used through an outer guide needle. With the double-needle technique, if the tip is inserted correctly into the placenta, maternal contamination should not occur. If a single needle is used, the aspirated tissue should be dissected under the microscope to exclude maternal contamination. Whatever technique is selected, the sample is placed in a suitable CVS medium before it is transferred to the cytogenetics laboratory.

Maternal contamination of chorionic cell cultures may lead to a false-negative diagnosis, particularly when polymerase chain reaction amplification is used and in some biochemical examinations. Operator experience reduces the risk of maternal cell contamination.

Transcervical CVS

This approach is less common now because of an apparent increased risk of fetal loss.[16,34,35] Some practitioners consider this approach useful in high-risk patients who require early diagnosis. It is also helpful when the uterus is retroverted and the placenta is posterior or when an anterior wall leiomyoma makes an abdominal approach difficult. A bendable polyethylene catheter with a metal obturator is introduced through the cervix and advanced into the placenta under ultrasound guidance. A syringe that is partially filled with saline is attached to the hub and a vacuum created to aspirate 10 to 50 mg of tissue, which is then rinsed into a Petri dish. Some units prefer curved biopsy forceps.[36]

Complications

Canadian, Danish, and American multicenter trials found no significant difference in procedure-related loss rates between the first and second trimesters. A 1% fetal loss rate is usually quoted for amniocentesis and CVS.[1] A rate of 0.25% is reported for CVS and amniocentesis.[20]

Some reports[37,38] suggested that first-trimester CVS (including those performed as early as 6–7 weeks) may be associated with severe limb defects. These defects were not observed in CVS performed after 11 weeks' gestation. The World Health Organization (WHO) International Registry for Limb Defects after CVS found no difference in the prevalence of limb defects after CVS compared with the background population.[39] Therefore, during counseling, it is standard practice to indicate that there is no increased incidence of limb defects after 10 weeks.

PLACENTAL MOSAICISM

Confined placental mosaicism occurs in approximately 1% of samples.[40] Analyzing several cultures makes it easier to detect in vitro changes, because they are usually present in a single culture (pseudomosaicism). However, the same finding in several or all of the cultures increases the likelihood of true mosaicism, either confined to the placenta or present in both placenta and fetus. In this case, another fetal tissue, such as blood or amniotic fluid, should be tested. The finding of markers or a structural abnormality on ultrasound is very important and makes it much less likely that the results are caused by confined placental mosaicism.

LATE PLACENTAL BIOPSY

Several small series indicate that late placental biopsy is both safe and reliable for diagnosis. The loss rate is similar to that of first-trimester CVS.[41,42]

Conclusion

CVS provides a rich source of fetal cells or DNA for analysis of karyotypic and genetic disorders. It is usually performed after 11 weeks, typically by a transabdominal route.

One advantage of first-trimester CVS is that an abnormal result allows surgical termination, if desired. Karyotypic analysis can be accomplished by direct preparation and culture. Placental mosaicism complicates 1% of samples.

SUMMARY OF MANAGEMENT OPTIONS

Chorionic Villus Sampling and Placental Biopsy

Management Options	Quality of Evidence	Strength of Recommendation	References
Indications			
Genetic	–	GPP	–
Fluorescent in situ hybridization karyotype, DNA			
Procedural Options			
Transabdominal (less commonly transcervical)	–	GPP	–
Aspiration or biopsy			
Complications			
Fetal loss	III	B	–
Fear of limb-reduction defects (gestation-dependent)	IIb	B	3–5,13
Placental mosaicism		GPP	–
Alloimmunization	III	B	–
Maternal contamination	III	GPP	–

Amniocentesis

Introduction

Amniotic fluid contains amniocytes in addition to fetal cells from the skin, genitourinary system, and gut, along with biochemical products that may be removed for analysis. Amniocentesis is performed only under continuous ultrasound guidance.[2]

Indications

GENETIC

Amniocentesis is usually performed to determine a fetal karyotype. Indications for fetal karyotyping include an abnormal screening test result for trisomy 21, advanced maternal age, a sonographically detected structural abnormality, previous aneuploidy, and known chromosomal translocation in either partner.

The amniotic fluid is labeled, the information is examined by the patient for accuracy, and the sample is sent promptly to the cytogenetics laboratory for analysis. The amniocytes are studied during the metaphase stage of cell division. Although standard culture techniques require 2 to 3 weeks, newer methods, with the cells grown on a cover slip, allow a complete analysis in 7 to 10 days.[43] Approximately 0.5% of cultures are unsuccessful; less often, maternal contamination complicates the diagnosis.[44] Fewer than 0.4% of cultures show evidence of pseudomosaicism or true mosaicism.[45,46] FBS may be helpful, but a normal result does not guarantee that all is well.

Direct DNA probing of interphase chromosomes by FISH can be used to detect known deletions, such as 22q in at-risk pregnancies, in addition to rapid diagnosis of trisomy 13, 18, and 21.[47,48] Although a positive test result is reliable, detecting 90% or more of chromosomal abnormalities, a normal FISH result should be confirmed by culture. Polymerase chain reaction (PCR)-based primers are now used with DNA from amniotic fluid samples to determine almost all potentially relevant fetal RBC and platelet genotypes.[49,50] Studies of free fetal DNA in maternal blood may further reduce the need for amniocentesis. In some countries, it is already used to detect fetal D status as part of routine prenatal care.[31]

BIOCHEMISTRY

Amniocentesis to diagnose inborn errors of metabolism and cystic fibrosis by measuring the activity of fetal enzymes and their byproducts has been largely replaced by molecular DNA analysis. Likewise, amniocentesis to measure α-fetoprotein and acetylcholinesterase to diagnose a neural tube defect is rarely necessary because of the reliability of ultrasonography.[51]

FETAL INFECTION

Cytomegalovirus is excreted in fetal urine, and fetal infection is reliably detected by culture of amniotic fluid.[52,53] However, PCR technology is the method of choice for the antenatal diagnosis of fetal viral infection, because many viruses grow poorly in clinical laboratories (see Chapter 27). PCR has replaced the traditional mouse inoculation test for toxoplasmosis because it can be used earlier in pregnancy and has greater sensitivity (see Chapter 33).[54] As with traditional methods, a false-negative result may occur if there has been insufficient time since the maternal infection for transplacental passage to occur.

CHORIOAMNIONITIS

Up to 97% of women with preterm premature rupture of the membranes (PPROM)[55] can be successfully sampled and the specimen assessed by direct microscopy, Gram stain, and culture. It is unclear whether the information gained in women with PPROM changes the clinical outcome. No randomized trial supports the use of routine amniocentesis to diagnose chorioamnionitis in women with either preterm labor or PPROM. Amniocentesis may be useful when the woman is asymptomatic and fetal infection is suspected. Between 17% and 34% of asymptomatic women with PPROM have positive culture findings,[55] allowing for earlier diagnosis and treatment.[56] However, most women with positive culture findings deliver within 48 hours, and there is inadequate information to guide antibiotic selection.

FETAL LUNG MATURITY

Improved gestational dating, appropriate use of corticosteroids, and a growing understanding of the timing of iatrogenic premature delivery has nearly eliminated the need for amniotic fluid analysis to assess fetal lung maturity.[57]

EARLY AMNIOCENTESIS

Some hoped that early amniocentesis (before 15 weeks) would be an alternative to CVS.[22,58,59] However, the risks of early amniocentesis, including spontaneous abortion, stillbirth, and neonatal death, are greater than those of CVS.[21] The CEMAT group concluded that early amniocentesis should be performed only in special circumstances because of the higher fetal loss rate and incidence of talipes with early versus second-trimester amniocentesis.[25] The risk of membrane rupture is particularly high when performed before 13 completed weeks, possibly because, at this stage, the amnion is not adherent to the chorion and so is more likely to rupture. Several other studies found an increased risk of oligohydramnios and associated orthopedic abnormalities, including talipes equinovarus.[21,60] Tenting of the amniotic membrane and the smaller amount of fluid in the amniotic sac before 15 weeks increase the incidence of a "dry" tap caused by tenting of the membranes.[61] The sample is smaller and there are fewer cells per milliliter, although a higher percentage of cells is dividing actively. Djalali and colleagues[62] reported that longer culture times were required after early amniocentesis.

PROCEDURE

AMNIOCENTESIS

Amniocentesis is performed under ultrasound guidance after 15 weeks' gestation. A typical karyotypic study requires the removal of 15 to 20 mL amniotic fluid.[2] Removal of larger volumes should be avoided unless necessary for specific tests.

Antiseptic and Anesthetic

Local anesthetic is not normally required for diagnostic amniocentesis.

Target Puncture

Under ultrasound guidance, the needle is advanced into the targeted pool of amniotic fluid, with care taken to avoid the fetus, placenta, and cord (see Fig. 10–2). If the freehand technique is used, the ultrasound beam is directed so that the length of the needle is visualized, allowing the operator to alter the course in response to fetal movements and contractions. When the tip of the needle reaches the targeted location, 1 to 2 mL amniotic fluid is aspirated and discarded to avoid maternal contamination. Approximately 15 to 20 mL fluid is aspirated and sent for analysis. To prevent maternal contamination, the syringe is removed from the hub before the needle is withdrawn from the patient.

Complications

Early studies, including CEMAT, reported a total loss rate of 3.2% after amniocentesis.[25,63] These losses are believed to reflect, at least in part, the large needles used (>19 gauge) as well as unsuccessful attempts. The British Working Party on Amniocentesis reported a 2.4% total fetal loss rate before 28 weeks (stillbirth rate of 1.2% vs. 0.8% in control subjects) and neonatal death (0.5% control subjects), but concluded that the loss rate attributed directly to amniocentesis was 1.5%.[4] A more randomized trial of low-risk women suggested a 1% risk of spontaneous abortion after amniocentesis.[1] Our study of fetal loss after amniocentesis (defined as the total loss rate minus known lethal condition minus losses beyond 2 weeks postprocedure) was 0.7%.[12] Perforating the placenta increases the relative risk of loss 2.6 times and increases the maternal serum α-fetoprotein level 8.3 times.[64] The transplacental route should be avoided unless no other option is available.

Although no randomized controlled trials assessed the procedure-related loss rate from amniocentesis in multiple pregnancies, case–control studies suggest that the loss rate is only slightly higher than the background rate.[12,65]

OLIGOHYDRAMNIOS

A report by the Medical Research Council[4] noted that 2% of amniocenteses are associated with chronic leakage of amniotic fluid. There are variable reports of an increased prevalence of neonatal respiratory morbidity after amniocentesis; the small risk of oligohydramnios after amniocentesis may contribute to this complication.[1,4,66] Similarly, talipes equinovarus is rarely attributable to amniocentesis, and only when there is oligohydramnios.

FETAL TRAUMA

Inadvertent puncture of the fetus during amniocentesis has not been not reported in a large series when the procedure was performed under continuous ultrasound guidance by experienced operators.[17] Several case reports suggest an association between amniocentesis and skin dimpling, fistulae, cord hematoma, and corneal perforation.[67–69] Because intended fetal puncture rarely leaves a mark and similar findings occur in neonates who did not undergo amniocentesis, the association is dubious.

Conclusion

Amniocentesis after 15 weeks is the most widely performed antenatal diagnostic technique. It is relatively simple to perform, and although a fetal karyotype is the most common reason for amniocentesis, the procedure has many indications. The use of FISH and PCR has steadily reduced the amount of material needed for testing and the time needed to obtain a result.

SUMMARY OF MANAGEMENT OPTIONS

Amniocentesis

Management Options	Quality of Evidence	Strength of Recommendation	References
Indications			
Chromosome analysis: fluorescent in situ hybridization, PCR, karyotype	–	GPP	–
DNA diagnosis: single-gene disorders (e.g., Huntingdon), X-linked disorders	–	GPP	–
Biochemistry: α-fetoprotein, acetylcholinesterase	–	GPP	–
Fetal infection: toxoplasmosis, cytomegalovirus	–	GPP	–
Chorioamnionitis	–	GPP	–
Lung maturity	–	GPP	–
Fetal therapy or amniodrainage	–	GPP	–
Complications			
Fetal loss			
Experience of operator increased with early amniocentesis	III	B	–
	IIb	A	–
Chorioamnionitis	III	C	3–5,16
Preterm premature rupture of the membranes, oligohydramnios	IIa	B	–
Alloimmunization	III	B	–
Maternal contamination	III	GPP	–

Fetal Blood Sampling (FBS)

Introduction

Fetal blood was first obtained during labor from the capillary circulation of the presenting part.[70] FBS in a continuing pregnancy was first undertaken transabdominally by fetoscopy to diagnose severe inherited diseases, with termination considered if the fetus was affected. Cordocentesis was first reported two decades ago.[71] The development of medical approaches to fetal disease has made the role of fetal phlebotomy (typically by cordocentesis) comparable to that in postnatal medicine.

Indications

Indications for FBS may be grouped into diagnostic and therapeutic areas. FBS is indicated when the potential benefit of a change in management outweighs the procedure-related risks.

Diagnostic Uses

CHROMOSOMAL ABNORMALITIES

The rapid rate at which white blood cells divide allows a high-quality karyotype with good chromosome banding to be obtained within 48 to 72 hours. The most common indication for a rapid karyotype is fetal malformation or early-onset fetal growth restriction detected by ultrasonography. Other problems that can be resolved by a fetal blood cytogenetic analysis include possible mosaicism, culture failure after either amniocentesis or placental biopsy, fetal karyotyping in a woman who seeks care late in pregnancy, and antenatal diagnosis of fragile X syndrome. For some indications, the application of FISH to amniocytes has replaced FBS.

SINGLE-GENE DEFECTS

FBS can diagnose hemoglobinopathies, coagulopathies, severe combined immunodeficiency, chronic granulomatous disease, and some metabolic disorders.[72] FBS is performed less often for antenatal diagnosis of single-gene disorders because many can be diagnosed earlier in gestation by applying various DNA techniques to amniocytes. FBS is important for at-risk patients who seek care late in pregnancy and when DNA analysis is not possible.

ANEMIA

Although various indirect methods are used to assess fetal anemia (see Chapter 14), the definitive test before and after birth is measurement of the hemoglobin concentration. This may be required in maternal red cell alloimmunization[72] and some cases of nonimmune hydrops.[73] The development of middle cerebral artery Doppler peak velocity greatly enhanced the likelihood of detecting anemia.[7]

THROMBOCYTOPENIA

Severe fetal thrombocytopenia as a result of alloimmune thrombocytopenia may lead to cerebral hemorrhage before, during, or after birth and may cause mental handicap or death (see Chapter 15). The fetal platelet count can be measured to guide diagnosis and treatment.

HYPOXIA AND ACIDOSIS

Fetal acidemia may be excluded by Doppler studies of the fetal vasculature (see Chapters 11 and 12). Suspected fetal hypoxia or acidemia can be confirmed or refuted by fetal blood gas analysis.[74] Increasing evidence shows that chronic fetal acidemia is associated with impaired long-term neurodevelopment.[75] However, no convincing evidence shows that the benefits of fetal acid–base status outweigh the risks of FBS, and it is rarely indicated.

INFECTION

Appropriate fetal blood tests (e.g., infection-specific fetal immunoglobulin M or detection of specific genomic material by PCR) can determine whether maternal infection has led to fetal infection. However, the difference between being "infected" and "affected" (i.e., damaged) must not be forgotten. Fetal blood tests may be unnecessary if the results of an amniotic fluid sample (e.g., a positive PCR result) agree with ultrasound findings (e.g., hydrocephalus).

MONITORING OF TRANSPLACENTAL THERAPY

Some fetal diseases are treated by drugs that are given to the mother, cross the placenta, and achieve therapeutic concentrations in the fetus. Examples include antiarrhythmic agents to correct fetal tachyarrhythmias and γ-globulin to improve low fetal platelet counts. An accurate assessment of placental transfer and monitoring of the success of therapy may require FBS.[76,77]

Procedure

The operator chooses the intended sampling site and guide technique from several options.

SAMPLING SITE

Umbilical Cord Vessels (Cordocentesis). FBS was first performed under fetoscopic guidance,[78] but fetoscopy carried a 2% to 5% risk of serious complications.[79] In addition, the maternal sedation that was used to facilitate the procedure affected fetal blood gas measurements.[80] Ultrasound-guided needling is considered safer than fetoscopy and is the preferred technique.[71,81]

The placental origin of the umbilical cord is often the easiest site to puncture. Many prefer this site because of its fixed location, which prevents movement of the needle. Others accept free loop puncture, but use pancuronium to minimize subsequent fetal movement. The relevant consideration is not the location, but the ease of access. The fetal origin of the umbilical cord is problematic because there is no length to buffer the effect of fetal movement after puncture. In addition, the proximal few centimeters of the umbilicus are sympathetically innervated, theoretically increasing the risk of bradycardia. Although cordocentesis is usually done after 18 weeks, success is reported as early as 12 weeks, at the cost of an increased fetal loss rate.[82,83]

Fetal Intrahepatic Vessels. Blood can also be obtained from vessels within the substance of the liver (Fig. 10–3).[76,84] This procedure is rarely done now, and usually after fetal paralysis with intramuscular injection of pancuronium,[85] but good results have been reported. However, fetal hepatic necrosis within 24 hours of intrahepatic vein blood sampling has been reported.[86]

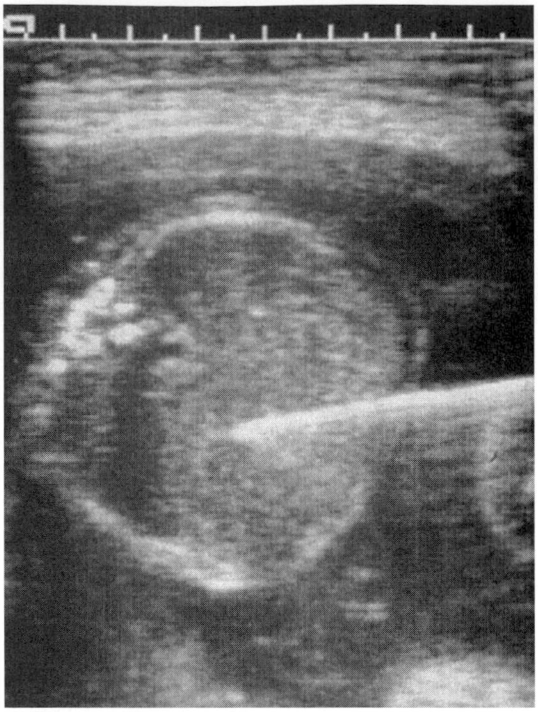

FIGURE 10–3
Fetal blood sampling by ultrasound-guided needling of the intrahepatic vein.

Intrahepatic blood sampling is an alternative when cordocentesis is difficult, but even then, many prefer to sample the heart.

Fetal Heart. The heart is larger than the umbilical cord, and puncture of the heart is relatively simple (Fig. 10–4). Despite fear of damage, cardiac puncture is relatively safe.[87] The heart can be used in the unusual event that the umbilical cord or hepatic vein cannot be punctured and fetal blood must be obtained. It can also be useful if an emergency blood transfusion is required (e.g., to treat procedure-related bleeding) or for feticide.

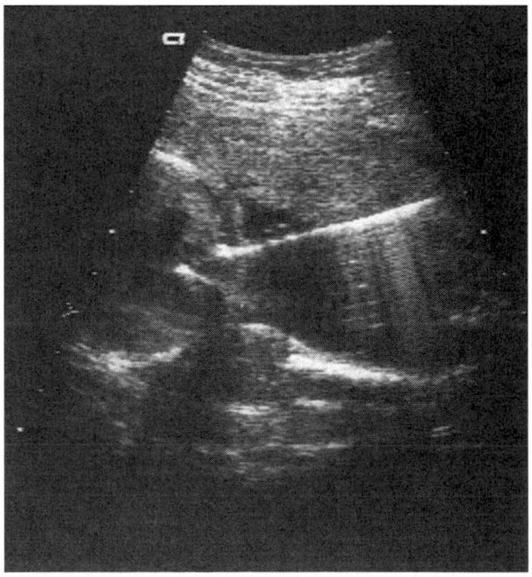

FIGURE 10–4
Fetal blood sampling by ultrasound-guided needling of the heart.

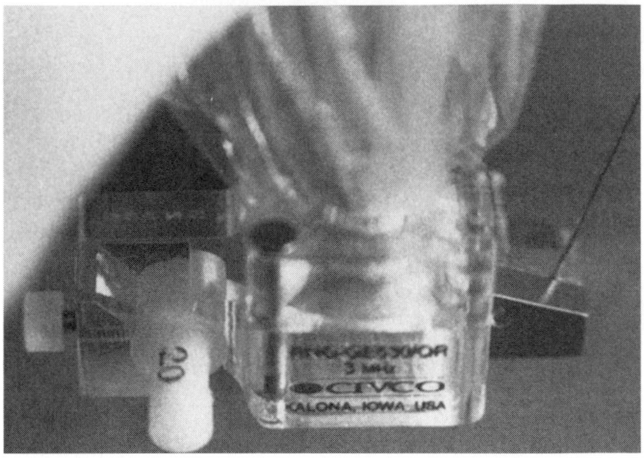

FIGURE 10–5
A, A typical needle guide used to perform cordocentesis. The small footprint allows the needle to enter the sonographic plane shortly after it penetrates the skin. *B*, The needle is seen as bright white echoes crossing the amniotic fluid diagonally. The predicted track of the needle is seen as a dotted line immediately adjacent to the needle.

Because the fetal heart contains blood from different circulatory origins, it may not be suitable for blood gas assessment.[88]

NEEDLING TECHNIQUE

A needle guide or freehand technique may be used (Figs. 10–5 and 10–6). The lowest loss rates for cordocentesis are reported with the use of a needle guide.[3]

PROCEDURE

FETAL BLOOD SAMPLING

The following elements are shared, regardless of whether FBS is performed freehand or with a needle guide. FBS should be performed only by physicians who have extensive experience with other obstetric, ultrasound-guided needle procedures (e.g., amniocentesis, transabdominal CVS). Units

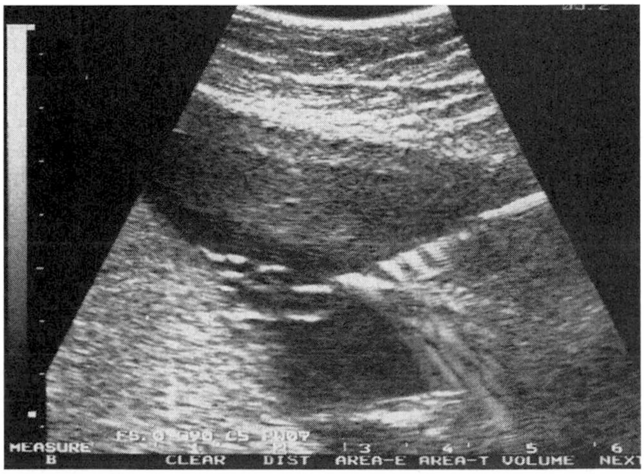

FIGURE 10–6
Cordocentesis with the freehand technique.

that offer this service must perform enough cases to maintain expertise; 20 procedures per year is a reasonable minimum. This typically requires a center with many referrals.[89]

Preparation

An urgent delivery may be required if the pregnancy is at a potentially viable gestation, and if the indication for the procedure does not indicate a conservative approach before the result is available (for example a major brain malformation). Therefore, the procedure must be performed at a site with easy and rapid access to an operative delivery room with an anesthetist immediately available. The mother should be positioned to avoid supine hypotension; hyperventilation and sedation should be avoided. A 12-cm needle is usually sufficient, but the distance should be measured on the ultrasound screen before starting.

Needle Path Selection

A transplacental approach usually provides the easiest route to the placental cord origin, unless the placenta is entirely posterior. However, in women with red cell alloimmunization, transplacental puncture boosts the maternal antibody titer as a result of fetal–maternal hemorrhage.[90] Therefore, it is best to avoid the placenta unless transfusion is anticipated in an alloimmunized woman (Fig. 10–7).

Target Puncture

Cordocentesis

Many operators prefer the placental origin of the umbilical cord, approximately 1 cm from the placenta, because the blood obtained from this site must be fetal. The needle is brought close to or even touching the umbilical vein, and then sharply advanced the remaining distance. A slow advance may push the tissues away, even at this relatively fixed site. After the needle tip is visualized within the lumen of the umbilical cord, the stylet is removed. If the needle is ideally sited, blood will fill the hub. A 1-mL syringe is applied tightly to the hub, and blood is withdrawn. After 20 weeks, 5 mL may be removed without concern. However, before 20 weeks, the volume removed should be the minimum necessary for the specific tests. Often, no blood is obtained initially and the operator must assess whether the needle tip has passed through the vessel lumen or perhaps is located in Wharton's jelly. The needle is sharply advanced or gently withdrawn, and the shaft is rotated 180° between the operator's finger and thumb while suction is maintained.

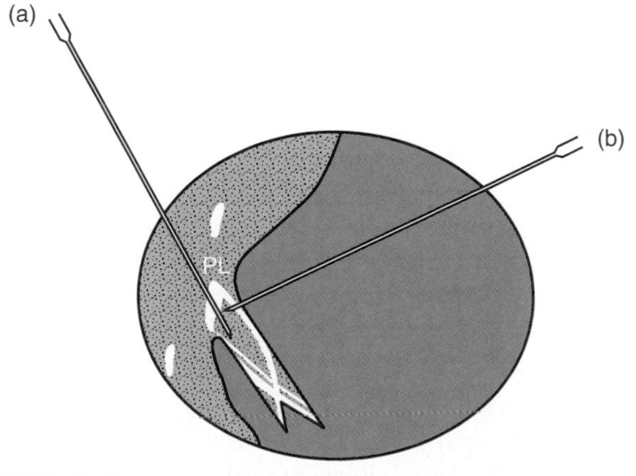

FIGURE 10–7
Transplacental (*A*) and transamniotic (*B*) fetal blood sampling from the placental insertion of the umbilical cord (cordocentesis). PL, placenta.

Occasionally, amniotic fluid is obtained when the needle tip appears intraluminal. With the freehand technique, the needle is moved side-to-side in search of cord movement. With a needle guide, an up-and-down movement of the needle produces the same result. Cord movement indicates that the needle has passed through the cord. It is withdrawn until no more amniotic fluid is aspirated, the syringe is changed (because even a small amount of amniotic fluid is a very powerful coagulant), and the procedure is continued. If the needle has passed through the side of the cord without entering a vessel lumen, it is withdrawn slightly and its path adjusted. If the tip is lateral to the umbilical cord, it is withdrawn and the needle used to touch the vein before the puncture attempt is repeated.

If blood gas results are to be interpretable, it is essential to identify the vessel that has been entered. If the puncture is performed at either the placental or the fetal origin of the umbilical cord, the vessel can usually be identified by the direction of turbulence after rapid injection of up to 1 mL normal saline.[81] If fetal paralysis is desired, intravascular administration of pancuronium (0.3 mg/kg estimated fetal weight) serves the same purpose as saline for identification.

Intrahepatic or Heart

If the intrahepatic vein or the heart is the intended sampling site, fetal paralysis with intramuscular pancuronium (0.2 mg/kg estimated fetal weight) may be used. The effect is rapid (within minutes) and lasts for 90 to 120 minutes. The techniques for needle path selection and guidance are similar to those described for the umbilical cord. However, the fetal chest or abdomen is entered first, the direction is checked, and the needle is advanced into the sampling site as a separate movement. The heart is best entered through the anterior chest, through the thick muscle of the ventricles, to reduce blood leakage and avoid damage to the valves or electrical conduction system.

A double-needle technique has also been described.[91] The first needle is used to puncture the fetal body cavity, and a second, finer needle is passed within the first to puncture the target. This technique offers no advantage and has several inherent weaknesses. The first needle is usually a larger gauge than otherwise required.

Postprocedure Monitoring

The puncture site is observed ultrasonically for bleeding after the needle is removed. Bleeding is common after transamniotic cordocentesis, but is usually brief and without clinical significance. After bleeding has stopped, the fetal heart rate is measured. Bradycardia is the most common complication of cordocentesis, but it is usually transient in the absence of fetal hypoxemia. If the fetus is previable, the woman should wait in the hospital until she feels well, and then return home. There are no special precautions or restrictions. If a local anesthetic is used, she should be warned to expect a bruised sensation in a few hours. Acetaminophen (paracetamol) or another nonprescription analgesic can be used safely. If the fetus is viable, the heart rate pattern is assessed by cardiotocography for at least 30 minutes before discharge. Pancuronium causes a nonreactive tracing, with mild fetal tachycardia. The mother should be warned that perceptible movement might not return for several hours.

In the rare event that bleeding from the puncture site is prolonged and heavy, maternal blood may be collected into heparinized syringes for an emergency fetal transfusion. This is most likely with alloimmune thrombocytopenia when the fetus is profoundly thrombocytopenic.

Laboratory Testing

Several laboratory techniques are available to rapidly confirm that the blood sample is fetal and pure. However, they may be unnecessary if the technique described above is used. Further, they may be usable if the fetal blood has been replaced by transfusion with adult blood. It is prudent to send a small sample of blood for a hematology profile to confirm that the mean cell volume is increased and that the hemoglobin concentration, white blood cell count, and platelet count are normal.

Complications and Risks

FETAL

The principal complications of FBS that threaten fetal well-being are hemorrhage or an obstructing hematoma at the puncture site,[92] fetal bradycardia (probably as a result of smooth muscle spasm after inadvertent puncture of the umbilical artery), and intrauterine infection.[93] Chorioamnionitis is often caused by *Staphylococcus epidermidis*. It typically causes myalgia, arthralgia, and a low fever 4 to 10 days after the procedure. There is no evidence to support prophylactic antibiotic administration. A case report of an abruption shortly after cordocentesis was published.[94] Premature membrane rupture is rare, and the expected frequency is similar to that of amniocentesis. There is a theoretical risk of transmitting infection from the mother's blood (e.g., hepatitis, human immunodeficiency virus) to the fetus, although it does not appear to have been documented. Nevertheless, invasive procedures should be avoided when a mother has a life-threatening viral illness, unless the fetal indication warrants the additional risk.[95]

POSTPROCEDURE LOSS RATES

Several well-recognized factors affect postprocedure loss rates. Loss and complication rates are clearly related to the indication for sampling and the final fetal diagnosis.[3,24,27,29,30,96] The background risk of intrauterine death is high when there is a severe structural malformation or a major chromosomal abnormality. The risk of profound bradycardia is significantly increased by fetal hypoxemia and arterial puncture. Gestational age at sampling is also an important determinant because a viable fetus can be delivered if a complication arises. Emergency cesarean section may prevent fetal death, but by the time the problem is recognized and delivery is accomplished, the neonate may survive permanently damaged or die in the neonatal period. Performing the procedure near the delivery suite minimizes these risks, if delivery can be accomplished within 15 minutes. Complications may not be seen until delivery occurs.

The literature must be interpreted carefully because postprocedure loss rates are described after the application of qualifiers. It is essential to control for the indication or final diagnosis when comparing loss rates. It is only by doing so and by limiting the comparison to healthy fetuses that the risk of the technique is shown. Reports of procedures performed freehand show a total procedure loss rate of approximately 1% to 2%, depending on the mix of indications. In one study of 202 pregnancies, the loss rate was 1 of 76 (1.5%) fetuses sampled for antenatal diagnosis, 5 of 76 (7%) sampled for an anomaly, 4 of 29 (14%) sampled for fetal assessment, and 9 of 35 (25%) sampled for nonimmune hydrops.[29] In our unit, the procedure-related loss rate for FBS is approximately 1.2% with the freehand method described.[12] Transfusion carries a considerably higher procedure-related risk than FBS.

MATERNAL

The main maternal risk associated with FBS is red cell alloimmunization. The fetal blood type should be tested in at-risk women, and anti-D immunoglobulin should be given if the fetus is Rhesus-positive. Chorioamnionitis or emergency cesarean section can create secondary maternal risks. When FBS or transfusion is undertaken and the fetus is considered viable, maternal aspects of emergency delivery should be considered. Needle injury to the maternal intra-abdominal organs, such as intestines, or vessels may be more common than recognized, but significant morbidity has not been reported after FBS. Maternal intra-abdominal infection and bleeding would be expected to occur at the same rate as that for amniocentesis.

Conclusion

FBS is indicated when the potential benefits of a change outweigh the procedure-related risks. The risks and benefits to both the fetus and the mother should be considered. Most prefer FBS by ultrasound-guided needling of the umbilical cord (cordocentesis). The fetal heart and intrahepatic vein are alternative sampling sites. None of these techniques should be attempted unless the operator has considerable experience with related procedures. The most important determinant of the fetal loss rate is the indication for sampling.

SUMMARY OF MANAGEMENT OPTIONS
Fetal Blood Sampling

Management Options	Quality of Evidence	Strength of Recommendation	References
Indications: Diagnostic			
Chromosomal abnormalities	–	GPP	–
DNA abnormality or single-gene defects	–	GPP	–
Fetal anemia	–	GPP	–
Fetal thrombocytopenia	–	GPP	–
Fetal hypoxia or acidosis	–	GPP	–
Fetal infection	–	GPP	–
Monitoring the effects of fetal therapy	–	GPP	–
Procedural Options			
Umbilical cord (cordocentesis)	–	GPP	–
Fetal heart	–	GPP	–
Intrahepatic vessels	–	GPP	–
Complications			
Fetal loss rate related to			
• Gestational age	III	B	–
• Operator experience	III	B	26,82,83
• Number of needle insertions	III	B	–
• Indication (e.g., intrauterine growth restriction, chromosomal abnormality)	III	B	–

Fetal Tissue Biopsy

Although progress in molecular biology allows more diseases to be diagnosed from fetal DNA, some conditions are diagnosable by testing of fetal tissue, such as skin, liver, and muscle. These tests are rarely indicated because the diseases are rare. Only experienced fetal medicine specialists should perform them. Rapid advances in the field mandate close contact with a clinical geneticist to stay abreast of advances.

Skin Biopsy

INDICATION

Histologic examination of a fetal skin biopsy specimen is useful for the diagnosis of some bullous disorders (congenital bullous epidermolysis, epidermolysis bullosa dystrophica, epidermolysis bullosa lethalis[79,97,98]) and hyperkeratotic disorders (congenital ichthyosiform erythroderma, epidermolytic hyperkeratosis, Harlequin ichthyosis) [Figs. 10–8 and 10–9].[99–101] A molecular understanding of these diseases will make early diagnosis by CVS possible.

PROCEDURE

Fetoscopy is rarely performed diagnostically, but the development of new fiberoptic scopes has decreased the pregnancy loss rate to less than the rate of 2% to 5% associated with classic fetoscopic methods.[97] These scopes are popular aids for some therapeutic fetal procedures (e.g., laser ablation). For skin sampling, this technique has been replaced by ultrasound-guided biopsy, commonly performed with a 20-gauge biopsy forceps introduced through a 16- to 18-gauge needle. Obtaining multiple small biopsy

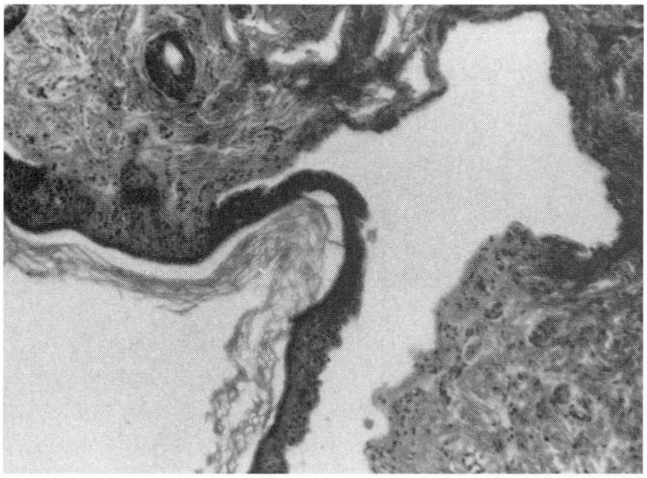

FIGURE 10–8
Histologic features of skin from a fetus with harlequin ichthyosis.

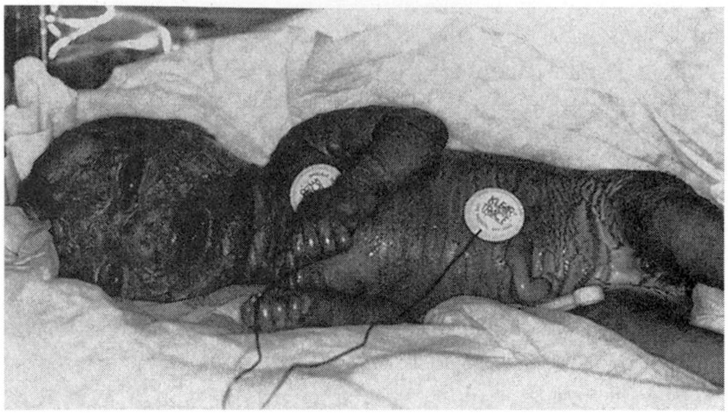

FIGURE 10–9
An infant with harlequin ichthyosis.

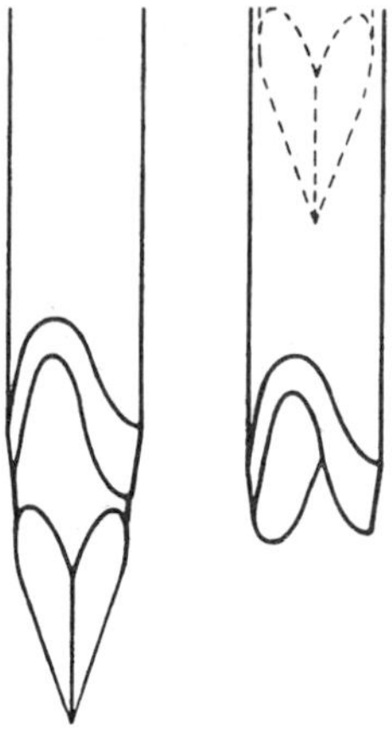

FIGURE 10–11
A cutting needle with an aspiration trocar.

specimens of skin from the scalp over the occiput or from the buttocks is recommended.[102,103] The fetal skin heals well after biopsy.

LABORATORY TECHNIQUES

Histologic and biochemical tools are used to diagnose skin conditions. Several ichthyoses and genetic conditions associated with ichthyoses are diagnosable with fetal cells obtained from CVS, amniocentesis, or FBS.[101]

Fetal Liver Biopsy

Amniotic fluid cells and placental tissue may be used to diagnose most fetal metabolic diseases.[104] However, some inheritable inborn errors of metabolism show defects in enzyme activity confined to the liver, and require a fetal liver biopsy.

PROCEDURE

Fetoscopic[97] and ultrasound-guided[105] procedures are used (Fig. 10–10). Either a hollow needle or a Tru-Cut biopsy needle is inserted through the skin, over the right upper quadrant of the fetal abdomen, and into the liver. (Fig. 10–11) The biopsy specimen is sent to a laboratory. Normal overall activity of a number of enzymes but low activity of a specific enzyme is considered evidence of disease.

Fetal Muscle Biopsy

The most common inheritable major muscular dystrophy is Duchene muscular dystrophy, which is caused by a defect in the gene for dystrophin.[106] Although it is often diagnosable antenatally from fetal DNA obtained by CVS, with molecular analysis seeking either a deletion

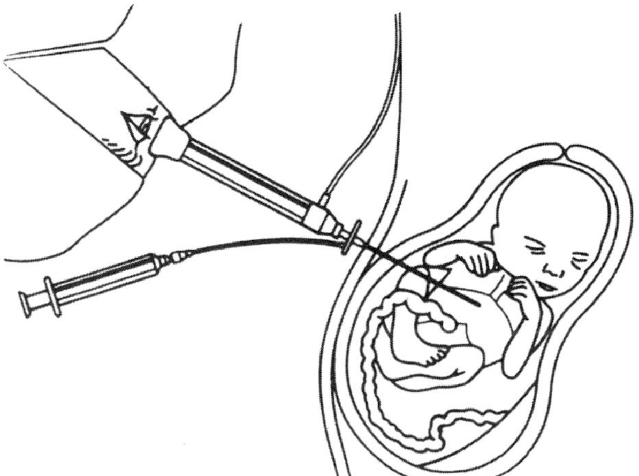

FIGURE 10–10
Fetal liver biopsy performed with a fetoscope.

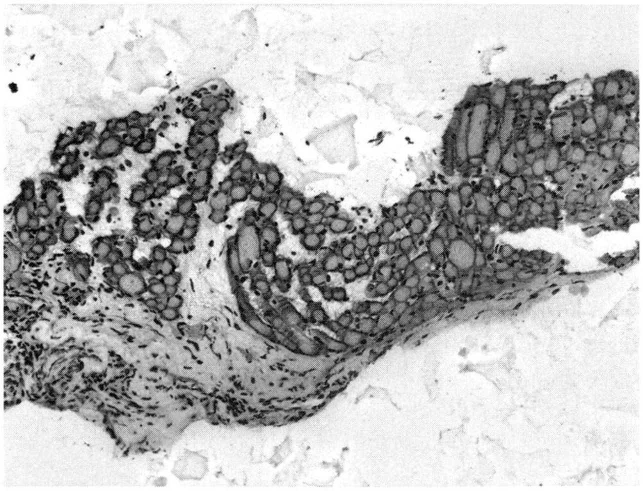

FIGURE 10–12
A fetal muscle biopsy specimen obtained at 22 weeks' gestation. The immunofluorescence of dystrophin indicates that the fetus is normal; this finding was confirmed at birth. (Courtesy of Prof S. Love, Department of Neuro-pathology, Bristol.)

mutation or linkage analysis, the gene is large, with many possible defect sites.[107] In some cases, no deletion is found and biopsy is the only recourse.[108]

LABORATORY TECHNIQUES

A wide range of studies is possible. For Duchenne muscular dystrophy, the biopsy specimen is examined to confirm the presence of muscle and treated with an immunofluorescent antibody for dystrophin protein (Fig. 10–12).[109]

PROCEDURE

These uncommon procedures should be performed only by experienced fetal medicine specialists.[110] The maternal abdominal skin is anesthetized, and a small nick is made with a scalpel to facilitate the entry of a Tru-Cut biopsy gun (Fig. 10–13).[108] Under ultrasound guidance, the tip is advanced into the fetal buttock or thigh in a down-and-out direction. The coring guide is extended, and the trigger is pulled to cut the biopsy specimen. Risks of the procedure include fetal bleeding, nerve damage, and pregnancy loss. There are reports of maternal contamination,[111] but this can be prevented with a double-needle technique.

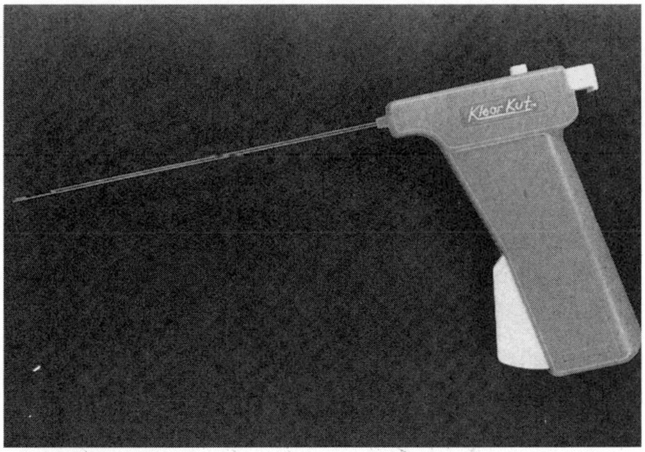

FIGURE 10–13
KlearKut biopsy gun.

Other Organ Biopsy

Histologic diagnosis of fetal tumors would be helpful in many cases, and there are reports of biopsy of fetal mediastinal and renal tumors.[112] However, biopsy of any tumor can cause uncontrollable bleeding, leading to severe fetal damage or death. In many cases, the histologic features vary in different locations. As a result, biopsy of a fetal mass is rarely advised.

Conclusion

Most antenatal fetal diagnoses are based on fetal DNA obtained by CVS, amniocentesis, or FBS. However, fetal skin, liver, and muscle biopsy specimens are required for some lethal or severely disabling conditions. These are complex procedures, with significant risk to the pregnancy, and they should be performed only in tertiary fetal medicine centers by experienced clinicians.

SUMMARY OF MANAGEMENT OPTIONS

Fetal Tissue Biopsy

Management Options	Quality of Evidence	Strength of Recommendation	References
Indications			
Possible or potential life-threatening disease in the fetal skin, liver, and muscle	–	GPP	–
Procedural Options			
Fetoscopy and biopsy	–	GPP	–
Ultrasound-guided aspiration	–	GPP	–
Ultrasound-guided Tru-cut biopsy	–	GPP	–
Complications			
Fetal loss	–	GPP	–
Fetal injury (scarring)	–	GPP	–
Preterm rupture of the membranes or oligohydramnios	–	GPP	–
Chorioamnionitis			

CONCLUSIONS

- The need for invasive procedures has decreased as the sophistication of ultrasound diagnosis has improved. However, indications for these procedures will continue, and they must be performed by specialists in fetal medicine who regularly audit their postprocedure complication rates.
- Training in these procedures must be well supervised and limited.
- Performing fetal invasive diagnostic procedures is a steppingstone to performing more complex invasive therapeutic procedures.

REFERENCES

1. Tabor A, Philip J, Bang J, et al: Safety of amniocentesis. Prenat Diagn 1988;8:167–168.
2. RCOG: Amniocentesis. London, 2000.
3. Weiner CP, Okamura K: Diagnostic fetal blood sampling-technique related losses. Fetal Diagn Ther 1996;11:169–175.
4. An assessment of the hazards of amniocentesis: Report to the Medical Research Council by their Working Party on Amniocentesis. Br J Obstet Gynaecol 1978;85(Suppl 2):1–41.
5. Murray JC, Karp LE, Williamson RA, et al: Rh isoimmunization related to amniocentesis. Am J Med Genet 1983;16:527–534.
6. Tabor A, Bang J, Norgaard-Pedersen B: Feto-maternal haemorrhage associated with genetic amniocentesis: Results of a randomized trial. Br J Obstet Gynaecol 1987;94:528–534.
7. Abdel-Fattah SA, Soothill PW, Carroll SG, Kyle PM: Middle cerebral artery Doppler for the prediction of fetal anaemia in cases without hydrops: A practical approach. Br J Radiol 2002;75(897):726–730.
8. Jeanty P, Shah D, Roussis P: Single-needle insertion in twin amniocentesis. J Ultrasound Med 1990;9:511–517.
9. Sebire NJ, Noble PL, Odibo A, et al: Single uterine entry for genetic amniocentesis in twin pregnancies. Ultrasound Obstet Gynecol 1996;7:26–31.
10. Nicolini U, Monni G: Intestinal obstruction in babies exposed in utero to methylene blue. Lancet 1990;336(8725):1258–1259.
11. Chen CP, Chern SR, Wang W: Rapid determination of zygosity and common aneuploidies from amniotic fluid cells using quantitative fluorescent polymerase chain reaction following genetic amniocentesis in multiple pregnancies. Hum Reprod 2000;15:929–934.
12. Nanal R, Kyle P, Soothill PW: A classification of pregnancy loss after invasive prenatal diagnostic procedures: An approach to allow comparison of units with a different case mix. Prenat Diagn 2003;23:488–492.
13. Silver RK, Russell TL, Kambich MP, et al: Midtrimester amniocentesis: Influence of operator caseload on sampling efficiency. J Reprod Med 1998;43:191–195.
14. Jahoda MGJ BH, Reuss A, Cohen-Overbeek TE, et al: Transcervical and transabdominal CVS for prenatal diagnosis in Rotterdam: Experience with 3611 cases. Prenat Diagn 1991;11:559–561.
15. Rhoads GG, Jackson LG, Schlesselman SE, et al: The safety and efficacy of chorionic villus sampling for early prenatal diagnosis of cytogenetic abnormalities. N Engl J Med 1989;320:609–617.
16. Jackson LG, Zachary JM, Fowler SE, et al: A randomized comparison of transcervical and transabdominal chorionic-villus sampling: The U.S. National Institute of Child Health and Human Development Chorionic-Villus Sampling and Amniocentesis Study Group [comment]. N Engl J Med 1992;327:594–598.
17. Tabor A, Philip J, Madsen M, et al: Randomised controlled trial of genetic amniocentesis in 4606 low-risk women. Lancet 1986;1(8493):1287–1293.
18. Multicentre randomised clinical trial of chorion villus sampling and amniocentesis: First report. Canadian Collaborative CVS-Amniocentesis Clinical Trial Group [comment]. Lancet 1989;1(8628):1–6.
19. Hanson FW, Zorn EM, Tennant FR, et al: Amniocentesis before 15 weeks' gestation: Outcome, risks, and technical problems. Am J Obstet Gynecol 1987;156:1524–1531.
20. Smidt-Jensen S, Permin M, Philip J, et al: Randomised comparison of amniocentesis and transabdominal and transcervical chorionic villus sampling [see comment]. Lancet 1992;340 (8830):1237–1244.
21. Nicolaides KH, Brizot ML, Patel F, Snjders R: Comparison of chorion villus sampling and early amniocentesis for karyotyping in 1,492 singleton pregnancies. Fetal Diagn Ther 1996;11:9–15.
22. Johnson A, Godmilow L: Genetic amniocentesis at 14 weeks or less. Clin Obstet Gynecol 1988;31:345–352.
23. Sundberg K, Bang J, Smidt-Jensen S, et al: Randomised study of risk of fetal loss related to early amniocentesis versus chorionic villus sampling [see comment]. Lancet 1997;350(9079):697–703.
24. Wilson RD, Farquharson DF, Wittmann BK, Shaw D: Cordocentesis: Overall pregnancy loss rate as important as procedure loss rate. Fetal Diagn Ther 1994;9:142–148.
25. Randomised trial to assess safety and fetal outcome of early and midtrimester amniocentesis: The Canadian Early and Midtrimester Amniocentesis Trial (CEMAT) Group [comment]. Lancet 1998;351(9098):242–247.
26. Medical Research Council European trial of chorion villus sampling: MRC working party on the evaluation pf chorion villus sampling [comment]. Lancet 1991;337(8756):1491–1499.
27. Anandakumar C, Annapoorna V, Chee WY, et al: Fetal blood sampling and its complications related to the indications for fetal blood sampling. Aust N Z J Obstet Gynaecol 1993;33:259–261.
28. Wapner RJ: Chorionic villus sampling. Obstet Gynecol Clin North Am 1997;24:83–110.
29. Maxwell DJ, Johnson P, Hurley P, et al: Fetal blood sampling and pregnancy loss in relation to indication [comment]. Br J Obstet Gynaecol 1991;98:892–897.
30. Ghidini A, Sepulveda W, Lockwood CJ, Romero R: Complications of fetal blood sampling [comment]. Am J Obstet Gynecol 1993; 168:1339–1344.
31. Finning KM, Martin PG, Soothill PW, Avent ND: Prediction of fetal D status from maternal plasma: Introduction of a new noninvasive fetal RHD genotyping service. Transfusion 2002;42: 1079–1085.
32. Smidt-Jensen S, Hahnemann N: Transabdominal fine needle biopsy from chorionic villi in the first trimester. Prenat Diagn 1984;4:163–169.
33. Nicolaides KH, Soothill PW, Rosevear S: Transabdominal placental biopsy. Lancet 1987;2(8563):855–856.
34. Smidt-Jensen S, Philip J: Comparison of transabdominal and transcervical CVS and amniocentesis: Sampling success and risk. Prenat Diagn 1991;11:529–537.
35. Young SR, Shipley CF, Wade RV, et al: Single-center comparison of results of 1000 prenatal diagnoses with chorionic villus

sampling and 1000 diagnoses with amniocentesis. Am J Obstet Gynecol 1991;165:255–261; discussion 261–263.
36. Vaughn JRC: Interventional procedures. In K Dewbury HM, Cosgrove D (eds): Clinical Ultrasound: A Comprehensive Text. Ultrasound in Obstetrics and Gynaecology. Edinburgh, Churchill Livingstone, 1992, p 463.
37. Firth HV, Boyd PA, Chamberlain P, et al: Severe limb abnormalities after chorion villus sampling at 56–66 days' gestation [comment]. Lancet 1991;337(8744):762–763.
38. Schloo R, Miny P, Holzgreve W, et al: Distal limb deficiency following chorionic villus sampling? Am J Med Genet 1992;42: 404–413.
39. Froster UG, Jackson L: Limb defects and chorionic villus sampling: Results from an international registry, 1992–94 [comment]. Lancet 1996;347(9000):489–494.
40. Holzgreve W, Miny P, Gerlach B, et al: Benefits of placental biopsies for rapid karyotyping in the second and third trimesters (late chorionic villus sampling) in high-risk pregnancies. Am J Obstet Gynecol 1990;162:1188–1192.
41. Nicolaides KH, Soothill PW, Rodeck CH, et al: Why confine chorionic villus (placental) biopsy to the first trimester? Lancet 1986;1(8480):543–544.
42. Hogdall CK, Doran TA, Shime J, et al: Transabdominal chorionic villus sampling in the second trimester. Am J Obstet Gynecol 1988;158:345–349.
43. Levett LJ, Liddle S, Meredith R: A large-scale evaluation of amnio-PCR for the rapid prenatal diagnosis of fetal trisomy. Ultrasound Obstet Gynecol 2001;17:115–118.
44. Thirkelson A: Cell culture and cytogenetic technique. In Murken JD S-RS, Schwinger EN (eds): Third European Conference on Prenatal Diagnosis of Genetic Disorders. Stuttgart, Ferdinand Enke, 1979, pp 258–270.
45. Bui TH, Iselius L, Lindsten J: European collaborative study on prenatal diagnosis: Mosaicism, pseudomosaicism and single abnormal cells in amniotic fluid cell cultures. Prenat Diagn 1984;4:145–162.
46. Worton RG, Stern R: A Canadian collaborative study of mosaicism in amniotic fluid cell cultures. Prenat Diagn 1984;4:131–144.
47. Van Opstal D, Van Hemel JO, Sachs ES: Fetal aneuploidy diagnosed by fluorescence in-situ hybridisation within 24 hours after amniocentesis. Lancet 1993;342(8874):802.
48. Isada NB, Hume RF Jr, Reichler A, et al: Fluorescent in situ hybridization and second-trimester sonographic anomalies: Uses and limitations. Fetal Diagn Ther 1994;9:367–370.
49. Bennett PR, Le Van Kim C, Colin Y, et al: Prenatal determination of fetal RhD type by DNA amplification [comment]. N Engl J Med 1993;329:607–610.
50. Bennett PR, Warwick R, Letsky E, Fisk NM: Determination of fetal RhD type by DNA amplification from fetal skin following massive fetomaternal haemorrhage and intrauterine fetal death. Br J Obstet Gynaecol 1994;101:636–637.
51. Sepulveda W, Donaldson A, Johnson RD, et al: Are routine alpha-fetoprotein and acetylcholinesterase determinations still necessary at second-trimester amniocentesis? Impact of high-resolution ultrasonography. Obstet Gynecol 1995;85:107–112.
52. Weiner CP, Grose C: Prenatal diagnosis of congenital cytomegalovirus infection by virus isolation from amniotic fluid. Am J Obstet Gynecol 1990;163(4 Pt 1):1253–1255.
53. Borg KL, Nordbo SA, Winge P, Dalen A: Detection of cytomegalovirus using "boosted" nested PCR. Mol Cell Probes 1995;9:251–257.
54. Antsaklis A, Daskalakis G, Papantoniou N, et al: Prenatal diagnosis of congenital toxoplasmosis. Prenat Diagn 2002;22: 1107–1011.
55. Dudley J, Malcolm G, Ellwood D: Amniocentesis in the management of preterm premature rupture of the membranes. Aust N Z J Obstet Gynaecol 1991;31:331–336.
56. Fisk NM: Modifications to selective conservative management in preterm premature rupture of the membranes. Obstet Gynecol Surv 1988;43:328–334.
57. James DK, Tindall VR, Richardson T: Is the lecithin/sphingomyelin ratio outdated? Br J Obstet Gynaecol 1983;90: 995–1000.
58. Benacerraf BR, Greene MF, Saltzman DH, et al: Early amniocentesis for prenatal cytogenetic evaluation. Radiology 1988; 169:709–710.
59. Rooney DE, MacLachlan N, Smith J, et al: Early amniocentesis: A cytogenetic evaluation [comment]. BMJ 1989;299(6690):25.
60. Sundberg K, Bang J, Smidt-Jensen S, et al: Randomised study of risk of fetal loss related to early amniocentesis versus chorionic villus sampling [comment]. Lancet 1997;350(9079):697–703.
61. Hackett GA, Smith JH, Rebello MT, et al: Early amniocentesis at 11–14 weeks' gestation for the diagnosis of fetal chromosomal abnormality: A clinical evaluation. Prenat Diagn 1991;11:311–315.
62. Djalali M, Barbi G, Kennerknecht I, Terinde R: Introduction of early amniocentesis to routine prenatal diagnosis. Prenat Diagn 1992;12:661–669.
63. Midtrimester amniocentesis for prenatal diagnosis: Safety and accuracy. JAMA 1976;236:1471–1476.
64. Kappel B, Nielsen J, Brogaard Hansen K, et al: Spontaneous abortion following mid-trimester amniocentesis: Clinical significance of placental perforation and blood-stained amniotic fluid. Br J Obstet Gynaecol 1987;94:50–54.
65. Ghidini A, Lynch L, Hicks C, et al: The risk of second-trimester amniocentesis in twin gestations: A case-control study. Am J Obstet Gynecol 1993;169:1013–1016.
66. Hunter AG: Neonatal lung function following mid-trimester amniocentesis. Prenat Diagn 1987;7:433–441.
67. Naylor G, Roper JP, Willshaw HE: Ophthalmic complications of amniocentesis. Eye 1990;4(Pt 6):845–849.
68. Rummelt V, Rummelt C, Naumann GO: Congenital nonpigmented epithelial iris cyst after amniocentesis: Clinicopathologic report on two children [comment]. Ophthalmology 1993;100: 776–781.
69. Eller KM, Kuller JA: Porencephaly secondary to fetal trauma during amniocentesis. Obstet Gynecol 1995;85(5 Pt 2):865–867.
70. Saling E: Foetal and neonatal hypoxia. In Loeffler TF (ed): London, Arnold, 1963.
71. Daffos F, Capella-Pavlovsky M, Forestier F: A new procedure for fetal blood sampling in utero: Preliminary results of fifty-three cases. Am J Obstet Gynecol 1983;146:985–987.
72. Nicolaides KH: Cordocentesis. Clin Obstet Gynecol 1988; 31:123–135.
73. Soothill P: Intrauterine blood transfusion for non-immune hydrops fetalis due to parvovirus B19 infection [comment]. Lancet 1990;336(8707):121–122.
74. Soothill PW: Cordocentesis: Role in assessment of fetal condition. Clin Perinatol 1989;16:755–770.
75. Soothill PW, Ajayi RA, Campbell S, et al: Fetal oxygenation at cordocentesis, maternal smoking and childhood neuro-development. Eur J Obstet Gynecol Reprod Biol 1995;59:21–24.
76. Nicolini U, Nicolaidis P, Fisk NM, et al: Fetal blood sampling from the intrahepatic vein: Analysis of safety and clinical experience with 214 procedures [comment]. Obstet Gynecol 1990;76:47–53.
77. Prentice ED, Rayburn WF: Research involving fetal drug therapy: Ethical, legal, and practical considerations. Clin Obstet Gynecol 1991;34:360–368.
78. Rodeck CH, Campbell S: Umbilical-cord insertion as source of pure fetal blood for prenatal diagnosis. Lancet 1979;1(8128): 1244–1245.
79. Soothill PW, Nicolaides KH, Rodeck CH: Invasive techniques for prenatal diagnosis and therapy. J Perinat Med 1987; 15:117–127.
80. Soothill PW, Nicolaides KH, Bilardo K, et al: Utero-placental blood velocity resistance index and umbilical venous pO_2, pCO_2, pH, lactate and erythroblast count in growth-retarded fetuses. Fetal Ther 1986;1:176–179.

81. Nicolaides KH, Soothill PW, Rodeck CH, Campbell S: Ultrasound-guided sampling of umbilical cord and placental blood to assess fetal wellbeing. Lancet 1986;1(8489):1065–1067.
82. Orlandi F, Damiani G, Jakil C, et al: The risks of early cordocentesis (12–21 weeks): Analysis of 500 procedures. Prenat Diagn 1990;10:425–428.
83. Levi Setti PE, Buscaglia M, Ferrazzi E, et al: [Evaluation of the fetal risk after echo-guided blood sampling from the umbilical cord in the 2d trimester of pregnancy]. Ann Ostet Ginecol Med Perinat 1989;110:98–104.
84. Bang J, Bock JE, Trolle D: Ultrasound-guided fetal intravenous transfusion for severe rhesus haemolytic disease. Br Med J Clin Res Ed 1982;284(6313):373–374.
85. Mouw RJ, Klumper F, Hermans J, et al: Effect of atracurium or pancuronium on the anemic fetus during and directly after intravascular intrauterine transfusion: A double blind randomized study. Acta Obstet Gynecol Scand 1999;78:763–767.
86. Sturgiss SN, Wright C, Davison JM, Robson SC: Fetal hepatic necrosis following blood sampling from the intrahepatic vein. Prenat Diagn 1996;16:866–869.
87. Westgren M, Selbing A, Stangenberg M: Fetal intracardiac transfusions in patients with severe rhesus isoimmunisation. Br Med J Clin Res Ed 1988;296(6626):885–886.
88. Soothill P: Blood gas studies in fetal heart blood [comment]. Am J Obstet Gynecol 1990;162:1636–1637.
89. Whittle MJ: Cordocentesis. Br J Obstet Gynaecol 1989;96: 262–264.
90. Weiner C, Grant S, Hudson J, et al: Effect of diagnostic and therapeutic cordocentesis on maternal serum alpha-fetoprotein concentration. Am J Obstet Gynecol 1989;161:706–708.
91. Bovicelli L, Orsini LF, Grannum PA, et al: A new funipuncture technique: Two-needle ultrasound- and needle biopsy-guided procedure. Obstet Gynecol 1989;73(3 Pt 1):428–431.
92. Jauniaux E, Donner C, Simon P, et al: Pathologic aspects of the umbilical cord after percutaneous umbilical blood sampling. Obstet Gynecol 1989;73:215–218.
93. Weiner CP: Cordocentesis for diagnostic indications: Two years' experience. Obstet Gynecol 1987;70:664–668.
94. Feinkind L, Nanda D, Delke I, Minkoff H: Abruptio placentae after percutaneous umbilical cord sampling: A case report. Am J Obstet Gynecol 1990;162:1203–1204.
95. Workman MR, Philpott-Howard J: Risk of fetal infection from invasive procedures. J Hosp Infect 1997;35:169–174.
96. Weiner CP, Wenstrom KD, Sipes SL, Williamson RA: Risk factors for cordocentesis and fetal intravascular transfusion. Am J Obstet Gynecol 1991;165(4 Pt 1):1020–1025.
97. Rodeck CH, Nicolaides KH: Fetal tissue biopsy: Techniques and indications. Fetal Ther 1986;1:46–58.
98. Nazzaro V, Nicolini U, De Luca L, et al: Prenatal diagnosis of junctional epidermolysis bullosa associated with pyloric atresia. J Med Genet 1990;27:244–248.
99. Holbrook KA, Dale BA, Williams ML, et al: The expression of congenital ichthyosiform erythroderma in second trimester fetuses of the same family: Morphologic and biochemical studies. J Invest Dermatol 1988;91:521–531.
100. Elias S, Mazur M, Sabbagha R, et al: Prenatal diagnosis of harlequin ichthyosis. Clin Genet 1980;17:275–280.
101. Dale BA, Perry TB, Holbrook KA, et al: Biochemical examination of fetal skin biopsy specimens obtained by fetoscopy: Use of the method for analysis of keratins and filaggrin. Prenat Diagn 1986;6:37–44.
102. Buckshee K, Parveen S, Mittal S, et al: Percutaneous ultrasound-guided fetal skin biopsy: A new approach. Int J Gynaecol Obstet 1991;34:267–270.
103. Adzick NS, Longaker MT: Scarless fetal healing: Therapeutic implications [comment]. Ann Surg 1992;215:3–7.
104. Evans MI, Moore C, Kolodny EH, et al: Lysosomal enzymes in chorionic villi, cultured amniocytes, and cultured skin fibroblasts. Clin Chim Acta 1986;157:109–113.
105. Holzgreve W, Golbus MS: Prenatal diagnosis of ornithine transcarbamylase deficiency utilizing fetal liver biopsy. Am J Human Genet 1984;36:320–328.
106. Hoffman EP, Brown RH Jr, Kunkel LM: Dystrophin: The protein product of the Duchenne muscular dystrophy locus. Cell 1987;51:919–928.
107. Hoffman EP: Genotype/phenotype correlations in Duchenne/Becker dystrophy. Mol Cell Biol Hum Dis 1993;3: 12–36.
108. Evans MI, Greb A, Kunkel LM, et al: In utero fetal muscle biopsy for the diagnosis of Duchenne muscular dystrophy. Am J Obstet Gynecol 1991;165:728–732.
109. Evans MI, Farrell SA, Greb A, et al: In utero fetal muscle biopsy for the diagnosis of Duchenne muscular dystrophy in a female fetus "suddenly at risk." Am J Med Genet 1993;46:309–312.
110. Evans MI, Hoffman EP, Cadrin C, et al: Fetal muscle biopsy: Collaborative experience with varied indications. Obstet Gynecol 1994;84:913–917.
111. Overton TG, Smith RP, Sewry CA, et al: Maternal contamination at fetal muscle biopsy. Fetal Diagn Ther 2000;15:118–121.
112. Golbus MS, McGonigle KF, Goldberg JD, et al: Fetal tissue sampling: The San Francisco experience with 190 pregnancies. West J Med 1989;150:423–430.

SECTION THREE

Late Prenatal—Fetal

CHAPTER 11

Critical Evaluation of Fetal Assessment Methods

Clare Gribbin / Jim Thornton

INTRODUCTION

Much of modern obstetric practice consists of fetal assessment to permit early delivery if it is considered safer than continued observation. However, little evidence supports much of this practice.

For the high risk fetus, in certain clear-cut cases, careful monitoring and timed delivery prevents fetal death. Some evidence from randomized controlled trials of fetal monitoring supports this belief. Whether timed delivery has an effect on fetal brain damage is not known.

For low risk pregnancies, there is little evidence that direct assessment of the fetus reduces adverse outcomes, and screening for fetal compromise may do more harm than good. In the few areas in which trials have been done, the results generally support this view. Conventional practice is to monitor the maternal condition by regular blood pressure screening and urine testing, and at most, to perform simple, indirect fetal assessment, such as reporting fetal movement and measuring fundal height. Other tests should be used only in the context of research trials.

Prenatal assessment of the fetal condition has the following two main phases:

- In the first half of pregnancy, assessment is done to exclude fetal abnormality and, in a limited way, fetal infection. These issues are discussed in Chapters 7, 8, and 27.
- In the second half of pregnancy, the priority is to monitor the condition of the presumed normal fetus, with a view to determining the optimum time for delivery.

Practical Problems

Much of our understanding of fetal compromise comes from animal studies in which the fetus was rendered chronically hypoxemic by narrowing of certain vessels. These models provide rough guidance for the management of the human fetus. However, even the best models do not mimic human diseases precisely, and obviously, there is no reliable animal model for human hypoxic brain damage. Policies for investigating and managing human pregnancy must be based on human research studies.

At least four problems arise in practice:

- Tests are rarely evaluated for the prediction of important endpoints, such as fetal death and brain damage. More often, an abnormal test result is related to another adverse outcome, such as fetal acidemia, a low Apgar score, or admission for neonatal care. Because the relation between these outcomes and fetal death or brain damage is weak, it is easy to be misled.
- To evaluate tests for the prediction of death or disability, the results should be concealed from the clinician to avoid treatment paradox. For example, if an abnormal test result correctly predicts fetal death but is revealed to the clinician, who administers an effective treatment (e.g., delivery), and the fetus survives, the test result will appear to have been false-positive. In contrast, if a false-positive result is revealed and the physician delivers the infant so early that the infant dies of complications of prematurity, the test will appear to have correctly predicted death. The only way to avoid this paradox is to conceal the results from the physicians who treat these patients. This has been done for the umbilical artery waveform,[1] but has rarely been done for other tests because of ethical concerns about concealing potentially important clinical information.
- The difficulty facing the physician who is attempting to interpret a specific test result, such as a biophysical score of 6, is that the meaning of the result for this patient depends on the population of pregnancies in which it is

being applied. In a woman who smokes, has had two previous stillbirths, and is hypertensive and bleeding, this result would predict a high risk of fetal death in the next week or so. However, in an asymptomatic, nonsmoking, normotensive woman in her first pregnancy who had an ultrasound scan because of anxiety, the same test result would be associated with a much better prognosis. Among women with low risk pregnancies, there is a relatively greater chance of a false-positive result. Physicians often neglect the effect of different previous risks on test interpretation (discussed later).

- Finally, timed delivery is the only effective treatment for the preterm fetus that is failing to thrive. However, timed delivery may do harm as well as good, and until recently, it had never been evaluated by a randomized controlled trial. The lack of clear evidence that one testing regimen is better than another is reflected in the different practice across the Atlantic Ocean. In North America, a biophysical profile is the most popular test for deciding the timing of delivery, whereas in Europe, a combination of cardiotocography (CTG) and Doppler findings is more common.

Clinical Judgment

The lack of hard evidence from randomized trials is not an argument for a nihilistic approach to testing in high-risk pregnancy. Few tests have been shown to be useless, and most have not been properly evaluated. Even adequately powered trials of good tests may give negative results if participating physicians do not know how to interpret the results or act on them wisely. The Growth Restriction Intervention Trial (GRIT)[2] provides reassuring evidence that at least the specialists who participated in the trial know how to interpret the results of these tests properly. When the obstetrician was uncertain, participants were randomly allocated to "deliver now" or "delay." Although more stillbirths occurred in the "delay" group, these were balanced by other deaths in the "deliver now" group. It is likely that when specialists were certain that delivery was indicated, they were usually correct.

INDICATIONS FOR FETAL ASSESSMENT

Pregnancies with No Risk Factors for Fetal Compromise ("Low Risk")

As discussed earlier, the most common and conventional methods of fetal assessment in low risk pregnancies are the following:

- Maternal monitoring of fetal movement
- Measurement of symphysis–fundal height
- Auscultation of the fetal heart

No evidence supports the use of routine ultrasound to screen for fetal compromise in low risk pregnancies.[3–5]

Pregnancies with Risk Factors for Fetal Compromise ("High Risk")

Disease in the Fetus (See also Chapter 12)

Triploidy is associated with severe asymmetrical growth restriction and abdominal measurement that lags many weeks behind the head measurement. The diagnosis is easily made by recognizing this and identifying the multicystic appearance of the placenta. The diagnosis is confirmed by placental biopsy. These fetuses are nonviable. Other aneuploidies, such as trisomy 13, trisomy 18, and to a lesser extent, trisomy 21, are associated with lesser degrees of growth restriction. These can be diagnosed by identifying the typical anatomic features on ultrasound and by placental biopsy (see Chapters 8, 9, and 10).

Confined placental mosaicism explains some cases of growth restriction.[6] Most specific syndromes associated with uniparental disomy (UPD), such as Prader-Willi syndrome (maternal UPD15). Angelman syndrome (paternal UPD15), Silver-Russell syndrome (mUPD7), and Beckwith-Wiedemann syndrome (pUPD11), are also characterized by growth restriction. Uniparental disomy of other chromosomes has been described in growth-restricted patients without additional phenotypic abnormalities. However, with current searching techniques, few cases can be explained by uniparental disomy, usually for chromosome 16.[7]

Growth restriction is a feature of intrauterine infection with toxoplasmosis, cytomegalovirus, and rubella. However, this type of infection accounts for few cases of isolated growth restriction.[8] In areas and settings in which they are prevalent, malaria and HIV infection are also important causes.

Multiple pregnancies are associated with an increased risk of fetal compromise from either uteroplacental vascular disease or twin–twin transfusion syndrome (see Chapter 24).

Disease in the Mother

Two types of patients can be identified:

- Those with a specific pathology
- Those with no known pathology, but a risk of adverse fetal outcome

RISK WITH SPECIFIC PATHOLOGY

Essential hypertension and preeclampsia and renal and autoimmune diseases, especially systemic lupus erythematosus, are associated with an increased risk of growth restriction in association with uteroplacental vascular disease (see Chapters 36 and 44). Many types of thrombophilia, such as lupus anticoagulant and factor V Leiden homozygosity, are associated with growth restriction.[9–12]

Maternal diabetes typically causes fetal macrosomia and risk of fetal death (probably from a combination of fetal hypoxia, acidemia, and hyperglycemia[13]), especially in women with microvascular complications (see Chapter 45).

Drugs and toxins can reduce fetal growth. Important examples include anticonvulsants, especially phenytoin; smoking; cocaine use; and excessive alcohol intake.

Other maternal factors associated with increased fetal risk are thyroid disease (transplacental transfer of thyroid-stimulating antibodies that cause fetal thyrotoxicosis), isoimmunization (fetal hemolytic anemia [see Chapter 14]), maternal cyanotic heart disease (see Chapter 37), and inadequate nutrition.

RISK WITH NO KNOWN PATHOLOGY

Risks with no known pathology include the following:

- Reduced fetal movements (discussed later)
- Vaginal bleeding (see Chapter 59)
- Prolonged pregnancy (see Chapter 66)
- Abdominal pain of uncertain cause
- Ruptured membranes (see Chapter 63)

In high-risk pregnancies, the following methods are often used to assess fetal health:

- Measurement of fetal growth
- Measurement of amniotic fluid volume
- Umbilical artery Doppler recordings
- Measurement of middle cerebral artery blood flow
- Measurement of ductus venosus blood flow
- Uterine artery Doppler recordings
- Fetal heart rate recordings
- Biophysical profile testing

The following methods, which are less commonly used, are also reviewed:

- Placental grading
- Biochemical testing

CRITICAL EVALUATION OF FETAL ASSESSMENT METHODS

Monitoring of Fetal Movements

Although it is easy for women to count fetal movements, obtaining a total daily count is time-consuming and unnecessary for most pregnancies in which movement is normal. A better method is for women to count 10 movements and to record how long it took for these movements to occur (the "count to 10" chart). Inability to count 10 movements in a 12-hour period is associated with an increased likelihood of fetal death, although randomized trials of this policy have not shown improvement in fetal outcome with this approach.

The authors of the largest randomized study suggested that the failure to reduce the death rate was mainly caused by false reassurances or inappropriate interpretation of subsequent studies, including fetal heart rate monitoring (discussed later) (cardiotocography, CTG; and nonstress testing, NST).[14]

Symphysis–Fundal Height Measurement

Inspection and informal palpation of the abdomen alone detect only 30% of fetuses that are small for gestational age.[15] Formal measurement of symphysis–fundal height (the distance in centimeters from the top of the uterus to the pubic bone) is not more effective and did not improve the perinatal outcomes measured in the one controlled trial found during systematic review.[16]

A controlled trial of fundal height measurement plotted on customized antenatal growth charts compared this practice with fundal height assessment by abdominal palpation (the usual management). The study group had a significantly higher antenatal detection rate of infants who were small for gestational age (48% vs. 29%; odds ratio, 2.2; 95% confidence interval, 1.1–4.5). There were no differences in perinatal outcome.[17] The United Kingdom National Institute of Clinical Excellence (NICE) guidance on antenatal care stated that pregnant women should be offered estimation of fetal size at each antenatal appointment.

Auscultation of Fetal Heart Sounds

No studies have examined whether auscultation of fetal heart sounds identifies fetuses at risk or improves fetal outcome. Nevertheless, it is recommended as standard practice. In theory, fetal arrhythmia, such as congenital heart block or tachyarrhythmia, could be identified, although detection of such rare conditions would require routine and regular documentation of fetal heart rate, which is not performed in routine practice.

Ultrasound Assessment of Fetal Growth

A systematic review showed no evidence from randomized trials that the use of fetal growth assessment reduces important adverse outcomes in either high-risk or low-risk pregnancies.[4] In low-risk pregnancies, most trials were of isolated measurement of fetal size (usually abdominal circumference). Because single measurements of abdominal circumference are poor predictors of fetuses with pathologic growth, serial measurements may be better. The trial of McKenna and associates[18] supports this approach. In this study, scans were performed at 30 to 32 weeks and at 36 to 37 weeks. The rates of intervention in the study and control groups were 31.3% and 16.9%, respectively. The authors concluded that introduction of an ultrasound scan at 30 to 32 weeks and at 36 to 37 weeks may reduce the risk of the delivery of a growth-restricted infant, but increase antenatal interventions.

In theory, serial measurements can show a decline in growth as a fetal measurement crosses percentile lines.

This approach may be superior to waiting until the absolute measurement is below a particular cutoff value. Measurements of abdominal circumference are relatively inaccurate, and using two measurements doubles the chance of measurement error. If the first measurement is randomly high and the second measurement is randomly low, a normal fetus can easily be classified as having falling growth.

Ultrasound measurements are the best predictors of fetal weight.[19] Few experts would consider not performing at least some measure of fetal size when managing a high-risk pregnancy.

Amniotic Fluid Volume

In the second half of pregnancy, the fetal kidneys produce most of the amniotic fluid. If the fetus redistributes blood flow away from them (discussed later), urine production and amniotic fluid volume decrease. Amniotic fluid volume cannot be measured accurately in clinical practice. Ultrasound measurement of amniotic fluid volume is the best reproducible method. There are two ways in which this can be measured with ultrasound: the single maximum pool diameter and the amniotic fluid index (the sum of the maximum vertical pool in each of four uterine quadrants, excluding those containing fetal limbs or cord [see also Chapter 13]).

A systematic review with a meta-analysis of 18 studies involving more than 10,000 pregnancies showed that oligohydramnios (defined as an amniotic fluid index below the third percentile) was associated with an increased risk of a 5-minute Apgar score of less than 7 (relative risk, 5.2; 95% confidence interval, 2.4–11.3).[20] However, a low Apgar score is considered a fairly poor outcome endpoint. In that systematic review, only one study looked at the predictive value of the amniotic fluid index for neonatal acidosis, and this study reported a poor correlation between the two.

Chamberlain and associates[21] and Bastide and associates[22] showed that pregnancies with reduced liquor volume were associated with increased perinatal mortality compared with control subjects with normal liquor volume. However, the predictive value of a low volume of amniotic fluid is not clear when it occurs in isolation (e.g, in the absence of an abnormal umbilical artery Doppler recording or abnormal growth velocity). Further, no randomized controlled trials have shown the effect on fetal outcome of the use of amniotic fluid volume in the management of high-risk pregnancies.

Pathophysiology of Fetal Blood Flow

Much can be inferred from Doppler ultrasound recordings of blood flow velocity waveform signals from the fetal circulation in normal and pathologic pregnancies as well as from experimental models of acute hypoxia in animals. The umbilical artery is the most commonly studied vessel.

Umbilical Artery

In the first half of a normal pregnancy, the fetal side of the placental circulation is of relatively high resistance. There is little or no forward blood flow in the umbilical artery at the end of diastole. Even as late as 28 weeks, nearly 1% of normal pregnancies have absent end diastolic flow velocities. However, as gestation advances, placental resistance decreases, and in the normal fetus, considerable forward movement of blood occurs in the umbilical artery throughout the cardiac cycle. Therefore, the systolic-to-diastolic ratio is low. In normal pregnancy, the actual values for the S/D ratio decrease with increasing gestational age. In placental insufficiency, the S/D ratio increases until forward flow ceases at the end of diastole (absent end diastolic flow) and flow reverses later (reversed end diastolic flow).

Regional Changes in Blood Flow

Animal models show a consistent increase in blood flow to the heart, brain, and adrenal glands with experimental hypoxia and redistribution of umbilical venous return, with an increased proportion of highly oxygenated blood bypassing the liver through the ductus venosus. Initially, this causes increased heart rate and cardiac output. With increasingly adverse conditions, progressive impairment of cardiac function occurs, leading to decreased cardiac output. Normally, right-sided cardiac output is higher than left-sided output by a factor of approximately 1.3. With redistribution, the ratio changes as the left ventricle (which mainly sends blood to the brain) afterload decreases and the right ventricle afterload increases. If the right side of the heart begins to fail, then the increased right atrial pressure causes marked reduction in flow velocities during the atrial systole phase of the cycle in the vena cava, ductus venosus, and umbilical vein. Atrial systole is timed by the "A wave" of the venous cycle, and reduced flow velocities are seen as an increase in the size of this inverted A wave. These venous pulsations are analogous to the pulsatile waveforms seen in the jugular vein in adults with left-sided heart failure.

As the afterload in the right ventricle increases and end diastolic pressure increases in the right atrium, impairing forward flow, the reduction in forward flow progresses to absence and then reversal of venous blood flow with atrial contractions. This reversal is initially restricted to the inferior vena cava, but as fetal compromise progresses, it is seen across the ductus venosus and umbilical vein. This distal progression reflects deterioration in myocardial function.

In humans, the flow velocity waveforms in fetal cerebral arteries show the development of low resistance patterns under hypoxic situations. This suggests that, as in animals, the human fetus is redistributing blood flow and giving preferential supply to the brain ("brain-sparing phenomenon" or "centralization" of flow). There is some evidence that, as in animals, redistribution of the umbilical venous return occurs, with an increased proportion of highly oxygenated blood bypassing the liver through the ductus venosus, although this has not been shown directly in humans.

Studies comparing Doppler circulatory changes with cord blood gas levels at cordocentesis suggest that fetal arterial and ductus venosus pulsatility provides a good estimate of the degree of fetal hypoxemia and acidemia.[23] Vasodilatation in the cerebral vasculature occurs during mild to moderate hypoxemia. With severe hypoxemia (2–4 standard deviations below the mean for gestation) and acidemia, the reduction in middle cerebral artery pulsatility index (PI) reaches a limit that may represent maximum vessel dilation. At this point, vital organs receive so much of the available cardiac output that the oxygen supply for nonessential organs is inadequate and leads to metabolic acidosis, myocardial hypoxia, and cardiac failure.

Fetal Umbilical Artery Doppler Recordings

Perinatal mortality and morbidity rates increase with the degree of abnormality of umbilical artery Doppler recording.[24–26] Karsdorp and associates[24] estimated that the odds ratios for perinatal mortality in pregnancies complicated by absent and reversed end diastolic flow were 4 and 11, respectively. Although most studies were susceptible to treatment paradox, these waveforms have been measured in studies in which the results were concealed. Those results confirm that the umbilical artery waveform is a good test for the prediction of fetal death.[1]

Fetal umbilical artery Doppler blood flow waveform is the only test that has been evaluated in randomized trials that included a reasonable number of pregnancies. These studies support the conclusion that its use in high risk pregnancies reduces the rates of perinatal morbidity (defined as admission to antenatal units and induction of labor) and mortality.[27] No data are available to guide clinicians about the optimum frequency of use.

However, studies of its use in low risk pregnancies showed more deaths in the groups allocated to Doppler.[5,28] The numbers were small, and the results are equally compatible with an important beneficial effect and an important adverse effect. It is unlikely that umbilical artery waveforms behave differently in low risk women. More likely, the clinicians did not recognize that the predictive value of a positive test result in a low risk population was lower than the predictive value of the same result in a high risk group. This would have resulted in an excessively high rate of unwise early delivery. Whatever the mechanism, Doppler cannot be recommended as a general screening tool in low risk populations.

Regional Blood Flow: Cerebral Artery

Measurement of Redistribution

The middle cerebral artery is the easiest fetal cerebral vessel to visualize. It is the main branch of the circle of Willis and the direct intracranial continuation of the internal carotid artery. It carries approximately 80% of blood to the ipsilateral hemisphere and is divided into the following four segments.

- M1, which extends from the origin by the internal carotid to the anterolateral side of the sphenoid bone, where the anterior temporal artery originates
- M2, which extends from this point to the origin of the frontal arteries (anterior and ascending)
- M3, the posterior temporal artery
- M4, the cortical segments

Because the PI in M2 is always higher than that in M1, measurement must be made in the same portion of the vessel to allow reliable comparisons. Conventionally, PI is measured in the most proximal segment of M1, at the origin by the internal carotid.

Definition of Arterial Redistribution

Redistribution is indicated by a low middle cerebral artery PI (or resistance index, RI). Usually, a cutoff value of less than 2 standard deviations from the mean for gestational age is used. However, cerebral redistribution of fetal blood flow during hypoxia is probably associated with peripheral vasoconstriction. Therefore, the ratio between cerebral arterial PI or RI and, say, umbilical artery PI may be a more sensitive indicator of redistribution. The ratio between blood flow velocity of the umbilical artery and that of the middle cerebral artery does not appear to depend on gestational age. A cerebroplacental ratio of less than 1 indicates redistribution.

Clinical Value

Several comparative studies examined high risk pregnancies with redistribution and correlated this finding with perinatal outcome. As with umbilical artery Doppler assessment, the fetus with small for gestational age (SGA) and middle cerebral artery PI in the normal range is at lower risk perinatally than the fetus with abnormal middle cerebral artery PI.[23,29,30]

Studies reporting longer-term outcome found no difference in neurodevelopmental assessment in infants up to 2 years of age.[31] However, by 5 years of age, some neurologic differences were detectable.[32] The inclusion of fetal cerebral artery velocimetry in the management of complicated pregnancies may improve the outcome.

No randomized controlled trials have tested the effect of including measurement of fetal cerebral artery velocimetry or venous waveforms (discussed later) in the management of even high risk pregnancies.

Fetal Anemia (See also Chapter 14)

The fetal middle cerebral artery has been the subject of research that has directly affected the clinical management of conditions that cause fetal anemia. Doppler peak velocity recording appears to correlate with fetal hemoglobin more precisely than the maternal antibody titer. Moderate and severe anemia can be detected noninvasively by Doppler ultrasonography on the basis of an increase in the peak velocity of systolic blood flow in the middle cerebral artery.[33,34] This should decrease the need for invasive procedures (e.g., amniocentesis, fetal blood sampling) and their associated complications. Reference ranges for middle cerebral artery peak systolic velocity and intervention zones have been developed to guide clinical practice.[35]

Regional Blood Flow: Venous Waveforms

The development of abnormal waveforms in the umbilical vain, inferior vena cava, and ductus venosus point to a late stage of progressive deterioration of the fetal condition and severe fetal compromise.[23,29,30] However, venous Doppler waveforms can be difficult to obtain, and in some series, evaluable waveforms were achieved in only approximately 75% of cases.

Uterine Artery Doppler Waveforms

The uterine artery waveform is used more often to predict disease in late pregnancy than to assess the fetal condition directly. An abnormal waveform at 11 to 14 weeks[36] or at 23 weeks[37,38] identifies a high proportion of cases of severe preeclampsia or fetal growth restriction. This may provide the basis for preventive therapy with either low-dose aspirin or vitamin supplements. After 34 weeks, abnormal uterine artery Doppler waveforms at diagnosis are associated with a fourfold increased risk of adverse neonatal outcome.[39]

Biophysical Measures of Fetal Assessment

*Fetal Heart Rate Patterns**

The normal fetal heart rate varies continuously as the vagal and sympathetic tone constantly adjust cardiac output to meet the demands of fetal activity. Regular acceleratory periods occur in response to movement and are superimposed on a lower level of baseline variability. As the fetus becomes hypoxic, both the baseline variability and the accelerations in response to movement decrease. At a late stage of hypoxemia, the fetus has intermittent periods of bradycardia in response to temporarily worsening hypoxia related to Braxton Hicks contractions.

The fetal heart rate pattern is easily measured noninvasively with an external Doppler device. These devices calculate the fetal heart rate every three to five beats and plot the rate on paper. Uterine contractions can be measured simultaneously with an external tocometer, and fetal movements may be recorded by the mother with a marker device. The normal fetal heart rate pattern varies with gestational age. Beyond 30 weeks, the normal baseline is between 120 and 160 beats/min, the baseline variability is more than 5 beats/min, and there is a 20- to 30-minute cycle of sleep activity. During the active phase of the cycle, the fetal heart rate accelerates in response to uterine contractions and fetal movement.

Computerized Analysis of Fetal Heart Rate

Short-term variation derived from fetal heart rate monitoring is a widely used indicator of fetal compromise. It correlates well with the development of metabolic acidemia and intrauterine death.[40] Dawes and associates[41] developed a computer program to assess variations in fetal heart rate. Short-term variation is best correlated with hypoxemia and increases with gestational age. The 2.5 percentile value is 4.4 msec at 26 weeks, 5 msec at 28 weeks, 5.4 msec at 30 weeks, 5.9 msec at 32 weeks, and 6 msec at 34 weeks and beyond. Acidemia is rare when the short-term variation is 4 msec or more. Administration of steroids causes a transient decrease in short-term variability.

Clinical Studies of the Value of CTG/NST

In a systematic review of four randomized controlled trials (involving fewer than 2000 pregnancies), the use of CTG/NST did not improve fetal outcome. There was a trend toward increased mortality in the group receiving CTG/NST compared with those who did not.[42] However, the trials did not have sufficient power to detect a significant effect on perinatal mortality rates. Computer analysis of CTG/NST had greater accuracy than clinical experts in predicting fetal acidosis and low Apgar scores.[43,44]

Biophysical Profile Score

The biophysical profile score predicts both acute and chronic outcome (the former more than the latter) and has very high negative predictive value.[45–47] In a systematic review, Alfirevic and Neilson[48] concluded that there were insufficient data to determine the value of the biophysical profile score in the management of high-risk pregnancies. However, only four poor-quality studies, with fewer than 3000 patients, were available for review.

Order of Changes

Four studies[29,30,49,50] attempted to describe the order in which these changes occur. This is difficult in humans because not all fetuses follow the same pattern, the results depend on how abnormality is defined, and because it is unethical to withhold delivery from sick human fetuses, whichever test is used to time delivery will appear to be the last result to change. Nevertheless, abnormalities in the umbilical artery waveform tend to appear first, followed by cerebral redistribution, early venous changes, and decreased breathing movements. Amniotic fluid volume starts to decrease, and then short-term variability in the fetal heart rate decreases.

*Cardiotocography (CTG) or non-stress testing (NST)

Abnormal umbilical venous pulsation, reversed umbilical artery pulsation, abnormal fetal movements and tone, and fetal bradycardia are late events.

Test Combinations

There is no accepted standard of practice for the surveillance and management of high risk fetuses. Many centers use a combination of fetal growth, umbilical artery Doppler recordings together with CTG, biophysical profile, and other Doppler studies[49,51,52] and give the mother steroids, if preterm delivery is considered. The optimum timing of delivery is unknown, although most would not continue the pregnancy beyond 34 weeks if Doppler recordings show persistent abnormality of the umbilical artery.[49]

Placental Grading

As the normal placenta ages, its ultrasound appearance changes. It becomes calcified, and the cotyledons become more clearly demarcated. These changes can be graded from I to IV. There has been only one randomized controlled trial of routine placental grading as a screening tool in a low risk population.[53] This trial showed improved perinatal outcome in the scanned group compared with those who were not scanned. However, several important points should be noted. The numbers in the study were smaller than would normally be expected to show a significant difference in fetal outcome measures. The group that did not have placental grading had a higher incidence of adverse fetal outcome than would normally be expected for a low risk population, and the improvement in outcome did not occur exclusively in those with abnormal placental grading. Further research on placental grading in low risk and high risk pregnancies is needed. Placental grading is not widely used in clinical practice.

Biochemical Tests

The most recent Cochrane review[54] found that the use of biochemical tests of placental function led to no obvious differences in perinatal mortality rates (relative risk, 0.88; 95% confidence interval, 0.36–2.13). Available trial data do not support the use of estriol estimation in high risk pregnancies. This review included only one eligible trial of poor quality. The only argument in favor of using a biochemical test in fetal assessment is the use of midtrimester elevated maternal serum α-fetoprotein levels as a predictor of later intrauterine growth restriction or preeclampsia.[55] There is no information about the ideal frequency of subsequent surveillance, nor is there evidence that this surveillance is associated with improved outcome.

CONCLUSIONS

- Maternal monitoring of fetal movements is useful for identifying fetuses at increased risk for fetal death.
- Further study is needed to determine the best method for subsequent fetal monitoring when women report reduced fetal movements.
- Symphysis–fundal height measurement has considerable limitations when used as the sole screening test for pathologic fetal growth. It has low sensitivity, a high false-positive rate, and significant intraobserver and interobserver variation. Customized serial measurements give a better clinical prediction.
- Auscultation of the fetal heart gives information only about fetal viability. There is no evidence that it identifies at-risk fetuses or improves fetal outcome.
- Routine recording of the fetal heart rate helps to identify fetal arrhythmias.
- Ultrasound assessment of fetal growth and size in a high risk pregnancy predicts fetal outcome, but there is no evidence that this strategy alters outcome.
- Amniotic fluid volume less than the third percentile is associated with an increased risk of poor perinatal outcome. It is not clear whether this association is valid if it is an isolated finding.
- Umbilical artery Doppler recordings in high risk pregnancies are a useful screening tool and reduce perinatal morbidity and possibly mortality rates. There is no agreement about the optimum frequency of use of this modality.
- No evidence supports the use of umbilical artery Doppler recordings in screening low risk pregnancies.
- There is no evidence that the use of regional blood flow recordings in patients with chronic hypoxia and anemia improves pregnancy outcome, although these recordings indicate the degree of fetal compromise.
- Uterine artery Doppler recordings obtained before 24 weeks can identify an increased risk of intrauterine growth restriction and preeclampsia. There is evidence that their use improves pregnancy outcome, although the degree of improvement needs further research.

CONCLUSIONS *(Continued)*

- A biophysical profile score is not recommended for routine screening in low risk pregnancies. However, it is a useful adjunct to umbilical artery Doppler recordings in high risk pregnancies, particularly because of its high negative predictive value.
- A biophysical profile score is predominantly an acute measure of fetal well-being, giving short-term information and reassurance. In high risk cases, an abnormal biophysical profile score usually predicts imminent fetal death.
- Cardiotocography analysis, especially by computer, predicts outcome. However, like the biophysical profile score, in most cases, cardiotocography provides information about the acute status of the fetus. The findings become grossly abnormal late in the process of fetal deterioration. Arguably, it should be used only in combination with tests of chronic fetal health (e.g., measurement of fetal growth, umbilical artery Doppler).
- The use of cardiotocography has not been shown to improve fetal outcome, but large enough studies have not been performed and none relate to computer analysis.
- Further randomized controlled trials with appropriate power should be conducted to determine whether placental grading is a valuable screening tool in low risk pregnancies.
- Biochemical testing has no place in fetal assessment, with the exception of midtrimester maternal serum α-fetoprotein levels, which may indicate an increased risk of intrauterine growth restriction and preeclampsia later in the pregnancy.

SUMMARY OF MANAGEMENT OPTIONS
Assessing Fetal Health

Management Options	Quality of Evidence	Strength of Recommendation	References
Indications			
Low risk patients: Implement a surveillance program to identify when the risk ceases to be low; this might include:	–	GPP	–
• Ultrasound in the first half of pregnancy: Insufficient evidence to show the value of routine ultrasound screening in pregnancy	Ia	A	3–5
• Fetal movement counting: Evidence suggests that this identifies fetuses at risk but does not improve outcome	Ib	A	14
• Fundal height measurement: Poor at identifying pathologically grown fetuses although measurements are better if they are serial and customized; insufficient evidence of value in improving fetal outcome	III IIa Ib	B B A	15 17 16
• Auscultation of fetal heart sounds: Recommended in practice, but no evidence of value; recording the rate may identify fetal arrythmias	–	GPP	–
High risk patients, where there is a risk of chronic hypoxemia:	III	B	9–13
• Maternal: cyanotic heart disease, diabetes, autoimmune disease, renal disease, hypertension, inadequate nutrition, smoking (often synergistic with other factors), alcohol and other drug abuse			
• Placental: idiopathic growth restriction, recurrent abruption, preeclampsia			
• Fetal: congenital anomalies (monitoring not likely to be implemented), acquired abnormalities (infection, anemia, hydrops, metabolic)			
• Combined: serum α-fetoprotein	III	B	55

SUMMARY OF MANAGEMENT OPTIONS
Assessing Fetal Health *(Continued)*

Management Options	Quality of Evidence	Strength of Recommendation	References
Principles			
Select the test that is appropriate for the pathology or problem if possible or known	–	GPP	–
Comprehensive assessment of mother and fetus	–	GPP	–
Multiple repeated fetal assessment methods are more likely to be informative than any single test	Ib	A	51
	III	B	49
	IV	C	52
Methods—Maternal			
Clinical (e.g., evaluation of hypertension, cardiac disease)	–	GPP	–
Laboratory (e.g., diabetes, Kleihauer, renal and liver function)	–	GPP	–
Methods—Fetal			
Ultrasound measurement of fetal growth:			
• Standard practice, but there is no randomized controlled trial of benefit in low or high risk pregnancy	Ia	A	4
• Serial measurements may be best in identifying fetal growth problems in apparently low risk pregnancy	Ib	B	18
• Ultrasound is the best method of estimating fetal weight	III	B	19
Amniotic fluid volume:			
• Low values are predictive of adverse fetal outcome; predictive value in the absence of other ultrasound abnormalities is uncertain	Ia	A	20
Umbilical artery Doppler velocimetry:	Ia	A	27
• The only test shown in randomized trials to reduce perinatal morbidity and mortality rates			
• No information about the optimum frequency of use			
Regional recordings of fetal blood flow:	III	B	23,29–35
• Indicate the degree of fetal compromise in chronic fetal hypoxia and anemia, but there is no evidence that their use improves outcome			
Uterine artery blood flow before 24 wk:	III	B	36–39
• Identifies pregnancies at risk for intrauterine growth restriction and preeclampsia; use may improve outcome			
CTG/NST:			
• Predicts short-term outcome; computerized assessment is more accurate	III	B	40,41,43,44,49
• No grade A evidence that use improves outcome	Ia	A	42
• Probably best in combination with other methods	Ia	A	51
	III	B	49
	IV	C	52
BPS:			
• Gives the best indication of acute and chronic fetal compromise	III	B	45–47
• No grade A evidence that use improves outcome	Ia	A	48
• Probably best in combination with other methods	Ia	A	51
	III	B	49
	IV	C	52

Continued

SUMMARY OF MANAGEMENT OPTIONS
Assessing Fetal Health *(Continued)*

Management Options	Quality of Evidence	Strength of Recommendation	References
Methods—Fetal			
Placental grading:			
• Only one study supports use in low risk population screening	Ib	A	53
• More research is needed			
Biochemical testing:			
• No evidence supports use in high risk pregnancies	Ia	A	54

REFERENCES

1. Thornton JG, Lilford RJ: Do we need randomised trials of antenatal tests of fetal wellbeing? Br J Obstet Gynaecol 1993;100: 197–200.
2. GRIT Study Group: A randomised trial of timed delivery for the compromised preterm fetus: Short term outcomes and Bayesian interpretation. Br J Obstet Gynaecol 2003;110:27–32.
3. Bucher H, Schmidt JG: Does routine ultrasound scanning improve outcome of pregnancy? Meta-analysis of various outcome measures. BMJ 1993;307:13–17.
4. Bricker L, Neilson JP: Routine ultrasound in late pregnancy (after 24 weeks): Cochrane Review. In The Cochrane Library, Issue 3. Oxford, UK, Update Software, 2003.
5. Bricker L, Neilson JP: Routine Doppler ultrasound in pregnancy: Cochrane Review. In: The Cochrane Library, Issue 3. Oxford, UK, Update Software, 2003.
6. Wilkins-Haug L, Roberts DJ, Morton CC: Confined placental mosaicism and intrauterine growth retardation: A case-control analysis of placentas at delivery. Am J Obstet Gynecol 1995;172:44–50.
7. Moore GE, Ali Z, Khan RU, et al: The incidence of uniparental disomy associated with intrauterine growth retardation in a cohort of thirty-five severely affected babies. Am J Obstet Gynecol 1997;176:294–299.
8. Khan NA, Kazzi SN: Yield and costs of screening growth-retarded infants for TORCH infections. Am J Perinatol 2000;17:131–135.
9. Kupferminc MJ, Eldor A, Steinman N, et al: Increased frequency of genetic thrombophilia in women with complications of pregnancy. N Engl J Med 1999;340:9–13.
10. Martinelli P, Grandone E, Colaizzo D, et al: Familial thrombophilia and the occurrence of fetal growth restriction. Haematologica 2001;86:428–431.
11. Grandone E, Margaglione M, Colaizzo D, et al: Lower birth-weight in neonates of mothers carrying factor V G1691A and factor II A(20210) mutations. Haematologica 2002;87:177–181.
12. Resnik R: Intrauterine growth restriction. Obstet Gynecol 2002;99:490–496.
13. Siddiqui F, James D: Fetal monitoring in type 1 diabetic pregnancies. Early Hum Dev 2003;72:1–13.
14. Grant A, Elbourne D, Valentin L, Alexander S: Routine formal fetal movement counting and risk of antepartum late death in normally formed singletons. Lancet 1989;ii:345–349.
15. Rosenberg K, Grant JM, Hepburn M: Antenatal detection of growth retardation: Actual practice in a large maternity hospital. Br J Obstet Gynecol 1982;89:12–15.
16. Neilson JP: Symphysis-fundal height measurement in pregnancy: Cochrane Review. In The Cochrane Library, Issue 3. Oxford, UK, Update Software, 2003.
17. Gardosi J, Francis A: Controlled trial of fundal height measurement plotted on customised antenatal growth charts. Br J Obstet Gynaecol 1999;106:309–317.
18. McKenna D, Tharmaratnam S, Mahsud S, et al: A randomized trial using ultrasound to identify the high risk fetus in a low-risk population. Obstet Gynecol 2003;101:626–632.
19. Chang TC, Robson SC, Boys RJ, Spencer JA: Prediction of the small for gestational age infant: Which ultrasonic measurement is best? Obstet Gynecol 1992;80:1030–1038.
20. Chauhan SP, Sanderson M, Hendrix NW, et al: Perinatal outcome and amniotic fluid index in the antepartum and intrapartum: A meta-analysis. Am J Obstet Gynecol 1999;181:1473–1478.
21. Chamberlain PF, Manning F, Morrison I, et al: Ultrasound evaluation of amniotic fluid volume: I. The relationship of marginal and decreased amniotic fluid volumes to perinatal outcome. Am J Obstet Gynecol 1984;150:245–249.
22. Bastide A, Manning F, Harman C, et al: Ultrasound evaluation of amniotic fluid: Outcome. Am J Obstet Gynecol 1986;154: 895–900.
23. Hecher K, Campbell S, Doyle P, et al: Assessment of fetal compromise by Doppler investigation of the fetal circulation. Circulation 1995;91:129–138.
24. Karsdorp VH, van Vugt JM, Van Geijn HP, et al: Clinical significance of absent or reversed end diastolic velocity waveforms in umbilical artery. Lancet 1994;344:1664–1668.
25. Pattinson RC, Norman K, Odendaal HJ: The role of Doppler velocity waveforms in the management of high risk pregnancies. Br J Obstet Gynaecol 1994;101:114–120.
26. Todros T, Ronco G, Fianchino O, et al: Accuracy of the umbilical arteries Doppler flow velocity waveforms in detecting adverse perinatal outcomes in a high risk population. Acta Obstet Gynecol Scand 1996;75:113–119.
27. Alfirevic Z, Neilson JP: Doppler ultrasonography in high-risk pregnancies: Systematic review with meta-analysis. Am J Obstet Gynecol 1995;172:1379–1387.
28. Goffinet F, Paris-Llado J, Nisand I, Breart G: Umbilical artery Doppler velocimetry in unselected and low risk pregnancies: A

review of randomised controlled trials. Br J Obstet Gynaecol 1997;104:425–430.

29. Ferrazi E, Bozzo M, Rigano S, et al: Temporal sequence of abnormal Doppler changes in the peripheral and central circulatory systems of the severely growth restricted fetus. Ultrasound Obstet Gynecol 2002;19:140–146.
30. Hecher K, Bilardo CM, Stighter RH, et al: Monitoring of fetuses with intrauterine growth restriction: A longitudinal study Ultrasound Obstet Gynecol 2001;18:564–570.
31. Scherjon SA, Smolders-DeHaas H, Kok JH, Zondervan HA: The "brain-sparing" effect: Antenatal cerebral Doppler findings in relation to neurologic outcome in very preterm infants. Am J Obstet Gynecol 1993;169:169–175.
32. Scherjon SA, Oosting H, DeWilde T, et al: Fetal "brain-sparing" is associated with accelerated shortening of visual evoked potential latencies during early infancy. Am J Obstet Gynecol 1996;175:1569–1575.
33. Mari G: Noninvasive diagnosis by Doppler ultrasonography of fetal anaemia due to maternal red-cell alloimmunization. N Engl J Med 2000;342:9–14.
34. Zimmerman R, Durig P, Carpenter RJ, Mari G: Longitudinal measurement of peak systolic velocity in the fetal middle cerebral artery for monitoring pregnancies complicated by red cell alloimmunisation: A prospective multicentre trial with intention-to-treat. Br J Obstet Gynaecol 2002;109:746–752.
35. Kurmanavicius J, Streicher A, Wright EM, et al: Reference values of fetal peak systolic blood flow velocity in the middle cerebral artery at 19–40 weeks gestation. Ultrasound Obstet Gynecol 2001;17:50–53.
36. Martin AM, Bindra R, Curcio P, et al: Screening for preeclampsia and fetal growth restriction by uterine artery Doppler at 11–14 weeks of gestation. Ultrasound Obstet Gynecol 2001;18:583–586.
37. Papageorghiou AT, Yu CK, Bindra R, et al: Multicentre screening for pre-eclampsia and fetal growth restriction by transvaginal uterine artery Doppler at 23 weeks of gestation. Ultrasound Obstet Gynecol 2001;18:441–449.
38. Becker R, Vonk R Vollert W, Entezami M: Doppler sonography of uterine arteries at 20–23 weeks: Risk assessment of adverse pregnancy outcome by quantification of impedence and notch. J Perinat Med 2002;30:388–394.
39. Vergani P, Roncaglia N, Andreotti C, et al: Prognostic value of uterine artery Doppler velocimetry in growth-restricted fetuses delivered near term. Am J Obstet Gynecol 2002;187:932–936.
40. Street P, Dawes GS, Moulden M, Redman CWG: Short-term variation in abnormal antenatal fetal heart rate records. Am J Obstet Gynecol 1991;165:515–523.
41. Dawes GS, Moulden M, Redman CWG: Short-term fetal heart rate variation, decelerations, and umbilical flow velocity waveforms before labor. Obstet Gynecol 1992;80:673–678.
42. Pattison N, McCowan L: Cardiotocography for antepartum fetal assessment: Cochrane Review. In The Cochrane Library, Issue 3. Oxford, UK, Update Software, 2003.
43. Nielsen PV, Stigsby B, Nickelsen C, Nim J: Computer assessment of the intrapartum cardiotocogram: II. The value of compared with visual assessment. Acta Obstet Gynecol Scand 1988;67:461–464.
44. Royal College of Obstetricians and Gynaecologists: The Use of Electronic Fetal Monitoring. Evidence-based Clinical Guideline No. 8. London, RCOG, 2001, pp 50, 109–110.
45. Manning FA, Morrison I, Harman CR, et al: Fetal assessment based on fetal biophysical profile scoring: Experience in 19,221 referred high risk pregnancies. Am J Obstet Gynecol 1987;157: 880–884.
46. Manning FA, Snijders R, Harman CR, et al: Fetal biophysical profile score: VI. Correlation with antepartum umbilical venous fetal pH. Am J Obstet Gynecol 1993;169:755–763.
47. Manning FA, Bondaji N, Harman CR, et al: Fetal assessment based on fetal biophysical profile scoring: VIII. The incidence of cerebral palsy in tested and untested perinates. Am J Obstet Gynecol 1998;178:696–706.
48. Alfirevic Z, Neilson JP: Biophysical profile for fetal assessment in high risk pregnancies: Cochrane Review. In The Cochrane Library, Issue 4. Oxford, UK, Update Software, 2003.
49. James DK, Parker MS, Smoleniec JS: Comprehensive fetal assessment with three ultrasonographic characteristics. Am J Obstet Gynecol 1992;166:1486–1495.
50. Baschat AA, Gembruch U, Harman CR: The sequence of changes in Doppler and biophysical parameters as severe fetal growth restriction worsens. Ultrasound Obstet Gynaecol 2001;18:571–577.
51. Tyrrell SN, Lilford RJ, Macdonald HN, et al: Randomized comparison of routine vs highly selective use of Doppler ultrasound and biophysical scoring to investigate high risk pregnancies. Br J Obstet Gynaecol 1990;97:909–916.
52. Harrington KF: Making best and appropriate use of fetal biophysical and Doppler ultrasound data in the management of the growth restricted fetus. Ultrasound Obstet Gynecol 2000;16: 399–401.
53. Proud J, Grant AM: Third trimester placental grading by ultrasonography as a test of fetal wellbeing. BMJ 1987;294: 1641–1647.
54. Neilson JP: Biochemical tests of placental function for assessment in pregnancy: Cochrane Review. In The Cochrane Library, Issue 1. Oxford, UK, Update Software, 2003.
55. Shipp TD, Wilkins-Haug L: The association of early-onset fetal growth restriction, elevated maternal serum alpha-fetoprotein and the development of severe pre-eclampsia. Prenat Diagn 1997;17:305–309.

CHAPTER 12

Fetal Growth Disorders

Ahmet Alexander Baschat

INTRODUCTION

Disturbance of normal fetal growth can result in abnormal weight, body mass, or body proportion at birth. The two principal fetal growth disorders are intrauterine growth restriction (IUGR) and macrosomia, both of which are associated with increased perinatal mortality rates and short- and long-term morbidity rates. Perinatal detection of fetal growth disorders has evolved dramatically over the last four decades. Before antenatal ultrasound assessment of fetal growth was clinically available, absolute birth weight was classified as either macrosomia (>4000g) or low birth weight, very low birth weight, or extremely low birth weight (<2500g, <1500g, and <1000g respectively). Growth is a dynamic process, and only the comparison of absolute measurements with gestational age reference ranges allows the detection of discrepancies between expected and actual growth. The landmark observations of Lubchenco and colleagues[1] in 1963 showed that the classification of neonates by birth weight percentile has a significant prognostic advantage because it improves the detection of neonates with IUGR who are at increased risk for adverse health events throughout life.[2–4] Neonates are now classified as very small for gestational age (below the third percentile), small for gestational age (below the 10th percentile), appropriate for gestational age (10th–90th percentile), or large for gestational age (above the 90th percentile).[5] The detection of a fetal growth disorder is further enhanced if the reference ranges for fetal biometric data and birth weight account for maternal height and race and fetal birth order and sex[6] (growth potential). A neonate may be of normal weight but still significantly lighter than its growth potential. Growth potential percentiles are superior to conventional reference ranges for the prediction of adverse perinatal outcome.[7,8]

The detection of abnormal body mass or proportions is based on anthropometric measurements and ratios that are relatively independent of sex, race, and to a certain extent, gestational age. The ponderal index [(birth weight (g)/crown–heel length^3) × 100][9] is one tool that has high accuracy for the identification of IUGR[10] and macrosomia,[11] independent of the birth weight percentile.[12] In one study, 40% of neonates with a birth weight below the 10th percentile did not have growth restriction based on the ponderal index.[10] From a clinical perspective, the ponderal index correlates more closely with perinatal morbidity and mortality than traditional birth weight percentiles, but may miss proportionally small and lean neonates with growth restriction.[13,14] Inappropriate fetal growth is also suggested by abnormal symmetry between head and abdominal measurements. Again, a different subset of neonates is identified with this descriptive approach.[15]

A gold standard for birth weight criteria that distinguishes between abnormal and physiologic growth patterns is highly desirable for any study of the relationship between neonatal size and outcome. Although the immediate effect of disturbed fetal growth is an abnormal expression of the growth potential, the effect on outcome and fetal programming is determined predominantly by the underlying condition.

REGULATION OF FETAL GROWTH

Fetal growth is regulated at multiple levels, and successful placentation is required for the coordination of key components within the maternal, placental, and fetal compartments. In the first trimester, placental adherence and implantation are prerequisites for placental vascular development, which is necessary for the delivery of nutrients and oxygen to the growing trophoblast beyond simple diffusion. Successful adherence permits differentiation of placental transport mechanisms and paracrine and endocrine signaling pathways between the mother, placenta, and fetus by the second trimester. These are essential for efficient and coordinated nutrient transfer and waste and gas exchange. These milestones promote exponential fetal growth and differentiation in the third trimester.

After fertilization, the cytotrophoblast migrates to form anchoring villi between the decidua and uterus through controlled breakdown of the extracellular matrix by metalloproteinases and localized expression of adhesion molecules, including integrins and collagen IV. Simultaneously, hypoxia-stimulated angiogenesis initiates vascular connections between the maternal circulation and the intervillous space. Once the maternal blood supply to the intervillous space is established, increasing quantities of placental secretory products appear in the maternal circulation. Concurrently, extravillous cytotrophoblasts infiltrate the maternal spiral arteries, progressively remodeling the vessel walls so that the musculoelastic media is lost[16,17] In parallel, continuous villous vascular branching and thinning of the cytotrophoblast occurs in the fetal compartment.[18] These processes result in low-resistance, high-capacitance vascular beds that allow increasing and matched perfusion of the maternal and fetal placental compartments. Intervillous blood flow is regulated mainly through paracrine factors, such as nitric oxide, endothelin, adenosine, released cyclic guanosine monophosphate, and fetal atrial natriuretic peptide.[18] After successful placentation, approximately 600 mL/min maternal cardiac output[19,20] is matched to 400 mL/kg/min fetal flow distributed over a term placental exchange area of 12 m.[2,21]

The design of the fetal circulation allows preferential streaming of nutrients that enter the circulation through the umbilical vein. Modulated by shunting in the ductus venosus, 70% to 80% of the returning blood continues on to the liver; the rest is distributed to the heart.[22] In the right atrium, the directionality of incoming bloodstreams ensures that nutrient-rich blood is distributed to the myocardium and brain, whereas venous return from the body is distributed to the descending aorta and ultimately to the placenta for reoxygenation and nutrient and waste exchange.[23,24] In addition, because of the preferential distribution of left- and right-sided cardiac output, several organs can modify local flow by autoregulation to meet oxygen and nutrient demands.[25]

Once the blood supply to the trophoblast and fetal circulation is established, placental transport capacity is the major determinant of maternal–fetal nutrient transport. All substances that traverse between the maternal and fetal circulation must pass through the villous trophoblast, a syncytial bilayer 4 μm thick that consists of a maternal microvillus and a fetal basal layer.[26] Its capacity for transport is enhanced by a growing membrane surface area and increased density and affinity of carrier proteins for glucose, amino acids (mainly), and fatty acids.[24,27–29] The sodium/hydrogen (Na/H^+) family of transport proteins maintains syncytiotrophoblast intracellular pH and cell volume homeostasis, ensuring proper function of the transplacental substrate carrier proteins.[30] By the second trimester, these placental activities consume 40% of the O_2 and 70% of the glucose entering the uterus, leaving the rest for fetal use.[31–33] This proportion decreases progressively until term.

With the establishment of placental transport systems, endocrine signaling between maternal, placental, and fetal compartments helps to coordinate placental and fetal growth. Maternal metabolic changes include postprandial hyperglycemia, lipolysis, and increased fasting levels of free fatty acids, triglycerides, and cholesterol. All of these enhance substrate availability to the placenta and fetus and are at least partly mediated by increases in placental levels of lactogen and leptin. Similarly, maternal intravascular volume expansion and its relative refractoriness to vasoactive agents promote steady nutrient delivery to the placenta.[34]

Placental and fetal growth is regulated by the combination of substrate availability and endocrine or paracrine signaling. Glucose and amino acids stimulate insulin release from the fetal pancreas, and the subsequent release of insulin-like growth factors I and II provides the major stimulus for fetal growth and differentiation.[35] Leptin stimulates fetal pancreatic growth and transplacental amino acid transport and affects fatty acid transport. Therefore, it may be an important modulator of fetal body fat content and body proportions.[36,37]

Normal placental and fetal growth across pregnancy is characterized by sequential cellular hyperplasia, hyperplasia plus hypertrophy, and finally, hypertrophy alone.[38] Placental growth follows a sigmoid curve, with a plateau occurring earlier in gestation than the fetal curve. Between 16 weeks and term, human fetal weight increases 20-fold.[27] The fetal growth curve is exponential. Maximal growth occurs in the third trimester, when significant body mass and particularly adipose tissue are accumulated.

FETAL GROWTH RESTRICTION

Etiology and Risk Factors

Several conditions may interfere with normal placentation and culminate in either pregnancy loss or IUGR. Broadly categorized into maternal, uterine, placental, and fetal disorders, these conditions affect either nutrient and oxygen delivery to the placenta, nutrient and oxygen transfer across the placenta, fetal uptake, or regulation of growth processes. When they are sufficiently abnormal, they produce growth restriction characterized by a reduction in fetal cell size, and when they are early and severe enough, cell number is also affected (Fig. 12–1). In clinical practice, considerable overlap occurs between conditions that determine the manifestation, progression, and outcome of growth restriction. Fetal

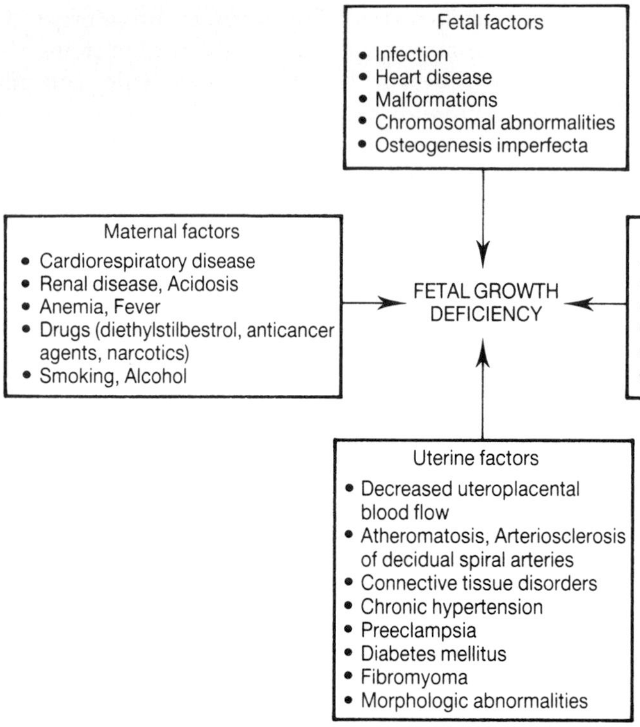

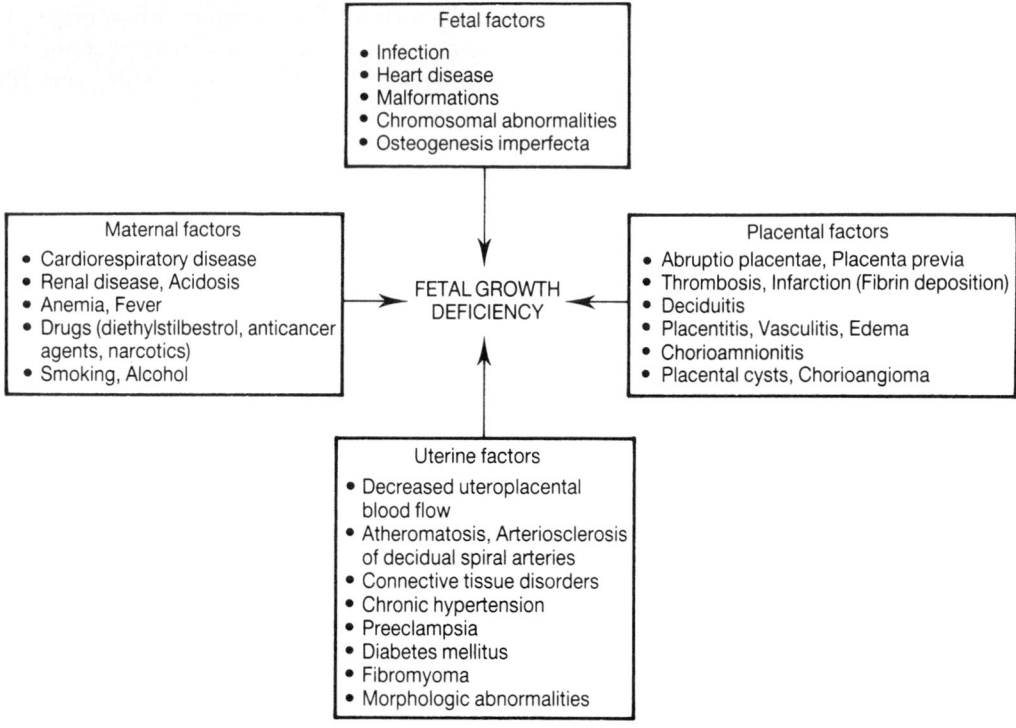

FIGURE 12–1
Causes of growth restriction by compartment.

abnormalities (both chromosomal and anatomic) and abnormal placental vascular development account for the vast majority of cases of IUGR in singleton pregnancies.[39–43] Usually, the earlier the onset of the disease process, the more likely the fetus is to be symmetrically small, with a reduced cell number, and the more likely the etiology is to be either a severe maternal vascular disorder, fetal infection, or a chromosome disorder.[44]

Maternal causes of growth restriction include chronic renal disease, collagen vascular disease, hypertension, and some thrombophilias. Aggravating circumstances include smoking, malnutrition, and drug use. Many risk factors can act synergistically. For example, the adverse effect of smoking is doubled in thin, white women and further potentiated by poor maternal weight gain.[45] Similarly, the possible benefits of low-dose aspirin therapy and the detrimental effects of excessive blood pressure reduction are also more apparent in this group of women.[46,47]

Pathophysiology

Our knowledge of the pathophysiology of IUGR was initially derived from animal experiments but has been greatly expanded by human studies with sophisticated epidemiologic analyses and by advanced ultrasound technology to elucidate the relationships between fetoplacental hemodynamic characteristics, fetal behavior, amniotic fluid production, and regulation of fetal heart rate.

Interference with the placental nutrient supply can affect all aspects of placental function. The gestational age at onset, the magnitude of injury, and the success of adaptive mechanisms determine the ultimate severity. Mild placental disease is more likely to affect organ function and maturation at the cellular level, with little perceivable growth delay perinatally, but may affect adult health by fetal programming. With more severe placental disease, fetal growth delay and adaptive organ responses become evident in utero. Exhaustion of the placental and fetal adaptive potential leads to decompensation, with variable progression and manifestations in the fetal organ systems. Adaptive responses that are intended to enhance fetal survival in a hypoxic environment may become destructive under conditions such as acute ischemia-reperfusion. Much of the long-term effect of growth restriction is unclear, as are the effects of obstetric intervention. As a result, severe disturbances of fetal growth pose a challenge to even the most experienced multidisciplinary team.

Mechanisms of Placental Dysfunction

Early interference with placentation affects all levels of placental and fetal development and culminates in the most severe clinical picture. Diffusion may be adequate to meet embryonic nutrient needs, but it compromises fetal survival and growth potential. Typically, the trophoblastic invasion is confined to the decidual portion of the myometrium, and the spiral and radial arteries do not transform into low-resistance vessels.[16,48,49] Altered expression of vasoactive substances increases vascular reactivity, and if hypoxia-stimulated angiogenesis is inadequate, placental autoregulation becomes deficient. Maternal placental floor infarcts and fetal villous obliteration and fibrosis increase placental blood flow resistance, producing a maternal–fetal placental perfusion mismatch that decreases the effective exchange area.[18,24,50,51] With progressive vascular occlusion, fetoplacental flow resistance is increased throughout the vascular bed, which is the metabolically active placental mass, and nutrient exchange decreases or is outgrown.

The severity of placental vascular dysfunction is clinically assessed in the fetal and maternal compartments with Doppler ultrasound. An early diastolic notch in the uterine arteries at 12 to 14 weeks (Fig. 12–2) suggests delayed trophoblast invasion,[52] whereas persistence of "notching" beyond 24 weeks provides confirmatory evidence.[16,51,53] A reduction of umbilical venous blood flow volume may be the earliest Doppler sign of subtle decreases in fetal villous perfusion.[54] Umbilical artery waveforms correlate with both the tertiary villous architecture and blood flow resistance. If villous damage is minimal, elevated blood flow resistance may be seen only with sophisticated Doppler techniques.[55] At least 30% of the fetal villous vasculature is abnormal when the umbilical artery end-diastolic velocities are low and Doppler resistance indices are elevated.[56] Absence or reversal of umbilical artery end-diastolic velocity suggests that 60% to 70% of the villous vascular tree is damaged (Fig. 12–3).[56,57] Abnormal flow patterns in the uterine

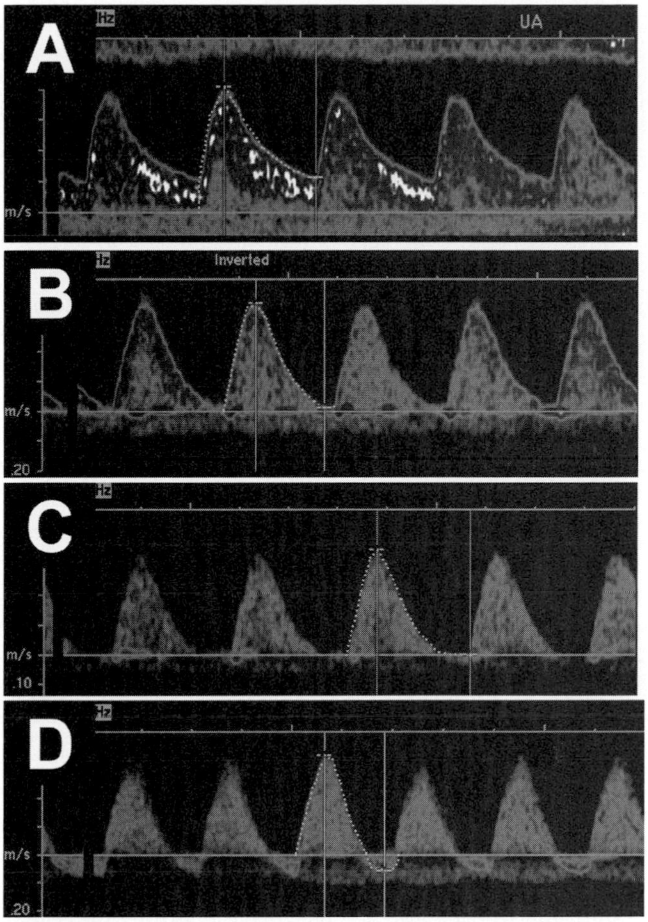

FIGURE 12–3
The normal umbilical artery flow velocity waveform has marked positive end-diastolic velocity that increases in proportion to systole toward term (*A*). Moderate abnormalities in the villous vascular structure increase blood flow resistance and are associated with a decrease in end-diastolic velocity (*B*). When a significant proportion of the villous vascular tree is abnormal, end-diastolic velocities may be absent (*C*) or even reversed (*D*).

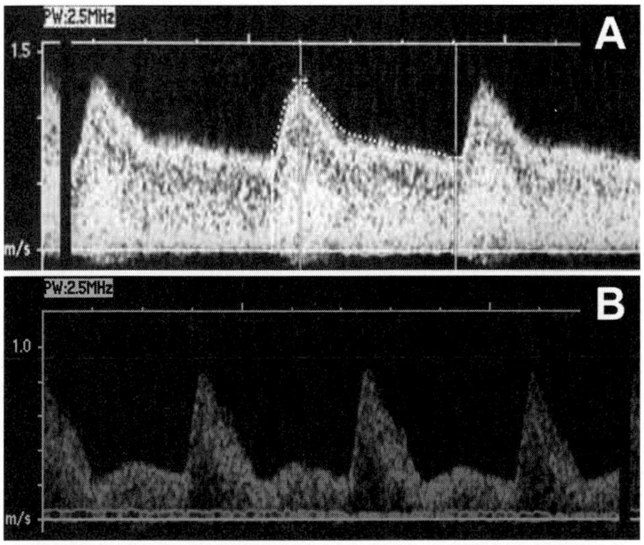

FIGURE 12–2
Flow velocity waveforms obtained from the uterine artery beyond 24 weeks' gestation. (*A*) High-volume diastolic flow is established, indicating successful trophoblast invasion. (*B*) Impaired trophoblast invasion of the spiral arteries is associated with elevated placental vascular resistance and persistence of an early diastolic notch in the uterine artery flow velocity waveform.

arteries are consistent with abnormal implantation and indicate an increased risk of preeclampsia, placental abruption, and IUGR.[58] Abnormal umbilical flow patterns indicate an increased risk of hypoxemia and acidemia proportional to the severity of Doppler abnormality.[18,59–61]

Metabolic and Cellular Effects of Placental Dysfunction

Oxygen and glucose consumption by the placenta is unaffected when nutrient delivery to the uterus is only mildly restricted and fetal demands can be met by increased fractional extraction. Fetal hypoglycemia occurs when uterine oxygen delivery (and likely substrate delivery) is less than a critical value (0.6 mmol/min/kg fetal body weight in sheep) and fetal oxygen uptake is reduced.[31,33,62] Insulin is an important fetal growth factor. Fetal pancreatic insulin responses are blunted by mild hypoglycemia, allowing gluconeogenesis from hepatic glycogen stores.[63–66] At this stage, fetal glucose stores and lactate are preferentially diverted to the placenta to maintain placental metabolic, endocrine, and nutrient transfer function.[24,29,31]

As the nutrient supply worsens, fetal hypoglycemia intensifies and secondary energy sources are required. Proteins are catabolized to gluconeogenic amino acids. However, limitations in placental amino acid transfer eventually result in hypoaminoacidemia.[27] Decreased transfer leads to relative deficiencies of circulating long-chain polyunsaturated fatty acids, whereas metabolic limitation leads to hypertriglyceridemia and the inability to estabish essential adipose stores. Even if provided adequate substrate, inadequate oxygen is available to maintain oxidative metabolism. Hypoglycemia, hyperlactic acidemia, and a growing base deficit correlate with the degree of fetal hypoxemia and protein energy malnutrition.[24,67–71] Down-regulation of several cellular transporters and the Na/H^+ pump affects placental cellular function and aggravates the condition further.[27,28,30,37] In this setting, the fetal brain and heart switch primary nutrients from glucose to lactate and ketones.[72] Cardiac metabolism may consume as much as 80% of the circulating lactate.[73,74]

Simultaneously, the principal endocrine growth axis (insulin and insulin-like growth factors I and II) as well as leptin-coordinated fat deposition is down-regulated.[75] As a result, the placenta and fetus do not reach their size potential. The combination of fetal starvation, a modified endocrine milieu, and deficient tissue stores limits fetal growth and affects cellular and functional differentiation in many target organs.

Fetal Response in Major Organ Systems

Vascular and metabolic disturbances within the placenta lead to alterations in many fetal organ systems. Cardiovascular and central nervous system functions are best studied and provide the most practicable clinical means to document the progression of disease and assess the fetal condition.

Changes in fetal blood flow are related to placental resistance, fetal oxygenation, organ autoregulation, and vascular reactivity. Because of the parallel arrangement of the fetal circulation, placental dysfunction has specific effects on the relative distribution of right and left ventricular output. Increase in the right, or decrease in the left ventricular afterload shifts cardiac output toward the left ventricle, supplying well-oxygenated umbilical venous blood to downstream organs. In the compensated hypoxemic state, fetal cardiac output is increased and organ autoregulation maintained.[76,77] The response of the fetal trunk and cerebral circulation to hypoxemia differ from each other. The peripheral arteries constrict and truncal resistance increases, as evident by the elevated umbilical, thoracic, and descending aorta Doppler resistance indices ("hind limb reflex") that account for most of the increase in right ventricular afterload.[78–81] The fetal cerebral circulation dilates in response to hypoxemia. Fetal cerebral vasodilatation is reflected in decreased Doppler indices (poorly described as "brain-sparing")[82,83] and reduces left ventricular afterload. This changing balance between right and left ventricular afterload decreases the cerebroplacental Doppler index ratio[84] and redistributes well-oxygenated left ventricular output to the heart and brain.[78,79,85,86]

Enhanced blood flow to individual organs is documented in the myocardium,[87] adrenal glands,[88] spleen,[89] and liver.[90] Conversely, blood flow resistance in the peripheral pulmonary arteries,[91] celiac axis,[92] mesenteric vessels,[93,94] kidneys,[95,96] and femoral and iliac arteries[97] increases. The overall effect is an improved distribution of well-oxygenated blood to vital organs, with preferential streaming of descending aorta blood flow to the placenta for reoxygenation. In contrast, blood flow to organs that are not vital for fetal survival is decreased. These Doppler-determined parameters are corroborated by direct measurements of cardiac output,[78] increases in umbilical venous volume flow,[54,98] and progressive decreases in amniotic fluid volume after long-standing redistribution.[96] Further, increased circulating levels of endothelin, arginine vasopressin, norepinephrine, epinephrine, vasoactive intestinal peptide, and atrial natriuretic peptide[99–101] are related directly to the severity of the acid–base disturbance. These adaptations are likely responsible for the enhanced vascular reactivity that may aggravate the patient's clinical status and increase the complication rate during cordocentesis.

The primary central nervous system effect of mild placental dysfunction is delayed maturation of several fetal behaviors. The normal behavioral sequence of development for the fetus proceeds from the appearance of movement, to coupling and cyclicity of behavior, and finally to integration of movement patterns into stable behavioral states. Likewise, the development of autonomic reflexes superimposed on intrinsic cardiac activity determines the characteristics of the fetal heart rate. These reflexes originate in the brain stem and are modulated by the ambient oxygen tension, signals from higher brain centers, the reticular activating system, and peripheral sensory inputs. Variations of heart rate and episodic accelerations coupled with fetal movement indicate normal functioning of these regulatory sites. Once organized behavioral states are established (typically by 28 weeks' gestation), diurnal and responsive cyclicity (e.g., to maternal glucose) and their coupling to heart rate variables (heart rate reactivity) are usually achieved.[102]

A delay occurs in all aspects of central nervous system maturation in fetuses with IUGR and chronic hypoxemia.[103–107] There is also a progressive decline in global fetal activity.[108] The combination of delayed central integration of fetal heart rate control, decreased fetal activity, and chronic hypoxemia results in a higher baseline heart rate, with lower short- and long-term variation (on computerized analysis) and delayed development of heart rate reactivity.[106,107,109–112] Computerized heart rate analyses show that the changes in characteristics are particularly evident between 28 and 32 weeks. Progressive fetal hypoxemia is associated with a gradual decline in amniotic fluid volume, fetal breathing, gross body movement, tone, and computerized and traditional fetal heart rate variables. This decline is determined by the central effects of hypoxemia or acidemia, independent of cardiovascular status.[113–117]

Placental dysfunction affects many other fetal organ systems. Hypoxemia-stimulated erythropoietin release increases red blood cell mass through both medullary and extramedullary hematopoiesis.[60,67,118–120] More complex interactions are observed with persistent hypoxemia and progressive degrees of placental vascular damage. Nucleated red blood cell precursors enter the peripheral circulation independent of erythropoietin levels.[121,122] Placental platelet aggregation and consumption increases the risk of thrombocytopenia.[123,124] Other organ-specific alterations of note include thyroid dysfunction, increased cortisol level, vitamin deficiency, and immune deficiency. The effect of these fetal manifestations on short- and long-term outcome is unknown.

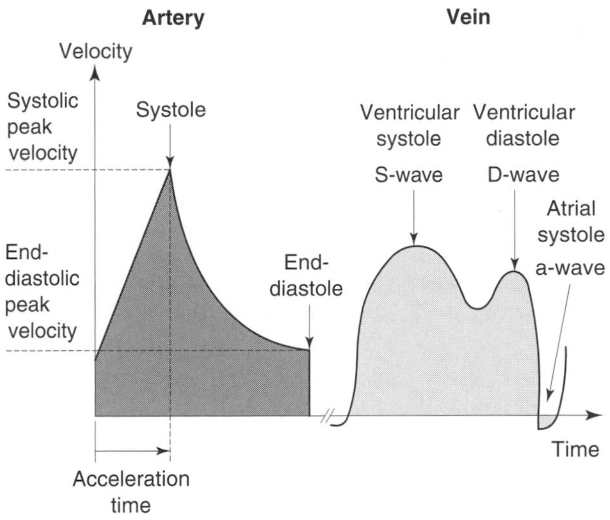

FIGURE 12–4
Arterial and venous flow velocity waveforms. Absolute measurements for arteries include peak systolic and end-diastolic velocities, acceleration time, and heart rate. The venous flow velocity waveform has a triphasic profile. During ventricular systole and diastole, blood flows toward the heart, with a slight decrease after systole as the arteriovenous ring ascends. With the opening of the arteriovenous valves in diastole, antegrade flow increases again and produces the second peak (D-wave). Atrial contraction is associated with a sharp increase in atrial pressure, which is transmitted retrograde to the venous system and may be associated with brief retrograde flow (A-wave).

Fetal Decompensation

If placental dysfunction is progressive or sustained, the adaptive mechanisms become exhausted and decompensation begins. Multiple-organ failure as a result of placental dysfunction is caused by the metabolic milieu and the regulatory loss of cardiovascular homeostasis. Metabolic abnormalities are exaggerated, acidemia worsens, and the risks of intrauterine damage or perinatal death increase dramatically.

Forward blood flow in the venous system is determined by cardiac compliance, contractility, and afterload. The normal venous flow velocity waveform is triphasic and therefore more complex than the arterial waveform. It consists of systolic and diastolic peaks (S-wave and D-wave) that are generated by the descent of the arterioventricular ring during ventricular systole and passive diastolic ventricular filling, respectively. The sudden increase in right atrial pressure with atrial contraction in late diastole causes a variable amount of reverse flow, producing a second trough after the D-wave (A-wave) (Fig. 12–4). A decrease in forward cardiac function marks the onset of cardiovascular decompensation[76–78,125] and causes decreased forward velocity during atrial systole (A-wave). Impaired preload handling, as evidenced by increased venous Doppler indices (discussed later),[126,127] is documented in the precordial veins (ductus venosus, inferior vena cava,[128] and superior vena cava[129]), hepatic veins (right, middle, and left hepatic[130,131]), and head and neck veins (jugular veins[132] and cerebral transverse sinus[133]). If the failure to accommodate preload is progressive, umbilical venous pulsations may be the ultimate reflection of increased central venous pressure (Fig. 12–5).[134] This finding is consistent with umbilical venous pressure measurements obtained at the time of cordocentesis. Simultaneously, autoregulation may be exaggerated in the coronary circulation[77,78] or may become dysfunctional in the cerebral and placental circulation.[135–137]

Progressive metabolic acidemia is associated with oligohydramnios and loss of fetal breathing, movement, and tone.[138,139] Abnormal fetal heart rate patterns, including overt late decelerations or a decrease in the short-term variation on computerized analysis, develop and appear to be related to metabolic status and concurrent worsening of cardiac function.[111,113,116,125,136,140] In the final stages of compromise, cardiac dilation with holosystolic tricuspid insufficiency, complete fetal inactivity, and spontaneous late decelerations may be seen before intrauterine demise.[141]

The sequence of deteriorating cardiovascular, biophysical, and heart rate parameters is reasonably predictable in 70% to 80% of fetuses with IUGR before 34 weeks.[114,142] Flow abnormalities confined to the umbilical or cerebral circulation are typically early changes.[143–145] The progressive decline in (computerized) heart rate variation and increasing venous Doppler indices are closely related.[133,146] Oligohydramnios, loss of fetal tone and or movement, abnormal venous flow, and overt heart rate decelerations are typically "late" changes.[145,146] Closer to term, the relationship between

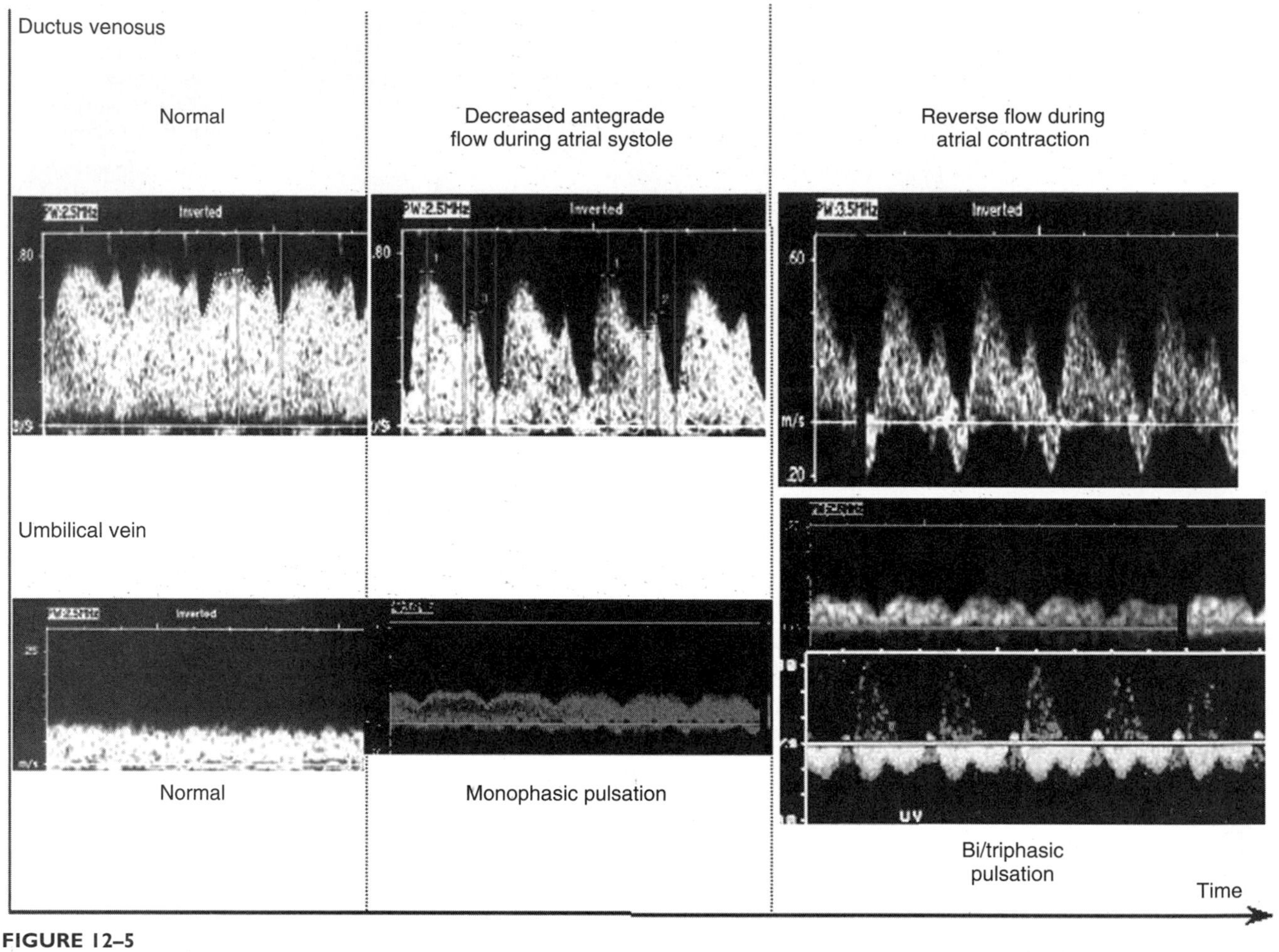

FIGURE 12–5
Progression of abnormal venous flow patterns. The *left panel* shows normal flow in the ductus venosus, with antegrade flow throughout the cardiac cycle. The umbilical vein equally shows constant flow. An increase in the retrograde flow component during atrial contraction is believed to be the hallmark of decreased cardiac function and reflects increased cardiac end-diastolic pressures. Flow in the umbilical vein may show a monophasic pulsatile pattern, with nadirs corresponding to atrial contraction (*center panel*). In the most severe form of cardiac dysfunction, reverse flow occurs during atrial contraction in the ductus venosus. Pulsations in the umbilical vein may show a biphasic profile, with systolic and diastolic peaks or even retrograde flow during atrial contraction (triphasic) (*right panel*).

cardiovascular and biophysical deterioration is weaker, largely because of less prominent Doppler abnormalities.[147–149] In contrast, the correlation (but not necessarily the slope of the regression) between the deterioration of biophysical parameters and acid–base status is relatively independent of gestational age (Fig. 12–6).[102,111]

Summary

Macrosomia and IUGR are the principal abnormalities of fetal growth. Although several definitions apply at birth, antenatal diagnosis is based on estimates of fetal size and weight. The regulation of fetal growth is complex and exists on multiple levels in the maternal, placental, and fetal compartments. Accordingly, IUGR results from several underlying factors that interfere with normal development to produce a complex, multisystem fetal disorder. Because outcome is strongly dependent on the cause, identifying the underlying disease is an essential step toward appropriate management. Several premonitory metabolic alterations affect long-term adult health. Fetal dynamic variables, Doppler parameters, and regulation of amniotic fluid volume reflect progressive deterioration and allow accurate antenatal detection of fetal hypoxemia and acidemia.

Screening Options for Growth Restriction

Clinical

The maternal uterine fundus is objectively measured and charted during each antenatal visit. After 20 weeks' gestation, the normal symphyseal fundal height in centimeters approximates the number of weeks gestation, after appropriate allowances for maternal height and fetal station. The reported sensitivity for the detection of IUGR ranges from 60% to 85%, and the positive

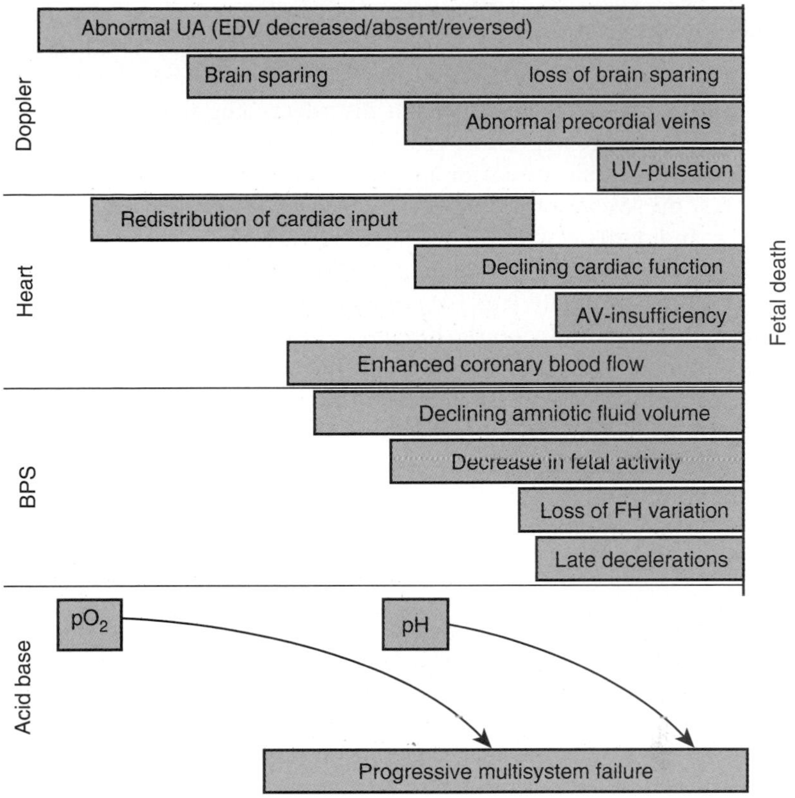

FIGURE 12–6
Progressive deterioration in fetal cardiovascular and behavioral variables seen with declining metabolic status. In most fetuses with intrauterine growth restriction, Doppler abnormalities progress from the arterial to the venous side of the circulation. Although cardiac adaptations and alterations in coronary blood flow dynamics may be operational for a variable period, overt abnormalities of cardiac function and evidence of markedly enhanced coronary blood flow usually are not seen until the late stages of disease. The decline in biophysical variables shows a reproducible relationship with the acid–base status. If adaptation mechanisms fail, stillbirth ensues. AV, atrioventricular; EDV, end-diastolic velocity; FH, fetal heart rate; UV, umbilical vein.

predictive values are 20% to 80%. Although measurement of the symphyseal fundal height is a poor screening tool for the detection of IUGR, the accuracy of subsequent ultrasound prediction of IUGR is enhanced if there is clinical suspicion of IUGR, based on lagging fundal height.

Biochemical

At least four hormone or protein markers measured in the maternal sera early in the second trimester are associated with subsequent IUGR. These include estriol, human placental lactogen, hCG, and α-fetoprotein (see Chapters 7 and 8). Clinically, maternal serum α-fetoprotein is the most useful as a marker of abnormal placentation. Most studies conclude that a single, unexplained elevated value increases the risk of growth restriction 5- to 10-fold, proportional to the magnitude of the elevation. As a result, some argue that α-fetoprotein measurement is clinically useful, even after earlier aneuploidy screening by nuchal translucency measurement.

Uterine Artery Doppler Studies

Deficient placentation is highly associated with gestational hypertensive disorders, IUGR, and fetal demise.[150,151] A uterine artery Doppler resistance profile that is high, persistently notched, or both, identifies women who are at high risk for preeclampsia and IUGR. Sensitivity is up to 85% when performed between 22 and 23 weeks' gestation.[152,153] Because low-dose aspirin treatment initiated this late in pregnancy improves neither placental function nor long-term outcome,[154] first-trimester screening tests are under investigation. They cannot be recommended clinically. The utility of first-trimester uterine artery screening appears to be profoundly affected by the target population. Although low risk patients derive little benefit, high risk patients (those with thrombophilia, hypertension, or a history of preeclampsia or a fetus with IUGR) who are given low-dose aspirin because of bilateral uterine artery notching at 12 to 14 weeks have an 80% reduction of placental disease compared with matched control subjects given placebo.[155] Although low-dose aspirin therapy initiated beyond the first trimester may have benefit in a highly select group of patients, uterine artery Doppler studies provide diagnostic and prognostic information beyond this point. The risk of complicating preeclampsia or HELLP affecting fetal outcome is increased more than 10-fold when abnormal umbilical artery Doppler findings are associated with bilateral uterine artery notching.[156] However, after 24 weeks, the response to an abnormal uterine artery Doppler waveform should be monitoring of blood pressure and not serial Doppler studies.

Ultrasound Assessment (See also Chapter 11)

Ultrasound biometry is the diagnostic tool of choice for the documentation of fetal growth disorders. The first step in the management of IUGR is the identification of fetuses that are truly at risk for an adverse outcome. This requires the exclusion of small, but normally grown fetuses and fetuses with IUGR that is caused by an underlying condition that cannot be altered through obstetric management (e.g., aneuploidy, nonaneuploid syndromes, viral infection). Because almost all fetal measurements change with gestation, accurate assessment of gestational age is a necessary first step so that percentile ranks of the absolute measurements can be derived. Once gestational age is assigned, the interpretation of an ultrasound growth study is based on the fetal anatomic survey, amniotic fluid volume, percentile rank of fetal size measurements, interval growth since the last study, and functional assessment of the fetoplacental unit with Doppler ultrasound (umbilical and uterine arteries).

The adequacy of fetal growth cannot be determined by a single sonographic examination without a preexisting estimate of gestational age. Even after several examinations, fetal growth assessment is facilitated by knowledge of the likely gestational age because the rate of growth for many parameters also varies with gestation. The traditional assessment of gestational age is based on the first day of the last menstrual period (LMP) (Naegle's rule). Yet, gestational age is uncertain in 20% to 40% of pregnant women who keep a written menstrual calendar.[157,158] This fact reflects both normal physiologic variation in the timing of ovulation and misinterpretation of implantation bleeding as menses by either the patient or the caregiver. Other potential and common variables that may explain an apparent discrepancy between sonographic and LMP-based gestational age include oral contraceptive use, increased cycle length, breast-feeding, and a limited number of coital exposures. Because all commonly used ultrasound tables are based on women with a known LMP rather than a known ovulation or conception date, they share the inaccuracy of menstrual dates (± 3 weeks). Because normal variation among fetuses also increases with advancing gestational age, the accuracy of the sonographic estimate of age diminishes. An estimated date of confinement (EDC) is based on the LMP when the sonographic estimate of gestational age is within the predictive error (7 days in the first semester, 10–11 days in the second trimester, and 21 days in the third trimester). Once the EDC is set by this method or a first-trimester ultrasound, it does not change, even if subsequent measurements deviate from the expected values. Repeated reassignments of the EDC are confusing to the physician and patient and interfere with the ability to diagnose fetal growth abnormalities.

After establishment of the best obstetric estimate of gestational age, the next critical step is the selection of appropriate reference ranges. Because the goal is to identify poorly growing fetuses, the reference tables for ultrasound measurements should not be population-based, but based on uncomplicated pregnancies delivered at term. Individualized reference ranges of growth potential that account for maternal, ethnic, and fetal variables provide the most accurate reference.[6]

Because fetal growth restriction has many underlying etiologies that affect the timing of onset and fetal features, no single sonographic method is adequate for diagnosis. Only a complete evaluation that includes the maternal history and fetal, placental, and amniotic fluid characteristics can direct an appropriate diagnostic workup and perinatal management.

Direct Measurements

BIPARIETAL DIAMETER

Although biparietal diameter is easy to measure, it is a poor tool for the detection of IUGR. The physiologic variation inherent with advancing gestation is high, cranial growth delay as a result of insufficient nutrition is relatively late, and the shape of the cranium is readily altered by external forces (e.g., oligohydramnios, breech presentation).[159] Further, a technically adequate biparietal diameter may be hard to determine if the fetal head is oriented in a direct anterior or posterior position.

HEAD CIRCUMFERENCE (Table 12–1)

Head circumference is not subject to the same extrinsic variability as biparietal diameter. The measurement technique is important because calculated head circumference measurements are systematically smaller than those directly measured. Thus, the table selected should be based on measurements obtained with the same method as your laboratory.

ABDOMINAL CIRCUMFERENCE (Table 12–2)

Abdominal circumference is the single best measurement for the detection of IUGR because it is related to liver size, which is a reflection of fetal glycogen storage.[160–162] The abdominal circumference percentile has the highest sensitivity and greatest negative predictive value for the sonographic diagnosis of IUGR, whether defined postnatally by birth weight percentile or by ponderal index.[10] Its sensitivity is further enhanced by serial measurements obtained at least 14 days apart.[163] Because of its high sensitivity, some type of abdominal measurement should be part of every sonographic growth evaluation. Because abdominal circumference reflects fetal nutrition, it should be excluded from the calculation of the composite gestational age after the early second trimester.

The most accurate abdominal circumference is the smallest value obtained at the level of the hepatic vein between fetal respirations because the smallest perimeter most closely approximates the plane perpendicular to the spine. The practice of averaging several measurements

TABLE 12-1

Normal Head Circumference Measurements across Gestation

	PERCENTILE RANKS OF HEAD CIRCUMFERENCE (CM)*				
WEEK†	10	25	50	75	90
18	14.0	16.5	16.0	17.0	17.5
19	15.0	16.0	17.0	17.5	18.0
20	16.0	17.0	18.0	18.5	19.0
21	17.0	18.0	19.0	19.5	20.0
22	18.0	19.0	20.0	20.5	21.0
23	19.5	20.0	21.0	21.5	22.0
24	21.0	21.5	22.0	22.5	23.0
25	22.0	22.5	23.0	23.5	24.0
26	23.0	23.5	24.0	24.5	25.0
27	24.0	26.0	26.0	26.5	27.0
28	25.5	26.0	27.0	27.5	28.0
29	26.5	27.0	28.0	29.0	29.5
30	27.0	27.5	28.5	29.0	30.5
31	27.0	28.0	29.0	30.0	31.0
32	27.5	28.0	29.0	30.0	31.5
33	28.0	28.5	29.5	30.5	32.0
34	28.5	29.0	30.5	31.5	32.5
35	29.5	30.0	31.5	32.0	33.0
36	30.0	31.0	32.0	33.0	34.0
37	30.5	31.5	32.5	33.5	35.0
38	30.5	31.5	32.5	34.0	35.0
39	31.0	32.0	33.0	34.5	35.0
40	31.5	32.5	33.5	34.5	35.5
41	32.0	33.0	34.0	34.5	36.0

*Measured directly from tracings in the screen of ultrasound machines or, alternatively, by digitizer from photographs.
†Menstrual weeks of pregnancy. (Adapted from).
From Sabbagha RE: Intrauterine growth retardation. In Sabbagha RE (ed): Diagnostic Ultrasound Applied to Obstetrics and Gynecology, 2nd ed. Philadelphia, Lippincott, 1987, pp 112–131.

only increases the error. A measured circumference is superior to either a calculated circumference or the sum of several diameters because the shape of the fetal abdomen is typically irregular.[164] Like bony measurements, the circumference of a healthy fetus grows within a fixed percentile range. An abrupt change in the percentile, especially an increase, suggests that the current measurement results from an oblique cut and should be repeated.

If a normal table based exclusively on healthy women delivering appropriately nourished neonates at term is used (see Table 12–2), an abdominal circumference above the percentile 2.5 for gestational age is inconsistent with IUGR.[10] If a table based on a cross-sectional population is used (i.e., including small for gestational age, appropriate for gestational age, preterm, and term newborns), the 10th percentile is more appropriate. The positive predictive value of a low abdominal circumference percentile for IUGR is approximately 50% in any given population. It is best not to label a fetus "growth-restricted" and trigger expensive fetal surveillance unless the circumference is far below normal or other ultrasound variables support the suspicion.

TRANSVERSE CEREBELLAR DIAMETER

Transverse cerebellar diameter is one of the few soft tissue measurements that correlates well with gestational age[165] in IUGR. This structure is relatively spared the effects of mild to moderate uteroplacental dysfunction. Whether its measurement offers an advantage over bony

TABLE 12-2

Normal Abdominal Circumference Measurements across Gestation

	PERCENTILE								
GESTATION (WK)	2.5	5	10	25	50	75	90	95	97.5
18	9.8	10.3	10.6	11.8	13.1	14.2	14.5	15.9	16.4
19	11.1	11.6	12.3	13.3	14.4	15.6	15.9	17.2	17.8
20	12.1	12.6	13.3	14.3	15.4	16.6	16.9	18.2	18.8
21	13.7	14.2	14.8	15.9	17.0	18.1	18.4	19.8	20.3
22	14.7	15.2	15.8	16.9	18.0	19.1	19.4	20.8	21.3
23	16.0	16.5	17.1	18.2	19.3	20.4	20.7	22.1	22.6
24	17.2	17.7	18.3	19.4	20.5	21.6	21.9	23.3	23.8
25	18.0	18.5	19.1	20.2	21.3	22.4	22.7	24.1	24.6
26	18.8	19.3	19.9	21.0	22.1	23.2	23.5	24.9	25.4
27	25.4	20.9	21.5	22.6	23.7	24.8	25.1	26.5	27.0
28	22.0	22.5	23.1	24.2	25.3	26.4	26.7	28.1	28.6
29	23.6	24.1	24.7	25.8	26.9	28.0	28.3	29.7	30.2
30	24.1	24.6	25.2	26.3	27.4	28.5	28.8	30.2	30.7
31	24.7	26.2	25.8	26.8	28.0	28.1	29.4	30.0	31.3
32	25.4	25.9	20.0	27.0	28.7	30.8	30.1	31.5	32.0
33	25.7	20.2	20.0	27.0	20.0	30.1	30.4	31.8	32.3
34	26.8	27.3	27.9	29.0	30.1	31.2	31.5	32.0	33.1
35	28.9	29.4	30.0	31.1	32.2	33.3	33.3	35.0	36.5
36	30.0	30.5	31.1	32.2	33.3	34.4	34.7	36.1	36.6
37	31.1	31.6	32.2	33.3	34.4	35.5	35.8	37.2	37.7
38	32.4	32.9	33.5	34.6	35.7	36.8	37.1	38.5	39.0
39	32.6	33.1	33.7	34.8	35.9	37.0	37.3	38.7	39.2
40	32.8	33.3	33.9	35.0	36.1	37.2	37.5	38.9	39.4

From Tamura RK, Sabbagha RE: Percentile ranks of sonar fetal abdominal circumference measurements. Am J Obstet Gynecol 1980; 138:475.

measurements in the assessment of compromised fetal growth is controversial.[166,167]

Measurement Ratios

Approximately 70% of neonates with asymmetrical growth restriction have a head circumference-to-abdominal circumference ratio two standard deviations above the norm.[168] However, both the sensitivity and the positive predictive value of this ratio for growth restriction are worse than that of either abdominal circumference percentile or sonographically estimated fetal weight (discussed later).[10,169]

The cephalic index is the ratio of the biparietal diameter to the occipitofrontal diameter. Proposed as an age-independent aid to identify dolichocephaly and brachycephaly,[170] it is of limited value. Dolichocephaly is rare before the third trimester, and the ability to measure head circumference easily eliminated the need to recognize mild degrees of either dolichocephaly or brachicephaly as it relates to the prediction of gestational age. This ratio has also been proposed as an aid for the diagnosis of trisomy 21. The sonographic signs of aneuploidy are reviewed in Chapters 7 and 8.

The femur length (FL)-to-head circumference ratio was proposed as a tool to identify short-limbed dwarfism, hydrocephaly, or microcephaly.[171] However, the greatly improved resolution of modern ultrasound equipment makes this measurement unnecessary for the diagnosis of hydrocephaly (see Chapter 18); dwarfism, because the length of the fetal limbs is well below the 10th percentile for gestation (see Chapter 21); or microcephaly, which is diagnosed when head circumference is more than three standard deviations below the mean.

It would be attractive if the sonographic FL could be used to generate an index of fetal mass because it correlates with neonatal crown–heel length. Unfortunately, no clinically useful results have been obtained. The FL-to-abdominal circumference ratio has lower sensitivity, specificity, and positive and negative predictive values for the diagnosis of IUGR than either the abdominal circumference percentile or sonographic estimate of fetal weight.[10,172,173]

Sonographic Estimate of Fetal Weight

Many general purpose and special application formulas have been devised; several are listed in Table 12–3. The accuracy of most (±2 standard deviations) is 10% or greater, and none has proven superior to the first devised by Warsof and reported by Sheppard. Although an estimate of fetal weight does not routinely add to the abdominal circumference percentile for the diagnosis of IUGR, it adds a graphic image that is easy for both patient and referring physician to conceptualize. Although its sensitivity is considerably lower than that of the abdominal circumference percentile, the positive predictive value of a fetal weight estimate below the 10th percentile is greater.

Arterial and Venous Doppler Studies

Quantification of blood flow volume with Doppler studies is prone to error because of variations in insonation angle and the measurement of vessel diameter. Consequently, Doppler waveform analysis with angle-independent Doppler indices is preferred for fetal surveillance. The most widely used arterial indices are the systolic-to-diastolic ratio,[174] resistance index,[175]and pulsatility index (Table 12–4).[176] A relative decrease in end-diastolic velocities elevates each of the indices and usually reflects increased downstream resistance. When end-diastolic flow is lost, the systolic-to-diastolic ratio approaches infinity and the resistance index becomes 1. The pulsatility index offers the advantage of a smaller measurement error, narrower reference limits, and the theoretical advantage of ongoing numerical analysis, even when end-diastolic velocity is lost.[177]

In the venous system, the magnitude of flow reversal during atrial contraction varies considerably in individual veins. Reverse flow may occur during atrial contraction in the inferior vena cava and hepatic veins. In contrast, normal blood flow in the ductus venosus is forward throughout the cardiac cycle. Because of the complex nature of the venous flow velocity waveform, several venous Doppler indices are described (see Table 12–4).[128,145,178–181] No venous Doppler index appears to

TABLE 12–3

Sample Formulas Validated Prospectively for Sonographic Estimates of Fetal Weight

PARAMETER	FORMULA	REFERENCE
BPD, AC	$\text{Log}_{10}\, BW = -1.7492 + (0.166/[BPD] + 0.46\,[AC] - 2 - 646(AC \times BPD)/1000$	278
AC, FL	$\text{Log}_{10}\, BW = 1.3598 + 0.051\,(AC) + 0.1844(FL) - 0.0037\,(AC \times FL)$	279
HC, AC, FL	$\text{Log}_{10}\, BW = 1.5662 - 0.0108(HC) + 0.0468(AC) + 0.171(FL) + 0.00034(HC)^2 - 0.003685(AC \times FL)$	278
		278
		<2200 g
HC, AC, FL	$\text{Log}_{10}\, BW = 1.6961 + 0.02253(HC) + 0.01645(AC) + 0.06439(FL)$	280

AC, abdominal circumference; BPD, biparietal diameter; BW, birthweight; FL, femur length; HC, head circumference.

TABLE 12-4

Doppler Indices for Arterial and Venous Flow Velocity Waveforms

DOPPLER INDICES	CALCULATION
Arterial Flow	
Pulsatility index	$\frac{\text{Systolic–end-diastolic peak velocity}}{\text{Time-averaged maximum velocity}}$
Resistance index	$\frac{\text{Systolic–end-diastolic peak velocity}}{\text{Systolic peak velocity}}$
Systolic-to-diastolic ratio	$\frac{\text{Systolic peak velocity}}{\text{Diastolic peak velocity}}$
Venous Flow	
Preload index	$\frac{\text{Peak velocity during atrial contraction}}{\text{Systolic peak velocity}}$
Pulsatility index for veins	$\frac{\text{Systolic–diastolic peak velocity}}{\text{Time-averaged maximum velocity}}$
Peak velocity index for veins	$\frac{\text{Systolic–atrial contraction peak velocity}}{\text{Diastolic peak velocity}}$
Percentage reverse flow	$\frac{\text{Systolic time-averaged velocity}}{\text{Diastolic time-averaged velocity}} \times 100$
Ductus venosus preload index	$\frac{\text{Systolic–diastolic peak velocity}}{\text{Diastolic peak velocity}}$

offer a significant advantage over the others.[182] Except for the descending aorta pulsatility index, all fetal arterial and venous indices change with gestational age. Thus, interpretation of Doppler findings requires accurate knowledge of gestational age.

In many locales, it is standard practice to perform ultrasound twice during pregnancy to enhance the identification of fetuses with IUGR and improve outcome.[169] Although the cost–benefit ratio of this practice is unclear,[183,184] the combination of fetal biometry and umbilical artery Doppler is the best available tool for the identification of a small fetus at risk for adverse outcome.[185–188] Randomized trials and meta-analyses confirm that the use of umbilical artery Doppler in this setting is associated with a significant reduction in perinatal mortality rates and less iatrogenic intervention, despite the lack of a standardized response in those trials.[189–191] Before 34 weeks, small fetal size associated with an elevated umbilical artery Doppler index is likely to reflect placental dysfunction. Near term, when umbilical artery Doppler findings may be subtler, a decrease in the middle cerebral artery Doppler index or the cerebroplacental ratio increases suspicion for fetal growth restriction, even if the umbilical artery blood flow resistance index remains within the normal range.[149,188]

Although the umbilical artery flow velocity waveform is primarily determined by the architecture of the villous vascular tree (and therefore placental blood flow resistance), study of other fetal arterial vessels is required to determine the effect on the fetus. Changes in Doppler studies of numerous arteries are described in association with IUGR. However, it seems logical to use vessels that represent a single vascular bed, are easy to sample at a low insonation angle, and provide the most information about the fetal response to hypoxemia. For example, flow in the fetal descending aorta is affected by changes in the placenta as well as by the peripheral fetal vasculature, and these changes may be difficult to detect at a small insonation angle. In contrast, the middle cerebral artery is easily identified and examined at a favorable angle. The examination technique and the reference ranges also require standardization because measurements may vary significantly in different portions of the same vessel. Similarly, measurements of the cerebroplacental ratio are affected by the indices used in calculation, and a standardized approach with gestational reference ranges rather than single cutoff values should be used.[192]

With ongoing compromise, little further change in the middle cerebral artery Doppler waveform occurs, with the notable exception of "normalization" of the Doppler indices. Therefore, the next step after identifying evidence of fetal hypoxemia is to monitor cardiac function through study of the venous system. The inferior vena cava and ductus venosus Doppler indices and umbilical venous pulsations correctly predict acid–base status in a significant proportion of neonates with IUGR. This combination, rather than single-vessel assessment, provides the best predictive accuracy. Although the choice of Doppler index is guided by operator preference, familiarity with the examination technique for all three vessels is encouraged to offer the greatest flexibility in clinical practice.[182]

Biophysical Profile Score

The biophysical profile score (BPS) applies categorical cutoffs for a composite of dynamic variables, such as fetal tone, breathing, gross body movement, and amniotic fluid volume, as well as traditional fetal heart rate analysis. The cutoffs were chosen to account for biologic variation and maturational differences; therefore, they produce a reliable relationship with fetal acid–base status, regardless of gestational age and underlying pathology.[139,193] Although a gradual decrease in all of these parameters precedes an overtly abnormal BPS, analysis of percent change in these variables offers no advantage for the prediction of acidemia.[108] A normal score is usually achieved within the first 10 minutes of study. One notable disadvantage of the BPS is that, apart from amniotic fluid volume, it lacks variables that allow useful longitudinal prediction of compromise in pregnancies affected by IUGR.[117] This limitation must be considered if BPS is selected as the sole monitoring tool (discussed later).

Summary

Several biochemical markers, the clinical history, and uterine artery Doppler screening are effective in identifying patients who are at risk for preeclampsia or IUGR. However, once lagging fetal growth is suspected, abdominal and head circumference measurements based on normal population reference ranges, in combination with umbilical artery Doppler studies, are most likely to separate constitutionally small fetuses from those with growth restriction. Repeat uterine artery study is of no clinical value. A complete anatomic survey and assessment of amniotic fluid volume is a critical component of the ultrasound evaluation that addresses possible other etiologies and directs appropriate management. Arterial and venous Doppler indices provide an assessment of placental function, fetal response to placental dysfunction, and the onset of fetal compromise. The BPS has a reproducible relationship with fetal status, but in isolation, it is of limited value for the longitudinal prediction of compromise.

Diagnosis and Evaluation of Fetal Growth Restriction

The diagnosis of fetal growth restriction is based on the measurement of objective fetal parameters. Diagnosis requires knowledge of the features of normal and abnormal growth as well as the basis for these standards. Ideally, the estimate of gestational age is not based solely on a recent sonographic estimate.

The postnatal definition of IUGR is of pragmatic concern because it affects the stated accuracy of antenatal diagnosis. For example, a thin fetus whose estimated weight is normal might be classified postnatally as growth-restricted by the ponderal index. Practitioners must understand the diagnostic criteria used in their hospitals, and neonatal caregivers should not rely solely on birth weight percentiles.

"Asymmetrical" and "symmetrical" growth restriction should be considered descriptive terms and not diagnoses. More relevant than symmetry is the timing of onset. Late-onset growth restriction of structurally normal fetuses after 32 weeks' gestation usually results from placental dysfunction. These fetuses are slender, with normal head circumference and body length. In contrast, early-onset growth restriction is often associated with aneuploidy, congenital infection, or more severe forms of placental dysfunction (Table 12–5). Although these fetuses may be symmetrically small when delivered weeks or months after the initial diagnosis, they are often asymmetrical when first identified.

Maternal History and Examination

In view of the many maternal disorders that affect placental development, thorough maternal medical, medication, and obstetric histories should be obtained. A family history of unexpected thromboembolic events or a history of a previous pregnancy affected by early-onset IUGR or fetal demise should be sought. Maternal studies for antiphospholipid antibodies and thrombophilia are more likely to have a diagnostic yield with such a history.[194]

Two-Dimensional Ultrasound Assessment of Fetal Size

The most accurate prediction of fetal growth delay can be achieved if fetal growth parameters are related to customized growth curves.[6] When population-based reference ranges are used, a fetus is considered "at risk" for growth restriction when the abdominal circumference percentile is less than percentile 2.5 (or the 10th percentile, depending on the table selected), but the estimated weight is above the 10th percentile. Suspicion is strengthened when both the abdominal circumference percentile and the estimated weight are abnormally low or when progressive growth delay occurs. Serial ultrasound examinations at least 14 days apart allow assessment of growth patterns and may provide additional diagnostic clues. Fetuses that are constitutionally small

TABLE 12–5

Causes of Severe Intrauterine Growth Restriction, University of Iowa, 1984–1992

DIAGNOSIS	N	%
Placental dysfunction	62	54.9
Chromosomal abnormality	22	19.5
Associated structural malformations	13	11.5
Congenital infection		
Proven	7	6.2
Likely	2	1.8
Miscellaneous	7	6.2
Total	**113**	

are more likely to show normal interval growth.[163] In contrast, fetuses with aneuploidy or placental dysfunction are more likely to show progressive growth delay and to "fall off" the growth curve.[39,163,195] Because fetuses with "suspected" and "diagnosed" IUGR are managed similarly, and because the accuracy of the diagnosis based on a small abdominal circumference alone is only approximately 50%, there is no need to worry the parents unnecessarily by basing the diagnosis on a single parameter. Once the suspicion of IUGR is raised, evaluation of fetoplacental blood flow and anatomy is required.

Two-Dimensional Ultrasound of Fetal Anatomy and Possible Invasive Testing

A thorough ultrasound examination to detect major anomalies and markers of aneuploidy is mandatory in all fetuses with IUGR. Fetal echocardiography to detect major cardiac anomalies (e.g., atrioventricular canal defect) and evaluate cardiac function should be included. Echogenic bowel or liver or increased amniotic fluid volume suggests an increased risk of either aneuploidy or viral infection,[196,197] particularly in patients with normal umbilical and uterine artery Doppler findings.[39] A chromosomal abnormality is associated with 20% of cases of severe, early-onset IUGR. Although half of these abnormalities are lethal, a fetus with trisomy 21 may pose philosophical problems for both the physician and the patient. Knowledge of a major anomaly, such as atrioventricular canal defect, can lead the parents in one direction or another in terms of pregnancy termination or cesarean delivery for fetal distress.

Doppler Velocimetry of Arterial and Venous Circulation

The fetal vascular responses to placental dysfunction were discussed earlier. There is now considerable knowledge about the relationship between Doppler findings and perinatal outcome variables that allow for an accurate noninvasive assessment of the presence and severity of fetal hypoxemia. Until recently, the clinical role of Doppler ultrasound in the overall evaluation of fetal growth disturbance was unclear. Part of the problem was the diverse nature of the published studies. Investigators sought to predict a variety of neonatal outcomes with disparate etiologies using a single parameter, such as umbilical artery index. Not surprisingly, the positive and negative predictive values were, as a whole, unsatisfactory.

Based on the current level of knowledge, we designed a clinical evaluation algorithm that uses "progressive" Doppler studies of fetal vasculature. Although Doppler findings in each of the examined vascular beds correlate with fetal acid–base status, there is a wide variation in fetal pH with abnormal results (Fig. 12–7). However, as with most obstetric tests, the negative predictive values are superb. A normal umbilical artery Doppler index is inconsistent with fetal acidemia as a result of uteroplacental dysfunction. Absence of umbilical artery end-diastolic velocity indicates significant villous abnormality; however, the relationship between placental pathology and

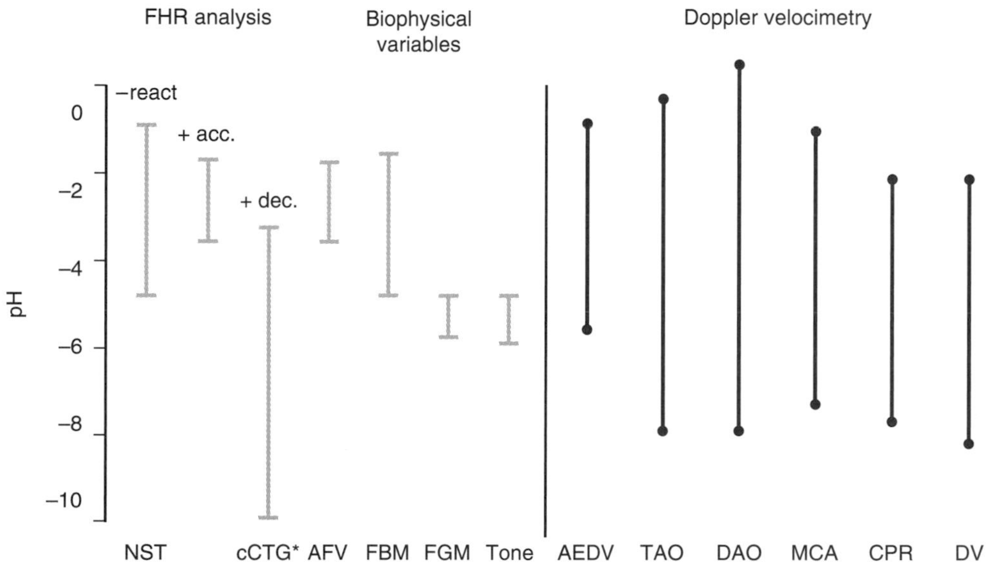

FIGURE 12–7
Deviation in pH from the gestational age mean (ΔpH) with abnormal results on various antenatal tests. These include fetal heart rate (FHR) analysis with traditional nonstress testing (NST) and computerized cardiotocogram (cCTG). The same relationships are expressed for umbilical artery absent end-diastolic velocity (AEDV) and deviation of the arterial or venous Doppler index more than two standard deviations from the gestational age mean for the thoracic aorta (TAO), descending aorta (DAO), middle cerebral artery (MCA), cerebroplacental ratio (CPR), and ductus venosus (DV). +acc, accelerations present; +dec, obvious decelerations present; −react, nonreactive; AFV, amniotic fluid volume; FBM, fetal body movement; FGM, fetal gross movement. (From Baschat AA: Integrated fetal testing in growth restriction: Combining multivessel Doppler and biophysical parameters. Ultrasound Obstet Gynecol 2003;21:1–8.)

fetal acidemia is inconsistent both at cordocentesis and at birth.[59,61,198–200] This inconsistency may occur because the oxygen demands of the fetus vary with gestational age. A 23-week fetus can withstand a much higher degree of placental dysfunction than a 32-week fetus. Thus, evaluation of other fetal blood flow is necessary to determine the fetal response to the level of hypoxemia present and to refine the prediction of fetal acid–base balance. Brain-sparing (cephalization, or centralization), elevation of the thoracic and abdominal aortic pulsatility index, and an abnormal cerebroplacental ratio are associated with fetal hypoxemia and a decrease in pH of at least two standard deviations.[61,81,201] Elevation of the precordial venous Doppler indices (inferior vena cava and ductus venosus) provides the most consistent relationship to a significant decrease in umbilical venous pH (approximately four standard deviations) in fetuses with IUGR.[128,201,202] Because not all fetuses with IUGR have abnormal venous flow, venous Doppler has sensitivity of approximately 70% and specificity of 60% to 70% for the identification of significant fetal acidemia.[182,201,202] Umbilical venous pulsations occur at a late stage of compromise, and if they are observed concurrently with an elevated venous Doppler index, they improve sensitivity in the prediction of birth pH of less than 7.20.[182] Normal fetal arterial pH in the absence of labor should be greater than 7.32 at term and even higher preterm (Fig. 12–8).

In preterm fetuses with IUGR, Doppler findings of progressive abnormality are associated with increased perinatal mortality and morbidity rates.[87,125,126,147] Although neonatal morbidity is determined primarily by the degree of prematurity, the risks of stillbirth and acidemia are significantly related to the extent of venous Doppler abnormality.[126,147] Therefore, multivessel Doppler studies that include the arterial and venous systems are required for the greatest prediction of critical outcomes in preterm infants with IUGR.[203]

Our understanding of the relationships between Doppler-derived flow measurements and short-term outcomes has become more refined. Unfortunately, there is relatively little information on the intermediate- and long-term relationships between Doppler measurements and outcome parameters in infancy and adult life. Elevated fetal aortic blood flow resistance is associated with neurodevelopmental delay in early childhood.[204,205] Similarly, adverse long-term neurologic development at school age appears most closely related to reversal of umbilical artery end-diastolic velocity.[206] Although

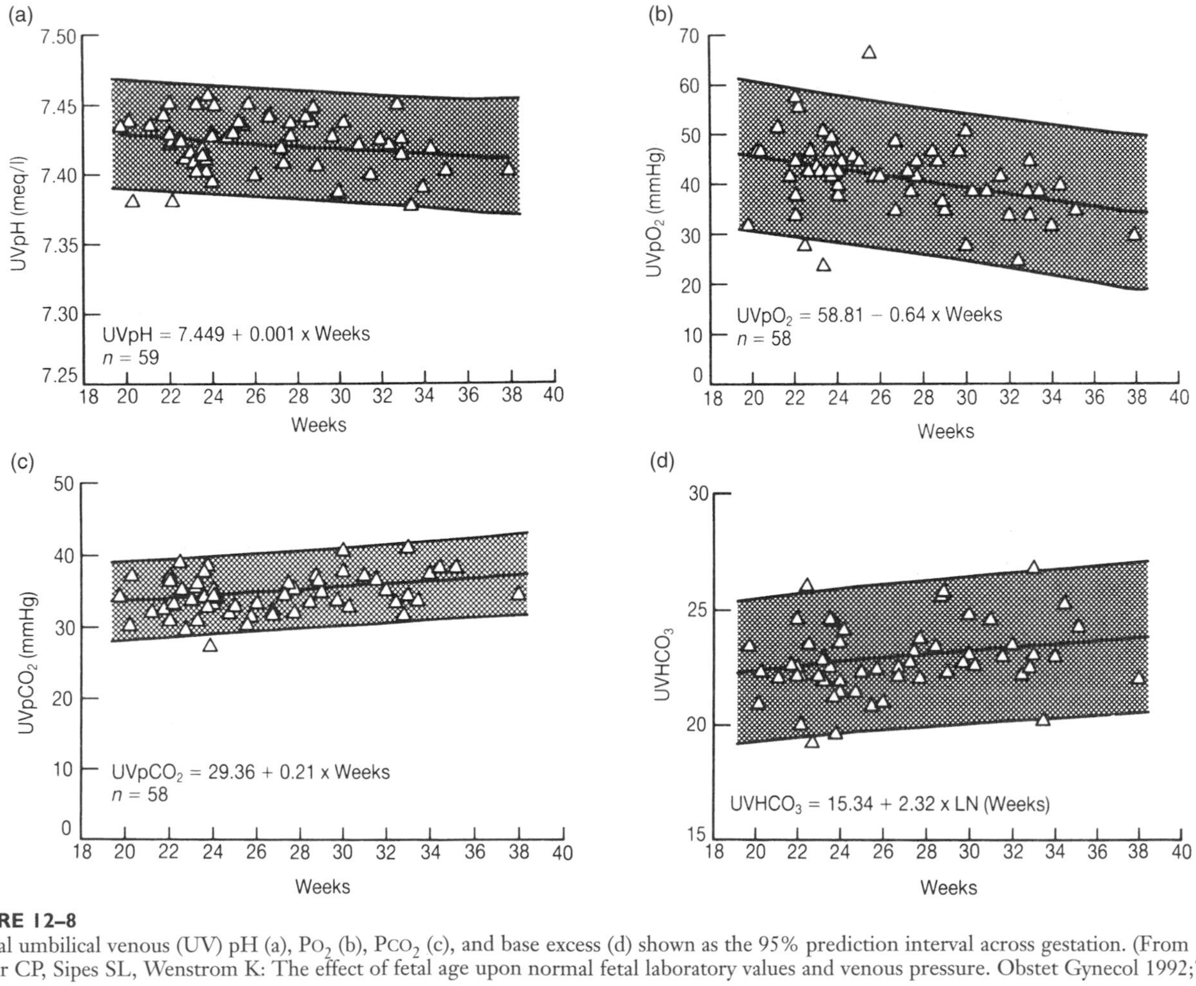

FIGURE 12–8
Normal umbilical venous (UV) pH (a), P_{O_2} (b), P_{CO_2} (c), and base excess (d) shown as the 95% prediction interval across gestation. (From Weiner CP, Sipes SL, Wenstrom K: The effect of fetal age upon normal fetal laboratory values and venous pressure. Obstet Gynecol 1992;79:71.)

studies suggested a protective effect of brain-sparing on cognitive outcome, 5-year follow-up showed no sustained benefit.[207] The phrase would seem a misnomer. Detailed studies clarifying these relationships are urgently needed before surrogate markers for long-term outcome can be incorporated into perinatal management decisions.

Computerized Cardiotocography and Biophysical Profile Score

Like the observations made with Doppler measurements, a progressive decline in acid–base status is also demonstrable by fetal heart rate analyses and the assessment of breathing, tone, gross body movement, and amniotic fluid volume. Each component of the BPS relates to fetal oxygenation, but the five-component BPS most effectively predicts fetal acid–base status. Although a reactive cardiotocogram, even by criteria graded for gestational age, virtually excludes hypoxemia, a nonreactive cardiotocogram is associated with a wide range of pH values.[138,193] The prediction of acidemia is improved by computerized fetal heart rate analysis. All computerized variables (e.g., short-term, long-term, and mean minute variations) and episodic or periodic changes are related to a range of normal and abnormal fetal pH values.[109,111,112] In fetuses with IUGR, short-term variation below 3.5 msec as a result of prolonged episodes of low variation appears to be the best predictor of an umbilical artery pH of less than 7.20.[140] Although it is clearly abnormal in a nonlaboring patient, the clinical relevance of this pH value is not clear. Loss of fetal breathing movements is associated with moderate hypoxemia and a wide range of pH values at the time of either cordocentesis or birth. In contrast, the absence of fetal tone and gross body movement is almost always associated with acidemia (see Fig. 12–7). By accounting for physiologic variability, the BPS maintains its relationship with fetal pH in fetuses with IUGR, independent of gestational age. However, the BPS has limited utility in the prediction of longitudinal deterioration in these fetuses.[117,142]

Long-term relationships between the BPS parameters and long-term outcome were studied in large cohorts of patients. A low BPS is associated with neonatal complications, cerebral palsy, cortical blindness, and attention deficit disorder.[208] Although randomized testing was not performed, application of the BPS management algorithm appears to have significantly decreased the frequency of cerebral palsy in the tested population.

Integrated Fetal Testing

The combined use of multiple testing modalities to monitor fetuses with IUGR has several advantages because of the wide clinical spectrum and the variance in the relationship between testing and outcome variables.[209] Because deterioration of cardiovascular and biophysical parameters is initially independent, the information gained by combining them may be additive. Doppler studies provide good longitudinal assessment, and the BPS refines the relationship with fetal pH. This combined approach provides the most accurate fetal assessment, particularly in preterm fetuses with growth restriction.[210–214] The management details are described later.

Summary

It is important to differentiate between early- and late-onset growth restriction. The former has a strong association with aneuploidy, fetal infection, and severe placental dysfunction. Ultrasound is central to the diagnosis of IUGR, but is greatly aided by an independent assessment of gestational age. The single most sensitive parameter for the detection of IUGR is the abdominal circumference percentile, although its positive predictive value is only 50%. Doppler ultrasound is an important adjunct that provides diagnostic and correlative information on fetal oxygenation. Current evidence supports a progression from arterial to venous flow abnormalities associated with deteriorating blood gas values in IUGR and worsening perinatal outcome. Because of variations in fetal response to placental dysfunction, the combined assessment of cardiovascular and biophysical parameters offers the most comprehensive assessment of fetal status. Fetal monitoring that integrates arterial and venous Doppler studies and biophysical parameters is most useful in the preterm fetus with IUGR, when the balance between in utero risk and prematurity is critical. The long-term implications of these findings need further study.

Prenatal Management Options

Diagnostic and therapeutic interventions often go hand in hand when IUGR is suspected, and management options may need to be reevaluated as gestation advances. The goal of the initial evaluation is to make a presumptive diagnosis of IUGR and then to use the clinical presentation to direct additional diagnostic workup. Subsequently, antenatal surveillance is instituted and tailored to the severity of the fetal condition, considering the strengths and weaknesses of the available tests. Therapeutic interventions are dictated by the maternal and fetal condition as well as by gestational age, while respecting the wishes of the parents.

Presumptive Diagnosis of IUGR

Fetuses with a small abdominal circumference percentile are at risk for IUGR. A flattening growth curve on two consecutive examinations at least 14 days apart (in the third trimester, preferably 21 days apart) heightens diagnostic suspicion. Individualized reference ranges are based on normal pregnancies, and maternal characteristics are probably the most accurate.[6] Beyond 24 weeks, an elevated umbilical artery Doppler index is strong corroborating evidence for IUGR as a result of placental dysfunction. A false-positive diagnosis is likely in a sonographically small fetus with normal findings on umbilical artery Doppler examination, and the risk of fetal distress in labor as a result of chronic hypoxia is low. After 34 weeks, the umbilical artery Doppler index may be within the normal range, and a decreased cerebroplacental ratio or middle cerebral artery Doppler index may be the only supporting evidence of placental-based IUGR.[149,187,215] After completion of the anatomic survey and assessment of amniotic fluid volume, the fetus is categorized as either likely or unlikely to have IUGR. Based on the combination of findings, the fetus may have evidence of one of four diagnoses: aneuploidy, viral infection, placental dysfunction, or nonaneuploid fetal syndromes.

Diagnostic Workup

It is important to determine the specific etiology of IUGR before delivery when possible. The wide availability of fluorescent in situ hybridization for fetal karyotyping for major chromosomal abnormalities from amniocytes offers the possibility of a result within 48 to 72 hours in many centers. Polymerase chain reaction of amniotic fluid samples can provide accurate and reproducible detection of the viral genome (see Chapter 27). Thus, amniocentesis should be offered to all patients with early-onset IUGR (<32 weeks) and those with symmetrical IUGR detected later in gestation UGR. In addition, women with known familial syndromes may be evaluated for single-gene mutations if appropriate gene probes are available. The relative ease of amniocentesis and the advances in antenatal surveillance that allow an accurate assessment of the fetal acid–base status have largely obviated the need for cordocentesis.

However, cordocentesis is the technique of choice if more in-depth diagnostic information is needed. For example, fetal blood sampling provides direct measurement of fetal acid–base status (of value, especially at the threshold of viability, where the variance of Doppler methods is much greater), hepatic transaminases, a complete blood count, serology, and polymerase chain reaction for evidence of fetal viremia, all of which increase the diagnostic yield. For example, although traditional serologic and culture techniques identify an infectious etiology in 5% of fetuses with IUGR,[216] the yield roughly doubles with polymerase chain reaction.[196] Although specific treatments for fetal infection are not available, antenatal diagnosis is important. First, the fetal response to infection is often transient; therefore, the opportunity for diagnosis is lost and the neonate is inappropriately excluded from specific follow-up if diagnostic efforts are delayed until delivery. Further, infected neonates typically shed virus. They should be isolated for the protection of pregnant staff and susceptible nursing mothers of other newborns. Finally, fetuses with IUGR caused by congenital infection are well oxygenated in the absence of placentitis. Extensive antenatal testing geared toward the diagnosis of hypoxemia is unnecessary, and the need for iatrogenic intervention is low in the absence of oligohydramnios.

Measurement of hematologic parameters can shed light on the etiology while final karyotyping is pending and may provide additional information about the severity of disease. Fetuses with IUGR and chronic hypoxemia are more likely to have elevated erythropoietin levels and polycythemia. Macrocytosis is more typical of trisomic and triploid fetuses.[217,218] Despite an elevated nucleated red blood cell count, fetal thrombocytopenia and anemia are signs of chronic compromise associated with poor perinatal outcome.[67,118,121,122,218,220]

The diagnostic benefits of cordocentesis must be weighed against the risks on a case-by-case basis. Early-onset growth restriction increases the risk of reactive fetal bradycardia after cordocentesis in proportion to the severity of fetal hypoxemia.[221] There is approximately a 1 in 5 chance that a fetus with severe IUGR will have bradycardia after cordocentesis. The higher the umbilical artery Doppler index, the greater the likelihood of bradycardia. The mother of a fetus of borderline viability should decide in advance whether emergency cesarean delivery should be performed in the event of sustained bradycardia. Cordocentesis must be performed in close proximity to a delivery suite and only by individuals trained in surgical delivery.

Once the diagnostic workup is initiated, management and outcome are largely determined by the underlying condition and the decisions made by the parents. If aneuploidy is the explanation, the cause and risk of recurrence are known. This knowledge may help to reduce the inevitable parental soul-searching and guilt feelings that accompany any perinatal loss. The diagnosis of a structural anomaly that is incompatible with survival eliminates both the need for extensive (and expensive) antenatal monitoring and the high likelihood of cesarean delivery for fetal indications. Documentation of infection allows precautions to be taken to minimize the risks of infection in the nursery as a result of viral shedding. Management is difficult in fetuses with early-onset IUGR as a result of placental dysfunction. In these otherwise normal fetuses, outcome is determined by the condition at birth and the degree of prematurity.[126,147,222]

Maternal and Fetal Therapy

Intrauterine therapeutic options are limited in pregnancies complicated by IUGR. The first step is to reduce or eliminate potential external contributors, such as stress or smoking, and to encourage maternal rest in a lateral position. Although their efficacy is unproven, these steps should maximize maternal uterine blood flow. In addition, bed rest in the hospital should be considered because it has theoretical advantages over rest at home. First, even the most motivated patient rests less and less as time passes. The family support structure may be poor, and the patient may not have any real opportunity to rest. Second, hospitalization facilitates daily fetal testing. The choice of inpatient versus outpatient management is based on the severity of the maternal or fetal condition and the local standard of care.

Although low-dose aspirin therapy (81 mg/day) does not help severe early-onset IUGR, it may help patients with mild placental dysfunction.[223,224] In view of its documented safety,[225,226] we typically consider low-dose aspirin therapy after the diagnosis of placental-based IUGR is made.

IUGR as a result of placental dysfunction is the most common fetal disorder that is potentially amenable to direct fetal therapy. To be a candidate for this therapy, the fetus must show a proportionate increase in fetal oxygen and substrate delivery. Techniques to achieve these goals are available. Maternal hyperoxygenation,[227,228] intravascular volume expansion,[229] and hyperalimentation[230] are reported. Many issues, such as the effect of therapy on outcome, patient selection, efficacy, and the requisite testing required to monitor the fetus during therapy remain to be resolved. Until these issues are clarified, this therapy is experimental.

Universally available therapeutic options that may improve outcome include antenatal administration of corticosteroids to hasten fetal lung maturity in the preterm fetus and delivery at an institution with a neonatal care unit that can carry out the complex management of the neonate with IUGR. Antenatal corticosteroids should be administered to any fetus with IUGR when delivery is anticipated before 34 weeks. The long-held belief that the "stress" of the intrauterine condition enhances maturation and protects against prematurity is not supported by large population studies of neonates with IUGR.[3,231]

Timing and Mode of Delivery

Because of the limited intrauterine treatment options and the possibility of continued fetal damage as a result of progressive metabolic deterioration, the timing of intervention is critical. Current recommendations are based on an incomplete understanding of background mortality and morbidity rates. Further, critical perinatal variables that affect short- and long-term quality of life must be better defined. Many fetuses with IUGR are hypoxemic before the onset of labor. Chronic in utero acidemia rather than chronic hypoxemia alone appears to be most strongly associated with intellectual impairment postnatally.[232] The gestational age at decompensation is the primary determinant of perinatal survival. Between 24 and 32 weeks, each day gained in utero may increase the neonatal survival rate by 1% to 2%.[117,222] After delivery, the condition of the neonate at birth as well as the degree of prematurity affect perinatal complication and mortality rates. In survivors, neonatal complications have an additional significant effect on long-term outcome.[233] In principle, the timing of delivery is straightforward. Delivery takes place either at term, when fetal lung maturity is documented, if fetal distress occurs, or if the maternal condition dictates delivery. Between the age of viability and 32 weeks, however, the risks of perinatal damage from fetal deterioration compete with the risks of iatrogenic prematurity.

Prenatal Surveillance Tests (See also Chapter 11)

In euploid fetuses with presumed uteroplacental dysfunction, the patterns of deterioration are characteristic, but variable, and place specific demands on antenatal surveillance. In addition to acute assessments of fetal well-being, the likelihood of clinical progression necessitates a plan for longitudinal surveillance. Traditional fetal heart rate analysis, assessment of fetal activity (tone, movement, breathing), and evaluation of fetoplacental blood flow (arterial and venous Doppler) allow the most precise assessment of fetal well-being. Computerized fetal heart rate analysis, serial amniotic fluid volume measurement, and knowledge of arterial and venous Doppler status allow a reasonably accurate prediction of longitudinal progression.[133,142,145,146]

Management of IUGR with Integrated Fetal Testing

At the University of Maryland, we use an approach that combines fetal heart rate analysis with Doppler and biophysical assessment initiated at 24 weeks' gestation. The management algorithm is guided by the severity of the maternal and fetal condition and by gestational age. It includes arterial and venous Doppler studies and determination of the BPS (Fig. 12–9).

Integrated fetal testing has three core elements: correct diagnosis of IUGR; assessment of fetal well-being; and prediction of fetal deterioration to time delivery. Delivery is indicated when the results of fetal testing are grossly abnormal, when fetal lung maturity is documented, or when maternal disease poses a serious risk to the mother. Before 34 weeks, a single course of betamethasone should be completed over 48 hours, when delivery is anticipated, to ameliorate neonatal respiratory disease and reduce the risk of intraventricular hemorrhage.

Although local preferences for antenatal surveillance and management vary, several guiding principles apply. First, the limits of viability and intervention dictated by the accepted standard of care must be discussed with the patient when management is initiated. Second, because cardiovascular deterioration is such a prominent feature of IUGR, Doppler assessment must be an integral part of antenatal surveillance. No other method effectively predicts deterioration prospectively. Third, the management of IUGR is too complex to rely on a single surveillance modality. If alternative surveillance methods

IUGR UNLIKELY		
Normal AC, AC growth rate and HC/AC ratio UA, MCA Doppler, BPS and AFV normal	Asphyxia extremely rare Low risk for intrapartum distress	Deliver for obstetric, or maternal factors only, follow growth

IUGR		
AC < 5th, low AC growth rate, high HC/AC ratio, abnormal UA and/or CPR; normal MCA and veins BPS 8/10, AFV normal	Asphyxia extremely rare Increased risk for intrapartum distress	Deliver for obstetric, or maternal factors only, fortnightly Doppler Weekly BPS
	With blood flow redistribution	
IGUR diagnosed based on above criteria, low MCA, normal veins BPS 8/10, AFV normal	Hypoxemia possible, asphyxia rare Increased risk for intrapartum distress	Deliver for obstetric, or maternal factors only, weekly Doppler BPS 2 times/week
	With significant blood flow redistribution	
UA A/REDV Normal veins BPS 6/10, oligohydramnios	Hypoxemia common, acidemia or asphyxia possible Onset of fetal compromise	> 34 weeks later: deliver < 32 weeks: antenatal steroids repeat all testing daily
	With proven fetal compromise	
Significant redistribution present Increased DV pulsatility BPS 6/10, oligohydramnios	Hypoxemia common, acidemia or asphyxia likely	> 34 weeks later: deliver < 32 weeks: admit, steroids, individualized testing daily vs. tid.
	With fetal decompensation	
Compromise by above criteria Absent or reversed DV a-wave, pulsatile UV BPS < 6/10, oligohydramnios	Cardiovascular instability, metabolic compromise, stillbirth imminent, high perinatal mortality irrespective of intervention	Deliver at tertiary care center with the highest level of NICU care

FIGURE 12–9
Management algorithm for pregnancies complicated by intrauterine growth restriction (IUGR) based on the ability to perform arterial and venous Doppler as well as a full five-component biophysical profile score (BPS). AC, abdominal circumference; AFV, amniotic fluid volume; A/REDV, absent/reversed end-diastolic velocity; CPR, cerebroplacental ratio; DV, ductus venosus; HC, head circumference; MCA, middle cerebral artery; NICU, neonatal intensive care unit; NST, nonstress test; tid, three times daily; UA, umbilical artery. (From Baschat AA, Hecher K: Fetal growth restriction in placental disease. Semin Perinatol 2004;28:67–80.)

are used, longitudinal monitoring should be tailored to the limitations of the surveillance test. For example, traditional nonstress testing analysis lacks the sensitivity and interobserver agreement needed to facilitate longitudinal monitoring. For this purpose, computerized heart rate monitoring offers superior accuracy. Similarly, if the BPS is the sole method of surveillance in severe IUGR, daily testing may be necessary to provide longitudinal assessment.[234]

Delivery Management Options

The premature neonate with IUGR requires the highest level of neonatal intensive care, and intrauterine transport to an appropriate institution is recommended in all cases of early-onset IUGR. The route of delivery is dictated by the severity of the fetal and maternal condition, along with other obstetric factors. Cesarean section without a trial of labor is indicated when the risks of vaginal delivery are unacceptable. These circumstances include prelabor evidence of fetal acidemia, spontaneous late decelerations, or late decelerations with minimal uterine activity. When fetal testing shows less serious conditions and gestational age is more advanced, the delivery route is tailored to the cervical Bishop score and preinduction oxytocin challenge testing may be required. Pharmacologic or mechanical ripening of the cervix, placement of the woman in the left lateral decubitus position, and the use of supplemental oxygen increase the likelihood of successful vaginal delivery.

Summary

The management of pregnancies with suspected IUGR is initiated with a diagnostic workup, including assessment of maternal and fetal risk factors. After aneuploidy, fetal anomalies, and infection are excluded, uteroplacental dysfunction is the most likely underlying cause. Because antenatal therapeutic options are limited, tailored surveillance and timed delivery are the primary management goals. A combination of surveillance tests, including arterial and venous Doppler and BPS, provides the most accurate assessment of fetal status and the best prediction of longitudinal progression. They are the surveillance techniques of choice for severe early-onset IUGR (integrated fetal testing). The timing, route, and acuity level of the medical center for delivery are determined by gestational age at delivery and the severity of the fetal or maternal condition.

CONCLUSIONS

- Normal fetal growth is a dynamic process that is regulated throughout gestation on multiple levels in the maternal, placental, and fetal compartments.
- Fetal growth restriction is a complex multisystem syndrome. Identification of the small fetus that is most likely to benefit from surveillance and interventions requires exclusion of those etiologies such as aneuploidy and viral syndromes where outcome is mostly predetermined by the underlying condition.
- A sonographically measured fetal abdominal circumference (AC) below the 10 percentile (reference ranges based on a mixed group of high and low risk pregnancies) or below the 2.5th percentile (reference ranges based on normal pregnancies only) is the most sensitive biometric parameter to detect growth delay. If found in an anatomically normal fetus with low, or normal amniotic fluid volume and abnormal umbilical artery Doppler the clinical picture is strongly suggestive of placental insufficiency. However, the possibility of aneuploidy, syndromes and viral infection should always be considered and fetal karyotyping should be offered.
- Progressive deterioration of fetal status is reflected in dynamic variables (tone, movement, breathing, and heart rate characteristics), Doppler parameters and regulation of amniotic fluid volume following a reasonable predictable pattern.
- As the prenatal therapeutic options are limited, tailored surveillance and timed delivery are the primary management goals. Because of the variations in fetal responses to placental dysfunction, the combined assessment of cardiovascular and biophysical parameters (integrated fetal testing) offers the most comprehensive assessment of fetal status and is the suggested surveillance technique of choice for severe early onset IUGR where the balance between in utero risk and prematurity is center stage.
- The timing, route, and acuity level of the medical center for delivery is determined by gestational age at delivery, and the severity of the fetal or maternal conditions. Severe early onset fetal growth restriction prior to 34 weeks' gestation delivery frequently requires experienced multidisciplinary perinatal effort and should be managed accordingly.

SUMMARY OF MANAGEMENT OPTIONS
Intrauterine Growth Restriction

Management Options	Quality of Evidence	Strength of Recommendation	References
Prenatal			
First Trimester			
Uterine artery Doppler in patients with thrombophilia, previous midtrimester loss, or previous IUGR. Give low-dose aspirin (81–100 mg/day) if bilateral notching occurs.	Ib	A	155
Second Trimester			
If bilateral uterine artery notching persists until 24 weeks, there is only a marginal benefit of low-dose aspirin in selected patients. There is no evidence of a harmful effect.	Ib	A	154,223–226
On Clinical Suspicion of IUGR			
Two abdominal circumference measurements are obtained at least 14 days apart, with umbilical and middle cerebral arteries, to distinguish between normally grown small and growth-restricted fetuses. Follow for IUGR if:	Ib, IIa	A, B	149,162,163, 187,189,190,215

SUMMARY OF MANAGEMENT OPTIONS

Intrauterine Growth Restriction *(Continued)*

Management Options	Quality of Evidence	Strength of Recommendation	References
Prenatal			
• Abdominal circumference <5th percentile or growth rate is <11 mm in 2 wk			
• Umbilical artery Doppler index is elevated			
• Cerebroplacental ratio is decreased			
• Middle cerebral Doppler index is decreased (centralization) even if uterine artery Doppler is normal (especially after 34 wk)			
With a Diagnosis of IUGR			
If the sole monitoring tool is biophysical profile scoring, up to daily testing is required.	IIa	B	234
In the preterm fetus with IUGR <37 wk, multivessel Doppler, including arterial and venous Doppler, provides the best assessment of disease severity.	III	B	126,145,147,203
The most accurate assessment of fetal status is obtained with combined Doppler and biophysical assessment.	III	B, C	117,211,213,214
The timing of delivery is still guided by local standards of care and expert opinion; clear indicators for delivery timing have not been tested in a randomized fashion.	Ib	A	222
Administer betamethasone when delivery is anticipated before 34 wk.	III	B	3,222,231
Labor and Delivery			
Route of delivery is determined by fetal status before the onset of labor as well as maternal and obstetric factors. Oxytocin challenge test may be useful before induction. The left lateral decubitus position is used during labor.	III	B	126,130,142,162

IUGR, intrauterine growth restriction.

FETAL MACROSOMIA

Fetal macrosomia is excessive fetal growth, which is the opposite of fetal growth restriction. Two terms are used to identify excessive fetal growth: large for gestational age (discussed earlier) and fetal macrosomia, implying a birth weight above 4000 or 4500 g, regardless of gestational age. Unlike in IUGR, the morbidity and mortality rates for macrosomic fetuses are more closely related to absolute birth weight than to birth weight percentile. The sharp increase in birthweight beyond 4500 g makes this a more suitable diagnostic cutoff.[235–238] In the United States, 10% of neonates have a birth weight greater than 4000 g and in 1.5%, it is more than 4500 g.[239] Macrosomia is associated with significant fetal, neonatal, and maternal risks that emphasize the need for antepartum detection and modified intrapartum management. Maternal diabetes mellitus is a common cause of excessive fetal growth (see Chapter 45).

Etiology and Risk Factors

Genetic factors, such as parental height and race, and the level of maternal hyperglycemia during pregnancy are important determinants of birth weight. In decreasing order of importance, recognized risk factors for macrosomia include a previous macrosomic infant, prepregnancy maternal obesity or excessive maternal weight gain, multiparity,[240] a male fetus, post-term gestation, Hispanic race,[241] present maternal height and weight at birth, and maternal age younger than 20 years.[242]

The positive relationship between maternal height, weight, and body mass index and neonatal birth weight is likely the expression of genetically predetermined growth potential[6] as well as maternal glycemic status.[243,244] Women who previously delivered a child larger than 4000 g are 5 to 10 times more likely than negative control subjects to deliver an infant larger than 4500 g in a subsequent pregnancy.[242,245] Women who themselves had a birth weight greater than 3600 g are twice as likely to deliver a neonate larger than 4000 g.[246] Male infants are typically heavier than female infants at any gestational age, and more males than females have a birth weight greater than 4500 g.[238] As fetal growth continues, the proportion of infants larger than 4500 g increases from 1.5% at 40 weeks to 2.5% at 42 weeks.[239]

TABLE 12–6

Genetic Causes of Macrosomia

SYNDROME	CLINICAL FEATURES	INHERITANCE
Perlman syndrome	Fetal macrosomia with visceromegaly, ascites, and polyhydramnios; bilateral renal hamartomas; Wilms' tumor; cryptorchidism; facial abnormalities; micrognathia; volvulus; ileal atresia; diaphragmatic hernia; interrupted aortic arch; corpus callosum agenesis	Autosomal recessive
Lethal macrosomia with micropthalmia	Macrosomia, microphthalmia, median cleft palate; associated with respiratory infection in early life and early infant death	Autosomal recessive
Macrosomia adipose congenita	Macrosomia, voracious appetite, precocious skeletal development; death in first year common	Autosomal recessive
MOMO syndrome	Macrocephaly, retinal coloboma, nystagmus, mental retardation, delayed bone maturation	Autosomal dominant
Cleft lip or palate, characteristic facies, intestinal malrotation, congenital heart disease	Macrosomia, bilateral cleft lip or palate, flat facial profile, lethal complex congenital heart defect, bifid thumbs	Autosomal recessive
ABCD syndrome	Macrosomia, defective intestinal innervation, neonatal fatal intestinal dysfunction	Autosomal recessive
Simpson-Golabi-Behmel syndrome	Macrosomia, macrocephaly, coarse facies, hypertelorism, cleft palate, ventricular septal defect, pulmonic stenosis, transposition of great vessels, patent ductus arteriosus, lung segmentation defects, cervical ribs, pectus excavatum, 13 pairs of thoracic ribs, diaphragmatic hernia, polysplenia, duplication of renal pelvis, postaxial polydactyly, syndactyly of the 2nd–3rd fingers, clubfoot, corpus callosum agenesis, cerebellar vermis hypoplasia, hydrocephalus, embryonal tumors, Wilms' tumor	X-linked recessive
Weaver-Smith syndrome	Macrosomia with predominant developmental features	Autosomal dominant
CHIME syndrome	Early-onset migratory ichthyosiform dermatosis, seizures, mental retardation, cleft palate, tetralogy of Fallot, transposition of the great vessels	Autosomal recessive
CANTU syndrome	Generalized congenital hypertrichosis, narrow thorax, cardiomegaly	Autosomal recessive
Marfan syndrome	Macrosomia, micrognathia, enophthalmos, predominant features postdelivery	Autosomal dominant
Beckwith-Wiedemann syndrome	Macrosomia, macroglossia, cardiomegaly, omphalocele, Wilms' tumor	Autosomal dominant

Environmental and genetic interactions are complex. Much birth weight variation is unexplained, and most infants with macrosomia have no identifiable risk factor.[235] Further, no risk factor predicts macrosomia accurately. Several inheritable syndromes that may be responsible for fetal macrosomia are listed in Table 12–6.

Pathophysiology

Excessive fetal growth may result from excess substrate availability, optimal placentation, and overstimulation of the fetal insulin–insulin-like growth factor–leptin axis. Maternal diabetes mellitus is the primary example of excessive substrate availability and subsequent fetal hyperinsulinemia. Maternal obesity and excessive maternal weight gain are associated with intermittent periods of hyperglycemia and thus may act by the same mechanism. Progressive immune recognition and improved placentation with successive pregnancies could explain the increased birth weight observed in the multipara. Overexpression of placental substrate transporters has not been evaluated systematically.

The fetal growth pattern and type of tissue overgrowth reflects the underlying etiology. Insulin-sensitive tissues, such as the heart, liver and spleen, thymus, adrenal gland, subcutaneous fat, and shoulder girdle, can show differential glycogen and fat deposition when insulin levels are high. As a result, total body fat, shoulder and upper-extremity circumference, upper-extremity skin-fold thickness, and liver size are disproportionately greater in macrosomic infants of diabetic women compared with those of women without diabetes.[247,248] These differences in growth patterns are at least partially responsible for the significant associated fetal, neonatal, and maternal risks.

Fetal and Neonatal Risks

Macrosomia is associated with increased perinatal mortality; intrapartum risks, including shoulder dystocia; brachial plexus injury; skeletal injuries; meconium aspiration; perinatal asphyxia; and postpartum complications, including respiratory distress syndrome and neonatal hypoglycemia.[235,236,249,250] The complication rates reflect the absolute birth weight. Perinatal morbidity rates are increased in infants larger than 4500 g, and mortality rates are increased in infants larger than 5000 g.[251] Rates of shoulder dystocia and associated clavicular fracture increase 10-fold.[252] Yet, only a small percentage of macrosomic fetuses have complicated deliveries. The risk of shoulder dystocia is significantly affected by the underlying cause of macrosomia. In women without diabetes, shoulder dystocia occurs in 9.8% to 24% of deliveries with a fetus weighing more than 4500 g. This prevalence is doubled in women with diabetes.[237,253,254] Clavicular fracture and brachial plexus injuries, including

Erb-Duchenne palsy, are most frequently associated with shoulder dystocia.[252,255] However, the risk of brachial plexus injury is increased independent of the mode of delivery or the clinical diagnosis of shoulder dystocia. This finding suggests an in utero origin for at least some brachial plexus injuries.[256] When birth weight exceeds 4500 g, the risk of shoulder dystocia is 18- to 21-fold higher than that in neonates with lower birth weight.[238,248,257]

Maternal Risks

Maternal complications of macrosomia are also related to neonatal birth weight. The incidences of cephalopelvic disproportion and prolonged labor increase at birth weights greater than 4500 g, and as a result, the cesarean delivery rate doubles.[236,257] The incidence of postpartum hemorrhage greater than 1000 ml increases with birth weights above 4000 g.[258] The rate of third- and fourth-degree laceration is especially increased when shoulder dystocia is diagnosed.[259] Thromboembolic events and anesthetic complications are increased in great part because of the increased need for operative intervention.

Summary

Excessive fetal growth is associated with fetal, neonatal, and maternal risks. These risks are proportional to the absolute, rather than relative, birth weight. Although macrosomia is variably defined, a birth weight greater than 4500 g is associated with the highest risk of morbidity, whereas a birth weight greater than 5000 g is associated with an increased risk of perinatal mortality. Maternal hyperglycemia is the most common risk factor for macrosomia; it also affects perinatal outcome by altering neonatal body proportions and increasing the risk of shoulder dystocia and related birth trauma.

Diagnosis

There are no useful, general-purpose screening tools for the detection of macrosomia. A history of obstetric and maternal risk factors (discussed earlier) heightens the clinical index of suspicion. In addition, an unexplained very low serum maternal serum α-fetoprotein level is associated with increased birth weight and an increased prevalence of obstetric complications.[260]

Clinical Examination

Mothers of infants with birth weight greater than 4500 g have greater symphyseal fundal height than expected.[261] However, several variables, including amniotic fluid volume and maternal body habitus, limit the usefulness of this measurement unless it is combined with clinical palpation or Leopold's maneuvers.[262] Prospective studies of fundal height measurement combined with Leopold's maneuvers report sensitivity of 10% to 43%, specificity of 99.0% to 99.8%, and positive predictive values of 28% to 53% for the detection of macrosomia.[263,264] Finally, the mother's subjective assessment of fetal weight can be as accurate as the clinical assessment by Leopold's maneuvers.[265]

Ultrasound

Ultrasound prediction of fetal weight loses accuracy above 4000 g does not exceed the diagnostic accuracy of clinical estimates.[265–267] Only 50% of fetuses larger than 4500 g weigh within 10% of the predicted weight.[268] In women without diabetes mellitus, the sensitivity of ultrasound for the detection of macrosomia (birth weight >4500 g) is 22% to 44%, with specificity of 99% and positive predictive values of 30% to 44%.[269,270] There are several reasons for these inaccuracies. First, even at lower weights, the typical error associated with sonographic estimates is 10%, a large error in a macrosomic fetus. Second, the accuracy of these formulas, when confined to macrosomic fetuses, is even lower, up to 13%.[271] Because the birth weight of macrosomic infants is largely determined by organ size and fat deposition, formulas that include abdominal circumference and exclude bony measurements perform better than those that do not.[269] Ultrasound methods that account for skin thickness[272] or incorporate algorithms to calculate fetal volume may have a role in the future.[273] Ultrasound can provide diagnostic information on fetal anatomy, organ size, and fat deposition. Further, ultrasound allows an objective assessment of amniotic fluid volume that may prompt further evaluation for underlying syndromes (see Table 12–6) or recommendation of a 3-hour glucose tolerance test when hydramnios is suspected. In women with diabetes mellitus, macrosomia may be a biologic indicator of suboptimal maternal metabolic control.

Management Options

In the absence of maternal diabetes mellitus, principal management considerations for suspected macrosomia focus on the timing and type of delivery and intrapartum management. Evidence suggests that labor induction for suspected macrosomia, defined as estimated fetal weight of 4000 to 4500 g,[274] increases the cesarean delivery rate without improving perinatal outcome.[275] Although seemingly logical, labor induction should not be undertaken in the absence of a high cervical Bishop's score.

Because perinatal and maternal risks increase with birth weight and cesarean section reportedly decreases the risks of birth trauma and brachial plexus injury,[236,248,252] it is logical to conclude that elective cesarean delivery should be offered beyond a certain estimated fetal weight. However, there is no adequate study to support this practice. No clinical studies show a significant reduction in the prevalence of birth injury by adopting such a practice, although arguably, a much larger sample size is needed. Cohort and case–control studies show that a trial of labor is safe and cost-effective at estimated fetal weights of 5000 g or less.[276] Although the predictive accuracy of fetal weight estimates is poor at greater than 5000 g, most authors agree that prophylactic cesarean section should be offered.[236,257] For suspected fetal macrosomia less than 5000 g, prophylactic cesarean section does not appear to reduce birth trauma significantly in the absence of maternal diabetes mellitus. In these women and those with other risk factors, such as a history of shoulder dystocia in a macrosomic infant, estimated weight is important when planning the delivery route.

During labor, special attention is given to the progress of labor and the uterine contraction pattern. Cesarean delivery is indicated when the estimated fetal weight exceeds 4500 g; the second stage is prolonged (>2 hours), with documented adequate uterine contractions (>200 Montevideo units); or descent is arrested. The risk of shoulder dystocia is increased by assisted vaginal delivery. A trial of vaginal delivery after a previous cesarean delivery appears safe for both infant and mother, with success rates of 58% when birth weight is less than 4500 g and 43% when birth weight is higher.[277]

Summary

Antenatal prediction of fetal macrosomia is unsatisfactory because most women with a macrosomic fetus lack characteristic risk factors. Further, the predictive accuracy of diagnostic ultrasound decreases with increasing fetal weight. Manual assessment of fetal weight supplemented with Leopold's maneuvers is just as efficient as assessment with ultrasound. The main role of ultrasound is detecting fetal anomalies and quantifying amniotic fluid volume. In the absence of maternal diabetes mellitus, little evidence supports elective induction or cesarean section with estimated fetal weight of less than 5000 g unless other obstetric factors (e.g., high Bishop's score) are present. With an estimated fetal weight of greater than 4500 g, a prolonged second stage of labor or arrest of descent in the second stage is an indication for cesarean delivery. Although the diagnosis of fetal macrosomia is imprecise, prophylactic cesarean delivery may be reasonable when estimated fetal weight is greater than 5000 g in women without diabetes or greater than 4500 g in women with diabetes mellitus. Suspected fetal macrosomia is not a contraindication to attempted vaginal birth after a previous cesarean delivery.

CONCLUSIONS

- Excessive fetal growth is associated with fetal, neonatal, and maternal risks that are proportional to the absolute rather than the birthweight percentile. A birthweight greater than 4500 g identifies pregnancies at highest risk for morbidity, while a birthweight above 5000 g identifies those at increased risk of a perinatal mortality.
- Maternal hyperglycemia is the greatest risk factor for macrosomia by promoting accelerated fetal growth as well as altered body proportions that escalate the risk for shoulder dystocia and related birth trauma.
- Prenatal prediction of macrosomia is unsatisfactory due to the lacking of characteristic risk factors in many women and the inadequate accuracy of diagnostic ultrasound with increasing fetal weight.
- In the absence of maternal diabetes mellitus unfavorable obstetric factors, prolonged, or arrested second stage are indications for cesarean delivery in fetuses with an estimated weight in excess of 4500 g.
- Prophylactic cesarean section may be offered to all women carrying a fetus with an estimated fetal weight greater than 5000 g and to diabetic women if the estimated fetal weight is greater than 4500 g.
- Suspected fetal macrosomia with an estimated fetal weight below 5000 g is not a contraindication to attempted vaginal birth after a previous cesarean delivery.

SUMMARY OF MANAGEMENT OPTIONS

Fetal Macrosomia

Management Options	Quality of Evidence	Strength of Recommendation	References
Prenatal			
On Clinical Suspicion of Macrosomia			
• Abdominal circumference 95th percentile, particularly if associated with increased amniotic fluid volume	III	B	278
• Exclude gestational diabetes	–	GPP	–
• Family history of inheritable disorders (see Table 12–6)	–	GPP	–

Continued

SUMMARY OF MANAGEMENT OPTIONS
Fetal Macrosomia *(Continued)*

Management Options	Quality of Evidence	Strength of Recommendation	References
Prenatal			
With Diagnosis of Macrosomia			
• Maternal glycemic control, if indicated		see Chapter 45	
Labor and Delivery			
Delivery indicated for maternal factors; induction vs. expectant management is associated with increased cesarean rate without improved outcome	IIb	B	274
Delivery Route • For estimated fetal weight <4500 g, offer vaginal delivery and vaginal birth after cesarean section • For estimated fetal weight >4500 g in a diabetic patient, offer elective cesarean delivery • For estimated fetal weight >5000 g in nondiabetic patient, offer cesarean delivery	III	B	276,277
Early detection of protraction disorder is made by failure to progress over 3 hr with >200 Montevideo units.	III	B, C	252–254,276

REFERENCES

1. Lubchenco LO, Hansman C, Boyd E: Intrauterine growth as estimated from live born birth-weight data at 24–42 weeks of gestation. Pediatrics 1963;32:793.
2. Battaglia FC, Lubchenco LO: A practical classification of newborn infants by weight and gestational age. J Pediatr 1967;71: 159–163.
3. Bernstein IM, Horbar JD, Badger GJ, et al: Morbidity and mortality among very-low-birth-weight neonates with intrauterine growth restriction: The Vermont Oxford Network. Am J Obstet Gynecol 2000;182:198–206.
4. Barker DJ: Fetal growth and adult disease. Br J Obstet Gynaecol 1992;99:275–276.
5. Hoffman HJ, Stark CR, Lundin FE, Ashbrook JD: Analysis of birthweight, gestational age, and fetal viability, U.S. births, 1968. Obstet Gynecol Surv 1974;29:651.
6. Gardosi J, Chang A, Kalyan B, et al: Customised antenatal growth charts. Lancet 1992;339:283–287.
7. Clausson B, Gardosi J, Francis A, Cnattingius S: Perinatal outcome in SGA births defined by customised versus population-based birthweight standards. Br J Obstet Gynaecol 2001;108: 830–834.
8. Bukowski R, Burgett AD, Gei A, et al: Impairment of fetal growth potential and neonatal encephalopathy. Am J Obstet Gynecol 2003;188:1011–1015.
9. Miller HC: Fetal growth and neonatal mortality. Pediatrics 1972;49:392.
10. Weiner CP, Robinson D: The sonographic diagnosis of intrauterine growth retardation using the postnatal ponderal index and the crown heel length as standards of diagnosis. Am J Perinatol 1989;6:380–383.
11. Lepercq J, Lahlou N, Timsit J, et al: Macrosomia revisited: Ponderal index and leptin delineate subtypes of fetal overgrowth. Am J Obstet Gynecol 1999;181:621–625.
12. Owen P, Farrell T, Hardwick JC, Khan KS: Relationship between customised birthweight centiles and neonatal anthropometric features of growth restriction. Br J Obstet Gynaecol 2002;109:658–662.
13. Walther FJ, Ramaekers LHJ: The Ponderal Index as a measure of the nutritional status at birth and its relation to some aspects of neonatal morbidity. J Perinat Med 1982;10: 42–47.
14. Ballard JL, Rosenn B, Khoury JC, Miodovnik M: Diabetic fetal macrosomia: Significance of disproportionate growth. Pediatrics 1993;122:115–119.
15. Dashe JS, McIntire DD, Lucas MJ, Leveno KJ: Effects of symmetric and asymmetric fetal growth on pregnancy outcomes. Obstet Gynecol 2000;96:321–327.
16. Pijnenborg R, Bland JM, Robertson WB, Brosens I: Uteroplacental arterial changes related to interstitial trophoblast migration in early human pregnancy. Placenta 1983;4:397–413.
17. Aplin J: Maternal influences on placental development. Semin Cell Dev Biol 2000;11:115–125.
18. Kingdom JC, Burrell SJ, Kaufmann P: Pathology and clinical implications of abnormal umbilical artery Doppler waveforms. Ultrasound Obstet Gynecol 1997;9:271–286.
19. Edman CD, Toofanian A, MacDonald PC, Gant NF: Placental clearance rate of maternal plasma androstenedione through placental estradiol formation: An indirect method of assessing uteroplacental blood flow. Am J Obstet Gynecol 1981;141: 1029–1037.
20. Maini CL, Rosati P, Galli G, et al: Non-invasive radioisotopic evaluation of placental blood flow. Gynecol Obstet Invest 1985; 19:196–206.
21. Luckhardt M, Leiser R, Kingdom J, et al: Effect of physiologic perfusion-fixation on the morphometrically evaluated dimensions of the term placental cotyledon. J Soc Gynecol Invest 1996;3:166–171.
22. Kiserud T: The ductus venosus. Semin Perinatol 2001;25:11–20.
23. Rudolph AM: Distribution and regulation of blood flow in the fetal and neonatal lamb. Circ Res 1985;57:811–821.

24. Pardi G, Marconi AM, Cetin I: Placental-fetal interrelationship in IUGR fetuses: A review. Placenta 2002;23(Suppl A): S136–S141.
25. Guyton AC, Cowley AW Jr, Young DB, et al: Integration and control of circulatory function. Int Rev Physiol 1976;9: 341–385.
26. Kaufmann P, Scheffen I: Placental development. In Polin RA, Fox WW (eds): Fetal and Neonatal Physiology. Philadelphia, Saunders, 1998, pp 59–70.
27. Battaglia FC, Regnault TR: Placental transport and metabolism of amino acids. Placenta 2001;22:145–161.
28. Haggarty P: Placental regulation of fatty acid delivery and its effects on fetal growth: A review. Placenta 2002;23:S28–S38.
29. Illsely NP: Glucose transporters in the human placenta. Placenta 2000;21:14–22.
30. Sibley CP, Glazier JD, Greenwood SL, et al: Regulation of placental transfer: The Na(+)/H(+) exchanger. A review. Placenta 2002;23:S39–S46.
31. Meschia G: Placenta respiratory gas exchange and fetal oxygenation. In Creasy RK, Resnik R (eds): Maternal Fetal Medicine: Principles and Practice. Philadelphia, Saunders, 1987, pp 274–285.
32. Meschia G, Battaglia FC, Hay WW, Sparks JW: Utilization of substrates by the ovine placenta in vivo. Fed Proc 1980;39: 245–249.
33. Carter AM: Placental oxygen consumption. Part I. In vivo studies: A review. Placenta 2000;21:S31–S37.
34. Lederman SA, Paxton A, Heymsfield SB, et al: Maternal body fat and water during pregnancy: Do they raise infant birth weight? Am J Obstet Gynecol 1999;180:235–240.
35. Reece EA, Wiznitzer A, Le E, et al: The relation between human fetal growth and fetal blood levels of insulin-like growth factors I and II, their binding proteins, and receptors. Obstet Gynecol 1994;84:88–95.
36. Hoggard N, Haggarty P, Thomas L, Lea RG: Leptin expression in placental and fetal tissues: Does leptin have a functional role? Biochem Soc Trans 2001;29:57–66.
37. Jansson N, Greenwood SL, Johansson BR, et al: Leptin stimulates the activity of the system A amino acid transporter in human placental villous fragments. J Clin Endocrinol Metab 2003;88:1205–1211.
38. Winick M, Noble A: Quantitative changes in DNA, RNA, and protein during prenatal and postnatal growth in the rat. Dev Biol 1965;12:451.
39. Snijders RJM, Sherrod C, Gosden CM, Nicolaides KH: Fetal growth retardation: Associated malformations and chromosome abnormalities. Am J Obstet Gynecol 1993;168:547–555.
40. Khoury MJ, Erickson D, Cordero JE, McCarthy BJ: Congenital malformations and intrauterine growth retardation: A population study. Pediatrics 1988;82:83–90.
41. Sickler GK, Nyberg DA, Sohaey R, Luthy DA: Polyhydramnios and fetal intrauterine growth restriction: Ominous combination. J Ultrasound Med 1997;16:609–614.
42. Odegard RA, Vatten LJ, Nilsen ST, et al: Preeclampsia and fetal growth. Obstet Gynecol 2000;96:950–955.
43. Kupferminc MJ, Peri H, Zwang E, et al: High prevalence of the prothrombin gene mutation in women with intrauterine growth retardation, abruptio placentae and second trimester loss. Acta Obstet Gynecol Scand 2000;79:963–967.
44. Weiner CP: Pathogenesis, evaluation, and potential treatments for severe, early onset growth retardation. Semin Perinatol 1989; 13:320.
45. Cliver SP, Goldenberg RL, Cutter GR, et al: The effect of cigarette smoking on neonatal anthropometric measurements. Obstet Gynecol 1995;85:625–630.
46. Goldenberg RL, Hauth J, Cutter GR, et al: Fetal growth in women using low-dose aspirin for the prevention of pre-eclampsia: Effect of maternal size. J Matern Fetal Med 1995;4:218–222.
47. Goldenberg RL, Cliver SP, Cutter GR, et al: Blood pressure, growth retardation and preterm delivery. In J Tech Assess Health Care 1992;8:82–90.
48. Brosens I, Dixon HG, Robertson WB: Fetal growth retardation and the arteries of the placental bed. Br J Obstet Gynaecol 1977;84:656–663.
49. Meekins JW, Pijnenborg R, Hanssens M, et al: A study of placental bed spiral arteries and trophoblast invasion in normal and severe pre-eclamptic pregnancies. Br J Obstet Gynaecol 1994; 101:669–674.
50. Aardema MW, Oosterhof H, Timmer A, et al: Uterine artery Doppler flow and uteroplacental vascular pathology in normal pregnancies and pregnancies complicated by pre-eclampsia and small for gestational age fetuses. Placenta 2001;22:405–411.
51. Ferrazzi E, Bulfamante G, Mezzopane R, et al: Uterine Doppler velocimetry and placental hypoxic-ischaemic lesion in pregnancies with fetal intrauterine growth restriction. Placenta 1999;20:389–394.
52. Harrington K, Carpenter RG, Goldfrad C, Campbell S: Transvaginal Doppler ultrasound of the uteroplacental circulation in the early prediction of pre-eclampsia and intrauterine growth retardation. Br J Obstet Gynaecol 1997; 104:674–681.
53. Bower S, Kingdom J, Campbell S: Objective and subjective assessment of abnormal uterine artery Doppler flow velocity waveforms. Ultrasound Obstet Gynecol 1998;12:260–264.
54. Rigano S, Bozzo M, Ferrazzi E, et al: Early and persistent reduction in umbilical vein blood flow in the growth-restricted fetus: A longitudinal study. Am J Obstet Gynecol 2001;185:834–838.
55. Yagel S, Anteby EY, Shen O, et al: Placental blood flow measured by simultaneous multigate spectral Doppler imaging in pregnancies complicated by placental vascular abnormalities. Ultrasound Obstet Gynecol 1999;14:262–266.
56. Morrow RJ, Adamson SL, Bull SB, Ritchie JW: Effect of placental embolization on the umbilical artery velocity waveform in fetal sheep. Am J Obstet Gynecol 1989;161:1055–1060.
57. Wilcox G, Trudinger B, Cook CM, et al: Reduced fetal platelet counts in pregnancies with abnormal Doppler umbilical flow waveforms. Obstet Gynecol 1989;73:639–643.
58. Papageorghiou AT, Yu CK, Cicero S, et al: Second-trimester uterine artery Doppler screening in unselected populations: A review. J Matern Fetal Neonatal Med 2002;12:78–88.
59. Weiner CP: The relationship between the umbilical artery systolic/diastolic ratio and umbilical blood gas measurements in specimens obtained by cordocentesis. Am J Obstet Gynecol 1990;162:1198–1202.
60. Weiner CP, Williamson RA: Evaluation of severe growth retardation using cordocentesis: Hematologic and metabolic alterations by etiology. Obstet Gynecol 1989;73:225–229.
61. Bilardo CM, Nicolaides KH, Campbell S: Doppler measurements of fetal and uteroplacental circulations: Relationship with umbilical venous blood gases measured at cordocentesis. Am J Obstet Gynecol 1990;162:115–120.
62. Jones CT, Ritchie JW, Walker D: The effects of hypoxia on glucose turnover in the fetal sheep. J Dev Physiol 1983;5:223–235.
63. Nicolini U, Hubinont C, Santolaya J, et al: Maternal-fetal glucose gradient in normal pregnancies and in pregnancies complicated by alloimmunization and fetal growth retardation. Am J Obstet Gynecol 1989;161:924–927.
64. Economides DL, Nicolaides KH: Blood glucose and oxygen tension levels in small-for-gestational-age fetuses. Am J Obstet Gynecol 1989;160:385–389.
65. Hubinont C, Nicolini U, Fisk NM, et al: Endocrine pancreatic function in growth-retarded fetuses. Obstet Gynecol 1991;77: 541–544.
66. Van Assche FA, Aerts L, DePrins FA: The fetal endocrine pancreas. Eur J Obstet Gynecol Reprod Biol 1984;18:267–272.
67. Soothill PW, Nicolaides KH, Campbell S: Prenatal asphyxia, hyperlacticaemia, hypoglycaemia, and erythroblastosis in growth retarded fetuses. Br Med J 1987;294:1051–1053.

68. Owens JA, Falconer J, Robinsin JS: Effect of restriction of placental growth on fetal uteroplacental metabolism. J Dev Physiol 1987;9:225–238.
69. Paolini CL, Marconi AM, Ronzoni S, et al: Placental transport of leucine, phenylalanine, glycine, and proline in intrauterine growth-restricted pregnancies. J Clin Endocrinol Metab 2001; 86:5427–5432.
70. Economides DL, Nicolaides KH, Gahl WA, et al: Plasma amino acids in appropriate and small-for-gestational-age fetuses. Am J Obstet Gynecol 1989;161:1219–1227.
71. Bernstein IM, Silver R, Nair KS, Stirewalt WS: Amniotic fluid glycine-valine ratio and neonatal morbidity in fetal growth restriction. Obstet Gynecol 1997;90:933–937.
72. Vannucci RC, Vannucci SJ: Glucose metabolism in the developing brain. Semin Perinatol 2000;24:107–115
73. Fisher DJ, Heymann MA, Rudolph AM: Fetal myocardial oxygen and carbohydrate consumption during acutely induced hypoxemia. Am J Physiol 1982;1242:H657–H661.
74. Spahr R, I Probst, HM Piper: Substrate utilization of adult cardiac myocytes. Basic Res Cardiol 1985;80(Suppl 1):53–56.
75. Fant ME, Weisoly D: Insulin and insulin-like growth factors in human development: Implications for the perinatal period. Semin Perinatol 2001;25:426–435.
76. Rizzo G, Arduini D: Fetal cardiac function in intrauterine growth retardation. Am J Obstet Gynecol 1991;165:876–882.
77. Baschat AA, Gembruch U, Gortner L, et al: Coronary artery blood flow visualization signifies hemodynamic deterioration in growth-restricted fetuses. Ultrasound Obstet Gynecol 2000;16:425–431.
78. Reed KL, Anderson CF, Shenker L: Changes in intracardiac Doppler flow velocities in fetuses with absent umbilical artery diastolic flow. Am J Obstet Gynecol 1987;157:774–779.
79. Al Ghazali W, Chita SK, Chapman MG, Allan LD: Evidence of redistribution of cardiac output in asymmetrical growth retardation. Br J Obstet Gynaecol 1987;96:697–704.
80. Griffin D, Bilardo K, Masini L, et al: Doppler blood flow waveforms in the descending thoracic aorta of the human fetus. Br J Obstet Gynaecol 1984;91:997–1006.
81. Akalin-Sel T, Nicolaides KH, Peacock J, Campbell S: Doppler dynamics and their complex interrelation with fetal oxygen pressure, carbon dioxide pressure, and pH in growth-retarded fetuses. Obstet Gynecol 1994;84:439–444.
82. Wladimiroff JW, Tonge HM, Stewart PA: Doppler ultrasound assessment of cerebral blood flow in the human fetus. Br J Obstet Gynaecol 1986;93:471–475.
83. Arbeille P, Maulik D, Fignon A, et al: Assessment of the fetal PO2 changes by cerebral and umbilical Doppler on lamb fetuses during acute hypoxia. Ultrasound Med Biol 1995;21:861–870.
84. Gramellini D, Folli MC, Raboni S, et al: Cerebral-umbilical Doppler ratio as a predictor of adverse perinatal outcome. Obstet Gynecol 1992;79:416–420.
85. Fouron JC, Skoll A, Sonesson SE, et al: Relationship between flow through the fetal aortic isthmus and cerebral oxygenation during acute placental circulatory insufficiency in ovine fetuses. Am J Obstet Gynecol 1999;181:1102–1107.
86. Makikallio K, Jouppila P, Rasanen J: Retrograde net blood flow in the aortic isthmus in relation to human fetal arterial and venous circulations. Ultrasound Obstet Gynecol 2002;19: 147–152.
87. Baschat AA, Gembruch U, Reiss I, et al: Demonstration of fetal coronary blood flow by Doppler ultrasound in relation to arterial and venous flow velocity waveforms and perinatal outcome: The "heart-sparing effect." Ultrasound Obstet Gynecol 1997;9: 162–172.
88. Tekay A, Jouppila P: Fetal adrenal artery velocimetry measurements in appropriate-for-gestational age and intrauterine growth-restricted fetuses. Ultrasound Obstet Gynecol 2000;16: 419–424.
89. Abuhamad AZ, Mari G, Bogdan D, Evans AT III: Doppler flow velocimetry of the splenic artery in the human fetus: Is it a marker of chronic hypoxia? Am J Obstet Gynecol 1995;172: 820–825.
90. Kilavuz O, Vetter K: Is the liver of the fetus the 4th preferential organ for arterial blood supply besides brain, heart, and adrenal glands? J Perinat Med 1999;27:103–106.
91. Rizzo G, Capponi A, Chaoui R, et al: Blood flow velocity waveforms from peripheral pulmonary arteries in normally grown and growth-retarded fetuses. Ultrasound Obstet Gynecol 1996;8:87–92.
92. Gamsu HR, Vyas S, Nicolaides K: Effects of intrauterine growth retardation on postnatal visceral and cerebral blood flow velocity. Arch Dis Child 1991;66:1115–1118.
93. Mari G, Abuhamad AZ, Uerpairojkit B, et al: Blood flow velocity waveforms of the abdominal arteries in appropriate- and small-for-gestational-age fetuses. Ultrasound Obstet Gynecol 1995;6:15–18.
94. Rhee E, Detti L, Mari G: Superior mesenteric artery flow velocity waveforms in small for gestational age fetuses. J Matern Fetal Med 1998;7:120–123.
95. Veille JC, Kanaan C: Duplex Doppler ultrasonographic evaluation of the fetal renal artery in normal and abnormal fetuses. Am J Obstet Gynecol 1989;161:1502–1507.
96. Arduini D, Rizzo G: Fetal renal artery velocity waveforms and amniotic fluid volume in growth-retarded and post-term fetuses. Obstet Gynecol 1991;77:370–373.
97. Mari G: Arterial blood flow velocity waveforms of the pelvis and lower extremities in normal and growth-retarded fetuses. Am J Obstet Gynecol 1991;165:143–151.
98. Boito S, Struijk PC, Ursem NT, et al: Fetal brain/liver volume ratio and umbilical volume flow parameters relative to normal and abnormal human development. Ultrasound Obstet Gynecol 2003;21:256–261.
99. Weiner CP, Robillard JE: Atrial natriuretic factor, digoxin-like immunoreactive substance, norepinephrine, epinephrine, and plasma are in activity in human fetuses and their alteration by fetal disease. Am J Obstet Gynecol 1988;159:1353–1360.
100. Rizzo G, Capponi A, Rinaldo D, et al: Release of vasoactive agents during cordocentesis: Differences between normally grown and growth restricted fetuses. Am J Obstet Gynecol 1996;175:563–570.
101. Rizzo G, Montuschi P, Capponi A, Romanini C: Blood levels of vasoactive intestinal polypeptide in normal and growth retarded fetuses: Relationship with acid-base and haemodynamic status. Early Hum Dev 1995;41:69–77.
102. Manning FA: Fetal biophysical profile. Obstet Gynecol Clin North Am 1999;26:557–577.
103. Arduini D, Rizzo G, Romanini C, Mancuso S: Computerized analysis of behavioural states in asymmetrical growth retarded fetuses. J Perinat Med 1988;16:357–363.
104. Arduini D, Rizzo G, Caforio L, et al: Behavioural state transitions in healthy and growth retarded fetuses. Early Hum Dev 1989;19:155–165.
105. Nijhuis IJ, ten Hof J, Nijhuis JG, et al: Temporal organisation of fetal behaviour from 24-weeks gestation onwards in normal and complicated pregnancies. Dev Psychobiol 1999;34:257–268.
106. Vindla S, James D, Sahota D: Computerised analysis of unstimulated and stimulated behaviour in fetuses with intrauterine growth restriction. Eur J Obstet Gynecol Reprod Biol 1999;83:37–45.
107. Yum MK, Park EY, Kim CR, Hwang JH: Alterations in irregular and fractal heart rate behavior in growth restricted fetuses. Eur J Obstet Gynecol Reprod Biol 2001;94:51–58.
108. Ribbert LS, Nicolaides KH, Visser GH: Prediction of fetal acidaemia in intrauterine growth retardation: Comparison of quantified fetal activity with biophysical profile score. Br J Obstet Gynaecol 1993;100:653–656.
109. Nijhuis IJ, ten Hof J, Mulder EJ, et al: Fetal heart rate in relation to its variation in normal and growth retarded fetuses. Eur J Obstet Gynecol Reprod Biol 2000;89:27–33.

110. Henson G, Dawes GS, Redman CW: Characterization of the reduced heart rate variation in growth-retarded fetuses.Br J Obstet Gynaecol 1984;91:751–755.
111. Ribbert LS, Snijders RJ, Nicolaides KH, Visser GH: Relation of fetal blood gases and data from computer-assisted analysis of fetal heart rate patterns in small for gestation fetuses. Br J Obstet Gynaecol 1991;98:820–823.
112. Smith JH, Anand KJ, Cotes PM, et al: Antenatal fetal heart rate variation in relation to the respiratory and metabolic status of the compromised human fetus. Br J Obstet Gynaecol 1988;95: 980–989.
113. Ribbert LS, Visser GH, Mulder EJ, et al: Changes with time in fetal heart rate variation, movement incidences and haemodynamics in intrauterine growth retarded fetuses: A longitudinal approach to the assessment of fetal well being. Early Hum Dev 1993;31:195–208.
114. Pillai M, James D: Continuation of normal neurobehavioural development in fetuses with absent umbilical arterial end-diastolic velocities. Br J Obstet Gynaecol 1991;98:277–281.
115. Rizzo G, Arduini D, Pennestri F, et al: Fetal behaviour in growth retardation: Its relationship to fetal blood flow. Prenat Diagn 1987;7:229–238.
116. Arduini D, Rizzo G, Capponi A, et al: Fetal pH value determined by cordocentesis: An independent predictor of the development of antepartum fetal heart rate decelerations in growth retarded fetuses with absent end-diastolic velocity in umbilical artery. J Perinat Med 1996;24:601–607.
117. Baschat AA: Integrated fetal testing in growth restriction: Combining multivessel Doppler and biophysical parameters. Ultrasound Obstet Gynecol 2003;21:8.
118. Thilaganathan B, Athanasiou S, Ozmen S, et al: Umbilical cord blood erythroblast count as an index of intrauterine hypoxia. Arch Dis Child Fetal Neonat Ed 1994;70:F192–F194.
119. Maier RF, Gunther A, Vogel M, et al: Umbilical venous erythropoietin and umbilical arterial pH in relation to morphologic placental abnormalities. Obstet Gynecol 1994;84:81–87.
120. Snijders RJM, Abbas A, Melby O, et al: Fetal plasma erythropoietin concentration in severe growth retardation. Am J Obstet Gynecol 1993;168:615–619.
121. Baschat AA, Gembruch U, Reiss I, et al: Neonatal nucleated red blood cell counts in growth-restricted fetuses: relationship to arterial and venous Doppler studies. Am J Obstet Gynecol 1999;181:190–195.
122. Bernstein PS, Minior VK, Divon MY: Nucleated red blood cell counts in small for gestational age fetuses with abnormal umbilical artery Doppler studies. Am J Obstet Gynecol 1997;177: 1079–1084.
123. Trudinger B, Song JZ, Wu ZH, Wang J: Placental insufficiency is characterized by platelet activation in the fetus. Obstet Gynecol 2003;101:975–981.
124. Baschat AA, Gembruch U, Reiss I, et al: Absent umbilical artery end-diastolic velocity in growth-restricted fetuses: A risk factor for neonatal thrombocytopenia. Obstet Gynecol 2000;96: 162–166.
125. Rizzo G, Capponi A, Rinaldo D, et al: Ventricular ejection force in growth-retarded fetuses. Ultrasound Obstet Gynecol 1995;5: 247–255.
126. Hecher K, Campbell S, Doyle P, et al: Assessment of fetal compromise by Doppler ultrasound investigation of the fetal circulation: Arterial, intracardiac, and venous blood flow velocity studies. Circulation 1995;91:129–138.
127. Kiserud T, Eik-Nes SH, Blaas HG, et al: Ductus venosus blood velocity and the umbilical circulation in the seriously growth retarded fetus. Ultrasound Obstet Gynecol 1994;4:109–114.
128. Rizzo G, Capponi A, Talone PE, et al: Doppler indices from inferior vena cava and ductus venosus in predicting pH and oxygen tension in umbilical blood at cordocentesis in growth-retarded fetuses. Ultrasound Obstet Gynecol 1996;7:401–410.
129. Fouron JC, Absi F, Skoll A, et al: Changes in flow velocity patterns of the superior and inferior venae cavae during placental circulatory insufficiency. Ultrasound Obstet Gynecol 2003; 21:53–56.
130. Hecher K, Campbell S: Characteristics of fetal venous blood flow under normal circumstances and during fetal disease. Ultrasound Obstet Gynecol 1996;7:68–83.
131. Hofstaetter C, Gudmundsson S, Hansmann M: Venous Doppler velocimetry in the surveillance of severely compromised fetuses. Ultrasound Obstet Gynecol 2002;20:233–239.
132. Weiner Z, Goldberg Y, Shalev E: Internal jugular vein blood flow in normal and growth-restricted fetuses. Obstet Gynecol 2000;96:167–171.
133. Senat MV, Schwarzler P, Alcais A, Ville Y: Longitudinal changes in the ductus venosus, cerebral transverse sinus and cardiotocogram in fetal growth restriction. Ultrasound Obstet Gynecol 2000;16:19–24.
134. Gudmundsson S, Tulzer G, Huhta JC, Marsal K: Venous Doppler in the fetus with absent end-diastolic flow in the umbilical artery. Ultrasound Obstet Gynecol 1996;7:262–267.
135. Rowlands DJ, Vyas SK: Longitudinal study of fetal middle cerebral artery flow velocity waveforms preceding fetal death. Br J Obstet Gynaecol 1995;102:888–890.
136. Arduini D, Rizzo G, Romanini C: Changes of pulsatility index from fetal vessels preceding the onset of late decelerations in growth-retarded fetuses. Obstet Gynecol 1992;79:605–610.
137. Sebire NJ, Talbert DG: The dynamic placenta: A closer look at the pathophysiology of placental hemodynamics in uteroplacental compromise. Ultrasound Obstet Gynecol 2001; 18:557–561.
138. Vintzileos AM, Fleming AD, Scorza WE, et al: Relationship between fetal biophysical activities and umbilical cord blood gas values. Am J Obstet Gynecol 1991;165:707–713.
139. Manning FA, Snijders R, Harman CR, et al: Fetal biophysical profile score: VI. Correlation with antepartum umbilical venous fetal pH. Am J Obstet Gynecol 1993;169:755–763.
140. Guzman ER, Vintzileos AM, Martins M, et al: The efficacy of individual computer heart rate indices in detecting acidemia at birth in growth-restricted fetuses. Obstet Gynecol 1996;87: 969–974.
141. Rizzo G, Capponi A, Pietropolli A, et al: Fetal cardiac and extracardiac flows preceding intrauterine death. Ultrasound Obstet Gynecol 1994;4:139–142.
142. Baschat AA, Gembruch U, Harman CR: The sequence of changes in Doppler and biophysical parameters as severe fetal growth restriction worsens. Ultrasound Obstet Gynecol 2001; 18:571–577.
143. James DK, Parker MJ, Smoleniec JS: Comprehensive fetal assessment with three ultrasonographic characteristics. Am J Obstet Gynecol 1992;166:1486–1495.
144. Harrington K, Thompson MO, Carpenter RG, et al: Doppler fetal circulation in pregnancies complicated by pre-eclampsia or delivery of a small for gestational age baby: 2. Longitudinal analysis. Br J Obstet Gynaecol 1999;106:453–466.
145. Ferrazzi E, Bozzo M, Rigano S, et al: Temporal sequence of abnormal Doppler changes in the peripheral and central circulatory systems of the severely growth-restricted fetus. Ultrasound Obstet Gynecol 2002;19:140–146.
146. Hecher K, Bilardo CM, Stigter RH, et al: Monitoring of fetuses with intrauterine growth restriction: A longitudinal study. Ultrasound Obstet Gynecol 2001;18:564–570.
147. Baschat AA, Gembruch U, Reiss I, et al: Relationship between arterial and venous Doppler and perinatal outcome in fetal growth restriction. Ultrasound Obstet Gynecol 2000;16: 407–413.
148. Beattie RB, Dornan JC: Antenatal screening for intrauterine growth retardation with umbilical artery Doppler ultrasonography. BMJ 1989;298:631–635.
149. Hershkovitz R, Kingdom JC, Geary M, Rodeck CH: Fetal cerebral blood flow redistribution in late gestation: Identification of

compromise in small fetuses with normal umbilical artery Doppler. Ultrasound Obstet Gynecol 2000;15:209–212.
150. Papageorghiou AT, Yu CK, Cicero S, et al: Second-trimester uterine artery Doppler screening in unselected populations: A review. J Matern Fetal Neonat Med 2002;12:78–88.
151. Soregaroli M, Valcamonico A, Scalvi L, et al: Late normalization of uterine artery velocimetry in high risk pregnancy. Eur J Obstet Gynecol Reprod Biol 2001;95:42–45.
152. Coleman MA, McCowan LM, North RA: Mid-trimester uterine artery Doppler screening as a predictor of adverse pregnancy outcome in high-risk women. Ultrasound Obstet Gynecol 2000;15:7–12.
153. Aquilina J, Barnett A, Thompson O, Harrington K: Comprehensive analysis of uterine artery flow velocity waveforms for the prediction of pre-eclampsia. Ultrasound Obstet Gynecol 2000;16:163–170.
154. Yu CK, Papageorghiou AT, Parra M, et al: Fetal Medicine Foundation Second Trimester Screening Group: Randomized controlled trial using low-dose aspirin in the prevention of pre-eclampsia in women with abnormal uterine artery Doppler at 23 weeks' gestation. Ultrasound Obstet Gynecol 2003;22:233–239.
155. Vainio M, Kujansuu E, Iso-Mustajarvi M, Maenpaa J: Low dose acetylsalicylic acid in prevention of pregnancy-induced hypertension and intrauterine growth retardation in women with bilateral uterine artery notches. Br J Obstet Gynaecol 2002; 109:161–167.
156. Joern H, Rath W: Comparison of Doppler sonographic examinations of the umbilical and uterine arteries in high-risk pregnancies. Fetal Diagn Ther 1998;13:150–153.
157. Drumm JE: The prediction of delivery date by ultrasonic measurement of fetal crown-rump length. Br J Obstet Gynaecol 1977;84:1.
158. Selbing A, Fjallbrant B: Accuracy of conceptual age estimation from fetal crown-rump length. J Clin Ultrasound 1984;12:343.
159. Hadlock FP, Deter RL, Carpenter RJ, Park SK: Estimating fetal age: Effect of head shape on BPD. Am J Roentgenol 1981;137:83–85.
160. Sabbagha RE: Intrauterine growth retardation. In RE Sabbagha (ed): Diagnostic Ultrasound Applied to Obstetrics and Gynecology, 2nd ed. Philadelphia, Lippincott, 1987, pp 112–131.
161. Tamura RK, Sabbagha RE: Percentile ranks of sonar fetal abdominal circumference measurements. Am J Obstet Gynecol 1980;138:475.
162. Baschat AA, Weiner CP: Umbilical artery Doppler screening for detection of the small fetus in need of antepartum surveillance. Am J Obstet Gynecol 2000;182:154–158.
163. Divon MY, Chamberlain PF, Sipos L, et al: Identification of the small for gestational age fetus with the use of gestational age-independent indices of fetal growth. Am J Obstet Gynecol 1986;155:1197–1201.
164. Tamura RK, Sabbagha RE, Pan WH, Vaisrub N: Ultrasonic fetal abdominal circumference: Comparison of direct versus calculated measurement. Obstet Gynecol 1986;67:833.
165. Smith PA, Johansson D, Tzannatos C, Campbell S: Prenatal measurement of the fetal cerebellum and cisterna cerebellomedullaris by ultrasound. Prenat Diagn 1986;6:133.
166. Reece EA, Goldstein I, Pilu G, Hobbins JC: Fetal cerebellar growth unaffected by intrauterine growth retardation: A new parameter for prenatal diagnosis. Am J Obstet Gynecol 1987;157:632.
167. Hill LM, Guzick D, Rivello D, et al: The transverse cerebellar diameter cannot be used to assess gestational age in the small for gestational age fetus. Obstet Gynecol 1990;75:329.
168. Campbell S, Thoms A: Ultrasound measurement of the fetal head to abdomen circumference ratio in the assessment of growth retardation. Br J Obstet Gynaecol 1977;84:165.
169. Warsof SL, Cooper DJ, Little D, Campbell S: Routine ultrasound screening for antenatal detection of intrauterine growth retardation. Obstet Gynecol 1986;67:33.
170. Gray DL, Songster GS, Parvin CA, Crane JP: Cephalic index: A gestational aged dependent biometric parameter. Obstet Gynecol 1989;74:600–603.
171. Hadlock FP, Harrist RB, Shah Y, Park SK: The femur length/head circumference relation in obstetric sonography. J Ultrasound Med 1984;3:439.
172. Sarmandal P, Grant JM: Effectiveness of ultrasound determination of fetal abdominal circumference and fetal ponderal index in the diagnosis of asymmetrical growth retardation. Br J Obstet Gynaecol 1990;97:118.
173. Hadlock FP, Deter RL, Harrist RB, et al: A data-independent predictor of intrauterine growth retardation: Femur length/abdominal circumference ratio. AJR 1983;141:979.
174. Stuart B, Drumm J, Fitzgerald DE, Diugnan NM: Fetal blood velocity wavefroms in normal pregnancy. Br J Obstet Gynaecol 1980;87:780.
175. Pourcelot L: Applications cliniques de l'examen Doppler. Ultrasonogr Doppler 1974;34:625–627.
176. Gosling RG, King DH: Ultrasound angiology. In Marcus AW, Adamson L (eds): Arteries and Veins, 2nd ed. Edinburgh, Churchill Livingstone, 1975, pp 61–98.
177. Thompson RS, Trudinger BJ, Cook CM: Doppler ultrasound waveform indices: A/B ratio, pulsatility index and Pourcelot ratio. Br J Obstet Gynaecol 1988;95:581–588.
178. Reed KL, Appleton CP, Anderson CF, et al: Doppler studies of vena cava flows in human fetuses. Circulation 1990;81: 498–505.
179. Hecher K, Campbell S, Snijders R, Nicolaides K: Reference ranges for fetal venous and atrioventricular blood flow parameters. Ultrasound Obstet Gynecol 1994;4:381–390.
180. Kanzaki T, Chiba Y: Evaluation of the preload condition of the fetus by inferior vena caval blood flow pattern. Fetal Diagn Ther 1990;5:168–174.
181. De Vore GR, Horenstein J: Ductus venosus index: A method for evaluating right ventricular preload in the second trimester fetus. Ultrasound Obstet Gynecol 1993;3:338–342.
182. Baschat AA, Güclü S, Kush ML, et al.: Venous Doppler in the prediction of acid-base status of growth-restricted fetuses with elevated placental blood flow resistance. Am J Obstet Gynecol 2004;191: 277–284.
183. Bakketeig LS, Jacobsen G, Brodtkorb CJ, et al: Randomized controlled trial of ultrasonographic screening in pregnancy, Lancet 1984;8396:207–211.
184. Saari-Kemppainen A, Karjalainen O, Ylostalo P, Heinonen OP: Ultrasound screening and perinatal mortality: Controlled trial of systematic one-stage screening in pregnancy. Lancet 1990; 336:387.
185. Ott WJ: Intrauterine growth restriction and Doppler ultrasonography. J Ultrasound Med 2000;19:661–665.
186. Strigini FA, De Luca G, Lencioni G, et al: Middle cerebral artery velocimetry: Different clinical relevance depending on umbilical velocimetry. Obstet Gynecol 1997;90:953–957.
187. Hecher K, Spernol R, Stettner H, Szalay S: Potential for diagnosing imminent risk for appropriate- and small for gestational fetuses by Doppler examination of umbilical and cerebral arterial blood flow. Ultrasound Obstet Gynecol 1995;5:247–255.
188. Severi FM, Bocchi C, Visentin A, et al: Uterine and fetal cerebral Doppler predict the outcome of third-trimester small-for-gestational age fetuses with normal umbilical artery Doppler. Ultrasound Obstet Gynecol 2002;19:225–228.
189. McGowan LM, Harding JE, Roberts AB, et al: A pilot randomized controlled trial of two regimens of fetal surveillance for small-for-gestational age fetuses with normal results of umbilical artery Doppler velocimetry. Am J Obstet Gynecol 2000;182:81–86.
190. Neilson JP, Alfirevic Z: Doppler ultrasound for fetal assessment in high risk pregnancies: Cochrane Review. In The Cochrane Library, Issue 1. Oxford, UK, Update Software, 2002.
191. Westergaard HB, Langhoff-Roos J, Lingman G, et al: A critical appraisal of the use of umbilical artery Doppler ultrasound in high-risk pregnancies: Use of meta-analyses in evidence-based obstetrics. Ultrasound Obstet Gynecol 2001;17:466–476.

192. Baschat AA, Gembruch U: The cerebroplacental Doppler ratio revisited. Ultrasound Obstet Gynecol 2003;21:124–127.
193. Ribbert LS, Snijders RJ, Nicolaides KH, Visser GH: Relationship of fetal biophysical profile and blood gas values at cordocentesis in severely growth-retarded fetuses. Am J Obstet Gynecol 1990;163:569–571.
194. Kupferminc MJ, Many A, Bar-Am A, et al: Mid-trimester severe intrauterine growth restriction is associated with a high prevalence of thrombophilia. Br J Obstet Gynaecol 2002;109: 1373–1376.
195. Doubilet PM, Benson CB, Wilkins-Haug L, Ringer S: Fetuses subsequently born premature are smaller than gestational age-matched fetuses not born premature. J Ultrasound Med 2003;22: 359–363.
196. Van den Veyver IB, Ni J, Bowles N, et al: Detection of intrauterine viral infection using the polymerase chain reaction. Mol Genet Metab 1998;63:85–95.
197. Baschat AA, Towbin J, Bowles NE, et al: Is adenovirus a fetal pathogen? Am J Obstet Gynecol 2003;189:758–763.
198. Gudmundsson S, Lindblad A, Marsal K: Cord blood gases and absence of end-diastolic blood velocities in the umbilical artery. Early Hum Dev 1990;24:231–237.
199. Yoon BH, Romero R, Roh CR, et al: Relationship between the fetal biophysical profile score, umbilical artery Doppler velocimetry, and fetal blood acid-base status determined by cordocentesis. Am J Obstet Gynecol 1993;169:1586–1594.
200. Nicolini U, Nicolaidis P, Fisk NM, et al: Limited role of fetal blood sampling in prediction of outcome in intrauterine growth retardation. Lancet 1990;336:768–772.
201. Hecher K, Snijders R, Campbell S, Nicolaides K: Fetal venous, intracardiac, and arterial blood flow measurements in intrauterine growth retardation: Relationship with fetal blood gases. Am J Obstet Gynecol 1995;173:10–15.
202. Rizzo G, Capponi A, Arduini D, Romanini C: The value of fetal arterial, cardiac and venous flows in predicting pH and blood gases measured in umbilical blood at cordocentesis in growth retarded fetuses. Br J Obstet Gynaecol 1995;102:963–969.
203. Baschat AA, Gembruch U, Weiner CP, Harman CR: Qualitative venous Doppler waveform analysis improves prediction of critical perinatal outcomes in premature growth-restricted fetuses. Ultrasound Obstet Gynecol 2003;22:240–245.
204. Ley D, Tideman E, Laurin J, et al: Abnormal fetal aortic velocity waveform and intellectual function at 7 years of age. Ultrasound Obstet Gynecol 1996;8:160–165.
205. Skrablin S, Kalafatic D, Banovic I, et al: Antenatal predictors of the neurologic sequelae at 3 years of age: A multivariate analysis. Eur J Obstet Gynecol Reprod Biol 2000;93:173–180.
206. Schreuder AM, McDonnell M, Gaffney G, et al: Outcome at school age following antenatal detection of absent or reversed end diastolic flow velocity in the umbilical artery. Arch Dis Child Fetal Neonatal Ed 2002;86:F108–F114.
207. Scherjon S, Briet J, Oosting H, Kok J: The discrepancy between maturation of visual-evoked potentials and cognitive outcome at five years in very preterm infants with and without hemodynamic signs of fetal brain-sparing. Pediatrics 2000;105:385–391.
208. Manning FA: Fetal biophysical profile: A critical appraisal. Clin Obstet Gynecol 2002;45:975–985.
209. Morrison I, Menticoglou S, Manning FA, et al: Comparison of antepartum test results to perinatal outcome. J Matern Fetal Med 1994;3:75–83.
210. Arabin B, Becker R, Mohnhaupt A, et al: Prediction of fetal distress and poor outcome in intrauterine growth retardation: A comparison of fetal heart rate monitoring combined with stress tests and Doppler ultrasound. Fetal Diagn Ther 1993;8: 234–240.
211. Ott WJ, Mora G, Arias F, et al: Comparison of the modified biophysical profile to a 'new' biophysical profile incorporating the middle cerebral artery to umbilical artery velocity flow systolic/diastolic ratio. Am J Obstet Gynecol 1998;178: 1346–1353.
212. Weiner Z, Farmakides G, Schulman H, et al: Surveillance of growth-retarded fetuses with computerized fetal heart rate monitoring combined with Doppler velocimetry of the umbilical and uterine arteries. J Reprod Med 1996;41:112–118.
213. Arabin B, Snijders R, Mohnhaupt A, et al: Evaluation of the fetal assessment score in pregnancies at risk for intrauterine hypoxia. Am J Obstet Gynecol 1993;169:549–554.
214. Baschat AA, Gembruch U, Weiner CP, Harman CR: Combining Doppler and biophysical assessment improves prediction of critical perinatal outcomes. Am J Obstet Gynecol 2002;187:S147.
215. Bahado-Singh RO, Kovanci E, Jeffres A, et al: The Doppler cerebroplacental ratio and perinatal outcome in intrauterine growth restriction. Am J Obstet Gynecol 1999;180:750–756.
216. Weiner CP, Grose CF, Naides SJ: Diagnosis of fetal infection in a patient with an abnormal ultrasound examination and without a positive clinical history. Am J Obstet Gynecol 1993;168:6–11.
217. Nicolaides KH, Snijders RJ, Thorpe-Beeston JG, et al: Mean red cell volume in normal, anemic, small, trisomic and triploid fetuses. Fetal Ther 1990;4:1–13.
218. Sipes SL, Weiner CP, Wenstrom KD, et al: The association between fetal karyotype and mean corpuscular volume. Obstet Gynecol 1991;165:1371–1376.
219. Thilaganathan B, Nicolaides KH: Erythroblastosis in birth asphyxia. Ultrasound Obstet Gynecol 1992;2:15–17.
220. Baschat AA, Gembruch U, Reiss I, et al: Neonatal nucleated red blood cell count and postpartum complications in growth restricted fetuses. J Perinat Med 2003;31:323–329.
221. Weiner CP, Wenstrom KD, Sipes SL, Williamson RA: Risk factors for cordocentesis and intravascular transfusion. Am J Obstet Gynecol 1991;165:1020–1023.
222. GRIT Study Group: A randomized trial of timed delivery for the compromised pre-term fetus: Short term outcomes and Bayesian interpretation. Br J Obstet Gynaecol 2003;110:27–32.
223. Trudinger BJ, Cook CM, Thompson RS, et al: Low-dose aspirin therapy improves fetal weight in umbilical placental insufficiency. Am J Obstet Gynecol 1988;159:681–685.
224. Newnham JP, Godfrey M, Walters BJ, et al: Low dose aspirin for the treatment of fetal growth restriction: A randomized controlled trial. Aust N Z J Obstet Gynaecol 1995;35:370–374.
225. CLASP: A randomised trial of low-dose aspirin for the prevention and treatment of pre-eclampsia among 9364 pregnant women: CLASP (Collaborative Low-dose Aspirin Study in Pregnancy) Collaborative Group. Lancet 1994;343:619–629.
226. Kozer E, Nikfar S, Costei A, et al: Aspirin consumption during the first trimester of pregnancy and congenital anomalies: A meta-analysis. Am J Obstet Gynecol 2002;187:1623–1630.
227. Nicolaides KH, Campbell S, Bradley RJ, et al: Maternal oxygen therapy for intrauterine growth retardation. Lancet 1987; 8539:942–945.
228. Battaglia C, Artini PG, D'Ambrogio G, et al: Maternal hyperoxygenation in the treatment of intrauterine growth retardation. Am J Obstet Gynecol 1992;167:430–435.
229. Karsdorp VH, van Vugt JM, Dekker GA, van Geijn HP: Reappearance of end-diastolic velocities in the umbilical artery following maternal volume expansion: A preliminary study. Obstet Gynecol 1992;80:679–683.
230. Ronzoni S, Marconi AM, Paolini CL, et al: The effect of a maternal infusion of amino acids on umbilical uptake in pregnancies complicated by intrauterine growth restriction. Am J Obstet Gynecol 2002;187:741–746.
231. Ley D, Wide-Swensson D, Lindroth M, et al: Respiratory distress syndrome in infants with impaired intrauterine growth. Acta Paediatr 1997;86:1090–1096.
232. Soothill PW, Ajayi RA, Campbell S, et al: Fetal oxygenation at cordocentesis, maternal smoking and childhood neuro-development. Eur J Obstet Gynecol Reprod Biol 1995;59:21–24.

233. Leitner Y, Fattal-Valevski A, Geva R, et al: Six-year follow-up of children with intrauterine growth retardation: Long-term, prospective study. J Child Neurol 2000;15:781–786.
234. Divon MY, Girz BA, Lieblich R, Langer O: Clinical management of the fetus with markedly diminished umbilical artery end-diastolic flow. Am J Obstet Gynecol 1989;161:1523–1527.
235. Boyd ME, Usher RH, McLean FH: Fetal macrosomia: Prediction, risks, proposed management. Obstet Gynecol 1983;61:715–722.
236. Spellacy WN, Miller S, Winegar A, Peterson PQ: Macrosomia-maternal characteristics and infant complications. Obstet Gynecol 1985;66:158–161.
237. Menticoglou SM, Manning FA, Morrison I, Harman CR: Must macrosomic fetuses be delivered by a cesarean section? A review of outcome for 786 babies > = 4,500 g. Aust N Z J Obstet Gynaecol 1992;32:100–103.
238. Lipscomb KR, Gregory K, Shaw K: The outcome of macrosomic infants weighing at least 4500 grams: Los Angeles county + University of Southern California experience. Obstet Gynecol 1995;85:558–564.
239. Ventura SJ, Mosher WD, Curtin SC, et al: Trends in pregnancies and pregnancy rates by outcome: Estimates for the United States, 1976–96. Vital Health Stat 2000;21:1–47.
240. Babinszki A, Kerenyi T, Torok O, et al: Perinatal outcome in grand and great-grand multiparity: Effects of parity on obstetric risk factors. Am J Obstet Gynecol 1999;181:669–674.
241. Dooley SL, Metzger BE, Cho NH: Gestational diabetes mellitus: Influence of race on disease prevalence and perinatal outcome in a U.S. population. Diabetes 1991;40:25–29.
242. Okun N, Verma A, Mitchell BF, Flowerdew G: Relative importance of maternal constitutional factors and glucose intolerance of pregnancy in the development of newborn macrosomia. J Matern Fetal Med 1997;6:285–290.
243. Cogswell ME, Serdula MK, Hungerford DW, Yip R: Gestational weight gain among average-weight and overweight women: What is excessive? Am J Obstet Gynecol 1995;172:705–712.
244. Ogunyemi D, Hullett S, Leeper J, Risk A: Prepregnancy body mass index, weight gain during pregnancy, and perinatal outcome in a rural black population. J Matern Fetal Med 1998;7:190–193.
245. Lazer S, Biale Y, Mazor M, et al: Complications associated with the macrosomic fetus. J Reprod Med 1986;31:501–505.
246. Klebanoff MA, Mills JL, Berendes HW: Mother's birth weight as a predictor of macrosomia. Am J Obstet Gynecol 1985;153: 253–257.
247. Nasrat H, Abalkhail B, Fageeh W, et al: Anthropometric measurements of newborns of gestational diabetic mothers: Does it indicate disproportionate fetal growth? J Matern Fetal Med 1997;6:291–295.
248. McFarland MB, Trylovich CG, Langer O: Anthropometric differences in macrosomic infants of diabetic and nondiabetic mothers. J Matern Fetal Med 1998;7:292–295.
249. Wollschlaeger K, Nieder J, Koppe II, Hartlein K: A study of fetal macrosomia. Arch Gynecol Obstet 1999;263:51–55.
250. Ferber A: Maternal complications of fetal macrosomia. Clin Obstet Gynecol 2000;43:335–339.
251. Boulet SL, Alexander GR, Salihu HM, Pass M: Macrosomic births in the United States: Determinants, outcomes, and proposed grades of risk. Am J Obstet Gynecol 2003;188:1372–1378.
252. Perlow JH, Wigton T, Hart J, et al: Birth trauma: A five-year review of incidence and associated perinatal factors. J Reprod Med 1996;41:754–760.
253. Acker DB, Gregory KD, Sachs BP, Friedman EA: Risk factors for Erb-Duchenne palsy. Obstet Gynecol 1988;71:389–392.
254. Ecker JL, Greenberg JA, Norwitz ER, et al: Birth weight as a predictor of brachial plexus injury. Obstet Gynecol 1997;89:643–647.
255. Chez RA, Carlan S, Greenberg SL, Spellacy WN: Fractured clavicle is an unavoidable event. Am J Obstet Gynecol 1994;171: 797–798.
256. Gherman RB, Goodwin TM, Ouzounian JG, et al: Brachial plexus palsy associated with cesarean section: An in utero injury? Am J Obstet Gynecol 1997;177:1162–1164.
257. Bérard J, Dufour P, Vinatier D, et al: Fetal macrosomia: Risk factors and outcome. A study of the outcome concerning 100 cases >4500 g. Eur J Obstet Gynecol Reprod Biol 1998;77:51–59.
258. Stones RW, Paterson CM, Saunders NJ: Risk factors for major obstetric haemorrhage. Eur J Obstet Gynecol Reprod Biol 1993;48:15–18.
259. el Madany AA, Jallad KB, Radi FA, et al: Shoulder dystocia: Anticipation and outcome. Int J Gynaecol Obstet 1990;34: 7–12.
260. Baschat AA, Harman CR, Farid G, et al: Very low second trimester maternal serum alphafetoprotein: Association with high birth weight. Obstet Gynecol 2002;99:531–536.
261. Wikstrom I, Bergstrom R, Bakketeig L, et al: Prediction of high birth weight from maternal characteristics, symphysis fundal height and ultrasound biometry. Gynecol Obstet Invest 1993; 35:27–33.
262. Neilson JP: Symphysis-fundal height measurement in pregnancy. Cochrane Database Syst Rev 2000;2:CD000944.
263. Gonen R, Spiegel D, Abend M: Is macrosomia predictable, and are shoulder dystocia and birth trauma preventable? Obstet Gynecol 1996;88:526–529.
264. Chauhan SP, Hendrix NW, Magann EF, et al: Limitations of clinical and sonographic estimates of birth weight: Experience with 1034 parturients. Obstet Gynecol 1998;91:72–77.
265. Chauhan SP, Sullivan CA, Lutton TD, et al: Parous patients' estimate of birth weight in postterm pregnancy. J Perinatol 1995;15:192–194.
266. Sherman DJ, Arieli S, Tovbin J, et al: A comparison of clinical and ultrasonic estimation of fetal weight. Obstet Gynecol 1998;91:212–217.
267. Chauhan SP, Cowan BD, Magann EF, et al: Intrapartum detection of a macrosomic fetus: Clinical versus 8 sonographic models. Aust N Z J Obstet Gynaecol 1995;35:3:266–270.
268. Benacerraf BR, Gelman R, Frigoletto FD Jr: Sonographically estimated fetal weights: Accuracy and limitation. Am J Obstet Gynecol 1988;159:1118–1121.
269. Smith GC, Smith MF, McNay MB, Fleming JE: The relation between fetal abdominal circumference and birth weight: Findings in 3512 pregnancies. Br J Obstet Gynaecol 1997;104: 186–190.
270. O'Reilly-Green CP, Divon MY: Receiver operating characteristic curves of sonographic estimated fetal weight for prediction of macrosomia in prolonged pregnancies. Ultrasound Obstet Gynecol 1997;9:403–408.
271. Alsulyman OM, Ouzounian JG, Kjos SL: The accuracy of intrapartum ultrasonographic fetal weight estimation in diabetic pregnancies. Am J Obstet Gynecol 1997;177:503–506.
272. Rigano S, Ferrazzi E, Radaelli T, et al: Sonographic measurements of subcutaneous fetal fat in pregnancies complicated by gestational diabetes and in normal pregnancies. Croat Med J 2000;41:240–244.
273. Combs CA, Jaekle RK, Rosenn B, et al: Sonographic estimation of fetal weight based on a model of fetal volume. Obstet Gynecol 1993;82:365–370.
274. Gonen O, Rosen DJ, Dolfin Z, et al: Induction of labor versus expectant management in macrosomia: A randomized study. Obstet Gynecol 1997;89:913–917.
275. Sanchez-Ramos L, Bernstein S, Kaunitz AM: expectant management versus labor induction for suspected fetal macrosomia: A systematic review. Obstet Gynecol 2002; 100: 997–1002.
276. Rouse DJ, Owen J, Goldenberg RL, Cliver SP: The effectiveness and costs of elective cesarean delivery for fetal macrosomia diagnosed by ultrasound. JAMA 1996;276:1480–1486.
277. Flamm BL, Goings JR: Vaginal birth after cesarean section: Is suspected fetal macrosomia a contraindication? Obstet Gynecol 1989;74:694–697.

278. Shepard MJ, Richards VA, Berkowitz RL, et al: An evaluation of two equations predicting fetal weight by ultrasound. Am J Obstet Gynecol 1982;142:47–54.

278. Hadlock FP, Harrist RB, Carpenter RJ, et al: Sonographic estimation of fetal weight: The value of femur length in addition to head and abdomen measurements. Radiology 1984;150:535–540.

280. Weiner CP, Sabbagha RE, Vaisrub N, Socol ML: Ultrasonic fetal weight prediction: Role of head circumference and femur length. Obstet Gynecol 1985;65:812–817.

CHAPTER 13

Hydramnios and Oligohydramnios

Myles J. O. Taylor / Nicholas M. Fisk

INTRODUCTION

Amniotic fluid (AF) provides the fetus a protective low resistance environment suitable for growth and development. Essentially, AF volume is the sum of the inflow and outflow of fluid into the amniotic space, and as such reflects fetal fluid balance. In addition, the constitution of AF also reflects maternal hydration because fluid shifts freely across the placenta, predominantly in response to osmotic gradients. The clinical assessment of AF volume, including bimanual palpation and symphyseal-fundal height measurements, is unreliable, although any utility is greater for hydramnios than for oligohydramnios. AF volume derangement is usually severe when hydramnios or oligohydramnios is suspected clinically. Direct quantification of AF by dye dilution is described but rarely used because it requires two amniocenteses with attendant risks and relies on the dubious assumption that complete mixing of the injected dye indicator occurs within a 15- to 30-minute interval.[1,2] On the other hand, ultrasonic estimates of amniotic volume correlate directly with the measured volume change at both amnioreduction and amnioinfusion procedures.[3–5]

Accordingly, definitions of increased and decreased AF volume are based on sonographic criteria. The prevalence of hydramnios and oligohydramnios varies with the diagnostic criteria used, fetal number, and whether a referral or hospital-based population is studied. Semiquantitative methods include estimates of the deepest vertical pool (DP) and the amniotic fluid index (AFI). AFI, which summates the DP in each of four quadrants and is a more sensitive estimate of AF volume throughout gestation,[6,7] is preferred by many to the DP, because DP does not allow for an asymmetrical fetal position within the uterus and because the regression curve between AFI and gestational age is similar in shape to that between AF volume and gestational age.[8] On the other hand, a recent prospective survey concluded that the single DP was more reliable than either AFI or two diameter pocket measurements of AF because it is least likely to lead to a false-positive diagnosis of either oligohydramnios or hydramnios.[9] Reference ranges for AFI and DP throughout gestation are available (Fig. 13–1).[7,9,10] The AFI is always less than that determined using gray-scale ultrasonography alone when color Doppler is employed to facilitate identification of the umbilical cord.[11] However, every method is influenced by transducer pressure, which may explain reported difficulties with reproducibility.[12] New methods for AF volume estimation such as three-dimensional (3D) ultrasound or magnetic resonance imaging may circumvent this problem.[13]

In multiple pregnancies, the assessment of AF volume should probably include an overall assessment of the AFI along with a DP measurement for each fetus. Attempts to measure AFI for each individual fetus are not feasible, particularly in monochorionic pregnancies in which the intertwin membrane is so thin as to hinder exact separate delineation and do not provide any additional information to the recommended technique.

HYDRAMNIOS

Definition

Hydramnios is variably defined as a DP of 8 cm or greater or an AFI above the 95th percentile for gestational age[7] (see Fig. 13–1). In older studies, hydramnios was reported to complicate 3.5%[14,15] of pregnancies, but a more recent study of a population undergoing routine anomaly scanning found the incidence to be much lower—0.2%.[16]

Etiology

Common causes of hydramnios are shown in Table 13–1. Hydramnios may be mild (DP 8 to 12 cm), moderate (12 to 15 cm), or severe (>15 cm). Severe hydramnios occurs in only 5% of cases.[15] Although impairment of fetal swallowing is implicated in anencephaly, only 65% develop hydramnios. Although this

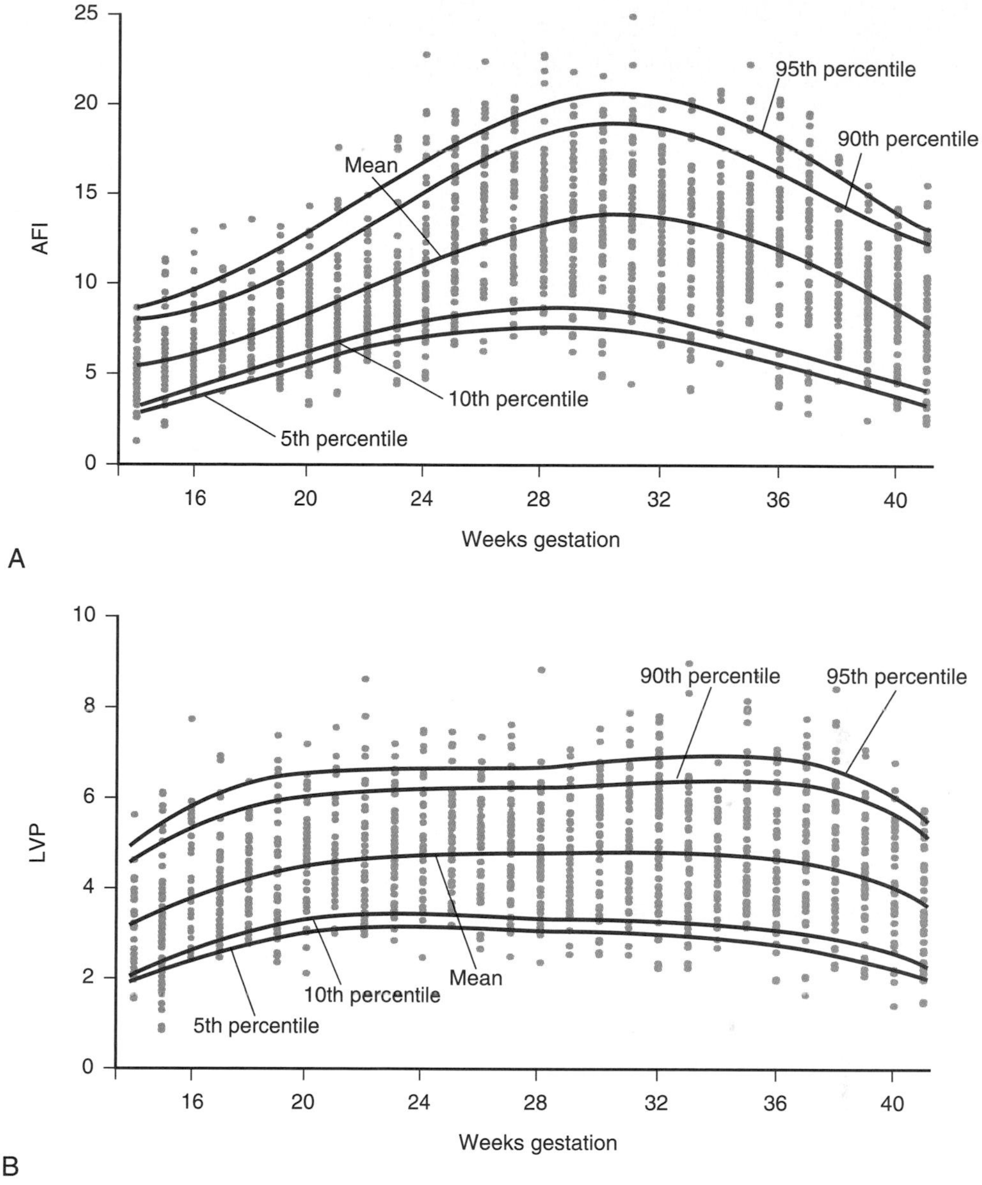

FIGURE 13–1
Normal range for amniotic fluid index, AFI (*A*), and single deepest pocket (lowest vertical pool, LVP) (*B*) from 14 to 41 weeks' gestation. (From Magann EF, Sanderson M, Martin JN, Chauhan S: The amniotic fluid index, single deepest pocket, and two-diameter pocket in normal human pregnancy. Am J Obstet Gynecol 2000;182(6):1581–1588.)[9]

association may reflect variation in the amount of brain tissue present, alternative mechanisms include fluid transudation across the meninges or vasopressin deficiency resulting in fetal polyuria.[17] The incidence of hydramnios secondary to maternal diabetes has declined from 26% to 22% in older series[1] to 13% to 5%[15] presumably as a result of tighter glucose control. Although fetal polyuria secondary to osmotic diuresis might seem an obvious mechanism in diabetes mellitus, Van Otterlo and associates[18] found normal fetal urine production rates in most diabetic pregnancies with mild hydramnios. However, Yasui and associates[19] observed increased fetal urine output during maternal fasting. On the other hand, fetal polyuria is clearly documented in recipient fetuses of twin-twin transfusion syndrome (TTTS) in association with increased atrial naturetic peptide levels.[20–23] These measurements are supported by histologic demonstration of enlarged glomeruli and dilated distal convoluted tubules.[17,22] Increased cardiac output may underlie hydramnos in TTTS and in some cases of hydrops and Rh alloimunization, although investigations in gravid sheep suggest this may be an oversimplification.[24] For example, an infusion of angiotensin I into fetal sheep with functional kidneys leads to hydramnios,[25] although the mechanism is poorly understood. Hydramnios in nonhydropic red blood cell (RBC) alloimmunization may in part be explained by a hypoxia-induced hyperlactinemia[26] as animal data reveal powerful osmotic effects as an elevated fetal plasma lactate draws fluid from the maternal into the fetal compartment.[24]

Rarer causes of hydramnios include substance abuse, in which the incidence of hydramnios is several times higher than in control subjects,[27] and maternal lithium

TABLE 13–1

Common Causes or Associations with Hydramnios

Maternal
Diabetes mellitus
Substance abuse
Lithium therapy
Fetal
Obstruction of fluid transit through the gastrointestinal tract
Intestinal atresias (commonly duodenal)
Esophageal compression secondary to thoracic or mediastinal masses (including diaphragmatic hernia)
Neurologic impairment of swallowing
Central nervous system lesions (e.g., anencephaly)
Chromosomal abnormalities (e.g., trisomy 18)
Muscular dystrophies
Fetal polyuria
Twin-twin transfusion syndrome
Bartter syndrome
High-output cardiac failure
Fetal anemia
Sacrococcygeal teratoma
Chorioangioma
Congenital infection (e.g., syphilis, viral hepatitis)

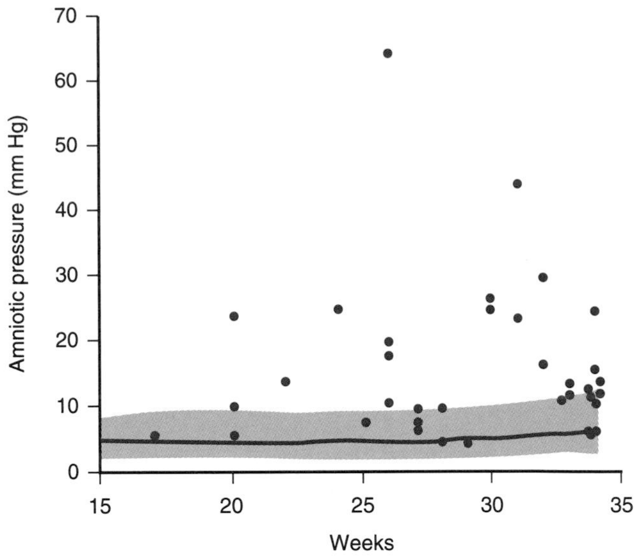

FIGURE 13–2
Amniotic fluid pressure in 36 pregnancies complicated by hydramnios shown against the normal pregnancy reference range with continuous line representing the mean and the upper and lower limits of the shaded area, the reference range. (From Fisk NM, Tannirandorn Y, Nicolini U, et al: Amniotic pressure in disorders of amniotic fluid volume. Obstet Gynecol 1990;76(2):210–214.)[55]

therapy.[28,29] Bartter syndrome, an autosomal recessive condition characterized by hypokalemic alkalosis and hypercalciuria, may also present with hydramnios.[30] Matsushita and associates[31] conducted biochemical tests of both the amniotic fluid and maternal urine for antenatal diagnosis and concluded that the latter parameters may allow prediction of fetal Bartter syndrome. Amniotic fluid electrolytes, except for potassium, are high in a fetus with Bartter syndrome. Urinary chloride, sodium, and calcium are very low.

The incidence of idiopathic hydramnios is related to severity, with a cause identified in 75% to 91% when the DP is greater than 12 cm, compared to 17% to 29% with a DP of 8 to 12 cm.[15,32] If the sonographic evaluation is normal, the risk of a major anomaly approximates 1% with mild hydramnios, 2% with moderate hydramnios, and 11% with severe hydramnios.[33] The term "acute hydramnios" refers to a sudden accumulation of amniotic fluid associated with maternal symptoms. Acute hydramnios is almost exclusively a manifestation of TTTS before 26 weeks' gestation when there is a rapid accumulation in the sac of the recipient.[1,34]

Maternal Risks

Maternal complications are mostly attributed to uterine distention[35,36] and include abdominal discomfort, uterine irritability, postpartum hemorrhage, and compromised respiratory function. Intra-amniotic pressure is markedly elevated in most women with severe hydramnios (Fig. 13–2).[37,38] The incidence of cesarean section is also increased as a result of unstable lie and placental abruption, which may occur with the rapid decrease in intrauterine pressure that accompanies membrane rupture.[39,40] The higher incidence of preeclampsia may be a manifestation of the "mirror syndrome" in association with fetal hydrops.[41] Ureteric obstruction occurs very rarely with gross uterine distention.[42,43]

Fetal Risks

Increased perinatal mortality rates (<5% in recent series[33,44]) associated with hydramnios are largely due to the presence of congenital malformations, preterm premature rupture of membranes, or preterm labor and delivery. Although the high incidence of fetal anomalies and multiple pregnancies makes the exact risk for spontaneous preterm labor difficult to determine, a 22% rate was reported after excluding malformations.[15] Hypoxic events secondary to cord prolapse, placental abruption and uteroplacental dysfunction also contribute to the high perinatal rates. Loss rates are lower when fetuses with structural defects are excluded,[1,15] but these associations do not entirely account for the high perinatal mortality rate. Six to14% of perinatal deaths occur antepartum in normally formed singletons.[1,15,45] One explanation may be an increased risk of hypoxemia and acidemia and raised intra-amniotic pressure observed in fetuses with hydramnios.[38] Based on the increased pressure, it is suggested uteroplacental perfusion can be impaired by extreme hydramnios. This hypothesis is supported by the observation that uterine blood flow increases substantially after amnioreduction in pregnancies complicated by severe hydramnios.[46–48] Further, multivariate analysis suggests hydramnios is an independent risk factor for intrapartum fetal death.[49]

Diagnosis

Objectives include an assessment of the following:

- Fetal number and chorionicity
- Degree of hydramnios
- Underlying etiology
- Presence of associated anomalies
- Karyotype
- Presence of viral infection

A recommended diagnostic approach is outlined in Table 13–2. Kirshon[50] observed that hourly fetal urine production rates (HFUPR) calculated by ultrasonic change in bladder dimensions over 20-min intervals[51] distinguished hydramnios secondary to fetal polyuria from that secondary to other causes. Unfortunately, the technique used may underestimate fetal urine production by more than 50%.[52] In multiple pregnancies, hydramnios can occur in dichorionic pregnancies as a consequence of any of the listed causes in singleton pregnancy, or alternatively, in monochorionic placentas secondary to TTTS or twin reversed arterial perfusion (TRAP) sequence. The bladder of recipient fetuses in TTTS remains chronically full, with its size at the upper limit of normal. Thus, there is little rationale in calculating HFUPR. In view of the up to 3%[53] association with chromosomal abnormalities, karyotyping was recommended in the past. However, more recent series generated when routine anomaly scanning was available suggest a much lower risk of aneuploidy (<1%)[33,44] if the fetus is sonographically normal.

Maternal diabetes mellitus should be excluded by carbohydrate tolerance testing, and alloimmunization excluded by maternal serologic testing. When fetal hydrops is present but unassociated with a structural malformation, fetal viral infection or anemia should be suspected (see Chapter 27).

TABLE 13–2

Diagnostic Evaluation of Hydramnios

History taking with emphasis on maternal symptoms, diabetes mellitus, red blood cell alloimmunization, maternal drug ingestion
High-resolution ultrasound to assess:
The degree of hydramnios (amniotic fluid index)
Presence of multiple gestation, growth deficiency, or macrosomia
Fetal thorax
Fetal central nervous system (midline structures, neural tube, tone)
Fetal gastrointestinal system (mouth, stomach, small bowel, abdominal wall)
Fetal bladder dynamics
Middle cerebral artery peak systolic velocity for suspected fetal anemia
Chorionicity in multiple pregnancy
Fetal specimens for karyotyping and viral infection

Management Options

General

The therapeutic aim is to relieve maternal symptoms and prolong gestation. Mild asymptomatic hydramnios is managed expectantly. There are no data to support dietary restriction of salts and fluids. Similarly, diuretics administered to the mother seem ineffective and may in fact reduce uteroplacental perfusion.[54]

Treatment is usually warranted only in moderate to severe hydramnios during the mid or early third trimester. The criteria for intervention include either excessive maternal symptoms or an AFI above 40 cm or DP over 12 cm (moderate hydramnios), above which thresholds intra-amniotic pressure may increase.[55] Although treatment should ideally be directed at the underlying etiology, this is possible only in a limited number of instances such as the correction of fetal anemia by transfusion, relief of obstructed cardiac return by drainage of pleural effusions, and more recently laser ablation of placental anastomoses in advanced stage TTTS.

Prostaglandin Synthase Inhibitors

INDOMETHACIN

Cifuentes and associates[56] first noted decreased urinary production rates in neonates receiving indomethacin for closure of the ductus arteriosus. Subsequently, maternally administered indomethacin was shown to reduce fetal urine production[57] and amniotic fluid volume.[58–60] The E class of prostaglandins antagonize the antidiuretic effect of arginine vasopressin on the collecting tubule of the kidney,[61] and prostaglandin inhibition enhances proximal tubular resorption of water and sodium.[62] Indomethacin is believed to decrease urine output by either or both of these mechanisms. Although decreased renal blood flow is postulated as a cause for the decreased urine production, Doppler flow studies do not reveal changes in the renal artery resistance indices during indomethacin therapy.[63] The dose of indomethacin varies between 50 and 200 mg/day, depending on the AF volume response assessed ultrasonically. The time interval between commencing treatment and achieving normal AF volume ranges from 4 to 20 days.[64,65] Amnioreduction prior to initiating indomethacin[66] may be beneficial by avoiding the delayed pharmacologic response should the maternal symptoms be severe, or there is concern for preterm delivery. AF volume is monitored to ensure that oligohydramnios does not ensue.

Most authors report that they discontinue treatment by 32 to 35 weeks because of reports of neonatal morbidity resulting from indomethacin use in late gestation.[58,60] Although the initial clinical experience was promising, there are concerns about the risks of:

- Premature closure of the ductus[66]
- Cerebral vasoconstriction in the fetus[67]
- Impaired renal function[68]

The need for caution in pregnancies less than 32 weeks is highlighted by a retrospective cohort study revealing an increased incidence of necrotizing enterocolitis (29% vs. 8%), intracranial hemorrhage (28% vs. 9%), and patent ductus arteriosus (62% vs. 44%) in infants treated with indomethacin in utero[69] compared to control infants. However, the conclusions of more recent studies suggest that neonatal complications after in utero exposure to indomethacin are inconsistent. Indeed, Abbassi and associates[70] and Panter and associates[71] observed no increased risk. Fetal echocardiography is recommended by some within 24 hours of starting treatment and weekly thereafter despite the fact the incidence of ductal constriction depends on gestation (approximately 5% before 27 weeks and increasing to nearly 50% by 32 weeks[72]). The indomethacin is discontinued if there is evidence of ductal constriction.[73] However, there is no definitive proof of an association between indomethacin and neonatal persistent fetal circulation and pulmonary hypertension.[74] Nor is there any evidence to suggest such monitoring is cost effective. Vermillion and associates reported that constriction of the fetal ductus arteriosus during indomethacin tocolysis may occur at any gestational age.[75] However, their study showed that ductal constriction was reversible with early identification and timely discontinuation of therapy; thus, they advised caution in its use over 31 weeks' gestation. Raised serum creatinine with or without renal failure has been described in neonates of women who received indomethacin antenatally but is usually a transient phenomenon. Treatment is also discontinued if oligohydramnios develops. Indomethacin is no longer used long term as renal failure and irreversible renal damage are observed in neonates with prolonged exposure to indomethacin in utero.[76] Its use is also contraindicated in TTTS because of the adverse effects on the oliguric donor twin.

The true safety of antenatally administered indomethacin requires a prospective randomized controlled trial. Until one is performed, the evidence indicates long-term indomethacin use should be avoided, but that cautious short-term use of indomethacin before 32 weeks of gestation will add minimal risks for neonatal complication.

SULINDAC

Sulindac is an alternative prostaglandin synthase inhibitor with similar structure to indomethacin. It appears to have a lesser effect on fetal urine output and the ductus arteriosus[77] and thus may be a safer alternative to indomethacin. Although the active form of sulindac (the sulfide metabolite) does cross the placenta,[78] fetal levels are half the maternal levels. This relationship contrasts with the inactive forms of sulindac, for which the fetal and maternal levels are similar. At a recommended dose of 200 mg every 12 hours, sulindac can reduce AF volume without evidence of ductal constriction during prolonged therapy in the second and early third trimester.[79] Any mild effect on the fetal ductus is transient,[80] which is advantageous in the longer term management of hydramnios or threatened preterm labor.

The finding that sulindac may have fewer fetal side effects than indomethacin is perhaps explained by its greater selectivity against cyclooxygenase enzyme 2 (COX-2) than COX-1 (16-fold more selective). In contrast, indomethacin is an equipotent inhibitor of COX-1 and COX-2. This prompted some authors to suggest that a highly selective COX-2 inhibitor such as nimesulide, which is 25-fold more COX-2 selective than indomethacin, may be safer yet. Unfortunately, this supposition was not substantiated, at least after short-term exposure, in a recent randomized controlled trial in which nimesulide had a similar fetal side effect profile to indomethacin and sulindac.[81] These results suggest that the use of newer COX-2 specific drugs, developed for the treatment of preterm labor, are unlikely to be advantageous as they too will be limited by their fetal oliguric side effects.

Therapeutic Amniocentesis (Amnioreduction)

Amnioreduction describes transabdominal aspiration of amniotic fluid under ultrasound control. Several studies suggest it prolongs gestation in both singleton and multiple pregnancies[1,82,83] and improves perinatal survival.[83–88] The risks of the procedure include preterm premature rupture of the membranes, chorioamnionitis, placental abruption, membranous detachment, which follows multiple procedures and which appears to precede membrane rupture by several weeks, and perforation of the amnion separating monochorionic twins.

PROCEDURE

AMNIOREDUCTION

Preprocedure

Counsel the mother about the 0.3% procedure-related fetal loss rate, although preterm labor and amniorrhexis risk is considerable if already complicated by contractions and cervical dilatation.

Procedure

Choose a skin entry site and track to target on scan to (i) avoid placenta, (ii) avoid lateral entry through thick myometrium, which may induce painful contractions during the procedure, and (iii) allow for a reduction in uterine volume and thus fundal height. The ideal entry is through midanterior uterine wall with needle pointing slightly cephalad, moving slightly caudal as uterine volume diminishes.

Infiltrate local anesthetic (i.e., 5–10 mL 1% lidocaine) into superficial maternal tissues. Some authors recommend prophylactic antibiotic (i.e., cefuroxime 750 mg IV), though there is no evidence of efficacy.

Use a larger wide-bore needle (18–20 gauge) with sterile technique. The methods are described in Chapter 10.

Confirm intra-amniotic location free of membrane tenting by aspiration of aliquot of amniotic fluid. Collect diagnostic samples.

Attach a three-way tap via wide-bore tubing to needle hub, and commence aspiration using two 50-mL syringes serially.

If the mother has difficulty tolerating the procedure owing to problematic contractions, reposition the mother on her side, let go of cannula, and wait until the contractions have passed.

Confirm correct intra-amniotic positioning, either by continuous or frequent intermittent ultrasound. If flow stops, desist aspiration, check location, and consider readjusting needle position, especially in twins, in which the flow may be occluded by septum.

Continue drainage until the DP is 5 to 8 cm (or AFI 10–20 cm).

Postprocedure

Check umbilical artery Doppler; demonstrate to parents.

Administer anti-D antibodies IM to RhD-negative women.

After 26 weeks, consider CTG, especially if the procedure was complicated or the fetus compromised.

Amniodrainage may need to be repeated, even serially. In our own unit, a repeat procedure is indicated if the AFI rises above 40 to 45 cm, or the DP is over 12 cm, above which the level AF pressure, and hence the risk of preterm labor and amniorrhexis, is known to exceed the reference range.[55] Instead of using syringes to aspirate AF at amniodrainage, Jauniaux and associates[89,90] suggested using a suction bottle system, which, by enabling as much AF to be removed as possible, reduced the total number of amnioreductions required from a mean of 5.6 to 1.5 procedures in a series of 30 TTTS patients. After 37 weeks, the risks of amniodrainage, particularly of abruption, outweigh the benefits of prolongation of pregnancy and are thus rarely performed.

The perinatal mortality rate with untreated TTTS complicated by hydramnios presenting prior to 28 weeks approaches 80%.[91] A recent meta-analysis of those presenting before 28 weeks and treated by serial amniodrainage showed an overall survival rate in the region of 60% (see Chapter 24). Amniotic fluid reaccumulation in the sac of the oligohyramniotic donor is reported. One explanation offered for this change is that the relief of raised intra-amniotic pressure in the hydramniotic recipient twin improves the circulation to the "stuck" donor twin, thus restoring its renal function.[84] However, there is no evidence to support this theory, which seems to violate known laws of fluid mechanics. A more likely explanation is leakage of fluid into the sac of the "stuck" twin through needle puncture. Intentional amniotic septostomy (creating a hole in the septa between the sacs of the donor and recipient twin) was associated with an 83% survival rate in one small series.[92] It leads to equilibration of AF volume between the two sacs and although the mechanism appears uncertain, it could improve hemodynamics in the donor twin through restitution of swallowing. In a recent randomized controlled trial comparing amniodrainage versus septostomy in the treatment of TTTS, the perinatal survival rate (65%) was no different between therapies. However, septostomy reduced the requirement for repeat procedure due to recurrent polyhydramnios from 70% to 40%.[93]

Septostomy, laser and occlusive fetocide for polyhydramnios in complicated monochorionic twins are dealt with in Chapter 24.

SUMMARY OF MANAGEMENT OPTIONS
Hydramnios

Management Options	Quality of Evidence	Strength of Recommendation	References
Identify Cause (if possible)			
Take detailed history, especially maternal diabetes, maternal lithium therapy, family history of myotonic dystrophy or past history of skeletal dysplasia/arthrogryposis, red blood cell alloimmunization, and diabetes insipidus. Arrange blood sugar series/glucose tolerance test.	–	GPP	–
Determine severity: Polyhydramnios defined as AFI >25 cm or DVP >8 cm. Mild: AFI 25–35 cm, DVP 8–10 cm; moderate: AFI 35–45 cm, DVP 10–12 cm; severe: AFI >45, DVP >12 cm.	III	B	55
Make detailed assessment of the fetal anatomy to determine cause. Chance of fetal abnormality or genetic condition is related to severity, with 90% of mild cases idiopathic vs. only 10% of severe cases. Look for markers of aneuploidy	III	B	54

SUMMARY OF MANAGEMENT OPTIONS
Hydramnios *(Continued)*

Management Options	Quality of Evidence	Strength of Recommendation	References
Identify Cause (if possible)—*Continued*			
and associated structural abnormalities, particularly those interfering with swallowing, intestinal transit, fetal movement, or venous return. Assess bladder dynamics qualitatively, with a chronically full, albeit normal-sized bladder suggestive of fetal polyuria as cause (mainly idiopathic, large baby, or volume overload, although rare renal defect/Bartter syndrome/diabetes insipidus is also possible).			
Aneuploidy risk depends on underlying cause, structural anomalies (1/3 for duodenal atresia), a priori risk, and severity. Karyotyping for isolated mild polyhydramnios controversial – only offer if increased a priori risk. Same probably applies to investigation for viral infection.	III	B	53
Treatment (relieve maternal symptoms; prolong gestation)			
If mild asymptomatic, manage expectantly; no evidence to suggest diuretics and salt or fluid restriction are of value.	–	GPP	–
Specific treatment depends on underlying cause (see relevant chapters).	–	GPP	–
Consider amnioreduction (see separate protocol) if AFI >40 cm or earlier if patient is symptomatic and prolongation of pregnancy indicated.	III	B	84
Consider sulindac (200 mg bid) in gestations <32 wk.	Ib	A	77,80
Avoid indomethacin because of adverse fetal affects.	Ib	A	77,80
Counsel patient about risks of PPROM (cord prolapse, infection) and preterm labor. If polyhydramnios persists, elective delivery at 38 wk in view of increased risk of unexplained stillbirth. Can deliver vaginally if singleton and stable cephalic presentation.	III III	B B	58 90
Alert pediatricians (need to assess upper gastrointestinal patency, risk of neonatal milk aspiration, etc.).	–	GPP	–

AFI, amniotic fluid index; DVP, deepest vertical pool; PPROM, preterum premature rupture of membranes.

OLIGOHYDRAMNIOS

Definition

Oligohydramnios has been defined as the DP devoid of cord or fetal limbs measuring less than 3, 2, or 1 cm,[94,95] the latter indicating moderate to severe oligohydramnios. An AFI below the 5th percentile for gestational age is a more popular definition today (see Fig. 13–1), though a recent study suggests this approach overdiagnoses oligohydramnios.[9] Likewise, the concurrent use of color Doppler may lead to the overdiagnosis of oligohydramnios.[96,97] Shipp and associates[98] noted a bimodal distribution in the diagnosis of severe oligohydramnios with more cases diagnosed at 13 to 21 weeks and at 34 to 42 weeks. Survival rate was lower when diagnosed during the second versus third trimester (10% vs. 85%), reflecting two different populations in terms of both etiology and prognosis.

The common causes of oligohydramnios are summarized in Table 13–3. Human data suggest that oligohydramnios associated with intrauterine growth restriction (IUGR) is secondary to fetal oliguria,[99] the degree of reduction in HFUPR correlating with the level of hypoxemia.[100] Doppler studies reveal increased resistance to flow through the renal artery.[101,102] HFUPR does decline after 40 weeks, but in contrast to IUGR, Doppler studies do not support a renovascular mechanism with redistribution of blood flow[102] away from the kidneys in postmature fetuses.

Prelabor rupture of the membranes (PROM) complicates 3% to 17% of pregnancies.[103] Although the clinical diagnosis is obvious in most cases, only 5% to 44% have ultrasonic evidence of oligohydramnios.[104, 105] The earlier the gestation, the lower the incidence of premature PROM (PPROM) as an explanation of oligohydramnios. In one series, PPROM complicated only 0.7% of pregnancies less than 25 weeks with oligohydramnios.[106]

TABLE 13–4

Diagnostic Evaluation of Oligohydramnios

History taking with an emphasis on maternal symptoms of hypertension, rupture of membranes, and congenital infection
High-resolution ultrasonography to assess:
Degree of oligohydramnios
Presence of growth deficiency
Presence and structure of the kidneys
Genitourinary malformations
Color Doppler ultrasonography
Visualize the fetal renal arteries
Determine the severity of oligohydramnios by excluding loops of cord
Amnioinfusion, if necessary, to improve ultrasonographic resolution
Fetal specimens for karyotyping and viral infection

PROCEDURE

AMNIOINFUSION

Preprocedure

Some clinicians recommend prophylactic antibiotic use (cefuroxime 750 mg IV), though no trials even suggest efficacy.

Procedure

Choose a skin entry site and track to the target on ultrasound. Plan a route to an accessible pool of amniotic fluid using color or power Doppler. If there is no cord-free pocket, aim for potential space in region of fetal limbs devoid of cord.

Infiltrate local anesthetic (5–10 mL 1% lidocaine) into superficial maternal tissues.

After assessing viability, plan response to possible major postprocedural bradycardia (usually from inadvertent or concomitant blood sampling).

Use a 20-gauge needle and sterile technique, with or without a needle guide; advance the needle under continuous ultrasound guidance. After guiding needle to target pool, locate space by aspiration of amniotic fluid. If no pool exists, use test dose 2 mL saline flush to confirm position. Confirm successful infusion by injecting 10 mL saline and observing for intra-amniotic blooming.

Attach a three-way tap with wide-bore tubing to needle hub, and commence infusion using 50-mL syringes of warmed isotonic fluid (0.9% saline or Hartmann's).

For diagnostic infusions (usually 150–350 mL, depending on gestation), continue until AFI qualitatively is at lower limit of normal. For therapeutic infusions, continue until the DP is 6 cm or the AFI is 20 cm.

Concomitant karyotyping can be done on the initial amniotic fluid aspirate, on chorionic villi aspirated on needle withdrawal, or on fetal blood deliberately or inadvertently aspirated from a free loop of cord. Others have had success culturing the cells withdrawn after the amnioinfusion has been completed.

Postprocedure

Check umbilical artery by Doppler.

Administer anti-D antibodies IM to RhD-negative women.

After diagnostic infusions, repeat the scan and arrange for pad checks. After test infusions, arrange for pad checks, and check the volume 24 to 48 hours later.

Some clinicians recommend repeating the therapeutic infusions weekly in the presence of recurrent severe oligohydramnios. The efficacy of this procedure in improving outcome remains to be clarified.

After 26 weeks, consider CTG if there are postprocedure complications or a compromised fetus.

The role of amnioinfusion has greatly diminished with the widespread availability and use of color Doppler to identify the renal arteries (Fig. 13–5). In 33 pregnancies referred with severe oligohydramnios to our center, absence of renal artery flow signals accurately predicted all cases of renal agenesis. The only false-positive diagnoses were in fetuses with severely dysplastic kidneys, and thus functionally similar to agenesis.[137] Doppler flow

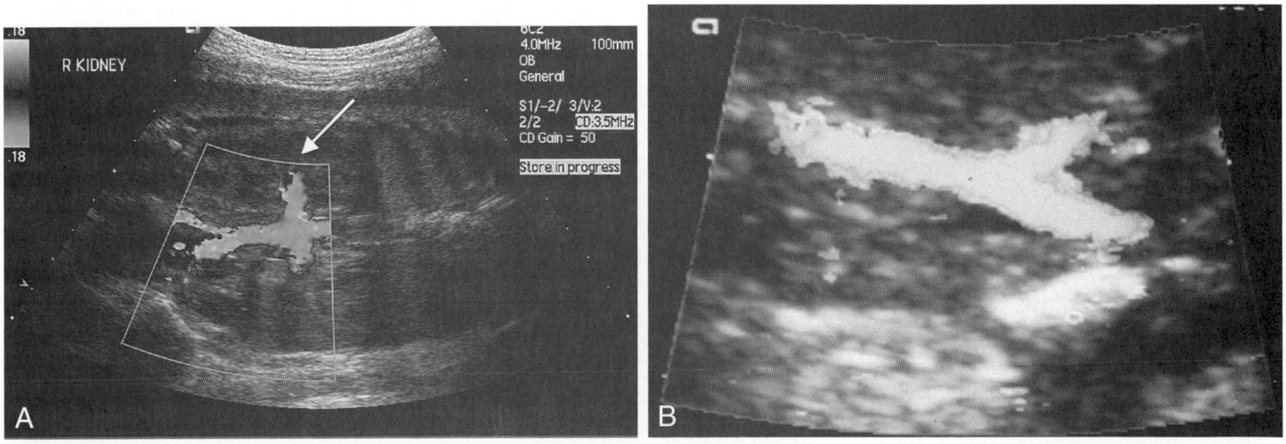

FIGURE 13–5
Color Doppler/power Doppler showing renal arteries in a normal fetus (*A*) but absent from a fetus with renal agenesis (*B*) (see Color Plate 2).

signals in renal arteries are an accurate, noninvasive way to predict the absence of renal function such as in renal agenesis or multicystic dysplastic kidney disease. In our experience, it has largely replaced amnioinfusion for the diagnosis of renal agenesis.

In contrast, lower urinary tract obstruction is relatively easy to diagnose because of the enlarged bladder or dilated upper collecting system. Visualization of other urinary structures such as the renal cortex and upper urethra has prognostic value. Visualization of extrarenal anatomy for associated anomalies remains suboptimal.

The severity of oligohydramnios is also assessed, not only for clues to etiology, but also for prognosis. Karyotyping should be considered; aneuploidy is detected in over 4%[98] of cases of severe oligohydramnios.

Therapeutic Options

Although the mechanism of oligohydramnios-related PH remains unknown, restoration of AF volume in animal models permits normal lung development.[138,139] Identification of fetuses at risk of pulmonary hypoplasia and who theoretically might benefit from AF replacement was previously based on ultrasonographic measurement of the fetal chest circumference,[140,141] lung length,[142] and Doppler studies[143] of the pulmonary vasculature. These parameters, however, are poorly reproducible in the absence of AF and seem predictive only after the end of the canalicular phase of lung development (~ 25 weeks), indicating established hypoplasia at a time too late for intervention.[140,144,145] Three-dimensional (3D) ultrasonography to assess lung volume[146] is becoming more widespread,[147] but its ability to predict pulmonary hypoplasia in the presence of oligohydramnios remains to be established.

Several treatments have been tried to maintain AF volume and thus promote lung development in pregnancies complicated by midtrimester oligohydramnios. These treatments include the following:

- Serial transabdominal amnioinfusions[132,148–152]
- Infusion of fluid via a transcervical catheter[153]
- Maternal hydration[154,155]
- Desmopressin (1- (3 mercaptoproprionic acid)- 8-D-arginine vasopression; dDAVP)[156]
- Cervical canal occlusion with fibrin gel[107,157]
- Intra-amniotic sealing techniques[158,159]
- Vesicoamniotic shunting in obstructive uropathies[160]
- Fetal cystoscopy[110,161]

SERIAL AMNIOINFUSIONS

Cohort series suggest amnioinfusion improves outcome. Fisk and associates[132] performed serial amnioinfusion weekly in women with PPROM until the end of the canalicular phase of lung development in nine at-risk pregnancies with severe oligohydramnios prior to 22 weeks. Pulmonary hypoplasia was found in two (22%), which compared favorably to the 60% reported for severe oligohydramnios diagnosed at or before 28 weeks.[162] Vergani and associates[149] observed that serial amnioinfusion in a population with PPROM at or before 25 weeks' gestation reduced the incidence of PH from 86% to 46%. Similarly, in the largest cohort study examining amnioinfusion, Locatelli and associates[150] found that amnioinfusion, if successful (when a pocket of AF >2 cm remained for at least 48 hours), reduced the rate of PH to that of so-called normal control subjects. In contrast, those with persistent oligohydramnios had a 62% incidence of PH. More recently, De Santis and associates found that amnioinfusion significantly increased the latency period between PPROM before 26 weeks and delivery (42 vs. 18 days), week of delivery (26 vs. 22 weeks), and neonatal weight (922 vs. 614 g). Unfortunately, there were no differences in overall survival or the incidence of PH compared to control subjects. Patients experiencing a slow loss of amniotic fluid between procedures seemed to benefit most. Thus, it is unlikely that amnioinfusion will prove advantageous in pregnancies that leak all the infused fluid immediately after the procedure.[151] In our center, we offer a test amnioinfusion first, as around 80% of patients with midtrimester oligohydramnios secondary to PPROM do not retain infused fluid after the procedure and would therefore not be candidates for serial amnioinfusion. Although serial amnioinfusion can prevent PH[163] in fetuses with renal agenesis, the ethics of such treatment remains controversial in the absence of successful neonatal or even infantile renal transplantation. In summary, there is mounting evidence of a role for amnioinfusion in the management of severe oligohydramnios in pregnancies with a structurally normal fetus. However, further research is needed, ideally in a context of a randomized controlled trial, to determine the following:

- The optimal gestation at which to commence and cease infusions
- The longevity of infused fluid within the amniotic cavity
- The optimal interval between infusions
- The optimal fluid to maintain AF volume

Studies should be directed toward identifying any particular subset of cases that will benefit from amnioinfusion.

TRANSCERVICAL FLUID REPLACEMENT, MATERNAL HYDRATION, AND DDAVP

Restoration of AF volume following infusion of normal saline through a cervical balloon catheter is performed in the third trimester but has not been evaluated for use earlier in pregnancy[153] for the prevention of PH.

Maternal hydration (drinking 2 L of water prior to ultrasound) increases the AFI in oligohydramnios and in normal[164] pregnancies by 2.01 cm (95% confidence interval 1.43 to 2.56) and 4.5 cm (95% confidence interval 2.92 to 6.08)[65] at term. These short-term improvements in AF volume persist into the longer term[166] when maternal hydration is continued (drinking at least 2 L/day for 1 week), suggesting a potential role in the management of oligohydramnios.

Ross and associates tested the hypothesis that[156] maintenance of maternal hypo-osmolality through a combination of maternal hydration and 1-deamino-8-D-arginine-vasopressin (DDAVP), a selective antidiuretic agonist, could increase AF volume in a series of 10 pregnancies at term. The AFI was increased at 8 hours (4.1 ± 0.6 to 8.2 ± 1.5 cm) and remained increased at 24 hours (8.2 ± 1.3 cm), suggesting a potential role for DDAVP in the prevention and treatment of oligohydramnios.

CERVICAL OCCLUSION

Cervical occlusion with fibrin gel was used in 12 patients with PPROM before 24 weeks.[157] In all instances, a reduction in the amount of amniotic leakage and an increase in AFI was observed. Larger trials are required to confirm the potential shown in this small series.

INTRA-AMNIOTIC SEALING TECHNIQUES

Intra-amniotic administration of gelatin sponge (Gelfoam) to 20 women with PPROM at an average of 18 weeks was associated with a 30% overall survival rate.[158] Similarly, endoscopic techniques have demonstrated some technical success in sealing the membranous defect but only after iatrogenic[167] rather than spontaneous PPROM. In seven pregnancies with iatrogenic PPROM, three did well with restoration of AF after intra-amniotic injection of platelets and cryoprecipitate (amniopatch), though two had sudden unexplained intrauterine death.[167] It is possible massive platelet degranulation of serotonin triggered severe vasospasm of fetal placental vessels. Case reports of using the amniopatch in patients with spontaneous PPROM note only limited success.[159,168] In vivo endoscopic visualization[169] in patients with spontaneous PPROM reveals that the size, location, and shape of the defect are such that it is unlikely to heal with an amniopatch.

VESICOAMNIOTIC SHUNTING

Despite the restoration of AF volume after vesicoamniotic shunting, perinatal mortality rates in obstructive uropathies remain high (see also Chapter 19). Complications occur in up to 45%[170] and include shunt blockage, shunt migration, preterm labor, urinary ascites, chorioamnionitis, and iatrogenic gastroschisis. A review of five large series involving[169] successfully placed shunts showed that the overall perinatal survival rate after intervention was only 47%.[110] Even in technically successful cases, end-stage renal disease occurred in 40% of survivors. If oligohydramnios was present before the shunt was placed, 56% of these babies died despite intervention. Failure to restore AF volume was associated with 100% mortality rate.

When intervention did improve the chances of postnatal survival, it did not appear to alter the renal outcome.[171] Freedman and associates[172] reviewed the long-term outcome of 34 fetuses that underwent vesicoamniotic shunt placement. Thirteen died, of which six deaths were due to PH. In the survivors, the ultimate diagnosis was mainly prune-belly syndrome or posterior urethral valves. Less than one third of the children needed ventilatory support in the neonatal period, and none of the children had pulmonary restriction to normal activities on follow-up. These children underwent a total of 62 surgical procedures, of which 47 were major (bladder augmentations and renal transplants). Six have maintained normal renal function, three have renal insufficiency, and five have progressed to renal failure. It appears that fetal therapy therefore only influences the outcome of fetuses with lower urinary tract obstruction that leads to midtrimester oligo- or anhydramnios by preventing PH, but does not seem to ameliorate the underlying kidney disease. This association is important, because parents need to be aware that there is still a 33% to 50% chance of renal failure in childhood.[173] They also need to be counseled that although affected children are expected to have normal cognitive abilities, participate in normal activities, and achieve a socially acceptable degree of continence, they will need considerable medical and surgical attention.

A retrospective review from the University of California, San Francisco,[174] of fetuses with posterior urethral valves who underwent fetal therapy (mainly vesicoamniotic shunting) after favorable urine analysis results confirmed a high fetal mortality rate of 42%. Chronic renal disease was diagnosed in 62% of the survivors, 25% of whom underwent renal transplantation. This study, like that of Freedman and associates,[172] suggests that fetal therapy does not cure fetuses with posterior urethral valves but may improve bladder function and decrease the morbidity rate of incontinence and recurrent infections.

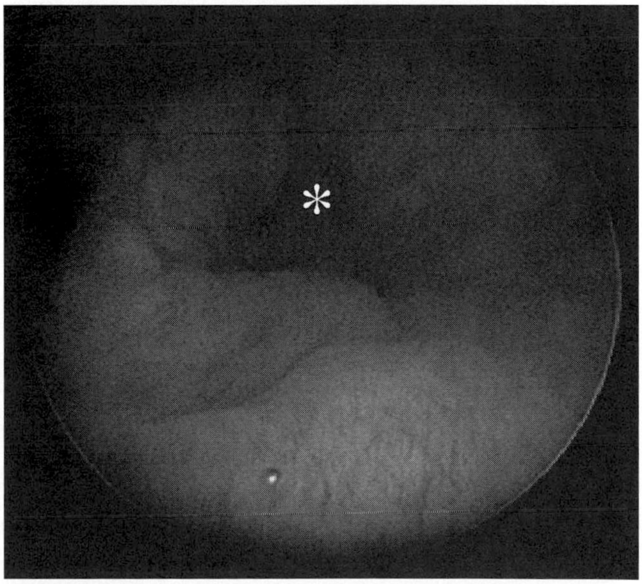

FIGURE 13–6
Fetal cystoscopic view of a fetal bladder and the proximal urethra (*) (see Color Plate 3).

FETAL CYSTOSCOPY

Fetal cystoscopy can be both diagnostic and therapeutic, and is currently undergoing evaluation as a management option in lower urinary tract obstruction.[161] It allows exploration of the bladder and the proximal part of the urethra under endoscopic vision (Fig.13–6). Obtaining a clear view of the bladder neck and urethra is facilitated by the use of flexible scopes to help overcome the problem of negotiating the urethrovesical angle. Posterior urethral valves, if present, can be disrupted by laser, although there may be damage the adjacent bowel and other structures. Alternatively, gentler techniques such as insertion of a guide wire or simple pressure saline injection may work in some instances.[175]

SUMMARY OF MANAGEMENT OPTIONS
Oligohydramnios

Management Options	Quality of Evidence	Strength of Recommendation	References
Identify Cause (if possible)			
Detailed history to include drug exposure (nonsteroidal anti-inflammatory drugs as angiotensin-converting enzyme inhibitors), prior aneuploidy screening, and history suggestive of preeclampsia, PPROM, including bleeding in pregnancy, which may obscure liquor loss.	–	GPP	–
Ultrasonography (transvaginal may be helpful) to assess: • Degree of oligohydramnios (AFI) • Presence of growth deficiency • Fetal and uterine blood flow studies • Presence and appearance of the kidneys • Genitourinary and other malformations In second trimester, PPROM accounts for 50%, fetal anomalies 15% (mainly renal tract), IUGR 20%, and idiopathic 5%. The more severe the oligohydramnios, the more likely it is secondary to a structural anomaly or PPROM.	III	B	133
Color/power Doppler ultrasonography to: • Visualize fetal renal arteries • Determine the severity of oligohydramnios by excluding loops of cord Oligohydramnios defined as AFI <5 cm or DVP <3 cm (<3 cm mild, <2 cm moderate, <1 cm severe).	III	B	96,137
Amnioinfusion may also have a role in diagnosing or confirming suspected PPROM.	III	B	132,153
If structural anomalies, or soft markers, or early onset IUGR (<24 wk), offer rapid karyotyping, possibly with concomitant amnioinfusion.		GPP	–
Prognosis depends on cause. In PPROM, prognosis poor due to risk of prematurity, and chorioamnionitis. Even if pregnancy progresses past viability, oligohydramnios beginning <25 wk with a DVP of <1 cm lasting >2 wk results in >90% perinatal mortality rate, primarily from pulmonary hypoplasia.	III	B	98
Skeletal deformities and contractures usually only complicate prolonged severe oligohydramnios, and rarely occur in the absence of pulmonary hypoplasia.	–	GPP	–
Management (depends on etiology)			
PPROM (see Chapter 63)			
Growth deficiency (see Chapters 11 and 12)			
Prolonged pregnancy (see Chapter 66)			
Fetal renal anomalies (see Chapter 19)			

Continued

SUMMARY OF MANAGEMENT OPTIONS
Oligohydramnios *(Continued)*

Management Options	Quality of Evidence	Strength of Recommendation	References
Management (depends on etiology)—*Continued*			
Treatments tried in midtrimester oligohydramnios to maintain amniotic fluid volume and promote lung development:			
• Serial transabdominal therapeutic amnioinfusions with PPROM <25 wk (after initial trial infusion to determine if retained)	III	B	132,148-152
• Transcervical infusion not evaluated in early pregnancy	III	B	153
• Vesicoamnioic shunting in obstructive uropathies	III	B	172
• Cervical canal occlusion with fibrin gel	III	B	107,157
• Maternal hydration possibly of value	Ib	A	155
• DDAVP needs further study	III	B	156

AFI, amniotic fluid index; DVP, deepest venous pool; IUGR, intrauterine growth restriction; PPROM, prenatal premature rupture of membranes.

CONCLUSIONS

- Abnormal amniotic fluid volume complicates up to 7% of pregnancies, although in many instances the alteration is mild, is idiopathic, occurs in the third trimester, and does not produce sequelae.
- In contrast, severe oligohydramnios and hydramnios in the midtrimester are associated with substantial perinatal morbidity and mortality rates, reflecting both the underlying etiology and the complications of disordered amniotic volume.
- The investigation of hydramnios involves detection of anomalies by ultrasonography, karyotyping, and exclusion of carbohydrate intolerance.
- Transplacental indomethacin reduces fetal urine output, but its use in severe hydramnios to prolong gestation is limited by fetal side effects.
- Sulindac may have fewer fetal side effects than indomethacin and is thus preferred for this purpose.
- Serial amnioreduction seems to improve perinatal survival in monochorionic twin pregnancies with midtrimester hydramnios secondary to TTTS by prolonging gestation, but it does not address the underlying pathophysiology like laser ablation.
- Severe oligohydramnios, whether secondary to ruptured membranes, growth restriction, absent renal function, or fetal urinary tract obstruction, poses a diagnostic challenge because it impairs ultrasonographic resolution.
- Transabdominal amnioinfusion facilitates visualization of fetal anatomy and determines membranous integrity.
- Color Doppler visualization of renal arteries aids both the diagnosis of renal agenesis and the determination of the severity of oligohydramnios by identifying loops in apparent pockets of amniotic fluid. Karyotyping and transvaginal ultrasonography may also be indicated in oligohydramnios.
- In order to prevent pulmonary hypoplasia, vesicoamniotic shunting, fetal cystoscopy, and serial amnioinfusion have been used to maintain AF volume in selected euploid fetuses with functioning renal tissue.
- Serial amnioinfusion appears to improve outcome in cohort series, but most patients with midtrimester oligohydramnios secondary to PPROM are unsuitable because all their fluid leaks out immediately.

REFERENCES

1. Queenan JT, Gadow EC: Polyhydramnios: Chronic versus acute. Am J Obstet Gynecol 1970;108(3):349–355.
2. Brans YW, Andrew DS, Dutton EB, et al: Dilution kinetics of chemicals used for estimation of water content of body compartments in perinatal medicine. Pediatr Res 1989;25(4):377–382.
3. Denbow ML, Sepulveda W, Ridout D, Fisk NM: Relationship between change in amniotic fluid index and volume of fluid removed at amnioreduction. Obstet Gynecol 1997;90(4): 529–532.
4. Sepulveda W, Flack NJ, Fisk NM: Direct volume measurement at midtrimester amnioinfusion in relation to ultrasonographic indexes of amniotic fluid volume. Am J Obstet Gynecol 1994;170(4):1160–1163.
5. Gramellini D, Piantelli G, Di Marino O, et al: Amniotic fluid index variations after amniocentesis, amnioinfusion and amnioreduction: Preliminary data. Clin Exp Obstet Gynecol 1997;24(2):70–73.

6. Moore TR: Superiority of the four-quadrant sum over the single-deepest-pocket technique in ultrasonographic identification of abnormal amniotic fluid volumes. Am J Obstet Gynecol 1990;163(3):762–767.
7. Moore TR, Cayle JE: The amniotic fluid index in normal human pregnancy. Am J Obstet Gynecol 1990;162(5):1168–1173.
8. Brace RA, Wolf EJ: Normal amniotic fluid volume changes throughout pregnancy. Am J Obstet Gynecol 1989;161(2): 382–388.
9. Magann EF, Sanderson M, Martin JN, Chauhan S: The amniotic fluid index, single deepest pocket, and two-diameter pocket in normal human pregnancy. Am J Obstet Gynecol 2000;182(6): 1581–1588.
10. Alley MH, Hadjiev A, Mazneikova V, Dimitrov A: Four-quadrant assessment of gestational age-specific values of amniotic fluid volume in uncomplicated pregnancies. Acta Obstet Gynecol Scand 1998;77(3):290–294.
11. Goldkrand JW, Hough TM, Lentz SU, et al: Comparison of the amniotic fluid index with gray-scale and color Doppler ultrasound. J Matern Fetal Neonatal Med 2003;13(5):318–322.
12. Flack NJ, Dore C, Southwell D, et al: The influence of operator transducer pressure on ultrasonographic measurements of amniotic fluid volume. Am J Obstet Gynecol 1994;171(1):218–222.
13. Hombo Y, Ohshita M, Takamura S, et al: Direct prediction of amniotic fluid volume in the third trimester by 3-dimensional measurements of intrauterine pockets: A tool for routine clinical use. Am J Obstet Gynecol 2002;186(2):245–250.
14. Chamberlain PF, Manning FA, Morrison I, et al: Ultrasound evaluation of amniotic fluid volume II. The relationship of increased amniotic fluid volume to perinatal outcome. Am J Obstet Gynecol 1984;150(3):250–254.
15. Hill LM, Breckle R, Thomas ML, Fries JK: Polyhydramnios: Ultrasonically detected prevalence and neonatal outcome. Obstet Gynecol 1987;69(1):21–25.
16. Thompson O, Brown R, Gunnarson G, Harrington K: Prevalence of polyhydramnios in the third trimester in a population screened by first and second trimester ultrasonography. J Perinat Med 1998;26(5):371–377.
17. Naeye RL, Milic AM, Blanc W: Fetal endocrine and renal disorders: Clues to the origin of hydramnios. Am J Obstet Gynecol 1970;108(8):1251–1256.
18. van Otterlo LC, Wladimiroff JW, Wallenburg HC: Relationship between fetal urine production and amniotic fluid volume in normal pregnancy and pregnancy complicated by diabetes. Br J Obstet Gynaecol 1977;84(3):205–209.
19. Yasuhi I, Ishimaru T, Hirai M, Yamabe T: Hourly fetal urine production rate in the fasting and the postprandial state of normal and diabetic pregnant women. Obstet Gynecol 1994; 84(1):64–68.
20. Nageotte MP, Hurwitz SR, Kaupke CJ, et al: Atriopeptin in the twin transfusion syndrome. Obstet Gynecol 1989;73(5 Pt 2): 867–870.
21. Wieacker P, Wilhelm C, Prompeler H, et al: Pathophysiology of polyhydramnios in twin transfusion syndrome. Fetal Diagn Ther 1992;7(2):87–92.
22. Rosen DJ, Rabinowitz R, Beyth Y, et al: Fetal urine production in normal twins and in twins with acute polyhydramnios. Fetal Diagn Ther 1990;5(2):57–60.
23. Bajoria R, Ward S, Sooranna SR: Atrial natriuretic peptide mediated polyuria: Pathogenesis of polyhydramnios in the recipient twin of twin-twin transfusion syndrome. Placenta 2001;22(8-9): 716–724.
24. Powell TL, Brace RA: Elevated fetal plasma lactate produces polyhydramnios in the sheep. Am J Obstet Gynecol 1991;165(6 Pt 1):1595–1607.
25. Faber JJ, Anderson DF: Hydrops fetalis in nephrectomized fetal lambs infused with angiotensin I. Am J Physiol 1994;267(6 Pt 2):R1522–1527.
26. Soothill PW, Nicolaides KH, Rodeck CH, et al: Relationship of fetal hemoglobin and oxygen content to lactate concentration in Rh isoimmunized pregnancies. Obstet Gynecol 1987;69(2): 268–271.
27. Panting-Kemp A, Nguyen T, Castro L: Substance abuse and polyhydramnios. Am J Obstet Gynecol 2002;187(3):602–605.
28. Krause S, Ebbesen F, Lange AP: Polyhydramnios with maternal lithium treatment. Obstet Gynecol 1990;75(3 Pt 2):504–506.
29. Ang MS, Thorp JA, Parisi VM: Maternal lithium therapy and polyhydramnios. Obstet Gynecol 1990;76(3 Pt 2):517–519.
30. Ohlsson A, Sieck U, Cumming W, et al: A variant of Bartter's syndrome. Bartter's syndrome associated with hydramnios, prematurity, hypercalciuria and nephrocalcinosis. Acta Paediatr Scand 1984;73(6):868–874.
31. Matsushita Y, Suzuki Y, Oya N, et al: Biochemical examination of mother's urine is useful for prenatal diagnosis of Bartter syndrome. Prenatal Diagn 1999;19(7):671–673.
32. Barkin SZ, Pretorius DH, Beckett MK, et al: Severe polyhydramnios: incidence of anomalies. AJR Am J Roentgenol 1987;148(1):155–159.
33. Dashe JS, McIntire DD, Ramus RM, et al: Hydramnios: Anomaly prevalence and sonographic detection. Obstet Gynecol 2002;100(1):134–139.
34. Duncan KR, Denbow M, Fisk NM: The aetiology and management of twin twin transfusion syndrome. Prenatal Diagn 1997;17:1227–1236.
35. Caldeyro-Barcia R: Uterine contractility in polyhydramnios and the effects of withdrawal of the excess of amniotic fluid. Am J Obstet Gynecol 1957;73:1238–1254.
36. Steinberg LH, Hurley VA, Desmedt E, Beischer NA: Acute polyhydramnios in twin pregnancies. Aust N Z J Obstet Gynaecol 1990;30(3):196–200.
37. Weiner CP, Heilskov J, Pelzer G, et al: Normal values for human umbilical venous and amniotic fluid pressures and their alteration by fetal disease. Am J Obstet Gynecol 1989;161(3): 714–717.
38. Fisk NM, Vaughan J, Talbert D: Impaired fetal blood gas status in polyhydramnios and its relation to raised amniotic pressure. Fetal Diagn Ther 1994;9:7–13.
39. Pritchard JA, Mason R, Corley M, Pritchard S: Genesis of severe placental abruption. Am J Obstet Gynecol 1970;108(1):22–27.
40. Panting-Kemp A, Nguyen T, Chang E, et al: Idiopathic polyhydramnios and perinatal outcome. Am J Obstet Gynecol 1999;181(5 Pt 1):1079–1082.
41. Midgley DY, Harding K: The Mirror syndrome. Eur J Obstet Gynecol Reprod Biol 2000;88(2):201–202.
42. Vintzileos AM, Turner GW, Campbell WA, et al: Polyhydramnios and obstructive renal failure: A case report and review of the literature. Am J Obstet Gynecol 1985;152(7 Pt 1):883–885.
43. Seeds JW, Cefalo RC, Herbert WN, Bowes W Jr: Hydramnios and maternal renal failure: Relief with fetal therapy. Obstet Gynecol 1984;64(3 Suppl):26S–29S.
44. Biggio JR Jr, Wenstrom KD, Dubard MB, Cliver SP: Hydramnios prediction of adverse perinatal outcome. Obstet Gynecol 1999;94(5 Pt 1):773–777.
45. Carlson DE, Platt LD, Medearis AL, Horenstein J: Quantifiable polyhydramnios: Diagnosis and management. Obstet Gynecol 1990;75(6):989–993.
46. Bower SJ, Flack NJ, Sepulveda W, et al: Uterine artery blood flow response to correction of amniotic fluid volume. Am J Obstet Gynecol 1995;173:502–507.
47. Guzman ER, Vintzileos A, Benito C, et al: Effects of therapeutic amniocentesis on uterine and umbilical artery velocimetry in cases of severe symptomatic polyhydramnios. J Matern Fetal Med 1996;5(6):299–304.
48. Fisk NM, Giussani DA, Parkes MJ, et al : Amnioinfusion increases amniotic pressure in pregnant sheep but does not alter

fetal acid-base status. Am J Obstet Gynecol 1991;165(5 Pt 1):1459–1463.
49. Sheiner E, Hallak M, Shoham-Vardi I, et al: Determining risk factors for intrapartum fetal death. J Reprod Med 2000;45(5):419–424.
50. Kirshon B: Fetal urine output in hydramnios. Obstet Gynecol 1989;73(2):240–242.
51. Campbell S, Wladimiroff JW, Dewhurst CJ: The antenatal measurement of fetal urine production. J Obstet Gynaecol Br Commonw 1973;80(8):680–686.
52. Hedriana H, Moore T: Ultrasonographic evaluation of human fetal urinary flow rate: Accuracy limits of bladder volume estimations. Am J Obstet Gynecol 1994;170(5 Pt 1):1250–1254.
53. Brady K, Polzin WJ, Kopelman JN, Read JA: Risk of chromosomal abnormalities in patients with idiopathic polyhydramnios. Obstet Gynecol 1992;79(2):234–238.
54. Boylan P, Parisi V: An overview of hydramnios. Semin Perinatol 1986;10(2):136–141.
55. Fisk NM, Tannirandorn Y, Nicolini U, et al: Amniotic pressure in disorders of amniotic fluid volume. Obstet Gynecol 1990;76(2):210–214.
56. Cifuentes RF, Olley PM, Balfe JW, et al: Indomethacin and renal function in premature infants with persistent patent ductus arteriosus. J Pediatr 1979;95(4):583–587.
57. Kirshon B, Moise K Jr, Wasserstrum N, et al: Influence of short-term indomethacin therapy on fetal urine output. Obstet Gynecol 1988;72(1):51–53.
58. Mamopoulos M, Assimakopoulos E, Reece EA, et al: Maternal indomethacin therapy in the treatment of polyhydramnios. Am J Obstet Gynecol 1990;162(5):1225–1229.
59. Lange IR, Harman CR, Ash KM, et al: Twin with hydramnios: Treating premature labor at source. Am J Obstet Gynecol 1989;160(3):552–557.
60. Cabrol D, Landesman R, Muller J, et al: Treatment of polyhydramnios with prostaglandin synthetase inhibitor (indomethacin). Am J Obstet Gynecol 1987;157(2):422–426.
61. Anderson RJ, Berl T, McDonald KD, Schrier RW: Evidence for an in vivo antagonism between vasopressin and prostaglandin in the mammalian kidney. J Clin Invest 1975;56(2):420–426.
62. Usberti M, Pecoraro C, Federico S, et al: Mechanism of action of indomethacin in tubular defects. Pediatrics 1985;75(3):501–507.
63. Mari G, Moise K Jr, Deter RL, et al: Doppler assessment of the renal blood flow velocity waveform during indomethacin therapy for preterm labor and polyhydramnios. Obstet Gynecol 1990;75(2):199–201.
64. Moise K Jr, Ou CN, Kirshon B, et al: Placental transfer of indomethacin in the human pregnancy. Am J Obstet Gynecol 1990;162(2):549–554.
65. Goldenberg RL, Davis RO, Baker RC: Indomethacin-induced oligohydramnios. Am J Obstet Gynecol 1989;160(5 Pt 1):1196–1197.
66. Kirshon B, Mari G, Moise K Jr: Indomethacin therapy in the treatment of symptomatic polyhydramnios. Obstet Gynecol 1990;75(2):202–205.
67. Cowan F: Indomethacin, patent ductus arteriosus, and cerebral blood flow. J Pediatr 1986;109(2):341–344.
68. Hendricks SK, Smith JR, Moore DE, Brown ZA: Oligohydramnios associated with prostaglandin synthetase inhibitors in preterm labour. Br J Obstet Gynaecol 1990;97(4): 312–316.
69. Norton ME, Merrill J, Cooper BA, et al: Neonatal complications after the administration of indomethacin for preterm labor. N Engl J Med 1993;329(22):1602–1607.
70. Abbasi S, Gerdes JS, Sehdev HM, et al: Neonatal outcome after exposure to indomethacin in utero: A retrospective case cohort study. Am J Obstet Gynecol 2003;189(3):782–785.
71. Panter KR, Hannah ME, Amankwah KS, et al: The effect of indomethacin tocolysis in preterm labour on perinatal outcome: A randomized placebo-controlled trial. Br J Obstet Gynaecol 1999;106(5):467–473.
72. Van den Veyver IB, Moise KJ Jr, Ou CN, Carpenter RJ Jr: The effect of gestational age and fetal indomethacin levels on the incidence of constriction of the fetal ductus arteriosus. Obstet Gynecol 1993;82(4 Pt 1):500–503.
73. Huhta JC, Cohen AW, Wood DC: Premature constriction of the ductus arteriosus. J Am Soc Echocardiogr 1990;3(1):30–34.
74. Respondek M, Weil SR, Huhta JC: Fetal echocardiography during indomethacin treatment. Ultrasound Obstet Gynecol 1995;5(2):86–89.
75. Vermillion ST, Scardo JA, Lashus AG, Wiles HB: The effect of indomethacin tocolysis on fetal ductus arteriosus constriction with advancing gestational age. Am J Obstet Gynecol 1997;177(2):256–259.
76. van der Heijden BJ, Carlus C, Narcy F, et al: Persistent anuria, neonatal death, and renal microcystic lesions after prenatal exposure to indomethacin. Am J Obstet Gynecol 1994;171(3): 617–623.
77. Carlan SJ, O'Brien WF, O'Leary TD, Mastrogiannis D: Randomized comparative trial of indomethacin and sulindac for the treatment of refractory preterm labor. Obstet Gynecol 1992;79(2):223–228.
78. Kramer WB, Saade G, Ou CN, et al : Placental transfer of sulindac and its active sulfide metabolite in humans. Am J Obstet Gynecol 1995;172(3):886–890.
79. Peek MJ, McCarthy A, Kyle P, et al: Medical amnioreduction with sulindac to reduce cord complications in monoamniotic twins. Am J Obstet Gynecol 1997;176(2):334–336.
80. Rasanen J, Jouppila P: Fetal cardiac function and ductus arteriosus during indomethacin and sulindac therapy for threatened preterm labor: A randomized study. Am J Obstet Gynecol 1995;173(1):20–25.
81. Sawdy RJ, Lye S, Fisk NM, Bennett PR: A double-blind randomized study of fetal side effects during and after the short-term maternal administration of indomethacin, sulindac, and nimesulide for the treatment of preterm labor. Am J Obstet Gynecol 2003;188(4):1046–1051.
82. Mahony BS, Petty CN, Nyberg DA, et al: The "stuck twin" phenomenon: Ultrasonographic findings, pregnancy outcome, and management with serial amniocenteses. Am J Obstet Gynecol 1990;163(5 Pt 1):1513–1522.
83. Chescheir NC, Seeds JW: Polyhydramnios and oligohydramnios in twin gestations. Obstet Gynecol 1988;71(6 Pt 1):882–884.
84. Elliott JP, Urig MA, Clewell WH: Aggressive therapeutic amniocentesis for treatment of twin-twin transfusion syndrome. Obstet Gynecol 1991;77(4):537–540.
85. Feingold M, Cetrulo CL, Newton ER, et al: Serial amniocenteses in the treatment of twin to twin transfusion complicated with acute polyhydramnios. Acta Genet Med Gemellol Roma 1986;35(1-2):107–113.
86. Saunders NJ, Snijders RJ, Nicolaides KH: Therapeutic amniocentesis in twin-twin transfusion syndrome appearing in the second trimester of pregnancy. Am J Obstet Gynecol 1992;166(3): 820–824.
87. Weiner CP, Ludomirski A: Diagnosis, pathophysiology, and treatment of chronic twin-to-twin transfusion syndrome. Fetal Diagn Ther 1994;9(5):283–290.
88. Pinette MG, Pan Y, Pinette SG, Stubblefield PG: Treatment of twin-twin transfusion syndrome. Obstet Gynecol 1993;82(5): 841–846.
89. Jauniaux E, Holmes A, Hyett J, et al: Rapid and radical amniodrainage in the treatment of severe twin-twin transfusion syndrome (dagger). Prenat Diagn 2001;21(6):471–476.
90. Leung WC, Jouannic JM, Hyett J, et al: Procedure-related complications of rapid amniodrainage in the treatment of polyhydramnios. Ultrasound Obstet Gynecol 2004;23(2):154–158.

91. Fisk N, Taylor M: The fetus(es) with twin twin transfusion syndrome. In Harrison M, Evans M, Adzick S, Holzgreve W (eds): The Unborn Patient: The Art and Science of Fetal Therapy. Philadelphia, WB Saunders, 2000, pp 341–355.
92. Saade GR, Belfort MA, Berry DL, et al: Amniotic septostomy for the treatment of twin oligohydramnios-polyhydramnios sequence. Fetal Diagn Ther 1998;13:86–93.
93. Saade GR, Moise K, Dorman K, et al : A randomized trial of septostomy versus amnioreduction in the treatment of twin oligohydramnios polyhydramnios sequence (TOPS). Am J Obstet Gynecol 2002;187(6):S54.
94. Crowley P: Nonquantitative estimation of amniotic fluid volume in suspected prolonged pregnancy. J Perinat Med 1980;8(5): 249–251.
95. Manning FA, Hill LM, Platt LD: Qualitative amniotic fluid volume determination by ultrasound: Antepartum detection of intrauterine growth retardation. Am J Obstet Gynecol 1981;139(3):254–258.
96. Bianco A, Rosen T, Kuczynski E, et al: Measurement of the amniotic fluid index with and without color Doppler. J Perinat Med 1999;27(4):245–249.
97. Magann EF, Chauhan SP, Barrilleaux PS, et al: Ultrasound estimate of amniotic fluid volume: Color Doppler overdiagnosis of oligohydramnios. Obstet Gynecol 2001;98(1):71–74.
98. Shipp TD, Bromley B, Pauker S, et al: Outcome of singleton pregnancies with severe oligohydramnios in the second and third trimesters. Ultrasound Obstet Gynecol 1996;7(2):108–113.
99. Wladimiroff JW, Campbell S: Fetal urine-production rates in normal and complicated pregnancy. Lancet 1974;1(849): 151–154.
100. Nicolaides KH, Peters MT, Vyas S, et al: Relation of rate of urine production to oxygen tension in small-for-gestational-age fetuses. Am J Obstet Gynecol 1990;162(2):387–391.
101. Vyas S, Nicolaides KH, Campbell S: Renal artery flow-velocity waveforms in normal and hypoxemic fetuses. Am J Obstet Gynecol 1989;161(1):168–172.
102. Arduini D, Rizzo G: Fetal renal artery velocity waveforms and amniotic fluid volume in growth-retarded and post-term fetuses. Obstet Gynecol 1991;77(3):370–373.
103. Beischer NA, Brown JB, Townsend L: Studies in prolonged pregnancy. 3. Amniocentesis in prolonged pregnancy. Am J Obstet Gynecol 1969;103(4):496–503.
104. Gonik B, Bottoms SF, Cotton DB: Amniotic fluid volume as a risk factor in preterm premature rupture of the membranes. Obstet Gynecol 1985;65(4):456–459.
105. Robson MS, Turner MJ, Stronge JM, O'Herlihy C: Is amniotic fluid quantitation of value in the diagnosis and conservative management of prelabour membrane rupture at term? Br J Obstet Gynaecol 1990;97(4):324–328.
106. Taylor J, Garite TJ: Premature rupture of membranes before fetal viability. Obstet Gynecol 1984;64(5):615–620.
107. Baumgarten K, Moser S: The technique of fibrin adhesion for premature rupture of the membranes during pregnancy. J Perinat Med 1986;14(1):43–49.
108. Watson WJ, Katz VL, Seeds JW: Fetal urine output does not influence residual amniotic fluid volume after premature rupture of membranes. Am J Obstet Gynecol 1991;164(1 Pt 1):64–65.
109. Moore TR, Longo J, Leopold GR, et al: The reliability and predictive value of an amniotic fluid scoring system in severe second-trimester oligohydramnios. Obstet Gynecol 1989;73(5 Pt 1):739–742.
110. Agarwal SK, Fisk NM: In utero therapy for lower urinary tract obstruction. Prenat Diagn 2001;21(11):970–976.
111. Thomas DF: Prenatal diagnosis: does it alter outcome? Prenat Diagn 2001;21(11):1004–1011.
112. Nicolini U, Fisk NM, Rodeck CH, Beacham J: Fetal urine biochemistry: an index of renal maturation and dysfunction. Br J Obstet Gynaecol 1992;99(1):46–50.
113. Dommergues M, Muller F, Ngo S, et al: Fetal serum beta2-microglobulin predicts postnatal renal function in bilateral uropathies. Kidney Int 2000;58(1):312–316.
114. Glick PL, Harrison MR, Golbus MS, et al: Management of the fetus with congenital hydronephrosis. II: Prognostic criteria and selection for treatment. J Pediatr Surg 1985;20(4):376–387.
115. Lipitz S, Ryan G, Samuell C, et al: Fetal urine analysis for the assessment of renal function in obstructive uropathy. Am J Obstet Gynecol 1993;168(1 Pt 1):174–179.
116. Berry SM, Lecolier B, Smith RS, et al: Predictive value of fetal serum beta 2-microglobulin for neonatal renal function. Lancet 1995;345(8960):1277–1278.
117. Guez S, Assael BM, Melzi ML, et al: Shortcomings in predicting postnatal renal function using prenatal urine biochemistry in fetuses with congenital hydronephrosis. J Pediatr Surg 1996;31(10):1401–1404.
118. Crowley P, O'Herlihy C, Boylan P: The value of ultrasound measurement of amniotic fluid volume in the management of prolonged pregnancies. Br J Obstet Gynaecol 1984;91(5):444–448.
119. Moberg LJ, Garite TJ, Freeman RK: Fetal heart rate patterns and fetal distress in patients with preterm premature rupture of membranes. Obstet Gynecol 1984;64(1):60–64.
120. Chauhan SP, Sanderson M, Hendrix NW, et al: Perinatal outcome and amniotic fluid index in the antepartum and intrapartum periods: A meta-analysis. Am J Obstet Gynecol 1999;181(6):1473–1478.
121. Locatelli A, Vergani P, Toso L, et al: Perinatal outcome associated with oligohydramnios in uncomplicated term pregnancies. Arch Gynecol Obstet 2004;269:130–133.
122. Moretti M, Sibai BM: Maternal and perinatal outcome of expectant management of premature rupture of membranes in the midtrimester. Am J Obstet Gynecol 1988;159(2):390–396.
123. Kilbride HW, Yeast J, Thibeault DW: Defining limits of survival: Lethal pulmonary hypoplasia after midtrimester premature rupture of membranes. Am J Obstet Gynecol 1996;175(3 Pt 1):675–681.
124. Shumway JB, Al-Malt A, Amon E, et al: Impact of oligohydramnios on maternal and perinatal outcomes of spontaneous premature rupture of the membranes at 18-28 weeks. J Matern Fetal Med 1999;8(1):20–23.
125. Winn HN, Chen M, Amon E, et al: Neonatal pulmonary hypoplasia and perinatal mortality in patients with midtrimester rupture of amniotic membranes—A critical analysis. Am J Obstet Gynecol 2000;182(6):1638–1644.
126. Wigglesworth JS, Desai R: Is fetal respiratory function a major determinant of perinatal survival? Lancet 1982;1(8266):264–267.
127. Knox WF, Barson AJ: Pulmonary hypoplasia in a regional perinatal unit. Early Hum Dev 1986;14(1):33–42.
128. Harrison MR, Ross N, Noall R, de-Lorimier AA: Correction of congenital hydronephrosis in utero. I. The model: Fetal urethral obstruction produces hydronephrosis and pulmonary hypoplasia in fetal lambs. J Pediatr Surg 1983;18(3):247–256.
129. Nimrod C, Varela-Gittings F, Machin G, et al: The effect of very prolonged membrane rupture on fetal development. Am J Obstet Gynecol 1984;148(5):540–543.
130. Rotschild A, Ling EW, Puterman ML, Farquharson D: Neonatal outcome after prolonged preterm rupture of the membranes. Am J Obstet Gynecol 1990;162(1):46–52.
131. Vergani P, Ghidini A, Locatelli A, et al: Risk factors for pulmonary hypoplasia in second-trimester premature rupture of membranes. Am J Obstet Gynecol 1994;170(5 Pt 1):1359–1364.
132. Fisk NM, Ronderos-Dumit D, Soliani A, et al: Diagnostic and therapeutic transabdominal amnioinfusion in oligohydramnios. Obstet Gynecol 1991;78(2):270–278.
133. Benacerraf BR: Examination of the second-trimester fetus with severe oligohydramnios using transvaginal scanning. Obstet Gynecol 1990;75(3 Pt 2):491–493.

134. Harman CR: Maternal furosemide may not provoke urine production in the compromised fetus. Am J Obstet Gynecol 1984;150(3):322–323.
135. Chamberlain PF, Cumming M, Torchia MG, et al: Ovine fetal urine production following maternal intravenous furosemide administration. Am J Obstet Gynecol 1985;151(6):815–819.
136. Gembruch U, Hansmann M: Artificial instillation of amniotic fluid as a new technique for the diagnostic evaluation of cases of oligohydramnios. Prenat Diagn 1988;8(1):33–45.
137. Sepulveda W, Stagiannis KD, Flack NJ, Fisk NM: Accuracy of prenatal diagnosis of renal agenesis with color flow imaging in severe second-trimester oligohydramnios. Am J Obstet Gynecol 1995;173(6):1788–1792.
138. Harrison MR, Nakayama DK, Noall R, de Lorimier AA: Correction of congenital hydronephrosis in utero. II. Decompression reverses the effects of obstruction on the fetal lung and urinary tract. J Pediatr Surg 1982;17(6):965–974.
139. Nakayama DK, Glick PL, Harrison MR, et al: Experimental pulmonary hypoplasia due to oligohydramnios and its reversal by relieving thoracic compression. J Pediatr Surg 1983;18(4): 347–353.
140. Nimrod C, Davies D, Iwanicki S, et al: Ultrasound prediction of pulmonary hypoplasia. Obstet Gynecol 1986;68(4):495–498.
141. Chitkara U, Rosenberg J, Chervenak FA, et al: Prenatal sonographic assessment of the fetal thorax: normal values. Am J Obstet Gynecol 1987;156(5):1069–1074.
142. Roberts AB, Mitchell JM: Direct ultrasonographic measurement of fetal lung length in normal pregnancies and pregnancies complicated by prolonged rupture of membranes. Am J Obstet Gynecol 1990;163(5 Pt 1):1560–1566.
143. van Eyck J, van der Mooren K, Wladimiroff JW: Ductus arteriosus flow velocity modulation by fetal breathing movements as a measure of fetal lung development. Am J Obstet Gynecol 1990;163(2):558–566.
144. Songster GS, Gray DL, Crane JP: Prenatal prediction of lethal pulmonary hypoplasia using ultrasonic fetal chest circumference. Obstet Gynecol 1989;73(2):261–266.
145. D'Alton M, Mercer B, Riddick E, Dudley D: Serial thoracic versus abdominal circumference ratios for the prediction of pulmonary hypoplasia in premature rupture of the membranes remote from term. Am J Obstet Gynecol 1992;166(2):658–663.
146. Lee A, Kratochwil A, Stumpflen I, et al: Fetal lung volume determination by three-dimensional ultrasonography. Am J Obstet Gynecol 1996;175(3 Pt 1):588–592.
147. Kalache KD, Espinoza J, Chaiworapongsa T, et al: Three-dimensional ultrasound fetal lung volume measurement: A systematic study comparing the multiplanar method with the rotational (VOCAL) technique. Ultrasound Obstet Gynecol 2003;21(2):111–118.
148. Garzetti GG, Ciavattini A, De Cristofaro F, et al: Prophylactic transabdominal amnioinfusion in oligohydramnios for preterm premature rupture of membranes: Increase of amniotic fluid index during latency period. Gynecol Obstet Invest 1997;44(4):249–254.
149. Vergani P, Locatelli A, Strobelt N, et al: Amnioinfusion for prevention of pulmonary hypoplasia in second trimester rupture of membranes. Am J Perinatol 1997;14(6):325–329.
150. Locatelli A, Vergani P, Di Pirro G, et al: Role of amnioinfusion in the management of premature rupture of the membranes at <26 weeks' gestation. Am J Obstet Gynecol 2000;183(4): 878–882.
151. Tan LK, Kumar S, Jolly M, et al: Test amnioinfusion to determine suitability for serial therapeutic amnioinfusion in midtrimester premature rupture of membranes. Fetal Diagn Ther 2003;18(3):183–189.
152. De Santis M, Scavo M, Noia G, et al: Transabdominal amnioinfusion treatment of severe oligohydramnios in preterm premature rupture of membranes at less than 26 gestational weeks. Fetal Diagn Ther 2003;18(6):412–417.
153. Imanaka M, Ogita S, Sugawa T: Saline solution amnioinfusion for oligohydramnios after premature rupture of the membranes. A preliminary report. Am J Obstet Gynecol 1989;161(1): 102–106.
154. Kilpatrick SJ, Safford KL, Pomeroy T, et al: Maternal hydration increases amniotic fluid index. Obstet Gynecol 1991;78(6): 1098–1102.
155. Flack NJ, Sepulveda W, Bower S, Fisk NM: Acute maternal hydration in third-trimester oligohydramnios: Effects on amniotic fluid volume, uteroplacental perfusion, and fetal blood flow and urine output. Am J Obstet Gynecol 1995;173(4):1186–1191.
156. Ross MG, Cedars L, Nijland MJ, Ogundipe A: Treatment of oligohydramnios with maternal 1-deamino-[8-D-arginine] vasopressin-induced plasma hypoosmolality. Am J Obstet Gynecol 1996;174(5):1608–1613.
157. Sciscione AC, Manley JS, Pollock M, et al: Intracervical fibrin sealants: a potential treatment for early preterm premature rupture of the membranes. Am J Obstet Gynecol 2001;184(3): 368–373.
158. O'Brien JM, Barton JR, Milligan DA: An aggressive interventional protocol for early midtrimester premature rupture of the membranes using gelatin sponge for cervical plugging. Am J Obstet Gynecol 2002;187(5):1143–1146.
159. Quintero RA, Morales WJ, Bornick PW, et al: Surgical treatment of spontaneous rupture of membranes: The amniograft—first experience. Am J Obstet Gynecol 2002;186(1):155–157.
160. Manning FA, Harrison MR, Rodeck C: Catheter shunts for fetal hydronephrosis and hydrocephalus. Report of the International Fetal Surgery Registry. N Engl J Med 1986;315(5):336–340.
161. Quintero RA, Johnson MP, Romero R, et al: In-utero percutaneous cystoscopy in the management of fetal lower obstructive uropathy. Lancet 1995;346(8974):537–540.
162. Harrison MR, Golbus MS, Filly RA, et al: Management of the fetus with congenital hydronephrosis. J Pediatr Surg 1982;17(6): 728–742.
163. Cameron D, Lupton BA, Farquharson D, Hiruki TP: Amnioinfusions in renal agenesis. Obstet Gynecol 1994;83(5 Pt 2):872–876.
164. Kilpatrick SJ, Safford KL: Maternal hydration increases amniotic fluid index in women with normal amniotic fluid. Obstet Gynecol 1993;81(1):49–52.
165. Hofmeyr GJ, Gulmezoglu AM: Maternal hydration for increasing amniotic fluid volume in oligohydramnios and normal amniotic fluid volume. Cochrane Database Syst Rev 2002(1): CD000134.
166. Fait G, Pauzner D, Gull I, et al: Effect of 1 week of oral hydration on the amniotic fluid index. J Reprod Med 2003;48(3): 187–190.
167. Quintero RA, Morales WJ, Allen M, et al: Treatment of iatrogenic previable premature rupture of membranes with intra-amniotic injection of platelets and cryoprecipitate (amniopatch): Preliminary experience. Am J Obstet Gynecol 1999;181(3): 744–749.
168. Quintero RA: New horizons in the treatment of preterm premature rupture of membranes. Clin Perinatol 2001;28(4):861–875.
169. Quintero RA, Morales WJ, Kalter CS, et al: Transabdominal intra-amniotic endoscopic assessment of previable premature rupture of membranes. Am J Obstet Gynecol 1998;179(1): 71–76.
170. Elder JS, Duckett J Jr, Snyder HM: Intervention for fetal obstructive uropathy: Has it been effective? Lancet 1987;2(8566):1007–1010.
171. Coplen DE: Prenatal intervention for hydronephrosis. J Urol 1997;157(6):2270–2207.

172. Freedman AL, Johnson MP, Smith CA, et al: Long-term outcome in children after antenatal intervention for obstructive uropathies. Lancet 1999;354(9176):374–377.
173. McLorie G, Farhat W, Khoury A, et al: Outcome analysis of vesicoamniotic shunting in a comprehensive population. J Urol 2001;166(3):1036–1040.
174. Holmes N, Harrison MR, Baskin LS: Fetal surgery for posterior urethral valves: Long-term postnatal outcomes. Pediatrics 2001;108(1):E7.
175. Welsh A, Agarwal S, Kumar S, et al: Fetal cystoscopy in the management of fetal obstructive uropathy: Experience in a single European centre. Prenat Diagn 2003;23(13):1033–1041.

CHAPTER 14

Fetal Hemolytic Disease

Carl P. Weiner

INTRODUCTION

Hydrops, anemia, and jaundice of the neonate were first recognized in 1932 as a single disease characterized by perinatal hepatosplenomegaly, extramedullary hematopoiesis, and nucleated red blood cells on the peripheral smear.[1] Levine and coworkers identified the cause of the anemia in 1941 when they found rhesus (Rh) antibodies on the red blood cells of affected but not unaffected neonates.[2] Seven years later, Chown proved transplacental fetal to maternal hemorrhage was a cause of maternal isoimmunization.[3] In 1961, hemolytic anemia became the first treatable fetal disease after Liley characterized its natural history and then successfully transfused ill fetuses intraperitoneally with adult red blood cells.[4,5] Freda and colleagues demonstrated in 1964 that passive immunization of Rh– individuals with Rh+ antibodies prior to purposeful exposure to Rh+ red blood cells prevented immunization.[6] In 1981, Rodeck and associates achieved a high survival rate for hydropic fetuses using intravascular transfusion.[7] And in 2000, Mari and coworkers demonstrated that the majority of moderately to severely anemic fetuses could be identified noninvasively by the measurement of the middle cerebral artery peak velocity.[8] Despite these landmark advances, fetal hemolytic disease remains a serious and common cause of perinatal illness and death.

INCIDENCE

Though antibodies to D antigen remain most common, the development of immunoprophylaxis has diminished its relative importance and enhanced that of the other antigen groups (Table 14–1). Yet, anti-D antibody remains the prototype for maternal red blood cell alloimmunization and is used for illustration throughout this chapter.

The incidence of Rh– individuals varies by race with a low of 1% in Chinese and Japanese to a high of 100% in the Basques, in whom the mutation likely originated.[9] In North American whites, the incidence of Rh– genotype is 15%, and in blacks it is 7% to 8%. Thus, the incidence of alloimmunization varies greatly among populations. The overall incidence of alloimmunization has declined dramatically over the last decade owing in part to immunoprophylaxis and smaller families.[10]

PATHOPHYSIOLOGY AND RISKS

Maternal red blood cell alloimmunization results from exposure and response to a foreign red blood cell antigen. Transplacental fetal to maternal hemorrhage is the most common cause of alloimmunization. Heterologous blood transfusion is the second most common cause overall, but the most common cause of sensitization to uncommon antigens (see Table 14–1). It is estimated that 75% of women have fetal red blood cells identified on a Kleihauer stained peripheral smear at some time during either pregnancy or delivery.[11] Both the frequency and magnitude of the bleed increase as pregnancy advances: from 3% and 0.03 mL, respectively, in the first trimester, up to 45% and 25 mL in the third trimester. Spontaneous abortion, too, is associated with fetal to maternal hemorrhage, but the incidence is less than 1% and the volume usually under 0.17 mL. In contrast, surgically induced abortion has a 20% to 25% risk of transplacental hemorrhage of a significantly greater volume.

There are three major nomenclatures for the rhesus blood group: Wiener and Wexler, Rosenfield, and Fisher and Race. The latter works best in clinical practice and has been confirmed genetically.[12] Three pairs of closely linked Rh antigens—Cc, Dd, and Ee—are inherited, one from each parent, as two sets of three alleles. An individual may be homozygous or heterozygous for each of the three alleles. The presence or absence of the D antigen site determines whether an individual is Rh+ or Rh–. Because certain combinations are more common than

TABLE 14–1

Antigens Causing Fetal Hemolytic Disease Requiring Treatment

Common
- rhesus family: D, C, E, c, e
- Kell

Uncommon
- JK^a (Kidd)
- Fy^a (Duffy)
- $Kp^{a \text{ or } b}$
- k
- S

Rare
- Do^a $Di^{a \text{ or } b}$, Fy^b, Hutch, Jk^b Lu^a M, N, s, U, yt

Never
- $Le^{a \text{ or } b}$, p

others, the D genotype can be predicted from the phenotype obtained using antibody specific sera for D, C, c, E, and e (Table 14–2). The d antigen has never been detected, and its existence is questionable. The genes for all other Rh alleles are sequenced, and the genotype can be determined directly using polymerase chain reaction (PCR) technology.

The Rh blood group includes more than 40 other antigens, of which the Du variant is most common. There are more than 16 recognized epitopes. The first (and most common) type is the Du+ variant. Here, the patient is actually Rh+, but the D expression is weakened by the presence of a C allele on the complementary chromosome (e.g., Cde/cDe). These women are not at risk for D alloimmunization. The second type is sometimes termed Du–. Here, part of the D antigen is missing. As such, these women are at risk for D alloimmunization and should receive immunoprophylaxis when otherwise indicated.[13]

The primary immune response to the D antigen occurs over 6 weeks to 12 months. It is usually weak, consisting predominantly of IgM that does not cross the placenta. As a result, the first pregnancy is not typically at great risk. Fifteen percent of Rh– volunteers will become sensitized after a 1 mL exposure of Rh+ erythrocytes. The proportion increases to 30% after 40 mL and 65% after 250 mL. Three percent of women with uncomplicated pregnancies become sensitized at delivery after a small amount of fetal to maternal hemorrhage (0.1 mL). A second antigen challenge generates an amnestic response that is both rapid and almost exclusively IgG. Bowman[14] observed that the longer the interval between challenges, the greater the increase in both the quantity of antibody and the avidity that it binds the red blood cell. These features increase the risk of severe fetal disease.

Fetal hematopoiesis consists of three overlapping phases corresponding to the major hematopoietic organ: mesoblastic, hepatic, and myeloid. Erythropoiesis begins in the fetal yolk sac by day 21, then moves to the liver, and finally reaches the bone marrow by 16 weeks' gestation.[15] The decreasing contribution of the liver is characterized by an exponential decrease in the number of circulating erythroblasts. Contrary to ABO antigens, which are weakly expressed on fetal red blood cells, the Rh antigens are well developed by day 30 of gestation. Anti-D antibody-triggered hemolysis is not complement mediated. Rather, the anti-D-coated fetal red blood cells are destroyed extravascularly by the reticuloendothelial system at a rate faster than normal. The response of the affected fetus is quite variable, reflecting the quantity and subclass of IgG antibody, the efficiency of placental passage, the avidity the antibody binds the antigen site, the maternal HLA make-up, the maturity and efficiency of

TABLE 14–2

Prediction of Rh (D) Zygosity based on Phenotype

PHENOTYPE	GENOTYPE	FREQUENCY (%)		WHITES – ZYGOSITY (%)		BLACKS–ZYGOSITY (%)	
CDE	CDE	WHITES	BLACKS	HOMO-	HETERO-	HOMO-	HETERO-
CcDe	*CDe/cde*	31.1	8.8				
	CDe/cDe	3.4	15.0	10	90	59	41
	CDe/cDe	0.2	1.8				
CDe	*CDe/CDe*	17.6	2.9	91	9	81	19
	CDe/Cde	1.7	0.7				
cDEe	*cDe/cde*	10.4	5.7	10	90	63	37
	cDe/cDe	1.1	9.7				
cDe	*CDE/cDE*	2.0	1.2	87	13	99	1
	cDE/cdE	0.3	<0.1				
CcDEe	*CDe/cDE*	11.8	3.7				
	CDe/cdE	0.8	<0.1	89	11	90	10
	Cde/cDE	0.6	0.4				
cDe	*cDe/cde*	3.0	22.9	6	94	46	54
	cDe/cDe	0.2	19.4				

Modified from Mourant AE, Kopec AC, Domaniewska-Sobazak K: The Distribution of Human Blood Groups and Other Polymorphisms, 2nd ed. London, Oxford University Press, 1976, pp 351–505.

the reticuloendothelial system, and perhaps even the fetal sex.[16] For example, IgG1 and IgG3 appear to be the important subclasses for fetal hemolytic disease, and the maternal to fetal placental transport of IgG3 is significantly greater in pregnancies at risk for hemolytic disease.[17] Further, there is a strong correlation between HLA-DQB1 allele *0201 and both an indirect Coombs titer greater than 512 and fetal anemia.[18]

Hemolytic anemia may occur whenever the erythrocyte lifespan declines below 70 to 90 days and the hematopoietic system can no longer meet the demands. Anemia may develop slowly over several months in association with a gestationally low reticulocyte count and a gestationally normal bilirubin, or within a week in association with reticulocytosis and hyperbilirubinemia.[19,20] Significant fetal anemia is associated with increased erythropoietin, but in the absence of labor, the concentrations are lower than those observed in adults with the same hemoglobin deficit (Widness and Weiner, unpublished observation). Erythropoiesis may occur anywhere in the fetal-placental unit. Both the fetal liver and spleen are enlarged secondary to extramedullary hematopoiesis and congestion. Nucleated red blood cell precursors (erythroblasts) are released into the peripheral circulation, hence the term erythroblastosis fetalis. The greater the number of erythroblasts, the greater the likelihood an antenatal transfusion therapy will be necessary.

All fetal sequelae of hemolytic disease relate to the development of anemia. In general, the fetus tolerates mild to moderate anemia well. However, other metabolic alterations develop as the anemia worsens. Because the red blood cell is the principal fetal buffer, a metabolic acidemia with hyperlactatemia occurs in fetuses with extreme anemia.[21] The precise mechanism underlying the development of hydrops is uncertain, but the elements are clear. First, the hemoglobin deficit for gestation must be extreme.[22] Because the hemoglobin concentration rises with advancing gestation, hydrops occurs at higher absolute hemoglobin levels during late compared to early pregnancy and is rare before 20 weeks.

Second, though hepatomegaly could hinder cardiac return or cause portal hypertension, it cannot be the sole cause of hydrops in light of the findings listed here. Nor is hypoalbuminemia secondary to liver failure a contributing factor, as once thought based on postnatal studies,[23] because the albumin concentration is normal for gestation in all but premoribund, hydropic fetuses.[19,20] Finally, cardiac dysfunction, probably secondary to insufficient oxygen-carrying capacity, occurs in at least 90% of hydropic fetuses. This dysfunction is detectable immediately prior to the development of hydrops and resolves rapidly after transfusion with an increase in the fetal oxygen-carrying capacity. It is characterized by an increase in the biventricular cardiac diameter, systolic atrioventricular valve regurgitation, and an elevated umbilical pressure for gestation[24] (Fig. 14–1*A*). Consistent with ventricular dysfunction, the umbilical venous pressure

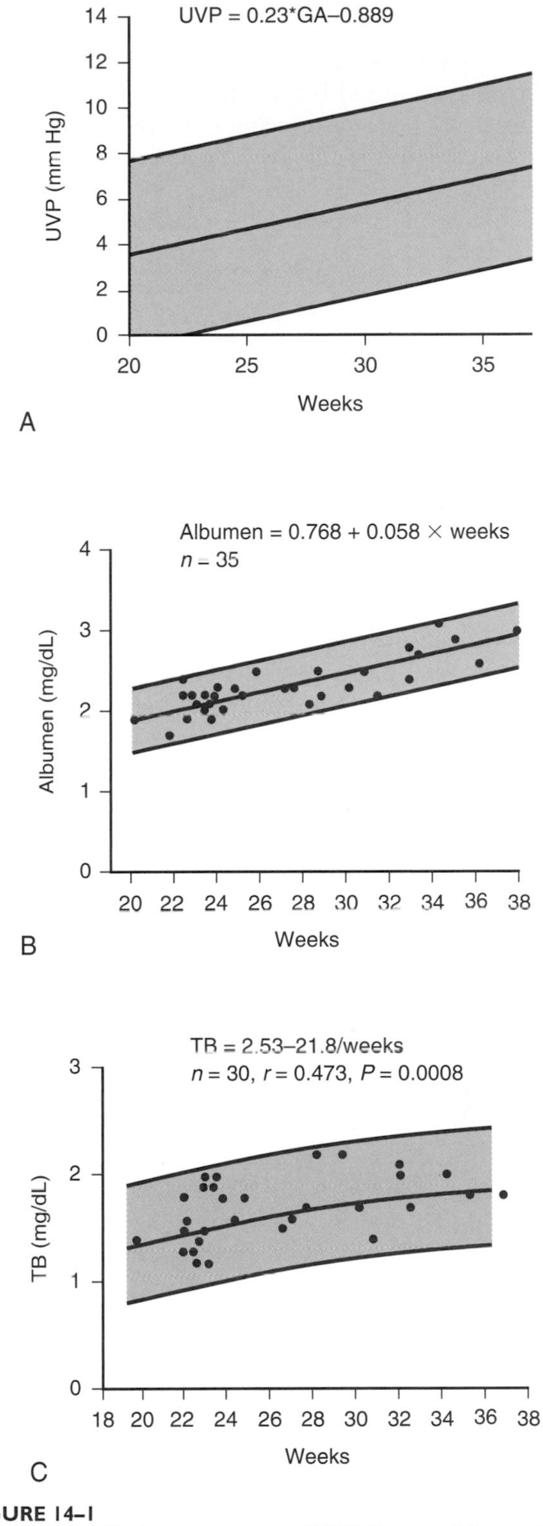

FIGURE 14–1
A, Normal umbilical venous pressure (UVP) (corrected for amniotic fluid pressure) across gestational age (GA) illustrated as the 95% prediction interval. (From Weiner CP, Heilskov J, Pelzer G, et al: Normal values for human umbilical venous and amniotic fluid pressures and their alteration by fetal disease. Am J Obstet Gynecol 1989;161:714–717, with permission). *B*, Normal fetal serum albumin concentration across gestation illustrated as the 95% prediction interval. (From Weiner CP, Heilskov J, Pelzer G, et al: Normal values for human umbilical venous and amniotic fluid pressures and their alteration by fetal disease. Am J Obstet Gynecol 1989;161:714–717, with permission). *C*, Normal fetal serum total bilirubin (TB) across gestation illustrated as the 95% prediction interval.

rises to a greater extent in the hydropic fetus after intravascular transfusion compared to nonhydropic fetus.[25,26] Within 48 hours of the first red blood cell (RBC) transfusion and before the hydrops resolves, the umbilical venous pressure declines into the normal range. This reversal is too rapid for the occurrence of hydrops to be explained solely by hepatosplenomegaly. Thus, cardiac dysfunction is probably the immediate cause of immune hydrops.

Hyperbilirubinemia secondary to erythrocyte hemolysis is an important part of alloimmune hemolytic disease. Heme pigment is first converted into biliverdin by heme oxygenase and then to a water-insoluble, lipid-soluble bilirubin (the indirect fraction) by biliverdin reductase. Both the fetus and neonate have reduced levels of glucuronyl transferase, the enzyme necessary for the production of the water-soluble diglucuronide. Indirect bilirubin unbound to albumin penetrates the lipid neuronal membrane, causing cell death. During normal pregnancy, both the fetal serum albumin and bilirubin concentrations rise linearly with advancing gestation (Fig. 14–1*B* and *C*).[20,27] Virtually all fetal bilirubin under normal and hemolytic conditions is indirect bilirubin; there is no need routinely to fractionate it. The normal fetal total bilirubin is 5 to 10 times above normal adult levels, suggesting placental bilirubin transport is limited. Bilirubin rises progressively as the severity of hemolysis increases. The total bilirubin concentration in fetuses with hemolytic disease often exceeds 3 mg/dL before the development of anemia.[20]

The neonate with severe hyperbilirubinemia is at risk to develop an encephalopathy (kernicterus). The concentration of bilirubin necessary to cause kernicterus also rises with advancing gestational age. Thus, whereas a term neonate can tolerate a total bilirubin of 25 mg/dL, the extremely preterm neonate is at risk for kernicterus when the total bilirubin level exceeds 12 mg/dL. Affected neonates are initially lethargic and then become hypertonic, lying with their neck hyperextended, their back arched, and their knees, wrists, and elbows flexed. They suck poorly and ultimately develop apneic episodes. Fortunately, bilirubin toxicity is rarely observed with current monitoring protocols and treatment. Neural tissue in the auditory center is particularly sensitive to indirect bilirubin. Survivors often have profound neurosensory deafness and choreoathetoid spastic cerebral palsy. When severe signs of toxicity are present, the mortality rate approximates 90%.

MANAGEMENT OPTIONS FOR THE DETECTION OF ALLOIMMUNIZATION

The identification and management of potential fetal hemolytic disease employs several methods for the detection of antibodies either in the maternal serum or bound to the fetal red blood cell.

Agglutination Tests

Saline

Rh+ red blood cells suspended in saline agglutinate when serum added to the slide contains IgM but not IgG. IgM does not cross the placenta.

Colloid

Rh+ red blood cells suspended in a colloid medium such as bovine albumin agglutinate if serum containing either IgM or IgG is added to the slide. Thus, if both saline and colloid tests are positive, the antibody may be either an IgM or an IgG. Pretreating the serum with dithiothreitol disrupts the sulfhydryl bonds of IgM and prevents its binding to the red blood cell. IgG is unaffected by dithiothreitol.

Antiglobulin or Coombs Tests

INDIRECT

Red blood cells of specific or mixed antigen type are incubated with the patient's serum. The addition of antihuman antiglobulin causes agglutination if the red blood cells adsorb antibody from the patient's serum. The reciprocal of the highest dilution that causes agglutination is the titer. Indirect antiglobulin titers are one to three times more sensitive for the detection of RBC alloimmunization than colloid agglutination.

DIRECT

Antihuman antiglobulin is added directly to the red blood cells from the patient. Agglutination indicates antibody is bound to the red blood cell. It may be eluted off and identified by performing an indirect test using type-specific antigen type cells.

ENZYME PRETREATMENT

Red blood cells are incubated with either a proteinase-like trypsin or with bromelin to reduce the negative electric potential between cells. Treated cells lie closer together in saline and more readily agglutinate by the IgG bound to them. These are the most sensitive manual methods for the detection of RBC alloimmunization. The technique can be automated, permitting detection of microgram quantities of antibody.[28] Unfortunately, the automated techniques also produce false-positive tests and as a result are not widely used.

Other Serum Tests

Two other tests have been suggested—the Marsh Score and the Monocyte Monolayer assay. Neither in comparative study performs significantly better than the Coombs titers.[29,30] Preliminary study with monocyte-mediated chemiluminescence suggested it may be advantageous for antibody quantification,[31] but the technique has not been pursued further.

MANAGEMENT OPTIONS FOR THE RH-NEGATIVE PATIENT IN PREGANCY

All women, regardless of past medical and obstetric history, should have on record at least two blood type determinations that are in agreement. Typically, blood is drawn in nulliparous women for the determination of her ABO and Rh blood type during the first prenatal visit and after delivery. All pregnant women should have a red blood cell antibody screen (both indirect and direct Coombs tests) performed at booking. This includes women previously typed as Rh– or found to have a negative antibody screen. Laboratory errors remain a significant contributing cause of anti-D prophylaxis failure. Further, almost 50% of patients managed by the author since 1983 have an RBC antibody directed against an antigen other than D.[19] Although there is controversy on how Rh+ women can be cost-effectively managed after an initial negative screen, the most complete approach is to repeat the antibody screen at 32 weeks in search of newly developed non-anti-D antibodies.

Nonsensitized Rh-Negative Women

Ideally, the indirect Coombs test is repeated monthly beginning at 18 to 20 weeks in at-risk Rh– women without evidence of sensitization. For financial and practical reasons, many units screen for new alloimmunization far less frequently. In some societies, it may be reasonable to test the father, and if he is Rh–, repeat the screen only once between 32 and 34 weeks' gestation. However, paternity is on occasion other than claimed or simply unknown. If the father is tested, the patient should be informed in private of the potential risk for management error should paternity be other than that stated. The decision how to approach paternity is best left to the physician's discretion.

Maternal-fetal ABO incompatibility reduces the risk of D alloimmunization.[14] If the father is heterozygous Rh+, there is a 50% chance the fetus will be Rh–. If the father is also ABO incompatible with the mother, there is a 60% chance that the fetus will be ABO incompatible. If the fetus is both Rh+ and ABO incompatible with the mother ($0.5 \times 0.6 = 0.3\%$ probability), than the risk of maternal Rh alloimmunization is reduced from approximately 16% to 2%.

Successful passive immunization for Rh factor isoimmunization with anti-D immunoglobulin was first achieved in 1964. The Food and Drug Administration approved its use in 1968 after confirming efficacy in male prisoners. Anti-D immunoglobulin is extracted by cold alcohol fractionation from the sera of individuals with high titers. This extraction process removes viral pathogens such as HIV and hepatitis B, and an infectious risk from anti-D immunoglobulin has not been substantiated. Anti-D immunoglobulin binds D antigen sites on fetal erythrocytes present in the maternal circulation. Presumably, blockade of these sites prevents immune recognition by B lymphocytes, and the transformation of activated B lymphocytes to IgG-producing plasma cells never occurs. Anti-D immunoglobulin has a half-life of 24 days, and a standard 300-μg dose provides 12 weeks of protection against exposure to up to 30 mL of blood, or 15 mL of erythrocytes. Before the introduction of anti-D immunoglobulin, 10% of susceptible pregnancies developed hemolytic disease of the fetus and newborn. Approximately 90% of these were due to fetomaternal hemorrhage at term. Administration of anti-D immunoglobulin within 72 hours of delivery reduces this incidence by 90%. The administration of an additional dose at 28 weeks produces a further decline in incidence from 2% to 0.1%. Although the 72-hour limit is based on the original study protocol evaluating the efficacy of anti-D immunoglobulin, beneficial effects may still be present with administration up to 28 days after delivery.

Current guidelines for management of Rh– women with uncomplicated pregnancy are focused on the prevention of isoimmunization from physiologic fetomaternal hemorrhage (Table 14–3). If a patient is Rh– and the antibody screen is negative on the first prenatal visit, the screen is repeated at 28 weeks and anti-D immunoglobulin administered if negative. Another antibody screen is repeated in labor. If the father is Rh– and there is no question on paternity, the prophylactic doses of anti-D immunoglobulin can be omitted.

Women with vaginal bleeding of unknown origin should receive anti-D immunoglobulin prophylaxis (see Table 14–3). Routine antenatal anti-D immunoglobulin therapy is cost effective and should be administered to all nonsensitized Rh– women at 28 weeks' gestation.[32] Anti-D immunoglobulin is also administered after amniocentesis if the fetal Rh genotype is unknown, as it carries a 2% risk of maternal sensitization even when performed under ultrasound guidance.[33] Umbilical cord blood is obtained at delivery from Rh– women to determine the neonatal ABO and Rh blood type and to seek red blood cell bound antibodies. Anti-D immunoglobulin (300 mg) prevents maternal sensitization secondary to fetal-maternal hemorrhage when the volume is less than 30 mL of Rh+ blood.[34,35] Maternal blood is screened by Kleihauer testing for evidence of a fetal-maternal hemorrhage in excess of 30 mL. This test exploits the relative resistance of fetal hemoglobin to acid denaturation. Acid citrate buffer is used to remove adult hemoglobin, leaving red blood cell ghosts. The maternal blood is examined on a counting chamber after fixation with 80% ethanol and hematoxylin-eosin staining. The amount of fetal blood in the maternal circulation can be

TABLE 14-3

Preventive Guidelines for Rh– Women in Pregnancy

TIME	TEST	ANTI-D-IG DOSE
First prenatal visit	ABO and Rh blood typing, direct and indirect Coombs test	None
28–29 wk	Direct and indirect Coombs test for newly developed antibodies	300 μg*
32 wk	Direct and indirect Coombs test for newly developed antibodies	None
At birth	Neonatal cord blood for ABO and Rh type as well as direct Coombs test for red blood cell bound antibodies	
Within 72 hr of delivery	Rosette test, Kleihauer-Betke estimate of fetoplacental hemorrhage	300 μg (individualize for Kleihauer-Betke result)
First trimester spontaneous miscarriage		50–200 μg
First trimester therapeutic abortion		300 μg
Following prenatal diagnosis by chorionic villous sampling of amniocentesis		300 μg
Other high risk situations—abdominal trauma, placental abruption, antepartum hemorrhage	Rosette test, Kleihauer-Betke estimate of fetoplacental hemorrhage	300 μg (individualize for Kleihauer-Betke result)

* Some protocols recommend the use of a lower dose of anti-D Ig at 28 weeks followed by a further dose at 34 weeks in nonimmunized Rh– women.
Anti-D Ig, anti-D immunoglobulin.

approximated from the number of fetal red blood cells per grid using this formula: fetal cells/number of maternal cells = estimated blood loss/estimated maternal blood volume in milliliters (85 mL/kg). About 1/400 women suffer a larger bleed and require more anti-D immunoglobulin.[35] Cesarean section and manual removal of the placenta each increase the risk and magnitude of fetal-maternal hemorrhage. In situations in which the estimated bleed exceeds 30 mL, 150% to 200% of the estimated anti-D immunoglobulin requirement is given.

Postpartum, anti-D immunoglobulin may be withheld if the last administration was given less than 21 days previously and passively acquired antibodies are still demonstrable on the antibody screen. The rosette test may also be performed in maternal blood to assess the need for further administration of anti-D immunoglobulin. Rosette formation indicates the presence of fetal red blood cells, and dosage of anti-D immunoglobulin may have to be adjusted, guided by the Kleihauer-Betke test.

Rh-Negative Sensitized Women

Noninvasive Evaluation

Once an alloimmunized woman is identified, the medical professional caring for the mother must make some estimate of the risk of fetal disease. The prediction of fetal risk by combining the maternal obstetric history and serologic examination is an imprecise art. The magnitude of fetal and neonatal disease typically progresses from one pregnancy to another. The risk of hydrops in the undiagnosed and untested pregnancy approximates 10% in the first sensitized pregnancy.[14]

If maternal indirect Coombs antibody titers are performed in the same hospital using constant techniques, the results are both reproducible and of clinical value in predicting the risk of severe fetal disease. In every laboratory, there is a titer below which severe fetal hemolytic disease does not occur. The practitioner must be familiar with the laboratory's threshold to avoid clinical error. When the maternal titer is below that threshold, it should be repeated at monthly intervals. In the absence of a relevant clinical history, the fetus may be followed noninvasively by the measurement of the peak middle cerebral artery velocities once that critical titer is exceeded. The utility of antibody titers above the threshold in predicting fetal risk is greatest during the first sensitized pregnancy. In subsequent pregnancies, titer and history are inadequate measures upon which to base management. Bowman reported in 1965 a lethal management error would occur in a third of severely sensitized fetuses if only maternal obstetric history and antibody titer were relied upon.[36]

One of the most important advances in the management of fetal hemolytic anemia over the last 5 years is the development and application of molecular tools to determine the fetal genotype for most of the offending RBC antigens. It is possible using polymerase chain reaction (PCR) to rapidly determine from either amniocytes or a placental biopsy specimen the fetal antigen status.[37–41] Determination of the fetal Rh genotype should be standard after any second trimester amniocentesis or chorionic villus sampling (CVS) in an at-risk woman. Though genetic heterogeneity can be problematic, the technique is as accurate as serologic testing.[42] A negative finding obviates the need for further follow-up. More exciting for Rh– women sensitized only to D for the future is the ability to determine fetal D status from fetal DNA extracted from the maternal blood. Sensitivities in excess of one-third are reported.[43]

Anticipation of the disease onset or ultrasound evidence of fetal anemia determines the timing of invasive fetal testing. The approach depends on the number of previously affected pregnancies. Brass and colleagues first observed in adults a relationship between the systolic flow velocity in the middle cerebral artery and hematocrit.[44] Subsequently, several investigators demonstrated that the development of fetal anemia is associated with increased middle cerebral artery peak systolic velocities (Fig. 14–2).[45–47] Though we found that at least half of anemic fetuses have normal peak velocities,[48] high peaks corrected for gestational age typically indicate anemia.

Other sonographic findings have been claimed to either precede the development of hydrops or predict fetal anemia, including amniotic fluid volume, liver and spleen length or thickness, placental thickness, increased bowel echogenicity, and the cardiac biventricular diameter.[21,49,50] Unfortunately, none of these sonographic markers has proved reliable. Further, the fetal hematocrit may change rapidly. We have observed fetuses with a normal hematocrit become hydropic over a 7-day period without a change in the maternal antibody titer. Each had a completely normal two-dimensional ultrasonographic examination 7 days before the detection of hydrops.

In summary, the measurement of middle cerebral artery peak velocities is an excellent noninvasive tool for the monitoring of fetal anemia. Other than that, ultrasonography is an adjunct to, not a replacement for, invasive fetal studies.

Invasive Evaluation

Two invasive methods are used to search for fetal anemia secondary to hemolytic disease:

- Indirect: spectrophotometry (the ΔOD450) using a specimen of amniotic fluid obtained by ultrasound-guided amniocentesis.
- Direct: fetal blood studies using a sample obtained by cordocentesis.

Each method has advantages and disadvantages, proponents and opponents. The method selected should reflect the facilities available and the physician's experience. Because the incidence of maternal alloimmunization is declining, so is the number of physicians experienced with its management. The author concurs with Craig, who opined that these services should be centralized.[51] The alloimmunized patient should be referred either to a fetal medicine specialist or to the individual in the geographic locale with the greatest experience in managing fetal hemolytic disease once RBC alloimmunization is confirmed.

AMNIOTIC FLUID SPECTROPHOTOMETRY

The fetus with hemolytic anemia frequently has an elevated serum bilirubin (Fig. 14–3).[20] By the middle of the second trimester, the amniotic fluid consists predominantly of fetal urine and tracheopulmonary effluent; thus, the amniotic fluid bilirubin is also elevated. Although William Liley was not the first to use amniotic fluid spectrophotometry for the management of rhesus disease, he standardized an approach that has remained essentially unchanged since first reported in 1961.[4] Although the ΔOD450 satisfactorily predicts the

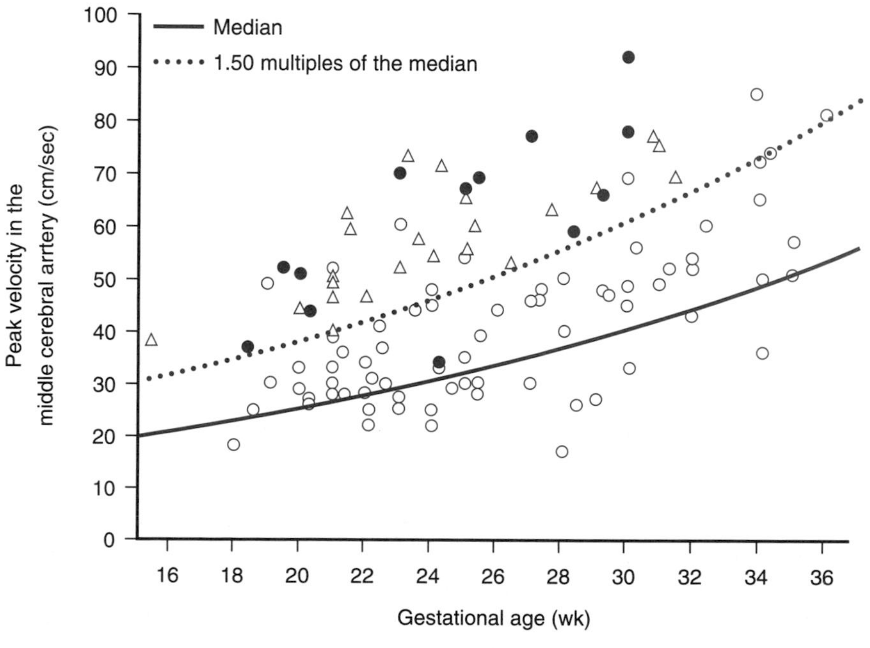

FIGURE 14–2
Peak velocity of systolic blood flow in the middle cerebral artery in 111 fetuses at risk for anemia due to maternal red-cell alloimmunization. Open circles indicate fetuses with either no anemia or mild anemia (≥0.65 multiples of the median hemoglobin concentration). Triangles indicate fetuses with moderate or severe anemia (<0.65 multiples of the median hemoglobin concentration). The solid circles indicate the fetuses with hydrops. The solid curve indicates the median peak systolic velocity in the middle cerebral artery, and the dotted curve indicates 1.5 multiples of the median. (From Mari G, Deter RL, Carpenter RL, et al: Noninvasive diagnosis by Doppler ultrasonography of fetal anemia due to maternal red-cell alloimmunization. Collaborative Group for Doppler Assessment of the Blood Velocity in Anemic Fetuses. N Engl J Med 2000;342(1):9–14.)

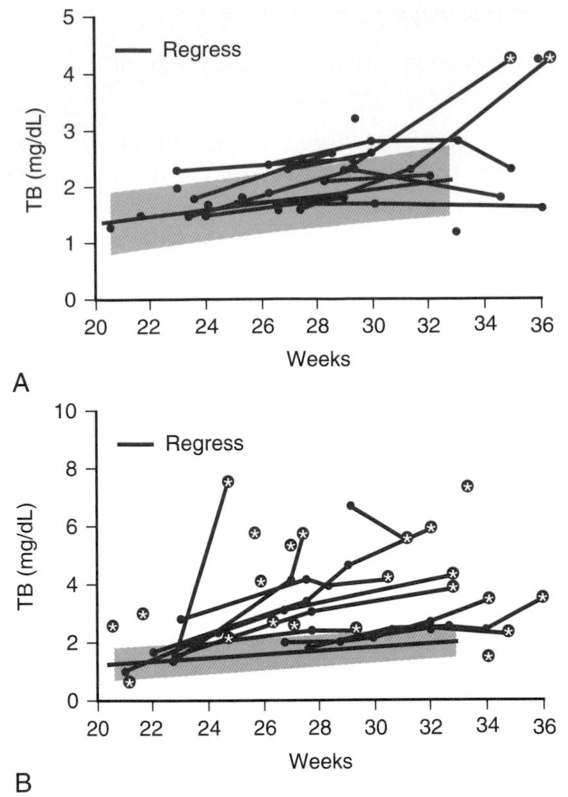

FIGURE 14–3
Effect of hemolytic disease on the fetal total bilirubin (TB) concentration comparing fetuses who do not (*A*) to those who do (*B*) develop anemia. *indicates at which point a hematocrit below 30% was first discovered. (From Weiner CP, Williamson RA, Wenstrom KD, et al: Management of fetal hemolytic disease by cordocentesis: I. Prediction of fetal anemia. Am J Obstet Gynecol 1991;165:546–553.)

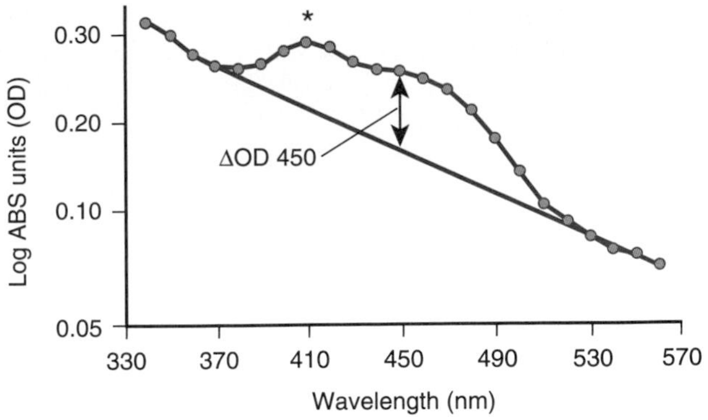

FIGURE 14–4
Semilogarithmic plot of an amniotic fluid ΔOD450. *illustrates a spike in the absorption of light produced by contaminating blood. (Courtesy of G. Snyder, University of Iowa.)

relative fetal hematocrit when used appropriately, it is best at predicting hydrops.

The principal advantage of amniocentesis is that most obstetricians are familiar with the technique and find it simple. Amniotic fluid is obtained by ultrasound-guided amniocentesis (see Chapter 10), transported to the laboratory in a light-resistant container to prevent degradation of bilirubin, centrifuged, and filtered. If the fetal blood type is unknown, an aliquot of the sample should be subjected to PCR to confirm the fetal genotype is antigen positive.

The optical density (OD) is measured between 700 and 350 nm and plotted on semilogarithmic graph paper with the wavelength on the *x*-axis. A line parallel to the *y*-axis is drawn through 450 nm, and the deviation from linearity of the absorption trace measured at that point. The result is plotted on semilogarithmic paper with gestational age on the *x*-axis and the ΔOD450 on the *y*-axis (Fig. 14–4). Based on the study of 101 amniotic fluid specimens obtained between 28 and 35 weeks' gestation, Liley observed that the ΔOD450 normally declines with advancing gestation (the opposite direction of the fetal serum bilirubin concentration) (Fig. 14–5).[4] The graph is divided into three ascending zones. Zone 1 represents mild or no fetal disease. Zone 3 indicates severe disease with the possibility of hydrops developing within 7 days. Zone 2 is intermediate, with the disease severity increasing as zone 3 is approached. Amniocentesis is repeated at 1-to 2-week intervals, depending on the gestational age, the zone of the ΔOD450, and the change from the preceding sample. Management is dictated by the trend revealed by serial values. A fetal blood sample is considered when either the ΔOD450 is in zone 3 or serial amniotic fluid specimens reveal a progressive and rapid rise of the ΔOD450 into the upper 80% of zone 2. Based on that result, the decision is made for either transfusion or delivery.

The determination of hemolytic disease severity by amniotic fluid spectrophotometry has several important disadvantages. First, its application requires serial invasive procedures over the space of several weeks. In a 20-year experience that included 1027 women, Bowman and associates[14] performed a mean of 3.1 procedures per patient. Each procedure carries a risk of enhanced maternal sensitization, as well as a loss from either amnionitis or premature rupture of the membranes. Though there are no large series reported of women undergoing amniocentesis after 22 weeks' gestation to document the frequency of such complications, some conclusions may be drawn from studies of second trimester genetic amniocenteses. Amniocentesis performed under ultrasound guidance is clearly associated with sensitization, amnionitis, and rupture of membranes (in our experience approximately 1 in 300). Simplicity of a procedure is not synonymous with safety.

Second, amniotic fluid spectrophotometry is an indirect test for fetal anemia. The natural history studies by Liley revealed a wide range of disease severity for a given ΔOD450 at any gestational age between 28 and 34 weeks (see Fig. 14–5).[4,5] Liley's postnatal observation is confirmed antenatally using cordocentesis. Though most obvious for zone 2, it is also true for zone 3 measurements. In a series of 11 fetuses with a ΔOD450 in zone 3 followed for several weeks, 30% had a clinically accept-

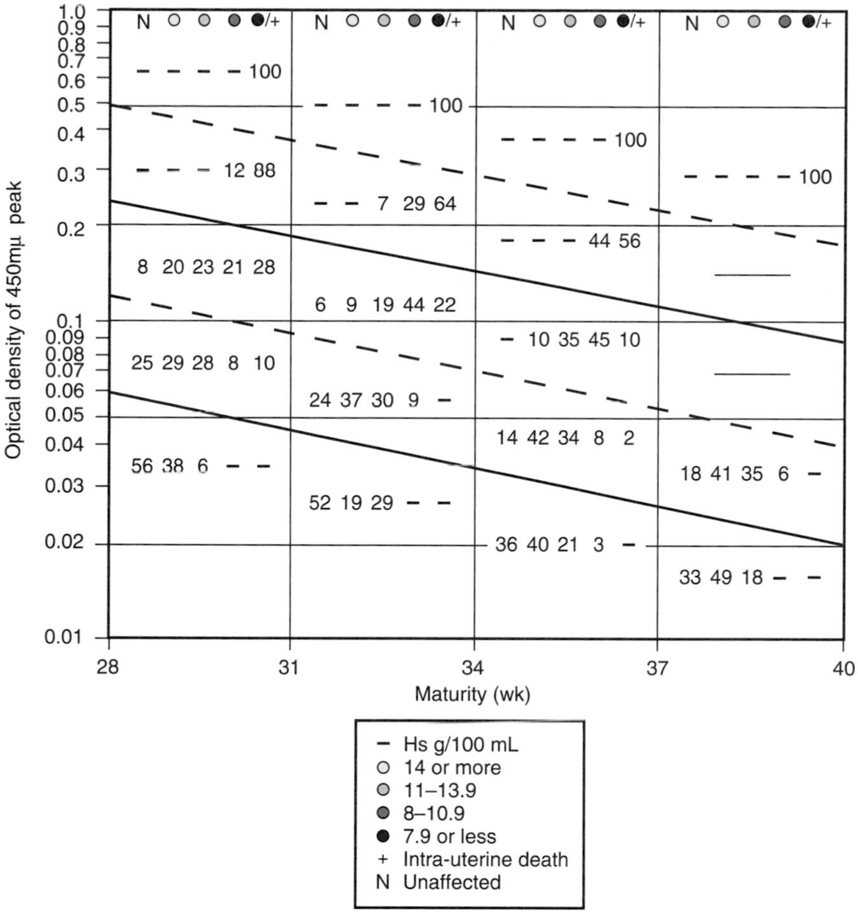

FIGURE 14–5
Relationship between the ΔOD450, hemoglobin, and gestational age. Note, for example, that of fetuses between 28 and 31 weeks and a ΔOD450 in low zone 2, 25% are unaffected, whereas 18% are either profoundly anemic or dead. (From Liley AW: Liquor amnii analysis and management of pregnancy complicated by rhesus immunization. Am J Obstet Gynecol 1961;82:1359–1368.)

able hematocrit at birth.[52] Gottval and Hilden[53] concluded that the maternal indirect Coombs titer was actually superior to the ΔOD450 for the prediction of fetal anemia, and yet the titers were useful only when less than 32 or more than 1000. Bowman opined that the "experience and judgment of the individual assessing the amniotic fluid findings were more important than the method used."[14] Yet, in their almost unparalleled experience, 9% of the predictions based on a zone 2 ΔOD450 (which comprised almost 50% of the measurements) were erroneous. Few clinicians in this era of anti-D immunoglobulin prophylaxis have a comparable breadth of experience with amniotic fluid spectrophotometry.

The third disadvantage of amniocentesis and the ΔOD450 is that the system was modeled on anti-D alloimmunization. This author and others[54–56] have shown that Kell alloimmunization has salient pathophysiologic differences that account for the very poor performance of the ΔOD450 reported in the past.[57] Fetuses with Kell alloimmunization have lower serum bilirubin concentrations, and lower reticulocyte levels for their degree of anemia compared to D-alloimmunized fetuses. Vaughan and associates[58] found that monoclonal IgG and IgM anti-Kell antibodies inhibit the growth of Kell-positive erythroid burst-forming units and colony-forming units in a dose-dependent fashion. This suggests that the fetal anemia secondary to Kell reflects erythroid suppression at the progenitor cell level.

The fourth disadvantage of amniocentesis is that the normal ΔOD450 in the second trimester is mid zone 2 of the Liley curve. Some have concluded that there is no clinically useful correlation between the ΔOD450 reading and the fetal hemoglobin before 28 weeks.[59] Yet, amniocentesis is often initiated weeks earlier. Experienced practitioners rely, in this situation, on the trend of several amniocenteses or the finding of an extraordinarily high ΔOD450 value (e.g., >0.400). Unfortunately, the published experience validating this practice is small.

The fifth disadvantage of the ΔOD450 measurement is that it is subject to a variety of extrinsic errors that can interfere with its laboratory measurement, for example, maternal hyperbilirubinemia and specimen contamination with blood or meconium.

Finally, the correlation between hemoglobin and the peak middle cerebral artery velocity has rendered amniocentesis for the measurement of the ΔOD450 an outdated tool because transfusion therapy should never be initiated without confirming fetal anemia.

FETAL BLOOD SAMPLING

The accuracy of cordocentesis for the evaluation of fetal anemia was never an issue. The concerns were safety (immediate vascular accidents and the longer-term risk of worsening sensitization) and how to decide if and when to repeat the cordocentesis. The safety of cordocentesis is detailed in Chapter 10. The loss rate reflects the indication for the procedure, the presence of hypoxemia, the vessel actually punctured, and the technique used (needle guide versus free hand).[60,61] It has been estimated that technique accounts for at least 30% of losses. Using a needle guide, the loss rate for alloimmunization is less than 0.3%, a rate similar to amniocentesis. Further, the size of the fetal-maternal bleed after cordocentesis when a needle guide is used and the placenta is not punctured is similar to that after amniocentesis.[62] In contrast, the magnitude of the bleed is much greater when the freehand technique is used.

The first cordocentesis is performed either a few weeks before the last sensitized fetus required transfusion, or when the peak middle cerebral artery velocity becomes elevated. Laboratory tests performed on the first and subsequent fetal blood samples are listed in Table 14–4. Either a strongly positive direct Coombs test or a manual reticulocyte count outside the 95% confidence interval (Fig. 14–6) are high risk factors for the development of antenatal anemia if the fetus is not anemic when sampled.

A sensitive and specific assessment of the risk for developing anemia can be made using direct fetal hematologic and serologic tests. A prospectively validated protocol for risk assessment and the timing of any repeat cordocentesis are shown in Table 14–5. There is a direct correlation between the reticulocyte count, the strength of the direct Coombs test, the risk of fetal anemia, and the trimester in which it occurs.[17] Approximately 50% of alloimmunized women require only one cordocentesis (Fig. 14–7). With ultrasonography as a backup, delivery may be safely deferred until 37 to 38 weeks with less than 2% risk of unexpected anemia (only twice in the experience of the author covering more than 400 alloimmunized pregnancies).[63] About 80% of pregnancies requiring more than one cordocentesis ultimately need a fetal transfusion for a hematocrit less than 30%. This protocol predicts antenatal anemia only and not postnatal hyperbilirubinemia. Untreated neonates remain at significant risk for postnatal complications (Table 14–6).[63]

Delivery of the nontransfused fetus is planned between 37 and 38 weeks' gestation in a medical center capable of caring for a neonate with potentially severe hyperbilirubinemia.

Direct testing of the fetus has several advantages over amniotic fluid testing. Both sensitivity and specificity for the diagnosis and the prediction of fetal anemia are much greater than the ΔOD450. Direct testing of the fetus for anemia has a zero false-positive rate and a very low false-negative rate. Fewer invasive procedures are necessary, reducing the overall risk of premature rupture of the membranes, amnionitis, and worsening of sensitization, especially if a needle guide is used.

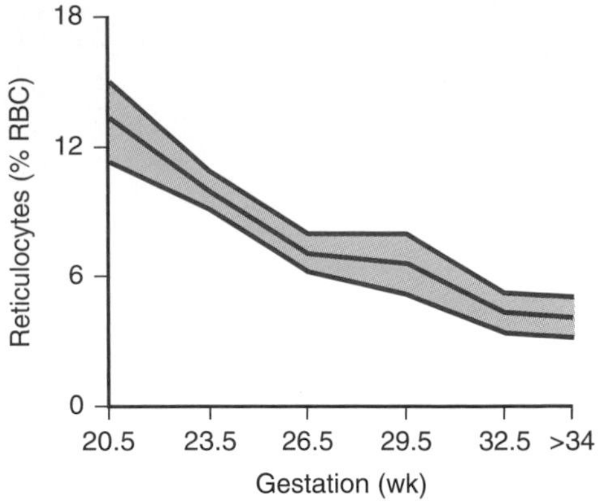

FIGURE 14–6
Normal fetal reticulocyte count across gestation illustrated as the 95% prediction interval. (From Weiner CP, Williamson RA, Wenstrom KD, et al: Management of fetal hemolytic disease by cordocentesis: I. Prediction of fetal anemia. Am J Obstet Gynecol 1991;165:546–553.)

TABLE 14–4

Fetal Hematologic and Serologic Testing for the Prediction of Anemia

First Specimen
ABO and Rh type
Direct Coombs test
Complete blood count (CBC)
Manual reticulocyte count (%RBCs)
Total bilirubin
Subsequent Specimens
Complete blood count (CBC)
Manual reticulocyte count (%RBCs)
Total bilirubin

Treatment Options

SUPPRESSION OF MATERNAL ANTIERYTHROCYTE ANTIBODIES

Several methods are used to suppress or ameliorate either the maternal antibody concentration or its effect on the fetus. None are of documented efficacy, and only two appear to have limited potential.

Plasmapheresis. Although plasmapheresis reduces antibody concentration by as much as 80%,[64] the decline is transient. Current information suggests plasmapheresis may delay the need for fetal transfusion by a few weeks. This costly procedure is indicated only when there is a history of hydrops prior to 20 to 22 weeks and the father is homozygous for the offending antigen. Plasmapheresis is begun at 12 weeks, removing 15 to 20 L

TABLE 14–5

Criteria for Repeat Cordocentesis with Affected Fetus

PATTERN	HEMATOCRIT	RETICULOCYTES	& OR DC	INTERVAL FOR CORDOCENTESIS	SCAN	COMMENTS
1	Normal	Normal	–/tr	–	4-wk interval	Repeat if initial maternal indirect Coombs <128 and twofold increase documented.
2	Normal	Normal or <2.5 per centile	J+/2+	5–6 wk	2-wk interval	Do not repeat after 32 wk if studies unchanged. Delivery at term.
3	Normal	>97.5 percentile	3+/4+	2 wk	1-wk interval	Continue through 34 weeks if hematocrit stable. Deliver at 37–38 wk if not transfused.
4	<2.5 per centile but >30%	Any	Any	1–2 wk	1-wk interval	Repeat as long as hematocrit criteria fulfilled. Deliver with pulmonary maturity if not transfused.

DC, direct Coombs.
Modified from Weiner CP, Heilskov J, Pelzer G, et al: Normal values for human umbilical venous amniotic fluid pressures and their alteration by fetal disease. Am J Obstet Gynecol 1989;161:714–717.

per week. It entails a risk of hepatitis and should not be undertaken lightly.

Immunoglobulin. The maternal intravenous infusion of immunoglobulin (400–500 mg/kg maternal weight every 4 weeks) reportedly reduces the severity of fetal hemolytic disease.[65] There are no prospective randomized trials. Rarely indicated alone in light of the currently available therapies, intravenous immunoglobulin may be effective as an adjunct to plasmapheresis.[66] Another option is to administer the immunoglobulin directly to the infused fetus. Several abstracts suggest that such fetal therapy has the potential to reduce the frequency of transfusion therapy. Yet, the interval between transfusions at those institutions is normally shorter than recommended here.

FETAL TRANSFUSION

Fetal transfusion therapy should not be undertaken in the absence of hydrops without first confirming that the fetus has significant anemia. The author has used a hematocrit below 30% because it is below the 2.5 percentile for all gestational ages greater than 20 weeks (see later discussion under Intravascular Transfusion). These procedures should be performed whenever possible only by individuals with considerable and regular experience, namely 8 to 10 transfusions per year as a minimum.

Intraperitoneal Injection. The original, but now least preferred method for fetal transfusion is the intraperitoneal injection of packed red blood cells. The protocol is shown in Table 14–7. The blood is absorbed via the lymphatic vessels and requires fetal respiration for absorption. Approximately 10% of the transfused cells are absorbed each day by the nonhydropic fetus. Absorption is poor in the hydropic fetus. The volume infused is a compromise between the amount necessary to correct the estimated hemoglobin deficit and the amount that will safely fit into the intra-abdominal cavity. The formula of Bowman is quite practical and recommended:

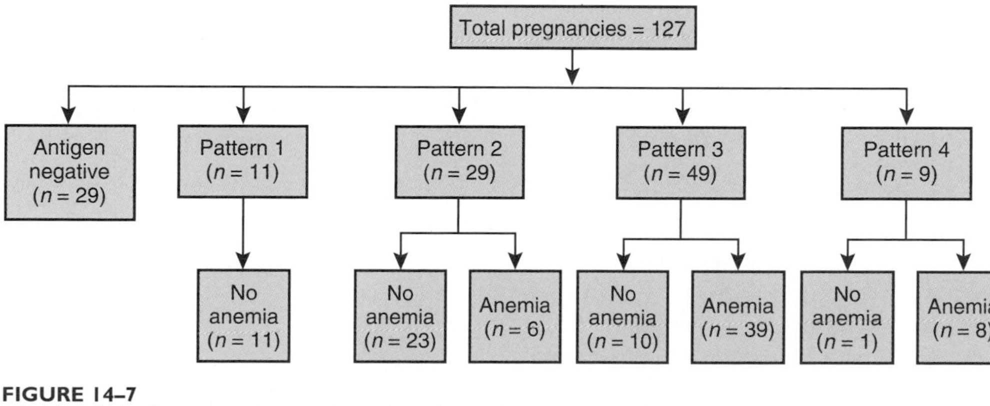

FIGURE 14–7
Likelihood of a fetus requiring transfusion based on its hematologic pattern. (From Weiner CP, Williamson RA, Wenstrom KD, et al: Management of fetal hemolytic disease by cordocentesis: I. Prediction of fetal anemia. Am J Obstet Gynecol 1991;165:546–553.)

TABLE 14-6

Neonatal Complications in Affected, Untreated, Pregnancies

	N	(%)	MEAN	(SD)	RANGE
Gestation (wk)	48	(100)	38	(2)	34–41
Birth weight (g)	48	(100)	3176	(552)	2010–4171
Hematocrit (%)	23	(47)	47	(9)	24–59
Reticulocytes	10	(21)	9.2	(7)	2.8–28
Maximum total bilirubin (mg/dL)	28	(58)	14.9	(5)	5–23
Phototherapy (hr)					
No	17	(36)	–	–	–
Yes	31	(64)	110	(60)	23–240
DVET	8	(17)	–	–	–
Late transfusion*	6	(13)			

DVET, double volume exchange transfusion.
*Late transfusion, performed in the first 3 weeks of life for anemia not present.
Modified from Weiner CP, Grant SS, Hudson J, et al: Effect of diagnostic and therapeutic cordocentesis upon maternal serum alpha fetoprotein concentration. Am J Obstet Gynecol 1989;161:706–708.

$$\text{Volume} = (\text{weeks gestation} - 20) \times 10\text{ mL}$$

Once absorption is complete, the residual hemoglobin concentration may be estimated by the following equation:

$$\text{Residual hemoglobin concentration} = ((0.8x)/(125y)) \times ((120 - z\text{ days})/120\text{ days})$$

where x is the amount of donor blood in grams transfused, y is the estimated fetal weight, z is the interval in days since the last transfusion, and 120 the estimated life (in days) of the transfused blood.

The second transfusion is performed when the first has been completely absorbed and thereafter at 3- to 4-week intervals. If the fetus is hydropic and survives the first intraperitoneal transfusion, the fetal abdomen is drained at the second transfusion to minimize pressure and maximize the amount of fresh packed cells infused. The last transfusion is performed no later than 32 weeks' gestation.

Intraperitoneal transfusion has many drawbacks. In addition to a slow correction of the hemoglobin deficit, there is a higher risk of trauma and the unique risk of obstructing cardiac return should the intra-abdominal pressure rise too high. Intraperitoneal transfusion has no advantage over intravenous transfusion except when percutaneous access to the fetal vasculature is problematic (e.g., prior to 18 weeks). Nor is there any advantage to combining intravascular and intraperitoneal transfusions. The intravascular route already allows routine spacing of 3 to 5 weeks (see later discussion), and a combined transfusion approach does not reduce the actual number of required needle punctures. Further, there is a lower risk of trauma and death for both hydropic and nonhydropic fetuses from the intravascular approach. The highest reported survival rates with intraperitoneal transfusion are well below those for intravascular transfusion[67–69] In a comparison of historical data from an experienced team in Winnipeg, Canada, the risk of death per transfusion was six times that of intravascular transfusion.[69] Intraperitoneal transfusion is rarely indicated in the modern practice of fetal medicine.

Intravascular Transfusion. In contrast to intraperitoneal transfusion, the goal of intravascular transfusion therapy is the delivery of a healthy, nonanemic neonate at term when it can better transition to ex utero life and withstand hyperbilirubinemia. Transfusions are begun

TABLE 14-7

Protocol for Fetal Intraperitonal Transfusion

Preparation

Confirm fetal hematocrit <30%
Prepare donor blood as fresh as possible and compatible with both mother and fetus
Buffy coat poor, washed in saline × 3, and irradiated
Final hematocrit 90% ideal
Prepare two sets of tubing with three-way valves for transfusion; filters are mandatory
Diazepam, 5–10 mg slow IV for maternal comfort
Lateral displacement of the uterus, support lower back
Acetone wipe to remove ultrasound contact gel from the skin
Popovidine or alcohol surgical preparation of the skin
Drape as desired and prepare surgical tray
  20 gauge Tuohy needle 25 cm long
  20 mL syringe
  5 mL normal saline
  gauge spinal needle
  pancuronium, 0.3 mg/kg estimated fetal weight
Sterile prepare ultrasound transducer

Transfusion

Target fetal abdomen between umbilicus and bladder; avoid liver
Administer pancuronium intramuscularly targeting the fetal buttock
Insert Tuohy needle into selected site
Confirm intra-abdominal, extravascular location by injecting saline
Infuse donor blood in 1 mL aliquots over 10 min checking the fetal heart rate after each aliquot
Continue transfusion until planned volume infused calculated by: volume = (wk gestation – 20) × 10 mL

Follow-up

Continuous heart rate monitoring until fetal movement resumes
Document complete absorption of donor blood by serial ultrasonography
Examinations every 2–3 days
Second transfusion after complete absorption; thereafter, repeat at 4-wk intervals

when the fetal hematocrit declines below 30%.[24] Though most fetuses tolerate a hematocrit of 25% or lower without clinically significant sequelae, this cutoff point has proved a pragmatic threshold for the following reasons:

- Hematocrit of 30% is below the 2.5th percentile after 20 weeks' gestation (Fig. 14–8).
- Women referred often travel great distances and cannot come either semiweekly or even weekly without great hardship.
- It is difficult to predict with certainty how fast the fetal hematocrit will decline.
- Treatment of anemia prevents the development of hydrops that would greatly increase the chance of an adverse outcome.

The protocol used for intravascular transfusion is shown in Table 14–8. Blood for the transfusion should be fresh when available, and compatible with both mother and fetus. Infectious agents routinely tested for include cytomegalovirus (CMV), hepatitis A through C, and human immunodeficiency virus. Some blood banks use a lymphocyte filter in lieu of serologic testing for CMV. This procedure has the added benefit of reducing the risk of graft versus host disease without irradiating the blood. The blood is prepared on the day of transfusion, rendered leukocyte poor, and washed several times in saline to remove particles associated with viral transmission infection. It is then resuspended in saline to a hematocrit between 70% and 80%. Blood with a higher hematocrit mixes poorly; that with a lower hematocrit unnecessarily increases the volume required.

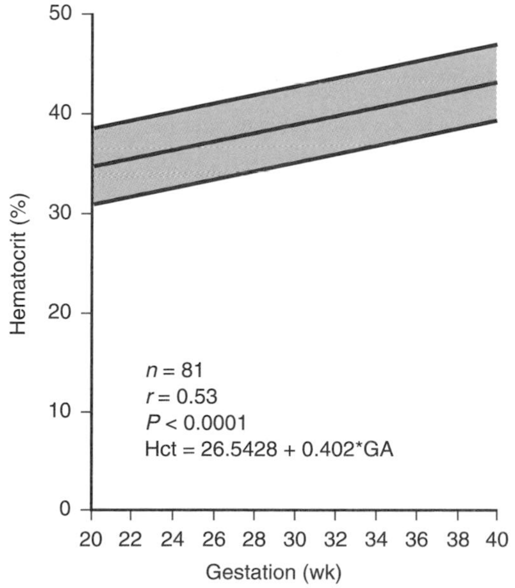

FIGURE 14–8
Normal fetal hematocrit across gestation illustrated as the 95% prediction interval. (From Weiner CP, Williamson RA, Wenstrom KD, et al: Management of fetal hemolytic disease by cordocentesis: I. Prediction of fetal anemia. Am J Obstet Gynecol 1991;165:546–553.)

The patient is made comfortable with pillows under her knees to take pressure off the lower back. The uterus is displaced laterally to avoid supine hypotension during the transfusion. Because the transfusion takes on average 25 to 30 minutes, diazepam 5 to 10 mg IV is given to enhance maternal comfort and cooperation. The abdomen is surgically prepared and draped, and the operator's hands are gloved. Neither a surgical mask nor cap is necessary. Nor is there evidence that prophylactic antibiotic administration is either effective or cost efficient. The skin is the main source of bacterial contamination. The operator must never touch the shaft of the needle. A new needle is used if one must be removed after insertion into the skin. With this protocol, our incidence of amnionitis is less than 0.5%. The skin is infiltrated with 1% lidocaine in light of the duration of time the needle is in situ.

The easiest approach to the umbilical vein is selected; 35% of the author's transfusions are performed in a free

TABLE 14–8

Protocol for Fetal Intravascular Transfusion

Preparation
Confirm fetal hematocrit <30%
Preparation of donor blood as fresh as possible and compatible with both mother and fetus
Buffy coat poor, washed in saline × 3, irradiated
Final hematocrit 70–80%
Preparation two sets of tubing for transfusion and measurement of umbilical venous pressure (UVP)
Filters are mandatory
Diazepam, 5–10 mg slow IV for maternal comfort
Lateral displacement of the uterus, support lower back
Acetone wipe to remove ultrasound contact gel from the skin
Popovidine or alcohol surgical preparation of the skin
Drape as desired and prepare surgical tray
Eight 1-mL tuberculin syringes
Flush three with heparin (100 U/mL); fill one with lidocaine (1%) and fill one with desired dose of pancuronium (0.3 mg/kg sonographically estimated fetal weight)
Three 3-way valves
One 5 22-gauge needle
Three 4 × 4 gauze sponges
Prepare transducer
Transfusion
Puncture vein at most accessible site
Immediately administer pancuronium — paralysis will be rapid
Aspirate 1 mL for complete blood count, Kleihauer stain and reticulocyte count; check hematocrit immediately
Aspirate 1 mL for venous blood gases
Measure pressure and confirm puncture is of umbilical vein
Begin infusion of packed red blood cells after double checking there is no air in the system
Infuse half the estimated requirement (see Table 14–9)
Repeat blood sampling and pressure measurement
Halt transfusion if the rise in the UVP has exceeded 10 mm Hg; check heart rate to rule out bradycardia as an explanation
If UVP acceptable, calculate remaining volume necessary to achieve a hematocrit of 50%; infuse that volume
Repeat blood sampling and pressure measurement; remove needle if UVP at acceptable level
Monitor fetus until spontaneous movement resumes

loop of cord. The vein is punctured with a 22-gauge needle. A larger gauge needle unnecessarily increases the risk of premature rupture of the membranes, and there is no significant hemolysis. Immediately following the free return of blood, the fetus is paralyzed with pancuronium (approximately 0.3 mg/kg of the estimated fetal weight [EFW], range 0.2 to 0.6 mg/kg), regardless of the puncture location because any fetal movement may lacerate the vessel or dislodge the needle. Should the latter occur during transfusion, a catastrophic Wharton's jelly hematoma with concomitant decrease in umbilical blood flow may result. There is no advantage in not paralyzing the fetus. Pancuronium, as opposed to other agents used for neuromuscular blockade, has the advantage of increasing heart rate secondary to catecholamine release. Without pancuronium, intravascular transfusion decreases both the fetal heart rate and cardiac output, prolonging the time required for the fetus to clear the acid contained in the preserved banked donor blood. With pancuronium, the fetal heart rate remains at or above the pretransfusion rate. The injection of the pancuronium, followed by the measurement of the umbilical venous pressure, allows the definitive identification of the vessel punctured. The needle is removed if the artery is inadvertently entered because the risk of fetal bradycardia can rise fivefold. Though furosemide is used (3 mg/kg EFW) by some, including the author, clinical and laboratory investigations have failed to show measurable benefit.[70]

The equipment for an intravascular transfusion is illustrated in Figure 14–9. The blood must be filtered immediately prior to transfusion to remove aggregates that may obstruct the microvasculature. Careful attention is paid to purge the system of air. With a series of three-way valves, an assistant injects the donor blood while the operator is free to concentrate on the fetus and needle placement. The assistant must remain poised to halt the infusion if there is any abrupt change in the resistance to flow. To minimize the time the needle is in place, the blood is infused with haste up to 5mL/minute.

Except for the first transfusion of a hydropic fetus, the target for the post-transfusion fetal hematocrit is 48% to 55%. The volume required depends on gestational age and the initial hematocrit. Assuming similar opening and closing hematocrit measurements, the volume infused is dependent on gestational age (Table 14–9). The volume required for correction frequently equals or exceeds the calculated total fetal-placental intravascular volume.

HYDROPS

Because most hydropic fetuses have myocardial dysfunction that prevents them from tolerating the required infusion volume,[26] the target hematocrit after their first transfusion is only 25% (see Pathophysiology). Twenty-four hours later, the hematocrit can be safely brought to 50% during a second transfusion. The decline in umbilical vein pH (UVpH) that normally occurs during transfusion is especially important to the severely anemic fetus. The red blood cell is the principal fetal buffer, and the pH of the citrated banked blood is 6.98 to 7.01. Our losses of hydropic fetuses after transfusion occurred even though the increase in their umbilical venous pressure during the procedure was acceptable and there was no acute bradycardia. All losses, however, were associated with a profound acidemia, and the deaths occurred hours after transfusion. The author believes the acidemia aggravated the myocardial failure and now infuses bicarbonate in 1-mEq increments to maintain the UVpH above 7.30. There have been no further losses since that practice was initiated in 1988. In point, the overall survival rate for hydropic fetuses using this protocol now exceeds 90%.

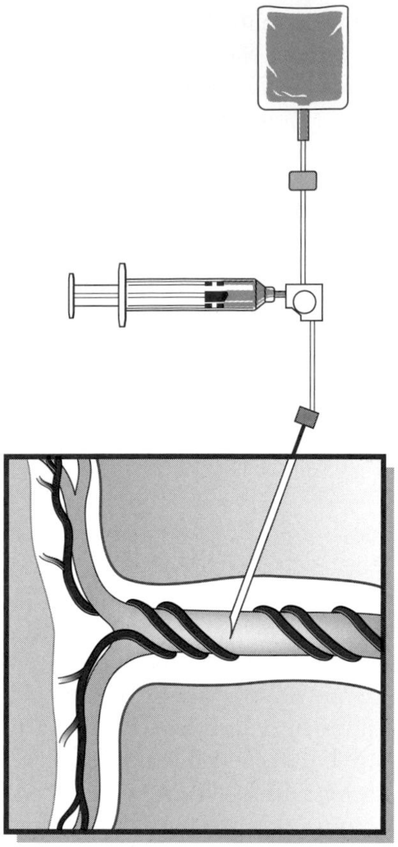

FIGURE 14–9
Set-up for an intravascular transfusion.

TABLE 14–9

Approximate Volumes of 72% Hematocrit Blood Required for Intravascular Transfusion after the First Transfusion

GESTATION (WK)	VOLUME (ML)
≤ 22.5	25–40
22.5–27.49	45–65
27.5–32.49	75–90
≥32.5	100–120

Several formulae have been proposed to calculate the volume of blood necessary to correct the hemoglobin deficit. Though reasonably accurate, none are reliable enough to remove the needle without first checking the hematocrit. Further, there is a possibility of overtransfusion when any formula is relied upon blindly. The author prefers to transfuse half the estimated total volume and then check the hematocrit. Based on the increase in hematocrit achieved following the first aliquot, the remaining volume necessary is rapidly and accurately calculated. Contrary to the adult or child, donor blood with a hematocrit below 80% equilibrates rapidly, perhaps because of the rapid fluid exchange across the placenta. On multiple occasions, the author has found that the hematocrit 24 hours after the transfusion is within a few percentage points of the closing hematocrit. However, transfused blood with a hematocrit higher than 80% is more viscous and does not equilibrate as rapidly.

The decline in hematocrit after transfusion is more rapid and variable between the first and second transfusions compared to subsequent procedures. This variability results from the differing rates of destruction of disparate amounts of fetal antigen positive and banked antigen negative red blood cells. Except for the hydropic fetus, the second transfusion is performed 2 weeks after the first. Subsequently, the decline in hematocrit per week is predictable for any given fetus (Fig. 14–10). The rate at which the hematocrit declines between transfusions with advancing gestation is such that by 34 to 35 weeks, delivery may be safely delayed 4 to 5 weeks without another transfusion. These findings have been confirmed.[71]

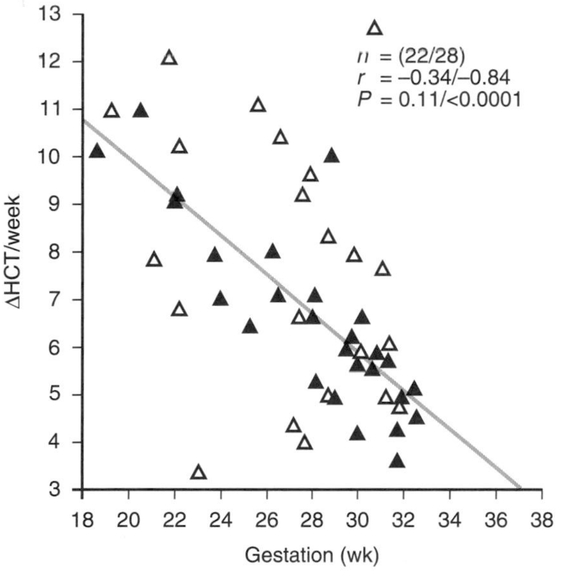

FIGURE 14–10
The rate at which the hematocrit (HCT) declines per week after a transfusion. Open triangles reflect the interval decline between the first and second transfusion. The solid black triangles and the regression line reflect the decline in hematocrit per week between subsequent transfusions. Thus, if the fetus was transfused to 50% hematocrit at 22 weeks, we would expect it to decline approximately 9% per week. Based on this estimate, the transfusion would be repeated in 2.5 weeks.

The fetus is monitored during transfusion using a variety of methods. Many prefer to image the fetal heart at periodic intervals to rule out bradycardia; although important, it is of limited value. A second option is umbilical venous pressure measurement, which has several advantages. First, an occasional nonhydropic fetus (frequescy of approximately 5% in the author's experience) with a low hematocrit does not tolerate the transfusion volume necessary to correct the hemoglobin deficit. An increase in the umbilical venous pressure of more than 10 mm Hg is associated with an increased perinatal mortality rate. The transfusion should either be halted, or an appropriate volume of blood removed to reduce preload if the pressure rises more than 10 mm Hg. Second, fetal bradycardia increases the umbilical venous pressure. The third option is pulsed Doppler, which can also help differentiate the two causes of an elevated umbilical venous pressure by dropping a Doppler gate on the umbilical artery. Whichever technique is selected, it is important to keep the needle in place because any resuscitative efforts necessitated by a fetal bradycardia are facilitated by access to the fetal circulation.

Intravascular transfusion has many effects on the fetus (Table 14–10) other than raising the hematocrit.[72–74] Some, such as the increases in atrial natriuretic peptide and prostacyclin, help the fetus tolerate a volume load that postnatally would be lethal. Prostaglandin synthetase inhibitors are contraindicated for two reasons: (1) an increase in fetal prostacyclin and prostaglandin E_2 (PGE_2) is part of the normal adaptive response to the abrupt increase in intravascular volume,[74] and (2) there is no evidence they are of any utility.

Adequate transfusion therapy rapidly suppresses fetal erythropoiesis. The fetal erythropoietin level declines, and the average reticulocyte count is less than 1% by the

TABLE 14–10

Acute Nonhematologic Effects of Intravascular Transfusion

Cardiovascular
Increased intravascular volume
Decreased heart rate (without pancuronium)
Decreased cardiac output (without pancuronium)
Increased umbilical venous pressure
Increased renal blood flow
Decreased placental resistance measured by Doppler
Decreased aortic resistance measured by Doppler
Biochemical
Acidemia (blood preservative, inadequate fetal buffer capacity)
Increased oxygen-carrying capacity
Increased viscosity
Increased atrial natriuretic peptide
Increased prostacyclin
Increased prostaglandin E_2
Increased iron stores (chronic)

third transfusion. It is advantageous to perform at least two transfusions 3 weeks apart prior to delivery because postnatal complications of hyperbilirubinemia are significantly less likely to occur after two or more antenatal transfusions.[25] In experienced hands, losses are uncommon and confined to the previable fetus. In the author's view there is no justification for routine preterm delivery. The last transfusion can be performed at 34 to 35 weeks' gestation and labor induced at 37 to 38 weeks.

DELIVERY

The obstetric philosophy need not be altered for the nonanemic, transfused fetus. Antenatal transfusion is not a reason to deny a vaginal birth after cesarean section. If the final hematocrit at the end of the last transfusion was 50%, it will be in the mid-30s in the umbilical cord at delivery. Typically, the neonatal hematocrit increases approximately 15% within 8 hours of delivery, reflecting a massive shift of extracellular and intravascular fluid. The hematocrit then declines to or below the delivery level over the next few days to weeks.

POSTNATAL CARE

Postnatally, infants who received in utero transfusion therapy do remarkably well with an average hospitalization stay of less than 7 days (unpublished data). Because they are delivered at term, a higher peak neonatal bilirubin concentration is tolerated and is normally manageable with just phototherapy. Double volume exchange transfusion is rarely needed when two or more antenatal transfusions are performed. Small, simple transfusions are frequently necessary, beginning at several weeks of age, because the banked blood transfused 5 weeks earlier is at the end of its life span. This anemia is typified by a low reticulocyte count. The neonatal hematocrit and reticulocyte count should be monitored weekly. If not, a severe anemia may escape detection with resulting high output failure and failure to thrive. The pediatric goal is to keep the neonate asymptomatic but with a modest anemia to maintain an erythropoietic stimulus. Newborns may be 16 weeks old before reticulocytes reappear on the peripheral smear. Once a reticulocytosis is noted, further transfusion therapy is generally not needed. The need for neonatal transfusion can be decreased significantly by the administration of recombinant human erythropoietin.[75]

Effect of Anemia and Treatment on the Fetus

It is remarkable how well the fetus tolerates all but the most severe anemia. Fetuses who have a mild, chronic anemia are neither growth deficient nor acidemic. Though mild to moderate anemia is not associated with dramatic antenatal sequelae, severe anemia clearly is. As dramatic as hydrops fetalis may be, it is for the most part preventable and completely reversible. Hydropic fetuses not yet severely acidemic recover quickly with appropriate transfusion therapy and on long-term follow-up appear without specific sequelae[76,77] (unpublished data).

Transfusion therapy has a predictable and desirable effect on fetal erythropoiesis. With adequate RBC replacement, the reticulocyte count and percentage of circulating red blood cells of fetal origin drops rapidly (Fig. 14–11). Part of this decline is due to consumption of newly formed fetal RBCs as they emerge from the fetal bone marrow and liver. However, after two transfusions correcting the hematocrit to 50%, smears of neonatal bone marrow reveal decreased erythrogenic precursors.[78] The greater the number of antenatal transfusions (i.e., the longer the period of fetal erythrocytic suppression) performed, the less severe the hyperbilirubinemia postnatally and the longer the suppression of erythropoiesis postnatally.[25] These findings coupled with the decrease in fetal plasma erythropoietin concentrations after several transfusions are indicative of marrow and liver suppression.

The long-term outcomes of the most severely affected fetuses have until recently been the subject of scant study. We conducted a case-control study of all 16 consecutive children born at the University of Iowa between July 1985 and August 1990 who as fetuses had intrauterine intravascular transfusion therapy for alloimmune hydrops fetalis.[79] Eight nonhydropic older siblings were control subjects. Hospital records were reviewed, and parents completed behavioral questionnaires and were interviewed. Affected children and their sibling controls

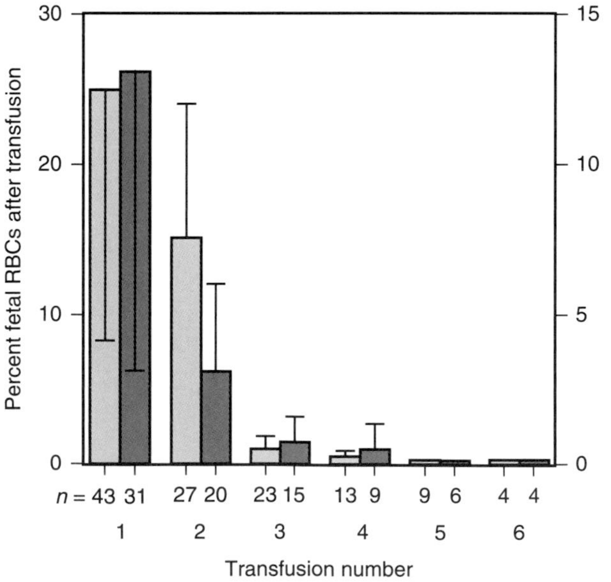

FIGURE 14–11
Effect of simple intravascular transfusion on the circulating fetal red blood cell (RBC) percentage (*M* left *x*-axis) and the percentage of RBCs that are reticulocytes ($\overline{M}$ right *x*-axis).

received comprehensive neuropsychological evaluations, hearing tests, and neurologic examinations. The hydrops children had cranial computed tomography (CT) scans for the measurement of brain and ventricular volumes. No significant differences were noted between the hydrops group and the sibling control group on neuropsychological measures (Table 14–11). Modest but statistically significant correlations were noted between the severity of anemia at the time of hydrops and composite standardized testing of nonverbal and computational skills at follow-up. The first child treated was electively delivered at 35 weeks. He suffered complications of kernicterus associated with a maximum bilirubin of 28 mg/dL. A second child who at 25 weeks' gestation experienced a prolonged fetal bradycardia (heart rate of 40 bpm for 5 minutes) due to technical difficulties during an intra-arterial transfusion followed by delivery had cerebral palsy. The remaining 13 children had physical, neurologic, and neuropsychological findings within the normal range. Of the 16 CT scans, 14 were normal, and 2 revealed minor structural abnormalities. Mean total intracranial volume was 1477 mL. All intracranial volumes were within published normative values.

ABO INCOMPATIBILITY AND MINOR BLOOD GROUP ANTIGENS

ABO incompatibility rarely causes fetal disease because the antibodies are often IgM and because these antigens are not strongly expressed on the fetal erythrocyte. Alloimmunization to minor blood group antigens is usually due to blood transfusion. Although Lewis antibodies are most common, they are almost always IgM and do not pose a risk for fetal disease. Further, the antigen is poorly expressed on the fetal erythrocyte. Therefore, the risk for hemolysis is low.

Kidd, Kell, and Duffy are the most common minor blood group antigens that cause perinatal hemolytic disease. Kell alloimmunization is of particular interest because the pathophysiology differs from the others. The clinical course is particularly unpredictable by indirect fetal assessment because the anti-Kell IgG antibodies damage or inhibit erythrocyte progenitors. Severe anemia and hydrops may develop rapidly with low antibody titers and ΔOD450 values. Management is similar to Rh isoimmunization with monitoring and intervention tailored to the individual circumstances.

OTHER CAUSES OF HEMOLYTIC DISEASE

Rare causes of fetal and neonatal hemolytic disease include hemoglobinopathies, RBC membrane defects, and RBC enzyme deficiencies. Because thallassemia can affect the α and β hemoglobin chains, it may result in disease in utero. Bart's hemoglobin (deletion of all four α chain genes) is the most severe form and causes hydrops fetalis. Hemoglobin H disease (deletion of three α chain genes) is less severe, but the affected patient requires lifelong transfusion treatment. In contrast, sickle cell disease (defective β chain) does not manifest in utero owing to the protective effect of fetal hemoglobin.

FUTURE PREGNANCIES, PREPREGNANCY CONSULTATION

Modern approaches to fetal hemolytic disease have drastically reduced the impact of this disease on the family. Though we may be cognizant that it may occur, we do not expect to lose a fetus to hemolytic disease. Several women under our care have, after presenting with a hydropic fetus in the first treated pregnancy, gone on to a second and a third treated pregnancy. Though not unreasonable to suggest, there is no reason to badger these women toward either an undesired surgical sterilization or a pregnancy by artificial insemination with an Rh– donor to avoid a recurrence. It is, however, essential they understand the time demands required of them, along with the costs and risks involved. This information is best supplied prior to conception.

TABLE 14–11

Long-Term Outcome of Consecutive Hydropic Fetuses Treated in Utero

GROUP	HEMOGLOBIN AT g/100mL	AGE F/U (YR)	COGNITIVE ACHIEVEMENT	VISUAL/MOTOR-SPATIAL	ATTENTIONAL PROBLEMS	MEMORY
Hydrops	3.5±1.5	9.43	99.33	100.25	40%	9.16
Sibcontrol	NA	11.93	107.50	107.37	25%	10.58

Dx, diagnosis; F/U, follow-up.
From Swingle HM, Harper DC, Bonthius D, et al: Long-term Neurodevelopmental Follow-up and Brain Volumes of Children Following Severe Fetal Anemia with Hydrops. American Academy of Cerebral Palsy and Developmental Medicine, Los Angeles, 9/29 to 10/1, 2004.

CONCLUSIONS

Pathophysiology and Risks

- Fetal hemolytic disease remains a major cause of perinatal morbidity.
- Maternal alloimmunization results either from fetal to maternal hemorrhage or heterologous blood transfusion.
- Only IgG class antibodies cross the placenta and bind to the fetal red blood cells. Anti-D alloimmunization remains the most common type
- All sequelae of the disease are secondary to hemolysis or severe anemia.
- Severe anemia leads to the development of hydrops fetalis, reflecting cardiac and hematologic events.
- There is clear evidence of cardiac dysfunction in most hydropic fetuses that precedes the development of hydrops and resolves promptly after fetal transfusion.
- Postnatally, the affected neonate is at risk for complications of hyperbilirubinemia that include neural deafness and encephalopathy.
- All complications of fetal hemolytic anemia are potentially preventable.

Options for Antibody Detection and Management of Non-Immunized Rh-Negative Women

- RBC alloimmunization is detected using a combination of indirect and direct methods.
- Unless previously documented on two or more occasions, all women should be tested on registration for prenatal care.
- Nonimmune Rh– women should be tested regularly (ideally monthly) throughout pregnancy for evidence of alloimmunization.
- Anti-D immunoglobulin effectively prevents maternal alloimmunization. It should be given after amniocentesis, episodes of vaginal bleeding, at 28 weeks' gestation, and after the delivery of a Rh+ child
- The recommended dose of anti-D immunoglobulin for these potential sensitization events varies among countries.

Management of Sensitized Rh-Negative Women

- The management of the pregnant alloimmunized woman utilizes both direct and indirect methods of maternal/fetal evaluation.
- Serial indirect Coombs tests are performed at monthly intervals after 18 weeks' gestation until the critical titer for the laboratory is exceeded.
- At that time, serial peak middle cerebral artery velocity measurements are performed weekly. The correlation between hemoglobin concentration and the peak middle cerebral artery velocity has rendered amniocentesis for the measurement of the ΔOD450 an outdated tool because transfusion therapy should never be initiated without confirming fetal anemia.
- Cordocentesis is performed when the peak middle cerebral artery velocity is elevated.
- The care of these pregnancies should be under the guidance of a consultant skilled in the area.
- During the first sensitized pregnancy, the Coombs titer correlates with the severity of fetal disease. However, these titers are poorly predictive after the first sensitized pregnancy.

Treatment of Hemolytic Fetal Anemia

- The treatment of significant fetal hemolytic anemia prior to 34 weeks' gestation is transfusion.
- Successful transfusion eliminates the antenatal and, largely, the postnatal complications of fetal hemolytic disease.
- Intravascular transfusion is the procedure of choice.
- However, whether the transfusion is intravascular or intraperitoneal, the most experienced person or team available should perform it.
- Delivery may be safely delaved until 37 to 38 weeks if intravascular transfusion is done.
- By maintaining the hematocrit at the high end, fetal erythropoiesis is minimized, reducing the risk of postnatal hyperbilirubinemia.

SUMMARY OF MANAGEMENT OPTIONS

Fetal Hemolytic Disease

Management Options	Quality of Evidence	Strength of Recommendation	References
Prevention of Rh Hemolytic Disease in Nonimmunized Women			
Routine screening in Rh– women at booking and regularly through pregnancy	III	B	19
Antenatal prophylaxis at delivery	Ib	A	34
Antenatal prophylaxis at 28–34 wk and at delivery	IIb	B	32
Prophylaxis after potential sensitizing events	III	B	33
Prediction of Disease Severity in Immunized Women			
Refer to experienced center when critical antibody titer reached	–	GPP	–
Prenatal determination of fetal RhD status	III	B	38
Measure maternal serum anti-D antibody concentration serially	III	B	19
Sonographic imaging to predict severity of disease—poor without evidence of frank hydrops	III	B	50
Middle cerebral Doppler appears to be reliable noninvasive technique to determine severity of anemia	III	B	45
Amniocentesis bilirubin/ΔOD450 from 27–41 wk—three zones helpful in managing patients (true level of anemia not known)	III	B	4
Liley curves of amniotic fluid bilirubin/ΔOD450 between 18–25 wk detected only 32% of fetuses with a Hb <6 g/dL (appropriate management and survival may not be directly correlated with Hb <6 g/dL)	III	B	59
An extrapolated Liley curve from 20–27 wk can be used to appropriately manage patients	III	B	80
Fetal blood sampling: variation exists in practice over which method to use and when to perform it	III	B	19
Treatment			
Fetal blood transfusion is treatment of choice; intravascular (Table 14–8) is preferable to intraperitoneal (Table 14–7)	IIa	B	69
Intravascular transfusion is associated with a >90% survival rate	III	B	25
	IIa	B	69
Fetal transfusion via the intrahepatic vein has similar success rates to intravascular transfusion	III	B	81
Decline in donor red blood cells is approximately 2% /day	III	B	71
The efficacy of intravenous immunoglobulin (IVIG) as a treatment for severe fetal hemolytic disease has not been established; the same is true for plasmapheresis; many reserve these for women with a history of early onset hydrops (?<22 wk)	IIb	B	65 82
Long-term neurodevelopmental outcome after intravascular transfusion is normal in most cases	III	B	76,77
Kell sensitization does not behave like Rh disease	IV	C	55
Kell sensitization is due to inhibition of erythroid progenitor cells by anti-Kell antibodies	III	B	58
Delivery Options			
In Nontransfused Fetus	–	GPP	–
At 37–38 wk			

Continued

SUMMARY OF MANAGEMENT OPTIONS
Fetal Hemolytic Disease *(Continued)*

Management Options	Quality of Evidence	Strength of Recommendation	References
Delivery Options			
In Transfused Fetus	–	GPP	–
Last intravascular transfusion at 34 weeks (unless dangerous or difficult) and deliver at 37 weeks			
32–34 wk (with prior maternal steroid therapy) for intraperitoneal transfusion			
Neonatal Care			
Pediatric surveillance from birth	–	GPP	–
Phototherapy			
Exchange transfusions if severe			
Top-up transfusions and long-term hematinic supplementation may be necessary			

REFERENCES

1. Diamond LK, Blackfan KD, Baty JM: Erythroblastosis fetalis and its association with universal edema of the fetus, icterus gravis neonatorum and anemia of the newborn. J Pediatr 1932;1:269–274.
2. Levine P, Katzin EM, Burnham L: Isoimmunization in pregnancy: its possible bearing on the etiology of erythroblastosis fetalis. JAMA 1941;116:825–830.
3. Chown B: Anemia from bleeding of the fetus into the mother's circulation. Lancet 1954;I:1213–1215.
4. Liley AW: Liquor amnii analysis and management of pregnancy complicated by rhesus immunization. Am J Obstet Gynecol 1961;82:1359–1368.
5. Liley AW: Errors in the assessment of hemolytic disease from amniotic fluid. Am J Obstet Gynecol 1963;86:485–494.
6. Freda VJ, Gorman JG, Pollack W: Successful prevention of experimental Rh sensitization in man with an anti-Rh gamma-2-globulin antibody preparation—A preliminary report. Transfusion 1964;4:26–31.
7. Rodeck CH, Holman CA, Karnicki J, et al: Direct intravascular fetal blood transfusion by fetoscopy in severe rhesus isoimmunization. Lancet 1981;I:652–654.
8. Mari G, Deter RL, Carpenter RL, et al: Noninvasive diagnosis by Doppler ultrasonography of fetal anemia due to maternal red cell alloimmunization. Collaborative Group for Doppler Assessment of the Blood Velocity in Anemic Fetuses. N Engl J Med 2000;342:9–14.
9. Mourant AE, Kopec AC, Domaniewska-Sobozak K: The Distribution of Human Blood Groups and Other Polymophisms, 2nd ed. London, Oxford University Press, 1976, pp 351–505.
10. Joseph KS, Kramer MS: The decline in Rh hemolytic disease: Should Rh prophylaxis get all the credit? Am J Publ Health 1998;88:209–215.
11. Bowman, JM, Pollock JM, Penston LE: Fetomaternal transplacental hemorrhage during pregnancy and after delivery. Vox Sang 1986;51:117–125.
12. Race RR: The Rh genotype and Fisher's theory. Blood 1948;3:27.
13. Tippett P, Sanger R: Observations on subdivisions of the Rh antigen D. Vox Sang 1962;7:9–14.
14. Bowman JM: Maternal alloimmunization and fetal hemolytic disease. In Reece EA, Hobbins JC, Mahoney MJ, Petrie RH (eds): Medicine of the Fetus and Mother. Philadelphia, JB Lippincott, 1992, pp 1152–1182.
15. Knibll W: Der gang der erythrophose beim menschlichen embryo. Acta Haematol 1949;2:369–377.
16. Ulm B, Ulm MR, Panzer S: Fetal sex and hemolytic disease from maternal red cell alloimmunization (letter). N Engl J Med 1998;338:1699–1700.
17. Palfi M, Hilden JO, Gottvall T, Selbing A: Placental transport of maternal immunoglobulin G in pregnancies at risk of Rh (D) hemolytic disease of the newborn. Am J Reprod Immunol 1998; 39:323–328.
18. Hilden JO, Gottvall T, Lindblom B: HLA phenotypes and severe Rh (D) immunization. Tissue Antigens 1995;46:313–315.
19. Weiner CP, Williamson RA, Wenstrom KD, et al: Management of fetal hemolytic disease by cordocentesis: I. Prediction of fetal anemia. Am J Obstet Gynecol 1991;165:546–553.
20. Weiner CP: Human fetal bilirubin and fetal hemolytic disease. Am J Obstet Gynecol 1992;116:1449–1454.
21. Soothill PW, Nicolaides KH, Rodeck CH, et al: Relationship of fetal hemoglobin and oxygen content to lactate concentration in sensitized pregnancies. Obstet Gynecol 1987;69:268–271.
22. Nicolaides KH, Warenski JC, Rodeck CH: The relationship of fetal protein concentration and haemoglobin level to the development of hydrops in rhesus isoimmunization. Am J Obstet Gynecol 1985;152:341–344.
23. Phibbs RH, Johnson P, Tooley WE: Cardio-respiratory status of erythroblastotic infants. II. Blood volume, hematocrit, and serum albumin concentration in relation to hydrops fetalis. Pediatrics 1974;53:13–26.
24. Weiner CP, Heilskov J, Pelzer G, et al: Normal values for human umbilical venous and amniotic fluid pressures and their alteration by fetal disease. Am J Obstet Gynecol 1989;161: 714–717.

25. Weiner CP, Williamson RA, Wenstrom KD, et al: Management of fetal hemolytic disease by cordocentesis: ii. Outcome of treatment. Am J Obstet Gynecol 1991;165:1302–1307.
26. Weiner CP, Pelzer GD, Heilskov J, et al: The effect of intravascular transfusion on umbilical venous pressure in anemic fetuses with and without hydrops. Am J Obstet Gynecol 1989;161:149E
27. Weiner CP, Sipes SL, Wenstrom KD: The effect of gestation upon normal fetal laboratory parameters and venous pressure. Obstet Gynecol 1992;79:713–718.
28. Moore EPL: Automation in the blood transfusion laboratory. I. Antibody detection and quantification in the Technicon AutoAnalyzer. Can Med J 1969;100:381–387.
29. Lucas GF, Hadley AG, Nance SJ, Garratty G: Predicting hemolytic disease of the newborn: A comparison of the monocyte monolayer assay and the chemiluminescence test. Transfusion 1993;33:484–487.
30. Moise KJ Jr, Perkins JT, Sosler SD, et al: The predictive value of maternal serum testing for detection of fetal anemia in red blood cell alloimmunization. Am J Obstet Gynecol 1995;172: 1003–1009.
31. Buggins AG, Thilaganathan B, Hambley H, Nicolaides KH: Predicting the severity of rhesus alloimmunization: Monocyte-mediated chemiluminescence versus maternal anti-D antibody estimation. Br J Haematol 1994;88:199–200.
32. Bowman JM, Chown B, Lewis M, Pollack JM: Rh-immunization during pregnancy: Antenatal prevention. Can Med J 1978;118:623–629
33. Bowman JM, Pollack JM: Transplacental fetal hemorrhage after amniocentesis. Obstet Gynecol 1985;66:749–755.
34. Chown B, Duff AM, James J, et al: Prevention of primary Rh immunization: First report of the Western Canadian Trial. Can Med J 1969;100:1021–1047.
35. Pollack W, Ascari WQ, Kochesky RJ, et al: Studies on Rh prophylaxis. I. Relationship between doses of anti-Rh and the size of the antigenic stimulus. Transfusion 1971;11:333–339.
36. Bowman JM, Pollack JM: Amniotic fluid spectrophotometry and early delivery in the management of erythroblastosis fetalis. Pediatrics 1965;35:815–821.
37. LeVanKim C, Mouro I, Brossard Y, et al: PCR-based determination of Rhc and RhE status of fetuses at risk of Rhc and RhE haemolytic disease. Br J Haematol 1994;88:193–195.
38. Bennet PR, LeVanKim C, Colin Y, et al: Prenatal determination of fetal RhD type by DNA amplification. N Engl J Med 1993;329:607–610.
39. Van Den Veyver IB, Subramanian SB, Hudson KM, et al: Prenatal diagnosis of the RhD fetal blood type on amniotic fluid by polymerase chain reaction. Obstet Gynecol 1996;87:419–422.
40. Fisk NM, Bennett P, Warwick RM, et al: Clinical utility of fetal RhD typing in alloimmunized pregnancies by means of polymerase chain reaction on amniocytes or chorionic villi. Am J Obstet Gynecol 1994;171:50–54.
41. Yankowitz J, Li S, Weiner CP: Polymerase chain reaction determination of RhC, Rhc, and RhE blood types: An evaluation of accuracy and clinical utility. Am J Obstet Gynecol 1997;176: 1107–1111.
42. Yankowitz J, Li S, Murray JC: Polymerase chain reaction determination of RhD blood type: An evaluation of accuracy. Obstet Gynecol 1995;86:214–217.
43. Hengstschlaeger M, Hoelzl G, Ulm B, Bernaschek C: Raising the sensitivity of fetal RhD typing and sex determination from maternal blood (letter). J Med Genet 1997;34:350–351.
44. Brass LM, Pavlakis SG, DeVivo D, et al: Transcranial Doppler measurements of the middle cerebral artery. Effect of hematocrit. Stroke 1988;19:1466–1469.
45. Mari G, Adrignolo A, Abuhamad AZ, et al: Diagnosis of fetal anemia with Doppler ultrasound in pregnancy complicated by maternal blood group immunization. Ultrasound Obstet Gynecol 1995;5:400–405.
46. Steiner H, Schaffer H, Spitzer D, et al: The relationship between peak velocity in the fetal descending aorta and hematocrit in rhesus isoimmunization. Obstet Gynecol 1995;85:659–662.
47. Vyas S, Nicolaides KH, Campbell S: Doppler examination of the middle cerebral artery in anemic fetuses. Am J Obstet Gynecol 1990;162:1066–1068.
48. Johnson MJ, Kramer WB, Alger LS, et al: Middle cerebral artery peak velocity and fetal anemia. 17th Annual Meeting of Society of Perinatal Obstetricians, Anaheim, CA, Jan. 22–25, 1997.
49. Vintzileos AM, Campbell WA, Storlazzi E, et al: Fetal liver ultrasound measurements in isoimmunized pregnancies. Obstet Gynecol 1986;68:162.
50. Nicolaides KH, Fontanarosa M, Gabbe SG, Rodeck CH: Failure of six ultrasonographic parameters to predict the severity of fetal anemia in Rhesus isoimmunization. Am J Obstet Gynecol 1988;158:920–926.
51. Craig JS, McClure BG, Tubman TR: Preventing RhD haemolytic disease of the newborn. Services should be centralised for pregnancies affected by RhD haemolytic disease. Br Med J 1998;316:1611.
52. Frigoletto FD, Greene MF, Benacerraf BR, et al: Ultramonographic fetal surveillance in the management of the isoimmunized pregnancy. N Engl J Med 1986;315:430–432.
53. Gottval T, Hilden JO: Concentration of anti-D antibodies in Rh(D) alloimmunized pregnant women, as a predictor of anemia and/or hyperbilirubinemia in their newborn infants. Acta Obstet Gynecol Scand 1997;76:733–738.
54. Weiner CP, Widness JA: Decreased fetal erythropoiesis and hemolysis in Kell hemolytic anemia. Am J Obstet Gynecol 1996;174:547–551.
55. Berkowitz RL, Beyth Y, Sadovsky E: Death in utero due to Kell sensitization without excessive elevation of the delta OD450 value in amniotic fluid. Obstet Gynecol 1982;60:746–749.
56. Bowman JM, Pollock JM, Manning FA, et al: Maternal Kell blood group alloimmunization. Obstet Gynecol 1992;79: 239–244.
57. Vaughan JI, Warwick R, Letsky E, et al: Erythropoietic suppression in fetal anemia because of Kell alloimmunization. Am J Obstet Gynecol 1994;171:247–252.
58. Vaughan JI, Manning M, Warick RM, et al: Inhibition of erythroid progenitor cells by anti-Kell antibodies in fetal alloimmune anemia. N Engl J Med 1998;338:798–803.
59. Nicolaides KH, Rodeck CH, Mibashan RS, Kemp JR: Have Liley charts outlived their usefulness? Am J Obstet Gynecol 1986;155:90–94.
60. Weiner CP, Wenstrom KD, Sipes SL, Williamson RA: Risk factors for cordocentesis and fetal intravascular transfusions. Am J Obstet Gynecol 1991;165:1020–1023.
61. Weiner CP, Okamura K: Diagnostic fetal blood sampling—Technique related losses. Fetal Diagn Ther 1996;11:169–175.
62. Weiner CP, Grant SS, Hudson J, et al: Effect of diagnostic and therapeutic cordocentesis upon maternal serum alpha fetoprotein concentration. Am J Obstet Gynecol 1989;161:706–708.
63. Weiner CP: Management of fetal hemolytic disease by cordocentesis: outcome of affected neonates not requiring transfusion. Fetal Diagn Ther 1996;11:176–178.
64. Graham-Pole J, Barr W, Willoughby ML: Continuous-flow plasmapheresis management of severe rhesus disease. Br Med J 1977;1:1185–1188.
65. Berlin G, Selbing A, Ryden G: Rhesus haemolytic disease treated with high dose intravenous immunoglobulin. Lancet 1985;I:1153.
66. Zhao L, Huang X, Wang Q: Antenatal treatment of maternal-fetal Rh incompatibility hemolysis disease. Zhonghua Fu Chan Ke Za Zhi 1998;33:406–408.
67. Watts DH, Luthy DA, Benedetti TJ, et al: Intraperitoneal fetal transfusion under direct ultrasound guidance. Obstet Gynecol 1988;71:84–88.

68. Frigoletto FD, Umansky I, Birnholz J, et al: Intrauterine fetal transfusion in 365 fetuses during fifteen years. Am J Obstet Gynecol 1981;139:781–786.
69. Harman CR, Bowman JM, Manning FA, Menticoglou SM: Intrauterine transfusion—Intraperitoneal versus intravascular approach: A case-control comparison. Am J Obstet Gynecol 1990;162:1053–1059.
70. Chestnut DH, Pollack KL, Weiner CP, et al: Does furosemide alter the hemodynamic response to rapid intravascular transfusion of the anemic fetal lamb. Am J Obstet Gynecol 1989;161:1571–1575.
71. Egberts J, van Kamp IL, Kanhai HH, et al: The disappearance of fetal and donor red blood cells in alloimmunized pregnancies: A reappraisal. Br J Obstet Gynaecol 1997;104:818–824.
72. Robillard JE, Weiner CP: Atrial natriuretic factor in the human fetus effect of volume expansion. Pediatrics 1988;113:552–555.
73. Weiner CP, Robillard JE: Arginine vasopressin and acute, intravascular volume expansion in the human fetus. Fetal Ther 1989;4:69–72.
74. Weiner CP, Robillard JE: Effect of acute intravascular volume expansion upon human fetal prostaglandin concentrations. Am J Obstet Gynecol 1989;161:1494–1497.
75. Ovali F, Samanci N, Dagoglu T: Management of late anemia in Rhesus hemolytic disease: use of recombinant human erythropoietin (a pilot study). Pediatr Res 1996;39:831–834.
76. Ellis MI: Follow-up study of survivors after intrauterine transfusion. Dev Med Child Neurol 1980;22:48–54.
77. White CA, Goplerud CP, Kisker CT, et al: Intrauterine fetal transfusion, 1965–1976, with an assessment of the surviving children. Am J Obstet Gynecol 1978;130:933–942.
78. Giller RH, Widness JA, Dealarcon PA, et al: Postnatal anemia following intravascular intrauterine transfusion for isoimmune hemolytic disease: Natural history and possible mechanisms. Pediatr Res 1990;27:265 (abstract 1571).
79. Swingle HM, Harper DC, Bonthius D, et al: Long-term Neurodevelopmental Follow-up and Brain Volumes of Children following Severe Fetal Anemia with Hydrops. American Academy of Cerebral Palsy and Developmental Medicine, Los Angeles 9/29 to 10/1, 2004.
80. Spinnato JA, Clark AL, Ralston KK, et al: Hemolytic disease of the fetus: A comparison of the Queenan and extended Liley methods. Obstet Gynecol 1998;92:441–445
81. Nicolini U, Nicolaidis P, Fisk NM, et al: Fetal blood sampling from the intrahepatic vein: Analysis of safety and clinical experience with 214 procedures. Obstet Gynecol 1990;76:47–53
82. Voto LS, Mathet ER, Zapaterio JL, et al: High-dose gammaglobulin (IVIG) followed by intrauterine transfusions (IUT): A new alternative for the treatment of severe fetal hemolytic disease. J Perinat Med 1997;25:85–88

CHAPTER 15

Fetal Thrombocytopenia

Humphrey H.H. Kanhai / Anneke Brand

INTRODUCTION

Thrombocytopenia is diagnosed in approximately 0.9% of newborns.[1] The incidence of thrombocytopenia during the neonatal period is 3% to 5%.[2] Pathologic conditions associated with fetal/neonatal thrombocytopenia include preterm birth, severe intrauterine growth restriction (IUGR), asphyxia, congenital malformations (e.g., TAR syndrome, trisomy 21), congenital infection, platelet iso- or alloimmunization, and red blood cell alloimmunization. Maternal disorders such as cocaine abuse, HIV (human immunodeficiency virus) infection, preeclampsia, and systemic lupus erythematosus (SLE) are associated with maternal, but not usually fetal, thrombocytopenia. Hemorrhagic disorders such as von Willebrand's disease and hemophilia may lead to coagulation disorders in the fetus/newborn other than thrombocytopenia. Thrombocytopenia secondary to either platelet allo- or isoimmunzation is found in 0.3% of newborns.[1] Alloimmune thrombocytopenia (AITP) (also known as neonatal alloimmune thrombocytopenia [NAIT] or fetal/neonatal alloimmune thrombocytopenia [FNAIT]) and isoimmune thrombocytopenia (ITP) (also known as idiopathic or autoimmune thrombocytopenic purpura) are immune-mediated thrombocytopenias. They are the focus of this chapter.

DEFINITIONS

Neonatal thrombocytopenia is defined as a platelet count below $150 \times 10^9/L$. It is further classified according to the severity:

- Mild thrombocytopenia ($100–150 \times 10^9/L$) generally does not require treament.
- Moderate thrombocytopenia ($50–99 \times 10^9/L$) also does not require treament, but both mild and moderate thrombocytopenias require careful observation for further deterioration and may trigger additional diagnostic tests.

Severe thrombocytopenia ($<50 \times 10^9/L$) generally mandates a diagnostic evaluation and some type of treatment. Very severe thrombocytopenia ($<20 \times 10^9/L$) is a serious condition that requires action, often including platelet transfusion.

Isoimmune thrombocytopenic purpura (ITP) (also known as autoimmune and previously as idiopathic thrombocytopenia) is an autoimmune process whereby the mother produces antibodies against her own platelets. IgG type antibodies may cross the placenta and lead to perinatal thrombocytopenia.

Alloimmune thrombocytopenia of the fetus/newborn (AITP) is caused by the placental transfer of maternal immunoglobulin G (IgG) antibodies that react with a paternal human platelet antigen (HPA) expressed on the fetal platelets.

ISOIMMUNE THROMBOCYTOPENIA

Incidence

Adult ITP has an annual incidence of 6 per 100,000 population[3,4] and most often affects young women. Consequently, a past or present history of ITP complicates 1 to 5 per 10,000 pregnancies.[5] Typically, the woman either has a history of ITP and presents with or without thrombocytopenia, or is currently being treated for ITP. Occasionally, asymptomatic ITP is accidentally discovered during pregnancy.

Risks

Maternal

Platelet counts in pregnant women with ITP tend to decrease, reaching their nadir during the third trimester.[6] Unless the counts are very low, the patient is either asymptomatic or experiences easy bruising. However, some patients do bleed despite platelet counts above $20 \times 10^9/L$ ("wet" thrombocytopenia). In these instances, it is assumed that the autoantibodies interact with functional receptors on the platelet surface. Women who do not respond to treatment are at risk for bleeding during pregnancy and delivery. The lowest maternal platelet count during the prior pregnancy is fairly predictive of the extent of thrombocytopenia in successive pregnancies.

Fetus and Newborn

The perinatal mortality rate is around 0.6% with virtually all losses secondary to related medical illnesses rather than fetal thrombocytopenia.[7] Severe in utero bleeding is not documented in ITP, which contrasts with alloimmune thrombocytopenia (see later discussion). It is the neonate who is at greatest risk. The chance of neonatal thrombocytopenia below 50×10^9/L ranges from 9% to 15%.[7–11,15] In large series, neonatal intracranial hemorrhage (ICH) is reported in 0% to 1.5%.[12,13] The nadir neonatal platelet count and the highest risk for hemorrhage occur 1 to 4 days after birth.[6,14,15]

Because the majority of patients with ITP during pregnancy have a benign course, several investigators sought to predict the risk of fetal thrombocytopenia. This information is of practical importance as it could dictate the center selected for delivery. In most studies, there was only a weak correlation between the maternal and newborn platelet counts, the presence of antibodies in the maternal serum, or a history of splenectomy.[3,7,8,12,16–18] A few studies reported a higher correlation between the newborn platelet count and a maternal history of splenectomy.[11,15,19] Perhaps the strongest predictive factor for neonatal thrombocytopenia is an older sibling with a platelet count below 50×10^9/L.[20] A report that HLA (DRB3*) type in the mother is protective requires confirmation.[21] Even though each of these factors is relatively weak alone, the combination of a prior sibling with thrombocytopenia and a mother with a history of splenectomy and thrombocytopenia less than 50×10^9/L during the current pregnancy creates a high probability (>50%) of neonatal thrombocytopenia and indicates the need for delivery in a tertiary hospital.[15]

Management Options (Fig. 15–1)

None of the published guidelines for the management of ITP in pregnancy and neonates[3,12,16,17] are based on a high level of evidence, and most are based on clinical cohort studies.

Prepregnancy

ITP is not a reason to avoid pregnancy, except perhaps for those women refractory to corticosteroids and splenectomy, and who cannot maintain a platelet count above 30×10^9/L despite immunosuppressive drugs.[12,17]

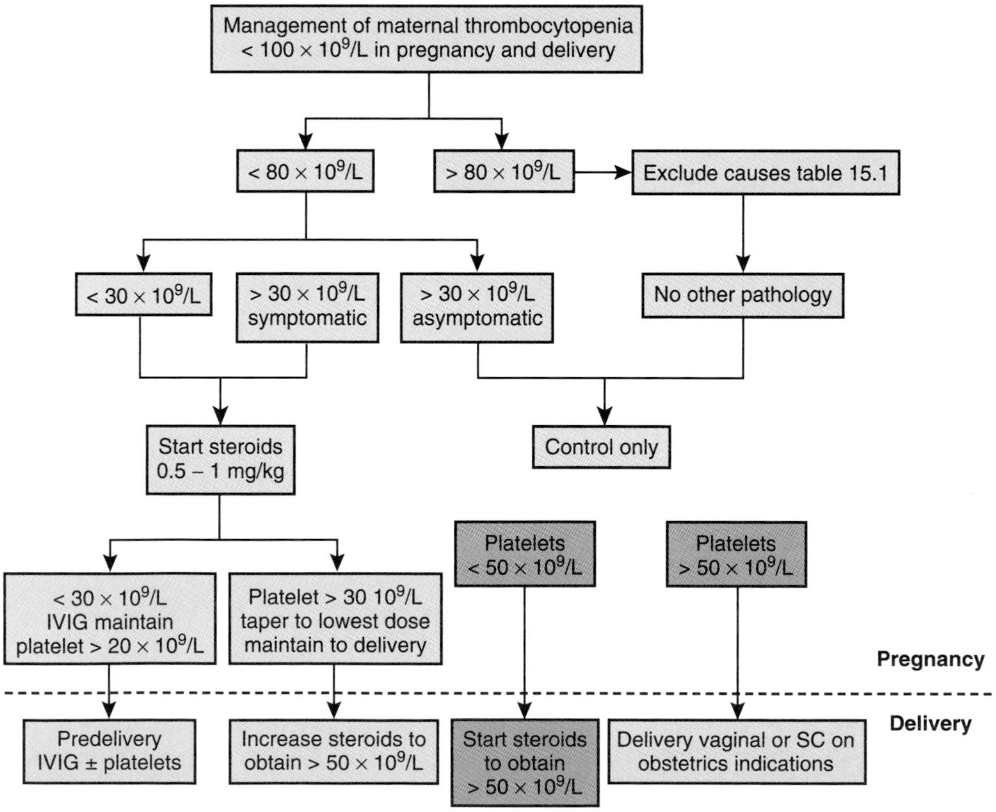

FIGURE 15–1
Management of maternal thrombocytopenia. IVIG, intravenous immunoglobulin.

Although the risk of fetal and neonatal thrombocytopenia cannot be predicted from the maternal platelet count, it approaches the background rate in asymptomatic women. A history of a thrombocytopenic older sibling enhances the likelihood of a thrombocytopenic child.[20,22]

Prenatal

LABORATORY INVESTIGATIONS

These studies are summarized in Table 15–1.

Women with No History of ITP. Thrombocytopenia below 100 × 10^9/L occurs in 1% to 2% of pregnant women.[6] The most common cause is gestational thrombocytopenia (GT), which has an overall frequency of 5% to 8%. In 95% of pregnant women, the platelet count is between 100 and 150 × 10^9/L.[6,14] Preeclampsia, HIV (human immunodeficiency virus), or rarer causes, such as von Willebrand's disease type IIB[23] and underlying systemic diseases such as SLE, antiphospholipid syndrome, thyroid dysfunction, and hematologic disease, must be excluded (see Table 15–1). No further analysis is indicated to distinguish GT from ITP after the aforementioned pathologic conditions are excluded as long as the maternal platelet count is above 80 × 10^9/L. As neither condition poses risks for mother or child, management decisions with respect to center and mode of delivery are unnecessary. The performance of a diagnostic bone marrow aspiration is reserved for special indications. There is little value in testing for maternal platelet-associated IgG antibodies because the rates of false-positive and false-negative results are high.[3,12,16–18] The platelet count should be monitored every 2 weeks. If the count falls below 80 × 10^9/L, the patient is managed based on the assumption she has ITP.

Women with a History of ITP. If a woman has a history of ITP (with or without prior splenectomy), the platelet count should be monitored at an interval dependent on the initial platelet count every 2 weeks if it is below 80 × 10^9/L. The need for antenatal therapy is based exclusively on maternal indications[3,17] with the goal of maintaining the count above 20 × 10^9/L (or higher in case of bleeding symptoms). The first line of treatment is the lowest effective dose of corticosteroids. Intravenous immunoglobulin (IVIG) is a second-line treatment, in case of corticosteroid refractoriness or side effects and because of its transient efficacy. The effect of IVIG lasts 2 to 3 weeks and often decreases or ceases with repetitive dosing. IVIG is best reserved for use late in pregnancy or immediately prior to delivery. Immunosuppressive drugs (azathioprine or vincristine—best avoided in the first trimester) and splenectomy (the second trimester is the best time) may rarely be needed. There is no demonstrable effect of maternal treatment such as corticosteroids[24,27] or IVIG on the fetal platelet count.[25] However, higher dosages of corticosteroids have not been investigated in controlled studies.

TABLE 15–1

Laboratory Investigations in a Pregnant Woman with Thrombocytopenia

TEST	AIM
Bloodfilm	Exclude spurious thrombocytopenia, HELLP, TTP, other hematologic diseases
Liver functions	
Proteinuria	
Coagulation tests	Exclude rare causes of thrombocytopenia
APTT – lupus anticoagulants	
SLE serology	Consider when indicated
HIV	
Thyroid function tests	

APPT, activated partial thromboplastin time; HELLP, hemolysis, elevated liver enzymes, liver function disturbances, low platelet count; TTP, thrombotic thrombocytopenic purpura.

Labor and Delivery

A history of splenectomy, current maternal thrombocytopenia or treatment for ITP, or thrombocytopenia in a sibling at birth dictates delivery at a center with expertise in maternal-fetal medicine. A maternal platelet count above 50 × 10^9/L is generally considered safe for either vaginal or cesarean delivery, though the factual basis for this recommendation is weak. Many members of a consensus panel consider a platelet count of >30 × 10^9/L, without bleeding, safe for vaginal delivery.[12] A low platelet count may in point be an argument against cesarean delivery. Should the count be below 50 × 10^9/L, either platelet transfusions or preferentially IVIG, or both may be given in time to raise the counts during labor and delivery. A maternal platelet count above 70 to 80 × 10^9/L is often recommended if epidural anesthesia is planned.[3,26]

The evidence is convincing that route of delivery does not alter the risk of severe perinatal internal hemorrhage,[3,6,12,16,17] and cesarean delivery is undertaken for traditional obstetric indications. However, it is prudent to avoid invasive manipulations such as fetal scalp blood sampling, or vacuum extraction or rotational forceps.[3,12,26]

Several investigators have suggested either cordocentesis or fetal scalp blood sampling to estimate the perinatal platelet count. However, this practice cannot be condoned because altering the route of delivery based on the perinatal platelet count does not change the outcome. Further, scalp blood samples are subject to technical errors, and the maternal and fetal risks of cordocentesis clearly exceed the risk of fetal hemorrhage from ITP.

Routine thrombosis prophylaxis in case of surgical delivery, immobilization, or individual risk factors should be undertaken unless there is either bleeding or severe thrombocytopenia (<50 × 10^9/L). When the platelet count is between 50 and 100 × 10^9/L, the risks of thrombosis and bleeding should be carefully weighed against each other.[3]

Postnatal

The maternal platelet counts generally improve over the first 6 weeks. Either tranexamic acid (1 g given three times daily) or hormonal therapy may help reduce excessive vaginal bleeding. Breastfeeding is not contraindicated.[12,24]

The newborn's platelet count, even if normal at birth, should be tested for at least the first 5 days, as one third develop a delayed thrombocytopenia.[7,15] Neonates with counts below 50 × 10^9/L may bleed, and the risk for intracranial hemorrhage is 0% to 1.5%.[12,13] IVIG, with or without corticosteroids, is the first-line treatment for the neonates whose counts are below 50 × 10^9/L and is combined with platelet transfusion if the counts are below 20 × 10^9/L or there is bleeding.[3,7,17,68] Brain imaging e.g., ultrasound is recommended in these cases.

Summary

The management of ITP during pregnancy is based on several large and well-designed clinical cohort studies that demonstrate that ITP runs a benign course in pregnancy for both mother and child. Severe fetal bleeding and in utero intracranial hemorrhage remain unreported. Should one be confronted with such a case, other bleeding disorders and alloimmune antibodies must be sought before assuming the explanation is ITP.

CONCLUSIONS

- ITP is relatively common during pregnancy, but in instances of thrombocytopenia above 80 × 10^9/L, gestational thrombocytopenia is 10 times more common.
- In pregnancies with a history of ITP, the likelihood of a nadir neonatal platelet count below 50 × 10^9/L is 9% to 15%, and the risk of major (intracranial) bleeding 0% to 1.5%. In a third of the cases, thrombocytopenia develops during the first 4 days postnatally.
- The probability of fetal thrombocytopenia is higher if a prior sibling was thrombocytopenic, or the mother has had splenectomy, or has severe thrombocytopenia and requires ITP treatment during pregnancy.
- Severe in utero bleeding has not been documented.
- Cesarean section is not indicated for presumed fetal thrombocytopenia.
- Cordocentesis is not recommended, and a scalp platelet count is unreliable.
- Minimize fetal blood sampling in labor and assisted vaginal delivery.

SUMMARY OF MANAGEMENT OPTIONS
Isoimmune Thrombocytopenia

Management Options (see Fig. 15–1)	Quality of Evidence	Strength of Recommendation	References
Prepregnancy			
Risk of neonatal thrombocytopenia is increased if there was a previously affected pregnancy.	III	B	20, 22
Avoidance of pregnancy arguably is an issue only in women refractory to splenectomy, steroids, and immunosuppression.	III	B	12
Prenatal			
Laboratory investigations:			
• Exclude other causes (see Table 15–1).	II	B	6,7
• Monitor maternal platelet counts fortnightly through pregnancy of history ITP or platelet count <80 × 10^9/L.	IV	D	3,12
Treatment:	III	B	3,17
• Threshold target titer varies between 30 and <50 × 10^9/L.			
• Corticosteroids are first-line therapy (<0.5–19/kg); toper to lowest dose.	IV	C	3,12
• IVIG (intravenous immunoglobulin) is best reserved for administration between 36 and 37 weeks (predelivery).	IV	D	3,12

SUMMARY OF MANAGEMENT OPTIONS

Isoimmune Thrombocytopenia *(Continued)*

Management Options (see Fig. 15–1)	Quality of Evidence	Strength of Recommendation	References
Prenatal—Continued			
• Consider splenectomy with severe ITP in early pregnancy with no response to steroids or IVIG; immunosuppressives (vincristine and azathiaprine) are options for refractory disease in late pregnancy.	–	GPP	–
Labor and Delivery			
Plan delivery in center with appropriate multidisciplinary expertise.	–	GPP	–
Aim for platelet count >50 × 10^9/L for delivery.	III	B	3,17,27
Maternal platelet transfusion is needed to cover delivery if the platelet count is <50 × 10^9/L.	–	GPP	–
Epidural anesthesia likely safe if platelet count >80×10^9/L	III	B	26
No evidence that cordocentesis at 38–39 weeks and fetal scalp blood sampling in labor are justified.	III	B	3,6,12,16,17
Cesarean section is performed entirely for obstetric indications; no evidence shows that any fetal/neonatal hemorrhage risk is lessened by elective cesarean section.	III	B	3,6,11,12,16, 17
Minimize (some advocate avoidance of) fetal scalp sampling and assisted vaginal delivery, especially by vacuum extraction.	III	B	3,12,16,17
Episiotomy should be avoided if possible with low maternal platelet counts.	–	GPP	–
Postnatal			
Monitor neonatal platelet counts for 5 days:	III	B	3,7,17
• IVIG if <50 × 10^9/L	IV	B	68
• Platelet transfusion if <20 × 10^9/L if clinically indicated			
Breastfeeding is not contraindicated.	III	B	24,27

ITP, isoimmune thrombocystic purpura; IVIG, intravenous immunoglobulin.

ALLOIMMUNE THROMBOCYTOPENIA

Incidence

Alloimmune thrombocytopenia in the perinate results from maternal antibodies directed against an alloantigen on the fetal platelet membrane, localized to glycoprotein (GP) IIIa (CD61) of the GP IIb/IIIa complex. The preferred terminology for these alloantigens is presently human platelet antigen (HPA), though other names linger in the literature. The first discovered antigen system was named Zw (Zw^a and Zw^b) after the first two letters of the patient's family name.[28] A few years later, the PL^A system, which appeared to be identical to Zw, was described.[29] The International Platelet Antigen Working Party suggests the name human platelet antigen (HPA).[30] The nomenclature is based on the chronologic numbering of alloantibodies in the order of their discovery. The letter "a" or "b" is assigned to the high- and low-frequency alleles, respectively. "W" marks an HPA system antigen of which only one allele is identified so far. Finally, a few "private" or family-restricted antigens are described that have been identified only on the platelets of members in one family, and thus do not qualify for an HPA number.

The incidence of a particular HPA varies by race.[31] In whites, 2% are negative for HPA-1a, which accounts for about 85% of FNAIT. Anti-HPA-1a antibodies are produced in approximately 11% of the HPA-1a negative mothers.[32,33] The other antigens most commonly involved in FNAIT among whites are the HPA-5b and HPA-3a.[31]

The development of anti-HPA-1a antibodies is strongly associated with the presence of the HLA class type II DRB3*0101. The absence of DRB3*0101 in a HPA-1a negative woman virtually precludes the development of antibodies. About a third of HPA-1a negative women who are DRB3*0101 positive develop antibodies.[32,34–40] The incidence of severe thrombocytopenia caused by anti HPA-1a antibodies approximates 1 in 1100 pregnancies.[32] Antenatal screening is not warranted.

Risks

In contrast to red blood cell immunization, platelet alloimmunization affects the first pregnancy in half of the cases.[41] Most infants with FNAIT are born either without symptoms or with petechiae or bleeding from puncture sites. The most serious complication of FNAIT is internal hemorrhage, such as gastrointestinal, lung, and intracranial bleeding, occurring in either the fetus or newborn. Intracranial hemorrhage (ICH) is the most common internal hemorrhage in FNAIT and causes serious perinatal morbidity and even death.[42,43] Serious bleeding, including ICH, is often associated with HPA-1a immunization. The risk of perinatal ICH as a result of HPA-1a incompability approximates 11% excluding and 15% including fetal deaths.[44] The results of two large, prospective antibody screening programs (25,000 women in Cambridge, England,[32] and 100,000 women in Norway [Husebekk, personal communication]) document in aggregate two severe ICH and one ICH without clinical consequence. Most cases of FNAIT are identified after the birth of an affected child. The degree of fetal thrombocytopenia reportedly remains similar or increases in 80% of subsequent pregnancies when the father is homozygous for the offending antigen.[45–51] Unfortunately, the predictive value of the antibody titer for the severity of fetal thrombocytopenia is inconsistent, though some studies observe that severe thrombocytopenia is associated with an anti–HPA-1a titer ≥1:32.[32,33] Antenatal screening is not practiced given the low prevalence of ICH in an unselected population and the appropriate reticence for unnecessary population-based screening.

The risk for ICH in a subsequent pregnancy of HPA-1a alloimmunized women depends on the obstetric history. In the large majority of FNAIT cases, the chance of an ICH in a subsequent pregnancy with an HPA-1a positive fetus, after the birth of a thrombocytopenic sibling without ICH, approximates 7%.[44] In contrast, the recurrence rate of ICH in subsequent offspring of women with a history of FNAIT and ICH in the older sibling approximates 75%.[44] In one review, ICH was reported to occur in utero in 80.5% of the at-risk pregnancies.[43] Most cases of ICH in utero occur in the third trimester, though ICH has been documented before 20 weeks.[52,53] ICH in utero may cause either fetal death or, if the fetus survives, fetal hydrops or hydrocephalus.

It is unknown why one fetus with AITP may experience severe antenatal (intracranial) bleeding in contrast to another fetus with a comparable degree of thrombocytopenia due to maternal ITP who does not suffer this complication. In addition, there is only mild bleeding in the majority of ITP patients when it does occur in the fetus/newborn, whereas in alloimmune (anti-HPA-1a) thrombocytopenic conditions, as in post-transfusion purpura, bleeding may be life-threatening. The GP IIb/IIIa complex on the platelet membrane carries not only the amino acid difference between HPA-1a (Leu[33]) and HPA-1b (Pro[33]) but also most of the autoantigens involved in ITP antibodies. The IIb/IIIa complex is expressed not only on platelets but also on vascular endothelium. Although no data are available, one may postulate that the density of antigenic molecules of HPA-1a and the autoantigens on IIb/IIIa may be different. Differences in antigen density or in the nature of the antibodies may result in antigen-antibody reactions initiating different immune-mediated cascades involving complement, coagulation activation, and cytokine induction. A severe bleeding risk in a fetus or neonate often affects cerebral vessels, whereas in adults other bleeding sites emerge.

Management Options (Fig. 15–2)

Prepregnancy

Prepregnancy management begins with an accurate diagnosis of FNAIT in the newborn with thrombocytopenia. Platelet alloimmunization should be part of the differential diagnosis in all cases of neonatal thrombocytopenia (platelet count $<100 \times 10^9$/L in term infants). The laboratory evaluation includes the following:

- Confirming the presence of anti-HPA autoantibodies against platelets in maternal serum.
- Cross-matching of the maternal serum with paternal platelets, both untreated and chloroquine-treated (to remove HLA antigens that may cause a "false positive" test).
- HPA pheno- or genotyping of mother and father.
- Exclusion of maternal thrombocytopenia.

When the diagnosis of FNAIT is established, and the couple is considering another pregnancy, careful prepregnancy counseling in a specialized center is advised. Counseling should include documentation of disease severity in the index case, the antibody specificity, and the hetero/homozygosity of the father. The option of artificial insemination with the sperm of a donor negative for the offending antigen should be discussed.

Prenatal

Antenatal diagnosis is feasible when the father is heterozygous for the offending antigen. Although fetal genotyping is possible using chorionic villi, amniocentesis in the early second trimester is generally preferable because of its lower risk of boosting sensitization and pregnancy loss. Genotyping for all-important HPAs is possible using polymerase chain reaction (PCR). In very severe instances, donor insemination or preimplantation diagnosis using single cell of the blastomere can be considered.[54] When the fetus is positive for the offending antigen and at risk for severe thrombocytopenia, the pregnancy should be managed in or in collaboration with

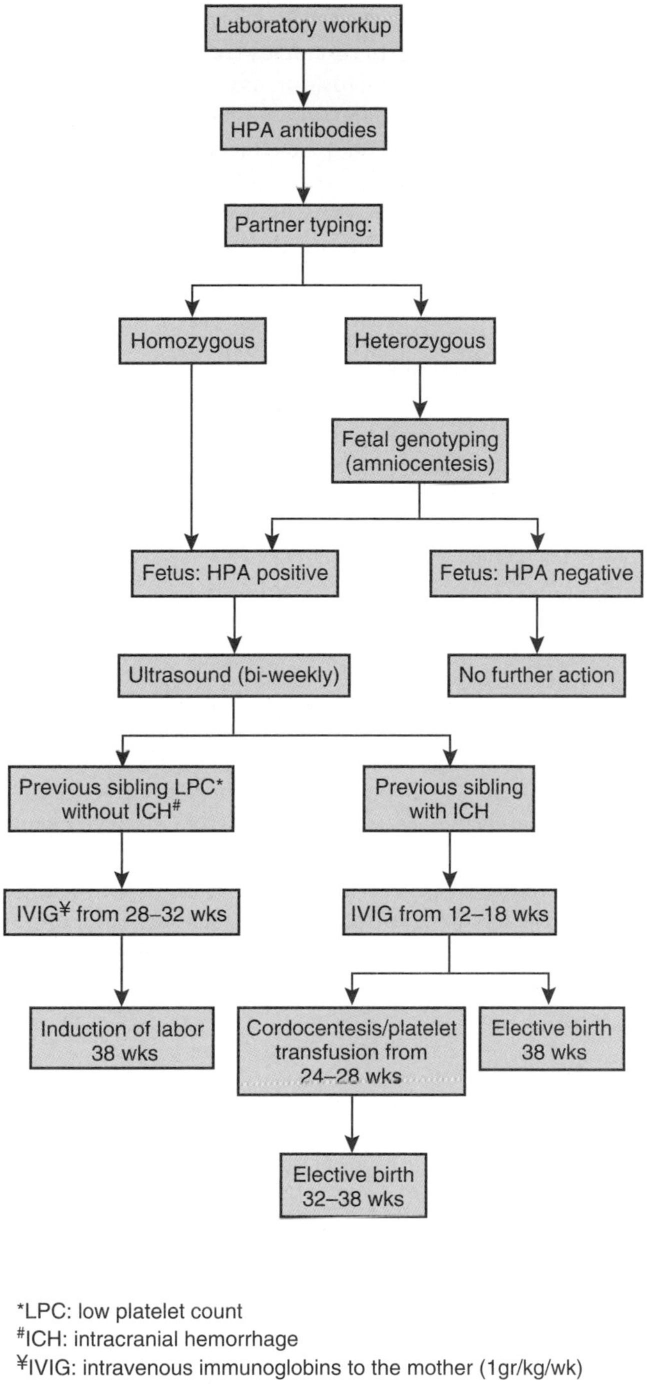

FIGURE 15–2
Management of platelet alloimmunization. Note that different options are controversial. HPA, human platelet antigen; ICH, intracranial hemorrhage; IVIG, intravenous immunoglobulin; LPC, low platelet count.

a specialized fetal medicine center. Monitoring of anti-HPA antibodies cannot accurately predict the severity of fetal thrombocytopenia,[55,56] but a high titer (>1:32) may imply severe thrombocytopenia.[32,33]

Several strategies can be used for the monitoring and treatment of pregnancies at risk for FNAIT,[45–51] including fetal blood sampling with platelet transfusion when indicated, and maternal treatment with high-dose intravenous immunoglobulin (IVIG) and corticosteroids. In one review of the literature, 26 different combinations of treatment were reported.[43] Unfortunately, no controlled trials compare intervention to nonintervention, and all recommendations are based on historical control subjects and natural history surveys. With these limitations, the current treatment of choice is a weekly maternal infusion of immunoglobulin at a dose of 1 g/kg of maternal weight. Several case series published since the initial report of Bussel and associates in 1988[57] confirm that weekly IVIG effectively increases the fetal platelet count to a variable degree.[58–61] The result of a multicenter, prospective randomized trial comparing IVIG with or without dexamethasone revealed a 70% response rate with IVIG alone,[62] and dexamethasone did not improve the effect when used routinely. Significantly, there were no instances of ICH in IVIG-treated perinates in this study and others,[61,63] even if they failed to respond with an increased platelet count.

Although cordocentesis is the only tool available to directly monitor the severity of fetal thrombocytopenia, its routine use is not advised. Fetal blood sampling has caused fatal hemorrhage from the umbilical cord puncture site in fetuses with a low platelet count. Special precautions may lower the risk of complications in these patients (Table 15–2). The published literature reports a mean fetal loss rate of cordocentesis in FNAIT pregnancies of 1.6% per procedure. In addition, there is a risk of procedure-related complications such as emergency cesarean section for fetal bleeding and bradycardia in 2.4% per procedure.[44,61,64,65] The reported complications might be method-related, as no increase was seen when a needle guide was used.[66] Platelet transfusion is problematic because the half-life of transfused platelets is only 4 to 5 days. Thus, fetal blood sampling and platelet transfusions are required frequently throughout pregnancy once initiated, introducing a cumulative risk for complications. The transfused platelets may degranulate and release serotonin, compounding the risk of a bradycardia. The cumulative risk of fetal loss with transfusion therapy approximates 6% per pregnancy.[66,67] Given the 70% likelihood that the initial fetal platelet count at cordocentesis between 20 and 28 weeks in FNAIT pregnancies with affected siblings is $\leq 50 \times 10^9/L$,[45] we suggest IVIG be begun as a precaution after the amniocentesis genotype results confirm an affected fetus.

TABLE 15–2

Extra Safety Precautions for Fetal Blood Sampling in Pregnancies at Risk for Severe Thrombocytopenia

The procedure should be performed by the most experienced members of a fetal medicine unit.
Sample in the umbilical vein and thus avoid puncturing the artery.
Use a hematologic cell counter in order to obtain the platelet count within 2 minutes.
If the fetal platelet count is $<50 \times 10^9/L$, compatible platelets should be infused before withdrawal of the needle.

The antenatal management protocols in FNAIT should be based on the following principles. First, the primary goal is the prevention of ICH and not just fetal thrombocytopenia per se. Second, the protocol should reflect the obstetric history. Given the fact that the large majority of patients have a sibling with a history of more or less severe thrombocytopenia, but without ICH, and the risk of ICH approximates the procedure-related complication rate of invasive therapy, it is best to avoid cordocenteses in these patients. Considering that the majority of in utero ICH occurs later in pregnancy and the cost of IVIG, treatment of pregnancies with no ICH history may be delayed to 28–32 weeks (see Fig. 15–2). We have seen no ICH or other serious morbidity applying this approach to 40 women in Leiden over the past few years.[67] In fetuses whose siblings experienced an ICH, IVIG should be initiated to 12 to 18 weeks followed by cordocentesis at 24 to 28 weeks to evaluate the response. When the anticipated risk of complication from cordocentesis is higher (e.g., less experienced operators), the IVIG can be continued until delivery without periodic cordocentesis (see Fig. 15–2). In recent years, we treated eight pregnancies in six women with an older sibling with ICH according to this less invasive protocol. Each received IVIG (median 20 weeks; range 8–24 weeks) without initial or follow-up cordocentesis. In four pregnancies, one fetal blood sampling, with platelet transfusion was performed at term. In these pregnancies labor was induced between 37 and 38 weeks, within 3 days of the intrauterine platelet transfusion. Elective cesarean section was performed in five pregnancies between 34 and 37 weeks. All perinates had a platelet count of less than 50×10^9/L (three were < 20×10^9/L), either at birth or in the predelivery cordocentesis sample. Four of the neonates received one platelet transfusion after birth. None of the neonates showed any signs of internal or external bleeding. In the very rare case, a patient with a history of ICH might benefit from either rescue corticosteroids or a higher dose of IVIG despite the early initiation of IVIG (1 g/kg/week).

Labor and Delivery

Ideally, labor should be planned by the obstetrician in close consultation with the fetal medicine and pediatric teams and the blood bank to assure compatible platelets are available shortly after birth. A term delivery can be achieved in almost all pregnancies treated with IVIG. If serial fetal platelet transfusions are necessary for local reasons, we suggest elective delivery after 32 weeks because of the risks of the procedure.

There is no consensus about the safety of vaginal birth in FNAIT infants. However, there is no evidence that a vaginal birth enhances the risk for ICH in a treated term infant with FNAIT. The preponderance of perinatal ICH in FNAIT occurs before the start of labor.[43,44] Similar to ITP, we suggest an instrumented vaginal delivery be avoided if the fetal platelet count is unknown. In Leiden, we perform cesarean delivery for obstetric indications only in women with platelet alloimmunization, whose prior child did not suffer ICH and who has been treated antenatally with IVIG. Last, cesarean delivery does not guarantee protection against the perinatal occurrence of ICH in a severe thrombocytopenic infant.

Postnatal

In platelet alloimmunized pregnancies, the newborn's platelets count should be tested daily for the first 5 to 7 days. In case of thrombocytopenia the neonate may respond to IVIG. In case of fetal thrombocytopenia, brain imaging should be performed. In severe cases and infants treated prenatally with at least 4 weeks with IVIG, transfusion with compatible platelets is the first-line treatment. Breastfeeding is not contraindicated in FNAIT newborns.

Summary

Severe platelet alloimmunization, leading to perinatal ICH is a rare but potentially disastrous condition. Management strategies should focus on the prevention of ICH and not thrombocytopenia per se. There is a lack of adequately sized, well-designed control studies regarding management. After the index pregnancy, the obstetric history is one of the important factors for risk estimation of ICH. The majority of ICH cases occur during fetal life. Maternally administered IVIG is the first line of therapy in pregnancies at risk for severe disease, and appears to significantly reduce the risk of ICH even when there has been no reponse in the fetal platelet count.

CONCLUSIONS

- Because there is no effective screening, the diagnosis of alloimmune thrombocytopenia is typically made after the birth of an affected child.
- Antenatally, the diagnosis of FNAIT should be considered in fetuses with ICH, hydrocephalus, hydrops, or tumor in cerebrum.
- Intravenous immunoglobulin given to the mother is first-line therapy, with steroids being used for the IVIG-resistant cases. Timing depends on obstetric history.

CONCLUSIONS (Continued)

- Cordocentesis can be avoided in women with no history of ICH in the older sibling.
- When there is an older sibling with ICH, IVIG may be given without cordocentesis, especially if the risk of the procedure is anticipated to be high.

SUMMARY OF MANAGEMENT OPTIONS
Alloimmune Thrombocytopenia

Management Options (see Fig. 15–2)	Quality of Evidence	Strength of Recommendation	References
Prepregnancy			
Review history of index case, including severity.	–	GPP	–
Investigate:	–	GPP	–
• Confirm human platelet antigen (HPA) antibodies in mother.			
• HPA genotyping of both parents is needed.			
• Exclude maternal thrombocytopenia.			
• Cross-match maternal serum with paternal platelets.			
Provide careful counseling of parents about risks (main risk is intracranial hemorrhage, ICH) and potential management (including donor insemination from HPA-negative donor).	–	GPP	–
In addition to the parents, members of the mother's family should be typed to establish whether her sisters are at similar risk during their pregnancies.	–	GPP	–
Prenatal			
Management requires specialist center.	–	GPP	–
With heterozygous father, perform amniocentesis early in second trimester to determine fetal genotype by polymerase chain reaction	III	B	55, 56
No further action is taken if the fetus types as HPA negative.	–	GPP	–
Maternal titer does not predict severity.	III	B	55, 56
Treatment regimen varies and is controversial:	IV	C	43
• Maternal administration of IVIG (intravenous immunoglobulin) weekly (1–2g/kg maternal weight) is the main approach; timing might be determined by severity in previous baby.	III	B	57, 58–62
• Fetal blood sampling for fetal platelet count might be reserved only for those with previous ICH; advisable to defer sampling until after IVIG regimen is under way because >70% of fetuses will be <50 × 10^9/L; timing also might be determined by severity in previous baby (see Table 15–2).	III	B	64
• No evidence shows that initial use of oral corticosteroids with IVIG yields any better response than using IVIG alone.	Ib	A	63
• Some reserve use of oral corticosteroids for IVIG-resistant cases.	III	B	57
• Repeated fetal platelet sampling and intravascular transfusions of fresh platelets are used only in those cases that fail to respond to maternal therapy.	III	B	57, 58–62
Regular ultrasound of fetal brain is needed.	–	GPP	–
Labor and Delivery			
Close liaison with pediatric staff is necessary.	–	GPP	–
Mode of delivery depends on the fetal platelet count. A trial of labor is reasonable if the count is >50 × 10^9/L.	III	B	43, 44

Continued

SUMMARY OF MANAGEMENT OPTIONS
Alloimmune Thrombocytopenia *(Continued)*

Management Options (see Fig. 15–2)	Quality of Evidence	Strength of Recommendation	References
Labor and Delivery			
Platelet transfusion just before delivery may be considered even if a cesarean section is contemplated; no evidence shows that abdominal delivery reduces risk of ICH; it is not always atraumatic.			
Postnatal			
Neonatal platelet count is monitored daily for the first 7 days; platelet transfusion and IVIG for 4 weeks if platelets are <50 × 10^9/L.	–	GPP	–
Breastfeeding is not contraindicated.	–	GPP	–

HPA, human plalelet antigen; ICH, intracranial hemorrhage; IVIG, intravenous immunoglobulin.

REFERENCES

1. Dreyfus M, Kaplan C, Verdy E, et al: Immune thrombocytopenia working group. Frequency of immune thrombocytopenia in newborns: A prospective study. Blood 1997;89:4402–4406.
2. Burrows RF, Kelton JG: Incidentally detected thrombocytopenia in healthy mothers and their infants. N Engl J Med 1988; 319:142–145.
3. Guidelines for the investigation and management of idiopathic thrombocytopenic purpura in adults, children and pregnancy. Br J Haematol 2003;120:574–596.
4. McMillan R: Therapy for adults with refractory chronic immune thrombocytopenic purpura. Ann Intern Med 1997;126:307–314.
5. Kessler I, Lancet M, Borenstein R, et al: The obstetrical management of patients with immunologic thrombocytopenic purpura. Int J Gynaecol Obstet 1982;20:23–28.
6. Burrows RF, Kelton JG: Fetal thrombocytopenia and its relation to maternal thrombocytopenia. N Engl J Med 1993;329:1463–1466.
7. Burrows RF, Kelton JG: Thrombocytopenia during pregnancy. In Greer IA, Turpie AGG, Forbes CD (eds): Haemostasis and Thrombosis in Obstetrics and Gynaecology. London, Chapman & Hall, 1992.
8. Samuels P, Bussel JB, Braitman LE, et al: Estimation of thrombocytopenia in the offspring of pregnant women with presumed immune thrombocytopenic purpura. N Engl J Med 1990;323: 229–235.
9. Kaplan C, Daffos F, Forestier F, et al: Fetal platelet counts in thrombocytopenic pregnancy. Lancet 1990;336:979–982.
10. Garmel SH, Craigo SD, Morin LM, et al: The role of percutaneous blood sampling in the management of immune thrombocytopenic purpura. Prenat Diagn 1995;15:439–445.
11. Payne SD, Resnik R, Moore TR, et al: Maternal characteristics and risk of severe neonatal thrombocytopenia and intracranial hemorrhage in pregnancies complicated by autoimmune thrombocytopenia. Am J Obstet Gynecol 1997;717:149–155.
12. George JN, Woolf SH, Raskob GE, et al: Idiopathic thrombocytopenic purpura: A practice guideline developed by explicit methods for the American Society of Hematology. Blood 1996;88:3–40.
13. Cook RL, Miller R, Katz VL, Cefalo RC: Immune thrombocytopenic purpura in pregnancy: A reappraisal of management. Obstet Gynecol 1991;78:578–583.
14. Burrows RF, Kelton JG: Thrombocytopenia at delivery: A prospective survey of 6715 deliveries. Am J Obstet Gynecol 1990;162:731–734.
15. Valat AS, Caulier MT, Devos P, et al: Relationships between severe neonatal thrombocytopenia and maternal characteristics in pregnancies associated with autoimmune thrombocytopenia. Br J Haematol 1998;103:397–401.
16. Letsky EA, Greaves M: Guidelines on the investigation and management of thrombocytopenia in pregnancy and neonatal alloimmune thrombocytopenia. Maternal and Neonatal Haemostasis and Thrombosis Task Force of the British Society for Haematology. Br J Haematol 1996;95:21–26.
17. George JN, Woolf SH, Raskob GE: Idiopathic thrombocytopenic purpura: A guideline for diagnosis and management of children and adults. American Society of Hematology. Ann Med 1998;30:38–44.
18. Boehlen F, Hohlfeld P, Extermann P, de Moerloose P: Maternal antiplatelet antibodies in predicting risk of neonatal thrombocytopenia. Obstet Gynecol 1999;93:169–173.
19. Mazzucconi MG, Petrelli V, Gandolfi GM, et al: Autoimmune thrombocytopenic purpura in pregnancy: Maternal risk factors predictive of neonatal thrombocytopenia. Autoimmunity 1993;16:209–214.
20. Christiaens GC, Nieuwenhuis HK, Bussel JB: Comparison of platelet counts in first and second newborns of women with immune thrombocytopenic purpura. Obstet Gynecol 1997;90:546–552.
21. Gandemer V, Kaplan C, Quelvennec E, et al: Pregnancy-associated autoimmune neonatal thrombocytopenia: Role of maternal HLA genotype. Br J Haematol 1999;104:878–885.
22. Sainio S, Joutsi L, Jarvenpaa AL, et al: Idiopathic thrombocytopenic purpura in pregnancy. Acta Obstet Gynecol Scand 1998;77:272–277.
23. Giles AR, Hoogendoorn H, Benford K: Type IIB von Willebrand's disease presenting as thrombocytopenia in pregnancy. Br J Haematol 1987;67:349–353.
24. Christiaens GCML, Nieuwenhuis HK, von dem Borne AE, et al: Idiopathic thrombocytopenic purpura in pregnancy: A randomized trial on the effect of antenatal low dose corticosteroids on neonatal platelet count. BJOG 1991;98:334–336.

25. Yamada H, Fugimoto S: Perinatal management of idiopathic thrombocytopenic purpura in pregnancy: Risk factors for passive immune thrombocytopenia. Ann Haematol 1994;68:39–42.
26. Beilin Y, Zahn J, Comerford M: Safe epidural analgesia in thirty parturients with platelet counts between 69,000 and 98,000 mm^{-3}. Anesth Analg 1997;85:385–388.
27. Owen PH: Idiopathic thrombocytopenic purpura in pregnancy: A randomised trial on the effect of antenatal low dose corticosteroids on neonatal platelet count. BJOG 1991;98:948.
28. van Loghem JJ, Dorfmeijer H, van der Hart M, Schreuder F: Serological and genetical studies on a platelet antigen. Vox Sang 1959;4:161–169.
29. Shulman NR, Nader VJ, Hiller MC, Collier EM: Platelet and leukocyte isoantigens and their antibodies. Serologic and clinical studies. Progr Hematol 1964;4:222.
30. von dem Borne AEGK, Decary I: ICSI / ISBT working party on platelet serology. Nomenclature of platelet-specific antigens. Vox Sang 1990;58:176.
31. Porcelijn L, Kanhai HHH: Diagnosis and management of fetal platelet disorders. In Rodeck CH, Whittle MJ (eds): Fetal Medicine: Basic Science and Clinical Practice. London, Churchill Livingstone, 1999, pp 805–815.
32. Williamson LM, Hacket G, Rennie J, et al: The natural history of fetomaternal alloimmunization to the platelet-specific antigen HPA-1a (PlA1, Zwa) as was determined by antenatal screening. Blood 1998;92:2280–2287.
33. Jaegtvik S, Husebekk A, Aune B, et al: Neonatal alloimmune thrombocytopenia due to anti-HPA1a antibodies; the level of maternal antibodies predicts the severity of thrombocytopenia in the newborn. BJOG 2000;107:691–694.
34. de Waal LP, van Dalen CM, Engelfriet CP, von dem Borne AEGK: Alloimmunization against the platelet-specific Zw(a) antigen, resulting in neonatal alloimmune thrombocytopenia or posttransfusion purpura, is associated with the supertypic DRw52 antigen including DR3 and DRw6. Hum Immunol 1986;17:45–53.
35. Valentin N, Vergracht A, Bignon JD, et al: HLA-DRw52a is involved in alloimmunization against PL-A1 antigen. Hum Immunol 1990;27:73–79.
36. Reznikoff-Etievant MF, Kaplan C, Muller JY, et al: Allo-immune thrombocytopenias, definition of a group at risk; a prospective study. Curr Stud Hematol Blood Transf 1988;55:119–124.
37. L'Abbé D, Tremblay L, Goldman M, et al: Alloimmunization to platelet antigen HPA-1a (Zwa): association with HLA-DRw52a is not 100%. Tansfus Med 1992;2:251.
38. Taaning E: HLA antigens and maternal antibodies in alloimmune neonatal thrombocytopenia. Tissue Antigens 1983;21:351–359.
39. Mueller-Eckhardt C, Mueller-Eckhardt G, Willen Ohff H, et al: Immunogenicity of an immune response to human platelet antigen Zw(a) is strongly associated with HLA-B8 and DR3. Tissue Antigens 1985;26:71–76.
40. Mueller-Eckhardt G, Mueller-Eckhardt C: Alloimmunization against the platelet specific Zw(a) antigen associated with HLA-DRw52 and/or DRw6? Hum Immunol 1987;18:181–182.
41. Reznikoff-Etievant MF: Management of alloimmune neonatal and antenatal thrombocytopenia. Vox Sang 1988;55:193–201.
42. Kaplan C, Daffos F, Forestier F, et al: Current trends in neonatal alloimmune thrombocytopenia: Diagnosis and therapy. In Kaplan-Gouet C, Schlegel N, Salmon C, McGregor J (eds): Platelet Immunology: Fundamental and Clinical Aspects. Paris, France, Colloque INSERM / John Libbey Eurotext, 1991, pp 206:267–278.
43. Spencer JA, Burrows RF: Feto-maternal alloimmune thrombocytopenia: A literature review and statistical analysis. Aust N Z J Obstet Gynecol 2001;41:45–55.
44. Radder CM, Brand A, Kanhai HHH: Will it ever be possible to balance the risk of intracranial haemorrhage in fetal or neonatal alloimmune thrombocytopenia against the risk of treatment strategies to prevent it? Vox Sang 2003;84:318–325.
45. Bussel JB, Zabusky MR, Berkowitz RL, McFarland JG: Fetal alloimmune thrombocytopenia. N Engl J Med 1997;337:22–26.
46. de Vries LS, Connell J, Bydder GM, et al: Recurrent intracranial haemorrhages in utero in an infant with alloimmune thrombocytopenia. Case report. BJOG 1988;95:299–302.
47. Herman JH, Jumbelic MI, Ancona RJ, Kickler TS: In utero cerebral hemorrhage in alloimmune thrombocytopenia. Am J Pediatr Hematol Oncol 1986;8:312–317.
48. Kanhai HH, Porcelijn L, van Zoeren D, et al: Antenatal care in pregnancies at risk of alloimmune thrombocytopenia: Report of 19 cases in 16 families. Eur J Obstet Gynecol Reprod Biol 1996;68:67–73.
49. Kaplan C, Daffos F, Forestier F, et al: Management of alloimmune thrombocytopenia: Antenatal diagnosis and in utero transfusion of maternal platelets. Br J Haematol 1988;72:340–343.
50. Murphy MF, Waters AH, Doughty HA, et al: Antenatal management of fetomaternal alloimmune thrombocytopenia—Report of 15 affected pregnancies. Transfus Med 1994;4:281–292.
51. Reznikoff-Etievant MF: Management of alloimmune neonatal and antenatal thrombocytopenia [review] [65 refs]. Vox Sang 1988;55:193–201.
52. Giovangrandi Y, Daffos F, Kaplan C, et al: Very early intracranial haemorrhage in alloimmune fetal thrombocytopenia. Lancet 1990;336:310.
53. Murphy MF, Metcalfe P, Waters AH, et al: Antenatal management of severe feto-maternal alloimmune thrombocytopenia: HLA incompatibility may affect responses to fetal platelet transfusions. Blood 1993;81:2174–2179.
54. van den Veyver IB, Chong SS, Kristjansson K: Molecular analysis of human platelet antigen on single cells can be applied to preimplantation genetic diagnosis for prevention of alloimmune thrombocytopenia. Am J Obstet Gynecol 1994; 170:807–812.
55. Proulx C, Filion MM, Goldman M, et al: Analysis of immunoglobulin class IgG subclass and titre of HPA-1a antibodies in alloimmunized mothers giving birth to babies with or without neonatal alloimmune thrombocytopenia. Br J Hematol 1994;87:813–817.
56. Kaplan C, Daffos F, Forestier F, et al: Management of alloimmune thrombocytopenia: Antenatal diagnosis and in utero transfusion of maternal platelets. Blood 1988;72:340–343.
57. Bussel JB, Richard MD, Berkowitz L, et al: Antenatal treatment of neonatal alloimmune thrombocytopenia. N Engl J Med 1988;319:1374–1378.
58. Bussel JB, Zabusky MR, Berkowitz RL, McFarland JG: Fetal alloimmune thrombocytopenia. N Eng J Med 1997;337:22–24.
59. Nicolini U, Tannirandorn Y, Gonzalez P, et al: Continuing controversy in alloimmune thrombocytopenia: Fetal hyperimmunoglobulinemia fails to prevent thrombocytopenia. Am J Obstet Gynecol 1990;163:1144–1146.
60. Mir N, Samson D, House MJ, Kovar IZ: Failure of antenatal high-dose immunoglobulin to improve fetal platelet count in neonatal alloimmune thrombocytopenia. Vox Sang 1988;55: 188–189.
61. Radder CM, Brand A, Kanhai HH: A less invasive treatment strategy to prevent intracranial hemorrhage in fetal and neonatal alloimmune thrombocytopenia. Am J Obstet Gynecol 2001; 185 :683–688.
62. Bussel JB, Berkowitz RL, Lynch L, et al: Antenatal management of alloimmune thrombocytopenia with intravenous gamma-globulin: A randomized trial of the addition of low-dose steroid to intravenous gamma-globulin. Am J Obstet Gynecol 1996;174:1414–1423.
63. Wenstrom KD, Weiner CP, Williamson RA: Antenatal treatment of fetal alloimmune thrombocytopenia. Obstet Gynecol 1992;80:433–435.
64. Birchall JE, Murphy MF, Kaplan C, Kroll H: European collaborative study of the antenatal management of feto-maternal alloimmune thrombocytopenia. Br J Hematol 2003;122:275–288.

65. Overton TG, Duncan KR, Jolly M, et al: Serial aggressive platelet transfusion for fetal alloimmune thrombocytopenia: Platelet dynamics and perinatal outcome. Am J Obstet Gynecol 2002;186:826–831.
66. Weiner CP: Fetal blood sampling and fetal thrombocytopenia. Fetal Diagn Ther 1995;10:173–177.
67. Engelfriet CP, Reesink HW, Kroll H, et al: Prenatal management of alloimmune thrombocytopenia of the fetus. International Forum. Vox Sang 2003;84:142–149.
68. Ballin A, Andrew H, Ling E, et al: High dose intravenous gammaglobulin therapy for neonatal autoimmune thrombocytopenia. J Pediatr 1988;112:789–792.

CHAPTER 16

Fetal Cardiac Arrhythmias: Diagnosis and Therapy

Christopher S. Snyder / Joshua A. Copel

INTRODUCTION

Clinical Significance

Fetal cardiac arrhythmias are common in clinical practice. Most reflect transient, isolated ectopic beats. However, sustained episodes can occur and, if not treated appropriately, can lead to congestive heart failure, nonimmune hydrops, and even fetal or neonatal demise. In this chapter we define fetal arrhythmias and review their frequency, the methods of detection, and their basic mechanisms. With this foundation, we will provide the recommendations for the detection and differentiation of arrhythmias as well as their management. We illustrate the importance of a team approach to fetal arrhythmia management, involving physicians from each subspecialty needed to care for mother, fetus, and the newborn.

History

Cremer first described fetal electrocardiography in 1906.[1] Fetal electrocardiography proved reliable for identifying tachycardias but was limited in its ability to determine the etiology. In the 1950s, Smyth described invasive electrocardiographic monitoring with an intra-amniotic electrode.[2] Despite this technologic advance, its use remained limited because it required ruptured membranes for access.

With the advent of echocardiography, and specifically M-mode, the field of fetal arrhythmia detection and differentiation blossomed. Robinson and Shaw-Dunn detailed the use of M-mode in the evaluation of fetal arrhythmias during the early 1970s.[3] As ultrasound technology expanded to include two-dimensional and both spectral and color Doppler modes, numerous authors described additional echocardiographic techniques for the identification and differentiation of fetal arrhythmias.

Definition

A fetal dysrhythmia is best defined as an irregularity in the fetal cardiac rhythm or a regular rhythm that remains outside the normal range. The currently accepted normal range in clinical practice is between 100 and 160 bpm, although no standard rate has been formally established, and somewhat higher rates may be seen during labor, especially with maternal fever. The American College of Obstetrics and Gynecology (ACOG) established a range at term as "usually 120–160 beats per minute."[4] This range does not exclude hypoxic fetuses. Davignon found the minimum heart rate for infants younger than 1 day of age was 88 bpm, the mean was 123 bpm, and the maximum was 168 bpm in a study of nearly 200 healthy children.[5] Any of these ranges may serve as a guide, and the identification of heart rate may be based on data collected for an extended period to assure that any deviations are not associated with uterine contractions, periodic decelerations, maternal fever, or physiologic fetal activity such as hiccupping.

Frequency

Fetal arrhythmias are relatively common at routine obstetric visits, with a frequency ranging from 1% to 3% of all pregnancies.[6,7] The most common causes of irregularities are either extrasystoles or respiratory sinus arrhythmia. Respiratory sinus arrhythmia is the variation in the heart rate related to respiration, increasing with inspiration and decreasing with expiration. It is not associated with symptoms or abnormalities and requires no further evaluation. Extrasystoles occur in upwards of 14% of term, healthy newborns[8] and account for 43% to 98% of fetal arrhythmia referrals.[9,10] The vast majority of the extrasystoles are atrial in origin, with premature ventricular contractions accounting for less than 4%.[9–11]

TABLE 16–1

Fetal Cardiac Arrhythmias

ARRHYTHMIA	NUMBER
Isolated extrasystoles	1213
Tachycardias	114
Supraventricular tachycardia	69
Atrial flutter	21
Sinus tachycardia	7
Ventricular tachycardia	7
Atrial fibrillation	4
Atrial ectopic tachycardia	4
Junctional tachycardia	2
Bradycardias	51
Complete AV block	39
Second-degree AV block	10
Sinus bradycardia	2

The fetal arrhythmias diagnosed in 1384 patients evaluated at our institution over 20 years are listed in Table 16–1. The experience reflects the general findings of others that extrasystoles are the most common cause of fetal arrhythmias and that tachycardias are more than twice as common as bradycardias.[7,10] The most common causes of fetal tachycardias are atrioventricular (AV) reentry supraventricular tachycardia (SVT), atrial flutter, and sinus tachycardia. Rare causes of SVT include atrial ectopy, atrial fibrillation, junctional tachycardia, and ventricular tachycardia, each constituting less than 1% of fetal arrhythmias.[9,10,12] The most common cause of fetal bradycardia is complete AV block, which accounts for more than three quarters of cases. Other, less frequent causes of bradycardia include isolated sinus bradycardia, advanced second-degree AV block, prolonged QT interval syndrome, and fetal toxicity.[13,14]

ASSESSMENT OF A FETAL ARRHYTHMIA

A variety of methods are available for the evaluation of fetal cardiac arrhythmias. The majority of techniques are noninvasive, though invasive techniques, such as scalp electrodes, are used occasionally. Herein, we focus on the commonly used noninvasive techniques, their advantages and disadvantages, and the future of fetal arrhythmia detection and differentiation.

When a fetal dysrhythmia is detected, the physician must determine the etiology of the abnormal rhythm. Multiple factors must be considered, given that fetal dysrhythmias can result from maternal connective tissue disorders, drugs, hyperthyroidism, or infection, or can be a sign of fetal compromise or an arrhythmia.[14–18] A complete maternal assessment should be made, including inquires regarding recent illnesses, medicinal and recreational drug use, caffeine intake, and signs of hyperthyroidism. A complete family history is essential with an emphasis on the presence of inherited causes of arrhythmia, such as prolonged QT interval syndrome, deafness (associated with prolonged QT interval syndrome), previous fetal demise, sudden unexplained death in family members younger than 50 years of age, and tuberous sclerosis. In addition, the fetus must be thoroughly evaluated for signs of hydrops, compromise, or structural cardiac disease.

Auscultation

The simplest method to detect a dysrhythmia is auscultation with a stethoscope. The technique is a quick, easy, and readily reproducible tool for ascertaining fetal heart rates. It was also the most common method of fetal heart rate assessment prior to electronic fetal monitoring (EFM).[19] Since the advent of EFM in the 1960s, the use of fetoscopic auscultation has dwindled. If a brady- or tachyarrhythmia is detected during auscultation, further investigation into the cause of the dysrhythmia is indicated.

Doppler

Doppler ultrasound is the most commonly used screening tool for fetal dysrhythmia detection. A beam of sound is directed toward fetal cardiac structures such as valves, walls, and aortic pulsations that is reflected back to the transducer at a slightly different frequency due to tissue or blood movement. Doppler principles are employed in two readily available devices; the handheld Doppler device, which is frequently used for routine office assessment of the fetal heart rate, and as part of cardiotocography. Both devices have proved to be highly effective tools for the detection of fetal dysrhythmias. The handheld devices can be used from the 12th week of gestation, while cardiotocography is not usually used before 24 weeks.

Fetal Electrocardiography

The fetal electrocardiogram (FECG) is another method for the detection of fetal dysrhythmia. It is similar in principle to standard electrocardiography, with the placement of electrodes on the maternal abdomen to record the differences in electrical potential arising from the fetal cardiac electrical activity. Most fetal QRS complexes are easily identified from the raw signal with FECG, and with signal averaging, the P waves can be located occasionally. T waves are rarely seen on these recordings. Fetal heart rate tracings can be obtained in approximately 60% of long-term (8–24 hours) recordings in late gestation.[20]

The advantage of FECG is that it is a reflection of the cardiac electrical and not the mechanical activity. When P waves are visible on the FECG, the exact cause of the arrhythmia can be deduced. In addition, FECG tracings can be obtained quickly, and because the units are small and simple, they can be used for long-term outpatient monitoring. The major problems are poorly reliability and limited signal acquisition. The fetal cardiac signal is attenuated by amniotic fluid, the distance from the electrical activity to recording surface, and the small size of the fetal heart. Because of limited signal acquisition, atrial activity is rarely recorded, limiting the FECG's current clinical use in arrhythmia diagnoses.

Magnetocardiography

Described by Kariniemi in 1974, fetal magnetocardiography (FMCG) has evolved from a research tool to an important clinical modality.[21] FMCG noninvasively records the cardiac magnetic activity of the fetal heart generated by electrical excitation, and with specialized offline analysis of the magnetic activity, an equivalent of the surface electrocardiogram (ECG) is created. Its use and reliability are documented from 20 weeks to birth.[22] Numerous studies demonstrate the accuracy of FMCG for the diagnosis of fetal arrhythmias such as atrial and ventricular ectopy, supraventricular tachycardia (SVT), atrial flutter, complete atrioventricular (AV) block, torsades de points, and ventricular tachycardia (VT).[23–25]

The advantages to FMCG over FECG include the following: it takes less time (seconds vs. minutes), it overcomes the assumption mechanical activity correlates with electrical activity, and it has greater reliability. And because FMCG is currently the only antenatal method of measuring cardiac repolarization, it is the only way to antenatally diagnose prolonged QT interval syndrome. Conversely, the disadvantages of FMCG are its size, high cost, and limited availability of the equipment, and these factors limit its use in current clinical practice.

Echocardiography

Fetal echocardiography is the current gold standard for the diagnosis and monitoring of fetal arrhythmias. Its status is due, in part, to its widespread availability and relative ease of use. A significant advantage of fetal echocardiography is its safety throughout pregnancy, starting as early as 11 weeks[26] with a transvaginal probe and 14 weeks transabdominally. Both fetal atrial and ventricular rates along with the AV activation sequence are readily seen. Knowledge of the activation sequence facilitates differentiation of the arrhythmia into ventricular or supraventricular and long or short AV tachycardia. In addition, fetal well-being, cardiac structure, and hemodynamics can be evaluated concurrently with the arrhythmia assessment.

In addition to a careful examination of the fetal heart and circulation, assessment of a fetal arrhythmia should result in a detailed, full sonographic examination of the fetus, looking for syndromic features, especially chromosomal.

The two most common echocardiographic methods of arrhythmia analysis are M-mode and spectral Doppler. Although either method alone is reliable in the majority of fetuses, comfort in performing and interpreting both techniques is essential in the event that fetal position or ultrasound window access limits the use of one or the other method. In the following sections, the methods, advantages, and disadvantages of the M-mode and Doppler techniques of fetal arrhythmia assessment are outlined.

M-mode

In M-mode echocardiography, the M-mode line is positioned by two-dimensional (2D) image guidance to transect one structure that represents atrial contraction (atrial wall) and one that represents ventricular contraction (ventricular wall, or aortic or pulmonary valve). Atrial systole is represented by the onset of atrial wall movement or the A peak of the mitral or tricuspid valve, and ventricular systole is represented by the onset of ventricular wall movement or the opening of either the aortic or pulmonary valve. The fetal cardiac mechanical movements are then plotted against time. From a hard copy of the M-mode tracing, a "ladder diagram" of atrial and ventricular activity can be constructed[27] (Fig. 16–1). Cardiac time intervals are then measured from the M-mode tracing along with the sequence of atrial and ventricular events and intervals (VA and AV).

The main limitations of M-mode echocardiography are technical (obtaining properly positioned and interpretable tracings) and the assumption that mechanical cardiac events reflect electrical events. The latter can lead to an errant diagnosis with junctional ectopic tachycardia, which occurs when the electrical focus originates in the AV node. By M-mode echocardiography, the mechanical activity of the ventricle precedes the atria, thus mimicking ventricular tachycardia. Atrial wall motion may be minimal in atrial fibrillation or in the setting of a dilated, poorly contractile atrium. Lastly, discerning the A waves of the mitral or tricuspid valve can be quite challenging.

Spectral Doppler

Spectral Doppler is the second echocardiographic method for fetal arrhythmia assessment. Similar to M-mode, the sample volume is placed under 2D image guidance in a location that allows for the simultaneous recording of flow events that represent atrial and ventricular systole. The sample volume can be placed in a number of locations, such as the left ventricular outflow tract, which will record mitral valve inflow and ventricular outflow, the pulmonary vein and pulmonary artery, the inferior vena cava and the aorta or the superior vena cava and aorta.[28–32] The simplest to obtain is left ventricular inflow and outflow from an apical 4-chamber view (see Fig. 16–1). After the appropriate sample volume position has been attained, a tracing of the flow velocity is recorded, a ladder diagram is constructed, and the sequence of atrial and ventricular events and intervals is

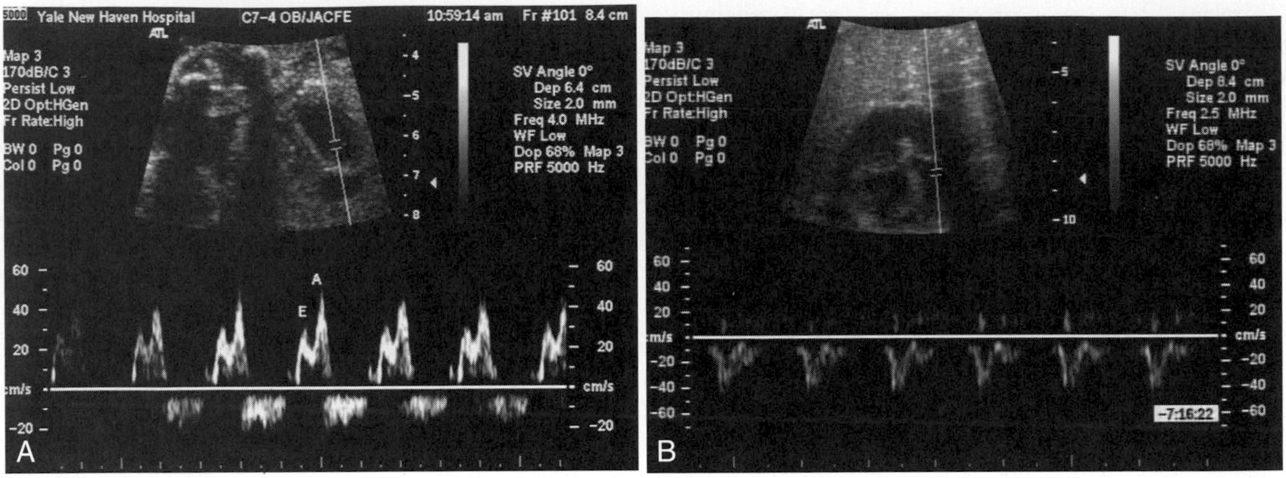

FIGURE 16–1
A, Doppler flow velocity waveform of normal flow across the mitral valve. Note that early ventricular filling (E) has a lower velocity than active atrial systole, reflecting the dependence of the fetal myocardium on atrial systole to overcome the inherent stiffness of the immature muscle. *B*, Doppler flow velocity waveform of flow across the mitral valve in a fetus with reentrant tachycardia. Note the reversal of the normal E:A ratio. Time scale is twice that shown in *A*.

deduced similar to M-mode. The main limitation is that this requires proper fetal positioning and the need to place the Doppler sample volume from an apical four-chamber view so as to maximize both inflow and outflow velocities.

MECHANISMS OF TACHYARRHYTHMIAS

Fetal arrhythmias are generally first detected during routine prenatal visits or ultrasound examinations. Transient fetal rhythm disturbances represent 20% to 30% of all indications for fetal cardiac evaluations at tertiary centers.[33] Frequently, the cause of these transient arrhythmias is extrasystoles. The incidence of malignant fetal arrhythmias, ventricular and supraventricular, is unknown but are felt to be rare. The most common causes of fetal tachycardias are AV reentry supraventricular tachycardias (SVT), atrial flutter, and sinus tachycardia. Rare causes of fetal tachycardia include atrial ectopy, atrial fibrillation, and junctional and ventricular tachycardia, which constitute less than 1% of fetal arrhythmias. Knowledge of the incidence, mechanism, and associated morbidity and mortality rates of the different arrhythmias is critical in determining the appropriate treatment for the fetus.

IRREGULAR HEART RATE

Premature Atrial Contractions

Premature atrial contractions (PACs) are the result of nonsinus atrial depolarization that occurs earlier than the expected sinus beat. PACs can originate from either the right or left atrium and are conducted through the AV node either in the normal fashion or aberrantly, or they may block at the level of the AV node. PACs are the most common fetal dysrhythmia, with a prevalence of 1% to 3% of all pregnancies.[34] PACs are associated with illicit drug use, trisomy 18, and hyperthyroidism.[35] It is also hypothesized that PACs are caused by an aneurysm of the flap valve of the foramen ovale.[36] Rarely, isolated PACs are reported to trigger episodes of sustained SVT. Fetal PACs are easily recognized either by their characteristic early atrial wall movement (M-mode) or mitral inflow (Doppler) pattern.

Management Options

Isolated PACs require no treatment, but because of their association with SVT, weekly auscultation of the fetal heart rate is prudent until the ectopic beats resolve. There is no increase in the incidence of structural heart disease in affected fetuses.[9] Patients are advised to avoid caffeine and medications that may increase ectopy, such as β-adrenergic drugs (e.g., terbutaline). Persistent postnatal ectopy warrants only a neonatal ECG and consideration for a 24-hour Holter monitor.

Premature Ventricular Contractions

Premature ventricular contractions (PVCs) are caused by early, nonsinus depolarization of the ventricles. A compensatory pause may be observed if the PVC is conducted retrogradely through the AV node to the atrium. PVCs produce a characteristic Doppler flow pattern with absence of diastolic flow across the AV (mitral) valve prior to the initiation of ventricular systole (aortic outflow). They account for approximately 2% to 4% of all fetal ectopy.

Management Options

PVCs are usually benign and generally warrant simple maternal avoidance of cardiac stimulants such as caffeine. Under rare circumstances, PVCs may be a harbinger of cardiomyopathy, myocarditis, structural cardiac malformations, or long QT interval syndrome.[37] Postnatal ectopy requires an ECG to evaluate the corrected QT interval and a 24-hour Holter monitor.

TACHYCARDIAS

Sinus Tachycardia

Sinus tachycardia in a fetus is defined as a sustained heart rate between 160 and 210 bpm. If the rate is greater than 210 bpm and is nonvariable, SVT should be considered. Persistent fetal sinus tachycardia may be secondary to acidosis, hypoxic ischemic encephalopathy, myocarditis, infection, maternal fever, and maternal drug ingestion.[38] Even though maternal thyroid hormone does not cross the placenta, prenatal thyrotoxicosis secondary to transplacental passage of thyroid-stimulating immunoglobulin (TSiG) with maternal Graves' disease has also been associated with fetal sinus tachycardia.[39] Management of persistent sinus tachycardia involves recognition and treatment of the underlying cause. Sinus tachycardia should be differentiated from ventricular tachycardia (see later discussion). In sinus tachycardia, atrial systole precedes ventricular contraction, whereas in ventricular tachycardia, ventricular contraction precedes the atrial systole. This can be difficult to distinguish in utero.

Supraventricular Tachycardia

Fetal SVT may present at any time after 15 weeks. SVT is a general term used to describe an arrhythmia originating at or above the bundle of His, and thus it is characterized by a narrow QRS complex (Fig. 16–2). The causes of SVT are categorized by their dependence on the AV node for propagation of the arrhythmia. Those that require the AV node to maintain the tachycardia (Wolff-Parkinson-White [W-P-W] syndrome, AV node reentry tachycardia [AVNRT], permanent junctional reciprocating tachycardia [PJRT], concealed accessory pathway [CAP] and Mahaim pathways) are referred to as AV node dependent. Those that do not (atrial fibrillation, atrial flutter, atrial and junctional ectopic tachycardia) are referred to as AV node independent tachycardias.

Based upon their mechanism of propagation, the AV node dependent SVTs are further divided into the short and long ventriculoatrial (VA) tachycardias. This distinction is important in determining the correct medication to control fetal tachycardia. The VA time in tachycardia is determined by simultaneous Doppler interrogation of either the SVC (A) and ascending aorta (V), or by measuring mitral (A) and aortic (V) flow in the left ventricular outflow. The VA time is considered long if it is greater than one half of the V-V interval.

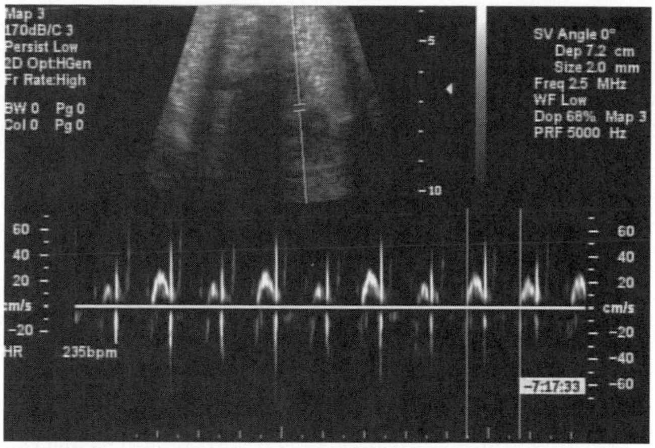

FIGURE 16–2
Doppler flow velocity waveform of flow into pulmonary artery in a fetus with reentrant supraventricular tachycardia. Typical rate of 235 bpm is shown.

AV Node Dependent SVT

SHORT VA TACHYCARDIA

The most common form of SVT is the short VA, AV node dependent SVT. This category includes concealed accessory pathways, W-P-W syndrome, and typical AV node reentry. Characteristics unique to these tachycardias include rates of 220 to 300 bpm (typically close to 240 bpm), little rate variability, and 1:1 VA concordance. Atrial and ventricular ectopies typically trigger abrupt initiation and secession of the tachycardia. The distinction between these arrhythmias generally cannot be made in utero. On rare occasions when a short VA SVT occurs in conjunction with structural cardiac disease (e.g., rhabdomyoma, ventricular inversion, or Ebstein's anomaly of the tricuspid valve), W-P-W syndrome should be suspected because of its known association with these lesions.

Management Options. In general these arrhythmias respond to transplacental digoxin or beta-blocker therapy. Occasionally, when digoxin or beta-blockers fail, second tier antiarrhythmic agents such as flecainide, sotalol, or amiodarone become necessary and are usually effective. Preterm delivery is rarely, if ever, indicated in nonhydropic patients with this form of SVT. When found close to term or with documented fetal lung maturity, delivery is preferable to attempts at in utero treatment. At a minimum, all patients should have a postnatal ECG to determine the etiology of the tachycardia, which will help guide further medication. If structural cardiac disease is suspected, a transthoracic echocardiogram should be performed. Usually, the antiarrhythmic medication(s) are continued up to a year postnatally to avoid recurrence.

LONG VA TACHYCARDIA

Incessant slow fetal SVT may be due to a slowly conducting accessory pathway found in the permanent form of junctional reciprocating tachycardia (PJRT). The incidence of this fetal tachycardia is extremely rare. It is characterized by long VA times, an incessant nature, and slower rates (180–220 bpm) which can be misdiagnosed as sinus tachycardia. Due in part to its incessant nature, it can be a relatively dangerous arrhythmia, causing severe cardiac dysfunction and hydrops fetalis.

Management Options. PJRT rarely responds to digoxin or beta-blockade, so flecainide or sotalol would be the appropriate choices.

AV Node Independent SVT

ATRIAL FLUTTER

Atrial flutter accounts for 30% to 40% of all fetal tachycardias.[35] This rapid, regular atrial reentrant rhythm is characterized by atrial rates of 400 to 550 bpm. Because the reentry cycle occurs within the atrium, propagation through the AV node is not necessary to maintain the tachycardia. The ventricular rates vary, depending on whether there is uniform conduction of atrial beats. The most common form of AV conduction in fetal atrial flutter is 2:1 AV block. The diagnosis of atrial flutter can be made by a fetal echocardiogram showing a fast atrial rate with variable AV conduction or the typical sawtooth appearance on a fetal magnetocardiography (Fig. 16–3). Atrial flutter is associated with structural cardiac defects that dilate the atrium, such as Ebstein's malformation, atrial septal defects, hypoplastic left heart syndrome, and cardiomyopathy as well as with W-P-W syndrome.[34]

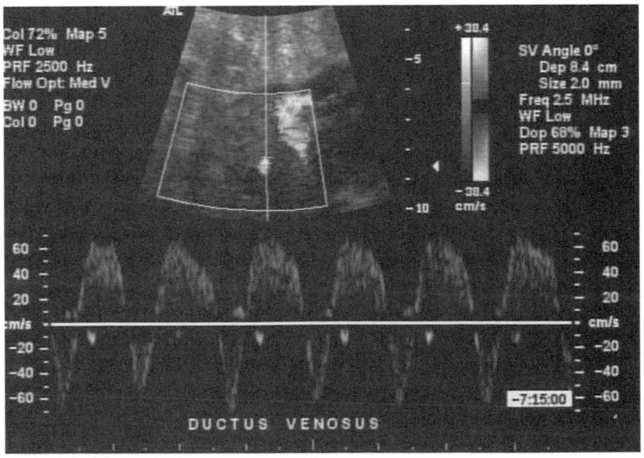

FIGURE 16–3
Flow in ductus venosus of a fetus with reentrant supraventricular tachycardia. Normal flow is unidirectional in contrast with bidirectional flow shown here (see Color Plate 4).

Hydrops occurs in upwards of 35% of the fetuses with incessant atrial flutter.

Management Options. The management of atrial flutter is based on either termination of the intra-atrial reentry, or by ventricular rate control. Ventricular rate control can be accomplished with the maternal administration of digoxin in the absence of hydrops fetalis. Sotalol has shown to be effective for termination of the arrhythmia in 80%.

It is prudent to continue transplacental treatment throughout pregnancy once the fetal rate is successfully converted, with careful attention to maternal drug levels, ECG, and symptoms to avoid adverse treatment effects. The prognosis for fetal atrial flutter is excellent if delivery is at term and there is no associated structural cardiac disease. After successful conversion to sinus rhythm, the majority of pediatric patients do not experience recurrence and require no treatment. Early delivery is indicated only if the fetus fails to respond to medications or has hydrops fetalis.

ATRIAL FIBRILLATION

Atrial fibrillation is a rare fetal arrhythmia with a reported incidence of 0.2%.[35] It is characterized by an extremely rapid, chaotic atrial rate of greater than 500 bpm with variable ventricular conduction. In cases of fine atrial fibrillation, the atria may appear to actually stand still during fetal echocardiography. Atrial fibrillation can occur in association with Ebstein malformation of the tricuspid valve, thyrotoxicosis, and cardiac tumors.

Management Options. No antiarrhythmic agent has to date been used to convert fetal atrial fibrillation to sinus rhythm. Ventricular rate control may be achieved with transplacental digoxin administration. The prognosis for atrial fibrillation is unknown, due in part to its relative rarity and the fact that the majority of cases are associated with structural and other conduction abnormalities. Postnatally, newborns are converted to a sinus rhythm through DC cardioversion. Atrial fibrillation is not an indication for early delivery unless hydrops fetalis develops, or fetal compromise is suspected based on biophysical testing.

ATRIAL TACHYCARDIA

Ectopic or chaotic atrial tachycardias are rare but are occasionally seen in the later stages of pregnancy. This arrhythmia is characterized by regular or irregular atrial and ventricular Doppler flow patterns depending on the atrial rate and AV conduction. It is typically well tolerated and hydrops fetalis is rare.

Management Options. Once the diagnosis is established, medical management should be initiated, but the arrhythmia is frequently resistant to basic drug therapies such as digoxin and beta-blockers.[40] Flecainide is the drug of choice for fetal atrial ectopic tachycardia. Postnatal recognition and treatment may be needed if the tachycardia is persistent.

JUNCTIONAL ECTOPIC TACHYCARDIA

Congenital junctional ectopic tachycardia (JET) is an extremely rare, incessant form of ectopic focus SVT. The focus is located within the AV node, resulting in near simultaneous electrical activation of the atria and ventricles, though dissociation of the ventricles from the atria can occur, mimicking ventricular tachycardia. This arrhythmia is unique in its inheritance pattern; approximately 50% have a close family member affected. JET is very difficult to diagnose in utero without magnetocardiography and is frequently resistant to conventional therapy. The mortality rate approaches 35% in infancy.[41]

Management Options. Fetuses with JET may respond to either amiodarone or sotalol.

VENTRICULAR TACHYCARDIA

Ventricular tachycardia (VT) is another relatively rare form of tachycardia with the focus originating in the ventricle(s). It may be associated with fetal myocarditis, myocardial dysfunction of any cause, or long QT interval syndrome. The most common form of VT is called slow ventricular tachycardia or accelerated idioventricular rhythm. The rate is between 160 and 200 bpm and does not warrant any intervention. Ventricular tachycardia is diagnosed when faster heart rates, greater than 200 bpm, are observed. In addition, AV dissociation is frequently seen, with the ventricular rate being faster than atrial rate.

Management Options. Sustained fast fetal ventricular tachycardia with or without hydrops fetalis is often refractory to treatment, which requires agents such as amiodarone or sotalol. Beta-blockers should be used in suspected long QT interval syndrome.

BRADYCARDIAS

Fetal bradycardia is defined as a persistent heart rate below 100 bpm not associated with uterine contractions or periodic decelerations. A thorough investigation into fetal well-being and cause of the dysrhythmia is warranted when fetal bradycardia is detected. First, extrinsic, noncardiac causes of fetal bradycardia such as drugs, maternal hypothermia, and mechanical compression of the umbilical cord must be excluded.[14,42] If the bradycardia persists and no obvious extrinsic causes are evident, the next step is to determine the exact rhythm (e.g., sinus bradycardia, partial or complete AV block) to facilitate appropriate management. As previously noted, a maternal history or screening for connective tissue disorders or drug use, along with a complete family history, probing for arrhythmias, pacemakers, and structural heart disease in close family members, is warranted.

Sinus Bradycardia

Sinus bradycardia can be differentiated from other causes of fetal bradycardia by Doppler or M-mode echocardiography. The hallmark of sinus bradycardia is the presence of a normal AV activation sequence. Confirmation that any slow heart rate is due to sinus bradycardia is mandatory to rule out advanced or complete AV block or blocked premature atrial ectopic beats. In addition to rhythm confirmation, a thorough fetal assessment is necessary to seek signs of fetal compromise, hydrops fetalis, or structural cardiac disease. Well-known causes of fetal sinus bradycardia include long QT interval syndrome and heterotaxy syndrome with left atrial isomerism, in which the fetus has two left atria, and thus lacks a true sinus node and right atrial structure.

Management Options

The management of a fetal sinus bradycardia depends on the cause, as well as the clinical status of the fetus. Close observation generally is all that is necessary if the fetus is not compromised, and all extrinsic causes of sinus bradycardia are removed. A postnatal ECG should be performed to rule out or confirm the presence of a prolonged QT interval.[43]

Atrioventricular Block

The designation AV block describes an abnormality in the conduction of atrial impulses through the AV node to the ventricles. This abnormality can range from a simple delay in impulse transmission, as in first-degree AV block, to a complete interruption of signal transmission, classified as complete or third-degree AV block. Each form of AV block has a distinct anatomic or physiologic cause for the electrical abnormality and can be either transient or permanent in nature. In utero, these abnormalities are diagnosed using either fetal echocardiography or FMCG with postnatal confirmation by ECG. The following sections focus on the definition, evaluation, and treatment of the more advanced forms of fetal AV block.

Second-Degree AV Block

Second-degree AV block is defined as the failure of at least one, nonpremature atrial impulse to be conducted to the ventricles. A number of different forms of second-degree AV block exist. Mobitz type I, or Wenckebach, is the most common, but least significant. Wenckebach is characterized by a progressive prolongation of the PR or AV interval with an eventual dropped ventricular beat. The delay occurs in the AV node, proximal to the bundle of His.[44] This conduction abnormality is generally transient in nature and is caused by vagal influence. In rare instances, it can be caused by digitalis toxicity or inflammatory disorders that affect the cardiac muscle. No treatment is necessary in asymptomatic fetuses. Mothers should be screened for presence of anti-Ro anti-La antibodies and the fetus should be observed closely.

The more pathologic forms of second-degree AV block include Mobitz type II and the advanced types.

Type II second-degree AV block is characterized by a constant P-P and PR intervals followed by a nonconducted atrial impulse. The anatomic site of block is at or below the bundle of His.[45] High-grade or advanced second-degree AV block is when two or more successive sinus atrial impulses are not propagated through the AV node. If either form of AV block is identified, the presence of prolonged QT interval syndrome or maternal connective tissue disorders must be investigated and the fetus followed closely for progression to pre- or postnatal complete AV block.[46]

Complete Atrioventricular Block

Fetal complete AV block (CAVB), or third-degree AV block is the complete failure of sinus atrial impulse conduction to the ventricles. In addition, the atrial rate must be faster than the ventricular rate to assure that the AV dissociation is not due to accelerated junctional or ventricular rhythm (e.g., sinus bradycardia with appropriate junctional response, or an accelerated junctional or ventricular rhythm). The prevalence of complete AV block in live born infants is 1 in 20,000.[47] The majority of affected fetuses fall into one of two distinct groups: those with structural cardiac disease and those with maternal connective tissue disorders.[48–50]

The association between fetal CAVB and maternal autoimmune disorders is well established.[17,18,51,52] It occurs in fetuses of women with systemic lupus erythematosus (SLE), Sjögren syndrome, rheumatoid arthritis, scleroderma, and undifferentiated connective tissue disorders.[53–55] Specifically, it is strongly associated with maternal autoantibodies designated anti-SS-A/Ro, anti-SS-B/La, or both.[55,56] Many women carrying a fetus with CAVB do not have symptoms of any connective tissue disorder at the time, with half demonstrating only serologic evidence of disease.[57] In addition, the vast majority of mothers with SLE do not have children with CAVB.[58] The risk of a woman with SSA/Ro and SSB/La antibodies having a fetus with heart block is 1% to 2%.[59] The risk of recurrence of CAVB in subsequent pregnancies after delivering an affected infant is 10% to 16%.[49,56]

The conduction system is damaged by maternal antibodies that cross the placenta and react with their corresponding antigens expressed on the surface of cells in the fetal cardiac conduction system, resulting in immunoglobulin deposition on the cells. The resulting local inflammatory reaction leads to permanent damage of the fetal cardiac conduction system due to localized cellular apoptosis.[60–64]

The second group of fetuses with CAVB have structural cardiac disorders. The etiology of nonimmune complete AV block was postulated by Lev to be the result of a developmental abnormality of the AV node. This abnormality can result from either the complete absence of the AV node, lack of union between the AV node and distal conduction system, or the presence of an aberrant, non- or poorly functioning system.[65] The most common structural cardiac abnormalities associated with CAVB are AV septal defects, both with and without associated left atrial isomerism, and AV discordance with ventriculoarterial discordance (corrected transposition of the great arteries).[48,50] Additional cardiovascular malformations (tetralogy of Fallot, atrial septal defects, transposition of the great vessels, and tricuspid atresia) are described, without any apparent association between the structural abnormality and the conduction defect.[48,50]

In addition to those with well-known immunologic and structural causes, a small group of patients were recently identified with a genetic mutation that results in CAVB. An autosomal dominant mutation in the cardiac transcription factor Nkx2.5 can result in familial atrial septal defects and AV node conduction abnormalities including Holt-Oram syndrome and atrial septal defects. There are also fetuses with structurally normal hearts but a mutation in SCN5A, a sodium ion channel, that is responsible for long QT interval and Brugada syndrome, who can have a range of AV conduction abnormalities including complete block.[66]

In contrast to the oft-quoted dogma that the majority of fetuses with CAVB without structural cardiac abnormalities have few if any problems with gestation and delivery, recent studies document an exceptionally high mortality rate among these perinates. The mortality rates range from 7% to 33% with structurally normal heart and as high as 86% for those with structural cardiac lesions.[48–50,57,67] Poor outcomes are associated with the presence of structural cardiac disease, hydrops, ventricular rates below 55 bpm, atrial rates below 120 bpm, AV valve regurgitation, a dilated cardiomyopathy, prolonged corrected QT interval, or delivery at or before 32 weeks' gestation.[48–50,57,67]

Management Options for Heart Block

Second-degree AV block (Mobitz type I/Wenckebach): No treatment is necessary in asymptomatic fetuses. Mothers should be screened for presence of anti-Ro anti-La antibodies and the fetus observed closely.

Second-degree AV block (Mobitz type II and advanced types): Management of these conduction abnormalities is similar to that of complete AV block (see next item).

Third-degree/complete AV block: The goal of management of a fetus with complete AV block is the birth of a healthy, viable infant. This outcome is best achieved through a two-tiered approach. First, early intervention(s) is required at the first sign of fetal compromise. Second, early identification of the fetus at risk for developing CAVB is extremely important, allowing for the initiation of therapies in an attempt to prevent the onset or progression of the conduction abnormality or its sequelae. These goals may be accomplished by increasing the fetal heart rate or contractility or by blunting or removing the inflammatory stimulus through immune suppression.

The maternal or direct fetal administration of sympathomimetic agents like ritodrine, terbutaline, isoproterenol, and salbutamol has shown some efficacy increasing both fetal chronotropy and ionotropy.[48,68–71] Reported fetal responses to these agents range from no improvement to complete resolution of hydrops and survival.[48,68,69,71,85] The applicability of these results is limited by the small number of patients treated, the highly variable clinical situations, and concomitant use of additional therapies. We believe it is unlikely this therapy works, as it does nothing to restore AV concordance. The relative stiffness of the fetal ventricular myocardium, and the consequent reliance of the fetus on atrial systole for normal ventricular filling, makes the fetus exquisitely sensitive to interruption of this relationship.

Another approach to increase the fetal heart rate is through ventricular pacing. Transvenous and epicardial ventricular pacing was accomplished in fetal animal models, and transuterine-transthoracic pacing is reported in a few human fetuses.[86–88] Despite the fact the pacing was successful, all treated fetuses died. With the advent of new, smaller (1.4 Fr), soft-tipped temporary pacing wires, transvenous ventricular pacing may become more feasible and less risky to mother and fetus in the future, although placement would require open fetal surgery with the pacemaker generator itself buried under the fetal skin, to avoid exposure of the fetus to entanglement in free-floating wires in the amniotic sac.

Reduction of the maternal antibody titer or the fetal inflammatory response to the antibodies is accomplished either through suppression or removal of the offending agents. Removal of the anti-SSA/Ro and SSB/La antibodies was reported in a few cases by plasmapheresis with variable results. Intravenous gamma globulin has also been reported to reduce the maternal anti-Ro antibody titer.[89] Despite their encouraging results, only a limited number of patients have undergone these therapies during pregnancy. Further studies are warranted.

Fluorinated steroids such as dexamethasone and betamethasone have been used for prevention and treatment of CAVB.[61,62,69,90–92] A recent retrospective case control investigation compared pregnancy outcomes of those treated with fluorinated steroids to those untreated. Although steroid use for fetuses with complete AV block failed to resolve the AV conduction defect, it was associated with some improvement in hydrops and other symptoms. Steroids administered early after the onset of early AV block (second degree) reversed the block and prevented its advancement in at least some fetuses.[93] These findings suggest that fluorinated steroids are a therapeutic option in fetuses with early forms of AV block to prevent progression and potentially cure the abnormality. Their use should also be considered in fetuses with hydrops.

In summary, fetal complete AV block is a relatively rare condition with rapidly evolving management. We recommend early fetal echocardiography in all mothers with anti-Ro and anti-La antibodies (SSA and SSB). Fetuses with structural cardiac disorders associated with CAVB should be closely observed for signs of arrhythmia. In the fetus of a mother with a connective tissue disorder, early detection of advanced AV conduction abnormalities should prompt the consideration of fluorinated steroids with the goal of preventing the progression of the inflammatory process. The presence of hydrops or ventricular rates below 55 bpm should prompt reconsideration of therapy with steroids. Additional studies on the benefits of plasmapheresis and intravenous immunoglobulins are needed. In addition, the patient should be referred to a center with expertise in high risk obstetrics and fetal cardiology, as well as pediatric and neonatal pacemaker implantation and management.

Management of Fetal Tachyarrhythmias—General

The management of a fetus with a dysrhythmia should involve a coordinated team approach including experts in obstetric imaging, maternal-fetal medicine, electrophysiology, and pediatric cardiology. Medications are often administered to pregnant women with hopes that the beneficial effects of the drug will be transferred to the fetus. In many instances, the kinetics of drug transfer are poorly studied. When transplacental antiarrhythmic therapy is to be administered, the authors feel an adult electrophysiologist should be available to guide dosage selection and assist in monitoring the mother for adverse events and side effects. In support, Strasburger and associates[72] observed a higher rate of cesarean section (84% vs. 18%) and lower gestational age at delivery (37 weeks vs. 39 weeks) in infants managed at nontertiary centers without prenatal pediatric cardiology support.

Hydrops Fetalis (See also Chapter 25)

Hydrops fetalis is an abnormal collection of fluid in at least two areas, such as ascites, pleural or pericardial effusions, polyhydramnios, or skin or placental edema. Cardiac reasons for the development of hydrops include structural cardiac defects and rhythm disturbances, which constitute up to 50% of all nonimmunologic hydrops.[73] Multiple risk factors for hydrops fetalis and subsequent poor outcome are suggested and include prematurity, sustained SVT exceeding 12 hours, structural cardiac defects, and ventricular rates exceeding 220 bpm.[74] In subsequent studies, the correlation between hydrops and ventricular rate or duration of the tachycardia was not substantiated.[75,76] Untreated hydrops fetalis can be associated with decreased fetal movement, fetal metabolic acidemia, myocardial dysfunction, and poor tolerance of labor. In addition, placental edema may contribute to decreased placental drug transfer requiring more drugs (two vs. one) or more days (12.5 vs. 3) to control their arrhythmia.[77] Mortality rate may be as high as 13% in a term, hydropic fetus and increases as gestation falls.[76]

Therapeutic Options

One must ask if it is worth the effort before initiating medical therapy for fetal tachyarrhythmia. We are currently unsure of the exact pharmacokinetics of many of the medicines used in transplacental treatments. All the drugs we might use have potentially dangerous side effects. They may not be effective, and there could be spontaneous resolution of the tachycardia even without treatment. Therefore, the treatment for fetal tachycardia depends on a multitude of factors, including the type of arrhythmia, gestational age of the fetus, maternal and fetal health, and the presence of either structural cardiac disease or hydrops.

Therapeutic options for a fetal tachyarrhythmia include monitoring without pharmacologic intervention, transplacental or direct administration of antiarrhythmic medications to the fetus, or delivery of the fetus with postnatal arrhythmia management. The management choice for most fetuses with tachycardia at or very near term (≥34–35 weeks) is delivery. The nonhydropic fetus with an intermittent tachyarrhythmia can often be safely and effectively induced with oxytocin for vaginal delivery as long as there are sufficient intervals of normal rhythm present to permit electronic fetal heart rate monitoring. Whether new techniques such as fetal pulse oximetry, which requires rupture of the membranes and sufficient cervical dilation to place the transducer, will permit adequate monitoring of the fetus with a sustained tachycardia remains speculative, but this approach is worth evaluating in selected pregnancies. In pregnancies with evidence of fetal compromise or impending cardiac dysfunction, a complete fetal and maternal assessment must be performed and the pros and cons of all available treatment options weighed by the treatment team and family.

When the treatment of a fetal arrhythmia is indicated, a number of options are available. Transplacental therapy is preferred for a stable arrhythmia when both the fetus and mother are in excellent health. If, for some reason, transplacental therapy is not an option, consideration must be given to direct fetal therapy with drug infusion into the umbilical vein, into the amniotic fluid, or by direct fetal intramuscular injection. The following sections will review the advantages as well as the risks of each of these therapeutic options and provide data and clinical scenarios that apply to each therapy.

When a fetal arrhythmia is detected, signs of fetal compromise must be sought. Delivery of infants less than 34 to 35 weeks' gestational age with hydrops is associated with very high mortality rate and is indicated only under exceptional circumstances, such as failed transplacental/direct therapy, worsening diastolic dysfunction, or a poor fetal biophysical profile.[78] When iatrogenic premature delivery is anticipated, documentation of fetal lung maturity by amniocentesis may help with the decision. If the pregnancy is at or before 34 weeks, appropriate doses of betamethasone or dexamethasone should be administered to hasten fetal lung maturation.

Pregnancies close to term should be delivered rather than exposing the mother to these potent medications. The aim of transplacental therapy is to use the normal function of the placenta as a fetal drug delivery mechanism. Transplacental therapy is indicated in fetuses with a stable biophysical profile and sustained tachycardia.[79] Those fetuses with tachycardia less than 30% of the time without hydrops can probably be left untreated and instead followed closely. This decision should be individualized and based on the ability to follow the patient closely. We believe twice weekly echocardiographic evaluation of nonhydropic infant is warranted. In contrast, almost all neonates with any episodes of nonsinus tachycardia will receive antiarrhythmic medications for up to 1 year of age to minimize their risk of developing congestive heart failure.

Antiarrhythmic medicines should be initiated under close supervision. With the exception of β-blockers, most antiarrhythmic drugs require close monitoring of both fetus and mother for side effects as well as a successful conversion to a sinus rhythm. We believe that when most antiarrhythmic drugs are used, the mothers should be monitored as inpatients on cardiac telemetry with consultation of an adult electrophysiologist to monitor the maternal ECG, electrolytes, and vital signs. Conversion can generally be achieved within a few days. Once control or steady state is achieved, the patients may be discharged with close follow-up. Successful conversion rates of fetal SVT range from 80% to 90%.[80] The resolution of hydrops after successful treatment of tachycardia may take several weeks. Acceleration of fetal maturity with corticosteroids should be considered if elective preterm delivery seems likely.[35]

Pharmacokinetics and Choice of Antiarrhythmic Agents

Transfer of any drug across the placental barrier is promoted by low molecular size, low ionization, and high lipid solubility.[81] The rate of diffusion is also dependent on fetal-maternal concentration gradient and the thickness of the placental membrane. Higher doses of drugs are often required to achieve therapeutic levels in pregnancy because of increased blood volume and distribution, increased protein binding of drugs, increased hepatic metabolism, and greatly increased glomerular filtration rate in the mother. The placenta is able to transfer, concentrate, and metabolize drugs to inactive metabolites. Fetal metabolism of drugs is primarily renal or placental because hepatic enzymes are immature (only 20%–50% active). The transplacental transfer of drugs is poor in the presence of hydrops fetalis, therefore making management of fetal SVT with associated hydrops more difficult. To circumvent mitigating factors that affect transplacental transfer, direct umbilical or fetal intramus-

TABLE 16–2

Pharmacologic Agents Used to Treat Fetal Arrhythmias

DRUG	ADVERSE EFFECT	DOSING RANGE	THERAPEUTIC LEVEL
Digoxin	Nausea, bradycardia, vision disturbance, first- and second-degree atrioventricular block, rhythm disturbances	Loading dose: 1200–1500 μg/24 hr IV; Maintenance: 375–875 μg/day po divided bid	1.5–2.5 ng/dL
Propranolol	Low birth weight, hypoglycemia, bradycardia, increased uterine tone	80–320 mg/day po in 3–4 divided doses	25–50 ng/mL
Flecainide	Fetal demise, conduction defects, QT interval prolongation, proarrhythmia	100–400 mg/day po divided bid	0.2–10 μg/mL
Sotalol	Tiredness, dizziness, nausea, QT interval prolongation, torsades de pointes	40 mg bid increasing to 160 mg po bid	Not known
Amiodarone	Nausea, thrombocytopenia, visual disturbances, QT interval prolongation, hypothyroidism	Loading dose: 600 mg po q6h; Maintainance: 100–200 mg/day po	0.7–2.8 μg/mL

cular administration of drugs has been used to treat the fetus directly.[82,83]

The proper diagnosis of the type of tachycardia is required to guide therapy. Based on a 1998 survey of 15 institutions treating fetal arrhythmias, the commonest drug used was digoxin (78%) followed by flecanide (18%), verapamil (7%), procainamide (6%), quinidine (6%), amiodarone (6%), propranolol (2%), and sotalol (2%).[81] Verapamil is contraindicated in newborns owing to the risk of profound hypotension and shock and should be used rarely and with extreme caution, if at all, in fetuses. In addition, quinidine has proarrhythmic effects and also should used rarely. Amiodarone is effective in 90% of the reentrant SVTs and 60% of the atrial flutter. However, the long half-life of amiodarone, measured in weeks, and the potential for profound fetal hypothyroidism, as a result of exposure and consequent goiter and even cretinism, mandates great caution when considering amiodarone. The maternal ECG and side effects should be monitored along with desired fetal effect and the dose titrated for optimal response. Standard doses and some common side effects of different drugs are listed in Table 16–2.

Prognosis

The perinatal mortality rate for fetal tachycardia with hydrops ranges from 3.5% to 30% in different studies. The differences may relate to use of different antiarrhythmic agents, some with proarrhythmic effects, the incidence of premature delivery, and fetal interventions including cordocentesis.[84] Marked acidosis, prematurity, and prolonged tachycardia may be associated with long-term postnatal sequelae. Postnatal pharmacologic therapy is needed in 50% of cases with SVT irrespective of the presence of hydrops, with over 75% having no clinical episodes after 1 year of age.

CONCLUSIONS

- Discovery of a fetal arrhythmia should lead to a careful ultrasound examination for
  - Nature of the arrhythmia (including M-mode)
  - Anatomy of heart and vascular connections
  - Exclusion of other abnormality and syndromes (with karyotyping if syndrome suspected)
- Maternal history and examination are necessary to exclude precipitating factors.
- Most conditions should be managed by a center with expertise in high risk obstetrics and fetal cardiology, as well as pediatric and neonatal pacemaker implantation and management.

SUMMARY OF MANAGEMENT OPTIONS
Fetal Cardiac Arrhythmias

Management Options	Quality of Evidence	Strength of Recommendation	References
Irregular Fetal Heart Rate			
Prenatal Diagnosis			
Careful history and examination to exclude	IV	C	35
Familial long QT interval syndrome			
Maternal illicit drug use			
Maternal hyperthyroidism			
Fetal echocardiography to confirm cardiac normality; detailed fetal sonography to exclude syndromes; consider karyotype if aneuploidy (especially trisomy 18) suspected	III IV	B C	9 35
Prenatal Treatment			
No treatment if isolated (as in the majority of cases)	–	GPP	–
Avoid caffeine and drugs that promote ectopy (e.g., beta-sympathomimetics)	–	GPP	–
Weekly ausculation to confirm no progression to supraventricular tachycardia (SVT)	–	GPP	–
Postnatal			
If ectopic beats persist in the neonatal period, perform electrocardiogram (ECG) and 24-h Holter monitor to exclude long QT interval syndrome.	IV	C	37,43
Tachycardias			
Prepregnancy			
Counseling of those with history of			
Wolff-Parkinson-White (W-P-W) syndrome	IV	C	35
Familial long QT interval syndrome	IV	C	37,43
Prenatal Diagnosis			
Auscultation and fetal echocardiography for sustained fetal rate > 180 bpm	–	GPP	–
Ultrasound evaluation of cardiac structure, function, presence of hydrops, and mechanism of arrhythmia (including M-mode and spectral Doppler)	III	B	6
Search for other abnormalities with ultrasound; consider karyotype if aneuploidy suspected.	–	GPP	–
Prenatal Treatment			
Depends on	–	GPP	–
Underlying mechanism/diagnosis			
Persistence of tachyarrythmia			
Presence of hydrops			
Gestational age			
Nonsustained tachycardia requires monitoring but no treatment unless hydrops is present.	–	GPP	–
Medical (Transplacental) control of sustained tachycardia; five drugs are commonly used:	III & IV	B,C	41,77,79,84
Digoxin			
Beta-blockers			

SUMMARY OF MANAGEMENT OPTIONS
Fetal Cardiac Arrhythmias *(Continued)*

Management Options	Quality of Evidence	Strength of Recommendation	References
Prenatal Treatment			
Flecainide			
Soltalol			
Amiodarone			
Sinus tachycardia—Treat cause (e.g., maternal thyrotoxicosis).			
Short VA SVT—preceding five drugs have been used.			
Long VA SVT—use flecainide, soltalol.			
Atrial flutter—digoxin, soltalol.			
Atrial fibrillation—no intrauterine drug is effective; DC after birth.			
Atrial tachycardia—flecainide.			
Junctional ectopic tachycardia—soltalol, amiodarone.			
Ventricular tachycardia—soltalol, amiodarone.			
Monitor maternal ECG and drug levels with use of these drugs.			
Therapy delivered directly to the fetus has been effective, particularly in the setting of hydrops.	III	B	82,83
Delivery is an option if close to term (34+ w); short trial of drug therapy before delivery if hydrops even if close to term is a controversial option because newborns with hydrops have poor prognosis.	–	GPP	–
Postnatal			
12-lead ECG to confirm W-P-W or long QT interval syndrome and precise diagnosis.	IV	C	37,43
Take local advice re prophylactic treatment for tachycardia—some will not use this routinely. Some centers will treat asymptomatic neonates for 6–12 months and review.	–	GPP	–
Treat recurrent tachycardia in infancy (medical therapy or ablation).	III	B	77,78
Bradycardias			
Prepregnancy			
Counseling of women with the following risk factors for complete atrioventricular block (CAVB):			
Previous child with CAVB	III	B	83
Maternal anti-SSA (Ro) or SSB (La) antibodies (1–2% risk)	III	B	55,59
Maternal heart block	–	GPP	–
Previous child with left atrial isomerism	–	GPP	–
Familial prolonged QT interval syndrome is a possible risk factor.	IV	C	37,43
Prenatal Diagnosis			
Detailed and serial echocardiography (every 1–2 weeks) of antibody-positive mothers and those with a positive family history.	–	GPP	–
Fetal echocardiography for persistent fetal rate <100 bpm.	–	GPP	–
Serial echocardiography (every 1–2 weeks) for emerging block (second- or third-degree heart block).	–	GPP	–

Continued

SUMMARY OF MANAGEMENT OPTIONS
Fetal Cardiac Arrhythmias *(Continued)*

Management Options	Quality of Evidence	Strength of Recommendation	References
Prenatal Diagnosis *(Continued)*			
Irregular rhythms	–	GPP	–
If occasional, clinical follow-up.			
If persistent, fetal echocardiography and intensify follow-up.			
Evaluation of asymptomatic mothers for anti-Ro and anti-La antibodies and autoimmune disease (rheumatoid arthritis, Sjögren syndrome, systemic lupus erythematosus, or undifferentiated autoimmune syndrome).	III	B	55,59
Prenatal Treatment			
Early steroids (dexamethasone/betamethasone) are common first-line treatment; no evidence of benefit of prophylactic steroids.	III	B	70,89,93
More research is needed into role of plasmapheresis and intravenous immunoglobulin (IVIG).	IV	C	70,89
Inotropic/chronotropic support is of limited benefit.	III	B	71,85
Fetal pacing has been attempted but without success.	IV	C	88,90
Consider early delivery in tertiary center if hydrops is evident, but generally try to avoid preterm delivery.	–	GPP	–
Mode of delivery—intrapartum monitoring of fetal distress may be difficult in CAVB.	–	GPP	–
Postnatal			
Temporary pacing may be necessary.	III	B	49,67
Permanent pacemaker for rate <60 bpm, symptoms, or structural disease.	III	B	49,67

Va SVT, ventriculoatrial supraventricular tachycardia.

REFERENCES

1. Cremer MV: Ueber die direkte ableitung der akionsstrome des menschlichen herzens vom oesophagus und uber das electrokardiogramm des foetus. Muench Med Wochensch 1906;53:811–813.
2. Smyth CN: Experimental electrocardiography of the foetus. Lancet 1953;1:1124–1126.
3. Robinson HP, Shaw-Dunn J: Fetal heart rates as determined during pregnancy and labour. Br J Obstet Gynaecol 1977;84:492–496.
4. American College of Obstetrics and Gynecology: Fetal heart rate patterns: Monitoring, interpretation and management. ACOG Technical Bulletin 207, July 1995.
5. Davignon A, Rautaharju P, Boisselle E, et al: Normal ECG standards for infants and children. Pediatr Cardiol 1979;1:123–152.
6. Cameron A, Nimrod C, Nicholson S, et al: Evaluation of fetal cardiac dysrhythmias with two-dimensional, M-mode, and pulsed Doppler ultrasonography. Am J Obstet Gynecol 1998;158:286.
7. Reed K: Fetal arrhythmias: Etiology, diagnosis, pathophysiology, and treatment. Semin Perinatol 1989;13:294.
8. Southall DP, Richards J, Mitchell P, et al: Study of cardiac rhythm in healthy newborn infants. Br Heart J 1980;43:14–20.
9. Copel J, Liang RI, Demasio K, et al: The clinical significance of the irregular fetal heart rhythm. Am J Obstet Gynnecol 2000;182:813–819.
10. Ferrer PL, Quetel T, Bezjian A, et al: Outcome of fetal and perinatal cardiac arrhythmias, an eight year experience. J Ultrasound Med 1991;10(suppl):13s.
11. Respondek M, Wloch A, Kaczmarek P, et al: Diagnostic and perinatal management of fetal extrasystole. Pediatr Cardiol 1997;18:361–366.
12. Kleinman C, Copel J: Fetal cardiac arrhythmias: Diagnosis and therapy. Proceedings of the 9th International Fetal Cardiology Symposium, Orlando, FL, 1996, pp 326–341.
13. Green DW, Ackerman NB, Lund G, et al: Prolonged QT syndrome presenting as fetal bradycardia. J Matern Fetal Med 1992;1:202–205.
14. Hamersley S, Landy H, O'Sullivan M: Fetal bradycardia secondary to magnesium sulfate therapy for preterm labor. A case report. J Reprod Med 1998;43(3):206–210.
15. Ferrer P, Quetel T, Mas M, et al: Diagnosis and outcome of fetal myocardial diseases. J Am Coll Cardiol 1996;27:158A.
16. Geggel R, McInerny J, Estes N: Transient neonatal ventricular tachycardia associated with maternal cocaine use. Am J Cardiol 1989;63(5):383–384

17. Chameides L, Truex R, Vetter V, et al: Association of maternal lupus erythematosus with congenital complete block. N Engl J Med 1977;297:1204–1207.
18. Hull D, Binns B, Joyce D: Congenital heart block and widespread fibrosis due to maternal lupus erythematosus. Arch Dis Child 1966:41:688–690.
19. Kubli FW, Hon EH, Khazin AF, et al: Observations on heart rate and pH in the human fetus during labor. Am J Obstet Gynecol 1969;104:1190.
20. Peters M, Crowe J, Pieri J, et al: Monitoring the fetal heart noninvasively: A review of methods. J Perinat Med 2001;29:408–416.
21. Kariniemi V, Ahopeto J, Karp PJ, Katila TE: The fetal magnetocardiogram. J Perinat Med 1974;2:214–216.
22. Quinn A, Weir A, Shahani U, et al: Antenatal fetal magnetocardiography: A new method for fetal surveillance? Br J Obstet Gynaecol 1994;10:866–870.
23. Menendez T, Achenbach S, Beinder E, et al: Usefulness of magnetocardiography for the investigation of fetal arrhythmias. Am J Cardiol 2001;88(3):334–336.
24. Wakai RT, Leuthold AC, Cripe L, Martin CB: Assessment of fetal rhythm in complete heart block by magnetocardiography. Pacing Clin Electrophysiol 2000;23(6):1047–1050.
25. Hosono T, Kanagawa T, Chiba Y, et al: Fetal atrial flutter recorded prenatally by magnetocardiography. Fetal Diagn Ther 2002;17(2):75–77.
26. Achiron R, Rotstein Z, Liptiz S, et al: First-trimester diagnosis of fetal congenital heart disease by transvaginal ultrasonography. Obstet Gynecol 1994;84:69–72.
27. DeVore G, Siassi B, Platt L: Fetal echocardiography. III. The diagnosis of cardiac arrhythmias using real-time directed M-mode ultrasound. Am J Obstet Gynecol 1983;146:792.
28. Strasburger J, Huta J, Carpenter R, et al: Doppler echocardiography in the diagnosis and management of persistent fetal arrhythmias. J Am Coll Cardiol 1986;7:1385–1391.
29. Kleinman C, Valdez-Cruz L, Weinstein E, Shan D: Two-dimensional Doppler echocardiographic analysis of fetal cardiac arrhythmias. Pediatr Res 1984;18:124A.
30. Devore G, Horenstein J: Simultaneous Doppler recording of the pulmonary artery and vein: A new technique for the evaluation of a fetal arrhythmia. J Ultrasound Med 1993;12:669–671.
31. Chan F, Woo S, Ghosh A, et al: Prenatal diagnosis of congenital fetal arrhythmias by simultaneous pulsed Doppler velocimetry of the fetal abdominal aorta and inferior vena cava. Obstet Gynecol 1990;76:200–205.
32. Fouron J, Proulx F, Gosselin J, Infante-Rivard C: Investigation of fetal arrhythmias by simultaneous recording of ascending aortic and superior vena caval blood flow. Arch Mal Coeur Vaiss 2001;94(10):1063–1071.
33. Copel JA, Liang RI, Demasio K, et al: The clinical significance of the irregular fetal heart rhythm. Am J Obstet Gynecol 2000;182:813–819.
34. Shenker L: Fetal cardiac arrhythmias. Obst Gynecol Surv 1979;34:561–572.
35. Ferrer PL: Fetal arrhythmias. In Deal BJ, Wolff GS, Gelband H (eds): Current Concepts in Diagnosis and Management of Arrhythmias in Infants and Children. Armonk, NY, Futura,1998, pp 17–63.
36. Fernandez-Pineda L, Maitre-Azcarte MJ, Lopez-Zea M, et al: Redundancy of the interatrial septum without associated congenital cardiopathy. Its prenatal echocardiographic diagnosis and follow-up. Rev Espanola Cardiol 1995;48:537–541.
37. Southhall DP, Arrowsmith WA, Oakley JRJ, et al: Prolonged QT interval and cardiac arrhythmias in 2 neonates: Sudden infant death syndrome in one case. Arch Dis Child 1979;54(10):776–779.
38. Gimovsky ML, Caritis SN: Diagnosis and management of hypoxic fetal heart rate patterns. Clin Perinatal 1982;9(2): 313–324.
39. Benson DW Jr, Dunnigan A, Benditt DG, et al: Transesophageal study of infant supraventricular tachycardia: Electrophysiologic characterstics. Am J Cardiol 1983;52:1002–1006.
40. Dodo H, Gow RM, Hamilton RM, et al: Chaotic atrial rhythm in children. Am Heart J 1995;129:990–995.
41. Villain E, Vetter VL, Garcia JM, et al: Evolving concepts in management of congenital junctional ectopic tachycardia. A multicenter study. Circulation 1990;81:1544–1549.
42. Hankins G, Leicht T, Van Hook J: Prolonged fetal bradycardia secondary to maternal hypothermia in response to urosepsis. Am J Perinatol 1997;14(4):217–219.
43. Beinder E, Grancay T, Menendez T, et al: Fetal sinus bradycardia and the long QT syndrome. Am J Obstet Gynecol 2001;185:743–747.
44. Denes P, Levy L, Pick A, Rosen K: The incidence of typical and atypical AV Wenckebach periodicity. Am Heart J 1975;89:26–31.
45. Rosen K, Gunnar R, Rahimtoola S: Site and type of second degree AV block. Chest 1972;61:99–100.
46. Geggel R, Tucker L, Szer I: Postnatal progression from second to third-degree heart block in neonatal lupus syndrome. J Pediatr 1988;113:1049–1052.
47. Michaelsson M, Engle M: Congenital complete heart block: An international study of the natural history. Cardiovasc Clin 1972;4:85–101.
48. Schmidt K, Ulmer H, Silverman N, et al: Perinatal outcome of fetal complete atrioventricular block: A multicenter experience. J Am Coll Cardiol 1991;17:1360–1366.
49. Eronen M, Siren M, Ekblad H, et al: Short-and long-term outcome of children with congenital complete heart block diagnoses in utero or as a newborn. Pediatrics 2000;106:86–91
50. Machado M, Tynan M, Curry P, Allan L: Fetal complete heart block. Br Heart J 1988;60:512–515.
51. McCue C, Mantakas M,Tingelstad J, Ruddy S: Congenital heart block in newborns of mothers with connective tissue disease. Circulation 1977;56:82–90.
52. Taylor P, Scott J, Gerlis L, et al: Maternal antibodies against fetal cardiac antigens in congenital complete heart block. N Engl J Med 1986;315:667–672.
53. Tan E: Antinuclear antibodies: Diagnostic markers for autoimmune diseases and probes for cell biology. Adv Immunol 1989;44:93–152.
54. Meilof J, Smeenk R: Autoantibodies and their target antigens in Sjogren's syndrome. Neth J Med 1992;40:140–147.
55. Waltuck J, Buyon J: Autoantibody-associated congenital heart block: Outcome in mothers and children. Ann Intern Med 1994;120:544–551.
56. Buyon J, Heibert R, Copel J, et al: Autoimmune-associated congenital heart block: Demographics, mortality, morbidity and recurrence rates obtained from a national neonatal lupus registry. J Am Coll Cardiol 1998;31:1658–1666.
57. Michaelsson M, Riesenfeld T, Jonzon A: Natural history of congenital complete atrioventricular block. Pacing Clin Electrophysiol 1997;20(8 Pt 2):2098–2101.
58. Goble M, Dick M, McCune J, et al: Atrioventricular conduction in children of women with systemic lupus erythematosus. Am J Cardiol 1993;71:94–98.
59. Brucato A, Frassi M, Franceschini F, et al : Risk of congenital complete heart block in newborns of mothers with anti-Ro/SSA antibodies detected by counterimmunoelectrophoresis: A prospective study of 100 women. Arthritis Rheum 2001;44(8):1832–1835.
60. Watson R, Lane A, Barnett N, et al: Neonatal lupus erythematosus. A clinical, serological and immunogenetic study with review of the literature. Medicine 1984;63:362–378.
61. Garcia S, Nascimento J, Bonfa E, et al: Cellular mechanism of the conduction abnormalities induced by serum from anti-Ro/SSA-positive patients in rabbit hearts. J Clin Invest 1994;93:718–724.

62. Horsfall A, Venables P, Taylor P, et al: Ro and La antigens and maternal anti-La idiotype on the surface of myocardial fibres in congenital heart block. J Autoimmun 1991;4:165.
63. Thomas J, Edwards M, Park W, Thomas L: Apoptosis as a possible cause of gradual development of complete heart block and fatal arrhythmias associated with absence of the AV node, sinus node and internodal pathways. Circulation 1996;93:1424–1438.
64. Tran H, Ohlsson M, Beroukas D, et al: Subcellular redistribution of la/SSb autoantigen during physiologic apoptosis in the fetal mouse heart and conduction system: A clue to the pathogenesis of congenital heart block. Arthritis Rheum 2002;46:202–208.
65. Lev M: Pathogenesis of congenital atrioventricular block. Progr Cardiovasc Dis 1972;15:146.
66. Probst V, Hoorntje T, Hulsbeek M, et al: Cardiac conduction defect associated with mutation in SCN5A. Nature Genet 1999;23:20–21.
67. Groves A, Allan L, Rosenthal E: Outcome of isolated congenital complete heart block diagnosed in utero. Heart 1996;75(2): 190–194.
68. Groves A, Allan L, Rosenthal E: Therapeutic trial of sympathomimetics in three cases of complete heart block in the fetus. Circulation 1995;92:3394–3396.
69. Lopez L, Cha S, Leone C, et al: Use of sympathomimetic agents in fetal atrioventricular block. Arg Bras Cardiol 1994;63: 297–298.
70. Bunyon J, Waltuck J, Kleinmaan C, Copel J: In utero identification and therapy of congenital heart block. Lupus 1995;4: 116–121.
71. Yoshida H, Iwamoto M, Sakakibara H, et al: Treatment of fetal congenital complete heart block with maternal administration of beta-sympathomimetics. Gynecol Obstet Invest 2001;52(2): 142–144.
72. Strasburger JF, Huhta JC, Carpenter RJ, et al: Doppler echocardiography in the diagnosis and management of persistent fetal arrhythmias. J Am Coll Cardiol 1986;7:1385–1391.
73. Campbell WA, Vintzilleos AM, Nochimson DJ: Intrauterine versus extrauterine management/resuscitation of the fetus/ neonate. Clin Obstet Gynecol 1986;29(1):33–41.
74. Naheed RJ, Strassburger JF, Deal BJ, et al: Fetal tachycardia mechanisms and predictors of hydrops fetalis. J Am Coll Cardiol 1996;27:1736–1740.
75. Newburber JW, Keane JF: Intrauterine supraventricular tachycardia. J Pediatr 1979;95:780–786.
76. Strasburger JF, Duffy E, Gidding SS: Abnormal Doppler flow patterns in atrial tachycardia in infants. Am J Cardiol 1997;80:27–30.
77. Van Engelen AD, Weitjens O, Brenner JI, et al: Management outcome and follow-up of fetal tachycardia. J Am Coll Cardiol 1994;24:1371–1375.
78. Casey F A, McCrindle BW, Hamilton RM, Gow RM: Neonatal atrial flutter: Significant early morbidity and excellent long term prognosis. Am Heart J 1997;133(3):302–306.
79. Allan LD, Crawford DC, Anderson RH, Tynan M: Evaluation and treatment of fetal arrhythmias. Clin Cardiol 1984;7:467–473.
80. Strasburger JF: Fetal arrhythmias. Progr Pediatr Cardiol 2000;11(1):1–17.
81. Polin RA, Fox WW (eds): Fetal and Neonatal Physiology. Philadelphia, WB Saunders, 2002.
82. Weiner CP, Thompson MIB: Direct fetal treatment of supraventricular tachycardia after failed transplacental therapy. Am J Obstet Gynecol 1988;158:570–573.
83. Parilla BJ, Strasburger JF, Sokol M: Fetal supraventricular tachycardia complicated by hydrops fetalis: A role for direct fetal intramuscular therapy. Am J Perinatol 1996;13(8):483–486.
84. Simpson JM, Sharland GK: Fetal tachycardias: Management and outcome of 127 cases. Heart 1998;79:576–581.
85. Koike T, Minakami H, Shiraishi H, Sato I: Fetal ventricular rate in case of congenital complete heart block is increased by ritrodrine. Journal Perinat Med, 1997;25(2):216–218.
86. Assad R, Jatene M, Moreira L, et al: Fetal heart block: A new experimental model to assess fetal pacing. Pacing Clin Electrophysiol 1994;17(7):1256–1263.
87. Kikuchi Y, Shiraishi H, Igarashi H, et al: Cardiac pacing in fetal lambs: Intrauterine transvenous cardiac pacing for fetal complete heart block. Pacing Clin Electrophysol 1995;18 (3 Pt 1): 417–423.
88. Carpenter R, Strasburger J, Garson A, et al: Fetal ventricular pacing for hydrops secondary to complete atrioventricular block. J Am Coll Cardiol 1986;8:1434–1436.
89. Kaaja R, Julkunen H, Ammala, et al: Congenital heart block: Successful prophylactic treatment with intravenous gamma globulin and corticosteroid therapy. Am J Obstet Gynecol 1993;82:11–16.
90. Copel JA, Buyon JP, Kleinman CS: Successful in utero therapy of fetal heart block. Am J Obstet Gynecol 1995;173:1384–1390.
91. Bierman F, Baxi L, Jaffe I, Driscoll J: Fetal hydrops and congenital complete heart block: Response to maternal steroid therapy. J Pediatr 1988:646–648.
92. Yamada H, Kato E, Ebina Y, et al: Fetal treatment of congenital heart block ascribed to anti-SSA antibody: Case reports with observation of cardiohemodynamics and review of the literature. Am J Reprod Immunol 1999;42(4):226–232.
93. Saleeb S, Copel J, Friedman D, Buyon J: Comparison of treatment with fluorinated glucocorticoids to the natural history of autoantibody-associated congenital heart block: Retrospective review of the research registry for neonatal lupus. Arthritis Rheum 1999;42:2335–2345.

CHAPTER 17

Fetal Cardiac Abnormalities

Giuseppe Rizzo / Alessandra Capponi

INTRODUCTION

Major advances in diagnostic ultrasonography incorporating echocardiographic techniques[1] such as pulsed and color Doppler allow the study of normal and abnormal cardiac anatomy and function. Structural and functional abnormalities do affect the development of the heart, and the importance of antenatal diagnosis is well recognized in modern perinatal practice. Congenital heart disease occurs in 0.4% to 1.1% of live births[2] and accounts for 35% of infant deaths secondary to congenital disease.[3] Cardiovascular anomalies are frequently associated with other anomalies.[4,5] In this chapter, the indication and the sonographic technique for assessing fetal cardiac status are reviewed, the principal structural cardiac diseases are described, and the management options available are discussed.

INDICATIONS FOR FETAL ECHOCARDIOGRAPHY

"Routine" Fetal Echocardiography

Despite the high incidence of congenital heart disease, "routine" fetal echocardiography (i.e., all pregnancies) remains unavailable because it requires sophisticated equipment, a skilled operator, and meticulous scanning. Thus, it is not presently practical to screen the entire obstetric population. Moreover, the pregnancies at greatest risk of congenital heart disease are those in which an abnormality of the fetal heart is suspected during the routine 18- to 22-week anatomic scan. This underscores the importance of a meticulous scanning of the fetal heart in all pregnancies at this gestational age in order to identify those who should be referred for fetal echocardiography.

Selective Fetal Echocardiography

Fetal echocardiography is performed in selected pregnancies at increased risk of carrying a fetus with a congenital heart disease. Risk factors can be divided into familial, maternal, and fetal (Table 17–1).

An association has been shown between increased nuchal translucency (NT) measured between 11 and 14 weeks and congenital heart disease (see Chapters 7 and 8).[6] Indeed, the risk of a congenital heart disease is 6% in fetuses with a NT above the 99th percentile (i.e., >3.5 mm) and a normal karyotype.[6] Further, abnormalities of cardiac function have also been demonstrated in fetuses with normal cardiac anatomy,[7] suggesting a pivotal role for NT measurement in the screening of fetuses who should undergo fetal echocardiography.

The sensitivity of screening for congenital heart diseases reported in the literature is incredibly wide—10% and 81%.[8,9] These differences may be explained in part by the characteristics of the study population (low or high risk), the study design (prospective and retrospective), training and experience of the operators, content of the examination (four-chamber view or four-chamber view plus outflow tract visualization), and quality of follow-up (postnatal clinical examination or postnatal echocardiography). Moreover, the technology has not been stagnant. With the latest technology and proper training of the examiners, demonstration of the four-chamber view allows for the detection of 40% to 50% congenital heart disease in low risk pregnancies. The addition of outflow tract visualization increases the sensitivity of detecting cardiac lesions to 65% to 70%. It is not likely sensitivity can improve much more, considering the evolving nature of cardiac lesions.

ULTRASONOGRAPHIC EXAMINATION OF THE FETAL HEART (Table 17–2)

Timing of Fetal Echocardiography

Women should be seen within 48 hours of referral when an anomaly is suspected to avoid growing parental anxiety during the interval between detection of the

TABLE 17-1

Indications for Fetal Echocardiography

Family history
- Previous affected fetus or child
- Maternal or paternal congenital heart disease
- History of a single-gene disorder (DiGeorge, Noonan, Marfan, William, Holt-Oram syndromes)

Maternal history
- Metabolic diseases
  - Insulin-dependent diabetic mother
  - Maternal phenylketonuria
  - Connective tissue disease
- Exposure to teratogens
  - Alcohol
  - Valproic acid
  - Phenytoin
  - Isoretinoin
  - Lithium
  - Hydantoin
- Infections
  - Rubella
  - Parvovirus
  - Coxsackievirus
  - Cytomegalovirus

Fetal history
- Arrhythmias
- Extracardiac anomalies
- Hydrops
- Hydramnios
- Growth restriction
- Chromosomal defects
- Increased nuchal translucency thickness at 11–14 weeks' gestation
- Abnormal heart at 18–20 weeks' routine scan (usually abnormal four-chamber view)

possible anomaly and the consultation. Planned fetal echocardiography is typically performed between 20 and 22 weeks. The maternal abdominal wall thickness, prior abdominal surgery, and the number of fetuses each influence the ideal time for study.

Transvaginal ultrasonography permits a detailed view of the fetal anatomy early in gestation, and some investigators believe fetal echocardiography can be performed well between 14 and 16 weeks of gestation.[10,11] We currently limit performance of these early scans to women with a prior affected child or with insulin-dependent diabetes.[12] Because the sensitivity of early transvaginal echocardiography is at a maximum 60%,[10,13] it should be repeated between 20 and 22 weeks even if the first finding was normal, as an additional 20% of the congenital heart defects will be evident later.[13]

General Principles

It is imperative that the mother be informed before the examination in a clear and considerate manner about the reason for the fetal cardiac evaluation and its efficacy and limitations. The findings of the scan should then be explained at the end of the examination. Fetal echocardiography consists of several steps:

TABLE 17-2

Schematic Approach to Scanning the Fetal Heart

Cardiac malformations
- **Make diagnosis**
- **Inform the patients** (possibilities and limitations)
- **Fetal position**
- **Fetal situs** (transverse section of the upper abdomen)

Real-time view of the fetal heart
- Apical four-chamber view
  - Size of the heart (1/3 of the thorax)
  - Two atria, approximately equal size
  - Two ventricles, equal size, normally contracting
  - Morphologically right ventricle on the right
  - Two opening atrioventricular valves
  - Pulmonary veins
- Lateral four-chamber view
  - Integrity of the interventricular septum (muscular portion)
  - Foramen ovale flap
- Left ventricle outflow tract, aortic arch
  - The aorta arise's from the left ventricle
  - Integrity of the interventricular septum (membranous portion)
  - Opening aortic valve
  - Regular size of aortic arch
- Right ventricle outflow tract, ductus arch
  - The pulmonary artery rises from the right ventricle
  - Opening of the pulmonary valve
  - Regular size of main pulmonary artery
  - Branching of the pulmonary artery and continuity with the ductus arteriosus
- Three-vessel view
  - Pulmonary artery, aorta, and superior vena cava visualization
  - Identification of trachea and thymus
- Systemic venous return
  - Transverse section of the upper abdomen position of aorta (left and posterior) and inferior vena cava (right anterior)
  - Parasagittal view of the fetal trunk (inferior and superior vena cava)
- Pulmonary venous return
  - From apical four-chamber view identify inlet in the left atrium

Color Doppler Echocardiography
- Apical four-chamber view
  - Normal ventricular filling
  - Absence of regurgitation
- Ventricles outflow tracts
  - Normal aortic and pulmonary artery color visualization
  - Absence of flow reversal
- Three-vessel view
  - Same color direction in pulmonary artery and aorta

Pulsed Doppler
- Apical four-chamber view
  - Mitral and tricuspid velocity waveforms flow only during diastole (E and A waves)
  - Ventricle outflow tract
  - Aortic and pulmonary velocity waveforms flow only during systole (peak velocity, time to peak velocity cardiac output?)
- Ductus arteriosus flow
  - Flow throughout all the cardiac cycle
  - Highest velocities in fetal circulation
  - Exclude ductal constriction (P1 < 2)
- Venous flow
  - Inferior vena cava reflects overall cardiac function
  - Poor cardiac function is associated with increased reverse flow during atrial contraction (high preload index)

- Determine the fetal cardiac orientation and position.
- Evaluate the cardiac anatomy.
- Evaluate the cardiac hemodynamics and function using color and pulsed Doppler techniques.

Fetal Cardiac Orientation and Position

The examination begins with identification of the fetal head and spine so that the fetal right and left sides are known. The fetal visceral orientation, known as situs, is easily identified by noting the location of the following landmarks while viewing a transverse section of the upper abdomen (Fig. 17–1):

1. The stomach and spleen are on the left.
2. The abdominal aorta is a circular, pulsating structure on the left, anterolateral to the spine without another vessel posterior.
3. The inferior vena cava is an elliptical structure on the right of the spine in a plane anterior to the aorta.
4. The umbilical vein bends to the right, continuing in the portal sinus.

The arrangement described here constitutes *situs solitus*. An abnormal visceral-vascular arrangement may be either *situs inversus* or *situs ambiguous*. In the former, the visceral-vascular arrangements are the mirror image of *situs solitus*, so that the stomach and aorta are on the right and the inferior vena cava and the liver are on the left side. *Situs ambiguous* refers to an abnormal arrangement of the abdominal and thoracic organs and is usually associated with cardiosplenic syndromes.

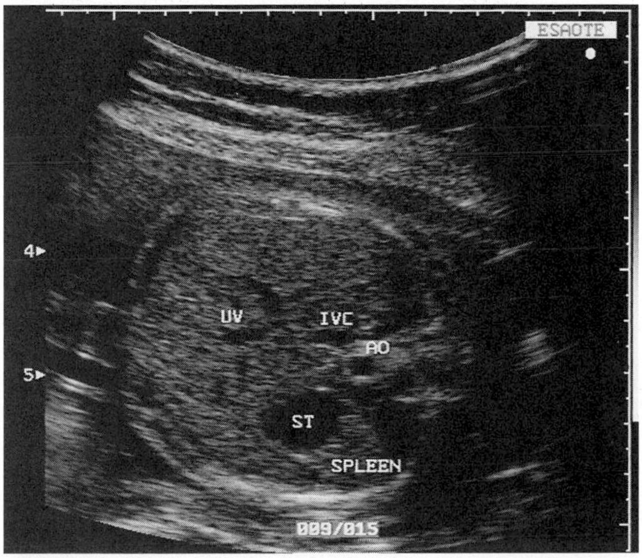

FIGURE 17–1
Transverse section of the upper fetal abdomen showing the spleen, the stomach (ST), aorta (AO), inferior vena cava (IVC), and umbilical vein (UV).

Normal Fetal Cardiac Anatomy

A sequential approach is applied to fetal echocardiography derived from the pathologic and angiographic examination of the heart.[14] The main steps include identification of the cardiac position within the body, identification of the cardiac chambers, study of atrioventricular connections, study of ventriculoarterial connections, and study of venous return to the atria. This is accomplished by examining the following standardized, echocardiographic planes.

Apical Four-Chamber View

The apical four-chamber view is found in a cross-sectional scan of the fetal thorax just above the level of the diaphragm where the normal heart is almost horizontal, mainly on the left side of the chest with the apex pointing left. *The apical four-chamber view is the single most important view of the heart and provides the following anatomic information* (Fig. 17–2):

1. The heart is correctly situated in the thorax with apex on the left, and it occupies about one third of the

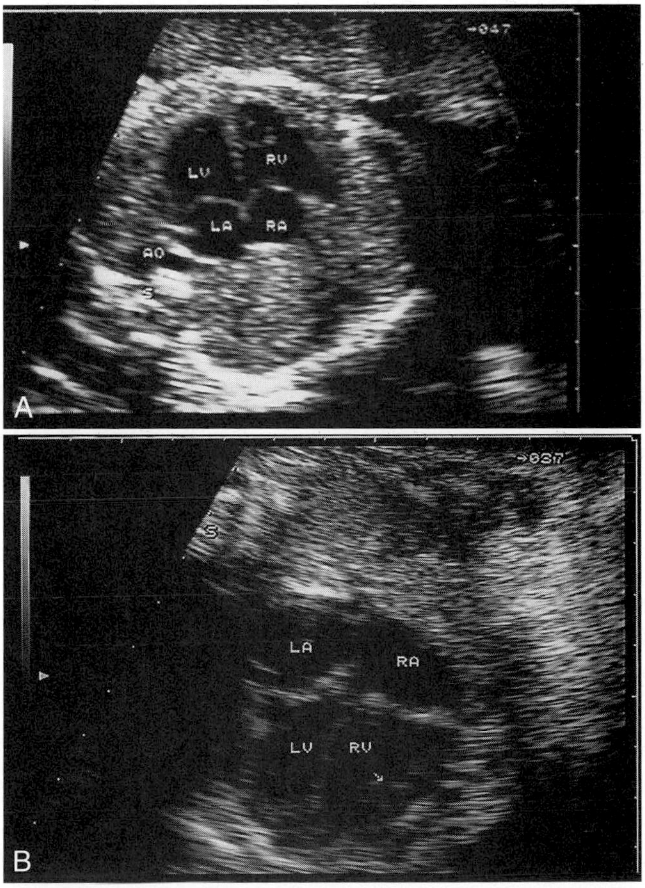

FIGURE 17–2
Apical four-chamber view of the fetal heart (*A*). In the magnified image (*B*) the arrow indicates the moderator band of the right ventricle. LA, left atrium; RA, right atrium; LV, left ventricle; RV, right ventricle.

thorax. The ratio between the cardiac and thoracic circumferences in this view during end diastole (i.e., while the atrioventricular valves are closed) is constant across gestation with an upper limit of 0.58.[15] Larger values suggest either cardiomegaly or a small chest.
2. There are two atria of equal size. The two ventricles are approximately equal in size and thickness, and in real time, their contractility appears similar.
3. The right ventricle is on the right and near the anterior thoracic wall. It has a septomarginal trabeculum, or moderator band, located near the apex in contiguity with the interventricular septum. The left ventricular cavity is smooth.
4. Two atrioventricular valves open in real time, and the insertion of the tricuspid valve is located more toward the apex than the mitral valve.
5. The interatrial septum, the foramen ovale, and the interventricular septum are visualized. The atria and ventricular septa meet at the level of atrioventricular valve, generating a crux.
6. The pulmonary veins enter the left atrium.

Although the four-chamber view is an essential component of any study of the fetal heart, it alone is insufficient, as less than a third of congenital defects are detectable.

Lateral Four-Chamber View

This view allows visualization with higher resolution of certain structures lying perpendicular to the line of ultrasound transmission. The artifactual dropout at the level of the high portion of the interventricular septum and of the atrium septum secundum common in the apical four-chamber view is avoided, and the integrity of the interventricular and interatrial septa is optimally demonstrated. This view also allows enhanced imaging of the foramen ovale and the movement of its valve into the left atrium (Fig. 17–3).

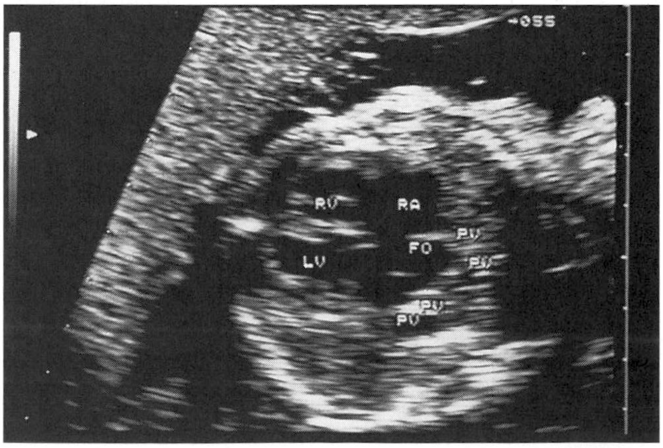

FIGURE 17–3
Transverse section of the fetal thorax showing the lateral four-chamber view. The muscular portion of the interventricular septum is visualized as well as the foramen ovale (FO). LA, left atrium; RA, right atrium; LV, left ventricle; RV, right ventricle; PV, pulmonary vein.

Left Ventricle Outflow Tract

It is possible to obtain a long axis view of the fetal heart in an oblique section of the fetal thorax. This section reveals the following landmarks (Fig. 17–4):

1. The mitral valve is seen between the left atrium and left ventricle, and the posterior leaflet is shorter than the anterior leaflet.
2. The anterior leaflet of the mitral valve is continuous with the posterior wall of the aorta.
3. The anterior wall of the aorta is continuous with the interventricular septum.
4. The aortic valve and its movement are seen at the base of the aorta. By orienting the transducer from the left shoulder to the right hemithorax, the aortic arch and the origin of the brachiocephalic vessels are fully visualized (Fig. 17–5).

Right Ventricle Outflow Tract

This view is a transverse cross section of the fetal thorax. The pulmonary artery is seen arising from the right ventricle anterior to and left of the ascending aorta (circle and sausage image) (Fig. 17–6). The movement of the pulmonary valve is seen. With slight movement of the transducer, the longitudinal view of the ductal arch is obtained. It is also possible to visualize the bifurcation of the main pulmonary artery and the ductus arteriosus connecting to the descending aorta in this section (Fig. 17–7).

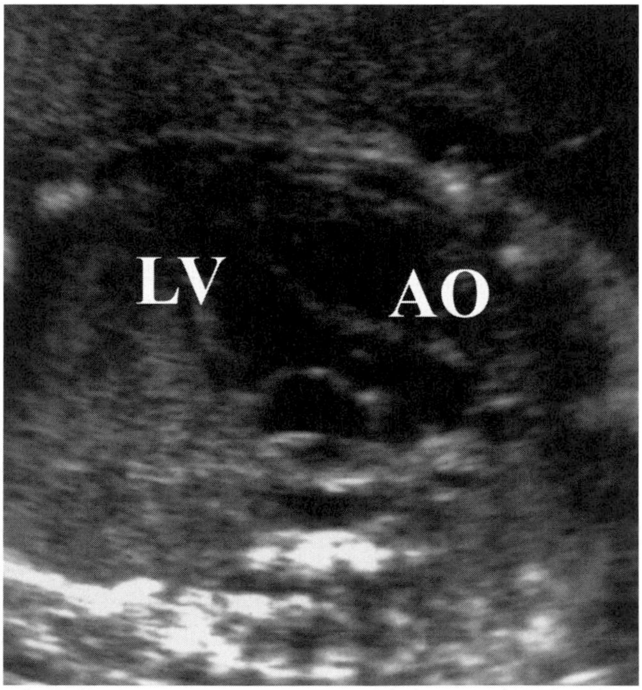

FIGURE 17–4
Long-axis view of the fetal heart showing the continuity between left ventricle (LV) and aorta (AO).

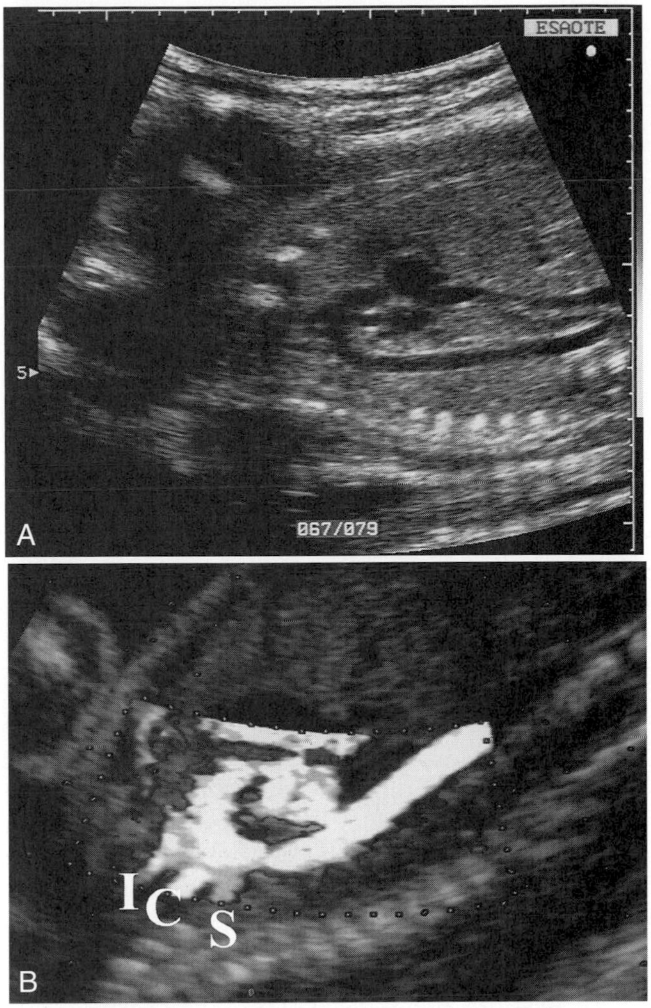

FIGURE 17–5
A, Longitudinal view of the aortic arch and of brachiocephalic vessels. *B*, Same section with power Doppler superimposed showing the arch with its three branches: innominate artery (I), left carotid artery (C) and subclavian artery (S) (see Color Plate 5).

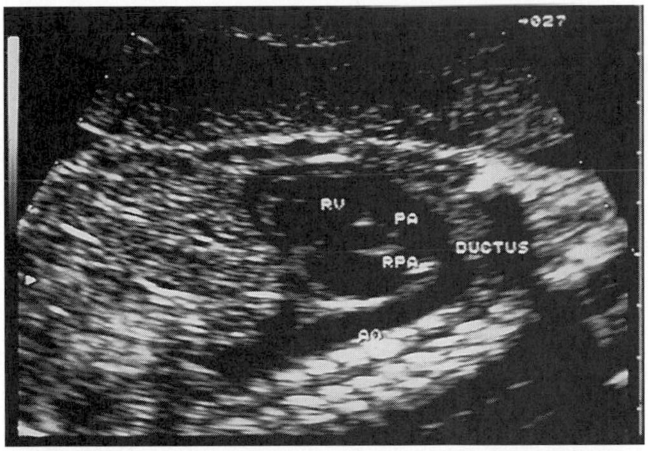

FIGURE 17–7
Longitudinal view of the ductus arteriosus arch. RV, right ventricle; PA, pulmonary artery; RPA, right pulmonary artery; DUCTUS, ductus arteriosus; AO, descending aorta.

Three-Vessel View

From the four-chamber view, the transducer is moved parallel in the direction of the upper thorax. In this view, the pulmonary trunk with the ductus arteriosus, the aortic arch with aortic isthmus, and the superior vena cava are seen. (Fig. 17–8). The aorta and pulmonary trunk are seen in a longitudinal view and form a V-shaped area in the posterior thorax on the left side of the spine.[16] In this section, the trachea is a circular structure with an echogenic wall adjacent and to the right of the aorta. In front of the trachea, the superior vena cava can be seen. The following landmarks are contained in this view:

1. Three vessels are seen from left to right: pulmonary artery, aorta, and superior vena cava.
2. These vessels are listed in descending order of size: pulmonary artery, aorta, superior vena cava.
3. Each vessel lies posterior to the other: pulmonary artery anterior to aorta, aorta anterior to superior vena cava.

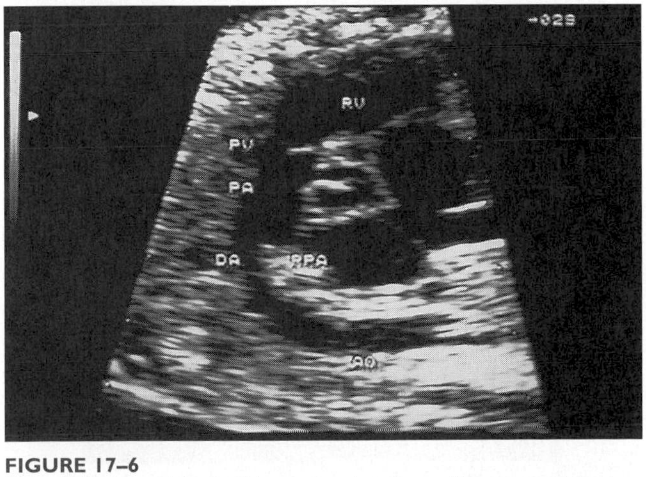

FIGURE 17–6
Short-axis view of the fetal heart showing the outflow tract of the right ventricle. PV, pulmonary valve; PA, main pulmonary artery; RPA, right pulmonary artery; DA, ductus arteriosus; AO, descending aorta.

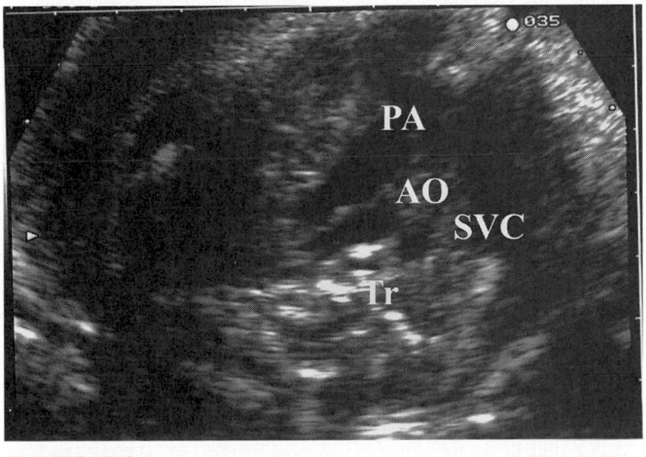

FIGURE 17–8
Transverse section of the fetal thorax at the level of the three-vessel view. The pulmonary artery (PA) is the largest of the three vessels, the aorta (AO) is between the PA and the superior vena cava (SVC), which is the smallest and most posterior vessel. The trachea (Tr) is visualized posterior to the aorta.

4. Pulmonary artery arises closest to the anterior chest wall.
5. Trachea and thymus can be visualized.

The position of the trachea in comparison to these vessels may be used to differentiate a normal, left-sided aortic arch from an abnormal right-sided aortic arch.[17] Furthermore, the thymus can be seen in front of these vessels (Fig 17–9*A*), and its absence is a possible marker of congenital heart disease associated with a microdeletion deletion of chromosome 22q11 (Fig 17–9*B*).[18]

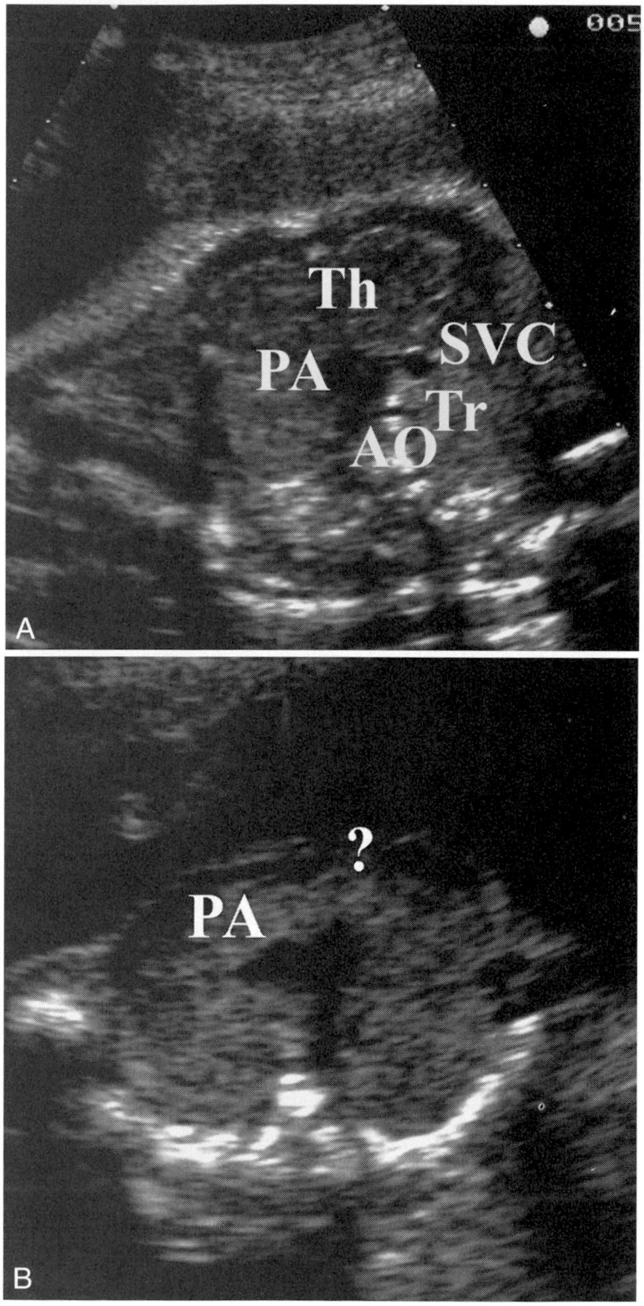

FIGURE 17–9
A, Three-vessel view of a normal fetus showing the fetal thymus (Th), trachea (Tr), pulmonary artery (PA), aorta (AO), and superior vena cava (SVC). *B*, Three-vessel view in a fetus with a microdeletion deletion of chromosome 22q11 with an absent pulmonary valve, resulting in a dilated pulmonary artery (PA) and absent thymus (?).

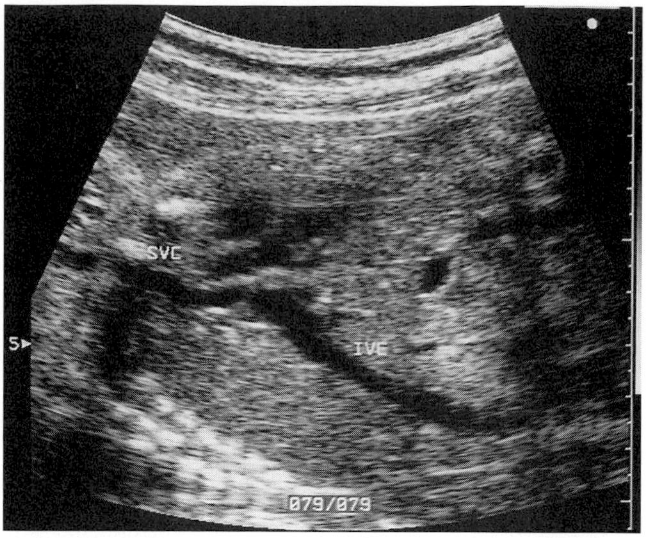

FIGURE 17–10
Parasagittal view of the fetal trunk showing the inlet in the right atrium of the superior vena cava (SVC) and inferior vena cava (IVC).

Venous Return

The systemic venous return is assessed using a right parasagittal scan of the fetal thorax to demonstrate the inferior and superior vena cava entering the right atrium (Fig. 17–10). The pulmonary veins are seen entering the left atrium from either the apical or lateral four-chamber views (Fig 17–11).

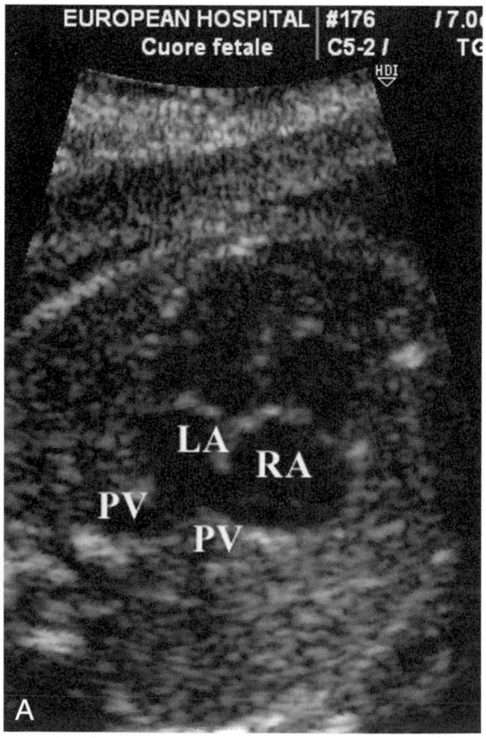

FIGURE 17–11
Apical four-chamber view of the fetal heart showing the inlet of the pulmonary veins (PV) in the left atrium in real time (*A*) (see Color Plate 6).

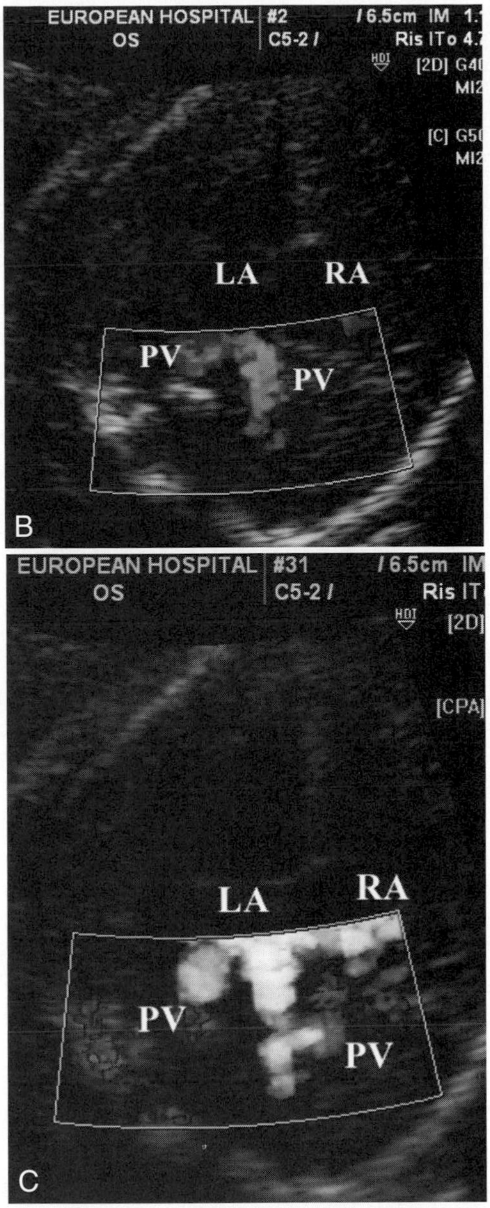

FIGURE 17–11 Contd (*B*) and power (*C*) Doppler (see Color Plate 6).

DOPPLER EXAMINATION OF THE FETAL HEART

General Principles

Although real-time imaging provides information on the structural integrity of the fetal heart, Doppler ultrasonography provides information that enhances both the definition of the presence and the severity of structural and functional cardiac disease. The parameters used to describe fetal cardiac velocity waveforms differ from those used to describe the peripheral fetal vessels. In the latter, pulsatility, resistance, or systole/diastole indices are used. They are derived from the relative ratios of systolic, diastolic, and mean velocities and are independent of the absolute velocity and the angle of insonation[19] (see also Chapter 11).

In contrast, the measurements at the cardiac level are absolute values and require knowledge of the angle of insonation, which may be difficult to obtain accurately. The error in the absolute velocity measurement resulting from angle uncertainty is strongly dependent on the magnitude of the angle itself. For example, the error is insignificant if the angle is less than about 20 degrees. However, when the angle is greater than 20 degrees, the cosine term in the Doppler equation converts the small uncertainty in the measurement to a large error in the velocity equations.[19] Thus, recordings should be obtained with the Doppler beam as parallel to the bloodstream as possible. All recordings with an estimated angle greater than 20 degrees should be rejected.

The use of color Doppler velocimetry can help solve many of these problems by revealing in real time the flow direction so that the beam can be properly aligned. Pulsed Doppler is generally preferred over continuous wave Doppler because of its superior range of resolution. The sample volume is placed immediately distal to the location to be studied (e.g., distal to the aortic semilunar valves to record the left ventricle outflow). The continuous wave Doppler may be useful when there are particularly high velocities (e.g., in the ductus arteriosus) because it avoids the aliasing effect.

Parameters Measured

The following parameters are commonly used to describe the cardiac velocity waveforms:

- The *peak velocity* (PV) is expressed as the maximum velocity at a given moment (e.g., systole, diastole) on the Doppler spectrum.
- The *time to peak velocity* (TPV) or acceleration time is expressed as the time interval between the onset of the waveform and its peak.
- The *time velocity integral* (TVI) is calculated by planimetering the area beneath the Doppler spectrum.

It is possible to calculate absolute cardiac flow from both atrioventricular valve and outflow tracts by multiplying as follows:

$$\text{TVI} \times \text{valve area} \times \text{fetal heart rate}$$

The calculation of the measurement valve area is also prone to inaccuracy. It is derived from the measurement of a valve diameter that is near the limit of ultrasonographic resolution. The measurement is then halved and squared in the calculation, amplifying potential errors. Despite these limitations, absolute cardiac flow can be used in longitudinal studies over a short duration during which the valve dimensions are assumed constant. It is also possible to calculate accurately the relative ratio between the right and left cardiac output (RCO/LCO) and avoid the valve measurement completely because the relative dimensions of the aortic and pulmonary valves remain similar through gestation in the absence of cardiac structural diseases.[1]

Site of Recordings; Velocity Waveform Characteristics and Their Significance

Blood flow velocity waveforms can be recorded at all cardiac levels including venous return, foramen ovale, atrioventricular valves, outflow tracts, pulmonary arteries, and ductus arteriosus. Factors affecting the morphology of the velocity waveforms include preload, afterload, myocardial contractility, ventricular compliance, and fetal heart rate.[1,19] As it is impossible to obtain simultaneous recordings of pressure and volume, these factors cannot be fully investigated in the human fetus. However, as each waveform parameter and the site of its recording are specifically affected by one of these factors, it is possible to elucidate indirectly the underlying pathophysiology by performing the measurements at various cardiac levels.

Venous Circulation

Blood flow velocity waveforms can be recorded in the superior and inferior vena cava, ductus venosus, and pulmonary, hepatic, and umbilical veins. The vessel most intensively studied to date is the inferior vena cava (IVC). Waveforms recorded just distal to the entrance of the ductus venosus[20,21] have a triphasic profile. There is a first forward wave concomitant with ventricular systole, a second forward wave of smaller dimension occurring in early diastole, and a third but reverse wave during atrial contraction (Fig. 17–12). Several indices have been proposed for the analysis of the IVC waveforms. We found that the preload index (PLI) expressed as the ratio between the peak velocities during atrial contraction and systole (PLI = A/S) is the most reproducible and efficient index.[22] This index is related to the pressure gradient between the right atrium and ventricle during end diastole, which is a function of both ventricular compliance and ventricular end-diastolic pressure.[23] Decreased cardiac function is associated with an increase in the A wave, and as a consequence, the PLI increases.

The ductus venosus (DV) is seen in a transverse section of the upper fetal abdomen at the level of its origin from the umbilical vein. Color Doppler is superimposed and the pulsed Doppler sample volume is placed just above its inlet (close to the umbilical vein) at the point of maximum flow velocity as expressed by color brightness. The DV flow velocity waveform has a biphasic pattern with a first peak concomitant with systole (S), a second peak concomitant with diastole (D), and a nadir during atrial contraction (A) (Fig. 17–13). Among the indices suggested to quantify DV velocity waveforms is the ratio of the S peak velocity to A peak velocity (S/A). This index is angle independent and describes DV hemodynamics efficiently.[24] The hemodynamic significance of the DV is similar to the IVC. In the presence of poor cardiac function, the A wave is reduced or negative and the S/A ratio increases.

Pulmonary vein velocity waveform is recorded at its entrance into the left atrium. The waveform morphology is similar to that of the DV and is characterized by positive velocities during atrial contraction (Fig. 17–14). The striking variation in the velocity waveform morphology between IVC and pulmonary vein reflects the different hemodynamic conditions of the fetal systemic and pulmonary venous circulations. Indeed, an abnormal pattern has been described in corrected transposition of the great

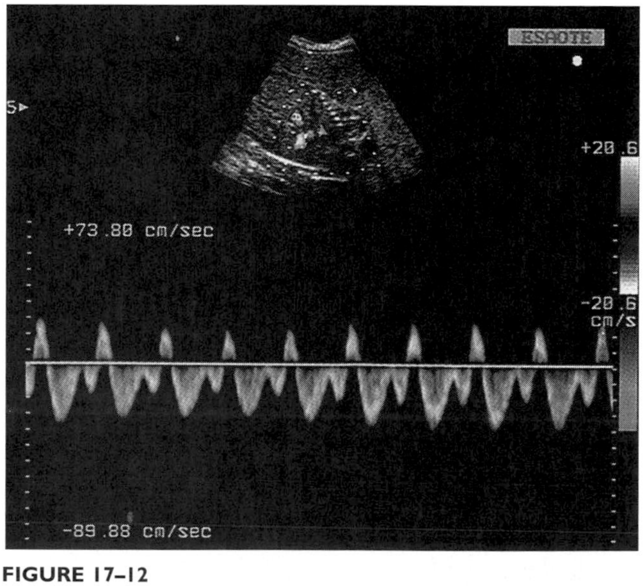

FIGURE 17–12
Parasagittal view of the fetal trunk with the sample volume placed on the inferior vena cava. Note the typical triphasic morphology with the reverse flow (upper channel) during atrial contraction (A wave) (see Color Plate 7).

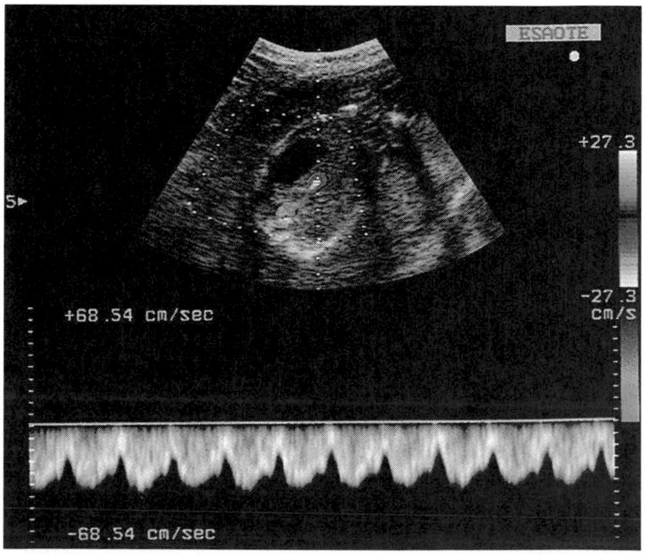

FIGURE 17–13
Transverse section of the upper fetal abdomen with the sample volume placed on the ductus venosus. Note the typical biphasic morphology (see Color Plate 8).

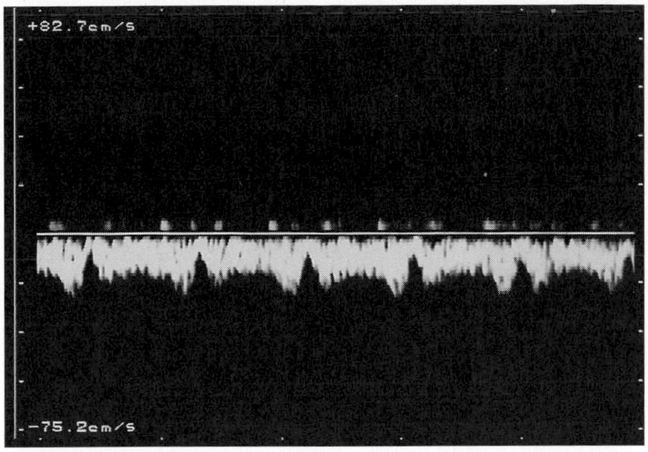

FIGURE 17–14
Velocity waveforms from the pulmonary vein showing the presence of forward flow for all the cardiac cycle.

arteries, a condition in which the afterload of the left ventricle is altered.[25]

Umbilical venous blood flow is usually continuous. However, pulsations in the umbilical venous flow reflecting the heart rate occur in the presence of a relevant amount of reverse flow in the inferior vena cava during atrial contraction. In normal pregnancies, these pulsations cease after the 12 weeks of gestation. Before 12 weeks, they are secondary to ventricular stiffness, which causes a high percentage of reverse flow into the inferior vena cava.[1] The presence of pulsations in the umbilical vein after 12 weeks indicates severe cardiac compromise.[1] *In clinical practice, the venous circulation is evaluated in sequence moving away from the heart. The further the pulsations are from the heart, the greater the stiffness/cardiac compromise.*

Atrioventricular Valves

Flow velocity waveforms at the level of mitral and tricuspid valves are recorded in the apical four-chamber view of the fetal heart. They are characterized by two diastolic peaks corresponding to early ventricular filling (the "E" wave) and active ventricular filling during atrial contraction (the "A" wave) (Fig. 17–15). The ratio between the E and A waves (E/A) is a widely accepted index of ventricular diastolic function and is an expression of both the cardiac compliance and preload conditions.[26,27]

Outflow Tracts

Flow velocity waveforms from the aorta and pulmonary artery are recorded respectively from the five-chamber and short-axis views of the fetal heart (Figs. 17–16 and 17–17). PV and TPV are the most commonly used indices. The former is influenced by several factors, including valve size, myocardial contractility, and afterload, whereas the latter is believed to reflect the mean arterial pressure.[26]

Pulmonary Vessels

Velocity waveforms may be recorded from the right and left pulmonary arteries or from peripheral vessels within the lung. The morphology of the waveforms varies according to the sample site, and their analysis has been used to study the normal development of the pulmonary circulation.[27]

Three-Vessel View

In this view, the pulmonary artery and ascending aorta have the same flow direction and thus have the same

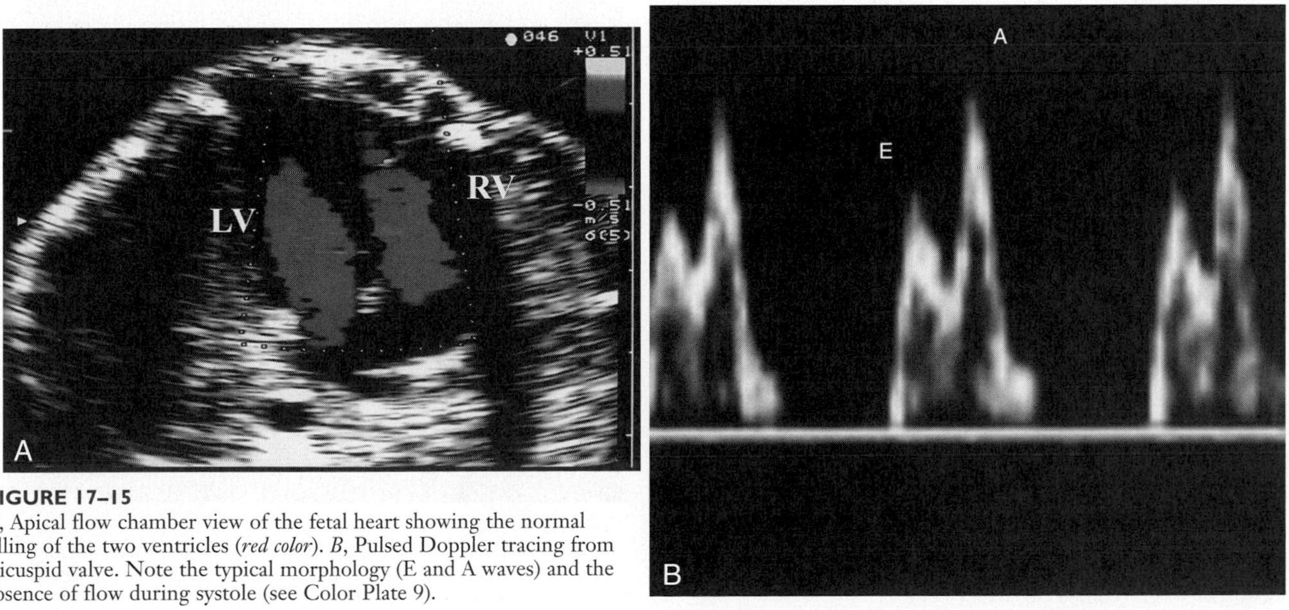

FIGURE 17–15
A, Apical flow chamber view of the fetal heart showing the normal filling of the two ventricles (*red color*). *B*, Pulsed Doppler tracing from tricuspid valve. Note the typical morphology (E and A waves) and the absence of flow during systole (see Color Plate 9).

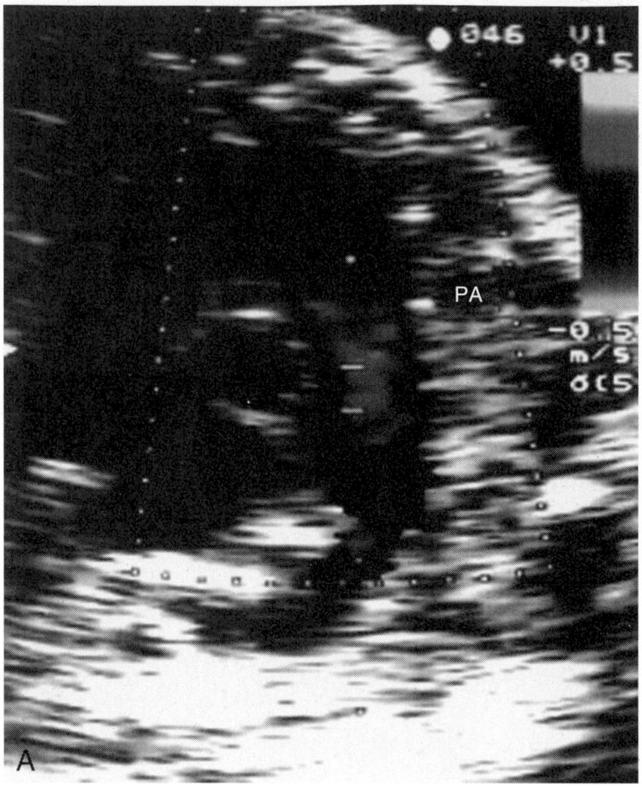

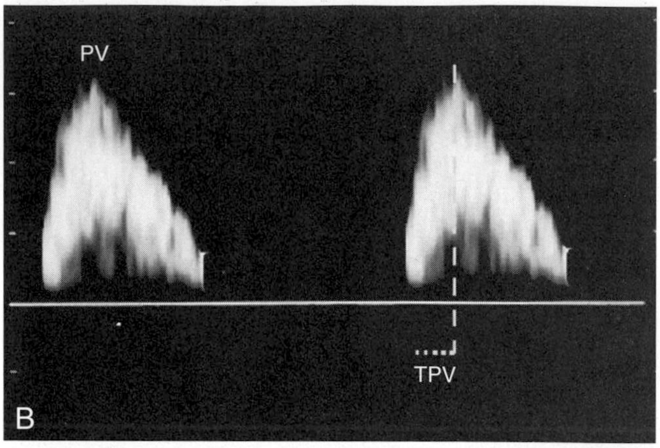

FIGURE 17–16
A, Short-axis view of the fetal heart with the color Doppler superimposed showing the outflow of the right ventricle (*blue*). *B*, Pulsed Doppler tracing at the level of the pulmonary valve and the typical velocity waveform recorded. PV, peak velocity; TPV, time to peak velocity (see Color Plate 10).

color when imaged with color flow Doppler (Fig. 17–18). Severe outflow obstruction to one of the ventricles leads to reverse flow in the pulmonary artery (right side obstruction) or in aorta (left side obstruction) (Fig. 17–19).

Ductus Arteriosus

Ductal velocity waveforms are recorded in a short-axis view showing the ductal arch. They are characterized by continuous forward flow throughout the cardiac cycle.[26]

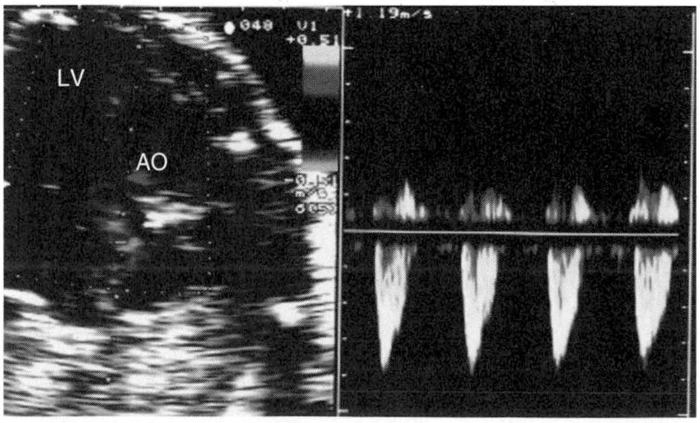

FIGURE 17–17
Long-axis view of the fetal heart with the color Doppler superimposed showing the outflow of the left ventricle (*blue*). The sample volume is placed at the level of the aorta and the typical velocity waveform recorded (see Color Plate 11).

The parameter most commonly analyzed is the PV during systole or, similarly to peripheral vessels, the pulsatility index[28]:

PI = (systolic velocity–diastolic velocity)/mean velocity

Normal Ranges of Doppler Cardiac Indices

The velocity waveforms are recordable from 11 weeks on.[29] The cardiovascular indices change dramatically at all levels up to 20 weeks. The PLI of the IVC decreases

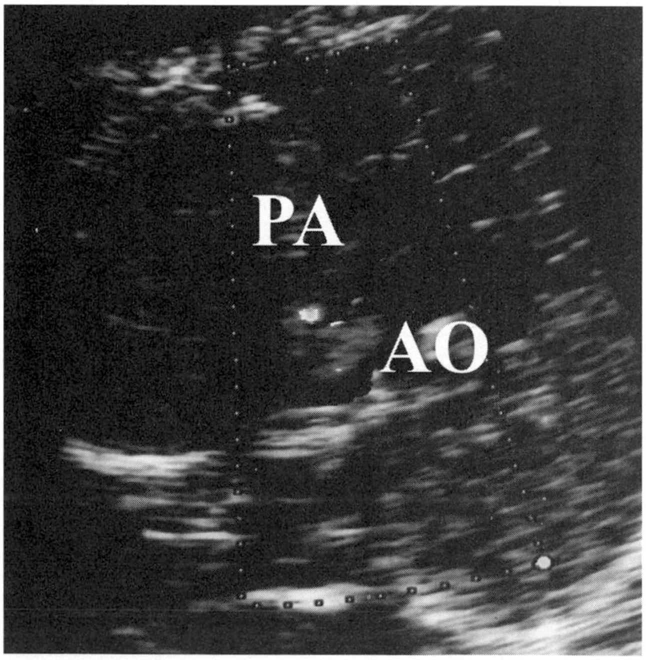

FIGURE 17–18
Three-vessel view with the color Doppler superimposed showing pulmonary artery (PA) and ascending aorta (AO) with the same flow direction (see Color Plate 12).

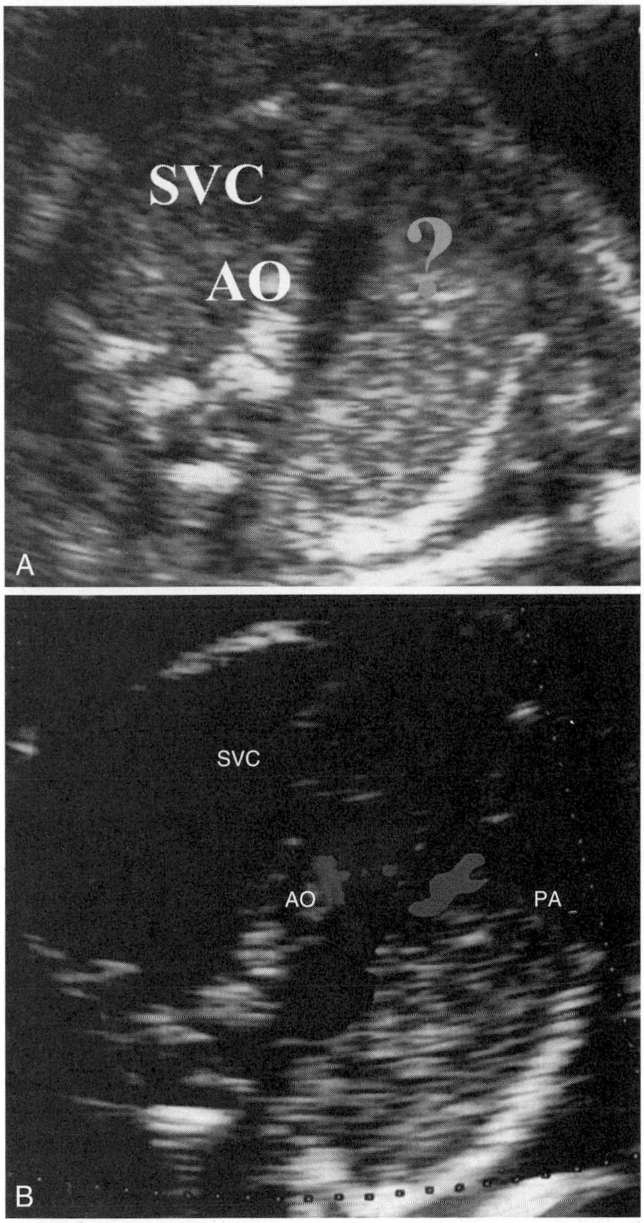

FIGURE 17–19
Three-vessel view in a fetus with pulmonary atresia. *A*, The pulmonary artery is not evidenced (?) in real-time image. *B*, With the color Doppler superimposed, a small caliber pulmonary artery is identified with reversal flow (*red*) indicating retrograde perfusion from the systemic circulation to pulmonary circulation (see Color Plate 13).

significantly,[1,24,26] the E/A ratio at both atrioventricular levels increases dramatically,[1,26] and the PV and TVI of the outflow tracts, particularly at the level of pulmonary valve, increase.[26] These changes are consistent with rapid development of ventricular compliance (explaining the decrease in the IVC PLI and the increase in the E/A) and a shift in the cardiac output toward the right ventricle as placental resistance falls, decreasing right ventricular afterload.

After 20 weeks, the IVC PLI declines less dramatically while there is a significant decline in the S/A ratio of the DV.[22] At the level of atrioventricular valves, the E/A ratios increase progressively, reaching a value near 1 at term.[19,20] Similarly, the PV increases linearly at the level of both the pulmonary and aortic valves.[26] The PV of the aortic valve is usually greater than at the pulmonary artery, and under normal conditions, it is always below 100 cm per second. The change in TPV is minimal.[26] TPV measurements at the level of pulmonary valve are lower than at the level of the aortic valve, suggesting the blood pressure in the pulmonary artery is slightly higher than in the ascending aorta.[26] Quantitative measurements reveal the right cardiac output (RCO) is higher than the left (LCO), and that the RCO/LCO ratio remains constant from 20 weeks onward, with a mean value of 1.3.[1,26] This is lower than that reported in fetal sheep (RCO/LCO = 1.8) and may reflect the higher brain weight of humans, requiring a higher left cardiac output.[26]

The ductus arteriosus PV increases linearly with advancing gestation, and its values represent the highest velocities in the fetal circulation under normal conditions.[26] Ductal constriction is suggested by a systolic velocity measurement above 140 cm per second in conjunction with a diastolic velocity greater than 35 cm per second or a pulsatility index value less than 2.[28]

CARDIAC STRUCTURAL ANOMALIES

Septal Defects

Septal defects are the most common congenital heart defects with an estimated incidence of about 0.5 per 1000 live births.[2] They are either atrial, ventricular, or atrioventricular septal in location.

Isolated atrial septal defects have been diagnosed in utero, but the diagnosis remains difficult because of the foramen ovale. Echocardiographic diagnosis requires demonstration of either the absence or reduction in the dimension of the foramen ovale valve flap (ostium secundum defect). Dropout of echoes at the level of the outlet of the atrial septum in a perpendicular view suggests the presence of an ostium primum defect or an incomplete form of atrioventricular canal.

Atrial septal defects do not impair fetal cardiac function and only rarely do so in the neonate. However, atrial septal defects are associated with other cardiac malformations (coarctation and conotruncal anomalies), an abnormal karyotype (e.g., trisomy 21), and genetic syndromes (e.g., Holt-Oram syndrome).

Ventricular septal defects are classified by their location in the septum: perimembranous, inlet, trabecular, and outlet. Perimembranous defects are most common (80%), and involve the membranous portion of the interventricular septum just below the aortic valve. They can extend a variable degree into the muscular portion. Septal defects are not responsible for fetal compromise.

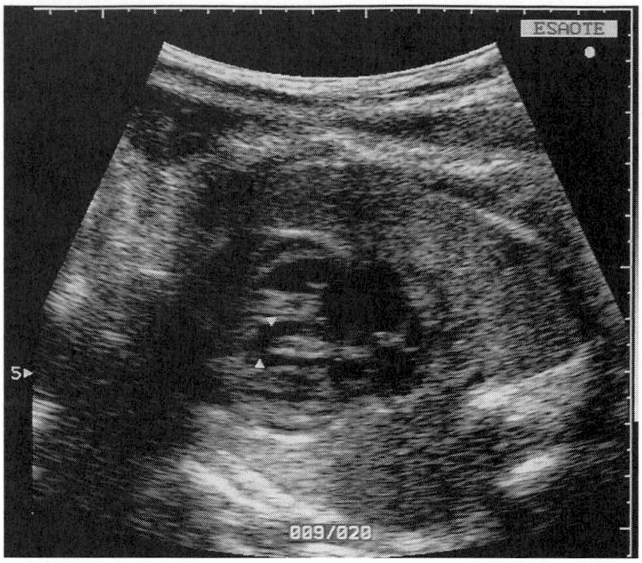

FIGURE 17–20
Lateral four-chamber view showing the interventricular septum with an evident defect (*arrows*) in the muscular portion.

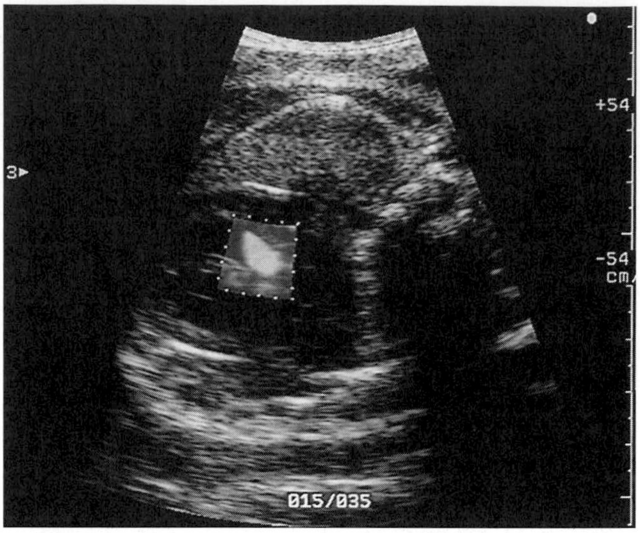

FIGURE 17–21
This small perimembranous septal defect is visualized with the help of color Doppler. High-velocity jet from the left to the right ventricle is due to the association of aortic stenosis (see Color Plate 14).

Because the pressure of both ventricular cavities is similar, even large defects cause only small bidirectional shunts that do not affect intracardiac hemodynamics. The vast majority of infants with interventricular septal defects are asymptomatic in the neonatal period. It is calculated that a quarter of the ventricular septal defects close spontaneously during intrauterine life,[31] and another third of the remaining defects close during the first year of life.[30]

Echocardiographic diagnosis relies on the demonstration of echo dropout in the interventricular septum. Care is necessary to avoid artifact due to the inherent limitations in the lateral resolution of ultrasound. The diagnosis is made only when the ultrasound beam is perpendicular to the septum (Fig. 17–20). Color Doppler is useful for demonstrating the shunt between ventricles. This is particularly clear when the outflow of one ventricle is obstructed (unidirectional shunt) (Fig. 17–21). The application of new generation equipment with high-resolution color and power energy Doppler (in which flows are independent of the angle of insonation) is also helpful for detection of isolated ventricular septal defects.[32] The prognosis for an infant with an isolated interventricular septal defect is good. However, it is essential that other cardiac and extracardiac anomalies be carefully excluded and a normal fetal karyotype documented.[4,5]

Abnormal development of both the atrial and ventricular septa is described as an atrioventricular septal defect; either the endocardial cushion or an atrioventricular canal forms. The typical appearance is of a single, atrioventricular valve opening above and bridging the two ventricles (Figs. 17–22 and 17–23). The common atrioventricular valve may be incompetent, with systolic regurgitation leading to fetal heart failure and hydrops. Atrioventricular septal defects are frequently associated with fetal aneuploidy (50% of the cases, particularly trisomy 21),[5] cardiac isomerism (cardiosplenic syndromes), and other extracardiac anomalies.[4]

Hypoplastic Left Ventricle

A small left ventricle secondary to mitral or aortic stenosis/atresia characterizes the hypoplastic left heart syndrome. Blood flow to the head and coronary artery is supplied by retrograde flow through the ductus arteriosus and the aortic arch. The incidence of hypoplastic left heart

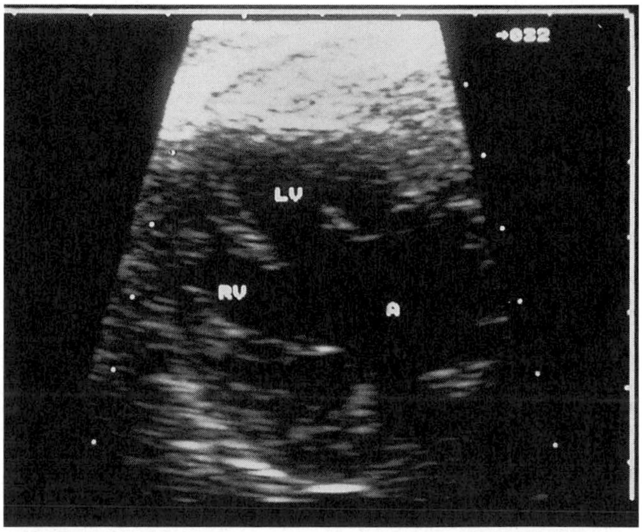

FIGURE 17–22
Apical four-chamber view showing a defect of the atrioventricular septum in a case of atrioventricular canal. A, atrium; LV, left ventricle; RV, right ventricle.

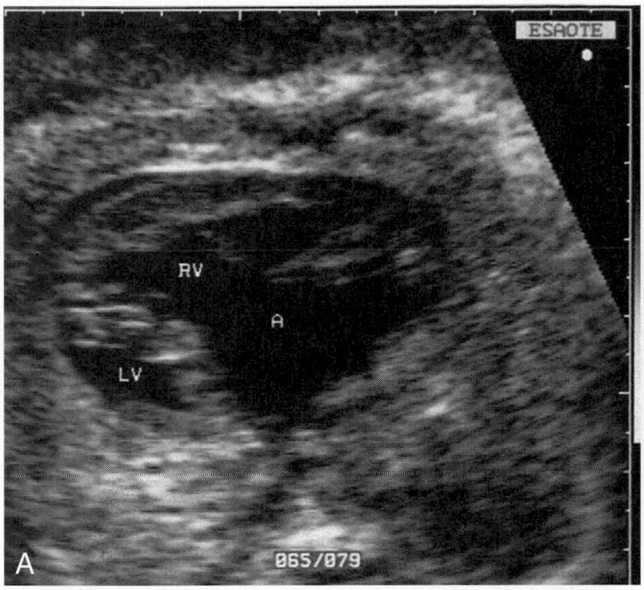

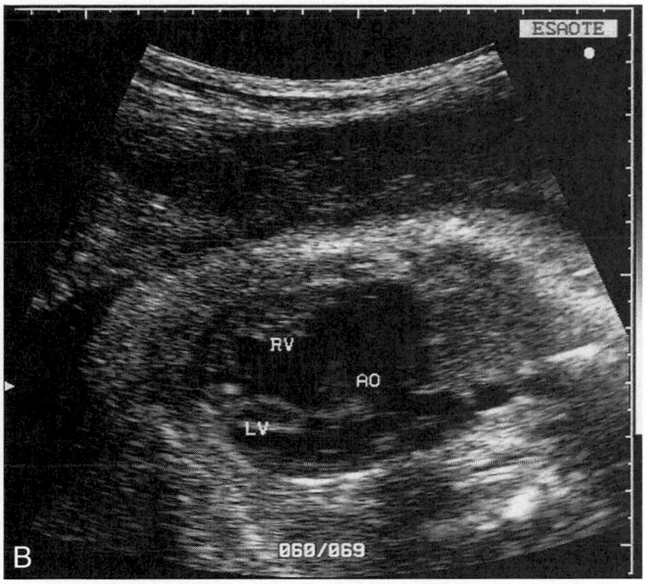

FIGURE 17–23
A, Lateral four-chamber view of the fetal heart showing a common atrium (A) with a huge defect of the atrioventricular septum and, *B*, the small dimensions of the left ventricle (LV) and aorta (AO) with respect to the right ventricle (RV), demonstrating the presence of an atrioventricular canal with right ventricle dominance.

syndrome approximates 0.16 per 1000 live births, and constitutes about 10% of infants with congenital heart diseases[33] and up to 20% of those detected in utero.[34]

Echocardiographic diagnosis begins with the demonstration of a small left ventricle (Fig. 17–24). The ascending aorta is severely hypoplastic, and the right atrium,

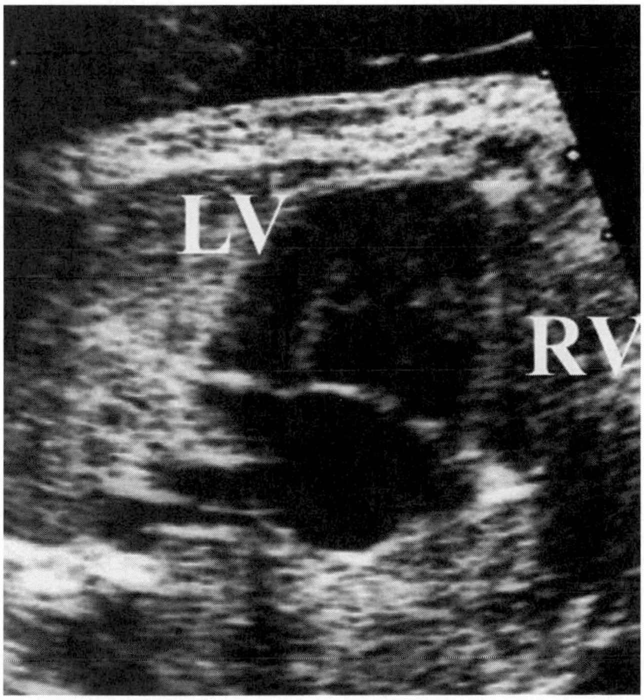

FIGURE 17–24
Lateral four-chamber view showing the hypoplasia of the left ventricle. LV, left ventricle; RV, right ventricle.

right ventricle, and pulmonary artery relatively enlarged. Color and pulsed Doppler flow examination may reveal absent flow from the left atrium to the left ventricle (mitral atresia) (Fig. 17–25) and retrograde flow in the aortic arch.

A hypoplastic left ventricle is well tolerated in utero, and congestive heart failure is unusual. However, the postnatal prognosis is poor. This lesion is responsible for 25% of cardiac deaths during the first week of life.[35,36] Surgical options are limited. Norwood's three-stage operation was developed to correct this disease. And even though the reported survival rate in selected centers reaches 60%, the long-term prognosis for these children after three procedures remains uncertain.[37] Cardiac transplant programs for the neonate have also been developed, but the long-term results of these, too, are disappointing.[38]

Pulmonary Atresia With Intact Ventricular Septum

Pulmonary atresia with intact ventricular septum makes up 3% to 4% of neonatal and prenatal series.[2,33] There are two forms of pulmonary atresia found in the fetus. In about 75%, the right ventricle is hypoplastic,[28] and in the remaining 25%, the right ventricle is enlarged (see Fig. 17–27).[33] In the former instance, the tricuspid valve is atretic (Fig. 17–26), and in the latter case, it is typically insufficient (Fig. 17–27). Echocardiographic diagnosis relies on the demonstration of a small pulmonary artery with an atretic pulmonary valve. The four-chamber view is abnormal and shows variable degrees of right ventricular hypoplasia.

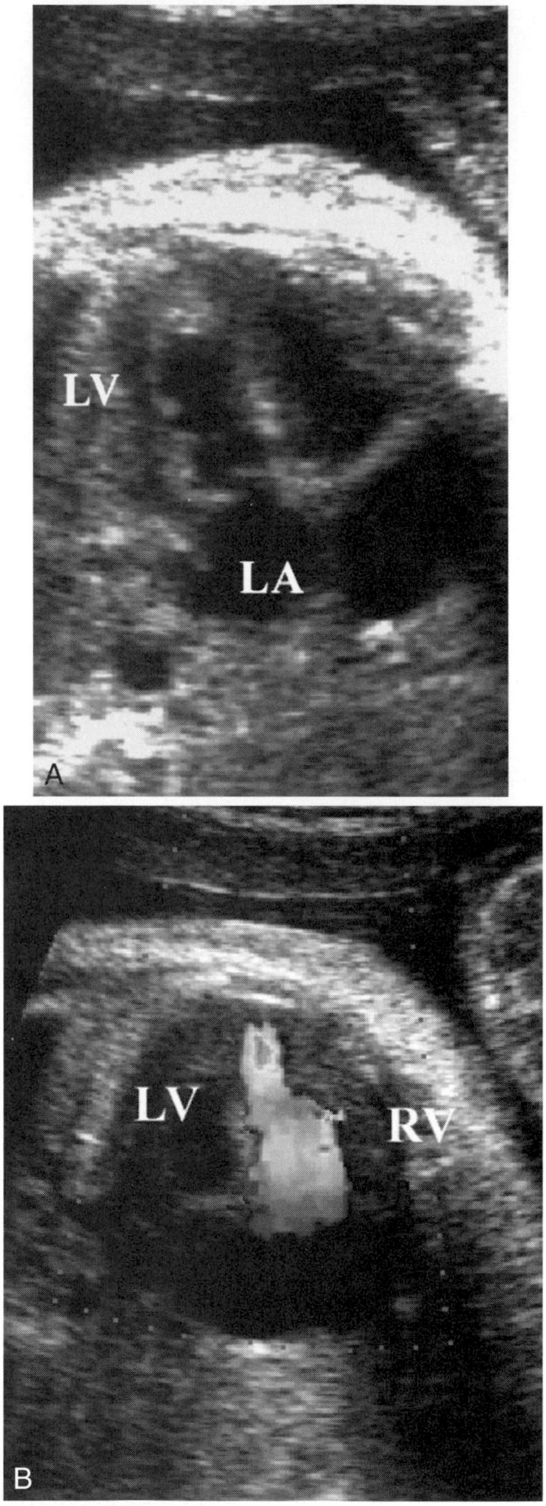

FIGURE 17–25
A, Apical four-chamber view of the fetal heart in a hypoplastic left ventricle. *B*, The color Doppler shows the normal filling of the right ventricle (*red*) and the absent filling of the left ventricle (mitral atresia) (see Color Plate 15). LV, left ventricle; RV, right ventricle.

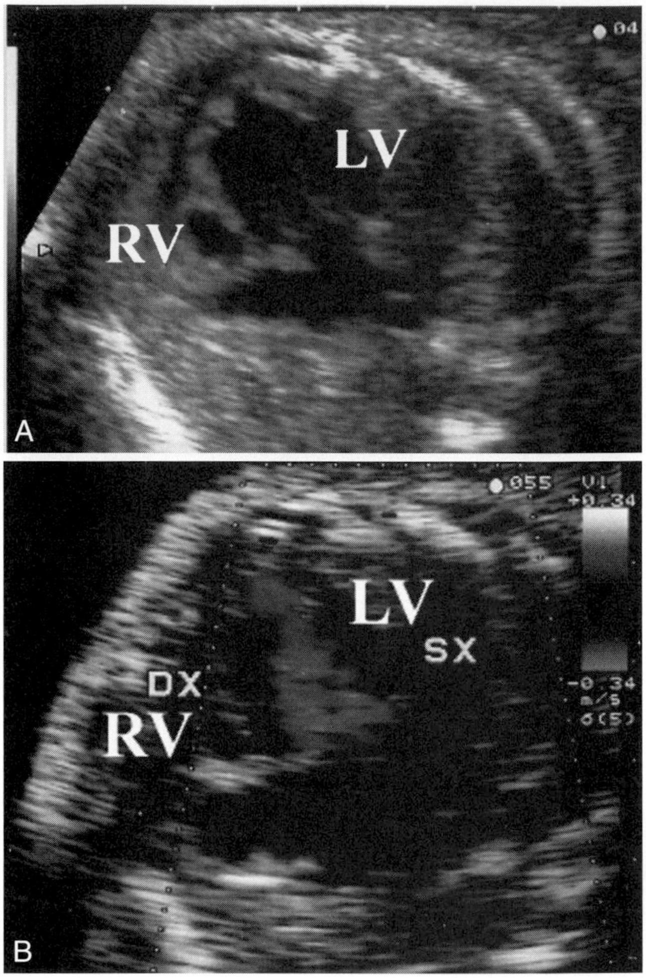

FIGURE 17–26
A, Four-chamber view of the fetal heart in the presence of a pulmonary atresia and intact septum. The right ventricular size is reduced, and the tricuspid valve is hyperechogenic. *B*, Color Doppler shows the absent filling of the right ventricle (tricuspid atresia) (see Color Plate 16). LV, left ventricle; RV, right ventricle.

Color and pulsed Doppler studies reveal retrograde flow in the pulmonary artery and either the absence (atresia) of or retrograde flow (insufficiency) across the tricuspid valve. Heart failure and hydrops often develop with tricuspid regurgitation. Anomalies of the coronary arteries are common and can complicate surgical correction. Extracardiac anomalies are unusual.

Factors that affect prognosis are strictly related to ventricular size and presence of coronary fistulas. If a postnatal two-ventricular repair can be achieved, the long-term outcome can be good. On the other hand, if the right ventricle is a severely hypoplastic right ventricle and addressed therapeutically with a Fontana procedure (placement of a circuit between the right atrium and the main pulmonary artery), the action is considered palliative, associated with several short- and long-term complications. Transplantation often becomes necessary during young adult life.[39,40]

Outflow Tract Obstructions

Aortic Stenosis and Coarctation of the Aortic Arch

Aortic stenosis is found in 0.04 per 1000 live births[2] and may be supravalvular, valvular, and subvalvular.[41] The

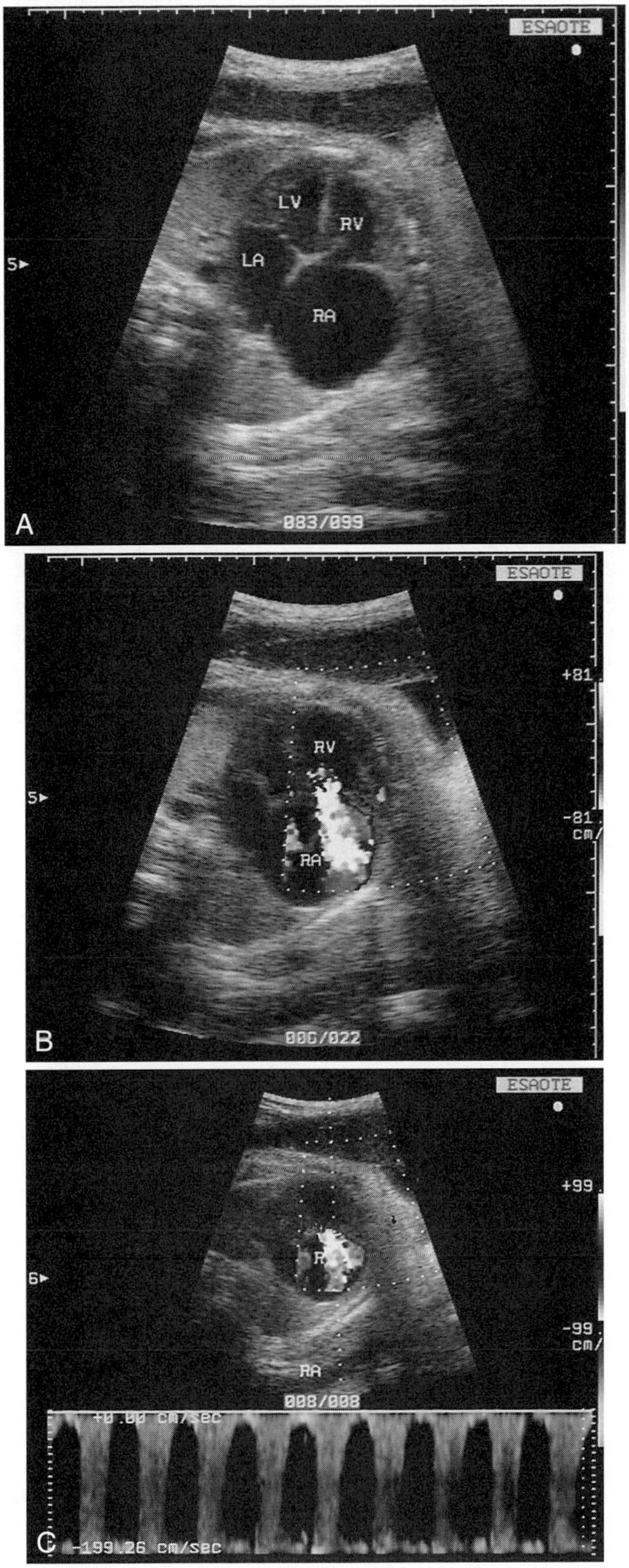

FIGURE 17–27
Apical four-chamber view in the presence of a pulmonary atresia and intact septum. The right ventricular size is normal and the right atrium is increased (*A*). When the color Doppler is superimposed a high-velocity retrograde jet is seen (*blue*) (*B*) and a holosystolic high velocity (>2 m/sec) tricuspid regurgitation is measured by pulsed Doppler (*C*) (see Color Plate 17). LA, left atrium; RA, right atrium; LV, left ventricle; RV, right ventricle.

pressure in the left ventricle is increased. In severe cases, the left ventricular pressure overload decreases coronary perfusion, leading to subendocardial ischemia, secondary endocardial fibroelastosis, and in utero congestive heart failure. The echocardiographic diagnosis requires demonstration of a small and abnormal aortic valve usually associated with an enlarged, poststenotic ascending aorta. Doppler examination will show increased flow velocities in the ascending aorta distal to the stenotic site (Fig. 17–28) and, in the severe cases, regurgitation across the mitral valve.

Several fetal medicine specialists have attempted in utero balloon dilation of the stenotic aortic valve by transthoracic puncture of the fetus. In several instances, the procedure was a technical success with a reduction in severity. Unfortunately, antenatal treatment has yet to produce a survivor past the neonatal period.[42,43]

Coarctation is a narrowing of a portion of aortic arch, usually between the left subclavian artery and the ductus arteriosus. In some cases, the narrowing encompasses the proximal aortic arch and is defined as a hypoplastic aortic arch or, if completely interrupted, an interrupted aortic arch. The incidence approximates 0.18 per 1000 live births and is frequently associated with other cardiac anomalies (up to 90%) including ventricular septal defect, aortic stenosis, and transposition of great arteries.[2,41] Extracardiac anomalies including diaphragmatic hernia, renal agenesis, esophageal atresia, Turner syndrome, and the chromosome 22q11 deletion syndrome are also frequent.

Coarctation has no significant impact on intrauterine hemodynamics because it is the right ventricle that mainly supplies the descending aorta via the ductus arteriosus. Symptoms develop in the neonatal period. The only in utero echocardiographic evidence of coarctation

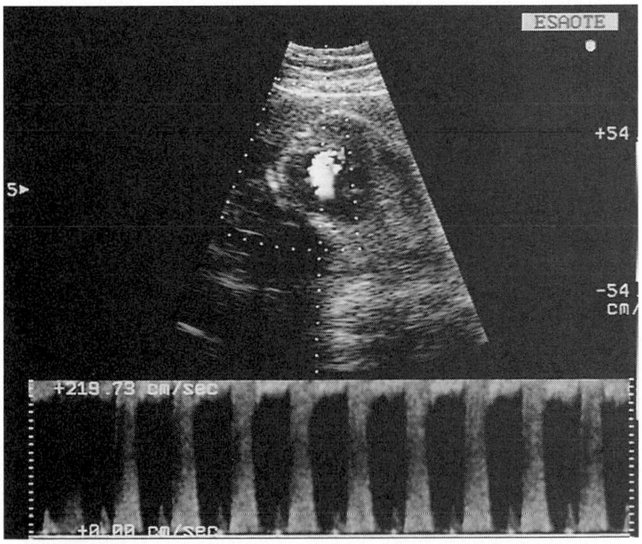

FIGURE 17–28
Color Doppler image with the pulsed Doppler sample placed on the aortic valve showing high velocities (PV > 220 cm/sec) suggestive of aortic stenosis (see Color Plate 18).

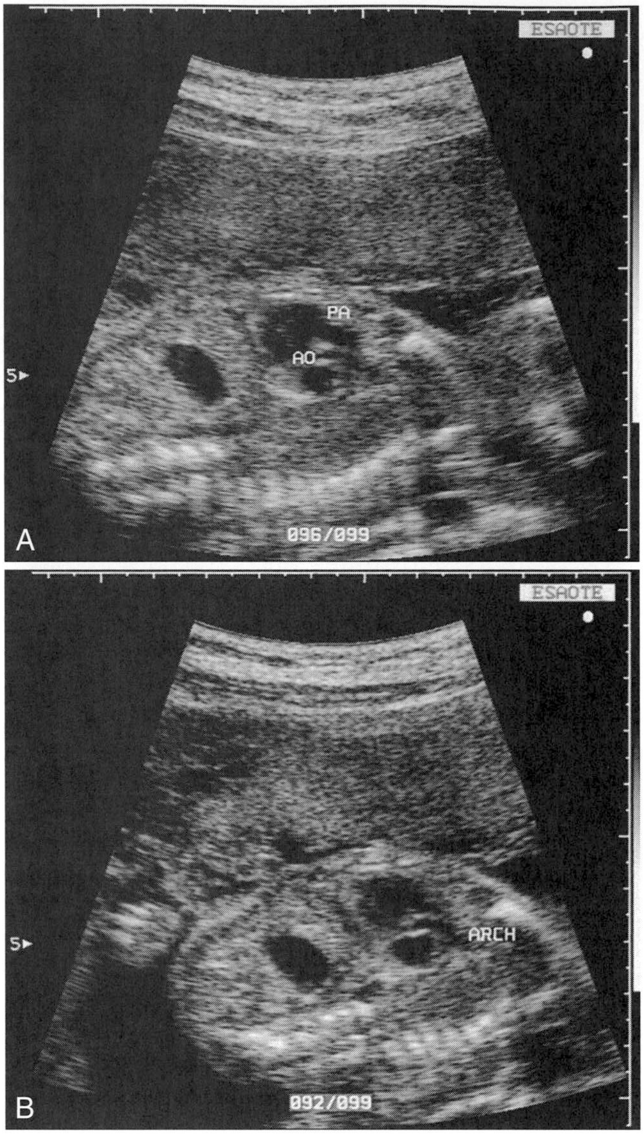

FIGURE 17–29
Short-axis view of the fetal heart showing the small size of the aorta (AO) with respect to pulmonary artery (PA) (*A*) and arch view showing severe hypoplasia of the aortic arch (*B*).

may be a relatively enlarged right ventricle compared to the left ventricle. Additional signs of coarctation include an echogenic shelf in the aortic lumen at the level of the isthmus, a relative decrease in the diameter of the aorta compared to the pulmonary artery (Fig. 17–29*A*), and a hypoplastic arch (Fig. 17–29*B*).[44] Hypoplasia of the left ventricle may develop in more severe cases (hypoplastic arch or interruption).[45] The surgical mortality rate reported for coarctation of the aorta is less than 10%. However, surgical mortality rate may be higher when there are additional lesions, particularly if there is a significant left-sided heart obstruction, and the surgical approach and thus morbidity overlaps with the correction of hypoplastic left heart syndrome.[46]

Pulmonary Stenosis

Pulmonary stenosis occurs in about 0.9 per 1000 live births and is generally thought to result from fusion of the pulmonary valve leaflets.[2] Associated cardiac and extracardiac anomalies are less common than they are with aortic stenosis but can include atrial septal defects and total anomalous pulmonary venous return. It is usually present in Noonan's syndrome.

The relevant hemodynamic concerns for pulmonary stenosis are the same as aortic stenosis. The right ventricular pressure is increased in proportion to the degree of stenosis. The resulting ventricular wall hypertrophy may cause tricuspid regurgitation. The echocardiographic diagnosis relies on identification of a small, sometimes thickened pulmonary valve with a characteristic abnormal movement (doming). A poststenotic enlargement of the pulmonary artery is common.[47] Doppler examination reveals increased velocities at the level of the pulmonary valve (Fig. 17–30) and tricuspid insufficiency. The progression from stenosis to atresia in utero is well documented.[48] The prognosis is usually good, and postnatal balloon valvuloplasty is usually the only treatment required.

Conotruncal Malformations

Conotruncal malformations are a heterogeneous group of defects affecting the connection between the ventricles and the great arteries. They constitute 20% to 30% of all cardiac anomalies.[2] Conotruncal malformations include the following four anomalies:

- Transposition of the great arteries
- Tetralogy of Fallot
- Double outlet right ventricle
- Truncus arteriosus

Unfortunately, they are commonly missed during the routine obstetric sonographic examination if limited to the four-chamber view, as the ventricles are usually similar in size. Undiagnosed conotruncal malformations can result in neonatal emergency with considerable morbidity and even death. However, the outcome is generally good if promptly recognized and early corrective surgery is undertaken.

Transposition of Great Arteries

The prevalence of transposition approximates 0.2 in 1000 live births.[2] The complete form, characterized by atrioventricular concordance and ventricular-arterial discordance is most common. The aorta arises from the right ventricle and the pulmonary artery from the left ventricle. Either a ventricular septal defect or pulmonary stenosis is present in about half, though complete transposition is only rarely associated with extracardiac anomalies or an abnormal karyotype. Echocardiographic diagnosis requires demonstration that the left ventricle in the long-axis view connects to a great vessel with a posterior course that bifurcates (pulmonary artery) (Fig. 17–31). In the short-axis view, the vessel originating from the right ventricle has an upward course and gives rise to the brachiocephalic vessels (Figs. 17–32 and 17–33).

The parallel circulatory model of the fetus permits normal development, and hemodynamic compromise is unusual. However, newborns may be cyanotic and deteriorate rapidly, depending on the size of the shunt at the level of the foramen ovale or across any associated ventricular septal defect. Identification of a small foramen ovale prenatally may be an indication for a balloon atrial septostomy (Rashkind procedure) immediately after birth. Cardiac surgery consists of switching the great arteries and is usually performed during the neonatal period. The survival rate ranges between 85% and 90%.[49]

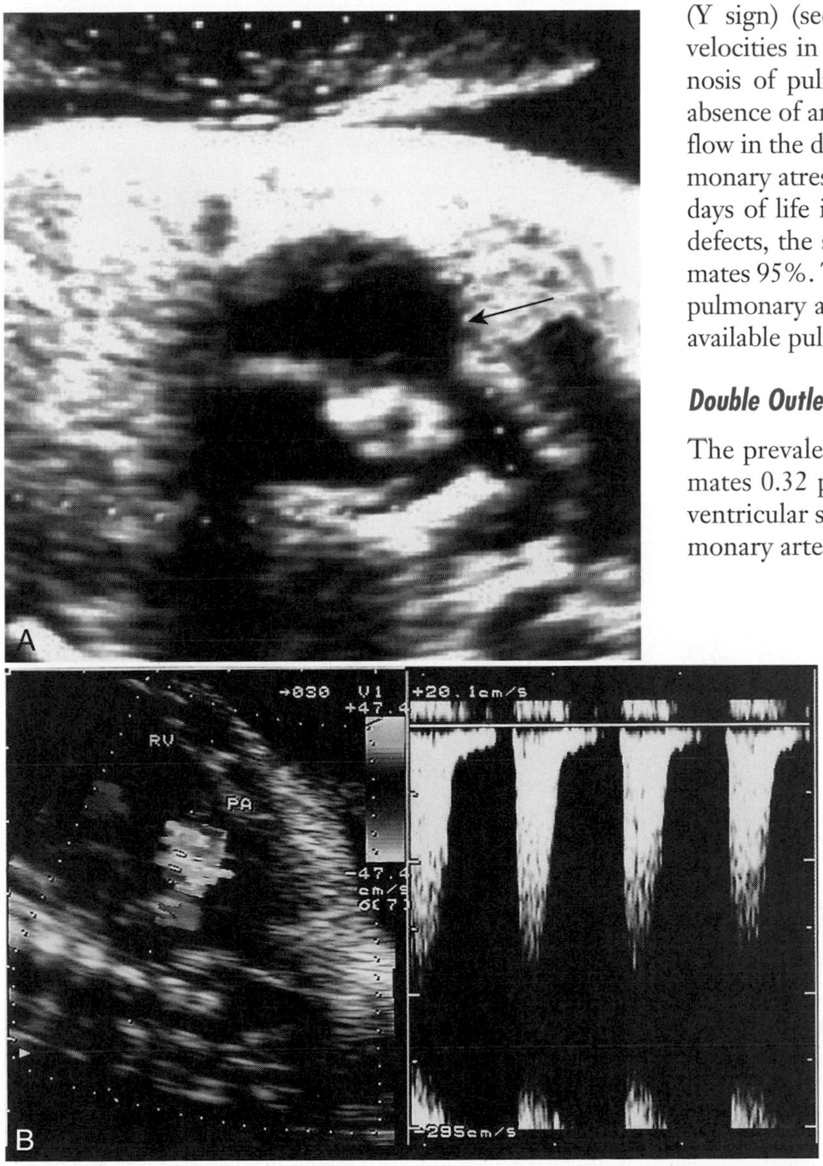

FIGURE 17–30
Short-axis view of the fetal heart in a fetus with pulmonary stenosis. *A*, Narrowing of the valve. *B*, Color Doppler superimposed showing high velocities in pulmonary artery (PA). Pulsed Doppler demonstrates high-velocity waveforms (180 cm/sec) consistent with pulmonary stenosis (see Color Plate 19).

Tetralogy of Fallot

Tetralogy of Fallot occurs in 0.4 in 1000 live births[2] and includes stenosis of the infundibulum of the pulmonary artery, a ventricular septal defect, an aortic valve overriding the interventricular septum, and hypertrophy of the right ventricle. The hypertrophy usually develops only after birth. In about 20%, the pulmonary valve is atretic, a condition usually described as pulmonary atresia with ventricular septal defect. Tetralogy of Fallot is associated with other cardiac defects such as an atrioventricular canal (4%) or pulmonary valve absence (1%). Extracardiac anomalies (particularly chromosomal) are frequent.

The echocardiographic diagnosis requires demonstration of an enlarged aortic root overriding the intraventricular septum (Fig. 17–34*A*),[50,51] an intraventricular septal defect (Fig. 17–35), and a small pulmonary valve. Color flow mapping will reveal systolic jets from both the right and left ventricles into the overriding aorta with a Y shape (Y sign) (see Fig. 17–34*B*). The presence of increased velocities in the pulmonary artery corroborates the diagnosis of pulmonary stenosis (see Fig. 17–35), while the absence of anterograde flow across the valve or retrograde flow in the ductus arteriosus supports the diagnosis of pulmonary atresia. Cardiac failure in utero or during the first days of life is uncommon. In the absence of extracardiac defects, the survival rate after corrective surgery approximates 95%. This percentage is lower when associated with pulmonary atresia.[50] In that instance, the diameter of any available pulmonary artery is crucial.

Double Outlet Right Ventricle

The prevalence of double outlet right ventricle approximates 0.32 per 1000 live births.[2] It is characterized by a ventricular septal defect associated with an aorta and pulmonary artery that arise from the right ventricle anterior

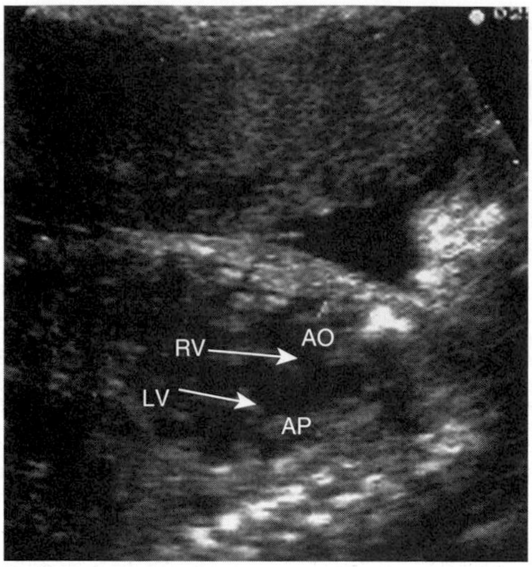

FIGURE 17–31
Example of correct transposition of great artery with intact septum. The heart is seen in long axis, and in contrast to normal, both great arteries are seen in this projection. They arise in parallel orientation with the aorta (AO) from the anterior right ventricle (RV) and the pulmonary artery (PA) from the posterior left ventricle (LV) (see Color Plate 20).

to the ventricular septum (Fig. 17–36). The position of the great arteries relative to each other may vary from normal to transposition. Associated anomalies include mitral valve atresia, atrioventricular canal, and pulmonary stenosis. Extracardiac and chromosomal anomalies are common. Distinguishing double outlet right ventricle from tetralogy of Fallot can be difficult when the relationship between the great arteries is normal and pulmonary artery stenosis is present.

The hemodynamic effects of this malformation are similar to tetralogy of Fallot. Cardiac decompensation is

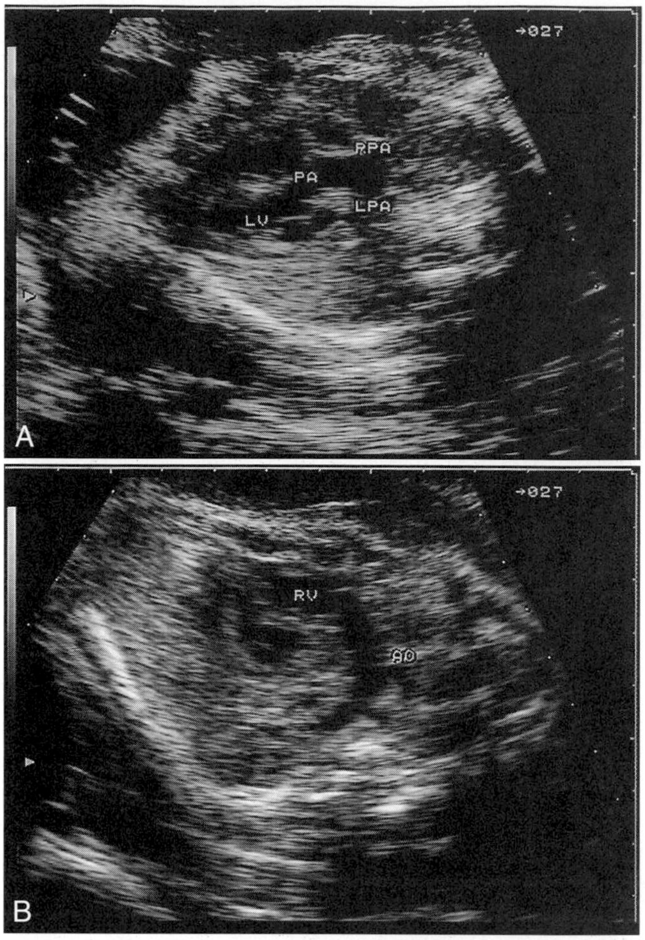

FIGURE 17–32
Example of correct transposition of great artery and intact septum. *A*, From the long-axis view the left ventricle (LV) is connected to the pulmonary artery (PA) that bifurcates into the right (RPA) and left (LPA) branches. *B*, The right ventricle (RV) is connected to the aorta (AO).

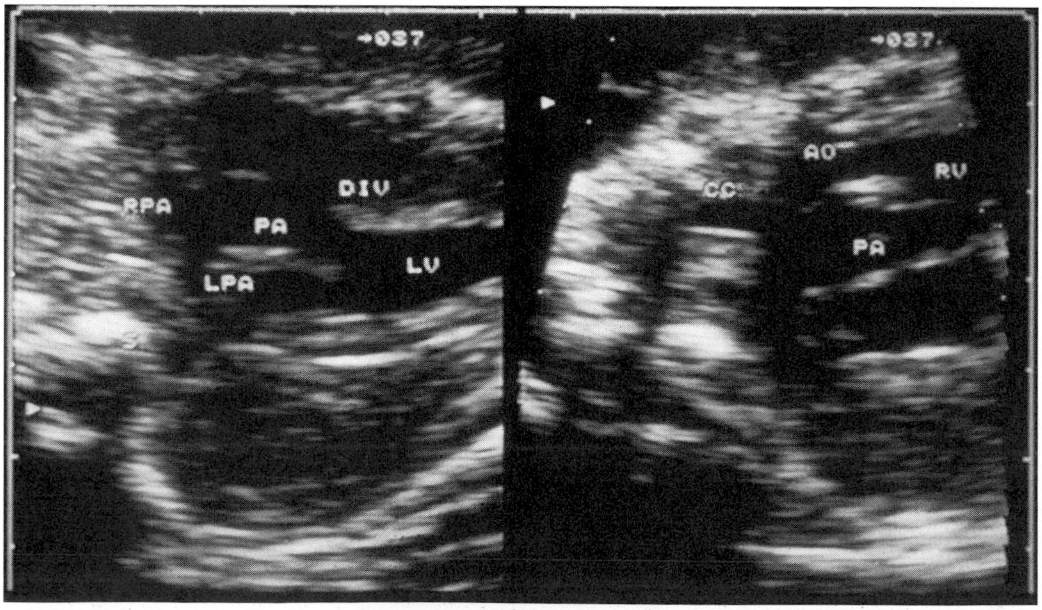

FIGURE 17–33
Example of correct transpotion of great artery associated with a ventricular septal defect (DV). From the long-axis view the left ventricle (LV) is connected to the pulmonary artery (PA), which bifurcates into the right (RPA) and left (LPA) branches (*left panel*). The right ventricle (RV) is connected to the aorta (AO) (*right panel*).

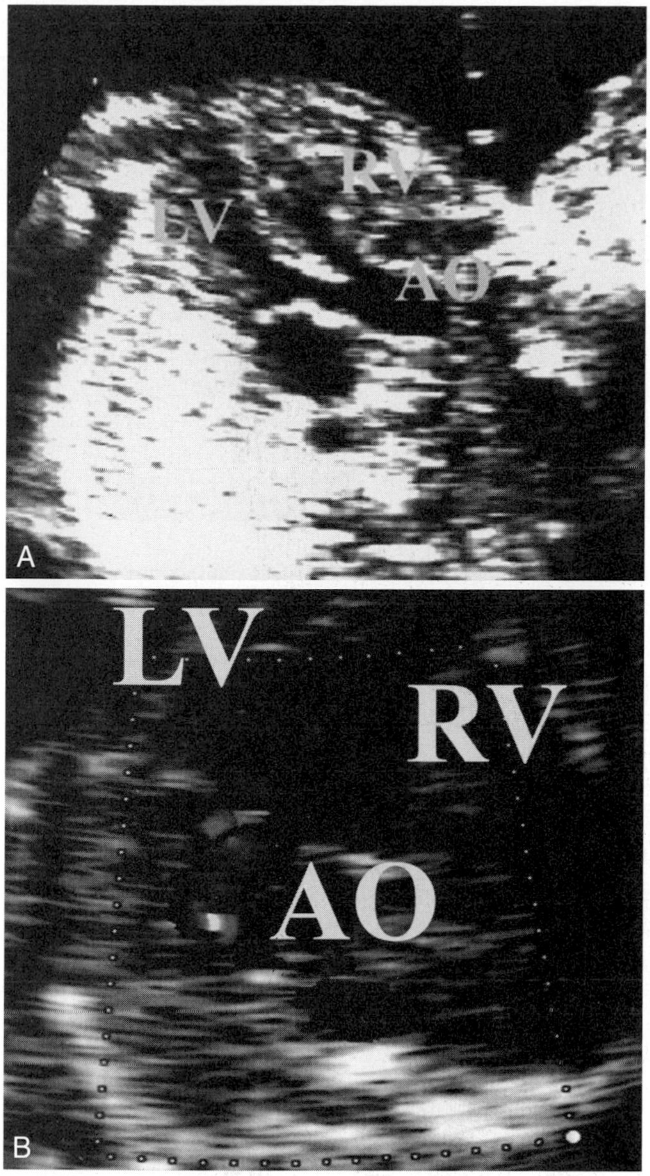

FIGURE 17–34
Long-axis view of the fetal heart in a fetus with tetralogy of Fallot. *A*, The aorta (AO) is overriding the left (LV) and right ventricles (RV) in real time. *B*, The color Doppler shows the perfusion during systole from the left (LV) and right (RV) ventricles into the overriding aorta (AO) (Y sign) (see Color Plate 21).

unusual in utero as well as in the early neonatal period. Long-term survival after corrective surgery is good (70%–80%) in the absence of associated anomalies.[52]

Truncus Arteriosus

Truncus arteriosus complicates approximately 0.01 of 1000 live births.[2] It is characterized by a single great artery, usually larger than the aorta, arising from both ventricles and overriding the ventricular septum. The truncus supplies the systemic, coronary, and pulmonary circulations. A ventricular septal defect may be present (type A) or absent (type B). Type A has four subclasses according to the origin of the pulmonary arteries.[31] Associated intracardiac anomalies are common and

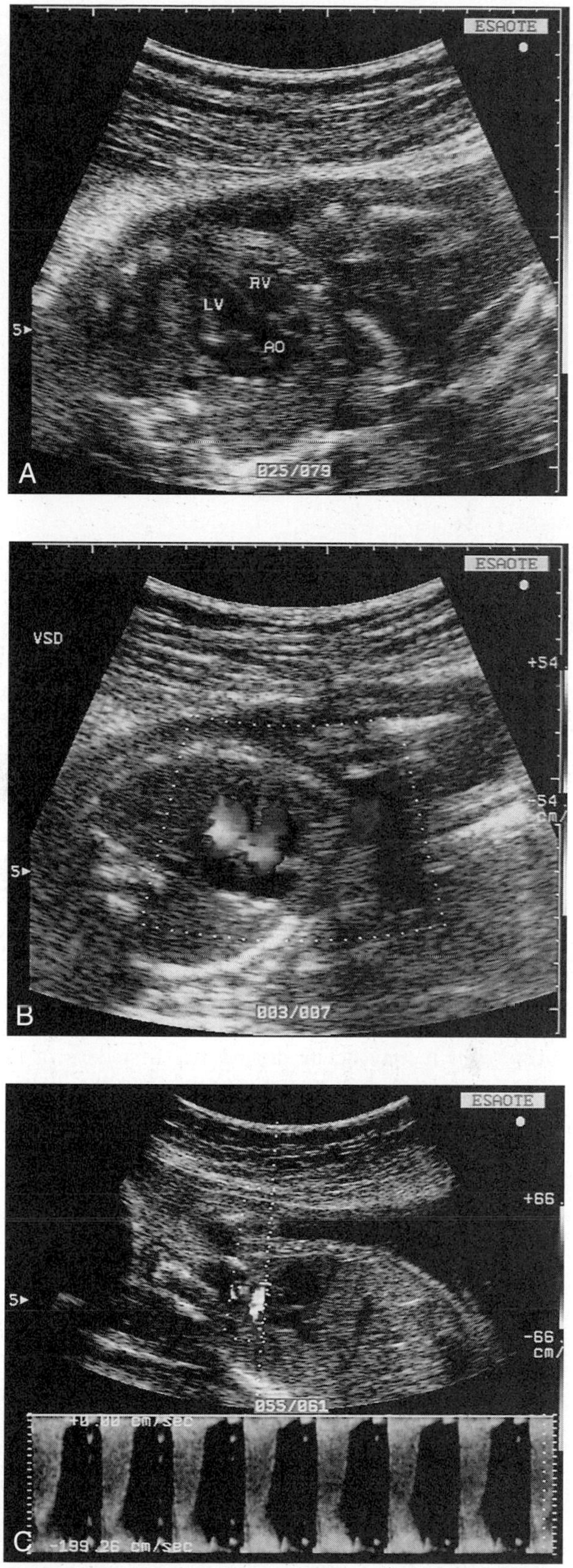

FIGURE 17–35
Tetralogy of Fallot. *A*, Presence of ventricular septal defect with the aorta (AO) overriding the right (RV) and left (LV) ventricles. Color Doppler demonstrates the presence of the ventricular septal defect (*B*) and pulsed Doppler placed at the level of pulmonary valve demonstrates the presence of high velocities (>2 m/sec) consistent with pulmonary stenosis (*C*) (see Color Plate 22).

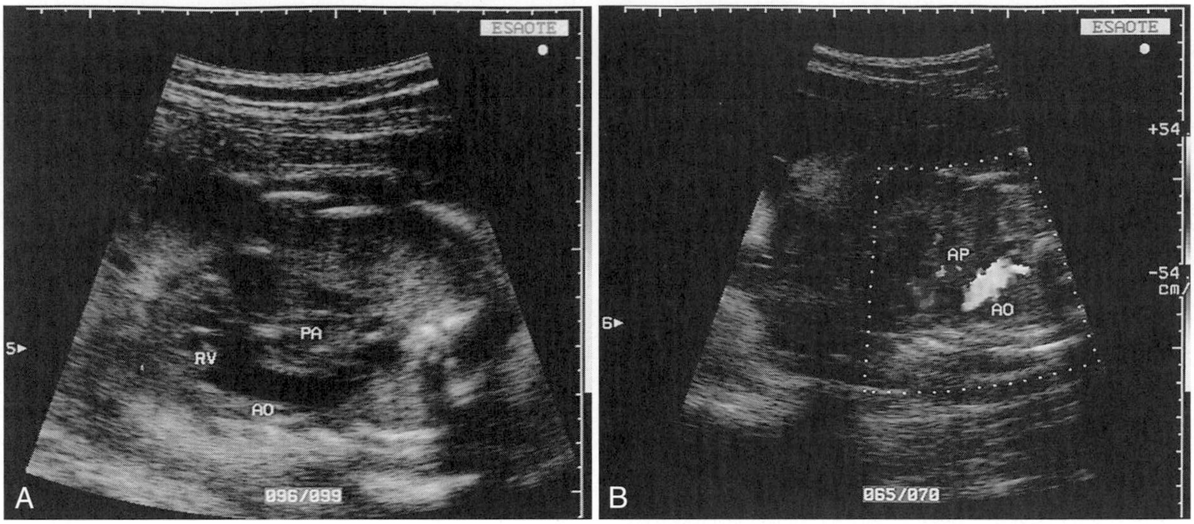

FIGURE 17–36
Double outlet right ventricle. Both great vessels originate from the right ventricle (RV). However, there is an associated transposition of the great vessels, and the aorta (AO) is posterior to pulmonary artery (PA) (*A*). Furthermore the PA is atretic and a retrograde flow (*blue*) is evident, suggesting that the pulmonary circulation depends on the aorta (*B*) (see Color Plate 23).

include mitral atresia and aortic arch hypoplasia and interruption (type A4). Extracardiac malformations are also common.

The echocardiographic diagnosis is based on the identification of a single great vessel overriding both ventricles whose dimensions are usually larger than the aorta (Fig. 17–37). The diagnosis requires that the pulmonary arteries originate from the truncus. Distinguishing truncus arteriosus from a tetralogy of Fallot with an atretic pulmonary valve may be difficult in utero.

As with other conotruncal malformations, truncus arteriosus is not associated with cardiac decompensation in utero, but it may occur during the first days of life. Surgical correction is often complex because the dysplastic truncal valve must be transformed into an aortic valve and a circuit created from the right ventricle to the pulmonary arteries. The reported survival rate at 10 years is less than 80%.[53]

Tumors of the Heart

Congenital tumors of the heart are extremely rare with an incidence estimated at 0.1 in 1000 live births. The most common is rhabdomyoma. They tend to be multiple and involve the septum. Cardiac tumors are usually isolated, but are present in 50% to 86% of fetuses with tuberous sclerosis. Frequently, they are the only detectable sign of tuberous sclerosis in utero.

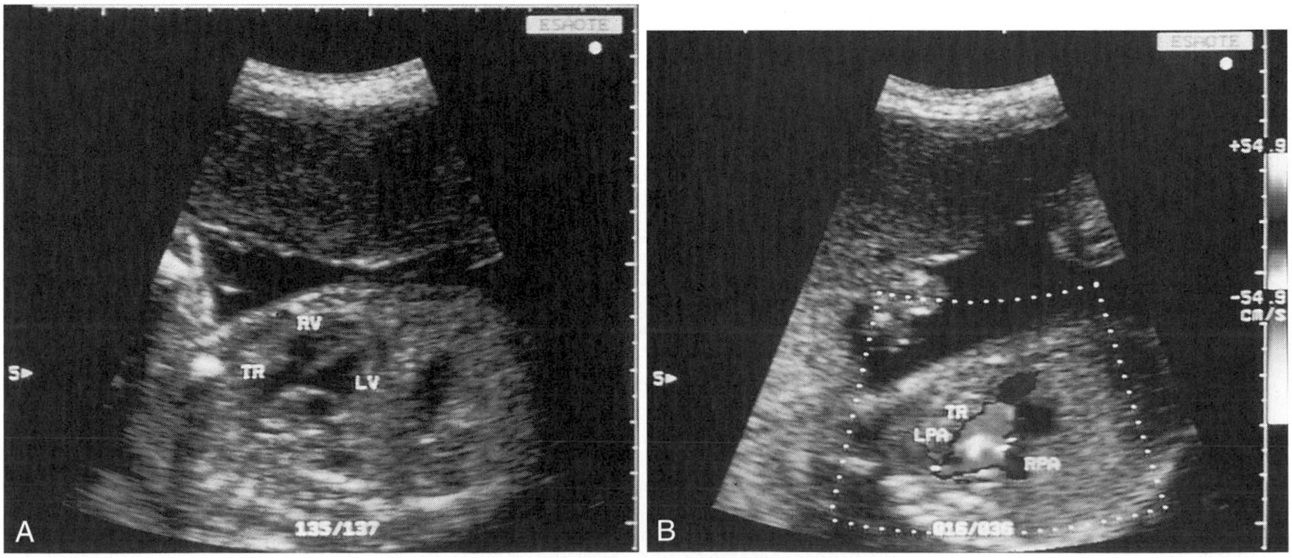

FIGURE 17–37
Truncus arteriosus. *A*, A single vessel (TR) overrides the two ventricles (RV, right ventricle; LV, left ventricle). *B*, Color Doppler allows the visualization of the origin of the right (RPA) and left (LPA) pulmonary arteries from the truncus (TR) (see Color Plate 24).

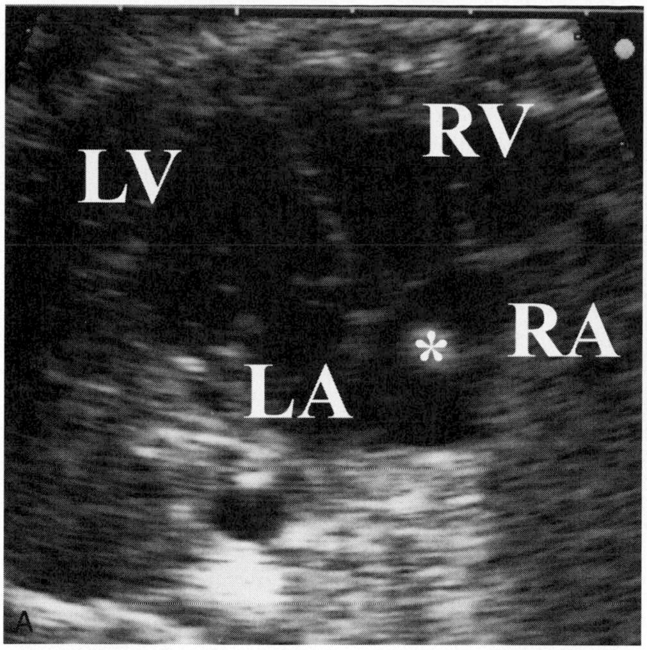

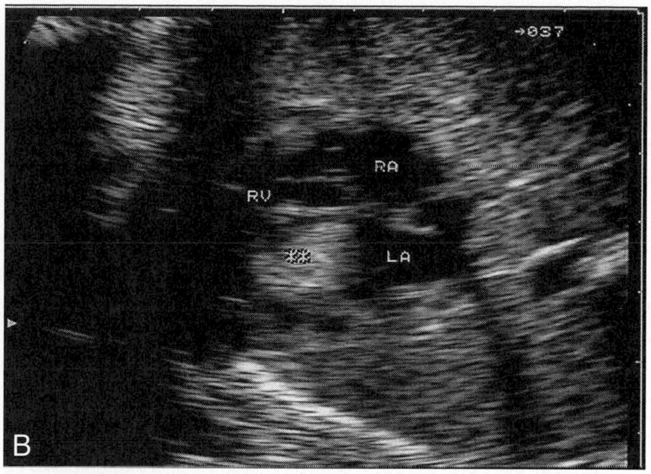

FIGURE 17–38
A, Apical four-chamber view showing a rhabdomyomas (*) in the right atrium (RA). *B*, Lateral four-chamber view of the fetal heart showing that the left ventricle is filled by rhabdomyomas (**). RV, right ventricle; RA, right atrium; LA, left atrium.

The echocardiographic diagnosis is based on finding one or more hyperechogenic masses within the heart (Fig. 17–38). They can create mechanical obstruction to ventricular inflow and outflow with the subsequent development of congestive heart failure. Cardiac dysrhythmias are also seen. The postnatal prognosis depends on the presence of tuberous sclerosis. Surgical excision is necessary in selected cases. Intracardiac tumors not associated with tuberous sclerosis may also shrink postnatally and remain asymptomatic.[54]

ABNORMAL DOPPLER EXAMINATION OF THE STRUCTURALLY NORMAL HEART

Real-time ultrasonography remains the primary tool for the examination of the fetal heart. However, color and pulsed Doppler flow studies are essential for a complete study. Demonstration of normal blood flow direction, a lack of turbulence, and normal velocity waveforms confirm "normal flow" in the cardiac structures and support the impression of an anatomically and functionally normal heart. On the other hand, Doppler studies may reveal abnormal flow patterns in a heart that on real-time ultrasonography appears to be structurally normal, indicating the need for additional study.

Valve Regurgitation

Valve regurgitation is characterized by bidirectional flow across the valve on Doppler interrogation. There is unidirectional flow from the atrium to the ventricle during diastole with regurgitant flow during systole. Regurgitation is uncommon across the fetal semilunar valves, but if it occurs, the regurgitation occurs during diastole.

Valve regurgitation may either be primary from valve dysplasia (e.g., tricuspid dysplasia)[52] or secondary due to increased ventricular pressure (e.g., pulmonary atresia or stenosis with intact septum) or papillary muscle dysfunction (cardiomyopathy).[56] The diagnosis of AV valve regurgitation requires demonstration of an abnormal color jet from the ventricle into the atrium during systole when imaged in the apical four-chamber view (see Fig. 17–27*B*). The amount of regurgitation is proportional to the peak velocity of the regurgitant jet. High velocities can cause frequency aliasing on pulsed Doppler. As a result, continuous wave Doppler is preferable when measuring the peak velocities. Although the amplitude of the jet is directly related to the pressure gradient across the valve by the Bernoulli equation ($P = 4V2$), it should not be used to quantify the severity of the disease because the pressure is influenced by both the severity of the obstruction and the ventricular contractility. A severe obstruction can be associated with a low amplitude jet if ventricular contractility is too impaired to generate an adequate pressure gradient. Analogously, a low-grade stenosis associated with a normally functioning ventricle can generate a high-velocity jet in the absence of hypertension.

The duration of the regurgitant jet is of particular clinical importance.[56] Regurgitation limited to early systole is usually benign, whereas a jet that is holosystolic suggests severe hemodynamic compromise (see Fig. 17–27*C*). Here, venous return is impaired and venous hypertension develops. Heart failure and hydrops may result.

Normal flow direction with high velocities

This pattern of flow may result from hemodynamic adaptation to a hypoplastic or atretic structure in the contralateral side. For example, the flow across the tricuspid and pulmonary valves is increased in the presence of a hypoplastic left ventricle. Likewise, the flow across the mitral and aortic valves is increased in the presence of pulmonary atresia. The diagnosis is made when pulsed Doppler interrogation reveals a normal velocity waveform associated with increased PV and TVI.

Increased velocities may also occur with stenotic lesions such as pulmonary or aortic stenosis. In this setting, the flow is turbulent and the velocities high. Color Doppler allows for the identification of turbulent flow, and the velocity waveforms obtained with pulsed or continuous wave Doppler reveal an irregular profile and a high PV. Again, the value of the PV is not used clinically to define the severity of the stenosis because it also reflects ventricular contractility.

Absent Filling

No flow in a cardiac chamber suggests atresia of either the mitral (left ventricle) (see Fig. 17–25*B*) or tricuspid (right ventricle) valves (see Fig. 17–26*B*). For accuracy, the equipment must have the correct settings and the angle of insonation must parallel the expected direction of flow (apical four-chamber view). Further, the gain, pulse repetition frequency, and filter must be set correctly to avoid artifact. Flow in the contralateral ventricle (apical four-chamber view) is proof of proper technique.

Abnormal Flow Direction

Because of the parallel nature of the fetal circulation, arterial blood can flow in a reverse direction if the flow from one ventricle is either absent or severely reduced. Examples include hypoplastic left heart syndrome or a severe aortic stenosis in which the aortic arch is perfused in a retrograde manner from the ductus arteriosus (Fig. 17–39). In this way, the right ventricle can supply the cerebral and coronary circulations. On the other hand, both pulmonary atresia and severe ductal stenosis are associated with reversed aortic arch flow as the pulmonary circulation depends on the left ventricle. Such abnormal hemodynamics are particularly important after birth.

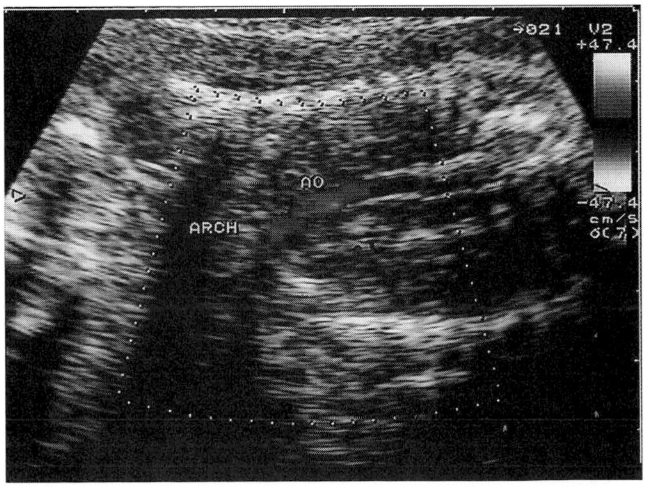

FIGURE 17–39
Arch view in presence of a hypoplastic left ventricle. The arch is perfused in the reverse direction (blue color is seen instead of red) suggesting that the brain and coronary circulation depend on the right ventricle. AO, aorta (see Color Plate 25).

Abnormal flow direction may be detected at the level of the foramen ovale or at the level of a ventricular septal defect. Visualization of these abnormal flow patterns suggests the presence of a malformation that alters the pressure equilibrium between the right and left heart chambers. Examples include reverse direction flow (left to right) through the foramen ovale with a hypoplastic left ventricle, or a unidirectional jet across an interventricular septal defect when there is an outflow tract lesion (see Fig. 17–21).

ADVANTAGES OF DOPPLER EXAMINATION FOR THE EVALUATION OF FETAL HEART DISEASES

An investigation of the cardiac flows helps the assessment of cardiac disease in several ways:

- *Define the nature of the cardiac malformation.* Copel and associates[57] observed retrospectively that color Doppler was essential for establishing the correct diagnosis in 29%, helpful in 47%, and neither helpful nor misleading in the remaining fetuses. We analyzed prospectively 145 fetuses with congenital heart disease, and found that the combination of color and spectral Doppler was essential for the diagnosis in 34 fetuses (23%, mainly outflow tract stenosis or complex heart diseases such as isomerism and double outlet right ventricle with atresia of one semilunar valve), useful in 62 fetuses (42%, mainly congenital heart disease complicated by valve atresia or outflow tract obstruction causing abnormal flow direction), and not helpful in the remaining 49 fetuses (34%, mainly complete atrioventricular canal and ventricular septal defects).
- *Evaluate the hemodynamic consequence of congenital heart disease.* The consequences of the sonographically same congenital heart disease may range in utero from no effect to cardiac failure and hydrops. This wide range of hemodynamic effects reflects the severity of the primary lesion, the presence of associated anomalies, the cardiac rhythm, and any impairment of ventricular function. The detection of regurgitation at the level of atrioventricular valve by Doppler is a particularly useful predictor of hydrops. The presence of holosystolic, tricuspid regurgitation either isolated or associated with mitral regurgitation predicts the development of hydrops fetalis with subsequent poor prognosis. Study of the systemic venous circulation also provides a valuable index of the overall cardiac performance. Although there is no general agreement on the significance of the venous indices and on the vessel of choice, it is our experience that the velocity waveforms from IVC show a higher correlation with cardiac function than either the DV or umbilical vein.[22] This information is helpful as the health care team formulates a plan, predicts prognosis, and counsels the parents (also see Chapters 11 and 12).

- *Monitor the evolution of congenital heart diseases.* Doppler echocardiography is not only helpful in establishing the correct diagnosis, but is also valuable longitudinally to follow the natural history and progression of a malformation. One example is the evolution of pulmonary stenosis or atresia in fetuses with primary tricuspid valve regurgitation, which is presumably due to the lack of forward flow in the pulmonary artery. This has been described in both fetuses with tricuspid regurgitation due to a dysplastic tricuspid valve and fetuses with presumed cardiac overload secondary to presumed twin-to-twin transfusion syndrome.[58] Similarly, a progressive increase in the severity of pulmonary stenosis of tetralogy of Fallot up to atresia is documented.[59,60] Knowledge of the pathologic evolution can be useful for timing delivery and for developing prenatal treatments such as balloon valvuloplasty in fetuses with deteriorating function.
- *Plan neonatal management.* The hemodynamic information gained from antenatal Doppler studies helps predict problems after birth. For example, the neonate with a critical stenosis or atresia at the level of the outflow tract (e.g., hypoplastic left ventricle, pulmonary atresia with intact septum) is ductal dependent after birth and will require continuous intravenous prostaglandin E_1. Closure of the ductus would have disastrous consequences because either systemic (left obstruction) or pulmonary (right obstruction) blood flow depends on ductal patency. Another example is the detection of a small (restrictive) foramen ovale in a fetus with complete transposition of the great arteries and an intact septum. Here, it can be anticipated that the shunt between the two circulations after birth will be insufficient, and cyanosis with rapid deterioration expected. A pediatric cardiologist should be present at delivery to promptly perform a balloon septostomy (Rashkind procedure) if needed. Advanced knowledge of these issues permits a planned delivery at a tertiary center where the facilities exist to optimize outcome.[61]

MANAGEMENT OPTIONS FOR THE FETUS WITH CONGENITAL HEART DISEASE

Cardiac malformations are the most common birth defects. Experienced fetal diagnosis units can detect a high percentage of major malformations (type 1 lesions, though typically requiring a surgical treatment). Once the diagnosis of a cardiac malformation is made, the following steps are recommended.

General

A plan of management should be formulated in concert with a multidisciplinary team that includes a perinatal obstetrician, a pediatric cardiologist, and where appropriate, a cardiac surgeon.

Define the Malformation and Search for Associated Anomalies

Extracardiac anomalies and a normal karyotype are common in fetuses with congenital heart defects (10% in our series). Consequently, a detailed ultrasonographic evaluation in an experienced fetal medicine center is mandatory. The presence of an associated anomaly may well influence the prognosis and postnatal management.

Search for Chromosomal Abnormalities

A karyotype is mandatory, as the result may alter management. The choice of the technique is based on the gestational age of the fetus and experience of the center (see Chapter 10). Chromosomal abnormalities are present in 10% to 40%.[5] In our prospective series of 489 fetuses with congenital heart diseases, autosomal trisomy (trisomy 18, 13, and 21) and Turner's syndrome (45XO) was the most common abnormality and accounted for 19.4% (Table 17–3). The incidence of aneuploidy varies with the type of malformation, being extremely high with some (e.g., atrioventricular canal) or unusual with others (e.g., transposition of a great artery). This information should be part of the patient counseling.

A detailed study of chromosome 22 is indicated in fetuses with a conotruncal malformation because a microdeletion at the critical region 22q11,2 occurs in high frequency of fetuses patients with this anomaly. The 22q11,2 syndrome (in the past also called CATCH 22)[63] consists of several genetic syndromes including velocardiofacial syndrome, DiGeorge syndrome, Opitz G/BBB syndrome, and conotruncal anomaly face syndrome. Patients with these syndromes have some or all of the following features:

- Mental retardation, learning disabilities, and psychiatric illness
- Congenital heart diseases, mainly conotruncal defects
- Palatal anomalies: overt and submucous cleft palate, velopharyngeal insufficiency
- Facial anomalies: long face with prominent nose, malar hypoplasia, retrognathia, and minor ear anomalies
- Thymus aplasia or hypoplasia associated with hypocalcemia and immunologic deficiency

The estimated prevalence of this deletion in the general population is 1 in 4500,[64] which makes the 22q11.2 deletion syndrome the second most common genetic condition after Down syndrome. The prevalence of this syndrome in fetuses with conotruncal anomaly approximates 20%,[18] and the syndrome cannot be detected by routine karyotypic analysis. It is necessary to use either quantitative hybridization or fluorescence in situ hybridization (FISH) techniques that are now standards in most genetic laboratories. It is also important to extend the genetic diagnosis of affected fetuses to the parents, because inherited microdeletions occur in 30%

TABLE 17-3

Incidence of Chromosomal Abnormalities in 167 Fetuses with Congenital Heart Disease Diagnosed at Fetal Medicine Center of Università of Roma "Tor Vergata" between 1992 and 1996

ANOMALY	NO.	NO. OF CHROMOSOMAL DEFECTS	PERCENT
Atrial septal defect	3	2	66.67
Ventricular septal defect	46	12	26.09
Atrioventricular canal	20	8	40.00
Hypoplastic left heart	14	0	0
Pulmonary atresia intact septum	4	0	0
Pulmonary stenosis	11	0	0
Aortic stenosis, coarctation, hypoplastic arch	16	1	6.25
Transposition of great artery	6	0	0
Tetralogy of Fallot	14	5	35.71
Double outlet right ventricle	8	3	37.50
Truncus arteriosus	2	0	0
Cardiac tumor	10	0	0
Others	16	1	6.25
Total	167	32	19.16

with the remainder being de novo. The transmission is autosomal dominant; thus, a parent with the syndrome has a 50% risk of transmitting the deletion to the offspring.[63,64]

Counseling the Parents

The parents are formally counseled by the care team after all useful information is acquired (correct and complete diagnosis of the malformation, presence or absence of associated structural and chromosomal abnormalities). It is essential the care team include, when possible, the perinatal obstetrician, the pediatric cardiologist, and the cardiac surgeon. They should describe the malformation, the possibility of surgical correction, the chance of short- and long-term survival, and the quality of life expected after the correction. Further, the parents should be provided information on the possible neurologic complications of the surgical procedures. Indeed, the correction of malformations requiring deep hypothermic cardiopulmonary bypass is associated with neurologic impairment in up to 10% of survivors.[65] After complete information is provided and all questions asked by the parents answered, the parents should be allowed freedom of choice to continue or end the pregnancy. It is particularly helpful to make an appointment a few days later to discuss their thought processes and decision and, when available, to offer psychological support.

Prenatal Monitoring

The development of the malformation should be followed serially, particularly by using Doppler ultrasonography every 2 to 4 weeks. The interval is based on the likelihood of an in utero complication developing (e.g., 4 weeks for a transposition of great artery, 2 weeks for tetralogy of Fallot). Furthermore, it is important in the third trimester to monitor fetal growth, amniotic fluid volume, Doppler velocity waveforms from peripheral fetal vessels, and fetal heart rate patterns, because the prevalences of suboptimal growth and acute fetal distress are increased.

Place, Timing, and Method of Delivery

The need to deliver in a tertiary referral center will vary with the diagnosis and upon the local resources and geographic constraints. It is important to anticipate before birth the type of assistance that may be needed. This may range from simple observation in the nursery (e.g., small ventricular septal defect), to assistance in neonatal intensive care unit or pediatric cardiology unit (e.g., ductal-dependent congenital heart disease, hydrops, immaturity), to immediate postnatal treatment (e.g., balloon septostomy in transposition of great artery with small foramen ovale).

Most fetuses with congenital heart disease tolerate labor well in the absence of uteroplacental dysfunction. There is no a priori indication for cesarean delivery. Further, it is rarely necessary for a cardiac reason to induce labor early, though it may facilitate postnatal management if the delivery is planned between 38 and 40 weeks.

Postnatal and Neonatal Management

Postnatal management includes further cardiac evaluation by the pediatric cardiologist to confirm the diagnosis and to assess the hemodynamic environment. The neonate is stabilized and the necessary treatments (interventional catheterization or surgery) are planned. Continued communication with the parents during the additional diagnostic steps and on the therapeutic strategies is extremely important.

CONCLUSIONS

- Although the prenatal identification of congenital heart disease is difficult, most cardiac anomalies can be identified by echocardiography.
- Prenatal recognition offers the chance to identify associated structural and chromosomal anomalies and to make prognostic statements about the evolution and treatability of these diseases.
- The use of appropriate antenatal and postnatal management protocols may positively impact on the care and outcome of fetuses with cardiac malformations.

SUMMARY OF MANAGEMENT OPTIONS
Fetal Cardiac Abnormalities

Management Options	Quality of Evidence	Strength of Recommendation	References
Prepregnancy			
All Women:	Ib	A	66
~1% risk of congenital heart defects (CHD) in pregnancy.	IIa	B	67
Most babies with CHD are born to mothers perceived to be low risk.			
Multifetal pregnancies are at increased risk of CHD (3%).			
Periconceptual folic acid and multivitamin preparations reduce risks of CHD as well as neural tube defects.			
High risk groups (see Table 17–1):	III	B	68, 69
Maternal/paternal CHD; sibling or relatives with CHD			
Maternal insulin-dependent diabetes mellitus			
Maternal illness (phenylketonuria, epilepsy, autoimmune antibodies [e.g., SLE], drugs [e.g., lithium])			
Possibility of multifetal pregnancy (assisted conception)			
Genetic study chromosome 22 in parents if previous child with conotruncal heart malformations			
Prenatal—Screening and Diagnosis			
Increased nuchal translucency with normal karyotype indicates higher risk of cardiac anomaly and need of careful cardiac scan in second trimester.	III	B	6,7
Routine level 2 anomaly scanning at 20 weeks should include situs and orientation, apical four-chamber view, lateral four-chamber view, left outflow tract, right outflow tract, three-vessel view, and venous return.	III	B	14, 15, 16
Refer all high risk groups for level 3 (tertiary) fetal echocardiography (see Tables 17–1 and 17–2).	–	GPP	–
Prenatal—Management			
Multidisciplinary team includes specialist obstetrician, pediatric cardiologist, and where appropriate, cardiac surgeon.	–	GPP	–
Establish clear plan of management.	–	GPP	–
Establish morphologic diagnosis and severity of circulatory compromise.	–	GPP	–
Search for other cardiac and extracardiac anomalies.	IV	C	4
	III	B	5
Offer fetal karyotyping including 22q deletion.	IV	C	4
	III	B	5
	III	B	70

Continued

SUMMARY OF MANAGEMENT OPTIONS
Fetal Cardiac Abnormalities *(Continued)*

Management Options	Quality of Evidence	Strength of Recommendation	References
Prenatal Management—*Continued*			
Multidisciplinary counseling and psychological support for parents:	–	GPP	–
Give full explanation of all findings.			
Discuss possible treatments (medical and surgical) and their implications and complications, prognosis (short- and long-term), and impact on neurodevelopment.			
Offer further meeting/discussions.			
In most cases the only options are to continue with pregnancy or termination.			
Continue monitoring defect (structural and functional) to document progression of disease.	–	GPP	–
Monitor fetal health generally in chromosomally normal fetuses (growth, amniotic fluid volume, behavior, Doppler of peripheral vessels).	–	GPP	–
Labor and Delivery			
Plan delivery in center with appropriate obstetric, pediatric, and cardiologic facilities (varies with abnormality and anticipated neonatal compromise).	III	B	71
Vaginal delivery is usually appropriate for isolated cardiac defects.	–	GPP	–
Fetal monitoring is advised in labor but may not be useful (e.g., in fetal complete heart block).	–	GPP	–
Elective delivery at 38–39 weeks may be appropriate for fetuses with complex defects such as hypoplastic left heart syndrome and for optimizing pediatric facilities.	III	B	72, 73
Postnatal and Neonatal			
Stabilize the neonate, confirm the diagnosis by detailed echocardiography, and manage accordingly.	–	GPP	–
After termination of pregnancy or perinatal death, obtain postmortem examination whenever possible and arrange for bereavement counseling and discussion of the full diagnosis and implications for future pregnancies.	–	GPP	–

REFERENCES

1. Arduini D, Rizzo G, Romanini C: Fetal Cardiac Function. Casterton Hall, UK, Parthenon Publishing, 1995.
2. Hoffman JIE: Congenital heart disease: Incidence and inheritance. Pediatr Clin North Am 1990;37:25–43.
3. Buskens E, Grobbee DE, Wladimiroff JW, Hess J: Routine screening for congenital heart disease: A prospective study in the Netherlands. In Wladimiroff JW, Pilu G (eds): Ultrasound and the Fetal Heart. Casterton Hall, UK, Parthenon Publishing, 1996, pp 71–80.
4. Copel JA, Pilu G, Kleiman GS: Congenital heart disease and extra-cardiac malformations: Associations and indications for fetal echocardiography. Am J Obstet Gynecol 1987;154: 1121–1130.
5. Allan LD, Sharland GK, Chita SK, et al: Chromosomal anomalies in fetal congenital heart disease. Ultrasound Obstet Gynecol 1991;1:8–11.
6. Hyett J, Perdu M, Sharland G, et al: Using fetala nuchal translucency to screen for major congenital cardiac defects at 10–14 weeks of gestation: Population based cohort study. Br Med J 1999;318:81–85.
7. Rizzo G, Muscatello A, Angelini E, Capponi A: Abnormal cardiac function in fetuses with increased nuchal translucency. Ultrasound Obstet Gynecol 2003;21;539–542.
8. Tegnander E, Eik Nes SH, Linker DT: Prenatal detection of heart defects at the routine fetal examination at 18 weeks in a nonselected population. Ultrasound Obstet Gynecol 1995;5:372–380.
9. Achiron R, Glaser J, Gelerenter I, et al: Extended fetal echocardiography examination for detecting cardiac malformations in low risk population. Br Med J 1992;404:671–674.
10. Bronshtein M, Siegler E, Esheoli Z, Zimmer EZ: Fetal cardiac abnormalities detected by transvaginal sonography at 12–16 weeks' gestation. Obstet Gynecol 1991;82:225–229.
11. Gembruch U, Knopfle G, Bald R, Hansmann M: Early diagnosis of fetal congenital heart disease by transvaginal echocardiography. Ultrasound Obstet Gynecol 1993;3:310–317.

12. Rizzo G, Capponi A, Scatigna L, et al: Is early second trimester transvaginal echocardiography useful in diagnosing congenital heart disease in fetuses of insulin dependent diabetic mothers? Ultrasound Obstet Gynecol 1995;4:205.
13. Yagel S, Weissman A, Rostein Z: Congenital heart defect: Natural course and in utero development. Circulation 1997;42: 641–647.
14. Shinebourne EA, Macartney FJ, Anderson RH: Sequential chamber localization: Logical approach to diagnosis in congenital heart disease. Br Heart J 1976;38:327–344.
15. Paladini D, Chita SK, Allan LD: Prenatal measurement of the cardiothoracic ratio in the evaluation of heart disease. Arch Dis Childhood 1990;65:20–23.
16. Yoo SL, Heling KS, Kim ES: Abnormal three vessel view on sonography: A clue to the diagnosis of congenital heart disease. Ultrasound Obstet Gynecol 1997;9:173–182.
17. Achiron R, Rostein Z, Heggesh J, et al: Anomalies of the fetal aortic arch: A novel sonographic approach to in-utero diagnosis. Ultrasound Obstet Gynecol 2002;20:553–557.
18. Chaoui R, Kalache KD, Heling KS, et al: Absent or hypoplastic thymus on ultrasound: A marker for deletion 22q11.2 in fetal cardiac defects. Ultrasound Obstet Gynecol 2002;20:546–557.
19. Burns PN: Doppler flow estimations in the fetal and maternal circulations: Principles, techniques and some limitations. In Maulik D, McNellis D (eds): Doppler Ultrasound Measurement of Maternal-Fetal Hemodynamics. Ithaca, NY, Perinatology Press, 1987, pp 43–78.
20. Reed KL, Appleton CP, Anderson CF, et al: Doppler studies of vena cava flows in human fetuses—Insights into normal and abnormal cardiac physiology. Circulation 1990;81:498–505.
21. Rizzo G, Arduini D, Romanini C: Inferior vena cava flow velocity waveforms in appropriate and small for gestational age fetuses. Am J Obstet Gynecol 1992;166:1271–1280.
22. Rizzo G, Capponi A, Talone PE, et al: Doppler indices from inferior vena cava and ductus venosus in predicting pH and oxygen tension in umbilical blood at cordocentesis in growth retarded fetuses. Ultrasound Obstet Gynecol 1996;7:401–410.
23. Rizzo G, Capponi A, Pasquini L, et al: Abnormal fetal pulmonary venous blood flow velocity waveforms in the presence of complete transposition of the great arteries. Ultrasound Obstet Gynecol 1996;7:299–300.
24. Reed KL, Sahn DJ, Scagnelli S, et al: Doppler echocardiographic studies of diastolic function in the human fetal heart: Changes during gestation. J Am Coll Cardiol 1986;8: 391–395.
25. Rizzo G, Arduini D, Romanini C, Mancuso S: Doppler echocardiographic assessment of atrioventricular velocity waveforms in normal and small for gestational age fetuses. BJOG 1988;95:65–69.
26. Rizzo G, Arduini D, Romanini C: Doppler echocardiographic assessment of fetal cardiac function. Ultrasound Obstet Gynecol 1992;2:434–445.
27. Rizzo G, Capponi A, Chaoui R, et al: Blood flow velocity waveforms from peripheral pulmonary arteries in normally grown and growth-retarded fetuses. Ultrasound Obstet Gynecol 1996;8:87–92.
28. Huhta JC, Moise KJ, Fisher DJ, et al: Detection and quantitation of constriction of the fetal ductus arteriosus by Doppler echocardiography. Circulation 1987;75:406–412.
29. Wladimiroff JW, Huisman TWA, Stewart PA, Stijnen TH: Normal fetal Doppler inferior vena cava, transtricuspid and umbilical artery flow velocity waveforms between 11 and 16 weeks' gestation. Am J Obstet Gynecol 1992;166:46–49.
30. Metha AV, Chidamabaradam B: Ventricular septal defect in the first year of life. Am J Cardiol 1992;70:364–366.
31. Paladini D, Palmieri S, Lamberti A, et al: Characterization and natural hystory of ventricular septal defetcs in the fetus. Ultrasound Obstet Gynecol 2000;16:118–122.
32. De Vore GR, Alfi O: The use of color Doppler ultrasound to identify fetuses at increased risk for trisomy 21: An alternative for high risk patients who decline genetic amniocentesis. Obstet Gynecol 1995;85:378–386.
33. Fyler DC, Buckley LP, Hellembrand WE, et al: Report of the New England Regional Cardiac program. Pediatrics 1980;65:375–461.
34. Allan LD, Crawford DC, Anderson RH, Tynann MJ: Prenatal screening of congenital heart disease. Br Med J 1986;292: 1717–1720.
35. Doty DB: Aortic atresia. J Thorac Cardiovasc Surg 1980;79:462–467.
36. Allan LD, Sharland GK, Tynan MJ: The natural hystory of the hypoplastic left heart syndrome. Int J Cardiol 1989;25:341–343.
37. Jonas RA, Hansen DD, Cook N, Wessel D: Anatomic subtype and survival after reconstructive operation for the hypoplastic left heart syndrome. J Thorac Cardiovasc Surg 1994;107: 1121–1128.
38. Bailey LL, Gundry SR, Razzouk AJ, et al and the Loma Linda University Pediatric Heart Transplant Group: Bless the babies; one hundred and fifteen late survivors of heart transplantion during the first year of life. J Thorac Cardiovasc Surg 1993;105: 805–815.
39. Fontan F, Kirklin JW, Fernandez G, et al: Outcome after a "perfect" Fontan operation. Circulation 1990;81:1520–1536.
40. Hanley FL, Sade RM, Blackstone EH, et al: Outcome in neonatal pulmonary atresia with intact ventricular septum: A multinstitutional study. J Thorac Cardiovasc Surg 1993;105:406–427.
41. Becker AE, Anderson RH: Pathology of Congenital Heart Disease. London, Butterworths, 1981.
42. Maxwell DJ, Allan LD, Tynan M: Balloon aortic valvuloplasty in the fetus report of two cases. Br Heart J 1991;65:256–258.
43. Khol T, Sharland G, Allan LD, et al: World experience of percutaneous ultrasound guided balloon valvuloplastic in human feuses with severe aortic valve obstruction. Am J Cardiol 2000;85:1230–1233.
44. Hornberger LK, Sahn DJ, Kleinman CS, et al: Antenatal diagnosis of coarctation of the aorta: A multicenter experience. J Am Coll Cardiol 1994;23:417–423.
45. Allan LD, Crawford DC, Tynan MJ: Evolution of coarctation of the aorta in intrauterine life. Br Heart J 1984;52:471–473.
46. Conte S, Lacour Gayest F, Serraf A: Surgical repair of coartation of the aorta in the neonate. J Thorac Cardiovasc Surg 1995;109: 663–674.
47. Hornberger LK, Benacerraf BR, Bromley BS, et al: Prenatal detection of severe right ventricular outflow tract obstruction: Pulmonary stenosis and pulmonary atresia. J Ultrasound Med 1994;13:743–750.
48. Rice MJ, McDonald RW, Reller MD: Progressive pulmonary obstruction in the fetus: Two cases report. Am J Perinatol 1983;10:424–427.
49. Vouhe PR, Tamiser D, Leca F, et al: Transposition of great arteries ventricular septal defect ventricular outflow obstruction. J Thorac Cardiovasc Surg 1993; 103:428–436.
50. De Vore GR, Siassi B, Platt LD: Fetal echocardiography. VIII. Aortic root dilatation—A marker for tetralogy of Fallot. Am J Obstet Gynecol 1988;159:129–136.
51. Paladini D, Rustico M, Todros T, et al: Conotruncal anomalies in prenatal life. Ultrasound Obstet Gynecol 1996;8:241–246.
52. Allan LD, Sharland GK: Prognosis in fetal tetralogy of Fallot. Pediatr Cardiol 1992;13:1–4.
53. Piccoli G, Pacifico AD, Kirklin JW: Changing results and concepts in the surgical treatment of double outlet right ventricle: Analysis of 137 operations in 126 patients. Am J Cardiol 1994;52:549–555.
54. Di Donato RM, Fyfe DA, Puga FJ: Fifteen years experience with surgical repair of truncus arteriosus. J Thorac Cardiovasc Surg 1982;89:414–421.

55. Holley DG, Martin GR, Brenner JI, et al: Diagnosis and management of fetal cardiac tumors: A multicenter experience and review of published reports. J Am Coll Cardiol 1995;26:516–520.
56. Hornenberg LK, Sahn DJ, Kleinmann CS, et al: Tricuspid valve disease with significant tricuspid insufficiency in the fetus: diagnosis and outcome. J Am Coll Cardiol 1991;17:167–173.
57. Respondek M, Kammermeier M, Hutha JC, Weil SR: Fetal tricuspid valve regurgitation in normal heart anomaly. Am J Obstet Gynecol 1995;171:1265–1270.
58. Copel JA, Morotti R, Hobbins JC, Kleinmann CS: The antenatal diagnosis of congenital heart disease using fetal echocardiography: Is color flow mapping necessary? Obstet Gynecol 1991;78:1–8.
59. Sharland GK, Chita SK, Allan LD: Tricuspid valve dysplasia or displacement in intrauterine life. J Am Coll Cardiol 1991; 17:944–949.
60. Todros T, Presbitero P, Gagliotti G, Demaria D: Pulmonary stenosis with intact ventricular septum: Documentation of the development of the lesion echocardiographically during fetal life. Int J Cardiol 1986;19:335–360.
61. Hornberger LK, Sanders SP, Sahn DJ, et al: In utero pulmonary artery and aortic growth and potential for progression of pulmonary outflow tract obstruction in tetralogy of Fallot. J Am Coll Cardiol 1995;25:739–745.
62. Bonnet D, Coltri A, Butera G: Detection of transposition of great arteries in fetuses reduces neonatal mortality and morbidity. Circulation 1999;99:916–918.
63. Puder KS, Humes RA, Gold RL, et al: The genetic implication for preceding generations of the prenatal diagnosis of interrupted aortic arch in association with unsuspected DiGeorge anomaly. Am J Obstet Gynecol 1995;175:239–241.
64. Driscoll DA, Salvin J, Sellinger B: Prevalence of 22q11 microdeletion in DiGeorge and velocardiofacial syndromes: Implication for genetic counselling and prenatal diagnosis. J Med Genet 1993;30:813–817.
65. Miller G, Eggli KD, Contant C, et al: Postoperative neurologic complications after open heart surgery on young infants. Arch Pediatr Adolesc Med 1996;150:560–561.
66. Czeizel AE: Reduction of urinary tract and cardiovascular defects by periconceptional multivitamin supplementation. Am J Med Genet 1996;62:179–183.
67. Botto LD, Mulinare J, Erickson JD: Occurrence of congenital heart defects in relation to maternal multivitamin use. Am J Epidemiol 2000;151:878.
68. Burn J, Brennan P, Little J, et al: Recurrence risks in offspring of adults with major heart defects: Results from first cohort of British collaborative study. Lancet 1998;351:311–316.
69. Gladman G, McCrindle BW, Boutin C, Smallhorn JF: Fetal echocardiographic screening of diabetic pregnancies for congenital heart disease. Am J Perinatol 1997;14:59–62.
70. Ryan AK, Goodship JA, Wilson DI, et al: Spectrum of clinical features associated with interstitial chromosome 22q11 deletions: A European collaborative study. J Med Genet 1997;34:798–804.
71. Bonnet D, Coltri A, Butera G, et al: Detection of transposition of the great arteries in fetuses reduces morbitidity and mortality in newborn infants. Circulation 1999;99:916–918.
72. Brackley KJ, Kilby MD, Wright JG, et al: Outcome after prenatal diagnosis of hypoplastic left-heart syndrome: A case series. Lancet 2000;356:1143–1147.
73. Tworetzky W, McElhinney DB, Reddy VM, et al: Improved surgical outcome after fetal diagnosis of hypoplastic left heart syndrome. Circulation 2001;103:1269–1273.

CHAPTER 18

Fetal Craniospinal and Facial Abnormalities

Robin B. Kalish / Jane Streltzoff / Frank A. Chervenak

INTRODUCTION

Craniospinal and facial defects are among the most commonly diagnosed congenital anomalies and have a profound impact on survival, physical appearance, and function in society. Because the central nervous system is the earliest organ system to form, and facial development completes near the end of embryogenesis, teratogenic exposures such as drug ingestion, maternal illness, and infection may cause craniospinal or facial malformations at any time during embryogenesis. Genetic syndromes and chromosomal abnormalities frequently affect the development of the neuraxis and face. Further, the fetal brain continues to develop throughout gestation. Consequently, it is vulnerable to disorders of growth, as well as vascular, infectious, and traumatic insults.

OPEN NEURAL TUBE DEFECTS: ANENCEPHALY, CEPHALOCELE, AND SPINA BIFIDA

General

Neural tube closure occurs in the third to fourth weeks after fertilization. Fusion begins in the region of the fourth somite and then extends both rostrally and caudally. Closure in the region of the developing head and sacrum is completed approximately 24 and 26 days after conception, respectively. Neural tube defects most likely result from either a primary overgrowth of neural tube tissue within the line of closure, or a failure of induction by adjacent mesodermal tissues that interrupt closure. Depending on the timing and the extent of the interruption, defects may occur at both cranial and caudal ends of the neural tube. Large or small and continuous or noncontinuous regions of the neuroaxis can be affected. Anencephaly is a lethal disorder in which the brain and the overlying calvarium are absent. It is thought to result from failure of the entire rostral portion of the neural tube to close. Less extensive failure of closure in the rostral region results in cephalocele. Failure of neural tube closure in the more caudad regions results in spina bifida.

Open neural tube defects (ONTDs) are multifactorial in origin, arising from a combination of genetic and environmental factors that exhibit a threshold effect. Thus, the incidence of ONTD is highly variable, depending on geographic location, ethnicity, and gender. In particular, the incidence of ONTD is reportedly higher in Hispanic patients,[1,2] in female fetuses,[3] and in areas with low maternal folic acid intake.[4] Additional at-risk groups include women with insulin-requiring diabetes[5] or obesity.[6,7] In addition, women with a seizure disorder taking anticonvulsants including valproic acid,[8] women consuming high doses of vitamin A,[9] and women with folate or vitamin B_{12} insufficiency may be at increased risk.[10] It is important to note that women who themselves are affected, or who have had an affected infant or sibling, have a higher incidence of ONTD than the general population. ONTD also may be associated with aneuploidy and other rare genetic syndromes.[11]

Diagnosis

Screening for ONTD may be either biochemical via measurement of the maternal serum α-fetoprotein (MS-AFP) concentration or sonographic (see Chapter 8). MS-AFP screening does not detect all cases of ONTD, as the MS-AFP concentration can be normal if the lesion is predominantly skin-covered. The definitive antenatal diagnosis is made by visualizing the defect using sonography, which can be accomplished as early as the first trimester.[12] Amniocentesis for the measurement of amniotic fluid AFP and the detection of acetylcholinesterase (AChE) is usually no longer required, but remains an adjunct to ultrasonography when the MS-AFP is elevated but no defect is visualized. However, most ONTDs can be definitively diagnosed sonographically and do not require amniocentesis for the measurement of amniotic fluid AFP or AChE.[13] The use of three-dimensional ultrasound and fetal magnetic resonance imaging (MRI) are reputed to assist in the detection and localization of ONTDs in high risk patients[12,14–16] but do not, at this time, have broad applicability.

Anencephaly

The antenatal sonographic diagnosis of anencephaly is based on the absence of the fetal calvaria, the domelike portion of the cranial vault. A mass of thin-walled channels, known as the area cerebrovasculosa, is often seen protruding from the base of the skull above the orbits (Fig. 18–1). Though easily diagnosed during the second and third trimesters, first-trimester diagnosis of anencephaly is sometimes difficult because the normal immature brain may be difficult to differentiate from the area cerebrovasculosa. However, the bony structures of the skull above the orbits should be visualized by 10 weeks' gestation. Other diagnoses should be excluded before finalizing the diagnosis of anencephaly. For example, in severe microcephaly, the bones of the skull are present but may be difficult to see sonographically. Also, constricting bands in the early amnion-rupture sequence may prevent the normal formation of the skull. In this instance, the malformation is usually asymmetrical and brain tissue is present. Amniotic bands may produce a spectrum of abnormalities from anencephaly to asymmetrical defects. Encephalocele may simulate anencephaly until a brain-filled sac is identified. Lastly, acrania, in which there is a normally formed brain with an absent skull, is often difficult to distinguish from anencephaly.

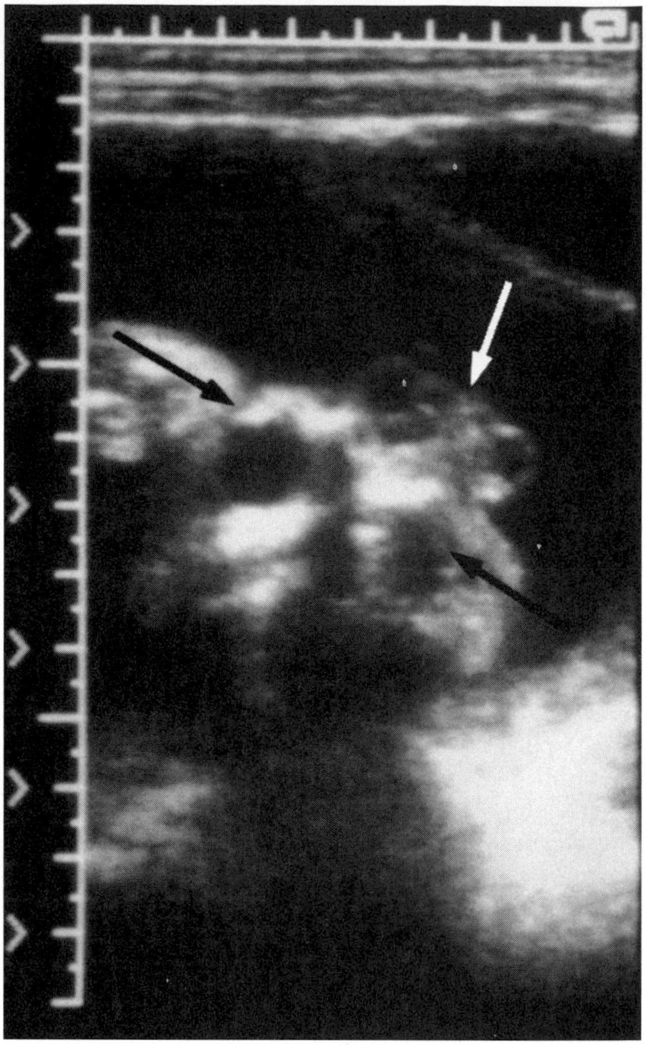

FIGURE 18–1
Coronal sonogram of fetal head demonstrating anencephaly. Black arrows point to orbits; white arrow points to area cerebrovasculosa.

Cephalocele

A cephalocele resembles a saclike protrusion from the head not covered with bone. The malformation is termed an encephalocele when the brain has herniated into the sac. In contrast, a cranial meningocele does not contain brain substance. Although large amounts of brain tissue are readily seen on ultrasound, the precise diagnosis can be difficult as smaller amounts may be undetectable by ultrasonography.[17] The contents of the herniated sac are typically heterogeneous (Fig. 18–2*A* and *B*). The position of the defect can be determined using the bony structures of the face, spine, and when possible, the midline echo of the brain for orientation. Most cephaloceles are occipital, but they may also be parietal, frontal, or nasopharyngeal.[18] The incidence of anterior lesions is considerably higher in Asia (Fig. 18–3).[19,20] Defects away from the midline or in other atypical locations are suggestive of the amnion-rupture sequence, rather than a failure of the neural tube closure. The diagnosis of cephalocele is certain only if the bony defect in the skull is detected. Otherwise, the diagnostic possibilities include cystic hygroma, teratoma, hemangioma, and subcutaneous cyst (Fig. 18–4).

Spina Bifida

Viewed longitudinally on ultrasound, the normal spine narrows progressively as the transducer is moved caudally. In defective vertebrae, the posterior ossification centers are more widely spaced than those in vertebrae above and below the defect. Whereas an ONTD is detectable on a longitudinal ultrasound image by the loss of skin continuity (Fig. 18–5), meticulous transverse examination of the entire vertebral column is

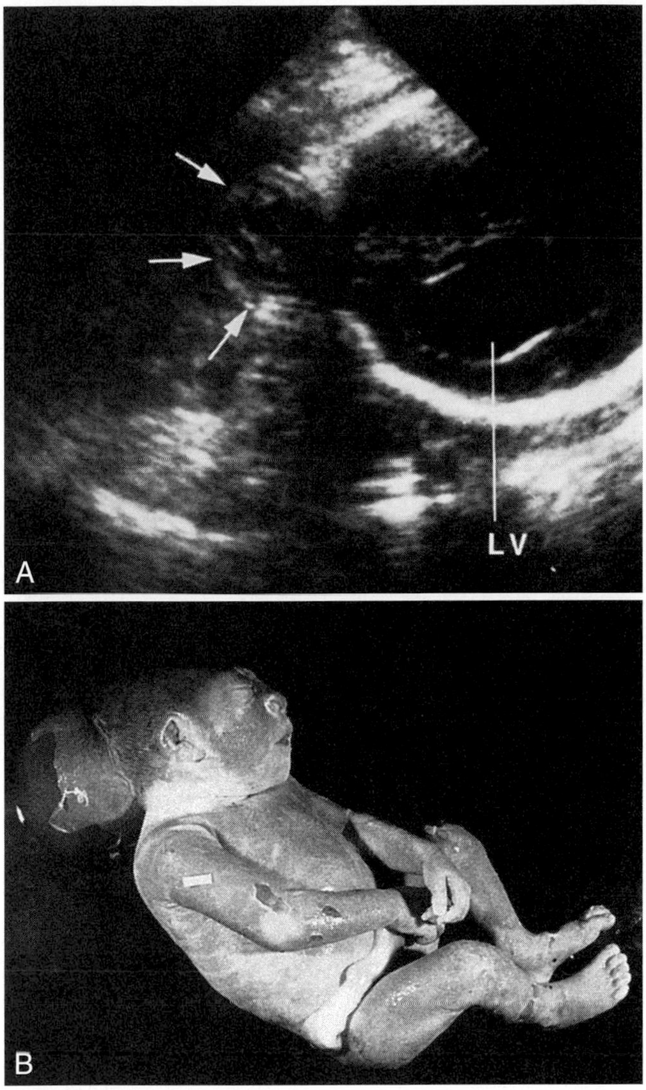

FIGURE 18–2
A, Transverse section of an occipital encephalocele (*arrows*). Note LV, dilated lateral ventricle. *B*, Neonate with large occipital encephalocele.

usually necessary to detect smaller defects. In the transverse view, spina bifida appears as a splaying of the posterior ossification centers (Fig. 18–6). In the second and third trimesters, posterior vertebral elements, including the laminae and spinous processes, are normally visible sonographically. Their absence supports the diagnosis of spina bifida. When the sonographic examination is not definitive, three-dimensional ultrasound and fetal MRI can be effective, noninvasive tools for the assessment of the fetal CNS, allowing precise localization of the lesion and evaluation of any associated hydrocephalus.[14–16] However, two-dimensional ultrasound remains the diagnostic tool of choice for evaluation of fetal anomalies including myelomeningocele.

The majority of cases of spina bifida are associated with the Arnold-Chiari malformation in which the cerebellar vermis, fourth ventricle, and medulla are displaced caudally. Nicolaides described the now classic sono-

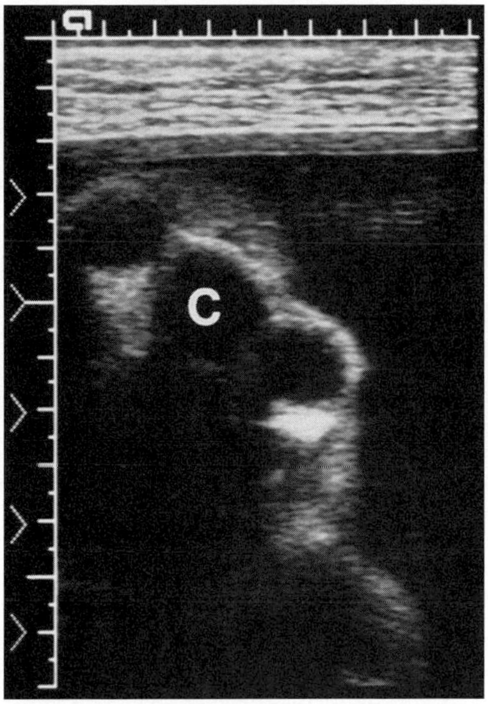

FIGURE 18–3
Transverse section of the fetal head demonstrating cephalocele (C) protruding between bony orbits, resulting in hypertelorism. (From Chervenak FA, Isaacson G, Rosenberg JC, et al: Antenatal diagnosis of frontal cephalocele in a fetus with atelosteogenesis. J Ultrasound Med 1986;5:111–113.)

graphic signs of the Arnold-Chiari malformation: the "lemon" and the "banana" signs (Fig. 18–7).[21] A lemon-like configuration is seen in axial section during the second trimester and is caused by scalloping of the frontal bones owing to caudal displacement of the cranial contents within a pliable skull (Fig. 18–8). As the cerebellar hemispheres are displaced into the cisterna magna, they are flattened rostrocaudally and the cisterna magna is

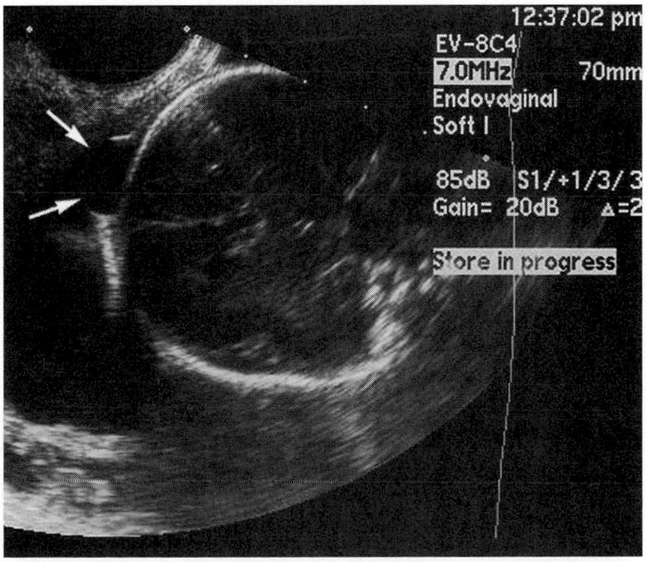

FIGURE 18–4
Fetal skull, coronal view, demonstrates a subcutaneous cystic structure (*arrows*), integrity of skull intact.

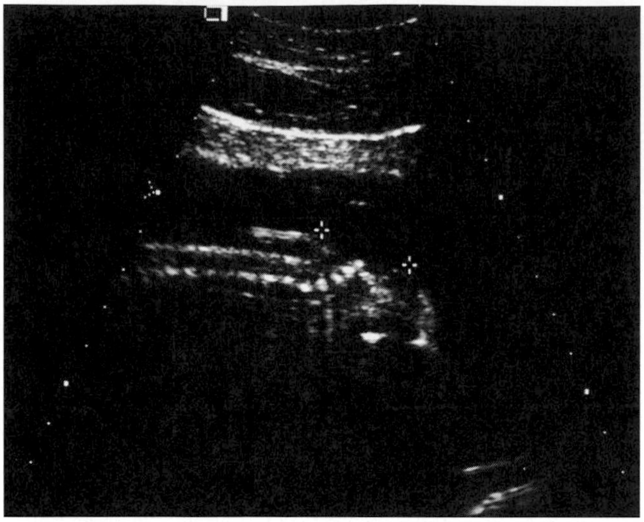

FIGURE 18–5
Longitudinal view of fetal spine with sacral spina bifida demonstrated by the loss of skin continuity caudally (calipers).

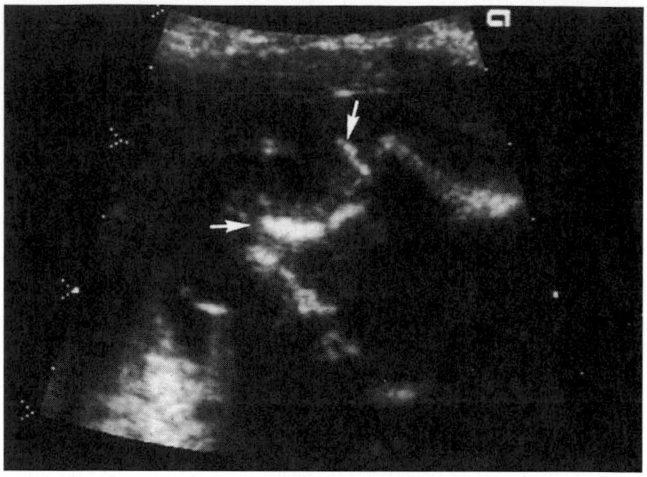

FIGURE 18–6
Transverse view through sacrum demonstrates splaying of posterior ossification elements (*arrows*).

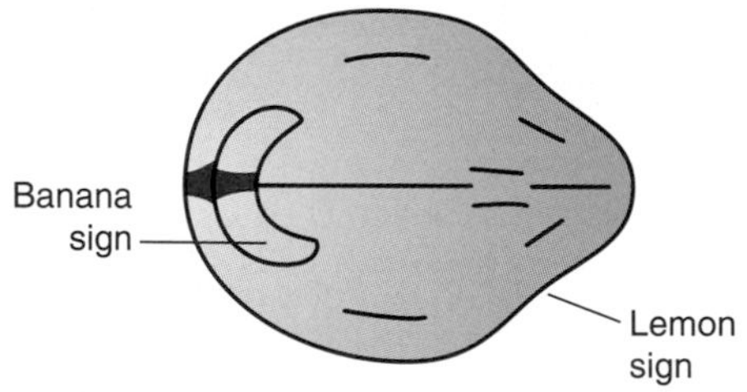

FIGURE 18–7
Schematic representation of the "lemon" and "banana" signs described by Nicolaides and associates. (From Nicolaides KH, Campbell S, Gabbe SG, Guidetti R: Ultrasound screening for spina bifida. Cranial and cerebellar signs. Lancet 1986;ii:72–74.)

obliterated, causing a flattened, centrally curved, banana-like sonographic appearance (Fig. 18–9). These ultrasound markers are present in over 95% of second trimester fetuses with open spina bifida.[22] Eventually, the flow of cerebrospinal fluid (CSF) becomes obstructed, causing some degree of ventriculomegaly/hydrocephalus in most cases.

Management Options

Prenatal

The management of pregnancies with ONTD depends on the severity of the lesion and parental wishes. A comprehensive survey of the entire anatomy must be undertaken in all fetuses with an ONTD by an experienced sonographer to exclude other structural anomalies. Ventriculomegaly is present in the majority of cases, and the degree of hydrocephalus and subsequent macrocephaly likely impacts on the prognosis.[23] ONTDs are also seen in association with a variety of genetic syndromes, some of whose features are detectable by ultrasonography. Thus, a fetal karyotype is recommended in all instances.

Anencephaly is lethal. Most affected fetuses are stillborn or die shortly after birth.[24] Because anencephaly can be diagnosed confidently by antenatal ultrasound with a high degree of accuracy, termination of pregnancy is an ethical option at any time in gestation.[25] If it is diag-

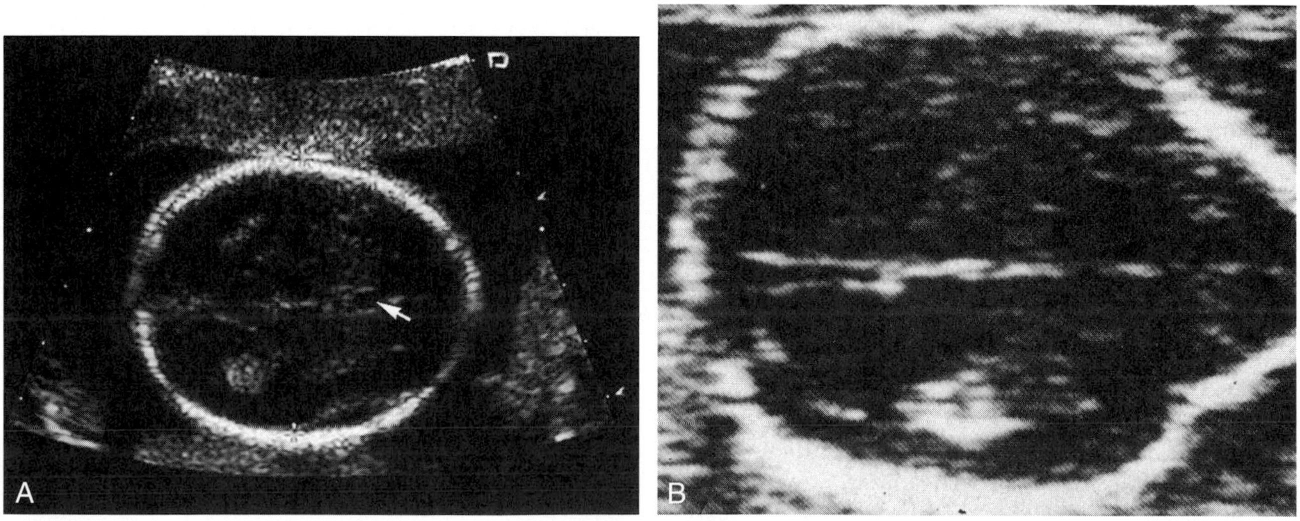

FIGURE 18–8
A, Transverse section of normal fetal head at the level of cavum septi pellucidi (*arrow*). *B*, Transverse section of fetal head in a fetus with open spina bifida showing "lemon" sign. (From Nicolaides KH, Campbell S, Gabbe SG, Guidetti R: Ultrasound screening for spina bifida. Cranial and cerebellar signs. Lancet 1986;ii:72–74.)

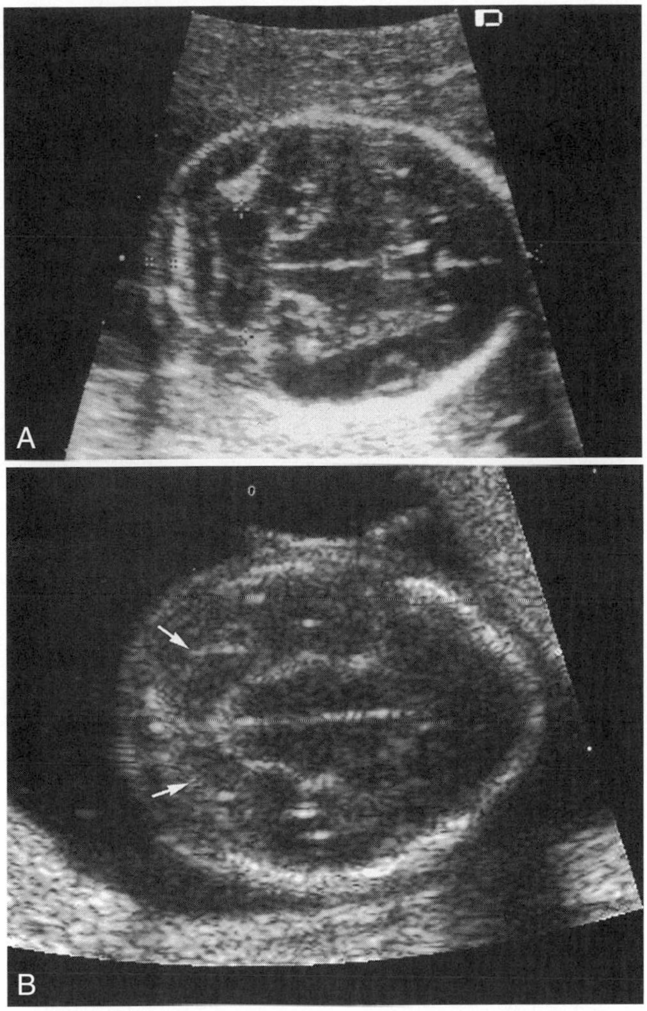

FIGURE 18–9
A, Suboccipital bregmatic view of fetal head in an 18-week fetus with normal cerebellum, callipers, and cisterna magna. *B*, Suboccipital bregmatic view of fetal head in an 18-week fetus with open spina bifida demonstrating "banana" sign (*arrow*).

nosed in the third trimester and the parents elect termination, a number of methods are available.

The most important prognostic indicators for a poor outcome with cephalocele are the presence of brain in the protruding sac and the presence of additional congenital abnormalities.[26–28] In several series, 50% to 65% of affected fetuses had additional anomalies. Burdick and associates observed that only two of eight liveborns survived infancy.[29] Brown and associates reviewed 34 cases of neonatal cephalocele and noted an overall mortality rate of 29%.[30] Perhaps the most optimistic report came from Martinez-Lage and associates, who reported an overall mortality rate of 36% in 46 newborns with cephalocele with 20 infants free of neurologic sequelae.[31] In general, about half the infants with an isolated occipital cephalocele develop normally after surgery. The outlook is dismal for children with microcephaly secondary to brain herniation. The impact of concurrent hydrocephalus has been reduced by modern shunt therapy, and thus, hydrocephalus has less impact than the presence and amount of brain herniation. Frontal cephaloceles have a better prognosis than those in other locations because they tend to be smaller with less brain herniation.[32] Further, the loss of frontal cortex may produce fewer or less significant neurologic deficits than other areas of cortical loss.

The prognosis for spina bifida is variable. The extent and severity of the neurologic deficits depend on the presence of neural tissue in the meningeal sac and the spinal level and length of the lesion, as the spinal cord below the lesion is dysplastic.[33,34] Generally, lower extremity paralysis and incontinence of bowel and bladder are common; intelligence may be affected from either the lesion itself or the impact of treatment (e.g., shunt placement). A comprehensive fetal ultrasound examination should be performed to exclude genetic syndromes associated with encephalocele. For example, Meckel-Gruber syndrome has a 25% recurrence risk. Overall, 75% of infants born with spina bifida survive long term.[35]

Twenty- to 25-year outcome was reported in one study of 118 children treated neonatally for the myelomeningocele. Of the 99 patients with follow-up, 28 had died.[35] Of the 71 survivors, 85% reached high school. One quarter suffered seizures. In another study of 117 patients born with open spina bifida, 54% had died within 38 years of closure.[36] The neurologic status of the survivors ranged from normal to severe disability. Thirty-nine of the 54 survivors had an IQ of 80 or higher; 16 could walk without assistance, 22 lived independently in the community, and only 11 were fully continent. Although improvements in the management of patients with open spina bifida have reduced the infant mortality rate, long-term disability is still significant, and late deterioration is common. Dise and Lohr examined the cognitive skills of adolescents born with spina bifida up to 23 years of age.[37] All patients, regardless of IQ, had significant impairments of mental flexibility, efficiency of processing, conceptualization, or problem-solving ability. There was a high degree of variability within profiles, all containing at least one area of dysfunction. These deficits may underlie the "motivational" and academic difficulties commonly observed in these patients.

Still, affected children can grow to be productive adults with normal intelligence. Early closure of the defect, ventriculoperitoneal shunting of any associated hydrocephalus, management of urinary and fecal incontinence by surgery, dietary management, and feedback techniques are in part responsible for these improvements. It is unclear whether cesarean delivery improves the prognosis.[38] A selection bias brought about by antenatal diagnosis with termination of the most severely affected fetuses may account at least in part for the reportedly improved outcomes. The prognosis for the severely affected newborn remains serious, with gross permanent multisystem defects. It is difficult to accurately predict the prognosis in the first half of pregnancy when the diagnosis is frequently made. The option for pregnancy termination should be included in counseling the patients.

Alternatively, in utero repair of myelomeningocele to stop or slow any progression in damage to the exposed spinal cord reportedly decreases the incidence of hindbrain herniation and shunt-dependent hydrocephalus.[39] The rationale for the procedure is that closure antenatally may decrease spinal cord dysplasia and preserve neurologic function by protecting it from potential insults such as amniotic fluid trauma. Although fetal surgery is promising on a theoretical basis, significant complications are associated with in utero repair, including prematurity and lethal pulmonary hypoplasia secondary to oligohydramnios. In addition, the evidence of long-term benefit including improved lower extremity motor function and bladder and bowel continence is at this time unclear.[40,41] To date, no prospective randomized trials comparing the outcomes of the antenatal versus postnatal surgical repair of meningomyelocele have been published. The American College of Obstetrics and Gynecology advised in 2000 that such surgery should be considered experimental until the availability of evidence that the benefits outweigh the risks to both mother and fetus. Currently, there is a multicentered randomized clinical trial under way in the United States in order to compare the outcomes of fetal surgery with postnatal management for spina bifida.[34]

When a meningomyelocele is diagnosed and the patient plans to continue the pregnancy, a multidisciplinary team consisting of a pediatric neurologist, neurosurgeon, obstetrician, and neonatologist assemble to discuss the implications with the family. An actively involved perinatal social worker can provide invaluable support to the family before and after birth. Fetal surveillance is recommended for all ongoing pregnancies with the exception of anencephaly, including serial sonography to assess fetal growth, head size, and severity of ventriculomegaly. Unless maternal or other obstetric indication takes precedence, delivery should occur at term or with documentation of fetal lung maturity.

Labor and Delivery

Postmaturity is common in pregnancies complicated by anencephaly. Cesarean delivery is not indicated for fetal distress, but may be necessary for maternal indications. Humane care is provided to the liveborn anencephalic infant until death. The use of anencephalic newborns as organ donors remains widely debated.[42,43] Pathologic examination of the fetus is important to confirm the diagnosis and to exclude conditions in which anencephaly is part of a genetic syndrome.

The optimal mode of delivery for the fetus with cephalocele is controversial. If a large amount of brain tissue is observed in the sac, and especially if one of the more grave prognostic factors (i.e., microcephaly or associated anomalies) is also present, the parents are counseled that the chance of a good outcome is remote, and cesarean delivery for fetal indications avoided. Decompression of a large sac or associated hydrocephalus may be necessary to allow vaginal delivery. However, cesarean delivery is an option in those rare instances when a cephalocele is very large and sufficiently solid to cause dystocia. There is no clear objective evidence that cesarean delivery reduces birth trauma and improves neonatal outcome when a cephalocele is present. However, this does not exclude the possibility that trauma during vaginal delivery could, in theory, worsen the prognosis for these children.

Similarly, no conclusive information demonstrates that the optimal route of delivery for the vertex fetus with a meningomyelocele is cesarean. One retrospective clinical study concluded that elective cesarean delivery prior to the onset of labor improved outcome in terms of the functional level of the spinal defect at age 2 years.[44] However, this study contained numerous sources of bias. Multiple subsequent studies, which have sought to eliminate some of the design flaws of the first, could identify no benefit from cesarean delivery.[45–48] A randomized trial to study this question is needed. Until then, in our view, cesarean delivery of a fetus with meningomyelocele remains the first choice.

Care must be taken during delivery to minimize traction on the spine regardless of the route of delivery. If there is an indication for cesarean delivery, a low transverse incision is acceptable if the lower uterine segment is well developed. Otherwise, a vertical incision should be performed. After the head is delivered, the bisacromial diameter is positioned horizontally. Both fetal flanks are grasped and gentle traction applied in an outward direction away from the uterine wall near the meningomyelocele. The assistant retracts the edge of the uterine incision as the body of the infant is delivered (Fig. 18–10).

Postnatal and Prepregnancy

The recurrence risk for any neural tube defect after one affected child may be as high as 3% to 5% in the United

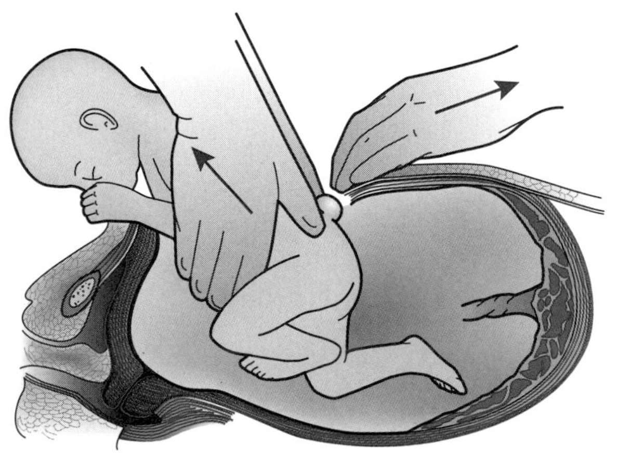

FIGURE 18–10
Fetus with a meningomyelocele is delivered through a low transverse uterine incision. Both fetal flanks are grasped, and gentle traction is applied in an outward direction. Assistant retracts edge of uterine incision as body is delivered. (From Chervenak FA, Duncan C, Ment LR, et al: Perinatal management of myelomeningocele. Obstet Gynecol 1984;63:376.)

States,[49,50] and up to 10% after having two affected offspring. The risk is greater in populations where ONTDs are more common. The recurrence risk is 4% to 5% if one parent is affected, and 25% when the ONTD is part of the Meckel-Gruber syndrome. A cephalocele may also occur as part of other autosomal recessive syndromes.

Randomized, placebo-controlled trials demonstrate that the likelihood of recurrence is reduced by periconceptual administration of folate (4 mg orally daily). This treatment should be offered to all women with a prior affected child. Antenatal ultrasonography should be performed in future pregnancies initially at 12 to 13 weeks in search of a recurrent ONTD.

SUMMARY OF MANAGEMENT OPTIONS

Open Neural Tube Defects: Anencephaly, Cephalocele, and Spina Bifida

Management Options	Quality of Evidence	Strength of Recommendation	References
Prenatal			
Search for skull defect in cephalocele and associated anomalies in all cases of open neural tube defects (especially hydrocephalus), including magnetic resonance imaging.	III	B	23, 87, 103
Prognosis for cephalocele depends on amount of herniated brain tissue; prognosis for spina bifida is difficult to predict early and depends on level and extent of lesion.	–	GPP	–
Advise karyotype in all cases.	–	GPP	–
Monitor for hydrocephalus.	–	GPP	–
Interdisciplinary approach is needed.	–	GPP	–
Termination may be chosen.	–	GPP	–
Monitor ongoing pregnancies (growth, umbilical artery Doppler recordings, amniotic fluid volume).	–	GPP	–
Fetal surgery for spina bifida should be regarded as experimental at present.	III	B	39, 40, 41
Labor and Delivery			
Deliver by vaginal route for anencephaly and humane neonatal care.	–	GPP	–
Mode of delivery for cephalocele is uncertain; some suggest that method should be determined by prognosis; no evidence suggests that cesarean section is beneficial.	–	GPP	–
Cephalocentesis is performed for encephaloceles if parents wish.	–	GPP	–
Optimal route of delivery is unknown for spina bifida.	III	B	45–48
Great care is needed with delivery of the back, regardless of delivery route.	–	GPP	–
Postnatal and Prepregnancy			
Necropsy is performed for abortuses/stillbirths/neonatal deaths.	–	GPP	–
Karyotype if not already done.	–	GPP	–
Assess for diabetes, teratogens (anticonvulsants, vitamin A).	–	GPP	–
Provide counseling.	–	GPP	–
Periconceptual high-dose folate is given to women with a history of neural tube defect.	Ia	A	113
Provide pediatric neurosurgical management.	–	GPP	–

HYDROCEPHALUS

General

Hydrocephalus is defined as ventriculomegaly and macrocephaly associated with increased intracranial pressure. As such, hydrocephalus is a description and not a disease diagnosis. It results from an abnormal increase in the cerebral ventricular volume compared to brain tissue. There are many causes of hydrocephalus. It may result from abnormal formation of central nervous system structures, as in hydrocephalus inherited along a mendelian pattern or hydrocephalus associated with a malformation syndrome. Hydrocephalus may result from defects acquired in utero, from infection with subsequent scarring, or inflammation and CSF obstruction, from intraventricular hemorrhage, or from intracranial tumors and mass lesions. Many cases of hydrocephalus cannot currently be assigned to any one specific etiologic category.

In general, there are four ways in which the ventricles grow to an abnormal size (Fig. 18–11):

- Obstruction to outflow (noncommunicating hydrocephalus), usually at a point of narrowing in the system (frequently the aqueduct of Sylvius or the foramina of either Lushka or Magendie)
- Impaired resorption of CSF by the arachnoid granulations (communicating hydrocephalus)
- Overproduction of CSF
- Underdevelopment or destruction of cortical tissue with a relative increase in the size of the ventricles (hydrocephalus ex vacuo)

Obstructive causes are the most common in both fetus and newborn.[51,52] Hydrocephalus is described as isolated when the fetus is otherwise free of anomalies and is not the direct result of the ventricular enlargement or increased intracranial pressure. Meningomyelocele is the most common abnormality associated with hydrocephalus. In the United States, the incidence of congenital hydrocephalus unassociated with a neural tube defect is 5.8 per 10,000 total births. This is likely an underestimate of the true incidence, as both spontaneous regression and antepartum death occur in some cases.[51]

Diagnosis

A variety of techniques are advocated for the diagnosis of ventriculomegaly. Measurement of the atrium of the lateral ventricles is most common (Fig. 18–12). This method is optimal because the width of the atrium of the lateral ventricle usually remains constant throughout the second and third trimesters despite the fact that there is a decrease in the proportion of the cross-section of the brain occupied by the lateral ventricles as pregnancy advances. Cardoza and associates[53] presented strong evidence that a single measurement of the lateral ventricle atrium accurately differentiates a normal ventricle system from one that is pathologically enlarged.

Evaluation of the choroid plexus can also be useful when ventriculomegaly in hydrocephalus is suspected.[54] The choroid plexus usually fills the posterior portion of the lateral ventricles and appears symmetrical bilaterally, regardless of the orientation of the fetal head. In ventriculomegaly and hydrocephalus, the choroid plexus assumes a dependent position in the enlarged ventricle and appears as a dangling structure (Fig. 18–13). Serial ultrasound examinations are especially important for at-risk pregnancies. The absence of hydrocephalus at one

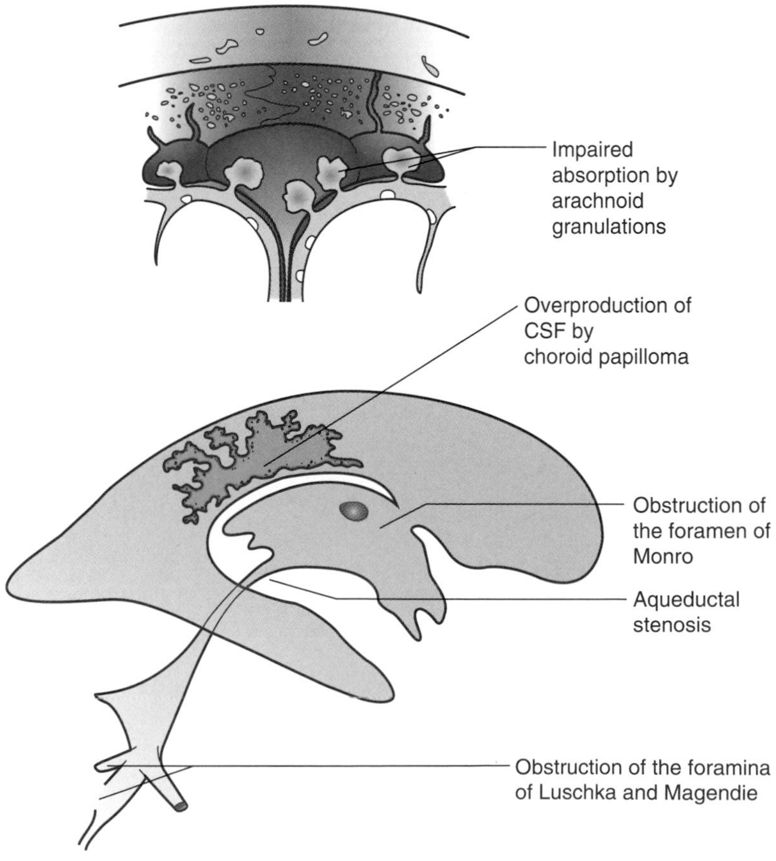

FIGURE 18–11
Diagrammatic representation of mechanisms of ventriculomegaly.

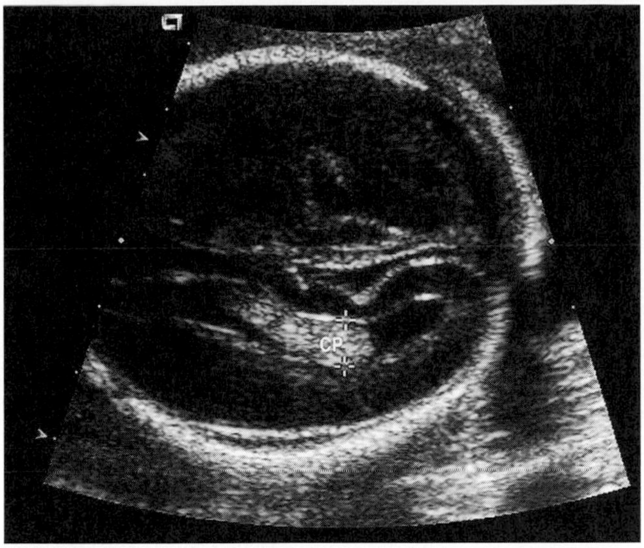

FIGURE 18–12
Transverse section demonstrating distal lateral ventricle with its atrial measurements (+). CP, choroid plexus.

point early in gestation does not preclude its development later in gestation. Once hydrocephalus is diagnosed as an isolated abnormality, serial scans are important to identify in utero progression. The differential diagnoses for severe hydrocephalus includes alobar holoprosencephaly, hydrancephaly, porencephaly, and arachnoid cyst (Fig. 18–14), which may be distinguished by the criteria listed later in this chapter. Another rare cause of large, intracranial fluid-like collection is an aneurysm of the vein of Galen, characterized by blood flow that can be visualized by color Doppler ultrasonography (Fig. 18–15).

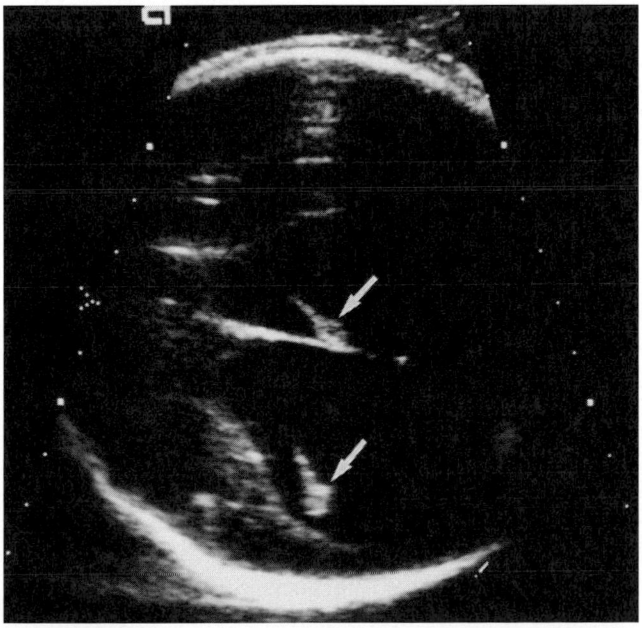

FIGURE 18–13
Transverse section of fetal head demonstrating hydrocephalus. Arrows point to dependent dangling of the choroid plexus within the dilated lateral ventricles.

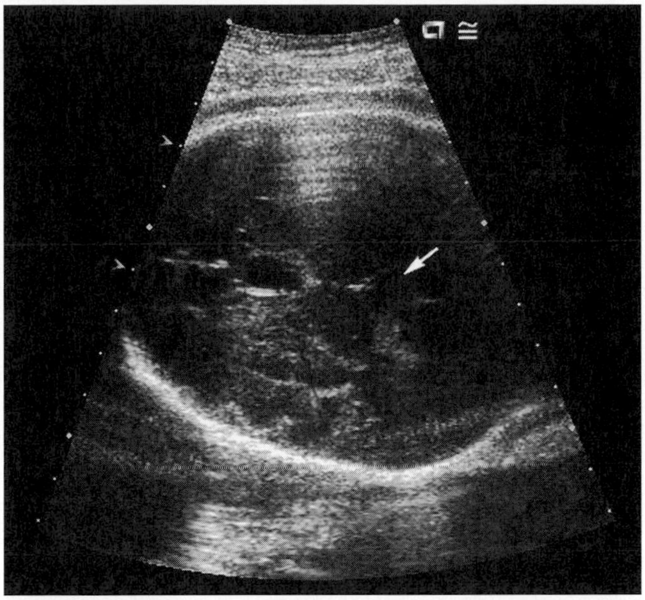

FIGURE 18–14
Transverse section through fetal head demonstrates an arachnoid cyst, cavum septum pellucidum anteriorly, and arachnoid cyst (*arrow*) posteriorly. Cyst with no flow on color Doppler and separate from CSP on all planes.

Management Options

Prenatal

Prior to the development of postnatal surgical shunting of the dilated ventricular system, the outlook for the infant with hydrocephalus was generally poor. Although some cases of unoperated obstructive hydrocephalus progressed slowly, or arrested spontaneously, massive head enlargement with blindness and mental retardation were far more common and still occur in the nonindustrialized world.[55]

After the development of postnatal surgical shunting, the prognosis of isolated hydrocephalus improved greatly. Most neonatal deaths are attributable to associated anomalies as well as obstetric trauma from cephalocentesis. Intellectual development is related to the etiology, and not necessarily to the severity of the hydrocephalus.[56,57] The association between the age at initial shunt placement and intellectual development is controversial.[58,59] Infants with associated central nervous system anomalies or secondary hydrocephalus related to other defects such as Dandy-Walker malformation or porencephaly have significantly lower IQs than infants with isolated hydrocephalus.[60,61] In addition, infants with congenital hydrocephalus have somewhat lower overall survival rates compared to infants who develop hydrocephalus in the neonatal period.[62] Recently, a 10-year follow-up study of 129 consecutive children with non–tumor-related hydrocephalus who underwent their first shunt insertion before age 2[63] had an overall mortality rate below 10%. However, motor deficits were found in 60%, visual or auditory deficits in 25%, and epilepsy

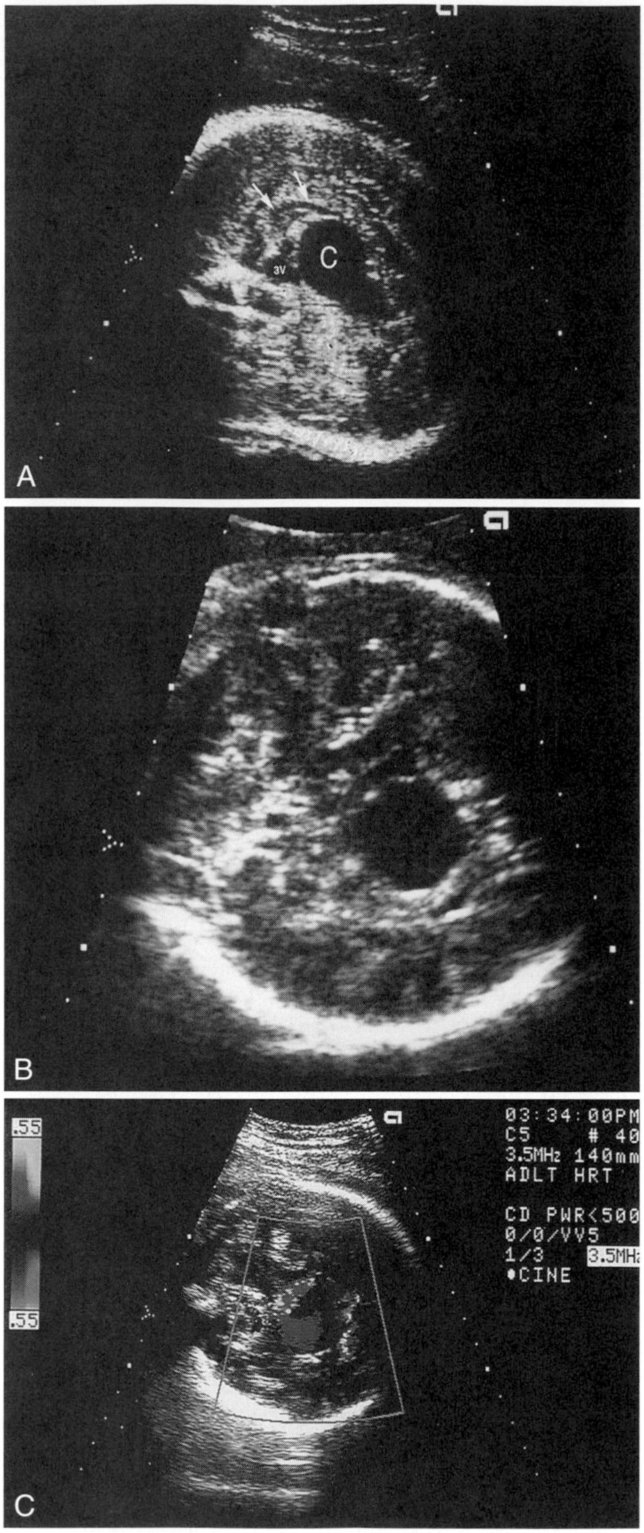

FIGURE 18–15
A, Midsagittal view of fetal head demonstrating large intracranial fluid-like collection (C), third ventricle (3V), and corpus callosum (*arrows*). *B*, Transverse section of fetal head demonstrating large intracranial fluid-like collection. *C*, Transverse section through fetal head using color Doppler demonstrating blood flow in cystic structure, vein of Galen (see Color Plate 26).

in 30%. Intellectual deficits were common and 40% had an IQ below 70. Only 32% of the children had an IQ above 90. Other studies have reported similar long-term intellectual prognosis.[64,65]

Once fetal hydrocephalus is identified, a careful sonographic search for associated fetal anomalies, including meningomyelocele, is mandatory. Because hydrocephalus is among the extracardiac anomalies associated with congenital heart disease, fetal echocardiography should also be performed. Up to 10% have a chromosomal aberration.[66,67] The obstetric management of fetal hydrocephalus reflects the gestational age at diagnosis, the presence of other anomalies, the results of the karyotype, and infectious studies and the views of the parents. If the diagnosis is made prior to fetal viability, the patient may consider pregnancy termination. If the karyotype is normal, and the parents wish to continue the pregnancy, serial ultrasound examinations are performed to identify progressive ventricular enlargement. In some cases, ventriculomegaly may regress in utero.

Although experimental placement of ventriculoamniotic shunts in fetal Rhesus monkeys yielded encouraging results, the experience in human pregnancies has to date been disappointing. A study of 39 fetal ventriculoamniotic shunt placements reported to the International Fetal Surgery Registry in 1993[68] listed 34 survivors: 14 had apparently normal neurodevelopment, and 18 had severe handicaps. The remaining two survivors had varying degrees of neurologic impairment. Children with intact intellectual development were all diagnosed with simple aqueductal stenosis. Of a total of seven deaths, four were directly attributed to the procedure. Many of the operated-on fetuses were misdiagnosed, errors that would be less likely to occur using MRI. Although most fetal medicine practitioners are not placing intrauterine ventriculoamniotic shunts, others believe it is time to revisit the issue.[69]

Labor and Delivery

Serial sonography may detect worsening hydrocephalus. In this situation, delivery should be considered as soon as pulmonary maturity in hopes of minimizing the potential ill effects of progressive ventricular enlargement. There is no clear indication for preterm delivery if the hydrocephalus is rapidly progressive prior to fetal lung maturity because respiratory distress syndrome, which would delay shunt placement, could actually worsen the final outcome. If delivery before fetal lung maturity is elected, maternal corticosteroids should be administered to hasten pulmonary maturity and reduce the risk and severity of respiratory distress syndrome. Fetuses with isolated disease and moderate to severe macrocephaly should be delivered by cesarean section to facilitate the atraumatic delivery of the enlarged fetal head. However, cesarean delivery is not necessary for all cases of fetal hydrocephalus. Attempted vaginal delivery is appropriate when the fetus is in vertex presentation and has only mild macrocephaly.

Fetal cortical mantle thickness correlates poorly with subsequent intelligence. Further, normal intelligence is possible for infants with hydrocephalus who receive optimal neonatal neurosurgical care. In cases of fetal hydrocephalus with associated anomalies that are either incompatible with life or associated with the severest forms of neurologic dysfunction (e.g., alobar holoprosencephaly, hydrancephaly, or thanatophoric dysplasia with cloverleaf skull), cephalocentesis and subsequent vaginal delivery are an acceptable alternative to cesarean delivery. Cephalocentesis is performed by passing a 14- to 18-gauge needle transabdominally or transvaginally under ultrasound guidance (Fig. 18–16), and removing sufficient cerebrospinal fluid to allow overlapping of the cranial sutures. This is a destructive procedure. In a recent series of three cases reported by Chasen and associates, all fetuses were stillborn with two delivering vaginally and one abdominally through a low transverse uterine incision.[70]

Postnatal and Prepregnancy

Hydrocephalus has diverse etiologies and the identification of its specific cause aids greatly the subsequent genetic counseling. A postmortem examination is essential. Several heritable patterns are recognized. X-linked recessive aqueductal stenosis carries a 1:4 risk of recurrence in future pregnancies, or 1:2 risk for male fetuses. Cerebellar agenesis with hydrocephalus is extremely rare, but also may be X-linked. Hydrocephalus is also associated with a variety of chromosomal abnormalities including triploidy, trisomies 13, 18, and 21, and certain balanced translocations. The risk of recurrence is relatively low for sporadic chromosomal abnormalities but is much higher for balanced translocations.

Additionally, hydrocephalus is associated with several syndromes that manifest dominant inheritance (e.g., achondroplasia and osteogenesis imperfecta).[71] The Dandy-Walker syndrome has been reported in siblings, suggesting the possibility of autosomal recessive inheritance. Several studies suggest an increased risk of uncomplicated hydrocephalus in families with neural tube defects. Lorber and De[72] studied uncomplicated congenital hydrocephalus and found an empiric risk of 4% for a central nervous system malformation and 2% for spina bifida or hydrocephalus in future pregnancies. Other causes of fetal hydrocephalus include prenatal infection (i.e., toxoplasmosis), intracranial tumors or cysts, and vascular malformations. Such causes are unlikely to result in an increased risk of hydrocephalus in future pregnancies.

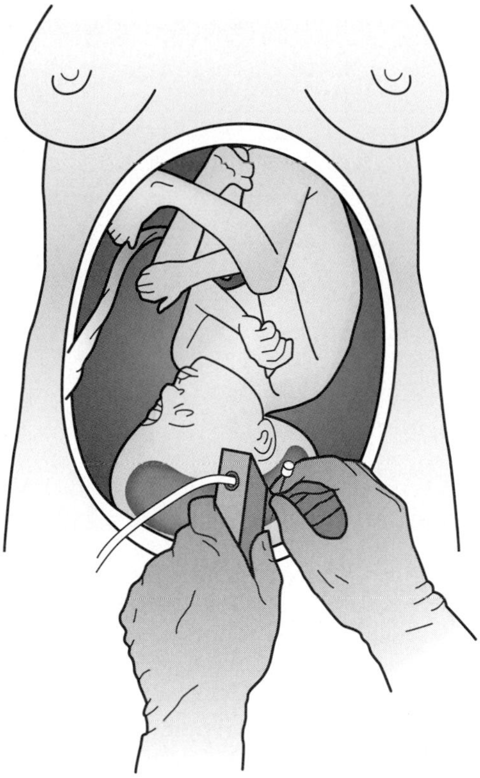

FIGURE 18–16
Sonographic guidance of the needle during cephalocentesis.

SUMMARY OF MANAGEMENT OPTIONS

Hydrocephalus

Management Options	Quality of Evidence	Strength of Recommendation	References
Prenatal			
Search for other anomalies including karyotype; magnetic resonance imaging often helps to clarify diagnosis; full workup is recommended for congenital infection.	III	B	66, 67, 87, 103
Provide cautious counseling regarding prognosis if isolated finding.	–	GPP	–
Interdisciplinary approach is indicated.	–	GPP	–
Termination remains an option.	–	GPP	–
In continuing pregnancy:			
Interdisciplinary care	–	GPP	–
Serial scans to identify progressive dilation of ventricles and head enlargement	–	GPP	–
No basis for fetal shunt placement	III	B	69

Continued

SUMMARY OF MANAGEMENT OPTIONS
Hydrocephalus *(Continued)*

Management Options	Quality of Evidence	Strength of Recommendation	References
Labor and Delivery			
No evidence supports preterm delivery with worsening ventriculomegaly; deliver fetus when risk of prematurity is low.	–	GPP	–
No evidence supports cesarean delivery a priori, but cesarean section with excessive ventriculomegaly is common.	–	GPP	–
Cephalocentesis is potentially destructive and not to be used if optimal survival is the aim.	III	B	70
Postnatal and Prepregnancy			
Establish cause and type.	–	GPP	–
Provide counseling.	–	GPP	–
Provide pediatric neurosurgical management.	–	GPP	–
Necropsy is performed for abortuses/stillbirths/neonatal deaths.	–	GPP	–

CRANIOFACIAL DISORDERS OF VENTRAL INDUCTION: THE HOLOPROSENCEPHALY SEQUENCE

General

The prechordal mesoderm, an embryonic connective mass between the undersurface of the neural tube and the oral cavity, is thought to be responsible for both the division of the prosencephalon, or forebrain, and the production of the nasofrontal process. The term holoprosencephaly includes several cerebral abnormalities that share incomplete cleavage of the primitive prosencephalon. Because of the underlying embryologic insult, various midline facial abnormalities are closely associated with holoprosencephaly, although the face can be normal (Fig. 18–17). The incidence of holoprosencephaly approximates 1 in 10,000 live births.[73] Holoprosencephaly is divided into alobar, semilobar, and lobar categories, based on the degree of separation of the cerebral hemispheres (Fig. 18–18). The alobar form is the most severe, with no evidence of cerebral cortical division.

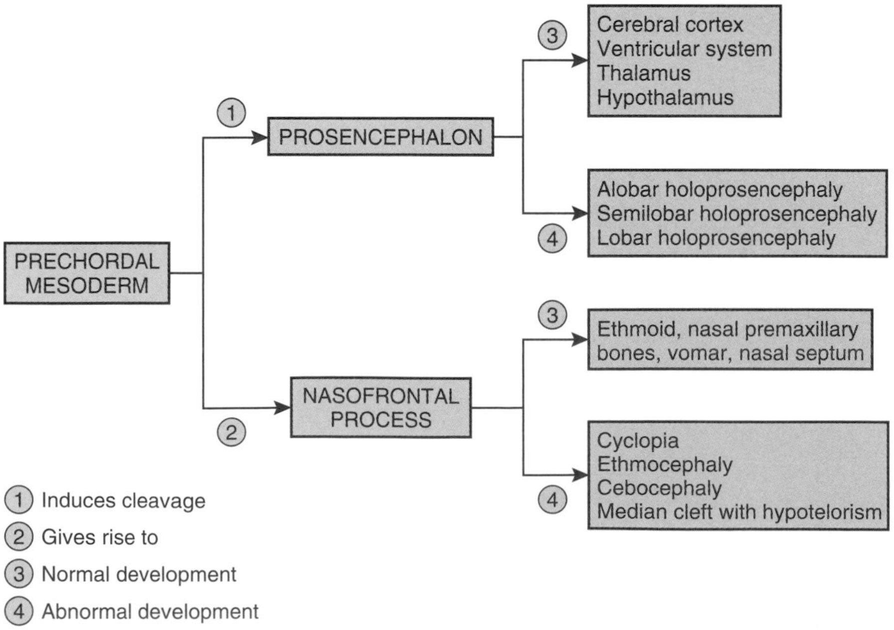

FIGURE 18–17
Embryology of holoprosencephaly and midline facial defects.

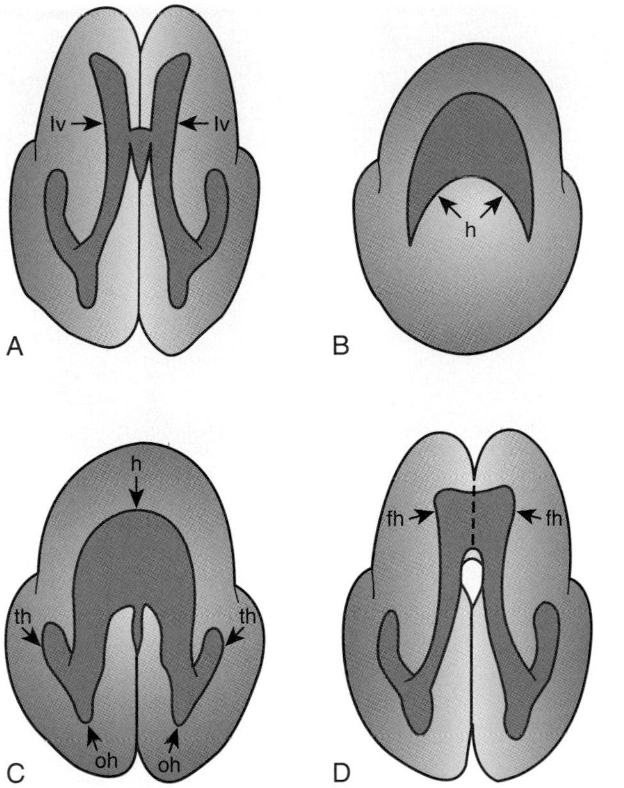

FIGURE 18–18
Schematic representation of the alobar, semilobar, and lobar forms of holoprosencephaly. *A*, Normal brain. Both the cerebral hemispheres and the lateral ventricles are separated. *B*, Alobar holoprosencephaly. The normal division of the cerebral hemispheres is absent, and there is a single ventricular cavity. *C*, Semilobar holoprosencephaly, showing an incomplete separation of the cerebral hemispheres in the occipital area and partial development of the occipital and temporal horns of the lateral ventricles. *D*, Lobar holoprosencephaly. Separation of the cerebral hemispheres and lateral ventricles is nearly complete except for the frontal portions. The frontal horns of the lateral ventricles are usually mildly dilated. (From Pilu G, Romero R, Rizzo N, et al: Criteria for the prenatal diagnosis of holoprosencephaly. Am J Perinatol 1987;4:41–49.)

The falx cerebri and the interhemispheric fissure are absent. There is a common ventricle with fused thalami. The semilobar and lobar forms represent a higher degree of brain development with the semilobar having partial separation of the hemispheres. Although there is much variability in the types of defects in the midline cerebral structures (corpus callosum, septum pellucidum, thalamus, etc.), the olfactory tracts and bulbs are usually absent, explaining the older term "arrhinencephaly."

The holoprosencephaly sequence results in the following characteristic facial findings (Fig. 18–19):

- Cyclopia with one median orbit, proboscis from the lower forehead, and absent nose
- Ethmocephaly with proboscis between two narrowly placed orbits and absent nose
- Cebocephaly with hypotelorism and rudimentary nose (single nostril)
- Hypotelorism (decreased intraorbital distance), median cleft lip, and flat nose
- Bilateral cleft lip

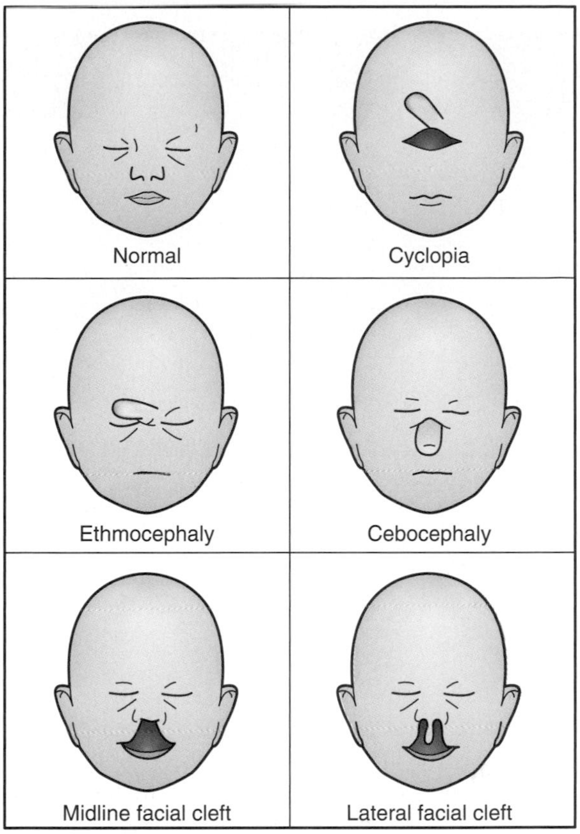

FIGURE 18–19
Schematic drawings of the facies associated with holoprosencephaly. (From Mahony BS, Hegge FN: The face and neck. In Nyberg DA, Mahony BS, Pretorius DH [eds]: Diagnostic Ultrasound of Fetal Anomalies: Text and Atlas. Chicago, Year Book, 1990, pp 203–261.)

Diagnosis

The dictum "the face predicts the brain" is often used to describe holoprosencephaly, as cyclopia, ethmocephaly, cebocephaly, and hypotelorism with midline cleft lip are commonly found in association with this central nervous system anomaly.[74] Sonographic markers include hypotelorism and a single common cerebral ventricle with absent midline echo (Fig. 18–20). The general appearance of the face, the position and configuration of the nose, and the integrity of the upper lip should be observed closely for clues. It may be impossible to differentiate semilobar from lobar holoprosencephaly before birth.

It is not sufficient to diagnose holoprosencephaly based solely on a central fluid collection in the brain, as this may also represent hydranencephaly or a midline porencephalic cyst. Other anatomic aberrations associated with holoprosencephaly detectable by ultrasonography include hydrocephalus, polydactyly, and hydramnios.

Management Options

Prenatal

The prognosis for alobar holoprosencephaly is uniformly poor. Most infants die shortly after birth, and the

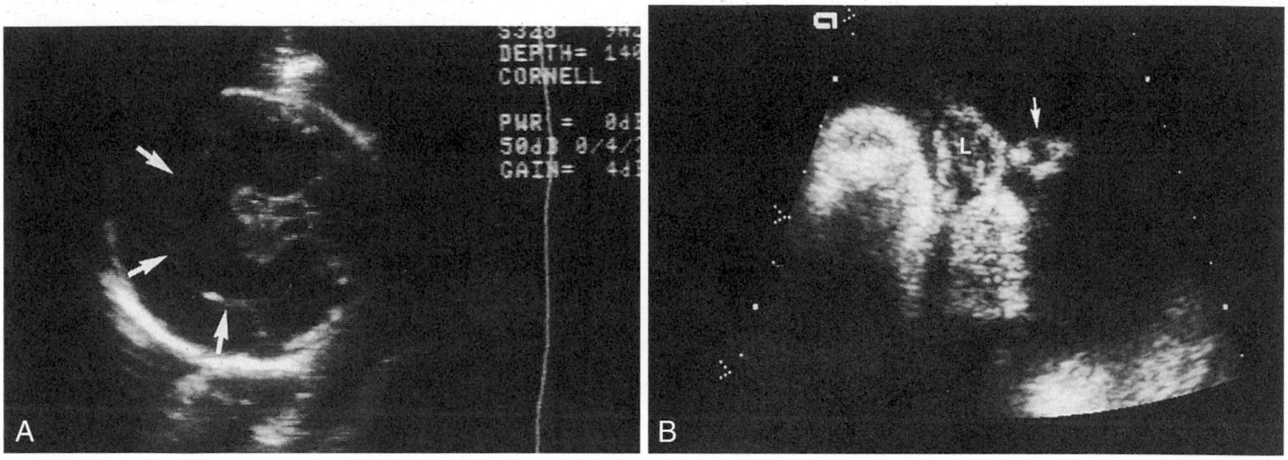

FIGURE 18–20
A, Transverse section demonstrating alobar holoprosencephaly with single ventricle (*arrows*), prominent fused thalamus, and compressed cerebral cortex. *B*, Coronal view of single nostril cebocephaly through lower face, upper lip, lower lip. Single nostril (*arrow*), lips (L).

survivors have profound mental retardation.[75] Less is known about the prognosis for lobar and semilobar varieties. A normal life span is reported, but many are severely mentally retarded. Subtle forms of lobar holoprosencephaly with little neurologic abnormality may exist. Karyotyping should be offered because of the association with aneuploidy (especially trisomy 13).

Labor and Delivery

The obstetric management of holoprosencephaly is dependent on gestational age at the time of diagnosis. Many patients opt for pregnancy termination when the diagnosis is made in the first or second trimester. Macrocephaly in the third trimester may obstruct labor, and cephalocentesis should be considered to avoid cesarean delivery. The destructive nature of this procedure must be explained to the parents.

Postnatal and Prepregnancy

The diagnosis of holoprosencephaly signals the need for a careful postmortem examination and a fetal karyotype to guide the management of future pregnancies. A chromosomal anomaly may predict either a recurrence risk less than 1% (as when a trisomy is demonstrated), or a much higher risk if there is a translocation in one of the parents.

Absent a chromosomal abnormality, the reported empiric risk for recurrence ranges from 6% to 14%,[76,77] although some families have a 25% risk associated with autosomal recessive inheritance. Rarely, autosomal dominant inheritance is present, predicting a 50% recurrence rate. A close examination of both parents for minor signs of midline facial abnormalities (e.g., hypotelorism) is essential to rule out this possibility. Last, maternal diabetes should be excluded, as it significantly increases the risk of holoprosencephaly.[78]

SUMMARY OF MANAGEMENT OPTIONS

Disorders of Ventral Induction: The Holoprosencephaly Sequence

Management Options	Quality of Evidence	Strength of Recommendation	References
Prenatal			
Scan and magnetic resonance imaging are used to clarify the extent of abnormalities.	III	B	87, 103
Karyotype is advised.	III	B	75
Provide counseling.	III	B	75
Interdisciplinary approach is warranted.	–	GPP	–
Offer pregnancy termination (prognosis poor) or induction of labor.	–	GPP	–

SUMMARY OF MANAGEMENT OPTIONS

Disorders of Ventral Induction: The Holoprosencephaly Sequence

Management Options	Quality of Evidence	Strength of Recommendation	References
Labor and Delivery			
Aim for vaginal delivery; cephalocentesis is ethically justified in cases of severe macrocephaly to avoid cesarean section, but warn parents that this is a destructive procedure.	III	B	70
Postnatal			
Necropsy is performed if abortus/stillbirth/neonatal death.	–	GPP	–
Karyotype if not already done.	III	B	75
Check family history.	–	GPP	–
Screen for diabetes.	III	B	78
Provide counseling.	–	GPP	–

FACIAL CLEFTS

General

Cleft lip or palate is the most common congenital facial deformity diagnosed at birth.[79] It results from failure of the nasofrontal prominence to fuse with the maxillary process. Clefts may be complete, incomplete, unilateral or bilateral, symmetrical or asymmetrical. Although more than 100 syndromes are associated with cleft lip or palate, these syndromes probably account for fewer than 10% of cases, as the majority are isolated. A multifactorial etiology is reflected in the varied incidences depending on race, sex, and geographic location. Similar to other lesions with a multifactorial etiology, the empiric recurrence risk increases with the number of previously affected siblings.

Diagnosis

The lower portion of the face must be anterior and clearly visualized in order to demonstrate a facial cleft on antenatal ultrasound (Fig. 18–21). The coronal, sagittal, and transverse planes are used to clearly assess the features of the lower face. Facial clefts may be suspected when either undulating tongue movements, hypertrophied tissue at the edge of the cleft, or hypertelorism is seen on ultrasound. An intact lip does not mean the palate is intact. Transverse sections may reveal a break in the maxillary ridge. Caution is necessary to avoid a false-positive diagnosis from a shadowing artifact produced by the maxillary bones. The availability of three-dimensional ultrasound may facilitate visualization of the precise location and extent of facial clefting.[80,81]

Management Options

It is important to search carefully for other anomalies after a facial cleft is identified. Fetal karyotyping should be offered. The prognosis and management depend on the presence of associated abnormalities and the severity of the defect. If the cleft appears isolated, then the prognosis is excellent. Staged plastic surgical correction is typically offered early in infancy, though the timing of the repairs remains controversial. Prior to surgery, the newborn may experience some difficulty feeding, but this is usually remedied with a specially designed artificial palate. Antenatal diagnosis of a cleft may help the parents prepare for a visually disturbing deformity that is typically correctable and allows the birth to occur with a treatment plan in place.

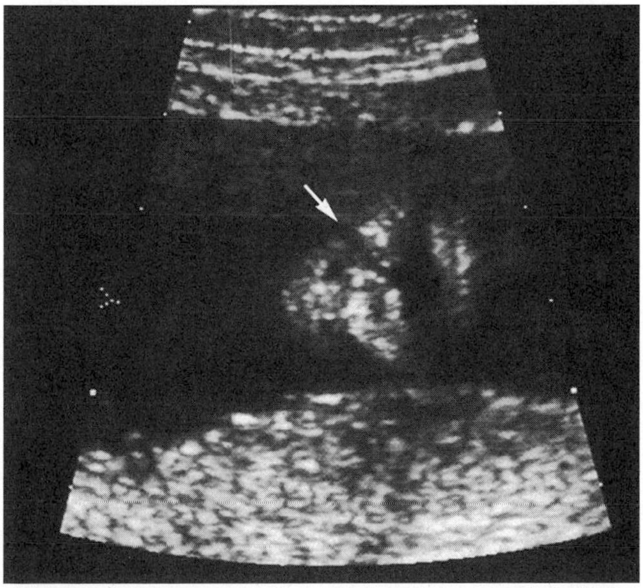

FIGURE 18–21
Coronal section through lower face demonstrating unilateral cleft lip (*arrow*).

SUMMARY OF MANAGEMENT OPTIONS
Facial Clefts

Management Options	Quality of Evidence	Strength of Recommendation	References
Prenatal			
Carefully search for other anomalies.	–	GPP	–
Karyotype.	–	GPP	–
Prognosis depends on cause and severity (good if isolated).	–	GPP	–
Provide counseling with interdisciplinary approach.	–	GPP	–
Postnatal			
Provide counseling.	–	GPP	–
Special measures are needed for infant feeding.	–	GPP	–
Early pediatric surgery is indicated.	–	GPP	–

DANDY-WALKER MALFORMATION

General

The Dandy-Walker malformation is characterized by the complete or partial absence of the cerebellar vermis and an enlarged posterior fossa cyst continuous with the fourth ventricle (Fig. 18–22). Hydrocephalus with ventriculomegaly is often present. Theories on pathogenesis include atresia of the foramina of Lushka and Magendie, and hypoplasia or gross alteration of the cerebellum. In addition to the classic Dandy-Walker malformation, a Dandy-Walker variant indicates a spectrum of anomalies classified by variable hypoplasia of the cerebellar vermis with or without enlargement of the posterior fossa. The Dandy-Walker malformation occurs in approximately 1 in 30,000 births, and is diagnosed in 4% to 12% of all cases of infantile hydrocephalus.[82] There is an increased risk of chromosomal anomalies and mendelian syndromes. In the absence of a genetic syndrome, the recurrence risk is probably about 1% to 5%.[83] The Dandy-Walker malformation occurs with increased frequency in families with a history of polycystic kidney disease and after the birth of a child with another central nervous system abnormality. Autosomal recessive inheritance is documented in some families.

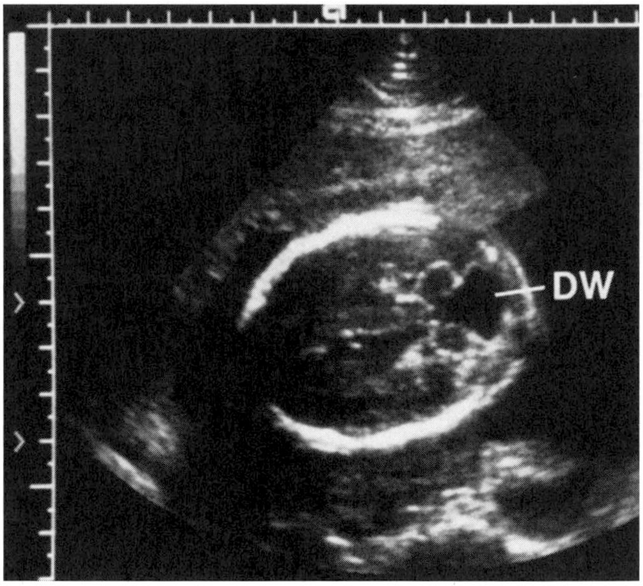

FIGURE 18–22
Suboccipital bregmatic view demonstrating Dandy-Walker cyst (DW) with defect in the cerebellar vermis and its communication with the fourth ventricle.

Diagnosis

Dandy-Walker cyst appears on ultrasound as an echo-spared area in the posterior fossa. The cerebellar vermis, a bright echogenic midline structure caudal to the fourth ventricle, is absent or defective. As a result, the Dandy-Walker cyst is seen communicating with the fourth ventricle. Hydrocephalus usually involves all four ventricles.

Management Options

The prognosis for infants with a Dandy-Walker malformation is quite variable. A relatively recent review of 50 cases of Dandy-Walker malformation and 49 cases of Dandy-Walker variant diagnosed by antenatal ultrasound[84] noted a frequent occurrence of associated anomalies and aneploidy. Of fetuses with a classic Dandy-Walker malformation, 85% had other anomalies (32% ventriculomegaly and 38% cardiac defects) and 46% were aneuploid. Of the fetuses with Dandy-Walker variant, 85% had other anomalies (27% ventriculomegaly and 41% cardiac defects) with a 36% aneuploidy rate. Fifty of the 99 women elected pregnancy termination. Of the remaining 49 fetuses, 16 survived the neonatal period with only 8 having a normal pediatric examination at 6 weeks, including 6 with an isolated finding of Dandy-Walker variant. Clearly, the overall prognosis is not good and the presence of other anomalies is associated with the worst prognosis.

Hydrocephalus and associated anomalies are more common in cases diagnosed in utero and the prognosis is less favorable. The option of pregnancy termination should be discussed with the parents. There is an increased risk of chromosomal anomalies and mendelian syndromes associated with the Dandy-Walker malformation, and it occurs at higher frequency in families with a history of polycystic kidney disease and after the birth of a previous child with Dandy-Walker malformation. Autosomal recessive inheritance is documented in some families. In the absence of a clear genetic syndrome, the recurrence risk is between 1% and 5%.[82]

SUMMARY OF MANAGEMENT OPTIONS

Dandy-Walker Malformation

Management Options	Quality of Evidence	Strength of Recommendation	References
Prenatal			
Careful detailed scan and magnetic resonance imaging are needed.	III	B	84, 87, 103
Interdisciplinary approach includes cautious counseling; prognosis is difficult to predict and largely influenced by other abnormalities.	III	B	10–12
Genetic counseling is needed if there is a family history.	III	B	82
Pregnancy termination remains an option.	–	GPP	–
Labor and Delivery			
No evidence contraindicates vaginal delivery.	–	GPP	–
Postnatal and Neonatal			
Careful neonatal review and follow-up are needed.	–	GPP	–

ANEURYSM OF THE VEIN OF GALEN

The cerebral veins may enlarge as a direct result of arterial fistula or adjacent arteriovenous malformation. Aneurysmal dilation of the great vein of Galen from an arteriovenous malformation is well documented. The dilated vein appears on ultrasound as a nonpulsatile, midcerebral tubular structure often seen behind the third ventricle (see Fig 18–15).[85,86] MRI and three-dimensional ultrasonography can be useful adjuncts to definitively diagnose an aneurysm of the vein of Galen antenatally.[87,88] The lesion may be isolated or associated with fetal hydrocephalus or other abnormalities. The increased intracranial blood flow to a low-resistance shunt can cause cardiomegaly and hydrops, and serial studies are indicated to monitor for the development of fetal hydrops. Traditionally, the prognosis for neonates with an aneurysm of the vein of Galen was considered poor, as many die from heart failure.[89] However, recent therapeutic advances may be improving outcome. In one study of 18 cases of antenatally diagnosed vein of Galen aneurysm, the neonatal mortality rate was 25% despite evidence of cardiac deterioration in 94%. All survivors required digoxin therapy. Neurologic development was normal in 67% of the surviving neonates.[90]

SUMMARY OF MANAGEMENT OPTIONS

Aneurysm of the Vein of Galen

Management Options	Quality of Evidence	Strength of Recommendation	References
Prenatal			
Color flow Doppler is used to differentiate from hydrocephalus and porencephalic cyst.	III	B	III
Three-dimensional ultrasound and magnetic resonance imaging help to elucidate the extent of the lesion.	III	B	87, 103
Provide counseling with interdisciplinary approach.	–	GPP	–
Prognosis is difficult to predict but is no longer uniformly poor.	III	B	90
Maintain vigilance for the development of hydrops, hydrocephalus, or other abnormalities.	–	GPP	–
Labor and Delivery			
No data guide the mode of delivery; many avoid vaginal delivery empirically to avoid cerebral (and hence aneurysm) trauma.	–	GPP	–
Delivery should take place in a tertiary center with facilities for all potential neonatal care options.	–	GPP	–
Postnatal and Neonatal			
Main significant therapeutic advance is in the use of embolization for occluding the aneurysm.	III	B	90

HYDRANENCEPHALY

General

Hydranencephaly is characterized by replacement of the cerebral hemispheres with fluid covered by leptomeninges such that no cerebral cortex is present. Only the basal ganglia and remnants of the mesencephalon remain within a normally formed skull above the tentorium cerebelli. The subtentorial structures are usually intact, and the falx cerebri is frequently present. Hydranencephaly is thought to result from a severe destructive insult, most likely bilateral occlusion of the internal carotid arteries.

Diagnosis

Ultrasonographic findings include a normal cranial vault filled with fluid. The cerebral cortex is absent, but a midline echo, the tentorium cerebelli, and cerebellum may be visible. This disorder is differentiated from hydrocephalus, holoprosencephaly, and porencephaly by the absence of cerebral cortex. In severe hydrocephalus, the thin cortical mantle may be hard to detect sonographically and MRI or less frequently used intrauterine computed tomography scanning may aid the diagnosis (Fig. 18–23).

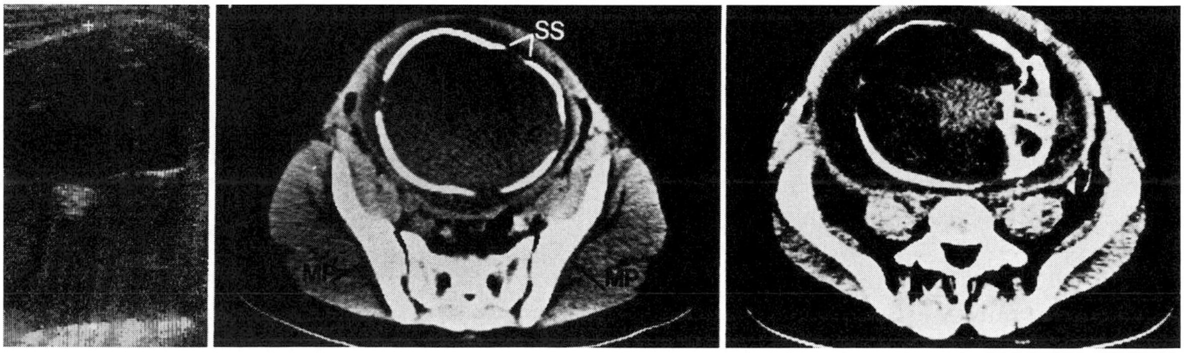

FIGURE 18–23
In utero computed tomogram showing widening of sutures of fetal calvarium. Skull is filled by homogeneous low-density fluid with no evidence of cortex present. MP, maternal pelvis; SS separated suture. (From Chervanak FA, Berkowitz RL, Romero R, et al: The diagnosis of fetal hydrocephalus. Am J Obstet Gynecol 1983;147:703–716.)

Management Options

Most infants with hydranencephaly die in the first year of life. Survivors are profoundly retarded. Sporadic familial recurrences are reported, but these are the exception. In general, the recurrence risk is negligible. The option for pregnancy termination should be offered to the parents when the diagnosis is firm.

SUMMARY OF MANAGEMENT OPTIONS

Hydranencephaly

Management Options	Quality of Evidence	Strength of Recommendation	References
Prenatal			
Karyotype.	–	GPP	–
Counsel parents about poor prognosis.	–	GPP	–
Offer termination or induction of labor.	–	GPP	–

MICROCEPHALY

General

Strictly translated, microcephaly means "small head." The clinical importance of the entity is its association with mental retardation. Some authors classify postnatal microcephaly as a head perimeter smaller than 2 standard deviations (SD) below the mean.[91] Alternatively, a definition of 3 SD below the mean for gender and age may correlate better with mental retardation.[92]

Diagnosis

The postnatal diagnosis of microcephaly is made simply by measuring the neonatal head circumference, but the antenatal diagnosis is more difficult. The head circumference is preferable to the biparietal diameter (BPD), which carries a high false-positive rate because of such normal variants as dolichocephaly. Serial ultrasound examinations are important in suspected cases, as significant microcephaly may not manifest until the third trimester.

Management Options

Prenatal

Because microcephaly is a part of many different malformation syndromes, a careful sonographic search for associated anomalies is mandatory. Cortical mass may be decreased in microcephaly, leading to ventriculomegaly in the absence of an obstructive process. A careful pedigree should be taken and a search made for causes, including possible teratogen exposure, alcohol abuse, and infection. The definitive diagnosis of fetal infection requires an invasive procedure: Amniocentesis and even cordocentesis are often necessary.

The majority of microcephalic children are mentally retarded, many severely so. As a rule, the smaller the head, the worse the prognosis. If microcephaly occurs as part of a genetic syndrome (e.g., Meckel-Gruber syndrome), the outcome is uniformly poor. However, children born with microcephaly may have normal intelligence despite their very small head size.

Labor and Delivery

Vaginal delivery of a microcephalic infant is appropriate. Shoulder dystocia due to incomplete dilation of the cervix by the small fetal head is a rare occurrence.

Postnatal and Prepregnancy

The risk of recurrence for microcephaly depends on the underlying etiology. The search for an etiology should include a physical examination of the infant, a maternal history for teratogenic exposure, a careful family pedigree, chromosomal, microbiologic, and serologic studies, and an autopsy should death occur. Alcohol abuse is a common cause of mental retardation, and often associated with microcephaly. Several patterns of inheritance are described within the subgroup of microcephaly without associated anomalies, which is termed "true" microcephaly. These patterns include autosomal recessive, autosomal dominant with incomplete penetrance, and sporadic patterns of inheritance.

SUMMARY OF MANAGEMENT OPTIONS
Microcephaly

Management Options	Quality of Evidence	Strength of Recommendation	References
Prenatal			
A careful ultrasound search for other anomalies is undertaken.	–	GPP	–
Magnetic resonance imaging is performed to elucidate the extent of cortical loss.	III	B	87,103
Karyotype and full workup needed for congenital infection.	–	GPP	–
Look for history of teratogens, alcohol use, family history, infection.	–	GPP	–
Exercise caution with counseling because prognosis is difficult to predict.	–	GPP	–
Labor and Delivery			
Aim for vaginal delivery; shoulder dystocia is very rare.	–	GPP	–
Postnatal and Prepregnancy			
Establish cause if not already done (teratogens, alcohol use, family history, karyotype, infection serology, necropsy).	–	GPP	–
Counseling will depend on cause.	–	GPP	–

AGENESIS OF THE CORPUS CALLOSUM

General

The corpus callosum is the great commissural plate of nerve fibers interconnecting the cortical hemispheres. It lies at the base of the interhemispheric fissure and curves in the midline, forming the roof of the third ventricle. Agenesis of the corpus callosum can occur as either an isolated anomaly or in association with other anomalies, such as hydrocephalus and holoprosencephaly. It is usually a sporadic occurrence, although it has been associated with various genetic syndromes, chromosomal abnormalities, and prenatal exposure to teratogens such as alcohol.

Diagnosis

Agenesis of the corpus callosum is diagnosed in utero on coronal and midline sagittal views of the fetal head, including the routine transverse planes. Transvaginal ultrasonography improves access to these planes by providing an acoustic window through the anterior fontanelle.

On a midsagittal ultrasound examination, the corpus callosum appears as a hypoechoic structure below the pericallosal artery, where it forms the roof of the cavum septum pellucidum and cavum vergae. (Fig. 18–24). Failure to image it suggests agenesis of the corpus callosum. However, it is quite difficult antenatally to be definitive. The pathognomonic "sunburst lesion" is seen on midsagittal section and represents the radial orientation of the gyri and sulci of the cerebral cortex to the third ventricle (Fig. 18–25). Normally, the gyri and sulci parallel the corpus callosum.[93] As the corpus callosum itself cannot be seen on transverse scan, it is necessary to

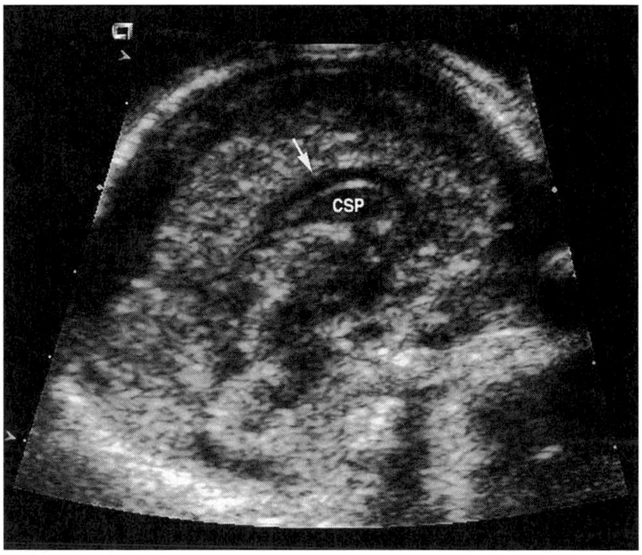

FIGURE 18–24
Midsagittal section through normal fetal cranium demonstrating the corpus callosum (*arrow*), the hypoechoic structure superior to the cavum septum pellucidum (CSP) (*arrows*).

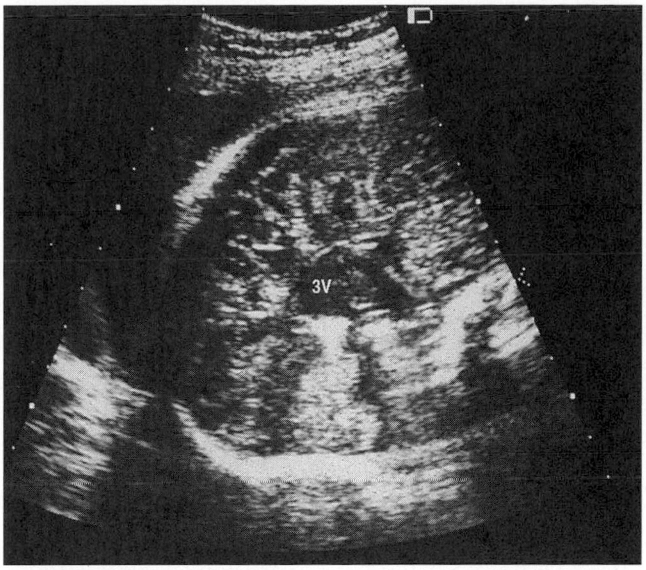

FIGURE 18–25
Midsagittal view of fetal head with agenesis of the corpus callosum demonstrating the pathognomonic "sunburst lesion" representing the radial orientation of the gyri and sulci of the cerebral cortex to the third ventricle (3V).

search for the anatomic alterations produced by its absence. These indications include lateral displacement of the bodies of the lateral ventricles, enlargement of the atria and occipital horns producing a characteristic tear-drop shape, and enlargement or upward displacement of the third ventricle (Fig. 18–26).

Management Options

The prognosis for a fetus with agenesis of the corpus callosum is highly variable and depends on the presence of associated defects. Management is based on these underlying anomalies. Agenesis of the corpus callosum has been reported as an incidental autopsy finding in intellectually normal adults[94] and caution should be exercised counseling patients when isolated agenesis of the corpus callosum is suspected. Three-dimensional ultrasonography and MRI may provide additional prognostic information.

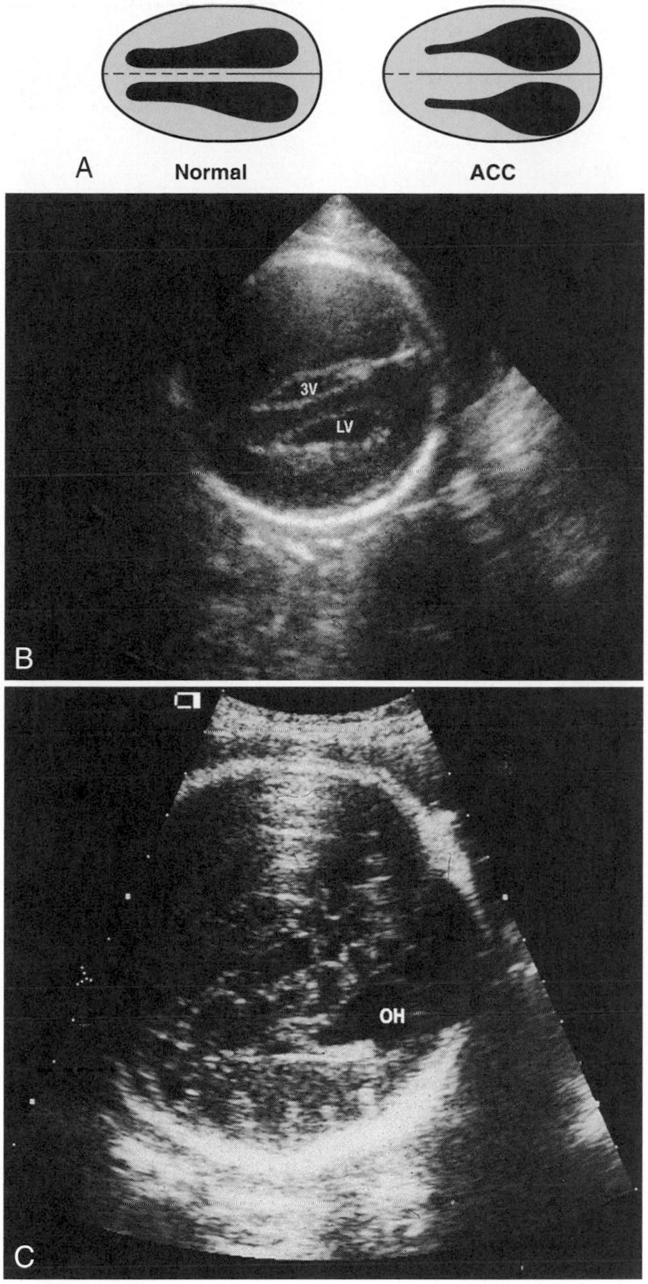

FIGURE 18–26
A, Schematic representation of agenesis of the corpus callosum in coronal view. *B*, Transverse section of a fetus in the second trimester with agenesis of the corpus callosum. Note the tear-drop shape of the lateral ventricle (LV) and the abnormal displacement of the third ventricle (3V). *C*, Transverse view of a fetus in the third trimester with agenesis of the corpus callosum with a tear-drop appearance of the lateral ventricle and prominent occipital horn (OH).

SUMMARY OF MANAGEMENT OPTIONS

Agenesis of the Corpus Callosum

Management Options	Quality of Evidence	Strength of Recommendation	References
Prenatal			
Make careful search for other anomalies.	–	GPP	–

Continued

SUMMARY OF MANAGEMENT OPTIONS

Agenesis of the Corpus Callosum *(Continued)*

Management Options	Quality of Evidence	Strength of Recommendation	References
Prenatal			
Magnetic resonance imaging may be helpful in further evaluation.	III	B	87, 103
Counseling depends on other lesions; prognosis for isolated condition is difficult to predict.	–	GPP	–
Pregnancy termination remains an option.	–	GPP	–

INTRACRANIAL HEMORRHAGE AND PORENCEPHALY

General

Bleeding within the head of the newborn is a well-recognized phenomenon. In particular, intraventricular hemorrhage is often associated with prematurity. When severe, it can produce obstructive hydrocephalus and intraparenchymal hemorrhage. On the other hand, the antenatal diagnosis of intracranial hemorrhage is uncommon. In most instances, hydrocephalus is first identified in association with echogenic areas of hemorrhage in the dilated ventricular system. Alloimmune thrombocytopenia may be the underlying cause of antenatally diagnosed intracranial hemorrhage (see Chapter 15).

Porencephaly describes a condition in which a portion of the cerebral cortex is replaced by a cystic cavity and is thought to represent the remains of a severe intrauterine insult. The cavity may communicate with the subarachnoid space or a ventricle (Fig. 18–27). Most cases result from a vascular lesion, either hemorrhagic or embolic. Areas of prior hemorrhage or tissue necrosis resorb, leaving behind porencephalic cysts. In rare cases, an infection or traumatic insult may result in porencephaly.

Diagnosis

Antenatal hemorrhage typically appears as an echogenic mass in the region of the germinal matrix or within the lateral ventricles (Fig. 18–28). Antenatal diagnosed intracranial hemorrhage is predominantly grade 3 or 4, using the established grading system for neonatal intracranial hemorrhage, which classifies grade 1 as isolated periventricular hemorrhage, grade 2 as intraventricular hemorrhage with normal ventricular size, grade 3 as intraventricular hemorrhage with acute ventricular dilation, and grade 4 as intraventricular hemorrhage with parenchymal involvement.[95] Consequently, these lesions are associated with a high perinatal mortality rate. These cases demonstrate that high-grade intraventricular hemorrhage can occur in the absence of birth trauma.

Porencephalic cysts appear sonographically as solitary or multiple echo-spared areas of variable size and location within the brain. The midline echo is present but may be displaced. Some cortical tissue may be preserved in each cerebral hemisphere. These distinctions help differentiate a large porencephalic cyst from unilateral hydrocephalus, holoprosencephaly, and hydranencephaly.

Although the prognostic validity of the grading system for neonatal intracranial hemorrhage is well estab-

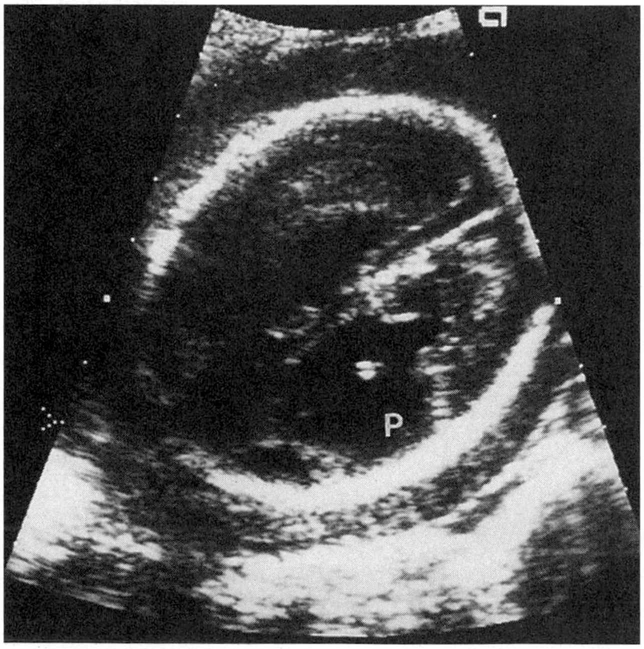

FIGURE 18–27
Transverse section of fetal head demonstrating porencephalic cyst (P) communicating with the ventricle.

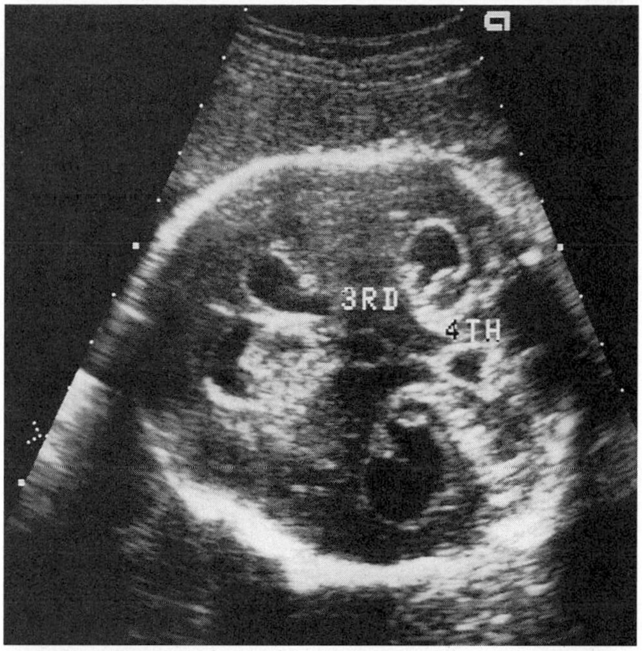

FIGURE 18–28
Transverse section of fetal head demonstrating an echogenic clot in the anterior horn of the lateral ventricle, the result of an intracranial hemorrhage. All the ventricles appear to be dilated. Third and fourth ventricles are shown.

lished, it has not been extensively evaluated in the antenatal period. Ghi and associates followed 109 cases of antenatally diagnosed intracranial hemorrhage and concluded that intracranial hemorrhage could be accurately identified and categorized by antenatal sonography.[96]

Management Options

When antenatal intracranial hemorrhage is diagnosed in the absence of an identifiable cause, a search for alloimmune thrombocytopenia is warranted. Serologic studies for intrauterine infection, a fetal karyotype for aneuploidy, and a workup for maternal infections including hepatitis and pancreatitis may also be of value.

The prognosis for porencephaly depends on the underlying etiology, location, and volume of tissue loss. The outcome in the majority of reported cases is poor.[97] Fortunately, there is no increased risk of recurrence unless alloimmune thrombocytopenia is diagnosed. Alloimmune thrombocytopenia carries a greater than 75% recurrence risk.[98]

SUMMARY OF MANAGEMENT OPTIONS
Intracranial Hemorrhage and Porencephaly

Management Options	Quality of Evidence	Strength of Recommendation	References
Prenatal			
These anomalies may be associated with severe maternal illness.	–	GPP	–
In absence of identifiable cause, workup for alloimmune thrombocytopenia and congenital infection; offer karyotype.	–	GPP	–
Prognosis is related to location and degree of tissue loss and is usually poor with larger lesions.	III	B	97
Postnatal and Prepregnancy			
Recurrence risk is relevant only for alloimmune thrombocytopenia.	III	B	98

CHOROID PLEXUS CYST

General

Small areas of cystic dilation are seen in the choroid plexus of the lateral ventricles in 1% to 2% of all fetuses (Fig. 18–29). They typically resolve before the end of the second trimester and lack clinical significance. Choroid plexus cysts may be associated with trisomy 18. However, the great majority of fetuses with trisomy 18 have other structural abnormalities detectable by ultrasonography.

Management Options

A karyotype is recommended for all fetuses with choroid plexus cysts associated with other structural abnormalities. However, the vast majority of isolated choroid

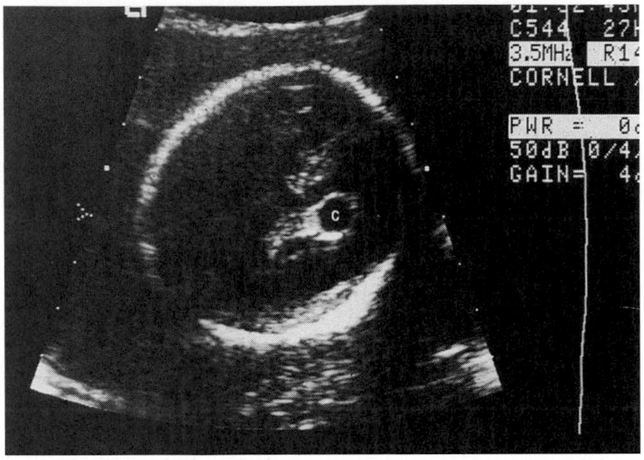

FIGURE 18–29
Transverse section demonstrating a choroid pexus cyst (C).

plexus cysts are clinically insignificant, and the need for genetic evaluation is controversial. A meta-analysis reported that the risk of trisomy 18 associated with an isolated choroid plexus cyst in all women was 1:374.[99] Another large study concluded an isolated choroid plexus cyst increased the midtrimester risk of trisomy 18 enough to justify genetic testing only in women over 35 years old.[100] Other large studies have concluded that isolated choroid plexus cysts in women under 35 years old do not increase the risk of trisomy 18 to a degree that amniocentesis is warranted.[101,102] We believe the presence of a choroid plexus cyst should be disclosed to the patient. However, counseling should take into account the presence of associated anomalies, the age of the patient, and the results of first- and second-trimester screening tests for aneuploidy.

SUMMARY OF MANAGEMENT OPTIONS

Choroid Plexus Cyst

Management Options	Quality of Evidence	Strength of Recommendation	References
Prenatal			
Make careful search for other structural abnormalities.	IIa	B	99
Karyotype if other anomalies are found	IIa	B	99
Risk of amniocentesis likely exceeds risk of aneuploidy in an otherwise low risk woman if isolated	III	B	100–102
Benign if isolated with normal chromosomes.	IIa	B	100–102

CYSTIC HYGROMA

General

Cystic hygromas are congenital malformations of the lymphatic system (Fig. 18–30). They appear as single or multiloculated, fluid-filled cavities lined by true epithelium. In fetal life, they are associated with a generalized disorder of lymphatic formation. Cystic hygromas may occur as isolated defects or as part of a variety of genetic syndromes (Fig. 18–31).

Diagnosis

Cystic hygromas can be diagnosed reliably by ultrasonography. Their posterolateral location and cystic appearance are characteristic. Larger hygromas are frequently divided by incomplete septa and often have a dense midline septum extending from the fetal neck across the full width of the hygroma (Fig. 18–32). Hydrops is often associated with cystic hygroma, as both may result from a defect in lymphatic formation. The sonographic features that differentiate a cystic hygroma from another craniocervical mass (e.g., cephalocele or other neural tube defects, cystic teratoma, or nuchal edema) include an intact skull and spinal column, lack of a solid component to the mass, a constant position of the mass relative to the fetal head, and the separation of cysts by septa.

Management Options

Prenatal

Once a cystic hygroma is detected, a careful search for skin edema, ascites, pleural or pericardial effusions, and cardiac or renal anomalies is indicated. A fetal karyotype is essential and may be performed by chorionic villus sampling in the first trimester or amniocentesis in the second trimester. When there is little fluid and the hygromas are large, the cyst can be aspirated and the karyotype obtained from the contained lymphocytes.

The prognosis and management depend on the underlying cause and any associated anomalies. The outlook is grave if there is hydrops and no treatable cause is identi-

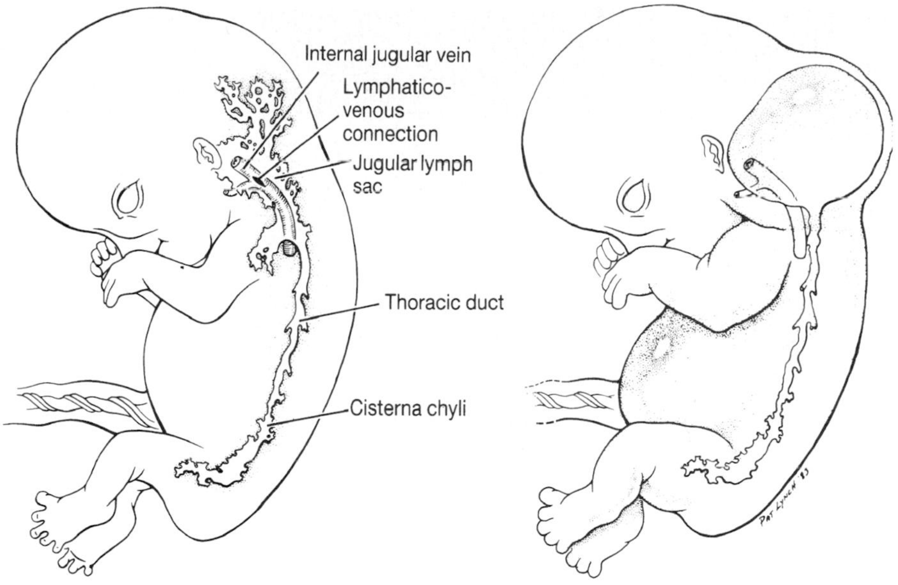

FIGURE 18–30
Lymphatic system in a normal fetus (*left*) with a patent connection between the jugular lymph sac and the internal jugular vein and a cystic hygroma and hydrops from a failed lymphaticovenous connection (*right*). (From Chervenak FA, Isaacson G, Blakemore KJ, et al: Fetal cystic hygroma. Cause and natural history. N Engl J Med 1983;309:822–825.)

fied. Isolated cystic hygromas may be surgically corrected postnatally and the prognosis for survival is then good. Some cystic hygroma regress in utero, leaving only a webbed neck. This may account for this physical feature in girls with Turner's syndrome.

Labor and Delivery

There is no evidence that cesarean delivery improves outcome.

Postnatal and Prepregnancy

A careful postmortem examination is recommended, and tissue for cytogenetic studies is obtained whenever there is an unstudied aborted or stillborn fetus. In live births, tissue samples may be taken from fetal membranes or from the newborn itself. Because these fetuses may have chromosomal mosaicism, several tissues should be studied before concluding they are euploid. The content of the postpartum counseling depends on the underlying cause.

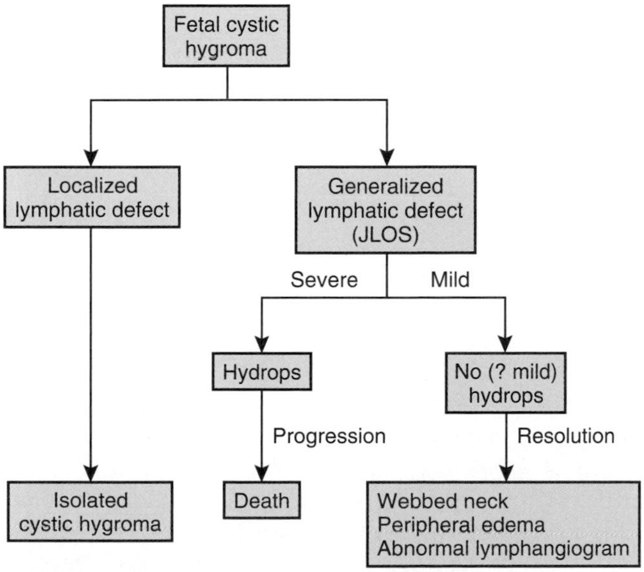

FIGURE 18–31
Natural history of fetal cystic hygroma. Generalized edema results from jugular-lymphatic-obstruction sequence (JLOS). (From Chervenak FA, Isaacson G, Blakemore KJ, et al: Fetal cystic hygroma. Cause and natural history. N Engl J Med 1983;309:822–825.)

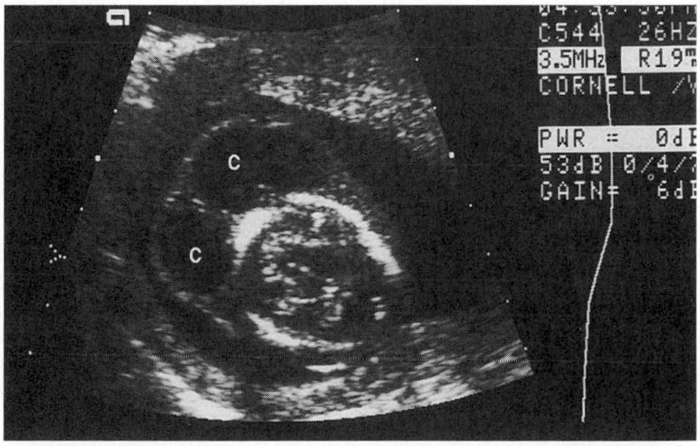

FIGURE 18–32
Sonogram demonstrating nuchal cystic hygroma (C) divided by a midline septum, nuchal ligament.

SUMMARY OF MANAGEMENT OPTIONS

Cystic Hygroma

Management Options	Quality of Evidence	Strength of Recommendation	References
Prenatal			
Make careful search for evidence of fetal hydrops and other anomalies.	–	GPP	–
Investigate as for nonimmune hydrops, including karyotype (see Chapter 25).	–	GPP	–
Prognosis and management depend on cause and other abnormalities.	–	GPP	–
Pregnancy termination is an option.	–	GPP	–
Labor and Delivery			
If pregnancy continues and cyst is massive, transabdominal aspiration of cyst fluid may allow vaginal delivery; cesarean section is rarely justified.	–	GPP	–
Postnatal			
Establish cause including necropsy if abortus/stillbirth/neonatal death.	–	GPP	–
Counseling depends on cause.	–	GPP	–
"Cosmetic" surgery may be needed if baby survives with "web neck."	–	GPP	–

CAUDAL REGRESSION SYNDROME

Caudal regression syndrome describes an embryologic malformation leading to structural defects in the caudal region. The severity is quite variable and may include incomplete development of the sacrum and lumbar vertebrae (Fig. 18–33) and disruption of the distal spinal cord, causing neurologic impairment. Caudal regression syndrome is strongly associated with maternal diabetes. Although this disorder was previously considered a severe form of sirenomelia, recent evidence suggests the two defects are pathogenetically unrelated.[70] The etiology of caudal regression syndrome is unknown and most likely heterogeneous.

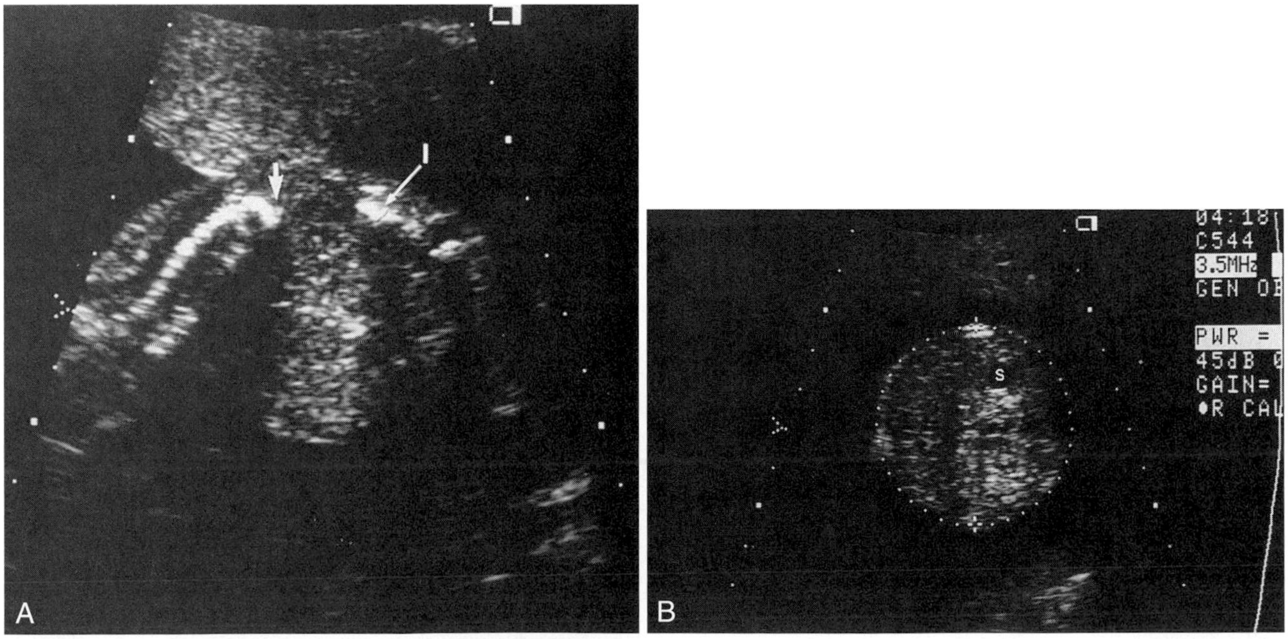

FIGURE 18–33
A, Longitudinal view of a fetus with caudal regression syndrome demonstrating the absence of vertebral bodies below the level of the thorax (*arrow*). I, iliac crest. *B*, Transverse view of a fetal abdomen at the level of the fetal stomach in a fetus with caudal regression syndrome demonstrating the absence of vertebral bodies below the level of the thorax.

SUMMARY OF MANAGEMENT OPTIONS

Caudal Regression Syndrome

Management Options	Quality of Evidence	Strength of Recommendation	References
Prenatal			
Determine degree of malformation.	–	GPP	–
Termination is an option.	–	GPP	–
Screen for diabetes.	–	GPP	–
Provide interdisciplinary counseling.	–	GPP	–
Postnatal			
Screen for diabetes.	–	GPP	–
Counseling is needed.	–	GPP	–

MAGNETIC RESONANCE IMAGING OF FETAL CENTRAL NERVOUS SYSTEM ANOMALIES

Ultrasonography is currently the primary imaging technique used for antenatal evaluation of fetal CNS anomalies when the ultrasonographic findings are not straightforward. The ability to make definitive diagnoses by ultrasound alone is often restricted by various factors, including reverberative artifacts from the bony calvarium, fetal position, oligohydramnios, and maternal body habitus. In addition, ultrasound often does not have the sensitivity to detect subtle abnormalities of fetal brain development.

MRI can enhance the diagnostic accuracy of ultrasound for the assessment of fetal brain abnormalities (Figs. 18–34 and 18–35).[87,103] MRI permits acquisition of multiplanar views of the fetal brain, allowing for a detailed evaluation of the CNS anatomy that is not possible using ultrasound alone. Additionally, MRI is not hindered by the same technical limitations of ultrasound, such as low amniotic fluid amount or fetal position. The use of ultrafast MRI techniques permits good quality brain images, even when there is fetal movement.[104,105] To date, there have been no reports of adverse fetal effects from MRI. Baker and associates evaluated children 3 years after prenatal MRI exposure and reported no deleterious effects.[106] The information obtained from the MRI may change management by enhancing the diagnostic accuracy. Sharma and associates recently described a series of pregnant patients with fetal brain abnormalities in whom MRI provided valuable additional information in all cases.[107] Ultrasound remains the standard modality for assessing fetal anatomy. Moreover, prenatal ultrasound allows for reliable detection of fetal brain abnormalities. However, MRI of the fetal CNS is evolving as a useful adjunct for obtaining additional information in cases in which confirmation of a suspected abnormality or further clarification is sought.

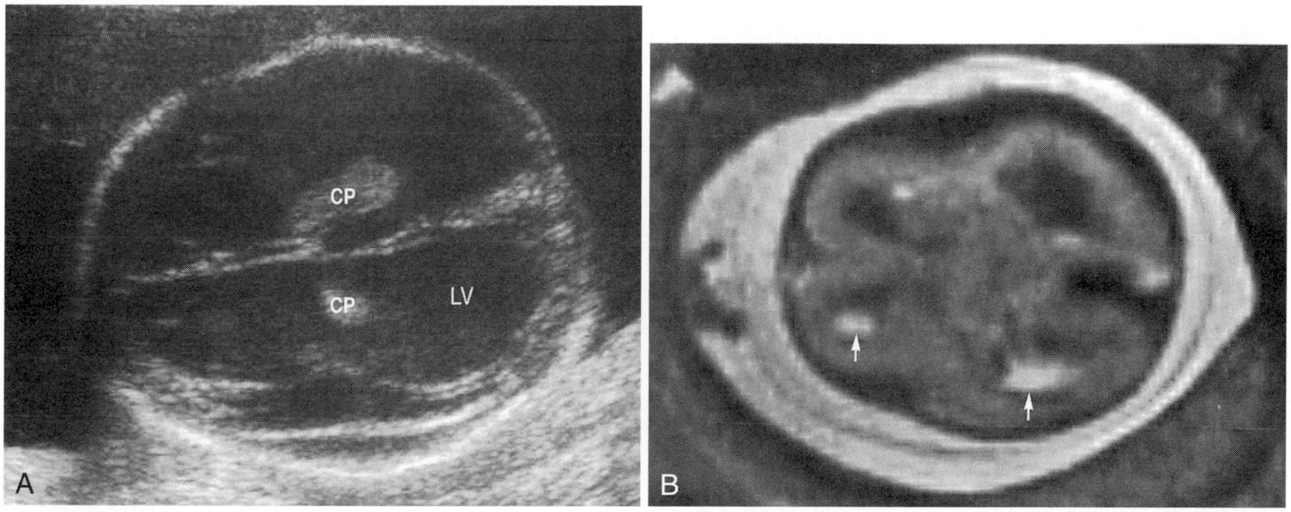

FIGURE 18–34
A, Transverse scan of fetal head demonstrating severe ventriculomegaly in an 18-week fetus. LV, lateral ventricle; CP, choroid plexus. *B*, T_1-weighted axial MRI of the same fetus demonstrating that a recent hemorrhagic event is causing the fetal ventriculomegaly. The bright areas represent hemorrhage within the ventricles (*arrows*).

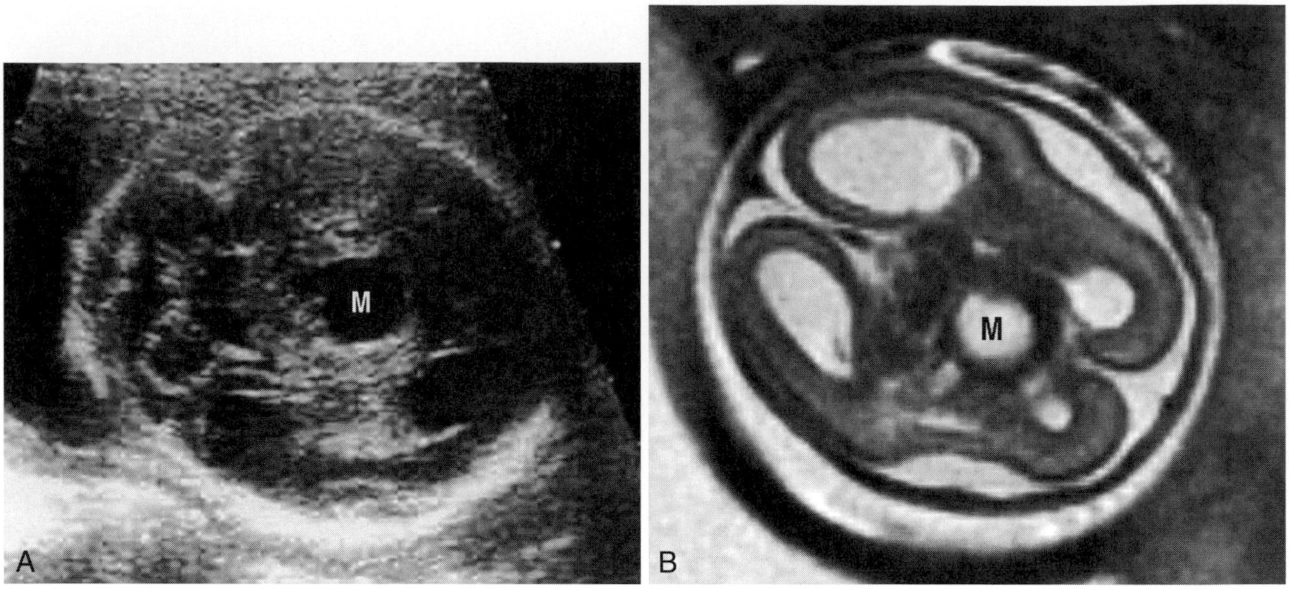

FIGURE 18–35
A, Suboccipital bregmatic view demonstrating an intracranial mass (M) of unclear etiology. *B*, T_2-weighted axial MRI demonstrating a well-marginated brain mass (M), probably representing a primary neoplasm.

CONCLUSIONS

- Craniospinal and facial abnormalities are among the more commonly detected fetal anomalies at the 20-week scan.
- Detailed ultrasound is required to elucidate the nature of the abnormality and to search for other anomalies.
- MRI may be a useful adjunct in the evaluation process.
- Karyotyping is indicated for many conditions.
- Interdisciplinary counseling is advisable.
- In utero therapeutic interventions are not currently of proven benefit, although clinical investigations are underway.

REFERENCES

1. Candfield MA, Annegers JF, Brender JD, et al: Hispanic origin and neural tube defects in Houston/Harris County Texas. II. Risk factors. Am J Epidemiol 1996;143:12–24.
2. Feuchtbaum LB, Currier RJ, Riggle S, et al: Neural tube defect prevalence in California (1990–1994): Eliciting patterns by type of defect and maternal race/ethnicity. Genet Test 1999;3:265–272.
3. Seller MJ: Sex, neural tube defects, and multisite closure of the human neural tube. Am J Med Genet 1995;158:332–336.
4. Ray JG, Meier C, Vermeulen MJ, et al: Association of neural tube defects and folic acid food fortification in Canada. Lancet 2002;360:2047–2048.
5. Hendricks KA, Nuno OM, Suarez L, Larsen R: Effects of hyperinsulinemia and obesity on risk of neural tube defects among Mexican Americans. Epidemiology 2001;12:630–635.
6. Shaw GM, Todoroff K, Finnell RH, Lammer EJ: Spina bifida phenotypes in infants or fetuses of obese mothers. Teratology 2000;61:376–381.
7. Watkins ML, Rasmussen SA, Honein MA, et al: Maternal obesity and risk for birth defects. Pediatrics 2003;111(5 Part 2):1152–1158.
8. Arpino C, Brescianini S, Robert E, et al: Teratogenic effects of antiepileptic drugs: Use of an International Database on Malformations and Drug Exposure (MADRE). Epilepsia 2000;41:1436–1443.
9. Yasuda Y, Konishi H, Kihara T, Tanimura T: Discontinuity of primary and secondary neural tube in spina bifida induced by retinoic acid in mice. Teratology 1990;41:257–274.
10. Ray JG, Blom HJ: Vitamin B12 insufficiency and the risk of fetal neural tube defects. Q J Med 2003;96:289–295.
11. Hume RF Jr, Drugan A, Reichler A, et al: Aneuploidy among prenatally detected neural tube defects. Am J Med Genet 1996;61:171–173.
12. Blaas HG, Eik-Nes SH, Isaksen CV: The detection of spina bifida before 10 gestational weeks using two- and three-dimensional ultrasound. Ultrasound Obstet Gynecol 2000;16:25–29.
13. Nadel AS, Green JK, Holmes LB, et al: Absence of need for amniocentesis in patients with elevated levels of maternal serum alpha-fetoprotein and normal ultrasonographic examinations. N Engl J Med 1990;323:557–567.
14. Bonilla-Musoles F, Machado LF, Osborne NG, et al: Two- and three-dimensional ultrasound in malformations of the medullary canal: Report of four cases. Prenat Diagn 2001;21:622–626.
15. Mangels KJ, Tulipan N, Tsao LY, et al: Fetal MRI in the evaluation of intrauterine myelomeningocele. Pediatr Neurosurg 2000;32:124–131.
16. Beuls EA, Vanormelingen L, van Aalst J, et al: In vitro high-field magnetic resonance imaging-documented anatomy of a fetal myelomeningocele at 20 weeks' gestation. A contribution to

the rationale of intrauterine surgical repair of spina bifida. J Neurosurg 2003;98:210–214.
17. Chervenak FA, Isaacson G, Mahoney MJ, et al: Diagnosis and management of fetal cephalocele. Obstet Gynecol 1984;64:86–91.
18. Goldstein RB, LaPidus AS, Filly RA: Fetal cephaloceles: Diagnosis with US. Radiology 1991;180:803–808.
19. Simpson DA, David DJ, White J: Cephaloceles: Treatment, outcome, and antenatal diagnosis. Neurosurgery 1984;15:14–21.
20. Mahapatra AK, Suri A: Anterior encephaloceles: A study of 92 cases. Pediatr Neurosurg 2002;36:113–118.
21. Nicolaides KH, Campbell S, Gabbe SG, Guidetti R: Ultrasound screening for spina bifida. Cranial and cerebellar signs. Lancet 1986;ii:72–74.
22. Van den Hof MC, Nicolaides KH, Campbell J, Campbell S: Evaluation of the lemon and banana signs in one hundred thirty fetuses with open spina bifida. Am J Obstet Gynecol 1990;162:322–327.
23. Brumfield CG, Aronin PA, Cloud GA, Davis RO: Fetal myelomeningocele. Is antenatal ultrasound useful in predicting neonatal outcome? J Reprod Med 1995;40:26–30.
24. Brackbill Y: The role of the cortex in orienting: Orienting reflex in an anencephalic infant. Dev Psychol 1971;5:195–203.
25. Chervenak FA, Farley MA, Walters LE, et al: When is termination of pregnancy during the third trimester morally justifiable? N Engl J Med 1984;310:501–504.
26. Bannister CM, Russell SA, Rimmer S, et al: Can prognostic indicators be identified in a fetus with an encephalocele? Eur J Pediatr Surg 2000;10(Suppl 1):20–23.
27. Mealy J, Ozenitis AJ, Hockley AA: The prognosis of encephaloceles. J Neurosurg 1970;32:209–218.
28. Field B: The child with an encephalocele. Med J Aust 1974;1:700–703.
29. Budorick NE, Pretorius DH, McGahan JP, et al: Cephalocele detection in utero: Sonographic and clinical features. Ultrasound Obstet Gynecol 1995;5:77–85.
30. Brown MS, Sheridan-Pereira M: Outlook for the child with a cephalocele. Pediatrics 1992;90:914–919.
31. Martinez-Lage JF, Poza M, Sola J, et al: The child with a cephalocele: Etiology, neuroimaging, and outcome. Childs Nerv Syst 1996;12:540–550.
32. Hoving EW: Nasal encephaloceles. Childs Nerv Syst 2000;16:702–706.
33. Peralta CF, Bunduki V, Plese JP, et al: Association between prenatal sonographic findings and postnatal outcomes in 30 cases of isolated spina bifida aperta. Prenat Diagn 2003;23:311–314.
34. Jobe AH: Fetal surgery for myelomeningocele. N Engl J Med 2002;347:230–231.
35. Bowman RM, McLone DG, Grant JA, et al: Spina bifida outcome: A 25-year prospective. Pediatr Neurosurg 2001;34: 114–120.
36. Hunt GM, Oakeshott P: Outcome in people with open spina bifida at age 35: Prospective community based cohort study. BMJ 2003;326:1365–1366.
37. Dise JE, Lohr ME: Examination of deficits in conceptual reasoning abilities associated with spina bifida. Am J Phys Med Rehab 1998;77:247–251.
38. Bensen JT, Dillard RG, Burton BK: Open spina bifida: Does cesarean delivery improve prognosis? Obstet Gynecol 1988;71:532–534.
39. Bruner JP, Tulipan N, Paschall RL, et al: Fetal surgery for myelomeningocele and the incidence of shunt-dependent hydrocephalus. JAMA 1999;282:1819–1825.
40. Tubbs RS, Chambers MR, Smyth MD, et al: Late gestational intrauterine myelomeningocele repair does not improve lower extremity function. Pediatr Neurosurg 2003;38:128–132.
41. Holmes NM, Nguyen HT, Harrison MR, et al: Fetal intervention for myelomeningocele: Effect on postnatal bladder function. J Urol 2001;166:2383–2386.
42. Truog RD, Fletcher JC: Anencephalic newborns: Can organs be transplanted before brain death? N Engl J Med 1989;321:388–390.
43. Medearis DN, Holmes LB: On the use of anencephalic infants as organ donors. N Engl J Med 1989;321:391–393.
44. Luthy DA, Wardinsky T, Shurtleff DB, et al: Cesarean section before the onset of labor and subsequent motor function in infants with meningomyelocele diagnosed antenatally. N Engl J Med 1991;324:662–666.
45. Hill AE, Beattie F: Does caesarean section delivery improve neurological outcome in open spina bifida? Eur J Pediatr Surg 1994;4:32–34.
46. Bensen JT, Dillard RG, Burton BK: Open spina bifida: Does cesarean section delivery improve prognosis? Obstet Gynecol 1988;71:532–534.
47. Merrill DD, Goodwin P, Burson JM, et al: The optimal route of delivery for fetal meningomyelocele. Am J Obstet Gynecol 1998;179:235–240.
48. Sakala EP, Andree I: Optimal route of delivery for meningomyelocele. Obstet Gynecol Surv 1990;45:209–212.
49. Carter CO: The inheritance of common congenital malformations. Prog Med Genet 1965;4:59–84.
50. Bonaiti-Pellie C, Smith C: Risk tables for genetic counseling in some common congenital malformations. J Med Genet 1974;11:374–377.
51. Drugan A, Krause B, Canady A, et al: The natural history of prenatally-diagnosed ventriculomegaly. JAMA 1989;261: 1785–1788.
52. Chervanak FA, Berkowitz RL, Romero R, et al: The diagnosis of fetal hydrocephalus. Am J Obstet Gynecol 1983;147:703–716.
53. Cardoza JD, Goldstein RB, Filly RA: Exclusion of fetal ventriculomegaly with a single measurement: The width of the lateral ventricular atrium. Radiology 1988;169:711–714.
54. Benacerraf BR, Birnholz JC: The diagnosis of fetal hydrocephalus prior to 22 weeks. J Clin Ultrasound 1987;15:531–536.
55. Laurence KM, Coates S: The natural history of hydrocephalus. Arch Dis Childhood 1962;37:345–362.
56. Futagi Y, Suzuki Y, Toribe Y, Morimoto K: Neurodevelopmental outcomes in children with fetal hydrocephalus. Pediatr Neurol 2002;27:111–116.
57. Bottcher K, Jacobsen S, Gyldensted C, et al: Intellectual development and brain size in 13 shunted hydrocephalic children. Neuropadiatrie 1978;9:369–377.
58. Kao CL, Yang TF, Wong TT, et al: The outcome of shunted hydrocephalic children. Zhonghua Yi Xue Za Zhi 2001;64:47–53.
59. Lumenta CB, Skotarczak U: Long-term follow-up in 233 patients with congenital hydrocephalus. Childs Nerv Syst 1995;11:173–175.
60. Raimondi AJ, Soare P: Intellectual development in shunted hydrocephalic children. Am J Dis Child 1974;127:664.
61. Op Heij CP, Renier WO, Gabreels FJ: Intellectual sequelae of primary non-obstructive hydrocephalus in infancy: Analysis of 50 cases. Clin Neurol Neurosurg 1985;87:247–253.
62. Lorber J: The results of early treatment of extreme hydrocephalus. Dev Med Child Neurol 1968;16:21–29.
63. Hoppe-Hirsch E, Laroussinie F, Brunet L, et al: Late outcome of the surgical treatment of hydrocephalus. Childs Nerv Syst 1998;14:97–99.
64. Kirkinen P, Serlo W, Jouppila P, et al: Long-term outcome of fetal hydrocephaly. J Child Neurol 1996;11:189–192.
65. Billard C, Santini JJ, Gillet P, et al: Long-term intellectual prognosis of hydrocephalus with reference to 77 children. Pediatr Neurosci 1985–1986;12:219–225.
66. Pretorius DH, David K, Manco-Johnson ML, et al: Clinical course of fetal hydrocephalus: 40 cases. Am J Radiol 1985;144:827–831.
67. Chervenak FA, Berkowitz RL, Tortora M, et al: Management of fetal hydrocephalus. Am J Obstet Gynecol 1985;151: 933–942.

68. Holzgreve W, Evans MI: Non-vascular needle and shunt placements for fetal therapy. West J Med 1993;159:333–340.
69. Cavalheiro S, Moron AF, Zymberg ST, Dastoli P: Fetal hydrocephalus—Prenatal treatment. Childs Nerv Syst 2003;19: 561–573.
70. Chasen ST, Chervenak FA, McCullough LB: The role of cephalocentesis in modern obstetrics. Am J Obstet Gynecol 2001;185:734–736.
71. Smith DW: Recognizable Patterns of Human Malformation, 3rd ed. Philadelphia, WB Saunders, 1982, p 617.
72. Lorber J, De NC: Family history of congenital hydrocephalus. Dev Med Child Neurol 1970;22:94–100.
73. Bullen PJ, Rankin JM, Robson SC: Investigation of the epidemiology and prenatal diagnosis of holoprosencephaly in the North of England. Am J Obstet Gynecol;184:1256–1262.
74. DeMeyer W, Zeman W, Palmer CG: The face predicts the brain: Diagnostic significance of median facial anomalies for holoprosencephaly (arhinencephaly). Pediatrics 1964;34:256.
75. Matsunaga E, Shiota K: Holoprosencephaly in human embryos: Epidemiologic studies of 150 cases. Teratology 1977;16:261–272.
76. Roach E, Demyer W, Conneally PM, et al: Holoprosencephaly: Birth data, genetic and demographic analyses of 30 families. Birth Defects Orig Artic Ser 1975;11:294–313.
77. Odent S, Le Marec B, Munnich A, et al: Segregation analysis in nonsyndromic holoprosencephaly. Am J Med Genet 1998;77: 139–143.
78. Cohen MM Jr, Shiota Kohei: Teratogenesis of holoprosencephaly. Am J Med Genet 2002;109:1–15.
79. Stewart RE: Craniofacial malformations: Clinical and genetic considerations. Pediatr Clin North Am 1978;25:485.
80. Mueller GM, Weiner CP, Yankowitz J: Three-dimensional ultrasound in the evaluation of fetal head and spine anomalies. Obstet Gynecol 1996;88:372–378.
81. Johnson DD, Pretorius DH, Budorick NE, et al: Fetal lip and primary palate: Three-dimensional versus two-dimensional US. Radiology 2000;217:236–239.
82. Osenbach RK, Menezes AH: Diagnosis and management of the Dandy-Walker malformation: 30 years of experience. Pediatr Neurosurg 1992;18:179–189.
83. Murray JC, Johnson JA, Bird TD: Dandy-Walker malformation: Etiologic heterogeneity and empiric recurrence risks. Clin Genet 1985;28:272–283.
84. Ecker JL, Shipp TD, Bromley B, Benacerraf B: The sonographic diagnosis of Dandy-Walker and Dandy-Walker variant: Associated findings and outcomes. Prenat Diagn 2000;20: 328–332.
85. Hirsch JH, Cyr D, Eberhardt H, Zunkel D: Ultrasonographic diagnosis of an aneurysm of the vein of Galen in utero by duplex scanning. J Ultrasound Med 1983;2:231.
86. Vintzeleos AM, Eisenfeld LI, Campbell WA, et al: Prenatal ultrasonic diagnosis of arteriovenous malformation of the vein of Galen. Am J Perinatol 1986;3:209.
87. Sepulveda W, Vanderyden T, Pather J, Pasquini L: Prenatal 3D color-Doppler angiography is superior to MRI in the evaluation of arteriovenous malformation of vein of Galen. Ultrasound Obstet Gynecol 2003;22:74.
88. Breysem L, Bosmans H, Dymarkowski S, et al: The value of fast MR imaging as an adjunct to ultrasound in prenatal diagnosis. Eur Radiol 2002;13:1538–1548.
89. Has R, Gunay S, Ibrahimoglu L: Prenatal diagnosis of a vein of galen aneurysm. Fetal Diagn Ther 2003;18:36–40.
90. Rodesch G, Hui F, Alvarez H, et al: Prognosis of antenatally diagnosed vein of Galen aneurismal malformations. Childs Nerv Syst 1994;10:79–83.
91. Avery GB, Menesses L, Lodge A: The critical significance of "measurement microcephaly." Am J Dis Child 1972;123:214–217.
92. Bell WE: Abnormalities in size and shape of the head. In Shaffer AJ, Avery ME (eds): Diseases of the Newborn, 4th ed. Philadelphia, WB Saunders, 1977, pp 717–719.
93. Cohen HL, Haller JO: Advances in perinatal neurosonography. Am J Radiol 1994;163:801–810.
94. Babcock DS: The normal, absent and abnormal corpus callosum: Sonographic findings. Radiology 1984;151:449–453.
95. Papile LA, Burstein J, Burstein R, Koffler H: Incidence and evolution of subependymal and intraventricular hemorrhage: A study of infants with birth weights less than 1500 g. J Pediatr 1978;92:529–534.
96. Ghi T, Simonazzi G, Perolo A, et al: Outcome of antenatally diagnosed intracranial hemorrhage: Case series and review of the literature. Ultrasound Obstet Gynecol 2003;22:121–130.
97. Pilu G, Rizzo N, Orsini LF, Bovicelli L: Antenatal recognition of cerebral anomalies. Ultraound Med Biol 1986;12:319–326.
98. Dickinson JE, Marshall LR, Phillips JM, Barr AL: Antenatal diagnosis and management of fetomaternal alloimmune thrombocytopenia. Am J Perinatol 1995;12:333–335.
99. Gross SJ, Shulman LP, Tolley EA, et al: Isolated fetal choroids plexus cysts and trisomy 18: A review and meta-analysis. Am J Obstst Gynecol 1995;172:83–87.
100. Gupta JK, Khan KS, Thorton JG, Lilford RJ: Management of fetal choroids plexus cysts. BJOG 1997;104:881–886.
101. Brown T, Kliewer MA, Hertzberg BS, et al: A role for maternal serum screening in detecting chromosomal abnormalities in fetuses with isolated choroids plexus cysts: A prospective multicentre study. Prenat Diagn 1999;19:405–410.
102. Sullivan A, Giudice T, Vavelidis F, Thiagarajah S: Choroid plexus cysts: Is biochemical testing a valuable adjunct to targeted ultrasonography? Am J Obstet Gynecol 1999;181:260–265.
103. Levine D, Barnes PD, Madsen JR, et al: Central nervous system abnormalities assessed with prenatal magnetic resonance imaging. Obstet Gynecol 1999;94:1011–1019.
104. Hubbard AM: Ultrafast fetal MRI and prenatal diagnosis. Semin Pediatr Surg 2003;12:143–153.
105. Wagenvoort AM, Bekker MN, Go AT, et al: Ultrafast scan magnetic resonance in prenatal diagnosis. Fetal Diagn Ther 2000;15:364–372.
106. Baker PN, Johnson IR, Harvey PR, et al: A three-year follow-up of children imaged in utero with echo-planar magnetic resonance. Am J Obstet Gynecol 1994;170:32–33.
107. Sharma G, Heier L, Troiano R, et al: Use of fetal magnetic resonance imaging in patients who elect the termination of pregnancy by dilation and evacuation. Am J Obstet Gynecol 2003;189:990–993.
108. Chervenak FA, Isaacson G, Rosenberg JC, et al: Antenatal diagnosis of frontal cephalocele in a fetus with atelosteogenesis. J Ultrasound Med 1986;5:111–113.
109. Chervenak FA, Duncan C, Ment LR, et al: Perinatal management of myelomeningocele. Obstet Gynecol 1984;63:376.
110. Pilu G, Romero R, Rizzo N, et al: Criteria for the prenatal diagnosis of holoprosencephaly. Am J Perinatol 1987;4:41–49.
111. Mahony BS, Hegge FN: The face and neck. In Nyberg DA, Mahony BS, Pretorius DH (eds): Diagnostic Ultrasound of Fetal Anomalies: Text and Atlas. Chicago, Year Book, 1990, pp 203–261.
112. Chervenak FA, Isaacson G, Blakemore KJ, et al: Fetal cystic hygroma. Cause and natural history. N Engl J Med 1983; 309:822–825.
113. Lumley J, Watson L, Watson M, Bower C: Periconceptional supplementation with folate and/or multivitamins for preventing neural tube defects. Cochrane Database Syst Rev 2000;1.

CHAPTER 19

Fetal Genitourinary Abnormalities

Marc Dommergues / Rodrigo Ruano / Marie-Cécile Aubry

INTRODUCTION

Genitourinary abnormalities consist of a wide spectrum of heterogeneous malformations. Urinary tract dilations and kidney abnormalities are relatively common with a prevalence ranging from 1/250 to 1/1000 deliveries.

The majority of genitourinary abnormalities are detected during routine screening sonography in the absence of any significant clinical or family history. Generally, the sensitivity of antenatal screening depends on the experience of the sonographer and on the timing of the onset of detectable consequences of the abnormality. Antenatal diagnosis of urinary malformations is facilitated by the often conspicuous, transonic image. The diagnosis of a lethal form may become evident with severe oligohydramnios and patent dilation of the urinary tract. In contrast, some urinary tract abnormalities, such as urinary reflux, may remain undetectable in utero. Urinary dilation above an incomplete obstruction may occur in the third trimester only after the urinary volume exceeds the obstructed capacity. These will be missed unless there is a policy of routine third-trimester ultrasound. Renal abnormalities without urinary tract dilation can be detected if examination of the fetal kidneys is included in the screening ultrasound.

In contrast to uronephrologic abnormalities, isolated genital malformations are rare disorders. There is no consensus on whether the structure of the fetal genitalia should be imaged as part of a screening ultrasound examination. Minor abnormalities are virtually impossible to identify, and counseling may be extremely difficult when ambiguous genitalia are identified.

FETAL UROPATHIES

Pathophysiology

Uropathies potentially detectable in utero may be classified according to their pathophysiology:

- Obstruction of the ureteropelvic junction: This abnormality is the most common lesion of the fetal urinary tract. The obstruction may result from compression by an ectopic vessel, or it may occur in the setting of duplication or ectopy.
- Megaureter: True megaureter is the result of a dysfunction at the ureterovesical junction. Spontaneous relief of megaureter with mild hydronephrosis often occurs during the first years of life, whereas major hydronephrosis or a retrovesical ureteral diameter greater than 1 cm tends to resolve slowly and may require surgery.[1,2]
- Ureterocele: This cystic dilation of the distal intravesical ureter arises most often from an abnormal location of the ureteral meatus in the bladder. Ureterocele is often associated with double ureter, in which the ureterocele at the lower ureteric orifice drains the upper pole of the duplicated kidney. The lesion is associated with obstruction, accounting for the dilation of the corresponding ureter and renal pelvis. A large ureterocele can even obstruct the bladder neck, and the disease resembles an infravesical obstruction. Antenatal diagnosis is important to plan postnatal management and to avoid future complications.[3]
- Bladder outlet obstruction: This obstruction usually occurs in the urethra, causing bladder dilation with muscle hypertrophy and hydronephrosis. The kidneys may be dysplastic, resulting in a variable degree of renal failure.[4] The most common cause of bladder outlet obstruction is posterior urethral valves. Urethral atresia is less common, causing lethal lesions with fetal anuria in the early second trimester. In spite of advances in antenatal care, posterior urethral valves may still result in postnatal renal failure.[5]
- Reflux: This common disorder is often suspected antenatally, but is rarely diagnosed definitively. Occasionally, it may be diagnosed based on the dynamic dilation of the upper urinary tract or of the bladder. Dynamic imaging of reflux is sometimes possible. In severe cases, the bladder and ureters appear dilated owing to

a functional increase in urinary outflow. Antenatal diagnosis permits the initiation of prophylactic antibiotic therapy to avoid postnatal urinary infection and subsequent kidney damage. Postnatal surgery may be required for severe forms.[6]

- Prune-belly sequence: This abnormality consists of deficient abdominal wall musculature, bladder distention with renal dysplasia, absence of prostatic tissue, and cryptorchidism.[7] A patent urachus is common. The uropathy usually consists of urethral obstruction and dysfunction resulting in megacystis and bilateral megaureter. Prostatic hypoplasia is common in males. It is rare in females in whom the uropathy and the abdominal wall defect are associated with vaginal atresia, rectovaginal or rectovesical fistula, and bicornuate uterus. The prognosis depends on the amount of functional renal tissue.

The antenatal diagnosis of fetal uropathies is rarely made before the second trimester. An intra-abdominal transonic mass in the first trimester suggests a dilated bladder. It may resolve spontaneously, and follow-up is needed to confirm the diagnosis of fetal urinary tract dilation. Most antenatal diagnoses of urinary tract dilation are made in the second trimester. Third-trimester ultrasound may reveal late onset uropathies. In a substantial number of cases, urinary dilation appears only late in gestation or during postnatal life and will not be amenable to antenatal screening.

Sonographic Assessment of Normal Development of the Fetal Kidneys, Urinary Tract, and Genitalia

The fetal bladder and kidneys are identifiable by 11 to 12 weeks of gestation (Figs. 19–1 and 19–2) when they appear as homogeneous echoes on each side of the spine. Between 18 and 24 weeks' gestation, the medulla becomes hypoechogenic and is distinguishable from the echogenic renal cortex (Fig. 19–3). The growth of fetal kidneys parallels the fetus and can be evaluated in a quantitative manner.[8–10]

The image of the genital tubercle should be interpreted carefully during the first trimester,[11] though it is possible to identify fetal gender at 12 to 14 weeks in 70% to 90% of cases.[12] In boys, the urethral canal can be seen at 26 to 27 weeks, but it is easier to see in the third trimester (Fig. 19–4). Undescended testes are physiologic until 32 weeks but should be intrascrotal near term. In girls, vulvar structure can be identified as early as 15 weeks and seen clearly by 22 weeks. However, a detailed analysis of a vulva anomaly is not usually feasible until 24 weeks (Fig. 19–5). In the third trimester, the external genitalia are large and easier to analyze.

It is not always possible to identify the uterus, even late in gestation. The fetal sacrum is an indirect but useful marker of the harmonious development of the fetal pelvis. It curves inward progressively during the second trimester (Fig. 19–6). The anal sphincter can also be seen (Fig. 19–7).

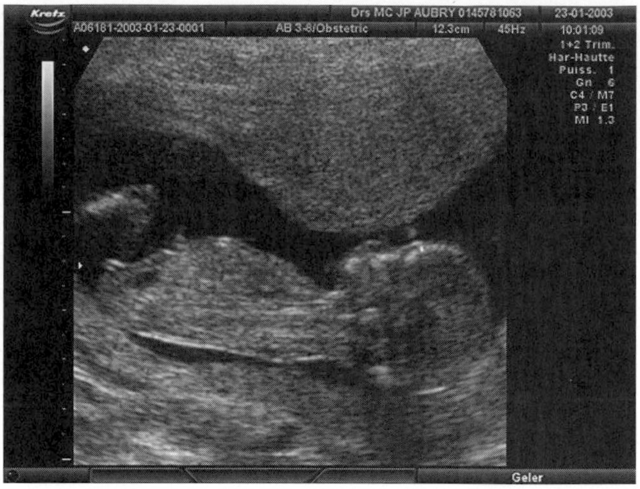

FIGURE 19–2
Bladder, sagittal view, at 12 weeks.

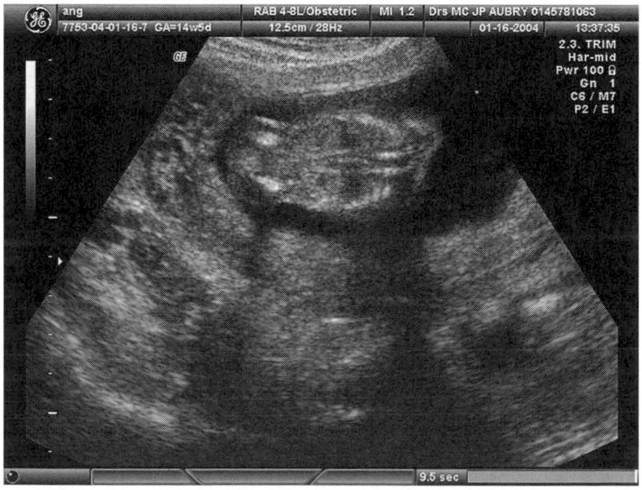

FIGURE 19–1
Kidneys, frontal view, at 12 weeks.

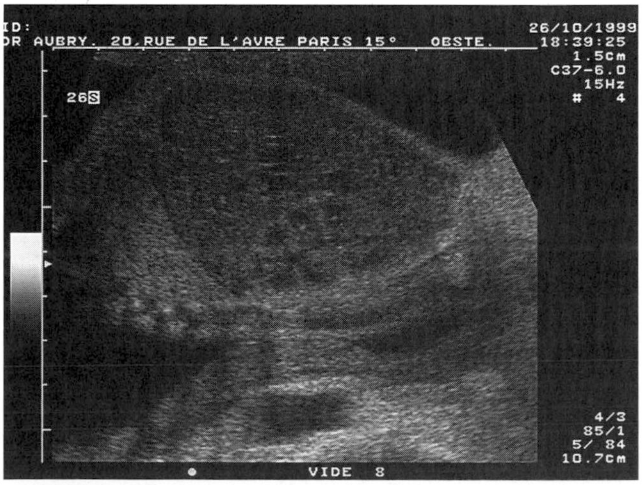

FIGURE 19–3
Renal parenchyma at 23 weeks, showing corticomedullary differentiation.

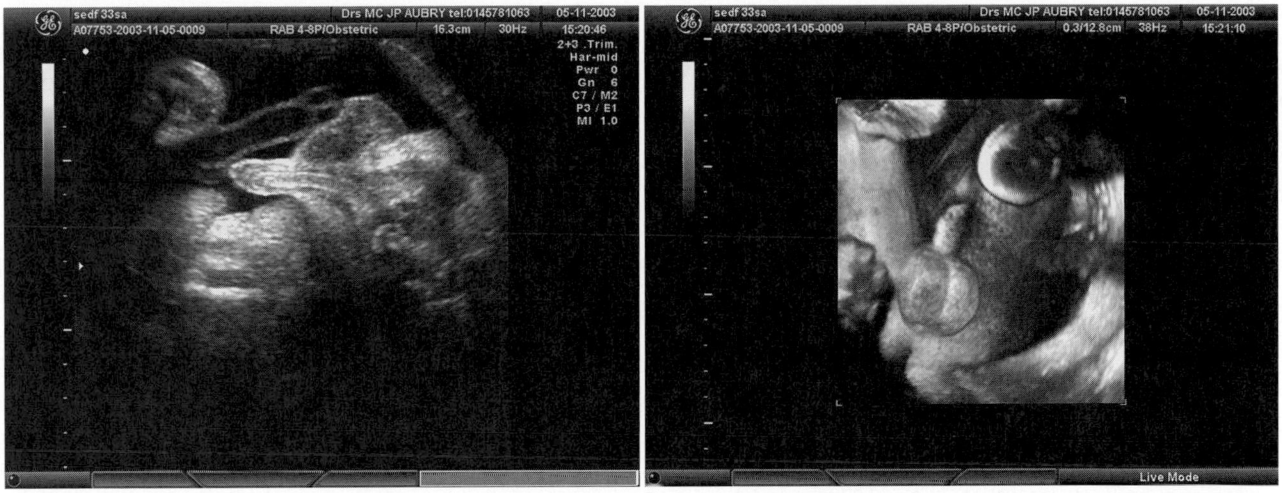

A B

FIGURE 19–4
Male external genitalia at 33 weeks. See urethral canal. Bidimensional (*A*) and three-dimensional (*B*) views are shown.

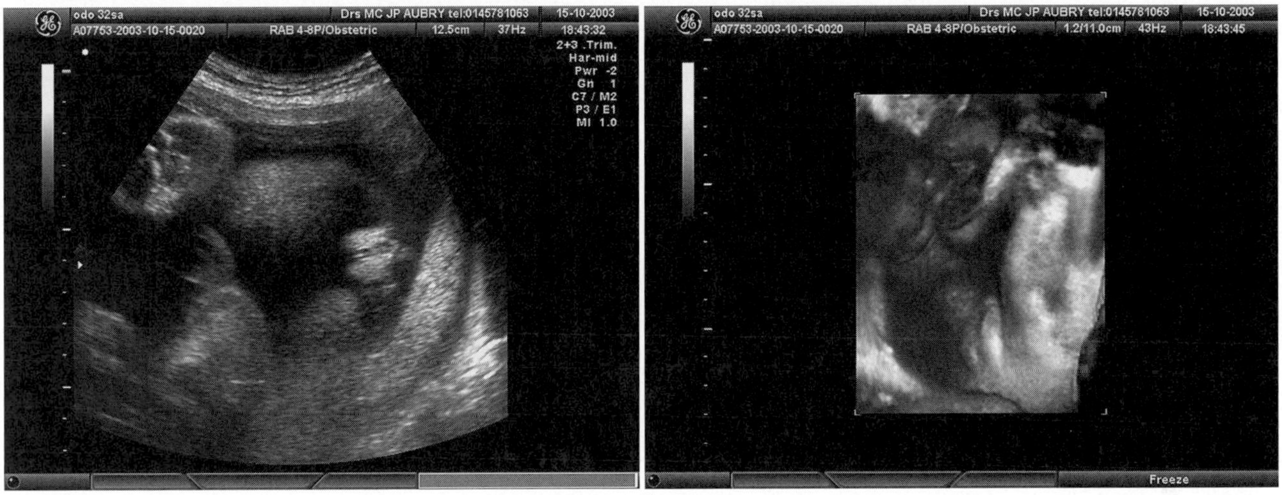

A B

FIGURE 19–5
Female external genitalia at 32 weeks. Bidimensional (*A*) and three-dimensional (*B*) views are shown.

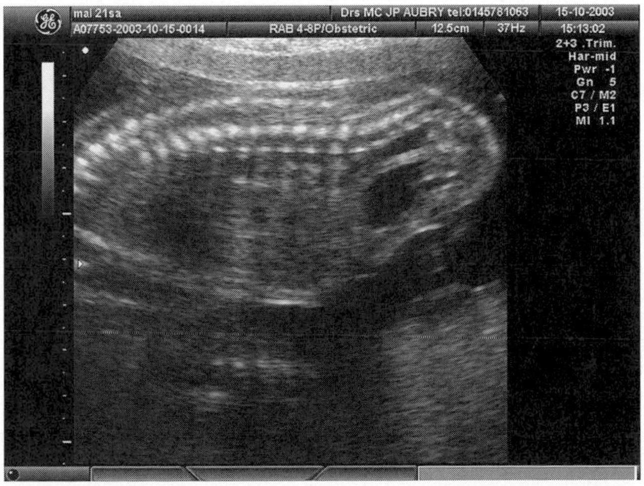

FIGURE 19–6
Normal curvature of the sacrum, sagittal view, at 21 weeks.

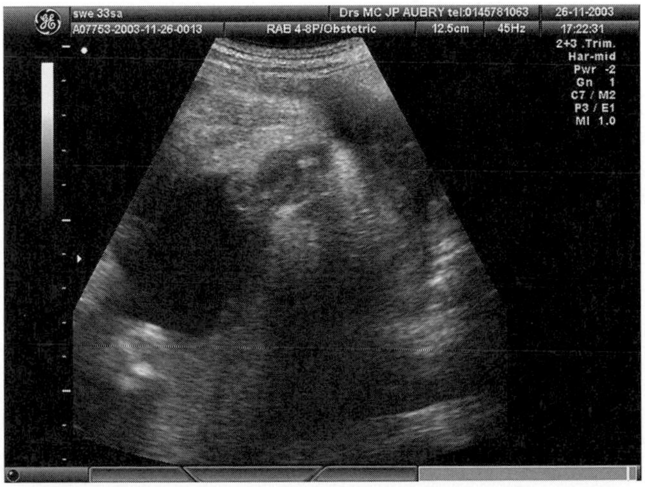

FIGURE 19–7
Normal anal margin, tangential view, at 30 weeks.

Management Options

Once fetal urinary tract dilation is detected, the following issues should be addressed rapidly:

1. The diagnosis should be confirmed.
2. Associated abnormalities should be ruled out, which requires a special expertise in the field of fetal ultrasound.
3. The risk of aneuploidy should be evaluated and weighed against the potential iatrogenic risks of performing an amniocentesis.
4. The risk of developing postnatal respiratory distress (due to severe oligohydramnios leading to pulmonary hypoplasia) should be evaluated.
5. The risk of developing postnatal renal failure should be evaluated.
6. A perinatal management plan should be established in collaboration with a pediatric urologist. The potential need for emergency neonatal surgery should be evaluated in order to plan the site of delivery.

Sonographic Diagnosis of Fetal Urinary Tract Abnormalities

Antenatal diagnosis of fetal urinary tract anomalies is relatively easy based on the identification of transonic images corresponding to the dilated urinary tract. However, it is not always possible to ascertain the mechanism of the uropathy in utero, because the obstructive lesion cannot be imaged directly, and because urinary tract dilations resulting from a vesicoureteral reflux can mimic the dilation of a true obstruction. Nevertheless, it is rarely important to recognize the exact cause of the dilation before birth. A satisfactory surgical repair can be achieved postnatally in most cases, resulting in a good pediatric outcome provided the renal function is not altered and there is no associated malformation.

Apparent Level of Urinary Dilation

Fetal uropathies can be classified by the level of dilation.[13–17] Only the renal pelves are dilated in upper dilations, whereas the ureters are also involved in midlevel dilations. Upper and midlevel dilations are also categorized as unilateral or bilateral, an important prognostic feature because postnatal renal function should be normal in unilateral cases. Dilation of the upper urinary tract may correspond to either ureteropelvic junction obstruction or to ureteropelvic reflux. Similarly, midlevel dilation may be a sonographic feature of vesicoureteral reflux as well as congenital megaureter.

The bladder is involved in low-level dilations, which are usually referred to as low urinary tract obstructions (LUTOs). They comprise mainly the posterior urethral valves. However, a dilated bladder may be the hallmark of major vesicoureteral reflux, which increases the urine output through the bladder. More complex urinary defects, for example, cloacal malformations, may appear as a bladder dilation, and occasionally, as a midlevel dilation associated with minor abnormalities of the fetal pelvis. Complex pelvic floor malformations are the most common LUTO diagnosed antenatally in females, and posterior urethral valves are the most frequent etiology of LUTO in males.

Upper Urinary Tract Dilation. There is no universally accepted definition and grading of fetal upper urinary tract dilation. Pyelectasis is defined by moderate dilation of the renal pelvis without associated dilated calyces, whereas hydronephrosis refers to kidneys with a variable degree of calyceal dilation.

Pyelectasis. The renal pelvis is measured in the anteroposterior (AP) plane on cross section. However, the upper size limit of a normal fetal renal pelvis remains controversial, partly because there is substantial overlap in renal pelvic sizes between normal fetuses and infants who later prove to have reflux or obstruction. Low thresholds tend to stimulate unnecessary and potentially dangerous intervention, and high threshold values will lead to false-negative conclusions.[18]

Pyelectasis is variously defined in the literature as an AP pelvic diameter exceeding 4 to 6 mm in the second trimester and 8 to 10 mm in the third.[19–25] Depending on the definition, pyelectasis (Figs. 19–8 and 19–9) occurs in 1% to 3 % of pregnancies. In most cases, isolated fetal pyelectasis is physiologic. However, it may correspond to a mild reflux or to an ureteropelvic junction syndrome. The likelihood of pyelectasis being associated with substantial morbidity requiring postnatal surgery increases with the degree of antenatal pelvic dilation.[6,26,27] Fetuses with pyelectasis should be followed serially to confirm the dilation does not increase with advancing gestational age.[18,28]

Postnatal evaluation is required but should not be performed immediately after delivery as the false-negative rate is increased. At-risk neonates should have a renal ultrasound between 1 and 3 weeks of age. There is no consensus on whether and when postnatal ultrasound should be repeated, and on which patients should be offered a retrograde cystogram and when. Whatever the

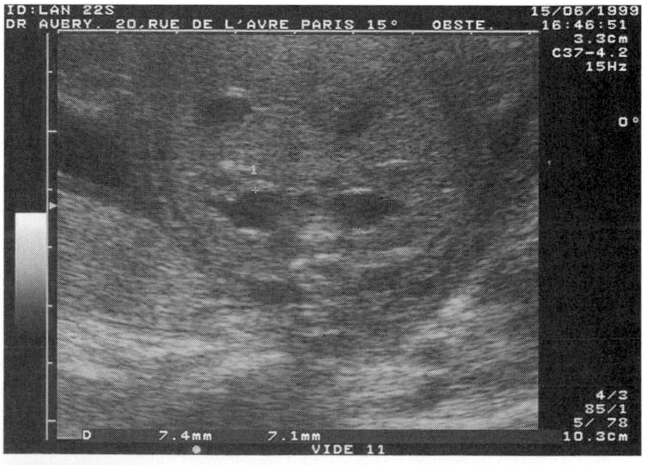

FIGURE 19–8
Mild pyelectasis, transverse view, at 22 weeks.

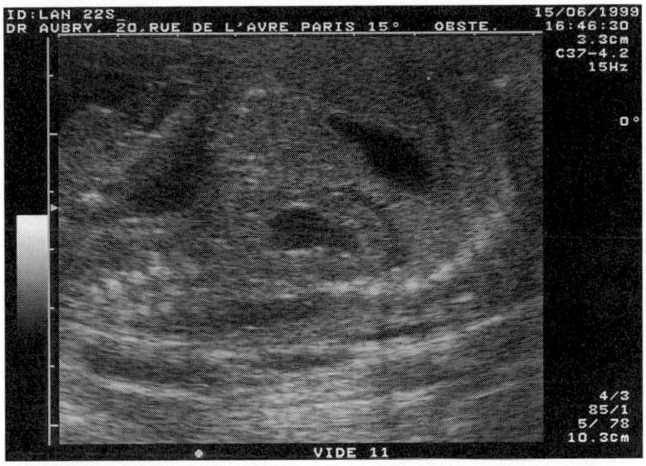

FIGURE 19–9
Mild pyelectasis, parasagittal view, at 22 weeks.

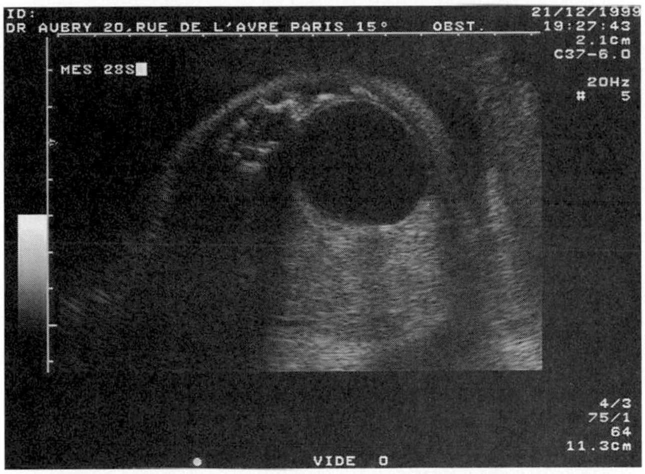

FIGURE 19–11
Large unilateral hydronephrosis, transverse view, at 28 weeks.

postnatal strategies for the diagnosis of reflux or for the prevention of urinary tract infections are, the prenatal history should be kept in mind when unexplained symptoms occur postnatally.[29–31] The sensitivity of antenatal ultrasound for the detection of clinically significant reflux remains low,[16,17] and most cases of reflux are discovered after postnatal symptoms.

Hydronephrosis. Hydronephrosis is defined by an AP pelvic size of more than 1.5 cm or calyceal involvement.[32–34] In mild hydronephrosis, the calyces are slightly dilated and retain their shape. With greater upper urinary tract dilation, the calyces become rounded (Fig. 19–10), but the transonic calyceal images are distributed regularly and are connected to the renal pelvis in contrast to the irregular pattern of a multicystic kidney in which the cysts are independent of the pelvis. In severe cases, the calyceal images are no longer identified separate from the pelvis, appearing instead as a large single transonic image (Fig. 19–11). The renal parenchyma is considered thinned when it is less than 3 mm thick. This finding is not always ominous, because large dilations with thin parenchyma can be associated with a normal renal function. At the parenchymal level, the presence or absence of a corticomedullary differentiation should be noted, as well as the echogenicity of the parenchyma and the presence of cysts. Although subjective,[35–39] the evaluation of the sonographic structure of the renal parenchyma may be a useful predictor of renal function, although it is less sensitive than urinalysis to predict postnatal survival with altered renal function.[40]

Midlevel Dilations. Hydroureter is a dilated ureter that appears as a convoluted transonic image, located between the kidney and the bladder (Figs. 19–12 and 19–13); normally, the ureter is unseen sonographically. Peristaltic activity suggests a megaureter, but a dilated ureter may also result from vesicoureteral reflux.[41]

A ureterocele can cause ureteric dilation. It appears as a round transonic image located inside the bladder and lined by a thin border (Figs. 19–14 and 19–15).

Low-Level Dilation (Low Urinary Tract Obstruction). A dilated bladder that does not empty over the course of the sonographic examination suggests an outlet obstruction.

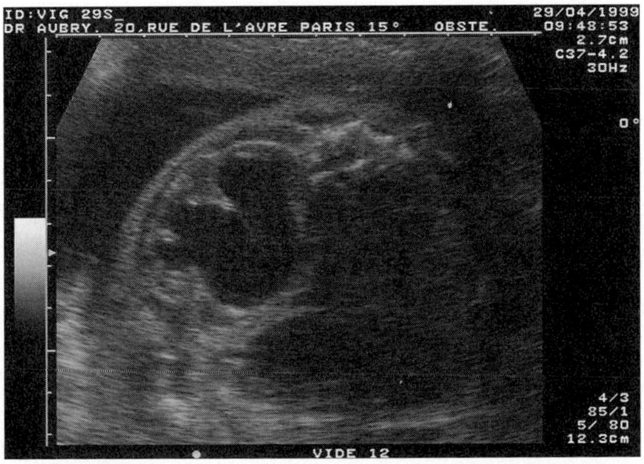

FIGURE 19–10
Unilateral hydronephrosis with rounded calyces, transverse view, at 22 weeks.

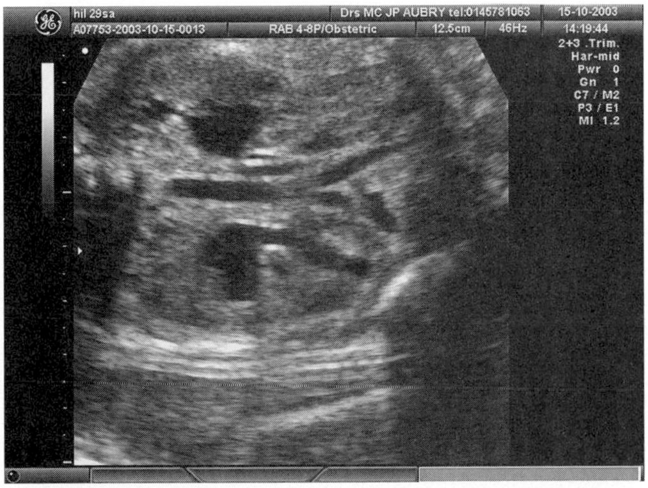

FIGURE 19–12
Dilated ureter, frontal view, at 29 weeks.

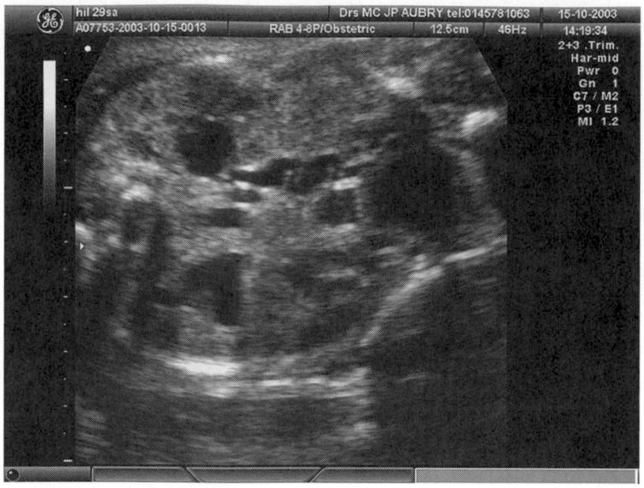

FIGURE 19–13
Dilated ureter, transverse view, at 29 weeks.

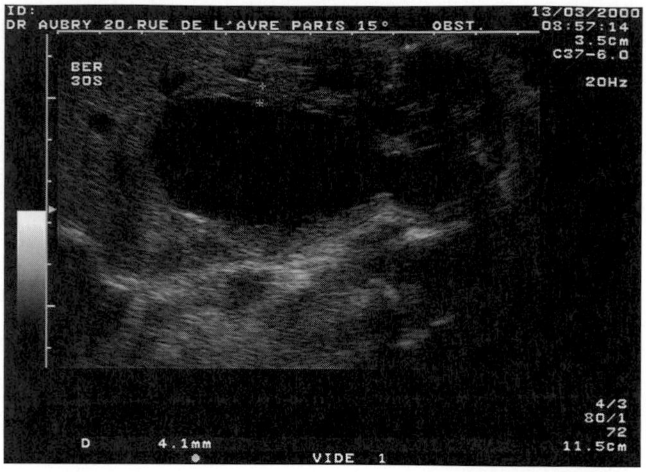

FIGURE 19–16
Enlarged bladder, frontal view, at 30 weeks. Note thickened bladder wall and infravesical image of the dilated urethra (posterior urethral valves).

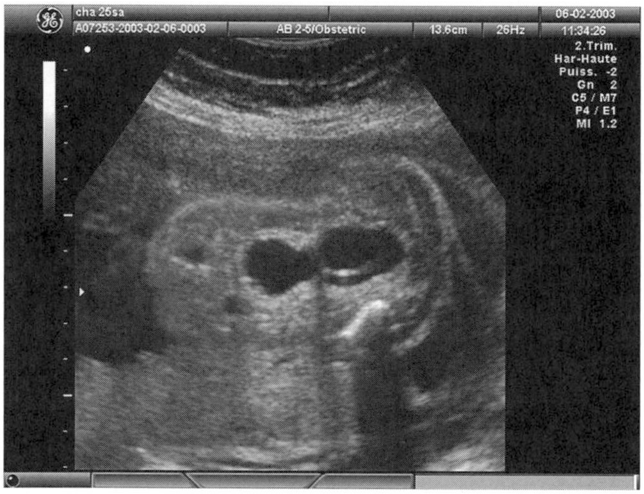

FIGURE 19–14
Ureterocele (bladder), frontal view, at 25 weeks.

The dilated bladder is usually round, but may be larger above the umbilical arteries than below, evoking the shape of the champagne bottle cork. The image of a dilated urethra is rather specific for posterior urethral valves, but is far from constant. At a later stage, bladder outlet obstruction can result in a muscular hypertrophy imaged as a bladder wall thicker than 3 mm (Figs. 19–16 and 19–17). Bladder diverticula may also form. Although posterior urethral valves are the most common cause of bladder dilation in males, other etiologies are possible. Urethral atresia is an almost universally lethal condition and cannot be directly imaged. Rather, it is usually diagnosed at pathologic postmortem examination (Fig. 19–18). Complex genitourinary anomalies should also be carefully sought and ruled out. Keep in mind that a low urinary tract obstruction, including posterior urethral valves, can present as a midlevel or even an upper-level obstruction with bladder enlargement becoming noticeable during subsequent sonographic examinations.

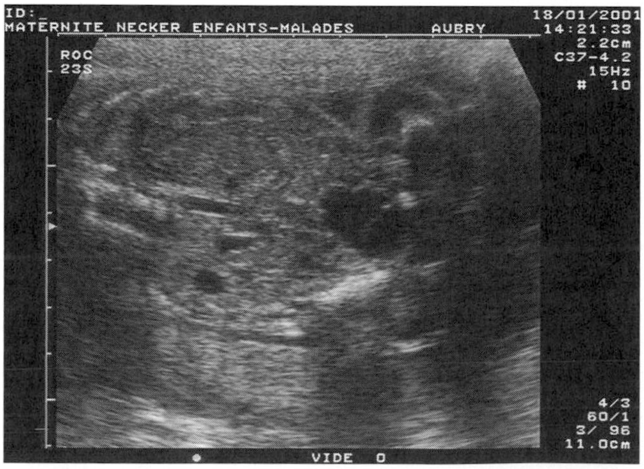

FIGURE 19–15
Ureterocele with renal duplication, frontal view, at 23 weeks.

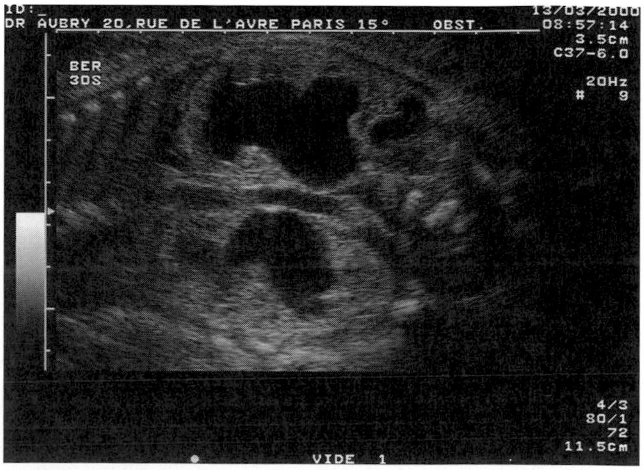

FIGURE 19–17
Hydronephrosis with hyperechogenic renal parenchyma (posterior urethral valves), frontal view, at 30 weeks.

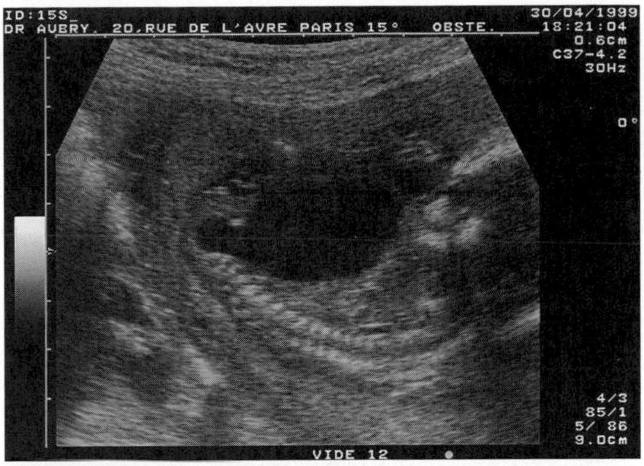

FIGURE 19–18
Enlarged bladder with infravesical image of the dilated urethra (urethral atresia), sagittal view, at 15 weeks.

Ascites and Urinoma

Urine may leak into the peritoneal cavity through minor and usually unidentifiable disruptions of the urinary tract wall, causing ascites. Urinous ascites is not specific for a given uropathy and is not necessarily an ominous finding. The urinary origin of the ascites is usually apparent. Similarly, disruption of the urinary tract in the retroperitoneal space may lead to a urinoma (Fig. 19–19), which appears as a transonic image surrounding the kidney and confined within Gerota's facia.[42] Urinomas are usually easy to differentiate from renal masses, lymphangioma, neuroblastoma, mesenteric cyst, and enteric duplications.

Once the antenatal sonographic diagnosis of a fetal uropathy is made, the most clinically relevant question is prognosis. Because virtually any isolated uropathy can be successfully repaired postnatally, the prognosis is based on the presence of additional birth defects and postnatal renal function.

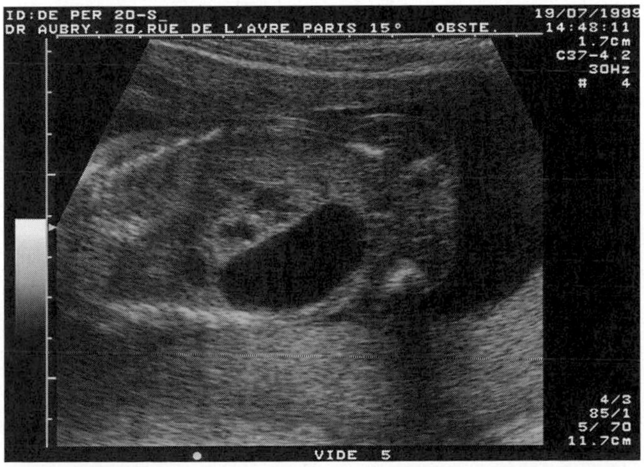

FIGURE 19–19
Urinoma, frontal view, at 20 weeks.

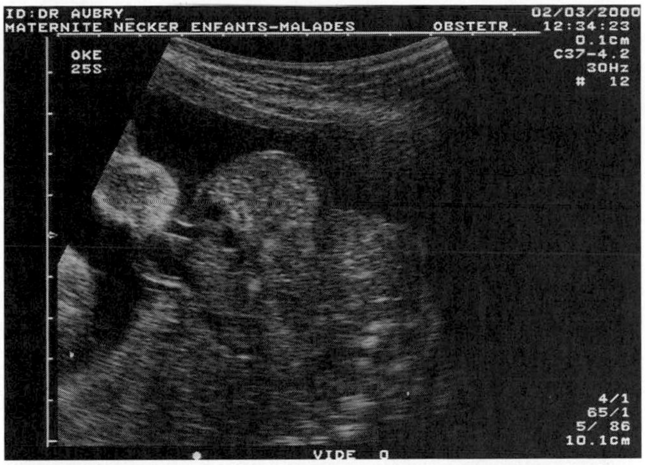

FIGURE 19–20
Bladder exstrophy. Note the abnormal appearance of the anterior abdominal wall, the absence of vesical image, and the low-lying fetal insertion of the umbilical cord, at 25 weeks.

Ruling Out Associated Anomalies Including Karyotyping

The first step in the management of a fetus with a urinary tract abnormality is to rule out extraurinary anomalies by a complete sonographic assessment performed by an experienced practitioner.[43–45] Soft markers suggestive of a chromosomal abnormality should be sought (see later discussion) Complex pelvic malformations should be sought.

Bladder exstrophy is characterized by the absence of a vesical image[46,47] and can sometimes be imaged directly (Fig. 19–20). The antenatal diagnosis on cloacal malformations is based on the association of a variety of relatively minor signs that may appear only in the third trimester.[48–52] Rectal atresia is suggested when the sacrum appears too straight (Fig. 19–21). A urodigestive fistula is suspected when the bowel is dilated with hyperechogenic material (Figs. 19–22 and 19–23). The image of an enlarged duplicated vagina is quite specific of a cloacal malformation[53] but may not appear until the third

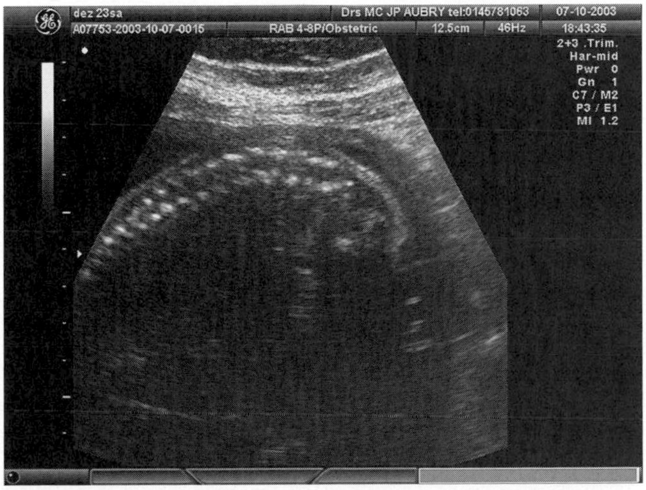

FIGURE 19–21
Straightened and shortened sacrum (cloacal abnormality), sagittal view, at 23 weeks.

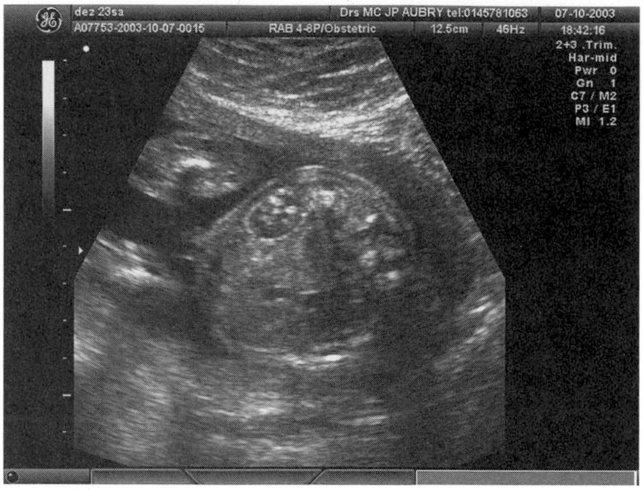

FIGURE 19–22
Hyperechogenic content of the small bowel (urodigestive fistula), transverse view, at 23 weeks.

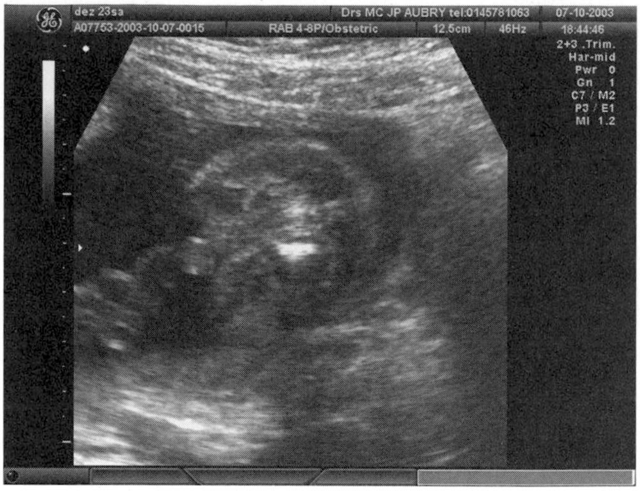

FIGURE 19–24
Absence of image of the anal margin, tangential view of the perineum, at 23 weeks.

trimester. Though it is possible to image the anal sphincter, this does not rule out the diagnosis of anal atresia (Fig. 19–24). The external genitalia should also be carefully imaged. They may appear as enlarged and fused labia "floating" in the amniotic fluid. Overall, the potential for surgical repair may be difficult to establish when a complex malformation of the pelvic floor is diagnosed in utero, and the procedure should be discussed with an expert pediatric surgeon. Magnetic resonance imaging may be helpful in some instances if the radiographer is comfortable and skilled.

The prune-belly syndrome is another complex malformation in which the prognosis may be difficult to establish. The diagnosis is suspected antenatally when a large bladder (Fig. 19–25) and substantial ureteral dilations (Fig. 19–26) are seen, in contrast to mild hydronephrosis (Fig. 19–27). Undescended testes are common. It is possible to depress the fetal abdomen with a moderate amount of pressure by the ultrasound probe.

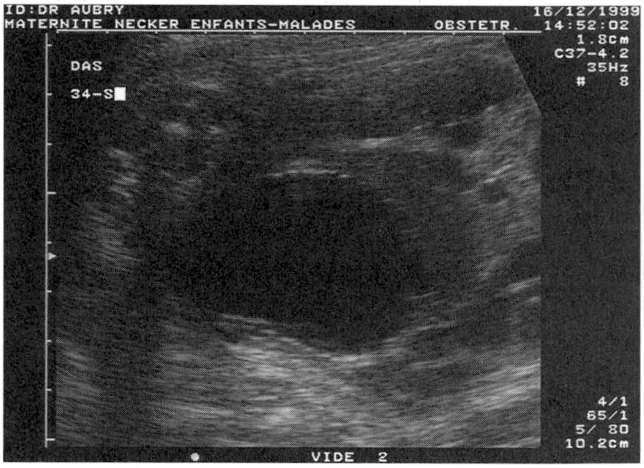

FIGURE 19–25
Enlarged bladder at 34 weeks. No infravesical urethral dilation. Normal bladder wall (prune-belly).

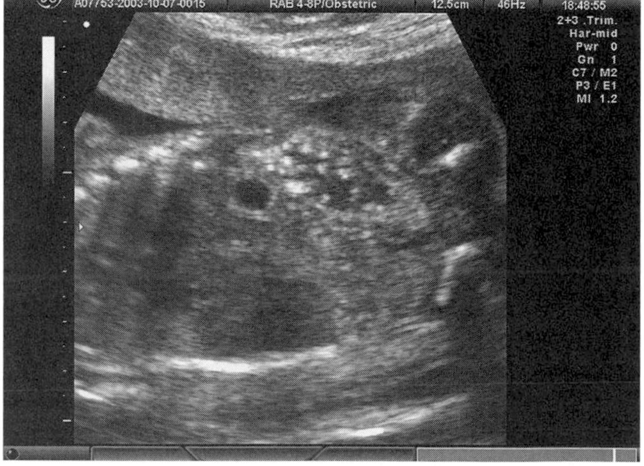

FIGURE 19–23
Hyperechogenic content of the small bowel (urodigestive fistula), frontal view, at 23 weeks.

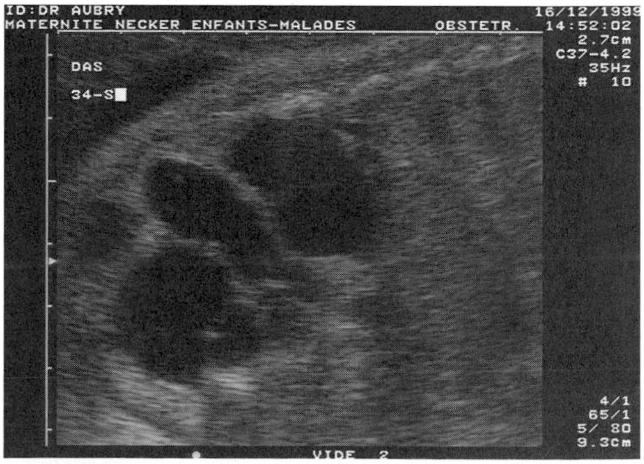

FIGURE 19–26
Oblique view showing bladder, ureter, and kidney (prune-belly), at 34 weeks.

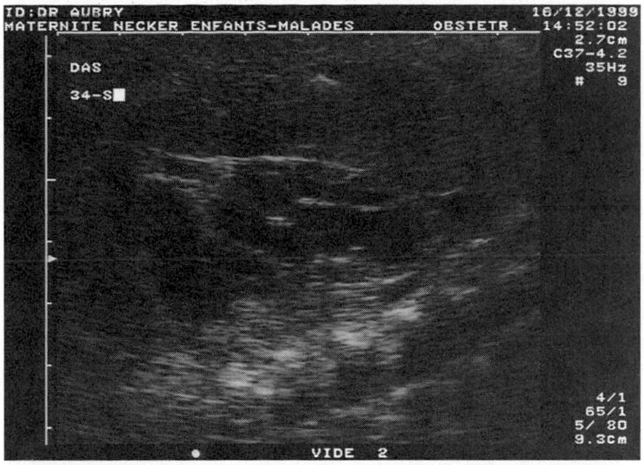

FIGURE 19–27
Mild pyelectasis (prune-belly), parasagittal view, at 34 weeks.

Some less common conditions are even more difficult to diagnose than the prune-belly sequence. For example, a microcolon megacystis syndrome[54,55] is suspected when there is a large bladder and bowel dilation. However, the bowel dilation may only occur late in the third trimester, explaining why this condition is often missed antenatally. It carries a poor postnatal prognosis owing to associated alterations in digestive function.

The second step of the diagnostic workup is to consider a fetal karyotyping. In pilot studies, the incidence of chromosomal abnormalities associated with genitourinary defects was 12%.[56] However, in many uropathies secondary to chromosomal abnormalities, additional extrarenal defects are sonographically detectable, reducing the prevalence of aneuploidy in truly isolated uropathies such as posterior urethral valves or hydronephrosis. Thus, the risk of aneuploidy should be evaluated and weighed against the potential risk of an amniocentesis.[57–60] When at least one soft ultrasound marker is associated with the uropathy, such as a short femur or humerus, a facial abnormality, or a minor anomaly of the fingers or toes, or when an additional malformation is found, the parents should be informed there is a high risk of aneuploidy. When previous aneuploidy screening tests such as nuchal translucency measurement or maternal serum makers yielded "borderline" risks, one should consider the finding of the fetal uropathy as raising the risk above the usual "action line." Unfortunately, large studies that would allow calculation of the likelihood ratio of aneuploidy associated with isolated unilateral hydronephrosis or posterior urethral valves in utero are lacking. Regardless of any attempt at estimating the risk of aneuploidy, some parents may wish to have a karyotype to maximize their opportunities of ruling out associated abnormalities in a baby for whom neonatal surgery and long-term uronephrologic follow-up are likely.

Whether or not pyelectasis is an indication for karyotyping has been a matter of some controversy owing to the high incidence of pyelectasis in normal children. When pyelectasis is associated with another fetal anomaly, even minor, the risk of aneuploidy is increased 10 to 20 times the baseline maternal rate,[61,62] and karyotyping is indicated. In contrast, the risk of aneuploidy is increased by only 1.5 times the baseline maternal rate in cases of isolated pyelectasis. This information should be considered as a part of the sequential screening process for aneuploidy using multiple parameters including maternal age, nuchal translucency measurement, and maternal serum markers (see Chapters 7 and 8).[21–24,60,63–70] The integrated risk of aneuploidy should then be weighed against the risks related with amniocentesis.[58]

Predicting Postnatal Pulmonary Function

Pulmonary hypoplasia (PH) is a disorder of impaired lung growth characterized by diminished size and generational branching and vasculature. Severe oligohydramnios from 16 weeks onward appears to preclude further pulmonary development. In contrast, oligohydramnios after the second trimester is unlikely to result in PH because the crucial canalicular phase of lung development (occurring between 16 and 25 weeks) has largely been completed by this stage. Predicting the likelihood of PH is difficult. Most studies that give predictive data have used cases with preterm premature membrane rupture (PPROM),[71–73] and it is not clear how applicable such data are to cases of olgohydramnios secondary to fetal uropathies. In the case of PPROM additional factors such as preterm delivery and infection contribute to the outcome, and one might speculate that they will worsen the prognosis in contrast to oligohydramnios alone. However, the PPROM data suggest the following:

- If there is a mean vertical pocket of amniotic fluid on ultrasound prior to 26 weeks of greater than 10 mm, PH is very unlikely to occur.[71]
- If the mean vertical pocket of amniotic fluid on ultrasound prior to 26 weeks is less than 10 mm, there is a 90% neonatal mortality rate.[71]
- If the mean vertical pocket of amniotic fluid on ultrasound after 26 weeks is less than 10 mm, PH is very unlikely to occur.[71–73]

Thus, in summary, although absence of severe oligohydramnios before 26 weeks probably means that PH is unlikely, predicting which fetus will develop PH after birth is more difficult. Alternative ultrasound measures, such as chest size, do not appear to produce reliable results.[71,74]

Predicting Postnatal Renal Function

The next goal, once associated abnormalities are ruled out, is to predict postnatal renal function. Unilateral uropathies are associated with a good functional outcome, and it is unnecessary to perform invasive fetal studies to obtain biochemical data from the abnormal kidney, regardless of its sonographic appearance. Serial examinations are required to ensure that contralateral lesions do not appear later in gestation.

The evaluation of fetal renal function with bilateral renal dilation or low urinary tract obstruction is based mainly on ultrasound and, in select cases, on fetal urine analysis or fetal blood sampling. Ultrasound permits assessment of the parenchyma and the amniotic fluid volume.[14,35,75] Fetal urinalysis assesses the ability of the renal tubule to reabsorb a variety of compounds, including sodium, β_2-microglobulin, calcium, phosphorus, and glucose.[32,45,76–84] The β_2-microglobulin level in the fetal serum is thought to reflect fetal glomerular function.[85–88]

Sonographic features related to terminal renal failure in utero include severe oligohydramnios and abnormal images of the renal parenchyma, such as loss of the normal corticomedullary differentiation, hyperechogenicity, and cortical cysts (see Fig. 19–17). In these instances, fetal urinalysis might confirm renal failure, showing high fetal urinary concentrations of sodium and β_2-microglobulin.[89] On the other hand, the functional prognosis is usually good and fetal urine sampling unnecessary in cases of upper obstruction with normal amniotic fluid volume and normal renal parenchyma throughout pregnancy.

In select cases, the functional prognosis cannot be established sonographically. These cases include fetuses with bilateral lesions and moderately decreased amniotic fluid, and fetuses with mild alterations of the renal parenchyma. Moreover, in cases in which the antenatal diagnosis of posterior urethral valves is almost certain, the relatively high incidence of postnatal renal failure could advocate in favor of fetal urine sampling, even in the absence of any ominous sonographic finding. For such cases, one of the most clinically relevant issues is to identify among the children expected to survive those who are at risk for developing postnatal renal failure from those whose renal function will remain normal after surgical repair. The establishment of prognostic values for any marker is complicated by the fact that renal failure may occur relatively late in life, for instance, during adolescence, which underscores the need for long-term follow-up of children in whom fetal urine analysis was performed in utero. Some studies show that fetuses with a normal urinary sodium but a urinary β_2-microglobulin above the 95th percentile are at increased risk of having a serum creatinine greater than one standard deviation (1 SD) above the mean by 1 year of age.[78] When both compounds are abnormally high, neonatal renal failure is likely. In contrast, a good postnatal outcome is anticipated when both compounds are within the normal range.[78] Others report higher thresholds for fetal urinary β_2-microglobulin to predict a postnatal serum creatinine greater than 2 SD above the mean, thereby increasing specificity.[83] To increase the accuracy of fetal urinalysis, it has been advocated that the apparently less affected kidney be sampled[40] or to repeat vesicocentesis serially as long as the values continue to improve or until they normalize.[83,90] In our experience, the results of fetal urinalysis should be interpreted with great care, because in the absence of ominous sonographic findings, only very high levels of urinary β_2-microglobulin (i.e., >10 mg/L) are error-proof predictors of renal failure at the age of 10 to 16 years (unpublished data).

Overall Management

GENERAL

Once the prognosis is decided, management options including termination of pregnancy, occasionally fetal therapy, and postnatal care and follow-up should be discussed with the parents. The option of pregnancy termination should be raised whenever there is terminal renal failure or multiple malformations. Fetal intervention is not indicated when there is unilateral disease or an isolated uropathy with normal renal parenchyma and normal renal function. In these instances, postnatal treatment is planned. It is important to refer the couple antenatally to the pediatric urologist who will be in charge of the baby.

IDENTIFICATION OF CONDITIONS REQUIRING EMERGENCY NEONATAL SURGERY

Some isolated uropathies in which postnatal renal function is anticipated to be reasonably good may require emergency postnatal surgery, requiring delivery in a tertiary care center with pediatric surgery facilities. These include posterior urethral valves, obstructive ureterocele, major bilateral hydronephrosis, and more generally cases with late onset oligohydramnios leading to the diagnosis of acute blockage of urinary output.

Fetal Therapy

Fetal therapy for uropathies is considered because although obstruction of the urinary tract may be treated by relatively simple postnatal procedures, they can be associated with severe renal lesions that manifest before birth. The lesions include severe renal dysplasia, severe oligohydramnios, and pulmonary hypoplasia, leading to either perinatal death or end-stage neonatal renal failure. Animal investigation suggested that intrauterine decompression of experimental urinary tract obstruction in the fetal lamb prevented renal dysplasia.[91–94] Unfortunately the positive impact of fetal urinary decompression on chronic renal disease has not been demonstrated in the clinical setting.[95–101]

Lower urinary obstruction in the human fetus has been treated by open fetal surgery, endoscopic ablation of posterior urethral valves, percutaneous vesicoamniotic shunting, or serial vesicocentesis. Some of these techniques can also be applied to upper tract obstruction. Open fetal surgery was abandoned with the development of percutaneous techniques. Endoscopic ablation of the posterior valves has to date yielded poor perinatal outcomes.[102–104] Serial vesicocentesis was performed as early as the first trimester,[105] but its efficacy remains unclear. Indeed, resolution of first-trimester urinary dilation following percutaneous needling may reflect the natural history rather than the intervention.[106]

Percutaneous ultrasound-guided vesicoamniotic shunting was first reported in the 1980s.[107] Briefly, a cannula is inserted percutaneously through the maternal abdomen under ultrasound guidance and after local analgesia into the dilated fetal bladder or kidney. A double pigtail catheter is inserted through the cannula, with the distal end placed into the dilated urinary tract and the proximal end left in the amniotic cavity. Complications are similar to most "needle"-type procedures and include chorioamnionitis, preterm labor, premature rupture of membranes, or preterm delivery in around 10% of cases.[108,109] Up to half of the shunts are displaced after a few days or weeks. Migration of the amniotic end into the peritoneal cavity can cause urinary ascites, which can be addressed with modest success by placing a peritoneoamniotic shunt.[110] Other complications include an iatrogenic gastroschisis.

A systematic review and meta-analysis published in 2003[111] concluded there is a lack of high-quality evidence to guide clinical practice regarding prenatal bladder drainage.[95,98,112–115] However, in utero drainage may improve survival in severely affected fetuses by improving lung function, but it is achieved at the expense of increasing pediatric morbidity. Long-term follow-up of shunted survivors reveals that some form of chronic renal disease is the rule. Many are ultimately transplanted.

SUMMARY OF MANAGEMENT OPTIONS

Fetal Uropathies/Dilation of the Renal Tract

Management Options	Quality of Evidence	Strength of Recommendation	References
Diagnosis			
Confirm diagnosis with more detailed ultrasound.	III	B	37
Search for other abnormalities.	III	B	44
Consider karyotype.	III	B	56
Management			
Assess risk of respiratory failure (pulmonary hypoplasia).	IIa	B	75, 76, 77
Assess risk of renal failure:			
Ultrasound	III	B	35
Urinalysis	IIa	B	78,79,82,84,87, 88,90
Interdisciplinary management and planning includes pediatric nephrologist/urologist.	–	GPP	–
Counsel parents.	–	GPP	–
Consider termination of pregnancy in severe cases.	–	GPP	–
Plan for delivery depends on likely need for early pediatric surgery.	–	GPP	–
Fetal therapy (decompression procedures) has an uncertain role at present; these procedures probably reduce fetal deaths from pulmonary hypoplasia but at the expense of long-term renal dysfunction in survivors.	Ia	A	111–115
Perform careful examination and assessment of baby after delivery or postmortem examination after perinatal death.	III	B	89

CONCLUSIONS

- Dilations of the urinary tract are common findings at the 20–22 week ultrasound scan with varying prognosis.
- Associated abnormalities should be sought using ultrasound; karyotype should be considered, but the risk of amniocentesis should be weighed against the risk of chromosomal anomaly, taking into account previous screening tests.

CONCLUSIONS *(Continued)*

- Evaluation of renal function by ultrasound (amniotic fluid volume and renal parenchyma) and, occasionally, fetal urinalysis or fetal blood sampling may help clarify prognosis; renal function is good with unilateral disease.
- In the most severe cases with bilateral disease, the option of pregnancy termination should be considered.
- In continuing pregnancies, perinatal management should be planned with a pediatric surgeon/pediatrician.
- Fetal urinary decompression should be considered with great caution; although it does improve prognosis, parents should be aware that even though it allows survival of a baby, it might carry the price of long-term renal dysfunction.

KIDNEY ABNORMALITIES

General

Fetal renal anomalies include those of number, location, size, and structure. These malformations are primarily renal and usually occur in the absence of a urinary tract defect. Some, such as renal agenesis or multicystic kidney disease, are rather common and easy to diagnose. The diagnosis and antenatal management can be more difficult when renal structural anomalies present as hyperechogenic or enlarged kidneys. The first step after a renal abnormality has been identified is to exclude associated anomalies and, if necessary, offer fetal karyotyping.

The prognosis of isolated unilateral renal abnormalities is uniformly good, whereas bilateral anomalies associated with severe oligohydramnios are lethal. In bilateral cases with normal amniotic fluid, the long-term postnatal morbidity is difficult to predict. Biochemical markers that have been proved predictive of postnatal morbidity in uropathies have not performed well in fetal nephropathies. Our personal experience suggests that neither the fetal urinary electrolytes nor the fetal serum β_2-microglobulin are reliable predictors of postnatal renal function in fetuses with bilaterally enlarged and hyperechogenic kidneys and normal amniotic fluid volume (unpublished data).

Anomalies of Number

Renal agenesis can be unilateral or bilateral. It may result from early degeneration of the ureteric bud, or from a failed interaction between the ureteric bud and the blastema (Figs. 19–28 to 19–31). The corresponding adrenal gland assumes a globoid shape and should not be mistaken for a hypoplastic kidney.[116] Bilateral agenesis is lethal, causing the oligohydramnios sequence (pulmonary hypoplasia, dysmorphic face, and limb deformities).[62,117] In contrast, fetuses with unilateral renal agenesis remain symptom-free during postnatal life in the absence of associated anomalies. Minor genital anomalies such as duplicated/hypoplastic uterus, absent fallopian tube, absent epididymis and vas efferens can be found ipsilateral to unilateral renal agenesis. They cannot be diagnosed in utero and would not alter the prognosis for survival.[118]

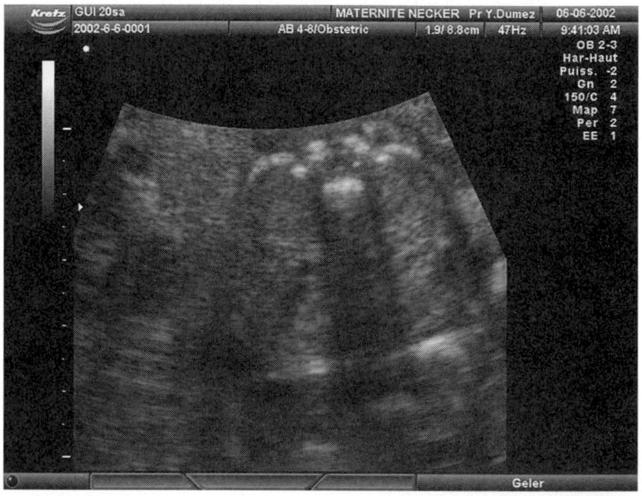

FIGURE 19–28
Bilateral renal agenesis, transverse view, at 20 weeks.

Duplication of the kidney is caused by the premature division of the ureteric bud before it connects to the nephrogenic mesoderm (Fig. 19–32). This explains its association with a double or bifid ureter. In the instance of a double ureter, the upper ureter typically enters the bladder more caudally, but may also connect ectopically to the urethra, vagina, seminal vesicle, or the rectum.

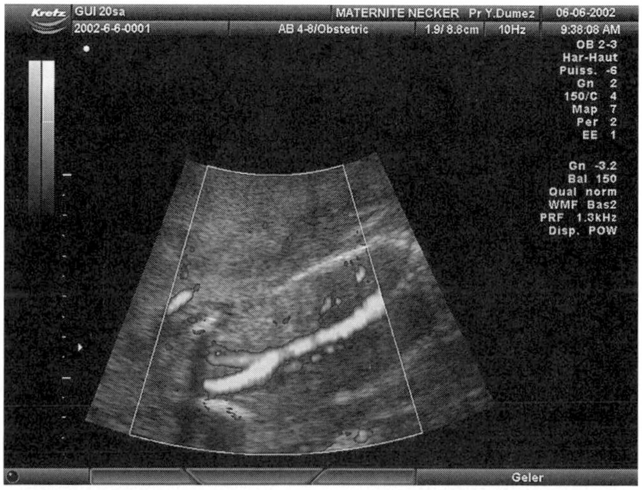

FIGURE 19–29
Bilateral renal agenesis, frontal view, at 20 weeks. Note the bilateral absence of renal vessels.

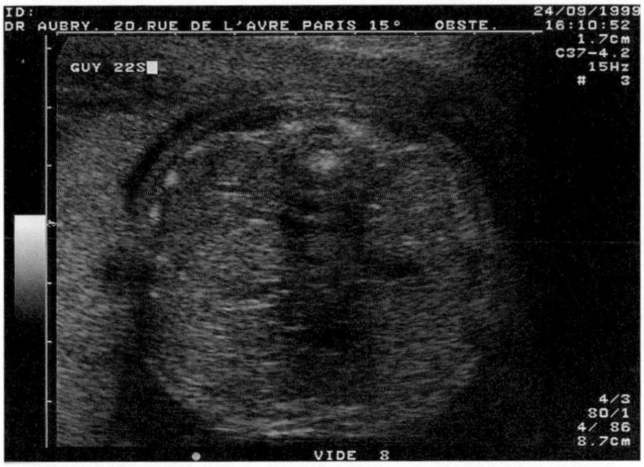

FIGURE 19–30
Unilateral renal agenesis, transverse view, at 22 weeks.

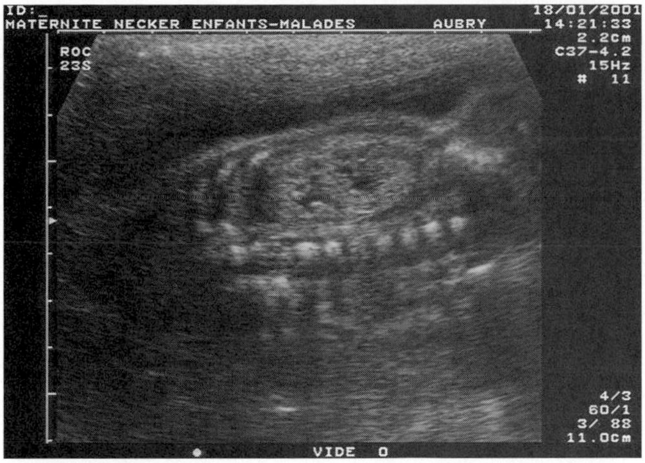

FIGURE 19–32
Renal duplication, frontal view, at 23 weeks.

The upper kidney usually shows some degree of outflow obstruction and parenchymal dysplasia. Therefore, a dilated pelvis or an abnormal structure in a dysplastic part of the kidney with a ureterocele at the connection of the distal ureter to the bladder may be a hallmark finding.[119] The accuracy of antenatal ultrasound for the diagnosis of fetal duplex kidney approximates 75%, based on two main sonographic features: identification of two separate poles in the affected kidney and the presence of a ureterocele.

Supernumerary kidney results from premature branching of the ureteric bud. The supernumerary kidney has its own ureter and blood supply, and frequently has complications such as obstruction or dysplasia.

Abnormalities of Position

Ectopic kidneys are usually displaced caudally. One or both kidneys may be involved, and the shape is abnormal due to malrotation. This condition is asymptomatic provided the renal parenchyma is well differentiated and free of dysplasia.[120] In crossed renal ectopia, both kidneys are located on the same side of the body and may be fused.

Horseshoe kidney results from the fusion of the kidneys, usually by their lower poles.[121] Fusion of both upper and lower poles produces the ring kidney. When isolated, horseshoe kidneys are usually asymptomatic. However, they are also associated with aneuploidy (trisomy 18, Turner syndrome, triploidy).

Isolated Abnormalities of Size and Structure

Renal hypoplasia is defined as kidney mass smaller than 2 SD below the mean. This condition is diagnosed postnatally except in its most severe form.

Multicystic dysplasia manifests antenatally as kidneys that have lost their normal shape (Figs. 19–33 and 19–34), containing a collection of macrocysts of variable diameter

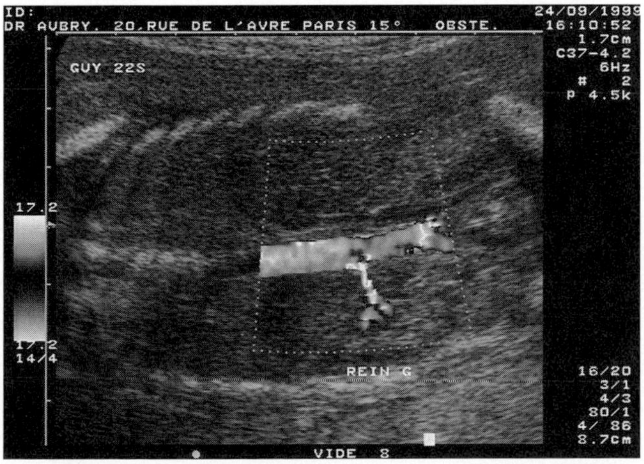

FIGURE 19–31
Unilateral renal agenesis, frontal view, at 22 weeks. Note the unilateral absence of renal vessels.

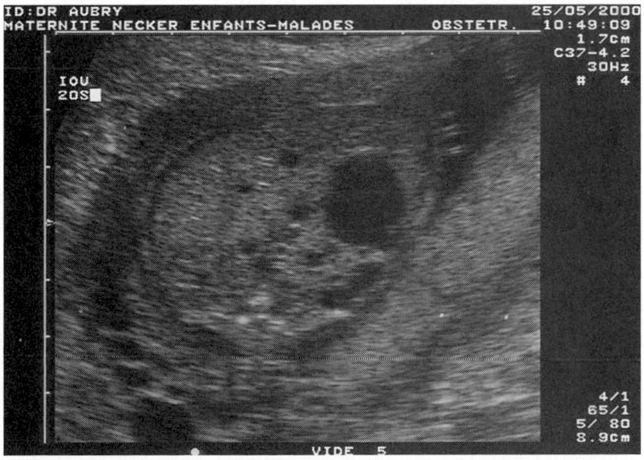

FIGURE 19–33
Unilateral multicystic kidney, transversal view, at 20 weeks.

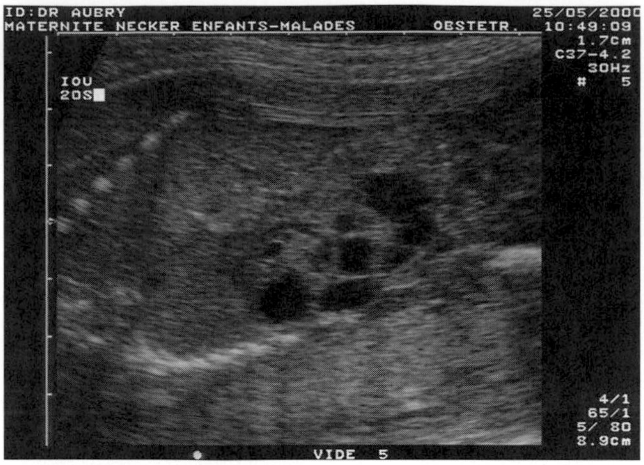

FIGURE 19–34
Unilateral multicystic kidney, frontal view, at 20 weeks.

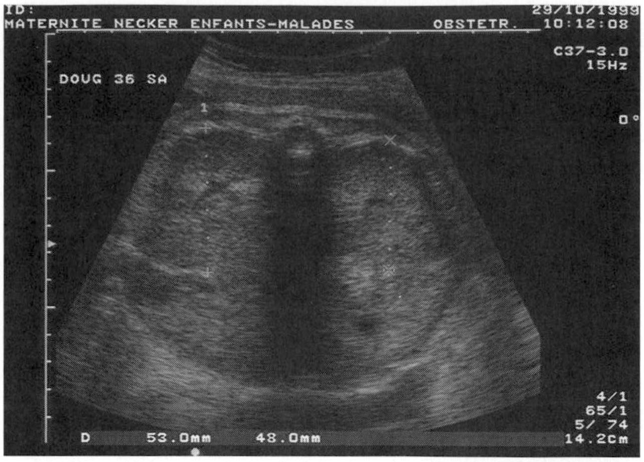

FIGURE 19–35
Enlarged hyperechogenic kidney (recessive autosomal polycystic kidney disease), transverse view, at 36 weeks.

(0.5–3 cm or more) that are connected neither to each other nor to the rest of the urinary tract. Some clusters of tubules, rudimentary glomeruli, primitive ducts, and bars of metaplastic cartilage may be irregularly distributed within the loose mesenchyme. It usually occurs in the absence of any obstructive uropathy. Whereas bilateral disease is lethal, unilateral forms have a good prognosis. Spontaneous involution of the multicystic kidney is usual during postnatal life and may on occasion occur in utero. The cyst size is usually constant throughout fetal life, but rarely extremely large cysts may compress the fetal abdomen or cause dystocia and therefore require intrauterine needling. These macrocystic lesions are easy to distinguish from polycystic kidney diseases, which present antenatally as enlarged hyperechoic kidneys. The sonographic pattern of the latter conditions is due to the microscopic cysts that fill the renal parenchyma.[122]

Autosomal recessive polycystic kidney disease is an inherited disorder and is also referred to as infantile polycystic kidney disease. It is characterized by enlarged kidneys that retain their shape. The cut surface has a spongy appearance due to elongated microcysts that have a radial orientation extending from the medulla to the cortical surface. These cysts correspond to dilated collecting ducts.[118] The liver is always involved with portal fibrosis and proliferation of bile ducts.[123,124] Postnatally, the diagnosis is easy to make based on typical anatomic features. The fetopathologic diagnosis, however, may be far more difficult in second trimester fetuses, underscoring the need for referring abnormal kidneys to pathologists familiar with fetal renal development.

Disease expression in utero is variable.[125–129] Some fetuses remain sonographically normal. In this instance, renal enlargement develops during infancy, and renal failure occurs relatively late in the second decade. At the other end of the spectrum, autosomal recessive polycystic kidney disease manifests in the second trimester as a premortem, anuric fetus with absent amniotic fluid and dramatically enlarged, hyperechogenic kidneys with no corticomedullary differentiation (Figs. 19–35 and 19–36). Intermediate forms are the norm, with a variable combination of renal enlargement and late-onset oligohydramnios.[128] The controlling gene has been mapped.[130]

Autosomal dominant polycystic kidney disease is also referred to as adult polycystic kidney disease because its clinical onset usually occurs in adulthood. This term, however, is misleading because autosomal dominant polycystic disease may manifest early and occasionally quite severely, including during fetal life. Autosomal dominant polycystic kidney is a common cause of enlarged hyperechogenic kidneys in the fetus because of the relatively high frequency of the mutation in the general population.[129,131–133] The diagnosis is easy when renal cysts are present in one of the parents. However, this hint may be lacking either because of the variability of disease expression or because the fetus has a new mutation.

In the adult, the kidneys are enlarged and their surface distorted by bulging macrocysts. During fetal life, however, the cysts are usually very small, producing a sonographic

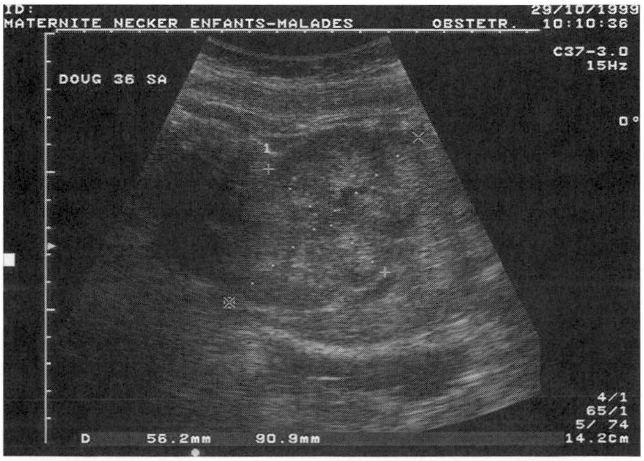

FIGURE 19–36
Enlarged hyperechogenic kidney (recessive autosomal polycystic kidney disease), parasagittal view, at 36 weeks. Note the absence of corticomedullary differentiation of the renal parenchyma.

pattern of enlarged, hyperechogenic kidneys similar in appearance to that of the recessive disease.[129] In the most severe cases, terminal renal failure occurs in utero. The diagnosis is made post mortem by showing both collecting tubules and nephrogenic cysts. Several mutations can result in disease. Known sites include chromosome 16 (PKD1 locus) and chromosome 4 (PKD2 locus).[134,135]

Transient nephromegaly is a poorly understood condition and can be defined as renal enlargement without any alteration of renal function. These patients may present as fetuses with moderately enlarged kidneys in which corticomedullary differentiation is usually retained. The kidneys may appear slightly hyperechogenic. The amniotic fluid volume remains normal. The sonographic abnormalities tend to regress during infancy, and the children remain symptom-free.[136] The uneventful postnatal course may be the only way to distinguish this condition from a true renal disease, such as polycystic kidney disease, or from less common causes of enlarged fetal kidneys.[129]

Prenatal Management of Isolated Hyperechogenic Kidneys

The counseling of a pregnant woman after sonographic diagnosis of isolated hyperechogenic fetal kidneys is challenging, because providing patients with overly pessimistic information leads to unnecessary pregnancy termination, whereas unrestricted reassurance may be unfair. Fetal sonography usually fails to provide an accurate etiologic diagnosis, and fetal hyperechogenic kidneys can result from a variety of etiologies, including recessive and dominant polycystic kidney disease and transient nephromegaly.[137] Further, there is a wide range of outcomes within each etiologic group. Postnatal series are likely to overlook the most severe cases leading to perinatal death, as well as the mildest ones, which may remain clinically undetectable over a long period.

The outcome can be predicted accurately in the most severe cases, in which terminal renal failure is certain with the discovery of severe oligohydramnios in the second trimester. If the pregnancy is terminated, it is crucial to obtain an accurate etiologic diagnosis and to store fetal DNA, because this information may lead to first-trimester molecular prenatal diagnosis at subsequent pregnancies, should autosomal recessive or dominant polycystic kidney disease be identified. A wrong histopathologic diagnosis might have dramatic consequences in terms of genetic counseling and prenatal diagnosis.

In less severe cases, antenatal counseling should be based on prospective studies with long postnatal follow-up. In our experience[129] of a continuous series of 45 fetuses with bilateral isolated hyperechogenic kidneys, there were 20 with autosomal recessive disease, 8 with autosomal dominant disease, 9 with other renal disorders, and 6 symptom-free survivors without etiologic diagnosis. There were 19 pregnancy terminations, 5 neonatal deaths, and 19 survivors, of whom 14 had normal renal function, 3 had mild renal failure, and 2 had end-stage renal failure. None of those with severe oligohydramnios and fetal kidneys greater than 4 SD survived (n = 14, 10 terminations, 4 neonatal deaths), whereas 13 of 16 with normal amniotic fluid volume and kidneys less than 4 SD survived; 9 were symptom-free with a follow-up of 34 to 132 months.

Rare Etiologies of Fetal Nephropathies

Renal tubular dysgenesis is a rare condition characterized by poorly developed or undeveloped proximal tubules, causing severe oligohydramnios.[138] It is thought due to an abnormality of the renin-angiotensin system because similar renal anomalies are reported after prenatal exposure to angiotensin-converting enzyme inhibitors. This lethal condition is probably inherited in an autosomal recessive disorder and should be recognized at fetal autopsy to provide adequate genetic counseling. Prolonged exposition to indomethacin may also induce renal failure, but probably by a different mechanism.[139]

Nephroblastomatosis is characterized by the presence of nephrogenic rests of metanephric blastema in both kidneys.[140] The kidneys may appear hyperechogenic and are associated with overgrowth syndromes such as Beckwith-Wiedemann syndrome. Affected patients are also at increased risk for developing Wilms' tumor (see Chapter 23).

Renal tumors that present during fetal life are rapidly growing solid heterogeneous masses.[141] They are easy to distinguish from single transonic cysts that can also be recognized in utero but remain asymptomatic postnatally. Mesoblastic nephroma are reported to have a typical "ring" sign on Doppler examination, which consists in an anechoic ring surrounding the tumor with a color Doppler signal.[142]

Fetal Nephropathies with Polyhydramnios

The Finnish type of congenital nephrotic syndrome may present antenatally with hydramnios, placentomegaly, and moderate growth restriction. Modest alterations in the renal parenchyma such as hyperechogenicity are inconstant, making the antenatal diagnosis difficult in the absence of an index case.[143–145] In practice, one should consider performing a biochemical analysis of amniotic fluid in cases of unexplained hydramnios, which may occasionally lead to the diagnosis of fetal proteinuria (high concentration of α-fetoprotein and other proteins). Inconsistently,[146] anomalies of electrolyte or aldosterone concentrations in the amniotic fluid may suggest Bartter's syndrome,[147–150] which is characterized by early-onset hydramnios and mild pyelectasis resulting from the fetal polyuria.

Cystic Kidneys and Multiple Malformation Syndromes

Cystic kidneys are part of several multiple malformation syndromes.[151] The autosomal recessive Meckel-Gruber syndrome is one of the most common and lethal. It is characterized by severe oligohydramnios during the second trimester with markedly enlarged kidneys whose normal structure has been replaced by multiple cysts.[152] Encephalocele and postaxial polydactyly are characteristic of the Meckel-Gruber syndrome but can be difficult to see once severe oligohydramnios has occurred.[153] Severe oligohydramnios and enlarged dysplastic kidneys can also be sonographic features of chromosomal abnormalities such as trisomy 13.

Horseshoe kidney is associated with trisomy 18, Turner syndrome, or triploidy.

The Laurence-Moon-Bardet-Biedl syndrome presents antenatally as hyperechogenic kidneys with polydactyly. Growth is usually normal during fetal life. In the Beckwith-Wiedemann syndrome the enlarged kidneys are part of a more generalized visceromegaly, occasionally associated with an omphalocele. DiGeorge syndrome may manifest as a heart defect associated with renal abnormalities. Zellweger syndrome appears as renal cortical cysts with cerebral periventricular pseudocysts. Smith-Lemli-Opitz syndrome is considered when dysplastic kidneys are associated with intrauterine growth restriction, abnormal fingers, and ambiguous genitalia.

Dysplastic kidneys are also found in a variety of other syndromes, but usually as a secondary finding (e.g., short rib polydactyly associations). This underscores the need for careful sonographic evaluation when abnormal kidneys are found. Fetal karyotyping is considered when the structure of the kidneys is abnormal (hyperechogenicity, suspected dysplasia). However, isolated multicystic kidneys, renal agenesis, and ectopic kidneys are not associated with an increased risk of aneuploidy.

SUMMARY OF MANAGEMENT OPTIONS
Kidney Abnormalities

Management Options	Quality of Evidence	Strength of Recommendation	References
When kidney anomaly is found, immediately examine to exclude other abnormalities.	III	GPP	137
Consider karyotype in specific conditions with risk of aneuploidy.	–	GPP	–
• Identify inherited disease based on family history and postnatal follow up, or postmortem examination.	–	GPP	–
• Store fetal DNA when appropriate	–	GPP	–
• Identify inherited disease based on family history and postnatal follow-up	–	GPP	–
Evaluation of fetal renal function is based on ultrasound (amniotic fluid volume). Renal function is good in unilateral cases.	III	GPP	129, 137
Organize prenatal sonographic follow-up.	–	GPP	–
In the most severe cases, the option of pregnancy termination should be considered.	III	GPP	129, 137
With ongoing pregnancies, and particularly in bilateral cases, plan perinatal management with pediatric nephrologist/pediatrician.	–	GPP	129, 137
Place for delivery is determined by anticipated immediate neonatal needs.	–	GPP	–
Perform careful examination and assessment of baby after delivery or postmortem examination after perinatal death.	–	GPP	–

CONCLUSIONS

- Fetal anomalies can vary in prognosis; the prognosis is generally good for unilateral lesions, poor for bilateral lesions with oligohydramnios, and difficult to predict with bilateral lesions with normal amniotic fluid volume; biochemical testing of urine is not helpful in predicting kidney function.
- Other abnormalities should be excluded; karyotyping will be indicated with specific abnormalities.
- Fetal DNA should be stored when a termination of pregnancy is performed for a suspected genetic renal abnormality, such as polycystic kidney disease.

ABNORMAL GENITALIA

General

Although fetal ultrasound is widely used to determine fetal gender, there is no consensus as to whether the structure of external genitalia should be part of standard screening ultrasound. Major genital abnormalities can have a devastating impact on postnatal life, and genital abnormalities may be the hallmark of a multiple malformation syndrome. Ambiguous genitalia can be a medical emergency in neonates with salt-wasting forms of congenital adrenal hyperplasia. An examination of the fetal genitalia is mandatory whenever a uronephrologic abnormality is found to rule out a complex malformation of the fetal pelvis (see previous section) (Fig. 19–37).

Sonographic Diagnosis

Abnormal fetal genitalia may be identified under different circumstances:

- A specific genetic risk based on family history. This includes 5α-reductase deficiency, androgen insensitivity, and congenital adrenal hyperplasia. However, in a growing number of cases, the molecular mechanism of the disease is established, allowing for first-trimester genetic diagnosis using chorionic villi.
- A discrepancy between the fetal gender established on routine ultrasound and fetal karyotyping.
- Abnormal or ambiguous genitalia found during routine ultrasound, either isolated or as part of a complex anomaly of the fetal pelvis or of a multiple malformation syndrome.

Undescended testis (Fig. 19–38) can be physiologic in the second trimester. Associated abnormalities, including uropathies and the prune-belly syndrome, should be ruled out.

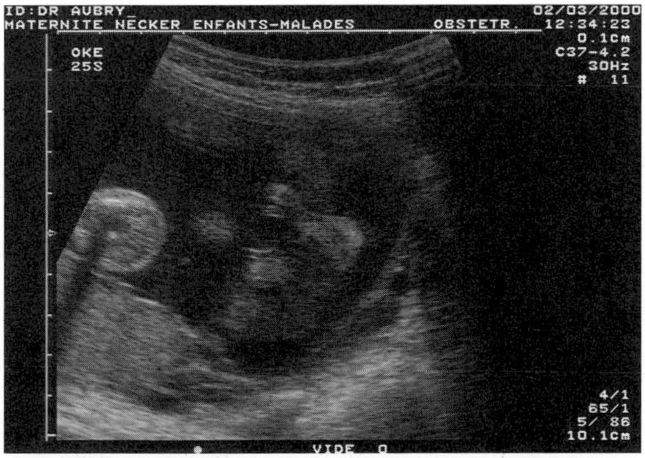

FIGURE 19–37
Bifidity of external genitalia in a girl with bladder exstrophy, Tangential view of the perineum, at 25 weeks.

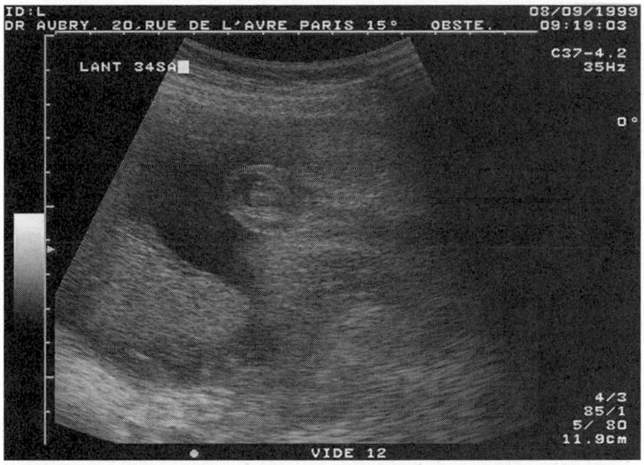

FIGURE 19–38
Unilateral undescended testes at 34 weeks.

The diagnosis of hypospadias is more often made during the third trimester than in the second. Even in experienced hands, the antenatal diagnosis of hypospadias can be impossible because of fetal position or technical limitations, including oligohydramnios. Anterior or middle hypospadias is rarely identified antenatally on ultrasound, although it is usually self-evident on examination of the neonate. Occasionally, the fetal penis is suspected to be shorter than usual, or to have a certain degree of abnormal curvature (Fig. 19–39). The tip of the penis may seem blunt. Ventral deflection of urinary stream can occasionally be seen using color Doppler.[154] Posterior hypospadias may be diagnosed antenatally based on the finding of a bifid scrotum, a short and curved penis, and no urethral canal (Fig. 19–40). The angulated penis located between the two scrotal folds is said to resemble a tulip flower.[155] When associated with undescended testis, posterior hypospadias may be difficult to differentiate from masculinized female genitalia with fused labia and an enlarged clitoris.[156]

Rare conditions identifiable antenatally by ultrasound include distal obstruction of the fetal urethra

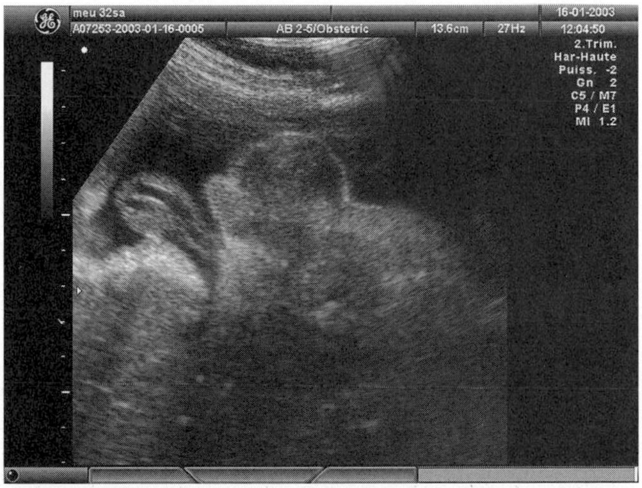

FIGURE 19–39
Short penis, sagittal view at 32 weeks.

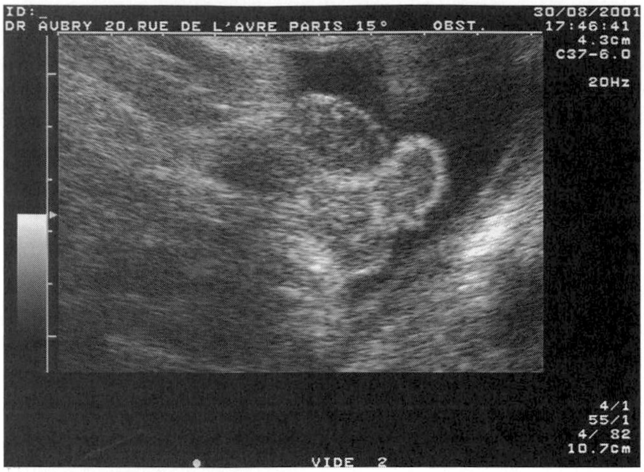

FIGURE 19–40
Short penis with abnormal curvature (hypospadias) at 32 weeks.

(Fig. 19–41), perineal tumors, congenital hernia, and penoscrotal transposition.[157]

Gender discrepancies may be explained by a variety of mechanisms.[158] A discrepancy between the phenotypic fetal gender and fetal karyotype may result from a labeling error of the amniotic fluid sample, a typing error in sonographic or genetic records, or maternal contamination of amniotic fluid cultures. The ultrasound examination should seek to establish whether the external genitalia seem structurally normal or ambiguous. Enlarged adrenal glands in the third trimester are suggestive of adrenal hyperplasia, and result more often in ambiguous virilized female genitalia than in a male phenotype with an abnormal scrotum (Fig. 19–42). The presence of a fetal uterus can occasionally be documented sonographically, but its absence can never be ascertained confidently. Conversely, when abnormal genitalia are first identified by ultrasound, fetal karyotyping is the first step toward an antenatal diagnosis.[156]

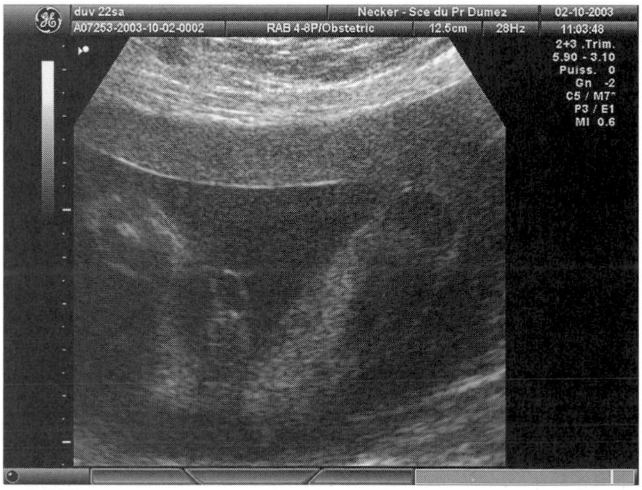

FIGURE 19–41
Distal urethral obstruction with dilated penile urethra, at 22 weeks.

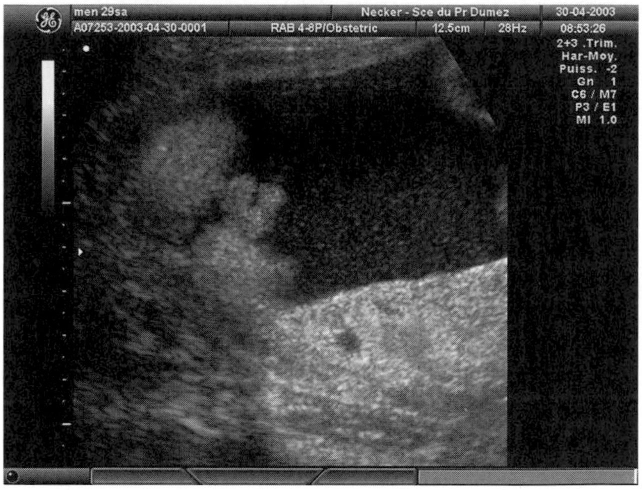

FIGURE 19–42
Ambiguous genitalia, showing virilization of an XX fetus (congenital adrenal hyperplasia) at 29 weeks.

Management Options

Parallel to establishing the anatomy of the fetal genitalia, associated abnormalities should be sought. A number of multiple malformation syndromes including Smith-Lemli-Opitz, CHARGE, Prader-Willi, and camptomelic dwarfism, can be associated with genital abnormalities. Complex cloacae malformations should also be sought (see previous section) and may be part of a more complex entity, such as the VATER association or a caudal regression syndrome. Fetuses with bladder exstrophy have abnormal genitalia. A bifid genital tubercle with epispadias may be found in males. The diagnosis is based on the absence of a fetal bladder associated with a low-lying fetal umbilical cord insertion and an abnormal bony pelvis. Cloacal exstrophy can produce bowel abnormalities suggestive of gastroschisis associated with vesical exstrophy.

The results of the fetal karyotype should be interpreted with great care, for the "genetic" gender may not be the "true" gender of the infant. For example, XX males bearing the *SRY* gene are unambiguously boys, and XY fetuses with complete androgen insensitivity present as females. Adrenal hyperplasia may be suspected by ultrasound and confirmed by measuring the amniotic fluid 17-OH progesterone concentration. Counseling after the antenatal diagnosis of an apparently isolated abnormality of external genitalia is challenging and may be devastating for the family. Identifying the mechanism of the anomaly is helpful. Determining the anatomy of the fetal genitalia is crucial to establish the prognosis in terms of the potential for surgical repair. Counseling by a pediatric surgeon and a pediatric endocrinologist having extensive experience of intersex states is warranted to provide the parents with information on postnatal management and gender assignment.

SUMMARY OF MANAGEMENT OPTIONS
Abnormal Genitalia

Management Options	Quality of Evidence	Strength of Recommendation	References
Exclude other abnormalities.	–	GPP	–
Karyotype for gender and to exclude other chromosomal abnormalities, but exercise care in assigning gender even after birth.	–	GPP	–
Organize prenatal sonographic follow-up.	–	GPP	–
Interdisciplinary approach: plan perinatal management with pediatric surgeon, pediatric endocrinologist, and geneticist.	–	GPP	–
Delivery is probably best in center where careful examination, assessment, and plans for management can be made after birth.	–	GPP	–

CONCLUSIONS

- Full extent of abnormalities not always clear before birth.
- Careful search for other abnormalities including chromosomal is advisable.
- Interdisciplinary management is manadatory.
- Care needs to be taken with gender assignment.

REFERENCES

1. Liu HY, Dhillon HK, Yeung CK, et al: Clinical outcome and management of prenatally diagnosed primary megaureters. J Urol 1994;152(2 Pt 2):614–617.
2. McLellan DL, Retik AB, Bauer SB, et al: Rate and predictors of spontaneous resolution of prenatally diagnosed primary nonrefluxing megaureter. J Urol 2002;168:2177–2180.
3. Upadhyay J, Bolduc S, Braga L, et al: Impact of prenatal diagnosis on the morbidity associated with ureterocele management. J Urol 2002;167:2560–2565.
4. Nakayama D, Harrison M, de Lorimier A: Prognosis of posterior urethral valves presenting at birth. J Pediatr Surg 1986;21: 43–45.
5. El-Ghoneimi A, Desgrippes A, Luton D, et al: Outcome of posterior urethral valves: To what extent is it improved by prenatal diagnosis? J Urol 1999;162:849–853.
6. Upadhyay J, McLorie GA, Bolduc S, et al: Natural history of neonatal reflux associated with prenatal hydronephrosis: Long-term results of a prospective study. J Urol 2003;169:1837.
7. Moerman P, Fryns JP, Godderis P, Lauweryns J: Pathogenesis of the prune belly syndrome: A functional urethral obstruction caused by prostatic hypoplasia. Pediatrics 1984;73:470–475.
8. Grannum P, Bracken M, Silverman R, Hobbins J: Assessment of fetal kidney size in normal gestation by comparison of ratio of kidney circumference to abdominal circumference. Am J Obstet Gynecol 1980;136:249–254.
9. Jeanty P, Dramaix-Wilmet M, Elkazen N, et al: Measurement of fetal kidney growth on ultrasound. Radiology 1982;144:159–162.
10. Whitlow BJ, Lazanakis MS, Economides DL: The sonographic identification of fetal gender from 11 to 14 weeks of gestation. Ultrasound Obstet Gynecol 1999;13:301–304.
11. Emerson DS, Felker RE, Brown DL: The sagittal sign—An early second trimester sonographic indicator of fetal gender. J Ultrasound Med 1989;8:293–297.
12. Mazza V, Falcinelli C, Paganelli S, et al: Sonographic early fetal gender assignment: A longitudinal study in pregnancies after in vitro fertilization. Ultrasound Obstet Gynecol 2001;17(6): 513–516.
13. Hayden SA, Russ PD, Pretorius DH, et al: Posterior urethral obstruction. Prenatal sonographic findings and clinical outcome in fourteen cases. J Ultrasound Med 1988;7(7):371–375.
14. Hobbins J, Romero R, Grannum P, et al: Antenatal diagnosis of renal anomalies with ultrasound. I Obstructive uropathy. Am J Obstet Gynecol 1984;148:868–877.
15. Wladimiroff J, Scholtmeijer R, Stewart P, et al: Prenatal evaluation and outcome of fetal obstructive uropathies. Prenat Diagn 1988;8:93–102.
16. Paduano L, Giglio L, Bembi B, et al: Clinical outcome of fetal uropathy. II. Sensitivity of echography for prenatal detection of obstructive pathology. J Urol 1991;146(4):1097–1098.
17. Paduano L, Giglio L, Bembi B, et al: Clinical outcome of fetal uropathy. I. Predictive value of prenatal echography positive for obstructive uropathy. J Urol 1991;146(4):1094–1096.
18. Chudleigh T: Mild pyelectasis. Prenat Diagn 2001;21:936–941.
19. Anderson N, Clautice-Engle T, Allan R, et al: Detection of obstructive uropathy in the fetus: Predictive value of sonographic measurements of renal pelvic diameter at various gestational ages. AJR Am J Roentgenol 1995;164:719–723.
20. Dremsek PA, Gindl K, Voitl P, et al: Renal pyelectasis in fetuses and neonates: Diagnostic value of renal pelvis diameter in pre-

and postnatal sonographic screening. AJR Am J Roentgenol 1997;168(4):1017–1019.
21. Corteville JE, Dicke JM, Crane JP: Fetal pyelectasis and Down syndrome: Is genetic amniocentesis warranted? Obstet Gynecol 1992;79(5 Pt 1):770–772.
22. Bronshtein M, Bar-Hava I, Lightman A: The significance of early second-trimester sonographic detection of minor fetal renal anomalies. Prenat Diagn 1995;15(7):627–632.
23. Adra AM, Mejides AA, Dennaoui MS, Beydoun SN: Fetal pyelectasis: Is it always "physiologic"? Am J Obstet Gynecol 1995;173:1263–1266.
24. Morin L, Cendron M, Crombleholme TM, et al: Minimal hydronephrosis in the fetus: Clinical significance and implications for management. J Urol 1996;155:2047–2049.
25. Ouzounian JG, Castro MA, Fresquez M, et al: Prognostic significance of antenatally detected fetal pyelectasis. Ultrasound Obstet Gynecol 1996;7(6):424–428.
26. Jaswon MS, Dibble L, Puri S, et al: Prospective study of outcome in antenatally diagnosed renal pelvis dilatation. Arch Dis Child Fetal Neonat Educ 1999;80:F135–F138.
27. Sairam S, Al-Habib A, Sasson S, Thilaganathan B: Natural history of fetal hydronephrosis diagnosed on mid-trimester ultrasound. Ultrasound Obstet Gynecol 2001;17(3):191–196.
28. Bobrowski RA, Levin RB, Lauria MR, et al: In utero progression of isolated renal pelvis dilation. Am J Perinatol 1997;14(7):423–426.
29. Barker AP, Cave MM, Thomas DF, et al: Fetal pelvi-ureteric junction obstruction: Predictors of outcome. Br J Urol 1995;76:649–652.
30. Thomas DF, Madden NP, Irving HC, et al: Mild dilatation of the fetal kidney: A follow-up study. Br J Urol 1994;74(2):236–239.
31. Persutte WH, Koyle M, Lenke RR, et al: Mild pyelectasis ascertained with prenatal ultrasonography is pediatrically significant. Ultrasound Obstet Gynecol 1997;10(1):12–18.
32. Glick PL, Harrison MR, Golbus MS, et al: Management of the fetus with congenital hydronephrosis II: Prognostic criteria and selection for treatment. J Pediatr Surg 1985;20(4):376–387.
33. Fernbach SK, Maizels M, Conway JJ: Ultrasound grading of hydronephrosis: Introduction to the system used by the Society for Fetal Urology. Pediatr Radiol 1993;23(6):478–480.
34. Grignon A, Filion R, Filiatrault, et al: Urinary tract dilatation in utero: Classification and clinical applications. Radiology 1986;160:645–647.
35. Mahony BS, Filly RA, Callen PW, et al: Fetal renal dysplasia: Sonographic evaluation. Radiology 1984;152(1):143–146.
36. Corteville JE, Gray DL, Crane JP: Congenital hydronephrosis: Correlation of fetal ultrasonographic findings with infant outcome. Am J Obstet Gynecol 1991;165(2):384–388.
37. Gunn TR, Mora JD, Pease P: Antenatal diagnosis of urinary tract abnormalities by ultrasonography after 28 weeks' gestation: Incidence and outcome. Am J Obstet Gynecol 1995;172(2 Pt 1):479–486.
38. Blachar A, Blachar Y, Livne PM, et al: Clinical outcome and follow-up of prenatal hydronephrosis. Pediatr Nephrol 1994;8(1):30–35.
39. Hutton KA, Thomas DF, Davies BW: Prenatally detected posterior urethral valves: Qualitative assessment of second trimester scans and prediction of outcome. J Urol 1997;158(3 Pt 2):1022–1025.
40. Muller F, Dommergues M, Mandelbrot L, et al: Fetal urinary biochemistry predicts postnatal renal function in children with bilateral obstructive uropathies. Obstet Gynecol 1993;82(5):813–820.
41. Caione P, Patricolo M, Lais A, et al: Role of prenatal diagnosis in the treatment of congenital obstructive megaureter in a solitary kidney. Fetal Diagn Ther 1996;11(3):205–209.
42. Adzick NS, Harrison MR, Flake AW, deLorimier AA: Urinary extravasation in the fetus with obstructive uropathy. J Pediatr Surg 1985;20:608–615.
43. Bois E, Feingold J, Benmaiz H, Briard ML: Congenital urinary tract malformations: Epidemiologic and genetic aspects. Clin Genet 1975;8:37–47.
44. Cocchi G, Magnani C, Morini MS, et al: Urinary tract abnormalities (UTA) and associated malformations: Data of the Emilia-Romagna registry. Eur J Epidemiol 1996;12:493–497.
45. Nicolaides KH, Cheng HH, Snijders RJ, Moniz CF: Fetal urine biochemistry in the assessment of obstructive uropathy. Am J Obstet Gynecol 1992;166(3):932–937.
46. Mirk P, Calisti A, Fileni A: Prenatal sonographic diagnosis of bladder extrophy. J Ultrasound Med 1986;5:291–293.
47. Barth R, Filly R, Sondheimer F: Prenatal sonographic findings in bladder extrophy. J Ultrasound Med 1990;9:359–361.
48. Nussbaum AR, Sanders RC, Gearhart JP: Obstructed uterovaginal anomalies: Demonstration with sonography. Part I. Neonates and Infants. Radiology 1991;179:79–83.
49. Jaramillo D, Lebowitz RL, Hendren WH: The cloacal malformation: Radiologic findings and imaging recommendations. Radiology 1990;177:441–448.
50. Petrikovsky BM, Walzak MP, D'Addario PF: Fetal cloacal anomalies: Prenatal sonographic findings and differential diagnosis. Obstet Gynecol 1988;72(3 Pt 2):464–469.
51. Mandell J, Blyth BR, Peters CA, et al: Structural genitourinary defects detected in utero. Radiology 1991;178(1):193–196.
52. Smith DP, Felker RE, Noe HN, et al: Prenatal diagnosis of genital anomalies. Urology 1996;47(1):114–117.
53. Mirk P, Pintus C, Speca S: Ultrasound diagnosis of hydrocolpos: Prenatal findings and postnatal follow-up. J Clin Ultrasound 1994;22(1):55–58.
54. Gillis DA, Grantmyre EB: Megacystis-microcolon-intestinal hypoperistalsis syndrome: Survival of male infant. J Pediatr Surg 1985;20(3):279–281.
55. Mandell J, Lebowitz RL, Peters CA, et al: Prenatal diagnosis of the megacystis-megaureter association. J Urol 1992;148(5): 1487–1489.
56. Nicolaides KH, Cheng HH, Abbas A, et al: Fetal renal defects: Associated malformations and chromosomal defects. Fetal Diagn Ther 1992;7:1–11.
57. Nicolaides K: Screening for chromosomal effects (editorial). Ultrasound Obstet Gynaecol 2003;21:313–321.
58. Smith-Bindman R, Hosmer W, Feldstein VA, et al: Second trimester ultrasound to detect fetuses with Down syndrome. A meta-analysis. JAMA 2001;285:1044–1455.
59. Bromley B, Lieberman E, Shipp TD, Benacerraf BR: The genetic sonogram, a method of risk assessment for Down syndrome in the second trimester. J Ultrasound Med 2002;21: 1087–1096.
60. Nyberg DA, Souter VL, El-Bastawissi A, et al: Isolated sonographic markers for detection of fetal Down syndrome in the second trimester of pregnancy. J Ultrasound Med 2001;20: 1053–1063.
61. Benacerraf BR, Nadel A, Bromley B: Identification of second-trimester fetuses with autosomal trisomy by use of a sonographic scoring index. Radiology 1994;193(1):135–140.
62. Bronstein M, Amit A, Achiron R, et al: The early prenatal sonographic diagnosis of renal agenesis: Techniques and possible pitfalls. Prenat Diagn 1994;14(4):291–297.
63. Snijders RJM, Sebire NJ, Faria M, et al: Fetal mild hydronephtosis and chromosomal defects: Relation to maternal age and gestation. Fetal Diagn Ther 1995;10:349–355.
64. Wickstrom EA, Thangavelu M, Parilla BV, et al: A prospective study of the association between isolated fetal pyelectasis and chromosomal abnormality. Obstet Gynecol 1996;88(3):379–382.
65. Vintzileos AM, Campbell WA, Guzman ER, et al: Second-trimester ultrasound markers for detection of trisomy 21: Which markers are best? Obstet Gynecol 1997;89(6):941–944.
66. Nyberg DA, Luthy DA, Cheng EY, et al: Role of prenatal ultrasonography in women with positive screen for Down syndrome

on the basis of maternal serum markers. Am J Obstet Gynecol 1995;173:1030–1035.
67. Verdin SM, Whitlow BJ, Lazanakis M, et al: Ultrasonographic markers for chromosomal abnormalities in women with negative nuchal translucency and second trimester maternal serum biochemistry. Ultrasound Obstet Gynecol 2000;16:402–406.
68. DeVore GR: The genetic sonogram: Its use in the detection of chromosomal abnormalities in fetuses of women of advanced maternal age. Prenat Diagn 2001;21:40–45.
69. Bromley B, Lieberman E, Shipp TD, Benacerraf BR: The genetic sonogram, a method of risk assessment for Down syndrome in the second trimester. J Ultrasound Med 2002;21:1087–1096.
70. Havutcu AE, Nikolopoulos G, Adinkra P, Lamont RF: The association between fetal pyelectasis on second trimester ultrasound scan and aneuploidy among 25,586 low risk unselected women. Prenat Diagn 2002;22:1201–1206.
71. Kilbride HW, Yeast J, Thibeault DW: Defining limits of survival: Lethal pulmonary hypoplasia after midtrimester premature rupture of membranes. Am J Obstet Gynecol 1996;175(3 Pt 1):675–681.
72. Nimrod C, Varela-Gittings F, Machin G, et al: The effect of very prolonged membrane rupture on fetal development. Am J Obstet Gynecol 1984;148(5):540–543.
73. Vergani P, Ghidini A, Locatelli A, et al: Risk factors for pulmonary hypoplasia in second-trimester premature rupture of membranes. Am J Obstet Gynecol 1994;170(5 Pt 1):1359–1364.
74. Nimrod C, Nicholson S, Davies D, et al: Pulmonary hypoplasia testing in obstetrics. Am J Obstet Gynecol 1988;158:277–280.
75. Silver RK, MacGregor SN, Cook WA, Sholl JS: Fetal posterior urethral valve syndrome: A prospective application of antenatal prognostic criteria. Obstet Gynecol 1990;76(5 Pt 2):951–955.
76. Adzick NS, Harrison MR, Flake AW, Laberge JM: Development of a fetal renal function test using endogenous creatinine clearance. J Pediatr Surg 1985;20:602–607.
77. Elder JS, O'Grady JP, Ashmead G, et al: Evaluation of fetal renal function: Unreliability of fetal urinary electrolytes. J Urol 1990;144(2 Pt 2):574–578.
78. Muller F, Dommergues M, Bussieres L, et al: Development of human renal function: Reference intervals for 10 biochemical markers in fetal urine. Clin Chem 1996;42(11):1855–1860.
79. Eugène M, Muller F, Dommergues M, et al: Evaluation of postnatal renal function in fetuses with bilateral uropathies by proton nuclear magnetic resonance spectroscopy. Am J Obstet Gyneol 1994;170:595–602.
80. Nicolini U, Fisk NM, Rodeck CH, Beacham J: Fetal urine biochemistry: An index of renal maturation and dysfunction. BJOG 1992;99:46–50.
81. Wilkins IA, Chitkara U, Lynch L, et al: The nonpredictive value of fetal urinary electrolytes: Preliminary report of outcomes and correlations with pathologic diagnosis. Am J Obstet Gynecol 1987;157(3):694–698.
82. Lipitz S, Ryan G, Samuell C, et al: Fetal urine analysis for the assessment of renal function in obstructive uropathy. Am J Obstet Gynecol 1993;168:174–179.
83. Johnson MP, Corsi P, Bradfield W, et al: Sequential urinalysis improves evaluation of fetal renal function in obstructive uropathy. Am J Obstet Gynecol 1995;173(1):59–65.
84. Tassis BM, Trespidi L, Tirelli AS, et al: In fetuses with isolated hydronephrosis, urinary beta2-microglobulin and *N*-acetyl-beta-*D*-glucosaminidase (NAG) have a limited role in the prediction of postnatal renal function. Prenat Diagn 1996;16(12):1087–1093.
85. Berry SM, Lecolier B, Smith RS, et al: Predictive value of fetal serum beta 2-microglobulin for neonatal renal function. Lancet 1995;345(8960):1277–1278.
86. Cobet G, Gummelt T, Bollmann R, et al: Assessment of serum levels of alpha-1-microglobulin, beta-2-microglobulin, and retinol binding protein in the fetal blood. A method for prenatal evaluation of renal function. Prenat Diagn 1996;16(4):299–305.
87. Tassis BM, Trespidi L, Tirelli AS, et al: Serum beta 2-microglobulin in fetuses with urinary tract anomalies. Am J Obstet Gynecol 1997;176(1 Pt 1):54–57.
88. Dommergues M, Muller F, Ngo S, et al: Fetal serum beta2-microglobulin predicts postnatal renal function in bilateraluropathies. Kidney Int 2000;58:312–316.
89. Daikha-Dahmane F, Dommergues M, Muller F, et al: Development of human fetal kidney in obstructive uropathy: Correlations with ultrasonography and urine biochemistry. Kidney Int 1997;52(1):21–32.
90. Evans MI, Sacks AJ, Johnson MP, et al: Sequential invasive assessment of fetal renal function and the intrauterine treatment of fetal obstructive uropathies. Obstet Gynecol 1991;77(4):545–550.
91. Vallancian G, Beurton D, Szemat R, et al: Etude expérimentale comparée des conséquences rénales du reflux vésico-urétéral et de l'obstruction urétérale chez le fœtus de brebis. J Urol 1982;88:27–30.
92. Harrison M, Nakayama D, Noall R, deLorimier A: Correction of congenital hydronephrosis in utero II. Decompression reverses the effects of obstruction on the fetal lung and urinary tract. J Pediatr Surg 1982;17:965–974.
93. Harrison M, Ross N, Noall R, de Lorimier A: Correction of congenital hydronephrosis in utero I the model: Fetal urethral obstruction produces hydronephrosis and pulmonary hypoplasia in fetal lamb. J Pediatr Surg 1983;18:247–256.
94. Glick PL, Harrison MR, Noall RA, Villa RL: Corrections of congenital hydronephrosis in utero III. Early mid-trimester ureteral obstruction produces renal dysplasia. J Pediatr Surg 1983;18(6):681–687.
95. Coplen DE, Hare JY, Zderic SA, et al: 10-year experience with prenatal intervention for hydronephrosis. J Urol 1996;156: 1142–1145.
96. Crombleholme TM, Harrison MR, Golbus MS, et al: Fetal intervention in obstructive uropathy: Prognostic indicators and efficacy of intervention. Am J Obstet Gynecol 1990; 162(5):1239–1244.
97. Elder JS, Duckett JW Jr, Snyder HM: Intervention for fetal obstructive uropathy: Has it been effective? Lancet 1987;2(8566):1007–1010.
98. Freedman AL, Bukowski TP, Smith CA, et al: Fetal therapy for obstructive uropathy: Diagnosis of specific outcomes. Urol 1996;156(2 Pt 2):720–723.
99. Grannum P: In utero therapy of fetal obstructive uropathy. Fetal Ther 1986;1(2–3):119–120.
100. Manning FA, Harrison MR, Rodeck C: Catheter shunts for fetal hydronephrosis and hydrocephalus. Report of the International Fetal Surgery Registry. N Engl J Med 1986;315(5):336–340.
101. Weiner C, Williamson R, Bonsib SM, et al: In utero bladder diversion—Problems with patient selection. Fetal Ther 1986;1:196–202.
102. Estes JM, MacGillivray TE, Hedrick MH, et al: Fetoscopic surgery for the treatment of congenital anomalies. J Pediatr Surg 1992;27(8):950–954.
103. Quinterro R, Hume R, Smith C, et al: Percutaneous fetal cystoscopy and endoscopic fulguration of posterior urethral valves. Am J Obstet Gynecol 1995;172:206–209.
104. Quintero RA, Shukla AR, Homsy YL, Bukkapatnam R: Successful in utero endoscopic ablation of posterior urethral valves: A new dimension in fetal urology. Urology 2000;55(5):774.
105. Wisser J, Kurmanavicius J, Lauper U, et al: Successful treatment of fetal megavesica in the first half of pregnancy. Am J Obstet Gynecol 1997;177(3):685–689.
106. Liao AW, Sebire NJ, Geerts L, et al: Megacystis at 10–14 weeks of gestation: Chromosomal defects and outcome according to bladder length. Ultrasound Obstet Gynecol 2003;21:338–341.
107. Rodeck CH, Nicolaides KH: Ultrasound guided invasive procedures in obstetrics. Clin Obstet Gynecol 1983;10:515–539.
108. Nicolini U, Rodeck C, Fisk N: Shunt treatment for fetal obstructive uropathy. Lancet 1987;2:1338–1339.

109. Bernaschek G, Deuntinger J, Hansman M, et al: Feto-amniotic shunting report of the experience of four European centers. Prenat Diagn 1994;14:821–833.
110. Johnson MP, Freedman AL: Fetal uropathy. Curr Opin Obstet Gynecol 1999;11:185–194.
111. Clark TJ, Martin WL, Divakaran TG, et al: Prenatal bladder drainage in the management of fetal lower urinary tract obstruction: A systematic review and meta-analysis. Obstet Gynecol 2003;102(2):367–382.
112. Johnson MP, Bukowski TP, Reitleman C, et al: In utero surgical treatment of fetal obstructive uropathy: A new comprehensive approach to identify appropriate candidates for vesicoamniotic shunt therapy. Am J Obstet Gynecol 1994;170(6): 1770–1776.
113. Mc Lorie G, Farhat W, Khoury A, et al: Outcome analysis of vesicoamniotic shunting in a comprehensive population. J Urol 2001;166:1036–1040.
114. Agarwal SK, Fisk NM: In utero therapy for lower urinary tract obstruction. Prenat Diagn 2001;21(11):970–976.
115. Holmes N, Harrison MR, Baskin LS: Fetal surgery for posterior urethral valves: Long-term postnatal outcomes. Pediatrics 2001;108(1):E7.
116. Sepulveda W, Stagiannis KD, Flack NJ, Fisk NM: Accuracy of prenatal diagnosis of renal agenesis with color flow imaging in severe second-trimester oligohydramnios. Am J Obstet Gynecol 1995;173(6):1788–1792.
117. Romero R, Cullen M, Grannum P, et al: Antenatal diagnosis of renal anomalies with ultrasounds III. Bilateral renal agenesis. Am J Obstet Gynecol 1985;151:38–43.
118. Thorner P, Berstein J, Landing BH: Kidneys and lower urinary tract. In Reed GB, Claireaux AE, Cockburn F (eds): Disease of the Fetus and Newborn. London, Chapman and Hall, 1995, pp 609–630.
119. Abuhamad AZ, Horton CE Jr, Horton SH, Evans AT: Renal duplication anomalies in the fetus: Clues for prenatal diagnosis. Ultrasound Obstet Gynecol 1996;7:174–177.
120. Meizner I, Yitzhak M, Levi A, et al: Fetal pelvic kidney: A challenge in prenatal diagnosis? Ultrasound Obstet Gynecol 1995; 5(6):391–393.
121. Sherer D, Cullen J, Thompson H, et al: Prenatal sonographic findings associated with a fetal horseshoe kidney. J Ultrasound Med 1990;9:477–479.
122. Fong C, Rahamani M, Rose T, et al: Fetal renal cystic disease: Sonographic-pathologic correlation. Am J Roentgenol 1986;146: 767–773.
123. Gagnadoux MF, Habib R, Levy M, et al: Cystic renal diseases in children. Adv Nephrol 1989;18:33–58.
124. Lieberman E, Salinas-Madriga L, Gwinn JL, et al: Infantile polycystic disease of the kidneys and liver: Clinical pathological and radiological correlations and comparison with congenital hepatic fibrosis. Medicine 1971;50:577–588.
125. Shenker L, Anderson C: Intrauterine diagnosis and management of fetal polycystic kidney disease. Obstet Gynecol 1982;59:385–389.
126. Reuss A, Wladimiroff JW, Stewart PA, Niermeijer MF: Prenatal diagnosis by ultrasound in pregnancies at risk for autosomal recessive polycystic kidney disease. Ultrasound Med Biol 1990;16(4):355–359.
127. Barth RA, Guillot AP, Capeless EL, Clemmons JJ: Prenatal diagnosis of autosomal recessive polycystic kidney disease: Variable outcome within one family. Am J Obstet Gynecol 1992;166(2): 560–561.
128. Wisser J, Hebisch G, Froster U, et al: Prenatal sonographic diagnosis of autosomal recessive polycystic kidney disease (ARPKD) during the early second trimester. Prenat Diagn 1995;15(9):868–871.
129. Tsatsaris V, Gagnadoux MF, Aubry MC, et al: Prenatal diagnosis of bilateral isolated hyperechogenic kidneys. Is it possible to predict long term outcome? BJOG 2002;109: 1388–1393.
130. Zerres K, Mücher G, Bachner L, et al: Mapping of the gene for autosomal recessive polycystic kidney disease (ARPKD) to chromosome 6p21-cen. Nature Genet 1994;7:132,429.
131. Pretorius D, Lee M, Manco-Johnson M, et al: Diagnosis of autosomal dominant polycystic kidney disease in utero and in the young infant. J Ultrasound Med 1987;6:242–255.
132. Fick GM, Johnson AM, Strain JD, et al: Characteristics of very early onset autosomal dominant polycystic kidney disease. J Am Soc Nephrol 1993;3(12):1863–1870.
133. Sinibaldi D, Malena S, Mingarelli R, Rizzoni G: Prenatal ultrasonographic findings of dominant polycystic kidney disease and postnatal renal evolution. Am J Med Genet 1996;65(4):337–341.
134. The European polycistic kidney disease consortium: The polycystic kidney disease 1 gene encodes a 14 Kb transcript and lies within a duplicated region on chromosome 16. Cell 1994;77:881–894.
135. The American PKD1 consortium: Analysis of the genomic sequence for the autosomal dominant polycystic kidney disease (PKD1) gene predicts the presence of a leucine-rich repeat. Hum Mol Genet 1995;4:575–582.
136. Howlett DC, Greenwood KL, Jarosz JM, et al: The incidence of transient renal medullary hyperechogenicity in neonatal ultrasound examination. Br J Radiol 1997;70:140–143.
137. Carr MC, Benacerraf BR, Estroff JA, Mandell J: Prenatally diagnosed bilateral hyperechoic kidneys with normal amniotic fluid: Postnatal outcome. J Urol 1995;153(2):442–444.
138. Allanson JE, Pantzar JT, MacLeod PM: Possible new autosomal recessive syndrome with unusual renal histopathological changes. Am J Med Genet 1983;16:57–60.
139. Gloor JM, Muchant DG, Norling LL: Prenatal maternal indomethacin use resulting in prolonged neonatal renal insufficiency. J Perinatol 1993;13(6):425–427.
140. Ambrosino M, Hernanz-Schulman M, Horii S, et al: Prenatal diagnosis of nephroblastomatosis in two siblings. J Ultrasound Med 1990;9:49–51.
141. Appuzion J, Unwin W, Adhate A, Nichols R: Prenatal diagnosis of fetal mesoblastic nephroma. Am J Obstet Gynecol 1986;154:636–637.
142. Kelner M, Droulle P, Didier F, Hoeffel JC: The vascular "ring" sign in mesoblastic nephroma: Report of two cases. Pediatr Radiol 2003;33:123–128.
143. Perale R, Talenti E, Lubrano G, et al: Late ultrasonographic pattern in congenital nephrotic syndrome of the Finnish type. Pediatr Radiol 1988;18:71.
144. Huttunen NP: Congenital nephrotic syndrome of the Finnish type. Arch Dis Child 1976;51:344–348.
145. Moore B, Pretorius D, Scioscia A, Reznik V: Sonographic findings in a fetus with congenital nephrotic syndrome of the Finnish Type. J Ultrasound Med 1992;11:113–116.
146. Shalev H, Ohaly M, Meizner I, Carmi R: Prenatal diagnosis of Bartter syndrome. Prenat Diagn 1994;14:996–998.
147. Sieck UV, Ohlsson A: Fetal polyuria and hydramnios associated with Bartter's syndrome. Obstet Gynecol 1984;63:22S.
148. Abramson O, Zmora E, Mazor M, Shinwell ES: Pseudohypoaldosteronism in a preterm infant: Intrauterine presentation as hydramnios. J Pediatr 1992;120:129–132.
149. Proesmans W, Massa G, Vandenberghe K, Van Assche A: Prenatal diagnosis of Bartter syndrome. Lancet 1987;i:394.
150. Al-Rasheed SA, Patel PJ, Kolawole TM, et al: Renal sonographic patterns in Bartter's syndrome. Pediatr Radiol 1996;26:116–119.
151. Welesley D, Howe D: Fetal renal anomalies and genetic syndromes. Prenat Diagn 2001;21:992–1003.
152. Rehder H, Labbé F: Prenatal morphology in Meckel's syndrome. Prenat Diagn 1981;1:161–172.
153. Dumez Y, Dommergues M, Gubler MC, et al: Meckel-Gruber syndrome: Prenatal diagnosis at 10 menstrual weeks using embryoscopy. Prenat Diagn 1994;14:141–144.
154. Devesa R, Munoz A, Torrents M, et al: Prenatal diagnosis of isolated hypospadias. Prenat Diagn 1998;18:779–788.

155. Meizner I, Mashiach R, Shalev J, et al: The 'tulip sign': A sonographic clue for in-utero diagnosis of severe hypospadias. Ultrasound Obstet Gynecol 2002;19:250–253.
156. Cheikhelard A, Luton D, Philippe-Chomette P, et al: How accurate is the prenatal diagnosis of abnormal genitalia? J Urol 2000;164:984–987.
157. Vijayaraghavan SB, Muruganand SK, Ravikumar VR, Marimuthu K: Prenatal sonographic features of penoscrotal transposition. J Ultrasound Med 2002;21:1427–1430.
158. Bretelle F, Salomon L, Senat MV, et al: Fetal gender: Antenatal discrepancy between phenotype and genotype. Ultrasound Obstet Gynecol 2002;20:286–289.

CHAPTER 20

Fetal Gastrointestinal Abnormalities

Peter Stone

INTRODUCTION

Fetal gastrointestinal and abdominal wall malformations are easily visualized by ultrasound and may be detected either during a second trimester scan for anomalies or by chance during an examination for an unrelated indication, such as the evaluation of poor fetal growth, abnormal amniotic fluid volume (usually hydramnios), or an increased maternal serum α-fetoprotein concentration. The most common gastrointestinal abnormalities detected antenatally are omphalocele, gastroschisis, and diaphragmatic hernia. The other malformations are both less common and less frequently diagnosed by ultrasonography. Upon detection, the abnormality should be managed in consultation with a multidisciplinary team that provides consistent advice and treatment. Team members typically include an obstetrician with expertise in fetal medicine, a neonatal pediatrician, pediatric surgeon, clinical geneticist, and anesthesiologist. The patient should meet before delivery with these people either on an individual basis or as a group as needed.

OMPHALOCELE (EXOMPHALOS)

General

Omphalocele is an extraembryonic hernia caused by the arrest of ventral medial migration of the dermatomyotomes (Fig. 20–1). It is associated with other malformations in 60% of cases. Omphalocele has an annual prevalence of 1:2500 to 1:5000 pregnancies. The annual prevalence is similar to gastroschisis, though recent publication suggests the latter is growing more common.[1] "Physiologic" herniation of abdominal contents into the base of the umbilical cord is normal up until around 11 weeks' gestation (Fig. 20–2) and must be distinguished from an omphalocele.

Diagnosis

An omphalocele contains abdominal contents enclosed in a membrane. The diagnosis is made after 11 weeks when an anterior, extra-abdominal mass is detected upon which the umbilical cord inserts rather than to the anterior abdominal wall (see Fig. 20–1). Defect size and type have some prognostic importance. Although the omphalocele contents are usually enclosed within a membrane, spontaneous rupture does occur. A less common variant is the "giant omphalocele" (Fig. 20–3) in which the abdominal wall defect is massive. Giant defects and those in which the membrane has ruptured are often associated with a small or defective thoracic cage associated with pulmonary hypoplasia and postnatal respiratory complications.[2] There may on rare occasion be difficulty distinguishing a ruptured omphalocele from gastroschisis. Omphalocele is commonly associated with other malformations (Table 20–1) and, like gastroschisis, may be associated with hydramnios. Intrauterine growth restriction is common, and approximately one of six fetuses with omphalocele are chromosomally abnormal. A small omphalocele may be missed on ultrasonography, especially if the fluid volume is reduced and the anterior abdominal wall cannot be clearly delineated. However, the sensitivity of ultrasound detection exceeds 86%.[3]

Both omphalocele and gastroschisis cause a very high maternal serum α-fetoprotein concentration during the second trimester. If an amniotic fluid sample is obtained, it will reveal a faint acetylcholinesterase band and a dense pseudocholinesterase band. This pattern is opposite that of a neural tube defect (see Chapter 18).[4]

Risks

Maternal

There are few obstetric risks to the mother apart from the rare complication of hydramnios. The recurrence risk reflects the underlying etiology.

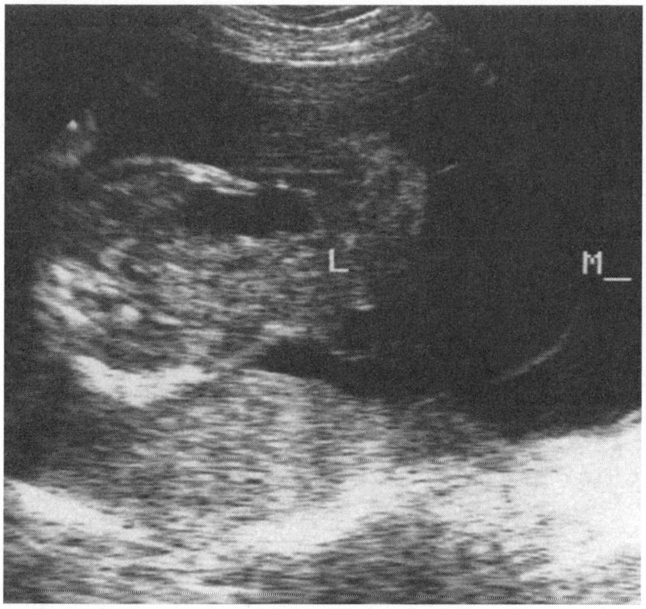

FIGURE 20–1
Characteristic ultrasound appearance of omphalocele. Note the membrane (M) surrounding the liver (L) and bowel.

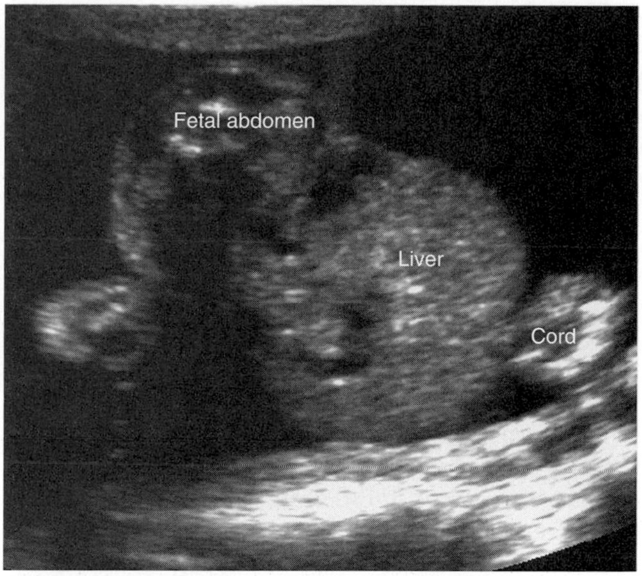

FIGURE 20–3
Ultrasound appearance of a giant omphalocele showing massive amount of extracorporeal tissue and cord insertion.

Fetal and Neonatal

Perinatal risks include those of invasive diagnostic testing, the implications of associated abnormalities, and postnatal surgery that may be complicated when there is extracorporeal liver.

Management Options

Antenatal

The first step is to exclude other abnormalities (found in at least 60% of cases).[5–7] This mandates a detailed ultrasonographic examination, including a fetal echocardiogram (see Chapter 17) and a fetal karyotype. Abnormal cardiac findings occur in 45% of fetuses with omphalocele.[8] The sonographic differentiation between

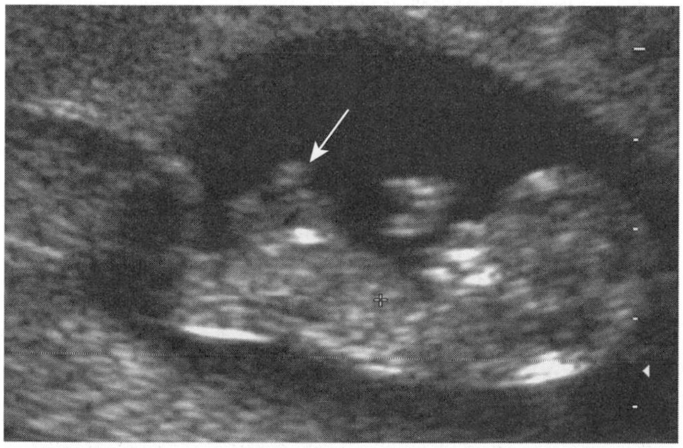

FIGURE 20–2
Normal appearance of abdominal contents outside the body cavity in the fetus at 11 to 12 weeks' gestation (indicated by the *arrow*).

TABLE 20–1

Associated Anomalies in Omphalocele

Pentalogy of Cantrell*
Diaphragmatic hernia
Pericardial defect
Distal sternal defect
Omphalocele
Cardiovascular malformations
Cloacal extrophy
Omphalocele
Bladder or cloacal extrophy
Other caudal abnormalities
Beckwith-Wiedemann syndrome
Omphalocele
Macroglossia
Generalized organomegaly (autosomal dominant)
Hypoglycemia
Trisomies
Trisomy 13
Trisomy 18
Trisomy 21
Other aneuploidy
Triploidy
Turner syndrome
Other abnormalities
Cardiac
Atrial septal defect
Ventricular septal defect
Patent ductus arteriosis
Pulmonary stenosis
Gastointestinal
Atresias
Meckel's diverticulum
Imperforate anus
Renal
Neurologic
Meningocele
Holoprosencephaly
Microphthalmos

*For a summary of the pentalogy of Cantrell, see *www.thefetus.net.*

omphalocele and gastroschisis is important and generally not difficult. The presence of a sac or membrane around the contents with the umbilical cord inserting upon it is pathognomonic. Difficulties arise when the sac has ruptured spontaneously, or when the relationship of the herniated tissue to the umbilical cord insertion is unclear. On occasion, thickened loops of bowel in the fetus with gastroschisis may appear as a covering membrane. The peritoneal membrane can also be difficult to visualize when there is oligohydramnios. In contrast to gastroschisis, extracorporeal liver is common (40%). Fetuses with intracorporeal liver are significantly more likely to have chromosomal abnormalities,[3] as are fetuses with other malformations and with mothers with advanced age. There is probably little prognostic significance of the omphalocele contents if the karyotype is normal, except for a worse prognosis with large defects.

Parental counseling after diagnosis stresses the importance of a fetal karyotype and that the prognosis is generally good if the chromosomes are normal and there are no associated malformations (though not all may be detected before birth). Even with postnatal diagnosis, the survival rate of otherwise normal infants exceeds 75%.[3] Large abdominal wall defects can pose particular problems for both neonatal respiratory management and surgical closure, and these issues should be covered during counseling with the neonatologist and pediatric surgeon. Death of the otherwise normal infant results from prematurity, sepsis, or problems with short gut syndrome, which is more common with gastroschisis than omphalocele. Long-term follow-up of adults with a congenital abdominal wall defect suggests the quality of life is similar to that of the general population, though common problems include disorders of the abdominal wall scar in 37% and functional gastrointestinal disorders in 51%.[9] Parents may benefit from illustrations showing typical defects before and after surgery (Fig. 20–4).

Labor and Delivery

Delivery should occur in a center with a neonatal medical and surgical team in attendance to optimize the transition to ex utero life and the preoperative care. There is no evidence elective cesarean delivery a priori confers any benefit to the fetus or neonate with omphalocele with or without a ruptured sac and irrespective of the contents of the sac.[10] Theoretical concerns for vaginal delivery—namely, visceral trauma, dystocia, and infection—are unsupported. In one series in which the diagnosis was known in only a minority of cases, cesarean delivery made no difference to neonatal outcome.[11] There are untested scenarios in which cesarean delivery might be considered, such as extracorporeal liver when torsion with obstructed cardiac return is a theoretical concern. Neonatal morbidity in all recent series relates to associated anomalies and prematurity. Isolated cases with late morbidity and death relate mostly to complications of bowel obstruction or short bowel syndrome in association with intestinal atresia.[12]

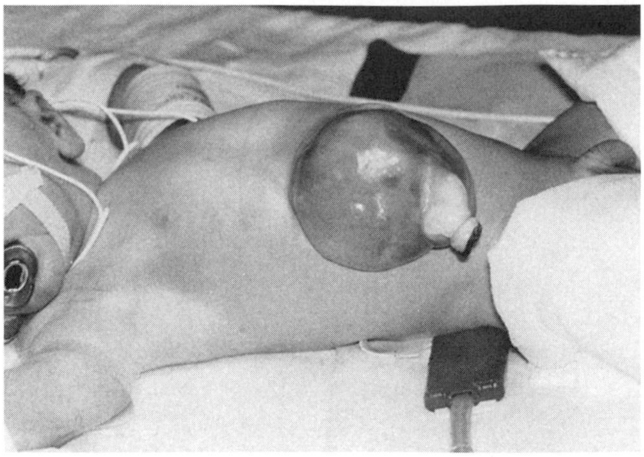

FIGURE 20–4
Omphalocele at delivery. Note that the lesion is epigastric and at the site of the umbilical cord insertion.

Postnatal

Prevention of heat and fluid loss and infection are the initial goals after delivery while the neonatal evaluation is completed and the surgery planned. These infants are at increased risk of hypothermia owing to the large surface area of exposed viscera. The neonate is immediately lowered into a sterile bag containing warm electrolyte (no warmer than 37.5°C), plasma solution, and antibiotics (e.g., Vi-Drape isolation bag). In emergencies, any sterile bag with warmed normal saline or lactated Ringer's solution and antibiotics will suffice. A suitable solution consists of 1 L lactated Ringer's solution, 500 mL stable plasma protein or similar solution, and 1 million units of penicillin. The bag is tied at the level of the axillae, and care is taken to avoid torsion of viscera (Fig. 20–5).

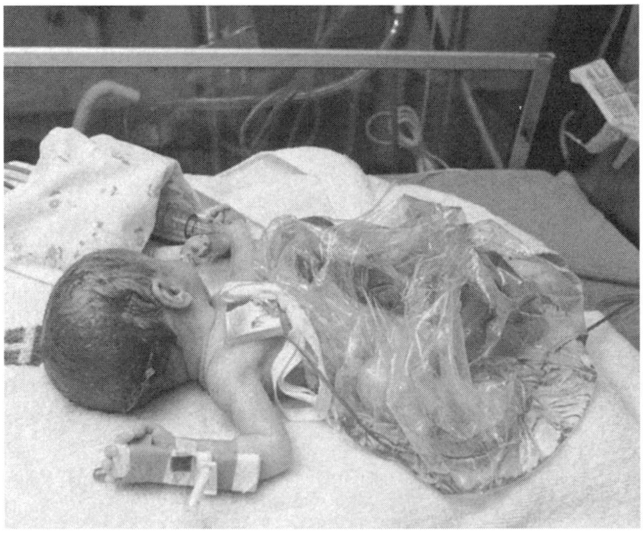

FIGURE 20–5
Neonate with an omphalocele showing bowel isolation bag tied above defect.

Alternatively, a sterile plastic bag without the fluid may be used. A nasogastric tube is passed to keep the bowel decompressed, and ventilatory support is provided when necessary.

Neonates with associated lethal structural malformations or trisomy 13 or 18 are typically managed nonsurgically. Untreated neonates generally die of dehydration or sepsis. There are two main options: either keep the neonate comfortable and provide supportive care only, or paint the unruptured omphalocele sac with 1% mercurochrome solution. Note that mercurochrome has been reported to be associated with renal failure.

All other infants are managed surgically with operative repair as soon as the general condition is stable. It is difficult to always predict antenatally whether a primary surgical closure is possible. Small defects less than 4 cm in diameter and without extracorporeal liver are almost always closed primarily. Large defects, or those containing liver, may not be closable during the first operation. When primary closure is not feasible, the defect and contents are covered with a Silastic silo sutured to the edge of the defect. Over the following days, the contents of the silo gradually enter the abdominal cavity under the influence of gravity coupled with the silo being compressed daily. Care must be taken to avoid respiratory or circulatory compromise during these maneuvers. Postoperative problems common to all abdominal wall defect repairs include respiratory embarrassment, pulmonary hypertension, small bowel perforation, bowel obstruction, and malrotation. The average neonatal hospital stay after a silo ranges from 3 to 4 weeks. Parenteral nutrition is often necessary for days or weeks postoperatively. It may be 3 months in some cases before satisfactory bowel function is achieved. Weakness of the anterior abdominal wall or a poor cosmetic result after the initial surgery may be corrected in a subsequent plastic surgical revision.

The long-term prognosis for surviving infants is generally very good, and in the absence of associated structural or chromosomal abnormalities, the risk of recurrence in a subsequent pregnancy is extremely low. The main recurrence risk is that for the associated abnormalities, although case reports of a familial recurrence have been recorded.[13]

SUMMARY OF MANAGEMENT OPTIONS

Exomphalos/Omphalocele

Management Options	Quality of Evidence	Strength of Recommendation	References
Antenatal			
Offer karyotyping.	III	B	3,6
Chromosomal abnormalities are more likely if liver is intra-abdominal.	III	B	3,6
Assess other structural defects (especially cardiac) with ultrasound.	III	B	5,6,7,8
Anticipate risk of prematurity.	III	B	2,13
Offer interdisciplinary counseling.	–	GPP	–
Delivery			
Mode of delivery does not affect outcome.	III	B	10,11,12
Delivery is recommended in a tertiary unit with neonatal surgical facilities.	–	GPP	–
Place abdominal contents in a sterile plastic bag with/without warm (37.5°C) isotonic solutions.	–	GPP	–
Respiratory distress may occur with ruptured or giant omphalocele.	IV	C	2
Neonatal Care			
Necrotizing enterocolitis is associated with increased mortality rate.	III	B	12
Primary closure minimizes morbidity.	III	B	18,24
Associated bowel malformations are possible.	III	B	30
Closure is performed in the neonatal unit in selected cases.	IIb	B	28,29

GASTROSCHISIS

General

Gastroschisis is a paraumbilical defect, usually on the right side of the anterior abdominal wall lateral to the umbilical vessels. Left-sided defects are rare. The annual prevalence of gastroschisis approximates 1:2500 to 1:3000 live births with an equal sex ratio.[5] It would appear that there is an increasing annual prevalence of gastroschisis not entirely explained by increased recognition of the problem. Population-based studies suggest an association with nonsteroidal anti-inflammatory drug use in the first trimester (see later discussion). Gastroschisis is generally considered a developmental accident whereby abnormal regression of usually the right umbilical vein weakens the abdominal wall, which then bursts. However, the precise etiology remains controversial.

Recent studies suggest an association between the ingestion of aspirin and other vasoactive substances.[14,15] These studies provide support for a vascular etiology. Iatrogenic abdominal wall defects have also resulted from placement of a vesicoamniotic shunt for obstructive uropathy. Perhaps the most important reason to distinguish from omphalocele is to emphasize the different incidence of associated abnormalities—less than 10% with gastroschisis compared to more than 60% with omphalocele.

Diagnosis

Antenatal detection is similar to that of omphalocele, either at "routine" ultrasonographic examination (Figs. 20–6, 20–7, and 20–8), because of a raised maternal serum α-fetoprotein, or during ultrasonographic examination for hydramnios when associated with intestinal atresia. The sonographic image is one of free-floating loops of bowel typically appearing like a clump of grapes.

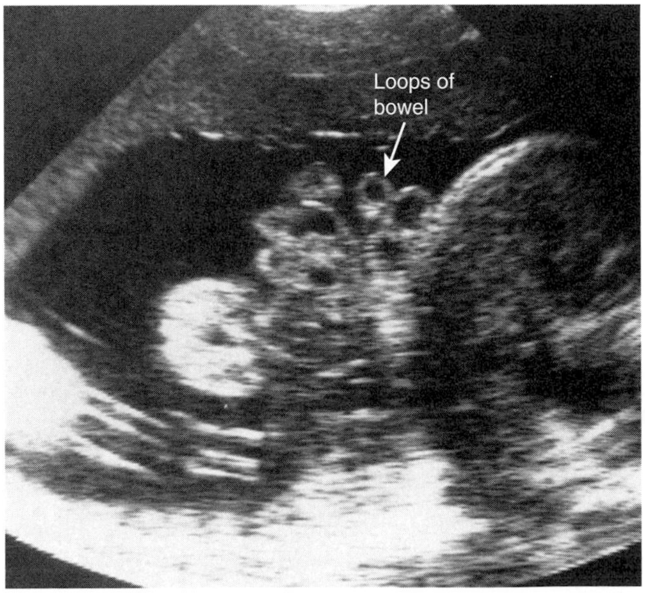

FIGURE 20–6
Typical appearance of gastroschisis: loops of bowel floating freely in the amniotic fluid (in this case, unusually, liver was also protruding through the defect).

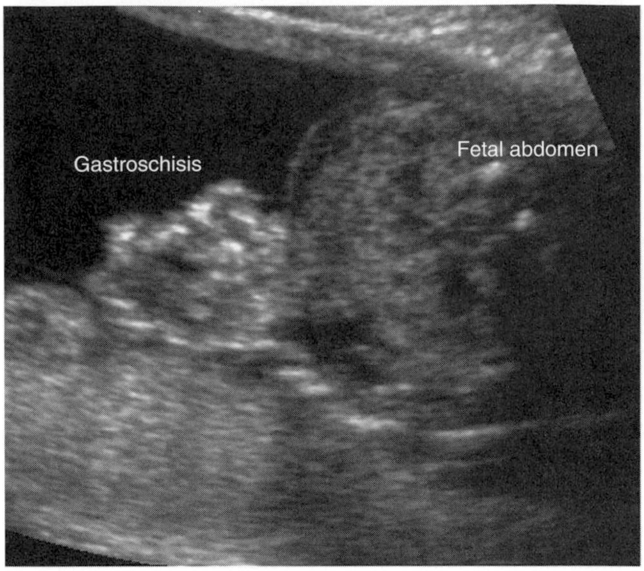

FIGURE 20–7
A transverse section through the fetal abdomen showing a gastroschisis. Note the absence of a membrane and the usual position, lower than omphalocele.

Risks

Maternal risks are similar to those for omphalocele, reflecting complications of the anomaly.

Fetal risks are associated with complications of bowel torsion that compromise the vascular supply or obstruction. It has also been theorized that exposure of the intestines to amniotic fluid may contribute to damage to the bowel serosa, though there are other explanations for the so-called "peel."

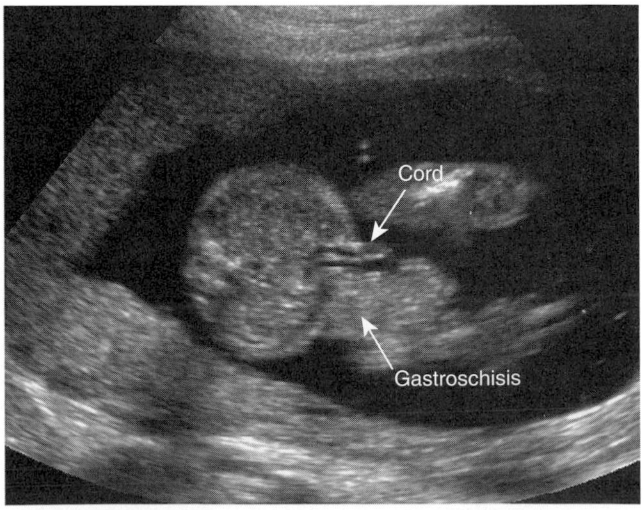

FIGURE 20–8
Ultrasound of gastroschisis showing the cord insertion adjacent to the abdominal wall defect.

Fetal growth restriction may also complicate gastroschisis but is not necessarily secondary to uteroplacental dysfunction.

Neonatal complications include not only difficulty reducing and closing the gastroschisis, but also complications due to atretic segments causing critical shortening of the bowel.

Management Options

Antenatal

Though the risk of associated structural abnormalities is lower than that for omphalocele, a detailed sonographic search by a skilled sonologist remains important. The risk of an abnormal karyotype is <1% and many physicians do not consider a karyotype necessary. One large review included only one case of trisomy 18.[13] The risk of an abnormal karyotype increases if other abnormalities are detected. Associated abnormalities include bowel stenosis or atresia (which are probably complications of the gastroschisis itself) and, less commonly, cleft palate and diaphragmatic hernia. On rare occasions, other viscera are contained within the gastroschisis: liver, uterus, and undescended testes each have been reported.

Serial ultrasonographic examination is recommended to assess fetal growth, amniotic fluid volume, and bowel appearance. However, any appraisal of fetal nutrition based on the abdominal circumference measurement is at best an approximation as any defect will artifactually reduce the circumference. Oligohydramnios may be associated with fetal growth restriction secondary to uteroplacental dysfunction (see Chapters 12 and 13). Polyhydramnios is the only antenatal sonographic finding correlated with severe neonatal bowel complications.[16] The appearance of the bowel and the diameter of the bowel loops are not of prognostic significance.[17,18] Increased echogenicity and apparent thickening of the bowel wall after 28 weeks may represent a fibrinous coating or "peel" covering and binding together loops of bowel. The etiology of the peel and interventions to prevent are debated. There is conflicting evidence for the hypothesis that amniotic fluid components cause a chemical peritonitis. Although there is evidence of intra-amniotic inflammation in human gastroschisis,[19] prolonged intestinal exposure to amniotic fluid does not invariably lead to peel formation.[20] Amnioinfusion or amnioexchange procedures are reported,[21] but there is little evidence of benefit.

An alternative explanation for peel formation is venous and lymphatic obstruction, a hypothesis supported by the observation that the intra-abdominal peritoneum does not always show a peel, although it too is exposed to amniotic fluid. Although the presence of peel can make the surgical closure more difficult, it has little correlation with outcome and resolves quickly after surgical closure (K. Pringle, personal communication). And though increasing dilation of bowel loops may appear worrisome, it is not an indication for delivery (Fig. 20–9).[22] Perhaps most important, no evidence suggests that early delivery to decrease exposure to amniotic fluid improves outcome. Term delivery at 37 weeks' gestation allows for an earlier, definitive closure of the defect, and shorter times to full oral feedings.[23]

Parental counseling should emphasize the high chance of a good outcome with over 80% survival (and a primary closure rate in the range of 52% to 80%). Prolonged hospitalization with durations of 47 to 75 days is recorded.[24] In the absence of ultrasonographic abnormalities of growth, amniotic fluid volume, umbilical artery Doppler recordings, or heart rate tracing abnormalities, the pregnancy may continue to term. However, close monitoring in the third trimester and especially after 34 weeks is recommended, as there appears to be a fairly high incidence of unexplained intrauterine death after 37 weeks, which may be due to either fetal growth restriction[25] or umbilical cord compression[26] (Fig. 20–10).

Labor and Delivery

Fetuses with a gastroschisis should be delivered at a referral center equipped with the appropriate facilities and staff. Like omphalocele, there is no evidence that cesarean delivery results in improved outcome. Large case series actually report a higher survival rate in fetuses subject to labor. Thus, vaginal delivery should be anticipated in the absence of other indications.

Postnatal

The immediate postnatal management is similar to that for omphalocele, but the preoperative workup and stabi-

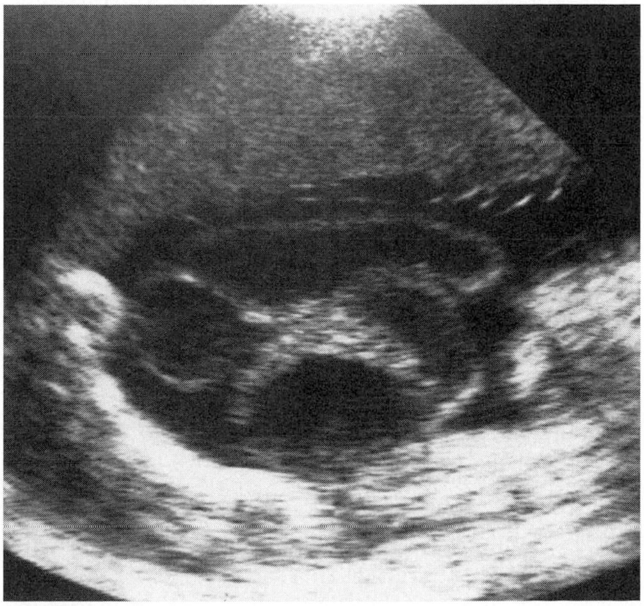

FIGURE 20–9
Gastroschisis: dilated loops of bowel. This fetus was delivered vaginally at term and primary abdominal wall closure was achieved.

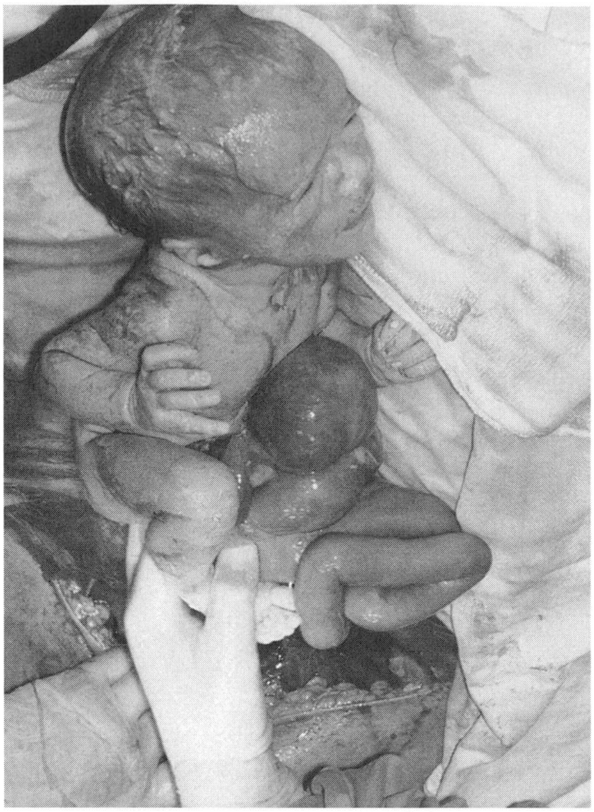

FIGURE 20–10
Gastroschisis at delivery, unusually containing the liver. Baby was delivered by cesarean section, the indications being a footling breech presentation.

lization of the newborn should be expedited, as there is no protecting membrane over the bowel. The neonate is immediately placed into the Lehey bag (or even a sterile plastic oven bag) containing the warmed electrolyte and antibiotic solution as described under omphalocele (see earlier discussion and Fig. 20–5). The bag is carefully tied at the axillae so not to kink or rotate the bowel, and a nasogastric tube is passed to keep the bowel decompressed.

Recently, reduction of the gastroschisis has been reported without general anesthesia or endotracheal ventilation.[27,28] The initial studies have been extended to develop selection criteria for safe application of the technique, and the current results reviewed.[29] Proposed contraindications are poor general condition, obvious gut atresia, significant vital organ anomaly, bowel to abdomen disproportion, and "at-risk" bowel circulation. The developments of distress or progressive metabolic acidosis during the procedure are indications to convert to a standard approach. There were two deaths in the original communication, but recent reports describe increased success. Ward reduction of umbilical hernia is also reported.[28] The role of ward reduction in routine management of abdominal wall defects remains to be determined by well-designed trials.[29]

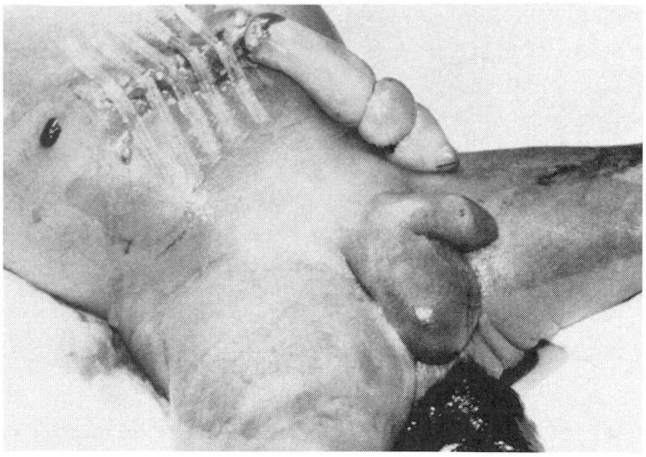

FIGURE 20–11
Abdominal wall closure in gastroschisis. Similar results are usually obtained with or without previous use of a silo.

Primary surgical closure is achieved in 52% to 85% of cases.[18,24] Postoperative ventilation is generally required for about 72 hours, and total parenteral nutrition is often required until oral feeding can commence. The surgical approach favored by the author's unit is a transverse incision at the level of the defect if required. The bowel is carefully examined for atretic segments. Any bowel incision made is closed transversely to minimize the risk of a subsequent stricture, and the abdominal wall defect is closed vertically with the umbilical cord left in place to produce a "normal" umbilicus (Fig. 20–11). When primary closure is not possible, a Silastic silo is created as with omphalocele (Figs. 20–12 and 20–13). Failure to pass stool by 28 days mandates a new search for atresia that will be found in up to 5%.[30]

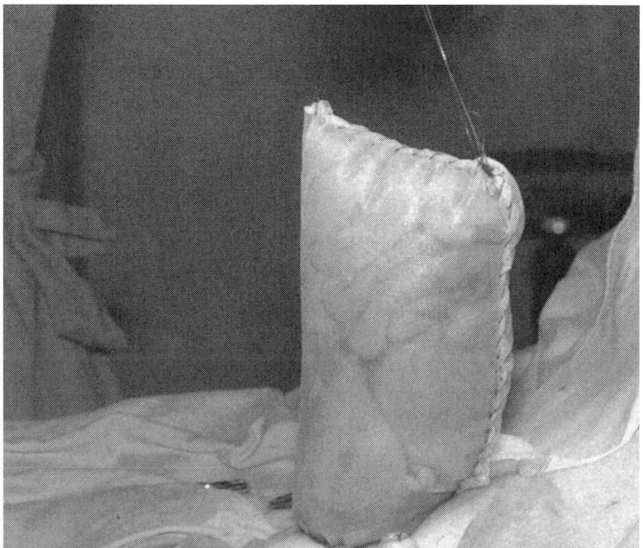

FIGURE 20–12
Silastic silo used to cover bowel.

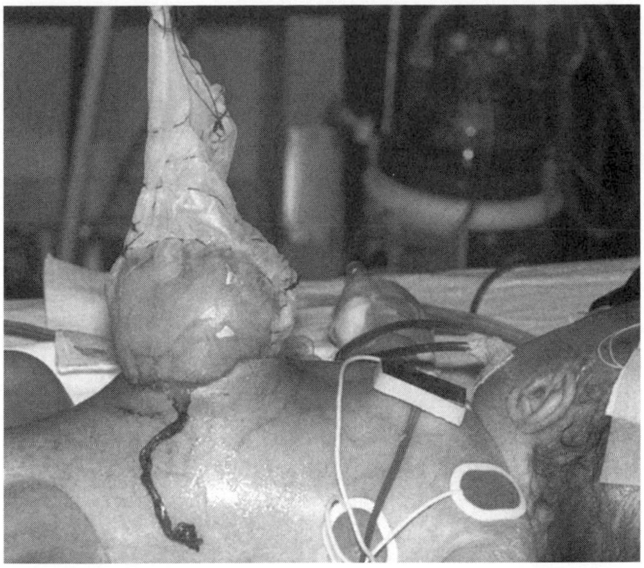

FIGURE 20–13
The silo is reduced in size over 7 days as its contents are returned to the abdomen.

The mortality rate is between 3% and 10% and reflects prematurity, intestinal ischemia or necrosis, late sepsis, or the effects of other associated abnormalities. Prolonged bowel dysfunction, especially motility disorders or malabsorption, occurs in a small percentage of cases, though short-term complications are very common. Fewer than 25% of neonates have a completely uncomplicated post-surgical course.[31] The few long-term studies of patients with gastroschisis[9,32] suggest that development beyond 5 years of age is normal when the lesion was isolated. Those with bowel atresia or complications requiring bowel resection have a higher frequency of long-term bowel problems or nonspecific abdominal complaints.

The risk of recurrence is very low, although isolated case reports suggest familial recurrence is possible.[33] Fear of recurrence of an abdominal wall defect may dominate the reproductive choices of couples.[34]

SUMMARY OF MANAGEMENT OPTIONS
Gastroschisis

Management Options	Quality of Evidence	Strength of Recommendation	References
Antenatal			
Scan for other anomalies, including fetal heart anomalies.	III	B	8
Need for karyotype is unclear, but risk of other abnormalities <10%.	III	B	5,10
No indication to deliver prematurely.	III	B	23
Increased surveillance to assess risk of death, risk of prematurity, and risk of intrauterine growth restriction.	III	B	25
Provide interdisciplinary counseling.	–	GPP	–
Delivery			
Mode of delivery does not affect outcome.	III	B	10,11
Monitor for intrapartum fetal distress.	III	B	25
Delivery should be in a center with neonatal surgical facilities.	–	GPP	–
Handle bowel carefully, and place contents in a sterile plastic bag with/without warm isotonic solutions.	–	GPP	–
Neonatal Care			
Primary early closure minimizes morbidity.	III	B	18, 24
At surgery, assess for associated bowel malformations.	III	B	18, 24
Prevent heat and fluid loss and early surgery.	–	GPP	–

CONGENITAL DIAPHRAGMATIC HERNIA

General

Congenital diaphragmatic hernia has several parallels to gastroschisis and omphalocele. Diaphragmatic hernia is a protrusion or herniation of the abdominal contents into the thoracic cavity. Herniation may occur through a posterolateral defect in the pleuroperitoneal canal (the most common is the hernia of the foramen of Bochdalek) (Fig. 20–14), defect in the sternocostal hiatus, a retrosternal or Morgagni hernia, a hiatus hernia, defect in

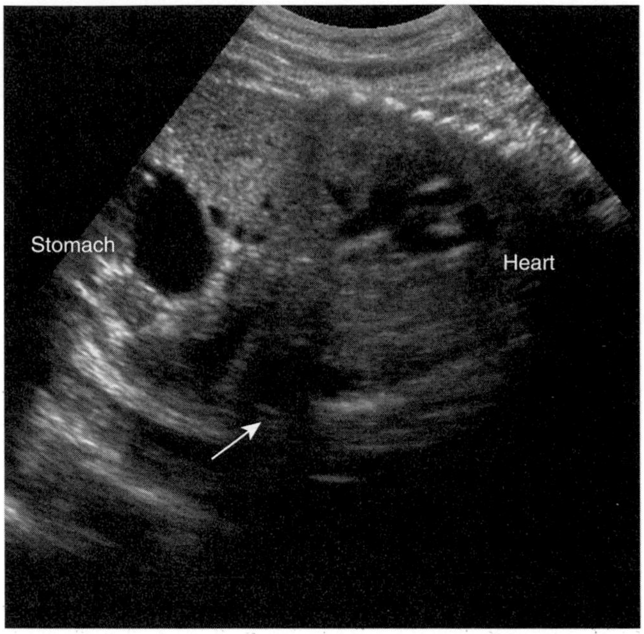

FIGURE 20–14
Prenatal ultrasound image of a posterior (Bochdalek) diaphragmatic hernia (shown by *arrow*). This was a late diagnosis despite earlier scans, possibly owing to the position of the stomach in the abdomen.

the central tendon of the diaphragm, and through complete eventration of the diaphragm. The reported annual prevalence is 1:3500 live births,[35] but this does not include terminations and stillbirths. Left-sided hernias are more common than right-sided ones. Up to 50% of antenatally diagnosed cases have associated abnormalities,[36] and diaphragmatic hernia is associated with a number of syndromes, including Beckwith-Wiedemann, Pierre Robin, Fryns, and chromosomal defects such as trisomy 13, trisomy 18, and deletion 9p. Lung hypoplasia, central to the poor prognosis of diaphragmatic hernia, may originate during embryogenesis and before the visceral herniation into the thoracic cavity.[37] Postnatally, pulmonary hypoplasia and pulmonary hypertension are often lethal.

Diagnosis

The most common postnatal presentation is cyanosis shortly after clamping the umbilical cord. Other signs include a scaphoid abdomen (Fig. 20–15), a barrel-shaped chest, and dextrocardia. Diaphragmatic hernia is the most common cause of dextrocardia diagnosed in the delivery suite.

The antenatal sonographic diagnosis can be difficult. A multinational study achieved an overall detection rate of 59%. Isolated diaphragmatic hernia was detected in 51% of cases, and in 72% when other malformations were present.[38] Small hernias may be missed by even the most thorough sonologists. A right-sided diaphragmatic hernia is extremely difficult to identify because liver and lung are of similar echogenicity in early pregnancy. As pregnancy advances, the lungs become more echogenic.

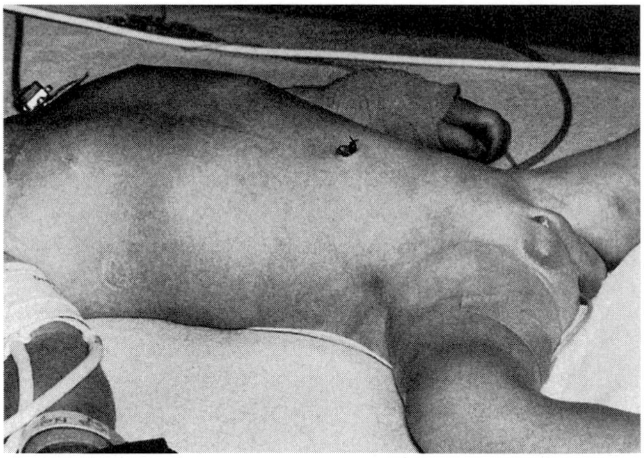

FIGURE 20–15
Neonate with congenital diaphragmatic hernia showing scaphoid abdomen.

The hypoechoic line seen on ultrasonography separating the thoracic from the abdominal cavities may appear present but is an unreliable sign for the exclusion of diaphragmatic hernia. The most sensitive sign is an abnormal thoracic location of the heart[39] (Fig. 20–16). Other signs, which are not necessarily prognostic, include hydramnios, visualization of the bowel or stomach at the level of the heart, and absence of the stomach in the abdomen. Hydramnios may result from either impaired swallowing (due to mediastinal compression) or obstruction of the upper gastrointestinal tract.

Several techniques can be used to facilitate the diagnosis of diaphragmatic hernia if there is uncertainty. The instillation of warmed normal saline into the fetal pleural or peritoneal cavities at the time of karyotyping or as a separate procedure is described.[40,41] Color and pulsed Doppler ultrasonography can help delineate the vascular anatomy when there is an echogenic mass in the fetal thorax.[42] Magnetic resonance imaging is especially helpful to confirm the location of the liver.

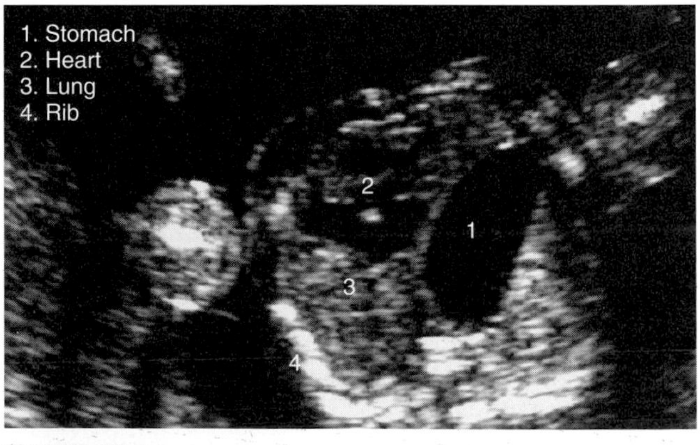

FIGURE 20–16
Ultrasound image of fetal thorax showing appearances of a diaphragmatic hernia. Note that the heart and stomach are visualized in the same imaging plane.

Management Options

Antenatal

The differential diagnosis of an intrathoracic ultrasonographic abnormality includes several possibilities:

- Diaphragmatic hernia
- Cystic adenomatoid malformation of the lung
- Extralobar sequestration (may be intra-abdominal)
- Bronchial atresia
- Other cystic and solid masses within the mediastinum

It is important to exclude the presence of other structural abnormalities notably in the cardiovascular (e.g., ventricular septal defect, tetralogy of Fallot), gastrointestinal, skeletal, and genitourinary systems because they may profoundly affect the prognosis. A karyotype is indicated. A summary of seven series revealed an overall 18% incidence of aneuploidy, only 2% when the diaphragmatic hernia is isolated, but up to 34% when other abnormalities are present.[43]

The option of pregnancy termination should be discussed with the parents if permissible, especially when other abnormalities are present, as the combination is generally fatal. The prognosis for isolated diaphragmatic hernia has in the past been controversial. Early reports of a less than 20% survival rate reflected a bias of ascertainment. Population-based studies confirm an overall survival rate of approximately 65%.[44] Although some units quote around 80% survival rate should postnatal management take place at a center with extracorporeal membrane oxygenation (ECMO) facilities,[45] others do not.[46] Thus, a definitive statement on the optimal management providing the highest survival rate cannot be made at present.

There is considerable debate on the accuracy of antenatal prediction of postnatal prognosis. The reported association between early diagnosis (<25 weeks) and poor prognosis (mortality rate as high as 58%)[47,48] is supported by recent study.[44] Hydramnios and the location of the fetal stomach do not appear to be prognostic factors,[48] nor do fetal echocardiographic variables in structurally normal hearts.[49] The presence of liver in the chest is a poor prognostic sign[48] and is associated with the triad of hydramnios, mediastinal shift, and intrathoracic stomach. The poor prognosis when liver is present in the chest is consistent with the finding of right-sided diaphragmatic hernia being an independent risk factor for decreased survival.[44] The estimation of lung size or volume has similarly proved difficult to measure reliably and correlate with prognosis. Fetuses with a left-sided hernia uncomplicated by liver herniation have a good prognosis, even in the presence of a low lung-to-heart ratio, which has been reported to be a poor prognostic sign.[50] Magnetic resonance imaging is used to estimate a lung volume.[51] A summary of the factors considered influential on outcome is shown in Table 20–2. None are accepted as completely reliable, as this condition has a spectrum of severity and fatality or morbidity due to varied factors, including pulmonary hypoplasia, pulmonary hypertension, morphologic and biochemical abnormalities of the lungs, and the longer-term sequelae of treatment.

TABLE 20–2

Factors Reported to Affect Prognosis in Diaphragmatic Hernia

Additional anomalies
Early diagnosis (<25 weeks' gestation)
Liver in the chest
Lung size
Bilateral hernias

As diaphragmatic hernia represents a wide spectrum of disease with multifactorial dysfunction as causes of death, some parents may accept this outcome and opt for termination of the pregnancy rather than the uncertainty of continuing with antenatal or postnatal treatments.

Recent experience has clarified the role of fetal surgery. There is no benefit from open fetal surgery for isolated congenital diaphragmatic hernia as the results are worse than conventional management after birth.[47] Investigative fetal treatments under study in some centers include a variety of tracheal occlusive[52] or plugging procedures[47] that prevent the egress of lung fluid with the aim of stimulating lung growth and development. The timing and duration of tracheal occlusion and the use of antenatal corticosteroids in congenital diaphragmatic hernia all require further investigation. Problems include chronic pulmonary dysfunction and direct complications of the procedures. An international trial is currently evaluating the effects of glucocorticoids in antenatally diagnosed congenital diaphragmatic hernia. Until the results of these treatments are fully evaluated, each remains experimental.[53]

Obstetrically, the pregnancy is monitored closely for the development of hydramnios and any of its sequelae. There is limited evidence that the antenatal administration of corticosteroids reduces the severity of lung disease and pulmonary surfactant deficiency.[54,55] Human trials are in progress. It is unknown whether amniotic fluid studies can define groups of fetuses with congenital diaphragmatic hernia most likely to benefit from corticosteroids or indeed postnatal surfactant therapy.

Where the parents elect to continue with the pregnancy, they should meet with a member of the surgical team before delivery who will explain that a period of preoperative stabilization after birth yields better results than immediate surgical repair. Poor ventilatory parameters that fail to improve with preoperative stabilization generally do not improve postoperatively and the prognosis is poor.

Labor and Delivery

There is no a priori indication for cesarean delivery. In the absence of massive hydramnios, labor and delivery are generally normal. However, these deliveries should be planned and occur at a referral center equipped for all likely complications.

Postnatal

Immediate intubation, ventilation, and paralysis of the newborn facilitate care, as the maintenance of good oxygenation is a good prognostic sign. Typically, the chest radiograph shows a mediastinal shift with abdominal contents in the thorax (Fig. 20–17). Maintenance of the mediastinum in a central position by preventing overdistention of the larger lung is associated with improved postoperative survival.[56] This suggests special care be taken during the resuscitation to avoid causing excessive mediastinal shift or lung overdistention. There is presently insufficient evidence to support either a policy of early (<24 hours) or late (>24 hours) repair after delivery.[57]

Extracorporeal membrane oxygenation (ECMO) is available in some centers for those neonates who cannot be adequately oxygenated using conventional ventilatory techniques. The criteria for ECMO vary among centers, as may the criteria for what constitutes good response. Early reports of ECMO responders (defined as a postductal Po_2 >100 mm Hg) noted a 90% survival rate compared with only 7% in nonresponders. The same series showed a similar high survival rate in those not requiring ECMO.[58] More recent reports support an increased survival rate in ECMO-treated groups, but the magnitude of the improvement is far more modest than first reported,[59] and others suggest similar survival rates are obtainable without ECMO.[46] ECMO complications include intracranial hemorrhage and vascular complications, and the survivors frequently experience long-term problems.[60] The place of ECMO along with other postnatal treatments including surfactant, partial liquid ventilation, pulmonary vasodilators, and lung transplantation remains to be settled.

A diaphragmatic hernia and its repair are illustrated in Figures 20–18 to 20–21.

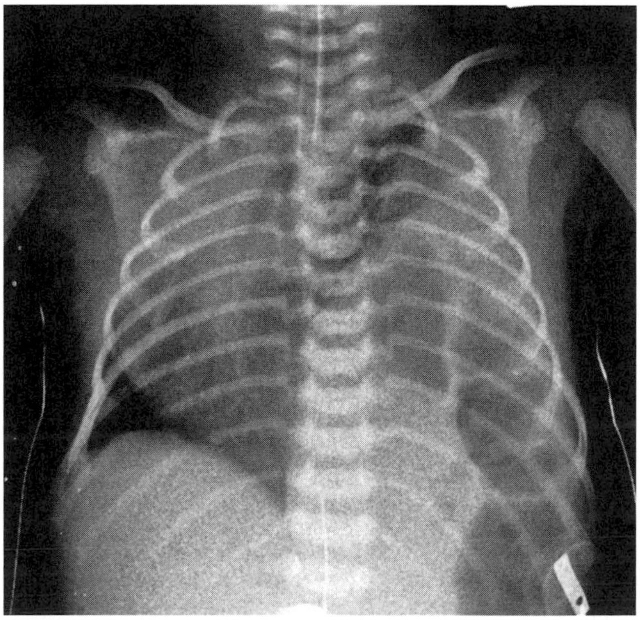

FIGURE 20–17
Diaphragmatic hernia. Neonatal chest radiograph showing the heart displaced to the right and abdominal contents in the left thorax.

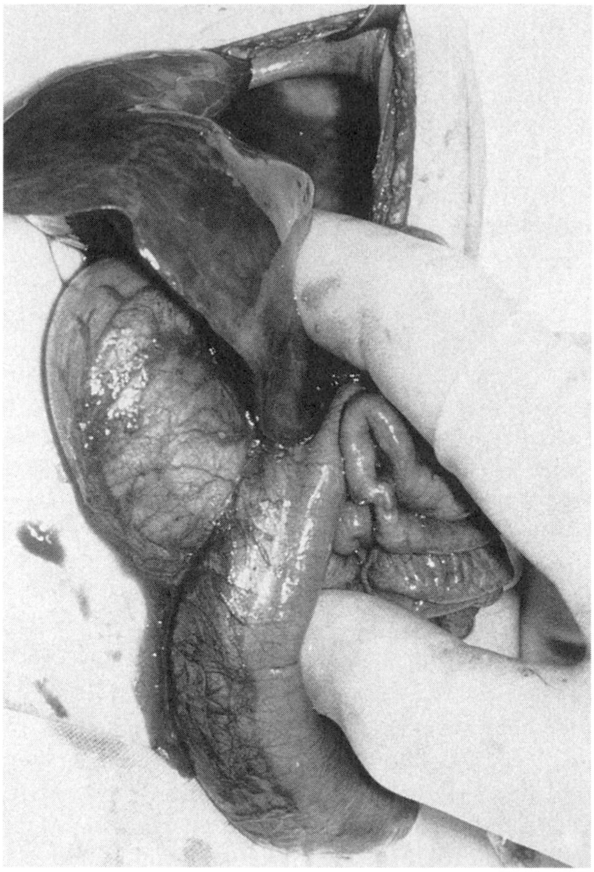

FIGURE 20–18
Diaphragmatic hernia. At surgery, the defect is shown as the contents of the hernia are being removed from the thorax.

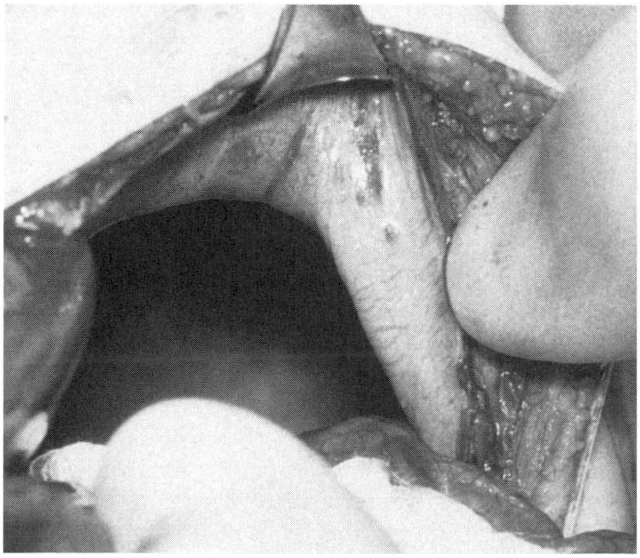

FIGURE 20–19
Diaphragmatic hernia. A large defect after the contents have been removed.

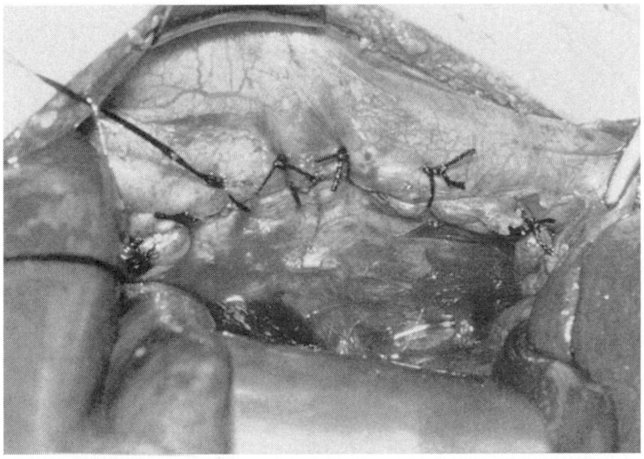

FIGURE 20–20
Diaphragmatic hernia illustrating closure of the defect.

Survivors of postnatal repairs may suffer long-term morbidity secondary to bronchopulmonary dysplasia or other lung degenerative disorders, such as emphysema. However, these problems occur in the minority of affected children. In general, the long-term prognosis is good if the neonate survives beyond surgery.

The recurrence risk is low, except where the defect occurs as part of a genetic syndrome such as Fryns syndrome, which is an autosomal recessive trait including diaphragmatic hernia, dysmorphic facies, and distal digital hypoplasia. A recent case report expanded the phenotype of Fryns syndrome to include microcephaly and midline defects.[61]

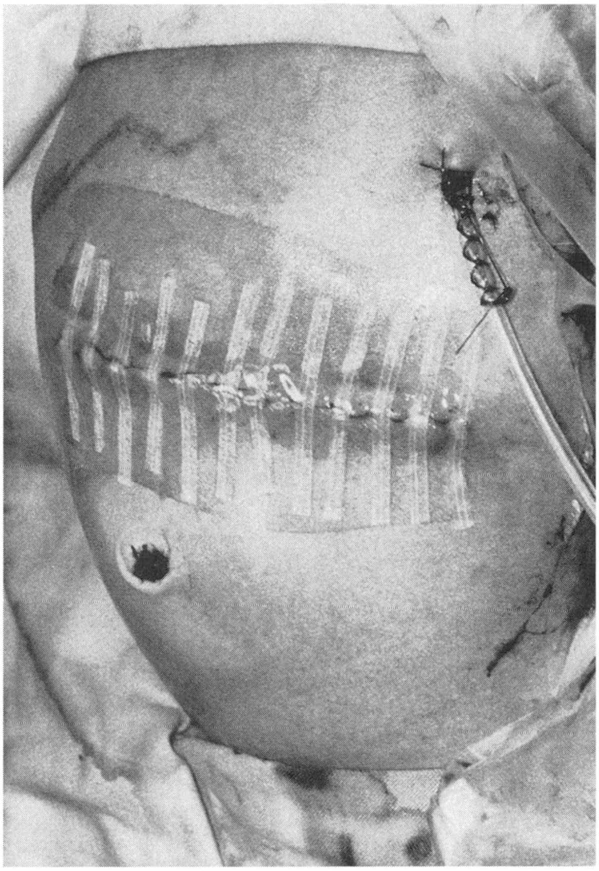

FIGURE 20–21
Diaphragmatic hernia showing wound closure and chest drain.

SUMMARY OF MANAGEMENT OPTIONS

Congenital Diaphragmatic Hernia

Management Options	Quality of Evidence	Strength of Recommendation	References
Antenatal			
Offer karyotyping.	III	B	43
Exclude other structural anomalies.	III	B	36
Prognosis is difficult to predict (see Table 20–2).	III	B	44, 45
Termination is an option before viability.	–	GPP	–
Provide interdisciplinary counseling.	–	GPP	–
Efficacy of fetal surgery not proved.	III	B	47
Labor and Delivery			
Normal management but conducted in a tertiary center.	–	GPP	–
Neonatal Management			
Provide immediate pediatric resuscitation and ventilation.	–	GPP	–
There is no clear evidence for optimal timing of repair.	IIb	B	57
There is limited evidence that ECMO (extracorporeal membrane oxygenation) improves survival; other managements have similar outcomes.	III	B	58, 59
Counsel parents that recurrence risk is low.	–	GPP	–

BODY STALK ANOMALY/LIMB BODY WALL COMPLEX

General

These rare abdominal wall defects have an annual prevalence of 1:14,000 births. The defect is considered to result from either maldevelopment of the body stalk or a disruption of part of the early amnion rupture sequence,[62] with the characteristic feature of unfused amnion and chorion such that the amnion forms a continuous sheet between the anterior abdominal wall and the placenta.[63]

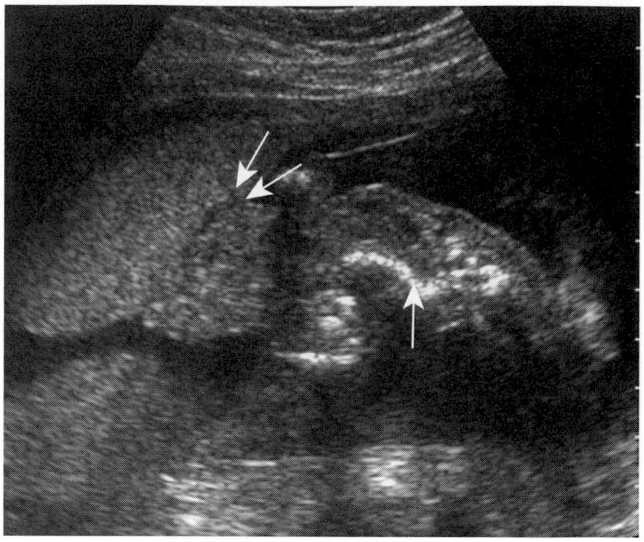

FIGURE 20–22
Body stalk anomaly showing abnormal fetal spine (*arrow*) and the appearance of the fetus being stuck to the placenta (*double arrows*).

Diagnosis

It is essential to differentiate a body stalk anomaly from other abdominal wall defects, as the former is incompatible with extrauterine life. Multiple organ system anomalies are present in most cases. Characteristically, there are neural tube and lower limb defects with scoliosis. The viscera of the fetus may appear either attached to the placenta (Fig. 20–22) or entangled with the fetal membranes. The umbilical cord is absent or abnormal.

Management Options

Antenatal

The option of pregnancy termination should be offered where legal. Vaginal delivery is the goal.

Postnatal

This defect is lethal. It is thought to be sporadic in occurrence, and thus, the recurrence risk is extremely low.

SUMMARY OF MANAGEMENT OPTIONS
Body Stalk Anomaly/Limb Body Wall Complex

Management Options	Quality of Evidence	Strength of Recommendation	References
Antenatal			
Be certain of diagnosis and exclude other abnormalities.	–	GPP	–
Discuss with parents the option of termination of pregnancy if that choice is appropriate.	–	GPP	–
Labor and Delivery			
Aim for vaginal delivery.	–	GPP	–
Neonatal Management			
Provide supportive/palliative care.	–	GPP	–

BLADDER AND CLOACAL EXSTROPHIES

General

Both exstrophies are rare, although bladder exstrophy is more common than cloacal exstrophy. The total annual prevalence approximates 1:200,000 live births, constituting less than 2% of anorectal malformations.[64] The primary defect is believed to be failure of the caudal fold of the anterior abdominal wall to develop. Failure of the urorectal septum to develop leads to a persistent cloaca with failure of the urogenital sinus to separate the bladder from the rectum.

Management Options

Antenatal

The antenatal diagnosis of cloacal exstrophy has been rarely reported. It is typically associated with severe oligohydramnios, probably due to the associated genitourinary abnormalities. The maternal serum α-fetoprotein may be high when associated with either a neural tube defect or an omphalocele. Ultrasound may show a lower than normal abdominal origin of the umbilical cord, with an infraumbilical abdominal wall defect that has a mass herniating through it. The bladder is absent from the normal position, but the pelvis may contain loops of bowel. These anomalies create difficult management issues, including gender assignment in neonates with cloacal exstrophy. The anomalies with these disorders (omphalocele, exstrophy, imperforate anus, and spina bifida) are grouped in the OEIS complex.

Termination of pregnancy is an option where legal in view of the associated genital abnormalities, the difficult surgical repair, and the long-term problems of achieving continence. The clinical management of the pregnancy is otherwise unaltered. The patient should meet with the neonatal surgical team prior to delivery to maximize understanding of the future medical requirements.[65]

Labor and Delivery

There is no a priori reason for cesarean delivery. Standard obstetric management is appropriate with delivery in a unit equipped with neonatal extensive care and surgical facilities.

SUMMARY OF MANAGEMENT OPTIONS

Bladder and Cloacal Extrophies

Management Options	Quality of Evidence	Strength of Recommendation	References
Antenatal			
Be certain of diagnosis and exclude other abnormalities.	–	GPP	–
Provide interdisciplinary counseling regarding prognosis and management.	–	GPP	–
Discuss termination of pregnancy if relevant and appropriate.	–	GPP	–
Labor and Delivery			
Normal management is sufficient.	–	GPP	–
Delivery is managed in a unit with appropriate neonatal medical and surgical facilities.	–	GPP	–
Neonatal Management			
Assessment and planning of surgery (often multiple operations) become the initial priority after birth.	–	GPP	–

ESOPHAGEAL ATRESIA WITH OR WITHOUT TRACHEOESOPHAGEAL FISTULA

General

The total annual prevalence of esophageal atresia and tracheoesophageal fistula is about 3:10,000 live births.[66] These abnormalities typically occur together because the esophagus and trachea develop from a common diverticulum of the primitive pharynx. The upper respiratory and gastrointestinal tracts separate between 3 and 5 weeks' gestation. The most common anomaly is esophageal atresia with a distal tracheoesophageal fistula (87% of cases). The variants of tracheoesophageal fistula are illustrated in Figure 20–23. Isolated esophageal atresia and isolated tracheoesophageal fistulas account for 8% and 4% of the cases, respectively.

Diagnosis

The most common antenatal presentation is hydramnios associated with preterm labor. Fetal swallowing begins around 16 weeks' gestation, and failure to visualize the stomach after this time is unusual. Failure to visualize the fetal stomach on serial scans from 20 weeks should alert the sonographer to the possibility.[67] The differential diagnosis for the sonographic absence of the stomach includes three possibilities:

- Esophageal atresia
- Congenital diaphragmatic hernia
- Impaired fetal swallowing from "neurologic" causes

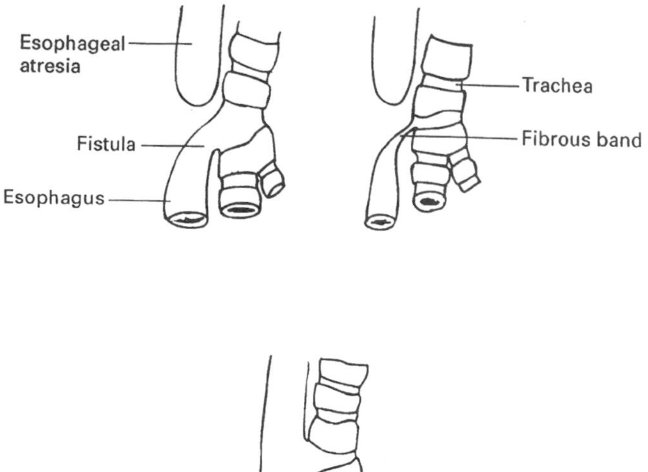

FIGURE 20–23
The main types of tracheoesophageal fistula.

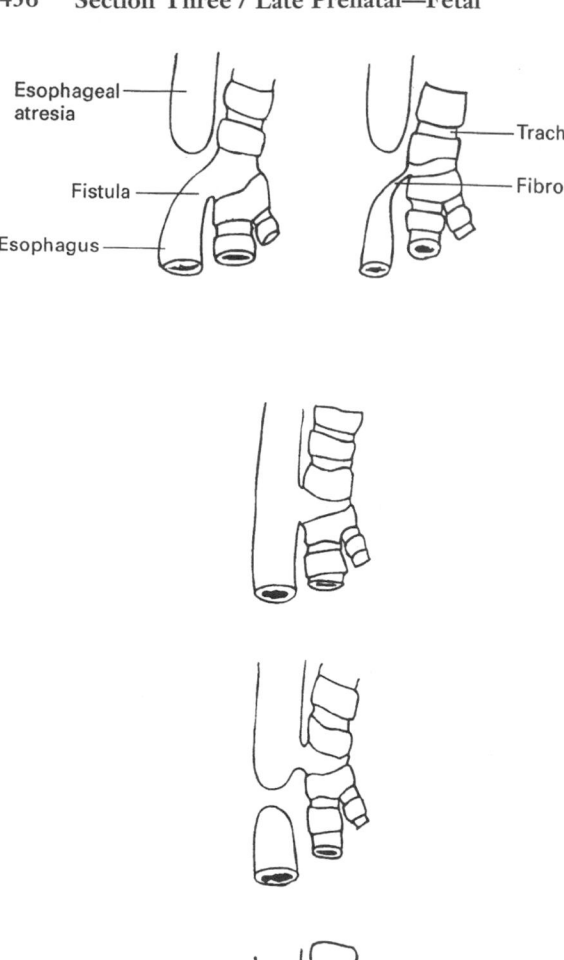

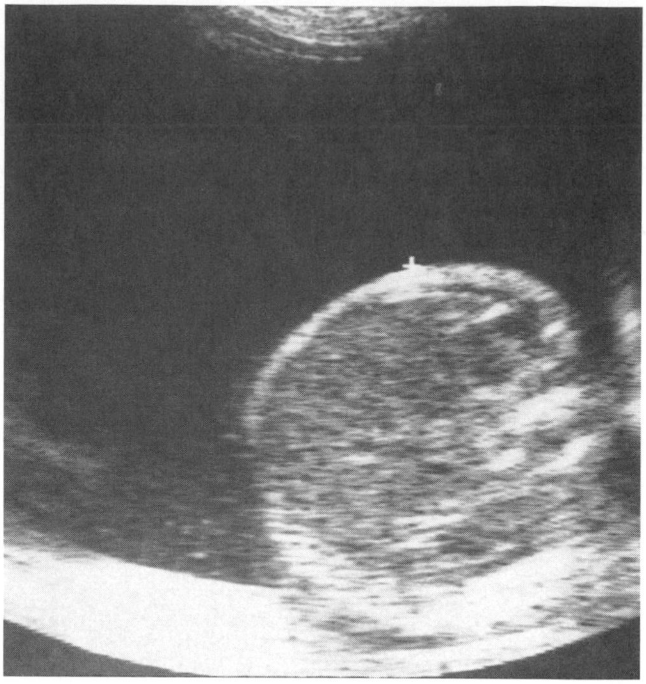

FIGURE 20–24
Esophageal atresia. Scan shows hydramnios and absent stomach in the imaging plane for the abdominal circumference measurement.

The stomach may simply be empty at the time of the scan, but after 20 weeks typically it will fill over the course of the examination. In the absence of other abnormalities, a repeat scan within a few days is warranted. The diagnosis is suspected in all cases of hydramnios (Fig. 20–24), and a targeted ultrasound examination should be part of the management of women with preterm labor (see Chapters 61 and 62). Esophageal atresia with tracheoesophageal fistula allows for the passage of amniotic fluid into the stomach and is not usually associated with either hydramnios or an absent stomach on examination. In point, the diagnosis may not be possible antenatally. A very small stomach in the presence of hydramnios suggests the diagnosis. The positive predictive value of hydramnios and an absent stomach for esophageal atresia approximates 50%.[68] A high number of fetuses have aneuploidy or other malformations. The prognosis for the fetus with esophageal atresia is markedly worse than for the neonate with esophageal atresia first suspected postnatally.

Occasionally, the proximal esophageal pouch can be imaged in the fetus with esophageal atresia when the stomach is absent. This has been referred to as the pouch sign, and can be seen as early as 23 weeks.[69] A blind pouch in the neck appears to have a worse outcome than a mediastinal pouch.[70] Magnetic resonance imaging has been successfully used when esophageal atresia was suspected but not confirmed on antenatal ultrasound.[71] Failure to demonstrate the stomach necessitates a careful search for other abnormalities including the VATER or VACTERL group of abnormalities. These abnormalities include vertebral, anal, cardiac (especially atrial and ventricular septal defects), renal and limb abnormalities, plus otocephaly, a major malformation of the mandible and temporal bones associated with abnormally placed ears.

Management Options

Antenatal

A karyotype should be obtained to rule out aneuploidy (particularly triploidy or trisomy 18), which is present in over 10% of cases.[72] Esophageal atresia may be part of the DiGeorge sequence identifiable by a characteristic deletion in chromosome 22.[73] More than half of the fetuses with esophageal atresia in one series had multiple malformations,[72] the VATER syndrome in either its complete or incomplete forms being the most common abnormality in another series.[74] The other cluster of abnormalities sufficiently different from the VATER complex to warrant distinction is the CHARGE association (Table 20–3). These infants usually have some degree of mental retardation. In contrast, the majority of neonates with VATER have normal intelligence (except those associated with either trisomy 18 or 13q deletion syndromes).

When the diagnosis is made before viability, parental counseling should include the influence of any associated abnormalities on neonatal outcome, the possible related problems during the pregnancy (e.g., hydramnios), and the short- and long-term prognosis after surgical repair. The latter has improved dramatically since the first recorded survival in 1939[75] owing to improvements in both surgical technique and neonatal intensive care. The option of pregnancy termination should be offered where legally possible, especially if there are multiple anomalies.

The most common anomaly is esophageal atresia with a distal tracheoesophageal fistula. This is usually managed by thoracotomy with division of the fistula and then end-to-end esophageal anastomosis. In the absence of other abnormalities, survival rates of up to 100% are reported.[75] However, this statistic may not represent the general experience, for a recent review of 176 repairs between 1985 and 1997 noted a perinatal and infant mortality rate of 22%, and a further 21% still had significant morbidity after 2 years of age.[76]

Continuing pregnancies are managed along standard obstetric lines. Hydramnios complicating esophageal atresia may prove to be difficult and is associated with preterm labor. Medical management of hydramnios using indomethacin has appeared to help in certain fetal abnormalities, but the one report with esophageal atresia was unsuccessful.[77] Other adverse fetal effects of indomethacin or cyclooxygenase inhibitors class II generally preclude their use in the third trimester of pregnancy. Therapeutic amniocentesis is an option after antenatal corticosteroids have been given to enhance pulmonary maturity if preterm labor occurs (see Chapters 61 and 62).

Labor and Delivery

Labor and delivery management are not influenced by the malformation.

Postnatal

Awareness of the potential for esophageal atresia in all cases of hydramnios and in any newborn with excessive oral secretions, particularly if there are breathing difficulties or possibly cyanosis, should lead to the same management as planned for the neonate diagnosed or suspected antenatally. Oral feedings are avoided until the diagnosis is clear to reduce the risk of aspiration pneumonia. Definitive surgery is offered once the infant's condition is stable.

TABLE 20–3

Components of the CHARGE Association Compared with VATER Complex

CHARGE	VATER
Colobomatous malformation	Vertebral defects
Heart defect	Anorectal (imperforate anus)
Atresia choanae	Tracheo
Retarded growth and CNS abnormalities	Esophageal fistula
Genital abnormalities and hypogonadism	Radial (and renal) aplasia (may have single umbilical artery)
Ear anomalies and deafness	
CHARGE association also includes	
Renal anomalies	
Tracheoesophageal fistula	
Facial palsy	
Micrognathia	
Cleft lip and palate	
Omphalocele	
Most have some degree of mental retardation	

The most important single determinant of outcome is the severity of the associated anomalies followed by ventilator dependence.[76,78–80] Prematurity and low birth weight are generally associated with a good outcome, especially if the birth weight is over 1500 g.[74,81] Immediate surgical complications include anastomotic leaks, tracheal perforation, and chest infection. Late complications are related either to the development of an esophageal stricture with obstruction to solids at the anastomotic site, or respiratory complications including pneumonia, tracheomalacia, and tracheal compression by the upper pouch. Only 10% have respiratory complications beyond the first year and 8% an esophageal stricture. A recent survey of the treatment results for over 370 consecutive neonates over 50 years revealed an 11% mortality rate, and incidences of 13% for tracheomalacia and 33% for gastroesophageal reflux.[82]

The less common types of esophageal atresia with or without fistula (the types producing an airless abdomen either because of blind upper and lower pouches and no fistula, or an atretic fistula) may require more complex surgery, and the prognosis, especially in terms of morbidity, is worse but improving.[76,80] In this group, gastrostomy feeding and delayed anastomotic repair until the child grows are more frequently required.

Although esophageal atresia is said to be a sporadic abnormality, a familial form is described.[83]

SUMMARY OF MANAGEMENT OPTIONS
Esophageal Atresia with/without Fistula

Management Options	Quality of Evidence	Strength of Recommendation	References
Antenatal			
Diagnosis by ultrasound during pregnancy is uncommon; raised alpha fetoprotein is a reported association.	III	B	67
Hydramnios is common.	III	B	68
Examine for associated abnormalities with ultrasound and karyotype.	III	B	72,74
Provide interdisciplinary counseling.	–	GPP	–
Labor and Delivery			
Normal management is provided in tertiary center with facilities for advanced neonatal resuscitation, intensive care, and surgery.	–	GPP	–
Postnatal			
Remove excess secretions at birth; place esophageal tube to maintain low pressure suction.	–	GPP	–
Early diagnostic imaging should include a chest x-ray.	–	GPP	–
Avoid oral feeding.	–	GPP	–
Check for other abnormalities.	–	GPP	–
The risk of recurrence is small.	–	GPP	–

ATRESIAS OF THE BOWEL

A wide variety of congenital anomalies can occur in perinates with either gut atresias or stenoses. The specific pattern of anomalies depends on the location of the atresia. For example, cardiac and renal atresias are associated with what may appear to be isolated esophageal atresia or duodenal atresia.[84] Other associations are discussed in the sections on the each abnormality.

DUODENAL ATRESIA

General

Atresia of the duodenum is generally considered to occur around 11 weeks' gestation after an insult to the duodenum, most commonly either just proximal or distal to the ampulla of Vater, causes failure of canalization. Occasionally, vascular accidents or midgut strangulation associated with omphalocele are implicated as causes. The annual prevalence of duodenal atresia approximates 1:6000 live births. Around 30% of cases of isolated duodenal atresia are associated with trisomy 21 or other aneuploidies.

Diagnosis

Hydramnios is common with upper intestinal atresias and implies total obstruction. Half the pregnancies complicated by duodenal atresia are associated with hydramnios. The sonographic diagnosis is made by the appearance of a "double bubble" (Fig. 20–25). Generally, this image appears late in the second trimester, but has been suspected as early as 12 weeks[85] and positively detected at 19 weeks.[86] Like all forms of gastrointestinal obstruction,

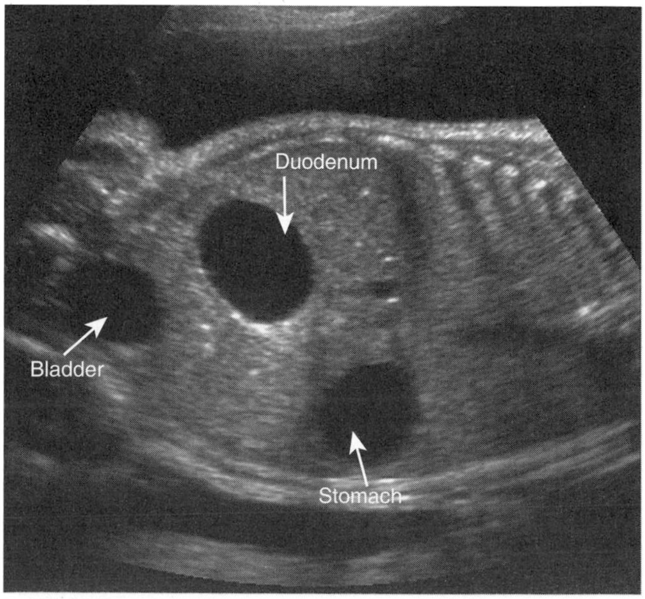

FIGURE 20–25
Duodenal atresia. Oblique longitudinal ultrasound image of fetal abdomen showing "double bubble" in a fetus with duodenal atresia.

duodenal atresia may not be diagnosable by ultrasonography until the third trimester. This may reflect the production of motilin, the hormone necessary for peristalsis, which begins in the mid to late second trimester. It is important that a true transverse section of the abdomen be obtained and that a connection between the two bubbles is seen (Fig. 20–26). This avoids the potential confusion of an oblique scan of the stomach artificially producing a double bubble, or confusing the stomach and a choledochal cyst with a duodenal atresia. Increased peristaltic waves may be seen during real-time imaging.

Management Options

Antenatal

Associated anomalies are present in over 50%. They include trisomy 21 in 30%, other gastrointestinal malformations in 25%, and cardiac, tracheal and esophageal, renal, hepatobiliary, and pancreatic ductal abnormalities in 48%. Apart from trisomy 21, other chromosomal abnormalities associated with duodenal atresia include abnormalities of chromosome 9. Other gastrointestinal abnormalities include malrotation (28%), annular pancreas (33%), esophageal atresia, imperforate anus, jejunal atresia, duplication of the duodenum, and Meckel's diverticulum.[87] Duodenal atresia may be associated with multiple atresias of the bowel. About half the infants have early onset growth deficiency.

This range of associated anomalies mandates a detailed ultrasonographic examination by experienced personnel for associated structural abnormalities and a karyotype. Fetuses with trisomy 21 have a high risk of cardiac abnormalities. They may also have heart rate abnormalities in labor not necessarily indicative of hypoxia and, in that circumstance, do not require cesarean delivery. Indomethacin (or similar cyclooxygenase inhibitors) has been given in an attempt to treat the hydramnios.[77] Few clinically adverse effects on the fetus are documented when given for a short time before 32 weeks, though a fetal pleural effusion is reported with maternal indomethacin therapy that resolved after stopping of therapy.[88] The main clinical risk is constriction of the ductus arteriosus. Therapeutic amniocentesis after antenatal corticosteroids represents a reasonable therapeutic option (see Chapter 10).

Labor and Delivery

There is no a priori indication for cesarean delivery because of duodenal atresia. As in any situation with gross hydramnios, delivery in a tertiary center is advised, both to manage the potential complications of the hydramnios and for access to neonatal surgical services. Similar to esophageal atresia in which the cause of the hydramnios may be in doubt, passage of a orogastric or nasogastric tube after delivery followed by radiographs of the neonate will help confirm the diagnosis. Because a double bubble is not absolutely diagnostic of duodenal atresia, other possibilities must be excluded after delivery. The differential diagnosis includes annular pancreas, peritoneal bands, and duodenal stenosis.

Postnatal

After delivery, a tube is passed into the stomach and abdominal radiographs taken. The diagnosis can be confirmed at this stage by examination of the gas pattern. The atretic area is excised (Fig. 20–27) when the infant is stable.

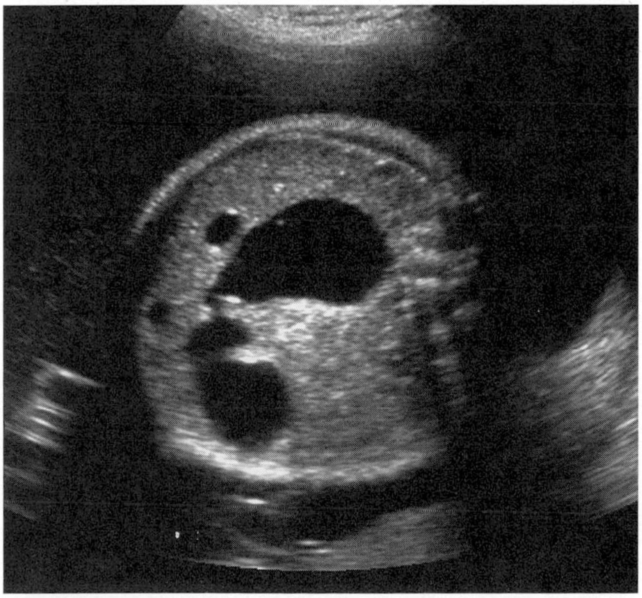

FIGURE 20–26
Duodenal atresia in true transverse section showing communication between stomach and duodenum. Increased amniotic fluid is noted.

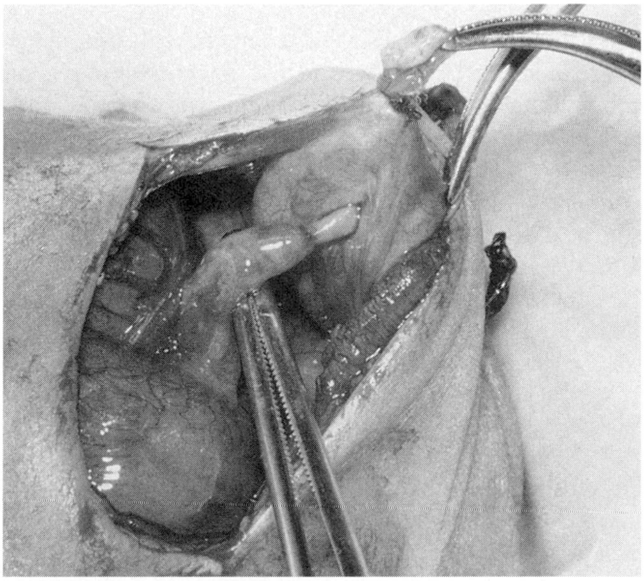

FIGURE 20–27
Duodenal atresia. Atretic segment as seen at neonatal surgery (segment above surgical forceps).

The prognosis for this condition, if recognized and isolated, is good, and the recurrence risk is low. Operative mortality rate is up to 4%, with long-term survival rate quoted as 86%. Cardiac lesions are one of the main contributors to long-term morbidity and death.[87]

SUMMARY OF MANAGEMENT OPTIONS

Duodenal Atresia

Management Options	Quality of Evidence	Strength of Recommendation	References
Antenatal			
Diagnosis is made by ultrasound: double-bubble with dilated stomach and proximal duodenum (usually detected latter part of second or third trimester).	III	B	86
Duodenal atresia is associated with polyhydramnios, annular pancreas, preterm labor, 20–30% incidence of Down syndrome, and higher incidence of other structural malformations.	III	B	87
Scan and karyotype for other anomalies.	III	B	87
Provide interdisciplinary counseling.	–	GPP	–
Labor and Delivery			
Normal management is given but at a tertiary center.	–	GPP	–
Vigilance is needed for complications of hydramnios.	–	GPP	–
Postnatal			
Pass nasogastric tube.	–	GPP	–
Confirm diagnosis by radiography.	–	GPP	–
Surgical correction is needed; search for other abnormalities at surgery.	–	GPP	–

JEJUNAL AND ILEAL ATRESIA

General

Jejunal and ileal atresia have an annual prevalence approximating 1:5000 live births. They are the second most common forms of neonatal bowel obstruction.[89] These atresias are thought to result from vascular compromise of a bowel segment after organogenesis is complete. Intestinal atresias are categorized according to the degree of occlusion or separation of the bowel on either side of the atretic segment.

Associated anomalies are less common than with duodenal atresia. Five cases of trisomy 21 were reported in one series of 589 perinates with jejunoileal atresia.[90] A special form, the "apple peel" deformity, is an autosomal recessive trait and may have a worse prognosis than the other forms of atresia.[91] Another review noted gastroschisis in 16% of cases, intrauterine volvulus in 27%, and meconium ileus in 11%.[87]

Diagnosis

The sonographic appearance of jejunal atresia is that of multiple distended bowel loops. Hydramnios is more common with upper gastrointestinal obstruction (duodenal and jejunal) than with lower obstructions. The development of ascites or an echogenic mass on scan is a sign of bowel perforation.

Detailed ultrasonographic examination of the wall of cystic or echogenic intra-abdominal structures for peristalsis is important, as it can be associated with bowel perforation and development of a meconium pseudocyst. Other features useful antenatally for diagnosing bowel obstruction are increased peristalsis, failure to detect a normal colon late in gestation, and a disproportionately large abdominal circumference for dates.

Management Options

Antenatal

Jejunal and ileal atresias are usually isolated from other gastrointestinal lesions. It is important to exclude other causes of echolucent structures within the abdomen, such as a urinary tract obstruction. It is suggested that serial measurements of the bowel loop diameter are of value, and tables of bowel diameter are available.[92] However, these measurements correlate with neither the diagnosis of bowel obstruction or prognosis. The appearance of the bowel is quite variable, particularly in the third trimester, and in our experience, mild bowel dilation is typically associated with a normal outcome (Fig. 20–28). However, a bowel obstruction should be suspected whenever the internal diameter of the small bowel is greater than 7 mm.[93] There is little evidence to support early delivery based on bowel loop diameter.

Labor and Delivery

Fetuses with a presumptive bowel obstruction should be delivered in a center with neonatal surgical facilities. Otherwise, obstetric management is unaltered by the presence of the abnormality. Hydramnios is not an indication for a cesarean delivery.

Postnatal

After delivery, the neonate is evaluated to determine the site of obstruction and the presence of any associated congenital anomalies or meconium peritonitis. The prognosis is very good following repair, with no losses in one series.[89] Even in the group with apple peel deformity, early diagnosis and prolonged parenteral nutrition has resulted in a dramatic improvement in survival.[94]

The risk of recurrence for jejunal and ileal atresia is small except in the group with apple peel syndrome, which would appear to follow autosomal recessive inheritance.[95]

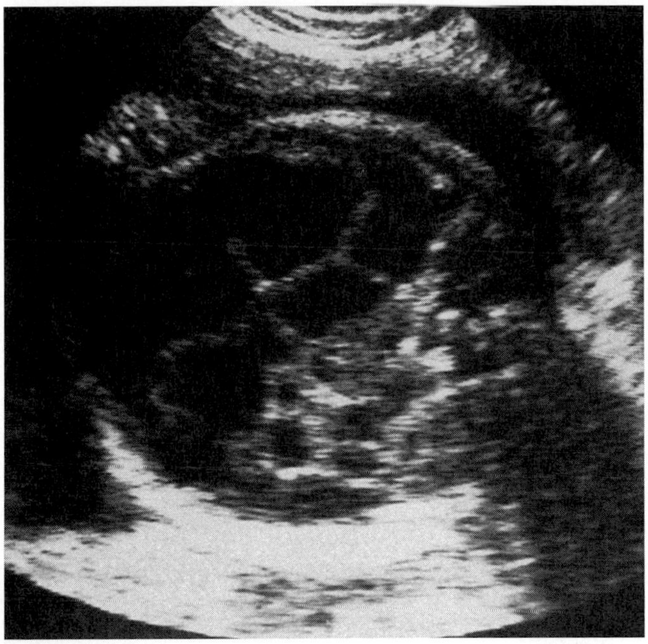

FIGURE 20–28
Dilated bowel on ultrasonography. This fetus had a normal outcome.

SUMMARY OF MANAGEMENT OPTIONS

Jejuno-ileal Atresia

Management Options	Quality of Evidence	Strength of Recommendation	References
Antenatal			
Diagnosis is made by ultrasound.	III	B	87
Hydramnios may develop.	III	B	87
Scan for other anomalies; value of karyotype is uncertain.	III	B	87
Serial ultrasound scans should recognize: perforation (ascites, echogenic mass).	–	GPP	–
Interdisciplinary counseling is needed.	–	GPP	–
Labor and Delivery			
Normal management is given but at a tertiary center.	–	GPP	–
Exercise vigilance for complications of hydramnios.	–	GPP	–
Postnatal			
Pass nasogastric tube.	–	GPP	–
Confirm diagnosis by radiography.	–	GPP	–
Surgical correction is needed; search for other abnormalities at surgery.	–	GPP	–
Recurrence risk is low (except for apple peel deformity with 1:4 risk).	–	GPP	–

LARGE BOWEL OBSTRUCTION, ANAL ATRESIA, AND IMPERFORATE ANUS

General

Colon atresia is rare and largely confined to the right colon.[89] The annual prevalence of imperforate anus is 1:2500 to 1:5000 live births. In the embryo, the distal colon develops a lumen beginning in the region of the descending colon. Anorectal malformations are complex, and there are several classifications. One is to classify them by the level of the defect and its association with fistula formation.[96] Anal anomalies may be part of multiple malformation syndromes, including the VATER and CHARGE complexes, and cloacal exstrophy and are often associated with spinal and genitourinary defects.[97] At least 25 such syndromes are defined.[98]

Presentation

Large bowel abnormalities are rarely diagnosed antenatally except when part of other multiple malformation syndromes. Apart from mechanical abnormalities such as malrotation or volvulus, other reasons for dilated large bowel or increased echogenicity are meconium ileus, aganglionosis (Hirschsprung's disease), and congenital syphilis. Generally, the ultrasound findings are nonspecific, and the diagnoses of these conditions are made postnatally. The fetal karyotype is generally normal.

SUMMARY OF MANAGEMENT OPTIONS

Large Bowel Obstruction, Anal Atresia and Imperforate Anus

Management Options	Quality of Evidence	Strength of Recommendation	References
Antenatal			
Assess for hydramnios (rare).	–	GPP	–
Provide interdisciplinary counseling.	–	GPP	–
Careful ultrasound examination is made for other abnormalities.	–	GPP	–
Labor and Delivery			
Normal management is given at a tertiary center.	–	GPP	–
Postnatal			
Do not give baby anything by mouth.	–	GPP	–
Pediatric assessment and management	–	GPP	–

MECONIUM ILEUS AND MECONIUM PERITONITIS, HYPERECHOGENIC BOWEL

General

Hyperechogenic bowel, defined sonographically as echogenicity at least equal to the surrounding bone, occurs in 0.1% to 1.8% of pregnancies in the second or third trimesters.[99] It may be transient. Meconium ileus is an obstruction of the lower ileum by thick meconium. Perforation can occur after bowel obstruction secondary to any cause, including meconium ileus producing meconium peritonitis, intestinal atresia, volvulus, and malrotation. These conditions are rare. Meconium ileus is most commonly associated with cystic fibrosis. In contrast, most cases of meconium peritonitis are not (though cystic fibrosis should be considered). Bayesian analysis of risk of prevalence of cystic fibrosis in a fetus with echogenic bowel yields a range of 3.3% to 13% in a mixed North American population.[100] In addition to cystic fibrosis, hyperechogenic bowel is associated with bowel obstruction, viral infection, aneuploidy, and fetal growth restriction. An echogenic mass in the stomach may be swallowed blood, for example, after an abruption or invasive procedure.

Diagnosis

Both meconium ileus and peritonitis have been diagnosed in the second trimester.[101] Meconium ileus presents as either a cluster of bright echoes, or the bowel may appear dilated and echogenic. Hyperechogenic bowel is present when the echogenicity is at least as bright as adjacent bone or liver. This definition overcomes variation in description due to ultrasound machine settings. Distinguishing it from normal, especially late in the third trimester, may be difficult (Fig. 20–29).

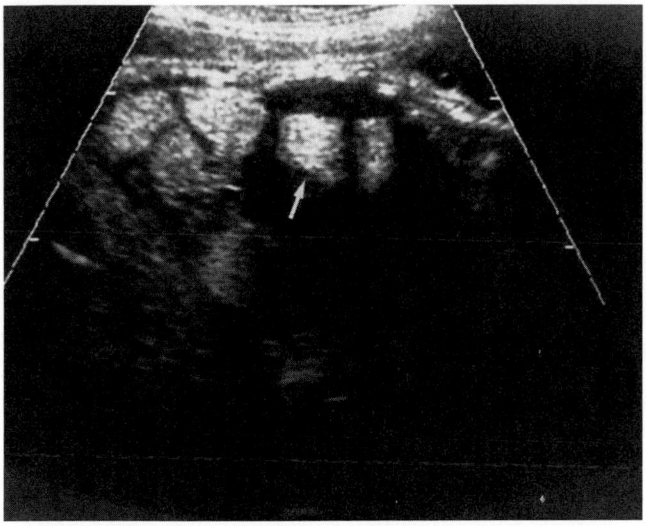

FIGURE 20–29
Ultrasound scan showing echogenic bowel (*arrow*) in the third trimester. This fetus had a normal outcome.

Fetal ascites and hydramnios are signs of perforation. A hyperechoic mass or diffuse hyperechoic deposits in the fetal abdomen suggest meconium peritonitis (Fig. 20–30). The thorax may be compressed if there is a volvulus or massive bowel distention.

Management Options

Antenatal

Suspected meconium ileus triggers a search for cystic fibrosis. The parents should be tested and if at least one is a carrier (not all mutations are known), the fetus should be tested either by amniocentesis or cordocentesis. Meconium ileus affects some 15% of neonates with cystic fibrosis.[102] Meconium peritonitis is a serious condition, and the guidelines for management are dictated by the ultrasonographic appearance. A discrete lesion within the fetal abdomen that appears unchanging and free of ascites or hydramnios does not warrant intervention. However, the presence of ascites, increasing abdominal distention, and hydramnios may warrant preterm delivery if the estimated risks of prematurity do not exceed the potential benefit of early intervention. There are no data to allow clear guidelines to be generated. In this situation, antepartum corticosteroid administration should be considered to hasten pulmonary maturation. Drainage of the ascites, especially if there is lung compression, has been associated with a good outcome, possibly by smoothing the transition to ex utero life. Appropriate study is lacking. Therapeutic amniocentesis is also an option for pronounced hydramnios (see Chapter 13), though indomethacin would be undesirable as a prostacyclin inhibitor. Unexplained death is reported in up to 5% of fetuses with echogenic bowel presenting in the second trimester in the absence of cystic fibrosis, aneuploidy, or infection.[99,103] Death was associated with fetal growth restriction and oligohydramnios.[103]

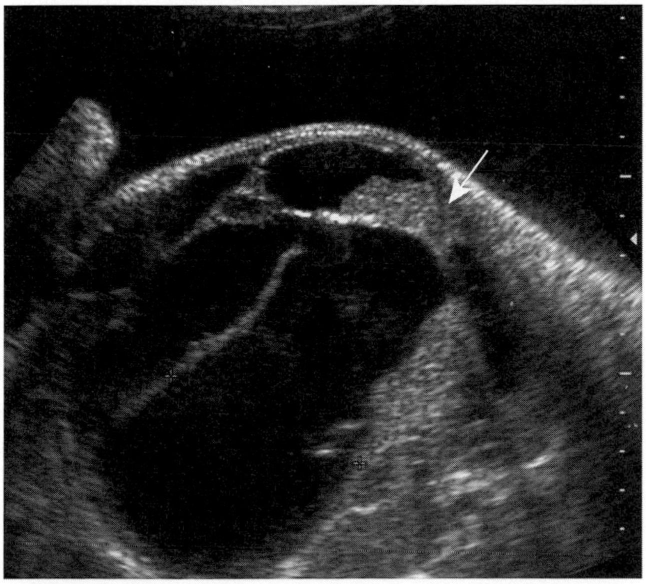

FIGURE 20–30
Longitudinal section of fetal abdomen showing massive bowel dilation. The bowel is surrounded by meconium (*arrow*) indicating the development of peritonitis in a fetus with cystic fibrosis. There is gross hydramnios.

Labor and Delivery

Expectant management is standard in the absence of perforation, though the neonatal intensive care team should be informed of the possible diagnosis. The management of meconium peritonitis in labor is determined by obstetric factors (e.g., the gestation and the ease of which labor can be induced). There is no information to suggest cesarean delivery a priori benefits the fetus with meconium peritonitis.

Postnatal

Infants with meconium ileus typically become symptomatic within the first 24 to 48 hours of life. Abdominal distention and delayed passage of the meconium plug are characteristic. Vomiting is a relatively late sign. The overall prognosis for the neonate with meconium ileus is determined in part by the success of either the Gastrografin enema or surgery in relieving the obstruction, but mainly by the severity of the cystic fibrosis if present. The prognosis for meconium peritonitis is not good, in part due to prematurity. The recurrence rate is low except when the condition is secondary to cystic fibrosis.

ECHOGENIC ('BRIGHT') LIVER AND HEPATIC CALCIFICATIONS

General

Echogenic ("bright") liver (Fig. 20–31) is an uncommon finding with a number of causes or associations, including liver tumors, congenital viral infection, and vascular congestion.

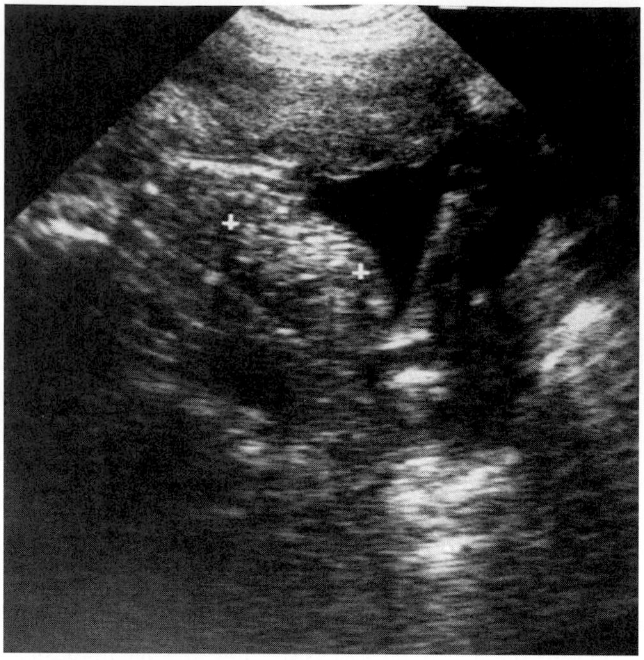

FIGURE 20–31
Longitudinal scan of fetus showing hyperechoic liver (*crosses*). This fetus had a normal outcome.

Hepatomegaly may occur in hemolytic disease or as part of a visceromegaly syndrome (e.g., Beckwith-Wiedemann syndrome).

Hepatic echogenic areas ("calcifications") may be on the surface or within the parenchyma (Fig. 20–32) or be associated with the vasculature. The cause of this ultrasound finding is not always known, and postnatal scanning does not invariably confirm their presence. Subcapsular calcifications may be seen with meconium peritonitis. Intrahepatic calcification is associated with fetal infection or thromboses.

Management Options

Antenatal

Management is directed toward making a diagnosis. The association of hepatic calcification with congenital viral or toxoplasmosis infection is well documented (see Chapters 27, 30, 31, and 33). Serologic screening is commonly employed to identify women at risk of having an affected child, but assumes one knows which infectious agent to screen for and that a maternal response has occurred. In one review, of 49 at-risk pregnancies for toxoplasmosis, fetal infection was diagnosed

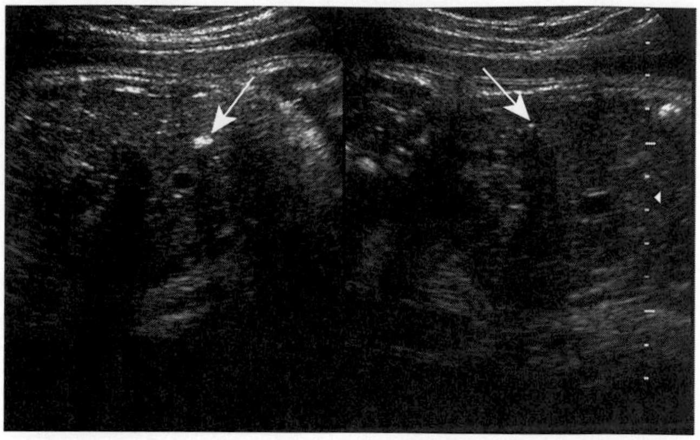

FIGURE 20–32
Hepatic calcifications in the fetal liver (*arrows*). Note the shadowing.

in 5. The diagnosis of fetal infection was based on the culture and detection of toxoplasmosis-specific immunoglobulin M (IgM) in blood obtained by cordocentesis. No abnormal fetal liver calcifications were recorded, but both hydrocephalus and intracranial calcifications were seen.[106]

Herpes virus, echovirus, varicella, coxsackie virus, and adenovirus all have similar hepatic manifestations of infection. Hepatitis leading to ascites is not rare. The ultrasonographic appearances are nonspecific, and invasive tests are usually necessary for a definitive diagnosis (see Chapters 27, 30, 31, and 33). In the case of toxoplasmosis, the risk of fetal transmission after proven maternal first-trimester infection is thought to be low (~4%),[107] but a negative result after fetal testing may provide reassurance.

Hepatic tumors including hepatoblastoma and hepatic adenoma[108] have been diagnosed *in utero*. Management involves observation until delivery, though the fetus may develop congestive heart failure as with any large tumor causing arteriovenous shunting.

A detailed search for markers of aneuploidy is indicated because there is an increased risk, but typically aneuploidy is associated with other findings.[109]

Labor and Delivery

Standard obstetric management is generally appropriate.

Postnatal

This care is determined by the likely diagnosis. Delivery in a center with pediatric surgical facilities as well as neonatal intensive care is advisable.

SUMMARY OF MANAGEMENT OPTIONS

Meconium Ileus/Peritonitis/Echogenic Bowel and Liver

Management Options	Quality of Evidence	Strength of Recommendation	References
Antenatal			
Diagnosis is made by ultrasound.	III	B	99,101
Use strict criteria for diagnosis of echogenic bowel/liver ("bone-white").			
For all, consider diagnosis of cystic fibrosis.	III	B	100,102
For echogenic bowel, consider diagnosis of cystic fibrosis, cytomegalovirus or parvovirus, aneuploidy, intestinal obstruction (meconium ileus), intra-amniotic bleeding, and increased risk of placental bleed, intrauterine growth restriction, and fetal death later in pregnancy.	III	B	101,102
Maintain vigilance for hydramnios and/or ascites.	–	GPP	–
No data support drainage or delivery if ascites or hydramnios develops.	–	GPP	–
Provide interdisciplinary counseling.	–	GPP	–
Labor and Delivery			
Timing depends on obstetric factors and/or presence of ascites/hydramnios.	–	GPP	–
Delivery is performed in a tertiary center with full pediatric resources but otherwise normal management.	–	GPP	–
Postnatal			
For meconium ileus and peritonitis, outcome is dependent upon surgical feasibility of repair, associated abnormalities, perforation, and gestation.	III	B	99,103
For echogenic bowel/liver, implement pediatric assessment and management.	–	GPP	–

ECHOLUCENT STRUCTURES WITHIN THE FETAL ABDOMEN

General

Echolucent or "cystic" structures separate from normal bowel or the urinary tract may be identified on ultrasonography. Differential diagnoses include the following possibilities:

- Omental cysts
- Mesenteric cysts
- Cysts of the ovary
- Urachal cysts
- Hepatic cysts
- Choledochal cysts
- Duplication cysts of the bowel
- Retroperitoneal cysts

Management Options

Antenatal

Intra-abdominal cysts are usually a chance finding on ultrasonography. The sonographer should attempt to determine the origin of the structure and exclude other fetal abnormalities. Massive intra-abdominal cysts, especially those detected early in pregnancy, seem to have a poor prognosis, but in many cases they remain unchanged or resolve.[104]

Hepatic cysts may be isolated or associated with adult type polycystic renal disease (see Chapter 19). Choledochal cysts (single or multiple) occur in the right upper quadrant, below the liver, and are intraperitoneal. Similar to most cystic lesions, their significance relates to postnatal management. Untreated, choledochal cysts can lead to biliary cirrhosis and portal hypertension.

The most common hypoechoic intra-abdominal lesion in the female fetus is an ovarian cyst. These cysts are best observed, as most resolve spontaneously over several weeks after delivery.

Labor and Delivery

Obstetric care is unaltered by these abnormalities.

Postnatal

Knowledge of the differential diagnosis is important. The neonate should undergo an ultrasound examination as soon after delivery as feasible. Duplications of the small and large bowel may rarely communicate with normal bowel lumen. In this instance, the neonate will present with signs of bowel obstruction. Intestinal duplications in association with spinal cord and vertebral body anomalies are reported.[105]

SUMMARY OF MANAGEMENT OPTIONS
Intra-abdominal Echolucent (Cystic) Structures

Management Options	Quality of Evidence	Strength of Recommendation	References
Antenatal			
Determine the organ of origin and diagnosis:	–	GPP	–
Omental cysts			
Mesenteric cysts			
Ovarian cysts			
Urachus			
Liver cysts			
Choledochal cysts			
Bowel duplication cysts			
Retroperitoneal cysts			
Exclude other fetal abnormalities.	–	GPP	–
Postnatal			
Implement pediatric assessment and management, including early neonatal ultrasonography.	–	GPP	–

CONCLUSIONS

- The fetal gastrointestinal and abdominal wall malformations most commonly identified prenatally are omphalocele, gastroschisis, and diaphragmatic hernia.
- They are detected either after an increased maternal serum α-fetoprotein concentration, at routine second-trimester ultrasound, or by chance in later pregnancy because a problem is detected (especially poor fetal growth or hydramnios).
- Management should involve a multidisciplinary team.
- Exclusion of other abnormalities is a priority for most conditions.
- Delivery should be in a tertiary center with full neonatal medical and surgical facilities.

Acknowledgments

I would like to acknowledge the following people for their assistance with the illustrations: Associate Professor Kevin Pringle, pediatric surgeon; Ms. Louise Goossens, medical photographer; and Ms. Jennie Flower and Mrs. Jenny Mitchell, ultrasonographers.

REFERENCES

1. Di Tanna GL, Rosano A, Mastroiacovo P: Prevalence of gastroschisis at birth: Retrospective study. Br Med J 2002; 325:1389–1390.
2. Kamata S, Ishikawa S, Usui N, et al: Prenatal diagnosis of abdominal wall defects and their prognosis. J Pediatr Surg 1996;31:267–271.
3. Salihu HM, Boos R, Schmidt W: Omphalocele and gastroschisis. J Obstet Gynaecol 2002;22:489–492.
4. Wald NJ, Cuckle RS: Neural tube defects: Screening and biochemical diagnosis. In Rodeck CH, Nicolaides KH (eds): Prenatal Diagnosis. Proceedings of the Eleventh Study Group of the Royal College of Obstetricians and Gynaecologists. London, Royal College of Obstetricians and Gynaecologists, 1983, p 234.
5. Raine PAM: Anterior abdominal wall defects. Curr Obstet Gynaecol 1991;1:147–153.

6. Nyberg DA, Fitzsimmons J, Mack LA, et al: Chromosomal abnormalities in fetuses with omphalocele: Significance of omphalocele contents. J Ultrasound Med 1989;8:299–308.
7. Vanamo K, Sairanen H, Louhimo I: The spectrum of Cantrell's syndrome. Pediatr Surg Int 1991;6:429–433.
8. Gibbin C, Touch S, Broth RE, Berghella V: Abdominal wall defects and congenital heart disease. Ultrasound Obstet Gynaecol 2003;21:334–337.
9. Koivusalo A, Lindahl H, Rintala RJ: Morbidity and quality of life in adult patients with a congenital abdominal wall defect: A questionnaire survey. J Pediatr Surg 2002;37:1594–1601.
10. Sipes SL, Weiner CP, Spies DR, et al: Gastroschisis and omphalocele: Does either antenatal diagnosis or route of delivery make a difference in perinatal outcome? Obstet Gynecol 1990;76:195–199.
11. Moretti M, Khoury A, Rodriquez J, et al: The effect of mode of delivery on the perinatal outcome in fetuses with abdominal wall defects. Am J Obstet Gynecol 1990;163:833–838.
12. Kohn MR, Shi ECP: Gastroschisis and exomphalos: Recent trends and factors influencing survival. Aust N Z J Surg 1990;60:199–202.
13. Baird PA, MacDonald EL: An epidemiologic study of congenital malformations of the anterior abdominal wall in more than half a million consecutive live births. Am J Hum Genet 1981;33: 470–478.
14. Kozer E, Nikfar S, Costei A, et al: Aspirin consumption during the first trimester of pregnancy and congenital anomalies: A meta-analysis. Am J Obstet Gynecol 2002;187:1623–1630.
15. Werler MM, Sheehan JE, Mitchell AA: Maternal medication use and risks of gastroschisis and small intestinal atresia. Am J Epidemiol 2002;155:26–31.
16. Japaraj RP, Hockey R, Chan FY: Gastroschisis: Can prenatal sonography predict neonatal outcome? Ultrasound Obstet Gynecol 2003;21:329–333.
17. Luton D, De Lagausie P, Guibourclenche J, et al: Prognostic factors of prenatally diagnosed gastroschisis. Fetal Diagn Ther 1997;12:7–14.
18. Babcook C, Hedrick MH, Goldstein RB, et al: Gastroschisis: Can sonography of the fetal bowel accurately predict postnatal outcome? J Ultrasound Med 1994;13:701–706.
19. Morrison JJ, Klein N, Chitty LS, et al: Intra-amniotic inflammation in human gastroschisis: Possible aetiology of postnatal bowel dysfunction. BJOG 1998;105:1200–1204.
20. Deans KJ, Mooney DP, Meyer MM, Shorter NA: Prolonged exposure to amniotic fluid does not result in peel formation in gastroschisis. J Pediatr Surg 1999;34:975–976.
21. Luton D, Lagausie P, Guibourdenche J, et al: Effect of amnioinfusion on the outcome of prenatally diagnosed gastroschisis. Fetal Diagn Ther 1999;14:152–155.
22. Sipes SL, Weiner CP, Williamson RA, et al: Fetal gastroschisis complicated by bowel dilation: An indication for imminent delivery? Fetal Diagn Ther 1990;5:100–103.
23. Huang J, Kurkchubasche AG, Carr SR, et al: Benefits of term delivery in infants with antenatally diagnosed gastroschisis. Obstet Gynecol 2002;100:695–699.
24. Sydorak RM, Nijagal A, Sbragia L, et al: Gastroschisis: Small hole, big cost. J Pediatr Surg 2002;37:1669–1672.
25. Blakelock R, Upadhyay V, Kimble R, et al: Is a normally functioning gastrointestinal tract necessary for normal growth in late gestation. Pediatr Surg Int 1998;13:17–20.
26. Kalache KD, Bierlich A, Hammer H, Bollmann R: Is unexplained third trimester intrauterine death of fetuses with gastroschisis caused by umbilical cord compression due to acute extra-abdominal bowel dilatation? Prenat Diagn 2002;22: 715–717.
27. Bianchi A, Dickson AP, Alizai NK: Elective delayed midgut reduction—No anesthesia for gastroschisis: Selection and conversion criteria. J Pediatr Surg 2002;37:1334–1336.
28. Kimble RM, Singh SJ, Bourke C, Cass DT: Gastroschisis reduction under analgesia in the neonatal unit. J Pediatr Surg 2001;36: 1672–1674.
29. Davies MW, Kimble RM, Woodgate PG: Ward reduction without general anaesthesia versus reduction and repair under general anaesthesia for gastroschisis in newborn infants. Cochrane Database Syst Rev 2002;cd003671.
30. Shah R, Woolley MM: Gastroschisis and intestinal atresia. J Pediatr Surg 1991;26:788–790.
31. Durfee SM, Downward CD, Benson CB, Wilson JM: Postnatal outcome of fetuses with the prenatal diagnosis of gastroschisis. J Ultrasound Med 2002;21:269–274.
32. Swartz KR, Harrison MW, Campbell JR, Campbell TJ: Long-term follow-up of patients with gastroschisis. Am J Surg 1986;151:546–549.
33. Lowry RB, Baird PA: Familial gastroschisis and omphalocele. Am J Hum Genet 1982;34:517–518.
34. Lunzer H, Menardi G, Brezinka C: Long term follow up of children with prenatally diagnosed omphalocele and gastroschisis. J Matern Fetal Med 2001;10:385–392.
35. Dillon E, Renwick M: Antenatal detection of congenital diaphragmatic hernias: The northern region experience. Clin Radiol 1993;48:264–267.
36. Bollman R, Kalache K, Mau H, et al: Associated malformations and chromosomal defects in congenital diaphragmatic hernia. Fetal Diagn Ther 1995;10:52–59.
37. Jesudason EC: Challenging embryological theories on congenital diaphragmatic hernia: Future therapeutic implications for paediatric surgery. Ann R Coll Surg Engl 2002;84:252–259.
38. Garne E, Haeusler M, Barisic I, et al: Congenital diaphragmatic hernia: Evaluation of prenatal diagnosis in 20 European regions. Euroscan Study Group. Ultrasound Obstet Gynecol 2002;19: 329–333.
39. Romero R, Pilu G, Jeanty P, et al: Prenatal Diagnosis of Congenital Anomalies. Norwalk, CT, Appleton & Lange, 1988, p 215.
40. Haeusler MCH, Ryan G, Robson S, et al: The use of saline solution as a contrast medium in suspected diaphragmatic hernia and renal agenesis. Am J Obstet Gynaecol 1993;168:1486–1492.
41. Meagher S, Fisk N, Boogert A: Utility of fetal intraperitoneal saline infusion in the prenatal evaluation of diaphragmatic hernia. Fetal Diagn Ther 1995;10:307–310.
42. Botash RJ, Spirt BA: Color Doppler imaging aids in the prenatal diagnosis of congenital diaphragmatic hernia. J Ultrasound Med 1993;12:359–361.
43. Snijders RJM, Nicolaides KH: Ultrasound Markers for Fetal Chromosomal Defects. London, Parthenon Publishing Group, 1996, p 28.
44. Skari H, Bjornland K, Frenckner B, et al: Congenital diaphragmatic hernia in Scandinavia from 1995 to 1998: Predictors of mortality. J Pediatr Surg 2002;37:1269–1275.
45. Screenan C, Etches P, Osiovich H: The western Canadian experience with congenital diaphragmatic hernia: Perinatal factors predictive of extracorporeal membrane oxygenation and death. Pediatr Surg Int 2001;17:196–200.
46. Al-Shanafey S, Giacomantonio M, Henteleff H: Congenital diaphragmatic hernia: Experience without extracorporeal membrane oxygenation. Pediatr Surg 2002;18:28–31.
47. Quinn TM, Adzick NS: Fetal surgery. Obstet Gynecol Clin North Am 1997;24:143–157.
48. Metkus AP, Filly RA, Stringer MD, et al: Sonographic predictors of survival in fetal diaphragmatic hernia. J Pediatr Surg 1996;31:148–151.
49. Van der Wall KJ, Kohl T, Adzick NS, et al: Fetal diaphragmatic hernia: Echocardiography and clinical outcome. J Pediatr Surg 1997;32:223–226.
50. Sbragia L, Paek BW, Filly RA, et al: Congenital diaphragmatic hernia without herniation of the liver: Does the lung-

to-head ratio predict survival? J Ultrasound Med 2000;19:845–848.
51. Paek BW, Coakley FV, Lu Y, et al: Congenital diaphragmatic hernia: Prenatal evaluation with MR lung volumetry—Preliminary experience. Radiology 2001;220:63–67.
52. Luks FI, Gilchrist BF, Jackson BT, Piasecki GJ: Endoscopic tracheal obstruction with an expanding device in a fetal lamb model: Preliminary considerations. Fetal Diagn Ther 1996;11:67–71.
53. Van Tuyl M, Hosgor M, Tibboel D: Tracheal ligation and corticosteroids in congenital diaphragmatic hernia: For better or worse? Pediatr Res 2001;50:441–444.
54. Moya FR, Thomas VL, Romaguera J, et al: Fetal lung maturation in diaphragmatic hernia. Am J Obstet Gynecol 1995;173:1401–1405.
55. Hedrick HL, Kaban JM, Pacheco BA, et al: Prenatal glucocorticoids improve pulmonary morphometrics in fetal sheep with congenital diaphragmatic hernia. J Pediatr Surg 1997;32:217–222.
56. Wiltshire E, Richardson VF, Pringle K: Congenital diaphragmatic hernia—Increased survival without ECMO. Proc Perinat Soc Aust N Z 1997;A67.
57. Moyer V, Moya F, Tibboel R, et al: Late versus early surgical correction for congenital diaphragmatic hernia in newborn infants. In The Cochrane Library, Issue 1. Oxford, Update Software, 2004.
58. Wilson JM, Lund DP, Lillehei CW, Vacant JP: Congenital diaphragmatic hernia: Predictors of severity in the ECMO era. J Pediatr Surg 1991;26:1028–1034.
59. Lessin MS, Thompson IM, Deprez MF, et al: Congenital diaphragmatic hernia with or without extracorporeal membrane oxygenation: Are we making progress? J Am Coll Surg 1995;181:65–71.
60. Bernbaum J, Schwartz IP, Gerdes M, et al: Survivors of extracorporeal membrane oxygenation at 1 year of age: The relationship of primary diagnosis with health and neurodevelopmental sequelae. Pediatrics 1995;96:907–913.
61. Arnold SR, Debich-Spicer DD, Opitz JM, Gilbert-Barness E: Documentation of anomalies not previously described in Fryns syndrome. Am J Med Genet 2003;116A:179–183.
62. Jones KL: Early amnion rupture sequence. In Smith's Recognizable Patterns of Human Malformation, 4th ed. Philadelphia, WB Saunders, 1988, pp 576–577.
63. Angtuaco TL: Fetal anterior abdominal wall defect. In Callen PW (ed): Ultrasonography in Obstetrics and Gynecology, 4th ed. Philadelphia, WB Saunders, 2000, p 507.
64. Rintala R, Lindahl H, Louhimo I: Anorectal malformations—Results of treatment and longterm follow up in 208 patients. Pediatr Surg Int 1991;6:36–41.
65. Paidas MJ, Crombleholme TM, Robertson FM: Prenatal diagnosis and management of the fetus with an abdominal wall defect. Semin Perinatol 1994;18:196–214.
66. Torfs CP, Curry CJ, Bateson TF: Population-based study of tracheoesophageal fistula and esophageal atresia. Teratology 1995;52:220–232.
67. Hill LM: Ultrasound evaluation of fetal gastrointestinal tract. In Callen PW (ed): Ultrasonography in Obstetrics and Gynecology, 4th ed. Philadelphia, WB Saunders, 2000, pp 460–461.
68. Stringer MD, McKenna KM, Goldstein RB, et al: Prenatal diagnosis of esophageal atresia. J Pediatr Surg 1995;30: 1258–1263.
69. Shulman A, Mazkereth R, Zalel Y, et al: Prenatal identification of esophageal atresia: The role of ultrasonography for evaluation of functional anatomy. Prenat Diagn 2002;22:669–674.
70. Kalache KD, Wauer R, Mau H, et al: Prognostic significance of the pouch sign in fetuses with prenatally diagnosed esophageal atresia. Am J Obstet Gynecol 2000;182:978–981.
71. Langer JC, Hussain H, Khan A, et al: Prenatal diagnosis of esophageal atresia using sonography and magnetic resonance imaging. J Pediatr Surg 2001;36:804–807.
72. Depaepe A, Dolk H, Lechat MF: The epidemiology of tracheo-oesophageal fistula and oesophageal atresia in Europe. EUROCAT working group. Arch Dis Childhood 1993;68:743–748.
73. Jones KL: Di George sequence. In Smith's Recognizable Patterns of Human Malformation, 4th ed. Philadelphia, WB Saunders, 1988, p 556.
74. Reys HM, Meller JL, Loeff DC: Management of esophageal atresia and tracheoesophageal fistula. Clin Perinatol 1989;16:79–84.
75. Myers NA: Evolution of the management of oesophageal atresia from 1948 to 1988. Pediatr Surg Int 1991;6:407–411.
76. Sparey C, Jawaheer G, Barrett AM, Robson SC: Esophageal atresia in the Northern Region Congenital Anomaly Survey, 1985–1997: Prenatal diagnosis and outcome. Am J Obstet Gynecol 2000;182:427–431.
77. Kirshon B, Mari G, Morse K: Indomethacin therapy in the treatment of symptomatic polyhydramnios. Obstet Gynecol 1990;75: 202–205.
78. Waterston DJ, Bonham-Carter RE, Aberdeen E: Oesophageal atresia: Tracheo-oesophageal fistula. A study of survival in 218 infants. Lancet 1962;ii:819–822.
79. Engum SA, Grosfeld JL, West KW, et al: Analysis of morbidity and mortality in 227 cases of esophageal atresia and/or tracheooesophageal fistula over two decades. Arch Surg 1995;130: 502–508.
80. Poenaru D, Laberge JM, Neilson IR, Guttman FM: A new prognostic classification for esophageal atresia. Surgery 1993;113:426–432.
81. Spitz L, Kiely FM, Morecroft JA, Drake DP: Oesophageal atresia: At risk groups for the 1990s. J Pediatr Surg 1994;29:723–725.
82. Deurloo JA, Ekkelkamp S, Schoorl M, et al: Esophageal atresia: Historical evolution of management and results in 371 patients. Ann Thorac Surg 2002;73:267–272.
83. Schimke RN, Leape LL, Holder TM: Familial occurrence of oesophageal atresia: A preliminary report. Birth Defects: Original Article Series 1972;8:22–23.
84. Kimble RM, Harding J, Kolbe A: Additional congenital anomalies in babies with gut atresia or stenosis: When to investigate and which investigation. Pediatr Surg Int 1997;12:565–570.
85. Dundas KC, Walker J, Laing IA: Oesophageal atresia and duodenal atresia suspected at the 12 week booking scan. BJOG 2001;108:225–226.
86. Romero R, Pilu G, Jeanty P, et al: Prenatal Diagnosis of Congenital Anomalies. Norwalk, CT, Appleton & Lange, 1988, p 237.
87. Dalla Vecchia LK, Grosfeld JL, West KW, et al: Intestinal atresia and stenosis: A 25-year experience with 277 cases. Arch Surg 1998;133:490–496.
88. Murray HG, Stone PR, Strand L, Flower J: Fetal pleural effusion following maternal indomethacin therapy. BJOG 1993;100:277–282.
89. Reyes HM, Meller JL, Loeff D: Neonatal intestinal obstruction. Clin Perinatal 1989;16:85–96.
90. De Lorimier AA, Fonkalsrud EW, Hays DM: Congenital atresia and stenosis of the jejunum and ileum. Surgery 1969;65: 819–827.
91. Seashore JH, Collins FS, Markowitz RI, Seashore MR: Familial apple peel jejunal atresia: Surgical, genetic and radiographic aspects. Pediatrics 1987;80:540–544.
92. Goldstein I, Lockwood C, Hobbins JC: Ultrasound assessment of fetal intestinal development in the evaluation of gestational age. Obstet Gynecol 1987;70:682–686.
93. Nyberg DA, Mack LA, Patten RM, Cyr DR: Fetal bowel. Normal sonographic findings. J Ultrasound Med 1987;6:3–6.
94. Manning C, Strauss A, Gyepes MT: Jejunal atresia with "apple peel" deformity: A report of eight survivors. J Perinatol 1989;9:281–286.
95. Smith MB, Smith L, Wells W, et al: Concurrent jejunal atresia with "apple peel" deformity in premature twins. Pediatr Surg Int 1991;6:425–428.

96. Santulli TV, Kiesmetter WB, Bill AH Jr: Anorectal anomalies: A suggested Int classification. J Pediatr Surg 1970;5: 281–287.
97. Martinez-Frias ML, Bermejo E, Rodriguez-Pinilla E: Anal atresia, vertebral, gental and urinary tract anomalies: A primary polytopic development field defect identified through an epidemiological analysis of associations. Am J Med Genet 2000;13:169–173.
98. de Sa DJ: The alimentary tract. In Wigglesworth JS, Singer DB (eds): Textbook of Fetal and Perinatal Pathology. Cambridge, MA, Blackwell Scientific Publications, 1991, pp 968–969.
99. Simon-Bouy B, Satre V, Ferec C, et al, and the French Collaborative Group: Hyperechogenic fetal bowel: A large French Collaborative study of 682 Cases. Am J Med Genet 2003;121A:209–213.
100. Monagham KG, Feldman GL: The risk of cystic fibrosis with prenatally detected echogenic bowel in an ethnically and racially diverse North American population. Prenat Diagn 1999;19:604–609.
101. Romero R, Pilu G, Jeanty P, et al: Prenatal Diagnosis of Congenital Anomalies. Norwalk, CT, Appleton & Lange, 1988, p 240.
102. Mushtaq I, Wright VM, Drake DP, et al: Meconium ileus secondary to cystic fibrosis. The East London experience. Pediatr Surg Int 1998;13:365–369.
103. Al-Kouatly HB, Chasen ST, Karam AK, et al: Factors associated with fetal demise in fetal echogenic bowel. Am J Obstet Gynecol 2001;185:1039–1043.
104. Zimmer EZ, Bronshtein M: Fetal intra-abdominal cysts detected in the first and early second trimester by transvaginal sonography. J Clin Ultrasound 1991;19:564–567.
105. de Sa DJ: The alimentary tract. In Wigglesworth JS, Singer DB (eds): Textbook of Fetal and Perinatal Pathology. Cambridge, MA, Blackwell Scientific Publications, 1991, p 933.
106. Foulon W, Naessens A, Mahler T, et al: Prenatal diagnosis of congenital toxoplasmosis. Obstet Gynecol 1990;76:769–772.
107. Daffos F, Forestier F, Capella-Pavlovsky M, et al: Prenatal management of 746 pregnancies at risk of congenital toxoplasmosis. N Engl J Med 1988;318:271–275.
108. Marks F, Thomas P, Lustig I, et al: In utero sonographic description of a fetal liver adenoma. J Ultrasound Med 1990;9:119–122.
109. Simchen MJ, Toi A, Bona M, et al: Fetal hepatic calcifications: Prenatal diagnosis and outcome. Am J Obstet Gynecol 2002;187:1617–1622.

CHAPTER 21

Fetal Skeletal Abnormalities

David R. Griffin

INTRODUCTION

The sonographic detection of a fetus with a skeletal disorder presents the clinician with challenging diagnostic dilemmas and management options. In some instances, the lethality of the disorder is apparent and a discussion of pregnancy interruption is appropriate. In other instances, the diagnosis, prognosis, and management options are far less evident, and require additional biochemical, genetic, or hematologic investigation. Consultation with a geneticist specializing in dysmorphology may be invaluable.

Women typically present for the prenatal diagnosis of a skeletal abnormality in one of three scenarios:

- A relevant family history
- An abnormality found during routine sonography
- A relevant maternal history—unfavorable intrauterine environment

Heritable Defect in Family

Inheritable skeletal disorders may be autosomal dominant, recessive, or sex-linked. The gene locations for an increasing number of conditions are now known, making antenatal diagnosis possible early in gestation in families at increased risk, often before any skeletal manifestation is evident sonographically. In this chapter, the gene, if known, is placed in parentheses at the heading for the appropriate syndrome. However, disease-related genes are being discovered at an astonishing rate. The reader is advised that the list will inevitably be incomplete by publication. In the remainder of disorders and in new presentations, sonography is the prime method for diagnosis.

Carriers of dominant disorders (Table 21–1) have a 50% offspring risk and are expressed in the heterozygous form. Some show variable expression and may be barely noticeable in a mildly affected individual (e.g., ectrodactyly, Holt-Oram syndrome). Many dominant conditions are new mutations and thus appear sporadically. In these cases, the risk of recurrence is low (about 1%). Recurrence is attributed to gonadal mosaicism in which some of the germ-line cells (but not the somatic cells) of one parent carry the mutation. Recent evidence suggests this may be the mechanism of recurrence in some types of osteogenesis imperfecta.

Recessive disorders (Table 21–2) are manifest in the homozygous form. They occur in the offspring of unaffected heterozygous carriers. The risk of a heterozygous couple having an affected child is 25%; 67% of unaffected children are carriers. Close relatives in the same family are more likely to carry the gene than members of the general population, so consanguineous unions increase the likelihood of two carriers coupling. The risk for a recessive disorder is such (up to 3% for first cousins) that it warrants a detailed ultrasonographic examination of the fetus.

Few X-linked disorders are in this group (X-linked chondrodysplasia punctata).

TABLE 21–1

Dominant Disorders
Achondroplasia
Cleidocranial dysostosis
Holt–Oram syndrome
Isolated polydactyly
Ectrodactyly
Ectrodactyly–ectodermal dysplasia–clefting syndrome
Spondylocostal dysplasia
Hypoglossia–hypodactyly syndrome
Distal dominant arthrogryposis
Dominant hypophosphatasia
Aase syndrome
Blackfan–Diamond syndrome

TABLE 21–2

Recessive Disorders
Most of the osteochondrodystrophies
Roberts syndrome
Jarcho–Levin syndrome
Fanconi pancytopenia syndrome
Thrombocytopenia–absent radius syndrome
Many polysyndactyly syndromes
Many multiple contracture syndromes

Chance Finding During a Routine Ultrasound Examination

The ultrasonographic abnormalities that may lead to the recognition of conditions with limb defects are listed in Table 21–3.

Unfavorable Intrauterine Environment

Factors associated with limb defects include insulin-dependent diabetes mellitus, drugs (e.g., sodium valproate), and oligohydramnios.

TABLE 21–3

Ultrasonographic Abnormalities and Skeletal Defects

	INHERITANCE	INCIDENCE	PROGNOSIS
Short Long Bones: Severe Symmetrical			
Achondrogenesis (types 1 and 2)	AR(1)/S(2)	1:75 000	Lethal
Thanatophoric dysplasia	AD/S	1:30 000	Lethal
Campomelic dysplasia	S	1:150 000	Mainly lethal
Osteogenesis imperfecta type 2	S	1:55 000	A + C: Lethal B/3: Often lethal
Hypophosphatasia (AR form)	AR or AD	1:110 000	AR: Lethal AD: Mild
Homozygous achondroplasia	AR	Very rare	Lethal
Schneckenbecken dysplasia[1]			
Atelosteogenesis[2]			
Grebe syndrome			
Short Long Bones: Moderate Symmetrical			
Hypochondrogenesis	S	Very rare	Lethal
Jeune thoracic dystrophy	AR	Rare	70% Lethal
Short-rib polydactyly syndromes	AR	Very rare	Lethal
Ellis–van Creveld syndrome	AR	Very rare	33% Lethal
Diastrophic dysplasia	AR	Rare	Variable
Rhizomelic chondrodysplasia punctata	AR	Rare	Poor
Kniest dysplasia	AD/AR	Rare	Variable
Spondyloepiphyseal dysplasia (severe form)	AD/AR	Very rare	Variable
Heterozygous achondroplasia	AD	1:66 000	Good
Noonan's syndrome	AD	Rare	Moderate
Down syndrome			
Dyssegmental dysplasia[3]			
Metatrophic dysplasia[4]			
Mesomelic dysplasia			
Fibrochondrogenesis			
Short Long Bones: Asymmetrical			
Isolated limb reductions			
Roberts' syndrome	AR	Rare	Poor
Femoral hypoplasia–unusual faces syndrome			
Femur–fibula–ulna syndrome			
Holt–Oram syndrome	AD	Rare	Variable
Thrombocytopenia–absent radius syndrome (TAR)	R	Very rare	Variable
Cleidocranial dysostosis (clavicles)	AD	Rare	Variable
Chromosomal abnormalities			
Phocomelias			
Congenital anemias[5] (e.g., Fanconi, Aase, Blackfan–Diamond)			
Bent Femur/Fractures	**Extra Bones**		
Campomelic dysplasia	Polydactyly		
Kyphomelic dysplasia	Short-rib polydactyly syndromes		
Osteogenesis imperfecta	Jeune thoracic dystrophy		
Hypophosphatasia	Joubert's syndrome		
Dyssegmental dysplasia			
Thanatophoric dysplasia (some)	**Positional Deformities**		
	Diastrophic dysplasia		
	Rhizomelic chondrodysplasia punctata		
Missing Bones/Limbs	Talipes		
Phocomelias	Rocker-bottom feet		
Syrenomelia	Multiple joint contractures		
Transverse reduction defects			
Thrombocytopenia–absent radius syndrome			

Continued

TABLE 21–3

Ultrasonographic Abnormalities and Skeletal Defects *(Continued)*

	INHERITANCE	INCIDENCE	PROGNOSIS
Missing Bones/Limbs *(Continued)*			
Syndactyly			
Ectrodactyly			
Fanconi pancytopenia syndrome			
Apert's syndrome			
Small Thorax	**Deformed Spine**		
Achondrogenesis syndromes	Isolated hemivertebrae		
Thanatophoric dysplasia	VACTERL association		
Schneckenbecken dysplasia	Jarcho-Levin syndrome		
Fibrochondrogenesis	Dyssegmental dysplasia		
Hypochondrogenesis	Spondyloepiphyseal dysplasia		
Short-rib polydactyly syndromes	Fibrochondrogenesis		
Jeune thoracic dystrophy	Atelosteogensis		
Osteogenesis imperfecta type 2			
Camptomelic dysplasia (some)	**Poor ossification**		
	Achondrogenesis		
Hydrops	Osteogenesis imperfecta type 2		
Hydramnios	Hypophosphatasia (severe form)		

AR, autosomal recessive; AD, autodominant recessive; S, sporadic.

ULTRASOUND SCANNING FOR FETAL LIMB ABNORMALITIES

A full examination of a fetus at risk for a skeletal abnormality requires a detailed study of the general fetal anatomy, which can provide important clues to the diagnosis.

Limbs

The long bones are measured in as near to the horizontal scanning plane as possible to avoid shadowing artifact (Fig. 21–1). As a result, the longest measurement of a technically adequate view is the true measurement. It is inappropriate to average limb measurements. The strongest reflections occur from the most proximal bone interface, so that a bone with thickened metaphysis may appear bowed. Hypomineralized long bones reflect less ultrasound at the proximal interface. Thus, they appear less echo-dense across the diaphysis and have reduced acoustic shadow. Minor degrees of hypomineralization are likely to go undetected. Several examples of actual femur length measurements from fetuses with skeletal dysplasia in the author's practice are plotted on the fetal size chart in Figure 21–2.

Head

Hypomineralization

Skull hypomineralization reduces the reflection of ultrasound and increases transmission. The net effect is to reduce both the echogenicity of the skull and the acoustic shadowing of tissues beyond it. The cranial contents are seen more clearly than normal. In severe cases of hypomineralization such as osteogenesis imperfecta types 2a and c, and achondrogenesis type 1, the cerebral hemispheres are almost anechoic, giving the appearance of ventriculomegaly. This is easily excluded by showing the choroid plexus, and the walls of the lateral ventricle antrum are normally situated within the hemisphere (see Fig. 21–6*A*). The skull bones are soft and can deform when subjected to pressure from the transducer. Hypomineralization may be less obvious in disorders such as hypophosphatasia or osteogenesis imperfecta types 2b and 3.

Skull Shape

The cloverleaf skull is characteristic of some forms of thanatophoric dysplasia. Other unusual skull shapes imply craniosynostosis, which occurs in some short-ribbed polydactyly syndromes.

Face

Cleft lip or palate (see Chapter 18) are features of short-rib polydactyly (SRP) type 2 (Majewski), fibrochondrogenesis, atelosteogenesis, ectrodactyly-ectodermal dysplasia-clefting (EEC) syndrome and a number of other dysplasias. Measurement of the intraorbital diameter[6,7] may reveal hypertelorism in some syndromes.

A facial profile in the sagittal plane may show frontal bossing (achondroplasia, thanatophoric dysplasia), a depressed nasal bridge (chondrodysplasia punctata), or micrognathia (campomelic dysplasia). The mandible is measured in the axial plane from the temporomandibular joint to the mental eminence.[8,9]

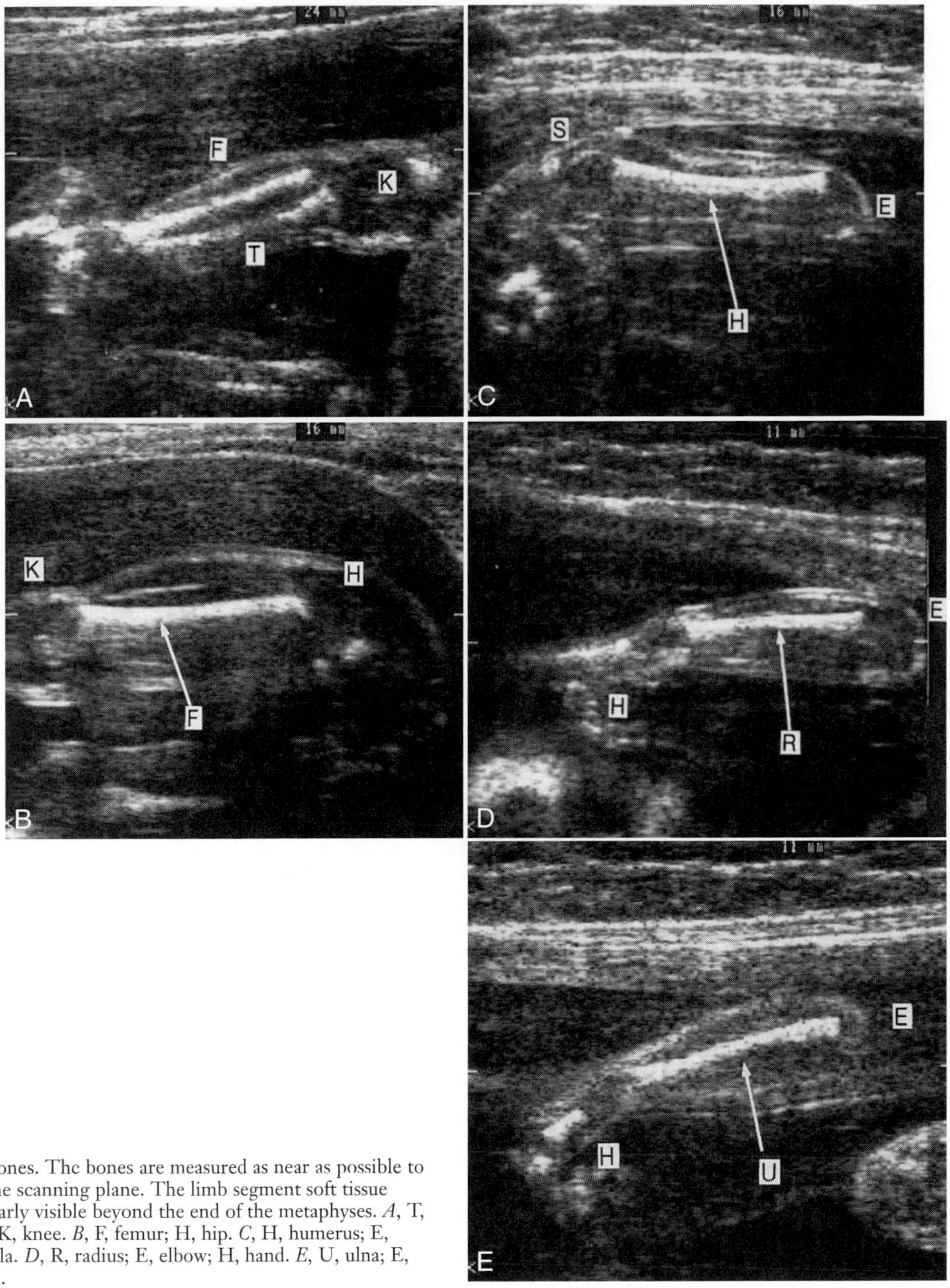

FIGURE 21–1
Normal long bones. The bones are measured as near as possible to horizontal in the scanning plane. The limb segment soft tissue extremity is clearly visible beyond the end of the metaphyses. *A*, T, tibia; F, fibula; K, knee. *B*, F, femur; H, hip. *C*, H, humerus; E, elbow; S, scapula. *D*, R, radius; E, elbow; H, hand. *E*, U, ulna; E, elbow; H, hand.

Thorax

The ribs may be short, thick, thin, beaded (i.e., fractured), flared, or irregular in shape, arrangement, or number. The thorax may be normal, constricted, short, or long. When constricted, the ratio of heart circumference to thoracic circumference (normally about 1:3)[10] is increased. Normal liver size and abdominal circumference cause the abdominal wall to protrude in the anteroposterior view, giving what is described as a "champagne cork" appearance. Pulmonary hypoplasia secondary to the restricted thorax is the major cause of death in neonates with this feature.

Congenital heart abnormalities can be found in Ellis–van Creveld syndrome (50%), SRP type 2, campomelic dysplasia, Holt-Oram syndrome, thrombocytopenia—absent radius (TAR) syndrome, Noonan's syndrome,

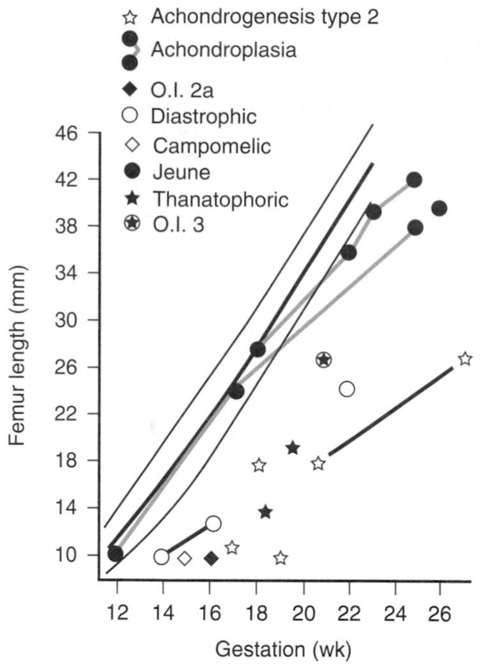

FIGURE 21–2
This diagram shows femur length measurements in many of the skeletal dysplasias described in the text set against a nomogram for femur length against postmenstrual age. (Modified from Griffin DR: Detection of congenital abnormalities of the limbs and face by ultrasound. In Chamberlain G (ed): Modern Antenatal Care of the Fetus. Oxford, Blackwell Scientific Publications, 1990, pp 389–427; Griffin DR: Skeletal dysplasias. In Brock DJH, Rodeck CH, Ferguson-Smith MA [eds]: Prenatal Diagnosis and Screening. Edinburgh, Churchill Livingstone, 1992, pp 257–313.)

Carpenter's syndrome, trisomies, and in fetuses of diabetic women.

Kidneys

Renal abnormalities may be a feature of Jeune thoracic dystrophy, some of the short-ribbed polydactyly syndromes, caudal regression syndrome, and the VACTERL (vertebral, anal, cardiac, tracheoesophageal, renal, and limb abnormalities) association.

TERMINOLOGY

Table 21–4 contains a list of terms employed in the text.

SHORT LONG BONES: SEVERE SYMMETRICAL

The prevalence of skeletal dysplasias is approximately 1:5000 live births and 1:500 stillbirths. The most common (achondroplasia) occurs with a frequency of about 1:20,000.[11]

TABLE 21–4

Terminology of Limb Defects

Acromelia—shortening predominantly of distal segments (hands and feet)
Amelia—absence of a limb
Campomelia—bent limbs
Diaphysis—central part of shaft of long bone
Epiphysis—bone ends with separate centers of ossification; may not be apparent prenatally
Hemimelia—absence or hypoplasia of longitudinal segment (e.g., radius)
Kyphoscoliosis—combination of lateral and convex curvature of the spine
Kyphosis—dorsally convex curvature of spine (as thoracic)
Lordosis—dorsally concave curvature of the spine (as lumbar)
Mesomelia—shortening predominantly in the intermediate long bones (radius/ulna, tibia/fibula)
Metaphysis—more recently developed growing extremities of shaft
Micromelia—severely shortened limb
Phocomelia (seal limb)—absence or hypoplasia of long bones with hands or feet attached to trunk
Platyspondyly—flattening of the vertebral body
Rhizomelia—shortening predominantly in proximal long bones (humerus, femur)
Scoliosis—lateral curvature of the spine

Achondrogenesis

This group of conditions is characterized by severe micromelia and hypomineralization. Fetal hydrops and hydramnios may appear late.

Diagnosis

TYPE 1 (PARENTI-FRACCARO SYNDROME) (5q31-5q34) DTDST

The long bones show extreme micromelia with very poor modeling (e.g., femur length of 10 mm at 19 weeks.[12] The calvarium and vertebral column are severely hypomineralized (Fig. 21–3*B*).

TYPE 2 (LANGER-SALDINO SYNDROME) (12q13-12q14) COL2AI

The long bones are better modeled than in type 1 but are still extremely short, thick, and straight (Fig. 21–3*A*). The calvarium is normally ossified, and although hypomineralization of the spine is variable, it can be striking (Fig. 21–3*B, C, D*).

HYPOCHONDROGENESIS (12q13-12q14) COL2AI

This condition is thought to represent the milder end of the spectrum of the achondrogenesis type 2/spondyloepiphyseal dysplasia group of conditions.[13] Spinal hypomineralization is seen only at the cervical and caudal portions of the spine.

Diagnosis

The condition is suspected when moderate long bone shortening (see Fig. 21–3) is associated with a constricted

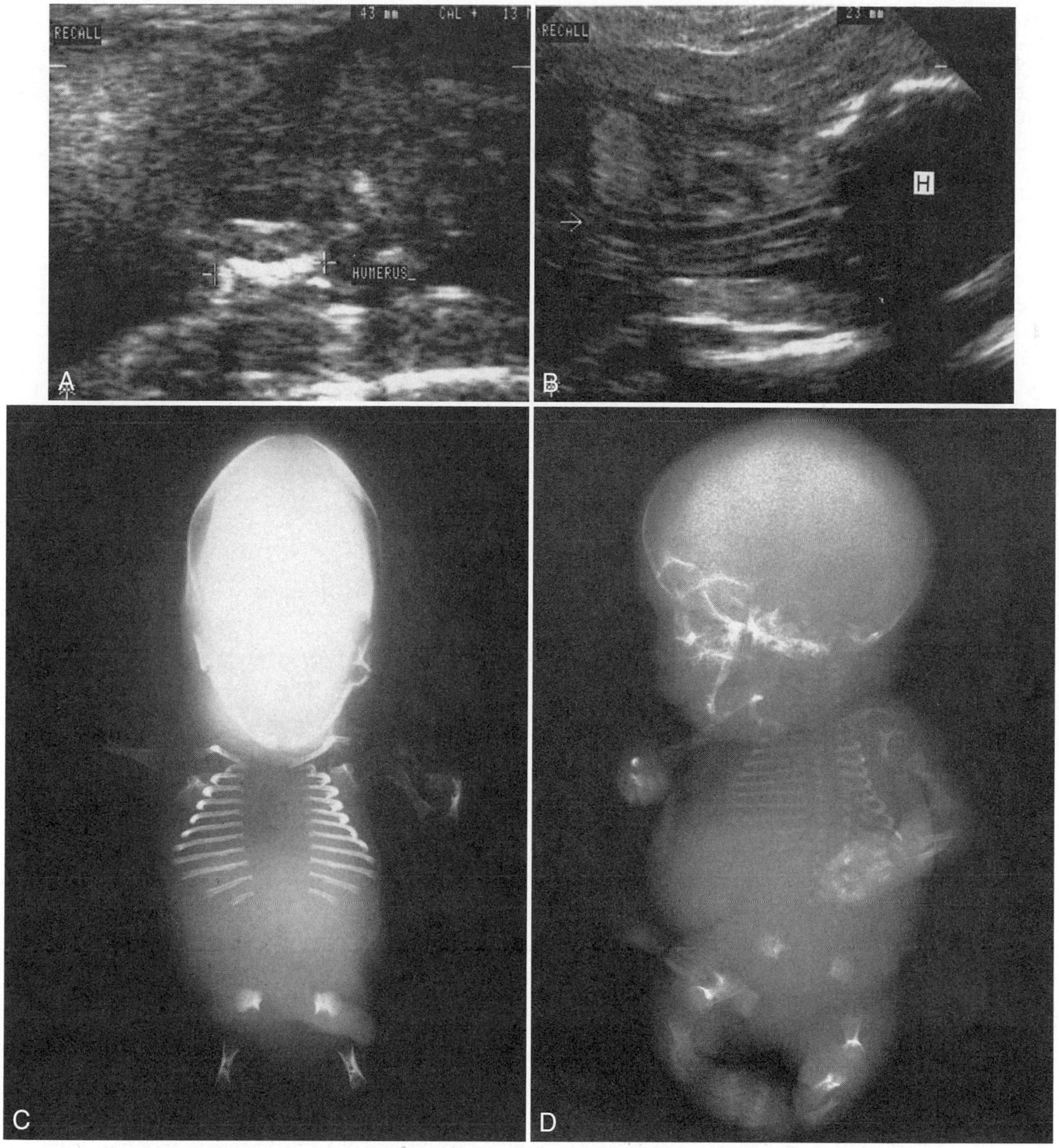

FIGURE 21–3
Achondrogenesis. *A*, Short (13 mm) humerus of a fetus with achondrogenesis type 2 at 18 weeks. *B*, Sonogram of the trunk and head (H) of the same fetus shown in *A*. The spinal column is shown (*arrow*) as an anechoic cartilaginous column. The skull shows some mineralization. *C*, Radiograph of the fetus in *A* showing total absence of ossification in all elements of the spinal column. The ribs are short and the thorax small. There is little mineralization of the skull. *D*, Postnatal radiograph of a different fetus with achondrogenesis type 2 at a similar gestation to that in *C*. In this case only the vertebral bodies show lack of calcification. Other features are similar to those in *C* with short, straight reasonably modeled long bones showing flared, cupped metaphyses. The ischial bones are unossified and the ilia small and halberd shaped. (*A* and *B* from Brock DJH, Rodeck CH, Ferguson-Smith MA [eds]: Prenatal Diagnosis and Screening. Edinburgh, Churchill Livingstone, 1992.)

thorax. The bones are straight and show some thickening of the metaphyses.

Risks and Management Options

Achondrogenesis types 1 and 2 and hypochondrogenesis are lethal conditions at or before birth. Termination of pregnancy should be included as an option during counseling. The diagnosis is supported by postnatal radiography and expert pathology. Where possible, it should be confirmed by DNA analysis. The recurrence risk is 1:4 for achondrogenesis type 1. Achondrogenesis and hypochondrogenesis are usually new, dominant mutations.

Thanatophoric Dysplasia (4p16) (*FGFR3*)

Thanatophoric dysplasia is the most common skeletal dysplasia encountered in obstetric practice.

Diagnosis

A definitive diagnosis is possible by 12 to 14 weeks, but is more commonly made at 18 to 20 weeks.[14,15] The femur and other limb-length measurements are well below the third percentile for menstrual age (Fig. 21–2) and display a characteristic thickening of the metaphyses. Measurements from 14 to 21 mm at 18 to 20 weeks to 26 mm at 32 weeks are reported.[16–19] The femurs may appear bowed in some cases and straight in others (Fig. 21–4*B*). The feet and hands are short. The short, splayed fingers are described as a "trident hand." Short stubby ribs produce a markedly small thorax (Fig. 21–4*C*). The cardiothoracic ratio is high (Fig. 21–4*C*), and the characteristic truncal champagne cork appearance is seen in the sagittal plane (Fig. 21–4*D*). Some cases show flattening of the vertebral bodies (platyspondyly) and a short spine. The skull is normally ossified and may be macrocephalic or brachycephalic. Some variants with straight, long bones show the cloverleaf (Fig. 21–4*A*) deformity produced by prominence of the parietal bones. This sign is more evident later in pregnancy. Lateral cerebral ventriculomegaly may occur. The facial profile shows a depressed nasal bridge and frontal bossing. Late in pregnancy, soft tissue folds can often be seen on the arms (the "Michelin man" appearance). Hydramnios is also a later feature.

Because the majority of cases result from a mutation at 4p16, it can be useful to test the index case. The recurrence risk is small (<1%), but confirmation by DNA extraction will allow for early prenatal diagnosis and reassurance in subsequent pregnancies, although a careful scan at 12 to 14 weeks could also exclude a recurrence.

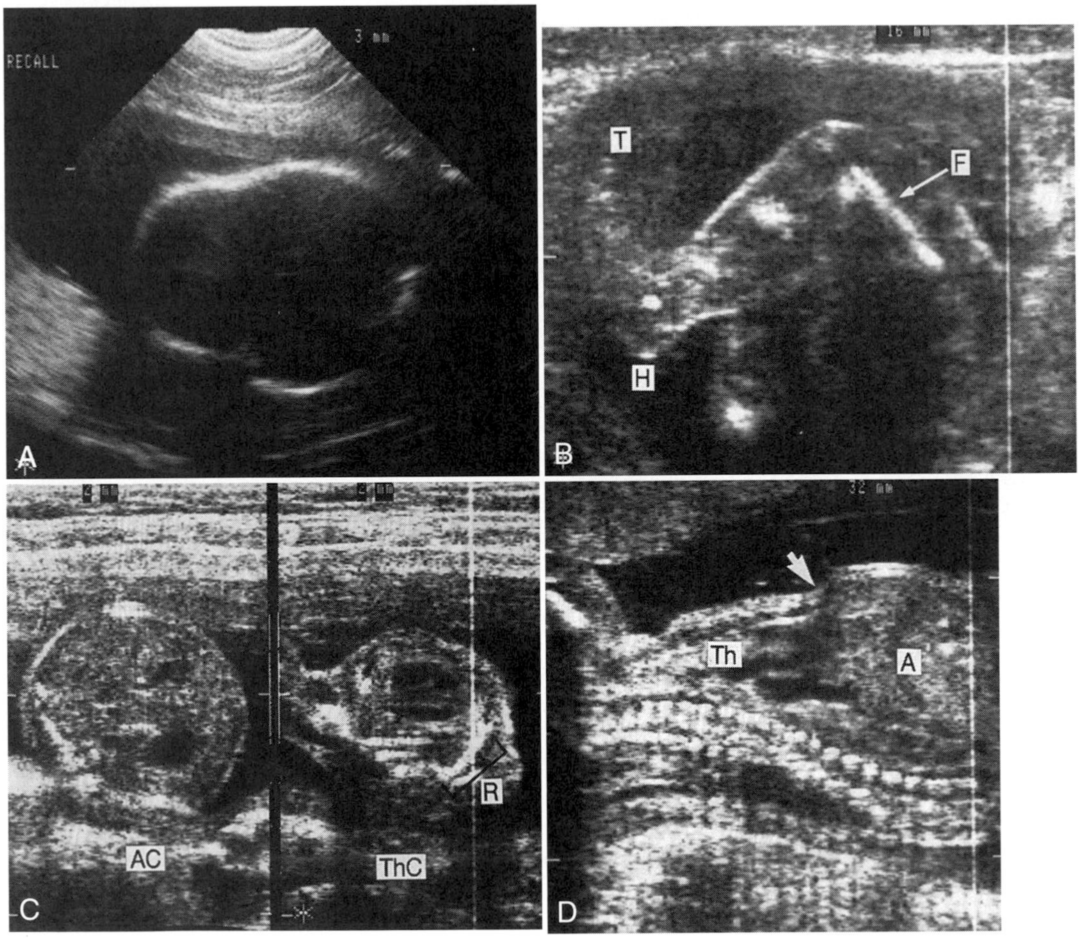

FIGURE 21–4
Thanatophoric dysplasia. *A*, Skull of a 20-week fetus showing the clover-leaf deformity. *B*, Lower limb of a fetus of 18 weeks showing short leg and femur (F) of 18 mm. H, heel; T, toes. *C*, Transverse sections of the trunk of the fetus in *B* at the level of the umbilical vein (AC) and the heart (ThC) showing marked reduction of the thoracic circumference and short ribs (R). *D*, Longitudinal anteroposterior sagittal scan of the trunk of the fetus in *B* showing the narrow thorax (Th) and abdomen (A) protruding anteriorly: the "champagne cork" appearance. A normally mineralized spine is posterior.

Risks and Management Options

Thanatophoric dysplasia is lethal and the option of pregnancy termination should be included in the counseling session. Support for the diagnosis by radiography or confirmation by DNA study is essential. Parents should be advised that recurrence risks are low because this is a dominant sporadic condition.

Campomelic Dysplasia (17q24-17q25) (*SOX9*)

Diagnosis

Early diagnosis is possible.[20–25] The characteristic midshaft bowing of the femur should be recognized during a routine ultrasound (Fig. 21–5), although there is considerable variation in presentation.[26] The tibia is short and bowed and the fibula hypoplastic. Marked talipes may cause the whole lower limb to be grossly bowed inward (campomelia). The ribs may be short and the thorax constricted. Brachycephaly, micrognathia, and short clavicles may be detected during a careful skeletal survey. Associated soft tissue anomalies are found in a third of cases and include atrial/ventricular septal defect (ASD/VSD), hydronephrosis, and ventriculomegaly. Hydramnios may occur late in pregnancy. Phenotypic sex reversal in males is common, but is detected only by a karyotype.

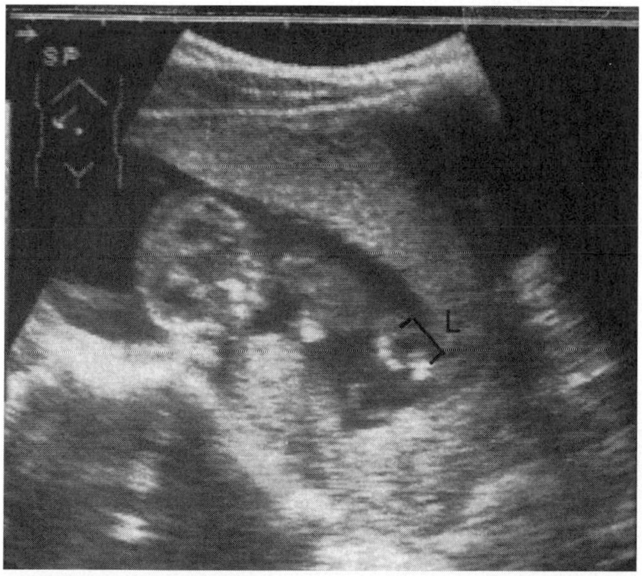

FIGURE 21–5
Sonogram of a 15-week fetus with camptomelic dysplasia. Note the short, bent leg (L). Micrognathia is evident in the facial profile. (From Griffin DR: Detection of congenital abnormalities of the limbs and face by ultrasound. In Chamberlain G [ed]: Modern Antenatal Care of the Fetus. Oxford, Blackwell Scientific Publications, 1990, pp 389–427.)

Risks and Management Options

Approximately three-quarters of newborns die during the neonatal period from pulmonary hypoplasia; 90% die by the age of 2 years. The prognosis depends on the severity of associated malformations. Survivors fail to thrive and can show neurologic impairment. The recurrence risk is around 5%; many cases are thought to be the result of a new dominant mutation.[26] The option of pregnancy termination should be offered when the diagnosis is made at a stage in gestation when termination is legal. Support for the diagnosis by pathologic examination and radiography is essential before counseling the parents about the recurrence risk. Antenatal ultrasonographic diagnosis should be offered in subsequent pregnancies.

Osteogenesis Imperfecta

Osteogenesis imperfecta is characterized by poor bone mineralization. Based on the clinical and pathoradiologic findings, it is divided into types 1 through 4; all are due to various mutations in the *COL1A1* gene. The overall incidence approximates to 1:10,000. Types 1 and 4 are probably not amenable to early ultrasound diagnosis, although diagnosis was reported in the second trimester for type 4 and the third trimester for type I. Types 2a, b, c, and type 3 have all been diagnosed before 22 weeks' gestation. Type 2 is usually sporadic, occurring in approximately 1:55,000 live births. Recent evidence suggests that recurrences are due to gonadal mosaicism and the recurrence risks should be quoted as around 5% to 7%. Both types 1 and 4 are autosomal dominant conditions. In type 3, recurrence is reported, and there is the possibility of autosomal recessive inheritance and again, gonadal mosaicism. Recurrence risks after an isolated case are around 7%.

Diagnosis

Osteogenesis imperfecta type 2a is the most common form. It is recognizable early in pregnancy by the characteristic hypomineralization of the skull and long bones with severe micromelia and apparent bowing or crumpling due to multiple fractures.[29-36] The usual bright echo of the skull bones is lost and there is no acoustic shadow (Fig. 21–6*A*). The orbits may be unusually prominent. The cerebral hemispheres take on a transsonic character. There may appear to be ventriculomegaly, though it can be excluded by identifying the choroid plexus within normal ventricular walls and a normal posterior horn measurement. The head is brachycephalic. It is easily deformed by pressure from the ultrasound transducer even late in pregnancy, yet anatomic details of cerebral structure remain prominent. The long bones are hypoechoic, irregularly bowed, and

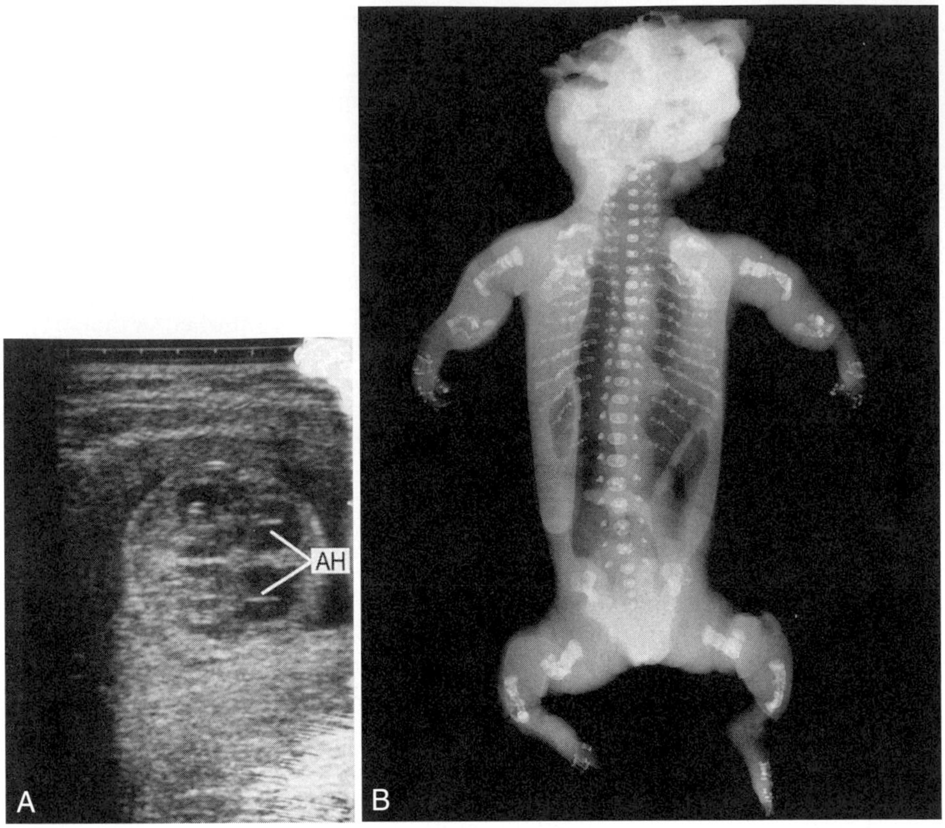

FIGURE 21–6
Osteogenesis imperfecta type 2a. *A*, Skull of a 20-week fetus showing the features of severe hypomineralization of the skull. The skull bones are poorly echogenic and they cast no acoustic shadow. The cerebral hemispheres are anechoic, giving the appearance of cerebral ventriculomegaly (pseudohydrocephaly). However, the echoes from the anterior horns (AH) are normally placed. *B*, Postnatal radiograph of fetus showing that the long bones are short, bowed, and crumpled by multiple intrauterine fractures. The lower limbs are held in a camptomelic (bent) posture. The ribs are "beaded" from fractures and hairline fractures are also evident in the vertebral bodies (the skull was lost in delivery). (From Griffin DR: Detection of congenital abnormalities of the limbs and face by ultrasound. In Chamberlain G [ed]: Modern Antenatal Care of the Fetus. Oxford, Blackwell Scientific Publications, 1990, pp 389–427.)

crumpled as a result of multiple fractures and callus formation (see Fig. 21–6*B*). The limbs show marked, fixed campomelia and talipes. Other features, such as beading of the ribs and a small thorax, may be recognized. Amniotic fluid abnormalities can occur later in pregnancy. Munoz and associates[36] report the reliable differentiation of osteogenesis imperfecta from other skeletal dysplasias using three criteria: multiple fractures, hypoechoic skull, and femoral length greater than 3 SD below the mean for gestation.

Type 2b shows features intermediate between type 2a and type 3. Type 2c has skeletal features similar to type 2a. Poor cranial ossification has the worst prognosis of this type.

Fetuses with type 2b or 3 rarely have a poorly calcified skull. The femurs may show bowing (Fig. 21–7) or fracture with mild to moderate shortening, but are generally well modeled. Typically, the tibias are bowed but the fibulas are straight.[33,37] Other long bones tend to be around or just less than the fifth percentile.

Type 1 has been diagnosed prenatally[21] but cannot reliably be excluded before viability. The author followed one affected case with normal limb growth and morphology through 24 weeks. However, bowed femurs were apparent at birth and fractures occurred shortly afterward. The clinical presentation and prognosis of types 1 and 4 are quite variable and can show considerable overlap. Expert advice is recommended before counseling. The antenatal diagnosis of type 4 has also been reported. The features are usually mild, with bowing of the femurs but preservation of limb growth in all other long bones.

Risks and Management Options

Types 2a and c are lethal. And although type 2b is often lethal, a child may survive to infancy. Children with type

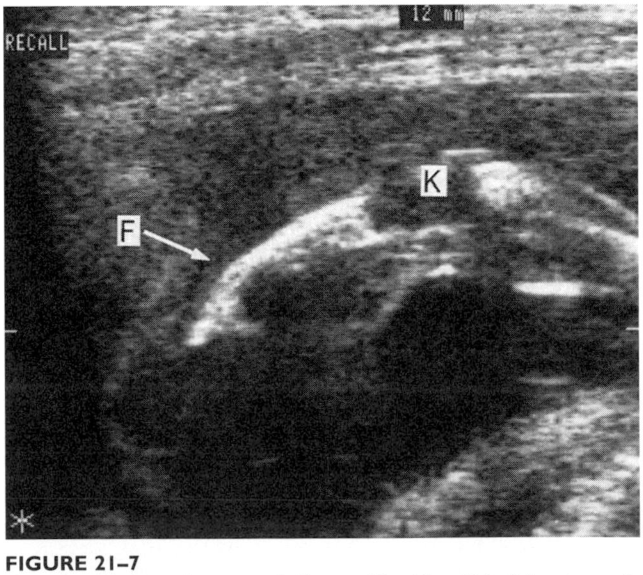

FIGURE 21–7
Osteogenesis imperfecta type 3. Femur (F) with midshaft bowing and poor mineralization. The cartilagenous epiphyses are evident at the knee (K).

3 can survive, but with significant physical handicap due to multiple deforming fractures. Types 1 and 4 overlap and are not often diagnosed during pregnancy.

The option of pregnancy termination should be discussed when the diagnosis of type 2 or 3 osteogenesis imperfecta is made at a time in gestation when it is still legal to act. It has been suggested that abdominal delivery might reduce the risk of either trauma or intracranial hemorrhage. Expert pathologic and radiologic examination is required to distinguish type 3 from 2b, as the genetic implications may be important.

Hypophosphatasia (1p34-1p36)

Bone hypomineralization results from a deficiency of alkaline phosphatase. This heterogeneous group of disorders varies from a lethal condition to milder forms, which become apparent only in childhood. The appearance of the lethal form is similar to that of osteogenesis imperfecta type 2. Although the bones are generally less "crumpled," they may show marked angulation.

Diagnosis

The diagnosis may be based on biochemical, ultrasonographic, or molecular tools, or a combination of the three. There are surprisingly few reports of the antenatal diagnosis of hypophosphatasia.[38,39] If cranial hypomineralization is marked, the skull appears similar to osteogenesis imperfecta type 2 with anechoic calvarium, with prominent intracranial structures and an easily deformed skull. The femurs and humeri are short and may be so bowed at the midshaft that full image and measurement of the shaft are difficult. Dislocations of the knees and elbows can occur.[39] The ribs are thin and may show fractures. The spine may be markedly demineralized, particularly in the area of the neural arch. In a case report of the milder form, the femoral bowing appeared to resolve during pregnancy.[40]

A biochemical diagnosis by measuring alkaline phosphatase (ALP) in amniotic fluid[41] or in cultured amniocytes is unreliable until after 20 weeks. Warren and associates[42] successfully diagnosed the condition in the first trimester of a high risk pregnancy by measuring cellular ALP in a chorion villous sample. Brock and Barron were successful making the diagnosis by measuring liver/bone/kidney (LBK) ALP.[43]

Risks and Management Options

The severe recessive form is lethal, and the option of pregnancy termination should be included in the counseling session. The osseous maldevelopment in the milder, autosomal dominant forms tends to improve with advancing age. The diagnosis must be confirmed by expert radiography and also by biochemical or genetic investigation of the parents. It is unclear whether milder forms should be delivered abdominally to avoid trauma.

Homozygous Achondroplasia

This form occurs only in the offspring of two heterozygous achondroplastic parents. Most fetuses perish in early pregnancy, as the condition is rarely seen among achondroplastic couples.

Diagnosis

The one case report[44] described severe micromelia and a small thorax, similar to thanatophoric dysplasia.

Risks and Management Options

This condition is lethal. The option of pregnancy termination should be included in the counseling session.

SHORT LONG BONES: MODERATE SYMMETRICAL

Jeune Thoracic Dystrophy (Asphyxiating Thoracic Dystrophy)

The severity of this condition and the degree of limb shortening are quite variable. Associated features include renal, hepatic, pancreatic, and pulmonary dysplasia and, occasionally, postaxial polydactyly.

Diagnosis

The reports of prenatal diagnosis of Jeune syndrome are based on the finding of a small thorax in high risk families.[45,46] The chest is reduced in the anteroposterior diameter with consequent protrusion of the anterior abdominal wall. Limb shortening may not be apparent until late in pregnancy (Fig. 21–8). Hydramnios may occur in late pregnancy.

Risks and Management Options

About 70% of live-born children die from respiratory failure during the neonatal period. Survivors are small in stature, and often succumb to respiratory, renal, hepatic, or pancreatic complications in childhood. Intelligence is normal. The option of pregnancy termination should be included in the counseling session if the diagnosis is made in a timely fashion, as the mortality and morbidity rates are high. This autosomal recessive disorder has a 25% recurrence risk.

Short-ribbed Polydactyly Syndromes (SRPS)

The main subdivisions of these conditions are characterized as follows:

- Type 1 (Saldino-Noonan syndrome) is associated with micromelia characterized by distinct, pointed ends to long bones, and associated urogenital and anorectal anomalies.

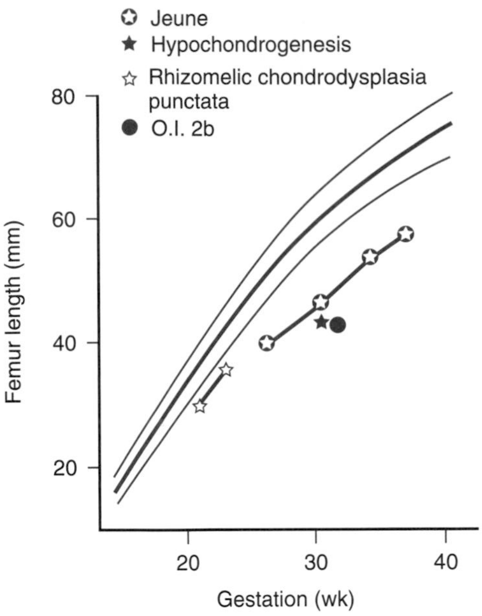

FIGURE 21–8
Diagram showing growth of the femur in a fetus with prenatal diagnosis (and postnatal confirmation) of Jeune thoracic dystophy against nomogram of fetal growth against postmenstrual age. Single measurements are also shown for fetuses with hypochondrogenesis and osteogenesis imperfecta type 2b.

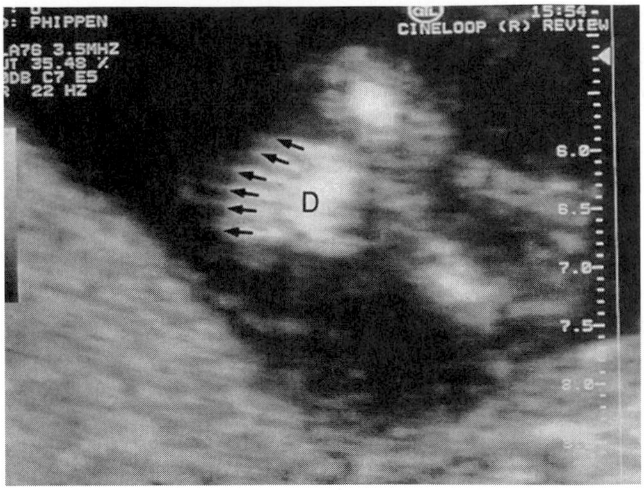

FIGURE 21–9
Scan of the foot of a fetus with short-rib polydactyly syndrome showing six digits (arrowed, D). (With thanks to Mr. P. Smith.)

- Type 2 (Majewski syndrome) is characterized by median cleft lip/palate and disproportionately short, ovoid tibiae. The differential diagnosis prenatally includes the orofacial digital syndrome (OFD) type 4.

Both syndromes can be associated with abnormalities of other organ systems. Fetal hydrops is common and may be a consequence of a cardiovascular anomaly. Phenotypic sex reversal (to apparent female) is a common finding and requires a karyotype for confirmation.

Diagnosis

Prenatal diagnosis is based on the identification of a small, narrow thorax with short ribs, short limbs, and polydactyly (Fig. 21–9) plus, occasionally, other distinguishing features. A number of other uncommon SRPSs have been described.

Risks and Management Options

SRPSs are lethal secondary to respiratory failure. The option of termination of pregnancy, if legal, should be included in the counseling session. These autosomal recessive disorders have a 25% recurrence risk.

Ellis–van Creveld Syndrome (Chondroectodermal Dysplasia) (4p16)

Diagnosis

Limb shortening is more pronounced in the forearm and lower leg (mesomelic) than in the remaining long bones. Polydactyly (hands more commonly than feet) is common.[47] The diagnosis should be considered when these findings are present in association with a small thorax.[48] A fetal echocardiogram is indicated, as half of these fetuses have congenital heart disease, typically an ASD.

Risks and Management Options

One-third of affected children succumb during infancy. Survivors have normal intelligence, but a final height of 3.5 to 5 ft (105–150 cm). The inheritance is autosomal recessive with a 25% chance of recurrence. DNA should be stored so that early, antenatal diagnosis can be offered in subsequent pregnancies. The option of pregnancy termination should be discussed if abortion is a legal option. Obstetric management of a continuing pregnancy is unaltered. Neonatal echocardiography is advisable.

Diastrophic Dysplasia (5q21-5q34) DTST

This condition has a variable presentation.

Diagnosis

Antenatal diagnosis is possible in severe cases based on the combination of rhizomelic limb shortening and bowing in association with the hitchhiker thumb and talipes (Fig. 21–10).[49–51] Other features may include micrognathia and cleft palate. It may be difficult to exclude the diagnosis before viability in milder cases of high risk families, as the degree of limb shortening can be minimal. Identification of normal thumbs is helpful in excluding the diagnosis.

Risks and Management Options

Diastrophic dysplasia is an autosomal recessive disorder with a 25% risk of recurrence. DNA should be stored so that early antenatal diagnosis can be offered in subsequent pregnancies. A significant number of newborns die

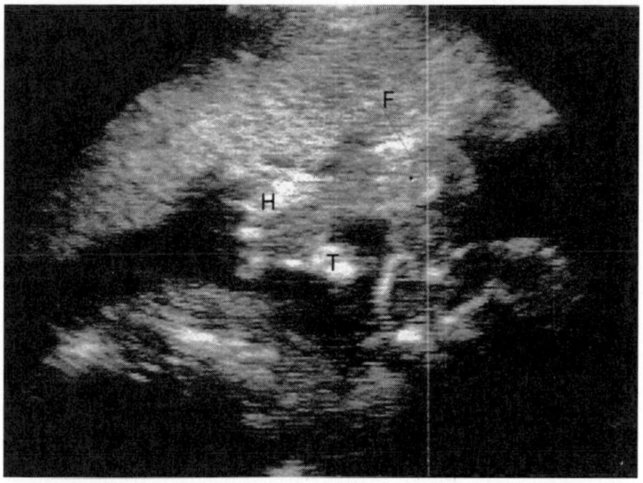

FIGURE 21–10
Scan of the hand (H) of a fetus with diastrophic dysplasia showing proximal displacement and abduction of the thumb (T) (the "hitchhiker" thumb). Femur length measurement from this fetus at 22 weeks is shown in Figure 21–2. F, forearm.

from respiratory failure and pneumonia. No specific measures are needed before birth in continuing pregnancies. Survivors have normal intellect, but suffer significant and progressive physical handicap coupled with limited mobility secondary to the kyphoscoliosis and arthropathy. They require considerable mobility and physiotherapy support. Surgical release of contractures is possible, but of limited value. In light of the disease severity, the option of pregnancy termination should be discussed when the diagnosis is made.

Chondrodysplasia Punctata

For this heterogeneous group of conditions definitive diagnosis can be impossible before birth, and indeed frequently after birth as well. Among the many forms the three most common are X-linked dominant (Conradi-Hunermann disease), X-linked recessive, and rhizomelic.

Diagnosis

X-LINKED DOMINANT CHONDRODYSPLASIA PUNCTATA (Xp11) (EBP)

This mildest form is seen only in females, as the heterozygous male form is lethal. Antenatal diagnosis is reported in high risk cases[52–54] when epiphyseal stippling and mild limb shortening was detected.

X-LINKED RECESSIVE FORM (Xp22) (ARSE)

The author has seen two cases diagnosed during the second trimester of high risk pregnancies. Affected males have generalized but moderate shortening of the long bones with epiphyseal echogenicities, particularly in the femurs. In each case, there was extensive, paravertebral epiphyseal stippling and a flat face with nasal depression. In one instance, echogenicities were seen in the larynx. This disorder also may be seen in association with cytogenetic deletions of the X chromosome, in which case it may also be associated with intellectual impairment.[55] Heterozygous female carriers are clinically normal, but tend to be slightly shorter than noncarrier relatives.

RHIZOMELIC FORM (6q22-6q24) (DHAPAT)

Individuals with rhizomelic chondrodysplasia punctata have rhizomelic shortening that is more pronounced in the humerus compared to other long bones. They may show sigmoid bowing. The characteristic feature on an ultrasound examination is stippled epiphyses.[52] There may also be stippling around the pelvic bones, the trachea, and larynx. Fixed flexion deformities of the limbs can be seen, more pronounced in the arm than the leg (Fig. 21–11). Cultured amniocytes and fibroblasts have low dihydroxyacetone phosphate transferase activity (DHAPT).[53]

Risks and Management Options

Many newborns with the rhizomelic chondrodysplasia punctata die from respiratory failure. Survivors fail to thrive and develop microcephaly associated with severely

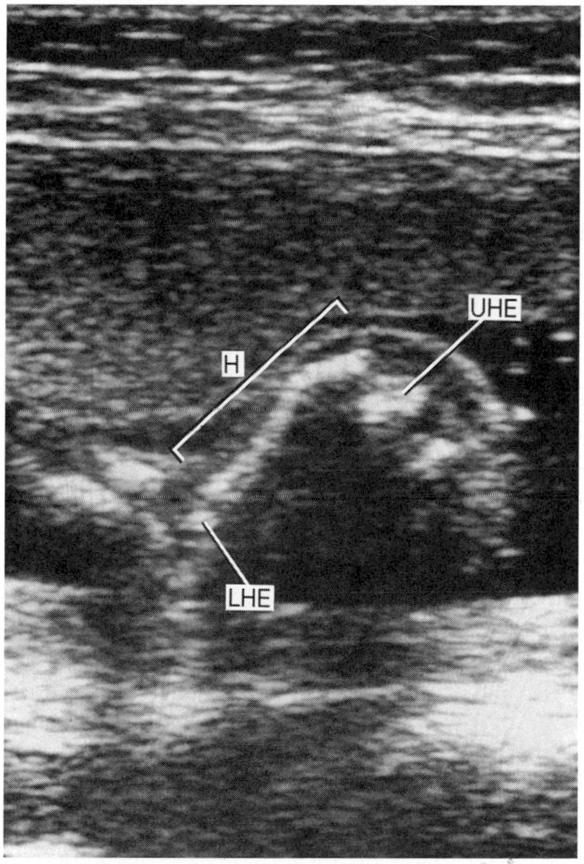

FIGURE 21–11
Scan of the arm and shoulder of a 21-week fetus with rhizomelic chondrodysplasia punctata. The humerus (H) is short (25 mm) and bowed. At both the upper (UHE) and lower (LHE) humeral epiphyses there are echogenic accumulations representing disorganized calcification. Movement of the upper limb was limited during examination.

retarded neurologic development. Survival beyond the first year is unusual; the longest reported survival is 5 years. Measurements of DHAPT activity in amniocytes or chromosome/molecular analysis are helpful adjuncts to the ultrasonographic diagnosis. The option of pregnancy interruption should be discussed.

Kniest Dysplasia (12q13-12q14) (*COL2A1*)

Diagnosis

Kniest dysplasia is characterized by moderately short, dumbbell-shaped long bones with metaphyseal flaring, restricted joint mobility, platyspondyly with vertebral clefts, and a flat face with depressed nasal bridge. Although the limbs are noticeably short at birth, antenatal diagnosis has been reported only once.[56] In this instance, the features were not evident at 16 weeks but were apparent at 31 weeks. In an unpublished case, the author noted features of metaphyseal flaring, micrognathia, mild frontal bossing, small chest, and talipes in a low risk pregnancy at 22 weeks. The diagnosis of Kniest dysplasia was made after interruption of the pregnancy.

Risks and Management Options

Affected children may survive with normal intelligence but are short (106–145 cm) and have limited mobility and severe orthopedic disabilities. Ophthalmic complications and deafness may occur in childhood.

Spondyloepiphyseal Dysplasia Congenita (12q13-12q14) (*COL2A1*)

Diagnosis

At the mild end of the hypochondrogenesis spectrum, the antenatal sonographic findings of spondyloepiphyseal dysplasia congenital was reported only once. There was moderate shortening of the femur at 16+ weeks followed by more marked rhizomelic shortening at 27 weeks.[57] No other distinguishing features were evident, and a definitive diagnosis was not made. The disorder is characterized by deficient ossification of the spine, pubis, talus, and calcaneum, and delayed appearance of the lower femoral and upper tibial epiphyses. Vertebrae show marked platyspondyly with ovoid vertebral bodies, the thorax is narrow and bell-shaped, and the long bones are moderately short. Cleft palate may also occur.

Risks and Management Options

This disorder is compatible with prolonged survival. Myopia and retinal detachment occur in about half the survivors. Hypotonic muscle weakness and restricted joint mobility reduce overall mobility, and the spinal deformities cause progressive kyphoscoliosis.

Heterozygous Achondroplasia (4p16) FGFR3

Achondroplasia is well recognized by the general population. Affected individuals have markedly short stature but normal intelligence and are generally well integrated members of society.

Diagnosis

The characteristic features are not usually evident until after 24 weeks' gestation, when the long bone shortening manifests[38,58] (see Fig. 21–2). Achondroplasia is characterized by predominantly acromesomelic limb shortening with stubby abducted fingers (trident hand). Typical facial features include a wide, prominent forehead (frontal bossing), depressed nasal bridge, hypertelorism, and a wide mandible. Thoracic dimensions may be reduced, but usually not enough to cause respiratory embarrassment. The spine is short and shows marked lumbar lordosis. Macrocrania and hydrocephalus can occur. The diagnosis can be confirmed by DNA analyses because the majority result from a single base substitution in the *FGFR3* gene.[59]

Risks and Management Options

Life expectancy and intellectual performance are good. Hydrocephaly secondary to partial obstruction of the restricted foramen magnum is usually mild and nonprogressive; surgical treatment is usually not needed. Progressive neurologic problems can result from spinal cord compression secondary to progressive narrowing of the interpedicular distance, particularly in the lumbar spine as the degree of lordosis increases. Corrective orthopedic surgery may be required to correct the spinal deformities and bowed legs.

Affected women usually require cesarean section because of a contracted pelvis. Cephalopelvic disproportion may also occur during the delivery of an affected fetus to a normal woman if the macrocephaly is marked. The recurrence risk for two unaffected parents is low, as achondroplasia usually results from a new mutation.

SHORT LONG BONES: ASYMMETRICAL

Isolated Limb Reductions

This heterogeneous group comprises disorders with asymmetrical reduction in limbs or portions of limbs.

Risks and Management Options

The majority of isolated limb reductions are nongenetic, but some may occur as part of a genetic syndrome or chromosomal abnormality.[60] Because of these associations, a detailed ultrasonographic examination is essential to exclude other markers. Karyotyping is recommended. The prognosis is generally good in the absence of associated physical or chromosomal abnormalities. Advances in prosthetics and orthopedics are such that much can be done to restore function and appearance of the reduced limbs. Parents should be encouraged to discuss these possibilities with appropriate professionals. There are, however, some specific syndromes associated with isolated or asymmetrical limb reductions.

Roberts' Syndrome (Pseudothalidomide Syndrome)

Diagnosis

Typically, all four limbs (tetraphocomelia) are affected, similar to the teratogenic effects of thalidomide. Median facial clefting, microcephaly, joint flexion deformities, talipes, syndactyly, and extremely short or missing fingers and toes are accompanying features. Other associated anomalies include hydrocephaly, encephalocele, and renal abnormalities such as polycystic or horseshoe kidneys. A similar condition of hypoglossia-hypodactyly syndrome involves asymmetrical limb reductions associated with micrognathia and microglossia. Facial clefting is uncommon in the latter. The two syndromes can be distinguished in utero by cytogenetic studies. In many cases of Roberts syndrome, premature separation of the centromeres produces a characteristic phenomenon of chromosome "puffing."

Risks and Management Options

Affected individuals have a high perinatal mortality rate (70%–80%) and severe growth restriction. Survivors are often profoundly mentally retarded. The option of pregnancy termination should be discussed. Survivors with hypoglossia-hypodactyly syndrome generally have satisfactory intellectual development, and the level of handicap depends on the severity of limb anomalies.

Femoral Hypoplasia: Unusual Faces Syndrome

This condition appears more common in the progeny of diabetic women. Cleft palate and micrognathia are associated with varying degrees of hypoplasia/aplasia of the femur. The tibia and fibula may be hypoplastic. Humeral reduction with a flexion deformity at the elbow can also be seen. Other associated abnormalities include vertebral anomalies of the lower spine, pelvic anomalies, and urogenital anomalies. The main differential diagnosis is caudal regression syndrome, but this syndrome is not associated with the facial dysmorphisms or humeral reduction. Most individuals have normal intelligence and are ambulatory.[5]

Femur-Fibula-Ulna Syndrome

This syndrome is characterized by femoral and fibula hypoplasia/aplasia and varying degrees of paraxial ulna hemimelia. It has been diagnosed antenatally.[61]

Holt-Oram Syndrome (12q21)–(*TXB5*)

Diagnosis

The cardinal features of Holt-Oram syndrome are congenital heart disease (usually ASD or VSD) associated with various upper limb and limb girdle reductions. The limb reductions are typically more severe in females and twice as common on the left than the right.[5,62,63] Abnormalities in the hand and forearm include aplastic, hypoplastic or triphalangeal (finger-like) thumb, syndactyly, and hypoplasia of the radius, ulna, humerus, clavicles, scapula, or sternum. This is a dominant condition and affected individuals have a 50% offspring risk. There is no consistent pattern, and expression is variable.

Risks and Management Options

Management options depend on the severity of the cardiac malformation and the skeletal deformities.

Thrombocytopenia–Absent Radius Syndrome

The skeletal manifestations of TAR syndrome are variable bilateral radial aplasia/hypoplasia sometimes associated with humeral or ulna reduction or bowing. The femurs can be affected, and cardiac anomalies are relatively common. Thrombocytopenia is a marker of an underlying hematopoietic abnormality. Antenatal diagnosis is based on both the sonographic findings and documentation of fetal thrombocytopenia in a blood sample obtained by cordocentesis. This is an autosomal recessive disorder with a 25% recurrence rate.

Cleidocranial Dysostosis (6p21)

Diagnosis

The characteristic findings of cleidocranial dysostosis are hypoplastic clavicles (Fig. 21–12*A*,*B*).[64] However, the clavicle is not generally included in routine prenatal surveys of the fetus. Further, they may be shadowed by the chin, arms, or scapulas. De novo presentations are frequently missed. Mild femoral shortening and a hypomineralized cranium with wide fontanelles may also be evident.

Risks and Management Options

Individuals with cleidocranial dysostosis are generally short. They may have respiratory difficulties in infancy if the thorax is restricted. Dental and hearing problems can present in later childhood. However, the absent or hypoplastic clavicles do not cause significant handicap, and intelligence is unimpaired. Poor skull ossification tends to improve with age. Affected mothers may require cesarean section because of a small pelvis.

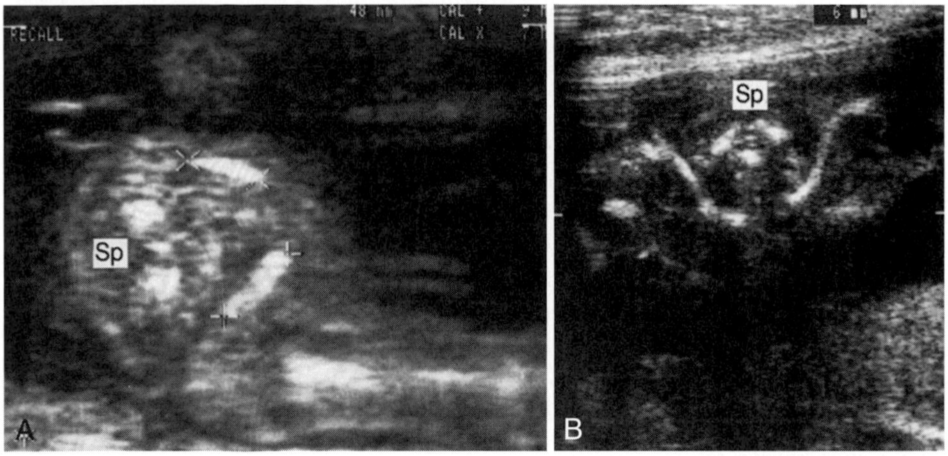

FIGURE 21–12
Cleidocranial dysostosis. *A*, Transverse scan of the clavicles of the fetus of a mother with cleidocranial dysostosis. The clavicles are short, thick, and straight. *B*, Similar posteroanterior scan of the clavicles of a normal 22-week fetus. Note the sigmoid form of the clavicle. Sp, spine.

CHROMOSOMAL ABNORMALITIES

Forearm reduction deformities can occur in fetuses with chromosomal abnormalities including 13q, trisomies 8, 13, and 18, triploidy and others.[60]

Polydactyly/Syndactyly

These conditions frequently coexist. The polydactyly can be either preaxial (on the radial side of the hand or medial side of the foot, including bifid thumb or great toe) or postaxial (on the ulnar side of the hand or lateral side of the foot). Polydactyly is associated with numerous genetic and chromosomal syndromes (Table 21–5). Isolated polydactyly can be inherited as an autosomal dominant trait with variable penetrance. The incidence of polydactyly is higher among some ethnic groups (e.g., Afro-Caribbean).

The syndactyly may be either osseous (fusion of the bones) or cutaneous (fusion of the digits by soft tissue). Some syndromes featuring syndactyly are listed in Table 21–6. Many are common to those with polydactyly.

Ectrodactyly

Ectrodactyly (split hand) is a variant of syndactyly in which the hands resemble a "lobster claw" (Fig. 21–13). It may occur either as an isolated phenomenon, or as part of several syndromes,[60] the most common of which is the ectrodactyly ectodermal dysplasia clefting (EEC) syndrome. Isolated ectrodactyly and EEC syndrome are both inherited as autosomal dominant traits with a 50% risk of recurrence.

Diagnosis

Isolated ectrodactyly may affect one or more limbs and has extremely variable penetrance. Parents of an affected child may show only minimal changes in the skin

TABLE 21–5

Syndromes Associated with Polydactyly

SYNDROME	ASSOCIATED FEATURES
Anocerebrodigital	CHD, renal agenesis, growth deficiency, anal atresia
Bloom	Growth deficiency, syndactyly
Carpenter	Craniosynostosis (acrocephaly)
C-trigonocephaly	Synostosis metopic suture, palate
Egger	Cerebellar anomalies (see Joubert)
Ellis–van Creveld	Mesomelic dysplasia (see above)
Fanconi pancytopenia	Forearm reductions (see above)
Fitch (Oto-palato-digital type 2)	Cleft palate, micrognathia, joint contractures, camptodactyly
Fuhrman	Polysyndactyly, fibula aplasia/hypoplasia, bowed femora
Golabi–Rosen	Prenatal macrosomia, extra ribs
Goltz	Syndactyly
Grebe	Short limbs (see above)
Greig cephalopolysyndactyly	Macrocephaly
Hydrolethalus	Hydrocephaly, micrognathia, CHD CL/CP (similar to Meckel's)
Jeune thoracic dystrophy	Short limbs, small thorax (see above)
Kaufman–McKusick	CHD, anal/vaginal atresia, urethral stenosis, intestinal malrotation
Klippel–Trenaunay–Weber	Asymmetrical limb hypertrophy, syndactyly, oligodactyly
Meckel–Grüber	Encephalocoele, polycystic kidney or liver, microcephaly, CP
Mohr	
(Orofacial-digital type 2)	Median CL/CP
(Orofacial-digital type 1)	Median CL/CP, porencephalic cysts
Robinow-Sorauf ACPS	Acrocephaly, bifid great toe
Sakati-Nyhan ACPS	Acrocephaly, CHD, short limbs, dysplastic ears
Trisomy 13, 3p-, dup(17q)	

Only those associated features which might be amenable to prenatal diagnosis have been included. For further details refer to Winter et al.[60]
CHD, Congenital heart disease; CL, cleft lip; CP, cleft palate.

TABLE 21–6

Syndromes Associated with Syndactyly

SYNDROME	ASSOCIATED FEATURES
Ablepharon-macrostomia (McCarthy)	Camptodactyly, cutaneous webs
Acrofacial dysostosis (Miller)	As Treacher Collins syndrome, postaxial defects
Acrocephalosyndactyly (Apert)	Coronal synostosis with brachycephaly, severe osseous syndactyly, CL/CP
(Pfeiffer)	2–3 Syndactyly, acrocephaly
Amniotic reduction	Oligohydramnios, CL/CP, limb reductions, abdominal wall defects (see text)
C-Trigonocephaly	As polydactyly
Carpenter	As polydactyly
Cenani-Lenz	Severe mesomelic limb hypoplasia. Complete syndactyly, radioulnar synostosis and severe hypoplasia
Cryptophthalmos	Renal agenesis, hypospadias
Ectrodactyly-ectodermal dysplasia-clefting	CL/CP, "split" hands and feet (see below)
Fitch	As polydactyly
Fuhrmann	As polydactyly
Greig	As polydactyly
Goltz	As polydactyly
Golabi–Rosen	As polydactyly
Hypoglossia–hypodactyly	Limb reductions, micrognathia (see Roberts syndrome)
Klippel–Trenauny–Weber	As polydactyly
Lenz–Majewski	Growth retardation
Moebius	Micrognathia, CL/CP, radial defects
Nager	
Neu–Laxova	Microcephaly, flexion deformities, agenesis corpus callosum
Oculodental-digital	4–5 syndactyly
Orofaciodigital (type I)	Median CL, CP, polydactyly, asymmetrical syndactyly, porencephalic cysts
Otopalatodigital	CP, "tree frog" hands and feet (clinodactyly of peripheral digits)
Popliteal pterygium (severe, lethal AR form)	Popliteal webs, CL/CP, microcephaly
Poland sequence	Hypoplasia of fingers or hand
Roberts	As polydactyly
Robinow–Sorauf	As polydactyly
TAR	Radial aplasia (see above)
Triploidy	Growth retardation, large placenta, umbilical hernia, talipes, micrognathia, CHD, hydrocephaly, holoprosencephaly, renal dysplasia, hydronephrosis
Yunis–Varon	Cleidocranial dysostosis + micrognathia, absent thumbs distal aphalangia

creases.[65] Although an antenatal diagnosis is possible in most severe cases, it may not be possible with mildly affected cases. In the EEC syndrome, ectrodactyly is associated with cleft lip or palate and skin, hair, and teeth dysplasia. Renal defects may also be present.

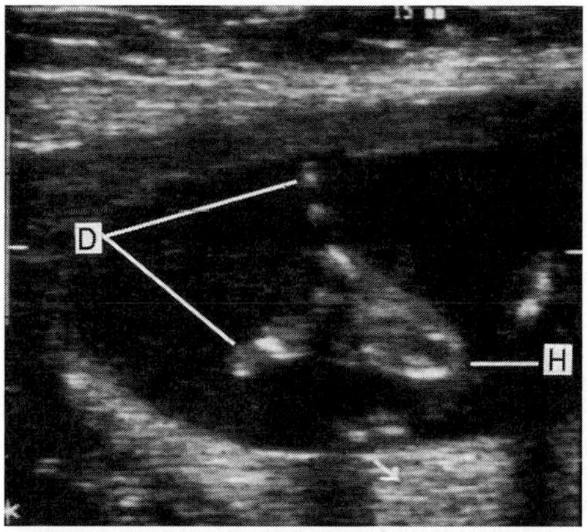

FIGURE 21–13
Scan of a fetal foot showing ectrodactyly. H, heel; D, digits. Reproduced with permission from Griffin (2). Griffin DR: Skeletal dysplasias. In Brock DJH, Rodeck CH, Ferguson-Smith MA (eds): Prenatal Diagnosis and Screening. Edinburgh, Churchill Livingstone, 1992, pp 257–313.

Risks and Management Options

Individuals with EEC syndrome have normal intelligence and can generally adapt to their deformities to lead productive lives. The facial clefting can be surgically corrected, as can some of the orthopedic deformities. Dentures and wigs may be of value, and it is important to assure lacrimal duct drainage from an early stage to prevent corneal scarring.

POSITIONAL DEFORMITIES

Positional deformities are found in several settings:

- In response to adverse intrauterine pressures (oligohydramnios, amniotic bands, or tumors)
- Diastrophic dysplasia
- Rhizomelic chondrodysplasia punctata
- Chromosomal disorders
- Generalized neuromuscular deficiencies
- As specific isolated phenomena

The deformities are generally ones of flexion, but extension and bizarre combinations can be seen in the legs.

Talipes

The most common positional deformity is talipes equinovarus, in which the foot is adducted and plantar inverted so that the sole points medially. In the equinovalgus (calcaneovalgus) deformity, the heel is elevated and the foot is plantar everted. Talipes occurs as an isolated phenomenon in about 1:1200 births with varying degrees of severity, or as a marker for chromosomal abnormalities or a number of genetic syndromes.

Diagnosis

Positional deformities of the feet are best sought in the sagittal and coronal scanning planes (Fig. 21–14). When

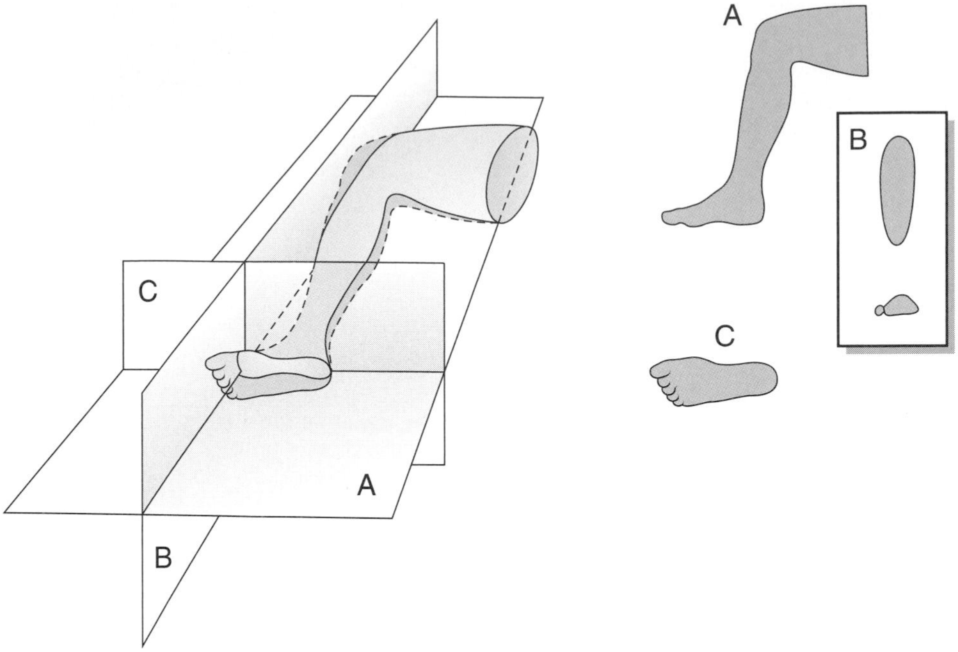

FIGURE 21–14
Diagram representing the scanning planes employed to visualize the foot. Plane A will show rocker-bottom feet; planes A and B will show talipes; planes B and C reveal polysyndactyly. (From Griffin DR: Skeletal dysplasias. In Brock DJH, Rodeck CH, Ferguson-Smith MA [eds]: Prenatal Diagnosis and Screening. Edinburgh, Churchill Livingstone, 1992, pp 257–313.)

severe talipes equinovarus is present, the plantar view of the foot is seen in continuity with the leg in sagittal section (Fig. 21–15). Because of the many associated syndromes, a careful search for other abnormalities is mandatory before counseling. The combination of talipes with polyhydramnios raises the suspicion of congenital myotonic dystrophy. The mother should be examined for evidence of mild disease.

Risks and Management Options

Isolated talipes is usually amenable to orthopedic correction. Karyotyping is recommended if other markers of aneuploidy or risk factors are present, as talipes is a marker of chromosomal anomalies. Management depends on the severity of any associated structural defects and the karyotype.

Rocker-bottom Feet

The typical appearance of rocker-bottom feet, usually caused by a vertical talus, is a posteriorly prominent heel and convexity of the normally concave contour of the plantar arch (Fig. 21–16). Rocker-bottom feet are associated with trisomy 18, 18q syndrome, trisomy 13, and Pena-Shokeir type 2 syndrome. Its finding requires a diligent search for other abnormalities. Karyotyping is indicated if other abnormalities are present.

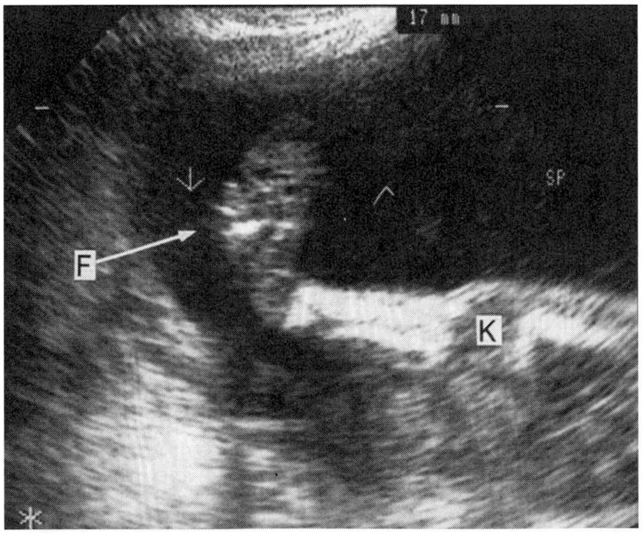

FIGURE 21–15
Positional deformities. Longitudinal sonogram of the leg showing the lower end of the femur, knee (K), tibia/fibula and foot with talipes. The plantar view of the foot would not normally be seen in this plane.

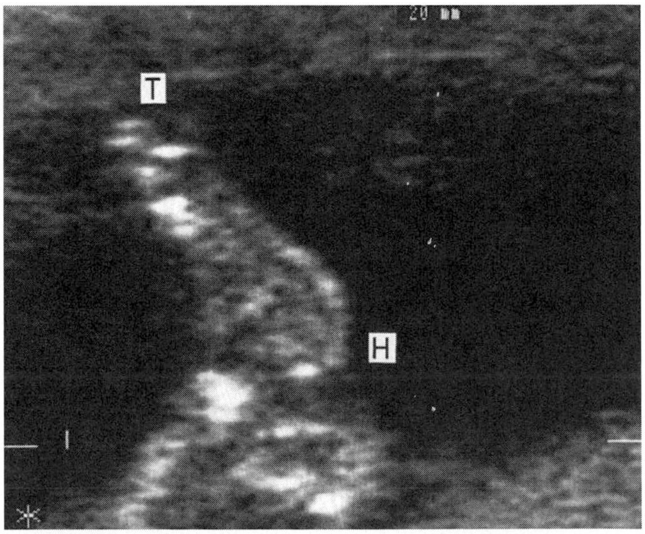

FIGURE 21–16
Rocker-bottom foot. Sagittal scan of the foot of a fetus with confirmed trisomy 18 showing prominent heel (H) and loss of the plantar arch. T, toe.

MULTIPLE JOINT CONTRACTURES

This heterogeneous group of disorders is characterized by multiple flexion deformities of the limbs, hands, and feet, resulting in fixed immobile limbs, sometimes with cutaneous webbing (pterygia) at joint flexures. The causes include the following:

- Central nervous system disease (55%)
- Peripheral neuromuscular disorder (8%)
- Connective tissue disease (11%)
- Miscellaneous skeletal or other abnormality (19%)[66]

Oligohydramnios is present in 7%.[66] Increased nuchal translucency in the first trimester and fetal hydrops in the second trimester are reported.[67,68] Deficient swallowing and fetal breathing may result in hydramnios and pulmonary hypoplasia. Within the spectrum of disease, the more severe forms, commonly designated arthrogryposis multiplex congenita, include congenital muscular dystrophy, lethal multiple pterygium syndrome, and Pena-Shokeir type 1 syndrome. Table 21–7 lists these and other syndromes with varying degrees of contractures that are potentially amenable to antenatal diagnosis.

TABLE 21–7

Syndromes Featuring Positional Deformities

SYNDROME	FEATURES
Aase-Smith-hydrocephalus-CP-joint contractures	CP, Dandy-Walker malformation (very variable presentation)
Amyoplasia	Multiple contractures with medial arm rotation (waiter's tip)
Bowed-Conradi	Like trisomy 18, rocker-bottom feet, micrognathia, camptodactyly
C-trigonocephaly	(see Polydactyly)
Cerebroarthrodigital	Digital hypoplasia, hydrocephalus microcephaly
Christian adducted thumbs	Craniosynostosis, micrognathia, CP adducted thumbs
Congenital myotonic dystrophy	More common with affected mother
Distal arthrogryposis	Camptodactyly of hands, talipes
Freeman–Sheldon	Ulnar deviation of hands, talipes
Marden-Walker	Camptodactyly, CHD, occ. CP
Multiple pterygium (Lethal type)	Severe webbing, cystic hygroma, hydrops, pulmonary and cardiac hypoplasia, CP
Neu–Laxova	(see Syndactyly)
Pena–Shokeir type I	Growth deficiency, pulmonary hypoplasia, camptodactyly, talipes
Syndesmoplastic dwarfism	No details
X-linked arthrogryposis	

Adapted from Winter RM, Knowles SAS, Bieber FR, Baraitser Mm: The malformed Fetus and Stillborth: A Diagnostic Approach. Chichester, John Wiley, 1988, pp 166–182.

Risks and Management Options

The more severe forms are associated with thoracic constriction, hydrops, and multiple deformities. Congenital muscular dystrophy, lethal multiple pterygium syndrome, and Pena-Shokeir type 1 syndrome are lethal or seriously handicapping. The choice of abortion should be discussed if it is a legal option. A definitive antenatal diagnosis of other syndromes may not be possible except in high risk families where detection or exclusion of relevant features is possible. Discussion with a geneticist prior to counseling is useful when there is uncertainty. The deformities can be severe enough to produce dystocia or trauma in continuing pregnancies with a vaginal delivery.

SPINAL DEFORMITIES

These deformities can occur as a consequence of neural tube defects, hemivertebrae, dysplasia or agenesis of the vertebrae, or asymmetrical muscle action (severe abdominal wall defects). Neural tube defects and abdominal wall defects are reviewed in Chapters 18 and 20.

Hemivertebrae

Hemivertebrae occur when one of the pair of chondrification centers that normally combine to form the vertebral body fails to appear. Only half of the vertebral body develops, and the result is lateral angulation of the spine (scoliosis). Hemivertebrae may be isolated or associated with cardiac, renal, radial, or digital anomalies, tracheoesophageal fistula, and anal atresia in the VACTERL association, or as a part of numerous other genetic syndromes.

Diagnosis

Hemivertebrae are recognized sonographically by spinal scoliosis and asymmetry in the vertebral echoes (Fig. 21–17). A careful search for associated abnormalities is essential. Hydramnios may be the only clue to tracheoesophageal atresia. A karyotype is indicated if other anomalies are seen, as a similar spectrum of deformities may be found in trisomy 18 and 13q syndromes.

Risks and Management Options

These options depend on the presence and severity of associated anomalies. The parents should meet with an orthopedic specialist to discuss the postnatal management including surgical correction of the spinal defor-

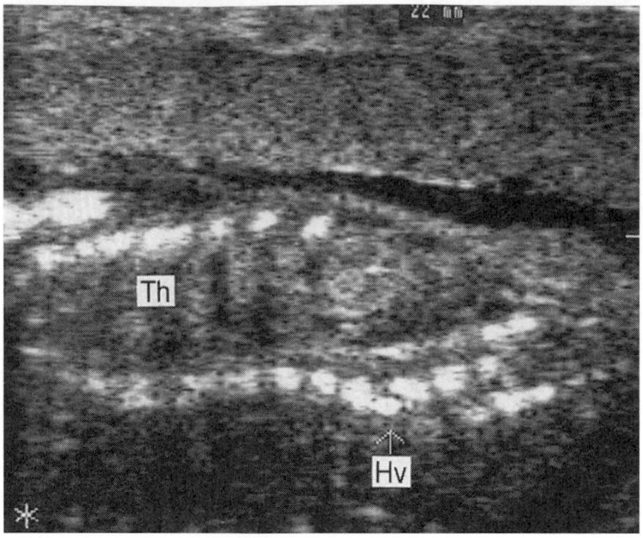

FIGURE 21–17
Longitudinal scan of the vertebral bodies of one of twin fetuses showing a midlumbar hemivertebra (HV). The spinal canal showed no evidence of narrowing on scan. Spinal deformity was minimal at birth. Th, thorax.

mity. Individuals with VACTERL association generally have normal intellectual potential.

Jarcho-Levin Syndrome

This autosomal recessive disorder is most common in the Puerto Rican population.

Diagnosis

The Jarcho-Levin syndrome is characterized by a grossly disorganized axial skeleton and thorax (Fig. 21–18). The spine may be missing or fused, and the hemivertebrae and ribs are frequently reduced in number with posterior fusion and anterior flaring (the "crab chest" deformity). Visceral and urogenital anomalies along with diaphragmatic hernia are also reported.[69,70]

Risks and Management Options

The majority of individuals with this condition die in the neonatal period or during early infancy as a result of respiratory insufficiency. The option of pregnancy termination should be discussed.

HYDROPS (See also Chapter 25)

Fetal hydrops may be a feature of the most severe forms of the following:

- Achondrogenesis types 1
- Short-rib polydactyly syndromes
- Multiple contracture syndromes (including Pena-Shokeir syndrome type 1)
- Noonan's syndrome

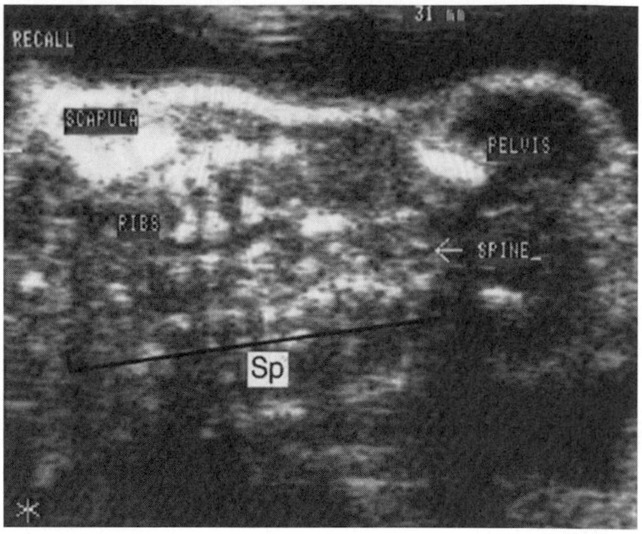

FIGURE 21–18
Longitudinal coronal scan of the trunk of a fetus with Jarcho-Levin syndrome. The ribs are thick and irregular and the spinal components (Sp) grossly disorganized. (From Griffin DR: Skeletal dysplasias. In Brock DJH, Rodeck CH, Ferguson-Smith MA [eds]: Prenatal Diagnosis and Screening. Edinburgh, Churchill Livingstone, 1992, pp 257–313.)

- Chromosomal abnormalities (Down syndrome, Turner's syndrome)

A karyotype is indicated.

HYDRAMNIOS (See also Chapter 13)

Many limb reduction deformities are associated with hydramnios and include the following:

- Achondrogenesis
- Asphyxiating thoracic dystrophy
- Chondrodysplasia punctata
- Dyssegmental dysplasia
- Roberts' syndrome
- VACTERL association
- Congenital myotonic dystrophy

Hydramnios generally presents late in pregnancy and may not be apparent at the time of a routine second trimester scan. As pregnancies complicated by diabetes mellitus may also develop hydramnios, spinal and lower limb deformities should also be sought.

UNFAVORABLE INTRAUTERINE ENVIRONMENT

Diabetes Mellitus

Patients with diabetes mellitus predating pregnancy have an 8% to 12% risk of fetal malformation (see Chapter 45). Skeletal malformations associated with diabetes mellitus include the caudal regression syndrome and femoral hypoplasia-unusual faces syndrome (discussed earlier).

Caudal Regression Syndrome

This syndrome is highly variable in severity and location of the malformation.

Diagnosis

The typical lesion is agenesis of the lower spine (Fig. 21–19) and may be associated with lower limb reductions or deformities including fusion of the legs (sirenomelia) (Fig. 21–20). Urogenital and anorectal organs of similar caudal origin are frequently malformed or atretic. Radial reduction and esophageal atresia may also occur similar to VACTERL. A single umbilical artery is usual.

Risks and Management Options

Survival and prognosis depend on the severity of the lesions. Minor degrees of sacral agenesis are compatible with normal life, whereas severe defects may cause considerable handicap or may be incompatible with life (e.g., renal agenesis). Karyotyping is recommended, as similar deformities may be associated with chromosomal abnormalities. The option of pregnancy termination, where it is legal, should be discussed in severe cases.

Early Amnion Rupture Sequence

This bizarre and sporadic group of disorders (1:2000 births) consists of asymmetrical anatomic disruptions associated in many cases with adherent bands or sheets of amnion. The current consensus view is that the deformities are secondary to early amnion rupture, the severity and site of the lesion being related to the stage of organogenesis at which rupture occurs. Vascular occlusion during organogenesis may be responsible for some of these anomalies. The abnormalities may not necessarily be associated with continued oligohydramnios.

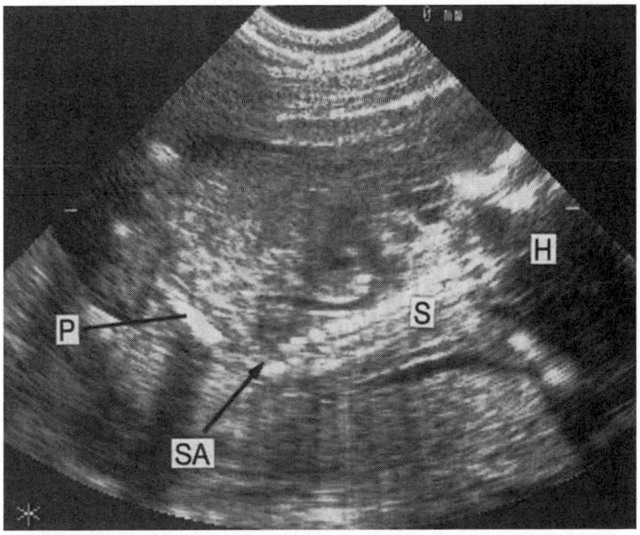

FIGURE 21–19
Caudal regression sequence. Longitudinal sagittal scan of the trunk and spine of a fetus with agenesis of the lumbosacral spine (S). The spine terminates at the lower thoracic region (SA). The pelvis (P) is present. H, head. (From Griffin DR: Skeletal dysplasias. In Brock DJH, Rodeck CH, Ferguson-Smith MA [eds]: Prenatal Diagnosis and Screening. Edinburgh, Churchill Livingstone, 1992, pp 257–313.)

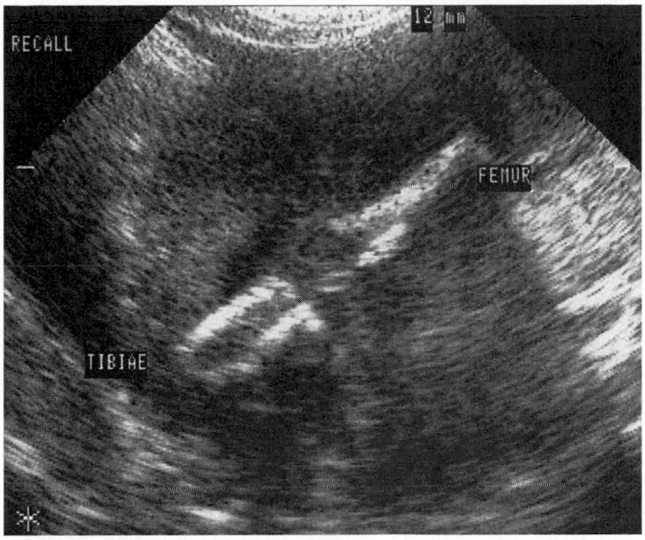

FIGURE 21–20
Sonogram of the lower "limb" of an 18-week fetus diagnosed as sirenomelia. The single femur arose from the midpelvis and the broadened lower metaphysis articulated with two bones, presumed to be the tibias.

Diagnosis

The diagnosis of early amnion rupture sequence is considered when transverse reduction defects or multiple asymmetrical disruptions are discovered. Manifestations include anencephaly, asymmetrical encephalocele, facial clefts and disruptions, abdominal wall defects (usually gastroschisis), and limb deformities, constrictions, or transverse reductions. Such malformations are reported after amniocentesis and chorionic villous sampling (CVS) before the 10th postmenstrual week.[71,72] Amniotic bands may be attached to deformed structures. In known cases of early amnion rupture or continued bleeding during the first trimester, such deformities should be excluded by a detailed second trimester ultrasonographic examination. Visualization may be difficult, if not impossible, when there is oligohydramnios. Amnioinfusion can be used to improve visualization.[73] The physician must bear in mind that amniotic band-like structures (synechiae) are commonly observed during routine sonographic examination. There is no evidence they cause deformities unless they are attached to the fetus, occasionally in a tourniquet fashion, or restrict mobility.

Risks and Management Options

These options depend on the severity of lesions. In instances of continuing severe oligohydramnios, preterm delivery and pulmonary hypoplasia threaten survival. The option of pregnancy termination should be discussed in nonviable or severely disrupted cases if abortion is legal. Karyotyping is indicated when deformities are seen.

Drugs in Early Pregnancy

Most drugs undergo extensive animal testing for evidence of teratogenicity before their release for human consumption. A detailed fetal scan is recommended for any pregnant individual who has ingested a significant medication during the first trimester. Some drugs specifically implicated in limb teratogenesis are thalidomide (whose distribution is now tightly controlled), coumadin, phenytoin, sodium valproate, alcohol, cytotoxic drugs, and lithium. The interested reader should consult a more extensive source.[74,75]

CONCLUSIONS

- Skeletal defects can be extremely difficult malformations to diagnose sonographically with accuracy.
- A multidisciplinary approach is essential.
- During the initial stages of diagnosis, the complex fetal deformities should be discussed with a geneticist who has a specific interest in dysmorphology.
- Thereafter, the diagnosis may be refined by further sonographic examination, karyotyping (if not already performed), biochemical, molecular biologic, or other ancillary test.
- Parents often find it useful to speak with relevant specialists who have experience with the disorder before deciding on further management.
- All relevant professionals who may encounter the mother during her pregnancy and labor should be informed of the diagnostic findings and their significance (if known).
- If the condition is lethal, the fetus or newborn should be photographed and xeroradiographed (mammography radiographs give excellent definition). Skin, blood, or placental samples should be obtained for karyotype/DNA analysis. When possible, the fetus should be examined by a perinatal pathologist. A pediatric radiologist should examine radiographs.
- It is only when all information has been gathered that the final consultation with the parents is arranged with the obstetrician, geneticist, or both. The parents are then informed of the recurrence risks in future pregnancies, and the offspring risks for their existing children or other family members. Management plans for antenatal diagnosis in a future pregnancy can then be discussed.

SUMMARY OF MANAGEMENT OPTIONS
Skeletal Abnormalities

Management Options	Quality of Evidence	Grade of Recommendation	References
Prepregnancy			
Ensure accuracy of diagnosis before counselling	–	GPP	–
Counseling (possibly interdisciplinary) about recurrence risks and prenatal diagnostic options	–	GPP	–
Prenatal			
Careful ultrasonography by experienced sonographer, including general examination of fetus for other anomalies	–	GPP	–
Consider a karyotype or other additional tests if other anomalies or suspicion of genetic condition with DNA probe	–	GPP	–
Interdisciplinary discussion before counselling parents (differential diagnosis rather than definitive diagnosis may be all that is possible)	–	GPP	–
Ongoing review of sonographic findings if pregnancy continues (further features may develop allowing definitive diagnosis)	–	GPP	–
Psychological support of parents	–	GPP	–

SUMMARY OF MANAGEMENT OPTIONS
Skeletal Abnormalities *(Continued)*

Management Options	Quality of Evidence	Grade of Recommendation	References
Labor and Delivery			
Consider pregnancy termination with severe and/or lethal anomalies	–	GPP	–
Psychological support of parents	–	GPP	–
Caesarean section for normal obstetric indications though severe forms of arthrogryposis may only deliver safely with caesarean section	–	GPP	–
Postnatal			
If lethal, encourage postmortem by experienced perinatal pathologist	–	GPP	–
Detailed postnatal examination including radiography	–	GPP	–
Tissue for karyotyping and other tests if not performed prenatally	–	GPP	–
Ensure accuracy of diagnosis before counseling	–	GPP	–
Counselling (possibly interdisciplinary) about recurrence risks and future prenatal diagnostic options	–	GPP	–

REFERENCES

1. Giedon A, Biedermann K, Briner J, et al: Case report 693 (Schneckenbecken dysplasia). Skeletal Radiol 1991;20:534–538.
2. Chervenak FA, Isaacson G, Rosenberg JC, Kardon NB: Antenatal diagnosis of frontal cephalocele in a fetus with atelosteogenesis. J Ultrasound Med 1986;5:111–113.
3. Kim HJ, Costales F, Bouzouki M, Wallach RC: Prenatal diagnosis of dysegmental dwarfism. Prenat Diagn 1986,6:143–150.
4. Nyberg DA, Mahony BS, Pretorius DH: Diagnostic Ultrasound of Fetal Anomalies: Text and Atlas. Chicago, Year Book, 1990, pp 196–197, 529.
5. Smith DW: Recognizable Patterns of Human Malformations: Genetic, Embryologic and Clinical Aspects. Philadelphia, WB Saunders, 1982.
6. Mayden KL, Tortora M, Berkowitz RL, et al: Orbital diameters: A new parameter for prenatal diagnosis and dating. Am J Obstet Gynecol 1982;144:289–297.
7. Jeanty P, Draimex-Wilmet M, Van Gansbeke D, et al: Fetal occular biometry by ultrasound. Radiology 1982;143: 513–516.
8. Otto C, Platt LD: The fetal mandible measurement: An objective determination of fetal jaw size. Ultrasound Obstet Gynecol 1991;1:12–17.
9. Chitty LS, Altman D, Campbell S: Fetal mandible measurement: Feasibility and development of centile charts. Prenat Diagn 1993;13:749–756.
10. Allen LD, Tynan MJ, Campbell S, Anderson RH: Normal fetal cardiac anatomy—A basis for the echocardiographic detection of abnormalities. Prenat Diagn 1981;1:131–139.
11. Orioli IM, Castilla EE, Barbosa-Neto JG: The birth prevalence rates for the skeletal dysplasias. J Med Genet 1986;23:328–332.
12. Glenn LW, Teng SSK: In utero sonographic diagnosis of achondrogenesis. J Clin Ultrasound 1985;13:195–198.
13. Borochowitz Z, Ornoy A, Lachman R, Rimoin DL: Achondrogenesis II—Hypochondrogenesis: Variability versus heterogeneity. Am J Med Genet 1986;24:273–288.
14. Chervenak FA, Blakemore KJ, Isaacson G, et al: Antenatal sonographic findings of thanatophoric dysplasia with cloverleaf skull. Am J Obstet Gynecol 1983;146:984–985.
15. Beetham FGT, Reeves JS: Early ultrasound diagnosis of thanatophoric dwarfism. J Clin Ultrasound 1984;12:43–44.
16. Burrows PE, Stannard MW, Pearrow J, et al: Early antenatal sonographic recognition of thanatophoric dysplasia with clover leaf skull deformity. Am J Roentgenol 1984;143:841–843.
17. Camera G, Dodero D, De Pascale S: Prenatal diagnosis of thanatophoric dysplasia at 24 weeks. Am J Med Genet 1984;18: 39–43.
18. Elejalde BR, de Elejalde MM: Thanatophoric dysplasia: Fetal manifestations and prenatal diagnosis. Am J Med Genet 1984;22:669–683.
19. Weiner CP, Williamson RA, Bonsib SM: Sonographic diagnosis of cloverleaf skull and thanatophoric dysplasia in the second trimester. J Clin Ultrasound 1986;14:463–465.
20. Fryns JP, van den Berghe K, van Assche A, van den Berghe H: Prenatal diagnosis of campomelic dwarfism. Clin Genet 1981;19:199–201.
21. Hobbins JC, Bracken MB, Mahoney MJ: Diagnosis of fetal dysplasias with ultrasound. Am J Obstet Gynecol 1982;142: 306–312.
22. Redon JY, Le Grevellec JY, Marie F, et al: Un diagnostic antenatal de dysplasie campomelique. J Obstet Gynecol Biol Reprod 1984;13:437–441.
23. Winter R, Rosenkranz W, Hofmann H, et al: Prenatal diagnosis of campomelic dysplasia by ultrasonography. Prenat Diagn 1985;5:1–8.
24. Gillerot Y, Vanheck C-A, Foulon M, et al: Campomelic syndrome: Manifestations in a 20-week fetus and case history of a five-year old child. Am J Med Genet 1989;34:589–592.
25. Cordone M, Lituania M, Zampatti C, et al: In utero ultrasonographic features of campomelic dysplasia. Prenat Diagn 1989;9:745–750.

26. Mansour S, Hall CM, Pembrey ME, Young ID: A clinical and genetic study of campomelic dysplasia. J Med Genet 1995;32:415–420.
27. Beluffy G, Fraccaro M: Genetic and clinical aspects of campomelic dysplasia. In Papadatos CJ, Bartsocas CS (eds): Skeletal Dysplasias. New York, Allan R. Liss, 1982, pp 53–65.
28. Houston CS, Opitz JM, Spranger JW, et al: The campomelic syndrome: Review, report of 17 cases and follow-up on the currently 17-year-old boy first reported by Maroteaux et al. in 1971. Am J Med Genet 1983;15:3–28.
29. Dinno ND, Yacuob US, Kadlec JF, Garver KL: Midtrimester diagnosis of osteogenesis imperfecta, type 11. Birth Defects 1982;18:125–132.
30. Milsom I, Mattsson L-A, Dahlen-Nilsson I: Antenatal diagnosis of osteogenesis imperfecta by real-time ultrasound: Two case reports. Br J Radiol 1982;55:310–312.
31. Shapiro JE, Phillips JA, Byers PH, et al: Prenatal diagnosis of lethal osteogenesis imperfecta (OI type II). J Paediatr 1982;100:127–133.
32. Elejalde BR, de Elejalde MM: Prenatal diagnosis of perinatally lethal osteogenesis imperfecta. Am J Med Genet 1983;14:353–359.
33. Aylsworth AS, Seeds JW, Guilford WB, et al: Prenatal diagnosis of a severe deforming type of osteogenesis imperfecta. Am J Med Genet 1984;19:707–714.
34. Brons JTJ, van der Harten JJ, Wladimiroff JW, et al: Prenatal ultrasonographic diagnosis of osteogenesis imperfecta. Am J Obstet Gynecol 1988;159:176–181.
35. Constantine G, McCormack J, McHugo J, Fowlie A: Prenatal diagnosis of severe osteogenesis imperfecta. Prenat Diagn 1991;11:103–110.
36. Munoz C, Filly R, Golbus MS: Osteogenesis imperfecta type 11: Prenatal sonographic diagnosis. Radiology 1990;174:181–185.
37. Robinson LP, Worthen NJ, Lachman RS, et al: Prenatal diagnosis of osteogenesis imperfecta type III. Prenat Diagn 1987;7:7–15.
38. Kurtz AB, Wapner RJ: Ultrasonographic diagnosis of second trimester skeletal dysplasias: A prospective analysis in a high risk population. J Ultrasound Med 1983;2:99–106.
39. Wladimiroff JW, Niermeijer MF, Van der Harten JJ, et al: Early prenatal diagnosis of congenital hypophosphatasia: Case report. Prenat Diagn 1985;5:47–52.
40. Walkinshaw SA, Burn J: The diagnosis and management of pregnancies complicated by fetal abnormality. In Dunlop W, Calder AA (eds): High Risk Pregnancy. Guildford, Surrey, Butterworths, 1991.
41. Mulivor RA, Mennuti M, Zackai EH, Harris H: Prenatal diagnosis of hypophosphatasia: Genetic, biochemical and clinical studies. Am J Hum Genet 1978;30:271–282.
42. Warren RC, McKenzie CF, Rodeck CH, et al: First trimester diagnosis of hypophosphatasia with a monoclonal antibody to the liver/bone/kidney isoenzyme of alkaline phosphatase. Lancet 1985;ii:856.
43. Brock JH, Barron L: First trimester prenatal diagnosis of hypophosphatasia: Experience with 16 cases. Prenat Diagn 1991;11:387–391.
44. Filly RA, Golbus MS: Ultrasonography of the normal and pathologic fetal skeleton. Radiol Clin North Am 1982;20:311–323.
45. Little D: Prenatal diagnosis of skeletal dysplasias. In Rodeck CH, Nicolaides KH (eds): Prenatal Diagnosis. London, Royal College of Obstetricians and Gynaecologists, 1984, pp 301–306.
46. Elejalde BR, de Elejalde MM, Pansch D: Prenatal diagnosis of Jeune syndrome. Am J Med Genet 1985;21:433–438.
47. Mahoney MJ, Hobbins JC: Prenatal diagnosis of chondroectodermal dysplasia (Ellis–van Creveld syndrome) with fetoscopy and ultrasound. N Engl J Med 1977;297:258–260.
48. Zimmer EZ, Weinraub Z, Raijman A, et al: Antenatal diagnosis of a fetus with an extremely narrow thorax and short-limbed dwarfism. J Clin Ultrasound 1984;12:112–114.
49. O'Brien GD, Rodeck C, Queenan JT: Early prenatal diagnosis of diastrophic dwarfism by ultrasound. Br Med J 1980;280:1300.
50. Mantagos S, Weiss RW, Mahoney M, Hobbins JC: Prenatal diagnosis of diastrophic dwarfism. Am J Obstet Gynecol 1981;139:111–113.
51. Gembruch U, Niesen M, Kehrberg H, Hansmann M: Diastrophic dysplasia: A specific prenatal diagnosis by ultrasound. Prenat Diagn 1988;8:539–545.
52. Duff P, Harlass FE, Milligan DA: Prenatal diagnosis of chondrodysplasia punctata by sonography. Obstet Gynecol 1990;76:497–500.
53. Hoefler S, Hoefler G, Moser AB, et al: Prenatal diagnosis of rhizomelic chondrodysplasia punctata. Prenat Diagn 1988;8:571–576.
54. Pryde PG, Bawle E, Brandt F, et al: Prenatal diagnosis of nonrhizomelic chondrodysplasia punctata (Conradi-Hunermann syndrome). Am J Med Genet 1993;47:426–431.
55. Curry CJR, Magenis RE, Brown M, et al: Inherited chondrodysplasia punctata due to a deletion of the terminal short arm of an X chromosome. N Engl J Med 1984;311:1010–1015.
56. Bromley B, Miller W, Foster SC, Benacerraf BR: The prenatal sonographic freatures of Kniest syndrome. J Ultrasound Med 1991;10:705–707.
57. Kirk JS, Comstock CH: Antenatal sonographic appearance of spondyloepithelial dysplasia congenita. J Ultrasound Med 1990;9:173–175.
58. Filly RA, Golbus MS, Cary JC, Hall JG: Short limbed dwarfism: Ultrasonographic diagnosis by mensuration of fetal femoral length. Radiology 1981;138:653–656.
59. Bellus GA, Hefferon TW, Oritz de Luna RI, et al: Achondroplasia is defined by recurrent G308R mutations of FGFR3. Am J Hum Genet 1995;56:363–373.
60. Winter RM, Knowles SAS, Bieber FR, Baraitser M: The Malformed Fetus and Stillbirth: A Diagnostic Approach. Chichester, John Wiley, 1988, pp 166–182.
61. Hirose K, Koyanagi T, Hara K, et al: Antenatal ultrasound diagnosis of the femur-fibula-ulna syndrome. J Clin Ultrasound 1988;16:199–203.
62. Muller LM, de Jong G, van Heerden KMM: The antenatal ultrasonographic detection of the Holt-Oram syndrome. South Afr Med J 1985;68:313–315.
63. Brons JTJ, Van Geijn HP, Wladimiroff JW, et al: Prenatal ultrasound diagnosis of the Holt-Oram syndrome. Prenat Diagn 1988;8:175–181.
64. Yarkoni S, Schmidt W, Jeanty P, et al: Clavicular measurement: A new biometric parameter for fetal evaluation. J Ultrasound Med 1985;4:467–470.
65. Penchaszadeh VB, Negrotti TC: Ectrodactyly-ectodermal dysplasia-clefting (EEC) syndrome: Dominant inheritance and variable expression. J Med Genet 1976;13:281–284.
66. Hageman G, Ippel EPF, Beemer FA, et al: The diagnostic management of newborns with congenital contractures: A nosologic study of 75 cases. Am J Med Genet 1988;30:883–904.
67. Shenker L, Reed K, Anderson C, et al: Syndrome of camptodactyly, ankyloses, facial anomalies and pulmonary hypoplasia (Pena-Shokeir syndrome): Obstetric and ultrasound aspects. Am J Obstet Gynecol 1985;152:303–307.
68. Kirkinen P, Herva R, Leisti J: Early prenatal diagnosis of a lethal syndrome of multiple congenital contractures. Prenat Diagn 1987;7:189–196.
69. Tolmie JT, Whittle MJ, McNay MB, et al: Second trimester prenatal diagnosis of the Jarcho-Levin syndrome. Prenat Diagn 1987;7:129–134.
70. Romero R, Ghidini A, Eswara MS, et al: Prenatal findings in a case of spondylocostal dysplasia type I (Jarco-Levin syndrome). Obstet Gynecol 1988;71:988–991.
71. Firth HV, Boyd PA, Chamberlain P, et al: Severe limb abnormalities after chorion villous sampling at 56–66 days gestation. Lancet 1991;337:762–763.

72 Burton BK, Schultz CJ, Burd LI: Limb abnormalities associated with chorionic villous sampling. Obstet Gynecol 1992;79: 726–730.
73. Gembruch U, Hansmann M: Artificial instillation of amniotic fluid as a new technique for the diagnostic evaluation of cases of oligohydramnios. Prenat Diagn 1988;8:33–45.
74. Koren G, Edwards MB, Miskin M: Antenatal sonography of fetal malformations associated with drugs and chemicals: A guide. Am J Obstet Gynecol 1987;176:79–85.
75. Weiner CP, Buhimschi C (eds): Drugs for Pregnant and Lactating Women. Philadelphia, Churchill Livingston, 2004.

CHAPTER 22

Fetal Thyroid and Adrenal Disease

Stephen Robson

FETAL THYROID DISEASE

Fetal Thyroid Function

The embryonic thyroid is derived from the endoderm of the buccal cavity. The gland enlarges and migrates to the lower neck by the seventh week of embryonic development. Thyroid hormone synthesis begins at 10 to 12 weeks, but appreciable amounts are only released from 14 to 16 weeks onward.[1,2] Prior to that time, all thyroid hormone comes from the mother. Thyroxine (T_4) concentrations increase thereafter, reaching adult values by term (total T_4 100–150 nmol/L, free T_4 15-25 pmol/L).[3] Thyroxine is converted locally to the active metabolite, triiodothyronine (T_3), by deiodinase enzymes. Free T_3 levels increase gradually, particularly after 28 weeks, but remain below adult values. Thyroid-stimulating hormone (TSH) is low until 15 to 18 weeks' gestation, and then increases to around 8 mU/L by term.[3] The fetal pituitary is capable of responding to thyrotropin-releasing hormone (TRH) after 20 weeks, but is relatively insensitive to negative feedback from T_3 and T_4 until late in the second trimester.

The placenta is freely permeable to iodide substrates, TRH, thionanides, and TSH receptor immunoglobulins, but is impermeable to TSH. Significant transfer of T_3 and T_4 occurs and is controlled by the action of placental deiodinase enzymes. Differential expression of deiodinases maintains a suitable maternal-fetal gradient.[2] The placenta also produces several peptides (including hCG) capable of stimulating the maternal thyroid. As a result, maternal free T_4 (FT_4) concentrations increase during early pregnancy.

Thyroid hormones are essential for optimal growth and development of the central nervous system (CNS), lung, gut, and liver and the regulation of carbohydrate, lipid, and protein metabolism. It is likely that several factors, including deiodinase activity and thyroid hormone receptor expression, maintain adequate local concentrations of thyroid hormone at different times during gestation (reviewed by Chan and Rovet[2]). Neural requirements for thyroid hormone vary across gestation. Because the maternal thyroid is the fetus' primary source of thyroid hormone in the first half of pregnancy, it can be anticipated that neurodevelopmental abnormalities associated with maternal thyroid disease reflect damage to different neural structures (e.g., brainstem) than those resulting from defective fetal gland development that impact development later in gestation and in the neonatal period (e.g., cortex, hippocampus, and cerebellum). Thus, the specific types of deficit reflect the timing and duration of thyroid hormone insufficiency, with prenatal hypothyroidism contributing to visual-spatial deficits, perinatal hypothyroidism to fine motor weakness, and hypothyroidism slightly later in infancy to memory and language deficits.[2,4]

Fetal Hyperthyroidism

Etiology (Table 22–1)

Fetal or neonatal hyperthyroidism affects less than 1 in 5000 pregnancies.[5] The disorder is almost invariably secondary to maternal autoimmune thyroid disorders, principally Graves' disease or less commonly Hashimoto's thyroiditis. Graves' disease complicates between 1 in 500 and 1 in 1700 pregnancies and is responsible for over 90% of cases of maternal hyperthyroidism.[6–7] Here, maternal IgG antibodies to the TSH receptor cross the placenta and stimulate the fetal thyroid. Transplacental passage of these thyroid-stimulating immunoglobulins (TSI) may also occur in euthyroid mothers who have undergone partial or complete thyroidectomy. Thyrotoxicosis occurs in 2% to 10% of neonates born to women with a history of Graves' disease, of which half require therapy.[7,9–11] Maternal Hashimoto's thyroiditis usually has no adverse effect on the fetal thyroid, even though antithyroid antibodies may be found in the newborn due to transplacental passage. Thyroid hormone concentrations are also

TABLE 22–1

Causes of Fetal Thyroid Dysfunction

Hyperthyroidism
Maternal autoimmune disease
Graves' disease
Hashimoto's thyroiditis
Anemia (secondary to alloimmunization)
Hypothyroidism
Dysgenesis
Athyreosis
Hypoplasia
Ectopic thyroid
Maternal TSH-receptor blocking antibodies
Defects in thyroid hormone synthesis and metabolism
TSH-receptor mutations
Thyroid hormone resistance
Hypothalamic-pituitary dysfunction
Iatrogenic
Inadvertent use of radioiodine in pregnancy
Excessive iodine/iodide
Antithyroid drugs
Iodine deficiency
Sick preterm infants
Hypoxic intrauterine growth restriction (IUGR)

TSH, thyroid-stimulating hormone.

increased in fetuses with anemia secondary to red blood cell alloimmunization.[12]

Presentation and Diagnosis

Fetal hyperthyroidism should be suspected in any woman with a history of active or treated Graves' disease or clinical features suggestive of hyperthyroidism. Most hyperthyroid fetuses are asymptomatic. Fetal tachycardia is the most common symptom, being much move common than growth restriction.[13]

MATERNAL THYROID FUNCTION AND ANTIBODY TESTS

Decreased TSH and increased FT_4 concentrations are diagnostic of maternal hyperthyroidism. However, maternal thyroid function does not predict fetal thyroid function. The value of measuring TSH-receptor immunoglobulins is controversial, and a variety of assays exist. Many studies report TSH binding inhibitory Ig (TBII) activity, measured by radioreceptor assay (elevated values >15%).[10,14] Assays are also available for both stimulating (TSI) and blocking (TBI) immunoglobulins.[14] TSI can be measured by immunoassay or more commonly by a biologic assay based on the release of cAMP by purified IgG from thyroid cell cultures (elevated values greater than 130% or greater than 1.3 index units [IU]).[13–15] Some 20% of women with Graves' disease have TSH-receptor immunoglobulins. Kung and Jones[15] reported a change from stimulatory to blocking Ig activity during pregnancy in Graves' disease; median levels of TSI fell from 280% in the first trimester to 130% at term while TBI increased from 16% to 43%. They postulate that this change contributes to the remission of Graves' disease during pregnancy.

The risk of fetal hyperthyroidism correlates with maternal TSI and TBII levels.[7,10,11] In one recent study, a TSI of 5 IU or more correctly predicted neonatal hyperthyroidism with a sensitivity of 100%, specificity of 76%, positive predictive value of 40%, and negative predictive value of 100%.[13] The risk of neonatal hyperthyroidism is very small if both TSI and TBII are negative and increases to 42% when both tests are positive.[9] Guidelines for the measurement of TSH-receptor immunoglobulins in pregnancy are suggested by the European Thyroid Association[11] (Table 22–2).

FETAL IMAGING

Ultrasound assessment of the thyroid may be of some value in at-risk fetuses. Very large goiters can be associated with esophageal/tracheal compression and hydramnios, and are reported to cause malpresentation or mechanical obstruction in labor owing to hyperextension of the neck.[16] The sonographic differential diagnosis of an anterior neck mass includes hygroma, teratoma, hamartoma, and hemangioma. Subtler degrees of thyroid enlargement are difficult to diagnose and require the measurement of thyroid size in a transverse section of the fetal neck. Reference ranges for midthyroid width and

TABLE 22–2

Guidelines for Measurement of TSH-Receptor Immunoglobulins in Pregnancy

1. **A euthyroid pregnant woman without medication, but who has previously received antithyroid drugs for Graves' disease**: the risk for fetal and neonatal hyperthyroidism is negligible. Measurements of TSH-receptor immunoglobulins are not necessary.
2. **A euthyroid pregnant women (with or without thyroid hormone substitution therapy) who has previously received radioiodine therapy or undergone thyroid surgery for Graves' disease**: the risk of fetal and neonatal hyperthyroidism reflects the level of TSH-receptor immunoglobulins in the mother. Immunoglobulins* should be measured early in pregnancy:
   - If absent or low, no further special evaluation is recommended.
   - If high,† the fetus should be followed carefully for signs of hyperthyroidism. Immunoglobulins should be measured again in the last trimester to evaluate the risk of neonatal hyperthyroidism.
3. **A pregnant women who takes antithyroid drugs for Graves' disease to keep thyroid function normal**: TSH-receptor immunoglobulins should be measured in the last trimester:
   - If absent or low, neonatal hyperthyroidism is unlikely.
   - If high,† evaluation for neonatal hyperthyroidism is needed (clinical evaluation and thyroid function tests on cord blood and again after 4–7 days).

*The generally available and technically simple assays measuring TSH-receptor immunoglobulins by competitive inhibition (not indicating whether the immunoglobulins are stimulating the thyroid) predicted nearly all cases of neonatal hyperthyroidism.

†In Europe a widely used method is TRAK (Brahms, Berlin, Germany). With this method levels >40 U/L are considered high enough to indicate risk of neonatal hyperthyroidism.

Source: Laurberg P, Nygaard B, Glinoer D, et al: Guidelines for TSH-receptor antibody measurements in pregnancy; results of an evidence-based symposium organized by the European Thyroid Association. Eur J Endocrinol 1998;139:584–586.

circumference are illustrated in Figure 22–1.[17] Other sonographic features of hyperthyroidism include fetal tachycardia, intrauterine growth restriction (IUGR), and hydrops fetalis.[13,16] Of six cases of fetal or neonatal thyrotoxicosis reported by Peleg and associates,[13] five had tachycardia, one of which was IUGR, and one had hydrops. Thyroid measurements were not made.

Serial fetal ultrasonography is generally recommended in women with hyperthyroidism.[18] Assessment of fetal heart rate, fetal growth, and thyroid size every 4 to 6 weeks is reasonable although more frequent scans may be prudent in women with high TSI. A recent study by Cohen and associates[19] suggests this approach does allow early detection of enlarged fetal thyroid (Fig. 22–2). Magnetic resonance imaging (MRI) has also been used to assess fetal thyroid size with a diffuse goiter showing homogeneously elevated signal on T_1-weighted images.[20] It remains to be determined whether MRI is more sensitive than ultrasound.

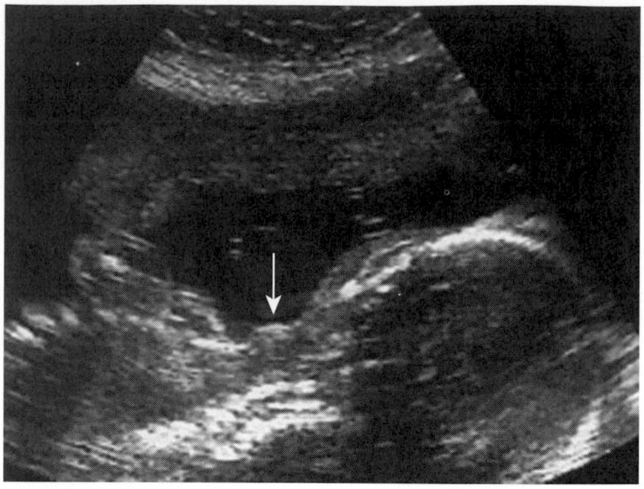

FIGURE 22–2
Sagittal scan of fetal neck at 24 weeks' gestation in woman with Graves' disease on propylthiouracil 1050 mg/week (FT_4 18.4 pmol/L, TSH 0 mU/mL). Arrow indicates enlarged fetal thyroid. (From Cohen O, Pinhas-Hamiel O, Sivan E, et al: Serial in utero ultrasonographic measurements of the fetal thyroid: A new complementary tool in the management of maternal hyperthyroidism in pregnancy. Prenat Diagn 2003;23:740–742.)

FETAL THYROID FUNCTION TESTS

Amniotic fluid thyroid hormone concentrations do not reliably predict fetal thyroid status.[21] Fetal blood sampling is the only method of directly assessing thyroid function.[3] TSH concentrations are low in fetal hyperthyroidism.[16] Cordocentesis is clearly justified in women with Graves' disease when there is evidence of fetal involvement (goiter, tachycardia, IUGR). Unclear is the role of cordocentesis in women with high TSI, in the abscence of other fetal ultrasonographic abnormalities.[7] In a series of nine women with Graves' disease undergoing cordocentesis, three of four fetuses with sonographic evidence of fetal involvement had abnormal thyroid function (one hyperthyroid and two hypothyroid) while only one of nine with "high" TSI (defined as bioassay levels of >160% or immunoassay levels >10 U/L) was hyperthyroid. This experience, though, is by no means uniform. Kilpatrick offered criteria for cordocentesis, which seem reasonable[22] (Table 22–3) if one assumes that either fetal hyperthyroidism or hypothyroidism (secondary to maternal antithyroid drug treatment) reliably results in sonographic abnormalities, or that fetal hypothyroidism will be compensated for by maternal transfer of hormone, and fetal hyperthyroidism not detectable by ultrasound has no morbidity. The evidence supporting these assumptions is weak.

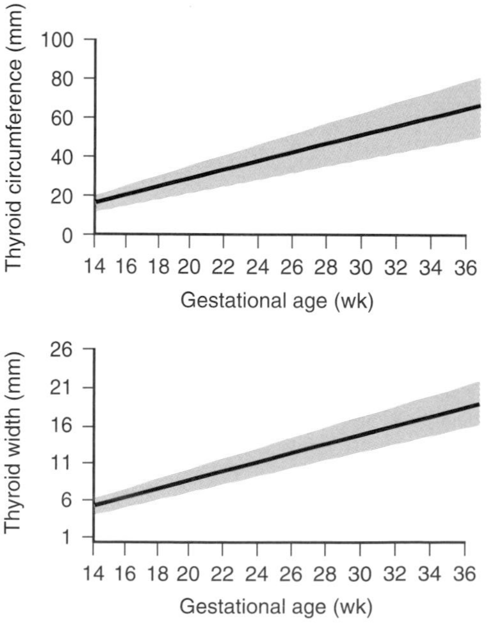

FIGURE 22–1
Ultrasound measurements of fetal thyroid circumference and width. Data are mean and 95% confidence limits based on 193 normal fetuses. (From Achiron R, Rotstein Z, Lipitz S, et al: The development of the foetal thyroid: In utero ultrasonographic measurements. Clin Endocrinol 1998;48:259–264.)

Risks

Perinatal risks of fetal hyperthyroidism include IUGR, hydrops, hydramnios, preterm delivery, and malpresentation. Overt neonatal thyrotoxicosis is associated with tachycardia, tachypnea, flushing, difficulty in feeding,

TABLE 22–3

Indications for Offering Fetal Blood Sampling and Measurement of Fetal FT_4 and TSH in Graves' Disease

1. Previously affected baby
2. History of maternal ^{131}I therapy and a high TSI level
3. Fetal tachycardia, growth restriction, goiter, hydrops, or cardiomegaly

TSH, thyroid-stimulating hormone; TSI, thyroid-stimulating immunoglobulin.

hyperirritability, and poor weight gain. There may be associated jaundice, hepatosplenomegaly, and a bleeding tendency due to thrombocytopenia and low prothrombin levels.[1] The half-life of antithyroid drugs in the neonate is shorter than the maternal immunoglobulin, and therefore, symptoms of neonatal thyrotoxicosis may not present until 5 to 10 days of age.

Early studies of perinatal thyrotoxicosis reported mortality rates up to 50%,[23] but more recent studies incorporating current standards of maternal and fetal surveillance suggest the risks are lower. In severely affected babies, mortality rate may still be as high as 25% due to cardiac arrhythmia or high output failure.[1] Autopsy findings include wasting, visceromegaly, pulmonary hypertension, and generalized adenopathy. Long-term sequelae include craniosynostosis and neurodevelopmental impairment.[24]

FETAL RISKS OF MATERNAL AND FETAL HYPERTHYROIDISM

The prognosis for mother and fetus is excellent for women who either become pregnant while their thyrotoxicosis is under control or in whom the condition is diagnosed and treated early.[6] However, untreated or poorly controlled maternal hyperthyroidism is associated with serious maternal and fetal sequelae. Most studies report increased early pregnancy loss[6] that may be partly explained by an increased incidence of structural and chromosomal abnormalities.[10,25] Heart failure occurs in up to 60% of untreated mothers and is often precipitated by an obstetric event (e.g., hemorrhage, sepsis, or hypertension).[26]

Maternal hyperthyroidism is associated with increased risks of IUGR and preeclampsia.[27–29] In one large study, the odds ratios (95% confidence intervals) in uncontrolled women were 9.2 (5.4–15.6) and 4.7 (1.1–19.7), respectively. Preterm delivery occurred in 33% (OR 16.5 [2.1–130]) while IUGR was present in 12% (OR 2.2 [0.4–11.5]).[28] Interestingly, the risk of IUGR was also doubled (OR 2.4 [1.4–4.1]) in women controlled during pregnancy (i.e., hyperthyroid at presentation but euthyroid at delivery). As a result, perinatal mortality rates as high as 37% are reported for uncontrolled maternal thyrotoxicosis, although more recent studies indicate much lower rates.[27–29] Thyrotoxicosis for 30 weeks or more of pregnancy, Graves' disease for 10 years or longer, onset of Graves' disease before 20 years of age, or a high TBII at delivery (>30%) are each associated with an increased risk of IUGR.[10] It is likely that the adverse outcomes associated with maternal Graves' disease reflect a combination of maternal and fetal hyperthyroidism.

Management Options (See also Chapter 46)

MATERNAL THIONAMIDE THERAPY

Treatment of fetal and maternal hyperthyroidism involves the use of antithyroid therapy. Effective treatment of maternal hyperthyroidism is associated with improved maternal and fetal outcomes.[10,19,28] Therapy ideally should be initiated before pregnancy. Women who remain euthyroid throughout gestation are not at increased risk of preeclampsia, preterm delivery, or IUGR.[28] However, neonatal complications are higher than in control subjects when euthyroidism is achieved only at the end of pregnancy.[28]

The thionamides inhibit the synthesis of thyroid hormone by preventing iodination of the tyrosine molecule. Propylthiouracil (PTU) and methimazole are widely used in the United States. Carbimazole, which is metabolized to methimazole, is popular in other countries. PTU has the advantage of crossing the placenta more slowly than carbimazole and methimazole.[30] Further, carbimazole and methimazole use are both associated with fetal scalp defects (aplasia cutis).[31] However, the incidence of major congenital malformations is comparable in offspring of women taking PTU and methimazole (2% to 3%),[32] and there is no evidence the use of PTU reduces the incidence of neonatal hyperthyroidism.[33] Umbilical cord FT_4 is low in 6% to 7% and TSH is elevated in 14% to 21% of women on thionamides.[33]

Carbimazole and methimazole are readily excreted in breast milk, achieving a milk-plasma ratio approaching unity. In contrast, PTU, which is highly bound by plasma proteins, is poorly excreted, with concentrations in milk approximating 10% of maternal serum.[34] Thus, PTU is the drug of choice in breastfeeding mothers and should be taken just after breastfeeding, allowing a 3- to 4-hour interval before feeding again.

In newly diagnosed cases of maternal hyperthyroidism, the initial dose of PTU is usually 150 mg every 8 hours. The equivalent dose of carbimazole is 20 mg twice daily. Clinical and biochemical improvement is usually evident after 2 to 4 weeks, although the fetal response may take longer. The dose should be halved once the maternal symptoms have improved and thyroid function is within normal range. Further reductions are possible because of the tendency of Graves' disease to ameliorate during the third trimester, and it is usually possible to reach a maintenance dose of 150 mg/day or less of PTU (or 15 mg/day or less of carbimazole). Side effects include nausea, arthralgia, skin rash, metallic taste, and fever. Leukopenia, agranulocytosis, and hepatitis can also occur. It is important to recognize that maternal euthyroidism does not mean the fetus is euthyroid.

Combined blocking-replacement regimens have been advocated, but there is no evidence they reduce the risk of fetal hypothyroidism, presumably because transplacental passage of T_4 is limited, and the maternal requirement for thionamides may increase.[35]

SURGERY

Subtotal thyroidectomy can successfully be performed during pregnancy. Maternal thyrotoxicosis must be adequately controlled preoperatively, which is most rapidly achieved with beta-blocking agents and iodide. Surgical complications include hemorrhage, recurrent laryngeal nerve palsy, hypoparathyroidism, and hypothyroidism. Although the incidence of complications is low in experienced hands, surgery is usually reserved for women who are allergic to antithyroid drugs or when adequate biochemical control cannot be attained with medical therapy. The optimal time for surgery is during the second trimester. Radioiodine is contraindicated in pregnancy, particularly after the 12th week of gestation when the fetal thyroid is able to concentrate iodine.[6] Inadvertent administration of ^{131}I in the first trimester causes perinatal hypothyroidism in 3%.[36]

MONITORING THIONAMIDE TREATMENT

Once control is achieved, the aim of therapy is to keep the mother and fetus euthyroid using the minimum amount of thionamide. Maternal thyroid function should be monitored every 4 weeks, aiming to keep the FT_4 at the upper end of the normal range. Although there is a correlation between maternal and umbilical cord FT_4 levels, normal maternal FT_4 levels do not preclude fetal hypothyroidism.[25] If the mother remains euthyroid despite a small dose of PTU (50–100 mg) or methimazole (5–10 mg), therapy should be discontinued. This may be possible in up to 30% of patients after 32 weeks.[6]

The effects of thionamides on fetal thyroid function are sometimes unpredictable and dose-independent. Correlation between maternal and fetal thyroid function is poor and in one series of 11 consecutive pregnancies, six fetuses were hyperthyroid and five were hypothyroid when the mother was euthyroid on stable drug therapy (Weiner C, personal communication). Accurate differentiation of thionamide-induced hypothyroidism from TSI-induced hyperthyroidism requires measurement of fetal FT_4 and TSH. Measurement of fetal thyroid function has also been used to modify the dose of thionamide.[37]

Fetal heart rate alone is unreliable for the detection of thyroid dysfunction; thionamide-induced hypothyroidism and TSI-induced hyperthyroidism may both occur in the absence of tachycardia.[7,38] In contrast, serial measurement of the fetal thyroid may allow early detection of thyroid dysfunction.[19,37] Cohen and associates[19] measured the thyroid in 20 women with Graves' disease on PTU (1050 mg/wk). Thyroid width and circumference were above the 95% percentiles in five fetuses; in three the thyroid size decreased concurrently with a decrease in maternal thionamide dosage and all were euthyroid at birth. In two fetuses, thyroid size was unaffected by a decrement in maternal PTU dose and both had thyrotoxicosis at birth. However, the variability of fetal thyroid measurements is unknown. This point is important because the absolute change in fetal thyroid size after a reduction in PTU was small. It remains to be determined whether serial ultrasound measurements can replace cordocentesis for monitoring thionamide dosage. Until these findings are confirmed in larger series, fetal thyroid status should be determined by cordocentesis when there is evidence of thyroid dysfunction, and umbilical cord blood obtained at birth for FT_4 and TSH levels. It is helpful to screen for TSI if these have not been measured previously.

SUMMARY OF MANAGEMENT OPTIONS

Fetal Hyperthyroidism

Management Options	Quality of Evidence	Strength of Recommendation	References
Prepregnancy			
Consider measurement of TSH-receptor immunoglobulins (TBII and TSI) in women with known autoimmune thyroid disease.	–	GPP	–
Check maternal thyroid function tests (TSH and FT_4) and optimize thionamide therapy.	III	B	28
Consider changing to propylthiouracil in preference to carbimazole/methimazole.	IIb	B	30
Prenatal			
Monitor maternal thyroid function tests every 4–6 weeks; aim to keep FT_4 at the upper end of the normal range on the minimum dose of thionamide.	–	GPP	–
Measure TSH-receptor immunoglobulins in women with Graves' disease who have previously received radioiodine therapy or undergone thyroid surgery or are taking antithyroid drugs to keep thyroid function normal.	III	B	11

SUMMARY OF MANAGEMENT OPTIONS

Fetal Hyperthyroidism *(Continued)*

Management Options	Quality of Evidence	Strength of Recommendation	References
Prenatal *(Continued)*			
Sonographic fetal surveillance every 4–6 weeks (more frequently in women with high thyroid-stimulating immunoglobulins) after 24 weeks looking for:	III	B	28
Goiter			
Cardiac hypertrophy			
Fetal tachycardia			
Growth restriction			
Hydrops			
Oligohydramnios			
Polyhydramnios			
Measure fetal thyroid function (TSH and FT_4) by fetal blood sampling if persistent tachycardia or goiter (poor correlation between maternal and fetal thyroid function tests) is found.	IV	C	38
If fetal hyperthyroidism is confirmed, adjust maternal thionamide dose to optimize maternal control.	III	B	29
Consider maternal beta-blockers if fetal tachycardia persists.	IV	C	108
Fetal thyroid assessment can be followed with color Doppler showing reduced vascularization under appropriate therapy.	IV	C	107
Postnatal			
Measure FT_4 and TSH in cord blood and at 7 days of age, and manage appropriately.	–	GPP	–
Give propylthiouracil if breastfeeding; Ensure that medication is taken immediately after feeding.	IIa	B	34

FETAL HYPOTHYROIDISM

Etiology (Table 22–1)

Congenital hypothyroidism occurs once in every 2500 to 4000 live births in nonendemic areas.[39,40] The condition can be permanent or transient. The most common cause of permanent hypothyroidism is thyroid dysgenesis, accounting for 80% to 90% of cases.[18] This term includes thyroid aplasia (40%), thyroid hypoplasia (20%), and ectopic thyroid (40%). Most cases are sporadic, nonfamilial embryologic defects, although familial cases are reported.[41]

Inborn defects of thyroid hormone synthesis and secretion (dyshormonogenesis) include iodine transport defects, organification defects, iodotyrosine deiodinase deficiency, and thyroglobulin abnormalities, all of which are inherited as autosomal recessive traits. Affected fetuses can develop large goiters. Thyroid dyshormonogenesis occurs in 1 in 40,000 births.[41]

Hypothalamic-pituitary disorders are associated with major and minor midline defects, including holoprosencephaly and septo-optic dysplasia, or with autosomal recessive genetic defects, including Pit-1 deficiency. These disorders, together with mutations in the TSH receptor and thyroid hormone resistance (due to mutations in the thyroid hormone receptor), have a prevalence of 1 in 60,000 to 1 in 100,000 births.[41]

TSH receptor immunoglobulins are responsible for about 2% of congenital hypothyroidism.[42] Reduced T_4 levels are transient and are more likely to be found in infants of women with high TBI levels.[43,44] Inadequate treatment of maternal Graves' disease is also associated with central congenital hypothyroidism (estimated prevalence 1/35,000).[45] The neonates have low FT_4 but variable TSH levels; TRH testing indicates pituitary dysfunction. It is suggested that a hyperthyroid fetal environment impairs maturation of the fetal hypothalamic-pituitary-thyroid axis.[45] The common thyroid autoantibodies (thyroperoxidase and antithyroglobulin), present in women with Hashimoto's thyroiditis, have little or no effect on fetal thyroid function.

Transient hypothyroidism may follow maternal administration of antithyroid drugs. In the series of 18 cases of maternal Graves' disease treated with PTU, Nachum and associates[7] observed that 4 (22%) developed fetal hypothyroidism, even with doses as low as 50 to 100 mg/day.[7] Hypothyroidism is also reported after maternal use of amiodarone and lithium, and after excessive maternal iodide intake. Inadvertent administration of radioiodine after 12 weeks' gestation invariably results in permanent fetal hypothyroidism.

All preterm infants have a fall in FT_4 during the first 2 weeks of life with a recovery to expected values by the third or fourth week.[46] Levels of FT_4 approximate 50% of those in utero, with around one-third of preterm neonates having T_4 levels greater than 3 SD below the term neonatal mean.[46] Acutely ill infants may also have lower levels of FT_4 and FT_3 due to decreased peripheral conversion. Hypoxic IUGR fetuses also have low FT_4 and FT_3 levels associated with a slightly elevated in TSH.[47] The contribution of early thyroid hormone deficiency to neurodevelopmental delay in these children is unclear.

Worldwide iodine deficiency is the most common cause of combined maternal-fetal hypothyroidism. Iodine deficiency leads to deficient thyroid hormone production, TSH hypersecretion and increased iodide trapping with goiter and a raised T_3:T_4 ratio. Such compensatory mechanisms can result in euthyroidism with goiter or varying degrees of goitrous hypothyroidism.[1] The problem is still common in some areas of Europe, Scandinavia, and the Middle East. In Zaire, where iodide intake is below 25 μg/day (recommended intake 200 μg/day), the frequency of fetal hypothyroidism, as evidenced by an elevated TSH at birth, is as high as 25%.[48]

In some areas of severe iodine deficiency, infants are born with endemic or neurologic cretinism characterized by severe mental retardation, deafness, squint, pyramidal signs, and extrapyramidal signs. These infants are euthyroid but frequently have a goiter. In other areas, notably Africa, the infants have hypothyroid cretinism with grossly impaired thyroid function, dwarfism, and delayed sexual maturation, but rarely a goiter. Variations in dietary ingestion of goitrogens, which inhibit thyroid function, and coexistent selenium deficiency are thought to account for the different phenotypes.[49]

Presentation and Diagnosis

Fetal hypothyroidism is usually unrecognized. The condition may be suspected because of a maternal history of thyroid disease or antithyroid medication. Features include IUGR, goiter, and reduced fetal movements. An abnormal fetal heart rate may occur, with both bradycardia and tachycardia reported.[8] In severe cases, there may be delayed skeletal development, congenital heart block, and cardiomegaly.[50] Malformations are reported in 8% of infants with hypothyroidism; 28% of these malformations are cardiac abnormalities.[51]

The classic neonatal features of congenital hypothyroidism are constipation, lethargy, poor feeding, and respiratory problems. Physical signs include macroglossia, dry mottled skin, "cretinoid" facies, abnormal cry, prolonged jaundice, enlarged fontanels, umbilical hernia, and mental retardation. Depending on the cause and severity, clinical features may be apparent for several weeks or months after birth.

MATERNAL THYROID FUNCTION AND IMMUNOGLOBULIN TESTS

Most women with known hypothyroidism have a history of thyroid disease that was either treated surgically or by radioiodine, and will be on thyroxine replacement. Women presenting with features of hypothyroidism in pregnancy (malaise, cold intolerance, dry skin, myalgia, excessive weight gain) often have discontinued or reduced their thyroxine intake. However, the symptoms may be subtle and a goiter may not be palpable. An elevated TSH and a reduced FT_4 confirm the diagnosis of maternal hypothyroidism. Women with Graves' disease previously treated with radioiodine or surgery should have their TSH-receptor immunoglobulins measured early in pregnancy[11] (Table 22–2).

FETAL ULTRASONOGRAPHY

Hypothyroidism is suspected if there is IUGR, reduced fetal movements, or an abnormal fetal heart rate. Unfortunately, and analogous to the sonographic findings associated with hyperthyroidism, none of these features are very sensitive.[7] Ultrasonic evidence of a fetal goiter suggests severe thyroid dysfunction. However, the majority of cases reflect sporadic, embryologic malformations not detectable by ultrasound. Serial ultrasound screening may detect a large goiter when there is a family history of congenital hypothyroidism due to a defect in thyroid hormone synthesis or metabolism.

FETAL THYROID FUNCTION TESTS

Definitive antenatal diagnosis requires fetal blood sampling and confirmation of an elevated TSH and low FT_4. Reported values of TSH in fetuses with goiter have ranged from 25 to 1640 mU/L,[52,53] but the development of a goiter or hydramnios does not closely correlate with the degree of fetal hypothyroidism.[7,53] In many countries, all newborns are screened for congenital hypothyroidism by the measurement of TSH on a blood spot.

Risks

In instances of congenital hypothyroidism, fetal thyroid hormone supply is deficient to varying degrees in utero and during early infancy. Transplacental passage of maternal thyroid hormones, along with compensatory deiodinase activity, ensure thyroid hormone sufficiency during the first half of pregnancy. However, the fetal contribution is reduced or totally lacking in the second half of gestation, and hypothyroxinemia persists until the diagnosis is made and treatment takes effect. As a result, children with congenital hypothyroidism manifest neuropsychological deficits with a mean IQ that is significantly lower than in control subjects, even with optimal neonatal thyroxine supplementation.[54] Infants with severe congenital hypothyroidism, particularly those with absent thyroid glands, or who show ultrasonographic or serum evidence of hypothyroidism in utero, have lower IQ scores than those with less severe hypothyroidism.[55-57] Perinatal hypothyroidism appears particularly to contribute to visual-spatial and fine motor weakness.[2] Disparity in performance is evident into adolescence.[2] The majority of athyrotic infants manifest systemic signs such as delayed skeletal maturation.[2]

FETAL RISKS OF MATERNAL HYPOTHYROIDISM (See also Chapter 46)

In iodine-sufficient areas, overt maternal hypothyroidism occurs in 5 to 10 per 1000 pregnancies[2,58] and is usually due to Hashimoto's thyroiditis or previous thyroid surgery. Subclinical hypothyroidism (normal FT_4 but elevated TSH) is reported in up to 2.5% of pregnancies,[59,60] and in areas of endemic iodine deficiency the incidence is even higher. Although thyroid hormone levels return to normal within 10 weeks in two-thirds of cases,[59] damage to the fetal CNS may already have occurred.

The rate of miscarriage is increased approximately twofold in women with overt hypothyroidism. This risk appears related more to the presence of circulating thyroid antibodies than thyroid function.[58] Recent reports do not reveal an increased rate of congenital anomalies.[58] Gestational hypertension, preeclampsia, and placental abruption are purportedly more common leading to an increased rate of preterm delivery.[60,61–63] Stillbirth rates range from 4% to 13%,[61,62] and severe maternal hypothyroidism in early pregnancy was in one study associated with a 56% rate of intrapartum cesarean section for fetal distress.[64] The risk appears related to the deficiency as the rate of adverse outcome improves with early therapy.[64]

Infants born to women who remain hypothyroid throughout pregnancy are at increased risk of neurologic impairment. Man and associates[65] initially reported that the mean IQ at 7 years of age was 13 points lower in children born to women who were hypothyroid during pregnancy compared to those born to women who were euthyroid on T_4 replacement. Several subsequent studies (reviewed by Chan and Rovet[2]) have reported on the effects of maternal hypothyroidism on offspring neurodevelopment. Klein and associates[66] initially measured maternal TSH levels at 15 to 18 weeks' gestation (from frozen samples obtained for Down syndrome screening) and found 2.5% had elevated TSH levels (≥6 mU/L), of which 12% (6 of 49) also had low FT_4 levels. Children of mothers who were hypothyroid scored lower than control subjects on all 15 of the neuropsychological tests and attained an average IQ that was 4 points below control subjects.[67] Children of untreated women performed less well than children of biochemically hypothyroid women who received T_4 treatment (albeit inadequate) during pregnancy.[67] The severity of maternal hypothyroidism, as assessed by TSH concentration, correlates with offspring IQ; in mothers with TSH concentrations below the 98th, 98th to 99. 85th, and above the 99. 85th percentiles, mean IQ at 8 years of age was reported to be 107, 102, and 97 respectively with the percentage of children with IQ above 1 SD below the control mean being 15%, 21%, and 50%.[68] The children of euthyroid women with increased thyroperoxidase autoantibodies are reported to have lower IQs than children of antibody-negative women.[69]

Evidence is accumulating that the key factor influencing neuropsychological development of the fetus is first trimester hypothyroxinemia, whether or not TSH is increased.[70] This is a consequence of decreased availability of maternal T_4 to the developing brain, its only source during the first trimester. Normal maternal T_3 concentrations do not appear to prevent the potential damage of a low supply of T_4, although they may prevent an increase in TSH (and detection of the hypothyroxinemia if only TSH is measured).[70] Pop and associates[71] reported recently that children of women with a FT_4 below the 10th percentile and a normal TSH (0.15–2.0 mIU/L) at 12 weeks' gestation had delayed mental and motor function (mean deficit of 8–10 points on Bayley scales of infant development) at 2 years of age compared to control subjects (FT_4 between 50th and 90th percentiles). However, the children had a lower risk of later impairment when FT_4 concentrations increased during pregnancy (at 24 and 32 weeks) in women hypothyroxinemic during early gestation.

As the body of information grows concerning the detrimental and long-term effects of maternal hypothyroidism on the fetus, many authorities have advocated screening all women as early as possible in pregnancy.[70] However, it is not certain whether FT_4 or TSH should be used, what cutoff point to adopt, nor what treatment should be instituted for screen positive women.[2] Ultimately the value of screening and treating mildly hypothyroid women in nonendemic areas can only be addressed in large trials with adequate follow-up.

Management Options

FETAL THERAPY

Fetal therapy is indicated in cases with confirmed fetal hypothyroidism because of the risk of neurologic damage. Direct fetal therapy is necessary because relatively little T_4 crosses the placenta, and the amount of T_4 needed to treat the fetus adequately would cause maternal hyperthyroidism. Van Herle and associates[72] reported fortnightly fetal intramuscular T_4 injections because the mother received radioiodine early in pregnancy. The fetus was severely hypothyroid at birth.

Weiner and associates[73] reported the first use of intra-amniotic T_4 in the treatment of fetal goiter. Subsequent reports confirm the effectiveness of this mode of administration with reduction in goiter size, resolution of hydramnios, and improvement in fetal thyroid function.[7,37,52] A weekly dose of 250 μg appears to be effective. This is consistent with the neonatal T_4 requirement of 10 μg/day and animal data suggesting that 90% of T_4 administered intra-amniotically is absorbed within 24 hours.[74] Whether this is the optimal dose and frequency is unclear, and larger doses (500–600 μg) given every 14 days may be as effective.[7,53] Fetal therapy should be started as early as possible once the diagnosis of fetal hypothyroidism is made.

In 2002 Agrawal and associates[75] reported the use of intra-amniotic T_3 (60–120 μg) and T_4 (150 μg) in a hypothyroid fetus with goiter and symptomatic hydramnios. They reasoned the more rapid onset of action of T_3 (4–8 hours) and its more potent effects compared to T_4, make it more suitable for "acute" management. However, more frequent intra-amniotic injections are needed because of its shorter half-life (1–2 days) compared to T_4 (6–7 days). Further research is needed to determine the value of combined therapy.

Repeat fetal blood sampling 1 to 2 weeks after starting therapy is justified to confirm that TSH and FT_4 have returned to normal.[37,76] Repeat sampling is particularly important if there is worsening of the fetal condition, failure of the goiter to resolve, or the development of hydramnios.[18,76] In women with Graves' disease and fetal hypothyroidism, assessing the fetal response to a reduction in maternal antithyroid therapy may be appropriate before considering direct fetal therapy.[7]

A possible noninvasive alternative to treat fetal hypothyroidism is maternal administration of 3′-triiodothyroacetic acid (Triac), a T_3-derived analogue that binds to thyroid hormone receptors with higher affinity than T_3. Triac crosses the placenta[77] and was used with apparent success to reduce TSH concentrations and goiter size in fetal hypothyroidism secondary to PTU therapy[53,77] and to reduce TSH concentrations in a fetus affected by a mutation in thyroid hormone receptor beta gene leading to resistance to thyroid hormones.[78] In both case reports, Triac was increased from a starting dose of 2.1 mg/day to 2.8 mg/day[53] and 3.5 mg/day,[78] respectively, in an attempt to normalize fetal TSH levels. Further experience is needed before this therapy can be recommended as a safe alternative to invasive therapy.

MATERNAL THERAPY (See also Chapter 46)

Most women with hypothyroidism already take T_4 prior to pregnancy. Adequate T_4 replacement eliminates or reduces the risk of an adverse pregnancy outcome. The serum FT_4 level should be kept at the upper normal range, necessitating increased T_4 in up to 75% of patients, usually during the first trimester.[79] Average T_4 requirements are increased by 25 to 100 μg/day during pregnancy.[79,80] However, the maternal dose should not be increased without objective proof of need. Maternal TSH and FT_4 should be measured at booking for prenatal care, at 16 to 20 weeks, and at 28 to 32 weeks (although it has been suggested that repeat testing is not necessary unless clinically indicated[81]). Ferrous sulfate reduces thyroxine absorption and ingestion of these drugs should be separated by at least 2 hours. After pregnancy, thyroxine is reduced to the prepregnancy dose. It is safe for women taking T_4 to breastfeed.

In cases of severe iodine deficiency, supplementation during pregnancy prevents the occurrence of hypothyroid cretinism and neonatal hypothyroidism, increases birth weight, reduces the chances of neonatal death, and improves developmental quotients.[48] Iodine can be given in the form of iodized salt, potassium iodide drips, or iodized oil.

NEONATAL THERAPY

Infants confirmed after screening to be hypothyroid should immediately be started on replacement thyroxine (10–15 μg/kg orally once daily). The dose is adjusted after 4 weeks according to the clinical response and serum T_4.[1] TSH often remains high in the presence of adequate replacement and normal T_4 levels. Therefore, TSH levels are not a useful guide to treatment.[1] Serum T_4 should be rechecked, and the dose of thyroxine adjusted, at 3 months, 6 months, and annually thereafter. The response to treatment varies with the etiology; athyrotic infants take longer to normalize their thyroid function and probably should be monitored more frequently in early life.[82]

Much attention has focused on the starting dose of thyroxine. One nonrandomized study indicated higher full scale and verbal IQ results at 7 to 8 years on the standard dose compared with lower doses, but treatment in the higher dose group was begun earlier.[83] In a recent study from Norway, young adults (mean age 20 years) with congenital hypothyroidism had lower scores than their sibling controls on intellectual, motor, and school-associated tests.[84] The initial thyroxine dose predicted their verbal IQ scores. Several studies investigated the value of higher starting doses of thyroxine on outcome, but the evidence currently for an effect on cognitive development, growth, or behavior is too weak to justify recommending a high or standard dose regimen.[85]

SUMMARY OF MANAGEMENT OPTIONS
Fetal Hypothyroidism

Management Options	Quality of Evidence	Strength of Recommendation	References
Prepregnancy			
Genetic counseling is needed if previous inborn errors of thyroid hormone biosynthesis that result in dyshormonogenesis.	III	B	39
Iodine supplementation is recommended in areas of iodine deficiency	IV	C	48

SUMMARY OF MANAGEMENT OPTIONS

Fetal Hypothyroidism *(Continued)*

Management Options	Quality of Evidence	Strength of Recommendation	References
Prepregnancy *(Continued)*			
In women with known hypothyroidism, check maternal TSH and FT_4 and optimize thyroxine replacement.	III	B	79,80
Prenatal			
In at-risk fetus, sonographic surveillance should look for:	IIb	B	7
Reduced movements			
Cardiomegaly			
Bradycardia; heart block			
Growth restriction			
Goiter			
Polyhydramnios			
Amniotic fluid thyroxine concentration does not correlate with fetal serum thyroxine.	IIb	B	7,53
Measure fetal TSH and FT_4 by fetal blood sampling if there is goiter or if there is growth restriction with bradycardia or reduced fetal movements in a fetus at risk.	IIb	B	7,37,52
If fetal hypothyroidism is confirmed, measure intra-amniotic T_4 with confirmation of response by repeat fetal blood sampling.	IIb	B	7,37,52,73,76
Reappraise T_4 replacement dose with TSH and FT_4 levels in women with hypothyroidism at booking and once during the second and third trimesters.	III	B	79,80
Postnatal			
Measure free T_4 and TSH in cord blood in at-risk fetuses.	–	GPP	–
Replace thyroxine to infants confirmed to be hypothyroid.	IV	C	1
When necessary, reduce maternal dose of T_4 to prepregnancy levels.	III	B	80
Sequelae of congenital hypothyroidism, including intellectual impairment, can be prevented with prompt treatment.	III	B	39,82

FETAL ADRENAL DISEASE

Fetal Adrenal Function

The adrenal cortex arises from the mesoderm of the mesonephros during the fifth week of embryonic development. The cells that form the medulla are derived from adjacent neural crest cells and come to be encapsulated by the fetal cortex, which rapidly increases in size from the end of the second trimester to occupy 80% of the adrenal cortex by term. The adult (or definitive) cortex, also derived from mesenchymal cells, forms a thin outer layer.

All adrenal steroids are formed from cholesterol (Fig. 22–3). In the zona fasciculate of the definitive cortex, steroid precursors are used to synthesize cortisol under the influence of 17α-hydroxylase. Fetal cortisol concentrations rise, particularly toward term, stimulating the maturation of several enzyme systems in the lungs and gastrointestinal tract. Glucocorticoid synthesis is under the control of pituitary adrenocorticotropic hormone (ACTH). Both hypothalamic corticotropin-releasing hormone (CRH) and AVP stimulate the release of ACTH, which is cleaved from a large prohormone pro-opiomelanocortin (POMC) containing the sequences of several other peptide hormones. 17α-Hydroxylase is inactive in the zona glomerulosa, and precursors are used to synthesize aldosterone under the control of the renin-angiotensin system. Adrenal androgen production is insignificant during fetal life.

The fetal adrenal gland provides precursors for maternal estrogen production. The cortex contains inactivated 3β-hydroxysteroid dehydrogenase. Therefore, pregnenolone is converted primarily into dehydroepiandrosterone sulfate (DHEAS), which appears in the fetal circulation from 8 weeks. DHEAS is hydroxylated in other fetal tissues, particularly the liver, to 16-hydroxy-DHEAS,

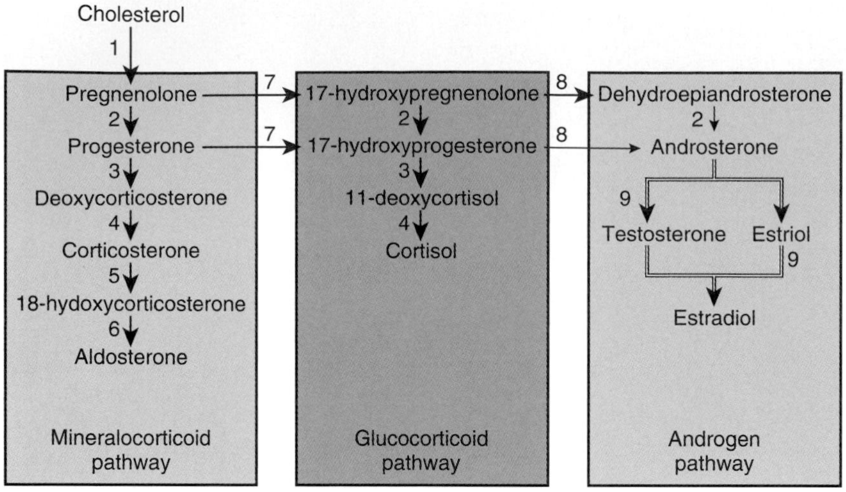

FIGURE 22–3
Pathways of adrenal hormone synthesis. Major pathways are indicated by thick arrows, minor ones by thin arrows. Extra-adrenal conversion of sex steroids is denoted by double arrows. Numbers indicate enzymatic steps as follows: 1, Cholesterol side chain cleaving system; 2, 3β-hydroxysteroid dehydrogenase; 3, 21-hydroxylase; 4, 11β-hydroxylase; 5, 18-hydroxylase; 6, 18-dehydrogenase; 7, 17α-hydroxylase; 8, 17,20-lyase; 9, 17β-hydroxysteroid dehydrogenase.

which then passes to the placenta, where it is converted into androstenedione and subsequently to estrogens.

CONGENITAL ADRENAL HYPERPLASIA

Etiology

Congenital adrenal hyperplasia (CAH) refers to a group of autosomal recessive disorders of adrenal steroidogenesis. The disorder may result from a defect in any of the five enzymes required to synthesize cortisol from cholesterol.

21-HYDROXYLASE (P450C21) DEFICIENCY

In 90% to 95% of cases, CAH is due to deficiency of 21-hydroxylase (21-OH), resulting in a blockade of the conversion of 17-hydroxyprogesterone into 11-deoxycortisol (see Fig. 22–3). Reduced synthesis of cortisol leads to increased ACTH and shunting of precursors into the pathways of androgen synthesis. A spectrum of phenotypes occurs: a severe form with a concurrent defect in aldosterone synthesis (salt-wasting type) and a simple virilizing form with apparently normal aldosterone synthesis. These two forms are responsible for classic CAH, which has a prevalence of approximately 1 in 15,000 whites.[86] There is also a mild, nonclassic form that may be asymptomatic or associated with signs of androgen excess.

Mutations in the *CYP21* (*CYP21A2*) gene, located in the polymorphic HLA histocompatibility complex on chromosome 6p21.3, along with a pseudogene, *CYP21P* (*CYP21A1P*), are responsible for CAH. The high degree of nucleotide sequence identity (98%) between *CYP21* and *CYP21P* permits two types of recombination events: (1) unequal crossing-over during meiosis, which results in complete deletions or duplications of *CYP21*, and (2) gene conversion events that transfer deleterious mutations present in the pseudogene to *CYP21*. Deletions generally account for 20% to 25% of classic 21-OH alleles; small deletions and point mutations make up the rest.[86,87] There are correlations between genotype and phenotype. Mutations that totally ablate enzyme activity are associated with the salt-wasting form, and those that produce enzymes with 1% to 2% normal activity, permitting adequate aldosterone synthesis, lead to simple virilizing disease. A third group of mutations produce enzymes retaining 20% to 60% normal activity and are responsible for the nonclassic form.[86]

OTHER FORMS

11β-Hydroxylase ($P450_c11$) deficiency accounts for 5% to 8% of CAH. 11-Deoxycortisol is not converted into cortisol, shunting precursors along the pathway for androgen synthesis. The enzymatic defect also leads to an accumulation of deoxycorticosterone within the aldosterone pathway. A mild, nonclassic form is also described. Two copies of the 11β-hydroxylase gene are present on chromosome 11q, and several mutations are known.[88] Deficiencies of 3β-hydroxysteroid dehydrogenase, 17α-hydroxylase, and cholesterol side chain cleavage enzyme account for less than 1% of CAH cases. Mild or partial defects may occur more frequently.[88]

Presentation and Diagnosis

Around 75% of patients with classic 21-OH deficiency have the salt-wasting form and can present in the early neonatal period with hyponatremic dehydration and shock.[86] Female fetuses with classic 21-OH deficiency are exposed to excess androgens from the seventh week of gestation onward, leading to virilization of the external genitalia ranging from clitoral hypertrophy to complete phallus formation and fusion of the labia (Fig. 22–4), causing erroneous assignment of gender. Affected males have normal external genitalia. Postnatally, androgen excess may manifest as progressive virilizing changes and accelerated growth and development. In the nonclassic form, virilizing symptoms appear postnatally. Females affected with 11β-hydroxylase deficiency also have

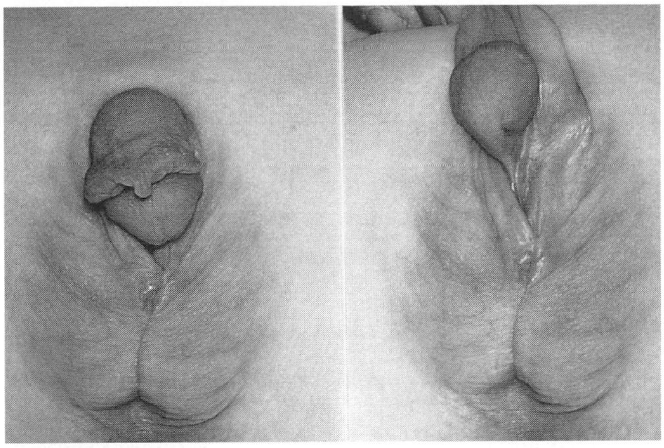

FIGURE 22–4
Severe virilization in two untreated female infants with 21-hydroxylase deficiency. There is almost complete formation of a phallus and scrotum.

ambiguous genitalia at birth. The excess deoxycorticosterone generally leads to hypertension and hypokalemia. Virilization of female fetuses is much less marked in 3β-hydroxysteroid dehydrogenase deficiency and in the other two forms, the male is incompletely masculinized.[88]

The diagnosis of 21-OH deficiency is confirmed by the measurement of neonatal plasma 17α-hydroxyprogesterone (17-OHP), which typically exceeds 10,000 ng/dL (300 nmol/L). Classic 21-OH deficiency is more common than phenylketonuria, and neonatal screening of blood spots is routine in many countries in view of the risks from salt wasting and late diagnosis.[89] Screening in the United Kingdom is generally considered uneconomical.[1] In 11β-hydroxylase deficiency, plasma deoxycorticosterone is elevated. The profile of urinary steroids by gas chromatography and mass spectrometry provides a definitive diagnosis.

Risks

Affected children require lifetime glucocorticoid replacement therapy (10–15 mg/m^2/day in three divided doses). Appropriate replacement will suppress androgen levels and allow normal growth, skeletal maturation, and puberty.[1] Mineralocorticoid replacement (fludrocortisone 0.1–0.2 mg daily) is necessary in salt-losing forms. The majority of female infants born with virilized genitalia require corrective surgery. Half require more than one operation. Clitoral reduction is best undertaken before 6 months of age, but the timing of vaginal reconstructive surgery is controversial. It was often delayed in the past until after puberty, but more recently, single-stage surgery at 2 to 6 months has been advocated.[90] In addition to progressive virilization, high androgens affect the hypothalamic-pituitary-gonadal axis in both sexes, leading to subfertility. Follow-up studies of adult females with CAH diagnosed in infancy or early childhood suggest that one-third are hirsute, and their ovulation rate is less than 50%.[91] After reconstructive surgery, about 75% have an adequate vaginal introitus; and in this group, pregnancy rates approximate 60%.[91] Early treatment with glucocorticoids improves fertility. It is suggested that prenatal exposure to excess androgens affects subsequent sexual behavior in adolescent and adult females.[92]

Management Options

PRENATAL DIAGNOSIS

All affected families should be offered genetic counseling. Ideally, this should be accomplished prior to conception. Subsequent offspring have a 1 in 4 chance of being affected and a 1 in 8 chance of being a virilized female. Prenatal diagnosis was initially accomplished by measuring 17-OHP in amniotic fluid, but is now mostly replaced by direct DNA analysis of the *CYP21* gene. Mutations can be identified in 95% of families by Southern blot analysis and selective amplification of the *CYP21B* gene by PCR followed by allele-specific hybridization with oligonucleotide probes for a panel of common *CYP21B* mutations.[93,94] The most common mutation (33–52%) is on intron 2.[87,93] In some families, direct DNA analysis provides limited information because of gene conversion or rearrangement between *CYP21* and *CYP21P* genes. In this instance, linkage analysis using informative marker loci (microsatellites) provides more comprehensive information.[95] Molecular diagnosis is possible for some families with other forms of CAH. Otherwise, antenatal diagnosis is dependent on the measurement of steroids in the amniotic fluid.[96]

MATERNAL DEXAMETHASONE THERAPY

The fetal adrenal gland can be pharmacologically suppressed by maternal administration of dexamethasone. Synthetic fluorinated steroids are poor substrates for placental 11β-hydroxysteroid dehydrogenase and readily cross the placenta to the fetus, suppressing ACTH. Because the external genitalia begin to differentiate around 7 weeks' gestation, dexamethasone (20 μg/kg prepregnancy weight per day given in three divided doses) should be begun before this time. Compared to their previously affected sisters, treated females have decreased virilization; 25%-50% require no genital surgery, and the extent of genital surgery for those who require it is reduced.[87,93,97] However, therapeutic failures occur[98] (Fig. 22–5), and although some failures are attributed to the late initiation or early cessation of therapy, noncompliance, or suboptimal dosing, there is no obvious explanation in others. The extent of virilization varies among affected females in the same family, even without treatment.[99]

Dexamethasone is discontinued if the fetus is male or an unaffected female (i.e., in seven of eight pregnancies initially treated). The success of therapy is monitored by the measurement of maternal urine estriol and amniotic fluid 17-OHP, though the interpretation can be difficult[100] and increasing the dose of dexamethasone can lead to side effects. Excessive weight gain, cutaneous striae, edema, hirsutism, and mood fluctuations are most com-

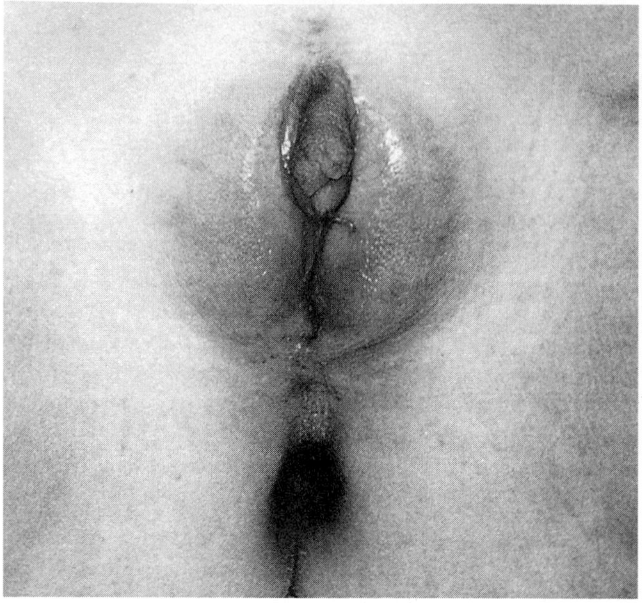

FIGURE 22–5
Partial virilization in a female infant with 21-hydroxylase deficiency treated prenatally with dexamethasone from 8 weeks' gestation. There is clitoromegaly with posterior labial fusion.

mon.[87,93] Hypertension and gestational diabetes develop in 15% and 8% of women, respectively.[87] Overall, side effects necessitate a reduction in the dexamethasone dose in up to 25% of women.[97] It is also reported that the dose of dexamethasone can be reduced later in pregnancy (to 5 µg/kg/day) and still maintain fetal and maternal adrenal suppression, as evidenced by urinary estriol and cortisol metabolites. The efficacy of this regimen in preventing virilization remains to be determined.[101]

Although the long-term safety of prenatal treatment remains uncertain, it is encouraging that no teratogenic effects are reported in fetuses treated to term with dexamethasone.[87] The administration of low doses of glucocorticoids to children has been reported to delay growth and cause diabetes and hypertension. Follow-up studies of prenatally treated CAH children suggest that growth and development are normal. However, the numbers are small and the duration of follow-up limited.[87,97] Concerns remain about the long-term implications of antenatal therapy with respect to hypertension and psychosexual/behavioral development. One small study suggested that although dexamethasone-treated children have cognitive abilities comparable to unexposed children, they have more behavior problems at 2 to 3 years of age.[102] Although antenatal dexamethasone appears justified, it is important to inform parents that the long-term safety and outcome of this therapy is not established.

DETERMINATION OF FETAL SEX

Fetal sex can be determined by ultrasound from 11 weeks' gestation, though a reliable assignment is not possible until 12 to 13 weeks[103] and a phenotypic male fetus can be a virilized female. Thus, ultrasound is of limited value in the management of an at-risk fetus, other than possibly for monitoring the success of prenatal therapy.[104]

Of far greater value is the determination of fetal sex from cell-free DNA in maternal blood. Using real-time PCR, the Y-chromosome-specific SRY sequence can be amplified from the plasma of women carrying a male fetus.[105] Rijnders and associates[106] reported detection of SRY as early as 5 weeks' gestation with correct fetal sex determined by 10 weeks in 13 of 13 cases. This group recently reported the largest experience of prenatal sexing using cell-free fetal DNA. The PCR result was negative in all 29 female fetuses using a protocol of duplicate DNA isolation from 2 mL of maternal plasma. In 35 of 36 male fetuses, SRY was amplified in both DNA isolations (positive predictive value 100%), and in one instance, only one SRY amplification was positive (negative predictive value 96.7%). Early fetal sexing avoids unnecessary dexamethasone treatment and invasive antenatal diagnosis when the fetus is male. Because clinical experience of prenatal sexing using fetal DNA is still limited in CAH, the optimal testing protocol remains to be determined. Rijnders and associates[105] suggest starting dexamethasone and weekly plasma SRY testing from 5 weeks' gestation. The dexamethasone can then be stopped if the SRY PCR is positive in two separate samples and male sex subsequently confirmed on ultrasound examination. When the SRY PCR is negative, testing should be repeated weekly until 10 weeks with a diagnostic CVS at 11 weeks. Dexamethasone can then be discontinued in unaffected females (and undetected males).

SUMMARY OF MANAGEMENT OPTIONS
Congenital Adrenal Hyperplasia

Management Options	Quality of Evidence	Strength of Recommendation	References
Prepregnancy			
Identify genetic mutation and feasibility of prenatal diagnosis by direct DNA analysis and linkage analysis.	III	B	93,94,95

SUMMARY OF MANAGEMENT OPTIONS
Congenital Adrenal Hyperplasia *(Continued)*

Management Options	Quality of Evidence	Strength of Recommendation	References
Prepregnancy (*Continued*)			
Counsel families regarding risks and options for prenatal diagnosis and treatment.	–	GPP	–
Prenatal			
Start maternal dexamethasone (20 µg/kg/day in three divided doses) once pregnancy is confirmed.	III	B	87,93,97
Weekly maternal blood sampling for fetal sexing using PCR amplification of Y-chromosome-specific SRY sequence.	IIa	B	105,106
If PCR amplification not available or negative, chorionic villus sampling is done at 11 weeks for karyotype and DNA analysis.	III	B	93,94,95
For noninformative affected families (no molecular diagnosis possible), diagnosis is by amniotic fluid steroid levels.	IV	C	96
For male fetus or unaffected female fetus stop maternal dexamethasone.	IIb	B	87,93,97,105
In affected female fetus continue dexamethasone.	II	B	87,93,97,105
Measure maternal serum estriol levels every 6–8 weeks to confirm compliance and adrenal suppression.	IIa	B	100
Ultrasonographic assessment of external genitalia: if there is evidence of virilization, measure amniotic fluid for 17-hydroxyprogesterone and androstenedione, and if elevated, increase the dose of dexamethasone.	III	B	87
Monitor for maternal side effects (hyperglycemia, hypertension, edema, and excessive weight gain) and, if necessary, reduce dose of dexamethasone.	III	B	87,93,97
Postnatal			
Examine child carefully after birth for evidence of virilization and salt-wasting disease.	IV	C	86,89
Corticosteroid/mineralocorticoid replacement are considered.	IV	C	86,89
Long-term developmental follow-up is required.	III	B	91

CONCLUSIONS

FETAL HYPERTHYROIDISM

- Suspected in at-risk women from ultrasound features (especially fetal heart rate), but diagnosis depends on fetal blood sampling.
- Treatment involves optimizing maternal thionamide therapy; maternal beta blockers are given if fetal thyrotoxicosis persists.
- Neonatal evaluation and management plan are important.

FETAL HYPOTHYROIDISM

- Key management is to optimize maternal thyroxine replacement.
- Fetal disease may be suspected with ultrasound, but diagnosis depends on fetal blood sampling.
- Treatment for affected fetuses is intra-amniotic thyroxine.
- Neonatal evaluation and management plan are important.

CONCLUSIONS *(Continued)*

CONGENITAL ADRENAL HYPERPLASIA

- Maternal dexamethasone therapy is begun as soon as pregnancy is diagnosed in at-risk pregnancies.
- Establish gender and molecular diagnosis if the patient is female.
- Continue dexamethasone therapy in affected females.
- Neonatal evaluation, management plan, and long-term follow-up are important.

REFERENCES

1. Kelnar CJH, Butler GE: Fetal endocrinology. In McIntosh N, Helms P, Smyth R (eds): Forfar & Arneil's Textbook of Pediatrics. Edinburgh, Churchill Livingstone, 2003, pp 443–559.
2. Chan S, Rovet J: Thyroid hormones in fetal central nervous system development. Fetal Maternal Med Rev 2003;14:1–32.
3. Thorpe-Beeston JG, Nicolaides KH, Butler J, McGregor AM: Maturation of the secretion of thyroid hormone and thyroid stimulating hormone in the fetus. N Engl J Med 1991;324: 532–536.
4. Song SI, Daneman D, Rovet J: The influence of etiology and treatment factors on intellectual outcome in congenital hypothyroidism. J Dev Behav Pediatr 2001;22:376–384.
5. Fisher DA: Neonatal thyroid disease in offspring of women with autoimmune thyroid disease. Thyroid Today 1986;9:1–7.
6. Mestman JH: Hyperthyroidism in pregnancy. Clin Obstet Gynaecol 1997;40:45–64.
7. Nachum Z, Rakover Y, Weiner E, Shalev E: Graves' disease in pregnancy: Prospective evaluation of a selective invasive treatment protocol. Am J Obstet Gynecol 2003;189:159–165.
8. McKenzie JM, Zakarija M: Fetal and neonatal hyperthyroidism and hypothyroidism due to maternal TSH receptor antibodies. Thyroid 1992;2:155–159.
9. Tamaki H, Amino N, Aozasa M, et al: Universal predictive criteria for neonatal overt thyrotoxicosis requiring treatment. Am J Perinatol 1988;5:152–158.
10. Mitsuda N, Tamaki H, Amnio N, et al: Risk factors for developmental disorders in infants born to women with Graves' disease. Obstet Gynecol 1992;80:359–364.
11. Laurberg P, Nygaard B, Glinoer D, et al: Guidelines for TSH-receptor antibody measurements in pregnancy; results of an evidence-based symposium organized by the European Thyroid Association. Eur J Endocrinol 1998;139:584–586.
12. Thorpe-Beeston JG, Nicolaides KH, Snijders RJM, Felton CV: Thyroid function in anaemic fetuses. Fetal Ther 1990;5:109–114.
13. Peleg D, Cada S, Peleg A, Ben-Ami M: The relationship between maternal serum thyroid-stimulating immunoglobulin and fetal and neonatal thyrotoxicosis. Obstet Gynecol 2002;99:1040–1043.
14. Kung AWC, Lau KS, Kohn LD: Epitope mapping of TSH receptor-blocking antibodies in Graves' disease that appear during pregnancy. J Clin Enocrinol Metab 2001;86:3647–3653.
15. Kung AWC, Jones BM: A change from stimulatory to blocking antibody activity in Graves' disease during pregnancy. J Clin Endocrinol Metab 1998;83:514–518.
16. Wenstrom KD, Weiner CP, Williamson RA, Grant SS: Prenatal diagnosis of fetal hyperthyroidism using funipuncture. Obstet Gynecol 1990;76:513–517.
17. Achiron R, Rotstein Z, Lipitz S, et al: The development of the foetal thyroid: In utero ultrasonographic measurements. Clin Endocrinol 1998;48:259–264.
18. Thorpe-Beeston JG, Nicolaides KH: Maternal and fetal hyper- or hypothyroidism. In Thorpe-Beetson JG, Nicolaides KH (eds.) Maternal and Fetal Thyroid Function in Pregnancy. New York, Parthenon, 1996, pp 47–49.
19. Cohen O, Pinhas-Hamiel O, Sivan E, et al: Serial in utero ultrasonographic measurements of the fetal thyroid: A new complementary tool in the management of maternal hyperthyroidism in pregnancy. Prenat Diagn 2003;23:740–742.
20. Karabulut N, Martin DR, Yang M, Boyd BK: MR imaging findings in fetal goiter caused by maternal Graves' disease. J Computer Assisted Imag 2002;26:538–540.
21. Hollingsworth DR, Alexander NM: Amniotic fluid concentrations of iodothyronines and thyrotropin do not reliably predict fetal thyroid status in pregnancies complicated by maternal thyroid disorders or anencephaly. J Clin Endocrinol Metab 1983;57:349–355.
22. Kilpatrick S: Umbilical blood sampling in women with thyroid disease in pregnancy: Is it necessary? Am J Obstet Gynecol 2003;189:1–2.
23. Pekonen F, Teramo K, Makinen T, et al: Prenatal diagnosis and treatment of fetal thyrotoxicosis. Am J Obstet Gynecol 1984;150:893–894.
24. Daneman D, Howard NJ: Neonatal thyrotoxicosis: Intellectual impairment and craniosynostosis in later years. J Pediatr 1980;97:257–262.
25. Momotani N, Noh J, Oyanagi H, et al: Antithyroid drug therapy for Graves' disease during pregnancy. Optimal regimen for fetal thyroid status. N Engl J Med 1986;315:24–28.
26. Sheffield JS, Cunningham FG: Thyrotoxicosis and heart failure that complicate pregnancy. Am J Obstet Gynecol 2004;190: 211–217.
27. Mestman JH: Hyperthyroidism complicating pregnancy. Clin Obstet Gynecol 1997;40:45–64.
28. Millar LK, Wing DA, Leung AS, et al: Low birth weight and preeclampsia in pregnancies complicated by hyperthyroidism. Obstet Gynecol 1994;84:946–949.
29. Phoojaroenchanachal M, Sriussadaporn S, Peerapatdit T, et al: Effect of maternal hyperthyroidism during late pregnancy on the risk of neonatal low birth weight. Clin Endocrinol 2001;54: 365–370.
30. Marchant B, Brownlie BEW, Hart DM, et al: The placental transfer of propylthiouracil, methimazole and carbimazole. J Clin Endocrinol Metab 1997;45:1187–1193.
31. Milham S: Scalp defects in infants of mothers treated for hyperthyroidism with methimazole and carbimazole during pregnancy. Teratology 1985;32:321.
32. Diav-Citrin O, Ornoy A: Teratogen update: Antithyroid drugs—methimazole, carbimazole, and propylthiouracil. Teratology 2002; 65: 38–44.
33. Momotani N, Noh JY, Ishikawa NB, Ito K: Effects of propylthiouracil and methimazole on fetal thyroid status in mothers with Graves' hyperthyroidism. J Clin Endocrinol Metab 1997;82: 3633–3636.
34. Gardener DF, Cruikshank DP, Hays PM, Cooper DS: Pharmacology of propylthiouracil (PTU) in pregnancy hyperthyroid women: Correlation of maternal PTU concentrations with cord serum thyroid function tests. J Clin Endocrinol Metab 1986;62:217–220.
35. Hall R, Richards CJ, Lazarus JH: The thyroid and pregnancy. Br J Obstet Gynaecol 1993;100:512–515.

36. Stoffer SS, Hamburger JI: Inadvertent ^{131}I therapy for hyperthyroidism in the first trimester of pregnancy. J Nucl Med 1976;17:146–149.
37. Van Loon AJ, Derksen JT, Bos AF, Rouwe CW: In utero diagnosis and treatment of fetal goitrous hypothyroidism, caused by maternal use of propylthiouracil. Prenat Diagn 1995;15:599–604.
38. Wallace C, Couch R, Ginsberg J: Fetal thyrotoxicosis: A case report and recommendations for prediction, diagnosis and treatment. Thyroid 1995;5:125–128.
39. Fisher DA, Dussault JH, Foley TP, et al: Screening for congenital hypothyroidism: Results of screening one million North American infants. J Pediatr 1979;94:700–705.
40. Kurinczuk JJ, Bower C, Lewis B, Byrne G: Congenital hypothyroidism in Western Australia 1981–1998. J Paediatr Child Health 2002;38:187–191.
41. Fisher DA: Fetal thyroid function: Diagnosis and management of fetal thyroid disorders. Clin Obstet Gynecol 1997;40:16–31.
42. Brown RS, Bellisaro RL, Botero D, et al: Incidence of transient congenital hypothyroidism due to maternal thyrotropin receptor–blocking antibodies in over one million babies. J Clin Endocrinol Metab 1996;81:1147–1151.
43. Matsura N, Harada S, Ohyama Y, et al: The mechanism of transient hypothyroxinemia in infants born to mothers with Graves' disease. Pediatr Res 1997;42:214–218.
44. Matsura N, Konishi J, Fujieda K, et al: TSH-receptor antibodies in mothers with Graves' disease and outcome in their offspring. Lancet 1988;i:14–17.
45. Kempers MJ, van Tijn DA, van Trotsenberg AS, et al: Central congenital hypothyroidism due to gestational hyperthyroidism: Detection where prevention failed. J Clin Endocrinol Metab 2003;88:5851–5857.
46. Fisher DA: The hypothyroxinemia [corrected] of prematurity. J Clin Endocrinol Metab 1997;82:1701–1703.
47. Thorpe-Beeston JG, Nicolaides KH, Snijders RJM, et al: Thyroid function in small for gestational age fetuses. Obstet Gynecol 1991;77:701–706.
48. Glinoer D: Maternal and fetal impact of chronic iodine deficiency. Clin Obstet Gynecol 1997;40:102–116.
49. Vanderpas JB, Contempre B, Duale NL, et al: Iodine and selenium deficiency associated with cretinism in northern Zaire. Am J Clin Nutr 1990;52:1087–1093.
50. Utiger RD: Recognition of thyroid disease in the fetus. N Engl J Med 1991;324:559–561.
51. Lazarus JH, Hughes IA: Congenital abnormalities and congenital hypothyroidism. Lancet 1988;ii:52.
52. Davidson KM, Richards DS, Schatz DA, Fisher DM: Successful in utero treatment of fetal goiter and hypothyroidism. N Engl J Med 1991;324:543–546.
53. Nicolini U, Venegoni E, Acaia B, et al: Prenatal treatment of fetal hypothyroidism: Is there more than one option? Prenat Diagn 1996;16:443–448.
54. Thyroid dysfunction in utero (editorial). Lancet 1992;i:155.
55. Tillotson SL, Fuggle PW, Smith I, et al: Relation between biochemical severity and intelligence in early treated congenital hypothyroidism: A threshold effect. Br Med J 1994;309:440–445.
56. Rovet JF: Congenital hypothyroidism: Long term outcome. Thyroid 1999;9:741–748.
57. Rovet JF, Ehrlich RM, Sorbara DL: Neurodevelopment in infants and preschool children with congenital hypothyroidism: Etiological and treatment factors affecting outcome. J Pediatr Psychol 1992;17:187–213.
58. Montoro MN: Management of hypothyroidism during pregnancy. Clin Obstet Gynecol 1997;40:65–80.
59. Kamijo K, Saito T, Sato M: Transient subclinical hypothyroidism in early pregnancy. Endocrinol Japan 1998;37:397–403.
60. Allan WC, Haddow JE, Palomaki GE, et al: Maternal thyroid deficiency and pregnancy complications: Implications for population screening. J Med Screening 2002;7:127–130.
61. Leung AS, Millar LK, Koonings PP, et al: Perinatal outcome in hypothyroid pregnancies. Obstet Gynecol 1993;81:349–353.
62. Davis LE, Leveno KH, Cunningham FG: Hypothyroidism complicating pregnancy. Obstet Gynecol 1988;72:108–112.
63. Buckshee K, Kriplani A, Kapil A, et al: Hypothyroidism complicating pregnancy. Aust NZ J Obstet Gynaecol 1992;32:240–242.
64. Wasserstrum N, Anania CA: Perinatal consequences of maternal hypothyroidism in early pregnancy and inadequate replacement. Clin Endocrinol 1995;42:353–358.
65. Man EB, Serunian SA: Thyroid function in human pregnancy. VIII. Retardation of progeny aged 7 years, relationships to maternal age and maternal thyroid function. Am J Obstet Gynecol 1976;125:949–957.
66. Klein RZ, Haddow JE, Faix JD, et al: Prevalence of thyroid deficiency in pregnant women. Clin Endocrinol 1991;35:41–46.
67. Haddow JE, Palomaki GE, Allan WC, et al: Maternal thyroid deficiency during pregnancy and subsequent neuropsychological development of the child. N Engl J Med 1999;341:549–555.
68. Klein RZ, Sargent JD, Larsen PR, et al: Relation of severity of maternal hypothyroidism to cognitive development of offspring. J Med Screening 2001;8:18–20.
69. Pop VJ, de Vries E, Van Baar AL, et al: Maternal thyroid peroxidase antibodies during pregnancy: A marker of impaired child development? J Clin Endocrinol Metab 1995;80:3561–3565.
70. Morreale de Escobar G, Obregon MJ, Escobar del Rey F: Is neuropsychological development related to maternal hypothyroidism or to maternal hypothyoxinemia? J Clin Endocrinol Metab 2000;85:3975–3987.
71. Pop VJ, Brouwers EP, Vader HL, et al: Maternal hypothyroxinaemia during early pregnancy and subsequent child development: A 3-year follow up study. Clin Endocrinol 2003;59: 282–288.
72. Van Herle AJ, Young RT, Fisher DA, et al: Intrauterine treatment of a hypothyroid fetus. J Clin Endocrinol Metab 1975;40:474–477.
73. Weiner S, Scharf JI, Bolognese RJ, Librizzi RJ: Antenatal diagnosis and treatment of a fetal goiter. J Reprod Med 1980;24:39–42.
74. Sack J, Fisher DA, Lam RW: Thyroid hormone metabolism in amniotic fluid and allantoic fluids of the sheep. Pediatr Res 1975;9:837–841.
75. Agrawal P, Ogilvy-Stuart A, Lees C: Intrauterine diagnosis and management of congenital goitrous hypothyroidism. Ultrasound Obstet Gynecol 2002;19:501–505.
76. Gruner C, Kollert A, Wildt L, et al: Intrauterine treatment of fetal goitrous hypothyroidism controlled by determination of thyroid-stimulating hormone in fetal serum. A case report and review of the literature. Fetal Diagn Ther 2001;16:47–51.
77. Cortelazzi D, Morpurgo PS, Zamperini P, et al: Maternal compound W serial measurements for the management of fetal hypothyroidism. Eur J Endocrinol 1999;141:570–578.
78. Asteria C, Rajanayagam O, Collingwood TN, et al: Prenatal diagnosis of thyroid hormone resistance. J Clin Endocrinol Metab 1999;84:405–410.
79. McDougall IR, Maclin N: Hypothyroid women need more thyroxine when pregnant. J Fam Pract 1995;41:238–240.
80. Kaplan MM: Monitoring thyroxine treatment during pregnancy. Thyroid 1992;2:147–152.
81. Girling JC, de Swiet M: Thyroxine dosage during pregnancy in women with primary hypothyroidism. Br J Obstet Gynaecol 1992;99:368–370.
82. Hanukoglu A, Perlman K, Shamis I, et al: Relationship of etiology to treatment in congenital hypothyroidism. J Clin Endocrinol Metab 2001;86:186–191.
83. Rovet J, Ehrlich RM: Longterm effects of L-thyroxine treatment for congenital hypothyroidism. J Pediatr 1995;126:380–386.
84. Oerbeck B, Sundet K, Kase BF, Heyerdahl S: Congenital hypothyroidism: Influence of disease severity and L-thyroxine treatment on intellectual, motor, and school-associated outcomes in young adults. Pediatrics 2003;112:923–930.

85. Hrytsiuk I, Gilbert R, Logan S, et al: Starting dose of levothyroxine for the treatment of congenital hypothyroidism: A systematic review. Arch Pediatr Adolesc Med 2002;156:485–491.
86. Speiser PW, White PC: Medical progress: Congenital adrenal hyperplasia. N Engl J Med 2003;349:776–788.
87. New MI, Carlson A, Obeid J, et al: Prenatal diagnosis for congenital adrenal hyperplasia in 532 pregnancies. J Clin Endocrinol Metabol 2001;86:5651–5657.
88. Cutfield WS: The adrenal cortex. In Gluckman PD, Heyman MA (eds): London, Edward Arnold, 1993, pp 319–329.
89. Kelnar CJ: Congenital adrenal hyperplasia (CAH) – The place for prenatal treatment and neonatal screening. Early Hum Devel 1993;35:81–90.
90. Schnitzer JJ, Donahoe PK: Surgical treatment of congenital adrenal hyperplasia. Endocrinol Metab Clin North Am 2001;30:137–154.
91. Premawardhana LD, Hughes IA, Read GC, Scanlon MF: Longer term outcome in females with congenital adrenal hyperplasia (CAH): The Cardiff experience. Clin Endocrinol 1997;46:327–332.
92. Dittman RW, Kappes ME, Kappes MH: Sexual behaviour in adolescent and adult females with congenital adrenal hyperplasia. Psychoneuroendocrinology 1992;17:153–170.
93. Mercado AB, Wilson RC, Cheng KC, et al: Prenatal treatment and diagnosis of congenital adrenal hyperplasia owing to steroid 21-hydroxylase deficiency. J Clin Endocrinol Metab 1995;80: 2014–2020.
94. Spiliotis BE: Prenatal diagnosis and treatment of congenital adrenal hyperplasia and consequences in adults. J Pediatr Endocrinol Metab 2001;14(Suppl 5):1299–1302.
95. Mao R, Nelson L, Kates R, et al: Prenatal diagnosis of 21-hydroxylase deficiency by gene conversion and rearrangements; pitfalls and molecular diagnostic solutions. Prenat Diagn 2002;22:1171–1176.
96. Mellon SH, Fleischer A, Abrams CA, et al: Prenatal diagnosis of congenital lipoid adrenal hyperplasia. J Clin Endocrinol Metab 1995;80:200–205.
97. Lajic S, Bui TH, Holst M, et al: Prenatal diagnosis and treatment of adrenogenital syndrome. Prevent virilization of female fetuses. Lakartidningen 1997;94:4781–4786.
98. Pang S, Pollack MS, Marshall RN, Immken L: Prenatal treatment of congenital adrenal hyperplasia due to 21-hydroxylase deficiency. N Engl J Med 1990;322:111–115.
99. Chin D, Speiser PW, Imperato-McGinley J, et al: Study of a kindred with classic congenital adrenal hyperplasia: Diagnostic challenge due to phenotype variance. J Clin Endocrinol Metab 1998;83:1940–1945.
100. Dorr HG, Sippell WG: Prenatal dexamethasone treatment in pregnancies at risk for congenital adrenal hyperplasia due to 21-hydroxylase deficiency: Effect on midgestational amniotic fluid steroid levels. J Clin Endocrinol Metab 1993;76:117–120.
101. Coleman MA, Honour JW: Reduced maternal dexamethasone dosage for the prenatal treatment of congenital adrenal hyperplasia. Int J Obstet Gynaecol 2004;111:176–178.
102. Trautman PD, Meyer-Bahlburg HFL, Postelnek J, New MI: The effects of early prenatal dexamethasone on the cognitive and behavioural development of young children. Psychoneuroendocrinology 1995;20:439–449.
103. Efrat Z, Akinfenwa OO, Nicolaides KH: First trimester determination of fetal gender by ultrasound. Ultrasound Obstet Gynecol 1999;13:305–307.
104. Bromley B, Mandell J, Gross G, et al: Masculinization of female fetuses with congenital adrenal hyperplasia may already be present at 18 weeks. Am J Obstet Gynecol 1994;171:264–265.
105. Rijnders RJP, Christiaens GCML, Bossers B, et al: Clinical applications of cell-free fetal DNA from maternal plasma. Obstet Gynecol 2004;103:157–164.
106. Rijnders RJP, van der Luijt RB, Peters EDJ, et al: Earliest gestational age for fetal sexing in cell free maternal plasma. Prenat Diagn 2003;23:1042–1044.
107. Luton D, Fried D, Sibony O, et al: Assessment of fetal thyroid function by colored Doppler echography. Fetal Diagn Ther 1997;12:24–27.
108. Thyroid disease in pregnancy. ACOG Tech Bull No. 181, 1993.

CHAPTER 23

Fetal Tumors

Joseph Biggio/Katharine Wenstrom

INTRODUCTION AND GENERAL APPROACH

Although fetal tumors are an uncommon, the use of sonography has made antenatal detection possible. Once a fetal neoplasm is identified or suspected, the physician and the family must formulate a management strategy based on the presumptive diagnosis and the prognosis for the specific lesion. An understanding of the sonographic appearance of specific lesions, the differential diagnosis, available treatment modalities, and overall prognosis is critical in providing families with accurate information at a time when difficult decisions may be required. A multidisciplinary team, with representatives from maternal-fetal medicine, neonatology, pediatric hematology-oncology, and pediatric surgery, provides an excellent source of information for the parents and allows for an integrated approach that minimizes maternal risk while maximizing fetal benefit.

The prevalence of fetal tumors is difficult to pinpoint because of imprecision defining what was a congenital tumor prior to the near universal application of ultrasonography. Historically, studies included only those tumors apparent at birth or diagnosed within the first 2 to 3 months of life.[1] Further, tumors found in stillbirths and nonmalignant tumors may not have been reported to cancer registries. A 30-year population study in the United Kingdom from 1960 to 1989 reported an incidence of 7.2 congenital tumors, both benign and malignant, per 100,000 live births. The incidence of malignancy in neonates is estimated at 36.5 per million live births.[2]

Although the histology of congenital tumors is similar to that in older children, the incidence, presentation, degree of differentiation, and biologic behavior frequently differ.[3] Teratomas and neuroblastomas are the most common solid tumors reported, but the behavior of these lesions in fetuses and neonates is markedly different from that observed in older children.[1,3,4] The prevalences of these and other neoplasms are listed in Table 23–1.

Prior to antenatal ultrasound, the first sign of a fetal tumor was often polyhydramnios due either to neurologic or mechanical interference with fetal swallowing. Frequently, the diagnosis was made in the perinatal period after dystocia, fetal hemorrhage, tumor rupture, or fetal hydrops. Modern ultrasonography and the availability of magnetic resonance imaging (MRI) now allow for a thorough antenatal investigation of suspected fetal masses. Harrison and Adzick[5] observed the natural history of several tumor types and found that in some cases the fetus tolerates the mass, while in others the fetus cannot and develops hydrops. Imaging does not provide a histologic diagnosis, but even if a biopsy were taken antenatally, the prognosis might still be obscure because the histologic appearance of malignancy in the fetus or neonate often reflects the immaturity of the patient and not tumor biology.[4] Moreover, even histologically benign lesions can cause fetal or neonatal death if the tumor mass disrupts other vital structures.[6] The location of the mass and the ability to predict the potential for impingement on vital structures is critical in assessing prognosis.

TABLE 23–1

Most Common Perinatal Tumors*

TUMOR TYPE	NUMBER	PERCENTAGE OF TOTAL
Teratoma	113	37%
Neuroblastoma	51	17%
Soft tissue	52	17%
Brain	20	6.6%
Renal	16	5.3%
Hepatic	13	4.3%

*Compiled from three large series of 302 tumors (Isaacs, 1985[4]; Werb et al., 1992[3]; Parkes et al., 1994[1]).

SUMMARY OF MANAGEMENT OPTIONS

Fetal Tumors—General

Management Options	Quality of Evidence	Strength of Recommendation	References
Uterine size greater than dates, hydramnios, and fetal hydrops are common presenting signs.	III	B	2–5
Diagnosis is most commonly made by ultrasonography, although adjunctive studies such as MRI may be helpful in some cases.	III	B	2–5
The possibility of genetic syndromes and associated malformations/deformations should be considered.	III	B	2–5
Multidisciplinary counseling and coordination of care with a team of specialty consultants are important in optimizing outcome for the neonate.	–	GPP	–
The development of hydrops is a poor prognostic sign.	III	B	2–5
If preterm delivery is contemplated, maternal steroids should be administered.	Ia	A	235

INTRACRANIAL TUMORS

Congenital brain tumors are extremely rare, with an estimated prevalence of 14 per 1 million live births.[2] Approximately 10% of all tumors diagnosed in the perinatal period arise in the brain.[7,8] While congenital tumors account for only 0.5% to 1% of all brain tumors diagnosed during childhood, they cause 5% to 20% of perinatal deaths due to neoplasms.[1,2,4,7–9]

There are several distinct differences between perinatal brain tumors and those occurring in older children. First, primary intracranial tumors in older children are mainly infratentorial (located in the cerebellum and brainstem), whereas the majority of those in the fetus and neonate are supratentorial.[4,7,8,10–12] Second, the initial clinical presenting sign in perinatal brain tumors is macrocephaly due to the tumor mass, hydrocephaly, or hemorrhage, with resulting dystocia and stillbirth. The lack of fusion of the calvaria and the patent fontanels permit expansion of the skull without increased intracranial pressure.[8,10] In contrast, older children develop signs of increased intracranial pressure, such as vomiting and focal neurologic changes. Third, intracranial teratomas are the most frequent intracranial neoplasms in the perinatal period, but they are highly unusual in older children. Finally, some tumor types behave differently in the perinatal period. For example, medulloblastoma is more aggressive in the perinatal period, while choroid plexus papilloma is more benign.[8] Discovery of a brain tumor in the perinatal period requires a careful search for additional defects, as 12% of congenital brain tumors result from a familial cancer syndrome.[8,13]

Teratomas

Teratomas are the most common congenital brain tumors, accounting for 26% to 50% of congenital intracranial masses.[8,10] They are thought to arise from any of several midline locations within the central nervous system, including the pineal gland, the hypothalamus, the suprasellar area, and the cerebral hemispheres. However, teratomas often become so large as to preclude determination of the exact site of origin.[8] Rapidly growing tumors have been reported to erode through the orbit, oral cavity, and skull, resulting in spontaneous rupture of the scalp and skull during delivery.[14,15]

Teratomas tend to appear as large cystic areas with solid components that frequently replace much of the normal brain architecture. Histologically, mature elements from all three germ layers are identified typically along with immature neuroglial components; these can easily give the impression of malignancy owing to their hypercellularity, high mitotic rate, and nuclear atypia.[8]

Diagnosis

Intracranial teratomas may present in a number of ways. Elevated midtrimester maternal serum α-fetoprotein (AFP) is reported in association with a fetal intracranial teratoma,[16] and some teratomas are seen on the midtrimester ultrasound examination. However, there are reports of normal ultrasound examinations and normal maternal serum AFP in pregnancies later found to be complicated by a massive fetal teratoma.[17] The most common presentation is rapid uterine growth. Macrocephaly, hydrocephaly, and an intracranial mass of mixed echogenicity with solid and cystic components are identifiable sonographically.[8,15,17] On occasion, there may be areas of calcification. The tumor mass can cause distortion or destruction of the normal intracranial architecture. Hydramnios occurs in 15% to 20% of cases.[8]

The differential diagnosis includes other intracranial neoplasms, hydrocephaly, hydranencephaly, porencephaly, holoprosencephaly, and encephalocele. Sonographic detection of a complex intracranial mass with the loss of normal intracranial architecture is highly suggestive of teratoma, but in cases in which the diagnosis is uncertain, MRI can be helpful (Fig. 23–1).

Risks

The frequent occurrence of uterine enlargement and hydramnios increases the risk of maternal respiratory compromise and preterm labor. In rare cases, the fetus may develop hydrops due to high-output cardiac failure secondary to arteriovenous shunting within the tumor,[18] which increases the maternal risk of preeclampsia (the "Mirror syndrome"). Perhaps the most significant maternal risk is dystocia due to macrocrania, and in most cases, cesarean section is required or cephalocentesis is necessary for vaginal delivery.[15,17,19] Although in some cases, a low transverse incision may be adequate, delivery of a breech fetus with macrocrania often requires a vertical uterine incision to minimize the risk of a broad ligament laceration. Regardless of the mode of delivery, the massive uterine distention markedly increases the risk of postpartum hemorrhage.

Management Options

The prognosis for a fetus with an intracranial teratoma is dismal. Most infants diagnosed antenatally are stillborn or die in the immediate perinatal period.[8,15,17,19] Although one case report described prolonged survival following tumor resection on the first day of life, that infant had severe motor and mental retardation.[17] Given the bleak prognosis, the patient should be counseled regarding her risks and the expected outcome, and the option of pregnancy termination offered. In ongoing pregnancies, the primary goal is to minimize maternal morbidity. Women who present in preterm labor should not be treated with tocolytic agents, as they do not improve the fetal prognosis and expose the mother to additional risk. Every effort should be made to avoid cesarean delivery, and cephalocentesis may be required to facilitate decompression of an enlarged fetal head and allow vaginal delivery.[15]

Other Intracranial Tumors

Neuroepithelial tumors predominate the miscellaneous group of other intracranial tumors. The most common types include astrocytomas, medulloblastomas, choroid plexus papillomas, and gliomas. Although less common, mesenchymal tumors such as meningioma and craniopharyngioma are also reported in the perinatal period.[8] These tumors are usually sporadic, and frequently are isolated. Some intracranial masses are associated with genetic syndromes such as neurofibromatosis or tuberous sclerosis. Neurofibromas and cortical tubers are reported on

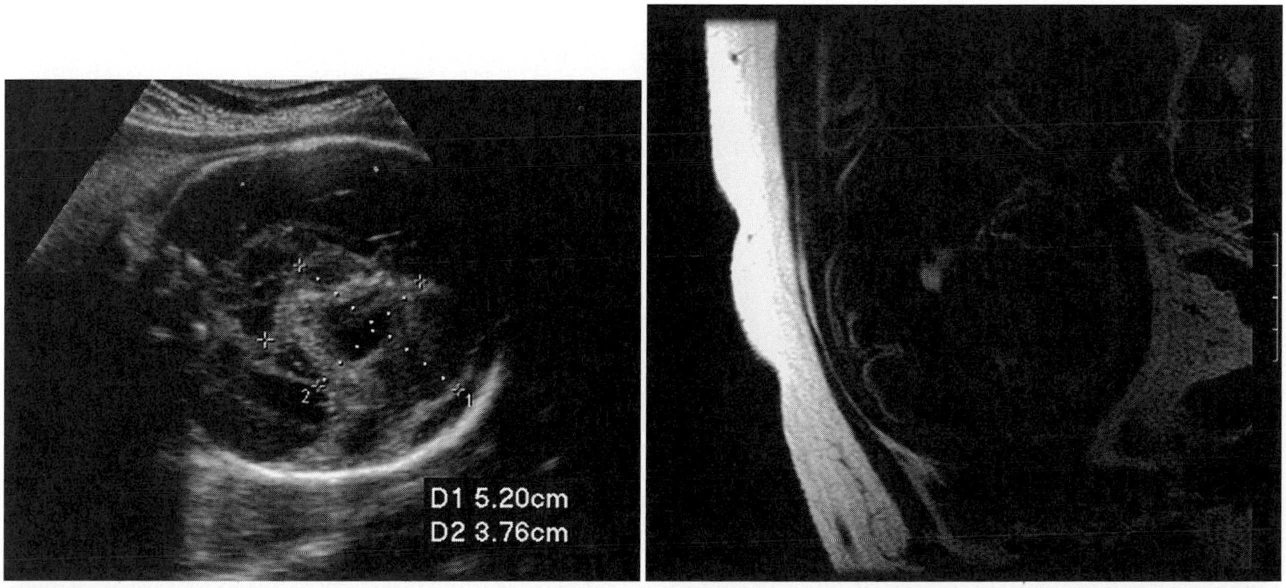

FIGURE 23–1
A large intrcranial mass with solid and cystic components, as well as calcification, was noted in this fetus at 28 weeks' gestation. The mass measured approximately 5 × 3 × 7 cm and caused compression of the ventricular system and development of ventriculomegaly. A fetal MRI was obtained to better define the extent of the lesion. The mass appeared to be arising from the base of the brain and was associated with disruption of normal architecture.

antenatal ultrasound[20–22] and, in the setting of a family history of these disorders, suggest an affected fetus. Both neurofibromatosis and tuberous sclerosis can also be the result of a new mutation, especially in cases of advanced paternal age. Hyperechoic areas with marked vascularity on Doppler interrogation suggest an AV malformation. Although the leptomeningeal angiomatosis associated with Sturge-Weber syndrome may appear hyperechoic, other vascular malformations,[23] such as a vein of Galen aneurysm, may appear as a hypoechoic, cystic structure until Doppler mapping is performed[24] (Fig. 23–2). A rare tumor, hypothalamic hamartoma, is closely associated with Pallister-Hall syndrome; identification of a tumor in the region of the hypothalamus should therefore prompt a search for associated anomalies including polydactyly, cardiac defects, and renal defects.[25,26]

Diagnosis

Although it is not possible to render a histologic diagnosis based on imaging studies alone, several of the more frequent intracranial neoplasms have a characteristic appearance that aids identification. The differential diagnosis for an intracranial mass includes neoplastic lesions, vascular malformations, parenchymal or intraventricular bleeding, and infarction.[27] Astrocytomas, the most common neuroglial tumor of the perinatal period, typically present as an intracranial mass associated with macrocrania. These tumors display a wide spectrum of cellular differentiation. The most poorly differentiated tumors (glioblastoma multiforme) generally appear as unilateral, echogenic, rapidly growing, solid masses that cause either a shift or destruction of the normal intracranial architecture and contralateral hydrocephalus.[8,9,28] Enlargement of the tumor over a short interval suggests hemorrhage, which occurs more frequently in the perinatal period than in childhood.[10] Medulloblastomas, a primitive cerebellar neuroendocrine tumor (PNET), are highly aggressive neoplasms that originate from the cerebellar vermis and grow into the fourth ventricle and cerebellar hemispheres, giving rise to the typical ultrasound findings of an echogenic cerebellar mass, hydrocephaly, and macrocrania.[8] Metastasis via the cerebrospinal fluid or vascular route occurs in up to 18%.

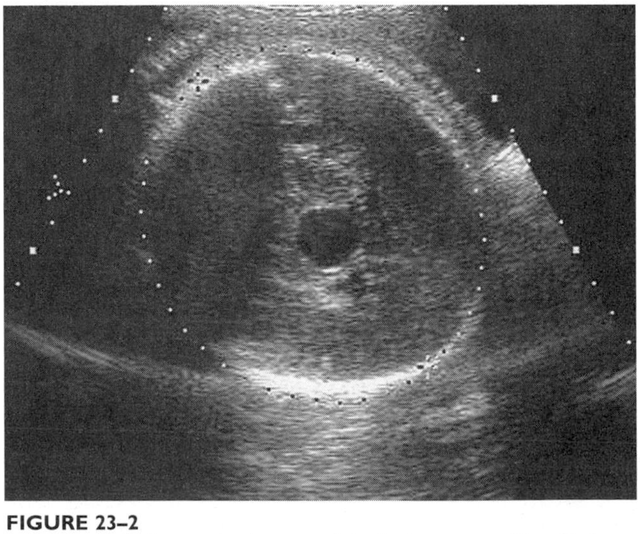

FIGURE 23–2
A cystic, anechoic mass in the area of the brainstem was identified at 22 weeks in this fetus. Using Doppler interrogation, the lesion was identified as a vein of Galen aneurysm.

Choroid plexus papillomas are histologically benign tumors in the ventricles composed of mature epithelial cells. They account for 5% of perinatal brain tumors.[7] Most commonly, choroid plexus papillomas appear sonographically as a nodular space-occupying lesion arising from the lateral ventricle, although third and fourth ventricle lesions are reported.[7,29,30] Tumor growth results in massive production of cerebrospinal fluid and severe dilation of the ventricular system.[7] These tumors have a more favorable prognosis than other intracranial neoplasms.

Although craniopharyngiomas are a relatively common tumor of childhood, they are rarely discovered perinatally. The most frequent ultrasound findings are hydramnios, a large, cystic, calcified mass in the suprasellar region, and macrocephaly. These tumors may grow quite large, replacing much of the normal brain tissue. The prognosis is poor.[7]

Neoplasms involving nearly all other intracranial tissues (e.g., meningiomas and ependymomas) are reported in the perinatal period as well, but their occurrence is less frequent.[7]

Several distinctive genetic syndromes can present with intracranial masses on the antenatal ultrasound. As noted, tuberous sclerosis is associated with multiple discrete echodense nodules in the cerebral cortex or ventricles. This finding or a family history of this disorder requires a careful search for other lesions, especially in the heart. Hypothalamic hamartomas are rare solid, echogenic tumors associated with Pallister-Hall syndrome. Other anomalies associated with this syndrome include holoprosencephaly, hydrocephaly, polydactyly, palatal abnormalities, renal and cardiac malformations, and imperforate anus. Identification of a tumor in the hypothalamic area mandates a search for these other defects.[26] Although typically not associated with antenatal cortical findings, rare patients with severe neurofibromatosis have diffuse tumor nodules throughout the entire CNS. The occurrence of multiple tumor nodules should prompt consideration of this disorder, especially if the family history is suggestive.[31]

Risks

The maternal risks are similar to those of a fetal intracranial teratoma (discussed previously). The propensity for the development of hydrocephaly and macrocrania predisposes to dystocia. The presence of hydramnios increases the risk of postpartum hemorrhage. The identification of an intracranial mass associated with a familial tumor syndrome (e.g., medulloblastoma and Gorlin syndrome or cerebellar hemangioblastoma and von Hippel–Lindau syndrome) suggests an increased risk of malignancy in family members.

Management Options

Because teratomas overall tend to destroy normal intracranial architecture, the prognosis is universally poor. The prediction of prognosis is more difficult with other intracranial neoplasms. Choroid plexus papillomas have a more favorable prognosis than most intracranial neoplasms, with a survival rate of 73%.[7] The prognosis for astrocytomas is highly dependent on the degree of cellular differentiation but overall is poor, with only 37% survival rate. Neonates with glioblastomas or anaplastic astrocytomas have a survival rate of only 14%.[7] Medulloblastomas have a propensity to spread throughout the CNS and bloodstream, and therefore have an extremely poor prognosis with less than 10% survival rate.[7] Intracranial lesions characteristic of phakomatoses, neurofibromatosis (NF), or tuberous sclerosis are in general not predictive of the severity of disease, and their presence alone cannot be used to make predictions on long-term outcomes.

Parents should be counseled on the full differential diagnosis of the intracranial mass, and the likely prognosis discussed. Because the ultrasound examination may not completely define the extent of the lesion, MRI can provide additional information to refine the counseling.[32] Many new MRI units are capable of rapid image acquisition, eliminating the need for fetal immobilization with a paralytic agent. In general, large or rapidly growing tumors that result in distortion of normal anatomy or massive hydrocephaly with macrocrania are more likely than not to be lethal. In these cases, the option of pregnancy termination should be offered, and cesarean section should be avoided wherever feasible.

SUMMARY OF MANAGEMENT OPTIONS

Intracranial Tumors

Management Options	Quality of Evidence	Strength of Recommendation	References
Intracranial Teratoma			
Supratentorial location and macrocephaly are common. Teratomas are the most common type of lesion; they cause destruction of normal brain tissue and have a dismal prognosis. Prognosis is variable for other tumor types.	III	B	8,10
MRI may be useful in evaluation of nature and extent of lesions.	III	B	32
Exercise vigilance for maternal respiratory compromise, preterm labor, premature rupture of membranes, and abruption in the presence of hydramnios, preeclampsia, or hydrops.	–	GPP	–
Counsel about poor prognosis. Most reported cases have been lethal. Consider termination.	III	B	8,15,17,19
Ongoing pregnancies should be managed with the goal of reducing maternal morbidity.	–	GPP	–
Cesarean delivery or cephalocentesis may be required if macrocephaly develops.	III	B	8,15,17,19
Other Intracranial Tumors			
Manage as for teratoma.	–	GPP	–
MRI may be helpful to further delineate intracranial anatomy.	III	B	32
Fetal prognosis is difficult to estimate. Large tumors associated with hydrocephalus or hemorrhage are likely to be lethal. Some tumors, however, have a fairly good prognosis. The prognosis of tumors associated with genetic syndromes depends on the syndrome itself.	III	B	7–10
Practical options for pregnancy are termination or continuation with vigilance for maternal respiratory compromise, preterm labor, premature rupture of membranes, and abruption in the presence of hydramnios, preeclampsia, or hydrops.	–	GPP	–
Cesarean section may be necessary, if macrocrania is found.	–	GPP	–

FACIAL TUMORS

Facial tumors most commonly involve the orbits, the paranasal sinuses, the tongue, the nasopharynx, and the oropharynx. Teratomas are the most frequent tumor type, but mesenchymal tumors are also encountered.

Orbital Tumors

The antenatal diagnosis of an orbital tumor is infrequent. The differential diagnosis includes a number of non-neoplastic entities such as encephalocele, vascular malformation, orbital cyst, and lesions of the conjunctiva, eyelid, and lacrimal apparatus. In addition, conditions that cause structurally shallow orbits, such as craniosynostosis, can cause proptosis and give the appearance sonographically of an orbital mass.

Diagnosis

An orbital teratoma presents as a unilateral mass arising within the orbit that both displaces the globe and enlarges the bony orbit. The globe may have degenerative changes and appear small because of compression by the tumor mass. As with other teratomas, both solid and cystic components are present, but there is no evidence of communication between cystic areas of the orbital tumor and the intracranial cavity.[33] These tumors occur twice as often in females and are more common on the left side.[34]

Retinoblastomas are the most frequent intraorbital tumors of childhood and usually present as intraocular tumors. Only rarely are these tumors large enough to visualize on an antenatal sonogram. However, giant congenital retinoblastomas protruding from the orbit are reported and can present as an exophytic, solid mass that may compress and destroy the normal ocular structures.[35]

Tumors arising within the ocular apparatus are also reported antenatally. Medulloepithelioma, a malignant tumor arising from the ciliary body, has an exophytic appearance and mixed cystic-solid composition that may mimic the appearance of a teratoma.[36] Massive retrobulbar orbital cysts, with subsequent orbital compression and microphthalmia, have also been diagnosed antenatally.[37]

In addition to intraocular tumors, epibulbar tumors can present as orbital masses. The most common epibulbar tumor is an epibulbar dermoid, a cystic lesion that contains pilosebaceous epithelial elements. Epibulbar dermoids are associated with Goldenhar syndrome and should raise the index of suspicion for this disorder.[38] Epibulbar vascular malformations are also reported.

Dacryocystocele secondary to obstruction of the lacrimal duct is reported antenatally; it has a characteristic cystic appearance and is located along the inferomedial border of the fetal orbit[39] (Fig. 23–3).

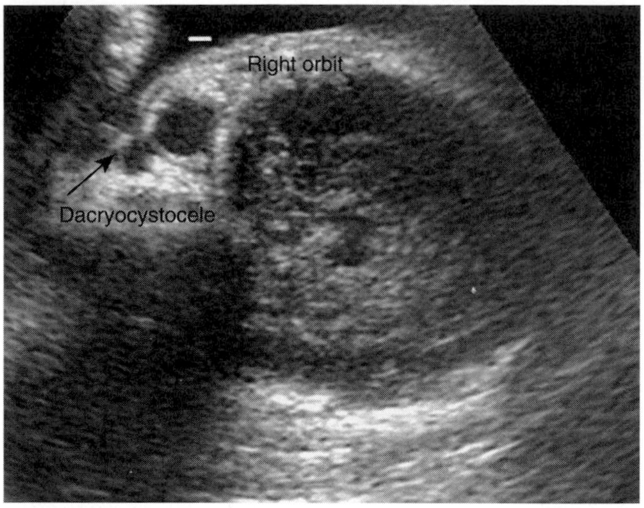

FIGURE 23–3
A cystic area between the nasal bone and the right orbit was identified on ultrasound in the midtrimester. The differential diagnosis included encephalocele, epibulbar dermoid, and dacryocystocele. At birth, the overlying skin had a bluish tinge characteristic of a dacryocystocele.

Risks

Orbital tumors are unlikely to result in a pregnancy complication or increased maternal risk. The degree of fetal risk depends on the nature of the lesion, as even some benign lesions can compromise future visual potential. Retinoblastomas diagnosed during the perinatal period are commonly due to a hereditary germline mutation in the retinoblastoma gene (a tumor suppressor gene) or a deletion of chromosome 13q; these mutations predispose to the development of other malignancies in addition to retinoblastoma.[40]

Management Options

The tumor type and size and degree of impingement on surrounding structures determine the prognosis of orbital tumors. In general, orbital teratomas have a favorable prognosis; even large lesions that require enucleation of the ipsilateral eye tend to have mature elements and an exceedingly low recurrence rate.[33,34] The prognosis for malignant orbital tumors such as retinoblastoma depends on the degree of spread outside the globe, and the presence of any associated anomalies or a chromosome disorder. A karyotype is indicated once the diagnosis of retinoblastoma is suspected.[35] In addition, parents should be counseled regarding the potential for postnatal treatment. Epibulbar tumors and abnormalities of the lacrimal apparatus have a favorable prognosis for survival and normal vision.[38,39] The management of pregnancy is unaltered, and cesarean delivery is reserved for the usual obstetric indications unless the lesion is large and exophytic and likely to cause dystocia or hemorrhage.

Nasal and Oral Tumors

Tumors of the nasal and oral cavities are rare and are most often teratomas.

Diagnosis

Teratomas of the nasopharynx and oropharynx originate from the sphenoid bone, the hard or soft palate, the jaw, or the tongue, and on ultrasound they typically appear as complex heterogeneous masses that protrude from the fetal mouth.[41–46] A subset of oropharyngeal teratomas are highly organized in appearance with recognizable organs suggestive of a parasitic twin; these tumors carry the special appellation of epignathus.[42,47] The location of these tumors can prevent fusion of the palatal shelves, resulting in a cleft palate, and up to 9% of cases are associated with other organ system anomalies.[41] The size and location of these tumors may cause hydramnios by occluding the pharynx or impeding fetal swallowing.[41,42,44,45] The maternal serum AFP was elevated in several cases.[41–44,46]

Other facial tumors in the nasal and oral regions are reported. There is one antenatal description of a nasal hemangiopericytoma, a rare tumor derived from the contractile cells of the capillary walls found in nasal tissues around the nasal cartilage and anterior skull base. The mass presented as an enlarging vascular mass visible on ultrasound examination.[48] Mesenchymal tumors of the paranasal sinuses are reported, as are granular cell tumors of the gingiva.[49,50] Leiomyoma of the tongue was reported in the neonatal period, and should be included in the differential diagnosis of oropharyngeal masses along with teratomas, hemangiomas, ectopic thyroid, and mesenchymal sarcoma.[51]

Risks

The majority of nasopharyngeal and oropharyngeal teratomas obstruct the oral cavity, interfere with fetal swallowing, and cause hydramnios.[41,42,44] Hydramnios increases the maternal risk of preterm labor, respiratory compromise, and postpartum hemorrhage. For fetuses with large teratomas, there is a significant risk of malposition of the fetal head and dystocia leading to cesarean section.[44]

Although these tumors may be massive in size at birth, most are benign and have a low risk of recurrence after appropriate surgical resection.[41,44] The greatest risk to the fetus is respiratory distress resulting from an inability to establish a patent airway. Arteriovenous shunting through the teratoma's large vascular bed is rare but reported with pharyngeal teratomas; shunting can lead to placentomegaly, high-output cardiac failure, and fetal hydrops with a maternal risk of Mirror syndrome.[44]

Management Options

A large tumor mass within the nasopharynx or oropharynx can impede normal gas exchange, and in some cases, tumor may extend into the trachea so that even if an oral airway is attainable, respiration is still impaired. In the case of large pharyngeal masses, especially if hydramnios is present, delivery coordination with a team including an anesthesiologist, neonatologist, and pediatric surgical specialist may prove lifesaving. The ex utero intrapartum treatment (EXIT) procedure, described and refined by a number of physicians since the early 1990s, allows either endotracheal intubation or tracheostomy to be performed while the placental and umbilical cord circulation is maintained.[42,47,52–54] General anesthesia is used to maximize uterine relaxation and fetal anesthesia, a hysterotomy is performed, and the fetus is partially delivered to the level of the shoulders to provide access to the fetal neck. Endotracheal intubation can then be attempted, either with a laryngoscope or fiberoptic endoscope; if unsuccessful, tracheostomy can be performed while the infant remains on placental support.[42,47,52–54] Some advocate having extracorporeal membrane oxygenation equipment in the operating suite in cases in which the tumor might distort the normal anatomic landmarks.[54,55] Fetoplacental circulation has been maintained for more than 50 minutes after delivery of the fetal head and shoulders, during which time fetal oxygen saturation is easily monitored with reflectance pulse oximetry.[52,53,56]

A substantial number of women will present in preterm labor associated with hydramnios. The presence of these tumors is not a contraindication to either therapeutic amniocentesis or tocolysis, as most of these infants have a favorable long-term prognosis if they survive the perinatal period and initial surgical resection. Prematurity is not a contraindication to the EXIT procedure.[52,53]

SUMMARY OF MANAGEMENT OPTIONS

Facial Tumors

Management Options	Quality of Evidence	Strength of Recommendation	References
Orbital Tumors			
Counseling depends on prognosis; orbital teratomas are most common; although the globe may be destroyed with loss of	IV	C	33, 34

Continued

SUMMARY OF MANAGEMENT OPTIONS
Facial Tumors *(Continued)*

Management Options	Quality of Evidence	Strength of Recommendation	References
Orbital Tumors—*Continued*			
ipsilateral eye, overall prognosis is favorable but depends on tumor type, size, and local pressure effects.			
Prognosis for orbital retinoblastoma depends on tumor stage, which cannot be determined antenatally. Parents should be counseled that neonatal management of retinoblastoma includes enucleation as well as radiotherapy and chemotherapy. With current treatment, survival rate may exceed 90%.	IV	C	35
Cesarean delivery is reserved for obstetric indications, or for those cases in which a large tumor is likely to cause dystocia.	–	GPP	–
DNA-based prenatal diagnosis is available for hereditary retinoblastoma.	IV	C	40
Nasal and Oral Tumors			
Vigilance is needed for maternal complications from hydramnios.	–	GPP	–
Discuss prognosis at counseling.	–	GPP	–
Greatest risk to the fetus is severe respiratory compromise at delivery. Coordination of delivery with appropriate specialists can significantly improve the outcome. If tracheal occlusion is anticipated, delivery should be by cesarean section in cooperation with pediatric and surgical consultants to assure prompt intubation, tracheostomy, or tracheoplasty. In some perinates, an ex utero intrapartum tracheoplasty (EXIT procedure) may be required. Some advocate ECMO (extracorporeal membrane oxygenation) to be available at the same time in theater.	III	B	42,47,52–54

NECK TUMORS

Masses in the fetal neck can be divided into those occurring anteriorly or posteriorly. The differential diagnosis depends on the location of the mass. Anteriorly, the most common diagnoses are goiter, thyroid/thyroglossal duct cyst, teratoma, nonseptated cystic hygroma, and branchial cleft cyst.[57] Posteriorly, the differential diagnosis includes nuchal edema, cystic hygroma, meningomyelocele, and rarely teratoma.[58] Structures in the anterior neck are usually small and barely discernible on antenatal ultrasound, so abnormalities involving the thyroid are often readily apparent. Most thyroid masses are solid and represent a goiter often associated with maternal Graves' disease and fetal thyrotoxicosis[57] (Fig. 23–4). The fetal neck is usually in a neutral position and freely mobile; any deviation, such as hyperextension, should prompt an investigation of possible etiologies because of the propensity for airway obstruction.[57] Nonseptated cystic hygromas are small cystic masses located in the antero-

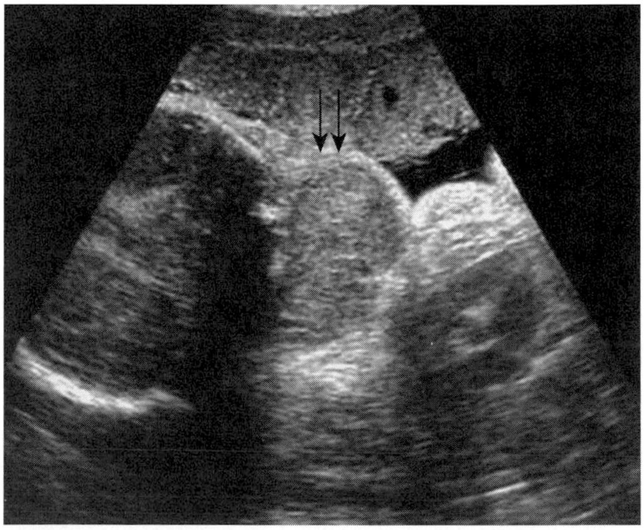

FIGURE 23–4
A large goiter identified in a fetus exposed to propylthiouracil for treatment of maternal Graves' disease.

lateral region of the fetal neck (Fig. 23–5). In contrast to posterior hygromas, they have no clear association with lymphatic abnormalities, and there is controversy regarding their association with anomalies and aneuploidy.[57] One report, however, documents an increased risk of aneuploidy and cardiovascular anomalies with both anterior and posterior hygromas.[59]

Teratoma

Although cervical teratomas are the most common fetal neck tumor, only about 5% of all teratomas are located in the fetal neck.[60,61] Extragonadal teratomas are believed to develop during early gestation when all three germ layers are in close approximation.[62] Historically, a distinction has been made between cervical and thyroid teratomas, depending on the presence or absence of thyroid tissue in the tumor and the presence of a normal thyroid gland, but this distinction is arbitrary.[63] These tumors can achieve a massive size prior to birth and significantly distort the anatomy in the neck, face and even thorax, but only rarely have malignant components or metastatic foci been reported.[64-69] When present, neuroglial cells are the most commonly identified immature elements.

Diagnosis

As with teratomas in other locations, derivatives of all three germ layers are present, and on antenatal ultrasound the lesion has a characteristic appearance with large solid and cystic areas extending from the anterior surface of the neck[64–69] (Fig. 23–6). Calcification within the mass occurs in 40% to 50%.[57,65,69] Although maternal serum AFP is not routinely helpful in diagnosis, those with endodermal sinus derivatives may produce AFP. Hydramnios complicates 25% to 55% of cases, especially those with large tumors causing esophageal and tracheal occlusion, and may provide a clue to the extent of the lesion.[57,64,69]

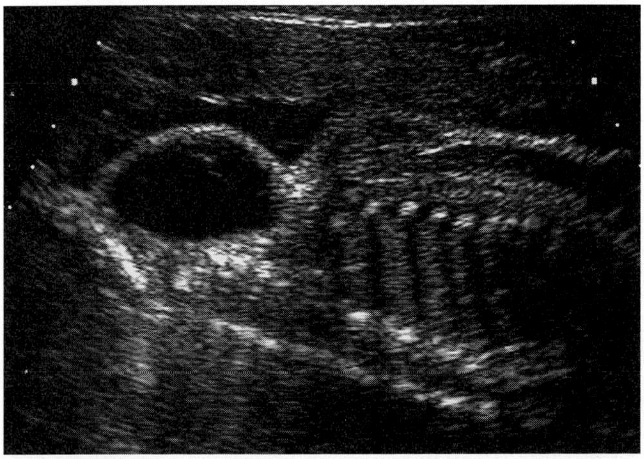

FIGURE 23–5
A large anterior cystic hygroma was identified as an isolated defect in this fetus. The lesion resolved as gestation progressed.

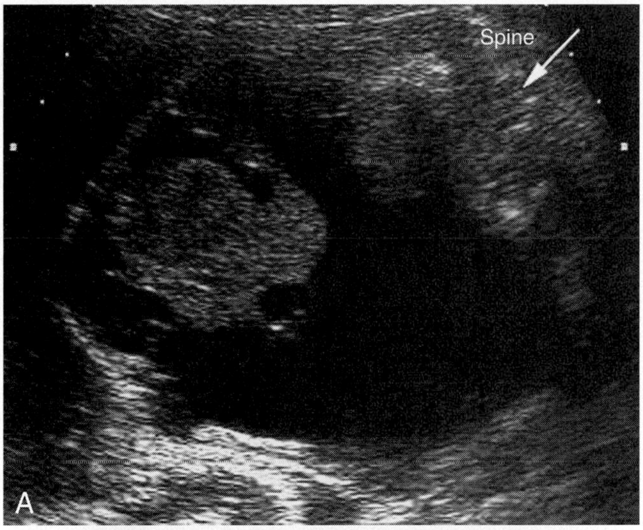

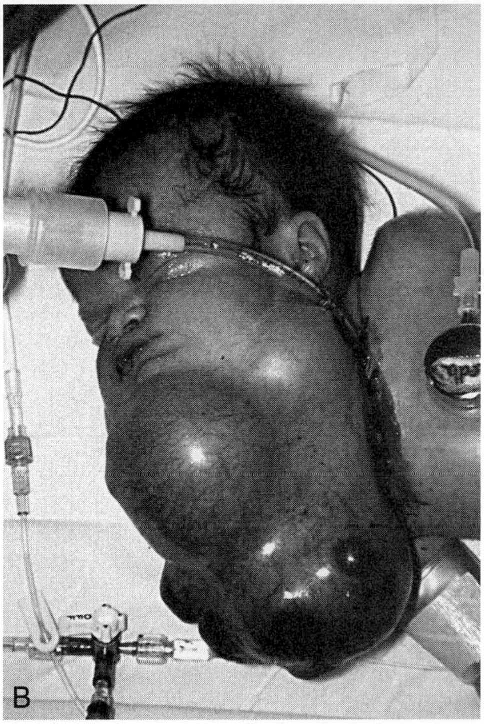

FIGURE 23–6
A, A large cervical teratoma was identified in this fetus at 22 weeks. Hydramnios developed and preterm labor ensued at 32 weeks. The fetus was delivered via the EXIT (ex utero intrapartum treatment) procedure. *B*, A postnatal image of the infant with an endotracheal tube in the left aspect of the neck demonstrating the distorted position of the trachea. (Photograph courtesy of Dr. John C. Hauth.)

Risks

As with pharyngeal tumors, the risk of hydramnios increases the maternal risk of preterm labor, respiratory compromise, and postpartum hemorrhage. The most substantial neonatal risk is respiratory distress due to an inability to obtain an airway, leading to hypoxia and resultant neurologic injury.[66] The overall survival rate with modern surgical care is 85% to 95%, even with large tumors. However, the most important prognostic factor is the ability to accomplish a complete surgical resection of the tumor,[66,69] which may not be possible in all cases owing to the involvement of vital structures. Although antenatal ultrasound can readily detect and identify these masses, a fetal MRI may allow better definition of involved structures. This information could be important for counseling and delivery management.[69,70]

Management Options

The size of the tumor and the resulting hyperextension of the fetal neck frequently cause dystocia and necessitate cesarean delivery. Because of the potential for airway complications, an EXIT procedure should be anticipated, and the delivery coordinated with a multidisciplinary team as described for pharyngeal tumors. Surgical resection is usually performed as soon after birth as possible to avoid loss of a previously secure airway. Although an operative mortality rate of 10% to 15% was reported in the past, more recent series note exceedingly low mortality rates.[65,66] The risk of morbidity due to operative injury to the thyroid and parathyroid glands, the neck vessels, and the recurrent laryngeal nerve remains significant, but an excellent functional and cosmetic result can be expected in 70% of cases.[66]

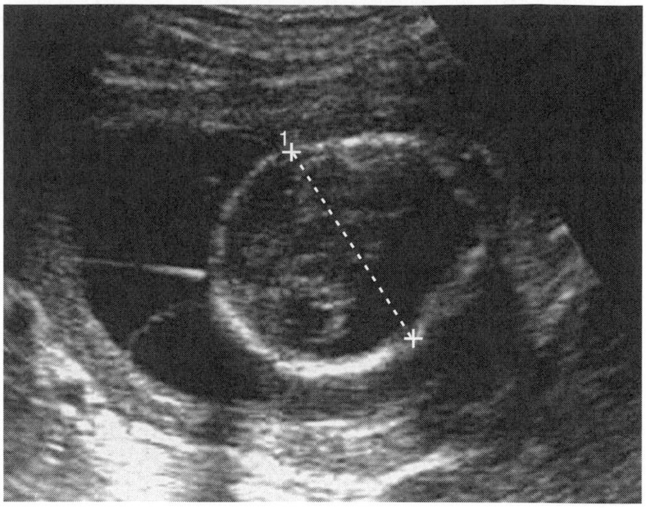

FIGURE 23–7
A multiseptated cystic hygroma was identified in this fetus at 17 weeks' gestation. The hygroma extended from the occiput to the level of the thoracic spine.

Cystic Hygroma

Cystic hygromas are malformations of the lymphatic system that appear as either single or multiloculated, fluid-filled, membranous cysts often in the occipitocervical area. The hygroma may be small, simple, and transient or may be large, multiseptated, and persistent. These lesions result from the jugular lymphatic obstruction sequence, in which either the normal communication between the jugular lymphatic sacs and the jugular veins fails to form by 40 days' gestation, or there is an overall lymphatic hypoplasia.[71,72] If the lymph sacs eventually connect with the venous system or an alternative route of lymphatic drainage develops, the cystic hygroma can spontaneously resolve. However, stigmata, such as low posterior hairline and neck-webbing, may persist.[71]

Diagnosis

Ultrasound allows ready diagnosis of cystic hygroma. Their location in the posterolateral portion of the neck and their cystic appearance are considered characteristic, but they must be distinguished from other potential abnormalities in this region. The differential diagnosis includes encephalocele, meningomyelocele, and the rare posterior teratoma[58,71] (Fig. 23–7). Nuchal translucency or edema may represent the most mildly affected end of the spectrum of the lymphatic obstruction sequence. It can be distinguished from a cystic hygroma by examining for a more subtle and continuous distribution of subcutaneous fluid (usually less than 10 mm in thickness) versus a larger and usually multiseptated process in cystic hygromas.[58] Cystic hygroma is associated with either an elevated maternal serum AFP or a multiple marker maternal serum test indicating an increased risk of trisomy 21, usually as the result of elevated human chorionic gonadotropin (hCG).[73,74] Other anomalies may be detected in part because of the association with fetal aneuploidy. Associated cardiac anomalies, particularly aortic coarctation and hypoplastic left ventricle, may occur as the enlarged thoracic duct impinges on the developing heart.[75] The development of hydramnios or hydrops may reflect fetal cardiac decompensation which lowers the chances for resolution or survival.[71]

Risks

Between 50% and 75% of fetuses with cystic hygromas are aneuploid; Turner syndrome (45,X and variants) accounts for 75% of the aneuploidies.[71,76] The remainder are autosomal trisomies, especially chromosomes 13, 18, and 21.[77] Noonan syndrome, multiple pterygium syndrome, and the Klippel-Feil sequence are each associated with cystic hygroma, as are abnormalities related to environmental exposures such as fetal alcohol syndrome.[71,77] Associated congenital heart defects are relatively common, as already noted.[77,78] Hydrops occurs in 50% to 90% of fetuses with cystic hygroma, and is associated with an exceedingly low survival rate.[77,79,80] Dysmorphic changes or structural abnormalities in adjacent organs may occur as the result of pressure from lymphatic dilation that alters normal morphogenesis. Dilated lymph sacs cause elevation, protrusion, and angulation of the ear, redundant skin in the nuchal region, and altered patterns of hair growth. Dilated lymphatic channels near the heart increase the resistance to blood flow through the ascending aorta, leading to left-sided hypoplastic cardiac lesions encountered with cystic hygromas.[75,77,78]

Management Options

Once a cystic hygroma is identified, a thorough anatomic survey including fetal echocardiography should be performed and a karyotype determination offered. Counseling and pregnancy management are guided by the presence of other malformations and the fetal karyotype. Because the prognosis for a fetus with a large, persistent cystic hygroma and hydrops is dismal, the option of pregnancy termination should be offered. If the hygroma decreases in size or resolves, the overall prognosis is more favorable. In general, nonseptated cystic hygromas are more likely to resolve than septated lesions (98% versus 44%) and have a higher survival rate (94% versus 12%).[80] Fetuses with persistent cystic hygromas should be scanned periodically for hydrops. Cesarean section should be avoided once a fetus with a cystic hygroma develops hydrops because of the poor prognosis.

SUMMARY OF MANAGEMENT OPTIONS

Neck Tumors

Management Options	Quality of Evidence	Strength of Recommendation	References
Teratomas			
Vigilance is needed for development of hydramnios and its complications.	–	GPP	–
Cesarean section may be necessary in cases of extreme dorsiflexion of fetal head or dystocia caused by large tumor.	–	GPP	–
Ex utero intrapartum treatment (EXIT procedure) may provide up to 1 hour of uteroplacental support to provide time to secure an airway.	III	B	42,47,52–54
Plans for intrapartum intubation, ex utero tracheoplasty or ECMO should be coordinated with pediatric and surgical specialists as described for oral tumors. Surgical resection is usually performed as soon as possible after stabilization to avoid loss of secure airway.	III	B	42,47,52–54
Prompt surgery for appropriate cases after delivery has reduced the mortality rate to 15%.	III	B	65, 66
Cystic Hygroma			
Manage as for fetal hydrops (see Chapter 25).	–	GPP	–
Search for other abnormalities including cardiac and chromosomal defects and development of hydrops.	IV	C	77
Prognosis for isolated hygromas without hydrops depends on whether the hygroma resolves.	IV	C	77

THORACIC TUMORS

Primary tumors of the fetal lung are rare, and most diagnoses are made during the neonatal period.[81] Primary pulmonary tumors reported in the perinatal period include pulmonary blastoma, fibrosarcoma, myofibromatosis, and hemangiomas. Metastatic lesions, especially from hepatoblastoma, neuroblastoma, or Wilms' tumor, are more frequently encountered.[82] Other mass lesions detected within the lung fields during the perinatal period include vascular malformations, congenital lobar emphysema, and bronchogenic cysts.[83]

Mediastinal and thoracic wall masses are also reported. The differential diagnosis of a mediastinal mass includes bronchogenic cyst, neurenteric cyst, esophageal duplication cyst, diaphragmatic hernia, pericardial cyst, lymphangioma, teratoma, and neuroblastoma.[84] Chest wall masses include hemangiomas, lymphangiomas, and mesenchymal tumors.

Diagnosis

Bronchogenic cysts result from abnormal budding of the bronchial tree between weeks 4 and 8 of gestation and usually lack a normal connection to the tracheobronchial tree.[85,86] Bronchogenic cysts typically appear sonographically as fluid-filled cystic areas located either within the pulmonary fields or the mediastinum, most commonly in the subcarinal area. The antenatal detection of a chest wall mesenchymal hamartoma is reported. The lesion had a heterogenous sonographic appearance and filled the right hemithorax.[87] With metastatic lesions, the primary tumor is often identifiable in another organ system. Approximately 15% of neuroblastomas (see later discussion) are located in either the thoracic cavity or mediastinum. On ultrasound, the lesions can appear either solid with calcification or cystic, which is more common, making the diagnosis problematic.[88–91] Thoracic neuroblastomas tend to be diagnosed at an earlier stage than their intra-abdominal counterparts, and therefore have a better prognosis. Chylothorax attributed to compression of pulmonary lymphatics by a mediastinal tumor is also reported.[88] Lymphangiomas can occur in either the anterior or posterior mediastinum.

Vascular malformations in the pulmonary tree may be part of a genetic syndrome that is associated with multiple hemangiomas such as Osler-Weber-Rendu syndrome. They appear similar to other vascular malformations, displaying hyperechogenicity on routine ultrasound with marked vascularity on Doppler interrogation.

Risks

Regardless of its etiology, any lesion that creates a mass effect within the fetal thorax has the potential to alter pulmonary development and cause hydrops by deviating the mediastinum and obstructing cardiac return. An intrathoracic mass can not only affect the ipsilateral lung by direct compression, but if large enough to cause a mediastinal shift, it may compress the contralateral lung.[92] Compression of the trachea and esophagus can cause hydramnios independent of cardiac function,[93] and hydramnios increases the risk of preterm labor. The ultimate prognosis for the infant depends on the nature of the tumor, its resectability, the degree of lung involvement, and the extent to which pulmonary development is impeded by the mass effect. One study concludes that hydramnios and mediastinal shift are poor prognostic indicators.[94]

Management Options

The progressive growth of a bronchogenic cyst can lead to hydrops as well as bronchial abnormalities.[85,86] Percutaneous drainage via repeated thoracentesis or thoracoamniotic shunt placement is reported.[95,96] The shunt will relieve hydrops only if secondary to mediastinal shift. It is unclear whether a shunt improves outcome in the absence of hydrops. MRI may assist the evaluation of large or atypical chest masses.[97] Because of the potential for respiratory compromise, fetuses with thoracic lesions should be delivered at a center prepared for appropriate fetal resuscitation and support.

TUMOR-LIKE CONDITIONS OF THE LUNG

Congenital Cystic Adenomatoid Malformation

Congenital cystic adenomatoid malformation (CCAM) is a developmental anomaly of the lung consisting of abnormal tertiary bronchioles. Most lesions are unilateral, but up to 15% have bilateral components.[98] These bronchioles display either hamartomatous changes, or an arrest in embryologic development with the formation of cystic lesions of various sizes.[93,98] They usually communicate with the bronchial tree. The blood supply for a CCAM derives from the pulmonary circulation.

Diagnosis

CCAM lesions are classified by their histologic appearance: type I lesions account for more than 50% and are composed of a small number of large cysts; type 2 lesions make up 40% and are composed of multiple small cysts; and type 3 lesions are microcystic, homogenous, solid-appearing masses[99] (Fig. 23–8). Recently, Adzick and associates proposed a simplified approach based on the antenatal sonographic findings. Macrocystic lesions contain single or multiple cysts that are at least 5 mm in diameter, whereas microcystic lesions have cysts less than 5 mm in diameter and appear more solid and echodense.[92,100] The differential diagnosis reflects whether there is a predominant cystic or solid component. For cystic lesions, the differential diagnosis includes diaphragmatic hernia, bronchogenic or enteric cysts, bronchial atresia, neuroblastoma, anterior meningomyelocele, and teratoma. While diaphragmatic hernia and neuroblastoma remain in the differential diagnosis for solid lesions, the most difficult distinction is often between a microcystic type 3 lesion and bron-

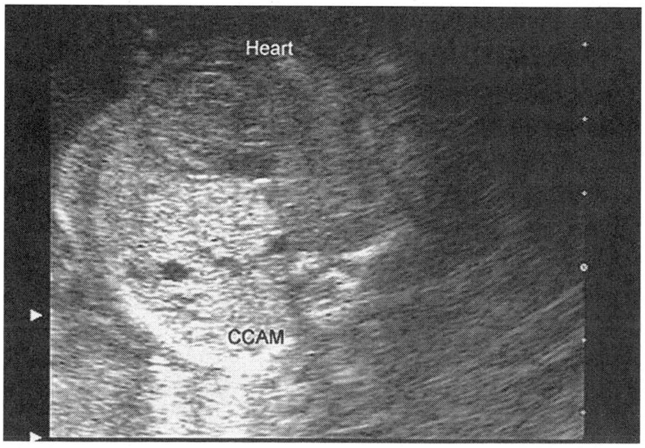

FIGURE 23–8
A type 2 CCAM was identified in this fetus. Although there was evidence of mediastinal shift and mild cardiac deviation, the CCAM decreased in size during gestation, and the fetus was asymptomatic at birth.

chopulmonary sequestration. Demonstration that the blood supply comes from the aorta is consistent with sequestration and excludes a diagnosis of CCAM.[76,92] Fetal MRI can provide additional anatomic detail to assist in achieving a definitive diagnosis, especially distinguishing CCAM from diaphragmatic hernia—two lesions often confused on ultrasound alone.[101,102]

Risks

The antenatal natural history of CCAM is variable, and the prognosis is guided by the size and type of the mass, the progression or regression of the mass, and the presence of cardiac axis deviation, hydrops, and associated anomalies. Although initial reports suggested that solid lesions have a worse prognosis than cystic lesions, more recent study suggests the overall size of the mass is more important than the composition of the mass.[76] However, the different composition may reflect a difference in cellular growth and thereby may influence lesion size. Large lesions that cause cardiac deviation and compression of the great vessels, esophagus, or trachea, leading to hydrops and hydramnios, clearly have a worse prognosis. Without antenatal intervention, the development of hydrops is a harbinger of fetal demise.[92,103] In addition, large lesions may cause compression of normal lung tissue and produce pulmonary hypoplasia. Up to 40% of fetuses develop hydrops, and up to 70% develop hydramnios. Crombleholme and colleagues described a technique for measuring the size of the CCAM that generates a volume ratio and then applied the ratio to predict the likelihood of hydrops developing.[103] Approximately 15% of CCAM lesions shrink in utero with resolution of any mediastinal shift. Although many of these lesions appear sonographically to involute or "disappear," this appearance may be due in part to changes in tissue echo texture, as postnatal radiographic or antenatal MRI studies confirm the persistence of at least some lesions.[92,97,102] In the absence of hydrops, more than 90% survive with most lesions resectable postnatally.[92,98]

Although 26% of fetuses had associated anomalies in Stocker's original report, a more recent series observed that only 2% of fetuses with CCAM had associated anomalies.[92,104] This raises questions regarding the diagnostic accuracy of the original series. The women whose fetuses develop hydrops or hydramnios are at increased risk for preterm delivery, Mirror syndrome, postpartum hemorrhage, and respiratory compromise.

Management Options

A complete anatomic survey is required to rule out associated malformations, determine the size and type of lesion, and detect any cardiac deviation or evidence of hydrops. Karyotype determination should be offered especially if there are associated structural malformations; otherwise, the yield is low. If multiple anomalies are detected or hydrops is identified, the family should be counseled regarding the poor prognosis and the option of pregnancy termination offered. In ongoing pregnancies, serial ultrasound studies to identify evolving hydramnios or signs of hydrops are indicated. Corticosteroids for pulmonary maturation followed by delivery are options after consultation with neonatal, pediatric surgery, and maternal-fetal medicine specialists should hydrops develop at a gestation when survival is possible. The delivery of any viable fetus with a persistent thoracic mass should occur at a tertiary center prepared for potential neonatal respiratory compromise.

The management of a pregnancy in which the fetus either develops hydrops at previable gestational age or whose large lesion is compressing the ipsilateral lung and therefore increasing the risk of pulmonary hypoplasia is more problematic. In fetuses with hydrops, the mortality rate is 100% with expectant management, so novel fetal therapy might be warranted. In a number of reports, decompression of large dominant cyst by thoracentesis or thoracoamniotic shunt placement has successfully reversed the mediastinal shift, pulmonary compression, and hydrops; survival rates of 80% to 90% after such a procedure are reported.[92,95,103] The initial procedure should be thoracentesis with cyst drainage, for in some cases the cyst resolves completely.[103] If the fluid rapidly reaccumulates, shunt placement can be considered (see Chapters 10 and 25). The utility of shunts is limited by occlusion or dislodgment, which occurs in up to 29% of cases.[105]

Thoracoamniotic shunt placement is ineffective for the treatment of multicystic and solid lesions. When these lesions are large and associated with hydrops, antenatal fetal surgery is an option. Adzick and associates described the outcomes of 13 hydropic fetuses with CCAM who underwent antenatal resection of an abnormal pulmonary lobe at 21 to 29 weeks' gestation.[92] Eight (62%) survived. Crombleholme and associates reported only two of seven (29%) similar fetuses surviving antenatal surgery.[103] Fetal surgery is limited to a few centers worldwide and is associated with considerable risks including chorioamnionitis, preterm premature rupture of the membranes, preterm labor, postoperative infection, pulmonary edema, and anesthetic complications, as well as an unstable uterine scar with the need for cesarean delivery in all subsequent pregnancies. As surgical techniques and the ability to identify fetuses at highest risk improve, the survival rate will likely improve.

Bronchopulmonary Sequestration

Bronchopulmonary sequestration is an isolated mass of lung tissue that lacks communication with the tracheobronchial tree and derives its blood supply from the systemic circulation, usually from the aorta or a major branch. The lesion is thought to result from a supernumerary lung bud that arose caudal to the normal lung bud and migrated with the esophagus.[93,106] Lesions that develop early in embryogenesis are surrounded by the adjacent lung tissue and covered by the same pleura. These are termed intralobar sequestrations. In contrast, those that develop later grow separately from the lung and become covered by their own pleura. These are termed extralobar sequestrations. The lesions are typically unilateral, with left-sided lesions being twice as common as right-sided. Although intralobar lesions typically involve the lower lobe of the lung, extralobar regions may be found between the lower lobe and the diaphragm, within the diaphragm, in the mediastinum, or below the diaphragm. Intralobar lesions are more common than extralobar in infants and children, but extralobar lesions predominate in the fetus and neonate.[107–110]

Diagnosis

Bronchopulmonary sequestration appears sonographically as a solid, highly echogenic, homogenous mass. Confirmation of a systemic vascular supply using color-flow Doppler is diagnostic.[111] It can be very difficult to distinguish a sequestration from a microcystic CCAM if the vascular supply cannot be identified. It is usually not possible to determine sonographically whether an intrathoracic sequestration is intralobar or extralobar. The differential diagnosis of an intrathoracic sequestration includes microcystic CCAM, diaphragmatic hernia, teratoma, and neuroblastoma. For extralobar lesions, the differential diagnosis includes neuroblastoma and renal tumors. Although it is usually possible to sonographically demonstrate the well-demarcated boundaries of sequestrations, an MRI can in some cases help to identify other conditions that can present with a solid echogenic mass in the lower thorax such as diaphragmatic hernia with liver herniation.[97]

Risks

The prognosis for bronchopulmonary sequestration is variable, although large sequestrations can cause pulmonary compression, mediastinal shift, and hydrops. The presence of hydrops is the most important prognostic sign. In one series published in the early 1990s, only 36% of fetuses survived, and all fetuses with hydrops (35% of all cases) died. The incidence of hydramnios was 80% and isolated pleural effusion 70%.[107] A more recent experience of 39 continuing pregnancies with bronchopulmonary sequestration reported 100% survival of nonhydropic fetuses.[92] Only four fetuses developed hydrops and the only death occurred in the one fetus not treated antenatally.[92] Significantly, 72% of sequestrations regressed or resolved spontaneously and were asymptomatic at birth.[92] Postnatal imaging revealed residual evidence of the lesions. Regression appears more common with extralobar sequestration, possibly because the separate pleural investment allows torsion on its vascular pedicle.[112, 113] Intra-abdominal extralobar bronchopulmonary sequestration is rarely associated with hydrops and has a better prognosis than intrathoracic lesions.

Even in the absence of a significant mediastinal shift, fetuses with bronchopulmonary sequestration may develop hydrothorax. This phenomenon is more common with extralobar lesions, possibly as the result of lymphatic and venous obstruction due to torsion.[107] The pressure gradient between the systemic artery and pulmonary vein and the resultant left-to-left shunting has been postulated as an explanation with intralobar lesions.[114]

Associated anomalies of the foregut are reported with bronchopulmonary sequestration, and reflect the embryologic derivation of this lesion from an abnormal outpouching of the foregut. These associated anomalies include tracheoesophageal fistula, esophageal duplication, diaphragmatic hernia, funnel chest, and cardiac defects. Additional malformations occur more commonly with extralobar lesions (58%) than with intralobar lesions (14%).[115–117]

Management Options

Once the diagnosis of bronchopulmonary sequestration is suspected, a complete anatomic survey to search for other anomalies and rule out any signs of incipient hydrops is required. Although the majority of intrathoracic lesions will regress to some degree, the possibility of hydrops justifies serial ultrasound examinations. If the lesion is large and associated with either hydrothorax or hydrops, antenatal therapy may be considered, given the otherwise dismal prognosis. Weekly thoracentesis and thoracoamniotic shunt placement are reported to effectively treat hydrops and pleural effusion when there is a mediastinal shift, but do not address the underlying lesion. Any fetus that fails to respond to these therapies, or has hydrops due to a large lesion without a significant pleural effusion, can be considered a candidate for in utero resection of the lesion. The maternal risks of such intervention should be carefully weighed against the potential fetal benefit.[92,93,106,118–120]

Isolated intra-abdominal bronchopulmonary sequestrations have a better prognosis than intrathoracic masses because these lesions do not cause pulmonary compression and hypoplasia. Like those above the diaphragm, regression occurs. Hydramnios may occur secondary to esophageal or gastric compression preventing fetal swallowing. All fetuses with bronchopulmonary sequestration should be delivered at a tertiary center equipped for appropriate resuscitative and treatment measures.

SUMMARY OF MANAGEMENT OPTIONS

Intrathoracic Tumors

Management Options	Quality of Evidence	Strength of Recommendation	References
Lung Tumors			
Exclude other malformations.	–	GPP	–
MRI may help delineate nature and size of lesion.	IV	C	97
Vigilance for hydramnios and hydrops is needed.	III	B	94
Interdisciplinary care is indicated.	–	GPP	–
Delivery should be in a tertiary care center with appropriate specialist consultants standing by.	–	GPP	–
Cystic Adenomatous Malformation			
Exclude other malformations.	–	GPP	–
MRI may help delineate nature and size of lesion.	IV	C	97
Vigilance for hydramnios and hydrops is needed.	III	B	94
Interdisciplinary care is indicated.	–	GPP	–
Cyst aspiration or placement of a cystoamniotic shunt in the setting of hydrops may relieve intrathoracic pressure and reverse hydropic changes. However, these procedures do not always provide long-term benefit.	III	B	95, 96
The place of antenatal fetal surgery is not clear and should be regarded as experimental at present.	III	B	92
Delivery should be in a tertiary care center with appropriate specialist consultants standing by.	–	GPP	–
Pulmonary Sequestration			
Exclude other malformations.	–	GPP	–
MRI may help delineate nature and size of lesion.	IV	C	97
Vigilance for hydramnios and hydrops is needed.	III	B	94
Interdisciplinary care is indicated.	–	GPP	–
Antenatal thoracoamniotic catheter placement to relieve pleural effusion and correct hydrops has been described with mixed results.	III	B	95, 96
The place of antenatal fetal surgery is not clear.	III	B	92
Delivery should be in a tertiary care center with appropriate specialist consultants standing by.	–	GPP	–

CARDIAC TUMORS

Primary cardiac tumors are rare, with a reported frequency of 2.7 per 10,000 infants and young children; the prevalence in utero is unknown.[121] Cardiac rhabdomyoma is the most common cardiac tumor detected in infancy, comprising 62% of cases, followed by teratoma in 21%, fibroma in 13%, and only rarely hemangioma, myxoma, or sarcoma.[122-124]

Diagnosis

Rhabdomyoma is thought to be a hamartoma and not a true neoplasm. It can be solitary or multiple, and located within any of the cardiac chambers or the myocardial wall (Fig. 23–9). The sonographic appearance of rhabdomyoma is of a discrete echogenic mass, but whether the mass is mobile or fixed depends on the location.[125,126] Rhabdomyomas can be isolated, but they are

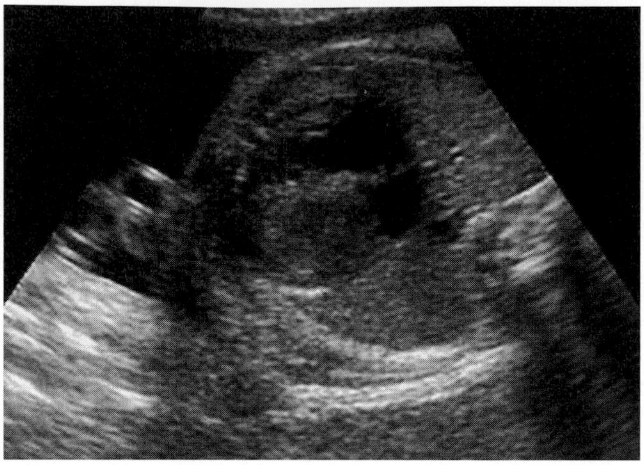

FIGURE 23–9
A cardiac lesion consistent with a rhabdomyoma was identified in this fetus at 24 weeks' gestation. The mass continued to grow during gestation, and at birth occupied most of the left ventricle. Several smaller lesions were noted in the myocardial wall on postnatal echocardiogram. Clinical examination revealed findings consistent with tuberous sclerosis.

more frequently found in association with tuberous sclerosis. Fifty-one percent to 86% of neonates born with cardiac rhabdomyomas will subsequently be diagnosed with tuberous sclerosis. Conversely, these lesions may be found in 50% to 60% of patients with tuberous sclerosis.[125,127,128] The tumors associated with tuberous sclerosis are typically multiple and range in size from 3 to 25 mm.[125] The differential diagnosis includes fibroma, myxoma, and sarcoma, although these lesions are less common in the fetus.

Pericardial teratomas appear sonographically similar to teratomas in other locations—a complex echogenic mass with cystic and solid components and occasional calcifications.[129] These tumors are located outside the heart, attach to the base of the heart and great vessels via a broad stalk, and are usually on the right. In nearly all cases, a pericardial effusion is present that assists in narrowing a differential diagnosis that includes mediastinal teratoma, extralobar bronchopulmonary sequestration, and CCAM. Pericardial effusion rarely occurs in isolation with the later conditions.

Risks

All cardiac tumors are space-occupying with the potential to cause hemodynamic compromise and hydrops due to obstruction of normal blood flow through either the cardiac chambers or the great vessels. This risk depends on the number, size, and location of the tumors.[122] The prognosis for fetuses with a cardiac tumor and hydrops is dismal. Pediatric patients with intramural tumors are at increased risk for cardiac arrhythmias such as ventricular tachycardia and Wolff-Parkinson-White syndrome. The tumor (especially rhabdomyomas, which have embryonal components and conductive capability) is believed to act as an accessory conduction pathway.[125,126,130,131] Whether fetuses have a similar risk is unstudied. Cardiac tumors are also associated with several genetic syndromes including Beckwith-Wiedemann syndrome, tuberous sclerosis, Gorlin (basal cell nevus) syndrome, and neurofibromatosis. A detailed sonographic anatomic survey by an expert should be performed to search for these stigmata.

Tuberous sclerosis is an autosomal dominant disorder, though approximately two thirds result from new mutations. Most mutations are in the *tuberin* or *hamartin* genes on chromosomes 16 or 9, respectively. Commercial testing for these mutations is not currently available, but consultation with a geneticist is recommended because a mutation can be identified in some families and commercial testing may become available in the future. Although the disorder has 95% penetrance, there is markedly variable expressivity, and evaluation by a geneticist can help confirm or refute the diagnosis. If a cardiac rhabdomyoma is identified or suspected, a professional familiar with the disease diagnostic criteria should carefully evaluate both parents and the fetus's siblings. Children diagnosed with tuberous sclerosis are at risk for mental retardation and seizures, but it is not possible to predict mental function accurately based on either the antenatal findings or the family history. It is suggested that children with cortical tubers or subependymal nodules are more likely to have unremitting seizures and severe mental retardation. Fetal MRI has been used to identify these findings which may not be visible on ultrasound.[132,133]

Management Options

The fetus with a cardiac mass should undergo serial sonographic examinations in search of either developing hydrops or an arrhythmia. If hydrops develops at a gestational age when survival is expected, the administration of antenatal corticosteroids followed by delivery should be considered. Should hydrops develop prior to viability, the option of pregnancy termination may be offered. Absent hydrops, the prognosis for the fetus with a cardiac mass is favorable, and the pregnancy should be managed expectantly. Delivery should be planned at a tertiary center capable of providing pediatric cardiac surgical intervention in the immediate perinatal period if necessary. Intrauterine pericardiocentesis is reported to relieve cardiac tamponade with a successful outcome of pregnancy in a fetus with pericardial teratoma and a pericardial effusion.[134,135] The majority of cardiac rhabdomyomas spontaneously regress after birth.[125,126,131] For this reason, intervention is considered only in the presence of hemodynamic compromise. All true cardiac tumors should be evaluated postnatally and surgical resection planned. Although malignant components have only rarely been identified in pericardial teratomas, all become symptomatic eventually, thus justifying surgical therapy.[129,136,137]

SUMMARY OF MANAGEMENT OPTIONS

Cardiac Tumors

Management Options	Quality of Evidence	Strength of Recommendation	References
Determine the tumor type and likely diagnosis; search for US markers of syndromes.	–	GPP	–
Because the most common fetal cardiac tumor is rhabdomyoma, the diagnosis of tuberous sclerosis must be strongly considered. Linkage studies may help to confirm a familial case, but no genetic test is available to diagnose cases due to a new mutation. Counseling is difficult. Fetal MRI may detect brain abnormalities that are not visible by ultrasonography. Referral to a geneticist for counseling is suggested.	III	B	132, 133
Serial sonographic surveillance is warranted to rule out hydrops and arrhythmias; in the absence of hydrops, prognosis is favorable, often with spontaneous regression.	III	B	122
If hydrops develops, timing affects response:			
Hydrops before fetal viability should prompt counseling and consideration of pregnancy termination.	–	GPP	–
If pericardial effusion with tamponade develops, pericardiocentesis is necessary.	III	B	134, 135
Preterm delivery with maternal steroids is indicated if early signs of hydrops and gestational age is acceptable.	–	GPP	–
Tumors can resolve after birth; surgery is indicated for those that persist with hemodynamic compromise.	III	B	125, 126

US, ultrasound.

ADRENAL TUMORS: NEUROBLASTOMA

Neuroblastoma is the most common malignant congenital tumor, with a prevalence of 0.6 to 2.0 per 100,000 live births. It originates from the neural crest cells that migrate along each side of the spine and give rise to the adrenal medulla and the sympathetic ganglia. Although tumor can begin anywhere along this path, the most common location is intra-abdominal, involving the adrenal gland. Other locations include the neck, thorax, and pelvis.[138] More than 90% of antenatally diagnosed neuroblastomas are adrenal in origin.[139]

Normal adrenal development can be difficult to distinguish in the fetus from neuroblastoma. Neuroblasts normally mature in the fetus to form ganglion cells referred to as neuroblastoma in situ, with a prevalence of 1 in 250 at term. The development of a clinical neuroblastoma represents a defect in the cellular maturation and differentiation. This defect is thought to be temporary in some cases and accounts for the 15% to 20% rate of spontaneous regression.[140]

Diagnosis

The sonographic appearance of adrenal neuroblastoma is variable, ranging from cystic with a thick-walled complex to solid with hyperechogenicity and foci of calcification.[89,139–142] Approximately 40% to 50% of antenatally diagnosed neuroblastomas have a cystic appearance, which may represent a stage of involution.[139] Doppler flow mapping may aid the diagnosis, as the nest of tumor cells is highly vascular, and the pulsatile flow observed in such tumors is suggestive of neovascularization.[143] Other lesions in the differential diagnosis include adrenal hemorrhage, renal mass, and intra-abdominal extralobar pulmonary sequestration. Adrenal hemorrhage is rare antenatally, and the neonatal diagnosis is frequently prompted by hemorrhage into nests of tumor cells.[89,140] Antenatal adrenal hemorrhage is also reported with Beckwith-Wiedemann syndrome, which is characterized by omphalocele and macroglossia.

Metastases occur frequently in utero and can be visualized with sonography. Hepatic metastases are most common, seen in up to 25% of fetuses with near total replacement of the hepatic parenchyma reported in some instances.[139,140] Other sites of metastasis include the retroperitoneal lymph nodes, bone marrow, umbilical cord, and skin. Although nearly 90% of children with neuroblastoma have elevated urinary levels of vanillylmandelic acid (VMA) or homovanillic acid (HVA), only 30% to 35% of prenatally diagnosed cases have elevated urinary levels when measured postnatally. Although the measurement of maternal urinary VMA or HVA has prompted diagnosis in a few instances, the yield is relatively low.[139]

Hydramnios or fetal hydrops is reported in association with neuroblastoma, and may be the findings that prompt the initial sonographic examination at which time the diagnosis is made. The precise mechanism is unknown, but possibilities include fetal anemia due to bone marrow infiltration, fetal arrhythmia due to catecholamine excess, placental vascular obstruction due to tumor metastases, and vena caval obstruction due to tumor compression.[138-140] In rare cases, the presenting complaints are maternal signs of catecholamine excess such as hypertension, coagulopathy, renal abnormality, or hepatic abnormality.[144,145] Several genetic disorders associated with abnormalities of neural crest derivatives—Beckwith-Wiedemann syndrome, DiGeorge syndrome, and CHARGE association—are associated with neuroblastoma. In addition, a familial form of neuroblastoma is described. Thus, a prior affected child should prompt antenatal screening of subsequent pregnancies.[82,146]

Risks

The prognosis for the fetus depends on tumor stage and the clinical manifestations of the disease. Although the survival rate in children older than 1 year at diagnosis is only 10% to 20%, the survival rate in neonates is greater than 90%.[89,138–140] The presence of fetal hydrops is strongly correlated with advanced disease and markedly increases the risk of the mother developing preeclampsia. In a series of 21 fetuses with an antenatal diagnosis of neuroblastoma collected from the literature, three fetuses developed hydrops. All had advanced stage disease, and all three mothers had preeclampsia. Two of the three died antenatally.[140]

The prognosis for a fetus with either stage I or stage IV tumors (metastases involving liver, skin, or bone marrow) is excellent with survival rates of 90% or better after resection of the primary lesion. The high survival rate reflects the tendency for these tumors to undergo spontaneous regression.[89,139] The prognosis for stages II and III disease is poor, but fortunately they are rare.

Tumor hemorrhage and rupture during labor are reported, but their occurrence is rare. Because dystocia can develop when the fetus has massive hepatomegaly, the abdominal circumference should be regularly monitored by ultrasound in fetuses with metastatic disease; cesarean section is an option should the abdominal circumference be markedly enlarged.[138,147–149]

Management Options

Most women whose fetus has neuroblastoma are relatively asymptomatic. Serial ultrasound examinations are indicated to assess tumor size, amniotic fluid volume, and fetal growth, and to seek evidence of developing hydrops. Careful surveillance for evidence of maternal hypertension is critical. In the setting of fetal hydrops, the decision to deliver is based on the gestation and the potential for survival. In fetuses younger than 32 weeks' gestation, antenatal corticosteroids may be administered to enhance pulmonary maturity prior to delivery. If maternal symptoms of preeclampsia develop, delivery should be seriously considered regardless of gestation. Any fetus suspected of having a neuroblastoma should be delivered at a tertiary center where the appropriate support staff is readily available. The appropriately grown fetus without evidence of fetal or maternal compromise may be delivered vaginally at term.

SUMMARY OF MANAGEMENT OPTIONS
Neuroblastoma

Management Options	Quality of Evidence	Strength of Recommendation	References
Evaluate for hydramnios, hydrops, maternal clinical features (hypertension/preeclampsia, hydramnios, abdominal distention); measurement of maternal urinary catecholamines may help confirm diagnosis.	III	B	140
Delivery may be the only effective treatment. The decision to deliver must include consideration of gestational age, the likelihood of fetal viability, and the maternal condition; use steroids if preterm.	–	GPP	–
Neuroblastomas have a high propensity for metastasis but a high rate of spontaneous regression postnatally.	III	B	139
Take serial measurements of fetal abdominal circumference: a very large renal mass may cause dystocia, necessitating cesarean delivery.	IV	C	138
Prognosis is based on tumor stage. Most cases of fetal neuroblastoma are stage I. Prognosis is generally good.	III	B	139

RENAL TUMORS

Although renal tumors in the neonate are rare, accounting for only 5% of all perinatal tumors, renal masses account for 70% of all abdominal masses in the perinatal period.[150] The majority of these masses are hydronephrotic or multicystic dysplastic kidneys.[4,150] Despite their low frequency, renal tumors are often identified antenatally because of the relative ease with which the kidneys are visualized sonographically. The most common renal tumors are congenital mesoblastic nephroma (renal hamartoma) and Wilms' tumor (nephroblastoma).

Diagnosis

Congenital mesoblastic nephroma is a benign renal lesion composed of spindle cell mesenchymal elements that grow between intact nephrons and replace normal renal parenchymal.[151] It is the most common renal tumor in neonates and is distinguished from Wilms' tumor by its benign clinical behavior.[4] Sonographically, these lesions usually appear as a solid mass without a distinct capsule. However, occasional cystic changes, nodular densities, or diffuse enlargement of one kidney are reported.[138] A fundal height larger than expected for dates may be the finding that initiates further evaluation, as the majority of the antenatal cases reported were associated with hydramnios.[3,4,151] The mechanism of the hydramnios is unclear, but increased renal blood flow, impaired renal concentrating ability, and impaired gastrointestinal motility due to a mass effect are all implicated.[138] The differential diagnosis includes hydronephrosis and multicystic dysplastic kidney (which can usually be excluded because of their predominantly cystic nature), Wilms' tumor, and metastasis from hepatic and adrenal gland malignancies. Wilms' tumor often cannot be distinguished from mesoblastic nephroma antenatally; a histologic examination may be required for diagnosis.[4,138,152] These tumors are isolated findings without associated anomalies.

Wilms' tumor appears sonographically very similar to congenital mesoblastic nephroma, except a distinct capsule may be identifiable. This tumor is believed to be derived from the metanephric blastema, which is the embryonic precursor of nephrons and the renal interstitium.[4] It typically is unilateral (95%) and does not cross the midline.[152] Associated congenital anomalies are common, and Wilms' tumor is described as a component of several genetic syndromes or associations, including WAGR (Wilms' tumor, aniridia, genitourinary malformations, and mental retardation) syndrome due to an 11p13deletion, and VATER (vertebral malformations, imperforate anus, tracheoesophageal fistula, limb abnormalities, and renal abnormalities) association.[153] It is also associated with several overgrowth syndromes including Beckwith-Wiedemann syndrome, Sotos (cerebral gigantism) syndrome, Perlman (nephromegaly, hydramnios, macrosomia, cardiac defects, and diaphragmatic hernia) syndrome, and Simpson-Golabi-Behmel (coarse facies, cardiac defects, islet cell hyperplasia, vertebral abnormalities, and vestigial tail) syndrome.[154,155] A sonographic suspicion of nephromegaly or the family history for any of these disorders requires a detailed sonographic examination and careful postnatal surveillance for the development of an obvious tumor mass (if not already present). Fewer than 1% of Wilms' tumor cases are familial with autosomal dominant inheritance. However, 20% of familial cases are bilateral, compared to only 3% of sporadic cases, thus warranting a thorough postnatal evaluation of both kidneys.[156]

Risks

Congenital mesoblastic nephroma is commonly associated with hydramnios. High renin levels are reported and hyper-reninism may precipitate fetal hypertension and rarely hydrops. Other potential causes of hydrops include obstruction of the portacaval circulation, arteriovenous shunting through the tumor, and hemorrhage into the tumor with resulting fetal anemia.[3,138,151] The prognosis for an affected fetus depends on the identity of the mass and the presence of hydrops or associated anomalies. Simple nephrectomy is usually curative with an isolated congenital mesoblastic nephroma. Fetuses with associated anomalies should be carefully evaluated to determine if the constellation of findings represents a defined genetic syndrome. An amniocentesis for karyotype may be warranted. The prognosis for Wilms' tumor depends on the stage of disease at diagnosis. Survival after surgery and adjuvant therapy is greater than 90% when disease is confined to the area of the kidney, as is usual for prenatally diagnosed tumors.[155] The prognosis for the hydropic fetus is more guarded.

Management Options

Because the majority of solid renal tumors are congenital mesoblastic nephromas with a benign clinical course, pregnancy should be allowed to go to term. Periodic sonographic examinations are indicated to monitor fetal growth and amniotic fluid volume and to rule out any signs of developing hydrops. Delivery should be contemplated if hydrops develops at a gestation when survival is expected. Before 32 weeks antenatal corticosteroids should be considered prior to delivery.[138] Dystocia is reported in cases with large renal masses. Cesarean section may be considered if the abdominal circumference is markedly enlarged.

SUMMARY OF MANAGEMENT OPTIONS

Renal Tumors

Management Options	Quality of Evidence	Strength of Recommendation	References
Assess for development of hydramnios or hydrops.	–	GPP	–
Renal tumors (majority are mesoblastic nephromas) are associated with hydramnios in contrast to dysplastic kidneys; prognosis overall is favorable.	Ib	A	155
Preterm delivery with maternal steroid therapy may be necessary if hydrops develops.	IV	C	138
If the abdominal circumference is enlarged, cesarean delivery may be required.	–	GPP	–

HEPATIC TUMORS

Primary liver tumors are rare in the fetus. Embryologically, the liver is derived from endodermal and mesodermal anlagen and is the potential site for a wide spectrum of neoplasms and other lesions that mimic neoplastic processes.[157] The most frequently identified lesions in the perinatal period are hemangioendothelioma, hemangioma, mesenchymal hamartoma, and hepatoblastoma. The differential diagnosis for hepatic mass lesions includes these lesions as well as metastatic lesions and polycystic liver disease.

Diagnosis

Hemangioendothelioma and hemangioma are vascular tumors derived from endothelial cells forming vascular channels. A hemangioendothelioma has focal or diffuse hypercellular areas, whereas a hemangioma contains flat, inconspicuous endothelium with dilated vascular spaces.[157] Hemangioendothelioma is the most common hepatic vascular lesion in the perinate, but hemangioma is the most common vascular lesion in all age groups. These lesions have a variable sonographic image, appearing hypoechogenic, hyperechogenic, or mixed, depending on the degree of fibrosis, hypercellularity, and the degree of involution.[138] Hepatomegaly and multifocal lesions are seen. Doppler study of the lesion provides confirmation of its vascular nature. Large vascular spaces within the mass are frequently seen with hemangioendotheliomas, and dominant feeding or draining vessels may also be identifiable.[158] Hydramnios is reported, and may be due to either arteriovenous shunting or gastrointestinal tract compression. Midtrimester maternal serum AFP levels are frequently elevated.[158]

Mesenchymal hamartomas are composed of connective tissue stroma, serous cysts, bile ducts, hepatocytes, and angiomatous components.[4,159] These lesions typically have a complex sonographic appearance, with irregular solid and cystic components that can become enlarged and calcified.[160] Hepatoblastoma is the most common hepatic malignancy in the first year of life when 50% to 60% of all hepatoblastomas present. Although hepatoblastoma is believed to develop in utero, fewer than 10% of tumors are detectable antenatally.[4] Sonographically, these lesions are solid-appearing with occasional calcifications. Approximately two thirds involve only one liver lobe, though occasionally only diffuse hepatic enlargement causing abdominal distention may be seen.[161] Although approximately 80% to 90% of childhood or adult patients with hepatoblastoma have an elevated AFP level, the maternal serum AFP levels are not apparently useful for a fetal diagnosis.[4,161]

Risks

Although hemangioendothelioma and hemangioma are benign tumors, they are associated with life-threatening perinatal complications such as hydrops secondary to high-output congestive heart failure and arteriovenous shunting, a consumptive coagulopathy due to platelet sequestration (Kasabach-Merritt syndrome), or hemoperitoneum from intrapartum hepatic rupture. Cutaneous hemangiomas and hemangiomas in other sites, such as the eye, are reported in 40% to 45% of children with hemangioendothelioma.[157,158] There also appears to be an association between hemangioendothelioma and placental chorioangioma, the latter often associated with hydramnios and hydrops.[162] Although the majority of lesions regress and involute during early infancy, the size of the lesion and the degree of arteriovenous shunting will determine the antenatal risk of complications such as hydramnios, hydrops, and preterm delivery. The prognosis for the fetus that remains free of hemodynamic compromise is excellent; the prognosis is poor if hydrops develops.[163]

Rapid growth of mesenchymal hamartomas characterized by enlargement of the cystic components is common and increases the risk of hydrops. Of 13 antenatally diagnosed cases in the literature, 5 were complicated by hydrops or maternal preeclampsia, necessitating delivery; the perinatal mortality rate was approximately 25%.[160] Intrauterine drainage of the cystic lesions has not proved beneficial because drainage into the abdominal or amniotic cavity does not decrease fluid production and may actually precipitate hemodynamic compromise. Further, most cysts are multiloculated and not amenable to a single drainage procedure. In the asymptomatic fetus delivered near term, the prognosis is favorable after surgical resection. Owing to a propensity for spontaneous regression, some pediatric surgeons recommend a conservative, observational strategy.[160]

Hepatoblastoma is a locally invasive tumor that can on occasion metastasize to the lung, brain, adrenal gland, and placenta. Large tumors are associated with hydramnios and hydrops due to a combination of factors including gastrointestinal obstruction, anemia from tumor hemorrhage, compression of the hepatic vasculature and inferior vena cava, and possibly decreased colloid oncotic pressure secondary to altered hepatic synthetic capabilities.[161] Hepatoblastoma, as well as adrenocortical and Wilms' tumors, can occur in association with Beckwith-Wiedemann syndrome; 1% of patients with this syndrome develop hepatoblastoma.[157] Other anomalies associated with hepatoblastoma include hemihypertrophy in 2% to 3%,[157] trisomy 18, Schinzel-Giedion syndrome (congenital heart defects, midface retraction, hypertrichosis, and embryonal malignancies), trisomy 21, and genitourinary abnormalities.[138] There are few reports of antenatally diagnosed hepatoblastoma, and the prognosis for these lesions is uncertain, but it appears dismal in the setting of hydrops.[161,164,165] Complete surgical resection is possible in 40% to 75% of patients, and the survival rate in this group is 60%. The prognosis is poor if complete resection is not possible due to infiltrative disease or metastatic lesions.[4,166]

Management Options

Once a hepatic mass is identified, serial sonographic studies are indicated to monitor fetal status, tumor size, and amniotic fluid volume. Although the ideal mode of delivery is unclear, there are case reports of intrapartum rupture of large hepatic masses with subsequent fetal death.[138,164] It seems reasonable to consider cesarean delivery in cases of marked hepatic enlargement leading to abdominal distention. However, the risks of operative delivery need to be carefully considered in the context of the fetal prognosis. If the fetus has no signs of decompensation, delivery occurs at term. The role of intratumor injection of corticosteroids is uncertain.[235]

SUMMARY OF MANAGEMENT OPTIONS

Hepatic Tumors

Management Options	Quality of Evidence	Strength of Recommendation	References
Assess for hydramnios and hydrops (high output failure).	–	GPP	–
Cesarean section may be considered for large tumors with possibility of dystocia or tumor rupture (vascular tumors are most common).	IV	C	138,164
Role of intratumor injections of corticosteroids with tumor enlargement and hydramnios is uncertain.	IV	C	236

INTRA-ABDOMINAL CYSTS

Although these cysts are not strictly tumors, the identification of a cyst or cysts in the fetal abdomen raises concern. A wide variety of cystic masses are detectable in the fetal abdomen including ovarian, mesenteric, urachal, choledochal, renal, hepatic, and splenic cysts. Enteric duplication, bowel obstruction, and meconium pseudocyst may also present as cystic lesions.[167] The location, size, and appearance of the cyst usually suggest the diagnosis.

Ovarian cysts are common. Approximately 95% are unilateral, and the majority are benign, functional cysts that occur in response to maternal hormones and resolve spontaneously after delivery. Sonographically, an ovarian cyst appears as a regular, hypoechoic structure in the lower abdomen. Septations or solid components may be seen if torsion or hemorrhage has occurred. Rarely, a cyst may become so large as to impinge on other organs, cause ovarian torsion and subsequent infarction, or result in dystocia. Ultrasound-guided in utero aspiration of large cysts is reported and may reduce these risks.[168,169]

Choledochal cysts represent a dilation of the common bile duct arising from either a weakness in the wall of the bile duct, or from a developmental anomaly and distal obstruction elsewhere in the biliary tree, especially at the junction of the pancreatic and common bile ducts.[170] These cysts have a prevalence of 1 in 2 million live births, and occur more frequently in females and Asians.[171,172] Sonographically, it appears as a simple, anechoic cyst in the upper abdomen, usually medial to the fetal gallbladder. Occasionally, a tubular structure is seen at the junction of the right and left hepatic ducts or the cystic and common bile ducts (Fig. 23–10). This lesion is not associated with an increased rate of either fetal or maternal complications.[173] However, the patency of the biliary tree must be evaluated in the neonate as it is impossible to distinguish biliary atresia from a choledochal cyst on ultrasound.[170,174,175] All infants with these lesions require surgical treatment and reconstructive surgery of the biliary connections. However, the long-term prognosis with appropriate surgical treatment is excellent.

Solitary cysts are occasionally identified in the hepatic parenchyma. These lesions are usually small and unilocular. Embryologically, they are thought reflect interruptions in the development of the intrahepatic biliary tree, and frequently resolve spontaneously.[167]

Bowel atresia or stenosis may produce cystic dilation of bowel segments proximal to the obstruction. Megacystis-microcolon-intestinal hypoperistalsis syndrome, an autosomal recessive disorder associated with vacuolation and degeneration of the smooth muscle in the bowel and bladder walls, may present as multiple cystic structures in the abdomen that represent dilated segments of proximal small intestine and bladder. No specific antenatal intervention is required. However, hydramnios may develop depending on the degree and level of obstruction. A pediatric surgical evaluation should be obtained after birth prior to the initiation of enteral feeding should bowel atresia be suspected.

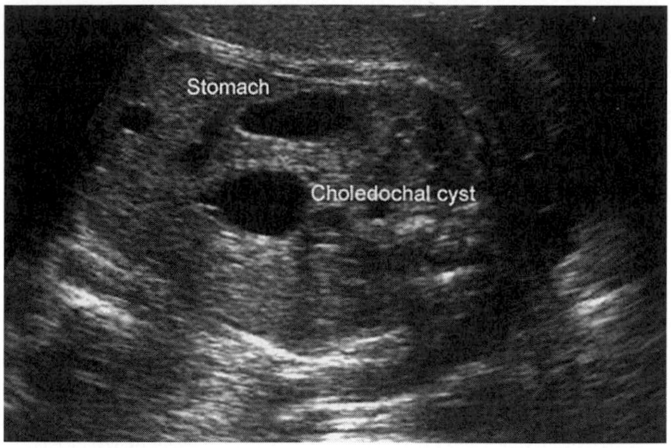

FIGURE 23–10
A choledochal cyst was identified in this fetus at 20 weeks' gestation. The cyst was located in the common bile duct.

Mesenteric and omental cysts represent the benign proliferation of ectopic lymphatic ducts that lack communication with normal lymphatic channels. They occur most commonly in the small bowel mesentery, but can occur anywhere in the gastrointestinal tract. Most of these lesions are asymptomatic antenatally and do not require specific intervention, although there is one report of an enteric cyst associated with hydrops (cause and effect unlikely).[176] Postnatally, enlarging lesions may cause partial bowel obstruction, but the prognosis following surgical resection is excellent.[177] Enteric duplication cysts have a similar sonographic appearance and can only be distinguished postnatally.

SUMMARY OF MANAGEMENT OPTIONS
Intra-Abdominal Cysts

Management Options	Quality of Evidence	Strength of Recommendation	References
Evaluate for cyst enlargement and pressure effects, hydramnios, and hydrops.	–	GPP	–
Rarely, an ovarian cyst impinges on other organs, causes an ovarian torsion, or results in dystocia. Transabdominal aspiration and decompression of the cyst may be preferable to cesarean delivery. The fluid is unlikely to be irritant or malignant.	III	B	168,169
Most cysts do not require intrauterine intervention.			
Delivery should be in a tertiary center because neonatal surgery may be required.	–	GPP	–

SACROCOCCYGEAL TERATOMA

Sacrococcygeal teratoma (SCT) is one of the most common tumors of the perinatal period with a prevalence of 1 in 35,000 to 40,000 live births. It is four to nine times more common in females than males.[60,138,178–181] Like teratomas in other locations, these tumors contain elements derived from all three germ cell layers. Sacrococcygeal tumors are believed to arise from either Hansen's node or from ectopic primordial germ cells.[179–181] The majority of sacrococcygeal teratomas diagnosed perinatally are benign, but malignant degeneration reportedly complicates up to 10%, especially when there is a delay in resection or when the tumor is not entirely resected.[179–181] Lesions with foci of immature cells are described in 10% to 15% of cases.[182,183]

The American Academy of Pediatrics (AAP) has adopted a staging system for sacrococcygeal teratomas that grades the involvement of intrapelvic structures and hence the complications associated with surgical resection.[184] Type I tumors, the most common type, are predominantly external and protrude from the perineal region with minimal, if any, presacral component. Type II lesions are primarily external, but have a significant intrapelvic portion, whereas type III lesions are primarily intrapelvic with a small external component. Type IV tumors are completely presacral with no external component.

Diagnosis

Teratomas have a similar gross appearance regardless of their site of origin, and are generally well circumscribed without direct invasion of adjacent tissues. The most common appearance is that of a complex mass, although predominantly solid or cystic masses are also described. The most common location is caudal and dorsal in close proximity to the coccyx[180] (Fig. 23–11). Teratomas with

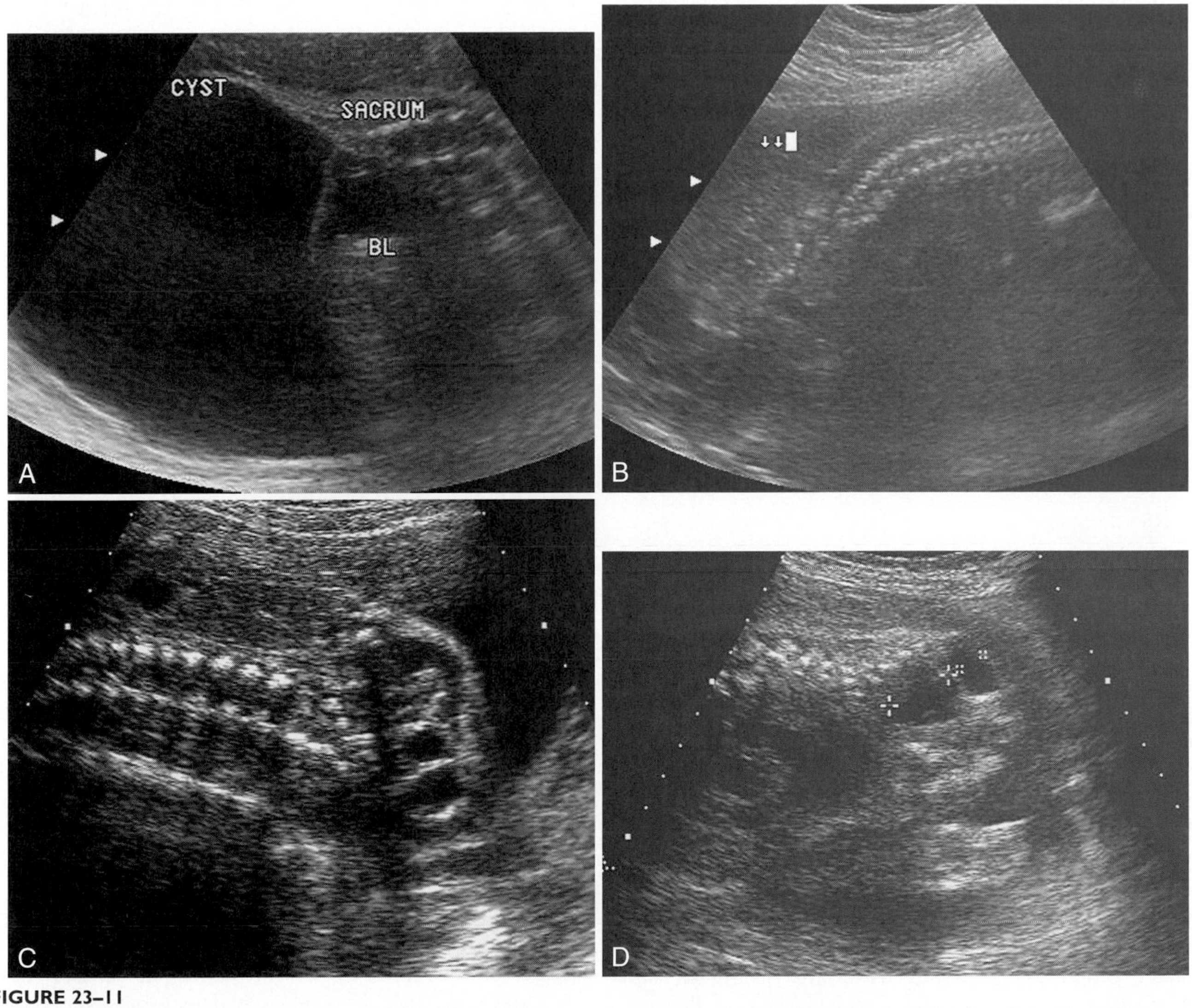

FIGURE 23–11
Different types of sacrococcygeal teratomas. *A*, Type 1 lesion—the tumor is entirely extrapelvic; this tumor is predominantly cystic. *B*, Type 1 lesion—although the tumor is entirely extrapelvic, it is more solid appearing. *C*, Type 2 lesion—the predominant portion of the tumor is extrapelvic, but intrapelvic portions are visible. *D*, Type 4 lesion—the tumor appears to be located entirely within the fetal pelvis with no external component evident.

a significant intrapelvic component can compress the urinary and gastrointestinal tracts. Fluid-filled anechoic areas may be visualized proximal to the obstruction. Immature teratomas tend to have a more solid than cystic appearance.[60] Doppler interrogation of the tumor confirms the highly vascular nature. The feeding vessels have blood flow velocities similar to the descending aorta and may have a diameter similar to the external iliac arteries.[185] The middle sacral artery and branches of the internal iliac artery are usually the main sources of blood and, because of the augmented blood flow, are often easily identified antenatally.[181,186,187] The differential diagnosis includes meningomyelocele, hemangioma, lipoma, and other rare soft tissue tumors. A lumbosacral meningomyelocele is differentiated from teratoma based on the presence of spinal dysraphism and intracranial changes that are typically absent with sacral teratoma. Hydramnios, placentomegaly, and fetal hydrops are associated with sacrococcygeal teratomas containing arteriovenous malformations.[179,185]

The incidence of associated anomalies is uncertain, and ranges in the literature from 0% to 35%.[3,178,184,188,189] Certainly, a detailed anatomic survey with special focus on skeletal/vertebral anomalies is obligatory. Defects in the area of the tumor, such as distal sacral agenesis, rectovaginal fistula, and imperforate anus, are reported and likely related to tumor growth during gestation.[189] Aneuploidy has not been reported with sacrococcygeal teratoma, and amniocentesis for a karyotype is not usually indicated.[138] Maternal serum AFP levels may be elevated, especially in those tumors with foci of endodermal sinus tumor. The amniotic fluid AFP and acetylcholinesterase levels may also be elevated.[190–192] MRI can aid ascertainment of intrapelvic involvement. This information is useful in both counseling the parents and planning surgical resection.[193,194]

Risks

The prognosis for antenatally diagnosed SCT differs from that of postnatally diagnosed lesions, with estimates of mortality rate ranging from 12% to 68%.[178,185,195–197] The main causes of perinatal death are hydrops, intrapartum trauma, and postnatally either difficulties with resection or hemorrhage secondary to tumor vascularity.[179] Hydrops may result from the inability of the heart to adequately perfuse the fetus, placenta, and tumor. An arterial steal syndrome often develops if the tumor contains arteriovenous malformations and blood is preferentially shunted to the tumor. The fetus may develop high-output failure due to limited cardiac pumping ability and anemia secondary to sequestration of blood volume in the tumor.[181,185] Because larger tumors require greater blood flow, fetuses with large, vascular, and especially solid tumors are more likely to develop hydrops[179,183,185] compared to those with predominantly cystic lesions associated with low blood flow.[182] The mortality rate is greater than 90% if hydrops develops.[178,179,185,197–199]

Other predictors of poor outcome include a second trimester diagnosis and delivery before 34 weeks' gestation.[179] The risk of preterm delivery correlates with the size of the tumor and the presence of hydramnios, both of which increase uterine distention.[182] In a compilation of 104 cases from the literature, Brace and associates noted that survival increased from 25% for fetuses delivered before 34 weeks' gestation to 88% for those born after 34 weeks' gestation. Survival was half as high when the diagnosis was made prior to 30 weeks' gestation (41% versus 84%).[179] Not only are large tumors associated with an increased risk of hydramnios, hydrops, and prematurity, but they are also associated with an increased risk of dystocia, intrapartum injury, hemorrhage, or rupture, regardless of the mode of delivery.[178–180,183]

The most important variable affecting long-term outcome is the adequacy of tumor removal.[60] The presence of a substantial presacral component is associated with a worse prognosis because of the complexity involved with resection. Optimal treatment consists of an en bloc removal of the tumor and coccyx, but with extensive presacral involvement, this cannot always be accomplished. Although both mature and immature teratomas are equally resectable, there is a greater risk of intraoperative hemorrhage with an immature teratoma, reflecting its increased vascularity. The identification of frankly malignant elements, especially endodermal sinus or embryonal cell tissue, markedly worsens the prognosis. If the primary tumor is not completely resected, there is an increased risk for recurrence, often with malignant components.[60]

Management Options

Counseling should be provided at the time of diagnosis when the evaluation including MRI is complete. If the tumor is identified at an early gestational age or is associated with hydrops, the option of termination of pregnancy should be offered. Serial antenatal sonographic examinations are indicated to assess fetal well-being and to evaluate tumor growth. If hydramnios develops, amnioreduction may improve maternal symptoms and delay the onset of preterm delivery. If preterm labor develops, tocolysis can be attempted. The efficacy of magnesium as a tocolytic is at best unclear, and in this setting coexistent hydramnios may intensify maternal side effects. Indomethacin may worsen the fetal cardiovascular function by reducing renal free water clearance and premature closure of the ductus arteriosus. A calcium-channel antagonist such as nifedipine may be a superior alternative. In the fetus without evidence of cardiac decompensation, delivery is planned at or near term in a tertiary center. If signs of fetal cardiac decompensation develop after 30 weeks, corticosteroids should be administered to improve postnatal pulmonary function and delivery effected. The optimal management for the fetus with hydrops at earlier gestational ages is unclear, but the prognosis for these fetuses is dismal.

Operative intervention to interrupt the vascular shunt in fetuses with hydrops, who are otherwise preterminal, has been attempted. Open fetal surgery with in utero debulking or complete resection of the tumor was reported in eight cases, with three long-term survivors.[200,201] Other techniques have been investigated to avoid the maternal morbidity associated with fetal surgery. Radiofrequency ablation via a percutaneously placed electrode was reported in four fetuses; two died after the procedure due to intratumor hemorrhage. The hydrops reversed in the two surviving fetuses, but both were found at birth to have large areas of soft tissue necrosis requiring reconstructive surgery.[186] Further refinement is needed.

Because of the risk of intrapartum traumatic injury, rupture, and hemorrhage, cesarean delivery prior to the onset of active labor is recommended for fetuses with a SCT greater than 5 to 10 cm in diameter.[178–180,182,183] A large vertical uterine incision is required to minimize delivery trauma which may trigger massive hemorrhage. Type O negative blood should be immediately available for the neonate. It has been suggested that a vaginal delivery may be considered if the tumor is smaller than 5 cm, with an emergent cesarean delivery should any evidence of fetal hemodynamic compromise develop.[180,187] Percutaneous aspiration of a large, predominantly cystic teratoma to facilitate vaginal delivery is reported.[202] Regardless of the mode of delivery, successful management requires the multidisciplinary efforts of maternal-fetal medicine specialists, neonatologists, anesthesiologists, and pediatric surgeons.

Neonates who are stable and have no complications of prematurity will typically undergo surgical resection within the first few days of life. Although in some, surgical trauma to the sacral and pelvic nerves results in urologic or bowel dysfunction, most neonates have excellent functional and cosmetic outcomes.[181–183] The long-term prognosis is determined by the extent of intrapelvic involvement and the ability to completely resect the tumor mass.

SUMMARY OF MANAGEMENT OPTIONS

Sacrococcygeal Teratoma

Management Options	Quality of Evidence	Strength of Recommendation	References
Search for other abnormalities.	III	B	178,184
Use of MRI as an adjunct may clarify anatomy and aid counseling.	IIb	B	193,194
Cystic lesions have better prognosis.	III	B	179,185
Early diagnosis, especially with development of hydrops, allows termination of pregnancy to be considered as a management option.	–	GPP	–
Serial sonographic surveillance is warranted because hydramnios and hydrops are common.	III	B	179,185
Amnioreduction with hydramnios may be indicated.	–	GPP	–
Delivery should be in tertiary center with multidisciplinary approach, especially at and after delivery.	–	GPP	–
Preterm delivery with maternal corticosteroid administration is an option if hydrops develops (prognosis poor).	–	GPP	–
In utero surgery should be regarded as experimental.	IV	C	200,201
Cesarean section (including a classical approach) may be required to facilitate atraumatic delivery, especially with larger lesions.	IV	C	180,187
Have O-negative blood standing by at delivery.	–	GPP	–
Neonatal stabilization and surgery may be indicated.	III	B	181–183

LIMB TUMORS

Limb masses are usually either soft tissue tumors (such as fibrous connective tissue tumors, lipomas), skeletal muscle tumors, or tumor-like conditions such as vascular or lymphatic anomalies or hamartomas.

Diagnosis

Soft tissue tumors are often identified at birth or during neonatal life, but rarely reported in the fetus. In the neonate, most soft tissue limb tumors are described as a palpable mass in fascia, muscle, or subcutaneous tissue, or a smooth, solid, asymmetrical enlargement of a digit or extremity.[4] Hemangiomas are the most common tumors diagnosed in the neonate, and although they may first appear in the late fetal period, they are rarely identified before birth.[203]

Infantile fibromatosis is a benign neoplasm of fibrous tissue that occurs in fascia, muscle, or periosteum. This lesion is a type of proliferative fibroblastic disorder difficult to distinguish from low-grade fibrosarcoma, and although locally aggressive and subject to recurrence, is not associated with metastases.[4] Digital fibromas are among the most common of these lesions, and are typically found on the medial side of digits.[203]

Fibrosarcoma and rhabdomyosarcoma are the two most common malignant soft tissue tumors. Fibrosarcoma is usually cured by local resection, but rhabdomyosarcoma has a propensity for early metastasis and has, therefore, a less favorable prognosis.[204,205]

Congenital lymphangiomas appear sonographically as multicystic masses with anechoic cyst cavities and often result in hypertrophy of the affected extremity. Because of an association with fetal aneuploidy, especially Turner syndrome, a fetal karyotype determination should be offered when a lymphangioma is suspected antenatally.[206]

Klippel-Trenaunay syndrome is a rare congenital syndrome with generalized mesodermal abnormalities including macular vascular nevus, skeletal and soft tissue hypertrophy, and venous varicosities due to abnormal small vessels.[207] Unilateral leg hypertrophy is the most frequent finding on ultrasound, but any extremity may be involved, as may an entire half of the body including the head and brain.[208,209] The finding of a complex mass in the subcutaneous tissue in the presence of hypertrophy of a limb or other body part is highly suggestive of Klippel-Trenaunay syndrome.[210] Proteus syndrome shares several features with Klippel-Trenaunay syndrome, including asymmetrical focal overgrowth, hemihypertrophy, and subcutaneous vascular abnormalities, but is distinguished by the presence of warty pigmented nevi and lipoid visceral tumors.[211] This distinction between the two conditions may not be antenatally possible if limb hypertrophy is the main clinical finding. Both syndromes have a variable prognosis.[211,212]

Risks

These tumors are unlikely to cause maternal symptoms, but vascular tumors are associated with an increased risk of fetal cardiac decompensation. Kasabach-Merritt syndrome, a consumptive coagulopathy due to intralesional clotting and platelet sequestration, occurs in superficial vascular malformations, and can be life-threatening. It is reported in the neonatal period.[207]

Management Options

Close antenatal sonographic monitoring is warranted once a lesion is suspected, not only to identify early signs of fetal compromise, but also to monitor the size of the affected area. A markedly enlarged extremity or body wall can lead to dystocia; cesarean delivery may be necessary.

SUMMARY OF MANAGEMENT OPTIONS

Limb Tumors

Management Options	Quality of Evidence	Strength of Recommendation	References
Serial surveillance is needed to assess growth of tumor and development of hydramnios and hydrops.	–	GPP	–
Obstetric care is usually unaffected, though occasionally cesarean section may be necessary to avoid dystocia.	–	GPP	–

PLACENTAL AND UMBILICAL CORD TUMORS

Tumors of the umbilical cord and placenta are rare. Most masses identified in these structures are vascular malformations or hematomas. Although the majority of lesions are asymptomatic, some can have significant impact on pregnancy outcome.

Diagnosis

Chorioangioma is the most common benign tumor of the placenta, and is thought to be either an angioma or hamartoma derived from primitive chorionic mesenchyme.[213,214] Small lesions are found in up to 1% of placentas examined pathologically, and larger lesions are much less common. Tumors ranging in size from a few millimeters to more than 10 cm have been reported.[213]

The sonographic appearance of a chorioangioma is that of a solid or complex mass on the fetal surface of the placenta (Fig. 23–12). Doppler interrogation will confirm the highly vascular nature of the mass and is typically required to distinguish these lesions from a placental or subchorionic hematoma.[213–216] The maternal serum AFP levels may also be elevated.[213,216]

Although exceedingly rare, placental teratomas are reported.[217–219] As with other teratomas, the cystic and solid components appear sonographically as a complex mass.

Other solid masses identified in placental tissue include metastases from fetal and maternal primary tumors, especially melanoma.[220,221] Although antenatal identification of such lesions has yet to be described, they should be considered in the differential diagnosis of solid placental masses when the clinical scenario warrants.

The most commonly identified umbilical cord masses are hematomas, true cysts, and pseudocysts. An umbilical cord hematoma appears sonographically as a cylindrical solid mass occluding the umbilical vein. Doppler studies may reveal turbulent flow in the area of the hematoma. True cysts in the umbilical cord are remnants of the omphalomesenteric duct or allantois, and are usually located near the fetal end of the umbilical cord (Fig. 23–13). Pseudocysts are more common, and represent localized degeneration and edema of Wharton's jelly. Although they can occur anywhere along the umbilical cord, they are usually near the fetal end.[222,223] The differentiation between pseudocysts and true cysts cannot be made on sonographic findings alone. Hemangiomas of the umbilical cord and varicosities of the umbilical vein are also seen antenatally, as are teratomas. Masses located at the fetal cord insertion site must be distinguished from omphalocele.[224–227]

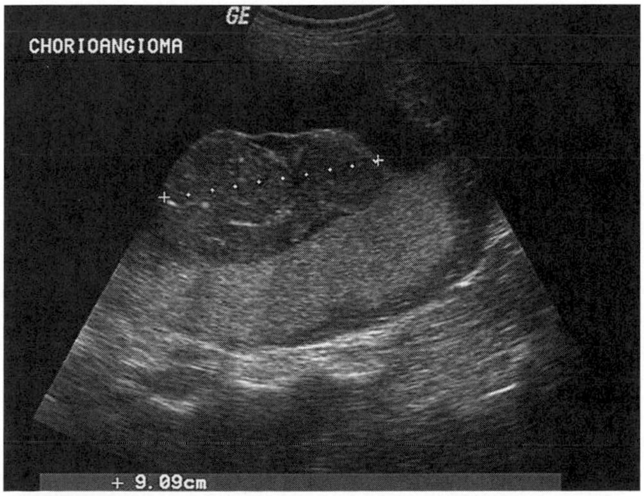

FIGURE 23–12
A large chorioangioma was diagnosed at 22 weeks' gestation. The tumor continued to grow over the next several weeks and the fetus developed severe hydramnios. Intractable preterm labor occurred at 29 weeks.

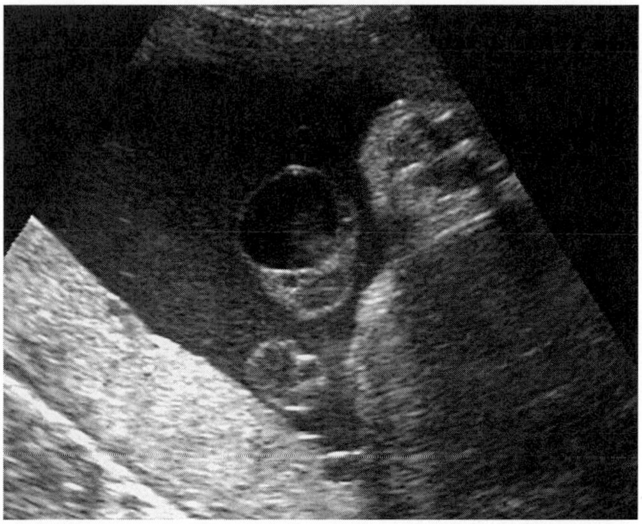

FIGURE 23–13
An isolated umbilical cord cyst was identified near the fetal end of the umbilical cord in this fetus. Doppler studies confirmed normal blood flow in the umbilical vessels.

Risks

If a chorioangioma is 4 cm or larger, the risk of hydramnios, and its attendant risks of preterm delivery and maternal morbidity, is at least 30%.[213] Large chorioangiomas contain significant arteriovenous shunts and are associated with an increased risk of high-output fetal cardiac failure due to sequestration of blood within the tumor. The prognosis is poor if the fetus develops hydrops.[213,214] The development of fetal hydrops increases the risk of the mother developing Mirror syndrome.[228] Chorioangioma of the placenta is often associated with cutaneous and visceral hemangiomas in the fetus.

Any umbilical cord mass that obstructs blood flow to the fetus can lead to heart failure and hydrops. Large umbilical cord hemangiomas may be associated with sequestration or shunting leading to hydrops. True cysts of the umbilical cord are associated with other anomalies including omphalocele, patent urachus, hydronephrosis, and mesenteric duct cysts.[223] Pseudocysts of the umbilical cord are also associated with multiple anomalies including omphalocele, hemangioma, and chromosome abnormalities, especially trisomy 18 (identified in two of seven fetuses with umbilical cord cysts in one study).[223] These conditions are thought to impair local fluid transport in the umbilical cord leading to edema and myxoid degeneration of Wharton's jelly.[223]

Management Options

Once a placental lesion is identified, close antenatal surveillance is essential to follow fetal well-being and observe for any evidence of cardiac decompensation. Delivery should be considered if fetal hydrops occurs after 32 weeks. At earlier gestational ages, antenatal corticosteroids should be administered and any further management individualized. Fetal intrauterine transfusion has been performed in several cases of fetal cardiac decompensation due to chorioangioma as a temporizing measure.[229,230] Large chorioangiomas are associated with a perinatal mortality rate of 40%, and interventions attempted to decrease the arteriovenous shunting include fetoscopic coagulation, alcohol injection, and microcoil embolization of feeding vessels.[231–234] Only alcohol injection met with reported success[232,233]; more investigation is needed.

If an umbilical vein hematoma is identified, careful antenatal surveillance is required to demonstrate regression of the lesion. If the hematoma appears to be growing, delivery may be required to prevent complete occlusion of venous flow. The identification of a cystic structure in the umbilical cord should prompt a detailed anatomic survey of the fetus. Although the true incidence of chromosome abnormalities in the presence of a cystic cord lesion is unknown, karyotype analysis should be offered, especially if other anomalies are present.

SUMMARY OF MANAGEMENT OPTIONS
Placental and Umbilical Cord Tumors

Management Options	Quality of Evidence	Strength of Recommendation	References
Carefully search for other abnormalities with umbilical cord cysts.	IIb	B	223
Vigilance for hydramnios and hydrops is needed.	IV	C	213
Role of transfusion or sclerosing/occlusive therapies when hydrops develops is uncertain.	IV	C	229, 231, 233

CONCLUSIONS

- Fetal tumors are uncommon but important causes of pregnancy pathology.
- Antenatal diagnosis creates the opportunity to alter antenatal care and optimize delivery.
- Interdisciplinary (obstetric, fetal medicine, pediatric surgery and medicine) management in a tertiary center is advisable.
- For each case, an individualized approach is required covering:
  - surveillance in pregnancy
  - intervention (if necessary) in pregnancy
  - timing and method of delivery
  - immediate neonatal care
  - definitive management of tumor

REFERENCES

1. Parkes SE, Muir KR, Southern L, et al: Neonatal tumours: A thirty-year population-based study. Med Pediatr Oncol 1994;22:309–317.
2. Bader JL, Miller RW: US cancer incidence and mortality in the first year of life. Am J Dis Child 1979;133:157–159.
3. Werb P, Scurry J, Ostor A, et al: Survey of congenital tumors in perinatal necropsies. Pathology 1992;24:247–253.
4. Isaacs H Jr: Perinatal (congenital and neonatal) neoplasms: A report of 110 cases. Pediatr Pathol 1985;3:165–216.
5. Harrison MR, Adzick NS: The fetus as a patient. Surgical considerations. Ann Surg 1991;213:279–291; discussion 277–278.
6. Wienk MA, Van Geijn HP, Copray FJ, Brons JT: Prenatal diagnosis of fetal tumors by ultrasonography. Obstet Gynecol Surv 1990;45:639–653.
7. Isaacs H Jr: II. Perinatal brain tumors: A review of 250 cases. Pediatr Neurol 2002;27:333–342.
8. Isaacs H Jr: I. Perinatal brain tumors: A review of 250 cases. Pediatr Neurol 2002;27:249–261.
9. Doren M, Tercanli S, Gullotta F, Holzgreve W: Prenatal diagnosis of a highly undifferentiated brain tumour—A case report and review of the literature. Prenat Diagn 1997;17:967–971.
10. Buetow PC, Smirniotopoulos JG, Done S: Congenital brain tumors: A review of 45 cases. AJNR Am J Neuroradiol 1990;11:793–799.
11. Di Rocco C, Iannelli A, Ceddia A: Intracranial tumors of the first year of life. A cooperative survey of the 1986–1987 Education Committee of the ISPN. Childs Nerv Syst 1991;7:150–153.

12. Raisanen JM, Davis RL: Congenital brain tumors. Pathology (Phila) 1993;2:103–116.
13. Wakai S, Arai T, Nagai M: Congenital brain tumors. Surg Neurol 1984;21:597–609.
14. Washburne JF, Magann EF, Chauhan SP, et al: Massive congenital intracranial teratoma with skull rupture at delivery. Am J Obstet Gynecol 1995;173:226–228.
15. DiGiovanni LM, Sheikh Z: Prenatal diagnosis, clinical significance and management of fetal intracranial teratoma: A case report and literature review. Am J Perinatol 1994;11:420–422.
16. Saiga T, Osasa H, Hatayama H, et al: The origin of extragonadal teratoma: Case report of an immature teratoma occurring in a prenatal brain. Pediatr Pathol 1991;11:759–770.
17. Ferreira J, Eviatar L, Schneider S, Grossman R: Prenatal diagnosis of intracranial teratoma. Prolonged survival after resection of a malignant teratoma diagnosed prenatally by ultrasound: A case report and literature review. Pediatr Neurosurg 1993;19: 84–88.
18. Sherer DM, Onyeije CI: Prenatal ultrasonographic diagnosis of fetal intracranial tumors: a review. Am J Perinatol 1998;15: 319–328.
19. ten Broeke ED, Verdonk GW, Roumen FJ: Prenatal ultrasound diagnosis of an intracranial teratoma influencing management: Case report and review of the literature. Eur J Obstet Gynecol Reprod Biol 1992;45:210–214.
20. Czechowski J, Langille EL, Varady E: Intracardiac tumour and brain lesions in tuberous sclerosis. A case report of antenatal diagnosis by ultrasonography. Acta Radiol 2000;41:371–374.
21. Durfee SM, Kim FM, Benson CB: Postnatal outcome of fetuses with the prenatal diagnosis of asymmetric hydrocephalus. J Ultrasound Med 2001;20:263–268.
22. Levine D, Barnes P, Korf B, Edelman R: Tuberous sclerosis in the fetus: Second-trimester diagnosis of subependymal tubers with ultrafast MR imaging. AJR Am J Roentgenol 2000;175: 1067–1069.
23. Sperner J, Schmauser I, Bittner R, et al: MR-imaging findings in children with Sturge-Weber syndrome. Neuropediatrics 1990;21:146–152.
24. Filly R: Ultrasound Evaluation of the Fetal Neural Axis. In Callen P (ed): Ultrasonography in Obstetrics and Gynecology. Philadelphia, WB Saunders, 1994.
25. Squires LA, Constantini S, Miller DC, Wisoff JH: Hypothalamic hamartoma and the Pallister-Hall syndrome. Pediatr Neurosurg 1995;22:303–308.
26. Gorlin RJ, Cohen MM, Hennekam RCM: Syndromes with Unusual Facies: Other Syndromes of the Head and Neck. Oxford, Oxford University Press, 2001.
27. Diguet A, Laquerriere A, Eurin D, et al: Fetal capillary haemangioblastoma: an exceptional tumour. A review of the literature. Prenat Diagn 2002;22:979–983.
28. Lee DY, Kim YM, Yoo SJ, et al: Congenital glioblastoma diagnosed by fetal sonography. Childs Nerv Syst 1999;15:197–201.
29. Costa JM, Ley L, Claramunt E, Lafuente J: Choroid plexus papillomas of the III ventricle in infants. Report of three cases. Childs Nerv Syst 1997;13:244–249.
30. Lippa C, Abroms IF, Davidson R, DeGirolami U: Congenital choroid plexus papilloma of the fourth ventricle. J Child Neurol 1989;4:127–130.
31. Drouin V, Marret S, Petitcolas J, et al: Prenatal ultrasound abnormalities in a patient with generalized neurofibromatosis type 1. Neuropediatrics 1997;28:120–121.
32. Wenstrom KD, Williamson RA, Weiner CP, et al: Magnetic resonance imaging of fetuses with intracranial defects. Obstet Gynecol 1991;77:529–532.
33. Mamalis N, Garland PE, Argyle JC, Apple DJ: Congenital orbital teratoma: A review and report of two cases. Surv Ophthalmol 1985;30:41–46.
34. Spinelli HM, Criscuolo GR, Tripps M, Buckley PJ: Massive orbital teratoma in the newborn. Ann Plast Surg 1993;31:453–458.
35. Zwaan CM, de Waal FC, Koole FD, et al: A giant congenital orbital tumor: An unusual presentation of retinoblastoma. Med Pediatr Oncol 1994;23:507–511.
36. Steinkuller PG, Font RL: Congenital malignant teratoid neoplasm of the eye and orbit: A case report and review of the literature. Ophthalmology 1997;104:38–42.
37. Yen MT, Tse DT: Congenital orbital cyst detected and monitored by prenatal ultrasonography. Ophthal Plast Reconstr Surg 2001;17:443–446.
38. Elsas FJ, Green WR: Epibulbar tumors in childhood. Am J Ophthalmol 1975;79:1001–1007.
39. Sherer DM, Eisenberg C, Schwartz BM, et al: Prenatal sonographic diagnosis of dacryocystocele: A case and review of the literature. Am J Perinatol 1997;14:479–481.
40. Schubert EL, Hansen MF, Strong LC: The retinoblastoma gene and its significance. Ann Med 1994;26:177–184.
41. Conran RM, Kent SG, Wargotz ES: Oropharyngeal teratomas: A clinicopathologic study of four cases. Am J Perinatol 1993;10:71–75.
42. Marras T, Poenaru D, Kamal I: Perinatal management of nasopharyngeal teratoma. J Otolaryngol 1995;24:310–312.
43. Smart PJ, Schwarz C, Kelsey A: Ultrasonographic and biochemical abnormalities associated with the prenatal diagnosis of epignathus. Prenat Diagn 1990;10:327–332.
44. Sagol S, Itil IM, Ozsaran A, et al: Prenatal sonographic detection of nasopharyngeal teratoma. J Clin Ultrasound 1999;27: 469–473.
45. McMahon MJ, Chescheir NC, Kuller JA, et al: Perinatal management of a lingual teratoma. Obstet Gynecol 1996;87: 848–851.
46. Papageorgiou C, Papathanasiou K, Panidis D, Vlassis G: Prenatal diagnosis of epignathus in the first half of pregnancy: A case report and review of the literature. Clin Exp Obstet Gynecol 2000;27:67–68.
47. Catalano PJ, Urken ML, Alvarez M, et al: New approach to the management of airway obstruction in "high risk" neonates. Arch Otolaryngol Head Neck Surg 1992;118:306–309.
48. Gotte K, Hormann K, Schmoll J, Hiltmann WD: Congenital nasal hemangiopericytoma: Intrauterine, intraoperative, and histologic findings. Ann Otol Rhinol Laryngol 1999;108:589–593.
49. McMahon MG, Mintz S: In utero diagnosis of a congenital gingival granular cell tumor and immediate postnatal surgical management. J Oral Maxillofac Surg 1994;52:496–498.
50. Nazeer T, Ro JY, Varma DG, et al: Chondromyxoid fibroma of paranasal sinuses: Report of two cases presenting with nasal obstruction. Skeletal Radiol 1996;25:779–782.
51. Kotler HS, Gould NS, Gruber B: Leiomyoma of the tongue presenting as congenital airway obstruction. Int J Pediatr Otorhinolaryngol 1994;29:139–145.
52. Wagner W, Harrison MR: Fetal operations in the head and neck area: current state. Head Neck 2002;24:482–490.
53. Bouchard S, Johnson MP, Flake AW, et al: The EXIT procedure: Experience and outcome in 31 cases. J Pediatr Surg 2002; 37:418–426.
54. Kelly MF, Berenholz L, Rizzo KA, et al: Approach for oxygenation of the newborn with airway obstruction due to a cervical mass. Ann Otol Rhinol Laryngol 1990;99:179–182.
55. Langer JC, Tabb T, Thompson P, et al: Management of prenatally diagnosed tracheal obstruction: Access to the airway in utero prior to delivery. Fetal Diagn Ther 1992;7:12–16.
56. Shih GH, Boyd GL, Vincent RD Jr, et al: The EXIT procedure facilitates delivery of an infant with a pretracheal teratoma. Anesthesiology 1998;89:1573–1575.
57. Suchet IB: Ultrasonography of the fetal neck in the second and third trimesters. Part 3. Anomalies of the anterior and anterolateral nuchal region. Can Assoc Radiol J 1995;46:426–433.
58. Suchet IB: Ultrasonography of the fetal neck in the first and second trimesters. Part 2. Anomalies of the posterior nuchal region. Can Assoc Radiol J 1995;46:344–352.

59. Zimmer EZ, Drugan A, Ofir C, et al: Ultrasound imaging of fetal neck anomalies: Implications for the risk of aneuploidy and structural anomalies. Prenat Diagn 1997;17:1055–1058.
60. Tapper D, Lack EE: Teratomas in infancy and childhood. A 54-year experience at the Children's Hospital Medical Center. Ann Surg 1983;198:398–410.
61. Bezuidenhout J, Schneider JW, Hugo F, Wessels G: Teratomas in infancy and childhood at Tygerberg Hospital, South Africa, 1973 to 1992. Arch Pathol Lab Med 1997;121:499–502.
62. Kountakis SE, Minotti AM, Maillard A, Stiernberg CM: Teratomas of the head and neck. Am J Otolaryngol 1994;15: 292–296.
63. Thompson LD, Rosai J, Heffess CS: Primary thyroid teratomas: A clinicopathologic study of 30 cases. Cancer 2000;88: 1149–1158.
64. Elmasalme F, Giacomantonio M, Clarke KD, et al: Congenital cervical teratoma in neonates. Case report and review. Eur J Pediatr Surg 2000;10:252–257.
65. Gundry SR, Wesley JR, Klein MD, et al: Cervical teratomas in the newborn. J Pediatr Surg 1983;18:382–386.
66. Azizkhan RG, Haase GM, Applebaum H, et al: Diagnosis, management, and outcome of cervicofacial teratomas in neonates: A Childrens Cancer Group study. J Pediatr Surg 1995;30:312–316.
67. Rothschild MA, Catalano P, Urken M, et al: Evaluation and management of congenital cervical teratoma. Case report and review. Arch Otolaryngol Head Neck Surg 1994;120:444–448.
68. Baumann FR, Nerlich A: Metastasizing cervical teratoma of the fetus. Pediatr Pathol 1993;13:21–27.
69. Kerner B, Flaum E, Mathews H, et al: Cervical teratoma: Prenatal diagnosis and long-term follow-up. Prenat Diagn 1998;18:51–59.
70. Hubbard AM, Crombleholme TM, Adzick NS: Prenatal MRI evaluation of giant neck masses in preparation for the fetal exit procedure. Am J Perinatol 1998;15:253–257.
71. Chervenak FA, Isaacson G, Blakemore KJ, et al: Fetal cystic hygroma. Cause and natural history. N Engl J Med 1983;309: 822–825.
72. Chitayat D, Kalousek DK, Bamforth JS: Lymphatic abnormalities in fetuses with posterior cervical cystic hygroma. Am J Med Genet 1989;33:352–356.
73. Saller D, Canick J, Schwartz S, Blitzer M: Multiple marker screening in pregnancies with hydropic and nonhydropic Turner syndrome. Am J Obstet Gynecol 1992;167:1021–1024.
74. Wenstrom KD, Williamson RA, Grant SS: Detection of fetal Turner syndrome with multiple-marker screening. Am J Obstet Gynecol 1994;170:570–573.
75. Berdahl LD, Wenstrom KD, Hanson JW: Web neck anomaly and its association with congenital heart disease. Am J Med Genet 1995;56:304–307.
76. Abramowicz JS, Warsof SL, Doyle DL, et al: Congenital cystic hygroma of the neck diagnosed prenatally: Outcome with normal and abnormal karyotype. Prenat Diagn 1989;9:321–327.
77. Allanson J: Lymphatic circulation. In Stevenson R, Hall J, Goodman R (eds): Human Malformations and Related Anomalies. New York, Oxford University Press, 1993.
78. Clark EB: Neck web and congenital heart defects: A pathogenic association in 45 X-O Turner syndrome? Teratology 1984;29: 355–361.
79. Brumfield CG, Wenstrom KD, Davis RO, et al: Second-trimester cystic hygroma: Prognosis of septated and nonseptated lesions. Obstet Gynecol 1996;88:979–982.
80. Bronshtein M, Bar-Hava I, Blumenfeld I, et al: The difference between septated and nonseptated nuchal cystic hygroma in the early second trimester. Obstet Gynecol 1993;81:683–687.
81. Hartman GE, Shochat SJ: Primary pulmonary neoplasms of childhood: A review. Ann Thorac Surg 1983;36:108–119.
82. Isaacs H Jr: Tumors of the Fetus and Infant: An Atlas. New York, Springer Verlag, 2002.
83. Vogt-Moykopf I, Rau B, Branscheid D: Surgery for congenital malformations of the lung. Ann Chir 1992;46:141–156.
84. Meizner I, Levy A: A survey of non-cardiac fetal intrathoracic malformations diagnosed by ultrasound. Arch Gynecol Obstet 1994;255:31–36.
85. DuMontier C, Graviss ER, Silberstein MJ, McAlister WH: Bronchogenic cysts in children. Clin Radiol 1985;36:431–436.
86. Dembinski J, Kaminski M, Schild R, et al: Congenital intrapulmonary bronchogenic cyst in the neonate—Perinatal management. Am J Perinatol 1999;16:509–514.
87. Jung AL, Johnson DG, Condon VR, et al: Congenital chest wall mesenchymal hamartoma. J Perinatol 1994;14:487–491.
88. Easa D, Balaraman V, Ash K, et al: Congenital chylothorax and mediastinal neuroblastoma. J Pediatr Surg 1991;26: 96–98.
89. Granata C, Fagnani AM, Gambini C, et al: Features and outcome of neuroblastoma detected before birth. J Pediatr Surg 2000;35:88–91.
90. Li AM, Chang J, Kumar A: Neonatal neuroblastoma presenting with respiratory distress. J Paediatr Child Health 2001;37: 203–205.
91. de Filippi G, Canestri G, Bosio U, et al: Thoracic neuroblastoma: Antenatal demonstration in a case with unusual post-natal radiographic findings. Br J Radiol 1986;59:704–706.
92. Adzick NS, Harrison MR, Crombleholme TM, et al: Fetal lung lesions: Management and outcome. Am J Obstet Gynecol 1998;179:884–889.
93. Devine PC, Malone FD: Noncardiac thoracic anomalies. Clin Perinatol 2000;27:865–899.
94. Bromley B, Parad R, Estroff JA, Benacerraf BR: Fetal lung masses: Prenatal course and outcome. J Ultrasound Med 1995; 14:927–936, 1378 (quiz).
95. Nicolaides KH, Azar GB: Thoraco-amniotic shunting. Fetal Diagn Ther 1990;5:153–164.
96. Blott M, Nicolaides KH, Greenough A: Pleuroamniotic shunting for decompression of fetal pleural effusions. Obstet Gynecol 1988;71:798–800.
97. Hubbard AM: Magnetic resonance imaging of fetal thoracic abnormalities. Top Magn Reson Imaging 2001;12:18–24.
98. Duncombe GJ, Dickinson JE, Kikiros CS: Prenatal diagnosis and management of congenital cystic adenomatoid malformation of the lung. Am J Obstet Gynecol 2002;187:950–954.
99. Stocker JT, Madewell JE, Drake RM: Congenital cystic adenomatoid malformation of the lung. Classification and morphologic spectrum. Hum Pathol 1977;8:155–171.
100. Adzick NS, Harrison MR, Glick PL, et al: Fetal cystic adenomatoid malformation: Prenatal diagnosis and natural history. J Pediatr Surg 1985;20:483–488.
101. Kasales CJ, Coulson CC, Meilstrup JW, et al: Diagnosis and differentiation of congenital diaphragmatic hernia from other noncardiac thoracic fetal masses. Am J Perinatol 1998;15:623–628.
102. Hubbard AM, Adzick NS, Crombleholme TM, et al: Congenital chest lesions: Diagnosis and characterization with prenatal MR imaging. Radiology 1999;212:43–48.
103. Crombleholme TM, Coleman B, Hedrick H, et al: Cystic adenomatoid malformation volume ratio predicts outcome in prenatally diagnosed cystic adenomatoid malformation of the lung. J Pediatr Surg 2002;37:331–338.
104. Stocker JT: An approach to handling pediatric liver tumors. Am J Clin Pathol 1998;109:S67–S72.
105. Bernaschek G, Deutinger J, Hansmann M, et al: Feto-amniotic shunting—Report of the experience of four European centres. Prenat Diagn 1994;14:821–833.
106. Becmeur F, Horta-Geraud P, Donato L, Sauvage P: Pulmonary sequestrations: Prenatal ultrasound diagnosis, treatment, and outcome. J Pediatr Surg 1998;33:492–496.
107. Dolkart LA, Reimers FT, Helmuth WV, et al: Antenatal diagnosis of pulmonary sequestration: A review. Obstet Gynecol Surv 1992;47:515–520.
108. Collin PP, Desjardins JG, Khan AH: Pulmonary sequestration. J Pediatr Surg 1987;22:750–753.

109. Felker RE, Tonkin IL: Imaging of pulmonary sequestration. AJR Am J Roentgenol 1990;154:241–249.
110. Buntain WL, Woolley MM, Mahour GH, et al: Pulmonary sequestration in children: A twenty-five year experience. Surgery 1977;81:413–420.
111. Hernanz-Schulman M, Stein SM, Neblett WW, et al: Pulmonary sequestration: Diagnosis with color Doppler sonography and a new theory of associated hydrothorax. Radiology 1991;180:817–821.
112. Morin L, Crombleholme TM, D'Alton ME: Prenatal diagnosis and management of fetal thoracic lesions. Semin Perinatol 1994;18:228–253.
113. Morin L, Crombleholme TM, Louis F, D'Alton ME: Bronchopulmonary sequestration: Prenatal diagnosis with clinicopathologic correlation. Curr Opin Obstet Gynecol 1994;6: 479–481.
114. Thilenius OG, Ruschhaupt DG, Replogle RL, et al: Spectrum of pulmonary sequestration: Association with anomalous pulmonary venous drainage in infants. Pediatr Cardiol 1983;4:97–103.
115. Sauerbrei E: Lung sequestration. Duplex Doppler diagnosis at 19 weeks gestation. J Ultrasound Med 1991;10:101–105.
116. Leithiser RE Jr, Capitanio MA, Macpherson RI, Wood BP: "Communicating" bronchopulmonary foregut malformations. AJR Am J Roentgenol 1986;146:227–231.
117. Savic B, Birtel FJ, Tholen W, et al: Lung sequestration: Report of seven cases and review of 540 published cases. Thorax 1979;34:96–101.
118. Adzick NS: Fetal thoracic lesions. Semin Pediatr Surg 1993;2:103–108.
119. Bratu I, Flageole H, Chen MF, et al: The multiple facets of pulmonary sequestration. J Pediatr Surg 2001;36:784–790.
120. Weiner C, Varner M, Pringle K, et al: Antenatal diagnosis and palliative treatment of nonimmune hydrops fetalis secondary to pulmonary extralobar sequestration. Obstet Gynecol 1986;68:275–280.
121. Nadas AS, Ellison RC: Cardiac tumors in infancy. Am J Cardiol 1968;21:363–366.
122. Sbragia L, Paek BW, Feldstein VA, et al: Outcome of prenatally diagnosed solid fetal tumors. J Pediatr Surg 2001;36:1244–1247.
123. Groves AM, Fagg NL, Cook AC, Allan LD: Cardiac tumours in intrauterine life. Arch Dis Child 1992;67:1189–1192.
124. Fenoglio JJ Jr, McAllister HAJ, Ferrans VJ: Cardiac rhabdomyoma: A clinicopathologic and electron microscopic study. Am J Cardiol 1976;38:241–251.
125. DiMario FJ Jr, Diana D, Leopold H, Chameides L: Evolution of cardiac rhabdomyoma in tuberous sclerosis complex. Clin Pediatr (Phila) 1996;35:615–619.
126. Bosi G, Lintermans JP, Pellegrino PA, et al: The natural history of cardiac rhabdomyoma with and without tuberous sclerosis. Acta Paediatr 1996;85:928–931.
127. Harding CO, Pagon RA: Incidence of tuberous sclerosis in patients with cardiac rhabdomyoma. Am J Med Genet 1990;37:443–446.
128. Webb DW, Thomas RD, Osborne JP: Cardiac rhabdomyomas and their association with tuberous sclerosis. Arch Dis Child 1993;68:367–370.
129. de Bustamante TD, Azpeitia J, Miralles M, et al : Prenatal sonographic detection of pericardial teratoma. J Clin Ultrasound 2000;28:194–198.
130. Takach TJ, Reul GJ, Ott DA, Cooley DA: Primary cardiac tumors in infants and children: Immediate and long-term operative results. Ann Thorac Surg 1996;62:559–564.
131. Nir A, Tajik AJ, Freeman WK, et al: Tuberous sclerosis and cardiac rhabdomyoma. Am J Cardiol 1995;76:419–421.
132. Mirlesse V, Wener H, Jacquemard F, et al: Magnetic resonance imaging in antenatal diagnosis of tuberous sclerosis. Lancet 1992;340:1163.
133. Inoue Y, Nakajima S, Fukuda T, et al: Magnetic resonance images of tuberous sclerosis. Further observations and clinical correlations. Neuroradiology 1988;30:379–384.
134. Benatar A, Vaughan J, Nicolini U, et al: Prenatal pericardiocentesis: Its role in the management of intrapericardial teratoma. Obstet Gynecol 1992;79:856–859.
135. Bruch SW, Adzick NS, Reiss R, Harrison MR: Prenatal therapy for pericardial teratomas. J Pediatr Surg 1997;32:1113–1115.
136. Paw PT, Jamieson SW: Surgical management of intrapericardial teratoma diagnosed in utero. Ann Thorac Surg 1997;64:552–554.
137. Burke AP, Rosado-de-Christenson M, Templeton PA, Virmani R: Cardiac fibroma: Clinicopathologic correlates and surgical treatment. J Thorac Cardiovasc Surg 1994;108:862–870.
138. Garmel SH, Crombleholme TM, Semple JP, Bhan I: Prenatal diagnosis and management of fetal tumors. Semin Perinatol 1994;18:350–365.
139. Acharya S, Jayabose S, Kogan SJ, et al: Prenatally diagnosed neuroblastoma. Cancer 1997;80:304–310.
140. Jennings RW, LaQuaglia MP, Leong K, et al: Fetal neuroblastoma: Prenatal diagnosis and natural history. J Pediatr Surg 1993;28:1168–1174.
141. Atkinson GO Jr, Zaatari GS, Lorenzo RL, et al: Cystic neuroblastoma in infants: Radiographic and pathologic features. AJR Am J Roentgenol 1986;146:113–117.
142. Saylors RL 3rd, Cohn SL, Morgan ER, Brodeur GM: Prenatal detection of neuroblastoma by fetal ultrasonography. Am J Pediatr Hematol Oncol 1994;16:356–360.
143. Goldstein I, Gomez K, Copel JA: The real-time and color Doppler appearance of adrenal neuroblastoma in a third-trimester fetus. Obstet Gynecol 1994;83:854–856.
144. Newton ER, Louis F, Dalton ME, Feingold M: Fetal neuroblastoma and catecholamine–induced maternal hypertension. Obstet Gynecol 1985;65:49S–52S.
145. Voute PA Jr, Wadman SK, van Putten WJ: Congenital neuroblastoma. Symptoms in the mother during pregnancy. Clin Pediatr (Phila) 1970;9:206–207.
146. Wagget J, Aherne G, Aherne W: Familia neuroblastoma: Report of two sib pairs. Arch Dis Child 1973;48:63–66.
147. Petit T, de Lagausie P, El Ghoneimi A, et al : Postnatal management of cystic neuroblastoma. Eur J Pediatr Surg 2001;11: 411–414.
148. Jaffa AJ, Many A, Hartoov J, et al: Prenatal sonographic diagnosis of metastatic neuroblastoma: Report of a case and review of the literature. Prenat Diagn 1993;13:73–77.
149. Ho PT, Estroff JA, Kozakewich H, et al: Prenatal detection of neuroblastoma: A ten-year experience from the Dana-Farber Cancer Institute and Children's Hospital. Pediatrics 1993;92:358–364.
150. McVicar M, Margouleff D, Chandra M: Diagnosis and imaging of the fetal and neonatal abdominal mass: An integrated approach. Adv Pediatr 1991;38:135–149.
151. Angulo JC, Lopez JI, Ereno C, et al: Hydrops fetalis and congenital mesoblastic nephroma. Child Nephrol Urol 1991;11:115–116.
152. Pinto E, Guignard JP: Renal masses in the neonate. Biol Neonate 1995;68:175–184.
153. Reinberg Y, Anderson GF, Franciosi R, et al: Wilms tumor and the VATER association. J Urol 1988;140:787–789.
154. Beckwith JB: Wilms' tumor and other renal tumors of childhood: A selective review from the National Wilms' Tumor Study Pathology Center. Hum Pathol 1983;14:481–492.
155. D'Angio GJ, Breslow N, Beckwith JB, et al: Treatment of Wilms' tumor. Results of the Third National Wilms' Tumor Study. Cancer 1989;64:349–360.
156. Matsunaga E: Genetics of Wilms' tumor. Hum Genet 1981;57:231–246.
157. Dehner LP: Hepatic tumors in the pediatric age group: A distinctive clinicopathologic spectrum. Perspect Pediatr Pathol 1978;4:217–268.
158. Meirowitz NB, Guzman ER, Underberg-Davis SJ, et al: Hepatic hemangioendothelioma: Prenatal sonographic findings and evolution of the lesion. J Clin Ultrasound 2000;28:258–263.

159. Smith WL, Ballantine TV, Gonzalez-Curssi F: Hepatic mesenchymal hamartoma causing heart failure in the neonate. J Pediatr Surg 1978;13:183–185.
160. Kamata S, Nose K, Sawai T, et al: Fetal mesenchymal hamartoma of the liver: Report of a case. J Pediatr Surg 2003;38:639–641.
161. Kazzi NJ, Chang CH, Roberts EC, Shankaran S: Fetal hepatoblastoma presenting as nonimmune hydrops. Am J Perinatol 1989;6:278–280.
162. Kanai N, Saito K, Homma Y, Makino S: Infantile hemangioendothelioma of the liver associated with anomalous dilated and tortuous vessels on the placental surface. Pediatr Surg Int 1998;13:175–176.
163. Gonen R, Fong K, Chiasson DA: Prenatal sonographic diagnosis of hepatic hemangioendothelioma with secondary nonimmune hydrops fetalis. Obstet Gynecol 1989;73:485–487.
164. van de Bor M, Verwey RA, van Pel R: Acute polyhydramnios associated with fetal hepatoblastoma. Eur J Obstet Gynecol Reprod Biol 1985;20:65–69.
165. Shih JC, Tsao PN, Huang SF, et al: Antenatal diagnosis of congenital hepatoblastoma in utero. Ultrasound Obstet Gynecol 2000;16:94–97.
166. Gonzalez-Crussi F, Upton MP, Maurer HS: Hepatoblastoma. Attempt at characterization of histologic subtypes. Am J Surg Pathol 1982;6:599–612.
167. Hackmon-Ram R, Wiznitzer A, Gohar J, Mazor M: Prenatal diagnosis of a fetal abdominal cyst. Eur J Obstet Gynecol Reprod Biol 2000;91:79–82.
168. Armentano G, Dodero P, Natta A, et al: Fetal ovarian cysts: Prenatal diagnosis and management. Report of two cases and review of literature. Clin Exp Obstet Gynecol 1998;25:88–91.
169. Kurjak A, Zalud I, Jurkovic D, et al: Ultrasound diagnosis and evaluation of fetal tumors. J Perinat Med 1989;17:173–193.
170. Saito S, Ishida M: Congenital choledochal cyst (cystic dilatation of the common bile duct). Prog Pediatr Surg 1974;6:63–90.
171. Dewbury KC, Aluwihare AP, Birch SJ, Freeman NV: Prenatal ultrasound demonstration of a choledochal cyst. Br J Radiol 1980;53:906–907.
172. Kim SH: Choledochal cyst: Survey by the surgical section of the American Academy of Pediatrics. J Pediatr Surg 1981;16: 402–407.
173. Benhidjeb T, Chaoui R, Kalache K, et al : Prenatal diagnosis of a choledochal cyst: A case report and review of the literature. Am J Perinatol 1996;13:207–210.
174. Bancroft JD, Bucuvalas JC, Ryckman FC, et al: Antenatal diagnosis of choledochal cyst. J Pediatr Gastroenterol Nutr 1994;18:142–145.
175. Mackenzie TC, Howell LJ, Flake AW, Adzick NS: The management of prenatally diagnosed choledochal cysts. J Pediatr Surg 2001;36:1241–1243.
176. Franzek DA, Strayer SA, Hull MT, et al: Enteric cyst as a cause of nonimmune hydrops fetalis: fetal thoracentesis with fluid analysis. J Clin Ultrasound 1989;17:275–279.
177. Egozi EI, Ricketts RR: Mesenteric and omental cysts in children. Am Surg 1997;63:287–290.
178. Gross SJ, Benzie RJ, Sermer M, et al: Sacrococcygeal teratoma: Prenatal diagnosis and management. Am J Obstet Gynecol 1987;156:393–396.
179. Brace V, Grant SR, Brackley KJ, et al: Prenatal diagnosis and outcome in sacrococcygeal teratomas: A review of cases between 1992 and 1998. Prenat Diagn 2000;20:51–55.
180. McCurdy CM Jr, Seeds JW: Route of delivery of infants with congenital anomalies. Clin Perinatol 1993;20:81–106.
181. Pringle KC, Weiner CP, Soper RT, Kealey P: Sacrococcygeal teratoma. Fetal Ther 1987;2:80–87.
182. Chisholm CA, Heider AL, Kuller JA, et al: Prenatal diagnosis and perinatal management of fetal sacrococcygeal teratoma. Am J Perinatol 1999;16:89–92.
183. Perrelli L, D'Urzo C, Manzoni C, et al: Sacrococcygeal teratoma. Outcome and management. An analysis of 17 cases. J Perinat Med 2002;30:179–184.
184. Altman RP, Randolph JG, Lilly JR: Sacrococcygeal teratoma: American Academy of Pediatrics Surgical Section Survey—1973. J Pediatr Surg 1974;9:389–398.
185. Bond SJ, Harrison MR, Schmidt KG, et al: Death due to high-output cardiac failure in fetal sacrococcygeal teratoma. J Pediatr Surg 1990;25:1287–1291.
186. Paek BW, Jennings RW, Harrison MR, et al: Radiofrequency ablation of human fetal sacrococcygeal teratoma. Am J Obstet Gynecol 2001;184:503–507.
187. Graf JL, Albanese CT: Fetal sacrococcygeal teratoma. World J Surg 2003;27:84–86.
188. Carney JA, Thompson DP, Johnson CL, Lynn HB: Teratomas in children: Clinical and pathologic aspects. J Pediatr Surg 1972;7:271–282.
189. Berry CL, Keeling J, Hilton C: Coincidence of congenital malformation and embryonic tumours of childhood. Arch Dis Child 1970;45:229–231.
190. Kirkinen P, Heinonen S, Vanamo K, Ryynanen M: Maternal serum alpha-fetoprotein and epithelial tumour marker concentrations are not increased by fetal sacrococcygeal teratoma. Prenat Diagn 1997;17:47–50.
191. Gonzalez-Crussi F, Winkler RF, Mirkin DL: Sacrococcygeal teratomas in infants and children: Relationship of histology and prognosis in 40 cases. Arch Pathol Lab Med 1978;102:420–425.
192. Grosfeld JL, Ballantine TV, Lowe D, Baehner RL: Benign and malignant teratomas in children: Analysis of 85 patients. Surgery 1976;80:297–305.
193. Kirkinen P, Partanen K, Merikanto J, et al: Ultrasonic and magnetic resonance imaging of fetal sacrococcygeal teratoma. Acta Obstet Gynecol Scand 1997;76:917–922.
194. Avni FE, Guibaud L, Robert Y, et al: MR imaging of fetal sacrococcygeal teratoma: Diagnosis and assessment. AJR Am J Roentgenol 2002;178:179–183.
195. Flake AW: Fetal sacrococcygeal teratoma. Semin Pediatr Surg 1993;2:113–120.
196. Sheth S, Nussbaum AR, Sanders RC, et al: Prenatal diagnosis of sacrococcygeal teratoma: Sonographic-pathologic correlation. Radiology 1988;169:131–136.
197. Holterman AX, Filiatrault D, Lallier M, Youssef S: The natural history of sacrococcygeal teratomas diagnosed through routine obstetric sonogram: a single institution experience. J Pediatr Surg 1998;33:899–903.
198. Nakayama DK: Survival in a fetus with sacrococcygeal teratoma and hydrops. Am J Obstet Gynecol 1990;163:682.
199. Nakayama DK, Killian A, Hill LM, et al: The newborn with hydrops and sacrococcygeal teratoma. J Pediatr Surg 1991;26: 1435–1438.
200. Graf JL, Paek BW, Albanese CT, et al: Successful resuscitation during fetal surgery. J Pediatr Surg 2000;35:1388–1389.
201. Adzick NS, Crombleholme TM, Morgan MA, Quinn TM: A rapidly growing fetal teratoma. Lancet 1997;349:538.
202. Kay S, Khalife S, Laberge JM, et al: Prenatal percutaneous needle drainage of cystic sacrococcygeal teratomas. J Pediatr Surg 1999;34:1148–1151.
203. Arceci R, Weinstein H: Neoplasia. In Avery G, Fletcher M, MacDonald M (eds): Neonatology: Pathophysiology and Managment of the Newborn, 4th ed. Philadelphia, JB Lippincott, 1994.
204. Dillon PW, Whalen TV, Azizkhan RG, et al: Neonatal soft tissue sarcomas: The influence of pathology on treatment and survival. Children's Cancer Group Surgical Committee. J Pediatr Surg 1995;30:1038–1041.
205. Ben Arush MW, Ben Arie Y, Bialik V, Meller I: Limb congenital fibrosarcoma: Report of two cases and review of the literature. Pediatr Hematol Oncol 1993;10:357–361.

206. Katz VL, Watson WJ, Thorp JM Jr, et al: Prenatal sonographic findings of massive lower extremity lymphangioma. Am J Perinatol 1992;9:127–129.
207. Samuel M, Spitz L: Klippel-Trenaunay syndrome: Clinical features, complications and management in children. Br J Surg 1995;82:757–761.
208. Cristaldi A, Vigevano F, Antoniazzi G, et al: Hemimegalencephaly, hemihypertrophy and vascular lesions. Eur J Pediatr 1995;154:134–137.
209. Yankowitz J, Slagel DD, Williamson R: Prenatal diagnosis of Klippel-Trenaunay-Weber syndrome by ultrasound. Prenat Diagn 1994;14:745–749.
210. Roberts RV, Dickinson JE, Hugo PJ, Barker A: Prenatal sonographic appearances of Klippel-Trenaunay-Weber syndrome. Prenat Diagn 1999;19:369–371.
211. Richards DS, Williams CA, Cruz AC, Hendrickson JE: Prenatal sonographic findings in a fetus with Proteus syndrome. J Ultrasound Med 1991;10:47–50.
212. Berry SA, Peterson C, Mize W, et al: Klippel-Trenaunay syndrome. Am J Med Genet 1998;79:319–326.
213. Hadi HA, Finley J, Strickland D: Placental chorioangioma: Prenatal diagnosis and clinical significance. Am J Perinatol 1993;10:146–149.
214. D'Ercole C, Cravello L, Boubli L, et al: Large chorioangioma associated with hydrops fetalis: Prenatal diagnosis and management. Fetal Diagn Ther 1996;11:357–360.
215. Zalel Y, Weisz B, Gamzu R, et al: Chorioangiomas of the placenta: Sonographic and Doppler flow characteristics. J Ultrasound Med 2002;21:909–913.
216. Bromley B, Benacerraf BR: Solid masses on the fetal surface of the placenta: Differential diagnosis and clinical outcome. J Ultrasound Med 1994;13:883–886.
217. Block D, Cruikshank S, Kelly K, Stanley M: Placental teratoma. Int J Gynaecol Obstet 1991;34:377–380.
218. Svanholm H, Thordsen C: Placental teratoma. Acta Obstet Gynecol Scand 1987;66:179–180.
219. Chandy RG, Korula A, Seshadri L: Teratoma of the placenta. Aust N Z J Obstet Gynaecol 2002;42:556–557.
220. Lynn AA, Parry SI, Morgan MA, Mennuti MT: Disseminated congenital neuroblastoma involving the placenta. Arch Pathol Lab Med 1997;121:741–744.
221. Baergen RN, Johnson D, Moore T, Benirschke K: Maternal melanoma metastatic to the placenta: A case report and review of the literature. Arch Pathol Lab Med 1997;121:508–511.
222. Clausen I, Thomsen SG: Pseudotumors of the umbilical cord and fetal membranes. Acta Obstet Gynecol Scand 1992;71: 148–150.
223. Ross JA, Jurkovic D, Zosmer N, et al: Umbilical cord cysts in early pregnancy. Obstet Gynecol 1997;89:442–445.
224. Miller KA, Gauderer MW: Hemangioma of the umbilical cord mimicking an omphalocele. J Pediatr Surg 1997;32:810–812.
225. Gramellini D, Pedrazzoli G, Sacchini C, et al: Color Doppler ultrasound in prenatal diagnosis of umbilical cord angiomyxoma. Case report. Clin Exp Obstet Gynecol 1993;20:241–244.
226. Satge DC, Laumond MA, Desfarges F, Chenard MP: An umbilical cord teratoma in a 17-week-old fetus. Prenat Diagn 2001;21:284–288.
227. Kamitomo M, Sueyoshi K, Matsukita S, et al: Hemangioma of the umbilical cord: Stenotic change of the umbilical vessels. Fetal Diagn Ther 1999;14:328–331.
228. Dorman SL, Cardwell MS: Ballantyne syndrome caused by a large placental chorioangioma. Am J Obstet Gynecol 1995;173:1632–1633.
229. Haak MC, Oosterhof H, Mouw RJ, et al: Pathophysiology and treatment of fetal anemia due to placental chorioangioma. Ultrasound Obstet Gynecol 1999;14:68–70.
230. Hubinont C, Bernard P, Khalil N, et al: Fetal liver hemangioma and chorioangioma: Two unusual cases of severe fetal anemia detected by ultrasonography and its perinatal management. Ultrasound Obstet Gynecol 1994;4:330–331.
231. Lau TK, Leung TY, Yu SC, et al: Prenatal treatment of chorioangioma by microcoil embolisation. Br J Obstet Gynecol 2003;110:70–73.
232. Nicolini U, Zuliani G, Caravelli E, et al: Alcohol injection: A new method of treating placental chorioangiomas. Lancet 1999;353:1674–1675.
233. Wanapirak C, Tongsong T, Sirichotiyakul S, Chanprapaph P: Alcoholization: The choice of intrauterine treatment for chorioangioma. J Obstet Gynaecol Res 2002;28:71–75.
234. Quintero RA, Reich H, Romero R, et al: In utero endoscopic devascularization of a large chorioangioma. Ultrasound Obstet Gynecol 1996;8:48–52.
235. Crowley P, Chalmers I, Keirse MJNC: The effects of corticosteroid administration before preterm delivery: An overview of the evidence from controlled trials. Br J Obstet Gynaecol 1990;97:11–25.
236. Mejides AA, Adra AM, O'Sullivan MJ, Nicholas MC: Prenatal diagnosis and therapy for a fetal hepatic vascular malformation. Obstet Gynecol 1995;85:850–853.

CHAPTER 24

Fetal Problems in Multiple Pregnancy

Liesbeth Lewi / Jan Deprest

INTRODUCTION

In the developed world, the incidence of multiple births has increased dramatically over the past few decades from 1/100 to about 1/60 to 1/70 deliveries, with a 40% increase in twinning rates and a three- to fourfold rise in higher-order multiple births. This rise in multiple births is largely attributable to the increased application of assisted reproductive techniques (ART), although advanced maternal age accounts for a slight increase in spontaneously conceived multiplets.[1]

In twins, about 30% are identical, or monozygotic, and 70% are fraternal, or dizygotic (Fig. 24–1). Monozygotic twins result from the fertilization of a single egg followed by early cleavage into two halves, which develop further separately. Monozygotic twins may be dichorionic diamniotic, monochorionic diamniotic, monochorionic monoamniotic, and even conjoined, depending on the time between fertilization and cleavage. The longer the time span, the more structures the fetuses will have in common. In terms of the presence of separate placentas for each twin, the time period around the third day is important. In 30% of monochorionic twins, cleavage occurs before the third day after fertilization, leading to a separate placenta for each twin (dichorionic); twins that have their own placentas are always in separate amniotic sacs and by definition diamniotic. However, in 70% of monozygotic twins, cleavage occurs after the third day, resulting in a single placenta for two fetuses (monochorionic). Rarely, cleavage takes place after the ninth day, resulting in monoamniotic, monochorionic twins. Finally, splitting after the 12th day results in conjoined twins. Dizygotic twins result from the fertilization of two different eggs, and by definition each twin has its own placenta and amniotic sac (dichorionic diamniotic) with some exceptional reports on dizygotic monochorionic twins due to fusion of two separate blastocysts, confirming the rule.[2,3] The incidence of dizygotic twins related to polyovulation has a hereditary component and also varies with ethnic group (up to five times higher in certain parts of Africa and half as high in parts of Asia), advanced maternal age (2% at 35 years), increasing parity (2% after four pregnancies), and method of conception. In contrast, the incidence of monozygotic twins is fairly constant throughout the world at 3 to 4 per 1000 births.[4] After assisted reproductive technology (ART), the overall majority of twins are dizygotic (85%), yet 15% are monozygotic.[1] Actually, ART increases the risk of monozygotic twinning fourfold, with about 1/50 of all conceptions being monozygotic compared with 3 to 4 per 1000 of natural conceptions. Several mechanisms have been put forward to explain why these techniques predispose to embryo cleavage, such as hardening of the zona pellucida with ovulation induction, extended culture and blastocyst transfer with in vitro fertilization, micromanipulations of the zona pellucida with intracytoplasmic sperm injection (ICSI) as well as assisted hatching.[5] As for triplets and higher-order multiplets, the overall majority now result from ART and are therefore usually polyzygotic and polychorionic/ polyamniotic. Nevertheless, 5% to 10% of multiple pregnancies after ART[6] and up to 50% of naturally conceived higher-order multiplets contain a monochorionic pair.[7]

Multiplets have a more complicated in utero stay compared to singletons, with higher incidences of growth restriction, congenital anomalies, and intrauterine demise; monozygotic twins are at higher risk for complications than dizygotic twins.[8] However, at closer look, it is chorionicity rather than zygosity that determines outcome.[9] The increased morbidity and mortality rates in monochorionic twins is primarily related to the angioarchitecture of the monochorionic placenta with its almost ever-present (96%) vascular anastomoses (Fig. 24–2),[10] which are virtually absent in dichorionic twin pregnancies. These vascular anastomoses are unpredictable and randomly distributed and can cause significant blood

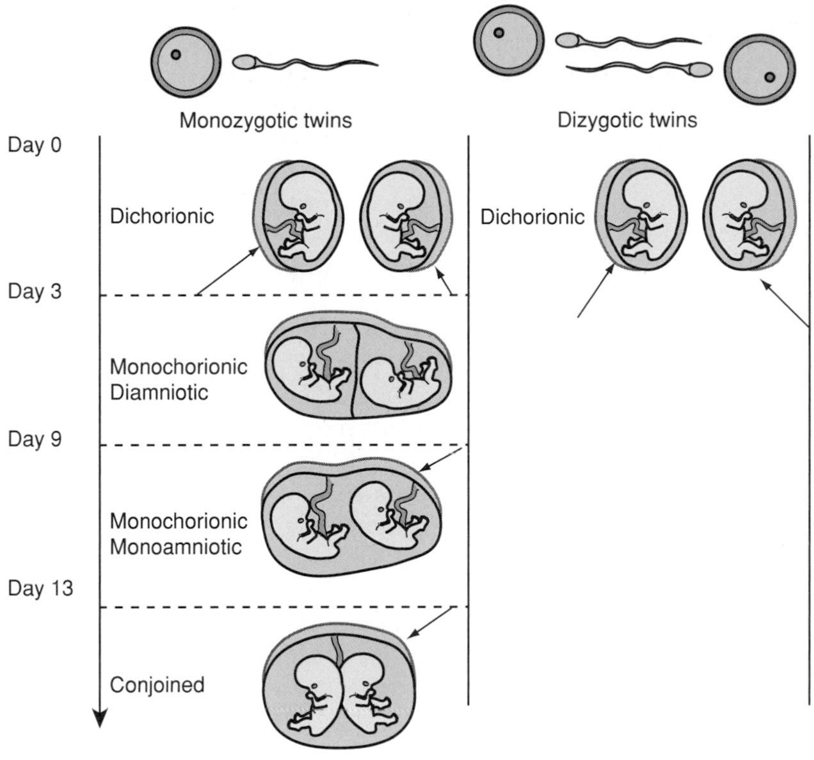

FIGURE 24–1
Zygocity and chorionicity in twin pregnancies. (Courtesy of T. Van den Bosch, H. Hart Hospital, Tienen, Belgium.)

volume shifts between the fetuses, leading to unique complications such as twin-to-twin transfusion syndrome, twin reversed arterial perfusion, and acute fetal transfusion after single intrauterine death.[11] Important to some selected situations, the shared circulation precludes the injection of potassium chloride for selective feticide into the target fetus' circulation. Furthermore, this single placenta, originally designed to support one fetus, has to care for two or more fetuses and is often not equally divided, explaining the increased incidence of poor growth in monochorionic compared to dichorionic multiplets. Consequently, the perinatal mortality rate in monochorionic twins is nearly twice as high as in dichorionic twins (2.8% versus 1.6%) and four times as high as in singletons (2.8 versus 0.7%). However, perinatal statistics underestimate the problem because the highest fetal loss rate is prior to viability. As such, monochorionic twins have a sixfold higher fetal loss rate (12%) between 10 and 24 weeks compared to dichorionic twins and singletons (2%), which is largely attributable to complications of the twin-to-twin transfusion syndrome.[12] Also, there is a direct relationship between the timing of embryo cleavage and the risk of adverse outcome, with monoamniotic and conjoined twins having the highest complication rates. Not only do multiplets pose more problems, management issues are also complicated by the fact that two or more fetuses have to be taken into account. This concern especially applies to monochorionic multiplets, in whom the well-being of one fetus crucially depends on that of the other, as their fates are invariably linked by the vascular anastomoses in the shared placenta.

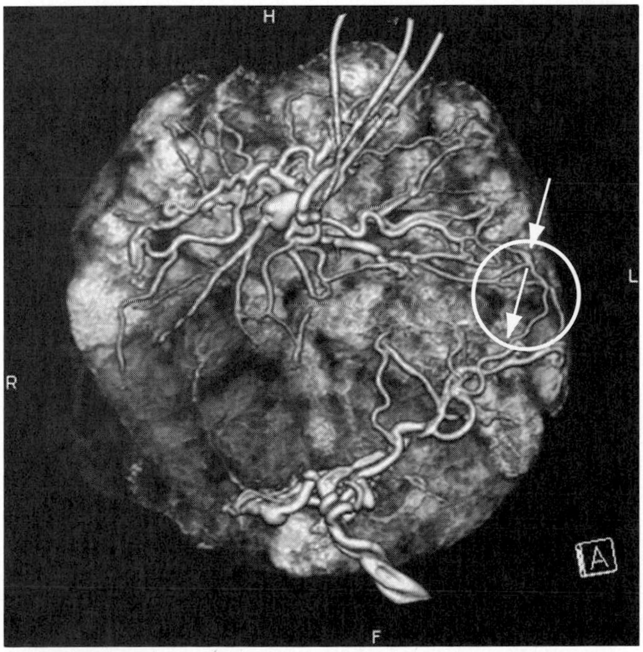

FIGURE 24–2
Three-dimensional reconstruction of a CT-angiogram of a monochorionic placenta at term, showing an equal distribution of the placental mass and a large arterioarterial and venovenous superficial anastomosis (*arrows*) (see Color Plate 27). (In collaboration with M. Cannie, UZ Leuven, Belgium.)

Correct determination of chorionicity is therefore of vital importance to identify this high-risk group, for which increased monitoring may improve outcome. Moreover, it is essential for genetic counseling and for the management of discordant anomalies, fetal compromise, and intrauterine death of one twin. Determination of chorionicity is highly accurate when performed prior to 14 weeks' gestation (100% sensitivity and 99% specificity).[13,14] At these early stages in pregnancy, the amniotic membrane is still separated from the chorion. Chorionicity determination is therefore simply a matter of counting the layers that separate the twins (Fig. 24–3). If there are two thin layers (two amniotic sacs) and two thick separate chorionic plates or one fused chorion (beyond 9 weeks) that forms a lambda at insertion on the placenta, then they are dichorionic diamniotic twins. However, if there are only two thin layers (two amniotic sacs) inserting as a T on the placental disk, then they are monochorionic diamniotic twins. Later on in pregnancy because of close apposition of the amnion and chorion and regression of the chorion laeve, it becomes far more difficult and often not possible at all to determine whether same-sex twins do or do not share a common placenta. Only examination of the placenta after birth will then give a definite answer. Therefore, failure to determine chorionicity in multiple pregnancies undergoing first-trimester scanning is considered substandard care. In contrast to chorionicity, it is not possible to determine zygosity of dichorionic same-sex twins on ultrasound scan: about 8 out of 10 will be dizygotic, but still 2 out of 10 will be monozygotic. Only genetic examination (DNA fingerprinting) can then determine zygosity, which prenatally would require an amniocentesis of both sacs, or cordocentesis of both umbilical cords. After birth, zygosity of same-sex dichorionic twins can be determined from umbilical cord blood.

POOR GROWTH

General

Multiplets are particularly prone to abnormal intrauterine growth, as the human uterus appears less capable of adequately nurturing more than one fetus to term.[15] Consequently, the percentage of small-for-gestational-age (SGA) babies (birth weight <10th percentile of singleton nomograms) is about 27% in twins[16] and 46% in triplets.[17] Growth curves for twins and triplets are similar to those of singletons up to 28 weeks' gestation, when the growth velocity of multiplets begins to fall. In twins

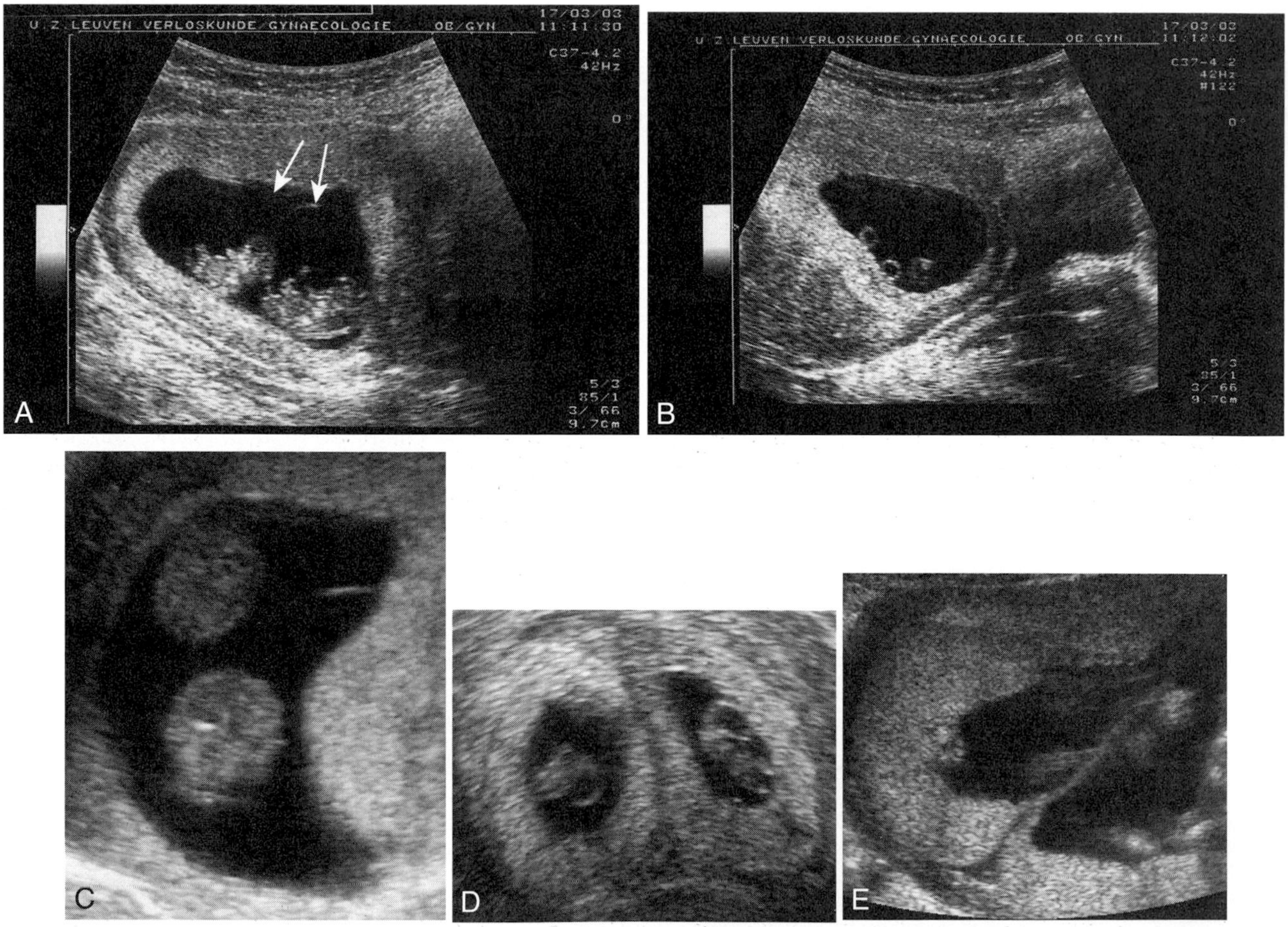

FIGURE 24–3
Chorionicity determination on the first trimester ultrasound scan. *A*, Monochorionic diamniotic twins: only two thin amniotic membranes (*arrows*) separate the two fetuses. *B*, Both yolk sacs are in a common coelomic cavity. *C*, The insertion of intertwin membrane on the chorionic surface is T-shaped; dichorionic diamniotic twins. *D*, the fetuses are separated by three layers (amnion, chorion-chorion, amnion), and the yolk sacs are in separate coelomic cavities. *E*, Where the placentas fuse, a wedge-shaped junction (Y sign) is seen.

and triplets the average birth weight crosses the 10th percentile for singletons after 38 and 35 weeks' gestation, respectively,[15] when the majority of twins and triplets actually have already delivered.[18] Some authors consider this growth restriction physiologic and therefore advocate for the use of twin[16] or triplet[17] specific nomograms. However, twins who are SGA according to singleton standards are at equal risk of perinatal death compared to SGA singletons.[19] Thus, the concept that being small is "normal" for twins creates a false sense of security with possible deleterious consequences in this high risk population. Because the impact of size on outcome is similar for singletons and multiplets, singleton growth charts should be used for the clinical management of twin pregnancies.

Accurate pregnancy dating and knowledge of the chorionicity are essential, and both are most reliably determined in the first trimester.[13,14] Two methods are used to describe growth in multiplets: the growth of each individual fetus and the difference (Δ) in sonographic estimated fetal weight (ΔEFW) between the individual fetuses (discordant growth). A fetus is considered SGA when both the abdominal circumference and EFW are below the 10th percentile. The EFW prediction is as accurate in twins as it is in singletons.[20] The chance of both fetuses being SGA is twice as high in monochorionic (17%) as in dichorionic (8%) twins, revealing that a single placenta is less efficient for two fetuses. The rate of delivery before 32 weeks is also greater in monochorionic twin gestations in great part because of the risks of twin-to-twin transfusion syndrome (TTTS). We currently scan monochorionic twins fortnightly for growth and amniotic fluid volume, whereas dichorionic twins are scanned on a monthly basis.

The degree of discordant growth, expressed in percentages, is determined as $(A - B) \times 100/A$, where A is the weight of the heavier fetus and B is the weight of the lighter fetus. Severe growth discordancy is usually defined as a weight difference of 25% or more. It occurs in about 12% of twins[12] and 34% of triplets[21] and more commonly affects primiparous women.[22] The most accurate parameter to detect growth discordance is to compare the abdominal circumferences: a difference of more than 20 mm after 24 weeks has a positive predictive value of 83% for a birth weight difference of greater than 20% (Fig. 24–4).[23] In each pair of discordant twins, the heavier twin is usually appropriate for gestional age (AGA), whereas the lighter twin eventually becomes growth restricted.[24]

Although severe growth discordancy complicates monochorionic (11.3%) as often as dichorionic (12.1%) twins,[12] the growth pattern and underlying pathophysiology are probably different. The onset of discordant growth in monochorionic twins is unpredictable and may present early as well as late in pregnancy, whereas in dichorionic twins, discordancy usually becomes apparent only later in pregnancy.[24] Monochorionic twins are by definition monozygotic and thus have the same genetic growth potential. Occasionally, unequal allocation of

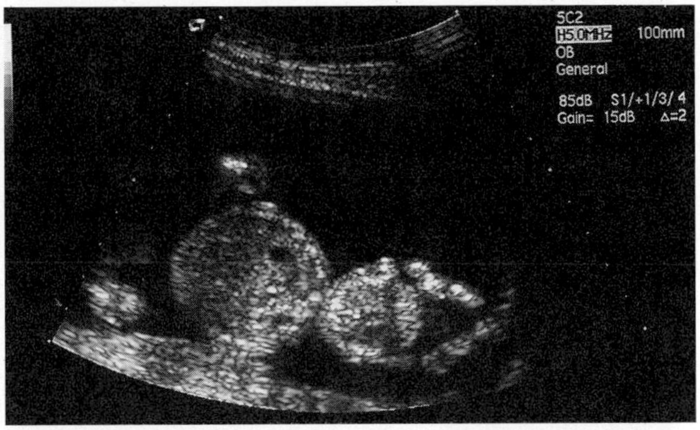

FIGURE 24–4
Ultrasound image illustrating the difference in abdominal circumference in a monochorionic twin pair with discordant growth at midgestation.

blastomeres may alter the growth potential of some monochorionic twins and account for very early discordant growth.[25]

Three factors seem to influence growth in monochorionic twins: the division of the single placenta between the fetuses, the vascular anastomoses,[26] and the effectiveness of invasion of each placental portion into the spiral arteries. These factors determine the magnitude of venous return upon which the fetus depends for its oxygen and nutritional supply. Although it remains impossible to adequately assess the venous return and functional placental territory for each individual twin antenatally, the umbilical cord insertion site provides a good estimate.[27] Placental studies reveal that the combination of a velamentous and normal cord insertion is three times more common in monochorionic than in dichorionic twins (18% and 6%, respectively). Additionally, nearly half of these monochorionic twins have a birth weight discordancy of 20% or more.[28] The site of the umbilical cord insertion can be determined sonographically between 18 and 20 weeks' gestation (Fig. 24–5)[29] and identifies a group of monochorionic twins at high risk for discordant growth. Vascular anastomoses also influence fetal growth in monochorionic twins. As such, an unbalanced net arteriovenous transfusion toward the twin with the smaller placental share may be advantageous to that smaller twin. This so-called "rescue" transfusion could explain the absence of discordant growth in some monochorionic twins with gross unequal placental sharing.[10] Finally, growth in monochorionic twins may be determined by suboptimal implantation of the placental portion of the smaller twin, as suggested by the increased resistance of the blood flow in the spiral arteries of the smaller twin's portion of the placenta.[30]

Dichorionic twins are dizygotic in about 90% of cases, and therefore a different genetic growth potential may account for discordant growth; one twin may be "normal" SGA, whereas the other may be "normal" AGA. Additionally, each twin has its own placenta without vascular anastomoses connecting the separate fetoplacental

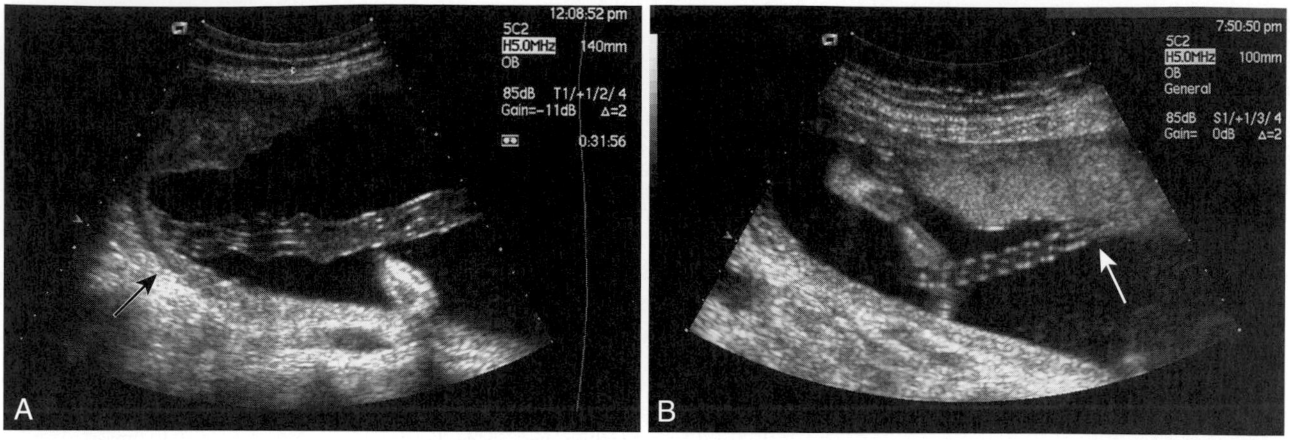

FIGURE 24–5
Ultrasound image of umbilical cord insertion at midgestation. *A*, Velamentous cord. *B*, Nonvelamentous cord inserting in the placenta.

circulations. Suboptimal trophoblastic invasion of placenta of the smaller twin may also account for growth restriction via similar mechanisms as in singletons.[31] Furthermore, growth discordance in dichorionic twins has been found to be greater when the placentas are fused compared to those with separate placentas.[32]

Several investigators have addressed the use of uterine artery Doppler velocimetry at 18 to 24 weeks of gestation to predict intrauterine growth restriction (IUGR) in twin pregnancies,[33,34] demonstrating a disappointing sensitivity of 10%. Mean uterine artery resistance is lower in twin compared to singleton pregnancies, probably because of a larger placental implantation area. Additionally, the normally implanted portion of the placenta supplying the AGA twin may attenuate the hemodynamic effects of suboptimal implantation of the portion of the placenta supplying the SGA twin.[35]

Fetal Risks

Fetal risks associated with IUGR for multiplets are similar to singletons (see Chapter 12) and include intrauterine fetal death (IUFD) and neurologic morbidity due to chronic oxygen and nutrient deprivation. Erythropoietin levels are elevated in SGA compared to AGA twins, and in twins with discordant growth, in the lighter of twins compared with the heavier.[36] Likewise, nucleated red blood cells tend to be higher in the lighter twin compared with the larger; the difference increasing with greater discordancy.[37] These findings further support the concept that poor growth in twins is not "physiologic" but indicative of chronic fetal hypoxia. SGA dichorionic twins have similar risks of perinatal death compared to singletons, whereas the perinatal mortality rate for SGA monochorionic twins is twice as high.[19]

Growth discordancy (birth weight difference ≥25%) as well as being SGA confers an increased risk for adverse perinatal outcome. Although most discordant pairs contain one or two SGA infants,[38] discordant pairs in which both are AGA still face elevated risks compared with nondiscordant pairs[39]; twins who are both SGA and discordant have the highest risks.[40] The same applies for triplets with higher degrees of discordancy associated with increasing rates of IUFD in the smaller and middle-sized fetuses.[41]

Growth discordant monochorionic twins are at higher risk of adverse outcome than growth discordant dichorionic twins.[42] Unfortunately, most of the data reported on discordant growth in monochorionic twins are a mixture of pregnancies with twin-to-twin transfusion syndrome (TTTS) and isolated discordant growth. Although TTTS is frequently associated with discordant growth, its distinction from isolated discordant growth is essential and based on the sonographic absence of hydramnios (deepest vertical pocket ≥8 cm prior to 20 weeks, ≥10 cm after 20 weeks) in the AGA twin in cases with discordant growth (Fig. 24–6). Whereas TTTS is extensively studied, little is known of the outcome of discordant growth in monochorionic twins. Large population-based studies indicate that the risk for IUFD for growth discordant same-sex twins (30% monochorionic and 70% dichorionic) is increased compared to growth discordant different-sex twins (100% dichorionic). In same-sex twins, both the lighter and heavier twins are at risk of IUFD with a threshold of discordancy of 10% and 20%, respectively. This is in contrast to different-sex twins, in which only the lighter twin is at risk of IUFD, provided the discordancy is at least 20%.[40] Small case series (N = 47)[43,44] of discordant growth (≥20%) without TTTS in

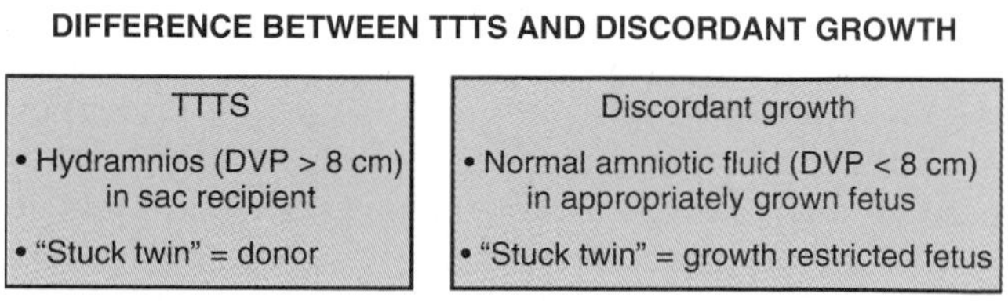
DIFFERENCE BETWEEN TTTS AND DISCORDANT GROWTH
TTTS
• Hydramnios (DVP > 8 cm) in sac recipient
• "Stuck twin" = donor
Discordant growth
• Normal amniotic fluid (DVP < 8 cm) in appropriately grown fetus
• "Stuck twin" = growth restricted fetus

FIGURE 24–6
Differential diagnosis of twin-to-twin transfusion syndrome and discordant growth. DVP, deepest vertical pocket.

monochorionic twins report an IUFD rate of about 25% in the lighter twin, with concomitant or subsequent IUFD of the larger twin occurring in 25%, or 6% overall. In a series of discordant dichorionic twins (N = 29) managed expectantly until 32 weeks, the IUFD rate of the smaller twin was 35%, with the larger twins surviving in all cases.[45]

After birth, twins with IUGR and discordant growth face increased risks of neonatal morbidity and death.[46,47] In discordant pairs, the lighter twin more frequently has a low 5-minute Apgar score and is at higher risk of neonatal death, whereas the heavier twin has more respiratory difficulties when delivered between 33 and 36 weeks.[39] The fear of an IUFD may prompt obstetric intervention, adding the complications of iatrogenic prematurity to the inherent complications of multiple gestation.[48] Clearly, any decision for iatrogenic preterm delivery to prevent IUFD must be weighed against the risks of death and handicap for each twin as determined by gestational age and EFW.

Finally, IUGR is associated with increased risks of cerebral palsy (CP).[49] Likewise, twins with discordant growth are at increased risk of neurodevelopmental morbidity and CP compared with nondiscordant twins. However, this increased risk may also be determined by their lower birth weight or their earlier delivery rather than the discordancy itself.[50] Nonetheless, in a recent series of preterm twin pregnancies (GA between 24 and 34 weeks), the CP rate was 19% in growth discordant monochorionic twins (N = 20) compared with 5% in dichorionic twins (N = 13). This incidence was actually higher than the 4% CP rate in the report's survivors of TTTS (N - 15)[51] and suggests that monochorionic twins with discordant growth are at especially high risk for adverse outcome. IUFD of one twin is a strong predictor of CP in the survivor, with population-based studies indicating a risk of CP of 30 per 1000 infant survivors of different-sex twins and as high as 106 per 1000 infant survivors in same-sex twins.[52] In the Adegbite series,[51] there were four instances of IUFD associated with discordant growth; three neonates survived and all had cerebral palsy.

Management Options

Similar to singletons, the goals of management are to prevent IUFD and long-term neurologic damage due to poor oxygen and nutritional supply. This discussion is, however, restricted to twins, as twins are far more common than triplets. Nevertheless, growth problems are more frequent and occur earlier in higher-order multiples, and the management issues are comparable to those of twins. Because of the different pathophysiology and prognosis, the management of IUGR in monochorionic and dichorionic twins is discussed separately. A small paragraph is also dedicated to the management of those twin pregnancies in which the opportunity for adequate chorionicity determination in the first trimester was missed.

Dichorionic Twins

Dichorionic twins are conceptually singletons who happen to occupy the same womb at the same time. Therefore, the diagnostic workup and follow-up are comparable to that of an IUGR in a singleton pregnancy (see Chapter 12).

ANTENATAL DIAGNOSIS

In instances of severe early-onset IUGR, it is important to exclude aneuploidy, structural anomalies, and congenital infection because these fetuses will not usually benefit from the intense antenatal surveillance and iatrogenic early delivery. Study of amniotic fluid and Doppler studies can help to differentiate the growth-restricted fetus from the constitutionally or abnormal SGA fetus.

FETAL SURVEILLANCE

Methods of fetal surveillance for IUGR in dichorionic twins include a combination of fetal growth and amniotic fluid assessment, nonstress test, biophysical profile score, and Doppler velocimetry. Similar to singletons, uteroplacental dysfunction is associated with a sequence of Doppler and fetal biophysical profile changes, suggesting progressive deterioration and hypoxia.

TREATMENT

The risk of IUFD with expectant management must be balanced against the risks of iatrogenic prematurity. When both twins are growth restricted to a similar degree (which is rare), the risks are similar for both. However, the most common scenario is discordant growth with one growth-restricted twin. The Doppler changes that allow the reliable identification of fetal hypoxemia are discussed in Chapters 11 and 12. Early delivery to rescue the hypoxemic twin may expose the AGA twin to the risks of prematurity. Therefore, it may be preferable in dichorionic twins with early-onset severe discordant growth to delay delivery until the risk of death and handicap due to iatrogenic prematurity are minimal for the AGA twin, irrespective of the condition of the SGA twin. Such an expectant management until 32 weeks or when EFW of the AGA twin was more than 1500 g resulted in a 35% rate of IUFD in the SGA twin but no deaths or handicaps in the AGA co-twins in one series.[45] The timing of any intervention depends on the clarity of the diagnosis in the SGA twin and the chances of survival and handicap for each fetus, and the initiation of intensive fetal surveillance must be planned accordingly. The efficacy of antenatal corticosteroid therapy to enhance maturation is insufficiently examined in twins. However, the available information suggests it is reasonable to administer corticosteroid agents to women whose pregnancies are complicated by discordant twins whenever early delivery is contemplated. Testing of fetal lung maturity can also be performed if there is a likelihood of a mature study. It is generally recommended in twins to sample both sacs, especially before 32 weeks.[53]

Monochorionic Twins

Monochorionic twins have an identical genetic constitution and share a single placenta, with their circulations connected through vascular communications in the placenta. Therefore, the management of IUGR in monochorionic twin pregnancies poses some unique challenges.

ANTENATAL DIAGNOSIS

The need to exclude aneuploidy, discordant structural anomalies, and congenital infection also applies to monochorionic twins. Monochorionic twins can be discordant for most common human aneuploidies.[25,54,55] Both amniotic sacs must be sampled in order to diagnose these rare heterokaryotypic monochorionic twins. Additionally, structural anomalies are more common in monochorionic twins[56] and usually only affect one fetus.[57] On the other hand, congenital infection typically affects both twins, although the degree of severity may vary. It is equally important to distinguish discordant growth from TTTS by the absence of hydramnios in the sac of the AGA twin in cases of discordant growth.

FETAL SURVEILLANCE

It is unclear as to what the best method is to monitor fetal well-being in growth-restricted monochorionic twins. Doppler velocimetry of the umbilical artery may not have the same prognostic value in monochorionic twins as it has in singletons and dichorionic twin gestations. Umbilical artery waveforms reflect downstream vascular resistance, which in monochorionic twins is determined not only by the adequacy of spiral artery invasion, but also by the direction and shunting across the vascular anastomoses. Large arterioarterial anastomoses can influence umbilical artery waveforms, leading to intermittent absent end-diastolic or even reversed flow.[58] This phenomenon occurs typically in the SGA twin of a monochorionic pair with severe growth discordance (Fig. 24–7).[59,60] IUFD may occur unexpectedly in these fetuses, without additional signs of deterioration of either the Doppler flow profile or the biophysical profile score (unpublished observations), as these large arterioarterial anastomoses may facilitate acute exsanguination or other hemodynamic aberrations. On the other hand, the SGA twin in some cases of discordant growth may have absent end-diastolic flow from early in pregnancy onward for up to 13 weeks, without any adverse effect on fetal survival.[10] Whether brain sparing and venous Doppler velocimetry are better means to assess fetal well-being in monochorionic twins remains to be determined. One recent study observed evidence of brain sparing in 70% of growth-restricted monochorionic twins, but its influence on outcome was not reported. Clearly, the potential role of Doppler velocimetry in growth-restricted monochorionic twins requires additional study. In the meantime, the biophysical profile score (including the nonstress test) seems the best method available.

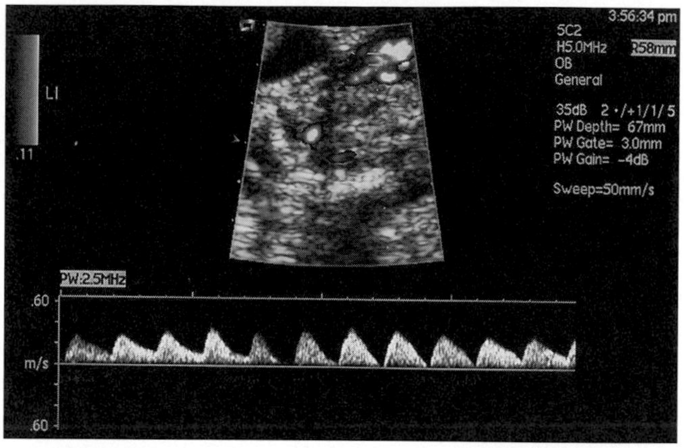

FIGURE 24–7
Doppler pattern of intermittent absent end-diastolic flow as typically seen in the smaller twin of a monochorionic pair with discordant growth (see Color Plate 28).

TREATMENT

In monochorionic twins, the management is complicated by the almost obligatory presence of a shared circulation. In dichorionic twins, single IUFD (sIUFD) is associated with perinatal death or handicap of the surviving twin in 5% to 10% and is largely due to extreme preterm delivery. In contrast, sIUFD in monochorionic twins leads to double IUFD in 10% to 25% and antenatal cerebral lesions in 25% to 45% of surviving co-twins. This extra morbidity and mortality is due to a combination of pressure instability as the first twin dies and acute exsanguination in the fetoplacental unit of the dead twin, all in addition to the effects of extreme preterm delivery.[61,62] Expectant management irrespective of the condition of the SGA fetus until 32 weeks is therefore not appropriate in monochorionic twins. Possible management options for severe, early discordant growth in monochorionic twins are expectant management with timely delivery, selective feticide by umbilical cord occlusion, or selective coagulation of the vascular anastomoses. The problems with expectant management are that IUFD may occur before viability, is difficult to predict, and may have major consequences. IUFD is especially dramatic once a viable stage of gestation has been reached. As a result, some advocate elective delivery of all monochorionic twins with a growth discordance of more than 25% at 32 weeks after the administration of maternal corticosteroids or at the latest after confirmation of fetal lung maturity.

Umbilical cord occlusion may be considered prior to viability when there are signs of imminent fetal death. The rationale for cord occlusion is that it may protect the surviving twin better against the adverse effects of spontaneous demise. However, a major drawback is that the maximum survival rate is 50%. Further, it is not always clear which signs predict impending IUFD in monochorionic twins, and it may be that the risks of co-twin death and neurologic damage are less with sIUFD of the SGA twin because of the smaller fetoplacental unit.

Selective photocoagulation of the vascular anastomoses performed before 26 weeks' gestation also seeks to protect the AGA twin against the adverse effect of IUFD of the SGA twin by "unlinking" the two fetal circulations and transforming the monochorionic placenta into a "functional" dichorionic placenta. However, a small case series comparing treated and expectantly managed cases series did not show any significant difference in survival or neurologic morbidity rates.[44,63] Several explanations for this apparent lack of benefit are possible. First, selective coagulation is technically more challenging for discordant growth than for TTTS owing to the absence of hydramnios. Second, unequal sharing is frequently the reason for discordant growth, and coagulation of the vascular anastomoses may diminish the already critical placental reserve of the SGA twin further. Third, circulatory instability may have already damaged the AGA twin. And finally, the natural history of monochorionic twins needs to be better understood because an overactive management plan may risk the loss of pregnancies that would have reached viability without IUFD of the SGA fetus. Clearly, management of these high risk pregnancies should be individualized after input from the parents, fetal medicine specialists, neonatologist, and obstetricians.

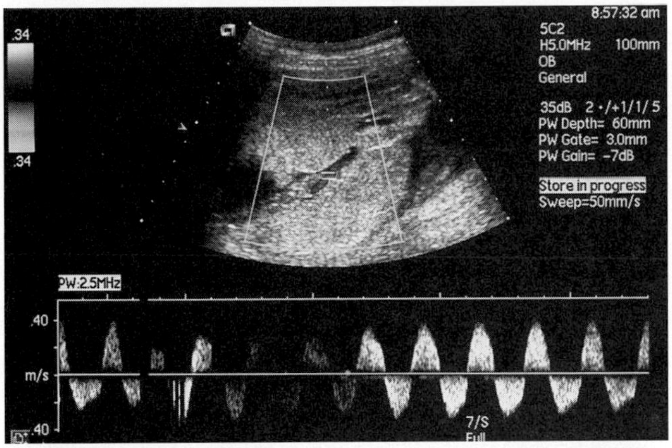

FIGURE 24–8
Characteristic bidirectional Doppler pattern in an arterioarterial anastomosis, which confirms monochorionicity. (see Color Plate 29)

Twins of Unknown Chorionicity

Determining chorionicity in same-sex twins with discordant growth in the second trimester can be challenging. Oligohydramnios with the intertwin membrane plastered around the SGA twin makes assessment of membrane thickness or the presence or absence of a lambda sign especially unreliable. It is estimated that just 3 out of 10 same-sex twins are monochorionic. In these instances, the detection of an arterioarterial anastomosis with its characteristic bidirectional waveform (Fig. 24–8) confirms monochorionicity with 100% reliability.[64] Also, DNA determination of zygosity by amniocentesis will rule out monochorionicity if dizygosity is confirmed.[65] In cases of persistent doubt, it is prudent to manage the pregnancy as a monochorionic twin gestation.

SUMMARY OF MANAGEMENT OPTIONS

Poor Fetal Growth in Twin Pregnancies

Management Options	Quality of Evidence	Strength of Recommendation	References
Dichorionic Twins			
Exclude aneuploidy, structural anomalies, and congenital infection.	–	GPP	–
Determine when to intervene upon signs of fetal distress of the SGA (small for gestational age) twin and plan fetal surveillance accordingly.	See Chapters 11 and 12		
In severe early discordant growth, it may be preferable not to intervene to maximize the chances of the AGA (appropriate for gestational age) twin at the expense of spontaneous demise of the SGA twin.	III	B	45
Fetal surveillance is usually done by a combination of fetal growth assessment, biophysical profile scoring, and Doppler velocimetry.	See Chapters 11 and 12		
Consider administration of corticosteroids and fetal lung maturity testing whenever early delivery is contemplated.	III	B	53

Continued

SUMMARY OF MANAGEMENT OPTIONS

Poor Fetal Growth in Twin Pregnancies *(Continued)*

Management Options	Quality of Evidence	Strength of Recommendation	References
Monochorionic Twins			
Exclude aneuploidy, structural anomalies, congenital infection, and TTTS (twin-to-twin transfusion syndrome).	IIa	B	54–56
Consider referral to a tertiary care center.	–	GPP	–
If spontaneous demise is presumed imminent and in the previable period, selective feticide by cord occlusion may protect the AGA twin better against the side effects of spontaneous demise.	IV	C	63
Consider elective preterm delivery at 32 weeks for cases with a growth difference of ≥25% after administration of corticosteriods or at the latest when lung maturity has been established.	–	GPP	–
Nonstress testing and biophysical profile score are currently the best methods to ascertain fetal well-being, although IUFD can occur unexpectedly, despite normal biophysical profile scoring.	III	B	58–60
Assess for TTTS.	–	GPP	–
Twins of Unknown Chorionicity			
Consider DNA fingerprinting to exclude monochorionicity.	III	B	65
Check for arterioarterial anastomoses to confirm monochorionicity.	III	B	64
If chorionicity remains unconfirmed, manage as monochorionic twins.	–	GPP	–

MONOAMNIOTIC TWINS

General

Splitting of the inner cell mass after day 9 after fertilization results in monochorionic monoamniotic twins. These twins share not only their placenta but also their amniotic sac. Monoamniotic twins are rare, occurring in 1 in 10,000 pregnancies and, as such, constitute 5% of monochorionic twins.[66] The umbilical cords insert usually close to each other midplacenta with multiple deep and superficial large-caliber (8–12 mm) anastomoses connecting the placental stem vessels of the twins (Fig. 24–9).[67]

The diagnosis of monoamniotic twin gestation is reliably made in the early first trimester by the presence of a single yolk sac,[68] one amniotic cavity containing two fetal poles, and a single placenta. Cord entanglement is diagnostic of monoamniotic twins and often already demonstrable in the first trimester by imaging two heart rates on pulsed Doppler in an entangled mass of umbilical cord vessels (Fig. 24–10).[69,70] Current ultrasound technology with sharper resolution usually permits the distinction between diamniotic and monoamniotic monochorionic twins. On occasion, transvaginal scanning at high frequencies will help confirm or refute any dividing membrane. "The stuck twin phenomenon" is regularly mistaken for a monoamniotic twin pregnancy because of the difficulty of seeing the dividing membrane. However, the fixed position of the stuck twin rules it out because in a monoamniotic gestation both fetuses move freely about.

Fetal Risks

Monoamniotic twins are at increased risk of congenital malformation and sudden IUFD. Although rare, conjoined twins must be excluded. Conjoined twins arise when the embryonic disk incompletely divides beyond the 12th day of fertilization and have an estimated incidence of 1 in 50,000 pregnancies. The diagnosis is possible as early as the first trimester by the close and fixed apposition of the fetal bodies with fusion of the skin lines at some point (Fig. 24–11).[71] IUFD occurs in 60% of conjoined twins, and of those that are live born, the majority die as a result of severe anomalies or as a consequence of surgery.[72] Except for conjoined twinning, congenital malformations occur in 38% to 50% monoamniotic twins, usually affecting only one twin.[66,73] At least one third of the perinatal deaths in monoamniotic twins are caused by congenital malformations.[74] Late embryonic splitting and hemodynamic imbalances due to the large and multiple anastomoses may account for the extremely high prevalence.

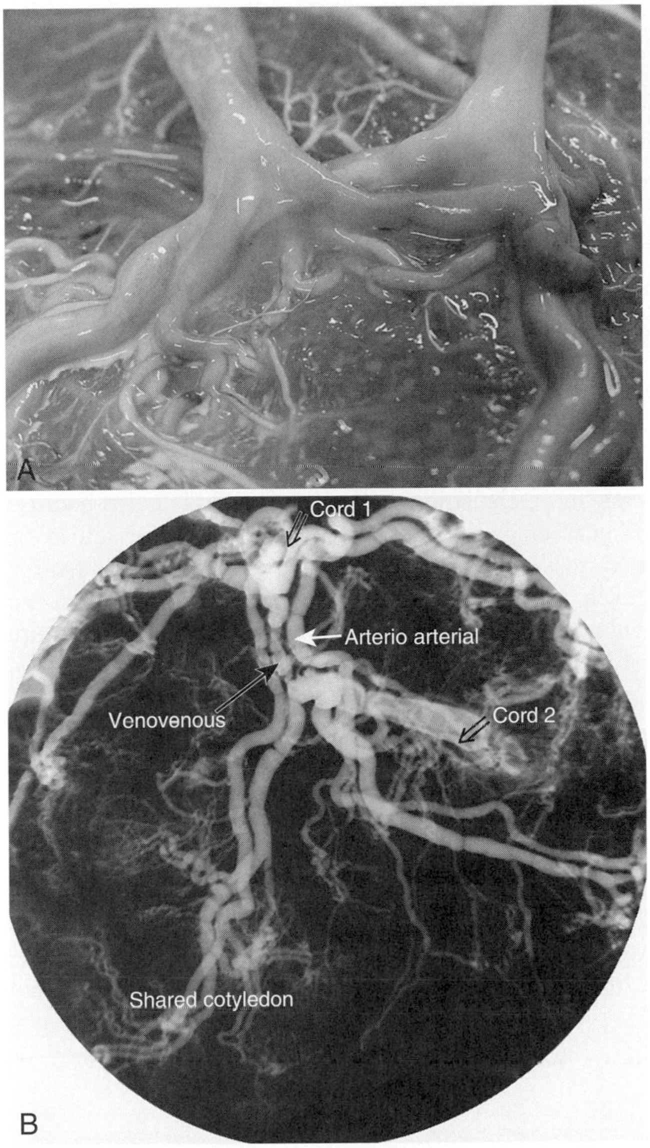

FIGURE 24–9
A, Macroscopic image of large-diameter anastomoses and side-to-side insertion of the umbilical cords as typically seen in a monoamniotic twin pregnancy (see Color Plate 30). *B*, Rx angiography where injection of the umbilical vessels of one twin was sufficient to visualize the placental vascularization of both twins due to the presence of a large arterioarterial and venovenous anastomosis. Furthermore, about half of the placenta consisted of shared cotyledons.

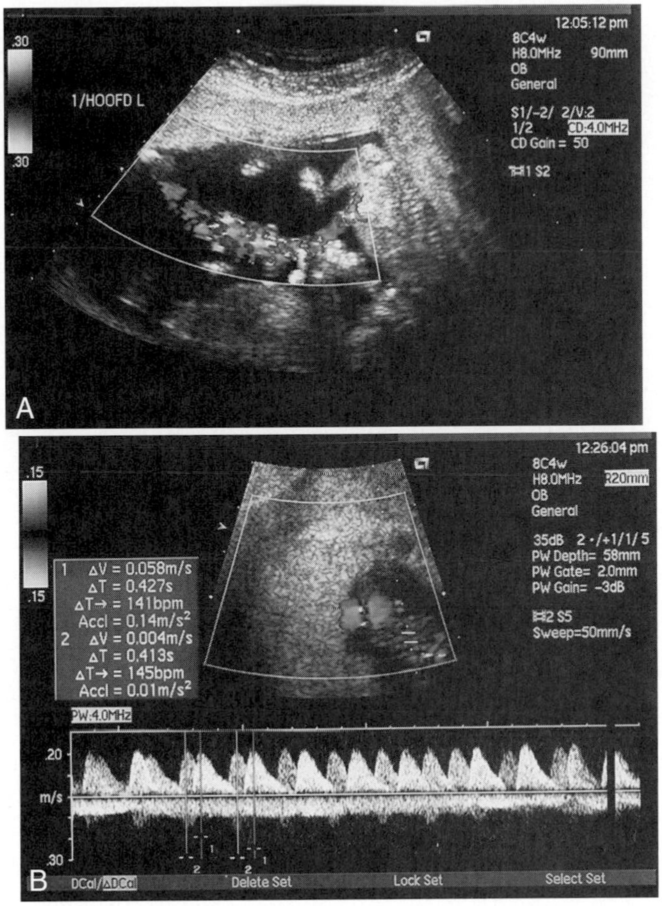

FIGURE 24–10
Ultrasound image of cord entanglement at 14 weeks' gestational age in monoamniotic twins. *A*, Color Doppler demonstrating cord entanglement. *B*, Pulsed Doppler of the entangled mass showing two different heart rates. (Courtesy of D. Van Schoubroeck, UZ Leuven, Belgium.)

In structurally normal monoamniotic twins, sudden IUFD is the most important cause of death. Recent series report rates of 2.4%[75] to 10%[74] with careful fetal surveillance and early delivery compared to previously quoted risks of 30% to 70%.[76,77] However, most pregnancies included in these series were diagnosed in the second trimester, and the IUFD rate is likely to be higher when cases diagnosed in the first trimester would be included.[66] Umbilical cord entanglement was long considered the only reason for the high mortality rate, but almost all monoamniotic twins have entangled cords at birth (Fig. 24–12) and usually from early in gestation. "Acute" TTTS may be an important contributing factor, perhaps triggered by cord compression. Acute hemodynamic imbalances across the large-caliber anastomoses may also explain the 70% rate of double IUFDs in monoamniotic twins[67] compared to 25% in diamniotic twins.[61] Indeed, chronic TTTS is only rarely reported in monoamniotic twins, probably

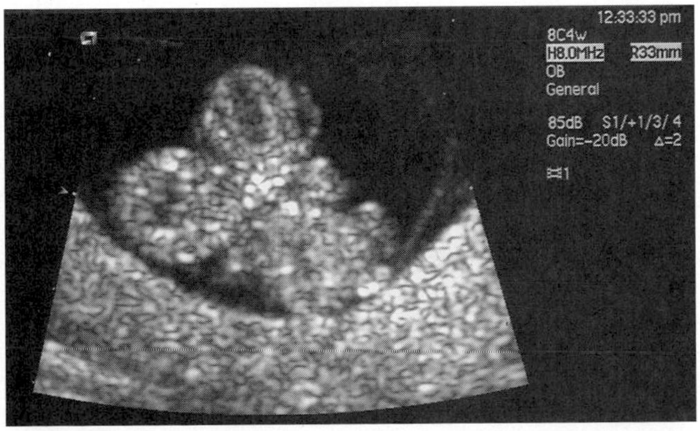

FIGURE 24–11
Ultrasound image of conjoined twins at 9 weeks' gestational age. (Courtesy of I. Witters, UZ Leuven, Belgium.)

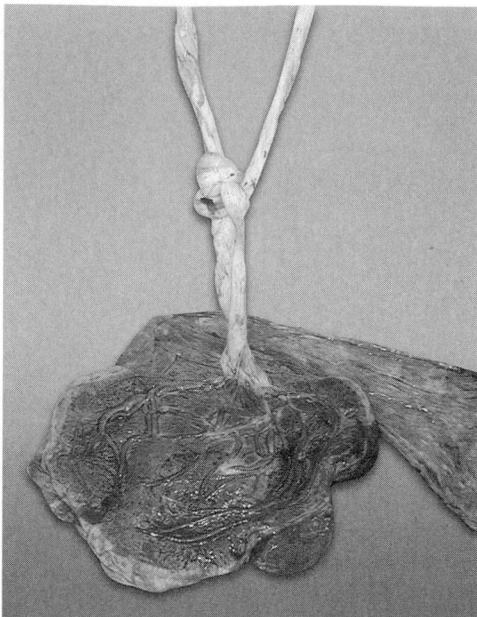

FIGURE 24–12
Cord entanglement and knotting at birth in a monoamniotic twin pregnancy. (Courtesy of S. Dobbelaere, H. Hart Hospital, Lier, Belgium.) (see Color Plate 31)

because volume shifts through the large-caliber anastomoses are not tolerated for long periods and are more likely to lead to sudden IUFD typically of both twins. The deaths usually occur within a short period of each other. However, cord entanglement may still cause IUFD[78] or asphyxia later in gestation if the co-twin survives.[79]

Management Options

The cornerstone of management is a detailed anomaly scan at 16 to 18 weeks to rule out associated anomalies, followed by scans every fortnight for growth and amniotic fluid volume, intense antenatal surveillance from 26 to 28 weeks onward, and timely delivery. It is the authors' opinion that delivery should be planned for 32 weeks or at the latest when lung maturity is established. However, others note extremely low loss rates after 32 weeks, possibly because there is little room for fetal movement.[80] Selective feticide for discordant anomalies in monoamniotic twins can be accomplished by fetoscopic/ultrasound-guided coagulation and laser transsection of the umbilical cord (Fig. 24–13). The procedure is technically more challenging than in diamniotic twins because of cord entanglement. An accessory port for fetoscopy may facilitate cord transsection and to a lesser degree helps to identify the correct cord, albeit with an unknown additional risk of preterm premature rupture of membranes (PPROM) when compared to single port procedures.

Although IUFD in monoamniotic twins may be sudden and unpredictable, careful antenatal surveillance and early elective delivery appear to improve perinatal survival rate to about 90%.[75] However, the best way to manage these cases is simply not known. Generally, it is agreed that intense fetal surveillance should be started from 26 to 28 weeks onward, with regular nonstress testing and ultrasound scans for biophysical profile score, Doppler, and growth checks. The recommended

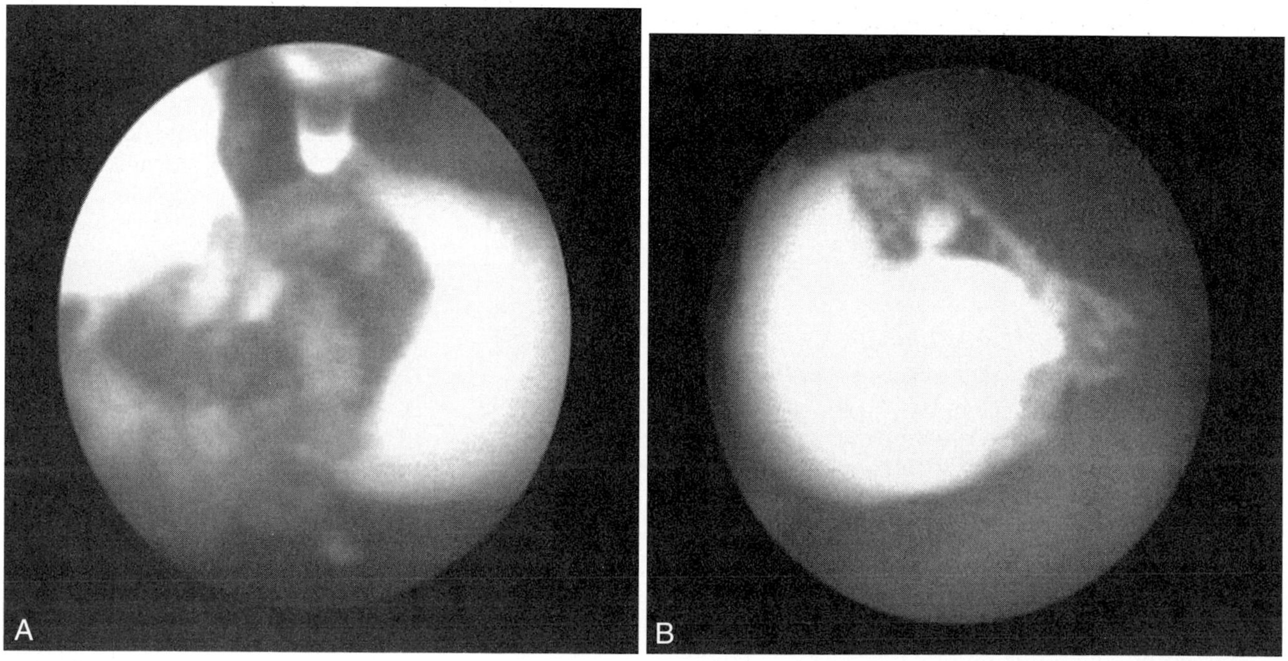

FIGURE 24–13
Fetoscopic image during (*A*) and after (*B*) umbilical cord transsection by laser in a monoamniotic twin pregnancy with a severe discordant anomaly (see Color Plate 32).

frequency is disputed, and in the literature nonstress testing varies from twice-weekly to several times daily. The high frequency of nonstress testing is justified by the suddenness of the events, but fetal death in between remains possible. Some advocate weekly ultrasound examinations with a biophysical profile score, yet these fetuses are likely lost because of acute events, and not because of chronic hypoxemia. Abnormal umbilical artery Doppler flow waveforms such as diastolic notch[81] or absent/reversed end-diastolic flow are reported to indicate cord compression. But similar to monochorionic twins in general, the predictive value of abnormal umbilical artery Doppler velocimetry may be different compared to singletons and, like biophysical profile scoring, requires additional validation.[82] The need for hospitalization is likewise controversial, and this decision should be individualized based on the results of the ultrasound scan and antenatal testing.[83] Sulindac was suggested as a "safe" means of medical amnioreduction in monoamniotic twins.[84] Yet, because acute transfusion seems to be an important cofactor, IUFD can still occur after 32 weeks[85] despite sulindac.[66] For these reasons, we advocate delivery at 32 weeks when feasible. Even though cases of successful vaginal delivery are reported, cesarean delivery is the preferred mode of delivery to avoid cord entanglement and inadvertent clamping of the cord of the second twin, which may be tightly around the neck of the first.[86]

SUMMARY OF MANAGEMENT OPTIONS

Monoamniotic Twins

Management Options	Quality of Evidence	Strength of Recommendation	References
Exclude structural anomalies.	–	GPP	–
Consider referral to tertiary care center.	–	GPP	–
Determine when to intervene upon signs of fetal distress and plan fetal surveillance accordingly.	III	B	74,75
Fetal surveillance consists of daily to twice weekly nonstress testing and biophysical profile scoring.	III	B	74,75
Value of hospitalization is uncertain.	III	B	83
Risk of fetal death does not decline after 32 weeks; thus, some advocate delivery at 32 weeks after maternal steroids are given. Others advocate delivery at term, or sooner if evidence of fetal compromise, but consider steroid administration.	IIa III	B B	83,84 85
Most advocate cesarean section; vaginal delivery requires continuous fetal heart rate monitoring of both twins and facilities for immediate cesarean section.	IIa	B	80,86
Color Doppler may predict cord entanglement.	III	B	79–82

IN UTERO DEATH OF ONE FETUS

General

Fetuses of multifetal pregnancies are more likely to die in utero than singletons.[87] Not unexpectedly, the risk grows with an increasing number of fetuses.[88] The rate of sIUFD in twins or higher-order multiplets is difficult to ascertain during the first trimester, as the loss may occur before the diagnosis of either a multifetal pregnancy or sIUFD is made. Also, the "vanishing embryo syndrome" may go unrecognized or may be wrongly diagnosed as a retromembranous blood collection (Fig. 24–14). The diagnosis of sIUFD should be made when fetal remnants are clearly identified or when a later ultrasound examination demonstrates the IUFD or disappearance of a previously known fetus. The risk of sIUFD in twin pregnancies resulting from in vitro fertilization (IVF), which are regularly followed throughout the first trimester, is maternal age–dependent and ranges from 10% to 20% with most cases occurring prior to 12 weeks.[89] These figures are currently the best estimates available for first-trimester sIUFD in dichorionic twins, as about 90% of IVF pregnancies are dichorionic.[90] In a general population scanned between 10 and 14 weeks of gestation, the prevalence of sIUFD is reportedly 4% in dichorionic twins and less than 1% in monochorionic twin pregnancies (compared with 2% in singletons), with double IUFD in 1.6% of dichorionic and 2% of monochorionic twin pregnancies.[91] Thus, double IUFD appears more common than sIUFD in monochorionic twins. Gross unequal placental sharing or hemodynamic imbalances in

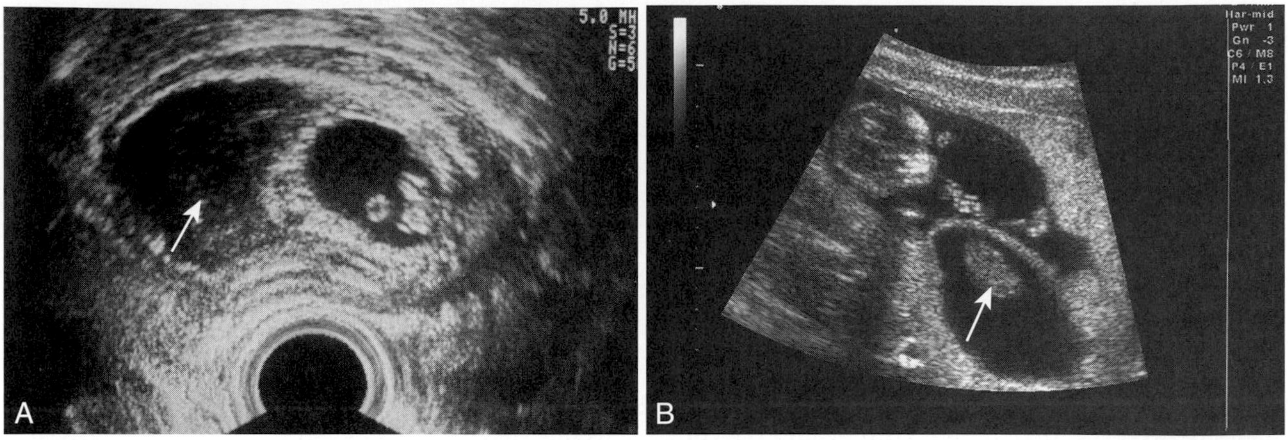

FIGURE 24–14
A, Ultrasound image of a retromembranous blood collection (*arrow*) in a singleton pregnancy, which must be differentiated from (*B*) "vanishing twin syndrome" in which felt remnants (*arrow*) can be clearly identified.

monochorionic twins may cause sIUFD, with the connected fetal circulations leading to double IUFD. Also, chromosomal abnormalities or an adverse maternal factor (infection, teratogens) will usually affect both fetuses similarly. In contrast, sIUFD in dichorionic twins is twice as common than double IUFD and may be explained by either a discordant chromosomal or structural anomaly or suboptimal placentation. Because each fetus has a separate fetoplacental circulation, sIUFD will not cause co-twin death per se. About 10% of dichorionic twins are monozygotic and therefore concordant for chromosomal anomalies. Double IUFD in dichorionic twins may also occur because of exposure to the same adverse maternal factor.

From 10 to 14 weeks onward, sIUFD occurs in about 2% of dichorionic but 4% of monochorionic twin pregnancies, and double IUFD occurs in 0.2% of dichorionic and in at least 6% of monochorionic twins. This extra fetal loss of monochorionic twins occurs before 24 weeks and is largely attributable to complications of the connected fetoplacental circulations.[12] Toward the end of gestation, the risk of IUFD in twins increases from 1/3333 at 33 weeks to 1/313 at 36 weeks and 1/69 beyond 39 weeks. IUFD rates of twins at 37 to 38 weeks equal those of postterm singleton pregnancies, and elective delivery at 37 to 38 completed weeks may be justified when uncomplicated twin pregnancies reach that milestone.[92] Data on the risk of IUFD toward term according to chorionicity are currently not available.

Fetal Risks

The prognosis of sIUFD for the surviving fetus depends first and foremost on chorionicity. To a lesser degree, outcome is determined by the gestational age of sIUFD. There is little evidence regarding the implications of sIUFD in the first trimester. Nonetheless, it seems most likely that sIUFD in a monochorionic twin pregnancy leads to either double IUFD or miscarriage. Rarely, the surviving co-twin may prevent "vanishing" of the dead twin by reversed perfusion along the vascular anastomoses—a twin reversed arterial perfusion (TRAP) sequence.[93] Color Doppler should be used to exclude TRAP whenever sIUFD occurs in a monochorionic twin pregnancy, and if there is any doubt, follow-up scans should be arranged. It is also hypothesized that unrecognized, early sIUFD in a monochorionic twin pregnancy may explain some cases of cerebral palsy and certain congenital anomalies such as renal agenesis and intestinal atresias in birth singletons, attributable to agonal hemodynamic events.[94] The outcome of sIUFD in the first trimester in dichorionic twins is usually favorable, although the rate of preterm delivery and subsequent miscarriage may be increased especially if the sIUFD occurs toward the end of the first trimester. In the case series of sIUFD diagnosed between 10 and 14 weeks, 18% (3/16) of dichorionic twins subsequently miscarried.[91]

sIUFD in dichorionic twins during the second to third trimester is associated with either death or handicap in 5% to 10% of survivors, presumably in great part secondary to extreme prematurity, though no doubt in some instances an adverse maternal event may cause demise of one twin but only damage the survivor. Conversely, in monochorionic twins, sIUFD results in a double IUFD in 10% to 25%, and cerebral damage in 25% to 45% due in part to acute TTTS plus the risks of extreme prematurity.[61,62] In dichorionic twins, survival is inversely related to the gestational age of the sIUFD, with infant survival rates improving from 71%, when the sIUFD occurs between 20 and 24 weeks, to 98% for sIUFD occurring beyond 37 weeks.[88] The reported rate of cerebral palsy (CP) after sIUFD in dichorionic twins is 30 per 1000 infant survivors with prematurity being the leading factor in this excess risk compared with 1 per 1000 in singletons.[52,95] In monochorionic twins, the influence of gestational age of sIUFD on outcome is less clear. It seems early sIUFD is more often associated with death of the co-twin. But, if the co-twin survives, severe morbidity is less common. In contrast, a late sIUFD more frequently results in the delivery of a live-born infant who is neurologically damaged.[62,96] Specific CP rates are not available for sIUFD in monochorionic twins. However, the CP rate in same-sex twins (30% monochorionic and 70% dichorionic) after sIUFD is 106 per 1000 survivors, which is about three times higher than different-sex twins (100% dichorionic).[52] In addition, most of the twins in the same-sex group with CP had monochorionic placentation.[95] Cerebral damage is often detectable sonographically but does not usually become apparent until weeks after the insult. Prenatal magnetic resonance imaging (MRI) may detect brain lesions earlier and with better definition.[97,98] Sonographic evidence of brain injury includes porencephaly, multicystic encephalomalacia, ventriculomegaly, cerebral atrophy, and cerebellar or cerebral infarcts. Less frequently reported complications include renal cortical necrosis, small bowel atresia, aplasia cutis, and limb infarction. Originally, thromboembolic phenomena with passage of thromboplastin from the dead to the living twin were thought to be responsible for these lesions.[99] A variety of studies have failed to find any such evidence, though perimortal circulatory instability and acute exsanguination are well documented.[100] Reversed perfusion of the dead twin has been demonstrated by Doppler interrogation of the chorionic plate vessels,[101] and fetal blood sampling within 24 hours of sIUFD has consistently revealed decreased hematocrits in survivors with normal coagulation profiles.[102] Further, fetoscopy within 3 hours of the demise of a donor twin has documented reversal of the transfusion with a plethoric donor and anemic recipient.[103] Outcome of the survivor may not only depend on the gestational age at sIUFD but also on the type and direction of vascular anastomoses and the fetoplacental mass of the demised twin. The presence of superficial arterioarterial anastomoses is associated with higher rates of death and neurologic damage.[61] However, significant anemia and co-twin death may occur, even in the absence of arterioarterial anastomoses.[96] The outcome of sIUFD associated with TTTS treated by amniodrainage does not differ from sIUFD unassociated with TTTS, and the risk of sIUFD is similar for donors and recipients. It was suggested that the risk of co-twin death and neurologic damage is lower with sIUFD of the donor compared with sIUFD of the recipient, because transfusion is more likely to be directed toward the recipient.[61] However, other small series show similar incidences of anemia and adverse outcome in surviving recipients and donors.[96,104] And even though TTTS treatment by laser coagulation of the vascular anastomoses more frequently results in sIUFD than amniodrainage, it consistently leads less often to a double IUFD.[105] Significantly, anemia in the survivor is rare in the event of sIUFD after laser[106] and the neurologic morbidity[107] less than after amniodrainage.[106,108] These findings provide further support for the concept that the vascular anastomoses are responsible for most of the adverse outcomes associated with sIUFD in monochorionic twins.

Management Options

Again, knowledge of chorionicity is fundamental to the management of sIUFD in multiple pregnancies. Because of the different pathophysiology and prognosis, management of sIUFD in monochorionic and dichorionic twins is discussed separately. Not to complicate matters unnecessarily, the discussion will be restricted to twins. Although sIUFD is more common in higher-order multiplets and management issues are more complex, they are based largely on the same principles as in twins. A small paragraph is dedicated to issues that are relevant to both groups of twins.

Dichorionic Twins

The main risks of sIUFD in dichorionic twins are miscarriage and severe preterm delivery. Therefore, conservative management is advocated with regular ultrasound scans to check growth and well-being of the survivor. Admittedly, parental anxiety may be an important factor in persuading the obstetrician to intervene, and these complex emotional responses should be adequately addressed.[109]

Monochorionic Twins

The main risks of sIUFD in monochorionic twins are death and ischemic brain lesions secondary to acute TTTS. Depending upon gestational age, there are additional risks of miscarriage or severe preterm delivery. It is presumed that death and especially ischemic brain damage in the survivor occurs during or soon after the death of its co-twin. Therefore, a pre-emptive preterm delivery is inappropriate once a sIUFD has been diagnosed, as this would only worsen the outcome of the surviving twin by adding the complications of prematurity. Further, a long death-to-delivery interval is associated with a better outcome compared to a short death-to-delivery interval, further supporting the benefit of conservative management.[62] Monochorionic twin pregnancies with a sIUFD should be managed in a tertiary referral center with sufficient neonatal support. Also, regular detailed (transvaginal if vertex) ultrasound examinations of the fetal brain are indicated to detect brain injury. Unlike hemorrhage, ischemic brain lesions are difficult to visualize in the early phase, and MRI scan may aid early detection.[97,98] Fetal blood sampling shortly after sIUFD may have prognostic value, as all nonanemic fetuses in one study had a good outcome and did not develop any brain injury.[96] Middle cerebral artery Doppler velocimetry is effective in predicting fetal anemia after sIUFD in cases complicated by TTTS and obviates the need of cordocentesis (Fig. 24–15). There is insufficient evidence a rescue intrauterine transfusion improves outcome. Whereas it may prevent co-twin death, it may not prevent brain injury.[96,104] As such, intrauterine transfusion may increase the survival of severely handicapped infants. Additional multicenter studies are necessary to determine whether rescue transfusion improves the outcome of survivors after sIUFD in monochorionic twins.

After birth, a thorough neonatal evaluation should be performed to detect any neurologic, renal, circulatory, and cutaneous defects. All survivors should undergo an early neonatal brain scan and be enrolled for long-term neurodevelopmental follow-up.

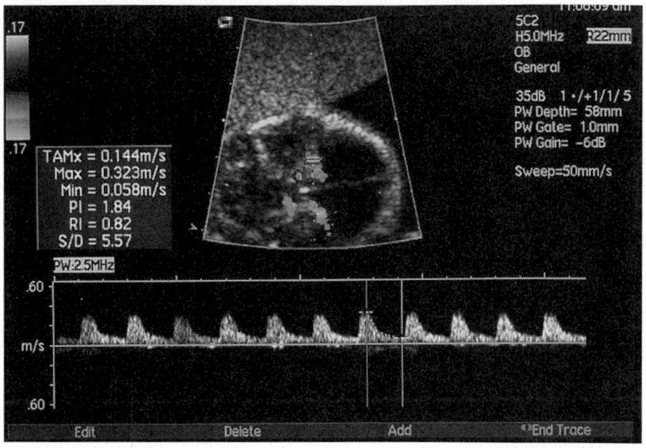

FIGURE 24–15
Doppler examination of the middle cerebral artery of the surviving twin of a monochorionic pair at 20 weeks' gestation, within 4 days after sIUFD of the growth-retarded co-twin (see Color Plate 33).

Issues Applicable to Dichorionic and Monochorionic Twins

It seems justified to administer Rhesus prophylaxis whenever a sIUFD is diagnosed in a Rhesus-negative woman. Maternal disseminated intravascular coagulation has been described in singletons after IUFD and retention of the fetus for more than 5 weeks. However, in twins its incidence with conservative management appears extremely low, and it can be treated with heparin when it does occur.[110,111] Vaginal delivery is not contraindicated after sIUFD, but labor may be obstructed, especially if the sIUFD occurs late and is presenting. A postmortem examination should be performed on the dead twin, and the placenta sent for histologic examination to confirm chorionicity.

The family will require both psychological support and counseling prior to, during, and after delivery. The grief experienced after a sIUFD equals that for a singleton loss, yet the parents rarely receive equal sympathy.[112] The death is also invisible for the parents and their immediate associates, which hampers the grieving process. Many parents worry the dead twin will have an adverse effect on the remaining fetus, and need reassurance that except for the possibility of an earlier delivery, no additional harm is expected. The delay between diagnosis and delivery permits some grieving, but sorrow resurfaces at birth.[113] It is important not to ignore the deceased twin; the parents may wish to see it during ultrasound examination and after birth. Demise after 12 to 15 weeks should end with an identifiable fetus at birth, though compressed and mummified, and parents should be prepared and told what to expect.[114]

SUMMARY OF MANAGEMENT OPTIONS

Single Fetal Death in Twins

Management Options	Quality of Evidence	Strength of Recommendation	References
Issues Applicable to All Twins			
Offer counseling and psychological support to patient and family.	III	B	112,113
Administer Rhesus prophylaxis if Rh negative.	–	GPP	–
Monitor maternal coagulation status.	IV	C	110
Give steroids if preterm delivery is contemplated.	Ia	A	222
Dichorionic Twins			
Check for signs of threatening miscarriage and severe preterm delivery.	III	B	109
If dichorionic pregnancy, continue fetal surveillance in survivor.	III	B	109
Monochorionic Twins			
Check for signs of threatening miscarriage and severe preterm delivery.	III	B	109
Continue fetal surveillance in surviving twin.	III	B	109

SUMMARY OF MANAGEMENT OPTIONS
Single Fetal Death in Twins *(Continued)*

Management Options	Quality of Evidence	Strength of Recommendation	References
Monochorionic Twins—Continued			
Consider Doppler of the middle cerebral artery to detect anemia, which may predict the risk of brain damage.	III	B	96,104
Check for brain injury by (transvaginal) ultrasound scan or MRI (magnetic resonance imaging).	III	B	97,98
Preemptive preterm delivery is no longer advocated.	III	B	62
Perform pediatric assessment and neurodevelopmental follow-up.	III	B	109

TWIN REVERSED ARTERIAL PERFUSION

General

The twin reversed arterial perfusion (TRAP) sequence, also known as acardiac twinning, is an anomaly unique to monochorionic multiple pregnancies that affects approximately 1 of 35,000 pregnancies and 1% of monochorionic twins.[115] In TRAP, blood flows from an umbilical artery of the pump twin in a reverse direction into the umbilical artery of the perfused twin, via an arterioarterial anastomosis. The perfused (or acardiac) twin is a true parasite. Its blood is poorly oxygenated, and the hypoxemia contributes to variable degrees of deficient development of the head, heart, and upper limb structures. The lower half of the body is usually better developed, which may be explained by the mechanism of transfusion of the acardiac twin. Blood enters the acardiac twin via the umbilical artery, and flows through the common iliac artery and aorta. What little oxygen is present is extracted in the lower part of the body, allowing at least partial development of the lower limbs and abdomen. By the time the blood reaches the upper body, most of the oxygen will already have been extracted, leading to poor development of upper body structures[111] (Fig. 24–16).

Two criteria must be fulfilled for the development of a TRAP sequence. The first is an arterioarterial anastomosis and the second is discordant development[116] or IUFD[101] in one of monochorionic twins, allowing for the blood flow reversal. Not infrequently, chromosomal abnormalities are identified in the acardiac twin, while the pump twin has a normal karyotype.[117,118] Embryos/fetuses with chromosome abnormalities have a high rate of spontaneous IUFD, which in dichorionic twins would lead to a "vanishing" twin. However, in monochorionic twins, the "vanishing" can be prevented by the occurrence of persistent, yet reversed, flow to the chromosomally abnormal twin via the vascular anastomoses. Therefore, whenever sIUFD is suspected in monochorionic twins on a first-trimester scan, the differential diagnosis or development of TRAP should be kept in mind and follow-up scans arranged.[93]

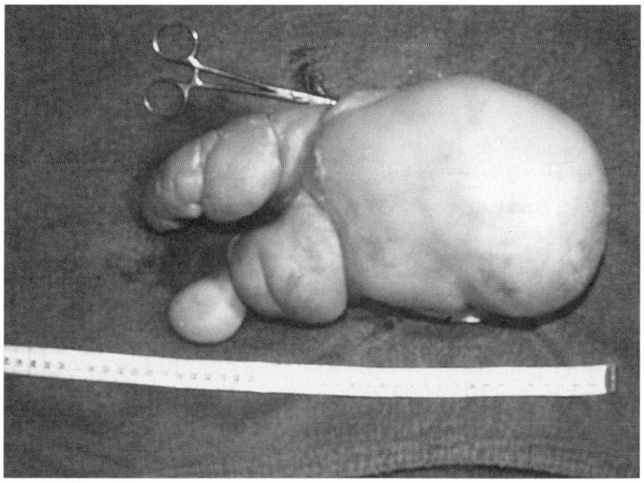

FIGURE 24–16
Macroscopic image of an acardiac twin with absent head and partial development of lower limbs and abdomen. This acardiac mass weighed about 4 kg and was not diagnosed until the third trimester. The patient delivered at 37 weeks, and the pump twin survived (see Color Plate 34).

The diagnosis can be reliably made on ultrasound scan in the first trimester.[119] TRAP sequence is characterized by a grossly abnormal fetus that grows, may even show movements, but has no functional cardiac activity of its own. Rarely, a rudimentary heart may show pulsatility (Fig. 24–17). Marked hydrops and cystic hygroma are frequently present, especially toward the end of pregnancy. Doppler studies reveal pathognomonic features of reversed arterial perfusion through an arterioarterial anastomosis (Fig. 24–18). TRAP can easily be distinguished from sIUFD by the presence of fetal movements and the typical retrograde perfusion.

Fetal Risks

Risks for the pump twin include heart failure secondary to the strain of perfusing the acardiac twin and extreme premature birth associated with hydramnios.[117,120] The

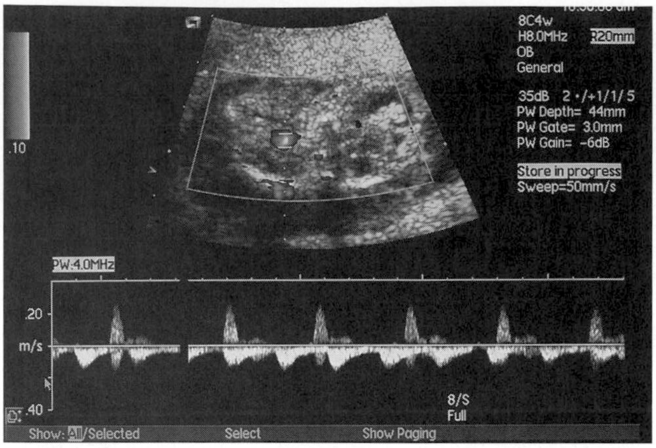

FIGURE 24–17
Doppler examination demonstrating cardiac activity in the rudimentary heart (70 bpm) of the acardiac twin, with flow in the opposite direction in the aorta (140 bpm) (see Color Plate 35).

pump twin may be chronically hypoxemic if the deoxygenated blood from the acardiac returns by a vein to vein anastomosis.

The natural history of TRAP is poorly documented due to the rarity of the disorder. Reported perinatal mortality rates for the pump twin vary between 35% and 50%[117,120] of cases diagnosed at birth, whereas some series of antenatally diagnosed cases report better,[121] similar,[122,123] and worse [124] outcomes. One explanation for a better outcome in antenatally diagnosed cases may be spontaneous resolution of the TRAP sequence following complete cessation of flow to the acardiac twin[121,123,125] Conversely, outcome may also be worse due to spontaneous demise of the pump twin leading to an early second-trimester loss not otherwise identified as a TRAP [121]. Long-term outcome data are not available for pump twins, although it is reasonable to speculate the risk of long-term cardiac and neurodevelopmental sequelae is high[126,127] due to vascular imbalances in utero.

Prognostic prediction of outcome of antenatally diagnosed TRAP is challenging. An acardiac/pump weight ratio above 70% at birth was associated with increased rates of congestive heart failure, hydramnios, and prematurity, suggesting a relatively small acardiac mass is a good sign. Certainly, a larger acardiac mass will put a greater hemodynamic strain on the pump twin. However, antenatal weight estimation of the acardiac mass is hampered by the absence of normal biometric structures, and the errors are likely large. Others suggest a rapid increase in the acardiac mass is indicative of poor prognosis.[122] Doppler velocimetry is probably the best tool to predict outcome. Large differences in the umbilical artery Doppler values suggest relatively little flow to the acardiac twin, thereby predicting a more favorable outcome.[122–124,128] In contrast, small differences in the umbilical artery Doppler values would signify similar flows, the presence of large anastomoses placing a greater hemodynamic strain on the pump twin. Additional factors thought predictive of poor outcome are congestive heart failure with hydrops, hydramnios,[117] and certain morphologic characteristics of the acardiac twin such as the presence of a head and upper limbs.[120] It remains unknown to what degree these parameters apply in the early second trimester, and spontaneous resolution as well as sudden death of the pump twin remains largely unpredictable.

Management Options

As the natural history of antenatally diagnosed TRAP has not been properly documented, its treatment is equally controversial and can be conservative, palliative, or invasive. Conservative management consists of close antenatal surveillance and timed delivery for signs of cardiac failure, whereas palliative treatment involves prolongation of pregnancy by serial amnioreduction and maternal administration of indomethacin for preterm labor and digoxin for cardiac failure. Reported perinatal mortality rates from conservative and palliative treatment vary widely between 10%[121] and 50%.[117] This range is not

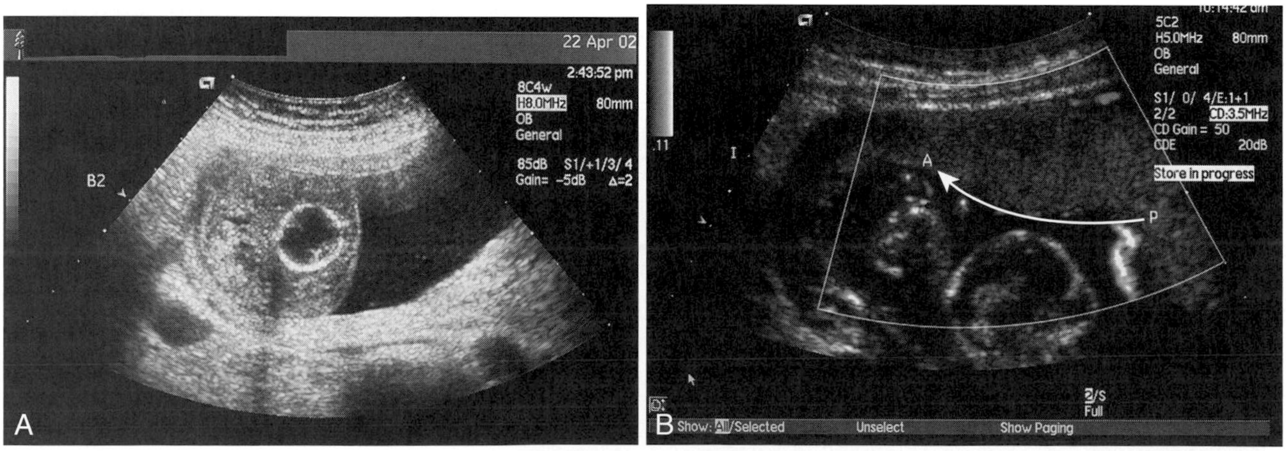

FIGURE 24–18
A, Ultrasound image of an acardiac twin at the level of the rudimentary head with typical, severe subcutaneous edema. *B*, Doppler examination at 15 weeks' gestation, demonstrating the typical, retrograde flow from the pump twin toward the acardiac twin over an arterioarterial anastomosis (*arrow*) (see Color Plate 36).

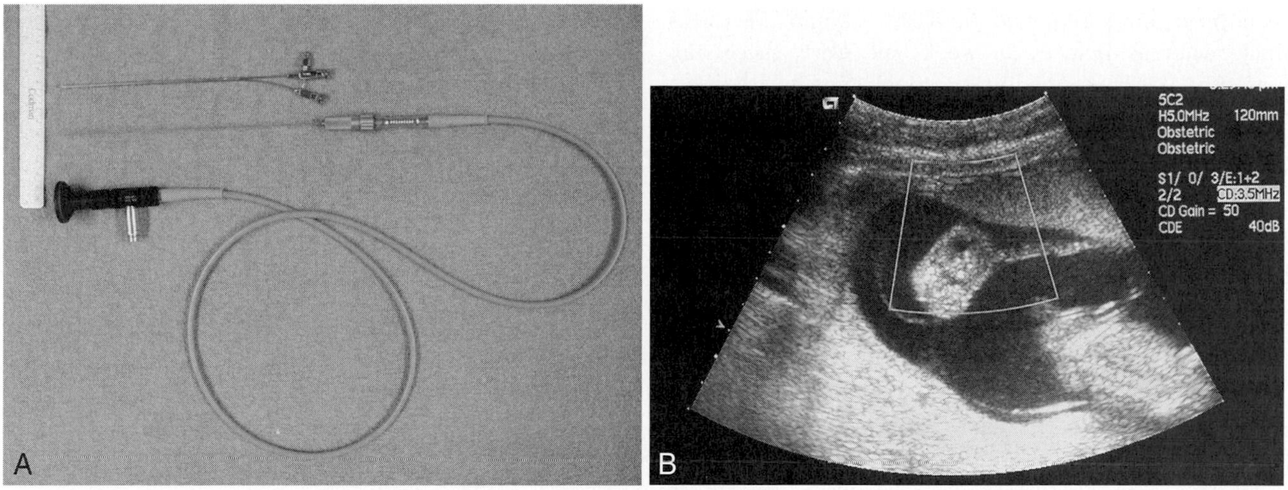

FIGURE 24–19
A, This 1.0-mm fetoscope is used for fetoscopic interventions early in the second trimester (Karl Storz). *B*, Doppler examination confirms arrest of flow after laser cord coagulation at 16 weeks' gestation.

surprising considering how poor the placental transport of digoxin is normally, much less when the fetus is hydropic. Also, little or no data are available on the long-term outcome of surviving pump twins, but as stated previously there is concern about long-term neurologic and cardiac sequelae.

Invasive treatment seeks to arrest the flow of blood to the acardiac twin. Several methods are proposed, ranging from hysterotomy and delivery of the acardiac twin[129] to embolization of the acardiac's circulation[130] to fetoscopic cord ligation[131] to ultrasound guided or fetoscopic coagulation of the umbilical cord[132,133] or intrafetal vessels.[134] Clearly, hysterotomy with selective delivery of the acardiac twin is unacceptable because of the high maternal morbidity risk. And embolization by the injection of thrombogenic substances into the acardiac twin's circulation (e.g., absolute alcohol, coils, and enbucrilate gel) is no longer advocated as a first-line treatment, as double IUFD is not uncommon owing to incomplete vascular occlusion or embolization of the product to pump twin.[135,136]

A number of minimally invasive techniques are now available to produce complete circulatory confinement of the acardiac twin. Fetoscopic cord ligation causes immediate and complete interruption of both arterial and venous flow, irrespective of umbilical cord size, but is cumbersome and has a high risk of PPROM. Although the published series are small, ultrasound or fetoscopic guided cord coagulation together with needle-based intrafetal coagulation appear to yield the most consistent results. The method of cord coagulation by laser is derived from that used for the coagulation of vascular anastomoses in TTTS.[133] It can be performed as early as 16 weeks using a double needle loaded with a 1.0-mm fetoscope and a 400-µm laser fiber (Fig. 24–19).[137] Fetoscopic laser coagulation is performed percutaneously under local or regional anesthesia using a single 1.3-mm operating sheath or 10 Fr (3.3 mm) trocar, depending on the gestation. Fetoscopically guided laser offers good visual control of the coagulation site but may fail if the umbilical cord diameter is large or more rarely if the amniotic fluid is stained. In these instances, bipolar cord coagulation with purpose-designed 2.4- to 3-mm bipolar forceps under ultrasound guidance is a secondary technique (Fig. 24–20). Needle-based coagulation techniques using laser,[138] monopolar technique,[134] or radiofrequency[139] each involve the insertion of a 14- to 18-gauge needle into the fetal abdomen under ultrasound aiming for the intra-abdominal rather than umbilical vessels. This technique is attractive for its simplicity, the smaller membrane defect produced, and the seemingly lower risks of PPROM. However, it may fail at gestations above 21 weeks. The four reported successful cases of intrafetal coagulation with laser were before 19 weeks. And with monopolar and radiofrequency coagulation, three out of

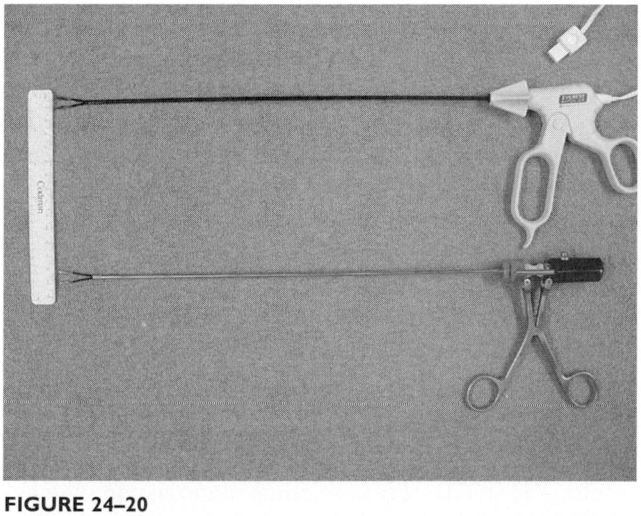

FIGURE 24–20
A, Disposable 3-mm bipolar forceps (Everest Medical). *B*, Reusable 2.4-mm bipolar forceps (Karl Storz).

seven procedures reported between 22 and 24 weeks failed, whereas before 21 weeks all were successful. Currently, it is not possible to conclude what the best management is for TRAP. The outcome may be good without treatment if spontaneous arrest of flow occurs. Conversely, the pump twin may die unexpectedly or sustain sequelae from very preterm delivery, cardiac failure, and chronic hypoxia. At present, cases of TRAP are usually diagnosed early in the second trimester when it is impossible to predict outcome. Early intervention may preclude the difficulties achieving an arrest of flow in larger and often hydropic acardiac masses, and it seems preferable awaiting signs of decompensation. We believe it is justifiable to offer prophylactic, minimally invasive intervention if no spontaneous arrest of flow has occurred by 16 weeks, recognizing that the pump twin may survive without any intervention in at least half of cases. The choice of technique will reflect gestational age and the size of the acardiac twin. These procedures should be performed in specialized units by surgeons familiar with different techniques in order to tailor therapy to the needs of each individual case.

SUMMARY OF MANAGEMENT OPTIONS

Twin Reversed Arterial Perfusion (TRAP) Sequence

Management Options	Quality of Evidence	Strength of Recommendation	References
Conservative with no hydramnios or hydrops–maintain surveillance in 'pump twin' for the development of hydramnios and/or hydrops and timely delivery	III	B	117
Palliative with hydramnios or cardiac failure (variable prognosis)– serial amniodrainage and tocolysis for hydramnios and digoxin for the cardiac failure. This is a backup option if intervention is not possible.	III	B	117,121
Intervention with hydramnios or cardiac failure (hydrops) – Arrest of flow toward the cardiac twin by a number of possible methods			
- coagulation of cord to acardiac twin	III	B	132,133
- ligation of cord to acardiac twin	III	B	131
- intrafetal (in acardiac twin) vessesl coagulation	III	B	134
- hysterotomy and removal of acardiac twin (supplanted by above)	III	B	129
For invasive treatment before 21 weeks, intrafetal coagulation and cord coagulation (laser and bipolar) are effective methods to arrest flow	III	B	132,133,135
Beyond 21 weeks and in cases with hydropic cord, bipolar cord coagulation may be more effective	III	B	132
It is justifiable to offer invasive treatment if no spontaneous arrest has occurred by 16 weeks	–	GPP	–
Mode of delivery depends on factors such as presentation and fetal health	III	B	117

TWIN-TO-TWIN TRANSFUSION SYNDROME

General

Twin-to-twin transfusion syndrome (TTTS) is a complication unique to monochorionic multiple pregnancies. In most monochorionic twin gestations, interfetal transfusion across the anastomoses is a constant, but balanced, phenomenon. However, in 10% to 15% of monochorionic twins, a chronic imbalance in net flow develops, resulting in TTTS. Hypovolemia, oliguria, and oligohydramnios develop in the donor twin, producing the "stuck twin" phenomenon. Hypervolemia, polyuria, and hydramnios evolve in the recipient twin, who can develop circulatory overload and hydrops (Fig. 24–21). TTTS usually occurs between 15 and 26 weeks and is a sonographic diagnosis based on the following criteria: hydramnios in the sac of the recipient twin (defined as deepest vertical pocket of ≥8 cm prior to 20 weeks and ≥10 cm between 20 and 26 weeks) believed secondary to polyuria, combined with oligohydramnios in the donor's sac (deepest vertical pocket ≤2 cm) presumably secondary to oliguria. Quintero and associates suggested a staging system[140] based on the sonographic time sequence of cases with progressive deterioration. Stage I cases include those with hydramnios in the recipient sac but the bladder of the donor twin still visible. In stage II, the bladder

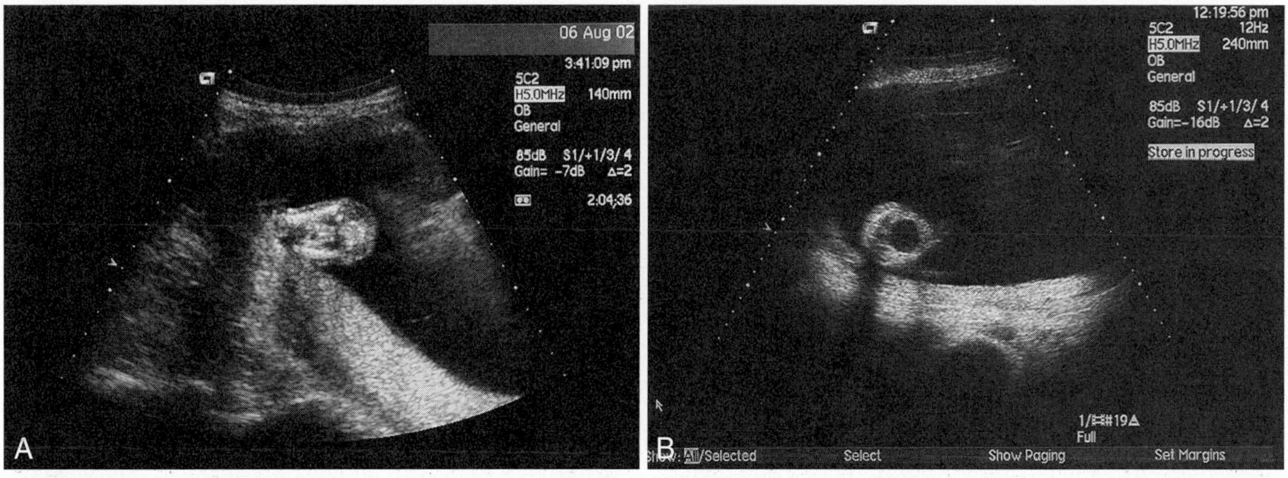

FIGURE 24–21
Ultrasound image of twin-to-twin transfusion syndrome. *A*, The donor is stuck to the uterine wall without bladder filling. *B*, There is hydramnios in the sac of the recipient, who has a distended bladder.

of the donor twin remains empty ("stuck twin"). Stage III is characterized by severely abnormal Doppler studies: absent or reversed end-diastolic flow in the umbilical artery of the donor fetus or abnormal venous Doppler pattern in the recipient, such as reverse flow in the ductus venosus or pulsatile umbilical venous flow. Fetal hydrops means stage IV and the end-stage V corresponds to fetal death of one or both twins. In medicine, the purpose of any classification system is to predict prognosis, to stratify therapy, and to predict the response to a given therapy. It is uncertain whether this staging does so. The onset of TTTS can be abrupt, and therefore, all monochorionic twins at our institution are scanned between 15 and 26 gestational weeks at 2-week intervals.

As already discussed, the differential diagnosis includes discordant growth, in which the growth-restricted twin may appear "stuck" due to oligohydramnios, but in which hydramnios is absent in the recipient twin. Likewise, the isolated presence of hydramnios in one sac with normal amniotic fluid in the other precludes the diagnosis of TTTS, and in that case other causes for hydramnios must be sought.

The pathophysiology of TTTS is most often explained on an angioarchitectural basis. Placental anastomoses can be arterioarterial (AA), arteriovenous (AV or VA), and venovenous (VV).[141] AA and VV anastomoses are typically superficial, bidirectional anastomoses on the surface of the chorionic plate, forming direct communications between the arteries and veins of the two fetal circulations. The direction of flow depends on the relative interfetal vascular pressure gradients. AV anastomoses are usually referred to as "deep" anastomoses. They occur at the capillary level deep within a shared cotyledon, receiving arterial supply from one twin and providing venous (well-oxygenated) drainage to the other twin. The supplying artery and draining vein of the AV anastomosis can be visualized on the placental surface as an unpaired artery and vein that pierce the chorionic plate at close proximity of each other and supply the underlying, shared cotyledon (Fig. 24–22). The AV anastomoses allow flow in one direction only, and hence may create an imbalance in the interfetal transfusion, leading to TTTS, unless balanced by an oppositely directed transfusion through other superficial or deep anastomoses.

Both postnatal injection studies[10] and in vivo fetoscopic observations[142,143] indicate the presence of at least one unidirectional AV anastomosis as an anatomic prerequisite for the development of TTTS. Although a TTTS case was recently reported with only superficial anastomoses (one AA and one VV),[143] this seems the exception confirming the rule. The presence of bidirectional AA anastomoses is believed to protect against the development of TTTS because most non-TTTS monochorionic placentas have AA anastomoses (84%) in contrast to TTTS placentas (20%–30%).[10,143]

Although vascular anastomoses are an anatomic prerequisite for the development of TTTS, other pathophysiologic mechanisms are likely involved. Because

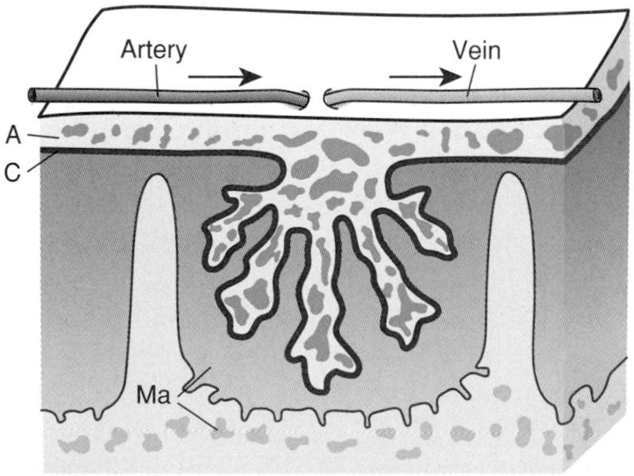

FIGURE 24–22
Schematic three-dimensional drawing of the human "shared" cotyledon. Artery and vein enter the chorionic plate very close to each other. A, amnion; C, chorion; Ma, maternal circulation; depicted as solid shading (Drawing by Luc Brullemans.)

75% of sonographically defined TTTS have an intertwin hemoglobin difference less than 15%,[144] this syndrome cannot be explained by the simple transfer of blood from one twin to the other. Further, there is no increased erythropoietin production in the donor[145] and no evidence of iron depletion/overload in the donor/recipient.[146] It is suggested that discordant placental function may offset TTTS, as placental dysfunction is associated with an increased fetoplacental resistance, which may promote transfusion from the growth-restricted donor twin to the recipient twin. Reduced insulin growth factor II[147] and decreased leptin levels[148] in donors compared to recipients may indicate discordant placental development rather than transfusion as a cause of the growth restriction. Other hormonal changes occur in donors and recipients. Raised endothelin-1 levels were observed in recipients, potentially causing increased peripheral vasoconstriction and hypertension. Recipients have increased levels of atrial natriuretic peptide (ANP),[149] and those with severe cardiac dysfunction have higher levels of brain natriuretic peptide (BNP), suggestive of cardiac remodeling. Increased renin gene and protein expression are found in donor kidneys, but the expression is virtually absent in the recipient kidneys,[150,151] implicating a role of the renin-angiotensin system in TTTS. Thus, the pathophysiology of sonographically defined TTTS is most likely multifactorial with vascular anastomoses providing the anatomic basis, while hemodynamic and hormonal factors contribute in varying degrees to its clinical development.

Identification of monochorionic twin pregnancies at increased risk of TTTS would assist patient counseling and planning of follow-up. Further, early diagnosis and treatment of TTTS might improve outcome, although the extent to which earlier treatment will lead to a better outcome has yet to be determined. It has also been suggested undiagnosed TTTS may trigger cervical ripening, which may be an important prognostic factor for adverse outcome, increasing the risk of PPROM before or after therapy.[152]

An increased nuchal translucency (NT) (>95th percentile) in at least one fetus during the 11 to 14 weeks' examination occurs in 13% of monochorionic twins (37/287) and is a marker for chromosomal anomalies, cardiac defects, and a wide range of genetic syndromes. In monochorionic twins, an increased NT may reflect early cardiac dysfunction due to hypervolemic congestion in the recipient and thus herald the subsequent development of TTTS. Indeed, fetuses of monochorionic twin pregnancies with increased NT have a higher likelihood for the subsequent development of TTTS (likelihood ratio: 3:5; 95% CI 1.9–6.2).[153] However, the sensitivity of the NT measurement for TTTS is only 28% with a positive predictive value of 33%. Because 72% of TTTS cases had NT measurements in the normal range, it is not an ideal screening test. Furthermore, it may not be possible to predict TTTS as early as 12 weeks, as TTTS may result from a random asymmetrical reduction in vascular anastomoses later in pregnancy.[154]

Folding of the intertwin membrane (Fig. 24–23) at 15 to 17 weeks may be a more promising sign for the prediction of TTTS. It is present in 32% of monochorionic twin pregnancies and believed to reflect oliguria and reduced amniotic fluid in the sac of the donor. It is associated with an increased likelihood for the development of TTTS (likelihood ratio: 4:2; 95% CI 3.0–6.0). Membrane folding is identified in 91% of TTTS cases with a positive predictive value of 43%.[153]

Another possible marker for the prediction of TTTS is the absence of AA anastomoses. These anastomoses can be detected by color flow mapping and pulsed Doppler[64] as early as 12 weeks, though the majority are detectable only after 18 weeks.[155] The difficulty with using the absence of AA anastomoses as a prognostic sign is that it is impossible in early pregnancy to ascertain whether they are truly absent or simply undetected. However, when an AA anastomosis is identified, only 15% of monochorionic twin pregnancies develop TTTS, compared to 61% when no AA anastomosis can be detected. Furthermore, the perinatal mortality rate is lower when AA anastomoses are present, whether or not TTTS develops.

Finally, a velamentous cord insertion increases the risk for TTTS and can be reliably detected by 18 weeks. Although this marker has not been evaluated antenatally, postnatal studies demonstrate that 60% of monochorionic twin gestations with a velamentous cord insertion develop TTTS, while 65% of those pregnancies that develop TTTS have a velamentous cord.[156]

Although none of the proposed markers are ideal for the prediction of TTTS, it is possible a combination of markers will improve risk stratification in the early second trimester. The performance of such a risk assessment system is currently being addressed by a prospective multicenter study funded by the European Commission (EuroTwin2Twin).[157]

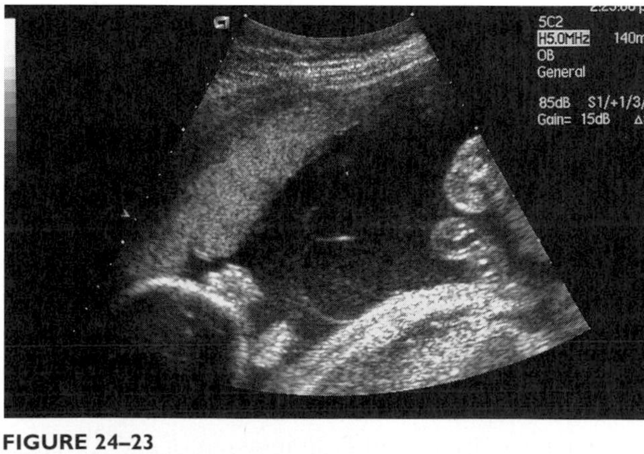

FIGURE 24–23
Ultrasound image of membrane folding in a monochorionic twin pregnancy, which reflects discordant amniotic fluid in a monochorionic twin pregnancy (see Color Plate 37).

Fetal Risks

Untreated, TTTS has been quoted to have a mortality rate of nearly 100%, although advances in neonatal care may have decreased that rate to 63%.[158] Spontaneous abortion and extreme preterm delivery are associated with hydramnios, and fetal death may result from cardiac failure in the recipient or poor perfusion in the donor. Substantial risks of cerebral and cardiac sequelae in survivors are due to the chronic hemodynamic imbalances. Both the donor and recipient are at risk of antenatally acquired cerebral white matter lesions with reported incidences of 35%[159] to 50%.[160] In donor twins, hypovolemia, hypotension, and anemia may induce cerebral hypoxia and brain damage, whereas in the recipient, hyperviscosity and cardiac failure may impair cerebral perfusion. Depending on the therapy used, the reported incidences of cerebral palsy and global developmental delay range from 4% to 26%.[108] The risks of neurologic damage are increased, especially after a sIUFD, presumably due to acute exsanguination of the survivor across the vascular anastomoses into the fetoplacental unit of the dead co-twin. Middle cerebral artery peak systolic velocity measurement seems a reliable noninvasive method to detect anemia after sIUFD in TTTS.[106] Though it is tempting to intervene based on this finding, it remains to be demonstrated whether a rescue transfusion decreases the risks of neurologic sequelae. Monochorionic twins with TTTS managed primarily by amniodrainage have a reported 7% prevalence of pulmonary valve stenosis in recipients.[161] Further, up to 48% of survivors have signs of transient oliguric renal failure affecting the donor as well as the recipient, although long-term renal impairment does not appear to be a problem.[162] More rarely, limb, gastrointestinal, and cerebral infarctions that preferentially affect the recipient are described, and may originate from hyperviscosity, hypoperfusion, or thromboembolic phenomena.[163]

Management Options

In view of the poor survival rates with conservative management, there is little disagreement that therapy should be offered. The four most commonly used therapies for midtrimester TTTS are amnioreduction, fetoscopic laser coagulation of the vascular anastomoses, septostomy, and selective feticide by cord occlusion.

Serial amnioreduction controls the amniotic fluid volume, is relatively simple, and is widely available. It may improve the fetal condition by reducing the amniotic fluid pressure and thus enhancing uteroplacental perfusion. Decompression also appears to prolong pregnancy.[164,165] However, amniodrainage does not address the vascular basis of TTTS, and in the event of a sIUFD, the surviving twin is at high risk for IUFD and neurologic damage. Amniodrainage techniques vary considerably in terms of the amount of fluid drained and whether the fluid is removed quickly or slowly. Denbow and associates advocate aggressive amniodrainage with the removal of 1 L for every 10 cm the amniotic fluid index (AFI) is raised, reducing the AFI to less than 25 cm.[166] An often-quoted fear of abruption following removal of such large volumes seems unfounded, because aggressive amniodrainage has a low complication rate (PPROM, abruption) (1.3%–3.8%).[167–169] Available data suggest that amnioreduction is effective only in mild cases of TTTS (stages I–II) and outright fails in a third. The overall perinatal survival rate in uncontrolled series with cases diagnosed prior to 26 weeks was 57%.[158] This rate was confirmed in a literature review compiled by Skupsi[170] (double survival, 50%; single survival rate 20%; total survival rate 61%). Further, amnioreduction is associated with a 16% to 26% risk of severe sequelae in survivors.[108,158]

Whereas amniodrainage is a palliative and repetitive measure, fetoscopic laser coagulation of the vascular anastomoses seeks to address the underlying cause of the disease through a single intervention. Provided the vascular hypothesis is correct and that anastomosing vessels can be visualized during fetoscopy, their occlusion will result in the arrest of intertwin transfusion. Most fetoscopic laser centers concur that coagulation of nonanastomosing vessels should be avoided, as this increases the number of nonfunctional cotyledons and therefore the risk of IUFD. In most centers, the technique of coagulating all vessels crossing the intertwin septum is no longer practiced.[171] The vascular equator does usually not coincide with the membranous equator, and coagulation along the intertwin septum will lead to unnecessary placental loss. Nevertheless, most groups coagulate all anastomoses visualized (Fig. 24–24). A "hyperselective" approach, as discussed by Feldstein and associates,[172] coagulating only the causative AV anastomosis is interesting only from a theoretical point of view. It is

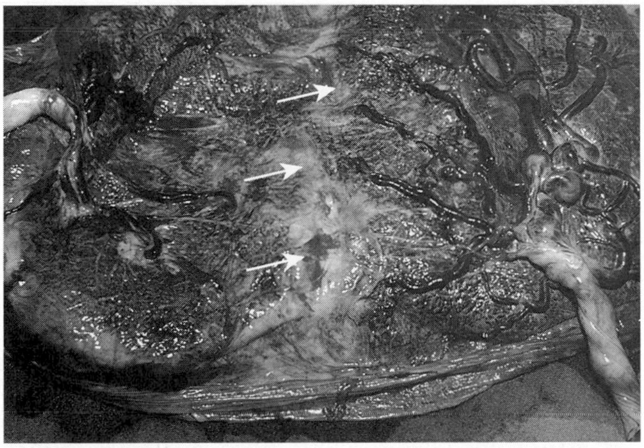

FIGURE 24–24
Macroscopic image of a placenta at birth demonstrating "bichorionization" and laser impact (*arrows*) on the monochorionic placenta after laser coagulation for twin-to-twin transfusion syndrome (see Color Plate 38).

simply not possible to identify this anastomosis in the presence of others. Also, leaving certain anastomoses open puts the remaining fetuses at risk for hypovolemic events in case of sIUFD, and may lead even to a reversal of transfusion. However, in some monochorionic pregnancies with unequal placental territories or large shared part of the placenta, coagulation of all anastomoses may leave too little unshared placenta for one or both fetuses, leading to single or even double IUFD.

In Europe, Canada, and some sites in the United States, laser coagulation is performed percutaneously (Fig. 24–25) under local or locoregional anesthesia. A cannula or fetoscopic sheath is inserted into the hydramniotic sac, and the placenta is inspected. For coagulation, the laser tip is directed toward the target vessels at as close to a 90-degree angle as possible, and with a nontouch technique a 1-cm section of the selected vessel is photocoagulated (Fig. 24–26). At the conclusion, amniodrainage is performed until the amniotic fluid pockets on ultrasound are normal. With an anterior placenta, the amniotic sac as well as the vessels on the placenta may be more difficult to access. Some instruments have been purposely developed, but it is yet unclear whether they improve performance. So far, placental localization does not appear to influence outcome.[173]

PPROM remains the most important complication of invasive antenatal procedures: the incidence after fetoscopic laser coagulation is estimated around 10%.[174] In contrast to amniodrainage, when the death of one or both fetuses often occurs remotely from the procedure, most deaths with laser are diagnosed within 48 hours. However, the surviving twin appears far less likely to be anemic after laser[106] or to sustain neurologic sequelae[107] when compared with survivors of amniodrainage where the anastomoses remain patent.[108] Apart from IUFD, other fetal complications are uncommon but include congenital skin loss, gangrenous limb lesions, amniotic bands, microphthalmia, and intestinal atresia. These anomalies have each been described in TTTS not treated by laser[163,175–180] and are more likely related to the disease process than to the treatment. Maternal safety should remain a priority, and serious maternal complications should be registered carefully in a registry, such as the one set up by Eurofoetus.[181] Transient maternal Mirror or Ballantyne syndrome with pulmonary edema,

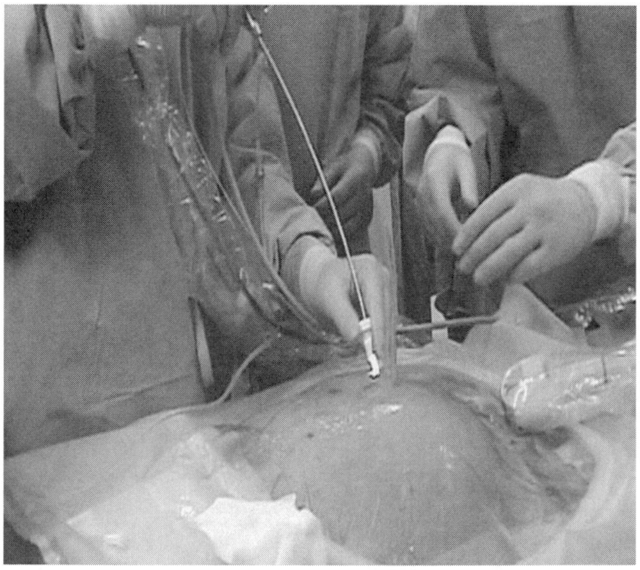

FIGURE 24–25
Image of the operative setup and percutaneous access used for fetoscopic interventions.

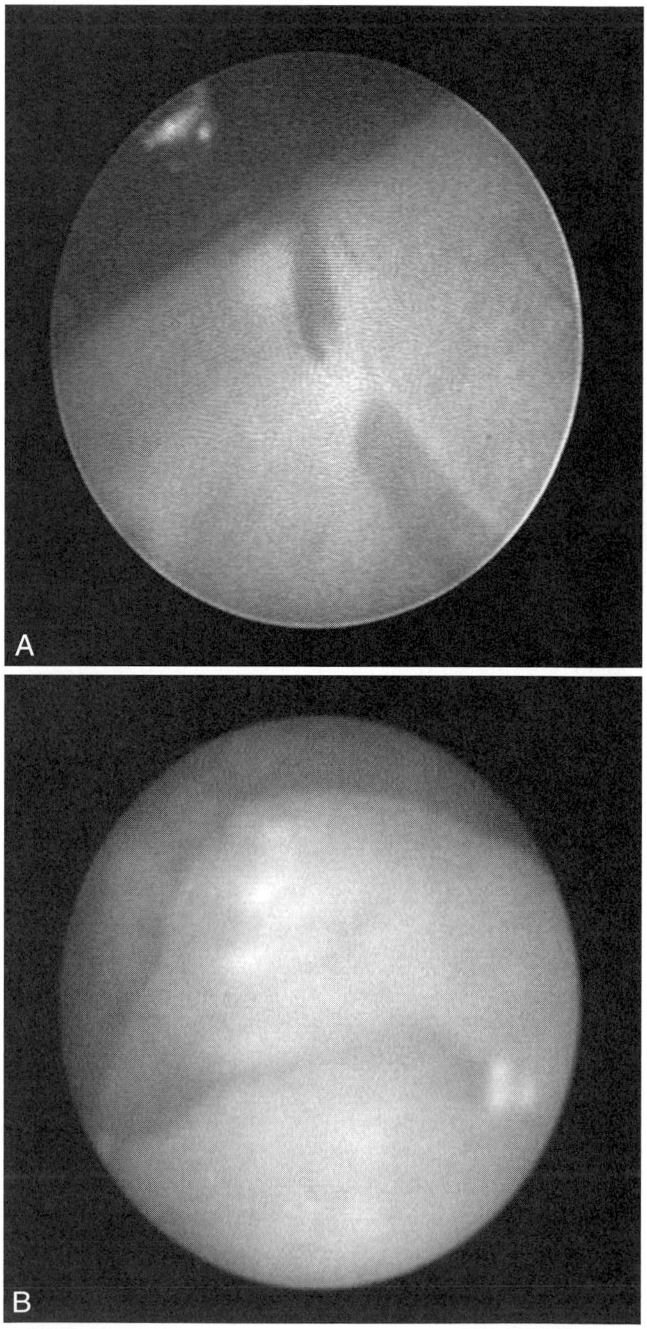

FIGURE 24–26
A, Fetoscopic image of laser coagulation of an arteriovenous anastomosis for twin-to-twin transfusion syndrome. *B*, Fetoscopic image of the hands of the donor twin, who is stuck behind the intertwin septum (see Color Plate 39).

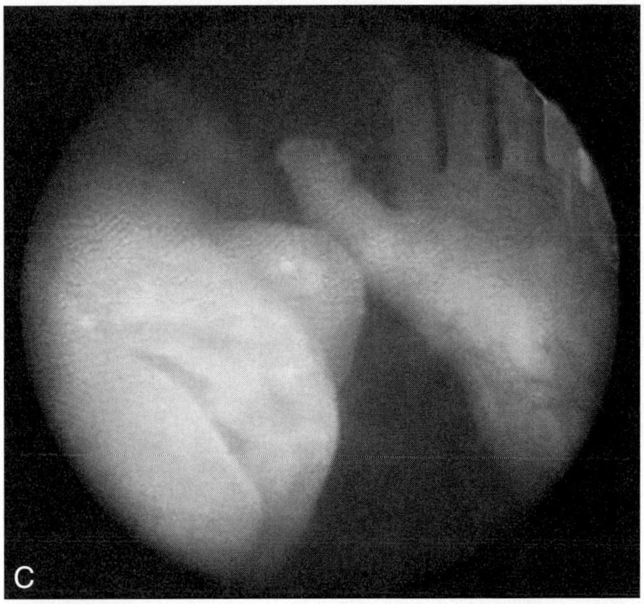

FIGURE 24–26 cont'd
C, Fetoscopic image of the face of the recipient, who moves freely in the hydramniotic sac.

placental abruption, chorioamnionitis, and bleeding requiring transfusion are reported but none yet leading to maternal death. Hecher and associates demonstrated a learning curve, arguing against scattering the experience over too many centers.[182]

In uncontrolled series, the overall fetal survival rate has consistently been between 55% and 68%, with a risk for neurologic morbidity in survivors of 2% to 11% (Jan Nakyken, personal communication). The Eurofoetus research consortium was granted by the European Commission to conduct a randomized trial comparing serial amnioreduction versus laser coagulation followed by amnioreduction as a primary therapy (i.e., no treatment of any form prior to enrollment) for severe TTTS prior to 26 weeks. The primary outcome measure was survival of at least one twin at 6 months of age, and the secondary outcome measure was intact neurologic survival.[183] The findings are in press at the time this chapter was written. No staging system had been defined when the trial was initiated, but the vast majority of pregnancies would now be considered either Quintero stage II or III (Table 24–1). The technique of percutaneous laser coagulation was standardized with coagulation of all visibly communicating vessels between the two fetuses, as well as the ones from which it could not be excluded that they were anastomosing. Amniodrainage was performed through an 18-gauge needle or the fetoscopic cannula, until normalization of amniotic fluid levels as measured by ultrasound. Further therapy after the primary therapy was left to the physician's discretion.

There was no severe maternal morbidity (no woman required ICU admission or blood transfusion), although three placental abruptions occurred at the end of the amniodrainage (two in the drainage and one in the laser group); all required immediate delivery. There was no significant difference in the pregnancy loss rate before 24 weeks (17% versus 11%, $P = 0.37$). The median gestational age at delivery was significantly higher in the laser than in the amnioreduction group (33.3 versus 29.0 weeks' gestation; $P = 0.004$), with 53% and 78% delivering before 32 weeks. The interval between randomization and delivery was longer in the laser group ($P = 0.006$). Among liveborns, the birth weight was higher in the laser group (1757 g versus 1359 g; $P < 0.001$); differences between groups were significant for both recipients ($P = 0.02$) and donors ($P = 0.01$). Compared to the amnioreduction group, the laser group had a higher likelihood of survival of at least one twin to 6 months (76.4% versus 51.4%; $P = 0.002$). The number of stage I and IV cases was too low for an analysis of outcome by stage. However, stratified analysis by Quintero stage I and II or III and IV showed a significantly higher survival rate for stage I and II (73%) than for III and IV (55%), but laser-treated patients did better than amnioreduction-treated patients for all Quintero stages. Survival rates were similar for donors and recipients.

Overall, a higher percentage of infants were alive without major neurologic morbidity at 6 months of age or older in the laser group. Infants in the drainage group had a higher incidence of periventricular leukomalacia diagnosed in utero or during the first 6 months of life (laser 0.6% versus drainage 14%; $P = 0.02$), in particular the recipients. This led to spontaneous neonatal death in three cases and withdrawal of intensive care support during the first 6 months of life in another nine babies. There was a trend for lower rates of intraventricular hemorrhage (IVH) in the laser group, but this trend was significant only for recipients. Eight of 144 (6%) and 20 of 140 (14%) infants in the laser and in the amnioreduction groups respectively, had overt cystic periventricular leukomalacia. Other major neurologic morbidity was present in two (grade 3 IVH and blindness, respectively) and eight (1% and 6%) of the survivors in the laser and in the amnioreduction group, respectively. In conclusion, children were more likely to be alive and without clinical neurologic morbidity at 6 months when treated by laser (52%) than with amniodrainage (31%; P=0.003). This is the first randomized trial comparing these popular treatment modalities. Presently, the children are being followed until 2 years of age (EuroTwin2Twin study, also supported by the European Commission[157]), and these results are eagerly awaited. A recent long-term follow-up study of children surviving an uncontrolled series managed by laser (ages between 14 and 44 months) observed major neurologic problems in 11% of survivors.[184]

Intentional puncturing of the intertwin septum ("septostomy") with or without amnioreduction was suggested to be beneficial, but there is little evidence to support this technique, and the pathophysiologic rationale remains unclear. It definitely increases the amniotic fluid volume in the donor's sac but also creates an iatrogenic monoamniotic state with possibility of cord entanglement. A small retrospective study comparing amnioreduction to septostomy ($N = 14$) failed to identify any survival benefit with septostomy.[185]

TABLE 24–1

Randomized Controlled Trial of Fetoscopic Laser Surgery versus Serial Amniodrainage*

	LASER (N = 72)	AMNIOREDUCTION (N = 70)	P VALUE
Gestational age at randomization (weeks)	20.6 (±2.4)	20.9 (±2.5)	ns
Quintero stage at randomization			
Stage 1	6 (8%)	5 (7%)	ns
Stage 2	31 (43%)	31 (44%)	ns
Stage 3	34 (47%)	33 (47%)	ns
Stage 4	1 (1%)	1 (1%)	ns
Number of procedures	1†	2.6 (±1.9)	–
Volume of amniotic fluid drained per procedure—ml**			–
Median	1725	2000	
Range	500-5500	243-4000	
Total volume of amniotic fluid drained—ml**			<0.001
Median	1725	3800	
Range	500–5500	600–18,000	
Pregnancy loss at or within 7 days of the initial procedure	8 (12%)	2(3%)	0.10
Premature rupture of membranes at or within 7 days of the first procedure	4 (6%)	1 (1%)	0.37
Premature rupture of membranes at or within 28 days of the first procedure	6 (9%)	6 (9%)	0.98
Intrauterine death within 7 days of the first procedure‡	16/138 (12%)	9/136 (7%)	0.23
At least one survivor at 6 months of life	55 (76%)	36 (51%)	0.002
No survivors	17 (24%)	34 (49%)	
One survivor	29 (40%)	18 (26%)	
Two survivors	26 (36%)	18 (26%)	
At least one survivor at 6 months stratified by stage			
Quintero stages I and II	32/37 (86%)	21/36 (58%)	0.007
Quintero stages III and IV	23/35 (66%)	15/34 (44%)	0.07
Gestational age at delivery - median (interquartile range)	33.3 (26.1–35.6)	29.0 (25.6–33.3)	0.004
Neonatal and infant death	12 (8%)	41 (29%)	
Intraventricular hemorrhage (grades III–IV)§	2 (1%)	8 (6%)	0.10
Donor	2 (3%)	2 (3%)	1.0
Recipient	0 (0%)	6 (9%)	0.02
Cystic periventricular leukomalacia¶	8 (6%)	20 (14%)	0.02†
Donor	2/72 (3%)	5/70 (7%)	0.27
Recipient	6/72 (8%)	15/70 (21%)	0.03

*Baseline characteristics according to group, results reported as number of pregnancies (n), percentage, means (SD).
†Two patients had two laser procedures.
‡With number of fetuses as denominator (P value adjusted for clustering).
§Severe intraventricular hemorrhage was defined as ventricular bleeding with dilatation of the cerebral ventricles (grade III) or parenchymal hemorrhage (grade IV).
¶Cystic periventricular leukomalacia was defined as periventricular densities evolving into extensive cystic lesions (grade III) or extending into the deep white matter evolving into cystic lesions (grade IV).
**The median in the laser group is the median volume drained at the end of a single procedure.

Selective feticide was suggested in 1993 to try to salvage at least one twin in complicated cases of TTTS.[186] Selective feticide by bipolar cord occlusion has been suggested for the treatment of stages III and IV of TTTS.[187] This approach is certainly open for debate and may lead to some difficult decisions. It is not necessarily easy to determine which fetus will have the worst outcome, a major drawback because the maximum survival rate is 50%. Selective feticide should in our opinion be reserved for instances of discordant anomalies (such as hydrocephaly), when imminent death of one twin is anticipated, or in cases in which full visualization of the vascular equator is likely to be technically impossible.

SUMMARY OF MANAGEMENT OPTIONS

Twin-Twin Transfusion Syndrome (TTTS)

Management Options	Quality of Evidence	Strength of Recommendation	References
Serial amniodrainage does prolong pregnancy and improves fetal condition by reduced intrauterine pressure, although it does not protect the surviving twin in the event of sIUFD (single intrauterine fetal death) and is only effective in mild cases of TTTS.	IIb	B	106,164,168

SUMMARY OF MANAGEMENT OPTIONS

Twin-Twin Transfusion Syndrome (TTTS) *(Continued)*

Management Options	Quality of Evidence	Strength of Recommendation	References
Laser coagulation, as compared to amniodrainage, has been shown to have better survival rates and neurologic outcome, and is therefore considered to be the best first-line treatment for TTTS in centers experienced in this technique.	Ib	A	184
Septostomy does not seem to have a survival benefit as compared to amniodrainage.	IIb	B	186
Selective feticide by cord occlusion does arrest the transfusion process and is indicated for TTTS with associated discordant anomalies or in rare cases of imminent fetal death, or when laser coagulation with full inspection of the vascular equator is technically not feasible.	III	B	187

CONGENITAL ANOMALIES IN TWINS

Structural Anomalies

Structural anomalies are 1.2 to 2 times more common in twins than in singletons. Unfortunately, most studies do not subgroup incidence by either zygosity or placentation. Nevertheless, it seems that the rate per fetus in dizygotic twins is the same as in singletons, whereas the rate is two to three times higher in the monozygotic twins.[56] Abnormalities associated with twins are neural tube defects, brain defects, facial clefts, gastrointestinal defects, anterior abdominal wall defects, and cardiac defects.[188] Even in monozygotic twins, concordance (both fetuses similarly affected) for a structural anomaly is rare (<20%).[57] Also, discordance for genetic diseases is frequently reported in monozygotic twins and may reflect variations in gene expression secondary to postzygotic mutation, parental imprinting effects, asymmetrical chromosome X inactivation,[25] and differential DNA methylation.[189] The exact mechanism of the increased prevalence of structural anomalies in monozygotic twins remains largely unknown, although several mechanisms are proposed. It is possible the twinning process itself is teratogenic owing to an unequal distribution of the inner cell mass or to splitting after laterality gradients have already been determined, resulting in abnormalities such as midline defects.[25] Vascular events in early embryogenesis and later fetal life might account for part of the observed discordant brain and heart anomalies. The prevalence of cardiac anomalies in monochorionic twins is reported to be 2.3% in those without TTTS and 7% in those with TTTS, compared to 0.6% in the general population. Pulmonary valve stenosis in recipients accounts for all the additional congenital heart defects found in TTTS cases, suggesting a causative role of the hemodynamic imbalance. The global prevalence of congenital heart defects in monochorionic twins (3.9%) is thus comparable to that in a family with a history of congenital heart disease (2.5%). Thus, detailed echocardiography is indicated both in second and third trimesters, because pulmonary artery stenosis is a dynamic process that may evolve until delivery.[161] Anomalies unique to monochorionic twins are the twin reversed arterial perfusion (TRAP) sequence and conjoined twinning as discussed earlier.

Chromosomal Anomalies

Risks of Chromosomal Abnormalities

In dizygotic twins, the age-related risk of Down syndrome for one twin is independent of the risk for the other and should be the same as in singletons. Therefore, the risk of at least one fetus having Down syndrome is double that in singletons. Whereas chorionicity can be accurately determined during the first trimester, there are no noninvasive means to establish zygosity antenatally. Nonetheless, dichorionic twins are dizygotic in about 90% of cases, and all dichorionic twins are for risk assessment considered to be dizygotic. In a dichorionic twin pregnancy, the age-related risk of at least one twin having Down syndrome can then be calculated by adding the age-related risks together (e.g. for a 40-year-old woman, $1/100 + 1/100 = 1/50$), whereas the risk of both fetuses being affected is obtained by multiplying the age-related risks ($1/100 \times 1/100 = 1/10{,}000$).

In a monochorionic (and by definition monozygotic) twin pregnancy, the age-related risk is the same for both twins and similar to that in singletons with usually both twins affected, although discordances in the phenotypic expression of the aneuploidy are frequently observed.[192,193] It is important to note that though rare, even monochorionic twins may be discordant for chromosomal anomalies and discordancy for nearly all common human aneuploidies (trisomy 13,[55] trisomy 21,[54] monosomy 45 X[54]) are reported. Most of these cases involve one twin with Turner syndrome and the other with either a female or male phenotype but usually a mosaic karyotype.[92] This rare phenomenon is called heterokaryotypic monozygotism and it reflects either a postzygotic mitotic event (nondisjunction or anaphase lag) or prezygotic meiotic errors. Several mechanisms may be involved. The zygote may initially have been karyotypically normal (46), but a trisomic (47) respectively monosomic cell line (45) develops because of a mitotic nondisjunction or anaphase lag. Conversely, the zygote may initially have been trisomic (47), but a diploid cell line (46) may be established as a result of a mitotic disjunction or anaphase lag, a phenomenon known as trisomic rescue. At the blastocyst stage, the embryo proper originates from only three to five progenitor cells and splitting at this stage will give rise to monochorionic twinning. If a mitotic error takes place in any of these cells, it may actually trigger the twinning process with the proliferative advantaged diploid cell line separating out the aneuploid progenitors (Fig. 24–27). If the aneuploidy is nonviable, then this aneuploid "twin" will vanish without leaving any detectable remnants.[194] However, if the aneuploidy is viable, then this may give rise to heterokaryotypic monochorionic twins.

Screening for Aneuploidies in Twins

Screening for aneuploidy is more complex in multiple pregnancies than in singletons, because although selective feticide is an option if only one fetus is affected, the procedures can cause the loss of the unaffected co-twin. It is therefore essential the parents be adequately counseled on the pros and cons of screening in multiple pregnancy. The screening tests should have good detection rates and an acceptably low false-positive rate, as invasive testing carries a higher risk and is technically more challenging in multiple pregnancy.

Second-trimester serum screening for aneuploidy has disappointingly low detection rates in twins (45% for a 5% screen positive rate),[191] presumably because the altered biochemical markers of the aneuploid fetoplacental unit are masked by the presence of an euploid co-twin.

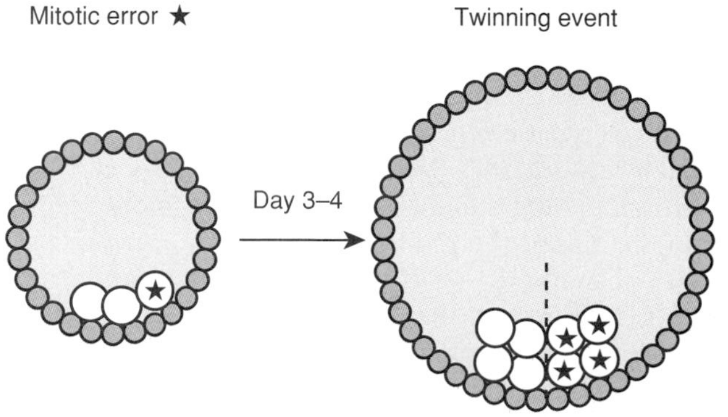

FIGURE 24–27
Illustration of mitotic error in an initially euploid zygote leading to a twinning event. (Courtesy of T. Van den Bosch.)

Also, serum screening provides only the risk of at least one affected fetus (pregnancy-specific risk) and does not give a feature to identify the fetus at increased risk (fetus-specific risk). In contrast, first-trimester nuchal translucency (NT) measurement has better detection rates, identifies the fetus at increased risk, and allows a selective feticide in the first trimester. It is therefore the preferred screening method in twins. The combination of NT with first-trimester serum biochemistry further increases the detection rate. In a three-year review of combined NT and serum screening in the first trimester on 230 twin pregnancies, detection rate of Down syndrome was 75%, with 7% of fetuses and 9% of pregnancies (with at least one fetus) having a risk above 1/300.[195]

Although combined NT and biochemical screening allow a fetus-specific risk, it seems logical to quote only one risk for monochorionic fetuses (pregnancy-specific risk) because both will be affected or both will be unaffected in nearly all cases. Quoting the risk of the fetus with the largest NT may overestimate the true risk, especially because increased NT in a monochorionic twin pair may be an early sign of unbalanced intertwin transfusion.[153] Alternatively, one may quote the average of the two NT measurements. Unfortunately, there is little data at present to guide clinical practice. Nevertheless, it is proposed for combined NT and first-trimester biochemistry in monochorionic twins to use the average of the two NT measurements for a combined risk calculation. For dichorionic twins, it makes sense to quote the fetus-specific risk, although it is probably more relevant to the parents to hear what the risk is that at least one fetus will be affected (pregnancy-specific), which is obtained by adding the two fetus-specific risks. The risk that both are affected is extremely rare and is obtained by multiplying the two fetus-specific risks.

Invasive Antenatal Testing in Twins

Fetal karyotyping requires invasive testing by amniocentesis or chorionic villous sampling (CVS). Because these procedures are technically more demanding in multiple pregnancies, it is generally advocated they be performed in tertiary referral centers. The choice of invasive technique(s) will depend on the procedure related risk, on the accuracy of obtaining a result from both fetuses and on technical circumstances. Although genetic amniocentesis is a well-accepted procedure, it remains unclear whether the postprocedural loss is higher in twins compared to singletons and whether the risk increases with increasing number of fetuses. Historically, amniocentesis in twin pregnancies was considered to have higher procedure related loss rates (2.7%–8.1%).[196] However, this may be largely attributable to the higher background risk of fetal loss in twins (6%),[197] rather than to the invasive procedure. As such, Ghidini and associates found that amniocentesis in experienced hands did not increase loss rates significantly.[198] Conversely, Yukobowich and associates reported loss rates within 4 weeks after the procedure that were five times higher in twins (2.6%) compared to singletons (0.6%) and unexposed twins (0.6%).[199]

Several techniques are used to ascertain that all fetuses are correctly sampled. No technique is shown to be superior, and the choice depends largely on operator preference. In any event, great care must be taken to note distinguishing features, such as gender, placental localization, umbilical cord insertion, and fetal positions. A diagram should be made to prevent the potentially disastrous consequence of incorrect sampling. Samples should also be meticulously labeled. Amniocentesis in twins can be done through a single or double uterine entry. With the double needling technique, each sac is sampled separately and consecutively. The injection of dyes after sampling of the first sac to ensure it is sampled only once is no longer recommended. Methylene blue is contraindicated because of well-documented fetal risks, such as intestinal atresia, hemolytic anemia, and fetal death.[200] Although no similar fetal risks are reported with indigo carmine, it has serotonergic properties[201] and may in theory lead to hypertension and bradycardia and is therefore best avoided. A less commonly used technique is the double needle simultaneous visualization technique.[202] An amniocentesis needle is advanced into the first cavity, while a second needle is introduced into the other amniotic cavity without altering the position of the transducer. This technique permits visualization of both needles simultaneously on either site of the septum but necessitates the presence of two operators. Finally, a single uterine entry technique is described[203] in which the needle is first advanced into the proximal sac and fluid aspirated. The stylet is replaced, and under direct visualization, the needle is advanced through the septum into the second sac. After discarding the first 1 mL of fluid to avoid contamination, a sample is aspirated from the second sac. This technique has the advantage of creating only one membrane defect, and to date, no cytogenetic errors have been reported, although there is the theoretic concern of contamination and the creation of an iatrogenic monoamniotic pregnancy.

CVS in multiple pregnancy can be performed using either the transabdominal approach, transcervical approach, or a combination of the two. In the hands of an experienced operator, the loss rate attributable to CVS in twins may be comparable to that after amniocentesis. However, cytogenetic results are incorrect in 1.5% to 2% of cases because of contamination of one sample with villi from the other, placental mosaicism, culture failure, or sampling the same fetus twice. As a result, the resampling rate approximates 2%. To reduce the rate of incorrect sampling, it is imperative placental sites are accurately mapped and the extreme ends of each placenta preferentially sampled. For example, in those cases with a lower and upper placenta, a combined technique with a transcervical approach for the lower placenta and transabdominal approach of the upper placenta may be used.

Which technique (amniocentesis or CVS) should be used in twins, and should both or rather one fetus be sampled? The answer largely depends on chorionicity and the risk of one or both being affected. For dichorionic twins, both CVS and amniocentesis are valuable options. As CVS can be performed in the first trimester, selective feticide can be done at an earlier stage in the event of discordant chromosomal anomaly with possibly lower risks for the healthy co-twin. On the other hand, because of the higher rates of contamination, it may be preferable to restrict CVS to fetuses at especially high risk (e.g., if the risk of first-trimester screening is greater than 1 in 50) and defer invasive testing to 15 weeks in lower risk cases for amniocentesis. It is generally recommended that both fetuses be sampled. Even though only one has an increased NT or anomaly, they can still be monozygotic. Amniocentesis is preferred to CVS in monochorionic twins, as rare heterokaryotypic monozygotic twins can only be diagnosed by sampling both sacs. Only if monochorionicity is accurately documented in the first trimester and none of the twins show any structural anomalies is it possibly justifiable to sample only one fetus (by CVS or amniocentesis). In heterokaryotypic monozygotic twins, CVS of the common placenta may show mosaicism, a normal or abnormal karyotype, depending on the type and timing of postzygotic event.[54] If trisomic rescue is the mechanism involved, then the diploid fetus will have a one in three risk of uniparental disomy (UPD) for the specific chromosomal pair that is trisomic in its co-twin. UPD, when both chromosomes in a pair are inherited from the same parent, will produce an abnormal phenotype if the involved chromosomal pair carries an imprinted region/gene or homozygous recessive mutation.[204] The presence of UPD should be excluded in heterokaryotic monozygotic twins. Counseling may be very difficult in hetorokaryotypic twins because it is not possible to exclude the presence of hidden, but phenotypically important, mosaicism in the twin with normal karyotype on amniotic fluid cells. Cordocentesis is of little help in monochorionic twins because blood chimerism is invariably present, making genotyping of lymphocytes unreliable.

Fetal Risks

In dichorionic twins, the presence of a discordant anomaly usually does not affect the well-being of the other twin unless associated with hydramnios (such as anencephaly, duodenal atresia) or spontaneous demise, which increases the risk of preterm delivery for the healthy co-twin. An ethical dilemma arises when elective preterm delivery for *ex utero* treatment or antenatal invasive procedures with risk of iatrogenic PPROM (such as shunt placement) to ameliorate the outcome for the affected twin places the normal co-twin at risk of iatrogenic prematurity. In contrast to dichorionic twins, the spontaneous death of the anomalous twin may have disastrous consequences in a monochorionic twin pregnancy, because in addition to the consequences of severe preterm delivery it may lead to an acute exsanguination of the healthy co-twin with double fetal death in about 10% to 25% and cerebral damage in 25% to 45%.

Management Options

There are essentially three management options for discordant structural and chromosomal anomalies:

- Conservative management
- Selective feticide
- Termination of the whole pregnancy

Paramount to safe management is an accurate determination of chorionicity in the first trimester because the methods for selective feticide differ between mono- and dichorionic twins.

Management in Dichorionic Twins

If the abnormality is nonlethal but may well result in serious handicap, parents must decide whether the burden of a handicapped child is enough to risk the loss of the healthy twin from feticide-related complications. If the abnormality is lethal, it may be best to avoid such risk, and conservative management is preferable unless the condition threatens the well-being of the healthy twin. Such a dilemma is illustrated by dichorionic twins discordant for anencephaly, which is always lethal, but the associated hydramnios place the healthy co-twin at risk of severe preterm delivery. However, expectant management in such cases has been shown to have a favorable outcome for the unaffected fetus in dichorionic twins, with less than half developing hydramnios and none delivering before 29 weeks (mean, 36 weeks).[205] Selective feticide in the second trimester is associated with a higher gestational age at delivery but carries the risk of procedure-related fetal loss.[206]

Selective feticide in dichorionic twins is performed by intracardiac or intrafunicular injection of potassium chloride under continuous ultrasound guidance. It is of utmost importance to ascertain that the correct fetus is terminated by identification of gender differences, obvious structural anomalies, placental localizations, and cord insertions. The risks of selective termination are loss of the entire pregnancy and premature delivery. The overall loss rate reported by the international selective feticide registry of 402 multiple pregnancies, including some higher-order multiple pregnancies, is 7.5%. A breakdown by gestation (5.4% at 9–12 weeks; 8.7% at 13–18 weeks and 6.8% at 19–24 weeks) reveals a nonsignificant trend toward higher loss rates for procedures performed after 13 weeks. Preterm delivery before 33 weeks occurred in 22%, with 6% delivering between 25 and 28 weeks.[207] One center with 200 selective feticides reported an overall loss rate of only 4%, with significantly higher loss rates in triplets or higher-order multiplets (11%) compared to twins (2.4%), with only 16% of patients delivering before 32 weeks. This underlines the importance of referring to experienced centers. In order to reduce loss rates, it has been proposed to defer selective feticide to 28 to 32 weeks, which is only an option in countries where late termination is legal and may be emotionally more difficult to accept for both parents and doctors. In a series on 23 in dichorionic twins with nonlethal anomaly, there were no fetal losses, and all patients delivered beyond 35 weeks.[208]

Selective Feticide in Monochorionic Twins

For selective feticide in monochorionic twins, the conventional techniques of potassium chloride injection used in multichorionic pregnancies cannot be used because the potassium can reach the other fetus by the obligatory anastomoses.[209] In addition, patent intertwin vessels may lead to acute fetofetal hemorrhage into the terminated twin's fetoplacental unit, putting the surviving twin at risk for central nervous system damage or co-twin death.[62] Therefore, the appropriate techniques arrest and isolate the terminated twin's circulation completely and permanently,[210] although all have considerably higher risks for fetal loss and very early PPROM compared with systemic injection of potassium chloride. Further, although expectant management may be preferable in dichorionic twins for discordant anomalies with an expected spontaneous demise of the anomalous twin, monochorionic twins specifically warrant a preventive selective feticide. This is particularly relevant for discordant chromosomal anomalies as aneuploidy has a high spontaneous IUFD rate.[211,212]

As discussed in the management of TRAP, the preferred method for selective feticide is cord occlusion by either laser/bipolar coagulation or cord ligation. The initially reported method of umbilical cord embolization using a variety of agents, including absolute alcohol, coils, and enbucrilate gel, is no longer recommended because of failure rates greater than 60%.[136] Anecdotal successes are reported, but double IUFD is unfortunately common, probably due to incomplete vascular obliteration or migration of the sclerosants or thrombogenic products to the co-twin.

Fetoscopic cord ligation is already a historical technique, although it does cause immediate, complete, and permanent interruption of both arterial and venous flow in the umbilical cord. Though co-twin survival rates are over 70%,[213] these procedures are quite cumbersome with a high risk for PPROM. In comparison, laser cord coagulation (Fig. 24–28) is a relatively simple and straightforward procedure and uses similar instruments and set-up as for coagulation of the vascular anastomoses in TTTS. It is the preferred method, especially before 21

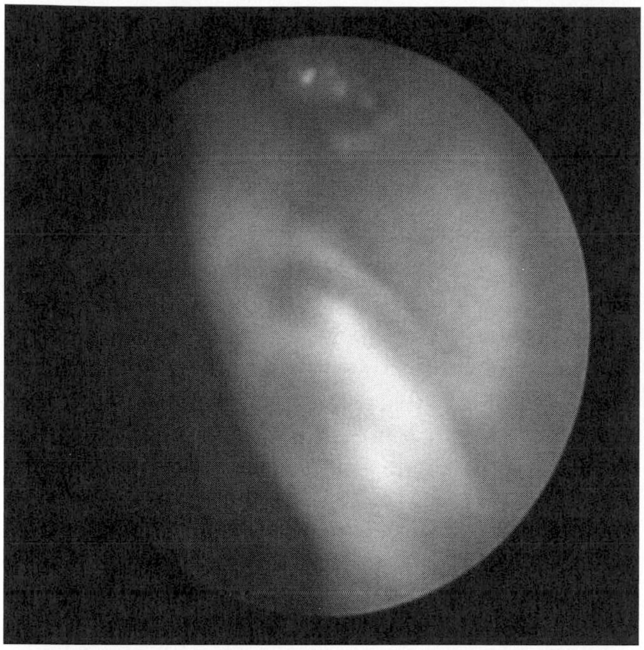

FIGURE 24–28
Fetoscopic image of laser cord coagulation (see Color Plate 40).

weeks. It can be performed as early as 16 weeks, using a double needle loaded with 1.0-mm fetoscope and a 400-μm laser fiber.[137] However, it may be difficult to coagulate the umbilical cord at later gestational ages. For this reason, bipolar energy was explored. Initially, a large-diameter forceps was used, but now purpose-designed devices of 3 mm or less are on the market as well as adapted cannulas and trocars. Most procedures can be done with a single port under ultrasound guidance (Fig. 24–29), but rarely an ancillary port is used for the fetoscope to identify the correct umbilical cord (e.g., monoamniotic twins). We always try to work within the sac of the target fetus and use amnioinfusion only where needed. In our initial series of 10 cases, two patients had PPROM and underwent a termination. The other eight patients delivered at a mean gestational age of 35 weeks (more than 15 weeks after the procedure).[63] Nicolini and associates reported their experience with 17 cases.[214] The survival rate was 81% (13 of 16 survivors; one patient had TOP because of an abnormality diagnosed later). There was one fetal hemorrhage caused by cord perforation, which is a complication of too much energy. We reported the outcome of 50 consecutive cord coagulations in complicated monochorionic twins by laser or bipolar coagulation performed between 16 and 28 weeks (mean 21 weeks).[215] Indications were TRAP (38%), discordant anomaly (38%), severe TTTS (20%), and selective IUGR (4%). In 75%, the laser was used as the primary technique; additional bipolar was necessary in about half of cases. Overall survival was 78% with normal outcome (range: 1–36 months, 100% follow-up), except for two children with mild developmental delay born after PPROM less than 28 weeks GA. Persistent PPROM before 30 weeks occurred in 21%, and if before 25 weeks, this was associated with a mortality rate of 80%. There were no serious maternal complications, except for one mild transient Mirror or Ballantyne syndrome. Four cases involved heterokaryotypic monochorionic twins (46,XY/47,XY,+21; 46,XX/47,XX,+13; 46,XY/45,X; 46,XX/45,X) and umbilical cord occlusion that resulted in a successful outcome in all four cases. All children were phenotypically normal at birth (range: 34–40 weeks GA) and are developing normally.[216] To avoid the risks of early PPROM for the healthy co-twin, it may be preferrable to defer selective feticide until after 26 weeks in highly selected cases of discordant anomaly when the risk of IUFD is small (such as in severe discordant CNS, genitourinary, skeletal anomaly). Bipolar coagulation can then be performed using the 3.0-mm forceps by over-

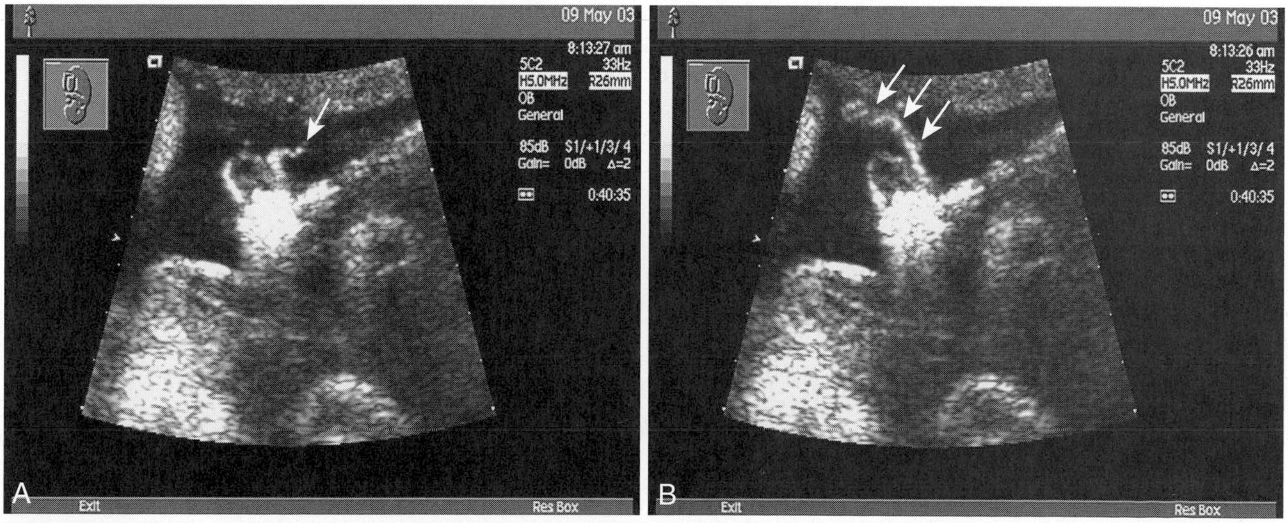

FIGURE 24–29
A, Ultrasound image of a bipolar cord coagulation in a monochorionic twin pregnancy. *B*, Ascending steam bubbles (*arrows*) confirm adequate coagulation impact.

stretching the blades whereupon the forceps opens more widely to accommodate for the larger cord diameter. We recently reported on a consecutive series of five cases in which selective feticide was performed between 26 and 30 weeks GA. All deliveries occurred beyond 31 weeks (range: 31–37 weeks). All infants survived, except for one unrelated neonatal death of a child born at 36 weeks due to a complication of failed therapy for pulmonary stenosis related to TTTS.[217] Needle-based intrafetal coagulation[218,219] does not appear to be an effective technique to achieve selective feticide in non-TRAP discordant monochorionic twins, and no successes have as yet been reported.

Currently, it is not possible to say what the single best method is for selective feticide in monochorionic pregnancies. The surgeon should be familiar with several techniques in order to tailor therapy to the individual requirements of each case. Generally, we recommend laser fetoscopic cord coagulation as a primary technique before 21 weeks, whereas beyond 21 weeks laser or bipolar coagulation can be used, depending on cord diameter.[220] Cord ligation should be available as backup if all other methods fail. These procedures should be performed in experienced tertiary referral centers to ensure a large enough caseload. Also, the surviving twin should be followed carefully throughout pregnancy and after birth with an early neonatal brain scan and developmental assessment at 1 year of age.

Issues Applicable to Monochorionic and Dichorionic Twins

As for singletons, Rhesus prophylaxis should be given in all instances of invasive prenatal procedures in Rhesus-negative women when the fetal genotype is unknown. As with sIUFD, the incidence of maternal disseminated intravascular coagulation appears to be rare after selective fetacide,[110,111] and routine checks of coagulation parameters may therefore be unnecessary. From 20 weeks onward, the use of fetal analgesia or anesthesia by administration of fentanyl or other opioid alternative should be considered prior to feticide to reduce fetal awareness and pain sensation.[221] To many people, any deliberate termination of a fetus is controversial, and the decision to proceed to selective feticide may be difficult. Therefore, psychological support and counseling for the family is strongly recommended before and after the selective feticide.

SUMMARY OF MANAGEMENT OPTIONS
Congenital Abnomalies in Twins

Management Options	Quality of Evidence	Strength of Recommendation	References
Issues Applicable to All Twins			
Options	–	GPP	–
Conservative management			
Selective feticide of the abnormal fetus			
Termination of the pregnancy			
Offer counseling and psychological support.	–	GPP	–
Accurate chorionicity determination is essential.	IIb	B	13,14
From 20 weeks onward, consider fetal analgesia or anesthesia.	III	B	222
Anti-D prophylaxis for procedures.	–	GPP	–
Serial surveillance of maternal coagulation status is often undertaken after feticide, but risks are low.	III	B	209
Dichorionic Twins			
Conservative management is usually preferred if the condition is lethal to avoid intervention loss rates (see below).	III	B	206
Selective feticide is performed by intracardiac or intrafunicular injection of KCl (potassium chloride).	III	B	208
Loss of the healthy fetus occurs in about 7.5% with delivery before 33 weeks in 22%.	III	B	207, 208

SUMMARY OF MANAGEMENT OPTIONS

Congenital Abnomalies in Twins *(Continued)*

Management Options	Quality of Evidence	Strength of Recommendation	References
Monochorionic Twins			
Conditions with a high risk of IUFD may indicate selective feticide.	–	GPP	–
Selective feticide is performed by cord occlusion (to avoid the loss of normal co-twin if KCl used).	III	B	210,217
Loss of the healthy fetus occurs in about 22% with preterm rupture of the membranes before 30 weeks occurring in 21%.	III	B	217
Careful follow-up of surviving normal twin.	–	GPP	–

CONCLUSIONS

- Multiplets have more problems during their *in utero* life than singletons.
- Management issues are complex, because more than one fetus has to be taken into account. This situation may pose some difficult dilemmas:
  - Should one save a distressed growth-retarded twin by conferring risks of iatrogenic prematurity to its nondistressed appropriately grown co-twin?
  - How does the burden of raising a multiplet with one handicapped child weigh against the risks of selective feticide for the nonaffected fetus?
- The shared circulation is responsible for the increased mortality rate in monochorionic multiplets and may lead to some unique complications.
- Chorionicity determination plays a key role in the management of multiple pregnancies and is accurately done in the first trimester. Correct determination of chorionicity is indispensable for the management of poor growth, intrauterine death of one twin, and discordant anomalies.
- Management issues are reasonably well-established for complicated dichorionic multiplets and recently also for TTTS. However, comparatively little is known about the natural history, best management, and long-term outcome of poor growth, sIUFD, TRAP, and monoamnionicity in monochorionic multiple pregnancies.
- Clearly, because of the rarity of these disorders, these questions can be addressed only by large multicenter prospective studies.

ACKNOWLEDGMENTS

Dr. L. Lewi is beneficent from a grant of the European Commission in its 5th Framework Programme (#QLG1-CT-2002-01632 EuroTwin2Twin). The other members of the EuroTwin2Twin Consortium are thanked for setting up the group: Y. Ville (Poissy), K. Hecher (Hamburg), E. Gratacos (Barcelona), R. Vlietinck (Leuven), M. van Gemert (Amsterdam), G. Barki (Tuttlingen), K. Nicolaides (London), R. Denk (Munchen), C. Jackson (London).

REFERENCES

1. Platt MJ, Marshall A, Pharoah PO: The effects of assisted reproduction on the trends and zygosity of multiple births in England and Wales 1974-99. Twin Res 2001;4(6):417–421.
2. Souter VL, Kapur RP, Nyholt DR, et al: A report of dizygous monochorionic twins. N Engl J Med 2003;349(2):154–158.
3. Quintero RA, Mueller OT, Martinez JM, et al: Twin-twin transfusion syndrome in a dizygotic monochorionic-diamniotic twin pregnancy. J Matern Fetal Neonat Med 2003;14(4):279–281.
4. Bulmer MG: The Biology of Twinning in Man. Oxford, Clarendon Press, 1970.
5. Alikani M, Cekleniak NA, Walters E, Cohen J: Monozygotic twinning following assisted conception: An analysis of 81 consecutive cases. Hum Reprod 2003;18(9):1937–1943.
6. Chow JS, Benson CB, Racowsky C, et al: Frequency of a monochorionic pair in multiple gestations: Relationship to mode of conception. J Ultrasound Med 2001;20(7):757–760.

7. De Catte L, Camus M, Foulon W: Monochorionic high-order multiple pregnancies and multifetal pregnancy reduction. Obstet Gynecol 2002;100(3):561–566.
8. Derom R, Orlebeke J, Eriksson A: The epidemiology of multiple births in Europe. In Keith LG, Papiernik E, Keith DM, Luke B (eds): Multiple Pregnancy: Epidemiology, Gestation and Perinatal Outcome. New York, Parthenon, 1995, pp 145–162.
9. Dubé J, Dodds L, Armson A: Does chorionicity or zygosity predict adverse perinatal outcomes in twins? Am J Obstet Gynecol 2002;186:479–583.
10. Denbow ML, Cox P, Taylor M, et al: Placental angioarchitecture in monochorionic twin pregnancies: Relationship to fetal growth, fetofetal transfusion syndrome, and pregnancy outcome. Am J Obstet Gynecol 2000;182:417–426.
11. Lewi L, Van Schoubroeck D, Gratacos E, et al: Monochorionic diamniotic twins: Complications and management options. Curr Opin Obstet Gynecol 2003;15(2):177–194.
12. Sebire N, Snijders R, Hughes K, et al: The hidden mortality of monochorionic twin pregnancies. BJOG 1997;104:1203–1207.
13. Stenhouse E, Hardwick C, Maharaj S, et al: Chorionicity determination in twin pregnancies: How accurate are we? Ultrasound Obstet Gynecol 2002;19:350–352.
14. Caroll SGM, Soothill PW, Abdel-Fattah SA, et al: Prediction of chorionicity in twin pregnancies at 10–14 weeks of gestation. BJOG 2002;109:182–186.
15. Blickstein I: Normal and abnormal growth of multiples. Semin Neonatol 2002;7(3):177–185.
16. Ananth CV, Vintzileos AM, Shen-Schwarz S, et al: Standards of birth weight in twin gestations stratified by placental chorionicity. Obstet Gynecol 1998;91:917–924.
17. Strauss A, Peak B, Genzl-Boroviczény, et al: Multifetal gestation—Maternal and perinatal outcome of 112 pregnancies. Fetal Diagn Ther 2002;17(4):209–217.
18. Alexander GR, Kogan M, Martin J, Papiernik E: What are the fetal growth patterns of singletons, twins, and triplets in the United States? Clin Obstet Gynecol 1998;41:114–125.
19. Hamilton EF, Platt RW, Morin L, et al: How small is too small in a twin pregnancy? Am J Obstet Gynecol 1998;179:682–685.
20. Lynch L, Lapinski R, Alvarez M, Lockwood CJ: Accuracy of ultrasound estimation of fetal weight in multiple pregnancies. Ultrasound Obstet Gynecol 1995;6(5):349–352.
21. Fountain SA, Morrison JJ, Smith SK, Winston RM: Ultrasonographic growth measurements in triplet pregnancies. J Perinat Med 1995;23:257–263.
22. Blickstein I, Jacques DL, Keith LG: A novel approach to intertriplet birth weight discordance. Am J Obstet Gynecol 2003;188:1026–1030.
23. Hill LM, Guzick D, Cheveney P, et al: The assessment of twin growth discordancy. Obstet Gynecol 1994;84:501–504.
24. Senoo M, Okamura K, Murotsuki J, et al: Growth pattern of twins of different chorionicity evaluated by sonographic biometry. Obstet Gynecol 2000;95:656–661.
25. Machin GA: Some causes of genotypic and phenotypic discordance in monozygotic twin pairs. Am J Med Genet 1996;61:216–228.
26. Machin G, Still K, Lalani T: Correlations of placental vascular anatomy and clinical outcomes. Am J Med Genet 1996;61(3): 229–236.
27. Machin GA: Velamentous cord insertion in monochorionic twin gestation: An added risk factor. J Reprod Med 1997;42:785–789.
28. Hanley ML, Ananth CV, Shen-Schwarz S, et al: Placental cord insertion and birth weight discordancy in twin gestations. Obstet Gynecol 2002;99:477–482.
29. Nomiyama M, Toyota Y, Kawano H: Antenatal diagnosis of velamentous umbilical cord insertion and vasa previa with color Doppler imaging. Ultrasound Obstet Gynecol 1998;12:426–429.
30. Matijevic R, Ward S, Bajoria R: Non-invasive method of evaluation of trophoblast invasion of spiral arteries in monochorionic twins with discordant birthweight. Placenta 2002;23:93–99.
31. Almog B, Fainaru O, Gamzu R, et al: Placental apoptosis in discordant twins. Placenta 2002;23(4):331–336.
32. Buzzard IM, Uchida IA, Norton JA, Christian JC: Birth weight and placental proximity in like sex twins. Am J Hum Genet 1983;35:318–323.
33. Geipel A, Berg C, Germer U, et al: Doppler assessment of the uterine circulation in the second trimester in twin pregnancies: Prediction of pre-eclampsia, fetal growth restriction and birth weight discordance. Ultrasound Obstet Gynecol 2002;20: 541–545.
34. Yu CKH, Papageorghiou AT, Boli A, et al: Screening for preeclampsia and fetal growth restriction at 23 weeks of gestation by transvaginal uterine artery Doppler. Ultrasound Obstet Gynecol 2002;20:535–540.
35. Sebire NJ: Opinion. Routine uterine artery Doppler screening in twin pregnancies. Ultrasound Obstet Gynecol 2002;20:532–534.
36. Maier RF, Bialobrzeski B, Gross A, et al: Acute and chronic hypoxia in monochorionic and dichorionic twins. Obstet Gynecol 1995;86:973–977.
37. Mori H, Mori K, Kojima Y, et al: Neonatal nucleated red blood cell counts in twins. J Perinat Med 2001;29:144–150.
38. O'Brein WF, Knuppel RA, Scerbo JC, Rattan PK: Birth weight in twins: An analysis of discordancy and growth retardation. Obstet Gynecol 1986;67:483–486.
39. Hartley RS, Hitti J, Irvin E: Size-discordant twin pairs have higher perinatal mortality rates than nondiscordant pairs. Am J Obstet Gynecol 2002;187:1173–1178.
40. Demissie K, Ananth CV, Martin J, et al: Fetal and neonatal mortality among twins gestations in the United States: The role of intrapartum birth weight discordance. Obstet Gynecol 2002;100:474–480.
41. Jacobs AR, Demissie K, Jain NJ, Kinzler WL: Birth weight discordance and adverse fetal and neonatal outcomes among triplets in the United States. Obstet Gynecol 2003;101:909–914.
42. Victoria A, Mora G, Arias F: Perinatal outcome, placental pathology, and severity of discordance in monochorionic and dichorionic twins. Obstet Gynecol 2001;97(2):310–315.
43. van Gemert MJ, Vandenbussche FP, Schaap AH, et al: Classification of discordant fetal growth may contribute to risk stratification in monochorionic twin pregnancies. Ultrasound Obstet Gynecol 2000;16:237–244.
44. Quintero RA, Bornick PW, Morales WJ, Allen MH: Selective photocoagulation of the communicating vessels in the treatment of monochorionic twins with selective growth retardation. Am J Obstet Gynecol 2001;185:689–696.
45. Sebire NJ, D'Ercole C, Hughes K, et al: Dichorionic twins discordant for intrauterine growth retardation. Arch Dis Child 1997;77:F235–F236.
46. Williams MC, O'Brien WF: Low birthweight/length ratio to assess risk of cerebral palsy and perinatal mortality in twins. Am J Perinat 1998;15(4):225–228.
47. Branum AM, Schoendorf KC: The effect of birthweight discordance on twin neonatal mortality. Obstet Gynecol 2003;101: 570–574.
48. Hollier LM, McIntire DD, Leveno KJ: Outcome of twin pregnancies according to intrapair birthweight differences. Obstet Gynecol 1999;94:1006–1010.
49. Williams MC, O'Brien WF: Cerebral palsy in infants with asymmetric growth restriction. Am J Obstet Gynecol 1997;14(4): 211–215.
50. Scher AI, Petterson B, Blair E, et al: The risk of mortality or cerebral palsy in twins: A collaborative population-based study. Pediatr Res 2002;52:671–681.
51. Adegbite AL, Castille S, Ward S, Bajoria R: Neuromorbidity in preterm twins in relation to chorionicity and discordant birth weight. Am J Obstet Gynecol 2004;190(1):156–163.
52. Pharoah PO, Adi Y: Consequences of in-utero death in a twin pregnancy. Lancet 2000;355:1597–1602.

53. Whitworth NS, Magann EF, Morrison JC: Evaluation of fetal lung maturity in diamniotic twins. Am J Obstet Gynecol 1999;180(6 Pt 1):1438–1441.
54. Nieuwint A, Van Zalen-Sprock R, Hummel P, et al: 'Identical' twins with normal karyotypes. Prenat Diagn 1999;19(1): 72–76.
55. Heydanus R, Santema JG, Stewart PA, et al: Preterm delivery rate and fetal outcome in structurally affected twin pregnancies: A retrospective matched control study. Prenat Diagn 1993;13(3):155–162.
56. Baldwin VJ: Anomalous development in twins. In Baldwin VJ (ed.): Pathology of Multiple Pregnancies. New York, Springer Verlag, 1994, pp 169–197.
57. Bryan E, Little J, Burn J: Congenital anomalies in twins. Baillieres Clin Obstet Gynecol 1987;1:697–721.
58. Erkine RL, Ritchie JW, Murnaghan GA: Antenatal diagnosis of placental anastomosis in a twin pregnancy using Doppler ultrasound. BJOG 1986;93:955–959.
59. Nakai Y, Ishoko O, Nishio J, et al: Cyclic changes in the umbilical arterial flow in monochorionic diamniotic twin pregnancy. Eur J Obstet Gynecol Reprod Biol 2002;101:135–138.
60. Wee LY, Taylor MJ, Vanderheyden T, et al: Transmitted arterio-arterial anastomosis waveforms causing cyclically intermittent absent/reversed end-diastolic umbilical flow in monochorionic twins. Placenta 2003;24(7):772–778.
61. Bajoria R, Wee LY, Anwar S, Ward S: Outcome of twin pregnancies complicated by single intrauterine death in relation to vascular anatomy of the monochorionic placenta. Hum Reprod 1999;14(8):2124–2130.
62. Nicolini U, Poblete A: Single intrauterine death in monochorionic twin pregnancies. Ultrasound Obstet Gynecol 1999;14:297–301.
63. Myers SA, Bennett TL: Selective photocoagulation of monochorionic twin pregnancy. Letter. Am J Obstet Gynecol 2002;187(1):258–259.
64. Joern H, Klein B, Schmid-Schoenbein H, Rath W: Antenatal visualization of vascular anastomoses in monochorionic twins using colour Doppler sonography: The protective function of these anastomoses and the phenomenon of interference beating. Ultrasound Obstet Gynecol 1999;14:422–425.
65. Norton ME, D'Alton ME, Bianchi DW: Molecular zygosity studies aid in the management of discordant multiple gestations. J Perinat 1997;17(3):202–207.
66. Sebire NJ, Souka A, Skentou H, et al: First trimester diagnosis of monoamniotic twin pregnancies. Ultrasound Obstet Gynecol 2000;16:223–225.
67. Bajoria R: Abundant vascular anastomoses in monoamniotic versus diamniotic placentas. Am J Obstet Gynecol 1998;179: 788–793.
68. Bromley B, Benacerraf B: Using the number of yolk sacs to determine amnionicity in early first trimester monochorionic twins. J Ultrasound Med 1995;14:415–419.
69. Arabin B, Laurini RN, Van Eyck J: Early prenatal diagnosis of cord entanglement in monoamniotic multiple pregnancies. Ultrasound Obstet Gynecol 1999;13:181–186.
70. Overton TG, Denbow ML, Duncan KR, Fisk NM: First trimester cord entanglement in monoamniotic twins. Ultrasound Obstet Gynecol 1999;13:140–142.
71. Lam YH, Sin SY, Lam C, et al: Prenatal sonographic diagnosis of conjoined twins in the 1st trimester: Two case reports. Ultrasound Obstet Gynecol 1998;11(4):289–291.
72. Spitz L, Kiely EM: Experience and management of conjoined twins. Br J Surg 2002;89:1188–1192.
73. Baldwin VJ: The pathology of monochorionic monozygosity. In Baldwin VJ (ed): Pathology of Multiple Pregnancy. New York, Springer Verlag, 1994, pp 199–214.
74. Allen VM, Windrim R, Barrett J, Ohlsson A: Management of monoamniotic twin pregnancies: A case series and systemic review of the literature. BJOG 2001;108: 931–936.
75. Rodis J, McIlveen P, Egan J, et al: Monoamniotic twins: improved perinatal survival with accurate prenatal diagnosis and antenatal fetal surveillance. Am J Obstet Gynecol 1997;177:1046–1049.
76. Quigley JK: Monoamniotic twin pregnancy. Am J Obstet Gynecol 1935;29:354–362.
77. Timmons JD, DeAlvarez RR: Monoamniotic twin pregnancy. Am J Obstet Gynecol 1963;86:875–881.
78. Mantoni M, Pedersen J: Monoamniotic twins diagnosed by ultrasound scan in the first trimester. Acta Obstet Gynecol Scand 1980;59:551–553.
79. Shahabi S, Donner C, Wallond J, et al: Monoamniotic twin cord entanglement: A case report with color flow Doppler ultrasonography for antenatal diagnosis. J Reprod Med 1997;42:740–742.
80. Tessen JA, Zlatnik FJ: Monoamniotic twins: A retrospective controlled study. Obstet Gynecol 1991;77:832–834.
81. Abuhamad AZ, Mari G, Copel JA, et al: Umbilical artery flow velocity waveforms in monoamniotic twins with cord entanglement. Obstet Gynecol 1995;86:674–677.
82. Rosemond RL, Hinds NE: Persistent abnormal umbilical cord Doppler velocimetry in a monoamniotic twin with cord entanglement. J Ultrasound Med 1998;17:337–339.
83. Su LL: Monoamniotic twins: Diagnosis and management. Acta Obstet Gynecol Scand 2002;81:995–1000.
84. Peek MJ, McCarthy A, Kyle P, et al: Medical amnioreduction with sulindac to reduce cord complications in monoamniotic twins. Am J Obstet Gynecol 1997;176:334–336.
85. Baisley E, Megerian G, Gerson A, Roberts NS: Monoamniotic twins: Case series and proposal for antenatal management. Obstet Gynecol 1999;93:130–134.
86. McLeod FN, McCoy DR: Monoamniotic twins with an unusual cord complication. Case Report. BJOG 1981;97:774–775.
87. Kiely JL: The epidemiology of perinatal mortality in multiple births. Bull NY Acad Med 1990;66:618–637.
88. Johnson CD, Zhang J: Survival of other fetuses after a fetal death in twin or triplet pregnancies. Obstet Gynecol 2002;99:698–703.
89. Tummers P, De Sutter P, Dhont M: Risk of spontaneous abortion in singleton and twin pregnancies after IVF/ICSI. Hum Reprod 2003;18(8):1720–1723.
90. Wenstrom KD, Syrop CH, Hammitt DG, Van Voorhis BJ: Increased risk of monochorionic twinning associated with assisted reproduction. Fertil Steril 1993;60:510–514.
91. Sebire NJ, Thornton S, Hughes K, et al: The prevalence and consequences of missed abortion in twin pregnancies at 10 to 14 weeks of gestation. BJOG 1997;104:847–848.
92. Sairam S, Costeloe K, Thilaganathan B: Prospective risk of stillbirth in multiple-gestation pregnancies: A population-based analysis. Obstet Gynecol 2002;100:638–641.
93. Petersen BL, Broholm H, Skibsted L, et al: Acardiac twin with preserved brain. Fetal Diagn Ther 2001;16:231–233.
94. Pharoah POD: Neurological outcome in twins. Semin Neonatol 2002;7:223–230.
95. Glinianaia SV, Pharoah POD, Wright C, et al: Fetal or infant death in twin pregnancy: Neurodevelopmental consequence for the survivor. Arch Dis Child Fetal Neonatal Ed 2002;86(1): F9–F15.
96. Tanawattanacharoen S, Taylor MJO, Letsky EA, et al: Intrauterine rescue transfusion in monochorionic multiple pregnancies with recent single intrauterine death. Prenat Diagn 2001;21:274–278.
97. Righini A, Salmona S, Bianchini E, et al: Prenatal magnetic resonance imaging evaluation of ischemic brain lesions in the survivors of monochorionic twin pregnancies: Report of 3 cases. J Comput Assist Tomogr 2004;28(1):87–92.
98. de Laveaucoupet J, Audibert F, Guis F, et al: Fetal magnetic resonace imaging (MRI) of ischemic brain injury. Prenat Diagn 2001;21(9):729–736.
99. Moore CM, McAdams AJ, Sutherland J: Intrauterine disseminated intravascular coagulation: A syndrome of multiple pregnancy with a dead twin fetus. J Pediatr 1969;74:523–528.

100. Fusi L, McParland P, Fisk N, et al: Acute twin-twin transfusion: A possible mechanism for brain-damaged survivors after intrauterine death of a monochorionic twin. Obstet Gynecol 1991;78:517–520.
101. Gembruch U, Viski S, Bagamery K, et al: Twin reversed arterial perfusion sequence in twin-to-twin transfusion syndrome after the death of the donor co-twin in the second trimester. Ultrasound Obstet Gynecol 2001;17:153–156.
102. Okamura K, Murotsuki J, Tanigawara S, et al: Funipuncture for evaluation of hematologic and coagulation indices in the surviving twin following co-twin's death. Obstet Gynecol 1993;82:841–846.
103. Quintero RA, Martinez JM, Bermudez C, et al: Picture of the month: Fetoscopic demonstration of perimortem feto-fetal hemorrhage in twin-twin transfusion syndrome. Ultrasound Obstet Gynecol 2002;20:638–639.
104. Senat M-V, Bernard J-P, Loizeau S, Ville Y: Management of single fetal death in twin-to-twin transfusion syndrome: A role for fetal blood sampling. Ultrasound Obstet Gynecol 2002;20:360–363.
105. Quintero RA, Dickinson JE, Morales WJ, et al: Stage-based treatment of twin-twin transfusion syndrome. Am J Obstet Gynecol 2003;188(5):1333–1340.
106. Senat MV, Loizeau S, Couderc S, et al: The value of middle cerebral artery peak systolic velocity in the diagnosis of fetal anemia after intrauterine death of one monochorionic twin. Am J Obstet Gynecol 2003;189(5):1320–1324.
107. Sutcliff AG, Sebire NJ, Pigott AJ, et al: Outcome of children born after in utero laser ablation therapy for severe twin-to-twin transfusion syndrome. BJOG 2001;108:1246–1250.
108. Lopriore E, Nagel HT, Vandenbussche FP, Walther FJ: Long-term neurodevelopmental outcome in twin-to-twin transfusion syndrome. Am J Obstet Gynecol 2003;189(5):1314–1319.
109. Woo HHN, Sin SY, Tang LCH: Single fetal death in twin pregnancies: Review of the maternal and neonatal outcomes and management. Hong Kong Medical Journal 2001;6:293–300.
110. Romero R, Duffy TP, Berkowitz RL, et al: Prolongation of a preterm pregnancy complicated by death of a single twin in utero and disseminated intravascular coagulation. Effects of treatment with heparin. N Engl J Med 1984;310:772–774.
111. Sebire NJ, Sepulveda W, Jeanty P, et al: Multiple gestations. In Nyberg DA, McGahan JP, Pretorius DH, Pilu G (eds): Diagnostic Imaging of Fetal Anomalies. Philadelphia, Lippincott Williams & Wilkins, 2003, pp 777–815.
112. Bryan E: Loss in higher multiple pregnancy reduction. Twin Res 2002;3:169–174.
113. Sainsburry MK: Grief in multifetal death. Acta Genet Med Gemellol (Roma) 1988;37(2):181–185.
114. Bryan E, Hallet F: Guidelines for Professionals: Bereavement. London, Multiple Births Foundation, 1997.
115. James WH: A note on the epidemiology of acardiac monsters. Teratology 1977;16:211–216.
116. Van Allen MI, Smith DW, Shephard TH: Twin reversed arterial perfusion (TRAP) sequence: A study of 14 twin pregnancies with acardiacus. Semin Perinatol 1983;7:285–293.
117. Moore TR, Gale S, Benirschke K: Perinatal outcome of forty-nine pregnancies complicated by acardiac twinning. Am J Obstet Gynecol 1990;163(3):907–912.
118. Chaliha C, Schwarzler P, Booker M, et al: Trisomy 2 in an acardiac twin in a triplet in-vitro fertilization pregnancy. Hum Reprod 1999;14(5):1378–1380.
119. Schwarzler P, Ville Y, Moscosco G, et al: Diagnosis of twin reversed arterial perfusion sequence in the first trimester by transvaginal color Doppler ultrasound. Ultrasound Obstet Gynecol 1999;13(2):143–146.
120. Healey MG: Acardia: Predictive risk factors for the co-twin's survival. Teratology 1994;50(3):205–213.
121. Sullivan AE, Varner MW, Ball RH, et al: The management of acardiac twins: A conservative approach. Am J Obstet Gynecol 2003;189(5):1310–1313.
122. Brassard M, Fouron JC, Leduc L, et al: Prognostic markers in twin pregnancies with an acardiac fetus. Obstet Gynecol 1999;94(3):409–414.
123. Dashe JS, Fernandez CO, Twickler DM: Utility of Doppler velocimetry in predicting outcome in twin reversed-arterial perfusion sequence. Am J Obstet Gynecol 2001;185(1):135–139.
124. Sogaard K, Skibsted L, Brocks V: Acardiac twins: Pathophysiology, diagnosis, outcome and treatment. Six cases and review of the literature. Fetal Diagn Ther 1999;14(1):53–59.
125. Meyberg H, Gross C: Increased nuchal translucency and pathological ductus venosus flow: Two cases of TRAP sequence with different outcomes. Ultrasound Obstet Gynecol 2002;20(1): 72–74.
126. Kosno-Kruszewska E, Deregowski K, Schmidt-Sidor B, et al: Neuropathological and anatomopathological analyses of acardiac and "normal" siblings in an acardiac-twin pregnancy. Folia Neuropathol 2003;41(2):103–109.
127. Chandra S, Crane JM, Young DC, Shah S: Acardiac twin pregnancy with neonatal resolution of donor twin cardiomyopathy. Obstet Gynecol 2000;96(5 Pt 2):820–821.
128. Sherer DM, Armstrong B, Shah YG, et al: Prenatal sonographic diagnosis, Doppler velocimetric umbilical cord studies, and subsequent management of an acardiac twin pregnancy. Obstet Gynecol 1989;74(3 Pt 2):472–475.
129. Robie GF, Payne GG Jr, Morgan MA: Selective delivery of an acardiac, acephalic twin. N Engl J Med 1989;320(8):512–513.
130. Holzgreve W, Tercanli S, Krings W, Schuierer G: A simpler technique for umbilical-cord blockade of an acardiac twin. N Engl J Med 1994;331(1):56–57.
131. Quintero RA, Reich H, Puder KS, et al: Brief report: Umbilical-cord ligation of an acardiac twin by fetoscopy at 19 weeks of gestation. N Engl J Med 1994;330(7):469–471.
132. Deprest J, Audibert F, Van Schoubroeck D, et al: Bipolar cord coagulation of the umbilical cord in complicated monochorionic twin pregnancy. Am J Obstet Gynecol 2000;182:340–345.
133. Ville Y, Hyett JA, Vandenbussche FP, Nicolaides KH: Endoscopic laser coagulation of umbilical cord vessels in twin reversed arterial perfusion sequence. Ultrasound Obstet Gynecol 1994;4(5):396–398.
134. Rodeck C, Deans A, Jauniaux E: Thermocoagulation for the early treatment of pregnancy with an acardiac twin. N Engl J Med 1998;339:1293–1294.
135. Tan TY, Sepulveda W: Acardiac twin: A systematic review of minimally invasive treatment modalities. Ultrasound Obstet Gynecol 2003;22(4):409–419.
136. Denbow ML, Overton TG, Duncan KR, et al: High failure rate of umbilical vessel occlusion by ultrasound guided injection of absolute alcohol or enbucrilate gel. Prenat Diagn 1999;19:527–532.
137. Hecher K, Hackeloer BJ, Ville Y: Umbilical cord coagulation by operative microendoscopy at 16 weeks' gestation in an acardiac twin. Ultrasound Obstet Gynecol 1997;10(2):130–132.
138. Jolly M, Taylor M, Rose G, et al: Interstitial laser: A new surgical technique for twin reversed arterial perfusion sequence in early pregnancy. BJOG 2001;108:1098–1102.
139. Tsao K, Feldstein VA, Albanese CT, et al: Selective reduction of acardiac twin by radiofrequency ablation. Am J Obstet Gynecol 2002;187(3):635–640.
140. Quintero RA, Morales WJ, Allen MH, et al: Staging of twin-twin transfusion syndrome. J Perinat 1999;19(8):550–555.
141. Campbell S: Opinion: Twin-to-twin transfusion syndrome—Debates on the etiology, natural history and management. Ultrasound Obstet Gynecol 2000;16:210–213.
142. Diehl W, Hecher K, Zikulnig L, et al: Placental vascular anastomoses visualized during fetoscopic laser surgery in severe mid-trimester twin-twin transfusion syndrome. Placenta 2001;22: 876–881.
143. Bermudez C, Becerra CH, Bornick PW, et al: Placental types and twin-twin transfusion syndrome. Am J Obstet Gynecol 2002;187(2):489–494.

144. Denbow ML, Fogliani R, Kyle P, et al: Haematological indices at fetal blood sampling in monochorionic pregnancies complicated by feto-fetal transfusion syndrome. Prenat Diagn Ther 1998;18:941–946.
145. Bajoria R, Ward S, Sooranna SR: Erythropoietin in monochorionic twin pregnancies in relation to twin-twin transfusion syndrome. Hum Reprod 2001;16(3):574–580.
146. Bajoria R, Lazda EJ, Ward S, Sooranna S: Iron metabolism in monochorionic twin pregnancies in relation to twin-twin transfusion syndrome. Hum Reprod 2001;16(3):567–573.
147. Bajoria R, Gibson MJ, Ward S, et al: Placental regulation of insulin-like growth factor axis in monochorionic twins with chronic twin-twin transfusion syndrome. J Clin Endocrinol Metab 2001;86:3150–3155.
148. Sooranna SR, Ward S, Bajoria R: Discordant fetal leptin levels in monochorionic twins with chronic midtrimester twin-twin transfusion syndrome. Placenta 2001;22:392–398.
149. Bajoria R, Ward S, Chatterjee R: Natriuretic peptides in the pathogenesis of cardiac dysfunction in the recipient fetus of twin-to-twin transfusion syndrome. Am J Obstet Gynecol 2002;186:121–127.
150. Mahieu-Caputo D, Dommergues M, Delezoide AL, et al: Twin-to-twin transfusion syndrome. Role of the fetal renin-angiotensin system. Am J Pathol 2001;156(2):629–636.
151. Kilby MD, Platt C, Whittle MJ, et al: Renin gene expression in fetal kidneys of pregnancies complicated by twin-twin transfusion syndrome. Pediatr Dev Pathol 2001;4(2):175–179.
152. De Lia JE, Carr MH: Pregnancy loss after successful laser surgery for previable twin-twin transfusion syndrome (Letter). Am J Obstet Gynecol 2002;187(2):517–518.
153. Sebire NJ, Souka A, Skentou H, et al: Early prediction of severe twin-to-twin transfusion syndrome. Hum Reprod 2000;15(9):2008–2010.
154. Sebire NJ, Talbert D, Fisk NM: Twin-to-twin transfusion syndrome results from dynamic asymmetrical reduction in placental anastomoses: A hypothesis. Placenta 2001;22:383–391.
155. Taylor MJ, Denbow ML, Tanawattanacharoen S, et al: Doppler detection of arterio-arterial anastomoses in monochorionic twins: Feasibility and clinical application. Hum Reprod 2000;15(7):1632–1636.
156. Fries MH, Goldstein RB, Kilpatrick SJ, et al: The role of velamentous cord insertion in the aetiology of twin-twin transfusion syndrome. Obstet Gynecol 1993;81:569–574.
157. Grant of the European Commission in its 5th Framework Programme (#QLG1-CT-2002-01632 EuroTwin2Twin).
158. van Gemert MJ, Umur A, Tijssen JG, Ross MG: Twin-twin transfusion syndrome: Etiology, severity and rational management. Curr Opin Obstet Gynecol 2001;13:193–206.
159. Denbow ML, Battin MR, Cowan F, et al: Neonatal cranial ultrasound findings in preterm twins complicated by severe fetofetal transfusion syndrome. Am J Obstet Gynecol 1998;178:479–483.
160. Bejar R, Vigliocco G, Gramajo H, et al: Antenatal origins of neurological damage in newborn infants. II. Multiple gestations. Am J Obstet Gynecol 1990;162:1230–1236.
161. Karatza AA, Wolfenden JL, Taylor MJO, et al: Influence of twin-twin transfusion syndrome on fetal cardiovascular structure and function: Prospective case-control study of 136 monochorionic twin pregnancies. Heart 2002;88:271–277.
162. Cincotta RB, Gray PH, Phythian G, et al: Long term outcome of twin-twin transfusion syndrome. Arch Dis Child Fetal Neonatal Ed 2000;83(3):F171–F176.
163. Luks FI, Carr SR, Tracy TF Jr: Intestinal atresia associated with twin-twin transfusion syndrome. J Pediatr Surg 2001;36(7):1105–1106.
164. Fisk NM, Vaughan J, Talbert D: Impaired fetal blood gas status in polyhydramnios and its relation to raised amniotic pressure. Fetal Diagn Ther 1994;9(1):7–13.
165. Bower SJ, Flack NJ, Sepulveda W, et al: Uterine artery blood flow response to correction of amniotic fluid volume. Am J Obstet Gynecol 1995;173:502–507.
166. Denbow M, Sepulveda W, Ridout D, Fisk NM: Relationship between change in AFI and volume of fluid removed at amnioreduction. Obstet Gynecol 1997;90:529–532.
167. Elliott JP, Sawyer AT, Radin TG, Strong RE: Large volume therapeutic amniocentesis in the treatment of hydramnios. Obstet Gynecol 1994;84:1025–1027.
168. Mari G, Roberts A, Detti L, et al: Perinatal morbidity and mortality rates in severe twin-twin transfusion syndrome: Results of the International Amnioreduction Registry. Am J Obstet Gynecol 2001;185:708–715.
169. Leung WC, Jouannic JM, Hyett J, et al: Procedure-related complications of rapid amniodrainage in the treatment of polyhydramnios. Ultrasound Obstet Gynecol 2004;23(2):154–158.
170. Skupski DW, Gurushanthaiah K, Chasen S: The effect of treatment of twin-twin transfusion syndrome on the diagnosis to delivery interval. Twin Res 2002;5:1–4.
171. Ville Y, Hyett J, Hecher K, Nicolaides K: Preliminary experience with endoscopic laser surgery for severe twin twin transfusion syndrome. N Engl J Med 1995;332:224–227.
172. Feldstein VA, Machin GA, Albanese CT, et al: Twin-twin transfusion syndrome: The "select" procedure. Fetal Diagn Ther 2000;15:257–261.
173. Quintero RA, Bornick PW, Allen MH, Johnson PK: Selective laser photocoagulation of communicating vessels in severe twin twin transfusion syndrome in women with an anterior placenta. Obstet Gynecol 2001;97(3):477–481.
174. Ville Y, Hecher K, Gagnon A, et al: Endoscopic laser coagulation in the management of severe twin transfusion syndrome. BJOG 1998;105:446–453.
175. Stone CA, Quinn MW, Saxby PJ: Congenital skin loss following Nd:YAG placental coagulation. Burns 1998;24:275–277.
176. De Lia JE, Lamboy M: Congenital skin loss following Nd:YAG placental coagulation. Burns 1998;24:366–367.
177. Luks F, Carr S, Tracy T: Intestinal complications associated with twin twin transfusion syndrome after antenatal laser treatment: Report of 2 cases. J Pediatr Surg 2001;36:1105–1106 (replying letter).
178. Lundvall L, Skibsted L, Graem N: Limb necrosis associated with twin twin transfusion syndrome treated with YAG laser coagulation. Acat Obstet Gynecol Scand 1999;78:349–350.
179. Scott F, Evans N: Distal gangrene in a polycythemic recipient fetus in twin-twin transfusion. Obstet Gynecol 1995;86:677–679.
180. Deprest JA, Van Schoubroeck D, Van Ballaer PP, et al: Ultrasound Obstet Gynecol 1999;12:347–352.
181. Gratacós E, Deprest J: Current experience with fetoscopy and the Eurofoetus registry for fetoscopic procedures. Eur J Obstet Gynecol Reprod Biol 2000;92(1):151–159.
182. Hecher K, Diehl W, Zikulnig L, et al: Endoscopic laser coagulation of placental anastomoses in 200 pregnancies with severe mid-trimester twin-to-twin transfusion syndrome. Eur J Obstet Gynecol Reprod Biol 2000;92(1):135–140.
183. Senat MV, Deprest J, Boulvain M, et al: A randomized trial of endoscopic laser surgery versus serial amnioreduction for severe twin-to-twin transfusion syndrome at midgestation. N Engl J Med 2004;35/(2):136–144.
184. Banek CS, Hecher K, Hackeloer BJ, Bartmann P: Long-term neurodevelopmental outcome after intrauterine laser treatment for severe twin-twin transfusion syndrome. Am J Obstet Gynecol 2003;188(4):876–880.
185. Johnson JR, Rossi KQ, O'Shaughnessy RW: Amnioreduction versus septostomy in twin-twin transfusion syndrome. Am J Obstet Gynecol 2001;185:1044–1047.
186. Mahone PR, Sherer DM, Abramowicz JS, Woods JR: Twin transfusion syndrome: Rapid development of severe hydrops of

the donor following selective fetocide of the recipient. Am J Obstet Gynecol 1993;169:166–168.
187. Taylor MJ, Shalev E, Tanawattanacharoen S, et al: Ultrasound-guided umbilical cord occlusion using bipolar diathermy for stage III/IV twin-twin transfusion syndrome. Prenat Diagn 2002;22(1):70–76.
188. Little J, Bryan E: Congenital anomalies in twins. Semin Perinatol 1986;10:50–64.
189. Singh SM, Murphy B, O'Reilly R: Epigenetic contributors to the discordance in monozygotic twins. Clin Genet 2002;62:97–103.
190. Cuckle H: Down's syndrome screening in twins. J Med Screen 1998;5(1):3–4.
191. Wald NJ, Rish S, Hackshaw AK: Combining nuchal translucency and serum markers in prenatal screening for Down syndrome in twin pregnancies. Prenat Diagn 2003;23(7):588–592.
192. Schlessel JS, Brown WT, Lysikiewicz A, et al: Monozygotic twins with trisomy 18: A report of discordant phenotype. J Med Genet 1990;27:640–642.
193. Loevy HT, Miller M, Rosenthal IM: Discordant monozygotic twins with trisomy 13. Acta Genet Med Gemellol 1985;34: 185–188.
194. Hall JH: Twins and twinning. Am J Med Genet 1996;61: 202–204.
195. Spencer K, Nicolaides KH: Screening for trisomy 21 in twins using first trimester ultrasound and maternal serum biochemistry in a one-stop clinic: A review of three years experience. BJOG 2003;110(3):276–280.
196. Rochon M, Stone J: Invasive procedures in multiple gestations. Curr Opin Obstet Gynecol 2003;15(2):167–175.
197. Yaron Y, Bryant-Greenwood PK, Dave N, et al: Multifetal pregnancy reductions of triplets to twins: Comparison with nonreduced triplets and twins. Am J Obstet Gynecol 1999;180(5): 1268–1271.
198. Ghidini A, Lynch L, Hicks C, et al: The risk of second-trimester amniocentesis in twin gestations: A case-control study. Am J Obstet Gynecol 1993;169(4):1013–1016.
199. Yukobowich E, Anteby EY, Cohen SM, et al: Risk of fetal loss in twin pregnancies undergoing second trimester amniocentesis. Obstet Gynecol 2001;98(2):231–234.
200. Kidd SA, Lancaster PA, Anderson JC, et al: Fetal death after exposure to methylene blue dye during mid-trimester amniocentesis in twin pregnancy. Prenat Diagn 1996;16(1):39–47.
201. Yang J, Monk T, White P: Acute hemodynamic effects of indigo carmine in the presence of compromised cardiac function. J Clin Anesthesiol 1991;3:320–323.
202. Bahado-Singh R, Schmitt R, Hobbins JC: New technique for genetic amniocentesis in twins. Obstet Gynecol 1992;79(2): 304–307.
203. Sebire NJ, Noble PL, Odibo A, et al: Single uterine entry for genetic amniocentesis in twin pregnancies. Ultrasound Obstet Gynecol 1996;7(1):26–31.
204. Kalousek DK: Pathogenesis of chromosomal mosaicism and its effect on early human development. Am J Med Genet 2000;91: 39–45.
205. Lipitz S, Meizner I, Yagel S, et al: Expectant management of twin pregnancies discordant for anencephaly. Obstet Gynecol 1995;86(6):969–972.
206. Sebire NJ, Sepulveda W, Hughes KS, et al: Management of twin pregnancies discordant for anencephaly. BJOG 1997;104(2): 216–219.
207. Evans MI, Goldberg JD, Horenstein J, et al: Selective termination for structural, chromosomal, and mendelian anomalies: International experience. Am J Obstet Gynecol 1999;181(4): 893–897.
208. Shalev J, Meizner I, Rabinerson D, et al: Improving pregnancy outcome in twin gestations with one malformed fetus by postponing selective fetacide in the third trimester. Fetal Steril 1999;72:257–260.
209. Olivennes F, Doumerc S, Senat MV, et al: Evidence of early placental vascular anastomosis during selective embryo reduction in monozygotic twins. Fertil Steril 2002;77(1):183–184.
210. Challis D, Gratacós E, Deprest J: Selective termination in monochorionic twins. J Perinat Med 1999;27:327–338.
211. Snijders RJM, Sebire NJ, Cuckle H, et al: Maternal age and gestational age-specific risks for chromosomal defects. Fetal Diag Ther 1995;10:356–367.
212. Snijders RJM, Sundberg K, Holzgreve W, et al: Maternal age and gestation-specific risk for trisomy 21. Ultrasound Obstet Gynecol 1999;13:167–170.
213. Deprest JA, Evrard VA, Van Ballaer PP, et al: Experience with fetoscopic cord ligation. Eur J Obstet Gynecol Reprod Biol 1998;81:157–164.
214. Nicolini U, Poblete A, Boschetto C, et al: Complicated monochorionic twin pregnancies: experience with bipolar cord coagulation. Am J Obstet Gynecol 2000;185:703–707.
215. Lewi L, Jani J, Gratacos E, et al: 50 consecutive cord coagulations in monochoronic twins. Ultrasound Obstet Gynecol 2003; 22(51):163.
216. Lewi L, Van Schoubroeck D, Gloning KP, et al: Selective feticide by cord occlusion in four sets of heterokarytypic monochorionic twins. J Soc Gynecol Investig 2003;10(suppl):97A, 405.
217. Deprest J, van Schoubroeck D, Senat M-V, et al: Cord coagulation in monochorionic multiplets late in gestation. Am J Obstet Gynecol 2003;S189.6:S612.
218. Soothill P, Sohan K, Carroll S, Kyle P: Ultrasound-guided, intra-abdominal laser to treat acardiac pregnancies. BJOG 2002; 109(3):352–354.
219. Holmes A, Jauniaux E, Rodeck C: Monopolar thermocoagulation in acardiac twinning. BJOG 2001;108: 1000–1002.
220. Ville Y: Selective feticide in monochorionic pregnancies: Toys for the boys or standard of care? Ultrasound Obstet Gynecol 2003;22(5):448–450.
221. Anand KJ, Maze M: Fetuses, fentanyl, and the stress response: Signals from the beginnings of pain? Anesthesiology 2001;95(4): 823–825.
222. Crowley P: Prophylactic corticosteroids for preterm birth (Cochrane Review). Cochrane Library Issue 4. Oxford. Update software, 2000.

CHAPTER 25

Fetal Hydrops

John Smoleniec

INTRODUCTION

Fetal hydrops is associated with high perinatal morbidity and mortality rates at all gestational ages (up to 100% in some series[1]). The reported incidence approximates 1:2500 to 1:3500 in neonates.[2] Traditionally, fetal hydrops was categorized into immune (IH) and nonimmune (NIH) disease. Although Rhesus (D) hemolytic disease was the most common cause of hydrops in the past (see Chapter 14), the widespread implementation of anti-D immunoglobulin prophylaxis and the improved antenatal management of at-risk fetuses has led to a remarkable decrease in its incidence and morbidity. At present, NIH is more prevalent than IH in most countries with adequate anti-D immunoglobulin prophylaxis supplies and fetomaternal expertise. A comparative incidence ratio of NIH to IH of 9:1 is reported.[3]

Advances in ultrasound make hydrops easy to diagnose. The pathogenesis of human fetal hydrops reflects the underlying etiology and as a result is often unclear. The "causes" or rather associations with NIH are many[4,5] (Table 25–1). Physiologic research using animal models[6–8] is providing some understanding of the complexity of fluid dynamics within the uterus (fetal, fetoplacental, fetoamniotic fluid, and between the uterine decidua and the placenta and membranes).

INCIDENCE

A prevalence of 1:1000[9] is reported, though the true incidence is regionally dependent. It is also subject to seasonal variation, for example, parvovirus B19 epidemics.[10,11] α-Thalassemia is the most common cause of fetal hydrops in Southeast Asia,[12] accounting for between 53% and 81% of cases.[13] Considering the population density in this region, it is probably the leading cause of NIH in the world. Population screening can reduce the incidence of thalassemia, as it has in Cyprus, providing the resources are available. The uptake of first trimester nuchal translucency screening is likely to have an impact on the incidence of hydrops associated with aneuploidy, which is normally identified in the second and third trimesters. In those fetuses with an increased nuchal translucency but a normal karyotype, there is an increased risk of hydrops fetalis and cardiac anomalies.[14,15]

DIAGNOSIS

Hydrops is defined as the excessive extravascular accumulation of fluid in the interstitial compartment secondary to the disruption of the normal intravascular interstitial fluid homeostatic mechanisms. The excessive accumulation of interstitial fluid, particularly in serous cavities (peritoneal, pleural, pericardial), placenta, and amniotic fluid, facilitate the sonographic diagnosis of fetal hydrops (Figs. 25–1 and 25–2). Classically, the sonographic diagnosis of hydrops requires the presence of generalized edema plus the accumulation of fluid within two or more serous cavities, though clearly, many of the pathologies leading to such a diagnosis go through phases in which fluid is recognized sonographically only in one site.

PATHOPHYSIOLOGY

Hydrops occurs when the microvascular fluid exchange regulatory system is disturbed. Microvascular fluid exchange mechanisms in the human fetus are complex, gestationally dependent, and poorly understood. The number of fluid exchange pathways in the fetus is greater than in either the infant or adult. They include transplacental, transmembrane, and transcutaneous pathways. Transplacental fluid exchange has a large influence on blood volume, as the placental blood volume accounts for

TABLE 25–1

Abnormalities Associated with Hydrops*

- Immune (see also Chapter 14)
  - Anti-D and c Rhesus antibodies
  - Antibodies to K in Kell system
  - Antibodies to Fya in the Duffy system
- Nonimmune
- Idiopathic/unknown
- Anemia (other than alloimmunization
  - α-Thalassemia major (Chapter 39)
  - Parvovirus B19 congenital infection (Chapter 30)
  - Fetomaternal transfusion
  - Twin-twin transfusion syndrome (TTTS) and variants (Chapter 24)
  - Erythroleukemia
  - Congenital erythropoietic porphyria (Gunther's disease)
- Cardiovascular (Chapters 16 and 17)
  - Severe congenital heart disease (atrial septal defect, ventriculoseptal defect, hypoplastic left heart, pulmonary valve insufficiency, Ebstein's anomaly, subaortic stenosis, atrioventricular canal defect, tetralogy of Fallot, premature closure of foramen ovale, large arteriovenous malformation)
  - Premature closure of ductus (? indomethacin therapy)
  - Myocarditis (coxsackie virus, cytomegalovirus, parvovirus B19 infections)
  - Tachyarrhythmias (supraventricular tachycardia, atrial flutter)
  - Bradyarrhythmias (heart block)
  - Wolff-Parkinson-White syndrome
  - Intracardiac tumors (teratoma, rhabdomyoma) (Chapter 17)
  - Cardiomyopathy (e.g., fibroelastosis)
  - Myocardial infarction
  - Arterial calcification
- Chromosomal (Chapter 2)
  - Trisomies
  - Turner syndrome (45 XO)
  - Triploidy
- Pulmonary
  - Congenital hydro-/chylothorax
  - Pulmonary lymphangiectasia
  - Congenital cystic adenomatous
  - Malformation of the lung (CCAM) (Chapter 20)
  - Pulmonary sequestration
  - Bronchogenic cysts and other tumors (Chapter 20)
  - Diaphragmatic hernia (Chapter 20)
  - Chondrodysplasia
  - Pulmonary hypoplasia
- Renal (Chapter 19)
  - Congenital nephrosis (Finnish type)
  - Renal vein thrombosis
  - Urethral obstruction (atresia, posterior valves)
  - Spontaneous bladder perforation
  - Cloacal malformation
  - Prune belly
- Infection (intrauterine) (Chapters 30, 31, 33)
  - Parvovirus B19 (either by anemia, myocarditis or hepatitis)
  - Syphilis
  - Cytomegalovirus
  - Toxoplasmosis
  - Herpes simplex
  - Leptospirosis
  - Chagas' disease
- Liver
  - Hepatic clacifications
  - Hepatic fibrosis
  - Congenital hepatitis (Chapter 28)
  - Cholestasis
  - Polycystic disease
  - Biliary atresia (Chapter 20)
  - Familial cirrhosis
- Genetic metabolic disease (many have their effect via the liver)
  - Gaucher disease
  - GM_1 gangliosidosis
  - Mucopolysaccharidosis (MPS), types VIa and VII†
  - Iron-storage disease
- Anomalies (many associated with fetal immobility)
  - Achondroplasia (Chapter 21)
  - Achondrogenesis type 2 (Chapter 21)
  - Thanatophoric dwarfism (Chapter 21)
  - Sacrococcygeal teratoma (Chapter 23)
  - Arthrogryphosis
  - Multiple pterygium syndrome
  - Neu-Laxova syndrome
  - Pena-Shokeir type 1 syndrome
  - Cerebro-oculofacioskeletal syndrome (COFS)
  - Noonan syndrome
  - Myotonic dystrophy
  - Neuronal degeneration
- Miscellaneous
  - Cystic hygroma (Chapters 2,18 and 23)
  - Meconium peritonitis
  - Fetal neuroblastosis
  - Tuberous sclerosis (Chapter 23)
  - Small bowel volvulus (Chapter 20)
  - Amniotic band syndrome
  - Torsion of ovarian cyst
  - Polysplenia syndrome
- Lymphatic: intestinal lymphatic hypoplasia
- Placental
  - Monochorionic twins—TTTS (Chapter 24)
  - Umbilical vein thrombosis
  - Chorioangioma
  - True cord knots
  - Umbilical cord cysts
- Maternal
  - Diabetes mellitus (Chapter 45)
  - Thyroid disease (Chapters 22 and 46)
  - Preeclampsia (Chapter 36)
  - Severe anemia (Chapter 39)
  - Hypoalbuminemia

*Chapter numbers in text refer the reader to detailed discussion of management options for specific conditions within a given group.
†Tokieda et al.[84]

approximately 40% of the total fetal circulation.[16] Fetal development is associated with the changing influence of the different fluid exchange pathways and forces. These routes of fetal fluid exchange may be important compensatory mechanisms when fluid homeostasis is disturbed, as shown by the common clinical association of hydramnios and placental edema with fetal hydrops. The fetal extracellular fluid volume (ECF) exceeds the intracellular fluid volume (ICF), though the ECF:ICF ratio declines progressively with gestation, becoming less than 1 only in the newborn period.[17] The interstitial:plasma volume ratio is therefore greatest in the fetus and declines into adulthood. The control of this relatively large interstitial fluid compartment is fundamental to the understanding of fetal hydrops. Unfortunately interstitial fluid control mechanisms are poorly understood because of the

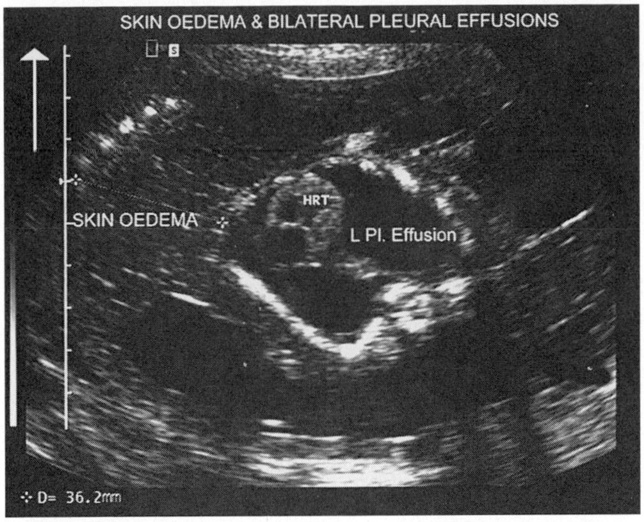

FIGURE 25–1
Skin edema and bilateral pleural effusions associated with a congenital heart defect.

difficulty of measuring plasma and interstitial volumes.[18] The many influences on fetal fluid homeostasis make it unlikely that there is a single or simple pathophysiologic explanation for all cases of fetal hydrops. The "Starling equation" does not provide pathophysiologic explanations in the fetus.[19] The fluid-dominated milieu of the fetus and the specific physiologic characteristics of the fetal heart and the lymphatic system make it particularly susceptible to hydrops. Animal research[6,7,20,21] coupled with clinical study[19,22,23] suggest that raised central venous pressure is a critical step in the pathophysiology of hydrops. The clinical use of umbilical venous pressure in the investigation and management of some cases of fetal hydrops is a vindication of the relatively recent physiologic research findings on the importance of the central venous pressure and the lymphatic system.[22,23] At the same time, some of the traditional pathophysiologic forces such as colloid oncotic pressure are being relegated to a lower tier of importance.

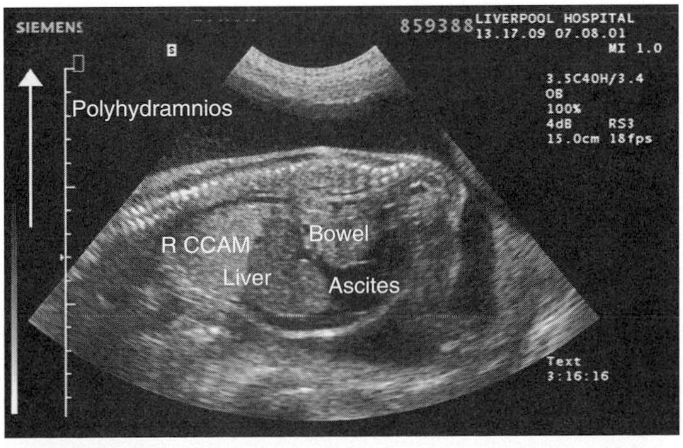

FIGURE 25–2
Ascites associated with a solid lung tumor.

MANAGEMENT OPTIONS

Once fetal hydrops is identified, the mother should be counseled regarding the following:

- Prognosis: namely, fetal risks in the short and long term, influenced by the diagnosis and may be unknown
- Diagnosis: based on maternal and fetal investigations (see Tables 25–2 and 25–3) and associated fetal risks from invasive procedures
- Treatment: if available and feasible in the circumstances

PROGNOSIS

Fetal Risks

The main fetal risks from hydrops are fetal death and infant morbidity:

- *Fetal death* may be the result of the underlying pathophysiology, invasive fetal investigations, or fetal treatment. The reported mortality rate ranges between 50% and 100%.[1] Complications of the various invasive diagnostic and therapeutic procedures include

TABLE 25–2

Maternal Investigations for Fetal Hydrops

Maternal History
Parvovirus B19 epidemic and close proximity to children
Previous fetal hydrops or diagnosis associated with hydrops
Previous baby with jaundice
Ethnic origin
Endocrine disorder
Maternal Blood
Complete blood count (e.g., microcytosis – alpha-thalassemia trait)
Electrophoresis (depending upon blood count result and ethnic background)
Blood group and antibody screen* (titer if antibodies present)
Glucose-6-phosphate dehydrogenase and pyruvate kinase carrier status
Alpha-fetoprotein
Serologic tests (of limited value, see Chapters 30–33)
Syphilis
Parvovirus B19
Toxoplasmosis
Cytomegalovirus
Herpes simplex virus
Coxsackievirus
Urate, urea, and electrolytes
Liver function including albumin
Kleihauer (-Betke) test
Test of glucose tolerance
Systemic lupus erythematosis (SLE), especially anti-Ro/SSA or anti-La/SSB antigens, if bradycardia/ heart block
Thyroid function tests including antibodies: thyroid stimulating hormone (TSH) and TSH, binding inhibitor IgG
IgG (Chapter)

*Data from references 3, 9, 23, 33, 39.

TABLE 25–3

Fetal Prenatal Investigations for Fetal Hydrops*

Ultrasound
Sites and severity of hydrops (see Figs. 25–1 to 25–4)
Detailed real-time ultrasound for congenital abnormality and abnormality of placenta and cord (cysts[85])
Fetal echocardiography, pulsed and color Doppler studies and M-mode
Amniotic fluid volume
Biophysical assessment (nonstress testing or biophysical profile score).
Invasive (mainly fetal blood)
Hematologic tests: full blood count, hemoglobin electrophoresis (depending on ethnic background); group and Coombs'
Infection: polymerase chain reaction, serologic tests for acute phase specific IgM antibodies for infection; culture
Blood gas analysis and pH estimation to provide an indication of the immediate well-being of the fetus
Karyotype (blood, placenta, amniotic fluid, ascitic or pleural fluids are suitable sources)
Umbilical venous pressure (UVP)
Liver function tests (albumin)
White blood cell enzymes (Gaucher's mucopolysaccharidoses)

*From references 3, 9, 31, 33, 85.

abortion, preterm delivery, intrauterine fetal death, and fetal trauma (see Chapters 10 and 24).

- *Infant morbidity*: The short- and long-term prognosis depends on the underlying diagnosis and treatment, such as terminal cardiac failure and heart transplantation associated with parvovirus B19 infection,[24] cardiac anomaly needing surgical correction; chromosomal abnormality; or persistent generalized edema as a result of protein-losing enteropathy associated with congenital intestinal lymphatic hypoplasia.[25]

Maternal Risks

- *Prenatal* causes of hydrops include preterm rupture of membranes—risk of chorioamnionitis, preeclampsia ("mirror" syndrome),[26] anemia, hydramnios, maternal red blood cell alloimmunization, and placental abruption from invasive fetal procedures. In the event of fetal surgery,[27] the maternal risks include anesthetic risks, fluid overload and electrolyte imbalance, uterine hemorrhage (during entry for fetal shunting and intrauterine laser procedures),[28] psychological stress and associated mental illness, and even maternal death.[28]
- *During labor and delivery:* Hydrops may be associated with preterm labor and tocolysis side effects, dystocia (e.g., large tumors), cesarean delivery (e.g., associated with malpresentation, cord prolapse), abruption associated with membrane rupture in cases with hydramnios, postpartum hemorrhage (primary and secondary), and retained placenta.

DIAGNOSIS

Presentation

Fetal hydrops presents clinically in one of several ways (Table 25–4). The fetal sites of fluid collection and the amount of fluid (severity) may be helpful in the management of the hydrops once the cause is ascertained. In general, the absence of amniotic fluid is a poor prognostic sign.

Investigations

A comprehensive search in the mother and fetus for the "cause" usually involves antenatal invasive procedures (Tables 25–2 and 25–3). The severity, gestational age, ultrasound identified anomalies, and the parents' consent will influence the decision to perform these procedures. The ultrasound scan (see Figs. 25–1 and 25–2) may identify an associative cause in more than 50% of cases.[5] The diagnosis may not be possible in 10%[1] to 26%.[5] The most common invasive procedures are fetal blood sampling and amniocentesis. Fetal blood sampling is preferred (Table 25–5), but the associated mortality rates are likely to be higher than when the invasive procedures are performed for nonhydropic indications,[29,30] especially if the fetus is thrombocytopenic (e.g., parvovirus B19 infection) and when it is technically more difficult.

It is important to optimize the information available when planning intrauterine procedures (amniocentesis or fetal blood sample). For example, in the case of severe lung compression with heart axis deviation associated with large pleural effusions, a pleural tap may be combined with either procedure to determine the effect of decompression on the lungs and the restoration of the heart to its normal midline position. Pleural fluid can be used for investigations (karyotype, infection screen). Intrathoracic pressure and umbilical vein pressure measurements (if vein cordocentesis is performed) before and after the drainage may be used prognostically. The measurement of umbilical venous pressure

TABLE 25–4

Presentation of Fetal Hydrops

By chance:
Ultrasound examination
Fetal heart rate recording
Ultrasound surveillance for twin-twin transfusion syndrome in monochorionic twin pregnancy
Large-for-dates/hydramnios
Reduced fetal movements
Placental abruption
Maternal diabetes
Maternal preeclampsia/mirror syndrome
Maternal parvovirus B19 infection or at risk for infection

TABLE 25-5

Comparative Diagnostic Value of Amniocentesis and Fetal Blood Sampling

Amniocentesis
Karyotyping (FISH for chromosomes 13, 18, 21, sex chromosomes, and culture may take 2 weeks for a result)
Infection screen
Congenital erythropoietic porphyria (CEP)—amniotic fluid is dark brown which fluoresces red under Wood's light; increase in type 1 uro- and coproporphyrin isomers*
Fetal blood sampling
Karyotyping (48–72 hours for a result in many centers)
Hematologic causes (anaemia; hemoglobinopathies)
Infection screen
Umbilical vein pressure (UVP)

*Pannier et al.[2]

(UVP) is a surrogate for fetal central venous pressure (CVP). However, it requires an additional invasive pro cedure (amniocentesis and pleural aspiration) while measuring the UVP.

Amniotic fluid may be used to karyotype and to diagnose most infections associated with hydrops, such as parvovirus B19, cytomegalovirus (CMV), syphilis, toxoplasmosis, and herpes simplex virus (HSV) (see Chapters 30, 31 and 33). It has also recently been shown to be useful in the diagnosis of the rare condition of congenital erythropoietic porphyria.[2] The advantage fetal blood sampling has over amniocentesis is that more information can be obtained (anemia, Coombs' test, umbilical venous pressure) along with quicker karyotyping of all 23 pairs of chromosomes. Furthermore, treatment can be administered at the time of the procedure in cases of anemia.[31] It is important to screen for rare antibodies (Coombs' test), which can only be comprehensively done in regional blood transfusion laboratories, before making the diagnosis of NIH.[32]

Polymerase chain reaction investigation has revolutionized the diagnosis of fetal infection. A maternal infection screen should be performed before the fetal screen in order to optimize the use of the relatively small fetal sample. An extra 2-mL aliquot should be stored at −20°C in case the need for additional tests becomes apparent after the preliminary laboratory results have been completed.

The optimal time for prognostic counseling is after the results of the maternal and fetal investigations are available. After multidisciplinary counseling, the patient may elect to undergo a termination of pregnancy, if this is an option.

Postmortem Examination

When prenatal treatment has not been possible or successful, a postmortem examination of the fetus and placenta is to be encouraged.

TREATMENT

General

The proportion of cases amenable to prenatal treatment varies in each reported series, as they are generally small in number and reflect variation in the local referral practices. It is likely that no more than 20% to 30% of hydropic fetuses are potential therapeutic candidates.[33]

To date, fetal hydrops has proved amenable to fetal therapy only when associated with the following:

- Anemia
- Arrhythmia
- Hydrothoraces
- Twin-twin transfusion syndrome (TTTS)
- Tumors (few case reports)

Infection, arrhythmia, and twin-twin transfusion syndrome are conditions in which spontaneously reversible hydrops is clearly documented. The management of twin-twin transfusion syndrome is discussed in Chapter 24.

Anemia

Fetal blood transfusion is the only therapeutic option for the treatment of hydrops secondary to anemia (for details see Chapter 14). However, the prognosis may be worse than that for hemolytic disease secondary to red blood cell alloimmunization (e.g., with homozygous α-thalassemia, CMV infection, parvovirus B19 infection, trisomy 21, Gunther's disease).[2] It is important, therefore, to try to discern before intrauterine transfusion the cause of the anemia (α-thalassemia or fetomaternal hemorrhage) and whether it is secondary to another condition causing hydrops (e.g., trisomy 21 usually causes mild anemia unless the fetus is acidotic and terminal). This may mean not transfusing the fetus (with the patient's agreement) before all investigations (especially the parents for α-thalassemia trait) and fetal karyotype are available. This point should be discussed at the initial counseling session; otherwise, ill-advised intrauterine transfusions for the fetus with homozygous α-thalassemia may result in lifelong transfusions, iron chelation, and the associated morbidity.[34]

In Southeast Asia α-thalassemia is the main cause of fetal hydrops.[13] α-Thalassemia major (no functional α genes) is incompatible with life. Most fetuses develop hydrops (Fig. 25–3) and, if born alive, die within hours. This is in contrast with other common causes of fetal anemia for which the prognosis is generally good. Antenatal diagnosis is an option for those pregnancies at risk. Preconceptual education, screening, and counseling are to be encouraged (Chapter 39). The prognosis may change with advances in intrauterine therapy.[35]

In fetomaternal hemorrhage associated with hydrops, one should screen the patient and the fetus (using

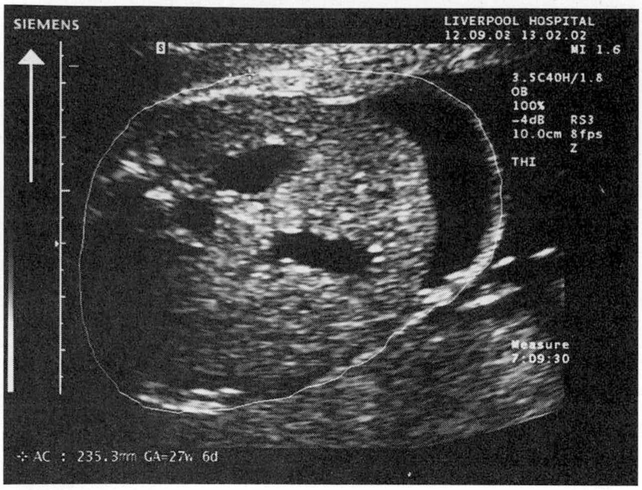

FIGURE 25–3
Fetal hydrops (ascites) associated with α-thalassemia major.

ultrasound parameters) regularly for further episodes, as they may be fatal. Under these conditions, delivery may be considered once the pregnancy has reached an appropriate gestation.

There are no effective antenatal treatments for glucose 6-phosphate dehydrogenase (G6PD) deficiency and erythroleukemia. Gene therapy may prove possible in the future, and interdisciplinary counseling including pediatric colleagues and clinical geneticists is advisable.

Twin-Twin Transfusion Syndrome with Hydrops

The management of hydrops associated with TTTS has included intrauterine placental vessel (ideally selective) laser ablation, amniodrainage (poorer results compared with selective laser), umbilical cord occlusion (e.g., previable weight of donor with hydropic recipient), delivery, and termination. The reader is referred to Chapter 24 for a detailed discussion of TTTS. In some instances, intrauterine fetal transfusion was deemed necessary after selective laser therapy.[28]

Cardiovascular Defects

Cardiac anomalies are the most common anatomic anomaly associated with fetal hydrops.[5] In general, hydrops associated with a structurally abnormal heart carries a poor prognosis, with a survival rate of 10% or less (Table 25–6).[36] Involvement of a pediatric cardiologist in the antenatal management (especially diagnosis and prognostic counseling) is advisable. The management options for these conditions are discussed in Chapters 16 and 17.

The majority of cases with a hydropic fetus associated with a tachyarrhythmia but a structurally normal heart respond to either transplacental (60%[37] to 95%[38] supraventricular tachycardia) or direct fetal therapy (see Chapter 16). Fetal tachycardia with hydrops associated with thyrotoxicosis in a patient with a history of Graves' disease can be treated with antithyroid medication in utero.[39] The prognosis is good in general with a survival rate of as high as 80%[37]; however, there may be neurologic morbidity associated with a long duration of hydrops.[40] Fetal myocarditis associated with congenital infection may unexpectedly have severe complications requiring perinatal heart transplantation.[24]

TABLE 25–6

Approximate Survival Rates for Major Treatable Causes of Fetal Hydrops

CAUSE	SURVIVAL RATES (%)
Anemia—parvovirus B19 infection	62.5[31] to 84%[74]
Cardiovascular—supraventricular tachyarrhythmia	60%[37] to 95%[38]
Pulmonary—primary hydrothorax	50%[51]

Pulmonary Defects

The prognosis for thoracic conditions associated with hydrops is generally poor and the number of successful therapeutic options limited. Diaphragmatic hernia is discussed in Chapter 20. The prognosis is better for drainage of fluid, cystic thoracic abnormalities (e.g., congenital cystic adenomatoid malformation [CCAM] type I; primary hydrothorax) as opposed to solid lesions (e.g., CCAM type III [Figs. 25–2 and 25–4] and some type II; pulmonary sequestration, see Chapter 23). The survival for solid CCAM masses ranges from as low as 0% with hydrops to 90% with no hydrops[41,42] and has led some to offer open fetal surgery to those with solid lesions and hydrops. It is associated with less than 50% survival and significant maternal and fetal morbidity.[43,44] There are case reports of other therapeutic options for solid lung lesions including percutaneous

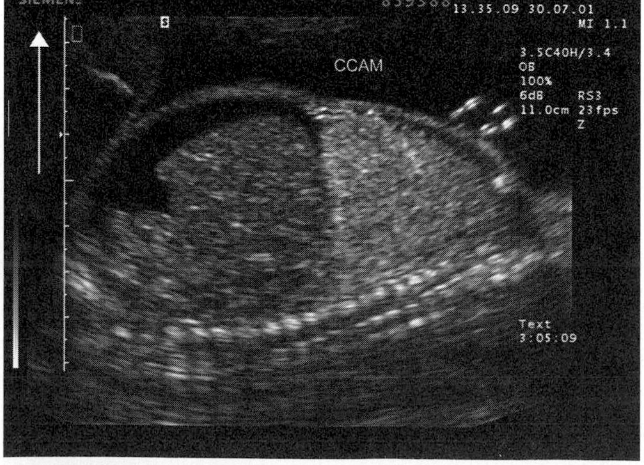

FIGURE 25–4
Fetal hydrops associated with congenital cystic adenomatoid malformation (CCAM).

ultrasound guided injection of a vascular sclerosant (alcohol)[45] and laser vaporization.[46,47] There are also rare reports of spontaneous resolution of fetal hydrops[48,49] associated with regression of the lesion. In contrast, a number of hydropic cases with CCAM type I and II have been treated successfully using pleuroamniotic shunts providing they have a single large predominant cyst.[44,50]

Fetal hydrops associated with isolated primary or congenital hydrothorax has a much improved prognosis in contrast to the poor prognosis with solid thoracic lesions. The survival rate in hydrops and pleural effusions treated conservatively approximates 12%; however, the survival rate in cases treated with a pleuroamniotic shunt is around 50%.[51] The pathogenesis is unknown, but is often attributed to abnormalities of the lymphatic system of the lung and thoracic duct. The diagnosis of congenital hydrothorax is a diagnosis of exclusion—excess pleural fluid in the absence of another detectable cause. The hydrothorax typically presents after 24 weeks when human lung development has entered the canalicular phase. The lymphocyte content of the fluid is not relevant to either the prognosis or the diagnosis.[52] Although it was known since the early 1980s that placement of a thoracoamniotic shunt could reverse the hydrops,[53] the rate of reported success rates are quite variable.[51] This suggests more than one mechanism underlies the hydrops. The effectiveness of pleuroamniotic shunting is thought to be due to the relief of an obstructive cardiac return secondary to mediastinal deviation[54] resulting in low cardiac output (Fig. 25–5). It is further believed that relief of lung compression prevents pulmonary hypoplasia (assuming onset of the hydrothorax before 24 weeks) (Fig. 25–6). An initially elevated UVP associated with elevated intrathoracic pressure, both of which normalize after the effusion(s) have been drained, suggests that an elevated intrathoracic pressure is associated with the

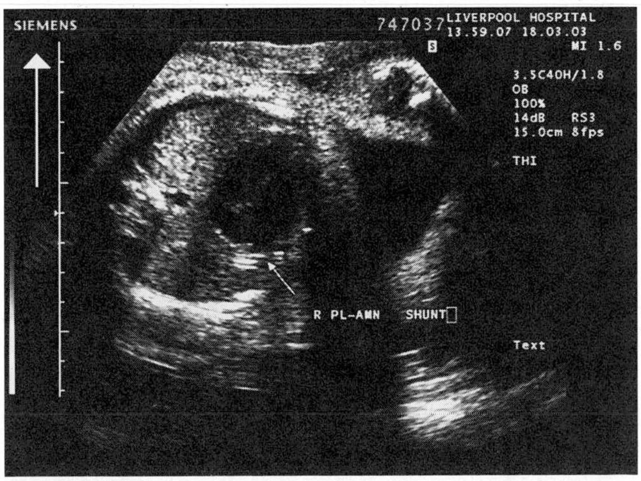

FIGURE 25–5
Pleuroamniotic shunt in-situ showing lung expansion associated with drainage of the pleural effusion i.e. used to treat a fetus with primary hydrothorax.

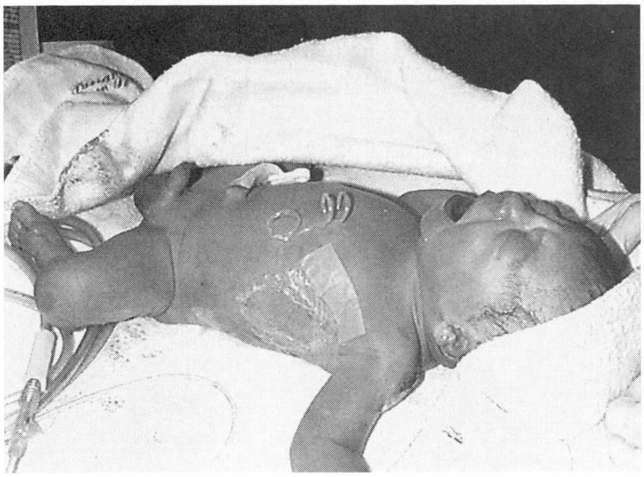

FIGURE 25–6
Infant at birth immediately after removal of pleuroamniotic shunt (see pigtail drain on chest) with no need for respiratory support.

pathophysiology. If the effusion recurs, placement of a thoracoamniotic shunt should be curative. On the other hand, if the UVP is normal prior to decompression of the chest, or remains elevated after the chest has been drained and the heart has returned to its normal midline position, the placement of a thoracoamniotic shunt will not be beneficial.

PROCEDURE: INSERTION OF FETAL THORACOAMNIOTIC SHUNT (FIG. 25–7)

METHOD

Hydramnios and iatrogenic oligohydramnios complicate the procedure. The usual preparations for a major invasive procedure (such as fetal blood transfusion) should be followed (see Chapter 14). The majority of procedures are performed under local anesthesia with the option of premedication. Maternal regional anesthesia[54] and rarely general anesthesia may be needed. The practice of using fetal paralysis varies. Fetal analgesia may also be used.[55]

In preparation for the procedure, the ultrasound transducer is positioned to give a transverse view of the fetal chest at the level of the maximal fluid collection. The optimal line of approach is chosen to avoid (if possible) the placenta and to avoid the broad ligament vessels (use color Doppler to identify) and to enter ideally the anterolateral aspect of the fetal chest. Once the line of approach is determined, the maternal abdomen is cleaned and draped and a local anesthetic instilled down to the uterine visceral peritoneum.

In order to overcome the problems with insertion of the pigtail catheter into the cannula, a guidewire and pusher are now available from the supplier. The double pigtailed catheter with its forming wire in place should be gently straightened. This can be done before inserting the introducer into the fetal chest to avoid delay. A stab incision (5 mm) is made with a blade into the abdominal wall to

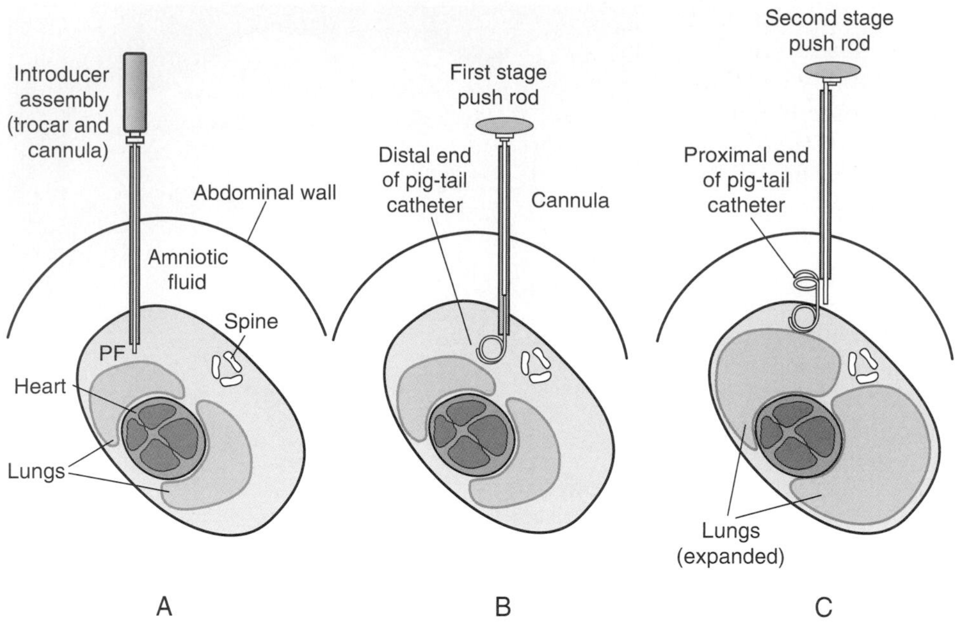

FIGURE 25–7
Procedure for the insertion of a pleuroamniotic shunt. *A*, The introducer (trocar and cannula) are sited under ultrasound guidance in the left side of the fetal chest. *B*, The trocar has been removed, the pigtail catheter sited into the cannula, and the "first stage push rod" (shorter rod) used to push the distal end of the pigtail catheter in the fetal chest. *C*, The tip of the cannula is withdrawn from the chest into the amniotic space and the "second stage punch rod" (longer rod) is inserted into the cannula and displaces the proximal/maternal end of the pigtail out of the end of the cannula into the aminotic space, resulting in a pleuralamniotic pigtail shunt.

minimize the resistance of insertion. The introducer (trocar and cannula) is inserted along the optimal line of approach into the amniotic cavity, taking care to minimize amnion separation and to avoid contact with the fetus. The line of entry into the fetal chest is then reviewed and adjusted if necessary. Once this secondary adjustment is made, the introducer is inserted into the pleural cavity with a sharp, stabbing motion, taking care not to traumatize intrathoracic organs and vessels. The trocar is removed, and the elongated double pigtailed catheter with introducing guidewire carefully slid down into the cannula by an assistant, taking care not to remove the guidewire before the proximal end of the pigtail is sited within the shaft of the cannula using the guidewire pusher (to prevent jamming). Once the guidewire is removed, pleural fluid will escape through the cannula. After checking that the end of the cannula is still within the fetal chest, the shorter of the two push rods (i.e., the "first stage" pusher rod) is used to advance the distal part of the catheter (fetal component) into the fetal chest, where it should be seen to adopt its natural coiled shape. The introducing cannula is withdrawn from the fetal chest, into the amniotic cavity, taking care (using ultrasound) not to withdraw the cannula too far away from the fetal chest wall, otherwise one may pull the distant end of the catheter out of the chest. Ensure (by ultrasound) the end of the cannula is still within the amniotic cavity and not in the uterine wall. The maternal component of the double pigtailed catheter is now pushed out of the cannula into the amniotic cavity using the longer "second stage" push rod. The correct position of the pigtail catheter is confirmed ultrasonically. The cannula is now removed from the uterus and the wound sutured and dressed. If there are bilateral large effusions, a second shunt is required because decompressing only one side can actually worsen cardiac displacement.

A sonographic examination is performed 8 to 24 hours postoperatively to assess shunt function (Fig. 25–5). Resolution of the majority of the effusion is expected if the shunt is working well. The hydrops itself (and hydramnios if still present) may take an additional 10 to 14 days to resolve. The shunt will continue to function for a variable time interval. In a series of 28 cases the median interval was 12 weeks (range = 1–14) for the survivors, and 3 weeks (range = 1–11) for the perinatal losses (Nicolini, personal communication). If the pleural fluid reaccumulates, it is due to either blockage or displacement. At this juncture, the decision is made whether to replace the shunt or to deliver the fetus, depending mainly on the severity of any residual hydrops, the duration of the functional shunt, and the current gestational age.

At delivery the pigtail drain must be immediately occluded and then removed to prevent a pneumothorax (Fig. 25–6).

COMPLICATIONS

Insertion of a pleuroamniotic shunt is not without complications, which need to be included in the counseling of parents. Maternal complications of shunt placement include those associated with maternal analgesia, anesthesia (+/– epidural), hemorrhage, broad ligament hematoma, abortion, preterm rupture of membranes, preterm labor and delivery, maternal trauma, and red blood cell alloimmunization. The fetal complications include death, prematurity, fetal injury to thoracic organs and vessels, fetal severe hypoproteinemia,[56] shunt displacement into the fetal chest or blockage (12%),[51] and even limb entanglement with the development of circulatory compromise.[57]

Other Treatments

Serial intrapleural injections of OK-432 were used to treat a hydropic fetus, resulting in a liveborn infant with right renal dysfunction.[58] Termination of pregnancy is also an option if there is no improvement in the hydrops after treatment.

Tumors (See Chapter 23)

In selected cases with a poor prognosis, open fetal surgery[59] has been used for a small number (three) of surgically correctable conditions, in particular, solid pulmonary and sacrococcygeal tumors. Only a few centers in the world are willing to attempt such novel therapy. Other, less invasive (percutaneous) therapeutic options for the treatment of tumors have been tried to circumvent many of the problems of open fetal surgery with varying success. These include percutaneous alcohol,[60] radiofrequency ablation,[61] thermocoagulation,[62] and percutaneous ultrasound-guided injection of alcohol for the treatment of sacrococcygeal teratoma and placental chorioangioma.

Chromosomal Abnormalities

Chromosomal anomalies are found in about 13% of cases,[5] some of which will be associated with structural fetal anomalies. It is important to exclude aneuploidy before offering therapy, especially in fetuses with hydrothorax. Aneuploidy with hydrops has a dismal prognosis, and the option of pregnancy termination should be offered the parents (also see Chapter 2).

Infection

Fetal infection may be the etiology in 8% of fetuses with nonimmune hydrops.[63] The application of polymerase chain reaction technologies has revealed a number of previously unsuspected fetal infections. Viral hepatitis is the most common cause of noncardiac hydrops in some populations (see Table 25–1) (Weiner, personal communication). Hydrops of noncardiac origin does not generally progress, and preterm delivery is not usually required.

The common infectious causes of hydrops include parvovirus B19, cytomegalovirus (CMV), syphilis, and toxoplasmosis. Apart from parvovirus induced fetal anemia, very little can currently be done antenatally to treat these conditions once they produce hydrops.

Parvovirus B19 infection (see Chapter 30) is a recognized cause of human fetal hydrops.[64] Most common among school-age children, it is also known as "slapped cheek" syndrome, erythema infectiosum, fifth disease, or academy rash.[65] Twenty percent to 50% of pregnant women are susceptible to parvovirus infection.[66,67] It often occurs regionally in 3- to 5-year epidemic cycles,[68] at which time it may be the leading cause of hydrops fetalis in the region.[10,11,69] The risk of fetal hydrops may be higher in mothers with asymptomatic infection.[10] Hydrops is mainly due to profound hypoplastic anemia, but can also be associated with myocarditis[24,69,70] and hepatitis.[31] The risk of fetal loss is greatest during the first half of pregnancy, with most reported cases of hydrops between 16 and 32 weeks.[71,72] However, the true incidence of first trimester losses due to parvovirus infection is unknown. The interval from maternal infection to fetal death is described between 1 and 16 weeks, with the majority occurring by 8 weeks.[72]

Management depends on the severity. Serial ultrasound examinations are used to assess severity.[73] Some suggest no fetal investigation is necessary with mild to moderate hydrops showing improvement on serial scans.[11,31] Of course, improvement can only be determined over time during which the fetus might also deteriorate. When longitudinal ultrasound studies are not possible, a fetal blood sample should be obtained. The finding of mild to moderate hydrops, coupled with the absence of severe thrombocytopenia, acidemia, and the presence of an increased reticulocyte count, suggests spontaneous recovery is under way. In severe cases without a reassuring hematologic or metabolic profile, intrauterine transfusion is indicated.[31,73] The risk of fetal blood sampling and therapy is increased because of the increased risk of associated thrombocytopenia. However, a successful outcome may be expected in the majority of cases (83.8%) (Table 25–6).[74] Myocarditis secondary to parvovirus is treated with fetal digitalization. Infant follow-up is mandatory in view of the risk of congenital red blood cell aplasia[75] and even the need for perinatal heart transplantation.[24]

Other Causes

Generalized lymphatic dysfunction (e.g., primary hydrothorax is believed to be a variant) can be associated with abnormal vascular development. The prognosis is guarded and may include significant infant morbidity.[25,76]

Recurrent idiopathic NIH is reported[33,77] and postulated to be related to a recessive gene. There are a few reports of familial hydrops consistent with autosomal recessive[78] and X-linked recessive[79] inheritance.

Fetal akinesia is another condition associated with fetal hydrops, with a large number of causes (cerebro-oculofacioskeletal, Pena-Shokeir, multiple pterygium, Neu-Laxova syndromes) that carry a poor prognosis. The risk of recurrence is generally low, but will be influenced by the cause if identified (e.g., Neu-Laxova syndrome has autosomal recessive inheritance[80]).

Renal associations with hydrops are discussed in detail in Chapter 19.

Few therapeutic options are available for antenatal treatment of other causes of fetal hydrops. Several case reports from Japan describe the localized injection of OK-432 into body cavities containing localized collections of excessive extravascular fluid (e.g., cystic hygroma[81]; pleural effusion[58]) with poor results to date.[81,82]

Role of Uterine Venous Pressure in Treatment

The uterine venous pressure (UVP) measurement is helpful in the management of fetal hydrops. If it is raised and therapy reduces it, then the prognosis is good. Hydrops characterized by an elevated UVP not remedied by either surgical or medical therapy is usually progressive, and the fetus either dies in utero or requires preterm delivery for postnatal therapy.[23] However, not all disorders that increase the UVP are associated with hydrops, and cardiac dysfunction does not necessarily mean cardiac decompensation. And although there are many reports of hydrops not associated with an elevated UVP, there are no reports of reproducibly effective therapy.[19] Limited human study suggests a good correlation between the fetal UVP and central venous pressure, but this relationship was not true in the anemic fetal sheep.[8] It seems, therefore, that measurement of the fetal UVP should be viewed as a guide to therapy when fetal blood sampling is planned but is not, in and of itself, an indication for the sampling.

Fetal Albumin Therapy

Fetal hypoproteinemia or hypoalbuminemia from the pathophysiology appears to be a secondary effect.[8,19] It may occur in a third of nonimmune hydrops fetuses, but is distributed with equal frequency in groups with a high and low UVP (the exception being twin-twin transfusion syndrome, which is discussed in Chapter 24). Clearly, the practice of giving the fetus albumin[83] in the absence of knowing its cardiac status and its albumin level cannot be recommended, although some advocate its use.[81] A more productive approach is to try to discover other causes of fetal hydrops and to reduce this "idiopathic" group.

CONCLUSIONS

- Fetal hydrops is an uncommon but serious condition with a complex pathophysiology; it is associated with a wide range of etiologies and carries a poor prognosis overall.
- Comprehensive antenatal and postnatal investigations (e.g., postmortem) are necessary if the cause is to be identified, as the diagnosis may not be made in as many as a quarter of cases.
- Antenatal therapy should be directed at a specific pathologic condition, but is possible in less than a third of cases.
- Research into the pathophysiology is needed to improve our understanding of the fetal fluid-regulating mechanisms.
- In the short term, the largest impact on the incidence of NIH is made by implementing screening programs both preconceptually (e.g., populations at risk for α-thalassemia) and antenatally (e.g., nuchal translucency; monochorionicity and TTTS surveillance; anomaly scans, especially cardiac scans; being alert to outbreaks of parvovirus B19 infection in the local community).

SUMMARY OF MANAGEMENT OPTIONS
Fetal Hydrops (see also Chapter 14)

Management Options	Quality of Evidence	Strength of Recommendation	References
Prevention			
Preconceptual and prenatal screening for:			
α-Thalassemia	III	B	13
Fetal aneuploidy	IIb	B	14,15
Fetal anomalies, especially severe cardiac disease	III	B	9
Monochorionicity screening for twin-twin transfusion syndrome	III	B	28
Diagnosis—Investigations			
Maternal (see Table 25–3)	III	B	3,4,5,9
Fetal (see Table 25–4)	III	B	3,4,5,9
Diagnosis will be made in 75–90% of cases.	III	B	3,4,5,9

SUMMARY OF MANAGEMENT OPTIONS
Fetal Hydrops (see also Chapter 14)

Management Options	Quality of Evidence	Strength of Recommendation	References
Diagnosis—Investigations—Continued			
Risks of fetal invasive procedures are increased in presence of hydrops.	III	B	29,30
Counseling and Prognosis			
Counseling is given before and after investigations.	–	GPP	–
Prognosis is determined by the underlying etiology.	III	B	3,4,5,9
The earlier it is detected, the worse the prognosis.	III	B	10,33
Earlier detection is more likely to be associated with chromosomal abnormality.	III	B	3,4,5,9
Presence of a congenital anomaly worsens the prognosis.	III	B	9
Bilateral pleural effusions are a poor prognostic sign.	III	B	14,15,17
Generally prognosis is good for psychomotor development in survivors.	III	B	17,18
Prevention of prematurity improves long-term outcome.	III	B	17
Management—Treatment			
In utero, therapy can be effective in selected cases (about one-third):			
Intrauterine transfusions for fetal anemia (hemolytic disease [see Chapter 14], fetal bleed, parvovirus)	III	B	33,83
Antiarrhythmic medication	III	B	33,38,83
Specific treatments for twin-twin transfusion syndrome (see Chapter 24)	III	B	52
Pleuroamniotic shunts for primary hydrothorax, cystic adenomatous malformation	III	B	28
Open surgery for chest lesions should be regarded as experimental.	III	B	59
Management—General			
Interdisciplinary approach is used for ongoing pregnancies.	–	GPP	–
Consider termination in those with severe hydrops at a pre-viable gestation with a condition for which there is no effective treatment.	–	GPP	–
Postnatal			
Perform postmortem examination in cases of fetal/neonatal death.	–	GPP	–
Pediatric follow-up and counseling are needed in survivors.	–	GPP	–

REFERENCES

1. Forouzan I: Hydrops fetalis: Recent advances. Obstet Gynecol Surv 1997;97:130–138.
2. Pannier E, Viot G, Aubry MC, et al: Congenital erythropoietic porphyria (Gunther's disease): Two cases with very early prenatal manifestation and cystic hygroma. Prenat Diagn 2003;23:25–30.
3. Warsof SL, Nicolaides KH, Rodeck C: Immune and non-immune hydrops. Clin Obstet Gynecol 1986;29:533–542.
4. Smoleniec JS, James D: Fetal hydrops—Is the prognosis always poor. J Obstet Gynaecol 1994;14:142–145.
5. Keeling JW: Fetal hydrops. In Keeling JW (ed): Fetal and Neonatal Pathology, 2nd ed. London, Springer Verlag, 1993, pp 253–271.
6. Brace RA: Effects of outflow pressure on fetal lymph flow. Am J Obstet Gynecol 1989;160:494–497.
7. Gest AL, Bair DK, Van der Straten MC: The effect of outflow pressure upon thoracic duct lymph flow rate in fetal sheep. Pediatr Res 1992;32:585–588.
8. Blair DK, Van der Straten MC, Gest AL: Hydrops in fetal sheep from rapid induction of anaemia. Pediatr Res 1994;35:560–564.
9. Machin GA: Hydrops revisited: Literature review of 1414 cases published in the 1980s. Am J Med Genet 1989;34:366–390.
10. Smoleniec JS, Pillai M, Caul EO, Usher J: Subclinical transplacental parvovirus B19 infection: An increased fetal risk? Lancet 1994;343:1100.
11. Kailasam C, Brennand J, Cameron AD: Congenital parvovirus B19 infection: Experience of a recent epidemic. Fetal Diagn Ther 2001;16:18–22.

12. Lorey F, Charoenkwan P, Witkowska HE, et al: HbH hydrops foetalis syndrome: A case report and review of literature. Br J Haematol 2001;115:1:72–78.
13. Liang ST, Wong VC, So WW, et al: Homozygous alpha-thalassaemia: Clinical presentation, diagnosis and management. A review of 46 cases. BJOG 1985;92:680–684.
14. Hyett J, Perdu M, Sharland G, et al: Using fetal nuchal translucency to screen for major congenital heart defects at 10–14 weeks of gestation: Population based cohort study. BMJ 1999;318:81–85.
15. Souka AP, Snijders J, Novakov A, et al: Defects and syndromes in chromosomally normal fetuses with increased nuchal translucency thickness at 10–14 weeks of gestation. Ultrasound Obstet Gynecol 1998;11:391–400.
16. Barcroft J: Researches on prenatal life. Oxford, Blackwell, 1946.
17. Friis-Hansen B: Body water compartments in children: Changes during growth and related changes in body composition. Pediatrics 1961;28:169.
18. Brace RA: Fluid distribution in the fetus and neonate. In Polin RA, Fox WW (eds): Fetal and Neonatal Physiology, Vol. II. London, WB Saunders, 1992, pp 1288–1298.
19. Moise KJ, Carpenter RJ, Hesketh DE: Do abnormal Starling forces cause fetal hydrops in red cell alloimmunisation? Am J Obstet Gynecol 1992;167:907–912.
20. Brace RA, Valenzuela GJ: Effects of outflow pressure and vascular volume loading on thoracic duct flow in the adult sheep. Am J Physiol 1990;258:R240.
21. Andres RL, Brace RA: The development of hydrops fetalis in the ovine fetus after lymphatic ligation or lymphatic incision. Am J Obstet Gynecol 1990;62:1331–1334.
22. Johnson P, Sharland G, Allan LD, et al: Umbilical venous pressure in nonimmune hydropis fetalis: Correlation with cardiac size. Am J Obstet Gynecol 1992;167:1309–1313.
23. Weiner CP: Umbilical pressure measurement in the evaluation of nonimmune hydrops fetalis. Am J Obstet Gynecol 1993;168:817–823.
24. Von Kaisenberg CS, Bender G, Scheewe J, et al: A case of fetal parvovirus B19 myocarditis, terminal cardiac heart failure and perinatal heart transplantation. Fetal Diagn Ther 2001; 16:427–432.
25. Stormon MO, Mitchell JD, Smoleniec JS, et al: Congenital intestinal lymphatic hypoplasia presenting as non-immune hydrops in utero, and subsequent neonatal protein-losing enteropathy. J Pediatr Gastroenterol Nutrition 2002;35:691–694.
26. Nicolaides K, Gainey H: Pseudotoxemic state associated with severe Rh isoimmunisation. Am J Obstet Gynecol 1964;89:41–45.
27. Howell L, Adzick N, Harrison M: The fetal treatment center. Semin Pediatr Surg 1993;2:143–146.
28. Ville Y, Hecher K, Gagnon A, et al: Endoscopic laser coagulation in the management of severe twin-to-twin transfusion syndrome. BJOG 1998;105:446–453.
29. Weiner CP, Wenstrom KD, Sipes SL, Williamson RA: Risk factors for cordocenteses and fetal intravascular transfusion. Am J Obstet Gynecol 1993;165:1020–1025.
30. Maxwell DJ, Johnson P, Hurley P, et al: Fetal blood sampling and pregnancy loss in relation to indication. BJOG 1991;98:892–897.
31. Smoleniec JS, Pillai M: Fetal hydrops associated with parvovirus B19 infection: Management. BJOG 1994;101: 1079–1081.
32. Smoleniec JS, Anderson N, Poole G: Hydrops fetalis caused by a blood group antibody usually undetected in routine screening. Arch Dis Child 1994;71:F216–F217.
33. Hansmann M, Gembruch U, Bald R: New therapeutic aspects in nonimmune hydrops fetalis based on 402 prenatally diagnosed cases. Fetal Ther 1989;4:29–36.
34. Yang Q, McDonnell SM, Khoury MK, et al: Hemochromatosis-associated mortality in the United States from 1979–1992: An analysis of multiple-cause mortality data. Ann Intern Med 1998;20:946–953.
35. Hayward A, Ambruso D, Battaglia F, et al: Microchimerism and tolerance following intrauterine transplantation and transfusion for α-thalassemia. 1. Fetal Diagn Ther 1998;13:8–14.
36. Sharland GK, Lokhart SM, Chita SK, Allan LD: Factors influencing the outcome of congenital heart disease detected prenatally. Arch Dis Child 1991;66:284–287.
37. Jouannic JM, Delahaye S, Fermont L, et al: Fetal supraventricular tachycardia: A role for amiodarone as second-line therapy? Prenat Diagn 2003;23:152–156.
38. Krapp M, Baschat AA, Gembruch U, et al: Flecainide in the intrauterine treatment of fetal supraventricular tachycardia. Ultrasound Obstet Gynecol 2002;19:158–164.
39. Ibrahim H, Asamoah A, Krouskop RW, et al: Congenital chylothorax in neonatal thyrotoxicosis. Source J Perinatol 1999;19:1:68–71.
40. Schade RP, Stoutenbeck P, de Vries LS, Meijboom EJ: Neurological morbidity after superventricular tachyarrhythmia. Ultrasound Obstet Gynecol 1999;13:43–47.
41. Bromley B, Parad R, Estroff JA, Benacerraf BR: Fetal lung masses: Prenatal course and outcome. J Ultrasound Med 1995;12:927–936.
42. Laberge JM, Flageole H, Pugash D, et al: Outcome of the prenatally diagnosed congenital cystic adenomatoid lung malformation: A Canadian experience. Fetal Diagn Ther 2001;16:3:178–186.
43. Adzick NS, Harrison MR, Crombleholme TM, et al: Fetal lung lesions. Management and outcome. Am J Obstet Gynecol 1998;179:884–889.
44. Crombleholme TM, Coleman B, Hedrick H, et al: Cystic adenomatoid malformation volume ratio predicts outcome in prenatally diagnosed cystic adenomatoid malformation of the lung. J Pediatr Surg 2002;37:331–338.
45. Nicolini U, Cerri V, Groli C, et al: A new approach to prenatal treatment of extralobar pulmonary sequestration. Prenat Diagn 2000;20:758–760.
46. Fortunato S, Lombardo S, Dantrell J, Ismael S: Intrauterine laser ablation of a fetal cystic adenomatoid malformation with hydrops. The application of minimally invasive surgical techniques to fetal surgery. Am J Obstet Gynecol 1997;S84:177.
47. Bruner JP, Jarnagin BK, Reinisch L: Percutaneous laser ablation of fetal congenital cystic adenomatoid malformation: Too little, too late? Fetal Diagn Ther 2000;15:359–363.
48. Taguchi T, Suita S, Yamanouchi T, et al: Antenatal diagnosis and surgical management of congenital cystic adenomatous malformation of the lung. Fetal Diagn Ther 1995;10:400–407.
49. Da Silva OP, Ramanan R, Romano W, Evans M: Nonimmune hydrops fetalis, pulmonary sequestration, and favourable neonatal outcome. Obstet Gynecol 1996;88:681–683.
50. Kitano Y, Adzick NS: New developments in fetal lung surgery. Curr Opin Pulm Med 1999;6:383–389.
51. Pettersen HN, Nicolaides KH: Pleural effusions. In Fisk NM, Moises KJ (eds): Fetal Therapy. Cambridge, UK, Cambridge University Press, 1997, pp 261–272.
52. Rodeck CH, Fisk NM, Fraser DI, Nicolini U: Long-term in utero drainage of fetal hydrothorax. N Engl J Med 1988;319: 1135–1138.
53. Weiner CP, Varner MW, Pringle KC, et al: Antenatal diagnosis and treatment of nonimmune hydrops fetalis secondary to pulmonary extralobar sequestration. Obstet Gynecol 1986;68: 275–280.
54. Grisaru-Granovsky S, Seaward PGR, Windrim R, et al: Midtrimester thoracoamniotic shunting for the treatment of fetal primary pleural effusions in a twin pregnancy. Fetal Diagn Ther 2000;15:209–211.
55. Glover V, Fisk NM: Fetal pain: Implications for research and practice. BJOG 1999;106:881–886.
56. Koike T, Minakami H, Kosuge S, et al: Severe hypoproteinemia in a fetus after pleuro-amniotic shunts with double-basket catheters for treatment of chylothorax. J Obstet Gynaecol Res 2000;26(5):373–376.

57. Chan FY, Borzi P, Cincotta R, et al: Limb constriction as a complication of intra-uterine vesico-amniotic shunt: fetoscopic release. Fetal Diagn Ther 2002;17(5):315–320.
58. Tanemura M, Nishikawa N, Kojima K, et al: A case of successful fetal therapy for congenital chylothorax by intrapleural injection of OK-432. Ultrasound Obstet Gynecol 2001;18(4):371–375.
59. Coleman BG, Adzick NS, Crombleholme TM, et al: Fetal therapy: State of the art. J Ultrasound Med 2002;21:1257–1288.
60. Nicolini U, Zuliani G, Caravelli E, et al: Alcohol injection: A new method of treating placental chorioangiomas. Lancet 1999;353:1674–1675.
61. Paek BW, Jennings RW, Harrison MR, et al: Radiofrequency ablation of human fetal sacrococcygeal teratoma. Am J Obstet Gynecol 2001;184(3):503–507.
62. Lam YH, Tang MH, Shek TW: Thermocoagulation of fetal sacrococcygeal teratoma. Prenat Diagn 2002;22(2):99–101.
63. Barron SD, Pass RF: Infectious causes of hydrops fetalis. Semin Perinatol 1995;19:493–501.
64. Brown T, Anand A, Ritchie LD, et al: Intrauterine parvovirus infection associated with hydrops fetalis. Lancet 1984; II:1033–1034.
65. Anderson MJ, Jones SE, Fisher-Hock SP, et al: Human parvovirus, the cause of erythema infectiosum (fifth disease). Lancet 1983;I:1378.
66. Mortimer PP, Cohen BJ, Buckley MM, et al: Human parvovirus and the fetus. Lancet 1985;2:1012.
67. Klopper PE, Morris DJ: Screening for viral and protozoal infections in pregnancy. A review. BJOG 1990;97: 974–983.
68. Anderson LJ: Human parvoviruses. J Infect Dis 1990;161: 603–608.
69. Porter HJ, Quantrill AM, Flemming KA: B19 parvovirus infection of the myocardium. Lancet 1988;I:535–536.
70. Naides SJ, Weiner CP: Antenatal diagnosis and palliative treatment of non-immune hydrops fetalis secondary to parvovirus B19 infection. Prenat Diagn 1989;9:105–114.
71. Public Health Laboratory Service Working Party on Fifth Disease: Prospective study of human parvovirus (B19) infection in pregnancy. BMJ 1990;300:1166–1170.
72. Rodis JF, Borgida AF, Wilson M, et al: Management of parvovirus infection in pregnancy and outcomes of hydrops: A survey of members of the Society of Perinatal Obstetricians. Am J Obstet Gynecol 1998;179(4):985–988.
73. Fairley CK, Smoleniec JS, Caul OE, Miller E: Observational study of effect of intrauterine transfusions on outcome of fetal hydrops after parvovirus B19 infection. Lancet 1995;346: 1335–1337.
74. Schild RL, Bald R, Plath H, et al: Intrauterine management of fetal parvovirus B19 infection. Ultrasound Obstet Gynecol 1999;13:161–166.
75. Brown KE, Green SW, de Mayolo JA, et al: Congenital anaemia after transplacental parvovirus infection. Lancet 1984;343: 895–896.
76. Windebank KP, Bridges NA, Ostman-Smith I, Stevens JE: Hydrops fetalis due to abnormal lymphatics. Arch Dis Child 1987;62:198–200.
77. Onwude JL, Thornton JG, Mueller RH: Recurrent idiopathic non-immunologic hydrops fetalis: A report of two families, with three and two affected siblings. BJOG 1992;99:854–856.
78. Scott-Emuakpor AB, Warren ST, Kapur S, et al: Familial occurrence of congenital pulmonary lymphangiectasias. Genetic implications. Am J Dis Child 1981;135:532–534.
79. Reece EA, Lockwood CJ, Rizzo N, et al: Intrinsic intrathoracic malformations of the fetus: Sonographic detection and clinical presentation. Obstet Gynecol 1987;70:627–632.
80. Shivarajan MA, Suresh S, Jagadeesh S, et al: Second trimester diagnosis of neu laxova syndrome. Prenat Diagn 2003;23:21–24.
81. Ogita K, Suita S, Taguchi T, et al: Outcome of fetal cystic hygroma and experience of intrauterine treatment. Prenat Diagn Ther 2001;16:105–110.
82. Negishi H, Yamada H, Okuyama K, et al: Outcome of non-immune hydrops fetalis and a fetus with hydrothorax and/or ascites: With some trials of intrauterine treatment. J Perinat Med 1997;25:71–77.
83. Maeda H, Koyanagi T, Nakano H: Intrauterine treatment of non-immune hydrops fetalis. Early Hum Dev 1994;29:241–249.
84. Tokieda K, Morikawa Y, Natori M, et al: Intrauterine growth acceleration in the case of a severe form of mucopolysaccharidosis type VII. [Review] [12 refs]. J Perinat Med 1998;26(3):235–239.
85. Sepulveda W, Sebire NJ, Harris R, Nyberg DA: The placenta, umbilical cord, and membranes. In Nyberg DA, McGraham JP, Pretorious DH, Pilu G (eds): Diagnostic Imaging of Fetal Anomalies. Philadelphia, Lippincott, Williams & Wilkins, 2003, p 85.
86. McCoy MC, Katz VL, Gould N, Kuller JA: Non-immune hydrops after 20 weeks' gestation: Review of 10 years' experience with suggestions for management. Obstet Gynecol 1995;85:578–582.
87. Smoleniec J, James D: Predictive value of pleural effusions in fetal hydrops. Fetal Diagn Ther 1995;10:95–100.
88. Castillo RA, Devoe LD, Hadi HA, et al: Non-immune hydrops fetalis: Clinical experience and factors related to a poor outcome. Am J Obstet Gynecol 1986;155:812–816.
89. Nakayama H, Kukita J, Hikino S, et al: Long-term outcome of 51 liveborn neonates with non-immune hydrops fetalis. Acta Paediatr 1999;88:24–28.
90. Haverkamp F, Noeker M, Gerresheim G, Fahnenstich H: Good prognosis for psychomotor development in survivors with non-immune hydrops fetalis. BJOG 2000;107: 282–284.

CHAPTER 26

Fetal Death

Carl P. Weiner

INTRODUCTION

The death of a fetus is a tragic loss. The known threat of an embryonic loss has passed, and both patient and caregiver are optimistic about the future. Whether the death occurs in a singleton or multiple gestation, it triggers a change in management and the patient's psychosocial needs. It also spurs a search for an explanation. The results of this search may be crucial for the successful management of any subsequent pregnancy.

MANAGEMENT OPTIONS

Evaluation

The investigation of a fetal death involves both the fetus and mother. It is essential to determine the cause of death whenever possible. Only then can the likelihood of a recurrence and the possibility of prevention be ascertained. Further, knowledge of the actual cause of death aids the grieving process by eliminating the natural tendency for self-recrimination. A thorough maternal past and current medical history should again be obtained and the physical examination repeated in search of an unsuspected preexisting or acquired systemic illness. If the fetus is still in utero, a targeted ultrasound examination of the uterus and contents is performed in search of fetal or placental malformations and evidence of fetal growth restriction.

The more common, known causes of fetal death are listed in Table 26–1. Over the last 30 years the fetal death rate has declined, and the causes of fetal death have changed.[1] For example, fetal death due to intrapartum asphyxia and Rh disease has all but disappeared in some centers, and the death rate from unexplained growth restriction has also declined.[1] Unless the history and physical examination pinpoint the cause, a basic group of laboratory tests (Table 26–2) should be performed until a cause is found. An amniocentesis to both search for fetal infection (see Chapter 10) and obtain a karyotype is recommended. A chromosome abnormality is the explanation in 15% of second-trimester stillbirths. The karyotype should be documented in most fetuses, even in the apparent absence of extrinsic structural malformations, because the usual dysmorphic features of aneuploidy may be obscured by postmortem changes. In contrast to fetal fascia, muscle, or subcutaneous tissue, amniocytes can be cultured successfully weeks after the death has occurred. Placental tissue is also more likely to be a viable source for karyotyping.

After delivery, photographs of the child are made for both the medical record and the parents. If the parents decline the photographs, a common grief/fear response, the photographs should be stored with the medical record in case the parents subsequently change their minds. A fetogram is made (xerography is an excellent modality) and permission requested for an autopsy. The performance of an autopsy significantly increases the likelihood of discovering a presumed cause.[2] Ideally, an individual with both an interest and experience in perinatal pathology should perform the autopsy. The placenta is an important component of that examination. The fetal organ cavities are cultured for both bacteria and viruses even if an infection workup was initiated antenatally. A growing understanding in the role of viral infection in poor fetal outcome suggests that in some instances, the search for an infectious etiology be coupled with a molecular biologic search for the nuclear fingerprint of the infectious agent. Maternal serology is, in general, not useful.[2]

Many stillborn fetuses are small for gestational age. However, customized fetal growth charts may be needed to demonstrate this because the use of preterm neonatal birth weight charts, derived from preterm newborns who are commonly growth restricted, may obscure this.[3] In the absence of another explanation, growth restriction increases the likelihood that severe placental dysfunction of some etiology is the explanation.[3]

TABLE 26–1

Causes of Fetal Death

Maternal systemic illness:
Diabetes mellitus
Hypertension—includes prepregnancy and pregnancy-associated connective tissue disorders
Any disorder causing septicemia with associated hypoperfusion—fetal malformations, structural and chromosomal
Fetal:
Infection—bacterial, viral
Fetal immune hemolytic disease
Cord accident—includes prolapse, thrombosis, strangulation
Bands or knots and torsion (likely to be greatly overdiagnosed)
Metabolic disorders
Placental dysfunction includes those associated with fetal growth restriction, postmaturity and abruption causing hypoxemia, placenta previa or infarction, twin-to-twin transfusion, fetal-to-maternal hemorrhage
Inherited disorders: thombophilias

Pregnancy Management

The approach to the pregnancy after a fetal loss depends on whether it is a single or multiple gestation, the gestational age at death, and the parents wishes.

Singleton Gestation

Prior to 15 weeks' gestation, a dilation and evacuation can be performed. This remains an option until 24 weeks, although the risk of maternal hemorrhage may be increased after fetal death.[4] Caution is indicated. The second and more common alternative after 15 weeks' gestation is an induction of labor. This has the advantage of preserving the fetus intact for a postmortem examination.

Prior to the introduction of prostaglandin analogues for the induction of labor, women were observed until the onset of spontaneous labor after a late demise. First, 90% or more of women with an intrauterine demise spontaneously labor within 3 weeks of its detection.[5,6] Second, oxytocin is frequently ineffective because of the associated early gestation. Consequently, prolonged induction time was the rule. Though the instillation of intra-amniotic hypertonic saline or glucose was said to shorten the time interval, it was also associated with several maternal deaths. Thus, despite the considerable social pressure for delivery, observation was the best medical approach.

The disadvantage to observation is that about a quarter of women who retain their dead fetus for 4 or more weeks (i.e., after 20 weeks' gestation) develop a chronic, consumptive coagulopathy. This is a true disseminated intravascular coagulopathy (DIC) state characterized by degrees of decreased fibrinogen, plasminogen, antithrombin III, and platelets and increased fibrin degradation products.[7–10] The etiology of the coagulopathy has never been conclusively determined. Using sensitive coagulation tests, pathologic activation of the clotting cascade is demonstrable within 48 hours of the demise. The incidence of the coagulopathy increases with the duration of the delay, but less than 2% of these women experience a hemorrhagic complication. Fortunately, this chronic, low-grade intravascular coagulopathy can be reversed by the administration of low-dose heparin.[11–13] Traditionally, labor was induced after treatment of the coagulopathy even if the cervix was unfavorable. The coagulopathy resolves within 48 hours of delivery.

Fortunately, the development of the prostaglandin E and F analogues for the induction of labor eliminated the need to wait. The efficacy of these agents for the induction of labor exceeds 90% (reviewed in Kochenour[14]). Delivery shortly after detection of the demise has several advantages. First, it brings an end to an emotionally painful event and allows the psychological healing process to begin. Second, any postmortem examination is more likely to yield useful information if done before the development of severe autolysis.

The various prostaglandin preparations may be administered via oral, vaginal, intracervical, extraovular, or intramuscular routes, depending on regional availability. Misoprostol (either per vaginam or by mouth) has a favorable cost profile and is at least as effective as other forms of prostaglandin. When used specifically for pregnancy termination in the second trimester, misoprostol administered orally is less effective (i.e., more failures) than the vaginal route (relative risk [RR] 3.00, 95% confidence interval [CI] 1.44 to 6.24), and side effects may be more common.[15] A commonly used dose is 400 μg every 6 to 8 hours. A priming dose of 800 μg per vaginam is also recommended.[5] Neither misoprostol nor prostaglandin E_2 (PGE_2) vaginal suppositories are yet approved by the U.S. Food and Drug Administration (FDA) for the termination of pregnancy after an intrauterine demise of a fetus older than 28 weeks. However,

TABLE 26–2

Routine Laboratory Evaluation and Follow-up of Fetal Death

Maternal (on detection)
Fasting blood glucose
Platelet count, fibrinogen
Indirect Coombs' test
Stain of a peripheral smear for fetal red blood cells (Kleihauer-Betke test)
Anticardiolipins, antinuclear antibodies, lupus anticoagulant
Fetal karyotype
Thrombophilia workup
Polymerase chain reaction studies of fetal products for evidence of viral infection
Amniotic fluid culture for cytomegalovirus, anaerobic and aerobic bacteria
Subsequent maternal weekly fibrinogen measurements and platelet counts if fetal death is of 4 weeks' duration or more
Fetal (at delivery)
Repeat infection workup (see Chapter 27)
Karyotype (if not done antenatally)
Postmortem examination
Fetogram (total body radiograph) if dysmorphic stigmata at postmortem examination

clinical experience supports both their reliability and safety.[14] Common complications include nausea and vomiting, fever, and tachycardia. Their prevalence is generally dependent on route of administration and dose and is greatly reduced by premedication.[17] Their use is further discussed in Chapter 68.

Multiple Gestation (See also Chapters 24 and 60)

The optimal management of the multiple gestation with a singleton demise is unclear. The incidence of this complication is low (<1% of all twin gestations), but the risk of prematurity, morbidity (especially neurologic), and neonatal death is high among antenatal survivors.[18,19] Several factors must be considered. First is the cause of death. Could the same stimulus, such as congenital infection or a maternal systemic illness, have caused a sublethal insult yielding a damaged survivor? If so, will continuation of the pregnancy worsen the outcome by prolonging the exposure? An informed decision requires knowledge of the cause and is a matter for individualization.

The second item to consider is whether the dead twin's continued presence poses a risk to the surviving twin. In monochorionic twin gestations, approximately half of the co-twins in an affected pregnancy will either die or experience serious morbidity[20] (see Chapter 24). Sequelae in survivors of monochorionic gestations with a single demise include bilateral renal cortical necrosis, multicystic encephalomalacia, gastrointestinal structural malformations, and even a disseminated intravascular coagulopathy.[21–26] It was previously suggested they result from the fetus-fetus transfer of necrotic, thromboplastic emboli through placental anastomoses. If this were true, delivery of the surviving twin as soon as possible would be prudent. However, there are no published reports of a fetal coagulopathy, and the evidence for necrotic emboli (as opposed to thrombotic phenomena) is weak. Further, the syndrome is also reported in monochorionic pregnancies uncomplicated by demise. Remembering that all monochorionic twins share placental vascular anastomoses, it seems more likely these sequelae share a vascular etiology. Most likely is an abrupt, hypotensive event either during the co-twin's death associated with extensive vascular anastomosis or after the death as the surviving twin acutely hemorrhages into the dead twin's placenta.[27] If this is, as it appears, the mechanism, preterm delivery may be too late to prevent the sequelae and may only add complications of prematurity. Thus, it seems prudent to observe the surviving co-twin very closely, if not continuously, for the first 7 days, should the gestation appear monochorionic. Survivors should be watched serially for evidence of multicystic encephalomalacia.

The course is clearer if the pregnancy is dizygotic because the risk of death to the surviving co-twin is less than 5%.[18] There is no reason for an iatrogenic delivery prior to 36 weeks solely for the indication of a dead co-twin.

The third and final concern after the death of a co-twin is the development of a maternal coagulopathy should the pregnancy continue. This is an uncommon but treatable event. Laboratory testing for hypofibrinogenemia and thrombocytopenia should be done biweekly after the first 4 weeks. Low-dose heparin, between 10,000 and 30,000 units given subcutaneously in divided doses, is usually adequate to reverse the hypofibrinogenemia.[28,29] There is no need to prolong the partial thromboplastin time. The amount of heparin necessary may seem quite high, reflecting the low antithrombin III concentration. Interestingly, the few reports suggest the need for heparin is temporary. It can usually be discontinued 6 to 8 weeks later without recurrence of the hypofibrinogenemia.[27–30]

Giving Bad News

Giving a patient bad news is one of the more difficult tasks most physicians face on a regular basis. Unfortunately, the act of teaching techniques for the breaking of bad news seem almost as awkward as the teaching of contraception must have been in the Victorian era. Yet, these techniques can be learned and applied in a busy clinical practice. The problem now is not whether it is necessary to tell the patient, but how to deliver it.

Why is it difficult to give bad news? There are a number of plausible explanations including the fear of causing pain, sympathetic pain, fear of being blamed for the poor outcome, fear of a therapeutic failure and all that it entails, fear of the medical-legal consequences, fear of eliciting a reaction, fear of saying "I don't know," and fear of expressing emotion.

Why are patients unhappy with the way they are given bad news? The most common complaints are that the physician is not listening, is using jargon, or is "talking down" to them. The process of informing a patient about bad news should follow the basic steps of the traditional medical interview: *prepare* for listening; *question*; *listen* actively; show verbally that you've *heard*; and *respond*. The necessary modifications and additions to the basic interview as they relate to fetal medicine include finding out how much the patient knows, how much misinformation must be corrected, and how much the patient wants to know before sharing the information in an unambiguous, plain-spoken fashion that minimizes the chance of denial; responding to the patient's feelings; and then presenting an appropriate action plan.

Perhaps the most difficult component of the interview arises when the patient starts reacting. It usually has begun by the time you enter the room. It is important to recall that people perceive bad news in a myriad of ways, some of which may not be clear to the health care provider. A mentally competent and informed patient has the right to accept or reject any treatment offered and to react to the news or express their feelings in any (legal) way they choose. Unexpected reactions often reflect a misunderstanding of the information presented. It is important to reinforce those parts of what the patient has said that are correct and then continue from there. Avoid jargon, use diagrams and written messages, and then look for evidence of understanding. Listen for and try to address the patient's concerns; do not dismiss them as irrelevant. Common reactions run the gamut and include disbelief, anger, blame, shock, guilt, denial, hope, despair, depression, displacement, fear and anxiety, crying, bargaining, awkward questions, relief, threats, and humor. There is no question that giving parents bad news tests the entire range of one's professional skills and abilities. But if it is done poorly, the family will never forgive. And if the interview is done well, they will never forget.

Parental Psychosocial Care

Many hospitals have a counselor or psychologist on the perinatal team to facilitate the grieving process. Frequently, there are local support groups consisting of women who have experienced an intrauterine demise. It may be helpful if a representative of one of these groups meets with the patient shortly after the diagnosis is made. Where appropriate, pastoral care may also be helpful. The woman's partner is encouraged to remain and provide support during labor and after delivery when the couple should be encouraged to view and hold the newborn. Too often, patients incorrectly assume they have conceived a monstrosity. They should also be informed that any bruising and facial marks are normal. Neonatal footprints and handprints are made, and the parents encouraged to name the child. Photographs are taken, and if the patient does not want any of these remembrance items, they should be stored. Many women change their mind and later write to request them.

Upon discharge from the hospital, the patient is given an appointment to return after an interval, which should be individualized to her needs. The results of all studies performed are reviewed and the parents given an opportunity to voice any questions they may have about their care.

Evaluation Prior to Conceiving Again

If the cause of death was ascertained, its implications (if any) to subsequent pregnancies should be discussed at their initial postpartum meeting, and again prior to conception if desired. The actions needed should be cause-specific. For example, the discovery of a maternal thrombophilia or connective tissue disorder coupled with the history of a prior stillbirth might warrant prophylactic anticoagulation (see Chapter 42). The practice of ordering a barrage of antenatal surveillance tests when the cause of death was not hypoxemia due to placental dysfunction cannot be supported. When the cause of death has escaped detection, it is important to again reinforce to both parents that these events are not usually under their control and that they bear no guilt for its occurrence.

CONCLUSIONS

- Death of a fetus, whether anticipated or not, inevitable or not is a tragedy
- The first and ongoing priority in management is emotional and psychological support of the parents and family
- The second priority is to find an explanation
- The third priority is to implement an appropriate management strategy for future pregnancies

SUMMARY OF MANAGEMENT OPTIONS
Fetal Death

Management Options—For Singleton Pregnancy Unless Stated Otherwise	Quality of Evidence	Strength of Recommendation	References
Singleton Fetal Death			
Psychosocial Support	III	B	31
	IV	C	32
Investigate for a Cause:	III	B	32–37
Maternal	IV	C	32
Fetal (see Tables 26–1 and 26–2)	IV	C	32
Screen for Maternal Coagulopathy			
if death of 4 weeks' duration or more	III	B	7–10

SUMMARY OF MANAGEMENT OPTIONS
Fetal Death *(Continued)*

Management Options—for singleton pregnancy unless stated otherwise	Quality of Evidence	Strength of Recommendation	References
Singleton Fetal Death—*Continued*			
Empty Uterus (see also Chapter 68)			
many options:			
<13–15 Weeks			
vacuum evacuation/curettage	–	GPP	–
oral mifepristone followed by oral or vaginal prostaglandin 48h later	Ia/Ib	A	15,40
13/15–22 Weeks			
Ripen cervix with laminaria and:	–	GPP	–
dilatation and evacuation (not been formally compared to contemporary medical methods but safer in comparison to older methods)	III	B	42
or			
high dose oxytocin induction	III	B	38
Prostaglandin E_2 vaginal pessaries	III	B	38
Oral mifepristone followed by oral or vaginal prostaglandin 48h later. This regimen may need to be supplemented by oxytocin infusion	Ib	A	40
Misoprostol is very effective.	Ib	A	16,40,41
22–28 Weeks			
Ripen cervix with laminaria and	–	GPP	–
oxytocin induction	III	B	38
Prostaglandin E_2 vaginal pessaries with oxytocin augmentation	III	B	17,39
Oral mifepristone followed by oral or vaginal prostaglandin 48h later. This regimen may need to be supplemented by oxytocin infusion	Ib	A	40
Misoprostol is very effective.	Ib	A	16,40,41
>28 Weeks			
Cervix favorable:	IV	C	14
oxytocin induction			
Cervix unfavorable:			
ripen cervix with low dose prostaglandin E_2 vaginal suppositories or misoprostol *without* concurrent oxytocin			
Overall vaginal prostaglandin E_2 is superior to oxytocin at inducing labor	Ia	A	43,44
Single Fetal Death in Twin Pregnancy		See Chapters 24 and 60	

REFERENCES

1. Fretts RC, Boyd ME, Usher RH, Usher HA: The changing pattern of fetal death, 1961–1988. Obstet Gynecol 1992;79: 35–39.
2. Incerpi MH, Miller DA, Samadi R, et al: Stillbirth evaluation: What tests are needed? Am J Obstet Gynecol 1998;178: 1121–1125.
3. Gardosi J, Mul T, Mongelli M, Fagan D: Analysis of birthweight and gestational age in antepartum stillbirths. Br J Obstet Gynaecol 1998;105:524–530.
4. Gerl D, Noschel H: Course of delivery in intrauterine fetal death with special reference to blood loss. Zentralb Gynakol 1968;90:1463–1466.

5. Dippel AL: Death of foetus in utero. Johns Hopkins Med J 1934;54:24–34.
6. Tricomi V, Kohl SG: Fetal death in utero. Am J Obstet Gynecol 1957;74:1092–1098.
7. Weiner AE, Read DE, Roby CC, Diamond LK: Coagulation defects with intrauterine death from Rh isoimmunization. Am J Obstet Gynecol 1950;60:1015–1018.
8. Pritchard JA: Fetal death in utero. Obstet Gynecol 1959;14:573–580.
9. Pritchard JA, Ratnoff OD: Studies of fibrinogen and other hemostatic factors in women with intrauterine death and delayed delivery. Surg Gynecol Obstet 1955;101:467–473.
10. Goldstein DP, Reid DE: Circulating fibrinolytic activity—A precursor of hypofibrinogenemia following fetal death in utero. Obstet Gynecol 1963;22:174–181.
11. Lerner R, Margolin M, Slate WG, et al: Heparin in the treatment of hypofibrinogenemia complicating fetal death in utero. Am J Obstet Gynecol 1967;97:373–381.
12. Jimenez JM, Prichard JA: Pathogenesis and treatment of coagulation defects resulting from fetal death. Obstet Gynecol 1968;32:449–459.
13. Waxman B, Gambrill R: Use of heparin in disseminated intravascular coagulation. Am J Obstet Gynecol 1972;112:434–439.
14. Kochenour NK: Management of fetal demise. Clinical Obstet Gynecol 1987;30:322–330.
15. Kulier R, Gulmezoglu A, Hofmeyr G, et al: Medical methods for first trimester abortion. Cochrane Database Syst Rev 2004;1:CD002855.
16. Feldman DM, Borgida AF, Rodis JF, et al: A randomized comparison of two regimens of misoprostol for second-trimester pregnancy termination. Am J Obstet Gynecol 2003;189:710–713.
17. Lauersen NH, Cederqvist LL, Wilson KH: Management of intrauterine death with prostaglandin E2 vaginal suppositories. Am J Obstet Gynecol 1980;137:753–764.
18. Hagay ZJ, Mazor M, Leiberman JR, Biale Y: Management and outcome of multiple pregnancies complicated by the antenatal death of one fetus. J Reprod Med 1986;31:717–720.
19. Litschgi M, Stucki D: Course of twin pregnancies after fetal death in utero. Z Geburtshilfe Perinatol 1980;184:227–239.
20. van Heteren CF, Nijhuis JG, Semmekrot BA, et al: Risk for surviving twin after fetal death of co-twin in twin-twin transfusion syndrome. Obstet Gynecol 1998;92:215–219.
21. Reisman LE, Pathak A: Bilateral renal necrosis in the newborn. Am J Dis Child 1966;111:541–555.
22. Moore CM, McAdams AJ, Sutherland J: Intrauterine disseminated coagulation: A syndrome with multiple pregnancy with a dead twin fetus. Pediatrics 1969;74:523–528.
23. Melnick M: Brain damage in a survivor after in utero death of monozygous co-twin. Lancet 1977;ii:1287–1289.
24. Yoshioka H, Kadomoto Y, Mino M, et al: Multicystic encephalomalacia in liveborn twin with a stillborn macerated co-twin. J Pediatr 1979;95:79.
25. Fusi L, Gordon H: Twin pregnancy complicated by single intrauterine death. Problems and outcome with conservative management. Br J Obstet Gynaecol 1990;97:511–516.
26. Anderson RL, Golbus MS, Curry CJ, et al: Central nervous system damage and other anomalies in surviving fetus following second trimester antenatal death of co-twin. Report of four cases and a review of the literature. Prenat Diagn 1990;10:513–518.
27. Fusi L, McParland P, Fisk N, et al: Acute twin-twin transfusion: A possible mechanism for brain-damaged survivors after intrauterine death of a monochorionic twin. Obstet Gynecol 1991;78:517.
28. Skelly H, Marivate M, Normal R, et al: Consumptive coagulopathy following fetal death in a triplet pregnancy. Am J Obstet Gynecol 1982;142:595–601.
29. Romero R, Duffy TP, Berkowitz RL, et al: Prolongation of a preterm pregnancy complicated by death of a single twin in utero and disseminated intravascular coagulation. N Engl J Med 1984;310:772–774.
30. Levine W, Rosengart M, Siegler A: Spontaneous correction of hypofibrinogenemia with fetal death in utero. Obstet Gynecol 1962;19:551–555.
31. Schapp AHP: Long-term impact of perinatal bereavement. Comparison of grief reactions after intrauterine versus neonatal death. Eur J Obstet Gynecol Reprod Biol 1997;75:161–167.
32. Pitkin RM: Fetal death: Diagnosis and management. Am J Obstet Gynecol 1987;157:583–589.
33. Saller DN, Lesser KB, Harrel U, Rogers B, Oya CE: The clinical utility of the perinatal autopsy. JAMA 1995;273:663–665.
34. Ahlenius I, Floberg, J, Thomassen, P: Sixty-six cases of intrauterine fetal death. Acta Obstet Gynecol Scand 1995;74: 109–117.
35. Ogunyemi D, Jackson, U, Buyske, S, Risk, A: Clinical and pathologic correlates of stillbirths in a single institution. Acta Obstet Gynecol Scand 1998;77:722–728.
36. Maslow AD, Breen TW, Sarna MC, Soni AK, Watkins J, Oriol NE: Prevalence of coagulation abnormalities associated with intrauterine fetal death. Can J Anaesth 1996;43:1237–1243.
37. Pauli RM, Reiser CA: Wisconsin stillbirth service program II. Analysis of diagnosis and diagnostic categories in the first 1,000 referrals. Am J Med Genet 1994;50:135–153.
38. Winkler CL, Gray SE, Hauth JC, Owen J, Tucker JM: Mid-second trimester labor induction: concentrated oxytocin compared with prostaglandin E_2 vaginal suppositories. Obstet Gynecol 1991;77:297–300.
39. Scher J, Jeng DY, Moshirpur Kerenyi, TD: A comparison between vaginal prostaglandin E_2 suppositories and intrauterine extra-amniotic prostaglandins in the management of fetal death. Am J Obstet Gynecol 1980;137:769–772.
40. Rodger MW, Baird DT: Pretreatment with mifepristone (RU 486) reduces interval between prostaglandin administration and expulsion in second trimester abortion. Br J Obstet Gynaecol 1990;97:41–45.
41. Frydman R, Fernandez H, Pons JC, Ulmann A: Mifepristone (RU486) and therapeutic late pregnancy termination: a double-blind study of two different doses. Hum Reprod 1988;3:803–806.
42. Peterson WF, Berry FN, Grace MR, Gulbranson CL: Second-trimester abortion by dilatation and evacuation: an analysis of 11,747 cases. Obstet Gynecol 1983;62:185–190.
43. Tan BP, Hannah ME. Prostaglandins versus oxytocin for prelabour rupture of membranes at term. Cochrane Database Syst Rev 2001;3
44. Tan BP, Hannah ME: Prostaglandins for prelabour rupture of membranes at or near term. Cochrane Database Syst Rev 2001;3

SECTION FOUR

Infection

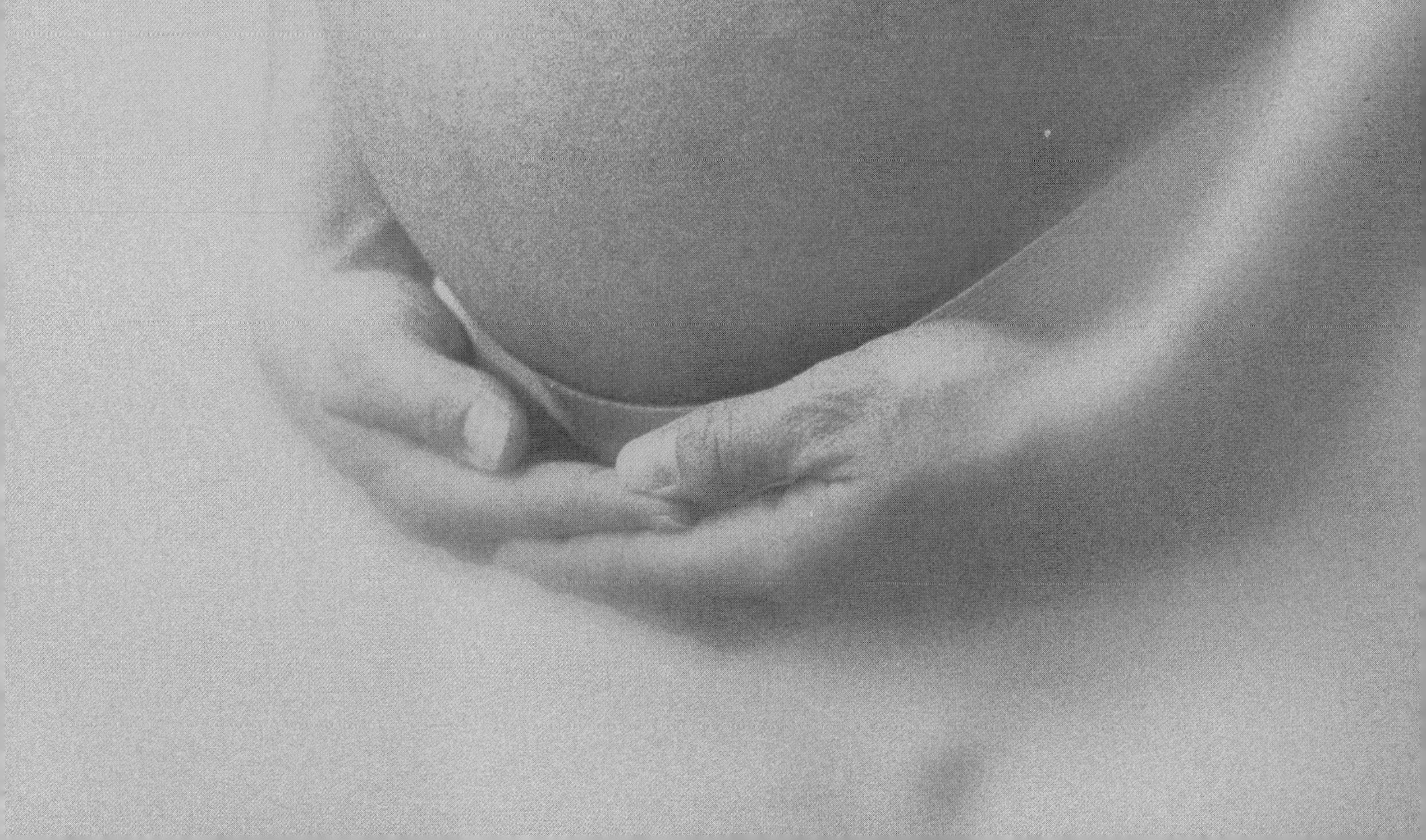

CHAPTER 27

Intrauterine Infection, Preterm Parturition, and the Fetal Inflammatory Response Syndrome

Luís F. Gonçalves / Tinnakorn Chaiworapongsa / Roberto Romero

INTRODUCTION

Infection has long been recognized as an important and frequent cause of preterm parturition.[1–8] Indeed, it is the only pathologic process for which both a firm causal link with prematurity has been established and a defined molecular pathophysiology is known.[9] Moreover, fetal infection/inflammation has been implicated in the genesis of fetal and neonatal injury[10,11] leading to cerebral palsy[12] and chronic lung disease.[13] In this chapter, we review the pathways of intrauterine infection, the microbiology and frequency of intra-amniotic infection, the fetal inflammatory response syndrome, and the contribution of fetal infection to short- and long-term neonatal morbidity. We conclude with the potential role of viral infection in adverse outcomes.

PATHWAYS OF INTRAUTERINE INFECTION

Microorganisms may gain access to the amniotic cavity and fetus using any of the following pathways: (1) ascending from the vagina and the cervix, (2) hematogenous dissemination through the placenta (transplacental infection), (3) retrograde seeding from the peritoneal cavity through the fallopian tubes, and (4) accidental introduction at the time of invasive procedures such as amniocentesis, cordocentesis, chorionic villus sampling, or shunting.[14–18] The most common pathway for intrauterine infection is the ascending route.[7,14,15,18] Evidence in support of this includes the following: (1) histologic chorioamnionitis is more common and severe at the site of membrane rupture than at other locations, such as the placental chorionic plate or umbilical cord[19]; (2) in virtually all cases of congenital pneumonia (stillbirths or neonatal), inflammation of the chorioamniotic membranes is present[14,16,18]; (3) bacteria identified in cases of congenital infections are similar to those found in the lower genital tract[15]; and (4) in twin gestations, histologic chorioamnionitis is more common in the firstborn twin and has not been demonstrated only in the second twin. This is taken as evidence favoring ascending infection, as the membranes of the first twin are generally opposed to the cervix.[15] This observation is consistent with those made during the course of microbiologic studies of the amniotic fluid in twin gestations. When infection is present, the presenting sac is always involved.[20]

STAGES OF ASCENDING INTRAUTERINE INFECTION

Ascending intrauterine infection has four stages (Fig. 27–1).[7] Stage I consists of a change in the vaginal/cervical microbial flora or the presence of pathologic organisms (i.e., *Neisseria gonorrhoeae*) in the cervix. Some forms of aerobic vaginitis[21] may be an early manifestation of this stage. Once microorganisms gain access to the intrauterine cavity, they reside in the decidua (stage II). A localized inflammatory reaction causes deciduitis initially and then chorionitis. Microorganisms may then reside in the chorion and amnion. The infection may invade the fetal vessels (choriovasculitis) or proceed through the amnion (amnionitis) into the amniotic cavity (stage III). Rupture of the membranes is not a prerequisite for intra-amniotic infection, as microorganisms are capable of

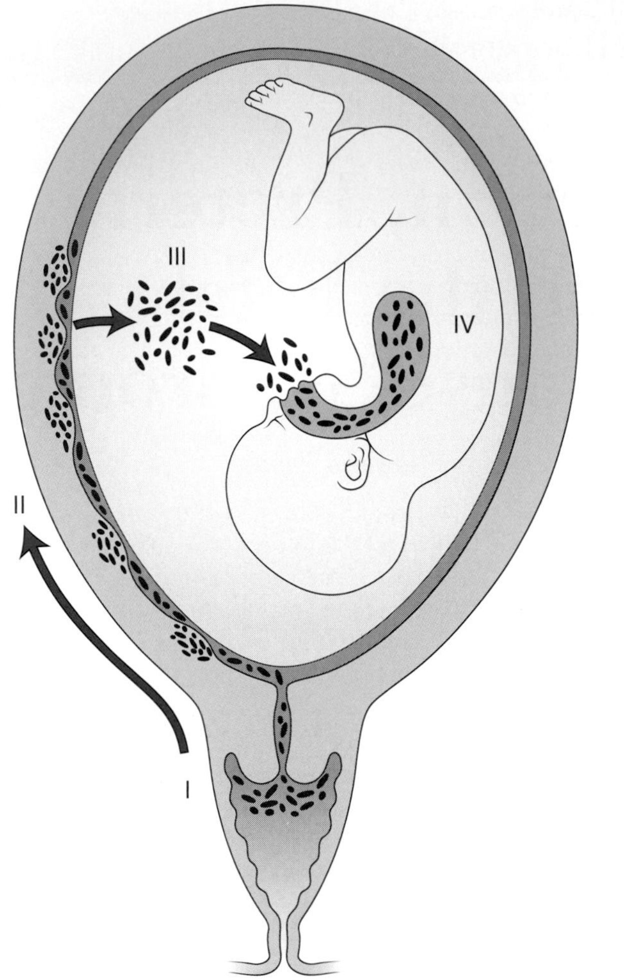

FIGURE 27–1
The stages of ascending infection (From Romero R, Mazor M: Infection and preterm labor: Pathways for intrauterine infections. Clin Obstet Gynecol 1988;31:558).

crossing intact membranes.[22] Once in the amniotic cavity, the bacteria may gain access to the fetus by several ports of entry (stage IV). Aspiration of the infected fluid by the fetus may cause congenital pneumonia. Otitis, conjunctivitis, and omphalitis are localized infections that occur by direct seeding of the microorganisms from infected amniotic fluid. Seeding from any of these sites to the fetal circulation results in bacteremia and sepsis.

The last stage of ascending intrauterine infection is fetal microbial invasion. Clinical and experimental evidence is now available that suggests that the fetus is exposed to microorganisms and their products (i.e., bacterial endotoxin)[23,24] in the amniotic cavity and then responds by mounting both a cellular and humoral immunoresponse.[25,26]

MICROBIOLOGY OF INTRAUTERINE INFECTION

The most common microbial isolates from the amniotic cavity of women with preterm labor and intact membranes are *Ureaplasma urealyticum*, *Fusobacterium* spp., and *Mycoplasma hominis*.[7,27–30] In patients with premature rupture of membranes (PROM), microbial invasion of the amniotic cavity by *U. urealyticum* is associated with a robust inflammatory response in the fetal, amniotic, and maternal compartments.[31] *U. urealyticum* is implicated in the genesis of clinical chorioamnionitis, puerperal endometritis, postoperative wound infections, neonatal sepsis, meningitis, and bronchopulmonary dysplasia.[31–33]

Other microorganisms found in the amniotic fluid include *Streptococcus agalactiae*, *Peptostreptococcus* spp., *Staphylococcus aureus*, *Gardnerella vaginalis*, *Streptococcus viridans*, and *Bacteroides* spp. Occasionally, *Lactobacillus* spp., *Escherichia coli*, *Enterococcus faecalis*, *N. gonorrhoeae*, and *Peptococcus* spp. are encountered. *Haemophilus influenzae*, *Capnocytophaga* spp., *Stomatococcus* spp., and *Clostridium* spp. are rarely identified.[34,35] In 50% of patients with microbial invasion, more than one microorganism is isolated from the amniotic cavity. The inoculum size varies considerably, and in 71% of the cases more than 10^5 colony-forming units per milliliter (cfu/mL) are found.[19]

FREQUENCY OF INTRA-AMNIOTIC INFECTION IN PRETERM GESTATION

Studies examining the clinical circumstances surrounding preterm delivery indicate that one third of all patients present with preterm labor and intact membranes and one third with preterm PROM. The remaining third are the result of delivery for maternal or fetal indications (e.g., preeclampsia, growth restriction).[36–39] We review the evidence supporting an association between intrauterine infection and spontaneous preterm labor (with or without intact membranes) to examine the relationship between microbial invasion of the amniotic cavity and preterm delivery.

Microbial Invasion of the Amniotic Cavity in Preterm Labor and Intact Membranes

The mean rate of positive amniotic fluid cultures for microorganisms in patients with preterm labor and intact membranes is approximately 12.8% (379/2963), based on a review of 33 studies.[30,40] Women with positive amniotic fluid cultures generally do not have clinical evidence of infection at presentation but are more likely to develop clinical chorioamnionitis (37.5% [60/160] vs. 9% [27/301]), be refractory to tocolysis (85.6% [101/118] vs. 16.3% [8/49]), and rupture their membranes spontaneously (40% [6/15] vs. 3.8% [2/52]) than women with negative amniotic fluid cultures. Several investigators have demonstrated higher rates of complications in neonates born to women with microbial invasion of the amniotic cavity than to those without infection.[28] Moreover, the earlier the gestational age at birth, the more likely microbial invasion of the amniotic cavity is present.[41]

Microbial Invasion of the Amniotic Cavity in Patients with Preterm PROM

The rate of positive amniotic fluid cultures for microorganisms is approximately 32.4% (47/142) in patients with preterm PROM.[30] Clinical chorioamnionitis is present in only 29.7% (49/165) of those with proven microbial invasion.[9,30] The rate of microbial invasion in preterm PROM is probably an underestimation of the true prevalence and reflects in part the sophisticated facilities required to make this determination. Further, available evidence indicates that women with PROM and a severely reduced volume of amniotic fluid have a higher incidence of intra-amniotic infection than those without oligohydramnios.[42,43] Since women with oligohydramnios are less likely to have an amniocentesis, there is an inherent bias to underestimate the prevalence of infection. Another bias stems from the fact that women with preterm PROM admitted in labor do not generally undergo amniocentesis. These patients have a higher rate of microbial invasion of the amniotic cavity than those admitted without labor (39% [24/61] vs. 25% [41/160], $p < 0.05$). Finally, 75% of women who are not in labor on admission have a positive amniotic fluid culture at the time of the onset of labor.[44] Clearly, studies restricted to women not in labor provide a lower rate of microbial invasion of the amniotic cavity than those including patients in labor.

Microbial Invasion of the Amniotic Cavity in Patients Presenting with Acute Cervical Incompetence

Women presenting with a dilated cervix, intact membranes, and few, if any, contractions before the 24th week are considered to have clinical cervical incompetence. In one study, 51.1% of these patients had a positive amniotic fluid culture for microorganisms.[45] The outcome of patients with microbial invasion was uniformly poor because these individuals developed subsequent complications (rupture of membranes, clinical chorioamnionitis, or pregnancy loss). Therefore, infection is frequently associated with acute cervical incompetence.[46] Whether intra-amniotic inflammation is the cause or consequence of cervical dilation remains unknown. It is possible that clinically silent cervical dilation with protrusion of the membranes into the vagina leads to a secondary intrauterine infection.

Microbial invasion of the amniotic cavity occurs in 11.9% of twin gestations presenting with preterm labor and delivering a preterm neonate.[20] This finding is in contrast to the 21.6% culture positive rate in singleton gestations with preterm labor and delivery.[19] These data suggest that intra-amniotic infection is a possible cause of preterm labor and delivery in twin gestation, but does not support the hypothesis that intra-amniotic infection is responsible for a large part of the excessive rate of preterm delivery observed.

Chorioamniotic Infection, Histologic Chorioamnionitis, and Preterm Birth

Inflammation of the placenta and chorioamniotic membranes is a nonspecific host response to a variety of stimuli, including infection. Acute inflammation of the chorioamniotic membranes has traditionally been considered an indicator of amniotic fluid infection,[14–18,47–49] a view based on indirect evidence. In the context of preterm birth, this seems reasonable. Several studies demonstrate an association between acute inflammatory lesions of the placenta and the recovery of microorganisms from the subchorionic plate[50,51] and chorioamniotic space.[47] Bacteria were recovered from the subchorionic plate of 72% of placentas with histologic evidence of chorioamnionitis.[47,50,52] Furthermore, there is a strong correlation between positive amniotic fluid cultures for microorganisms and histologic chorioamnionitis.[48,49] Cassell and colleagues reported an association between positive microbial cultures obtained from the chorioamniotic interface and histologic chorioamnionitis.[32,53] The presence of inflammation in the umbilical cord (funisitis) represents evidence of a fetal inflammatory response.[54,55] In contrast, histologic chorioamnionitis reflects a maternal inflammatory response.

Several studies investigated the prevalence of inflammation in placentas from women delivering preterm infants. Collectively, the evidence indicates an association between preterm birth and the occurrence of acute chorioamnionitis; it also indicates that the lower the gestational age at birth, the higher the frequency of histologic chorioamnionitis and funisitis.[52]

Fetal Infection

The most advanced stage of ascending intrauterine infection is fetal infection (stage IV) (see Fig. 27–1). The overall mortality rate of neonates with congenital neonatal sepsis ranges from 25% to 90%.[56–63] The wide range may reflect the effect of gestational age on the likelihood of survival. In one study, which focused on infants born before 33 weeks' gestation, the mortality rate was 33% for infected and 17% for noninfected fetuses.[63] Carroll and coworkers reported fetal bacteremia in 33% of fetuses with positive amniotic fluid culture and in 4% of those with negative amniotic fluid culture.[64] Clearly, subclinical fetal infection is far more common than traditionally recognized.

INTRAUTERINE INFECTION/ INFLAMMATION AS A CHRONIC PROCESS

Although intrauterine infection is traditionally considered an acute complication of pregnancy, accumulating evidence suggests that it may be a chronic condition. The evidence in support of this view is derived from studies of the microbiologic state of the amniotic fluid, as well as the concentration of inflammatory mediators at the time of genetic amniocentesis.

Microbial Invasion of the Amniotic Cavity at the Time of Genetic Amniocentesis

Cassel and colleagues[32] recovered genital mycoplasmas from 6.6% (4/61) of amniotic fluid samples collected by amniocentesis between 16 and 21 weeks. Two cultures were positive for *M. hominis* and two for *U. urealyticum*. Patients contaminated with *M. hominis* delivered at 34 and 40 weeks without neonatal complications, whereas those with *U. urealyticum* had premature delivery, sepsis, and neonatal death at 24 and 29 weeks. Subsequently, Gray and colleagues[65] reported a 0.37% prevalence (9/2461) of positive cultures for *M. hominis* or *U. urealyticum* in amniotic fluid samples obtained at the time of second-trimester genetic amniocentesis. Except for one individual who had a therapeutic abortion, all patients (8/8) with a positive amniotic fluid culture had either a fetal loss within 4 weeks of the amniocentesis ($n = 6$) or preterm delivery ($n = 2$). Furthermore, all had histologic evidence of chorioamnionitis. These observations suggest that microbial invasion may be clinically silent in the midtrimester of pregnancy and that pregnancy loss/preterm delivery can take weeks to occur. Similar observations are reported by Horowitz and coworkers,[66] who detected *U. urealyticum* in 2.8% (6/214) of amniotic fluid samples obtained between 16 and 20 weeks' gestation. The rate of adverse pregnancy outcome (fetal loss, preterm delivery, and low birth weight) was significantly higher in patients with a positive amniotic fluid culture than in those with a negative culture (3/6 [50%] vs. 15/123 [12%], $p = 0.035$). Of note, women with a positive amniotic fluid culture were more likely to have an obstetric history that included >3 previous abortions than those with a negative culture (2/6 [33.3%] vs. 5/123 [4.0%]), $p = 0.034$).[66]

Chronic Intra-amniotic Inflammation/Infection and Preterm Birth

Amniotic fluid interleukin-6 (IL-6) concentration is a marker of intra-amniotic inflammation and is frequently associated with microbiologic infection in either the amniotic fluid or chorioamniotic space.[67–70] Romero and colleagues[71] conducted a case-control study in which IL-6 was measured in the stored amniotic fluid of women who had a pregnancy loss after a midtrimester amniocentesis and compared them to a control group who delivered at term. Patients who lost their pregnancies had a significantly higher median amniotic fluid IL-6 concentration than those with a normal outcome. Similar findings were reported by Wenstrom and colleagues.[72] In contrast, maternal plasma IL-6 concentration is not associated with adverse pregnancy outcome. Chaiworapongsa and colleagues[73] compared amniotic fluid monocyte chemotactic protein-1 (MCP-1) concentration at the time of genetic amniocentesis in 10 patients who had a pregnancy loss after the procedure to a control group of 84 patients. MCP-1 concentrations were higher among those who had a spontaneous pregnancy loss after the procedure compared to those with a normal pregnancy outcome. An amniotic fluid MCP-1 concentration >765 pg/mL was strongly associated with pregnancy loss (odds ratio, 7.35; 95% confidence interval, 1.7–31.0).

An association can also be demonstrated between markers of inflammation in the midtrimester amniotic fluid of asymptomatic women and preterm delivery. The concentrations of matrix metalloproteinase (MMP-8),[74] IL-6,[75] tumor necrosis factor alpha (TNFα),[76] angiogenin,[77] and C-reactive protein[78] in amniotic fluid samples obtained at midtrimester amniocentesis were each elevated in patients who subsequently delivered preterm.

Collectively, the evidence suggests that a chronic intra-amniotic inflammatory process is associated with both spontaneous abortion and spontaneous preterm delivery. Whether intra-amniotic inflammation is detectable noninvasively remains to be determined. Goldenberg and colleagues[79] demonstrated that the maternal plasma concentration of granulocyte colony-stimulating factor (G-CSF) at 24 and 28 weeks' gestation was associated with early preterm birth. To the extent that G-CSF may reflect an inflammatory process, this finding suggests that a chronic inflammatory process identifiable in the maternal compartment is associated with early preterm birth.

Is the Relationship Between Intrauterine Infection and Spontaneous Premature Birth Causal?

An association does not mean infection *causes* preterm delivery. Indeed, it has been argued that microbial invasion of the amniotic cavity is merely a consequence of labor.[80–83] Determining whether or not this relationship is causal is critical because it has major clinical and therapeutic implications. The evidence supporting a causal role for infection in preterm parturition includes: (1) biologic plausibility, (2) temporal relationship, (3) consistency and strength of association, (4) dose-response gradient, (5) specificity, and (6) human experimentation.

Animal experimentation reveals that the administration of bacterial products or microorganisms to pregnant animals can lead to premature labor and delivery.[84–93] Three sets of observations suggest that infection precedes the spontaneous onset of preterm labor and delivery: (1) subclinical microbial invasion of the amniotic cavity or intrauterine inflammation in the midtrimester of pregnancy leads to either spontaneous abortion or premature delivery (see preceding section on intrauterine inflammation/infection as a chronic process); (2) patients with preterm PROM who had a positive amniotic fluid culture for mycoplasmas (*U. urealyticum* or *M. hominis*, neither of which are visible on Gram stain) on admission have a significantly shorter amniocentesis-to-delivery interval than those with sterile amniotic fluid, suggesting that patients with preterm PROM and microbial invasion of the amniotic cavity are more likely to initiate preterm labor than those with a negative amniotic fluid culture[94]; and (3) abnormal colonization of the lower genitourinary tract with microorganisms is a risk factor for preterm delivery. These conditions include asymptomatic bacteriuria, bacterial vaginosis, and infection with *N. gonorrhoeae*.[95–106] The consistency and strength of association between infection and preterm delivery is demonstrated by the many studies in which amniotic fluid was cultured for microorganisms in women with preterm PROM and preterm labor with intact membranes. Moreover, the relative risk for preterm delivery in patients with preterm labor and intact membranes and microbial invasion of the amniotic cavity is high (>2) and the hazard ratio for the duration of pregnancy after preterm PROM is also high.

The likelihood of a causal relationship is increased if a dose-response gradient can be demonstrated. Is there a dose-response gradient between the severity of the infection and the likelihood of preterm delivery? Evidence supporting the existence of this gradient includes: (1) The median concentration of bacterial endotoxin is higher in patients in preterm labor than in patients not in labor.[107] (2) The microbial inoculum is significantly greater in patients with preterm PROM admitted with preterm labor than in those admitted with preterm PROM but not in labor.[44] Specifically, the proportion of patients with an inoculum $<10^5$ cfu/mL was 41.6% in patients with preterm labor and only 15% in patients not in labor ($p = 0.03$).[44] (3) Lastly, the rate of abortion/preterm delivery after the administration of *E. coli* bacterial endotoxin to pregnant mice exhibits a clear dose-response gradient.

One criterion for causality that is not met is specificity. Although intrauterine infection appears sufficient to induce preterm labor and delivery, it is not specific because many patients have a preterm delivery in the absence of evidence of intrauterine infection/inflammation. However, a high degree of specificity is rare in biologic systems. Although the causal relationship between smoking and lung cancer is widely accepted, it is also nonspecific. Lung cancer occurs in nonsmokers and, of course, smoking can cause diseases other than lung cancer, such as emphysema and chronic bronchitis. Second, the formulation of "the necessary and sufficient cause" can inappropriately restrict the conceptualization of cause. In the case of premature labor, microbiologic, cytologic, biochemical, immunologic, and pathologic data indicate that preterm labor is a syndrome and infection is but one of its causes.[9,108]

An important criterion for causation is whether eradication of the agent decreases the frequency of outcome or illness. Many trials of antimicrobial treatment for the prevention of preterm birth have been conducted. There is evidence that treatment of patients with asymptomatic bacteriuria will reduce the rate of prematurity/low birth weight[103] and that antibiotic treatment of patients with preterm PROM prolongs the latency period and reduces the rate of maternal and neonatal infection.[109] However, treatment of patients with preterm labor and intact membranes has not yielded positive results in most trials.[110–112] The reasons for this are complex and have been reviewed elsewhere but are probably related to the syndromic nature of preterm parturition, the chronic nature of the process, and the inclusion in the clinical trials of many patients who do not have intrauterine infection and thus cannot benefit from antimicrobial treatment. This applies to patients presenting with preterm labor as well as those with bacterial vaginosis.[113,114]

Detection of Microbial Footprints in the Amniotic Fluid with Sequence Based Techniques

Estimates of the frequency and type of microorganisms participating in intrauterine infections are based on standard microbiologic techniques (e.g., culture). These estimates are likely to change with the introduction of more sensitive methods for microbial recovery and identification. For example, surveys of terrestrial and aquatic ecosystems indicate that more than 99% of existing microorganisms may not be cultivated in the laboratory and that only molecular diagnosis can provide identification of these microorganisms.[115] In fact, the identification of the infectious agents for the following disorders became possible only recently with the aid of molecular diagnosis: hepatitis C virus for non-A, non-B hepatitis[116]; *Bartonella henselae* for bacillary angiomatosis[117]; *Tropheryma whippelii* for Whipple's disease[115,118]; and Sin Nombre virus for hantavirus pulmonary syndrome.[119]

Sequenced-based methodologies are likely to demonstrate how insensitive conventional microbiology methods are for the detection of already known and potentially "new" microorganisms in perinatal medicine. However, application of these techniques to clinical practice poses clinical, technologic, and conceptual questions and challenges. For example, when does the detection of microbial footprints in a biologic fluid by sequence-based methods represent true microbial invasion rather than contamination? What criteria should be used to determine causality between the presence of a microorganism and an infectious disease, as it is now possible to identify with sequence-based methods bacteria that cannot be cultured in diseased tissues and therefore, Koch's postulates cannot be met?[120]

These questions were explored in two studies[121,122] comparing the outcome of patients in preterm PROM or preterm labor with intact membranes who had cultures and polymerase chain reaction (PCR) performed for

U. urealyticum. Patients with microbial invasion of the amniotic cavity with *U. urealyticum*, as determined by sequence-based methods for microbial detection, had adverse outcomes with the same frequency as patients with positive amniotic fluid cultures.[121,122]

Two strategies have been used to detect microorganisms in the amniotic fluid with PCR. The first, also known as broad-range PCR, uses primer pairs designed to anneal with highly conserved DNA regions of all bacteria, such as the 16S ribosomal DNA. A positive result indicates the presence of bacteria, but identification of the specific organism requires subsequent sequencing of the PCR products. The second approach is to use specific primers for a particular microorganism. At the time of this writing, three studies used primers for the conserved sequence,[35,123,124] five used specific primers to recover bacterial DNA from amniotic fluid,[121,122,125–127] while one applied both approaches.[128]

Blanchard and colleagues[125] were the first to report the recovery of *U. urealyticum* from amniotic fluid samples using specific primers for the urease structural genes. They collected 293 amniotic fluid samples by amniocentesis at cesarean section. The samples were cultured for bacteria, mycoplasmas, and chlamydia and had PCR performed for *U. urealyticum*. Among the 10 PCR-positive amniotic fluid samples, only 4 were also culture-positive. Subsequently, Jalava and colleagues,[123] Hitti and colleagues,[35] and Markenson and colleagues[124] applied broad-spectrum bacterial 16S rDNA PCR for the detection of bacteria in the amniotic fluid. Jalava and coworkers[123] studied 20 amniotic fluid samples from patients with PROM and 16 control samples: PCR detected five microorganisms (*U. urealyticum* [n = 2], *H. influenzae* [n = 1], *Streptococcus oralis* [n = 1], and *Fusobacterium* spp. [n = 1]), but only two were positive in a routine bacterial culture. The two patients who developed infectious complications were correctly identified by PCR, and amniotic fluid glucose levels were lower in PCR-positive compared to PCR-negative patients. Hitti and coworkers[35] studied 69 women in preterm labor with intact membranes. PCR was positive in 94% of the culture-positive amniotic fluid samples (15/16) and in 36% of the patients with a negative culture. Five of the 14 women with an elevated IL-6 concentration had bacteria detected by PCR. In Markenson's study,[124] 55.5% of the amniotic fluid samples from 54 women in preterm labor but no clinical evidence of infection were PCR-positive, whereas only 9.2% of the cultures recovered a microorganism ($p < 0.05$). Two thirds (6/9) of the amniotic fluid samples with an elevated IL-6 were also PCR-positive.

Oyarzun and colleagues[126] described a PCR amplification technique aimed at detecting the 16 microorganisms most commonly cultured from the amniotic fluid of patients in preterm labor (*U. urealyticum*, *M. hominis*, *Gardnerella vaginalis*, *E. coli*, *Fusobacterium* spp., *Peptostreptococcus anaerobius*, *Bacteroides fragilis*, *Chlamydia trachomatis*, *H. influenzae*, *N. gonorrhoeae*, and *Streptococcus* spp.). Amniotic fluid samples were examined with bacterial culture and PCR in 50 patients with preterm labor and intact membranes and 23 patients not in labor. All control samples were both culture- and PCR-negative. A higher proportion of samples were positive by PCR compared to culture (46% [23/50] vs. 12% [6/50], $p < 0.05$). The sensitivity of PCR for the prediction of preterm labor before 34 weeks was better than culture (64% [7/11] vs. 18% [2/11, $p < 0.05$). However, there were patients with positive PCR who delivered at term without maternal or neonatal complications.

The clinical implications of detecting *U. urealyticum* by PCR in patients with preterm PROM[121] or preterm labor and intact membranes[122] were evaluated by Yoon and colleagues. Patients with a positive PCR assay of amniotic fluid but a negative culture had a stronger amniotic fluid inflammatory reaction (higher amniotic fluid white blood cell count and IL-6), a shorter interval to delivery, as well as a higher rate of histologic chorioamnionitis, funisitis, and neonatal morbidity than those with a negative amniotic fluid culture and negative amniotic fluid PCR assay for *U. urealyticum*. These studies reveal that patients with preterm PROM or preterm labor with intact membranes and a positive PCR assay for *U. urealyticum* (but a negative culture) have worse pregnancy outcomes than those with a sterile amniotic fluid culture and negative PCR.

Gerber and coworkers[127] used PCR to detect *U. urealyticum* DNA in the amniotic fluid of 254 asymptomatic patients undergoing genetic amniocentesis. Test results were positive in 11.4% of the pregnancies (29/254) and, among these, 58.6% (17/29) delivered preterm. In contrast, only 4.4% (10/225) of the PCR-negative patients delivered prematurely ($p < 0.0001$). This study is consistent with the premise of chronic *U. urealyticum* infection since women with a positive *U. urealyticum* DNA in the amniotic fluid had a higher frequency of preterm births in previous pregnancies compared to women with PCR-negative amniotic fluid (20.7% [6/29] vs. 2.7% [6/225], $p = 0.0008$). In a smaller study of 78 patients undergoing genetic amniocentesis, bacterial 16S ribosomal DNA was detected in 18% (14/78) of the amniotic fluid samples.[128] In this study, no samples tested positive for *Mycoplasma* spp. DNA although it was specifically sought using a PCR/enzyme-linked immunosorbent assay. No association was found between the recovery of bacteria at the time of amniocentesis and either increased IL-6 concentration in the amniotic fluid or preterm delivery. Thus, further studies will be necessary to clarify this issue.

MOLECULAR MECHANISMS FOR PRETERM PARTURITION IN THE SETTING OF INTRAUTERINE INFECTION

A considerable body of evidence supports a role for inflammatory mediators in the mechanisms of preterm parturition associated with infection. These factors may also play a part in spontaneous labor at term, although the evidence for this is less compelling. Much attention has been placed on proinflammatory cytokines such as IL-1β, tumor necrosis factor alpha (TNFα), and chemokines such as IL-8. However, other proinflammatory and anti-inflammatory cytokines may be relevant, including platelet activating factor, prostaglandins, and arachidonate lipoxygenase metabolites.[9] The current understanding of the pathophysiology of preterm parturition in the context of intrauterine infection is summarized here. The interested reader is referred to the references for a comprehensive discussion.[9]

Prostaglandins and Lipoxygenase Products

Intrauterine prostaglandins are considered by many to be the key mediators of the biochemical mechanisms regulating the onset of labor. They can induce myometrial contractility,[129–132] as well as changes in the extracellular matrix metabolism associated with cervical ripening,[133–137] and are thought to participate in decidual/fetal membrane activation.[9]

The evidence traditionally invoked in support of a role for prostaglandins in the initiation of human labor includes the following: (1) administration of prostaglandins induces early and late termination of pregnancy (abortion or labor)[138–146]; (2) treatment with indomethacin or aspirin delays the spontaneous onset of parturition in animals[147–149]; (3) concentrations of prostaglandins in plasma and amniotic fluid increase during labor[150–156]; and (4) intra-amniotic injection of arachidonic acid can induce abortion.[157] Infection can increase prostaglandin production by amnion, chorion, or decidua through the activity of bacterial products, proinflammatory cytokines, growth factors, and other inflammatory mediators. Indeed, amniotic fluid concentrations of the prostaglandins PGE_2 and $PGF_{2\alpha}$ and their stable metabolites, PGEM and PGFM, are significantly higher in women with preterm labor and microbial invasion of the amniotic fluid cavity than in women with preterm labor without infection. Similar observations have been made in patients with labor and high concentrations of proinflammatory mediators in the amniotic cavity (i.e., IL-1β, TNF, IL-6). Moreover, amnion obtained from women with histologic chorioamnionitis produces higher amounts of prostaglandins than amnion from patients without histologic chorioamnionitis.

Metabolites of arachidonic acid derived through the lipoxygenase pathway, including leukotrienes (LTs) and hydroxyeicosatetraenoic acids (HETEs), are also implicated in the mechanisms of spontaneous preterm and term parturition. Concentrations of 5-HETE, LTB_4, and 15-HETE are increased in the amniotic fluid of women with preterm labor and microbial invasion of the amniotic fluid cavity. Similarly, amnion from patients with histologic chorioamnionitis releases more LTB_4 in vitro than amnion from women delivering preterm without inflammation. However, the precise role of arachidonate lipoxygenase metabolites in human parturition remains to be determined. 5-HETE and LTB_4 can stimulate uterine contractility, and LTB_4 is thought to play a role in the recruitment of neutrophils to the site of infection and regulation of specific arachidonic acid metabolites of the cyclooxygenase pathway. Additionally, LTB_4 can act as a calcium ionophore in human intrauterine tissues (i.e., it increases phospholipase activity and enhances the rate of prostaglandin biosynthesis).[158] Oxygen-derived free radicals are also proposed to have a role in the mechanism of preterm parturition.[159,160] Exposure of chorioamniotic membranes to superoxide anion in vitro results in increased activity of MMP-9, a matrix-degrading enzyme involved in the pathogenesis of PROM. Administration of the antioxidant N-acetylcysteine inhibits MMP-9 activity and the generation of superoxide within the membranes.[159]

Inflammatory Cytokines

Evidence for the participation of IL-1 and TNFα in preterm parturition includes the following: (1) IL-1β and TNFα stimulate prostaglandin production by amnion, decidua, and myometrium,[161–163] while prostaglandins are considered a central mediator for the onset of labor; (2) human decidua produces IL-1β and TNFα in response to bacterial products[161,164,165]; (3) amniotic fluid IL-1β and TNFα bioactivity and concentrations are elevated in women with preterm labor and intra-amniotic infection[166–169]; (4) in women with preterm PROM and intra-amniotic infection, IL-1β and TNFα concentrations are higher in the presence of labor[158,161–163]; (5) IL-1β and TNFα induce preterm parturition when administered systemically to pregnant animals[85,170]; (6) pretreatment with the natural IL-1 receptor antagonist prior to the administration of IL-1 to pregnant animals prevents preterm parturition[171]; (7) fetal plasma IL-1β is elevated in the context of preterm labor with intrauterine infection[172]; and (8) placental tissue obtained from patients with labor, particularly those with chorioamnionitis, produces larger amounts of IL-1β than that obtained from women not in labor.[173]

However, there is considerable redundancy in the cytokine network, and it remains unclear whether a particular cytokine signals the onset of labor. Experimental studies in which anti-TNF and the natural IL-1 receptor antagonist were administered to pregnant animals with intrauterine infection did not prevent preterm delivery.[174] The results of knockout animal experiments suggest that infection-induced preterm labor and delivery occurs in animals that lack a particular cytokine.[175]

The precise mechanisms by which IL-1 and TNF participate in the activation of the myometrium have been the subject of intensive research, and there is evidence that they involve the participation of cytosolic phospholipase A_2 (PLA_2), cyclooxygenase-2,[176,177] MAP kinases,[178] and nuclear factor kappa B (NFκB). A role for thrombin (an enzyme with oxytocin-like properties generated during the course of inflammation) is also postulated to have a role.[179–183] A novel observation is that labor is associated with increased activity of NFκB, a transcription factor responsible for many of the actions of IL-1 and TNFα. NFκB may affect uterine function by generating a functional progesterone withdrawal.[184]

Matrix Degrading Enzymes

Preterm PROM accounts for 30% to 40% of all preterm deliveries. The mechanisms responsible for PROM are only partially understood. Since the tensile strength and elasticity of the chorioamniotic membranes are attributed to extracellular matrix proteins, matrix-degrading enzymes have been implicated in preterm PROM. There is now compelling evidence that preterm PROM is associated with increased availability of MMP-1,[185] MMP-8,[186–188] MMP-9,[189–191] and neutrophil elastase,[192] but not MMP-2,[193,194] MMP-3,[195] MMP-7,[196] and MMP-13.[197] Proposed mechanisms to regulate the expression and activity of matrix-degrading enzymes in fetal membranes include programmed cell death (apoptosis)[198] and increased availability of superoxide anions (redox state),[159] respectively.

Because intrauterine infection is present in 30% of patients with preterm PROM and proinflammatory cytokines can stimulate the production of MMP-1, MMP-9, and MMP-8, a genetic predisposition to overproduction of MMPs in response to microorganisms has been implicated in the genesis of PROM. Fetal carriage of two functional polymorphisms for MMP-1 and MMP-9 has been associated with preterm PROM.[199,200]

A polymorphism at nt-1607 in the MMP-1 promoter (an insertion of a guanine [G]) creates a core Ets binding site and increases promoter activity.[200] The 2G promoter has more than two-fold greater activity compared to the 1G allele in amnion mesenchymal cells and a cloned amnion cell line. Phorbol 12-myristate 13-acetate (PMA) increased mesenchymal cell nuclear protein binding, with greater affinity to the 2G allele. Induction of MMP-1 mRNA by PMA is significantly greater in cells with a 1G/2G or 2G/2G genotype than in cells homozygous for the 1G allele. After treatment with PMA, the 1G/2G and 2G/2G cells produce greater amounts of MMP-1 protein than 1G/1G cells. A significant association was found between the presence of a 2G allele in the fetus and preterm PROM. Thus, the 2G allele has stronger promoter activity in amnion cells, and confers increased responsiveness of amnion cells to stimuli that induce MMP-1. Carriage of this polymorphism augments the risk of preterm PROM.[200]

A second polymorphism implicated in preterm PROM is located within the MMP-9 gene.[199] Functional studies of the 14 CA-repeat allele indicate that the allele is a stronger promoter than the 20 CA-repeat allele in both amnion epithelial cells and WISH amnion-derived cells (yet the 14 and 20 CA-repeat alleles have similar activities in monocyte/macrophage cell lines). A case-control study concluded that the 14 CA-repeat allele was more common in newborns delivered to mothers who had preterm PROM than in those delivered at term. Thus, differences in MMP-9 promoter activity related to the CA-repeat number as well as fetal carriage of the 14 CA-repeat allele appear associated with preterm PROM.[199]

THE FETAL INFLAMMATORY RESPONSE SYNDROME

The term *fetal inflammatory response syndrome* (FIRS) was coined to define a subclinical condition originally described in fetuses of women presenting with preterm labor and intact membranes as well as those presenting with preterm PROM.[10,11] The operational definition was an elevation of fetal plasma IL-6 concentration above 11 pg/mL.[11] IL-6, a major mediator of the host response to infection and tissue damage, is capable of eliciting biochemical, physiologic, and immunologic changes in the host, including stimulation of the production of C-reactive protein by liver cells, the acute phase plasma protein response, and activation of T and natural killer cells. Fetuses with FIRS have a higher rate of neonatal complications[12,13] and are frequently born to mothers with subclinical microbial invasion of the amniotic cavity.[10]

Fetal microbial invasion or other insults result in a systemic fetal inflammatory response that can progress toward multiple organ dysfunction, septic shock, and perhaps death in the absence of timely delivery. Evidence of multisystem involvement in cases of FIRS includes increased concentrations of fetal plasma MMP-9,[201] an enzyme involved in the digestion of type IV collagen. In addition, these fetuses have neutrophilia, a higher number of circulatory nucleated red blood cells, and higher plasma concentrations of G-CSF than fetuses without inflammation.[202] FIRS is also associated with changes in markers of monocyte and neutrophil activation.[203] Fetuses with elevated concentrations of IL-6 in the umbilical cord blood have decreased amniotic fluid volume.[42] There is also evidence that FIRS is associated with cardiac dysfunction and neonatal hypotension.[204–206]

The original work describing FIRS was based on fetal blood samples obtained by cordocentesis.[10,11] Many of the findings have since been confirmed by studying umbilical cord blood at the time of birth, including the elevation of proinflammatory cytokines, and the relationship between these cytokines and the likelihood of clinical and suspected sepsis.[13]

Pathologic examination of the umbilical cord is an easy approach to determine whether fetal inflammation was present before birth. Funisitis and chorionic vasculitis are the histopathologic hallmark of FIRS.[55] Another approach is to measure C-reactive protein concentration in umbilical cord blood, which was shown to be elevated in patients with amniotic fluid infection, funisitis, and congenital neonatal sepsis.[207] Neonates with funisitis are at increased risk for neonatal sepsis,[54] as well as long-term handicap such as bronchopulmonary dysplasia[13] and cerebral palsy.[12] Neutrophils in the amniotic fluid are predominantly of fetal origin.[208] Thus, the amniotic fluid white blood cell count is an indirect index of fetal inflammation.[208] Intra-amniotic inflammation is a risk factor for impending preterm delivery and adverse perinatal outcome in women with preterm PROM, even in the absence of documented intra-amniotic infection.[209]

Among women with preterm PROM, FIRS is associated with the impending onset of preterm labor, regardless of the inflammatory state of the amniotic fluid (Fig. 27–2).[10] This suggests that the human fetus plays a role in initiating the onset of labor. However, maternal cooperation must be present for parturition to occur. Fetal inflammation is linked to the onset of labor in association with ascending intrauterine infection. Systemic fetal inflammation may occur in the absence of labor when the inflammatory process does not involve the chorioamniotic membranes and decidua. Such instances occur in the context of hematogenous viral infections or other disease processes (i.e., alloimmunization).

Three approaches can be used to interrupt the course of FIRS: (1) delivery; (2) antimicrobial treatment of women in whom the FIRS is due to microbial invasion of susceptible bacteria; and (3) administration of agents that down-regulate the inflammatory response. Preterm delivery places the unborn child at risk for complications of prematurity. Therefore, the risks of prematurity and intrauterine infection must be balanced.

The administration of antimicrobial agents may eradicate microbial invasion of the amniotic cavity in cases of preterm PROM.[201,210] The results of the ORACLE I trial suggest that antibiotic administration may not only delay the onset of labor but also improve neonatal outcome.[109] These findings are supported by recent experimental evidence in pregnant rabbits inoculated with *E. coli*.[211] Antibiotic administration within 12 hours of microbial inoculation (but not after 18 hours) effectively prevented maternal fever, reduced the rate of preterm delivery, and improved neonatal survival. It is tempting to postulate that this was accomplished by improving or preventing a fetal inflammatory response.

Agents that down-regulate the inflammatory response, such as anti-inflammatory cytokines (i.e., IL-10),[212,213] antibody to macrophage migration inhibitory factor (MIF),[214,215] and antioxidants, may also play a role in preventing preterm delivery, neonatal injury, and long-term perinatal morbidity.[210,216,217] A combination of antibiotics and immunomodulators (dexamethasone and indomethacin) given to nonhuman pregnant primates was effective in eradicating infection, suppressing the inflammatory response, and prolonging gestation in experimental premature labor induced by intra-amniotic inoculation with group B streptococci.[218]

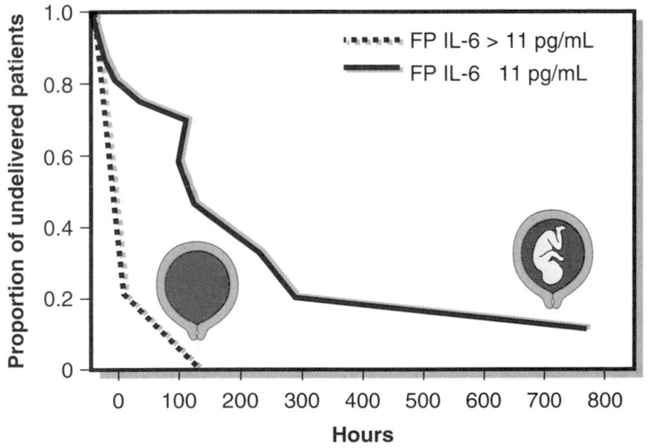

FIGURE 27–2
Fetuses with fetal plasma IL-6 levels >11 pg/mL have a shorter cordocentesis-to-delivery interval than those with plasma IL-6 concentrations ≤11 pg/mL (median, 0.8 days [range, 0.1 to 5 days] vs. median, 6 days [range, 0.2 to 33.6 days], respectively; $P < 0.05$) (From Romero R, Gomez R, Ghezzi F, et al: A fetal systemic inflammatory response is followed by the spontaneous onset of preterm parturition. Am J Obstet Gynecol 1998;179:186–193).

CONTRIBUTION OF FETAL INFECTION/ INFLAMMATION TO LONG-TERM HANDICAP

Cerebral Palsy

Cerebral palsy (CP) is a symptom complex characterized by the aberrant control of movement or posture that appears in early life and can lead to costly lifelong disability.[219] The estimated annual prevalence of CP ranges from 1.5 to 2.5 per 1000 live births, depending on the cohort studied.[220,221]

Prematurity has a strong association with CP[222]; approximately one third of all neonates who later have signs of CP weigh less than 2500 g.[223] Newborns with birth weights <1500 g have a rate of CP 25 to 31 times higher than those with a normal birth weight. The most common form of CP affecting preterm babies is spastic diplegia.[223] In turn, preterm babies that subsequently develop spastic diplegia have a high rate of periventricular leukomalacia (PVL).[222,224–232]

Strong evidence links brain injury and infant exposure to perinatal infection and inflammation.[219,233–236] In 1955, Eastman and DeLeon observed that intrapartum maternal fever was associated with a seven-fold increase in the risk of CP.[237] In 1978, Nelson and Ellenberg[238] showed, using data from the Collaborative Perinatal Project, that among low birth weight infants, chorioamnionitis increased the risk of CP from 12 per 1000 to 39 per 1000 live births. These observations were independently confirmed by several other studies.[225,233,239–241] The general view is that an initiator event (either prepregnancy infection or intrauterine infection) leads to maternal and fetal inflammatory responses, which, in turn, contribute to adverse outcomes such as preterm delivery, intraventricular hemorrhage (IVH), white matter damage (WMD), and neurodevelopmental disability (mainly CP).[242] The following evidence supports this concept: (1) a fetal inflammatory response precedes spontaneous preterm delivery; (2) white matter lesions are associated with spontaneous preterm labor[222,240,243–246]; (3) chorioamnionitis is associated with an increased risk of CP[219,225,233,239–241,247,248]; (4) infection is causally linked to WMD[222,225,234,240]; (5) fetal cytokinemia is associated with IVH, WMD, and CP[235,242,249–255]; and (6) chorionic and umbilical cord vessel inflammation (fetal vasculitis) is associated with an increased risk for IVH, WMD, and cerebral palsy.[12,256–259]

Periventricular leukomalacia describes foci of coagulation necrosis of the white matter near the lateral ventricles. This condition is frequently associated with the subsequent development of CP,[260–262] is more common in infants born between 28 and 31 weeks, and 9 times more common among those with documented bacteremia.[222] Among preterm neonates, the frequency of IVH and PVL is significantly higher for those born after spontaneous preterm labor or PROM when compared to those infants delivered for fetal or maternal indications.[240,246]

Chorioamnionitis Is Associated with an Increased Risk of White Matter Damage and Cerebral Palsy

Maternal infection is also implicated as a significant risk factor for CP in term neonates. Grether and Nelson[219] investigated maternal infection during admission for delivery as a possible risk factor for CP in infants weighing 2500 g or more. In a cohort of 155,636 children in four Northern California counties, 46 children with disabling spastic CP who had no recognized prenatal brain lesions and survived to age 3 years were compared to 378 randomly selected controls. Maternal fever exceeding 38°C in labor or a clinical diagnosis of chorioamnionitis were strongly associated with subsequent development of CP (odds ratio, 9.3; 95% confidence interval, 2.7–31.0), as was histologic evidence of placental infection (odds ratio, 8.9; 95% confidence interval, 1.9–40.0). Twenty-two percent of children with CP had one or more indicators of maternal infection. Newborns exposed to maternal infection had signs attributed to birth asphyxia more often than those unexposed: 5-minute Apgar scores below 6, hypotension, need for intubation, neonatal seizures, and more clinical diagnoses of hypoxic-ischemic encephalopathy. A subsequent larger study by the same group confirmed that clinical chorioamnionitis is a significant independent risk factor for the development of CP in term or near-term infants.[263]

That the fetus is involved in clinical chorioamnionitis is strongly suggested by a study comparing plasma concentrations of IL-6 in umbilical venous blood obtained from pregnancies with (n = 26) and without (n = 111) clinical chorioamnionitis.[264] The median concentration of venous plasma IL-6 was higher in neonates born to mothers with clinical chorioamnionitis than in those born to women in the control group. Sixty-two percent (16/26) of the neonates born to women with clinical chorioamnionitis had elevated plasma concentrations of IL-6 >11 pg/mL in the umbilical vein. The observation that the concentration of IL-6 was higher in the blood from the umbilical artery than in the umbilical vein suggests a fetal origin of the excess plasma IL-6.

Experimental Evidence Linking Infection with White Matter Brain Damage

White matter damage is more common among children of pregnancies complicated by chorioamnionitis[240] and purulent amniotic fluid,[225] as well as among neonates with bacteremia.[222] Experimental evidence indicates that intrauterine infection results in WMD and neuronal lesions.[234,265–270] The reader is referred to the review by Hagberg and colleagues[269] for details. Yoon and coworkers[234] experimentally induced ascending intrauterine infection with *E. coli* in 31 pregnant rabbits; 14 controls were inoculated with sterile saline solution. Histologic evidence of WMD was identified in 12 fetuses born to 10 *E. coli*-inoculated rabbits compared to none in the control group ($p < 0.05$). All cases with WMD had evidence of intrauterine inflammation. Similar findings were reported by DeBillon et al.[266,267]

Fetal Cytokinemia Is Associated with Intraventricular Hemorrhage, White Matter Damage, and Long-Term Disability

Leviton[252] proposed that inflammatory cytokines (TNFα) released during the course of intrauterine infection could play a central role in the pathophysiology of brain WMD. TNF could participate in the pathogenesis of PVL by four different mechanisms: (1) induction of fetal hypotension and brain ischemia[253]; (2) stimulation of tissue factor production and release, which activates the hemostatic system and contributes to coagulation necrosis of white matter[271]; (3) induction of the release of platelet activating factor, which could act as a membrane detergent causing direct brain damage[254]; and (4) a direct cytotoxic effect of TNFα on oligodendrocytes and myelin.[250,251]

The hypothesis that fetal inflammation is linked to brain injury is supported by studies documenting higher concentrations of IL-6 in the umbilical cord plasma[246] and amniotic fluid[235] of fetuses who subsequently develop WMD. Moreover increased expression of TNFα and IL-6 is observed in hypertrophic astrocytes and microglia cells obtained from subjects with PVL.[249] Yoon and colleagues[235] advanced one mechanism to explain how inflammatory cytokines might lead to WMD and CP. According to their theory, microbial invasion of the amniotic cavity (which occurs in approximately 25% of preterm births) results in congenital fetal infection/inflammation that stimulates fetal mononuclear cells to produce IL-1β and TNFα. These cytokines increase the permeability of the blood-brain barrier, facilitating the passage of microbial products and cytokines into the brain.[272] Microbial products then stimulate the human fetal microglia to produce IL-1 and TNFα, with subsequent activation of astrocyte proliferation and production of TNFα. TNFα damages the oligodendrocyte, which is the cell responsible for the deposition of myelin.

Fetal Vasculitis, Intraventricular Hemorrhage, White Matter Damage, and Cerebral Palsy

Yoon and colleagues[12] observed in a study of 123 preterm infants followed to age 3 years that the odds of developing CP were higher in the presence of funisitis (odds ratio, 5.5; 95% confidence interval, 1.2–24.5), increased amniotic fluid IL-6 concentrations (odds ratio, 6.4; 95% confidence interval, 1.3–33.0), and increased amniotic fluid IL-8 concentrations (odds ratio, 5.9; 95% confidence interval, 1.1–30.7). All 14 children who subsequently developed CP had evidence of WMD, and 11 had evidence of intrauterine inflammation. Fifty percent of the children (7/14) had positive amniotic fluid cultures. Although histologic chorioamnionitis was associated with subsequent development of CP, this association disappeared after adjusting for gestational age at birth. The findings of this study suggest that it is the fetal, rather than maternal, inflammatory response that predisposes to CP. Nonetheless, neither infection nor inflammation were considered sufficient causal factors for WMD or CP, as the latter did not develop in 82% (23/28) of fetuses with documented microbial invasion of the amniotic cavity and in 76% (34/45) of those with evidence of intrauterine inflammation. Factors implicated in the genesis of brain injury include: (1) gestational age; (2) virulence of the microorganisms; (3) fetal attack rate; (4) the nature of the fetal immunoresponse; and (5) vulnerability of the central nervous system. It is likely that genes coding for proinflammatory and anti-inflammatory cytokines as well as neurotrophic agents regulate the intensity of the inflammatory response and, therefore, the host response to infection and tissue injury.[256–259]

Bronchopulmonary Dysplasia

Bronchopulmonary dysplasia (BPD) is one of the most frequent and clinically significant complications of prematurity; there is evidence of an association between fetal inflammatory responses and BPD.[13,273–275]

Watterberg and coworkers[274] studied the association between lung inflammation and chorioamnionitis in 53 low birth weight infants who required intubation. Lung inflammation was evaluated on days 1, 2, and 4 of intubation by measuring the concentration of IL-1β, thromboxane B_2, leukotriene B_4, and prostaglandin E_2 in tracheal lavage samples. Infants exposed to chorioamnionitis had a higher concentration of IL-1β in their tracheal fluid from day 1 of intubation forward and were more likely to develop BPD.

Antenatal exposure to proinflammatory cytokines is also a risk factor for the development of BPD.[273] Ghezzi and colleagues[273] measured IL-8 in the amniotic fluid of women with preterm labor with intact membranes or preterm PROM ($n = 47$) who delivered between 24 and 28 weeks of gestation. BPD was diagnosed in 23.4% (11/47). The prevalence of a positive amniotic fluid culture was 44.7% (21/47). IL-8 concentrations were higher in the amniotic fluid of neonates who subsequently developed BPD compared to those who did not. The majority of mothers whose fetuses developed BPD had an amniotic fluid IL-8 level greater than 11.5 ng/mL, and this relationship remained significant even after correction for the effect of gestational age and birth weight (odds ratio: 11.9; $p < 0.05$). The relationship between amniotic fluid IL-6, TNFα, IL-1β, and IL-8 and the occurrence of BPD was further examined in a subsequent study[276] of 69 neonates delivered preterm (≤33 weeks) within 5 days of amniocentesis. BPD was diagnosed in 19% (13/69), and the median amniotic fluid concentrations of IL-6, IL-1β, and IL-8 were each significantly higher in the amniotic fluid of infants who developed BPD compared to those who did not.

Yoon and colleagues[13] studied the relationship between IL-6 concentration in umbilical cord plasma at birth and the occurrence of BPD in 203 preterm births (25 to 34 weeks' gestation). BPD was diagnosed in 17% (34/203). Neonates who developed BPD had a significantly higher median IL-6 concentration in umbilical cord plasma at birth than those in whom BPD did not develop (median 68.3 pg/mL [0.3–6150.0 pg/mL] vs. median 6.9 pg/mL [0–19, 230.0 pg/mL], $p < 0.001$). This difference remained significant after adjustment for gestational age at birth (odds ratio, 4.2; 95% confidence interval, 1.6–11.2). This same group[275] has also observed an association between a fetal inflammatory response (defined as the presence of funisitis or umbilical cord plasma IL-6 concentration >17.5 pg/mL or amniotic fluid MMP-8 concentration >23 ng/mL) and the development of atypical chronic lung disease (defined as chronic lung disease in the absence of respiratory distress syndrome). Chronic lung disease was diagnosed in 70 newborns. A fetal inflammatory response was present in 76% (53/70) and was more common among those with atypical chronic lung disease (90% [27/30] vs. 65% [26/40]; $p < 0.05$).

Perinatal Death

Infectious diseases, birth asphyxia, and prematurity are considered the major causes of neonatal death worldwide.[277] In one review of 27 hospital-based studies evaluating the impact of infection as a cause of neonatal death, Stohl[277] observed that infection was associated with 7% to 54% of early neonatal deaths and 30% to 73% of late neonatal deaths. Even in the absence of a suggestive clinical history, infection and inflammation can still contribute significantly to perinatal mortality. In a study of 94 autopsies performed in fetuses and neonates, evidence of an infectious or inflammatory condition was present 48% (45/94) of the time.[278] In 58% (26/45) of cases, no previous signs or symptoms of infection/inflammation were present. The most common diagnosis was chorioamnionitis (79.1% [38/48]), followed by acute villitis (4.2% [2/48]), chronic villitis (4.2% [2/48]), disseminated cytomegalovirus infection (4.2% [2/48]), disseminated herpes simplex virus infection (2.1% [1/48]), pneumonia (4.2% [2/48]), and mixed placental infection (2.1% [1/48]). The reader is referred to a review by Goldenberg and Thompson[279] for a comprehensive summary.

Blackwell and colleagues[280] proposed that failure of the fetus to mount an inflammatory response sufficient to signal the onset of preterm labor might account for some cases of fetal death. Indeed, histologic chorioamnionitis (a maternal host response) is nine times more frequent than funisitis (20.9% [9/43] vs. 2.3% [1/43], $p = 0.008$) in cases of fetal death. Changes in the adaptive limb of the maternal immune response are also associated with unexplained fetal death. Evidence in support of this concept includes the finding that an increased proportion of "memory-like" T cells (CD45RO+ isoform) was observed in the maternal blood of pregnancies complicated by unexplained fetal death, suggesting that prior maternal exposure to microbial products (bacterial or viral) or other unidentified antigens occurred in these cases.[281]

THE ROLE OF VIRUSES IN FETAL INFECTION

Viral infections acquired during pregnancy are associated with a variety of severe but nonspecific outcomes, including spontaneous abortion, fetal growth disorders, microcephaly, hydrocephaly, congenital cataract, myocarditis, pericardial effusion, liver calcifications, ascites, and nonimmune hydrops. The consequences of fetal infection by rubella, cytomegalovirus (CMV), varicella zoster virus, parvovirus B19, herpes simplex virus (HSV), and lymphocytic choriomeningitis virus are detailed elsewhere (see Chapters 30 and 31). The detection of viral genome in the amniotic fluid, either in low risk pregnancies or pregnancies at risk for fetal infection, has expanded the list of potential fetal pathogens to include adenovirus, coxsackievirus, human papillomavirus, influenza, and respiratory syncytial virus (RSV). The list may grow with the application of novel diagnostic tools.[282] In addition to the well-known teratogenic effects, viral infection during pregnancy may also be implicated in the pathogenesis of abnormal placentation[283–286] and in the etiology of neuropsychiatric disorders.[287–291]

Detection of Viral Genome in the Amniotic Fluid and Other Tissue Samples

Viral genome is detected in the amniotic fluid of up to 15% of asymptomatic low risk pregnancies[292–295] and 41% of pregnancies at risk for viral infection.[296–298] The most common viral DNA isolates, in both low and high risk pregnancies, are adenovirus, CMV, and enterovirus.[292,293,295–298]

Viral Genome in the Amniotic Fluid of Low Risk Pregnancies

Viral genomes have been detected in the amniotic fluid of asymptomatic low risk pregnancies at the time of midtrimester amniocentesis.[292,293,296] McLean and colleagues[294] were the first to report the detection of viral genome in the amniotic fluid of patients at low risk for viral infection at the time of genetic amniocentesis. Amniotic fluid samples were analyzed by polymerase chain reaction (PCR) for the presence of adenovirus, CMV, parvovirus, or HSV. Two hundred and forty-three samples had detectable DNA by β-globin chain amplification but none had detectable viral DNA. In three subsequent studies, however, the prevalence of viral genome in the amniotic fluid of asymptomatic low risk patients ranged from 2.6% to 15%.[292,293,295] The largest study conducted to date[292] reported a prevalence of viral genome in 6.4% (44/686) of amniotic fluid samples obtained at midtrimester amniocentesis. The most prevalent viral genome was adenovirus (37/44), followed by CMV (5/44), Epstein-Barr virus (EBV) (2/44), enterovirus (2/44), and RSV (1/44). Another finding of this study was a bimodal seasonal variation in prevalence of viral DNA in the amniotic fluid, with the highest detection rate observed during the summer and winter months.

Detection of Viral Genome in Biological Specimens of Pregnancies at Risk for Fetal Infection

Viral genome can be detected in the amniotic fluid of 12% to 41% of pregnancies at risk for fetal infection.[292,296] Van den Veyver and colleagues[296] analyzed amniotic fluid ($n = 233$) and other biologic samples (fetal blood at cordocentesis [$n = 42$], cord blood at the time of delivery [$n = 18$], ascitic fluid [$n = 8$], pleural fluid [$n = 10$], and other tissue samples [$n = 40$]) in 303 pregnancies at risk for viral infection. Risk factors included nonimmune fetal hydrops, pleural effusion, twin-to-twin transfusion syndrome, fetal ventriculomegaly, fetal intracranial calcification/microcephaly, fetal hepatic calcification or echogenic bowel, fetal myocarditis, maternal exposure to virus, polyhydramnios, oligohydramnios, intrauterine growth restriction, or a combination of these. Amniotic fluid from 154 controls was obtained at the time of genetic amniocentesis. PCR was used to detect the presence of viral DNA or RNA (reverse transcriptase-PCR) for the following viruses: CMV, HSV, parvovirus B19, adenovirus, enterovirus, EBV, and RSV. When all samples were considered in the analysis, viral genome was detected in 41% (124/303) of the cases. Among the high risk pregnancies, ascitic fluid was positive for one or more viral genomes in 50% (10/20), amniotic fluid in 41% (95/233), pleural fluid in 33% (6/18), and fetal blood in 22% (13/60). Fifty-five percent (50/91) of the fetuses with nonimmune hydrops had a viral infection. The most commonly recovered viral genome was adenovirus (24% [74/303]), which was also the most prevalent virus in cases of nonimmune fetal hydrops (60% of the positive samples [30/50]). CMV was present in 9.9% of the samples obtained from high risk pregnancies (30/303) and was frequently associated with the recovery of other viral genomes (such as adenovirus and enterovirus), as well as with the presence of several fetal abnormalities, including nonimmune hydrops, hepatic calcification, growth restriction, stuck twin syndrome, and fetal ascites. Enterovirus was present in 7.3% (22/303) of the cases and was associated with stuck twin syndrome, myocarditis, fetal ascites with pericardial effusion, hydramnios, and nonimmune hydrops. RSV and parvovirus were present in 3% (9/303) and 2.6% (8/303) of the high risk pregnancies, respectively, mainly those complicated by nonimmune hydrops (parvovirus and HSV) or stuck twin syndrome (HSV). Among low risk pregnancies, 2.6% (4/154) had positive viral genome in the amniotic fluid (adenovirus $n = 3$; CMV $n = 1$), and this finding was unassociated with fetal complications.

Baschat and coworkers[297] compared the prevalence of viral genome in amniotic fluid of normal pregnancies (genetic amniocentesis, $n = 240$) and amniotic fluid, fetal blood, or pleural fluid in pregnancies complicated by fetal anomalies, small-for-gestational age fetuses, or proven maternal infection ($n = 138$). The overall detection of viral genome was 12.4% (47/378). The most frequently isolated viral genome was adenovirus (10.3% [39/378], followed by enterovirus (1.3% [5/378]), CMV (0.8% [3/378]), RSV (0.3% [1/378]), EBV (0.3% [1/378]), and parvovirus B19 (0.3% [1/378]). The prevalence of viral genome was higher in pregnancies with an adverse outcome than in patients with a normal outcome (19.6% [27/138] vs. 8.3% [20/240], $p < 0.005$).

Detection of Viral Genome in the Amniotic Fluid and Adverse Pregnancy Outcome

Reddy and coworkers[298] found an association between detection of a viral genome in the amniotic fluid and adverse pregnancy outcome. PCR was conducted for CMV, parvovirus B19, adenovirus, enterovirus, HSV, EBV, and RSV in 147 pregnancies. One hundred thirty-eight fetuses were chromosomally normal; among these, 25 (18%) had a positive amniotic fluid PCR. These fetuses were more likely to deliver prematurely, have preterm PROM, nonimmune hydrops, low birth weight, or an intrauterine fetal demise. When only structurally normal fetuses were analyzed, those with a positive amniotic fluid PCR for viral genome were more likely to die in utero and have both a lower gestational age and lower birth weight at delivery.

Detection of Viral Genome in the Amniotic Fluid and Pregnancy Loss

Wenstrom and colleagues[293] investigated the prevalence of viral DNA and measured IL-6 levels in the amniotic fluid of 62 patients who had a pregnancy loss within 30 days of genetic amniocentesis. Sixty control pregnancies delivering uneventfully at term were matched for the year that the amniocentesis was performed, indications for the procedure, gestational age, and maternal age. Amniotic fluid was studied by PCR for the presence of adenovirus, parvovirus, CMV, EPV, and HSV, and by reverse transcriptase PCR for enterovirus and influenza A. The prevalence of viral DNA was not significantly different between cases and controls (8% [5/62] vs. 15% [9/60], respectively; $p = 0.27$). Adenovirus was the most frequently recovered viral genome (64% [9/14]), followed by CMV (21% [3/14]), HSV (7% [1/14]), and parvovirus (7% [1/14]). Although IL-6 concentration was significantly higher in patients who lost their pregnancies within 30 days of genetic amniocentesis, no association between the detection of viral genome and the concentration of IL-6 in amniotic fluid was demonstrated. In summary, a developing body of work suggests that fetal viral infection can induce an inflammatory response. Most fetuses with evidence of viral infection do well. The response is likely altered by gestational age and genetic factors.

CONCLUSIONS

- Intrauterine infection/inflammation contributes significantly to pregnancy pathology:
  - Preterm labor/late miscarriage
  - Premature rupture of membranes
  - Chorioamnionitis
  - Neurodevelopmental disability after birth
  - Chronic lung disease
  - Perinatal death

CONCLUSIONS *(Continued)*

- Molecular genetic techniques have allowed a greater understanding of the pathophysiologic processes.
- Although bacteria were thought to be the main trigger for intrauterine infection/inflammation, a role of viral infection is now emerging.
- Application of this knowledge has yet to change practice and improve outcome, though such mechanistic knowledge should ultimately do so.

SUMMARY OF MANAGEMENT OPTIONS

Intrauterine Infection, Preterm Parturition, and the Fetal Inflammatory Response Syndrome

Management Options	Quality of Evidence	Strength of Recommendation	References
Diagnosis of Intra-amniotic Infection/Inflammation			
Perform Amniocentesis to retrieve amniotic fluid	III	B	29
• **Rapid tests:** Gram stain, amniotic fluid wbc count, amniotic fluid glucose, and IL-6 concentration			
• **Culture:** Aerobic, anaerobic bacteria and genital mycoplasmas			
• **PCR** with specific primers for the detection of organisms in patients with intra-amniotic inflammation and negative culture			
Diagnosis of a Fetal Inflammatory Response Syndrome			
General			
• The diagnosis of fetal inflammatory response syndrome suggests antenatal exposure to an agent that promoted inflammation.	–	GPP	–
• It may have medicolegal value, as there is no current evidence that treatment can modify the natural history and the risk for adverse outcome (short- and long-term) conferred by fetal systemic inflammation.	–	GPP	–
Take levels from umbilical cord blood obtained at the time of delivery:	III	B	54, 55, 69, 207, 246, 299, 300–303, 308, 310
CBC and differential, platelet count			
C-reactive protein; elevated C-reactive protein is associated with:			
• Histologic chorioamnionitis			
• Funisitis			
• Neonatal sepsis			
IL-6 concentration; elevated IL-6 level associated with:			
• Positive amniotic fluid cultures (MIAC)			
• Histologic chorioamnionitis[55,300-302]			
• Funisitis			
• Neonatal sepsis			
• Congenital pneumonia			
• Necrotizing enterocolitis			
• Intracranial hemorrhage			

SUMMARY OF MANAGEMENT OPTIONS

Intrauterine Infection, Preterm Parturition, and the Fetal Inflammatory Response Syndrome *(Continued)*

Management Options	Quality of Evidence	Strength of Recommendation	References
• Central nervous system white matter damage			
• Impaired neurologic outcome (lower Bayley psychomotor developmental index scores)			
Examine the placenta	III	B	51, 52, 54, 55
• Histologic chorioamnionitis is a maternal host response.			
• Funisitis is a marker of fetal inflammation.			
For Premature Neonates, After Birth			
Perform pathologic examination of the placenta	III	B	12, 225, 309, 311, 312
Specifically seek for evidence supporting the following diagnoses:			
Histologic chorioamnionitis associated with intracranial hemorrhage			
Funisitis associated with:			
• Neonatal sepsis			
• Intracranial hemorrhage			
• White matter damage			
• Cerebral palsy			

REFERENCES

1. Brocklehurst P: Infection and preterm delivery. BMJ 1999;318:548–549.
2. Gibbs RS, Romero R, Hillier SL, et al: A review of premature birth and subclinical infection. Am J Obstet Gynecol 1992;166:1515–1528.
3. Goldenberg RL, Hauth JC, Andrews WW: Intrauterine infection and preterm delivery. N Engl J Med 2000;342:1500–1507.
4. Ledger WJ: Infection and premature labor. Am J Perinatol 1989;6:234–236.
5. Minkoff H: Prematurity: Infection as an etiologic factor. Obstet Gynecol 1983;62:137–144.
6. Naeye RL, Ross SM: Amniotic fluid infection syndrome. Clin Obstet Gynecol 1982;9:593–607.
7. Romero R, Mazor M: Infection and preterm labor. Clin Obstet Gynecol 1988;31:553–584.
8. Romero R, Mazor M, Wu YK, et al: Infection in the pathogenesis of preterm labor. Semin Perinatol 1988;12:262–279.
9. Romero R, Mazor M, Munoz H, et al: The preterm labor syndrome. Ann NY Acad Sci 1994;734:414–429.
10. Gomez R, Romero R, Ghezzi F, et al: The fetal inflammatory response syndrome. Am J Obstet Gynecol 1998;179:194–202.
11. Romero R, Gomez R, Ghezzi F, et al: A fetal systemic inflammatory response is followed by the spontaneous onset of preterm parturition. Am J Obstet Gynecol 1998;179:186–193.
12. Yoon BH, Romero R, Park JS, et al: Fetal exposure to an intra-amniotic inflammation and the development of cerebral palsy at the age of three years. Am J Obstet Gynecol 2000;182:675–681.
13. Yoon BH, Romero R, Kim KS, et al: A systemic fetal inflammatory response and the development of bronchopulmonary dysplasia. Am J Obstet Gynecol 1999;181:773–779.
14. Blanc WA: Amniotic and neonatal infection: Quick cytodiagnosis. Gynaecologia 1953;136:100–110.
15. Benirschke K: Routes and types of infection in the fetus and the newborn. Am J Dis Child 1960;99:714–721.
16. Benirschke K, Clifford SH: Intrauterine bacterial infection of the newborn infant: Frozen sections of the cord as an aid to early detection. J Pediatr 1959;54:11–18.
17. Driscoll SG: Pathology and the developing fetus. Pediatr Clin North Am 1965;12:493–514.
18. Blanc WA: Pathways of fetal and early neonatal infection. Viral placentitis, bacterial and fungal chorioamnionitis. J Pediatr 1961;59:473–496.
19. Romero R, Sirtori M, Oyarzun E, et al: Infection and labor. V. Prevalence, microbiology, and clinical significance of intraamniotic infection in women with preterm labor and intact membranes. Am J Obstet Gynecol 1989;161:817–824.
20. Romero R, Shamma F, Avila C, et al: Infection and labor. VI. Prevalence, microbiology, and clinical significance of

intraamniotic infection in twin gestations with preterm labor. Am J Obstet Gynecol 1990;163:757–761.
21. Donder GG, Vereecken A, Bosmans E, et al: Definition of a type of abnormal vaginal flora that is distinct from bacterial vaginosis: Aerobic vaginitis. BJOG 2002;109:34–43.
22. Galask RP, Varner MW, Petzold CR, Wilbur SL: Bacterial attachment to the chorioamniotic membranes. Am J Obstet Gynecol 1984;148:915–928.
23. Romero R, Kadar N, Hobbins JC, Duff GW: Infection and labor: The detection of endotoxin in amniotic fluid. Am J Obstet Gynecol 1987;157:815–819.
24. Romero R, Roslansky P, Oyarzun E, et al: Labor and infection. II. Bacterial endotoxin in amniotic fluid and its relationship to the onset of preterm labor. Am J Obstet Gynecol 1988;158:1044–1049.
25. Kramer BW, Kramer S, Ikegami M, Jobe AH: Injury, inflammation, and remodeling in fetal sheep lung after intra-amniotic endotoxin. Am J Physiol Lung Cell Mol Physiol 2002;283: L452–L459.
26. Newnham JP, Moss TJ, Kramer BW, et al: The fetal maturational and inflammatory responses to different routes of endotoxin infusion in sheep. Am J Obstet Gynecol 2002;186:1062–1068.
27. Altshuler G, Hyde S: Clinicopathologic considerations of fusobacteria chorioamnionitis. Acta Obstet Gynecol Scand 1988;67:513–517.
28. Hillier SL, Krohn MA, Kiviat NB, et al: Microbiologic causes and neonatal outcomes associated with chorioamnion infection. Am J Obstet Gynecol 1991;165:955–961.
29. Leigh J, Garite TJ: Amniocentesis and the management of premature labor. Obstet Gynecol 1986;67:500–506.
30. Goncalves LF, Chaiworapongsa T, Romero R: Intrauterine infection and prematurity. Ment Retard Dev Disabil Res Rev 2002;8:3–13.
31. Yoon BH, Romero R, Park JS, et al: Microbial invasion of the amniotic cavity with *Ureaplasma urealyticum* is associated with a robust host response in fetal, amniotic, and maternal compartments. Am J Obstet Gynecol 1998;179:1254 –1260.
32. Cassell GH, Davis RO, Waites KB, et al: Isolation of *Mycoplasma hominis* and *Ureaplasma urealyticum* from amniotic fluid at 16-20 weeks of gestation: Potential effect on outcome of pregnancy. Sex Transm Dis 1983;10:294–302.
33. Chaim W, Horowitz S, David JB, et al: *Ureaplasma urealyticum* in the development of postpartum endometritis. Eur J Obstet Gynecol Reprod Biol 2003;109:145–148.
34. Alanen A: Polymerase chain reaction in the detection of microbes in amniotic fluid. Ann Med 1998;30:288–295.
35. Hitti J, Riley DE, Krohn MA, et al: Broad-spectrum bacterial rDNA polymerase chain reaction assay for detecting amniotic fluid infection among women in premature labor. Clin Infect Dis 1997;24:1228–1232.
36. Kimberlin DF, Hauth JC, Owen J, et al: Indicated versus spontaneous preterm delivery: An evaluation of neonatal morbidity among infants weighing </=1000 grams at birth. Am J Obstet Gynecol 1999;180:683–689.
37. Meis PJ, Goldenberg RL, Mercer BM, et al: The preterm prediction study: Risk factors for indicated preterm births. Maternal-Fetal Medicine Units Network of the National Institute of Child Health and Human Development. Am J Obstet Gynecol 1998;178:562–567.
38. Meis PJ, Michielutte R, Peters TJ, et al: Factors associated with preterm birth in Cardiff, Wales. II. Indicated and spontaneous preterm birth. Am J Obstet Gynecol 1995;173:597–602.
39. Arias F, Tomich P: Etiology and outcome of low birth weight and preterm infants. Obstet Gynecol 1982;60:277–281.
40. Romero R, Gomez R, Chaiworapongsa T, et al: The role of infection in preterm labour and delivery. Pediatr Perinat Epidemiol 2001;15 Suppl 2:41–56.
41. Watts DH, Krohn MA, Hillier SL, Eschenbach DA: The association of occult amniotic fluid infection with gestational age and neonatal outcome among women in preterm labor. Obstet Gynecol 1992;79:351–357.
42. Yoon BH, Kim YA, Romero R, et al: Association of oligohydramnios in women with preterm premature rupture of membranes with an inflammatory response in fetal, amniotic, and maternal compartments. Am J Obstet Gynecol 1999;181:784–788.
43. Vintzileos AM, Campbell WA, Nochimson DJ, et al: Qualitative amniotic fluid volume versus amniocentesis in predicting infection in preterm premature rupture of the membranes. Obstet Gynecol 1986;67:579–583.
44. Romero R, Quintero R, Oyarzun E, et al: Intraamniotic infection and the onset of labor in preterm premature rupture of the membranes. Am J Obstet Gynecol 1988;159:661–666.
45. Romero R, Gonzalez R, Sepulveda W, et al: Infection and labor. VIII. Microbial invasion of the amniotic cavity in patients with suspected cervical incompetence: Prevalence and clinical significance. Am J Obstet Gynecol 1992;167:1086–1091.
46. Mays JK, Figueroa R, Shah J, et al: Amniocentesis for selection before rescue cerclage. Obstet Gynecol 2000;95:652–655.
47. Chellam VG, Rushton DI: Chorioamnionitis and funiculitis in the placentas of 200 births weighing less than 2.5 kg. BJOG 1985;92:808–814.
48. Hillier SL, Witkin SS, Krohn MA, et al: The relationship of amniotic fluid cytokines and preterm delivery, amniotic fluid infection, histologic chorioamnionitis, and chorioamnion infection. Obstet Gynecol 1993;81:941–948.
49. Romero R, Salafia CM, Athanassiadis AP, et al: The relationship between acute inflammatory lesions of the preterm placenta and amniotic fluid microbiology. Am J Obstet Gynecol 1992;166: 1382–1388.
50. Aquino TI, Zhang J, Kraus FT, et al: Subchorionic fibrin cultures for bacteriologic study of the placenta. Am J Clin Pathol 1984;81:482–486.
51. Pankuch GA, Appelbaum PC, Lorenz RP, et al: Placental microbiology and histology and the pathogenesis of chorioamnionitis. Obstet Gynecol 1984;64:802–806.
52. Hillier SL, Martius J, Krohn M, et al: A case-control study of chorioamnionic infection and histologic chorioamnionitis in prematurity. N Engl J Med 1988;319:972–978.
53. Cassell GH, Andrews WW, Hauth JC, Cutter G: Chorioamnion colonization: Correlation with gestational age in women delivered following spontaneous labor versus indicated delivery. Am J Obstet Gynecol 1993;168:425.
54. Yoon BH, Romero R, Park JS, et al: The relationship among inflammatory lesions of the umbilical cord (funisitis), umbilical cord plasma interleukin 6 concentration, amniotic fluid infection, and neonatal sepsis. Am J Obstet Gynecol 2000;183: 1124–1129.
55. Pacora P, Chaiworapongsa T, Maymon E, et al: Funisitis and chorionic vasculitis: The histological counterpart of the fetal inflammatory response syndrome. J Matern Fetal Neonatal Med 2002;11:18–25.
56. Boyer KM, Gadzala CA, Burd LI, et al: Selective intrapartum chemoprophylaxis of neonatal group B streptococcal early-onset disease. I. Epidemiologic rationale. J Infect Dis 1983;148: 795–801.
57. Ohlsson A, Vearncombe M: Congenital and nosocomial sepsis in infants born in a regional perinatal unit: Cause, outcome, and white blood cell response. Am J Obstet Gynecol 1987;156: 407–413.
58. Philip AG: Diagnosis of neonatal bacteraemia. Arch Dis Child 1989;64:1514.
59. Philip AG: The changing face of neonatal infection: Experience at a regional medical center. Pediatr Infect Dis J 1994;13: 1098–1102.
60. Philip AG: Sepsis + C-reactive protein. Pediatrics 1994;93: 693–694.
61. Placzek MM, Whitelaw A: Early and late neonatal septicaemia. Arch Dis Child 1983;58:728–731.

62. Seo K, McGregor JA, French JI: Preterm birth is associated with increased risk of maternal and neonatal infection. Obstet Gynecol 1992;79:75–80.
63. Thompson PJ, Greenough A, Gamsu HR, et al: Congenital bacterial sepsis in very preterm infants. J Med Microbiol 1992;36:117–120.
64. Carroll SG, Papaioannou S, Ntumazah IL, et al: Lower genital tract swabs in the prediction of intrauterine infection in preterm prelabour rupture of the membranes. BJOG 1996;103: 54–59.
65. Gray DJ, Robinson HB, Malone J, Thomson RB, Jr: Adverse outcome in pregnancy following amniotic fluid isolation of *Ureaplasma urealyticum*. Prenat Diagn 1992;12:111–117.
66. Horowitz S, Mazor M, Romero R, et al: Infection of the amniotic cavity with *Ureaplasma urealyticum* in the midtrimester of pregnancy. J Reprod Med 1995;40:375–379.
67. Romero R, Avila C, Santhanam U, Sehgal PB: Amniotic fluid interleukin 6 in preterm labor. Association with infection. J Clin Invest 1990;85:1392–1400.
68. Romero R, Sepulveda W, Kenney JS, et al: Interleukin 6 determination in the detection of microbial invasion of the amniotic cavity. Ciba Found Symp 1992;167:205–220.
69. Romero R, Yoon BH, Kenney JS, et al: Amniotic fluid interleukin-6 determinations are of diagnostic and prognostic value in preterm labor. Am J Reprod Immunol 1993;30:167–183.
70. Yoon BH, Romero R, Kim CJ, et al: Amniotic fluid interleukin-6: A sensitive test for antenatal diagnosis of acute inflammatory lesions of preterm placenta and prediction of perinatal morbidity. Am J Obstet Gynecol 1995;172:960–970.
71. Romero R, Munoz H, Gomez R, et al: Two thirds of spontaneous abortion/fetal deaths after genetic amniocentesis are the result of a preexisting subclinical inflammatory process of the amniotic cavity. Am J Obstet Gynecol 1995;172:S261.
72. Wenstrom KD, Andrews WW, Tamura T, et al: Elevated amniotic fluid interleukin-6 levels at genetic amniocentesis predict subsequent pregnancy loss. Am J Obstet Gynecol 1996;175:830–833.
73. Chaiworapongsa T, Romero R, Tolosa JE, et al: Elevated monocyte chemotactic protein-1 in amniotic fluid is a risk factor for pregnancy loss. J Matern Fetal Neonatal Med 2002;12:159–164.
74. Yoon BH, Oh SY, Romero R, et al: An elevated amniotic fluid matrix metalloproteinase-8 level at the time of midtrimester genetic amniocentesis is a risk factor for spontaneous preterm delivery. Am J Obstet Gynecol 2001;185:1162–1167.
75. Wenstrom KD, Andrews WW, Hauth JC, et al: Elevated second trimester amniotic fluid interleukin-6 levels predict preterm delivery. Am J Obstet Gynecol 1998;178:546–550.
76. Ghidini A, Eglinton GS, Spong CY, et al: Elevated midtrimester amniotic fluid tumor necrosis alpha levels: A predictor of preterm delivery. Am J Obstet Gynecol 1996;174:S307.
77. Spong CY, Ghidini A, Sherer DM, et al: Angiogenin: A marker for preterm delivery in midtrimester amniotic fluid. Am J Obstet Gynecol 1997;176:415–418.
78. Ghezzi F, Franchi M, Raio L, et al: Elevated amniotic fluid C-reactive protein at the time of genetic amniocentesis is a marker for preterm delivery. Am J Obstet Gynecol 2002;186:268–273.
79. Goldenberg RL, Andrews WW, Mercer BM, et al: The preterm prediction study: Granulocyte colony-stimulating factor and spontaneous preterm birth. National Institute of Child Health and Human Development Maternal-Fetal Medicine Units Network. Am J Obstet Gynecol 2000;182:625–630.
80. Cox SM, King MR, Casey ML, MacDonald PC: Interleukin-1β, -1α, and -6 and prostaglandins in vaginal/cervical fluids of pregnant women before and during labor. J Clin Endocrinol Metab 1993;77:805–815.
81. Cox SM, Casey ML, MacDonald PC: Accumulation of interleukin-1β and interleukin-6 in amniotic fluid: A sequela of labour at term and preterm. Hum Reprod Update 1997;3:517–527.
82. MacDonald P: Parturition: Biomolecular and physiologic processes. In Cunningham FG, MacDonald PC, Leveno KJ, Gilstrap LC (eds): Williams Obstetrics. Norwalk, Conn., Appleton and Lange, 1993, pp 297–361.
83. MacDonald PC, Casey ML: The accumulation of prostaglandins (PG) in amniotic fluid is an aftereffect of labor and not indicative of a role for PGE_2 or $PGF_{2\alpha}$ in the initiation of human parturition. J Clin Endocrinol Metab 1993;76:1332–1339.
84. Witkin SS, Gravett MG, Haluska GJ, Novy MJ: Induction of interleukin-1 receptor antagonist in rhesus monkeys after intraamniotic infection with group B streptococci or interleukin-1 infusion. Am J Obstet Gynecol 1994;171:1668–1672.
85. Romero R, Mazor M, Tartakovsky B: Systemic administration of interleukin-1 induces preterm parturition in mice. Am J Obstet Gynecol 1991;165:969–971.
86. McDuffie RS Jr, Sherman MP, Gibbs RS: Amniotic fluid tumor necrosis factor-alpha and interleukin-1 in a rabbit model of bacterially induced preterm pregnancy loss. Am J Obstet Gynecol 1992;167:1583–1588.
87. Katsuki Y, Kaga N, Kakinuma C, et al: Ability of intrauterine bacterial lipopolysaccharide to cause in situ uterine contractions in pregnant rabbits. Acta Obstet Gynecol Scand 1997;76:26–32.
88. Gravett MG, Witkin SS, Haluska GJ, et al: An experimental model for intraamniotic infection and preterm labor in rhesus monkeys. Am J Obstet Gynecol 1994;171:1660–1667.
89. Gravett MG, Haluska GJ, Cook MJ, Novy MJ: Fetal and maternal endocrine responses to experimental intrauterine infection in rhesus monkeys. Am J Obstet Gynecol 1996;174:1725–1731.
90. Gibbs RS, Davies JK, McDuffie RS Jr, et al: Chronic intrauterine infection and inflammation in the preterm rabbit, despite antibiotic therapy. Am J Obstet Gynecol 2002;186:234–239.
91. Fidel PI Jr, Romero R, Maymon E, Hertelendy F: Bacteria-induced or bacterial product-induced preterm parturition in mice and rabbits is preceded by a significant fall in serum progesterone concentrations. J Matern Fetal Med 1998;7:222–226.
92. Brown MB, Peltier M, Hillier M, et al: Genital mycoplasmosis in rats: A model for intrauterine infection. Am J Reprod Immunol 2001;46:232–241.
93. Baggia S, Gravett MG, Witkin SS, et al: Interleukin-1β intra-amniotic infusion induces tumor necrosis factor-alpha, prostaglandin production, and preterm contractions in pregnant rhesus monkeys. J Soc Gynecol Invest 1996;3:121–126.
94. Romero R, Yoon BH, Gonzalez R, et al: The clinical significance of microbial invasion of the amniotic cavity with mycoplasmas in patients with preterm PROM. J Soc Gynecol Invest 1993.
95. Carey JC, Blackwelder WC, Nugent RP, et al: Antepartum cultures for *Ureaplasma urealyticum* are not useful in predicting pregnancy outcome. The Vaginal Infections and Prematurity Study Group. Am J Obstet Gynecol 1991;164:728–733.
96. Amstey MS, Steadman KT: Asymptomatic gonorrhea and pregnancy. J Am Vener Dis Assoc 1976;3:14–16.
97. Gravett MG, Hummel D, Eschenbach DA, Holmes KK: Preterm labor associated with subclinical amniotic fluid infection and with bacterial vaginosis. Obstet Gynecol 1986;67:229–237.
98. Handsfield HH, Hodson WA, Holmes KK: Neonatal gonococcal infection. I. Orogastric contamination with *Neisseria gonorrhoeae*. JAMA 1973;225:697–701.
99. Layton R: Infection of the urinary tract in pregnancy: An investigation of a new routine in antenatal care. J Obstet Gynaecol Br Commonw 1964;71:927–933.
100. Minkoff H, Grunebaum AN, Schwarz RH, et al: Risk factors for prematurity and premature rupture of membranes: A prospective study of the vaginal flora in pregnancy. Am J Obstet Gynecol 1984;150:965–972.
101. Patrick MJ: Influence of maternal renal infection on the foetus and infant. Arch Dis Child 1967;42:208–213.
102. Robertson JG, Livingstone JR, Isdale MH: The management and complications of asymptomatic bacteriuria in pregnancy.

Report of a study on 8,275 patients. J Obstet Gynaecol Br Commonw 1968;75:59–65.
103. Romero R, Oyarzun E, Mazor M, et al: Meta-analysis of the relationship between asymptomatic bacteriuria and preterm delivery/low birth weight. Obstet Gynecol 1989;73:576–582.
104. Sarrel PM, Pruett KA: Symptomatic gonorrhea during pregnancy. Obstet Gynecol 1968;32:670–673.
105. Wren BG: Subclinical renal infection and prematurity. Med J Aust 1969;2:596–600.
106. Leitich H, Bodner-Adler B, Brunbauer M, et al: Bacterial vaginosis as a risk factor for preterm delivery: A meta-analysis. Am J Obstet Gynecol 2003;189:139–147.
107. Romero R, Roslansky P, Oyarzun E, et al: Labor and infection. II. Bacterial endotoxin in amniotic fluid and its relationship to the onset of preterm labor. Am J Obstet Gynecol 1988;158: 1044–1049.
108. Romero R, Sepulveda W, Baumann P, et al: The preterm labor syndrome: Biochemical, cytologic, immunologic, pathologic, microbiologic, and clinical evidence that preterm labor is a heterogeneous disease. Am J Obstet Gynecol 1993; 168:288.
109. Kenyon SL, Taylor DJ, Tarnow-Mordi W: Broad-spectrum antibiotics for preterm, prelabour rupture of fetal membranes: The ORACLE I randomised trial. ORACLE Collaborative Group. Lancet 2001;357:979–988.
110. Cox SM, Bohman VR, Sherman ML, Leveno KJ: Randomized investigation of antimicrobials for the prevention of preterm birth. Am J Obstet Gynecol 1996;174:206–210.
111. King J, Flenady V: Antibiotics for preterm labour with intact membranes. Cochrane Database Syst Rev 2000;CD000246.
112. Romero R, Sibai B, Caritis S, et al: Antibiotic treatment of preterm labor with intact membranes: A multicenter, randomized, double-blinded, placebo-controlled trial. Am J Obstet Gynecol 1993;169:764–774.
113. Klebanoff MA, Regan JA, Rao AV, et al: Outcome of the Vaginal Infections and Prematurity Study: Results of a clinical trial of erythromycin among pregnant women colonized with group B streptococci. Am J Obstet Gynecol 1995;172:1540–1545.
114. Koumans EH, Markowitz LE, Hogan V: Indications for therapy and treatment recommendations for bacterial vaginosis in nonpregnant and pregnant women: A synthesis of data. Clin Infect Dis 2002;35:S152–S172.
115. Relman DA, Schmidt TM, MacDermott RP, Falkow S: Identification of the uncultured bacillus of Whipple's disease. N Engl J Med 1992;327:293–301.
116. Choo QL, Kuo G, Weiner AJ, et al: Isolation of a cDNA clone derived from a blood-borne non-A, non-B viral hepatitis genome. Science 1989;244:359–362.
117. Relman DA, Loutit JS, Schmidt TM, et al: The agent of bacillary angiomatosis. An approach to the identification of uncultured pathogens. N Engl J Med 1990;323:1573–1580.
118. Wilson KH, Blitchington R, Frothingham R, Wilson JA: Phylogeny of the Whipple's disease-associated bacterium. Lancet 1991;338:474–475.
119. Nichol ST, Spiropoulou CF, Morzunov S, et al: Genetic identification of a hantavirus associated with an outbreak of acute respiratory illness. Science 1993;262:914–917.
120. Fredericks DN, Relman DA: Sequence-based identification of microbial pathogens: A reconsideration of Koch's postulates. Clin Microbiol Rev 1996;9:18–33.
121. Yoon BH, Romero R, Kim M, et al: Clinical implications of detection of *Ureaplasma urealyticum* in the amniotic cavity with the polymerase chain reaction. Am J Obstet Gynecol 2000;183:1130–1137.
122. Yoon BH, Romero R, Lim JH, et al: The clinical significance of detecting *Ureaplasma urealyticum* by the polymerase chain reaction in the amniotic fluid of patients with preterm labor. Am J Obstet Gynecol 2003;189:919–924.
123. Jalava J, Mantymaa ML, Ekblad U, et al: Bacterial 16S rDNA polymerase chain reaction in the detection of intra-amniotic infection. BJOG. 1996;103:664–669.
124. Markenson GR, Martin RK, Tillotson-Criss M, et al: The use of the polymerase chain reaction to detect bacteria in amniotic fluid in pregnancies complicated by preterm labor. Am J Obstet Gynecol 1997;177:1471–1477.
125. Blanchard A, Hamrick W, Duffy L, et al: Use of the polymerase chain reaction for detection of *Mycoplasma fermentans* and *Mycoplasma genitalium* in the urogenital tract and amniotic fluid. Clin Infect Dis 1993;17 Suppl 1:S272–S279.
126. Oyarzun E, Yamamoto M, Kato S, et al: Specific detection of 16 microorganisms in amniotic fluid by polymerase chain reaction and its correlation with preterm delivery occurrence. Am J Obstet Gynecol 1998;179:1115–1119.
127. Gerber S, Vial Y, Hohlfeld P, Witkin SS: Detection of *Ureaplasma urealyticum* in second-trimester amniotic fluid by polymerase chain reaction correlates with subsequent preterm labor and delivery. J Infect Dis 2003;187:518–521.
128. Markenson GR, Adams LA, Hoffman DE, Reece MT: Prevalence of *Mycoplasma* bacteria in amniotic fluid at the time of genetic amniocentesis using the polymerase chain reaction. J Reprod Med 2003;48:775–779.
129. Bennett PR, Elder MG, Myatt L: The effects of lipoxygenase metabolites of arachidonic acid on human myometrial contractility. Prostaglandins 1987;33:837–844.
130. Carraher R, Hahn DW, Ritchie DM, McGuire JL: Involvement of lipoxygenase products in myometrial contractions. Prostaglandins 1983;26:23–32.
131. Ritchie DM, Hahn DW, McGuire JL: Smooth muscle contraction as a model to study the mediator role of endogenous lipoxygenase products of arachidonic acid. Life Sci 1984;34:509–513.
132. Wiqvist N, Martin JN, Bygdeman M, Green K: Prostaglandin analogues and uterotonic potency: A comparative study of seven compounds. Prostaglandins 1975;9:255–269.
133. Calder AA:. Pharmacological management of the unripe cervix in the human. In Naftolin F, Stubblefield P (eds): Dilatation of the Uterine Cervix. New York, Raven Press, 1980, p. 317.
134. Greer I: Cervical ripening. In Drife J, Calder AA (eds): Prostaglandins and the Uterus. London, Springer Verlag, 1992, p. 191.
135. Ellwood DA, Mitchell MD, Anderson AB, Turnbull AC: The in vitro production of prostanoids by the human cervix during pregnancy: Preliminary observations. BJOG 1980;87:210–214.
136. Rajabi M, Solomon S, Poole AR: Hormonal regulation of interstitial collagenase in the uterine cervix of the pregnant guinea pig. Endocrinol 1991;128:863–871.
137. Calder AA, Greer IA: Pharmacological modulation of cervical compliance in the first and second trimesters of pregnancy. Semin Perinatol 1991;15:162–172.
138. Karim SM, Filshie GM: Therapeutic abortion using prostaglandin $F_{2\alpha}$. Lancet 1970;1:157–159.
139. Embrey MP: Induction of abortion by prostaglandins E1 and E2. BMJ 1970;1:258–260.
140. Husslein P: Use of prostaglandins for induction of labor. Semin Perinatol 1991;15:173–181.
141. Macer J, Buchanan D, Yonekura ML: Induction of labor with prostaglandin E_2 vaginal suppositories. Obstet Gynecol 1984;63:664–668.
142. MacKenzie IZ: Prostaglandins and midtrimester abortion. In Drife J, Calder AA (eds): Prostaglandins and the Uterus. London, Springer-Verlag, 1992, p 119.
143. World Health Organization Task Force: Repeated vaginal administration of 15-methyl $PGF_{2\alpha}$ for termination of pregnancy in the 13th to 20th week of gestation. Contraception 1977;16:175.
144. World Health Organization Task Force: Comparision of intra-amniotic prostaglandin $F_{2\alpha}$ and hypertonic saline for second trimester abortion. BMJ 1976;1:1373.

145. World Health Organization Task Force: Termination of second trimester pregnancy by intra-muscular injection of 16-phenoxy-w-17,18,19,20-tetranor PGE methyl sulfanilamide. Int J Gynaecol Obstet 1982;20:383.
146. Ekman G, Forman A, Marsal K, Ulmsten U: Intravaginal versus intracervical application of prostaglandin E_2 in viscous gel for cervical priming and induction of labor at term in patients with an unfavorable cervical state. Am J Obstet Gynecol 1983;147:657–661.
147. Giri SN, Stabenfeldt GH, Moseley TA, et al: Role of eicosanoids in abortion and its prevention by treatment with flunixin meglumine in cows during the first trimester of pregnancy. Zentralbl Veterinarmed A 1991;38:445–459.
148. Keirse MJ, Turnbull AC: E prostaglandins in amniotic fluid during late pregnancy and labour. J Obstet Gynaecol Br Commonw 1973;80:970–973.
149. Harper MJ, Skarnes RC: Inhibition of abortion and fetal death produced by endotoxin or prostaglandin $F_{2\alpha}$. Prostaglandins 1972;2:295–309.
150. Romero R, Wu YK, Mazor M, et al: Increased amniotic fluid leukotriene C_4 concentration in term human parturition. Am J Obstet Gynecol 1988;159:655–657.
151. Sellers SM, Mitchell MD, Anderson AB, Turnbull AC: The relation between the release of prostaglandins at amniotomy and the subsequent onset of labour. BJOG 1981;88:1211–1216.
152. Romero R, Emamian M, Quintero R, et al: Amniotic fluid prostaglandin levels and intra-amniotic infections. Lancet 1986;1:1380.
153. Romero R, Emamian M, Wan M, et al: Prostaglandin concentrations in amniotic fluid of women with intra-amniotic infection and preterm labor. Am J Obstet Gynecol 1987;157:1461–1467.
154. Romero R, Wu YK, Mazor M, et al: Amniotic fluid prostaglandin E2 in preterm labor. Prostaglandins Leukot Essent Fatty Acids 1988;34:141–145.
155. Keirse MJ: Endogenous prostaglandins in human parturition. In Keirse MJ, Anderson AB, Bennebroek-Gravenhorst J,(eds): Human Parturition. Kluwer Academic Press, Dordrecht, Netherlands, 1979, p. 101.
156. Romero R, Wu YK, Mazor M, et al: Amniotic fluid concentration of 5-hydroxyeicosatetraenoic acid is increased in human parturition at term. Prostaglandins Leukot Essent Fatty Acids 1989;35:81–83.
157. MacDonald PC, Schultz FM, Duenhoelter JH, et al: Initiation of human parturition. I. Mechanism of action of arachidonic acid. Obstet Gynecol 1974;44:629–636.
158. Serhan CN, Fridovich J, Goetzl EJ, et al: Leukotriene B_4 and phosphatidic acid are calcium ionophores. Studies employing arsenazo III in liposomes. J Biol Chem 1982;257:4746–4752.
159. Buhimschi IA, Kramer WB, Buhimschi CS, et al: Reduction-oxidation (redox) state regulation of matrix metalloproteinase activity in human fetal membranes. Am J Obstet Gynecol 2000;182:458–464.
160. Buhimschi IA, Buhimschi CS, Pupkin M, Weiner CP: Beneficial impact of term labor: nonenzymatic antioxidant reserve in the human fetus. Am J Obstet Gynecol 2003;189:181–188.
161. Romero R, Wu YK, Brody DT, et al: Human decidua: A source of interleukin-1. Obstet Gynecol 1989;73:31–34.
162. Romero R, Mazor M, Manogue K, et al: Human decidua: A source of cachectin-tumor necrosis factor. Eur J Obstet Gynecol Reprod Biol 1991;41:123–127.
163. Romero R, Durum SK, Dinarello CA, et al:. Interleukin-1: A signal for the initiation of labor in chorioamnionitis. Paper presented at the 33rd Annual Meeting for the Society for Gynecologic Investigation, 1986, Toronto.
164. Casey ML, Cox SM, Beutler B, et al: Cachectin/tumor necrosis factor-alpha formation in human decidua. Potential role of cytokines in infection-induced preterm labor. J Clin Invest 1989;83:430–436.
165. Gauldie J, Richards C, Harnish D, et al: Interferon beta 2/B-cell stimulatory factor type 2 shares identity with monocyte-derived hepatocyte-stimulating factor and regulates the major acute phase protein response in liver cells. Proc Natl Acad Sci USA 1987;84:7251–7255.
166. Romero R, Manogue KR, Mitchell MD, et al: Infection and labor. IV. Cachectin-tumor necrosis factor in the amniotic fluid of women with intraamniotic infection and preterm labor. Am J Obstet Gynecol 1989;161:336–341.
167. Romero R, Brody DT, Oyarzun E, et al: Infection and labor. III. Interleukin-1: A signal for the onset of parturition. Am J Obstet Gynecol 1989;160:1117–1123.
168. Romero R, Mazor M, Sepulveda W, et al: Tumor necrosis factor in preterm and term labor. Am J Obstet Gynecol 1992;166:1576–1587.
169. Romero R, Mazor M, Brandt F, et al: Interleukin-1 alpha and interleukin-1 beta in preterm and term human parturition. Am J Reprod Immunol 1992;27:117–123.
170. Silver RM: Tumor necrosis factor-alpha mediates LPS-induced abortion: Evidence from the LPS-resistant murine strain C3H/HeJ. J Soc Gynecol Invest 40th Annual Meeting 1993:P218.
171. Romero R, Tartakovsky B: The natural interleukin-1 receptor antagonist prevents interleukin-1-induced preterm delivery in mice. Am J Obstet Gynecol 1992;167:1041–1045.
172. Gomez R, Ghezzi F, Romero R, et al: Two thirds of human fetuses with microbial invasion of the amniotic cavity have a detectable systemic cytokine response before birth. Am J Obstet Gynecol 1997;176:514.
173. Taniguchi T, Matsuzaki N, Kameda T, et al: The enhanced production of placental interleukin-1 during labor and intrauterine infection. Am J Obstet Gynecol 1991;165:131–137.
174. Fidel PL Jr, Romero R, Cutright J, et al: Treatment with the interleukin-I receptor antagonist and soluble tumor necrosis factor receptor Fc fusion protein does not prevent endotoxin-induced preterm parturition in mice. J Soc Gynecol Invest 1997;4:22–26.
175. Hirsch E, Muhle RA, Mussalli GM, Blanchard R: Bacterially induced preterm labor in the mouse does not require maternal interleukin-1 signaling. Am J Obstet Gynecol 2002;186: 523–530.
176. Molnar M, Romero R, Hertelendy F: Interleukin-1 and tumor necrosis factor stimulate arachidonic acid release and phospholipid metabolism in human myometrial cells. Am J Obstet Gynecol 1993;169:825–829.
177. Hertelendy F, Rastogi P, Molnar M, Romero R: Interleukin-1 β-induced prostaglandin E_2 production in human myometrial cells: Role of a pertussis toxin-sensitive component. Am J Reprod Immunol 2001;45:142–147.
178. Molnar M, Rigo J Jr, Romero R, Hertelendy F: Oxytocin activates mitogen-activated protein kinase and up-regulates cyclooxygenase-2 and prostaglandin production in human myometrial cells. Am J Obstet Gynecol 1999;181:42–49.
179. Elovitz MA, Saunders T, Ascher-Landsberg J, Phillippe M: Effects of thrombin on myometrial contractions in vitro and in vivo. Am J Obstet Gynecol 2000;183:799–804.
180. Elovitz MA, Ascher-Landsberg J, Saunders T, Phillippe M: The mechanisms underlying the stimulatory effects of thrombin on myometrial smooth muscle. Am J Obstet Gynecol 2000; 183:674–681.
181. Elovitz MA, Baron J, Phillippe M: The role of thrombin in preterm parturition. Am J Obstet Gynecol 2001;185:1059–1063.
182. Phillippe M, Elovitz M, Saunders T: Thrombin-stimulated uterine contractions in the pregnant and nonpregnant rat. J Soc Gynecol Invest 2001;8:260–265.
183. Chaiworapongsa T, Espinoza J, Yoshimatsu J, et al: Activation of coagulation system in preterm labor and preterm premature rupture of membranes. J Matern Fetal Neonatal Med 2002;11: 368–373.

184. Allport VC, Pieber D, Slater DM, et al: Human labour is associated with nuclear factor-kappa B activity which mediates cyclooxygenase-2 expression and is involved with the "functional progesterone withdrawal." Mol Hum Reprod 2001;7: 581–586.
185. Maymon E, Romero R, Pacora P, et al: Evidence for the participation of interstitial collagenase (matrix metalloproteinase 1) in preterm premature rupture of membranes. Am J Obstet Gynecol 2000;183:914–920.
186. Maymon E, Romero R, Pacora P, et al: Human neutrophil collagenase (matrix metalloproteinase 8) in parturition, premature rupture of the membranes, and intrauterine infection. Am J Obstet Gynecol 2000;183:94–99.
187. Maymon E, Romero R, Chaiworapongsa T, et al: Value of amniotic fluid neutrophil collagenase concentrations in preterm premature rupture of membranes. Am J Obstet Gynecol 2001;185:1143–1148.
188. Maymon E, Romero R, Chaiworapongsa T, et al: Amniotic fluid matrix metalloproteinase-8 in preterm labor with intact membranes. Am J Obstet Gynecol 2001;185:1149–1155.
189. Maymon E, Romero R, Pacora P, et al: Evidence of in vivo differential bioavailability of the active forms of matrix metalloproteinases 9 and 2 in parturition, spontaneous rupture of membranes, and intra-amniotic infection. Am J Obstet Gynecol 2000;183:887–894.
190. Athayde N, Edwin SS, Romero R, et al: A role for matrix metalloproteinase-9 in spontaneous rupture of the fetal membranes. Am J Obstet Gynecol 1998;179:1248–1253.
191. Athayde N, Romero R, Gomez R, et al: Matrix metalloproteinases-9 in preterm and term human parturition. J Matern Fetal Med 1999;8:213–219.
192. Helmig BR, Romero R, Espinoza J, et al: Neutrophil elastase and secretory leukocyte protease inhibitor in prelabor rupture of membranes, parturition and intra-amniotic infection. J Matern Fetal Neonatal Med 2002;12:237–246.
193. Maymon E, Romero R, Pacora P, et al: Evidence of in vivo differential bioavailability of the active forms of matrix metalloproteinases 9 and 2 in parturition, spontaneous rupture of membranes, and intra-amniotic infection. Am J Obstet Gynecol 2000;183:887–894.
194. Maymon E, Romero R, Pacora P, et al: A role for the 72 kDa gelatinase (MMP-2) and its inhibitor (TIMP-2) in human parturition, premature rupture of membranes and intraamniotic infection. J Perinat Med 2001;29:308–316.
195. Park KH, Chaiworapongsa T, Kim YM, et al: Matrix metalloproteinase 3 in parturition, premature rupture of the membranes, and microbial invasion of the amniotic cavity. J Perinat Med 2003;31:12–22.
196. Maymon E, Romero R, Pacora P, et al: Matrilysin (matrix metalloproteinase 7) in parturition, premature rupture of membranes, and intrauterine infection. Am J Obstet Gynecol 2000;182:1545–1553.
197. Fortunato SJ, LaFleur B, Menon R: Collagenase-3 (MMP-13) in fetal membranes and amniotic fluid during pregnancy. Am J Reprod Immunol 2003;49:120–125.
198. Fortunato SJ, Menon R, Bryant C, Lombardi SJ: Programmed cell death (apoptosis) as a possible pathway to metalloproteinase activation and fetal membrane degradation in premature rupture of membranes. Am J Obstet Gynecol 2000;182:1468–1476.
199. Ferrand PE, Parry S, Sammel M, et al: A polymorphism in the matrix metalloproteinase-9 promoter is associated with increased risk of preterm premature rupture of membranes in African Americans. Mol Hum Reprod 2002;8:494–501.
200. Fujimoto T, Parry S, Urbanek M, et al: A single nucleotide polymorphism in the matrix metalloproteinase-1 (MMP-1) promoter influences amnion cell MMP-1 expression and risk for preterm premature rupture of the fetal membranes. J Biol Chem 2002;277:6296–6302.
201. Romero R, Athayde N, Gomez R, et al: The fetal inflammatory response syndrome is characterized by the outpouring of a potent extracellular matrix degrading enzyme into the fetal circulation. Am J Obstet Gynecol 1998;178:S3.
202. Berry SM, Gomez R, Athayde N, et al: The role of granulocyte colony stimulating factor in the neutrophilia observed in the fetal inflammatory response syndrome. Am J Obstet Gynecol 1998;178:S202.
203. Berry SM, Romero R, Gomez R, et al: Premature parturition is characterized by in utero activation of the fetal immune system. Am J Obstet Gynecol 1995;173:1315–1320.
204. Rounioja S, Rasanen J, Glumoff V, et al: Intra-amniotic lipopolysaccharide leads to fetal cardiac dysfunction. A mouse model for fetal inflammatory response. Cardiovasc Res 2003;60:156–164.
205. Romero R, Gomez R, Ghezzi F, et al: A novel form of fetal cardiac dysfunction in preterm premature rupture of membranes. Am J Obstet Gynecol 1999;180:S27.
206. Yanowitz TD, Jordan JA, Gilmour CH, et al: Hemodynamic disturbances in premature infants born after chorioamnionitis: Association with cord blood cytokine concentrations. Pediatr Res 2002;51:310–316.
207. Yoon BH, Romero R, Shim JY, et al: C-reactive protein in umbilical cord blood: A simple and widely available clinical method to assess the risk of amniotic fluid infection and funisitis. J Matern Fetal Neonatal Med 2003;14:85–90.
208. Sampson JE, Theve RP, Blatman RN, et al: Fetal origin of amniotic fluid polymorphonuclear leukocytes. Am J Obstet Gynecol 1997;176:77–81.
209. Shim SS, Yoon BH, Romero R, et al: The frequency and clinical significance on intra-amniotic inflammation in patients with preterm premature rupture of the membranes. Am J Obstet Gynecol 2003;189:S83.
210. Ben Haroush A, Harell D, Hod M, et al: Plasma levels of vitamin E in pregnant women prior to the development of preeclampsia and other hypertensive complications. Gynecol Obstet Invest 2002;54:26–30.
211. Fidel P, Ghezzi F, Romero R, et al: The effect of antibiotic therapy on intrauterine infection-induced preterm parturition in rabbits. J Matern Fetal Neonatal Med 2003;14:57–64.
212. Rodts-Palenik S, Barrilleaux P, Thigpen B, et al: Intravenous interleukin-10/antibiotic therapy prolongs gestation, improves birthweight, and reduces fetal wastage in *E. coli*-mediated preterm labor. Am J Obstet Gynecol 2002;186:S65.
213. Terrone DA, Rinehart BK, Granger JP, et al: Interleukin-10 administration and bacterial endotoxin-induced preterm birth in a rat model. Obstet Gynecol 2001;98:476–480.
214. Chaiworapongsa T, Espinoza J, Kim YM, et al: A novel mediator of septic shock, macrophage migration inhibitory factor, is increased in intra-amniotic infection. Am J Obstet Gynecol 2002;187:S73.
215. Calandra T, Echtenacher B, Roy DL, et al: Protection from septic shock by neutralization of macrophage migration inhibitory factor. Nat Med 2000;6:164–170.
216. Buhimschi IA, Buhimschi CS, Weiner CP: Protective effect of N-acetylcysteine against fetal death and preterm labor induced by maternal inflammation. Am J Obstet Gynecol 2003;188: 203–208.
217. Buhimschi IA, Kramer WB, Buhimschi CS, et al: Reduction-oxidation (redox) state regulation of matrix metalloproteinase activity in human fetal membranes. Am J Obstet Gynecol 2000;182:458–464.
218. Gravett MG, Sadowsky D, Witkin M, Novy M: Immunomodulators plus antibiotics to prevent preterm delivery in experimental intra-amniotic infection (IAI). Am J Obstet Gynecol 2003;189:S56.
219. Grether JK, Nelson KB: Maternal infection and cerebral palsy in infants of normal birth weight. JAMA 1997;278:207–211.

220. Paneth N, Kiely J: The frequency of cerebral palsy: A review of population studies in industrialized nations since 1950. In Stanley F, Alberman E (eds): The Epidemiology of the Cerebral Palsies. Oxford, Blackwell Scientific, 1984, pp 46–56.
221. Stanley FJ, Watson L: Trends in perinatal mortality and cerebral palsy in Western Australia, 1967 to 1985. BMJ 1992;304: 1658–1663.
222. Leviton A, Paneth N: White matter damage in preterm newborns—an epidemiologic perspective. Early Hum Dev 1990;24:1–22.
223. Hagberg B, Hagberg G, Olow I, von Wendt L: The changing panorama of cerebral palsy in Sweden. V. The birth year period 1979-82. Acta Paediatr Scand 1989;78:283–290.
224. Weindling AM, Wilkinson AR, Cook J, et al: Perinatal events which precede periventricular haemorrhage and leukomalacia in the newborn. BJOG 1985;92:1218–1223.
225. Bejar R, Wozniak P, Allard M, et al: Antenatal origin of neurologic damage in newborn infants. I. Preterm infants. Am J Obstet Gynecol 1988;159:357–363.
226. Trounce JQ, Shaw DE, Levene MI, Rutter N: Clinical risk factors and periventricular leucomalacia. Arch Dis Child 1988;63:17–22.
227. Costello AM, Hamilton PA, Baudin J, et al: Prediction of neurodevelopmental impairment at four years from brain ultrasound appearance of very preterm infants. Dev Med Child Neurol 1988;30:711–722.
228. Shortland D, Levene MI, Trounce J, et al: The evolution and outcome of cavitating periventricular leukomalacia in infancy. A study of 46 cases. J Perinat Med 1988;16:241–247.
229. Levene MI: Cerebral ultrasound and neurological impairment: Telling the future. Arch Dis Child 1990;65:469–471.
230. Pidcock FS, Graziani LJ, Stanley C, et al: Neurosonographic features of periventricular echodensities associated with cerebral palsy in preterm infants. J Pediatr 1990;116:417–422.
231. Fazzi E, Lanzi G, Gerardo A, et al: Correlation between clinical and ultrasound findings in preterm infants with cystic periventricular leukomalacia. Ital J Neurol Sci 1991;12:199–203.
232. Graziani LJ, Mitchell DG, Kornhauser M, et al: Neurodevelopment of preterm infants: Neonatal neurosonographic and serum bilirubin studies. Pediatrics 1992;89:229–234.
233. Murphy DJ, Sellers S, MacKenzie IZ, et al: Case-control study of antenatal and intrapartum risk factors for cerebral palsy in very preterm singleton babies. Lancet 1995;346:1449–1454.
234. Yoon BH, Kim CJ, Romero R, et al: Experimentally induced intrauterine infection causes fetal brain white matter lesions in rabbits. Am J Obstet Gynecol 1997;177:797–802.
235. Yoon BH, Jun JK, Romero R, et al: Amniotic fluid inflammatory cytokines (interleukin-6, interleukin-1β, and tumor necrosis factor-α), neonatal brain white matter lesions, and cerebral palsy. Am J Obstet Gynecol 1997;177:19–26.
236. Nelson KB, Dambrosia JM, Grether JK, Phillips TM: Neonatal cytokines and coagulation factors in children with cerebral palsy. Ann Neurol 1998;44:665–675.
237. Eastman NJ, DeLeon M: The etiology of cerebral palsy. Am J Obstet Gynecol 1955;69:950-61.
238. Nelson KB, Ellenberg JH: Epidemiology of cerebral palsy. Adv Neurol 1978;19:421-35.
239. O'Shea TM, Klinepeter KL, Dillard RG: Prenatal events and the risk of cerebral palsy in very low birth weight infants. Am J Epidemiol 1998;147:362–369.
240. Verma U, Tejani N, Klein S, et al: Obstetric antecedents of intraventricular hemorrhage and periventricular leukomalacia in the low birth weight neonate. Am J Obstet Gynecol 1997;176:275–281.
241. Alexander JM, Gilstrap LC, Cox SM, et al: Clinical chorioamnionitis and the prognosis for very low birth weight infants. Obstet Gynecol 1998;91:725–729.
242. Dammann O, Leviton A: Role of the fetus in perinatal infection and neonatal brain damage. Curr Opin Pediatr 2000;12:99–104.
243. DeReuck J, Chattha AS, Richardson EP Jr: Pathogenesis and evolution of periventricular leukomalacia in infancy. Arch Neurol 1972;27:229–236.
244. Johnston MV, Trescher WH, Taylor GA: Hypoxic and ischemic central nervous system disorders in infants and children. Adv Pediatr 1995;42:1–45.
245. Tamisari L, Vigi V, Fortini C, Scarpa P: Neonatal periventricular leukomalacia: Diagnosis and evolution evaluated by real-time ultrasound. Helv Paediatr Acta 1986;41:399–407.
246. Yoon BH, Romero R, Yang SH, et al: Interleukin-6 concentrations in umbilical cord plasma are elevated in neonates with white matter lesions associated with periventricular leukomalacia. Am J Obstet Gynecol 1996;174:1433–1440.
247. Nelson KB: The epidemiology of cerebral palsy in term infants. Ment Retard Dev Disabil Res Rev 2002;8:146–150.
248. Shea KG, Coleman SS, Carroll K, et al: Pemberton pericapsular osteotomy to treat a dysplastic hip in cerebral palsy. J Bone Joint Surg Am 1997;79:1342–1351.
249. Yoon BH, Romero R, Kim CJ, et al: High expression of tumor necrosis factor-alpha and interleukin-6 in periventricular leukomalacia. Am J Obstet Gynecol 1997;177:406–411.
250. Selmaj KW, Raine CS: Tumor necrosis factor mediates myelin and oligodendrocyte damage in vitro. Ann Neurol 1988;23: 339–346.
251. Robbins DS, Shirazi Y, Drysdale BE, et al: Production of cytokine profile in plasma of baboons challenged with lethal and sublethal *Escherichia coli*. Circ Shock 1992;33:84–91.
252. Leviton A: Preterm birth and cerebral palsy: Is tumor necrosis factor the missing link? Dev Med Child Neurol 1993;35: 553–558.
253. Iida K, Takashima S, Takeuchi Y: Etiologies and distribution of neonatal leukomalacia. Pediatr Neurol 1992;8:205–209.
254. Camussi G, Bussolino F, Salvidio G, Baglioni C: Tumor necrosis factor/cachectin stimulates peritoneal macrophages, polymorphonuclear neutrophils, and vascular endothelial cells to synthesize and release platelet-activating factor. J Exp Med 1987;166:1390–1404.
255. Benett JC: Approach to the patient with immune disease. In Benett JC, Plum F (eds): Cecil Textbook of Medicine. Philadelphia, WB Saunders, 1996, p. 1993–1998.
256. Stuber F, Petersen M, Bokelmann F, Schade U: A genomic polymorphism within the tumor necrosis factor locus influences plasma tumor necrosis factor-alpha concentrations and outcome of patients with severe sepsis. Crit Care Med 1996;24:381–384.
257. McGuire W, Hill AV, Allsopp CE, et al: Variation in the TNF-αpromoter region associated with susceptibility to cerebral malaria. Nature 1994;371:508–510.
258. Monzon-Bordonaba F, Parry S, Holder J, et al: A genetic marker for preterm delivery. J Soc Gynecol Invest 1998;5:71A.
259. Wilson AG, Symons JA, McDowell TL, et al: Effects of a polymorphism in the human tumor necrosis factor alpha promoter on transcriptional activation. Proc Natl Acad Sci USA 1997;94:3195–3199.
260. Graham M, Levene MI, Trounce JQ, Rutter N: Prediction of cerebral palsy in very low birthweight infants: Prospective ultrasound study. Lancet 1987;2:593-96.
261. Han TR, Bang MS, Lim JY, et al: Risk factors of cerebral palsy in preterm infants. Am J Phys Med Rehabil 2002;81:297–303.
262. Lewis DB, Wilson CB: Developmental immunology and role of host defenses in fetal and neonatal susceptibility to infection. In Remington JS, Klein JO (eds): Infectious Diseases of the Fetus and Newborn Infant. Philadelphia, WB Saunders, 2001, p. 27.
263. Wu YW, Escobar GJ, Grether JK, et al: Chorioamnionitis and cerebral palsy in term and near-term infants. JAMA 2003;290:2677–2684.
264. Chaiworapongsa T, Romero R, Kim JC, et al: Evidence for fetal involvement in the pathologic process of clinical chorioamnionitis. Am J Obstet Gynecol 2002;186:1178–1182.

265. Bell MJ, Hallenbeck JM: Effects of intrauterine inflammation on developing rat brain. J Neurosci Res 2002;70:570–579.
266. Debillon T, Gras-Leguen C, Verielle V, et al: Intrauterine infection induces programmed cell death in rabbit periventricular white matter. Pediatr Res 2000;47:736–742.
267. Debillon T, Gras-Leguen C, Leroy S, et al: Patterns of cerebral inflammatory response in a rabbit model of intrauterine infection-mediated brain lesion. Brain Res Dev Brain Res 2003;145:39–48.
268. Duncan JR, Cock ML, Scheerlinck JP, et al: White matter injury after repeated endotoxin exposure in the preterm ovine fetus. Pediatr Res 2002;52:941–949.
269. Hagberg H, Peebles D, Mallard C: Models of white matter injury: Comparison of infectious, hypoxic-ischemic, and excitotoxic insults. Ment Retard Dev Disabil Res Rev 2002;8:30–38.
270. Mallard C, Welin AK, Peebles D, et al: White matter injury following systemic endotoxemia or asphyxia in the fetal sheep. Neurochem Res 2003;28:215–223.
271. van der PT, Buller HR, ten Cate H, et al: Activation of coagulation after administration of tumor necrosis factor to normal subjects. N Engl J Med 1990;322:1622–1627.
272. Sharief MK, Thompson EJ: In vivo relationship of tumor necrosis factor-alpha to blood-brain barrier damage in patients with active multiple sclerosis. J Neuroimmunol 1992;38:27–33.
273. Ghezzi F, Gomez R, Romero R, et al: Elevated interleukin-8 concentrations in amniotic fluid of mothers whose neonates subsequently develop bronchopulmonary dysplasia. Eur J Obstet Gynecol Reprod Biol 1998;78:5–10.
274. Watterberg KL, Demers LM, Scott SM, Murphy S: Chorioamnionitis and early lung inflammation in infants in whom bronchopulmonary dysplasia develops. Pediatrics 1996;97:210–215.
275. Yoon BH, Romero R, Shim JY, et al: "Atypical" chronic lung disease of the newborn is linked to fetal systemic inflammation. Am J Obstet Gynecol 2002;187:S129.
276. Yoon BH, Romero R, Jun JK, et al: Amniotic fluid cytokines (interleukin-6, tumor necrosis factor-alpha, interleukin-1 beta, and interleukin-8) and the risk for the development of bronchopulmonary dysplasia. Am J Obstet Gynecol 1997;177: 825–830.
277. Stoll BJ: Neonatal infections: A global perspective. In Remington JS, Klein JO (eds): Infectious Diseases of the Fetus and Newborn Infant. Philadelphia, WB Saunders, 2001, pp 139–168.
278. Bonds LA, Gaido L, Woods JE, et al: Infectious diseases detected at autopsy at an urban public hospital, 1996-2001. Am J Clin Pathol 2003;119:866–872.
279. Goldenberg RL, Thompson C: The infectious origins of stillbirth. Am J Obstet Gynecol 2003;189:861–873.
280. Blackwell S, Romero R, Chaiworapongsa T, et al: Maternal and fetal inflammatory responses in unexplained fetal death. J Matern Fetal Neonatal Med. 2003;14:151–157.
281. Blackwell S, Romero R, Chaiworapongsa T, et al: Unexplained fetal death is associated with changes in the adaptive limb of the maternal immune response consistent with prior antigenic exposure. J Matern Fetal Neonatal Med 2003;14:241–246.
282. Wang D, Coscoy L, Zylberberg M, et al: Microarray-based detection and genotyping of viral pathogens. Proc Natl Acad Sci USA 2002;99:15687–15692.
283. Fisher S, Genbacev O, Maidji E, Pereira L: Human cytomegalovirus infection of placental cytotrophoblasts in vitro and in utero: Implications for transmission and pathogenesis. J Virol 2000;74:6808–6820.
284. Koi H, Zhang J, Makrigiannakis A, et al: Differential expression of the coxsackievirus and adenovirus receptor regulates adenovirus infection of the placenta. Biol Reprod 2001;64: 1001–1009.
285. Arechavaleta-Velasco F, Koi H, Strauss JF III, Parry S: Viral infection of the trophoblast: Time to take a serious look at its role in abnormal implantation and placentation? J Reprod Immunol 2002;55:113–121.
286. Chan G, Hemmings DG, Yurochko AD, Guilbert LJ: Human cytomegalovirus-caused damage to placental trophoblasts mediated by immediate-early gene-induced tumor necrosis factor-alpha. Am J Pathol 2002;161:1371–1381.
287. Lipkin WI: The search for infectious agents in neuropsychiatric disorders: Lessons from multiple sclerosis. Mol Psychiatry 1997;2:437–438.
288. Yolken RH, Torrey EF: Viruses, schizophrenia, and bipolar disorder. Clin Microbiol Rev 1995;8:131–145.
289. Hornig M, Weissenbock H, Horscroft N, Lipkin WI: An infection-based model of neurodevelopmental damage. Proc Natl Acad Sci USA 1999;96:12102–12107.
290. Patterson PH: Maternal infection: Window on neuroimmune interactions in fetal brain development and mental illness. Curr Opin Neurobiol 2002;12:115–118.
291. Shi L, Fatemi SH, Sidwell RW, Patterson PH: Maternal influenza infection causes marked behavioral and pharmacological changes in the offspring. J Neurosci 2003;23:297–302.
292. Baschat AA, Towbin J, Bowles NE, et al: Prevalence of viral DNA in amniotic fluid of low risk pregnancies in the second trimester. J Matern Fetal Neonatal Med 2003;13:381–384.
293. Wenstrom KD, Andrews WW, Bowles NE, et al: Intrauterine viral infection at the time of second trimester genetic amniocentesis. Obstet Gynecol 1998;92:420–424.
294. McLean LK, Chehab FF, Goldberg JD: Detection of viral deoxyribonucleic acid in the amniotic fluid of low-risk pregnancies by polymerase chain reaction. Am J Obstet Gynecol 1995;173:1282–1286.
295. Yankowitz J, Weiner CP, Henderson J, et al: Outcome of low-risk pregnancies with evidence of intraamniotic viral infection detected by PCR on amniotic fluid obtained at second trimester genetic amniocenteses. J Soc Gynecol Invest 1996;3:132A.
296. Van denVeyver I, Ni J, Bowles N, et al: Detection of intrauterine viral infection using the polymerase chain reaction. Mol Genet Metab 1998;63:85–95.
297. Baschat AA, Harman CR, Towbin JA, Weiner CP: Fetal sonographic abnormalities and intrauterine viral infection. Am J Obstet Gynecol 2000;182:S95.
298. Reddy U, Zlatnik M, Baschat AA, et al: Detection of viral deoxyribonucleic acid in amniotic fluid: Predictor of abnormal pregnancy (abstract # 408). Am J Obstet Gynecol 2001; 185:S192.
299. Yoon BH, Romero R, Moon J, et al: Differences in the fetal interleukin-6 response to microbial invasion of the amniotic cavity between term and preterm gestation. J Matern Fetal Neonatal Med 2003;13:32–38.
300. Dollner H, Vatten L, Halgunset J, et al: Histologic chorioamnionitis and umbilical serum levels of pro-inflammatory cytokines and cytokine inhibitors. BJOG 2002;109: 534–539.
301. Rogers BB, Alexander JM, Head J, et al: Umbilical vein interleukin-6 levels correlate with the severity of placental inflammation and gestational age. Hum Pathol 2002;33:335–340.
302. Kashlan F, Smulian J, Shen-Schwarz S, et al: Umbilical vein interleukin 6 and tumor necrosis factor alpha plasma concentrations in the very preterm infant. Pediatr Infect Dis J 2000;19:238–243.
303. Naccasha N, Hinson R, Montag A, et al: Association between funisitis and elevated interleukin-6 in cord blood. Obstet Gynecol 2001;97:220–224.
304. Messer J, Eyer D, Donato L, et al: Evaluation of interleukin-6 and soluble receptors of tumor necrosis factor for early diagnosis of neonatal infection. J Pediatr 1996;129:574–580.
305. Dollner H, Vatten L, Linnebo I, et al: Inflammatory mediators in umbilical plasma from neonates who develop early-onset sepsis. Biol Neonate 2001;80:41–47.
306. Smulian JC, Bhandari V, Campbell WA, et al: Value of umbilical artery and vein levels of interleukin-6 and soluble intracellular

adhesion molecule-1 as predictors of neonatal hematologic indices and suspected early sepsis. J Matern Fetal Med 1997;6:254–259.

307. Krueger M, Nauck MS, Sang S, et al: Cord blood levels of interleukin-6 and interleukin-8 for the immediate diagnosis of early-onset infection in premature infants. Biol Neonate 2001;80:118–123.
308. Weeks JW, Reynolds L, Taylor D, et al: Umbilical cord blood interleukin-6 levels and neonatal morbidity. Obstet Gynecol 1997;90:815–818.
309. Tauscher MK, Berg D, Brockmann M, et al: Association of histologic chorioamnionitis, increased levels of cord blood cytokines, and intracerebral hemorrhage in preterm neonates. Biol Neonate 2003;83:166–170.
310. Mittendorf R, Montag AG, MacMillan W, et al: Components of the systemic fetal inflammatory response syndrome as predictors of impaired neurologic outcomes in children. Am J Obstet Gynecol 2003;188:1438–1434.
311. Martius JA, Roos T, Gora B, et al: Risk factors associated with early-onset sepsis in premature infants. Eur J Obstet Gynecol Reprod Biol 1999;85:151–158.
312. Grafe MR: The correlation of prenatal brain damage with placental pathology. J Neuropathol Exp Neurol 1994;53:407–415.

CHAPTER 28

Hepatitis Virus Infections

Neil S. Silverman

HEPATITIS A

General

Although person-to-person contact resulting in "infectious jaundice" was described in a review of hepatitis epidemics published by Blumer in 1923,[1] the hepatitis A virus was not identified until 1973, when Feinstone and colleagues, using immunofluorescent electron microscopy, described virus-like particles in filtered stool samples that stained positively when mixed with hepatitis A virus (HAV) convalescent serum.[2] These investigators also demonstrated a lack of cross-reactivity between HAV-specific antibodies and both hepatitis B virus and Norwalk particles, proving HAV to be a distinct infectious viral entity. Subsequent work by this group then demonstrated a temporal link between detectable shedding of the HAV antigen in feces and symptomatic illness in experimentally infected subjects.[3] HAV has subsequently been identified as a positive-strand RNA virus, with intact virions carrying the messenger RNA strand, and is classified in the family Picornaviridae. As a picornavirus, HAV is nonenveloped and is resistant to organic solvent dissolution owing to its lipid-poor coating.

HAV produces little to no typical cytopathic effect in cell culture and is difficult to propagate in tissue culture.[4] Compared to other picornaviruses such as poliovirus, HAV is relatively resistant to heat, surviving 60°C for 1 hour[5]; it is also resistant to inactivation by drying for up to 1 month.[6] Autoclaving, ultraviolet (UV) radiation, and heat extremes (>100°C), however, do prevent viral infectivity, as does chlorination.[7] This latter effect helps explain the ready propagation of HAV in areas of poor sanitation. All human HAV strains studied to date are extremely similar antigenically, if not identical.[8] Antigenic cross-reactivity has not been demonstrated between HAV and any other vectors producing viral hepatitis.

Because HAV produces a self-limited illness and does not result in a chronic carrier state, prevalence studies have been mostly limited to adult hospitalized populations. In these, HAV was responsible for approximately 20% of cases of acute hepatitis, with hepatitus B virus producing 50% and the remainder attributed to non-A, non-B hepatitis (now hepatitis C).[9]

The distribution of HAV is global, though outbreaks are typically seen in areas with crowded conditions or poor hygiene and sanitation. The virus can be isolated from the feces of all infected patients, which facilitates the fecal-oral route of transmission, not uncommonly via contamination of water or food. Parenteral transmission is rare, for the virus is present only transiently in serum.

Serologic evidence of past infection is nearly universal by age 10 in developing countries, whereas in industrialized countries, lower rates of infection in early life are seen.[10] Major risk factors for HAV infection in pregnant women in developed countries would include (1) travel to developing countries (especially Southeast Asia, Africa, central America, Mexico, and the Middle East), (2) household or sexual contact with infected individuals, and (3) contact with infected food or water. In the United States, sewage contamination of public and private water supplies (and the food products they supply) has been most frequently implicated in outbreaks of HAV.[11,12] Bivalve mollusks such as clams and oysters can act as reservoirs for HAV within contaminated waters; crustaceans such as shrimp do not seem to carry the same infectious risk. Infected food handlers have also been implicated in HAV outbreaks, especially when they are from global areas with endemic HAV infection rates.[13] In the United States, the incidence of hepatitis A in pregnancy is approximately 1 in 1000.

Although HAV infection tends to be clinically less severe than infection with other viral hepatitides, and serious complications are uncommon, distinction between infection with HAV and other viruses can only be made serologically. Conversely, not all HAV infections are symptomatic. Before immunoglobulin was available for preventive passive immunization, 80% to 95% of infected adults in HAV epidemics were symptomatic, two thirds of whom were icteric.[14] Severity of illness with HAV infection appears to be directly related to the patient's age (older patients are more severely ill), as well as to the size of the viral inoculum. Viral load also can accelerate the incubation period from infection to illness[15]; usually the mean incubation period is 28 to 30 days, with a range of 15 to 50 days.

Diagnosis

The initial clinical symptoms of acute HAV infection are nonspecific, consisting of fatigue, malaise, fever, nausea, and anorexia. Significant weight loss may be a presenting complaint in pregnant women. Arthralgias may be present, but frank arthritis or vasculitis is unusual.[16,17] The classic picture of icteric illness becomes apparent within 10 days of the generalized symptoms and is usually preceded by palpable hepatosplenomegaly. Liver function abnormalities, typically characterized by elevations in serum alanine aminotransferase (ALT) higher than aspartate aminotransferase (AST), peak prior to the appearance of jaundice. They may remain elevated for over a month in adults. Prolonged illness, with elevations in liver functions tests (LFTs) lasting over 12 months, has been reported in 8% to 10% of older patients, and jaundice and pruritus may persist despite an overall improving trend in symptoms and LFTs. Corticosteroids are usually not given to ameliorate symptoms because of the overall benign nature of HAV infection. Fulminant hepatitis, resulting in death, occurs in fewer than 1% of cases.[18]

HAV-specific immunoglobulin M (IgM) is the serologic marker for acute infection and can be reliably identified with an automated enzyme-linked immunosorbent assay (ELISA).[19] By the time a patient is symptomatic, she will almost uniformly be seropositive for IgM anti-HAV. IgM levels drop below the detectable range within 3 to 6 months in 85% to 90% of patients and parallel a concomitant normalization of LFTs in 80% to 85% of cases.[20] HAV-specific immunoglobulin G (IgG), however, will remain positive for years after acute infection.

Maternal and Fetal Risks

As an almost entirely self-limited illness, acute HAV infection does not confer an increased risk of adverse outcome to an infected pregnant woman. Supportive care for the patient is essential, and in areas where the virus may be endemic as the result of sanitation or housing issues, the availability of such care might not be assumed to exist. Poor maternal nutritional status has been linked to adverse pregnancy outcome in the context of viral hepatitis in general.[21] A chronic carrier state for HAV does not appear to exist. Perinatal transmission of the virus has failed to be identifiable in a number of published series,[22,23] and pregnant women with acute HAV infection should be reassured overall as to fetal risks and status. Administration of immunoglobulin is recommended for neonates born within 2 weeks of acute maternal illness with HAV; the globulin does not appear to be effective if given after 2 weeks after a known exposure.[23]

Management Options

No specific antiviral treatment of hepatitis A is currently available. However, both preventive vaccination and postexposure prophylaxis with immunoglobulin are available. The current HAV vaccine is available as either a single-agent vaccine (Havrix and Vaqta) or as one combined with hepatitis B virus vaccine (Twinrix). HAV vaccine is given as two doses, 6 to 12 months apart. As an inactivated-virus vaccine, there is no contraindication to the use of HAV vaccine during pregnancy. Women at risk for HAV infection, such as those traveling to endemic areas, should be vaccinated.[24]

Individuals who have close personal or sexual contact with an HAV-infected person should receive immunoglobulin if they have not been immunized, concomitant with also starting the HAV immunization series. Immunoglobulin is not contraindicated during pregnancy, and it should be administered, if indicated, to avoid potential illness in the woman. For postexposure prophylaxis, a single intramuscular dose of 1 mL should be given as soon as possible after contact with the infected individual, but not after 2 weeks. With the existence of a safe, effective HAV-specific vaccine, pre-exposure prophylaxis with immunoglobulin prior to travel is no longer a preferred option unless the time before travel (at least 2 weeks) does not permit initial protective impact of the vaccine. In such a case, both immunoglobulin and HAV vaccine should be administered.

HEPATITIS B

General

Infection with the hepatitis B virus (HBV) has been accepted as a health concern of worldwide importance because 5% to 10% of those infected become chronic HBV carriers,[25] and 25% to 30% of those carriers die as a result of long-term sequelae of HBV-related disease.[26] Workers in an endemic area in Asia (Taiwan) found more than 15% of subjects screened in a general program to be HBsAg (hepatitis B surface antigen) positive; deaths in 54% of the carriers were attributable to primary hepatocellular carcinoma (PHC) and cirrhosis compared with 1.5% of deaths among noncarriers.[27] Since that initial linkage, the virus has been shown to be the cause of approximately 80% of all cases of PHC globally.[28]

In areas endemic for HBV, up to 20% of the general population is chronically infected, with perinatal/neonatal and childhood infections existing as a primary route for perpetuating the reservoir of carriers. This finding is especially significant because the risk of chronic HBV infection for a child infected in the newborn period, in the absence of prophylactic therapy, is 70% to 90%.[29,30]

In areas of low endemicity for HBV carriage, however, such as the United States, screening programs for the general population have been targeted to decrease household, transfusion, sexual, and perinatal transmission risks among contacts of Hepatitis B surface antigen (HBsAg)-positive individuals. Population subsets have been identified that are at increased risk for HBV acquisition, and HBV vaccination is recommended for individuals within those groups who are serologically negative for HBsAg and Hepatitis B surface antibody (HBsAb). The efficacy of a serum-derived HBV vaccine was demonstrated initially on a large scale in a cohort of more than 1000 homosexual men in the United States; this trial showed an antibody (HBsAb) response in 96% of those vaccinated, with an overall protective efficacy of 88% against all HBsAg-positive events for vaccine compared with placebo.[31] More recently, a recombinant vaccine consisting of purified HBsAg particles derived from yeast cells was licensed in the United States,[32] eliminating even the theoretical (but never proved) risk of transmitting other viral agents with a serum-based vaccine. Controlled trials in homosexual men showed an equivalent prevalence of acquired immunodeficiency syndrome (AIDS) in groups receiving either placebo or the serum-derived HBV vaccine.[33]

Estimates in the United States tabulate approximately 200,000 new primary cases of HBV infection per year, only 25% of which are associated with acute symptomatic infection.[34] Interestingly, the dose of initial viral infection appears to correlate negatively with the risk of development of persistent disease. Survivors of fulminant hepatitis rarely have chronic infection, whereas experimental infections with low doses of virions result in longer incubation periods, milder clinical disease, and persistent antigenemia.[35]

Blood and blood products are the most thoroughly established sources of hepatitis B infection, although HBsAg has been demonstrated in a variety of body fluids. Of those, however, only serum, saliva, and semen have been associated consistently with transmission in experimental models.[36]

Percutaneous transfer of the virus is the most obvious route of transmission in the medical setting, either through blood products or needle-stick accidents. Contact of infectious material with broken skin or mucous membranes also can result in effective transmission. Recent surveys, however, show that up to 50% of health care workers at risk of contracting HBV have not been vaccinated against the virus.[37]

Compared with other transmissible viruses, such as the human immunodeficiency virus (HIV), HBV is a fairly stable virus and remains infectious on household surfaces that may then contact mucous membranes, such as toothbrushes, baby bottles, razors, and eating utensils.[38] Although transmission in households is more common through sexual contact than through fomite contact,[39] nonsexual household transmission has been established as a route for HBV infection.[40] In areas of the world with higher HBV carrier rates than the United States, nonparenteral transmission would be expected to constitute the major route of person-to-person HBV infection. Vertical transmission is a major source; investigators in Taiwan estimated that 40% to 50% of HBsAg carriers became infected in the perinatal period.[29,41]

Children born to carrier mothers who escape the neonatal period without evidence of infection are still at risk for childhood acquisition of HBV. One of the early vaccine trials conducted in Senegal showed that among children seronegative at the beginning of a randomized HBV vaccination trial, almost 10% acquired HBV infection in the absence of vaccination by the end of a 12-month follow-up period.[42]

Diagnosis

Hepatitis B is distinguished from the other viral hepatitides by its long incubation period (1–6 months), by the presence of extra hepatic symptoms in up to 20% of patients (arthralgia, rash, and myalgia thought to be a result of antigen-antibody complex deposition),[43] and, eventually, by the detection of HBV-specific serum markers.

The appearance of hepatitis B surface antigen (HbsAg) usually predates any clinical symptoms by 4 weeks on average and remains detectable for 1 to 6 weeks in most patients.[44] In the 90% to 95% of patients in whom chronic infection does not develop, HBsAg titers decrease as symptoms diminish. The appearance of hepatitis B surface antibody (HbsAb) defines the absence of the carrier state; titers increase slowly during the clinical recovery period and may continue to increase up to 10 to 12 months after HBsAg is no longer detectable. In most patients with self-limited, acute hepatitis B, HBsAb is detectable only after HBsAg titers in serum disappear.[45] A "window" of time has been described in which a patient still with clinical hepatitis is negative both for HBsAg and HBsAb. During this time, HBV infection still can be diagnosed by the detection of hepatitis B core antibody (HBcAb), which begins to appear 3 to 5 weeks after HBsAg does. HBcAb titers may drop off in the first 1 to 2 years after infection, although the antibody is still detectable years after acute disease in most patients.[45] The appearance of hepatitis Be antigen (HBeAg) parallels that of HBsAg; in self-limited infections, HBeAb is detectable shortly after the time that HBeAg disappears.

The chronic HBV carrier state usually can be predicted by HBsAg seropositivity for 20 weeks or longer. HBcAb is detectable in the serum of carriers at levels higher than those seen in either acute or recovering self-limited infections, and e-antigen markers are variable. HBeAb develops, with the disappearance of HBeAg, in one half to three quarters of carriers,[46] and its presence is inversely related to the relative infectivity index of a patient's serum.[47]

Maternal and Fetal Risks

Risks During Pregnancy

Acute HBV infection during pregnancy is treated mainly by supportive measures, as in the nonpregnant state. An increase in fulminance and mortality rates with acute HBV infection during pregnancy has been demonstrated in some HBV-endemic areas,[48] although other investigators in Western countries have suggested that these adverse outcomes were related more to health care conditions and maternal malnutrition.[49] No teratogenic association has been established for maternal HBV infections,[49,50] even though evidence of HBV infection at birth in children of HBV-carrier women has suggested the possibility of transplacental leakage of HBV-infected blood from mother to fetus in utero.[51,52] Encouragement is necessary to maintain adequate nutrition during the early symptomatic phase, and liver-metabolized drugs, if not avoidable, need to be monitored carefully through blood levels. Phenothiazines may be used, if needed, to control nausea and vomiting. In addition, household and sexual contacts of patients should be offered passive immunization with Hepatits B immunoglobulin (HBIG) after their HBsAg seronegativity is established.

Universal screening protocols for prenatal patients have been advocated by a number of groups. Routine screening with HBsAg testing detects both chronic carriers and asymptomatic, acutely infected patients. A positive HBsAg result in early pregnancy should be followed up by tests for liver function, as well as HBeAg and HBeAb; HBcAb is not helpful in distinguishing acute from chronic disease, and HBsAb rarely is present if HBsAg is still circulating. Repeating the tests for HBsAg and liver function later in pregnancy, however, does help to make the diagnosis and guide the need for perinatal prophylaxis of the neonate.

Hepatitis B Screening in Pregnancy

The unique opportunity to provide almost complete protection against perinatally acquired HBV infection makes antenatal identification of HBV carriers critical so that combined neonatal prophylaxis can be administered in a timely fashion. In nonendemic areas such as the United States, screening protocols were organized initially to test pregnant women who fell into HBV risk groups, as defined by the U.S. Public Health Service (Table 28–1).[53] Such recommendations, however, were not without problems. Reports from a number of groups working in geographically diverse areas around the country found that using risk groups alone for prenatal HBV screening would miss 40% to 60% of all HBsAg-positive parturients.[54–56] Overall, in these studies, the HBsAg-positive rate ranged from 0.3% to 1.5%. Even if risk factors were to be used to identify these women, however, evidence from one survey shows that only 60% of obstetricians could name more than two HBV risk groups, and less than 30% knew the recommended treatment for infants born to carrier mothers.[57]

TABLE 28–1

Public Health Service Risk Groups for Prenatal Hepatitis B Virus (HBV) Screening Protocols (1984)

Asian, Pacfic-Island, or Alaskan Eskimo descent, whether immigrant or born in the United States
Born in Haiti or sub-Saharan Africa
History of acute or chronic liver disease
Rejection as a blood donor
Staff or patient in a hemodialysis unit
Staff or patient in an institution for the mentally retarded
Occupational exposure to blood in medical/dental settings
Repeated blood transfusions
Household contact with HBV carrier or hemodialysis patient
Multiple episodes of venereal disease
Percutaneous use of illicit drugs

From Centers for Disease Control and Prevention: Protection Against viral hepatits: Recommendations of the Immunization Practices Advisory Committee. MMWR 1990;39 (RR-Z): 1–26.

Such findings led to recommendations by the Public Health Service[58] and, most recently, by the American College of Obstetricians and Gynecologists[59] that HBsAg screening be performed as part of routine prenatal testing in all pregnant women. An elegant cost-analysis study by Arevalo and Washington[60] shows that such a program, taking into account both acute and long-term costs of neonatally acquired HBV disease, is cost effective at a prenatal population prevalence for HBsAg of only 0.06%. In countries in which HBsAg carriage is endemic, funding for medical screening programs tends to be limited. In these settings, especially as the cost for HBV vaccine begins to decline, workers have advocated consideration of empiric vaccination for all newborns.[61]

However, protocols establishing prenatal HBsAg screening policies do not address the problematic issue of deliveries in inner-city populations among women with minimal to no prenatal care. Maternal HBsAg status, in the absence of prenatal testing, then can only be known in the 1 to 2 days after delivery, and the newborn may miss out on maximally effective HBV prophylaxis. Investigators have recognized this problem because most hospital laboratories perform HBsAg testing at best on a daily basis.[62] This fact is particularly important because evidence suggests that HBIG given as perinatal prophylaxis may have limited efficacy if it is not given as soon as possible after birth.[63] A study from Philadelphia showed the rate of HBsAg carriage to be significantly higher among such unregistered women than in a comparison group enrolled in an inner-city clinic (7.8% vs. 0.8%), and that the increase was specifically related to substance abuse. Among unregistered women with positive urine drug screens, moreover, the HBsAg-positive rate was 15%, and a maternal urine drug screen was suggested as a rapid screening test to target neonates at highest risk for HBV infection for prophylaxis, before the 24 to 48 hours usually required to await maternal HBsAg status.[64]

Management Options

Prevention of HBV Infection

Immunoprophylaxis regimens to prevent HBV transmission in the perinatal period were a direct extension of the success of these therapies in high risk adult populations. Postexposure immunization was first demonstrated through the use of immunoglobulin preparations with high titers of HBsAb, when given within 4 hours of experimental infection with HBV.[65] Before the development of an effective HBV-specific vaccine, transient preexposure prophylaxis was demonstrated using hyperimmunoglobulin (HBIG),[66] although such use of HBIG is now of purely historical interest in terms of understanding the evolution of therapeutic standards. Currently, postexposure treatment consists of a single dose of HBIG administered as temporally as possible to the exposure. Immediate therapy is, of course, optimal for maximal protection, although 75% efficacy has been shown when HBIG is given within 7 days of exposure.[67] Although it does not increase the efficacy of HBIG therapy, a series of HBV vaccination also should be initiated if the exposure was within a setting of ongoing risk, such as a health care or institutional setting. This regimen consists of injections at 0, 1, and 6 months and results in high antibody titers in more than 90% of those younger than 60 years of age.[68] Administration of HBV vaccine simultaneously with HBIG does not diminish the immunologic response to the vaccine.[69] Still, the currently available HBV vaccine's efficacy is conferred by stimulating production of HBsAb by exposure to HBsAg; vaccine-related immunity can be distinguished from natural immunity in most cases by the absence of HBcAb in the serum of successfully vaccinated patients.

Preventing Perinatal HBV Transmission

Discussion of perinatal HBV infection focuses on the following three major areas:

- The transmissibility of the virus from mother to fetus
- The sequelae of neonatal infection
- The effectiveness of currently available modalities for prophylaxis

Finally, the extensive variance in prevalence rates worldwide requires that the feasibility of prenatal screening programs to identify carrier mothers be addressed.

The potential for vertical transmission of HBV at birth is significant. Most infants born to carrier mothers are HBsAg negative at birth but seroconvert in the first 3 months after delivery, suggesting acquisition of the virus at birth.[70] Mothers positive for both HBsAg and HBeAg are at highest risk for transmitting the virus; 85% to 100% of their offspring become infected, with 70% to 90% becoming chronic carriers. Mothers who are HBsAg positive but HBeAg negative, presumably indicating lower levels of replicating virus, do have a lower risk of transmitting the virus, but up to 35% of their children still will become carriers in the absence of neonatal therapy.[71,72] In addition to the long-term risks of HBV-related sequelae in chronic carriers, such as cirrhosis and hepatocellular carcinoma, fulminant fetal neonatal hepatitis[73] has been described in children born to HBsAg-positive mothers.

Early attempts at interrupting the perinatal transmission cycle employed HBIG alone, administered in the neonatal period. Globulin alone had a protective efficacy against the carrier state of 70% to 75%, although the protection was not permanent, and many children eventually became infected after the passively acquired antibody was cleared, undoubtedly through household contact.[74,75] With the advent of the hepatitis B vaccine, trials were established to test its efficacy when administered in the newborn period, both alone and in conjunction with HBIG. A combination of HBIG and vaccine in the newborn period conferred significantly greater protection against perinatally transmitted HBV than even the vaccine alone, increasing efficacy from a range of 75% to 85% up to 90% to 95%.[42,74–76] The small but identifiable percentage of babies who become infected, despite even combined HBV therapy at birth, is believed to represent in utero infection.[77,78] Still, combination HBV-specific immunotherapy provides the best opportunity to prevent the chronic carrier state in the offspring of HBsAg-positive mothers. In the United States alone, approximately 16,500 births occur to HBsAg-positive women each year, about 4300 of whom are also HBeAg positive.[58] Infants born to these women should receive HBIG (0.5 mL) intramuscularly (IM), ideally within 12 hours of birth. HBV vaccine should be administered concurrently at a different site (0.5 mL IM), or can be given up to 7 days after birth if it is not immediately available.[58] The timing of HBIG appears to be more critical than that of vaccine in achieving maximal effectiveness of passive–active therapy. Subsequent vaccination is performed, also 0.5 mL IM, at 1 month and 6 months of age. Follow-up for these infants is crucial, as one recent study confirms the concern that in the United States, groups at highest risk for HBV infection are also least likely to be compliant with follow-up care.[79]

Impact of Perinatal Hepatitis B Virus Vaccination Programs

The efficacy of perinatal HBV vaccination programs in preventing infection in children born to carrier mothers has led to the inclusion of the HBV vaccine series in the American Academy of Pediatrics' current recommendations for childhood vaccines for the general population.[80] Still, investigators have demonstrated that, even in high risk groups for perinatal HBV transmission, appropriate neonatal surveillance is critical. Among 426 children born to HBsAG-positive mothers in one longitudinal series, only 68% were completely vaccinated with the full three-dose sequence. Among the children followed, it was shown that the third vaccine dose was least likely to be received (64%). Serologic evaluation of the children in this well-conceived surveillance program showed 4% to have acquired chronic carrier status, with an additional 10% having evidence of resolved natural infection, as demonstrated by positive tests for anti-HBc. Not surprisingly, incompletely vaccinated children were more likely to be HBsAG positive than those completing the series (12% vs. 1%; relative risk 7.9 [confidence interval = 1.5–41.2]).[81] These findings underscore the need for reinforcement of complete vaccination for all children enrolled in the HBV vaccine series, particularly those born to carrier or other high risk mothers.

The beneficial impact of adequate childhood vaccination for HBV recently has been demonstrated dramatically in reports from Taiwan, where large-scale mass vaccination programs were begun in 1984. Researchers there have conclusively proved a link between HBV and hepatocellular carcinoma (HCC) by showing a significant decrease in the average annual incidence of childhood HCC since the institution of the program.[82,83] The decline in the rate of childhood HCC was also paralleled by a drop in the rate of HBsAg carriage among children born before the vaccination program was started, suggesting a herd immunity effect from the mass inoculation of children in the much more infectious younger birth cohorts, and resulting in a lower rate of horizontal HBV infection among the older unvaccinated children.[82] These researchers had demonstrated previously that 5 years into the institution of the vaccination program in Taipei, the HBsAg carrier rate in children younger than 5 years of age had decreased from 9.3% in 1984 to 2% in 1989.[84] These results even further bolster the need to identify HBsAg carrier mothers and provide timely and complete HBV vaccination to their children.

HEPATITIS C VIRUS

General

The term "non-A, non-B hepatitis" (NANBH) traditionally was used to describe the clinical picture of post-transfusion hepatitis in the absence of positive serologic markers for either hepatitis A or hepatitis B viral infections. Molecular investigation of the serum of such affected patients led to the reporting in 1989 of the identification of a novel viral agent, named hepatitis C (hepatitis C virus [HCV]), with a uniquely sequenced viral genome.[85]

Soon after HCV was identified, a number of studies employed screening with the first-generation assays for anti-HCV to describe seroprevalence rates for groups perceived to be both at high and low risks for HCV infection. Among presumably low risk volunteer blood donors in the general population, rates of 0.5% to 1.4% for anti-HCV seropositivity were described.[86] Higher risk groups, using HBV infection patterns as a model, were shown to have higher rates of HCV antibody positivity also. These high risk groups have included patients in sexually transmitted disease clinics (seroprevalence 1.5%–6.2%), prostitutes (2%–10%), hemophiliacs (64%–86%), and patients with drug abuse histories (56%–86%).[87–89]

Overall, the principal risk factors for HCV transmission are blood and blood products transfusion and use of intravenous drugs. At least 90% of reported cases of post-transfusion hepatitis can be traced to HCV, usually within 5 to 10 weeks of the transfusion.[90] Although mass screening of banked blood products for HCV antibodies has reduced the risk of transfusion-associated HCV substantially, up to 10% of donors later implicated in transfusion-related HCV may be seronegative carriers at the time of blood donation.[91,92] Current estimates place the risk of transfusion-associated HCV infection at approximately 1 in 100,000 per unit transfused (range 1 in 28,000 to 1 in 288,000).[92] This rate is significantly lower than was reported from the period before the use of HCV-specific assays for screening donated blood, when only surrogate markers of NANBH, such as elevated liver function tests, were employed. Still, it is higher than current estimates of transmission risks by transfusion for other viral vectors, specifically HIV (1 in 500,000 per transfused unit) and HTLV-1 (1 in 641,000 per unit).[92,93] In contrast, the risk of HBV transmission is approximately 1 in 63,000 per unit, so that HBV and HCV together account for 88% of the aggregate risk of transfusion-related infection of 1 in 34,000.[92] As the risk of HCV infection resulting from blood transfusions has diminished, a direct result of mass screening of blood products, the proportion of HCV infections attributable to drug use has markedly increased, from 20% to 60%.[94]

Sexual transmission of HCV has been variably implicated, though the overall rate of infection between HCV-discordant sexual partners appears to be relatively low, on the order of 0% to 4%.[95] In addition, an interaction increasing the risk of concomitant transmission of HCV and HIV has been described. With heterosexual sexual activity, men with evidence of infection with both HCV and HIV were five times more likely to transmit both viruses to a female partner than would have been expected by chance.[96] This potential interaction of HIV and HCV to increase transmissibility of either or both agents also has become important in describing issues surrounding maternal-fetal HCV transmission.

Acute HCV infection occurs after an incubation period of 30 to 60 days. Asymptomatic infection occurs in 75% of patients; the remaining 25% of infected individuals present with the typical manifestations of other viral hepatitides. Fulminant hepatitis and hepatic failure attributable to HCV, as compared with that from other viral hepatitis agents, are uncommon.

Chronic liver disease occurs frequently after acute HCV infection; at least 50% of patients progress to chronicity, regardless of the mode of acquisition or severity of initial infection.[97] Chronic HCV infection has also been associated with an increased risk of developing both B-cell lymphomas and cryoglobulinemia.[98] HCV antibody has been detected in serum from patients with both cryptogenic cirrhosis and HCC, although a linkage between the latter and HCV is controversial and geographically may be quite variable.[99] Evidence also exists that coexisting HIV and HCV infections may accelerate progression of hepatic injury.[100]

TABLE 28–2

Risk Factors Warranting Hepatitis C Screening: CDC Guidelines

Individuals who should be screened routinely
1. Persons who ever injected illegal drugs (even once)
2. Persons notified that they received blood/blood products from a donor who later tested positive for hepatitis C virus
3. Recipients of transfusions or organ transplants, particularly if received before July 1992
4. Persons ever on long-term hemodialysis
5. Persons with persistently elevated alanine aminotransferase (ALT) levels or other evidence of liver disease
Individuals for whom routine testing is of uncertain need
1. Recipients of tissue transplants (e.g., corneal, skin, sperm, ova)
2. Users of intranasal cocaine or other illegal noninjected drugs
3. Persons with a history of tattooing or body piercing
4. Persons with a history of sexually transmitted diseases or multiple sexual partners
5. Long-term steady sex partner of an HCV-infected individual

From CDC: Recommendations for prevention and control of hepatitis C virus (HCV) infection and HCV-related chronic disease. MMWR 1998; 47(RR-19):1-33.

Diagnosis

Although anti-HCV testing includes initial screening with an enzyme-linked immunoassay (ELISA), the false-positive rate of approximately 1%, especially for a low risk patient, raises the possibility of an improper diagnosis being given without appropriate confirmatory testing. In contrast to serologic diagnosis of hepatitis B infection, for which certified laboratories are required to perform supplemental confirmatory testing before issuing a positive HbsAg test result, no such automatic "reflex" testing has been mandated for HCV antibody screening. In a patient at high risk for HCV infection with a positive anti-HCV test result, the chance of a false-positive ELISA is exceedingly low. However, recognizing that the majority of laboratories report positive anti-HCV results using screening assays alone[101] despite previous recommendations,[94] the CDC expanded its HCV testing algorithm to include an option for supplemental testing based on "signal-to-cutoff (s/co)" ratios of positive assay results.[101] Because pregnant women do not constitute a high risk group requiring HCV screening by CDC guidelines unless other risk factors exist (Table 28–2), both the importance of understanding the limitations of even the most currently available screening assays and the ability to interpret test results for patients is critical for clinicians who might be ordering HCV screening tests.

Diagnosis of HCV infection also has been assisted by the use of the polymerase chain reaction (PCR) to amplify and detect extremely small amounts of HCV-RNA in serum, with both qualitative and quantitative tests currently available commercially.[102] PCR is still a technically demanding procedure, however, with a need to maintain stringent testing conditions to assure both accuracy and precision. Heparinized samples interfere with the polymerase in the assay, and sample storage techniques can have great impact on detectable viral particles. Prolonged sample storage at room temperature, for example, reduces PCR signal detection, as do repeated freeze-thaw cycles, even when the sample is otherwise stored appropriately at –70°C.

At least six distinct HCV genotypes have been identified with broad geographic variation,[103] and this mutability may limit the reproducibility of results from laboratory to laboratory, and from study to study, if primer standardization is not verified. Genotype prevalence of HCV infection varies widely by geographic location; variants of genotype 1 are the most prevalent types seen among infected individuals in the United States and Japan, for example.[104] This genotypic variability has been found to have a significant impact on disease progression and response to therapy for infected individuals, with genotype 1 associated with poorer outcomes and responses overall.[105] Despite this fact, HCV genotype has not been determined to be an independent risk factor for perinatal HCV transmission.[106]

Maternal and Fetal Effects

Seroprevalence data describing HCV antibody status among pregnant women or women of reproductive age emerged quickly as HCV testing became more readily available. In Taiwan, for example, where HBV infection is endemic, the prevalence of anti-HCV among a cohort of pregnant women was reported as 0.6%.[95]

A number of studies to date have looked specifically at HCV antibody seroprevalence in prenatal populations in the United States. One, designed as a vertical transmission study, reported a 4.5% positive rate in a county hospital in New York; 74% reported a parenteral source of exposure, and 17% reported no risk factors. Of these, 17% (14 of 23) were also HIV positive.[107] Investigators in Dallas, Texas studied 1013 obstetric patients and found 2.3% to be positive for anti-HCV. Risk factors for infection were specifically studied, with history of intravenous drug use, prior sexually transmitted disease, substance-abusing partner, and more than three lifetime sexual partners being significantly associated with HCV antibody positivity.[108] A study from Philadelphia detected anti-HCV antibodies in 4.3% of pregnant women screened, which was significantly higher than infection rates for HIV (0.5%), HTLV-1 (0.8%), and HBV (0.8% HBsAg). The relative risk of other coexisting viral infections was significantly higher among anti-HCV positive women than for those who were antibody negative. Risk-factor–targeted screening would have failed to detect half the anti-HCV–positive women in the study.[109] A follow-up study from this group, using a larger cohort of more than 1400 women from a heterogenous socioeconomic sample, showed an HCV seropositive rate of 3.2%, with only 19% having HCV-RNA positive test results in newborn cord blood samples. Women who were antibody positive were also more likely to need to undergo cesarean section, suggesting an increased risk of other coexisting obstetric complications in that subpopulation.[110]

Information regarding the maternal-fetal transmission of HCV has continued to steadily accumulate. Although reported rates of transmission have been variable, overall it is encouraging that most series show the risk to be generally less than 5%. However, the definition of which mothers are most infectious dramatically alters the relative risks of vertical transmission. Surveillance of mothers and their newborns using HCV-specific antibodies in published reports has, on the whole, demonstrated low rates of transmission from anti-HCV–positive mothers to their offspring.[95] The designs of these earlier studies, however, were mostly retrospective, with limited neonatal follow-up. Subsequent work has used HCV-RNA as a marker of neonatal infection rather than antibody seropositivity only, with rates of newborn RNA retrieval averaging 5% to 10% when the mother is also HCV-RNA positive.[107,111,112]

More recent studies from Asia and Europe have established what appears to be a correlation between maternal viral titer of HCV near delivery and the risk of neonatal infection. These studies have used newer technologies to determine quantitative, rather than qualitative, PCR results. One team in Japan showed significantly higher (2 logs) HCV-RNA titers in transmitting mothers than in those whose infants remained uninfected.[113] Using similar techniques, another group in China drew similar conclusions, also demonstrating that perinatal transmission occurred only in those women whose serum was HCV-RNA positive.[114] A group from the United States, however, failed to establish a similar viral burden correlation in their series, suggesting a possible role for geographic variability in genotype and virulence in explaining the variance in results.[112] More recent reports have continued to confirm clearly that maternal viremia (usually defined as HCV-RNA detected in maternal blood) is a key determinant for vertical HCV transmission, regardless of maternal HIV status. Still, the independent impact of quantitative maternal viremia ("viral load") on vertical transmission remains less uniformly established across the studies than the presence of viremia at all,[115–118] in direct contrast to previous experience with vertical HIV transmission.

Recent investigators also have confirmed earlier reports that women coinfected with HCV and HIV had significantly higher rates of perinatal infection than women infected with HCV alone. Earlier, smaller series suggested rates ranging from 15% to 87% in the face of maternal coinfection.[119,120] The more recent series have narrowed but not lowered the risk range to 23% to 44%.[112,115,121,122]

The interaction between maternal and fetal humoral and immunologic factors is thought to be a critical contributor to both the occurrence and persistence of perinatally acquired neonatal HCV infection. The fact that maternal or neonatal coinfection with HIV increases the risk of vertical HCV infection suggests that HIV-infected infants, who are known to have early deficits in cell-mediated and humoral immunity, may be less able to clear small amounts of perinatally presented HCV than HIV-uninfected infants.[121,122] Although no large-scale longitudinal follow-up studies exist into the natural history of perinatal HCV infection through childhood, at least one published case report has documented clearance of neonatally documented HCV-RNA by 24 months of age in a child born to an HIV-negative, HCV-RNA-positive mother.[123] Therefore, an intact neonatal immune system may allow for HCV clearance in early infancy, as can occur in HIV-uninfected adults.

The impact of maternal HCV infection on perinatal HCV transmission has been extensively studied, but the potential impact of pregnancy on maternal infection and HCV-related illness is less well documented. One large study of over 15,000 HCV-infected pregnant women in northern Italy, however, demonstrated a downward trend (almost 50% lower) in transaminase levels as pregnancy progressed, with no concomitant change in the proportion of women with documented viremia. The authors hypothesized that a favorable immunomediated positive effect of pregnancy on liver cell necrosis might be one explanation for these findings, though liver biopsy samples were not a routine prospective component of their study.[118]

Management Options

Optimal route of delivery, if, in fact, one exists, remains an area of controversy in the context of maternal HCV infection. This debate, to some degree, parallels the one that evolved regarding maternal HIV infection.

However, unlike with HCV infection, maternal HIV viral load was a clearly established independent predictor of vertical transmission[124] and had a direct bearing on the current guidelines regarding route of delivery and maternal HIV infection, specifically when maternal HIV viral load is durably suppressed to greater than 1000 RNA copies/mL.[125] Route of delivery appears to be much less clearly associated with an increased risk of HCV transmission, however.[115,117,118,121] Although the rate of cesarean section in HCV-infected mothers is higher than that for uninfected women, this increase is thought to be more related to the higher rates of obstetric complications and comorbidities in a subgroup of women whose primary risk factor for HCV infection is illicit drug use.[109,117,118] Current consensus opinions, therefore, recommend cesarean delivery in HCV-infected women only for usual obstetric indications.[126,127]

The experience with antiretroviral treatment in decreasing both maternal viral load and the risk of neonatal HIV infections[128] raises the question of potential comparable treatment options in the context of maternal HCV infection. Recent advances in combination therapy of HCV infection in nonpregnant adults have made sustained normalization of transaminase levels and clearance of HCV-RNA a reality, even in individuals with the less-favorable HCV genotype 1.[105] More recently, the modification of interferon alfa-2a via a branched-chain polyethylene glycol moiety has produced a compound, peginterferon alfa-2a, with prolonged absorption, slower clearance, and a longer half-life than standard interferon, with once-weekly dosing possible.[129] Randomized trials have shown peginterferon to be superior to standard interferon, either alone or combined with ribavirin, for the treatment of chronic hepatitis C infection in adults.[130] Even though the use of ribavirin is contraindicated during pregnancy,[131] interferon has been used safely for the treatment of T-cell leukemias during pregnancy,[132,133] and its potential role as an anti-HCV therapy for both maternal and fetal/neonatal benefits warrants further exploration.

Finally, questions surrounding the safety of breastfeeding frequently arise from HCV-infected women. Many of these women have other risk factors, such as ongoing substance addiction or coexisting HIV infection, which preclude breastfeeding in general and override concerns about transmission of HCV through breast milk. For those women who have no other obstetric or medical issues that prevent nursing, limited data have failed to demonstrate breast milk as an effective route for HCV transmission. Although most of these studies were not designed to specifically address this topic, the authors' evaluation of mother-infant pairs enrolled in some of the published vertical HCV transmission studies failed to document any neonatal HCV infection in breast-fed infants, even when the mother was HCV-RNA positive. One study from China that did look at breast milk specifically found a correlation between maternal HCV serum titer and detection of HCV by means of PCR in breast milk; however, no infants in this small series ($n = 15$) became infected with HCV.[134] More recent studies from Australia,[135] United Arab Emirates,[136] and Switzerland[137] have studied an additional 100 pregnancies in HCV-infected women who breast-fed (up to two thirds of whom were HCV-RNA-positive in sera), with no detectable impact of breastfeeding on the risk of neonatal infection. As a result of the currently available supporting data, consensus opinions do not view maternal HCV infection as a contraindication to breastfeeding except, perhaps, in cases in which a mother experiences cracked or bleeding nipples.[126,127] A recently published survey study, in fact, did demonstrate that that the majority of community-based obstetricians are questioning patients about issues that could relate to HCV infection risk. However, the authors showed that HCV screening practices and counseling provided were discrepant with CDC recommendations up to 53% of the time, particularly in the area of counseling against breastfeeding in the face of maternal HCV infection.[138]

CONCLUSIONS

- Viral hepatitis is one of the more serious infections that can occur during pregnancy, with risks for both the woman and her newborn.
- Hepatitis A tends to be self-limited and produces no chronic carrier state. Risks to the fetus and newborn are minimal.
- Hepatitis B can cause serious long-term sequelae in the woman, and carries significant (90%–95%) perinatal transmission risks for the newborn in the absence of appropriate, timely neonatal prophylaxis.
- Hepatitis C, while more difficult to acquire than hepatitis B, carries much higher long-term risks of chronic liver disease. Perinatal transmission rates of up to 10% have been reported in the absence of maternal HIV coinfection.

SUMMARY OF MANAGEMENT OPTIONS

Hepatitis Virus Infections

Management Options	Quality of Evidence	Strength of Recommendation	References
Hepatitis A			
Prenatal			
• Supportive care	–	–	–
Intrapartum/neonatal			
• Newborn Ig if acute maternal infection occurs proximate to delivery	IV	C	127
Prevention			
• Hepatitis A vaccine available; not contraindicated during pregnancy	IV	C	59
• Women traveling to endemic areas during pregnancy should be vaccinated	III	C	24
Hepatitis B			
Prenatal			
• Supportive care	–	–	–
• 20% rate of extrahepatic symptoms	–	–	–
Intrapartum/Neonatal			
• Newborns of chronic carrier mothers should all receive HBV immunoglobulin (HBIG) within 12 hours of birth and HBV vaccine within 72 hours of birth	Ib	A	75,76
Prevention			
• Universal screening of pregnant women (HbsAg), not risk-factor based	IIa	B	55,57,60
• No contraindications to HBV vaccine during pregnancy	IV	C	59
Hepatitis C			
Prenatal			
• Primary source currently illicit drug use	IIa	B	86,89
• Most cases asymptomatic; supportive care for clinical illness			
Intrapartum/Neonatal			
• No need to alter delivery route for maternal HCV infection	IV	C	126,127
• Risk of neonatal transmission up to 10%, only if mother is viremic	IIa	B	107,111,112
• No neonatal measures available to lower risk of transmission			
• Breastfeeding not contraindicated	IIa	B	134,136,137
Prevention			
• Screen pregnant women only if in high risk groups			
• No vaccine or passive (Ig) prevention available			
• Blood product screening has lowered risk of infection from that source	IIa	B	91,92

REFERENCES

1. Blumer G: Infectious jaundice in the United States. JAMA 1923;81:353–358.
2. Feinstone SM, Kapakian AZ, Purcell RH: Hepatitis A: Detection by immune electron microscopy of a viruslike antigen associated with acute illness. Science 1973;182:1026–1028.
3. Dienstag JL, Feinstone SM, Kapikian AZ, et al: Faecal shedding of hepatitis A antigen. Lancet 1975;1:765–767.
4. Provost PJ, Hilleman MR: Propagation of human hepatitis A virus in cell culture in vitro. Proc Soc Exp Biol Med 1979;160:213–221.
5. Provost PJ, Ittensohn OL, Villarejos VM, et al: Etiologic relationship of marmoset-propagated CR326 hepatitis A virus to hepatitis in man. Proc Soc Exp Biol Med 1973;142:1257–1267.
6. McCaustland KA, Bond WW, Bradley DW, et al: Survival of hepatitis A virus in feces after drying and storage for one month. J Clin Microbiol 1982;16:957–958.
7. Provost PJ, Wolanski BS, Miller WJ, et al: Physical, chemical and morphologic dimensions of human hepatitis strain CR326. Proc Soc Exp Biol Med 1975;148:532–539.
8. Ping LH, Lemon SM: Antigenic structure of human hepatitis A virus defined by analysis of escape mutants selected against murine monoclonal antibodies. J Virol 1992;66:2208–2216.
9. Hoofnagle JH, Ponzetto A, Mathiesen LR, et al: Serologic diagnosis of acute viral hepatitis. Dig Dis Sci 1985;30:1022–1027.
10. Gust ID: Comparison of the epidemiology of hepatitis A and B. In Szmuness W, Alter HJ, Maynard JE (eds): Viral Hepatitis. Philadelphia, Franklin Institute Press, 1982, pp 129–143.
11. Mosley JW: Water-borne infectious hepatitis. N Engl J Med 1959;261:703–708, 748–753.
12. Mosley JW, Schrack WD Jr, Densham TW, et al: Infectious hepatitis in Clearfield County, Pennsylvania. I. A probable water-borne epidemic. Am J Med 1959;26:555–558.
13. Meyers JD, Roman FJ, Tihen WS, et al: Food-borne hepatitis A in a general hospital: Epidemiologic study of an outbreak attributed to sandwiches. JAMA 1975;231:1049–1053.
14. Lemon SM: Type A viral hepatitis. New developments in an old disease. N Engl J Med 1985;313:1059–1067.
15. Krugman S, Ward R, Giles JP: The natural history of infectious hepatitis. Am J Med 1962;32:717–728.
16. Routenberg JA, Dienstag JL, Harrison WO, et al: A food borne outbreak of hepatitis A: Clinical and laboratory features of acute and protracted illness. Am J Med Sci 1979;278:123–137.
17. Inman RD, Hodge M, Johnston MEA, et al: Arthritis, vasculitis, and cryoglobulinemia associated with relapsing hepatitis A virus infection. Ann Intern Med 1986;105:700–703.
18. Gust ID: The epidemiology of viral hepatitis. In Vyas GN, Dienstag JL, Hoofnagle JH (eds): Viral Hepatitis and Liver Disease. Orlando, FL, Grune & Stratton, 1984, pp 415–418.
19. CDC: Protection against viral hepatitis. Recommendations of the Immunization Practices Advisory Committe (ACIP). MMWR 1990;39(RR-2):1–26.
20. Duermeyer W, Wielaard F, van der Veen J: A new principle for the detection of specific IgM antibodies applied in an ELISA for hepatitis A. J Med Virol 1979;4:25–32.
21. Borhanmanesh F, Haghig P, Hekmat K, et al: Viral hepatitis during pregnancy: Severity and effect on gestation. Gastroenterology 1973;64:304–312.
22. Tong MJ, Thursby M, Rakela J, et al: Studies on the maternal-infant transmission of the viruses which cause acute hepatitis. Gastroenterology 1981;80:999–1004.
23. Zhang RL, Zeng JS, Zhang HZ: Survey of 34 pregnant women with hepatitis A and their neonates. Chin Med J (Engl) 1990;103:552–555.
24. Totos G, Gizaris V, Papaevangelou G: Hepatitis A vaccine: Persistence of antibodies 5 years after the first vaccination. Vaccine 1997;15:1252–1253.
25. Hoofnagle JH: Toward universal vaccination against hepatitis B virus. N Engl J Med 1989;321:1333.
26. Beasley RP, Hwang LY: Epidemiology of hepatocellular carcinoma. In Vyas GN, Dienstag JL, Hoofnagle JH (eds): Viral Hepatitis and Liver Disease. Proceedings of the 1984 International Symposium on Viral Hepatitis. Orlando, Grune & Stratton, 1984, pp 209–224.
27. Beasley RP, Hwang LY, Lin CC, Chien CS: Hepatocellular carcinoma and hepatitis B virus. Lancet 1981;2:1129.
28. World Health Organization: Prevention of liver cancer: Report of a WHO meeting. WHO Tech Rep Ser 1988;691:8.
29. Stevens CE, Beasley RP, Tsui J, Lee W-C: Vertical transmission of hepatitis B antigen in Taiwan. N Engl J Med 1975;292:771.
30. Stevens CE, Toy PT, Tong MJ, et al: Perinatal hepatitis B virus transmission in the United States: Prevention by passive-active immunization. JAMA 1985;253:1740.
31. Szmuness W, Stevens CE, Harley EJ, et al: Hepatitis B vaccine: Demonstration of efficacy in a controlled clinical trial in a high-risk population in the United States. N Engl J Med 1980;303:833.
32. Scolnick EM, McLean AA, West DJ, et al: Clinical evaluation in healthy adults of a hepatitis B vaccine made by recombinant DNA. JAMA 1984;251:2812.
33. Stevens CE: No increased incidence of AIDS in recipients of hepatitis B vaccine. N Engl J Med 1983;308:1163.
34. CDC: Inactivated hepatitis B virus vaccine. MMWR 1982;31:318.
35. Barker LF, Murray R: Relationship of virus dose to incubation time of clinical hepatitis and time of appearance of hepatitis-associated antigen. Am J Med Sci 1972;263:27.
36. Bancroft WH, Snitbhan R, Scott RM, et al: Transmission of hepatitis B virus to gibbons by exposure to human saliva containing hepatitis B surface antigen. J Infect Dis 1977;135:79.
37. CDC: Update on hepatitis B prevention. MMWR 1989;36:353.
38. Gocke DJ: Type B hepatitis: Good news and bad news. N Engl J Med 1974;291:1409.
39. Hersh T, Melnick JL, Goyal RK, Hollinger FB: Nonparenteral transmission of viral hepatitis type B (Australia antigen-associated serum hepatitis). N Engl J Med 1971;285:1363.
40. Bernier RH, Sampliner R, Gerety R, et al: Hepatitis B infection in households of chronic carriers of hepatitis B surface antigen: Factors associated with prevalence of infection. Am J Epidemiol 1982;116:199.
41. Beasley RP, Hwang LY, Lin CC, et al: Incidence of hepatitis B virus infections in preschool children in Taiwan. J Infect Dis 1982;146:198.
42. Maupas P, Chiron JP, Barin F, et al: Efficacy of hepatitis B vaccine in prevention of early HBsAg carrier state in children: Controlled trial in an endemic area (Senegal). Lancet 1981;1:289.
43. Gocke JD: Immune complex phenomena associated with hepatitis. In Vyas GN, Cohen SN, Schmidt R (eds): Viral Hepatitis: A Contemporary Assessment of Etiology, Epidemiology, Pathogenesis, and Prevention. Philadelphia, Franklin Institute Press, 1978, p 277.
44. Shulman RN: Hepatitis-associated antigen. Am J Med 1971; 49:669.
45. Krugman S, Overby LR, Mushahwar IK, et al: Viral hepatitis, type B: Studies on natural history and prevention reexamined. N Engl J Med 1979;300:101.
46. Aldershvile J, Skinhoj P, Frosner GG, et al: The expression pattern of hepatitis B e antigen and antibody in different ethnic and clinical groups of hepatitis B surface antigen carriers. J Infect Dis 1980;142:18.
47. Scullard G, Greenberg HB, Smith JL, et al: Antiviral treatment of chronic hepatitis B virus infection: Infectious virus cannot be detected in patient serum after permanent responses to treatment. Hepatology 1982;2:39.

48. Borhanmanesh F, Haghighi P, Hekmat K, et al: Viral hepatitis during pregnancy: Severity and effect on gestation. Gastroenterology 1973;64:304.
49. Hieber JP, Dalton D, Shorey J, Combes B: Hepatitis and pregnancy. J Pediatr 1977;91:545.
50. Towers CV, Keegan KA: The many forms of viral hepatitis. Contemp Ob/Gyn 1987;8:39.
51. Lin HH, Lee TY, Chen DS, et al: Transplacental leakage of HBeAg-positive maternal blood as the most likely route in causing intrauterine infection with hepatitis B virus. J Pediatr 1987;111:877.
52. Ohto H, Lin HH, Kawana T, et al: Intrauterine transmission of hepatitis B virus is closely related to placental leakage. J Med Virol 1987;21:1.
53. Immunization Practices Advisory Committee: Post-exposure prophylaxis of hepatitis B. MMWR 1984;33:285.
54. Malecki JM, Guarin O, Hulbert A, Brumback CL: Prevalence of hepatitis B surface antigen among women receiving prenatal care at the Palm Beach County Health Department. Am J Obstet Gynecol 1986;154:625.
55. Jonas MM, Schiff ER, O'Sullivan MJ, et al: Failure of Centers for Disease Control criteria to identify hepatitis B infection in a large municipal obstetrical population. Ann Intern Med 1987;107:335.
56. Butterfield CR, Shockley M, San Miguel G, Rosa C: Routine screening for hepatitis B in an obstetric population. Obstet Gynecol 1990;76:25.
57. Kane MA, Hadler SC, Margolis HS, Maynard JE: Routine prenatal screening for hepatitis B surface antigen. JAMA 1988; 259:408.
58. CDC: Recommendations of the Immunization Practices Advisory Committee. Prevention of perinatal transmission of hepatitis B virus: Prenatal screening of all pregnant women for hepatitis B surface antigen. MMWR 1988;37:341.
59. ACOG Committee Opinion: Guidelines for hepatitis B virus screening and vaccination during pregnancy. Washington DC, American College of Obstetricians and Gynecologists, January 1990.
60. Arevalo JA, Washington AE: Cost-effectiveness of prenatal screening and immunization for hepatitis B virus. JAMA 1988;259:365.
61. Maynard JE, Kane MA, Hadler SC: Global control of hepatitis B through vaccination: Role of hepatitis B vaccine in the expanded programme on immunization. Rev Infect Dis 1989;11(S3):S574.
62. Kane MA, Hadler SC, Margolis HS: Prenatal screening for hepatitis B antigen: Reply. JAMA 1989;261:1727.
63. Beasley RP, Stevens CE. Vertical transmission of HBV and interruption with globulin. In Vyas GM, Cohen SN, Schmid T (eds): Viral Hepatitis: A Contemporary Assessment of Etiology, Epidemiology, Pathogenesis and Prevention. Philadelphia, Franklin Institute Press, 1978, pp 333–345.
64. Silverman NS, Darby MJ, Ronkin SL, Wapner RJ: Hepatitis B prevalence in an unregistered prenatal population—Implications for neonatal therapy. JAMA 1991;266:2852.
65. Krugman S, Giles JP: Viral hepatitis, type B (MS-2 strain): Further observations on natural history and prevention. N Engl J Med 1973;288:755.
66. Iwarson S, Ahlmen J, Erickson E, et al: Hepatitis B immune serum globulin and standard gamma globulin in prevention of hepatitis B infection among hospital staff: A preliminary report. Am J Med Sci 1975;270:385.
67. Grady GF: Viral hepatitis passive prophylaxis with globulins: State of the art in 1978. In Vyas GN, Cohen SN, Schmidt R (eds): Viral Hepatitis: A Contemporary Assessment of Etiology, Epidemiology, Pathogenesis, and Prevention. Philadelphia, Franklin Institute Press, 1978, pp 467–476.
68. Dienstag JL, Werner BG, Polk BF, et al: Hepatitis B vaccine in health-care personnel: A randomized, double-blind, placebo-controlled trial. Hepatology 1982;2:696.
69. Szmuness W, Stevens CE, Oleszko WR, Goodman A: Passive-active immunization against hepatitis B: Immunogenicity studies in adult Americans. Lancet 1981;1:575.
70. Lee AKY, Ip HMH, Wong VCW: Mechanisms of maternal-fetal transmission of hepatitis B virus. J Infect Dis 1978;138:668.
71. Okada K, Kamiyama I, Inomata M, et al: The e antigen and anti-e in the serum of asymptomatic carrier mothers as indicators of positive and negative transmission of hepatitis B virus to their infants. N Engl J Med 1976;294:746.
72. Beasley RP, Trepo C, Stevens CE, Szmuness W: The e antigen and vertical transmission of hepatitis B surface antigen. Am J Epidemiol 1977;105:94.
73. Delaplane D, Yogev R, Crussi F, Shulman ST: Fatal hepatitis B in early infancy: The importance of identifying HBsAg-positive pregnant women and providing immunoprophylaxis to their newborns. Pediatrics 1983;72:176.
74. Reesink HW, Reesink-Brongers EE, Lafeber-Schut BJT, et al: Prevention of chronic HBsAg carrier state in infants of HBsAg-positive mothers by hepatitis B immunoglobulin. Lancet 1979;1:436.
75. Beasley RP, Hwang LY, Lee GC, et al: Prevention of perinatally transmitted hepatitis B virus infections with hepatitis B immune globulin and hepatitis B vaccine. Lancet 1983;2:1099.
76. Wong VCW, Ip HMH, Reesink HW, et al: Prevention of the HBsAg carrier state in newborn infants of mothers who are chronic carriers of HBsAg and HBeAg by administration of hepatitis-B vaccine and hepatitis-B immunoglobulin. Double-blind randomized placebo-controlled study. Lancet 1984;2:921.
77. London WT, O'Connell AP: Transplacental transmission of hepatitis B virus. Lancet 1986;1:1037.
78. Tang SX, Yu GL: Intrauterine infection with hepatitis B virus. Lancet 1990;335:302.
79. Jonas MM, Reddy RK, DeMedina M, Schiff ER: Hepatitis B infection in a large municipal obstetrical population: Characterization and prevention of perinatal transmission. Am J Gastroenterol 1990;85:277.
80. Advisory Committee on Immunization Practices, American Academy of Pediatrics, American Academy of Family Physicians: Recommended childhood vaccination schedule: United States, January–June 1996. Pediatrics 1996;97:145.
81. Kohn MA, Farley TA, Scott C: The need for more aggressive follow-up of children born to hepatitis B surface antigen-positive mothers: Lessons from the Louisiana Perinatal Hepatitis B Immunization Program. Pediatr Infect Dis J 1996;15:535.
82. Chang MH, Chen CJ, Lai MS, et al: Universal hepatitis B vaccination in Taiwan and the incidence of hepatocellular carcinoma in children. N Engl J Med 1997;336:1855.
83. Lee CL, Ko YC: Hepatitis B vaccination and hepatocellular carcinoma in Taiwan. Pediatrics 1997;99:351.
84. Tsen YJ, Chang MH, Hsu HY, et al: Seroprevalence of hepatitis B virus infection in children in Taipei, 1989: Five years after a mass hepatitis B vaccination program. J Med Virol 1991;34:96.
85. Choo QL, Kuo G, Weiner AJ, et al: Isolation of a cDNA clone derived from a blood-born non-A, non-B hepatitis genome. Science 1989;244:359.
86. Stevens CE, Taylor PE, Pindyck J, et al: Epidemiology of hepatitis C virus. A preliminary study in volunteer blood donors. JAMA 1990;263:49.
87. Widell A, Hanson BG, Berntop E, et al: Antibody to a hepatitis C virus related protein among patients at high risk for hepatitis. B Scand J Infect Dis 1991;10:19.
88. Brettler DB, Alter HJ, Dienstag JL, et al: Prevalence of hepatitis C virus antibody in a cohort of hemophilia patients. Blood 1990;76:254.
89. Van den Hoek JAR, van Haastrecht HJA, Goudsmit J, et al: Prevalence, incidence, and risk factors of hepatitis C virus infection among drug users in Amsterdam. J Infect Dis 1990;162:823.
90. Japanese Red Cross Non-A, Non-B Hepatitis Research Group: Effect of screening for hepatitis C virus antibody and hepatitis B

virus core antibody on incidence of post-transfusion hepatitis. Lancet 1991;338:1040.
91. Donahue JG, Munoz A, Ness PM, et al: The declining risk of post-transfusion hepatitis C virus infection. N Engl J Med 1992;327:369.
92. Schreiber GB, Busch MP, Kleinman SH, et al: The risk of transfusion transmitted viral infections. N Engl J Med 1996;334:1685.
93. Vyas GN, Rawal BD, Busch MP: The risk of HIV transmission by screened blood. N Engl J Med 1996;334:992.
94. CDC: Recommendations for prevention and control of hepatitis C virus (HCV) infection and HCV-related chronic disease. MMWR 1998;47(RR-19):1–33.
95. Lin HH, Hsu HY, Chang MH, et al: Low prevalence of hepatitis C virus and infrequent perinatal or spouse infections in pregnant women in Taiwan. J Med Virol 1991;35:237.
96. Eyster ME, Alter HJ, Aledort LM, et al: Heterosexual co-transmission of hepatitis C virus (HCV) and human immunodeficiency virus (HIV). Ann Intern Med 1991;115:764.
97. Brown J, Dourakis S, Karayyiannis P, et al: Seroprevalence of hepatitis C virus nucleocapsid antibodies in patients with cryotogenic chronic liver disease. Hepatology 1992;15:175.
98. Zignego AL, Ferri C, Giannini C, et al: Hepatitis C virus genotype analysis in patients with type II mixed cryoglobulinemia. Ann Intern Med 1996;124:31–34.
99. Jeffers LJ, Hasan F, deMedina M, et al: Prevalence of antibodies to hepatitis C virus among patients with cryptogenic chronic hepatitis and cirrhosis. Hepatology 1992;15:187.
100. Martin P: Hepatitis C: More than just a liver disease. Gastroenterology 1993;104:320.
101. CDC: Guidelines for laboratory testing and result reporting of antibody to hepatitis C virus. MMWR 2003;52(RR-3):1–13.
102. Inchauspe G, Abe K, Zebedee S, et al: Use of conserved sequences from hepatitis C virus for the detection of viral RNA in infected sera by polymerase chain reaction. Hepatology 1991; 14:595.
103. vanderPoel CL, Cuypers HT, Reesink HW: Hepatitis C virus six years on. Lancet 1994;344:1475–1479.
104. McOmish F, Yap PL, Dow BC, et al: Geographical distribution of hepatitis C virus genotypes in blood donors: an international collaborative survey. J Clin Microbiol 1994;32:884–892.
105. Poynard T, Marcellin P, Lee SS, et al: Randomised trial of interferon alpha2b plus ribavirin for 48 weeks or for 24 weeks versus interferon alpha2b plus placebo for 48 weeks for treatment of chronic infection with hepatitis C virus. Lancet 1998;352: 1426–1432.
106. Resti M, Azzari C, Mannelli F, et al: Mother to child transmission of hepatitis C virus: Prospective study of risk factors and timing of infection in children born to women seronegative for HIV-1. BMJ 1998;317:437–441.
107. Reinus JF, Leikin EL, Alter HJ, et al: Failure to detect vertical transmission of hepatitis C virus. Ann Intern Med 1992;117:881.
108. Bohman VR, Slettler W, Little BB, et al: Seroprevalence and risk factors for hepatitis C virus antibody in pregnant women. Obstet Gynecol 1992;80:609.
109. Silverman NS, Jenkin BK, Wu C, et al: Hepatitis C virus in pregnancy: Seroprevalence and risk factors for infection. Ann J Obstet Gynecol 1993;169:583.
110. Silverman NS, Snyder M, Hodinka RL, et al: Detection of hepatitis C virus antibodies and specific hepatitis C virus ribonucleic acid sequences in cord bloods from a heterogeneous prenatal population. Am J Obstet Gynecol 1995;173:1396.
111. Wejstal R, Widell A, Mansson AS, et al: Mother-to-infant transmission of hepatitis C virus. Ann Intern Med 1992;117:887.
112. Silverman NS, Jaffee FN, Hodinka RL: Hepatitis C virus infection in pregnancy: Is maternal viral burden related to vertical transmission? Infect Dis Obstet Gynecol 1996;4:357.
113. Ohto H, Terazawa S, Sasaki N, et al: Transmission of hepatitis C virus from mothers to infants. N Engl J Med 1994;330:744.
114. Lin HH, Kao JH, Hsu HY, et al: Possible role of high-titer maternal viremia in perinatal transmission of hepatitis C virus. J Infect Dis 1994;169:638.
115. Thomas DL, Villano SA, Riester KA, et al: Perinatal transmission of hepatitis C virus from human immunodeficiency virus type 1-infected mothers. Women and Infants Transmission Study. J Infect Dis 1998;177:1480–1488.
116. Giacchino R, Tasso L, Timitilli A, et al: Vertical transmission of hepatitis C virus infection: Usefulness of viremia detection in HIV-seronegative hepatitis C virus-seropositive mothers. J Pediatr 1998;132:167–169.
117. Hillemanns P, Dannecker C, Kimmig R, Hasbargen U: Obstetric risks and vertical transmission of hepatitis C virus in pregnancy. Acta Obstet Gynecol Scand 2000;79:543–547.
118. Conte D, Fraquelli M, Prati D, et al: Prevalence and clinical course of chronic hepatitis C virus (HCV) infection and rate of HCV vertical transmission in a cohort of 15,250 pregnant women. Hepatology 2000;31:751–755.
119. Giovannini M, Tagger A, Ribero ML, et al: Maternal-infant transmission of hepatitis C virus and HIV infections: A possible interaction. Lancet 1990;335:1216.
120. Thaler MM, Park CK, Landers DV, et al: Vertical transmission of hepatitis C virus. Lancet 1991;338:17.
121. Papaevangelou V, Pollack H, Rochford G, et al: Increased transmission of vertical hepatitis C virus (HCV) infection to human immunodeficiency virus (HIV)-infected infants of HIV- and HCV-coinfected women. J Infect Dis 1998;178:1047–1052.
122. Borkowsky W, Rigaud M, Krasinski K, et al: Cell-mediated and humoral responses in children infected with human immunodeficiency virus during the first four years of life. J Pediatr 1992; 120:371–375.
123. Padula D, Rodella A, Spandrio M, et al: Spontaneous recovery from perinatal infection due to hepatitis C virus. Chronic Infect Dis 1999;28:141–142.
124. Garcia PM, Kalish LA, Pitt J, et al: Maternal levels of plasma human immunodeficiency virus type 1 RNA and the risk of perinatal transmission. Women and Infants Transmission Study Group. N Engl J Med 1999;341:394–402.
125. ACOG: Scheduled cesarean delivery and the prevention of vertical transmission of HIV infection. ACOG Committee Opinion 234, May 2000.
126. Burns DN, Minkoff H: Hepatitis C: Screening in pregnancy. Obstet Gynecol 1999;94:1044–1048.
127. ACOG: Viral hepatitis in pregnancy. Educational Bulletin No. 248, July 1998.
128. Cooper ER, Chaurat M, Mofenson L, et al: Combination antiretroviral strategies for the treatment of pregnant HIV-1-infected women and the prevention of perinatal HIV-1 transmission. J Acquir Immune Defic Syndr 2002;29:484–494.
129. Lindsay KL, Trepo C, Heintges T, et al: A randomized, double-blind trial comparing pegylated interferon alfa-2b to interferon alfa-2b as initial treatment for chronic hepatitis C. Hepatology 2001;34:395–403.
130. Fried MW, Shiffman ML, Reddy R, et al: Peginterferon alfa-2a plus ribavirin for chronic hepatitis C virus infection. N Engl J Med 2002;347:975–982.
131. Briggs GG, Freeman RK, Yaffe SJ (eds): Drugs in Pregnancy and Lactation, 5th ed. Baltimore, Williams & Wilkins, 1998, pp 942–943.
132. Hiratsuka M, Minakami H, Koshizuka S, Sato I: Administration of interferon-alpha during pregnancy: Effects on fetus. J Perinat Med 2000;28:372–376.
133. Crump M, Wang XH, Sermer M, Keating A: Successful pregnancy and delivery during alpha-interferon therapy for chronic myeloid leukemia. Am J Hematol 1992;40:238–239.
134. Lin HH, Kao JH, Hsu HY, et al: Absence of infection in breast-fed infants born to hepatitis C virus-infected mothers. J Pediatr 1995;126:589.

135. Garland SM, Tabrizi S, Robinson P, et al: Hepatitis C—Role of perinatal transmission. Aust NZ J Obstet Gynecol 1998;38: 424–427.
136. Kumar RM, Shahul S: Role of breast-feeding in transmission of hepatitis C virus to infants of HCV-infected mothers. J Hepatol 1998;29:191–197.
137. Zimmermann R, Perucchini D, Fauchere JC, et al: Hepatitis C virus in breast milk. Lancet 1995;345:928.
138. Boaz K, Fiore AE, Schrag SJ, et al: Screening and counseling practices reported by obstetricians-gynecologists for patients with hepatitis C infection. Infect Dis Obstet Gynecol 2003;11:39–44.

CHAPTER 29

Human Immunodeficiency Virus*

D. Heather Watts

INTRODUCTION

The management of human immunodeficiency virus (HIV) infection continues to evolve rapidly. Amazing advances have been made in therapy of primary infection, prevention of opportunistic infections, and prevention of perinatal transmission since the first cases of acquired immunodeficiency syndrome (AIDS) were described in 1981. Perinatal transmission rates have decreased from 20% to 30% early in the epidemic to 1% to 2% in developed countries with the use of antiretroviral therapy and scheduled cesarean delivery. While reducing transmission, these interventions have increased the complexity of prenatal care for HIV-infected women. As standards of care evolve rapidly, providers are urged to access resources available on the Internet such as www.aidsinfo.nih.gov or www.WHO.int/hiv/topics/arv/ for the most recent update.

Women represent the fastest growing group of persons with new HIV infections. In the United States, over 100,000 women are estimated to be infected, and worldwide, the number is over 19 million.[1] Approximately 6000 HIV-infected women deliver annually in the United States, with approximately 280 to 370 infants acquiring HIV infection compared to 2 million deliveries to HIV-infected women worldwide resulting in over 600,000 HIV-infected infants.[1,2] Improvements in availability of prenatal care, HIV counseling and testing, antiretroviral therapy, and strategies to reduce HIV transmission through breastfeeding are vitally needed in areas of the world most affected by HIV to improve maternal health and survival and reduce perinatal transmission.[3] This chapter will focus on interventions currently available to maximize maternal health and minimize perinatal transmission in developing countries.

DIAGNOSIS

All pregnant women should be tested for HIV infection to allow optimal care for maternal health and prevention of perinatal transmission. A policy of universal HIV testing, with patient notification and right of refusal, is recommended.[2] All pregnant women should be encouraged to be tested regardless of perceived risk factors or local seroprevalence, as many HIV-infected women were infected heterosexually and are unaware of their risk. If women decline testing, the reasons for declining should be explored and further education regarding the benefits and risks of testing provided. Federal policy recommends universal HIV testing along with other prenatal laboratory studies unless the woman refuses testing, and state laws may require detailed pretest counseling and written informed consent. Providers should be aware of their own local and state requirements while striving for universal testing for pregnant women.

The recommended algorithm for HIV testing consists of initial screening with an FDA-licensed enzyme immunoassay (EIA) followed by confirmatory testing with an FDA-licensed supplemental test, usually a Western blot (WB), if the EIA is repeatedly reactive.[2] If the EIA is repeatedly reactive and the WB is positive, HIV infection is confirmed, as false-positive WB results are rare.[4] However, given the implications of a positive HIV test result, repeat testing on a separate blood sample is recommended to rule out any possibility of mislabeling or other clerical error. A more common, though still infrequent, event is an indeterminate WB. Indeterminate WB results can be caused by incomplete antibody response to HIV seen with recent infection or late stage disease or by nonspecific reactions in uninfected persons, possibly related to recent immunizations or current or previous pregnancy. Although indeterminate results are more common among pregnant or parous women, they are estimated to occur during pregnancy at a rate of less than 1 per 4000 samples based on a study of over 1 million specimens.[5,6] Pregnant women with indeterminate WB results should be queried regarding recent exposures to HIV through occupational, sexual, or needle-sharing activity; have repeat testing to evaluate for evolving infection versus resolution of nonspecific reactivity; and consider testing of sexual partners to clarify risk. For women with repeatedly indeterminate testing, alternate testing for HIV itself using an approved HIV RNA test may be helpful, although these tests are not approved for diagnosis of HIV infection. If no recent high risk exposures are identified, women with repeatedly indeterminate WB results should be reassured that HIV infection is unlikely.

Women delivering with no prenatal care represent a group at high risk for perinatal HIV transmission. During the period 1993–1996, approximately 15% of HIV-infected pregnant women in the United States received no prenatal care, compared to 2% in the general population.[7] Thirty-five percent of HIV-infected pregnant women who used illicit drugs had no prenatal care compared to 6% of HIV-infected women who did not use drugs. Given the reduction in transmission achieved with several different intrapartum/neonatal prophylaxis regimens[8–11] and the increased risk of HIV infection among women presenting without prenatal care, rapid HIV testing should be offered to all pregnant women presenting in labor without prenatal care or documentation of previous testing during pregnancy.[2] Testing should be done only after pretest counseling, including discussion of the need for confirmatory testing if rapid assays are positive, and informed consent. Rapid testing may be done using the recently approved OraQuick Rapid HIV antibody test, other rapid tests as they become approved, the more complex Single Use Diagnostic System for HIV-1, or EIA testing.[12] The OraQuick test has been granted a Clinical Laboratory Improvement Amendments waiver, allowing its use as a point of care test.[13] Because of the relatively low prevalence of HIV even in this setting, the negative predictive value of a single negative rapid test is high, so no further testing is required to confirm a negative rapid test.[2,12] All positive rapid tests should be confirmed by supplemental testing with either a WB or immunofluorescence assay,[2] but decisions regarding use of antiretrovirals for prevention of perinatal transmission may need to be made pending confirmatory test results because initiation of therapy during labor or shortly after birth is required to reduce risk of transmission.[9] Use of a second, different screening test, such as EIA, can improve the positive predictive value of a single reactive rapid test. In studies done outside the United States, specific combinations of two or more rapid tests provided results as reliable as those from a combination of EIA and WB.[14] Thus, as more rapid tests are approved for use in the United States, combinations with enhanced specificity may become available, allowing more certain decision-making.

MATERNAL AND FETAL RISKS

Disease Progression

Studies in the United States and Europe have been consistent in not demonstrating an effect of pregnancy on HIV disease progression.[15–17] More recently, a report from the Women and Infants Transmission Study (WITS) did not show a difference in CD4+ lymphocyte count or HIV RNA trajectory or clinical AIDS rate between women with one or multiple pregnancies after HIV diagnosis.[18] Studies in developing countries suggest that pregnancy may enhance disease progression, but they included small numbers and may have had selection bias in HIV testing.[19,20]

Increased Toxicity of Antiretroviral Therapy

The hormonal effects of pregnancy may increase the risk of toxicity of antiretroviral therapy, especially the nucleoside reverse transcriptase inhibitors. Several cases of lactic acidosis and hepatic failure, some resulting in maternal deaths, have been reported among women on long-term nucleoside therapy during pregnancy, most frequently stavudine and didanosine in combination.[21,22] Clinical findings were similar to those seen in acute fatty liver of pregnancy, which occurs more frequently among women with heterozygous defects of mitochondrial fatty acid metabolism carrying fetuses homozygous for the defect.[23] Similar enhancement of mitochondrial toxicity due to reduced fatty acid oxidation has been shown in pregnant mice and in mice treated with high doses of estrogen and progesterone to simulate pregnancy.[24,25] The potential for lactic acidosis and hepatic failure is present with the use of any nucleoside agent, with the binding affinity for mitochondrial polymerase gamma, the key enzyme, highest for zalcitabine, then decreasing for didanosine, stavudine, lamivudine, zidovudine, and abacavir.[26] Thus, all pregnant women on nucleoside antiretroviral therapy should be educated regarding the signs and symptoms of lactic acidosis and hepatic dysfunction including nausea, vomiting, fatigue, tachycardia, dyspnea or hyperventilation, and abdominal pain, and clinicians should be vigilant for these signs and symptoms that may be difficult to distinguish from normal pregnancy symptoms.

Impact on Future Therapy

Another potential impact of pregnancy on HIV infection is the effect of short duration therapy during pregnancy for prevention of perinatal transmission on development of resistance and response to future therapy. Current indications for initiation of antiretroviral therapy in nonpregnant adults are an HIV RNA level above 55,000 copies/mL or a CD4+ lymphocyte count below 350 cells/μL.[27] Many women do not meet these criteria for therapy but will take antiretrovirals to reduce the risk of perinatal transmission and stop therapy after delivery. As will be discussed in more detail later, these women should receive highly active therapy with a combination of three or more drugs to minimize HIV RNA levels and risk of transmission.[28] Although aggressive combination therapy with suppression of HIV RNA to undetectable levels during pregnancy should minimize the risk of resistance, the impact of short-term therapy on future response to therapy has not been well studied. In addition, the use of the two-dose nevirapine regimen (one dose intrapartum to the mother and one dose to the neonate) for women without prior antiretroviral therapy during pregnancy was associated with a 19% rate of nevirapine resistance at 6 weeks post partum, which did not persist at 1 year.[29] Nevirapine resistance was also observed among 14 (15%) of 95 women tested after exposure to the same regimen among women on established antiretroviral therapy at delivery in the Pediatric AIDS Clinical Trials Group (PACTG) 316 study.[30] The significance of these mutations for response to future therapy is unknown.

Pregnancy Complications

The effect of HIV infection and antiretroviral therapy on pregnancy outcome is another issue for consideration. The majority of, but not all, studies in developed countries done before the availability of antiretroviral therapy did not demonstrate an increased rate of adverse pregnancy outcomes among HIV-infected women compared to uninfected women with similar risk profiles.[31–33] Conversely, most studies in developing countries have suggested an increased risk of preterm birth, low birth weight, intrauterine growth restriction, stillbirth, and infant death among infants born to HIV-infected women, with increasing risk with more advanced HIV infection.[31,34] Factors associated with an increased risk of preterm birth and low birth weight among HIV-infected women included previous adverse pregnancy outcome, hypertension, multiple gestation, smoking, bleeding, alcohol use, low maternal weight, *Trichomonas vaginalis* infection, and other sexually transmitted infections, similar to risk factors in HIV-uninfected women.[33,36,37] Low CD4+ percentage was an additional risk factor for adverse outcome among women not receiving antiretroviral therapy,[36] but neither CD4+ lymphocyte count nor HIV RNA levels were associated with adverse outcomes among women receiving zidovudine therapy.[37]

Zidovudine monotherapy has not been associated with an increased risk of preterm birth or low birth weight in any study to date, but the potential impact of combination antiretroviral therapy on pregnancy outcome is unclear.[38,39] A small study from Europe and an analysis of the European Collaborative Study found an increased risk of preterm birth with increasing numbers of drugs, with the highest rate occurring among women receiving protease inhibitor therapy.[40,41] An analysis of several cohorts in the United States did not find an increased risk of preterm delivery among women on dual therapy or regimens including protease inhibitors, although there was a slight increase in risk of very low birth weight infants born to women receiving protease inhibitor therapy compared to those on no therapy or zidovudine.[42] Clinicians should be aware of a possible increased risk of preterm birth with protease inhibitor use, but given the clear benefits for maternal health and reduction in perinatal transmission, these agents should not be withheld because of these concerns.

Perinatal Transmission

A major concern with HIV infection in pregnancy is the risk of perinatal transmission of HIV to the infant. Among untreated women who do not breastfeed, transmission will occur in 20% to 30%.[43] Estimates are that about two thirds of transmissions from untreated women occur at delivery and one third occur in utero, many late in pregnancy.[44] An additional transmission risk of 15% to 20% occurs during breastfeeding.[45] Maternal HIV RNA levels appear to be the factor most predictive of transmission.[46,47] Antiretroviral therapy during pregnancy and in the neonatal period is clearly beneficial by reducing the risk of perinatal transmission of HIV. The first study demonstrating this benefit was the PACTG 076 study with a transmission rate of 8.3% among those receiving oral antepartum, intravenous intrapartum, and oral neonatal zidovudine for 6 weeks compared to 25.5% among those receiving placebo.[38] The PACTG 185 trial found no benefit from addition of HIV immunoglobulin to the PACTG 076 regimen but demonstrated benefit of zidovudine among women with CD4+ lymphocyte counts under 500 cells/μL at enrollment, with a transmission rate of 4.6%.[48] Subsequent trials have demonstrated benefit from shorter courses of antepartum/intrapartum or antepartum/intrapartum/neonatal zidovudine or zidovudine/lamivudine compared to placebo, but no benefit was seen from intrapartum zidovudine/lamivudine alone.[10,49–54] In addition, the HIVNET 012 trial demonstrated the benefit of a two-dose nevirapine regimen (one dose intrapartum to the mother and one dose to the infant at 48 hours of age) compared to oral intrapartum and 1 week of neonatal zidovudine.[8] A subsequent trial demonstrated that intrapartum and 1 week of neonatal zidovudine/lamivudine therapy was similar in efficacy to the HIVNET 012 nevirapine regimen.[11] These trials provide data for implementation of shorter, less complex regimens for reduction of transmission of HIV in resource limited settings or for women diagnosed in the peripartum period as being HIV-infected.

A trial in the United States, Europe, and Latin America (PACTG 316) evaluating addition of the HIVNET 012 nevirapine regimen to established antiretroviral therapy demonstrated no benefit of adding nevirapine to ongoing therapy.[55] However, this trial provides the most current data regarding transmission of HIV with the use of combination antiretroviral therapy. The transmission rate overall was 1.5%, with rates of 2.1% for women on zidovudine alone, 1.1% with combination nucleoside therapy, and 1.6% with combination with protease inhibitor.[55] Similarly, an analysis from WITS, including women enrolled from 1990 through 2000, observed transmission rates of 20.0% for women not receiving antiretroviral agents, 10.4% for women receiving zidovudine monotherapy (not necessarily the complete 076 regimen), 3.8% for those receiving dual nucleoside therapy, and 1.2% for those receiving highly active antiretroviral regimens.[43] These low rates of transmission with highly active regimens occurred despite potential confounding by indication in which women with the highest HIV RNA levels and lowest CD4+ lymphocyte counts were most likely to be treated with highly active regimens, especially early in the period of availability. Thus, current data demonstrate significant fetal benefit from combination antiretroviral regimens, which would require significant evidence of harm to negate.

Antiretroviral Therapy

Teratogenesis

Another concern with the use of antiretroviral drugs in pregnancy is the potential for birth defects, especially with first-trimester exposure. Limited data from animal studies are available for most of the drugs (Table 29–1). Of concern, birth defects, including anencephaly, microophthalmia, and cleft palate, were seen in 3 (20%) of 15 monkeys exposed to efavirenz in the first trimester.[28] One case of meningomyelocele has been reported in the literature after first-trimester efavirenz exposure.[56,57] Too few cases of first-trimester efavirenz exposure have been reported to the Antiretroviral Pregnancy Registry to assess risk thus far.[58] Other drugs with concerning animal data (see Table 29–1) include delavirdine and hydroxyurea, which are of limited utility for HIV therapy. No increase in birth defects was detected among infants born to women enrolled in the European Collaborative Study with first-trimester (compared to later or no) antiretroviral exposure.[59] No clear increase in birth defects associated with antiretroviral therapy has been noted among prospective cases reported to the Antiretroviral Pregnancy Registry, although adequate numbers to rule out a twofold or greater increased risk have been reported for only a limited number of drugs (zidovudine, lamivudine, stavudine, nelfinavir, nevirapine).[58] Providers caring for pregnant women receiving antiretroviral drugs are urged to report cases as early in pregnancy as possible to the Registry (1-800-258-4263 or http://www.apregistry.com) to allow better assessment of risks.

Mitochondrial Toxicity in Offspring

Another concern, potential mitochondrial toxicity in the children of women treated with antiretrovirals, has been suggested by French researchers. Eight children with clinical or laboratory abnormalities, including two who died, were reported from a cohort of 1754 HIV-uninfected children exposed to zidovudine or zidovudine/lamivudine during pregnancy and the neonatal period.[60,61] Subsequently, an increased risk of febrile seizures was reported among infants born to HIV-infected women with perinatal antiretroviral exposure (11/1000 by 18 months) compared to those without exposure (4.1/1000, $P = 0.02$) in the same cohort.[62] In a review of over 16,000 children born to HIV-infected women in several cohorts in the United States, no increase in death rate was found in children exposed to nucleoside reverse transcriptase inhibitors compared to those with no antiretroviral exposure.[63] No deaths definitely related to mitochondrial toxicity were noted. Monitoring for symptoms among living children is ongoing. In a follow-up of 395 children born to women randomized to zidovudine or placebo in Thailand, five children exposed to zidovudine experienced febrile seizures, compared to one in the placebo group. No other signs or symptoms of possible mitochondrial toxicity were noted in either group through 18 months of age.[64] No association was found between clinical findings suggestive of mitochondrial abnormalities and antiretroviral exposure among 2414 children followed in the European Collaborative Study, 1008 of whom had antiretroviral exposure.[65] Among infants enrolled in the PETRA study, which included three zidovudine/lamivudine arms with up to 5 weeks of treatment or placebo, the rate of symptoms potentially related to mitochondrial toxicity was low, 5 (0.28%) of 1798, and did not differ by treatment arm.[66] The French cases are concerning in light of recent studies demonstrating reduced levels of mitochondrial DNA among placentas and cord blood[67] and through 2 years of age[68] among infants exposed to nucleoside reverse transcriptase inhibitors during pregnancy and the neonatal period compared to infants born to HIV-negative or untreated women. Of note, infants born to HIV-infected women but not exposed to nucleosides had intermediate levels of mitochondrial DNA depletion.[68] Clinical correlation is lacking. The risk of clinically apparent mitochondrial toxicity related to antiretroviral therapy appears to be low and must be balanced against the known benefits in reduction of perinatal transmission. However, long-term follow-up of children exposed to antiretrovirals is required to assess for toxicity.

Transplacental Carcinogenesis

Another concern requiring long-term surveillance of children exposed to antiretrovirals is transplacental carcinogenesis. One study in rats treated with zidovudine in utero at about 30 times the human dose found an increase in liver, lung, and reproductive system tumors, yet a similar study using lower doses did not find an increased rate.[69,70] Among 727 children enrolled in the PACTG 076 study or WITS, no tumors occurred with over 1100 person-years of follow-up.[71] No tumors were identified among the 395 Thai infants followed for 18 months.[64] A recent study of HIV-infected children with

TABLE 29–1

Preclinical and Clinical Data Relevant to the use of Antiretroviral Drugs in Pregnancy[27,28]

DRUG	FDA PREGNANCY CATEGORY*	NEWBORN: MATERNAL DRUG RATIO	ANIMAL STUDIES	MAJOR TOXICITIES	HUMAN STUDIES; CONCERNS SPECIFIC TO PREGNANCY
Nucleoside/Nucleotide Reverse Transcriptase Inhibitors				**Class Effect: Rare, but Potentially Fatal, Lactic Acidosis with Hepatic Steatosis**	
Zidovudine (Retrovir, AZT, ZDV)	C	~0.8 human	No effect on rodent fertility, but cytotoxic to mouse embryos. Positive teratogenicity in rodents only at near-lethal doses.	Bone marrow suppression, myopathy	ARV agent most used in pregnancy, safe in short term. See discussion of rodent tumors, mitochondrial toxicity in text.
Zalcitabine (HIVID, ddC)	C	0.3–0.5 rhesus monkey	No effect on rodent fertility, but cytotoxic to mouse embryos. Hydrocephalus in rats at 1000× human dose, skeletal defects and decreased weight at moderate doses.	Peripheral neuropathy, stomatitis	No studies.
Didanosine (Videx, ddI)	B	0.5 human	No effect on rodent fertility or mouse embryos. No teratogenicity in mice, rats, rabbits.	Pancreatitis, peripheral neuropathy, nausea, diarrhea	Pk study (n = 14) shows no need for dose modification, well tolerated.
Stavudine (Zerit, d4T)	C	0.76 rhesus monkey	No effect on rodent fertility, but cytotoxic to mouse embryos. No evidence of teratogenicity. Ossification delay at high doses in rats.	Peripheral neuropathy	Phase I/II study indicated no change in pk in pregnancy; well-tolerated.
Lamivudine (Epivir, 3TC)	C	~1.0 human	No effect on rodent fertility or mouse embryos. No teratogenicity.	Pancreatitis increased in children	Pk study (n = 20) shows no need for dose modification, well tolerated.
Abacavir (Ziagen, ABC)	C	Passage in rats	No effect on fertility in rodents. Anasarca, skeletal abnormalities at 35× human dose in rodents, not seen in rabbits.	Potentially fatal hypersensitivity reactions, symptoms: fever, rash, fatigue, nausea, vomiting, diarrhea, abdominal pain.	No studies.
Tenofovir (Viread)	B	0.17 monkeys	No effect on fertility. No birth defects, but growth restriction, reversible bone changes with chronic use in monkeys.	Asthenia, nausea, vomiting, diarrhea, headache, flatulence	No studies in human pregnancy thus far.
Non-Nucleoside Reverse Transcriptase Inhibitors				**Class Effects: Rash with Rare Cases of Stevens-Johnson Syndrome; Increased Transaminase Levels**	
Nevirapine (Viramune)	C	~0.9 human	Impaired fertility in female rats. Not teratogenic in rats, rabbits.	Rash, drug interactions, potential for fulminant hepatitis and hepatic failure	Increased risk of potentially fatal hepatotoxicity, in women starting therapy with CD4+ lymphocyte count >250 cells/µl. Single dose in labor and the neonate decreased transmission in otherwise untreated women. See text.
Delavirdine (Rescriptor)	C	Unknown	No effect on fertility in rodents. Embryotoxic in rabbits. VSD in rats, maternal toxicity, developmental delay, decreased pup survival.	Rash, drug interactions	No studies.
Efavirenz (Sustiva)	C	~1.0 cynomolgous monkey	Increased fetal resorptions in rats. Anencephaly, anophthalmia, or cleft palate in 3/20 monkeys treated with human doses.	Rash, drug interactions, CNS symptoms such as dizziness, insomnia, confusion	None planned. Use in pregnancy should be avoided because of primate teratogenicity.

Protease Inhibitors				**Class Effects: Hyperglycemia, Possible Fat Redistribution and Lipid Abnormalities, Increased Bleeding Episodes in Hemophiliacs**	
Indinavir (Crixivan)	C	Minimal	No effect on fertility in rodents. No teratogenicity in rats, rabbits, or dogs. Extra ribs in rats.	Kidney stones, hyperbilirubinemia, drug interactions, nausea	Phase I/II study in progress; suggests lower AUC in pregnancy. Theoretical concerns re: kidney stones, hyperbilirubinemia in neonate from maternal exposure.
Ritonavir (Norvir)	B	Minimal	No effect on fertility in rodents at half the human dose. Hepatotoxicity at higher doses. Developmental toxicity at toxic doses but no teratogenicity in rats, rabbits.	Nausea, vomiting, diarrhea; increased triglycerides, transaminases; drug interactions, paresthesias	Phase I/II study in progress.
Saquinavir (Fortovase)	B	Minimal	No effect on fertility in rodents. Negative teratogenicity.	Nausea, diarrhea, elevated transaminases	Insufficient levels in pregnancy with 1200 mg TID; adequate levels with SQV 800 mg/ritonavir 100 mg, both BID.
Nelfinavir (Viracept)	B	Minimal	No effect on fertility in rodents. Studies negative in rats, rabbits.	Diarrhea, drug interactions	Phase I/II study showed low AUC with 750 TID, adequate levels with 1250 mg BID.
Amprenavir (Agenerase)	C	Unknown	No effect on fertility in rodents. Negative teratogenicity studies but deficient ossification and thymic elongation in rats, rabbits.	Nausea, vomiting, diarrhea, rash, oral paresthesias, increased liver function tests	No studies. Liquid formulation should not be used in pregnancy because of high propylene glycol content.
Lopinavir/ritonavir (Kaletra)	C	Minimal for ritonavir, unknown for lopinavir	No effects on fertility. No teratogenicity in rats, rabbits.	Nausea, vomiting, diarrhea, asthenia, elevated transaminase levels	Oral solution contains 42% alcohol so not recommended in pregnancy. Pk studies in pregnancy in progress.
Atazanavir (Reyataz)	B	Unknown	No effect on fertility. No teratogenicity in rats, rabbits.	Drug interactions, prolonged PR interval, hyperbilirubinemia, rash	No studies in human pregnancy. Theoretical concern of hyperbilirubinemia in neonate from maternal exposure.
Fusion Inhibitors					
Enfurvirtide (Fuzeon, T-20)	B	Unknown	No effect on fertility. No teratogenicity in rats, rabbits.	Injection site reactions, eosinophilia, rare systemic hypersensitivity	No studies in human pregnancy.
Other Agents					
Hydroxyurea	D	Crosses in animals	Testicular atrophy and decreased spermatogenesis in rats. Teratogenic with multiple defects seen in rats, rabbits, hamsters, cats, monkeys.	Bone marrow suppression, rash, fever, stomatitis, vomiting, diarrhea	Reported use in 16 women, 13 in first trimester. No anomalies seen. Because of unclear efficacy in HIV therapy and potential teratogenicity based on animal studies, use should be avoided during pregnancy.

*Food and Drug Administration pregnancy categories: A, adequate and well-controlled studies of pregnant women fail to demonstrate a risk to the fetus during the first trimester of pregnancy (and there is no evidence of risk during the later trimesters); B, animal reproduction studies fail to demonstrate a risk to the fetus and adequate and well-controlled studies of pregnant women have not been conducted; C, safety in human pregnancy has not been determined, animal studies are either positive for fetal risk or have not been conducted, and the drug should not be used unless the potential benefit outweighs the potential risk to the fetus; D, positive evidence of human fetal risk based on adverse reaction data from investigational or marketing experiences, but the potential benefits from the use of the drug in pregnant women may be acceptable despite its potential risks; X, studies in animals or reports of adverse reactions have indicated that the risk associated with the use of the drug for pregnant women clearly outweighs any possible benefit.

ARV, antiretroviral; AUC, area under the curve; BID, twice daily; CNS, central nervous system; Pk, pharmacokinetic; SQV, Saquinavir; TID, three times daily; VSD, ventricular septal defect.

malignancies did not identify zidovudine exposure, either in utero or after birth, as a risk factor for developing cancer.[72] Thus, human data thus far do not support zidovudine use as a risk factor for carcinogenesis, but long-term follow-up of exposed children is required.

MANAGEMENT OPTIONS

Prepregnancy

Ideally, all HIV-infected women would have a preconceptional visit to optimize their status before pregnancy.[28] Issues to be discussed include current maternal status and indications for antiretroviral therapy and opportunistic infection prophylaxis, choice of antiretroviral drugs to minimize risk of birth defects and toxicity, risk of perinatal transmission and strategies to reduce transmission, immunization status, optimal nutritional status and use of folate supplements, and assessment of other preconceptional issues such as family history pertinent to genetic screening, screening for other infectious diseases, and assessment for other medical or psychological conditions. The risk of perinatal transmission is most strongly related to HIV RNA levels, with the lowest transmission risk associated with undetectable HIV RNA.[46,47] For women currently on antiretroviral therapy or with indications for antiretrovirals based on current guidelines (HIV RNA level > 55,000 copies/mL or CD4+ lymphocyte count <350 cells/μL), a highly active regimen that does not include efavirenz should be used. Pregnancy should be delayed until HIV RNA levels are undetectable, if possible. For women not meeting criteria for therapy for their own health, initiation of therapy to prevent transmission after the first trimester should be discussed. Need for opportunistic infection prophylaxis should be assessed.[73] Ideally, if CD4+ lymphocyte counts are in the range where opportunistic infection prophylaxis is indicated, highly active antiretroviral therapy should be initiated to enhance immunity and obviate the need for prophylaxis during pregnancy. Pregnancy should be delayed until sustained CD4+ lymphocyte counts over 200 cells/μL are achieved to minimize the number of drugs needed during pregnancy. Any indicated immunizations should be provided before pregnancy to avoid the theoretical risk of increased transmission risk related to HIV RNA rebound after immunization. If the HIV-infected woman has not previously been tested for antibodies to *Toxoplasma gondii*, hepatitis C virus, or cytomegalovirus, antibody status should be documented at the preconceptional visit to establish risk for seroconversion or reactivation. Tuberculin skin testing should be done if not done within the past year. The range of transmission risks based on maternal HIV RNA levels and antiretroviral therapy should be discussed, and the woman must understand that although the risk is now low, there is no guarantee that transmission will not occur.

Prenatal

The same principles as outlined for preconceptional care should be followed for HIV-infected women presenting already pregnant. Women newly diagnosed with HIV infection during pregnancy should be assessed for any signs or symptoms suggestive of acute HIV infection or opportunistic infection and undergo laboratory testing (HIV RNA and CD4+ lymphocyte testing) to establish the stage of HIV infection. HIV infection should be confirmed by repeat testing if not previously done. In general, highly active combination antiretroviral therapy is indicated during pregnancy to prevent perinatal transmission and may also be indicated for maternal health.[28] A regimen recommended as first-line therapy for nonpregnant adults, generally including two nucleoside reverse transcriptase inhibitors with either one or more protease inhibitors or a non-nucleoside reverse transcriptase inhibitor, should be chosen.[27] However, nevirapine should not be initiated in women with CD4+ lymphocyte counts over 250 cells/μL as the risk of potentially fatal hepatotoxicity is greatly increased in this group compared to women with lower CD4+ lymphocyte counts.[28] Highly active antiretroviral therapy is indicated to lower HIV RNA levels to undetectable levels to minimize transmission risk and also minimize the risk of development of resistant virus. Extensive discussions with the woman should emphasize the importance of complete adherence to the regimen to prevent development of resistance. Unless contraindicated or not tolerated, the regimen should include zidovudine, which has the most data on efficacy in reducing transmission. Intravenous zidovudine should be given during labor, and the infant should receive zidovudine for 6 weeks after birth. For women with HIV RNA levels below 1,000 copies/mL who want to minimize their exposure to antiretrovirals, monotherapy with the PACTG 076 zidovudine regimen can be offered. In an analysis of data from several studies, transmission among women with HIV RNA levels below 1000 copies/mL during pregnancy was 9.8% among 368 untreated women and 1% among 834 women receiving zidovudine.[74] Zidovudine monotherapy during pregnancy was not associated with a difference in disease progression post partum among women in several studies.[75–77] The risk of developing resistance to zidovudine among women with HIV RNA below 1000 copies/mL is expected to be low given limited viral replication. The option of stopping therapy after delivery should be discussed with women who initiate therapy solely for prevention of perinatal transmission.

Indications for resistance testing during pregnancy should be the same as for nonpregnant adults.[28] Technical aspects of resistance testing and a more thorough discussion of the implications for pregnant women and their infants have been reviewed elsewhere.[44,78] The use of resistance testing to optimize therapy during pregnancy and to reduce the rate of perinatal transmission has not been studied specifically. Resistance testing in adults has been most useful in the setting of a failing regimen to help guide the choice of the next regimen.[78] Because current resistance testing will detect resistant virus only if it constitutes at least 20% of the viral population, testing is unlikely to be useful in the therapy-naïve pregnant patient without acute infection, as wild-type virus will predominate in the absence of selective pressure from antiretroviral agents. For therapy-naïve women initiating therapy before the third trimester, a highly active regimen can be selected, and the response to therapy monitored with serial HIV RNA determinations.[28] If the expected response of at least a one log drop in HIV RNA in the first 8 weeks is not obtained, specimens for resistance testing should be obtained while the woman is on therapy before switching to an alternate regimen. For women initiating therapy late in pregnancy with high HIV RNA levels, consideration could be given to obtaining resistance testing either before starting or shortly after starting therapy to have results sooner to guide a switch in therapy if indicated.

The majority of studies evaluating the impact of resistance on risk of perinatal transmission have not found the presence of zidovudine, lamivudine, or nevirapine resistance to increase the risk of transmission.[78] One study, including women on zidovudine for their own health but not including intrapartum or neonatal zidovudine, found zidovudine resistance was not associated with an increased risk of transmission on univariate analysis but, after adjustment for total lymphocyte count and duration of membrane rupture, was a factor.[79] The women included in this study had low $CD4^+$ lymphocyte counts and would now be recommended to receive highly active combination therapy during pregnancy. Given the currently observed rates of transmission of under 2% among women on highly active antiretroviral therapy during pregnancy, antiretroviral resistance does not appear to be a major issue in perinatal transmission. However, as the prevalence of resistant HIV increases among those with recent infection[80] and as women have repeat pregnancies, the chance of coexistent resistant HIV and pregnancy will increase and may become a larger problem. Resistance patterns among pregnant women and among infected infants must be monitored to allow adaptation of treatment guidelines.

For women presenting during pregnancy already taking antiretroviral therapy, management will depend on gestational age, regimen, HIV levels before starting therapy and time to response, and current symptoms such as nausea that may interfere with adherence during pregnancy. Women presenting after the first trimester should continue on their current regimen as long as HIV RNA levels are below the level of detection. Women presenting early in the first trimester should be counseled regarding the potential teratogenic risks of antiretroviral exposure in the first trimester versus the competing risk of rebound in HIV RNA levels if therapy is stopped, with potential risk for perinatal transmission. Women on efavirenz-containing regimens should be switched to alternate regimens if they choose to continue therapy in the first trimester. Hydroxyurea should not be used during pregnancy. If a woman chooses to discontinue therapy during the first trimester, she should stop and restart all agents concurrently to minimize the risk of development of resistance.

If not previously documented, antibody status for *T. gondii*, hepatitis C, and cytomegalovirus should be obtained. Tuberculin skin testing should be performed if not done within the past year. Prophylaxis and treatment of opportunistic infection in pregnant women is generally the same as for nonpregnant women.[77] Ideally, use of highly active antiretroviral therapy should optimize the immune status so that prophylaxis is not indicated. For more detailed information regarding prophylaxis of opportunistic infections in pregnancy, providers should consult current guidelines at http://aidsinfo.nih.gov/guidelines.

HIV-infected pregnant women should receive counseling regarding issues of HIV and pregnancy and should be provided with psychosocial support during pregnancy and the postpartum period. Women can be reassured that pregnancy per se does not appear to have an impact on the progression of HIV infection. Women should be educated regarding signs and symptoms such as rash, nausea, vomiting, extreme fatigue, and muscle aches that may indicate toxicity related to antiretroviral drugs. The risks of perinatal transmission of HIV and the evaluation of the infant for infection should be discussed. The need for careful adherence to therapy to maximize response and minimize the development of resistance should be emphasized.

In addition to use of antiretroviral therapy to lower HIV RNA levels and reduce transmission, performance of cesarean delivery before the onset of labor and membrane rupture has been shown to reduce transmission among women on no antiretrovirals or on zidovudine.[81,82] In a meta-analysis of data from 15 cohorts, the adjusted odds ratio (AOR) for transmission was 0.43 (95% confidence interval [CI] 0.33–0.56) for those with cesarean delivery before labor or membrane rupture compared to those with other modes of delivery.[81] A similar benefit was seen among the subset receiving zidovudine. In a randomized trial of planned cesarean section compared to vaginal delivery, transmission occurred in 1.8% of infants assigned to planned cesarean group and 10.5% of 200 who delivered vaginally ($P < 0.001$).[82] A similar magnitude in reduction of transmission was seen among the subset receiving zidovudine, although small numbers did not reach statistical significance. Given transmission rates of under 2% among women receiving highly active antiretroviral therapy or with HIV RNA below 1000 copies/mL receiving zidovudine, it is difficult to assess for any additional benefit of planned cesarean delivery. Of note in the WITS analysis was the suggestion of benefit in reduction of transmission from planned cesarean compared to vaginal delivery, even after adjustment for maternal HIV RNA level and level of antiretroviral therapy (AOR 0.27, 95% CI 0.06–1.12, P = 0.07).[43] Similarly in the European Collaborative Study, the AOR was 0.42 (95% CI 0.27–0.67) for transmission with elective cesarean compared to other modes of delivery, adjusting for maternal treatment group and $CD4^+$ cell count.[59] Currently, cesarean delivery before labor or membrane rupture is recommended for women with HIV RNA levels above 1000 copies/mL in the third trimester.[83] Women with HIV RNA levels below 1000 copies/mL should have the option of planned cesarean delivery discussed with them, along with the lack of clear data regarding benefit in this setting. All HIV-infected pregnant women should be informed of the increased risks, primarily infectious, associated with cesarean compared to vaginal delivery. Despite early case-control studies suggesting increased rates of morbidity among HIV-infected compared to uninfected women undergoing cesarean delivery (reviewed by the CDC[28]), more recent cohort studies suggest that the increased risk is similar in magnitude to that observed in similar HIV-uninfected women.[84–87] Cesarean delivery may be scheduled at 38 weeks of gestation without amniocentesis, rather than the usually recommended 39 weeks, to minimize the risk of labor or membrane rupture, although this increases the risk of respiratory distress in the newborn.[88] To minimize risks of perioperative infection, genital infections such as bacterial vaginosis should be treated, and the use of antibiotic prophylaxis should be considered, although these interventions have not been specifically evaluated in HIV-infected women. Scheduled cesarean delivery also appears to confer a reduced risk of hepatitis C transmission to the infant among HIV-infected women with detectable hepatitis C viremia.[89]

HIV-infected women should undergo baseline testing of renal and hepatic function. The schedule of testing for drug toxicity will vary with drugs chosen. In general, visits for assessment for any new symptoms and laboratory testing should occur about every 2 to 4 weeks during the first 1 to 2 months of therapy. An optimal schedule of testing for early diagnosis of such complications as hepatic toxicity or lactic acidosis has not been established, but clinicians should consider evaluating hepatic function and electrolytes monthly in the third trimester and certainly in the presence of any new symptoms. Accurate blood lactate levels are difficult to obtain, and normal values in pregnancy have not been established. Routine testing of lactate levels is not recommended, but may be helpful during pregnancy if values are elevated above nonpregnant adult levels in the presence of suggestive symptoms. $CD4^+$ lymphocyte counts should be done every 3 months during pregnancy. HIV RNA levels should be monitored as per guidelines in nonpregnant adults (i.e. every 4 weeks after initiating or changing therapy until undetectable, then every 3 months on stable therapy).[27] A drop of at least one log on HIV RNA levels should be seen after 4 to 8 weeks of therapy.

Protease inhibitor therapy has been associated with an increased risk of glucose intolerance and diabetes in nonpregnant adults.[90] Small studies in pregnancy have not shown an increased risk of gestational diabetes among pregnant women on protease inhibitors compared to those on no therapy or zidovudine monotherapy, but a review of women in the PACTG 316 study has suggested that long-term protease inhibitor use in pregnancy may increase the risk of gestational diabetes.[91] Clinicians may consider early 50g glucose load testing in pregnant women on protease inhibitor therapy with repeat testing at 24 to 28 weeks of gestation if earlier testing is normal.

Clinicians caring for HIV-infected pregnant women on methadone should be aware of potential drug interactions when initiating or changing therapy. Nevirapine, efavirenz, and protease inhibitors other than indinavir may decrease methadone levels and precipitate drug withdrawal so pregnant women should be monitored for symptoms in this setting.[27]

Counseling regarding options for prenatal diagnosis is complicated by HIV infection. Amniocentesis and other invasive procedures such as scalp electrode placement increased the risk of transmission by two- to fourfold in early studies among women not receiving antiretrovirals.[92,93] In more recent cohort studies among women receiving antiretroviral therapy, invasive testing has not been identified as a risk factor for transmission, but amniocentesis is uncommon and chorionic villus sampling rare among HIV-infected women. Thus, specific risk figures are not available to use in counseling. Further complicating the discussion is the recent suggestion that median serum human chorionic gonadotropin and α fetoprotein values may be higher among HIV-infected women and elevations may correlate with increasing disease severity, although confirmation is needed.[94] Women should be counseled regarding the unknown but potential risk of transmission of HIV infection with invasive testing that would be indicated in the event of an abnormal result on a screening serum marker or nuchal translucency test. If she would not undergo amniocentesis with an abnormal screening result, then such screening may be more anxiety-provoking than helpful. On the other hand, the woman must understand that only invasive testing can definitively rule out chromosomal abnormalities. If an invasive prenatal diagnostic procedure is planned for an HIV-infected woman, she should be on optimal antiretroviral therapy with an undetectable HIV RNA level beforehand to minimize the risk of transmission.

Labor and Delivery

Ideally, the decision regarding mode of delivery should be made after discussions throughout pregnancy, based on

HIV RNA results obtained at 34 to 36 weeks of gestation. If the decision is made to attempt vaginal delivery, zidovudine infusion at a dose of 2 mg/kg of body weight over 1 hour, followed by a continuous infusion of 1 mg/kg/hour should be given until delivery.[38] Other antiretroviral drugs should be continued as scheduled during labor, except stavudine, which may antagonize zidovudine and should be discontinued when zidovudine infusion is begun. If the woman is unable to tolerate zidovudine, then stavudine may be continued during labor. During labor, artificial rupture of membranes should be avoided if possible, and labor should be augmented as needed to minimize the duration of ruptured membranes. Fetal scalp electrodes, scalp blood sampling, and instrumented delivery should be avoided to limit fetal exposure to maternal blood. Infants should be washed before undergoing blood draws, injections, or other procedures.

If cesarean delivery is planned, it should be scheduled at or after 38 weeks of gestation.[83] Infusion of intravenous zidovudine as described earlier should be begun at least 3 hours before surgery and continued until cord clamping. Other medications should be continued as scheduled. For women who had planned on a scheduled cesarean delivery presenting with ruptured membranes, management must be individualized based on HIV RNA levels, time since rupture, stage of labor, and patient preference. The benefit of cesarean delivery shortly after rupture of membranes or onset of labor is unclear. Among women not receiving antiretrovirals or receiving zidovudine monotherapy, transmission rates increase with increasing duration of rupture before delivery.[95,96] However, in most studies, transmission rates were similar among women delivering vaginally and those delivering by cesarean after labor or rupture. Women with a short duration of ruptured membranes and an unripe cervix in whom a prolonged labor is anticipated may benefit from urgent cesarean delivery, and those progressing rapidly in labor may be less likely to benefit. In the setting of ruptured membranes without labor before 32 weeks of gestation, expectant management with continuing antiretroviral therapy, potentially including intravenous zidovudine, should be offered to attempt to prolong gestation and reduce complications of prematurity. HIV-infected women with preterm labor should be treated the same as HIV-negative women, with a decision regarding delivery mode based on obstetric considerations and recent HIV RNA levels once delivery is deemed to be inevitable.

For HIV-infected women presenting or diagnosed in labor or post partum without antiretroviral therapy during pregnancy, several options are available. Observational data from Wade and associates demonstrated transmission rates of 6.1% with zidovudine begun prenatally and continued intrapartum and to the neonate for 6 weeks, 10.0% given intrapartum and to the neonate for 6 weeks, 9.3% when started within 48 hours of birth and continued for 6 weeks, 18.4% when started after 48 hours, and 26.6% with no zidovudine for mother or infant.[9] Subsequent studies have demonstrated transmission rates at 14 to 16 weeks of 13.1% with the a single dose of 200 mg nevirapine to mother and 2 mg/kg to the infant compared to 25.1% with oral zidovudine during labor and for 1 week for the infant,[8] a rate at 6 weeks of 10.8% with oral zidovudine/lamivudine in labor and for 1 week in mother and infant compared to 17.2% for placebo,[10] and a rate at 8 weeks of 13.3% with the maternal/infant nevirapine regimen compared to 10.9% for zidovudine/lamivudine orally in labor and for 1 week in the infant.[11] The latter three trials were done in predominantly breastfeeding populations. Thus, any of these three regimens (intravenous zidovudine in labor and oral for the infant for 6 weeks; the maternal/infant nevirapine dosing; or oral zidovudine/lamivudine in labor and for 1 week in the infant) could be used for women presenting in labor without therapy during pregnancy. Some clinicians would choose to use a combination of zidovudine and nevirapine in this setting, although this regimen has not been studied specifically. No trials have been reported evaluating postpartum therapy alone for prevention of transmission, although by extrapolation, any of these regimens could be given. Some clinicians might choose to add additional drugs to these regimens to mimic postexposure prophylaxis recommendations, although formulations and dosing recommendations for neonates are limited.

Postnatal

The postpartum period is a very demanding period for all women, but HIV-infected women have the added stresses of administering medication to the infant and waiting to discern the infant's infection status. Additional psychosocial support is needed during this period. If she plans to continue antiretroviral therapy after delivery, measures to enhance adherence are indicated.[27] For women stopping antiretroviral therapy, all drugs should be stopped simultaneously to minimize the development of resistance. HIV-infected women should be counseled against breastfeeding as it increases the risk of transmission by 15% to 20%, based on studies of women not receiving antiretrovirals.[45]

Follow-up care for the woman, both reproductive and HIV-specific, and her infant should be assured before hospital discharge. During prenatal care, women should be counseled regarding contraceptive options. Condom use should be reinforced. Hormonal contraceptives may be used by HIV-infected women, although estradiol levels are reduced by nevirapine, ritonavir, nelfinavir, rifampin, rifabutin, and possibly amprenavir.[27] The impact on contraceptive efficacy of these interactions is unknown, although these changes may increase the risk of irregular bleeding. Possible pharmacokinetic interactions between depomedroxyprogesterone acetate and antiretrovirals are under study, although given the high dose of progesterone used, contraceptive efficacy should be maintained. Studies in HIV-infected women suggest that intrauterine contraceptive devices may be used safely by HIV-infected women with a low risk of sexually transmitted infections without severe immune compromise.[97]

Infants born to HIV-infected women require HIV-specific as well as routine pediatric care. Infants should receive zidovudine syrup 2 mg/kg of body weight every 6 hours, or equivalent dosing schedule, for 6 weeks after birth.[28] A complete blood count should be obtained from the neonate before starting zidovudine as anemia is the primary side effect of the zidovudine. Use of additional antiretrovirals in the infant may be considered in some situations, such as for an infant born to women not receiving antiretrovirals during pregnancy.[28] Observational data suggest that transmission is reduced with 6 weeks of oral zidovudine in the infant if started within 24 hours of birth.[9] Infants should be started on prophylaxis for *Pneumocystis carinii* pneumonia at 4 to 6 weeks of age, with prophylaxis continued until the infant is confirmed to be HIV-uninfected.[98] Testing of the infant should be done within 48 hours of birth, at 2 weeks, 1 to 2 months, and 3 to 6 months of age or as soon as any positive result is obtained. HIV DNA PCR is the preferred method for infant diagnosis. Using this method, over 90% of infected children will be identified by 14 days of age.[99] HIV RNA PCR may also be useful for diagnosis in infants, but this methodology has not been studied as extensively. Infants with two positive HIV virologic tests on separate samples are considered to be HIV-infected. Infants with two or more negative virologic tests, with at least two different samples drawn at or after age 1 month and at least one sample at age 4 months or more can be considered to be HIV-uninfected if not exposed through ongoing breast-feeding. HIV-exposed children should be managed by or in consultation with a specialist in pediatric HIV infection.

Summarized here are recommendations for appropriate care for HIV-infected pregnant women to maximize maternal health and minimize the risk of perinatal transmission. Although huge advances have been made in management of HIV infection and prevention of transmission in developed countries, the greater challenge is to translate these interventions into practical and sustainable interventions throughout the world. Ultimately, the goal must be to prevent transmission of HIV to avoid the coexistence of HIV infection in pregnancy.

CONCLUSIONS

- A policy of universal HIV testing of pregnant women, with patient notification and right of refusal is recommended.
- All women presenting in labor without prenatal care or without documentation of HIV testing during pregnancy should be offered rapid HIV testing in the peripartum period.
- Pregnancy does not appear to enhance HIV disease progression among women in industrialized countries.
- Pregnancy may enhance the mitochondrial toxicity of nucleoside analogues, producing a syndrome similar to acute fatty liver of pregnancy.
- Use of combination antiretroviral therapy, especially regimens including protease inhibitors, has been associated with an increased risk of preterm birth in European but not U.S. studies.
- Rates of perinatal transmission of under 2% have been achieved with use of zidovudine and scheduled cesarean delivery or highly active antiretroviral therapy.
- Birth defects including anencephaly, microophthalmia, and cleft palate were seen in 3 (20%) of 15 monkeys after first-trimester exposure to efavirenz. Use of this drug in pregnancy should be avoided.
- In utero and neonatal exposure to nucleoside analogues may rarely cause mitochondrial toxicity in infants, but the risk is outweighed by the benefits in reduction of HIV transmission.
- Current guidelines for treatment of HIV infection during pregnancy, treatment of adults and children, and prevention of opportunistic infections can be found at *http://aidsinfo.nih.gov/guidelines*.
- Cesarean section done before labor and membrane rupture reduces the risk of perinatal HIV transmission among women not on antiretrovirals or on zidovudine. Scheduled cesarean delivery is recommended for women with HIV RNA levels over 1000 copies/mL late in pregnancy. The benefit for women with HIV RNA levels below 1000 copies/mL is unclear.
- Women should receive intravenous zidovudine in labor or before scheduled cesarean delivery.
- Regimens recommended for prophylaxis of transmission for women not treated with antiretrovirals during pregnancy include intravenous zidovudine in labor and oral zidovudine for the infant for 6 weeks; oral zidovudine/lamivudine in labor and for 1 week in the infant; single dose nevirapine in labor and to the infant at 48 hours of age; or a combination of the zidovudine and nevirapine regimens.
- HIV-infected women should not breastfeed if safe alternatives are available.
- Infants should be managed by or in consultation with an HIV expert, should receive zidovudine for 6 weeks, prophylaxis against *Pneumocystis carinii* pneumonia beginning at 4 to 6 weeks of age, and be tested for HIV using a DNA PCR assay.

SUMMARY OF MANAGEMENT OPTIONS
Human Immunodeficiency Virus

Management Options	Quality of Evidence	Strength of Recommendation	References
Prepregnancy			
Careful counseling and offer of screening for at-risk women	–	GPP	–
Assess indications for antiretroviral therapy and opportunistic infection prophylaxis with HIV RNA, and $CD4^+$ cell counts. Initiate highly active antiretroviral therapy if HIV RNA level >55,000 copies/mL or $CD4^+$ cell count <350/µL. Avoid regimens containing efavirenz because of teratogenicity concerns.	Ia	A	27
Recommend against conception until HIV RNA level undetectable and no indication for opportunistic infection prophylaxis ($CD4^+$ cell count above 200/mm^3 for >6 months)	IIa	B	28
Complete other routine preconception assessments such as genetic screening, evaluation for other medical conditions.	IIa	B	28
Recommend folate supplementation.	Ia	A	28
Prenatal Screening Policy			
Screening practices vary—options: Most centers offer screening to ALL women Counseling and offer of selective screening for at-risk women; most centers require informed consent before testing can occur	–	GPP	–
All unscreened at-risk women should be managed as if they were HIV positive in terms of infection control measures with blood and other body products (preventative measures should be employed when handling blood from all women in pregnancy)	–	GPP	–
Prenatal—HIV Positive Patients			
Assess immunization status and update as needed for pneumococcus, influenza, hepatitis A and B, tetanus.	IIa	B	73
Assess antibody status to hepatitis C, *Toxoplasma gondii*, and CMV if not previously documented.	IIa	B	73
Perform tuberculin skin test if not done in past year.	IIa	B	73
Counsel regarding risk of transmission, methods to minimize risk (antiretroviral therapy with scheduled cesarean delivery if HIV RNA >1,000 copies/ml after 34 weeks), lack of impact of pregnancy on maternal disease progression, symptoms of drug toxicity, possible effects of therapy on infant, evaluation of infant after birth for HIV status.	Ia	A	28,31,100
Review antiretroviral therapy and opportunistic infection prophylaxis with HIV RNA level, $CD4^+$ lymphocyte count. For women already on therapy, discuss risks/benefits of continuing or stopping. Modify regimen if first trimester and on efavirenz. If not on therapy, recommend highly active antiretroviral regimen including zidovudine for all women starting after first trimester, regardless of HIV RNA and $CD4^+$ cell count, with option of zidovudine monotherapy discussed if HIV RNA level <1, 000 copies/ml not on therapy. Provide opportunistic infection prophylaxis according to adult guidelines.	Ia	A	28,31,100
Monitor HIV RNA levels monthly after changing or initiating therapy. Level should drop by ≥1 log in first 4–8 weeks.	IIa	B	27
Monitor $CD4^+$ lymphocyte counts each trimester.	IIa	B	28

SUMMARY OF MANAGEMENT OPTIONS
Human Immunodeficiency Virus *(Continued)*

Management Options	Quality of Evidence	Strength of Recommendation	References
Prenatal—HIV Positive Patients			
Perform complete blood count, liver enzymes, renal function frequently (every 2–4 weeks) on new regimen, monthly in third trimester.	III	B	28
Perform HIV resistance testing if not responding to regimen or confirmed rebound on previously suppressive regimen.	IIa	B	27
Perform ultrasound at 18–20 weeks of gestation to rule out anomalies and confirm dates.	–	GPP	–
Discuss risks versus benefits of scheduled cesarean delivery; advise cesarean section. Recommend for HIV RNA levels >1,000 copies/mL after 34 weeks. Schedule at or after 38 weeks of gestation if dating criteria adequate.	Ia	A	28,31,100
Routine prenatal care. If indicated, discuss unknown risk of transmission with amniocentesis or chorionic villus sampling. Perform only if on antiretroviral therapy with undetectable HIV RNA.	III	B	27, 28
Labor and Delivery			
Cesarean section reduces vertical transmission and should be advised	Ia	A	28,31,100
Start intravenous zidovudine infusion	Ia	A	28,31,38,100
a. For those choosing vaginal delivery 2 mg/kg over one hour followed by 1 mg/kg/hour until delivery with onset of labor			
b. Same regimen at least 3 hours before scheduled cesarean delivery.			
Continue other medications orally except stavudine, which may antagonize zidovudine.			
If vaginal delivery minimize duration of ruptured membranes as much as possible.	IIa	B	28,95,96
Avoid scalp electrodes, scalp sampling, instrumented delivery. Wash infant before blood draws, injections.	III	B	92,93
Postnatal			
Discuss option of stopping or continuing antiretroviral therapy if initiated solely for transmission prophylaxis. Reinforce adherence if continuing therapy.	IIa	B	28
Counsel against breastfeeding.	Ia	A	28
Provide contraception (condom preferred) and assure continued HIV and reproductive health care.	II	A	28
Provide psychosocial support as infant infection status assessed.	III	B	28
Assure routine and HIV specific care for infant including zidovudine 2 mg/kg every six hours or equivalent until six weeks of age, HIV DNA PCR testing, initiation of prophylaxis against *Pneumocystis carinii* pneumonia beginning at 4–6 weeks of age.	Ia	A	98

REFERENCES

1. UNAIDS/WHO-AIDS epidemic update, December 2002, available at *www.unaids.org*.
2. Centers for Disease Control and Prevention: Revised recommendations for HIV screening of pregnant women. MMWR 2001;50(RR19):59–86.
3. DeCock KM, Fowler MG, Mercier E, et al: Prevention of mother-to-child HIV transmission in resource-poor countries: Translating research into policy and practice. JAMA 2000;283:1175–1182.
4. MacDonald KL, Jackson JB, Bowman RJ, et al: Performance characteristics of serologic tests for human immunodeficiency virus type 1 (HIV-1) antibody among Minnesota blood donors: Public health and clinical implications. Ann Intern Med 1989;110:617–621.
5. Celum CL, Coombs RW, Jones ME, et al: Risk factors for repeatedly reactive HIV-1 EIA and indeterminate Western blots: A population-based case-control study. Arch Intern Med 1994;154:1129–1137.
6. Gwinn M, Redus MA, Granade TC, et al: HIV-1 serologic test results for one million newborn dried-blood specimens: assay performance and implications for screening. J Acquir Immune Defic Syndr 1992;5:505–512.
7. Centers for Disease Control and Prevention: Success in implementing Public Health Service guidelines to reduce perinatal transmission of HIV—Louisiana, Michigan, New Jersey, and South Carolina, 1993, 1995, and 1996. MMWR 1998;47:688–691.
8. Guay LA, Musoke P, Fleming T, et al: Intrapartum and neonatal single-dose nevirapine compared with zidovudine for prevention of mother-child transmission of HIV-1 in Kampala, Uganda: HIVNET 012 randomised trial. Lancet 1999;354:795–802.
9. Wade NA, Birkhead GS, Warren BL, et al: Abbreviated regimens of zidovudine prophylaxis and perinatal transmission of the human immunodeficiency virus. N Engl J Med 1998;339:1409–1414.
10. The Petra Study Team: Efficacy of three short-course regimens of zidovudine and lamivudine in preventing early and late transmission of HIV-1 from mother to child in Tanzania, South Africa, and Uganda (Petra study): A randomised double-blind placebo-controlled trial. Lancet 2002;359:1178–1186.
11. Moodley D, Moodley J, Coovadia H, et al for the South African Intrapartum Nevirapine Trial (SAINT) Investigators: A multicenter randomized controlled trial of nevirapine versus a combination of zidovudine and lamivudine to reduce intrapartum and early postpartum mother-to-child transmission of human immunodeficiency virus type 1. J Infect Dis 2003;187:725–735.
12. Centers for Disease Control and Prevention: Notice to readers: Approval of a new rapid test for HIV antibody. MMWR 2002;51:1051–1052.
13. U.S. Department of Health and Human Services: HHS extends use of rapid HIV test to new sites nationwide. Press release available at *http://www.hhs.gov/news/press/2003pres/20030131b.htm*.
14. Stetler HC, Granade TC, Nunez CA, et al: Field evaluation of rapid HIV serologic tests for screening and confirming HIV-1 infection in Honduras. AIDS 1997;11:369–375.
15. Saada M, Le Chenadec J, Berrebi A, et al: Pregnancy and progression to AIDS: Results of the French prospective cohorts. AIDS 2000;14:2355–2360.
16. Burns DN, Landesman S, Minkoff H, et al: The influence of pregnancy on human immunodeficiency virus type 1 infection: Antepartum and postpartum changes in human immunodeficiency virus type 1 viral load. Am J Obstet Gynecol 1998;178:355–359.
17. Weisser M, Rudin C, Battegay M, et al: Does pregnancy influence the course of HIV infection? Evidence from two large Swiss cohort studies. J Acquir Immune Defic Syndr Hum Retrovirol 1998;15:404–410.
18. Minkoff H, Hershow R, Watts DH, et al: The relationship of pregnancy to HIV disease progression. Am J Obstet Gynecol 2003;189:552–559.
19. Deschamps MM, Pape JW, Desvarieux M, et al: A prospective study of HIV-seropositive asymptomatic women of childbearing age in a developing country. J Acquir Immune Defic Syndr 1993;6:446–551.
20. Kumar RM, Uduman SA, Khurrana AK: Impact of pregnancy on maternal AIDS. J Reprod Med 1993;42:429–434.
21. Bristol-Myers Squibb: Dear Health Care Provider letter, January 5, 2001. Available at *www.fda.gov/medwatch/safety/2001/zerit&videx_letter.htm*.
22. Hill JB, Sheffield JS, Zeeman GG, Wendel GD Jr: Hepatotoxicity with antiretroviral treatment of pregnant women. Obstet Gynecol 2001;98:909–911.
23. Ibdah JA, Yang Z, Bennett MJ: Liver disease in pregnancy and fetal fatty acid oxidation defects. Mol Genet Metab 2000;71:182–189.
24. Grimbert S, Fromenty B, Fisch C, et al: Decreased mitochondrial oxidation of fatty acids in pregnant mice: Possible relevance to development of acute fatty liver of pregnancy. Hepatology 1993;17:628–637.
25. Grimbert S, Fisch C, Deschamps D, et al: Effects of female sex hormones on mitochondria: Possible role in acute fatty liver of pregnancy. Am J Physiol 1995;268:G107–115.
26. Brinkman K, Ter Hofstede HJM, Burger DM, et al: Adverse effects of reverse transcriptase inhibitors: Mitochondrial toxicity as common pathway. AIDS 1998;12:1735–1744.
27. Centers for Disease Control and Prevention: Report of the NIH panel to define principles of therapy of HIV infection and guidelines for the use of antiretroviral agents in HIV-infected adults and adolescents. MMWR 1998;47(RR-5):1–82. Updated February 4, 2002, available at *http://aidsinfo.nih.gov/guidelines/*.
28. Centers for Disease Control and Prevention: USPHS task force recommendations for the use of antiretroviral drugs in pregnant women infected with HIV-1 for maternal health and for reducing perinatal HIV-1 transmission in the United States. MMWR 1998;47(RR-2):1–30. Updated June 16, 2003. Available at *http://aidsinfo.nih.gov/guidelines/*.
29. Eshelman S, Mracna M, Guay L, et al: Selection and fading of resistance mutations in women and infants receiving nevirapine to prevent HIV-1 vertical transmission (HIVNET012). AIDS 2001;15:1951–1957.
30. Cunningham CK, Chaix ML, Rekacewicz C, et al: Development of resistance mutations in women receiving standard antiretroviral therapy who received intrapartum nevirapine to prevent perinatal human immunodeficiency virus type 1 transmission: A substudy of Pediatric AIDS Clinical Trials Group protocol 316. J Infect Dis 2002;186:181–188.
31. Brocklehurst P, French R: The association between maternal HIV infection and perinatal outcome: A systematic review of the literature and meta-analysis. Br J Obstet Gynaecol 1998;105:836–848.
32. Bucceri A, Luchini L, Rancilio L, et al: Pregnancy outcome among HIV positive and negative intravenous drug users. Eur J Obstet Gynecol Reprod Biol 1997;72:169–174.
33. Ellis J, Williams H, Graves W, Lendsay MK: Human immunodeficiency virus infection is a risk factor for adverse perinatal outcome. Am J Obstet Gynecol 2002;186:903–906.
34. Leroy V, Ladner J, Nyiraziraje M, et al: Effect of HIV-1 infection on pregnancy outcome in women in Kigali, Rwanda, 1992-1994. AIDS 1998;12:643–650.
35. Embree JE, Braddick M, Datta P, et al: Lack of correlation of maternal human immunodeficiency virus infection with neonatal malformations. Pediatr Infect Dis J 1989;8:700–704.
36. Stratton P, Tuomala RE, Abboud R, et al: Obstetric and newborn outcomes in a cohort of HIV-infected pregnant women: A report of the Women and Infants Transmission Study. J Acquir Immune Defic Syndr 1999;20:179–186.

37. Lambert JS, Watts DH, Mofenson L, et al for the Pediatric AIDS Clinical Trials Group 185 Team: Risk factors for preterm birth and low birth weight in infants born to HIV-infected pregnant women receiving zidovudine. AIDS 2000;14: 1389–1399.
38. Connor EM, Sperling RS, Gelber R, et al: Reduction of maternal-infant transmission of human immunodeficiency virus type 1 with zidovudine treatment: Pediatric AIDS Clinical Trials Group Protocol 076 Study Group. N Engl J Med 1994;331: 1173–1180.
39. European Collaborative Study: Is zidovudine therapy in pregnant HIV-infected women associated with gestational age and birth weight? The European Collaborative Study. AIDS 1999;13:119–124.
40. Lorenzi P, Spicher VM, Laubereau B, et al: Antiretroviral therapies in pregnancy: Maternal, fetal and neonatal effects. Swiss HIV Cohort Study, the Swiss Collaborative HIV and Pregnancy Study, and the Swiss Neonatal HIV Study. AIDS 1998;12: F241–247.
41. The European Collaborative Study and the Swiss Mother+Child HIV Cohort Study: Combination antiretroviral therapy and duration of pregnancy. AIDS 2000;14:2913–2920.
42. Tuomala RE, Shapiro DE, Mofenson LM, et al: Antiretroviral therapy during pregnancy and the risk of an adverse outcome. N Engl J Med 2002;346:1863–1870.
43. Cooper ER, Charurat M, Mofenson L, et al: Combination antiretroviral strategies for the treatment of pregnant HIV-1-infected women and prevention of perinatal HIV-1 transmission. J Acquir Immune Defic Syndr 2002;29:484–494.
44. Minkoff H: Human immunodeficiency virus infection in pregnancy. Obstet Gynecol 2003;101:797–810.
45. Dunn DT, Newell ML, Ades AE, et al: Risk of human immunodeficiency virus type 1 transmission through breastfeeding. Lancet 1992;340:585–588.
46. Mofenson LM, Lambert JS, Stiehm ER, et al: Risk factors for perinatal transmission of human immunodeficiency virus type 1 in women treated with zidovudine. N Engl J Med 1999;341: 385–393.
47. Garcia PM, Kalish LA, Pitt J, et al: Maternal levels of plasma human immunodeficiency virus type 1 RNA and the risk of perinatal transmission. N Engl J Med 1999;341:394–402.
48. Stiehm ER, Lambert JS, Mofenson L, et al: Efficacy of zidovudine and human immunodeficiency virus (HIV) hyperimmune immunoglobulin for reducing perinatal HIV transmission from HIV-infected women with advanced disease: Results of Pediatric AIDS Clinical Trials Group protocol 185. J Infect Dis 1999;179: 567–575.
49. Shaffer N, Chuachoowong R, Mock PA, et al: Short-course zidovudine for perinatal HIV-1 transmission in Bangkok, Thailand: A randomized controlled trial. Lancet 1999;353:773–780.
50. Lallemant M, Jourdain G, Le Coeur S, et al: A trial of shortened zidovudine regimens to prevent mother-to-child transmission of human immunodeficiency virus type 1. Perinatal HIV Prevention Trial (Thailand) Investigators. N Engl J Med 2000;343: 982–991.
51. Wiktor SZ, Ekpini E, Karon J, et al: Short-course zidovudine for prevention of mother-to-child transmission of HIV-1 in Abidjan, Cote d'Ivoire: A randomised trial. Lancet 1999;353:781–785.
52. Dabis F, Msellati P, Meda N, et al: 6-month efficacy, tolerance and acceptability of a short regimen of oral zidovudine to reduce vertical transmission of HIV in breastfed children in Cote d'Ivoire and Burkina Faso: A double-blind placebo-controlled multicentre trial. Lancet 1999;353:786–792.
53. DITRAME ANRS 049 Study Group: 15-month efficacy of maternal oral zidovudine to decrease vertical transmission of HIV-1 in breastfed African children. Lancet 1999;354:2050.
54. Dabis F, Elenga N, Meda N, et al for the DITRAME Study Group: 18-month mortality and perinatal exposure to zidovudine in West Africa. AIDS 2001;15:771–779.
55. Dorenbaum A, Cunningham CK, Gelber RD, et al: Two-dose intrapartum/newborn nevirapine and standard antiretroviral therapy to reduce perinatal HIV transmission: A randomized trial. JAMA 2002;288:189–198.
56. De Santis M, Carducci B, De Santis L, et al: Periconceptional exposure to efavirenz and neural tube defects. Arch Intern Med 2002;162;355.
57. Fundaro C, Genovese O, Rendeli C, et al: Myelomeningocele in a child with intrauterine exposure to efavirenz. AIDS 2002;16:299–300.
58. The Antiretroviral Pregnancy Registry: Interim report. 1/1/89–1/31/03; issued May 2003.
59. European Collaborative Study: HIV-infected pregnant women and vertical transmission in Europe since 1986. AIDS 2001;15: 761–770.
60. Blanche S, Tardieu M, Rustin P, et al: Persistent mitochondrial dysfunction and perinatal exposure to antiretroviral nucleoside analogues. Lancet 1999;354:1084–1089.
61. Mandelbrot L, Landreau-Mascaro A, Rekacewicz C, et al: Lamivudine-zidovudine combination for prevention of maternal-infant transmission of HIV-1. JAMA 2001;285:2129–2131.
62. French Perinatal Cohort Study Group: Risk of early febrile seizure with perinatal exposure to nucleoside analogues. Lancet 2002;359:583–584.
63. The Perinatal Safety Review Working Group: Nucleoside exposure in the children of HIV-infected women receiving antiretroviral drugs: absence of clear evidence for mitochondrial disease in children who died before 5 years of age in five United States cohorts. J Acquir Immune Defic Syndr 2000;25:261–268.
64. Chotpitayasunondh T, Vanprapar N, Simonds RJ, et al: Safety of late in utero exposure to zidovudine in infants born to human immunodeficiency virus-infected mothers: Bangkok. Pediatrics 2001;107:1–6.
65. European Collaborative Study: Exposure to antiretroviral therapy in utero or early life: The health of uninfected children born to HIV-infected women. J Acquir Immune Defic Syndr 2003;32:380–387.
66. Lange J, Stellato R, Brinkman K, et al: Review of neurological adverse events in relation to mitochondrial dysfunction in the prevention of mother to child transmission of HIV: PETRA study. Second Conference on Global Strategies for the Prevention of HIV Transmission from Mothers to Infants. September 1–6, 1999, Montreal, Canada, abstract 250.
67. Shiramizu B, Shikuma KM, Kamemoto L, et al: Placenta and cord blood mitochondrial DNA toxicity in HIV-infected women receiving nucleoside reverse transcriptase inhibitors during pregnancy. J Acquir Immune Defic Syndr 2003;32:370–374.
68. Porier MC, Divi RL, Al-Harthi L, et al: Long-term mitochondrial toxicity in HIV-uninfected infants born to HIV-infected mothers. J Acquir Immune Defic Syndr 2003;33:175–183.
69. Olivero OA, Anderson LM, Diwan BA, et al: Transplacental effects of 3′-azido-2′3′-dideoxythymidine (AZT): Tumorigenicity in mice and genotoxicity in mice and monkeys. J Natl Cancer Inst 1997;89:1602–1608.
70. Ayers KM, Torrey CE, Reynolds DJ: A transplacental carcinogenicity bioassay in CD-1 mice with zidovudine. Fundament Appl Toxicol 1997;38:195–198.
71. Hanson IC, Antonelli TA, Sperling RS, et al: Lack of tumors in infants with perinatal HIV-1 exposure and fetal/neonatal exposure to zidovudine. J Acquir Immune Defic Syndr Hum Retrovirol 1999;20:463–467.
72. Pollock BH, Jenson HB, Leach CT, et al: Risk factors for pediatric human immunodeficiency virus-related malignancy. JAMA. 2003;289:2393–2399.
73. Centers for Disease Control and Prevention: 2001 USPHS/IDSA guidelines for the prevention of opportunistic infection in persons infected with human immunodeficiency virus: U.S. Public Health Service (USPHS) and Infectious Diseases Society of America (IDSA). MMWR 1999;48:1–66.

Available at *http://aidsinfo.nih.gov/guidelines/*. Updated November 28, 2001.
74. Ioannidis JPA, Abrams EJ, Ammann A, et al: Perinatal transmission of human immunodeficiency virus type 1 by pregnant women with RNA virus loads <1,000 copies/ml. J Infect Dis 2001;183:539–545.
75. Bardeguez A, Shapiro DE, Mofenson LM, et al: Effect of cessation of zidovudine prophylaxis to reduce vertical transmission on maternal disease progression and survival. J Acquir Immune Defic Syndr 2003;32:170–181.
76. Watts DH, Lambert J, Stiehm ER, et al for the PACTG 185 Study Team: Progression of HIV disease among women following delivery. J Acquir Immune Defic Syndr 2003;33:585–593.
77. Ekpini R-A, Nkengasong JN, Sibailly T, et al: Changes in plasma HIV-1-RNA viral load and CD4+ cell counts, and lack of zidovudine resistance among pregnant women receiving short-course zidovudine. AIDS 2002;16:625–630.
78. Nolan M, Fowler MG, Mofenson LM: Antiretroviral prophylaxis of perinatal HIV-1 transmission and the potential impact of antiretroviral resistance. J Acquir Immune Defic Syndr 2002;30: 216–229.
79. Welles SL, Pitt J, Colgrove R, et al: HIV-1 genotypic zidovudine drug resistance and the risk of maternal-infant transmission in the women and infants transmission study. The Women and Infants Transmission Study Group. AIDS 2000;14:263–271.
80. Grant RM, Hecht FM, Warmerdam M, et al: Time trends in primary HIV-1 drug resistance among recently infected persons. JAMA 2002;288:181–188.
81. The International Perinatal HIV Group: The mode of delivery and the risk of vertical transmission of human immunodeficiency virus type 1: A meta-analysis of 15 prospective cohort studies. N Engl J Med 1999;340:977–987.
82. The European Mode of Delivery Collaboration: Elective caesarean-section versus vaginal delivery in prevention of vertical HIV-1 transmission: A randomised clinical trial. Lancet 1999;353:1035–1039.
83. American College of Obstetricians and Gynecologists Committee Opinion: Scheduled cesarean delivery and the prevention of vertical transmission of HIV infection. Number 234, May 2000.
84. Watts DH, Lambert JS, Stiehm ER, et al for the Pediatric AIDS Clinical Trials Group 185 Team: Complications according to mode of delivery among HIV-infected women with CD4+ lymphocyte counts of 500 or less. Am J Obstet Gynecol 2000;173: 100–107.
85. Read J, Kpamegan E, Tuomala R, et al: Mode of delivery and postpartum morbidity among HIV-infected women: The Women and Infants Transmission Study (WITS). J Acquir Immun Defic Syndr 2001;26:236–245.
86. Rodriquez EJ, Spann C, Jamieson D, Lindsay M: Postoperative morbidity associated with cesarean delivery among human immunodeficiency virus-seropositive women. Am J Obstet Gynecol 2001;184:1108–1111.
87. Marcollet A, Goffinet F, Firtion G, et al: Differences in postpartum morbidity in women who are infected with the human immunodeficiency virus after elective cesarean delivery, emergency cesarean delivery, or vaginal delivery. Am J Obstet Gynecol 2002;186:784–789.
88. Madar J, Richmond S, Hey E: Surfactant-deficient respiratory distress after elective delivery at "term." Acta Paediatr 1999;88: 1244–1248.
89. Newell ML, Pembrey L: Mother-to-child transmission of hepatitis C virus infection. Drugs Today 2002;38:321–337.
90. Dube MP: Disorders of glucose metabolism in patients infected with human immunodeficiency virus. Clin Infect Dis 2000;31: 1467–1475.
91. Watts DH, Balasubramanian R, Maupin RT, et al for the PACTG 316 study team: Maternal toxicity and pregnancy complications in HIV-infected women receiving antiretroviral therapy: PACTG 316. Am J Obstet Gynecol 2004;190:506–516.
92. Mandelbrot L, Mayaux MJ, Bongain A, et al: Obstetric factors and mother-to-infant transmission of human immunodeficiency virus type 1: The French perinatal cohorts. SEROGEST French Pediatric HIV Infection Study Group. Am J Obstet Gynecol 1996;175:661–667.
93. Tess BH, Rodrigues LC, Newell ML, et al: Breastfeeding, genetic, obstetric and other risk factors associated with mother-to-child transmission of HIV-1 in Sao Paulo State, Brazil. Sao Paulo Collaborative Study for Vertical Transmission of HIV-1. AIDS 1998;26:513–520.
94. Gross S, Castillo W, Crane M, et al: Maternal serum alpha-fetoprotein and human chorionic gonadotropin levels in women with human immunodeficiency virus. Am J Obstet Gynecol 2003;188:1052–1056.
95. Landesman SH, Kalish LA, Burns DN, et al: Obstetrical factors and the transmission of human immunodeficiency virus type 1 from mother to child. N Engl J Med 1996;334:1617–1623.
96. International Perinatal HIV Group: Duration of ruptured membranes and vertical transmission of HIV-1: A meta-analysis from 15 prospective cohort studies. AIDS 2001;15:357–368.
97. Sinei SK, Morrison CS, Sekadde-Kigondu C, et al: Complications of use of intrauterine devices among HIV-1-infected women. Lancet 1998;351:1238–1241.
98. Centers for Disease Control and Prevention: Guidelines for the use of antiretroviral agents in pediatric HIV infection. MMWR 1998;47(RR-4):1–43. Updated June 25, 2003. *Available at http://www.aidsinfo.nih.gov/guidelines.*
99. Dunn DT, Brandt CD, Krivine A, et al: The sensitivity of HIV-1 DNA polymerase chain reaction in the neonatal period and the relative contributions of intra-uterine and intrapartum transmission. AIDS 1995;9:F7–11.

CHAPTER 30

Rubella, Measles, Mumps, Varicella, and Parvovirus

Laura E. Riley

RUBELLA

Maternal and Fetal Risks

Rubella (German measles or third disease) is an exanthematous disease caused by a single-stranded RNA virus of the togavirus family.[1] Like rubeola, rubella is acquired via respiratory droplet exposure. After a 2- to 3-week incubation period, symptomatic patients develop a rash that spreads from the face to the trunk and extremities lasting about 3 days. Fever, arthralgias, and postauricular and suboccipital lymphadenopathy are characteristic. Severe complications such as encephalitis, bleeding diathesis, and arthritis are rare. Overt clinical symptoms occur in only 50% to 75% of rubella-infected patients, and thus, clinical history is not a useful marker of prior illness.[2]

Rubella infection is usually a mild illness in both adults and children. However, fetal infection may be devastating. Congenital rubella syndrome (CRS) may produce transient abnormalities, including purpura, splenomegaly, jaundice, meningoencephalitis, and thrombocytopenia or permanent anomalies such as cataracts, glaucoma, heart disease, deafness, microcephaly, and mental retardation. Long-term sequelae may include diabetes, thyroid abnormalities, precocious puberty, and progressive rubella panencephalitis.[2,3] Defects involving virtually every organ have been reported (Table 30–1).[4] A 50-year follow-up of 40 survivors of CRS born between 1939 and 1943 revealed that all had hearing impairment; 23 had eye defects related to the rubella.[5]

The results of one large survey of maternal rubella infection in pregnancy are summarized in Table 30–2.[6] The rate of fetal infection is highest at 11 weeks and greater than 36 weeks. However, the overall rate of congenital defects is greatest in the first trimester (90%) and declines steadily in the second and third trimesters.

Rubella vaccine became available in the United States in 1969. Vaccination given as a trivalent preparation of measles, mumps, and rubella (MMR) vaccine produces long-term immunity in 95% of vaccinees. The rates of rubella dropped precipitously after introduction of the vaccine. Ten years later, the annual incidence of rubella infections, including CRS, had decreased by 99.6%.[7] However, in the 1990s there were several outbreaks in groups of adults with unknown vaccination status living in close quarters.[8] The largest outbreak in the United States occurred in Nebraska in 1999 and involved 125 cases; 87% of these patients were born in Latin America.[9] In this outbreak, seven pregnant women were infected and one child was born with CRS. Almost half of these women had prior births in the United States and had missed prior vaccination opportunities.

Diagnosis

The clinical diagnosis of rubella infection is difficult. Most infections are subclinical, and the rash is nonspecific. Serologic testing is the primary mode of diagnosis using enzyme-linked immunoassay (ELISA). In a woman with exposure or suspected illness, seroconversion demonstrated by paired acute and convalescent specimens is indicative of acute infection. Acute infection may also be diagnosed by isolation of virus from the blood, nasopharynx, urine, or cerebrospinal fluid. Serologic testing for immunity is based on the assumption that rubella-specific antibodies of the IgG class are present for life after natural infection or vaccination.

Management Options

Prepregnancy

Vaccination of all children and susceptible adults will help prevent outbreaks of rubella. All children should

TABLE 30–1

Abnormalities in Congenital Rubella: Triad of Gregg

ABNORMALITY	DESCRIPTION
Eye	
Cataract	Usually bilateral and present at birth
Retinopathy	"Salt and pepper" appearance, may have a delayed onset, frequently bilateral, visual acuity is not affected
Microphthalmia	Often associated with cataract
Glaucoma	Is rare but leads to blindness if not recognized
Heart	
Patent ductus arteriosus	Common, often associated with persistence of the foramen ovale
Pulmonary valvular stenosis	Common, due to intimal proliferation and arterial elastic hypertrophy
Pulmonary artery stenosis	
Coarctation of the aorta	Infrequent
Ventricular septal defects	Rare
Atrial septal defects	Rare
Ear	
Commonly damaged	Injury of cells of the middle ear leading to sensorineural deafness may also have a central origin
Bilateral and progressive	May be present at birth or develop later in childhood. Severe enough for the child to need education at a special school; rare when maternal rubella occurs after the fourth month of pregnancy

Adapted from Freij BJ, South MA, Sever JL, et al: Maternal rubella and the congenital rubella syndrome. Clin Perinatol 1988;15:247–257.

receive a single dose of live, attenuated rubella vaccine at 12 to 15 months of age in a trivalent preparation of MMR strains. The second dose of MMR may be administered at least 1 month after the first dose but before 6 years of age. Susceptible young women should be vaccinated and refrain from pregnancy for 1 month following vaccination.[10] Evidence of immunity is required of health care workers and women of childbearing age.[11] According to ongoing studies, antibody to rubella virus should be detectable for up to 16 years after vaccination.[12] However, individuals with low levels of antibody after vaccination may be susceptible to viremia and clinical infection.[13] CRS after previous maternal rubella vaccination has been rarely reported.[14]

The rubella vaccine is a live virus preparation, which may cross the placenta; thus, it should not be administered to pregnant women. However, the Centers for Disease Control have monitored inadvertent rubella vaccination during pregnancy, collecting over 500 cases. No case of CRS due to vaccination was documented, although virus was isolated from the conceptus in several cases.[15] Thus, patients inadvertently vaccinated during pregnancy, or becoming pregnant shortly after vaccination, should be reassured and counseled that the risk of fetal infection is negligible.[16,17]

Prenatal

A pregnant woman infected with rubella is at little risk. However, depending on the gestational age at infection, the fetus may be at great risk for congenital anomalies. Methods for in utero diagnosis include fetal blood sampling measurement of rubella-specific IgM,[18] rubella-specific reverse transcription polymerase chain reaction (RT-PCR), and virus isolation from amniotic fluid or products of conception.[19,20] RT-PCR can detect the presence of viral RNA even when the fetal rubella virus-specific IgM obtained by fetal blood sampling is negative.[21] Although these tests may indicate fetal infection, the counseling is largely based on the gestational age related risk of congenital abnormalities due to CRS. No treatment other than pregnancy termination is available.

TABLE 30–2

Fetal Consequences of Symptomatic Maternal Rubella during Pregnancy

STAGE OF PREGNANCY (WEEKS)	INFECTION: NO. TESTED	INFECTION: NO. POSITIVE	DEFECTS: NO. FOLLOWED	DEFECTS: RATE (%)	OVERALL RISK OF DEFECT (RATE OF INFECTION × RATE OF DEFECTS) (%)
<11	10	9 (90%)	9	100	90
11–12	6	4 (67%)	4	50	33
13–14	18	12 (67%)	12	17	11
15–16	36	17 (47%)	14	50	24
17–18	33	13 (39%)	10	0	0
19–22	59	20 (34%)			
23–26	32	8 (25%)			
27–30	31	11 (35%)			
31–36	25	15 (60%)	53	0	0
>36	8	8 (100%)			
Total	258	117 (45%)	102	20	9

From Miller E, Cradock-Watson JE, Pollock TM: Consequences of confirmed maternal rubella at successive stages of pregnancy. Lancet 1982;2:781–784.

Treatment for acute maternal rubella is generally symptomatic. Rarely, patients who develop thrombocytopenia or encephalitis may benefit from glucocorticoids or platelet transfusion. Immunoglobulin for pregnant women with acute infection is controversial. Furthermore, no data suggest that immunoglobulin will prevent fetal anomalies.

Labor, Delivery, and Postnatal

Acute infection during these time periods is unlikely. If suspected, appropriate infection control measures should be instituted. The neonate should be evaluated for infection following birth.

SUMMARY OF MANAGEMENT OPTIONS

Rubella

Management Options	Quality of Evidence	Strength of Recommendation	References
Prepregnancy			
Prevent by childhood vaccination.	III	B	24
Vaccination programs for girls in their early teens contribute to prevention.	III	B	11,24
Serologic evaluation and, if negative, vaccination of woman inquiring about status.	III	B	11,24
Prenatal			
Routine check of rubella immunity status at first visit for all women is standard practice in many centers.	III	B	17,24
Accidental vaccination in early pregnancy is not an indication for termination.	IIb	B	14–16
If suspected exposure in woman with immunity: • Confirm presence of rubella-specific IgG (if immediately after exposure). • Confirm failure of appearance of IgM (acute phase) antibodies with two serum samples 2–3 weeks apart. • Reassure patient.	–	GPP	–
If suspected exposure in susceptible woman:			
• Establish validity of diagnosis serologically in index case if possible.	III	B	11,24
• Check for appearance of IgM (acute phase) antibodies.	III	B	11,24
• If there is no serologic evidence of infection, reassure patient.	–	GPP	–
If maternal infection is confirmed serologically, options will depend on gestation at time of infection:			
• In early pregnancy, termination should be discussed; it may be performed immediately or only after confirmation by invasive procedure.	IIb	B	5,6
• In late pregnancy, confirmation of fetal infection by invasive procedure can be considered; fetal growth and health should be monitored if infection is suspected or confirmed.	–	GPP	–
Labor, Delivery, and Postnatal			
If fetal infection is suspected, cord blood should be sent for serologic confirmation.	III	C	24
If fetal infection is confirmed, careful pediatric assessment and follow-up are needed.	–	GPP	–

RUBEOLA

Maternal and Fetal Risks

Rubeola (red measles or first disease), caused by a paramyxovirus, is highly infectious, and commonly attacks children. The illness is spread by respiratory droplet and may include high fever, rash, cough and rhinorrhea, conjunctivitis, and the pathognomonic Koplik's spots on the oral buccal epithelium. The incubation period is generally 10 to 14 days. The infection is usually self-limited in children.[22] Rarely, the disease may be severe and may be complicated by bronchopneumonia, hepatitis, otitis media, diarrhea, or death.[23,24] Encephalitis occurs in 1 of every 1000 reported cases and may lead to permanent brain damage and mental retardation. Death, usually due to pneumonia or encephalitis, is reported to occur in 1 to 2 per 1000 cases in the United States. The fatality rate is greater in infants, young children, and adults. Additionally, subacute sclerosing panencephalitis, an extremely rare degenerative disease of the central nervous system, is caused by this virus presenting years after the initial measles infection.

The number of cases of measles in the United States and other industrialized countries has decreased markedly since the introduction of an effective vaccine in 1963.[24,25] Still, in 1990, there were 55,000 cases and 120 measles-related deaths. This resurgence was largely due to an increase in unvaccinated preschool children, particularly in urban areas.[25]

Some report that measles during pregnancy is not associated with increased maternal or fetal death rates.[26] Others find higher rates of measles-related hospitalization, pneumonia, and death for infected pregnant women.[27] Placental damage from the infection has been implicated in stillbirths.[28] Furthermore, measles infection of mothers in developing countries is associated with an increase in the perinatal mortality rate.[29] As with any febrile illness, measles infection may precipitate premature uterine activity and lead to premature delivery.[30]

No specific syndrome is attributed to intrauterine measles infection. However, the newborn delivered to a woman with active disease is at high risk for severe neonatal measles. Pneumonia is the primary cause of death and is more common in the premature newborn. Recent reports suggest an association between in utero measles infection and postnatal development of Crohn's disease.[31] This potential relationship has yet to be confirmed and does not warrant prenatal diagnosis in the fetus.

Diagnosis

The clinical diagnosis of rubeola is based on the presence of a maculopapular rash occurring 1 to 2 days after a specific exanthematous rash (Koplik's spots), photophobia, and upper respiratory symptoms. Serologic tests can provide a definitive diagnosis and include testing for hemagglutination inhibition antibody, which is present by the onset of the rash and remains positive for life, and a complement fixation antibody that rises slightly later but becomes undetectable after approximately a decade[32] (Fig. 30–1).

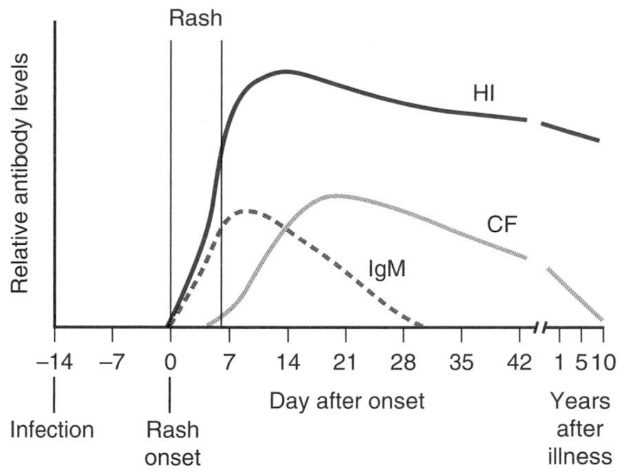

FIGURE 30–1
Immune response to an acute rubeola infection. HI, Hemagglutination inhibition antibody; CF, complement fixation antibody. (From Centers for Disease Control and Prevention: Update on adult immunization: Recommendations of the Immunization Practices Advisory Committee (ACIP). MMWR 1991,40(RR-12):1–52.)

Management Options

Prepregnancy

Prevention is the best available mechanism to protect against measles. All children should receive one dose of the live measles virus vaccine as part of MMR between 12 and 15 months of age followed by a second dose at age 6. Vaccination results in long-lasting immunity in over 95% of recipients.

Likewise, immunity to natural infection is lifelong and the high infectivity of the virus during childhood leaves few susceptible adults. Women contemplating pregnancy with a negative or questionable history of measles illness or vaccination, or laboratory evidence of susceptibility, should receive the live, attenuated virus vaccine followed by a second dose not less than 1 month later. Women vaccinated before 1967 (and likely to have received a heat-killed viral vaccine), or who were vaccinated before 1 year of age, should also receive two doses of vaccine.[24] Pregnancy should be delayed 1 month after receiving MMR vaccine.

Prenatal

The upper respiratory symptoms of acute measles can be ameliorated with cough suppressants. Fever, especially if high, should be treated aggressively with antipyretics. Measles pneumonia may require respiratory support, and if superimposed bacterial pneumonia develops, antibiotic therapy is required. Even when there is no life-threatening disease, pregnant women should be closely monitored during the acute illness for evidence of uterine activity.

Although pregnant women are not candidates for vaccination with any live virus vaccine, accidental vaccination with rubeola vaccine is not a cause for alarm or an indication for pregnancy termination. Immune serum globulin (ISG) may be given to susceptible pregnant women exposed to rubeola in an attempt to prevent or modify the clinical expression of the disease.[33] The intramuscular preparation (0.25 mL/kg, maximum 15 mL) should be given within 6 days of exposure.[11]

Labor, Delivery, and Postnatal

There are no specific management recommendations for these intervals, because acute disease is unlikely. Clinicians, however, should be aware of appropriate isolation precautions instituted for rubeola in the hospital. Observation of the neonate for infection is mandatory.

SUMMARY OF MANAGEMENT OPTIONS

Measles (Rubeola)

Management Options	Quality of Evidence	Strength of Recommendation	References
Prepregnancy			
Prevent by childhood vaccination.	III	B	24
Serologic evaluation and, if negative, vaccination of woman inquiring about status.	III	B	11, 24
Prenatal			
Treat acute infection symptomatically.	–	GPP	–
Antibiotics are given if secondary bacterial infection is suspected.	–	GPP	–
Observe and monitor for uterine activity for termination.	–	GPP	–
Immunoglobulin should be considered for the susceptible woman exposed to the infection.	III	B	24
Inadvertent vaccination is not an indication for termination.	III	B	24
Labor, Delivery, and Postnatal			
Appropriate isolation precautions must be taken when in hospital.	–	GPP	–

MUMPS

Maternal and Fetal Risks

Mumps is a contagious acute viral illness caused by a paramyxovirus, primarily infecting children and young adults. Human beings are the only recognized natural host for this pathogen. The classic presenting symptom for mumps is either unilateral or bilateral parotitis, which usually develops 14 to 18 days after exposure. Respiratory droplets typically transmit the virus. Prodromal symptoms include fever, chills, malaise, and myalgias. The disease can also remain asymptomatic in 20% of cases. Persons are considered infectious from 2 days before the onset of symptoms to approximately 9 days after the parotitis is noted.

Although generally a self-limited disease with symptoms resolving within 5 to 7 days, mumps can result in significant complications, particularly in the adult population. Orchitis occurs in up to 38% of cases in postpubertal males and may lead to infertility.[24] On the other hand, mastitis and oophoritis have been reported in women, but infertility is rare.[34] Other complications include aseptic meningitis, pancreatitis, and thyroiditis. Mumps meningoencephalitis can cause permanent sequelae such as sensorineural hearing loss, seizures, nerve palsies, and hydrocephalus.[24]

There are limited data on mumps in pregnancy. In a cohort study of measles, mumps, and rubella, Siegel reported an increased incidence of first-trimester pregnancy loss with acute mumps infection.[35] No data suggest mumps specifically increases the incidence of stillbirths or preterm deliveries. There were early studies that suggested an association between endocardial fibroelastosis and mumps virus antigen; however, a clear relationship of mumps to this or other congenital malformations has not been confirmed.[36]

The number of reported cases of mumps in the United States has decreased dramatically since the broad institution of effective vaccination. In 1968, over 180,000 cases of mumps were reported in the United States compared to 266 cases reported in 2001.[37] Most cases occurred in persons younger than 20 years of age. Although the presumption was that these outbreaks were due to failure to vaccinate, more recent surveillance data suggest that there may be a waning of vaccine-induced immunity over time, allowing for susceptibility to wild virus infection.[38] Current recommendations, which were enacted in 1989, include a second dose of MMR vaccine given at age 6 years. This practice has resulted in a further decline in mumps infection.[39] A remaining concern is that only 38% of countries worldwide use routine mumps vaccination. Therefore, the importation of mumps into previously protected communities has become increasingly recognized.

Diagnosis

The diagnosis of mumps is usually suspected based on presenting features of the disease in the appropriate clinical setting. Although the virus can be isolated in culture or by RT-PCR detection from a clinical specimen (saliva, CSF, urine, or other infected organ system), the diagnosis is more typically established by serologic techniques. Enzyme immunoassay is the most widely used methodology and is more sensitive than complement fixation or hemagglutination inhibition. Both IgM and IgG antibody testing is available. A positive mumps-specific IgM result from a reliable laboratory or a significant rise between acute and convalescent titers of IgG antibody helps establish the diagnosis of acute infection. After acute infection, it is presumed that one has lifelong immunity and persistent IgG titers.

Management Options

Prepregnancy

Two doses of mumps vaccine in combination with measles and rubella (MMR) are routinely recommended for children in the United States. Therefore, adequate protection against infection should be established prior to a woman reaching her reproductive years. There are no current routine recommendations to test for mumps immunity prior to conception. However, if there is reasonable concern that prior vaccination is not adequate, IgG testing can be obtained. If susceptible, a dose of MMR vaccine should be administered at least 1 month prior to attempting pregnancy.[40]

Prenatal

Because the mumps component in MMR is a live attenuated virus, the vaccine is contraindicated in pregnancy. Because there are no data indicating that mumps vaccination is associated with congenital malformations or other specific adverse outcomes, the inadvertent administration of the vaccine during pregnancy is not an indication for pregnancy termination.

During pregnancy, if exposure to an infected individual is reported, immediate testing for IgG antibody will in most cases confirm immunity and can be used to reassure the patient. In those individuals who lack proven immunity, postexposure immunoglobulin has not been shown to be beneficial as a prophylactic agent. Careful surveillance and symptomatic care should be instituted. Appropriate infection control procedures should be undertaken. These procedures can be rapidly procured from hospital infection-control authorities and via the Centers for Disease Control and Prevention (CDC) website.

Labor, Delivery, and Postpartum

There are no specific recommendations for these periods of time, because an acute outbreak is unlikely to occur. However, in suspected cases in the laboring gravida, the above-mentioned infection control measures should be started as the diagnostic workup is begun. The neonate should be carefully observed for early signs of infection manifested by parotitis or aseptic meningitis. Pediatric infectious disease consultation should be sought.

SUMMARY OF MANAGEMENT OPTIONS

Mumps

Management Options	Quality of Evidence	Strength of Recommendation	References
Prepregnancy			
Prevent by childhood vaccination.	III	B	24
Prenatal			
Accidental vaccination is not an indication for termination.	III	B	11,24
If suspected exposure in woman with "immunity," confirm presence of mumps-specific IgG.	III	B	24
Labor, Delivery, and Postnatal			
Observe neonate for parotitis or aseptic meningitis.	–	GPP	–

VARICELLA

Maternal and Fetal Risks

Varicella-zoster virus (VZV) is a member of the herpesvirus family and is the causative agent of varicella (chickenpox) and herpes zoster (shingles). Varicella is generally a mild, self-limited illness in healthy children. It is transmitted by infected secretions from the nasopharynx, by direct contact with vesicular fluids, or by airborne spread of the virus. This is followed by viral replication in regional lymph nodes and the tonsils. Viral replication continues for approximately 4 to 6 days. Primary viremia develops and virus spreads to internal organs. When the virus replicates again and is released into the bloodstream, it invades the skin, resulting in the classic viral exanthem by 14 days. Therefore, patients are infectious 1 to 2 days prior to developing this rash.

The incubation period of chickenpox is 10 to 12 days. Many patients have a prodrome of fever, malaise, or myalgia a few days prior to the rash, which is vesicular and erupts in crops over the trunk, face, oropharynx, and scalp. Several crops erupt every 2 to 3 days and last 6 to 10 days. Complications are rare but may include bacterial superinfection of vesicles, pneumonia, arthritis, glomerulonephritis, myocarditis, ocular disease, adrenal insufficiency, and central nervous system abnormalities.[41]

In the 1960s varicella pneumonia was reported in up to 50% of adult varicella cases.[42] Retrospective studies suggest that varicella pneumonia in pregnant women is more severe than in nonpregnant adults.[43] In a recent case-control study, smoking and the occurrence of 100 or more skin lesions were risk factors for developing pneumonia.[44] A pregnant woman with varicella and cough, dyspnea, fever, or tachypnea warrants immediate attention. Pneumonia generally develops within a week of the rash and may rapidly progress to hypoxia and respiratory fever. The mortality rate in untreated varicella pneumonia in pregnancy exceeds 40%.[45] If treated aggressively with intravenous acyclovir and supportive measures, reported mortality rates are less than 15%.[42]

Congenital varicella syndrome (CVS) is characterized by dermatomal scarring; ocular abnormalities such as cataracts, chorioretinitis, and microphthalmia; low birth weight; cortical atrophy; and mental retardation (Table 30–3). Most cases occur in infants whose mothers were infected between 8 and 20 weeks' gestation. However, the number of cases is low. Data compiled from multiple retrospective cohort studies have determined the rate of embryopathy is approximately 2%.[46–49] In fact, in a recent, prospective study of 347 varicella-infected mothers, the incidence of CVS was 3 per 231 births (1.3%, 95% CI 0.3 to 0.7) where followup was complete.[50]

Neonatal varicella generally occurs in neonates born to mothers who are infected with varicella within 2 weeks of delivery.[51] It is a serious illness characterized by fever and vesicular rash, which resolves, but in some cases disseminated disease or visceral involvement may ensue. In the latter, the mortality rate may be as high as 25%.

Herpes zoster or shingles, which arises from reactivated VZV, which had been dormant in the dorsal root ganglia, does not lead to congenital varicella syndrome.

TABLE 30–3

Fetal Abnormalities Associated with Congenital (Intrauterine) Varicella Infection

Cutaneous scarring
Limb hypoplasia
Missing/hypoplastic digits
Limb paralysis/muscle atrophy
Psychomotor retardation
Convulsions
Microcephaly
Cerebral cortical atrophy
Chorioretinitis
Cataracts
Chorioretinal scarring
Optic disk hypoplasia
Horner syndrome
Early childhood zoster

Diagnosis

Varicella is usually diagnosed clinically based on the characteristic exanthem. Culture of the vesicular fluid is a lengthy process. Serologic tests are useful to document immunity (when IgG is present) in a patient immediately following exposure. IgM antibody specific to VZV may be identified as soon as 3 days after the onset of symptoms in an acutely infected gravida. IgG seroconversion can be seen as of 7 days after VZV symptom onset. Paired sample analysis for IgG may be useful to establish the diagnosis of primary infection.

Prenatal diagnosis of varicella is possible. Ultrasonography may detect limb abnormalities, and fetal blood or amniotic fluid may be tested for VZV antibody or DNA.[52,53] However, despite detection of virus, the presence of embryopathy cannot be predicted.

Management Options

Prepregnancy

Varivax, a live attenuated varicella vaccine is recommended for susceptible children under age 13 and susceptible adults.[54] The vaccine is given in two doses 4 to 8 weeks apart, and approximately 82% of adults will seroconvert. Women should avoid pregnancy for at least 1 month after vaccination. Results from a voluntary registry of Varivax administered early pregnancy revealed no cases of CVS among 56 live births.[55] Thus, inadvertant Varivax exposure should not prompt medical recommendations for pregnancy termination.

Pregnancy

Varicella zoster immunoglobulin (VZIG) prepared from donors with high levels of VZV should be administered to pregnant women who are susceptible to VZV and are exposed to varicella or herpes zoster. VZIG should be administered with 48 hours of exposure but may be effective up to 96 hours. Although VZIG diminishes the severity of maternal disease, there is no evidence that VZIG prevents congenital varicella.

If a pregnant woman becomes infected with chickenpox, she may be offered oral acyclovir to decrease the number of febrile days and shorten the duration of active lesions.[56] As previously noted, parenteral antiviral therapy may be needed in cases of varicella complicated by pneumonia or central nervous system involvement.

Labor, Delivery, and Postnatal

There are no specific management recommendations for labor. Infected pregnant women should be placed in a negative pressure room for labor, delivery, and the postpartum period in accordance with infection control protocols. Neonates should be given VZIG after birth and monitored closely because the neonate at greatest risk for chickenpox is born within 4 days prior to or 2 days after maternal chickenpox.[57] A recent small study of 24 prenatally infected newborns suggests that VZIG in conjunction with intravenous acyclovir is a more effective prevention strategy than VZIG alone.[58]

SUMMARY OF MANAGEMENT OPTIONS

Varicella-Zoster (VZ) Infection

Management Options	Quality of Evidence	Strength of Recommendation	References
Prepregnancy			
Prevent by childhood vaccination.	III	B	11
Vaccinate susceptible adults.	IV	C	11
Prenatal			
If mother exposed to VZ virus, check immunity status.	–	GPP	–
If mother is IgG negative (susceptible), give VZIG within 96 hours of exposure.	IV	C	54,57
If mother develops chickenpox:			
• Counsel about minimal fetal risks.	IIa	B	46–51
• Offer acyclovir to decrease lesions.	IIa	B	56
• Monitor for dissemination to pneumonia or severe illness.	III	C	42–45
Labor, Delivery, and Postnatal			
Take appropriate infection control measures.	–	GPP	–
Evaluate newborn clinically and serologically.	–	GPP	–
Administer active or passive immunization to neonate if not infected.	IV	C	57, 58

PARVOVIRUS B19

Maternal and Fetal Risks

Human parvovirus B19 (erythema infectiosum, fifth disease) is an infectious exanthematous childhood illness transmitted by droplet. B19 viremia occurs 6 to 8 days after exposure and may persist for up to a week. An infected individual is contagious before the onset of symptoms, and the virus can be detected in the blood or secretions as early as 5 to 10 days after exposure. Parvovirus B19 infection is characterized by fever, rash, and arthropathy. The rash has a "slapped cheek" appearance on the face and a "lace-like" appearance on the trunk and extremities. The arthropathy may affect the joints of the hands, wrist, knees, and ankles. In addition, the virus may cause aplastic crisis in patients with sickle cell disease[59] and other hemolytic states,[60] chronic bone marrow failure in patients with immunodeficiency,[61] a chronic arthropathy,[62] and the childhood illness fifth disease (erythema infectiosum).[63]

Parvovirus B19 infection preferentially infects rapidly dividing cells and is cytotoxic for erythroid progenitor cells.[64,65] As a result, B19 virus also may stimulate a cellular process involving programmed cell death.[66] B19 infection during pregnancy may rarely be associated with fetal loss or hydrops fetalis. The risk of fetal loss appears highest in the first 20 weeks of pregnancy. In a prospective study of 186 pregnancies with confirmed parvovirus B19 infection, there were 27 first-trimester spontaneous abortions versus 7 abortions or fetal deaths in the second trimester and only one death in the third trimester.[67] There have been several additional series of parvovirus infection in pregnancy reported. When these series are summarized, the risk of fetal loss among pregnancies infected prior to 20 weeks' gestation is approximately 10%.[67–71] The risk of loss after 20 weeks' gestation is less than 1% and the risk of hydrops is 0.3%.[71] A prospective study of 618 exposed pregnancies showed no hydrops or fetal death attributable to B19 in 52 babies born to infected mothers.[72] The hydrops may develop rapidly within 7 to 14 days and can lead either to fetal death or can resolve spontaneously.[73,74]

Although B19 infection appears to be teratogenic in fetal animals (cerebellar hypoplasia and ataxia in cats and anencephaly, microcephaly, facial defects, and ectopic hearts in hamsters have been described), epidemiologic studies do not suggest that B19 infection is teratogenic in human fetuses.[75] Furthermore, long-term follow-up of offspring of women with B19 infections suggests the children are normal.[76,77]

Parvovirus B19 infection is distributed worldwide. Antibody to B19 virus occurs in 30% to 60% of adults.[78,79] Secondary attack rates for household contacts may be as high as 50% but as low as 20% to 30% for classroom contacts.[80] Serologic surveys of pregnant women revealed that 35% to 65% are B19 seropositive.[69,72] In one large study during an epidemic, the risk of seroconversion for pregnant women was highest in those with the greatest exposure to young children.[81]

Diagnosis

B19 virus is difficult to culture and clinical manifestations are often lacking. Serology is the easiest method to detect infection using either IgM antibody capture radioimmunoassay or enzyme-linked immunosorbent assay (ELISA). These tests will detect between 80% and 90% of B19 seropositive individuals.[82] IgM, indicating acute infection, can be detected approximately 10 days after exposure and can last for 3 months or longer.[83,84] IgG antibodies may be detected several days after IgM and can persist for years as markers of past infection. Polymerase chain reaction (PCR) to detect small amounts of B19 virus is useful to diagnose in utero infection from amniotic fluid.[85–87] Additional methods such as electron microscopy, detection of viral DNA, and hybridization assays for nucleic acids may be useful for pathologic specimens in the evaluation of stillbirths.

Management Options

Prepregnancy

Immunocompetent adults rarely need treatment; however, patients at risk for hemolysis may need multiple transfusions.

Prenatal

Pregnant women following exposure to B19 virus should have immediate serologic testing. Presence of IgG and absence of IgM suggests prior exposure to B19 virus and that the fetus is protected from infection. If the IgG is negative or positive and the IgM is positive, this finding is consistent with acute infection. Women should be counseled about the low risk of fetal loss in the first trimester and low risks of hydrops or stillbirth in the second and third trimesters. Prior to 20 weeks' gestation, no further action is required. However, after 20 weeks' gestation, periodic ultrasound examinations may be useful to identify hydrops. In addition, Doppler studies of the fetal middle cerebral artery peak velocity may yield an accurate reflection of fetal anemia.[88] In some reported cases hydrops did not appear until 8 weeks following maternal infection; hence the recommendation to continue monitoring for 8 to 12 weeks after infection.[89] If hydrops is noted, percutaneous umbilical blood sampling may be warranted to determine fetal hematocrit and provide transfusion.[90,91] Although some small series show improvement following transfusion, other reports note spontaneous resolution in the absence of intervention.[92,93]

The pregnant woman who is IgG negative and IgM negative is susceptible to infection. She should be counseled that repeat testing may be required if her serologic results were obtained within 2 weeks of her exposure. Preventive measures include minimizing contact with known parvovirus infection and good contact precautions. According to the CDC, there is no proven benefit to removing seronegative women from high risk employment for the duration of the pregnancy.

Labor, Delivery, and Postpartum

Onset of signs and symptoms suggesting acute infection during these time periods requires appropriate infection control measures. The neonate should be carefully observed for vertical transmission of the infection. Neonatal IgG levels immediately after birth reflect transplacentally passed maternal immunoglobulin.

SUMMARY OF MANAGEMENT OPTIONS
Parvovirus B19 Infection

Management Options	Quality of Evidence	Strength of Recommendation	References
Prepregnancy			
If the diagnosis is confirmed before pregnancy, avoid contraception until clinical cure and antibody response.	–	GPP	–
Prenatal			
If mother is exposed to B19 parvovirus or symptoms are noted, check immunity status.	–	GPP	–
If mother is IgG negative/IgM negative (susceptible), repeat testing in 3–4 weeks.	–	GPP	–
If mother is IgG negative/IgM positive:			
• Counsel that risks are minimal.	IIb	B	67–72
• If greater than 20 weeks, screen with serial ultrasound for hydrops.	III	B	67–71
• If hydrops is detected, consider intrauterine fetal transfusion.	III	B	90, 91
Labor, Delivery, and Postnatal			
Take appropriate infection control measures.	–	GPP	–
Evaluate newborn clinically and serologically.	–	GPP	–

CONCLUSIONS

RUBELLA

- Outbreaks are sporadic but occur predominantly in unvaccinated individuals.
- Maternal infection is mild, but fetal malformations may be devastating, depending on the gestational age at infection.
- Inadvertent rubella vaccination does not lead to congenital rubella syndrome.

RUBEOLA (MEASLES)

- Severe disease caused by measles is rare.
- Measles during pregnancy may be associated with increased maternal or fetal morbidity.
- Prevention using MMR vaccine is the optimal mechanism to avoid infection.

MUMPS

- Mumps is generally a self-limited disease.
- Mumps infection during pregnancy is not associated with pregnancy complications or congenital malformations.

VARICELLA

- Varicella pneumonia is a rare but potentially serious disease in pregnant women.
- Congenital varicella syndrome occurs in less than 2% of pregnancies complicated by primary varicella before 20 weeks' gestation.
- Varicella immunoglobulin should be administered to susceptible pregnant women following exposure.

PARVOVIRUS B19

- Maternal infection is frequently asymptomatic.
- Following maternal infection before 20 weeks' gestation, the risk of fetal loss is approximately 10%.
- Fetal hydrops is rare but may be treated with in utero transfusions.

REFERENCES

1. Gershon AA: Rubella virus (german measles). In Mandell GL, Douglas RG, Bennett JE (eds): Principles and Practice of Infectious Diseases, 3rd ed. New York, Churchill Livingstone, 1990, pp 1242–1247.
2. Cochi SL, Edmonds LE, Dyer K, et al: Congenital rubella syndrome in the United States, 1970–1985. Am J Epidemiol 1989;129:349–361.
3. Grossman JH: Why congenital rubella continues to occur. Contemp Obstet Gynecol 1990;36:50–54.
4. Freij BJ, South MA, Sever JL, et al: Maternal rubella and the congenital rubella syndrome. Clin Perinatol 1988;15:247–257.
5. McIntosh EDG, Menser MA: A fifty-year follow-up of congenital rubella. Lancet 1992;340:414–415.
6. Miller E, Cradock-Watson JE, Pollock TM: Consequences of confirmed maternal rubella at successive stages of pregnancy. Lancet 1982;2:781–784.
7. Centers for Disease Control and Prevention: Rubella and congenital rubella syndrome—United States, 1994–1997. MMWR 1997;46:350–353.
8. Centers for Disease Control and Prevention: Rubella outbreak—Westchester County, New York, 1997–1998. MMWR 1999;48:560.
9. Danovaro-Holliday MC, LeBaron CW, Allensworth C, et al: A large rubella outbreak with spread from workplace to the community. JAMA 2000;284:2773–2779.
10. Centers for Disease Control and Prevention: Notice to readers. Revised ACIP recommendation for avoiding pregnancy after receiving a rubella-containing vaccine. MMWR 2001;50(49): 1117.
11. Centers for Disease Control and Prevention: Update on adult immunization: Recommendations of the Immunization Practices Advisory Committee (ACIP). MMWR 1991;40(RR-12):1–52.
12. Chu SY, Bernier RH, Stewart JA, et al: Rubella antibody persistence after immunization. Sixteen-year follow-up in the Hawaiian islands. JAMA 1988;259:3133–3136.
13. O'Shea S, Best JM, Banatvala JE: Viremia, virus excretion, and antibody responses after challenge in volunteers with low levels of antibody to rubella virus. J Infect Dis 1983;148:639–647.
14. Enders G, Calm A, Shaub J: Rubella embryopathy after previous maternal rubella vaccination. Infection 1984;12:96–98.
15. Bart SW, Stetler HC, Preblud SR, et al: Fetal risk associated with rubella vaccine: An update. Rev Infect Dis 1985;7(Suppl 1): S95–102.
16. Centers for Disease Control and Prevention: Rubella vaccination during pregnancy—United States, 1971–1988. MMWR 1989;38:289–291.
17. Immunization during pregnancy. ACOG committee opinion No. 282. Am Cell Obstet Gynecol. Obstet Gynecol 2003; 101:207–212.
18. Daffos F, Forestier F, Grangeot-Keros L, et al: Prenatal diagnosis of congenital rubella. Lancet 1984;2:1–3.
19. Bosma TJ, Corbett KM, O'Shea S, et al: PCR for detection of rubella virus RNA in clinical samples. J Clin Microbiol 1995;33:1075–1079.
20. Ho-Terry L, Terry GM, Londesborough P: Diagnosis of foetal rubella virus infection by polymerase chain reaction. J Gen Virol 1990;71(Pt 7):1607–1611.
21. Tanemura M, Suzumori K, Yagami Y, Katow S: Diagnosis of fetal rubella infection with reverse transcription and nested polymerase chain reaction: A study of 34 cases diagnosed in fetuses. Am J Obstet Gynecol 1996;174:578–582.
22. Modlin JF: Measles virus. In Belshe RB (ed): Human Virology. Littleton, MA, PSG Publishing, 1984, pp 333–360.
23. Gavish D, Kleinman Y, Morag A, Chajek-Shaul T: Hepatitis and jaundice associated with measles in young adults. An analysis of 65 cases. Arch Intern Med 1983;143:674–677.
24. Centers for Disease Control and Prevention: Measles, mumps and rubella. Vaccine use and strategies for elimination of measles, rubella, and congenital rubella syndrome and control of recommendations of the Advisory Committee on Immunization Practices (ACIP). MMWR 1998;44(RR-8):1–57.
25. Hersh BS, Markowitz LE, Maes EF, et al: The geographic distribution of measles in the United States, 1980–1989. JAMA 1992;267:1936–1941.
26. Young NA, Gershon AA: Chickenpox, measles and mumps. In Remington JS, Klein JO (eds): Infectious Diseases of the Fetus and Newborn Infant, 2nd ed. Philadelphia, WB Saunders, 1983, pp 375–427.
27. Eberhart-Phillips JE, Frederick PD, Baron RC, Mascola L: Measles in pregnancy: A descriptive study of 58 cases. Obstet Gynecol 1993;82:797–801.
28. Moroi K, Saito S, Durata T, et al: Fetal death associated with measles virus infection of the placenta. Am J Obstet Gynecol 1991;164:107–1108.
29. Aaby P, Bukh J, Lisse IM, et al: Increased perinatal mortality among children of mothers exposed to measles during pregnancy. Lancet 1988;1:516–519.
30. Stein SJ, Greenspoon JS: Rubeola during pregnancy. Obstet Gynecol 1991;78:925–929.
31. Ekbom A, Daszak P, Kraaz W, Wakefield AJ: Crohn's disease after in utero measles virus exposure. Lancet 1996;348:515–517.
32. Centers for Disease Control and Prevention: Serologic diagnosis of measles. MMWR 1982;31(29):396–402.
33. Amstey MS: Measles. In Gleicher N (ed): Principles and Practice of Medical Therapy in Pregnancy, 2nd ed. Norwalk, CT, Appleton & Lange, 1992, pp 659–661.
34. Korones SB: Uncommon virus infections of the mother, fetus, and newborn: Influenza, mumps, and measles. Clin Perinatal 1988; 15(2): 259–272.
35. Siegel M: Congenital malformations following chickenpox, measles, mumps, and hepatitis: Results of a cohort study. JAMA 1993;226:1521–1524.
36. Nahmias AJ, Armstrong G: Mumps virus and endocardial fibroelastosis. N Engl J Med 1966;275:1448–1450.
37. Centers for Disease Control and Prevention: Summary of notifiable disease—United States, 2001. MMWR 2001;50(53): 1–108.
38. Hersh BS, Fine PE, Kent WK: Mumps outbreak in a highly vaccinated population. J Pediatr 1991;119:187–193.
39. Van Loon FP, Holmes SJ, Sirotkin BI: Mumps surveillance—United States, 1988–1993. MMWR 1995;44:1–14.
40. Bakshi SS, Cooper LZ: Rubella and mumps vaccines. Pediatr Clin 1990;37:651–668.
41. Whitley RJ: Varicella-zoster virus. In Mandell GL, Douglas RG, Bennett JE (eds): Principles and Practice of Infectious Diseases, 3rd ed. New York, Churchill Livingstone, 1990, pp 1153–1159.
42. Smego RA, Asperilla MO: Use of acyclovir for varicella pneumonia during pregnancy. Obstet Gynecol 1991;78:1112–1116.
43. Harris RE, Rhoades ER: Varicella pneumonia complication pregnancy: Case report and review of the literature. Obstet Gynecol 1965;25:734–736.
44. Harger JH, Ernest JM, Thurnau GR, et al: Risk factors and outcome of varicella-zoster virus pneumonia in pregnant women. J Infect Dis 2002;185:422–427.
45. Haake DA, Zakowski PC, Haake DL, et al: Early treatment for varicella pneumonia in otherwise healthy adults: Retrospective controlled study and review. Rev Infect Dis 1990;12:788–798.
46. Balducci J, Rodis JR, Rosengren S, et al: Pregnancy outcome following first-trimester varicella infection. Obstet Gynecol 1992;79:5–6.
47. Pastuszak AL, Levy M, Schick B, et al: Outcome after maternal varicella infection in the first 20 weeks of pregnancy. N Engl J Med 1994;330:901–905.

48. Paryani SG, Arvin AM: Intrauterine infection with varicella-zoster virus after maternal varicella. N Engl J Med 1986;314:1542–1546.
49. Enders G, Miller E, Cradock-Watson J, et al: Consequences of varicella and herpes zoster in pregnancy: Prospective study of 1739 cases. Lancet 1994;343:1547–1550.
50. Harger JH, Ernest JM, Thurnau GR, et al: Frequency of congenital varicella syndrome in prospective cohort of 347 pregnant women. Obstet Gynecol 2002;100:260–265.
51. Meyers JD: Congenital varicella in term infants: Risk reconsidered. J Infect Dis 1974;129:215–217.
52. Cuthbertson G, Weiner CP, Giller RH, et al: Prenatal diagnosis of second trimester congenital varicella syndrome by virus-specific immunoglobulin. J Pediatr 1987;111:592–595.
53. Isada NB, Paar DP, Johnson MP, et al: In utero diagnosis of congenital varicella-zoster virus infection by chorionic villus sampling using polymerase chain reaction. Am J Obstet Gynecol 1991;165:1727–1730.
54. Centers for Disease Control and Prevention: Prevention of varicella: Recommendations of the Advisory Committee on Immunization Practices (ACIP). MMWR 1996;45(RR-11):1–36.
55. Shields KE, Galilk, Seware J, et al: Varicella vaccine exposure during pregnancy: Data from first 5 years of the pregnancy registry. Obstet Gynecol 2001;98:14–19.
56. Balfour HH, Kelly JM, Suarez CS, et al: Acyclovir treatment of varicella in otherwise healthy children. J Pediatr 1990;116:633–639.
57. Centers for Disease Control and Prevention: Varicella-zoster immune globulin for the protection of chickenpox. MMWR 1984;33:84–90, 95–100.
58. Huang YC, Lin Ty, Lin YJ, et al: Prophylaxis of intravenous immunoglobulin and acyclovir in perinatal varicella. Eur J Pediatr 2001;160:91–94.
59. Serjeant GR, Topley JM, Mason K, et al: Outbreak of aplastic crises in sickle cell anemia associated with parvovirus-like agent. Lancet 1981;2:595–597.
60. Thurn J: Human parvovirus B19: Historical and clinical review. Rev Infect Dis 1988;10:1005–1011.
61. Kurtzman GJ, Ozawa K, Cohen B, et al: Chronic bone marrow failure due to persistent B19 parvovirus infection. N Engl J Med 1987;317:287–294.
62. White DG, Woolf AD, Mortimer PP, et al: Human parvovirus arthropathy. Lancet 1985;1:419–421.
63. Anderson MJ, Lewis E, Kidd IM, et al: An outbreak of erythema infectiosum associated with human parvovirus infection. J Hyg 1984;93:85–93.
64. Brown KE, Anderson SM, Young NS: Erythrocyte P antigen: Cellular receptor for B19. Science 1993;262:114–117.
65. Young N, Mortimer P: Viruses and bone marrow failure. Blood 1984;63:729–737.
66. Morey AL, Ferguson DJ, Fleming KA: Ultrastructural features of fetal erythroid precursors infected with parvovirus B19 in-vitro: Evidence of cell death by apoptosis. J Pathol 1993; 169:213–220.
67. Public Health Laboratory Service Working Party on Fifth Disease: Prospective study of human parvovirus (B19) infection in pregnancy. Br Med J 1990;300:1166–1170.
68. Gratacos E, Torres PJ, Vidal J, et al: The incidence of human parvovirus B19 infection during pregnancy and its impact on perinatal outcome. J Infect Dis 1995;171:1360–1363.
69. Rodis JF, Quinn DL, Gary W, et al: Management and outcomes of pregnancies complicated by human B19 parvovirus infection: A prospective study. Am J Obstet Gynecol 1990;163:1168–1171.
70. Guidozzi F, Ballot D, Rothberg A: Human B19 parvovirus infection in an obstetric population: A prospective study determining fetal outcome. J Reprod Med 1994;39:36–38.
71. Markenson GR, Yancey ML: Parvovirus B19 infections in pregnancy. Semin Perinatol 1998;22:309–317.
72. Harger JH, Adler SP, Koch WC, Harger GF: Prospective evaluation of 618 pregnant women exposed to parvovirus B19. Risks and symptoms. Obstet Gynecol 1998;91:413–420.
73. Miller E, Fairley CK, Cohen BJ, Seng C: Immediate and long term outcome of human parvovirus B19 infection in pregnancy. BJOG 1998;105:174–178.
74. Rodis JF, Borgida AF, Wilson M, et al: Management of parvovirus infection in pregnancy and outcomes of hydrops: A survey of members of the Society of Perinatal Obstetricians. Am J Obstet Gynecol 1998;179:985–988.
75. Kinney J, Anderson L, Farrar J, et al: Risk of adverse outcomes of pregnancy after human parvovirus B19 infection. J Infect Dis 1988;157:663–667.
76. Rodis JF, Rodner C, Hansen AA, et al: Long-term outcome of children following maternal human parvovirus B19 infection. Obstet Gynecol 1998;91:125–128.
77. Dembinsk J, Haverkamp F, Maara H, et al: Neurodevelopmental outcome after intrauterine red cell transfusion for parvovirus B19–induced fetal hydrops. BJOG 2002;109:1232–1234.
78. Koch WC, Adler SP: Human parvovirus B19 infections in women of childbearing age and within families. Pediatr Infect Dis J 1989;8:83–87.
79. Woolf AD, Campion GV, Chishick A, et al: Clinical manifestations of human parvovirus B19 in adults. Arch Intern Med 1989;149:1153–1156.
80. Gillespie SM, Cartter ML, Asch S, et al: Occupational risk of human parvovirus B19 infection for school and daycare personnel during an outbreak of erythema infectiosum. JAMA 1990;263:2061–2065.
81. Valeur-Jensen AK, Pedersen CB, Westergaard T, et al: Risk factors for parvovirus B19 in pregnancy. JAMA 1999;281:1099–1105.
82. Schwarz TF, Jager G, Gilch S: Comparison of seven commercial tests for the detection of parvovirus B19-specific IgM. Zentralbl Bakteriol 1997;285:525–530.
83. Torok T: Human parvovirus B19. In Remington J, Klein J (eds): Infectious Diseases of the Fetus and Newborn Infant. Philadelphia, WB Saunders, 1995, pp 668–702.
84. Rotbart HA: Human parvovirus infections. Annu Rev Med 1990;41:25–34.
85. Torok TS, Wang QY, Gary GW, et al: Prenatal diagnosis on intrauterine infection with parvovirus B19 by the polymerase chain reaction technique. Clin Infect Dis 1992;14:149–155.
86. Clewley JP: Polymerase chain reaction assay of parvovirus B19 DNA in clinical specimens. J Clin Microbiol 1989;27: 2647–2651.
87. Yamakawa Y, Oka H, Hori S, et al: Detection of human parvovirus B19 DNA by nest polymerase chain reaction. Obstet Gynecol 1995;86:126–129.
88. Cosmi E, Mari G, Delle-Chiaie L, et al: Noninvasive diagnosis by Doppler ultrasonography of fetal anemia resulting from parvovirus infection. Am J Obstet Gynecol 2002;187: 1290–1293.
89. Mielke G, Enders G: Late onset of hydrops fetalis following intrauterine parvovirus B19 infection. Fetal Diagn Ther 1997;12:40–42.
90. Fairley C, Smoleniec J, Caul O, Miller E: Observational study of effect of intrauterine transfusions on outcome of fetal hydrops after parvovirus B19 infection. Lancet 1995;346:1335–1337.
91. Schild RL, Bald R, Plath H, et al: Intrauterine management of fetal parvovirus B19 infection. Ultrasound Obstet Gynecol 1999;13:161–166.
92. Sheikh AU, Ernest JM, O'Shea M: Long-term outcome in fetal hydrops from parvovirus B19 infection. Am J Obstet Gynecol 1992;167:337–341.
93. Humphrey W, Magoon M, O'Shaughnessy R: Severe nonimmune hydrops secondary to parvovirus B19 infection: Spontaneous reversal in-utero and survival of a term infant. Obstet Gynecol 1991;78:900–902.

CHAPTER 31

Cytomegalovirus, Herpes Simplex Virus, Adenovirus, Coxsackievirus, and Human Papillomavirus

Thomas Roos

INTRODUCTION

Viral infections can pose a serious threat to the fetus and the newborn. In the healthy adult, infections might be asymptomatic or cause only mild unspecific symptoms. Consequently, the virus may reside dormant for prolonged periods, and asymptomatic virus shedding may occur unnoticed. Virus can be transmitted by trivial interpersonal contacts such as occurs when handling a baby (cytomegalovirus, herpes simplex virus, adenovirus, coxsackievirus) or in a swimming pool (adenovirus). Sexual activities with multiple partners confer a high risk for infection with viruses associated with severe disease in the adult and in the infant. Pregnancy is associated with decreased maternal cell-mediated immunity to viral infections; thus, the pregnant woman and her fetus are theoretically at increased risk for serious illness. Depending on gestational age, transplacental viral infection may range from asymptomatic to severe, causing fetal or neonatal death, or long-term sequelae in the survivors. Intrauterine growth restriction (IUGR), nonimmune hydrops, isolated ascites, intracranial calcifications, microcephaly, and hydrocephaly are common ultrasound findings associated with in utero viral infection. The possible severe impact of viral infections and the lack of specific antiviral treatment options in the fetus and newborn available to date imply that prevention is the most important approach to disease containment. The development of antiviral drugs and vaccines in progress holds the promise of a reduced incidence of fetal viral infections and of their sequelae in the future.

CYTOMEGALOVIRUS

General

Cytomegalovirus (CMV), a DNA virus, is a member of the herpes family of viruses, which causes a number of infectious syndromes in humans. However, because CMV is highly efficient in remaining dormant or silent in the host, the most common manifestation of CMV infection in humans is the lack of demonstrable disease. Three disease states are particularly important: intrauterine and neonatal infection, heterophil-negative mononucleosis, and infection in the immunocompromised patient.

Diagnosis

Human CMV is readily grown in cell lines of human fibroblasts. In patients with symptoms suggestive of acute CMV infection, viral culture from urine, nasopharynx, or blood may document the presence of the organism. Direct immunofluorescence tests in combination with a limited culture can detect the virus more rapidly. More recently, nucleic acid amplification systems using polymerase chain reaction (PCR) techniques have been used to identify the virus in amniotic and other fluid samples.[1–3] High numbers of virus copies in the amniotic fluid can possibly signal a fetus at risk for severe CMV disease; however, this relationship needs further study. Tissue specimens (biopsy, necropsy) may also be evaluated for virus by immunofluorescence, in situ hybridization, or PCR techniques; these specimens may also reveal the characteristic histologic changes associated with CMV infection.[4]

Because many previously infected patients excrete CMV intermittently throughout their lives depending on certain circumstances (e.g., pregnancy, AIDS), the presence of CMV in a specimen does not guarantee that the illness in question is caused by this particular virus. The physician must be extremely careful with the interpretation of these results.

Approximately 50% of reproductive age women have antibody to CMV. Thus, paired specimens are necessary, if seroconversion from negative to positive has not been documented. A significant rise in titer is usually consistent with a primary infection. Immunoglobulin M (IgM)-specific antibody is usually present 4 to 8 weeks after a primary infection but can increase periodically or persist at a low titer for years. IgM and less frequently IgA are of use in distinguishing transplacental transfer of maternal antibodies in the diagnosis of congenital infection.[5]

Serologic testing consists of the older complement fixation test or the more current indirect fluorescent antibody and anticomplement immunofluorescent tests. In a primary infection, these tests become positive sooner than the complement fixation test.[6] Enzyme immunoassay (EIA) methods also have been used to detect CMV-specific IgG, IgM, IgA, and IgE antibodies.[7] This is important because reactivation of latent CMV during pregnancy may not be accompanied by either an increase or reappearance of IgM antibodies (depending on the methodology used), which theoretically would help differentiate it from new infection.[8] Recently, more labor-intensive EIA assays have been used to detect low avidity IgG antibodies that are produced early in infection.[9–11] In a recent study, CMV immediate-early messenger RNA in maternal blood was detected only in cases of primary CMV infection and not in immune subjects; thus, EIA has been suggested to be helpful in differentiating primary from recurrent infection.[12]

Isolation of the virus or DNA from amniotic fluid and demonstration of viral DNA, immunologic response, or nonspecific markers in fetal blood collected by cordocentesis have all been used to supplement antenatal diagnosis.[13–16] A prospective evaluation of 1771 pregnant Belgian women by serial serology and culture of urine, saliva, and cervical secretions at each prenatal visit revealed a seronegative rate of 49%. Of this group, seroconversion occurred in 20 susceptible women (2.3%). Five of the seven who agreed to cordocentesis and amniocentesis had positive amniotic fluid cultures for CMV; three had a positive fetal IgM for CMV. The presence of CMV in fetal tissue was confirmed after termination, supporting the authors' contention that amniotic fluid culture is superior to fetal IgM in diagnosing fetal infection.[17] Others have reported either a lack of fetal CMV seropositivity for IgM in culture-positive fetuses or the failure of the fetus to sustain the IgM response. Thus, amniotic fluid culture or PCR analysis of amniotic fluid is superior to fetal CMV-specific IgM.[18,19] There have been a few reports of false-negative amniotic fluid cultures, as ascertained by neonatal shedding, but the relationship of these apparently negative results to the timing of infection and to long-term sequelae is unclear. Culture failure may be related to performance of amniocentesis too close to the time of initial maternal infection or too early in gestation; that is, before the fetal kidneys produce sufficient amounts of urine containing shedded virus.[20,21] The best results for detecting congenital CMV infection by testing amniotic fluid samples occur when amniocentesis is performed after 21 weeks' gestation and after an interval of at least 6 weeks from the first diagnosis of maternal infection.[22,23] Sensitivity to CMV can be enhanced using PCR or nested PCR assays.[9,24] Since all of these techniques can produce false-negative results, a negative diagnostic workup does not guarantee absence of infection.

Detection of specific IgM in the fetal blood has been found to be associated with severe CMV disease.[22] Some, but not all, infected fetuses have sonographic abnormalities (e.g., intracranial calcifications, growth restriction), anemia, thrombocytopenia, and elevated liver function test results.[13,25] The natural history of the disease was followed antenatally by serial ultrasound and cordocentesis in at least one reported case.[26] Hyperechoic bowel may precede development of ventriculomegaly, IUGR, nonimmune hydrops, and fetal death in infected fetuses.[27] In a group of 50 pregnant women (51 fetuses) with primary CMV infection and confirmed in utero transmission, abnormal fetal ultrasound findings could be demonstrated in 22% (11 out of 51 fetuses). In the same study, however, 3 out of 16 newborns (19%) with normal ultrasound findings had neurologic abnormalities.[28] Thus, normal ultrasound findings in infected fetuses at 22 weeks' gestation can neither exclude an abnormal ultrasound later in pregnancy and the birth of a severely damaged child nor the birth of neonates afflicted by single manifestations at birth or later in life, of the kind not detectable by currently available ultrasonographic techniques.

Maternal and Fetal Risks

Approximately 10% of healthy adults infected with CMV for the first time may develop a syndrome of fever, atypical lymphocytosis, malaise, and mild lymphadenopathy, which generally follows a benign course. This illness is clinically indistinguishable from Epstein-Barr virus (EBV) mononucleosis, save that the heterophil-antibody test is negative in patients with CMV infection. Patients with CMV mononucleosis tend to be slightly older than patients with EBV infection. This syndrome is generally self-limiting, although the fever may last for over a month. Serious complications of the acute infection rarely occur, including interstitial pneumonitis, hepatitis, Guillain-Barré syndrome, meningoencephalitis, myocarditis, thrombocytopenia, and hemolytic anemia.[29] The virus may be excreted in tears, saliva, breast milk, cervical secretions, and urine for weeks, months, or years after a primary infection. A latency period eventually occurs, but reinfection and reactivation are common.[30]

Cytomegalovirus infection in the immunosuppressed patient can be serious, depending on the type and degree of immunosuppression. Patients on immunosuppressive drugs because of organ transplantation or patients with AIDS most commonly exhibit the mononucleosis syndrome. The next most frequent manifestation is interstitial pneumonia, which may progress rapidly from asymptomatic to fatal disease (often in association with *Pneumocystis* infection in AIDS patients). A large percentage of persons suffering primary CMV infection exhibit hepatitis; severely immunosuppressed patients may develop clinical symptoms, including malaise, nausea, and vomiting. Gastrointestinal disease, including ulceration leading to hemorrhage and perforation, is another effect of CMV in the immunocompromised patient. The AIDS patient may suffer coexistent CMV infection with other infections such as cryptosporidiosis and *Mycobacterium avium-intracellulare*. In fact, endoscopic examination of the AIDS patient with colitis due to CMV may demonstrate lesions that resemble Kaposi's sarcoma. Finally, in the AIDS patient specifically, CMV infection of the eye may produce retinitis, typically noted in neonates with the disease, and miscellaneous effects on endocrine organs, including adrenals, pancreas, parathyroids, pituitary, and ovaries.[6]

Venereal spread of CMV is conceptually attributed to presence of virus in the semen and to cervical shedding. CMV has been isolated from semen of both homosexual and heterosexual men.[31] Heterosexual transmission has been demonstrated by outbreaks of CMV mononucleosis among populations of sexual partners.[32] Aside from the fact that differences in rates of cervical shedding are noted in different patient groups throughout the world, it is fairly clear that sexual activity, in particular higher numbers of sexual partners and earlier age at onset of sexual activity, is positively correlated with CMV isolation from the cervix.[33]

Whereas CMV is transmitted by such routes as transfused blood[34] and bone marrow,[35] a common route of acquisition is through perinatal transmission. The fetus may be infected either transplacentally or by exposure to the virus from the cervix and birth canal. The neonate may also be infected by virus excreted in breast milk.[36] Another source of childhood infection is exposure to other babies in nurseries and day-care centers,[37,38] since infected children tend to shed virus from the urine and respiratory tract for a prolonged time (unlike infected but otherwise healthy adults).

The rate of seropositivity varies by age and multiple demographic factors. The rate increases steadily after the first year or two of life. The prevalence is higher in underdeveloped countries[39] and in lower socioeconomic patient populations.[40] One study of over 21,000 women attending a prenatal clinic in London revealed marked variation by race (white, 46%; Asian, 88%; black, 77%), parity (increasing seropositivity with increasing parity), and socioeconomic status.[41,42] Among most middle-income women in Alabama, 54% were seropositive, with whites having a lower rate than blacks.[40] The incidence of seroconversion in women of childbearing age approximates 2% in high socioeconomic groups and up to 6% in lower socioeconomic groups. The higher infection rate in young adults (hence mothers) does not necessarily lead to higher congenital infection rates.[43]

Primary infection occurs in 1% to 3% during pregnancy, with approximately 40% to 50% of women of childbearing age being serologically determined to be susceptible to such primary infection.[40,44] Serologic or culture evidence of in utero CMV infection is present in 0.2% to 2.2% of all liveborns. Thus, congenital CMV infection is a major health problem; CMV is still thought to be the most common congenital infection in the United States based on serologic study.[30,45,46]

Unlike other viral infections, CMV, on the basis of its latency and intermittent shedding from the female genital tract, may infect a fetus or neonate despite the presence of maternal antibody. Virus is shed from the cervix more readily as gestation progresses and occurs in approximately 0% to 2% of women in the first, 6% to 10% in the second, and 11% to 28% in the third trimester.[6] The infection rates at birth are higher in newborns whose mothers excrete virus. The most severe neonatal disease usually occurs in children born to women who experience primary infection during pregnancy. Vertical transmission of CMV occurs in 21% to 50% of fetuses following primary maternal infection.[22,23,47] A study of preconceptional and periconceptional primary CMV infection in 25 women identified a 9% risk for congenital fetal infection in the preconceptional group (1 out of 12 newborns) and a 31% risk in the periconceptional group (4 out of 13 newborns).[48]

Naturally acquired immunity results in a 69% reduction in the risk of congenital CMV infection in future pregnancies.[49] In addition, severe transplacental infection is not usually seen in children of women with preexisting antibody.[50]

Cytomegalovirus is found in roughly 1% of all newborn infants. In the United States, this results in an estimated 33,000 infected newborns annually[29]; in the United Kingdom CMV causes much more neonatal disease than rubella.[45] Approximately 5% to 10% of infected newborns are clinically symptomatic at birth. This is one of the classic TORCH syndromes, consisting of hepatosplenomegaly, hyperbilirubinemia, petechiae, thrombocytopenia, intracranial calcifications, microcephaly, and often growth restriction. In primary infection, mortality may be as high as 20% to 30%, with 90% of survivors suffering late complications (Fig. 31–1) using "averaged" published data.[51] Of the asymptomatic infected neonates, 5% to 15% develop some abnormality attributable to CMV before their second birthday, primarily sensorineural hearing loss.[46,52] Vertical transmission may also occur in recurrent CMV infection[53]; however, the

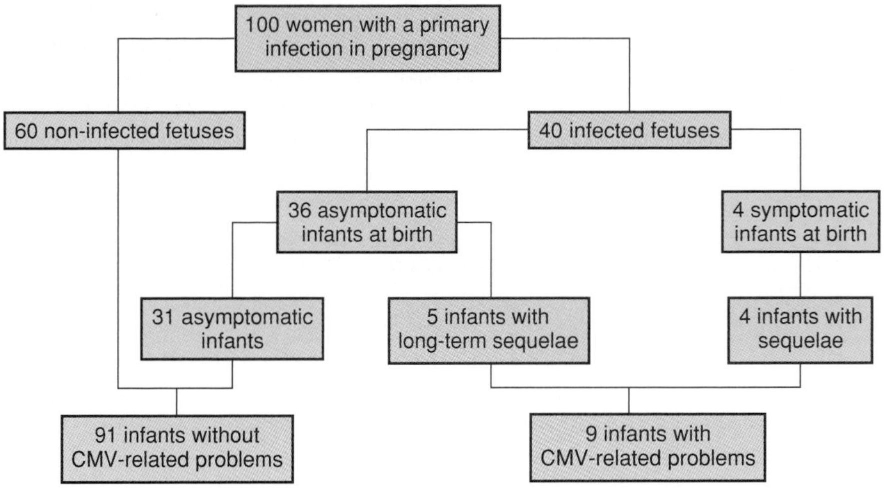

FIGURE 31–1
Infant outcome following primary CMV maternal infection in pregnancy. (Adapted from Greenough A, Osborne J, Sutherland S [eds]: Congenital, Perinatal and Neonatal Infections. Edinburgh, Churchill Livingstone,1992, p 124.)

percentage of symptomatic children at birth or of those developing sequelae is much lower (Table 31–1).[54]

Cytomegalovirus is the most common cause of congenital sensorineural hearing loss, developing in 30% of neonates symptomatic at birth.[55] Hepatosplenomegaly is the most common clinical finding. Microcephaly, frequently associated with paraventricular cerebral calcifications, is also common.[56] Chorioretinitis, optic atrophy, mental and psychomotor delay, learning disabilities, and dental abnormalities are reported.

Management Options

Treatment of acute, symptomatic CMV infection in the immunocompetent normal individual is palliative. The vast majority of infections are asymptomatic; the remainder are mild. Currently, eradication of the virus is beyond the capacity of modern medicine. In the patient with compromised immunity, such as the transplant patient or the patient with AIDS, the antiviral drug ganciclovir provides temporary relief from such severe effects as retinitis.[6] To date, there is no accepted therapy for acute maternal or neonatal infection.[57]

There is progress in the development of a specific CMV vaccine,[58] although a number of real and theoretic obstacles remain.[59] Even though complete eradication of the virus may appear unlikely, antibody presence similar to that after primary human infection could reduce the rate of congenital fetal infection and its sequelae. Thus, an effective CMV vaccine will be a significant step forward. Passive immunization with specific anti-CMV immunoglobulins appears useful as prophylaxis only in cases of renal and marrow transplantation.[60] Thus, prevention of maternal infection is clearly the strategy to avert intrauterine infection. Three different areas offer potential to reduce the likelihood of maternal CMV infection in pregnancy: patient education, physician education, and vaccine development. CMV is typically spread by interpersonal contact with transmission of infected secretions from person to person, so, in particular, pregnant women working in high-risk situations (e.g., day-care centers) should be counseled to wash their hands carefully after changing diapers and after any contact with children's secretions (saliva, etc.).[57,61] Mouth-to-mouth kissing with children should be discouraged. Physicians need to be aware of the risk of transfusion-related CMV transmission.[62] Thus, when transfusing women of childbearing age who could potentially be or soon become pregnant, CMV-negative blood products should be used whenever possible. Any fetal transfusion in utero must use CMV-negative washed packed cells to avoid fetal CMV contamination. It is not appropriate, however, to screen all pregnant women either for anti-CMV IgG or viral excretion with the aim of isolating them for the duration of the pregnancy. The most reasonable course is to serologically screen all women in high risk areas (e.g., day-care workers) and recommend to susceptible individuals that they pay attention to hygiene measures. For prevention of CMV as well as other sexually transmitted diseases (STDs), all women with nonmonogamous relationships should be strongly encouraged to use condoms during sexual contact.[57]

TABLE 31–1

Sequelae in Children with Congenital Cytomegalovirus Infection According to Type of Maternal Infection

	PRIMARY	RECURRENT
Symptomatic disease at birth	24/132 (18%)	0/65 (0%)
Any sequelae	31/125 (25%)	5/64 (8%)
More than one sequela	7/125 (6%)	0/64 (0%)
Sensorineural hearing loss	18/120 (15%)	3/56 (5%)
Bilateral hearing loss	10/120 (8%)	0/56 (0%)
Microcephaly	6/125 (5%)	1/64 (2%)
Seizures	6/125 (5%)	0/64 (0%)
IQ <70	9/68 (13%)	0/32 (0%)
Death	3/125 (2%)	0/64 (0%)

From Fowler KB, Stagno S, Pass RF, et al.: The outcome of congenital cytomegalovirus infection in relation to maternal antibody status. N Engl J Med 1992;326:663–667.

No effective fetal therapy is yet available. Ganciclovir has been administered into the umbilical vein of a fetus at about 27 weeks. Dosage was 10 mg/day for 5 days, 15 mg/day for 3 days, and 20 mg/day for 4 days. Several episodes of bradycardia were noted after administration. Although the viral load in amniotic fluid decreased dramatically over the time of treatment and liver function tests improved, a fetal demise was noted at 32 weeks.[63] Whether direct administration of antiviral agents to the fetus to treat CMV will be an acceptable treatment awaits more work.

SUMMARY OF MANAGEMENT OPTIONS

Cytomegalovirus

Management Options	Quality of Evidence	Strength of Recommendation	References
Prepregnancy			
Advise women working in high risk environment (e.g., child care) about risks.	III	B	57, 61
Counsel pregnancy planning in women with history of proven CMV infection; establishing their "shedding status" may help.	–	GPP	–
Encourage use of condoms in nonmonogamous relationships.	IV	C	57
Use CMV-negative blood products in transfusions.	IV	C	62
Prenatal			
Advise women working in high risk environment (e.g., child care) about risks.	III	B	57, 61
Use CMV-negative blood products in transfusions.	IV	C	62
If patient is diagnosed to have CMV infection in pregnancy:	–	GPP	–
• offer careful counseling about fetal risks			
• consider invasive procedure to establish fetal risk			
• check fetal growth and health			
• consider pregnancy termination (if early gestational age)			
• no effective treatment, although acyclovir has been used in severe retinitis	IV	C	6
Labor, Delivery, and Postnatal			
If patient is diagnosed to have CMV infection in pregnancy:	–	GPP	–
• put infection control measures in place			
• conduct clinical and serologic evaluation of the newborn with pediatric follow-up if infection confirmed			

HERPES SIMPLEX VIRUS

General

The herpes simplex virus (HSV) is a DNA virus of the herpes family. HSV-1 has classically been considered the cause of orolabial herpes, referred to commonly as *fever blisters;* HSV-2 has been considered the cause of genital herpes infection, a well-known STD. Although these two types of HSV are generally thought to be segregated in this way, there is a great deal of overlap; that is, of HSV-2 causing oral disease and HSV-1 causing genital infection. In fact, up to a third of genital infections may be due to HSV-1. However, HSV-1 is somewhat less prone to produce recurrent infection than HSV-2. Generally, the two viruses may be considered identical in the clinical circumstance of a patient with characteristic ulcerative lesions.[64]

Diagnosis

Herpes simplex virus is relatively easy to culture; viral culture is the preferred test of genital HSV infection in patients who present with genital ulcers. The sensitivity of culture declines rapidly as lesions begin to heal, usually within a few days of onset. When more rapid diagnosis is desirable, fluorescent antibody (FA) staining performed on short-incubation tissue culture slides allows identification within 48 hours, especially when the original specimen contains large numbers of virus. In high inocula situations, direct FA staining of the original specimen may give the diagnosis, though it is neither as sensitive nor as specific as tissue culture.[65,66] More recently, enzyme-linked immunosorbent assay (ELISA) tests directed toward virus antigens have been developed that provide rapid diagnosis of viral shedding, including asymptomatic shedding from the cervix, with reasonable sensitivity.[67,68] PCR assays for HSV DNA are highly sensitive and can be used to rapidly detect HSV DNA in pregnant women.[69]

Both type-specific and nonspecific antibodies to HSV develop during the first 6 to 8 weeks after infection and persist indefinitely. Antibodies can be detected using immunofluorescence, EIA, or immunoblot methods. Accurate type-specific assays must be based on the HSV-1 specific glycoprotein G1 for diagnosis of infection with HSV-1 and on the HSV-2 specific glycoprotein G2 for diagnosis of infection with HSV-2.[70] Sensitivity of serology tests vary between 80% and 90%, and false-negative results may occur, especially at early stages of infection. Specificity is >96%, and false-positive results can occur. Thus, repeat testing may be indicated in some settings. Type-specific serology in combination with HSV DNA testing by PCR might prove helpful in confirming a clinical diagnosis of genital herpes, especially in patients with healing sores or recurrent episodes of genital herpes when HSV culture provides false-negative results.[71] Clinical examination is likely to miss many cases of genital herpes,[72] and antepartum cultures may not accurately predict viral shedding at the time of delivery.[73] There are three stages of HSV infection based on clinical presentation and serology. Primary HSV infection is confirmed when no HSV-1 or HSV-2 IgG antibodies are present. In nonprimary first-episode disease, HSV-1 antibodies are present in the woman who has HSV-2 infection or HSV-2 antibodies are present in the woman who has HSV-1 infection. In recurrent infections, homologous antibodies are present.[74] Routine screening in the general population appears not to be cost-effective[75] and is not recommended.[70] However, identification of seronegative women provides the opportunity to properly address the risk of primary transmission during pregnancy and counsel serologically discordant couples, in particular.[76]

Maternal and Fetal Risks

Primary orolabial herpes is mainly a disease of childhood, children acquiring the infection from family members through close contact. Although 90% to 95% of primary oral infections are asymptomatic, a few may consist of a rather florid vesiculoulcerative outbreak in the oropharynx and lips about a week after exposure. Adenopathy and viremia, along with fever and malaise, may persist for a week or two, with viral shedding for up to 6 weeks. Thereafter, antibody production limits the virus such that it remains dormant, occasionally flaring up as localized blisters on the lips in times of stress, sunburn, or febrile systemic illness (hence the term *fever blisters*). During recurrent disease, viral shedding lasts up to a week.[77] HSV-1 infection is common in children, whereas HSV-2 is more common in sexually active adolescents and adults. Epidemiologic studies are hampered by the fact the two viruses cross-react in a number of serologic tests used. Confounding this technical difficulty is the latency of the virus. As a result, patients who have been infected and who may be infectious are for the most part asymptomatic. It should be noted that adults with recurrent oral herpes may transmit the illness through orogenital contact, causing infections typically thought to arise from sexual contact.

Genital herpes may occur after sexual contact, either genital-genital or orogenital, with an infected person. The incubation period is less than a week. Persons transmitting the virus may be asymptomatic themselves,[78] confusing identification of the origin of the infection. In one study, 10% of pregnant women were at risk of contracting primary HSV-2 infection from their HSV-2 seropositive husbands.[76] Subclinical cervical and vulvar shedding following a primary HSV infection occurs in 2.3% of women with HSV-2 infection and 0.65% with HSV-1 infection.[79] If the infected person possesses preexisting anti-HSV antibody, perhaps from HSV-1 infection acquired early in life, there are fewer constitutional symptoms, lesions, and complications, and the duration of the lesions and the time of viral shedding are reduced.[64] In the absence of circulating antibody, primary HSV genital infection can be severe, with symptoms of fever, malaise, myalgias, and aseptic meningitis. HSV encephalitis[80] and hepatitis[81] have proven fatal. Lower motor neuron and autonomic dysfunction may lead to bladder atony and urine retention. Extragenital lesions are present in a quarter of women with primary disease, possibly by autoinoculation rather than viremia. Increased viral shedding occurs for nearly 3 weeks in severe cases. Local disease may recur weeks or months later if the offending virus is HSV-2, in particular, which recurs much more frequently than does HSV-1, especially in the genital area.[82]

Genital herpes infection is common in the United States, with 45 million people ages 12 and older, or one out of five of the total adolescent and adult population, infected with HSV-2.[83] Since the late 1970s, the number of people in the United States with genital herpes infection has increased by 30%. HSV-2 infection is more common in women (approximately 1 out of 4) than in men (almost 1 out of 5), and more in blacks (45.9%) than in whites (17.6%). The largest increase is now occurring in young white teens. HSV-2 infection is now five times more common in 12- to 19-year-old whites, and it is twice as common in young adults ages 20 to 29 than it was 20 years ago.[83] Among sexual partners discordant for HSV infection, the annual risk of acquisition of genital HSV infection was 31.9% among women who were both HSV-1 and HSV-2 negative versus 9.1% among women who were HSV-1 positive.[84] Approximately 1.6 million new HSV-2 infections are acquired yearly, and approximately 2% of women seroconvert to HSV-2 during pregnancy.[85,86]

Herpes simplex virus infection during pregnancy has two important components: primary infection of the mother and transmission of infection (either primary or recurrent) to the fetus/neonate and subsequent disseminated infection. Because of the relative immunosuppression during pregnancy,[87] dissemination of HSV may lead to death from hepatitis, encephalitis, and general viral dissemination.[88] Primary infection early in pregnancy, perhaps due to a viral endometritis ascending from cervical infection, may end in spontaneous abortion. However, there are no consistent reports of a congenital syndrome due to intrauterine infection with HSV. The spectrum of fetal/neonatal infection includes abortion, prematurity, and intrapartum infection with resultant disseminated HSV infection.[89] Primary HSV infection in the second or third trimesters increases the risk for preterm delivery as well as the risk of virus transmission to the newborn.[90] The fetus acquiring HSV, especially if the mother suffers an acute, primary infection, may sustain severe neonatal morbidity, including chorioretinitis, meningitis, encephalitis, mental retardation, seizures, and death.[91]

Nonspecific tests for HSV (i.e., not differentiating between HSV-1 and HSV-2) demonstrate 90% seropositivity by the fourth decade of life.[92] Over the past decade or two, industrialized countries have reported a decrease in seropositivity rates of HSV-1, due perhaps to increasing sanitation measures, and increasing rates of HSV-2, due to increasingly permissive sexual behavior.[93] The rates of clinical genital HSV infection have risen dramatically since the 1960s in the United States,[94] United Kingdom, and other parts of Europe.[93]

The incidence of a positive culture in laboring women is 0.5% in the general population.[95] Rates of 0.96%[73] to 2.4%[96] have been reported in asymptomatic women with known histories of genital HSV infection. The rate of neonatal disease is in the range of 0.01% to 0.05%. The variability is due to differences in maternal antibody (and thus passively acquired fetal antibody) levels and the size of the viral inoculum (i.e., primary, severe infection versus mild, recurrent infection in the mother). The majority of infants developing neonatal HSV infection are born to mothers without symptoms or even a history of genital herpes infection and who test seronegative for specific HSV antibodies.[73,95,97] In Seattle, a prospective study was conducted in a cohort of 58,362 pregnant women, of whom 40,023 had genital HSV cultures at the time of labor and 31,663 had HSV specific serology; 202 women (0.5%) had a positive HSV culture, of whom 10 (5%) had neonates with HSV infection.[95] Women without a history of genital herpes were more likely to shed HSV subclinically than women with such a history. However, women with a history of genital herpes were more likely to have cesarean deliveries. The rate of vertical HSV transmission was 31.3% (5/16) in HSV-1 culture-positive mothers, and 2.7% (5/186) in HSV-2 positive mothers. Neonatal HSV infection rates per 100,000 live births were 54 among HSV-seronegative women, 26 among women who were HSV-1 seropositive only, and 22 among all HSV-2 seropositive women. Thus, the highest rate of neonatal HSV infection occurred in women who were seronegative and had no specific HSV antibodies. Heterologous antibody in this study did not seem to protect against transmission for primary versus nonprimary first-episode as, in contrast, did homologous antibody. The results emphasize the need for counseling seronegative women, in particular, to reduce the risk of neonatal HSV infection.

Most neonatal HSV infection is the consequence of delivery of a neonate through an infected birth canal. Most infants have localized skin, eye, and mouth disease, which usually is a mild illness. However, localized disease may progress to encephalitis or disseminated disease. Disseminated disease is associated with a 57% mortality rate, and CNS disease has 15% mortality; localized disease shows no mortality.[98] In a group of 202 women from whom HSV was isolated, HSV transmission occured in 9 out of 117 (7.7%) infants after vaginal delivery, and in 1 out of 85 (1.2%) newborns delivered by cesarean section.[95] Thus, cesarean section could reduce the rate of HSV transmission from mother to infant, but cannot completely prevent HSV infection in the newborn.

Management Options

Prepregnancy

The consistent, correct use of latex condoms can help protect against infection, particularly in women.[99] However, condoms do not provide complete protection because the condom may not cover the herpes sore(s) and viral shedding may nevertheless occur, which makes this STD difficult to prevent. In case of symptomatic genital herpes, it is best to abstain from sex and to use latex condoms between outbreaks. Pivotal efficacy trials of an experimental vaccine to prevent genital herpes indicated that the vaccine was effective in more than 70% of HSV-1 and HSV-2 seronegative women whose sexual partners were known to be infected.[100] However, for reasons not identified, it had no efficacy in men.

Prenatal

It is important that women avoid contracting herpes during pregnancy because a primary infection during pregnancy causes a greater risk of transmission to the newborn. All pregnant women should be asked whether they have a history of genital herpes. Women without known genital herpes should be counseled to avoid intercourse during the third trimester, in particular, with partners known or suspected of having genital herpes. In addition, women with no history of orolabial herpes should be advised to avoid cunnilingus during the third trimester with partners known or suspected to have orolabial herpes.[70] In case a women's sex partner has a history of HSV infection, serologic testing for HSV-1 and HSV-2 antibodies might prove to be helpful to identify and consequently counsel seronegative women at risk for primary HSV infection during pregnancy. Pregnant women with a significant primary HSV infection should be hospitalized and monitored closely for evidence of sequelae. Premature labor should be appropriately treated when necessary. Evidence of severe, disseminated disease such as hepatitis (elevated hepatic transaminase levels) and encephalitis (abnormal neurologic testing) should trigger the administration of intravenous acyclovir to prevent serious morbidity.[88] Treatment of primary genital herpes with oral acyclovir reduces viral shedding, reduces pain, and heals lesions faster.[101] Different studies have demonstrated that the use of acyclovir is safe during pregnancy and does not impose an increased risk to the developing fetus during the first trimester.[101,102] A first clinical episode of genital herpes may be effectively treated by oral acyclovir, 200 mg five times a day (or 400 mg three times a day) for 7 to 14 days, or until clinical resolution.[70,103] Recurrent HSV infection may be treated with the same dosage of oral acyclovir as in primary infection for 5 days.[103] Daily suppressive oral acyclovir (400 mg twice a day) has demonstrated significant reduction of symptomatic recurrences and subclinical virus shedding.[104,105] No induction of acyclovir-resistant HSV strains was noted in immunocompetent patients.[106] However, the extent to which suppressive therapy prevents HSV transmission to the infant is unknown.[70] In severe HSV disease, intravenous acyclovir is given at 5 to 10 mg/kg bodyweight every 8 hours for 2 to 7 days or until clinical improvement is observed. Oral acyclovir therapy should follow to complete at least 10 days total therapy.[70] Oral or intravenously administered acyclovir reaches therapeutic concentrations in the breast milk, the amniotic fluid, and the fetus.[107] Topical treatment with acyclovir offers minimal clinical benefit and is not recommended.[70] Newer antiherpetic drugs, valacyclovir and famciclovir, demonstrate increased bioavailability over acyclovir and thus require less frequent dosing. In the treatment of a first clinical episode of genital herpes valacyclovir is effective at 1000 mg orally twice a day for 7 to 14 days, and famciclovir at 250 mg three times a day for the same period.[103,108] Recurrent episodes of genital herpes may be treated orally with either valacyclovir (500 mg twice a day for 3–5 days) or famciclovir (125 mg twice a day for 5 days). Suppressive therapy requires oral valacyclovir at 500 mg once a day (9 or fewer recurrences per year) or 1000 mg once a day (>9 recurrences per year). Famciclovir is efficient in suppressive therapy at 250 mg twice a day. However, experience with prenatal exposure to valacyclovir and famciclovir is too limited to provide sufficient information on pregnancy outcome.

The management of pregnancy in the woman with active or historic herpes is aimed at preventing neonatal infection and subsequent dissemination. It was previously recommended that such women have weekly genital cultures for HSV in the latter weeks of pregnancy and be delivered abdominally if the most recent culture was positive.[109] However, it is now recognized that there is little correlation between prenatal HSV shedding and shedding at delivery,[73] and that most women whose infants develop HSV infection have no lesions or history.[73,97] Thus, weekly cultures are no longer recommended.[70]

Labor and Delivery

On admission to the delivery suite, all women should be questioned carefully about symptoms of genital herpes, and all women should be examined carefully for herpetic lesions.[70] In the absence of visible lesions in the genital area at the onset of labor vaginal delivery is permitted. If active genital lesions or prodromal symptoms of vulvar pain or burning (which may indicate an impending outbreak) are present, cesarean delivery is indicated. The incidence of infection in newborns whose mothers have recurrent infection is low, but cesarean delivery is warranted because of the serious nature of the disease.

The extent to which maternal antibodies will protect a neonate from an infection during a recurrence has not been determined with certainty. Cesarean delivery is not recommended in women with a history of HSV infection, but no active lesions, during labor.[70,103]

In women with premature rupture of membranes (PROM) near term and active HSV infection, cesarean delivery should be performed as soon as possible. It should not, however, be assumed the fetus is infected just because of prolonged rupture of membranes. Women with preterm PROM and active lesions are considered individually, taking into account gestational age and other relevant factors. Remote from term, expectant management and use of glucocorticoids is increasingly supported, and antiviral therapy is indicated because premature neonates are at greatest risk of infection.[103]

Lastly, fetal HSV infection has been attributed to the use of fetal scalp electrodes even in the absence of active lesions.[95,110] Thus, fetal scalp monitoring should be used cautiously even in women with a history of recurrent HSV and no active lesions. In case vesicular lesions develop at the site of the electrode, quick, accurate diagnosis should be followed immediately by the start of systemic antiviral therapy in the neonate.[103]

Postnatal

Postpartum, endometritis due to HSV infection has been reported,[111] and is responsive to acyclovir. Postnatally acquired HSV infections in the newborn can be severe, and mothers with skin or oropharyngeal lesions should use caution when handling their babies. HSV-1 is more likely to cause nosocomial infections in the infant than is HSV-2. Breast-feeding is unlikely to cause infection in the infant; only in the case of an obvious lesion on the breast is breast-feeding contraindicated.[103]

SUMMARY OF MANAGEMENT OPTIONS
Herpes Simplex Virus

Management Options	Quality of Evidence	Strength of Recommendation	References
Prepregnancy and Prenatal			
Inform about nature of the disease and that sexual transmission can occur during asymptomatic periods; counsel about condom protection during asymptomatic intervals and sexual abstinence during active disease.	IV	C	70, 99
Perform HSV-type specific serology testing; allows more specific advice by identifying seronegative women at risk for HSV acquisition.	IV	C	70
• Advise HSV-2 negative women to abstain from intercourse during third trimester with men who have genital herpes.			
• Advise HSV-1 negative women to avoid intercourse with a partner who has genital HSV-1 infection; no cunnilingus with a partner who has orolabial herpes.			
Vaccine being developed; not available for clinical use.	Ib	A	100
Provide symptomatic treatment of infections (primary and recurrent); hospitalize for severe cases.	–	GPP	–
Give acyclovir for active disease:			
• Oral (7-14d) for primary local infection	Ib	A	101
• IV (for 2-7d then oral) for primary systemic disease	IV	C	88
• Oral (5d) for recurrent disease	III	B	103
Provide prophylactic acyclovir (400 mg bid) for last trimester in patients with previous HSV to reduce recurrence risk (no known effect on fetal/neonatal transmission).	Ib	A	104, 105
No information about newer anti-HSV drugs; not recommended for pregnancy.	–	GPP	–
Remain vigilant for dissemination.	–	GPP	–
Remain vigilant for preterm uterine activity.	–	GPP	–
Serial viral cultures are no longer recommended in the last trimester for patients who are asymptomatic; culture only to document a new case.	IV	C	70
Consider delivery with septicemic cases.	–	GPP	–
Labor and Delivery			
Enquire and inspect perineum, vagina, and cervix for HSV in all women at onset of labor (especially those with history of HSV).	IV	C	70
Allow vaginal delivery if no active lesions and no prodromal symptoms at time of labor.	–	GPP	–
Active lesions at time of labor is considered an indication for cesarean section by most obstetricians, though the risk of fetal infection is less with recurrent disease.	–	GPP	–
Counseling about the benefits of cesarean section in preventing fetal infection with membrane rupture is controversial, although most would still advise cesarean section. Expectant approach with suspected preterm labor and PROM is reasonable.	–	GPP	–
Avoid fetal electrodes and fetal scalp sampling.	Ib	A	95, 110
Postnatal			
Maintain infection control measures if mother has active lesions.	–	GPP	–
Treat maternal infection; reduces dissemination and morbidity.	III	B	103
Perform clinical, microbiologic, and serologic evaluation of the newborn if active maternal lesions are present.	–	GPP	–
Give IV acyclovir to HSV-infected newborns.	III	B	103

ADENOVIRUS

General

Adenoviruses are medium-sized (90 to 100 nm) double-stranded DNA viruses. There are 6 subgenera (A through F) with 49 immunologically distinct types that can cause infection in the human. Most commonly, in the healthy adult adenovirus infection causes gastrointestinal and respiratory tract illness with a wide range of symptoms.

In recent years, there has been considerable interest in developing adenoviruses as defective vectors to deliver and express foreign genes for therapeutic purposes.[112–114] Adenovirus is relatively easy to manipulate in vitro and the coupled genes are effectively expressed in large amounts. Direct administration of adenovirus gene vectors to the fetus can be achieved by fetoscopy or ultrasonographic guidance.[115,116] However, repeated prenatal exposure to an adenovirus vector was associated with pulmonary inflammation as reported in newborn sheep.[117] Alternatively, selective placental and maternal intravenous adenovirus vector application has demonstrated only low numbers of adenovirus replication in the fetus, thus reducing the risk of fetal exposure to the virus.[118] In addition, intraplacental adenovirus-mediated gene delivery showed only low numbers of virus in the mother, thus possibly providing a suitable strategy for basic studies of placental function or even a method of correcting placental dysfunctions in the future.

Diagnosis

Conventional virus culture, electronmicroscopy and serology tests,[119,120] and modern laboratory techniques such as antigen detection by immunofluorescence tests[121] and PCR assay[16] are all suitable means to identify adenovirus disease. Adenovirus typing requires the use of type-specific antisera in hemagglutination-inhibition and/or neutralization tests.[119,120] Adenovirus infection in tissues or cell smears can be identified using in situ hybridization technique.[122] The presence of adenovirus does not necessarily mean disease because viruses can be shed for a prolonged time. Adenovirus genome could be identified in amniotic fluid of 30 out of 91 (33%) fetuses with ultrasound evidence of nonimmune hydrops. However, concomitant infection with parvovirus, cytomegalovirus (CMV), enterovirus, HSV, and respiratory syncytial virus was found in the majority of cases by PCR technique.[16]

Maternal and Fetal Risks

In healthy adults, adenoviruses commonly cause respiratory illness with symptoms that range from the common cold to pneumonia, croup, and bronchitis. However, depending on the serotype or route of infection (inhalation or ingestion), adenoviruses might cause febrile disease and keratoconjunctivitis, rash illness, gastroenteritis, or cystitis. Immunocompromised patients are susceptible to severe complications of adenovirus infections.

Transmission is by direct contact and the fecal-oral route. Adenoviruses are unusually stable in adverse conditions. Occasionally, waterborne transmission occurs, often centering around swimming pools and small lakes. Infection is usually acquired during childhood and at a higher incidence in late winter, spring, and early summer. Depending on the serotype, adenovirus infection can persist in either the tonsils, adenoids, or intestines of infected patients. Virus shedding can continue for years. Adenovirus types 40 and 41 are known to cause gastroenteritis, primarily in children. Inhalation of adenovirus type 7 is known to cause severe lower respiratory tract infection, and acute respiratory disease is most often associated with types 4 and 7.[119,120]

Adenovirus infection of the infant might occur transplacentally or at delivery via birth canal or contact with feces.

Amniotic fluid obtained from 303 pregnancies with abnormal ultrasound findings tested positive for adenovirus infection in 124 cases (41%).[16] PCR technique could demonstrate adenovirus to be the only viral genome present in the amniotic fluid of oligohydramnios in 18% (2/11; 2 additional patients positive for CMV), hydrothorax/pleural effusion in 22% (4/18; 2 additional patients positive for enterovirus and CMV), ventriculomegaly in 23% (6/26; 1 additional patient positive for CMV), microcephaly in 20% (1/5), and echogenic bowel in 5% (1/22; 5 additional patients positive for CMV and HSV). In the control group of 154 structurally normal fetuses, viral infection of the amniotic fluid was detected in 4 cases (3%), and adenovirus was the only microorganism in 2% (3/154; 1 additional patient positive for CMV). Intrauterine adenovirus infection might cause fetal myocarditis with tachyarrhythmia, dilated cardiac chambers, poor ventricular function, and subsequent hydrops fetalis.[123,124]

Severe neonatal adenovirus illness is rare, but is most often manifested as necrotizing pneumonitis.[121,122,125,126] Within 10 days of birth, infected infants demonstrate rapidly progressing pneumonia, thrombocytopenia, disseminated intravascular coagulopathy, hepatomegaly, and hepatitis. Respiratory failure might require extracorporeal membrane oxygenation in the newborn.[127] Case fatality might be as high as 84% and death often occurs around day 16.[125,128,129] Neonatal infection may also be seen in epidemic proportions in neonatal nurseries.[130] Severity of the disease in newborns seems to be less pronounced in the presence of maternal antibodies.

Management Options

Prepregnancy and Prenatal

To date, there is no specific therapy available for adenovirus infections in pregnancy or for the infected newborn, although new antiviral drugs (cidofovir, ribavirin) show promising results in pediatric patients.[131,132] Thus, the best treatment of adenovirus infection is prevention. Women should be counseled on proper hygiene measures to avoid fecal-oral transmission. Also, inadequately chlorinated swimming pools should be avoided. Most infections are mild and require no therapy.

Severe adenovirus infection can be managed only by treatment of symptoms and complications. Fetal tachyarrythmia and associated fetal hydrops may be treated by maternal oral digoxin. Maternal therapy with oral digoxin at 0.5 mg loading, and 0.125 to 0.25 mg/day maintenance dose has shown to convert fetal tachyarrhythmia to normal sinus rhythm and to produce spontaneous resolution of hydrops. Transplacental transfer ratio of digoxin is at an estimated rate of 60% to 100%. Maternal digoxin levels or persistent fetal tachyarrhythmia might require adjustment of the daily administered digoxin dosage. Vaccines for adenovirus types 4 and 7 were developed for military use only. Risk to the general population is so low that vaccination is not a viable proposition.

Labor, Delivery, and Postnatal

Strict attention to good infection control practices is effective in stopping nosocomial outbreaks of adenovirus disease, such as epidemic keratoconjunctivitis.

SUMMARY OF MANAGEMENT OPTIONS

Adenovirus

Management Options	Quality of Evidence	Strength of Recommendation	References
Prepregnancy and Prenatal			
Route of transmission is fecal-oral and waterborne; thus, transmission can be prevented by • personal hygiene • public hygiene (chlorinated swimming pools).	–	GPP	–
Treat adenovirus infections symptomatically because there is no proven therapy for maternal infection.	–	GPP	–
If hydrops develops due to fetal tachyarrhythmia, see Chapters 16 and 25.	–	–	–
Labor, Delivery, and Postnatal			
Strictly implement infection control policies.	–	GPP	–
No neonatal therapy other than symptomatic and supportive.	–	GPP	–
Severe pneumonitis in the newborn might require extracorporeal oxygenation.	–	GPP	–

COXSACKIEVIRUS

General

Coxsackievirus is a single-strand RNA virus, a member of the picornaviridae, which includes human enteroviruses and rhinoviruses. The enterovirus serotypes are determined by type-specific antisera and are traditionally grouped into four classes: poliovirus, group A coxsackievirus, group B coxsackievirus, and echovirus. Newly discovered serotypes are assigned enteroviral numbers (e.g., hepatitis A virus: enterovirus 72).

In northern latitudes enterovirus infections are more firmly associated with a seasonal periodicity (pronounced in summer and fall) than can be observed in more tropical climates. However, infections may occur at any time of the year. Group B coxsackievirus serotypes 2 to 5 are isolated more frequently, whereas other serotypes are rarely reported. Group A coxsackievirus infections have been identified less frequently, possibly due to poor growth in routine cell culture.

Enteroviruses are transmitted by direct contact with nose and throat discharge or feces of infected humans. Because many infections are clinically inapparent, spread of coxsackievirus infection may occur accidentally; the incubation period is 3 to 5 days (range, 2 to 15 days).[133]

In healthy, nonpregnant adults, enterovirus infections are either asymptomatic or cause simple febrile illness with or without signs of upper respiratory tract infection or rash. However, some clinical syndromes are characteristically associated with enterovirus infection, including aseptic meningitis, pleurodynia, and the hand-foot-and-mouth disease. The rate of infection is higher in young children than among older children and adults.

Diagnosis

Coxsackievirus infection can be identified by virus culture from the oropharynx, stool, blood, urine, cerebrospinal fluid, and amniotic fluid. After virus isolation by culture, virus typing is performed by conventional neutralization tests. More rapid specific virus identification techniques using immunofluorescence assay (IFA) or ELISA have not proven to be useful because of the large number of different serotypes.[134] However, development of monoclonal group-specific antibodies that can be used for rapid identification of enterovirus groups by IFA and ELISA is in progress.[135–137] Modern laboratory methods provide accurate and fast diagnosis of coxsackievirus infection by PCR technique.[16,138] In addition, PCR seems to be more suitable for detection of Group A coxsackievirus that grows poorly in culture, which has led to a possible clinical underrecognition of this virus as a cause of disease.

Serology using hemagglutination-inhibition, complement fixation, and ELISA tests can readily identify IgG, IgM, IgA, and IgE classes of specific antibodies; however, the large number of different enterovirus type-specific antigens require the performance of large numbers of serologic tests. Recently, gene-sequencing technology has identified a common epitope in a number of enteroviruses, which might prove to be helpful for serology tests in the future.[137] When case serology is performed, paired specimens should be obtained to ensure proper diagnosis.

Tissue samples can be examined for specific enteroviral antigens by immunofluorescence or PCR technique.[139]

Maternal and Fetal Risks

The prevalence of enterovirus infection is inversely related to socioeconomic status and age, whereas individual factors, including age, sex, immune status, and pregnancy, are important determinants of the severity of infection.[140]

In pregnancy, most maternal coxsackievirus infections are either inapparent or cause only minimal symptoms similar to a viral upper respiratory tract infection or viral gastroenteritis[141]; however, hepatic failure has been reported.[142] The exact incidence of coxsackievirus infections in pregnancy is not known. There is no direct virologic evidence available that suggests that coxsackievirus infections in pregnancy may result in miscarriage.[134] However, an increased frequency of coxsackievirus IgM in women with spontaneous abortion has been reported.[143] In a collaborative study serologic evidence of coxsackievirus B (types 1 to 6) infection during pregnancy was demonstrated in 9% of 198 women[144]; during peak enterovirus season a seroconversion rate of 25% was noted during the last 2 to 6 weeks of pregnancy among 55 women.[145] Most women were either asymptomatic or had only mild symptoms, and no newborn had signs of severe enterovirus infection. The incidence of neonatal coxsackievirus B infection, based on laboratory records, was estimated at a minimum of 50 per 100,000 liveborn children.[146] Thus, enterovirus infection during late pregnancy might be a rather common event; however, most infections did not produce a significant maternal or neonatal morbidity. Alternatively, in women delivering newborns with evidence of group B coxsackievirus infection, 59% to 65% had symptomatic illness during the perinatal period with febrile disease and upper respiratory symptoms, pleurodynia, myocarditis, and aseptic meningitis.[140,146]

In animal studies, pregnant mice experimentally infected with different strains of enterovirus have a shorter incubation period, develop higher titers in blood and various organs, and remain viremic longer. Susceptibility increases with advancing gestation and rapidly reverts to that of nonpregnant animals within days of delivery. In nonpregnant female mice, administration of corticosterone or estrogen reduced the resistance to encephalomyocarditis virus infection, but this resistance was not altered by exogenous progesterone. Group B coxsackievirus infection of the pregnant mouse may also result in infection of the fetus before delivery or in infection of the mouse intrapartum.[140]

In humans, in vitro experiments demonstrated that vertical infection from mother to fetus rarely happens through transplacental passage.[147] However, 22% to 25% of neonatal group B coxsackievirus infections have been attributed to antepartal transmission.[141,146] The mechanisms of intrauterine coxsackievirus infection are poorly understood. Evidence of congenital disease is inconsistently related to recovery of virus from the placenta and the respective fetus,[134,145,148] and it is assumed that besides hematogeneous transmission involving the placenta, a number of fetuses might be infected by ingesting coxsackievirus contained in the amniotic fluid.[149] Transplacental infection of the fetus occurs in the absence of maternal immunity and is unrelated to the clinical severity of the disease in the mother. Viral shedding from the cervix has been reported; however, ascending viral infection seems to be a rare event.[150] At the time of delivery infection of the infant might occur by cervical or fecal contamination. Fecal carriage rates of coxsackievirus was reported to range from 0% to more than 6% in different population groups.[134,145]

In a study of 630 infants with 778 anomalies of different organ systems, intrauterine infection with coxsackievirus B2 and B4 was associated with urogenital anomalies, and coxsackievirus B3 and B4 with cardiovascular anomalies. The likelihood of congenital heart disease was increased by maternal infection with two or more coxsackievirus B serotypes rather than one. Also, first-trimester infection with coxsackievirus B4 occurred more frequently in mothers of infants with any anomaly than in the control group.[151] In 28 newborns with severe congenital defects of the central nervous system, neutralizing antibody to coxsackievirus B6 was demonstrated in 4 cases (14%); 2 had hydranencephaly, 1 had occipital meningocele, and 1 had aqueductal stenosis.[152] In a stillborn infant with calcific pancarditis and hydrops fetalis, coxsackievirus B3 antigen could be demonstrated.[148]

Newborns who acquire coxsackievirus infection in the immediate peripartum period are more likely to experience severe disease in the absence of protecting maternal antibodies. Neonatal infection might range from asymptomatic viral shedding to severe and rapidly fatal illness. Infection that occurs more than 5 days before delivery is likely to induce production of maternal IgG that can cross the placenta and protect the newborn from severe disease, but not necessarily from infection. In the newborn coxsackievirus infection may cause benign neonatal arrhythmias,[153] fever,[146] oral vesicular lesions,[154] vesiculopapular rash,[155] severe respiratory failure,[156] pneumonitis,[141] fatal pulmonary hemorrhage,[146,157] hepatitis, hepatomegaly, jaundice, bleeding diatheses, hepatic failure and necrosis,[134,146] aseptic meningitis,[146] meningoencephalitis, fatal encephalomyocarditis and encephalohepatomyocarditis,[141,158] acute aseptic and interstitial myocarditis,[159] and result in heart disease.[160] A study of 16 neonates with enterovirus hepatitis and coagulopathy demonstrated hemorrhagic complications in 10 out of 16 cases (63%); 5 infants had intracranial bleeding.[161] The overall fatality rate was 31% (5/16). In the group of 5 neonates with intracranial bleeding, 4 (80%) died. Overall, mortality rates are highest in children with myocarditis, encephalitis, or sepsis-like illness with liver involvement. In addition, prognosis seems to be related to the infecting viral strain. In general, infection with coxsackievirus B1 to B4 seems to carry the most ominous prognoses. Long-term sequelae are mostly reported with regard to heart and CNS-related impairment. Animal studies of coxsackievirus myocarditis demonstrated a T cell-mediated immunopathic process and a virus-induced autoimmunity. In a study of 7 newborn infants with neurodevelopmental delays, coxsackievirus was retrieved from the respective placenta in 6 of the 7 cases (86%).[156] A 28-year follow-up study of 145 patients, particularly those with coxsackievirus B5 CNS infection during childhood, demonstrated an increased risk for adult onset of schizophrenia or other psychoses.[162] In a group of 15 children who had meningoencephalitis due to coxsackievirus B5, 2 were reported to have developed spasticity, and their intelligence was low.[163] Epidemiologic and serologic studies suggest a role for intrauterine coxsackievirus infection for the onset of insulin-dependent diabetes mellitus in childhood (IDDM).[164–166] However, conflicting serologic data exist that do not indicate an association of coxsackievirus infections during pregnancy with the development of islet autoantibodies; these results do not support a major role of fetal coxsackievirus infection in the development of IDDM.[167,168]

Infection with coxsackievirus A in neonates has been reported less frequently than with coxsackievirus B. Coxsackievirus A infection has been associated with small-for-gestational-age newborns,[141] sudden infant death,[169–171] anorexia, fever, bronchopneumonia, pericarditis and meningitis.[134]

A number of reports have confirmed that coxsackieviruses may be responsible for outbreaks of apparent infections with fatalities among neonates in obstetrical wards and maternity homes.[172–174] Most commonly, mild nonspecific febrile illness is observed in full-term infants. A careful history frequently reveals a trivial illness in a family member. Feeding difficulties are frequently observed, and short periods of vomiting and diarrhea may occur. The most consistent source of original nursery infection is coxsackievirus transmission from mother to her child, but introduction of the virus into the nursery by personnel also occurs. After infection of the pharynx and lower alimentary tract, minor viremia with spread to regional lymph nodes and secondary infection sites (CNS, heart, liver, pancreas, respiratory tract, skin) occurs on the third day. Major viremia ceases with the appearance of antibodies on day 7. Infection can continue in the lower intestinal tract for prolonged periods, and isolation measures are warranted.[134]

Management Options

Prenatal, Labor, and Delivery

Coxsackievirus infections during late pregnancy seem to be a common event, in particular during late summer and early autumn in temperate climates. Epidemics in the region may be signaled by the occurrence of aseptic meningitis, pleurodynia, or Bornholm disease (myalgia epidemica). Unseasonal respiratory tract infection or symptoms of fever, muscle pain, neck stiffness, skin rashes, and vesicular lesions (mouth, hand, foot) are suggestive of an enteroviral infection. Ultrasound examination in some cases may reveal an enlarged fetal heart with dilated chambers and unusually thick myocardium. Fetal arrythmias and congestive heart failure in combination with nonimmune hydrops may be treated by maternal digoxin (oral digoxin at 0.5 mg loading, and 0.125 to 0.25 mg/day maintenance dose). Conversion of fetal arrhythmia to normal sinus rhythm and, consequently, spontaneous resolution of hydrops may be observed. If a woman is suspected of having an acute coxsackievirus infection, she is a potential risk for transmitting coxsackievirus in the obstetrical wards. Isolation measures for delivery, newborn care, and postpartum care are warranted.[134] Coxsackievirus infection in the adult usually takes a benign course. If delivery occurs within 4 days of maternal infection, the newborn is at risk for severe disease.

Postnatal

No specific therapy is available to treat coxsackievirus infection in the newborn. Commercially available immune serum globulin contains titers of antibodies to coxsackievirus; however, no beneficial clinical effect has been observed when administered to an infected infant.[175,176] However, viremia and viruria ceased earlier in treated infants than in the control group. Recent studies with new antiviral drugs (e.g., pleconaril) seem promising.[177]

In most cases, transmission of coxsackievirus occurs by direct contact from mother or staff members to the newborn or by mouth and gavage feeding. Coxsackievirus B and echoviruses have been recovered from specimens obtained from nurses and physicians caring for infected patients.[174] Rigorous attention to hygienic measures and handwashing after handling each baby are imperative to avoid the transmission of enteroviruses. Infected newborns should be isolated, and closure on the neonatal unit to new admissions has been advocated.[134]

In sudden and virulent nursery outbreaks passive immunization by intramuscular or intravenous immunoglobulin can be useful in preventing disease.[175,178]

A vaccine to prevent coxsackievirus infection is not available. However, an experimental attenuated vaccine has been developed.[179] Because of the considerable morbidity and mortality associated with coxsackievirus B infection in neonates (and in older persons as well), these agents should be candidates for vaccine development.

SUMMARY OF MANAGEMENT OPTIONS

Coxsackievirus

Management Options	Quality of Evidence	Strength of Recommendation	References
Prenatal, Labor, and Delivery			
Suspect coxsackievirus infection if unseasonal respiratory tract infection and/or clinical signs of meningitis.	–	GPP	–
Treat infections symptomatically (hospitalize severe cases).	–	GPP	–
Evaluate hydropic fetuses for tachyarrhythmia, congestive heart failure; see Chapters 16, 17, and 25 for management options.	–	–	–
Deliver women suspected for acute coxsackievirus infection in an isolated unit.	IV	C	134
Postnatal			
Isolate women known to have coxsackievirus infection during postpartum care.	IV	C	134
Maintain strict attention to infection control measures.	IV	C	134
Provide clinical, microbiologic, and serologic evaluation of the newborn if acute maternal infection is present within the peripartum period.			
Isolate newborns of mothers suspected of having coxsackievirus infection.	IV	C	134
Consider passive immunization of newborns in case of sudden virulent coxsackievirus infection outbreak.	III	B	175, 178

HUMAN PAPILLOMAVIRUS

General

Human papillomavirus (HPV) is a double-stranded DNA virus that can persist as a latent provirus in epithelial cells after infection. Nucleotide sequencing of the DNA has identified more than 100 genotypes of HPV associated with epithelial neoplasias of the skin and mucosa. More than 30 different HPV types can infect the genital tract, and 8 HPV types are predominantly identified in the most common HPV-associated genital diseases.

HPV types 6 and 11 are detected in more than 90% of condylomata acuminata (genital warts), and also in laryngeal papillomatosis, and conjunctival, oral, and nasal warts. HPV types 16, 18, 31, 33, 51, and 54 have been designated high risk HPV types because they have been strongly associated with cervical intraepithelial neoplasia (CIN) and cervical cancer.[180] Genital warts are contagious and are spread during oral, genital, or anal sex. About two-thirds of people who have sex with a partner with genital warts will develop warts, usually within 3 months after contact.

Diagnosis

The diagnosis of condylomata acuminata can be made visually by the appearance of white or pink verrucous friable growths. However, most cases of HPV infection are subclinical. Cytologic evaluation of the Papanicolaou (Pap) smear may reveal evidence of infection in 10% to 30% of cases. If koilocytosis is noted on the Pap smear, liberal use of colposcopy is warranted, given the association of HPV infection and CIN. Colposcopy may identify up to 70% of infected cases. Directed biopsies can support diagnostic evaluation in certain cases (e.g., unresponsiveness to therapy, uncertain clinical diagnosis); however, it is not mandatory.[70] HPV isolation in culture is difficult to accomplish. Highly specific and sensitive DNA methods utilizing type-specific HPV gene probes can identify HPV infection in vaginal washings, Pap smears, and amniotic fluid. In situ hybridization technique is useful to demonstrate type-specific HPV infection in tissues and cervical cell scrapings. PCR methods can identify even the lowest levels of HPV infection in blood and other kinds of fluids or in tissue samples. The usefulness of DNA technology in the clinical diagnosis of genital warts is not supported by any data.[70] However, identification of high risk HPV types might prove helpful for follow-up strategies of women in whom cervical cytology has demonstrated atypical squamous cells of undetermined significance (ASCUS). Screening for subclinical HPV infection by DNA or RNA tests is not recommended.[70]

Maternal and Fetal Risks

Epidemiologic data suggest that HPV infection is the most prevalent STD. Although the occurence of grossly visible genital warts is infrequent, sensitive detection tests utilizing dot blot DNA analysis or PCR for detection of HPV DNA indicate that as many as 30% of sexually active adults in the United States may be infected,[181] with a similar rate seen in pregnancy.[182] The highest rates of genital HPV infection are detected in adults age 18 to 28. Major risk factors to acquiring genital HPV infection include multiple sex partners, younger age at first intercourse and first pregnancy, oral contraceptive use, pregnancy, and impairment of cell-mediated immunity.[181,183] Estimates indicate that approximately 1% of the sexually active population have clinically apparent genital warts.[181] Controversial data exist on a possible increase in the prevalence of HPV infections during pregnancy. An up to threefold increase in HPV DNA-positive women during the third trimester as compared to nonpregnant controls has been reported.[184,185] Possible underlying reasons to facilitate HPV infection during late pregnancy could involve hormonal changes inducing virus transcription and the transient immunosuppression experienced by pregnant women.

Genital HPV infections in pregnant women have long been suspected to cause genital warts or laryngeal papillomatosis in the respective infants.[186] Juvenile laryngeal papillomatosis represents the most common neoplasm of the larynx in infants and young children and usually occurs by age 5.[187] The symptoms range from hoarseness to complete upper airway obstruction. A history of genital warts can be obtained from over 50% of women whose infants subsequently develop laryngeal papillomatosis.[188] However, the absolute risk of laryngeal papillomatosis following exposure to maternal infection is extremely low. Conservative estimates suggest the risk of papillomatosis developing in an offspring of a mother with HPV genital infection is approximately 1 in 400.[187] Surgical excision is the mainstream therapy, and most afflicted patients experience spontaneous remission. However, some endure several hundred surgical procedures. Further development of new antiviral drugs (e.g., cidofovir) and preventive and therapeutic vaccines hold promise for eliminating the virus in cases of recurrent respiratory papillomatosis.[189,190] Genital warts in children show spontaneous resolution in up to 75% of cases. In a cohort of 41 children overall resolution of condylomata was noted in 31 infants (76%) with spontaneous resolution in 22 of 41 (54%); girls were affected three times more often than boys.[191]

Vertical transmission and persistence of high risk cancer-associated HPV in the infant is of great concern. Amniotic fluid samples of 37 women with cervical lesions tested positive for HPV in 24 cases (65%) using PCR technique.[192] HPV type 16 amniotic fluid infection was present in 54% (13/24), and HPV type 18 was detected in 21% (5/24). A correlation was noted between viral DNA amplification and grade of the cervical lesions. In a group of 11 women carrying HPV type 16, 7 infants out of 11 (64%) tested positive for HPV type 16.[193] Viruses were detected in buccal or genital swabs collected 24 hours after delivery, demonstrating infection rather than contamination. Persistence of HPV type 16 infection after a 6-month interval was noted in 83% of infants. In 270 healthy children between age 3 and 11, 131 (49%) buccal swabs tested positive for HPV type 16. Serologic study performed on 229 children demonstrated IgM seropositivity rates indicative of acute infection that peaked between age 2 and 5, and again between age

13 and 16.[193] Thus, given the lack of demonstrable disease in children, consequences of perinatal high risk HPV transmission need to be clarified in long-term studies to establish whether perinatal acquisition of high risk HPV types predisposes for an increased risk of cervical neoplasia later in life.

The frequency of perinatal HPV transmission is a controversial subject. Transmission rates may be as low as 5.3%, whereas other studies demonstrate vertical transmission in up to 73% of newborns.[193,194] Discrepancies in infection rates of the newborn may be due to different PCR techniques with up to a 100-fold difference in sensitivity, differences in study population (e.g., concomitant STDs), sampling technique (nasopharyngeal, buccal, genital), and timing (immediately after birth, contamination versus infection). HPV is thought to cause infection in the infant by direct contact during the passage through the birth canal. However, several studies have shown infants being infected with different strains of HPV despite being delivered by cesarean section.[195,196] In a study of 68 HPV-positive women, 35 delivered vaginally and 33 by cesarean section.[197] At 3 to 4 days of age buccal and genital swabs were collected. In the group of vaginally born infants 18 out of 35 (51%) had a positive HPV test, whereas in 9 out of 33 (27%) infants delivered by cesarean section HPV was detected. Although the study did show a lower incidence of HPV infection in infants delivered by cesarean section, the study also demonstrated that cesarean section did not consistently protect from vertical HPV transmission. In addition, the presence of HPV has been demonstrated in amniotic fluid, placenta, and cord blood; thus, the fetus is at risk for exposure to the virus prior to delivery.[192,196,198]

Management Options

Prepregnancy

Patients should be counseled on the nature of genital warts and advised on using protection (e.g., latex condoms) when having sex with an infected partner. Some genital warts may resolve spontaneously; however, treatment should be considered for expanding genital warts. Treatment for genital warts reduces but does not eradicate infectivity. In nonpregnant women, podophyllum resin 10% to 25% antimitotic solution, podofilox 0.5% solution, and 5-fluorouracil are commonly used for topical treatment; however, they should not be applied during pregnancy because of the potential for fetal toxicity. All treatments show a 10% to 40% probability of recurrence. Intralesional injections of different types of interferon have demonstrated comparable efficacy to other modalities for the treatment of genital warts; however, use of interferons has been frequently associated with systemic adverse effects. Interferons should not be used during pregnancy. Although some HPV types are associated with CIN and cervical cancer, HPV infection does not necessarily progress to cancer. It is important for women with a history of abnormal Pap smears to receive appropriate cytologic testing on a regular basis so that early treatment, if necessary, can be instituted.

Prenatal

There is no single definitive treatment for HPV infection in pregnancy. Treatment is dependent on the size, location, and number of identified lesions and entails the removal or ablation of all visible warts. Due to the subclinical and multifocal nature of HPV infection, recurrences are common. Certain treatment modalities that are effective in the nonpregnant patient are contraindicated during pregnancy.

In pregnant women topical application of 80% to 90% trichloroacetic acid (TCA) can be used for small lesions and is the least expensive treatment. TCA is not absorbed systemically and can be used in pregnancy. However, it has a cure rate of only 20% to 30% after a single application; therefore, weekly applications may be required until the lesions are resolved. TCA solutions have a low viscosity and can spread rapidly, thus, damaging adjacent tissues. If an excess amount is applied, the treated area should be powdered with talc, sodium bicarbonate, or liquid soap preparations to remove unreacted acid.[70] Cryotherapy with liquid nitrogen has also been successfully used in pregnancy and is a reasonable first-line treatment option. Cryotherapy is not recommended for use in the vagina because of the risk of vaginal perforation and fistula formation.[70] Surgical removal by tangential scissor excision, tangential shave excision, curettage, or electrosurgery has the advantage of eliminating warts at a single visit in most cases. Carbon dioxide laser vaporization has been used successfully in pregnancy, although recurrence rates of 10% to 14% have been reported. In particular, laser therapy is recommended for those patients with large or multiple lesions or with lesions refractory to TCA application or cryotherapy. Recurrences usually occur during the first 3 months after treatment, and a follow-up evaluation should be offered.

Imiquimod 5% cream, an immune-response modulator that induces host TH1 cytokines, including interferon-γ, has been demonstrated to be effective in eradicating genital warts when applied topically three times weekly in nonpregnant patients. Although not yet recommended in pregnancy, imiquimod may represent an effective alternative to other topical or destructive therapies during pregnancy. New antiviral drugs (e.g., cidofovir) have not been evaluated for safety and efficacy during pregnancy.[199]

Labor and Delivery

Elective debulking of genital warts should not be done at the time of delivery for two reasons: first, these lesions may be very vascular and obstetric hemorrhage may ensue; second, most lesions regress to some extent after delivery.

Because of the lack of substantial evidence for the preventive value of cesarean delivery, cesarean section should not be performed solely to prevent transmission of HPV infection to the newborn.[70] However, cesarean section may be indicated in women with genital warts obstructing the pelvic outlet or when vaginal delivery would result in excessive bleeding.

SUMMARY OF MANAGEMENT OPTIONS
Human Papillomavirus

Management Options	Quality of Evidence	Strength of Recommendation	References
Prepregnancy			
Identify and treat lesions:	–	GPP	–
• Topical therapy (podophyllum, podofilox, 5-fluorouracil)			
• Ablation (e.g., cryocautery)			
• Removal			
Counsel about risks (infectious condition) and use of condoms if partner infected.	IIa	B	201, 202
Advise that treatment does not eradicate infectivity.	–	GPP	–
Implications from cervical smear screening programs:	–	GPP	–
If Pap smear reports ASCUS but no other types of abnormalities:			
• Consider HPV testing			
If Pap smear reports ASCUS, and high risk HPV types are detected:			
• Perform colposcopy, consider biopsy			
• Perform pelvic exam, Pap smear on a regular basis			
Screening for subclinical HPV infection is not recommended.			
Prenatal			
Topical 80% TCA	III	B	203
Cryotherapy	IV	C	204
Electrodiathermy	IV	C	204
Laser vaporization (carbon dioxide)	III	B	203
Excision (tangential scissors, excision, curettage)	IV	C	204
Contraindicated preparations:			
• Podophyllum	IV	C	204
• Podofilox	–	GPP	–
• 5-fluorouracil	–	GPP	–
• Interferon	IV	C	205
Counsel about low newborn risk, and about nature of HPV infection in the infant.	–	GPP	–
Labor and Delivery			
Avoid treatment at delivery, especially debulking, because of risk of hemorrhage.	–	GPP	–
Cesarean section may be indicated in women with genital warts obstructing labor or vaginal delivery that would result in excessive bleeding; not recommended solely to prevent HPV transmission to the infant.	III	B	70
Postnatal			
Maintain vigilance for secondary infection, especially in episiotomy site.	–	GPP	–
Offer sitz baths.	–	GPP	–

Postnatal

Large lesions should be observed for secondary infection, if they involve an episiotomy site. Sitz baths may be particularly useful in comforting and cleansing the perineal area with multiple HPV lesions.

Currently, preventive and therapeutic vaccine development is in progress to possibly reduce HPV infection in the future.[200]

CONCLUSIONS

- Viral infections with cytomegalovirus, herpes simplex virus, adenovirus, coxsackievirus, and human papillomavirus pose a serious threat to the fetus and the newborn.
- Specific antiviral treatment options are scarce and cannot reduce the incidence of viral infection during pregnancy. Therefore, counseling patients and physicians about the infectious nature and on how to avoid viral transmission is the most viable and effective treatment modality to reduce congenital virus infections to date.
- Careful questioning and examination of pregnant women and subsequent use of specific diagnostic procedures are the most important methods to identify and counsel pregnant women at risk for viral infections.
- Perinatal and postpartum attention to infection control measures can greatly reduce the risk of severe neonatal infection.
- Progress in the development of new antiviral drugs for the treatment of the fetus and the newborn can possibly reduce the sequelae of congenital viral infection in the future.
- However, the development of vaccines and vaccination programs holds the most promising option to reduce congenital viral disease.

REFERENCES

1. Gouarin S, Gault E, Vabret A, et al: Real-time PCR quantification of human cytomegalovirus DNA in amniotic fluid samples from mothers with primary infection. J Clin Microbiol 2002;40:1767–1772.
2. Lazzarotto T, Varani S, Guerra B, et al: Prenatal indicators of congenital cytomegalovirus infection. J Pediatr 2000;137:90–95.
3. Revello MG, Zavattoni M, Furione M, et al: Quantification of human cytomegalovirus DNA in amniotic fluid of mothers of congenitally infected fetuses. J Clin Microbiol 1999;37: 3350–3352.
4. Kumazaki K, Ozono K, Yahara T, et al: Detection of cytomegalovirus DNA in human placenta. J Med Virol 2002;68:363–369.
5. Nigro G, Marria S, Midulla M: Simultaneous detection of specific serum IgM and IgA antibodies for rapid serodiagnosis of congenital or acquired cytomegalovirus infection. Serodiagn Immunother 1989;3:355–361.
6. Crumpacker CS: Cytomegalovirus. In Mandell GL, Douglas RG, Bennett JE (eds): Principles and Practice of Infectious Diseases, 5th ed. New York, Churchill Livingstone, 2000, pp 1586–1599.
7. Demmler G, Six H, Hurst M, Yow M: Enzyme-linked immunosorbent assay for the detection of IgM-class antibodies against cytomegalovirus. J Infect Dis 1986;153: 1152–1155.
8. Griffiths PD, Stagno S, Pass RF, et al: Infection with cytomegalovirus during pregnancy: Specific IgM antibodies as a marker of recent primary infection. J Infect Dis 1982;145:647–653.
9. Ruellan-Eugene G, Barjot P, Campet M, et al: Evaluation of virological procedures to detect fetal human cytomegalovirus infection: Avidity of IgG antibodies, virus detection in amniotic fluid and maternal serum. J Med Virol 1996;50:9–15.
10. Lazzarotto T, Varani S, Spezzacatena P, et al: Maternal IgG avidity and IgM detected by blot as diagnostic tools to identify pregnant women at risk of transmitting cytomegalovirus. Viral Immunol 2000;13:137–141.
11. Bodeus M, Van Ranst M, Bernard P, et al: Anticytomegalovirus IgG avidity in pregnancy: A 2-year prospective study. Fetal Diagn Ther 2002;17:362–366.
12. Revello MG, Lilleri D, Zavattoni M, et al: Human cytomegalovirus immediate-early messenger RNA in blood of pregnant women with primary infection and of congenitally infected newborns. J Infect Dis 2001;184: 1078–1081.
13. Azam AZ, Vial Y, Fawer CL, et al: Prenatal diagnosis of congenital cytomegalovirus infection. Obstet Gynecol 2001;97: 443–448.
14. Nigro G, Mazzocco M, Anceschi MM, et al: Prenatal diagnosis of fetal cytomegalovirus infection after primary or recurrent maternal infection. Obstet Gynecol 1999;94:909–914.
15. Grose C, Weiner CP. Prenatal diagnosis of congenital cytomegalovirus infection: Two decades later. Am J Obstet Gynecol 1990;163:447–450.
16. Van den Veyver IB, Ni J, Bowles N, et al: Detection of intrauterine viral infection using the polymerase chain reaction. Mol Genet Metab 1998;63:85–95.
17. Lamy ME, Mulango KN, Gadisseux J-F, et al: Prenatal diagnosis of fetal cytomegalovirus infection. Am J Obstet Gynecol 1992;166:91–94.
18. Hogge WA, Buffone GJ, Hogge JS: Prenatal diagnosis of cytomegalovirus (CMV) infection: A preliminary report. Prenat Diagn 1993;13:131–136.
19. Xu W, Sundqvist V-A, Brytting M, Linde A: Diagnosis of cytomegalovirus infections using polymerase chain reaction, virus isolation and serology. Scand J Infect Dis 1993;25: 311–316.

20. Catanzarite V, Dankner WM. Prenatal diagnosis of congenital cytomegalovirus infection: False-negative amniocentesis at 20 weeks' gestation. Prenat Diagn 1993;13:1021–1025.
21. Conner C, Liesnard C, Brancart F, Rodesch F: Accuracy of amniotic fluid testing before 21 weeks' gestation in prenatal diagnosis of congenital virus infection. Prenat Diagn 1994;14:1055–1059.
22. Enders G, Bäder U, Lindemann L, et al: Prenatal diagnosis of congenital cytomegalovirus infection in 189 pregnancies with known outcome. Prenat Diagn 2001;21:362–377.
23. Liesnard C, Donner C, Brancart F, et al: Prenatal diagnosis of congenital cytomegalovirus infection: Prospective study of 237 pregnancies at risk. Obstet Gynecol 2000;95:881–888.
24. Revello MG, Baldanti F, Furione M, et al: Polymerase chain reaction for prenatal diagnosis of congenital human cytomegalovirus infection. J Med Virol 1995;47:462–466.
25. Lynch L, Daffos F, Emanuel D, et al: Prenatal diagnosis of fetal cytomegalovirus infection. Am J Obstet Gynecol 1991;165: 714–718.
26. Watt-Morse ML, Laifer SA, Hill LM: The natural history of fetal cytomegalovirus infection as assessed by serial ultrasound and fetal blood sampling: A case report. Prenat Diagn 1995;15:567–570.
27. Peters MT, Lowe TW, Carpenter A, Kole S: Prenatal diagnosis of congenital cytomegalovirus infection with abnormal triple-screen results and hyperechoic fetal bowel. Am J Obstet Gynecol 1995;173:953–954.
28. Lipitz S, Achiron R, Zalel Y, et al: Outcome of pregnancies with vertical transmission of primary cytomegalovirus infection. Obstet Gynecol 2002;100:428–433.
29. Stagno S, Pass RF, Dworsky ME, Alford CA: Congenital and perinatal cytomegalovirus infection. Semin Perinatol 1983;7:31–42.
30. Raynor BD: Cytomegalovirus infection in pregnancy. Semin Perinatol 1993;17:394–402.
31. Lang DJ, Kummer JF: Demonstration of cytomegalovirus in semen. N Engl J Med 1972;287:756–758.
32. Chretien JH, McGinnis CG, Muller A: Venereal causes of cytomegalovirus mononucleosis. JAMA 1977;238:1644–1645.
33. Chandler SH, Handsfield HH, Mc Dougall JK: Isolation of multiple strains of cytomegalovirus from women attending a clinic for sexually transmitted diseases. J Infect Dis 1987;155: 655–660.
34. Yeager AS, Grumet FC, Hafleigh EB, et al: Prevention of transfusion-acquired cytomegalovirus infections in newborn infants. J Pediatr 1981;98:281–287.
35. Hersman J, Meyers JD, Thomas ED, et al: The effect of granulocyte transfusions on the incidence of cytomegalovirus infection after allogenic marrow transplantation. Ann Intern Med 1982;96:149–152.
36. Stagno S, Reynolds DW, Pass RF, Alford CA: Breast milk and the risk of cytomegalovirus infection. N Engl J Med 1980;302:1073–1076.
37. Gurevich I, Cunha BA: Nonparenteral transmission of cytomegalovirus in a neonatal intensive care unit. Lancet 1981;ii:222–224.
38. Pass RF, Little EA, Stagno S, et al: Young children as a probable source of maternal and congenital cytomegalovirus infection. N Engl J Med 1987;316:1366–1370.
39. Krech U: Complement-fixing antibodies against cytomegalovirus in different parts of the world. Bull WHO 1973;49: 103–106.
40. Stagno S, Pass RF, Cloud G, et al: Primary cytomegalovirus infection in pregnancy. Incidence, transmission to the fetus, and clinical outcome. JAMA 1986;256:1904–1908.
41. Tookey PA, Ades AE, Peckham CS: Cytomegalovirus prevalence in pregnant women: The influence of parity. Arch Dis Child 1992;67:779–783.
42. Peckham CS, Coleman JC, Hurley R, et al: Cytomegalovirus infection in pregnancy: Preliminary findings from a prospective study. Lancet 1983;i:1352–1355.
43. Preece PM, Tookey P, Ades A, Peckham CS: Congenital cytomegalovirus infection: Predisposing maternal factors. J Epidemiol Community Health 1986;40:205–209.
44. Yow MD, Williamson DW, Leeds LJ, et al: Epidemiologic characteristics of cytomegalovirus infection in mothers and their infants. Am J Obstet Gynecol 1988;158:1189–1195.
45. Griffiths PD, Campbell-Benzie A, Heath RB: A prospective study of primary cytomegalovirus infection in pregnant women. BJOG 1980;87:308–314.
46. Stagno S, Whitley RJ: Herpesvirus infections of pregnancy. Part I: Cytomegalovirus and Epstein-Barr virus infections. N Engl J Med 1985;313:1270–1274.
47. Stagno S: Cytomegalovirus. In Remington JS, Klein JO (eds): Infectious Diseases of the Fetus and Newborn Infant, 5th ed. Philadelphia, WB Saunders, 2001, pp 389–424.
48. Revello MG, Zavattoni M, Furione M, et al: Diagnosis and outcome of preconceptional and periconceptional primary human cytomegalovirus infections. J Infect Dis 2002; 186:553–557.
49. Fowler KB, Stagno S, Pass RF: Maternal immunity and prevention of congenital cytomegalovirus infection. JAMA 2003;289:1008–1011.
50. Fowler KB, Stagno S, Pass RF, et al: The outcome of congenital cytomegalovirus infection in relation to maternal antibody status. N Engl J Med 1992;326:663–667.
51. Greenhough A, Osborne J, Sutherland S (eds): Congenital, Perinatal and Neonatal Infections. Edinburgh, Churchill Livingstone, 1992.
52. Demmler GJ: Infectious Diseases Society of America and Centers for Disease Control summary of a workshop on surveillance for congenital cytomegalovirus disease. Rev Infect Dis 1991;13:315–329.
53. Boppana SB, Rivera LB, Fowler KB, et al: Intrauterine transmission of cytomegalovirus to infants of women with preconceptional immunity. N Engl J Med 2001;344:1366–1371.
54. Fowler KB, Stagno S, Pass RF, et al: The outcome of congenital cytomegalovirus infection in relation to maternal antibody status. N Engl J Med 1992;326:663–667.
55. Hicks T, Fowler K, Richardson M, et al: Congenital cytomegalovirus infection and neonatal auditory screening. J Pediatr 1993;123:779–782.
56. Ahlfors K, Ivarsson SA, Bjerre I: Microcephaly and congenital cytomegalovirus infection: A combined prospective and retrospective study of a Swedish infant population. Pediatrics 1986;78:1058–1063.
57. Piper J, Wen TS: Perinatal cytomegalovirus and toxoplasmosis: Challenges of antepartum therapy. Clin Obstet Gynecol 1999;42:81–96.
58. Griffith PD, McLean A, Emery VC: Encouraging prospects for immunisation against primary cytomegalovirus infection. Vaccine 2001;19:1356–1362.
59. Plotkin SA: Is there a formula for an effective CMV vaccine? J Clin Virol 2002;25:S13–S21.
60. Center for Disease Control: Update on adult immunization: Recommendation of the Immunization Practices Advisory Committee (ACIP). MMWR 1991;40:69.
61. Adler SP: Cytomegalovirus and child day care. Evidence for an increased infection rate among day-care workers. N Engl J Med 1989;321:1290–1296.
62. McGregor JA, Rubright G, Ogle JW: Congenital cytomegalovirus infection as a preventable complication of maternal transfusion. A case report. J Reprod Med 1990;35:61–64.
63. Revello MG, Rercivalle E, Baldanti F, et al: Prenatal treatment of congenital human cytomegalovirus infection by fetal intravascular administration of ganciclovir. Clin Diagn Virol 1993;1:61–67.
64. Landy HJ, Grossman JH: Herpes simplex virus. Obstet Gynecol Clin North Am 1989;16:495–515.

65. Volpi A, Lakeman AD, Pereira L, Stagno S: Monoclonal antibodies for rapid diagnosis and typing of genital herpes infections during pregnancy. Am J Obstet Gynecol 1983;146:813–815.
66. Nerukar LS, Namba M, Sever JL: Comparison of standard tissue culture, tissue culture plus staining, and direct staining for detection of genital herpes simplex virus infection. J Clin Microbiol 1984;19:631–633.
67. Warford AL, Levy RA, Rdkrut KA, Steinberg E: Herpes simplex virus testing of an obstetric population with an antigen enzyme-linked immunosorbent assay. Am J Obstet Gynecol 1986;154:21–28.
68. Baker DA, Gonik B, Milch PO, et al: Clinical evaluation of a new herpes simplex virus ELISA: A rapid diagnostic test for herpes simplex virus. Obstet Gynecol 1989;73:322–325.
69. Cone RW, Hobson AC, Brown ZA, et al: Frequent detection of genital herpes simplex virus DNA by polymerase chain reaction among pregnant women. JAMA 1994;272:792–796.
70. Centers for Disease Control: Sexually transmitted diseases treatment guidelines. MMWR 2002;51:1–80.
71. Brown ZA: Case study: Type-specific HSV serology and the correct diagnosis of first-episode genital herpes during pregnancy. Herpes 2002;9:24–26.
72. Koutsky LA, Stevens CE, Holmes KK, et al: Underdiagnosis of genital herpes by current clinical and viral-isolation procedures. N Engl J Med 1992;326:1533–1539.
73. Arvin AM, Hensleigh PA, Prober CG, et al: Failure of antepartum maternal culture to predict the infant's risk of exposure to herpes simplex virus at delivery. N Engl J Med 1986;315:796–800.
74. Riley LE: Herpes simplex virus. Semin Perinatol 1998;22: 284–292.
75. Rouse DJ, Stringer JSA: An appraisal of screening for maternal type-specific herpes simplex virus antibodies to prevent neonatal herpes. Am J Obstet Gynecol 2000;183:400–406.
76. Kulhanjian JA, Soroush V, Au DS, et al: Identification of women at unsuspected risk of primary infection with herpes simplex virus type 2 during pregnancy. N Engl J Med 1992; 326:916–920.
77. Baker DA, Amstey MS: Herpes simplex virus: Biology, epidemiology, and clinical infection. Semin Perinatol 1983;7:1–8.
78. Rooney JF, Felser JM, Ostrove JM, Straus SE: Acquisition of genital herpes from an asymptomatic sexual partner. N Engl J Med 1986;314:1561–1564.
79. Koelle DM, Benedetti J, Langenberg A, Corey L: Asymptomatic reactivation of herpes simplex virus in women after the first epsiode of genital herpes. Ann Intern Med 1992;116:433–437.
80. Whitley RJ, Soong S-J, Linneman C, et al: Herpes simplex encephalitis. Clinical assessment. JAMA 1982;247:317–320.
81. Rubin MH, Ward DM, Painter CJ: Fulminant hepatic failure caused by genital herpes in a healthy person. JAMA 1985;253:1299–1301.
82. Laffery WE, Coombs RW, Benedetti J, et al: Recurrences after oral and genital herpes simplex virus infection. Influence of site of infection and viral type. N Engl J Med 1987;316:1444–1449.
83. Fleming DT, McQuillan GM, Johnson RE, et al: Herpes simplex virus type 2 in the United States, 1976 to 1994. N Engl J Med 1997;16:1105–1011.
84. Mertz GL, Benedetti J, Ashley R, et al: Risk factors for the sexual transmission of genital herpes. Ann Intern Med 1992;116:197–202.
85. Amstrong GL, Schillinger J, Markowitz L, et al: Incidence of herpes simplex virus type 2 infection in the United States. Am J Epidemiol 2001;153:912–920.
86. Brown ZA, Selke S, Zeh J, et al: The acquisition of herpes simplex virus during pregnancy. N Engl J Med 1997;337: 509–515.
87. Gonik B, Loo LS, West S, Kohl S. Natural killer cell cytotoxicity and antibody-dependent cellular cytotoxicity to herpes simplex virus-infected cells in human pregnancy. Am J Reprod Immunol Microbiol 1987;13:23–26.
88. Lagrew DC, Furlow TG, Hager WD, Yarrish RL. Disseminated herpes simplex virus infection in pregnancy. Successful treatment with acyclovir. JAMA 1984;252:2058–2059.
89. Whitley RJ, Corey L, Arvin A, et al: Changing presentation of herpes simplex virus infection in neonates. J Infect Dis 1988; 158:109–116.
90. Brown ZA, Benedetti J, Ashley R, et al: Neonatal herpes simplex virus infection in relation to asymptomatic maternal infection at the time of labor. N Engl J Med 1991;324:1247–1252.
91. Brown ZA, Vontver LA, Benedetti J, et al: Effects on infants of a first episode of genital herpes during pregnancy. N Engl J Med 1987;317:1246–1251.
92. Nahmias AJ, Roizman B: Infection with herpes simplex virus 1 and 2. N Engl J Med 1973;289:667-74, 719-25, 781–789.
93. Corey L, Spear PG: Infections with herpes simplex virus. N Engl J Med 1986;314:686–691.
94. Becker TM, Blount JH, Guinan ME: Genital herpes infections in private practice in the United States. JAMA 1985;253: 1601–1603.
95. Brown ZA, Wald A, Morrow A, et al: Effect of serologic status and caesarean delivery on transmission rates of herpes simplex virus from mother to infant. JAMA 2003;289:203–209.
96. Catalono PM, Meritt AO, Mead PB: Incidence of genital herpes simplex virus at the time of delivery in women with known risk factors. Am J Obstet Gynecol 1991;164:1303–1306.
97. Stone KM, Brooks CA, Guinan ME, Alexander ER: National surveillance for neonatal herpes simplex virus infections. Sex Transm Dis 1989;16:152–156.
98. Whitley R, Arvin A, Prober C, et al: Predictors of morbidity and mortality in neonates with herpes simplex infections. The National Institute of Allergy and Infectious Diseases Collaborative Antiviral Study Group. N Engl J Med 1991;324:450–454.
99. Casper C, Wald A: Condom use and the prevention of genital herpes acquisition. Herpes 2002;9:10–14.
100. Stanberry LR, Spruance SL, Cunningham AL, et al: Glycoprotein-D-adjuvant vaccine to prevent genital herpes. N Engl J Med 2002;347:1652–1661.
101. Scott LL, Sanchez PJ, Jackson GL, et al: Acyclovir suppression to prevent cesarean delivery after first-episode genital herpes. Obstet Gynecol 1996;87:69–73.
102. Centers for Disease Control and Prevention: Pregnancy outcomes following systemic acyclovir exposure. June 1, 1984–June 30, 1993. MMWR 1993;42:806–809.
103. American College of Obstetricians and Gynecologists (ACOG): Management of herpes in pregnancy: Clinical management guidelines for obstetrician-gynecologists. ACOG Practice Bulletin. No 8. Int J Gynaecol Obstet 2000;165–174.
104. Goldberg LK, Kaufman R, Kurtz TO, et al: Long-term suppression of recurrent genital herpes with acyclovir. A 5-year benchmark. Acyclovir Study Group. Arch Dermatol 1993;129: 582–587.
105. Wald A, Zeh J, Barnum G, et al: Suppression of subclinical shedding of herpes simplex virus type 2 with acyclovir. Ann Intern Med 1996;124:8–15.
106. Fife KH, Crumpacker CS, Mertz GJ, et al: Recurrence and resistance patterns of herpes simplex virus following cessation of ≥6 years of chronic suppression with acyclovir. Acyclovir Study Group. J Infect Dis 1994;169:1338–1341.
107. Frenkel LM, Brown ZA, Bryson YJ, et al: Pharmacokinetics of acyclovir in the term human pregnancy and neonate. Am J Obstet Gynecol 1991;164:569–576.
108. Baker DA: Antiviral therapy for genital herpes in nonpregnant and pregnant women. Int J Fert 1998;43:243–248.
109. Boehm FH, Estes W, Wright PF, Growdon JF: Management of genital herpes simplex virus infection occurring during pregnancy. Am J Obstet Gynecol 1981;141:735–740.
110. Goldkrand JW: Intrapartum inoculation of herpes simplex virus by fetal scalp electrode. Obstet Gynecol 1982;59:263–265.

111. Hollier LM, Scott LL, Murphree SS, et al: Postpartum endometritis caused by herpes simplex virus. Obstet Gynecol 1997;89:836–838.
112. Larson JE, Morrow SL, Happel L, et al: Reversal of cystic fibrosis phenotype in mice by gene therapy in utero. Lancet 1997;349:619–620.
113. Kita Y, Li X-K, Ohba M, et al: Prolonged cardiac allograft survival in rats systemically injected adenoviral vectors containing CTLA4IG-gene. Transplantation 1999;68:758–766.
114. Schneider H, Muehle C, Douar AM, et al: Sustained delivery of therapeutic concentrations of human clotting factor IX—a comparison of adenoviral and AAV vectors administered in utero. J Gene Med 2002;4:46–53.
115. Sylvester KG, Yang EY, Cass DL, et al: Fetoscopic gene therapy for congenital lung disease. J Pediatr Surg 1997;32:964–969.
116. Baumgartner TL, Baumgartner BJ, Hudon L, Moise KJ: Ultrasonographically guided direct gene transfer in utero: Successful induction of beta-galactosidase in a rabbit model. Am J Obstet Gynecol 1999;181:848–852.
117. Iwamoto HS, Trapnell BC, McConnell CJ, et al: Pulmonary inflammation associated with repeated, prenatal exposure to an E1, E3-deleted adenoviral vector in sheep. Gene Ther 1999;6:98–106.
118. Xing A, Boileau P, Caüzac M, et al: Comparative in vivo approaches for selective adenovirus-mediated gene delivery to the placenta. Hum Gene Ther 2000;11:167–177.
119. Horwitz MS: Adenoviruses. In Fields BN, Knipe DM, Howley PM (eds): Fields Virology, 3rd ed. Philadelphia, Lippincott-Raven, 1995, 2149–2171.
120. Foy HM: Adenoviruses. In Evans A, Kaslow R (eds): Viral Infection in Humans: Epidemiology and Control, 4th ed. New York, Plenum, 1997, pp 119–138.
121. Matsuoka T, Naito T, Kubato Y, et al: Disseminated adenovirus (type 19) infection in a neonate: Rapid detection of the infection by immunofluorescence. Acta Paediatr Scand 1990;79:568–571.
122. Montone KT, Furth EE, Pietra GG, Gupta PK: Neonatal adenovirus infection: A case report with in situ hybridization confirmation of ascending intrauterine infection. Diagn Cytopathol 1995;12:341–344.
123. Ranucci-Weiss D, Uerpairojkit B, Bowles N, et al: Intrauterine adenoviral infection associated with fetal nonimmune hydrops. Prenat Diagn 1998;18:182–185.
124. Towbin JA, Griffin LD, Martin AB, et al: Intrauterine adenoviral myocarditis presenting as nonimmune hydrops fetalis: Diagnosis by polymerase chain reaction. Pediatr Infect Dis J 1994;13:144–150.
125. Abzug MJ, Levine MJ: Neonatal adenovirus infection: Four patients and review of the literature. Pediatrics 1991; 87:890–896.
126. Angella JJ, Connor JD: Neonatal infection caused by adenovirus type 7. J Pediatr 1968;72:474–478.
127. Kinney JS, Hierholzer JC, Thibault DW: Neonatal pulmonary insufficiency caused by adenovirus infection successfully treated with extracorporeal membrane oxygenation. J Pediatr 1994;125:110–112.
128. Brown M, Rossier E, Carpenter B, Anand CM: Fatal adenovirus type 35 infection in newborns. Pediatr Infect Dis J 1991;10:955–956.
129. Meyer K, Girgis N, McGravey V: Adenovirus associated with congenital pleural effusions. J Pediatr 1985;107:433–435.
130. Finn A, Anday E, Talbot GH: An epidemic of adenovirus 7a infection in a neonatal nursery: Course, morbidity, and management. Infect Control Hosp Epidemiol 1988;9:398–404.
131. Carter BA, Karpen SJ, Quiros-Tejeira RE, et al: Intravenous cidofovir therapy for disseminated adenovirus in pediatric liver transplant recipient. Transplantation 2002;74:1050–1052.
132. Arav-Boger R, Echavarria M, Forman M, et al: Clearance of adenoviral hepatitis with ribavirin therapy in a pediatric liver transplant recipient. Pediatr Infect Dis J 2000;19:1097–1100.
133. Tindall JP, Callaway JL: Hand-foot-and-mouth disease—It's more common than you think. Am J Dis Child 1972;124: 372–375.
134. Cherry JD: Enteroviruses. In Remington JS, Klein JO (eds): Infectious Diseases of the Fetus and Newborn Infant, 4th ed. Philadelphia, WB Saunders, 1995, pp 404–446.
135. Yagi S, Schnurr D, Lin J: Spectrum of monoclonal antibodies to coxsackievirus B-3 includes type- and group-specific antibodies. J Clin Microbiol 1992;30:2498–2501.
136. Trabelsi A, Grattard F, Nejmeddine M, et al: Evaluation of an enterovirus group-specific anti-VP-1 monoclonal antibody, 5-D8/1, in comparison with neutralization and PCR for rapid identification of enteroviruses in cell culture. J Clin Microbiol 1995;33:2454–2457.
137. Shin SY, Kim KS, Lee YS, et al: Identification of enteroviruses by using monoclonal antibodies against a putative common epitope. J Clin Microbiol 2003;41:3028–3034.
138. Zoll GJ, Melchers WJG, Kopecka H, et al: General primer-mediated polymerase chain reaction for detection of enteroviruses: Application for diagnostic routine and persistent infections. J Clin Microbiol 1992;30:160–165.
139. Redline R, Genest D, Tycko B: Detection of enteroviral infection in paraffin-embedded tissue by the RNA polymerase chain reaction technique. Am J Clin Pathol 1991;96:568–571.
140. Modlin JF: Perinatal echovirus and group B coxsackievirus infections. Clin Perinatol 1988;15:233–246.
141. Baker DA, Phillips CA: Maternal and neonatal infection with coxsackievirus. Obstet Gynecol 1980;55 Suppl 3:12S–15S.
142. Archer JS: Acute liver failure in pregnancy. J Reprod Med 2001;46:137–140.
143. Frisk G, Diderholm H: Increased frequency of coxsackie B virus IgM in women with spontaneous abortion. J Infect 1992;24: 141–145.
144. Sever JL, Huebner RJ, Costellano GA, et al: Serologic diagnosis "en masse" with multiple antigens. Am Rev Respir Dis 1963;88:342–349.
145. Cherry JD, Soriano F, Jahn CL: Search for perinatal virus infection. A prospective, clinical, virologic and serologic study. Am J Dis Child 1968;116:245–250.
146. Kaplan MH, Klein SW, McPhee J, Harper RG: Group B coxsackievirus infection in infants younger than three months of age: A serious childhood disease. Rev Infect Dis 1983;5:1019–1032.
147. Amstey MS, Miller KR, Menegus AM, di Sant'Agnese PA: Enterovirus in the pregnant women in the perfused placenta. Am J Obstet Gynecol 1988;158:775–782.
148. Bates HR: Coxsackievirus B3 calcific pancarditis and hydrops fetalis. Am J Obstet Gynecol 1970;106:629–630.
149. Strong BS, Young SA: Intrauterine coxsackievirus group B type 1 infection: Viral cultivation from amniotic fluid in the third trimester. Am J Perinatol 1995;12:78–79.
150. Reyes MP, Zalenski D, Smith F, et al: Coxsackievirus-positive cervices in women with febrile illness during the third trimester in pregnancy. Am J Obstet Gynecol 1986;155:159-61.
151. Brown GC, Karunas RS: Relationship of congenital anomalies and maternal infection with selected enteroviruses. Am J Epidemiol 1972;95:207–217.
152. Gauntt CJ, Gudvangen RJ, Brans YW, Marlin AE: Coxsackievirus group B antibodies in the ventricular fluid of infants with severe anatomic defects in the central nervous system. Pediatrics 1985;76:64–68.
153. Nathenson G, Spigland I, Eisenberg R: Benign neonatal arrhythmias and coxsackie B virus infection. J Pediatr 1975;86:152–153.
154. Murray D, Altschul M, Dyke J: Aseptic meningitis in a neonate with an oral vesicular lesion. Diagn Microbiol Infect Dis 1985;3:77–80.
155. Theodoridou M, Kakourou T, Laina I, et al: Vesiculopapular rash as a single presentation in intrauterine coxsackie virus infection. Eur J Pediatr 2002;161:412–413.

156. Euscher E, Davis J, Holzman I, Nuovo GJ: Coxsackie virus infection of the placenta associated with neurodevelopmental delays in the newborn. Obstet Gynecol 2001;98:1019–1026.
157. Hurley R, Norman AP, Pryse-Davies J: Massive pulmonary haemorrhage in the newborn associated with coxsackie B virus infection. BMJ 1969;3:636 637.
158. Gear JHS: Coxsackievirus infections in Southern Africa. Yale J Biol Med 1961/1962;34:289–296.
159. Burch GE, Sunn SC, Chu KC, et al: Interstitial and coxsackievirus B myocarditis in infants and children. A comparative histologic and immunofluorescent study of 50 autopsied hearts. JAMA 1968;203:1–8.
160. Overall JC: Intrauterine virus infections and congenital heart disease. Am Heart J 1972;84:823–833.
161. Abzug MJ: Prognosis for neonates with enterovirus hepatitis and coagulopathy. Pediatr Infect Dis J 2001;20:758–763.
162. Rantakallio P, Jones P, Moring J, von Wendt L: Association between central nervous system infections during childhood and adult onset schizophrenia and other psychoses: A 28-year follow-up. Int J Epidemiol 1997;26:837–843.
163. Farmer K, MacArthur BA, Clay MM: A follow-up study of 15 cases of neonatal meningoencephalitis due to coxsackie virus B5. J Pediatr 1975;87:568–571.
164. Drash A: The etiology of diabetes mellitus. Editorial. N Engl J Med 1979;300:1211–1213.
165. Dahlquist GG, Ivarsson S, Lindberg B, Forsgren M: Maternal enteroviral infection during pregnancy as a risk factor for childhood IDDM. Diabetes 1995;44:408–413.
166. Hyöty H, Hiltunen M, Knip M, et al: A prospective study of the role of coxsackie B and other enterovirus infections in the pathogenesis of IDDM. Diabetes 1995;44:652–657.
167. Füchtenbusch M, Irnstetter A, Jäger G, Ziegler A-G: No evidence for an association of coxsackievirus infections during pregnancy and early childhood with development of islet autoantibodies in offspring of mothers or fathers with type 1 diabetes. J Autoimmun 2001;17:333–340.
168. Viskari HR, Roivainen M, Reunanen A, et al: Maternal first-trimester enterovirus infection and future risk of type 1 diabetes in the exposed fetus. Diabetes 2002;51:2568–2571.
169. Balduzzi PC, Greendyke RM: Sudden unexpected death in infancy and viral infection. Pediatrics 1966;38:201–206.
170. Gold E, Carver DH, Heineberg H, et al: Viral infection: A possible cause of sudden, unexpected death in infants. N Engl J Med 1961;264:53–55.
171. Valdes-Dapena MA, Hummeler K: Sudden and unexpected death in infants. II. Viral infections as causative factors. J Pediatr 1963;63:398–401.
172. Lapinleimu K, Kaski U: An outbreak caused by coxsackie B5 among newborn infants. Scand J Infect Dis 1987;4:27–30.
173. Borulf S, Walder M, Ulmsten U: Outbreak of coxsackie virus A14 meningitis among newborns in a maternity hospital ward. Acta Paediatr Scand 1987;76:234–238.
174. Brightman VJ, McNair STF, Westphal M, Boggs TR: An outbreak of coxsackie B5 virus infection in a newborn nursery. J Pediatr 1966;69:179–192.
175. Hammond GW, Lukes H, Wells B, et al: Maternal and neonatal neutralizing antibody titers to selected enteroviruses. Pediatr Infect Dis 1985;4:32–35.
176. Abzug MJ, Keyserling HL, Lee ML, Rotbart HA: Neonatal enterovirus infection: Virology, serology, and effect of intravenous immune globulin. Clin Infect Dis 1995;20: 1201–1206.
177. Abzug MJ, Cloud G, Bradley J, et al: Double blind placebo-controlled trial of pleconaril in infants with enterovirus meningitis. National Institute of Allergy and Infectious Diseases Collaborative Antiviral Study Group. Pediatr Infect Dis J 2003;22:335–341.
178. Nagington J, Gandy G, Walker J, Gray JJ: Use of normal immunoglobulin in an echovirus 11 outbreak in a special-care baby unit. Lancet 1983;2:443–446.
179. Chapman NM, Ragland A, Leser JS, et al: A group B coxsackievirus/poliovirus 5′ nontranslated region chimera can act as an attenuated vaccine strain in mice. J Virol 2000;74: 4047–4056.
180. zur Hausen H: Molecular pathogenesis of cancer of the cervix and its causation by specific human papillomavirus types. Curr Top Microbiol Immunol 1994;186:131–156.
181. Koutsky L: Epidemiology of genital human papillomavirus infection. Am J Med 1997;102:3–8.
182. Kemp EA, Hakenewerth AM, Laurent SL, et al: Human papillomavirus prevalence in pregnancy. Obstet Gynecol 1992;79: 649–656.
183. Smith EM, Johnson SR, Cripe T, et al: Perinatal transmission and maternal risks of human papillomavirus infection. Cancer Detect Prev 1995;19:196–205.
184. Schneider A, Hotz M, Gissmann L: Increased prevalence of human papillomaviruses in the lower genital tract of pregnant women. Int J Cancer 1987;40:198–201.
185. Rando RF, Lindheim S, Hasty L, et al: Increased frequency of detection of human papillomavirus DNA in exfoliated cervical cells during pregnancy. Am J Obstet Gynecol 1989;161: 50–54.
186. Sedlaceck TV, Lindheim S, Eder C: Mechanism for human papillomavirus transmission at birth. Am J Obstet Gynecol 1989;161:55–59.
187. Kashima HK, Shah K: Recurrent respiratory papillomatosis: Clinical overview and management principles. Obstet Gynecol Clin North Am 1987;14:581–588.
188. Hallden C, Majmudar B: The relationship between juvenile laryngeal papillomatosis and maternal condylomata acuminata. J Reprod Med 1986;31:804–807.
189. Milczuk HA: Intralesional cidofovir for the treatment of severe juvenile recurrent respiratory papillomatosis: Long-term results in 4 children. Otolaryngol Head Neck Surg 2003;128:788–794.
190. Auborn KJ: Therapy for recurrent respiratory papillomatosis. Antivir Ther 2002;7:1–9.
191. Allen AL, Siegfried EC: The natural history of condylomas in children. J Am Acad Dermatol 1998;39:951–955.
192. Armbruster-Moraes E, Ioshimoto LM, Leao E, Zugaib M: Presence of human papillomavirus DNA in amniotic fluids of pregnant women with cervical lesions. Gynecol Oncol 1994;54:152–158.
193. Cason J, Kaye JN, Jewers RJ, et al: Perinatal infection and persistence of human papillomavirus 16 and 18 in infants. J Med Virol 1995;47:209–218.
194. Watts DH, Koutsky LA, Holmes KK, et al: Low risk of perinatal transmission of human papillomavirus: Results from a prospective cohort study. Am J Obstet Gynecol 1998;178: 365–373.
195. Smith EM, Johnson SR, Cripe TP, et al: Perinatal vertical transmission of human papillomavirus and subsequent development of respiratory tract papillomatosis. Ann Otol Rhinol Laryngol 1991;100:479–483.
196. Favre M, Majewski S, De Jesus N, et al: A possible vertical transmission of human papillomavirus genotypes associated with epidermodysplasia verruciformis. J Invest Dermatol 1998; 111:333–336.
197. Tseng CJ, Liang CC, Soong YK, Pao CC: Perinatal transmission of human papillomavirus in infants: Relationship between infection rate and mode of delivery. Obstet Gynecol 1998;91:92–96.
198. Tseng CJ, Lin CY, Wang RL, et al: Possible transplacental transmission of human papillomavirus. Am J Obstet Gynecol 1992;166:35–40.
199. Snoeck R, Bossens M, Parent D, et al: Phase II double-blind, placebo-controlled study of the safety and efficacy of cidofovir topical gel for the treatment of patients with human papillomavirus infection. Clin Infect Dis 2001;33: 597–602.
200. Pinto LA, Edwards J, Castle PE, et al: Cellular immune responses to human papillomavirus (HPV)-16 L1 in healthy volunteers immunized with recombinant HPV-16 L1 virus like particles. J Infect Dis 2003;188:327–338.

201. Kjellberg L, Hallmans G, Ahren AM, et al: Smoking, diet, pregnancy and oral contraceptive use as risk factors for cervical intraepithelial neoplasia in relation to human papillomavirus infection. Br J Cancer 2000; 82:1332–1338.
202. Tenti P, Zappatore R, Migliora P, et al: Perinatal transmission of human papillomavirus from gravidas with latent infections. Obstet Gynecol 1999; 93:475–479.
203. Schwartz DB, Greenberg MD, Daoud Y, Reid R: Genital condylomas in pregnancy: Use of trichloroacetic acid and laser therapy. Am J Obstet Gynecol 1988;158:1407–1416.
204. Eskelinen A, Mashkilleyson N: Optimum treatment of genital warts. Drugs 1987;34:599–603.
205. Piper JM, Wen TT, Xenauis EM, et al: Interferon therapy in primary care. Prim Care Update Obset Gynecol 2001;8: 163–169.

CHAPTER 32

Other Infectious Conditions

Breton C. Freitag / Michael G. Gravett

INTRODUCTION

Infections are an important contributor to maternal and perinatal morbidity and mortality rates. Maternal immunosuppression that occurs during pregnancy, may alter the natural course of many infectious diseases. Higher attack rates are seen in pregnancy for a variety of bacterial and viral infections. Furthermore, many of these infections are associated with adverse outcomes of pregnancy, including preterm birth, low birth weight, and stillbirth. This chapter addresses a large group of infectious diseases not discussed in other chapters, including streptococcal infections, listeriosis, common sexually transmitted infections, and vaginitis.

GROUP A STREPTOCOCCUS

Group A streptococcus (*Streptococcus pyogenes*) has been associated with obstetric and neonatal infections since the 16th century. It is probable that group A streptococcus was responsible for much of puerperal sepsis, or "childbed fever," described by Semmelweis in 19th century Vienna.[1] However, with the advent of the antibiotic era, group A streptococcal (GAS) infections became increasingly infrequent until the 1980s, when GAS infections dramatically increased again for poorly understood reasons.[2] Group A streptococcus causes a broad spectrum of invasive and noninvasive diseases, including bacterial pharyngitis, impetigo, scarlet fever, necrotizing fasciitis, and the more recently recognized streptococcal toxic shock syndrome (STSS), as outlined in Table 32–1.[2,3]

Streptococcus pyogenes, the etiologic agent for GAS infections, was first described by Louis Pasteur in 1879. The *Streptococcus* genus is classified into groups, based upon polysaccharide capsular antigens and the cell wall M protein, as first described by Lancefield.[4] *Streptococcus pyogenes* is divided into serotypes according to the M protein, and to date more than 80 M protein serotypes have been identified. Different serotypes are associated with different forms of infection, and M1 and M3 have been the most common serotypes identified in serious infection in recent years.[5]

M protein is also important as a virulence factor because of its antiphagocytic properties. Other significant virulence factors are the streptococcal pyrogenic exotoxins (SPE), which act as superantigens. Superantigens are able to bind to T-cell receptors and the class II major histocompatibilty complex (MHC) without first undergoing antigen processing and presentation. The cross-linking of a T-cell receptor with a class II MHC molecule by a superantigen stimulates the proliferation and activation of T cells and macrophages, causing them to release large amounts of cytokines, which can cause shock or inflammation and tissue damage.[2,6] A large number of SPE superantigens have been identified, but SPE A, SPE B, SPE C, SPE F, and streptococcal super-

TABLE 32–1

Classification of Group A Streptococcal Infections

1. Streptococcal toxic shock syndrome (streptococcal TSS)
2. Other invasive infections (isolation of *S. pyogenes* from a normally sterile site in patients not fulfilling criteria from streptococcal TSS)
   a. Bacteremia with no identifiable focus
   b. Focal infection with or without bacteremia (meningitis, pneumonia, peritonitis, puerperal sepsis, osteomyelitis, septic arthritis, necrotizing fasciitis, surgical wound infections, erysipelas, cellulitis)
3. Scarlet fever
4. Noninvasive infections (recovery of *S. pyogenes* from a nonsterile site)
   a. Mucous membranes (pharyngitis, tonsillitis, otitis media, sinusitis, vaginitis)
   b. Cutaneous (impetigo)
5. Nonsuppurative sequelae (specific clinical findings with evidence of a recent group A streptococcal infection)
   a. Acute rheumatic fever
   b. Acute glomerulonephritis

Adapted from The Working Group on Severe Streptococcal Infections: Defining the group A streptococcal toxic shock syndrome. JAMA 1993; 269:390.

antigen (SSA) are among the best characterized. By stimulating cytokine production these streptococcal exotoxins likely play an important role in the pathogenicity of invasive GAS infections by exacerbating the onset of clinical signs and symptoms of infection.

Maternal and Fetal Risks

Group A streptococcus may be recovered from skin or mucous membrane of asymptomatic colonized patients. GAS may gain entry to the body via the skin, mucosa, pharynx, and vagina and cause infections with both suppurative and nonsuppurative complications.[2,7] During pregnancy, the most notable GAS infections are bacteremia without a focus of infections and endometritis, but invasive infections including streptococcal toxic shock syndrome (STSS) and necrotizing fasciitis also occur (Table 32–2). The reasons for the increased susceptibility seen during the puerperium include the breach of integrity in the integumentary system associated with either vaginal delivery or cesarean section. Invasive infections are characterized by hypotension and shock, multiple organ failure, systemic toxicity, severe local pain, rapid necrosis of subcutaneous tissues and skin, renal dysfunction, and fever.[2,7] GAS invasive disease is characterized by a rapid, often fatal course and by difficulties in the early diagnosis, when intervention may be more successful.

Postpartum invasive group A streptococcal infection occurs in approximately 1 in 11,000 to 1 in 17,000 births, with an average of 220 cases occurring in the United States every year.[8,9] The rate of invasive GAS infection is 1.6- to 2.0-fold greater among black patients compared to white patients.[8] Maternal case fatality rate ranges from 3.5% to 30% in postpartum invasive GAS. Maternal GAS disease has also been associated with stillbirth.

Neonatal invasive GAS has also been reported and has a case fatality rate of up to 30%.[9–11] Although the neonate may be colonized following horizontal transmission within the nursery, vertical transmission from a colonized mother has been demonstrated.[10,12] Furthermore, 50% of neonatal cases of invasive GAS disease occur within the first week of life, suggesting that vertical transmission from a colonized parturient may be the most important route of infection. The most frequent manifestation of neonatal GAS disease is omphalitis, but cellulitis, meningitis, sepsis, and fasciitis also occur. Fortunately, neonatal GAS disease is rare, with an estimated incidence of 1 in 18,000 births.

TABLE 32–2

Diseases Seen among Patients with Postpartum Group A Streptococcus Infection

INFECTION	NUMBER (%) OF PATIENTS (N = 87)
Bacteremia without focus	40 (46%)
Endometritis	24 (28%)
Peritonitis	7 (8%)
Septic abortion	6 (7%)
Cellulitis	3 (3%)
Septic arthritis	3 (3%)
Necrotizing fasciitis	3 (3%)
Streptococcal toxic shock syndrome	3 (3%)
Chorioamnionitis	3 (3%)
Pneumonia	1 (1%)
Other	3 (3%)

Adapted from Chuang I, Van Beneden C, Beall B, Schuchat A: Population-based surveillance for postpartum invasive group A streptococcus infections, 1995–2000. Clin Infect Dis 2002;35:665–670.

Diagnosis

Group A streptococci can be readily recovered from most patients with evidence of GAS disease. Group A streptococci are catalase-negative gram-positive cocci that are beta-hemolytic on blood agar. The colonies may appear as highly mucoid to nonmucoid, and the organisms are usually 1 to 2 mm in diameter. Although cultures may be helpful in confirming the diagnosis of GAS disease, they are seldom available when considering the initial diagnosis. Group A streptococcal disease may progress rapidly, and therapy must be initiated before cultures are generally available.

Therefore, the diagnosis of GAS disease depends upon a high index of suspicion. Fever is the most common presenting sign, and 20% of patients have a flu-like syndrome with fever, chills, myalgia, nausea, vomiting, and diarrhea.[13] Confusion or altered mental status is present in over one half of patients. Renal dysfunction occurs in 80% of patients and may precede hypotension or shock. The presence of hemaglobinuria or an elevated serum creatinine are evidence of renal involvement. Hemoconcentration, as a result of a fluid shift to the extravascular compartment, and leukocytosis (often $>20,000/mm^3$), with a predominance of immature neutrophils, are common. Respiratory failure and adult respiratory distress syndrome occur in approximately 50% of patients but usually develop after the onset of clinically recognized shock. Criteria for the diagnosis of STSS are outlined in Table 32–3.

Eighty percent of patients have evidence of soft tissue infection characterized by induration and erythema, which progress to necrotizing fasciitis in 70% of cases.[13] The hallmark of these soft tissue infections is the abrupt onset of severe pain, which usually precedes physical findings or is out of proportion to physical findings. Any patient suspected of having GAS-associated necrotizing fasciitis must have the diagnosis confirmed by immediate wound exploration and debridement. A purulent discharge is usually not present, and a limited wound inspection may fail to confirm the diagnosis. Upon opening the wound, a thin, watery, nonmalodorous discharge is frequently present. The diagnosis of necrotizing fasciitis can be easily confirmed by the bloodless blunt dissection of the superficial fascia and by pathologic frozen section.

TABLE 32–3

Diagnostic Criteria for Streptococcal Toxic Shock Syndrome

I. Isolation of *Stcptococcus pyogcncs*
  A. From a normally sterile site
  B. From a nonsterile site (throat, sputum, vagina, superficial skin lesion)
II. Clinical evidence of severity
  A. Hypotension (systolic blood pressure ≤90 mm Hg in adults or ≤*5th* percentile for age in children) and
  B. Two or more of the following:
    1. Renal impairment (serum creatinine ≥2.0 mg/dL or a twofold elevation over baseline level in patients with preexisting renal impairment)
    2. Coagulopathy (platelets ≤100 × 10^6/L or disseminated intravascular coagulation)
    3. Liver involvement (AST, ALT, or total bilirubin ≥ two times upper limits of normal)
    4. Adult respiratory distress syndrome
    5. Generalized erythematous macular rash
    6. Soft tissue necrosis (necrotizing fasciitis, myositis, or gangrene)

Adapted from The Working Group on Severe Streptococcal Infections: Defining the group A streptococcal toxic shock syndrome. JAMA 1993;269:390.

In summary, the diagnosis of GAS disease should be considered in any patient with the sudden onset of hypotension and shock, or the abrupt onset of severe pain in a wound, or systemic signs and symptoms such as confusion, renal impairment, or respiratory distress in a patient with a wound or episiotomy infection. Aggressive intravenous fluid resuscitation, antibiotic therapy, and wound debridement are necessary in these patients.

Management Options

Prepregnancy

No current evidence suggests that the identification of GAS carriers prior to pregnancy is predictive of either subsequent pregnancy outcome or in reducing puerperal infectious morbidity. Therefore, prepregnancy screening is not recommended.

Prenatal

A high index of suspicion is necessary for the early diagnosis of GAS infection. Unfortunately, diagnosis may be difficult in the early stages of GAS infection, and delays in therapy may be associated with increased morbidity and mortality rates. Many patients die within 24 to 48 hours of infection.[13] In general, treatment must be directed at hemodynamic stabilization with intravenous fluids and vasopressors, antibiotic therapy, and in the case of soft tissue infections, surgical exploration and aggressive debridement of involved tissues. Massive amounts of intravenous crystalloids, in the range of 10 to 20 L/day, are often necessary to maintain blood pressure and tissue perfusion. Vasopressors such as dopamine are also frequently required. In soft tissue GAS infections such as necrotizing fasciitis antibiotic therapy alone, without surgical debridement, usually results in maternal death. Intraoperative Gram stain and histologic frozen section may be necessary to fully delineate the extent of involved tissues. Hyperbaric oxygen therapy has no role in the treatment of necrotizing fasciitis but may be a useful adjunct in delineating necrotic tissue that must be surgically debrided.

Broad-spectrum parenteral antibiotics should be administered promptly. Penicillin G (200,000 to 400,000 U/kg/day) is the drug of choice for GAS invasive infections. However, studies in mice have demonstrated that even a short delay of 2 hours after initiation of infection dramatically reduces the efficacy of penicillin G.[14] Recent studies indicate that clindamycin may be more efficacious than penicillin when therapy is delayed. In an experimental model with mice, survival was 70% even when initiated 16 hours after GAS infection.[14] Several potential advantages to clindamycin therapy (900 mg intravenously every 8 hours) have recently been summarized.[7] First, in contrast to penicillins, clindamycin is not affected by bacterial inoculum size or rate of growth. Second, clindamycin suppresses the synthesis of bacterial toxins. Third, clindamycin facilitates phagocytosis of *S. pyogenes* by inhibition of M protein synthesis. Fourth, clindamycin has a longer postantibiotic effect than does penicillin. Last, clindamycin suppresses lipopolysaccharide-induced monocyte synthesis of tumor necrosis factor-alpha (TNF-α), a cytokine that contributes to hypotension and shock. However, a small proportion of GAS infections are resistant to clindamycin, and clindamycin should not be used alone until the organism is demonstrated to be susceptible by susceptibility testing. Therefore, initial therapy usually includes a combination of penicillin G and clindamycin.

Recent data also indicate that intravenous immunoglobulin (IVIG) (1–2 g/kg given once) may be a useful adjunct to antibiotic therapy in the treatment of GAS toxic shock syndrome. Commercial preparations of IVIG have been shown to contain neutralizing antibodies to several streptococcal virulence factors.[15] Recently, investigators reported a significant reduction in mortality rate among patients with GAS disease treated with IVIG when compared to a historical cohort.

Thus, the optimal treatment for invasive GAS disease includes a high index of suspicion, aggressive fluid resuscitation and hemodynamic support, surgical exploration and aggressive debridement, parenteral antibiotics including penicillin G and clindamycin, and possibly intravenous immunoglobulin.

Labor and Delivery

Group A streptococcus may be associated with intra-amniotic infection and with stillbirth. However, most patients with invasive GAS disease usually present in the postpartum period, frequently within the first 24 to 48 hours. Treatment should follow the general guidelines provided previously.

Postnatal

There are no current recommendations for screening for or treating asymptomatic parturients colonized with group A streptococcus. However, careful attention should be given to any parturient with the sudden onset of systemic signs such as hypotension or shock or to parturients with severe pain out of proportion of physical findings or rapidly progressive soft tissue infections, as noted earlier. Although these findings, which are consistent with necrotizing fasciitis, usually suggest a polymicrobial infection, group A streptococcus should be considered in the diagnosis, and broad-spectrum antibiotics including penicillin and clindamycin should be utilized in the initial management.

SUMMARY OF MANAGEMENT OPTIONS

Group A Streptococcal Infection

Management Options	Quality of Evidence	Strength of Recommendation	References
Prepregnancy			
No benefit to screening and treatment.	–	GPP	–
Prenatal, Labor, and Delivery			
No benefit to screening and treatment.	–	GPP	–
May cause intra-amniotic infection.	–	GPP	–
Diagnosis requires a high index of suspicion:	III	B	13
Severe pain			
Hypotension or shock			
Altered mental status			
Renal or respiratory impairment			
Treatment requires prompt intervention:	Ib	A	14, 15
IV antibiotics (penicillin G, clindamycin)			
IV fluids and circulatory support including vasopressors			
IVIG in nonresponsive cases			
Surgical debridement if appropriate			
Postnatal			
Infection may cause toxic shock syndrome or soft tissue infection.	–	GPP	–
Diagnosis requires a high index of suspicion:	III	B	13
Severe pain			
Hypotension or shock			
Altered mental status			
Renal or respiratory impairment			
Therapy	Ib	A	14, 15
Broad-spectrum antibiotics (penicillin and clindamycin)			
Surgical wound exploration and debridement			

GROUP B STREPTOCOCCUS

Group B streptococcus *(Streptococcus agalactiae)* has become recognized over the past 2 decades as one of the most important causes of neonatal infection and is currently considered one of the leading infectious causes of neonatal morbidity and death. Although early reports in the 1930s and 1940s linked group B streptococcus (GBS) with postpartum infections and neonatal meningitis, it was not until the early 1960s that the scope of perinatal and neonatal GBS infections became evident.[16] Initial case series reported case fatality rates as high as 50%. In the 1980s, trials of empiric intrapartum antibiotics to women at risk of transmitting infection to their newborns demonstrated a protective benefit against neonatal infection in the first week of life (early-onset disease). In the 1990s, these efforts led to the implementation of guidelines for intrapartum antibiotic prophylaxis of at-risk mothers, endorsed and issued by the American College of Obstretricians and Gynecologists (ACOG),[17] the Centers for Disease Control (CDC),[18] and the American Academy of Pediatrics (AAP).[19] This practice has resulted in a significant reduction in early-onset disease, as well as a smaller impact on maternal morbidity. Based upon these results, in 2002 updated guidelines were issued by the CDC to recommend optimization of screening and treatment of pregnant women in an attempt to improve upon the success already demonstrated.[20]

Group B streptococci are one of many serologically distinct species within the genus *Streptococcus*. Streptococci are facultatively anaerobic gram-positive cocci, usually arranged in chains on Gram stain. The most important pathogenic streptococcal species for humans include group A (*Streptococcus pyogenes*), group B (*Streptococcus agalactiae*), group D (enterococci), *Streptococcus pneumoniae*, and *Streptococcus viridans*. Definitive identification is based on the presence of a polysaccharide group-specific antigen common to all group B streptococcal strains as determined by serologic testing. Group B streptococci can be further subdivided into eight distinct serotypes (Ia, Ib, Ia/c, II, III, IV, V, and VI) on the basis of distinctive type-specific polysaccharide antigens. About 99% of strains can be typed into one of these six antigen types. Group B streptococci can be recovered from the vagina or cervix in 10% to 30% of pregnant women at some point during gestation.[21] The colonization may be transient, chronic, or intermittent, and the rate of colonization does not vary with gestational age. There is evidence that the gastrointestinal tract is the major primary reservoir and that vaginal or cervical contamination and colonization occur from a gastrointestinal source. The frequency of GBS isolation increases as one proceeds from the cervix to the introitus, and GBS can be recovered twice as frequently from rectal cultures as from vaginal cultures. Group B streptococci can also be recovered from the urethra of 45% to 63% of the male consorts of female carriers, implying that sexual transmission may also occur.

Neonatal GBS colonization may occur either by vertical transmission from a colonized mother as the neonate passes through the birth canal or by horizontal transmission, including both nosocomial spread in the nursery from colonized nursery personnel or other colonized neonates and acquisition from community sources. Overall, 3% to 12% of all neonates are colonized with GBS in the first week of life. Forty percent to 70% of neonates born to colonized mothers become colonized, usually with the same serotype that is present in the mother. In contrast, only 1% to 12% of neonates born to noncolonized mothers will become culture positive. Several additional factors may modify or enhance the risk of GBS vertical transmission. Higher neonatal transmission rates occur when women are persistently culture-positive carriers or when women are heavily colonized with GBS as demonstrated by semiquantitative vaginal cultures.[22] The site of maternal carriage is also important; vertical transmission is more likely to occur with cervical GBS carriage than with rectal carriage.

The most important determinant of susceptibility to invasive infection after colonization may be maternal antibodies directed against the capsular polysaccharide antigens of GBS. Immunity to GBS is mediated by antibody-dependent phagocytosis. Mothers of infants with type III GBS invasive disease have lower serum levels of type-specific antibodies than women giving birth to asymptomatically colonized infants. This antibody, which has some broad reactivity to all group B streptococcal types, is an IgG that readily crosses the placenta. When measured in mother-infant pairs, an excellent correlation exists between maternal and cord antibody levels. Baker and associates demonstrated that 73% of 45 GBS-colonized mothers with healthy neonates had high serum levels of type III antibody in contrast to only 19% of 32 GBS-colonized mothers whose neonates developed early-onset septicemia or meningitis ($P < 0.001$).[23] Strain virulence is also an important determinant of disease. Although type III strains of GBS represent approximately one third of isolates from symptomatically colonized infants, they account for over 85% of the isolates from early-onset meningitis or late-onset disease. Overall, type III strains account for more than 60% of isolates from infants with all varieties of invasive GBS infections.

Maternal and Fetal Risks

Although most research has focused on GBS neonatal infection, GBS is also an important pathogen for maternal intrapartum, postpartum, and occasionally prenatal infections. Data from an earlier report suggest puerperal septicemia due to GBS occurs with an incidence of approximately 1 to 2 per 1000 deliveries and accounts for up to 15% of positive blood cultures from postpartum patients.[24] Postpartum endometritis is reported to be more frequently observed among GBS-colonized parturients than among noncolonized parturients. GBS is also associated with clinical intra-amniotic infection, and is a frequent isolate from amniotic fluid of patients with intra-amniotic infection. Finally, GBS has been isolated from the urine of pregnant women, with or without symptoms of urinary tract infection.

GBS has also been associated with premature rupture of the membranes and with preterm delivery prior to the 32nd gestational week in some, but not all, studies.[25] Previous studies have indicated that this association may be strongest for patients with GBS bacteriuria.[26] Thomsen and associates have demonstrated significant reductions in premature rupture of the membranes and preterm labor among patients with asymptomatic GBS bacteriuria who were treated with penicillin.[27] However, antepartum antibiotic treatment to eradicate GBS from patients with asymptomatic vaginal colonization without bacteriuria has not been demonstrated to alter pregnancy outcome. Thus, a causal relationship between GBS colonization and prematurity still remains to be established.

In the past three decades, GBS has become a leading cause of septicemia and meningitis during the first 3 months of life in neonates. Early surveillance data in the 1990s suggested an incidence of 1.8 cases per 1000 live births. Two distinct clinical syndromes occur among neonates with GBS infections. These differ in the age at onset, pathogenesis, and outcome. The first clinical syndrome, early-onset infection, occurs within the first 7 days of life, and represent nearly three fourths of all cases in infants under 3 months age. The mean age at onset is 20 hours of life, and 72% will present within the first 24 hours of life.[28] A significant portion of these infections are apparent at birth or become symptomatic within the first 90 minutes of life, indicating that in utero GBS exposure and infection often occur. Early infection attack rates were estimated at 1.5 per 1000 for all live births prior to widespread use of intrapartum antibiotics. Among offspring of maternal GBS carriers, however, the attack rate is much higher, ranging from 10 to 60 per 1000.

Early neonatal infection is presumed to result from vertical transmission of GBS from a colonized mother. There is a direct relationship between neonatal attack rates and the size of the inoculum and number of colonized neonatal sites. In a recent epidemiologic review, early-onset infection presented as bacteremia (80%), pneumonia (7%), or meningitis (6%). Eighty-three percent of cases were in term infants (≤37 weeks' gestation). The overall case fatality rate was approximately 4% but was significantly higher in preterm infants, approaching 30% in infants of 33 weeks' gestation or less.[28]

The second type of disease (late-onset infection) occurs in infants after the first week of life until 3 months of age, with a typical range of 3 to 4 weeks. The overall attack rate is estimated to be 0.5 case per 1000 live births, and these cases represent 28% of infections in infants under 3 months of age.[28] In contrast to early-onset infection, nosocomial transmission may be as important as vertical transmission, although it is believed that some infants are colonized at birth, with subsequent development of invasive disease. The serotype distribution of strains recovered from late-onset infection does not reflect the serotypes present in the maternal genital tract; over 90% of late-onset infection is caused by type III GBS. Late-onset disease also presents most commonly as bacteremia (63%), but may appear as meningitis (24%, relative risk 4.3 versus early-onset disease, $P < 0.001$) and may demonstrate other sites of infection, such as septic arthritis or osteomyelitis. The overall case fatality rate for late-onset disease is 2.8%.[28] Approximately 50% of meningitis survivors will have neurologic sequelae, including cortical blindness, diabetes insipidus, deafness or other cranial nerve deficits, and spasticity.

Diagnosis

Group B streptococci can be easily grown on selective or nonselective media. Most group B streptococcal colonies appear on blood plates as small, 1 mm to 2 mm, gray-white colonies surrounded by a zone of beta-hemolysis, although 2% of strains are nonhemolytic. Preliminary identification and distinction of GBS from other streptococci is based on biochemical reactions including resistance to bacitracin, hydrolysis of sodium hippurate, and the production of a soluble hemolysin that acts synergistically with B-lysin of *Staphylococcus aureus* to produce hemolysis (CAMP test). Although GBS can be recovered after overnight growth on nonselective media, such as blood agar, the use of a selective broth medium such as Todd-Hewitt broth or Lim broth greatly enhances the isolation rate of GBS from any culture site.

A major limitation of cultures is the length of time necessary for growth and identification. A number of more rapid screening tests have been developed to directly detect GBS in either body fluids or in cervical-vaginal secretions. These culture-independent tests include Gram stain, latex particle agglutination (LPA), and enzyme immunoassay. A large number of studies have evaluated the ability of these indirect tests to rapidly detect GBS colonization of the maternal lower genital tract. Such identification is important to interrupt maternal-to-neonatal vertical transmission that leads to early-onset neonatal disease. However, subsequent studies have not confirmed initially encouraging results.[29,30] More recently, a study from Quebec reported a fluorogenic polymerase chain reaction (PCR) assay that demonstrated excellent sensitivity and specificity compared to traditional culture methods, but this assay awaits further testing to determine feasibility of widespread application.[31] In addition, only culture techniques currently allow for antibiotic sensitivity profiling of positive cultures, which is particularly important in cases of maternal penicillin hypersensitivity.

Management Options

Prepregnancy

No current evidence suggests that the identification of GBS carrier status prior to pregnancy is predictive of subsequent pregnancy outcome. Similarly, treatment of asymptomatic women found to be colonized with GBS prior to pregnancy does not impart any recognized benefit, with the possible exception of women with asymptomatic bacteruria.

Prenatal, Labor, and Delivery

Group B streptococcus rarely causes maternal symptoms in the prenatal period, but is an infrequent cause of urinary tract infection symptoms. However, GBS bacteriuria (whether symptomatic or not) provides a significant risk factor for neonatal disease, as previously mentioned. When detected, group B streptococcal bacteriuria should be treated according to current standard of care for urinary tract infections during pregnancy. Pregnant women with documented group B streptococcal bacteriuria at any time during their prenatal course will not require screening cultures to be performed and should receive intrapartum antibiotics, which will be discussed in further detail.

Although, in general, the attack rate for neonatal GBS infection is low, a variety of prevention strategies have been advocated because of the high mortality and morbidity rates seen in neonatal GBS disease. These strategies have involved chemoprophylaxis, aimed at eradicating the organism from the mother or the neonate, or immunoprophylaxis, aimed at inducing humoral immunity.

Antibiotic chemoprophylaxis has been advocated for the pregnant patient in either the antepartum or intrapartum period, or for the neonate in the immediate neonatal period. Attempts to eradicate GBS colonization with antepartum treatment have been unsuccessful, and early neonatal prophylaxis is also frequently unsuccessful because many neonates are already septic at birth as a result of in utero infection.[32] Initial chemoprophylactic prevention strategies released in the 1990s focused upon selective intrapartum treatment based upon either the presence of risk factors associated with neonatal infection, maternal genital tract colonization, or both.

Major risk factors for neonatal early-onset GBS disease include low birth weight (<2500 g), premature delivery (<37 weeks of gestation), prolonger duration of rupture of membranes (≥18 hours), and intrapartum fever (≥38.0°C). Boyer and associates have demonstrated that 74% of neonates with early-onset infection and 94% of those infections with a fatal outcome occur among those neonates with one or more of these risk factors.[32] Additional risk factors include having previously had a neonate with invasive GBS disease and maternal GBS bacteriuria during the current pregnancy. A study in 1985 documented that the overall attack rate for early-onset neonatal GBS disease increased from the then observed 3.0 per 1000 births in the total population to 8.4 per 1000 births among those pregnancies in which risk factors were present.[33] The attack rate rose even more dramatically to 40.8 per 1000 births if risk factors were present and the mother was colonized with GBS.

Several studies utilizing the presence of risk factors, maternal colonization status, or both, as a determinant for prophylaxis have documented the efficacy of intrapartum chemoprophylaxis in reducing neonatal early-onset GBS disease.[34–40] A meta-analysis of these studies demonstrated a 30-fold reduction in early-onset disease with intrapartum chemoprophylaxis.[41] The two alternative approaches to intrapartum chemoprophylaxis were proposed in the United States by the CDC in 1996[18] and have been endorsed by both ACOG[17] and the AAP.[19] The first approach is based upon universal screening for maternal GBS colonization at 35 to 37 weeks of gestation. Intrapartum chemoprophylaxis is offered to all pregnant women identified as GBS carriers. In addition, intrapartum chemoprophylaxis is offered to women with a previous neonate with GBS infection, or GBS bacteriuria during the current pregnancy, or delivering prior to 37 weeks of gestation, regardless of maternal colonization status. Women with an unknown carrier status are offered prophylaxis in the event of an intrapartum fever of 38.0°C or higher, or rupture of membranes at 18 hours or before. It was estimated this screening-based approach would result in intrapartum chemoprophylaxis of 26.7% of all deliveries and prevent 86% of early-onset neonatal GBS disease (Table 32–4).[18]

An alternative prophylactic strategy, also initially endorsed by the CDC, is based upon offering intrapartum chemoprophylaxis only in the presence of risk

TABLE 32–4

Intrapartum Chemoprophylaxis (ICP) Trials for the Prevention of Neonatal Early-onset GBS Disease

STUDY	CASE SELECTION*	COMPARISON GROUP	EARLY-ONSET DISEASE ICP	EARLY-ONSET DISEASE NO ICP	P VALUE
Allardice[131]	I	Nonrandom	0/57	9/136	0.06
Boyer[35]	PC	Random	0/85	5/79	0.02
Morales[36]	PC	Random	0/135	3/128	0.2
Morales[37]	I	Nonrandom	0/36	13/48	0.002
Tuppurainen[38]	PC	Random	1/88	10/111	0.03
Matorras[39]	I	Random	0/60	3/65	0.14
Garland[40]	PC	Nonrandom	16/30,197	27/26,915	0.04

*I, intrapartum colonization; PC, prenatal colonization.
Adapted from American Academy of Pediatrics: Revised guidelines for prevention of early-onset group B streptococcus (GBS) infection. Pediatrics 1997;99:489–496.

factors. In this risk-factor approach, prophylaxis would be offered only to those women with delivery prior to 37 weeks' gestation, rupture of membranes at or before 18 hours, an intrapartum fever at or above 38.0°C, a previously infected neonate, or with GBS bacteriuria in the current pregnancy. With this approach, 18.3% of pregnancies were estimated to merit chemoprophylaxis and 68.8% of early-onset neonatal disease would be potentially prevented.[18]

The impact of implementing these guidelines has been studied extensively in the period following their initial recommendation. In the surveillance areas studied, the incidence of early-onset disease declined from 1.7 per 1000 in 1993 to 0.6 per 1000 in 1998, a 65% reduction, with the steepest decline occurring in 1996 following the initial release of consensus guidelines from the CDC. Schrag and associates recently published the first comprehensive study directly comparing the two management strategies, and found that the screening-based approach was greater than 50% more effective in preventing perinatal GBS disease.[42] This result was felt to stem from two main factors. First, the screening-based approach identified mothers who were GBS positive but did not exhibit risk factors during pregnancy or labor, a group representing 18% of all parturients during the study period. Second, women identified as being GBS positive were more likely to receive intrapartum antibiotics than women who qualified on the basis of risk factors (89% versus 61%, $P < 0.001$), indicating improved compliance with the guidelines utilizing the screening-based approach. In this study, similar numbers of patients (24%) in each group received intrapartum prophylaxis, negating previous concerns that the screening-based approach would result in a significant increase in the use of antibiotics and potential contribution to antibiotic resistance. Also, other studies have suggested that the increased cost of performing routine cultures on all eligible pregnant women would be offset by the impact of disease prevention.[20] This idea led to the release of new guidelines by the CDC in 2002, recommending a universal screening-based approach (Fig. 32–1). In addition, a new algorithm is provided for the management of women with preterm delivery, summarized in Figure 32–2.

Intravenous penicillin G (5 million units IV initially, then 2.5 million units every 4 hours until delivery) is preferred for intrapartum chemoprophylaxis. Ampicillin (2 g IV initial dose, then 1 g every 4 hours until delivery) is an acceptable alternative, but penicillin G is preferable because its narrower spectrum of activity may be less likely to select for antibiotic-resistant microorganisms. Previous debate had centered on the minimum duration of therapy for effective prophylaxis, in terms of length of therapy versus number of doses of antibiotics administered prior to delivery. Recent evidence has confirmed that an initial dose of antibiotics at least 4 hours prior to delivery is as effective as two or more doses of antibiotics in preventing GBS transmission[43] and early-onset disease,[44] and this emphasis is maintained in the current guidelines.

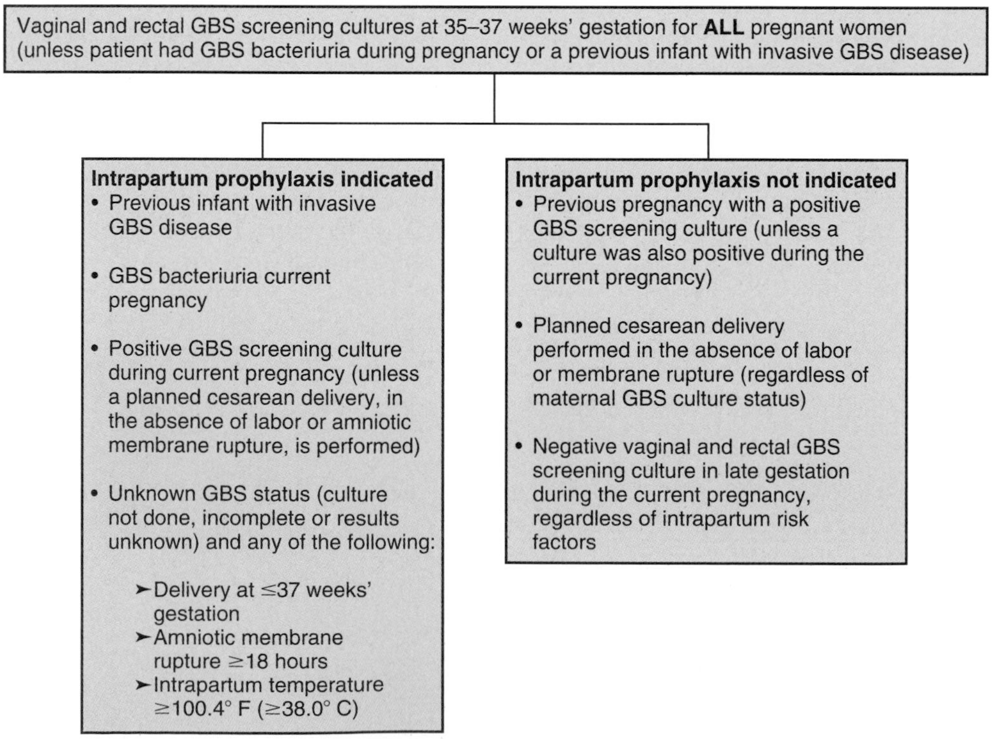
Vaginal and rectal GBS screening cultures at 35–37 weeks' gestation for ALL pregnant women
(unless patient had GBS bacteriuria during pregnancy or a previous infant with invasive GBS disease)
Intrapartum prophylaxis indicated
• Previous infant with invasive GBS disease
• GBS bacteriuria current pregnancy
• Positive GBS screening culture during current pregnancy (unless a planned cesarean delivery, in the absence of labor or amniotic membrane rupture, is performed)
• Unknown GBS status (culture not done, incomplete or results unknown) and any of the following:
➢Delivery at ≤37 weeks' gestation
➢Amniotic membrane rupture ≥18 hours
➢Intrapartum temperature ≥100.4° F (≥38.0° C)
Intrapartum prophylaxis not indicated
• Previous pregnancy with a positive GBS screening culture (unless a culture was also positive during the current pregnancy)
• Planned cesarean delivery performed in the absence of labor or membrane rupture (regardless of maternal GBS culture status)
• Negative vaginal and rectal GBS screening culture in late gestation during the current pregnancy, regardless of intrapartum risk factors

FIGURE 32–1
Indications for intrapartum antibiotic prophylaxis to prevent prenatal GBS disease under a universal prenatal screening strategy based on combined vaginal and rectal cultures collected at 35 to 37 weeks' gestation from all pregnant women. (From CDC: Prevention of perinatal group B streptococcal disease: Revised guidelines from CDC. MMWR 2002;51(RR-11):1–18.)

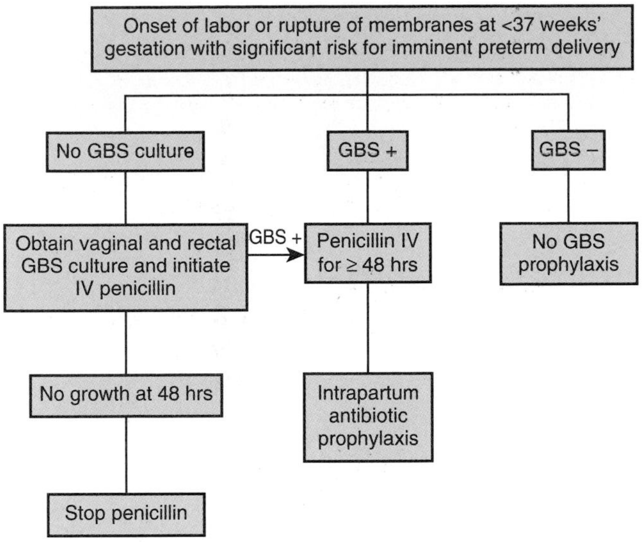

FIGURE 32–2
Sample algorithm for GBS prophylaxis for women with threatened preterm delivery. This algorithm is not an exclusive course of management. Variations that incorporate individual circumstances or institutional preferences may be appropriate. (From CDC: Prevention of perinatal group B streptococcal disease: Revised guidelines from CDC. MMWR 2002;51(RR-11):1–18.)

If pencillin resistance is documented but the risk of anaphylaxis is judged to be low, cefazolin (2 g IV initial dose, then 1 g every 8 hours) may be used. Clindamycin (900 mg IV every 8 hours) or erythromycin (500 mg IV every 6 hours) may be used in the severely penicillin-allergic patient. However, increasing resistance in GBS to both of the agents has led to the recommendation of routine susceptibility testing of positive cultures if penicillin allergy is suspected or documented. In cases of resistant organisms (or unknown susceptibility) and high risk for anaphylaxis to penicillins and cephalosporins, vancomycin (1 g every 12 hours) is the preferred treatment. This underscores the need to accurately determine true beta-lactam allergy as well as risk for anaphylaxis.

An alternative approach to intrapartum chemoprophylaxis is to immunize pregnant women. As noted previously, women delivering neonates with invasive early-onset disease usually have very low (less than 2 μg/mL) serum concentrations of type III GBS antibody.[23] Recent preliminary trials have been conducted among nonpregnant adults utilizing monovalent protein-conjugate vaccines containing capsular polysaccharide antigens against serotypes Ia and Ib,[45] type II,[46] and type III.[47] Further work is needed in this area prior to the implementation of a vaccination strategy toward women of childbearing age and pregnant women.

Postnatal

In thc asymptomatic parturient receiving intrapartum chemoprophylaxis, there is no need to continue antibiotics following delivery. Conversely, in the symptomatic patient with intra-amniotic infection, therapy should be continued as described previously. Because GBS may also be associated with postpartum endometritis, known carriers should be observed closely for this and treated accordingly. Of note, Schrag and associates reported a modest but significant reduction in invasive GBS disease, including postpartum endometritis, among pregnant women following implementation of the original guidelines for intrapartum prophylaxis, from 0.29 cases per 1000 live births in 1993, to 0.23 per 1000 in 1998 ($P < 0.03$).[42] It should be recognized that postpartum endometritis is frequently a polymicrobial infection and broad-spectrum antibiotics should be utilized, even among those patients known to be colonized with GBS.

SUMMARY OF MANAGEMENT OPTIONS
Group B Streptococcal Infection

Management Options	Quality of Evidence	Strength of Recommendation	References
Prepregnancy			
Treatment of GBS carrier before pregnancy has no benefit.	–	GPP	–
Immunization strategies currently are being evaluated.	–	GPP	–
Prenatal, Labor, and Delivery			
Treat symptomatic bacteriuria during prenatal period.	–	GPP	–
Recommended universal screening–based approach:	III	B	18,42
Perform rectal and vaginal cultures on all pregnant women at 35–37 weeks' gestation. (Exception: women with documented GBS bacteriuria during current pregnancy or history of previous GBS-infected infant warrant intrapartum prophylaxis and do not require screening.)			

Continued

SUMMARY OF MANAGEMENT OPTIONS
Group B Streptococcal Infection *(Continued)*

Management Options	Quality of Evidence	Strength of Recommendation	References
Prenatal and Delivery			
Intrapartum antibiotic prophylaxis (IAP) is recommended for all women with positive culture unless delivery by cesarean section prior to rupture of membranes and onset of labor.			
If culture status is unknown at time of delivery, administer IAP for gestation <37 weeks, rupture of membranes = 18 hours, or intrapartum temperature = 38.0°C.			
Suggested management of threatened preterm delivery:	III	B	18
No culture done: obtain cultures and initiate IAP for 48 hours until results obtained or delivery occurs.			
Culture positive prior to or during labor: IAP for 48 hours or until delivery occurs.			
Culture negative prior to labor (or after 48 hours): no IAP (or stop IAP).			
Recommended prophylaxis regimens:	Ia	A	41,43,44
Penicillin G 5 million U IV followed by 2.5 mU IV every 4 hours until delivery (ampicillin 2 g IV initially followed by 1 g IV every 4 hours until delivery is acceptable but less preferred due to broader spectrum activity).			
For penicillin allergic (low anaphylaxis risk), cefazolin 2 g IV initial dose followed by 1 g IV every 8 hours until delivery.			
For penicillin allergic (high anaphylaxis risk, documented susceptibility of GBS), clindamycin 900 mg IV every 8 hours, or erythromycin 500 mg IV every 6 hours.			
For penicillin allergic (high anaphylaxis risk and resistance to clindamycin and erythromycin or susceptibility unknown), vancomycin 1 g IV every 12 hours.			
Immunization strategies currently are being evaluated.	–	GPP	–
Postnatal			
Antibiotic prophylaxis need not be continued after delivery.	–	GPP	–
Diagnosis of postpartum endometritis in a GBS-positive woman should be treated with broad-spectrum antibiotics.	–	GPP	–

LISTERIOSIS

Listeriosis is a relatively uncommon infection, caused by the organism *Listeria monocytogenes*, an aerobic and facultatively anaerobic, non-spore-forming, motile, gram-positive bacillus. However, the infection shows a predilection for populations with relative immunosuppression, including infants, the elderly, and the pregnant woman, with the latter group demonstrating an incidence of 12 per 100,000 (compared to 0.7 per 100,00 in the general population, a 17-fold increase).[48] Most cases of human listeriosis during pregnancy are sporadic with occasional epidemic common-source outbreaks, mostly attributed to contaminated food substances, particularly soft cheeses, other milk products, or processed meats.

Maternal and Fetal Risks

Listeria exhibits an unusual life cycle, demonstrating obligate intracellular replication and spread, without significant exposure to the extracellular environment and its defense mechanisms. Thus, cell-mediated immunity is the primary host defense, and this may explain the unique susceptibility of humans to this infection during periods of relative suppression of cell-mediated immunity, including pregnancy.[49]

Listeria infection is well established as a cause of pregnancy loss in domestic and wild animals. Subsequently, it has been implicated as a possible cause for recurrent spontaneous abortion in pregnant women. An Israeli study reported a significantly increased rate of multiple positive cervical cultures for *Listeria* in women with a history of recurrent losses, compared to a control group without such history.[50] However, subsequent studies failed to replicate this association, and at this time the association is controversial.[51–53] Multiple gestation pregnancies may also be at increased risk for listeriosis, as reported by Mascola and associates.[54]

Pregnant women with listeriosis most commonly suffer from a flu-like illness, with fever, general malaise, and other nonspecific symptoms. Rarely it may cause meningoencephalitis or sepsis-like manifestations. In one large series, 65% of patients had fever (defined usually as temperature at or above 38.2°C), 32% a "flu-like" illness, 21.5% abdominal or back pain, and less commonly headache, myalgia, or sore throat.[55] The average duration of symptoms prior to diagnosis was 6.6 days. Of note, 29% of patients were asymptomatic.

The primary mode of transmission to the fetus or newborn has not been proved, but is suspected to occur via either ascending infection through the vaginal canal, or transplacentally secondary to maternal bacteremia.[48] Neonatal listeriosis may present as respiratory distress, fever, neurologic symptoms, or skin rash, or it may be asymptomatic. Rarely, the infant may present with granulomatosis infantisepticum, which classically exhibits disseminated granulomatous reaction in the lung, skin, liver, and other locations. Similar to group B streptococcal infection in the neonate, there is a bimodal distribution of disease. Early-onset infection (usually defined as less than 5 days of life) is more commonly associated with maternal illness and produces a sepsis-like illness, with onset of disease exhibited within hours of birth. Late-onset disease presents more commonly as meningitis, is less commonly associated with maternal symptoms or positive *Listeria* cultures, and may be associated with nosocomial or environmental acquisition.[56]

Outcomes of pregnancies complicated by listeriosis vary. In the study by Mylonakis amd associates, 1 in 5 pregnancies resulted in spontaneous abortion or stillbirth.[55] In the remainder, 68.3% of the infants demonstrated infection with a positive culture from one or more sites. Of these infants for which follow-up was available, 62.8% recovered completely, 24.5% died, and 12.7% recovered with neurologic sequelae or other long-term complications. The worst prognosis occurred in patients with meningeal involvement. Similar data were reported in a British review of 248 perinatal cases of listeriosis from 1967 to 1985 in which 19% of cases in which the outcome was known resulted in abortion or stillbirth.[56] Of the remaining infants in which gestational age was known, 58% were delivered prematurely (defined as <38 weeks). The overall neonatal mortality rate in known outcome cases was 35%.

Diagnosis

Listeria grows well on most routine media, although the use of selective media may be required when cultures are obtained from sites of heavy bacterial colonization such as vagina or rectum. Owing to morphologic similarity, it may be confused with nonpathogenic diphtheroids. However, the organism produces a characteristic tumbling motion when viewed on wet preparation, allowing it to be distinguished. Of the four serotypes, subtypes 1/2a, 1/2b, and 4b are responsible for the vast majority of infections, and serotype analysis may be useful in epidemic settings.[48]

The diagnosis depends upon clinical suspicion and isolation of the organism from a culture of appropriate source. In the large series mentioned previously, *Listeria* was most commonly isolated from cultures of the blood (43%), cervix/vagina (34%), and placenta (12%). It may also be cultured from amniotic fluid obtained by amniocentesis performed for suspected intra-amniotic infection. Staining of amniotic fluid by meconium, especially in the preterm infant, may increase clinical suspicion for listeriosis, as this was observed in 12 of 23 infants in a reported series from Australian authors.[57]

Management Options

Prepregnancy

Treatment of listeriosis in the nonpregnant woman is identical to that of other adult patients and dependent on the site of the infection (i.e., bacteremia versus meningitis or other location). As mentioned, the possibility of *Listeria* colonization or carriage as a risk factor for subsequent pregnancy loss has been previously evaluated with inconclusive results. Thus, the role of *Listeria* as a cause of poor obstetric outcome in asymptomatic patients is questionable, and routine screening is not recommended at this time.[48]

Prenatal, Labor, and Delivery

Prevention of maternal listeriosis has been targeted as a primary objective following epidemiologic data confirming the role of contaminated food products as a major source for listeriosis, both in epidemic and sporadic cases. A large outbreak occurred in 1985 in the Los Angeles area, in which 65.5% of all cases were pregnant women or their offspring.[58] A surveillance project followed,

TABLE 32–5

Dietary Recommendations for Pregnant Women

Do not eat hot dogs, luncheon meats, or deli meats **unless they are reheated** until steaming hot.
Do not eat soft cheeses such as feta, brie, camembert, blue-veined cheeses, and Mexican-style cheeses such as "queso blanco fresco." Hard cheeses, semisoft cheeses such as mozzarella, pasteurized processed cheese slices and spreads, cream cheese, and cottage cheese can be safely consumed.
Do not eat refrigerated pâté or meat spreads. Canned or shelf-stable pâté and meat spreads can be eaten.
Do not eat refrigerated smoked seafood **unless** it is an ingredient in a **cooked** dish such as a casserole. Examples of refrigerated smoked seafood include salmon, trout, whitefish, cod, tuna, and mackerel, which are most often labeled as "nova-style," "lox," "kippered," "smoked," or "jerky." This fish is found in the refrigerated section or sold at deli counters of grocery stores and delicatessens. Canned fish such as salmon and tuna or shelf-stable smoked seafood may be safely eaten.
Do not drink raw (unpasteurized) milk **or eat** foods that contain unpasteurized milk.

beginning in 1986, coordinated between the Food and Drug Administration (FDA) and CDC over multiple diverse demographic areas throughout the United States. This effort led to identification of many at-risk food sources and implementation of more stringent regulations for these food groups over the next several years.[59] In 1992, multiple agencies including the CDC, FDA, and FSIS (Food Safety and Inspection Service) issued dietary recommendations for persons at increased risk, including pregnant women. Results of this project resulted in a decrease of perinatal listeriosis in the surveillance areas from 17.4 per 100,000 (1989) to 8.6 per 100,000 (1993, $P < 0.003$).[59] A list of at-risk food substances has been summarized in a handout for pregnant women on the FSIS website and may be viewed in Table 32–5.[60]

For women with suspected or confirmed listeriosis during pregnancy, intravenous antibiotics are indicated. Multiple cases have been reported of successful antepartum treatment of listeriosis with normal neonatal outcome, including cases diagnosed in the first and second trimesters.[60–62] First-line therapy consists of ampicillin 2g given every 6 hours for 10 to 14 days. The addition of gentamicin for synergistic activity has been recommended in some cases but lacks adequate study to determine a conclusive advantage. Because of its bactericidal activity and excellent intracellular concentration, trimethoprim/sulfamethoxazole (20 mg/kg/day TMP component IV divided into four daily doses) is the recommended second-line therapeutic agent in cases of penicillin-allergic patients.[49] However, because of fetal effects, its utility must be evaluated in each case individually, weighing the potential risks and benefits. This underscores the necessity of accurately determining true penicillin-allergy status and consideration of desensitization therapy. Other second-line considerations include erythromycin, vancomycin, or the carbapenems, but experience is limited. Cephalosporins are not effective against *Listeria*.

Postnatal

For mothers with proven listeriosis, antibiotic therapy should be continued for a total of 10 to 14 days for bacteremia or superficial infections, or 14 to 21 days for meningitis. Care of the neonate should involve obtaining blood and CSF cultures to assess potential infection, and empiric treatment with ampicillin and gentamicin pending culture results. Antibiotic therapy is recommended for a minimum of 14 days in cases of bacteremia or pneumonia, and 21 days in cases involving the CNS.

SUMMARY OF MANAGEMENT OPTIONS

Listeriosis Monocytogenes

Management Options	Quality of Evidence	Strength of Recommendation	References
Prepregnancy			
No benefit to screening and treatment.	III	B	48
Treatment of documented infection depending on the site (see below)	IV	C	60, 61, 62
Prenatal, Labor, and Delivery			
Avoid unpasteurized dairy products and certain meat products (see Table 32–5)	III	B	59, 60
Culture appropriate sites if listeriosis suspected (blood, CSF, cervix, amniotic fluid).	–	GPP	–
Treatment	IV	C	60, 61, 62
First-line therapy: IV ampicillin 200 mg/kg/day (divided into four doses), max = 12/g/Day			

SUMMARY OF MANAGEMENT OPTIONS
Listeriosis Monocytogenes *(Continued)*

Management Options	Quality of Evidence	Strength of Recommendation	References
Prenatal, Labor, and Delivery			
For penicillin-sensitive patients: trimethoprim/sulfamethoxazole (20 mg/kg/day in three or four doses).			
Other antibiotics: erythromycin, vancomycin. *Note*: cephalosporins not effective.			
Duration of therapy: 10–14 days for superficial infection/bacteremia; 14–21 days for meningitis.			
Postnatal			
Evaluate neonate with blood and CSF cultures.	–	GPP	–

SEXUALLY TRANSMITTED DISEASES

Gonorrhea

Gonorrhea is a common sexually transmitted disease caused by *Neisseria gonorrhoeae*, a gram-negative diplococcus. The prevalence of gonococcal infection in pregnancy varies, depending upon the population studied, from 0.5% to 7.4% in the United States.[63,64] Risk factors for gonococcal infection include multiple sexual partners, young age, nonwhite race, low socioeconomic status, and being unmarried.

Maternal and Fetal Risks

The most prevalent type of gonococcal infection in pregnancy is asymptomatic infection of the cervix. *N. gonorrhoeae* may also cause acute cervicitis, proctitis, pharyngitis, and disseminated systemic infection. The rate of pharyngeal gonococcal infection increases during pregnancy, possibly as a result of altered sexual practices.[65] Disseminated gonococcal infection (DGI) also occurs more frequently in pregnant than nonpregnant women.[66] DGI is characterized by a bacteremic phase associated with malaise, fever, and a pustular hemorrhagic rash, a secondary septic arthritis stage usually with asymmetrical involvement of the knees, wrists, or ankles. Acute salpingitis secondary to gonococcal infection may rarely occur during the first trimester but is rare after the 12th week of gestation because obliteration of the endometrial cavity by the pregnancy prevents ascending infection. In pregnancy, gonococcal cervicitis has been associated with premature rupture of the membranes, premature delivery, chorioamnionitis, and both postabortion and postpartum endometritis.[67,68] In addition, gonococcal ophthalmia neonatorum may develop in up to 40% of newborns exposed to maternal infection and who did not receive ocular prophylaxis.

Diagnosis

It is estimated that up to 80% of women with gonococcal infection of the cervix are asymptomatic; for this reason, prevention of sequelae of gonorrhea depends upon prenatal screening to detect infected parturients. Diagnosis depends upon the demonstration of gram-negative intracellular diplococci within leukocytes of a smear obtained from an exudate, if present, or upon culture. Cultures should be inoculated immediately after collection onto a selective medium such as Thayer-Martin. Culture-independent identification of *N. gonorrhoeae* by immunoassay or DNA detection assays, are also available and have been demonstrated to be highly specific and sensitive for the detection of gonococcal infections.

Management Options

PREPREGNANCY

Guidelines are similar for most STDs with regard to the identification and treatment of these diseases prior to pregnancy. Test of cure cultures should be done, as well as partner notification and treatment.

PRENATAL

Uncomplicated gonorrhea in pregnancy should be treated with cefixime 400 mg orally in a single dose, ceftriaxone 125 mg intramuscularly in single dose, or spectinomycin, 2 g intramuscularly in a single dose (Table 32–6). Because concurrent cervical infection with *Chlamydia trachomatis* occurs frequently,[69] azithromycin 1 g orally in a single dose or erythromycin base 500 mg orally four times daily for 7 days should also be administered, unless specific testing for *C. trachomatis* has been done. For disseminated gonococcal infection, hospitalization and parenteral therapy are recommended for initial therapy. Recommended regimens include ceftriaxone 1 g intramuscularly or intravenously once daily, ceftizoxime 1 g intravenously every 8

TABLE 32-6

Treatment of Uncomplicated Gonococcal or Chlamydial Infections in Pregnancy

Gonococcal infection
- Recommended:
  - Cefixime 400 mg orally in a single dose, or
  - Ceftriazone 125 mg IM in a single dose
- Alternative:
  - Spectinomycin 2 g IM
  - Aqueous procaine penicillin G, 4.8 million units IM or Amoxicillin 3 g orally, both with probenecid 1 g orally*
  - All regimens followed by erythromycin 1 g orally in a single dose or base 500 mg orally four times daily for 7 days, or amoxicillin 500 mg orally three times daily for 7 days

Chlamydial infections
- Recommended:
  - Azithromycin 1 g orally in a single dose, or
  - Erythromycin base 500 mg orally four times daily for 7 days
- Alternative:
  - Erythromycin base 250 mg orally four times daily for 14 days
  - Amoxicillin 500 mg orally three times daily for 7 days
  - Clindamycin 450 mg orally four times daily for 7 days

*Recommended only if infection source known not to have penicillin-resistant gonorrhea.

hours, or cefotaxime 1 g intravenously every 8 hours. Parenteral therapy should be continued until 24 to 48 hours after symptoms resolve and then converted to oral therapy for a total of 1 week of antibiotics. In areas where penicillin-resistant strains are uncommon, parenteral ampicillin, 1 g intravenously every 6 hours, may be used. Identification, screening, and treatment of sexual contacts of patients with gonococcal infection is recommended.

Tetracyclines and the quinoline antibiotics are also highly effective in gonococcal infections but are contraindicated in pregnancy because of potential adverse fetal effects.

LABOR AND DELIVERY

Rapid diagnostic screening tools such as Gram stain, immune-based assays, and DNA detection assays are available. These tests can be useful in evaluating the intrapartum patient at risk for infection. Intrapartum treatment of the mother may reduce the neonate's risk for infection, although specific treatment and ocular prophylaxis of the infant after delivery is usually done.

POSTNATAL

Treatment guidelines for the postpartum patient are similar to those outlined previously. However, doxycyline or the quinolone antibiotics may be used in nonlactating women.

Chlamydia Trachomatis

Chlamydia trachomatis is the cause of one of the most prevalent sexually transmitted bacterial infections in the world and is the most prevalent sexually transmitted bacterial organism in the United States.[70] Chlamydiae are obligate intracellular organisms. *Chlamydia trachomatis* may be differentiated into 15 serotypes. Serotypes A, B, and C cause endemic trachoma, a chronic ocular infection considered to be the leading cause of blindness in the world. Serotypes L1, L2, and L3 cause lymphogranuloma venereum, discussed later in this chapter. Serotypes D through K cause genital and ocular infections, discussed in this section. The prevalence of genital infection in pregnant women in the United States has been reported as between 2% and 37%, with an average estimate of 5% to 7%.[71–73] Risk factors for cervical infection include young age, single marital status, multiple sexual partners, and previous history of sexually transmitted disease.[70]

Maternal and Fetal Risks

The majority of infected patients have asymptomatic cervical infection. In the nonpregnant female, chlamydial infections may cause mucopurulent cervicitis, endometritis, acute salpingitis, infertility and ectopic pregnancy, and acute urethral syndrome. The role of maternal chlamydial infection in pregnancy is more controversial. Several studies have found an association between maternal cervical infection and preterm delivery, premature rupture of the membranes, low birth weight, perinatal death, and late-onset postpartum endometritis.[74–77] Two prospective studies have found that only those women with recently acquired infection, as detected by the presence of IgM serum antibody to *C. trachomatis*, are at increased risk for premature rupture of membranes, preterm delivery, and low birth weight.[73,78] Treatment and eradication of maternal cervical chlamydial infection reduce the risk of premature rupture of the membranes and premature delivery.[79–81] Thus, the available data suggest an association between maternal chlamydial infection and adverse pregnancy outcome and that screening and treatment in pregnancy is warranted.

Maternal chlamydial infection also poses significant risk to the neonate. Approximately 50% to 60% of the neonates delivered vaginally to a women with chlamydial cervicitis will be colonized with *C. trachomatis*.[72] The most common manifestations of neonatal infection are inclusion conjunctivitis and pneumonia. Eighteen percent to 50% of exposed infants develop conjunctivitis within the first 2 weeks of life, and 11% to 18% will develop pneumonia in the first 4 months of life.

Diagnosis

The diagnosis of chlamydial infections is based upon isolation of the organism, or culture-independent detection by immunoassay, DNA detection by PCR and serologic testing. Because chlamydiae are obligatory intracellular bacteria, isolation by culture requires inoculation onto a susceptible tissue culture cell line. Cell cultures are both labor intensive and expensive and are not readily available to most clinicians. Antigen detection kits are widely available to detect chlamydia and represent a less costly alternative to culture. More recently, detection of *C. trachomatis* DNA from the genital tract, or from urine, by PCR or LCR has been demonstrated to be greater than 90% sensitive and specific for the detection of *C. trachomatis* and has largely replaced cultures and antigen detection assays. A serum microimmunofluorescent antibody test is also available to detect recent or past infection but is more useful as a research tool than for the clinical diagnosis of chlamydial infection.

Management Options

PREPREGNANCY

Chlamydia trachomatis is susceptible to a wide range of antibiotics including azithromycin, erythromycin, doxycycline, tetracycline, and ofloxacin. For the nonpregnant patient azithromycin 1 g orally in a single dose, erythromycin base 500 mg orally four times daily for 7 days, doxycycline 100 mg orally two times a day, or tetracycline 500 mg orally four times a day for 7 days is recommended. Ofloxacin, a quinoline antibiotic, given as 300 mg orally twice a day, is also highly effective in the nonpregnant patient.

PRENATAL

In pregnancy, azithromycin 1 g orally in a single dose, erythromycin base 500 mg orally four times a day for 7 days, or erythromycin ethylsuccinate 800 mg orally four times a day for 7 days is recommended (see Table 32–6). If gastrointestinal intolerance occurs, these doses may be reduced in half, and therapy extended to 14 days. Erythromycin estolate should probably not be used because it may be associated with hepatotoxicity when given during pregnancy. Because erythromycin therapy is frequently associated with gastrointestinal intolerance in pregnancy, alternative regimens have been proposed. Therapy with either amoxicillin, 500 mg orally three times a day for 7 days, or clindamycin, 450 mg orally four times a day for 14 days, results in cure rates (98% and 93%, respectively) comparable to cure rates with erythromycin base therapy, and are better tolerated by the patient.[82,83] Sexual contacts should be examined and treated.

LABOR AND DELIVERY

See the section on gonorrhea.

POSTNATAL

The incidence of neonatal inclusion conjunctivitis can be reduced by ocular prophylaxis at birth with 0.5% erythromycin ocular ointment or 1% tetracycline ointment, but not as well by 1% silver nitrate drops. Conjunctivitis that does occur, or pneumonia, should be treated with oral erythromycin for 2 weeks.

Genital Mycoplasmas

Maternal and Fetal Risks

Mycoplasmas are a ubiquitous group of microorganisms that inhabit the mucosa of the genital and respiratory tracts. They differ from bacteria in that they lack a cell wall, but they are susceptible to antibiotics that inhibit protein synthesis. The two most common genital mycoplasmas are *Mycoplasma hominis* and *Ureaplasma urealyticum*. The prevalence of these two microorganisms in the lower genital tract in sexually active women has been reported as 40% to 95% for *U. urealyticum* and 15% to 70% for *M. hominis*. Their high prevalence rates among otherwise healthy women make it difficult to determine their role in adverse pregnancy outcomes. In general, *M. hominis* has been associated in some, but not all, studies with septic abortion, postpartum endometritis, and postpartum fever.[78,84,85] *Ureaplasma urealyticum* has been associated with histologic chorioamnionitis, low birth weight, and perinatal death.[86–89]

Serologic evidence of infection with *M. hominis* has been found in 50% of febrile abortions versus 17% of afebrile abortions.[84] In a recent study of early postpartum endometritis among women, genital mycoplasmas, including *M. hominis*, accounted for 30% of the total endometrial isolates and 19% of the total blood isolates, but were usually recovered in association with other pathogenic bacteria, suggesting a mixed infection.[85] *M. hominis* has also been isolated from amniotic fluid of patients with amniotic fluid infection, but almost always in association with other bacteria, again implying a mixed infection.[24] Significantly, infected patients from whom *M. hominis* is recovered almost always respond to therapy with beta-lactam antibiotics, which have no activity against genital mycoplasmas.

A number of studies have found an association between *U. urealyticum* and chorioamnionitis[87,88] and with perinatal death.[88,90] In one study, *U. urealyticum* was isolated as the sole isolate from fetal lungs in 24 (8%) of 290 perinatal deaths.[90] Twenty-two of these deaths occurred in utero and all but one were associated with pneumonia and chorioamnionitis, implying an ascending intrauterine infection. Some studies have also found decreased birth weight among offspring of women colonized with *U. urealyticum*,[86] but this association has not been confirmed by others.[78] Intervention treatment trials have also been inconclusive. McCormack and associates demonstrated an increase in birth weight among the offspring of women colonized with *U. urealyticum* treated with erythromycin in the third trimester when compared to colonized women treated with placebo.[91] Because the presence of potential genital pathogens was not ascertained, their potentially confounding influence upon birth weight cannot be excluded. In contrast, Eschenbach and associates found no beneficial effect of erythromycin taken for up to 14 weeks by a large cohort of women colonized for *U. ureaplasma* upon birth weight, gestational age at delivery, frequency of premature rupture of membranes, or in neonatal outcome.[92] In this study, women also colonized with either *Chlamydia trachomatis* or group B streptococci were excluded from analysis, eliminating any potential confounding bias from coinfection.

Management Options

Taken collectively, the data linking either *M. hominis* or *U. urealyticum* to adverse pregnancy outcome are inconclusive. At present, antenatal vaginal cultures for either of these mycoplasmas cannot be recommended. Current evidence does not support the treatment of colonized patients for the prevention of adverse pregnancy outcomes. If treatment is deemed necessary, tetracycline is effective against both *M. hominis* and *U. urealyticum* but should not be used in pregnancy. *Ureaplasma urealyticum* is also sensitive to erythromycin but is resistant to clindamycin; *M hominis* is resistant to erythromycin but sensitive to clindamycin. Because the mycoplasmas lack a cell wall, they are resistant to beta-lactam antibiotics.

Chancroid

Maternal and Fetal Risks

Chancroid is an acute ulcerative disease, usually of the genitals, caused by infection with *Haemophilus ducreyi*, a facultative gram-negative bacillus. Although rare in North America and Europe, it remains an important public health concern in developing countries. Chancroid is spread only through sexual contact and is much more prevalent in men than women. The incubation period after transmission is usually between 4 and 7 days. A chancre then develops at the site of entry, beginning as a small papule that, over the course of 1 to 2 days, becomes eroded and ulcerated. Although the ulcer is usually quite painful in men, it is frequently not painful in women. In women, the majority of ulcers are on the fourchette, vestibule, or labia minora. The classic ulcer of chancroid is shallow with an irregular border surrounded by erythema. The base of the ulcer is frequently covered with a necrotic exudate. Painful inguinal adenopathy develops in about 50% of cases and may lead to suppuration and spontaneous rupture if untreated. These buboes appear 7 to 10 days after the initial ulcer and are unilateral in two thirds of cases. *Haemophilus ducreyi* has not been shown to cause systemic infection or spread to distant sites and poses no special risk to pregnancy.

Management Options

The diagnosis of chancroid is based upon clinical characteristics and Gram stain and culture of the ulcer or aspirated bubo. The Gram stain may reveal gram-negative rods that form chains but has a sensitivity of only 50%.[93] Cultures should be taken from the base of the ulcer and placed on selective media. Cultures are both sensitive and specific in the diagnosis of *H. ducreyi* infection, but may not be readily available. An enzyme-linked immunosorbent assay has been developed that is both sensitive and specific and may represent a good alternative when culture is not available.

H. ducreyi is susceptible to a variety of antibiotics, although resistance to sulfonamides and tetracycline has emerged which precludes their use. Quinolones, which are very active against *H. ducreyi*, are contraindicated during pregnancy. Current recommended regimens which may be given in pregnancy include (1) azithromycin 1 g orally in a single dose; (2) erythromycin base 500 mg four times daily for 7 days; (3) ceftriaxone 250 mg intramuscularly as a single dose; and (4) trimethoprim/sulfamethoxazole 160/800 mg orally two times daily for 7 days. Azithromycin and ceftriaxone offer the advantage of single-dose therapy. Although evidence of fetal toxicity is lacking, trimethoprim/sulfamethoxazole is generally not recommended for use in pregnancy if other alternatives are available because it is a folic acid antagonist. Treatment of sexual partners is recommended.

Lymphogranuloma Venereum

Maternal and Fetal Risks

Lymphogranuloma venereum (LGV) is a sexually transmitted disease caused by *Chlamydia trachomatis* serotypes L1, L2, and L3. It is characterized by inguinal lymphangitis, anogenital lesions, and fibrosis with gross distortion of the perineal tissues. Although LGV occurs sporadically in North America, Europe, and Australia, it is endemic in Africa, India, Southeast Asia, and parts of South America.[94] LGV is predominantly a disease of lymphatic tissue characterized by thrombolymphangitis and spread of the inflammatory process into the adjacent tissues. Three stages of infection are recognized: primary, secondary, and tertiary. The primary lesion is characterized by a small shallow genital ulcer that appears at the site of infection after an incubation period of 3 to 12 days and heals rapidly and is associated with few symptoms. The secondary stage occurs 10 to 30 days later and is characterized by inguinal lymphadenitis, buboes, inflammatory mats of contiguous lymph nodes, and loculated abscesses. The tertiary stage is characterized by a chronic inflammatory response with progressive tissue destruction, ulceration, fistula formation, and lymphatic obstruction. Antibiotic treatment during the secondary stage will prevent these tertiary complications.

The course of the disease is not dramatically altered by pregnancy, and transmission to the fetus does not occur. However, infection may be acquired during birth and passage through the infected birth canal.

Management Options

The diagnosis of LGV is based upon clinical appearance, serologic test, and recovery of *C. trachomatis* from infected tissue or its identification by the direct immunofluorescent antibody test. The Frei intradermal antigen test, formerly used in the diagnosis of LGV, has now largely been replaced by the complement fixation test for *Chlamydia* group antibodies. This test is very sensitive and titers greater than 1:64 are diagnostic of infection.

A variety of antibiotics have been used to treat LGV. Nonpregnant patients and sexual partners of pregnant patients should be treated with tetracycline (500 mg orally four times a day) or doxycycline (100 mg orally two times a day) for 21 days. An alternative regimen that may be used in pregnancy is erythromycin base 500 mg orally four times a day for 21 days. Late sequelae such as fistulas or strictures may require subsequent surgical repair.

Granuloma Inguinale (Donovanosis)

Maternal and Fetal Risks

Granuloma inguinale (GI) is a rare, chronic genital infection characterized by granulomatous ulcers. It is common in tropical climates and developing countries, but extremely rare in temperate climates.[95] Granule inguinale is caused by infection with Calymmatobacterium granulomatis, a facultative, gram-negative bacillus. Although most infections probably result from sexual transmission, autoinoculation and nonsexual transmission also occur. The infection is only mildly contagious, and repeated close physical contact is necessary for transmission.[96] Following infection, the incubation period varies from 8 to 80 days. The disease begins as a subcutaneous nodule that erodes through the skin and slowly enlarges to form an exuberant, granulomatous heaped ulcer, which is usually painless. Redundant, beefy-red granulation tissue may be present, giving an exophytic appearance to the lesion. In the female, these lesions are most commonly on the labia.

Pregnancy may accelerate the growth of these lesions. The effects of GI upon the fetus are not completely understood, but perinatal transmission at the time of birth through an infected birth canal has been reported.[97]

Management Options

The diagnosis of GI is based upon the clinical appearance of the disease. The diagnosis is readily confirmed by examination of a smear of a crushed tissue preparation of the lesion. The smear is stained with Wright or Giemsa stain and examined for Donovan bodies. Donovan bodies are the darkly stained organisms within cytoplasmic inclusions contained in infected mononuclear cells. Their presence is diagnostic for GI. Neither cultures nor serologic tests are available.

The treatment of GI for nonpregnant patients is tetracycline 500 mg orally four times a day for a minimum of 3 weeks. Chloramphenicol and gentamicin have been used successfully for resistant cases. In pregnancy, erythromycin base (500 mg orally four times a day) for at least 3 weeks or trimethoprim-sulfamethoxazole (two tablets orally twice a day) are effective. Azithromycin (1 g orally per week for at least 3 weeks) may also be effective. The addition of a parenteral aminoglycoside should be considered if improvement is not evident within the first few days of therapy. Treatment should continue for a minimum of 3 weeks and until lesions are completely healed to prevent recurrence. Treatment of asymptomatic sexual partners is generally not recommended.

SUMMARY OF MANAGEMENT OPTIONS

Sexually Transmitted Diseases

Management Options	Quality of Evidence	Strength of Recommendation	References
Gonorrhea			
Prepregnancy			
Identify and treat prior to pregnancy.	III	B	67
Contact tracing and treatment.	III	B	67
Confirm response with follow-up swabs.	III	B	67
Prenatal			
Give antibiotics (see Table 32–6).	III	B	67
Contact tracing and treatment.	III	B	67
Exclude chlamydia infection.	III	B	69
Postnatal			
Screen newborn for infection, although most units treat anyway.	–	GPP	–

Continued

SUMMARY OF MANAGEMENT OPTIONS
Sexually Transmitted Diseases *(Continued)*

Management Options	Quality of Evidence	Strength of Recommendation	References
Chlamydia			
Prepregnancy			
Identify and treat with doxycycline or ofloxacin.	Ia	A	80,82,83
Contact tracing and treatment.	Ia	A	80,82,83
Prenatal-Treatment			
If diagnosed, give antibiotics (see Table 32–6).	Ia	A	80,82,83
Contact tracing and treatment.	Ia	A	80,82,83
Mycoplasma			
Prenatal			
If treatment necessary, use erythromycin.	Ia	A	92
Chancroid			
Prenatal			
Treatment of patient and partner with either erythromycin, a cephalosporin, or ampicillin/clavulonate.	IV	C	94
Lymphogranuloma Venereum			
Prenatal			
Erythromycin if diagnosed in pregnancy.	IV	C	94
Fistulas or strictures may need repair after pregnancy.	IV	C	94
Granuloma Inguinale			
Prenatal			
Erythromycin, azithromycin, or cotrimoxazole for a minimum of 3 weeks.	IV	C	95,96

VAGINITIS

Vaginal discharge is one of the most common complaints of pregnant patients. The discharge may be the result of normal physiologic adaptations of pregnancy or may result from infectious vaginitis, with possible increased risk for pregnancy complications. The vagina has both a nutrient-rich biochemical mileau and a complex microbial flora. A normal vaginal discharge consists of water (primarily as a serum transudate), desquamated epithelial cells, microorganisms, electrolytes, and organic compounds including organic acids, fatty acids, proteins, and carbohydrates (primarily glycogen).[98] Normal vaginal fluid contains two to nine species of facultative and anaerobic bacteria in concentrations of 10^9 colony-forming units/mL.[99] Normally, facultative lactobacillus species account for the majority of the total organisms present. These microorganisms utilize the available glycogen, producing lactic acid, which serves to acidify the vaginal pH to less than 4.5, inhibiting the growth of non-acid-tolerant potentially pathogenic microorganisms. They also produce hydrogen peroxide, a potent antimicrobial toxin to other microorganisms including *Candida albicans*, *Gardnerella vaginalis*, and anaerobic bacteria.[99,100] When this complex relationship is changed, potentially pathogenic microorganisms indigenous to the vagina such as *C. albicans* or *G. vaginalis* and the anaerobes, may proliferate and cause vaginal discharge. Alternatively, sexually transmitted exogenous microorganisms, such as *Trichomonas vagi-*

nalis, may disrupt the normal vaginal ecosystem and lead to vaginitis.

Pregnancy may also lead to physiologic changes of the lower genital tract, which may predispose to vaginitis. During pregnancy, the vaginal walls become engorged with blood, leading to increased transudation, and the glycogen content of the vagina increases.[99] Elevated levels of progesterone seen during pregnancy enhance the adherence of *C. albicans* to vaginal epithelial cells. Finally, cell-mediated immunity is impaired during pregnancy, predisposing to candidal infections.

The three most commonly occurring causes of infectious vaginitis in pregnancy are bacterial vaginosis, candidiasis, and trichomoniasis. Although frequently asymptomatic, these infections have been implicated in a variety of adverse pregnancy outcomes. Bacterial vaginosis has been associated with premature rupture of the membranes, preterm labor and delivery, amniotic fluid infection, chorioamnionitis, and postpartum endometritis.[75,85,89,101,102] *Trichomonas vaginalis* has been associated with premature rupture of the membranes and a reduction in gestational age at delivery,[71,103] and *Candida albicans* has been associated with intraamniotic infection.[102]

The diagnosis of vaginitis is based in large part upon the appearance of the discharge and microscopic examination of the discharge. However, microscopic examination is somewhat insensitive and accurately identifies only 60% to 70% of women with symptomatic infection. Cultures for *Candida* species and *T. vaginalis* are both highly sensitive and specific but are not widely available, and vaginal cultures for anaerobes or *G. vaginalis* are not useful in the identification of bacterial vaginosis. Other adjunctive diagnostic tests, as described later, are therefore frequently utilized in confirming the diagnosis of vaginitis.

Bacterial Vaginosis

Maternal and Fetal Risks

Bacterial vaginosis is the most common vaginal infection of sexually active women. Bacterial vaginosis occurs in approximately 20% of pregnant women.[75,101,102] In contrast to other vaginal infections, bacterial vaginosis cannot be attributed to a single pathogenic microorganism. Rather, the symptoms associated with bacterial vaginosis result from an increase in the prevalence and concentration of certain facultative and anaerobic bacteria normally found as part of the vaginal microflora. Specifically, there is an increased prevalence of *Gardnerella vaginalis*, selected anaerobes (*Bacteroides*, *Peptostreptococcus*, and *Mobiluncus*), and *Mycoplasma hominis*, and a decreased prevalence of hydrogen peroxidase–producing *Lactobacillus*.[100,104] Additionally, there is a 100-fold increase in the intravaginal concentration of *G. vaginalis* and a 1000-fold increase in the concentration of the anaerobes.[104] Thus, the diagnosis of bacterial vaginosis does not depend upon the recovery or identification of any single microorganism from the vagina, but rather requires the recognition of the altered vaginal microbial milieu. An association between bacterial vaginosis and adverse pregnancy outcome has been reported in several studies. Bacterial vaginosis has been associated with preterm labor or delivery, amniotic fluid infection, chorioamnionitis, and postpartum endometritis. This association is based upon the following:

- Case-control and cohort studies demonstrating an approximate twofold increase in preterm labor or delivery among women with bacterial vaginosis (Table 32–7)
- The recovery of bacterial vaginosis–associated microorganisms from the amniotic fluid of 30% of women with intact fetal membranes in preterm labor and subclinical amniotic fluid infection (see Martius and Eschenbach[101] for a review)
- The frequent recovery of bacterial vaginosis–associated microorganisms from amniotic fluid of women with overt clinical amniotic fluid infection[105] or from the chorioamnion of women with histologic chorioamnionitis or preterm delivery[89]
- The recovery of *Gardnerella vaginalis* or anaerobes associated with bacterial vaginosis from the endometrium in over 60% of women with early postpartum endometritis[106]

Little is known about the mechanisms by which bacterial vaginosis may cause prematurity. The increased intravaginal concentrations of bacteria may simply overwhelm the local host defenses, allowing for ascending infection. Alternatively, these bacteria could also produce protease or phospholipases, which weaken the membranes or stimulate prostaglandin production.[107] Although the magnitude of the increased risk for prematurity noted in

TABLE 32–7

Association between Bacterial Vaginosis and Preterm Labor or Preterm Birth

STUDY	RISK RATIO OR ODDS RATIO	95% CONFIDENCE INTERVAL
Case-control		
Eschenbach, 1984[100]	3.1	1.6–6.0
Gravett, 1986[102]	3.8	1.2–11.6
Martius, 1988[101]	2.3	1.1–5.0
Prospective cohort		
Minkoff, 1984[103]	2.3	0.96–5.5
Gravett, 1986[75]	2.0	1.1–3.7
McGregor, 1990[123]	2.6	1.1–6.5
McDonald, 1991[124]	1.8	1.01–3.2
Kurki, 1992[125]	6.9	2.5–18.8
Riduan, 1993[126]	2.0	1.0–3.9
McGregor, 1994[127]	3.3	1.2–9.1
Hay, 1994[128]	5.2	2.0–13.5
McGregor, 1995[129]	1.9	1.2–3.0
Meis, 1995[130]	1.8	1.15–2.95
Hillier, 1995[108]	1.4	1.1–1.8

these studies is modest (approximately a twofold increased risk compared to patients without bacterial vaginosis), the total impact upon prematurity may be much greater given the high prevalence of 20% for bacterial vaginosis in pregnancy. It has been estimated that as many as 6% of preterm deliveries of infants with low birth weight may be attributable to bacterial vaginosis.[108]

Thus, bacterial vaginosis represents an important, and potentially preventable cause of prematurity. Two recent studies have demonstrated significant reductions of 40% to 50% in preterm deliveries among pregnant women with bacterial vaginosis, who were otherwise identified as at high risk for preterm delivery, treated with metronidazole.[109,110]

However, routine prenatal screening for bacterial vaginosis and treatment of asymptomatic cases among low risk obstetric populations has not been well studied and cannot yet be recommended until adequate randomized prospective treatment trials have been performed to ascertain whether treatment reduces the risk of an adverse outcome of pregnancy.

Diagnosis

The most common symptom among women with vaginosis is thin, watery nonpruritic discharge with a fishy odor. However, one half of women with bacterial vaginosis are asymptomatic.

Criteria for the clinical diagnosis of bacterial vaginosis are well established.[106] These criteria include (1) the presence of a thin, homogeneous discharge, which adheres to the vaginal walls; (2) a vaginal pH above 4.5; (3) the release of a fishy odor upon alkalinization with 10% potassium hydroxide; and (4) clue cells on a saline wet mount. The diagnosis of bacterial vaginosis requires the presence of three of these four criteria. The diagnosis of bacterial vaginosis can also be made by direct Gram stain of the vaginal discharge. The Gram stain is both highly sensitive (97%) and specific (79%) when compared to the clinical diagnosis and offers the advantages of being easily performed, readily available, and inexpensive with high interobserver reproducibility.[106]

Management Options

The treatment of choice for symptomatic bacterial vaginosis is metronidazole given orally in a dose of 250 mg three times daily for 7 days, or 375 mg or 500 mg twice daily for 7 days. This results in cure rates of 90%. A single 2-g oral dose of metronidazole is also effective. Oral clindamycin, 300 mg twice a day for 7 days, may be used an an alternative. In pregnancy, it is usually recommended that treatment with these systemic regimens be deferred until the beginning of the second trimester, when fetal organogenesis is complete. There has been some concern about the use of nitroimidazoles in pregnancy. Nitroimidazoles cross the placenta and are mutogenic in bacteria and carcinogenic in some animals. However, human studies have not revealed any increase in the expected frequency of congenital anomalies among the offspring of mothers treated with metronidazole during the pregnancy.[111] Further, long-term surveillance studies of women treated for trichomoniasis have not found any increase in the occurrence of cancer attributable to metronidazole.[112] Although evidence of fetal or maternal harm is lacking, the nitromidazoles should probably be avoided during the first trimester. Cure rates utilizing topical therapy with metronidazole vaginal gel 0.75%, given intravaginally once daily for 5 days, or clindamycin cream 2.0%, given intravaginally once daily for 7 days, are comparable to systemic therapy and may safely be utilized at any gestational age. However, topical therapy may not be adequate to reduce the risk of preterm delivery. Further studies are necessary to address this important consideration. Treatment with other antimicrobial agents, including sulfa cream, amoxicillin or ampicillin, and erythromycin has resulted in disappointing cure rates of 14% to 56% and cannot be recommended.

Candida Vaginitis

Maternal and Fetal Risks

Candida vaginitis may be caused by many species of *Candida*, but the predominant species is *Candida albicans*, which is responsible for 80% to 90% of infections. The remainder are caused by *Candida (Torulopsis) glabrata* and other *Candida* species. These organisms are saprophytic fungi, which may be recovered from the vagina in 25% to 40% of asymptomatic women. *Candida* also accounts for approximately 25% of all symptomatic vaginitis among nonpregnant patients and up to 45% of vaginitis in pregnancy. In pregnancy, alterations in the vaginal microflora, glycogen availability, and a depression in maternal cellular immunity may all contribute to increase the risk of *Candida* overgrowth leading to vaginitis. Although infrequent, *C. albicans* has been reported as a cause of amniotic fluid infection.[102]

Diagnosis

Women with vaginal candidiasis experience vulvar and vaginal pruritus, external dysuria, and a nonmalodorous flocculent discharge. Examination usually reveals an erythematous vulvar rash and a characteristic white "cottage cheese" discharge that adheres to the vaginal walls. The vaginal pH is usually lower than 4.5 and no odor is present. Microscopic examination of material suspended in 10% potassium hydroxide reveals typical mycelial forms and pseudohyphae in 80% of patients with symptomatic infection. Because *Candida* species may exist in the vaginal flow in low concentrations among normal asymptomatic patients, cultures are usually not indicated. Cultures should be limited to women in whom candidiasis is suspected but cannot be confirmed by microscopic examination.

Management Options

Treatment by local application of antifungals results in relief of symptoms and eradication of the yeasts in 70% to 90% of patients. The mainstay of treatment has been with imidazoles. These broad-spectrum antifungals include miconazole, clotrimazole, teraconazole, and butaconazole. These agents inhibit fungal ergosterol synthesis, resulting in disruption of the cell membrane. They may be given as a one-time intravaginal suppository or as either 3-day or 7-day courses of intravaginal suppositories or creams given once daily at bedtime. In recognition of the immunosuppression of pregnancy, most clinicians prefer a 7-day course of either suppositions or cream. These imidazoles are not absorbed systemically and are safe to use in pregnancy. Boric acid powder, in 600-mg capsules, placed intravaginally daily for 14 days is also 90% effective in eradicating symptomatic vaginal candidiasis and has the advantage of being very inexpensive.[113] Although borate is poorly absorbed systemically in nonpregnant women, its absorption during pregnancy is uncertain. Thus, boric acid should probably not be used during pregnancy if alternative therapies with topical imidazoles are available. Two other antifungal agents that are systemically absorbed after oral or intravenous administration are ketoconazole, an imidazole, and fluconazole, a triazole. These both have superb activity against *Candida* species and are useful in the treatment of systemic fungal infections or chronic, recurrent vaginal candidiasis in nonpregnant women.

Trichomoniasis

Maternal and Fetal Risks

Trichomoniasis is caused by *Trichomonas vaginalis*, a sexually transmitted anaerobic protozoa. *T. vaginalis* may be recovered from 40% of women screened in sexually transmitted disease clinics, and from the prostatic fluid of 70% of the male contacts of the women with symptomatic trichomoniasis.[114,115] The prevalence of trichomoniasis in pregnancy ranges from 6% to 22%. Risk factors associated with *T. vaginalis* colonization include black race, cigarette smoking, greater number of sexual partners, and a history of gonorrhea.[116] It is estimated that approximately 50% of women harboring *T. vaginalis* are asymptomatic.[114]

In addition to vaginitis, *T. vaginalis* may also cause other infections of the lower genitourinary tract including bartholinitis, urethritis, periurethral gland infection, and cystitis. Although risk of infection to the neonate is low (less than 1%), vaginitis and cystitis may occur as manifestations of neonatal disease. *T. vaginalis* has also been rarely suspected as a cause of neonatal pneumonitis. Although the relationship between vaginal trichomoniasis and adverse pregnancy outcome has not been well studied, two prospective studies have found a decrease in mean gestational age at delivery and an increase in premature rupture of membranes among women infected with *T. vaginalis*.[71,103] Further studies are necessary to confirm these relationships.

Diagnosis

Women with trichomoniasis characteristically complain of a profuse and sometimes frothy malodorous, pruritic vaginal discharge. Dysuria and lower abdominal tenderness may also be present. On examination, a gray or yellow-green purulent discharge is frequently present. The pH of the discharge is usually higher than 4.5 and may have an amine odor after addition of 10% potassium hydroxide. Small submucosal punctate hemorrhages of the cervix, the so-called "strawberry cervix" are present inconsistently. Microscopically, motile trichomonads may easily be identified on a saline wet mount by their characteristic pear shape, flagella, and rapid, jerking motility. Polymorphonuclear leukocytes are also present on saline wet mount microscopy and may be so abundant that they obscure the trichomonads. The sensitivity of the saline wet mount, when compared to culture, is 60%, but its specificity is near 100%.[117] *Trichomonas* cultures are easily performed utilizing Diamond's medium and are highly sensitive (92%– 95%) and specific. However, cultures have limited practicality in the clinical setting because 3 to 7 days are needed for growth before the diagnosis can be confirmed. Trichomonads can also be seen on a Papanicolaou smear with a similar sensitivity to the wet mount, but with a higher rate of false positive results. Other sensitive and specific rapidly performed diagnostic tests have recently been developed, including direct immunofluorescence assay, enzyme-linked immunoassay, and latex particle agglutination. These are not, however, in widespread use currently. All women with trichomoniasis, whether symptomatic or not, should have a culture taken for *Neisseria gonorrhoeae* because of the frequency of coinfection.

Management Options

Because *T. vaginalis* resides not only in the vagina but also in the urethra and bladder, systemic therapy is necessary for treatment. The only effective therapy for trichomoniasis are the nitroimidazole antibiotics, including metronidazole, ornidazole, and tinidazole. Standard treatment with metronidazole consists of either 250 mg orally three times daily for 7 days, 375 mg or 500 mg orally twice daily for 7 days, or alternatively, a single 2-g oral dose. These regimens result in a 90% cure rate and the choice of regimen depends upon the physician and patient. With tinidazole, a single 1.5-g oral dose is usually adequate to eradicate *T. vaginalis*. Patients should be advised not to drink ethanol for 24 hours after the last dose because of a disulfiram-like effect of the medication. Simultaneous treatment of the male consort is required to prevent recurrent trichomoniasis in the female.

The treatment for patients who do not respond to the initial therapy is controversial. Metronidazole-tolerant and metronidazole-resistant strains of *T. vaginalis* do occur, but infrequently. Low to moderate levels of resistance (metronidazole-tolerant strains) occur in 1 of every 200 to 400 cases of trichomoniasis and highly metronidazole-resistant strains occur in 1 in every 2000 to 3000 cases.[117] Most cases associated with strains that have low to moderate resistance can be cured by oral administration of 2 to 2.5 g metronidazole per day, in divided doses, for 7 days. Most cases caused by highly resistant strains can be cured by increasing the dose of metronidazole to 3 g daily, orally, in divided doses, for 14 days. Alternatively, cures have been reported with the use of intravenous metronidazole, 2 g given every 6 to 8 hours for 3 days.[118] Metronidazole-associated neurotoxicity may occur with longer courses of therapy.

Although cross-resistance to other nitroimidazoles among metronidazole-resistance strains occurs, it is usually incomplete. Sixty-five percent to 70% of metronidazole highly resistant strains are susceptible to tinidazole. For those cases, treatment with oral tinidazole, 2 g daily for 7 to 14 days, has been highly effective in eradicating *T. vaginalis*.[117]

There has been concern regarding the use of nitroimidazoles in pregnancy, as noted previously. Although evidence of fetal or maternal harm is lacking,[119] systemic nitroimidazoles should probably be avoided during the first trimester. As an alternative treatment in the first trimester, treatment with intravaginal 100-mg clotrimazole suppositories (a chemically related nonabsorbed imidazole antifungal) daily for 14 days provides symptomatic relief in approximately 50% of patients with trichomoniasis.[120,121]

Ideally, treatment should be given prior to pregnancy, because treatment during pregnancy has not been demonstrated to reduce the occurrence of adverse pregnancy outcomes[108] and has been associated with an increased risk of spontaneous preterm birth in recent studies.[109,120,122]

SUMMARY OF MANAGEMENT OPTIONS

Bacterial Vaginosis, Candidiasis, Trichomonas

Management Options	Quality of Evidence	Strength of Recommendation	References
Bacterial Vaginosis			
Prepregnancy, Prenatal, and Postnatal			
Treat with oral metronidazole.	IV	C	110
Give intravaginal metronidazole gel or clindamycin cream.	IV	C	110
Candidiasis			
Prepregnancy, Prenatal, and Postnatal			
Treat topically with an imidazole (miconazole, clotrimazole, teraconazole, butaconazole).	–	GPP	–
Ketoconazole and fluconazole are best avoided in pregnancy except for severe systemic infection.	–	GPP	–
Trichomonas			
Prepregnancy, Prenatal, and Postnatal			
Treat patient and partner systemically with a nitroimidazole antibiotic (metronidazole, ornidazole, tinidazole).	IV	C	117,118

CONCLUSIONS

- GAS infection can result in a potentially fatal infection in the mother requiring intensive therapy in the form of parenteral broad-spectrum antibiotics, inotropic support, immunoglobulin, and possible surgical debridement; the fetus is at risk of preterm delivery, chorioamnionitis, and stillbirth.
- GBS is largely asymptomatic in the mother but can produce a profound neonatal illness with a high mortality rate; routine screening at 35 to 37 weeks to identify GBS carriers and subsequent use of peripartum antibiotics will reduce this risk significantly.
- Listeriosis is a rare infection with an increased risk of miscarriage or fetal death; preventive measures should be directed at food handling.
- Sexually transmitted diseases are mainly a risk to the mother and are amenable to antibiotic therapy.
- Bacterial vaginosis is important because of its association with preterm labor and delivery; effective treatment can reduce this risk.
- *Candida* and *Trichomonas* infections produce troublesome symptoms for the mother, but they are very responsive to treatment.

REFERENCES

1. Adriaanse AH, Pel M, Bleker OP: Semmelweis: The combat against puerperal fever. Eur J Obstet Gynecol Reprod Biol 2000;90:153–158.
2. Cunningham MW: Pathogenesis of group A streptococcal infections. Clin Microbiol Rev 2000;13:470–511.
3. The Working Group on Severe Streptococcal Infections: Defining the group A streptococcal toxic shock syndrome. Rationale and consensus definition. JAMA 1993;269:390–391.
4. Lancefield R: A serological differentiation of human and other groups of hemolytic streptococci. J Exp Med 1933;57:574–595.
5. Efstratiou A: Group A streptococci in the 1990s. J Antimicrob Chemother 2000;45(Suppl):3–12.
6. Bannan J, Visvanathan K, Zabriskie JB: Structure and function of streptococcal and staphylococcal superantigens in septic shock. Infect Dis Clin North Am 1999;13:387–396.
7. Stevens DL: The flesh-eating bacterium: What's new? J Infect Dis 1999;179(Suppl 2):s366–374.
8. Chuang I, Van Beneden C, Beall B, Schuchat A: Population-based surveillance for postpartum invasive group a streptococcus infections, 1995–2000. Clin Infect Dis 2002;35:665–670.
9. Barnham MR, Weightman NC: Bacteraemic Streptococcus pyogenes infection in the peri-partum period: Now a rare disease and prior carriage by the patient may be important. J Infect 2001;43:173–176.
10. Greenberg D, Leibovitz E, Shinnwell ES, et al: Neonatal sepsis caused by Streptococcus pyogenes: Resurgence of an old etiology? Pediatr Infect Dis J 1999;18:479–481.
11. Verboon-Maciolek MA, Krediet TG, van Ertbruggen I, et al: Severe neonatal group A streptococcal disease. Eur J Pediatr 2000;159:450–452.
12. Panaro NR, Lutwick LI, Chapnick EK: Intrapartum transmission of group A streptococcus. Clin Infect Dis 1993;17:79–81.
13. Stevens DL, Tanner MH, Winship J, et al: Severe group A streptococcal infections associated with a toxic shock-like syndrome and scarlet fever toxin A. N Engl J Med 1989;321:1–7.
14. Stevens DL, Gibbons AE, Bergstrom R, Winn V: The Eagle effect revisited: Efficacy of clindamycin, erythromycin, and penicillin in the treatment of streptococcal myositis. J Infect Dis 1988;158:23–28.
15. Norrby-Teglund A, Kaul R, Low DE, et al: Evidence for the presence of streptococcal-superantigen-neutralizing antibodies in normal polyspecific immunoglobulin G. Infect Immun 1996;64:5395–5398.
16. Eickhoff T, Klein J, Daly A, et al: Neonatal sepsis and other infections due to group B beta-hemolytic streptococci. N Engl J Med 1964;271:1221–1228.
17. Committee on Obstetric Practice: Prevention of early-onset group B streptococcal disease in newborns. Am Coll Obstet Gynecol 1996;173:1–8.
18. Centers for Disease Control and Prevention: Prevention of perinatal group B streptococcal disease: A public health perspective. MMWR 1996;45:1–24.
19. American Academy of Pediatrics: Revised guidelines for prevention of early-onset group B streptococcal (GBS) infection. Pediatrics 1997;99:489–496.
20. Centers for Disease Control and Prevention: Prevention of perinatal group B streptococcal disease. MMWR 2002;51(RR-11):1–18.
21. Regan JA, Klebanoff MA, Nugent RP, et al: Colonization with group B streptococci in pregnancy and adverse outcome. VIP Study Group. Am J Obstet Gynecol 1996;174:1354–1360.
22. Hoogkamp-Korstanje JA, Gerards LJ, Cats BP: Maternal carriage and neonatal acquisition of group B streptococci. J Infect Dis 1982;145:800–803.
23. Baker CJ, Edwards MS, Kasper DL: Role of antibody to native type III polysaccharide of group B streptococcus in infant infection. Pediatrics 1981;68:544–549.
24. Blanco JD, Gibbs RS, Castaneda YS: Bacteremia in obstetrics: Clinical course. Obstet Gynecol 1981;58:621–625.
25. Romero R, Mazor M, Oyarzun E, et al: Is there an association between colonization with group B streptococcus and prematurity? J Reprod Med 1989;34:797–801.
26. Moller M, Thomsen AC, Borch K, et al: Rupture of fetal membranes and premature delivery associated with group B streptococci in urine of pregnant women. Lancet 1984;2:69–70.
27. Thomsen AC, Morup L, Hansen KB: Antibiotic elimination of group-B streptococci in urine in prevention of preterm labour. Lancet 1987;1:591–593.
28. Schrag SJ, Zywicki S, Farley MM, et al: Group B streptococcal disease in the era of intrapartum antibiotic prophylaxis. N Engl J Med 2000;342:15–20.
29. Yancey MK, Armer T, Clark P, Duff P: Assessment of rapid identification tests for genital carriage of group B streptococci. Obstet Gynecol 1992;80:1038–1047.
30. Walker CK, Crombleholme WR, Ohm-Smith MJ, Sweet RL: Comparison of rapid tests for detection of group B streptococcal colonization. Am J Perinatol 1992;9:304–308.

31. Bergeron MG, Ke D, Menard C, et al: Rapid detection of group B streptococci in pregnant women at delivery. N Engl J Med 2000;343:175–179.
32. Boyer KM, Gadzala CA, Burd LI, et al: Selective intrapartum chemoprophylaxis of neonatal group B streptococcal early-onset disease. I. Epidemiologic rationale. J Infect Dis 1983;148:795–801.
33. Boyer KM, Gotoff SP: Strategies for chemoprophylaxis of GBS early-onset infections. Antibiot Chemother 1985;35:267–280.
34. Allardice JG, Baskett TF, Seshia MM, et al: Perinatal group B streptococcal colonization and infection. Am J Obstet Gynecol 1982;142:617–620.
35. Boyer KM, Gotoff SP: Prevention of early-onset neonatal group B streptococcal disease with selective intrapartum chemoprophylaxis. N Engl J Med 1986;314:1665–1669.
36. Morales WJ, Lim DV, Walsh AF: Prevention of neonatal group B streptococcal sepsis by the use of a rapid screening test and selective intrapartum chemoprophylaxis. Am J Obstet Gynecol 1986;155:979–983.
37. Morales WJ, Lim D: Reduction of group B streptococcal maternal and neonatal infections in preterm pregnancies with premature rupture of membranes through a rapid identification test. Am J Obstet Gynecol 1987;157:13–16.
38. Tuppurainen N, Hallman M: Prevention of neonatal group B streptococcal disease: Intrapartum detection and chemoprophylaxis of heavily colonized parturients. Obstet Gynecol 1989;73:583–587.
39. Matorras R, Garcia-Perea A, Omenaca F, et al: Intrapartum chemoprophylaxis of early-onset group B streptococcal disease. Eur J Obstet Gynecol Reprod Biol 1991;40:57–62.
40. Garland SM, Fliegner JR: Group B streptococcus (GBS) and neonatal infections: The case for intrapartum chemoprophylaxis. Aust N Z J Obstet Gynaecol 1991;31:119–122.
41. Allen UD, Navas L, King SM: Effectiveness of intrapartum penicillin prophylaxis in preventing early-onset group B streptococcal infection: Results of a meta-analysis. Can Med Assoc J 1993;149:1659–1665.
42. Schrag SJ, Zell ER, Lynfield R, et al: A population-based comparison of strategies to prevent early-onset group B streptococcal disease in neonates. N Engl J Med 2002;347:233–239.
43. de Cueto M, Sanchez MJ, Sampedro A, et al: Timing of intrapartum ampicillin and prevention of vertical transmission of group B streptococcus. Obstet Gynecol 1998;91:112–114.
44. Lin FY, Brenner RA, Johnson YR, et al: The effectiveness of risk-based intrapartum chemoprophylaxis for the prevention of early-onset neonatal group B streptococcal disease. Am J Obstet Gynecol 2001;184:1204–1210.
45. Baker CJ, Paoletti LC, Wessels MR, et al: Safety and immunogenicity of capsular polysaccharide-tetanus toxoid conjugate vaccines for group B streptococcal types Ia and Ib. J Infect Dis 1999;179:142–150.
46. Baker CJ, Paoletti LC, Rench MA, et al: Use of capsular polysaccharide-tetanus toxoid conjugate vaccine for type II group B streptococcus in healthy women. J Infect Dis 2000;182:1129–1138.
47. Kasper DL, Paoletti LC, Wessels MR, et al: Immune response to type III group B streptococcal polysaccharide-tetanus toxoid conjugate vaccine. J Clin Invest 1996;98:2308–2314.
48. Silver HM: Listeriosis during pregnancy. Obstet Gynecol Surv 1998;53:737–740.
49. Southwick FS, Purich DL: Intracellular pathogenesis of listeriosis. N Engl J Med 1996;334:770–776.
50. Rappaport F, Rabionovitz M, Toaff R, et al: Genital listeriosis as a case of repeated abortion. Lancet 1960;1:1273–1275.
51. MacNaughton M, Glasg M: Listeria monocytogenes in abortion. Lancet 1962;2:484–486.
52. Anasbacher R, Borchchardt K, Hannegan M, et al: Clinical investigation of Listeria monocytogenes as a possible cause of human fetal wastage. Am J Obstet Gynecol 1966;94:386–390.
53. Lawler F, Wood W, King S, et al: Listeria monocytogenes as a cause of fetal loss. Am J Obstet Gynecol 1964;89:915–923.
54. Mascola L, Ewert DP, Eller A: Listeriosis: A previously unreported medical complication in women with multiple gestations. Am J Obstet Gynecol 1994;170:1328–1332.
55. Mylonakis E, Paliou M, Hohmann EL, et al: Listeriosis during pregnancy: A case series and review of 222 cases. Medicine (Baltimore) 2002;81:260–269.
56. McLauchlin J: Human listeriosis in Britain, 1967–85, a summary of 722 cases. 1. Listeriosis during pregnancy and in the newborn. Epidemiol Infect 1990;104:181–189.
57. Simon C, Craig S, Permezel M, et al: Perinatal infection with Listeria monocytogenes. Aust N Z J Obstet Gynaecol 1996;36:286–290.
58. Linnan MJ, Mascola L, Lou XD, et al: Epidemic listeriosis associated with Mexican-style cheese. N Engl J Med 1988;319:823–828.
59. Tappero JW, Schuchat A, Deaver KA, et al: Reduction in the incidence of human listeriosis in the United States. Effectiveness of prevention efforts? The Listeriosis Study Group. JAMA 1995;273:1118–1122.
60. Listeriosis and Pregnancy: What is Your Risk? Safe Food Handling for a Healthy Pregnancy (Web site). Available at http://www.fsis.usda.gov/OA/pubs/lm_tearsheet.htm. 2001.
61. Cruikshank DP, Warenski JC: First-trimester maternal Listeria monocytogenes sepsis and chorioamnionitis with normal neonatal outcome. Obstet Gynecol 1989;73:469–471.
62. Fleming AD, Ehrlich DW, Miller NA, Monif GR: Successful treatment of maternal septicemia due to Listeria monocytogenes at 26 weeks' gestation. Obstet Gynecol 1985;66:52S–53S.
63. Charles AG, Cohen S, Kass MB, Richman R: Asymptomatic gonorrhea in prenatal patients. Am J Obstet Gynecol 1970;108:595–599.
64. Spence MR: Gonorrhea in a military prenatal population. Obstet Gynecol 1973;42:223–226.
65. Corman LC, Levison ME, Knight R, et al: The high frequency of pharyngeal gonococcal infection in a prenatal clinic population. JAMA 1974;230:568–570.
66. Holmes KK, Counts GW, Beaty HN: Disseminated gonococcal infection. Ann Intern Med 1971;74:979–993.
67. Edwards LE, Barrada MI, Hamann AA, Hakanson EY: Gonorrhea in pregnancy. Am J Obstet Gynecol 1978;132:637–641.
68. Burkman RT, Tonascia JA, Atienza MF, King TM: Untreated endocervical gonorrhea and endometritis following elective abortion. Am J Obstet Gynecol 1976;126:648–651.
69. Christmas JT, Wendel GD, Bawdon RE, et al: Concomitant infection with Neisseria gonorrhoeae and Chlamydia trachomatis in pregnancy. Obstet Gynecol 1989;74:295–298.
70. Centers for Disease Control and Prevention: Ten leading nationally notifiable infectious diseases—United States. MMWR 1996;45:883–884.
71. Hardy PH, Hardy JB, Nell EE, et al: Prevalence of six sexually transmitted disease agents among pregnant inner-city adolescents and pregnancy outcome. Lancet 1984;2:333–337.
72. Schachter J, Grossman M, Sweet RL, et al: Prospective study of perinatal transmission of Chlamydia trachomatis. JAMA 1986;255:3374–3377.
73. Sweet RL, Landers DV, Walker C, Schachter J: Chlamydia trachomatis infection and pregnancy outcome. Am J Obstet Gynecol 1987;156:824–833.
74. Martin DH, Koutsky L, Eschenbach DA, et al: Prematurity and perinatal mortality in pregnancies complicated by maternal Chlamydia trachomatis infections. JAMA 1982;247:1585–1588.
75. Gravett MG, Nelson HP, DeRouen T, et al: Independent associations of bacterial vaginosis and Chlamydia trachomatis infection with adverse pregnancy outcome. JAMA 1986;256:1899–1903.

76. Alger LS, Lovchik JC, Hebel JR, et al: The association of Chlamydia trachomatis, Neisseria gonorrhoeae, and group B streptococci with preterm rupture of the membranes and pregnancy outcome. Am J Obstet Gynecol 1988;159:397–404.
77. Wager GP, Martin DH, Koutsky L, et al: Puerperal infectious morbidity: Relationship to route of delivery and to antepartum Chlamydia trachomatis infection. Am J Obstet Gynecol 1980;138:1028–1033.
78. Harrison HR, Alexander ER, Weinstein L, et al: Cervical Chlamydia trachomatis and mycoplasmal infections in pregnancy. Epidemiology and outcomes. JAMA 1983;250:1721–1727.
79. Ryan GM Jr, Abdella TN, McNeeley SG, et al: Chlamydia trachomatis infection in pregnancy and effect of treatment on outcome. Am J Obstet Gynecol 1990;162:34–39.
80. Rastogi S, Das B, Salhan S, Mittal A: Effect of treatment for Chlamydia trachomatis during pregnancy. Int J Gynaecol Obstet 2003;80:129–137.
81. Cohen I, Veille JC, Calkins BM: Improved pregnancy outcome following successful treatment of chlamydial infection. JAMA 1990;263:3160–3163.
82. Crombleholme WR, Schachter J, Grossman M, et al: Amoxicillin therapy for Chlamydia trachomatis in pregnancy. Obstet Gynecol 1990;75:752–756.
83. Alger LS, Lovchik JC: Comparative efficacy of clindamycin versus erythromycin in eradication of antenatal Chlamydia trachomatis. Am J Obstet Gynecol 1991;165:375–381.
84. Harwick HJ, Purcell RH, Iuppa JB, Fekety FR Jr: Mycoplasma hominis and abortion. J Infect Dis 1970;121:260–268.
85. Watts DH, Eschenbach DA, Kenny GE: Early postpartum endometritis: The role of bacteria, genital mycoplasmas, and Chlamydia trachomatis. Obstet Gynecol 1989;73:52–60.
86. Braun P, Lee YH, Klein JO, et al: Birth weight and genital mycoplasmas in pregnancy. N Engl J Med 1971;284:167–171.
87. Shurin PA, Alpert S, Bernard Rosner BA, et al: Chorioamnionitis and colonization of the newborn infant with genital mycoplasmas. N Engl J Med 1975;293:5–8.
88. Kundsin RB, Driscoll SG, Monson RR, et al: Association of Ureaplasma urealyticum in the placenta with perinatal morbidity and mortality. N Engl J Med 1984;310:941–945.
89. Hillier SL, Martius J, Krohn M, et al: A case-control study of chorioamnionic infection and histologic chorioamnionitis in prematurity. N Engl J Med 1988;319:972–978.
90. Tafari N, Ross S, Naeye RL, et al: Mycoplasma T strains and perinatal death. Lancet 1976;1:108–109.
91. McCormack WM, Rosner B, Lee YH, et al: Effect on birth weight of erythromycin treatment of pregnant women. Obstet Gynecol 1987;69:202–207.
92. Eschenbach DA, Nugent RP, Rao AV, et al: A randomized placebo-controlled trial of erythromycin for the treatment of Ureaplasma urealyticum to prevent premature delivery. The Vaginal Infections and Prematurity Study Group. Am J Obstet Gynecol 1991;164:734–742.
93. Hammond GW, Lian CJ, Wilt JC, Ronald AR: Comparison of specimen collection and laboratory techniques for isolation of Haemophilus ducreyi. J Clin Microbiol 1978;7:39–43.
94. Willcox RR: International aspects of the venereal diseases and nonvenereal treponematoses. Clin Obstet Gynecol 1975;18: 207–222.
95. Kuberski T: Granuloma inguinale (Donovanosis). Sex Transm Dis 1980;7:29–36.
96. Sowmini CN: Donovanosis. In Holmes KK, Mardh PA (eds.) International Perspectives on Neglected Sexually Transmitted Diseases. Washington, Hemisphere Publishing Corp., pp 205–217.
97. Scott C, Harper G, Jason R, et al: Neonatal granuloma inguinale. Am J Dis Child 1953;85:308–315.
98. Huggins GR, Preti G: Vaginal odors and secretions. Clin Obstet Gynecol 1981;24:355–377.
99. Redondo-Lopez V, Cook RL, Sobel JD: Emerging role of lactobacilli in the control and maintenance of the vaginal bacterial microflora. Rev Infect Dis 1990;12:856–872.
100. Eschenbach DA, Davick PR, Williams BL, et al: Prevalence of hydrogen peroxide-producing Lactobacillus species in normal women and women with bacterial vaginosis. J Clin Microbiol 1989;27:251–256.
101. Martius J, Eschenbach DA: The role of bacterial vaginosis as a cause of amniotic fluid infection, chorioamnionitis and prematurity—A review. Arch Gynecol Obstet 1990;247:1–13.
102. Gravett MG, Hummel D, Eschenbach DA, Holmes KK: Preterm labor associated with subclinical amniotic fluid infection and with bacterial vaginosis. Obstet Gynecol 1986;67:229–237.
103. Minkoff H, Grunebaum AN, Schwarz RH, et al: Risk factors for prematurity and premature rupture of membranes: A prospective study of the vaginal flora in pregnancy. Am J Obstet Gynecol 1984;150:965–972.
104. Spiegel CA, Amsel R, Eschenbach D, et al: Anaerobic bacteria in nonspecific vaginitis. N Engl J Med 1980;303:601–607.
105. Silver HM, Sperling RS, St Clair PJ, Gibbs RS: Evidence relating bacterial vaginosis to intraamniotic infection. Am J Obstet Gynecol 1989;161:808–812.
106. Eschenbach DA, Hillier S, Critchlow C, et al: Diagnosis and clinical manifestations of bacterial vaginosis. Am J Obstet Gynecol 1988;158:819–828.
107. Bejar R, Curbelo V, Davis C, Gluck L: Premature labor. II. Bacterial sources of phospholipase. Obstet Gynecol 1981;57: 479–482.
108. Hillier SL, Nugent RP, Eschenbach DA, et al: Association between bacterial vaginosis and preterm delivery of a low-birth-weight infant. The Vaginal Infections and Prematurity Study Group. N Engl J Med 1995;333:1737–1742.
109. Morales WJ, Schorr S, Albritton J: Effect of metronidazole in patients with preterm birth in preceding pregnancy and bacterial vaginosis: A placebo-controlled, double-blind study. Am J Obstet Gynecol 1994;171:345–349.
110. Hauth JC, Goldenberg RL, Andrews WW, et al: Reduced incidence of preterm delivery with metronidazole and erythromycin in women with bacterial vaginosis. N Engl J Med 1995;333:1732–1736.
111. Burtin P, Taddio A, Ariburnu O, et al: Safety of metronidazole in pregnancy: A meta-analysis. Am J Obstet Gynecol 1995;172: 525–529.
112. Beard CM, Noller KL, O'Fallon WM, et al: Lack of evidence for cancer due to use of metronidazole. N Engl J Med 1979;301: 519–522.
113. Van Slyke KK, Michel VP, Rein MF: Treatment of vulvovaginal candidiasis with boric acid powder. Am J Obstet Gynecol 1981;141:145–148.
114. McLellan R, Spence MR, Brockman M, et al: The clinical diagnosis of trichomoniasis. Obstet Gynecol 1982;60:30–34.
115. Block E: Occurrence of trichomonas in sexual partners of women with trichomoniasis. Acta Obstet Gynecol Scand 1959;38:398–401.
116. Cotch MF, Pastorek JG 2nd, Nugent RP, et al: Demographic and behavioral predictors of Trichomonas vaginalis infection among pregnant women. The Vaginal Infections and Prematurity Study Group. Obstet Gynecol 1991;78:1087–1092.
117. Lossick JG, Kent HL: Trichomoniasis: Trends in diagnosis and management. Am J Obstet Gynecol 1991;165:1217–1222.
118. Dombrowski MP, Sokol RJ, Brown WJ, Bronsteen RA: Intravenous therapy of metronidazole-resistant Trichomonas vaginalis. Obstet Gynecol 1987;69:524–525.
119. Caro-Paton T, Carvajal A, Martin de Diego I, et al: Is metronidazole teratogenic? A meta-analysis. Br J Clin Pharmacol 1997;44:179–182.
120. Klebanoff MA, Carey JC, Hauth JC, et al: Failure of metronidazole to prevent preterm delivery among pregnant women with asymptomatic Trichomonas vaginalis infection. N Engl J Med 2001;345:487–493.
121. Gulmezoglu AM: Interventions for trichomoniasis in pregnancy. Cochrane Database Syst Rev 2002;CD000220.

122. Kigozi GG, Brahmbhatt H, Wabwire-Mangen F, et al: Treatment of trichomonas in pregnancy and adverse outcomes of pregnancy: A subanalysis of a randomized tiral in Rakai, Uganda. Am J Obstet Gynecol 2003;189:1398–1400.
123. McGregor JA, French JI, Richter R, et al: Antenatal microbiologic and maternal risk factors associated with prematurity. Am J Obstet Gynecol 1990;163:1465–1473.
124. McDonald HM, O'Loughlin JA, Jolley P, et al: Vaginal infection and preterm labour. Br J Obstet Gynaecol 1991;98:427–435.
125. Kurki T, Sivonen A, Renkonen OV, et al: Bacterial vaginosis in early pregnancy and pregnancy outcome. Obstet Gynecol 1992;80:173–177.
126. Riduan JM, Hillier SL, Utomo B, et al: Bacterial vaginosis and prematurity in Indonesia: Association in early and late pregnancy. Am J Obstet Gynecol 1993;169:175–178.
127. McGregor JA, French JI, Jones W, et al: Bacterial vaginosis is associated with prematurity and vaginal fluid mucinase and sialidase: Results of a controlled trial of topical clindamycin cream. Am J Obstet Gynecol 1994;170:1048–1059.
128. Hay PE, Lamont RF, Taylor-Robinson D, et al: Abnormal bacterial colonisation of the genital tract and subsequent preterm delivery and late miscarriage. BMJ 1994;308:295–298.
129. McGregor JA, French JI, Parker R, et al: Prevention of premature birth by screening and treatment for common genital tract infections: Results of a prospective controlled evaluation. Am J Obstet Gynecol 1995;173:157–167.
130. Meis PJ, Goldenberg RL, Mercer B, et al: The preterm prediction study: Significance of vaginal infections. National Institute of Child Health and Human Development Maternal-Fetal Medicine Units Network. Am J Obstet Gynecol 1995;173:1231–1235.
131. Allardice JG, Baskett TF, Seshia MMK, Bowman N, Molazdrewicz R: Perinatal group B streptococcal colonization and infection. American Journal of Obstetrics and Gynecology 1982;142:617–620.

CHAPTER 33

Parasitic Infections

J. M. Ernest

INTRODUCTION

In the developing world, pregnant women frequently experience a cycle of undernutrition and parasitic infections, resulting in adverse pregnancy outcomes, including abortion, malformation, and neonatal death. Although malnutrition in general and parasitic infections specifically are less common in developed countries, no society is immune from their potential effects during pregnancy. Five parasitic infections that have major health, financial, or combined consequences worldwide are Lyme disease, malaria, tuberculosis, syphilis, and toxoplasmosis.

LYME DISEASE

General

In the early 1970s, a mysterious clustering of juvenile rheumatoid arthritis-like cases occurring in children in and around Lyme, Connecticut, was subsequently recognized as a distinct disease and named Lyme disease. Further investigation revealed that tiny deer ticks infected with a spirochetal bacteria later named *Borrelia burgdorferi* were responsible for the outbreak.[1] Subsequent research has discovered additional vectors, three distinct stages of the disease, and multiple therapy options.

Ticks, obligate blood-sucking members of the order *Acarina* and class *Arachnida*, are the most common agents of vector-borne diseases in the United States.[2] Black-legged ticks *(Ixodes scapularis)* are responsible for transmitting *B. burgdorferi* to humans in the northeastern and north central United States; on the Pacific Coast, the bacteria are transmitted to humans by the western black-legged tick *(Ixodes pacificus)*. The life cycle of ticks is 2 years and includes egg, larva, nymph, and adult. *I. scapularis* nymphs appear to be the most important vector for transmission of *B. burgdorferi*. Ixodes ticks are much smaller than common dog and cattle ticks and usually feed and mate on deer during the adult part of their life cycle. The larvae (or seed ticks) are six-legged, whereas adult and nymphs are eight-legged. In their larval and nymphal stages, these ticks are no bigger than a pinhead. According to laboratory studies, a minimum of 36 to 48 hours of attachment of the tick is required for transmission,[3] presumably because of the time required for the bacteria to travel from the midgut of the tick to its salivary glands.

In the United States, Lyme disease is mostly localized to states in the northeastern, mid-Atlantic, and upper north central regions and to several counties in northwestern California, although it has been reported in 49 of the 50 states. In 2000, 17,730 cases of Lyme disease were reported to the Centers for Disease Control and Prevention (CDC), making it the most common vector-borne illness in the United States.[4] Ninety-two percent of these were from the states of Connecticut, Rhode Island, New York, Pennsylvania, Delaware, New Jersey, Maryland, Massachusetts, and Wisconsin. Most cases occur in the United States between May and August, corresponding with increased outdoor human activity and nymphal activity.

Diagnosis

Clinically, Lyme disease has three stages:

- early-localized
- early-disseminated
- late-stage disease.

Only the early-localized stage contains a hallmark unique to Lyme disease—the erythema migrans rash—which is present in 60% to 80% of patients at the site of the bite.[5] Adding to this difficulty in diagnosis is the frequent absence of notable tick bite in many individuals who subsequently have symptoms of Lyme disease.

Although the gold standard for diagnosis of an infectious disease is isolation of the causative organism, this confirmation is often difficult in Lyme disease and the reliability of other methods currently available is questionable.[6] The diagnosis of Lyme disease is therefore based on the history of a tick bite in an endemic area and on characteristic clinical findings. Serology using enzyme-linked immunosorbent assay (ELISA) is the most common laboratory test to screen for antibodies to *B. burgdorferi*, but the test is not standardized and results may vary between laboratories, with false-negatives and false-positives commonly seen.[7] If obtained, a positive or equivocal ELISA should be followed by an immunoblot on the same specimen to detect IgM and IgG antibodies. If positive, the diagnosis is confirmed.[6] In patients with only cutaneous disease, laboratory testing is neither necessary nor recommended; in suspected cases of extracutaneous Lyme diseases, laboratory studies are essential.

Diagnosis of Early-Localized Disease

The hallmark of Lyme disease—the erythema migrans rash—typically occurs within 1 week of infection, but can develop as late as 16 weeks after the tick bite. The rash develops centrifugally as an erythematous, annular, round to oval, well-demarcated plaque and can reach a diameter of more than 30 centimeters. Occasionally, the lesion might be hemorrhagic or nonmigratory. The rash may be accompanied by constitutional symptoms such as myalgia, arthralgia, low-grade fever, and regional lymphadenopathy. Untreated, the lesions usually resolve within 3 to 4 weeks. Within days to a few weeks after the infection, hematogenous and lymphatic dissemination of the organism to distant sites occurs, leading to the early-disseminated stage.

Diagnosis of Early-Disseminated Disease

The most characteristic manifestations of this stage occur in the skin, musculoskeletal system, and neurologic system.[8] Skin manifestations during this stage include the development of other annular plaques resembling erythema migrans, found in up to half of patients. About 6 months after infection, approximately 60% of patients develop musculoskeletal symptoms, including arthralgias and myalgias early in the process, and asymmetrical, oligoarticular arthritis primarily of the large joints (especially the knee) later in the disease. The most common neurologic feature is cranial neuropathy, including unilateral or bilateral facial paralysis. Cardiac involvement, a less common component of this stage, may include atrioventricular block (in up to 8% of patients), left ventricular dysfunction, pericarditis, or fatal pancarditis.[9]

Diagnosis of Late-Stage Disease

Manifestations of late-stage disease can occur months to years after the initial infection and most commonly involve the skin, musculoskeletal system, and neurologic system. Localized scleroderma-like lesions may involve the skin, and approximately 10% of patients in the United States with untreated disease will develop chronic Lyme arthritis, an asymmetrical oligoarticular or monoarticular arthritis. Permanent joint disease is unusual. The central and peripheral nervous system can be affected, most commonly with intermittent distal paresthesias or radicular pain.[7]

Maternal and Fetal Risks

Although transplacental transmission of *B. burgdorferi* has been reported, it seems to be infrequent.[10,11] In a report by Markowitz and colleagues, in which 19 cases of Lyme disease were collected retrospectively, 5 had adverse outcomes, including syndactyly, cortical blindness, intrauterine fetal death, prematurity, and rash. Neither trimester of acquisition nor therapy administered seemed to be associated with the outcome.[12] Weber and Pfister collected 58 cases from Slovenia, including 13 in the first trimester, 27 in the second trimester, and 18 in the third trimester, and concluded that the outcomes of one missed abortion and five preterm infants revealed no causal connection between the organism and adverse fetal effects.[13] Likewise, Williams and Strobino divided a group of 463 infants after birth into those serologically positive and negative to *B. burgdorferi* and found no difference in the incidence of malformations based on the infant's serology or geographic location.[14] Therefore, recommendations for therapy during pregnancy are similar to those of nonpregnant individuals, with the exception of avoidance of tetracyclines and doxycycline in pregnancy.

Management Options

Prepregnancy and Prenatal

With the exception of the avoidance of tetracyclines during pregnancy, management options are similar before and during pregnancy. Four clinical situations can occur during which the practitioner may need to consider Lyme disease and the need for therapy:

- tick bites without signs of infection
- early-localized
- early-disseminated
- late-stage disease.

TICK BITES WITHOUT SIGNS OF INFECTION

Although some practitioners routinely treat patients who have been bitten by *I. scapularis*, a meta-analysis pooling over 600 patients estimated that if amoxicillin rather than doxycycline were used, 8 cases of drug-associated rash (including 1 severe life-threatening reaction) would occur for every 10 cases of early Lyme disease that were prevented. The authors concluded that routine prophylaxis is not indicated in this situation.[15] Due to the current limitations of the techniques, routine serologic tests after a tick bite are also not recommended. Persons who remove attached ticks should be monitored closely for signs and symptoms of tick-borne diseases for up to 30 days and should be especially observant for the occurrence of a skin lesion at the site of the tick bite (which may suggest Lyme disease) or a temperature >38°C (which may suggest other tick-related illnesses). Persons who develop a skin lesion or other illness within 1 month after removing an attached tick should promptly seek medical attention.

EARLY-LOCALIZED STAGE

Identification of the bulls-eye rash of erythema migrans should prompt early oral treatment for nonpregnant adults with doxycycline 100 mg PO twice a day for 10 to 21 days. Pregnant women should be given amoxicillin 500 mg PO three times a day for 21 days. If allergic to penicillin, cefuroxime axetil 500 mg PO twice a day for 21 days or erythromycin 250 to 500 mg PO four times a day for 21 days may be substituted.[16] More than 90% of infected individuals respond to antibiotic therapy; when prompt and complete response is not seen the practitioner should consider a later or underdiagnosed stage of disease (such as unsuspected neurologic disease) or co-infection with other tick-borne infections, such as ehrlichiosis or babesiosis.

A Jarisch-Herxheimer–type reaction may occur in the first 24 hours of treatment, consisting of fever, chills, myalgia, headache, tachycardia, increased respiratory rate, and mild leukocytosis.[17] Defervescence usually takes place within 12 to 24 hours, and the patient can be managed by bed rest and appropriate antipyretics.

EARLY-DISSEMINATED AND LATE-STAGE DISEASE

In the absence of neurologic involvement or third-degree atrioventricular heart block, oral doxycycline or amoxicillin are recommended for early disseminated disease. Cefuroxime axetil is an acceptable alternative when the patient is unable to take either doxycycline or amoxicillin. Parenteral antibiotics such as ceftriaxone 2 grams IV daily for 14 to 28 days may be used for acute neurologic disease and third-degree atrioventricular heart block.

Labor and Delivery

No specific recommendations apply to the intrapartum period.

Postnatal

Women who develop Lyme disease during pregnancy should be monitored for up to 1 year for symptoms that may represent late-stage disease. These include localized scleroderma-like lesions of the skin, chronic Lyme arthritis involving single large joints such as the knee, and intermittent distal paresthesias or radicular pain.

SUMMARY OF MANAGEMENT OPTIONS

Lyme Disease

Management Options	Quality of Evidence	Strength of Recommendation	References
Prepregnancy and Prenatal			
Avoid tick-infested areas when possible and carefully remove all ticks as soon as recognized.	IV	C	16
Observe skin after tick bites for up to 30 days for signs of infection.	IIb	B	16
Prophylactic antibiotics are usually not warranted in absence of infection.	Ib	A	15
Doxycycline 100 mg po bid for 10 to 21 days for nonpregnant or amoxicillin 500 mg po tid for 21 days for pregnant adults are comparable therapies for early-stage disease.	Ib	A	13,16
Intravenous therapy should be considered for late-stage disease.	III	B	13,16
Postnatal			
Observe the patient for up to 12 months for signs of chronic Lyme disease.	IV	C	13,16

TUBERCULOSIS

General

Tuberculosis (TB) is a disease with enormous worldwide implications; the World Health Organization (WHO) estimates that approximately one third (1.9 billion people) of the world's population is infected with *Mycobacterium tuberculosis*. The disease is thought to cause at least 3 million deaths each year, and the annual number of new cases is now nearly 8 million.[18-20]

Tuberculosis may be caused by any one of three mycobacterial pathogens: *M. tuberculosis* (the most common), *Mycobacterium bovis*, and *Mycobacterium africanum. Mycobacterium microti*, also a tubercle bacilli, does not cause disease in humans.

Tuberculosis is spread from person to person through the air by droplet nuclei, particles 1 to 5 µm in diameter that contain *M. tuberculosis* complex.[21] Droplet nuclei are produced when persons with pulmonary or laryngeal TB cough, sneeze, speak, or sing. Droplet nuclei, containing two to three *M. tuberculosis* organisms, are so small that air currents normally present in any indoor space can keep them airborne for long periods of time.[22] These particles are small enough to reach the alveoli within the lungs, where the organisms replicate.[23] Organisms deposited on intact mucosa or skin do not invade tissue. After inhalation, the droplet nuclei are carried down the bronchial tree, where the tubercle bacilli are ingested by alveolar macrophages. The organisms can multiply there, growing for 2 to 12 weeks until a critical number of 10^3 to 10^4 is reached, which is sufficient to elicit a cellular immune response that can be detected by a reaction to the tuberculin skin test (TST).[24]

Before the infected individual develops cellular immunity, tubercle bacilli spread via the lymphatics to the hilar lymph nodes and through the bloodstream to more distant sites. After cellular immunity develops, granulomas are formed that limit multiplication and further spread.

Diagnosis

In non-HIV-infected patients, the majority of reported TB cases are limited to the lungs. Advanced infection with HIV, however, results in extrapulmonary involvement over 60% of the time.[25]

Systemic effects of tuberculosis include fever (present in up to 80% of patients),[26] weight loss, increases in peripheral leukocyte count and anemia (present in approximately 10% of patients),[27] and hyponatremia, occurring in as many as 11% of patients.[28]

Cough is the most common symptom of pulmonary tuberculosis, beginning as nonproductive but subsequently becoming sputum-producing. Hemoptysis is uncommon early in the disease process. Physical findings in pulmonary TB are generally unhelpful, although the chest film almost always reveals abnormalities, generally seen as a middle or lower lung zone infiltrate, often associated with ipsilateral hilar adenopathy when the disease is primary and is occurring as a result of a recent infection. TB that develops as a result of endogenous reactivation of latent infection usually causes abnormalities in the upper lobes of one or both lungs and may also involve cavitation.[29]

Pending confirmatory cultures, which may take several weeks, pulmonary TB can be diagnosed with sputum samples that show the presence of acid-fast bacilli (AFB), identified in 50% to 80% of patients with pulmonary TB.[29] A series of at least three single specimens should be collected on different days. Specimens should be transported to the laboratory and processed as soon as possible. If delay is inevitable, the specimen should be refrigerated until prompt delivery can be assured. No fixative or preservative agents should be used. Direct amplification tests using gene probes or PCR testing and high-performance liquid chromatography may also be useful in some circumstances in evaluating the patient. Regardless of the method used to diagnosis TB, cultures of the organism are essential for confirmation and to allow for drug susceptibility testing, a critical component of TB infection management.

Extrapulmonary tuberculosis can present as a disseminated form or in the lymph nodes, pleural cavity, genitourinary system, skeleton, CNS, abdomen, or pericardium. The ease and accuracy of diagnosis of extrapulmonary TB depend on the system involved.

In addition to symptomatic tuberculosis, patients who may have asymptomatic latent infection require careful consideration and thoughtful diagnosis as well. Current recommendations discourage screening of low risk populations because of false-positive results and subsequent inappropriate and potentially hazardous drug administration.

When screening for latent infection is considered, the preferred skin test for *M. tuberculosis* is the intradermal, or Mantoux, method. It is administered by injecting 0.1 mL of 5 tuberculin units (TU) PPD (purified protein derivative) intradermally into the dorsal or volar surface of the forearm. Tests should be read 48 to 72 hours after test administration, and the transverse diameter of induration (not inflammation) should be recorded in millimeters. Multiple puncture tests (Tine and Heaf) and PPD strengths of 1 TU and 250 TU are not sufficiently accurate and should not be used.

Three cutoff levels have been recommended for defining a positive tuberculin reaction: ≥5mm, ≥10mm, and ≥15mm of induration, depending on the risk group in which the patient resides. For persons who are at highest risk for developing TB disease if they become infected with *M. tuberculosis*, a cutoff level of ≥5mm is recommended. This group contains immunosuppressed patient and those with recent close contact with a patient with infectious TB. A reaction of ≥10mm of induration should be considered positive for those persons with an increased probability of recent infection or with other clinical conditions that increase the risk of TB, such as recent immigrants from endemic areas, IV drug users, or those with normal or mildly impaired immunity including groups with poor access to health care. This level is reasonable for pregnant patients. A reaction of ≥15mm of induration should be used for groups at low risk for latent infection, should that group be tested.[30] In most individuals, PPD skin test sensitivity persists throughout life. Over time, however, the size of the skin test may diminish or disappear. If a PPD test is administered in this situation, the initial test result may be small or nonidentifiable. However, there may be accentuation of response on repeated testing. This is called the *booster effect* and does not represent a skin test conversion. This two-step method is commonly used in healthcare workers who undergo repeated tests and involves an initial test that, if negative, is followed in 1 to 3 weeks by a second and similar TB skin test, administered at a different site. The second test should be considered the "correct" one and the results from its induration measurement used. Because of the small amount of antigen administered, repeated skin testing with tuberculin will not induce a positive skin test reaction in individuals who have no cellular immunity to the antigens in PPD.[31]

Previous immunization with bacillus Calmetté-Guerin (BCG) has been shown to protect against disseminated TB and meningitis in children, but has not been conclusively demonstrated to have protective effects against pulmonary disease in children or adults.[32] Millions of people around the world have been vaccinated with this attenuated strain of *M. bovis*, which frequently causes a false-positive Mantoux skin test. However, to avoid undertreatment of those truly infected, it is considered prudent by many experts to consider induration of more than 5 mm as indicating infection with *M. tuberculosis*, even with a history of BCG immunization.

Maternal and Fetal Risks

Tuberculosis during pregnancy appears to progress in a similar fashion as in the nonpregnant individual. There appears to be no risk to the fetus with maternal exposure or positive skin testing in the absence of active pulmonary or extrapulmonary disease, although the tubercle bacillus has been reported to cross the placenta and granulomas rarely are found in the placenta.[33–35] Because of these reassuring findings, risks to mother are similar to those of the nonpregnant individual, and both mother and fetus share potential medication side effect risks.

Management Options

Prepregnancy and Prenatal

The main points about prepregnancy and prenatal care in patients with TB are the following:

- Pregnancy does not affect the course of tuberculosis.[30,34]
- Tuberculosis is unlikely to have fetal effects, and maternal effects of latent disease are primarily related to side effects of medications.[34]
- Latent disease should be treated with isoniazid and pyridoxine during pregnancy or immediately postpartum.[30,34]
- Active disease should be treated aggressively during pregnancy, with a combination of isoniazid, rifampin, and ethambutol.[34]
- Streptomycin should be avoided during pregnancy.[34]

Labor and Delivery

Factors that should be considered when managing an intrapartum patient with TB include the following:

- Masks worn by persons exposed to an infectious source are less effective than are masks worn by patients, because most airborne droplet nuclei are much smaller than their parent droplets.
- Droplet nuclei do not settle but remain suspended in the air for long periods of time.[22]
- Within 2 days of therapy that includes isoniazid, there is a 2 log/mL reduction of colony counts in sputum, with an additional 1 log/mL reduction within the next 12 days.[36]

Asymptomatic patients under appropriate medical therapy do not pose a risk to healthcare providers. However, patients with untreated or undiagnosed disease may pose a serious threat to the healthcare team. In labor and delivery, any coughing patient who comes in contact with the healthcare team should immediately be provided a surgical mask, tissues, and a container to collect tissues. Patients with any of the following symptoms should be evaluated for the presence of TB: persistent cough for 3 weeks or more, bloody sputum, night sweats, weight loss, or fever. If any of these are noted, a chest x-ray should be obtained and sputum sent for AFB. If active TB is suspected, use of an isolation room with airborne transmission precautions should be implemented until further workup is complete. Healthcare workers should wear respirators capable of filtering particles to 1 μm in diameter with facial leak of 10% or less. Healthcare workers exposed to patients with active disease should have a PPD administered immediately and again in 12 weeks. Nursery personnel should be alerted when a newborn has an actively infected mother.

Postpartum

Patients with recent skin test conversion who have not been treated during pregnancy should be considered for therapy in the postpartum period. Although antituberculous drugs can be measured in breast milk, breastfeeding is safe during therapy for TB.

SUMMARY OF MANAGEMENT OPTIONS

Tuberculosis

Management Options	Quality of Evidence	Strength of Recommendation	References
Prepregnancy and Prenatal			
Pregnancy does not affect the course of tuberculosis.	III	B	30, 34
Tuberculosis is unlikely to have fetal effects, and maternal effects of latent disease are primarily related to side effects of medications.	III	B	34
Latent disease should be treated with isoniazid and pyridoxine during pregnancy or immediately postpartum.	III	B	30, 34
Active disease should be treated aggressively during pregnancy, with a combination of isoniazid, rifampin, and ethambutol.	III	B	34
Streptomycin should be avoided during pregnancy.	III	B	34
Labor and Delivery			
Take special anesthetic precautions if general anesthesia is necessary.	–	GPP	–
Place patients suspected of having active TB on respiratory isolation.	III	B	22
Postnatal			
Continue treatment until course completed.	–	GPP	–
Breastfeeding is not contraindicated.	III	B	34
If mother has been treated, give baby isoniazid-resistant BCG and a course of prophylactic isoniazid.	III	B	34
Treat any untreated patients with recent TB skin test conversions after delivery.	III	B	34
Notify nursery personnel about the neonate exposed to active disease.	III	B	34
Some antituberculous agents may reduce efficacy of oral contraceptives.	–	GPP	–

MALARIA

General

Malaria is produced by intraerythrocytic parasites of the genus *Plasmodium* that are transmitted by the bite of the infective female anopheline mosquito. One billion people worldwide are estimated to carry parasites at any one time,[37] and estimates for annual malaria mortality range from 0.5 to 3.0 million people.[38] Its name is derived from the belief of the ancient Romans that *mal-aria* was due to the bad air of the marshes surrounding Rome.

Four plasmodia produce malaria in humans: *Plasmodium falciparum*, *Plasmodium vivax*, *Plasmodium ovale*, and *Plasmodium malariae*. Most deaths are the result of *P. falciparum* and occur in children under age 5 years, although pregnant women are also at increased risk for severe disease. Early treatment usually results in cure without recurrence, although *P. ovale* and *P. vivax* may remain dormant and recur months or years after the initial infection. Once infected, partial immunity may develop.

Human infection begins when sporozoites in the salivary gland of the female *Anopheles* mosquito are inoculated into the human host as the insect feeds. These parasites infect human hepatocytes within 30 minutes of entering the human body.[39] In the hepatocyte, each sporozoite divides and differentiates to form up to 30,000 merozoites, which rupture the hepatocyte and enter the bloodstream to infect erythrocytes.[40] Sporozoites of *P. vivax* and *P. ovale* may also form hypnozoites, dormant forms that remain in hepatocytes and may lead to recurrent infection months or years later. Merozoites actively enter the host erythrocytes, where they differentiate into ring-shaped trophozoites. These trophozoites develop into a schizont, which fills with merozoites, subsequently rupturing the erythrocyte and infecting other red blood cells (RBCs). Periodically, merozoites differentiate into male or female gametocytes, sexual forms that are ingested by *Anopheles* mosquitoes feeding on the infected human host. In the mosquito midgut, gametocytes merge to form a diploid zygote that differentiates into a motile ookinete that enters the gut wall to form an oocyst.

Sporozoites released from the oocyst migrate to the salivary glands of the mosquito to repeat the cycle.[39]

Rupture of erythrocytes by proliferating merozoites occurs with a periodicity related to the species of plasmodia. This cycle repeats every 72 hours for *P. malariae (quartan malaria)* and every 48 hours for other malaria species *(tertian malaria)*. Fever greater than 40°C is lethal to schizonts; consequently, the life cycle tends to be synchronized over the course of the infection, leading to periodic fever spikes rather than continuous fever.[41] Anemia develops in the infected human as a result of erythrocyte rupture by merozoite proliferation and by sequestration of normal uninfected RBCs by an engorged liver and spleen. Iron stores are depleted as hemoglobin from lysed RBCs is lost in urine.

Renal failure can result from a number of causes, including the rigidity of RBCs filled with merozoites that fail to pass through venules and capillaries, leading to microvascular sludging and ischemia in the kidneys. Cerebral malaria (the most common cause of death in this disease) occurs only with *P. falciparum* infection, as clumps of erythrocytes occlude the cerebral microvasculature, causing diffuse cerebral ischemia.

Acutely ill patients with malaria typically have either *P. falciparum* or *P. vivax* infections.[41] Partial resistance to malaria occurs in the presence of sickle cell trait (due to decreased intra-erythrocytic ATPase activity, which decreases surplus energy available to support parasite proliferation[39]) and in the absence of the Duffy antigen (due to the propensity of merozoites of *P. vivax* to invade erythrocytes by binding to that antigen).

Diagnosis

Fevers, chills, and headaches are the hallmark of malarial infection. The chills can last for periods of 1 to 2 hours. Concomitant with lysis of RBCs, the febrile stage is characterized by rigors, flushing, headache, and muscle aches with temperatures of 39° to 42°C. This stage can last for up to 6 hours, followed by profuse sweating and, as these symptoms disappear, excessive fatigue. Although most cases of malaria are classified as mild or uncomplicated, as the degree of parasitemia in patients with *P. falciparum* rises above 2%, the risk of severe malaria grows. Severe malaria is characterized by renal failure (sometimes accompanied by gross hemoglobinuria from lysed RBCs, termed *black-water fever*), noncardiogenic pulmonary edema, severe anemia, jaundice, seizures, parasitemia of greater than 5%, coma, circulatory collapse, or hypoglycemia, in the presence of either recent exposure to malaria or *P. falciparum* on smear.[42]

For the past 100 years, confirmation of the diagnosis of malaria has been made with the demonstration of intraerythrocytic parasites by Giemsa-stained thick and thin smears of fresh fingerprick blood. All four *Plasmodium* species may be identified in this fashion. Although the thin smear is easier to read, the thick smear is 10 to 40 times more sensitive and can detect as few as 50 parasites/μL.[43] Detectable parasitemia may lag behind aches, fevers, and chills by 2 days. If malaria is suspected, thick and thin smears should be done every 8 to 12 hours on at least three occasions, the collection of which should not be tied to fever spikes. Persistently negative smears after this time period argue against the presence of malaria.[41]

Several alternative laboratory methods have been developed, including the quantitative buffy-coat centrifugal hematology system, immunofluorescence, ELISA tests for the detection of the *P. falciparum* antigen, and the polymerase chain reaction (PCR) technique. Because of cost and complexity, none of these tests are used routinely.[44] Rapid blood tests using a dipstick or test strip with monoclonal antibodies directed against the target parasite antigen histidine-rich protein 2 (Pf HRP2) or parasite-specific lactate dehydrogenase (pLDH) are currently commercially available. Limitations in these methods include persistent Pf HRP2 antigenemia despite microscopic and clinical cure and positivity of pLDH only when viable parasites are present.[41]

Maternal and Fetal Risks

Pregnant women have an increased risk of malarial infection compared to their nonpregnant adult counterparts,[45] the difference being most marked during the first pregnancy. In one study in Malawi, the incidence of parasitemia in primigravidas was 66%, falling to 29% in second and 20.9% in subsequent pregnancies.[46] This increased susceptibility may be due to a number of reasons. Pregnant women seem to be more attractive to the female *Anopheles* mosquito than nonpregnant women and incur a significantly greater number of bites.[47] Sequestration of *P. falciparum* in the placenta may be another; in one case in which a woman's peripheral blood parasitemia was 3% at presentation (and presumably less after treatment), her placenta at delivery showed a local parasitemia of 70%.[48]

Although the major adverse effect of malaria in pregnancy on the mother is anemia, the risk of developing severe and complicated malaria is three times higher in pregnancy[49] and that of developing hypoglycemia is seven times more likely.[50] Both *P. falciparum* and *P. vivax* have been associated with an increased incidence of low birth weight.[51] Studies have demonstrated an increased incidence of intrauterine growth restriction when parasitemia is found during the antenatal period and an increased incidence of premature birth when cord blood parasitemia (probably reflecting recent active infection) is seen.[52,53]

Management Options

Prepregnancy

Malaria chemoprophylaxis and therapy before pregnancy is similar to that administered to other adults, and can be reviewed at www.cdc.gov. Management principles are similar to those discussed in the following sections, with the exception that additional drugs are available to the nonpregnant adult that are not appropriate for the pregnant woman.

Prenatal

Management of the pregnant patient involves two components: prevention of infection and treatment of disease. To prevent serious infection in pregnancy, pregnant women should be advised to avoid travel into areas where there is chloroquine-resistant *P. falciparum* malaria. However, when travel is unavoidable into these regions, use of pyrethroid-containing flying-insect spray in living and sleeping areas during evening and nighttime hours is advisable. Bednets, especially those sprayed with the insecticide permethrin, are effective in limiting mosquito bites, and use of the insecticide DEET is a safe and effective means to minimize bites during pregnancy as well.[55] Recommended chemoprophylaxis in areas *without* chloroquine-resistant *P. falciparum* is chloroquine phosphate (Aralen) 500 mg/week (300 mg chloroquine base) once weekly beginning 2 weeks before travel and during exposure and for 4 weeks after leaving the endemic area. Recommended chemoprophylaxis in areas *with* chloroquine-resistant *P. falciparum* is mefloquine (Lariam) 250 mg/week following the same schedule as chloroquine. It is critical that the patient continue the medication for 4 weeks after leaving the endemic area because infection is not prevented by the chemoprophylaxis, since sporozoites released into the bloodstream by the biting mosquito still reach the liver even in the presence of these medications. As the developing merozoites are released into the bloodstream, the infection succumbs to the drugs at this point.[55]

Before treating a pregnant patient with malaria, one should consider the place where the infection occurred, the trimester of pregnancy, and whether the clinical and parasitologic situation is severe. Consideration of the place where the infection occurred allows the clinician to use drugs that should meet with the least chance of resistance in the parasite. Consideration of the trimester of pregnancy allows the clinician to use drugs with the least chance of fetal toxicity, and consideration of the clinical and parasitologic situation allows the clinician to determine the aggressiveness and length of therapy. The drug or drugs chosen should be effective in the reduction of the asexual forms in the blood and in the placenta in order to prevent or reduce the severe clinical forms. Although the latest recommendations regarding specific treatment from certain regions may be obtained from the CDC, we review concepts of malaria therapy and drugs useful in the pregnant patient.

CHLOROQUINE

Although in many areas of the world, 80% or more of *P. falciparum* infections exhibit a high degree of chloroquine resistance,[56] chloroquine is still considered one of the safest antimalarials. It is not considered to be a cause of spontaneous abortion or teratogenesis when used for chemoprophylaxis or in recommended dosages for treatment,[57] but when given in large doses, has been reported to cause alterations of the eighth cranial nerve and retinal pigmentation in the fetus.[58]

QUININE AND QUINIDINE

Quinine and quinidine remain effective therapies for malaria, and a quinine-tetracycline combination cures nearly 100% of *P. falciparum* infections no matter in which region of the world the disease is contracted.[41] Unfortunately, although quinine may be used during pregnancy, tetracyclines should be avoided because of adverse fetal effects. Quinine may cause cinchonism (headache, tinnitus, nausea, vision disturbances) and, if glucose-6-phosphate dehydrogenase deficiency is present, hemolysis. Quinidine may be used intravenously with caution, because of its cardiosuppressant effects and its tendency to cause severe hypotension when administered rapidly. It can also cause hypoglycemia in the pregnant patient because of its tendency to stimulate the beta cells to produce insulin.[42]

Quinine has been shown to be safe in therapeutic doses in the first trimester of pregnancy.[59]

ANTIFOLATE DRUGS

The drug combinations sulfadoxine/pyrimethamine and sulfamethoxazole/trimethoprim work synergistically on two enzymes of the *Plasmodium* organism: dihydropteroate synthase and dihydrofolate reductase. Pyrimethamine has produced a teratogenic effect in laboratory test animals (which can be avoided by the administration of folinic acid), and sulfa administration to the mother near delivery has a theoretical risk to the fetus of kernicterus. Because of these concerns, these combinations should be limited to second or early third trimesters.

MEFLOQUINE

Mefloquine is critical for chemoprophylaxis or therapy in areas of chloroquine-resistant *P. falciparum*. Studies have not shown significant adverse effects on mother or fetus when mefloquine is administered in the second or third trimester of pregnancy. Observations made on a group of 1133 women who used mefloquine before conceiving or during pregnancy failed to show any toxic or teratogenic effects on the embryo.[60] Side effects in general may include the induction of neuropsychiatric alterations including anxiety, affective disorders, hallucinations, psychosis, and convulsions.[61]

CLINDAMYCIN

Clindamycin is useful in the treatment of resistant *P. falciparum* and is an alternative to tetracycline or doxycycline, because it does not produce important adverse effects in the pregnant patient or fetus. Clindamycin in combination with quinine has been used for over 20 years in Brazil and has been found to be an effective therapy for multiresistant strains of malaria, with no observed significant side effects in mother or fetus.[45]

ARTEMISININS

These antimalarials, isolated by Chinese scientists from *Artemisia annua*, currently are the fastest acting of all antimalarial drugs and have not shown significant toxicity.[62]

Resistance is rare, and while experimental studies with laboratory animals showed that doses above 10 mg/kg weight cause fetal resorption,[63] preclinical studies did not show any mutative or teratogenic effects.[64] Therefore, use should be limited to the second or third trimesters of pregnancy.

Labor and Delivery

No specific recommendations are needed for labor and/or delivery in these patients.

Postpartum

Breastfeeding patients should use the same chemoprophylaxis schedule and medication regimen for therapy as the pregnant patient.

Malaria Vaccines

Due to the various life cycles of the protozoan and other features of the infection, development of a malaria vaccine remains elusive.[65]

SUMMARY OF MANAGEMENT OPTIONS

Malaria

Management Options	Quality of Evidence	Strength of Recommendation	References
Prepregnancy			
If possible, women trying to conceive should avoid travel to endemic areas.	IV	C	45
If such travel is unavoidable, prophylaxis should be taken.	Ib	A	54
Consult www.cdc.gov for appropriate chemoprophylaxis and therapy; significant resistance exists in various regions of the world.	–	GPP	–
Advise patient that use of pyrethroid-containing insect spray and permethrin-impregnated bednets with liberal use of DEET insect spray topically will reduce frequency of mosquito bites.	Ib	A	54
Currently, no effective vaccines are available.	IV	C	44, 65
Prenatal–General			
If possible, women trying to conceive should avoid travel to endemic areas, especially those with drug-resistant strains.	IV	C	45
If such travel is unavoidable, prophylaxis should be taken and spray and nets used as recommended.	Ib	A	54
Prenatal–Treatment			
Chemoprophylaxis should begin 2 weeks *before* travel and continue for 4 weeks *after* leaving the endemic area.	III	B	43
Chloroquine is a safe, effective chemoprophylactic drug for susceptible strains of *Plasmodium*.	IIa	B	45,59
Quinine, mefloquine, and clindamycin are also appropriate and safe therapies in pregnancy.	IIa	B	45,59
Monitor electrolytes, renal and liver function, and hematology.	–	GPP	–
After therapy, maintain vigilance/surveillance for IUGR and preterm labor.	IIb	B	52
Labor and Delivery			
No specific recommendations are necessary for labor and delivery.	–	–	–

Continued

SUMMARY OF MANAGEMENT OPTIONS
Malaria (Continued)

Management Options	Quality of Evidence	Strength of Recommendation	References
Postnatal			
Breastfeeding is not contraindicated, but the same chemotherapeutic regimens should be used as in pregnancy.	III	B	43
Consider malaria for as long as 1 year after travel to endemic areas when evaluating a patient with fever or other signs that may indicate malaria.	III	B	43

SYPHILIS

General

Syphilis is a complex systemic illness caused by the spirochete *Treponema pallidum*. Debate about the origin of syphilis has continued for nearly 500 years, with sixteenth century Europeans blaming each other, referring to it variously as the Venetian, Naples, or French disease. Recent evaluations of several hundred skeletons from archaeological sites in the United States and Ecuador ranging in age from 400 to 6000 years favor a New World origin.[66] Syphilis currently is a worldwide malady that can lead to serious maternal and fetal complications. The nickname "lues" came from the Latin *lues venereum*, which means "disease," "sickness," or "pestilence" and originally was loosely applied to any venereal disease. It became a synonym for syphilis at the beginning of the 20th century.

Despite continued declines among African Americans and women of all races, overall rates of primary and secondary syphilis have recently increased for the first time in more than a decade. Primary and secondary syphilis in the United States rose by 2% between 2000 and 2001 (from 5979 cases in 2000 to 6103 cases in 2001). The overall syphilis rate in the United States increased from 2.1 per 100,000 people to 2.2 per 100,000 people, the first such increase since 1990.[67]

The causal agent of syphilis is *T. pallidum* spp. *pallidum*, which belongs to the family Spirochaetaceae. Other members of the genus *Treponema* that can infect humans are *Treponema pallidum* spp. *pertenue* (yaws), *Treponema carateum* (pinta), and *Treponema pallidum* spp. *endemicum* (bejel, nonvenereal, or endemic syphilis). A number of nonpathogenic treponemes have also been isolated from humans, particularly from the oral cavity. Other pathogenic organisms of the family Spirochaetaceae belong to the genera *Borrelia* and *Leptospira*.[68]

Syphilis can be acquired by sexual contact, by the fetus during pregnancy or birth, by kissing or other close contact with an active lesion, by transfusion of fresh human blood (banked less than 24 to 48 hours), or by accidental direct inoculation. The overwhelming majority of cases of syphilis are transmitted by sexual intercourse, but for all practical purposes a patient cannot spread syphilis by sexual contact 4 years or more after acquiring the disease.[68] Clinically, syphilis can be divided into five stages: incubating, primary, secondary, latent, and late syphilis. Diagnosis, therapy, and risk to the fetus vary with the stage of the disease.

Within hours or days after *T. pallidum* penetrates the intact mucous membrane or gains access through abraded skin, it enters the lymphatics or bloodstream and disseminates through the body. Virtually any organ, including the CNS, may be invaded. The minimum dose for human infection is not known, but in rabbits, an inoculum containing as few as four spirochetes can establish an infection. The incubation period is directly related to the size of the inoculum.[69] The median incubation period is 21 days, but can range from 3 to 90 days. During this stage, a spirochetemia develops that sets the stage for subsequent multiple organ invasion. The first symptomatology to develop occurs in the primary stage, which can last for 4 to 6 weeks (range, 2 to 8 weeks), and which usually includes development of the chancre. This painless ulcer (which may be slightly tender to the touch) occurs at the site of inoculation. A small inoculum produces only a papular lesion; a larger inoculum produces the ulcerative chancre. Persons with a history of previous syphilitic infection fail to develop any lesion or develop only a small, darkfield-negative papule.[69] Multiple chancres may occur.[70] Chancres heal spontaneously in 3 to 6 weeks (range, 1 to 12 weeks), leaving no trace or a thin atrophic scar. The manifestations of secondary syphilis often develop while the chancre is still present,[71] especially in HIV-infected patients.

The secondary or disseminated stage becomes evident 2 to 12 weeks (mean, 6 weeks) after contact. The generalized nature of this stage becomes evident as parenchymal, constitutional, and mucocutaneous manifestations may develop. The greatest number of treponemes is present in the body during this stage, and the classic and most commonly recognized lesions involve the skin. Macular, maculopapular, papular, or pustular lesions, and combinations and variations thereof, all may occur.[71] Vesicular lesions are notably absent. In warm, moist intertriginous areas, the papules enlarge, coalesce, and erode to produce painless, broad, moist, gray-white to erythematous, highly infectious plaques called *condylomata lata*. Constitutional symptomatology is also frequently present during the secondary stage and may include low-grade fever, malaise, pharyngitis, laryngitis, anorexia, weight loss, arthralgias, and generalized painless lymphadenopathy. The CNS may be involved in up to 40% of patients—headache and meningismus are common. The differential diagnosis of secondary syphilis is extensive—hence the name "The Great Imitator."

Latent syphilis is by definition that stage of the disease during which a specific treponemal antibody test is present but during which there are no clinical manifestations of syphilis. It does not imply a lack of progression of disease. Early latent syphilis distinguishes the first year of that period, and late latent syphilis begins after 1 year. Only during the first 4 years of latent syphilis may a relapse occur; thus, the patient must continue to be considered infectious during those 4 years. After 4 years of late latent syphilis, the patient develops host resistance to reinfection and to infectious relapse. However, a pregnant woman with late latent syphilis can transmit the infection vertically to her fetus.

Late or tertiary syphilis is a slowly progressive, inflammatory disease that may affect any organ system and is usually subdivided into neurosyphilis, cardiovascular syphilis, and gummatous syphilis.

Diagnosis

Unlike many nonpathogenic treponemas, the virulent treponemes, including *T. pallidum*, cannot be cultivated in vitro.

Direct Examination for Spirochetes

In primary, secondary, and early congenital syphilis, the darkfield examination (a wet-preparation method for direct visualization of living *T. pallidum* spirochetes) or immunofluorescence staining of mucocutaneous lesions are the quickest and most direct laboratory methods of establishing the diagnosis.[72] Examination of a serous transudate from moist lesions such as a primary chancre or condyloma latum is productive because these lesions contain the largest number of treponemes. *T. pallidum* may be demonstrated from dry skin lesions or from lymph nodes by saline aspiration, if the saline is free of bactericidal additives. Specimens from mouth lesions are not accurate because *T. pallidum* cannot be distinguished from nonpathogenic treponemes with certainty.

Serologic Tests

Two different types of antibodies are measured in the evaluation of syphilis: the *nonspecific* nontreponemal reaginic antibody and the *specific* antitreponemal antibody.

Syphilis reaginic antibodies are immunoglobulin G (IgG) and IgM directed against a lipoidal antigen resulting from the interaction of host tissues with *T. pallidum* or from the organism itself. The earliest antigens used to measure reaginic antibody were phospholipid extracts made from beef livers and subsequently from beef hearts (hence the name *cardiolipin*). The standard nontreponemal test is the VDRL (Venereal Disease Research Laboratories) slide test, although most laboratories have adopted a modification for routine screening called the rapid plasma reagin (RPR) test or other similar method. The quantitative RPR test should become nonreactive 1 year after successful therapy in primary syphilis and 2 years after successful therapy in secondary syphilis.[73] A patient with late syphilis should have a negative response after 5 years.[74] However, the longer the disease has been present before treatment, the longer the VDRL takes to become nonreactive. In many cases after the secondary stage, it will never become nonreactive, even with adequate treatment (this is called *Wasserman fastness*). A prozone phenomenon occurs in about 2% of infected patients, especially in secondary syphilis and pregnancy, and appropriate dilutions should be performed whenever the index of suspicion is high.[75]

The principal specific antitreponemal antibody tests done today are the fluorescent treponemal antibody absorption test (FTA-abs), the *T. pallidum* particle agglutination (TPPA) test, *T. pallidum* hemagglutination assay (TPHA), and the microhemagglutination assay—*T. pallidum* (MHA-TP) test. The FTA-abs is a standard indirect immunofluorescent antibody test that uses *T. pallidum* harvested from rabbit testes as the antigen. Because of the difficulty with standardization between labs and with quantifying results and the meticulousness with which the test must be performed, the TPHA, which uses a sorbent for increased specificity, or the MHA-TP, an adaptation of the TPHA, are commonly used today. Once positive, the patient usually remains positive for life, although patients treated early may revert to a nonreactive state in up to 10% of cases.[68] Acute or transient false-positive nontreponemal reaginic test reactions may occur whenever there is a strong immunologic stimulus, such as with an acute bacterial or viral infection, vaccination, or early HIV infection. Positive reactions that last for months may occur with parenteral drug abuse, in those with autoimmune or connective tissue diseases, and in patients in hypergammaglobulinemic states. Syphilis may be excluded if a biologic false-positive (BFP) test is suspected by obtaining a negative specific treponemal antibody test, such as the FTP-abs or MHA-TP. Other spirochetal illnesses, such as relapsing fever (*Borrelia* spp.), yaws, pinta, leptospirosis, or rat-bite fever (*Spirillum minus*) may also yield a positive nontreponemal test. Infection with *Borrelia burgdorferi* (Lyme disease) results in a positive FTA-abs test but does not cause a positive nontreponemal reaginic reaction with either the VDRL or RPR.

Because of expense and ease of performance, screening large numbers of patients such as in pregnancy is usually done with reaginic antibody tests (RPR, VDRL), and confirmation is done with the specific treponemal tests (FTA-abs or MHA-TP).

Ultrasound

The prenatal diagnostic test with the greatest potential for identifying the severely infected fetus is ultrasound. Ultrasound findings suggestive of in utero infection include placentomegaly, intrauterine growth restriction, microcephaly, hepatosplenomegaly, anemia, and hydrops.

Maternal and Fetal Risks

Maternal risks of syphilis acquired during pregnancy are similar to those for acquisition in the nonpregnant state. However, because up to 75% of infants born to mothers with active syphilitic infections will become infected in utero,[76] it is critical to identify infections as early in pregnancy as possible to reduce this risk. Although vertical transmission can occur during any stage of infection in the untreated or inadequately treated gravida, infection of the fetus before 16 weeks' gestation is rare; therefore, early abortion is unlikely to be the result of syphilis. Treatment of the mother during that period usually ensures that the fetus will not be infected. Later in pregnancy, depending on the severity of the maternal infection, abortion, stillbirth, neonatal death, neonatal disease, or latent infection may be seen.[72] Recent evidence indicates that these manifestations appear to be caused largely by dysfunction of the maternal-fetal endocrine axis, resulting in decreased levels of dehydroepiandrosterone produced by the fetal adrenal glands.[77] Neonatal manifestations of congenital syphilis include rhinitis (snuffles), which may be followed by a diffuse maculopapular, desquamative rash with extensive sloughing of the epithelium, particularly on the palms, on the soles, and around the mouth and anus. Hepatic involvement with associated splenomegaly, anemia, thrombocytopenia, and jaundice are also common findings. Neonatal death is usually caused by liver failure, severe pneumonia, or pulmonary hemorrhage. Renal involvement and a generalized osteochondritis and perichondritis may be seen as well.

Management Options

Prepregnancy

Although the efficacy of penicillin in the treatment of syphilis is well established, there remains uncertainty regarding optimal dose and duration of therapy, especially during pregnancy.[78] Therefore, treatment regimens must be viewed with this in mind and with the understanding that treatment failures do occur and must be recognized and re-treated. From work with experimental infections, it is known that penicillin concentrations as low as 0.018 μg/mL sustained for 7 days in the nonpregnant adult results in almost 100% treponemicidal activity.[79] It has also been recognized that *T. pallidum* has been isolated from the cerebrospinal fluid (CSF) of patients with only a chancre.[80] Therefore, to adequately treat this infection that may affect the CNS, one must treat the parasite in the CSF. However, despite the fact that benzathine penicillin does not reliably achieve treponemicidal levels in the CSF[81] and that re-treatment may be required in as many as 1 in 33 cases,[82] clinical experience continues to suggest that benzathine penicillin remains a mainstay of therapy. When an early diagnosis is made, fewer treponemes exist and the likelihood of a complete cure is greatly enhanced. Because of the high risk of infection, treatment should be given to anyone exposed to infectious syphilis within the preceding 3 months. Serologic studies must be done to establish the diagnosis and monitor success of therapy.

Prenatal

Pregnant patients should receive penicillin in the same dosage schedules as nonpregnant adults for comparable stages of the disease. When a well-documented penicillin allergy exists, desensitization (which can be accomplished in as few as 3 to 4 hours) is recommended.[83,84]

For primary and secondary syphilis and for early latent syphilis, administer benzathine penicillin G 2.4 million units IM once. For late latent syphilis or for latent syphilis of unknown duration, administer benzathine penicillin G 7.2 million units total, as three doses of 2.4 million units IM each at 1-week intervals. Regimens for syphilis in pregnancy that do not include penicillin have not been documented to be adequate therapy to prevent congenital syphilis. Pregnant patients with concomitant HIV infections should be considered for treatment as if they have neurosyphilis, regardless of their clinical findings.[85]

All women should be screened serologically for syphilis at the first prenatal visit. In populations in which prenatal care is not optimal, RPR test screening and treatment (if the RPR test is reactive) should be performed at the time a pregnancy is confirmed. For communities and populations in which the prevalence of syphilis is high or for patients at high risk, serologic testing in addition to routine early screening should be performed twice during the third trimester: at 28 weeks' gestation and at delivery.

The fetus with hepatomegaly or ascites is more likely to fail prenatal therapy and may benefit from a more extended course than usual and more intense monitoring throughout the remainder of the pregnancy.[86]

The Jarisch-Herxheimer reaction is a systemic reaction that occurs 1 to 2 hours after the initial treatment of syphilis with effective antibiotics. It consists of the abrupt onset of fever, chills, myalgia, headache, tachycardia, hyperventilation, vasodilation with flushing, and mild hypotension. Additional findings at or beyond 24 weeks' gestation include uterine contractions (42%) and recurrent variable fetal heart rate decelerations (38%).[87] It lasts for 12 to 24 hours and may be treated in pregnancy with antipyretics or prednisone, although no studies have documented a clearly effective prophylaxis.

Labor and Delivery

In the United States some states mandate screening for syphilis at delivery for all women. Any woman who delivers a stillborn infant after 20 weeks' gestation should be tested for syphilis.

Postpartum

No infant should leave the hospital if maternal serologic status has not been determined at least once during pregnancy and preferably again at delivery. All patients with early or congenital syphilis should have repeat quantitative nontreponemal tests at 3, 6, and 12 months. All patients with secondary syphilis or syphilis of more than 1 year's duration should also have a nontreponemal serologic test 24 months after treatment. Many experts recommend examination of the CSF for those patients treated with benzathine penicillin because of its poor ability to penetrate the CSF. Re-treatment should be considered whenever clinical signs and symptoms of syphilis persist or recur, whenever there is a sustained level or an increase in the titer on the nontreponemal test, or whenever a positive RPR reaction persists beyond 12 months in primary syphilis, 24 months in secondary or latent syphilis, or 5 years in late syphilis.[68]

SUMMARY OF MANAGEMENT OPTIONS

Syphilis

Management Options	Quality of Evidence	Strength of Recommendation	References
Prepregnancy			
Identify and treat with penicillin (provided not allergic) before pregnancy.	IV	C	78
Initiate contact tracing and treatment.	–	GPP	–
Confirm response with serial serology.	–	GPP	–
Prenatal			
Provide routine serologic screening in early pregnancy.	IV	C	78
Treat with penicillin (provided not allergic) all with *T. palladum*–positive lesions (rare).	IV	C	78
Probably safer to treat all women with positive serology with penicillin (provided not allergic) even if history suggests they have been treated in the past; treatment before 16 weeks will usually prevent congenital syphilis.	IV	C	78
If significant penicillin allergy is determined, the pregnant patient should be desensitized, because only penicillin will adequately treat the fetus.	III	B	83, 84
Initiate contact tracing and treatment.	–	GPP	–
Confirm response with serial serology.	IV	C	78
Labor and Delivery			
Some states in the U.S. require testing of all women at delivery.	–	GPP	–
Evaluate all cases of stillbirth >20 weeks for the presence of syphilis.	IV	C	68
Inform pediatricians.	IV	C	86
Postnatal			
Alert pediatricians to the presence of syphilis during pregnancy so that they can properly evaluate the neonate for early (snuffles, rash, hepatosplenomegaly, jaundice) and late (deafness, hydrocephalus, optic nerve atrophy, mental retardation) manifestations of congenital syphilis.	IV	C	86
Follow-up tests should occur up to 2 years after treatment, with concomitant fall in titers during that period.	III	B	68, 76

TOXOPLASMOSIS

General

Toxoplasmosis is caused by the obligate intracellular parasite *Toxoplasma gondii*. Its name is derived from "toxon" (Greek for *arc*, the shape of the parasite during its acute infectious phase in humans) and "gundi" (the North African rodent from which the parasite was originally identified). Infections in immunocompetent individuals are frequently subclinical and innocuous unless the individual is pregnant, during which time vertical transmission can occur and lead to significant disease and possibly death in the fetus or neonate. The organism has three distinct forms: the tachyzoite, or arc form, found in the parasitemic or acute phase of infection; the tissue cyst, found in the quiescent or latent phase in many organs of humans and animals; and the oocyst, which originates only in the digestive tract of members of the family *Felidae* (including domestic and feral cats).

Toxoplasmosis can be transmitted to humans by three principal routes. It is estimated that approximately 50% of the toxoplasmosis cases in the United States are caused by eating inadequately cooked meat[88] (especially pork, mutton, and wild game meat) containing the tissue cyst form of the organism.[89] A second means of acquiring toxoplasmosis is by inadvertently ingesting the oocysts that cats have passed in their feces, either from a cat litter box, from infected soil where a cat has defecated, or from unwashed fruits or vegetables that have contacted infected soil. Under favorable conditions (i.e., in warm, moist soil), oocysts can remain infectious for approximately 1 year. A third means of transmission is transplacentally, when a primary infection occurs during pregnancy. Other than vertical transmission and the rare incidence of blood or organ donation between individuals, it is not possible to acquire toxoplasmosis from either a neonate or another adult. In adults, the incubation period ranges from 10 to 23 days from ingestion of undercooked meat, and from 5 to 20 days from ingestion of oocysts from cat feces.[90]

Since the 1960s, rates of infection with *Toxoplasma* in the United States appear to have declined from 14% (in a study of U.S. military recruits at that time) to a seroprevalence of 9.6% in a second study of recruits in 1989.[91,92] In the Third National Health and Nutrition Examination Survey (NHANES III) conducted in the United States from 1988 to 1994, 17,658 individuals were tested for *Toxoplasma*-specific IgG antibodies; 23% were found to be positive. Of 5988 women of childbearing age (12 to 49 years) in that series, 14% were seropositive.[93]

Determining the number of cases of congenital toxoplasmosis is more difficult than estimating seroprevalence, although prospective studies in the United States from the 1970s[94,95] and from the period 1986 to 1992[96] indicate an infection rate of between 1 in 10,000 to 10 in 10,000 live births. With an estimated 4 million births annually in the United States, 400 to 4000 neonates yearly will be born with congenital toxoplasmosis.

Although some studies identify cleaning the cat litter box[97] or owning a cat[98] as risk factors, the presence of a cat has not been a consistent risk factor for *T. gondii* infection. Owning a cat was not shown to be a risk factor for *T. gondii* infection in two studies of pregnant women[99,100] and in a study of HIV-infected persons.[101] Cats generally only shed oocysts for several weeks during their lives if they become infected with *T. gondii*. Cats kept indoors that do not hunt prey or are not fed raw meat are not likely to acquire *T. gondii* infection and therefore pose little risk. Because of their grooming habits, fecal matter has not been found on the fur of clinically normal cats, and adult cats are not diarrheal during the period in which they are shedding oocysts.[88] Therefore, the possibility of transmission to human beings via touching cats is minimal to nonexistent.[88] Because cats may not develop antibodies to *T. gondii* during the oocyst-shedding period, serologic examination of cats does not provide useful information regarding the ability of a particular cat to transmit the infection.[88]

Outbreaks of toxoplasmosis in humans have been attributed to ingestion of raw or undercooked ground beef, lamb, pork, venison,[102–107] unpasteurized goat's milk,[108] contaminated unfiltered drinking water,[109–110] soil exposure,[111] and aerosolized soil exposure.[112]

Diagnosis

Because most acute *Toxoplasma* infections are relatively asymptomatic, a universal challenge for obstetricians is how to identify acute infections during pregnancy. In France and Austria, where the incidence of toxoplasmosis is much higher than in the United States, universal screening is mandatory.[113] In the United States, although universal screening has frequently been discussed, it is not generally practiced. A recent article using decision analysis estimated that universal screening with medical treatment would result in 18.5 additional pregnancy losses for each case of toxoplasmosis avoided (12.1 additional pregnancy losses were estimated to occur if infected pregnancies underwent termination rather than treatment).[114]

When screening is performed or when a pregnant woman's clinical presentation leads the practitioner to suspect acute toxoplasmosis, the diagnosis may be established by serologic tests, amplification of specific nucleic acid sequences (using PCR), histologic demonstration of the parasite and/or its antigens (immunoperoxidase stain), or isolation of the organism. Ultrasound also has an important role in the evaluation of this infection.

Serologic Tests

The use of serologic tests for demonstration of specific antibody to *T. gondii* in maternal blood is the initial and primary method of diagnosis. IgG antibodies usually appear within 1 to 2 weeks of acquisition of an infection, peak within 1 to 2 months, decline at various rates, and usually persist for life. The most common methods of measurement of IgG include the Sabin-Feldman dye test, the ELISA, the immunofluorescence assay (IFA), and the modified direct agglutination test.[115] IgM antibodies, on the other hand, may appear earlier and decline more rapidly than IgG antibodies. They are measured by ELISA, IFA, and the immunosorbent agglutination assay.[115] False-positive results for the presence of IgM may occur when rheumatoid factor or antinuclear antibodies are present. Commercial kits often have low specificity, and positive results must be interpreted with great caution. Although IgM antibodies usually decline rapidly after the onset of infection, they may persist for years in some individuals, further complicating the interpretation of a positive serologic test.

A combination of serologic tests is usually required to establish whether an individual has most likely been infected in the distant past (which should pose minimal to no risk to an ongoing pregnancy) or has been recently infected. The traditional acute and convalescent titers of IgM and IgG are most helpful when either both are negative in two samples 3 or more weeks apart (no acute or chronic infection) or IgG is positive and IgM is negative in both samples (distant infection but no acute infection). When IgM is positive in either (especially when titers are drawn after the first trimester of pregnancy), or when IgG is negative in the first and positive in the second (or with a greater than fourfold rise in IgG antibody titer from the first sample) with or without positive IgM, concern about a recent infection must be raised. A combination of tests that has demonstrated value in pregnancy to distinguish acute from chronic infection includes the Sabin-Feldman dye test (for the presence of IgG antibodies), double sandwich IgM ELISA, IgA ELISA, IgE ELISA, and differential agglutination test.[116] IgA antibodies may be detected in the sera of acutely infected adults and congenitally infected infants, and IgE antibodies have a briefer duration in the sera than IgM or IgA. The differential agglutination test uses the differential amount of agglutination that occurs when fixing *Toxoplasma* organisms with acetone and with formalin and reacting those antigens to sera that contains IgM antibodies and allows the laboratory to distinguish IgM antibodies that are acute from those that are chronic. An example of results from sera of a patient infected in the distant past would include a positive dye test; negative IgM, IgA, and IgE; and a chronic pattern in the differential agglutination test. On the other hand, an acute infection should be suspected with high titers of the dye test; positive IgM, IgA, and IgE; and an acute pattern with the differential agglutination test. Because indeterminate results may occur even with this combination, follow-up samples may be required. Ideally, when duplicate samples of these or any acute and convalescent titers are requested, they should be run by the same laboratory in parallel with the earlier sample for greatest accuracy in interpretation. When done by an appropriate reference laboratory, this combination of tests allows great precision in differentiating acute from chronic infections. Another recently reported means by which acute and chronic infections may be distinguished is by measuring the binding strength of specific IgG antibodies to multivalent *Toxoplasma* antigen. This binding strength, or IgG avidity, increases as the duration of infection lengthens. Thus, higher IgG avidity indicates a more long-standing infection and may be useful in early pregnancy when other tests are inconclusive.[117]

PCR

Polymerase chain reaction amplification for detection of *T. gondii* DNA in amniotic fluid has been used to accurately and rapidly diagnose intrauterine infection with the parasite. The sensitivity is high (81% to 88%),[118,119] and the overall accuracy is comparable to or better than fetal blood testing by cordocentesis[118,119] with less risk to the fetus.

Histology

Demonstration of tachyzoites in amniotic fluid or placental tissue establishes the diagnosis of an acute infection. This is best accomplished with the immunoperoxidase technique with antisera to *T. gondii*.[120]

Isolation of *T. gondii*

Isolation of the organism from tissue or fluid establishes the infection as acute. Mouse inoculation coupled with PCR analysis of amniotic fluid has sensitivities of 91% to 94%.[118,121]

Ultrasound

Ultrasound findings of fetal infection with *T. gondii* are generally nonspecific; however, ventricular dilation (the most common finding), intracranial calcifications, increased placental thickness, hepatic enlargement, and ascites may be seen in over one-third of cases of fetal infection and may be useful in evaluation.[122] In highly suspicious cases in which serology or PCR is nonconclusive, follow-up ultrasound has been found to be valuable in confirming a diagnosis of congenital toxoplasmosis.[123]

Maternal and Fetal Risks

Maternal risks of toxoplasmosis in the immunocompetent gravida are minimal, and 90% of infections are asymptomatic and self-limited. Symptoms most commonly resemble infectious mononucleosis with posterior cervical or axillary lymphadenopathy that is discrete, nontender, and nonsuppurative. Other maternal symptoms may include malaise and muscle pain.

Fetal risks, on the other hand, vary widely, depending on the trimester of acquisition and presence or absence of maternal treatment. In general, the earlier the infection is acquired, the lower the risk of fetal transmission, but the greater the risk of serious sequelae to the fetus when congenital infection does develop.[124] Maternal seroconversion occurring at or before 5 weeks' gestation has been reported to have minimal to no risk of fetal infection, whereas seroconversion in the third trimester may result in congenital infections in as many as 60% of neonates.[125] As many as 85% of congenitally infected neonates have subclinical infections that will later surface as chorioretinitis, hearing loss, or developmental delays. Serious sequelae noted at or after birth, including intrauterine death, neurologic abnormalities, hydrocephalus and cerebral calcifications, and chorioretinal scars with or without severe visual impairment, may be reduced by the use of prenatal antibiotic therapy even though the rate of congenital infection may not change.[118,126]

Management Options

Prepregnancy

Preconception infection with toxoplasmosis generally conveys immunity to subsequent pregnancies against congenital toxoplasmosis. Reports exist describing preconception seroconversion and subsequent fetal infection, but these are extremely rare,[127] and gravidas with IgG positivity at the onset of pregnancy should be considered at low risk for subsequent congenital infection.

Prenatal

Prevention of acute infection during pregnancy is much preferred to treatment of toxoplasmosis.

Pregnant women, especially those determined to be IgG-negative during pregnancy, should be advised of appropriate preventive measures to use. When acute toxoplasmosis is suspected during pregnancy, appropriate laboratory testing is critical (see "Diagnosis"). If serologic testing confirms acute *maternal* toxoplasmosis, amniocentesis with PCR testing of amniotic fluid should be performed to document presence of *fetal* infection. Mouse inoculation may also be considered along with PCR testing of the fluid. Cordocentesis is no longer considered an essential component of the evaluation of fetal infection, having been replaced by PCR due to its simplicity and relative safety. Spiramycin 3 g/day should be administered as soon as maternal infection is documented, adding pyrimethamine/sulfadiazine if fetal infection is confirmed by PCR testing or mouse inoculation studies of amniotic fluid. Doses and dosing schedules and the addition of folinic acid with pyrimethamine vary, taking into consideration the trimester and local preferences.[128,129] In the United States, spiramycin may be obtained from the Food and Drug Administration after confirmation of acute maternal infection by a reputable reference laboratory.

Labor and Delivery

Patients with ongoing or recent toxoplasmosis infection pose a transmission risk only to their fetus and do not require isolation for themselves or for their newborn. The pediatrician caring for the neonate should be alerted to the possibility of congenital toxoplasmosis so appropriate follow-up studies can be performed on the infant. Congenital infection can be excluded if IgG does not persist in the infant beyond age 12 months.

Postpartum

After delivery, the parturient may be managed routinely, again emphasizing to the healthcare team that neither she nor the newborn poses a risk of transmission to others.

SUMMARY OF MANAGEMENT OPTIONS

Toxoplasmosis

Management Options	Quality of Evidence	Strength of Recommendation	References
Prepregnancy			
Toxoplasmosis infection before conception (documented by the presence of IgG antibodies) conveys a relative immunity to the gravida and makes congenital infection extremely unlikely.	III	B	127
Prenatal–Prevention			
Teach patient to prevent *Toxoplasma* infection: • Cook meat to well done (industrial deep-freezing also seems to destroy parasites efficiently). • When handling raw meat, avoid touching mouth and eyes. • Wash hands thoroughly after handling raw meat or vegetables soiled by earth.	–	GPP	–

SUMMARY OF MANAGEMENT OPTIONS
Toxoplasmosis *(Continued)*

Management Options	Quality of Evidence	Strength of Recommendation	References
Prenatal–Prevention *(Continued)*			
• Wash kitchen surfaces that come into contact with raw meat.			
• Wash fruit and vegetables before consumption.			
• Avoid contact with things that are potentially contaminated with cat feces.			
• Wear gloves when gardening or handling cat litter box.			
• Disinfect cat litter box for 5 min with boiling water.			
The policy of routine screening for toxoplasmosis varies between countries; it is not practiced universally in the United States.	III	B	114
Prenatal–Diagnosis			
Maternal infection should be confirmed by an appropriate lab using reliable testing, which may include Sabin-Feldman dye test for IgG and ELISA; testing for IgM, IgA, and IgE along with IgG avidity testing; or differential agglutination test for chronicity of infection.	III	B	116
IgM antibodies for toxoplasmosis are frequently false-positive or may represent chronic infection, and should *always* be confirmed by a reference lab.	IIb	B	116
Prenatal–Treatment			
When maternal infection is confirmed, begin spiramycin as soon as possible.	IIa	B	122,129
Fetal infection may be diagnosed by PCR testing of amniotic fluid, obviating the need for cordocentesis (though not possible to determine prognosis).	IIa	B	118,121
Documented fetal infection necessitates addition of pyrimethamine/sulfadiazine.	IIa	B	122,129
Serial ultrasound will give an identification of signs of fetal infection.	IIa	B	121,123
Labor and Delivery; Postpartum			
Neither the mother nor infant is infectious to the healthcare team and may be handled in routine fashion.	IV	C	120

CONCLUSIONS

LYME DISEASE

- The diagnosis of Lyme disease is based on history of a tick bite in an endemic area and characteristic clinical findings rather than isolation of the organism or serology.
- Observe skin after tick bites for up to 30 days for signs of infection.
- Prophylactic antibiotics are usually not warranted in the absence of Lyme disease infection.

TUBERCULOSIS

- Droplet nuclei, containing two to three *M. tuberculosis* organisms, are so small that air currents normally present in any indoor space can keep them airborne for long periods of time.
- Although experts disagree about the most appropriate management of pregnant patients with latent nonclinical TB, isoniazid 300 mg daily for 6 to 9 months with pyridoxine 50 mg daily and baseline and serial liver function tests is the preferred treatment.

Continued

CONCLUSIONS (Continued)

MALARIA

- Although the major adverse effect of malaria in pregnancy on the mother is anemia, the risk of developing severe and complicated malaria is three times higher in pregnancy and that of developing hypoglycemia is seven times more likely.
- Use of pyrethroid-containing insect spray and permethrin-impregnated bednets with liberal use of DEET insect spray topically will reduce frequency of mosquito bites.
- Consult www.cdc.gov for appropriate chemoprophylaxis and therapy for malaria, because significant resistance exists in various regions of the world.
- Chloroquine is a safe, effective chemoprophylactic drug for susceptible strains of *Plasmodium*.
- Quinine, mefloquine, and clindamycin are also appropriate and safe therapies for malaria in pregnancy.
- Chemoprophylaxis for malaria should begin 2 weeks *before* travel and continue for 4 weeks *after* leaving the endemic area.

SYPHILIS

- Benzathine penicillin G is the treatment of choice for syphilis.
- If significant penicillin allergy is determined, the pregnant patient should be desensitized, because only penicillin will adequately treat the fetus.
- The Jarisch-Herxheimer reaction is a systemic reaction that occurs 1 to 2 hours after the initial treatment of syphilis with effective antibiotics. In addition to the abrupt onset of fever, chills, myalgias, headache, and other systemic symptoms, at or beyond 24 weeks' gestation the gravida may also experience uterine contractions and recurrent variable fetal heart rate decelerations.

TOXOPLASMOSIS

- Toxoplasmosis infection prior to conception (documented by the presence of IgG antibodies) conveys a relative immunity to the gravida and makes congenital infection extremely unlikely.
- False-positive serology for toxoplasmosis with IgM testing is frequent and must be confirmed with an appropriate reference laboratory.
- Fetal infection with toxoplasmosis may be confirmed by amniotic fluid testing with PCR or mouse inoculation, making cordocentesis unnecessary.
- Spiramycin for maternal toxoplasmosis infection and pyrimethamine/sulfadiazine for fetal infection will reduce neonatal sequelae of the disease.
- Neither the pregnant woman nor her fetus/neonate are infectious to the healthcare team and require no special handling during treatment.

REFERENCES

1. Burgdorfer WA, Barbour AG, Hayes SF, et al: Lyme disease—a tick-borne spirochetosis? Science 1982;216:1317–1319.
2. Sonenshine DE: Biology of Ticks. New York, Oxford University Press, 1991.
3. Singh-Behl D, LaRosa SP, Tomecki KJ: Tick-borne infections. Dermatol Clin 2003;21:237–244.
4. Lyme Disease—United States, 2000. MMWR 2002;51:29–31.
5. Steere AC: Lyme disease. N Engl J Med 1989;321:586–596.
6. Nadelman RB, Wormser GP: Lyme borreliosis. Lancet 1998; 352:557–565.
7. Spach DH, Liles WC, Campbell GL, et al: Tick-borne diseases in the United States. N Engl J Med 1993;329:936–947.
8. Steere AC, Bartenhagen NH, Craft J, et al: The early clinical manifestations of Lyme disease. Ann Intern Med 1983;99: 76–82.
9. Pfister HW, Wilske B, Weber K: Lyme borreliosis: Basic science and clinical aspects. Lancet 1994;343:1013–1016.
10. Schlesinger PA, Duray PH, Burke BA, et al: Maternal-fetal transmission of the Lyme disease spirochete, *Borrelia burgdorferi*. Ann Intern Med 1985; 103:67–69.
11. Weber K, Bratzke HJ, Neubert U, et al: *Borrelia burgdorferi* in a newborn despite oral penicillin for Lyme borreliosis during pregnancy. Pediatr Infect Dis J 1988;7:286–289.
12. Markowitz LE, Steere AC, Benach JL, et al: Lyme disease during pregnancy. JAMA 1987;255:3394–3396.
13. Weber K, Pfister HW: Clinical management of Lyme borreliosis. Lancet 1994;343:1017–1020.
14. Williams CL, Strobino BA: Lyme disease transmission during pregnancy. Contemp Ob/Gyn 1990;35:48–64.
15. Warshafsky S, Nowakowski J, Nadelman RB, et al: Efficacy of antibiotic prophylaxis for prevention of Lyme disease. J Gen Intern Med 1996; 11:329–333.
16. Wormser GP, Nadelman RB, Dattwyler RJ, et al: Practice guidelines for the treatment of Lyme diseases. Clin Infect Dis 2000; 31(pp 1):1–14.
17. Moore JA: Jarish-Herxheimer reaction in Lyme disease. Cutis 1987;39:397.
18. Raviglione MR, Snider DE Jr, Kochi A: Global epidemiology of tuberculosis—Morbidity and mortality of a world-wide epidemic. JAMA 1995;273:220–226.

19. World Health Organization: Global Tuberculosis Control: WHO Report 1998. WHO Global Tuberculosis Programme. WHO/TB/98.237. Geneva, World Health Organization, 1998.
20. Dye C, Scheele S, Dolin P, et al: Consensus statement. Global burden of tuberculosis: Estimated incidence, prevalence, and mortality by country. WHO Global Surveillance and Monitoring Project. JAMA 1999;282:677–686.
21. Edwards K, Kirkpatrick CH: The immunology of mycobacterial diseases. Am Rev Respir Dis 1986;134:1062–1071.
22. Riley R: Airborne infection. Am J Med 1974;57:466–475.
23. Murray J: Defense mechanisms. In J. J. Murray (ed): The Normal Lung: The Basis for Diagnosis and Treatment of Pulmonary Disease. Philadelphia, WB Saunders, 1986, pp 313–338.
24. Smith D, Wiengeshaus E: What animal models can teach us about the pathogenesis of tuberculosis in humans. Rev Infect Dis 1989;11:S385–S393.
25. Small PM, Schecter GF, Goodman PC, et al: Treatment of tuberculosis in patients with advanced human immunodeficiency virus infection. N Engl J Med 1991; 324:289–294.
26. Arango L, Brewin AW, Murray JF: The spectrum of tuberculosis as currently seen in a metropolitan hospital. Am Rev Respir Dis 1978;108:805–812.
27. Carr WPJ, Kyle RA, Bowie EFW: Hematologic changes in tuberculosis. Am J Med Science 1964;248:709–714.
28. Chung DK, Hubbard WW: Hyponatremia in untreated active pulmonary tuberculosis. Am Rev Respir Dis 1969;99:592–597.
29. Dunlap NE, Bass J, Fujiwara P, et al: Diagnostic standards and classification of tuberculosis in adults and children. Am J Respir Crit Care Med 2000;161:1376–1395.
30. Targeted tuberculin testing and treatment of latent tuberculosis infection. MMWR. 2000;1–54: No RR-6.
31. Menzles D: Interpretation of repeated tuberculin tests. Am J Respir Crit Care Med 1991;159:15–21.
32. Wilson ME, Fineberg HV, Colditz GA: Geographic latitude and the efficacy of bacillus Calmetté-Guerin vaccine. Clin Infect Dis 1995;20:982–991.
33. Jana N, Vasishta K, Jindal SK, et al: Perinatal outcome in pregnancies complicated by pulmonary tuberculosis. Int J Gynaecol Obstet 1994;44:119.
34. Riley L: Pneumonia and tuberculosis in pregnancy. Infect Dis Clin North Am 1997;11:119.
35. Jana N, Vasishta K, Saha SC, et al: Obstetrical outcomes among women with extrapulmonary tuberculosis. N Engl J Med 1999; 341:645.
36. Jindani A, Aber VR, Edwards EA: The early bactericidal activity of drugs in patients with pulmonary tuberculosis. Am Rev Respir Dis 1980;121:939–949.
37. Breman JG: The ears of the hippopotamus: Manifestations, determinants, and estimates of the malaria burden. Am J Trop Med Hyg 2001;64:1–11.
38. Marsh K: Malaria disaster in Africa. Lancet 1998;352:924–925.
39. Levinson W, Jawetz E: Blood and tissue protozoa. In Levinson W, Jawetz E (eds): Medical Microbiology and Immunology, 4th ed. Norwalk, Conn., Appleton and Lange, 1996, pp 274–276.
40. Samuelson J, von Lichtenberg F: Infectious disease. In Cotran R, Kumar V, Robbins S (eds): Pathologic Basis of Disease, 5th ed. Philadelphia, WB Saunders, 1994, pp 362–363.
41. Jerrard DA, Broder JS, Hanna JR, et al: Malaria: A rising incidence in the United States. J Emerg Med 2002;23:23–33.
42. Warrell D, Molyneaux M, Beales P: Severe and complicated malaria. Trans R Soc Trop Med Hyg 1990;84(suppl):1–65.
43. Centers for Disease Control and Prevention: Recommendations for the prevention of malaria among travelers. MMWR 1990;39:1–10.
44. Guerin PJ, Olliaro P, Nosten F, et al: Malaria: Current status of control, diagnosis, treatment, and a proposed agenda for research and development. Lancet Infect Dis 2002;2:564–573.
45. Alecrim WD, Espinosa FE, Alecrim MG: Emerging and reemerging diseases in Latin America: *Plasmodium falciparum* infection in the pregnant patient. Infect Dis Clin North Am 2000;14:83–95.
46. Steketee R, Wirima J, Slutsker L, et al: Objectives and methodology in a study of malaria treatment and prevention in pregnancy in rural Malawi: The Mangochi malaria research project. Am J Trop Med Hyg 1996;55:17–23.
47. Ansell J, Hamilton KA, Pinder M, et al: Short-range attractiveness of pregnant women to Anopheles gambiae mosquitoes. Trans R Soc Trop Med Hyg 2002;96:113–116.
48. Procop N, Jessen R, Hyde S, et al: The persistence of *Plasmodium falciparum* in the placenta after apparently effective quinidine/clindamycin therapy. J Perinatol 2001;21:128–130.
49. Luxemburger C, Ricci F, Nosten F, et al: The epidemiology of severe malaria in an area of low transmission in Thailand. Trans R Soc Trop Med Hyg 1997;91:256–262.
50. Saeed BO, Atabani GS, Nawwfaf A, et al: Hypoglycaemia in pregnant women with malaria. Trans R Soc Trop Med Hyg 1990;84:349–350.
51. Brabin B, Piper C: Anaemia and malaria-attributable low birthweight in two populations in Papua New Guinea. Ann Hum Biol 1997;24:547–555.
52. Steketee RW, Wirima JJ, Hightower AW, et al: The effect of malaria and malaria prevention in pregnancy on offspring birthweight, prematurity, and intrauterine growth retardation in rural Malawi. Am J Trop Med Hyg 1996;55(suppl 1):33–41.
53. Sullivan AD, Nyirenda T, Cullinan T, et al: Malaria infection during pregnancy: Intrauterine growth retardation and preterm delivery in Malawi. J Infect Dis 1999;179:1580–1583.
54. McGready R, Hamilton KA, Simpson JA, et al: Safety of the insect repellent N,N-dimethyl-M-toluamide (DEET) in pregnancy. Am J Trop Med Hyg 2001;65:285–289.
55. Kain K: Chemotherapy and prevention of drug-resistant malaria. Wilderness Env Med 1995;6:307–324.
56. Bloland P, Lackritz E, Kazembe P, et al: Beyond chloroquine: Implications for evaluating malaria therapy efficacy and treatment policy in Africa. J Infect Dis 1993;167:932–937.
57. World Health Organization: Advances in malaria chemotherapy. WHO Tech Rep Ser 1984:711:71–78.
58. Hart C, Naughton R: The ototoxicity of chloroquine phosphate. Arch Otolaryngol Head Neck Surg 1964;80:407–410.
59. McGready R, Thwai KL, Cho T, et al: The effects of quinine and chloroquine antimalarial treatments in the first trimester of pregnancy. Trans R Soc Trop Med Hyg 2002;96:180–184.
60. World Health Organization: Management of uncomplicated malaria and the use of antimalarial drugs for the protection of travelers: Report of an informed consultation. WHO/MAL/96. 1996;1075:19–22.
61. Phillips-Howard PA, Ter Kuile FO: CNS adverse events associated with antimalarial agents: Fact or fiction? Drug Saf 1995; 12:370–383.
62. White N: Artemisinin: Current status. Trans R Soc Trop Med Hyg (Suppl) 1994;88:3–4.
63. Qinghaosu Antimalarial Coordinating Committee: Antimalarial studies on qinghaosu. Chin Med J (Engl) 1979;92:811–816.
64. World Health Organization: The use of artemisinin and its derivatives as antimalarial drugs. Report of a joint CTD/DMP/TDR informal consultation. Geneva, 10–12 June 1998. WHO/MAL/ 98. 1998;1086:1–27
65. Moore SA, Surgey EGE, Cadwgan AM: Malaria vaccines: Where are we and where are we going? Lancet Infect Dis 2002; 2:737–743.
66. Rose M: Origins of syphilis. Archaeol 1997;50:24–25.
67. Heffelfinger JD, Weinstock HS, Berman SM, et al: Primary and secondary syphilis—United States, 2000–2001. MMWR 2002;51(43):971–973.
68. Tramont EC: *Treponema pallidum* (syphilis). In Mandell GL, Bennett JE, Dolin R (eds): Principles and Practice of Infectious Diseases, 5th ed. Philadelphia, Churchill Livingstone, 2000, pp 2474–2490.

69. Magnuson HJ, Thomas EW, Olansky S, et al: Inoculation syphilis in human volunteers. Medicine (Baltimore), 1956;35:33–42.
70. Chapel TA: The variability of syphilitic chancres. Sex Transm Dis 1978;5:68–72.
71. Chapel TA: The signs and symptoms of secondary syphilis. Sex Transm Dis 1980;7:161–167.
72. Kampmeier RH: Essentials of Syphilology, 3rd ed. Philadelphia, JB Lippincott, 1943.
73. Brown St, Akbar Z, Larsen SA, et al: Serological response to syphilis treatment. JAMA 1985;253:1296–1299.
74. Fiumara NJ: Serologic responses to treatment of 128 patients with late latent syphilis. Sex Transm Dis 1979;6:243–246.
75. Berkowitz K, Baxi L, Fox HE: False-negative syphilis screening: The prozone phenomenon, nonimmune hydrops, and diagnosis of syphilis during pregnancy. Am J Obstet Gynecol 1990;163: 975–977.
76. Ravel R: Spirochetal and rickettsial infections. In Ravel R (ed): Clinical Laboratory Medicine, 6th ed. St Louis, Mosby, 1995, pp 226–236.
77. Parker CR, Wendel GD: The effects of syphilis on endocrine function of the fetoplacental unit. Am J Obstet Gynecol 1988; 159:1327–1331.
78. Walker GJA: Antibiotics for syphilis diagnosed during pregnancy. [Systematic Review] Cochrane Pregnancy and Childbirth Group. Cochrane Database of Systematic Reviews. 2004;4.
79. Nathan L, Bawdon RE, Sidawi JE, et al: Penicillin levels following the administration of benzathine penicillin G in pregnancy. Obstet Gynecol 1993;82:338–342.
80. Lukehart S, Hook EW, Baker-Zander SH, et al: Invasion of the central nervous system by *Treponema pallidum*: Implications for diagnosis and therapy. Ann Intern Med 1988;109:855–862.
81. Mohr JA, Griffiths W, Jackson R, et al: Neurosyphilis and penicillin levels in cerebrospinal fluid. JAMA 1976;236:2208.
82. Schroeter AL, Lucas JB, Price EV, et al: Treatment for early syphilis and reactivity of serologic tests. JAMA 1972;221:471–476.
83. Wendel GD Jr, Stark BJ, Jamison RB, et al: Penicillin allergy and desensitization in serious infections during pregnancy. N Engl J Med 1985;312:1229–1232.
84. Ziaya PR, Hankins GD, Gilstrap LC, Halsey AB: Intravenous penicillin desensitization and treatment during pregnancy. JAMA 1986; 256:2561–2562.
85. Workowski KA, Levine WC: Sexually Transmitted Diseases Treatment Guidelines—2002. MMWR 2002;51(No. RR-06): 1–77.
86. Hollier LM, Harstad TW, Sanchez PJ, et al: Fetal syphilis: Clinical and laboratory characteristics. Obstet Gynecol 2001;97: 947–953.
87. Myles TD, Elam G, Park-Hwang E, Nguyen T: The Jarisch-Herxheimer reaction and fetal monitoring changes in pregnant women treated for syphilis. Obstet Gynecol 1998;92:859–864.
88. Dubey JP: Toxoplasmosis. J Am Vet Med Assoc 1994;205: 1593–1598.
89. Roghmann MC, Faulkner CT, Lefkowitz A, et al: Decreased seroprevalence for *Toxoplasma gondii* in Seventh Day Adventists in Maryland. Am J Trop Med Hyg 1999;60;790–792.
90. Jones JL, Lopez A, Wilson M, et al: Congenital toxoplasmosis: A review. Obstet Gynecol Survey 2001;56:296–305.
91. Feldman HA: A nationwide serum survey of United States military recruits, 1962. VI. *Toxoplasma* antibodies. Am J Epidemiol 1965;81:385–391.
92. Smith KL, Wilson M, Hightower AW, et al: Prevalence of *Toxoplasma gondii* antibodies in U.S. military recruits in 1989: Comparison with data published in 1965. Clin Infect Dis 1996;23:1182–1183.
93. Hughes JM, Colley DG: Preventing congenital toxoplasmosis. MMWR 2000;49(No.RR-02):57–75.
94. Alford CA, Stagno S, Reynolds DW: Congenital toxoplasmosis: Clinical, laboratory, and therapeutic considerations, with special reference to subclinical disease. Bull NY Acad Med 1974;50: 160–181.
95. Kimball AC, Kean BH, Fuchs F: Congenital toxoplasmosis: A prospective study of 4,048 obstetric patients. Am J Obstet Gynecol 1971;111:211–218.
96. Guerina NG, Hsu H-W, Meissner H, et al: Neonatal serologic screening and early treatment for congenital *Toxoplasma gondii* infection. N Engl J Med 1994;330:1858–1863.
97. Kapperud G, Jenum PA, Stray-Pedersen B, et al: Risk factors for *Toxoplasma gondii* infection in pregnancy: Results of a prospective case-control study in Norway. Am J Epidemiol 1996;144:405–412.
98. Baril L, Ancelle T, Goulet V, et al: Risk factors for *Toxoplasma* infection in pregnancy: A case-control study in France. Scand J Infect Dis 1999;31:305–309.
99. Cook AJ, Gilbert RE, Buffolano W, et al: Sources of *Toxoplasma* infection in pregnant women. European multicentre case-control study. European Research Network on Congenital Toxoplasmosis. BMJ 2000;321:142–147.
100. Stray-Pedersen B, Lorentzen-Styr AM: Epidemiological aspects of *Toxoplasma* infections among women in Norway. Acta Obstet Gynecol Scand 1980;59:323–326.
101. Wallace MR, Rossetti RJ, Olson PE: Cats and toxoplasmosis risk in HIV-infected adults. JAMA 1993;269:76–77.
102. Kean BH, Kimball AC, Christenson WN: An epidemic of acute toxoplasmosis. JAMA 1969;208:1002–1004.
103. Centers for Disease Control: Toxoplasmosis—Pennsylvania. MMWR 1975;24:285–286.
104. Masur H, Jones TC, Lempert JA, et al: Outbreak of toxoplasmosis in a family and documentation of acquired retinochoroiditis. Am J Med 1978;64:396–402.
105. Fertig A, Selwyn S, Tibble MJ: Tetracycline and toxoplasmosis. BMJ 1977;2:192.
106. Choi WY, Nam HW, Kwak NH, et al: Foodborne outbreaks of human toxoplasmosis. J Infect Dis 1997;175:1280–1282.
107. Sacks JJ, Delgato DG, Lobel HO, et al: Toxoplasmosis infection associated with eating undercooked venison. Am J Epidemiol 1983;118:832–838.
108. Sacks JJ, Roberto RR, Brooks NF: Toxoplasmosis infection associated with raw goat's milk. JAMA 1982;248:1728–1732.
109. Benenson MW, Takafuji ET, Lemon SM, et al: Oocyst-transmitted toxoplasmosis associated with ingestion of contaminated water. N Engl J Med 1982;307:666–669.
110. Bowie WR, King AS, Werker DH, et al: Outbreak of toxoplasmosis associated with municipal drinking water. Lancet 1997; 350:173–177.
111. Stagno S, Dykes AC, Amos CS, et al: An outbreak of toxoplasmosis linked to cats. Pediatrics 1980;65:706–712.
112. Teutsch SM, Juranek DD, Sulzer A, et al: Epidemic toxoplasmosis associated with infected cats. N Engl J Med 1979;300:695–699.
113. Jeannel D, Costagliola D, Niel G, et al: What is known about the prevention of congenital toxoplasmosis? Lancet 1990;336: 359–361.
114. Bader TJ, Macones GA, Asch DA: Prenatal screening for toxoplasmosis. Obstet Gynecol 1997;90:457–464.
115. Montoya J: Laboratory diagnosis of *Toxoplasma gondii* infection and toxoplasmosis. J Infect Dis 2002;185:S73–S82.
116. Liesenfeld O, Montoya JG, Tathineni MJ, et al: Confirmatory serologic testing for acute toxoplasmosis and rate of induced abortions among women reported to have positive *Toxoplasma* immunoglobulin M antibody titers. Am J Obstet Gynecol 2001;184:140–145.
117. Liesenfeld O, Montoya JG, Kinney S, et al: Effect of testing for IgG avidity in the diagnosis of *Toxoplasma gondii* infection in pregnant women: Experience in a US reference laboratory. J Infec Dis 2001;183:1248–1253.
118. Foulon W, Pinon JM, Stray-Pedersen B, et al: Prenatal diagnosis of congenital toxoplasmosis: A multicenter evaluation of different diagnostic parameters. Am J Obstet Gynecol 1999;181: 843–848.

119. Fricker-Hidalgo H, Pelloux H, Muet F, et al: Prenatal diagnosis of congenital toxoplasmosis: Comparative value of fetal blood and amniotic fluid using serological techniques and cultures. Prenat Diag 1997;17:831–835.
120. Remington JS, McLeod R, Thulliez P, Desmonts G: Toxoplasmosis. In Remington JS, Klein J (eds): Infectious Diseases of the Fetus and Newborn Infant, 5th ed. Philadelphia, WB Saunders, 2001, pp 205–346.
121. Antsaklis A, Daskalakis G, Papantoniou N, et al: Prenatal diagnosis of congenital toxoplasmosis. Prenat Diagn 2002;22: 1107–1111.
122. Daffos F, Forestier F, Capella-Pavlovsky M, et al: Prenatal management of 746 pregnancies at risk for congenital toxoplasmosis. N Engl J Med 1988;318:271–275.
123. Gay-Andrieu F, Marty P, Pialat J, et al: Fetal toxoplasmosis and negative amniocentesis: Necessity of an ultrasound follow-up. Pren Diagn 2003;23:558–560.
124. Hohlfeld P, Daffos F, Thulliez P, et al: Fetal texoplasmosis: Outcome of pregnancy and infant followup after in utero treatment. J Pediatr 1989;115:765–769.
125. Forestier F, Daffos F, Hohlfeld P, Lynch L: Infectious fetal diseases. Prevention, prenatal diagnosis, practical matters. Presse Medicale 1991;20:1448–1454.
126. Gilbert RE, Gras L, Wallon M, et al: Effect of prenatal treatment on mother to child transmission of *Toxoplasma gondii*: Retrospective cohort study of 554 mother-child pairs in Lyon, France. Int J Epidemiol 2001;30:1303–1308.
127. Chemla C, Villena I, Aubert D, et al: Preconception seroconversion and maternal seronegativity at delivery do not rule out the risk of congenital toxoplasmosis. Clin Diagn Lab Immunol 2002;9:489–490.
128. European Multicentre Study on Congenital Toxoplasmosis: Effect of timing and type of treatment on the risk of mother to child transmission of *Toxoplasma gondii*. BJOG 2003;110:112–120.
129. Foulon W, Villena I, Stray-Pedersen B, et al: Treatment of toxoplasmosis during pregnancy: A multicenter study of impact on fetal transmission and children's sequelae at age 1 year. Am J Obstet Gynecol 1999;180:410–415.
130. Hughes JM, Colley DG, Lopez A, et al: Preventing congenital toxoplasmosis. MMWR 2000;49(RR02):57–75.

SECTION FIVE

Late Prenatal—Maternal

CHAPTER 34

Substance Abuse

James J. Walker / Ann Walker

INTRODUCTION AND OVERVIEW

Substance abuse during pregnancy is an increasing problem that is associated with significant maternal and fetal morbidity. The complication for the clinician is that the mother is the cause of the problem that potentially harms both herself and her unborn child. Abuse is often further complicated by associated legal, social, and environmental problems[1] that can interfere with both the provision of care and the patient's ability to care for her child after delivery. The aim of the obstetrician is to provide an environment that is nonjudgmental and supportive to minimize the risk to the mother and infant, not only during pregnancy and the neonatal period, but also in the long term. To achieve this goal, the caregivers must be multidisciplinary and tolerant.[2]

The aim of antenatal care is to reduce risk, but this does not necessarily mean that the mother must abstain from drug use. The ultimate goal is to keep her within the care system and encourage her to take responsibility for herself and her child. No one should be turned away or denied help; doing so ultimately is harmful to the mother and infant.

Because the care required includes support during pregnancy, preparation for labor and delivery and the neonatal period, and long-term follow-up and social support, the obstetrician needs help and support from others, including midwives, addiction counselors, social workers, neonatologists, and general practitioners. The structure of the health care system in the United Kingdom lends itself to this approach, but it is more difficult in other parts of the world, where health care provision is more fragmented. However, programs of comprehensive antenatal care that provide social and behavioral support along with medical care do not universally improve maternal health and pregnancy outcome.[3] The specifics of the care provided are probably less important than the quality of care given and the degree of engagement of the individual.[4]

Major life events, such as pregnancy, can be a turning point in a woman's life, allowing her to take control of her life to the benefit of herself and her infant. It is often the first time she has been given any responsibility. She may not be interested in harm reduction for herself, but she is likely to wish to protect her infant. Unfortunately, the associated social problems of poor hygiene, poor nutrition, and social deprivation are responsible for much of the risk, rather than the abuse itself. The use of drugs or alcohol is a symptom of these problems. Because most users abuse more than one substance and have multiple social complications, it is difficult to evaluate the risk of any given substance. However, this chapter will attempt to do this by discussing each one in turn.

TOBACCO SMOKING

Background

Smoking is a legal and socially tolerated form of substance abuse. Although it is accepted that smoking is harmful to general health and to pregnancy in particular, the incidence of smoking in the pregnant population has increased in recent decades to between 16.3% and 52%, depending on the characteristics of the patient group.[5–8] However, there is evidence that it is declining in some populations.[6,8] Smoking is more common in the socially deprived population and varies with race. It is also heavily dependent on family and partner influences.[9] The incidence of smoking in pregnancy is higher if the mother's mother smoked, suggesting a possible inherited factor. However, because the incidence is higher still if the patient's mother smoked during pregnancy, there is a potential intrauterine influence.[7] The incidence of smoking decreases throughout pregnancy because of voluntary cessation.[5]

Maternal and Fetal Risks

Maternal smoking increases almost all placental complications. These include placental abruption,[10,11] placental insufficiency,[12,13] placenta previa,[10,11] and low birth weight.[8,12,13] Many of these infants are admitted to the neonatal unit,[8] and they have a higher incidence of neonatal death and sudden infant death syndrome.[7,8] However, the increased risk is eliminated when women with proven placental pathology are excluded from data analysis, suggesting that smoking produces most of its effects through placental damage.[14]

Interestingly, smoking in pregnancy is a significant protective factor against preeclampsia, reducing the incidence by up to 50%[15]; however, the harmful consequences of smoking on pregnancy outcome far outweigh this risk reduction.[11] There is also an increased risk of preterm delivery, partly as a result of placental disease and also because of preterm premature rupture of the membranes.[11] Data on miscarriage are contradictory. Some studies suggest an increased incidence with smoking,[16] but recent large cohort studies found no link.[17,18] However, there is an increased risk of ectopic pregnancy.[11] There are also varied data on the role of smoking and cleft lip and palate, with some studies suggesting no effect[19]; others showing a possible effect, especially with heavy use[20]; and others showing a definite effect.[21] No evidence links maternal smoking to childhood cancer.[22]

The risk of growth restriction increases with the number of cigarettes smoked per day, and heavy smokers deliver babies up to 458 g lighter than nonsmokers.[23] The effect of smoking on birth weight also increases with maternal age. Passive smoking produces risks similar to those seen in women who smoke 1 to 5 cigarettes/day. Women who stop smoking during pregnancy deliver babies that are, on average, 120 g larger than babies of those who do not stop smoking, although these infants are still 39 g smaller than infants of those who never smoked. The difference in birth weight between infants of those who never smoked and infants of those who are still smoking is 153 g.[24] The main effect of smoking appears to occur in the latter part of pregnancy, presenting a compelling argument for smoking cessation interventions that emphasizes the risk of smoking late in pregnancy.

Complications do not stop at delivery, with neonatal neurobehavioral abnormalities[25] and reduced arousal reflexes seen in infants of mothers who smoke, which may explain the increase in sudden infant death syndrome in these infants. There is evidence that children whose mothers smoked during pregnancy have early neurodevelopmental impairment and behavioral problems,[26] but these effects appear to decrease with age.[27] However, some long-term effects remain, with maternal smoking increasing the risk of conduct disorders and criminal behavior in male offspring.[28] This effect can be alleviated if the mother is responsive to the child in infancy,[29] suggesting that at least some of these changes depend on the social environment and not just the effect of intrauterine exposure to smoking.

Management Options

Prepregnancy and Prenatal

Although the strategy appears simple, it can work only if the women are aware of the risks to the unborn child and willing to stop smoking. These women need support from their partners and caregivers. This was shown in a study in England in which a mass media campaign on smoking and pregnancy was targeted at high risk women.[30] After the campaign, more people understood the risks to the unborn child, but there was no significant change in smoking prevalence or consumption. Therefore, information itself does little to change practice, and more active intervention is required.

Few centers appear to offer specific programs to reduce smoking. A mail survey in Australia showed that although smoking advice was rated an essential activity at the first antenatal visit by 69% of caregivers, only 12% of clinics offered relevant staff training and only 4% had written policies.[31] A narrow array of strategies to promote cessation was used, and almost one third of respondents said that they advised smokers to cut down rather than stop smoking completely. Some of this lack of effort comes from skepticism about the success of intervention programs.

Various studies of the role of a specially designed self-help manual to help stop smoking show that some women had already stopped before recruitment. Although there was an increase in the number of those stopping and reducing smoking compared with a control group, the percentages of patients who stopped were small, ranging from 10% to 20%.[32,33] Better results (38%) occurred with a more intensive program. Therefore, although smoking cessation is beneficial, intervention programs have limited effect because some women do not comply,[34] partly because of environmental factors.[35]

These studies used patient histories to assess smoking habits. If smoking status in pregnancy is determined by a serum cotinine assay, the rate correlates well with declared smoking.[36] However, in studies in which the percentage of self-reported quitting was higher with intervention programs compared with control groups, cotinine-verified quit rates were not significantly different. These results suggest that biochemical verification of quitting is essential to evaluate smoking cessation interventions because self-reported cessation is overstated[37] and that previously reported successful intervention programs may have overrated the number of quitters.

In a high risk group of working mothers attending a large public hospital in Valencia, Spain, 62% smoked before pregnancy. Of these, 28% gave up smoking during pregnancy. Cessation was more common among women 26 to 30 years of age, those with secondary education, and those who were originally lighter smokers.[38] This and other studies suggest that approximately 25% of women stop smoking voluntarily during pregnancy. However, these women are usually lighter smokers from a higher socioeconomic group and therefore at lower risk for complications.[35,39] If smoking cessation programs are going to be cost-effective, it is in the high risk group of heavy smokers where most benefits can be achieved, but where intervention programs appear to fail.

Pregnant women are less able to quit smoking than nonpregnant women, possibly because pregnant women cannot use nicotine replacement therapy.[40] However, recent studies suggest that this therapy may be safe because the amount of nicotine transferred to the baby may be reduced compared with smoking itself,[41] and the FDA no longer states pregnancy as a contraindication to its use.[42] However, it should still be used with caution because studies in nonpregnant patients show that cessation rates may still be only 17%,[40] which is similar to that achieved by existing pregnancy smoking cessation programs. Despite the obvious difficulties and relatively low success rates, smoking cessation programs should be encouraged. Evidence shows increased long-term cessation. This benefits future pregnancies because cessation before conception has the greatest effect.[43]

If people stop smoking, what is the relapse rate? In a randomized trial, fewer women in the intervention group (8.8%) reported restarting smoking by 36 weeks compared with the usual care group (16.9%), a nonsignificant difference. Similarly, no significant difference in relapse rates was observed with urinary cotinine-to-creatinine ratios, but these rates, 29.5% and 27.9%, respectively, were substantially higher than those based on self-reporting. Long-term postpartum relapse rates were not significantly different, 50.9% and 50.0%, respectively. However, individual smoking relapse prevention counseling increased the interval to relapse. No particular advice appears to prevent smoking relapse during pregnancy, but repeated support and encouragement provided to women who quit early in pregnancy may be beneficial.[44] The effect of family and peer pressure is important, with increasing success occurring when there is family or peer support.[45]

Because randomized trials of antismoking advice did not affect the outcome of pregnancy compared with studies of women who stopped voluntarily, maternal smoking may merely be an index of another factor that retards growth, such as social deprivation. Greater benefits may be achieved by programs to prevent nicotine addiction among adolescent girls or by encouraging cessation before pregnancy, when cessation is easier. There is evidence that this is occurring because smoking in pregnancy appears to be decreasing.[46]

Labor and Delivery

Women who smoke are more likely to have preterm premature rupture of the membranes and premature delivery, possibly because of increased oxytocin sensitivity,[47] but there is no difference in treatment. Because the risk of placental insufficiency is increased, the infant may have growth restriction, with an increased possibility of fetal distress. Therefore, close vigilance in labor is recommended, with assessment of the fetal heart rate on admission and again near the end of labor, when the risks to the fetus are greatest. Interestingly, because of the effect on fetal growth, smoking is protective against macrosomia.

If a general anesthetic is required, women who smoke are at increased risk. Normally, smokers are asked to stop at least 24 hours before the anesthetic is administered, but labor is not predictable. Women should be told not to smoke once contractions have started.

Postnatal

Cigarette smoking during pregnancy is a significant health risk to the fetus, but most women continue to smoke during pregnancy, and most who quit relapse postpartum. This can have a significant effect on the future health of the child as well as on subsequent pregnancies.[9] Smoking cessation is easier in the nonpregnant state, but cessation appears to be more closely related to environmental and social factors than to any medical intervention. Failure to stop smoking also has a detrimental effect on long-term maternal health. A follow-up study in northern Finland showed that the mortality ratio, adjusted for age, place of residence, years of education, and marital status, in women who smoked during pregnancy was more than twice that in nonsmokers. The difference was related to an increase in expected smoking-related diseases.[48]

SUMMARY OF MANAGEMENT OPTIONS

Cigarette Smoking

Management Options	Quality of Evidence	Strength of Recommendation	References
Train staff to give advice and support.	III	B	171

Continued

SUMMARY OF MANAGEMENT OPTIONS

Cigarette Smoking *(Continued)*

Management Options	Quality of Evidence	Strength of Recommendation	References
Advice to be given			
• Tell women that smoking puts their baby at risk, although other confounders may also play a role.	III	B	172
• Stopping smoking by midpregnancy will improve the outcome.	III	B	74,172
• Reducing smoking is better than not reducing but not as good as stopping.	III	B	172
• Repeated encouragement and specially designed programs increase the chance of success and reduce relapse.	Ia	A	173
Factors affecting success			
• Low risk, more educated, lighter smokers are more likely to stop.	III	B	38,174
• Specific targeted intervention programs have benefit for both the mother and the newborn.	Ia	A	174,175
• Women underreport failure to stop smoking and smoking relapse.	Ia	A	176
• Nicotine patches can be beneficial.	IIa	B	42

ALCOHOL

Background

Alcohol is a natural substance with body enzymes designed to metabolize it. Therefore, it is unlikely that alcohol is in itself toxic. However, the consumption of excessive amounts of alcohol is detrimental. After many historical references to the harmful effects of alcohol consumption in pregnancy, Lemoine and colleagues[49] described defects in fetal growth and development associated with maternal alcohol abuse in 1968. Further studies described the range of fetotoxicity attributed to both heavy and social maternal alcohol consumption.[50] Although the risk depends on the level and frequency of alcohol use, therapy is dependent on the degree of maternal dependency. In women who are not dependent, there is a high success rate with simple educational and motivational methods.[51] However, those who are dependent need greater supportive input and often require pharmacologic intervention.[52]

Maternal and Fetal Risks

Excessive Consumption

Jones and Smith[53] were the first to coin the phrase "fetal alcohol syndrome" to describe the features associated with heavy maternal alcohol consumption, but the signs had been described before.[54] The main features include the following:

- Growth deficiency, both prenatally and postnatally
- Central nervous system disturbance that affects intellect and behavior
- Abnormal facial characteristics, particularly low-set, unparallel ears; a short, flattened philtrum; an elongated midface; a small head; and a short, upturned nose
- Malformation of major organs, especially the heart, and skeletal deformities

Newborns with the syndrome may be irritable, with hypotonia, severe tremors, and withdrawal symptoms. The main physical and cerebral signs are usually apparent at birth. Mild mental retardation, the most common and serious deficit, and other anomalies may accompany fetal alcohol syndrome, and the degree of facial abnormality is directly related to the long-term physical and intellectual deficits.[55] Sensory deficits include optic nerve hypoplasia, poor visual acuity, hearing loss, and receptive and expressive language delays. Atrial and ventricular septal defects as well as renal hypoplasia, bladder diverticula, and other genitourinary tract abnormalities may occur. Only complete abstinence during pregnancy is considered safe. Alcohol consumption in each trimester is associated with abnormalities, and the lowest innocuous dose of alcohol is not known.[56] However, abnormal facial features are apparent only at the highest levels of exposure.[56]

Fetal alcohol syndrome is relatively rare, with an incidence of less than 1 in 1000 live births, increasing to 4.3% among "heavy" drinkers. The general incidence is more than 20 times higher in the United States (1.95 in 1000) compared with Europe and other countries (0.08 in 1000).[57] Relatively few women who drink alcohol during pregnancy give birth to children with fetal alcohol syndrome, and various theories have been suggested.[58] In the United States, the incidence is higher in lower socioeconomic groups, suggesting that the problem is multifactorial and includes genetic factors, social deprivation, nutritional deficiencies, and tobacco and other drug abuse.[58]

Intrauterine growth restriction is also more frequent in women who drink alcohol during pregnancy. This effect is aggravated by maternal smoking.[56] Maternal alcohol intake of more than 20 g/day is associated with an increase in preterm delivery and neonatal jaundice.[59] Excessive consumption, especially when accompanied by a poor diet and smoking, can lead to significant fetal effects.

Social Alcohol Consumption

The evidence against more moderate consumption is controversial. Although effects are seen at all intake levels, the results are not conclusive.[60] Approximately 50% of women consume alcohol on a moderate and occasional basis during pregnancy, although more abstain in the first trimester.[61] This behavior is socially acceptable and considered normal. The consequences on pregnancy are difficult to assess because quantification of alcohol consumption is difficult to assess accurately. In addition, there are confounding factors, particularly socioeconomic group and tobacco consumption.

Far more studies have reported no significant effects of mild alcohol intake than have reported problems. The effect of smoking on birth weight is three times greater than the effect of alcohol.[56] When data are stratified by smoking status, moderate maternal alcohol consumption usually has no significant effect on birth weight in nonsmokers, but among smokers, there is a significant linear trend, with a threshold for decreased birth weight at an average of approximately two drinks per day (14 units/wk).[62] Lower consumption levels are associated with an increase in birth weight, suggesting an inverted J-shaped function between drinking during pregnancy and birth weight.[63] On its own, moderate intake of alcohol during pregnancy of less than 12 to 14 units/wk has no apparent detrimental effect on fetal growth.[63]

Although some studies show that children exposed to alcohol prenatally had significantly lower weight, height, head circumference, and palpebral fissure width at 6 years,[64] most show that the effect on growth is transient and the differences are not measurable after 8 months of age.[65]

Although most studies suggest that low alcohol intake in pregnancy does not have a substantial effect on child development, there is concern about the long-term neurodevelopment of exposed offspring. Dose-dependent effects on neurobehavioral function from birth to 14 years have been established and are described as fetal alcohol effects.[66] Specific problems include attention deficit, slower information processing, and learning problems, especially with arithmetic,[67] as well as slower reaction times, suggesting an alcohol-related deficit in "speed of central processing." Reaction time deficits were dose-dependent,[68] as were attention and memory deficits. The number of drinks per occasion was the strongest predictor of deficits. Fluctuating attention states, problems with response inhibition, and spatial learning also showed a strong association.[67] The higher the average number of drinks per occasion, the poorer the performance of the adolescent offspring on tasks believed to underlie numeric problem-solving and reading proficiency.[69] As with fetal alcohol syndrome, not all exposed offspring studied showed neurodevelopmental deficits. The effects appear to increase with advancing maternal age.[70]

Management Options

Prepregnancy and Prenatal

Because most women are not addicted to alcohol, they often take a "better safe than sorry" approach and reduce or stop drinking in pregnancy.[61] A successful previous pregnancy experience or a previous alcohol-related problem can influence this decision.[71] However, it is not the social drinker who concerns the obstetrician because these patients are relatively easily educated about risks and tend to reduce their intake.[61] The few heavy drinkers, either dependent or binge drinkers, are more likely to harm their unborn child and are difficult to manage. Smokers and older women are particularly at risk because of the associated additive effects.

Formalized questionnaires on alcohol use can be used to screen either the entire population or targeted at-risk groups. The T-ACE questionnaire has been validated and appears to be accurate in detecting women who drink more than 1 oz absolute alcohol/day (approximately 25 g, or 2.5 units). Screening is most sensitive during the first 15 weeks of pregnancy.[72]

T-ACE is an acronym for the following:

- T: TOLERANCE

  How many drinks does it take to make you feel "high"?

- A: ANNOYED

  Have people ANNOYED you by criticizing your drinking?

- C: CUT DOWN

  Have you felt you should CUT DOWN on your drinking?

- E: EYE OPENER

  Have you ever had a drink first thing in the morning?

Scoring of the test is straightforward. If the answer to the tolerance question is more than 2, a score of 2 is given. A score of 1 is assigned to a positive answer to all of the other questions. A total score of more than 2 is considered positive for problem drinking, and this score correctly identifies more than 70% of women who drink heavily during pregnancy. Although this questionnaire is better than traditional alcohol questionnaires, its sensitivity can be improved with the use of a further test.[73]

An alternative is the Leeds Dependence Questionnaire, which is a 10-item, self-completion questionnaire designed to measure dependence on a variety of substances. It is understood by users of alcohol and opiates. The questionnaire is sensitive to changes over time from severe to mild dependence. Test–retest reliability is 0.95.[74]

Biochemical markers, such as blood γ-glutamyltransferase, alcohol concentration, thiocyanate, and mean corpuscular volume, can be used as surrogates of excessive alcohol consumption, but they are not accurate and can be used only to identify potential at-risk women. Abnormalities of liver enzymes in women who drink heavily should be taken into account if these tests are used during pregnancy to monitor other diseases, such as preeclampsia.

As with smoking, studies show that approximately one third of women who drink alcohol before pregnancy stop drinking during pregnancy and those who continue to drink tend to reduce their consumption.[61] A few women continue high levels of alcohol intake, and if they can be identified, preventive efforts should be focused on this group.[75] In contrast to smoking, many of these women are in higher socioeconomic groups.[76]

Adults have a significantly higher average daily intake of alcohol than adolescents. However, adults are more likely to reduce their intake in pregnancy and have a reduced incidence of binge drinking during the first trimester, which puts the offspring of adolescents at greater risk.[77]

If intervention programs are established, help from outside agencies, such as the local addiction unit, is invaluable. As with smoking, these programs are more likely to be successful in women who want to stop and when supportive care is provided. Motivational intervention with close monitoring of alcohol consumption with a planned reduction program is of benefit, often with the help of friends, family, and organizations such as Alcoholics Anonymous, with their 12-step program.[78] Because the effects of alcohol are associated with dietary deficiencies, the importance of a good diet and vitamin supplementation should be discussed.[79] Many complications of alcohol abuse may be attenuated by these measures.

If there is continued dependent drinking and the patient is motivated to stop, planned detoxification should be considered, possibly with hospitalization or regular daily monitoring of withdrawal symptoms. Sudden withdrawal can lead to acute maternal symptoms, including convulsions, which may be detrimental to the fetus. Detoxification is normally undertaken with benzodiazepines, such as chlordiazepoxide, with the possible addition of phenobarbitone, if required, to manage convulsions.[80] These are given by reducing the regimen over 7 to 10 days. Benzodiazepines given in the first trimester may be associated with cleft palate abnormalities.[81] However, the benefits of stopping alcohol use outweigh this risk because alcohol is by far the greater teratogen. If delivery is likely within the next few days, benzodiazepines should be given with care because neonatal sedation and "floppy baby syndrome" can occur.[82] Disulfiram (Antabuse) should not be used because it is considered a potential teratogen, although the evidence is conflicting.[83] These patients should also be given vitamin B supplementation.

Labor and Delivery

There are no problems with labor and delivery, except for the occasional need for higher levels of opiate analgesia or problems with general anesthesia because of induced liver enzymes. Alcohol withdrawal occurs after 48 hours and may be a problem postnatally. Appropriate sedation can be used with vitamin, particularly thiamine, supplementation. Symptoms subside after a few days. Women may appear agitated and have difficulty caring for the infant during this time.

If alcohol abuse continues after delivery, breastfeeding should be discouraged. Alcohol crosses over to the baby, and there may be continued effects of alcohol on the neonate.[56] Alcohol abuse during breastfeeding can cause drowsiness in the baby and may aggravate existing nutritional problems, increasing the need for dietary supplementation. However, alcohol may interfere with milk production, necessitating artificial feeding.

Postnatal

In most follow-up studies, a significant percentage of women relapsed. In one study of adolescents, more than 30% reported using alcohol within 3 months of delivery. These women are more depressed, are under greater stress, and report a greater need for social support. Therefore, the use of alcohol, as with other drugs of abuse, may be a marker for other problems that would benefit from intervention.

There is increasing concern about children of parents who abuse alcohol. These children have a higher risk of psychiatric disorders, cognitive deficits, and substance abuse that may be genetic or a long-term effect of in utero alcohol exposure.[84] Significant alcohol use affects family functioning, and children of alcohol-abusing parents are at risk for abuse and neglect.[85] Family drinking patterns are associated with adolescent alcohol abuse.[84] Children of alcohol-abusing parents have a higher incidence of emotional and behavioral disturbances and are at risk for future adult morbidity other than alcoholism. Therefore, women who abuse alcohol during pregnancy require careful follow-up from the appropriate agencies.

SUMMARY OF MANAGEMENT OPTIONS

Alcohol Abuse

Management Options	Quality of Evidence	Strength of Recommendation	References
Obstetric risks are related to exposure as well as other associated social factors.	III	B	50,177
	IIa	B	35,178
A multidisciplinary approach is valuable in the care of these families.	III	B	51
Cessation help should be given to all "at-risk" groups.	III	B	77
	IIa	B	179
Some heavy alcohol users require specific counseling, with support from outside agencies.	IIa	B	179
	III	B	180
Some heavy alcohol users require pharmacologic support.	III	B	80
Dietary advice and vitamin supplementation should be given.	III	B	79
Breastfeeding should be discouraged if the woman is still drinking heavily because there can be ongoing neonatal damage.	III	B	56

DRUG ABUSE: GENERAL

The effects of maternal drug abuse on the mother and infant are controversial. Much of the research comes from the United States and involves low-income women with multiple drug use and social problems.[86] When matched for social factors, mothers who use heroin have similar birth outcomes to non-drug-using mothers.[2] Therefore, many effects attributed to maternal drug abuse may be related to socioeconomic deprivation or associated factors, such as smoking, rather than to in utero drug exposure. The only effects that can be definitely blamed on drug abuse are neonatal withdrawal. However, specific complications are associated with particular substances (discussed later).

The social factors are made worse by the fact that the drugs used are illegal. The women often live in a subculture of illegal behavior, including theft and prostitution.[87] Many mothers attempt to hide their lifestyle and claim fictitious support. They are often reluctant to be honest and may fear criticism, legal action, or removal of the child. They may resist antenatal care and must believe that the care is beneficial.[88] The service must be flexible and understanding enough to cope with these problems. In Glasgow, Scotland, a multidisciplinary approach was used to provide economic, social, and antenatal care during pregnancy.[2] This model has been copied elsewhere.[89] Because these problems persist after delivery, support for issues related to social problems and substance misuse must be continued after pregnancy to maximize the outcome for the mother and infant. This requires close collaboration with local addiction services.[90]

Care programs that have been developed attempt to modify the external influences as much as possible to stabilize the mother's substance misuse.[89] Some women can stabilize their habit, detoxify, leave the drug culture, become healthy and responsible, and keep and care for their infant. However, others struggle to stay within the system, and care should be directed at the best possible outcome for each individual rather than optimal outcome. These care systems may change the pattern of abuse, but not necessarily the neonatal outcome.[91]

The systems that work best are multidisciplinary, with input from obstetricians, midwives, pediatricians, community-based health workers, social workers, drug abuse counselors, and others who can offer support.[2,89]

Caregivers should not be judgmental, although they must establish boundaries and maintain discipline. It is important to keep the trust of women and encourage them to obtain care, regardless of whether they are using drugs. A system based on rewards structure is better than one based on punishment. The ultimate reward is being able to keep and care for the infant after delivery. Care programs are more successful when friends and family are supportive.[92]

It is difficult to believe addicts, and urine screening is beneficial to assess program compliance.[93] Inpatient care can be useful to detoxify the patient; remove her from an unhealthy, stressful street environment; and provide adequate nutrition. However, these patients may be disruptive, cause stress in other patients, and continue to abuse substances. In an attempt to overcome these problems, some hospitals have a segregated area for the care of addicts.[94] However, in Leeds, we believe that it is important to treat them as normally as possible and to house them in the regular areas.[89,90] Protocols must be in place and sympathetic staff available.

Establishing a Special Clinical Service for the Pregnant Addict

In Leeds, a special pregnancy addiction service was set up within an antenatal clinic.[90] This allows patients to have all of their needs met at a single site. The clinic is coordinated by a liaison midwife with an obstetrician and an addiction worker. This ensures access to necessary antenatal care and addiction advice. The service provides a regular clinic that is available by appointment as well as on a drop-in basis. Providing care at a single site avoids the potential stigma of a separate clinic as well as possible loss of confidentiality. The availability of the service is promoted in health centers, hospitals, and local relevant organizations.

To achieve this, a close working relationship was developed between the obstetric and addiction services, with links with community midwives, general practitioners, pediatricians, health visitors, child protection services, social services, and general support services, such as housing, probation, and community care projects. With so many individuals involved, regular monthly meetings are held to exchange information and discuss concerns. Treatment protocols are available for all staff, particularly those who share responsibility with other services.

Regular reviews of the women are important. The Standing Conference on Drug Addiction guidelines are followed.* An initial assessment is performed at presentation, and a full review of progress made and work outstanding is completed at 32 weeks. By that time, a plan should be in place to deal with outstanding issues. Other professionals, usually social services or housing authorities, can be contacted at that time. This process occurs with the consent of the woman, unless the infant is considered "at risk." In this case, authorities must be involved, even without the mother's consent. When significant concern is present, a full prebirth assessment by social services may be needed. A postnatal review at 3 months is scheduled to assess the progress of the mother and infant.

*Standing Conference on Drug Abuse (SCODA) 1997 "Drug using parents: Policy Guidelines for Inter-Agency working." Local government forum and association, United Kingdom.

Labor and Delivery

The labor and delivery unit must be prepared to provide the care required at delivery. As with alcohol, problems include issues of drug withdrawal and complications with analgesia, but also include the possibility of HIV and hepatitis infection. Specific problems depend on the drugs used.

Postnatal

The neonatal unit should be ready to care for an infant with withdrawal symptoms. The incidence and severity of these symptoms are related largely to the type and amount of drug used. In the past, babies of drug-using women were usually admitted routinely to the special care nursery and often treated for, or in anticipation of, withdrawal symptoms. These symptoms are a source of distress to the mother, but separation can cause further distress. In the United Kingdom, most infants do not require admission to a neonatal unit and can be cared for in a transitional care area, where the mother is directly involved.[89]

Drug abuse was formerly considered incompatible with adequate child care, but it is now realized that drug cessation and postnatal abstinence is largely unachievable. An attempt to enforce drug cessation is likely to drive the women away from the supportive environment that was carefully established during pregnancy. However, harm reduction and stabilization should be the goal, and this goal is compatible with maternal and child health. In the United Kingdom, methadone maintenance is the main treatment for opiate addicts who are unable or unwilling to stop using drugs.[90] This approach may allow the women to live a reasonably stable life and care for her children. Many studies show that infants who remain with their biologic parents do better than those who do not.[95] To achieve these outcomes, a good working relationship with the local addiction unit is necessary to ensure that adequate follow-up and support is available.[89,90]

The success of these policies is varied. More than 50% of women who stop abusing drugs resume drug use within 6 months of delivery. Many of their infants are cared for by extended family members on a voluntary basis, and others enter foster care or are adopted. This outcome may be upsetting to staff working in this area, but one success can lead to long-term benefit to at least two people (i.e., the mother and her child), and even a temporary success may reduce the long-term effects on the infant.

SUMMARY OF MANAGEMENT OPTIONS

Drug Abuse, General

Management Options	Quality of Evidence	Strength of Recommendation	References
Provide accurate rather than alarmist information.	IV	C	89
General guidelines include assessing the patient's living environment and	III	B	2,89,181

SUMMARY OF MANAGEMENT OPTIONS

Drug Abuse, General *(Continued)*

Management Options	Quality of Evidence	Strength of Recommendation	References
whether her partner uses drugs, encouraging the woman to take some responsibility for herself, making sure that she understands what is expected of her, improving her general health, and working toward achievable goals.			
A multidisciplinary approach may be beneficial.	III	B	2,3
Wear gloves to take blood from all patients (not just addicts).	–	GPP	
The increased risk of sexually transmitted disease, including HIV, should be discussed.	III	B	182
Screen for fetal normality and growth with ultrasonography.	III	B	183
Babies should be assessed for neonatal abstinence syndrome.	III	B	111

HEROIN ADDICTION: SPECIFIC PROBLEMS

Background

Heroin is processed from morphine, a naturally occurring substance extracted from the seedpod of the Asian poppy plant. Heroin usually appears as a white or brown powder. Street names for heroin include "smack," "H," "skag," and "junk." Other names refer to types of heroin produced in a specific geographic area, such as "Mexican black tar."

Heroin is a highly physically addictive drug, and its use is a serious worldwide problem. It can be injected, snorted, or smoked, and like many drugs of abuse, the ritual of preparation is an important part of the attraction. After heroin injection, there is a surge of euphoria ("rush") accompanied by warm flushing of the skin, dry mouth, and a heavy sensation of the extremities. A drowsy state occurs, and mental functioning becomes clouded as a result of central nervous system depression. This leads to a lack of motivation and reduced social interaction.

The management approaches discussed earlier are particularly relevant to the care of the patient who uses heroin in pregnancy. Outcome of the mother and infant is greatly enhanced by her attendance at an appropriate support clinic. The mother must know the risks of heroin addiction to her infant, particularly the risks of street heroin, which is of variable strength and quality and produces unpredictable results. The benefits of methadone maintenance or detoxification should be emphasized.[90,96] This support, including methadone maintenance treatment, should be provided within a multidisciplinary clinic, with regular follow-up.[90,96] In this environment, there is a reduction in supplementary drug use and an associated reduction in harm. Although the doses of methadone used in the United States tend to be higher than those used in the United Kingdom, the success of maintenance therapy is largely independent of either methadone dose or plasma concentration and relates to the degree of ongoing support.[93]

Maternal and Fetal Risks

The main clinical problems related to heroin use are direct drug effects on the fetus and neonate and the reduced ability of the mother to care for the child.[95] Opiates are not teratogenic.[97] However, their use is associated with intrauterine growth restriction and premature delivery,[95,98] a higher incidence of fetal distress, and a greater need for neonatal care.[99] Although other factors, such as poor antenatal attendance, poor nutrition, mixed drug use, and cigarette smoking, are undoubtedly involved, it is important to realize that these pregnancies are at risk, regardless of whether the drug is primarily responsible. Longitudinal studies found an increased incidence of deficits in cognitive development and more behavioral problems but no differences in motor development. It is difficult to separate the effects of in utero exposure to heroin from the problems of deficient child care.[100] Children who are adopted at an early age into nurturing families develop normally, suggesting that there is no inherent problem in these babies, and if the mother is stabilized and succeeds in changing her lifestyle, the long-term outcome for the infant can be good. However, these mothers have child care problems, and there is an increased risk of sudden infant death syndrome, with a risk ratio of nearly 3.[101] Pregnancy care is only the starting point, and there is a need for ongoing support after delivery, requiring collaboration with addiction services.[90]

Management Options

Prepregnancy and Prenatal

The main aim of care for the pregnant drug-abusing woman is engagement. With this, the rest of the care follows. She can be cared for by a multidisciplinary team (including addiction service), with the goal of risk reduction.[89,90] The core of risk reduction is the drug substitution program; methadone is the therapy most often used.

METHADONE USE IN PREGNANCY

Methadone use in pregnancy varies. In the United States, higher doses are used to block opiate receptors and reduce cravings, whereas in the United Kingdom, the approach is often to find the lowest dose to prevent withdrawal symptoms. Studies show that reducing the dose to a minimum improves birth weight and prolongs gestation.[102] It is difficult to determine whether these benefits result from the use of methadone, the reduction of other drug use, an improved lifestyle, or a combination of these factors.[102] However, the risk and severity of neonatal abstinence syndrome (NAS) appear to be increased by methadone compared with heroin,[103] but methadone stabilization has considerable overall benefits for the mother and infant. The purpose of substitution therapy is to reduce illegal heroin use as well as the crime, disease, and other consequences of street use. Reducing intravenous injection has the added benefit of reducing the risk of HIV infection and hepatitis B and C infection and well as other health risks. Because methadone, at therapeutic levels, does not create euphoria, sedation, or analgesia and has no adverse effects on motor skills, mental capability, or employability, it is compatible with a reasonably normal lifestyle. Therefore, it is suitable for stabilization during pregnancy and for short- to medium-term use after delivery to maintain stability. Although many patients reduce their opiate use, only a few (10%–25%) become drug-free,[97,98] and many of these return to heroin use after delivery.

The amount of methadone required should be assessed in the usual way. Women who are not regular (daily) users do not need substitution therapy. Those who are given methadone should have a clear history of daily use, withdrawal symptoms, and positive urine toxicology findings. The amount of methadone required can be assessed by the declared amount of heroin used or the amount of money spent per day. However, because the cost and purity of street heroin vary considerably, this guidance can only be approximate. Dosage is then titrated against withdrawal scores until stabilization is achieved. The aim is to find the lowest dose of methadone that is compatible with an absence of withdrawal symptoms or cravings. The dosage regimens in pregnancy are the same as those used in the nonpregnant user. The maximum dose of methadone used in the Leeds service is 80 mg/day. Because the metabolism of methadone is increased in pregnancy, leading to a shorter half-life, the dose may need to be split into a twice-daily dose in later pregnancy to maintain a satisfactory steady state.[104] This dosing can increase compliance without the need to increase the total dose.[105] Methadone maintenance treatment is more successful within a supportive environment and is largely independent of methadone dose or plasma concentration.[93] Therefore, the supportive nature of the service is more important than the drug regimen used.[87]

Once stabilization is achieved and lifestyle issues are addressed, if the woman is motivated, gradual dose reduction can begin. The main goal is stability. Because of the danger of miscarriage, this is more safely carried out between 12 and 30 weeks' gestation. After this point, it is better simply to stabilize the patient at the lowest possible dose in preparation for labor and delivery. Because of the changes in maternal metabolism, the maintenance dose may need to be increased to sustain maternal stability. Reduction should be done slowly, by decreasing the daily dosage by 5 mg, no more often than every 2 weeks, and then, from 20 mg/day, by 2 mg every 2 weeks, to achieve the lowest sustainable dose without the mother resorting to street heroin or suffering withdrawal symptoms.[102] It is important to aim for the lowest maternal dose to reduce the possibility of NAS. Although not strictly dose-related, a dose of less than 20 mg is not usually associated with significant NAS, unless there is concurrent street drug use. Regular urine toxicology testing allows accurate assessment of the success of the treatment program and assists in the planning of dose adjustments.[93]

ALTERNATIVES TO METHADONE

Because of the well-recognized limitations of methadone treatment, alternatives have been sought. Buprenorphine appears to be a potential option,[106] but the safety to the fetus is unknown. Early studies showed that stabilization is possible, and the risk of NAS appeared low.[107,108] However, more recent studies show that NAS occurs in 40% to 60% of cases, usually within 12 to 48 hours, peaks at approximately 72 to 96 hours, and lasts for 5 to 7 days.[109,110] However, NAS appears to be of less duration and severity than methadone and is related to polydrug use in at least 40% of cases.[110] The children are followed closely, with regular monitoring of physical and psychological development. So far, no clear detrimental effects have been found. Buprenorphine taken at the time of conception has been reported with no teratogenic effects.[107] If these results are confirmed by randomized trials, buprenorphine would offer a real alternative to methadone, with a reduced risk profile.

Labor and Delivery

The attendant staff must be trained in the care of pregnant drug users and treat them in the same way as other women in labor. On admission, a history of recent drug use (i.e., before admission) must be obtained. Many mothers use heroin before hospital admission to help them tolerate labor.

No specific problems are associated with labor or delivery, except for maternal analgesia. Methadone should be continued, with additional opiate analgesia as required. Because high doses of narcotic analgesia may be necessary, epidural analgesia has advantages. At delivery, the infant should not be given naloxone (Narcan) because it causes a severe withdrawal reaction.

Postnatal

After delivery, normal support should be continued, ideally in a transitional unit. This allows the mother and infant to be together, which is important for bonding and establishment of parenting skills. This is the ideal time for staff to promote support and assess possible risk.

The incidence and severity of NAS are partially related to the type and amount of drug used.[111,112] However, polydrug use can influence this, particularly street heroin, benzodiazepines, and cocaine.[111] Both benzodiazepines and cocaine delay the onset of NAS, but cocaine also appears to reduce the severity of symptoms.[112] The pediatric unit should be alerted to the potential clinical problems and involved in the case discussion and the development of management protocols.

In Leeds, a modified Finnegan scale is used to monitor the infant for signs of NAS.[113] This is initially carried out every 4 hours and monitoring is reduced when appropriate. Three scores of 8 or more should be used for the diagnosis. It is useful for the mother to be involved in these assessments because many drug-using mothers have strong feelings of guilt and want to feel that they can make a useful contribution. They can also improve the continuity of assessment. Withdrawal from heroin occurs over 1 to 3 days, whereas methadone has a longer clearance time, and symptoms in the newborn may not occur for up to 7 days after delivery. Assessment should last at least 7 days, although some centers advocate earlier discharge if there are no signs by 72 hours.[114] The classic symptoms are restlessness, jitteriness, failure to feed, tremors, a high-pitched cry, arching of the back, yawning, sneezing, and sweating.[113] Convulsions may also occur. Narcotics, either morphine or methadone, are the best drugs for the treatment of NAS, although phenobarbitone may be required if convulsions occur.[114,115] Although most babies show some withdrawal symptoms, fewer than 50% require treatment and most can be safely cared for in a transitional unit.[89,114] Of 200 babies born in Glasgow in the 1980s and early 1990s to mothers using illicit drugs or legal methadone, only 7% required treatment for withdrawal and even fewer required admission to the special care nursery.[94] However, other centers, including more recent figures from Glasgow, quote incidences of 10% to 80% of cases, depending on the amount of antenatal drug used and the success of the clinic maintenance program.[99,111,112,114]

Continuing supportive care, including methadone maintenance, may allow the new mother to live a reasonably stable life and care for her child, which is the best outcome for the child.[95] This requires a continued good working relationship with general practitioners, health visitors, community pediatricians, and the local addiction service. However, many babies are eventually cared for by extended family members, placed in foster care, or released for adoption.[116]

BREASTFEEDING

If the mother is stable on methadone, is not supplementing with street drugs, and is believed to be HIV-negative, breastfeeding should be encouraged. The secretion of methadone in breast milk is variable,[117] but it may help to reduce withdrawal symptoms.[118] A stable lifestyle helps successful breastfeeding. However, if the mother is still injecting street heroin, is known to be or is at risk for being HIV-positive, or is using other street drugs (e.g., cocaine), breastfeeding is not advisable.

HIV AND OTHER INFECTIOUS DISEASES

HIV infection is associated with drug abuse because of needle sharing and heterosexual spread from associated prostitution. The danger, particularly in the United Kingdom, has been overstated, although in some areas, the incidence of HIV infection is particularly high. In Edinburgh, in 290 at-risk pregnancies, 93 (32%) of the women were HIV-positive. However, of these 93 pregnancies, only 8 (8.7%) resulted in an HIV-infected child.[119] Since then, the prevalence of HIV has declined from 0.5% of all pregnancies in 1986 to 0.1% in 1992. This figure has not changed.[120] The risk of vertical transmission has been significantly reduced by the use of antiviral drugs and obstetric intervention.[121] However, although the incidence is decreasing in Scotland, the medical authorities knew most of the HIV-positive women in 1990, but by 1992, only 30% were identified.[122,123] This makes the targeting of antiviral treatment more difficult.

Because many HIV-positive patients are not known to the service, single-tier management of all pregnant women is important to minimize the risk of transmission to health care workers. This also helps to reduce discrimination against substance-misusing women. In the United Kingdom, HIV testing is offered to all pregnant women after appropriate counseling. The benefits of testing must be explained to the mother. Current therapy improves maternal health and significantly reduces vertical transmission to the baby.[121]

Intravenous drug users are also at risk for hepatitis B and C infection, and screening is routinely offered. The most common infection found is hepatitis C, which is found in approximately 40% to 60% of women who abuse intravenous drugs. Evidence suggests that hepatitis C does not adversely affect the pregnancy and the pregnancy does not worsen the viral load or prognosis of the disease, although many women have a slight rise in alanine aminotransferase levels postpartum.[124] Vertical transmission of hepatitis C infection occurs in approximately 1% to 6% of cases and is partly dependent on maternal viral load and concurrent HIV infection.[125,126] Transmission is also increased in longer labors, but breastfeeding does not influence it because hepatitis C virus RNA is not detected in breast milk. Infants who are hepatitis C virus-positive should be followed up for at least 1 year because some become seronegative and others have hepatitis. No treatment or vaccination is available.

Less frequently, women are hepatitis B-positive. Pregnancy does not appear to affect the course of the disease in the mother, but the rate of vertical transmission without intervention is 80% to 90%.[127] Of these patients, more than 85% become clinical carriers of the virus. Infection in the baby usually occurs at or directly after delivery, so the babies are candidates for postexposure prophylaxis. An at-risk infant should be given HepB immunoglobulin within 12 hours of delivery while concurrently being given the first dose of HepB vaccination.[128] This should be completed with follow-up vaccinations at 1 month and at 6 months. This intervention is safe and provides 90% protection against infection. One study suggested that maternal lamivudine treatment may also help to reduce neonatal infection.[129]

COCAINE ADDICTION: SPECIFIC PROBLEMS

Background

Cocaine is a vasoactive drug and can cause specific problems in the baby as a result of placental damage[130] and direct fetal vascular effects. Unlike alcohol, cocaine has no specific associated syndrome or cluster of signs.[131] Its effects are varied and may be more closely related to other drug use and associated social problems.[130,132]

It comes in the following two forms:

- Pure cocaine, or "coke," which is a white powder that is generally snorted through the nasal mucosa.
- "Crack," which is more addictive and dangerous. Crack is produced by mixing cocaine crystal or powder with water and baking soda or sodium bicarbonate. The mixture is boiled until the water evaporates, leaving brown and white rocks. It is usually smoked with special glass pipes or silver foil, although it can be injected after a solution is made with water.

Cocaine is absorbed rapidly into the bloodstream, producing a high in approximately 6 to 8 minutes. Unlike the physical addiction of heroin, cocaine addiction is more psychological. Cocaine and crack users are difficult to identify and treat. There are no suitable substitute drugs.

Many studies, particularly in the United States, found higher rates of cocaine abuse than of heroin abuse, with an incidence of 0.8% to 16%.[130,133,134] Radioimmunoassay of hair samples obtained immediately postpartum show much underreporting of cocaine use. Underreporting is more common among women who are unmarried, African American, and multiparous.[135, 136]

Maternal and Fetal Risks

Cocaine users often do not eat or sleep while under the influence of the drug and often become dehydrated. Although these effects may not present problems with occasional use, heavy use may be associated with exhaustion, dehydration, and poor nutrition. Some people use heroin to "come down" from cocaine highs, further complicating the medical problems. Because crack can be smoked, it can affect other people nearby; this has implications for children and babies in the room with a user.

Heavy usage of cocaine is associated with an increase in preterm delivery, low birth weight, the need for resuscitation at birth, and prolonged postnatal stay.[99,137] The effect of cocaine on birth weight may be related to shorter gestation and poor maternal nutrition. Women who use cocaine use prenatal care less often, smoke more cigarettes, and drink more alcohol, all of which are associated with poor growth.[138] When these variables are excluded, identifiable differences in birth weight between cocaine-using mothers and control subjects are no longer present.[132] However, peripartum exposure to cocaine is associated with an increased frequency of abruptio placentae; thick, meconium-stained amniotic fluid; and premature rupture of the membranes.[130] There is also an association with fetal abnormalities, including genitourinary anomalies and abdominal wall defects.[130]

Cocaine-exposed infants with very low birth weight had an increased incidence of mild intraventricular hemorrhage. However, the incidence of developmental delay was significantly higher, even after controlling for the effects of intraventricular hemorrhage and gestational age.[139] Cocaine-exposed infants with very low birth weight were also more likely to be living with relatives or in foster homes, which further affects their development.[139] Long-term assessment showed reduced head circumference, low Stanford-Binet Intelligence Scale (SBIS) verbal reasoning, and low SBIS abstract/visual reasoning. These children were also more aggressive.[140] These findings are similar to those associated with alcohol.

Binge cycles are a particular problem and reflect the chaotic lifestyle of many drug abusers. Binges range from 26.4 to 34.4 hours.[141] Bingeing is associated with premature delivery and an increased incidence of acute problems, such as vaginal bleeding (21.8%), abruptio placentae (14.3%), and stillbirth (20.5%). Erratic use of cocaine or crack results in perinatal complications that are as severe as those occurring with daily use.[141]

Like heroin, maternal cocaine exposure during pregnancy is associated with acceleration of amniotic fluid and fetal lung maturity, which may reflect increased fetal stress.[142]

Not all substance-exposed children have the same poor prognosis, suggesting that maternal and environmental factors modify the damage.[140] Surveys show that most cocaine users also use alcohol.[138] Comparison with alcohol shows that alcohol is the more potent teratogen. Those who use both agents are more likely to have troubled backgrounds, indulge in antisocial behavior, and drop out of treatment programs than those who use only alcohol. Good nutrition is very important in preventing congenital anomalies and fetal death, and cocaine use during pregnancy is more dangerous to the street person who uses multiple drugs and alcohol than to the middle-class woman who takes antenatal vitamins.[143]

ANIMAL STUDIES

Animal studies have been used to assess the direct effect of cocaine in pregnancy. Rhesus monkeys that were exposed to cocaine during pregnancy were compared with matched nonexposed control subjects. There was no difference in infant outcome, as measured by body weight, overall length, crown–rump length, rump–heel length, biparietal diameter, and crown circumference.[144]

Pregnant Sprague-Dawley rats were fed diets with differing protein content and exposed to cocaine. Cocaine was associated with reduced food intake, and this difference was greater in the group with low protein intake. This diet affected weight gain in pregnancy as well as skeletal maturation of the pups. Litter size was significantly reduced with higher doses of cocaine across all diet groups, suggesting a fetotoxic effect. Gestation length was unaffected. Therefore, cocaine may produce poor fetal growth by reducing dietary intake.[145]

Animal studies suggest that cocaine can cause functional problems. Perinatal cocaine exposure led to decreased responsiveness to inotropic drugs during the early neonatal period in rats[146] as well as to cognitive impairment in some male offspring, without apparent postnatal physical abnormalities or adverse effects on maternal health.[147]

In pregnant baboons, intravenous cocaine increased plasma oxytocin concentrations.[148] A similar study in rats produced a marked increase in uterine activity and arterial blood pressure.[149] These studies suggest that cocaine use may increase uterine activity in pregnancy and may increase the risk of premature labor. This may explain the chemically observed relationship between acute cocaine use and abruptio placentae.

Management Options

Prepregnancy and Prenatal

Again, the basis of care is trust between the woman and her caregivers. The true nature of cocaine or crack abuse may not be easily divulged, and support may be rejected. The risk to the fetus must be made clear and the particular risk of binge use emphasized. No substitute drug is available to help with stabilization in pregnancy. However, sudden cessation is not associated with adverse fetal effects. Although the desire for a healthy baby may be an incentive to stop using cocaine, success is rare because psychological addiction is usually strong. If a woman wishes to stop using cocaine or crack, hospital admission may be beneficial to remove her from her usual environment. Constant social support and encouragement increases the chance of success. If use is stopped at any time during pregnancy, the outcome is improved.

Labor and Delivery

There is no major problem with labor or delivery, other than an increased need for narcotic analgesia. There can be specific problems in anesthetizing a patient who uses cocaine or crack.[150] As noted earlier, drug-related hypertension may mimic preeclampsia. Excessive uterine activity may result in fetal compromise or acute separation of the placenta.

Postnatal

After delivery, the symptoms of fetal cocaine withdrawal may not reach a peak until 3 days of life, and they may persist for 2 to 3 weeks. Many babies are discharged home before symptoms occur, so community midwives should be vigilant. Common signs are irritability, tremulousness, mood alterations, and hypertonia; in addition, the infants may be difficult to console.

As with heroin, relapse to drug abuse may occur in the postpartum period. Close community support from the relevant agencies can help women to stay drug-free and develop parenting skills.

CANNABIS: SPECIFIC PROBLEMS

Background

Marijuana is the most prevalent illicit drug used in pregnancy (4%–30%).[134,151,152] Despite this, there are few reports on fetal effects.

Maternal and Fetal Risks

Studies suggest that there is no increase in the rate of morphologic anomalies, low birth weight, preterm delivery, or abruptio placentae.[64,99,134,153]

A study in Jamaica assessed newborns exposed to marijuana antenatally in a blinded fashion and compared them with nonexposed babies from socioeconomically matched mothers. At 1 month, marijuana-exposed infants scored higher on autonomic stability, reflexes, general irritability, and weight. No ill effects from marijuana were found, and there may have been dose-related positive effects. The Jamaican mothers reported that cannabis increased their appetite during pregnancy and relieved pregnancy-related nausea.[134]

Therefore, the use of marijuana is not a problem and may even be beneficial in pregnancy. However, some may see marijuana as a gateway drug that potentially leads to harder drugs because of its association with the drug culture. Users should be warned against progression to drugs that are more harmful.

Management Options

No management problems are specifically associated with cannabis use.

BENZODIAZEPINES: SPECIFIC PROBLEMS

Background

Benzodiazepines are commonly used as anxiolytics and sedatives.[154] Their legitimate use in pregnancy has varied over the years, including the management of preeclampsia.[155] However, because of the fear of harmful effects, many women and their physicians recommend stopping their medication acutely, often with adverse maternal effects.[156] There are no apparent fetal effects, although the fetus may be at risk if the mother has a convulsion. These substances are also taken as part of polydrug abuse,[157] making assessment of their risk difficult.

Maternal and Fetal Risks

Large epidemiologic studies show no teratogenic effects and no obvious problems related to withdrawal from various benzodiazepines.[158,159] However, some abnormalities, particularly cleft palate,[81] are associated with its use. This finding is not conclusive, and other studies found no link.[160] Further, cleft palate is a common abnormality that occurs with other drug use.[161] However, there is evidence of hypotonia and problems with feeding because of its sedative effect when taken immediately before delivery.[82]

Management Options

No specific management in pregnancy is needed, except to discourage its use or stabilize the patient to the lowest level tolerated. Further reduction and cessation is possible in motivated patients. Stopping suddenly can produce maternal side effects, but is safe for the baby, apart from the risk of maternal convulsion. Benzodiazepines are excreted in breast milk, but the levels are low and should not cause neonatal problems.[82]

AMPHETAMINES: SPECIFIC PROBLEMS

Amphetamines are synthetic amines that are similar to the body's own adrenaline (epinephrine). They exaggerate the normal reaction to emergency or stress. Common slang terms for amphetamines include "speed," "wizz," "crystal," "meth," "bennies," "dexies," "A," "uppers," "pep pills," "diet pills," "jolly beans," "truck drivers," "co-pilots," "eye openers," "wake-ups," "hearts," and "footballs." The stimulating effects of amphetamines have been widely used to counteract fatigue. These drugs are also used by athletes to increase performance and by others for general stimulation, pleasure, or fun. Their use in pregnancy varies but is usually less than 1%.[162] In the younger age group, approximately 9% describe past use.[152]

The drug is usually taken orally but can be injected or sniffed. It is sometimes used interchangeably with cocaine. Because amphetamine use produces undesirable personality changes, "speed freaks" are highly unpopular with other addicts. They may be aggressive and violent. Most drug users consider amphetamines extremely dangerous and do not use them.

After continued administration of moderate doses, recovery is associated with fatigue, drowsiness, and often depression. The increased energy produced by the drug merely postpones the need for rest. Regular users rely on the drug when fatigued and often do not get proper rest for long periods. Near the end of such a "run" (usually <1 week), toxic symptoms dominate and the effects become intolerable. If the drug is discontinued, fatigue sets in and prolonged sleep follows, sometimes lasting days. After wakening, the user feels lethargic, sometimes depressed, and extremely hungry. These effects can be overcome by further drug use, which restarts the cycle. To stop runs, "downers" or opiates are sometimes used. Amphetamines do not produce a physical dependence, and psychological and environmental factors appear to be the motivating factors in the addiction.

Maternal and Fetal Risks

The effect on the baby is not well documented, but it appears to be associated with congenital abnormalities, particularly an increased occurrence of cleft palate.[163] Because amphetamine use is associated with hypertension, the incidence of preeclampsia and convulsions is also increased, with associated intrauterine growth restriction and death. Premature labor is also more common, but this may be due to associated lifestyle factors. The long-term growth of infants born to mothers who were addicted to amphetamines during pregnancy was found to be impaired.[164] This reduction appeared to be global, suggesting symmetrical growth impairment, which is usually associated with direct injury to the developing fetus rather than placental insufficiency.

Management Options

Amphetamines are dangerous and should be discontinued. There is no drug substitute. Success in stopping the use of this drug is poor, and these addicts are probably the most difficult and problematic to treat. They value their sick appearance and often claim that they will die. Death as a result of amphetamine use is relatively rare. The best approach is to provide close, supportive care and constant encouragement to stop using the drug. The problem is that stopping is relatively easy, but so is restarting.

LSD: SPECIFIC PROBLEMS

Background

D-lysergic acid diethylamide-25 is an unusual, controversial drug better known as "LSD" or simply "acid." It is usually taken orally but may be sniffed or injected. LSD is one of the most potent biologically active substances known. It is well absorbed from the gastrointestinal tract, is distributed in the blood, easily diffuses into the brain, and crosses the placental barrier.

The psychological effects are not predictable and are affected by the user's personality and current thoughts. However, its use is compatible with a reasonably normal life and is not necessarily associated with the normal drug culture. In the younger age group, approximately 7% describe past use.[152]

Maternal and Fetal Risks and Management Options

High doses of LSD given to pregnant animals produce deformities in the offspring of some species and not others[165,166] There are little data on LSD use in human pregnancy.[167] Until more information is known, the most sensible approach is to recommend that pregnant women avoid LSD use. No other particular care is required.

BARBITURATES: SPECIFIC PROBLEMS

Background

The incidence of barbiturate use in pregnancy is relatively low.[168] There do not appear to be specific fetal effects, except for fetal dependence. Acute withdrawal during pregnancy can affect the fetus in utero and is not recommended, although the precise risk is unknown. Gradual withdrawal can be achieved with reducing doses of short-acting barbiturates, such as pentobarbitone.

Maternal and Fetal Risks

The main risk to the mother and neonate is associated with withdrawal. This can be alleviated with a gradually reducing regimen that includes supplementary drugs. Acute withdrawal is associated with seizures and mental instability, usually occurring approximately 48 hours after the last dose. The neonate may take longer to show symptoms because the clearance of barbiturates is slower in the newborn.

Management Options

Slow reduction and cessation of drug use is the mainstay of management.

SOLVENT ABUSE: SPECIFIC PROBLEMS

Background

Solvent abuse is extremely common, and up to 19% of schoolchildren in parts of the United States have used them. Along with alcohol, marijuana, and tobacco, they are considered gateway drugs. There are many types of inhalants, including spray paint, liquid correction fluid, hair spray, nail polish remover, paint thinners, felt-tip markers, air fresheners, octane booster, glues and adhesives, fabric protectors, acetone products, carburetor cleaner, gasoline, propane gas, gas inside Ping-Pong balls, VCR head cleaner, and vegetable cooking sprays. Other examples are butyl nitrates, called "locker room" or "rush," and amyl nitrate capsules, called "snappers" or "poppers."

Maternal and Fetal Risks

Solvent abuse produces clinical signs, such as irritation and sores around the mouth and nose, nausea and headache, coughing, memory loss, lack of concentration and coordination, and odd behavior or irritability.

Sniffing leads to rapid entry of the drugs into the brain and organ systems, producing a high that lasts 15 to 45 minutes. Inhaling from a plastic or paper bag ("bagging") or inhaling from a soaked rag placed in the mouth ("huffing") greatly increases these effects. Damage can occur to the brain, liver, kidneys, blood, and bone marrow, and unconsciousness is common. In a study in pregnant solvent users, renal tubular acidosis was diagnosed in 5.3%, and 3.6% had adverse neurologic sequelae. One patient was diagnosed with brain damage, including expressive aphasia. The incidence of premature delivery was 21.4%.

The substances in solvents can cross the placenta and enter the fetal bloodstream. In the same study, 16.1% of infants had major anomalies. Most of these had facial abnormalities similar to those seen in fetal alcohol syndrome, and a further 10.7% had hearing loss.[169]

In another study of infants exposed to toluene, there was a 10% incidence of neonatal death as well as an increased incidence of prematurity (42%), low birth weight (52%), and microcephaly (32%). In addition, some infants had craniofacial features similar to those seen in fetal alcohol syndrome as well as other minor anomalies.[170]

Management Options

Solvent use is associated with erratic behavior, is dangerous for the mother and fetus, and should be strongly discouraged. Close observation and monitoring is required because of the high incidence of premature delivery and intrauterine growth restriction. Because there is evidence of neonatal abnormalities similar to those seen with alcohol and there may be developmental problems, the babies require close long-term follow-up.

SUMMARY OF MANAGEMENT OPTIONS
Specific Drugs of Abuse (e.g., heroin, cocaine, barbiturates)

Management Options	Quality of Evidence	Strength of Recommendation	References
Use a multidisciplinary approach.	IIb	B	93,181
Explain the risks of low birth weight, intrauterine growth restriction, and preterm delivery, and the need for neonatal care, especially if withdrawal symptoms occur.	III	B	99
Explain the risk of developmental abnormality in infants.	III	B	95
	IIb	B	184
In women using heroin, encourage detoxification or substitution with methadone or buprenorphine.	III	B	95
Encourage cessation with cocaine and amphetamines.	IIb	B	184
Solvent abuse produces effects similar to those of alcohol.	III	B	170
Screen for fetal abnormality, growth, and well-being.	III	B	99
The patient may need an increased dose of narcotic analgesia (an epidural is preferable).	IV	C	185
Provide fetal monitoring if intrauterine growth restriction occurs.	–	GPP	–
If the patient is HIV-positive or is still injecting, discourage breastfeeding.	IV	C	121
Watch for symptoms of withdrawal in the infant (starting at 3 days with heroin, cocaine, and solvents; 7 days with methadone, barbiturates, and amphetamines)	IV	C	114, 186
Provide follow-up by an addiction team.	IV	C	187, 188

CONCLUSIONS

- Of all abused substances, tobacco has the greatest effect on fetal growth and development.
- Alcohol is the worst teratogen of all abused substances.
- Women who abuse recreational drugs are probably at increased risk because of social and environmental factors.
- Substance abuse is as much a sign of risk as the cause of the risk itself.
- A multidisciplinary team approach is required.
- Pregnancy is a life event that may give a woman the opportunity and motivation to change her lifestyle for hers and the baby's long-term benefit.

REFERENCES

1. Haller DL, Miles DR: Victimization and perpetration among perinatal substance abusers. J Interpers Violence 2003;18:760–780.
2. Hepburn M: Drug use in pregnancy: A multidisciplinary responsibility. Hosp Med 1998;59:436.
3. Hodnett ED, Fredericks S: Support during pregnancy for women at increased risk of low birthweight babies. Cochrane Database Syst Rev 2003:CD000198.
4. Aaronson LS: Perceived and received support: Effects on health behavior during pregnancy. Nurs Res 1989;38:4–9.
5. Ioka A, Tsukuma H, Nakamuro K: Lifestyles and pre-eclampsia with special attention to cigarette smoking. J Epidemiol 2003;13:90–95.
6. Ventura SJ, Hamilton BE, Mathews TJ, Chandra A: Trends and variations in smoking during pregnancy and low birth weight: Evidence from the birth certificate, 1990–2000. Pediatrics 2003;111(5 Part 2):1176–1180.
7. Tuthill DP, Stewart JH, Coles EC, et al: Maternal cigarette smoking and pregnancy outcome. Paediatr Perinat Epidemiol 1999;13:245 253.
8. Zotti ME, Replogle WH, Sappenfield WM: Prenatal smoking and birth outcomes among Mississippi residents. J Miss State Med Assoc 2003;44:3–9.
9. Lieb R, Schreier A, Pfister H, Wittchen HU: Maternal smoking and smoking in adolescents: A prospective community study of adolescents and their mothers. Eur Addict Res 2003;9:120–130.
10. Ananth CV, Smulian JC, Vintzileos AM: Incidence of placental abruption in relation to cigarette smoking and hypertensive disorders during pregnancy: A meta-analysis of observational studies. Obstet Gynecol 1999;93:622–628.
11. Castles A, Adams EK, Melvin CL, et al: Effects of smoking during pregnancy: Five meta-analyses. Am J Prev Med 1999;16:208–215.
12. Savitz DA, Dole N, Terry JW Jr, et al: Smoking and pregnancy outcome among African-American and white women in central North Carolina. Epidemiology 2001;12:636–642.
13. Secker-Walker RH, Vacek PM: Relationships between cigarette smoking during pregnancy, gestational age, maternal weight gain, and infant birthweight. Addict Behav 2003;28:55–66.
14. Ashfaq M, Janjua MZ, Nawaz M: Effects of maternal smoking on placental morphology. J Ayub Med Coll Abbottabad 2003;15:12–15.
15. Lindqvist PG, Marsal K: Moderate smoking during pregnancy is associated with a reduced risk of preeclampsia. Acta Obstet Gynecol Scand 1999;78:693–697.
16. Shiverick KT, Salafia C: Cigarette smoking and pregnancy: I. Ovarian, uterine and placental effects. Placenta 1999;20:265–272.
17. Rasch V: Cigarette, alcohol, and caffeine consumption: Risk factors for spontaneous abortion. Acta Obstet Gynecol Scand 2003;82:182–188.
18. Wisborg K, Kesmodel U, Henriksen TB, et al: A prospective study of maternal smoking and spontaneous abortion. Acta Obstet Gynecol Scand 2003;82:936–941.
19. Werler MM, Lammer EJ, Rosenberg L, Mitchell AA: Maternal cigarette smoking during pregnancy in relation to oral clefts. Am J Epidemiol 1990;132:926–932.
20. Lieff S, Olshan AF, Werler M, et al: Maternal cigarette smoking during pregnancy and risk of oral clefts in newborns. Am J Epidemiol 1999;150:683–694.
21. Chung KC, Kowalski CP, Kim HM, Buchman SR: Maternal cigarette smoking during pregnancy and the risk of having a child with cleft lip/palate. Plast Reconstr Surg 2000;105:485–491.
22. Pang D, McNally R, Birch JM: Parental smoking and childhood cancer: Results from the United Kingdom Childhood Cancer Study. Br J Cancer 2003;88:373–381.
23. Roquer JM, Figueras J, Botet F, Jimenez R: Influence on fetal growth of exposure to tobacco smoke during pregnancy. Acta Paediatr 1995;84:118–121.
24. Frank P, McNamee R, Hannaford PC, Kay CR: Effect of changes in maternal smoking habits in early pregnancy on infant birthweight. Br J Gen Pract 1994;44:57–59.
25. Law KL, Stroud LR, LaGasse LL, et al: Smoking during pregnancy and newborn neurobehavior. Pediatrics 2003;111(6 Pt 1):1318–1323.
26. Batstra L, Hadders-Algra M, Neeleman J: Effect of antenatal exposure to maternal smoking on behavioural problems and academic achievement in childhood: Prospective evidence from a Dutch birth cohort. Early Hum Dev 2003;75:21–33.
27. MacArthur C, Knox EG, Lancashire RJ: Effects at age nine of maternal smoking in pregnancy: Experimental and observational findings. BJOG 2001;108:67–73.
28. Piquero AR, Gibson CL, Tibbetts SG, et al: Maternal cigarette smoking during pregnancy and life-course-persistent offending. Int J Offender Ther Comp Criminol 2002;46:231–248.
29. Wakschlag LS, Hans SL: Maternal smoking during pregnancy and conduct problems in high-risk youth: A developmental framework. Dev Psychopathol 2002;14:351–369.
30. Campion P, Owen L, McNeill A, McGuire C: Evaluation of a mass media campaign on smoking and pregnancy. Addiction 1994;89:1245–1254.
31. Walsh RA, Redman S, Brinsmead MW, Arnold B: Smoking cessation in pregnancy: A survey of the medical and nursing directors of public antenatal clinics in Australia. Aust N Z J Obstet Gynaecol 1995;35:144–150.
32. Hjalmarson AI, Hahn L, Svanberg B: Stopping smoking in pregnancy: Effect of a self-help manual in controlled trial. Br J Obstet Gynaecol 1991;98:260–264.
33. Valbo A, Nylander G: Smoking cessation in pregnancy: Intervention among heavy smokers. Acta Obstet Gynecol Scand 1994;73:215 219.
34. Lawrence T, Aveyard P, Evans O, Cheng KK: A cluster randomised controlled trial of smoking cessation in pregnant women comparing interventions based on the transtheoretical (stages of change) model to standard care. Tobacco Control 2003;12:168–177.
35. Wakschlag LS, Pickett KE, Middlecamp MK, et al: Pregnant smokers who quit, pregnant smokers who don't: Does history of problem behavior make a difference? Soc Sci Med 2003;56:2449–2460.
36. Tappin DM, Ford RP, Nelson KP, Wild CJ: Prevalence of smoking in early pregnancy by census area: Measured by anonymous cotinine testing of residual antenatal blood samples. N Z Med J 1996;109:101–103.
37. Webb DA, Boyd NR, Messina D, Windsor RA: The discrepancy between self-reported smoking status and urine continine levels among women enrolled in prenatal care at four publicly funded clinical sites. J Public Health Manag Pract 2003;9:322–325.
38. Mas R, Escriba V, Colomer C: Who quits smoking during pregnancy? Scand J Soc Med 1996;24:102–106.
39. Pickett KE, Wakschlag LS, Rathouz PJ, et al: The working-class context of pregnancy smoking. Health Place 2002;8:167–175.
40. Diefenbacher LJ, Smith PO, Nashelsky J: What is the most effective nicotine replacement therapy? J Fam Pract 2003;52:492–494; discussion 494.
41. Ilett KF, Hale TW, Page-Sharp M, et al: Use of nicotine patches in breast-feeding mothers: Transfer of nicotine and cotinine into human milk. Clin Pharmacol Ther 2003;74:516–524.
42. Windsor R, Oncken C, Henningfield J, et al: Behavioral and pharmacological treatment methods for pregnant smokers: Issues for clinical practice. J Am Med Womens Assoc 2000;55:304–310.

43. Secker-Walker RH, Vacek PM, Flynn BS, Mead PB: Estimated gains in birth weight associated with reductions in smoking during pregnancy. J Reprod Med 1998;43:967–974.
44. Secker-Walker RH, Solomon LJ, Flynn BS, et al: Smoking relapse prevention during pregnancy: A trial of coordinated advice from physicians and individual counseling. Am J Prev Med 1998;15:25–31.
45. Malchodi CS, Oncken C, Dornelas EA, et al: The effects of peer counseling on smoking cessation and reduction. Obstet Gynecol 2003;101:504–510.
46. Arias E, MacDorman MF, Strobino DM, Guyer B: Annual summary of vital statistics: 2002. Pediatrics 2003;112(6 Pt 1):1215–1230.
47. Egawa M, Yasuda K, Nakajima T, et al: Smoking enhances oxytocin-induced rhythmic myometrial contraction. Biol Reprod 2003;68:2274–2280.
48. Rantakallio P, Laara E, Koiranen M: A 28 year follow up of mortality among women who smoked during pregnancy. BMJ 1995;311:477–480.
49. Lemoine P, Harousseau H, Borteyru JP, Menuet JC: Children of alcoholic parents: Observed anomalies. Discussion of 127 cases. Ther Drug Monit 2003;25:132–136.
50. O'Callaghan FV, O'Callaghan M, Najman JM, et al: Maternal alcohol consumption during pregnancy and physical outcomes up to 5 years of age: A longitudinal study. Early Hum Dev 2003;71:137–148.
51. Ingersoll K, Floyd L, Sobell M, Velasquez MM: Reducing the risk of alcohol-exposed pregnancies: A study of a motivational intervention in community settings. Pediatrics 2003;111(5 Part 2):1131–1135.
52. Bogenschutz MP, Geppert CM: Pharmacologic treatments for women with addictions. Obstet Gynecol Clin North Am 2003;30:523–544.
53. Jones KL, Smith DW: Recognition of the fetal alcohol syndrome in early infancy. Lancet 1973;2:999–1001.
54. Jones KL: From recognition to responsibility: Josef Warkany, David Smith, and the fetal alcohol syndrome in the 21st century. Birth Defects Res Part A Clin Mol Teratol 2003;67:13–20.
55. Streissguth AP, Clarren SK, Jones KL: Natural history of the fetal alcohol syndrome: A 10-year follow-up of eleven patients. Lancet 1985;2:85–91.
56. Streissguth AP, Martin DC, Martin JC, Barr HM: The Seattle longitudinal prospective study on alcohol and pregnancy. Neurobehav Toxicol Teratol 1981;3:223–233.
57. King JC, Fabro S: Alcohol consumption and cigarette smoking: Effect on pregnancy. Clin Obstet Gynecol 1983;26:437–448.
58. Abel EL: An update on incidence of FAS: FAS is not an equal opportunity birth defect. Neurotoxicol Teratol 1995;17: 437–443.
59. Lazzaroni F, Bonassi S, Magnani M, et al: Moderate maternal drinking and outcome of pregnancy. Eur J Epidemiol 1993;9:599–606.
60. Testa M, Quigley BM, Eiden RD: The effects of prenatal alcohol exposure on infant mental development: A meta-analytical review. Alcohol Alcohol 2003;38:295–304.
61. Waterson EJ, Murray-Lyon IM: Drinking and smoking patterns amongst women attending an antenatal clinic: II. During pregnancy. Alcohol Alcohol 1989;24:163–173.
62. Shu XO, Hatch MC, Mills J, et al: Maternal smoking, alcohol drinking, caffeine consumption, and fetal growth: Results from a prospective study. Epidemiology 1995;6:115–120.
63. Whitehead N, Lipscomb L: Patterns of alcohol use before and during pregnancy and the risk of small-for-gestational-age birth. Am J Epidemiol 2003;158:654–662.
64. Day NL, Richardson GA, Geva D, Robles N: Alcohol, marijuana, and tobacco: Effects of prenatal exposure on offspring growth and morphology at age six. Alcohol Clin Exp Res 1994;18:786–794.
65. Sampson PD, Bookstein FL, Barr HM, Streissguth AP: Prenatal alcohol exposure, birthweight, and measures of child size from birth to age 14 years. Am J Public Health 1994;84:1421–1428.
66. Olson HC, Streissguth AP, Sampson PD, et al: Association of prenatal alcohol exposure with behavioral and learning problems in early adolescence. J Am Acad Child Adolesc Psychiatry 1997;36:1187–1194.
67. Streissguth AP, Sampson PD, Olson HC, et al: Maternal drinking during pregnancy: Attention and short-term memory in 14-year-old offspring. A longitudinal prospective study. Alcohol Clin Exp Res 1994;18:202–218.
68. Jacobson SW, Jacobson JL, Sokol RJ: Effects of fetal alcohol exposure on infant reaction time. Alcohol Clin Exp Res 1994;18:1125–1132.
69. Streissguth AP, Barr HM, Olson HC, et al: Drinking during pregnancy decreases word attack and arithmetic scores on standardized tests: Adolescent data from a population-based prospective study. Alcohol Clin Exp Res 1994;18:248–254.
70. Jacobson JL, Jacobson SW, Sokol RJ: Increased vulnerability to alcohol-related birth defects in the offspring of mothers over 30. Alcohol Clin Exp Res 1996;20:359–363.
71. Testa M, Reifman A: Individual differences in perceived riskiness of drinking in pregnancy: Antecedents and consequences. J Stud Alcohol 1996;57:360–367.
72. Russell M, Martier SS, Sokol RJ, et al: Screening for pregnancy risk: Drinking. Alcohol Clin Exp Res 1994;18:1156–1161.
73. Russell M, Martier SS, Sokol RJ, et al: Detecting risk drinking during pregnancy: A comparison of four screening questionnaires. Am J Public Health 1996;86:1435–1439.
74. Raistrick D, Bradshaw J, Tober G, et al: Development of the Leeds Dependence Questionnaire (LDQ): A questionnaire to measure alcohol and opiate dependence in the context of a treatment evaluation package. Addiction 1994;89:563–572.
75. Bolumar F, Rebagliato M, Hernandez-Aguado I, Florey CD: Smoking and drinking habits before and during pregnancy in Spanish women. J Epidemiol Community Health 1994;48:36–40.
76. Counsell AM, Smale PN, Geddis DC: Alcohol consumption by New Zealand women during pregnancy. N Z Med J 1994;107:278–281.
77. Cornelius MD, Richardson GA, Day NL, et al: A comparison of prenatal drinking in two recent samples of adolescents and adults. J Stud Alcohol 1994;55:412–419.
78. Humphreys K: Alcoholics Anonymous and 12-step alcoholism treatment programs. Recent Dev Alcohol 2003;16:149–164.
79. Kaiser LL, Allen L: Position of the American Dietetic Association: Nutrition and lifestyle for a healthy pregnancy outcome. J Am Diet Assoc 2002;102:1479–1490.
80. Wiseman EJ, Henderson KL, Briggs MJ: Individualized treatment for outpatients withdrawing from alcohol. J Clin Psychiatry 1998;59:289–293.
81. Dolovich LR, Addis A, Vaillancourt JM, et al: Benzodiazepine use in pregnancy and major malformations or oral cleft: Meta-analysis of cohort and case-control studies. BMJ 1998;317: 839–843.
82. McElhatton PR: The effects of benzodiazepine use during pregnancy and lactation. Reprod Toxicol 1994;8:461–475.
83. Helmbrecht GD, Hoskins IA: First trimester disulfiram exposure: Report of two cases. Am J Perinatol 1993;10:5–7.
84. Baer JS, Sampson PD, Barr HM, et al: A 21-year longitudinal analysis of the effects of prenatal alcohol exposure on young adult drinking. Arch Gen Psychiatry 2003;60:377–385.
85. Christoffersen MN, Soothill K: The long-term consequences of parental alcohol abuse: A cohort study of children in Denmark. J Subst Abuse Treat 2003;25:107–116.
86. Little BB, Snell LM, Gilstrap LD III, Johnston WL: Patterns of multiple substance abuse during pregnancy: Implications for mother and fetus. South Med J 1990;83:507–509, 518.

87. Lejeune C, Floch-Tudal C, Montamat S, et al: [Management of drug addict pregnant women and their children]. Arch Pediatr 1997;4:263–270.
88. Hepburn M: Social problems. Baillieres Clin Obstet Gynaecol 1990;4:149–168.
89. Wright A, Walker J: Drugs of abuse in pregnancy. Best Pract Res Clin Obstet Gynaecol 2001;15:987–998.
90. Walker AM, Walker JJ: A methadone programme for substance-misusing pregnant women. In Tober GS, SJ (eds): Methadone Matters. London, Martin Dunit, 2003.
91. Martin Mardomingo MA, Solis Sanchez G, Malaga Guerrero S, et al: [Drug abuse in pregnancy and neonatal morbidity: Epidemiologic changes in the last ten years]. Ann Pediatr 2003;58:574–579.
92. Tuten M, Jones HE: A partner's drug-using status impacts women's drug treatment outcome. Drug Alcohol Depend 2003;70:327–330.
93. Wolff K, Hay AW, Vail A, et al: Non-prescribed drug use during methadone treatment by clinic- and community-based patients. Addiction 1996;91:1699–1704.
94. Hepburn M: Drug use in pregnancy. Br J Hosp Med 1993;49:51–55.
95. Soepatmi S: Developmental outcomes of children of mothers dependent on heroin or heroin/methadone during pregnancy. Acta Paediatr Suppl 1994;404:36–39.
96. Sarman I: [Methadone treatment during pregnancy and its effect on the child: Better than continuing drug abuse, should be monitored by a specialized antenatal care center]. Lakartidningen 2000;97:2182–2184, 2187–2188, 2190.
97. Schneider C, Fischer G, Diamant K, et al: [Pregnancy and drug dependence]. Wien Klin Wochenschr 1996;108:611–614.
98. Boer K, Smit BJ, van Huis AM, Hogerzeil HV: Substance use in pregnancy: Do we care? Acta Paediatr Suppl 1994;404:65–71.
99. Nair P, Rothblum S, Hebel R: Neonatal outcome in infants with evidence of fetal exposure to opiates, cocaine, and cannabinoids. Clin Pediatr 1994;33:280–285.
100. Ornoy A, Michailevskaya V, Lukashov I, et al: The developmental outcome of children born to heroin-dependent mothers, raised at home or adopted. Child Abuse Negl 1996;20:385–396.
101. Kandall SR, Gaines J, Habel L, et al: Relationship of maternal substance abuse to subsequent sudden infant death syndrome in offspring. J Pediatr 1993;123:120–126.
102. McCarthy JE, Siney C, Shaw NJ, Ruben SM: Outcome predictors in pregnant opiate and polydrug users. Eur J Pediatr 1999;158:748–749.
103. Johnson K, Greenough A, Gerada C: Maternal drug use and length of neonatal unit stay. Addiction 2003;98:785–789.
104. Jarvis MA, Wu-Pong S, Kniseley JS, Schnoll SH: Alterations in methadone metabolism during late pregnancy. J Addict Dis 1999;18:51–61.
105. DePetrillo PB, Rice JM: Methadone dosing and pregnancy: Impact on program compliance. Int J Addict 1995;30:207–217.
106. Robinson SE: Buprenorphine: An analgesic with an expanding role in the treatment of opioid addiction. CNS Drug Rev 2002;8:377–390.
107. Schindler SD, Eder H, Ortner R, et al: Neonatal outcome following buprenorphine maintenance during conception and throughout pregnancy. Addiction 2003;98:103–110.
108. Marquet P, Chevrel J, Lavignasse P, et al: Buprenorphine withdrawal syndrome in a newborn. Clin Pharmacol Ther 1997;62:569–571.
109. Lacroix I, Berrebi A, Chaumerliac C, et al: Buprenorphine in pregnant opioid-dependent women: First results of a prospective study. Addiction 2004;99:209–214.
110. Johnson RE, Jones HE, Fischer G: Use of buprenorphine in pregnancy: Patient management and effects on the neonate. Drug Alcohol Depend 2003;70(2 Suppl):S87–S101.
111. Berghella V, Lim PJ, Hill MK, et al: Maternal methadone dose and neonatal withdrawal. Am J Obstet Gynecol 2003;189: 312–317.
112. Dashe JS, Sheffield JS, Olscher DA, et al: Relationship between maternal methadone dosage and neonatal withdrawal. Obstet Gynecol 2002;100:1244–1249.
113. Finnegan LP, Connaughton JF Jr, Kron RE, Emich JP: Neonatal abstinence syndrome: Assessment and management. Addict Dis 1975;2:141–158.
114. Chapman JP, Galea P: Neonatal abstinence syndrome at Glasgow Royal maternity hospital. Health Bull 1999;57:247–251.
115. Johnson K, Gerada C, Greenough A: Treatment of neonatal abstinence syndrome. Arch Dis Child Fetal Neonatal Ed 2003;88:F2–F5.
116. Fabris C, Prandi G, Perathoner C, Soldi A: Neonatal drug addiction. Panminerva Med 1998;40:239–243.
117. Wojnar-Horton RE, Kristensen JH, Yapp P, et al: Methadone distribution and excretion into breast milk of clients in a methadone maintenance programme. Br J Clin Pharmacol 1997;44:543–547.
118. Ballard JL: Treatment of neonatal abstinence syndrome with breast milk containing methadone. J Perinat Neonatal Nurs 2002;15:76–85.
119. Ross A, Raab GM, Mok J, et al: Maternal HIV infection, drug use, and growth of uninfected children in their first 3 years. Arch Dis Child 1995;73:490–495.
120. Goldberg D, Smith R, MacIntyre P, et al: Prevalence of HIV among pregnant women in Dundee 1988–1997: Evidence to gauge the effectiveness of HIV prevention measures. J Infect 2000;41:39–44.
121. Mussi-Pinhata MM, Kato CM, Duarte G, et al: Factors associated with vertical HIV transmission during two different time periods: The impact of zidovudine use on clinical practice at a Brazilian reference centre. Int J STD AIDS 2003;14:818–825.
122. Johnstone FD, Brettle RP, Burns SM, et al: HIV testing and prevalence in pregnancy in Edinburgh. Int J STD AIDS 1994;5:101–104.
123. Tappin DM, Johnstone FD, Smith R, et al: Spread of maternal HIV infection in Scotland from 1990 to 1992. Scott Med J 1995;40:12–14.
124. Latt NC, Spencer JD, Beeby PJ, et al: Hepatitis C in injecting drug-using women during and after pregnancy. J Gastroenterol Hepatol 2000;15:175–181.
125. Armstrong GL, Perz JF, Alter MJ: Perinatal hepatitis C virus transmission: Role of human immunodeficiency virus infection and injection drug use. J Infect Dis 2003;187:872, author reply 872–874.
126. Dinsmoor MJ: Hepatitis C in pregnancy. Curr Womens Health Rep 2001;1:27–30.
127. Soderstrom A, Norkrans G, Lindh M: Hepatitis B virus DNA during pregnancy and post partum: Aspects on vertical transmission. Scand J Infect Dis 2003;35:814–819.
128. van Steenbergen JE, Leentvaar-Kuijpers A, Baayen D, et al: Evaluation of the hepatitis B antenatal screening and neonatal immunization program in Amsterdam, 1993–1998. Vaccine 2001;20:7–11.
129. Su GG, Pan KH, Zhao NF, et al: Efficacy and safety of lamivudine treatment for chronic hepatitis B in pregnancy. World J Gastroenterol 2004;10:910–912.
130. Little BB, Snell LM, Trimmer KJ, et al: Peripartum cocaine use and adverse pregnancy outcome. Am J Human Biol 1999;11: 598–602.
131. Vidaeff AC, Mastrobattista JM: In utero cocaine exposure: A thorny mix of science and mythology. Am J Perinatol 2003;20: 165–172.
132. Frank DA, Augustyn M, Knight WG, et al: Growth, development, and behavior in early childhood following prenatal cocaine exposure: A systematic review. JAMA 2001;285:1613–1625.

133. Martinez Crespo JM, Antolin E, Comas C, et al: The prevalence of cocaine abuse during pregnancy in Barcelona. Eur J Obstet Gynecol Reprod Biol 1994;56:165–167.
134. Shiono PH, Klebanoff MA, Nugent RP, et al: The impact of cocaine and marijuana use on low birth weight and preterm birth: A multicenter study. Am J Obstet Gynecol 1995;172(1 Pt 1):19–27.
135. Kline J, Ng SK, Schittini M, et al: Cocaine use during pregnancy: Sensitive detection by hair assay. Am J Public Health 1997;87:352–358.
136. Grant T, Brown Z, Callahan C, et al: Cocaine exposure during pregnancy: Improving assessment with radioimmunoassay of maternal hair. Obstet Gynecol 1994;83:524–531.
137. Kuhn L, Kline J, Ng S, et al: Cocaine use during pregnancy and intrauterine growth retardation: New insights based on maternal hair tests. Am J Epidemiol 2000;152:112–119.
138. Jacobson JL, Jacobson SW, Sokol RJ: Effects of prenatal exposure to alcohol, smoking, and illicit drugs on postpartum somatic growth. Alcohol Clin Exp Res 1994;18:317–323.
139. Singer LT, Yamashita TS, Hawkins S, et al: Increased incidence of intraventricular hemorrhage and developmental delay in cocaine-exposed, very low birth weight infants. J Pediatr 1994;124(5 Pt 1):765–771.
140. Griffith DR, Azuma SD, Chasnoff IJ: Three-year outcome of children exposed prenatally to drugs. J Am Acad Child Adolesc Psychiatry 1994;33:20–27.
141. Burkett G, Yasin SY, Palow D, et al: Patterns of cocaine binging: Effect on pregnancy. Am J Obstet Gynecol 1994;171:372–378, discussion 378–379.
142. Hanlon-Lundberg KM, Williams M, Rhim T, et al: Accelerated fetal lung maturity profiles and maternal cocaine exposure. Obstet Gynecol 1996;87:128–132.
143. Snodgrass SR: Cocaine babies: A result of multiple teratogenic influences. J Child Neurol 1994;9:227–233.
144. Morris P, Binienda Z, Gillam MP, et al: The effect of chronic cocaine exposure during pregnancy on maternal and infant outcomes in the rhesus monkey. Neurotoxicol Teratol 1996;18: 147–154.
145. Tonkiss J, Shultz PL, Shumsky JS, et al: The effects of cocaine exposure prior to and during pregnancy in rats fed low or adequate protein diets. Neurotoxicol Teratol 1995;17:593–600.
146. Sun LS, Takuma S, Lui R, Homma S: The effect of maternal cocaine exposure on neonatal rat cardiac function. Anesth Analg 2003;97:878–882.
147. Choi SJ, Mazzio E, Soliman KF: The effects of gestational cocaine exposure on pregnancy outcome, postnatal development, cognition and locomotion in rats. Ann N Y Acad Sci 1998;844:324–335.
148. Morgan MA, Honnebier MB, Mecenas C, Nathanielsz PW: Cocaine's effect on plasma oxytocin concentrations in the baboon during late pregnancy. Am J Obstet Gynecol 1996;174: 1026–1027.
149. Nakahara K, Iso A, Chao CR, et al: Pregnancy enhances cocaine-induced stimulation of uterine contractions in the chronically instrumented rat. Am J Obstet Gynecol 1996;175: 188–193.
150. Campbell D, Parr MJ, Shutt LE: Unrecognized "crack" cocaine abuse in pregnancy. Br J Anaesth 1996;77:553–555.
151. Ebrahim SH, Gfroerer J: Pregnancy-related substance use in the United States during 1996–1998. Obstet Gynecol 2003;101: 374–379.
152. Turner C, Russell A, Brown W: Prevalence of illicit drug use in young Australian women: Patterns of use and associated risk factors. Addiction 2003;98:1419–1426.
153. Fergusson DM, Horwood LJ, Northstone K: Maternal use of cannabis and pregnancy outcome. BJOG 2002;109:21–27.
154. Iqbal MM, Sobhan T, Aftab SR, Mahmud SZ: Diazepam use during pregnancy: A review of the literature. Del Med J 2002;74: 127–135.
155. Hutton JD, James DK, Stirrat GM, et al: Management of severe pre-eclampsia and eclampsia by UK consultants. Br J Obstet Gynaecol 1992;99:554–556.
156. Einarson A, Selby P, Koren G: Abrupt discontinuation of psychotropic drugs during pregnancy: Fear of teratogenic risk and impact of counselling. J Psychiatry Neurosci 2001;26:44–48.
157. Garretty DJ, Wolff K, Hay AW, Raistrick D: Benzodiazepine misuse by drug addicts. Ann Clin Biochem 1997;34(Pt 1):68–73.
158. Eros E, Czeizel AE, Rockenbauer M, et al: A population-based case–control teratologic study of nitrazepam, medazepam, tofisopam, alprazolum and clonazepam treatment during pregnancy. Eur J Obstet Gynecol Reprod Biol 2002;101:147–154.
159. Weinstock L, Cohen LS, Bailey JW, et al: Obstetrical and neonatal outcome following clonazepam use during pregnancy: A case series. Psychother Psychosom 2001;70:158–162.
160. Ornoy A, Arnon J, Shechtman S, et al: Is benzodiazepine use during pregnancy really teratogenic? Reprod Toxicol 1998;12:511–515.
161. Thomas DB: Cleft palate, mortality and morbidity in infants of substance abusing mothers. J Paediatr Child Health 1995;31:457–460.
162. Buchi KF, Zone S, Langheinrich K, Varner MW: Changing prevalence of prenatal substance abuse in Utah. Obstet Gynecol 2003;102:27–30.
163. Plessinger MA: Prenatal exposure to amphetamines: Risks and adverse outcomes in pregnancy. Obstet Gynecol Clin North Am 1998;25:119–138.
164. Eriksson M, Jonsson B, Steneroth G, Zetterstrom R: Cross-sectional growth of children whose mothers abused amphetamines during pregnancy. Acta Paediatr 1994;83:612–617.
165. Emerit I, Roux C, Feingold J: LSD: No chromosomal breakage in mother and embryos during rat pregnancy. Teratology 1972;6: 71–73.
166. Bogdanoff B, Rorke LB, Yanoff M, Warren WS: Brain and eye abnormalities: Possible sequelae to prenatal use of multiple drugs including LSD. Am J Dis Child 1972;123:145–148.
167. von Mandach U, Rabner MM, Wisser J, Huch A: [LSD and cannabis abuse in early pregnancy with good perinatal outcome: Case report and review of the literature]. Gynakol Geburtshilfliche Rundsch 1999;39:125–129.
168. Sloan LB, Gay JW, Snyder SW, Bales WR: Substance abuse during pregnancy in a rural population. Obstet Gynecol 1992;79:245–248.
169. Scheeres JJ, Chudley AE: Solvent abuse in pregnancy: A perinatal perspective. J Obstet Gynaecol Can 2002;24:22–26.
170. Pearson MA, Hoyme HE, Seaver LH, Rimsza ME: Toluene embryopathy: Delineation of the phenotype and comparison with fetal alcohol syndrome. Pediatrics 1994;93:211–215.
171. DiClemente CC, Dolan-Mullen P, Windsor RA: The process of pregnancy smoking cessation: Implications for interventions. Tob Control 2000;Suppl 3:III16–III21.
172. Nordstrom ML, Cnattingius S: Smoking habits and birthweights in two successive births in Sweden. Early Human Development 1994;37:195–204.
173. Lumley J, Oliver S, Waters E: Interventions for promoting smoking cessation during pregnancy. Cochrane Database Syst Rev 2000:CD001055.
174. Gielen AC, Windsor R, Faden RR, et al: Evaluation of a smoking cessation intervention for pregnant women in an urban prenatal clinic. Health Educ Res 1997;12:247–254.
175. Dolan-Mullen P, Ramirez G, Groff JY: A meta-analysis of randomized trials of prenatal smoking cessation interventions. Am J Obstet Gynecol 1994;171:1328–1334.
176. Haddow JE, Knight GJ, Kloza EM, et al: Cotinine-assisted intervention in pregnancy to reduce smoking and low birthweight delivery. Br J Obstet Gynaecol 1991;98:859–865.
177. Kaskutas LA, Graves K: Pre-pregnancy drinking: How drink size affects risk assessment. Addiction 2001;96:1199–1209.

178. Kesmodel U, Olsen SF, Secher NJ: Does alcohol increase the risk of preterm delivery? Epidemiology 2000;11:512–518.
179. Wilk AI, Jensen NM, Havighurst TC: Meta-analysis of randomized control trials addressing brief interventions in heavy alcohol drinkers. J Gen Intern Med 1997;12:274–283.
180. Pirie PL, Lando H, Curry SJ, et al: Tobacco, alcohol, and caffeine use and cessation in early pregnancy. Am J Prev Med 2000;18:54–61.
181. Scholl TO, Hediger ML, Belsky DH: Prenatal care and maternal health during adolescent pregnancy: A review and meta-analysis. J Adolesc Health 1994;15:444–456.
182. Johnstone F, Goldberg D, Tappin D, et al: The incidence and prevalence of HIV infection among childbearing women living in Edinburgh city, 1982–1995. AIDS 1998;12:911–918.
183. Little BB, Snell LM, Van Beveren TT, et al: Treatment of substance abuse during pregnancy and infant outcome. Am J Perinatol 2003;20:255–262.
184. Elk R, Mangus L, Rhoades H, et al: Cessation of cocaine use during pregnancy: Effects of contingency management interventions on maintaining abstinence and complying with prenatal care. Addict Behav 1998;23:57–64.
185. Kuczkowski KM: Labor analgesia for the drug abusing parturient: Is there cause for concern? Obstet Gynecol Surv 2003;58:599–608.
186. Elliott MR, Cunliffe P, Demianczuk N, Robertson CM: Frequency of newborn behaviours associated with neonatal abstinence syndrome: A hospital-based study. J Obstet Gynaecol Can 2004;26:25–34.
187. Schuler ME, Nair P, Kettinger L: Drug-exposed infants and developmental outcome: Effects of a home intervention and ongoing maternal drug use. Arch Pediatr Adolesc Med 2003;157:133–138.
188. Kaltenbach K, Berghella V, Finnegan L: Opioid dependence during pregnancy: Effects and management. Obstet Gynecol Clin North Am 1998;25:139–151.

CHAPTER 35

Medication

Bertis B. Little

INTRODUCTION

The safety of approximately one half of medications for the mother and embryo or fetus remains unknown. Most pregnant women (40%–90%) are exposed to medications during gestation. These medications include a range of agents, such as vitamins, minerals, antibiotics, laxatives, antiemetics, sedatives, antacids, diuretics, and antihistamines (Table 35–1).[1,2] Medications are frequently used without a physician's advice or before pregnancy is recognized. In a small fraction of pregnant women, medications are needed to treat serious or life-threatening medical conditions, making it necessary to formulate a clinical plan to manage the chronic disease and the acute physiology of pregnancy. Pharmacokinetics are profoundly affected by pregnancy-associated physiologic changes (e.g., renal clearance, metabolism, blood volume, cardiac output), and dose adjustments are usually needed to optimize the clinical outcome.[3]

FREQUENCY OF MEDICATION USE IN PREGNANCY

Many women use medications during gestation. In studies, approximately 90% to 97% of pregnant women took medications prescribed by their physician, and two thirds took over-the-counter medications without medical advice.[4,5] The percentage of pregnant women who used medication during gestation appeared considerably lower in the United Kingdom compared with the United States (e.g., fewer than 10% of pregnant women in the United Kingdom used medications other than prenatal vitamins and iron supplements during the first trimester).[6]

DRUGS THAT ARE POTENTIALLY HARMFUL TO THE EMBRYO OR FETUS

An unborn child may be harmed by medications through either teratogenic or fetal effects, depending on the timing of exposure. Teratogenic effects are traditionally considered to occur during the period of organogenesis (embryonic period), with vulnerability encompassing the second through eighth weeks after conception by embryonic age. Embryonic age is estimated from the day of conception. Menstrual age is approximately 2 weeks greater than embryonic age because the former is calculated from the first day of the last menstrual period. A teratogen may cause a malformation in the unborn child when given during the embryonal period (organogenesis).[2] The fetal period is classically counted from 9 weeks after conception to delivery. Fetal effects are alterations in the structure or function of organ systems that are normally formed during organogenesis or organ systems that develop during the fetal period.[2] Medications with suspected or known teratogenic effects are listed in Table 35–2.

Thalidomide

Thalidomide is a sedative and hypnotic agent that is also used to treat leprosy, tuberculosis, and HIV. It is the most notorious of all human teratogens. Thalidomide taken between 27 and 42 days after conception produced phocomelia (absence of the long bones from the upper or lower limbs).[7] Other congenital anomalies were observed when the drug was taken outside the critical period for limb formation, including defects of the external ear and heart. Thalidomide is commercially available for use, as in South America, to treat leprosy. It is also used to treat tuberculosis and HIV. Alternate antituberculosis and antileprosy drug regimens are indicated for the treatment of women of reproductive age. In the mid- to late 1990s, another epidemic of thalidomide embryopathy was reported in South America that continues unabated.[8]

Retinoids

Vitamin A is an essential nutrient that is the lipid-soluble parent compound of retinoic acids (retinoids). Nutritional

TABLE 35–1

Medications Frequently Used by Pregnant Women[1,2]

Vitamins
Iron
Analgesics
Diuretics
Antiemetics
Antimicrobials
Antihistamines
Hypnotics and sedatives
Laxatives

TABLE 35–2

Medications Known or Suspected to Be Human Teratogens or to Have Adverse Fetal Effects[2]

Retinoids
High-dose vitamin A
Isotretinoin
Etretinate
Acitretin
Hormones
Androgens
Diethylstilbestrol
Danazol
Anticoagulants
Warfarin
Other coumarin anticoagulants
Antineoplastics
Aminopterin and methylaminopterin
Methotrexate
Busulfan
Cyclophosphamide
Anticonvulsants
Phenytoin and other hydantoins
Trimethadione and paramethadione
Valproic acid
Carbamazepine
Phenobarbital
Primidone
Trimethadione and paramethadione
Antibiotics
Fluconazole
Tetracycline
Other drugs
Angiotensin-converting enzyme inhibitors
Amiodarone
Aminopterin
Cocaine
Danazol
Lithium
Methimazole
Misoprostol
Methotrexate
Penicillamine
Quinine
Radioiodine
Thalidomide
Trimethoprim

guidelines recommend that pregnant women consume approximately 10,000 IU vitamin A daily, through a combination of dietary intake and nutritional supplementation. A recent study showed that higher intake, including dietary intake and nutritional supplementation, is associated with an increased risk of malformations, beginning at 15,000 IU daily.[9]

Isotretinoin and etretinate are synthetic derivatives of retinoic acid (vitamin A). Isotretinoin (Accutane) is the primary medical therapy for intractable cystic acne, a dermatologic disorder that is common in women of reproductive age. Despite the serious warning in the manufacturer's package insert that isotretinoin use during pregnancy is a known cause of very severe congenital anomalies of the brain, ears, heart, and thymus, clinicians who provide health care for pregnant women are likely to encounter use of this medication during early pregnancy. Scientific studies support the manufacturer's warning that isotretinoin is a very harmful teratogen that causes serious congenital anomalies (Table 35–3). Among nearly 100 fetuses exposed to isotretinoin during early pregnancy, one third had an adverse outcome.[2,9–16] Nineteen percent had spontaneous abortion, and 28% had malformations.[16,17] Mental retardation occurred in more than 85% of children who did not have major congenital anomalies.[18] Isotretinoin has a terminal half-life of approximately 96 hours, but even if the medication is discontinued within days before conception, the risk of congenital anomalies is still increased.[19]

Etretinate (Tegison) is used to treat psoriasis and is associated with central nervous system, craniofacial, and skeletal anomalies in progeny of pregnant women who received this medication before or during pregnancy.[17,20] This medication has an unusually long half-life. Newborns with central nervous system and craniofacial abnormalities were born to women who discontinued etretinate use up to 12 months before conception, according to several published reports.[21,22] Serum etretinate levels persist in the therapeutic range for more than 5 years after the cessation of therapy (personal communication from the manufacturer). Psoriasis is not common during pregnancy and usually does not require systemic therapy. Topical agents should be used to treat psoriasis

TABLE 35–3

Fetal Anomalies Associated with Maternal Isotretinoin (Accutane) Use[2,10–16]

Microtia
Anotia
Micrognathia
Cleft palate
Heart defects
Eye anomalies
Brain anomalies
Hydrocephalus
Thymic agenesis
Limb-reduction defects

in pregnant women and probably women of reproductive age because these medications are poorly absorbed and are primarily metabolized in the skin (i.e., topical therapy with steroids or retinoids results in insignificant serum concentrations).

Acitretin is an active metabolite of etretinate and is another retinoid that is given systemically to treat dermatologic conditions. The terminal half-life of acitretin is only a few days (approximately 3) compared with the parent compound etretinate, whose terminal half-life is putatively 3 months or longer. Two cases of human malformation (one electively terminated fetus, one liveborn infant) were reported with acitretin exposure during the first trimester, but exposure to acitretin before conception does not seem to be associated with an increased frequency of congenital anomalies. No congenital anomalies occurred among 52 infants born to women who discontinued acitretin therapy more than 14 days before conception.[20]

Antineoplastics

Most antineoplastics are teratogenic in humans because the medications usually impede or halt cell replication (see Table 35–2). Folate antagonists (e.g., aminopterin, methotrexate) have long been recognized as potent human teratogens. Aminopterin and methotrexate are also used as abortifacients. Congenital anomalies associated with fetal aminopterin syndrome are summarized in Table 35–4.[2,23–25] Similar congenital anomalies were observed when methotrexate was used during the first trimester.[26,27]

Busulfan (Myleran) is an alkylating agent used to treat some forms of leukemia. One infant whose mother received this antineoplastic during the first trimester had fetal growth retardation, cleft palate, and eye defects.[27] These findings were similar to defects reported in animal teratology studies.[2] Another alkylating agent, cyclophosphamide (Cytoxan), is used to treat certain forms of leukemia and other forms of cancer (ovarian, cervical, endometrial, and breast carcinomas). First-trimester cyclophosphamide use is associated with cleft palate, absence of digits (thumbs, great toes), imperforate anus, and fetal growth retardation.[28,29] Nonhuman primates whose mothers were given this cyclophosphamide during organogenesis had craniofacial anomalies[30] similar to those observed in exposed human fetuses.[31]

TABLE 35–4

Features of Fetal Aminopterin Syndrome[2,23–25]
Short stature
Craniosynostosis
Calvarial ossification delay
Hydrocephalus
Hypertelorism
Micrognathia
Cleft palate

Available anecdotal data are not sufficient to quantitate the teratogenic risk of alkylating agents to the human fetus. Fourteen percent of offspring exposed to alkylating agents in the first trimester had major congenital anomalies,[32] and the other 86% were apparently normal.

Anticonvulsants

Anticonvulsant agents (phenytoin, trimethadione, carbamazepine, and valproic acid) are associated with an increased risk of congenital anomalies.[2] Hydantoin agents, phenytoin (Dilantin, Diphenylan), ethotoin (Peganone), and mephenytoin (Mesantoin) are teratogens long recognized for their association with a constellation of congenital anomalies known as fetal hydantoin syndrome (Table 35–5).[33] In a summary of studies that included more than 450 infants born to women who received hydantoin anticonvulsants during pregnancy, approximately 10% of infants exposed to phenytoin during gestation had major congenital anomalies (cardiac defects, cleft lip or palate), and one third had minor anomalies (craniofacial and digital).[34]

Paramethadione (Paradione) and trimethadione (Tridione) are known as dione anticonvulsants and are primarily used to treat petit mal seizures. Fetal dione syndrome has long been recognized. Its constellation of abnormalities is strikingly similar to fetal hydantoin syndrome.[35]

Carbamazepine (Tegretol) was considered relatively safe for use during pregnancy. It was the drug of choice to treat pregnant women with seizure disorders,[36] supported in part by one report that the frequency of congenital anomalies was not increased among fewer than 100 infants born to women who took carbamazepine during early pregnancy.[37] In 1989, however, it was reported that carbamazepine use during early pregnancy was associated with a pattern of malformations very similar to that caused by phenytoin (i.e., craniofacial abnormalities, minor limb defects, growth retardation, mental retardation) as well as with neural tube defects.[38] A 1991 U.S. Food and Drug Administration (FDA) report warned that the risk of neural tube defects is approximately 1% among carbamazepine-exposed offspring, compared with approximately 1 in 1000 in the general population.

TABLE 35–5

Features of Fetal Hydantoin Syndrome
Craniofacial abnormalities
Cleft lip on palate
Hypertelorism
Broad nasal bridge
Hypoplasia of the distal phalanges and nails
Growth deficiency
Mental deficiency

(Adapted from Hanson JW, Smith DW: The fetal hydantoin syndrome. J Pediatr 1975;87:285–290.)

A major difficulty with ascribing a specific risk of birth defects to anticonvulsant therapy is that epilepsy per se is a risk factor for congenital anomalies. Hence, it is unclear whether the anticonvulsant medication, the disease being treated (epilepsy), or a combination of factors causes the birth defects.[36] Pharmacogenetic evidence shows that deficits in maternal epoxide hydrolase enzyme activity are probably associated with birth defects, whereas normal enzyme activity is associated with normal infants after gestational phenytoin exposure.[39,40] This enzyme is essential for the elimination of a toxic phenytoin epoxide metabolite that is believed to be responsible for the teratogenicity of several anticonvulsant medications that share this metabolic pathway.[39,41]

Valproic acid (Depakene) is the most commonly prescribed medication for petit mal seizures. It is associated with a 1% to 2% risk of neural tube defects, which is 8 to 10 times greater than that in the general population.[42,43] Fetal valproate syndrome is a constellation of facial and digital anomalies associated with the use of valproic acid in early pregnancy.[44–46]

Anticoagulants

Warfarin is a coumarin anticoagulant. It is a small molecule that readily crosses the placenta.[36] Warfarin embryopathy is a distinct pattern of anomalies and occurs among 15% to 25% of infants and children whose mothers used warfarin during the first trimester.[47,48] Nasal hypoplasia and stippling of the epiphyses or malformed vertebral bodies are the most common features; other features also occur (Table 35–6).[47] When used during the second or third trimester, warfarin and other coumarin anticoagulants are associated with adverse fetal effects, including intracerebral hemorrhage, microcephaly, cataracts, blindness, and mental retardation.[47]

Hormones

Androgen therapy (i.e., testosterone) during pregnancy resulted in virilized external genitalia of female fetuses, including clitoromegaly and labioscrotal fusion.[49] Most hormone-induced fetal defects, short of actual fusion, usually resolve spontaneously during infant growth and development. Hormone-induced genital tract abnormalities that persist can be surgically corrected, and normal female pubertal development can be anticipated.[2]

Danazol, a drug used to treat endometriosis, is a testosterone derivative with weak androgenic activity. Female fetal exposure in utero may result in clitoromegaly or labial fusion.[50–53] However, the exact risk of this complication is unknown, and no apparent adverse effects were seen in male fetuses.

Diethylstilbestrol (DES), a nonsteroidal synthetic estrogen, causes vaginal clear cell adenocarcinoma in the progeny of women exposed to the drug during late embryogenesis.[54] The number of pregnant women actually exposed to this hormone during gestation is unknown. Other nonmalignant anomalies were also reported in female and male offspring of mothers exposed to this agent during early pregnancy (Table 35–7).[2,54–64] Women whose mothers used DES during pregnancy had an increased frequency of preterm labor, spontaneous abortion, and ectopic pregnancy.[59] Importantly, DES-exposed female progeny are in the reproductive or postreproductive years in 2004. DES is clearly contraindicated during pregnancy.

Antibiotics

The only antibacterial agents with known teratogenic effects are tetracyclines, and the effect is cosmetic and transient. The adverse effect caused by tetracyclines is yellow-brown discoloration of the deciduous teeth. The permanent teeth, the frequency of dental caries, and bone growth are unaffected by tetracycline exposure.[65–67] Tetracycline use during pregnancy is not associated with an increased frequency of structural congenital anomalies.[68–70] Tetracyclines should be given during pregnancy to treat life-threatening infections (e.g., syphilis) in patients who are allergic to penicillin. Otherwise, tetracyclines are not recommended for use during pregnancy because of the adverse effects on the deciduous teeth.

TABLE 35–6

Characteristic Features of Fetal Warfarin Syndrome

Nasal hypoplasia
Stippled bone epiphyses and malformed vertebral bodies
Hydrocephaly
Microcephaly
Growth retardation
Ophthalmologic anomalies
Postnatal developmental delay

(Adapted from Hall JG, Pauli RM, Wilson K: Maternal and fetal sequelae of anticoagulation during pregnancy. Am J Med 1980;68:122–140.)

TABLE 35–7

Abnormalities in the Offspring of Pregnant Women Exposed to Diethylstilbestrol[2,54–64]

Female Offspring
Clear cell adenocarcinoma of the vagina or cervix
Vaginal adenosis
T-shaped uterus
Uterine hypoplasia
Paraovarian cyst
Incompetent cervix
Male Offspring
Epididymal cyst
Hypoplastic testes
Cryptorchidism

Psychotropics

Lithium is used to treat affective mental disorders.[36] An increased risk of cardiovascular anomalies is observed in offspring born to women who used lithium during early gestation.[71] A meta-analysis of published data indicated that previous estimates of the association of lithium exposure and Ebstein's anomaly (3%–12%) were too high.[72] Ebstein's anomaly occurs in approximately 1 in 20,000 live births. Although the exact risk of cardiovascular anomalies as a result of maternal exposure to lithium during embryogenesis is unknown,[36,71] data show that 1% of infants exposed to lithium during gestation may have Ebstein's anomaly. In addition, the risk of noncardiovascular congenital anomalies does not appear to be increased substantially above background rates.[72] Prenatal diagnosis (fetal echocardiogram) is indicated to evaluate possible fetal tricuspid valve regurgitation. Possible secondary complications of lithium use during the second and third trimesters include polyhydramnios and fetal diabetes insipidus. If possible, first-trimester exposure to this agent should be avoided. Patients who use lithium during the second and third trimesters should be routinely evaluated for increased amniotic fluid volume.

Other Drugs

Penicillamine is used to treat rheumatoid arthritis and cystinuria.[2] It is also used as a chelating agent for heavy metal poisoning (e.g., lead). Penicillamine is putatively associated with connective tissue disorders in the offspring of exposed mothers,[73] although the risk is quantitatively unknown.[74] Therefore, penicillamine is contraindicated during pregnancy.

USE OF OTHER MEDICATIONS DURING PREGNANCY

Most currently available medications are not proven to be human teratogens, although fewer than 50% have been adequately studied for use in human pregnancy. Further, in the last 20 years, few advances in clinical teratology have occurred.[75] The use of medications during pregnancy is discussed later in the context of medical indications for their use. It is important to remember that absence of evidence is not evidence of absence.

Dermatologic Drugs

Tretinoin (Retin-A) is a retinoic acid analogue used topically to treat acne. Minimal systemic absorption occurs because tretinoin is poorly absorbed from the skin and partly metabolized by the skin. The frequency of congenital anomalies was not increased in two studies in which 212 and 86 infants were exposed to tretinoin during the first trimester.[76,77]

Anticonvulsants

Anticonvulsants long recognized to be associated with teratogenic effects (i.e., phenytoin, carbamazepine, valproic acid, trimethadione) were discussed earlier. The benefits of anticonvulsant therapy during pregnancy often outweigh the risks, such as birth defects and other adverse effects. A major confounder is that seizure activity in the pregnant patient with untreated epilepsy may itself be teratogenic (e.g., from hypoxia). Therefore, continuation of anticonvulsant therapy is usually recommended, as necessary, to control seizures in pregnant patients with epilepsy.

Some anticonvulsant agents (i.e., hydantoins and barbiturates) may cause hemorrhage as a result of drug-induced vitamin K deficiency. The need for vitamin K supplementation is controversial in pregnant women who take these medications and possibly in their newborns. Phenobarbital and ethosuximide are two anticonvulsants that were not discussed previously.

Phenobarbital

Scientific data are not clear on the potential teratogenicity of phenobarbital. In more than 1000 mother–infant pairs in which phenobarbital was used during the first trimester, there was no increased frequency of malformations detected at birth compared with control subjects.[69] However, a recent review of clinical teratology indicated that facial clefts, congenital heart disease, and nail hypoplasia were more common in infants of women who took phenobarbital in pregnancy.[75,78,79] Phenobarbital was not associated with an increased frequency of congenital anomalies when taken for nonseizure indications during pregnancy.

Ethosuximide

Ethosuximide (Zarontin) is a succinimide anticonvulsant used primarily to treat petit mal seizures. Ethosuximide was studied in 57 pregnancies exposed in the first trimester, and the frequency (2, or 3.5%) of congenital anomalies was not increased over the background risk.[80] However, a recent review classified ethosuximide as a teratogen.[75]

Antimicrobials

Health-threatening infections are common during pregnancy, and antimicrobial agents often must be prescribed. These include antibacterials, antifungals, antivirals, and antiparasitics.

Antibacterials

The third most frequently prescribed medication during pregnancy is antimicrobials, and the most frequently prescribed antimicrobials are antibacterial agents. Most antimicrobials are safe for use during pregnancy.

Antibiotics associated with adverse fetal effects are summarized in Table 35–8. Except for patients who are allergic to penicillin-based antibiotics, all penicillins are safe for use during pregnancy. The use of amoxicillin, penicillin, and ampicillin was studied. Congenital anomalies and other adverse effects were not increased in frequency with exposure during pregnancy. More recently developed broad-spectrum penicillins (e.g., piperacillin, mezlocillin) and those combined with the β-lactamase inhibitors, such as clavulanic acid (Timentin, Augmentin) and sulbactam (Unasyn), are not adequately studied during pregnancy, although a significant risk for adverse effects seems unlikely. Maternal serum levels of all penicillins are significantly lower in pregnant women compared with nonpregnant patients because the volume of distribution is increased during pregnancy (i.e., blood volume is increased approximately 40% during pregnancy).[79] In addition, renal clearance is increased during pregnancy, which contributes to lower serum drug levels.[81] All penicillins cross the placenta and result in fetal levels near adult therapeutic levels, as summarized in Table 35–9.[82,83] Therefore, the penicillin family of drugs is the first-line maternal therapy for syphilis during pregnancy and for prevention of congenital syphilis. In contrast, erythromycin does not cross the placenta in sufficient quantity to treat or protect the fetus in cases of maternal syphilis.

The three major classes of cephalosporins are first-, second-, and third-generation derivatives. Cephalosporins cross the placenta to achieve fetal levels similar to those in the mother.[81–83] No controlled scientific studies of cephalosporin use during pregnancy and congenital anomalies are published, but many pregnant women were prescribed these drugs to treat serious conditions. A theoretical risk of second- and third-generation cephalosporins is testicular hypoplasia in experimental animals exposed to the drugs during gestation.[84] Second- and third-generation cephalosporins contain the *N*-methylthiotetrazole side chain, which is putatively the cause of testicular hypoplasia in newborn animals,[84] but this finding has not been reported in humans. Cefoxitin, a second-generation cephalosporin that does not contain this side chain, appears to be the rational choice when broad-spectrum cephalosporin therapy is indicated during pregnancy.

TABLE 35–8

Antibiotics with Potentially Adverse Fetal Effects

ANTIBIOTIC	ADVERSE EFFECT
Tetracyclines	Yellow-brown discoloration of the deciduous teeth
Aminoglycosides	Ototoxicity (VIIIth cranial nerve damage)
Sulfonamides	Hyperbilirubinemia, transient
Nitrofurantoin	Hemolytic anemia, transient
Fluoroquinolones	Irreversible arthropathy
N-methyl thiotetrazole-containing cephalosporins	Testicular hypoplasia*

*Theoretical risk; adverse effect described only in animals.
(Adapted from Gilstrap LC, Little BB, Cunningham FG: Medication use during pregnancy: Part 2. Special considerations. In Cunningham G, Mac Donald P, Grant N (eds.). Williams Obstetrics, 18th ed, Appleton and Lange; Norwalk, CT. Supplement 11, 1991.)

TABLE 35–9

Ratio of Cord Blood to Maternal Blood for Some Penicillins and Cephalosporins

DRUG	RATIO
Ampicillin	0.7
Mezlocillin	0.4
Ticarcillin plus clavulanic acid	0.8
Ampicillin plus sulbactam	1.0

(Adapted in part from Gilstrap LC, Little BB, Cunningham FG: Medication use during pregnancy: Part 2. Special considerations. In Cunning G, Mac Donald P, Grant N (eds.). Williams Obstetrics, 18th ed, Appleton and Lange; Norwalk, CT. Supplement 11, 1991.)

Erythromycin is a macrolide antibiotic. It does not cross the placenta in quantities great enough to reach therapeutic levels in the fetal compartment. Erythromycin is not associated with adverse fetal effects or congenital anomalies, except when the drug is used to treat the fetus. For example, congenital syphilis was reported among the offspring of penicillin-allergic mothers who received erythromycin for syphilis during pregnancy.[85] An efficacious strategy for the treatment of penicillin-allergic pregnant women is to desensitize those who are infected with syphilis and treat the mother and fetus with penicillin. A less desirable approach is to treat pregnant women with syphilis with tetracycline, but many clinicians may not choose this strategy because of the risk of discoloration of the deciduous teeth.[86,87]

Azithromycin is used to treat bacterial and chlamydial infections. No information was published on its use during pregnancy, but it is closely related to erythromycin (discussed earlier). Clarithromycin is used to treat respiratory tract and other infections. More than 100 infants were born after first-trimester exposure to clarithromycin, and the frequency of congenital anomalies was not increased. Azithromycin and clarithromycin are probably safe for use during pregnancy because of their well-studied "cousin," erythromycin.

Aminoglycosides cross the placenta[82,88,89] and reach nearly therapeutic levels in the fetal compartment. Streptomycin, an aminoglycoside, was associated with eighth cranial nerve damage (sensorineural deafness) in fetuses whose mothers were exposed to multiple, high doses during pregnancy.[90,91] The risk of fetal ototoxicity from aminoglycosides is not known but appears to be 1% to 2%, a frequency approximately 20-fold greater than the background risk for sensorineural hearing loss.

Aztreonam (Azactam) is a monobactam antibiotic with a spectrum of activity similar to that of the aminoglycosides. No well-controlled studies are published on its use during pregnancy, but the U.S. FDA granted it risk category B status. Unlike the aminoglycosides, monobactam antibiotics are not associated with renal toxicity or ototoxicity in adults,[36] but it is important to remember that absence of evidence is not evidence of absence.

Clindamycin is used to treat anaerobic infections. It crosses the placenta sufficiently to reach therapeutic levels in the fetal compartment.[88] There are no scientific studies of its use during the first trimester. Its use in pregnant women is rarely indicated, and the effect of clindamycin on the developing conceptus is virtually unknown.

Chloramphenicol crosses the placenta and reaches higher than therapeutic concentrations in the fetus, causing perinatal complications. Evidence is not sufficient to exclude chloramphenicol as a human teratogen,[36] but its teratogenic potential seems very unlikely. Adverse neonatal effects with high doses administered to the mother near the time of delivery include the risk of maternal aplastic anemia and "gray baby syndrome" in the newborn. Because less potentially harmful medications are available, chloramphenicol is rarely used.

Sulfonamides and trimethoprim are often used in combination, primarily to treat urinary tract infections. Sulfonamides cross the placenta, and in the fetus, they compete with bilirubin for binding in the fetus. If given during late gestation, they may cause neonatal hyperbilirubinemia.[81] Trimethoprim is a weak folate antagonist. Despite reassurances from an early study that included more than 200 infants whose mothers used trimethoprim during the first trimester with no increased frequency of birth defects,[92] three recent studies presented evidence to the contrary. In these studies, the absolute risk of neural tube defects associated with folate deficiency or folate antagonist medications was estimated to be 1%,[93–95] approximately 10-fold greater than the risk for the general population.

Nitrofurantoin is used primarily to treat urinary tract infections, some of which occur during pregnancy. Its use during pregnancy was not associated with an increased risk of congenital anomalies in one small study, and there are no reports of adverse effects after its use in pregnancy.[36,96] The U.S. FDA gave nitrofurantoin a risk category rating of B based on limited information, and it seems unlikely to pose a risk when used as medically indicated during pregnancy.

Fluoroquinolones (ciprofloxacin and norfloxacin) are antibiotics that are frequently used to treat urinary tract infections in women who are not pregnant. In six studies of data from teratogen and manufacturer registries, the overall frequency of congenital anomalies was not increased in more than 300 infants whose mothers took these drugs during pregnancy.[97–102] The manufacturer reported that these agents were associated with irreversible arthropathy in dogs whose mothers were given the drug during pregnancy,[36] but other studies in rats, mice, and rabbits did not replicate these findings.[103] Moreover, the teratogen registry study data did not find a pattern of congenital anomalies or a consistently increased frequency of any class of congenital anomalies.

Antituberculotics (rifampin, isoniazid, ethambutol) were not associated with an increased frequency of congenital anomalies in summarized case reports[104] or among the offspring of 85 women who took isoniazid during pregnancy.[69] In a smaller study of fewer than 50 infants whose mothers used isoniazid during the first trimester, the frequency of congenital anomalies appeared increased, but the birth defects were so heterogeneous that no conclusions can be drawn about causality.[105]

Among 320 infants whose mothers used ethambutol during the first trimester, malformations were not increased in frequency.[104] No controlled epidemiologic studies are published of the use of antituberculotics during pregnancy, and many case series involved polydrug therapy. In life-threatening diseases, therapeutic agents often have benefits that outweigh any theoretical risk, depending on the stage of disease.

Antifungals

Medications prescribed to treat fungal infections during pregnancy include clotrimazole, miconazole, and nystatin. In infants born to women who used these drugs during pregnancy, the frequency of congenital anomalies was not increased above that in the general population in two large studies.[70,106] No epidemiologic studies of congenital anomalies in infants whose mothers took butoconazole during pregnancy were published, but the U.S. FDA assigned this drug a pregnancy risk category rating of C.

Fluconazole is used to treat mycotic infections and is given either parenterally or orally. Fluconazole requires special mention because high-dose parenteral administration during pregnancy was associated with a distinct pattern of birth defects (brachycephaly, abnormal facies and calvarial development, cleft palate, and congenital heart disease).[107–109] In contrast, oral doses do not appear to be associated with an increased frequency of congenital anomalies or with a pattern of birth defects among more than 500 infants exposed during the first trimester.[110–112]

Amphotericin B is used to treat systemic mycotic infections.[36] In one study, it was not associated with an increased frequency of malformations in infants whose mothers used the drug during pregnancy.[113] The little information available on the use of amphotericin B during pregnancy is confounded because this drug is part of a polydrug regimen (e.g., with flucytosine). Flucytosine is an antifungal used to treat severe systemic mycotic infections, and there is no information available on its use during pregnancy. Griseofulvin is also used to treat mycotic infections of the skin and nails. No scientific studies of griseofulvin use during human pregnancy are published. However, there are reports of increased frequency of central nervous system and skeletal anomalies in animal studies.[30,36] One case report implicated griseofulvin use during early pregnancy with conjoined twinning,[114] but a Hungarian case–control study of 86 conjoined twins did not confirm this anecdotal finding.[2]

Antivirals

Frequently prescribed antiviral agents include zidovudine, acyclovir, amantadine, rimantadine, ribavirin, idoxuridine, and vidarabine. Other antiviral agents include citreoviridin, ganciclovir, indinavir, saquinavir, valacyclovir, viridofulvin, lamivudine, nevirapine, and trifluridine.

Zidovudine is the primary agent used to treat HIV infection. In one large epidemiologic study that included more than 1800 infants, the frequency of congenital anomalies after first-trimester exposure was not increased.[115] In more than 470 infants exposed to zidovudine during the first trimester who were examined prospectively, the frequency of congenital anomalies was not increased.[116] In 10 infants whose mothers took zidovudine in the first trimester, there were no birth defects.[117] It is reasonable to conclude that the benefits of its use to treat the fatal disease caused by this virus, AIDS, far outweigh any theoretical risks. Importantly, this drug may prevent congenital HIV infection because it significantly reduces the HIV titer and decreases the risk of vertical infection.[118]

Acyclovir is the drug of choice in the treatment of herpes viruses, such as primary genital herpes and varicella. The registry maintained by the manufacturer of acyclovir indicates no increase in the frequency of congenital anomalies or adverse fetal effects in almost 600 pregnancies with first-trimester exposure.[119] Acyclovir is recommended for routine use in pregnant women with active genital herpes. It is also effective in treating overwhelming varicella infection. Topical acyclovir resulted in negligible systemic concentrations of the drug and poses no known risks of adverse effects in the developing embryo or fetus. Valacyclovir is an acyclovir analogue designed to lengthen the half-life. Although no studies are available on its use during pregnancy, its close relationship to acyclovir may reassure patients. Unpublished drug registry data include 14 normal infants born after first-trimester exposure.

Amantadine was not associated with an increased frequency of congenital anomalies in one anecdotal uncontrolled report of 20 patients who used the drug during early pregnancy.[36] Similarly, in 64 infants born to women who took amantadine during the first trimester, five malformations occurred (7.8%). This rate is slightly higher than expected (5%).[119] There are no reports of amantadine use during pregnancy.

Ribavirin is administered as an aerosol to treat respiratory syncytial viral infections in infants, and systemic regimens are available. No human studies are published on the use of this agent during pregnancy, but it was teratogenic in animals. It seems to be a potent teratogen because a high frequency of a constellation of malformations occurred among the offspring of rodents given the drug at human therapeutic doses and several times the human therapeutic dose during embryogenesis.[120] Therefore, it should not be prescribed for use during pregnancy. Inadvertent occupational exposure is probably not a clinically significant risk factor because the amount absorbed is so small. If the patient requests prenatal diagnosis for the limited reassurance it can provide, routine screening should assess central nervous system, craniofacial, eye, body wall, and skeletal development.

No scientific studies of the use of idoxuridine, vidarabine, citreoviridin, ganciclovir, indinavir, saquinavir, viridofulvin, lamivudine, nevirapine, or trifluridine during human pregnancy have been undertaken.

Antiparasitics

A commonly prescribed antiparasitic agent is metronidazole, a nitroimidazole. Metronidazole is prescribed primarily as an antiparasitic agent to treat vaginal trichomoniasis. This drug was not teratogenic in more than 60 offspring of women who took it during the first trimester.[36,121] Among more than 9000 infants exposed to metronidazole during the first trimester, the frequency of congenital anomalies was not increased.[122] In a case–control study of more than 20,000 infants, the frequency of congenital anomalies was not increased in those exposed to metronidazole.[123] Although the drug is carcinogenic in rats and mutagenic in certain bacteria, it appears safe for use during pregnancy.

Lindane is a topical agent indicated for the treatment of *Pediculosis pubis* and scabies. No epidemiologic studies of its use during human pregnancy were published, but it was not teratogenic in experiments of pregnant animals.[36] Toxicity of the central nervous system may occur if this agent is absorbed systemically. Some clinicians recommend a combination of pyrethrins and piperonyl butoxide as an alternative to lindane for the initial treatment of *P. pubis* during pregnancy. Topical application of lindane over limited skin surface areas apparently results in minimal systemic absorption.

Chloroquine is a first-line antimalarial agent. When used for chemoprophylaxis against malaria in pregnant women who travel to areas where malaria is endemic, the risk of congenital anomalies was not increased.[124] Prophylactic low-dose weekly use of chloroquine for malaria appears to pose no teratogenic risk.[36] Quinine is the prototypical antimalarial agent and is used to treat chloroquine-resistant *Plasmodium falciparum* malaria. No epidemiologic studies of the use of this agent during pregnancy were published. One report suggested an increased risk of congenital anomalies with the use of quinine in large doses as an abortifacient, but there is little information on its use in therapeutic doses.[125] Anecdotal data suggest that large doses may cause otolithic agenesis, eye defects, and vestibular abnormalities in infants born to mothers who took therapeutic, large doses during the first trimester.[2]

Pyrimethamine is an antiparasitic agent that is effective in the treatment of malaria and toxoplasmosis. This drug is a folic acid antagonist, although in one report of 64 offspring of women who took this drug in early pregnancy, the frequency of malformations was not increased.[126] However, special precautions should be taken. Concurrent dietary supplementation with folinic acid (*not* folic acid)[127] should be administered with pyrimethamine. Two other agents, spiramycin and sulfadiazine, are used to treat toxoplasmosis. No studies of the effect of spiramycin on the developing embryo have been published. Sulfadiazine was not associated with an increased frequency of congenital anomalies among more than 90 infants whose mothers took the drug during the first trimester.[128]

Mebendazole is an antiparasitic agent that is used primarily to treat helminthic infections, including enterobiasis (pinworms), trichuriasis (whipworm), ascariasis (roundworm), and necatoriasis (hookworm). Mebendazole is teratogenic in laboratory animals given the drug during gestation at many times the human therapeutic dose.[36] The frequency of congenital anomalies was not increased in more than 400 infants whose mothers took mebendazole during the first trimester.[129] Thiabendazole is another antihelminthic agent, but no human studies of its use during pregnancy have been published. Findings in animal studies were equivocal, with dose-related effects occurring in mice but not in three other experimental animal species. Pyrantel pamoate is another antihelminthic agent that is used to treat ascariasis and enterobiasis. The drug was not teratogenic in animal studies, and no human studies have been published. The relevance, if any, of animal teratology studies to human exposure is unknown.

Cardiovascular Drugs

Approximately 3% to 5% of pregnant women have cardiovascular disease. Many pregnant women require cardiovascular drugs for the treatment of life-threatening disorders. With few exceptions, cardiovascular medications may be given during pregnancy with minimal risk to the fetus. Cardiovascular agents with potentially adverse embryonic or fetal effects are summarized in Table 35–10 and were discussed earlier.[47,130–147]

Anticoagulants

Fetal warfarin syndrome, caused by the use of coumarin anticoagulants during gestation, was discussed previously (see Table 35–6).

High-molecular-weight heparin does not cross the placenta.[36] Heparin use during pregnancy is not associated with an increased frequency of congenital anomalies. Protracted use of this drug is associated with osteoporosis and thrombocytopenia in adults, including pregnant women. Calcium supplements should be given to patients who require long-term heparin therapy. Low-molecular-weight heparin does not cross the placenta but is associated with maternal complications similar to those of high-molecular-weight heparin.

Antihypertensives

Methyldopa (Aldomet) is used to treat chronic hypertension in pregnant women. No studies of congenital anomalies and the use of this agent during early pregnancy were published. Hydralazine (Apresoline) is another antihypertensive agent that is commonly used to treat pregnant women. Most clinical experience with this drug has been with its use during the latter half of pregnancy to treat acute, severe, pregnancy-induced hypertension; it is not usually prescribed for chronic hypertension. First-trimester experience is limited to eight patients.

Many β-adrenergic-blocking agents are commercially available to treat hypertension. β-Blockers commonly prescribed for use during pregnancy include propranolol (Inderal), labetalol (Normodyne, Trandate), metoprolol (Lopressor), nadolol (Corgard), and atenolol (Tenormin). No epidemiologic studies of congenital anomalies in infants whose mothers took any of these agents during pregnancy are published in peer-reviewed journals. However, reports of Franz Rosa's research (see preface, Briggs GG et al. Drugs in Pregnancy and Lactation, Fifth edition) in unreviewed book format suggest that the frequency of congenital anomalies was not increased in infants exposed to β-blockers during early pregnancy. Although some investigators reported an increased frequency of fetal growth retardation among infants born to

TABLE 35–10

Cardiovascular Agents with Possible Adverse Fetal Effects*

AGENT	POTENTIAL ADVERSE EFFECTS
Warfarin (see Table 35–6)	Fetal warfarin syndrome
Verapamil and other calcium channel blockers	Decrease in uterine blood flow, myocardial depression and fetal cardiac arrest
Propranolol and other β-adrenergic blockers	Intrauterine growth retardation, bradycardia, respiratory depression, and hypoglycemia
Diazoxide	Alopecia and abnormalities of body hair, and hyperglycemia
Sodium nitroprusside	Cyanide toxicity in animals
Furosemide	Decrease in uterine blood flow, hyperbilirubinemia
Spironolactone	Feminization of male animal genitalia
Thiazide diuretics	Neonatal thrombocytopenia
Angiotensin-converting enzyme inhibitors	Anuria and renal malformations, hypocalvaria

*Some of these effects have been described only in animals and are theorized to occur in humans.

women who used these agents on a long-term basis during pregnancy,[132,148] others reported no association.[149] However, the effect of the drug is difficult to differentiate from that of the disease state, pregnancy-induced hypertension, which causes fetal growth retardation. Previously observed adverse fetal or neonatal effects include transient bradycardia, respiratory depression, and hypoglycemia.[132–135] Based on available data, the benefits of β-adrenergic blockers appear to outweigh any theoretical risks associated with their use during pregnancy.

Clonidine (Catapres) is an α-adrenergic blocker antihypertensive that has been given to pregnant women without apparent adverse fetal effects.[150,151] However, no epidemiologic studies of the frequency of congenital anomalies in infants whose mothers used the drug during the first trimester were published.

Diazoxide (Hyperstat), a thiazide, is used as both an antihypertensive and a tocolytic agent. No epidemiologic studies of congenital anomalies among infants born to women who took this drug during the first trimester were published. Thiazide use during pregnancy is associated with body hair abnormalities (alopecia) and transient neonatal hypoglycemia.[136,137]

Sodium nitroprusside (Nipride, Nitropress) is a potent antihypertensive that is used to treat serious, life-threatening hypertension. In experimental animals, this agent caused fetal cyanide toxicity.[138] However, the human fetus does not appear to be at risk for this complication when therapeutic doses are used.[152] Nonetheless, it is prudent to avoid this drug during pregnancy unless it is needed to treat a life-threatening condition in which other medications have not proven effective.

Captopril (Capoten) and enalapril (Vasotec) are angiotensin-converting enzyme (ACE) inhibitors. No human studies of the use of these agents during pregnancy were published. However, highly convincing case series and case reports show an association of oligohydramnios, neonatal anuria, congenital hypocalvaria, renal anomalies, and nephrotoxicity with ACE inhibitor use during the second and third trimesters.[143–147] Therefore, ACE inhibitors are contraindicated during pregnancy and are considered human teratogens.

Diuretics

Diuretics are used to treat chronic hypertension and pulmonary edema associated with heart disease in pregnant women. The major classes of diuretics are thiazides, loop diuretics, potassium-sparing diuretics, and carbonic anhydrase inhibitors.

Thiazide diuretics are most commonly prescribed to pregnant women. Chlorothiazide (Diuril) and hydrochlorothiazide (HydroDIURIL, Esidrix, Hydro-Chlor) were not associated with an increased frequency of congenital anomalies among fewer than 70 exposed infants.[69] However, thiazides pose a risk of transient neonatal thrombocytopenia.[142] In the latter half of pregnancy, these drugs may also be associated with reduced maternal blood volume and decreased uteroplacental perfusion.

The use of loop diuretics, such as ethacrynic acid (Edecrin) and furosemide (Lasix, Myrosemide), during pregnancy has not been studied to identify an increased risk of congenital anomalies. Unreviewed data on furosemide from the Franz Rosa database suggested no increased risk of congenital anomalies among 350 infants whose mothers took the drug during the first trimester. Loop diuretics may interfere with the normal pregnancy-associated expansion of blood volume and may decrease placental perfusion. In addition, maternal use of furosemide seems to displace bilirubin from albumin, possibly causing neonatal hyperbilirubinemia.[140]

Spironolactone (Aldactone), a potassium-sparing diuretic, acts as a competitive inhibitor of aldosterone. Its effect on the developing human conceptus has not been studied, but it has mild antiandrogenic effects and was associated with feminization of male rat fetuses born to mothers given large doses of this drug during gestation.[141] For this reason, spironolactone is not recommended for use during pregnancy. However, two case reports suggest normal virilization of male infants whose mothers took the drug throughout pregnancy.

Acetazolamide is a carbonic anhydrase inhibitor diuretic. Inadequate data are published to allow an evaluation of possible human teratogenic effects. However, it is associated with a characteristic and replicable pattern of limb abnormalities in animals born to mothers given the drug during pregnancy.[153] Therefore, this diuretic should be avoided during pregnancy.

Antiarrhythmics

The cardiac glycoside digoxin is used as an antiarrhythmic agent to treat atrial fibrillation and flutter and to treat congestive heart failure. In more than 190 infants, the frequency of congenital anomalies was not increased after first-trimester exposure.[68,69] It has also been successfully used to treat fetal cardiac arrhythmias because it readily crosses the placenta.[154,155]

Quinidine is another agent that is commonly used to treat arrhythmias (supraventricular tachycardia and ventricular arrhythmia). No epidemiologic studies were published on the use of quinidine during pregnancy. Some clinicians believe that it is probably relatively safe for use during pregnancy,[156] but this opinion is not based on evidence.

Many local anesthetics are used as antiarrhythmic agents. The best known are probably lidocaine (Xylocaine), also known as lignocaine in the United Kingdom, and procainamide (Pronestyl, Rhthmin, Promine). Related agents include encainide (Enkaid), flecainide (Tambocor), tocainide (Tonocard), and mexiletine (Mexitil). These agents probably cross the placenta to an appreciable degree, but maternal concentrations from local administration are low. In one study, the frequency of congenital anomalies was not increased in 293 offspring of mothers who were given lidocaine for acute illness in early pregnancy.[6] However, a distinction must be made between short-term use of the drug as a local anesthetic and long-term use to treat cardiac arrhythmias. No studies have reported the possible association of malformations with the use of related agents during pregnancy. However, in most cases, the benefit of their use clearly outweighs any theoretical risk because cardiac arrhythmias may be life-threatening.

Disopyramide (Norpace) is an antiarrhythmic whose action is similar to that of quinidine. It is used to treat supraventricular and ventricular arrhythmias.[157] No studies of its use during human pregnancy and the frequency of congenital anomalies were published. However, the drug caused uterine contractions when administered during the third trimester.[155,156] Therefore, other treatment regimens should be used during gestation.

Bretylium (Bretylol) is used to treat ventricular tachycardia and fibrillation. The risk of congenital anomalies after its use in human pregnancy is unknown because no studies have been published. If this agent is clearly indicated for the treatment of life-threatening arrhythmias when other agents have been ineffective, it should be used, regardless of the stage of pregnancy.

Amiodarone (Cordarone) is another agent used to treat life-threatening arrhythmias, ventricular tachycardia, and fibrillation. Case reports are the only data available on the use of this agent,[158] and no published epidemiologic studies of its use during pregnancy are available. As with bretylium, it seems reasonable to use this agent during pregnancy, if indicated, to treat serious ventricular arrhythmias, when other agents have not been effective. Based on case reports, neonatal thyroid dysfunction or goiter is a risk associated with amiodarone therapy after 10 weeks' gestation because of the iodine content of the drug.[159,160] In addition, learning deficits were associated with its use during pregnancy.[161]

Antianginals

Organic nitrites are the most commonly used antianginal agents and include nitroglycerin, amyl nitrate, erythrityl tetranitrate (Cardilate), isosorbide dinitrate (Isordil, Sorbitrate), and pentaerythritol tetranitrate (Pentritol, Peritrate). Nitroglycerin has also been used to "blunt" the hypertensive effect of intubation during general anesthesia in the pregnant patient with hypertension or cardiac disease. No epidemiologic studies of the use of organic nitrites during human pregnancy have been published, but it is prudent to use these agents in patients with life-threatening conditions.

A variety of calcium-channel-blocking agents have antianginal effects. Some of these agents are also used to treat supraventricular tachycardia and hypertension. Verapamil (Clan, Isoptin) is the best known of this group of drugs. It has been given to many pregnant women without apparent adverse fetal effects, but it was associated with decreased uterine blood flow in experimental animals.[130] In addition, it may cause cardiac depression or even cardiac arrest in neonates whose mothers received it peripartum for supraventricular tachycardia associated with heart failure.[131] Theoretically, other calcium antagonists may be associated with similar adverse effects. As a group, calcium-channel-blocking agents are indicated for use during pregnancy only when life-threatening conditions exist and other therapeutic agents have been ineffective.

Dipyridamole (Persantine) is a selective coronary vasodilator that inhibits platelet aggregation. It is used as an adjunct to prevent thromboembolism, myocardial infarction, and transient ischemic events. The frequency of congenital anomalies was not increased in more than 190 infants whose mothers were treated with dipyridamole during the last two trimesters.[162–164] According to the manufacturer, dipyridamole was not teratogenic in animal studies, but the relevance of this finding to humans is unknown.

Asthma Drugs

Approximately 1% to 4% of pregnant women have clinically diagnosed asthma.[36] The two major classes of medications used to treat asthma, bronchodilators and immunosuppressants, seem to be safe for use during pregnancy.

Bronchodilators

Theophylline salts are the most frequently prescribed bronchodilators for treating both pregnant and nonpregnant patients with asthma. Aminophylline is the parenteral form, and numerous oral forms are available. This agent has been used extensively in pregnant women without apparent adverse effects.

Epinephrine is another bronchodilator that is reserved for the treatment of acute asthmatic attacks and is usually given at a dose of 0.3 to 0.5 mL subcutaneously in a 1:1000 dilution.[36] An increased frequency of heterogeneous, nonmajor malformations was reported in the Collaborative Perinatal Project.[69] However, it is unclear whether the effects were related to the maternal illness or to the drug itself. It seems very unlikely that epinephrine is a human teratogen. However, its use should be reserved for treatment of acute asthma attacks, and it should not be given on a long-term basis. Another agent, terbutaline (Brethaire, Brethine, Bricanyl) has significant activity as a bronchodilator. No reports have been published on congenital anomalies in infants whose mothers used this agent during early pregnancy. In one study of protracted maternal use of terbutaline during the second and third trimesters, no adverse effects were noted among offspring.[165] In 149 women, terbutaline use was reported during the first trimester, and the frequency of congenital anomalies was not increased.[166] However, these data were not reported in a peer-reviewed journal.

Albuterol (Proventil, Ventolin) and metaproterenol (Alupent, Metaprel) are β-adrenergic-blocking bronchodilators that are self-administered inhalation aerosols. Systemic concentrations resulting from inhalation are small. In a non-peer-reviewed publication, the frequency of congenital anomalies was not increased in more than 1000 infants who were exposed to albuterol during the first trimester.[166] These agents are commonly used to treat asthma in pregnant patients.

Immunosuppressants

Cromolyn sodium (Nasalcrom, Rynacrom) is an agent that inhibits mast cell histamine release and is given through nasal insufflation. It has little benefit during an acute asthmatic attack and is used primarily for prophylaxis in chronic asthma.[36] Among more than 350 infants born to women who used cromolyn during pregnancy, the frequency of congenital anomalies was not increased.[167,168] According to the manufacturer, this drug was not teratogenic in several animal species given several times the usual human dose during gestation.

Several glucocorticoids are used to treat pregnant women with asthma. The most commonly used agents are beclomethasone, betamethasone, cortisone, and prednisone. Therapeutic doses of these glucocorticoids for the treatment of asthma are unlikely to be associated with an increased frequency of congenital anomalies. Beclomethasone (Vanceril, Beclovent) is used primarily as an inhalational aerosol or nasally. Dexamethasone (Decadron, Respihaler, Turbinaire) is also used in this fashion. In some pregnant women, it is occasionally necessary to use large doses of parenterally administered corticosteroids to treat a life-threatening acute asthmatic attack. Some women may also need long-term steroid maintenance therapy to prevent exacerbation of respiratory symptoms.

An acute asthmatic attack may be life-threatening. These agents should be used because the potential risks are clearly outweighed by the potential benefit of saving the mother's life.

The American College of Obstetrics and Gynecology recommendations[169] for the treatment of asthma are outlined in Table 35–11.

Psychotropics

Psychiatric illnesses occur in approximately 1% to 2% of pregnant women, but some studies estimate much higher prevalences.[170] Treatment of most psychiatric disorders should continue during pregnancy for the benefit of the patient. Abrupt discontinuation of psychotropic therapy may have adverse effects, including suicide attempts.

Sedatives, Hypnotics, and Tranquilizers

A variety of sedatives, hypnotics, and tranquilizers are available and belong to several pharmacologic categories. Common agents include phenobarbital, secobarbital, butalbital, diazepam, chlordiazepoxide, chloral hydrate, and meprobamate.

Phenobarbital was implicated when used with other anticonvulsant agents in causing congenital anomalies.[36] It is unclear whether the anticonvulsant medication, the seizure disorder, or a combination of both was associated with an increased risk of congenital anomalies, as previously discussed. Phenobarbital has been prescribed to pregnant women as a sedative, and recent evidence suggests that it is teratogenic when used for this indication.[75] Among more than 1000 offspring exposed to this agent during the first trimester, the frequency of malformations

TABLE 35–11

ACAAI-ACOG Recommendations for the Pharmacologic Step Therapy of Chronic Asthma During Pregnancy

CATEGORY	STEP THERAPY
Mild intermittent	Inhaled beta-2 agonists as needed. (For all categories, most published human data obtained with albuterol, metaproterenol, or terbutaline)
Mild persistent	Inhaled cromolyn; continue inhaled nedocromil in patients showed a response before pregnancy; substitute inhaled corticosteroids if above treatment is not adequate.
Moderate persistent	Inhaled corticosteroids; beclomethasone or budesonide if treatment is initiated during pregnancy; continue the original inhaled corticosteroid if the patient was well controlled before pregnancy; consider budesonide if the patient requires high-dose inhaled corticosteroids for adequate control. Continue inhaled salmeterol in patients who showed a very good response before pregnancy. Add oral theophylline or inhaled salmeterol for patients who do not achieve adequate control with medium-dose inhaled corticosteroids.
Severe persistent	Above, plus oral corticosteroids (burst for active symptoms, alternate-day or daily therapy if necessary) [Anon, 2000].

From American College of Obstetrics and Gynecology, 2000; American College of Allergy, Asthma, and Immunology, 2000. (Adapted from ACAAI-ACOG Recommendations for the Pharmacologic Step Therapy of Chronic Asthma During Pregnancy. American College of Obstetrics and Gynecology, 2000.)

was not increased.[69] However, recent information suggests that phenobarbital use during organogenesis was associated with facial clefting, congenital heart defects, facial dysmorphism, nail hypoplasia, learning deficits, and mental retardation.[78,79] Another risk associated with barbiturates is maternal drug dependence and possible transient neonatal withdrawal.

Secobarbital (Seconal) is a short-acting barbiturate given primarily as a sleep medication. There is no scientific evidence that this agent is teratogenic in humans. It seems to be relatively safe for use during pregnancy, based on the findings in more than 370 infants whose mothers used it during the first trimester and 4200 whose mothers used it throughout pregnancy.

Butalbital is a short-acting barbiturate that is found in combination with a variety of other medications, such as aspirin (e.g., Fiorinal), acetaminophen (e.g., Fioricet, Rogesic), and codeine. Among more than 100 pregnant women exposed to this agent during the first trimester, the frequency of malformations among exposed offspring was not statistically increased compared with control subjects.[69]

Diazepam (Valium, Vazepam, Meval) and chlordiazepoxide (Librium, Librax, Lipoxide, Medilium, Novopoxide) are benzodiazepines commonly used as minor tranquilizers and sedatives. Diazepam is also used as an amnesic and anticonvulsant. In the 1970s, diazepam was believed to be associated with an increased risk of facial clefts.[171–173] However, this finding was not confirmed in several other large studies,[174–176] some of which were a reanalysis of previously reported data. In addition, there are reports of an association of maternal diazepam and cardiovascular anomalies in offspring exposed in utero,[177,178] but these findings were not confirmed in subsequent studies.[179,180] Available information does not support the idea that diazepam is a human teratogen. However, it may cause transient hypotonia, hypothermia, and respiratory depression ("floppy infant syndrome") in neonates chronically exposed to diazepam near delivery. These symptoms are not life-threatening when managed medically.

Chlordiazepoxide was associated with an increase in congenital anomalies in one study,[181] although this association was not confirmed in a much larger study of more than 250 offspring whose mothers used the drug during early pregnancy.[69] Similarly, the frequency of malformations was not increased in several other studies of infants whose mothers used the drug in the first trimester.[182–184]

Meprobamate (e.g., Equanil, Miltown) is a minor tranquilizer and muscle relaxant. Whether it is causally associated with congenital anomalies is controversial. Two groups of investigators reported an association of congenital anomalies with the use of this drug during gestation,[70,181] but a third group did not show this effect.[69] In one study of more than 350 offspring, meprobamate exposure during pregnancy was not associated with an increased frequency of malformations.[69] It is prudent to avoid prescribing this agent during all stages of pregnancy because of inconsistencies in the available data. However, if a patient has inadvertent exposure, the reassurance provided by an ultrasound study targeting the lip and palate is appropriate.

Chloral hydrate is a minor sedative that is sometimes prescribed as a sleep medication. The frequency of congenital anomalies in the offspring of 71 pregnant women who took chloral hydrate in early pregnancy was not increased compared with control subjects.[69] The chance of this agent being causally associated with congenital anomalies is remote.

Antidepressants

Antidepressants are generally divided into tricyclic and nontricyclic agents. Tricyclic antidepressants were the most commonly used agents until fluoxetine (Prozac) was introduced. These agents are summarized in Table 35–12.

Although limb-reduction defects have been reported with one of the tricyclic agents, amitriptyline,[185,186] during early pregnancy, this association was not confirmed by other studies.[69,187,188] This risk seems very unlikely. No information on the safety of other tricyclic antidepressants during pregnancy was published, but several are metabolites of amitriptyline. Therefore, their risks may be assumed to be similar to those of amitriptyline (i.e., negligible).

Tranylcypromine (Parnate), isocarboxazid (Marplan), and phenelzine (Nardil) are monoamine oxidase inhibitors that are used as antidepressants. No information was published on the safety of these agents for use during pregnancy.

Fluoxetine is one of the most frequently prescribed antidepressants. In one report by the manufacturer that included 485 offspring born to mothers who took this drug during pregnancy,[189] the frequency of congenital anomalies was not increased above the expected or background risk of congenital anomalies in humans (28 of 483, or 5.8%). In another study, the frequency of congenital anomalies was not increased among 98 infants whose mothers took the drug throughout pregnancy.[190] In a third study, the frequency of congenital anomalies

TABLE 35–12

Commonly Used Tricyclic Antidepressants

Imipramine (Tofranil, Janimine, Tipramine)
Amitriptyline (Amitril, Elavil, Endep, Emitrip, Enovil)
Desipramine (Norpramin, Pertofrane)
Doxepin (Adapin, Sinequan)
Nortriptyline (Aventyl, Pamelor)
Protriptyline (Vivactil)
Amoxapine (Asendin)
Clomipramine (Anafranil)

was not increased among 101 infants whose mothers took fluoxetine during the first trimester.[191]

Sertraline (Zoloft) is a popular antidepressant. Among 150, 112, and 28 infants born to women whose mothers took sertraline during pregnancy, the frequency of congenital anomalies was not increased.[192–194]

Antipsychotics

Phenothiazines are the largest pharmacologic class of antipsychotics. Several phenothiazines are also prescribed as antiemetics during pregnancy (chlorpromazine, perphenazine, prochlorperazine, and triflupromazine).

For several decades, chlorpromazine (Thorazine) has been prescribed to pregnant women as an antipsychotic. This agent was not associated with an increased risk of congenital anomalies in two studies of more than 4000 patients who took the drug during the first trimester for various indications.[69,195] Two of the most common side effects in adults are hypotension and extrapyramidal tract symptoms. Similar transient effects were seen in neonates exposed to the drug during late gestation.

Among more than 800 infants born to women who took prochlorperazine (Compazine) during early pregnancy, as reported in the Collaborative Perinatal Project,[69] the frequency of congenital anomalies was not increased above the background risk. Likewise, no increase in the frequency of malformations was found in the offspring of 63 pregnant women who took perphenazine (Trilafon) during the first trimester compared with control subjects.[69]

There are no epidemiologic studies of the safety of the use of thioridazine (Mellaril) or trifluoperazine (Stelazine) during pregnancy. Maternal use of thioridazine during the first trimester was reported in 23 infants who had no congenital anomalies, but there was no control group.[196] The frequency of congenital anomalies was not increased in 42 infants born to women who used trifluoperazine during the first trimester.[69]

Other antipsychotic drugs include haloperidol (Haldol, Decanoate), thiothixene (Navane), loxapine (Loxitane, Daxolin), clozapine (Clozaril), molindone (Moban, Lidone), and chlorprothixene (Taractan). The frequency of congenital anomalies was not increased in 90 infants whose mothers took haloperidol during the first trimester.[197] First-trimester exposure to thiothixene was not associated with an increased risk of congenital anomalies in 38 infants, but this was not a peer-reviewed study.[117] There is no relevant scientific information on the safety of the other agents during pregnancy.

Analgesics

Analgesics are the medications that are most commonly prescribed to pregnant women. Most analgesics can be administered to pregnant women with relative safety.

Nonsteroidal Anti-inflammatory Drugs

A variety of nonsteroidal anti-inflammatory drugs (NSAIDs) are commercially available for use as analgesics. Frequently prescribed NSAIDs are summarized in Table 35–13. Indomethacin is a commonly used NSAID that also acts as a tocolytic in perceived premature labor.[198] The frequency of congenital anomalies was not increased in one study of 50 patients who received this agent during the first trimester.[68] The major concern with NSAIDs is the possible association with premature closure of the ductus arteriosus when given during the latter half of pregnancy. There have been reports of fetal and newborn premature ductal arteriosus closure and subsequent pulmonary hypertension as a result of maternal use of these agents,[199–201] although other studies did not confirm this association.[198,202] These agents are also associated with decreased amniotic fluid volume.[203] NSAIDs usually are not recommended for use in pregnant women after 34 weeks' gestation because of the theoretical risk of these adverse effects. These agents are probably safe if used before this gestational age, especially for short-term use.

Salicylates and Acetaminophen

Salicylates and acetaminophen are non-narcotic analgesics that are commonly used by pregnant women. In one report of more than 1500 pregnant women, approximately half used aspirin and 41% used acetaminophen.[204]

Aspirin is also an NSAID and has been available for more than a century. Although there are reports of an association with malformations in humans,[205] this association was not confirmed in other studies.[206,207] Like other NSAIDs, aspirin is a prostaglandin synthetase inhibitor and is associated with premature closure of the ductus arteriosus and pulmonary hypertension in the newborn[201,208] as well as with oligohydramnios.[208] Large doses of aspirin may also be associated with hemorrhagic disorders in both mother and fetus as a result of reduced platelet activity. Low-dose adult aspirin probably poses little risk to the fetus. However, this drug should be avoided in late pregnancy because safer medications are available (i.e., acetaminophen).

TABLE 35–13

Commonly Used Nonsteroidal Anti-inflammatory Drugs

Indomethacin (Indocin)
Ibuprofen (Advil, Motrin)
Fenoprofen (Fenoproten, Nalfon)
Meclofenamate (Meclamen)
Naproxen (Naprosyn, Anaprox)
Tolmentin (Tolectin)
Diflunisal (Dolobid)
COX-2 inhibitors

Acetaminophen is the preferred analgesic for use in pregnancy. In one report of more than 300 offspring born to mothers who took this agent during pregnancy, the frequency of malformations was not increased.[68] Findings were similar in more than 200 offspring included in the Collaborative Perinatal Project database.[69] However, this analgesic may result in fetal liver toxicity when used in excessive amounts (e.g., attempted suicide late in pregnancy).[209] Acetaminophen apparently is not associated with premature ductal closure or oligohydramnios.

None of the selective COX-2 inhibitors have been studied for possible adverse effects in pregnancy. Hence, the risks associated with them are unknown, despite their widespread use.

Narcotic Analgesics

Many narcotic analgesic agents are available. Narcotic analgesics may be abused, and this section discusses only use according to therapeutic guidelines. Frequently prescribed drugs in this class include codeine, meperidine (Demerol), morphine, pentazocine (Talwin), butorphanol (Stadol), hydrocodone (Vicodin), nalbuphine (Nubain), hydromorphone (Dilaudid), and propoxyphene (Darvon).

Meperidine and morphine, as with all opioid narcotic agents, may cause a transient withdrawal syndrome in the newborn when used on a long-term basis during pregnancy. However, none of these analgesics was associated with an increased frequency of malformations in offspring after maternal use in early pregnancy.[69] Morphine in particular may be associated with newborn respiratory depression when given in large doses near the time of delivery. Codeine was not teratogenic in one study of more than 500 patients with first-trimester exposure.[69] Similarly, the frequency of malformations was not increased compared with unexposed control subjects in more than 700 newborns whose mothers used propoxyphene during early pregnancy.[69,70] There have been isolated case reports of malformations associated with propoxyphene use. The association was probably serendipitous and not causal.[36] Similarly, pentazocine use in early pregnancy was not associated with an increased frequency of congenital anomalies.[36]

Forty infants born to women who used hydrocodone during the first trimester had no increased frequency of congenital anomalies.[210] No epidemiologic studies of congenital anomalies in infants whose mothers used butorphanol or hydromorphone during the first trimester were published, although these drugs are potentially associated with neonatal withdrawal if abused or used for a protracted period during late pregnancy.

Thyroid Drugs

Hypothyroidism rarely occurs during pregnancy, but it is common to encounter pregnant women who received thyroid replacement therapy before pregnancy was recognized. Hyperthyroidism is infrequent during pregnancy.[36]

Thyroid Deplacement Drugs

Thyroxine does not cross the placenta measurably[36] and is not associated with congenital anomalies.[62]

Antithyroid Drugs

Agents used to treat hyperthyroidism include propylthiouracil (Propyl-Thyracil), methimazole (Tapazole), potassium iodide, and propranolol. Propranolol use during pregnancy was discussed previously.

The other three antithyroid agents readily cross the placenta. Propylthiouracil may result in fetal hypothyroidism and goiter formation, although clinically significant effects are uncommon with the usual therapeutic regimens. There is no firm scientific evidence that propylthiouracil is related to an increased risk of malformations, although the data are largely inconclusive. Methimazole was associated with scalp defects in the offspring of mothers who used this agent,[211,212] but other studies during pregnancy have not confirmed this association.[213,214]

Potassium iodide and sodium iodide block the release of thyroid hormone. Long-term use may result in fetal hypothyroidism and goiter formation. It is highly unlikely that short-term use of iodide medication results in such adverse effects when given to treat thyroid crisis ("thyroid storm") with intravenous sodium iodide or when used for prophylaxis before thyroid surgery (oral potassium iodide). Most adverse effects result from long-term iodine therapy.

Antineoplastics

Malignancy occurs in approximately 0.1% of pregnant women.[215] Breast carcinoma, melanoma, and Hodgkin's lymphoma are the most common malignancies in pregnant women.[215–218]

Chemotherapeutic agents can be grouped into alkylating, antimetabolite, plant alkaloid, antibiotic, and miscellaneous types. Antineoplastics are often associated with fetal growth retardation and congenital anomalies, and causality seems plausible because most chemotherapeutic agents are designed to impede cell division and growth.

When used after the first trimester, most chemotherapeutic agents are not associated with significant fetal risk, except for growth retardation. The potential life-saving benefits of these therapies always outweigh the fetal risk. Some conditions, such as acute leukemia, mandate chemotherapy immediately on confirmation of the diagnosis, even during the first trimester.

Alkylating Agents

Common alkylating agents include busulfan (Myleran), cyclophosphamide (Cytoxan), chlorambucil (Leukeran), melphalan (Alkeran), trimethylene thiophosphoramide (Thiotepa), and carmustine (BCNU).

There are no epidemiologic studies of congenital anomalies or fetal effects in infants whose mothers used melphalan, trimethylene thiophosphoramide, or carmustine during pregnancy. Based on the mode of pharmacologic action, these agents should be considered teratogenic.

Busulfan and cyclophosphamide were discussed earlier and are associated with an increased risk of congenital anomalies. In a report of 44 infants whose mothers received one of several alkylating agents during pregnancy, 6 (14%) had a major congenital anomaly, indicating an apparently increased risk of malformation.[219]

Antimetabolites

Antimetabolites used to treat neoplasia include methotrexate (Folex, Mexate), mercaptopurine (Purinethol), thioguanine, cytarabine (Cytosan), and fluorouracil (Efudex, Fluoroplex). Methotrexate was discussed earlier and is associated with an increased risk of congenital anomalies, similar to those associated with another folate antagonist, aminopterin.[23–27] Although there are only case reports of the possible association of congenital anomalies with the use of other antimetabolites during early pregnancy, common mechanisms of action suggest that the case reports represent a causal relationship. In a review by Doll and associates,[219] 15 of 77 offspring (19%) exposed to antimetabolites in utero had major congenital anomalies. Of these 15 infants, 13 were exposed to folate antagonists. Obviously, these agents should be avoided during pregnancy if possible, especially in the first trimester.

Plant Alkaloids

The two major plant alkaloids are vinblastine (Velban, Velsan) and vincristine (Oncovin, Vincasar, Vincrex). Although there are reports of a possible association of malformations with first-trimester exposure,[220] there are also reports of normal infants born to women who used this class of drugs during pregnancy.[221,222] In a review by Doll and associates,[223] 1 of 14 infants (7%) exposed to this group of agents had a major congenital anomaly. These agents are used to treat life-threatening malignancies (i.e., acute leukemia), and should be given when indicated, even during the first trimester.

Antibiotics

Antineoplastic antibiotics include daunorubicin (Cerubidine), doxorubicin (Adriamycin), bleomycin (Blenoxane), and dactinomycin (Cosmegen). No epidemiologic studies of the use of any of these agents during pregnancy have been published. However, anthracycline antibiotics (daunorubicin and doxorubicin) may be needed during the first trimester to treat acute leukemia because potentially life-saving therapy should not be withheld.

Miscellaneous Antineoplastics

Agents in this category include cisplatin (Platinol), procarbazine, and hydroxyurea (Hydrea). No controlled studies in human pregnancies involving any of these agents have been published. Treatment with these agents should ideally be avoided during the first trimester, but should not be withheld when clearly needed to treat life-threatening conditions.

Immunosuppressants

Immunosuppressants are used to treat autoimmune diseases (rheumatoid arthritis, systemic lupus) and for maintenance therapy in organ transplant recipients. The most frequently prescribed agents include glucocorticoids, azathioprine (Imuran), and cyclosporine (Sandimmune). Glucocorticoids were discussed earlier.

Azathioprine

A derivative of 6-mercaptopurine, azathioprine is given as an adjunct in the suppression of cell-mediated immunity. There are no controlled studies of the use of this agent in pregnant women. However, in two case series involving a total of 154 pregnant women who took azathioprine and prednisone throughout pregnancy,[221,224,225] malformations were reported in 11 infants (7.1%). It is impossible to differentiate the effects of monotherapy with this agent from the effects of multiple immunosuppressant medications and from the disease process itself. In one case series of 33 infants born to women who received azathioprine during the first trimester, the frequency of congenital anomalies was not increased.[226] Azathioprine is usually given to prevent organ rejection (a life-threatening condition) in renal transplant recipients. It should not be withheld from the pregnant patient.

Cyclosporine

Cyclosporine is used primarily to treat and prevent allograft rejection. Six hundred infants have been born after exposure to cyclosporine during gestation; however, it is unknown how many were exposed during organogenesis.[227] It should be used when indicated, even in pregnant women, because it is usually prescribed for potentially life-threatening conditions.

Antihistamines and Decongestants

Allergic disorders (rhinitis, hay fever, nasal congestion), upper respiratory infections, and sinusitis occur frequently during pregnancy. The "common cold" is the most common respiratory disorder in pregnant women and the most frequent reason for antihistamine, decongestant, or expectorant use.[228] No effective therapy against rhinoviruses exists, but the symptoms can be treated while the illness runs its course.

A wide selection of antihistamines is available, and many are used in combination with a sympathomimetic amine (e.g., pseudoephedrine) that is a decongestant. These drugs are used for symptomatic relief in pregnant women. Some commonly prescribed agents are discussed later. An important aspect of prescribing these medications is dose and systemic effects. Intranasal administration is as effective as oral administration and more effective in some instances. Intranasal administration dramatically reduces the dose delivered to the fetus and treats the symptoms effectively.[228]

Decongestants

PSEUDOEPHEDRINE

Pseudoephedrine hydrochloride is the preferred decongestant for pregnant women.[228] It is one of the most frequently used sympathomimetic decongestants used to treat "common cold" or "sinus" symptoms. In more than 1000 women who used this drug in the first trimester, the risk of congenital anomalies among offspring was not increased.[68–70]

PHENYLEPHRINE AND PHENYLPROPANOLAMINE

Phenylephrine and phenylpropanolamine are decongestants that are used in combination with antihistamines. The manufacturer cautions that these agents may interfere with uterine blood flow and should be avoided in pregnant women with conditions associated with decreased uterine blood flow (e.g., hypertension), but no reports in the peer-reviewed literature substantiate this claim. A weak association of phenylephrine and phenylpropanolamine with congenital anomalies was found in 1249 and 726 pregnancies, respectively,[69] but it was likely not causal. In more than 225 infants exposed to phenylephrine during the first trimester, the risk of congenital anomalies was not increased.[68,70] Phenylephrine (Neo-Synephrine, 4-Way) is also used in popular nasal sprays.

OXYMETAZOLINE, XYLOMETAZOLINE, AND NAPHAZOLINE

Oxymetazoline, xylometazoline, and naphazoline are sympathomimetic decongestants found in long-acting nasal sprays (Afrin, Allerest, Dristan, 4-Way). The frequency of congenital anomalies was not increased in more than 250 infants whose mothers used oxymetazoline during the first trimester[68,70] or in 432 infants whose mothers used xylometazoline in the first trimester.[68,70] No published studies were available on the use of naphazoline during pregnancy.

Antihistamines

Antihistamines act primarily by competing with histamine for H_1 receptors and are chemically related to local anesthetics. Effects of some older antihistamines include sedation, antiemesis, anti-motion sickness, and antidyskinesia. For convenience of discussion, antihistamines are best grouped according to their chemical derivation.

One report suggested that antihistamines may be associated with increased frequency of retrolental fibroplasia in premature infants.[229] This effect was substantiated in 2004.

PROPYLAMINE DERIVATIVES

Propylamine derivatives include brompheniramine, chlorpheniramine, dexchlorpheniramine, and triprolidine. Brompheniramine was weakly, and likely not causatively, associated with birth defects in a small sample of 65 offspring with first-trimester exposure.[69] The risk of congenital anomalies was not increased in 270 infants born after first-trimester exposure.[68,70] A summary meta-analysis of all data on brompheniramine strongly suggests that it is not a human teratogen.[233]

Chlorpheniramine and dexchlorpheniramine were not associated with an increased frequency of congenital anomalies after first-trimester exposure in two large epidemiologic studies.[69,70]

Similarly, triprolidine was not associated with an increased frequency of birth defects in offspring of 628 women who took this drug in the first trimester.[68,70]

ETHANOLAMINE AND ETHYLAMINE DERIVATIVES

No human epidemiologic studies of first-trimester use of bromodiphenhydramine, carbinoxamine, and clemastine were published. First-trimester diphenhydramine use was not associated with an increased frequency of congenital anomalies in 865 pregnancies.[69,70] No large epidemiologic studies of bromodiphenhydramine use during pregnancy were published, but no malformations occurred in 10 children whose mothers were exposed to bromodiphenhydramine during the first trimester.[69] Caution should be exercised with parenteral use of ethylamine derivatives because these drugs are reported to have oxytocic effects.[230–232]

Doxylamine has received considerable attention because it was one of the main components of the popular antinausea drug Bendectin (along with pyridoxine and dicyclomine). Reports of an association of Bendectin use and diaphragmatic hernias,[234] congenital heart disease, and pyloric stenosis[68,235] were published. Other studies of thousands of infants found no such association. Millions of women used Bendectin during the first trimester without scientific evidence of adverse fetal effects. The U.S. FDA concluded that either doxylamine or another component of this medication was a human teratogen. Unfortunately, it appears that the Bendectin component was a significant "litogen" (i.e., lawsuit-inducing agent).[236] It is well established that doxylamine is a safe drug for use during pregnancy. Bendectin will be reintroduced for the treatment of nausea after the U.S. FDA republishes its findings that the drug was not a teratogen.[237]

PIPERIDINE DERIVATIVES

No studies of the risk of congenital anomalies in the offspring of mothers who took azatadine, cyproheptadine, or diphenylpyraline during pregnancy were published.

ETHYLENEDIAMINE DERIVATIVES

Tripelennamine exposure during the first trimester was not associated with an increased frequency of congenital anomalies in 100 infants. Similarly, the risk of birth defects was not increased in 112 infants born to mothers who used pyrilamine during the first trimester.[69]

BUTYROPHENONE DERIVATIVES

First-trimester terfenadine (Seldane) exposure was not associated with an increased risk of birth defects in 134 infants.[238] According to the manufacturer, terfenadine is not recommended for use by nursing mothers because it was associated with decreased pup weight in rats.

PIPERAZINE DERIVATIVES

Cyclizine, buclizine, and meclizine have antihistamine actions, but are used primarily as antiemetics. Meclizine use by mothers during the third trimester was not associated with an increased frequency of fetal effects among exposed infants.[69] In more than 1000 offspring whose mothers used meclizine in the first trimester, the risk of birth defects was not increased. Further information indicating that meclizine is not teratogenic in humans was published in one cohort study and three case–control studies.[239–242] Similarly, in 111 infants with first-trimester exposure to cyclizine, the risk of congenital anomalies was not increased.[241]

PHENINDAMINE

No animal or human studies of the risk of congenital anomalies with phenindamine exposure during pregnancy were published. However, phenindamine is closely related to chlorpheniramine, which was studied during pregnancy and did not increase the risk of birth defects after exposure during organogenesis.

Nonsedating Antihistamines

Recently marketed nonsedating antihistamines include loratadine (Claritin), cetirizine (Zyrtec), Fexofenadine (Allegra), astemizole (Astemizol, which is not available in the United States), cromolyn (Intal), and ebastine (Ebast, Ebastel, Kestine). All but one of these agents, cromolyn, is a H_1 receptor antagonist.

LORATADINE

No studies of loratadine use during pregnancy were published that adequately address its safety. In one small study of fewer than 20 infants born to women who took loratadine during pregnancy, no congenital anomalies were observed.[243] However, the clinical and epidemiologic significance of this case series is questionable.

CETIRIZINE

Cetirizine is an oral H_1 antihistamine that is used to treat allergies. In 49 infants whose mothers took cetirizine during pregnancy, the frequency of congenital anomalies was not increased.[243,244] The data are tenuous, but suggest that the risk of congenital anomalies with this drug is low.

FEXOFENADINE

Fexofenadine is an oral H_1 receptor antagonist that is used to treat seasonal allergies and rhinitis. Although no studies of the risk of congenital anomalies in infants born to women who used fexofenadine during pregnancy were published, terfenadine is metabolized to fexofenadine. Terfenadine is not associated with an increased risk of birth defects after first-trimester exposure.

ASTEMIZOLE

Astemizole, a long-acting H_1 receptor antagonist, is used to treat allergic conditions. It is not available in the United States, but is available in Europe, Canada, and Mexico. It may be obtained by international mail order in the United States. In more than 100 infants exposed to astemizole during the first trimester, the risk of birth defects was not increased above background levels.[245]

CROMOLYN SODIUM

Cromolyn sodium is a mast cell inhibitor that is used prophylactically to treat chronic allergic conditions. In more than 440 infants whose mothers used cromolyn during the first trimester, the risk of congenital anomalies was not increased.[246,247]

IPRATROPIUM BROMIDE

No studies of first-trimester human exposure to ipratropium were published. One animal study found no increased frequency of congenital anomalies after exposure during organogenesis. However, this finding may be irrelevant to the risk of birth defects in humans.

EBASTINE

No studies of ebastine exposure during the first trimester of human pregnancy were published. In one animal study of exposure during organogenesis, the frequency of congenital anomalies was not increased. However, the relevance of these findings to the risk in humans is unknown.

Expectorants and Antitussives

Expectorants

Guaifenesin is the leading expectorant in current use and is a major component of most cough medications, both prescribed and over the counter. The risk of birth defects was not increased in more than 1000 infants born after first-trimester exposure.[68–70] Other mucolytic or expectorant medications contain iodide (potassium iodide, iodinated glycerol), and should not be used after 10 weeks' gestation. Iodide in iodide-containing medications crosses the placenta and may cause fetal goiter. Therefore, iodide-containing agents are contraindicated during pregnancy after formation of the fetal thyroid.

Antitussives

Dextromethorphan is available by prescription and over the counter as an antitussive. Among 300 infants born to women who used dextromethorphan during the first trimester, the frequency of congenital anomalies was not increased.[69] Several narcotics are used in cough preparations, such as codeine, hydrocodone, and hydromorphone. Long-term use, tantamount to abuse, of narcotic-containing antitussives may result in neonatal addiction, withdrawal, and respiratory depression. However, the risk of congenital anomalies is not increased by the narcotics commonly used in these formulations. Opiates were discussed previously.

Benzonatate (Tessalon) is an antitussive that anesthetizes stretch receptors in the respiratory smooth muscle. No human studies were published with which to assess the risk of birth defects or adverse fetal effects after exposure during gestation.

Many cough preparations contain alcohol (ethanol). The alcohol content of typical cough preparations is 15% to 26%. It is unlikely that short-term use is associated with a significant risk. However, according to case reports, long-term abuse of alcohol-containing cough medicines is associated with fetal alcohol syndrome.

Gastrointestinal Drugs

Gastrointestinal disorders occur frequently during pregnancy. Nausea, with or without vomiting, is the most common gastrointestinal disorder of early pregnancy. In the extreme form (i.e., hyperemesis gravidarum), vomiting may cause significant weight loss and dehydration. Another common gastrointestinal disorder in pregnancy is pyrosis, or "heartburn," which is related to increased gastroesophageal reflux as a result of decreased muscular tone in the lower esophagus and hypersecretion of gastric acid. Medications used to treat gastrointestinal disorders include antacids, histamine H_2 receptor antagonists, proton pump inhibitors, antiemetics, and corticosteroids (discussed earlier).

Antacids

Antacids are divided into five categories based on their metal salt content: aluminum, calcium, magnesium, magaldrate, sodium bicarbonate, and combinations of these. Antacids are the most frequently used over-the-counter and prescribed gastrointestinal medications among pregnant women. Aluminum hydroxide and magnesium hydroxide combinations are used in many commercial preparations, including Maalox, Mylanta, Riopan, and Gelusil. Calcium carbonate is a very popular antacid and is contained in such proprietary preparations such as Tums, Titralac, Rolaids, and Chooz.[103]

No teratology studies were published on antacids. Antacids are believed to be associated with little significant risk when used in moderation during pregnancy. However, long-term, high-dose use may be associated with adverse effects, such as maternal or fetal hypercalcemia, hypermagnesemia, or hypocalcemia.

H_2 Receptor Antagonists

H_2 receptor antagonists reduce gastric acidity through systemic action on histamine H_2 receptors. Time for absorption and distribution is needed before the patient experiences relief. Preparations include cimetidine, famotidine, nizatidine, and ranitidine. These agents are used as prophylaxis against aspiration and are given before general anesthesia. Long-term administration of systemic antacids is used to treat peptic ulcer disease, an uncommon ailment in pregnant women, and gastroesophageal reflux disease that is unresponsive to the usual antacids, such as the calcium and other metal salts mentioned earlier. These agents cross the placenta.[248,249]

Among more than 400 infants born to women treated with various histamine H_2 receptor antagonists during the first trimester, the risk of congenital anomalies was not increased.[250–252] The frequency of congenital anomalies in 237 infants whose mothers used cimetidine during the first trimester was not increased above that in control subjects.[253] The risk of congenital anomalies was not increased in 58 infants born to women who took famotidine during the first trimester.[252] No studies of nizatidine use during human pregnancy were published when this topic was researched in 2004. In more than 500 infants born to mothers who used ranitidine during the first trimester, the frequency of congenital anomalies was not increased above the expected background rate.[252,253]

Findings suggest that first-trimester use of histamine H_2 antagonists is not associated with an increased risk of congenital anomalies. Data on ranitidine are compelling because the sample sizes are large. Data on famotidine are less compelling because the sample size is much smaller.[254] Little information was published about nizatidine use during human pregnancy. In the latter half of pregnancy, histamine H_2 antagonists apparently can be used safely. No adverse maternal or fetal effects were noted.

Proton Pump Inhibitors

Proton pump inhibitors were recently developed to treat gastric hyperacidity. They act systemically by directly inhibiting the production of H^+,K^+-ATPase and related ions.[254]

OMEPRAZOLE

The first proton pump inhibitor used to treat ulcers and gastric reflux was omeprazole (Prilosec). This agent blocks the production and secretion of gastric acid. It has been used during organogenesis and the fetal periods of pregnancy. The frequency of major congenital anomalies was no greater than expected. In 91 infants of women who were treated with omeprazole during the first trimester, the frequency of congenital anomalies was not increased above the rate expected for the general population.[255] No adverse effects on newborns were noted when women were given omeprazole in preparation for delivery by elective cesarean section.[256,257]

ESOMEPRAZOLE

There are no epidemiologic studies of esomeprazole use during pregnancy. Esomeprazole is the sinister racemate of omeprazole. The clinical advantage of esomeprazole compared with omeprazole is that the sinister racemate isomer is cleared from the body more slowly, decreasing dose periodicity.[258] It is tempting to assume that esomeprazole is safe because a closely related drug (omeprazole) is apparently safe based on fewer than 100 first-trimester exposures. However, an isomer of thalidomide, the most notorious human teratogen ever discovered, was not associated with birth defects.

Antiemetics

Most pregnant women experience nausea during the first trimester. Most are managed comfortably without medication. However, some patients who have nausea and emesis require therapy because of protracted or health-threatening vomiting that causes dehydration. In serious cases of protracted vomiting during pregnancy, or hyperemesis gravidarum, inpatient treatment may be necessary.

PHENOTHIAZINES

Phenothiazines are used for several indications, including nausea and vomiting, psychotic disorders, and mild pain. They are also used as antidyskinetics and mild sedatives. The phenothiazine derivatives prochlorperazine, chlorpromazine, and promethazine are the most commonly used agents for the treatment of nausea and vomiting during pregnancy. Phenothiazine use during pregnancy may be associated with extrapyramidal symptoms in the mother and fetus, but these adverse effects are rare.[259,260] Phenothiazine use during gestation is not associated with an increased frequency of congenital anomalies.

PROMETHAZINE

Promethazine is marketed under many trade names. Phenergan is the most well known to obstetricians. It is also used as an adjuvant to meperidine during labor and for pain relief after cesarean delivery. In more than 100 infants born to women who took promethazine in the first trimester, the frequency of birth defects was not increased.[69] Similarly, the risk of congenital anomalies was not increased in two other studies that included several hundred women who used the drug during the first trimester[68,195] and later in pregnancy.[195] When promethazine was used to treat hyperemesis, the frequency of congenital anomalies was lower than expected.[195]

CHLORPROMAZINE

The risk of congenital anomalies was not increased in the offspring of more than 400 women who took this drug during the first trimester.[69,195]

PROCHLORPERAZINE

In more than 1000 infants whose mothers took prochlorperazine during the first trimester, the frequency of congenital anomalies was not increased above the background risk. In addition, in more than 2000 women who used prochlorperazine during the second and third trimesters, no adverse maternal or fetal adverse effects were observed.[69,70,241,261]

PIPERAZINE DERIVATIVES

Cyclizine, buclizine, and meclizine are piperazine derivatives that are used as antiemetics and antihistamines. The risk of congenital anomalies was not increased in several hundred infants whose mothers used piperazine derivatives during the first trimester[69] or in more than 100 infants whose mothers used cyclizine during the first trimester.[241]

DOXYLAMINE-PYRIDOXINE

Doxylamine-pyridoxine (Bendectin) was wrongly classified as a teratogen more than 20 years ago. Until it was taken off the market, Bendectin was the most commonly prescribed antiemetic for hyperemesis during pregnancy. It was reportedly very efficacious. After the drug combination was withdrawn from the market, many obstetricians prescribed the components of Bendectin separately to be taken concomitantly. Flawed studies associated Bendectin use with diaphragmatic hernias, congenital heart disease, and pyloric stenosis. Better-designed studies refuted the association of Bendectin with birth defects. Epidemiologic studies of first-trimester use of the individual components of Bendectin also show the safety of the drug combination.

Millions of women used Bendectin during the first trimester, and by chance alone, 3.5% would be expected to have infants with birth defects. In 2002, it was clear that Bendectin was not a teratogen. The U.S. FDA elected to republish its exonerative findings, and Brent reported that the drug would become available again.[237] Unfortunately, it appears that Bendectin was a significant "litogen" (i.e., capable of inducing nonmeritorious lawsuits).[236,262,263] Until Bendectin is reintroduced, obstetricians will likely prescribe doxylamine and pyridoxine under separate labels to be taken together as an antinauseant.

5-HT_3 RECEPTOR AGONISTS

Ondansetron. Ondansetron (Zofran) is a 5-HT_3 receptor agonist and a very potent antiemetic. It is most often used for severe nausea and vomiting associated with chemotherapy. It has also been used successfully to treat severe hyperemesis gravidarum. No human epidemiologic studies have been published, but this agent was not teratogenic in animal studies, according to its manufacturer. It is classified as U.S. FDA risk category B, although, as noted earlier, this classification does not provide reliable reassurance.

Prokinetic Agents. Prokinetic agents stimulate motility of the upper gastrointestinal tract. They are used primarily to treat gastrointestinal reflux disease. Metoclopramide (Reglan) is also used as an antiemetic, especially for postoperative nausea. No adequate human reproduction studies of cisapride (Propulsid) or metoclopramide were published. Neither drug was teratogenic in animal studies. Cisapride is listed as U.S. FDA risk category C, and metoclopramide is listed as U.S. FDA risk category B.

MANAGEMENT OF THE PREGNANT PATIENT WITH MEDICATION EXPOSURE

Management of the pregnant patient who has been exposed to medication during pregnancy, especially during the critical period of organogenesis, is a challenge. Several important questions must be answered. Is the medication or substance a known teratogen? Are there potential adverse fetal or neonatal effects? What is the risk to the mother if the medication is used or withheld? Are there other important factors to consider, such as the disease being treated? What are the available sources of information about medication use during pregnancy? How should the patient be counseled?

Etiology of Malformations

In most cases of congenital malformations (65%–70%) the cause is unknown. It was estimated that 20% to 25% are caused by genetic abnormalities 3% to 5% are caused by intrauterine infection and 4% are associated with maternal diseases, such as diabetes mellitus, phenylketonuria, or epilepsy.[264] Fewer than 1% of cases are causally related to prescribed medications. However, many patients, physicians, and lawyers often suspect that a medication caused a malformation in an exposed infant.[265]

Evaluating Risk

Few medications are known human teratogens. However, for most medications, perhaps more than 60%, inadequate data are available to allow an assessment of the risks of congenital anomalies or adverse fetal effects.

Sources of Information

Where can this information be found? Several major textbooks can provide a starting point. In addition, computerized databases, such as TERIS,[2] provide useful information for the assessment of potential risks (Table 35–14). Ultimately, referral to a tertiary care center with a clinical teratologist on staff is the preferred approach.

TABLE 35–14

Sources of Information on Drugs and Medications During Pregnancy

Databases

TERIS, Department of Pediatrics, University of Washington, Seattle, WA; 206-543-4365; http://depts.washington.edu/~terisweb/

Note: Individual summaries may be purchased for clinical use.

REPROTOX, An independent non-profit agency; reprotox@reprotox.org http://reprotox.org/

Hotlines

MotheRisk Program: 416-813-6780

Teratogen Information Service (TIS) 800-532-3749 or 619-294-6084

Organization of Teratology Information Services (OTIS) 888-285-3410

Textbooks

Shepard TH: *Catalog of Teratogenic Agents*, 10th ed. Baltimore, Johns Hopkins University Press, 2001.

Briggs GG, Freeman RK, Yaffe SJ (eds): *Drugs in Pregnancy and Lactation: A Reference Guide to Fetal and Neonatal Risk*, 6th ed. Philadelphia, Lippincott Williams & Wilkins, 2002.

Schardein JL: *Chemically Induced Birth Defects*, 3rd ed. New York, Marcel Dekker, 2002.

Gilstrap LC, Little BB: *Drugs and Pregnancy*, 2nd ed. New York, Chapman and Hall, 1998.

Yonkers KA, Little BB: *Management of Psychiatric Disorders in Pregnancy*. London, Arnold Press, 2001.

Friedman JM, Polifka JE: *The Effects of Neurologic and Psychiatric Drugs on the Fetus and Nursing Infant: A Handbook for Health Care Professionals*. Baltimore, Johns Hopkins University Press, 1998.

Friedman JM, Polifka JE: *Teratogenic Effects of Drugs: A Resource for Clinicians*, 2nd ed. Baltimore, Johns Hopkins University Press, 2000.

Weiner C, Buchimschi C: *Drugs for Pregnant and Lactating Women*. New York, Churchill Livingstone, 2004.

U.S. Food and Drug Administration Fetal Risk Categories

In 1979, the U.S. FDA established a risk category system to classify drugs with potential adverse fetal effects.[1,2,266] Category A drugs are considered relatively safe for use during pregnancy. Category B drugs have no known risks, but there are no controlled human studies. Category C agents are those for which little or no information is available. Most new drugs are placed in this category. Category D agents have a definite risk, but may be deemed necessary for use during pregnancy based on a risk–benefit assessment (i.e., anticonvulsants). Category X drugs pose a definite risk. Their use during pregnancy is contraindicated because the potential risks outweigh the benefits. Few medications are listed as category A (e.g., some prenatal vitamins). Ampicillin is an example of a category B drug (i.e., no controlled human studies). Isotretinoin (Accutane) is a category X drug. These categories usually do not reflect current scientific information on the potential teratogenic risk of a specific medication.[267] Therefore, they should not be considered primary directives for prescribing medication during pregnancy.

Counseling the Patient

It is important to take a detailed medical history and to perform a physical examination before counseling the patient and her family. The history should include gestational dating criteria, such as the date of the last menstrual period. In addition, detailed information should be obtained about drug exposure (class, dose, route of administration, timing, disease being treated). It is important to obtain information on concomitant medication use and ionizing radiation exposure as well as a detailed family history and genetic pedigree. Finally, it is necessary to review other medical conditions that may affect the risk of malformations.[2]

Determining the gestational age and the timing of exposure is of paramount importance. Ultrasound evaluation for dates should be done if the gestational age is questionable or is not confirmed by the findings on physical examination. If it can be determined that a medication was taken before conception or after organogenesis, for most medications, counseling may consist of simply reassuring the patient. Perhaps the most important information obtained during the counseling session is the gestational age at which exposure occurred. It is important to differentiate between embryonic age and menstrual age because menstrual age includes 2 weeks when the patient was not actually pregnant. It is important to determine whether the specific agent is absorbed from the maternal gastrointestinal tract, which may result in significant serum levels in the mother and possibly in the fetus. Some agents, such as stool softeners, have a local effect with no systemic absorption. These agents are expected to cause negligible embryonic or fetal exposure.

It is also necessary to determine whether significant amounts of a specific agent cross the placenta. For example, both low-molecular-weight and high-molecular-weight forms of heparin cross the placenta poorly and have no known direct adverse fetal effects. However, most drugs (99%) cross the placenta.

For known teratogens, such as isotretinoin, with reasonably established risk figures, the patient can be counseled that there are definite risks associated with exposure during a given gestational period. Therapeutic options include pregnancy termination. After the appropriate information is gathered during a cordial clinical interview, all counseling sessions should begin with an explanation of the background risk of congenital anomalies in the general population (3%–5%). The age-associated risk of chromosomal abnormalities should be elucidated if the patient is 35 years old or older.

No scientific studies on the use of approximately half of the currently available agents during pregnancy are available. Polifka and Friedman[75] point out that during the last 20 years research in clinical teratology has slowed significantly. When data are available, the counselor may explain the risk as follows: "Although a small risk cannot be 'ruled out,' the risk of spontaneous anomalies (3%–5%) is probably greater than any risk that can be estimated from available information for most medications that have been studied."[265] The counselor might continue to say: "For certain medical illnesses, such as diabetes or seizure disorders, the risk of the condition itself, especially if untreated, generally far outweighs any known or theoretical risk of medications to the fetus. These medications should not be withheld from a woman because she is pregnant." Obviously, preconception counseling is preferred, but this opportunity is rare.

Finally, when medications are being considered for a woman who is already pregnant, it is important to consider whether the initiation of therapy can be delayed until after the completion of the first trimester (i.e., embryogenesis). If a delay is unsafe, treatment should be initiated when needed, even if risk is involved. For example, chemotherapy for acute leukemia should be initiated as soon as the diagnosis is confirmed, regardless of gestational age.

CONCLUSIONS

- During pregnancy, many women take medication not all of which is prescribed.
- A detailed medication history should be taken at the beginning of pregnancy.
- Most drugs do not have proven adverse fetal effects, but they should be avoided in the first trimester, if possible.
- Medication should be used or continued in pregnancy only if the benefits outweigh the risks.
- When counseling patients about drug exposure in pregnancy, whether intended or inadvertent, it is important to obtain comprehensive and up-to-date data about known risks.

SUMMARY OF MANAGEMENT OPTIONS
Medication During Pregnancy

Management Options	Quality of Evidence	Strength of Recommendation	References
Inadvertent Exposure to Medication			
Obtain accurate details about exposure, especially gestational age	–	GPP	–
Check for confounding family or medical history	–	GPP	–
Obtain up-to-date information about published risks of the specific drug in humans	–	GPP	–
Emphasize "background" risks in counseling	–	GPP	–
Be clear about what is known, but do not assume that absence of data means no risk	–	GPP	–
Considering Initiating or Continuing Medication			
Medication should be used only if the expected benefits (usually to mother) are greater than the risks (usually to fetus)	–	GPP	–
Try to avoid first-trimester use	–	GPP	–
Use drugs that have been used extensively in pregnancy rather than new or untried drugs	–	GPP	–
Use the minimum dose to obtain the desired effect	–	GPP	–
Absence of data does not imply safety	–	GPP	–
Medications Known or Suspected to Be Human Teratogens or to Have Serious Adverse Fetal Effects (see Table 35–2)			
Retinoids			
High-dose vitamin A	IV	C	9
Isotretinoin (see Table 35–3)	III	B	19
Etretinate	IV	C	20
Acitretin	III	B	21
Hormones			
Danazol	III	B	50–53
Androgens	III	B	49
Diethylstilbestrol (see Table 35–7)	IIa	B	57
Anticoagulants			
Warfarin and other coumarin anticoagulants (see Table 35–6)	III	B	47
Antineoplastics			
Aminopterin and methylaminopterin (see Table 35–4)	IV	C	23–25
Methotrexate	IV	C	23–25

SUMMARY OF MANAGEMENT OPTIONS
Medication During Pregnancy *(Continued)*

Management Options	Quality of Evidence	Strength of Recommendation	References
Busulfan	IV	C	27
Cyclophosphamide	IV	C	28,29
Anticonvulsants			
Phenytoin and other hydantoins (see Table 35–5)	III	B	33,34
Carbamazepine	III	B	38
Valproic acid	III	B	44–46
Trimethadione and paramethadione	III	B	35
Primidone	III	B	35
Phenobarbital	III	B	75,78,79
Antibiotics (see also Table 35–8)			
Tetracycline	III	B	65–67
Aminoglycosides	III	B	90,91
Fluconazole administered parenterally (not orally)	III	B	107–109
Others			
Cocaine	IV	C	22
Lithium	III	B	71,72
Penicillamine	III	B	73,74
Thalidomide	III	B	7
Angiotensin-converting enzyme inhibitors	IIa	B	143–147
Amiodarone	IV	C	158–161
Nonsteroidal anti-inflammatory drugs	III	B	198–202

REFERENCES

1. Gilstrap LC, Cunningham FG: Drugs and medications during pregnancy. In Pritchard J, MacDonald P, Grant N (eds.) Williams Obstetrics, 17th ed, Appleton and Lange; Norwalk, CT. Supplement 13, 1987.
2. Little BB, Gilstrap LC, Cunningham FG: Medication use during pregnancy: Part 1. Concepts of human teratology. In Cunningham G, MacDonald P, Grant N (eds.) Williams Obstetrics, 18th ed, Appleton and Lange; Norwalk, CT. Supplement 10, 1991.
3. Little BB: Pharmacokinetics during pregnancy: Evidence-based maternal dose formulation. Obstetrics and Gynegology Gynecol 1999;93:858–868.
4. Nelson MM, Forfar JO: Association between drugs administered during pregnancy and congenital abnormalities of the fetus. Br Med J 1971;1:523–527.
5. Centers for Disease Control: Use of supplements containing high-dose vitamin A: New York. MMWR 1987;336:80.
6. Rubin PC: Prescribing in pregnancy. Br Med J 1986;293: 1415–1417.
7. McBride WG: Thalidomide embryopathy. Teratology 1977;16: 79–82.
8. Castilla EE, Ashton-Prolla P, Barreda-Mejia E, et al: Thalidomide, a current teratogen in South America. Teratology 1996;54:273–277.
9. Hathcock JN, Hattan DG, Jenkins MY, et al: Evaluation of vitamin A toxicity. Am J Clin Nutr 1990;52:183–202.
10. Lammer EJ, Chen DT, Hoar RM, et al: Retinoic acid embryopathy. N Engl J Med 1985;313:837–841.
11. Rosa FW, Wilk AL, Kelsey FO: Teratogen update: Vitamin A congeners. Teratology 1986;33:355–364.
12. Strauss JS, Cunningham WJ, Leyden JJ, et al: Isotretinoin and teratogenicity. J Am Acad Dermatol 1988;19:353–354.
13. Thomson EJ, Cordero JF: The new teratogens: Accutane and other vitamin-A analogs. MCN 1989;14:244–248.
14. Chen DT, Jacobson MM, Kuntzman RG: Experience with the retinoids in human pregnancy. In Volans GN (ed): Basic Science in Toxicology. London, Taylor and Francis, 1990, pp 473–482.
15. Lynberg MC, Khoury MJ, Lammer EJ, et al: Sensitivity, specificity, and positive predictive value of multiple malformations in isotretinoin embryopathy surveillance. Teratology 1990;42: 513–519.

16. Khoury MJ, James LM, Lynberg MC: Quantitative analysis of associations between birth defects and suspected human teratogens. Am J Med Genet 1991;40:500–505.
17. Teratology Society: Recommendations for isotretinoin use in women of childbearing potential. Teratology 1991;44:1–6.
18. Adams J: High incidence of intellectual deficits in 5 year old children exposed to isotretinoin "in utero." Teratology 1990;41:614.
19. Dai WS, LaBraico JM, Stern RS: Epidemiology of isotretinoin exposure during pregnancy. J Am Acad Dermatol 1992;26:599–606.
20. Verloes A, Dodinval P, Koulischer L, et al: Etretinate embryotoxicity 7 months after discontinuation of treatment. Am J Med Genet 1990;37:437–438.
21. Geiger JM, Baudin M, Saurat JH: Teratogenic risk with etretinate and acitretin treatment. Dermatology 1994;189:109–116.
22. Lammer EJ: Embryopathy in infant conceived one year after termination of maternal etretinate. Lancet 1988;2:1080–1081.
23. Char F: Denoument and discussion: Aminopterin embryopathy syndrome. Am J Dis Child 1979;133:1189–1190.
24. Reich EW, Cox RP, Becker MH, et al: Recognition in adult patients of malformations induced by folic-acid antagonists. Birth Defects 1977;14(6B):139–160.
25. Warkany J: Aminopterin and methotrexate: Folic acid deficiency. Teratology 1978;17:353–358.
26. Milunsky A, Graef JW, Gaynor MF: Methotrexate-induced congenital malformations. J Pediatr 1968;72:790–795.
27. Diamond I, Anderson MM, McCreadie SR: Transplacental transmission of busulfan (Myleran) in a mother with leukemia: Production of fetal malformations and cytomegaly. Pediatrics 1960;25:85–90.
28. Kirshon B, Wasserstrum N, Willis R, et al: Teratogenic effects of first trimester cyclophosphamide therapy. Obstet Gynecol 1988;72:462–464.
29. Murray CL, Reichert JA, Anderson J, Twiggs LB: Multimodal cancer therapy for breast cancer in first trimester of pregnancy. JAMA 1984;252:2607–2608.
30. McClure HM, Wilk AL, Horigan EA, Pratt RM: Induction of craniofacial malformations in rhesus monkeys (*Macaca mulatta*) with cyclophosphamide. Cleft Palate J 1979;16:248–256.
31. Greenberg LH, Tanaka KR: Congenital anomalies probably induced by cyclophosphamide. JAMA 1964;188:423–426.
32. Doll DC, Ringenberg S, Yarbro JW: Management of cancer during pregnancy. Arch Intern Med 1988;148:2058–2064.
33. Hanson JW, Smith DW: The fetal hydantoin syndrome. J Pediatr 1975;87:285–290.
34. Kelly TE: Teratogenicity of anticonvulsant drugs: I. Review of the literature. Am J Med Genet 1984;19:413–434.
35. Zackai EH, Mellman WJ, Neiderer B, Hanson JW: The fetal trimethadione syndrome. J Pediatr 1975;87:280–284.
36. Gilstrap LC, Little BB, Cunningham FG: Medication use during pregnancy: Part 2. Special considerations. In Cunningham G, MacDonald P, Grant N (eds.) Williams Obstetrics, 18th ed, Appleton and Lange; Norwalk, CT. Supplement 11, 1991.
37. Niebyl JR, Blake DA, Freeman JM, Luft RD: Carbamazepine levels in pregnancy and lactation. Obstet Gynecol 1979;53: 139–140.
38. Jones KL, Lacro RV, Johnson KA, Adams J: Pattern of malformations in the children of women treated with carbamazepine during pregnancy. N Engl J Med 1989;320:1661–1666.
39. Buehler BA, Delimont D, van Waes M, Finnell RH: Prenatal prediction of risk of the fetal hydantoin syndrome. N Engl J Med 1990;22:1567–1572.
40. Finnell RH, Gelineau-vanWaes J, Eudy JD, Rosenquist TH: Molecular basis of environmentally induced birth defects. Annu Rev Pharmacol Toxicol 2002;42:181–208.
41. Strickler SM, Dansky LV, Miller MA, et al: Genetic predisposition to phenytoin-induced birth defects. Lancet 1985;2:746–749.
42. Centers for Disease Control: Valproate: A new cause of birth defects. Report from Italy and follow-up from France. MMWR 1983;32:348.
43. Robert E, Robert JM, Lapras C: Is valproic acid teratogenic? Rev Neurol 1983;139:445–447.
44. Dalens B, Raynaud EJ, Gaulme J: Teratogenicity of valproic acid. J Pediatr 1980;97:332–333.
45. DiLiberti JH, Farndon PA, Dennis NR, Curry CJR: The fetal valproate syndrome. Am J Med Genet 1984;19:473–481.
46. Jager-Roman E, Deichl A, Jakob S, et al: Fetal growth, major malformations, and minor anomalies in infants born to women receiving valproic acid. J Pediatr 1986;108:997–1004.
47. Hall JG, Pauli RM, Wilson K: Maternal and fetal sequelae of anticoagulation during pregnancy. Am J Med 1980;68:122–140.
48. Stevenson RE, Burton M, Ferlauto GJ, Taylor HA: Hazards of oral anticoagulants during pregnancy. JAMA 1980;243: 1549–1551.
49. Schardein JL: Chemically Induced Birth Defects. New York, Marcel Dekker, 1985.
50. Kingsbury AC: Danazol and fetal masculinization: A warning. Med J Aust 1985;143:410–411.
51. Quagliarello J, Greco MA: Danazol and urogenital sinus formation in pregnancy. Fertil Steril 1985;43:939–942.
52. Rosa FW: Virilization of the female fetus with maternal danazol exposure. Am J Obstet Gynecol 1984;149:99–100.
53. Shaw RW, Farquhar JW: Female pseudohermaphroditism associated with danazol exposure in utero: Case report. Br J Obstet Gynaecol 1984;91:386–389.
54. Herbst AL, Hubby MM, Azizi F, Makii MM: Reproductive and gynecologic surgical experience in diethylstilbestrol-exposed daughters. Am J Obstet Gynecol 1981;141:1019–1028.
55. Herbst AL, Poskanzer DC, Robboy SJ, et al: Prenatal exposure to stilbestrol: A prospective comparison of exposed female offspring with unexposed controls. N Engl J Med 1975;292: 334–339.
56. Bibbo M: Transplacental effects of diethylstilbestrol. In Grundman E (ed): Perinatal Pathology. New York, Springer-Verlag, 1979, pp 191–211.
57. Robboy SJ, Szyfelbein WM, Goellner JR, et al: Dysplasia and cytologic findings in 4589 young women enrolled in Diethylstilbestrol-Adenosis (DESAD) project. Am J Obstet Gynecol 1981;140:579–586.
58. Robboy SJ, Noller KL, O'Brien P, et al: Increased incidence of cervical and vaginal dysplasia in 3980 diethylstilbestrol-exposed young women: Experience of the National Collaborative Diethylstilbestrol Adenosis Project. JAMA 1984;252:2979–2983.
59. Stillman RJ: In utero exposure to diethylstilbestrol: Adverse effects on the reproductive tract performance in male and female offspring. Am J Obstet Gynecol 1982;142:905–921.
60. Kaufman RH, Noller K, Adam E, et al: Upper genital tract abnormalities and pregnancy outcome in diethylstilbestrol-exposed progeny. Am J Obstet Gynecol 1984;148:973–984.
61. Barnes AB, Colton T, Gunderson J, et al: Fertility and outcome of pregnancy in women exposed in utero to diethylstilbestrol. N Engl J Med 1980;302:609–613.
62. Herbst AL: Clear cell adenocarcinoma and the current status of DES-exposed females. Cancer 1981;48:484–488.
63. Herbst AL, Hubby MM, Blough RR, Azizi F: A comparison of pregnancy experience in DES-exposed and DES-unexposed daughters. J Reprod Med 1980;24:62–69.
64. Sandberg EC, Riffle NL, Higdon JV, Getman CE: Pregnancy outcome in women exposed to diethylstilbestrol in utero. Am J Obstet Gynecol 1981;140:194–205.
65. Rendle-Short TJ: Tetracycline in teeth and bone. Lancet 1962;1:1188.
66. Kutscher AH, Zegarelli EV, Tovell HM, et al: Discoloration of deciduous teeth induced by administration of tetracycline antepartum. Am J Obstet Gynecol 1966;96:291–292.

67. Genot MG, Golan HP, Porter PJ, Kass EH: Effect of administration of tetracycline in pregnancy on the primary definition of the offspring. J Oral Med 1970;25:75–79.
68. Aselton P, Jick H, Milunsky A, et al: First-trimester drug use and congenital disorders. Obstet Gynecol 1985;65:451–455.
69. Heinonen OP, Slone D, Shapiro S: Birth Defects and Drugs in Pregnancy. Littleton, Mass, Publishing Sciences Group, 1977.
70. Jick H, Holmes LB, Hunter JR, et al: First trimester drug use and congenital disorders. JAMA 1981;246:343–346.
71. Yonkers KA, Little BB, March D: Lithium use during pregnancy: A controversy. CNS Drugs 1998;9:261–269.
72. Cohen LS, Friedman JM, Jefferson JW, et al: A reevaluation of risk of in utero exposure to lithium. JAMA 1994;271:146–150.
73. Harpey JP, Jaudon MC, Clavel JP, et al: *Cutis laxa* and low serum zinc after antenatal exposure to penicillamine. Lancet 1983;2:858.
74. Rosa FW: Teratogen update: Penicillamine. Teratology 1986;33: 127–131.
75. Polifka JE, Friedman JM: Medical genetics: 1. Clinical teratology in the age of genomics. CMAJ 2002;167:265–273.
76. Jick SS, Terris BZ, Jick H: First trimester topical tretinoin and congenital disorders. Lancet 1993;341:1181–1182.
77. Johnson KA, Chambers CD, Felix R, et al: Pregnancy outcome in women prospectively ascertained with Retin-A exposures: An ongoing study. Teratology 1994;49:375.
78. Waters CH, Belai Y, Gott PS, et al: Outcomes of pregnancy associated with antiepileptic drugs. Arch Neurol 1994;51: 250–253.
79. Koch S, Jager-Roman E, Losche G, et al: Antiepileptic drug treatment in pregnancy: Drug side effects in the neonate and neurological outcome. Acta Paediatr 1996;84:739–746.
80. Samren EB, van Duijn CM, Koch S, et al: Maternal use of antiepileptic drugs and the risk of major congenital malformations: A joint European prospective study of human teratogenesis associated with maternal epilepsy. Epilepsia 1997;38:981–990.
81. Landers DV, Green JR, Sweet RL: Antibiotic use during pregnancy and the postpartum period. Clin Obstet Gynecol 1983;26: 391–406.
82. Gilstrap LC, Bawdon RE, Burris JS: Antibiotic concentration in maternal blood, cord blood and placental membranes in chorioamnionitis. Obstet Gynecol 1988;72:124–125.
83. Maberry M, Trimmer K, Bawdon R, et al: Antibiotic concentrations in maternal blood, cord blood and placental membranes in women with chorioamnionitis. St. Louis, Society for Gynecologic Investigation, 1990, p A543.
84. Martens MG: Cephalosporins. Obstet Gynecol North Am 1989;16:291–304.
85. Fenton LG, Light LJ: Congenital syphilis after maternal treatment with erythromycin. Obstet Gynecol 1976;47:492–494.
86. Kline AH, Blattner RJ, Lunin M: Transplacental effects of tetracyclines on teeth. JAMA 1964;188:178–180.
87. Rendle-Short TJ: Tetracycline and teeth and bone. Lancet 1962;1:1188.
88. Weinstein AJ, Gibbs RS, Gallasher M: Placental transfer of clindamycin and gentamicin in term pregnancy. Obstet Gynecol 1976;124:688–691.
89. Yoshioka H, Monma T, Matsuda S: Placental transfer of gentamicin. J Pediatr 1972;80:121–123.
90. Conway N, Birt DN: Streptomycin in pregnancy: Effect on the foetal ear. BMJ 1965;2:260–263.
91. Donald PR, Doherty E, Van Zyl FJ: Hearing loss in the child following streptomycin administration during pregnancy. Cent Afr J Med 1991;37:268–271.
92. Colley DP, Kay J, Gibson GT: A study of the use in pregnancy of co-trimoxazole and sulfamethizole. Aust J Pharm 1982;63: 570–575.
93. Czeizel A: A case-control analysis of the teratogenic effects of co-trimoxazole. Reprod Toxicol 1990;4:305–313.
94. Hernandez-Diaz S, Werler MM, Walker AM, Mitchell AA: Folic acid antagonists during pregnancy and the risk of birth defects. N Engl J Med 2000;343:1608–1614.
95. Hernandez-Diaz S, Werler MM, Walker AM, Mitchell AA: Neural tube defects in relation to use of folic acid antagonists during pregnancy. Am J Epidemiol 2001;153:961–968.
96. Lenke RR, VanDorsten JP, Schifrin BS: Pyelonephritis in pregnancy: A prospective randomized trial to prevent recurrent disease evaluating suppressive therapy with nitrofurantoin and close surveillance. Am J Obstet Gynecol 1983;146:953–957.
97. Berkovitch M, Pastuszak A, Gazarian M, et al: Safety of the new quinolones in pregnancy. Obstet Gynecol 1994;84:535–538.
98. Bomford JAL, Ledger JC, O'Keeffe BJ, Reiter C: Ciprofloxacin use during pregnancy. Drugs 1993;45(Suppl 3):461–462.
99. Koren G: Use of the new quinolones during pregnancy. Can Fam Physician 1996;42:1097–1099.
100. Loebstein R, Addis A, Ho E, et al: Pregnancy outcome following gestational exposure to fluoroquinolones: A multicenter prospective controlled study. Antimicrob Agents Chemother 1998; 42:1336–1339.
101. Pastuszak A, Andreou R, Schick B, et al: New postmarketing surveillance data supports a lack of association between quinolone use in pregnancy and fetal and neonatal complications. Reprod Toxicol 1995;9:584.
102. Schaefer C, Amoura-Elefant E, Vial T, et al: Pregnancy outcome after prenatal quinolone exposure: Evaluation of a case registry of the European Network of Teratology Information Services (ENTIS). Eur J Obstet Gynecol Reprod Biol 1996;69:83–89.
103. USP DI: USP Dispensing Information, Vol. I. Drug Information for the Health Care Professional, 21st ed. Englewood, Colo, Micromedex Thomson Healthcare, 2001.
104. Snider DE Jr, Layde PM, Johnson MW, Lyle MA: Treatment of tuberculosis during pregnancy. Am Rev Respir Dis 1980;122: 65–79.
105. Varpela E: On the effect exerted by first-line tuberculosis medicines on the foetus. Acta Tuberc Scand 1964;35:53–69.
106. Rosa FW, Baum C, Shaw M: Pregnancy outcomes after first trimester vaginitis drug therapy. Obstet Gynecol 1987;69: 751–755.
107. Lee BE, Feinberg M, Abraham JJ, Murthy ARK: Congenital malformations in an infant born to a woman treated with fluconazole. Pediatr Infect Dis J 1992;11:1062–1064.
108. Pursley TJ, Blomquist IK, Abraham J, et al: Fluconazole-induced congenital anomalies in three infants. Clin Infect Dis 1996;22:336–340.
109. Reardon W, Smith A, Honour JW, et al: Evidence for digenic inheritance in some cases of Antley-Bixler syndrome? J Med Genet 2000;37:26–32.
110. Sorensen HT, Nielsen GL, Olesen C, et al: Risk of malformations and other outcomes in children exposed to fluconazole in utero. Br J Clin Pharmacol 1999;48:234–239.
111. Jick SS: Pregnancy outcomes after maternal exposure to fluconazole. Pharmacotherapy 1999;19:221–222.
112. Mastroiacovo P, Mazzone T, Botto LD, et al: Prospective assessment of pregnancy outcomes after first-trimester exposure to fluconazole. Am J Obstet Gynecol 1996;175:1645–1650.
113. Ismail MA, Lerner SA: Disseminated blastomycosis in a pregnant woman: Review of amphotericin B usage during pregnancy. Am Rev Respir Dis 1982;126:350–353.
114. Rosa FW, Hernandez C, Carlo WA: Griseofulvin teratology, including two thorapagus conjoined twins. Lancet 1987; 1:171.
115. Newschaffer CJ, Cocroft J, Anderson CE, et al: Prenatal zidovudine use and congenital anomalies in a medicaid population. J Acquir Immun Defic Syndr 2000;24:249–256,
116. Antiretroviral Pregnancy Registry: Antiretroviral Pregnancy Registry Interim Report for Abacavir (ZIAGEN(R)), Abacavir/

Lamivudine/Zidovudine (TRIZIVIR(R), TZV), Amprenavir (AGENERASE(R), APV), Delavirdine Mesylate (RESCRIPTOR(R)), Didanosine (VIDEX(R), ddI), Efavirenz (SUSTIVA, STOCRIN(R)), Indinavir (CRIXIVAN(R), IDV), Lamivudine (EPIVIR(R), 3TC), Lamivudine/Zidovudine (COMBIVIR(R)), Lopinavir/Ritonavir (KALETRA), Nelfinavir (VIRACEPT(R)), Nevirapine (VIRAMUNE(R)), Ritonavir (NORVIR(R), RTV), Saquinavir (FORTOVASE(R), SQV-SGC), Saquinavir Mesylate (INVIRASE(R), SQV-HGC), Stavudine (ZERIT(R), d4T), Zalcitabine (HIVID(R), ddC), and Zidovudine (RETROVIR(R), ZDV), 1 January 1989 through 31 July 2001. Wilmington, NC, 2001.
117. Sperling RS, Stratton P, O'Sullivan MJ, et al: A survey of zidovudine use in pregnant women with human immunodeficiency virus infection. N Engl J Med 1992;326:857–861.
118. Minkoff H: Prevention of mother to child transmission of HIV. Clin Obstet Gynecol 2001;44:210–215.
119. Reiff-Eldridge R, Heffner CR, Ephross SA, et al: Monitoring pregnancy outcomes after prenatal drug exposure through prospective pregnancy registries: A pharmaceutical company commitment. Am J Obstet Gynecol 2000;182:159–163.
120. TERIS: Department of Pediatrics, University of Washington, Seattle, WA (206/543-4365) http://depts.washington.edu/~terisweb/
121. Hammill HA: Metronidazole, clindamycin, and quinolones. Obstet Gynecol North Am 1989;16:317–328.
122. Rosa F: Personal communication, 1993. Cited in Briggs GG, Freeman RK, Yaffe SJ (eds): Drugs in Pregnancy and Lactation: A Reference Guide to Fetal and Neonatal Risk, 6th ed. Philadelphia, Lippincott Williams & Wilkins, 2002, p 1394.
123. Caro-Paton T, Carvajal A, Martin de Diego I, et al: Is metronidazole teratogenic? A meta-analysis. Br J Clin Pharmacol 1997; 44:179–182.
124. Wolfe MS, Cordero JF: Safety of chloroquine in chemosuppression of malaria during pregnancy. Br Med J 1985;290:1466–1467.
125. Nishimura H, Tanimura T: Clinical Aspects of the Teratogenicity of Drugs. Amsterdam, Excerpta Medica, 1976.
126. Hengst P: Investigations of the teratogenicity of Daraprim (pyrimethamine) in humans. Zentralbl Gynakol 1972; 94: 551–555.
127. Wong S-Y, Remington JS: Toxoplasmosis in pregnancy. Clin Infect Dis 1994;18:853–862.
128. Heinonen OP, Slone D, Shapiro S: Birth Defects and Drugs in Pregnancy. Littleton, Mass, John Wright-PSG, 1977, pp 298, 301, 435.
129. de Silva NR, Sirisena JLGJ, Gunasekera DPS, et al: Effect of mebendazole therapy during pregnancy on birth outcome. Lancet 1999;353:1145–1149.
130. Murad SH, Tabsh KM, Shilyanski G, et al: Effects of verapamil on uterine blood flow and maternal cardiovascular function in the awake pregnant ewe. Anesth Analg 1985;64:7–10.
131. Kleinman CS, Copel JA: Electrophysiological principles and fetal antiarrhythmic therapy. Ultrasound Obstet Gynecol 1991; 1:286–297.
132. Pruyn SC, Phelan JP, Buchanan GC: Long-term propranolol therapy in pregnancy: Maternal and fetal outcome. Am J Obstet Gynecol 1979;135:485–489.
133. Tunstall ME: The effect of propranolol on the onset of breathing at birth. Br J Anaesth 1969;41:792.
134. Habib A, McCarthy JS: Effects on the neonate of propranolol administered during pregnancy. J Pediatr 1977;91:808–811.
135. Rubin PC: Current concepts: Beta-blockers in pregnancy. N Engl J Med 1981;305:1323–1326.
136. Milner RD: Neonatal hypoglycaemia: A critical reappraisal. Arch Dis Child 1972;255:679–682.
137. Milsap RL, Auld PAM: Neonatal hyperglycemia following maternal diazoxide administration. JAMA 1980;243:144–145.
138. Lewis PE, Cefalo RC, Naulty JS, Rodkey FL: Placental transfer and fetal toxicity of sodium nitroprusside. Gynecol Invest 1977;8:46.
139. Gant NF: Lupus erythematosus, the lupus anticoagulant, and the anticardiolipin antibody. In Pritchard J, Mac Donald P, Grant N (eds.) Williams Obstetrics, 17th ed. Appleton and Lange; Norwalk, CT. Supplement 6, 1986.
140. Turmen T, Thom P, Louridas AT, et al: Protein binding and bilirubin displacing properties of bumetanide and furosemide. J Clin Pharmacol 1982;22:551–556.
141. Hecker A, Hasan SH, Neumann F: Disturbances in sexual differentiation of rat foetuses following spironolactone treatment. Acta Endocrinol 1980;95:540–545.
142. Rodriguez SU, Leikin SL, Hiller MC: Neonatal thrombocytopenia associated with antepartum administration of thiazide drugs. N Engl J Med 1964;270:881–884.
143. Boutroy MJ, Vert P, Hurault de Ligny BH, Miton A: Captopril administration in pregnancy impairs fetal angiotensin converting enzyme activity and neonatal adaptation. Lancet 1984;2: 935–936.
144. Boutroy MJ: Fetal effects of maternally administered clonidine and angiotensin-converting enzyme inhibitors. Dev Pharmacol Ther 1989;13:199–204.
145. Rothberg AD, Lorenz R: Can captopril cause fetal and neonatal renal failure? Pediatr Pharmacol 1984;4:189–192.
146. Barr M, Cohen MM: ACE inhibitor fetopathy and hypocalvaria: The kidney-skull connection. Teratology 1991;44:485–495.
147. Rosa F, Bosco L: Infant renal failure with maternal ACE inhibitors. Am J Obstet Gynecol 1991;164:273.
148. Sibai BM, Gonzales AR, Mabie WD, Moretti M: A comparison of labetalol plus hospitalization versus hospitalization alone in the management of preeclampsia remote from term. Obstet Gynecol 1987;70:323–327.
149. Rotmensch HH, Elkayam U, Frishman W: Antiarrhythmic drug therapy during pregnancy. Ann Intern Med 1983;98:487–497.
150. Horvath JS, Phippard A, Korda A, et al: Clonidine hydrochloride: A safe and effective antihypertensive agent in pregnancy. Obstet Gynecol 1985;66:634–638.
151. Raftos J, Bauer GE, Lewis RG, et al: Clonidine in the treatment of severe hypertension. Med J Aust 1973;1:786–793.
152. Shoemaker CT, Meyers M: Sodium nitroprusside for control of severe hypertensive disease of pregnancy: A case report and discussion of potential toxicity. Am J Obstet Gynecol 1984;149: 171–173.
153. Hirsch KS, Wilson JG, Scott WJ, O'Flaherty EJ: Acetazolamide teratology and its association with carbonic anhydrase inhibition in the mouse. Teratogenesis Carcinog Mutagen 1983;3:133–144.
154. Lingman G, Ohrlander S, Ohlin P: Intrauterine digoxin treatment of fetal paroxysmal tachydardia: Case report. Br J Obstet Gynaecol 1980;87:340–342.
155. Harrigan JT, Kangos JJ, Sikka A, et al: Successful treatment of fetal congestive failure secondary to tachycardia. N Engl J Med 1981;304:1527–1529.
156. Rotmensch HH, Rotmensch S, Elkayam U: Management of cardiac arrhythmias during pregnancy: Current concepts. Drugs 1987;33:623–633.
157. Rotmensch HH, Elkayam U, Frishman W: Antiarrhythmic drug therapy during pregnancy. Ann Intern Med 1983;98:487–497.
158. Pinsky WW, Rayburn WF, Evans MI: Pharmacologic therapy for fetal arrhythmias. Clin Obstet Gynecol 1991;34:304–309.
159. Bartalena L, Bogazzi F, Braverman LE, Martino E: Effects of amiodarone administration during pregnancy on neonatal thyroid function and subsequent neurodevelopment. J Endocrinol Invest 2001;24:116–130.
160. Magee LA, Downar E, Sermer M, et al: Pregnancy outcome after gestational exposure to amiodarone in Canada. Am J Obstet Gynecol 1995;172:1307–1311.

161. Magee LA, Nulman I, Rovet JF, Koren G: Neurodevelopment after in utero amiodarone exposure. Neurotoxicol Teratol 1999;21:261–265.
162. Beaufils M, Uzan S, Donsimoni R, Colau JC: Prevention of preeclampsia by early antiplatelet therapy. Lancet 1985;1:840–842.
163. Beaufils M, Uzan S, Donsimoni R, Colau JC: Prospective controlled study of early antiplatelet therapy in prevention of preeclampsia. Adv Nephrol 1986;15:87–94.
164. Wallenburg HCS, Rotmans N: Prevention of recurrent idiopathic fetal growth retardation by low-dose aspirin and dipyridamole. Am J Obstet Gynecol 1987;157:1230–1235.
165. Wallace RL, Caldwell D, Ansbacher R, Otterson W: Inhibition of premature labor by terbutaline. Obstet Gynecol 1978;51: 387–392.
166. Rosa F: Personal communication, 1993. Cited in Briggs GG, Freeman RK, Yaffe SJ (eds): Drugs in Pregnancy and Lactation: A Reference Guide to Fetal and Neonatal Risk, 6th ed. Philadelphia, Lippincott Williams & Wilkins, 2002, pp 1317–1318.
167. Schatz M, Zeiger RS, Harden K, et al: The safety of asthma and allergy medications during pregnancy. J Allergy Clin Immunol 1997;100:301–306.
168. Wilson J: Utilisation du cromoglycate de sodium au cours de la grossesse: Resultats sur 296 femmes asthmatiques. Acta Ther 1982;8(Suppl):45–51.
169. ACAAI-ACOG Recommendations for the Pharmacologic Step Therapy of Chronic Asthma During Pregnancy. American College of Obstetrics and Gynecology, 2000.
170. Little BB, Yonkers KA: Epidemiology of psychiatric disorders and the importance of gender. In Yonkers KA, Little BB (eds): Management of Psychiatric Disorders in Pregnancy. London, Arnold Press, 2001.
171. Aarskog D: Association between maternal intake of diazepam and oral clefts. Lancet 1975;2:921.
172. Safra MJ, Oakley BP Jr: An association of cleft lip with or without cleft palate and prenatal exposure to diazepam. Lancet 1975;2:478–480.
173. Saxen I, Saxen L: Association between maternal intake of diazepam and oral clefts. Lancet 1975;2:498.
174. Czeizel A: Lack of evidence of teratogenicity of benzodiazepine drugs in Hungary. Reprod Toxicol 1988;1:183–188.
175. Rosenberg L, Mitchell A, Parsells JL, et al: Lack of correlation of oral clefts to diazepam use during pregnancy. N Engl J Med 1983;309:1982–1985.
176. Shiono PH, Mills JL: Oral clefts and diazepam use during pregnancy. N Engl J Med 1984;311:919–920.
177. Rothman KJ, Fyler DC, Goldblatt A, Kreidberg MB: Exogenous hormones and other drug exposures of children with congenital heart disease. Am J Epidemiol 1979;109:433–439.
178. Bracken MB, Holford TR: Exposure to prescribed drugs in pregnancy and association with congenital malformations. Obstet Gynecol 1981;58:336–344.
179. Bracken MB: Drug use in pregnancy and congenital heart disease in offspring. N Engl J Med 1986;314:1120.
180. Zierler S, Rothman KJ: Congenital heart disease in relation to maternal use of Bendectin and other drugs in early pregnancy. N Engl J Med 1985;313:347–352.
181. Milkovich L, van den Berg BJ: An evaluation of the teratogenicity of certain antinauseant drugs. Am J Obstet Gynecol 1976;125:244–248.
182. Crombie DL, Pinsent RJ, Fleming DM, et al: Fetal effects of tranquilizers in pregnancy. N Engl J Med 1975;293:198–199.
183. Kullander S, Kallen B: A prospective study of drugs and pregnancy. Acta Obstet Gynecol Scand 1976;55:25–33.
184. Hartz SC, Heinonen OP, Shapiro S, et al: Antenatal exposure to meprobamate and chlordiazepoxide in relation to malformations, mental development and childhood. N Engl J Med 1975;292:726–728.
185. McBride WG: Limb deformities associated with iminodibenzyl hydrochloride. Med J Aust 1972;1:492.
186. Morrow AW: Imipramine and congenital abnormalities. N Zeal Med J 1972;75:228–229.
187. Crombie DL, Pinsent R, Fleming D: Imipramine in pregnancy. Br Med J 1972;1:745.
188. Scanlon FJ: Use of antidepressant drugs during the first trimester. Med J Aust 1969;2:1077.
189. Goldstein DJ, Marvel DE: Psychotropic medications during pregnancy: Risk to the fetus. JAMA 1993;270:2177.
190. Pastuszak A, Schick-Boschetto B, Zuber C, et al: Pregnancy outcome following first-trimester exposure to fluoxetine (Prozac). JAMA 1993;269:2246–2248.
191. Chambers CD, Johnson KA, Dick LM, et al: Birth outcomes in pregnant women taking fluoxetine. N Engl J Med 1996;335: 1010–1015.
192. Chambers CD, Dick LM, Felix RJ, et al: Pregnancy outcome in women who use sertraline. Teratology 1999;59:376.
193. Kulin NA, Pastuszak A, Sage SR, et al: Pregnancy outcome following maternal use of the new selective serotonin reuptake inhibitors: A prospective controlled multicenter study. JAMA 1998;279:609–610.
194. Wilton LV, Pearce GL, Martin RM, et al: The outcomes of pregnancy in women exposed to newly marketed drugs in general practice in England. Br J Obstet Gynaecol 1998;105: 882–889.
195. Farkas G, Farkas G Jr: Teratogenic effects of hyperemesis gravidarum and of the customary drugs used in its therapy. Zentralbl Gynakol 1971;10:325–330.
196. Scanlan FJ: The use of thioridazine (Melleril) during the first trimester. Med J Aust 1972;1:1271–1272.
197. van Waes A, van de Velde E: Safety evaluation of haloperidol in the treatment of hyperemesis gravidarum. J Clin Pharmacol 1969;9:224–227.
198. Niebyl J, Blake D, White R, et al: The inhibition of premature labor with indomethacin. Am J Obstet Gynecol 1980;136: 1014–1019.
199. Manchester D, Margolis HS, Sheldon RE: Possible association between maternal indomethacin therapy and primary pulmonary hypertension in the newborn. Am J Obstet Gynecol 1976;126: 467–469.
200. Csaba I, Sulyok FE, Ertl T: Relationship of maternal treatment with indomethacin to persistence of fetal circulation syndrome. J Pediatr 1978;92:484.
201. Levin DL, Fixler DE, Morriss FC, Tyson J: Morphologic analysis of the pulmonary vascular bed in infants exposed in utero to prostaglandin synthetase inhibitors. J Pediatr 1978;92: 478–483.
202. Dudley DKL, Hardie MJ: Fetal and neonatal effects of indomethacin used as a tocolytic agent. Am J Obstet Gynecol 1985;151:181–184.
203. Hickok DE, Hollenbach KA, Reilley SD, Nyberg DA: The association between decreased amniotic fluid volume and treatment with nonsteroidal anti-inflammatory agents for preterm labor. Am J Obstet Gynecol 1989;160:1525–1531.
204. Streissguth AP, Treder RP, Barr HM, et al: Aspirin and acetaminophen use by pregnant women and subsequent child IQ and attention decrements. Teratology 1987;35:211–219.
205. Agapitos M, Georgiou-Theodoropoulou M, Koutselinis A, Papacharalampus N: Cyclopia and maternal ingestion of salicylates. Pediatr Pathol 1986;6:309–310.
206. Slone D, Siskind V, Heinonen OP, et al: Aspirin and congenital malformations. Lancet 1976;1:1373–1375.
207. Turner G, Collins E: Fetal effects of regular salicylate ingestion in pregnancy. Lancet 1975;2:338–339.
208. Sibai B, Amon EA: How safe is aspirin use during pregnancy? Contemp Obstet Gynecol 1988;32:73–79.

209. Haibach H, Akhter JE, Muscato MS, et al: Acetaminophen overdose with fetal demise. Am J Clin Pathol 1984;82:240–246.
210. Schick B, Hom M, Tolosa J, et al: Preliminary analysis of first trimester exposure to oxycodone and hydrocodone. Reprod Toxicol 1996;10:162.
211. Milham S, Elledge W: Maternal methimazole and congenital defects in children (letter). Teratology 1972;5:125.
212. Mujtaba Q, Burrow GN: Treatment of hyperthyroidism in pregnancy with propylthiouracil and methimazole. Obstet Gynecol 1975;46:282–286.
213. Momotani N, Ito K, Hamada N, et al: Maternal hyperthyroidism and congenital malformations in the offspring. Clin Endocrinol 1984;20:695–700.
214. Van Dijke CP, Heydendael RJ, De Kleine MJ: Methimazole, carbimazole, and congenital skin defects. Ann Intern Med 1987;106:60–61.
215. Donegan WL: Cancer and pregnancy. CA 1983;33:194–197.
216. Donegan WL: The influence of pregnancy on the management of cancer. Cancer Bull 1986;38:278–284.
217. Parente JT, Amsel M, Lerner R, Chinea F: Breast cancer associated with pregnancy. Obstet Gynecol 1988;71:861–864.
218. Yazigi R, Cunningham FG: Cancer and pregnancy. In Cunningham G, MacDonald P, Grant N (eds.) Williams Obstetrics, 17th ed. Appleton and Lange; Norwalk, CT. Supplement 4, 1990.
219. Doll DC, Ringenberg S, Yarbro JW: Management of cancer during pregnancy. Arch Intern Med 1988;148:2058–2064.
220. Metz SA, Day TG, Pursell SH: Adjuvant chemotherapy in a pregnant patient with endodermal sinus tumor of the ovary. Gynecol Oncol 1989;32:371–374.
221. Caliguri MA, Mayer RJ: Pregnancy and leukemia. Semin Oncol 1989;16:388–396.
222. Briggs G, Freeman R, Yafee S: Drugs in Pregnancy and Lactation, 6th ed. Lippincott, Williams, and Wilkins; Philadelphia, PA, 2002.
223. Witter FR, Niebyl JR: Inhibition of arachidonic acid metabolism in the perinatal period: Pharmacology, clinical application, and potential adverse effects. Semin Perinatol 1986;20:316–333.
224. Penn I, Makowski EL, Harris P: Parenthood following renal transplantation. Kidney Int 1980;18:221–233.
225. Registration Committee of the European Dialysis and Transplant Association: Successful pregnancies in women treated by dialysis and kidney transplantation. Br J Obstet Gynaecol 1980;87:839–845.
226. Kallen B: Drug treatment of rheumatic diseases during pregnancy: The teratogenicity of antirheumatic drugs. What is the evidence? Scand J Rheumatol 1998;27(Suppl 107):119–124.
227. Friedman JM, Polifka JE: The Teratogen Information System, Online Knowledgebase, Seattle, University of Washington, 2004.
228. Hornby PJ, Abrahams TP: Pulmonary pharmacology. Clin Obstet Gynecol 1996;39:17.
229. Zierler S, Purohit D: Prenatal antihistamine exposure and retrolental fibroplasia. Am J Epidemiol 1986;123:192.
230. Hara GS, Carter RP, Krantz KE: Dramamine in labor: Potential boon or a possible bomb? J Kans Med Soc 1980;81:134.
231. Klieger JA, Massart JJ: Clinical and laboratory survey into the oxytocic effects of dimenhydrinate in labor. Am J Obstet Gynecol 1965;92:1.
232. Rotter CW, Whitaker JL, Yared J: The use of intravenous Dramamine to shorten the time of labor and potentiate analgesia. Am J Obstet Gynecol 1958;75:1101.
233. Seto A, Einarson T, Koren G: Evaluation of brompheniramine safety in pregnancy. Reprod Toxicol 1993;7:393.
234. Bracken MB, Berg A: Bendectin (Debendox) and congenital diaphragmatic hernia. Lancet 1983;1:586.
235. Eskenazi B, Bracken MB: Bendectin (Debendox) as a risk factor for pyloric stenosis. Am J Obstet Gynecol 1982;144:919.
236. Brent RR: The Bendectin saga: Another American tragedy (editorial). Teratology 1983;27:283.
237. Brent RR: Medical, social, and legal implications of treating nausea and vomiting of pregnancy. Am J Obstet Gynecol 2002;186(5 Suppl):S262–S266.
238. Schick B, Hom M, Librizzi R, et al: Terfenadine (Seldane) exposure in early pregnancy (abstract). Teratology 1994;49:417.
239. Greenberg G, Inman WHW, Weatherall JAC, et al: Maternal drug histories and congenital anomalies. Br Med J 1977;2:853.
240. Mellin GW: Drugs in the first trimester of pregnancy and the fetal life of *Homo sapiens*. Am J Obstet Gynecol 1964;90:1169.
241. Milkovich L, van den Berg BJ: An evaluation of the teratogenicity of certain antinauseant drugs. Am J Obstet Gynecol 1976;125:244.
242. Nelson MM, Forfar JO: Associations between drugs administered during pregnancy and congenital abnormalities of the fetus. Br Med J 1971;1:523.
243. Wilton LV, Pearce GL, Martin RM, et al: The outcomes of pregnancy in women exposed to newly marketed drugs in general practice in England. Br J Obstet Gynaecol 1998;105:882–889.
244. Einarson A, Bailey B, Jung G, et al: Prospective controlled study of hydroxyzine and cetirizine in pregnancy. Ann Allergy Asthma Immunol 1997;78:183–186.
245. Pastuszak A, Schick B, D'Alimonte D, et al: The safety of astemizole in pregnancy. J Allergy Clin Immunol 1996;98:748–750.
246. Schatz M, Zeiger RS, Harden K, et al: The safety of asthma and allergy medications during pregnancy. J Allergy Clin Immunol 1997;100:301–306.
247. Wilson J: Utilisation du cromoglycate de sodium au cours de la grossesse: Résultats sur 296 femmes asthmatiques. Acta Ther 1982;8(Suppl):45–51.
248. Howe JP, McGowan WAW, Moore J, et al: The placental transfer of cimetidine. Anaesthesia 1981;36:371.
249. Schenker S, Dicke J, Johnson RF, et al: Human placental transport of cimetidine. J Clin Invest 1987;80:1428.
250. Koren G, Zemlickis DM: Outcome of pregnancy after first trimester exposure to H2 receptor antagonists. Am J Perinatol 1991;8:37–38.
251. Magee LA, Inocencion G, Kamboj L, et al: Safety of first trimester exposure to histamine H2 blockers: A prospective cohort study. Dig Dis Sci 1996;41:1145–1149.
252. Kallen B: Delivery outcome after the use of acid-suppressing drugs in early pregnancy with special reference to omeprazole. Br J Obstet Gynaecol 1998;105:877–881.
253. Ruigomez A, Garcia-Rodriguez LA, Cattaruzzi C, et al: Use of cimetidine, omeprazole, and ranitidine in pregnant women and pregnancy outcomes. Am J Epidemiol 1999;150:476–481.
254. Gilstrap L, Little B: Gastrointestinal medications during pregnancy. In Gilstrap L, Little B (eds.) Drugs and Pregnancy. Oxford University Press; Cambridge, MA, 1999.
255. Lalkin A, Loebstein R, Addis A, et al: The safety of omeprazole during pregnancy: A multicenter prospective controlled study. Am J Obstet Gynecol 1998;179:727–730.
256. Moore J, Flynn RJ, Sampaio M, et al: Effect of single-dose omeprazole on intragastric acidity and volume during obstetric anaesthesia. Anaesthesia 1989;44:559–562.
257. Stuart JC, Kan AF, Rowbottom SJ, et al: Acid aspiration prophylaxis for emergency Caesarean section. Anaesthesia 1996;51: 415–421.
258. Kendall MJ: Review article: Esomeprazole: The first proton pump inhibitor to be developed as an isomer. Aliment Pharmacol Ther 2003;17:1365–2036.
259. Hill RM, Desmond MM, Kay JL: Extrapyramidal dysfunction in an infant of a schizophrenic mother. J Pediatr 1966;69:589.
260. Levy W, Wiseniewski K: Chlorpromazine causing extrapyramidal dysfunction in newborn infant of psychotic mother. NY State J Med 1974;74:684.

261. Kullander S, Kallen B: A prospective study of drugs and pregnancy: II. Anti-emetic drugs. Acta Obstet Gynecol Scand 1976;55:105.
262. Brent RR: Editorial comment or comments on "Teratogen Update: Bendectin™." Teratology 1985;31:429.
263. Holmes LB: Bendectin update. Teratology 1983;27:27.
264. Beckman DA, Brent RL: Mechanism of teratogenesis. Ann Rev Pharmacol Toxicol 1984;24:483–500.
265. Brent RL: Drugs and pregnancy: Are the insert warnings too dire? Contemp Obstet Gynecol 1982;20:42–49.
266. Federal Drug Administration: Pregnancy Labeling. FDA Drug Bull 1979;9:23–24.
267. Friedman JM, Little BB, Brent RL, et al: Potential human teratogenicity of frequently prescribed drugs. Obstet Gynecol 1990;75:594–599.

CHAPTER 36

Hypertension

Asnat Walfisch / Mordechai Hallak

INTRODUCTION

Hypertensive disorders of pregnancy are responsible for significant maternal and perinatal morbidity and are the second leading cause, after embolism, of maternal mortality.[1] Kaunitz and associates[2] reviewed the causes of maternal mortality in the United States and found that 421 (20%) of 2067 maternal deaths between 1974 and 1978 were related to hypertensive diseases. The clinical course of gestational hypertension is progressive and is characterized by continuous deterioration that is ultimately stopped only by delivery. Early detection and appropriate management of the pregnancy may improve the outcome for both the mother and the fetus.

Hypertensive disorders of pregnancy complicate approximately 12% to 22% of all pregnancies[3,4] and are directly responsible for 17.6% of maternal deaths in the United States. Gestational hypertension, which includes preeclampsia and eclampsia, is responsible for 70% of cases, whereas chronic hypertension represents 30% of hypertensive disorders in pregnancy.[5] Gestational hypertension is mainly a disease of young primigravidae, and accordingly, its incidence is higher in this group. The exact incidence of preeclampsia is unknown, but is approximately 5% to 8%.[6,7] The incidence was 14.1% in primigravidae versus 5.7% in multiparas among 2434 singleton pregnancies reported by Long and Oats.[8] The increased incidence of gestational hypertension in patients older than 35 years probably reflects undiagnosed chronic hypertension with superimposed gestational hypertension. The incidence of gestational hypertension is also increased in patients pregnant with twins (25.9%)[8] and in patients who had gestational hypertension in a previous pregnancy.[9] Other risk factors include pregestational diabetes, vascular or connective tissue disease, nephropathy, antiphospholipid antibody syndrome, obesity, positive family history, and African American race.[6,10–14]

The etiology of gestational hypertension is unknown, despite intensive research worldwide, and there is confusion about its classification, diagnosis, and treatment. More than 100 names have been given to the disease.[15] However, great advances in the understanding of the pathophysiology of gestational hypertension allow clinicians to better evaluate and manage patients. This progress is primarily responsible for the recent decline in maternal and perinatal mortality and morbidity rates.[16] This chapter emphasizes the most widely accepted knowledge about maternal and fetal risks and the management of the pregnant patient with hypertension.

DEFINITIONS

Several systems of classification of hypertensive disorders of pregnancy are used around the world. In 1972, the Committee on Terminology of the American College of Obstetricians and Gynecologists prepared a classification and definitions.[17] Table 36–1 shows a slight modification of this classification.[18] The modifications include eliminating edema from the diagnostic criteria and abandoning the use of changes in blood pressure as diagnostic.[19] Korotkoff phase V (disappearance), as opposed to phase IV (muffling), was chosen to determine the diastolic blood pressure because substantial data support its use.[20] The following definitions are proposed[19]:

Hypertension

Hypertension is defined as diastolic blood pressure of at least 90 mm Hg or systolic pressure of at least 140 mm Hg. Diastolic blood pressure is the pressure at which the sound disappears (Korotkoff phase V). These blood pressures must be recorded on at least two occasions 6 hours or more apart. Elevation of more than 30 mm Hg systolic

TABLE 36–1

Classification of Hypertensive Disorders in Pregnancy

Gestational hypertension
Preeclampsia
Mild
Severe
Eclampsia
Chronic hypertension before pregnancy (any etiology)
Chronic hypertension (any etiology) with superimposed gestational hypertension
Superimposed preeclampsia
Superimposed eclampsia

or more than 15 mm Hg diastolic above the patient's baseline is no longer part of the criteria and has not proved to be a good prognostic indicator.

Preeclampsia

Preeclampsia is defined as the development of hypertension, proteinuria, or both, after week 20 in a woman with previously normal blood pressure. It may be associated with many other signs and symptoms, such as edema, visual disturbances, headache, and epigastric pain. Preeclampsia may develop before week 20 in patients with extensive hydatidiform changes in the chorionic villi or in the presence of lupus anticoagulant. The following two types are recognized:

- Mild preeclampsia. No criterion for severe preeclampsia is present.
- Severe preeclampsia. One or more of the criteria shown in Table 36–2 are present.

Proteinuria

Proteinuria is defined as the presence of 300 mg/L or more protein in a 24-hour urine specimen. This finding usually correlates with a finding of +1 or greater, but should be confirmed with a random urine dipstick evaluation and 24-hour urine collection.

TABLE 36–2

Criteria for Severe Preeclampsia

Blood pressure reading, with the patient at rest, of at least 160 mm Hg systolic or 110 mm Hg diastolic pressure on two occasions at least 6 hours apart. In practice, after a diastolic pressure reading of 110 mm Hg, the clinician should not wait 6 hours for diagnosis and treatment.
Proteinuria levels of at least 5 g in 24-hour urine collection or 3+ to 4+ on semiquantitative assay collected at least 4 hours apart
Oliguria. 24-hour urinary output of less than 500 mL
Cerebral or visual disturbances, altered consciousness, headache, scotomata, or blurred vision
Pulmonary edema or cyanosis
Epigastric or right upper quadrant pain caused by stretching of Glisson's capsule. Occasionally, pain precedes hepatic rupture.
Impaired liver function of unclear etiology
Thrombocytopenia (postulated to be caused by platelet adherence to collagen exposed at sites of disrupted vascular endothelium)
Intrauterine growth restriction

Eclampsia

Eclampsia is defined as new-onset grand mal seizures in a woman whose condition also meets the criteria for preeclampsia when a coincidental neurologic disease, such as epilepsy, does not cause the convulsions.

Chronic Hypertension

Chronic hypertension is defined as persistent hypertension, of any cause, before week 20 in the absence of hydatidiform mole or persistent hypertension beyond 6 weeks postpartum.

Superimposed Preeclampsia or Eclampsia

Superimposed preeclampsia or eclampsia is defined as new-onset proteinuria in a woman with hypertension before 20 weeks' gestation. Other criteria include a sudden increase in proteinuria (if already present), a sudden increase in hypertension, and the development of hemolysis, elevated liver enzymes, and low platelet count (HELLP) syndrome in a woman with chronic hypertensive vascular or renal disease. Women with chronic hypertension who have headache, scotomata, or epigastric pain also may have superimposed preeclampsia.

PREECLAMPSIA AND ECLAMPSIA

Pathophysiology and Maternal and Fetal Risks

Although the etiology of preeclampsia is unknown, much of the literature focused on the degree of trophoblastic invasion by the placenta, which appears to be incomplete in preeclampsia.[21–23]

Cardiovascular System

The main feature of preeclampsia and eclampsia is hypertension. Blood pressure is a product of cardiac output and total peripheral resistance. Cardiac output increases in the first trimester of normal pregnancy, reaching a peak of 30% to 50% above the nonpregnant level. This increased output is maintained for the rest of the pregnancy.[24,25] This increase is maintained and rises further in patients with preeclampsia.[26,27] During normal pregnancy, total peripheral resistance decreases by 25%,[25,28] whereas in gestational hypertension, it increases.[26,27] This increase in peripheral vascular resistance appears to be the main cause of the elevation in blood pressure that is seen in gestational hypertension. Table 36–3 shows a comparison of the hemodynamic

TABLE 36-3

Comparison of the Hemodynamic Profile of Normal Nonpregnant Patients, Normal Pregnant (36–38 Weeks' Gestation) Patients, and Patients with Severe Pregnancy-Induced Hypertension (Mean, 35.4 Weeks' Gestation)

PARAMETER	NONPREGNANT PATIENT $N = 10$ MEAN (± SD)	% CHANGE	PREGNANT PATIENT $N = 10$ MEAN (± SD)	% CHANGE	SEVERE PIH $N = 45$ MEAN (± SD)
Heart rate (beats/min)	71 (10)	+17	83 (10)	+14	95 (13.4)
Cardiac output (L/min)	4.3 (0.9)	+43	6.2 (1)	+21	7.5 (1.5)
Mean arterial pressure (mm Hg)	86.4 (7.5)	NS	90.3 (5.8)	+53	138 (20)
Central venous pressure (mm Hg)	3.7 (2.6)	NS	3.6 (2.5)	NS	4 (6.7)
Pulmonary capillary wedge pressure (mmHg)	6.3 (2.1)	NS	7.5 (1.8)	+33	10 (6.7)
Colloid oncotic pressure (mm Hg)	20.8 (1)	−14	18 (1.5)	NS	19 (3.3)
Systemic vascular resistance (dyne × cm × sec^{-5})	1530 (520)	−21	1210 (266)	+24	1496 (428)
Pulmonary vascular resistance (dyne × cm × sec^{-5})	119 (47)	−34	78 (22)	NS	70 (33)
Left ventricular stroke work index (gm × m^{-2})	41 (8)	NS	48 (6)	+68	81 (13)

(The % change is significant at $p < 0.05$ in all values except when indicated as NS.)

profile of normal nonpregnant and pregnant women and patients with severe gestational hypertension, as measured by pulmonary artery catheterization.[25,26] Hemoconcentration, in addition to hypertension, is a significant vascular change because women with preeclampsia or eclampsia may not have the normal hypervolemia associated with pregnancy.[29]

Endocrine System

Alterations in vascular sensitivity to endogenous hormones (angiotensin II, catecholamines, and vasopressin) may have an important role in the increase in vascular resistance and elevated blood pressure seen in preeclampsia. In normal pregnancy, there is refractoriness to the pressor effect of angiotensin II.[30] Increased vascular reactivity to these pressor hormones is seen in patients with preeclampsia.[31,32] The abnormal sensitivity is acquired between week 17 and the clinical onset of gestational hypertension. Gant and colleagues[33] showed that loss of refractoriness to angiotensin II occurs 8 to 12 weeks before the appearance of the clinical manifestations of gestational hypertension.

The control of vascular tone and blood pressure achieved by angiotensin II is probably mediated by vascular endothelial synthesis of prostaglandins. The vascular response to angiotensin II is decreased by the use of prostaglandin inhibitors, indomethacin, and aspirin.[34,35] During normal pregnancy, production of prostacyclin and thromboxane A_2 increases, with a delicate balance that favors prostacyclin.[36] Prostacyclin, which is produced by the vascular endothelium, is a potent vasodilator and antiplatelet aggregant. Thromboxane A_2, which is produced by platelets and trophoblasts, is a potent vasoconstrictor and platelet aggregator. In preeclampsia, the ratio of thromboxane A_2 to prostacyclin is increased, with significantly decreased placental production of prostacyclin and significantly increased production of thromboxane A_2.[37] In addition, in gestational hypertension, a decreased amount of the prostacyclin metabolite 6-keto-prostaglandin $F_{1\alpha}$ was seen in maternal, placental, and umbilical vessels.[38,39] In patients with gestational hypertension, damaged endothelial cells may lead to decreased prostacyclin production in vessel walls and increased platelet activation, which in turn releases thromboxane A_2. This may result in an increased ratio of thromboxane A_2 to prostacyclin and may increase vascular tone and elevate blood pressure.

Hematologic System

During normal pregnancy, total blood volume increases by 50% by the end of the second trimester.[29] More of the increase is caused by the expansion of plasma than by erythrocytes, leading to the physiologic anemia of pregnancy. In gestational hypertension, the expansion in blood volume is reduced (16%).[29] The hemoconcentration seen in gestational hypertension can result in decreased regional perfusion. In these patients, in the absence of hemorrhage, the intravascular compartment is not underfilled because of the increase in vascular tone and vasospasm. Clinically, hematocrit increases with increased severity of gestational hypertension.[29] Vasospasm and subsequent hemoconcentration are associated with contraction of the intravascular space. Attempts to expand the intravascular space with fluid therapy may increase pulmonary wedge pressure and cause pulmonary edema as a result of associated capillary leak.[40]

The vasospasm that is part of the pathophysiology of gestational hypertension is likely to result in endothelial injury. Dadak and associates[41] found marked damage to the endothelium of the umbilical arteries of mothers with gestational hypertension. The injury to the endothelium could be the cause of the microangiopathic hemolysis that accompanies gestational hypertension. It causes thrombocytopenia, anemia, and fragmentation of red blood cells.

Gestational hypertension is also associated with high levels of fibronectin, low levels of antithrombin III, and low levels of α_2-antiplasmin.[42,43] These changes may reflect endothelial damage (high fibronectin levels),[44] clotting (low antithrombin III levels), and fibrinolysis (low α_2- antiplasmin levels). Changes in the levels of these factors can aid in the diagnosis of preeclampsia and help to differentiate it from chronic hypertension.[45–47]

Thrombocytopenia and hemolysis may occur as part of the HELLP syndrome. Thus, interpretation of hematocrit levels should take this into consideration. Lactate dehydrogenase is present in erythrocytes in high concentration, and when elevated, may be a sign of hemolysis.

Kidney

Renal blood flow and the glomerular filtration rate increase considerably during normal pregnancy. In women with gestational hypertension, renal perfusion decreases by an average of 20% and the glomerular filtration rate decreases by an average of 32% compared with normal pregnant women near term.[48] Oliguria, commonly defined as less than 500 mL in 24 hours, may occur as a result of hemoconcentration and decreased renal blood flow. Rarely, persistent oliguria reflects acute tubular necrosis.

Some consider the microscopic changes seen in renal biopsy specimens from women with preeclampsia to be pathognomonic of the disease. Characteristic changes include glomerular capillary endothelial swelling accompanied by deposits of fibrinogen derivatives within and under the endothelial cells.[49] This constellation of lesions was designated by Spargo and colleagues[50] as glomerular capillary endotheliosis. The swollen endothelial cells block the capillary lumens. Resolution of the glomerular changes occurs within several weeks postpartum.

Liver

In preeclampsia accompanied by HELLP syndrome, an elevation in liver function test results is noted. Alanine aminotransferase and aspartate aminotransferase levels may be elevated. Hyperbilirubinemia may occur, especially in the presence of hemolysis. Periportal hemorrhagic necrosis in the periphery of the liver lobule is probably the lesion that causes elevated serum liver enzyme levels. Bleeding from these lesions or from the liver capsule can lead to subcapsular hematomas. Hemorrhage under the liver capsule can be so severe that the capsule ruptures and causes life-threatening intraperitoneal bleeding. In this case, laparotomy with packing and drainage may prove lifesaving.[51]

Brain

Cerebral blood flow and cerebral oxygen metabolism are usually unaltered by gestational hypertension, whereas cerebral vascular resistance is significantly increased in gestational hypertension compared with normal pregnancy.[52] Cerebral blood volume response, measured noninvasively by near-infrared spectroscopy, provided additional evidence of altered cerebral hemodynamics in women with preeclampsia.[53] Approximately one-third of patients who died of eclampsia had cerebral hemorrhage, ranging from petechiae to large hematomas.[54] Sibai and associates[55] reported nonspecific, transient abnormal electroencephalographic findings in 75% of patients after eclamptic convulsion. Hypodense cortical areas corresponding to hemorrhages and local edema were the most common findings in computed topographic head scans of patients with eclampsia.[56] Although it is uncommon, temporary, and even permanent,[57] blindness may accompany severe preeclampsia.[58] Other central nervous system manifestations include headache, blurred vision, and hyper-reflexia.

Uteroplacental Circulation

In normal human pregnancy, the spiral arteries in the placental bed progressively lose their musculoelastic tissue by migration of trophoblasts into their walls. These trophoblast-induced changes involve the entire length of the spiral artery, from the intervillous space to its origin in the inner third of the myometrium. This process widens the spiral arteries and creates a low-resistance, low-pressure, high-flow system that allows the increased blood supply to reach the pregnant uterus.[59] The first stage of these changes may involve the decidual part of the spiral arteries and occurs in the first trimester. The second stage starts at 16 weeks' gestation, and the process progresses to the myometrium.[59]

In women with gestational hypertension, small-for-gestational-age fetuses, and diabetes mellitus, trophoblast-induced changes are restricted to the decidual arteries. Myometrial segments of the spiral arteries are left with their musculoelastic architecture, which make them sensitive to vasomotor influences.[59] This process may account for the twofold to threefold decrease in uteroplacental perfusion seen in hypertensive patients compared with normotensive women.[60]

Some histologic changes in the uteroplacental vessels that are seen in gestational hypertension are considered pathognomonic and termed "acute atherosis."[61] Microscopic vascular findings include endothelial cell damage, basement membrane disruption, platelet deposition, mural thrombi, fibrinoid necrosis, proliferation of intimal cells and myointimal hyperplasia, hyperplasia of smooth muscle cells, extensive lipid necrosis of myointimal and smooth muscle cells, and an increase in smooth muscle cells with vasospasm that leads to a decreased vessel lumen.[61–63]

Perinatal Mortality

The perinatal mortality rate is increased in preeclampsia, especially in patients with severe preeclampsia. Individual contributing factors include preterm delivery, uteroplacental insufficiency, abruptio placentae, and unexplained fetal death.

Preterm delivery is often necessitated because definitive treatment of preeclampsia mandates termination of pregnancy, regardless of gestational age. The uteroplacental bed is not spared the vasoconstrictive effects of preeclampsia. Therefore, this decrease in perfusion can result in fetal growth restriction, reduced amniotic fluid volume, and an inability to tolerate the in utero environment. Abruptio placentae also may occur. This complication is more common in pregnancies complicated by severe preeclampsia, HELLP syndrome, and superimposed preeclampsia.[64]

Management Options

Prenatal

PREDICTION

Many clinical and laboratory parameters have been used to predict preeclampsia, with varying degrees of success. The ideal predictive test should be simple, noninvasive, rapid, inexpensive, easy to perform early in pregnancy, and reproducible, with high sensitivity and predictive value. No single screening test for preeclampsia is reliable and cost-effective.[65–67] The "rollover" test was introduced more than 20 years ago to predict the development of preeclampsia as early as 28 to 32 weeks, but it did not have high specificity.[68] Increased vascular reactivity to intravenous infusion of angiotensin II, as shown by an increased pressure response, is predictive as early as 26 weeks' gestation.[33,69] In the 1980s, high plasma cellular fibronectin levels showed promise, but the test has not developed into a useful clinical tool.[70–72] Increased platelet angiotensin II receptors,[73] increased platelet intracellular calcium levels when exposed to arginine vasopressin,[74] decreased urinary calcium excretion,[75] higher fasting insulin levels,[76] increased mean arterial pressure early in pregnancy,[77] positive isometric exercise testing,[78] microalbuminuria, decreased platelet count, elevated hematocrit,[79–81] high second-trimester plasma homocysteine concentrations,[82] and low maternal serum pregnancy-associated plasma protein A (PAPP-A) or β human chorionic gonadotropin (βhCG)[83] have been used to predict preeclampsia. Increased serum uric acid level[84] is one of the most commonly used tests, but has a positive predictive value of only 33%.[85] Campbell and associates[86] reported that Doppler velocimetry of the uterine and umbilical vessels can predict preeclampsia as early as 18 weeks. Patients with preeclampsia had a characteristic notching of the diastolic waveform, suggesting increased peripheral vascular resistance. Doppler may be useful to monitor the course of hypertensive disorders of pregnancy and the treatment effect, but is not useful for screening pregnant women at low risk.[65,87] None of these predictive tests is used in clinical practice, primarily because they do not meet the criteria for a good predictor.

PREVENTION

The lack of understanding of the underlying pathophysiology of preeclampsia impeded attempts at prevention. Several empiric approaches have been studied, with varying degrees of success. These include dietary supplementation, antioxidants, diuretics, antihypertensives, and low-dose aspirin.

Manipulations of sodium, magnesium, and calcium intake have received interest. However, prospective trials have not produced consistent results. Supplementation with calcium, the best studied cation, shows the most promise. Epidemiologic data show an inverse relationship between calcium intake and eclampsia.[88] Animal and human data suggest that calcium supplementation can significantly reduce blood pressure. Studies in pregnant women are limited, but suggest that calcium can lower blood pressure and reduce the incidence of preeclampsia.[89] A meta-analysis of several small trials of calcium supplementation showed a significant reduction in the incidence of preeclampsia.[90] Calcium supplementation given in pregnancy to high-risk nulliparas (angiotensin II-sensitive patients) reduced the incidence of pregnancy-induced hypertension in a double-blind trial.[91] However, calcium did not prevent preeclampsia in healthy nulliparas in a prospective study of 4589 patients.[92] Additional data and reliable predictive tests are needed before calcium can be recommended to prevent preeclampsia in a high-risk population.

Recently, antioxidant therapy with vitamin C 1000 mg/day and vitamin E 400 mg/day showed promise in preventing preeclampsia.[93] These results need confirmation in larger randomized trials. Prophylactic administration of diuretics or antihypertensives did not prevent preeclampsia.[94] However, one report showed a decreased incidence of proteinuria in hypertensive gravidas treated with atenolol.[95] This preliminary finding requires additional study. A meta-analysis of randomized studies of antihypertensives given to women with chronic hypertension showed no effect on the incidence of superimposed preeclampsia.[96]

Aspirin inhibits the enzyme cyclooxygenase, which is essential for the synthesis of prostaglandins, such as thromboxane A_2 and prostacyclin.[97] Low-dose aspirin (60–80 mg/day) selectively inhibits platelet thromboxane A_2 release, but does not affect endothelial cell production of prostacyclin. On this basis, recent clinical trials focused on low-dose aspirin as a preventive agent.

Several large randomized multicenter clinical trials evaluated the safety and effectiveness of low-dose aspirin in preventing preeclampsia. The National Institute of

Health sponsored the Maternal-Fetal Medicine Network study of 2985 healthy, normotensive, nulliparous women who were randomized to receive aspirin versus placebo at 13 to 26 weeks' gestation.[98] The results showed a decreased incidence of preeclampsia in nulliparous patients (by 26%), no decrease in perinatal morbidity, and an increased risk of abruptio placentae. The authors recommended against the routine use of low-dose aspirin in healthy nulliparous women. In a recent study, the same group concluded that aspirin therapy did not reduce the incidence of preeclampsia in high-risk women.[99] The CLASP study included 9364 patients in 213 centers located in 16 countries, including patients at risk for preeclampsia.[100] The findings did not support the routine prophylactic or therapeutic use of low-dose aspirin to all women at increased risk for preeclampsia. The current literature does not support the routine use of low-dose aspirin to prevent preeclampsia. However, a recent randomized double-blind placebo-controlled trial showed some benefit of low-dose aspirin in reducing the incidence of preeclampsia in women with bilateral uterine artery notching.[101]

DIAGNOSIS

Signs.

Blood Pressure. High blood pressure is the hallmark of gestational hypertension. Blood pressure is taken with the patient in an upright position, after a 10-minute rest period. A mercury sphygmomanometer is preferred.[3] Sibai[4] suggested that blood pressure should be taken in a sitting position in ambulatory patients and in a semireclining position in hospitalized patients. The right arm should be used for the measurement, and the arm should be placed in a horizontal position at heart level. The increase in blood pressure reflects the arteriolar vasospasm that is basic to preeclampsia.

Proteinuria. In early preeclampsia, proteinuria is minimal. Proteinuria develops as the disease progresses and usually occurs after the development of hypertension and weight gain.[102,103] However, proteinuria accompanied by hypertension is the most reliable indicator of fetal morbidity and mortality.[104] Urine protein levels are affected by several factors and fluctuate in the same patient from hour to hour.[4] Therefore, a semiquantitative assay is unreliable, and a definitive diagnosis of proteinuria depends on the total amount of protein excreted in a 24-hour urine collection period.

Edema. Edema is an early, nonspecific sign of preeclampsia. Rapid weight gain of 5 pounds or more in 1 week is considered a warning sign.[18] However, edema occurs in 35% of normotensive patients.[105] Chesley[106] reviewed the literature and concluded that most women with rapid weight gain do not have preeclampsia and that preeclampsia occurs in the absence of this finding. Moreover, in one series, rapid weight gain of 5 pounds or more in 1 week occurred in only 10% of patients with eclampsia.[106] Therefore, only generalized edema that involves the body and face after 12 hours of bed rest is considered clearly abnormal.[18] Some investigators preclude edema as a prerequisite for the diagnosis of preeclampsia.[4]

Deep Tendon Reflexes. Hyper-reflexia is not considered a sign of preeclampsia or eclampsia. Although normal women may have hyper-reflexia and eclamptic seizures can occur in the absence of hyper-reflexia,[107] it is a common clinical impression that increased reflexes and clonus are signs of imminent eclampsia.

Retinal Changes. Spasm of the retinal arterioles is the physical finding that correlates best with the renal biopsy changes associated with preeclampsia.[108] It occurred in 85% of patients reported by Pollak and Nettles.[108] Segmental arteriolar spasm or generalized narrowing is usually seen.

Symptoms.

Cerebral. Headache, dizziness, tinnitus, drowsiness, and altered consciousness are common in severe preeclampsia and almost invariably precede an eclamptic convulsion. These symptoms indicate poor cerebral perfusion.

Visual. Symptoms may include blurred vision, diplopia, scotomata, blindness as a result of retinal arterial spasm, edema, and retinal detachment. The pathophysiology of these symptoms can also be vasospasm, ischemia, and hemorrhage in the occipital cortex.[56]

Gastrointestinal. Nausea, vomiting, and epigastric or right upper quadrant pain and hematemesis are caused by distention of Glisson's capsule by edema and hemorrhage. These are symptoms of severe preeclampsia and can precede hepatic rupture and convulsions.

Renal. Oliguria, anuria, and hematuria are symptoms of severe preeclampsia that may be caused by renal artery vasospasm.

Laboratory Findings and Clinical Tests.

Renal Function. Creatinine clearance is used to detect changes in glomerular filtration. Creatinine clearance decreases as the severity of preeclampsia increases. The serum uric acid concentration also predicts preeclampsia and perinatal outcome.[109] Serum creatinine concentration and blood urea nitrogen are also valuable tests to evaluate renal function.

Liver Function. Serum glutamic oxaloacetic transaminase (SGOT), serum glutamic pyruvic transaminase (SGPT), and lactate dehydrogenase (LDH) levels are increased in severe gestational hypertension and HELLP syndrome.[110,111] Elevated liver function test results may also indicate subcapsular hematoma and imminent liver rupture.

Hematologic Findings and Hemostasis. As the severity of gestational hypertension increases, hemoconcentration and hypoalbuminemia develop. The serum fibrinogen level, prothrombin time, and partial thromboplastin time are usually normal. Fibrinogen degradation products are increased, and thrombin time is usually prolonged. Thrombocytopenia is another sign of severe preeclampsia.[18] A decreased platelet count (<100,000/mm^3) is also part of HELLP syndrome.[110] Intravascular hemolysis is another feature of HELLP syndrome and is detected by evaluation of the peripheral smear and by elevated bilirubin, SGOT, and LDH levels.

Rollover Test. A positive rollover test result is defined as an increase in diastolic blood pressure of 20 mm Hg or more when measured 5 minutes after a gravida is "rolled" from the lateral to the supine position between 28 and 32 weeks' gestation.[68] Gant found that 93% of primigravid women with a positive rollover test result later had gestational hypertension and 91% of women who had a negative test result did not have hypertension during that pregnancy.[68] However, the value of this test as a clinical screening tool is debatable. In a study by Phelan and colleagues,[112] the rollover test predicted gestational hypertension in 78% of patients who subsequently had the disease, but the false-positive rate was 60%. Andersen[113] studied 191 patients and concluded that the test is not sufficiently reliable, sensitive, or specific for clinical use as a screening test.

Angiotensin II Test. A normal pregnant patient requires mean angiotensin II doses of 13.5 to 14.9 ng/kg/minute to increase diastolic blood pressure by 20 mm Hg. Ninety-one percent of women who require more than 8 ng/kg/minute to achieve this blood pressure elevation remained normotensive throughout pregnancy.[38] Conversely, normotensive primigravidae who later had gestational hypertension responded at doses of less than 8 ng/kg/minute as early as 28 to 32 weeks' gestation. Ninety percent of these patients later had overt gestational hypertension.[38]

DIFFERENTIAL DIAGNOSIS

Patients with preeclampsia, liver involvement, and epigastric or right upper quadrant abdominal pain can be misdiagnosed. Alternative diagnoses include hepatitis, gallbladder disease, peptic ulcer, gastroenteritis, pyelonephritis, nephrolithiasis, Reye's syndrome, acute fatty liver of pregnancy (AFLP), thrombotic thrombocytopenic purpura (TTP), and hemolytic uremic syndrome (HUS).

TTP is an uncommon entity characterized by fever, neurologic and renal abnormalities, thrombocytopenia, and hemolytic anemia.[114] The patient may have abnormal bleeding from mucous membranes, headache, visual disturbances, seizures, syncope, paresis, altered consciousness, other neurologic symptoms, jaundice, and fever.[114] The peripheral blood smear indicates microangiopathic hemolysis that includes anemia, with fragmented erythrocytes, reticulocytosis, and thrombocytopenia. These changes lead to elevation of indirect serum bilirubin and LDH levels as well as slight elevation of serum blood urea nitrogen and creatinine concentrations. Differentiating between TTP in pregnancy and the postpartum period and preeclampsia or eclampsia is difficult. Some investigators suggest that every case should be treated as preeclampsia unless the diagnosis of TTP was made before pregnancy or there is no evidence of pregnancy-induced hypertension.[115] New treatment modalities for TTP that include plasmapheresis or plasma infusion can be given during pregnancy and the postpartum period when the diagnosis of TTP is secure.[116] When the differential diagnosis between TTP and severe preeclampsia or eclampsia is difficult, it is reasonable to use both plasmapheresis and standard preeclampsia treatment. However, with available data, this approach cannot be recommended with certainty.

Microangiopathic hemolysis, thrombocytopenia, renal failure, and altered consciousness and seizures are also hallmarks of HUS (see also Chapters 41 and 80). However, these patients usually have a history of viral or bacterial gastrointestinal infection. Renal failure occurs early in the course of disease and is usually severe, whereas thrombocytopenia and bleeding are less severe than in TTP. The neurologic symptoms are less remarkable and usually correlate with the severity of renal failure and hypertensive encephalopathy. HUS is more common in children, although cases during pregnancy and postpartum are reported.[117] Finally, because HUS is being treated with plasma exchange, in the same way as TTP, the absolute diagnosis is less important and the same considerations should be applied in pregnancy and the postpartum period.[118]

AFLP (see Chapter 48) is an uncommon, potentially fatal disorder that may complicate the third trimester.[119] If it is unrecognized or untreated, AFLP may progress to fulminant hepatic failure, with jaundice, encephalopathy, disseminated intravascular coagulation, uncontrollable gastrointestinal and uterine bleeding, and death.[120] Early recognition of the disorder, rapid termination of pregnancy once the diagnosis was made, and intensive supportive treatment decreased fetal and maternal mortality rates considerably.[120] The differentiation of gestational hypertension with liver involvement from AFLP is difficult and sometimes impossible, and some investigators wonder whether these conditions are variants of the same disease.

Both conditions occur in primigravidae, mostly in the third trimester. They are common in twin gestations, improve with delivery, and include liver involvement, with elevated serum transaminase levels, low platelet counts, coagulopathy, hyperuricemia, hypoglycemia, and low antithrombin III levels. The elevated blood pressure and proteinuria that characterize preeclampsia may be present in patients with AFLP, and the liver histology is similar in some patients.[121,122] The management of severe preeclampsia with liver involvement is similar to the management of AFLP, making the differentiation between the two less important. Both conditions require prompt delivery and maternal supportive care.[119]

Acute cholecystitis, choledocholithiasis, and cholangitis may occur in pregnancy, leading to right upper quadrant pain, but are not associated with hepatic failure, coagulopathy, or other signs and symptoms of gestational hypertension. Ultrasonography of the right upper quadrant detects gallstones and a dilated bile duct.

Viral hepatitis[123] is the most common cause of hepatic dysfunction in pregnancy,[124] but is not usually associated with liver failure, disseminated intravascular coagulation, or hypertension and proteinuria. Acute hepatitis can be diagnosed by serologic tests. Fulminant viral hepatitis, which can cause hypoglycemia, disseminated intravascular coagulation,[125] and encephalopathy, may be difficult to distinguish from severe preeclampsia and AFLP.[123] Peak levels of SGOT and SGPT vary from 400 to 4000 IU; much lower levels are seen in pregnancy-induced hypertension.[126] The absence of thrombocytopenia and hyperuricemia, which coexist with pregnancy-induced hypertension, can also help with the differential diagnosis. Drug-induced hepatitis is usually identified from the clinical history. Drugs that are associated with hepatitis include halothane, diphenylhydantoin, α-methyldopa, isoniazid, and chlorothiazide. Tetracycline can also cause fatty liver syndrome.[127]

Reye's syndrome also causes fatty liver and hepatic encephalopathy, but it usually occurs in children. Twelve cases were reported in adults.[128] These patients had hypouricemia, and their hepatic histologic features differed from those in patients with gestational hypertension.[128]

Patients with peptic ulcer disease, gastroenteritis, pyelonephritis, and nephrolithiasis may have epigastric or abdominal pain, but the absence of other signs of gestational hypertension should help with the differential diagnosis.

Management Options

The goals of therapy are the following:

- Prevent convulsions
- Prevent complications, such as cerebrovascular hemorrhage, pulmonary edema, renal failure, abruptio placentae, and fetal death
- Deliver a surviving child with minimal trauma to the mother

Prenatal

Management of the patient with mild gestational hypertension is shown in Table 36–4. Induction of labor is reserved for patients who have reached 37 weeks' gestation when the fetus is mature and the cervical condition is favorable.[18] If the cervix is unfavorable, results of fetal evaluation are normal, and maternal blood pressure is stable, the patient may be followed beyond 37 weeks. For an immature fetus, watchful observation may be indicated until fetal maturity is documented and the cervix is favorable. If observation is indicated for pregnancy-induced hypertension, several parameters should be evaluated because their deterioration may be an indication

TABLE 36–4

Management of Mild Preeclampsia

COMPLIANT, IMPROVING PATIENT	NONCOMPLIANT OR NONIMPROVING PATIENT
Preterm or Immature Fetus: Expectant Management	
Ambulatory management:	Hospitalization:
See the patient twice weekly	Measure urine protein daily
Fetal surveillance	Fetal surveillance
Bed rest	Bed rest
Educate the patient about the increasing severity of the disease	Regular diet, with no salt restriction
Weigh the patient daily	Weigh the patient daily
Monitor blood pressure	Obtain blood pressure 4 times daily
FAVORABLE CERVIX	**UNFAVORABLE CERVIX AND NORMAL FINDINGS ON FETAL SURVEILLANCE***
Term or Mature Fetus	
Definitive management:	Expectant management:
Prevent convulsions	Hospitalization
Induce labor	

*Fetal surveillance includes tests of fetal well-being, including but not limited to fetal movement charts, contraction stress tests, nonstress tests, and biophysical profiles.

for delivery (Table 36–5). No randomized controlled trials have shown the best test for fetal evaluation.

Several antihypertensive drugs are used to treat the preterm patient with mild preeclampsia in an attempt to prolong the pregnancy and improve neonatal outcome. These include β-blockers, including β_1-selective and nonselective agents; α_1-antagonists, α_2-agonists; calcium channel blockers; vasodilators; and diuretics.[4] The use of

TABLE 36–5

Parameters That Indicate Delivery in a Patient with Gestational Hypertension

PARAMETER	INDICATION FOR DELIVERY
Maternal	
Blood pressure	≥160/110 mm Hg
Platelet count	<100,000 mm^3
Serum fibrinogen	<150 mg/dL
Serum glutamic-oxaloacetic transaminase, Serum glutamic pyruvic transaminase	Any elevation
Blood urea nitrogen	≥30 mg/dL
Creatinine	≥1.2 mg/dL
Creatinine clearance	<50 mL/min
Fetal	
Nonstress test, oxytocin challenge test, BPP (weekly or twice weekly for suspected intrauterine growth restriction or oligohydramnios)	Nonreactive nonstress test with positive oxytocin challenge test or abnormal BPP
Ultrasonic biometry (every 3 wks)	Severe intrauterine growth restriction

BPP, biophysical profile.

these drugs for the preterm patient with mild preeclampsia is controversial. However, studies of perinatal outcome in hospitalized patients with or without treatment show no advantage of long-term antihypertensive therapy in preeclampsia.[129]

Hospitalization is often initially recommended for women with new-onset preeclampsia. After the initial assessment, subsequent management of mild gestational hypertension or preeclampsia remote from term may be continued in an outpatient setting or at home. If this management is selected, it should include frequent maternal and fetal evaluation and access to health care providers. Admission to an outpatient unit instead of hospitalization for nonproteinuric hypertension reduces the time spent in the hospital and the proportion of women with induced labor.[130] If the patient's condition worsens, hospitalization is indicated. Management of the patient with severe gestational hypertension is best accomplished in a tertiary care setting (Table 36–6). Controversy surrounds the treatment of the patient with severe gestational hypertension when the fetus is immature but is not growth-restricted or in jeopardy. Some institutions follow the mother and fetus conservatively until maturity is achieved or maternal or fetal jeopardy develops. However, the perinatal and maternal outcome of these pregnancies is extremely poor.[131,132] Jenkins and associates[133] retrospectively reviewed maternal and neonatal outcome in patients with severe preeclampsia before 25 weeks' gestation. They concluded that delivery was associated with minimal short-term maternal morbidity, although the rates of neonatal morbidity and death were appreciable (only 10% survival, all with severe handicaps).

Labor and Delivery

FLUID THERAPY

During labor, patients with preeclampsia should remain in the left lateral position, with continuous electronic fetal heart rate monitoring. After rupture of the membranes, a scalp electrode and an internal uterine pressure catheter should be placed. Intravenous fluids, consisting of a balanced salt solution, should be infused at a rate of 75 to 125 mL/hour. Strict attention should be paid to urine output, and a Foley catheter may be needed, especially if preeclampsia is severe.

TABLE 36–6

Management of Severe Preeclampsia

MATURE FETUS OR IMMATURE FETUS WITH GROWTH RETARDATION OR FETAL JEOPARDY
Definitive Management
Prevent convulsions (magnesium sulfate)
Control blood pressure (hydralazine)
Deliver by vaginal or cesarean birth, depending on fetal and maternal conditions

Oliguria is defined as less than 0.5 mL/kg/hour over 2 consecutive hours. Oliguria is usually treated by prompt delivery. Under controlled conditions, a bolus of 500 to 1000 mL balanced salt solution can be administered. Careful attention is given to symptoms and signs of pulmonary edema. It may be necessary to follow blood oxygen saturation with a pulse oximeter when a fluid challenge is initiated without invasive monitoring to predict and prevent incipient pulmonary edema.

A fluid bolus of 1000 mL should be given at the time of vasodilator therapy. This results in a smoother and more gradual reduction in blood pressure and prevents the abrupt and profound drops in blood pressure that may be seen with vasodilator therapy in hypovolemic patients.[134] If a marked intake–output imbalance is noted, restriction of fluids to 50 mL/hour is advisable.

PREVENTION OF CONVULSIONS WITH MAGNESIUM SULFATE

Magnesium sulfate is considered the standard agent for the prevention and treatment of eclamptic convulsions in North America. The American College of Obstetricians and Gynecologists recommends the use of magnesium sulfate in every woman with a diagnosis of preeclampsia or eclampsia during labor and the postpartum period.[18] Although there is no unanimity of opinion on the prophylactic use of magnesium sulfate to prevent seizures in women with mild preeclampsia or gestational hypertension, a significant body of evidence attests to its efficacy in severe preeclampsia and eclampsia.[135–138] Two accepted regimens for parenteral magnesium sulfate therapy are shown in Table 36–7. Magnesium sulfate has a dual action. It interferes with transmission at the neuromuscular junction and also affects the central nervous system. Magnesium sulfate had central anticonvulsant

TABLE 36–7

Prevention and Treatment of Convulsions with Magnesium Sulfate

Pritchard Protocol
Loading Dose
Give 4 g (20 mL of 20%) IV over 4 minutes (only in severe preeclampsia or eclampsia), immediately followed by 10 g (20 mL of 50%) IM, 5 g in each buttock
If convulsions persist after 15 minutes, give 2 g (10 mL of 20%) IV over 2 minutes (if the woman is large, give 4 g)
Maintenance
Give 5 g (10 mL of 50%) IM every 4 hours, on alternate sides
Sibai Protocol
Loading Dose
Give 6 g IV over 20 minutes
Maintenance
Give 2–3 g/hr IV
At the time of convulsion, give 2 to 4 g by IV bolus over 5 minutes
If convulsion recurs, give amobarbital sodium 250 mg IV over 3 minutes
As a last measure, give a paralyzing agent and perform intubation

activity in an animal model, inhibiting the *N*-methyl-D-aspartate receptor in the brain.[139–142] These objective data and a vast amount of clinical experience support the use of magnesium sulfate for seizure prophylaxis.

The hypotensive effect of magnesium sulfate is transient and related to bolus administration and rapid infusion.[143] Continuous infusion does not maintain hypotension, and the dosages used for gestational hypertension do not depress myocardial work. Therefore, they do not usually contribute to myocardial compromise.[143–145]

To continue magnesium sulfate treatment, the patient should have a patellar reflex, urine flow greater than 30 mL/hour, respiratory rate greater than 12 beats/minute, and magnesium blood levels of 4 to 8 mg/dL, if obtained.[18] Table 36–8 shows the relationship between blood levels of magnesium sulfate and symptoms and signs. Magnesium toxicity can be reversed by slow intravenous administration of 10% calcium gluconate and nasal administration of oxygen. If toxicity is not reversed, respirations must be supported until plasma magnesium levels decrease.

Alternative anticonvulsant drugs have been recommended. Recently, phenytoin was mentioned as the drug of choice, but its safety and efficacy in eclampsia are not proven.[144] In the United States, magnesium sulfate is the standard drug used to treat and prevent eclamptic convulsions.

CONTROL OF HYPERTENSION

Careful control of hypertension must be achieved to prevent complications, such as maternal cerebrovascular accidents and placental abruption. Although no large randomized clinical trials compared treatment with placebo, antihypertensive therapy is usually recommended when systolic blood pressure exceeds 180 mm Hg or diastolic blood pressure exceeds 110 mm Hg.[6,19,145,146] A recent meta-analysis investigated the benefits of oral antihypertensives for mild to moderate gestational hypertension and concluded that treatment-induced decreases in maternal blood pressure may adversely affect fetal growth. Therefore, this treatment should be used cautiously.[147] Although many antihypertensive agents are available, this discussion focuses on the agents that are most commonly used to treat acute hypertensive crises in pregnancy. Hydralazine is the most widely accepted drug to treat hypertension in severe preeclampsia.[18] A method of administration is shown in Table 36–9.[148] Hydralazine increases heart rate and cardiac output and decreases mean arterial pressure and systemic vascular resistance.[134] Hydralazine carries the risk of a potentially harmful effect on the fetoplacental unit in the face of hypovolemia. It causes abrupt, profound decreases in blood pressure unless a fluid bolus is administered concomitantly.[139] Hypertension refractory to hydralazine therapy warrants central hemodynamic monitoring and the use of more potent antihypertensive agents.[149,150]

Labetalol is a combined α- and β-adrenoreceptor antagonist that may be used to induce a controlled, rapid decrease in blood pressure through decreased systemic vascular resistance in patients with severe hypertension. Reports on the efficacy and safety of labetalol in the treatment of hypertension during pregnancy are favorable.[151–154] Mabie and colleagues[152] compared bolus intravenous labetalol with intravenous hydralazine in the acute treatment of severe hypertension and found that labetalol had a more rapid onset of action and did not result in reflex tachycardia. Labetalol may exert a positive effect on early fetal lung maturation in patients with severe hypertension who are remote from term.[151] Lunell and associates[153] studied the effects of labetalol on uteroplacental perfusion in pregnant women with hypertension and noted increased uteroplacental perfusion and decreased uterine vascular resistance.

Labetalol can be administered parenterally by repeated intravenous injection or slow continuous infusion. An initial dose of 20 mg is administered, followed by additional doses of 40 or 80 mg at 10-minute intervals, until the desired effect is achieved or a total of 220 mg has been given. If a continuous infusion is used, labetalol is initiated at a dose of 2 mg/minute. Maximum effect is seen approximately 5 minutes after intravenous administration. Oral dosage of labetalol begins at 100 mg twice daily and can be increased to a maximum of 2400 mg/day.

Sodium nitroprusside is another potent antihypertensive agent that may be used to control severe hypertension. A dilute solution may be started at 0.25 mg/kg/minute and titrated to the desired effect by increasing the dose by 0.25 mg/kg/minute every 5 minutes. The solution is light-sensitive and should be covered in foil and changed every 24 hours. Arterial blood gases should be monitored to watch for developing metabolic acidosis, which may be an early sign of cyanide toxicity. Treatment

TABLE 36–8

Magnesium Sulfate Blood Levels

BLOOD LEVELS	SYMPTOMS AND SIGNS
4–8 mg/dL	Therapeutic
9–12 mg/dL	Nausea, warmth, flushing, somnolence, double vision, slurred speech, weakness, loss of patellar reflexes
15–17 mg/dL	Muscular paralysis and respiratory arrest
30–35 mg/dL	Cardiac arrest

TABLE 36–9

Control of Blood Pressure with Hydralazine

Give hydralazine intermittently as a bolus to patients with diastolic blood pressure greater than 110 mm Hg

Give 5 to 10 mg as an intravenous bolus with dosage intervals no less than every 20 minutes until blood pressure is controlled

Monitor blood pressure every 2 to 5 minutes

The goal of therapy is to decrease diastolic blood pressure to 90 to 100 mm Hg time should be limited because of the potential for fetal cyanide toxicity.[155] Hypovolemia must be corrected before the initiation of nitroprusside infusion to avoid abrupt and often profound decreases in blood pressure.

Nifedipine is administered at an initial oral dose of 10 mg, which may be repeated after 30 minutes, if necessary, for the acute management of severe hypertension; then 10 to 20 mg may be administered orally every 6 to 8 hours, as needed. Care must be taken when nifedipine is administered to patients who are receiving concomitant magnesium sulfate because an exaggerated hypotensive response may occur.[156] Nifedipine appears safe for the treatment of hypertensive crisis in pregnancy, but further controlled clinical trials are needed before the drug is accepted for general clinical use.

Nitroglycerin relaxes predominantly venous, but also arterial, vascular smooth muscle. It decreases preload at low doses and afterload in high doses. It is a rapidly acting, potent antihypertensive agent with a very short hemodynamic half-life. Using invasive hemodynamic monitoring, Cotton and associates[150] noted that the ability to control blood pressure precisely was dependent on volume status. Nitroglycerin is administered through an infusion pump at an initial rate of 10 mg/minute and titrated to the desired pressure by doubling the dose every 5 minutes. Methemoglobinemia may result from high-dose (>7 mg/kg/minute) intravenous infusion. Patients with normal arterial oxygen saturation who appear cyanotic should be evaluated for toxicity, which is defined as a methemoglobin level greater than 3%.[157]

MODE OF DELIVERY

A patient with preeclampsia at term whose intake and output are balanced and whose blood pressure is controlled should have a trial of vaginal delivery. No randomized clinical trials have evaluated the optimal method of delivery for women with severe preeclampsia or eclampsia. Cesarean section is reserved for cases in which the maternal and fetal conditions are adverse and deteriorating and for patients with preterm gestation and an unripe cervix. Nevertheless, in retrospective studies comparing induction of labor with cesarean delivery in women with severe preeclampsia remote from term, induction was a reasonable alternative.[158,159] Therefore, the decision to perform cesarean delivery should be individualized. If cesarean delivery is performed, the clinician should inspect and gently palpate the liver, especially if liver enzyme abnormalities are present, to exclude liver hematoma.[51] Regional anesthesia is the preferred technique for both labor and delivery in women with severe preeclampsia or eclampsia.[19] It provides superior pain relief compared with intravenous analgesia but apparently no additional therapeutic benefits.[160] General anesthesia carries more risk to pregnant women than does regional anesthesia.[161] However, regional anesthesia is generally contraindicated in the presence of coagulopathy. If general endotracheal anesthesia is used, then antihypertensive therapy should be used before intubation to prevent further increases in blood pressure during intubation. Agents used by anesthesiologists include hydralazine, nitroprusside, nitroglycerin, trimethaphan, fentanyl-droperidol, and labetalol.[143,162–165]

CONTROVERSIES IN THE MANAGEMENT OF SEVERE PREECLAMPSIA

Role of Invasive Monitoring. The American College of Obstetricians and Gynecologists[166] does not list severe preeclampsia or eclampsia as an indication for pulmonary artery catheterization. Others recommend invasive monitoring in patients with severe preeclampsia because of associated hypovolemia.[167] No prospective studies validated the use of invasive monitoring in severe pregnancy-induced hypertension. Invasive hemodynamic monitoring may be helpful in patients with pulmonary edema of uncertain etiology,[166] oliguria that is unresponsive to initial fluid challenge,[166] hypertension that is refractory to hydralazine, and other medical indications for hemodynamic monitoring.[166] The range of values obtained from invasive hemodynamic monitoring studies in normal nonpregnant patients, normal pregnant patients, and patients with pregnancy-induced hypertension are listed in Table 36–3.[25,26] There are several clinical recommendations for treatment in invasively monitored patients. They include maintaining pulmonary capillary wedge pressure between 10 and 15 mm Hg with discrete fluid challenges, vasodilators, or diuretics; treating oliguria on the basis of the patient's hemodynamic findings[168]; restricting fluids to 75 to 125 mL/hour and treating hypovolemia with 500- to 1000-mL boluses; and correcting colloid osmotic pressure only when the patient has a prolonged negative colloid osmotic pressure–pulmonary capillary wedge pressure gradient or a colloid osmotic pressure of 12 mm Hg or less.[169]

Conduction Anesthesia. The use of conduction anesthesia in preeclampsia is controversial. Decreases in blood pressure that lead to late decelerations in fetal heart rate can occur if volume contraction is not corrected before epidural placement.[102,170,171] Patients with gestational hypertension and associated hypovolemia are even more susceptible to hypotension during epidural anesthesia. Moore and associates[172] studied the safety of epidural anesthesia in patients with pregnancy-induced hypertension. They compared fetal and maternal outcomes in 285 patients with gestational hypertension delivered with epidural, general, or local anesthesia and found that continuous lumbar epidural anesthesia was safe and effective for patients with pregnancy-induced hypertension and also for their fetuses. Epidural anesthesia avoids the dramatic increase in blood pressure and central pressures seen with general anesthesia.[173] If volume loading is used, fetal well-being is evident, and the maternal coagulation profile is normal, in many studies, conduction anesthesia appears to be safe and efficacious.[172,174,175]

Postnatal

Magnesium sulfate should be continued postpartum for 24 hours while the patient is closely observed in the recovery area. Close monitoring and treatment with magnesium sulfate may continue beyond 24 hours postpartum in the patient with severe preeclampsia who is not improving or the patient with HELLP syndrome who continues to deteriorate. Efforts should be made to prevent pulmonary edema as a result of fluid shifts in patients with impaired renal function. If central hemodynamic monitoring was used intrapartum, it is continued until diuresis occurs.

If blood pressure remains greater than 150/100 mm Hg 2 to 3 days postpartum, oral antihypertensive therapy is usually initiated. Calcium channel blockers are most commonly used; however, α-methyldopa, hydralazine, or β-blockers may also be considered. Blood pressure is monitored one to two times per week. If hypertension persists beyond 6 weeks postpartum, the patient is classified as having chronic hypertension[18] and referred to a specialist.

HELLP SYNDROME

General

HELLP syndrome is considered a complication of severe preeclampsia and eclampsia. Weinstein,[111,176] who gave the syndrome its current name, specified that it should be considered an additional independent criterion for severe preeclampsia. The incidence of HELLP syndrome was 9.7% among 1153 pregnancies complicated by preeclampsia or eclampsia.[110] Martin and associates[177] reported an overall recurrence risk of 25% among 94 liveborn infants.

In another study, HELLP syndrome occurred in approximately 20% of women with severe preeclampsia.[178] HELLP syndrome develops antepartum in 70% of patients and after delivery in the rest.[4] As with severe preeclampsia, HELLP syndrome is associated with an increased risk of many adverse outcomes, including placental abruption, renal failure, preterm delivery, and maternal or infant death.[178,182]

The diagnosis of HELLP syndrome is based on laboratory findings and includes the following:

- Hemolysis. Microangiopathic hemolytic anemia is characterized by burr cells, schistocytes, and polychromasia on the peripheral smear. An increased bilirubin level, most of it indirect (>1.2 mg/dL), and an increased LDH level (>600 IU/L) confirm the diagnosis.
- Elevated liver enzyme levels. Levels of SGOT, SGPT, and LDH are increased. Right upper quadrant pain may be associated with hepatic cell damage, which also causes an elevation in liver enzymes. The hepatic lesion is parenchymal necrosis, in which deposits of fibrin-like material are seen in the sinusoids. In severe parenchymal necrosis, bleeding can extend to the subcapsular region, leading to a hematoma that stretches Glisson's capsule and eventually may rupture.
- Low platelet count. The platelet count is less than 100,000/mm^3.

According to Weinstein[111] and Sibai and colleagues,[110] the signs and symptoms, by incidence, are as follows:

- Right upper quadrant or epigastric pain (86%–90%)
- Nausea or vomiting (45%–84%)
- Headache (50%)
- Right upper quadrant tenderness on palpation (86%)
- Diastolic blood pressure greater than 110 mm Hg (67%)
- Proteinuria greater than 2+ on dipstick (85%–96%)
- Edema (55%–67%)

Management Options

Management of the patient with HELLP syndrome includes the same principles of treatment as management of severe preeclampsia or eclampsia. The first step is assessing and correcting maternal coagulation abnormalities. Platelets should be transfused when the platelet count is less than 20,000/mm^3, and blood products should be given if hypovolemia and coagulopathy must be corrected. Because of continued hemolysis in the postpartum period, packed red blood cell transfusions are often necessary.[111] Fetal status should be also evaluated. Maternal and fetal status should be considered to decide whether to pursue immediate delivery by cesarean section or attempt vaginal delivery. Patients who meet the criteria for HELLP syndrome should be delivered at any gestational age. Patients with overt HELLP syndrome and an immature fetus rarely benefit from steroid injections and delayed delivery. The patient should be monitored very closely before delivery with repeated clinical and laboratory studies. Conservative approaches to the treatment of gestational hypertension associated with HELLP syndrome have been reported.[111,183,184] These include plasma exchange transfusions and antithrombin III transfusions. Although reports are encouraging, this mode of treatment is considered experimental.

Expectant management before 32 weeks' gestation is undertaken only in tertiary care centers or as part of randomized clinical trials with appropriate safeguards and consent.[19]

The time between delivery and recovery was as long as 11 days in severely affected patients with HELLP syndrome.[185] These patients should be followed with repeated measurements of platelet count and LDH serum concentration, until the platelet count is increased to more than 100,000/mm^3 and effective diuresis is achieved. Neiger and associates[186] found that most patients with preeclampsia and thrombocytopenia reached nadir levels 27 hours after delivery. The mean time required for the platelet count to return to greater than 100,000/mm^3 was 60 hours; recovery time was inversely related to the severity of thrombocytopenia.

ECLAMPSIA

General

Eclampsia is defined as the occurrence of convulsions, not caused by coincidental neurologic disease (e.g., epilepsy), in a woman whose condition meets the criteria for preeclampsia.[18] The incidence of eclampsia is approximately 1 in 1600 pregnancies.[4] Eclampsia is much more common as term approaches; approximately 50% of cases develop before delivery.[4,187] The remaining 50% of cases are divided equally between the intrapartum and postpartum periods.[4,187] When the first convulsion occurs more than 48 hours postpartum, other causes should be excluded.[102]

Clinical Course

The initial presentation of the patient with preeclampsia is similar to that of the patient with preeclampsia. Sibai[188] reported that only 40% of patients with eclampsia had severe hypertension, and 20% had systolic blood pressure less than 140 mm Hg or diastolic blood pressure less than 90 mm Hg. The presence of edema and proteinuria among patients with eclampsia is variable. The signs and symptoms of severe preeclampsia may precede convulsions; however, they are not necessary for the development of convulsions.[189] Laboratory findings in patients with eclampsia are similar to those in patients with preeclampsia of varying degrees of severity.

Differential Diagnosis

When convulsions occur during pregnancy, delivery, or the puerperium, the diagnosis of eclampsia is made until proven otherwise. Other conditions that can cause convulsions and coma should be considered. These include epilepsy, intracranial hemorrhage and thrombosis, rupture of a cerebral aneurysm, meningitis, encephalitis, cerebral tumors, and hyperventilation syndrome.[102]

Management Options

Definitive treatment of eclampsia includes the following:

- Controlling convulsions and preventing their recurrence with magnesium sulfate
- Providing ventilation and correcting hypoxia and acidosis
- Using hydralazine to control diastolic blood pressure to 90 to 100 mm Hg to prevent maternal cerebrovascular accidents and congestive heart failure
- Prompt delivery of the fetus and placenta

Sibai[4] recommends cesarean delivery for patients with an unripe cervix at less than 32 weeks' gestation because of the high incidence of intrapartum complications in these patients. Pritchard and colleagues[29] advocate delivery as soon as the convulsions are controlled and the patient is conscious, certainly within 48 hours of the onset of seizures. Some investigators advocate more conservative management attempts to achieve fetal lung maturity before delivery.[190] This approach, if confirmed to be safe, applies only to the rare patient with eclampsia. No specific contraindications to labor induction are associated with eclampsia. Indications for cesarean delivery are based on obstetric issues, if the patient's condition is not rapidly deteriorating. The rate of cesarean delivery in patients with eclampsia is 11% to 57%.[191]

Most women with severe preeclampsia can be managed without invasive hemodynamic monitoring. No randomized controlled trials support the routine use of pulmonary artery catheters, although this approach may benefit women with severe cardiac or renal disease, oliguria, or pulmonary edema.[6,192–194]

Prognosis

Severe preeclampsia and eclampsia are responsible for considerable maternal morbidity and mortality. Maternal morbidity includes severe bleeding from abruptio placentae, with resultant coagulopathy, pulmonary edema, aspiration pneumonia, acute renal failure, cerebrovascular hemorrhage, liver rupture, and retinal detachment. The maternal mortality rate is 2% to 4% in patients with HELLP syndrome and 10% in patients with pulmonary edema.[195] The maternal mortality rate associated with eclampsia is still 0.4% to 5.8%, even in institutions with much experience.[4,29,196] Transient hypertension only, without the development of preeclampsia, does not appear to alter maternal or fetal outcome and is of limited clinical significance.[197]

The recurrence rate of pregnancy-induced hypertension in future pregnancies and the chance of later development of chronic hypertension are unclear from the literature. Chesley[198] reviewed several of these reports and concluded that the incidence of recurrent eclampsia is 10.3% (range, 0%–21%) and the average chance of a hypertensive disorder in a subsequent pregnancy is 33%. The incidence of chronic hypertension is highly variable in different reports and ranged from 0% to 78%, with an average of 23.8%.

SUMMARY OF MANAGEMENT OPTIONS
Preeclampsia

Management Option	Quality of Evidence	Strength of Recommendation	References
Prepregnancy			
Advise early prenatal care	–	GPP	–
Prepregnancy control of diabetes	–	GPP	–
Prepregnancy control of hypertension	–	GPP	–
Good nutrition for those at risk	–	GPP	–
Prenatal Prediction			
Increased risk and vigilance in patients with:	–	GPP	–
• Preexisting hypertension			
• Renal disease			
• Connective tissue disorder			
• Diabetes mellitus			
• Previous preeclampsia			
Prenatal Prevention			
Calcium supplements result in a modest reduction in risk and severity	Ia	A	207
No apparent benefit from magnesium supplements	Ia	A	208
No clear benefit from dietary sodium restriction	Ia	A	209
No evidence of benefit from fish liver oil	Ib	A	210
Diuretic therapy may reduce blood pressure but does not improve perinatal mortality	Ia	A	211
Antihypertensives for mild to moderate hypertension reduces severity of preeclampsia	Ia	A	212
Low-dose aspirin significantly reduces risk in women at high risk for early preclampsia	Ia	A	213
Antioxidants: Vitamin C and E supplements appear to benefit those at high risk	Ib	A	93
Prenatal Early Detection or Prediction			
Rollover test has a poor predictive value	III	B	214
Plasma cellular fibronectin is increased in pregnancy-induced hypertension but is not a predictor	III	B	215
Platelet angiotensin II receptors are a poor predictor of preeclampsia	III	B	216
Low urinary calcium excretion has poor predictive value	III	B	217
Elevated mean arterial pressure is a poor predictor of preeclampsia	IIb	B	218
Value of the isometric exercise test is inconsistent	III	B	219
Serum uric acid is an unreliable predictor	III	B	84
Microalbuminuria is increased in women who have preeclampsia, but its predictive value is poor	III	B	220
Corrected platelet aggregability may have good predictive value	III	B	221
Doppler velocimetry of the uterine artery may be an early predictor	III	B	222
Prenatal Management			
Diagnosis at term mandates delivery	–	GPP	–

Continued

SUMMARY OF MANAGEMENT OPTIONS
Preeclampsia *(Continued)*

Management Option	Quality of Evidence	Strength of Recommendation	References
Prenatal Management *(Continued)*			
Mild preeclampsia remote from term can be managed conservatively with fetal surveillance and monitoring for disease progression	Ib	A	129
Severe preeclampsia or eclampsia near or remote from term requires delivery; expectant management is unusual and requires careful patient and family counseling	III	B	223
Principles of expectant management:			
• Reduce blood pressure	Ia	A	224,225
• Prevent convulsions	Ia	A	226
• Use IV fluids carefully to avoid fluid overload	–	GPP	–
Laboratory studies during expectant management:	–	GPP	–
• 24-hr urine collection for quantitative protein and creatinine clearance			
• Platelet count			
• Liver function tests			
• Serum fibrinogen			
• Clotting studies			
Fetal assessment (see Chapters 11 and 12): growth, umbilical artery Doppler, biophysical profile testing	–	GPP	–
Give steroids if preterm	Ia	A	227
Consider in utero transfer if the neonatal facilities are not appropriate	–	GPP	–
Labor and Delivery			
Mode of delivery depends on maternal and fetal factors	–	GPP	–
Epidural is frequently advocated, but no benefit is demonstrated and care is needed to avoid fluid overload	IIb	B	228
Consider assisted second stage if the goal is vaginal delivery	–	GPP	–
Oxytocin for the third stage	–	GPP	–
Judicious use of fluid therapy	–	GPP	–
Frequent assessment of maternal vital signs	–	GPP	–
Continuous electronic fetal heart rate monitoring during labor	–	GPP	–
Magnesium sulphate for seizure prophylaxis	Ia	A	226
Antihypertensive medication to maintain blood pressure below 160/110 mm Hg	Ia	A	225
Vigilance for potential complications, including oliguria, pulmonary edema, HELLP syndrome, and seizures	–	GPP	–
Invasive monitoring is infrequently needed; it provides specific hemodynamic data to influence management if the patient is unstable or the volume status is uncertain	III	B	229
Postnatal			
Continue seizure prophylaxis for approximately 24 hours postpartum	–	GPP	–
In patients with severe disease, close monitoring and seizure prophylaxis continue for 2 to 4 days until the disease resolves:	–	GPP	–

SUMMARY OF MANAGEMENT OPTIONS

Preeclampsia *(Continued)*

Management Option	Quality of Evidence	Strength of Recommendation	References
Postnatal *(Continued)*			
• Blood pressure			
• Fluid balance			
• Renal function			
• Pulmonary function			
• Neurologic status			
• Coagulation status			
Patients who require antihypertensive medication at discharge should remain under surveillance	–	GPP	–
Further studies are needed in patients who are hypertensive at or more than 6 weeks postpartum	–	GPP	–

SUMMARY OF MANAGEMENT OPTIONS

Eclampsia

Management Option	Quality of Evidence	Strength of Recommendation	References
Prepregnancy			
Discuss the relatively low recurrence risk	–	GPP	–
Counsel about prevention	–	GPP	–
Prenatal Prediction			
Maintain vigilance in patients with preeclampsia, previous eclampsia, or hypertension	–	GPP	–
Prenatal Prevention			
Low-dose aspirin, as for preeclampsia, but there is no direct evidence of benefit	–	GPP	–
Antihypertensive therapy	–	GPP	–
Prompt action with warning clinical features	–	GPP	–
No evidence of benefit from prophylactic anticonvulsants in women with preeclampsia	Ia	A	226
Prenatal Management			
General measures: Resuscitate, maintain airway, give oxygen, and nurse semiprone	–	GPP	–
Transfer to high-dependency area	–	GPP	–
Control and prevent further convulsions with magnesium sulfate (some use diazepam for immediate control of convulsions)	–	–	84,219,220
Control blood pressure	Ia	A	224,225
Assess renal function and fluid balance; avoid fluid overload	–	GPP	–
Assess liver function	–	GPP	–
Assess clotting status	–	GPP	–

Continued

SUMMARY OF MANAGEMENT OPTIONS

Eclampsia *(Continued)*

Management Option	Quality of Evidence	Strength of Recommendation	References
Prenatal Management *(Continued)*			
Assess pulmonary function	–	GPP	–
Assess fetal health	–	GPP	–
Deliver when stable	–	GPP	–
Labor and Delivery			
Mode of delivery depends on the maternal status and fetal viability	–	GPP	–
If labor occurs:	–	GPP	–
• Continuous monitoring of fetal heart rate			
• Assisted second stage			
• Oxytocin for the third stage			
• Avoid prolonged labor			
Regional analgesia is contraindicated if the patient has a clotting abnormality	–	GPP	–
Postnatal			
Maintain high-dependency care for 24 to 48 hours	–	GPP	–
Stop anticonvulsants 24 hours after the last episode	–	GPP	–
Use antihypertensives as necessary (oral after 24 hours)	–	GPP	–
Reduce intensive monitoring when recovery is seen	–	GPP	–
Counsel about the risks of recurrence	–	GPP	–
Long-term follow-up:	–	GPP	–
• Neurologic assessment if atypical episodes occur			
• Monitor blood pressure and proteinuria and consider studies if values remain abnormal			

CHRONIC HYPERTENSION

General

Chronic hypertension is defined as persistent elevation in blood pressure of 140/90 mm Hg or greater before 20 weeks' gestation or persistent hypertension beyond 6 weeks postpartum. Because of the physiologic decrease in blood pressure that is seen in midpregnancy, patients with chronic hypertension may have pressures in the normotensive range for a good portion of pregnancy. This makes the diagnosis difficult in those with little prenatal care.

In chronic hypertension, elevated blood pressure is the cardinal pathophysiologic feature, whereas in preeclampsia, increased blood pressure is a sign of the underlying disorder. Thus, the effects of the two conditions on the mother and the fetus are different, and management differs as well.

The literature on chronic hypertension in pregnancy is clouded by inconsistencies in the criteria used to select study patients. Americans tend to use the definition given earlier, whereas Europeans and Australians tend to include patients with all forms of hypertension. Classification schemes also vary. In this chapter, patients with mild chronic hypertension include those with systolic blood pressure between 140 and 159 mm Hg and diastolic pressure between 90 and 109, whereas those with systolic blood pressure 160 mm Hg or greater or diastolic pressure 110 mm Hg or greater are classified as having severe chronic hypertension.

Depending on the population studied and the criteria used, the incidence of chronic hypertension in pregnancy is 0.5% to 3%. Essential hypertension is responsible for 90% of cases of chronic hypertension associated with pregnancy. Causes of secondary hypertension include renal disease (glomerulonephritis, nephropathy, renovascular disease), endocrinologic disorders (diabetes with vascular involvement, thyrotoxicosis, pheochromocytoma), and collagen vascular disease (systemic lupus erythematosus, scleroderma).

Maternal and Fetal Risks

Maternal and perinatal morbidity and mortality rates are not generally increased for patients with uncomplicated mild chronic hypertension. However, risks to the mother and fetus increase dramatically when the pregnancy is complicated by severe disease or superimposed preeclampsia. Other risk factors include maternal age older than 40 years, hypertension lasing longer than 15 years, blood pressure greater than 160/110 mm Hg early in pregnancy, diabetes classes B through F, renal disease, cardiomyopathy, connective tissue disease, and coarctation of the aorta.[199]

Maternal risks include exacerbation of hypertension, superimposed preeclampsia, congestive heart failure, intracerebral hemorrhage, acute renal failure, abruptio placentae with disseminated intravascular coagulation (DIC), and death as a result of any of these. Of these, superimposed preeclampsia and abruptio placentae are the two most common complications. Superimposed preeclampsia complicates approximately 5% to 50% of pregnancies of women with chronic hypertension, depending on whether the diagnosis of preeclampsia was made simply on the basis of exacerbation of hypertension or if significant proteinuria was included. In patients with risk factors, the incidence of superimposed preeclampsia is 25% to 50%. The incidence of abruptio placentae is 0.5% to 2% in patients with mild, uncomplicated hypertension and 3% to 10% in those with severe hypertension. The incidence of superimposed preeclampsia or abruption is not affected by antihypertensives.[199]

Fetal morbidity and mortality rates are directly related to the severity of hypertension. They are particularly high in patients with superimposed preeclampsia and abruptio placentae. Decreased uteroplacental perfusion can lead to fetal growth restriction. Spontaneous or intentional interruption of pregnancy adds the compounding complications of prematurity. The risk of midtrimester death in utero is higher in patients with chronic hypertension, especially those who do not receive prenatal care. Perinatal complications are not increased in those with mild, uncomplicated hypertension.

Management Options

Prepregnancy

Women with severe hypertension who desire pregnancy should be encouraged to receive prepregnancy care. The cause and severity of chronic hypertension should be established, if possible. Antihypertensives with potential adverse effects on the fetus, such as angiotensin-converting enzyme inhibitors and diuretics, should be discontinued under strict physician supervision. At times, these medications are continued into pregnancy, despite the potential fetal risk, because of difficulty controlling hypertension otherwise. Adequate time must be allowed preconceptionally to gauge the patient's response to new medications to control hypertension. Renal function should be assessed in more severe cases by measuring serum creatinine and performing 24-hour urine collection to determine creatinine clearance and protein concentrations. Once conception occurs, early prenatal care in an appropriate setting is important.

Prenatal

Early and frequent prenatal care is essential to optimize perinatal outcome in patients with hypertension. During the initial visits, a detailed evaluation of the etiology and severity of chronic hypertension should be made. Careful attention must be given to a history of cardiac or renal disease, diabetes, or thyroid disease and to the outcome of previous pregnancies. Baseline laboratory studies evaluating organ systems that are likely to be affected include urinalysis and culture; measurement of electrolytes, uric acid, and blood sugar; and 24-hour urine collection to measure creatinine clearance and protein concentrations. Patients with severe hypertension or proteinuria in the first trimester should have a chest x-ray, electrocardiogram, antinuclear antibody testing, and when indicated, serum complement studies. In those with severe, long-standing hypertension, an echocardiogram should be performed to evaluate cardiac function. Those with recurrent pregnancy loss or recent thromboembolic disease should be evaluated for lupus anticoagulant and anticardiolipin antibodies.

Women who are at low risk (those with mild, chronic hypertension and none of the listed risk factors) should be seen every 2 to 4 weeks in the first two trimesters, and then weekly. Sibai and colleagues[200] recommend discontinuation of all antihypertensives at the first prenatal visit in low-risk women. Only half require subsequent medication; treatment of patients who need antihypertensives can be tailored to their individual needs. Fetal evaluation includes serial ultrasound examinations to document adequate fetal growth and weekly antepartum fetal testing, beginning at approximately 34 weeks' gestation. If there is no superimposed preeclampsia or if fetal well-being cannot be documented, routine induction of labor before 41 weeks' gestation probably is not warranted.

Pregnancy in women with hypertension and additional risk factors is associated with increased maternal and perinatal complications. These pregnancies should be managed in consultation with appropriate specialists (e.g., maternal–fetal medicine, nephrology). Very close monitoring is essential, and multiple hospitalizations may be necessary to control maternal hypertension and associated medical complications. Severe hypertension mandates an aggressive pharmacologic approach. Carefully selected antihypertensives may benefit those with mild hypertension who have additional complicating factors, such as diabetes, renal disease, or cardiac dysfunction.

Intensive fetal surveillance is critical to optimize fetal outcome. Serial ultrasonography for fetal growth and weekly (or more frequent, depending on the fetal condition) antepartum fetal testing, beginning as early as 26 weeks, should be used. The pregnancy may be continued until term, until the onset of superimposed preeclampsia, or until fetal growth restriction or other signs of fetal decompensation occur. The development of severe, superimposed preeclampsia places the patient at highest risk for maternal and perinatal complications. This development after 28 weeks is an indication for delivery. Before 28 weeks, the pregnancy may be followed conservatively in a tertiary center with daily evaluation of the maternal and fetal condition, although this approach is controversial.[201]

Although the maternal and fetal benefits of antihypertensives are well documented in the treatment of pregnancies complicated by severe hypertension, the benefits of these drugs in pregnant patients with mild, uncomplicated hypertension is much less clear. There are no randomized trials of the treatment of severe hypertension. However, the general consensus is to start therapy when diastolic blood pressure reaches 110 mm Hg, to prevent cerebrovascular accident, the largest cause of maternal death in patients with hypertension. In the United States, methyldopa is the first-line agent because of the extensive experience with its use and the lack of known fetal effects. Labetalol, which was first popularized in European studies, is a reasonable second-line antihypertensive for use in these women.[200, 202]

The treatment of gravidas with mild to moderate chronic hypertension is more controversial. The many reports of antihypertensive use in this group of patients are difficult to evaluate because of differences in definitions, populations, and treatments. The trials are more limited by sample size, selection bias, and frequent initiation of therapy late in the second or third trimester. Nevertheless, a few generalizations can be made.[200,202] The use of methyldopa or labetalol in women with mild, uncomplicated hypertension does not significantly improve gestational age at delivery, birth weight, rates of intrauterine growth retardation, or the perinatal death rate over these measures in women who were untreated or received placebo. Trials comparing the efficacy of methyldopa with a β-blocker in mild hypertension showed few significant differences.[152,203,204] The use of these agents does not reduce the incidence of superimposed preeclampsia or abruptio placentae, the conditions responsible for most adverse perinatal outcomes in patients with mild, chronic hypertension.

Labor and Delivery

The goal of intrapartum management is to avoid acute maternal and fetal complications. Maternal blood pressure can be controlled with oral or intravenous hydralazine or labetalol (see). Judicious use of intravenous fluids and close attention to noninvasive hemodynamic parameters (e.g., blood pressure, pulse oximetry) are crucial. Fetuses may be compromised by long-standing growth restriction and hypoxemia before the onset of labor. Therefore, continuous electronic fetal monitoring and intermittent fetal scalp pH sampling, as needed, are important to assess the ability of the fetus to tolerate labor.

Postnatal

High risk patients with chronic hypertension should be monitored closely for at least 48 hours after delivery because they are at risk for hypertensive encephalopathy, pulmonary edema, and renal failure. Oral or intravenous hydralazine, methyldopa, labetalol, or calcium channel blockers can be used to control severe hypertension. Diuretic therapy is used in patients with evidence of circulatory congestion or pulmonary edema. These women must be evaluated after the postpartum period to detect deterioration in cardiac or renal function and to adjust antihypertensive medication.

After delivery, oral antihypertensives usually must be continued to control hypertension. Minute amounts of all antihypertensives are found in breast milk. Limited data suggest that there are no short-term effects on breastfeeding infants who are exposed to methyldopa, hydralazine, β-blockers, or calcium channel blockers.[205] However, thiazide diuretics inhibit adequate breast milk production.[206]

SUMMARY OF MANAGEMENT OPTIONS

Chronic Hypertension

Management Option	Quality of Evidence	Strength of Recommendation	References
Prepregnancy			
Establish the cause and severity of hypertension	–	GPP	–
Evaluate renal function	–	GPP	–
In those with mild to moderate hypertension, stop medication or switch to medication with few fetal side effects	–	GPP	–

SUMMARY OF MANAGEMENT OPTIONS
Chronic Hypertension *(Continued)*

Management Option	Quality of Evidence	Strength of Recommendation	References
Prepregnancy *(Continued)*			
In those with severe or difficult-to-control hypertension, medication may be needed despite the potential fetal risks	–	GPP	–
Encourage early prenatal care in an appropriate setting	–	GPP	–
Prenatal			
Early and frequent prenatal care	IV	C	230
Discontinue antihypertensive medication unless maternal diastolic pressure exceeds 100 to 110 mm Hg	Ia	A	212
Use oral medication in severe hypertension (methyldopa, hydralazine, calcium channel blockers) and in those with mild hypertension complicated by risk factors	Ia	A	224
Laboratory studies (where appropriate): • 24-hr collection for creatinine clearance and protein • Uric acid • Platelet count and clotting studies • Electrolytes • Antinuclear and antiphospholipid antibodies and serum complement • Blood sugar	–	GPP	–
Fetal surveillance with serial ultrasound for growth, umbilical artery Doppler, and biophysical profile testing: • Start at 26 weeks in women with severe hypertension or risk factors • Start later in women with mild, uncomplicated hypertension	IV	C	230
Maintain vigilance for superimposed preeclampsia	IV	C	230
Labor and Delivery			
Continuous electronic fetal monitoring	IV	C	230
Use antihypertensives to maintain blood pressure below 160/110 mm Hg	Ia	A	225
Monitor for potential complications (e.g., abruption, superimposed preeclampsia)	IV	C	230
Postnatal			
Monitor closely in the first 48 hours to anticipate hypertensive encephalopathy, pulmonary edema, or renal failure	IV	C	230
Use oral or intravenous medication to control hypertension	IV	C	230
Evaluate for deterioration in cardiac or renal status	IV	C	230
Most patients with hypertension are safe during lactation; avoid thiazide diuretics	IV	C	230

CONCLUSIONS

- Hypertensive disorders complicate approximately 12%–22% of all pregnancies.
- Established criteria are available to classify and differentiate preexisting hypertension, preeclampsia, and superimposed preeclampsia.
- Although the etiology of preeclampsia is undetermined, the maternal and fetal consequences of this condition have been thoroughly studied and documented.
- Preeclampsia cannot be accurately predicted. Prevention strategies are currently suboptimal.
- Management goals of preeclampsia focus on prevention of convulsions, minimization of adverse events, and, if possible, delivery of a surviving and intact child.
- The complications of HELLP syndrome and eclampsia generally require rapid stabilization of the mother and prompt delivery of the fetus.
- Complications and adverse events related to chronic hypertension in pregnancy can be minimized by careful blood pressure management, observation for evidence of superimposed preeclampsia, and diligent fetal surveillance.

REFERENCES

1. Koonin LM, MacKay AP, Berg CJ, et al: Pregnancy-related mortality surveillance: United States, 1987–1990. Morbid Mortal Wkly Rep CDC Surveill Summ 1997;46:17–36.
2. Kaunitz AM, Hughes MJ, Grimes DA, et al: Causes of maternal mortality in the United States. Obstet Gynecol 1985;65:605–612.
3. American College of Obstetricians and Gynecologists: Diagnosis and management of preeclampsia and eclampsia: ACOG Practice Bulletin No. 33. Obstet Gynecol 2002;99:159–167.
4. Sibai BM: Preeclampsia-eclampsia. Curr Prob Obstet Gynecol Fertil 1990;13:1–45.
5. Sibai BM: Chronic hypertension during pregnancy. In Sciarra J (ed): Gynecology and Obstetrics. Philadelphia, JB Lippincott, 1989, pp 1–8.
6. Cunningham FG, Gant NF, Leveno KJ, et al: Hypertensive disorders in pregnancy. In Williams Obstetrics, 21st ed. New York, McGraw-Hill, 2001, pp 567–618.
7. Hauth JC, Ewell MG, Levine RJ, et al: Pregnancy outcomes in healthy nulliparas who developed hypertension: Calcium for Preeclampsia Prevention Study Group. Obstet Gynecol 2000;95: 24–28.
8. Long PA, Oats JN: Preeclampsia in twin pregnancy: Severity and pathogenesis. Aust N Z J Obstet Gynecol 1987;27:1–5.
9. Campbell DM, Macgillivray I, Carr-Hill R: Pre-eclampsia in second pregnancy. Br J Obstet Gynaecol 1985;92:131–140.
10. Walker JJ: Pre-eclampsia. Lancet 2000;356:1260–1265.
11. Sibai BM, Ewell M, Lervine RJ, et al: Risk factors associated with preeclampsia in healthy nulliparous women: The Calcium for Preeclampsia Prevention (CPEP) Study Group. Am J Obstet Gynecol 1997;177:1003–1010.
12. Sibai BM, Hauth J, Caritis S, et al: Hypertensive disorders in twin versus singleton gestations: Nastional Institute of Child Health and Human Development Network of Maternal-Fetal Medicine Unit. Am J Obstet Gynecol 2000;182:938–942.
13. Conde-Agudelo A, Belizan JM: Risk factors for preeclampsia in a large cohort of Latin American and Caribbean women. BJOG 2000;107:75–83.
14. Salonen Ros H, Lichtenstein P, Lipworth L, Cnattingius S: Genetic effects on the liability of developing pre-eclampsia and gestational hypertension. Am J Med Genet 2000;91:256–260.
15. Davey DA, MacGillivray I: The classification and definition of the hypertensive disorders of pregnancy. Clin Exp Hypertens (B) 1986;51:97–133.
16. Rochat RW, Koonin LM, Atrash HK, Jewett JF: Maternal mortality in the United States: Report from the Maternal Mortality Collaborative. Obstet Gynecol 1988;72:91–97.
17. Hughes EC (ed): Obstetric-Gynecologic Terminology. Philadelphia, FA Davis, 1972, pp 422–423.
18. American College of Obstetrics and Gynecologists: Management of preeclampsia. Technical Bulletin 1986; No 91.
19. Report of the National Blood Pressure Education Program Working Group on High Blood Pressure in Pregnancy. Am J Obstet Gynecol 2000;183:S1–S22.
20. Brown MA, Buddle ML, Farrell T, et al: Randomised trial of management of hypertensive pregnancies by Korotkoff phase IV or phase V. Lancet 1998;352:777–781.
21. Zhou Y, Fisher SJ, Janatpour M, et al: Human cytotrophoblast adopt a vascular phenotype as they differentiate: A strategy for successful endovascular invasion? J Clin Invest 1997;99: 2139–2151.
22. Zhou Y, Damsky CH, Chiu K, et al: Preeclampsia is associated with abnormal expression of adhesion molecules by invasive cytotrophoblasts. J Clin Invest 1993;91:950–960.
23. Fox H: The placenta in pregnancy hypertension. In Rubin PC (ed): Handbook of Hypertension, vol. 10. Hypertension in Pregnancy. New York, Elsevier, 1988, pp 16–37.
24. DeSwiet M: The cardiovascular system. In Hytten FE, Chamberlain GVP (eds): Clinical Physiology in Obstetrics. Oxford, Blackwell, 1980, pp 3–42.
25. Clark SL, Cotton DB, Lee W, et al: Central hemodynamic assessment of normal term pregnancy. Am J Obstet Gynecol 1989;161:1439–1442.
26. Cotton DB, Lee W, Huhta JC, Dorman KF: Hemodynamic profile of severe pregnancy-induced hypertension. Am J Obstet Gynecol 1988;158:523–529.
27. Groenendijk R, Trimbos JBMJ, Wallenburg HCS: Hemodynamic measurements in preeclampsia: Preliminary observations. Am J Obstet Gynecol 1984;150:232–236.
28. Kirshon B, Cotton DB: Invasive hemodynamic monitoring in the obstetric patient. Clin Obstet Gynecol 1987;30:579–590.
29. Pritchard JA, Cunningham FG, Pritchard SA: The Parkland Memorial Hospital protocol for treatment of eclampsia: Evaluation of 245 cases. Am J Obstet Gynecol 1984;148: 951–963.
30. Abdul-Karim R, Assali NS: Pressor response to angiotonin in pregnant and nonpregnant women. Am J Obstet Gynecol 1961;82:246–251.
31. Talledo OE, Chesley LC, Zuspan FP: Renin-angiotensin system in normal and toxemic pregnancies: III. Differential sensitivity to angiotensin II and norepinephrine in toxemia of pregnancy. Am J Obstet Gynecol 1968;100:218–221.

32. Browne FJ: Sensitization of the vascular system in the pre-eclamptic toxemia and eclampsia. J Obstet Gynaecol Br Emp 1946;53:510–518.
33. Gant NF, Daley GL, Chand S, et al: A study of angiotensin II pressor response throughout primigravid pregnancy. J Clin Invest 1973;52:2682–2689.
34. Everett RB, Worley RJ, MacDonald PC, Gant NF: Effect of prostaglandin synthetase inhibitors on pressor response to angiotensin II in human pregnancy. J Clin Endocrinol Metab 1978;46:1007–1010.
35. Sanchez-Ramos L, O'Sullivan MJ, Garrido-Calderone J: Effect of low-dose aspirin on angiotensin II pressor response in human pregnancy. Am J Obstet Gynecol 1987;156:193–194.
36. Friedman SA: Preeclampsia: A review of the role of prostaglandins. Obstet Gynecol 1988;71:122–137.
37. Walsh SW: Preeclampsia: An imbalance in placental prostacyclin and thromboxane production. Am J Obstet Gynecol 1985;152: 335–340.
38. Remuzzi G, Marchesi D, Zoja C, et al: Reduced umbilical and placental vascular prostacyclin in severe pre-eclampsia. Prostaglandins 1980;20:5–10.
39. Moodley J, Norman RJ, Reddi K: Central venous concentrations of immunoreactive prostaglandins E, F and 6-keto-prostaglandin F_1 in eclampsia. BMJ 1984;288:1487–1489.
40. Hankins GD, Wendel GD Jr, Cunningham FG, Leveno KJ: Longitudinal evaluation of hemodynamic changes in eclampsia. Am J Obstet Gynecol 1984;150:506–512.
41. Dadak C, Ulrich W, Sinzinger H: Morphological changes in the umbilical arteries of babies born to pre-eclamptic mothers: An ultrastructural study. Placenta 1984;5:419–426.
42. Saleh AA, Bottoms SF, Welch RA, et al: Preeclampsia, delivery, and the hemostatic system. Am J Obstet Gynecol 1987;157: 331–336.
43. Saleh AA, Bottoms SF, Norman G, et al: Hemostasis in hypertensive disorders of pregnancy. Obstet Gynecol 1988;71: 719–722.
44. Stubbs TM, Lazarchick J, Horger EO III: Plasma fibronectin levels in preeclampsia: A possible biochemical marker for vascular endothelial damage. Am J Obstet Gynecol 1984;150: 885–887.
45. Eriksen HO, Kern Hansen P, Brocks V, Jensen BA: Plasma fibronectin concentration in normal pregnancy and pre-eclampsia. Acta Obstet Gynecol Scand 1987;66:25–28.
46. Weiner CP, Brandt J: Plasma antithrombin III activity: An aid in the diagnosis of preeclampsia-eclampsia. Am J Obstet Gynecol 1982;142:275–281.
47. Weiner CP, Kwaan HC, Xu C, et al: Antithrombin III activity in women with hypertension during pregnancy. Obstet Gynecol 1985;65:301–306.
48. Chesley LC, Duffus GM: Preeclampsia, posture and renal function. Obstet Gynecol 1971;38:1–5.
49. Pirani CL, Pollak VE, Lannigan R, Folli G: The renal glomerular lesions of pre-eclampsia: Electron microscopic studies. Am J Obstet Gynecol 1963;87:1047–1070.
50. Spargo B, McCartney CP, Winemiller R: Glomerular capillary endotheliosis in toxemia of pregnancy. Arch Pathol 1959;68:593–599.
51. Smith LG Jr, Moise KJ Jr, Dildy GA III, Carpenter RJ Jr: Spontaneous rupture of liver during pregnancy: Current therapy. Obstet Gynecol 1991;77:171–175.
52. McCall ML: Cerebral circulation and metabolism in toxemia of pregnancy: Observations on the effects of *Veratrum viride* and Apresoline (1-hydrazinophthalazine). Am J Obstet Gynecol 1953;66:1015–1030.
53. Chipchase J, Peebles D, Rodeck C: Severe preeclampsia and cerebral blood volume response to postural change. Obstet Gynecol 2003;101:86–92.
54. Sheehan HL: Pathological lesions in the hypertensive toxemias of pregnancy. In Hammond J, Browne FJ, Wolstenholme GEW (eds): Toxemias of Pregnancy: Human and Veterinary. Philadelphia, Blakiston, 1950, pp 16–22.
55. Sibai BM, Spinnato JA, Watson DL, et al: Eclampsia: IV. Neurological findings and future outcome. Am J Obstet Gynecol 1985;152:184–192.
56. Brown CEL, Purdy P, Cunningham FG: Head computed tomographic scans in women with eclampsia. Am J Obstet Gynecol 1988;159:915–920.
57. Moseman CP, Shelton S: Permanent blindness as a complication of pregnancy induced hypertension. Obstet Gynecol 2002;100: 943–945.
58. Cunningham FG, Fernandez CO, Hernandez C: Blindness associated with preeclampsia and eclampsia. Am J Obstet Gynecol 1995;172:1291–1298.
59. Brosens IA: Morphological changes in the uteroplacental bed in pregnancy hypertension. Clin Obstet Gynecol 1977;4:573–593.
60. Browne JCM, Veall N: The maternal placental blood flow in normotensive and hypertensive women. J Obstet Gynaecol Br Emp 1953;60:141–147.
61. Zeek PM, Assali NS: Vascular changes in the decidua associated with eclamptogenic toxemia of pregnancy. Am J Clin Pathol 1950;20:1099–1109.
62. De Wolf F, Robertson WB, Brosens I: The ultrastructure of acute atherosis in hypertensive pregnancy. Am J Obstet Gynecol 1975;123:164–174.
63. Shanklin DR, Sibai BM: Ultrastructural aspects of preeclampsia: I. Placental bed and uterine boundary vessels. Am J Obstet Gynecol 1989;161:735–741.
64. Abdella TN, Sibai BM, Hays JM, Anderson GD: Relationship of hypertensive disease to abruptio placentae. Obstet Gynecol 1984;63:365–370.
65. Friedman SA, Lindheimer MD: Prediction and differential diagnosis. In Lindheimer MD, Roberts JM, Cunningham FG (eds): Chesley's Hypertensive Disorders in Pregnancy, 2nd ed. Stamford, Conn, Appleton & Lange, 1999, pp 201–227.
66. Stamilio DM, Sehdev HM, Morgan MA, et al: Can antenatal clinical and biochemical markers predict the development of severe preeclampsia? Am J Obstet Gynecol 2000;182:589–594.
67. Helewa ME, Burrows RF, Smith J, et al: Report of the Canadian Hypertension Society Consensus Conference: 1. Definitions, evaluation and classification of hypertensive disorders in pregnancy. CMAJ 1997;157:715–725.
68. Gant NF, Chand S, Worley RJ, et al: A clinical test useful for predicting the development of acute hypertension of pregnancy. Am J Obstet Gynecol 1974;120:1–7.
69. Talledo OE, Chesley LC, Zuspan FP: Renin-angiotensin system in normal and toxemic pregnancies: III. Differential sensitivity to angiotensin II and norepinephrine in toxemia of pregnancy. Am J Obstet Gynecol 1968;100:218–221.
70. Lazarchick J, Stubbs TM, Remein L, et al: Predictive value of fibronectin levels in normotensive gravid women destined to become preeclamptic. Am J Obstet Gynecol 1986;154: 1050–1052.
71. Lockwood CJ, Peters JH: Increased plasma levels of $ED1^+$ cellular fibronectin precede the clinical signs of preeclampsia. Am J Obstet Gynecol 1990;162:358–362.
72. Stubbs TM, Lazarchick J, Horger EO III: Plasma fibronectin levels in preeclampsia: A possible biochemical marker for vascular endothelial damage. Am J Obstet Gynecol 1984;150: 885–887.
73. Baker PN, Broughton Pipkin F, Symonds EM: Platelet angiotensin II binding sites in normotensive and hypertensive women. BJOG 1991;98:436–440.
74. Zemel MB, Zemel PC, Berry S, et al: Altered platelet calcium metabolism as an early predictor of increased peripheral vascular resistance and preeclampsia in urban black women. N Engl J Med 1990;323:434–438.
75. Sanchez-Ramos L, Jones DC, Cullen MT: Urinary calcium as an early marker for preeclampsia. Obstet Gynecol 1991;77: 685–688.

76. Sowers JR, Saleh AA, Niyogi T, et al: Mid-gestational hyperinsulinemia and development of preeclampsia. Am J Obstet Gynecol 1992;166:294.
77. Fallis NE, Langford HG: Relation of second trimester blood pressure to toxemia of pregnancy in the primigravid patient. Am J Obstet Gynecol 1963;87:123.
78. Degani S, Abinader E, Eibschitz I, et al: Isometric exercise test for predicting gestational hypertension. Obstet Gynecol 1985;65:652–654.
79. Konstantin-Hansen KF, Hesseldahl H, Pedersen SM: Microalbuminuria as a predictor of preeclampsia. Acta Obstet Gynecol Scand 1992;71:343–346.
80. Ballegeer VC, Spitz B, De Baene LA, et al: Platelet activation and vascular damage in gestational hypertension. Am J Obstet Gynecol 1992;166:629–633.
81. Walker JJ, Cameron AD, Bjornsson S, et al: Can platelet volume predict progressive hypertensive disease in pregnancy? Am J Obstet Gynecol 1989;161:676–679.
82. Hogg BB, Tamura T, Johnston KE, et al: Second-trimester plasma homocysteine levels and pregnancy-induced hypertension, preeclampsia, and intrauterine growth restriction. Am J Obstet Gynecol 2000;183:805–809.
83. Ong CY, Liao AW, Spencer K, et al: First trimester maternal serum free beta human chorionic gonadotrophin and pregnancy associated plasma protein A as predictors of pregnancy complications. BJOG 2000;107:1265–1270.
84. Redman CW, Williams GF, Jones DD, Wilkinson RH: Plasma urate and serum deoxycytidylate deaminase measurements for the early diagnosis of pre-eclampsia. BJOG 1977;84:904–908.
85. Lim KH, Friedman SA, Ecker JL, et al: The clinical utility of serum uric acid measurements in hypertensive disease of pregnancy. Am J Obstet Gynecol 1998;178:1067–1071.
86. Campbell S, Pearce JM, Hackett G, et al: Qualitative assessment of uteroplacental blood flow: Early screening test for high-risk pregnancies. Obstet Gynecol 1986;68:649–653.
87. Irion O, Masse J, Forest JC, Moutquin JM: Prediction of preeclampsia, low birthweight for gestation and prematurity by uterine artery blood flow velocity waveform analysis in low risk nulliparous women. BJOG 1998;105:422–429.
88. Belizan JM, Villar J: The relationship between calcium intake and edema-, proteinuria-, and hypertension-gestosis: An hypothesis. Am J Clin Nutr 1980;33:2202–2210.
89. Villar J, Repke JT: Calcium supplementation during pregnancy may reduce preterm delivery in high-risk populations. Am J Obstet Gynecol 1990;163:1124–1131.
90. Carroli G, Duley L, Belizan JM, Villar J: Calcium supplementation during pregnancy: A systematic review of randomised controlled trials. BJOG 1994;101:753–758.
91. Sanchez-Ramos L, Briones DK, Kaunitz AM, et al: Prevention of pregnancy-induced hypertension by calcium supplementation in angiotensin II-sensitive patients. Obstet Gynecol 1994;84: 349–353.
92. Levine RJ, Hauth JC, Curet LB, et al: Trial of calcium to prevent preeclampsia. N Engl J Med 1997;337:69–76.
93. Chappell LC, Seed PT, Briley AL, et al: Effect of antioxidants on the occurrence of preeclampsia in women at increased risk: A randomized trial. Lancet 1999;354:810–816.
94. Collins R, Yusuf S, Peto R: Overview of randomised trials of diuretics in pregnancy. BMJ 1985;290:17–23.
95. Rubin PC, Butters L, Clark DM, et al: Placebo-controlled trial of atenolol in treatment of pregnancy-associated hypertension. Lancet 1983;1:431–434.
96. Duley L: Any hypertensive therapy in chronic hypertension. In Keirse MJNC, Renfrew MJ, Neilson JP, Crowther C (eds): Pregnancy and Childbirth Module. Cochrane Pregnancy and Childbirth Database: The Cochrane Collaboration, Issue 2 Oxford, Update Software, 1995. London, BMJ Publishing Group.
97. Walsh SW: Preeclampsia: An imbalance in placental prostacyclin and thromboxane production. Am J Obstet Gynecol 1985;152: 335–340.
98. Sibai BM, Caritis SN, Thom E, et al: Prevention of preeclampsia with low-dose aspirin in healthy, nulliparous pregnant women. N Engl J Med 1993;329:1213–1218.
99. Caritis SN for the NICHD network of Maternal-Fetal Medicine Units: Low dose aspirin does not prevent preeclampsia in high-risk women. Am J Obstet Gynecol 1997;176:S3.
100. CLASP (Collaborative Low-dose Aspirin Study in Pregnancy) Collaborative Group: CLASP: A randomised trial of low-dose aspirin for the prevention and treatment of pre-eclampsia among 9364 pregnant women. Lancet 1994;343:619–629.
101. Vainio M, Kujansuu E, Iso-Mustajarvi M, Maenpaa J: Low dose acetylsalicylic acid in prevention of pregnancy-induced hypertension and intrauterine growth retardation in women with bilateral uterine artery notches. BJOG 2002;109:161–167.
102. Cunningham FG, Grant NF, Leveno KJ, et al (eds): Hypertensive disorders in pregnancy. In Williams Obstetrics, 21st ed. New York, McGraw-Hill, 2001, pp 567–618.
103. MacGillivray I: Some observations on the incidence of preeclampsia. J Obstet Gynaecol Br Commonw 1958;65:536–539.
104. Tervila L, Goecke C, Timonen S: Estimation of gestosis of pregnancy (EPH-gestosis). Acta Obstet Gynecol Scand 1973;52: 235–243.
105. Thomson AM, Hytten FE, Billewicz WZ: The epidemiology of oedema during pregnancy. J Obstet Gynaecol Br Commonw 1967;74:1–8.
106. Chesley LC: Preeclampsia: Early signs and development. In Chesley LC (ed): Hypertensive Disorders in Pregnancy. New York, Appleton-Century-Crofts, 1978, pp 277–308.
107. Sibai BM, Lipshitz J, Anderson GD, Dilts PV Jr: Reassessment of intravenous $MgSO_4$ therapy in preeclampsia-eclampsia. Obstet Gynecol 1981;57:199–202.
108. Pollak VE, Nettles JB: The kidney in toxemia of pregnancy: A clinical and pathologic study based on renal biopsies. Medicine 1960;39:469–526.
109. Redman CWG, Beilin LJ, Bonnar J, Wilkinson RH: Plasma-urate measurements in predicting fetal death in hypertensive pregnancy. Lancet 1976;1:1370–1373.
110. Sibai BM, Taslimi MM, El-Nazer A, et al: Maternal-perinatal outcome associated with the syndrome of hemolysis, elevated liver enzymes, and low platelets in severe preeclampsia-eclampsia. Am J Obstet Gynecol 1986;155:501–509.
111. Weinstein L: Preeclampsia/eclampsia with hemolysis, elevated liver enzymes, and thrombocytopenia. Obstet Gynecol 1985;66: 657–660.
112. Phelan JP, Everidge GJ, Wilder TL, Newman C: Is the supine pressor test an adequate means of predicting acute hypertension in pregnancy? Am J Obstet Gynecol 1977;128:173–176.
113. Andersen GJ: The roll-over test as a screening procedure for gestational hypertension. Aust N Z J Obstet Gynaecol 1980;20: 144–146.
114. Bukowski RM: Thrombotic thrombocytopenic purpura: A review. Prog Hemost Thromb 1982;6:287–337.
115. Schwartz ML, Brenner WE: The obfuscation of eclampsia by thrombotic thrombocytopenic purpura. Am J Obstet Gynecol 1978;131:18–24.
116. Weiner CP: Thrombotic microangiopathy in pregnancy and the postpartum period. Semin Hematol 1987;24:119–129.
117. Segonds A, Louradour N, Suc JM, Orfila C: Postpartum hemolytic uremic syndrome: A study of three cases with a review of the literature. Clin Nephrol 1979;12:229–242.
118. Anderson HM: Maternal hematologic disorders. In Creasy RK, Resnik R (eds): Maternal-Fetal Medicine: Principles and Practice. Philadelphia, WB Saunders, 1989, pp 890–924.
119. Snyder RR, Hankins GDV: Etiology and management of acute fatty liver of pregnancy. Clin Perinatol 1986;13:813–825.

120. Watson WJ, Seeds JW: Acute fatty liver of pregnancy. Obstet Gynecol Surv 1990;45:585–593.
121. Minakami H, Oka N, Sato T, et al: Preeclampsia: A microvesicular fat disease of the liver? Am J Obstet Gynecol 1988;159:1043–1047.
122. Rolfes DB, Ishak KG: Liver disease in toxemia of pregnancy. Am J Gastroenterol 1986;81:1138–1144.
123. Brown MS, Reddy KR, Hensley GT, et al: The initial presentation of fatty liver of pregnancy mimicking acute viral hepatitis. Am J Gastroenterol 1987;82:554–557.
124. Douvas SG, Meeks GR, Phillips O, et al: Liver disease in pregnancy. Obstet Gynecol Surv 1983;38:531–536.
125. Shabot JM, Jaynes C, Little HM, et al: Viral hepatitis in pregnancy with disseminated intravascular coagulation and hypoglycemia. South Med J 1978;71:479–481.
126. Dienstag JL, Wands JR, Isselbacher KJ: Acute hepatitis. In Wilson JD, Braunwald E, Isselbacher KJ, et al (eds): Harrison's Principles of Internal Medicine. New York, McGraw-Hill, 1991, pp 1322–1337.
127. Schiffer MA: Fatty liver associated with administration of tetracycline in pregnant and nonpregnant woman. Am J Obstet Gynecol 1966;96:326–332.
128. Nesbitt JAA, Minuk GY: Adult Reye's syndrome. Ann Emerg Med 1988;17:155–158.
129. Sibai BM, Gonzalez AR, Mabie WC, Moretti M: A comparison of labetalol plus hospitalization versus hospitalization alone in the management of preeclampsia remote from term. Obstet Gynecol 1987;70:323–327.
130. Kroner C, Turnbull D, Wilkinson C: Antenatal day care units versus hospital admission for women with complicated pregnancy. Cochrane Database Syst Rev 2001:CD001803.
131. Sibai BM, Taslimi M, Abdella TN, et al: Maternal and perinatal outcome of conservative management of severe preeclampsia in midtrimester. Am J Obstet Gynecol 1985;152:32–37.
132. Odendaal HJ, Pattinson RC, Du Toit R: Fetal and neonatal outcome in patients with severe preeclampsia before 34 weeks. S Afr Med J 1987;71:555–558.
133. Jenkins SM, Head BB, Hauth JC: Severe preeclampsia at <25 weeks of gestation: Maternal and neonatal outcomes. Am J Obstet Gynecol 2002;186:790–795.
134. Cotton DB, Gonik B, Dorman KF: Cardiovascular alterations in severe pregnancy-induced hypertension seen with intravenously given hydralazine bolus. Surg Gynecol Obstet 1985;161:240–244.
135. The Eclampsia Trial Collaborative Group: Which anticonvulsant for women with eclampsia? Evidence from the Collaborative Eclampsia trial. Lancet 1995;345: 1455–1463.
136. Coetzee EJ, Dommisse J, Anthony J: A randomized controlled trial of intravenous magnesium sulphate versus placebo in management of women with severe preeclampsia. BJOG 1998;105:300–303.
137. Witlin AG, Sibai BM: Magnesium sulfate therapy in preeclampsia and eclampsia. Obstet Gynecol 1998;92:883–889.
138. Lucas MJ, Leveno KJ, Cunningham FG: A comparison of magnesium sulfate with phenytoin for the prevention of eclampsia. N Engl J Med 1995;333:201–205.
139. Hallak M, Berman RF, Irtenkauf SM, et al: Peripheral magnesium sulfate enters the brain and increases the threshold for hippocampal seizures in rats. Am J Obstet Gynecol 1992;167:1605–1610.
140. Cotton DB, Hallak M, Janusz C, et al: Central anticonvulsant effects of magnesium sulfate on *N*-methyl-D-aspartate-induced seizures. Am J Obstet Gynecol 1993;168:974–978.
141. Hallak M, Berman RF, Irtenkauf SM, et al: Magnesium sulfate treatment decreases *N*-methyl-D-aspartate receptor binding in the rat brain: An autoradiographic study. J Soc Gynecol Invest 1994;1:25–30.
142. Hallak M, Irtenkauf SM, Cotton DB: Effect of magnesium sulfate on excitatory amino acid receptors in the rat brain: I. *N*-methyl-D-aspartate receptor-channel complex. Am J Obstet Gynecol 1996;175:575–581.
143. Cotton DB, Gonik B, Dorman KF: Cardiovascular alteration in severe pregnancy-induced hypertension: Acute effects of intravenous magnesium sulfate. Am J Obstet Gynecol 1984;148:162–165.
144. Slater RM, Wilcox FL, Smith WD, et al: Phenytoin infusion in severe pre-eclampsia. Lancet 1987;1:1417–1420.
145. Lubbe WF: Hypertension in pregnancy: Whom and how to treat. Br J Clin Pharmacol 1987;24:15S–20S.
146. Sibai BM: Treatment of hypertension in pregnant women. N Engl J Med 1996;335:257–265.
147. von Dadelszen P, Ornstein MP, Bull SB, et al: Fall in mean arterial pressure and fetal growth restriction in pregnancy hypertension: A meta-analysis. Lancet 2000;355:87–92.
148. Pritchard JA: Management of severe preeclampsia and eclampsia. Semin Perinatol 1978;2:83–97.
149. Clark SL, Cotton DB: Clinical indications for pulmonary artery catheterization in the patient with severe preeclampsia. Am J Obstet Gynecol 1988;158:453–458.
150. Cotton DB, Longmire S, Jones MM, et al: Cardiovascular alterations in severe pregnancy-induced hypertension: Effects of intravenous nitroglycerin coupled with blood volume expansion. Am J Obstet Gynecol 1986;154:1053–1059.
151. Michael CA: The evaluation of labetalol in the treatment of hypertension complicating pregnancy. Br J Clin Pharmacol 1982;13:127S–131S.
152. Mabie WC, Gonzalez AR, Sibai BM, Amon E: A comparative trial of labetalol and hydralazine in the acute management of severe hypertension complicating pregnancy. Obstet Gynecol 1987;70:328–333.
153. Lunell NO, Lewander R, Mamoun I, et al: Uteroplacental blood flow in pregnancy induced hypertension. Scand J Clin Lab Invest Suppl 1984;169:28–35.
154. Magee LA, Elran E, Bull SB, et al: Risks and benefits of beta-receptor blockers for pregnancy hypertension: Overview of the randomized trials. Eur J Obstet Gynecol Reprod Biol 2000;88:15–26.
155. Pasch T, Schulz V, Hoppelshauser G: Nitroprusside-induced formation of cyanide and its detoxication with thiosulfate during deliberate hypotension. J Cardiovasc Pharmacol 1983;5:77–85.
156. Waisman GD, Mayorga LM, Cámera MI, et al: Magnesium plus nifedipine: Potentiation of hypotensive effect in preeclampsia? Am J Obstet Gynecol 1988;159:308–309.
157. Herling IM: Intravenous nitroglycerin: Clinical pharmacology and therapeutic considerations. Am Heart J 1984;108:141–149.
158. Nassar AH, Adra AM, Chakhtoura N, et al: Severe preeclampsia remote from term: Labor induction or elective cesarean delivery? Am J Obstet Gynecol 1998;179:1210–1213.
159. Alexander JM, Bloom SL, McIntire DD, Leveno KJ: Severe preeclampsia and the very low birth weight infant: Is induction of labor harmful? Obstet Gynecol 1999;93:485–488.
160. Lucas MJ, Sharma SK, McIntire DD, et al: A randomized trial of labor analgesia in women with pregnancy-induced hypertension. Am J Obstet Gynecol 2001;185:970–975.
161. Hawkins JL, Konnin LM, Palmer SK, Gibbs CP: Anesthesia-related deaths during obstetric delivery in the United States, 1979–1990. Anesthesiology 1997;86:277–284.
162. Hood DD, Dewan DM, James FM III, et al: The use of nitroglycerin in preventing the hypertensive response to tracheal intubation in severe preeclampsia. Anesthesiology 1985;63:329–332.
163. Connell H, Dalgleish JG, Downing JW: General anesthesia in mothers with severe pre-eclampsia/eclampsia. Br J Anaesth 1987;59:1375–1380.
164. Lawes EG, Downing JW, Duncan PW, et al: Fentanyl-droperidol supplementation of rapid sequence induction in the presence of severe pregnancy-induced and pregnancy-aggravated hypertension. Br J Anaesth 1987;59:1381–1391.

165. Ramanathen J, Sibai BM, Mabie WC, et al: The use of labetalol for attenuation of the hypertensive response to endotracheal intubation in preeclampsia. Am J Obstet Gynecol 1988;159: 650–654.
166. American College of Obstetricians and Gynecologists: Invasive hemodynamic monitoring in obstetrics and gynecology. Technical Bulletin 1988; No 121.
167. Benedetti TJ, Cotton DB, Read JC, Miller FC: Hemodynamic observations in severe pre-eclampsia with a flow-directed pulmonary artery catheter. Am J Obstet Gynecol 1980;136: 465–470.
168. Clark SL, Greenspoon JS, Aldahl D, Phelan JP: Severe preeclampsia with persistent oliguria: Management of hemodynamic subsets. Am J Obstet Gynecol 1986;154:490–494.
169. Kirshon B, Moise KJ, Cotton DB, et al: Role of volume expansion in severe pre-eclampsia. Surg Gynecol Obstet 1988;167: 367–371.
170. Asling JH: Hypotension after regional anesthesia. In Shnider SM (ed): Obstetrical Anesthesia: Current Concepts and Practice. Baltimore, Williams & Wilkins, 1970, pp 158–163.
171. Clark RB, Thompson DS, Thompson CH: Prevention of spinal hypotension associated with cesarean section. Anesthesiology 1976;45:670–674.
172. Moore TR, Key TC, Reisner LS, Resnik R: Evaluation of the use of continuous lumbar epidural anesthesia for hypertensive pregnant woman in labor. Am J Obstet Gynecol 1985;152: 404–412.
173. Hodgkinson R, Husain FJ, Hayashi RH: Systemic and pulmonary blood pressure during cesarean section in parturients with gestational hypertension. Can Anaesth Soc J 1980;27: 389–393.
174. Newsome LR, Bramwell RS, Curling PE: Severe preeclampsia: Hemodynamic effects of lumbar epidural anesthesia. Anesth Analg 1986;65:31–36.
175. Wheeler AS, Harris BA: Anesthesia for pregnancy-induced hypertension. Clin Perinatol 1982;9:95–111.
176. Weinstein L: Syndrome of hemolysis, elevated liver enzymes, and low platelet count: A severe consequence of hypertension in pregnancy. Am J Obstet Gynecol 1982;142:159–167.
177. Martin JN Jr, Perry KG Jr, Blake PG, et al: Recurrence risk of severe preeclampsia/eclampsia associated with HELLP syndrome. Proc Soc Gynecol Invest 1990;10:101.
178. Sibai BM, Ramadan MK, Usta I, et al: Maternal morbidity and mortality in 442 pregnancies with hemolysis, elevated liver enzymes, and low platelets (HELLP syndrome). Am J Obstet Gynecol 1993;169:1000–1006.
179. Sibai BM, Ramadan MK, Chari RS, Friedman SA: Pregnancies complicated by HELLP syndrome (hemolysis, elevated liver enzymes, and low platelets): Subsequent pregnancy outcome and long term prognosis. Am J Obstet Gynecol 1995;172:125–129.
180. Barton JR, Sibai BM: Hepatic imaging in HELLP syndrome (hemolysis, elevated liver enzymes, and low platelets). Am J Obstet Gynecol 1996;174:1820–1825.
181. Sullivan CA, Magann EF, Perry KG Jr, et al: The recurrence risk of the syndrome of hemolysis, elevated liver enzymes, and low platelets (HELLP) in subsequent gestations. Am J Obstet Gynecol 1994;171:940–943.
182. Isler CM, Rinehart BK, Terrone DA, et al: Maternal mortality associated with HELLP (hemolysis, elevated liver enzymes, and low platelets) syndrome. Am J Obstet Gynecol 1999;181:924–928.
183. Kris M, White DA: Treatment of eclampsia by plasma exchange. Plasma Ther 1981;2:143–147.
184. Buller HR, Weenink AH, Treffers PE, et al: Severe antithrombin III deficiency in a patient with pre-eclampsia: Observations on the effect of human AT III concentrate transfusion. Scand J Haematol 1980;25:81–86.
185. Martin JN Jr, Blake PG, Lowry SL, et al: Pregnancy complicated by preeclampsia-eclampsia with the syndrome of hemolysis, elevated liver enzymes, and low platelet count: How rapid is postpartum recovery? Obstet Gynecol 1990;76:737–741.
186. Neiger R, Contag SA, Coustan DR: The resolution of preeclampsia-related thrombocytopenia. Obstet Gynecol 1991; 77:692–699.
187. Sibai BM, Abdella TN, Spinnato JA, Anderson GD: Eclampsia: V. The incidence of nonpreventable eclampsia. Am J Obstet Gynecol 1986;154:581–586.
188. Sibai BM: Eclampsia. In Rubin PC (ed): Handbook of Hypertension: Hypertension in Pregnancy. Amsterdam, Elsevier, 1988, pp 320–340.
189. Sibai BM, McCubbin JH, Anderson GD, et al: Eclampsia: I. Observations from 67 recent cases. Obstet Gynecol 1981;58: 609–613.
190. Andersen WA, Harbert GM Jr: Conservative management of pre-eclamptic and eclamptic patients: A re-evaluation. Am J Obstet Gynecol 1977;129:260–267.
191. Dildy GA, Cotton DB, Phelan JP: Complications of pregnancy-induced hypertension. In Clark SL, Cotton DB, Hankins GDV, Phelan JP (eds): Critical Care Obstetrics, 2nd ed. Oxford, Blackwell, 1991, pp 251–288.
192. Clark SL, Cotton DB, Hankins GD, Phelan JP: Critical Care Obstetrics, 3rd ed. Malden, Mass, Blackwell, 1997.
193. Hallak M: Hypertension in pregnancy. In James DK, Steer PJ, Weiner C, Gonik B (eds): High Risk Pregnancy: Management Options, 2nd ed. London, Saunders, 1999, pp 639–663.
194. Easterling TR, Benedetti TJ, Schumacker BC, Carlson KL: Antihypertensive therapy in pregnancy directed by noninvasive hemodynamic monitoring. Am J Perinatol 1989;6:86–89.
195. Sibai BM: Preeclampsia-eclampsia: Maternal and perinatal outcomes. Contemp Obstet Gynecol 1988;32:109–118.
196. Gedekoh RH, Hayashi TT, MacDonald HM: Eclampsia at Magee-Womens Hospital, 1970–1980. Am J Obstet Gynecol 1981;140:860–866.
197. Terrone DA, Rinehart BK, May WL, et al: The myth of transient hypertension: Descriptor or disease process? Am J Perinatol 2001;18:73–77.
198. Chesley LC: Remote prognosis. In Chesley LC (ed): Hypertensive Disorders in Pregnancy. New York, Appleton-Century-Crofts, 1978, pp 421–444.
199. Sibai BM: Chronic hypertension in pregnancy. Clin Perinatol 1991;18:833–844.
200. Sibai BM: Diagnosis and management of chronic hypertension in pregnancy. Obstet Gynecol 1991;78:451–461.
201. Sibai BM, Akl S, Fairlie F, Moretti M: A protocol for managing severe preeclampsia in the second trimester. Am J Obstet Gynecol 1990;163:733–738.
202. Weitzc C, Khouzami V, Maxwell K, Johnson JW: Treatment of hypertension in pregnancy with methyldopa: A randomized double blind study. Int J Gynaecol Obstet 1987;25:35–40.
203. Sibai BM, Mabie WC, Shamsa F, et al: A comparison of no medication versus methyldopa or labetalol in chronic hypertension during pregnancy. Am J Obstet Gynecol 1990;162:960–967.
204. Plouin PF, Breart G, Maillard F, et al: Comparison of antihypertensive efficacy and perinatal safety of labetalol and methyldopa in the treatment of hypertension in pregnancy: A randomized controlled trial. BJOG 1988;95:868–876.
205. American Academy of Pediatrics Committee on Drugs: Transfer of drugs and other chemicals in human milk. Pediatrics 1989;84:924–936.
206. Healy M: Suppressing lactation with oral diuretics. Lancet 1961;1:1353–1354.
207. Atalah AN, Hofmeyer GJ, Duley L, et al: Calcium supplementation during pregnancy for preventing hypertensive disorders and related problems (Cochrane Review). In Cochrane Library, Issue 2. Oxford, Update Software, 2001.
208. Makrides M, Crowther CA: Magnesium supplementation in pregnancy (Cochrane Review). In Cochrane Library, Issue 2. Oxford, Update Software, 2001.
209. Duley L, Henderson-Smart D: Reduced salt intake compared to normal dietary salt, or high intake, in pregnancy (Cochrane

Review). In Cochrane Library, Issue 2. Oxford, Update Software, 2001.
210. Onwude JL, Lilford RJ, Hjartardottir H, et al: A randomised double blind placebo controlled trial of fish oil in high risk pregnancy. BJOG 1995;102:95–100.
211. Collins R, Yusuf F, Peto R: Overview of randomised trials of diuretics in pregnancy. BMJ 1985;290:17–23.
212. Abalos E, Duley L, Steyn DW, et al: Antihypertensive drug therapy for mild to moderate hypertension during pregnancy (Cochrane Review). In Cochrane Library, Issue 2. Oxford, Update Software, 2001.
213. Knight M, Duley L, Henderson-Smart DJ, et al: Antiplatelet agents for preventing and treating pre-eclampsia (Cochrane Review). In Cochrane Library, Issue 2. Oxford, Update Software, 2001.
214. Mahomed K, Lasiende OO: The roll over test is not of value in predicting pregnancy induced hypertension. Paediatr Perinat Epidemiol 1990;4:71–75.
215. Islami D, Shoukir Y, Dupont P, et al: Is cellular fibronectin a biological marker for pre-eclampsia? Eur J Obstet Gynecol Reprod Biol 2001;97:40–45.
216. Masse J, Forrest JC, Moutquin JM, et al: A prospective longitudinal study of platelet angiotensin II receptors for the prediction of preeclampsia. Clin Biochem 1998;3:251–255.
217. Suarez VR, Trelles JG, Miyahira JM, et al: Urinary calcium in asymptomatic primigravidas who later developed preeclampsia. Obstet Gynecol 1996;87:79–82.
218. Atterbury JL, Groome LJ, Baker SL, et al: Elevated midtrimester mean arterial blood pressure in women with severe preeclampsia. Appl Nurs Res 1996;9:161–166.
219. Tomoda S, Kitanaka T, Ogita S, et al: Prediction of pregnancy-induced hypertension by isometric exercise. Asia Oceania J Obstet Gynaecol 1994;20:249–255.
220. Shaarawy M, Salem ME: The clinical value of microtransferrinuria and microalbuminuria in the prediction of pre-eclampsia. Clin Chem Lab Med 2001;39:29–34.
221. Felfernig-Boehm D, Salat A, Vogl SE, et al: Early detection of preeclampsia by determination of platelet aggregability. Thromb Res 2000;98:139–146.
222. Coleman MA, McGowan LM, North RA: Mid-trimester uterine artery Doppler screening as a predictor of adverse pregnancy outcome in high-risk women. Placenta 2000;21:115–121.
223. Hall DR, Odendaal HJ, Steyn DWL: Expectant management of severe pre-eclampsia in the mid-trimester. Eur J Obstet Gynecol Reprod Biol 2001;96:168–172.
224. Magee LA, Duley L: Oral beta-blockers for mild to moderate hypertension during pregnancy (Cochrane Review). In Cochrane Library, Issue 2. Oxford, Update Software, 2001.
225. Duley L, Henderson-Smart DJ: Drugs for rapid treatment of very high blood pressure during pregnancy (Cochrane Review). In Cochrane Library, Issue 2. Oxford, Update Software, 2001.
226. Duley L, Gulmezoglu AM, Henderson-Smart DJ: Anticonvulsants for women with pre-eclampsia (Cochrane Review). In Cochrane Library, Issue 2. Oxford, Update Software, 2001.
227. Crowley P: Prophylactic corticosteroids for preterm birth (Cochrane Review). In Cochrane Library, Issue 2. Oxford, Update Software, 2001.
228. Hogg B, Hauth JC, Caritis SN, et al: Safety of labor epidural anesthesia for women with severe hypertensive disease: National Institute of Child Health and Human Development Maternal-Fetal Medicine Units Network. Am J Obstet Gynecol 1999;181:1096–1101.
229. Clark SL, Greenspoon JS, Aldahl D: Severe pre-eclampsia with persistent oliguria: Management of hemodynamic subsets. Am J Obstet Gynecol 1986;154:490–494.
230. Sibai BM: Diagnosis and management of chronic hypertension in pregnancy. Obstet Gynecol 1991;78:451–461.

CHAPTER 37

Cardiac Disease

Mark W. Tomlinson

INTRODUCTION

Maternal and Fetal Risks

Serious maternal cardiac disease complicating pregnancy is relatively uncommon; however, it can have a significant adverse effect on maternal and fetal outcomes, despite modern cardiac care. The overall incidence of serious heart disease complicating pregnancy is approximately 1%.[1,2] With a decrease in maternal death as a result of the classic causes of hemorrhage, hypertension, and infection, the relative importance of cardiac disease increased.[1–3] During the last few decades, the etiology of heart disease changed from primarily rheumatic to predominately congenital.[1,2,4]

Despite the potential for significant maternal morbidity, in most patients with cardiac disease, a satisfactory outcome can be expected with careful antenatal, intrapartum, and postpartum management.[1,2,4,5] Serious complications during pregnancy and the postpartum period include congestive heart failure, arrhythmias, and stroke. In a series reported by Siu and associates,[5] of 221 women with either congenital or acquired conditions, 18% of patients had one of these complications. No maternal deaths occurred. The rate of complications was related to several factors, including maternal functional status, myocardial dysfunction, significant aortic or mitral valve stenosis, and history of arrhythmias or a cardiac event.

Although maternal mortality is uncommon, several conditions are associated with a high risk of maternal death. Table 37–1 shows the estimated qualitative risk of maternal mortality associated with various cardiac conditions. Contemporary literature quantifying the risk of maternal mortality is limited for a number of reasons. Most congenital lesions are diagnosed early, allowing appropriate surgical repair. The significant decrease in the incidence of rheumatic heart disease limits the number of patients with acquired lesions who are seen for the first time because of the physiologic stresses of pregnancy. Patients who are at greatest risk for cardiac decompensation are offered sterilization or termination.

TABLE 37–1

Risk of Maternal Morbidity and Mortality Associated with Pregnancy

Low Risk
Atrial and ventricular septal defect previously repaired or without pulmonary hypertension
Pulmonic or tricuspid disease
Mitral valve prolapse
Patent ductus arteriosus
Corrected congenital heart disease without residual cardiac dysfunction
Mitral stenosis: New York Heart Association Class I or II
Moderate Risk
Mitral stenosis with atrial fibrillation
Aortic stenosis
Artificial valve
Moderate to severe systemic ventricular dysfunction
History of peripartum cardiomyopathy with no residual ventricular dysfunction
Coarctation of the aorta
Tetralogy of Fallot; uncorrected or with residual disease
Previous myocardial infarction
Marfan's syndrome with normal aorta
High Risk
Pulmonary hypertension
Coarctation of the aorta, complicated
Marfan's syndrome with aortic involvement
Any condition with New York Heart Association class III or IV
History of peripartum cardiomyopathy with residual ventricular dysfunction

Normal physiologic changes that occur during pregnancy can aggravate underlying cardiac disease, leading to the associated morbidity and mortality. Beginning in early pregnancy, total body water increases progressively by 6 to 8 L because an additional 500 to 900 mEq sodium is retained.[6–8] As a result, plasma volume increases steadily throughout the first two trimesters and into the early third trimester, reaching a plateau at approximately 32 weeks.[9] In a singleton pregnancy at term, plasma volume is nearly 50% greater than that seen in nonpregnant women.[10] Maternal cardiac output starts to increase at approximately 10 weeks and reaches a plateau near the end of the second trimester, at levels 30% to 50% above nonpregnant values.[11–15] This increased output results from increases in stroke volume and heart rate. The increase in heart rate peaks in the third trimester, at 10 to 15 beats/minute over baseline.[15,16] These physiologic changes increase the demand on the already compromised heart.

The pregnancy-related decrease in blood pressure may offset some of the increased work resulting from increased plasma volume. In some cases, a significant decrease may be deleterious. Normally, systolic and diastolic pressures fall throughout the first two trimesters, reaching a nadir between 24 and 28 weeks, before increasing to nonpregnant levels at term.[17] Systolic pressure decreases an average of 5 to 10 mm Hg, and diastolic pressure decreases 10 to 15 mm Hg.[18] Blood pressure and cardiac output may be further affected by maternal posture. Late in pregnancy, the gravid uterus may mechanically obstruct the aorta and vena cava in the supine position, leading to hypotension.[19,20] In addition, changes in cardiac output and blood pressure cause an initial decrease in systemic vascular resistance, followed by an increase toward nonpregnant values near term.[17]

Colloid oncotic pressure is another important variable that is affected by pregnancy. Both plasma and interstitial colloid oncotic pressure decrease throughout gestation, with the latter decreasing to a greater extent.[21] There is an accompanying increase in capillary hydrostatic pressure.[22] An increase in hydrostatic pressure or a decrease in plasma colloid oncotic pressure may overcome the delicate balance that favors edema formation, especially in late pregnancy. After delivery, a further decrease in plasma colloid oncotic pressure occurs, reaching a nadir between 6 and 16 hours, with a return toward intrapartum levels after 24 hours.[23,24] These changes can lead to the dependent edema that is commonly seen in normal pregnant patients, thus complicating the diagnosis of cardiac decompensation.

Fetal complications in pregnancies complicated by maternal cardiac disease commonly include growth restriction and prematurity. Despite the risk of low birth weight, overall perinatal mortality is not significantly greater than that in the general population. When a pregnant patient has congenital heart disease, the fetus is at increased risk for this disease. The incidence is 0% to 10%, depending on the specific lesion. When the fetus is affected, approximately 50% have the same anomaly as the mother.[2,25] The risk of a cardiac lesion in the fetus is also increased when other first-degree family members have a congenital heart lesion.[26,27]

Management Options

Prepregnancy

Ideally, in patients with significant heart disease, pregnancy is a planned event. This assumes regular and reliable use of an effective contraceptive method. Before discontinuation of contraception, preconception evaluation and counseling should take place. The patient's cardiologist should be an active participant in this process. Maternal disease status should be determined. An echocardiogram can be used not only to define the cardiac anatomy, but also to describe ventricular function and estimate intracardiac pressure gradients.[28] Nuclear medicine scans, although helpful in the nonpregnant state, should be avoided during pregnancy.

A careful history is obtained to identify previous cardiac complications, including arrhythmias. The patient's functional status should also be established. The New York Heart Association (NYHA) functional classification system[29] (Table 37–2) is commonly used. Ninety percent or more of patients are categorized as having class I or II disease.[4] Outcomes are favorable in these two groups, but deterioration may occur. The reported frequency of adverse cardiac events varies, depending on patient selection, from 13% to 79%.[1,4,5] Although few patients have class III or IV disease, historically, nearly 85% of maternal deaths occur in these groups.[30]

The risk of maternal cardiac complications during pregnancy was quantified by Siu and colleagues[5] with a combination of five echocardiographic and historical factors that could be obtained and evaluated at the initial evaluation. The complications studied include pulmonary edema, symptomatic arrhythmias, and stroke or transient ischemic attack of cardiac origin. The five predictive indicators were NYHA classification greater than II or cyanosis, left ventricular obstruction, cardiac dysfunction, previous arrhythmia, and previous cardiac complication. Left ventricular outflow obstruction was defined as aortic valve stenosis with a valve area less than 1.5 cm^2, mitral stenosis with a valve area of 2.0 cm^2, or a

TABLE 37–2

New York Heart Association Cardiac Functional Classification

Class I	No limitations of physical activity; ordinary physical activity does not cause undue fatigue, palpitation, dyspnea, or anginal pain
Class II	Slight limitation of physical activity; ordinary physical activity results in fatigue, palpitation, dyspnea, or anginal pain
Class III	Marked limitation of physical activity; less than ordinary activity causes fatigue, palpitation, dyspnea, or anginal pain
Class IV	Inability to perform any physical activity without discomfort; symptoms of cardiac insufficiency or anginal syndrome may be present, even at rest; any physical activity increases discomfort

peak left ventricular outflow tract gradient greater than 30 mm Hg. Myocardial dysfunction was defined as an ejection fraction less than 40%, restrictive or hypertrophic cardiomyopathy, or complex congenital heart disease. A significant history of arrhythmia was defined as symptomatic bradyarrhythmia or tachyarrhythmia requiring therapy. If no predictive factors were present at the beginning of pregnancy, only 3% of patients had a cardiac complication. When one factor was present, 30% of patients had a complication, and when two or more predictors were present, 66% of patients had a complication. This information can be useful in counseling patients.

Medical management of the patient's cardiac condition should be optimized. During maternal drug therapy, potential fetal effects must be considered. Table 37–3 shows a fetal risk factor classification scheme that is helpful when choosing optimal medical therapy.[31] The corresponding risk factor category is listed, with medications discussed in the next section. Coexisting conditions that may aggravate preexisting heart disease, such as anemia, arrhythmias, and hypertension, should be appropriately treated and controlled. Ideally, necessary cardiac surgery is carried out before conception.

Prenatal

Few patients are seen for prepregnancy evaluation. Therefore, evaluation and counseling should be initiated at the first prenatal visit. Cardiac surgery, although not contraindicated, is usually not required during pregnancy.[2] If possible, it is best delayed until postpartum. When the maternal mortality rate is excessive, as in Eisenmenger's syndrome, termination should be discussed.

During prenatal care, the patient should be routinely questioned and examined for signs or symptoms of cardiac failure. Vital signs and weight gain should be closely monitored. When there is an increased risk of intrauterine growth restriction, serial ultrasound examinations every 2 to 4 weeks in the third trimester allow assessment of interval fetal growth. Antenatal testing may begin at 32 to 34 weeks unless earlier surveillance is indicated because of compromised maternal or fetal status. Future fertility desires and contraceptive plans should be addressed in the antepartum period. Topics should include a discussion of sterilization, depending on future fertility desires, the maternal risk of pregnancy, and the long-term prognosis.

Labor and Delivery

Labor should proceed with the patient in the lateral position to avoid aortocaval compression and possible hypotension. Intrapartum fluid balance should be followed closely. Continuous electrocardiographic monitoring may be used, as necessary, to detect arrhythmias. Invasive hemodynamic monitoring with a pulmonary artery catheter (PAC) and an arterial line may be considered in particularly high risk conditions or in patients with deteriorating cardiovascular status. Although its use has not been rigorously evaluated during pregnancy, some question the safety and utility of the PAC in critically ill and high risk surgical patients.[32–34] Until more information is available on its safety and efficacy, a PAC should be used cautiously during pregnancy. Close fetal surveillance is needed throughout labor. Operative vaginal delivery is indicated in some patients to shorten the second stage of labor and avoid blood pressure changes associated with pushing. Cesarean delivery is usually reserved for obstetric indications.

An understanding of the principles of and indications for bacterial endocarditis antibiotic prophylaxis in pregnant patients is important. In patients with an uncomplicated labor and delivery, bacterial endocarditis is rare. In two series with a total of 906 pregnant women with cardiac disease, routine prophylactic antibiotics were not used and no cases of bacterial endocarditis were identified.[1,2]

TABLE 37–3

Classification System for Fetal Risk Associated with Medications used During Pregnancy

Category A	Controlled studies in women show no risk to the fetus in the first trimester (and no evidence of risk in later trimesters); the possibility of fetal harm appears remote
Category B	Either animal reproduction studies show no fetal risk but there are no controlled studies in pregnant women or animal reproduction studies show an adverse effect (other than a decrease in fertility) that was not confirmed in controlled studies in women in the first trimester (and there is no evidence of a risk in later trimesters)
Category C	Either studies in animals show adverse fetal effects (teratogenic, embryocidal, or other) and there are no controlled studies in women or studies in women and animals are not available; drugs should be given only if the potential benefit justifies the potential risk to the fetus
Category D	There is positive evidence of human fetal risk, but the benefits from use in pregnant women may be acceptable despite the risk (e.g., if the drug is needed in a life-threatening situation or for a serious disease for which safer drugs cannot be used or are ineffective)
Category X	Studies in animals or humans show fetal abnormalities or there is evidence of fetal risk based on human experience, or both, and the risk of the use of the drug in pregnant women clearly outweighs any possible benefit; the drug is contraindicated in women who are or may become pregnant

TABLE 37–4

American Heart Association Recommendations for Endocarditis Prophylaxis

Cardiac Conditions
Endocarditis prophylaxis recommended
High risk
Prosthetic cardiac valves, including bioprosthetic and homograft valves
Previous bacterial endocarditis
Complex cyanotic congenital heart disease (e.g., single ventricle states, transposition of the great arteries, tetralogy of Fallot)
Surgically constructed systemic pulmonary shunts or conduits
Moderate risk
Most other congenital cardiac malformations (other than those listed above and below)
Acquired valvar dysfunction (e.g., rheumatic heart disease)
Hypertrophic cardiomyopathy
Mitral valve prolapse with valvar regurgitation or thickened leaflets
Endocarditis prophylaxis not recommended
Negligible risk (no greater risk than in the general population)
Isolated secundum atrial septal defect
Surgical repair of atrial septal defect, ventricular septal defect, or patent ductus arteriosus (without residua beyond 6 months)
Previous coronary artery bypass graft surgery
Mitral valve prolapse without valvar regurgitation
Physiologic, functional, or innocent heart murmur
Previous Kawasaki disease without valvar dysfunction
Previous rheumatic fever without valvar dysfunction
Cardiac pacemaker (intravascular and epicardial) or implanted defibrillator
Surgical Procedures
Endocarditis prophylaxis not recommended
Genitourinary tract
Vaginal hysterectomy
Vaginal delivery*
Cesarean section
In uninfected tissue
Urethral catheterization
Uterine dilation and curettage
Therapeutic abortion
Sterilization procedure
Insertion or removal of intrauterine device

*Prophylaxis is optional for high-risk patients.
Adapted from Dajani AS, Taubert KA, Wilson, W, et al: Prevention of bacterial endocarditis: Recommendations of the American Heart Association. JAMA 1997;277:1794-1801.

Prophylactic antibiotics are not necessary in all patients with cardiac disease. Prophylaxis is indicated when the cardiac condition puts the patient at risk for endocarditis or when the planned procedure is likely to produce bacteremia with an organism that can cause endocarditis. The incidence of positive blood cultures is low after uncomplicated vaginal delivery, with a reported range of 1% to 5%.[35] Bacteremia is more common with dental procedures, in which positive blood cultures are obtained in 60% to 90% of patients, depending on the procedure.[36] The American Heart Association[37] guidelines for endocarditis prophylaxis are shown in Table 37–4. The Endocarditis Working Party of the British Society for Antimicrobial Chemotherapy[38] recommends antibiotic prophylaxis during obstetric and gynecologic procedures only for patients with prosthetic heart valves. Table 37–5 shows the drug regimens recommended by the American Heart Association[37] and the Endocarditis Working Party of the British Society for Antimicrobial Chemotherapy.[38]

TABLE 37–5

Recommended Antibiotic Regimens for Genitourinary Procedures

American Heart Association Recommendations
High-risk patients
Ampicillin 2.0 g IM or IV plus gentamicin 1.5 mg/kg (not to exceed 120 mg) within 30 minutes of starting the procedure: 6 hours later, ampicillin 1 g orally
Ampicillin-, amoxicillin-, or penicillin-allergic patient regimen
Vancomycin 1.0 g IV over 1 to 2 hr plus gentamicin 1.5 mg/kg IV or IM (not to exceed 120 mg); complete injection or infusion within 30 minutes of starting the procedure
Endocarditis Working Party of the British Society for Antimicrobial Chemotherapy Recommendations
Patients who are not allergic to penicillin and who have not had penicillin more than once in the previous month
1 g amoxycillin IM in 2 to 5 mL 1% lignocaine hydrochloride plus 120 mg gentamicin IM just before induction, then 0.5 g amoxycillin orally 6 hours later
Patients who are allergic to penicillin or who have had penicillin more than once in the previous month
Vancomycin 1.0 g by slow IV infusion over 60 minutes followed by gentamicin 120 mg IV just before induction or 15 minutes before the surgical procedure

Adapted from Dajani AS, Taubert KA, Wilson, W, et al: Prevention of bacterial endocarditis: Recommendations of the American Heart Association. JAMA 1997;277:1794-1801.

Postnatal

In the postpartum period, fluid balance must be monitored carefully. During the first 24 to 72 hours, significant fluid shifts occur and can lead to congestive heart failure in patients with cardiac disease. Careful attention should be paid to patients who do not have brisk spontaneous diuresis. In these patients, progressive reduction in oxygen saturation monitored by pulse oximetry often heralds the onset of clinical pulmonary edema. Previously developed contraceptive plans should be reviewed and implemented.

SUMMARY OF MANAGEMENT OPTIONS
Cardiac Disease: General

Management Options	Quality of Evidence	Strength of Recommendation	References
Prepregnancy			
Obstetrician and cardiologist in collaboration	III	B	1
Discussion of maternal and fetal risks	III	B	4,5,29
Discussion of safe and effective contraception	–	GPP	–
Evaluate current cardiac status	IV	C	28,29
Optimize medical and surgical management	III	B	1,2,31
Advise against pregnancy with certain conditions	III	B	4,5,29
Prenatal			
Assess functional class of heart disease (see Table 37–2)	III	B	4,5,29
Termination is an option with some conditions	III	B	4,5,29
Joint management with a cardiologist	III	B	1
Optimize medical management	III	B	1,2,31
Avoid or minimize aggravating factors	III	B	4,5
Anticoagulation for certain conditions; discuss the risks and benefits of continued warfarin therapy vs. changing to subcutaneous heparin	IV	C	126,127
Anesthesiology consultation	IV	C	30
Prophylactic antibiotics with certain conditions (see Tables 37–4 and 37–5)	IV	C	37,38
Fetal surveillance:			
• Growth and fetal surveillance (especially if left-to-right shunt)	III	B	1,2,4,5
• Detailed fetal cardiac ultrasonography if the patient has congenital heart disease	III	B	1,2,4,5
Labor and Delivery			
Elective induction may be necessary for maternal or fetal indications	III	B	1,2,4,5
Prophylactic antibiotics with certain conditions (see Tables 37–4 and 37–5)	IV	C	3,7,38
Avoid mental and physical stress; consider epidural	III	B	4,5
Labor in the left lateral and upright position	III	B	1,2,4,5
Monitor electrocardiogram; more invasive monitoring is needed with certain conditions	Ib	A	30
Administer extra oxygen with certain conditions	–	GPP	–
Full resuscitation facilities should be available	–	GPP	–
Provide continuous fetal heart rate monitoring	–	GPP	–
Assisted second stage with certain conditions	–	GPP	–
Avoid ergotamine for the third stage	–	GPP	–
Postnatal			
Vigilance for cardiac failure	III	B	1,2,4,5
Avoid fluid overload	III	B	1,2,4,5
Continued intensive care	–	GPP	–
Discuss safe and effective contraception	–	GPP	–

CARDIAC MURMUR

Maternal and Fetal Risks

Cardiac murmurs result from turbulent blood flow that causes vibration of the cardiac structures. Systolic murmurs are very common during pregnancy, with the reported incidence exceeding 90%.[39,40] Typically, the murmur is early to midsystolic and soft (grade I–II). The left sternal border area is usually the area of maximal intensity, followed by the aortic and pulmonic areas.[41] These murmurs are rarely associated with cardiac pathology and are likely secondary to the increased intravascular volume and cardiac output.

Echocardiographic studies of pregnant patients who are referred for evaluation of nonspecific systolic murmurs show normal structure and function in more than 90% of examinations. Most patients had the clinical characteristics of a benign flow murmur.[41–45] Most abnormalities were mild and were associated with a history suggesting pathology.[41–44] Clinically significant murmurs differ from the typical benign flow murmur. Systolic murmurs that are "loud or long" are suspicious and are more frequently associated with cardiac pathology. Late systolic, pansystolic, and diastolic murmurs are abnormal and require further evaluation.[42]

Management Options

Echocardiography adds little to the clinical evaluation of nonspecific systolic murmurs, because most significant cardiac conditions seen during pregnancy are diagnosed before conception. Unsuspected mild cardiac disease may initially present during pregnancy or the puerperium. A common benign flow murmur must be differentiated from a pathologic condition. Unfortunately, the accuracy of clinical evaluation of systolic murmurs by noncardiologists is unknown.[45] A history that suggests cardiac disease or a pathologic murmur (late systolic, pansystolic, or diastolic) heard on physical examination should prompt evaluation with echocardiography. When a suspicious systolic murmur is noted, either a cardiologist's clinical examination or echocardiogram can reliably identify significant pathology.[45] The method of choice depends on institutional resources.

MITRAL VALVE PROLAPSE

Maternal and Fetal Risks

Mitral valve prolapse (MVP) represents a range of valvular abnormalities that allow one or both mitral valve leaflets to extend above the plane that separates the atria and ventricle. The condition is common, with a prevalence of 2% to 4% in the general population.[46–48] There is a wide range in the reported prevalence, however, depending on the method of diagnosis, the diagnostic criteria, and the population studied. Females are affected twice as often as males. The condition is most common in women of reproductive age, with prevalence rates as high as 21%.[46]

Auscultation or echocardiography may be used to diagnose MVP. A midsystolic click, with or without a midsystolic to late systolic murmur, is the clinical hallmark. With M-mode or two-dimensional echocardiography, the diagnosis is made when the mitral valve is seen prolapsing into the left atrium.[47] Postural maneuvers are sometimes used to aid in the auscultatory diagnosis. Activities that decrease left ventricular volume increase the degree of prolapse. Hydration affects the auscultatory findings of MVP.[49] Pregnancy may have similar effects, with changes in the timing of the click and shortening or softening of the murmur. Serial echocardiograms during pregnancy showed disappearance of MVP during pregnancy in a significant number of patients.[50]

Palpitations, arrhythmias, chest pain, syncope, fatigue, and panic attacks are reported in association with MVP. Together they comprise MVP syndrome,[47] although the existence of a distinct syndrome has been questioned. The symptoms associated with MVP syndrome are very common and are seen with near equal frequency in patients with and without an echocardiographic diagnosis of MVP.[48,51]

Severe mitral regurgitation requiring surgery, infective endocarditis, cerebral ischemia, and sudden death are serious complications associated with MVP. Of the risk factors associated with these complications, only a holosystolic mitral regurgitant murmur is likely to be seen in pregnant patients.[52,53] Even mitral regurgitation is more likely to be seen in males and patients older than 45 years of age than in women of reproductive age.[54] In an examination of offspring of the Framingham Heart Study participants, with an average age of 54 years, the occurrence of severe complications in association with MVP was only minimally greater than that in those without the diagnosis.[48] The risk of serious complications in women younger than 45 years of age with uncomplicated MVP is estimated to be 0.2% per year.[53]

Management Options

Prepregnancy

Prepregnancy management should document associated mitral regurgitation by either echocardiography or evaluation by a cardiologist.

Prenatal

Patients should be observed for cardiac arrhythmias, particularly supraventricular tachycardia. Although these occur very infrequently, the patient should be counseled to avoid caffeine, alcohol, tobacco, and betamimetic drugs.

When necessary, digoxin (category C) or β-blockers (most category C) may be used.[47]

Labor and Delivery and Postnatal

In addition to continued observation for arrhythmias, some recommend endocarditis prophylaxis for high risk procedures in patients with MVP and associated mitral regurgitation.[47]

CONGENITAL HEART DEFECTS

Atrial Septal Defect

Maternal and Fetal Risks

Ostium secundum atrial defect is one of the most common congenital heart defects seen in pregnancy, and women are more commonly affected than men. Pregnancy is generally well tolerated and uncomplicated, especially in patients with normal systolic function shown by echocardiography and NYHA functional class I or II.[55] Significant complications can be associated with uncorrected atrial septal defect (ASD), but these are uncommon before 40 years of age.[56] Supraventricular arrhythmias are more frequent with advancing age and may aggravate right-sided heart failure. Paradoxical emboli from the venous to the systemic circulation can follow right-sided heart failure as a result of increased peripheral edema and venous stasis. Pulmonary hypertension is uncommonly associated with ASD and is typically found in older patients.[56] In fetuses born to mothers with an ASD, the risk of congenital heart disease is 3% to 10%.[25,27,56]

Management Options

PREPREGNANCY

The goal of preconception management is to identify secondary complications, such as supraventricular arrhythmias or pulmonary hypertension. Pregnancy should be discouraged and effective contraception initiated when significant pulmonary hypertension is present.

PRENATAL

Prenatal care is routine in the absence of supraventricular arrhythmias, right-sided heart failure, and pulmonary hypertension.

LABOR AND DELIVERY

Labor is generally well tolerated. Patients are monitored for arrhythmias. Blood pressure is carefully monitored, and fluid is restricted. Use of a PAC is considered only in the presence of pulmonary hypertension. In addition to pain control, epidural anesthesia reduces systemic vascular resistance and may reduce the left-to-right shunt.

POSTNATAL

In patients without secondary complications, postpartum management is routine. Postpartum management encourages ambulation to decrease the risk of deep venous thrombosis and paradoxical embolization.

Ventricular Septal Defect

Maternal and Fetal Risks

Ventricular septal defects (VSDs) are uncommon in adults. Small defects either close spontaneously or are corrected in childhood. Maternal morbidity is related to the size of the VSD and the presence of pulmonary hypertension. Small defects and those that are repaired in childhood usually present no problem during pregnancy. Some asymptomatic patients with a repaired VSD have significant, but unrecognized, pulmonary hypertension, which is manifested clinically in association with the hemodynamic stresses of pregnancy.[57,58] As with ASD, however, patients with good functional status and normal systolic ventricular function usually have a normal outcome.[55] Occasionally, an uncorrected VSD is complicated by congestive heart failure during pregnancy.[26] These patients are at risk for paradoxical systemic emboli. Infants born to mothers with a VSD have a 6% to 10% risk of congenital heart disease.[26,56]

Management Options

PREPREGNANCY

Before pregnancy, patients with a VSD (corrected or uncorrected) should be evaluated for pulmonary hypertension. Pregnancy is discouraged in patients with pulmonary hypertension. In the absence of pulmonary hypertension, repair of uncorrected lesions should be considered. Patients should be counseled about the increased risk of congenital heart disease in their offspring.

PRENATAL

Patients should be evaluated and followed with serial echocardiography. The size of the lesion, the degree of the shunt, and the presence of pulmonary hypertension should be determined. Termination should be offered to patients with pulmonary hypertension.

LABOR AND DELIVERY

Hypotension should be avoided to prevent shunt reversal. Endocarditis prophylaxis is indicated in patients with infection or a complicated delivery.

POSTNATAL

Volume status should be monitored during the postpartum period because of fluid shifts and the potential for congestive heart failure. Ambulation is encouraged to avoid the risk of deep venous thrombosis and paradoxical embolization.

Pulmonary Hypertension

Maternal and Fetal Risks

Pulmonary hypertension associated with pregnancy is a grave condition, and the maternal mortality rate is as high as 50%.[59] Primary pulmonary hypertension is an idiopathic disease of the pulmonary vasculature that is seen primarily in women. Secondary pulmonary hypertension can result from long-standing increases in pulmonary pressure as a result of underlying cardiac disease, such as ASD or VSD, mitral stenosis, or patent ductus arteriosus (PDA).[60]

With primary pulmonary hypertension, the most dangerous times are labor, delivery, and the early postpartum period. Intravascular volume changes are not well tolerated because of the fixed pulmonary vascular resistance. Increases in cardiac output during labor or as a result of postpartum fluid shifts may lead to sudden right-sided heart failure. At delivery, excessive blood loss decreases preload, resulting in an inability to overcome high pulmonary vascular resistance. Both situations lead to a decrease in left ventricular preload and a dramatic decrease in left ventricular output. A direct consequence is myocardial ischemia, leading to arrhythmias, ventricular failure, and sudden death. Pulmonary thromboembolic events are usually fatal. Even small thrombi in the lungs can dramatically aggravate pulmonary hypertension.[60] In the fetus, chronic maternal hypoxia can lead to intrauterine growth restriction. Despite this, the neonatal survival rate is nearly 90%.[59]

Management Options

PREPREGNANCY

Despite improvements in maternal outcome with a comprehensive team approach,[60] maternal morbidity and mortality are significant risks. As a result, pregnancy should be discouraged and permanent sterilization should be considered.

PRENATAL

If pregnancy occurs, termination should be offered because of maternal risks. If pregnancy is discovered in the second trimester and termination is chosen, dilation and evacuation is preferred over induction. In a continuing pregnancy, the cardiologist, critical care specialist, and obstetrician must work closely together. An obstetric anesthesiologist should be consulted early in the pregnancy. The use of calcium channel blockers is reported in some patients, with improvement in maternal cardiac output and successful pregnancy outcome. Nifedipine in doses of 90 to 120 mg daily was used.[61] Heparin (category C) thromboembolism prophylaxis is initiated early, with doses of 5000 to 10,000 units given subcutaneously twice daily. Patients with more severe disease, manifested by chest pain or oxygen saturation of 80% or less, are at higher risk and full heparin anticoagulation has been used. In the early third trimester, in-hospital bed rest with oxygen therapy (up to an FiO_2 of 0.4) and frequent monitoring with pulse oximetry is advocated. Late diagnosis and late admission to the hospital were associated with an increased risk of maternal mortality.[59] Lack of improvement in SaO_2 with oxygen suggests further increased maternal risk.[60]

LABOR AND DELIVERY

Close monitoring during labor is essential to achieve a good outcome. Spontaneous labor is preferred to prevent the increased risk of cesarean section associated with induction. When indicated, however, Pitocin or E series prostaglandins can safely be used for induction. Oxygen flow is increased to 5 to 6 L/minute. Oxygen saturation is monitored continuously with pulse oximetry. A radial artery line is placed to allow continuous blood pressure monitoring and facilitate frequent blood gas sampling. Maintenance of stable blood pressure is important. Adequate preload is essential to maintain cardiac output. Routine use of a pulmonary artery catheter (PAC) is discouraged.[59] An alternative is to place a central venous pressure (CVP) catheter early in labor. Arguments against the use of a PAC stem from the fact that information from the right side of the heart can be obtained from the CVP line. Left-sided heart pressure may not be accurately reflected due to elevated pulmonary artery pressures. Potential complications, such as arrhythmias, thrombosis, and pulmonary artery rupture, must be considered when deciding on PAC use. Despite these concerns, in some patients, cardiac output data obtained from a PAC is useful. The decision to use invasive hemodynamic monitoring should be made on an individual basis, after the risks and benefits are considered.

Several case reports described the use of intravenous prostacyclin or inhaled nitric oxide therapy during labor.[62–64] Both drugs cause vascular dilation and inhibit platelet aggregation, leading to improved oxygenation, decreased pulmonary vascular resistance, and a decreased risk of thromboembolism. Improvement in pulmonary hypertension is similar between the two drugs in nonpregnant patients, and there seems to be no added benefit to a combination of the two agents. Inhaled nitric oxide avoids systemic hemodynamic changes, is easy to administer, and may cost less than other agents. Nitric oxide is typically used at a dose of 5 to 20 ppm. Elevated methemoglobin levels are a potential toxicity, but this effect has not been reported at these doses.[65]

An epidural catheter is placed early in labor and carefully activated when contractions become painful, to avoid hypotension. Intrathecal narcotics can be added to decrease the hypotensive effect of local anesthetics. During labor and delivery, the patient is placed in the left lateral position to avoid supine hypotension. Vaginal delivery, with shortening of the second stage with forceps or a vacuum to decrease the need for pushing, is desirable. Blood loss at delivery is carefully monitored. Crystalloid solution can be used to replace volume and maintain preload if blood loss is greater than normal. Cesarean delivery is associated with increased maternal morbidity and mortality and should be reserved for obstetric indications.[59,60]

POSTNATAL

Antepartum and intrapartum management principles are continued into the postpartum period. Thromboembolism prophylaxis and oxygen therapy are continued. Excessive blood loss or right-sided heart failure as a result of fluid shifts can lead to sudden death. The patient must be monitored closely during the first 48 to 72 hours. During this time, nitric oxide is slowly weaned.[64] If prostacyclin is used, long-term therapy can continue, if necessary, through a central venous catheter.[63] Controlled diuresis is important during postpartum fluid mobilization to control preload and prevent worsening right-sided heart function.[61] Pulmonary edema may develop rapidly in patients who do not have brisk spontaneous diuresis. Permanent sterilization should be considered in patients with severe pulmonary hypertension.

Eisenmenger's Syndrome

Maternal and Fetal Risks

Eisenmenger's syndrome is defined as pulmonary hypertension as a result of uncorrected left-to-right shunt of a VSD, ASD, or PDA, with subsequent shunt reversal and cyanosis. Pulmonary hypertension is defined as mean pulmonary artery pressure greater than 25 mm Hg. The increase in blood volume and decrease in systemic vascular resistance can lead to right ventricular failure, with a decrease in cardiac output and sudden death. Maternal mortality with Eisenmenger's syndrome is as high as 40% in pregnancies that continue past the first trimester.[59,66] In contrast, the 15-year survival rate is more than 75% in nonpregnant patients.[67] Postoperative fluid shifts associated with cesarean delivery pose an even greater risk, with mortality rates approaching 70%. Although maternal risk remains high, a recent report emphasizing a team approach, with close follow-up and careful attention to detail, achieved a more optimistic outcome.[60] Intrauterine growth restriction is a common fetal complication. Preterm delivery is also frequent, occurring in up to 85% of pregnancies.[66] Despite the maternal and fetal complications, the neonatal survival rate approaches 90%.[59]

Management Options

PREPREGNANCY

Pregnancy should be discouraged and reliable contraception, preferably permanent sterilization, advised because of the extreme maternal risk associated with pregnancy. Even first-trimester termination is associated with a maternal mortality rate of 5% to 10%.[60]

PRENATAL, LABOR AND DELIVERY, AND POSTNATAL

Echocardiography is helpful in evaluating shunting, right ventricular function, and pulmonary hypertension. Cardiac catheterization may be necessary to quantify pulmonary hypertension. Pregnancy complications and outcome are related to the degree of pulmonary hypertension. Management of pulmonary hypertension associated with Eisenmenger's syndrome follows the same principles discussed in the section on pulmonary hypertension. Nitric oxide use is described in two case reports that showed improvement in pulmonary hypertension and maternal oxygenation during labor and delivery. Unfortunately, despite continued use, progressive deterioration occurred postpartum, and neither patient survived.[68,69] In one case, doses as high as 80 ppm were used, and an elevated methemoglobin level occurred.[68]

Coarctation of the Aorta

Maternal and Fetal Risks

Coarctation of the aorta complicating pregnancy is relatively uncommon, accounting for only 6% to 11% of cases of congenital heart disease in pregnant patients in older series. Most of these lesions were corrected before pregnancy.[1,2,4] When the lesions are corrected, maternal and fetal outcomes are not significantly different from those in the general obstetric population.[70] Several cardiovascular anomalies are associated with coarctation of the aorta. Aneurysms of the circle of Willis, intercostal arteries, and distal aorta may be present. Bicuspid aortic valve is also seen.[71] Although most patients complete pregnancy without complication, the risk of significant maternal morbidity exists, particularly if other anomalies are present. Surgical repair can reduce, but not eliminate, the risk of aortic rupture or dissection.[72] Bicuspid aortic valve increases the risk of bacterial endocarditis.[56] Aneurysms may rupture, with those involving the circle of Willis resulting in subarachnoid hemorrhage. Maternal hypertension is common, particularly if the lesion is not repaired.[72] In these patients, the risk of fetal congenital heart disease is 4% to 7%.[27,56,72]

Management Options

PREPREGNANCY

Coarctation of the aorta should be repaired before conception. Appropriate imaging studies should be done to identify aneurysms or aortic valve disease. If they are identified, elective surgical management should be considered.

PRENATAL

Termination may be considered in patients with uncorrected coarctation of the aorta, especially if it is associated with other anomalies, because of the increase in maternal morbidity and mortality.

LABOR AND DELIVERY AND POSTNATAL

Hypertension should be controlled in both the intrapartum and postpartum periods. Epidural anesthesia is encouraged because it effectively controls pain and decreases systemic vascular resistance.[73] Endocarditis prophylaxis is indicated for complicated deliveries with coexisting aortic valvular disease.

Tetralogy of Fallot

Maternal and Fetal Risks

Tetralogy of Fallot is a complex cyanotic heart disease that consists of VSD, overriding aorta, pulmonary stenosis, and right ventricular hypertrophy. Although survival to adulthood is possible, uncorrected tetralogy of Fallot is rarely seen in pregnancy for several reasons. Most patients undergo surgical correction early in life. In those who do not have surgery, life expectancy is shortened and fertility is impaired. After surgical correction, cardiac arrhythmias are seen in some patients, although these are not usually a severe problem.[4,74] Patients without residual defects who have normal functional status after surgical correction tolerate pregnancy well.[55,74,75]

In patients with uncorrected tetralogy of Fallot, pregnancy presents serious risks, including maternal mortality (see Table 37–1). Preexisting pulmonary hypertension is a concern.[74] In addition, increased cardiac output leads to increased venous return to the hypertrophic right ventricle. These changes, together with decreased systemic vascular resistance, increase the right-to-left shunt. Oxygenation decreases, hematocrit increases, and cyanosis worsens, further stressing an already compromised system.[56] Risk factors that worsen the prognosis include prepregnancy hematocrit exceeding 65%, a history of congestive heart failure or syncope, cardiomegaly, right ventricular pressure exceeding 120 mm Hg or strain pattern on electrocardiogram, or oxygen saturation less than 80%.[76]

A good neonatal outcome can be expected in patients with corrected tetralogy of Fallot and no residual defects.[74,75] Neonatal outcome is often poor in patients with an uncorrected lesion because of increased rates of spontaneous abortion, prematurity, and intrauterine growth restriction. Congenital heart disease affects approximately 5% of infants of mothers with tetralogy of Fallot.[25]

Management Options

PREPREGNANCY

Surgery is advocated for patients with uncorrected lesions. Patients who underwent previous corrective surgery should be evaluated for residual defects, such as VSD. If defects are found, repair should be considered.[75]

PRENATAL

After surgical correction, activity is restricted only to the point of preventing fatigue. Patients with uncorrected tetralogy of Fallot should be offered termination. Hematocrit should be followed. Supplemental oxygen may be of benefit. Serial obstetric ultrasound examinations are used to detect intrauterine growth restriction. Antenatal testing is started during the third trimester, as indicated.

LABOR AND DELIVERY

In patients with uncorrected defects, careful fluid management and maintenance of blood pressure are the main features of intrapartum care. Central hemodynamic monitoring may be used, but there is a risk of exacerbating arrhythmias. Hypotension should be prevented to avoid shunt reversal. Epidural anesthesia can be used if the patient is adequately hydrated and it is carefully administered. To prevent decreases in venous return with bearing down, operative vaginal delivery may be used to shorten the second stage of labor. This strategy is often applied in patients with corrected tetralogy of Fallot, although it probably is not necessary.[74,75]

POSTNATAL

In patients with uncorrected tetralogy of Fallot, volume status should be monitored during the early postpartum period. A reliable contraceptive plan should be made, with permanent sterilization a good alternative.

Transposition of the Great Arteries

Maternal and Fetal Risks

Transposition of the great arteries is a congenital heart disease consisting of discordance between the ventricles and the great arteries, in which the aorta arises from the right ventricle and the pulmonary artery originates from the left ventricle. Two types exist, depending on the concordance of the ventricles and the atria. In the first type, complete transposition, there is atrial concordance. Two parallel circulations exist. The systemic venous return enters the right atrium, proceeds to the right ventricle, and exits through the aorta, bypassing the pulmonary circulation. The pulmonary venous return enters the left atrium, continues into the left ventricle, and returns to the lungs through the pulmonary artery. Thus, no oxygenated blood reaches the systemic circulation. Without an additional congenital shunt lesion or a surgical procedure to redirect blood flow more appropriately, this condition is not compatible with life. Although several procedures are used to repair the condition, an atrial switch procedure, the Mustard operation, is most commonly used. In this procedure, a baffle is placed between the right and left atria. Systemic venous return is redirected to the left side of the heart and to the lungs, whereas the oxygenated pulmonary venous blood is shunted to the right ventricle and on to the systemic circulation. Surgery allowed these patients to reach adulthood and contemplate pregnancy.

The second type is congenitally corrected transposition. Both arterioventricular and atrioventricular discordance are present. The right atrium empties its systemic venous blood into the morphologic left ventricle. Oxygenated pulmonary venous blood returns to the left atrium and empties into the morphologic right ventricle. Additional cardiac anomalies are often present, including VSD, pulmonary stenosis, and valve abnormalities.[77,78] Patients with congenitally corrected transposition and no associated anomalies may be completely asymptomatic and remain undiagnosed into adulthood.[78]

The major concern in both types of transposition is the ability of the morphologic right ventricle to continue to support the systemic circulation as well as the increased cardiac output occurring during gestation. Several small series and case reports described the outcome of pregnancy in women with both complete[4,79–82] and congenitally corrected transposition of the great vessels.[4,77,78,83,84] In these patients, maternal mortality was rare, with only one death noted in the 78 patients who were followed. Morbidity was common, however, occurring in approximately 30% of patients. Not surprisingly, heart failure was seen most often. Other complications included arrhythmias, worsening cyanosis, cerebrovascular accident, and left atrioventricular (AV) valve regurgitation.

The incidence of miscarriage was high, approaching 40%. The increased risk was primarily related to maternal cyanosis.[83,84] The rate of preterm birth was 10% to 20%, and the incidence of growth restriction was infrequently reported. The risk of congenital heart disease in offspring of these women does not appear to be increased above that in the general population, although the number of patients evaluated was small.[25,82]

Management Options

PREPREGNANCY

As with all cardiac conditions in pregnancy, it is important to determine the patient's functional status. Echocardiography to evaluate the function of the systemic right ventricle is necessary. The patient should also be evaluated for arrhythmias. A cardiologist with experience in treating congenital heart disease in adults should be included in the initial evaluation and throughout pregnancy. Often, this role is filled by the patient's pediatric cardiologist because these physicians often follow patients into adulthood.

PRENATAL

Decreased activity is advised to minimize further stress on the right ventricle. Patients should have serial echocardiography to evaluate cardiac function. Symptoms of congestive heart failure should be evaluated quickly and treated with diuretics and digoxin, as indicated. An anesthesiologist should evaluate the patient before labor.

LABOR, DELIVERY, AND POSTNATAL

Maternal cardiac monitoring is used to detect arrhythmias. Supplemental oxygen is given, as necessary. Volume overload should be avoided during labor and thoughout the postpartum period. Adequate analgesia is important and can be provided with an epidural. Shortening of the second stage with forceps or a vacuum should be considered. Cesarean delivery is reserved for the usual obstetric indications.

Patent Ductus Arteriosus

Maternal and Fetal Risks

Surgical correction of PDA is usually accomplished in childhood. Uncorrected lesions have traditionally accounted for fewer than 5% of pregnancies complicated by congenital heart disease.[1,2] Maternal complications depend on the size of the ductus. Asymptomatic patients with a small PDA generally tolerate pregnancy without difficulty. Left-to-right shunting may decrease during pregnancy as a result of decreased systemic vascular resistance. A large lesion with a long-standing left-to-right shunt can lead to pulmonary hypertension.[85] In this situation, the normal decrease in systemic vascular resistance during pregnancy can cause shunt reversal, with an increase in maternal mortality.[56] The risk of congenital heart disease in the fetus is approximately 4%.[56]

Management Options

PREPREGNANCY

Before pregnancy, evaluation includes echocardiography to determine the size of the PDA and identify pulmonary hypertension.

PRENATAL

Antenatal management consists of echocardiography to detect pulmonary hypertension. If pulmonary hypertension develops, bed rest and supplemental oxygen should be instituted.

LABOR, DELIVERY, AND POSTNATAL

Intrapartum volume status should be monitored with care to avoid hypotension, which can result in shunt reversal. Use of a PAC may be indicated in patients with pulmonary hypertension. Endocarditis prophylaxis is indicated, except in uncomplicated deliveries. Careful attention to volume status should continue through the postpartum period.

RHEUMATIC HEART DISEASE: GENERAL

Maternal and Fetal Risks

Over the last several decades, a significant decline in the incidence and severity of rheumatic heart disease occurred in developed countries. A similar pattern was seen with rheumatic heart disease complicating pregnancy.[2,86] In a recent multicenter report of 562 women with heart disease managed during pregnancy, only 14% had acquired valvular lesions.[4] The changes were attributed in part to improved socioeconomic conditions. In many parts of the world, rheumatic heart disease is a significant public health problem. Asia, Africa, and South America have high prevalence rates.[87,88] Some positive trends were noted in developing nations. Sri Lanka, for example, saw an increase in the age at presentation and a decrease in the severity and resultant morbidity and mortality associated with mitral stenosis.[89] Despite the dramatic decline in developed countries, rheumatic heart disease will continue to be seen because of immigration from high-prevalence areas.[90]

Rheumatic heart disease is a complication of rheumatic fever. Cardiac valve damage results from an immunologic injury initiated by a group A β-hemolytic streptococcal infection.[91] During pregnancy, the increased maternal blood volume and heart rate can lead to heart failure and pulmonary edema. Arrhythmias also frequently complicate pregnancy. In a series of 64 women followed in Los Angeles, California, congestive heart failure occurred in 38% and arrhythmias occurred in 15%.[92] Not surprisingly, poor maternal functional class (NYHA class III or IV) is associated with worse maternal and fetal outcomes.[92] Rates of intrauterine growth retardation and prematurity are increased with complicated rheumatic heart disease.[92,93]

Management Options

General management principles for patients with rheumatic heart disease are aimed at preventing cardiac failure and bacterial endocarditis. Volume status is monitored, and activity should be limited. Antibiotics should be given in association with high-risk procedures (see Table 37–4). Specific valvular lesions are discussed individually.

Mitral Stenosis

Maternal and Fetal Risks

Mitral stenosis, either alone or in combination with other lesions, is the most common valvular disorder associated with rheumatic heart disease.[1,2,93] In a 12-year review of 486 pregnant patients in India through 1999, 63% of lesions affected a single valve. Mitral stenosis was the abnormality in 90% of these women.[93] Although in the past mitral stenosis was the most common rheumatic lesion associated with maternal mortality, death rarely occurs today.[1,2,89,94,95] Hemodynamically, mitral stenosis is a state of fixed cardiac output caused by left atrial outflow obstruction. Pressures in the left atrium and pulmonary vasculature are increased. Long-standing severe disease may be complicated by secondary pulmonary hypertension and atrial fibrillation. In pregnancy, the increased intravascular volume can further elevate pressures and lead to pulmonary edema and arrhythmias, even in previously asymptomatic patients.[95] Increased maternal heart rate and decreased left ventricular filling time may result in a decrease in cardiac output.[94] If maternal decompensation can be avoided, a good fetal outcome can be expected.[1,2,89,94]

Management Options

PREPREGNANCY

The goal of preconception care is to define the severity of cardiac compromise. Two-dimensional echocardiography and color flow Doppler are used to determine cardiac function and the degree of stenosis. Together, these modalities allow noninvasive evaluation of these patients and decrease the need for cardiac catheterization.[96] In symptomatic patients or those with severely stenotic valves, surgical correction should take place before conception. Surgical commissurotomy is the traditional treatment modality. Recently, percutaneous mitral valve commissurotomy emerged as an alternative. The percutaneous method is safe and as effective as the surgical approach. In addition, it is less invasive, less expensive, and even preferred as first-line therapy in some patients.[90,97] Satisfactory results persisted beyond 5 years in these reports, delaying and potentially avoiding the risks associated with prosthetic valves.[98]

PRENATAL

The goal of prenatal care is to avoid cardiac decompensation. Special attention should be paid to volume status. Weight gain should be closely monitored. Symptoms or physical findings associated with heart failure should be reported and evaluated promptly. Maternal tachycardia should be avoided to prevent a decrease in cardiac output. Restriction of physical activity can aid in this objective. β-Blockade may be used to control heart rate. It is used empirically in mitral stenosis during pregnancy to prevent the development of tachycardia, with good maternal and fetal outcome.[99] Atrial fibrillation can be managed with digoxin (category C) or cardioversion, as necessary.

Serial echocardiography is indicated to follow cardiac function objectively. Cardiac catheterization may be necessary to further evaluate and even treat patients with refractory pulmonary edema, despite optimal medical management. Several series showed successful treatment and good maternal and neonatal outcome in patients managed with balloon valvulotomy for severe symptomatic mitral stenosis during pregnancy.[100–103]

LABOR AND DELIVERY

During the intrapartum and postpartum periods, volume status and cardiac output are critical concerns. In patients with NYHA class III or IV disease, central hemodynamic monitoring may be considered. Pulmonary pressures and cardiac output can be measured reliably. Although pulmonary capillary wedge pressure (PCWP) can warn of the potential for pulmonary edema, it does not accurately reflect left ventricular preload. The pressure gradient across the stenotic valve may necessitate a high normal or even elevated PCWP to allow adequate left ventricular filling and maintain cardiac output. To prevent pulmonary edema after delivery as a result of postpartum fluid shifts, PCWP should be maintained as low as possible without compromising cardiac output. Fluid restriction or careful diuresis, with attention to cardiac output, may be used to obtain desirable pressures. Decreased diastolic filling time associated with tachycardia may also decrease cardiac output. Careful intravenous administration of β-blockers (most category C) may be necessary to control heart rate and maintain cardiac output during labor.[94]

Similar considerations accompany analgesia and anesthesia during labor and delivery. Epidural analgesia is both safe and effective. Careful administration of the anesthetic agent is necessary to avoid hypotension. Control of labor pain removes a stimulus for tachycardia. The increased venous capacitance can also moderate postpartum fluid shifts. Drugs such as atropine, pancuronium, and meperidine can cause tachycardia and should be avoided.

Cesarean delivery is reserved for obstetric indications. If abdominal delivery is necessary, epidural is the anesthetic method of choice. Although forceps delivery is advocated to shorten the second stage of labor and reduce bearing down, it is not always required.[94] Endocarditis antibiotic prophylaxis should be given when a complicated delivery is anticipated. Because these deliveries cannot always be predicted, routine antibiotic prophylaxis is recommended.[104]

POSTNATAL

Postpartum fluid shifts increase the risk of pulmonary edema. Clark and colleagues[94] noted a mean increase in PCWP of 10 mm Hg between the second stage of labor and the postpartum period in eight patients with functionally severe mitral stenosis. Because frank pulmonary edema is unlikely at a PCWP of less than 30 mm Hg, maintaining the PCWP at 14 mm Hg or lower should prevent this complication.[94]

Mitral Regurgitation

Maternal and Fetal Risks

Although mitral stenosis is almost exclusively caused by rheumatic heart disease, mitral regurgitation has several causes. In addition to rheumatic disease, floppy mitral valves in association with MVP, papillary muscle dysfunction, and ruptured chordae tendineae can result in mitral regurgitation.[105] In women of reproductive age, however, rheumatic heart disease is the most common cause of hemodynamically significant regurgitation. It is the dominant lesion in approximately one-third of patients with rheumatic heart disease, but it is often associated with mitral stenosis.[1,2] In patients without severe mitral regurgitation or ventricular dysfunction, pregnancy is generally well tolerated. The decrease in systemic vascular resistance associated with pregnancy has a beneficial effect. Atrial fibrillation may develop because of the effect of increased volume on a dilated atrium.

Management Options

PREPREGNANCY

NYHA functional status should be determined (see Table 37–2). The degree of regurgitation, atrial size, and ventricular function should be established with echocardiography. If required, digoxin (category C) therapy should be optimized. Although uncommon, if valve replacement is necessary, surgery should be performed before pregnancy. Valve replacement is indicated in asymptomatic patients with mild to moderate ventricular dysfunction and in those with atrial fibrillation, pulmonary hypertension, or symptoms such as dyspnea at rest or orthopnea.[106]

PRENATAL

In patients with NYHA class I or II disease, restriction of activity to prevent fatigue should be all that is required. In patients who have symptoms, serial echocardiography is indicated. Digoxin, diuresis, and afterload reduction should be instituted if left ventricular failure develops.

If medical therapy is unsuccessful, cardiac surgery during pregnancy can proceed, if necessary. Although small case series suggested that maternal mortality is not increased compared with nonpregnant women,[107] a recent review of the literature suggests that surgery for valvular disease during pregnancy and the early postpartum period is associated with a mortality rate of approximately 9%, roughly four times that of the nonpregnant population.[108] The fetal survival rate typically exceeds 70%.[107,108] Factors that affected survival were gestational age at hospital admission and the degree of emergency necessitating the procedure. During cardiac bypass, fetal bradycardia and prolonged loss of fetal heart tones can occur as a result of maternal hypotension.[109] Fetal risks are minimized with high flow to maintain a mean maternal blood pressure greater than 70 mm Hg. Fetal heart rate can be monitored during the procedure and used as a guide to adjust flow rates. Hypothermia is also a concern and is associated with fetal bradycardia. Uterine contractions are common, further complicating fetal heart rate abnormalities. Perfusion temperatures greater than 30°C are generally well tolerated.[107] In the larger review, neonatal outcome was not related to the evaluated variables associated with cardiac bypass, including duration of bypass, hypothermia versus normal temperature, and lowest temperature.[108]

LABOR, DELIVERY, AND POSTNATAL

Volume status should be monitored, and increases in blood pressure should be avoided to prevent worsening of regurgitant flow. When the left atrium is enlarged, cardiac monitoring may aid in the early identification of atrial fibrillation. Regional anesthesia is the method of choice for pain control during labor and delivery because of the decrease in systemic vascular resistance. Endocarditis prophylaxis should be used when indicated (see Table 37–4). Monitoring for congestive heart failure and atrial fibrillation should continue into the postpartum period.

Aortic Stenosis

Maternal and Fetal Risks

Aortic stenosis is the most common cardiac valve lesion in the United States. It can be congenital or rheumatic in origin, or it may be due to an age-related calcification of the aortic valve. All of these etiologies are uncommon in women of reproductive age. Both congenital aortic stenosis and age-related lesions more commonly affect men.[110] In addition, aortic stenosis of rheumatic origin is typically progressive and tends to be less severe in patients of reproductive age.[111] Aortic stenosis accounts for only 5% to 10% of cases of rheumatic heart disease in pregnancy and is usually seen in conjunction with mitral valve disease.[1,2]

The normal aortic valve area is 3 to 4 cm. The pressure gradient across the valve increases rapidly as the valve area is reduced to less than 2 cm, and this increase is associated with left ventricular outflow obstruction.[110] Mild to moderate stenosis (valve area >1 cm) is relatively well tolerated in pregnancy, with no cardiac complications reported in a recent case series of patients with congenital aortic stenosis. Even patients with severe aortic stenosis generally do well, with no maternal mortality and only a 10% rate of cardiac complications reported in the same series. During 2-year follow-up, 36% of patients had progression of the cardiac condition that required surgery.[112] In these patients, cardiac output is fixed. Increased left ventricular pressure leads to hypertrophy and subsequent atrial enlargement. Tachyarrhythmias may further complicate the condition. A decrease in cardiac output may result in inadequate coronary artery and cerebral perfusion, followed by sudden death. Patients with congenital stenosis are also at increased risk for endocarditis.[56] Despite the maternal risks, recent series reported a generally good outcome.[26,111,113,114] Decreased disease severity may be one factor.[111]

With severe stenosis, the fetus is at risk for intrauterine growth restriction. If maternal disease is congenital, the incidence of congenital heart disease in the fetus is 4% to 12%.[27]

Management Options

PREPREGNANCY

Before pregnancy, the severity of aortic stenosis should be determined by echocardiography and catheterization, if necessary. Severe disease should be corrected surgically before conception.

PRENATAL

Physical activity should be limited. Patients should be observed for signs of congestive heart failure or arrhythmias. Serial fetal ultrasounds should be scheduled to detect evidence of growth restriction. Antenatal testing is initiated, as indicated.

LABOR, DELIVERY, AND POSTNATAL

Fluid management is the critical component of intrapartum care. Volume overload can lead to pulmonary edema. Of greater concern, however, is hypovolemia or hypotension, with decreased venous return and cardiac output. Use of a PAC may aid in monitoring volume status. Patients should labor and deliver in the lateral position to avoid aortocaval compression. Regional anesthesia is administered slowly and cautiously, after adequate volume loading, to avoid hypotension. A narcotic epidural can decrease the chance of hypotension. Blood loss should be monitored closely and replaced as necessary. If pulmonary edema develops, aggressive diuresis is avoided to prevent a decrease in preload. Oxygen, morphine (category B), and inotropic agents, such as dopamine (category C) or dobutamine (category C), are used to maintain cardiac output. Bacterial endocarditis prophylaxis is used, as indicated (see Table 37–4). Close monitoring of volume status is essential in the postpartum period.

Continued follow-up after the postpartum period is important because the condition is progressive. Many patients require surgical intervention within 2 years of pregnancy.[112]

Aortic Regurgitation

Maternal and Fetal Risks

Like aortic stenosis, aortic regurgitation is uncommon in women of childbearing age. Although it is most likely of rheumatic origin, aortic regurgitation is an infrequent rheumatic lesion. Less common etiologies include Marfan's syndrome and syphilitic aortitis. Regurgitation in both is a consequence of aortic root dilation.

With progressive aortic insufficiency, cardiac output is usually maintained by left ventricular dilation and hypertrophy as a result of increased preload and stroke volume. Because the condition is progressive, severe disease, with ventricular dilation, hypertrophy, and widened pulse pressure, is not likely to be seen in pregnancy.[115] The decreased systemic vascular resistance and increased heart rate associated with pregnancy may improve the hemodynamics of aortic insufficiency because of decreased resistance to forward flow and decreased time for regurgitant flow to occur during diastole. As a result, pregnancy is generally well tolerated.[86]

Management Options

PREPREGNANCY

Preconceptually, the extent of disease should be defined by echocardiogram and catheterization, if necessary. In symptomatic patients, cardiac function should be optimized with digoxin (category C) and afterload reduction, as necessary. If indicated, valve replacement is done before pregnancy.

PRENATAL

Cardiac status should be optimized, as in the nonpregnant state, and patients should be followed for signs of congestive heart failure. If medical management is inadequate, valve replacement can be performed during pregnancy with relative safety.[107]

LABOR, DELIVERY, AND POSTNATAL

Volume status should be followed in the postpartum period while the patient is observed for congestive heart failure. Invasive hemodynamic monitoring is usually unnecessary unless other valvular disease is present. Pain control is best achieved with lumbar epidural anesthesia, which decreases regurgitant flow by reducing afterload.

PROSTHETIC HEART VALVES

Maternal and Fetal Risks

Surgical valve replacement allowed many patients with severe valvular heart disease to survive and lead near-normal lives. There are two broad categories of replacement valves, each with advantages and disadvantages. Mechanical valves are made of nonbiologic materials. Bioprosthetic valves are either heterografts, made of bovine or porcine valves or pericardium, or homografts, which are human aortic valves.[116] The different characteristics of these valves make the optimal choice in women of reproductive age difficult and controversial. Mechanical valves have the advantage of durability, but the risk of thrombosis requires long-term anticoagulation. Bioprosthetic valves do not require anticoagulation, but valve failure often occurs within 10 to 15 years.[116] To reduce the need for replacement, mechanical valves are recommended for young patients.[116] On the other hand, bioprosthetic valves are advocated to decrease the risk of thrombosis during pregnancy and the risk of bleeding complications as a result of anticoagulation. Bioprosthetic valves also eliminate the significant fetal risks associated with oral anticoagulants.[117]

The incidence of major thromboembolism in nonpregnant patients with mechanical valves averages 8%. Anticoagulation reduces this risk by 75%.[118] Valve thrombosis causes pulmonary congestion, poor perfusion, and systemic embolization. Rapid clinical deterioration often follows. Most embolization involves the cerebral vessels. Patients with atrial fibrillation or left ventricular dysfunction are at increased risk for embolic events. In addition, increased rates of pregnancy loss,[119,120] prematurity, and low birth weight[121] were reported in patients with mechanical valves compared with those with bioprosthetic valves.

Bioprosthetic valve dysfunction is often related to rupture or tearing of a leaflet. Progressive dyspnea and congestive heart failure suggest bioprosthetic valve deterioration. Failure in these valves is more common with a mitral valve prosthesis and in patients younger than 40 years old.[116] Pregnancy accelerated valve deterioration in one series,[119] although this finding was not confirmed by others.[122,123] In a recent report by Salazar and associates,[123] the need for bioprosthetic valve replacement was associated with the patient's age at the time of initial surgery and not with pregnancy. Bioprosthetic valve dysfunction occurred at a rate of 3.5% per patient-year in the pregnancy group compared with 3.4% per patient-year in the nonpregnant control group. Endocarditis complicates both types of prostheses equally. Reported rates vary from 3% to 6%[116] to as high as 10% to 22%.[122]

North and colleagues[122] reviewed their experience with valve replacement in a population of more than 230 patients 12 to 35 years of age, with nearly 1500 woman-years of follow-up. The report covered a 20-year period beginning in 1972. Of these women, 71 had a total of 132 pregnancies. Patients with bioprosthetic valves had a significantly lower incidence of thrombosis and bleeding complications as well as greater 10-year survival compared with those with mechanical valves. Not surprisingly, there was an increased need for replacement of the bioprosthetic valve within 10 years (Table 37–6).

In patients with mechanical valves, anticoagulation is required throughout pregnancy, and there is controversy about the method of choice. Heparin use was associated with an increased incidence of valve thrombosis compared with warfarin (category D).[120] This finding may be explained by inadequate heparin dosing.[124] On the other hand, warfarin is associated with increased risk in pregnancy, both early and late, compared with heparin.[120] In addition, a specific embryopathic pattern is seen when warfarin is used between weeks 6 and 9. Fetal warfarin syndrome is characterized by nasal hypoplasia and stippled epiphyses.[31] The incidence of fetal complications appears to be related to the warfarin dose, with a substantially increased risk noted in patients requiring more than 5 mg/day.[125] Because it crosses the placenta, warfarin can also cause fetal anticoagulation and bleeding, particularly if used within 2 weeks of labor.[124] Despite

TABLE 37–6

Comparison of Outcomes Associated with Mechanical and Prosthetic Valves in Young Women

OUTCOME	MECHANICAL (N = 178)	BIOPROSTHETIC (N = 73)	HOMOGRAFT (N = 72)	P
10-year survival (%)	70	84	96	0.12
Thrombotic complications (%)	45	13	1	<0.01
Bleeding complications (%)	15	4		0.05
10-year valve replacement (%)	29	82	28	<0.01

the potential fetal consequences associated with oral anticoagulation, a committee of the European Society of Cardiology Working Group on Valvular Heart Disease[126] advocates continued use of oral anticoagulation, with a switch to heparin (category C) during the final 2 to 3 weeks of gestation, as an acceptable treatment approach. Another acceptable regimen uses heparin during the first trimester, with a change to warfarin until 37 weeks, and a change back to heparin until after delivery. In both regimens, antenatal use of warfarin is advocated over heparin because of a decreased risk of valve thrombosis.[126] To prevent warfarin embryopathy, another option is to substitute heparin at therapeutic doses preconceptually or before week 6 and to continue its use until after delivery. This method is used successfully, with heparin given subcutaneously every 8 to 12 hours at a dose sufficient to maintain the activated partial thromboplastin time at greater than two times the control value.[116,124] The addition of low-dose aspirin was suggested as an adjunct to either heparin or warfarin to further reduce the risk of thrombosis; however, it is associated with a slight increase in the incidence of bleeding complications.[127] Osteoporosis and fractures are potential risks of long-term heparin therapy. Antiplatelet agents and low-dose heparin (5000 units given subcutaneously every 12 hours) do not adequately protect against thrombotic complications.[128]

The use of low-molecular-weight heparin for both prophylaxis and therapeutic anticoagulation during pregnancy increased in recent years. In 2002, Aventis issued a warning that enoxaparin should not be used for anticoagulation in patients with artificial heart valves because of reports of valve thrombosis associated with its use. Although this decision was criticized because of inadequate evidence,[127] until more data are available, it seems prudent not to use low-molecular-weight heparin for this purpose.

Management Options

Prepregnancy

As with other cardiac lesions, NYHA functional status is determined. Baseline echocardiography is indicated. Patients with bioprosthetic valves should be informed of the symptoms of valve deterioration, although the relationship with pregnancy is controversial. Warfarin embryopathy must be discussed with patients who have a mechanical valve. An informed decision about the potential use, timing, and duration of heparin treatment should be made.

Prenatal

Patients with bioprosthetic valves should be followed for signs of valve deterioration. Those with mechanical valves must maintain adequate anticoagulation. In patients who continue treatment with warfarin, the International Normalized Ratio is maintained between 2.0 and 4.9, depending on the valve type.[116,126] If heparin is used, the activated partial thromboplastin time is followed. Thrombocytopenia is associated with heparin therapy and has two types, early and late. The early type is seen during the first 5 days of therapy. Platelet counts usually return to normal within 72 hours.[129] Late-onset thrombocytopenia occurs after more than 5 days of heparin use and is associated with heparin-dependent immunoglobulin G antibodies. Immunoglobulins can cause platelet aggregation and activation, with subsequent paradoxical arterial or venous thrombosis.[129,130] A baseline platelet count should be obtained, and serial platelet counts are followed. The finding of late-onset thrombocytopenia requires heparin discontinuation. At term, if warfarin has been used, it is discontinued and heparin initiated.

Labor and Delivery

Clear recommendations for heparin use during labor and delivery are not available. Intravenous heparin at therapeutic doses may be given until 6 hours before delivery. This approach has the advantage of preventing thrombotic complications. The benefit is small, however, because the risk of valve thrombosis during the relatively short time of subtherapeutic anticoagulation is low.[118] If necessary, protamine can be used to reverse intravenous heparin anticoagulation at a dose of 1 mg/100 units heparin up to a maximum dose of 50 mg. The dose is decreased as the time since heparin withdrawal increases. Another approach is to give prophylactic doses of heparin (5000–7500 units every 12 hours) subcutaneously.

In some patients, endocarditis prophylaxis is indicated (see Tables 37–4 and 37–5). Patients with bioprosthetic valves may benefit from operative vaginal delivery to shorten the second stage of labor and avoid the additional hemodynamic stresses of pushing.

Postnatal

Warfarin is initiated in the postpartum period in patients with mechanical valves. Anticoagulation with intravenous heparin while awaiting therapeutic levels of warfarin is probably not warranted. The risk of bleeding, particularly after cesarean delivery, exceeds the risk of thrombotic complications.[118] Subcutaneous heparin in prophylactic doses may be used. Breast-feeding during anticoagulation with warfarin is not contraindicated.[131]

MARFAN'S SYNDROME

Maternal and Fetal Risks

Marfan's syndrome is a connective tissue disorder with characteristic findings in the skeletal, ocular, and cardiovascular systems. Cardiac manifestations include MVP and aortic root dilation. Aortic pathology is associated with increased morbidity and mortality. The pathophysiologic changes seen in the aorta result from decreased smooth muscle and abnormal connective tissue, leading to decreased distensibility.[132] Significant aortic root involvement is a particular problem because of the potential for aortic regurgitation, dissection, or rupture. In pregnant patients, morbidity and mortality rates increase when the aortic root diameter exceeds 40 mm.[133–135] With aortic root involvement, mortality rates as high as 25% to 50% are seen. Even with a normal aorta, significant maternal mortality is reported. The elevated risk seen in pregnancy may be related to the increased cardiac output, placing additional stress on the relatively stiff aorta. Pregnancy-associated hypertension may further aggravate the condition.[132] Recent reports suggested a better prognosis with minimal cardiovascular involvement. These patients had no increase in adverse maternal outcome and no accelerated dilation of the aorta compared with similar patients with Marfan's syndrome who did not become pregnant. Patients without aortic root dilation usually tolerate pregnancy well.[133–135] The syndrome is inherited by autosomal dominant transmission, so there is a 50% chance that the fetus may be affected.

Management Options

Prepregnancy

Genetic counseling is an essential part of family planning in Marfan's syndrome because of the 50% risk of transmission. If pregnancy is desired, echocardiographic evaluation of the aorta is performed to define maternal risk status. Pregnancy is discouraged in patients with significant aortic root dilation. Even when the aortic root size is normal, a risk-free pregnancy cannot be guaranteed.[135,136] If cardiac involvement is minimal, however, pregnancy may be cautiously planned. In this group of patients, initiation of β-blockade therapy should be considered if not already used. Although information on its use in pregnancy complicated by Marfan's syndrome is limited, long-term use outside of pregnancy slows the progression of aortic dilation.[137]

Prenatal

Serial echocardiography should be performed every 6 to 10 weeks throughout pregnancy to follow the aortic root size.[134] If not initiated preconceptually, the addition of β-blocker therapy should be considered. Little information is available to guide management in patients with progressive aortic root dilation during pregnancy. Patients should be kept at rest to minimize hemodynamic stresses. Hypertension should be avoided because of the increased risk of aortic dissection. Although it is best postponed until postpartum, prophylactic aortic root repair may be considered in extreme cases. In nonpregnant adults, 55 mm is the critical aortic root diameter at which prophylactic repair is undertaken.[137]

Prenatal diagnosis is available in some families through linkage analysis or mutation detection.[132]

Labor, Delivery, and Postnatal

Epidural anesthesia during labor should be considered. Adequate oxygenation must be maintained, and hypertension should be avoided. Vaginal delivery is desirable, with shortening of the second stage of labor with the use of a vacuum or forceps.[134] Some authors recommend elective cesarean delivery in patients who are at significant risk for aortic dissection.[135] Both patient and physician must remain vigilant because the risk of aortic dissection persists for 6 to 8 weeks postpartum.[134]

DILATED CARDIOMYOPATHY

Maternal and Fetal Risks

Dilated cardiomyopathy is uncommon in women of reproductive age. Peripartum cardiomyopathy is a subset of dilated cardiomyopathy that occurs in association with 1 in 1300 to 1 in 15,000 pregnancies.[138,139] Traditional diagnostic criteria include onset of heart failure in the last month of pregnancy or the first 5 months postpartum, with no other etiology of heart failure identified and no history of cardiac disease. A work group convened in 1997 by the National Institutes of Health and the National Heart Lung and Blood Institute added echocardiographic evidence of left ventricular dysfunction to the diagnostic criteria. The dysfunction may be documented by a reduced ejection fraction or decreased fractional shortening.[140] Patients with peripartum heart failure are typically older than 30 years of age, multiparous, and of African descent.[138,141,142] The condition is also more common in patients with preeclampsia, gestational hypertension, and those pregnant with twins.[140] The existence of peripartum cardiomyopathy as a distinct pathologic entity is debated. Clustering of cases in late pregnancy and the puerperium suggests a unique condition.[138] Others argue that pregnancy leads to unmasking and decompensation of preexisting heart disease.[139] To minimize confounding by exacerbation of unrecognized preexisting heart disease, the National Institutes of Health work group emphasized the importance of limiting the diagnosis to heart failure occurring within the defined 6-month window.[140]

Regardless of the etiology, cardiomyopathy during pregnancy is associated with significant morbidity and mortality. Reported complication rates vary widely and likely reflect different patient populations and variations in diagnostic criteria. Persistent cardiac dysfunction is seen in 45% to 90% of patients.[141,142] Life-threatening arrhythmias may occur.[139] Embolic complications, either pulmonary or systemic, are seen in as many as 50% of patients.[138] Maternal mortality was reported in 4% to 80% of patients, with recent estimates near 20%.[141,143] Survivors often require cardiac transplant.[140,141] The rate of recurrence in subsequent pregnancies is as high as 85%.[140] Pregnancy is poorly tolerated in patients with persistent ventricular dilation and dysfunction.[138,141] In this group of patients, mortality rates are 20% to 60%. Those with normal cardiac function 6 to 12 months postpartum are at risk for heart failure and a recurrent decrease in ejection fraction that may not recover after pregnancy. Mortality rates in these patients are lower, ranging from 0% to 15%.[138,144] Patients whose cardiomyopathy clinically resolved had decreased contractile reserve with provocative testing.[142] This lack of reserve may cause cardiac decompensation as a result of the hemodynamic stress of a subsequent pregnancy and may contribute to the morbidity after a previous return to normal cardiac function.

Management Options

Prepregnancy

Pregnancy is strongly discouraged in patients with a history of peripartum cardiomyopathy, particularly those with residual cardiac dysfunction. In those with normal cardiac function, pregnancy may be attempted cautiously. The patient should be informed of the potential for worsening cardiac function during pregnancy, which may not completely resolve postpartum.[145] Reliable contraception should be provided, with permanent sterilization considered.

Prenatal

If pregnancy occurs, echocardiography should be performed to document ventricular size and function as well as the presence of mural thrombi. Termination should be offered, especially to patients who have persistent echocardiographic abnormalities because of the high associated maternal morbidity and mortality. If the pregnancy is continued, a multidisciplinary team, including a cardiologist, a perinatologist, an anesthesiologist, and a neonatologist, should collaborate to optimize outcome. Decreased activity and potentially bed rest are recommended, along with salt restriction. Diuretics, digoxin (category C), and afterload reduction with hydralazine (category B) should be used, as necessary. Because of the risk of embolic phenomena, heparin (category C) may be given. Both prophylactic and therapeutic doses are used.[141]

Labor and Delivery

Patients are watched closely for signs of heart failure and pulmonary edema. Cardiac monitoring is instituted early in labor. Fluids are restricted, and central hemodynamic monitoring should be available if decompensation occurs. If a flow-directed PAC is necessary, care must be taken during insertion. Positioning may be difficult because of dilated chambers and decreased ejection fraction. Arrhythmias may also be precipitated during insertion. Heparin can be discontinued during early labor and resumed in the early postpartum period. Adequate pain control is important, and epidural anesthesia works well. Patients with significant cardiac dysfunction may need to labor in a sitting position to reduce or prevent shortness of breath.

Postnatal

Monitoring of volume status must continue through the postpartum period, with fluid restriction as necessary. Diuretics may be used as necessary, and the patient should be given an angiotensin-converting enzyme inhibitor (category D) for afterload reduction.[140] A reliable and effective plan for contraception should be discussed. Although uncommonly performed, endomyocardial biopsy is recommended to exclude treatable causes of cardiomyopathy. Some patients with myocarditis found on biopsy respond favorably to immunosuppressive therapy.[140,143]

CARDIAC ARRHYTHMIAS

Maternal and Fetal Risks

Cardiac arrhythmias are relatively common during pregnancy. Most are benign and include sinus bradycardia, sinus tachycardia, and atrial and ventricular premature contractions. These patients are often asymptomatic, but may have palpitations, although the correlation between symptoms and arrhythmia is poor. Shotan and associates[146] evaluated symptomatic pregnant patients who were referred to a cardiac clinic and compared them with asymptomatic pregnant patients who were referred for evaluation of a cardiac murmur. The incidence of premature atrial and ventricular contractions was 50% to 60% in each group. Although the frequency of arrhythmias was higher in symptomatic patients, only 10% of symptoms occurred in conjunction with arrhythmia. Healthy, asymptomatic patients without underlying pathology can often be managed with observation and rest.[147] Normal labor and delivery do not seem to increase the incidence or type of arrhythmias identified.[148]

Pregnancy may be associated with an increase in the incidence and severity of arrhythmias.[146,149,150] Supraventricular tachycardia is often seen in pregnancy. Ventricular tachycardia and multiform premature ventricular complexes are much less common but may be recognized for the first time during gestation. Atrial fibrillation is usually associated with underlying cardiac disease. An increase in cardiac complications as a result of long QT syndrome was noted, particularly during the postpartum period.[149] Serious maternal complications are rare, but include cardiac failure and sudden death. Fetal risk is primarily associated with exposure to drugs used for maternal therapy.

Management Options

Prepregnancy

All patients with a sustained arrhythmia should undergo a baseline electrocardiogram to determine whether the rhythm abnormality originates from the atrium or the ventricle. This is followed by a search for an underlying etiology. Patients with unexplained sinus tachycardia or premature atrial or ventricular contractions are questioned about tobacco, caffeine, and illicit drug use. They are also evaluated for anemia and hyperthyroidism. If a contributing factor is identified, behavior modification is attempted, as appropriate. Medical conditions should be treated before conception. Ambulatory monitoring is considered when patients have symptoms that suggest a rhythm disturbance but no objective evidence on examination. Patients who may benefit from ablative therapy should be identified and treated before conception.

Symptomatic and sustained arrhythmias often require appropriate antiarrhythmic therapy. Most antiarrhythmic agents are classified as category C, except when otherwise noted. β-Blockers can be used in patients with sinus tachycardia or frequent premature atrial or ventricular contractions when symptoms persist after conservative management.[150] In patients with long QT syndrome, β-blockers are continued to reduce the incidence of cardiac events.[149] Digoxin can be used safely to control the ventricular rate in atrial fibrillation and flutter and some supraventricular tachycardias.[147] Adenosine has a rapid onset and very short duration of action. It is used during pregnancy to treat supraventricular tachycardia and is the drug of choice.[150–152] Esmolol and intravenous verapamil can be used intravenously in the acute management of supraventricular tachycardia. Quinidine is used for some atrial and ventricular arrhythmias, when clinically indicated. Lidocaine (category B) is used acutely to control ventricular arrhythmias. Procainamide is a second-line agent because of maternal side effects, including cardiac rhythm disturbances, lupus-like syndrome, and blood dyscrasia.[153] Amiodarone (category D) is used to treat life-threatening ventricular arrhythmias when first-line agents are unsuccessful. It is associated with neonatal hypothyroidism, hyperthyroidism, and possibly intrauterine growth restriction, fetal bradycardia, and neurologic abnormalities.[154]

Prenatal, Labor, Delivery, and Postnatal

Management during pregnancy consists of maintenance therapy to control arrhythmias. Drug levels should be monitored, as indicated, because of pregnancy-associated changes in volume of distribution and protein binding. Vagal maneuvers can be tried initially in tachyarrhythmias with first onset in pregnancy. Cardioversion can be used safely during pregnancy in unstable patients or when medical therapy is unsuccessful.[147] Continuous cardiac monitoring may be necessary intrapartum and postpartum for symptomatic or complex arrhythmias.

MYOCARDIAL INFARCTION

Maternal and Fetal Risks

Myocardial infarction is very uncommon in women of reproductive age.[155] Most events occur in the third trimester, with a maternal mortality rate of approximately 20%. Labor occurring within 2 weeks of an acute myocardial infarction increases the risk of maternal death.[156] A coronary thrombus, with or without associated atherosclerotic changes, is seen in no more than 50% of patients.[155] No cardiac risk factors are present in 40% of cases.[157] Nearly 30% of patients have normal coronary arteries.[156] Fetal outcome is related to maternal status and outcome.

Diagnosis is difficult because the index of suspicion is low. Physiologic changes of pregnancy may mimic the symptoms of myocardial infarction and delay the diagnosis. During labor, the diagnosis is further complicated by the fact that creatinine phosphokinase and the cardiac-specific MB fraction may be normally elevated.[158] Troponin I is a specific marker for cardiac injury that does not increase during normal labor and delivery, making it a potentially useful tool in the diagnosis of myocardial infarction in the pregnant woman.[159] A few case reports described the utility of troponin I in the diagnosis of myocardial infarction during pregnancy.[160,161]

Management Options

Prepregnancy

Because the underlying condition is rare, pregnancy after myocardial infarction is uncommon. Unfortunately, it is even more uncommon for these patients to seek preconception counseling.[162] When possible, cardiac evaluation should be done, including stress testing and echocardiography. If the patient has no cardiac dysfunction, pregnancy can be planned cautiously.[162]

Prenatal

Patients should rest and avoid strenuous activity. They should also be monitored for evidence of arrhythmias or congestive heart failure. If a myocardial infarction occurs during pregnancy, management principles are similar to those for nonpregnant patients.[156,163,164] Most drugs used in the medical management of myocardial infarction are category C, except where otherwise noted. Nitroglycerin, oxygen supplementation, morphine (category B), heparin, and continuous cardiac monitoring are initiated. Lidocaine (category B), dopamine, calcium channel blockers, and β-blockers can be used, as indicated. Coronary angiography is also used during pregnancy.[163] Favorable pregnancy outcomes are reported after coronary angioplasty[164] and bypass surgery[165] during gestation. Pregnancy is a relative contraindication to thrombolytic therapy because of the theoretical increased risk of maternal and fetal bleeding.[156,163] However, safe and effective use is reported during pregnancy.[166]

In cases of cardiac arrest, cardiopulmonary resuscitation proceeds as in the nonpregnant patient, except that the gravid uterus is displaced laterally to prevent compression of the vena cava and improve venous return.[167] Successful cardioversion of ventricular fibrillation has been reported.[165] If initial attempts at resuscitation are unsuccessful, perimortem cesarean section is indicated to save the viable fetus. Optimal neonatal outcomes are seen when delivery occurs within 5 minutes of cardiac arrest. Alterations in maternal hemodynamics after delivery may improve maternal outcome.[167,168]

Labor and Delivery

External cardiac monitoring is necessary. Supplemental oxygen should be given, and epidural anesthesia is used for pain control. Operative vaginal delivery to shorten the second stage of labor is also advocated.[163,165,169] Labor can often be managed without invasive monitoring. Use of a PAC is reserved for unstable patients. Cesarean delivery is empirically advocated in patients who start labor within 4 days of an acute myocardial infarction.[163,169]

Postnatal

Volume status is monitored in the postpartum period, and the patient should avoid exertion. A reliable plan for contraception should be made. Combination oral contraceptives are usually contraindicated. Although the risk of atherosclerosis is not increased, estrogen increases thrombotic risk, especially when other risk factors are present. If permanent sterilization is not desired, reasonable alternatives include long-acting progestins or an intrauterine device.[170,171]

HYPERTROPHIC CARDIOMYOPATHY

Maternal and Fetal Risks

Hypertrophic cardiomyopathy is an autosomal dominant condition characterized by left ventricular hypertrophy without chamber dilation or another etiology to explain the hypertrophy. It is classically associated with left ventricular outflow obstruction, but this is not found in most patients. As a result, older names for this condition, such as idiopathic hypertrophic subaortic stenosis and hypertrophic obstructive cardiomyopathy, have been generally replaced. In the general population, the frequency of this condition is approximately 1 in 500.[172]

The presentation and prognosis are clinically variable. Most patients have a normal life expectancy without limitations; however, hypertrophic cardiomyopathy is a common cause of sudden cardiac death in young people. The annual mortality rate is estimated at 1%, substantially less than the rate reported in older series, primarily because of the identification and inclusion of patients with more benign forms of the disease.[172,173] Clinical risk factors for sudden death include a family history of sudden cardiac death, previous syncope, and documented ventricular tachycardia. Maki and associates[173] identified an inadequate increase in systolic blood pressure associated with exercise, defined as less than 24 mm Hg on treadmill testing, as a risk factor in patients younger than 50 years of age. Left ventricular wall thickness greater than 30 mm may be a risk factor in young adults.[172] Implantable cardiac defibrillators are used successfully in high-risk patients and can be used in pregnant patients.[174]

Physiologic changes associated with pregnancy have variable effects on the condition. Adequate preload and systemic vascular resistance are important factors in maintaining end-diastolic volume and cardiac output. A decrease in end-diastolic volume increases outflow obstruction. The increased blood volume associated with pregnancy has a beneficial effect, whereas the decrease in systemic vascular resistance can worsen outflow obstruction. The increased heart rate can also adversely affect maternal condition as a result of decreased diastolic filling time. Despite these concerns, maternal complications are uncommon and are confined primarily to women with specific risk factors.[175] The autosomal inheritance pattern gives the fetus a 50% chance of having the condition.

Management Options

Prepregnancy

Genetic counseling is indicated if either parent is affected. A careful history should be taken to identify patients with historical risk factors. An echocardiogram should be done. Patients should also be seen by a cardiologist who has experience with patients who have this condition to determine the need for exercise testing and the role of Holter monitoring.

Prenatal

Activity is limited to avoid tachycardia. Adequate hydration should be maintained. Although it is not necessary in all patients, β-blockade may be used in symptomatic patients.[172,176]

Labor, Delivery, and Postnatal

Volume status is monitored to avoid dehydration and hypotension during labor. Regional anesthesia may be used, but should be administered with care after adequate volume loading, again, to prevent hypotension. If tachycardia develops and the patient becomes symptomatic, β-blocking agents (mostly category C) may be used to control the heart rate. Esmolol, a short-acting β-blocker, is used successfully during labor to control symptoms.[176] Endocarditis prophylaxis is used, as indicated (see Table 37–4). The patient should be observed for excessive blood loss and tachycardia in the postpartum period. Volume replacement is given, as indicated.

SUMMARY OF MANAGEMENT OPTIONS

Cardiac Disease: Specific

Management Options	Quality of Evidence	Strength of Recommendation	References
Cardiac Murmur			
Echocardiogram for patients with a significant history or a pathologic murmur (late systolic, pansystolic, diastolic)	III	B	42,43
Cardiology referral if an echocardiogram is abnormal	IIb	B	45
Mitral Valve Prolapse			
Cardiology and echocardiogram evaluation prenatally for mitral regurgitation	IV	C	47
Surveillance and treatment of arrhythmias in pregnancy	IV	C	47
Atrial Septal Defect			
Pregnancy			
Screen for arrhythmias or pulmonary hypertension; manage accordingly both before and during pregnancy (if undertaken)	III	B	55,56
Prenatal			
Routine unless the patient has arrhythmias or Pulmonary hypertension	III	B	55,56
Screen fetus for congenital heart defect	IIb	B	25
Labor and Delivery			
Screen for arrhythmias, monitor blood pressure, and avoid fluid overload	III	B	55,56
Postnatal			
Encourage early mobilization	III	B	55,56
Screen newborn for congential heart defect	IIb	B	25

SUMMARY OF MANAGEMENT OPTIONS
Cardiac Disease: Specific *(Continued)*

Management Options	Quality of Evidence	Strength of Recommendation	References
Ventricular Septal Defect			
Prepregnancy			
Screen for pulmonary hypertension and manage accordingly; consider repair of uncorrectedlesions and counseling about the risk of congenital heart disease	III	B	57,58
Prenatal			
Obtain serial echocardiograms, and manage accordingly	III	B	57,58
Screen fetus for congenital defect	IIb	B	25
Labor and Delivery			
Avoid hypertension; provide antibiotic prophylaxis unless the patient has a normal delivery or if the defect has been repaired	III	B	57,58
Postnatal			
Provide careful fluid balance and early ambulation	III	B	57,58
Screen newborn for congenital heart defect	IIb	B	25
Pulmonary Hypertension			
Prepregnancy			
Counsel against pregnancy; offer sterilization if requested	III	B	59,60
Prenatal			
Consider termination	III	B	59,60
Joint obstetric and cardiology care and early anesthesiology consultation	III	B	60
Thromboembolism prophylaxis	III	B	59,60
Consider hospital admission and monitor SaO_2	III	B	59,60
Provide fetal surveillance	III	B	59,60
Use of calcium channel blocker has been reported	III	B	61
Labor and Delivery			
Intensive care setting (degree of invasive monitoring varies); dilemma over induction (to end the pregnancy) vs. spontaneous onset of labor (because of shorter labor); oxytocic or E series prostaglandins are safe; O_2 is given at 5 to 6 L/min; SaO_2 is monitored continuously; monitor blood pressure and maintain fluid balance; epidural analgesic is preferable (reduce or stop anticoagulation for a few hours for delivery)	III	B	59,60
IV Prostacyclin or inhaled nitric oxide	III	B	63,64
Postnatal			
Maintain intensive care monitoring; give O_2 therapy and thromboembolism prophylaxis; maintain vigilance for fluid retention and consequences; inhaled nitric oxide and IV prostacyclin may be continued or initiated; consider sterilization	III	B	59–61,63,64
Eisenmenger's Complex			
As for primary pulmonary hypertension	III	B	66–69
Echocardiography may be helpful in evaluation, shunt, right ventricular function, and pulmonary hypertension	III	B	66–69

Continued

SUMMARY OF MANAGEMENT OPTIONS
Cardiac Disease: Specific *(Continued)*

Management Options	Quality of Evidence	Strength of Recommendation	References
Coarctation of the Aorta			
Prepregnancy			
Screen for aneurysms or aortic valve disease, and manage appropriately (i.e. repair) before conception	III	B	70
Prenatal			
Consider termination in patients with severe uncorrected disease	III	B	71–73
Labor, Delivery, and Postnatal			
Avoid hypertension; provide antibiotic prophylaxis except for patients who are having normal delivery; screen the newborn for congenital heart disease	III	B	71–73
Tetralogy of Fallot			
Prepregnancy			
Surgical correction and evaluation of cardiac status after corrective surgery	III	B	74,75
Prenatal			
Consider termination in patients with uncorrected lesions; monitor maternal SaO_2 and exercise tolerance; consider rest and supplemental O_2 fetal surveillance	III	B	74,75
Labor and Delivery			
Provide careful fluid management; monitor the patient's blood pressure, SaO_2, and electrocardiogram; epidural use requires careful preloading, the need to shorten the second stage, and fetal monitoring; avoid fluid overload, maintain blood pressure	III	B	74,75
Postnatal			
Maintain maternal monitoring and discuss effective contraception	III	B	74,75
Transposition of the Great Arteries			
Prepregnancy			
Consultation with a cardiologist specializing in adults with congenital heart disease; evaluation of cardiac status with attention to the right (systemic ventricle); monitor for arrhythmias	III	B	77–82
Prenatal			
Decrease activity; monitor for heart failure and arrhythmias; perform serial echocardiography	III	B	77–82
Labor and Delivery			
Provide careful fluid management; give oxygen as necessary; perform an electrocardiogram; use an epidural, shorten the second stage, and provide fetal monitoring	III	B	77–82
Postnatal			
Monitor volume status, and discuss effective contraception	III	B	77–82
Patent Ductus Arteriosus			
Prepregnancy			
Screen for pulmonary hypertension, and manage appropriately before and during pregnancy (if undertaken).	III	B	56,85

SUMMARY OF MANAGEMENT OPTIONS

Cardiac Disease: Specific *(Continued)*

Management Options	Quality of Evidence	Strength of Recommendation	References
Patent Ductus Arteriosus—*(Continued)*			
Prenatal			
Screen for pulmonary hypertension.	III	B	56,85
Labor, Delivery, and Postnatal			
Monitor blood pressure and fluid balance; provide antibiotic prophylaxis except for normal deliveries.	III	B	56,85
Rheumatic Heart Disease: General			
Principles			
• Prevent heart failure	IV	C	87,88
• Prevent bacterial endocarditis	IV	C	87,88
• Use a team approach, including a cardiologist and an anesthesiologist	IV	C	87,88
Mitral Stenosis			
Prepregnancy			
Assess cardiac function, optimize medical therapy, and consider surgical correction.	III	B	96–98
Prenatal			
Avoid excess weight gain; provide tachycardia and serial echocardiography; treat tachycardia or arrhythmias; perform percutaneous commissurotomy or surgery for symptomatic severe disease; provide fetal surveillance.	III	B	99,100–103
Labor and Delivery			
Intensive care setting; consider central invasive monitoring, epidural analgesia, and antibiotic prophylaxis for complicated deliveries; provide fetal surveillance.	III	B	94
Mitral Regurgitation			
Prepregnancy			
As for stenosis	III	B	106
Prenatal			
Restrict activity; perform serial echocardiography; adjust medical control; consider surgery for symptomatic severe disease; perform fetal surveillance	III	B	106–108
Labor, Delivery, and Postnatal			
Avoid fluid overload and hypertension; provide maternal cardiac monitoring and endocarditis prophylaxis for complicated deliveries.	–	GPP	–
Aortic Stenosis			
Prepregnancy			
Determine severity by echocardiography and callretengation	III	B	110–114
Correct severe disease surgically before conception.	–	–	–
Prenatal			
Limit physical activity; maintain vigilance for heart failure and arrhythmias.	III	B	110–114
Fetal surveillance	–	–	–

Continued

SUMMARY OF MANAGEMENT OPTIONS
Cardiac Disease: Specific *(Continued)*

Management Options	Quality of Evidence	Strength of Recommendation	References
Labor, Delivery, and Postnatal			
Avoid fluid overload, hypovolemia, and hypertension.	III	B	110–114
Some would use pulmonary artery catheter.	–	–	–
Implement prophylaxis for bacterial endocaditis Cardiologic follow-up as risk of determination over the next 1–2 years.	–	–	–
Aortic Regurgitation			
Prepregnancy			
As for mitral disease, i.e. echocardiography; cardiac catheterization; optimistic medical control (Digoxin); value replacement if indicated	III	B	115
Prenatal			
Surveillance for cardiac failure; surgery for failed medical therapy; fetal surveillance	III	B	107
Labor, Delivery, and Postnatal			
Avoid fluid overload; invasive monitoring is usually unnecessary; epidural is beneficial; provide fetal surveillance	III	B	115
Prosthetic Valves			
Prepregnancy			
Assess cardiac status; provide counseling about valve function and risks associated with warfarin	III	B	122
Prenatal			
If the patient has biosynthetic valves, provide vigilance for deterioration; if the patient has mechanical valves, provide adequate anticoagulation; vigilance for thrombocytopenia when using heparin	III	B	116,126,129
Labor and Delivery			
Adjust anticoagulation and provide endocarditis prophylaxis	III	B	122,126
Postnatal			
Readjust anticoagulation	III	B	122,126
Marfan's Syndrome			
Prepregnancy			
Genetic counseling, and echocardiography (especially aortic root); counsel against pregnancy	III	B	135–137
Prenatal			
Serial aortic root echocardiography; give β-blockers; avoid hypertension; encourage rest; surgery in extreme cases	III	B	132,134,137
Labor, Delivery, and Postnatal			
Epidural is beneficial; avoid hypertension; ensure adequate oxygenation; shorten the second stage of labor; maintain vigilance for aortic root dissection for at least 8 weeks postnatally	III	B	134,135
Dilated Cardiomyopathy			
Prepregnancy			
Counsel against pregnancy if the patient has a history of peripartum cardiomyopathy	III	B	145

SUMMARY OF MANAGEMENT OPTIONS

Cardiac Disease: Specific *(Continued)*

Management Options	Quality of Evidence	Strength of Recommendation	References
Prenatal			
Echocardiography. Consider termination in patients with an abnormal echocardiogram; if the patient is symptomatic, provide medical therapy and anticoagulation	III	B	141,145
Multidiscliplinary team care			
Labor and Delivery			
Monitor for heart failure; avoid fluid overload; possibly use pulmonary artery catheter, vigilance for arrhythmias; adequate analgesia	III	B	141,143–145
Postnatal			
Avoid fluid overload; discuss contraception	III	B	141,143–145
Cardiac Arrhythmias			
Prepregnancy			
Investigate and treat	III	B	147,149–152
Prenatal, Labor, Delivery, and Postnatal			
Maintenance of therapy to control arrhythmia; cardioconversion can be used as indicated	III	B	147,149–152
Myocardial Infarction			
Prepregnancy			
Assess cardiac function (especially echocardiography and stress testing); counsel on the basis of results; give low-dose aspirin	III	B	162
Prenatal			
Avoid strenuous activity; provide surveillance for failure and arrhythmias; management as for a nonpregnant patient; surgery can be performed in pregnancy	III	B	156,163–165
Thrombolytic therapy has been used	III	B	156,163–165
Labor and Delivery			
Monitor electrocardiogram; provide supplementary oxygen; epidural is beneficial; consider cesarean section if labor occurs within 4 days of an acute myocardial infarction	III	B	156,165,169
Postnatal			
Avoid fluid overload and exertion; discuss contraception (avoid combination oral preparations)	III	B	165,170,171
Hypertrophic Cardiomyopathy			
Prepregnancy			
Genetic counseling; evaluate cardiac status with echocardiography	III	B	172
Prenatal			
Limit activity; give β-blockers for symptomatic patients	III	B	172,176
Labor, Delivery, and Postnatal			
Avoid dehydration or hypotension; give β-blockers for tachycardia and endocarditis prophylaxis for complicated deliveries	III	B	172,176

CONCLUSIONS

- Cardiac disease complicating pregnancy is not rare. Although both the incidence and the severity of rheumatic heart disease are decreasing, because of advances in cardiac surgery, more patients with repaired congenital heart disease are reaching reproductive age and choosing to become pregnant.
- The age at which women become pregnant is increasing, as is the incidence of diabetes and hypertension in the population, potentially leading to an increase in the incidence of ischemic heart disease during pregnancy.
- Physicians who treat these patients must understand the physiologic changes associated with pregnancy and their effect on specific cardiac conditions.
- With a complete diagnostic evaluation, optimization of cardiac function, and close follow-up throughout pregnancy and the puerperium, favorable maternal and fetal outcomes can be expected in most cases.

REFERENCES

1. Sugrue D, Blake S, MacDonald D: Pregnancy complicated by maternal heart disease at the National Maternity Hospital, Dublin, Ireland, 1969–1978. Am Obstet Gynecol 1981;139:1–6.
2. McFaul PB, Dornan JC, Lamki H, Boyle D: Pregnancy complicated by maternal heart disease: A review of 519 women. BJOG 1988;95:861–867.
3. Högberg U, Innala E, Sandström A: Maternal mortality in Sweden, 1980–1988. Obstet Gynecol 1994;84:240–244.
4. Siu S, Sermer M, Colman J, et al: Prospective multicenter study of pregnancy outcome in women with heart disease. Circulation 2001;104:515–521.
5. Siu S, Sermer M, Harrison D, et al: Risk and predictors for pregnancy-related complications in women with heart disease. Circulation 1997;96:2789–2794.
6. Seitchik J: Total body water and total body density of pregnant women. Obstet Gynecol 1967;29:155–156.
7. Theunissen IM, Parer JT: Fluid and electrolytes in pregnancy. Clin Obstet Gynecol 1994;37:3–15.
8. Lindheimer MD, Katz AI: Sodium and diuretics in pregnancy. N Engl J Med 1973;288:891–894.
9. Scott DE: Anemia during pregnancy. Obstet Gynecol Annu 1972;1:219–243.
10. Pritchard JA, Baldwin RM, Dickey JC, Wiggins KM: Changes in the blood volume during pregnancy and delivery. Am J Obstet Gynecol 1962;84:1271–1282.
11. Katz R, Karliner JS, Resnik R: Effects of a natural volume overload state (pregnancy) on left ventricular performance in normal human subjects. Circulation 1978;58:434–441.
12. Bader RA, Bader MG, Rose JD, et al: Hemodynamics at rest and during exercise in normal pregnancy as studied by cardiac catheterization. J Clin Invest 1955;34:1524–1536.
13. Walters WAW, MacGregor WG, Hills M: Cardiac output at rest during pregnancy and the puerperium. Clin Sci 1966;30:1–11.
14. Lees MM, Taylor SH, Scott DB, et al: A study of cardiac output at rest throughout pregnancy. J Obstet Gynecol Br Commonw 1967;74:319–328.
15. Ueland K, Novy MJ, Peterson EN, et al: Maternal cardiovascular dynamics: IV. The influence of gestational age on the maternal cardiovascular response to posture and exercise. Am J Obstet Gynecol 1969;104:856–864.
16. Sadaniantz A, Kocheril AG, Emaus SP, et al: Cardiovascular changes in pregnancy evaluated by two-dimensional and Doppler echocardiography. Am J Soc Echocardiogr 1992;5:253–258.
17. Wilson M, Morganti AA, Zervodakis I, et al: Blood pressure, the renin-aldosterone system, and sex steroids throughout normal pregnancy. Am J Med 1980;68:97.
18. MacGillivray I, Rose GA, Row B: Blood pressure survey in pregnancy. Clin Sci 1969;37:395–407.
19. Bieniarz J, Crottogini JJ, Curuchet E, et al: Aortocaval compression by the uterus in late human pregnancy: II. An arteriographic study. Am J Obstet Gynecol 1968;100:203–217.
20. Kerr MG: Cardiovascular dynamics in pregnancy and labour. Br Med Bull 1968;24:19–24.
21. Oian P, Maltau JM, Noddeland H, et al: Oedema-preventing mechanisms in subcutaneous tissue of normal pregnant women. BJOG 1985;92:1113–1119.
22. Oian P, Maltau JM: Calculated capillary hydrostatic pressure in normal pregnancy and preeclampsia. Am J Obstet Gynecol 1987;157:102–106.
23. Cotton DB, Gonik B, Spillman T, et al: Intrapartum to postpartum changes in colloid osmotic pressure. Am J Obstet Gynecol 1984;149:174–177.
24. Gonik B, Cotton D, Spillman T, et al: Peripartum colloid osmotic changes: Effects of controlled fluid management. Am J Obstet Gynecol 1985;151:812–815.
25. Burn J, Brennan S, Little J, et al: Recurrence risks in offspring of adults with major heart defects: Results from first cohort of British collaborative study. Lancet 1998;351:311–316.
26. Whittemore R, Hobbins JC, Engle MA: Pregnancy and its outcome in women with and without surgical treatment of congenital heart disease. Am J Cardiol 1982;50:641–651.
27. Rose V, Gold RJM, Lindsay G, Allen M: A possible increase in the incidence of congenital heart defects among the offspring of affected parents. J Am Coll Cardiol 1985;6:376–382.
28. Popp R: Echocardiography (first of two parts). N Engl J Med 1990;323:101–109.
29. Criteria Committee of the New York Heart Association: Nomenclature and Criteria for Diagnosis of Disease of the Heart and Great Vessels, 6th ed. Boston, Little, Brown, 1964.
30. Ostheimer GW, Alper MH: Intrapartum anesthetic management of the pregnant patient with heart disease. Clinical Obstet Gynecol 1975;18:81–97.
31. Briggs GG, Freeman RK, Yaffe SJ (eds): Drugs in Pregnancy and Lactation, 5th ed. Baltimore, Williams & Wilkins, 1998.
32. Bernard G, Sopko G, Cerra F, et al: Pulmonary artery catheterization and clinical outcomes: National Heart, Lung, and Blood Institute and Food and Drug Administration Workshop Report. JAMA 2000;283:2568–2572.
33. Sandham JD, Hull RD, Brant RF, et al: A randomized, controlled trial of the use of pulmonary-artery catheters in high-risk surgical patients. N Engl J Med 2003;348:5–14.
34. Parson PE: Progress in research on pulmonary-artery catheters. N Engl J Med 2003;348:66–68.
35. Seaworth BJ, Durack DT: Infective endocarditis in obstetrics and gynecologic practice. Am J Obstet Gynecol 1986;154:180–188.

36. Durack DT: Prevention of infective endocarditis. N Engl J Med 1995;332:38–44.
37. Dajani AS, Taubert KA, Wilson W, et al: Prevention of bacterial endocarditis: Recommendations of the American Heart Association. JAMA 1997;277:1794–1801.
38. Endocarditis Working Party of the British Society for Antimicrobial Chemotherapy: Antibiotic prophylaxis of infective endocarditis. Lancet 1990;335:88–90.
39. Goldberg LM, Uhland H: Heart murmurs in pregnancy: A phonocardiographic study and their development, progression and regression. Dis Chest 1967;52:381–386.
40. Harvey WP: Alterations of the cardiac physical examination in normal pregnancy. Clin Obstet Gynecol 1975;18:51–63.
41. Northcote RJ, Knight PV, Ballantyne D: Systolic murmurs in pregnancy: Value of echocardiographic assessment. Clin Cardiol 1985;8:327–328.
42. Mishra M, Chambers JB, Jackson G: Murmurs in pregnancy: An audit of echocardiography. BMJ 1992;304:1413–1414.
43. Xu M, McHaffie DJ: Nonspecific systolic murmurs: An audit of the clinical value of echocardiography. N Z Med J 1993;106:54–56.
44. Tan J, deSwiet M: Prevalence of heart disease diagnosed de novo in pregnancy in a West London population. BJOG 1998;105:1185–1188.
45. Etchells E, Bell C, Robb K: Does this patient have an abnormal systolic murmur? JAMA 1997;277:564–571.
46. Levy D, Savage D: Prevalence and clinical features of mitral valve prolapse. Am Heart J 1987;113:1281–1290.
47. Boudoulas H: Mitral valve prolapse: Etiology, clinical presentation and neuroendocrine function. J Heart Valve Dis 1992;1:175–188.
48. Freed LA, Levy D, Levine RA, et al: Prevalence and clinical outcome of mitral-valve prolapse. N Engl J Med 1999;341:1–7.
49. Lax D, Eicher M, Goldberg SJ: Effects of hydration on mitral valve prolapse. Am Heart J 1993;126:415–418.
50. Rayburn WF, LeMire MS, Bird JL, Buda AJ: Mitral valve prolapse. J Reprod Med 1987;32:185–187.
51. Retchin SM, Fletcher RH, Earp JA, et al: Mitral valve prolapse. Arch Intern Med 1986;146:1081–1084.
52. Devereux RB, Kramer-Fox R, Kligfield P: Mitral valve prolapse: Causes, clinical manifestations, and management. Ann Intern Med 1989;111:305–317.
53. Zuppiroli A, Rinaldi M, Kramer-Fox R, et al: Natural history of mitral valve prolapse. Am J Cardiol 1995;75:1028–1032.
54. Fukuda N, Oki T, Iuchi A, et al: Predisposing factors for severe mitral regurgitation in idiopathic mitral valve prolapse. Am J Cardiol 1995;76:503–507.
55. Zuber M, Gautschi N, Oechslin E, et al: Outcome of pregnancy in women with congenital shunt lesions. Heart 1999;81: 271–275.
56. Pitkin RM, Perloff JK, Koos BJ, Beall MH: Pregnancy and congenital heart disease. Ann Intern Med 1990;112:445–454.
57. Jackson GM, Dildy GA, Varner MW, Clark SL: Severe pulmonary hypertension in pregnancy following successful repair of ventricular septal defect in childhood. Obstet Gynecol 1993;82:680–682.
58. Alahuhta S, Jouppila P: Pregnancy after cardiac surgery in patients with secondary pulmonary hypertension due to a ventricular septal defect. Acta Obstet Gynecol Scand 1994;73: 836–838.
59. Weiss BM, Zemp L, Seifert B, Hess OM: Outcome of pulmonary vascular disease in pregnancy: A systemic overview from 1978 through 1996. J Am Coll Cardiol 1998;31:1650–1657.
60. Smedstad KG, Cramb R, Morison DH: Pulmonary hypertension and pregnancy: A series of eight cases. Can J Anaesth 1994;41:502–512.
61. Easterling TR, Ralph DD, Schmucker BC: Pulmonary hypertension in pregnancy: Treatment with pulmonary vasodilators. Obstet Gynecol 1999;93:494–498.
62. Robinson JN, Banerjee R, Landzberg MJ, Thiet M: Am J Obstet Gynecol 1999;180:1045–1046.
63. Stewart R, Tuazon D, Olson G, Duarte AG: Pregnancy and primary pulmonary hypertension. Chest 2001;119:973–975.
64. Lam GK, Stafford RE, Thorp J, et al: Inhaled nitric oxide for primary pulmonary hypertension in pregnancy. Obstet Gynecol 2001;98:895–898.
65. Hart CM: Nitric oxide in adult lung disease. Chest 1999;115:1407–1417.
66. Yentis SM, Steer PJ, Plaat F: Eisenmenger's syndrome in pregnancy: Maternal and fetal mortality in the 1990's. BJOG 1998;105:921–922.
67. Vongpatanasin W, Brickner E, Hillis LD, Lange RA: The Eisenmenger syndrome in adults. Ann Intern Med 1998;128: 745–755.
68. Goodwin TM, Gherman RB, Hameed A, Elkayam U: Favorable response of Eisenmenger syndrome to inhaled nitric oxide during pregnancy. Am J Obstet Gynecol 1999;180:64–67.
69. Lust KM, Boots RJ, Dooris M, Wilson J: Management of labor in Eisenmenger syndrome with inhaled nitric oxide. Am J Obstet Gynecol 1999;181:419–423.
70. Saidi AS, Bezold LI, Altman CA, et al: Outcome of pregnancy following intervention for coarctation of the aorta. Am J Cardiol 1998;82:786–788.
71. Deal K, Wooley CF: Coarctation of the aorta and pregnancy. Ann Intern Med 1973;78:706–710.
72. Beauschesne LM, Connolly HM, Ammach NM, Warnes CA: Coarctation of the aorta: Outcome of pregnancy. J Am Coll Cardiol 2001;38:1728–1733.
73. Barash PG, Hobbins JC, Hook R, et al: Management of coarctation of the aorta during pregnancy. J Thorac Cardiovasc Surg 1975;69:781–784.
74. Singh H, Bolton PJ, Oakley CM: Pregnancy after surgical correction of tetralogy of Fallot. BMJ 1982;285:168–170.
75. Nissenkorn A, Friedman S, Schonfeld A, Ovadia J: Fetomaternal outcome in pregnancies after total correction of the tetralogy of Fallot. Int Surg 1984;69:125–128.
76. Patton DE, Lee W, Cotton DB, et al: Cyanotic maternal heart disease in pregnancy. Obstet Gynecol Surv 1990;45:594–600.
77. Connolly HM, Grogan M, Warnes CA: Pregnancy among women with congenitally corrected transposition of great arteries. J Am Coll Cardiol 1999;33:1692–1695.
78. Harkness CB, Serfas DH, Imseis HM: L-transposition of the great arteries presenting as severe preeclampsia. Obstet Gynecol 1999; 94:851.
79. Lynch-Salamon DI, Maze SS, Combs A: Pregnancy after Mustard repair for transposition of the great arteries. Obstet Gynecol 1993;82:676–679.
80. Lao TT, Sermer M, Colman JM: Pregnancy following surgical correction for transposition of the great arteries. Obstet Gynecol 1994;83:865–868.
81. Megerian G, Bell JB, Huhta JC, et al: Pregnancy following Mustard procedure for transposition of the great arteries. Obstet Gynecol 1994;83:512–516.
82. Genoni M, Jenni R, Hoerstrup SP, Turina M: Pregnancy after atrial repair for transposition of the great arteries. Heart 1999;81:276–277.
83. Therrien J, Barnes I, Somerville J: Outcome of pregnancy in patients with congenitally corrected transposition of the great arteries. Am J Cardiol 1999;84:820–824.
84. Presbitero P, Somerville J, Stone S, et al: Pregnancy in cyanotic congenital heart disease: Outcome of mother and fetus. Circulation 1994;89:2673–2676.
85. Friedman WF, Heiferman MF: Clinical problems of postoperative pulmonary vascular disease. Am J Cardiol 1982;50:631–636.
86. Szekely P, Turner R, Snaith L: Pregnancy and the changing pattern of rheumatic heart disease. Br Heart J 1973;35:1293–1303.
87. Stollerman GH: Global strategies for the control of rheumatic fever. JAMA 1983;249:931.

88. Eisenberg MJ: Rheumatic heart disease in the developing world: Prevalence, prevention, and control. Eur Heart J 1993;14:122–128.
89. Stephen SJ: Changing patterns of mitral stenosis in childhood and pregnancy in serotonin reuptake inhibitor Lanka. J Am Coll Cardiol 1992;19:1276–1284.
90. Carroll JD, Feldman T: Percutaneous mitral balloon valvotomy and the new demographics of mitral stenosis. JAMA 1993;270:1731–1736.
91. Gray ED, Regelmann EW, Abdin Z, et al: Compartmentalization of cells surface antigens in peripheral blood and tonsils in rheumatic heart disease. J Infect Dis 1987;155:247.
92. Hameed A, Karaalllp IS, Tummala PP, et al: The effect of valvular heart disease on maternal and fetal outcome of pregnancy. J Am Coll Cardiol 2001;37:893–899.
93. Sawhney H, Aggarwal N, Srui V, et al: Maternal and perinatal outcome in rheumatic disease. Int J Gynecol Obstet 2003;80:9–14.
94. Clark SL, Phelan JP, Greenspoon J, et al: Labor and delivery in the presence of mitral stenosis: Central hemodynamic observations. Am J Obstet Gynecol 1985;152:984–988.
95. Silversides CK, Colman JM, Sermer M, Siu SC: Cardiac risk in pregnant women with rheumatic mitral stenosis. Am J Cardiol 2003;91:1382–1385.
96. Lee RT, Bhatia SJS, St. John Sutton MG: Assessment of valvular heart disease with Doppler echocardiography. JAMA 1989;262:2131–2135.
97. Hung JS, Chern MS, Wu JJ, et al: Short- and long-term results of catheter balloon percutaneous transvenous mitral commissurotomy. Am J Cardiol 1991;67:854–862.
98. Fawzy ME, Kinsara AJ, Stefadouros M, et al: Long-term outcome of mitral balloon valvotomy in pregnant women. J Heart Valve Dis 2001;10:153–157.
99. Al Kasab SM, Sabag T, Al Zailbag M, et al: β-Adrenergic receptor blockade in the management of pregnant women with mitral stenosis. Am J Obstet Gynecol 1990;163:37–40.
100. Esteves CA, Ramos AIO, Braga SLN, et al: Effectiveness of percutaneous balloon mitral valvotomy during pregnancy. Am J Cardiol 1991;68:930–934.
101. Ribeiro PA, Fawzy ME, Awad M, et al: Balloon valvotomy for pregnant patients with severe pliable mitral stenosis using the Inoue technique with total abdominal and pelvic shielding. Am Heart J 1992;124:1558–1562.
102. Wu JJ, Chern MS, Yeh KH, et al: Urgent/emergent percutaneous transvenous mitral commissurotomy. Catheterization and Cardiovascular Diagnosis 1994; 31:18–22.
103. Farhat M, Gamra H, Betbout F, et al: Percutaneous balloon mitral commissurotomy during pregnancy. Heart 1997;77: 564–567.
104. Siu SC, Colman JM: Heart disease and pregnancy. Heart 2001;85:710–715.
105. Waller BF, Howard J, Fess S: Pathology of mitral valve stenosis and pure mitral regurgitation: Part I. Clin Cardiol 1994; 17:330–336.
106. Otto CM: Evaluation and management of chronic mitral regurgitation. N Engl J Med 2001;345:740–746.
107. Rossouw GJ, Knott-Craig CJ, Barnard PM, et al: Intracardiac operation in seven pregnant women. Ann Thorac Surg 1993;55:1172–1174.
108. Weiss BM, von Sefesser LK, Seifert B, Turina MI: Outcome of cardiovascular surgery and pregnancy: A systematic review of the period 1984–1996. Am J Obstet Gynecol 1998;179:1643–1653.
109. Mahli A, Izdes S, Coskun D: Cardiac operations during pregnancy: Review of factors influencing fetal outcome. Ann Thorac Surg 2000;69:1622–1626.
110. Carbello BA: Aortic stenosis. N Engl J Med 2002;346:677–682.
111. Presbitero P, Prever SB, Brusca A: Interventional cardiology in pregnancy. Eur Heart J 1996;17:182–188.
112. Silversides CK, Colman JM, Sermer M, et al: Early and intermediate-term outcomes of pregnancy with congenital aortic stenosis. Am J Cardiol 2003;91:1386–1389.
113. Shime J, Mocarski EJM, Hastings D, et al: Congenital heart disease in pregnancy: Short- and long-term implications. Am J Obstet Gynecol 1987;156:313–322.
114. Lao TT, Sermer M, Magee L, et al: Congenital aortic stenosis and pregnancy: A reappraisal. Am J Obstet Gynecol 1993;169:540–545.
115. Spagnuolo M, Kloth H, Taranta A, et al: National history of rheumatic aortic regurgitation. Circulation 1971;44:368–380.
116. Vongpatansin W, Hillis LD, Lange RA: Prosthetic heart valves. N Engl J Med 1996;335:407–416.
117. Badduke AR, Jamieson WRE, Miyagishima RT, et al: Pregnancy and childbearing in a population with biologic valvular prostheses. J Thorac Cardiovasc Surg 1991;102:179–186.
118. Kearon C, Hirsh J: Management of anticoagulation before and after elective surgery. N Engl J Med 1997;336:1506–1511.
119. Lee CN, Wu CC, Lin PY, et al: Pregnancy following cardiac prosthetic valve replacement. Obstet Gynecol 1994;-83:353–356.
120. Sadler L, McCowan L, White H, et al: Pregnancy outcomes and cardiac complications in women with mechanical, bioprosthetic and homograft valves. BJOG 2000;107:245–253.
121. Born D, Martinez EE, Almeida PAM, et al: Pregnancy in patients with prosthetic heart valves: The effects of anticoagulation on mother, fetus, and neonate. Am Heart J 1992;124:413–417.
122. North R, Sadler L, Stewart AW, et al: Long-term survival and valve-related complications in young women with cardiac valve replacements. Circulation 1999;99:2669–2676.
123. Salazar E, Epinola N, Roman L, Casanova JM: Effect of pregnancy on the duration of bovine pericardial bioprostheses. Am Heart J 1999;137:714–720.
124. Ginsberg JS, Hirsch J: Use of antithrombotic agents during pregnancy. Chest 1998;114:524S–530S.
125. Vitale N, DeFeo M, De Santo LS, et al: Dose-dependent fetal complications of warfarin in pregnant women with mechanical heart valves. J Am Coll Cardiol 1999;33:1637–1641.
126. Ad Hoc Committee of the Working Group on Valvular Heart Disease, European Society of Cardiology: Guidelines for prevention of thromboembolic events in valvular heart disease. J Heart Valve Dis 1993;2:398–410.
127. Ginsberg JS, Chan WS, Bates SM, Kaatz S: Anticoagulation of pregnant women with mechanical heart valves. Arch Intern Med 2003;163:694–698.
128. Salazar E, Zajarias A, Gutierrez N, Iturbe E: The problem of cardiac valve prostheses, anticoagulants and pregnancy. Circulation 1984;70(Suppl I):1-169–1-177.
129. Warkentin TE, Levine M, Hirsh J, et al: Heparin-induced thrombocytopenia in patients treated with low-molecular-weight heparin or unfractionated heparin. N Engl J Med 1995;332: 1330–1335.
130. Aster RH: Heparin induced thrombocytopenia and thrombosis. N Engl J Med 1995;332:1374–1376.
131. American Academy of Pediatrics, Committee on Drugs: The transfer of drugs and other chemicals into human milk. Pediatrics 1994;93:137–150.
132. Dean JCS: Management of Marfan syndrome. Heart 2002;88:97–103.
133. Pyeritz RE: Maternal and fetal complications of pregnancy in the Marfan syndrome. Am J Med 1981;71:784–790.
134. Rossiter JP, Repke JT, Morales AJ, et al: A prospective longitudinal evaluation of pregnancy in the Marfan syndrome. Am J Obstet Gynecol 1995;173:1599–1606.
135. Lipscomb KJ, Smith JC, Clarke B, et al: Outcome of pregnancy in women with Marfan's syndrome. BJOG 1997;104:201–206.
136. Elkayam U, Ostrzega E, Shotan A, Mehra A: Cardiovascular problems in pregnant women with the Marfan syndrome. Annu Intern Med 1995;123:117–122.
137. Shores J, Berger KR, Murphy EA, Pyeritz RE: Progression of aortic dilatation and the benefit of long-term β-adrenergic blockade in Marfan's syndrome. N Engl J Med 1994;330: 1335–1341.

138. Veille JC: Peripartum cardiomyopathies: A review. Am J Obstet Gynecol 1984;148:805–818.
139. Cunningham FG, Pritchard JA, Hankins GDV, et al: Peripartum heart failure: Idiopathic cardiomyopathy or compounding cardiovascular events? Obstet Gynecol 1986;67: 157–168.
140. Pearson GD, Veille JC, Rahimtoola S, et al: Peripartum cardiomyopathy. JAMA 2000;283:1183–1188.
141. Witlin AG, Mabie WC, Sibai BM: Peripartum cardiomyopathy: An ominous diagnosis. Am J Obstet Gynecol 1997;176: 182–188.
142. Lampert MB, Weinert L, Hibbard J, et al: Contractile reserve in patients with peripartum cardiomyopathy and recovered left ventricular function. Am J Obstet Gynecol 1997;176: 189–195.
143. Homans DC: Peripartum cardiomyopathy. N Engl J Med 1985;312:1432–1436.
144. Elkayam U, Tummala PP, Rao K, et al: Maternal and fetal outcomes of subsequent pregnancies in women with peripartum cardiomyopathy. N Engl J Med 2001;344:1567–1571.
145. Elkayam U: Pregnant again after peripartum cardiomyopathy: To be or not to be? Eur Heart J 2002;23:753–756.
146. Shotan A, Ostrzega E, Mehra A, et al: Incidence of arrhythmias in normal pregnancy and relation to palpitations, dizziness, and syncope. Am J Cardiol 1997;79:1061–1064.
147. Page RL: Treatment of arrhythmias during pregnancy. Am Heart J 1995;130:871–876.
148. Berlinerblau R, Yessian A, Lichstein E, et al: Maternal arrhythmias of normal labor and delivery. Gynecol Obstet Invest 2001;52:128–131.
149. Rashba EJ, Zareba W, Moss AJ, et al: Influence of pregnancy on the risk for cardiac events in patients with hereditary long QT syndrome. Circulation 1998;97:451–456.
150. Tan HL, Lie KI: Treatment of tachyarrhythmias during pregnancy and lactation. Eur Heart J 2001;22:458–464.
151. Elkayam U, Goodwin TM: Adenosine therapy for supraventricular tachycardia during pregnancy. Am J Cardiol 1995;75:521–523.
152. Mason BA, Ricci-Goodman J, Koos BJ: Adenosine in the treatment of maternal paroxysmal supraventricular tachycardia. Obstet Gynecol 1992;80:478–480.
153. Olin ER: Antiarrhythmic agents. In Olin ER (ed): Facts and Comparisons. St. Louis, JB Lippincott, 1992, pp 144–150.
154. Magee LA, Downar E, Sermer M, et al: Pregnancy outcome after gestational exposure to amiodarone in Canada. Am J Obstet Gynecol 1995;172:1307–1311.
155. Pelitti DB, Sidney S, Quesenberry CP Jr, Bernstein A: Incidence of stroke and myocardial infarction in women of reproductive age. Stoke 1997;28:280–283.
156. Roth A, Elkayam RA: Acute myocardial infarction associated with pregnancy. Ann Intern Med 1996;125:751–762.
157. Badui E, Enciso R: Acute myocardial infarction during pregnancy and puerperium: A review. Angiology 1996;47:739–756.
158. Abramov Y, Abramov D, Abrahamov A, et al: Elevation of serum creatine phosphokinase and its MB isoenzyme during normal labor and early puerperium. Acta Obstet Gynecol Scand 1996;75:255–260.
159. Shivvers SA, Wians FH, Keffer JH, Ramin SM: Maternal cardiac troponin I levels during normal labor and delivery. Am J Obstet Gynecol 1999;180:122–127.
160. Krahenmann F, Huch A, Atar D: Troponin I measurement in the diagnosis of myocardial injury during pregnancy and delivery: Two cases. Am J Obstet Gynecol 2000;183:1308–1310.
161. Shade GH, Ross G, Bever FN, et al: Troponin I in the diagnosis of acute myocardial infarction in pregnancy, labor, and postpartum. Am J Obstet Gynecol 2002;187:1719–1720.
162. Vinatier D, Virelizier S, Depret-Mosser S, et al: Pregnancy after myocardial infarction. Eur J Obstet Gynecol Reprod Biol 1994;56:89–93.
163. Sheikh AU, Harper MA: Myocardial infarction during pregnancy: Management and outcome of two pregnancies. Am J Obstet Gynecol 1993;169:279–284.
164. Ascarelli MH, Grider AR, Hsu HW: Acute myocardial infarction during pregnancy managed with immediate percutaneous transluminal coronary angioplasty. Obstet Gynecol 1996;88:655–657.
165. Garry D, Leikin E, Fleisher AG, Tejani J: Acute myocardial infarction in pregnancy with subsequent medical and surgical management. Obstet Gynecol 1996;87:802–804.
166. Schumacher B, Belfort MA, Card RJ: Successful treatment of acute myocardial infarction during pregnancy with tissue plasminogen activator. Am J Obstet Gynecol 1997;176:716–719.
167. Kloeck W, Cummins RO, Chamberlain D, et al: Special resuscitation situations: An advisory statement from the International Liaison Committee on Resuscitation. Circulation 1997;95: 2196–2210.
168. Katz VL, Dotters DJ, Droegemueller W: Perimortem cesarean delivery. Obstet Gynecol 1986;68:571–576.
169. Mabie WC, Anderson GD, Addington MB, et al: The benefit of cesarean section in acute myocardial infarction complicated by premature labor. Obstet Gynecol 1988;71:503–506.
170. Sullivan JM, Lobo RA: Considerations for contraception in women with cardiovascular disorders. Am J Obstet Gynecol 1993;168:2006–2011.
171. Cardiovascular Disorders in Clinical Challenges in Contraception: A program on women with special medical conditions. ARHP Clinical Proceedings, 7, 1994.
172. Maron BJ: Hypertrophic cardiomyopathy: A systematic review. JAMA 2002;287:1308–1320.
173. Maki S, Ikeda H, Muro A, et al: Predictors of sudden cardiac death in hypertrophic cardiomyopathy. Am J Cardiol 1998;82: 774–778.
174. Natale A, Davidson T, Geiger M, Newby K: Implantable cardioverter-defibrillators and pregnancy: A safe combination? Circulation 1997;96:2808–2812.
175. Autore C, Conte MR, Piccininno M, et al: Risk associated with pregnancy in hypertrophic cardiomyopathy. J Am Coll Cardiol 2002;40:1864–1869.
176. Fairley CJ, Clarke JT: Use of esmolol in a parturient with hypertrophic obstructive cardiomyopathy. Br J Anaesth 1995;74: 801–804.

CHAPTER 38

Respiratory Disease

Raymond Powrie

INTRODUCTION

A variety of biologic adaptations occur in the maternal respiratory system in pregnancy. Resting ventilation increases, oxygen consumption rises, and residual lung volume decreases. Generally, these physiologic changes are well tolerated by the pregnant woman. Their interrelationship with various pulmonary diseases is less well understood, despite the common occurrence of these conditions during pregnancy. It is advisable to include a respiratory physician, preferably one with particular interest in pregnancy, in the management of these disorders. This is critically important in acute severe asthma, the severity of which may be underestimated by both doctor and patient, in severe pneumonia, in cystic fibrosis, and in tuberculosis, where guidelines for therapy change frequently. Acute pulmonary edema is one of the more common reasons that pregnant or postpartum women are transferred to critical care facilities, and its management requires understanding and addressing of the underlying precipitating causes most commonly seen in pregnancy.

BREATHLESSNESS OF PREGNANCY

General

Pregnancy is associated with several significant changes in respiratory function. Pregnant women increase their minute ventilation by nearly 50% in pregnancy. This is achieved not by increasing respiratory rate but by increasing the volume of each breath. This increased "depth" of breathing is an effect of progesterone. Increased ventilation leads to a drop in arterial P_{CO_2} to 27 to 32 mmHg. Pa_{O_2} is increased to 95 to 105 mmHg at sea level. A compensatory renal excretion of bicarbonate occurs in response to respiratory alkalosis, and serum bicarbonate decreases by 4 mEq/L.

Pulmonary function test results and peak expiratory flow rates (PEFR) remain largely unchanged in pregnancy. The main difference is a 20% drop in functional residual capacity (FRC, that portion of a breath that can still be exhaled after normal resting exhalation) due to a decrease in both expiratory reserve volume and residual volume.[1,2] Although the diaphragm will rise 4 cm above its usual position by term, this does not have a significant effect on respiratory function because diaphragmatic excursion is not altered.[3]

Breathlessness is a common symptom in normal pregnancy and therefore does not necessarily indicate cardiorespiratory disease. Up to 70% of pregnant women will report some level of dyspnea. The most typical description of this would be "air hunger."[2,4] This symptom can start during the late first or early second trimester. The peak gestation for the onset of breathlessness is 28 to 31 weeks. Often the breathlessness occurs spontaneously at rest and not in association with exertion. The etiology has not been clearly elucidated, although the hormonal effect of progesterone on ventilation and the associated fall in arterial carbon dioxide tension seem to be central features. It does not appear to be explained by increases in abdominal girth. Studies have suggested that the presence of dyspnea during pregnancy appears to correlate with a low P_{CO_2}. Those women most likely to experience dyspnea during pregnancy appear to be those with a relatively high baseline nonpregnant P_{CO_2}.[5,6]

Management Options

It can be difficult to differentiate benign breathlessness of pregnancy from the more serious causes of chronic dyspnea in pregnancy, such as asthma, pulmonary embolism, and cardiomyopathy. Initial evaluation should be based on a careful history and examination. A previous history of asthma, the presence of cough or wheezing, or an obstructive pattern on pulmonary function testing may point to asthma as a cause. Pulmonary embolism is typically characterized by the sudden onset of dyspnea or chest pain. Dyspnea attributable to pregnancy is generally insidious in onset and should not be associated with any chest discomfort, cough, or sudden exacerbation. Cardiac disease in pregnancy may present as dyspnea. This may be due to previously existing cardiac conditions that have been unmasked by the increased cardiac work of pregnancy. It may also be due to new onset peripartum cardiomyopathy. Findings on physical examination of tachypnea, tachycardia, an elevated jugular venous pulse, a concerning murmur, respiratory crackles on auscultation, or an abnormal chest x-ray can point to a cardiac cause of dyspnea. Suspicion of a cardiac cause should lead to evaluation with transthoracic echocardiography.

History and physical examination can be supplemented with a complete blood count (CBC), oxygen saturation measurement (SaO_2) with exercise, and, if necessary, a chest x-ray. CBC can be used to identify those cases of dyspnea attributable to severe anemia. Measurement of SaO_2 (by pulse oximeter) with moderate exertion can be used to help rule out serious causes of dyspnea in pregnancy. If the SaO_2 remains normal (>95%) on exercise, it is unlikely that the patient has a major problem. Demonstrating to the patient that oxygenation is maintained despite the feeling of dyspnea can also help alleviate a patient's anxiety about her symptoms. Measurement of arterial blood gases (ABGs) will not be necessary in most patients presenting with a complaint of mild dyspnea of insidious onset in pregnancy.

When clinical evaluation leads the clinician to suspect that a patient's dyspnea is due to more than just the pregnancy, the clinician should be confident that all relevant diagnostic imaging procedures for investigating other causes of dyspnea can be safely performed during pregnancy. This includes chest x-rays, computed tomography (CT) scans of the chest, ventilation-perfusion scans, and pulmonary angiography.[7]

Most often, if other causes of dyspnea do not appear to be present, management of breathlessness in pregnancy is limited to educating the patient regarding these physiologic changes and providing reassurance.

CONCLUSIONS

BREATHLESSNESS

- Most breathlessness in pregnancy is common and is due to physiologic changes.
- A careful history and physical examination should be performed on all patients with this complaint, with specific emphasis on trying to identify evidence of thromboembolism, cardiac disease, or asthma.
- Specific concern should be focused on those patients who report dyspnea that is sudden in onset or occurs at rest.
- Investigate if pathologic cause suggested from clinical features; tests might include:
  - oxygen saturation at rest and with exercise (ABGs in severe cases)
  - hemoglobin
  - chest x-ray
  - ventilation-perfusion scan and/or CT angiogram
  - echocardiography

SUMMARY OF MANAGEMENT OPTIONS
Breathlessness in Pregnancy

Management Options	Quality of Evidence	Strength of Recommendation	References
Ask about wheezing, nocturnal worsening, and cough to distinguish from asthma.	IV	C	8
Ask about orthopnea and paroxysmal dyspnea, and perform cardiac exam to distinguish from heart failure.	IV	C	9
Ask about sudden onset of dyspnea, presence of chest pain, personal or family history of thrombosis and look for tachypnea and tachycardia to distinguish from pulmonary embolism. Consider lung scan if any of the above present.	IV	C	10

Continued

SUMMARY OF MANAGEMENT OPTIONS
Breathlessness in Pregnancy *(Continued)*

Management Options	Quality of Evidence	Strength of Recommendation	References
Key investigations: • SaO_2 is the simplest, quickest test of oxygenation in presence of breathlessness (at rest and with exercise; ABGs in severe cases) • hemoglobin • chest x-ray • ventilation-perfusion scan or CT angiogram or MRI when pulmonary embolism suspected • echocardiography when cardiac causes suspected	IV	C	6

ASTHMA

General

Asthma is probably the most common potentially life-threatening medical disorder to occur in pregnancy. The worldwide prevalence of asthma has been steadily increasing such that it now occurs in approximately 1% to 4% of pregnant women.[8,11]

Asthma is defined as a chronic inflammatory disease of the airways that is manifest as a hyperresponsiveness of the airway to a wide variety of stimuli. It tends to be an episodic disease with exacerbations of reversible airway narrowing that are characterized clinically by coughing, wheezing, and shortness of breath. Precipitating factors for asthma exacerbations may include allergens, upper respiratory tract infections, medications (such as aspirin and beta blockers), environmental pollutants, occupational exposures, exercise, cold air, and emotional stress. The condition is more common in atopic individuals.

Maternal and Fetal Risks

Present data suggest that pregnancy does not have a consistent effect on the frequency or severity of asthma. In one prospective study of 330 asthmatic women, asthma was unchanged in 33%, improved in 28%, and worse in 35%.[12] Although it is not clear whether the severity of asthma before pregnancy predicts its course during pregnancy,[13] it does appear that women tend to have similar courses with their asthma in successive pregnancies.[14] Some investigators suggest that asthma tends to be less severe in the last 4 weeks of pregnancy and that if it does worsen, it tends to do so between 29 and 36 weeks' gestation.[15] Asthma exacerbations in labor appear to be very rare.

The usual reason asthmatic patients deteriorate in pregnancy is the mistaken belief that treatment for asthma is harmful to the fetus. Medical attendants as well as patients and their relatives are likely to promote this dangerous fallacy. A National Institutes of Health (NIH) Consensus Conference has concluded that "undertreatment of pregnant asthmatics, particularly because of unfounded fears of adverse pharmacologic effects on the developing fetus, remains the major problem in the management of asthma during pregnancy in the United States."[16] Other treatable reasons why asthma may worsen in pregnancy in individual women include pregnancy-related gastroesophageal reflux disease and pregnancy rhinitis. These precipitating factors should be considered and treated as possible contributors in pregnant women with difficult-to-control asthma.

In studies concerning the interaction between pregnancy and asthma, the only risks that are well established are those of preterm delivery [17,18] and maternal hypertension,[19] and even these risks have not been shown consistently.[20] Associations with hyperemesis, vaginal hemorrhage, complicated labor, neonatal mortality, placenta previa, prematurity and low birth weight infants have also been noted in some studies but not in others.[18,27] It is not clear if the possible relationship between asthma and these perinatal outcomes represents a direct effect of hypoxia and hypocapnia on the developing pregnancy, the effects of medication use, or a fundamental abnormality of smooth muscle in asthmatics manifest as increased contractile tone in the uterus, airways, and vasculature.[28] If indeed any of these associations exist, the effect is small. Asthma should in no way be considered a contraindication to pregnancy, and good asthma control may minimize the incidence of many of these complications.

The risk of the child developing asthma in later life varies between 6% and 30%, depending on whether or not the mother is atopic and whether or not the father also is atopic and has asthma.[29]

Management Options

Prepregnancy

Pregnancy counseling should be given based on the preceding information. Overall it should be anticipated that pregnancy will be well tolerated. Patient education as to maintenance and rescue medications, peak expiratory flow rate (PEFR) use, proper use of inhalers, asthma prevention, and an asthma management plan as described in the following section is important before and during pregnancy. Pulmonary function testing is rarely needed in the management of established asthmatics. Patients should be educated not to stop necessary medications when they find out they are pregnant.

Prenatal

Ideally asthma care should be optimized before conception. Close monitoring of the patient's status and adjustment of treatment as necessary are essential to ensuring the best outcome for mother and child. It is worth reviewing here in some detail the present management of asthma in pregnancy.

ASTHMA MANAGEMENT: GENERAL PRINCIPLES

Present thinking emphasizes that asthma is a chronic inflammatory airway disease and treatment therefore focuses on avoidance of triggers and the use of inhaled corticosteroids to decrease the underlying airway inflammation that leads to symptoms. Use of bronchodilators continues but is perceived of as a method of obtaining symptomatic relief rather than disease control. The underlying principle for treatment of asthma during pregnancy is that, aside from a few exceptions, the same drugs and dosages that would be used outside pregnancy should be used in pregnancy for a given clinical situation.[30] Whenever possible, treatment should be by inhalation rather than oral agents, since this reduces systemic effects.[22,31] It also reduces any possible effects on the fetus.

ASTHMA MANAGEMENT: PREVENTION AND EDUCATION

Essential to the successful pharmacologic management of asthma is vigorous patient education. Against the background of this patient education, medication prescribing for asthma will be far more effective, and severe asthmatic exacerbations may be avoided. This education may be most effective if initiated before pregnancy. Key concepts emphasized by present clinical guidelines are as follows[32]:

- Patients should be taught to measure their PEFR twice daily to allow early detection of deterioration in pulmonary function before they become symptomatic. PEFR is best measured on awakening and approximately 12 hours later. PEFR can be especially helpful to pregnant asthmatic patients in determining if their dyspnea is due to breathlessness of pregnancy or an asthmatic exacerbation.
- Patients need to have proper inhaler use reviewed with them repeatedly. Proper use includes using a spacer to improve delivery of medication to the lungs, help avoid local side effects of inhaled steroids (such as oral thrush), and decrease unnecessary systemic absorption of medication through the buccal mucosa.
- All patients should be given a written asthma management plan that directs the patient in adjusting medication according to their PEFR and guides them about when to seek medical advice. In general action plans are based on the best PEFR that a patient has ever obtained. A typical action plan for a patient would tell her that if the PEFR drops transiently by 20% from her personal best that her therapy needs "stepping up"; the patient should have instructions at home as to how to do this. The patient should be told that sustained drops in PEFR of more than 20% from the previous personal best warrants a call to the physician. A PEFR drop >50% from the previous personal best warrants a trip to the emergency department (ED). Patients should be taught to avoid triggers. This advice includes the use of impermeable pillow and mattress covers to minimize contact with dust mites, removal of pets from the home (or at least the bedroom), removal of carpets in the bedroom, and avoidance of cigarette smoke.
- Patients should be clearly informed that present evidence suggests that well-controlled asthma does not appear to increase pregnancy risk but poorly controlled asthma does.[11,12,25] This information may help enhance compliance and alleviate the patient's fears about medication use in pregnancy.

ASTHMA MANAGEMENT: SPECIFIC ASTHMA MEDICATIONS

Asthma medications are classified as either rescue agents or maintenance agents. *Rescue agents* are those medications used to treat acute bronchospasm and provide symptomatic relief but do not treat the underlying inflammation that causes bronchospasm. Rescue agents include all the inhaled β_2 agonists and ipratropium. The data regarding their effectiveness and safety in pregnancy is reviewed in Table 38–1. *Maintenance agents* are those medications that help to control airway hyperreactivity and generally treat the underlying inflammation of the airway. The inhaled steroids are the keystones of present asthma maintenance. Other maintenance agents include systemic steroids, leukotriene antagonists, and cromolyn. The data regarding their effectiveness and safety in pregnancy is reviewed in Table 38–2.[16,40]

ASTHMA MANAGEMENT: DAILY ASTHMA MANAGEMENT WITH STEPWISE PLAN

Asthma medications are presently prescribed in a "stepwise" manner with adjustments in medication being

TABLE 38–1

Summary of Pregnancy Data on Rescue Agents Commonly Used to Treat Asthma[33–36]

CLASS	AGENT	EFFECT ON EMBRYO AND FETUS
Short-acting inhaled β_2-adrenergic agonists	albuterol, isoproterenol, isoetharine biltolterol, pirbuterol, metaproterenol, terbutaline	Published experience with these drugs in animals and humans suggests that β-sympathomimetics do not increase the risk of congenital anomalies.[37,38] Albuterol is the most studied of these agents. Metaproterenol is the second most studied.
Long-acting inhaled β_2-adrenergic agonists	salmeterol	Animal data about intravenously administered salmeterol have not been reassuring, but this agent is still felt to probably be safe in humans when administered by inhalation. However, no human data about this agent have been published at this point; therefore, its use should be reserved for patients who have failed low-potency steroids and/or cromolyn alone.
Inhaled anticholinergic	ipratropium	Reassuring animal studies but no published human data. Poorly absorbed by the bronchial mucosa so fetal exposure is likely minimal.[39] Efficacy in acute asthma attack presenting to the ED makes its short-term use seem justifiable, however.

From Powrie RO: Drugs in pregnancy. Respiratory disease. Best Pract Res Clin Obstet Gynaecol 2001;15(6):913–936.

made either upward or downward in intensity in response to the severity of the individual patient's asthma at that particular point in time. Table 38–3 reviews the criteria for classification of asthma into four separate classes of severity and summarizes the treatment recommended during pregnancy for each classification. This stepwise approach is recommended by both the United States National Asthma Education and Prevention Program[32] and the British Thoracic Society.[60]

Once control has been established and is maintained for several months, consideration of stepping down the treatment to a regimen appropriate for the next lower level of asthma severity should occur. However, if asthma fails to be controlled or worsens, stepping up a treatment level is advisable. In any class of asthma a rescue course of 5 to 10 days of oral prednisone may be used to gain control from a prolonged or severe exacerbation. This is particularly true in the setting of an asthma exacerbation secondary to the common cold. In pregnancy, gastroesophageal reflux disease,[61,62] vasomotor rhinitis of pregnancy, and noncompliance should always also be considered as possible causes of difficult-to-control asthma.

ASTHMA MANAGEMENT: TREATMENT OF ACUTE ASTHMA EXACERBATIONS

Patients with worsening asthma not improving on home management by the stepwise approach will need to be seen in an ED for evaluation. Treatment in the ED is reviewed in Table 38–4. Acute severe asthma (status asthmaticus) is a very dangerous condition that should be managed with a respiratory physician in an intensive care environment. High-dose intravenous steroids are the cornerstone of treatment for asthmatic exacerbations requiring admission to hospital. Even in the absence of acute severe asthma, there should be a very low threshold for admission, because patients with asthma can deteriorate very quickly.[21] General guidelines for admission to hospital include a sustained drop in PEFR to less than 60% of baseline, a P_{O_2} <70 mmHg at sea level, a P_{CO_2} >35 mmHg, a heart rate of >120/minute, or a respiratory rate >22/minute. It is important to remember that a P_{CO_2} >40 mmHg in a pregnant women with an asthmatic exacerbation suggests impending respiratory failure, because the normal P_{CO_2} in pregnancy is 27 to 32 mmHg.

Clinical predictors of mortality from asthma include marked circadian variation in lung function, a large bronchodilator response, psychosocial instabilities, use of three or more medications, frequent visits to the ED, recurrent hospitalizations, and previous life-threatening attacks.

Asthma exacerbation is not an indication for elective delivery, though if there are other maternal or fetal problems, induction should not be withheld.

Labor and Delivery

Asthma exacerbations during labor are rare, presumably due to the natural outpouring of endogenous steroids and epinephrine associated with the stress of delivery. Exacerbations occurring at this time should always be approached with a differential diagnosis that includes pulmonary edema (from cardiac causes or noncardiac ones such as preeclampsia, tocolysis, and sepsis), pulmonary embolism, and aspiration. Although asthma is rarely a problem in labor, if readers wish to use a protocol for such cases, they are referred to the National Asthma Education Program Working Group on Asthma and Pregnancy guidelines.[30]

TABLE 38–2

Summary of Pregnancy Data on Maintenance Medications Commonly Used to Treat Asthma[38,41]

CLASS	AGENTS	PREGNANCY DATA
Inhaled corticosteroids	Low potency: beclomethasone dipropionate Medium potency: triamcinolone acetonide High potency: fluticasone propionate budesonide flunisolide mometasone furoate	Inhaled corticosteroids are the most important pharmacologic agents in maintaining asthma control in and out of pregnancy. Only 4% of 257 patients taking inhaled glucocorticoids from the start of pregnancy had acute attacks of asthma during pregnancy, in contrast with 17% of 177 patients who were not.[42] Beclomethasone[38,43,44] and budesonide are the most widely studied of the inhaled corticosteroids in pregnancy and should be considered the preferred inhaled steroids in pregnancy. Relatively little of these agents is absorbed, and human data have not suggested any teratogenic effects of these agents.[45–47] Triamcinolone is the next most studied inhaled steroid in pregnancy, with this limited experience suggesting no adverse pregnancy effects. Fluticasone has not been studied in pregnancy; however, its minimal systemic absorption and the safety of the other steroids in pregnancy make its use in pregnancy generally felt to be justifiable.[48]
Mast cell stabilizers	disodium cromoglycate (cromolyn) sodium nedocromil	Human and animal data suggest these agents are not teratogens. These agents are virtually not absorbed through mucosal surfaces, and the swallowed portion is largely excreted in the feces. These agents are best in mild cases of asthma in which the decision not to use inhaled steroids has been made. Cromolyn[38,43,49] has been better evaluated in human pregnancy than nedocromil and should be considered the preferred agent of this class.
Leukotriene antagonists	zileuton zafirlukast montelukast	The leukotriene antagonists represent an important exception to the general rule that asthma treatment is largely unchanged in pregnancy. Zafirlukast and montelukast both have favorable animal data, but data about their safety in human pregnancy are extremely limited at this point. Zileuton has concerning animal data. Their use should be limited in pregnancy to those unusual cases in which a woman has had significant improvement in asthma control with these medications before becoming pregnant, control that was not obtainable through other methods.
Sustained-release methylxanthines	theophylline	Theophylline and its intravenous form aminophylline do not appear to be human teratogens.[37,38,50] The safety of aminophylline therapy in the second and third trimester has been demonstrated in a large group of 212 gravidas in Finland.[50] The clearance of aminophylline is increased in pregnancy in a rather variable way.[51] Any patient who is taking more than 700 mg of aminophylline per day should have blood measurements made for optimal dosing. Their present role in treating asthma is generally felt to be as second- or third-line agents; they do not appear to be of benefit in an acute exacerbation.[52]
Systemic steroids	Oral: prednisone Intravenous: methylprednisolone hydrocortisone	Most data suggests that systemic steroids do not present a teratogenic risk in human pregnancy. In doses equivalent to prednisone 25 mg/day, they do not cross the placenta because of placental metabolism[53–55] (the same is not true for betamethasone or dexamethasone). Even in higher doses, the effect of hydrocortisone or prednisone on the fetus in terms of suppression of the hypothalmic-pituitary-adrenal axis is minimal. However, a recent case-control study found a significant association with first-trimester use and oral clefts (OR=6.55, 95% CI=1.44–29.76).[55,56] However, even if this association is real, the benefits of controlling a life-threatening disease make steroid use, when indicated, in the first trimester still generally justifiable.
Immunotherapy	Administering gradually increasing quantities of an allergen extract to an allergic subject to down-regulate response	Human data from small trials suggest safety of continuing immunotherapy in pregnancy, but present practice usually avoids initiation in pregnancy because of fear of provoking anaphylaxis.[57–59]

Adapted from Powrie RO: Drugs in pregnancy. Respiratory disease. Best Pract Res Clin Obstet Gynaecol 2001;15(6):913–936.

Prostaglandin E_2 compounds and oxytocin can be safely used in asthmatics. 15-Methyl prostaglandin $F_{2\alpha}$ should not be used in asthmatic patients because it can cause bronchoconstriction.[64,65] Ergonovine and other ergot derivatives should also not be used in asthmatics as they too have caused severe bronchospasm in asthmatic patients, particularly in association with general anesthesia. Although morphine and meperidine may theoretically cause bronchoconstriction through histamine release, in practice this is not generally a problem. Many asthmatic women will have been given morphine and meperidine in labor without harm. Nonetheless, some

TABLE 38–3

Classification of Asthma and Stepwise Management in Pregnancy[41]

CATEGORY	CRITERIA	STEP THERAPY
Mild intermittent	• Symptoms up to twice a week • Nighttime symptoms up to twice a month • Exacerbations last only hours to a few days • Asymptomatic between episodes • PEFR >80% predicted and day-to-day variability <20%	• No daily treatment necessary • Inhaled β_2-adrenergic agonists as needed
Mild persistent	• Symptoms more than twice a week but not daily • Nighttime symptoms more than twice a month • Exacerbations may affect activity • PEFR >80% predicted and day-to-day variability 20%–30%	• Inhaled β_2-adrenergic agonists as needed *and* • Daily treatment with inhaled cromolyn or nedocromil *or* inhaled low-dose corticosteroid (preferably beclomethasone or budesonide) *or* theophylline preparation
Moderate persistent	• Daily symptoms • Nighttime symptoms more than once a week • PEFR 60%–80% and day-to-day variability >30%	• Inhaled β_2-adrenergic agonists as needed *and* • Daily treatment with inhaled low- to medium-dose corticosteroid *and* • Daily treatment with salmeterol or theophylline preparation
Severe persistent	• Continual symptoms that limit activity • Frequent nighttime symptoms and acute exacerbations • PEFR <60% predicted and day-to-day variability >30%	• Inhaled β_2-adrenegic agonists as needed *and* • Daily treatment with inhaled high-dose corticosteroid *and* • Daily treatment with salmeterol or theophylline preparation *and* • Daily or alternate-day treatment with systemic prednisone

Adapted from Powrie RO: Drugs in pregnancy. Respiratory disease. Best Pract Res Clin Obstet Gynaecol 2001;15(6):913–936.

experts prefer to use butorphanol or fentanyl as alternatives in pregnant asthmatics because these agents are less likely to cause histamine release. If anesthesia is required, an epidural is preferable to general anesthesia because of the risks of chest infection and atelectasis with general anesthesia. For those patients who do require a general anesthetic, bronchodilatory agents such as ketamine and halogenated anesthetics are preferred.

It is known that daily doses of systemic steroids given for as little as several weeks may suppress the hypothalamic-pituitary-adrenal (HPA) axis for up to 1 year and thereby blunt the normal physiologic outpouring of adrenal corticosteroids that occurs with stressors such as illness, surgery, and labor. The practical significance of this in pregnancy remains unstudied. To avoid precipitating an adrenal crisis, many centers give empiric stress-dose steroids (hydrocortisone 100 mg IV every 8 hours on the day of delivery followed by 50 mg IV every 8 hours on day 1 after delivery and then back to the baseline dose) to any woman in labor who has received systemic steroids for longer than 2 to 4 weeks in the preceding year. Other centers will only do so if steroids have been used in the prior 4 weeks. Still other centers would advocate the use of a cosyntropin stimulation test to test the HPA axis prior to labor and delivery. If stress-dose steroids are not given, it is advisable to watch the patient for signs of adrenal insufficiency (anorexia, nausea, vomiting, weakness, hypotension, hyponatremia, and hyperkalemia) postpartum.

TABLE 38–4

Management of the Acute Asthma Exacerbation Presenting to the Emergency Department[41]

1. Place patient on oxygen to keep Sa_{O_2} >95%.
2. Administer inhaled β_2-adrenergic agonist until improvement obtained or toxicity is noted; e.g., albuterol metered-dose inhaler (MDI) with spacer 3 to 4 puffs *or* albuterol nebulizer every 10–20 minutes.
3. Administer methylprednisolone 125 mg IV acutely and then 40–60 mg IV q6h *or* hydrocortisone 60–80 mg IV q6h. When the patient improves, she can be switched to a tapering oral regimen of prednisone (usually 60 mg once daily slowly reduced to nothing over the next 2 weeks).
4. Consider use of ipratropium MDI (2 puffs of 18 μg/spray q6h) or nebulizer (one 62.5-mL vial by nebulizer q6h) in first 24 hours after presentation.[63]
5. Avoid use of subcutaneous epinephrine in the pregnant asthmatic.

Adapted from Powrie RO: Drugs in pregnancy. Respiratory disease. Best Pract Res Clin Obstet Gynaecol 2001;15(6):913–936.

Postnatal

Patients should have their medications continued postpartum and their PEFR monitored in the days following delivery. Breastfeeding is not contraindicated in patients taking any form of asthma treatment, including oral prednisone. Indeed breastfeeding for between 1 and 6 months reduces the prevalence of atopy in 17-year-olds who were breastfed by about 30% to 50%.[66]

CONCLUSIONS

ASTHMA

- Optimal control of asthma with prevention and management of medications in a stepwise manner will help ensure the best possible outcome for mother and fetus.
- All patients with asthma should have a peak flow monitor and an asthma action plan and should be able to demonstrate good technique in the use of their inhaler with a spacer.
- Most commonly used asthma medications can be safely administered in pregnancy. Human data about the leukotriene inhibitors are limited, so their routine use as a first line agent in pregnancy is not recommended at this time.
- In labor, the use of prostaglandin $F_{2\alpha}$ and ergonovine should be avoided, and patients who received steroids for more than 2 weeks in the past year should receive stress-dose steroids with delivery.
- Breastfeeding will decrease the risk of atopy in the offspring of mothers with asthma.

SUMMARY OF MANAGEMENT OPTIONS
Asthma

Management Options	Quality of Evidence	Strength of Recommendation	References
Prepregnancy			
Adjust maintenance medication stepwise to optimize respiratory function.	IV	C	30,32,60
Educate patient to minimize precipitating factors, if possible by timing of pregnancy (seasonal) and avoidance of allergens.	IV	C	30,32,60
Educate patient about use of peak expiratory flow meters.	IV	C	30,32,60
Provide patient with asthma action plan.	IV	C	30,32,60
Advise early referral for prenatal care.	IV	C	30,32,60
Prenatal			
Use same drugs as outside pregnancy, especially steroids, beta-sympathomimetics, and theophylline.	IV III	C B	30,32,60 22, 31
Regulate peak flow with adjustment of asthma medication as needed to control symptomatology and minimize need for rescue therapy.	IV	C	30
Use inhalation therapy rather than oral.	IV	C	30,32,60
Ensure adequate fetal oxygenation with acute exacerbation by keeping SaO_2 >95%.	IV	C	30,32,60
If theophylline used, monitor blood levels, since blood volume expansion in pregnancy may mandate higher doses of the drugs.	IV	C	30,32,60
In the stable patient, antepartum nonstress testing is not necessary. If concerns over fetal well-being arise, begin antepartum testing in the late second or early third trimester.	IV	C	30,32,60
Seek anesthesiology consultation in preparation for delivery if general anesthesia is anticipated.	IV	C	30,32,60
Labor and Delivery			
Maintain adequate maternal oxygenation.	IV	C	30,32,60
Avoid prostaglandin $F_{2\alpha}$ and ergometrine.	Ib	A	64
Avoid general anesthesia if possible.	IV	C	30,32,60
Use parenteral stress-dose steroids for patients on chronic oral therapy or in those who have received more than 2 weeks of systemic steroids in the past year.	IV	C	30,32,60
Encourage respiratory therapy to minimize atelectasis.	IV	C	30,32,60
Continue maintenance drug therapy.	IV	C	30,32,60

Continued

SUMMARY OF MANAGEMENT OPTIONS
Asthma *(Continued)*

Management Options	Quality of Evidence	Strength of Recommendation	References
Postnatal			
Perform physiotherapy to maintain adequate pulmonary toilet.	IV	C	30,32,60
Encourage respiratory therapy to minimize atelectasis.	IV	C	30,32,60
Restart maintenance drug therapy.	IV	C	30,32,60
Encourage breastfeeding.	IV	C	30,32,60

SARCOIDOSIS

General

Sarcoidosis is a noncaseating granulomatous condition typically affecting the lung with bilateral hilar adenopathy and/or pulmonary infiltrates. It is seen most commonly in women of reproductive age. It usually regresses spontaneously, although very occasionally lung disease is progressive.

The exact prevalence of sarcoidosis in the general population is difficult to establish because a large number of cases may be asymptomatic or go undiagnosed. The prevalence is estimated to be 10 to 20 per 100,000 population, with a lifetime risk of 0.85% among whites. It is three to four times more common in blacks.[67]

The etiology and pathogenesis of sarcoidosis remains unknown. The granulomas seen in this condition are focal chronic inflammatory reactions. Infectious agents such as mycobacterium or propionibacterium may produce this condition in genetically predisposed patients. Malignancy, tuberculosis, HIV infection, collagen vascular disease, and occupational lung disease should be ruled out before a diagnosis of sarcoidosis is made. Tissue biopsy should be obtained for all but the most classic presentations.

The lung is the most likely organ to be affected. Over one half of cases are detected incidentally on routine chest x-rays. When symptomatic, sarcoidosis may present as cough, dyspnea, chest pain, fatigue, malaise, weakness, fever, and weight loss. Chest x-ray may reveal the classic bilateral hilar adenopathy and/or interstitial or alveolar infiltrates. The classification of pulmonary involvement in sarcoidosis is based on the radiographic stage of disease. Stage I is defined by the presence of bilateral hilar adenopathy, which is often accompanied by right paratracheal node enlargement. Seventy-five percent of such patients will show spontaneous regression in 1 to 3 years. Stage II consists of bilateral hilar adenopathy and interstitial infiltrates. Two thirds of such patients undergo spontaneous resolution; the remainder either have progressive disease or display little change over time. Stage III disease consists of interstitial disease with shrinking hilar nodes. Stage IV disease is defined by advanced fibrosis. Both stage III and IV disease are more likely to lead to progressive lung impairment without treatment.

Other organ systems that may be affected include skin (maculopapular eruptions, skin nodules, and erythema nodosum), lymphatic system (lymphadenopathy), eye (iridocyclitis, chorioretinitis, and keratoconjunctivitis), and liver. Fatigue is also a common complaint in patients with sarcoidosis. Less common manifestations can occur in the spleen (splenomegaly), the neurologic system, the salivary glands, the bone marrow, the ear nose and throat, heart, kidneys, bone, joint, or muscle.[68,69] Calcium homeostasis (hypercalciuria and hypercalcemia) can be also affected in sarcoidosis. The frequencies of different extrapulmonary manifestations of sarcoidosis seem to vary with ethnic origin and gender.

Treatment for sarcoidosis is reserved for those with significant symptoms or pulmonary compromise. Systemic steroids are the cornerstone of treatment for sarcoidosis. Two studies have shown that corticosteroid therapy is also of benefit in mild cases with chest x-ray evidence of parenchymal disease. The degree of improvement averaged 10%. Whether the risks of long-term corticosteroids are worth the modest benefit seen in these studies of asymptomatic patients remains unclear.[70,71] Chloroquine, hydroxychloroquine, methotrexate, azathioprine, pentoxifylline, thalidomide, cyclophosphamide, cyclosporine, and infliximab have all also been used to treat chronic or steroid-unresponsive sarcoidosis with variable success.[72]

Maternal Risks

Sarcoidosis rarely involves the female reproductive organs. However, sarcoidosis of the endometrium, ovary, and leiomyoma have all been reported.[73,74] Systemic sarcoidosis, in the absence of significant cardiopulmonary compromise, does not appear to affect fertility and does not increase the incidence of fetal or obstetrical complications.[75]

Although relatively few studies have been published about sarcoidosis in pregnancy, the general observation is that pregnancy does not influence the natural history of the disorder.[76] In some cases it will improve during pregnancy, possibly due to increases in maternal free cortisol.

Some patients with sarcoidosis develop progressive pulmonary fibrosis and hypoxemia and proceed to cor pulmonale and pulmonary hypertension. Pulmonary hypertension has a very poor prognosis in pregnancy, whatever the cause. Patients with evidence of moderate to severe pulmonary hypertension should be discouraged from proceeding with pregnancy because of the significant risk of maternal mortality (see Chapter 37).

Fetal Risks

There are no specific risks aside from the uncommon circumstance in which a mother has severe systemic disease that is a threat to maternal health and thereby leads to fetal compromise. Severe disease unresponsive to steroids may also lead to consideration of treatments with pharmacologic agents less well studied in pregnancy than steroids. Untreated maternal hypercalcemia could theoretically lead to neonatal hypocalcemia and tetany, although the hypercalcemia associated with sarcoidosis is usually mild and unlikely to cause neonatal problems. Sarcoid granulomas have been found in the placenta[77] but not in the fetus.

Management Options

Prepregnancy

Prepregnancy counseling can be given, incorporating the above information. It is generally advisable to obtain a baseline $Sa\text{O}_2$ (both resting and with exercise), pulmonary function testing (including a diffusing capacity for carbon monoxide—DLco—as a measurement of gas exchange that is sensitive to the presence of interstitial lung disease), a chest x-ray, CBC, liver function tests, blood urea nitrogen, creatinine, and serum calcium. Patients with stage I or II disease and minor extrapulmonary manifestations should anticipate a good outcome. Patients with more severe disease should be warned that their disease progression and treatment may complicate the course of their pregnancy but will not usually have a direct adverse effect on the fetus.

Prenatal

Breathlessness is common in the normal pregnancy but can also be seen in stage II sarcoidosis. Obtaining the results of the baseline investigations listed will help in interpretation of additional testing if the patient with sarcoidosis reports new or worsening symptoms. Testing liver enzymes, creatinine, calcium, and CBC once a trimester can be helpful in identifying hypercalcemia before delivery and establishing a baseline that may help prevent the inappropriate attribution of abnormalities in creatinine or liver tests to preeclampsia later in pregnancy.

Complaints of increased dyspnea in women with known sarcoidosis will require evaluation with $Sa\text{O}_2$ (both resting and with exercise), chest x-ray, and pulmonary function testing, including DLco. Distinguishing the normal dyspnea of pregnancy from progression of disease will be difficult without these objective tests. In some circumstances a high-resolution CT scan may be needed to define the extent of disease; there is no reason why this test cannot be carried out during pregnancy.

Painful joints and erythema nodosum are also manifestations of sarcoidosis that may be seen in normal pregnancies and need to be interpreted cautiously as a manifestation of disease progression in the setting of pregnancy.

Symptomatic disease attributable to sarcoidosis should generally be treated with systemic steroids under the supervision of a pulmonologist experienced in treating this disease. The safety of steroids in pregnancy is well established and is discussed in the preceding section on asthma. Symptomatic disease unresponsive to steroids may require treatment with other agents that are less well studied in pregnancy and will require careful consideration of both risk and potential benefits of treatment.

Patients with sarcoidosis can develop hypercalcemia, particularly in the setting of vitamin D supplementation.[78] Even in a patient with a normal serum calcium level, sarcoidosis-associated hypercalciuria can lead to nephrocalcinosis. Pregnant patients with sarcoidosis may do well to avoid both vitamin D and calcium supplementation. The contents of their prenatal vitamins should be reviewed to prevent unintended supplementation of both vitamin D and calcium.

The level of angiotensin-converting enzyme has been advocated by some experts as an index of disease activity in sarcoidosis. This may be invalid in pregnancy where angiotensin-converting enzyme levels seem to change independently of sarcoid activity.[79]

Labor and Delivery

If there is any degree of parenchymatous lung disease, an epidural block would be better than general anesthesia. Women who have been on steroids for more than 2 weeks of the preceding year should be given stress-dose steroids around the time of labor and delivery, as discussed in the preceding section on asthma.

Postnatal

No specific recommendations are needed for postpartum management of the parturient with sarcoidosis.

CONCLUSIONS

SARCOIDOSIS

- Sarcoidosis usually does not impact maternal or fetal outcome in pregnancy unless there is preexisting evidence of pulmonary fibrosis, hypoxemia, or pulmonary hypertension.
- Pulmonary function testing (with DLCO) and echocardiography can help assess severity of disease and the possibility of pulmonary hypertension.
- Women with sarcoidosis in pregnancy should be watched for signs and symptoms of progressive pulmonary disease. Steroid therapy should be instituted with evidence of significant disease advancement.
- Hypercalcemia can be a problem in sarcoidosis. Serum calcium should be checked periodically in women with sarcoidosis, and women with sarcoidosis should not take vitamin D supplementation. They should also not take a prenatal vitamin with vitamin D in it.

SUMMARY OF MANAGEMENT OPTIONS

Sarcoidosis

Management Options	Quality of Evidence	Strength of Recommendation	References
Prepregnancy			
Reassure patient about benign nature of sarcoidosis during pregnancy (unless there is preexisting evidence of pulmonary fibrosis, hypoxemia, or pulmonary hypertension).	IV III	C B	75 76
Baseline pulmonary function studies may assist in the evaluation of the patient's lung status prior to pregnancy.	IV III	C B	75 76
If lung disease significant, evaluate by exam and echocardiogram for pulmonary hypertension. Discourage pregnancy in presence of pulmonary hypertension.	IV III	C B	75 76
Prenatal			
Avoid multivitamins containing vitamin D.	IV III	C B	75 76
Consider checking serum calcium once a trimester because of neonatal toxicities with maternal hypercalcemia.	IV III	C B	75 76
Watch for signs and symptoms of progressive pulmonary disease; institute steroid therapy with evidence of significant disease advancement.	IV III	C B	75 76
Labor and Delivery			
With substantial parenchymal disease, avoid inhalation anesthesia.	IV III	C B	75 76
Recognize that high block conduction anesthesia may cause significant respiratory compromise.	IV III	C B	75 76
Obtain early anesthesiology consultation in patients with severe disease.	IV III	C B	75 76
Use parenteral stress-dose steroids for patients on chronic oral therapy or in those who have received 2 weeks of systemic steroids in the past year.	IV III	C B	75 76
Postnatal			
Watch for neonatal tetany if mother has hypercalcemia.	IV	C	75
No other specific disease-related needs	III	B	76

TUBERCULOSIS

General

After a resurgence of tuberculosis (TB) in the western world in the early 1990s, the incidence of TB is once again declining in the resource-rich nations. In the year 2000, the United States reported the lowest rate of new TB infection in U.S. history, at 5.8 cases per 100,000 population.[80] However, there remain a large number of unidentified latent and active cases of TB in the western world.[81,82] This is particularly true among inner city minority populations and among immigrants from countries with a high prevalence of TB.

The global perspective on TB is much more daunting. It is estimated that one third of the world population has been infected with TB and that worldwide there are 8 million new cases of TB and 2 million deaths caused by TB each year.[81] Pregnancy offers a unique opportunity for identification and treatment of TB among young women to the benefit of a mother, her child, and the general public.

Maternal and Fetal Risks

Although pregnancy is not associated with an increased risk of tuberculosis, management of TB in pregnancy does require some additional considerations related to concerns about drug safety in pregnancy. In all cases, tubercular infections should be managed in conjunction with a physician specifically trained in the care of tubercular infections.

Maternal Risks

Tuberculosis used to have a sinister reputation in pregnancy,[83] but with the advent of modern chemotherapy, immunocompetent patients should make a complete recovery even if TB is first diagnosed in pregnancy.[84] Some concern exists that the hepatotoxicity of one of the key agents in antituberculous therapy—isoniazid—is increased in pregnancy and warrants increased monitoring.

Fetal Risks

Tuberculosis that is confined to the thorax or limited to lymphadenitis poses little risk to the fetus. Adverse fetal outcomes may be more frequent with extrapulmonary disease.[85] One small study that compared pregnancy outcomes in pregnant women with extrapulmonary TB versus healthy controls found significantly higher frequencies of low birth weight infants and infants with low Apgar scores among mothers with extrapulmonary TB.[86]

Tubercle bacilli very rarely cross the placenta,[87] though granulomata may be found in the placenta. True congenital infection is therefore exceptionally uncommon. Perhaps this is because congenital TB is almost invariably associated with genital tract TB, which in itself usually is a cause of infertility. Criteria for congenital TB have recently been re-evaluated and include a primary focus in the fetal liver.[88]

In practice the only risk to the fetus is the very questionable teratogenicity of antituberculous drugs. The neonate is only at risk of postnatally acquired infection if the mother still has active TB at the time of delivery. Then the risk is high.[89] Only under these most unusual circumstances should the mother be separated from her newborn. Any remote risks of neonatal infection may be reduced by giving the neonate bacille Calmette-Guérin (BCG) and prophylactic isoniazid.

Management Options

Prepregnancy

The main problem concerning the management of tuberculosis in pregnancy is the possible teratogenicity of some antituberculous drugs. Prepregnancy counseling may be given, incorporating the information on risks. Women undergoing treatment for active TB might consider delaying pregnancy until their treatment course is complete, but present data suggests that the most commonly used agents are safe in pregnancy. For those women who have completed an adequate course of chemotherapy, previous TB is no contraindication to pregnancy, and TB is no more likely to be reactivated in pregnancy than at any other time.

Prenatal

Screening is not justified in pregnancy except in high risk populations.[90] However, all pregnant women from populations at risk for tuberculosis (i.e., inner city minority populations and people who have recently emigrated from an area of the world with a high prevalence of TB) should undergo a tuberculin skin test (TST) unless documentation of recent TST status is available. TST is both safe and reasonably sensitive throughout pregnancy.[91,92] Positive skin test reactors (and women with symptoms suggestive of TB regardless of their TST results) should have a chest x-ray performed to look for active pulmonary TB.[93] If the chest x-ray is suggestive of TB, sputum examination for *Mycobacteria* should be performed and if positive (on smear, PCR testing, or culture), treatment should be initiated. Susceptibility testing for isoniazid, rifampin, and ethambutol should be performed on a positive initial culture. For all patients beginning antituberculous treatment, baseline measurements of serum aminotransferases, bilirubin, alkaline phosphatase, serum creatinine, and a platelet count should be obtained. Routine HIV testing of all patients with TB is also recommended. Testing of visual acuity and red-green color discrimination should be obtained when ethambutol is to be used.

Active tuberculosis can be treated successfully in pregnancy; the benefits of treatment dramatically outweigh any concerns about potential drug toxicity. Directly observed therapy, in which patients are observed to ingest each dose of antituberculous medications, is highly recommended because it helps maximize compliance. The current recommendation in the United Kingdom[93] and by the World Health Organization (WHO) and the International Union against Tuberculosis and Lung Disease (IUATLD) for uncomplicated TB in a pregnant individual is an initial phase of a 2-month course of ethambutol, pyrazinamide, rifampin, and isoniazid, followed by a continuation phase of a further 4 months of rifampin and isoniazid (i.e., a total of 6 months' treatment).[94] Such therapy can be given in various regimens. The most commonly used regimens entail either 7 days a week therapy in both phases or a modified regimen of 5 days a week in the initial phase and 5 days a week (or even twice weekly) in the continuation phase. Less frequent dosing makes directly observed therapy more feasible. An initial four-drug regimen has become increasingly important as multidrug-resistant TB has become more common. Although this standard regimen is effective in most cases, treatment may need to be adjusted once formal antibacterial susceptibility patterns are established.

Pregnancy data about the commonly used antimycobacterial agents is reviewed in Table 38–5.[69,95–98] Among the commonly used antituberculous drugs, streptomycin is the only one that is clearly contraindicated in pregnancy. It has been shown to cause both

TABLE 38–5

Pregnancy Data Regarding Commonly Used Antimycobacterial Agents[41]

AGENT AND USUAL DOSE	ADVERSE EFFECTS IN GENERAL	PREGNANCY DATA	ADDITIONAL NOTES
Isoniazid (INH) • 5 mg/kg, up to a maximum of 300 mg daily • Dispensed in the USA as 50, 100, and 300 mg tabs and 50 mg/5 mL syrup	• Hepatitis • Peripheral neuropathy • Drug interaction with many agents, especially anticonvulsants • Cutaneous hypersensitivity	• FDA pregnancy classification C • High lipid solubility; easily passes into fetal circulation • Fair data to suggest this agent is safe in human pregnancy and any risk is outweighed by potential benefit. However, concerns about potential increase in INH hepatotoxicity in pregnancy make its routine use for prophylaxis in pregnancy in low risk cases not advisable.	• Always administer with 25–50 mg/day of pyridoxine (vitamin B_6) to decrease the risk of neurotoxicity in the mother. • Give vitamin K to mother near birth (10 mg PO daily from 36 weeks on) and infant at birth to decrease risk of postpartum hemorrhage and hemorrhagic disease of the newborn. • Check transaminases monthly while on the medication
Rifampin • 10 mg/kg, up to a maximum of 600 mg daily • Dispensed as 150 and 300 mg scored tablets in the USA	• Fever • Nausea • Hepatitis • Purpura • Flulike symptoms at high doses • Orange secretions • Increased metabolism of many agents	• FDA pregnancy classification C • Limited data suggest no adverse fetal effects.	• Give vitamin K to mother near birth (10 mg PO daily from 36 weeks on) and infant at birth to decrease risk of postpartum hemorrhage and hemorrhagic disease of the newborn.
Ethambutol • 15–25 mg/kg, up to a maximum of 2500 mg daily • Dispensed as 100 and 400 mg tablets in the USA	• Retrobulbar neuritis in 1% of patients • Peripheral neuropathy	• FDA pregnancy classification B • Limited data suggest no adverse fetal effects.	• At each monthly visit patients taking this agent should be questioned regarding possible visual disturbances, including blurred vision or scotomata; monthly testing of visual acuity and color discrimination is recommended for patients receiving the drug for longer than 2 months.
Pyrazinamide • 15-30 mg/kg PO daily, up to a maximum of 3000 mg daily	• Thrombocytopenia • Hepatotoxicity • Interstitial nephritis • Nephrotoxicity	• FDA pregnancy classification C • Human data extremely limited	• Use in pregnancy supported by international recommendations in all pregnant patients with active TB after the first trimester; particularly essential for multidrug-resistant TB and HIV-positive patients.
Streptomycin • Dose varies	• Ototoxicity	• FDA pregnancy classification D • Reports of fetal ototoxicity preclude use.	• Avoid use in pregnancy.

Adapted from Powrie RO: Drugs in pregnancy. Respiratory disease. Best Pract Res Clin Obstet Gynaecol 2001;15(6):913–936.

vestibular and auditory eighth nerve damage,[99] leading to deafness in the newborn. Although detailed human pregnancy safety data are not available for pyrazinamide, most official recommendations now support its use in pregnancy. If pyrazinamide is not included in the initial treatment regimen, the minimum duration of therapy is 9 months.

Isoniazid should always be given in conjunction with pyridoxine 25 to 50 mg daily to minimize the risk of neuropathy.[100,101] The amount of pyridoxine in multivitamins is variable but generally less than the needed amount. Vitamin K should probably also be given to the mother from 36 weeks' gestation onward in a dose of 10 mg daily to decrease the risk of hemorrhagic disease of the newborn.[102] Drug-induced hepatitis is the most serious common adverse effect of isoniazid. Symptoms of hepatotoxicity (e.g., nausea, abdominal pain, hepatic tenderness) in association with hepatic transaminase elevations greater than three times the normal range or asymptomatic elevations in transaminases greater than five times the normal range should lead to discontinuation of therapy and consideration of the use of an alternative regimen. There is some evidence to suggest that pregnant women are at a higher risk of developing isoniazid-related hepatotoxicity; therefore, testing of hepatic transaminases at initiation of treatment and at monthly intervals thereafter is advisable.[103–105] During treatment of patients with pulmonary TB, a sputum specimen for microscopic examination and culture should be obtained at a minimum of monthly intervals until two consecutive specimens are negative on culture.

Management of HIV-related tuberculosis is complex and requires expertise in the management of both HIV disease and TB. Because HIV-infected patients are often taking numerous medications, some of which interact with antituberculous medications, it is strongly encouraged that experts in the treatment of HIV-related TB be consulted.

TB PROPHYLAXIS

The role of prophylaxis for positive tuberculin skin testing varies with the size of the patient's TST response, HIV status, and immune status and whether or not the patient has had recent contact with an active case of TB. The standard TST is a Mantoux test of 5 tuberculin units (TU) injected into the skin and reviewed at 48 to 72 hours by measuring the maximum area of induration. All HIV-infected women exposed to an active case of TB and all HIV-infected patients with a TST result >5 mm should receive prophylactic therapy even during pregnancy. Although some controversy around this issue exists, the pregnant woman with a normal immune status and a positive TST who has not been previously treated should probably only receive prophylaxis during pregnancy if there has been a recent contact with an active TB case and the patient has a TST that is >5 mm. Otherwise prophylaxis for TB in the asymptomatic immunocompetent pregnant woman can generally be delayed until the postpartum period.[106,107]

The preferred tuberculosis prophylaxis regimen is isoniazid 5 mg/kg (up to a maximum of 300 mg) daily for 9 months. A 6-month course may also be used but is less preferred than the 9-month regimen. Twice-weekly doses of 15 mg/kg (up to a maximum of 900 mg) for 9 months may also be used as an alternative but only if therapy is directly observed. Administration of pyridoxine 25 to 50 mg daily should occur, similar to what is done when treating active TB. Again, monthly clinical reassessment and monitoring of liver function tests should occur in pregnancy. Symptoms of hepatotoxicity (e.g., nausea, abdominal pain, hepatic tenderness) in association with hepatic transaminase elevations greater than three times the normal range or asymptomatic elevations in transaminases greater than five times the normal range should lead to discontinuation of therapy and consideration of the use of rifampin as an alternative regimen.

Labor and Delivery

No specific recommendations are needed for labor and delivery except as they relate to infection control issues. Transmission of infection from the mother to the infant can occur after delivery; thus the mother should be carefully evaluated for potential infectiousness at the time of delivery.[108]

Postnatal

After delivery, patients with sputum-positive tuberculosis (i.e., tubercular bacilli in their sputum) should be separated from their babies until they are no longer overtly infective. Because pyrazinamide renders the sputum sterile in 10 days, this situation should occur infrequently. In addition, the neonate should be given isoniazid to prevent it acquiring infection from its mother and should be given isoniazid-resistant BCG to boost its immunity.[109]

Breastfeeding should not be discouraged for women being treated with isoniazid, pyrazinamide, ethambutol, and/or rifampin. These agents are found in only small concentrations in breast milk and are not known to produce toxicity in the nursing newborn. These concentrations are also not significant enough to provide any protection to the nursing infant from infection with TB.[110]

CONCLUSIONS

TUBERCULOSIS

- All women from inner city minority populations and women from high risk areas of the world should be screened for TB in the setting of pregnancy with tuberculin skin testing.

Continued

CONCLUSIONS *(Continued)*

- Women with active TB should have cultures sent for antibiotic sensitivity testing and be started on a four-drug regimen of isoniazid, rifampin, ethambutol, and pyrazinamide.
- Hepatic transaminases should be measured monthly in pregnant women on isoniazid because of an increased risk of hepatotoxicity. All patients on isoniazid should receive daily pyridoxine.
- Infants should be separated from mothers with active TB as demonstrated by mycobacterium seen in their sputum. Ten days of treatment with a typical regimen will sterilize most patients' sputum.
- HIV testing in all women who have a positive TST or who have TB is strongly recommended.
- Women with a positive TST who have a known recent exposure or who are HIV infected should receive isoniazid prophylaxis in pregnancy. Other patients may have prophylaxis delayed until after delivery.

SUMMARY OF MANAGEMENT OPTIONS
Tuberculosis

Management Options	Quality of Evidence	Strength of Recommendation	References
Prepregnancy			
Establish the diagnosis and treat the condition prior to pregnancy.	IV	C	111,112
Screening of at-risk populations is advised.			
Counsel regarding the potential teratogenesis of streptomycin if being used (it is not standard therapy).	III	B	99
Prenatal			
Perform tuberculin skin testing on all women from inner city minority populations and women from high risk areas of the world.	IV	C	111,112
Recommend HIV testing to all women with a positive TST.	IV	C	111,112
Administer isoniazid prophylaxis during pregnancy to TST-positive mothers without active TB if they have a known recent exposure or are HIV infected.	IV	C	111,112
Send sputum cultures with antibiotic sensitivity testing on women with active TB and start a four-drug regimen of isoniazid, rifampin, ethambutol, and pyrazinamide.	IV	C	95,96,97
Give pyridoxine when using isoniazid.	III	B	100,101
Measure hepatic transaminases monthly in pregnant women on isoniazid.	IV	C	103
Labor and Delivery			
No specific recommendations except institute infection precautions with active disease.	IV	C	111,112
Postnatal			
Only separate mother from baby if open TB present and until no longer infective (approximately 10 days into therapy).	IV	C	108,111,112
Administer BCG and BCG-resistant isoniagid to neonate.	III	B	109
Advise mother that she can breastfeed.	IV	C	110
Be aware that oral contraceptive efficacy is impaired by antituberculous drugs.	IV	C	111,112

KYPHOSCOLIOSIS

General

The term *kyphosis* refers to spinal deformity with anteroposterior angulation; *scoliosis* refers to lateral displacement or curvature of the spine. Most commonly the disorder is idiopathic (80%) and begins in childhood. The degree of spinal deformity correlates well with the degree of lung function impairment. A restrictive pattern is seen on pulmonary function testing, with decreased total lung capacity (TLC) and vital capacity (VC) and preserved residual volume (RV). Chest wall compliance decreases with age and increases the work of breathing. Pulmonary hypertension develops in some patients as a result of persistent hypoxemia.

Mild disease has a good prognosis and requires supportive care only. Patients with cor pulmonale have a life expectancy of less than 1 year. Surgical treatment has little role in adults with kyphoscoliosis. Medical therapy is the mainstay of management and can include pulmonary rehabilitation, supplemental oxygen, and use of negative- or positive-pressure ventilators.[111]

The prevalence of kyphoscoliosis in pregnancy depends on the criteria used for the definition. However, kyphoscoliosis will not affect pregnancy unless there is some degree of respiratory impairment; such circumstances prevail in less than 0.1% of pregnancies. It is remarkable that patients can achieve successful pregnancy despite so much deformity; the abdominal cavity often appears so contracted that there should be insufficient room for a fetus to develop normally. Nevertheless, babies can and do grow normally in these adverse surroundings.

Maternal and Fetal Risks

The risks to the mother are those of cardiac failure and cor pulmonale in the very few patients with pulmonary hypertension. To develop pulmonary hypertension, the condition has to be severe enough to produce hypoxemia at rest. If the VC is <1.5 L, the patient is at risk of respiratory failure, especially so if it is <1 L.[112,113] The risks to the fetus are intrauterine growth restriction (IUGR) caused by maternal hypoxemia and preterm delivery,[114] which is often elective because of concern about maternal well-being. Very severe hypoxia in a single patient with kyphoscoliosis (maternal $Pa{O_2}$ <59 mmHg) has been associated with brain damage in the fetus.[115]

Management Options

Prepregnancy

Prepregnancy counseling should be given, incorporating the previously stated information. Pulmonary function testing should be obtained. If VC is >2 L, patients will generally tolerate pregnancy and delivery. If it is <2 L, patients will be at increased risk for pulmonary complications with pregnancy. An ABG analysis should also be obtained in all patients with a VC of <2 L. If the resting $Pa{O_2}$ is decreased, the fetus is at risk of growth deficiency. If the $Pa{CO_2}$ is increased, the risk of pulmonary complications is very high.

In the setting of significant compromise in pulmonary function testing—hypoxia or hypercapnia—the patient should be evaluated for pulmonary hypertension. Because of the distortion of the chest, the electrocardiogram is particularly poor at estimating right ventricular hypertrophy in kyphoscoliosis. Therefore, an estimate of the pulmonary circulation should be made by echocardiography, preferably with Doppler ultrasonography. Moderate to severe pulmonary hypertension is a relative contraindication to pregnancy (see Chapter 37). However, before such a drastic recommendation is made, the physician may want to perform a direct assessment of pulmonary vascular resistance by measurement of pulmonary artery pressure and cardiac output either by formal right sided cardiac catheterization.

Prenatal

Patients who have significantly increased pulmonary vascular resistance should be offered termination because of the maternal risk. All other patients require optimal medical care directed toward diagnosing and treating respiratory infection and bronchospasm and any cardiac failure. In addition, supplementary domiciliary oxygen therapy to prevent growth deficiency should be considered in those who are hypoxemic. This form of therapy has not been evaluated for this indication; however, it is successful in preventing the development of pulmonary hypertension in nonpregnant patients, and granted the association between growth deficiency and maternal hypoxia, it seems worth pursuing.

Patients may require hospital admission from about 30 weeks' gestation either because of concern about impending respiratory failure or simply because they get so tired. Nasal positive-pressure ventilation has been used to help in some patients who have deteriorated in the third trimester.[116,117] Obstetric prenatal care relates to detecting IUGR. Elective preterm delivery may be necessary for maternal reasons, increasing hypoxemia or frank respiratory failure, or because of the signs of fetal hypoxia either with or without IUGR.

Labor and Delivery

Many patients with severe kyphoscoliosis are delivered by cesarean section because of associated pelvic deformity.[118] This is better performed with epidural block rather than with general anesthesia. Surprisingly, epidural puncture and catheterization is often possible in these patients. This is because the defect in kyphoscoliosis is often in the upper part of the spine.

Postnatal

No special measures are necessary after delivery apart from a continuation of optimal medical and obstetric care, including early mobilization and physiotherapy.

CONCLUSIONS

KYPHOSCOLIOSIS

- Kyphoscoliosis will usually only represent a significant risk in pregnancy if the mother has hypoxia and/or pulmonary hypertension.
- Obtaining an ABG and pulmonary function testing will help assess the degree of pulmonary compromise from the skeletal abnormality.

SUMMARY OF MANAGEMENT OPTIONS
Kyphoscoliosis

Management Options	Quality of Evidence	Strength of Recommendation	References
Prepregnancy			
Counsel regarding risk for increase in pulmonary compromise as pregnancy advances, and risks for IUGR and preterm delivery.	III	B	118
Assess pulmonary vital capacity and obtain ABGs to assess O_2 and CO_2 levels.	III	B	118
Assess for evidence of pulmonary hypertension (unlikely); if present, advise against pregnancy.	IV	C	119
Prenatal			
Monitor respiratory function clinically and with Sao_2.	III	B	118
Discuss pregnancy termination if pulmonary hypertension present.	III	B	118
If severe cardiorespiratory compromise, begin prenatal surveillance for IUGR and fetal well-being in early third trimester.	III	B	118
Administer supplementary oxygen when hypoxemia present. Consider use of nasal intermittent nasal positive-pressure ventilation if respiratory status deteriorating.	IV	C	116,117
May need early delivery for frank respiratory failure.	III	B	118
Labor and Delivery			
Provide supplementary oxygen if Sao_2 low.	III	B	118
Perform cesarean section if associated pelvic deformities; vaginal delivery possible with most cases; regional anesthesia possible in many cases.	III	B	118
Postnatal			
Provide physiotherapy, especially if general anesthesia used.	–	GPP	–

CYSTIC FIBROSIS

General

Cystic fibrosis (CF) is an autosomal recessive multisystem disorder. The incidence of CF is between 1 in 2000 to 1 in 3000 live births. One in 20 whites are heterozygous for the CF gene. Although CF remains a fatal disease associated with a significant decrease in life expectancy, treatment of CF has undergone a rapid evolution in the past two decades that has lead to a substantial improvement in patient survival. Increasing numbers of women with CF are now surviving to an age at which pregnancy is possible.[119]

Cystic fibrosis is caused by mutations of the cystic fibrosis transmembrane conductance regulator (CFTR) gene located on chromosome 7.[120] This gene codes for a complex chloride channel found in all exocrine tissues. Mutations in this gene cause deranged chloride transport that leads to thick, viscous secretions in the lungs, pancreas, liver, intestine, and reproductive tract. It also leads to increased salt content in sweat gland secretions.[121]

The usual presenting symptoms and signs of CF include persistent pulmonary infection, pancreatic insufficiency, and elevated sweat chloride levels. Pulmonary disease is the leading cause of morbidity and mortality in patients with CF. Pulmonary involvement is characterized by recurrent pneumonias, chronic bronchitis with or without bronchiectasis, and an obstructive pattern on pulmonary function testing. Digital clubbing is common among adults with this disease.

Abnormal lung secretions permit colonization of the airway and sinuses with pathogenic bacteria. *Staphylococcus aureus* and *Haemophilus influenzae* are common pathogens during early childhood, but *Pseudomonas aeruginosa* is ultimately isolated from the respiratory secretions of most patients. Greater than 70% of adults with CF are chronically infected with these bacteria. Persistent infection with *Burkholderia cepacia* is associated with an accelerated decline in pulmonary function and shortened survival. This organism induces airway injury and often demonstrates a high level of antibiotic resistance.[122]

Antibiotics are routinely prescribed when patients with CF develop acute or subacute increases in cough, sputum production, fever, and/or shortness of breath. Spirometry usually demonstrates worsened airflow obstruction during these episodes, although chest radiographs may not show significant changes over baseline. Low-grade fevers may or may not be present. Oral antibiotics are appropriate if the exacerbation is relatively mild, providing all pathogens identified are sensitive. Treatment is usually continued for 2 to 3 weeks. Intravenous antibiotics are used if the exacerbation is severe or a previous course of oral antibiotics has failed. Nebulized antibiotics are often used as well. Dosing of antibiotics often requires alteration, as medication pharmacokinetics are greatly altered in patients with CF.

Most physicians prescribe aerosolized beta-adrenergic agents to CF patients, particularly those who have manifestations of asthma. Ipratropium bromide is also occasionally prescribed, but theophylline use has declined in parallel with its less frequent use in asthma. The nebulized endonuclease DNase I is often used in CF patients with persistent productive cough. It can decrease the viscosity of expectorated sputum by cleaving long strands of DNA into smaller segments and can be given on an alternate-day dosing schedule.

All patients who produce sputum should be instructed in some form of chest physiotherapy for secretion clearance. Because patients vary in their responses to different modes of therapy, several techniques should be introduced to each patient. Inhaled corticosteroids and/or daily azithromycin therapy are also sometimes used in the long-term management of this disease.

Pancreatic insufficiency is common in CF, leading to malabsorption of fat and protein. These problems can often be reversed with oral supplementation of pancreatic enzyme extracts. Many patients may remain significantly underweight. Diabetes mellitus can also be seen, particularly in adults. Less commonly cholelithiasis and biliary cirrhosis can be seen in patients with CF.

Advancements in the treatment of CF lung disease have delayed disease progression but have not stopped it. Premature death from respiratory failure still occurs in the majority of patients. As in other progressive lung diseases, lung transplantation provides an additional, albeit imperfect, management option for CF. Thirty-three percent of all double lung transplants in adults are performed for CF.[123]

Because of the complex nature of this disease, care for patients with cystic fibrosis is best accomplished in a multidisciplinary clinic with chest therapists, nutritionists, and social workers lead by a physician experienced in the care of CF.

Maternal and Fetal Risks

Maternal Risks

Fertility may be decreased among women with CF. This is likely due both to malnutrition-related amenorrhea and to the production of an abnormally tenacious cervical mucus.[124] Data from the United States[125] and the United Kingdom[126] suggest a pregnancy rate for women with CF over age 16 of 40/1000 per year (compared with 80/1000 for healthy women in the United Kingdom). Up to 70% to 80% of pregnancies in patients with CF will result in a delivery. In those pregnancies that continue beyond the first trimester, the likelihood of delivering a live infant is high.

Early reports of poor outcome in mothers with CF have been discounted by studies demonstrating the safety of pregnancies in women with CF with good lung function.[127–130] When patients with CF become pregnant, it is now known that maternal and fetal outcomes are generally favorable if the prepregnancy forced expiratory volume in 1 second (FEV_1) on pulmonary function testing exceeds 50% to 60% of the predicted value. However, if the mother has any evidence of pulmonary hypertension, her prognosis is much more guarded. Pulmonary hypertension in pregnancy from any cause carries with it a significant risk of right ventricular decompensation and maternal mortality.

In a retrospective study of 92 pregnancies in 54 women with CF, 49 women gave birth to 74 children and were followed for a mean of 11 years. Maternal deaths usually occurred in those with the most severe lung disease, with a cumulative mortality rate of 7.9% at 6 months after delivery and 13.6% at 2 years. Absence of *Burkholderia cepacia*, pancreatic sufficiency, and prepregnancy FEV_1 greater than 50% of predicted value were all associated with better survival rates. Pregnancy did not appear to affect the decline in FEV_1 survival as compared to the entire adult female CF population.[131]

Pregnancy puts an additional nutritional demand on the mother with CF, and women who enter a pregnancy underweight may become emaciated if unable to keep up with the nutritional demands of the fetoplacental unit.

Diabetes is also associated with an increased risk of adverse pregnancy outcome in women with CF. In those patients with CF who do not have diabetes, glucose tolerance is often already impaired and the risk of gestational diabetes may be high.

Fetal Risks

For the most part well-nourished mothers with reasonably preserved lung function can expect a good pregnancy outcome. However, IUGR and premature labor can result from chronic hypoxia. Acute severe hypoxia during delivery may also result in fetal loss. Pneumonia is associated with an increased risk of preterm delivery and pregnancy loss. Malnutrition can also lead to growth restriction. Although most medications used for treatment of CF are safe for use in pregnancy, infection with some multidrug-resistant organisms may require use of agents with less extensive pregnancy data.

Careful genetic counseling is necessary to explain the risk of having an affected child, as determined by the partner's carrier status, and to clarify the intentions of the couple with regard to testing the partner, antenatal diagnosis, and whether to terminate if a high risk pregnancy or affected fetus is identified. Any child of a mother with CF will be at least heterozygous and has a considerable risk of being a homozygote in view of the high prevalence of the CF gene in the community. Identification of the specific gene mutation in the mother will help in screening her partner and fetus if this is desired. At the time of writing, 90% of CF mutations can be identified by the screening typically employed for the 20 to 30 most prevalent mutations.[132] Screening for the remaining 10% is impractical because there are now over 900 identified mutations of the CFTR gene. If a mutation is identified in both mother and father, prenatal diagnosis with chorionic villus sampling or amniocentesis can be used to exclude CF in the fetus.[133] Prenatal diagnosis does carry a small risk of pregnancy loss. Parents should be aware that because there is no cure for CF, prenatal diagnosis should be performed either to help the couple emotionally prepare for an affected child or to guide them toward termination if the fetus is found to be affected.[134]

Management Options

Prepregnancy

Counseling, including detailed genetic counseling, should be given, acting on the preceding information. The patient's nutritional status should be assessed and optimized. The presence of pulmonary vascular disease should be accurately determined if this is to be a reason for precluding or terminating the pregnancy. Examination for evidence of pulmonary hypertension (elevated jugular venous pulse, right ventricular heave, and/or a loud or palpable second heart sound), obtaining current pulmonary function tests, ABGs, and an echocardiographic estimation of pulmonary artery pressures would all be advisable to help assess a women's pregnancy risk. Pulmonary hypertension and cor pulmonale should lead the clinician to strongly discourage pregnancy because of the high maternal risk.[135,136] Pregnancy should also be strongly discouraged when FEV_1 is <50% of predicted; completed pregnancies have been reported, but outcomes have been poor, with prematurity, infant complications, and maternal death.[137] A BMI <18 kg/m^2 should also be considered a relative contraindication to pregnancy.[108]

Medical care and drug treatment should be optimized before conception. In addition, the fact that a future child is at risk of being left without a mother at a relatively young age needs to be tactfully raised and future child care issues considered. The 10-year mortality rate among pregnant women with CF is 20%. Although heart and lung transplantation may be possible for some patients with CF, it will not be possible for the majority, if only because of the shortage of donors. Patients who are already significantly malnourished should be warned of the further weakness and emaciation that pregnancy may cause.

Prenatal

The principles of management of patients with CF in pregnancy are optimization of pulmonary and nutritional status. Patients with severe lung impairment and/or pulmonary hypertension should be informed of the substantial personal risk of a pregnancy to their own health and should be offered a termination of pregnancy.

Patients who are continuing with pregnancy require optimal medical care for their respiratory condition. Most patients who survive to become pregnant are giving themselves chest physiotherapy on a daily basis, and they or their partners should be encouraged to continue and increase this treatment. Pulmonary exacerbations should be treated as they would be outside of pregnancy. Pulmonary exacerbations can lead to hypoxia and increase the risk of preterm delivery. There should be no hesitation in arranging hospital admission either because of exacerbation of respiratory infection or because of malnutrition. Antibiotic dosing may need adjustments because of the altered pharmacokinetics of both CF and pregnancy. Use of penicillins, cephalosporins, and aminoglycosides for episodes of deterioration in pulmonary status is safe and readily justifiable in pregnancy for this indication.[138,139] Limited data have not shown quinolones to increase teratogenic risk in humans, and these agents should be used when indicated in pregnancy for the management of CF.[140,141] Use of trimethoprim/sulfamethoxazole may be necessary in pregnancy to treat *Burkholderia cepacia.* Nearly all bronchodilator drugs can be used safely in pregnancy. For patients with hypoxia, use of supplemental oxygen is routine. However, large-scale studies of supplemental oxygen have not been performed on CF patients.

Malnutrition may be the cause of IUGR. The healthy 10- to 12-kg weight gain usually associated with pregnancy can be a challenge for the pregnant woman with CF. Most patients with CF need to eat 120% to 150% of their recommended daily requirements to maintain their body weight even when not pregnant. Normal pregnancy weight gain requires them to eat a further 300 kcal/day.[142] Significantly underweight women may become emaciated in pregnancy because of the additional nutritional demands of the fetoplacental unit. However, even in those patients with normal weight, several factors may complicate weight gain. Pregnancy-related dyspepsia, reflux, nausea and vomiting, and constipation may lead to a decrease in caloric intake. The additional calorie requirements needed for pregnancy may then be difficult to match without resorting to enteral feeding. In some cases complicated by hyperemesis gravidarum, enteral feeding may be required.

Patients with diabetes will require the usual tight control of blood glucose to optimize pregnancy outcome. Because many women with CF will have impaired glucose tolerance, screening for gestational diabetes should occur early. Most CF patients identified to have gestational diabetes will require insulin therapy.

Intrauterine growth restriction, decreasing maternal weight, and deteriorating respiratory function despite optimal medical treatment in hospital are all indications that should prompt consideration of preterm delivery late in gestation.

Labor and Delivery

At delivery, the aim should be for a vaginal delivery to decrease the risk of postoperative pneumonia associated with surgery. The patient should be encouraged to receive an epidural to decrease maternal oxygen requirements associated with pain and avoid the need for general anesthesia should an urgent cesarean delivery be needed. Forceps or vacuum delivery should be considered early in the second stage of labor to avoid or relieve maternal exhaustion.

Postnatal

Most patients with cystic fibrosis should be encouraged to breast-feed. Most medications needed for the treatment of CF are safe to take during breastfeeding. Breastfeeding is not advisable, however, where maternal nutrition is a problem. Furthermore, if the mother's general health is very poor, bottle feeding has the advantage that somebody else can do it at night and thus allow the mother to rest. The breast milk of mothers with CF has normal electrolyte content but a slightly lower fat content than normal, specifically for essential fatty acids, although it has enough to nourish the child.[143–145]

Infants of mothers with CF will often be screened for CF by their pediatrician.

CONCLUSIONS

CYSTIC FIBROSIS

- Prepregnancy counseling of women with CF should include tactful discussions about her shortened life expectancy and the risk of CF in the patient's offspring.
- Obtaining pulmonary function testing, ABGs, and an echocardiographic estimation of pulmonary artery pressures is important in helping the woman with CF prepare for pregnancy.
- Women with CF who have a good nutritional status, an FEV_1 that exceeds 50% of the predicted value, no evidence of pulmonary hypertension, and have not been colonized by *Burkholderia cepacia* are most likely to have good pregnancy outcomes.
- A BMI <19, an FEV_1 <50% of predicted, and infection with *Burkholderia cepacia* all are predictors of poor outcome in pregnant women with CF. The presence of pulmonary hypertension is associated with a significant risk of maternal mortality.

SUMMARY OF MANAGEMENT OPTIONS
Cystic Fibrosis (Maternal)

Management Options	Quality of Evidence	Strength of Recommendation	References
Prepregnancy			
Document baseline/prepregnancy respiratory function.	III	B	126,137,138
Counsel for maternal risks of respiratory failure and congestive heart failure and preterm delivery if prepregnancy FEV_1 is <50% and/or pulmonary hypertension is present.	III	B	135,136
Counsel for fetal risks of having CF or being a carrier.	IV	C	134
Assess patient weight, and encourage patient to obtain optimal nutritional status.	III	B	126,137,138
Optimize medical management.	III	B	126,137,138
Prenatal			
Care for patient with multidisciplinary team led by individual with expertise in CF management.	–	GPP	–
Counsel for fetal risks of having CF or being a carrier.	III	B	126,137,138
Optimize medical management:	III	B	126,137,138
• physiotherapy	III	B	126,137,138
• bronchodilators	III	B	126,137,138
• treat pulmonary exacerbations as when nonpregnant with antibiotics (common antibiotics are safe; uncertainty with quinolones).	III	B	138,139,140,141
Increase caloric intake in pregnancy.	III	B	126,137,138
Institute screening and vigilance for IUGR and preterm delivery.	III	B	126,137,138
Labor and Delivery			
Monitor respiratory function (Sao_2).	III	B	126,137,138
Provide supplemental oxygen if Sao_2 is low.	III	B	126,137,138
Provide central hemodynamic monitoring if severe pulmonary hypertension present.	III	B	126,137,138
Assisted vaginal delivery may be necessary.	III	B	126,137,138
Avoid general anesthesia for cesarean section.	III	B	126,137,138
Postnatal			
Monitor respiratory function.	III	B	126,137,138
Breastfeeding is not contraindicated.	III	B	143,144,145

PNEUMONIA

General

Pneumonia remains the leading cause of infectious death in the United States[146] but is relatively infrequent in pregnancy. At the Sloan Hospital in New York, Berkowitz[147] found that the incidence of pneumonia in 1988–1989 was 1:3670 deliveries and in 1992 was 1:2288 deliveries. The mothers who developed pneumonia usually had coexisting medical problems, including drug abuse, anemia, and HIV infection.

In managing cases of pneumonia in pregnancy, perhaps the most important role for physicians is to carefully review the differential diagnosis. Pulmonary embolism is the leading cause of maternal mortality in the United States and the United Kingdom and can present identically to an acute pneumonia with dyspnea, cough, chest pain, fever, and chest x-ray infiltrates. Aspiration chemical pneumonitis, amniotic fluid embolism, and pulmonary edema related to sepsis, tocolysis, or preeclampsia can also present in a similar fashion.

Rigorous investigation into the specific etiology and treatment of pneumonia in pregnancy has not occurred.

However, the pathogens responsible for severe community-acquired pneumonia are likely similar in pregnant and nonpregnant patients. Importantly, the reduction in cell-mediated immunity associated with pregnancy does place women at an increased risk of severe pneumonia and disseminated disease from some atypical pathogens such as herpes virus, influenza,[148] varicella,[149] and coccidioidomycosis.[150] Pathogens known to cause pneumonia in pregnancy are reviewed in Table 38–6.

Maternal and Fetal Risks

The risks to the fetus are those of miscarriage and preterm labor; these are nonspecific risks associated with any febrile illness in pregnancy. In addition, the organism causing pneumonia may present specific risks to the fetus, particularly if it is a virus (e.g. varicella).[155] However, most cases of pneumonia in pregnancy are caused by organisms that do not affect the fetus. The fetus may also be at risk from maternal conditions that predispose to pneumonia (e.g., HIV infection), and all women who present with pneumonia in pregnancy should be offered HIV testing.

Effective antibiotic therapy has removed the excess maternal risk that pregnancy might have added to bacterial pneumonia. Even though the patients in Berkowitz's series from New York were seriously ill and required aggressive treatment, it is likely that this was because of their other underlying conditions rather than because of pregnancy.

TABLE 38–6

Causes of Community-Acquired Pneumonia[41]

ORGANISM	PERCENTAGE OF CAUSES OF COMMUNITY-ACQUIRED PNEUMONIA	COMMENTS
Streptococcus pneumoniae	20–60%	Currently believed that many culture-negative cases of pneumonia are caused by pneumococcus
Haemophilus influenzae	3–10%	More common in smokers or patients with underlying lung disease such as asthma
Staphylococcus aureus	3–5%	Rare in healthy young people, except in the setting of postinfluenza pneumonia
Gram-negative bacilli	3–10%	Unusual as a cause of pneumonia in the absence of underlying disease; therefore, rare in a young healthy pregnant population
Aspiration	6–10%	In the past aspiration pneumonia often associated with cesarean deliveries and general anesthesia. Typical case of aspiration pneumonia in obstetric populations is abrupt-onset chemical pneumonitis in which infection plays a limited, if any, role. Modern anesthetic management appears to have greatly decreased its occurrence. Treatment generally supportive. Bacterial aspiration pneumonia usually has a more insidious onset. Mouth anaerobes are the typical pathogens.
Legionella	2–8%	Not frequently seen in young patients without underlying disease
Mycoplasma pneumoniae	1–6%	Common cause of pneumonia in young adults but usually presents indolently
Chlamydia pneumoniae	4–6%	Similar indolent presentation as *Mycoplasma*
Viruses	2–15%	Among the many causes of viral pneumonia, pregnant women appear to be particularly susceptible to herpes, varicella, and influenza pneumonia. Altogether, 10% of cases of maternal varicella infection may be complicated by pneumonia, which can be very severe. In one series, two patients required ventilation and one died. In influenza epidemics, half the cases of maternal mortality have been due to pneumonia,[151] though this has not been a problem recently.
Miscellaneous	3–5%	Includes *Neisseria meningitidis, Moraxella catarrhalis, Streptococcus pyogenes* (group A streptococcus), psittacosis (from exposure to birds), tularemia (from exposure to rabbits), and *Coxiella burnetti* (from exposure to parturient animals or cats) *Mycobacterium tuberculosis* is an important and increasing cause of pneumonitis that should be particularly considered among inner city and new immigrant populations. *Pneumocystis carinii* always warrants consideration in patients with HIV infection. Coccidioidomycosis ("desert fever") is usually a mild pneumonia associated with arthralgias and erythema nodosum but can lead to disseminated disease, including meningitis, in pregnant women. It should be suspected in patients with a history of travel to the American Southwest.[150,152] In a series of 50 cases of coccidioidomycosis from North America, 22 became disseminated during pregnancy, with a maternal mortality of 100% in patients not treated with amphotericin B.[153,154]

Adapted from Powrie RO: Drugs in pregnancy. Respiratory disease. Best Pract Res Clin Obstet Gynaecol 2001;15(6):913–936.

Management Options

Prepregnancy

Prepregnancy counseling is usually not relevant, since pneumonia presents as an acute event without warning. However, in HIV-infected individuals with low CD4 cell counts requiring pneumocystis prophylaxis, patients should be counseled to continue this therapy into pregnancy. Additionally, based on recently revised recommendations from the Centers for Disease Control and Prevention (CDC) and the American College of Obstetricians and Gynecologists, women anticipating pregnancy should be advised that they should routinely receive influenza vaccination during the influenza season.[156] Pneumococcal vaccine is recommended before or during pregnancy for women with high risk conditions such as diabetes mellitus, asthma, chronic cardiac or pulmonary disease, or immune compromise disease. It is mandatory postsplenectomy and in women with functional hyposplenism (e.g., sickle cell disease). It is also recommended for women living in long-term care facilities or prisons.[157]

Prenatal

The patient with community-acquired pneumonia typically presents with the sudden onset of rigors followed by fever, pleuritic chest pain, and cough productive of purulent sputum. Physical examination shows tachycardia, tachypnea, fever, and crackles on lung auscultation, but any of these features may be absent at the time of presentation. Pneumonias caused by agents such as *Mycoplasma*, *Legionella*, *Chlamydia*, and viruses are likely to have a more indolent presentation, but the clinical utility of this observation when making treatment decisions is questionable as evidence suggests that all etiologies may present either acutely or subacutely.[158]

The presence of an infiltrate on chest x-ray is considered the "gold standard" for diagnosing pneumonia and should be obtained in most patients.[159] There should be no hesitation about performing chest radiology in pregnancy for patients who are suspected of having pulmonary disease. The radiation to the fetus is minimal (about equal to one day's background radiation), and the likelihood of harm to the fetus from missing a diagnosis such as pneumonia is far greater than the likelihood of harm from radiation. Despite traditional teaching to the contrary, studies have shown that radiologists cannot reliably differentiate bacterial from nonbacterial pneumonia on the basis of the x-ray appearance.[160] The role of routine cultures of sputum and blood and/or serologic studies in all individuals with pneumonia before initiation of therapy is controversial because an etiologic agent is found in only about half of cases investigated.[161–163]

In patients who present with high fever, purulent sputum, chest pain, and clinical and radiologic signs of consolidation, the diagnosis is not a problem. But patients who have only modest pyrexia, no sputum, and indeterminate physical and radiologic signs may well have pulmonary infarction rather than infection. They should be treated for both conditions simultaneously (if there is no contraindication to anticoagulation; see Chapter 43) until the diagnosis is best established, usually by radioisotope ventilation-perfusion scans or CT angiography.

TREATMENT

A synthesis for the pregnant patient based on present empiric therapy recommendations of the Infectious Disease Society of America (IDSA),[164] British Thoracic Society (BTS),[165] and the American Thoracic Society (ATS) is reviewed in Table 38–7. Treatment differs with the severity of illness (as reflected by whether the patient is being treated as an inpatient or an outpatient) and reflects the prevalence of drug-resistant pneumococcus. Patients initially treated with intravenous antibiotics can be switched to oral agents once the patient is afebrile. With appropriate antibiotic therapy, some improvement in the clinical course should be seen within 72 hours. Continuation of therapy for a total of 10 to 14 days is recommended for all agents except azithromycin, which can be given for only a 5-day course because of its extended half-life.

These recommendations need a few additional words of caution. First, although reasonable data exists that erythromycin is not a human teratogen, the use of the estolate ester of erythromycin has been associated with a relatively high incidence of subclinical, reversible hepatotoxicity when used during pregnancy[166] and should be avoided in favor of other formulations of this agent. Second, published human data regarding azithromycin safety in pregnancy is surprisingly small despite the widespread use of this agent. It is also considerably more expensive than erythromycin. For these two reasons, this author believes azithromycin

TABLE 38–7

Empiric Antibiotic Regimens for the Treatment of Community-Acquired Pneumonia in Pregnancy[41]

- For uncomplicated pneumonia in patients who do not require hospitalization:

Standard: erythromycin 250 mg qid PO for 10–14 days
Alternate: azithromycin 500 mg PO on day 1 followed by 250 mg daily for 4 days

- For uncomplicated pneumonia in patients requiring hospitalization:

Ceftriaxone 2 g IV once daily with erythromycin 500 mg IV q6h (azithromycin 500 mg IV daily may be used as an alternative to erythromycin if erythromycin is poorly tolerated). Once patient is afebrile and stable, switch to erythromycin 250–500 mg PO qid with cefuroxime axetil 500 mg PO bid for a total antibiotic course of 14 days
If patient has been treated with azithromycin instead of erythromycin, this antibiotic can be administered for a 5-day course only (500 mg the first day and then 250 mg daily for days 2 through 5) because of its long half-life.

Adapted from Powrie RO: Drugs in pregnancy. Respiratory disease. Best Pract Res Clin Obstet Gynaecol 2001;15(6):913–936.

should remain a second-line choice for women unable to tolerate or comply with erythromycin therapy.

Although clarithromycin and levofloxacin are often recommended for the treatment of possible resistant pneumococci in the nonpregnant population, these drugs should be avoided in pregnancy. Clarithromycin appears to be a teratogen in some animals and should only be used in humans in situations where it is the drug of choice. Although fluoroquinolones do not appear to be fetotoxic or teratogenic in animals, their use in pregnancy and pediatrics has been discouraged because of the ability of ciprofloxacin and ofloxacin to cause an irreversible arthropathy in immature experimental animals. Although recently published human data has been reassuring, these agents should still be considered relatively contraindicated in pregnancy at this point.[140,141] Tetracyclines should not be used in pregnancy because of their effects on fetal bones and teeth.

Dosage of antibiotics should be toward the upper range of therapeutic doses in pregnancy[51] because of increased renal clearance. Patients should receive acetaminophen as an antipyretic. Those that are very sick may require assisted ventilation as judged by deteriorating ABG status. Respiratory failure is one of the leading reasons for ICU admission of pregnant patients; pneumonia is responsible for some portion of these cases.[167,168]

The CDC recommends that all nonpregnant women of childbearing age who are not immune to varicella be vaccinated for it. If exposure to varicella occurs in pregnancy in a woman without immunity, varicella zoster immune globulin should be administered within 96 hours in an attempt to prevent maternal infection. Varicella embryopathy may occur as a result of maternal infection, particularly in the first half of pregnancy, with an incidence of 1% to 2%. Varicella of the newborn is a life-threatening illness that may occur when a newborn is delivered within 5 days of the onset of maternal illness or after postdelivery exposure to varicella. Because of the high prevalence and morbidity of pneumonia associated with varicella infection in pregnancy, parenteral acyclovir should be given to all varicella nonimmune patients who develop respiratory symptoms within 10 days of exposure to varicella.[169–173]

CONCLUSIONS

PNEUMONIA

- Pneumonia in the absence of fever, crackles on lung auscultation, and tachypnea is rare.
- Diagnosis is based on clinical presentation and chest x-ray. Chest x-rays are safe and readily justifiable in pregnancy.
- Pneumonia in pregnancy should only be diagnosed after careful consideration of the differential diagnosis of pulmonary embolism, pulmonary edema, and asthma.
- Treatment of community-acquired pneumonia can be done as an outpatient with erythromycin and with ceftriaxone and erythromycin in an inpatient.
- All women who are pregnant or anticipating a pregnancy should be offered influenza vaccine if they will be pregnant during influenza season.
- Varicella exposures in pregnancy in nonimmune individuals require prophylaxis with varicella zoster immune globulin and initiation of acyclovir treatment with the onset of any symptoms.

SUMMARY OF MANAGEMENT OPTIONS
Pneumonia

Management Options	Quality of Evidence	Strength of Recommendation	References
Prepregnancy			
None specifically related to pneumonia; in patients with underlying conditions (e.g., HIV), counsel regarding this possible complication.	–	GPP	–
Administer influenza vaccine during flu season.	IV	C	156
Administer pneumococcal vaccine if high risk conditions or population (e.g., splenectomy).	IV	C	157
Prenatal			
Differentiate from other conditions, especially pulmonary embolus.	IV	C	174
Do not avoid chest x-ray if pulmonary disease suspected.	IV	C	159

Continued

SUMMARY OF MANAGEMENT OPTIONS

Pneumonia *(Continued)*

Management Options	Quality of Evidence	Strength of Recommendation	References
Prenatal			
Use standard techniques for microbiologic assessment, though sputum culture unrewarding in many cases.	IV	C	161,162,163
Begin appropriate antimicrobial therapy based on underlying conditions and presentation; avoid tetracyclines in pregnancy. Avoid fluoroquinolones unless specifically indicated. Continue treatment for 10 to 14 days.	IV	C	164,165
Treat varicella infection in a pregnant woman with acyclovir.	IV	C	175
Provide oxygen therapy if $Sa{O_2}$ values are low.	–	GPP	–
Labor and Delivery			
None specific	–	–	–
Postnatal			
None specific	–	–	–

PULMONARY EDEMA, ACUTE LUNG INJURY, AND ACUTE RESPIRATORY DISTRESS SYNDROME

General

Pregnant women are known to develop pulmonary edema more frequently than nonpregnant women. The incidence of pulmonary edema in pregnancy is estimated to be 80 per 100,000.[174]

Pulmonary edema is due to the movement of excess fluid into the alveoli as a result of alteration in one or more of Starling's forces. Pulmonary edema can be cardiogenic or noncardiogenic. In cardiogenic pulmonary edema, a high pulmonary capillary wedge pressure (PCWP) is responsible for the movement of fluid into the alveoli. This phenomenon is commonly known as *congestive heart failure*. The causes and treatment of cardiogenic pulmonary edema are discussed in Chapter 37. Noncardiogenic pulmonary edema can be caused by a variety of disorders in which factors other than elevated PCWP are responsible for protein and fluid accumulation in the alveoli. For the diagnosis of noncardiogenic pulmonary edema to be made, the PCWP should be <18 mmHg and there should be no evidence of a cardiac cause.[176]

It is not always possible to make the distinction between cardiogenic and noncardiogenic causes, because the clinical syndrome may represent a combination of several different disorders. Determining which is the most important contributor is important, however, because treatment varies considerably depending on the underlying pathophysiologic mechanisms.

The major causes of noncardiogenic pulmonary edema are acute lung injury and the acute respiratory distress syndrome (ARDS). These two entities are defined in Table 38-8. ARDS has an incidence in the general population of 13.5 per 100,000 per year.[177] These entities generally represent diffuse damage to the alveoli, require mechanical ventilation, and run a protracted course associated with a significant mortality. Precipitants of acute lung injury/ARDS include sepsis, aspiration, pneumonia, severe trauma and burns, massive blood transfusion, sudden relief of upper airway obstruction, lung and bone marrow transplants, medications (especially aspirin, cocaine, narcotics, and nitrofurantoin), leukoagglutination reactions in the lungs after a blood transfusion, venous

TABLE 38–8

Diagnostic Criteria for Acute Lung Injury and Acute Respiratory Distress Syndrome[181]

1) Acute onset
2) Bilateral chest radiographic infiltrates
3) A pulmonary artery occlusion pressure of <18 mmHg or no evidence of left atrial hypertension
4) Impaired oxygenation manifested by a $Pa{O_2}/Fi{O_2}$ of <300 mmHg (<40 kPa) for acute lung injury and <200 mmHg (<27 kPa) for ARDS

Adapted and updated from material used with permission from Powrie RO: Acute lung injury. In Lee RV, Rosene-Montella K, Barbour LA, et al. (eds): Medical Care of the Pregnant Patient. Philadelphia, American College of Physicians, 2000, pp. 397–411.

air embolism with central venous catheter insertion, and neurocardiogenic (associated with a intracerebral bleed or seizure).[176,178]

Although many of the cases of noncardiogenic pulmonary edema seen in pregnancy will meet the strict diagnostic criteria set for acute lung injury/ARDS, the majority of the pregnancy-related cases will not run the protracted course typically seen with true ARDS. In fact, the majority of pregnancy related cases will improve rapidly with treatment and/or removal of the inciting factor and will not require mechanical ventilation. Experts suggest that such cases might better be termed *permeability pulmonary edema* rather than acute lung injury/ARDS. However, although the course of pregnancy-associated permeability pulmonary edema and ARDS may be different, the initial clinical presentations are often indistinguishable and the causes remain the same.[168,175,180–184]

Physiologic Changes in Pregnancy That Predispose Pregnant Women to Pulmonary Edema

The unique predisposition that pregnant women have to permeability pulmonary edema is attributable to a number of normal physiologic changes that occur in pregnancy. These changes can be viewed as "contributing" factors that increase the likelihood that a pregnant woman with a particular insult or condition will go into pulmonary edema, but do not, in and of themselves, cause pulmonary edema. These changes are summarized in Table 38–9 and discussed in the following.

Pregnancy-Associated Drop in Plasma Colloid Osmotic Pressure

Pregnancy is associated with a significant expansion of blood volume that occurs predominantly through an increase in plasma free water. This increase in plasma free water leads to a progressive decrease in the concentration of plasma proteins manifested by the dropping serum albumin seen with advancing gestation. Plasma protein concentration is the main determinant of plasma colloid osmotic pressure (PCOP), one of the forces that in Starling's law limits net filtration across the capillary wall, so its decrease may partly explain the increased propensity in pregnant women for fluid to move out of the intravascular spaces and into the interstitium.

TABLE 38–9

Normal Physiologic Changes of Pregnancy That Predispose to and May Exacerbate Pulmonary Edema

20% decrease in colloid osmotic pressure
50% increase in blood volume and cardiac output
Decreased FRC in pregnancy means end-expiratory volumes closer to critical closing volumes

Adapted and updated from material used with permission from Powrie RO: Acute lung injury. In Lee RV, Rosene-Montella K, Barbour LA, et al. (eds): Medical Care of the Pregnant Patient. Philadelphia, American College of Physicians, 2000, pp. 397–411.

The pregnancy-associated decrease in PCOP seen throughout gestation has been shown to drop further in the puerperium. The mechanism for this further decrease is multifactorial but normal peripartum blood loss, "autotransfusion" of blood into the circulation with each uterine contraction, and the sudden increase in preload that occurs when the gravid uterus' compression of the inferior vena cava is released all contribute to it. Preeclampsia is also associated with an additional drop in PCOP, which partially explains the increased risk of pulmonary edema seen with this entity.[185-192]

Pregnancy-Associated Increase in Blood Volume and Cardiac Output

The normal pregnancy is characterized by a progressive increase in blood volume and cardiac output (CO), which reaches a maximum at 26 to 32 weeks' gestation. Fever, pain, preeclampsia, and multiple gestations can further increase cardiac work and lead to a rise in pulmonary artery occlusion pressure (PCOP) that, although within the "normal" (<18 mmHg) range, can, in the setting of low PCOP and/or endothelial damage, lead to pulmonary edema.

Pregnancy-Associated Decrease in Functional Residual Capacity

Third, increased minute ventilation and elevation of the diaphragm by the gravid uterus decreases the FRC in pregnant women by around 18% as compared with nonpregnant individuals. Therefore, at end-expiration the pregnant woman is closer to her *critical closing volume* (the volume at which alveoli collapse upon themselves) than the nonpregnant woman. Some investigators believe that this decreased FRC increases the ease with which small airways and alveoli collapse when small amounts of pulmonary edema are present and may thereby contribute to a progressive worsening of oxygenation when intra-alveolar fluid is present.

Precipitating Causes of Pulmonary Edema

Despite the predisposition of the pregnant women to develop pulmonary edema due to low colloid osmotic pressure and increased cardiac work, the occurrence of pulmonary edema still requires an inciting agent or event to "tip the balance" and allow fluid to move into the interstitial spaces of the lung. All of the conditions described as causes of ARDS can cause pulmonary edema in pregnant women. Table 38–10 lists those causes of pulmonary edema most likely to be seen in pregnancy. The most common precipitants seen in pregnancy are reviewed in more detail in the text that follows. Some of these inciting agents or events have clear, causative relationships, but for others the link is not

TABLE 38–10

Some Causes of Noncardiogenic Pulmonary Edema in Pregnancy

Pulmonary edema more likely in the setting of multiple gestation, anemia, and fluid overload

- Tocolytic therapy
- Preeclampsia/eclampsia
- Sepsis
  - Especially pyelonephritis, chorioamnionitis, endometritis, septic abortion, and appendicitis
- Aspiration (Mendelson's syndrome)
- Severe hemorrhage, especially related to systemic inflammatory response, low PCOP, and rarely leukoagglutination in the lung
- Amniotic fluid embolism
- Venous air embolism
- Cocaine and high-dose opiates in susceptible patients
- Neurogenic pulmonary edema after eclamptic seizure

Adapted and updated from material used with permission from Powrie RO: Acute lung injury. In Lee RV, Rosene-Montella K, Barbour LA, et al. (eds): Medical Care of the Pregnant Patient. Philadelphia, American College of Physicians, 2000, pp. 397–411.

readily apparent. Some are unique to pregnancy; others are common to both the pregnant and nonpregnant populations. In all cases, it would appear that the presence of anemia and/or multifetal gestations further increases the risk that a particular inciting event will lead to pulmonary edema. In addition, the routine administration of generous amounts of crystalloid fluids to provide hydration during labor may have ill effect, because those patients with some other predisposition toward pulmonary edema may not be able to compensate for this excess volume.

Tocolysis

A relatively common cause of permeability pulmonary edema is the use of β-adrenergic agonists (such as terbutaline) and magnesium for tocolysis. Although β-adrenergic agonists have been used extensively in the treatment of asthma in nonpregnant patients without this complication, there is a clear association in the obstetric literature between these agents and pulmonary edema, the etiology of which remains unclear. Possible contributing factors include a primary cardiogenic component related to barometric-induced myocardial fatigue or altered capillary permeability. Fluids routinely given in association with tocolysis may be responsible for some cases; the β-adrenergic agonists themselves can cause further decreases in PCWP beyond the normal physiologic drop seen in pregnancy. The altered physiology of normal pregnancy must contribute to the effects of β-adrenergic agonists because this complication is not seen in nonpregnant individuals who receive β-adrenergic agonists for other indications.[193–200]

Preeclampsia

Preeclampsia is an important cause of pulmonary edema in pregnancy. Three percent of patients with preeclampsia will develop pulmonary edema during the course of their illness. Thirty percent of pulmonary edema associated with preeclampsia will occur antepartum and 70% will occur postpartum, usually within the first 72 hours after delivery. Maternal mortality from pulmonary edema may be as high as 10%; perinatal mortality may be as high as 50% in the presence of pulmonary edema associated with preeclampsia. This alarmingly high fetal mortality rate may be related to placental abruptions and therefore may be more reflective of the severity of the preeclampsia than the presence of the pulmonary edema itself.

Preeclampsia is believed to cause pulmonary edema by a variety of mechanisms. In some cases, the pulmonary edema is attributable to the additional drop in PCOP that occurs in pregnancy-induced hypertension (PIH) and is in excess of the normal PCOP drop in pregnancy. This additional decrease in PCOP may be enough in some cases to allow fluid to move into the interstitial spaces of the lungs. In other cases, there is evidence that the endothelial damage characteristic of severe PIH may disrupt the normal endothelial barrier in the lungs, as occurs with early sepsis or leaky capillary syndromes, thereby allowing the escape of fluid into the alveoli and interstitium. In some cases, a stiff left ventricle from chronic hypertension with significant diastolic dysfunction may be an important factor contributing to pulmonary edema in women with preeclampsia who have a sudden and dramatic increase in afterload due to the intense vasospasm and increased systemic vascular resistance. Last, a significant number of cases of pulmonary edema occurring in the setting of preeclampsia can be attributable to left ventricular systolic dysfunction. The occurrence of left ventricular dysfunction in preeclampsia has been well described but is poorly understood. Presumably the intense vasospasm and endothelial damage that characterizes preeclampsia have a significant impact on myocardial oxygen supply and thereby myocardial contractility.[201–206]

Sepsis

Sepsis is also a very important cause of pulmonary edema in pregnancy. Pneumonia can progress to acute lung injury and ARDS and is an important cause of prolonged mechanical ventilation in pregnant women (see Pneumonia). However, it would appear that any systemic bacterial infection can lead to pulmonary edema in pregnant women. This increased incidence of sepsis-related pulmonary edema in pregnancy seems to be related to a combination of decreased PCOP, altered capillary permeability, and increased sensitivity of pregnant women to endotoxins. The most well-described example of this is the occurrence of pulmonary edema in as many as 10% of cases of pyelonephritis during pregnancy. The greatly increased incidence of pyelonephritis in pregnancy makes this infection a particularly important cause of pulmonary edema and argues against routine outpatient management of pyelonephritis in pregnancy.[207-211]

Aspiration Syndromes: Mendelson's Syndrome and Bacterial Aspiration Pneumonia

Aspiration syndromes are seen in pregnancy because of the delayed gastric emptying and decreased lower esophageal sphincter pressure seen in all pregnant women. In the setting of altered mental status from drugs, anesthesia, or seizures, stomach contents can be aspirated and lead to Mendelson's syndrome and/or bacterial aspiration pneumonia.

Mendelson's syndrome usually occurs in association with a difficult intubation or during the postanesthesia period when the gag reflex may be depressed, but it may also occur de novo in pregnant women. Gastric juice is aspirated into the lungs and leads to intense pulmonary inflammation that can proceed with rapidity to a full acute lung injury/ARDS picture over 8 to 24 hours. The patient becomes tachypneic, hypoxic, and febrile. Chest x-ray changes classically show a complete "white out." Despite this rapid and marked deterioration, this syndrome generally resolves without antibiotics within 48 to 72 hours unless bacterial superinfection intervenes.[212] Modern anesthetic management has thankfully made this a far less common event than it was in the past.

Bacterial aspiration pneumonia usually has a more insidious onset than Mendelson's syndrome, with clinical manifestations presenting 48 to 72 hours after aspiration with persistent fever, sputum, and leukocytosis. Classically chest x-ray findings are localized to the basilar segments if the patient aspirated while upright and to the posterior segment of the upper lobe or the superior segment of the lower lobe if the patient aspirated while supine. The bacterial infection is generally polymicrobial, with mouth anaerobes predominating, so treatment with penicillin or clindamycin is advisable.

Massive Hemorrhage

Massive red cell transfusion for antepartum or postpartum hemorrhages can result in pulmonary edema. The mechanism for this is often multifactorial and can include volume overload, decrease in PCOP from replacement of whole blood loss with packed red cells and crystalloids, endothelial damage from a systemic inflammatory response to the massive hemorrhage, and, rarely, leukoagglutination in the lung.

Amniotic Fluid Embolism (Anaphylactoid Lung of Pregnancy)

Amniotic fluid embolism is a rare but catastrophic complication of pregnancy that may present as pulmonary edema but often proceeds to full ARDS. Its incidence is variably quoted as being between 1 in 8000 and 1 in 80,000 pregnancies. Prolonged labor, multiparity, increased maternal age, meconium staining of the amniotic fluid, and use of forceps are risk factors for this catastrophic complication. It almost always occurs at the time of delivery but has been reported to occur antepartum. It has a mortality rate that has been recently estimated to be between 26% and 60%[213] and is responsible for 10% of maternal deaths in the United States.[214-217] Amniotic fluid embolism usually presents with a sudden onset of agitation and dyspnea that is followed by symptomatic hypotension, hypoxia, and disseminated intravascular coagulation (DIC) resulting in massive obstetric hemorrhage. Seizures can also be seen with acute amniotic fluid embolism. The diagnosis is difficult to establish with certainty but should be considered in any woman near term (and especially in labor) who presents with sudden cardiorespiratory failure. Although the entry of amniotic fluid into the maternal circulation through the endocervical veins or uterine tears is an important prerequisite of the amniotic fluid embolism syndrome, it would appear from animal studies that it is not enough in itself to cause the catastrophic reaction seen in patients with this diagnosis. For this reason, some researchers would prefer that the diagnosis *anaphylactoid lung of pregnancy* be used to describe the syndrome of amniotic fluid embolism, thereby emphasizing the importance of the maternal immunologic response in this syndrome.

Presentation of Pulmonary Edema in Pregnancy

Clinical Features

The symptoms and signs of pulmonary edema in pregnancy are very similar to those seen in the general medical population. Early signs and symptoms of pulmonary edema may be few and mild; therefore, it can be difficult to distinguish pulmonary edema from other causes of cardiopulmonary complaints seen in pregnancy. One of the most common mistakes is a delay in diagnosis when the mild symptoms of pulmonary edema in pregnancy are attributed to less serious and more common causes of dyspnea such as respiratory tract infections, asthma, or dyspnea of pregnancy. This may be because the absence of comorbid conditions in the majority of pregnant women makes patients "look" better and maintain respiratory and cardiovascular stability longer than the typical medical patient with pulmonary edema.

Tachypnea is an important clinical sign that a woman's complaints are more than just the normal increased shortness of breath on exertion seen in pregnancy. The chest may initially be clear to auscultation early in the course of evolving pulmonary edema, especially in the otherwise well pregnant woman. The patient will often display some degree of anxiety related to mild dyspnea or hypoxia. Eventually, as the condition progresses and alveoli fill with fluid, diffuse crackles, wheezing, and cough will be present. Tachycardia is common, but heart rate should be interpreted with the knowledge that a resting pulse of 100 beats/minute is not unusual in normal pregnancies.

Arterial Blood Gas, Chest X-Ray, and Electrocardiogram Findings

Arterial blood gases in patients with pulmonary edema typically initially show a decrease in both $Pa{O_2}$ and $Pa{CO_2}$. As the condition worsens, $Pa{O_2}$ will decrease further, but $Pa{CO_2}$ will increase as the patient is no longer able to maintain adequate ventilation and respiratory failure ensues. (It is worth emphasizing again that a $Pa{O_2}$ of 70 mmHg or a $Pa{CO_2}$ of 40 mmHg in a pregnant woman is very abnormal and highly suggestive of ventilatory failure.)

The chest x-ray in pulmonary edema may initially be normal. Subsequently, pulmonic infiltrates, and in some cases pleural effusions, will become manifest. Although classically pulmonary edema is associated with diffuse chest x-ray changes, in some cases of pulmonary edema the damage may be patchy or unilateral, particularly if a patient has spent prolonged periods in the left lateral decubitus position. The radiation exposure necessary to obtain a proper chest film is well below the recommended maximal levels of radiation for pregnancy; therefore, an indicated chest x-ray should never be withheld due to concerns about fetal effects.

Additional tests that should be routinely obtained in the setting of suspected pulmonary edema are CBC, creatinine, and BUN, because anemia and renal failure may be contributing factors. "Preeclampsia labs" (aspartate aminotransferase, uric acid, and urinalysis in addition to CBC and creatinine) should also be obtained.

Treatment of Pulmonary Edema in Pregnancy

Pulmonary edema in pregnancy is a medical emergency. Irrespective of the etiology, the immediate goal is to maintain adequate maternal oxygenation ($Pa{O_2} \geq 70$ mm Hg) to avoid hypoxia in the fetus.[218–220] Therefore, it is recommended that maternal $Sa{O_2}$ be kept >95%. The second goal is to treat the underlying causes of the edema. Third, relief of symptoms leading to improved patient comfort must be instituted.

Careful monitoring of fluid balance should be initiated. Intravenous morphine sulfate is safe when used cautiously to reduce maternal anxiety and decrease pulmonary congestion. Clear, reassuring communication with both the patient and her support person is also important in decreasing maternal distress. Lastly, although the majority of patients with pulmonary edema in pregnancy will not be volume overloaded, diuresis to try to achieve the lowest possible PCWP that will still support normal blood pressure is advisable. Data from the treatment of ARDS in nonpregnant patients tell us that decreasing the PAWP by 25% with diuretics and fluid restriction can improve pulmonary function and perhaps outcome.[221–223] It is our experience that many of the patients with pulmonary edema in pregnancy who do not have cardiac or renal disease will still respond dramatically to intravenous doses of furosemide as low as 10 mg. Using the lowest possible dose of diuretics has an additional importance in the setting of preeclampsia in which patients are relatively volume contracted despite having massive amounts of peripheral edema and pulmonary edema. Overdiuresis in these patients can lead to intravascular hypovolemia that can impair placental perfusion and lead to fetal distress.

Differential Diagnosis of Pulmonary Edema in Pregnancy

Other causes of respiratory failure in pregnancy that should be routinely considered as part of the differential diagnosis of pulmonary edema are listed in Table 38–11. Differentiating the diagnosis of noncardiogenic pulmonary edema from cases of peripartum cardiomyopathy, ischemic heart disease, or occult valvular heart disease should begin with a careful history, cardiac examination, and electrocardiogram. When any doubt exists however, an echocardiogram is indicated to discern whether the pulmonary edema is actually congestive heart failure. A prospective study of 45 pregnant pulmonary edema patients found that echocardiography identified an unsuspected cardiac abnormality in 47% of cases and should probably be considered routine for these patients.[203] If pulmonary edema is persistent and severe without a clear precipitant and there appears to be no cardiac cause, a bronchoscopic alveolar lavage or lung biopsy can be necessary in cases of full ARDS.

A drug screen should be done for cocaine and heroin in most patients, although the vast majority of patients with cocaine-associated pulmonary edema will be notable for their severe hypertension.

Likewise, consideration of the possibility of acute infectious pneumonia should also occur. Features suggestive of pneumonia include the presence of a prodrome, fever, purulent sputum, chills, rigors, and pulmonary edema; consideration of use of empiric antibiotics pending cultures is often advisable in the initial 48 hours.

A careful drug history should be obtained because drug-induced pneumonitis is a rare but reversible cause of

TABLE 38–11

Causes of Respiratory Failure in Pregnancy to Be Considered in the Differential Diagnoses of Pulmonary Edema[41]

Cardiac disease	Peripartum cardiomyopathy Ischemic heart disease Valvular heart disease
Pneumonia	*Streptococcus*, *Haemophilus*, *Klebsiella*, *Staphylococcus*, bacterial aspiration pneumonia, *Mycoplasma*, *Legionella*, influenza A, varicella, measles
Drug-related pneumonitis	Nitrofurantoin, commonly used as urinary tract infection prophylaxis in pregnancy, can cause an acute pulmonary reaction

Adapted and updated from material used with permission from Powrie RO: Acute lung injury. In Lee RV, Rosene-Montella K, Barbour LA, et al. (eds): Medical Care of the Pregnant Patient. Philadelphia, American College of Physicians, 2000, pp. 397–411.

respiratory failure and has been reported to occur with the antibiotic nitrofurantoin, commonly used as a prophylactic agent for urinary tract infections during pregnancy.

Remove or Treat the Underlying Cause

TOCOLYTIC-RELATED PULMONARY EDEMA

Most important to the management of pulmonary edema in pregnancy is to treat the underlying cause. If the underlying cause is tocolytic agents, the tocolytic agents should be removed. This can be a difficult decision to make if the patient is in labor at a very early gestation. However, this decision can be made more comfortably when one recognizes that (1) fetal well-being is dependent on maternal well-being; and (2) tocolytics are of limited proven efficacy for prolongation of gestation beyond 48 hours.

PREECLAMPSIA-RELATED PULMONARY EDEMA

If the etiology is related to preeclampsia, delivery is the treatment of choice. Even in the absence of typical feature of preeclampsia, consideration of preeclampsia as a possible etiology of pulmonary edema is required. Blood pressure should be brought down below 160/100 in the setting of preeclampsia-associated pulmonary edema because a decrease in afterload may help decrease pulmonary edema. The intravenous infusion of magnesium sulfate (used for seizure prophylaxis in the setting of preeclampsia) requires high doses of fluids; this medication should be administered in the smallest volume considered safe with close following of total fluid balance.

INFECTION-RELATED PULMONARY EDEMA

Sepsis-related pulmonary edema is indicated by the presence of fever and should be treated with broad-spectrum antibiotics. As is the case for suspected pneumonia, it is generally advisable to initiate empiric antibiotic coverage pending cultures. Any abdominal pain and tenderness should prompt consideration of the possible diagnoses of appendicitis and chorioamnionitis/endometritis. Pyelonephritis should be considered in any cases of pulmonary edema associated with fever and a urinalysis and urine culture obtained.

AMNIOTIC FLUID EMBOLISM/ANAPHYLACTOID SYNDROME

Amniotic fluid embolism has no specific treatment other than supportive management. There is no pathognomonic finding or diagnostic test to prove this diagnosis, but there are few conditions present so suddenly with such severe manifestations aside from acute pulmonary embolism. Tests for DIC must be carried out when this diagnosis is considered. Treatment is supportive and should begin with aggressive volume administration to maintain blood pressure but will almost always require intubation, mechanical ventilation, and vasopressor support. Hemorrhage should be treated with fresh frozen plasma and cryoprecipitate as needed.

Endotracheal Intubation

If oxygenation cannot be maintained above a PaO_2 of 70 mmHg or the patient shows evidence of "tiring out" (either by subjective evidence based on the findings of accessory muscle use, intercostal indrawing, and abdominal breathing or on the basis of a rising $PaCO_2$), a trial of spontaneous breathing with supplemental oxygen and positive end-expiratory pressure (PEEP) administered through a tight-fitting mask should be attempted. Noninvasive nasal intermittent positive-pressure ventilation (NIPPV) may also be used, but concerns about its use in the setting of pregnancy-associated upper airway edema and the propensity of pregnant women to aspiration pneumonia may limit its use in critical care obstetrics.

Intubation is generally required if the patient is unresponsive to therapy and has signs of respiratory failure (PaO_2 <70 mmHg or $PaCO_2$ >45 mmHg on 100% oxygen administered through a tight-fitting mask and a nonrebreathing mask). In borderline cases it is worth remembering that it is always preferable to intubate a patient electively rather than delay intubation until it is required emergently. This is particularly true of pregnant women for several reasons. First, the upper airway in pregnant women is often difficult to visualize because of soft tissue swelling related to physiologic hyperemia of mucosal tissues during gestation. Second, pregnant women are at high risk for aspiration because of lower gastroesophageal sphincter tone and delayed gastric emptying, also a normal physiologic occurrence in pregnancy. Third, because pregnant women have decreased FRC, there is less available oxygen in their lungs to maintain PaO_2 between periods of "bagging." Preoxygenation with 100% oxygen should therefore always be done prior to and between any attempts to intubate a pregnant woman. Last, there is reason to believe that the fetus tolerates maternal hypoxia poorly and that a prolonged period off the manual inflation bag and supplemental oxygen necessary for intubation may harm the fetus. It is therefore paramount that intubation of the pregnant woman always be performed by the most experienced individual available and that every effort is made to ensure that all equipment is readily available and functioning properly before beginning an attempt at intubation (see Table 38–12). The rate of failed elective intubation attempts in pregnant patients is eight times greater than that seen in general surgical patients.

Mechanical Ventilation

Mechanical ventilation for the pregnant woman with pulmonary edema should be done in the same manner as for the nonpregnant patient. A reasonable method to start with would be volume-cycled ventilation in the assist control mode with PEEP added in increments of 3 to 5 cm H_2O to improve arterial oxygenation. Tidal volumes should be set at 10 to 12 mL/kg. Patients with decreased lung compliance may need lower volumes (6 to 8 mL/kg) to minimize peak airway pressures. The fraction of

TABLE 38-12

Equipment and Medications Necessary for the Intubation of a Pregnant Woman[41]

Continuous ECG monitoring
Blood pressure monitor on patient's arm
Pulse oximeter
High-flow oxygen source
Large-bore intravenous access secured in place
Intubation to be performed by most experienced individual available, with assistant at his/her side; the incidence of failed intubation in pregnancy is 1 in 200 to 1 in 300 cases, almost 10 times as high as for nonpregnant patients[226,227]
Mask (that fits patient securely) and manual bag-valve inflation device
Oropharyngeal suction equipment
Endotracheal tubes (with tested inflatable cuff) for oral intubation (rather than nasal intubation) with smaller endotracheal tube (6–6.5) than would be used with similar nonpregnant patient preferable due to upper airway narrowing in pregnancy[228]
Laryngoscope with light
Stylet
Medications for sedation and (if necessary) paralysis of patient, usually thiopental 3–5 mg/kg IV for sedation, and succinylcholine 1–1.5 mg/kg, up to 150 mg IV, for paralysis
Etomidate 0.3 mg/kg IV over 60 seconds may be needed in certain circumstances for muscle relaxation
Method readily available to assess that endotracheal placement is not esophageal (listener with stethoscope or CO_2 detector*)
Self-inflating bulbs or syringes have been found to be unreliable in pregnant women
Chest x-ray to be done shortly after intubation to ensure endotracheal tube is properly placed 4–7 cm above the carina
Gloves, mask, goggles, and gown available to intubater
Plan in place for next step if intubation attempt fails. Use of the laryngeal mask has been described in pregnancy and should be available in this circumstance.[229]

Adapted and updated from material used with permission from Powrie RO: Acute lung injury. In Lee RV, Rosene-Montella K, Barbour LA, et al. (eds): Medical Care of the Pregnant Patient. Philadelphia, American College of Physicians, 2000, pp. 397–411.

inspired oxygen (FIO_2) should be kept less than 60% if possible. There is little reason to use PEEP at greater than 15 to 20 cm H_2O. $PaCO_2$ should ideally be kept at 28 to 32 mmHg to mimic the physiologic changes in respiratory function seen in the normal pregnancy. Respiratory alkalosis from overventilation should be avoided, however, because alkalemia can have adverse effect on uterine blood flow. Some advocates in critical care suggest use of smaller tidal volumes (<6 mL/kg), pressure-limited ventilation (rather than volume cycled), PEEP at levels of 17 cm H_2O, and "permissive hypercapnia" for patients with ARDS, but the experience with such an approach among pregnant women is limited and there are theoretical reasons to believe that the fetus may not tolerate the acidosis necessary to this approach. Inverse-ratio ventilation has also been used in pregnant women. Clinicians should be aware that the degree of sedation or paralysis necessary for this mode of ventilation will make fetal testing uninterpretable.

Positive-pressure ventilation in pregnancy-associated pulmonary edema often results in a marked and rapid improvement in these patients, because the positive pressure helps to move fluid out of the interstitium. If a patient requires intubation it is important to correct the underlying cause before extubation because patients prematurely extubated may simply slip back into pulmonary edema once they are no longer under the therapeutic effects of positive-pressure ventilation.

Role of Pulmonary Artery Occlusion Pressure Monitoring in Pulmonary Edema/ARDS in Pregnancy

In the majority of cases of pulmonary edema in pregnancy, central hemodynamic monitoring will not be necessary for diagnostic purposes. In the absence of preeclampsia, and in the absence of history, physical examination, or ECG findings suggestive of cardiac disease, it can generally be assumed that the PCWP is unlikely to be >18 mmHg in a young pregnant woman. Preeclampsia is an exception because severe preeclampsia may be associated with either diastolic or systolic dysfunction. In cases where cardiac dysfunction is suspected, a bedside echocardiogram can be extremely useful in deciding if PCWP monitoring may be helpful.

In the absence of prompt clinical response to oxygen, diuresis, and morphine, invasive hemodynamic monitoring may be indicated to aid management. The goal of invasive monitoring in pulmonary edema in pregnancy is to reduce the PCWP and improve and optimize left ventricular performance. In general, however, it must be remembered that a PCWP that is normal for a nonpregnant patient may represent too high a level in the setting of preeclampsia or during the postpartum period. Since the most important factor is not the absolute number of the PCWP but the relationship of PCWP to the colloid osmotic pressure, therapeutic decisions may be difficult in some circumstances. If colloid osmotic pressure is very low, as it is in PIH and in the postpartum period, then a "normal" PCWP can still be associated with significant pulmonary edema. In general, trends in the PCWP may be more useful to follow than absolute numbers. However, it has been the experience of our group that in the absence of cardiac disease or sepsis, hemodynamic monitoring in the setting of pulmonary edema in pregnancy is not generally necessary.[228–242]

Use of Vasoactive and Inotropic Medications

Use of vasoactive substances to help maintain cardiac output at a lower PCWP may be helpful in some cases of pulmonary edema in pregnancy where cardiac dysfunction is present. In the setting of critical illness it is important not to withhold any potentially beneficial treatment from a pregnant woman because of concerns about possible fetal effects. However, the paucity of human data on the effects of most of these medications on placental blood flow should caution against their use to fine-tune maternal hemodynamic parameters.[242]

CONCLUSIONS

PULMONARY EDEMA, ACUTE LUNG INJURY, AND ACUTE RESPIRATORY DISTRESS SYNDROME

- Pregnancy predisposes women to pulmonary edema, particularly in the setting of tocolysis, sepsis, and preeclampsia.
- Pulmonary edema in pregnancy often responds to treatment or removal of the inciting agent, fluid restriction, and a small dose of intravenous diuretic.
- Endotracheal intubation in pregnancy is more difficult and should be done by an experienced anesthesiologist with the proper equipment readily available whenever possible.

SUMMARY OF MANAGEMENT OPTIONS

Pulmonary Edema, Acute Lung Injury, and Acute Respiratory Distress Syndrome

Management Options	Quality of Evidence	Strength of Recommendation	References
General care: communicate with patient and family, relieve anxiety, administer analgesia if appropriate.	–	GPP	–
High or intensive care setting; place patient at 45-degree angle if possible.	–	GPP	–
Provide supplemental oxygen to maintain PaO_2 >65 mmHg and SaO_2 >95%.	III	B	218, 219, 220
If patient is maintaining blood pressure and placental perfusion is not in question, consider administration of intravenous furosemide (at a dose of 10 mg if patient has not received furosemide in past).	IV	C	221, 222, 223
Consider possibility of primary pneumonia by questioning patient regarding presence of a prodromal illness, fever, chills, rigors, sputum, and by reviewing chest x-ray for focal pulmonary findings more suggestive of pneumonia. Treat empirically if significant suspicion of pneumonia entertained.	IV	C	207
Consider possibility of cardiogenic causes (ischemic heart disease, peripartum cardiomyopathy, and valvular heart disease) by careful review of history, cardiac exam, and ECG. Obtain echocardiogram in most cases to rule out cardiogenic causes.	III	B	175
Monitor fluid balance and avoid fluid overload; minimize intravenous fluids.	III	B	223
Remove or treat underlying causes of pulmonary edema in pregnancy:	–	GPP	–
• Discontinue tocolytics.			
• Evaluate for presence of preeclampsia and begin active efforts toward delivery of fetus if patient has preeclampsia.			
• Evaluate for presence of infection (especially pyelonephritis) and treat if present.			
• Protect airway if aspiration is suspected.			
• Check INR, aPTT, and CBC if amniotic fluid embolism suspected.			
If oxygenation cannot be maintained, consider use of nasal intermittent positive-pressure ventilation or semielective intubation.	IV	C	241, 242
Consider placement of central hemodynamic monitoring line if:	IV	C	228–233
• cardiac cause suspected and patient unresponsive to diuretics			
• poor urine output despite diuretic administration			
• hypotension present.			
Consider use of inotropic and vasoactive agents to maximize cardiac output in the minority of cases. Therapy should be guided in this setting by central hemodynamic monitoring.	IV	C	241, 242

REFERENCES

1. Cugell DW, Frank NR, Gaensler EA, Badger TL: Pulmonary function in pregnancy. I. Serial observations in normal women. Am Rev Tuberc 1953;67:568.
2. Prowse CM, Gaensler EA: Respiratory and acid-base changes during pregnancy. Anesthesiol 1965;26:381.
3. Weinberger SE, Weiss ST: Pulmonary diseases. In Burrow GN, Ferris TF (eds): Medical Complications During Pregnancy, 4th ed. Philadelphia, Saunders, 1995.
4. Simon PM, Schwartzstein RM, Weiss JW, et al: Distinguishable types of dyspnea in patients with shortness of breath. Am Rev Respir Dis 1990;142:1009.
5. Hytten FE, Leitch I: Respiration. In The Physiology of Human Pregnancy. Oxford, Blackwell Scientific Publications, 1971.
6. Weinberger S: Dyspnea during pregnancy. In Rose BD (ed): UpToDate. Wellesley, Mass, UpToDate, 2003.
7. Ponto JA: Fetal dosimetry from pulmonary imaging in pregnancy: Revised estimates. Clin Nucl Med 1986;11:108.
8. Tan KS, Thomson NC: Asthma in pregnancy. Am J Med 2000;109:727.
9. Gei AF, Hankins GD: Cardiac disease and pregnancy. Obstet Gynecol Clin North Am 2001;28:465–512.
10. Goldhaber SZ: Pulmonary embolism. N Engl J Med 1998;339:93.
11. Alexander S, Dodds L, Armson BA: Perinatal outcomes in women with asthma during pregnancy. Obstet Gynecol 1998;92:435–440.
12. Gluck JC, Gluck P: The effects of pregnancy on asthma: A prospective study. Ann Allergy 1976;37:164.
13. Williams DA: Asthma and pregnancy. Acta Allergol 1967;22:311.
14. Schatz M, Hoffman C: Interrelationships between asthma and pregnancy: Clinical and mechanistic considerations. Clin Rev Allergy 1987;5:301.
15. Weinberger S: Pregnancy in patients with asthma. In Rose BD (ed): UpToDate, Wellesley, Mass, 2003.
16. National Asthma Education Program: Report of the Working Group on Asthma and Pregnancy. Management of Asthma During Pregnancy (NIH publication no. 933279A), Bethesda, Md, National Institutes of Health, 1993.
17. Doucette JT, Bracken MB: Possible role of asthma in the risk of preterm labor and delivery. Epidemiol 1993;2:143–150.
18. Perlow JH, Montgomery D, Morgan MA, et al: Severity of asthma and perinatal outcome. Am J Obstet Gynecol 1992;167: 963–967.
19. Lehrer S, Stone J, Lapinski R, et al: Association between pregnancy-induced hypertension and asthma during pregnancy. Am J Obstet Gynecol 1993;168:1463–1466.
20. Schatz M, Zeiger RS, Hoffman CP, et al: Perinatal outcomes in the pregnancies of asthmatic women: A prospective controlled analysis. Am J Respir Crit Care Med 1995;151:1170–1174.
21. Gordon M, Niswander KR, Berendes H, Kantor AG: Fetal morbidity following potentially anoxigenic obstetric conditions. VII. Bronchial asthma. Am J Obstet Gynecol 1970;106:421–429.
22. Bahna SL, Bjerkedal T: The course and outcome of pregnancy in women with bronchial asthma. Acta Allergol 1972;27:397.
23. Schatz M, Zeiger RS, Hoffman CP: Intrauterine growth is related to gestational pulmonary function in pregnant asthmatic women. KaiserPermanente Asthma and Pregnancy Study Group. Chest 1990;98:389.
24. Minerbi-Codish I, Fraser D, Avnun L, et al: Influence of asthma in pregnancy on labor and the newborn. Respiration 1998;65:130.
25. Demissie K, Breckenridge MB, Rhoads CG: Infant and maternal outcomes in the pregnancies of asthmatic women. Am J Respir Crit Care Med 1998;158:1091–1095.
26. Liu S, Wen SW, Demissie K, et al: Maternal asthma and pregnancy outcomes: A retrospective cohort study. Am J Obstet Gynecol 2001;184:90.
27. Schatz M: Asthma and pregnancy. Lancet 1999;353:1202.
28. Landau R, Xie HG, Dishy V, Stein CM: β2-Adrenergic receptor genotype and preterm delivery. Am J Obstet Gynecol 2002; 187:1294.
29. Sibbald B: A Family Study Approach to the Genetic Basis of Asthma.[PhD thesis]. University of London, 1981.
30. Clark SL: Asthma in pregnancy. National Asthma Education Program Working Group on Asthma and Pregnancy. National Institutes of Health, National Heart, Lung and Blood Institute. Obstet Gynecol 1993;82:1036–1040.
31. Schatz M, Patterson R, Zeitz S: Corticosteroid therapy for the pregnant asthmatic patient. JAMA 1975;233:804–807.
32. National Asthma Education and Prevention Program: Expert Panel Report 2. Guidelines for the Diagnosis and Management of Asthma. (NIH Publication NO. 97-4051). Bethesda, Md, National Institutes of Health. National Heart, Lung, and Blood Institute, 1997.
33. Luskin AT: An overview of the recommendations of the Working Group on Asthma and Pregnancy. National Asthma Education and Prevention Program. J Allerg Clin Immunol 1999;103: S350–S353.
34. Schatz M, Zeigler RS: Asthma and allergy in pregnancy. Clin Perinatol 1997;350(suppl II):10–13.
35. Dombrowski MP: Pharmacologic therapy of asthma during pregnancy. Obstet Gynecol Clin North Am 1997;24:559–574.
36. ACOG and ACAAI: Position statement: The use of newer asthma and allergy medications during pregnancy. Ann Allerg Immunol 2000;84:475–480.
37. Greenberger PA: Management of asthma in pregnancy. Clin Immunother 1996;6:97–107.
38. Schatz M, Zeiger RS, Harden K, et al: The safety of asthma and allergy medications during pregnancy. J Allerg Clin Immunol 1997;100:301–306.
39. Wood CC, Fireman P, Grossman J, et al: Product characteristics and pharmacokinetics of intranasal ipratropium bromide. J Allerg Clin Immunol 1995;95:1111–1116.
40. Nelson-Piercy C: Asthma in pregnancy. Thorax 2001;56:325.
41. Powrie RO: Drugs in pregnancy. Respiratory disease. Best Pract Res Clin Obstet Gynaecol 2001;15:913–936.
42. Stenius-Aarniala B, Hedman J, Terama K: Acute asthma during pregnancy. Thorax 1996;51:411–414.
43. Briggs GC, Freeman RJK, Yaffe SJ: Drugs in Pregnancy and Lactation—A Reference Guide to Fetal and Neonatal Risk, 8th ed. Baltimore, Williams & Wilkins, 1998.
44. Greenberger PA, Patterson R: Beclomethasone diproprionate for severe asthma during pregnancy. Ann Intern Med 1983;98: 478–480.
45. Norjaara E, de Verdier MG: Normal pregnancy outcomes in a population-based study including 2968 pregnant women exposed to budesonide. J Allerg Clin Immunol 2003;111:736–742.
46. Morrow-Brown H, Storey G: Treatment of allergy of the respiratory tract with beclomethasone dipropionate steroid aerosol. Postgrad Med J 1975;51(Suppl 4):59–94.
47. Greenberger P, Patterson R: Safety of therapy for allergic symptoms during pregnancy. Ann Intern Med 1978;89:234–237.
48. Dombrowski M, Thom E, McNellis D: Maternal-Fetal Medicine Units (MFMU) studies of inhaled corticosteroids during pregnancy. J Allerg Clin Immunol 1999;103:S356–S359.
49. Wilson J: Use of sodium cromoglycate during pregnancy. Acta Ther 1982;8:S45–S51.
50. Stenius-Aarniala B, Riikonen S, Teramo K: Slow-release theophylline in pregnant asthmatics. Chest 1995;107:642–647.
51. Rubin PC: Prescribing in pregnancy: General guidelines. Br Med J Anaesth 1986;293:1415–1417.
52. Wendel PJ, Ramin SM, Barnett-Hamm C, et al: Asthma treatment in pregnancy: A randomized controlled study. Am J Ostet Gynecol 1996;175:150.

53. Ballard PL, Granverg P, Ballard RA: Glucocorticoid levels in maternal and cord serum after prenatal beclomethasone therapy in pregnancy near term. J Pediatr 1975;56:1548–1554.
54. Beitins R, Baynoard F, Anaes IG, et al: The transplacental passage of prednisone and prednisolone in pregnancy near term. J Pediatr 1972;81:936–945.
55. Rodriguez-Pinilla E, Martinez-Frias ML: Corticosteroids during pregnancy and oral clefts: A case-control study. Teratol 1998;58:2–5.
56. Park-Wyllie L, Mazzotta P, Pastuszak A, et al: Birth defects after maternal exposure to corticosteroids: Prospective cohort study and meat-analysis of epidemiological studies. Teratol 2000;62: 385–392.
57. Bousquet J, can Cauwenberge P, Khaltaev N, and the WHO panel members: Allergic Rhinitis and its Impact on Asthma (ARIA). J Allerg Clin Imunol 2001;108:S1–S315.
58. Metzger WJ, Turner E, Patterson R: The safety of immunotherapy during pregnancy. J Allerg Clin Immunol 1978;61:268–272.
59. Gotzsche PC, Hammarquist C, Burr M: House dust mite control measures in the management of asthma: Meta-analysis. BMJ 1998;317:1105–1110.
60. British Thoracic Society, Scottish Intercollegiate Guidelines Network (SIGN): British guidelines on the management of asthma. Thorax 2003;58(Suppl 1):31–94.
61. Theodoropoulos DS, Lockey RF, Boyce HW Jr, Bukantz SC: Gastroesophageal reflux and asthma: A review of pathogenesis, diagnosis, and therapy. Allergy 1999;54:651–661.
62. Samuelson WM, Kopita JM: Management of the difficult asthmatic. Gastroesophageal reflux sinusitis, and pregnancy. Respir Care Clin North Am 1995;1:287–308.
63. Stoodley RG, Aaron SD, Dales RE: The role of ipratropium bromide in the emergency management of acute asthma exacerbation: A meta-analysis of rendomized clinical trials. Ann Emerg Med 1999;34:8–18.
64. Smith AP: The effects of intravenous infusion of graded doses of prostaglandins $F_{2\alpha}$ and E_2 on lung resistance in patients undergoing termination of pregnancy. Clin Science 1973;44:17–25.
65. Weiner CP, Buhimschi C (eds): Drugs for Pregnant and Lactating Women. Philadelphia, Churchill Livingstone, 2004; pp.115–116.
66. Saarinen UM, Kajosaari M: Breastfeeding as prophylaxis against atopic disease: Prospective follow-up study until 17 years old. Lancet 1995;346:1065–1069.
67. Rybicki BA, Major M, Popovich J Jr, et al: Racial differences in sarcoidosis incidence: A 5-year study in a health maintenance organization. Am J Epidemiol 1997;145:234.
68. Baughman RP, Teirstein AS, Judson MA, et al: Case Control Etiologic Study of Sarcoidosis (ACCESS) research group. Clinical characteristics of patients in a case control study of sarcoidosis. Am J Respir Crit Care Med 2001;164:1885–1889.
69. Baughman RP, Lower EE, du Bois RM: Sarcoidosis. Lancet 2003;361:1111–1118.
70. Pietinalho A, Tukiainen P, Haahtela T, et al: Finnish Pulmonary Sarcoidosis Study Group. Oral prednisolone followed by inhaled budesonide in newly diagnosed pulmonary sarcoidosis: A double-blind, placebo-controlled, multicenter study. Chest 1999; 116:424–431.
71. Pietinalho A, Tukiainen P, Haahtela T, et al: Finnish Pulmonary Sarcoidosis Study Group. Early treatment of stage II sarcoidosis improves 5-year pulmonary function. Chest 2002;121:24–31.
72. King TE Jr: Overview of sarcoidosis. In Rose BD (ed): UpTo Date, Wellesley, Mass, 2003.
73. Menzin AW, You TT, Deger RB, et al: Sarcoidosis in a uterine leiomyoma. Int J Gynaecol Obstet 1995;48:79.
74. DiCarlo FJ, DiCarlo JP, Robboy SJ, Lyons MM: Sarcoidosis of the uterus. Arch Pathol Lab Med 1989;113:941.
75. Selroos O: Sarcoidosis and pregnancy: A review with results of a retrospective survey. J Intern Med 1990;227:221.
76. Agha FP, Vade A, Amendola MA, Cooper RF: Effects of pregnancy on sarcoidosis. Surg Gynecol Obstet 1982;155:817–822.
77. Keleman JT, Mandl L: Sarcoidose in der placenta. Zentralblatt fur Allgemeine Pathologie und Pathologische Anatomie 1969;281:520–522.
78. James DG: Sarcoidosis. Dis Mon 1970;1:43.
79. Erskine KJ, Taylor KS, Agnew RAL: Serial estimation of serum angiotensin converting enzyme activity during and after pregnancy in a woman with sarcoidosis. BMJ 1985;290:269–270.
80. Centers for Disease Control and Prevention, Division of Tuberculosis Elimination. Surveillance reports: Reported tuberculosis in the United States, 2000. Atlanta, 2001. (Accessed 31 July 2003 at *http://www.cdc.gov/hchstp/tb/surv/surv2000.*)
81. Dye C, Scheele S, Dolin P, et al: Consensus statement: Global burden of tuberculosis: Estimated incidence, prevalence, and mortality by country: WHO Global Surveillance and Monitoring Project. JAMA 1999;282:677–686.
82. Small PM., Fujiwara PI: Management of tuberculosis in the United States. N Engl J Med 2001;345:189–200.
83. Cohen JD, Patton EA, Badger TL: The tuberculous mother. Am Rev Tubercul 1952;65:1–23.
84. de March P: Tuberculosis and pregnancy: Five-in-ten year review of 215 patients in their fertile age. Chest 1975;68: 800–880.
85. Bass JB: Tuberculosis in pregnancy. In Rose BD (ed): UpToDate, Wellesley, Mass, 2003.
86. Jana N, Vasishta K, Saha SC, Ghosh K: Obstetrical outcomes among women with extrapulmonary tuberculosis. N Engl J Med 1999;341:645.
87. Ormerod P: Tuberculosis in pregnancy and the puerperium. Thorax 2001;56:494.
88. Cantwell MF, Shehab ZM, Costello AM, et al: Brief report: Congenital tuberculosis. N Engl J Med 1994;330:1051–1054.
89. Jana N, Vasishta K, Jindal SK, et al: Perinatal outcome in pregnancies complicated by pulmonary tuberculosis. Int J Gynaecol Obstet 1994;44:119–124.
90. Davidson PT: Managing tuberculosis during pregnancy. Lancet 1995;346:199.
91. Montgomery WP, Young RC Jr, Allen MP: The tuberculin test in pregnancy. Am J Obstet Gynecol 1968;100:829–831.
92. Present PA, Comstock GA: Tuberculin sensitivity in pregnancy. Am Rev Respir Dis 1975;112:413–415.
93. British Medical Association and Royal Pharmaceutical Society of Great Britain: British National Formulary, no. 22P. 210 London, BMA, 1991.
94. American Thoracic Society/Centers for Disease Control and Prevention/Infectious Diseases Society of America: Treatment of tuberculosis. Am J Respir Crit Care Med 2003;167:603–662.
95. Carter EJ, Mates S: Tuberculosis during pregnancy: The Rhode Island experience, 1987 to 1991. Chest 1994;106:1466–1470.
96. Snider DE, Layde PM, Johnson MW, Lyle MA: Treatment of tuberculosis during pregnancy. Am Rev Respir Dis 1980;122: 65–78.
97. Scheinhorn DJ, Angelillo VA: Antituberculous therapy in pregnancy: Risks to the fetus. West J Med 1977;127:195–198.
98. Llewelyn M, Cropley I, Wilkinson RJ, Davidson RN: Tuberculosis diagnosed during pregnancy: A prospective study from London. Thorax 2000;55:129.
99. Conway N, Birt BD: Streptomycin in pregnancy: Effect on the foetal ear. BMJ 1965;2:260–263.
100. Atkins NA: Maternal plasma concentration of pyridoxal phosphate during pregnancy: Adequacy of vitamin B6 supplementation during isoniazid therapy. Am Rev Respir Dis 1982;126: 714–716.
101. Brummer DL: Letter to the editor. Am Rev Respir Dis 1972;106:145–185.
102. Eggermont EN, Logghe W, Van De Casseye M, et al: Hemorrhagic disease of the newborn in the offspring of rifampin and isoniazid treated mothers. Acta Paediatr Belg 1976;29:87–89.

103. Snider DE, Caras GJ: Isoniazid-associated hepatitis deaths: A review of available information. Am Rev Respir Dis 1992;145: 484.
104. Brost BC, Newman RB: The maternal and fetal effects of tuberculosis therapy. Obstet Gynecol Clin North Am 1997;24:659.
105. Franks AL, Binkin NJ, Snider DE Jr, et al: Isoniazid hepatitis among pregnant and postpartum Hispanic patients. Publ Health Rep 1989;104:151–155.
106. American Thoracic Society/Centers for Disease Control and Prevention Statement Committee on Latent Tuberculosis Infection: Targeted tuberculin testing and treatment of latent tuberculosis infection. Am J Respir Crit Care Med 2000;161:S221.
107. Centers for Disease Control and Prevention: 1999 guidelines for the prevention of opportunistic infections in persons infected with human immunodeficiency virus: U.S. Public Health Service (USPHS) and Infectious Diseases Society of America (IDSA). MMWR 1999;48(No. RR-10):13–14.
108. Adhikari M, Pillay T, Pillay DG: Tuberculosis in the newborn: An emerging disease. Pediatr Infect Dis J 1997;16:1108.
109. Gaisford W, Griffiths MI: A freeze-dried vaccine from isonized-resistant BCG. BMJ 1961;1:1500–1501.
110. Snider DE, Powell KE: Should women taking antituberculosis drugs breast-feed? Arch Intern Med 1984;144:589.
111. Baron RM, Schwartzstein RM: Diseases of the chest wall. In Rose BD (ed): UpToDate, Wellesley, Mass, 2003.
112. Sawicka EH, Spencer GT, Branthwaite MA: Management of respiratory failure complicating pregnancy in severe kyphoscoliosis: a new use for an old technique? Br J Dis Chest 1986;80:191–196.
113. King TE Jr: Restrictive lung disease in pregnancy. Clin Chest Med 1992;13(4):607–622.
114. Lao TT, Yeung S, Leung BF: Kyphoscoliosis and pregnancy. J Obstet Gynecol 1986;7:11–15.
115. Barrett JFR, Dear PRF, Lilford RJ: Brain damge as a result of chronic intrauterine hypoxia in a baby born of a severely kyphoscoliotic mother. J Obstet Gynecol 1991;11:260–261.
116. Restrick LJ, Clapp BR, Mikelsons C, Wedzicha JA: Nasal ventilation in pregnancy: Treatment of nocturnal hypoventilation in a patient with kyphoscoliosis. Eur Respir J 1997;10(11):2657–2658.
117. Kahler CM, Hogl B, Habeler R, et al: Management of respiratory deterioration in a pregnant patient with severe kyphoscoliosis by noninvasive positive pressure ventilation. Wien Klin Wochenschr 2002;114:874–877.
118. To WW, Wong MW: Kyphoscoliosis complicating pregnancy. Int J Gynaecol Obstet 1996;55(2):123–128.
119. Matthews LW, Drotar D: Cystic fibrosis—a challenging long term chronic disease. Pediatr Clin North Am 1984;31:133–152.
120. Rommens JM, Iannuzzi MC, Kerem B, et al: Identification of the cystic fibrosis gene: Chromosome walking and jumping. Science 1989;245:1059.
121. Katkin JP: Clinical manifestations and diagnosis of cystic fibrosis In Rose BD (ed): UpToDate, Wellesley, Mass, 2003.
122. Simon RH: Treatment of cystic fibrosis lung disease. In Rose BD (ed): UpToDate, Wellesley, Mass, 2003.
123. Bennett LE, Keck BM, Daily OP, Novick RJ: Worldwide thoracic organ transplantation: A report from the UNOS/ISHLT International Registry for Thoracic Organ Transplantation. Clin Transpl 2000;31–44.
124. Lyon A, Bilton D: Fertility issues in cystic fibrosis. Paediatr Respir Rev 2002;3(3):236–240.
125. Hilman BC, Aitken M, Constantinescu M: Pregnancy in patients with cystic fibrosis. Clin Obstet Gynecol 1996;39:70–86.
126. Edenborough FP, Stableforth DE, Mackenzie WE: The outcome of 72 pregnancies in 55 women with cystic fibrosis in the United Kingdom 1977–1996. BJOG 2000;107:254–261.
127. Edenborough FP, Stableforth DE, Webb AK, et al: Outcome of pregnancy in women with cystic fibrosis. Thorax 1995;50: 170–174.
128. Kent NE, Farquaharson DF: Cystic fibrosis in pregnancy. Can Med Assoc J 1993;149:809–813.
129. Frangolias DD, Nakielna EM, Wilcox PG: Pregnancy and cystic fibrosis. Chest 1997;111:963–969.
130. Jankelson D, Robinson M, Parsons S, et al: Cystic fibrosis and pregnancy. Aust NZ J Obstet Gynaecol 1998;38:180–184.
131. Gilljam M, Antoniou M, Shin J, et al: Pregnancy in cystic fibrosis. Fetal and maternal outcome. Chest 2000;118(1):85–91.
132. Briard ML, Mattei JF: Cystic fibrosis: Preimplantation diagnosis, prenatal diagnosis and medical ethics, a successful combination. Pediatr Pulmonol Suppl 1997;16:65.
133. Super M, Ivinson A, Schwartz M, et al: Clinic experience of prenatal diagnosis of cystic fibrosis by use of linked DNA probes. Lancet 1997;2:782–784.
134. Wenstrom KD: Cystic fibrosis: Prenatal genetic screening. In Rose BD (ed): UpToDate, Wellesley, Mass, 2003.
135. Kotloff RM, FitzSimmons SC, Fiel SB: Fertility and pregnancy in patients with cystic fibrosis. Clin Chest Med 1992;13:623–635.
136. Larsen JW: Cystic fibrosis and pregnancy. Obstet Gynecol 1972;39:880–883.
137. Edenborough FP: Women with cystic fibrosis and their potential for reproduction. Thorax 2001;56(8):649–655.
138. Liaschko A, Koren G: Cystic fibrosis during pregnancy. Can Fam Physician 2002;48:463–467.
139. Koren G, Pastuszak A, Ito S: Drugs in pregnancy. N Engl J Med 1998;338:1128–1137.
140. Loebstein R, Addis A, Ho E, et al: Pregnancy outcome following gestational exposure to fluoroquinolones: A multicenter prospective controlled study. Antimicrob Agents Chemother 1998;42(6):1336–1339.
141. Larsen H, Nielsen GL, Schonheyder HC, et al: Birth outcome following maternal use of fluoroquinolones. Int J Antimicrob Agents 2001;18(3):259–262.
142. Dowsett J: An overview of nutritional issues for the adult with cystic fibrosis. Nutrition 2000;16:566–570.
143. Whitelaw A, Butterfield A: High breast milk sodium in cystic fibrosis. Lancet 1977;2:1988.
144. Alpert SE, Cormier AD: Normal electrolyte and protein content in milk from mothers with cystic fibrosis: An explanation for the initial report of elevated milk sodium concentration. J Pediatr 1983;102:77–80.
145. Bitman J, Hamosh M, Wood DL, et al: Lipid composition of milk from mothers with cystic fibrosis. Pediatr 1987;80:927–932.
146. Bartlett JG, Mundy LM: Community-acquired pneumonia. N Engl J Med 1995;333:1618–1624.
147. Berkowitz K, LaSAla A: Risk factors associated with the increasing prevalence of pneumonia during pregnancy. Am J Obstet Gynecol 1990;163:981–985.
148. Larsen JW Jr: Influenza and pregnancy. Clin Obstet Gynecol 1982;25:599.
149. Esmonde TF, Herdman G, Anderson G: Chickenpox pneumonia: An association with pregnancy. Thorax 1989;44:812.
150. Wack EE, Ampel NM, Galgiani JN, Bronnimann DA: Coccidioidomycosis during pregnancy. Chest 1988;94:376.
151. Freeman DW, Barno A: Death from Asian influenza associated with pregnancy. Am J Obstet Gynecol 1959;78:1172–1175.
152. Peterson CM, Schuppert K, Kelly PC, Pappagianis D: Coccidioidomycosis and pregnancy. Obstet Gynecol Surv 1993;48:149.
153. Harris RE: Coccidioidomycosis complicating pregnancy: Report of three cases and review of the literature. Obstet Gynecol 1966; 28:401– 405.
154. Moya F, Morishiama HO, Shnider SM, James LS: Influence of maternal hyperventilation on the newborn infant. Am J Obstet Gynecol 1975;91:76–84.
155. Parayani SG, Arvin AM: Intrauterine infection with varicella-zoster virus after maternal varicella. N Engl J Med 1986;314: 1542–1546.
156. Centers for Disease Control and Prevention: Prevention and control of influenza: Recommendations of the Advisory Committee on Immunization Practices (ACIP). MMWR 1998;47(RR-6):5.

157. Centers for Disease Control and Prevention: Prevention of pneumococcal disease: Recommendations of the Advisory Committee on Immunization Practices (ACIP). MMWR 1997; 46(RR-08):1.
158. Adelson-Mitty J, Zaleznik DF: UptoDate [serial on line]. 19 March 2003. Available at http://www.uptodate.com. Accessed 30 June 2003.
159. Bartlett JG, Breiman RF, Mandell LA, File TM Jr: Community-acquired pneumonia in adults: Guidelines for management. Guidelines from the Infectious Disease Society of America. Clin Infect Dis 1998;26:811.
160. Metlay JP, Kapoor WN, Fine MJ: Does this patient have community-acquired pneumonia? Diagnosing pneumonia by history and physical examination. JAMA 1997;278:1440.
161. Bates JH, Campbell GD, Barron AL, et al: Microbial etiology of acute pneumonia in hospitalized patients. Chest 1992;101:1005.
162. Niederman MS, Bass JB Jr, Campbell GD, et al: Guidelines for the initial management of adults with community-acquired pneumonia: Diagnosis, assessment of severity, and initial antimicrobial therapy. American Thoracic Society. Medical Section of the American Lung Association. Am Rev Respir Dis 1993;148: 1418–1426.
163. Marrie TJ: Community-acquired pneumonia. Clin Infect Dis 1994;18:501.
164. Bartlett JG, Dowell SF, Mandell LA, et al: Practice guidelines for the management of community-acquired pneumonia in adults. Infectious Diseases Society of America. Clin Infect Dis 2000;31(2):347–382.
165. British Thoracic Society: Guidelines for the management of community-acquired pneumonia in adults admitted to hospital. Br J Hosp Med 1993;49:346.
166. McCormack WM, George H, Donner A, et al: Hepatotoxicity of erythromycin estolate during pregnancy. Antimicrob Agents Chemother 1977;12: 630–635.
167. Kilpatrick SJ, Matthay MA: Obstetric patients requiring critical care. Chest 1992;101:1407.
168. Hollingsworth HM, Irwin RS: Acute respiratory failure in pregnancy. Clin Chest Med 1992;13:723.
169. Boyd K, Walker E: Use of acyclovir to treat chickenpox in pregnancy. BMJ 1988;296:393–394.
170. Glaser JB, Loftus J, Ferragamo V, et al: Varicella-zoster infection in pregnancy. N Engl J Med 1986;5:1416.
171. Haddad J, Simeoni U, Messner J, Willard D: Acyclovir in prophylaxis and perinatal varicella. Lancet 1987;1:161.
172. Cox SM, Cunningham FG, Luby J: Management of varicella pneumonia complicating pregnancy. Am J Perinatol 1990;7: 300–301.
173. Chapman SJ: Varicella in pregnancy. Semin Perinatol 1998;22: 339–346.
174. Sciscione AC, Ivester T, Largoza M, et al: Acute pulmonary edema in pregnancy. Obstet Gynecol 2003;101:511–515.
175. Catanzarite V, Willms D, Wong D, et al: Acute respiratory distress syndrome in pregnancy and the puerperium: Causes, courses, and outcomes. Obstet Gynecol 2001;97:760–764.
176. Kollef MH, Schuster DP: The acute respiratory distress syndrome. N Engl J Med 1995;332:27–44.
177. Luhr DR, Antonsen K, Karlsson M, et al: Incidence and mortality of pulmonary edema after acute respiratory failure and acute respiratory distress syndrome in Sweden, Denmark and Iceland. The ARF Study Group. Am J Respir Crit Care Med 1999;159: 1849.
178. Siegel MD, Hansen-Flaschen J: Acute respiratory distress syndrome: Definition, diagnosis, and etiology. In Rose BD (ed): UpToDate, Wellesley, Mass, 2003.
179. Powrie RO: Acute lung injury. In Le RV, Rosene-Montella K, Barbour LA, et al. (eds): Medical Care of the Pregnant Patient. Philadelphia, American College of Physicians, 2000, pp 397–411.
180. Hook JW: Acute respiratory distress syndrome in pregnancy. Semin Perinatol 1997;21(4):320–327.
181. Tan SN: Peripartum pulmonary edema. Anesth Intens Care 1991;19:111–113.
182. Phelan JP: Pulmonary edema in obstetrics. Obstet Gynecol Clin North Am 1991;18:319–331.
183. Hankins GDV, Nolan TE: Adult respiratory distress syndrome in obstetrics. Obstet Gynecol Clin North Am 1991;18:273–287.
184. Deblieux PM, Summer WR: Acute respiratory failure in pregnancy. Clin Obstet Gynecol 1996;39:143–152.
185. Wiederhielm CA: Dynamics of transcapillary fluid exchanges. J Gen Physiol 1968;52(Suppl 1):29S–63S.
186. Weil MH, Morissette M, Michaels S, et al: Routine plasma colloid osmotic pressure measurements. Crit Care Med 1979;2: 229–234.
187. Ian P, Maltau JM, Noddeland H, Fadnes HO: Oedema-preventing mechanisms in subcutaneous tissue of normal pregnant women. BJOG 1985;92:1113–1119.
188. Cotton DB, Gonik B, Spillmann T, Dorman KF: Intrapartum to postpartum changes in colloid osmotic pressure. Am J Obstet Gynecol 1984;149(2):174–177.
189. Gonik B, Cotton DB: Peripartum colloid osmotic pressure changes: Influence of intravenous hydration. Am J Obstet Gynecol 1984;150(1):99–100.
190. Weil MH, Henning RJ, Puri VK: Colloid oncotic pressure: Clinical significance. Crit Care Med 1979;7:113–116.
191. Nguyen HN, Clark SL, Greenspoon J, et al: Peripartum colloid osmotic pressure: Correlation with serum proteins. Obstet Gynecol 1986;68(6):807–810.
192. Benedetti TJ, Carlson RW: Studies of colloid osmotic pressure in pregnancy induced hypertension. Am J Obstet Gynecol 1978;135(3):308–311.
193. Bienrarz J, Ivankovich A, Scommegma A: Cardiac output during ritodrine treatment in preterm labor. Am J Obstet Gynecol 1974;118(7):910–920.
194. Pisani RJ, Rosenow EC III: Pulmonary edema associated with tocolytic therapy. Ann Intern Med 1989;110:714–718.
195. Benedetti TJ, Hargrove JC, Rosene KA: Maternal pulmonary edema during premature labor inhibition. Obstet Gynecol 1982; 59(6 Suppl):33S–37S.
196. Ingemarsson I, Arulkomoran S, Kottegoda SR: Complications of beta mimetic therapy in preterm labour. Aust NZ J Obstet Gynecol 1985;25(3):182–189.
197. Yeast JD, Halberstadt C, Meyer BA, et al: The risk of pulmonary edema and colloid osmotic pressure changes during magnesium sulfate infusion. Am J Obstet Gynecol 1993;169(6):1566–1571.
198. Kirkpatrick C, Quenon M, Desir D: Blood anions and electrolytes during ritodrine infusion in preterm labor. Am J Obstet Gynecol 1980;139:523–527.
199. Hatjis CG, Swain M: Systemic tocolysis for premature labor is associated with an increased incidence of pulmonary edema in the presence of maternal infection. Am J Obstet Gynecol 1988;159:723.
200. Nimrod CA, Beresford P, Frais M, et al: Hemodynamic observations on pulmonary edema associated with a β-mimetic agent. J Reprod Med 1984;29(5):341–344.
201. Zinaman M, Rubin J, Lindheimer MD: Serial plasma oncotic pressure levels and echoencephalography during and after delivery in severe pre-eclampsia. Lancet 1985;1(8440):1245–1247.
202. Sibai BM, Mabie BC, Harvey CJ, Gonzalez AR: Pulmonary edema in severe preeclampsia-eclampsia: Analysis of thirty-seven consecutive cases. Am J Obstet Gynecol 1987;156:1174.
203. Mabie WC, Hackman BB, Sibai BM: Acute pulmonary edema associated with pregnancy: Echocardiographic insights and implications for treatment. Obstet Gynecol 1993;81:227–234.
204. Benedetti TJ, Kates R, Williams V: Hemodynamic observations in severe pre-eclampsia complicated by pulmonary edema. Am J Obstet Gynecol 1985;152:330–334.

205. Mabie WC, Ratts TE, Ramanathan KB, Sibai BM: Circulatory congestion in obese hypertensive women: A subset of pulmonary edema in pregnancy. Obstet Gynecol 1988;72:553–558.
206. Gottlieb JE, Darby MJ, Gee MH, Fish JE: Recurrent noncardiac pulmonary edema accompanying pregnancy-induced hypertension. Chest 1991;100:1730–1732.
207. Goodrun LA: Pneumonia in pregnancy. Semin Perinatol 1997;21:276–283.
208. Cunningham FG, Lucas MJ, Hankins GDV: Pulmonary injury complicating antepartum pyelonephritis. Am J Obstet Gynecol 1987;156:797–807.
209. Pruett K, Faro S: Pyelonephritis associated with respiratory distress. Obstet Gynecol 1987;69:444–446.
210. Elkington KW, Greb LC: Adult respiratory distress syndrome as a complication of acute pyelonephritis during pregnancy: Case report and discussion. Obstet Gynecol 1986;67:18S–20S.
211. de Veciana M, Towers CV, Major CA, et al: Pulmonary injury associated with appendicitis in pregnancy; who is at risk ? Am J Obstet Gynecol 1994;171(4):1008–1013.
212. Soreide E, Bjornstad E, Steen PA: An audit of perioperative aspiration pneumonia in gynecological and obstetric patients. Acta Anaesth Scand 1996;40(1):14–19.
213. Gilbert WM, Danielsen B: Amniotic fluid embolism: Decreased mortality in a population-based study. Obstet Gynecol 1999;93(6):973–977.
214. Clark SL: Amniotic fluid embolism. Crit Care Clin 1991;7:877.
215. Clark SL, Hankins GDV, Dudley DA, et al: Amniotic fluid embolism: Analysis of the national registry. Am J Obstet Gynecol 1995;172:1158–1169.
216. Martin RW: Amniotic fluid embolism. Clin Obstet Gynecol 1996;39:101–106.
217. Burrows A, Khoo SK: The amniotic fluid embolism syndrome: 10 years experience at a major teaching hospital. Aust NZ J Obstet Gynaec 1995;35(3):245–250.
218. Metcalfe J: Oxygen supply and fetal growth. J Reprod Med 1985;30(4):301–307.
219. Meschia G: Safety margin of fetal oxygenation. J Reprod Med 1985;30(4):308–311.
220. Meschia G: Supply of oxygen to the fetus. J Reprod Med 1979;23(4):160–165.
221. Humphrey H, Hall J, Sznaider I, et al: Improved survival in ARDS patients associated with a reduction in pulmonary capillary wedge pressure. Chest 1990;97:1176.
222. Simmons RS, Berdine GG, Seidenfeld JJ, et al: Fluid balance and the adult respiratory distress syndrome. Am Rev Respir Dis 1987;135:924.
223. Mitchell JP, Schuller D, Calandrino FS, et al: Improved outcome based on fluid management in critically ill patients requiring pulmonary artery catheterization. Am Rev Respir Dis 1992; 145:990.
224. Barnardo PD, Jenkins JG: Failed tracheal intubation in obstetrics: A 6-year review in a UK region. Anaesth 2000;55: 690–694.
225. Hawthorne L, Wilson R, Lyon G, Dresner M: Failed intubation revisited: 17-year experience in a teaching maternity unit. Br J Anaesth 1996;76:680–684.
226. Baraka A, Pascale JK, Siddik SS, et al: Efficacy of the self-inflating bulb in differentiating esophageal from tracheal intubation in the parturient undergoing cesarean section. Anesth Analg 1997;84:533–537.
227. Han TH, Brimacombe J, Lee EJ, Yang HS: The laryngeal mask airway is effective (and probably safe) in selected healthy parturients for elective cesarean section: A prospective study of 1067 cases. Can J Anaesth 2001;48:1117–1121.
228. Nolan TE, Wakefield ML, Devoe LD: Invasive hemodynamic monitoring in obstetrics, a critical review of its indications, benefits, complications, and alternatives. Chest 1992;101:1429–1433.
229. Wallenburg HCS: Invasive hemodynamic monitoring in pregnancy. Eur J Obstet Gynecol Reprod Biol 1991;42:S45–S51.
230. Kirshon B, Cotton DB: Invasive hemodynamic monitoring in the obstetric patient. Clin Obstet Gynecol 1987;30(3):579–590.
231. Cotton DB, Benedetti TJ: Use of Swan Ganz catheter in obstetrics and gynecology. Obstet Gynecol 1980;56(5):641–645.
232. Clark SL, Horenstein JM, Phelan JP, et al: Experience with the pulmonary artery catheter in obstetrics and gynecology. Am J Obstet Gynecol 1985;152:374–378.
233. Clark SL, Cotton DB, Lee W, et al: Central hemodynamic assessment of normal term pregnancy. Am J Obstet Gynecol 1989;161:1439–1442.
234. Weil MH, Henning RJ, Morissette M, Michaels S: Relationship between colloid osmotic pressure and pulmonary artery wedge pressure in patients with acute cardiorespiratory failure. Am J Med 1978;64:643–650.
235. Clark SL, Cotton DB: Clinical indications for pulmonary artery catheterization in the patient with severe pre-eclampsia. Am J Obstet Gynecol 1988;158(3):453–459.
236. Strauss RG, Keefer R, Burke T, Civetta JM: Hemodynamic monitoring of cardiogenic pulmonary edema complicating toxemia of pregnancy. Obstet Gynecol 1980;55(2):170–174.
237. Cotton DB, Gonik B, Dorman K, Harrist R: Cardiovascular alterations in severe pregnancy-induced hypertension: Relationship of central venous pressure to pulmonary capillary wedge pressure. Am J Obstet Gynecol 1985;151:762–764.
238. Keefer JR, Strauss RG, Civetta JM, Burke T: Noncardiogenic pulmonary edema and invasive cardiovascular monitoring. Obstet Gynecol 1981;58:46–51.
239. Matthay MA, Chatterjee K: Bedside catheterization of the pulmonary artery: Risks compared with benefits. Ann Intern Med 1988;109:826–834.
240. Lapinsky SE, Kruczynski K, Seaward GR, et al: Critical care management of the obstetric patient. Can J Anaesth 1997;44(3): 325–329.
241. Lapinsky SE, Kruczynski K, Slutsky AS: Critical care in the pregnant patient. Am J Respir Crit Care Med 1995;152:427–455.
242. Rizk N, Kalassian KG, Gilligan T, et al: Obstetric complications in pulmonary and critical care medicine. Chest 1996;110:791–809.

CHAPTER 39

Anemia and White Blood Cell Disorders

Jane Strong

ANEMIA: OVERVIEW

Anemia is defined as a hemoglobin value that is lower than the threshold of two standard deviations below the median value for a healthy matched population. The World Health Organization defines anemia in pregnancy as a hemoglobin concentration of less than 11g/dL.[1] The cutoff point suggested by the United States Centers for Disease Control is 10.5g/dL in the second trimester.[2]

Marked physiologic changes in the composition of the blood occur in healthy pregnancy. Increased total blood volume[3] and hemostatic changes[4] help to combat the hazard of hemorrhage at delivery. Plasma volume increases dramatically (50%), and red cell mass increases as well (18%–25%, depending on iron status). These changes cause a physiologic dilution in hemoglobin concentration that is greatest at 32 weeks' gestation. In iron-replete women, hemoglobin returns to normal by 1 week postpartum.

Worldwide, pathologic anemia is the most common medical disorder of pregnancy. Deficiency of essential hematinics usually arises from increased requirements and inadequate intake. Iron deficiency is the most common hematinic deficiency in pregnancy, followed by folate deficiency. Vitamin B_{12} deficiency rarely causes anemia in pregnancy. Addisonian pernicious anemia does not usually occur in the reproductive years, and when it does, it is usually associated with infertility. Pregnancy occurs only when vitamin B_{12} deficiency is corrected. Only vegans and those from very poor communities are likely to have a diet that is deficient in vitamin B_{12} (i.e., containing no animal protein). In nonindustrialized countries, anemia is responsible for 40% to 60% of maternal deaths.[5] In industrialized countries, approximately 18% of women are anemic during pregnancy. The average prevalence is 56% in nonindustrialized countries.[6]

ANEMIA: IRON DEFICIENCY

Maternal Risks

To replenish losses, an adult man must absorb approximately 1 mg/day iron. Women of reproductive age require larger quantities of iron to compensate for menstrual losses. During an average menstrual cycle, a woman loses 10 to 15 mg iron. To maintain iron balance, women of reproductive age require 2 mg iron daily. Pregnancy further stresses iron balance. The iron requirements in pregnancy are approximately 900 mg.[7] The main demands for iron arise from expansion of the red cell mass (approximately 500–600 mg), and the fetus and placenta require approximately 300 mg. The daily iron requirement in pregnancy is approximately 4 mg (2.5 mg/day in early pregnancy, increasing to 6 to 8 mg/day from week 32 onward).[8] These requirements can be achieved only by maximizing dietary iron absorption and mobilizing iron stores.[9,10] If a woman enters pregnancy with depleted iron stores, the effects of iron deficiency develop. Vegetarians are at an additional disadvantage because heme iron (derived from meat) is more readily absorbed than non-heme iron, and heme iron also facilitates the absorption of non-heme iron in a mixed diet. Absorption of iron is less than 10%, so an average of 40 mg dietary iron is required daily. For many women, especially in nonindustrialized countries, where diets are low in iron bioavailability, sufficient iron is not supplied by diet alone.

As iron deficiency develops, the ferritin level decreases first and then the serum iron level. A decrease in hemoglobin concentration is a late development.[11] Iron-dependent enzymes in every cell are affected, and there is a profound effect on body functions (e.g., impaired muscle function, neurotransmitter activity, exercise tolerance, epithelial changes, alteration in gastrointestinal function).[12]

Tissue enzyme malfunction occurs, even in the early stages of iron deficiency. The various effects of iron deficiency on cellular function may be responsible for the reported association between anemia during pregnancy and preterm birth and the anecdotal evidence that blood loss at delivery is greater in women with anemia.[13,14]

In normal pregnancy, hypervolemia modifies the response to blood loss.[4] Blood volume decreases after the acute loss at delivery but remains relatively stable as long as the loss does not exceed 25% of predelivery volume. No compensatory increase in blood volume occurs, and plasma volume decreases gradually, primarily because of diuresis. The overall result is that hematocrit gradually increases and blood volume returns to nonpregnant values.

The average blood loss that can be tolerated without causing a significant decrease in hemoglobin concentration is 1000 mL, but this depends on a healthy increase in blood volume before delivery and on iron status.

Fetal Risks

The fetus obtains iron from maternal transferrin, regardless of maternal iron stores. The placenta traps maternal transferrin, removes the iron, and actively transports it to the fetus, mainly in the last 4 weeks of pregnancy.[7] If maternal iron stores are depleted, the fetus obtains iron from erythrocyte breakdown or maternal intestinal absorption. Most fetal iron is found in fetal hemoglobin, but one third is stored in the fetal liver as ferritin.

When maternal iron stores are depleted, the fetus cannot accumulate as much iron and there is a decrease in fetal iron stores.[15] This may have an important bearing on iron stores and the development of anemia during the first year of life, when oral iron intake is very poor.[16–18]

Studies suggest that behavioral abnormalities occur in children with iron deficiency. These abnormalities are related to changes in the concentration of chemical mediators in the brain.[18] Iron deficiency in the absence of anemia is associated with poor performance on the Bayley Mental Development Index.[19] Development delays in iron-deficient infants can be reversed by treatment with iron.[20] Cognitive function can also be improved with iron supplementation, as was shown in a randomized study in nonanemic, iron-deficient adolescent girls.[21]

Recent studies suggest that prophylaxis of iron deficiency during pregnancy may have an important role in the prevention of adult hypertension.[22,23] High blood pressure in adults appears to originate in fetal life and is associated with lower birth weight and high ratios of placenta to birth weight. Placental size at term was shown to be inversely proportional to serum ferritin concentrations at initial evaluation.

Diagnosis

Hemoglobin Concentration

A reduction in the concentration of circulating hemoglobin is a relatively late development in iron deficiency and is preceded by depletion of iron stores, reduction in serum iron levels, and detectable decrements in hemoglobin. However, measuring hemoglobin concentration is the simplest noninvasive practical test available. Hemoglobin values of less than 10.5 g/dL in the second and third trimesters are probably abnormal and require further investigation.

Red Cell Indices

The increased drive to erythropoiesis, resulting in a higher proportion of young large red cells, appears to mask the effect of iron deficiency on mean corpuscular volume (MCV) in pregnancy, even when anemia is established. Healthy, iron-replete pregnancy is associated with a small physiologic increase in red cell size, on average 4 fl*, but in some women, the increase may be as high as 20 fl.[24] MCV is a poor indicator of iron deficiency that develops during pregnancy.[25] Some women enter pregnancy with established anemia as a result of iron deficiency or with grossly depleted iron stores, and florid anemia quickly develops, with reduced MCV, mean corpuscular hemoglobin (MCH), and MCH concentration. These do not present diagnostic problems. Those who enter pregnancy with a precarious iron balance and a normal hemoglobin value present the most difficult diagnostic problems. Recognition of iron deficiency before a decrease in hemoglobin or an effect on red cell indices depends on several noninvasive laboratory tests.

Serum Iron and Total Iron-Binding Capacity

Serum iron level and total iron-binding capacity (TIBC) provide an estimate of transferrin saturation. Reduced transferrin saturation indicates a deficient iron supply to the tissues and the development of iron deficiency. At this early stage, erythropoiesis is impaired and iron-dependent tissue enzymes are adversely affected.

In health, the serum iron of adult nonpregnant women shows considerable diurnal variation and can fluctuate from hour to hour. TIBC rises in association with iron deficiency and decreases in chronic inflammatory states. It is increased in pregnancy because of the increase in plasma volume. In nonanemic patients, TIBC is approximately one third saturated with iron.

In pregnancy, most reports describe a decrease in both serum iron and percentage saturation of TIBC, which can be largely prevented by iron supplements. Serum iron,

* fl = femtoliters (10^{-15}L)

even in combination with TIBC, is not a reliable indicator of iron stores, because it fluctuates widely and is affected by recent ingestion of iron and other factors that are not directly involved in iron metabolism, such as infection.

Zinc Protoporphyrin

Zinc protoporphyrin increases when there is a defective iron supply to the developing red cell. Although zinc protoporphyrin may increase in patients with chronic inflammatory disease, malignancy, or infection, the increase usually is not as marked as the increase in ferritin.

Ferritin

Ferritin is a high-molecular-weight glycoprotein that is stable and is not affected by recent ingestion of iron. It appears to reflect iron stores accurately and quantitatively in the absence of inflammation, particularly in the lower range associated with iron deficiency, which is so important in pregnancy. In the development of iron deficiency, a low serum ferritin level is the first abnormal laboratory test result.

Transferrin Receptor

Serum transferrin receptor (TfR) is a relatively new method for assessing cellular iron status.[26] It is present in all cells as a transmembrane protein that binds transferrin-bound iron and transports it to the cell interior. A reduction in the iron supply increases TfR synthesis. Sensitive immunologic techniques show that TfR, like ferritin, circulates in small amounts in the plasma of all individuals, and the concentration is proportional to the total body mass of TfR. In patients with iron deficiency anemia, the plasma receptor is elevated threefold. This elevation is accompanied by an increase in the density of surface TfR in iron-deficient cells. Little or no change in the serum TfR concentration occurs during the early stages of storage iron depletion, but as soon as tissue iron deficiency is established, the serum TfR concentration increases in direct proportion to the degree of iron deficiency. This change, which precedes the reduction in MCV and the increase in zinc protoporphyrin, is a valuable measurement of early tissue iron deficiency. This measurement is particularly helpful in identifying iron deficiency in pregnancy.[27] It differentiates truly iron-deficient women from those who have a low serum ferritin level as a result of storage iron mobilization or those who have a low hemoglobin concentration as a result of hemodilution. It also helps to distinguish those with a normal or high serum ferritin level as a result of chronic inflammatory disease from those who have low stores that lead to genuine cellular iron deficiency. TfR accurately reflects tissue iron deficiency, both in pregnancy and in anemia of chronic disease, in which serum ferritin may be inappropriately elevated because of release from cells. In combination with serum ferritin, TfR gives a complete picture of iron status. Serum ferritin reflects iron stores (in the absence of chronic inflammatory disease), and TfR reflects tissue iron status.[26]

Marrow Iron

The most rapid and reliable method of assessing iron stores in pregnancy is by examination of an appropriately stained preparation of a bone marrow sample. Without iron supplementation, there is no detectable, stainable iron in more than 80% of women at term.[28] No stainable iron (hemosiderin) may be visible once serum ferritin has decreased to less than 40 mg/L,[29,30] but other signs of iron deficiency in developing erythroblasts, particularly late normoblasts, confirm that anemia is caused by iron deficiency in the absence of stainable iron. The effects of folate deficiency, which often accompanies iron deficiency, are also apparent (discussed later). Iron incorporation into hemoglobin *is blocked* if there is acute or chronic inflammation, particularly if it is caused by urinary tract infection, even if iron stores are replete. This problem is shown by examination of the marrow aspirate stained for iron and can be predicted by simultaneous assessment of serum ferritin and TfR and an indicator of chronic inflammatory disease, such as C-reactive protein.

With the development of noninvasive tests of iron status (described earlier), bone marrow examination is reserved for the differential diagnosis of severe anemia during pregnancy when the cause cannot be determined by any other means and for the investigation of other hematologic abnormalities that arise de novo during the index pregnancy.

Management Options

Prenatal

PROPHYLACTIC IRON SUPPLEMENTATION

Iron supplementation is used to prophylactically treat women with low iron stores or those at risk for low iron levels in pregnancy. Women with iron deficiency anemia are a different group and they require treatment doses of iron (discussed later).

Iron supplementation in pregnancy is controversial. Despite increased iron absorption from the gastrointestinal tract,[31] physiologic iron requirements in pregnancy often are not met by diet alone. In addition, many women enter pregnancy with depleted iron stores. The goal of prophylactic iron administration is to maintain maternal iron stores during the time of increased physiologic iron demand; it may also prevent anemia in infancy.[15] Studies found no improvement in maternal hemoglobin levels with iron prophylaxis, and it does not appear to benefit fetal growth or pregnancy outcome.[32] According to the

Cochrane library database, routine supplementation with iron or iron and folate had no detectable effect on substantive measures of fetal or maternal outcome.[33,34]

Other studies suggested that iron supplementation improves maternal iron status and increases neonatal iron reserves, preventing iron deficiency in the first year of life.[35] In pregnant women who did not receive supplementation, iron deficiency persisted many months after delivery.[36,37] Iron supplementation may prevent reduced or absent iron stores after pregnancy and reduce the risk of iron deficiency in subsequent pregnancies.[38]

Iron supplementation has few adverse effects. The dosage is generally low enough to avoid the gastrointestinal side effects seen with treatment doses. Iron supplements may interfere with the absorption of other trace elements, such as zinc.[39] Zinc depletion may be associated with fetal growth restriction.[40] A study of the effects of oral iron supplementation on zinc and magnesium levels during pregnancy concluded that decreases in the concentration of these elements were physiologic and unaffected by iron supplementation.[41]

High maternal hemoglobin concentrations are associated with poor pregnancy outcome.[42,43] This has led to concerns about iron prophylaxis. However, iron supplementation in iron-replete women does not increase hemoglobin level.[44] In iron-replete pregnancies, the hemoglobin concentration is largely dependent on the increase in plasma volume. Ineffective plasma volume expansion increases the rate of poor pregnancy outcome.

The other concern about iron prophylaxis is that excess iron can result in the production of free radicals and oxidative damage and may be implicated in cardiovascular disease and cancer.[45,46] Concerns about iron overloading in women with hemochromatosis have been raised. Approximately 12% of western white women are heterozygous for the common mutation of the hemochromatosis gene, and 0.5% are homozygous. A recent study of hemochromatosis and iron stores in pregnancy suggested that heterozygosity for the hemochromatosis mutation did not affect iron storage levels in reproductive-age women. One woman in the study who had markedly reduced iron stores was homozygous for the gene.[47]

Iron supplementation can be given on a selective or routine basis. Selective administration is appropriate for women with low or depleted iron stores, usually based on ferritin levels in early pregnancy. Ferritin cutoff levels for action vary between publications. A serum ferritin level less than 50 μg/L in early pregnancy is an indication for iron supplements. Some groups further stratify the starting time of these supplements, depending on ferritin levels.[48]

This approach avoids unnecessary supplementation in women with adequate iron stores. It identifies those who are at risk for iron depletion and anemia and targets these women with prophylactic or treatment doses of iron. The need for routine iron supplementation is debatable in western countries, but supplementation is recommended in nonindustrialized countries.[49,50] Various official bodies made recommendations for routine iron supplementation. The World Health Organization recommends universal oral iron supplementation with 60 mg elemental iron daily for 6 months in pregnancy in areas where the prevalence of iron deficiency is less than 40%. In areas where the prevalence is greater than 40%, the recommendation is to continue supplementation for 3 months postpartum.[51] The Centers for Disease Control and Prevention recommends supplementation with 30 mg elemental iron daily, as does the American College of Obstetricians and Gynecologists.[52,53] Some consider universal supplementation a practical and cost-effective approach.[32,54] The debate is ongoing, and the decision to choose universal or selective prophylaxis depends on the prevalence of iron deficiency in the obstetric population served, along with nutritional, economic, and social factors.

Prevention of iron deficiency also requires education about diet. Dietary iron has two forms, heme and non-heme iron. Heme iron is the most bioavailable form of iron in the diet and comes from food containing heme molecules, essentially animal meat, viscera, and blood. Non-heme iron is obtained from cereals, vegetables, milk, and eggs. Absorption of non-heme iron is enhanced by ascorbic acid, proteins, and heme, and inhibited by phytates, tea, coffee, and calcium. Many countries now fortify food products with iron compounds.[55] In nonindustrialized countries, other actions to prevent iron deficiency include iron prophylaxis in nonpregnant women[51] and treatment of hookworm infestation.[56]

Prophylaxis of iron deficiency is generally provided with oral iron. Various iron salts are available in tablet or syrup form (ferrous fumarate, gluconate, sulfate, and succinate). The elemental iron content of the different salts varies slightly. Compound preparations with folic acid are available, as are modified-release preparations, which release iron into the gastrointestinal tract slowly. However, these preparations may carry iron past the first part of the duodenum, where absorption is optimal, to areas of the gut where iron absorption is poor.

The frequency of oral dosing with iron supplementation has been questioned. Intermittent weekly or twice-weekly dosing schedules are as effective as daily dosing schedules.[57–59] In nonindustrialized countries, intermittent intramuscular iron dextran injections are used to ensure compliance and maintenance of adequate iron stores.[60] Compliance is a major problem with iron supplementation and may be as low as 36%.[61] In oral intermittent iron supplementation, compliance may be an even larger issue than with daily dosing schedules.[62] Iron-rich natural mineral water may be an acceptable alternative to oral iron prophylaxis. For example, Spatone Iron-Plus contains ferrous sulfate 0.20 mg/mL, which is highly bioavailable and maintains ferritin levels more effectively than placebo.[63]

MANAGEMENT OF IRON DEFICIENCY

Iron deficiency anemia is usually treated with oral iron preparations. The oral dose of elemental iron required to treat iron deficiency is 100 to 200 mg daily. Ferrous sulfate 200 mg three times daily is equivalent to 195 mg elemental iron daily. Many iron preparations are available, and no scientific evidence suggests that one brand is superior. Treatment doses of iron should continue until hemoglobin normalizes and should be followed with prophylactic or maintenance doses until 3 months postpartum to ensure that iron stores are replenished. Side effects with oral iron are common. Iron salts cause gastrointestinal irritation, with dose-related nausea and epigastric discomfort. Altered bowel habits (constipation or diarrhea) and abdominal cramping are common and have a less clear dose relationship. If side effects occur, reducing the dose or taking the tablets before meals (absorption can be reduced up to 50% if the dose is taken with meals) may help. Alternative iron salts can be tried, but tolerance is often related to reducing the dose of elemental iron. The addition of laxatives should overcome problems with constipation. The response to treatment doses of elemental iron is rapid. Reticulocyte counts increase within 5 to 10 days of initiation, and hemoglobin should rise 0.8 g/dL/wk (1.0 g/dL/wk in nonpregnant women). If no clinical or hematologic response is seen after 3 to 4 weeks of oral iron therapy, diagnostic reevaluation is required. Patients who do not respond to oral iron should be evaluated for ongoing blood loss, concomitant infection, additional hematinic deficiency, noncompliance, and other causes of anemia.

Parenteral iron therapy can be administered intravenously as an infusion or injection and also intramuscularly. It has no advantage over oral therapy if oral iron is well tolerated and absorbed. The response rate to parenteral iron is similar to that with oral preparations.[64] The advantage of parenteral therapy over oral therapy is the certainty of its administration.[65] Parenteral iron is given when oral iron therapy is unsuccessful because of patient intolerance, noncompliance, or malabsorption. Parenteral forms of iron include iron dextran and iron sucrose. Iron dextran is a complex of ferric hydroxide that contains 50 mg/mL iron and can be given intravenously. Dosage is calculated according to body weight and iron deficit. A small test dose is given, and the patient is observed for 1 hour for evidence of anaphylaxis. If the test dose is tolerated, the total dose can be administered in a 0.9% sodium chloride infusion over several hours. The product is licensed in the United Kingdom in the second and third trimesters but contraindicated in patients with a history of allergy. Anaphylactic reactions have been reported, and facilities for cardiopulmonary resuscitation must be available when these drugs are administered. Patients require close monitoring during and after administration, and treatment should be given in a hospital setting.

Iron dextran is now also available by deep intramuscular injections. Total dosage is calculated according to body weight and iron deficit. It is administered as a series of undiluted injections of up to 100 mg iron each. As with the intravenous preparation, anaphylactic emergency treatment should be available.

Preparations of iron sucrose complex contain 20 mg/mL iron and used in pregnancy as 5- to 10-mL aliquots up to three times per week in the second and third trimesters.[67]

Blood transfusions are rarely indicated in pregnant women with iron deficiency anemia. With vigilant antenatal care and appropriate iron prophylaxis and treatment, severe anemia should not be detected late in pregnancy. If a woman has severe anemia beyond 36 weeks' gestation and there is not time to achieve a reasonable hemoglobin concentration before delivery, blood transfusion is considered.

Recombinant human erythropoietin has also been used in difficult cases. Most experience has been with Jehovah's Witnesses.

Treatment of iron deficiency anemia in pregnancy was the subject of a recent Cochrane review.[68] Of 54 identified studies, only 5 met the inclusion criteria. Most studies evaluated laboratory outcome data rather than clinical outcome and did not address the question of whether treatment of iron deficiency anemia alters maternal or neonatal outcome. The review concluded that it was not possible to give evidence-based guidelines for the treatment of iron deficiency anemia in pregnancy.

Labor and Delivery

There are no specific recommendations for the management of iron-deficient patients during labor. Crossmatching should be carried out for women who are anemic on admission for labor. Blood transfusion may be necessary if significant blood loss occurs because these women have little reserve to tolerate bleeding.

Postnatal

As the physiologic effects of pregnancy diminish, hemoglobin levels rise during the puerperium. Patients who have clear evidence of iron deficiency anemia should continue oral supplementation for at least 3 months.

ANEMIA: FOLATE DEFICIENCY

Folic acid, together with iron, has assumed a central role in the nutrition of pregnancy. At a cellular level, folic acid is reduced first to dihydrofolate and then to tetrahydrofolate, which is fundamental to cell growth and division, through linkage with L-carbon fragments. The more active a tissue is in reproduction and growth, the more dependent it is on the efficient turnover and supply of folate coenzymes.

Maternal Risks

Megaloblastic anemia in pregnancy is nearly always secondary to folate deficiency. Plasma folate levels decrease as pregnancy advances, reaching approximately half of nonpregnant values at term.[24] Explanations for the reduction in folate levels include reduced dietary folate intake because of loss of appetite,[69] increased plasma clearance of folate by the kidneys (believed to play a minor role),[70, 71] transfer of folate from the mother to the fetus (approximately 800 μg at term), and uterine hypertrophy and expanded red cell mass. As pregnancy proceeds, increased folate catabolites are excreted in maternal urine.[72]

Worldwide, folic acid deficiency may complicate one third of pregnancies. The incidence is higher in multiple pregnancies and closely spaced successive gestations.[73] Folate is readily available in most diets. Good sources include broccoli, Brussel sprouts, and spinach. Folate is often lost in the cooking process. It is heat-labile and rapidly destroyed by boiling or steaming.

Body stores of folate are found predominantly in the liver and total approximately 10 mg. When body reserves of folate are low, stores last approximately 4 to 5 months before symptomatic anemia develops. A survey of reports from the United Kingdom suggests that the incidence of folate deficiency is 0.2% to 5.0%, but more women have megaloblastic changes in their bone marrow that are not suspected based on examination of peripheral blood alone.[74] The incidence of megaloblastic anemia in other parts of the world is considerably greater and is believed to reflect the nutritional standards of the population. There is controversy about the requirement for folate, particularly during pregnancy. In the past, the World Health Organization recommended daily folate intake of up to 800 μg in the prenatal period and 600 μg during lactation.[75] Current recommendations advise folic acid intake of 400 μg daily with 60 mg iron for 6 months during pregnancy and continuing for 3 months postpartum in areas of the world with poor nutrition.[51]

The maternal risk of folate deficiency appears to be megaloblastic anemia. This condition usually has an insidious onset, with gradually progressive symptoms and signs of anemia. It can be abolished with routine use of folic acid supplements during pregnancy.[76]

Fetal Risks

The risk of megaloblastic anemia is increased in the neonate of a folate-deficient mother, especially if delivery is preterm. Data also suggest an association between periconceptional folic acid deficiency and harelip, cleft palate, and most important, neural tube defects.[77,78] This subject was well reviewed in the past,[79] and the association between periconceptional folate deficiency and the recurrence of neural tube defects was confirmed in a multicenter controlled trial of prepregnancy folate supplementation.[80] Periconceptional folic acid reduces the recurrence of neural tube defects.[81]

A large randomized controlled trial in Hungary showed that periconceptional supplementation with 800 μg folic acid in a combined vitamin preparation prevented the first occurrence of neural tube defects.[82]

It is not known how folate supplements reduce the incidence of neural tube defects. Women who have children with this disorder do not appear to differ hematologically from those who have children who are unaffected. Terathanasia (selective spontaneous abortion of fetuses with birth defects) may explain the protective effect of folic acid supplements,[83] but many authorities dispute this.

Diagnosis

Outside of pregnancy, the hallmark of megaloblastic hemopoiesis is macrocytosis. This can be more difficult to interpret in pregnancy when there is a physiologic increase in red cell size and the possibility of a masking iron deficiency anemia. Examination of the blood film with oval macrocytes and hypersegmented neutrophil nuclei can provide useful diagnostic clues. The reticulocyte count is also low in relation to the hemoglobin. To diagnose folate deficiency, red cell folate assay is performed. Plasma folate levels fluctuate substantially from day to day, and postprandial increases are noted, limiting the use of serum folate as a diagnostic test. Red cell folate is believed to give a better indication of overall body tissue levels. However, the turnover of red blood cells is slow, and there is a delay before significant reductions in the folate concentration of red cells is evident. Patients who have a low red cell folate concentration at the beginning of pregnancy have megaloblastic anemia in the third trimester.[24] Folate deficiency in pregnancy is not always accompanied by significant hematologic changes. In the absence of changes, megaloblastic hemopoiesis is suspected when the expected response to adequate iron therapy is not achieved. Ultimately, the diagnosis of folate deficiency may depend on bone marrow examination and the finding of large erythroblasts and giant, abnormally shaped metamyelocytes. This test is usually reserved for patients with pancytopenia rather than isolated anemia.

Management Options

Prepregnancy

As with other anemias, a careful diagnostic evaluation should be undertaken, followed by prompt therapy before conception. The risks (described in earlier and later sections) should be discussed before pregnancy, and dietary advice about folate-rich foods should be given. Women who are contemplating pregnancy should be advised to take folate supplements 400 μg daily.[84,85] Targeted fortification of food is under consideration in the United Kingdom and United States. The plan includes adding folate to basic foods in an effort to ensure that women of reproductive age have adequate dietary folate to prevent neural tube defects.[86]

Prenatal

PROPHYLAXIS

The case for giving prophylactic folate supplementation throughout pregnancy is strong,[87,88] particularly in countries where nutritional and megaloblastic anemia is common. Folate should be given in combination with iron supplements. The folic acid content must be approximately 200 to 300 μg daily. The concern about routine folate supplementation is the risk to a woman with undiagnosed vitamin B_{12} deficiency. Folate treatment can worsen neuropathy in patients with vitamin B_{12} deficiency. The risk is low in pregnancy, and patients with severe vitamin B_{12} deficiency are usually infertile. Pernicious anemia is generally a disease of older people. Not one case of subacute combined degeneration of the spinal cord was reported among the thousands of women receiving folate supplements during pregnancy.[24]

MANAGEMENT OF ESTABLISHED FOLATE DEFICIENCY

Severe megaloblastic anemia is uncommon in the United Kingdom and the United States, largely as a result of prophylaxis and prompt treatment. Once megaloblastic hematopoiesis is established, treatment of folic acid deficiency is more difficult, presumably as a result of megaloblastic changes in the gastrointestinal tract that impair absorption. If the diagnosis is made prenatally, initial treatment is with folic acid 5 mg once daily continued for several weeks postpartum.

ANTICONVULSANTS AND FOLIC ACID

Outside of pregnancy, folate deficiency can develop in patients who take anticonvulsants. Folate status is further compromised in pregnancy.[87] Interference with epilepsy control by folate supplementation may be overestimated.[89] Anticonvulsant therapy is associated with an increased incidence of congenital abnormalities,[90] prematurity, and low birth weight.[91] Hence, folate supplements should be given to all pregnant epileptic women who take anticonvulsants.

DISORDERS THAT MAY AFFECT FOLATE REQUIREMENTS

Women with hemolytic anemia, particularly hereditary hemolytic conditions, such as hemoglobinopathy and red cell membrane and enzyme disorders, require extra folate supplements from early pregnancy onward, if megaloblastic anemia is to be avoided. The recommended supplementation is 5 to 10 mg orally daily. Anemia as a result of thalassemia trait is not strictly caused by hemolysis, but by ineffective erythropoiesis. However, the increased abortive marrow turnover results in folate depletion, and these women would probably benefit from routine administration of folic acid, 5.0 mg orally daily, from early pregnancy onward.

Labor and Delivery

There are no specific management recommendations for folate-associated anemia during labor and delivery, as long as the patient is hemodynamically stable and blood replacement therapy is available, if needed.

Postnatal

In the 6 weeks after delivery, indices of folate metabolism return to nonpregnant values. However, if folate deficiency develops and remains untreated in pregnancy, it may be seen clinically for the first time in the puerperium. Lactation provides an added folate stress. A folate content of 5 μg/100 mL human milk and a yield of 500 mL daily implies a loss of 25 μg folate daily in breast milk. Red cell folate levels in lactating women are significantly lower than those in infants during the first year of life.

SUMMARY OF MANAGEMENT OPTIONS

Iron and Folate Deficiency Anemia

Management Option	Quality of Evidence	Strength of Recommendation	References
At any Time			
Studies if hemoglobin <10.5 g/dL (opinions vary; ranges 10.0–11.0 g/dL) • Complete blood count • Blood film • Red cell indices • Reticulocyte count • Iron status (e.g., ferritin) • Red cell folate • Serum vitamin B_{12}	–	GPP	–

Continued

SUMMARY OF MANAGEMENT OPTIONS

Iron and Folate Deficiency Anemia *(Continued)*

Management Option	Quality of Evidence	Strength of Recommendation	References
At any Time *(Continued)*			
• Other studies as indicated by clinical findings and laboratory results			
Prepregnancy			
Dietary advice and iron therapy to ensure satisfactory hemoglobin status before pregnancy	–	GPP	–
Public health measures to prevent periconceptual folate deficiency	Ia	A	82
Use of folic acid periconceptually reduces the risk of neural tube defects	Ia	A	82,91
Prenatal			
Prophylactic use of iron or folate is controversial in industrialized countries, but important for pregnant women in developing countries to maintain or increase predelivery hemoglobin levels	Ia	A	33,34
When iron or folate is prescribed, selective use is better than routine use if women can have their hemoglobin status assessed and followed up reliably	Ia	A	33,34
Oral iron preparations are preferred; different compounds are used to minimize side effects	–	GPP	–
Side effects related to dose and weekly oral iron administration may be an alternative to improve compliance without losing efficacy	Ib	A	58,59
Parenteral iron therapy is given if oral iron treatment is unsuccessful because of noncompliance, poor follow-up, or poor absorption	IIa	B	65
Blood transfusion may be considered in patients with severe symptomatic anemia close to delivery	–	GPP	–
Folate prophylaxis with anticonvulsants	–	GPP	–
Continue routine oral folate therapy in cases of autoimmune hemolytic anemia	–	GPP	–
Parenteral folate therapy can be given if deficiency is severe	–	GPP	–
Labor and Delivery			
Crossmatch blood if anemia is severe	–	GPP	–
Postnatal			
Continue iron therapy for patients with iron deficiency	–	GPP	–

ANEMIA: VITAMIN B_{12} DEFICIENCY

Muscle, red cell, and serum vitamin B_{12} concentrations decrease during pregnancy.[92,93] Women who smoke tend to have lower serum vitamin B_{12} levels, which may account for the positive correlation between birth weight and serum levels in women without deficiency.

Maternal and Fetal Risks

Vitamin B_{12} absorption is unaltered in pregnancy,[94] but tissue uptake is increased under the influence of estrogens. Oral contraceptives also cause a decrease in serum vitamin B_{12} levels. This decrease in pregnancy is related to preferential transfer of absorbed vitamin B_{12} to the fetus at the expense of maintaining maternal serum concentration. The vitamin B_{12}-binding capacity of plasma increases in pregnancy because of the increased levels of transcobalamin II, which is derived from the liver and affects vitamin B_{12} transport. Cord blood serum vitamin B_{12} levels are higher than maternal vitamin B_{12} levels. Pregnancy does not greatly affect maternal vitamin B_{12} stores. Adult stores are 3000 μg or more, and stores in newborns are approximately 50 μg. Minimal amounts of vitamin B_{12} are required for fetal development, which may account for the few fetal problems seen in pregnancies complicated by vitamin B_{12} deficiency. A deficiency syndrome is described in breast-fed neonates of mothers with significant vitamin B_{12} deficiency. It is usually apparent by 6 months of age and is characterized by failure to thrive, developmental regression, and anemia.[95] Addisonian pernicious anemia is unusual during the reproductive years and is usually associated with infertility. Pregnancy is likely only if the deficiency is corrected.

Dietary deficiency of vitamin B_{12} is possible in strict vegans who consume no animal products. Other disorders associated with vitamin B_{12} deficiency include tropical and nontropical sprue, Crohn's disease, and surgical resection of the distal ileum.

Management Options

Prepregnancy

Women with vitamin B_{12} deficiency should have their therapy optimized and their anemia corrected before they become pregnant. This approach may be needed to restore fertility.

Prenatal

The recommended intake of vitamin B_{12} is 2.0 μg daily in the nonpregnant patient and 3.0 μg daily during pregnancy.[96] This intake is met by almost any diet that contains animal products. Strict vegans, who do not eat any animal-derived substances, may have a deficient intake of vitamin B_{12}, and this type of diet should be supplemented in pregnancy.

Difficulties can arise when interpreting vitamin B_{12} levels measured in pregnancy because many women have lower values than those quoted as the normal range outside of pregnancy.[97] This decline in vitamin B_{12} levels is not believed to represent a true deficiency. There is a minimal increase in vitamin B_{12} requirements in pregnancy, and this is unlikely to cause a significant decrease in vitamin B_{12} levels. Interestingly, supplementation in pregnancy does not prevent the progressive decrease in vitamin B_{12} levels.[98] These levels return to normal in the puerperium. Care must be taken in the interpretation of vitamin B_{12} levels in pregnancy. If deficiency is suspected, the etiology should be considered. A Schilling test is contraindicated because of the risks of radiation exposure. Intrinsic factor antibodies may be useful if the results are positive. Therapy is instituted empirically if there is clinical concern, especially if neurologic findings are consistent with vitamin B_{12} deficiency. The earliest symptoms are numbness and paraesthesia of the fingers and toes, followed by weakness, ataxia, and poor concentration. Patients may have changes in mental status that range from forgetfulness to dementia and possible psychosis.

Treatment of vitamin B_{12} deficiency is generally parenteral because patients usually have absorptive problems. Cyanocobalamin or hydroxycobalamin 1 mg is given three times a week for 2 weeks, and then every 3 months. In patients who have neurologic involvement, the dosage is higher. These patients are given 1 mg on alternate days until no further improvement is noted, and then 1 mg every 2 months. Oral vitamin B_{12} can be used in patients with dietary deficiency.

Labor, Delivery, and Postnatal

There are no specific measures for patients with genuine vitamin B_{12} deficiency, apart from continuing maintenance therapy.

SUMMARY OF MANAGEMENT OPTIONS

Vitamin B_{12} Deficiency

Management Option	Quality of Evidence	Strength of Recommendation	References
Prepregnancy			
Deficiency is rare	–	GPP	–
Prenatal			
Continue treatment if it was instituted before conception	–	GPP	–
Consider oral supplementation and other components for strict vegans and women with diets deficient in animal protein	–	GPP	–
Consider checking intrinsic factor antibodies if the diet is adequate	–	GPP	–
Labor and Delivery			
Continue treatment if already instituted	–	GPP	–
Postnatal			
Continue treatment if already instituted; if the patient is not receiving treatment, check vitamin B_{12} levels postpartum	–	GPP	–

HEMOGLOBINOPATHIES

Hemoglobinopathies are inherited disorders of hemoglobin. Hemoglobin is composed of heme (a combination of iron and porphyrin) and four globin chains. The type of globin chain determines many of the characteristics of the hemoglobin. Several types of globin chains are present at different times in embryonic development, in fetal life, and through to adulthood (Fig. 39–1 and Table 39–1). Abnormalities of the quantity or quality of the globin chains produced result in conditions known as hemoglobinopathies.

Hemoglobinopathies can be divided into two subgroups:

- Sickling disorders, which are qualitative abnormalities. An amino acid substitution in an α-globin or a β-globin chain results in the synthesis of an abnormal hemoglobin. Many types of hemoglobin can sickle.
- Thalassemia syndromes are usually quantitative problems of globin chain synthesis. They result in impaired production and imbalance of globin chains. α-Thalassemia is caused by reduced α-chain production, and β-thalassemia is caused by reduced or abnormal β-chain production.

Women with major sickling and thalassemic conditions require specialized multidisciplinary team management preconception and throughout pregnancy. Timely screening programs must be in place to identify women and their partners who are carriers of these conditions and couples who are at risk for having an infant affected with a major hemoglobinopathy. The chance of being a carrier is dependent on ancestry. Tables are available that show the prevalence of traits in different countries and ethnic groups.[99]

It is useful to be aware of the changes in complete blood count that are caused by these traits and the effects of superimposed conditions, including the physiologic changes of pregnancy.

TABLE 39–1

Composition of Adult Hemoglobin

FEATURE	HEMOGLOBIN A	HEMOGLOBIN F	HEMOGLOBIN A_2
Structure	$\alpha_2\beta_2$	$\alpha_2\gamma_2$	$\alpha_2\delta_2$
Normal (%)	96–98	0.5–0.8	1.5–3.7

Sickle Cell Syndromes

More than 300 abnormal (variant) hemoglobins are recognized. These qualitative defects are often caused by a single amino acid substitution in the globin chain. Sickle cell disease caused by homozygosity of hemoglobin S (i.e., HbSS) is the most common sickling disorder. It is caused by a point mutation in the β-globin gene on chromosome 11 that produces an amino acid change at position 6, changing valine to glutamic acid. This enhances the polymerization of hemoglobin S in the deoxygenated state and causes increased red cell rigidity and sickling. Increased blood viscosity and tissue hypoxia occur as sickled cells occlude the microcirculation. Clinical consequences of sickling include the following:

- Vaso-occlusive crises (micro- and macro-infarcts, leading to a painful crisis and organ damage)
- Anemic crises as a result of severe hemolysis, red cell aplasia, or splenic sequestration
- Chest and girdle syndrome
- Neurologic events

Maternal and Fetal Risks

Sickling occurs in the homozygous condition (HbSS) or in compound heterozygous states (e.g., HbSC or HbS β-thalassemia, HbSD-Punjab, HbSE, HbSLepore,

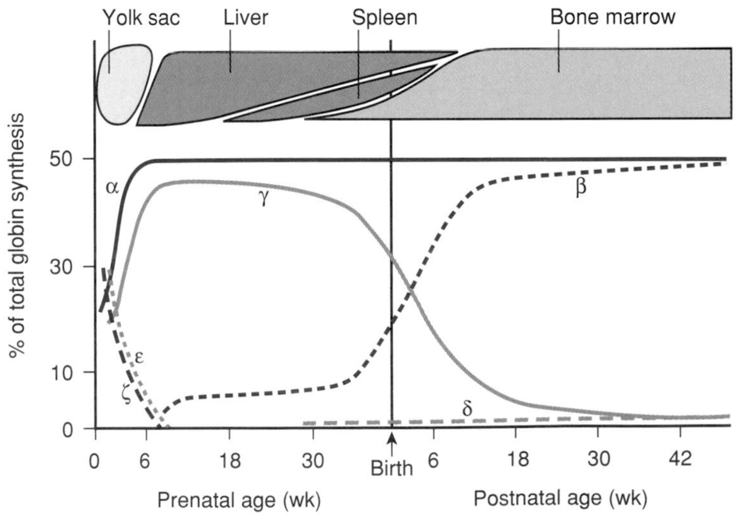

FIGURE 39–1
Production of different globin chains (From Hoffbrand AV, Pettit J: Essential Haematology, 3rd ed. Oxford, 1993, Blackwell, p 95.)

HbSO-Arab). Hemoglobin C, D-Punjab, E, and O-Arab are variant hemoglobins with mutations in the B globin gene. Hemoglobin Lepore is a variant hemoglobin that behaves like β-thalassemia.

The heterozygous state, or sickle cell trait (HbAS), is essentially a benign condition that is believed to have no particular antenatal sequelae. However, women with sickle cell trait are slightly more prone to renal papillary necrosis and urinary tract infection.[100] Their hemoglobin levels are similar to those of other pregnant women and should be managed similarly. Their sickle cell trait should be noted on their records, and the anesthesiologist should be informed of this condition if a general anesthetic is required. A recent study showed an increased incidence of preeclampsia in women with sickle cell trait.[101] Women with sickle cell trait should be identified by antenatal hemoglobinopathy screening. The goal of screening is to detect pregnancies in which there is a risk of a major hemoglobinopathy. Partners must be tested as well. If the partner of a woman with sickle cell trait also carries the trait, there is a 1 in 4 chance that the offspring will be affected by homozygous sickle cell disease. These couples require counseling and the opportunity for antenatal diagnosis. Termination is an option if a fetus is diagnosed as having a major hemoglobinopathy. This should be fully discussed with parents prior to prenatal diagnosis.

Pediatricians must be alerted to the possibility of sickle cell disease in neonates because antipneumococcal vaccines can now be given from 2 months of age and infants with sickle cell disease require long-term prophylactic penicillin treatment and regular evaluation.

People with major sickling disorders start life relatively protected from crises for 3 to 6 months because of the ongoing production of fetal hemoglobin. When hemoglobin A production becomes predominant, chronic hemolytic anemia develops. The severity and complications of the disease vary widely between patients. Many have debilitating chronic disease and frequent crises that require hospital admission. Others appear to be free of complications but have progressive organ damage. The life expectancy of these patients is still 25 to 30 years less than that of the general population, even in the developed world, with access to medical care.[102]

There are increased risks involved in pregnancy for the mother with sickle cell disease and her fetus.[103] These risks are not so great as to prohibit pregnancy. The importance of good prenatal care, with a multidisciplinary team, must be emphasized.

Maternal risks include exacerbated sickle cell disease phenomena,[104] such as anemia, vaso-occlusion, ischemic injury, and organ damage as a result of the physiologic stress of pregnancy. These patients have greater susceptibility to infection (chest and urinary tract), hypertensive disorders of pregnancy, and thromboembolic complications.

Risks to the fetus include increased frequency of miscarriage, intrauterine growth retardation, preterm labor, and premature delivery.[105,106] Perinatal morbidity and mortality rates vary widely in different regions of the world[107–109] but are higher than in the general poulation.

Diagnosis and Management Options

PREPREGNANCY

Before an affected woman becomes pregnant, a number of issues should be addressed.

Sickle Cell Disease. The frequency and management of crises outside of pregnancy is a useful starting point and may indicate the likelihood of crises throughout pregnancy. The patient's transfusion history and red cell antibody values should be documented. Discussion of hydroxyurea is important. Hydroxyurea is a disease-modifying drug that increases hemoglobin F, improves red cell hydration, and decreases the rate of polymerization of hemoglobin S. Its use decreases the frequency of crises.[110] However, it should be discontinued in women who are planning to conceive because it is teratogenic in animal models. Although there is little information about its effect on the human fetus, there are case reports in which hydroxyurea was taken throughout pregnancy with no reported adverse fetal effects.[111,112]

Contraception. Discussion of contraception and pregnancy planning is useful in women who have a chronic debilitating disease. They should be reassured about contraceptive choices. None are excluded on the grounds of sickle cell disease. The risks of pregnancy outweigh those of contraception.

Maternal and Fetal Complications. The patient's obstetric history is important, including a discussion of maternal and fetal risks associated with sickle cell disease. Strategies to reduce these risks require discussion, as does the part the women plays in reducing risk. Patients should be told that active prenatal management significantly affects pregnancy outcome, and the importance of attending visits should be emphasized.

Multidisciplinary Team Approach. The community sickle cell service and midwifery team, along with hospital obstetric, hematology, anesthetic, and pediatric teams, play an important role in the care of the pregnant woman and fetus.

Partner's Hemoglobinopathy Status. It is important to establish the partner's hemoglobinopathy status, ideally, before pregnancy. This information facilitates appropriate, timely, and nondirective counseling about antenatal diagnosis.

PRENATAL

These women should be seen early in pregnancy. Ideally, they should be seen by an obstetrician with experience in this area and also by the hematology team. Partner screening should be carried out if it has not been done. A discussion about prenatal diagnosis should take place, if appropriate, and time should be taken to review the patient's obstetric history and history of sickle cell disease, including a drug history and the typical management of crises.

Laboratory evaluation should include a complete blood count, hemoglobin electrophoresis (if not previously done or available), reticulocyte count, ferritin level, folate level, urea and electrolyte levels, liver function tests, blood typing, and red cell antibody screen. The red cell antibody screen serves two purposes: to identify women whose fetuses and newborns may be at risk for hemolysis because of red cell antibodies and to ensure screening for the most common minor red cell antigens so that phenotypically matched blood will be available for transfusion. This is especially important because the donor population differs in ethnic origin, carries different minor cell antigens, and may sensitize this group of patients. As a result, it may be difficult to obtain suitable blood for transfusion. Blood tests should be performed to determine hepatitis A, B, and C, HIV, and rubella antibody status. Urine dipstick and culture allow identification and treatment of women with asymptomatic bacteruria. This group is more susceptible to urinary tract infections.

People with homozygous sickle cell disease may have a hemoglobin concentration of 5 to 12 g/dL, but concentrations are typically 6 to 10 g/dL. Hemoglobin S has a lower affinity for oxygen, and symptoms of anemia are decreased by the increased delivery of oxygen to the tissues. The reticulocyte count is elevated in patients with sickle cell disease, reflecting increased red cell turnover. The bilirubin level also indicates the rate of hemolysis. Other abnormal liver function test results may indicate chololithiasis or acute cholecystitis as a result of chronic hemolysis or chronic hepatitis.

Pregnancy outcome appears to be similar in women who undergo prophylactic transfusion compared with those who undergo selective transfusion for clinical reasons.[113] No improvement in obstetric outcome was seen in a retrospective multicenter study in the United Kingdom.[114]

There is debate about the use of blood transfusions throughout pregnancy. Prophylactic versus selective blood transfusions was the subject of a recent Cochrane review.[115] This review found that there was not enough evidence to reach conclusions about the use of prophylactic blood transfusions. The development of atypical red cell antibodies is a real concern.[116] Transfusion is generally given before anesthesia or as an exchange procedure in severe crises, but no data suggest that transfusions should be given prophylactically.

Red cell indices in patients with sickle cell disease alone should be normal, but low MCV and MCH may indicate iron deficiency or an associated thalassemia trait. The blood film shows variable numbers of sickle cells and features of hyposplenism (Howell-Jolly bodies, target cells, and increased platelet and white cell counts). Hemoglobin electrophoresis and high-performance liquid chromatography can separate out the various hemoglobins and allow detection and characterization of variant hemoglobins. In homozygous sickle cell disease, hemoglobins S, F, and A_2 are seen. Hemoglobin S is usually the predominant hemoglobin, making up 90% to 95% of total hemoglobin. Hemoglobin A is absent. In compound heterozygous states, other hemoglobins are found, except in hemoglobin S β-thalassemia, in which hemoglobin S level is lower than that in homozygotes.

A sickle solubility test is a quick screening test for sickling hemoglobin, but it does not elucidate the type or quantity of sickling hemoglobin. In other words, it does not distinguish between a person with homozygous sickle cell disease and a person with sickle cell trait.

The antenatal care plan should be outlined, with a discussion of the risks for both mother and fetus and strategies to reduce these risks. The patient should be advised to avoid precipitating factors that may cause sickle crises, including education about the signs and symptoms of infection and appropriate analgesics.

Return visits are recommended every 2 to 3 weeks to allow early detection of maternal or fetal complications. The purpose of these visits is to monitor the course of the pregnancy, with regular monitoring of blood pressure and urine and assessment of fetal growth and development at appropriate intervals. Patients with sickle cell disease also should be asked about pain and crises and should undergo laboratory assessment, including complete blood counts, reticulocyte counts, and bilirubin measurements.

COMPLICATIONS OF SICKLE CELL DISEASE

Vaso-occlusive or Painful Crisis.[117,118] Crises occur when rigid sickle cells obstruct blood vessels in the microvasculature. This obstruction leads to tissue hypoxia, infarction, and pain. It is the most common type of crisis and the reason for most hospital admissions. Factors that may precipitate or exacerbate a crisis include cold, infection, dehydration, exercise, and stress. The pain is usually bony, although it may occur in the chest or abdomen. Systemic markers include low-grade fever, tachycardia, and mild leukocytosis.

As a result of sickling in the splenic circulation, most patients become hyposplenic at a young age, increasing their susceptibility to encapsulated organisms, such as *Streptococcus pneumoniae* and *Haemophilus influenzae*. This increased susceptibility is the rationale for pneumococcal, *H. influenzae* B, and meningococcal vaccination and prophylactic penicillin administration.

Treatment and evaluation are as for nonpregnant women. Most pain occurs in the third trimester and the postpartum period. Underlying precipitants of pain, such as infection and toxemia, should be sought. The management hinges on good rehydration, with careful fluid balance and adequate analgesia. The pain normally requires opioid analgesia as an infusion or patient-controlled analgesia. Nonsteroidal anti-inflammatory drugs are a useful adjunct but should be avoided in the second half of pregnancy because of the risk of patent ductus arteriosus.

Oxygen supplementation and intravenous antibiotics covering encapsulated organisms may be required. If intravenous antibiotics are not required, penicillin prophylaxis should be ongoing. Folic acid supplementation (5 mg daily) also should be ongoing. The patient should be kept warm. All of the relevant teams must be involved, including obstetricians, hematologists, and obstetric anesthesiologists. In women who have frequent sickling crises and heavy narcotic use, fetal growth must be monitored carefully because of the risk of intrauterine growth retardation. Pediatricians must be made aware of the risk of opiate dependence in the newborn and the need for opiate tapering. Blood testing must be performed frequently. On admission, the patient should have a complete blood count, reticulocyte count, biochemistry testing, blood typing, blood cultures, arterial gases and/or pulse oximetry. Potential sites of infection require culturing (e.g., throat swab, midstream urine, sputum, blood). Hemoglobin requires regular monitoring. Transfusion is generally given if hemoglobin is less than 5 g/dL. Review is required at regular intervals to assess the response to pain relief and look for evidence of infection, girdle or chest syndrome, splenic or hepatic sequestration, and complications of pregnancy, such as preeclampsia.

Acute Anemia. When a precipitate decrease in hemoglobin occurs, the differential diagnosis includes blood loss, bone marrow suppression secondary to infection, hyperhemolysis, and sequestration. Careful examination and basic blood tests are useful in determining the cause. A reticulocyte count will determine whether the bone marrow is responding appropriately to the anemia. If the count is low or absent, parvovirus B19 infection should be considered. This infection causes red cell aplasia, and transfusion is required. It can also cause miscarriage or hydrops, so careful fetal monitoring is required.

Prompt transfusion in splenic sequestration can be lifesaving when the decrease in hemoglobin is precipitous and hazardous for the mother and fetus. Patients have acute abdominal pain, with rapid enlargement of the spleen. This situation is rare because most patients with homozygous sickle cell disease are hyposplenic. Approximately 5% have splenomegaly, but it is more common in compound heterozygote sickling states, such as HbSC and HbS β^+ thalassemia.

Acute Chest Syndrome.[119] Acute chest syndrome is a form of acute lung injury that is distinct from pneumonia. It is believed to be caused by fat emboli from the bone marrow along with red cell sequestration. It does not resolve with antibiotics but may become secondarily infected. It usually causes clinical or radiologic evidence of consolidation, with elevated temperature, cough, and pleuritic chest pain. Hypoxemia, which may be severe, and leukocytosis are also features. Treatment is the same as for a crisis, as discussed earlier, with early recourse to top up or exchange transfusion, depending on the baseline hemoglobin. Oxygen saturation and blood gas values must be monitored carefully, and antibiotics and bronchodilators are useful. An intensive care setting is often the best place to monitor these patients.

Neurologic Events. Neurologic events are common in patients with sickle cell disease. Thrombotic cerebrovascular accidents and seizures are the main concern. The differential diagnosis (including metabolic disturbances, toxemia, subarachnoid or intracerebral hemorrhage, ischemic stroke, cerebral veneus thrombosis, meningitis, cerebral abscess, epilepsy, or tumor) must be considered, and studies may include neuroimaging, examination of the cerebrospinal fluid if fever is present, and assessment for toxemia. Sickle-related central nervous system events should be treated with exchange transfusion to reduce the sickle hemoglobin percentage to less than 30%. This value should be maintained by transfusions to keep hemoglobin levels between 10 and 11 g/dL.

LABOR AND DELIVERY

Close supervision is required during labor. The risk of sickle cell crisis in labor increases if the woman is dehydrated or has hypoxia, acidosis, or infection. Care should be taken to prevent these complications.

Labor is also a time of increased cardiac output, exacerbated by the pain of uterine contractions. Cardiac function may be reduced by chronic hypoxemia and long-standing anemia. Pain relief is important in reducing cardiac work, and epidural is particularly effective.[120] Prolonged labor should be avoided. The woman should be kept warm, well-hydrated, and oxygenated. Continuous intrapartum monitoring should take place. The timing and mode of delivery must be determined by obstetric factors.

Transfusion is considered if the hemoglobin is less than 8g/dL.[121]

Thromboprophylaxis is given to women who are immobilized or experiencing a sickle crisis at the time of delivery. Routine thromboprophylaxis for women with sickle cell disease is controversial. There are no randomized controlled trials, and efficacy has not been conclusively shown.

Patients who have cesarean delivery should have chest physiotherapy, and early mobilization is encouraged.

Cord blood can be sent to the laboratory for hemoglobinopathy screening. Those who interpret the results must be aware of the possibility of maternal contamination. Universal neonatal screening for sickle cell disorders has recently been introduced in England as part of the newborn blood spot test.

POSTPARTUM

The heightened risks of sickle crisis persist after delivery, and vigilance must be maintained. Adequate oxygenation and hydration must be ensured, and findings must be monitored closely for the first 24 hours. Patients must be monitored for infection and crises, and thromboprophylaxis may be considered, depending on the degree of mobility and individual risk assessment. Contraception can be discussed at this time (discussed earlier).

The results of neonatal screening and follow-up arrangements with the pediatrician should be confirmed before discharge.

SUMMARY OF MANAGEMENT OPTIONS

Sickle Cell Syndromes

Management Option	Quality of Evidence	Strength of Recommendation	References
Prepregnancy			
Counsel against conception until disease status is optimized; assess renal and liver function	–	GPP	–
Counsel about the risks of pregnancy	–	GPP	–
Screen partner; if the result is positive, counsel about prenatal diagnosis	–	GPP	–
Prenatal			
Hemoglobin electrophoresis screening of the entire population or high-risk groups	–	GPP	–
Screen partner; if the result is positive consider counseling and prenatal diagnosis			
Prompt treatment of crises (adequate hydration, oxygen, screening for infection) may include exchange transfusion	–	GPP	–
Prenatal fetal surveillance and tests for fetal well-being	–	GPP	–
Screen for: • Urinary infection • Hypertension or preeclampsia • Renal and liver function • Pathologic fetal growth and umbilical artery blood flow	–	GPP	–
Labor and Delivery			
Ensure adequate hydration	–	GPP	–
Avoid hypoxia	–	GPP	–
Continuous cardiotocography	–	GPP	–
Postnatal			
Use of prophylactic antibiotics is controversial	–	GPP	–
Maintain good hydration and oxygenation, especially for the first 24 hours	–	GPP	–
Contraceptive counseling	–	GPP	–
Testing of the neonate for hemoglobinopathies	–	GPP	–

Thalassemia Syndromes

Thalassemia syndromes are usually quantitative disorders of globin chain production that affect either the α- or the β-globin chain.

α-THALASSEMIA

There are normally two pairs (i.e., four) functional α-globin genes. If one or two of these genes are missing, the result is an α-thalassemia trait. The type of thalassemia trait is an important factor to consider when offering antenatal counseling and diagnosis. These traits are not detected on hemoglobin electrophoresis because no abnormal hemoglobin is made. In addition, there is neither excess nor lack of any normal hemoglobins.

Deletion of three α-globin genes results in hemoglobin H disease, a chronic hemolytic anemia, with normal life expectancy. This condition can be detected by hemoglobin electrophoresis.

In α-thalassemia major, there is no α-chain production and no synthesis of hemoglobin F, A, or A_2. Tetramers of fetal gamma chains (γ_4) form because no α chains are present. This condition is known as hemoglobin Barts. Patients have severe anemia, failure of oxygen delivery to tissues, cardiac failure, and abnormal organogenesis. The condition is incompatible with life and causes intrauterine hydrops. Serious obstetric complications often occur, including preeclampsia and delivery difficulties because of the large fetus and placenta. Experimental fetal treatment may be available if the condition is detected early in pregnancy. Antenatal screening for α-thalassemia is directed at preventing hemoglobin Barts hydrops. To prevent this condition, women and their partners who have a cis-(2) α-gene deletion (i.e., genotype- -/αα, or α_0-thalassemia trait) must be identified. These couples have a one in four chance of having a fetus with hydrops. In practice, these couples are identified on the basis of otherwise unexplained hypochromic, microcytic red cell indices. An MCH of less than 25 pg suggests the genotype - -/αα or - α/-α. Hemoglobin electrophoresis does not detect α-thalassemia traits, and definitive diagnosis requires DNA analysis. This diagnostic procedure is undertaken only if both the woman and her partner have indices and test results that suggest α_0-thalassemia trait. Persons particularly at risk for α_0-thalassemia trait are those of Chinese, Southeast Asian, and Mediterranean descent.

DIAGNOSIS AND MANAGEMENT OPTIONS

Prepregnancy. Women who have α_0-thalassemia trait should be identified before pregnancy so that they can be alerted to the one in four chance of having a hydropic fetus if their partner carries the same trait. Early screening of partners is strongly encouraged. If the woman and her partner are at risk, the possibility and techniques of antenatal diagnosis can be discussed. Women with hemoglobin H disease should be encouraged to take regular folate supplementation outside of pregnancy to meet the demands of increased bone marrow turnover. They may require transfusion to meet the demands of pregnancy. Partner screening specifically for α_0-thalassemia trait is an important aspect of management.

Prenatal. Prenatally, the main issues are antenatal diagnosis (if required) and maintenance of adequate hemoglobin. In women with indices that suggest α_0-thalassemia trait or hemoglobin H disease, partner carrier status should be sought early in pregnancy to determine risk, especially in affected racial groups. At-risk couples should be counseled about the risks and offered antenatal diagnosis.

In hemoglobin H disease, folate supplementation (5 mg daily) is recommended, and transfusion may be needed.

Labor, Delivery, and Postpartum. There are no specific management recommendations.

β-THALASSEMIA

MATERNAL AND FETAL RISKS

β-thalassemia has three phenotypic presentations: the trait, intermedia, and major.

β-thalassemia trait, or heterozygote state, is important to detect for antenatal screening purposes. It does not affect the mother's health, but causes hypochromic, microcytic red cell indices. Iron therapy must be based on hematinic measurements rather than the complete blood count.

Partner screening should be performed to determine the risk of having a child affected with a major hemoglobinopathy. If the partner carries a sickle cell trait, a β-thalassemia trait, or hemoglobin E, and the mother carries a β-thalassemia trait, there is a one in four risk of having a child with a major hemoglobinopathy. Sickle cell/β-thalassemia is a major sickling disorder, whereas hemoglobin E/β-thalassemia and homozygous β-thalassemia are transfusion-dependent states, with the associated problems of iron overload and iron chelation therapy.

Couples at risk for having a child with a major hemoglobinopathy need timely, nondirective counseling, with education about the possibility and techniques available for antenatal diagnosis.

Partners of women with β-thalassemia or hemoglobin E/β-thalassemia need antenatal screening to determine the risk of major hemoglobinopathy. If the partner has a relevant heterozygous condition, the risk of having an affected fetus increases to one in two. Although fertility is reduced in women with transfusion-dependent thalassemia, pregnancy has been reported.[122–124]

There are important considerations during pregnancy for both the mother and the fetus. The physiologic stress of pregnancy may exacerbate symptoms of thalassemia. The transfusion regimen must be monitored carefully because blood requirements tend to increase in pregnancy. Iron chelation therapy also needs to be reviewed. Outside of pregnancy, iron chelation is usually performed with deferoxamine mesylate (Desferal), which is given as a subcutaneous infusion over 12 hours 5 to 7 days per week. Continuing this treatment periconceptually and during pregnancy may put the fetus at risk for skeletal anomalies. This finding was noted in animal studies at doses equivalent to human dosages. The small number of reported cases in pregnant women is not sufficient to establish the safety of deferoxamine mesylate in this setting. There are case reports of desferrioxamine mesylate use in early pregnancy,[125] but ideally, iron status is optimized prepregnancy and chelation is discontinued periconceptually, at least for the first trimester, but ideally, throughout pregnancy. A risk–benefit assessment of continuing iron chelation in pregnancy is required, and the results will depend on the degree of iron overload at the start of pregnancy. At conception, various organs may already be affected by iron overload, particularly the heart, liver, and endocrine system. These patients require careful evaluation prepregnancy and monitoring throughout gestation.

Patients with β–thalassemia major are often small in stature, and affected women have small pelvic bones. This finding may be the reason for the increased rate of cesarean delivery reported in these women.[124]

The fetus is primarily at risk if the transfusion regimen is inadequate and the mother is anemic. Fetal hypoxia may occur and has been associated with intrauterine growth retardation, pregnancy loss, and preterm labor. These complications do not occur when maternal anemia is managed well. Women with iron overload are at increased risk for maternal diabetes, which can lead to an increased risk of birth defects and prenatal and maternal complications.

DIAGNOSIS AND MANAGEMENT OPTIONS

Prepregnancy and Prenatal. β-Thalassemia trait is indicated by hypochromic, microcytic red cell indices and usually is seen with a finding of increased hemoglobin A_2 on hemoglobin electrophoresis. Complications in diagnosis can arise in patients with iron deficiency anemia because it can falsely decrease hemoglobin A_2.

Racial groups at greatest risk include those of Mediterranean origin and some Asian populations, but it can occur in any racial group. The overall carrier rate in the United Kingdom is approximately 1 in 10,000 compared with 1 in 7 in Cyprus.

Women who are carriers of β-thalassemia trait need early education about the advisability of partner testing and the availability of antenatal diagnosis.[126,127]

In most cases, women with β-thalassemia intermedia or major are identified well before pregnancy and are receiving regular follow-up. Fertility is reduced in women with transfusion-dependent thalassemia major, but pregnancy is possible for some. Many require regular transfusion programs and iron chelation therapy. Unnecessary iron loading should be avoided. Oral and intravenous iron supplements are contraindicated. If possible, iron chelation therapy is discontinued during pregnancy. Assessment of the function of organs affected by iron overload (heart, liver, and endocrine system) should be carried out regularly throughout medical follow-up. Assessment includes evaluation of cardiac status, liver function tests, thyroid and parathyroid function tests, and glucose testing. If pregnancy was achieved spontaneously, (i.e., without fertility treatment) the pituitary axis is likely to be functioning, but thyroid function should be evaluated.

Involvement of a hematologist is essential in monitoring the transfusion regimen, which tends to increase in pregnancy. The fetomaternal medicine team should monitor the health of the mother and the growth and well-being of the fetus. Partner screening should be performed.

Labor, Delivery, and Postpartum. There are no specific management recommendations. As discussed earlier, issues relating to pelvis size, diabetes, and cardiac function may require assessment on an individual basis.

SUMMARY OF MANAGEMENT OPTIONS
Thalassemia Syndromes

Management Option	Quality of Evidence	Strength of Recommendation	References
β-Thalassemia Major			
Prepregnancy and Prenatal			
Pregnancy is rare	–	GPP	–
Avoid iron	–	GPP	–
Give folate	–	GPP	–
Regular transfusions for anemia	–	GPP	–
Screen partner; if the result is positive, consider counseling and prenatal diagnosis	–	GPP	–
Labor and Delivery			
Cord sample	–	GPP	–
Postnatal			
Neonatal follow-up	–	GPP	–
β-Thalassemia Minor			
Prepregnancy and Prenatal			
Give folate	–	GPP	–
Give oral (not parenteral) iron if ferritin level is low	–	GPP	–
Screen the patient's partner; if the result is positive, consider counseling and prenatal diagnosis	–	GPP	–

SUMMARY OF MANAGEMENT OPTIONS

Thalassemia Syndromes *(Continued)*

Management Option	Quality of Evidence	Strength of Recommendation	References
Labor and Delivery			
Obtain a cord sample if the patient has an at-risk pregnancy	–	GPP	–
Postnatal			
Provide neonatal follow-up if the patient has an at-risk pregnancy	–	GPP	–
α-Thalassemia (Hemglobin-H)			
Prepregnancy and Prenatal			
Give folate	–	GPP	–
Transfusion for severe anemia	–	GPP	–
Screen partner; if the result is positive, consider counseling and prenatal diagnosis	–	GPP	–
Labor and Delivery			
Crossmatch blood if anemia is severe	–	GPP	–
Postnatal			
Hematologic follow-up	–	GPP	–
α-Thalassemia (Hemoglobin Bart's Hydrops)			
Prenatal			
No treatment for fetal hydrops (incompatible with life)	–	GPP	–
Labor and Delivery			
Problems related to large fetus	–	GPP	–
Postnatal			
Counseling about events and approaches to future pregnancy	–	GPP	–
α-Thalassemia Minor/Trait			
Prepregnancy and Prenatal			
Provide iron and folate supplementation	–	GPP	–
Screen partner; if the result is positive, consider counseling and prenatal diagnosis	–	GPP	–

HEMOLYTIC ANEMIAS

Hemolytic anemias are characterized by accelerated red cell destruction, which typically results in an increased unconjugated bilirubin level, increased urobilinogen excretion, and an increased lactate dehydrogenase level. The reticulocyte count increases as the bone marrow responds. If intravascular hemolysis is present, free plasma hemoglobin and absent serum haptoglobins are characteristic findings.

Clinically, patients may have anemia, jaundice, splenomegaly, and pigment gallstones.

It is useful to think of hemolytic anemias as being caused by something intrinsic or extrinsic to the red blood cell. Intrinsic causes of hemolysis include abnormalities in hemoglobin structure or function (i.e., hemoglobinopathies), the red cell membrane (e.g., hereditary spherocytosis), or red cell metabolism (e.g., pyruvate kinase, glucose-6-phosphate dehydrogenase [G6PD] deficiency). Extrinsic causes may be the result of a red-cell-directed antibody (i.e., autoimmune hemolytic anemia), altered intravascular circulation (e.g., disseminated intravascular coagulation, thrombotic thrombocytopenic purpura) [see Chapters 79 and 80], or infection.

Red Cell Membrane Disorders

Hereditary spherocytosis occurs in approximately 1 in 2000 individuals of Northern European descent.[128] The inheritance pattern is autosomal dominant. The red cells are spherocytic and osmotically fragile. The condition is caused by defects in red cell membrane proteins and is clinically and genetically heterogeneous. Diagnosis is made by a combination of nonimmune hemolysis and typical blood film findings, with spherocytes and either osmotic fragility testing, or more recently, the use of an eosin-5-maleimide probe. This probe is a flow cytometric test that measures the fluorescence intensity of intact red cell membrane labeled with the dye eosin-5-maleimide. This fluorescent label binds to a component of the red cell membrane known as band 3. Binding is significantly reduced in hereditary spherocytosis.[129] A pregnant woman with this condition should be monitored for anemia and should receive folic acid supplementation (at least 5 mg daily). Patients must be aware of the symptoms and signs of the aplastic and hyperhemolytic crises that may occur. Aplastic crises are usually caused by parvovirus B19, which switches off erythropoiesis and causes a dramatic decrease in hemoglobin.[130] The virus may also affect fetal erythropoiesis and development. Hyperhemolysis is characterized by increased jaundice and splenic enlargement. Treatment with blood transfusion may be necessary.

Splenectomy ameliorates hemolytic anemia and reduces gallstone formation, but does not alter the underlying red cell defect. After splenectomy, women should ensure that their presplenectomy vaccinations (pneumococcal, *H. influenzae* B, and meningococcal) are current preconception and should take prophylactic penicillin V. Some small case series suggest that maternal morbidity and fetal outcome may be more favorable after splenectomy.[131] Pediatricians should be made aware of infants who are born to these women because there is a 50% chance that these children will be affected with hereditary spherocytosis, which may cause neonatal jaundice. Affected infants require long-term follow-up.

Red Cell Metabolism Disorders

The mature red cell has two principal pathways of glucose metabolism, the glycolytic pathway and the hexose monophosphate shunt. The glycolytic pathway provides the red cell with ATP as an energy source. Other products include the reduced form of nicotinamide adenine dinucleotide to reduce methemoglobin and 2,3-diphosphoglyceric acid to regulate the oxygen affinity of hemoglobin.

Pyruvate kinase deficiency is the most common defect of the glycolytic pathway. It is inherited in an autosomal recessive fashion and is clinically and genetically heterogeneous.[132] Varying degrees of anemia are seen. The need for transfusion of red cells must be assessed throughout pregnancy. Folic acid supplements are important for these patients, especially during pregnancy. Patients who have had splenectomy should be current with their vaccinations and are probably receiving prophylactic penicillin.

Metabolism of glucose through the hexose monophosphate shunt produces the reduced form of nicotinamide adenine dinucleotide phosphate to maintain the antioxidative activity of the red cell. G6PD deficiency is the most common abnormality of red cell metabolism.[133] Worldwide, it affects more than 200 million people and offers a survival advantage in the face of *Plasmodium falciparum* malaria.[134]

G6PD deficiency is X-linked. More than 300 genetic variants occur, and they are categorized according to the variant enzyme activity. The severity of hemolytic anemia depends on the type of defect, the level of enzyme activity, and the oxidative challenge (typically, drugs and fava beans). The G6PD A variant is an unstable enzyme, and enzyme activity decreases as the red cells age. This variant is found in approximately 10% to 15% of African American men. Women with this condition usually are only mildly anemic. The G6PD B variant (also known as G6PD Mediterranean) is found in up to 5% of people with Mediterranean or Asian ancestry and is clinically more severe. Men and heterozygous women may have severe hemolysis. The responsible agent must be removed because even the reticulocytes have low enzyme levels and are prone to hemolysis. Some variants cause congenital hemolytic anemia with persistent splenomegaly.

In more severe variants, women must be monitored for anemia throughout pregnancy, should avoid oxidant stresses, should take folic acid, and may need transfusion. The pediatrician must be alerted to the risk of hemolysis and neonatal jaundice because affected patients need careful monitoring and early therapy. Hepatic G6PD deficiency is probably an important factor in neonatal jaundice.

Autoimmune Hemolytic Anemia

Autoimmune hemolytic anemia may be primary or secondary to drugs, infection, autoimmune disease (typically systemic lupus erythematosus), neoplasia, or other hematologic disorders.

Usually, the antibodies are of the immunoglobulin G class, and antibody-coated red cells are cleared by the spleen. Symptoms of autoimmune hemolytic anemia are indistinguishable from those of other causes of hemolysis. The positive direct antiglobulin test (Coombs' test) is the mainstay of diagnosis.

Treatment is usually with glucocorticoids, but some patients have undergone splenectomy or are taking other immunosuppressive agents, such as cyclophosphamide, azathioprine, and cyclosporine. Transfusion may be required in patients who do not respond to treatment, but the autoantibodies may cause difficulties with crossmatching and close liaison with the blood bank is advisable.

Women who have autoimmune hemolytic anemia should have prepregnancy counseling, and treatment should be optimized. Careful antenatal supervision to assess maternal hemoglobin and markers of hemolysis, with adjustment of steroid therapy, is required.[135] Transplacental antibody transfer may occur, and hemoglobin levels in the newborn should be evaluated. Some infants require exchange transfusion,[136] but usually, no treatment is necessary.[137]

Autoimmune hemolytic anemia has been reported specifically associated with pregnancy, with remission occurring after delivery. This condition tends to recur in subsequent pregnancies. The anemia responds to steroids, and most infants are not affected.[138]

ANEMIA: BONE MARROW APLASIA

Aplastic Anemia

Aplastic anemia is a syndrome of bone marrow failure that is defined by pancytopenia and bone marrow hypocellularity. Normal hematopoietic tissue in the marrow is replaced by fat. Causative agents include infection, medications, and toxins, but most cases are idiopathic. Patients have pallor and fatigue as a result of anemia and bruising and bleeding as a result of thrombocytopenia. Infection is a risk because of neutropenia. Musculoskeletal abnormalities may indicate an inherited syndrome of bone marrow failure. The patient should be examined carefully for organomegaly and lymphadenopathy. These findings suggest viral infection or another underlying disease.

In patients with pancytopenia, testing should be directed by a hematologist and will include bone marrow aspirate and trephine with cytogenetic analysis and chromosome fragility tests.

Treatment of aplastic anemia is initially supportive, with blood products and growth factors. For younger patients with matched sibling donors, bone marrow transplantation is the treatment of choice. Immunosuppressive therapy with antilymphocyte globulin in combination with cyclosporin is also effective.

There are sporadic case reports of aplastic anemia in pregnancy[139–142] and reports of pregnancy occurring in women with underlying aplastic anemia.[143–145]

Aplastic anemia in pregnancy is rare. The relationship between aplastic anemia and pregnancy is uncertain, but the literature suggests that there is not a strong association in most cases.[146] In a few women, however, pregnancy may play an etiologic role. There are case reports of aplastic anemia that are diagnosed for the first time in pregnancy, with spontaneous remission occurring after cessation of pregnancy.[147]

Pregnancy may exacerbate bone marrow depression and cause clinical deterioration.[148]

If severe aplastic anemia occurs in the first trimester, early termination should be considered. If spontaneous recovery does not occur after termination, bone marrow transplantation is performed as soon as possible in women who have a histocompatible sibling donor. In women with severe aplastic anemia later in pregnancy and those who refuse termination, intensive hematologic support with red cells and platelet transfusions is required until delivery. After delivery, bone marrow transplantation should be considered if spontaneous recovery does not occur. There are case reports of the use of antilymphocyte globulin in pregnancy,[147] but each case requires individual assessment and close liaison between obstetricians and hematologists.

NEUTROPHILS

Neutrophilia

The neutrophil count increases throughout pregnancy. The increase is more marked during labor and immediately postpartum. Occasional band forms and myelocytes in the peripheral blood may be a normal finding during pregnancy. Neutrophilia may be associated with the following:

- Bacterial infection
- Acute or chronic inflammatory disorders
- Tissue damage or infarction
- Preeclampsia
- Hemorrhage
- Malignant disease, either hematologic (e.g., chronic myeloid leukemia) or nonhematologic

Neutropenia

The finding of neutropenia on an automated complete blood count should be verified by examination of the peripheral blood film. Aged samples may show spurious neutropenia or neutrophil clumping. A repeat count should be obtained to ensure that the findings are reproducible. Ethnic origin affects the neutrophil count; persons of African and Caribbean descent tend to have a lower peripheral blood neutrophil count because of an increase in the marginating pool. Neutropenia may be acute or chronic and isolated or part of generalized pancytopenia. It may be caused by peripheral destruction or underlying bone marrow disease. A summary of the causes of nonmalignant neutropenia is shown in Table 39–2. The investigation of neutropenia in the pregnant woman is identical to that outside pregnancy. Drugs that may be implicated should be discontinued immediately, especially if neutropenia is severe. If clinical assessment and examination of the blood film do not show the cause of neutropenia, bone marrow examination is indicated.

Maternal and Fetal Risks

In severe neutropenia, the principal maternal risk is sepsis. A patient with moderate or severe neutropenia (neutrophil count $<1.0 \times 10^9$/L) and fever should have prompt cultures of blood, urine, and sputum, if available, followed immediately by empirical treatment with broad-spectrum intravenous antibiotics, according to local policy. Antifungal therapy is considered if the fever does not resolve after 48 to 72 hours, especially when neutropenia is prolonged.

TABLE 39-2

Nonmalignant Neutropenia

TYPE	CAUSES
Acute	Drug-induced bone marrow suppression
	Agranulocytosis
	Viral infection
	Vitamin B_{12} or folate deficiency
Chronic	Race
	Immune neutropenia
	Primary
	Associated with connective tissue disorder or autoimmune disease
	Felty's syndrome
	Congenital neutropenia
	Kostmann's neutropenia
	Associated with other congenital disorders
	Chronic idiopathic neutropenia
	Cyclical neutropenia
	Aplastic anemia

There are many case reports of pregnancy in patients with cyclic neutropenia.[149,150] This disorder is characterized by cyclic fluctuations of the neutrophil count, with a periodicity of approximately 21 days. At its nadir, neutropenia is usually severe and is often associated with clinical infection. The onset is usually in childhood, but adult-onset cyclic neutropenia is also described. Pregnancy in cyclic neutropenia is associated with premature labor and stillbirth, possibly because of chorioamnionitis associated with the neutropenia. There are also reports of improvements in symptoms and neutrophil counts during pregnancy in patients with cyclic neutropenia, possibly because of the production of neutrophil growth factors, such as granulocyte-macrophage colony-stimulating factor, by the placenta.[151] In approximately one third of cases, cyclic neutropenia appears to be inherited in an autosomal dominant fashion; therefore, the fetus may be affected.

Management Options

Recombinant granulocyte colony-stimulating factor is successfully used to treat patients with severe chronic neutropenia of differing etiologies, including cyclic and congenital types.[152] A few pregnancies have occurred in patients treated with granulocyte colony-stimulating factor for severe chronic or cyclic neutropenia.[153] Pregnancy outcome was normal in some, but fetal abnormality, including bilateral hydronephrosis, occurred in others. Data on the safety of the use of granulocyte colony-stimulating factor during pregnancy are inconclusive. Risks and benefits should be evaluated individually.

For a patient with severe neutropenia, prophylactic antibiotics should be considered to cover invasive procedures for labor and delivery.

Some viral infections that cause neutropenia have implications for fetal development and congenital infection (e.g., rubella, parvovirus, cytomegalovirus) or hepatitis. Maternal autoimmune neutropenia may lead to transfer of antineutrophil antibodies across the placenta, resulting in fetal neutropenia.[154,155]

SUMMARY OF MANAGEMENT OPTIONS

White Cell Disorders

Management Options	Quality of Evidence	Strength of Recommendation	References
Neutrophilia			
Prenatal			
Increase in values for pregnancy	–	GPP	–
Search for pathology and treat if the count is above normal	–	GPP	–
Neutropenia			
Prepregnancy and Prenatal			
Give antibiotics for fever (and antifungals if fever persists)	–	GPP	–
For severe cases, consider recombinant granulocyte colony-stimulating factor; experience in pregnancy limited to case reports	Ib	A	152
Labor and Delivery			
Consider prophylactic antibiotics	IV	C	149

CONCLUSIONS

IRON DEFICIENCY ANEMIA

- The condition is common.
- Prophylactic iron treatment should be considered before deficiency develops.
- Oral, intramuscular, and intravenous forms of iron are equally effective.
- Treatment should continue into the postpartum period and be monitored by the full blood count and ferritin levels.

FOLATE DEFICIENCY ANEMIA

- Folate prophylaxis should be considered in patients who are at risk. The condition is more common in patients who take anticonvulsants or have a high turnover state, such as hemolytic anemia. Folate prophylaxis is indicated in these groups.
- Periconceptual use of folic acid is advised to reduce the incidence of neural tube defects.

VITAMIN B_{12} DEFICIENCY ANEMIA

- This condition is rare.
- Vitamin B_{12} levels decrease in pregnancy, but a decrease does not usually indicate deficiency.
- Intrinsic factor antibodies may be helpful if positive.

HEMOGLOBINOPATHIES

- Women should be screened for the trait or disease. If the results are positive, their partners should be screened. Counseling about prenatal diagnosis is appropriate.
- Patients with major hemoglobinopathy should be treated by senior obstetric and hematology teams throughout pregnancy.

REFERENCES

1. World Health Organization: Report of a WHO group of experts on nutritional anemias. Technical report series no. 503. Geneva, WHO, 1972.
2. Centers for Disease Control: Criteria for anemia in children and childbearing-aged women MMWR 1989;38:400–404.
3. Hytten F: Blood volume changes in normal pregnancy. In Letsky EA (ed): Hematological Disorders in Pregnancy. London, WB Saunders, 1985, pp 601–612.
4. Letsky EA: The Haematological System. In Broughton Pipkin F, Chamberlain GVP (eds): Clinical Physiology in Obstetrics. 3rd ed. Oxford, Blackwell, 1998, pp 71–110.
5. Bhatt R: Maternal Mortality in India: FOGSI. WHO Study. J Obstet Gynecol Ind 1997;47:207–214.
6. WHO Global Database: Geneva, WHO, 1997.
7. McFee JG: Iron metabolism and iron deficiency during pregnancy. Clin Obstet Gynecol 1979;22:799–808.
8. Turmen T, Abouzahr C: Safe motherhood. Int J Gynecol Obstet 1994;46:145–153.
9. Svanberg B: Absorption of iron in pregnancy. Acta Obstet Gynecol Scand Suppl 1975;48:100–108.
10. Fenton V, Cavill I, Fisher J: Iron stores in pregnancy. Br J Haematol 1977;37:145–149.
11. Thompson WG: Comparison of tests for the diagnosis of iron depletion in pregnancy. Am J Obstet Gynecol 1998;159: 1132–1134.
12. Finch CA, Cook JD: Iron deficiency. Am J Clin Nutr 1984;39:471–477.
13. Klebanoff MA, Shiono PH, Selby JV, et al: Anemia and spontaneous pre-term births. Am J Obstet Gynecol 1991; 164:59–63.
14. Scholl TO, Hediger ML, Fischer RL, Shearer JW: Anemia versus iron deficiency: Increased risk of pre-term delivery in a prospective study. Am J Clinical Nutr 1992;55:985–988.
15. Milman N, Agger AO, Nielson OJ: Iron status markers and serum erythropoietin in 120 mothers and newborn infants: Effect of iron supplementation in normal pregnancy. Acta Obstet Gynecol Scand 1994;73:200–204.
16. Colomer J, Colomert C, Gutierrez D, et al: Anemia during pregnancy as a risk factor for infant deficiency: Report from the Valencia Infant Anemia Cohort (VIAC) Study. Paediatr Perinat Epidemiol 1990;4:196–204.
17. Walter T: Effect of iron-deficiency anemia on cognitive skills in infancy and childhood. Ballieres Clin Hematol Poiesisatol 1994;7:815–827.
18. Lozoff B, Jimenz E, Wolf AW: Long-term developmental outcome of infants with iron deficiency. N Engl J Med 1991; 325:687–694.
19. Oski FA: Iron deficiency: Facts and fallacies. Pediatr Clinic North Am 1985;32:493–497.
20. Idjradinata P, Pollitt E: Reversal of developmental delays in iron-deficient anaemic infants treated with iron. Lancet 1993; 341:1–4.
21. Bruner AB, Joffee A, Duggan AK, et al: Randomised study of cognitive effects of iron supplementation in non-anaemic iron-deficient adolescent girls. Lancet 1996;348:992–996.
22. Hindmarsh PC, Geary MPP: Effect of early maternal iron stores on placental weight and structure. Lancet 2000;356:719–723.
23. Barker DJP, Bull AR, Osmand C, et al: Fetal and placental size and risk of hypertension in adult life. BMJ 1990; 301:259–262.
24. Chanarin I: Folate and cobalamin. Clinics in Haematology 1985;14:629–641.

25. Thompson WG: Comparison of tests for diagnosis of iron depletion in pregnancy. Am J Obstet Gynecol 1988; 159: 1132–1134.
26. Cook JD: Iron deficiency anemia. Baillieres Clin Haematology 1994;7,787–804.
27. Carriaga MT, Skikne BS, Finley B, et al: Serum transferrin receptor for the detection of iron deficiency in pregnancy Am J Clin Nutr 1991;54:1077–1081 .
28. De Leeuw NK, Lowenstein L, Hsieh YS: Iron deficiency and hydremia in normal pregnancy. Medicine (Baltimore) 1966; 45:291–315.
29. Krause JR, Stolc V: Serum ferritin and bone marrow iron stores: Correlation with absence of iron in biopsy specimens. Am J Clin Pathol 1979;72:817–820.
30. Baumann Kurer S, Seifert B, Michel B, et al: Prediction of iron deficiency in chronic inflammatory rheumatic disease anemia. Br J Haematol 1995;91:820–826.
31. Barrett JF, Whittaker PG, Williams JG, Lind T: Absorption of non-hemopoiesis iron from food during normal pregnancy. BMJ 1994;309:79–84.
32. Hemminki E, Starfield B: Routine administration of iron and vitamins during pregnancy: Review of clinical trials. Br J Obstet Gynaecol 1978;85:404–410.
33. Mahomed K: Iron and folate supplementation in pregnancy. Cochrane Database Syst Rev 2000;2:CD001135.
34. Mahomed K: Iron supplementation in pregnancy. Cochrane Database Syst Rev 2000;2:CD00017.
35. Blot I, Diallo D, Tchernia G: Iron deficiency in pregnancy: Effects on the newborn. Curr Opin Hematol 1999;6(2):65–70.
36. Allen LH: Pregnancy and iron deficiency in pregnancy: Unresolved issues. N Nutr Rev 1997;55:91–101.
37. Harris ED: New insights into placental iron transport. Nutr Rev 1992;50:329–331.
38. Allen LH: Anemia and iron deficiency: Effects on pregnancy outcome. Am J Clin Nutr 2000;71:12805–12845.
39. Meadows NJ, Grainger SL, Ruse W, et al: Oral iron and bioavailability of zinc. Br Med J Clin Res Ed 1983; 287:1013–1014.
40. Meadows NJ, Ruse W: Zinc and small babies. Lancet 1981;2:1135–1137.
41. Sheldon WL, Aspillaga MO, Smith PA, Lind T: The effects of oral iron supplementation on zinc and magnesium levels during pregnancy. BJOG 1985;92:892–898.
42. Murphy JF, O'Riordon J, Newcombe RG, et al: Relation of hemoglobin levels in first and second trimester to outcome of pregnancy. Lancet 1986;1:992–995.
43. Steer P, Alan MA, Wandsworth J, Welch A: Relation between maternal hemoglobin concentration and birth weight in different ethnic groups. BMJ 1995;310:489–491.
44. Taylor DJ, Mallen C, McDongall N, Lind T: Effect of iron supplementation on serum ferritin levels during and after pregnancy. BJOG 1982;89:1011–1017.
45. Gutteridge JMC: Iron and free radicals. In Hallberg L, Asp N-G (eds): Iron Nutrition in Health and Disease. London, John Libby, 1996, pp 239–246.
46. Beard JL: Are we at risk for heart disease because of normal iron status? Nutr Rev 1993;51:7–10.
47. Jackson HA, Worwood M, Beatley DP: Hemochromatosis mutations and iron stores in pregnancy. Br J Haematol 1998;101(Suppl):25.
48. Haram K, Nilsen ST, Ulvik RJ: Iron supplements in pregnancy: Evidence and controversies. Acta Obstet Gynecol Scand 2001;80:683–688.
49. Milman N, Bergholt T, Byg KE, et al: Iron status and iron balance during pregnancy: A critical re-appraisal of iron supplementation. Acta Obstet Gynecol Scand 1999;78:749–757.
50. Sharma JB: Iron deficiency anemia in pregnancy: Still a major cause of maternal mortality and morbidity in India. Obstet Gynaecol Today 1999;IV:693–701.
51. Stoltzfis R, Dreyfuss ML: Guidelines for the use of iron supplements to prevent and treat iron deficiency anemia. Washington, Geneva INAGG, WHO, UNICEF International Life Sciences Institute Press, 1998.
52. Allen LH: Pregnancy and iron deficiency: Unresolved issues. Nutr Rev 1997;55:91–101.
53. Lops VR, Hunter LP, Dixon LR: Anemia in pregnancy. Am Fam Physician 1995;51:1189–1197.
54. Horn E: Iron and folate supplements during pregnancy: Supplementing everyone treats those at risk and is cost effective. BMJ 1998;297:1325–1327.
55. Hurrell RF: Preventing iron deficiency through food fortification. Nutr Rev 1996;55:210–222.
56. Atukorala T, de Silva LD, Dechering WH, et al: Evaluation of effectiveness of iron folate supplementation and anthelminthic therapy against anemia in pregnancy study in the plantation of Sri Lanka. Am J Clin Nutr 1994;60:286–292.
57. Ridwin E, Schuttink W, Angeles I, et al: The effects of weekly iron supplementation on pregnant Indonesian women are similar to those of daily supplementation. Am J Clin Nutr 1996;63:884–890.
58. Young MW, Lupafya E, Kapenda E, et al: The effectiveness of weekly iron-supplementation in pregnant women of rural northern Malawi. Trop Doct 2000;30:84–88.
59. Lopes MC, Reffeira LO, Batista Filho M, et al: Use of daily and weekly ferrous sulphate to treat anaemic childbearing-age women. Cad Saude Publica 1999;15:799–808.
60. Bhatt RV: Poor iron compliance: The way out. J Obstet Gynecol Ind 1997;47:185–190.
61. Schultink JW, Van der Ree M, Matulessi P, Gross R: Low compliance with an iron supplementation program: A study among pregnant women in Jakarta, Indonesia. Am J Clin Nutr 1993;57:135–139.
62. Cook JD, Reddy M: Efficacy of weekly compared with daily iron supplementation. Am J Clin Nutr 1995;62:117–120.
63. McKenna D, Spence D, Haggan SE, et al: A randomized trial investigating an iron-rich natural mineral water as prophylaxis against iron deficiency in pregnancy. Clin Lab Hematol 2003;25:99–103.
64. Pritchard JA: Hemoglobin regeneration in severe iron deficiency anemia: Response to orally parenterally administered iron preparations JAMA 1996;195:717–720.
65. Singh K, Fon YF, Kuperan P: A comparison between intravenous iron polymaltose complex (Ferram Hausmann) and oral ferrous fumarate in the treatment of iron deficiency anemia in pregnancy. Eur J Hematol 1998;60:119–124.
66. Scott JM: Toxicity of iron sorbitol citrate. BMJ 1962;2:480–481.
67. Al-Momen AK, Al-Meshari A, Al-Nuaim L_5 et al: Intravenous iron sucrose complex in the treatment of iron deficiency during pregnancy. Eur J Obstet Gynecol Reprod Biol;1996;69:121–124.
68. Cuervo LG, Mahomed K: Treatments for iron deficiency anemia during pregnancy. Cochrane Database Syst Rev 2001;2: CD003094.
69. Bailey LB: Folate requirements and dietary recommendations. In Bailey LB (ed): Folate in Health and Disease. New York, Dekker 1995, pp 123–151.
70. Landon MJ: Folate metabolism in pregnancy. Clin Obstet Gynaecol 1975;2:413.
71. Fleming AF: Urinary excretion of folate in pregnancy. J Obstet Gynaecol Br Commonw 1972;79: 916–920.
72. McPartlin J, Halligan A, Scott JM, et al: Accelerated folate breakdown in pregnancy. Lancet 1993;341:148–149.
73. Chanarin I: Folate deficiency in pregnancy. In Chanarin I (ed): The Megaloblastic Anemias, 3rd ed. Oxford, Blackwell, 1990, pp 140–148.
74. Lowenstein L, Brunton L, Hsieh YJ: Nutritional anemia and megaloblastosis in pregnancy. Can Med Assoc J 1966; 94:636–645.

75. World Health Organization: Nutritional Anemias. Geneva, WHO, 1972.
76. Fletcher J, Gurr A, Fellingham FR, et al: The value of folic acid supplements in pregnancy. J Obstet Gynaecol Br Commonw 1971;75:781–785.
77. Laurence KM, James N, Miller MH, et al: Double-blind randomized controlled trial of folate treatment before conception to prevent recurrence of neural tube defects. Br Med J Clin Res Ed 1981;282:1509–1511.
78. Swithells RW, Sheppard S, Schorah CJ, et al: Possible prevention of neural tube defects by periconceptual vitamin supplementation. Lancet 1980;1:339–340.
79. Elwood JM: Can vitamins prevent neural tube defects? Can Med Assoc J 1983;129:1088–1092.
80. Prevention of neural tube defects: Results of the Medical Research Council Vitamin Study. MRC Vitamin Study Research Group. Lancet 1991;228:131–137.
81. Berry RJ, Li Z, Erickson JD, et al: Prevention of neural-tube defects with folic acid in China. N Engl J Med: 1991;341: 1485–1490.
82. Czeizel AE, Dudas I: Prevention of the first occurrence of neural-tube defects by periconceptional vitamin supplementation. N Engl J Med 1992;327:1832–1835.
83. Hook EB, Czeizel AE: Can terathanasia explain the protective effect of folic acid supplements on birth defects? Lancet 1997;350:513–515.
84. Editorial: Folic acid and neural tube defects. Lancet 1991;338:153–154.
85. Rosenberg IH: Folic acid and neural-tube defects: Time for action. N Engl J Med 1992;327:1875–1877.
86. Alberman E, Noble JM: Food should be fortified with folic acid: Commentary. BMJ 1999;319:93.
87. Chanarin I: Megaloblastic anemia associated with pregnancy. In The Megaloblastic Anemias. Oxford, Blackwell, 1971, p 466.
88. Giles CJ: An account of 335 cases of megaloblastic anemia of pregnancy and the puerperium. Clin Pathol 1966;19:1–11.
89. Hiilesmaa VK, Teramo K, Granstrom ML, Bardy AH: Serum folate concentrations during pregnancy in women with epilepsy: Relation to anti-epileptic drug concentrations, numbers of seizures and fetal outcome. BMJ 1983;287:577–579.
90. Hill RM, Verniaud WM, Horning MG, et al: Infants exposed in utero to anti epileptic drugs. Am J Dis Child 1974;127:645–653.
91. Bjerkedal T, Bahna SL: The course and outcome of pregnancy in women with epilepsy. Obstet Gynaecol Scand 1973; 52(Suppl):245–248.
92. Etelstein T, Metz J: Correlation between vitamin B12 concentration in serum and muscle in late pregnancy. J Obstet Gynaecol Br Commonw 1969;76:545–548.
93. Temperley IJ, Meehan MJ, Gatenby PB: Serum vitamin B12 levels in pregnant women. J Obstet Gynaecol Br Commonw 1968;75:511–516.
94. Cooper BA: Folate and vitamin B12 in pregnancy. Clin Hematol 1973;2:461–466.
95. Grange DK, Finlay JL: Nutritional vitamin B12 deficiency in a breastfed infant following maternal gastric bypass. Pediatr Hematol Oncol 1994;11:311.
96. World Health Organization: Nutritional Anemias. Geneva, WHO, 1972.
97. Ball EW, Giles CJ: Folic acid and vitamin B12 levels in pregnancy and their relation to megaloblastic anemia. Clin Pathol 1964;17:165.
98. Metz J, Festenstein H, Welch PAM: Effect of folic acid and vitamin B12 supplementation on tests of folate and vitamin B12 nutrition in pregnancy. J Clin Nutr 1965;16:472.
99. Bain B: The α, β, δ and γ thalassaemias and related conditions (Ch.3); Sickle cell haemoglobin and its interactions with other variant haemoglobins and with thalassaemias (Ch. 4). In Bain B (ed.) Haemoglobinopathy Diagnosis. Blackwell, 2001.
100. Tuck SM, Studd JWW, White JM: Pregnancy in women with sickle cell trait. BJOG 1983;90:108–111.
101. Larrabee K, Monga M: Women with sickle cell trait are at increased risk of preeclampsia. Am J Obstet Gynecol 1997;177:425–428.
102. Platt OS, Brambilla DJ, Rose WF, et al: Mortality in sickle cell disease: Life expectancy and risk factors for early death. N Engl J Med 1994;330:1639–1644.
103. Smith JA, Espeland M, Bellevue R, et al: Pregnancy in sickle cell disease: Experience of the co-operative study of sickle cell disease. Obstet Gynecol 1996;87:199–203.
104. Adam S: Caring for the pregnant woman with sickle cell crisis: Professional care of mother and child. 1996;6:34–36.
105. Tuck SM, Studd JWW, White JM: Pregnancy in sickle cell disease in the United Kingdom. BJOG 1983; 90:112–117.
106. Brown AK, Sleeper LA, Pegelow CH, et al: The influence of infant and maternal sickle cell disease on birth outcome and neonatal course. Arch Pediatr Adolesc Med 1994;148:156–162.
107. Horger EO: Sickle cell and sickle cell-hemoglobin C disease during pregnancy. Obstet Gynecol 1972;39:873–879.
108. Poddar D, Maude G, Plant M, et al: Pregnancy in Jamaican women with homozygous sickle cell disease: Fetal and maternal outcome. BJOG 1986;93:727–732.
109. Howard RJ, Lillis C, Tuck SM: Contraceptives, counselling and pregnancy in women with sickle cell disease. BJOG 1995;102: 947–951.
110. Charache S, Terrin ML, Moore RD, et al: Effect of hydroxyurea on the frequency of painful crises in sickle cell anemia. N Engl J Med 1995;332:1317–1322.
111. Diav-Citrin O, Hunnisett L, Sher GD, Koren G: Hydroxyurea use during pregnancy: A case report in sickle cell disease and review of the literature. Am J Hematol 1999;60:148–150.
112. Byrd DC, Pitts SR, Alexander CK: Hydroxyurea in two pregnant women with sickle cell anemia. Pharmacotherapy 1999; 19:1459–1462.
113. Koshy M, Burd L, Wallace D, et al: Prophylactic red cell transfusions in pregnant patients with sickle cell disease. N Engl J Med 1988;319:1447–1452.
114. Howard RJ, Tuck SM, Pearson TC: Pregnancy in sickle cell disease in the UK: Results of a multicentre survey on the effect of prophylactic blood transfusion on maternal and fetal outcome. BJOG 1995;102:947–951.
115. Mahomed K: Prophylactic versus selective blood transfusion for sickle cell anemia during pregnancy. Cochrane Database Syst Rev 2000;CD000040.
116. Rosse WF, Gallagher D: Transfusion and alloimmunisation in sickle cell disease: The co-operative Study of Sickle Cell Disease. Blood 1990;76:1431–1437.
117. Rees DC, Olujohungbe AD, Parker NE, et al: Guidelines for the management of the acute painful crisis in sickle cell disease. Br J Haematol 2003;120:744–752.
118. Koshy M, Burd L, Dorn L, Huff G: Frequency of painful crisis during pregnancy. Prog Clin Biol Res 1987;240:305–311.
119. Vichinsky EP, Neumayr LD, Earles AN, et al: Causes and outcomes of the acute chest syndrome in sickle cell disease: National Acute Chest Syndrome Study Group. N Engl J Med 2000; 342:1855–1865.
120. Finer P, Blair, Rowe P: Epidural analgesia in the management of labor pain and sickle cell crisis. Anesthesiology 1988;68:799.
121. Vichinsky EP, Haberkern CM, Neumayr L, et al: A comparison of conservative and aggressive transfusion regimens in the perioperative management of sickle cell disease: The Pre-operative Transfusion in Sickle Cell Disease Study Group. N Engl J Med;1995;333:206–213.
122. Jenson CE, Tuck SM, Wonke B: Fertility in β thalassaemia major: A report of 16 pregnancies, preconceptual evaluation and review of the literature. BJOG 1995; 102:625–629.
123. Kilpatrick SJ, Laros RK: Thalassaemia in pregnancy. Clin Obstet Gynecol 1995;38:485–496.

124. Aessopos A, Karabatsos F, Farmakis D, et al: Pregnancy in patients with well-treated beta-thalassaemia: Outcome for mothers and newborn infants. Am J Obstet Gynaecol 1999; 180:360–365.
125. Vaskaridou EM, Konstantopoulos K, Kyriakou D, et al: Desferrioxamine treatment during early pregnancy: Absence of teratogenicity in two cases. Haematologica 1993;78:183–184.
126. Model B, Harris R, Lane B, et al: Informed choice in genetic screening for thalassaemia during pregnancy: Audit from a national confidential inquiry. BMJ 2000;320:337–341.
127. Oliveiri NF: Medical progress: The β thalassaemias. N Engl J Med 1999; 341:99–109.
128. Bolton-Maggs PH: The diagnosis and management of hereditary spherocytosis. Best Pract Res Clin Hematol 2000;327–342.
129. King MJ, Behrens J, Rogers C, et al: Rapid flow cytometric test for the diagnosis of membrane cytoskeleton-associated hemo lytic anemia. Br J Hematol 2000;111:924–933.
130. Kudielka I, Nagele F, Chalubinski K, et al: B19 parvovirus infection in primipara with congenital spherocytosis. Acta Obstet Gynecol Scand 1998;77:785–786.
131. Pajor A, Lehoczky D, Szakacs Z: Pregnancy and hereditary spherocytosis: Report of 8 patients and a review. Arch Gynecol Obstet 1993;253:37–42.
132. Zanella A, Bianchi P: Red cell pyruvate kinase deficiency: From genetics to clinical manifestations. Best Pract Res Clin Hematol 2000;13:57–81.
133. Beutler: G6PD deficiency. Blood 1994;84:3613–3636.
134. Magill AJ: The prevention of malaria. Primary care; Clinics in Office Practice 2002;29:815–842.
135. Chaplin H, Cohen R, Bloomberg G, et al: Pregnancy and idiopathic autoimmune hemolytic anemia. Br J Haematol 1973; 24:219–239.
136. Lawe JE: Successful exchange transfusion of an infant for AIHA developing late in the mother's pregnancy. Transfusion 1982; 22:66–68.
137. Sokol RJ, Hewitt S, Stamps BK: Erythrocyte auto antibodies, autoimmune haemolysis and pregnancy. Vox Sang 1982; 43:169–176.
138. Benraad CEM, Scheerder HAJM, Overbeeke MAM: Autoimmune hemolytic anemia during pregnancy. Eur J Obstet Gynecol Reprod Biol 1994;55:209–211.
139. Ang HY, Ho HK, Linn YC: A case of aplastic anemia in pregnancy. Aust N Z J Obstet Gynecol 1999;39:102–105.
140. Van Besien, Trico G, Golichowski A, et al: Pregnancy associated aplastic anemia: Report of 3 cases. Eur J Hematol 1991; 47:253–256.
141. Ohba T, Yoshimura T, Araki M, et al: Aplastic anemia in pregnancy: Treatment with cyclosporine and granulocyte-colony stimulating factor. Acta Obstet Gynecol Scand 1999; 78:458–461.
142. Huter O, Brezinka C, Schiller L, et al: Successful treatment of pregnancy associated severe aplastic anemia by immunosuppression: A case report and review of the literature. J Matern Fetal Invest 1996;6:175–178.
143. Eliyahu S, Shalev E: A successful pregnancy after bone marrow transplantation for severe aplastic anemia with pre-transplant conditioning of total lymph-node irradiation and cyclophosphamide. Br J Haemopoiesisatol 1994;86:649–650.
144. Pajor A, Kelement E, Szakacs Z, Lehoczky D: Pregnancy in idiopathic aplastic anemia: Report of 10 patients. Eur J Obstet Reprod Biol 1992;45:19–25.
145. Calmard-Oriol P, Dauriac C, Vu Van H, et al: Successful pregnancy following allogeneic bone marrow transplantation after conditioning by thoraco-abdominal irradiation. Bone Marrow Transplant 1991;8:229–230.
146. Oosterkamp HM, Brand A, Kluin-Nelemans JC, Vandenbrioucke JP: Pregnancy and severe aplastic anemia: Causal relation or coincidence? Br J Haematol 1998; 103:315–316.
147. Aitchison RGM, Marsh JCW, Hows JM, et al: Pregnancy associated aplastic anemia: A report of five cases and a review of current management Br J Haematol 1989;73:541–545.
148. Van Besien, Tricot G, Golichowski A, et al: Pregnancy associated aplastic anemia: Report of 3 cases Eur J Hematol 1991; 47:253–256.
149. Yoshida Y, Ueda K, Tomimatsu T, et al: A case of pregnancy associated with cyclic neutropenia. Acta Obstet Gynecol Scand 1995;74:836–857.
150. Dicato M, Ries F, Richard J: Treatment of cyclic neutropenia with GCSF during pregnancy. Blood 1993;10:A497.
151. Bailie KEM, Irvine AE, Bridges JM, McClure BG: Granulocyte and granulocyte-macrophage colony stimulating factors in cord and maternal serum at delivery. Pediatr Res 1994;735:164–168.
152. Dale DC, Bonilla MA, Davis MW, et al: A randomized controlled phase III trial of recombinant human granulocyte colony-stimulating factor (filgrastim) for treatment of severe chronic neutropenia Blood 1993;81:2496–2502.
153. Boxer L, Dale DC, Bonilla MA, et al: Administration of r-mettlu G-GCSF during pregnancy in patients with severe chronic neutropenia (SCN). Blood 1995;86:2020.
154. Levine DH, Madyastha PR: Isoimmune neonatal neutropenia. Am J Perinatol 1986;3:231–233.
155. Kemeoka J, Funato T, Miura T, et al: Autoimmune neutropenia in pregnant women causing neonatal neutropaenia. Br J Haematol 2001;114:198–200.

CHAPTER 40

Malignancies of the Hematologic and Immunologic Systems

John Maelor Davies / Lucy Kean

INTRODUCTION

Fortunately, malignancy complicating pregnancy is uncommon. Hematologic disorders account for most malignancies in women of reproductive age. The incidence of acute leukemia complicating pregnancy is approximately 1 in 75,000, and lymphoma complicates 1 in 5000 pregnancies.[1,2] Hematologic malignancy is an important consideration in pregnancy because it threatens life and is potentially curable. This chapter discusses acute myeloblastic leukemia (AML), acute lymphoblastic leukemia (ALL), chronic myeloid leukemia (CML), lymphoma (both Hodgkin's disease and non-Hodgkin's lymphoma), chronic lymphocytic leukemia (CLL), and myeloma and the myeloproliferative disorders. The classification of tumors of the hemopoietic and lymphoid tissues is complex and subject to change. The World Health Organization classification[3] provides the major framework for categorizing these disorders. Much of the literature on these conditions in pregnancy predates the introduction of effective modern management. In some areas, data are limited, but as far as possible, the management principles discussed later are evidence-based.

ACUTE LEUKEMIA

Acute leukemia is caused by malignant changes in the hemopoietic precursor cells. Acute leukemia is traditionally subdivided into AML and ALL, depending on the cell lineage. Further subdivision of AML and ALL provides additional prognostic and therapeutic information. Both AML and ALL are usually acute and lead to progressive bone marrow failure, with symptoms and signs of anemia, neutropenia, and thrombocytopenia. More rarely, ALL, in particular, may cause extramedullary involvement.

Maternal Risks

Pregnancy does not appear to affect either the development or the course of acute leukemia. Patients who have symptoms or signs of abnormalities in the complete blood count suggesting bone marrow failure or infiltration should undergo appropriate testing. Studies in pregnant patients with acute leukemia do not differ from those in nonpregnant patients. They include bone marrow aspiration, trephine biopsy, and examination of the cerebrospinal fluid, as appropriate. Newer cytogenetic and molecular diagnostic techniques should be used because they provide additional prognostic information rapidly.[3] Renal and hepatic function should be monitored. Infection and bleeding are major risks in uncontrolled acute leukemia, particularly in some types, such as acute promyelocytic leukemia. Laboratory assessment of the degree of thrombocytopenia and evidence of coagulation factor depletion and disseminated intravascular coagulation should be undertaken.

Supportive care, with blood and platelet transfusions and antibiotic administration, should be instituted early. However, chemotherapy offers the only prospect for long-term maternal survival. If delivery is contemplated before complete remission is achieved, then infection and bleeding pose a major risk to maternal survival. These patients require antibiotic administration and appropriate coagulation factor and platelet replacement.

The outcome in both AML and ALL depends on a number of prognostic factors. The prognosis is determined by the response to treatment and the type of treatment offered. For example, when patients with acute promyelocytic leukemia are treated with modern protocols, the prognosis is relatively favorable,[3] whereas patients with Philadelphia-chromosome-positive ALL present significant management problems. This disease is essentially incurable with current chemotherapy regimens alone.[4] Discussion of the prognosis should be highly individualized and undertaken only when all necessary information is available. Fertility is likely to be maintained in many patients with AML and ALL treated with conventional chemotherapy, and future pregnancy outcome in survivors of AML and ALL is also likely to be favorable. Counseling and contraceptive advice should include these considerations.

Increasing numbers of patients have been treated with both autologous and allogeneic hemopoietic stem cell transplantation for acute leukemia. Although successful pregnancy has been reported, in most patients, this procedure impairs fertility.[5,6]

Fetal Risks

The main risks to the fetus are growth restriction, which occurs in both treated and untreated pregnancies, and chemotherapy-induced effects, both reversible and irreversible. Historically, fetal growth restriction and spontaneous preterm delivery occurred in approximately 40% to 50% of cases and appeared to be multifactorial.[7] With modern chemotherapy and the attainment of remission in most patients within 4 to 6 weeks, the fetal survival rate has improved significantly.[8] Congenital leukemia is rare and can essentially be discounted. The fetal risks associated with chemotherapy depend, in part, on the timing of the treatment in terms of gestational age and also on the agents used. Although data are limited, general conclusions can be drawn about the fetal risks of chemotherapy.

First, adverse fetal events may occur at any point in gestation, although congenital malformation is more likely to occur with first-trimester exposure to chemotherapy. The literature suggests that the risk of major fetal abnormality is 10% to 30%, depending on the degree of exposure and the agents used.[9,10] When a patient has known first-trimester exposure to cytotoxic agents, a careful fetal ultrasound should be performed at 18 to 22 weeks. However, not all teratogenic effects are detectable by ultrasound examination, and parents should be carefully counseled.

Second, some chemotherapeutic agents are more likely than others to produce adverse fetal effects. For example, first-trimester use of high-dose methotrexate produces adverse fetal effects.[11] Data on newer agents used to treat acute leukemia are limited. For example, when administered early in gestation, fludarabine, now widely used to treat AML, produces skeletal malformation in both rats and rabbits. The agent is not recommended for use at any stage in human pregnancy, and there are no adequate, well-controlled studies in pregnant women. Similarly, all-trans-retinoic acid, which is used to treat acute promyelocytic leukemia, is related to other retinoids that are potent human teratogens. These agents are contraindicated in women of childbearing age. There are single case reports of the use of all-trans-retinoic acid in the later stages of pregnancy. Maternal versus fetal risk must be balanced at all stages in patient management.[12]

Finally, many chemotherapeutic agents are associated with markers of chromosomal damage. The significance of this observation is not clear, and data on long-term effects in surviving infants exposed to chemotherapeutic agents in utero are encouraging. However, this observation may reflect a lack of good information rather than a true lack of adverse events. Chemotherapy-induced malignancies are the major potential concern.[13]

Management Options

Prepregnancy

Women who undergo chemotherapy for acute leukemia should be counseled and advised against conception until remission is achieved and chemotherapy is discontinued. Oral contraceptives are not contraindicated.

A much more common scenario is a woman who is in complete remission. As a result of the 1994 European Registration of Congenital Anomalies (EUROCAT) study of policies for karyotyping in pregnancy, patients began to seek invasive prenatal testing because of maternal anxiety about exposure to chemotherapy or radiation therapy.[14] Prepregnancy counseling should include a discussion of the prognosis in terms of the disease and the effect of the disease and its treatment on pregnancy. Although chemotherapy may cause chromosome breaks, there does not appear to be an increase in the risk of chromosomal or genetic problems in offspring. Previous chemotherapy does not appear to increase the risk of miscarriage, growth restriction, or stillbirth.[15,16]

Large studies have not determined whether the incidence of childhood cancer is increased in the offspring of patients who have undergone chemotherapy. However, smaller studies suggest that there is no increased risk. Given the lack of evidence suggesting an increase in the risk of chromosomal abnormalities in the fetus, invasive prenatal diagnosis should be based on normal criteria in relation to age and screening test results. Women who have undergone pelvic radiation therapy have a significantly increased risk of growth restriction in the fetus and should be counseled that increased surveillance is needed in pregnancy.

Prenatal

A pregnant woman with acute leukemia should be treated aggressively, with full supportive care and combination chemotherapy. Untreated acute leukemia is fatal to both mother and fetus. When possible, standard treatment is given, with appropriate counseling about fetal risk. No good data are available on the need for dosage modifications of chemotherapeutic drugs in pregnancy. In some cases, agents that are less likely to cause fetal abnormalities can be used (e.g., intrathecal cytarabine rather than intrathecal methotrexate for central nervous system prophylaxis in ALL). However, nonstandard regimens of unproven efficacy should not be substituted on the basis of fetal risk without full and informed discussion of maternal risks.

Counseling about the teratogenic risks of treatment should be provided, and fetal and maternal well-being should be monitored throughout pregnancy by a hemato-oncologist and an obstetrician.

Labor and Delivery

Delivery should be expedited for normal obstetric indications. The goal of management is to deliver a viable infant while the mother is in hematologic remission. This approach offers the best prospect for uncomplicated delivery and infant survival. There is no contraindication to the use of steroids before delivery to enhance fetal surfactant production. Early assessment of the infant should be undertaken to detect complications from in utero exposure to chemotherapy. This evaluation includes assessment of potential abnormalities and hematologic testing to exclude short-term effects (e.g., neutropenia as a result of recent in utero exposure to cytotoxic agents administered to the mother). If the mother recently received chemotherapy, a cord blood sample should be sent for a complete blood count.

Postnatal

If delivery is inevitable in a patient who is not in remission, vigorous supportive care should be continued. If the disease is in remission at the time of delivery, counseling and appropriate contraceptive advice should be given after delivery. Data on the excretion of cytotoxic drugs in breast milk are variable; however, patients who are receiving active treatment with cytotoxic drugs should not breastfeed.

SUMMARY OF MANAGEMENT OPTIONS

Hematologic Malignancies: Acute Leukemia

Management Options	Quality of Evidence	Strength of Recommendation	References
Prepregnancy			
Counsel about the prognosis	–	GPP	–
Advise against conception until the patient is in remission and not on chemotherapy	IV III	C B	9,11 10
Prenatal			
Interdisciplinary approach	–	GPP	–
Start chemotherapy as for a nonpregnant patient if the disease is diagnosed in pregnancy	IV	C	8
Supportive therapy (e.g., blood, platelets, antibiotics)	–	GPP	–
Careful counseling, especially if treatment commenced in the first trimester	IV	C	9,11
Monitor fetal growth and health	IV	C	8
Labor and Delivery			
Expedite for normal obstetric indications (ideally when the patient is in remission and the fetus is mature)	–	GPP	–
Give steroids if preterm delivery is contemplated	–	GPP	–
Postnatal			
Provide contraceptive advice	III IV	B C	10 9,11
Counseling about the long-term prognosis	–	GPP	–
Avoid breastfeeding if the patient is receiving cytotoxic treatment	III	B	35
Examination and follow-up of the newborn	–	GPP	–

CHRONIC LEUKEMIA

Chronic Myeloid Leukemia

CML is a triphasic disease (chronic phase, accelerated phase, and blast crisis) that is usually diagnosed in the chronic (early) phase. It accounts for 15% to 20% of cases of leukemia, and the median age at diagnosis is in the fifth and sixth decades. CML arises from a cytogenetic abnormality that results in production of the Philadelphia chromosome. As a result, the BCR/ABL fusion gene is produced and encodes for a protein with tyrosine kinase activity. CML causes systemic symptoms, such as weight loss, fatigue, and splenomegaly. Laboratory findings include marked leukocytosis, and as discussed earlier, a specific marker chromosome that is detectable in blood and bone marrow. Hyperleukocytosis with ocular and other central nervous system effects may occur.

Management Options Outside Pregnancy

The management of CML was revolutionized by the introduction of the specific tyrosine kinase inhibitor imatinib mesylate.[17] This agent is superior to α-interferon, either alone or in combination with cytarabine.[17] When imatinib is available, few patients are treated with the older treatment options of hydroxyurea and α-interferon. The role of related or unrelated allogeneic hemopoietic stem cell transplantation, which traditionally has been used to treat this condition, is under reevaluation. The practical management of patients with CML in the imatinib era has been reviewed.[18]

Maternal and Fetal Risks

There is no evidence that the behavior of CML is altered in pregnancy. Control of the maternal white count may be achieved in a number of ways. The risk to the fetus is probably secondary to exposure to maternal therapy, and control of the maternal white count with physical means, such as leukapheresis, should be considered. Successful pregnancies have been reported after the use of alkylating agents in pregnancy.[19] However, these agents should be avoided, at least in the first trimester. Successful pregnancy is also reported in patients treated with α-interferon, although data in pregnancy are limited.[20] Patients treated with imatinib should be counseled against becoming pregnant because there are no good data on its use in pregnancy.

Management Options

PREPREGNANCY

The implications and risks of pregnancy should be fully explained, and appropriate contraceptive advice should be given.

PRENATAL

Regular hematologic review is required to determine the need for active treatment. As discussed earlier, leukapheresis may be an effective method to control the white cell count, particularly in the first trimester. This approach may be continued throughout pregnancy. Successful pregnancies are described in patients treated with hydroxyurea and α-interferon, although cumulative data are insufficient to allow an estimate of the real risk of fetal abnormality. Patients who become pregnant while taking imatinib should be counseled about the risk of fetal abnormality, which is essentially unquantifiable. Careful ultrasonographic examination of the fetus should be performed in women who wish to continue the pregnancy. Patients in the early chronic phase who become pregnant while taking imatinib are advised to discontinue use of the agent; other methods to control the white cell count may be instituted.

Hematologic abnormalities that suggest disease progression, such as signs of the accelerated phase or blast crisis, should lead to management review. In the accelerated phase, delivery is expedited. Maternal options include reintroduction of imatinib and referral for hemopoietic stem cell transplantation, which is the only likely curative option. Blast crisis in pregnancy may be treated with imatinib, if the patient is not already receiving this agent, or with combination chemotherapy, as for other forms of acute leukemia. However, the maternal outlook is poor, and particularly if a second chronic phase occurs, urgent consideration should be given to early delivery and referral of the mother, if appropriate, for hemopoietic stem cell transplantation.[21]

Chronic Lymphocytic Leukemia

CLL is a disease of older populations[5] and rarely occurs in pregnancy. A "wait and watch" approach is often appropriate, and the patient may need treatment only if symptoms occur. When treatment is required, standard therapies include corticosteroids, alkylating agents, and fludarabine. Given the usual indolent course of CLL, most pregnancies can be managed without fetal exposure to potentially teratogenic agents and with no detriment to maternal outcome.

Myeloma

Myeloma is also a disease of older age groups and is rare in pregnancy. It presents a unique set of management problems and may cause significant skeletal damage, bone marrow failure, extended risk of infection, and renal failure. When treatment is required, standard therapies, as for nonpregnant patients, should be used.

SUMMARY OF MANAGEMENT OPTIONS

Hematologic Malignancies: Chronic Leukemia (Mainly Myeloid in Pregnancy)

Management Options	Quality of Evidence	Strength of Recommendation	References
Prepregnancy			
Counsel about the prognosis for pregnancy and in the long term	IV	C	19
Give contraceptive advice	–	GPP	–
Prenatal			
Interdisciplinary approach	–	GPP	–
Regular hematologic monitoring	–	GPP	–
Consider leukapheresis	–	GPP	–
Control with hydroxyurea or alpha interferon (avoid cytotoxics in the first trimester); data on imatinib are insufficient; current recommendation is not to use in pregnancy	IV	C	20
Manage accelerated phase and blast crisis as for nonpregnant patients, and expedite delivery if possible (to allow for the possibility of bone marrow transplantation)	IV	C	21
Postnatal			
As for acute leukemia	–	GPP	–

LYMPHOMA

Lymphomas are a heterogeneous group of disorders that arise in lymphoid tissue. The major histologic subdivision of lymphoma is into the following categories:

- Hodgkin's disease
- Non-Hodgkin's lymphoma[3]

Hodgkin's Disease

Hodgkin's disease is an uncommon lymphoid malignancy.[22] However, because of the age distribution of patients with Hodgkin's disease, it is the most common type of lymphoma seen in pregnancy. Hodgkin's disease causes nodal enlargement, classically in the neck, and diagnosis requires biopsy of the affected tissue. Further management depends on the stage of disease. Early-stage or localized Hodgkin's disease is amenable to treatment and may be cured with either radiation therapy alone or a combination of chemotherapy and radiation therapy in modified dosage. Intermediate- or late-stage disease requires combination chemotherapy for cure. The Ann Arbor system is still the most commonly used staging system, but staging may be refined anatomically with the Cotswolds revision.[23] Additionally, information available from laboratory tests (e.g., lymphocyte count, erythrocyte sedimentation rate, serum albumin level) may be used to produce a prognostic index that may affect management. However, in pregnancy, laboratory findings are of less value.

Maternal Risks

Hodgkin's disease in pregnancy does not appear to differ from that in nonpregnant patients, although interestingly, Hodgkin's disease is less common in multiparous women. Diagnosis is made by biopsy. Further studies in the pregnant patient are associated with specific problems, particularly with regard to computed tomography; however, magnetic resonance imaging, which is generally safe in pregnancy, may be used.[24] Staging laparotomy has largely been abandoned.[25] The outlook for cure in patients with early-stage disease treated with radiation therapy, with or without a short course of chemotherapy, is excellent.[26] The long-term disease-free survival rate in patients with advanced disease treated with combination chemotherapy is 70% to 80%.[26] After relapse, high-dose therapy may produce additional long-term survivors.[27]

Most patients who are successfully treated for Hodgkin's disease return to a normal or very near normal quality of life on cessation of treatment. Many women who receive combination chemotherapy for Hodgkin's disease remain fertile, although there is a risk of premature menopause.[28] No apparent increase in the complications of pregnancy or fetal abnormality in subsequent pregnancy is seen after combination chemotherapy for Hodgkin's disease.[29]

Fetal Risks

The risks to the fetus stem chiefly from the effects of either radiation therapy or chemotherapy. The risks to the fetus of diagnostic radiation have been reviewed.[30,31] Exposure of pregnant women to the radiation doses used in abdominal and pelvic computed tomography appears to have no substantial effect on the risk of fetal death or malformation. The risk of childhood cancer is more than doubled after fetal irradiation. When possible, irradiation of the fetus in utero should be avoided, but staging should be sufficient to determine the correct modality of treatment. Magnetic resonance imaging is the preferred tool for staging evaluation and avoids exposure to ionizing radiation.[24]

The use of therapeutic irradiation depends on whether early-stage Hodgkin's disease involves the abdomen or pelvis. Supradiaphragmatic irradiation with heavy lead shielding of the uterus resulted in no congenital abnormalities in one series.[32] When high-dose irradiation cannot be avoided by field manipulation, infradiaphragmatic radiation therapy with appropriate shielding carries a substantial risk of spontaneous miscarriage and fetal abnormality. Under these circumstances, chemotherapy rather than radiation therapy should be considered, with delivery before therapeutic irradiation. The fetal effects of combination chemotherapy used to treat Hodgkin's disease are unlikely to be substantially different from those seen in acute leukemia. The teratogenic risk is greatest with first-trimester exposure. However, some series found no apparent adverse effects with first-trimester exposure to the current "gold standard" treatment of doxorubicin (Adriamycin), bleomycin, vincristine, and dacarbazine (ABVD).[33]

Management Options

PREPREGNANCY

Women with active Hodgkin's disease should be counseled about the risks of pregnancy and should take appropriate contraceptive measures. Pregnancy outcome is good in patients who have been successfully treated for Hodgkin's disease, and routine amniocentesis is not recommended, as it is for leukemia (discussed earlier).

PRENATAL

The outlook for patients treated for Hodgkin's disease is good to excellent. Diagnosis and testing (discussed earlier) are as for the nonpregnant patient. Patients diagnosed in the first trimester should be counseled about the risks of continuing with the pregnancy. Early-stage supradiaphragmatic disease can be successfully treated with radiation therapy alone, with little fetal risk. Historically, early-stage intra-abdominal disease presented a management problem. The options were therapeutic abortion and early delivery, followed by local radiation therapy. Both supradiaphragmatic and infradiaphragmatic disease may be treated with a short course of combination chemotherapy until delivery, with radiation therapy given after delivery. Management decisions are complex, and discussion should include the patient, hemato-oncologist, obstetrician, and radiation oncologist.

Patients with more extensive disease should be counseled about the risks of proceeding with pregnancy. Some women continue with the pregnancy and opt for combination chemotherapy on evidence of disease progression. The optimum management in this context is not clear, but early in pregnancy, patients should receive standard chemotherapy, currently ABVD or an equivalent. Late in pregnancy, the mother can be treated with steroids alone or with single-agent vinblastine, which is not associated with a teratogenic risk at this point in gestation.[34] After delivery, patients may be treated with more aggressive combination chemotherapy, such as ABVD, as appropriate.

POSTNATAL

Careful counseling about the prognosis for both long-term disease-free survival and preservation of fertility should be given. Patients who are undergoing active treatment for Hodgkin's disease with combination chemotherapy should not breastfeed.[35]

SUMMARY OF MANAGEMENT OPTIONS

Hematologic Malignancies: Hodgkin's Disease

Management Options	Quality of Evidence	Strength of Recommendation	References
Prepregnancy			
Counsel about risks and prognosis	IIa	B	29
Give contraceptive advice	III	B	34
Prenatal			
Interdisciplinary approach	–	GPP	–

SUMMARY OF MANAGEMENT OPTIONS

Hematologic Malignancies: Hodgkin's Disease *(Continued)*

Management Options	Quality of Evidence	Strength of Recommendation	References
Prenatal *(Continued)*			
Diagnosis by lymph node biopsy	–	GPP	–
Staging by clinical assessment and magnetic resonance imaging; counsel about the prognosis and risks to the fetus	IV	C	30
Treatment			
Stage Ia/IIa (localized disease):			
• Extra-abdominal:	III	B	32,34
• Radiation therapy with shielding with or without abbreviated chemotherapy	Ib	A	46
• Intra-abdominal (depends on gestation and the patient's wishes):	III	B	32,34
	Ib	A	46
• Delivery and radiation therapy with or without abbreviated chemotherapy			
• Continue pregnancy with chemotherapy only and supportive care			
Stage III/IV (end-stage disease):	IIa	B	47
• Chemotherapy with supportive care			
Postnatal			
As for acute leukemia	–	GPP	–

Non-Hodgkin's Lymphomas

Non-Hodgkin's lymphomas comprise a heterogeneous group of malignancies. Unlike in Hodgkin's disease, extranodal presentation of non-Hodgkin's lymphoma is not uncommon. The increase in the incidence of non-Hodgkin's lymphomas is partly attributable to an aging population, but an unexplained real increase in incidence has been noted. As reflected in the literature, non-Hodgkin's lymphomas are uncommon in the reproductive years. The subclassification of non-Hodgkin's lymphomas is complex and changing. However, in general, three types of biologic behavior are seen.[3]

Low-grade, or indolent, lymphomas that are slow-growing do not threaten life and may be treated either on a wait and watch basis or with single-agent chemotherapy or local radiation therapy.[36] More aggressive lymphomas, such as diffuse large B cell lymphoma, have a much shorter clinical history and may cause early life-threatening complications. These are treated with combination chemotherapy in concert with a monoclonal antibody directed against CD20 (rituximab).[37] Some lymphomas, such as lymphoblastic lymphoma, behave biologically in a similar fashion to ALL. These must be treated with aggressive combination chemotherapy, the nature of which depends on the histologic subtype.

Maternal Risks

Diagnosis is made on biopsy, and testing and staging are as for Hodgkin's disease, although advanced disease is more common in non-Hodgkin's lymphomas. Treatment must be highly individualized and may, as discussed earlier, vary from a wait and watch policy to administration of intermediate- or high-dose combination chemotherapy. In these patients, the management and outlook are similar to those in nonpregnant patients.

Fetal Risks

The disease does not appear to affect the outcome of pregnancy, and the risks to the fetus are those of treatment. In terms of exposure to cytotoxic agents, fetal risk should not be substantially different from that seen in acute leukemia and Hodgkin's disease. The recent introduction of rituximab into the management of diffuse large B cell lymphoma poses an additional complication.[37] Insufficient data are available on the effects of rituximab on pregnancy to allow formal risk stratification. Rituximab is contraindicated in pregnancy. The introduction of an agent such as rituximab, which clearly improves outcome but has limited data in pregnancy, illustrates the dilemma that many physicians face.

Management Options

PREPREGNANCY

Women who have active non-Hodgkin's lymphoma should be counseled about the outlook for the particular subtype of disease and receive appropriate contraceptive advice. Patients who are receiving active treatment for non-Hodgkin's lymphoma should be advised against becoming pregnant.

PRENATAL

Management depends on the histologic subtype and extent of disease (discussed earlier).

POSTNATAL

Although data are limited, patients undergoing active treatment for non-Hodgkin's lymphoma should be advised against breastfeeding.

SUMMARY OF MANAGEMENT OPTIONS

Hematologic Malignancies: Non-Hodgkin's Lymphoma

Management Options	Quality of Evidence	Strength of Recommendation	References
Prepregnancy			
As for Hodgkin's disease	–	GPP	–
Prenatal			
Interdisciplinary approach	–	GPP	–
Comments about staging and diagnosis as for Hodgkin's disease	–	GPP	–
Treat as for a nonpregnant patient; options vary from "wait and watch" to aggressive combination chemotherapy with supportive care; termination and preterm delivery before chemotherapy are options	Ib III	A C	48 49
Counsel about the prognosis and risk to the fetus	III	C	49
Postnatal			
As for acute leukemia	–	GPP	–

MYELOPROLIFERATIVE DISORDERS

Essential Thrombocythemia

Diagnosis, Assessment, and Risks

Essential thrombocythemia is a myeloproliferative disorder that usually occurs in the elderly. Occasional cases complicating pregnancy are reported in the literature. Causes of reactive thrombocytosis are much more common and should be carefully excluded. Common causes of reactive thrombocytosis include iron deficiency, hemorrhage, infection, and inflammatory conditions. In essential thrombocythemia, the platelet count is consistently elevated in the absence of an apparent underlying cause. Samples obtained on bone marrow biopsy usually have a characteristic appearance. Cytogenetic studies should be carried out on bone marrow aspirate material to exclude CML. Essential thrombocythemia may be complicated by abnormal bleeding as a result of defective platelet function or small vessel thrombosis. The incidence of these complications in younger patients is unknown, and thrombosis may be less common. The literature on pregnancy includes small series and case reports. Spontaneous abortion, intrauterine death, and intrauterine growth restriction are possible risks, because placental infarction may occur.[38,39] However, others reported good pregnancy outcomes in small series of asymptomatic women.[40,41]

Management Options

If the patient is asymptomatic and the platelet count is only moderately increased, an expectant approach is reasonable.[38] If thrombosis or hemorrhage occurs, however, treatment is necessary. Because of a reluctance to use cytotoxic agents in pregnancy, plateletpheresis has been used.[38] However, this treatment is a very short-term measure, and it is virtually impossible to achieve good platelet control over longer periods. Aspirin may be used to treat thrombotic complications,[39] but routine use should be avoided because it may aggravate an underlying platelet function defect. Aspirin may have a role in patients with essential thrombocythemia and a history of previous pregnancy failure or growth restriction, but few data are available.[40] There are anecdotal reports of the use of hydroxyurea in essential thrombocythemia in pregnancy.[39] Most experience with this agent in pregnancy is with CML, when hydroxyurea has been used for prolonged periods. Because teratogenicity is reported in animals, however, first-trimester use of hydroxyurea and other cytotoxic agents should be avoided. The safety profile is good in the second and third trimesters. More recently, α-interferon has been used successfully throughout pregnancy in patients with essential thrombocythemia, without adverse effects.[42,43] More data are needed on the safety of α-interferon in pregnancy, but early reports are encouraging. It may emerge as the agent of choice if treatment of essential thrombocythemia is necessary in a pregnant woman.

Similarly, data on the safety of anagrelide, a new agent used to treat essential thrombocythemia, are limited. This agent should be avoided in pregnancy, and alternative methods should be used to control the platelet count, when necessary.

Because data are inconsistent, increased surveillance is appropriate when assessment of growth and umbilical artery Doppler recordings show intrauterine growth restriction and placental infarction.

Platelet dysfunction may lead to an increased risk of primary and secondary postpartum hemorrhage. Secondary hemorrhage is exacerbated by the risk of retained placental fragments from an infarcted placenta.

Polycythemia

Polycythemia occurs when hemoglobin, hematocrit, and the red cell mass are increased above the upper limit of normal for the patient's age and sex. Polycythemia may be relative or true. Relative, or stress, polycythemia occurs when plasma volume is reduced with no increase in the red cell mass. In true polycythemia, the red cell mass is greater than 32 mL/kg for women and 36 mL/kg for men. True polycythemia may be primary or secondary. Secondary polycythemia occurs in conditions associated with either chronic hypoxia or inappropriate erythropoietin production (e.g., renal cysts or tumors). Primary proliferative polycythemia, or polycythemia rubra vera, is caused by unchecked proliferation of erythroid precursors in the bone marrow. Primary polycythemia is believed to arise as a result of a clonal defect in a pluripotent stem cell. Polycythemia rubra vera is usually a disease of the elderly, but rare cases are described in women of childbearing age.[44]

The diagnosis of polycythemia is difficult during pregnancy because physiologic changes in plasma volume may decrease hemoglobin and hematocrit. Further, isotopic techniques used to determine the red cell mass and plasma volume are contraindicated in pregnancy. Definitive testing and diagnosis usually must be postponed until after delivery. In women who have a high hematocrit in pregnancy, secondary causes should be excluded. Preeclampsia and intrauterine growth restriction are associated with failure of normal plasma volume expansion. In these conditions, hematocrit may be relatively increased compared with levels in normal pregnancy, but an increase above the normal range in nonpregnant women usually does not occur. Features such as splenomegaly, increased white cell and platelet counts, and high serum vitamin B_{12} levels suggest primary polycythemia. If erythropoietin levels are available, a low level suggests primary proliferative polycythemia. However, erythropoietin levels increase physiologically during pregnancy,[45] and a normal or high level is difficult to interpret.

Maternal and Fetal Risks

In a series of patients with polycythemia rubra vera, 13 pregnancies were identified in 8 women.[44] Maternal outcome was good, but fetal outcome was adversely affected. Abortion, preterm delivery, and stillbirth were more common than expected. The risk of pregnancy-induced hypertension may also be increased. A relationship between pregnancy outcome and maternal red cell count was suggested, but the numbers in this study were too small to allow firm conclusions to be drawn. In some patients, hematocrit decreased significantly during pregnancy.

Management Options

Venesection may be performed to maintain the hematocrit below 0.45. Myelosuppressive therapy should be avoided but may be necessary in patients with associated marked thrombocytosis. Management principles are similar to those outlined for essential thrombocythemia. Thrombosis prophylaxis in the puerperium should be considered and should include compression stockings and early mobilization. Peripartum treatment with subcutaneous low-molecular-weight heparin is also an option, although there are no data in this patient group. Short-term treatment with low-molecular-weight heparin has a good safety profile for other indications, and the balance of risks is probably in favor of peripartum low-molecular-weight heparin prophylaxis in women with primary polycythemia.

SUMMARY OF MANAGEMENT OPTIONS
Myeloproliferative Disorders

Management Options	Quality of Evidence	Strength of Recommendation	References
Essential Thrombocythemia			
Prenatal			
Expectant approach in asymptomatic patients with moderate elevation of platelets	III	B	38
If the patient is symptomatic (thrombosis or bleeding), consider plasmapheresis	III	B	38
Give low-dose aspirin if the patient has thrombosis; no evidence supports use in all cases	III	B	39,40
Hydroxyurea has been used, but most experience is with chronic myeloid leukemia	III	B	39
Limited experience with alpha interferon	III	B	42,43
No experience with anagrelide; avoid	–	GPP	–
Serial fetal growth and umbilical artery Doppler recordings	–	GPP	–
Labor and Delivery			
Vigilance for PPH	–	GPP	–
Polycythemia			
Prenatal			
Vigilance for hypertensive disease	III	B	44
Serial fetal growth and umbilical artery Doppler recordings	III	B	44
Some advocate regular venisection to keep hematocrit <0.45; no evidence supports this practice	III	B	44
Postnatal			
Prophylactic low-molecular-weight heparin	–	GPP	–

PPH, postpartum hemorrhage

CONCLUSIONS

- Pregnancy should be deferred until the patient is in remission.
- When malignancy is diagnosed in pregnancy, the available options should be discussed with the patient.

Options include:
- Initiating treatment and continuing with the pregnancy
- Terminating pregnancy and initiating treatment
- First-trimester chemotherapy carries the risk of teratogenicity to the fetus.
- After the first trimester, the main fetal risk associated with chemotherapy is growth restriction.
- Radiation therapy is contraindicated in pregnancy.

REFERENCES

1. McClain CR: Leukaemia in pregnancy. Clin Obstet Gynaecol 1974;17:185–194.
2. Ward FT, Weiss RB: Lymphoma in pregnancy. Semin Oncol 1989;16:397–409.
3. WHO Classification of Tumours: Pathology and genetics of tumours of haemopoietic and lymphoid tissues. In Jaffe E, Harris NL, Stein H, Vardiman JW (eds): Lyon, IARC Press, 2001.
4. Fletcher JA, Lynch EA, Kimball VM, et al: Translocation 9;22 is associated with extremely poor prognosis in intensively treated children with acute lymphoblastic leukaemia. Blood 1991;77: 435–440.

5. Sanders JE, Buckner CD, Amos D, et al: Ovarian function following marrow transplantation for aplastic anaemia or leukaemia. J Clin Oncol 1988;6:813–818.
6. Milliken S, Powles R, Parikh P, et al: Successful pregnancy following bone marrow transplantation for leukaemia. Bone Marrow Transplant 1990;1:135–137.
7. Nicholson HO: Cytotoxic drugs in pregnancy: Review of reported cases. J Obstet Gynaecol Br Commonw 1968;75:307–312.
8. Colbear TN, Nagman A, Gorin NC, et al: Acute leukaemia during pregnancy: Favourable course of pregnancy in two patients treated with cytosine arabinoside and anthracyclines. Nouv Presse Med 1980;9:19–178.
9. Kirshond B, Wasserstrum N, Willis R, et al: Teratogenic effects of first trimester cyclophosphamide therapy. Obstet Gynecol 1988;72:462–464.
10. Selevan SG, Lindbohm ML, Hiornum GRW, et al: Study of occupational exposure to antineoplastic drugs and fetal loss in nurses. N Engl J Med 1985;313:1173–1178.
11. Powell HR, Ekert H: Methotrexate induced congenital malformation. Med J Aust 1971;2:1076–1077.
12. Fenaux P, Chomienne C, Degos L: Acute promyelocytic leukaemia: Biology and treatment. Semin Haematol 1987;33: 127–133.
13. Schleuning M, Clemm C: Chromosomal aberrations in a newborn whose mother received cytotoxic treatment during pregnancy. N Engl J Med 1987;317:166–167.
14. Cornel MC: Variation in prenatal cytogenetic diagnosis: Policies in 13 European countries, 1989–1991. EUROCAT Working Group: European Registration of Congenital Anomalies. Prenat Diagn 1994;14:337–344.
15. Byrne J, Rasmussen SA, Steinhorn SC, et al: Genetic disease in offspring of long-term survivors of childhood and adolescent cancer. Am J Hum Genet 1998;62:45–52.
16. Green DM, Whitton JA, Stovall M, et al: Pregnancy outcome of female survivors of childhood cancer: A report from the Childhood Cancer Survivor Study. Am J Obstet Gynecol 2002; 187:1070–1080.
17. O'Brien SG, Guilhot F, Larson RA, et al: Imatinib compared with interferon and low-dose cytarabine for newly diagnosed chronic-phase chronic myeloid leukaemia. N Engl J Med 2003;348:994–1004.
18. Deininger MWN, O'Brien SG, Ford JM, Druker BJ: Practical management of patients with chronic myeloid leukaemia receiving imatinib. J Clin Oncol 2003;21:1637–1647.
19. Ozumba BC, Obi GO: Successful pregnancy in a patient with chronic myeloid leukaemia following therapy with cytotoxic drugs. Int J Gynecol Obstet 1992;38:49–53.
20. Reichel RP, Linkesch W, Schetitska D: Therapy with recombinant interferon alpha 2c during unexpected pregnancy in a patient with chronic myeloid leukaemia. Br J Haematol 1992;82:472–473.
21. Goldman J: The management of chronic myeloid leukaemia. In Treleaven J, Barrett J (eds): Bone Marrow Transplantation in Practice. London, Churchill Livingstone, 1992, pp 19–31.
22. Macfarlane GJ, Evstifeeva T, Boyle P, et al: International patterns in the occurrence of Hodgkin's disease in children and young adult males. Int J Cancer 1995;61:165–169.
23. Lister TA, Crowther D, Sutcliff SP, et al: Report of a committee convened to discuss the evaluation of staging with patients with Hodgkin's disease: Cotswolds Meeting. J Clin Oncol 1989;6:1630–1636.
24. Nicklas AH, Baker ME: Imaging strategies in the pregnant cancer patient. Semin Oncol 2000;27:623–632.
25. Carde P: Diagnostic procedures in Hodgkin's disease. In Diehl V (ed): Clinical Haematology, Hodgkin's Disease. London, Bailliere Tindall 1996;9:479–501.
26. Joshing A, Wolf J, Diehl V: Hodgkin's disease: Prognostic factors and treatment strategies. Curr Opin Oncol 2000;12:403–411.
27. Anderson JE, Litzow MR, Appelbaum FR, et al: Allogeneic, syngeneic and autologous marrow transplantation for Hodgkin's disease: The twenty one year Seattle experience. J Clin Oncol 1993;11:2342–2350.
28. Clarke ST, Radford JA, Crowther D, et al: Gonadal function following chemotherapy for Hodgkin's disease: A comparative study of MVPP and a seven drug hybrid regime. J Clin Oncol 1995;130:134–139.
29. Aisner J, Wiernik PH, Pearl P: Pregnancy outcome in patients treated for Hodgkin's disease. J Clin Oncol 1993;11:507–512.
30. Statement by the National Radiological Protection Board: Diagnostic medical exposures. Advice and exposure to ionising radiation during pregnancy. Doc NRPB (Oxon) 1993;4:1–14.
31. Greskovich JF Jr, Macklis RM: Radiation therapy in pregnancy: Risk calculation and risk minimization. Semin Oncol 2000;27:633–645.
32. Woo SY, Fuller LM, Cundiff JH, et al: Radiotherapy during pregnancy for clinical stage JA-IIA Hodgkin's disease. Int J Radiat Oncol Biol Phys 1992;23:407–412.
33. Aviles A, Diaz-Maqueo JC, Talavera A, et al: Growth and development of children of mothers treated with chemotherapy during pregnancy: Current status of 43 children. Am J Hematol 1991;36:234–248.
34. Jacobs C, Donaldson SS, Rosenberg SA, et al: Management of the pregnant patient with Hodgkin's disease. Ann Intern Med 1981;95:669–675.
35. Committee on drugs, American Academy of Pediatrics: Transfer of drugs and other chemicals into human milk. Pediatrics 1994;93:137–150.
36. Horning SJ, Rosenberg SA: The natural history of initially untreated low grade non-Hodgkin's lymphomas. N Engl J Med 1994;311:1471–1475.
37. Coffier B, Lepage E, Briere J, et al: CHOP chemotherapy plus Rituximab compared with CHOP alone in elderly patients with diffuse large B cell lymphoma. N Engl J Med 2000;546: 235–238.
38. Mercer B, Drouin J, Jolly E, et al: Primary thrombocythemia in pregnancy: A report of two cases. Am J Obstet Gynecol 1988;159:127–128.
39. Beressi AH, Tefferi A, Silverstein MN, et al: Outcome analysis of 34 pregnancies in women with essential thrombocythemia. Arch Intern Med 1995;155:1217–1222.
40. Beard J, Hillmen P, Anderson CC, et al: Primary thrombocythaemia in pregnancy. Br J Haematol 1990;77:371–374.
41. Randi ML, Barnone E, Rossi C, et al: Essential thrombocythemia and pregnancy: A report of six normal pregnancies in five untreated patients. Obstet Gynecol 1994;83:915–917.
42. Williams JM, Schlesinger PE, Gray AG: Successful treatment of essential thrombocythaemia and recurrent abortion with alpha interferon. Br J Haematol 1994;88:647–648.
43. Delage R, Demers C, Cantin G, et al: Treatment of essential thrombocythemia during pregnancy with interferon-alpha. Obstet Gynecol 1996;87:814–817.
44. Ferguson II JE, Ueland K, Aronson WJ: Polycythemia rubra vera and pregnancy. Obstet Gynecol 1983;62:16S–20S.
45. Hytten F: Blood volume changes in normal pregnancy. Clin Haematol 1985;14:601–612.
46. Hoppe RT, Colman CN, Cox RS, et al: The management of stage I–II Hodgkin's disease with irradiation alone or combined modality therapy: The Stanford experience. Blood 1982;59: 445–446.
47. Cullen MH, Stuart NS, Woodroffe C, et al: ChlVPP/PABlOE and radiotherapy in advanced Hodgkin's disease. J Clin Oncol 1994;12:779–787.

48. Linch DC, Vaughan Hudson B, et al: A randomised comparison of a third generation regimen (PACEBOM) with a standard regimen (CHOP) in patients with histologically aggressive non-Hodgkin's lymphoma: A British National Lymphoma Investigation report. Br J Cancer 1996;74:318–322.

49. Aviles A, Diaz-Maqueo JC, Torras, et al: Non-Hodgkin's lymphomas and pregnancy: Presentation of 16 cases. Gynecol Oncol 1990;37:335–337.

CHAPTER 41

Thrombocytopenia and Bleeding Disorders

Elizabeth Helen Horn / Lucy Kean

THROMBOCYTOPENIA

Introduction

The normal range for peripheral blood platelet count in nonpregnant individuals is generally reported as 150 to 400 × 10^9/L. If a low platelet count is seen on an automated complete blood count, spurious thrombocytopenia should be excluded. This condition may occur because of a small clot in the blood sample or because of platelet clumping caused by the addition of the anticoagulant EDTA to the sample. A repeat count for confirmation and examination of the peripheral blood film can ascertain whether the thrombocytopenia is genuine. If the blood film shows platelet clumps, a repeat complete blood count in a sample anticoagulated with citrate may resolve the problem.

Studies of platelet counts during normal pregnancy differed in their conclusions, with some suggesting no overall effect of pregnancy on platelet count[1–3] and others showing a modest reduction in late pregnancy.[4–6] One study of platelet counts in 6715 consecutive patients delivering in a single Canadian center showed that thrombocytopenia (platelet count <150 × 10^9/L) occurred in 7.6% of women, and most (65.1%) had no associated pathology.[7] From a practical point of view, any pregnant woman with a platelet count of less than 100 × 10^9/L should undergo further clinical and laboratory assessment. No pathology is found in most women with mild thrombocytopenia.[8] Pregnant women with platelet counts between 100 and 150 × 10^9/L should be evaluated further if there has been a rapid decline in the platelet count.

Causes of Thrombocytopenia in Pregnancy

Causes of thrombocytopenia in pregnancy are summarized in Table 41–1. They can be broadly divided into the following categories:

- Platelet destruction or consumption
- Splenic sequestration of platelets
- Failure of platelet production in the bone marrow

Platelet destruction or consumption is much more common than bone marrow failure in obstetric practice. Causes with management implications in pregnancy are discussed in detail.

Investigation of Thrombocytopenia in Pregnancy

As discussed earlier, spurious thrombocytopenia should be excluded. In assessing pregnant women with genuine thrombocytopenia, close liaison is required between the obstetrician and the hematologist. Patients should be assessed clinically to obtain clues to the diagnosis. In patients with severe thrombocytopenia, the clinical severity of hemorrhagic problems should be assessed. In the history, current or previous bleeding problems or a family history of a hemorrhagic disorder should be noted. Other medical or obstetric problems, a drug and alcohol history, and a recent transfusion history should be noted. For example, a history of recurrent miscarriage suggests antiphospholipid syndrome. On examination, important features include petechiae and signs of mucosal bleeding. Blood pressure should be measured, and the clinician should look for clinical features that suggest underlying autoimmune disease, chronic liver disease, or splenomegaly. Urinalysis should be performed, and proteinuria should be quantified. Careful examination of the blood film is mandatory because it may give important clues to the diagnosis. For example, red cell fragmentation narrows the differential diagnosis to thrombotic microangiopathies (discussed later) (Table 41–2). Hypersegmented neutrophils and oval macrocytes suggest folate deficiency, and other red and white cell

TABLE 41–1

Causes of Thrombocytopenia in Pregnancy

Platelet Consumption or Destruction

- Gestational thrombocytopenia
- Autoimmune thrombocytopenia
  - Primary
  - Secondary
    - Antiphospholipid syndrome
    - Systemic lupus erythematosus and connective tissue disorders
    - Drug-induced
    - HIV-associated
    - Other viral infection (e.g., Epstein-Barr virus)
    - Lymphoma
  - Nonimmune
    - Disseminated intravascular coagulation
    - Preeclampsia or HELLP syndrome
    - Thrombotic thrombocytopenia purpura or hemolytic uremic syndrome
    - Acute fatty liver of pregnancy
    - Heparin-induced thrombocytopenia
    - Large vascular malformations

Splenic Sequestration

- Splenomegaly
- Portal hypertension
- Liver disease
- Portal or hepatic vein thrombosis
- Myeloproliferative disorders
- Lymphoproliferative disorders
- Storage disease (e.g., Gaucher's disease)
- Infection (e.g., tropical splenomegaly or malaria)

Failure of Platelet Production

- Bone marrow suppression
  - Drug-induced
  - Aplastic anemia
  - Paroxysmal nocturnal hemoglobinuria
  - Infection (e.g., parvovirus B19)
  - Bone marrow infiltration
    - Hematologic malignancy
    - Nonhematologic malignancy
- Severe vitamin B_{12} or folate deficiency

abnormalities may suggest underlying bone marrow disease. In gestational thrombocytopenia and autoimmune thrombocytopenia (AITP), the blood film is normal except for the apparent reduction in platelet count. The results of coagulation screening tests and D-dimer may be abnormal in thrombocytopenia associated with consumptive coagulopathy. Renal and liver function should be routinely checked. The serum urate level may be increased in preeclampsia, HELLP (hemolysis, elevated liver enzymes, low platelets) syndrome, or acute fatty liver of pregnancy. The lactate dehydrogenase level is usually elevated in microangiopathic hemolysis. The pattern of development of thrombocytopenia should be determined if previous platelet counts are available. Bone marrow examination is necessary only when the diagnosis is unclear after initial clinical and laboratory assessment or if features suggest underlying bone marrow disease. However, bone marrow examination may be carried out in suspected AITP if thrombocytopenia is severe or if treatment with steroids is contemplated.[8]

After initial assessment, further tests may be indicated, including antinuclear factor, specific tests for lupus anticoagulant and anticardiolipin antibodies, or tests for the diagnosis and typing of von Willebrand's disease (vWD). Platelet antibody testing by standard techniques is of little value both diagnostically and prognostically in suspected cases of AITP.[8–11] In cases of suspected thrombotic thrombocytopenic purpura (TTP), some specialized laboratories carry out von Willebrand factor (vWf) multimer analysis and assay of ADAMTS 13 (a member of the ADAMTS family), a vWf cleaving protease (discussed later), in plasma. These tests can be helpful but are not necessary in the differential diagnosis of thrombotic microangiopathy with typical clinical fea-

TABLE 41–2

Variation in the Features and Management of Thrombotic Microangiopathic Hemolytic Anemia

DIAGNOSIS	CLASSIC THROMBOTIC THROMBOCYTOPENIC PURPURA	POSTPARTUM HEMOLYTIC URENIC SYNDROME	HELLP SYNDROME	PREECLAMPSIA OR ECLAMPSIA
Time of onset	Usually < 24 weeks	Postpartum	After 20 weeks, Most >34 weeks	After 20 weeks, Most >34 weeks
Hemolysis	+++	++	++	+
Thrombocytopenia	+++	++	++	++
Coagulopathy	–	–	±	±
Central nervous system symptoms	+++	±	±	±
Liver disease	±	±	+++	±
Renal disease	±	+++	+	+
Hypertension	Rare	±	±	+++
Effect on fetus	Placental infarct can lead to intrauterine growth restriction and mortality	None, if maternal disease is controlled	Associated with placental ischemia and increased neonatal mortality	Intrauterine growth restriction; occasional mortality
Effect of delivery on disease	None	None	Recovery, but may worsen transiently	Recovery, but may worsen transiently
Management	Early plasma exchange is imperative	Supportive ± plasma exchange	Supportive; consider plasma exchange if persists	Supportive; plasma exchange rarely required; consider if persists

tures. There is no one diagnostic test for TTP or any microangiopathic syndrome. If specialized tests are considered, they should be discussed with a hematologist.

Gestational Thrombocytopenia

Gestational thrombocytopenia, or incidental thrombocytopenia of pregnancy, accounts for approximately 70% of cases of maternal thrombocytopenia at delivery.[7,12] The cause is unknown. There is evidence of a degree of physiologic platelet activation in vivo during pregnancy; platelet lifespan is reduced, and the site of platelet activation is believed to be the placental circulation.[13,14] These mechanisms may contribute to gestational thrombocytopenia.

Thrombocytopenia usually develops in the third trimester and is usually mild to moderate. Results of other studies are normal. The platelet count is usually greater than 80×10^9/L, and counts of 40 to 50×10^9/L are attributed to gestational thrombocytopenia.[7,15,16] The platelet count rapidly returns to normal after delivery, usually within 7 days.[7,15] Gestational thrombocytopenia is a diagnosis of exclusion. Antenatally, it can be difficult to distinguish from mild AITP. The diagnosis is suggested by a late decrease in platelet count in a patient with no history of this disorder. Certainty often rests on observations of platelet counts in the puerperium.

Maternal and Fetal Risks

Gestational thrombocytopenia has no pathologic significance for the mother or fetus.[7,8,12,15–17] When gestational thrombocytopenia and AITP cannot be distinguished, if the diagnosis is AITP, a potential concern is the transfer of antiplatelet antibodies across the placenta, leading to fetal and neonatal thrombocytopenia. However, neonatal thrombocytopenia is uncommon in women in whom thrombocytopenia is incidentally detected in pregnancy and in whom there is no history of AITP. The incidence of neonatal thrombocytopenia in these patients is approximately 4%,[16,18] which is not statistically different from the incidence of thrombocytopenia in infants of nonthrombocytopenic mothers. Further, no infants in these studies had cord platelet counts less than 50×10^9/L, and none had clinical hemostatic impairment.[16,18]

Management Options

PREPREGNANCY AND PRENATAL

If a woman with previous gestational thrombocytopenia seeks prepregnancy counseling, the most important issue is the exclusion of alternative diagnoses. This is also the case when thrombocytopenia is detected incidentally in the antenatal period. The maternal platelet count should be monitored at a frequency determined by the platelet count, rate of decline, and expected date of delivery.[8] No treatment is necessary for gestational thrombocytopenia. Invasive approaches to fetal monitoring, such as fetal blood sampling to determine the fetal platelet count, are not indicated because the risks are not justifiable (discussed later).[8,17]

LABOR AND DELIVERY

Because the fetus is not at risk for hemorrhage, the mode of delivery is determined by obstetric considerations, and

SUMMARY OF MANAGEMENT OPTIONS

Gestational Thrombocytopenia

Management Options	Quality of Evidence	Strength of Recommendation	References
Prepregnancy and Prenatal			
Exclude pathologic causes	IV	C	1
Monitor platelet count	IV	C	8
Fetal blood sampling not indicated	III	B	17
Observe if $>100 \times 10^9$/L	III	B	18
If rapid fall or $<50 \times 10^9$/L, reevaluate for pathologic causes	III	B	18
Labor and Delivery			
Avoid fetal blood sampling and traumatic vaginal delivery if autoimmune thrombocytopenia purpura not excluded	IV	C	8
Epidural anesthesia is considered safe if platelet count $>80 \times 10^9$/L	IV	C	8
Obtain cord blood or neonatal blood at delivery to check neonatal platelet count	III	B	18
Postnatal			
Verify that maternal count returns to normal after delivery to confirm the diagnosis	III	B	18

invasive fetal blood sampling to determine the fetal platelet count is not indicated. Epidural anesthesia is considered safe if the maternal platelet count is greater than 80×10^9/L.[8]

If AITP has not been excluded, traumatic delivery, the use of fetal scalp electrodes, and fetal scalp blood sampling for acid–base status should be avoided.[8]

POSTNATAL

If it is difficult to distinguish between gestational thrombocytopenia and AITP, a cord platelet count should be obtained. If this count is low, serial counts should be obtained in the neonate (discussed later). Maternal platelet counts should also be followed postnatally. A rapid return to normal confirms the diagnosis of gestational thrombocytopenia, whereas continued thrombocytopenia after pregnancy should prompt reassessment of the patient.

Autoimmune Thrombocytopenia

AITP is relatively common in women of childbearing age. AITP occurs in approximately 0.14% of pregnant women at delivery and accounts for 3% of cases of thrombocytopenia at that time.[15] AITP is caused by autoantibodies, which are usually directed against platelet surface glycoproteins, particularly glycoprotein IIb/IIIa and glycoprotein Ib/IX.[19,20] These antibodies adhere to the platelet membrane, causing platelet destruction through Fc receptors in the reticuloendothelial system. The major site of platelet destruction is usually the spleen. AITP may cause purpura and self-limited mucosal bleeding. This pattern of acute AITP, often after a viral infection, is most commonly seen in children. On the other hand, AITP in adults is usually chronic. The symptoms are variable and are often insidious. Although fluctuations in the platelet count may occur, the condition is not self-limiting, and continuing thrombocytopenia is the usual course. Chronic AITP may be asymptomatic and may be found by routine testing, such as the testing that is performed during pregnancy.

AITP may be primary or idiopathic or may be secondary to another disorder (see Table 41–1). In primary AITP, the clinical examination may show purpura, bruising, or signs of mucosal bleeding, but findings are otherwise normal. Other than a reduced platelet count, findings on the blood film are normal, and the bone marrow is normal, with normal or increased numbers of megakaryocytes. In primary or idiopathic AITP, all other test results are normal. Secondary causes of AITP may be associated with antinuclear antibodies or increased levels of anticardiolipin antibodies. HIV testing should be carried out if the patient is in an at-risk group, if this testing was not already performed as a routine antenatal check.

Previously, in AITP, the platelet antibody tests that were used depended on the finding of platelet-associated immunoglobulin G. However, this test has a high frequency of false-positive and false-negative results.[20] More recently, glycoprotein-specific antibodies have been detected in AITP by antigen immobilization assays.[20] These assays show improved specificity but are unreliable as diagnostic tools in individual patients.[20] Further, no assay of platelet antibodies has predictive value for maternal or fetal outcome.[8–11]

Maternal Risks

The risk of maternal bleeding relates to the severity of thrombocytopenia. In AITP, clinical bleeding is often less severe for a given platelet count than in conditions in which thrombocytopenia is caused by an underlying bone marrow disorder.

Women with severe thrombocytopenia (platelet count $<20 \times 10^9$/L) are at risk for spontaneous bleeding antenatally as well as at delivery, and they generally require treatment. Women with platelet counts less than 50×10^9/L may be at risk for increased bleeding at delivery[8,21]; therefore, treatment may be required in late pregnancy to ensure a safe platelet count for delivery in asymptomatic women. A platelet count of greater than 80×10^9/L is considered safe for epidural anesthesia.[8] These figures are generally accepted by clinicians but are somewhat arbitrary. There is no evidence that bleeding time is helpful in predicting hemorrhagic problems in AITP.

Fetal Risks

In mothers with AITP, immunoglobulin G antiplatelet antibodies may cross the placenta and cause fetal thrombocytopenia, resulting in fetal or neonatal bleeding. Maternal findings, such as platelet count and platelet-associated immunoglobulin G level, are of no value in predicting fetal thrombocytopenia.[10,22,23]

In the early 1990s, large prospective studies helped to clarify that in maternal AITP, the risk to the fetus and neonate of bleeding as a result of thrombocytopenia is extremely low. In these series, the overall incidence of fetal or neonatal thrombocytopenia was 10% to 30%, but severe thrombocytopenia was less common and intracranial hemorrhage was rare.[9,12,16,23] The largest study,[12] which was conducted over 7 years and included more than 15,000 mothers and infants, showed that among 46 mothers with AITP, 4 (8.7%) had cord platelet counts of 20 to 50×10^9/L. No infant whose mother had AITP had a platelet count of less than 20×10^9/L, and none had an adverse outcome, despite vaginal delivery in three of the four cases.[12] In this study, all of the neonates with clinically severe bleeding had alloimmune thrombocytopenia (see Chapter 15). Another study showed that 18 of 88 neonates (20%) born to women with AITP before the index pregnancy had platelet counts of less than 50×10^9/L. Five had clinically important bleeding, and two of these had intracranial hemorrhage.[16] In contrast, in this study, no infants born to women with incidentally detected thrombocytopenia in pregnancy had platelet counts of less than 50 × 10^9/L, and none had clinical bleeding. This study led to the suggestion that the only clear predictor of neonatal thrombocytopenia in pregnant woman with thrombocytopenia is a history of AITP, and even then, the incidence of neonatal bleeding is low. Limited data suggest that in women with AITP, the outcome of a previous pregnancy with respect to neonatal thrombocytopenia is a reasonable guide to the likely outcome of a current pregnancy, if there have been no significant changes in the course or management of AITP in the mother.[9,24] Another salient point is the time course of thrombocytopenia and bleeding complications in the fetus and neonate in a pregnancy affected by AITP. Bleeding in utero in maternal AITP is rare.[25] Other studies concluded that after birth, the platelet count continues to decrease in affected neonates, reaching a nadir 2 to 5 days after delivery.[10]

Management Options

PREPREGNANCY

In women known to have AITP before pregnancy, therapy should be optimized before pregnancy is planned. In patients with chronic AITP, decisions about splenectomy are best made before the patient becomes pregnant. In general, pregnancy does not affect the clinical course of AITP; however, there is anecdotal evidence of worsening of AITP during pregnancy, with improvement after delivery.[26] Some women of childbearing age have refractory AITP. In these women, if thrombocytopenia is severe, pregnancy may be hazardous and should be avoided. However, the potential hazards of pregnancy must be individually assessed, and patients should be counseled carefully. In addition to the risk of bleeding in the mother and fetus, the risks of third-line therapy in pregnancy (discussed later) must be reviewed. There is considerable experience in the use of azathioprine in pregnancy in clinical settings other than AITP.[27,28] When splenectomy is ineffective and ongoing treatment is needed, this may be a suitable third-line agent if pregnancy is a future consideration.

PRENATAL

In the prenatal period, the aims of management are as follows:

- To treat maternal symptoms of hemorrhage at any stage of pregnancy
- To achieve a safe platelet count for delivery

There is no evidence that any available modalities of treatment administered to the mother affect the platelet count in the fetus or neonate. The frequency of monitoring of platelet counts should be based on the initial count and the rate of decline. Closer surveillance is required in the last trimester to ensure a safe count for delivery. Treatment is generally required in symptomatic patients if the maternal platelet count is less than 20 × 10^9/L. Treatment is also required in late pregnancy, in the absence of symptoms, to raise the platelet count to 50 × 10^9/L or more for delivery.[8] Discussion about analgesia for labor should take place, preferably in the early part of the third trimester, because some women may consider regional analgesia. Alternatives should be discussed, but in some cases, it may be necessary to aim for a count of 80 × 10^9/L to allow regional analgesia to proceed. Balancing the risks requires particular assessment in these women, and treatment purely to allow for regional analgesia is discouraged.

Options for the treatment of AITP in pregnancy include corticosteroids and high-dose intravenous immunoglobulin (IVIG). Conventionally, steroids are used by many as the treatment of choice. When steroid therapy is chosen, prednisolone is usually given initially at a dose of 1 mg/kg daily (based on nonpregnant body weight). A response is obtained in most patients, allowing the dose to be tapered gradually to achieve the minimum dose at which a safe platelet count is achieved. Potential disadvantages of steroid therapy during pregnancy are the precipitation or exacerbation of hypertension, excessive weight gain, gestational diabetes, osteoporosis, and psychiatric disorders.[8,21] These considerations are particularly relevant when prolonged therapy is required and when high doses are required to control symptoms. From the fetal point of view, there is no evidence that corticosteroids are teratogenic, and fetal adrenal suppression is unlikely because prednisolone is extensively metabolized in the placenta.[29]

Concerns about potential adverse maternal effects of steroids have led some to use IVIG as first-line therapy in pregnancy.[15] Others reserve this treatment for patients who do not respond to steroids and patients in whom the maintenance dose of steroids is unacceptably high. IVIg is usually given in doses of 0.4 g/kg daily for 3 to 5 days.[30–38] Alternatively, 1 g/kg daily may be given for 1 or 2 days.[34] These regimens increase the platelet count in most cases, but the response to immunoglobulin is temporary in adult AITP. On average, responses are seen by the fifth day of infusion, with a peak response occurring approximately 4 to 5 days after the end of the infusion.[30] Responses tend to be sustained for only 2 to 4 weeks,[21] but the duration of response is extremely variable.[30] When IVIG is used to increase the platelet count before delivery, treatment is initiated approximately 10 days before delivery is planned. In mothers who need treatment for symptomatic AITP, courses of IVIG may be repeated at intervals to prevent symptoms and ensure a safe platelet count for delivery. One study outside the context of pregnancy showed that approximately one-third of patients who require repeated infusions eventually stop responding to immunoglobulin.[35]

IVIG is a pooled blood product. IVIG preparations that have been virally inactivated have an excellent safety record, but there is a small risk of transmission of infection.[8,33]

Other adverse effects include allergic reactions, and occasional cases of anaphylaxis have occurred in immunoglobulin A-deficient patients. Aseptic meningitis is well documented, and there are a few reports of thrombotic complications, mainly in elderly patients.[33] Renal failure may be precipitated by IVIG preparations with a high sucrose content.[36] IVIG is well tolerated in most patients. Other side effects tend to be mild.[33]

The placenta contains Fc receptors; therefore, immunoglobulins can cross the placenta. This finding led to hopes that maternal treatment with high-dose IVIG would improve the fetal platelet count.[31,32] There are no controlled studies, but fetal and neonatal thrombocytopenia has been reported with maternal use of IVIG.[33] Evidence does not show a substantial effect of IVIG on fetal platelet counts in maternal AITP.

Patients with severe hemorrhage associated with profound thrombocytopenia require aggressive management. In an emergency situation, 1g methylprednisolone given daily for 3 days has been advocated, perhaps combined with IVIG.[8,21] Although platelet transfusion has little efficacy prophylactically in AITP, platelets should be administered in large doses to patients with life-threatening bleeding.[8]

If a pregnant woman with AITP does not respond to standard treatment with steroids and IVIG, decisions about further therapy must be considered. Factors such as gestation and hemorrhagic symptoms should be taken into account. If the woman is not hemorrhagic, an observant approach is the best option. Platelet transfusion may be required at delivery, even if the patient is asymptomatic prenatally. If the patient is hemorrhagic, several options are available, but supporting evidence is anecdotal. Splenectomy was previously considered hazardous in pregnancy, but more recent literature suggests that, with modern supportive care, successful splenectomy may be carried out in pregnancy, preferably in the second trimester.[37] Splenectomy is commonly performed laparoscopically in nonpregnant patients. In pregnancy, the laparoscopic approach may also be preferable, if technically feasible. The enlarging uterus, however, is likely to cause difficulties with laparoscopic splenectomy after 20 weeks' gestation. Conventional splenectomy in the third trimester may precipitate premature labor, but in some cases, when the fetus is mature, splenectomy is combined with cesarean delivery in late pregnancy.[37] Approximately two thirds of patients have a useful response to splenectomy. Prophylaxis against infections with organisms such as pneumococci, *Haemophilus*, and *Neisseria meningitidis* is necessary. When splenectomy is performed during pregnancy, penicillin V prophylaxis should be given in the prenatal period, and vaccination against these organisms should be performed.

Patients in whom splenectomy is unsuccessful are extremely problematic. Several third-line therapies, such as danazol, vincristine, and cyclophosphamide, are unsuitable for use during pregnancy. In very severe refractory cases, when third-line therapy is necessary, azathioprine is probably the safest treatment. Experience with renal transplant recipients suggests that teratogenicity is rare in humans, but intrauterine growth restriction may occur.[27,28]

Collaboration with an obstetric anesthetist is necessary for all women with platelet counts low enough to affect delivery. Alternatives to regional analgesia, such as patient-controlled analgesia, can be offered when epidural analgesia is considered unsafe.

LABOR AND DELIVERY

From the maternal point of view, when possible, vaginal delivery is preferred in mothers affected by AITP. If the maternal platelet count remains low at the time of delivery, despite optimal antenatal treatment, platelet transfusion may be required to treat maternal bleeding. Platelets should be available for women who have a platelet count of less than $50 \times 10^9/L$ at delivery, but platelet transfusion given for purely prophylactic reasons is usually unnecessary and ineffective.

Epidural anesthesia should be avoided if the platelet count is less than $80 \times 10^9/L$,[8] although there is little concrete supporting evidence. The entire clinical scenario as well as the course of the decrease in platelet count should be considered.[8] Thrombocytopenic women are at risk for bleeding from surgical incisions. Judicious administration of platelets during operative procedures is reasonable in women with severe thrombocytopenia. Nonsteroidal anti-inflammatory drugs should be avoided for postpartum analgesia. AITP should not exclude women from consideration for peripartum thrombosis prophylaxis. Risk assessment should be carried out and should consider constitutional and acquired thrombotic risk factors as well as the risk of bleeding. Prophylactic doses of low-molecular-weight heparin are generally safe if the platelet count is greater than $50 \times 10^9/L$.[8] Graduated compression stockings may be used for women who require specific thrombosis prophylaxis if the platelet count is less than $50 \times 10^9/L$.

As discussed earlier, large, well-conducted studies show that the risk to the fetus and neonate of bleeding as a result of thrombocytopenia is low in maternal AITP.[12,16] No maternal findings are of value in predicting fetal thrombocytopenia. There is no role for measuring fetal platelet count in late pregnancy or during labor. Fetal scalp sampling is often inaccurate and can cause significant scalp bleeding or hematoma formation in thrombocytopenic fetuses. Intrauterine fetal blood sampling cannot be justified as a routine practice in maternal AITP because the associated risks outweigh the risk of serious neonatal hemorrhage.[8,9] In contrast, determining the fetal platelet count by intrauterine fetal blood sampling in the antenatal period has a role in the management of pregnancies potentially affected by neonatal alloimmune thrombocytopenia. In this situation, this sampling allows concomitant administration of therapeutic fetal platelet transfusion (see Chapter 15).[8,9]

In AITP, it was previously assumed that cesarean section may protect the fetus from bleeding as a result of head trauma. However, no difference was seen between vaginal delivery and cesarean section in bleeding complications in 474 infants born to mothers with AITP.[38] As the nadir of the platelet count often occurs several days after delivery,[10] peripartum events may not have a major effect on neonatal bleeding complications.[39]

The low incidence of neonatal bleeding in modern studies and the data on the mode of delivery and time course of thrombocytopenia support a conservative approach to the management of the fetus in pregnancies complicated by AITP, both antenatally and during labor and delivery. Traumatic delivery, delivery by Ventouse extraction, and the use of high-cavity rotational forceps should be avoided. Decisions about cesarean section should be made on obstetric grounds, without determining the fetal platelet count. Most authors recommend avoiding the use of fetal scalp electrodes and scalp blood sampling to determine acid–base status.[8]

POSTNATAL

Mothers with thrombocytopenia are unlikely to bleed from the uterine cavity after the third stage of labor, provided that there are no retained products of conception. However, bleeding may occur from surgical wounds, episiotomies, or perineal tears. Prompt suturing and close observation of these sites are required.

Immediately after delivery, a cord blood sample should be taken. If the infant is thrombocytopenic but not hemorrhagic, a complete blood count should be obtained daily because the platelet count often continues to decrease over the first few days of life. If the infant has signs of skin or mucosal bleeding or has severe thrombocytopenia (platelet count $<20 \times 10^9$/L, or $<50 \times 10^9$/L in a premature sick neonate), cranial ultrasound should be carried out and treatment instituted. IVIG 1 g/kg is the preferred treatment in neonates[8,9] and increases the platelet count in most infants affected by maternal AITP. Platelet transfusion is rarely necessary, but is indicated if bleeding is life-threatening (e.g., intracranial hemorrhage). Products that are known to be cytomegalovirus-negative should be used.[40] Products that are leukodepleted at the source, however (now standard in the United Kingdom), are generally free from cytomegalovirus.[40] Premature infants with very low birth weight (<1.5 kg) are at greater risk for transfusion-transmitted cytomegalovirus infection than are healthy term infants.

SUMMARY OF MANAGEMENT OPTIONS
Autoimmune Thrombocytopenia

Management Options	Quality of Evidence	Strength of Recommendation	References
Prepregnancy			
Optimize management and consider splenectomy or azathiprine	–	GPP	–
Discuss risks in pregnancy if the patient is not responsive to all therapy	–	GPP	–
Prenatal			
Monitor platelet count (frequency determined by initial values)	IV	C	8,9
Treat if symptoms occur or platelet count $<20 \times 10^9$/L at any stage in pregnancy	IV	C	21
Treat if $<50 \times 10^9$/L in late pregnancy even if the patient is asymptomatic:			
Treatment option 1: Prednisolone. Debate whether to use as first-line therapy vs. intravenous immunoglobulin G	IV III	C B	8,9 23
Treatment option 2: High-dose intravenous immunoglobulin G. Debate whether to use as first line vs prednisolone	IV Ib	C A	15,21,33 34
Treatment option 3: Splenectomy may be performed in refractory cases in the second trimester or occasionally in the third trimester at the time of cesarean section	IV	C	21,37
Treatment option 4: Azathioprine is used in nonresponsive cases. It is safe in pregnancy but beware of intrauterine growth restriction	III	B	28
Inform anesthetists and pediatricians of impending delivery	–	GPP	–

Continued

SUMMARY OF MANAGEMENT OPTIONS

Autoimmune Thrombocytopenia *(Continued)*

Management Options	Quality of Evidence	Strength of Recommendation	References
Labor and Delivery			
Platelets should be available if count <50 × 10^9/L, but use only if the patient is bleeding	IV	C	8,9
Avoid epidural if platelet count <80 × 10^9/L	IV	C	8,9
Avoid traumatic delivery, fetal scalp electrodes, and fetal blood sampling	IV	C	8,9,39
	III	B	12
Cesarean delivery has no benefit over vaginal delivery	III	B	12,38
Postnatal			
Because of the risk of bleeding, repair perineal trauma promptly	–	GPP	–
Obtain a cord blood platelet count	IV	C	8,9
Obtain a platelet count daily for a few days if count is initially low (nadir = day 2–5)	IV	C	8,9
If count <20 × 10^9/L or symptoms occur, perform ultrasound scan of brain and treat with intravenous immunoglobulin G	IV	C	8,9
	III	B	39
Administer platelets if bleeding is life-threatening	IV	C	8,9

Special Considerations in Secondary Autoimmune Thrombocytopenia: Risks and Management Options

Antiphospholipid Syndrome (See Chapter 44)

Primary antiphospholipid syndrome includes the reproducible presence of antiphospholipid antibodies (either lupus anticoagulant or anticardiolipin antibody) and one of the following clinical features: venous thrombosis, arterial thrombosis, recurrent fetal loss, or thrombocytopenia.[41,42]

Primary antiphospholipid syndrome is associated with thrombocytopenia in 20% to 40% of cases.[43] In these cases, thrombocytopenia is autoimmune, although antiphospholipid antibodies may not be the cause of the immune platelet destruction. Thrombocytopenia is rarely severe and usually does not require treatment. Outside the context of pregnancy, responses to the treatment of AITP are similar in patients with and without antiphospholipid antibodies.[44] In terms of thrombocytopenia, management options during pregnancy are similar to those for primary AITP. However, a diagnosis of primary antiphospholipid syndrome has other implications for pregnancy. In addition to recurrent spontaneous abortion, women with antiphospholipid syndrome are at risk for other complications, such as intrauterine fetal death, intrauterine fetal growth restriction, preeclampsia, and maternal thrombosis.[41,42,45] The mechanism of fetal loss is complex. Thrombosis in the placental vasculature is a contributory factor, but there is also evidence of inadequate trophoblastic invasion, induced by antiphospholipid antibodies.[46,47]

A combination of low-dose aspirin and low-dose subcutaneous heparin is helpful in preventing recurrent spontaneous abortions in antiphospholipid syndrome.[48]

Close maternal supervision and fetal monitoring are required antenatally. Antenatal and postnatal thrombosis prophylaxis is indicated in women with antiphospholipid syndrome and a history of thrombosis.[49,50] Moderate thrombocytopenia should not alter decisions about antiplatelet or antithrombotic therapy in antiphospholipid syndrome.[43] In unusual patients who have more marked thrombocytopenia, decisions should be made on an individual basis, taking account of the risks and potential benefits of various management options (see Chapter 44).

Systemic Lupus Erythematosus (See Chapter 44)

Immune platelet destruction may occur in systemic lupus erythematosus because of antiplatelet antibodies or immune complexes. Thrombocytopenia is not usually severe, but if treatment is required, management is governed by the principles outlined for primary AITP. Women with systemic lupus erythematosus are also at risk for preeclampsia, which may be complicated by thrombocytopenia. Other management issues are discussed in Chapter 44.

HIV-Associated Thrombocytopenia (See Chapter 29)

Thrombocytopenia may be associated with HIV infection. A survey of HIV-positive pregnant women showed that 3.2% were thrombocytopenic, and in most cases, thrombocytopenia was believed to be directly related to HIV infection.[5] Slightly fewer than half of the thrombocytopenic women in this series had platelet counts of less than 50 × 10^9/L, and 20% had hemorrhagic complications. Of 28 infants, only 1 had thrombocytopenia.[51]

Thrombocytopenia associated with HIV is multifactorial. In advanced disease, drugs and infection may lead to marrow dysfunction that results in thrombocytopenia. However, thrombocytopenia is relatively common in otherwise asymptomatic HIV-positive individuals. Immune platelet destruction by antiplatelet antibodies or immune complexes is the likely mechanism of thrombocytopenia in these patients.[52] TTP (discussed later) may also be associated with HIV.[53]

Suppression of viral replication by antiretroviral therapy increases the platelet count in HIV-positive patients with thrombocytopenia, but some antiretroviral drugs may also cause thrombocytopenia. Zidovudine improves platelet counts in HIV-positive thrombocytopenic women and reduces vertical transmission of HIV from mother to infant.[54] Combinations of antiretroviral drugs are much more effective at suppressing HIV viral load than monotherapy, and treatment is usually unaltered in pregnancy.[55] Careful evaluation of trends in platelet counts that correspond to changes in therapy and viral load is helpful in assessing thrombocytopenia in HIV-infected patients. Blood film examination (for red cell fragmentation associated with TTP and other cytopenias that may be associated with disease, infection, or therapy) and bone marrow examination to assess whether thrombocytopenia is caused by peripheral consumption are often useful.

When immune destruction is believed to be a significant component of thrombocytopenia, IVIG may be required to treat hemorrhagic symptoms or to increase the platelet count before delivery in thrombocytopenic HIV-positive women.[51] Corticosteroids are also effective in HIV-associated immune thrombocytopenia, but prednisolone is associated with oral candidiasis and reactivation of herpes simplex.[52] Many physicians avoid the use of steroids because of the risk of further immunosuppression and infection. Cesarean delivery reduces the risk of transmission of HIV from mother to fetus, although the benefit is less clear in women with an undetectable viral load.[56]

Drug-Induced Thrombocytopenia

Drugs may cause thrombocytopenia through immune destruction or through suppression of platelet production in the bone marrow. Both are uncommon in pregnancy, but drug-induced causes should be considered and excluded.

One type of drug-induced thrombocytopenia merits further discussion. Heparin-induced thrombocytopenia (HIT) occurs in 1% to 5% of patients receiving unfractionated heparin. HIT is caused by an antibody directed against the heparin–platelet factor 4 complex, which can induce platelet activation and aggregation in vivo.[57] The incidence of HIT in patients treated with low-molecular-weight heparin is considerably lower than that in patients treated with unfractionated heparin.[58] Cross-reactivity of antibodies is common, and low-molecular-weight agents are not suitable once HIT has occurred.[59] The recognition of HIT is important because the condition may be complicated by thrombosis. Thrombosis in HIT may be venous or arterial and may be life-threatening.[57] HIT has been reported in pregnancy,[60,61] although it may be less common in pregnancy than in nonpregnant individuals.[62] Fetal thrombocytopenia does not occur because heparin does not cross the placenta. Heparin should be withdrawn immediately on clinical suspicion of HIT. Laboratory tests are available to confirm the diagnosis. Some tests aid in identification of the cross-reactivity pattern of the antibody.[63] If ongoing anticoagulation is urgently required, the heparinoid danaparoid may be used in most patients.[64] Danaparoid has been used successfully to treat HIT in pregnancy.[61] Hirudin is an alternative in nonpregnant patients, but experience is limited in pregnancy and its use is not recommended unless there is no suitable alternative.[65,66] Ancrod has been used in HIT,[65] but great caution should be used in pregnancy. Platelet transfusion should be avoided in patients with HIT.

Because HIT is potentially life-threatening, all women must have a platelet count before treatment with heparin begins. The count must be repeated 5 to 7 days after the start of therapy and then at least weekly for the first 3 weeks.

Thrombocytopenia with Microangiopathy

Several syndromes are associated with thrombocytopenia as a result of platelet activation, red cell fragmentation, and a variable degree of hemolysis (microangiopathic hemolytic anemia). Some syndromes are unique to obstetric practice. The differential diagnosis is particularly pertinent for obstetricians and is important because management options differ. The differential diagnosis is summarized in Table 41–2.

DISSEMINATED INTRAVASCULAR COAGULATION (See Chapter 79)

Risks and Management Options. Platelet consumption and consequent thrombocytopenia occur as part of the process of disseminated intravascular coagulation (DIC). DIC, particularly if chronic, may also be associated with microangiopathic features on the blood film. DIC is discussed briefly in the section on acquired coagulation disorders.

PREECLAMPSIA AND HELLP SYNDROME (See Chapters 36 and 80)

Risks and Management Options. Preeclampsia is a multisystem disorder unique to pregnancy. Its pathophysiologic basis lies in widespread damage to the vascular endothelium.[67] The platelet count decreases as a result of platelet activation.[13] A decrease in the platelet count often precedes clinical signs of disease,[68] but thrombocytopenia is rarely severe and although there may be evidence of consumptive coagulopathy, severe DIC is unusual.[69] The extent and rate of the decrease in the platelet count indicate the severity of preeclampsia,[61] and together with other aspects of clinical and laboratory assessment, these findings may be used to guide the timing of delivery. HELLP syndrome is a variant of preeclampsia that is characterized by microangiopathic hemolysis, elevated liver enzyme levels, and a low platelet count.[70] Hypertension may be minimal. HELLP syndrome carries a particularly bad prognosis for pregnancy outcome if delivery is postponed, so recognition is important. Platelet transfusion is infrequently required in preeclampsia or HELLP[71] but may be needed if bleeding occurs or if thrombocytopenia is severe and cesarean delivery is planned.[72] In both preeclampsia and HELLP, delivery of the fetus and placenta is the only effective treatment, and delivery results in resolution of hematologic and other features of the condition. Regional analgesia is an option if the maternal platelet count is greater than 80×10^9/L and the results of coagulation screening tests are normal. If severe thrombocytopenia, hemolysis, or organ dysfunction persists after delivery, plasma exchange may be considered,[73] but the diagnosis should also be reviewed.

THROMBOTIC THROMBOCYTOPENIC PURPURA (See Chapter 80)

TTP is a rare disorder associated with platelet activation that leads to thrombocytopenia and the formation of platelet thrombi in the microcirculation. The clinical features of TTP consist of a classic pentad of thrombocytopenia, microangiopathic hemolysis, renal impairment, neurologic features, and fever.[74] Many patients do not have all of the features. Results of coagulation screening tests are normal, and D-dimer levels are normal or minimally elevated.[74] TTP may be related to infection (including HIV), drugs, underlying malignancy, or pregnancy; may occur after bone marrow transplant; or may have no clear trigger. Chronic relapsing TTP may be congenital.

Ultra-large vWf multimers that are not normally present in plasma have been found in convalescent plasma in patients with TTP who subsequently relapsed.[75] More recently, deficiency of a novel vWf cleaving metalloproteinase was recognized in patients with both congenital and acquired forms of TTP.[76,77] This metalloproteinase is a member of the ADAMTS family (ADAMTS 13) [78] and can cleave ultralarge vWf multimers. ADAMTS 13 deficiency may occur constitutionally[78] or may be caused by an inhibitory autoantibody.[77] Deficiency of ADAMTS 13 does not seem to be specific to TTP and is seen in other conditions, such as DIC, malignancy, and liver and renal impairment.[79] Further, ADAMTS 13 deficiency is not seen in some cases of secondary TTP.[80] Levels of ADAMTS 13 decrease in the third trimester.[79] The diagnostic role of ADAMTS 13 deficiency in microangiopathic syndromes is unclear. When the diagnosis is difficult, measurement of antithrombin may help to differentiate TTP from preeclampsia because the antithrombin level is reduced in preeclampsia but not in TTP.[81]

TTP associated with pregnancy tends to occur in the antenatal period, with more than half of cases occurring before 24 weeks' gestation.[82] In contrast, preeclampsia usually occurs later in pregnancy, and hemolytic uremic syndrome mainly occurs postnatally.[81]

Maternal and Fetal Risks. Untreated TTP is almost uniformly fatal for the mother and fetus. However, treatment with plasma exchange with fresh frozen plasma (FFP) markedly improves the outlook.[83] When treated with plasma exchange, the outlook for patients with TTP in pregnancy is similar to that in nonpregnant individuals.[84] Fetal risks include intrauterine growth restriction and intrauterine fetal death, but normal fetal growth may be sustained if the condition is quickly recognized and treated and there is a good response to plasma exchange. Relapse of TTP may occur in subsequent pregnancies.

Management Options. A randomized controlled study in more than 100 patients with TTP of differing etiologies showed that plasma exchange with FFP produced a better clinical response than infusion of FFP.[83] This improvement in response was still evident after 6 months. Plasma exchange with FFP should be instituted as soon as possible after the diagnosis of TTP (within 24 hours). Daily plasma exchange should continue until at least 48 hours after complete remission is obtained. Exchange is often tapered (e.g., to alternate-day treatments). In pregnancy, repeated plasma exchange cycles are usually maintained until delivery. Cryosupernatant may be superior to FFP as an exchange replacement fluid,[85] but in practice, the use of cryosupernatant is usually reserved for patients with a poor response to exchange with FFP. Steroids are often given concomitantly with plasma exchange in TTP, but there is no firm evidence of their benefit. However, recent guidelines in the United Kingdom recommended the use of adjuvant steroids in idiopathic TTP.[81] Similarly, antiplatelet therapy with aspirin is controversial. The use of low-dose aspirin has been advocated when the platelet count increases to more than 50×10^9/L.[81] Platelet transfusion is contraindicated and may lead to rapid worsening of the condition.[86] Red cell transfusion should be given as required, and folic acid is administered as requirements are increased in hemolytic states. Unlike in preeclampsia, delivery does not necessarily cause rapid resolution, but delivery should be considered in pregnant women with TTP when the response to standard therapy is poor.[81]

HEMOLYTIC UREMIC SYNDROME (See Chapter 80)

Hemolytic uremic syndrome is characterized by microangiopathic hemolytic anemia, renal impairment, and a variable degree of thrombocytopenia. Hemolytic uremic syndrome usually occurs after infection, particularly with verotoxin-producing *Escherichia coli* in children. Pregnancy-associated hemolytic uremic syndrome usually occurs postpartum with acute renal failure.[81,82] Subsequent chronic renal failure is common. Management is supportive and includes renal dialysis and red cell transfusion. Plasma exchange has no proven benefit.

SUMMARY OF MANAGEMENT OPTIONS

Secondary Autoimmune Thrombocytopenia

Management Options	Quality of Evidence	Strength of Recommendation	References
Antiphospholipid Syndrome and Systemic Lupus Erythematosus			
Manage thrombocytopenia as for autoimmune idiopathic thrombocytopenic purpura	IV	C	43
Thromboprohylaxis	IV	C	50
See Chapter 44 for a more detailed discussion of screening, diagnosis, and management of other complications			
HIV Thrombocytopenia			
Platelet count may be improved by the use of intravenous intravenous immunoglobulin G, antiretroviral therapy, or steroids	III	B	51
For cesarean section, consider platelet cover, as with autoimmune idiopathic thrombocytopenic purpura, if platelet count is low	–	GPP	–
Drug-Induced Thrombocytopenia			
Stop use of the drug, and choose an alternative	–	GPP	–
Alternatives for heparin-induced thrombocytopenia include danaparoid	III	B	60,61
Check maternal platelet count weekly for the first 3 weeks after commencing heparin therapy in pregnancy	–	GPP	–
Nonimmune Platelet Consumption			
Disseminated intravascular coagulation		See below and Chapter 79	
Preeclampsia or HELLP syndrome		See Chapters 36 and 80	
Thrombotic thrombocytopenic purpura (see also Chapter 80)	III	B	83
• Plasma exchange with fresh frozen plasma is the first-line treatment	IV	C	85
• Plasma exchange with cryosupernatant is the second-line treatment	IV	C	81
• Aspirin and steroids may have a role	III	B	86
• Avoid platelet transfusion	III	B	86
Hemolytic Uremic Syndrome (see also Chapter 80)			
Supportive care	IV	C	81,82
Renal dialysis	IV	C	81,82
Red cell transfusion	IV	C	81,82

COAGULATION DISORDERS

Congenital Coagulation Disorders

Von Willebrand's Disease

The primary function of vWf, which is a large, multimeric protein, is to promote platelet adhesion to the subendothelium. It also binds to and stabilizes plasma factor VIII. A common bleeding disorder that arises as a result of inherited vWf deficiency, vWD is divided into several types and subtypes.[87] Identification of the type of vWD has implications for management. Broadly speaking, patients may have a quantitative (type 1) or qualitative (type 2) defect in vWf. Some patients have little or no vWf in terms of measurable antigen and function, and these patients have associated marked reductions in factor VIII activity (type 3 vWD). Most types of vWD are inherited in an autosomal dominant fashion, but the pattern of inheritance in type 3 disease is autosomal recessive.

Patients with type 1 or 2 vWD usually have a mild to moderate bleeding disorder characterized by skin and mucosal bleeding and bleeding after surgery or trauma. Patients with type 3 disease have severe bleeding diathesis, with deep joint and intramuscular bleeding resembling the pattern seen in hemophilia, in addition to skin and mucosal bleeding.

Laboratory tests in patients with vWD show a long bleeding time and may show a prolonged activated partial thromboplastin time (APTT). More definitive diagnostic tests depend on the finding of reduced plasma vWf activity measured by ristocetin cofactor activity (vWf:RCo) or collagen binding assay (vWf:CB), accompanied by variable reductions (depending on the type) in vWf antigen and factor VIII (FVIII:C).[88] Several further tests that aid in classification include analysis of ristocetin-induced platelet aggregation, vWf multimer analysis, and assay of factor VIII binding to vWf.[88] Stress, inflammation, physical exercise, recent surgery, and pregnancy increase plasma vWf and factor VIII levels, and diagnosis may be difficult in these circumstances. A subtype of type 2 vWD, type 2B vWD, is associated with thrombocytopenia.

MATERNAL RISKS

Levels of vWf and factor VIII tend to increase during pregnancy. This increase results in improvement in the bleeding tendency in most patients with type 1 vWD.[89] In type 2 vWD, vWf antigen and factor VIII levels may increase, but this increase is not accompanied by clinical improvement.[90,91] The platelet count may decrease further in patients with type 2B vWD during pregnancy, causing diagnostic problems.[92,93] In type 3 vWD, no improvement occurs in either laboratory parameters or clinical severity.[94]

The risk of bleeding in patients with vWD is usually greatest postpartum.[91,94,95] Levels of factor VIII and vWf may decrease rapidly after delivery.[96] One series showed an 18.5% incidence of primary postpartum hemorrhage (PPH) and a 20% incidence of secondary PPH in vWD.[97] In type 1 vWD, factor VIII levels are a good predictor of the risk of bleeding at delivery (minimal if the factor VIII level is >0.5 IU/mL).[98] Invasive procedures during the first trimester (e.g., chorionic villus sampling) may also carry a risk of bleeding in all types of vWD because vWf and factor VIII levels do not start to increase until late in the first trimester.[99]

FETAL RISKS

There is very little literature on fetal risk in vWD. Two case series suggest a possible increased rate of spontaneous miscarriage, but others disagree.[95,97,100,101] A recent survey of risk factors for antenatal fetal intracranial hemorrhage listed maternal vWD as a predisposing factor.[102] General experience, however, is that fetal or neonatal hemorrhage is rarely encountered in infants with vWD. This observation is supported by a retrospective case series that showed no neonatal hemorrhagic complications after pregnancies affected by vWD.[97] In infants with type 3 vWD, the risk of bleeding during traumatic delivery is similar to that in those with severe hemophilia A. However, identification of these infants before birth is difficult because there is usually no history and mothers are asymptomatic carriers.

MANAGEMENT OPTIONS

Prepregnancy. One important aspect of pregnancy management in patients with vWD is its recognition. Patients with vWD may have menorrhagia. Recognition and treatment of vWD may allow a more conservative approach.[100,103]

In women diagnosed with vWD, counseling should be given about its inheritance, which is autosomal dominant in most cases. Vaccination against hepatitis A and B should be carried out before pregnancy. The type of vWD should be characterized to plan optimal management of pregnancy and delivery.[99] In patients with type 1 vWD, it is often useful to carry out a trial of therapy with intravenous desmopressin (DDAVP) to determine the patient's response.[99] This agent may help to prevent or control mild to moderate PPH. A synthetic analogue of vasopressin, DDAVP increases factor VIII and vWf levels in plasma.[104] Its major advantage is the avoidance of exposure to pooled blood products. If menorrhagia has been problematic, iron deficiency anemia should be corrected before pregnancy. For women with vWD who stopped using a combined oral contraceptive to become pregnant, alternative therapies to control menorrhagia may be required (e.g., tranexamic acid[99] if pregnancy can be excluded at the time of use).

Prenatal. Close liaison between the obstetrician and hematologist is necessary. Factor VIII, vWf antigen, and vWf:RCo levels should be monitored[99] and management plans determined individually, depending on the patient's hemostatic response to pregnancy. As discussed earlier, in patients with type 1 vWD, hemostatic values are more likely to normalize as pregnancy progresses. If hemostasis has not resolved, treatment may be required to cover invasive procedures (particularly in the first trimester) or episodes of antenatal bleeding. Outside of pregnancy, options for the treatment or prevention of bleeding in vWD include DDAVP (in responsive patients, mainly those with vWD type 1) and factor VIII concentrates that contain sufficient quantities of vWf.[99] The use of DDAVP is controversial in pregnancy. Some consider it to be contraindicated because of concerns that it may cause premature labor and concerns about water retention that may lead to hyponatremia. Others reported the use of DDAVP in pregnancy, particularly early pregnancy, without adverse effect,[104] and a case series reported the use of DDAVP to treat diabetes insipidus in pregnant women, without adverse pregnancy outcome.[105] No data have been reported on the incidence of neonatal hyponatremia, which is a theoretical concern.

DDAVP is contraindicated in type 2B vWD because it may worsen thrombocytopenia.[104] Patients with type 2A vWD have a variable response to DDAVP, and patients with type 3 vWD are unresponsive. When DDAVP is considered unsuitable, patients are treated with a factor VIII concentrate that contains sufficient vWf. Recombinant factor VIII concentrates do not contain vWf; therefore, suitable products are plasma-derived factor VIII concentrates that have undergone viral inactivation.[104] A high-purity, plasma-derived vWf concentrate is also available, but it must be administered initially with factor VIII.[106]

Labor and Delivery. For patients whose von Willebrand profile has normalized in pregnancy, no specific hemostatic support is required. Regional analgesia may proceed in these patients after discussion with an obstetric anesthetist. Although neonatal bleeding is rare, Ventouse delivery and high-cavity forceps should be avoided. The third stage of labor should be managed to ensure adequate uterine contraction. Careful and prompt repair of episiotomy wounds or perineal tears is advisable.

For patients whose vWf activity (vWf:RCo) has not normalized, decisions about regional analgesia should be individualized.[107] After treatment, laboratory values do not always reflect clinical hemostasis in vWD, and caution should be used in proceeding with epidural or spinal anesthesia. Patient-controlled analgesia with the short-acting opioid remifentanil can be useful when regional analgesia is contraindicated. Hemostatic supportive therapy should be given to cover delivery or cesarean section if the factor VIII level is less than 0.5 IU/mL or if vWf:RCo has not normalized.[99,104] Considerations about the choice of therapy before the umbilical cord is clamped are similar to those described earlier. After the cord is clamped, DDAVP is less controversial and is the treatment of choice for most responsive patients for prophylaxis or treatment of mild to moderate postpartum bleeding.[108] Because of the high incidence of secondary PPH in patients with vWD, effort should be made to ensure that the placenta is complete. A low threshold for antibiotics should be adopted if the uterine cavity is opened or explored.

Postnatal. All patients should be observed closely for PPH. Uncorrected hemostatic defects should be treated after delivery. In suitable responsive patients, DDAVP is the treatment of choice to prevent and treat mild to moderate postpartum bleeding. Factor VIII and vWf:RCo levels should be checked a few days after delivery because they may fall rapidly after delivery.[96] FVIII:C and vWf:RCo levels should be maintained in the normal range for at least 3 to 7 days after cesarean section.[94,104,108] It is difficult and unnecessary to diagnose vWD in the neonate, except when type 3 vWD is suspected. Generally, diagnosis can be postponed until later in childhood.

Carriers of Hemophilia A and B

Hemophilia A (deficiency of factor VIII) is the most common severe heritable bleeding disorder, with a prevalence of approximately 1 in 10,000 in the population. Hemophilia B (deficiency of factor IX) is approximately five times less prevalent. The conditions are inherited in an X-linked fashion and are clinically identical. Affected males have a bleeding disorder that correlates in severity with the reduction in the level of factor VIII or IX. Severely affected males have spontaneous bleeding into muscles and joints; mildly affected patients may bleed only after surgery or trauma. Females in families with a history of hemophilia may be obligate, potential, or sporadic carriers, depending on the details of the pedigree.[109] An obligate carrier is a woman whose father has hemophilia, a woman who has a family history of hemophilia and who has given birth to a hemophiliac son, or a woman who has more than one child with hemophilia. A potential carrier of hemophilia is a woman who has a maternal relative with the disorder. A woman with one affected child and no family history may be a sporadic carrier.[109] Carriers of hemophilia usually have factor VIII or IX levels that are approximately 50% of normal, because of lyonization. Abnormal bleeding does not occur at this level of factor VIII activity. Some carriers have lower factor VIII or IX levels, and these individuals have a bleeding disorder that varies according to the coagulation factor level.[110]

MATERNAL RISKS

As discussed earlier, factor VIII levels tend to increase during pregnancy.[111] This increase usually, but not invariably, occurs in carriers of hemophilia A. The risk of bleeding in carriers of hemophilia A is greatest in the postpartum period because factor VIII levels may decrease rapidly after delivery.[91,94,112] Invasive procedures during the first trimester, such as chorionic villus sampling, also carry a risk of bleeding. No substantial increase in factor VIII occurs at this early stage in pregnancy.[94]

There is usually no substantial increase in factor IX levels during pregnancy.[94,112,113] Consequently, compared with carriers of hemophilia A, carriers of hemophilia B who have low factor IX levels are more likely to require treatment to prevent bleeding complications during delivery.

Treatment with a coagulation factor concentrate often is not required in pregnancy.[113] However, the possible need for this treatment should be pointed out when counseling women who are carriers of hemophilia. The risks of pregnancy and the safety and potential risks of available treatments should be discussed. This is best carried out by medical and nursing staff with expertise in the management of bleeding disorders.

FETAL RISKS

If the mother is a definite carrier of hemophilia A or B, a male fetus has a 50% chance of being affected. Spontaneous fetal and neonatal bleeding is unusual, even in severe hemophilia, but there are well-documented cases after traumatic delivery.[112,114] The most serious risk is that of intracranial hemorrhage.

Cephalhematoma may also lead to serious bleeding. The incidence of such complications is poorly defined. One retrospective series reported a combined incidence of 3.58% for intracranial hemorrhage and cephalhematoma in newborns with hemophilia A and B.[115,116] Other reported areas of bleeding in hemophilic neonates are at puncture sites, the umbilical stump, and during circumcision.[116]

If the parents seek a prenatal diagnosis of hemophilia, counseling should cover the fetal risks associated with chorionic villus sampling. This procedure carries a 1% to 2% risk of miscarriage.[117]

MANAGEMENT OPTIONS

Prepregnancy. All women who are potential or obligate carriers of hemophilia require prepregnancy counseling, including genetic counseling. Arrangements for genetic counseling vary from one area to another, but there is general agreement that a genetic counselor and a physician who is responsible for the management of patients with hemophilia should be involved.[118] It should be established that there is truly a history of hemophilia in the family (not, for example, another bleeding disorder). The pedigree should be established and the possibility of hemophilia carriership determined. Counseling of obligate and potential carriers should include a discussion of the nature and management of hemophilia.[118] Carrier identification studies with molecular genetic techniques should be offered to all potential carriers of hemophilia A and B. Informed consent should be obtained before blood samples are collected for molecular analysis.[118] Advances in molecular genetics have made accurate diagnosis of carriership possible in most cases.[118,119] Hemophilia A and B are genetically heterogeneous. The starting point is identification of the mutation responsible for hemophilia in an affected male member of the family (direct mutation detection).[120] Potential carriers may be screened for this mutation. Approximately 20% of cases of severe hemophilia A are caused by an inversion in intron 22 of the factor VIII gene.[120,121] If an affected male is not available and there is a family history of severe hemophilia A, a potential carrier should be screened for this common molecular defect. Direct mutation detection is otherwise extremely difficult if there is no available affected male. Linkage analysis is now less commonly used, but may still be useful if the mutation responsible for hemophilia cannot be identified.[120] Blood from an affected male family member is required, and more extensive family testing is needed for successful linkage analysis. Linkage analysis will be unsuccessful if the potential carrier is homozygous (uninformative) for common intragenic polymorphisms.[120] The availability of a molecular marker in the family is necessary if prenatal diagnosis is required later.

Coagulation studies should also be carried out to identify carriers with low factor VIII or IX levels. Phenotypic data may be helpful in assessing the statistical risk of carriership if molecular diagnosis is not possible. However, normal levels of factor VIII or IX do not exclude carriership.[119] Women with low levels of factor VIII or IX should be offered vaccination against hepatitis A and B. The immunity status should be checked if the patient has been vaccinated. Women who have low levels of factor VIII may have a useful hemostatic response to DDAVP.[122] To establish whether this response is occurring, a trial of intravenous DDAVP can be attempted, with measurement of the response in factor VIII levels over the next 24 hours. DDAVP is not useful for women with low factor IX levels.

Once carriership has been established, careful planning of pregnancies should be encouraged. Partners of hemophilia carriers should be encouraged to attend prepregnancy counseling sessions.[109,113] Couples should be informed that hemophilia "breeds true" in families. In other words, its severity is predictable by the family history.[113] Couples should be counseled in a nondirective manner about all reproductive options, including the availability of prenatal diagnosis. They should be encouraged to consider the matter in advance of pregnancy,[109,118] although circumstances may change and final decisions must be made given the circumstances in each pregnancy. Prepregnancy counseling may need to be repeated in subsequent pregnancies. Discussion of the techniques and risks associated with prenatal diagnosis is appropriate during preconception counseling sessions.[109] Carriers should be encouraged to seek care early in pregnancy, especially if prenatal diagnosis is being considered or has not been excluded.

A new technique for preimplantation diagnosis is potentially useful for carriers of hemophilia who, after counseling, do not wish to contemplate bringing up a hemophilic child, but would not consider termination. Preimplantation diagnosis is possible only in in vitro fertilization and is available only in a few specialized centers. In the United Kingdom, each new test requires a license from the Human Fertilisation and Embryology Authority.

Prenatal. Identification and counseling of carriers should be carried out before pregnancy, but may be necessary in early pregnancy if a woman with a family history of hemophilia does not seek care until pregnancy is diagnosed. General practitioners, midwives, and obstetricians should refer these patients for specialized counseling as early as possible.[118]

Pregnancies in patients who are carriers of congenital bleeding disorders should be managed in a hospital with hemophilia expertise.[94,112] Close liaison between the obstetrician and the hemophilia team is necessary. Factor VIII or IX levels should be monitored regularly throughout pregnancy. It is particularly important to measure coagulation factor levels toward the end of the third trimester (34–36 weeks) to plan management of delivery.[112,113]

If prenatal diagnosis is requested and a suitable marker exists, testing is usually carried out by chorionic villus sampling at 11 to 14 weeks. Alternatives are amniocentesis from 14 weeks onward and fetal blood sampling by cordocentesis for phenotypic diagnosis of severe deficiencies. Risks associated with these procedures should be fully discussed with the patient. Chorionic villus sampling and amniocentesis carry a 1% to 2% risk of miscarriage. Fetal bleeding sufficient to result in death is a recognized risk of cordocentesis. This option is rarely used in the developed world because the risks are great, the causative mutation can be identified in most families, and the procedure may produce invalid or indeterminate results.

The use of prenatal diagnosis is decreasing in developed countries. As hemophilia care improves, more couples are willing to contemplate bringing up a child with hemophilia.[113]

If prenatal diagnosis is requested, treatment with a coagulation factor concentrate may be necessary to increase maternal factor VIII or IX levels if they are less than 0.5 IU/mL. Laboratory measurement of coagulation factor levels should be used to monitor treatment. The use of DDAVP is controversial in the prenatal period, although it has been used both prenatally and postpartum for women with reduced factor VIII levels.[104,105,112,113] If coagulation factor concentrates are used, a recombinant factor VIII or IX concentrate should be chosen[123] for a pregnant carrier of hemophilia who needs hemostatic support in the antenatal period. Many patients are previously untreated, and even a minimal risk of transmission of infection from plasma-derived products is unacceptable. Further, parvovirus B19, which can cause fetal hydrops, may be transmitted by plasma-derived concentrate, and no method of viral inactivation seems to be effective in eradicating this virus.[124] In countries where recombinant coagulation factor concentrates are not available, a plasma-derived concentrate that has undergone viricidal treatment, preferably by dual methods, should be used if hemostatic support is required.

When prenatal diagnosis has not been carried out, but there is a risk that the child may have hemophilia, fetal sex should be diagnosed by ultrasonography.[94,112,113] This information is necessary for the obstetrician and hematologist, even if the parents do not wish to know the sex of the infant.

Labor and Delivery. If maternal factor VIII or IX levels remain low at 34 to 36 weeks in hemophilia carriers, treatment to correct maternal hemostasis is necessary for delivery.[94,112,113] A factor VIII or IX plasma level of 0.4 IU/mL is safe for vaginal delivery, and a level of 0.5 IU/mL or greater is safe for cesarean section. Considerations similar to those discussed earlier govern the choice of treatment. Recombinant factor VIII or IX or DDAVP (for carriers of hemophilia A only) should be used. Full laboratory monitoring of hemostatic replacement therapy is necessary. Epidural anesthesia may be used if coagulation defects have been corrected.[112]

If the fetus is a known hemophiliac, is male and of unknown hemophilia status, or is of unknown sex, care should be taken to avoid traumatic vaginal delivery.[112–114,116] When possible, obstetric problems should be identified before the expected date of delivery, and the mode of delivery should be planned. Routine cesarean delivery is unnecessary,[113,114,116] but cesarean delivery should be carried out if obstetric complications are anticipated. Ventouse delivery is absolutely contraindicated because major cephalhematoma and intracranial bleeding have been documented after this procedure.[113,114,116] Midcavity rotational forceps delivery should be avoided, but simple lift-out forceps delivery may be preferable to a difficult cesarean section if the fetal head is impacted.[113] Maternal perineal trauma should be minimized, with suturing performed promptly after delivery. Fetal scalp sampling and scalp electrodes should not be used if the fetus may have hemophilia.[112,113]

Postnatal. Most bleeding problems in carriers of hemophilia occur postpartum. As discussed earlier, replacement therapy should be given immediately after delivery to mothers with an uncorrected hemostatic defect. Coagulation factor levels should be rechecked urgently if postpartum bleeding occurs. Options at this stage include DDAVP for mothers who are carriers of hemophilia A and recombinant coagulation factor concentrates for carriers of hemophilia A or B. Supportive therapy to maintain hemostasis should be continued for 3 to 4 days after vaginal delivery and for 5 to 10 days after cesarean section.[94] All hemostatic parameters must be normal before epidural catheters are removed. All mothers who are carriers, regardless of whether they need peripartum hemostatic support, should be observed for signs of PPH. Coagulation factor levels should be checked a few days after delivery because they may decrease quickly.[113]

In the infant, intramuscular injections (including vitamin K) should be avoided until hemophilia has been excluded.[113] Vitamin K may be given orally.[116] Cord blood should be obtained for appropriate factor assays.[113,116] Except for very mild cases, hemophilia A can be diagnosed easily in the neonatal period. Difficulties may arise with mild or moderate hemophilia B because of the physiologic reduction in factor IX levels that occurs in the newborn.[116,125] However, severe hemophilia B is usually easily identified. There has been debate about the routine administration of coagulation factor concentrates to neonates with hemophilia.[126] The majority view is that this is unnecessary if delivery has been atraumatic and there are no clinical signs of hemorrhage.[126] If a diagnosis of hemophilia has been made and if there has been an instrumental or traumatic delivery, prophylactic recombinant factor VIII or IX should be considered.[126] Prompt coagulation factor support is needed if there is clinical evidence of intracranial hemorrhage or significant bleeding from other sites.[116] Routine cranial ultrasound should be considered in all infants with severe hemophilia to detect intracranial hemorrhage as early as possible.[116]

The hemophilia team should be involved from the outset in counseling parents of infants with newly diagnosed congenital bleeding disorders. A clear follow-up plan should be discussed with the parents at discharge.[116]

Other Congenital Bleeding Disorders

Occasionally women have rare deficiencies of coagulation factors or congenital platelet function disorders. Detailed description is beyond the scope of this chapter. As with all bleeding disorders, close liaison between the obstetrician and hematologist is required. The principles of management revolve around assessment of the risk of bleeding for the mother and infant. The risks of hemostatic supportive therapy must be taken into account. Many (but not all) disorders are inherited in a recessive manner; therefore, the risk of fetal or neonatal bleeding is often negligible unless there is a consanguineous partnership. For rarer congenital coagulation factor deficiencies, clinical bleeding does not always correlate with coagulation factor levels. Women with coagulation factor deficiencies or abnormalities may have recurrent fetal loss.[127,128] Placental abruption is reported in congenital afibrinogenemia. Appropriate replacement therapy can help to maintain pregnancy.[127,128]

SUMMARY OF MANAGEMENT OPTIONS
Congenital Coagulation Disorders

Management Options	Quality of Evidence	Strength of Recommendation	References
Von Willebrand's Disease			
Prepregnancy			
Establish type of von Willebrand's disease	IV	C	87
Genetic counseling (usually dominant)	III	B	97,99
Hepatitis A and B immunization	III	B	97,99
For type I von Willebrand's disease, perform a DDAVP trial to establish efficacy (contraindicated in type 2B von Willebrand's disease)	III	B	105
Prenatal			
Combined or interdisciplinary team approach (obstetric and hemophilia team)	III	B	97,99
Monitor vWf:Ag, vWf:RCO, FVIII:C, platelet count (in many cases, parameters improve)	III	B	97,99
Treatment is unlikely to be required unless invasive procedures are performed or an episode of antenatal bleeding	III	B	97,99
Labor and Delivery			
Maternal hemostatic support is needed if FVIII:C <0.5 Iu/mL or if vWf:RCO significantly reduced	III	B	97,99
DDAVP is used in responsive patient (except in type 2B von Willebrand's disease), or a plasma-derived concentrate containing vWf may be used	III	B	94,105,106
Aim for atraumatic delivery (vaginal delivery if uncomplicated delivery is anticipated, but avoid fetal scalp electrode's and fetal scalp sampling)	III	B	97,99,103
Active management of the third stage	–	GPP	–
Prompt repair of perineal trauma	–	GPP	–
Postnatal			
Vigilance for postpartum hemorrhage	–	GPP	–
Cord samples are not indicated unless type 3 von Willebrand's disease is suspected in the newborn	III	B	97,99,103
Avoid neonatal intramuscular injections until status is known	III	B	97,99
Recheck maternal FVIII:C, vWf:Ag, and vWf:RCO for a few days after delivery. If parameters fall or if the patient is bleeding, give hemostatic supportive therapy. Maintain support for an operative delivery	III	B	94

SUMMARY OF MANAGEMENT OPTIONS

Congenital Coagulation Disorders *(Continued)*

Management Options	Quality of Evidence	Strength of Recommendation	References
Carriers of Hemophilia A or B			
Prepregnancy			
Genetic evaluation and counseling	III	B	109
Establish mutation, if possible; if not, define whether linkage analysis is of use	III	B	120
If maternal factor VIII or IX is reduced, obtain baseline virology (including hepatitis B and C, HIV, and immunity vs. hepatitis A and parvovirus)	III	B	97,99
Hepatitis A and B immunization if the patient is not immune	III	B	97,99
For carriers of hemophilia A with low factor VIII levels, perform a trial of DDAVP to establish efficacy	III	B	105
Prenatal			
Combined or interdisciplinary team approach (obstetric and hemophilia team)	III	B	97,99
Offer prenatal diagnosis (chorionic villus sampling) at 11 to 14 weeks (cover with factor concentrate if level of factor VIII or IX <0.5 iu/mL); use recombinant products, if available, or DDAVP	III	B	104,105,112, 113,123
Obtain maternal serial clotting factor levels, especially in the third trimester	III	B	112,113
Perform fetal sexing by ultrasonography at 16 to 20 weeks if invasive prenatal diagnosis is not requested	III	B	94,112,113
Labor and Delivery			
Consider further concentrate cover for labor and delivery if factor VIII or IX level is <0.5 iu/mL	III	B	94,112,113
For hemophilia A carriers, consider DDAVP alone if the patient is known to be responsive, if normal vaginal delivery is anticipated, and if the coagulation defect is mild	III	B	94,112,113
If high risk fetus, aim for atraumatic unassisted (no ventouse or forceps) delivery (vaginal delivery if uncomplicated delivery is anticipated, but avoid fetal scalp electrodes and fetal scalp sampling)	III	B	112–114,116
Postnatal			
Obtain cord blood for neonatal evaluation if risk of hemophilia A or B	III	B	116
Avoid neonatal intramuscular injections until status is known	III	B	116
Give vitamin K orally if status of neonate is unknown	III	B	116
Obtain cranial ultrasound if neonate has severe hemophilia	III	B	116
A clear follow-up plan is needed for the parents and child	III	B	116
Vigilance for postpartum hemorrhage	–	GPP	–
Provide maternal hemostatic support for 3 to 4 days if vaginal delivery and for 5 to 10 days if cesarean delivery	III	B	94

Acquired Coagulation Disorders

Disseminated Intravascular Coagulation (DIC) (See Chapter 79)

DIC occurs in a wide variety of obstetric complications. It is triggered by vascular endothelial damage, release of procoagulant substances as a result of tissue damage or liquor entering the circulation, or cytokine-mediated up-regulation of tissue factor expression on monocytes and endothelial cells.[129,130] These triggers lead to the generation of thrombin, cause defects in inhibitors of coagulation, and suppress fibrinolysis. These hemostatic changes result in deposition of fibrin in the microcirculation and consumption of coagulation factors and platelets, leading to a bleeding tendency. In obstetrics, DIC often develops acutely, for example, in placental abruption that results in rapid defibrination with hemostatic failure. Very long clotting times and marked thrombocytopenia usually occur. At the other end of the spectrum, chronic DIC may cause minimal or no abnormality on standard coagulation screening tests. No single test is diagnostic of DIC; the diagnosis depends on a combination of clinical findings and laboratory test results.[130] Thrombocytopenia and a decreasing platelet count are sensitive indicators. In most cases of DIC, whether acute or chronic, the plasma D-dimer level is elevated. In interpreting the results of coagulation screening tests in suspected DIC in pregnant women, it is prudent to note that normal baseline values are altered by physiologic changes. The plasma fibrinogen level is elevated and factor VIII levels increase in pregnancy, leading to an acceleration of APTT.[111,131] Normal fibrinogen levels and APTT in late pregnancy should be regarded suspiciously.

MATERNAL RISKS

Maternal risks arise as a result of the underlying disorder, but there are also risks of bleeding and small vessel occlusion as a direct result of DIC.

FETAL RISKS

Fetal risks in DIC are associated with the underlying cause.

MANAGEMENT OPTIONS

Management of DIC includes treatment of the underlying cause and appropriate resuscitative measures to maintain tissue perfusion. Hemostatic replacement therapy is indicated if there is significant hemorrhage or if invasive procedures are required. When clinically indicated, replacement therapy with FFP, platelet transfusions, and in some cases, a source of fibrinogen, such as cryoprecipitate, is based on the results of laboratory tests and clinical findings.[132] Prothrombin time and APTT provide a guide for FFP usage, and the fibrinogen level can be used to guide the use of both FFP and cryoprecipitate. The goal is to increase the fibrinogen level to 1 g/L. Platelet transfusion is required if the platelet count is less than 20×10^9/L or if bleeding occurs in a patient with a platelet count of less than 50×10^9/L. However, the goal is not simply to correct laboratory defects. Important concerns include addressing the clinical features and treating the underlying cause.[129]

The use of heparin is controversial, but it should be reserved for cases in which microvascular occlusion rather than hemorrhage is the predominant clinical problem. The cautious use of heparin may also have a place alongside replacement therapy in the management of amniotic fluid embolism. The rationale is that the underlying cause cannot be removed, and because of the rate of consumption, it is difficult to keep pace with replacement therapy unless thrombin generation is inhibited concomitantly.[129,130]

Concentrates of anticoagulant proteins, such as antithrombin, protein C, and activated protein C, have been used mainly in DIC that is caused by severe sepsis. Promising results in improvement in hemostatic parameters have been obtained, particularly with the use of activated protein C in patients with severe sepsis.[133] Recombinant activated protein C reduced mortality rates in a large clinical trial of patients with severe sepsis.[134] There are only preliminary data on DIC associated with complications of pregnancy.[135] Antithrombin concentrates are used in amniotic fluid embolism and may have a role.[136]

Massive Blood Loss (See Chapters 59 and 79)

Causes of massive obstetric hemorrhage are discussed elsewhere (see Chapters 59 and 79). Massive bleeding in obstetric practice (e.g., as a result of placental abruption) is often accompanied by DIC. Bleeding as a result of placenta previa is not necessarily associated with DIC, but may be massive. Resuscitative measures and red cell transfusion are the first considerations. However, dilutional effects on coagulation and platelets occur, and bank blood does not provide platelets and labile clotting factors, such as factors V and VIII.

MANAGEMENT OPTIONS

The underlying cause should be treated. Resuscitative measures and red cell transfusion are paramount concerns. Blood should be warmed when rapid transfusion is required.

Coagulation defects should be corrected with FFP, and thrombocytopenia is treated with platelet transfusion. Treatment should be guided by the findings on complete blood count, coagulation screening tests, and fibrinogen measurements. Reasonable aims are to keep the platelet count above 50×10^9/L and to keep the fibrinogen level above 0.8 g/L.[94,132] In some cases, cryoprecipitate may be required as a source of fibrinogen.

In intractable major hemorrhage, recombinant factor VIIa may be used to stem bleeding when all other measures have failed. This treatment, which was originally developed for the management of bleeding in hemophiliac patients with inhibitors, has been used successfully in a variety of clinical situations associated with major bleeding and is becoming viewed as a "universal" hemostatic agent.[137] DIC is not a contraindication to the use of recombinant factor VIIa if massive bleeding is occurring. However, caution should be used in patients with major DIC because there are occasional reports of thrombosis and DIC after the use of recombinant factor VIIa.[138] There are several reports of the successful use of recombinant factor VIIa to control massive hemorrhage in obstetric patients.[139,140]

Liver Disease (See Chapter 48)

MATERNAL RISKS AND MANAGEMENT OPTIONS

Patients with liver disease, especially if it is advanced, often have significant hemostatic impairment. Several mechanisms contribute to this impairment, including thrombocytopenia as a result of splenic enlargement or alcohol use, impaired production of coagulation factors in the liver, impaired polymerization of fibrin, platelet dysfunction, and hyperfibrinolysis.[141] In pregnant women with liver disease, a complete blood count should be obtained and coagulation parameters monitored. Coagulation screening tests and measurement of fibrinogen levels are indicated. In some cases, screening for DIC or coagulation factor assays is helpful. The risk of bleeding is greatest during and after surgery or invasive procedures. Hemostatic supportive therapy may be required in these situations or if bleeding occurs during labor or delivery. Standard therapy is with FFP and platelets. Efficacy may be limited in patients with liver disease, and large volumes of FFP may be required.

Acquired Inhibitors of Coagulation (Acquired Factor VIII Inhibitor)

MATERNAL RISKS

Rarely, pregnancy is associated with the development of an antibody that inhibits factor VIII activity. Most reported cases occur postpartum.[142,143] This antibody may lead to postpartum hemorrhage or postsurgical bleeding. The timing of the development of these inhibitors is highly variable. One series reported identification of acquired hemophilia between 3 and 150 days postpartum.[142] Postpartum factor VIII inhibitors may disappear spontaneously, but the usual pattern is persistent for months or even years.[142,143] The more common pattern seems to be that inhibitors do not recur in subsequent pregnancies.[142] In the laboratory, a factor VIII inhibitor is associated with prolonged APTT, with normal prothrombin time and fibrinogen levels. The addition of normal plasma in vitro does not correct APTT. Factor VIII inhibitors must be differentiated from a lupus inhibitor by specific tests because the clinical implications are profoundly different.

FETAL RISKS

Most inhibitors occur postpartum, so there are generally no fetal risks. However, inhibitors that arise antenatally have been reported. These antibodies may cross the placenta and persist for up to 3 months in the neonate.[143] Bleeding complications have not usually occurred, but intracranial hemorrhage has been reported.[143] The management of these pregnancies should be based on the assumption that the fetus potentially is phenotypically hemophiliac, regardless of the sex. Delivery plans and immediate neonatal management are as described earlier.

MANAGEMENT OPTIONS

Specialized management by a hematologist with expertise in hemophilia is required. Various coagulation factor concentrates are available for immediate control of bleeding in patients with factor VIII inhibitors. Detailed discussion is outside the scope of this chapter. In a young woman with bleeding as a result of acquired hemophilia, recombinant factor VIIa offers many advantages over other preparations. Disadvantages include the cost and the need for administration every 2 hours. In the longer term, therapy is given to encourage disappearance of the inhibitor. Steroids and immunosuppressive therapy have been used. Combination therapy is more efficacious in reducing the time to disappearance of the inhibitor.[142]

SUMMARY OF MANAGEMENT OPTIONS

Acquired Coagulation Disorders

Management Options	Quality of Evidence	Strength of Recommendation	References
Disseminated Intravascular Coagulation (DIC)			
See also Chapter 79			
Interdisciplinary approach (obstetric and hematology)	IV	C	129
Treat the cause	IV	C	129
Resuscitation volume replacement to maintain tissue perfusion	IV	C	129
Replace fresh frozen plasma, cryoprecipitate, and platelets on the basis of laboratory results and clinical condition	IV	C	132
Consider heparin in severe DIC due to amniotic fluid embolism	IV III	C B	129,130
Concentrates of anticoagulant proteins, such as antithrombin, protein C, and activated protein C, may be useful in DIC due to severe sepsis	III	B	133
Recombinant activated protein C is very effective in severe DIC due to sepsis outside pregnancy; limited experience in pregnancy	III IV	B C	134,135

Continued

SUMMARY OF MANAGEMENT OPTIONS
Acquired Coagulation Disorders

Management Options	Quality of Evidence	Strength of Recommendation	References
Massive Hemorrhage			
See also Chapters 59 and 79			
Treat the cause	IV	C	129
Resuscitation with volume replacement to maintain tissue perfusion	IV	C	129
Replace fresh frozen plasma, cryoprecipitate, and platelets on the basis of laboratory results and clinical condition	IV	C	132
Consider recombinant factor VIIa if massive bleeding continues despite correction of surgical hemostasis and adequate conventional product replacement; most experience is outside pregnancy, although it is increasing in pregnancy	III	B	137,139,140
Liver Disease			
See also Chapter 48			
Replace fresh frozen plasma, cryoprecipitate, and platelets on the basis of laboratory results and clinical condition	IV	C	132
Acquired Factor VIII Inhibitor			
Interdisciplinary approach (obstetric and hematology)	IV	C	129
Specific clotting factor (e.g., factor VIII) concentrates (individualized management)	III	B	142
Recombinant factor VIIa if severe acute bleeding is nonresponsive to other therapy			
Immunosuppressive therapy (better in combination)	III	B	142

CONCLUSIONS

Thrombocytopenia

- Thrombocytopenia requires further testing if the platelet count decreases to less than 100×10^9/L.
- Autoimmune thrombocytopenia does not substantially increase the risk of neonatal bleeding.
- A safe maternal platelet count for delivery is 50×10^9/L or greater.
- A safe maternal platelet count for regional analgesia is 80×10^9/L or greater.
- The neonatal platelet count should be obtained on cord blood in women with autoimmune thrombocytopenia. If the initial count is low, the count should be repeated daily.
- All women who receive heparin should have a complete blood count weekly for 3 weeks after the start of therapy.

Coagulation Disorders

- Coagulation disorders should be managed by a team of obstetricians and hematologists.
- Genetic diagnosis of hemophilia may require extensive workup before pregnancy to offer the best chance for prenatal testing.
- Women who may benefit from DDAVP should undergo a trial before pregnancy.
- Coagulation must be optimized before delivery in women with bleeding disorders. Support may need to be continued for approximately 1 week postnatally.
- Women with von Willebrand's Disease have an increased risk of secondary postpartum hemorrhage. They should report abnormal bleeding early.

CONCLUSIONS *(Continued)*

Disseminated Intravascular Coagulation

- Disseminated intravascular coagulation has several obstetric causes, but the management principles of replacement of blood volume, coagulation factors, and platelets remain the same, regardless of the cause.
- Laboratory test results and clinical findings should guide replacement therapy.
- Simultaneous treatment of the underlying cause is of paramount importance.
- When large volumes of blood are replaced, they must be warmed.

REFERENCES

1. Giles C: The platelet count and mean platelet volume. Br J Haematol 1981;48:31–37.
2. Tygart SG, McRoyan DK, Spinnato JA, et al: Longitudinal study of platelet indices during normal pregnancy. Am J Obstet Gynecol 1986;154:883–887.
3. Sill PR, Lind T, Walker W: Platelet values during normal pregnancy. Br J Obstet Gynaecol 1985;92:480–483.
4. Fay RA, Hughes AO, Hughes O, et al: Platelets in pregnancy: Hyperdestruction in pregnancy. Obstet Gynecol 1983;61:238–240.
5. O'Brien JR: Platelet counts in normal pregnancy. J Clin Pathol 1976;29:174.
6. Pitkin RM, Witte DL: Platelet and leukocyte counts in pregnancy. JAMA 1979;242:24.
7. Burrows RF, Kelton JG: Thrombocytopenia at delivery: A prospective survey of 6715 deliveries. Am J Obstet Gynecol 1990;162:731–734.
8. British Committee for Standards in Haematology: General Haematology Task Force Guidelines for the Investigation and Management of Idiopathic Thrombocytopenic Purpura in Adults, Children and in Pregnancy. Br J Haematol 2003;120: 574–596.
9. Bussel J, Kaplan C, McFarland J, et al: Recommendations for the evaluation and treatment of neonatal autoimmune and alloimmune thrombocytopenia. Thromb Haemost 1991;65:631–634.
10. Kelton JG, Inwood MJ, Barr RM, et al: The prenatal prediction of thrombocytopenia in infants of mothers with clinically diagnosed immune thrombocytopenia. Am J Obstet Gynecol 1982; 144:449–454.
11. Lescale KB, Eddleman KA, Cines DB, et al: Antiplatelet antibody testing in thrombocytopenic pregnant women. Am J Obstet Gynecol 1996;174:1014–1018.
12. Burrows RF, Kelton JG: Fetal thrombocytopenia and its relation to maternal thrombocytopenia. N Engl J Med 1993;329: 1463–1466.
13. Horn EH: Platelets in normal and hypertensive pregnancy: A review. Platelets 1991;2:138–195.
14. Douglas JT, Shah M, Lowe GDO, et al: Plasma fibrinopeptide A and beta-thromboglobulin in pre-eclampsia and pregnancy hypertension. Thromb Haemost 1982;47:54–55.
15. Crowther MA, Burrows RF, Ginsberg J, et al: Thrombocytopenia in pregnancy: Diagnosis, pathogenesis and management. Blood Rev 1996;10:8–16.
16. Samuels P, Bussel JB, Braitman LE, et al: Estimation of the risk of thrombocytopenia in the offspring of pregnant women with presumed immune thrombocytopenic purpura. N Engl J Med 1990;323:229–235.
17. Aster RH: 'Gestational' thrombocytopenia: A plea for conservative management. N Engl J Med 1990;323:264–266.
18. Burrows RF, Kelton JG: Incidentally detected thrombocytopenia in healthy mothers and their infants. N Engl J Med 1988; 319:142.
19. Van Leeuwen EF, van der Ven JTH, Engefriet CP, et al: Specificity of autoantibodies in autoimmune thrombocytopenia. Blood 1982;59:23.
20. Kelton JG: The serological investigation of patients with autoimmune thrombocytopenia. Thromb Haemost 1995;74: 228–233.
21. George JN, Woolf SH, Raskob GE, et al: Idiopathic thrombocytopenic purpura: A practice guideline developed by explicit methods for the American Society of Hematology. Blood 1996;88:3–40.
22. Scott JR, Rote NS, Cruikshank DP: Antiplatelet antibodies and platelet counts in pregnancies complicated by autoimmune thrombocytopenia. Am J Obstet Gynecol 1983;145:932.
23. Kaplan C, Daffos F, Forestier F, et al: Fetal platelet counts in thrombocytopenic pregnancy. Lancet 1990;336:979–982.
24. Skupski DW, Bussel JB: Further insights into autoimmune thrombocytopenia in pregnancy. Am J Obstet Gynecol 1996; 174:1944–1945.
25. Hohlfeld P, Forestier F, Kaplan C: Fetal thrombocytopenia: A retrospective survey of 5,194 fetal blood samplings. Blood 1994;84:1851–1856.
26. McCrae KR, Samuels P, Schreiber AD: Pregnancy-associated thrombocytopenia: Pathogenesis and management. Blood 1992;80:2697–2714.
27. Davison JM, Lindheimer MD: Pregnancy in renal transplant recipients. J Reprod Med 1982;27:613–621.
28. Alstead ME, Ritchie JK, Lennard-Jones JE, et al: Safety of azathioprine in pregnancy in inflammatory bowel disease. Gastroenterology 1990;99:443–446.
29. Smith BT, Torday JS: Steroid administration in pregnant women with autoimmune thrombocytopenia. N Engl J Med 1982;306: 744–745.
30. Newland AC, Treleaven JG, Minchinton RM, et al: High-dose intravenous IgG in adults with autoimmune thrombocytopenia. Lancet 1983;i:84–87.
31. Newland AC, Boots MA, Patterson KG: Intravenous IgG for autoimmune thrombocytopenia in pregnancy. N Engl J Med 1984;310:261–262.
32. Morgenstern GR, Measday B, Hegde UM: Autoimmune thrombocytopenia in pregnancy: New approach to management. BMJ 1983;287:584.
33. Clark AL, Gall SA: Clinical uses of intravenous immunoglobulin in pregnancy. Am J Obstet Gynecol 1997;176:241–253.
34. Godeau B, Lesage S, Divine M, et al: Treatment of adult chronic autoimmune thrombocytopenic purpura with repeated high-dose intravenous immunoglobulin. Blood 1993;82:1415.
35. Bussel JB, Pham LC, Aledort L, et al: Maintenance treatment of adults with chronic refractory immune thrombocytopenic purpura using repeated intravenous infusions of gammaglobulin. Blood 1988;72:121.
36. Sati HI, Ahya R, Watson HG: Incidence and associations of acute renal failure complication of high dose intravenous immunoglobulin therapy. Br J Haematol 2001;113:556–557.
37. Martin JN Jr, Morrison JC, Files JC: Autoimmune thrombocytopenic purpura: Current concepts and recommended practices. Am J Obstet Gynecol 1984;150:86.

38. Cook RL, Miller RC, Katz VL, et al: Immune thrombocytopenic purpura in pregnancy: A reappraisal of management. Obstet Gynecol 1991;78:578.
39. Silver RM, Branch DW, Scott JR: Maternal thrombocytopenia in pregnancy: Time for a reassessment. Am J Obstet Gynecol 1995;173:479–482.
40. BCSH Blood Transfusion Task Force: Guidelines for the use of platelet transfusions. Br J Haematol 2003;122:10–23.
41. Harris EN: A reassessment of the antiphospholipid syndrome. J Rheumatol 1990;17:733–735.
42. Wilson WA, Gharaui AE, Kolke T, et al: International consensus statement on preliminary classification criteria for definite antiphospholipid syndrome. Arthritis Rheum 1999;42:1309–1311.
43. Galli M, Finazzi G, Barrbui T: Thrombocytopenia in the antiphospholipid syndrome. Br J Haematol 1996;93:1–5.
44. Stasi R, Stipa E, Masi E et al: Longterm observation of 208 adults with chronic idiopathic thrombocytopenic purpura. Am J Med 1995;98:436–442.
45. Ware Branch D, Scott JR, Kochenour NK, et al: Obstetric complications associated with the lupus anticoagulant. N Engl J Med 1985;313:1322–1326.
46. Di Simone N, Castellini R, Caliandro D, Caruso A: Antiphospholipid antibodies regulate the expression of trophoblast cell adhesion molecules. Fertil Steril 2002;77:805–811.
47. Sebire NJ, Fox H, Backos M, et al: Defective endovascular trophoblast invasion in primary antiphospholipid syndrome: Associated early pregnancy failure. Hum Reprod 2002;17: 1067–1071.
48. Rai R, Cohen H, Dave M, et al: Randomized controlled trial of aspirin and aspirin plus heparin in pregnant women with recurrent miscarriage associated with phospholipid antibodies (or antiphospholipid antibodies). BMJ 1997;314:253–257.
49. Greaves M: Anticoagulants in pregnancy. Pharmacol Ther 1993;59:311–327.
50. Royal College of Obstetricians and Gynaecologists: Guidelines: Thromboprophylaxis during pregnancy, labour and after vaginal delivery. Guidelines No 37. London, RCOG Press, 2004.
51. Mandelbrot L, Schlienger I, Bongain A, et al: Thrombocytopenia in pregnant women infected with human immunodeficiency virus: Maternal and neonatal outcome. Am J Obstet Gynecol 1994;171:252–257.
52. Karpatkin S: Immunologic thrombocytopenic purpura in patients at risk for AIDS. Blood Rev 1987;1:119–125.
53. Ucar A, Fernandez HF, Byrnes JJ, et al: Thrombotic microangiopathy and retroviral infections: A 13 year experience. Br J Haematol 1994;45:304–309.
54. Connor EM, Sperling RS, Gelber R, et al: Reduction of maternal-infant transmission of human immunodeficiency virus type 1 with zidovudine treatment. N Engl J Med 1994;331:1173–1180.
55. Report of the NIH Panel to Define Principles of Therapy of HIV Infection. Ann Intern Med 1998;128:1057–1078.
56. Peckham C, Gibb D: Mother to child transmission of the human immunodeficiency virus. N Engl J Med 1995;333:298–302.
57. Aster RH: Heparin-induced thrombocytopenia and thrombosis. N Engl J Med 1995;332:1374–1376.
58. Warkentin TE, Levine MN, Hirsh J, et al: Heparin-induced thrombocytopenia in patients treated with low-molecular weight heparin or unfractionated heparin. N Engl J Med 1995;332: 1330–1335.
59. Greinacher A, Michels I, Mueller-Eckhardt C: Heparin-associated thrombocytopenia: The antibody is not heparin specific. Thromb Haemost 1992;67:545–549.
60. Van Besien K, Hoffman R, Golichowski A: Pregnancy associated with lupus anticoagulant and heparin induced thrombocytopenia: Management with a low molecular weight heparinoid. Thromb Res 1990;62:23–29.
61. Greinacher A, Eckhardt T, Mussmann J, et al: Pregnancy complicated by heparin-associated thrombocytopenia: Management by a prospectively in vitro selected heparinoid (Org 10172). Thromb Res 1993;71:123–136.
62. Fausset MB, Vogtlander M, Lee RM, et al: Heparin-induced thrombocytopenia is rare in pregnancy. Am J Obstet Gynaecol 2001;185:148–152.
63. Sheridan D, Carter C, Kelton JG: A diagnostic test for heparin-induced thrombocytopenia. Blood 1986;67:27–30.
64. Magnani HN: Heparin-induced thrombocytopenia (HIT): An overview of 230 patients treated with Orgaran (Org 10172). Thromb Haemost 1993;70:554–561.
65. Hirsh J, Warkentin TE, Shaughnessy SG, et al: Heparin and low molecular weight heparin: Mechanisms of action, pharmacokinetics, dosing, monitoring, efficacy, and safety. Chest 2001; 119:258S–275S.
66. Huhle G, Geberth M, Hoffman U, et al: Management of heparin-associated thrombocytopenia in pregnancy with subcutaneous r-hirudin. Gynaecol Obstet Invest 2000;49:67–69.
67. Roberts JA, Taylor RN, Muse TJ, et al: Preeclampsia: An endothelial cell disorder. Am J Obstet Gynecol 1989;161:1200–1204.
68. Redman CWG, Bonnar J, Beilin L: Early platelet consumption in preeclampsia. BMJ 1978;i:467–469.
69. Davies JA, Prentice CRM: Coagulation changes in pregnancy-induced hypertension and growth retardation. In Greer IA, Turpie AGG, Forbes CD (eds): Haemostasis and Thrombosis in Obstetrics and Gynaecology. London, Chapman and Hall, 1992, pp 143–162.
70. Weinstein L: Syndrome of hemolysis, elevated liver enzymes and low platelet count: A severe consequence of hypertension in pregnancy. Am J Obstet Gynecol 1978;142:159–167.
71. Romero R, Mazor M, Lockwood FJ: Clinical significance, prevalence and natural history of thrombocytopenia in pregnancy-induced hypertension. Am J Perinatol 1989;6:32–38.
72. Roberts WE, Perry KG Jr, Woods JB, et al: The intrapartum platelet count in patients with HELLP (hemolysis, elevated liver enzymes, and low platelets) syndrome: Is it predictive of later hemorrhagic complications? Am J Obstet Gynecol 1994;171: 799–804.
73. Martin JN, Files JC, Blake PG, et al: Plasma exchange for preeclampsia: Post-partum use for persistently severe pre-eclampsia-eclampsia with HELLP syndrome. Am J Obstet Gynecol 1990;162:126–137.
74. Kwaan HC: Clinicopathologic features of thrombotic thrombocytopenic purpura. Semin Hematol 1987;24:71–81.
75. Moake JL, Rudy CK, Troll JH, et al: Unusually large plasma factor VIII: Von Willebrand factor multimers in chronic relapsing thrombotic thrombocytopenic purpura. N Engl J Med 1982;307: 1432–1435.
76. Furlan M, Robles R, Solenthar M, et al: Deficient activity of von Willebrand factor-cleaving protease in chronic relapsing thrombotic thrombocytopenic purpura. Blood 1997;89:3097–3103.
77. Furlan M, Robles R, Galbusera M, et al: Von Willebrand Factor-cleaving protease in thrombotic, thrombocytopenic purpura and the hemolytic anemia syndrome. N Engl J Med 1998;399: 1578–1584.
78. Levy GG, Nichols WC, Lian EC, et al: Mutations in a member of the ADAMTS gene family cause thrombotic thrombocytopenic purpura. Nature 2001;413:488–494.
79. Manucci PM, Canciani MT, Forza I, et al: Changes in health and disease of the metalloprotease that cleaves Von Willebrand Factor. Blood 2001;98:2730–2735.
80. Vander Plas RM, Schiphorst ME, Huizinga EG, et al: Von Willebrand factor proteolysis is deficient in classic, but not in bone marrow transplantation associated, thrombotic thrombocytopenic purpura. Blood 1999;93:3798–3802.
81. BCSH Haemostasis and Thrombosis Task Force: Guidelines on the diagnosis and management of the thrombotic microangiopathic haemolytic anaemias. Br J Haematol 2003;120:556–573.
82. Weiner CP: Thrombotic microangiopathy in pregnancy and the postpartum period. Semin Hematol 1987;24:119–129.

83. Rock GA, Shumak KH, Buskard NA, et al: Comparison of plasma exchange with plasma infusion in the treatment of thrombotic thrombocytopenic purpura. N Engl J Med 1991;325:393–397.
84. Hayward CP, Sutton DM, Carter WH, et al: Treatment outcomes in patients with adult thrombotic thrombocytopenic purpura-haemolytic uraemic syndrome. Arch Intern Med 1994;154:982–987.
85. Rock G, Shumak KH, Sutton DMC, et al: Cryosupernatant as replacement fluid for plasma exchange in TTP. Br J Haematol 1996;94:383–386.
86. Gordon LI, Kwaan HC, Rossi EC: Deleterious effects of platelet transfusions and recovery thrombocytosis in patients with thrombotic microangiopathy. Semin Hematol 1987;24:194–201.
87. Sadler JE: A revised classification of von Willebrand disease. Thromb Haemost 1994;71:520–525.
88. Favorolo EJ: Laboratory assessment as a critical component of the appropriate diagnosis and sub-classification of von Willebrand's disease. Blood Rev 1999;13:185–204.
89. Greer IA, Lowe GDO, Walker JJ, et al: Congenital coagulopathies in obstetrics and gynaecology. In Greer IA, Turpie AGG, Forbes CD (eds): Haemostasis and Thrombosis in Obstetrics and Gynaecology. London, Chapman and Hall, 1992, pp 459–486.
90. Ramsahoye BH, Davies SV, Dasani H, et al: Pregnancy in von Willebrand's disease. Clin Pathol 1994;47:569–571.
91. Greer IA, Lowe GOD, Walker JJ, et al: Haemorrhagic problems in obstetrics and gynaecology in patients with congenital coagulopathies. Br J Obstet Gynaecol 1991;98:909–918.
92. Giles AR, Hoogendoorn H, Benford K: Type IIB von Willebrand's disease presenting as thrombocytopenia during pregnancy. Br J Haematol 1987;67:349–353.
93. Rick ME, Williams SB, Sacher RA, et al: Thrombocytopenia associated with pregnancy in a patient with type IIB von Willebrand's disease. Blood 1987;69:786–789.
94. Walker ID, Walker JJ, Colvin BT, et al: Investigation and management of hemorrhagic disorders in pregnancy. J Clin Pathol 1994;47:100–108.
95. Foster PA: The reproductive health of women with von Willebrand disease unresponsive to DDAVP: Results of an international survey. Thromb Haemost 1995;74:784–790.
96. Krishnamurthy M, Miotti AB: Von Willebrand's disease and pregnancy. Obstet Gynecol 1977;49:244–247.
97. Kadir RA, Lee CA, Sabin CA, et al: Pregnancy in women with von Willebrand's disease or factor XI deficiency. BJOG 1998;105:314–321.
98. Conti M, Mari D, Conti E, et al: Pregnancy in women with different types of von Willebrand disease. Obstet Gynecol 1986;68:282–285.
99. Federici AB, Mannucci PM: Diagnosis and management of von Willebrand disease. Haemophilia 1999;5 (Suppl 2):28–37.
100. Kirtava A, Drews C, Lally C, et al: Medical reproductive and psychosocial experiences of women diagnosed with vWD receiving care in haemophilia treatment centres: A case control study. Haemophilia 2003;9:292–297.
101. Lak M, Peyvandi F, Mannucci PM: Clinical manifestations and complications of childbirth replacement therapy in 385 Iranian patients with type 3 von Willebrand's Disease. Br J Haematol 2000;111:1236–1240.
102. Sherer DM, Anyaegbunam A, Onyeiye C: Antepartum fetal intracranial haemorrhage, predisposing factors and prenatal sonography: A review. Am J Perinatol 1998;15:431–441.
103. Kouides PA: Obstetric and gynaecological aspects of vWD. Ballieres Best Pract Clin Haematol 2001;14:381–399.
104. Mannucci PM: How I treat patients with von Willebrand's disease. Blood 2001;97:1915–1919.
105. Ray JG: DDAVP use during pregnancy: An analysis of its safety for mother and child. Obstet Gynecol Surv 1998;53:450–455.
106. Goudemard J, Negrier C, Ounnoughene O, Sultan Y: Clinical management of patients with vWD with a VHP VWF concentrate: The French experience. Haemophilia 1998;4:48–52.
107. Stedeford JC, Pittman JA: Von Willebrand's disease and neuraxial anaesthesia. Anaesthesia 2001;56:397.
108. Battle J, Noya MS, Giangrande P, Lopez-Fernandez MF: Advances in the therapy of von Willebrand's disease. Haemophilia 2002;8:301–307.
109. Miller R: Counselling about diagnosis and inheritance of genetic bleeding disorders: Haemophilia A and B. Haemophilia 1999;5:77–83.
110. Lusher JM, McMillan CW: Severe factor VIII and factor IX deficiency in females. Am J Med 1978;65:637–648.
111. Stirling Y, Woolf L, North WRS, et al: Haemostasis in normal pregnancy. Thromb Haemost 1984;52:176–182.
112. Econamides DL, Kadir RA, Braithwaite JM, et al: The obstetric experience of carriers of haemophilia. BJOG 1997;104:803–810.
113. Giangrande PLF: Management of pregnancy in carriers of haemophilia. Haemophilia 1998;4:779–784.
114. Ljung R, Lindgren A-C, Petrini P, et al: Normal vaginal delivery is to be recommended for haemophilia carrier gravidae. Acta Paediatr 1994;83:609–611.
115. Kulkarni R, Lusher JM: Intracranial and extracrainal haemorrhages in newborns with haemophilia: A review of the literature. J Paediatr Haematol Oncol 1999;21:289–295.
116. Kulkarni R, Lusher J: Perinatal management of newborns with haemophilia. Br J Haematol 2001;112:264–274.
117. Medical Research Council European trial of chorion villus sampling. MRC working party on the evaluation of chorion villus sampling. Lancet 1991;337:1491–1499.
118. Ludlam CA on behalf of the UKHCDO Genetics Working Party: Clinical Genetics Services for Haemophilia (submitted).
119. Peake IR, Lillicrap DP, Boulyjenkov V, et al: Report of a joint WHO/WFH meeting on the control of haemophilia: Carrier detection and prenatal diagnosis. Blood Coagul Fibrinolysis 1993;4:313–344.
120. Goodeve AC: Advances in carrier detection in haemophilia. Haemophilia 1998;4:358–364.
121. Naylor J, Brinke A, Hassock S, et al: Characteristic mRNA abnormality found in half of the patients with severe haemophilia A is due to large DNA inversions. Hum Mol Genet 1993;11:1773–1778.
122. Manucci PM: Desmopressin (DDAVP) in the treatment of bleeding disorders: The first 20 years. Blood 1997;90:2515–2521.
123. UKHCDO Guidelines: Guidelines on therapeutic products to treat haemophilia and other hereditary coagulation disorders. Haemophilia 1997;3:63–77.
124. Mannucci PM: The choice of plasma derived clotting factor concentrates. Baillieres Clin Haematol 1996;9:273–290.
125. Andrew M, Paes B, Milner R, et al: Development of the human coagulation system in the full-term infant. Blood 1987;70:165–172.
126. Kulkarni R, Lusher JM, Henry RC, Kaleen DJ: Current practices regarding newborn intracranial haemorrhage and obstetric care and mode of delivery of pregnant haemophilia carriers: A survey of obstetricians, neonataologists and haematologists in the United States. On behalf of the National haemophilia Foundation's Medical and Scientific Advisory Council. Haemophilia 1999;5:410–415.
127. Kobayashi T, Kanayama N, Tokunaga N, et al: Prenatal and peripartum management of congenital afibrinogenaemia. Br J Haematol 2000;109:364–366.
128. DiPaola J, Nugent D, Young G: Current therapy for rare factor deficiencies. Haemophilia 2001;7 (Suppl 1):16–22.
129. Giles AR: Disseminated intravascular coagulation. In Bloom AL, Forbes CD, Thomas DP, Taddenham EGD (eds): Haemostasis and Thrombosis, 3rd ed. Vol. 2. Edinburgh, Churchill Livingstone, 1994.

130. Levi M, TenCate H: Disseminated intravascular coagulation. N Engl J Med 1999;341:586–592.
131. Forbes CD, Greer IA: Physiology of haemostasis and the effect of pregnancy. In Greer IA, Turpie AGG, Forbes CD (eds): Haemostasis and Thrombosis in Obstetrics and Gynaecology. London, Chapman and Hall, 1992, pp 1–25.
132. Blood Transfusion Task Force: Guidelines for the use of fresh frozen plasma. Transfus Med 1992;2:57–67.
133. Matthay MD: Severe sepsis: A new treatment with both anticoagulant and anti-inflammatory properties. N Engl J Med 2001;344:759–762.
134. Bernard GR, Vincent J-L, Laterre PF, et al: Efficacy and safety of recombinant human activated protein C for severe sepsis. N Engl J Med 2001;344:699–709.
135. Kobayashi T, Terao T, Maki M, Ikenaie T: Activated protein C is effective for DIC associated with placental abruption (letter). Thromb Haemost 1999;82:1363.
136. Bick RL: DIC: A review of etiology, pathophysiology, diagnosis and management: Guidelines for care. Clin Appl Thromb Haemost 2002;8:1–31.
137. O'Connell NM, Perry DJ, Hodgson AJ, et al: Recombinant factor VIIa in the management of uncontrolled haemorrhage. Transfusion 2003;43:1649–1651.
138. Ludlam CA: The evidence behind inhibitor treatment with recombinant factor VIIa: Pathophysiology of haemostasis and thrombosis. 2002;32 (Supp 1):13–18.
139. Zupancic SS, Sokolic V, Viskovic T, et al: Successful use of recombinant factor VIIa for massive bleeding after cesaerean section due to HELLP syndrome. Acta Haematol 2002;108:162–163.
140. Moscardo F, Perez F, de la Rubia J, et al: Successful treatment of severe intraabdominal bleeding associated with disseminated intravascular coagulation using recombinant activated factor VIIa. Br J Haematol 2001;114:174–176.
141. Ratnoff OD: Haemostatic defects in liver and biliary disease and disorders of vitamin K metabolism. In Ratnoff OD, Forbes CD (eds): Disorders of Haemostasis, 3rd ed. Philadelphia, WB Saunders, 1996, pp 422–443.
142. Hauser I, Schneider B, Lechner K: Post-partum factor VIII inhibitors: A review of the literature with special reference to the value of steroid and immunosuppressive treatment. Thromb Haemost 1995;73:1–5.
143. Baudo F, deCataldo F: Italian Association of Haemophilia Centres (AICE): Register of acquired factor VIII inhibitors (RIIA). Acquired factor VIII inhibitors in pregnancy: Data from the Italian Haemophilia Register relevant to clinical practice. BJOG 2003;110:311–314.

CHAPTER 42

Clotting Disorders

Robert D. Auerbach / Charles J. Lockwood

INTRODUCTION

Disorders of coagulation are a major cause of maternal morbidity and mortality. Pregnancy and the puerperium present a significant challenge to the hemostatic system. Maintaining an intact vascular compartment requires coordination of platelet function, soluble coagulation and fibrinolytic products, and the vascular endothelium. Pregnancy poses paradoxical challenges to the hemostatic system. During implantation and early placentation, syncytiotrophoblasts penetrate the endothelium of uterine vessels to establish the primordial or lacunar-type uteroplacental circulation. High-volume, low-resistance flow is established in the intervillous space after endovascular cytotrophoblast invasion of the uterine spiral arteries. As this process progresses, thrombosis must be avoided to maintain normal fetal growth and viability, and hemorrhage must be avoided to ensure maternal and fetal well-being. During the third stage of labor, 140 placental bed spiral arteries, denuded of their muscular layer, must quickly thrombose during puerperal contractions to avoid fatal maternal hemorrhage. Dramatic changes in local and systemic clotting and fibrinolytic factors are needed to meet this complex hemostatic challenge.

Because both thrombosis and hemorrhage are more common in pregnancy, the physician must understand the normal homeostatic mechanisms involved in the coagulation system and how they are affected by pregnancy and specific pathologic conditions. Stasis, hypercoagulability, and vascular trauma (Virchow's triad) occur in pregnancy, enhancing the risk of thrombosis. Stasis of the lower extremities is a direct result of compression through the enlarging uterus and a hormone-mediated increase in deep vascular capacitance. Estrogen drives endothelium-derived nitric oxide production, inducing vessel dilation.[1] In addition, positional uterine compression (which is greatest in the supine position and least in the left lateral decubitus position) can lead to varying degrees of progressive deep vein dilation.[2] Associated hypercoagulability is a result of increases in the levels of fibrinogen, prothrombin, and clotting factors VII, VIII, IX, and X; a decrease in the level of protein S[3–5]; a progressive increase in resistance to activated protein C[6]; and an increase in the levels of antifibrinolytic types 1 and 2 plasminogen activator inhibitor (PAI-1 and PAI-2).[7,8] This hemostatic change likely reduces the risk of antepartum, intrapartum, and postpartum hemorrhage, but is responsible for the dramatic 10-fold increase in pregnancy-associated venous thromboembolic disease (VTE). The risk of VTE is further increased in patients with acquired or inherited thrombophilias.[9,10] Delivery, especially operative vaginal and cesarean delivery, and puerperal infections are associated with vascular damage.[4] This chapter discusses the regulation of hemostasis, the associated pregnancy-induced changes, and various coagulation abnormalities and their diagnosis, clinical consequences, and treatment.

CLOTTING SYSTEM

Tissue factor (TF) is a cell-membrane-bound glycoprotein that is responsible for initiating hemostasis.[11,12] After vascular disruption, perivascular cell TF comes into contact with plasma factor VII. The TF–factor VII complex either directly activates factor X or generates factor Xa by initially activating factor IX, which complexes with its cofactor (factor VIIIa) to activate factor X. The conversion of factor VII to factor VIIa by thrombin or factor IXa, Xa, or XIIa results in a 100-fold increase in activity. Once activated, factor Xa complexes with factor Va to convert factor II (prothrombin) to factor IIa (thrombin). Thrombin then cleaves fibrinogen to produce fibrin. A stable hemostatic plug is formed as fibrin monomers self-polymerize and are cross-linked by thrombin-activated factor XIIIa. Thrombin induces platelets to aggregate in the fibrin clot. Factor XI binds to the surface of activated platelets, is activated by factor XIIa, and in turn, activates factor IX.[12]

Thrombin cleaves fibrinogen to fibrin and amplifies the hemostatic system by activating factors V, VII, and XIII as well as platelets.[13] Thrombotic disease is caused by excess thrombin generation. To prevent this action, the endogenous anticoagulant system inhibits thrombin and factor Xa activity. This system is composed of heparin cofactor II, α_2-macroglobulin, and antithrombin. The thrombin–factor Xa complex binds to each of the inhibitors and to vitronectin.[14] The result is a conformational change that facilitates binding to heparin, augmenting the rate of thrombin inactivation several 1000-fold.[15–17] Thrombin–antithrombin is the most physiologically active complex of this group. The increase in thrombin generation in normal pregnancy is mirrored by the increase in thrombin–antithrombin complexes.[18]

Thrombin also binds to thrombomodulin, and the resultant complex activates protein C, which binds to protein S to inactivate factors VIIIa and Va.[19] Levels of free protein S and protein S activity decrease 40% during pregnancy, in part because of increases in the complement 4b binding protein, which acts as a protein S carrier protein.[20]

Fibrinolysis aids in the prevention of pathologic thrombosis. Fibrin degradation products are the result of the ability of plasmin to cleave fibrin. Plasmin is created by its conversion from plasminogen by tissue-type plasminogen activator (tPA) embedded in fibrin. Because it inactivates tPA, PAI-1 is the primary inhibitor of fibrinolysis. Sources of PAI-1 and PAI-2, respectively, include epithelium decidua[21] and the placenta.[22] Thrombin-activatable fibrinolysis inhibitor is another inhibitor of fibrinolysis. This inhibitor is also activated by the thrombin–thrombomodulin complex.[23] Thus, thrombomodulin inhibits both excessive clotting (through the generation of activated protein C) and premature fibrinolysis (by generating an inhibitor of tPA).

RISK FACTORS FOR VENOUS THROMBOEMBOLIC DISEASE IN PREGNANCY (See Chapter 43)

Pregnancy-associated changes in hemostatic and fibrinolytic proteins establish a hypercoagulable state. Endogenous anticoagulant levels increase minimally (tissue factor pathway inhibitor [TFPI] α_2-macroglobulin), remain constant (antithrombin, heparin cofactor II, and protein C), or decrease significantly (protein S) in pregnancy. In addition, levels of fibrinogen and factors II, VII, VIII, X, and XII increase.[18] A twofold to threefold increase in PAI-1 concentrations is noted.[24] The result is the promotion of clot formation and stability. Clinical risk factors for VTE include increased parity (which is associated with venous valvular insufficiency), cesarean delivery, and postpartum endomyometritis (which are associated with increases in the complement 4b binding protein). Independent risk factors include trauma, infection, obesity, nephrotic syndrome, age older than 35 years, bed rest, orthopedic surgery, and a history of VTE.

ACQUIRED THROMBOPHILIAS

Pregnant patients with acquired or inherited thrombophilia are at increased risk for VTE. Antiphospholipid antibodies constitute the acquired thrombophilias, accounting for 14% of VTE events in pregnancy.[9,10] In addition, these antibodies are associated with thrombocytopenia and various adverse obstetric outcomes. Two distinct classes are described: lupus anticoagulants and anticardiolipin antibodies.[25–27] Although antiphospholipid antibodies may arise from conditions associated with VTE and poor pregnancy outcomes (e.g., systemic lupus erythematosus), the antibodies directly promote placental and vascular thrombosis by interfering with a variety of anionic phospholipid-associated anticoagulant proteins, such as annexin V.[28,29] For a more detailed discussion of acquired thrombophilias, see Chapter 44.

INHERITED THROMBOPHILIAS

Maternal and Fetal Risks

Inherited thrombophilias also predispose pregnant women to VTE.[30] In addition to maternal deep vein thrombosis and pulmonary embolism, inherited thrombophilias are implicated in fetal loss (spontaneous abortion and stillbirth), intrauterine growth restriction, placental abruption, and preeclampsia.[31,32] Some studies also report an increased frequency of ischemic cerebrovascular events.[33] In addition to the variable risk of individual inherited thrombophilias, modifying factors (surgery, age >35 years, parity >4, obesity, smoking, immobility, and oral contraceptive use) contribute significantly to the overall risk of VTE.[34] The following are the most common inherited thrombophilias:

Heterozygosity for the following:

- Activated protein C resistance as a result of factor V Leiden (FVL) mutation
- G20210A mutation of the prothrombin gene

Homozygosity for the following:

- The thermolabile variant of methylenetetrahydrofolate reductase (MTHFR) that increases homocysteine levels, particularly in folate-deficient patients
- 4G/4G polymorphism in the promoter region of the PAI-1 gene that causes an increase in this antifibrinolytic agent

Rarer causes of inherited thrombophilias include autosomal dominant antithrombin, protein S, and protein C deficiencies. More than 70% of cases of pregnancy-associated VTE are related to these conditions, even though they are present in only approximately 10% to 15% of the population.[34,35] This chapter describes several individual inherited thrombophilias and discusses their clinical manifestations and treatment options.

Activated Protein C Resistance and Factor V Leiden Mutation

Present in 5% to 9% of the European population and 3% of African Americans and virtually absent in African blacks and the Chinese and Japanese populations, FVL is the most common heritable coagulopathy.[36] The condition arises from a point mutation in factor V at its site of inactivation by protein C (substitution of glutamine for arginine at position 506). This abnormality is inherited in an autosomal dominant fashion.[37] Patients with a single mutation have a 5- to 10-fold increased risk of VTE. Homozygous patients have a greater than 100-fold increased risk of VTE.[31,38] Although FVL is present in 40% of pregnant patients with VTE, given the low incidence of thrombosis in pregnancy (1 in 1400) and the high incidence of the mutation in the European-derived population, the estimated risk of VTE among heterozygous pregnant patients is only 0.2%.[32] As in pregnancy, the risk of VTE increases several-fold in women with FVL who take oral contraceptives.[40] Although clinical laboratories can screen for activated protein C resistance in pregnancy, polymerase chain reaction is the optimal method to confirm the presence of the FVL mutation in pregnancy.

Other adverse pregnancy outcomes have been reported in FVL carriers. Particularly at risk are homozygous patients and patients with a combined defect. Associated conditions include severe preeclampsia,[41] placental abruption,[42] fetal thrombosis as a result of fetal thrombophilia,[43] and fetal loss.[44] In a meta-analysis, both heterozygous and homozygous patients with a FVL mutation were at increased risk for recurrent first-trimester loss (odds ratio [OR], 2.01; 95% confidence interval [CI], 1.13–3.58), recurrent loss (>22 weeks) (OR, 7.83; 95% CI, 2.83–21.67), and nonrecurrent loss after 19 weeks' gestation (OR, 3.26; 95% CI, 1.82–5.83).[44]

Prothrombin Gene Mutation

A mutation in the promoter of the prothrombin gene (G20210A) leads to overexpression of prothrombin. Although it is present in only 2% to 3% of the European population, it accounts for 13% to 17% of women with an initial VTE.[31,32] Because of the low incidence of VTE in pregnancy, the actual risk of clotting in a carrier of this mutation is 0.5%.[31] Patients who are homozygous for the prothrombin gene mutation are at increased risk for VTE in pregnancy. A 4.6% risk of VTE occurs with compound heterozygotes for FVL and the prothrombin gene mutation.[32] Data suggest that placental dysfunction and pregnancy loss may be related to the prothrombin gene mutation. A meta-analysis that included women with the prothrombin gene mutation reported an increased risk of fetal loss prior to 28 weeks (OR, 2.56; 95% CI, 1.04–6.29), recurrent first-trimester loss (OR, 2.32; 95% CI, 1.12–4.79), and late nonrecurrent fetal loss (OR, 2.30; 95% CI, 1.09–4.87).[44]

Hyperhomocysteinemia

Homozygosity for the thermolabile variant of MTHFR results in hyperhomocysteinemia, particularly in folate-deficient patients. An increased prevalence of the thermolabile variant of MTHFR is seen in women with certain complications (VTE, recurrent abortion, fetal neural tube defects, preeclampsia, placental abruption, fetal growth restriction, stillbirth).[45–48] Little or no increase in early fetal loss was noted in three meta-analyses in carriers of the MTHFR mutation.[44,47,49] It is unknown whether folate supplementation reduces or prevents any complications except neural tube defects.

Protein C and Protein S Deficiencies

Protein C and protein S deficiencies occur with a frequency of 0.2% to 0.5% in the general population and account for 10% to 25% of VTE in pregnancy.[50] Protein C or protein S deficiency carries a less than 5% risk of VTE during pregnancy but a 10% to 20% risk in the puerperium.[51] Pregnancy loss also appears to be increased in this population. In one study, loss rates were 28% for protein C deficiency and 17% for protein S deficiency. The control group had a loss rate of 11%.[52] A meta-analysis found that women with protein S deficiency had an odds ratio of 7.39 (95% CI, 1.28–42.83) for fetal loss.[44]

Antithrombin Deficiency

An autosomal dominant condition, antithrombin deficiency is the most thrombogenic heritable coagulopathy. Antepartum VTE rates are 12% to 60%, with puerperium rates of 11% to 33%.[50] Antithrombin deficiency is associated with a twofold risk of miscarriage and a fivefold risk of stillbirth.[53]

Other Heritable Coagulopathies

In patients who are homozygous for the 4G/4G allele in PAI-1, the presence of four instead of five consecutive guanine nucleotides in the PAI-1 promoter produces a site that is too small to allow binding of repressors. As a result, gene transcription and circulating levels of PAI-1 are increased.[54] A modest increase in VTE occurs as well as an increased risk of preeclampsia, fetal growth restriction, fetal loss, and premature delivery.[55] Several reports link VTE with elevated levels of factors VII, VIII, IX, and XI.[56–59] Dysfibrinogenemia may be associated with VTE as well as hemorrhage. Other inherited abnormalities, including decreased tPA, factor XII deficiency, hypoplasminogenemia or dysplasminogenemia, and heparin cofactor II deficiency, are not associated with adverse pregnancy outcomes.[60]

Management Options

Diagnosis

Patients with a history of VTE, a strong family history of VTE, or a history of adverse pregnancy outcomes may be candidates for evaluation of acquired and heritable thrombophilias. Adverse pregnancy outcomes include stillbirth associated with intrauterine growth restriction and placental infarction or abruption and severe or recurrent preeclampsia in the second or early third trimester. Screening of an unselected population is not recommended.[61]

Laboratory evaluation of activated protein C resistance can be obtained; however, antiphospholipid antibodies, low levels of protein S, and elevated levels of factor VIII may produce a false-positive report in pregnancy.[10] Therefore, the FVL mutation should be determined by polymerase chain reaction. Other studies include evaluation for the following:

- Polymerase chain reaction to detect prothrombin 20210A and MTHFR mutations
- Activity assays for antithrombin, protein C, and protein S (with consideration of the normally reduced protein S levels in pregnancy)
- Fasting homocysteine levels
- Thrombocythemia (discussed later; see Chapter 40)
- Antiphospholipid studies (see Chapter 44)

Although genotyping for the 4G/4G PAI-1 mutation is not widely available, assays for plasma PAI-1 protein with a greater than threefold elevation is presumptive evidence of homozygosity. Laboratory evaluation of these disorders is best performed in the nonpregnant patient who is not receiving hormonal or anticoagulation therapy and is remote (>6 months) from a history of VTE.[34]

Treatment

Several small observational studies suggest a benefit of anticoagulation to prevent adverse pregnancy outcomes in patients with thrombophilia.[62,63] Gris et al. randomized 160 patients with FVL, prothrombin 20210A, or protein S deficiency and a history of one unexplained loss after 10 weeks to either low dose asprin or enoxaparin (40 mg SQgd).[64] They observed a significant increase in live born rates in the enoxaparin group (86.2% vs. 28.8%) (OR 1515; 95% CI, 7–34). Women with VTE during a current pregnancy should receive therapeutic anticoagulation for at least 4 months during the pregnancy, followed by prophylactic therapy for at least 6 weeks postpartum. Women with a history of VTE associated with nonrecurrent risk factors (e.g., surgery, orthopedic immobilization), but without acquired or inherited thrombophilia, appear to be at very low risk for a repeat event. Although anticoagulation during the antepartum period appears unnecessary in these patients, prophylaxis should be used during the higher-risk postpartum period.[65] Women with high-risk (more thrombogenic) thrombophilias (antithrombin deficiency and homozygosity for the FVL and prothrombin G20210A mutations) should be treated with full therapeutic anticoagulation during pregnancy and for at least 6 weeks postpartum, regardless of the history.

Pregnant women who have low-risk (less thrombogenic) thrombophilias (e.g., those who are heterozygous for the FVL and prothrombin G20210A mutations as well as protein C or protein S deficiency or those with hyperhomocysteinemia that does not respond to folate and vitamin B_{12} therapy) and no personal history of VTE have a low incidence of VTE in pregnancy (<5%). These patients do not appear to need antepartum anticoagulation.[66] However, they should receive postpartum prophylaxis if they require a cesarean section because most fatal pulmonary emboli occur during this period.[67] Some experts also recommend postpartum prophylaxis if the patient has an affected first-degree relative or another thrombotic risk factor (e.g., obesity or immobilization). In contrast, patients with these less thrombogenic thrombophilias and a history of VTE require prophylactic anticoagulation, as indicated, during the antepartum and postpartum periods.

Given the lack of consistent evidence of an association between maternal thrombophilia and recurrent early first-trimester loss (<10 weeks), anticoagulant therapy does not appear justified.[68] Women with less thrombogenic thrombophilias and a history of fetal loss (>10 weeks), unexplained abruption, severe early-onset preeclampsia, or severe fetal growth restriction pose a therapeutic conundrum. Definitive recommendations await further clinical trials of anticoagulation in this population.[64,69,70] As discussed earlier, patients in the high-risk thrombophilia group require therapy, regardless of their obstetric history. Vitamin B_{12} and folic acid should be supplemented if hyperhomocysteinemia is diagnosed.

HEPARIN (See Chapter 43)

During pregnancy, unfractionated heparin and low-molecular-weight heparin (LMWH) are the anticoagulants of choice, given their efficacy and safety profile.[71,72] Postpartum, oral anticoagulation with warfarin may be used and is considered safe in breast-feeding mothers.

Heparin enhances antithrombin activity, increases the level of factor Xa inhibitor,[73] and inhibits platelet aggregation.[74] Heparin does not cross the placenta or enter breast milk.[75,76] Side effects include hemorrhage, osteoporosis, and thrombocytopenia. Osteoporosis is more common with doses of heparin greater than 15,000 U daily for longer than 6 months.[77] All patients who are treated with heparin should receive calcium supplementation of

1500 mg daily. Heparin-induced thrombocytopenia occurs in 3% of patients. An early-onset, transient form of platelet aggregation does not require interruption of therapy. However, the immunoglobulin G-mediated thrombotic thrombocytopenia form requires cessation of therapy.[78] Platelet counts should be followed within 3 days of the initiation of therapy, and then weekly for 3 weeks. Heparin-induced thrombocytopenia appears to be far less common with LMWH, and LMWH also exerts lesser osteopenic effects.[79,80] The goals of therapy for a patient with acute VTE are to maintain anti-factor Xa activity between 0.6 and 1.0 U/mL or activated partial thromboplastin time (aPTT) between 1.5 and 2.5 times the control value. The dose required may vary as a result of differences in heparin-binding proteins in pregnancy.[78] During the initial phase of therapy, aPTT, the heparin level, or the anti-factor Xa level should be evaluated every 4 hours, with adjustments made in dosage as needed. Intravenous therapeutic unfractionated heparin administration should be continued for at least 5 days or until clinical improvement is seen.[81] Unfractionated heparin may then be administered subcutaneously every 8 to 12 hours to maintain aPTT at 1.5 to 2 times the control value 6 hours after the injection.[82]

As an alternative, LMWH (dalteparin, enoxaparin) is effective and safe when used during pregnancy.[83] For therapeutic dosing, the anti-factor Xa level should be 0.6 to 1.0 U/mL 4 to 6 hours after injection. Because regional anesthesia is contraindicated within 18 to 24 hours of LMWH administration, the recommendation is to switch to unfractionated heparin at 36 weeks' gestation, or earlier, if preterm delivery is expected. Patients with antithrombin deficiency and those who are homozygous for the FVL or prothrombin G20210A mutation require therapeutic anticoagulation throughout pregnancy. When only prophylactic therapy is required, unfractionated heparin or LMWH should be titrated to maintain the anti-factor Xa level at 0.1 to 0.2 U/mL 6 (unfractionated heparin) and 4 (LMWH) hours after injection. Administration of LMWH should be discontinued at 36 weeks, and treatment with unfractionated heparin at a prophylactic dose should be initiated, as indicated.

If vaginal or cesarean delivery occurs more than 4 hours after a prophylactic dose of unfractionated heparin, the patient is not at significant risk for hemorrhagic complications. Protamine sulfate may be administered to patients with increased aPTT who are receiving prophylactic or therapeutic unfractionated heparin and are about to deliver vaginally or by cesarean section. Anticoagulation-related problems with delivery are unlikely to occur 12 hours from prophylactic or 24 hours from therapeutic doses of LMWH. Antithrombin concentrates can be used in antithrombin-deficient patients in the peripartum period. Unfractionated heparin or LMWH can be used 6 hours after vaginal delivery or 8 to 12 hours after cesarean delivery. In patients who require therapy in the postpartum period, unfractionated heparin, LMWH, or warfarin (discussed later) may be prescribed.

WARFARIN

The anticoagulant activity of warfarin is a result of its inhibition of vitamin K, which is a cofactor in the synthesis of factors VII, IX, and X, and prothrombin II. Carrying a 33% risk of embryopathy (i.e., nasal hypoplasia, stippled epiphyses, central nervous system abnormalities) when exposure occurs between 7 and 12 weeks' gestation, it is loosely bound to albumin and crosses the placenta. Fetal and placental bleeding is also a serious complication of warfarin use throughout pregnancy. Vitamin K or fresh frozen plasma can be used to reverse its effect. Although its use during pregnancy is normally contraindicated,[84] warfarin use during the second trimester may be warranted in patients with mechanical heart valves because current studies suggest an increase in thrombogenic complications with heparin (unfractionated or LMWH).[85,86] Because the risk of fatal maternal valve thrombosis may outweigh the risk of warfarin exposure between 12 and 36 weeks' gestation, the risks and benefits should be discussed with these patients. Warfarin does not accumulate in breast milk or have an anticoagulant effect on the infant and is not contraindicated in breastfeeding mothers. Heparin should be continued for the initial 4 days of warfarin therapy and until a therapeutic international normalized ratio is achieved to avoid skin necrosis and paradoxical thromboembolus.

Maternal and Fetal Surveillance

Inherited thrombophilias present significant risk of maternal VTE and possibly adverse pregnancy outcomes after 10 weeks' gestation. Initiation of therapy, when indicated, and close maternal and fetal surveillance are mandated in this population. Patients with inherited thrombophilias should be educated about the signs and symptoms of thromboembolic disease. Standard screening for preeclampsia should continue (e.g., maternal weight, blood pressure, urine protein), and renal function, liver function, and platelet counts should be monitored with evolving signs or symptoms of preeclampsia. Fetal growth may be followed by establishing a definitive estimated date of confinement by first-trimester ultrasound and serial ultrasound examinations (every 4–6 weeks), beginning at 20 weeks' gestation. Doppler flow examination of the umbilical artery and middle cerebral artery may be used for assessment in fetal growth restriction. Nonstress testing and biophysical profiles may begin at 36 weeks or earlier, as clinically indicated. Taking into consideration gestational age, early delivery may be indicated if the maternal or fetal condition is deteriorating.

SUMMARY OF MANAGEMENT OPTIONS
Inherited Thrombophilias

Management Options (See also Chapter 43)	Quality of Evidence	Strength of Recommendation	References
Prepregnancy			
Consider evaluation in patients with venous thromboembolic disease, a strong family history of venous thromboembolic disease, and adverse pregnancy outcomes (fetal loss, intrauterine growth restriction, severe or recurrent preeclampsia).	III	B	132
Prenatal			
Consider evaluation in patients with venous thromboembolic disease, a strong family history of venous thromboembolic disease, and adverse pregnancy outcomes (fetal loss, intrauterine growth restriction, severe or recurrent preeclampsia).	IIb	B	133
Population screening is not recommended.	III	B	61
Laboratory testing includes polymerase chain reaction for factor V Leiden, prothrombin 20210A, and methylene tetrahydrofolate reductase; activity assays for antithrombin and proteins C and S; and a fasting homocysteine level.	IV	C	34
Unclear benefit of treatment for a history of adverse pregnancy outcome with anticoagulation; maternal and fetal surveillance empirically recommended	IIa	B	69, 70
Therapeutic heparin or low-molecular-weight heparin with venous thromboembolic disease during pregnancy	IV	C	67
Prophylactic or therapeutic heparin or low-molecular-weight heparin for a history of venous thromboembolic disease, depending on the level of risk and recurrent features	IV	C	66
Folate and vitamin B_{12} supplementation for hyperhomocysteinemia	III	B	66
Labor and Delivery			
Reduce or stop heparin for labor and delivery; restart after 6 hours.	III	B	134
Postnatal			
Switching to warfarin postpartum is an option.	III	B	135

ESSENTIAL THROMBOCYTHEMIA (See Chapter 40)

Maternal and Fetal Risks

Essential thrombocythemia is a nonreactive chronic myeloproliferative disorder. As a result of the effect of this process on the hemopoietic stem cells, patients show excessive proliferation of megakaryocytes and sustained elevation of the platelet count.[87] Although previously considered a malady of middle age, increasingly, elevated platelet counts are noted in the younger population. A slight female preponderance is noted, especially in the younger population, with 20% of those affected younger than 40 years of age. Mesa and colleagues[88] reported a prevalence rate of 2.38 patients per 100,000 population in southern Minnesota.

Typical criteria used in the diagnosis of essential thrombocythemia include the following:

- Platelet count greater than 600,000/mm^3
- Megakaryocyte hyperplasia
- Splenomegaly
- Clinical course complicated by hemorrhagic or thrombotic episodes

Although the cause of increased platelet production by megakaryocytes is unclear, the result is thrombocytosis. Proposed theories include increased sensitivity to cytokines, decreased inhibition of platelet inhibitory factors, and decreased accessory cell microenvironment or autonomous production.[89] The major cause of morbidity and mortality is complications of VTE. Complications are more common in the older population and in those with a history of thrombosis. Hemorrhagic complications are seen in patients with very high platelet counts. The evolution of essential thrombocythemia into leukemia is rare, but the incidence may be increased by some chemotherapeutic agents.[90]

Patients with essential thrombocythemia may have occlusive disease in the microvascular or macrovascular system (arterial or venous). Microvascular disease may involve transient cerebral ischemia, migraine, visual dysfunction, digital ischemia, and erythromelalgia.[91,92] Arterial thrombosis may include occlusion of the lower extremity, coronary, or renal arteries. Venous thrombosis of the splenic, hepatic, or pelvic veins may occur. Pulmonary hypertension may result from pulmonary vascular occlusion.[93,94] Hemorrhagic complications may include bruising of the skin and bleeding of the mucous membranes or digestive tract. These complications are most common in patients with platelet counts greater than 1,000,000/mm^3 and are considered a result of acquired deficiency of von Willebrand factor.[95,96] The elevated platelet count may affect the concentration of von Willebrand multimers and thus compromise hemostasis.

Essential thrombocythemia in pregnancy is associated with a 50% risk of obstetric complications, including recurrent abortion, premature delivery, intrauterine fetal growth restriction, and placental abruption. The proposed mechanism of pathogenesis is placental infarction.

Management Options

Diagnosis

Weight loss, sweating, low-grade fever, and pruritus may occur in up to 20% of patients. Although 40% to 50% of patients have splenomegaly and 20% have hepatomegaly, most patients have unremarkable findings on physical examination. Ultrasound or computed tomography scan may be used if splenomegaly is undetectable on physical examination.

The hallmark of essential thrombocythemia is sustained unexplained thrombocytosis. A complete blood count may show leukocytosis, erythrocytosis, and anemia (associated with hemorrhagic complications). Large platelets are typically identified on a peripheral blood smear. Some patients have spontaneous platelet aggregation. Typically, prothrombin time and aPTT are unaffected. One-fourth of patients have elevated uric acid and vitamin B_{12} levels. Levels of potassium, phosphorus, and acid phosphatase may be falsely elevated. Elevated levels of acute-phase reactant C-reactive protein, fibrinogen, and interleukin-6 suggest secondary thombocytosis.[97]

Polymerase chain reaction or Southern genomic blotting may be used to exclude chronic myelogenous leukemia. A normal red cell mass can be used to exclude polycythemia vera. In affected patients, the results of platelet aggregation studies are abnormal and show impaired aggregation to epinephrine, adenosine diphosphate, and collagen, but not to ristocetin and arachidonic acid. Bone marrow aspirate and biopsy may be useful, and most patients show increased bone marrow cellularity and megakaryocytic hyperplasia. Hyperplasia of the granulocytes and reticulocytes is also common. The level of bone marrow reticulin is usually increased, but collagen fibrosis is uncommon.[98]

General Management Guidelines

The risk of thrombotic or hemorrhagic complications as a result of essential thrombocythemia has been categorized into low risk and high risk populations, as follows[99]:

LOW RISK

- Age younger than 60 years
- No history of thrombosis
- Platelet count less than 1.5 million/μL

HIGH RISK

- Age older than 60 years
- History of thrombosis
- Platelet count greater than 1.5 million/μL

Most authorities recommend that myelosuppressive therapy for essential thrombocythemia should be reserved for high risk patients (defined earlier) because the risk of fatal thrombotic complications in low risk patients is rare and cytotoxic drugs have the potential for developing leukemia.[100] Aspirin may be used in both subsets of patients to reduce the microvascular symptoms of erythromelalgia and transient cerebral or ocular ischemia.[91,92] Acute management of these conditions usually requires 100 to 300 mg aspirin daily. In patients with high risk essential thrombocythemia, cytoreductive agents often relieve these symptoms; however, aspirin may be indicated for patients who have a normal platelet count and continue to be symptomatic. In addition, a dose of 75 to 100 mg aspirin daily may provide prophylaxis against major arterial thrombosis. A slightly increased risk of bleeding complications may be associated with this disorder.[101,102]

High risk patients with essential thrombocythemia are candidates for therapy with cytoreductive agents. Although a complete discussion of this therapeutic category is beyond the scope of this chapter, representative agents are discussed briefly. Hydroxyurea emerged as the treatment of choice because of its efficacy and limited toxicity. Neutropenia and macrocytic anemia are the major short-term toxic effects. Long-term follow-up studies show an increased rate of acute leukemia.[100] Busulfan is an alkylating agent that controls megakaryocyte proliferation. Intermittent doses can be given after initial normalization of the platelet count is achieved. Although busulfan was not found to induce leukemia, concerns continue about its possible relation to malignancy because other alkylating agents are associated with malignant transformation.[103,104] Interferon-α is a cytoreductive agent with little mutagenic potential. It antagonizes platelet-derived growth factor and is associated with a dose-dependent reduction in platelet count.

A 90% reduction in the platelet count (<600,000/µL) has been obtained after 3 months of therapy, with an average dose of 3 million IU daily. Interferon-α does not cross the placenta and is listed as a *Physician's Desk Reference* category C drug. It has been used in some pregnant patients without apparent harm.[105,106] If cytoreductive therapy is required before or during pregnancy, interferon-α is the agent of choice. Anagrelide is an imidazoquinolin that causes the suppression of megakaryocytes and thus decreases platelet counts without affecting other hematopoietic cell lines. No association with leukemia is noted. Significant complications include palpitations, tachycardia, cardiac arrhythmias, and congestive heart failure. Although it is listed as a category C drug, its use in pregnancy is not defined.[106]

Treatment in Pregnancy

Some authors recommend treatment during pregnancy with aspirin or subcutaneous heparin.[107,108] Current recommendations for treatment have yet to be defined, as illustrated by a Mayo Clinic study that showed no therapeutic benefit of treatment in 18 women (34 pregnancies) with essential thrombocythemia.[109] In this study, 45% of pregnancies ended in spontaneous abortion. The authors also could not predict the occurrence of spontaneous abortion based on the platelet count or course of disease. No other significant adverse events were noted. Because the outcome was the same in patients who received no therapy and in those treated with aspirin, treatment is not recommended in asymptomatic low risk patients with essential thrombocythemia. Thus, the use of aspirin or interferon-α in these low risk patients is of unproven benefit. Interferon-α has been used successfully in pregnant patients with essential thrombocythemia who are at increased risk for thrombosis.[110] Given the limited experience with this drug in pregnancy, its use is limited to patients in whom the potential benefits outweigh the theoretical risks. Appropriate counseling should be provided.

SUMMARY OF MANAGEMENT OPTIONS

Essential Thrombocythemia

Management Options	Quality of Evidence	Strength of Recommendation	References
Prenatal			
Interdisciplinary approach	III	B	100
Expectant approach in symptomatic patients with only moderate elevation of platelets	III	B	38
In symptomatic patients (thrombosis or bleeding), consider plasmapheresis in first instance	III	B	38
Low-dose aspirin and heparin if thrombosis occurs; evidence does not support use in all cases	III	B	39, 40
Hydroxyurea has been used, but most experience is with chronic myelogenous leukemia	III	B	39
Limited experience with α-interferon	III	B	42, 43
No experience with anagrelide; avoid	III	B	106
Serial fetal growth and umbilical artery Doppler recordings	III	B	109, 110
Labor and Delivery			
Vigilance for postpartum hemorrhage	III	B	95, 96

THROMBOTIC THROMBOCYTOPENIC PURPURA-HEMOLYTIC UREMIC SYNDROME (See Chapter 80)

Maternal and Fetal Risks

Although they were previously described as distinct entities, thrombotic thrombocytopenic purpura (TTP) and hemolytic uremic syndrome (HUS) are now considered a single syndrome.[115] Historically, the diagnosis of TTP-HUS was made only if the patient had the classic pentad of thrombocytopenia, hemolytic anemia, neurologic abnormalities, renal abnormalities, and fever. Because of the ability of plasma exchange to improve the survival rate from less than 10% to approximately 80%, the diagnostic criteria have been eased.[116,117] Thrombocytopenia coupled with microangiopathic hemolytic anemia without an alternative diagnosis is sufficient to define TTP-HUS and possibly begin plasma exchange.[117] Because the diagnosis of TTP-HUS is not precise, an alternative diagnosis may become apparent later in the clinical course. Relapse and chronic renal failure are long-term risks after recovery.

Damage to the microvascular endothelial cell is the current hypothesis to explain the pathogenesis of TTP-HUS.[118] Plasma from patients diagnosed with TTP can cause apoptosis of microvascular endothelial cells.[119] After endothelial damage occurs, release of unusually large von Willebrand factor occurs.[120] Typically, these large multimers are cleaved to a normal size by a plasma protease specific to von Willebrand factor.[121] Patients with TTP may have an inherited or acquired deficiency of this cleaving protease. Although this deficiency is clinically indistinguishable, it could differentiate TTP from HUS. Accumulation of these multimers is associated with the promotion of platelet aggregation.[122] Because these multimers may be noted in patients with disseminated malignancy without the clinical manifestations of TTP, they are not specific to this disease.[123] Less pronounced reductions in protease levels are also noted in patients with disseminated intravascular coagulation, idiopathic thrombocytopenic purpura, severe sepsis, systemic lupus erythematosus, cirrhosis, or heparin-induced thrombocytopenia. On occasion, this deficiency is noted in a patient without disease. In pregnancy, these protease levels decline with advancing gestation. Thus, an asymptomatic pregnant patient with decreased baseline levels of cleaving protease may not seek care until the peripartum period. This delay may account for the increased frequency of TTP-HUS in late pregnancy.[124]

Most patients with TTP-HUS are women, and a significant number are pregnant at the time of diagnosis. This tendency was shown by Hayward and associates, who reported that 69% (36 of 52) patients with TTP-HUS were women and 25% (9 of 36) were pregnant at the time of diagnosis.[124]

Management

Diagnosis

As discussed earlier, the diagnostic criteria for TTP-HUS are thrombocytopenia (typically <30,000 × 10^9/L) and microangiopathic hemolytic anemia (evidence of increased red cell production and destruction, red cell fragmentation, and negative findings on an antiglobulin test) in a patient with no other apparent clinical diagnosis. Other features that support the diagnosis of TTP-HUS, but are not required to make this diagnosis, include renal abnormalities (proteinuria and hematuria), changes in mental status, and abdominal symptoms (pain, nausea, diarrhea, and vomiting). In contrast, acute renal failure, seizures, fever with chills, and extensive purpura suggest an alternative diagnosis.[125] Patients with this syndrome have various clinical presentations, some of which may make the diagnosis suspect. TTP-HUS may be triggered by pregnancy, bloody diarrhea as a result of pathogenic bacteria, autoimmune disease, drugs (allergic reaction or dose-related toxicity), allogenic bone marrow transplantation, HIV, disseminated malignancy, or malignant hypertension. It may also occur without another current diagnosis.

Preeclampsia and HELLP syndrome (hemolysis, elevated liver function test results, low platelet count) may make the diagnosis of TTP-HUS difficult because both conditions may have associated thrombocytopenia, microangiopathic hemolytic anemia, and neurologic symptoms (visual changes or seizures). The criteria that are most often used to distinguish these processes are clinical recovery and lack of recovery after delivery. In preeclampsia and HELLP syndrome, thrombocytopenia may occur before or after delivery and typically reaches a nadir soon after delivery. Postpartum, the platelet count returns to normal. Hemolytic anemia is much less common in patients with preeclampsia (2%).[126] In contrast, patients with HELLP syndrome may have hemolytic anemia that is significantly slower to recover than thrombocytopenia.[127] The changes in mental status that are typical in TTP-HUS are rarely seen in patients with preeclampsia or HELLP syndrome. In these patients, neurologic symptoms usually include blurred vision, headache, visual scotomata, and rarely, eclamptic seizures. Although proteinuria is a diagnostic hallmark of preeclampsia, renal failure is rare unless the process is complicated by severe hypertension, disseminated intravascular coagulation, hypotension, or sepsis.[128]

Treatment

Plasma exchange is an empirical and effective treatment for TTP-HUS. With this procedure, the patient's blood is withdrawn through a large-bore central venous catheter. Initially, the plasma is separated from the cells, which are then retransfused with fresh plasma. The response to treatment is varied. Changes in mental status may be the first to resolve, with slower recovery of more severe neurologic symptoms, thrombocytopenia, hemolytic anemia, and renal failure. Increasing the frequency of plasma exchange may be required in patients who show a poor response. If plasma exchange is not available, plasma infusion and platelet transfusion have been advocated. This therapy is considered inferior to plasma exchange.[129] Although controversial, occasional supplemental treatment with glucocorticoids, vincristine, splenectomy, intravenous immunoglobulin, immunosuppressive agents, and antiplatelet drugs have been anecdotally recommended.[130] The number of treatments required to achieve a lasting remission is variable (days to months). To reduce the risk of relapse, plasma exchange is usually tapered. Complications of plasma exchange include those related to central venous catheter placement and the administration of large volumes of plasma.

When TTP-HUS occurs early in pregnancy, it is easily distinguished from preeclampsia or HELLP syndrome. With plasma exchange, pregnancy may be uninterrupted.[130] When the diagnosis is made later in pregnancy, the distinction from preeclampsia or HELLP syndrome becomes more difficult and the timing of delivery becomes more important. Observation may be appropriate in a clinically stable patient who is remote from term. Deterioration of clinical status should prompt treatment (plasma exchange) or delivery. If the patient's symptoms do not resolve after delivery, the clinician must consider the diagnosis of TTP-HUS, especially if symptoms persist beyond the third postpartum day. In patients with severe thrombocytopenia and microangiopathic anemia, possibly coupled with renal failure or changes in mental status, plasma exchange should be considered. TTP-HUS may recur in subsequent pregnancies; however, at least 50% have an uncomplicated pregnancy.[131]

SUMMARY OF MANAGEMENT OPTIONS

Thrombocytopenic Purpura and Hemolytic Uremic Syndrome

Management Options	Quality of Evidence	Strength of Recommendation	References
Plasmapheresis is the treatment of choice	IV	C	130
Fresh frozen plasma and platelet transfusions are secondary approaches	IV	C	130
High-dose steroids	III	B	121
Appropriate supportive therapy for renal failure and neurologic features	III	B	125, 127
Critical care setting and interdisciplinary approach	III	B	117

CONCLUSIONS

- Clotting disorders remain a leading cause of maternal morbidity and mortality.
- In addition to maternal disease, thrombosis may have a direct effect on fetal health.
- Pregnancy-associated changes in the hemostatic and antifibrinolytic systems predispose women to pathologic clotting disorders.
- In addition, various pregnancy-dependent and independent risk factors contribute to the overall risk of venous thromboembolic disease.
- Acquired and inherited thrombophilias augment this baseline risk.
- The principal clinical consequence is thrombosis. In some cases, thrombosis may cause adverse pregnancy outcomes, including fetal loss, severe preeclampsia, placental abruption, and fetal growth restriction.
- An interdisciplinary approach is advisable.
- Heparin is the anticoagulant of choice in pregnancy.
- Surveillance of fetal health is mandatory in these pregnancies.

REFERENCES

1. Goodrich S, Wood JE: Peripheral venous distensibility and velocity of venous blood flow during pregnancy or during oral contraceptive therapy. Am J Obstet Gynecol 1964;90:740.
2. Macklon NS, Greer IS, Bowman A: An ultrasound study of gestational and postural changes in the deep venous system of the leg in pregnancy. BJOG 1997;104:191.
3. Lockwood CJ, Krikun G, Schatz F: The decidua regulates hemostasis in the human endometrium. Semin Reprod Endocrinol 1999;17:45–51.
4. McColl MD, Ramsay JE, Tait RC, et al: Risk factors for pregnancy associated venous thromboembolism. Thromb Haemost 1997;78:1183–1188.
5. Hellgren M, Blomback M: Studies on blood coagulation and fibrinolysis in pregnancy, during delivery and in the puerperium. Gynecol Obstet Invest 1981;12:141–154.
6. Walker MC, Garner EJ, Keely EJ, et al: Changes in activated protein C resistance in normal pregnancy. Am J Obstet Gynecol 1997; 177:162–169.
7. Kruithof EK, Tran-Thang C, Gudinchet A, et al: Fibrinolysis in pregnancy: A study of plasminogen activator inhibitors. Blood 1987;69:460–466.
8. Gerbasi FR, Bottoms S, Farag A, et al: Increased intravascular coagulation associated with pregnancy. Obstet Gynecol 1990;75:385–389.

9. Barbour LA: ACOG committee on practice bulletins—Obstetrics. ACOG practice bulletin. Thromboembolism in pregnancy. Int J Gynecol Obstet 2001; 75:203–212.
10. Ginsberg JS, Wells PS, Brill Edwards P, et al: Antiphospholipid antibodies and venous thromboembolism. Blood 1995;86: 3685–3691.
11. Nemerson Y: Tissue factor and hemostasis. Blood 1988;71:1–8.
12. Rapaport SJ: Regulation of the tissue factor pathway. Ann N Y Acad Sci 1991;614:51–62.
13. Dennington PM, Berndt MC: The thrombin receptor. Clin Exp Pharmacol Physiol 1994;21:349–358.
14. Preissner KT, DeBoer H, Pannekoek H, DeGroot PG: Thrombin regulation by physiological inhibitors: The role of vitronectin. Semin Thromb Hemost 1996;22:223–232.
15. Ill CR, Rusolahti E: Association of thrombin-antithrombin III complex with vitronectin in serum. J Biol Chem 1985;260: 15610–15615.
16. Preissner KT, Zwicker L, Muller-Berhaus G: Formation, characterization and detection of a ternary complex between protein S, thrombin and antithrombin III in serum. Biochem J 1987; 243:105–111.
17. deBoer HC, deGroot PG, Bouma BN, Preissner KT: Ternary vitronectin-thrombin-antithrombin III complexes in human plasma: Detection and mode of association. J Biol Chem 1993; 257:3243–3248.
18. Delmore MA, Burrows RF, Ofosu FA, Andrew M: Thrombin regulation in mother and fetus during pregnancy. Semin Thromb Hemost 1992;18:81–90.
19. Esmon CT: Molecular events that control the protein C anticoagulant pathway. Thromb Haemost 1993;70:29–35.
20. Comp PC, Thrurnau GR, Welsh J, Esmon CT: Functional and immunologic protein S levels are decreased during pregnancy. Blood 1986;68:881–885.
21. Schatz F, Lockwood CJ: Progestin regulation of plasminogen activator inhibitor type-1 in primary cultures of the endometrial stromal and decidual cells. Clin Endocrinol Metab 1993; 77:621–625.
22. Estelles A, Gilabert J, Anar J, et al: Changes in plasma levels of type 1 and type 2 plasminogen activator inhibitors in normal pregnancy and in patients with severe preeclampsia. Blood 1989;74:1332–1338.
23. Booth NA: TAFI meets sticky ends. Thromb Haemost 2001;85:1–2.
24. Van Meijer M, Gebbink RK, Preissner KT, Pannekoek H: Determination of the vitronectin binding site on plasminogen activator inhibitor 1 (PAI-1). FEBS Lett 1994;352:342–346.
25. Conley CL, Hartman RC: Haemorrhagic disorder caused by circulating anticoagulant in patients with disseminated lupus erythematosus. J Clin Invest 1952;31:621–622.
26. Feinstein DI, Rapaport SI: Acquired inhibitors of blood coagulation. Prog Hemost Thromb 1972;1:75–95.
27. Harris EN, Gharavi AE, Boey ML, et al: Anticardiolipin antibodies: Detection by radioimmunoassay and association with thrombosis in systemic lupus erythematosus. Lancet 1983;2: 1211–1214.
28. Lockwood CJ, Rand JH: The immunobiology and obstetrical consequences of antiphospholipid antibodies. Obstet Gynecol Surv 1994;49:432–441.
29. Rand JH, Wu XX, Andree HA, et al: Pregnancy loss in the antiphospholipid-antibody syndrome: A possible thrombogenic mechanism. N Engl J Med 1997;337:154–160.
30. Lockwood CJ: Heritable coagulopathies in pregnancy. Obstet Gynecol Surv 1999;54:754–765.
31. Grandone E, Margaglione M, Colaizzo D, et al: Genetic susceptibility to pregnancy-related venous thromboembolism: Roles of factor V Leiden, prothrombin G20210A, and methylenetetrahydrofolate reductase mutations. Am J Obstet Gynecol 1998;179: 1324–1328.
32. Gerhardt A, Scharf RE, Beckmann MW, et al: Prothrombin and factor V mutations in women with a history of thrombosis during pregnancy and the puerperium. N Engl J Med 2000;342:374–380.
33. Kupferminc MJ, Yair D, Bornstein NM, et al: Transient focal neurological deficits during pregnancy in carriers of inherited thrombophilia. Stroke 2000;31:892–895.
34. Walker ID, Greaves M, Preston FE: Guideline investigation and management of heritable thrombophilia. Br J Haematol 2001;114:512–528.
35. Greer IA: The challenge of thrombophilia in maternal-fetal medicine. N Engl J Med 2000;342:424–425.
36. Dizon-Townson DS, Nelson LM, Jang H, et al: The incidence of the factor V Leiden mutation in an obstetric population and its relationship to deep vein thrombosis. Am J Obstet Gynecol 1997;176:883–886.
37. Bertina RM, Koeleman BPC, Koster T, et al: Mutation in blood coagulation factor V associated with resistance to activated protein C. Nature 1994;369:64–67.
38. Vandenbrocke JP, Koster T, Breit E, et al: Increased risk of venous thrombosis in oral-contraceptive users who are carriers of the factor V Leiden mutation. Lancet 1994;344:1453–1457.
39. Girling JC, deSwiet M: Thromboembolism in pregnancy: An overview. Current Opin Obstet Gynecol 1996;8:458–463.
40. Hellgren M, Svensson PJ, Dahlback B: Resistence to activated protein C as a basis for venous thromboembolism associated with pregnancy and oral contraceptives. Am J Obstet Gynecol 1995;173:210–213.
41. Dizon-Townson DS, Nelson LM, Easton K, Ward K: The factor V Leiden mutation may predispose women to severe preeclampsia. Am J Obstet Gynecol 1996;175:902–905.
42. Kupferminc MJ, Eldor A, Steinman N, et al: Increased frequency of genetic thrombophilia in women with complications of pregnancy. N Engl J Med 1999;340:9–13.
43. Thorarensen O, Ryan S, Hunter J, Younkin DP: Factor V Leiden mutation: An unrecognized cause of hemiplegic cerebral palsy, neonatal stroke, and placental thrombosis. Ann Neurol 1997;42:372–375.
44. Rey E, Kahn SR, David M, Shier I: Thrombophilic disorders and fetal loss: A meta-analysis. Lancet 2003;361:901–908.
45. Molloy AM, Daly S, Mills JL, et al: Thermolabile variant of 5,10-methylenetetrahydofolate reductase associated with low red-cell folates: Implications for folate intake recommendations. Lancet 1997;349:1591–1593.
46. van der Put NM, Eskes TK, Blom HJ: Is the common 677→T mutation in the methylenetetrahydrofolate reductase gene a risk factor for neural tube defects? A meta-analysis QJM 1997;90:111–115.
47. Wouters MG, Boers GH, Blom HJ, et al: Hyperhomocysteinemia: A risk factor in women with unexplained recurrent early pregnancy loss. Fertil Steril 1993;60:820–825.
48. Ray JG, Laskin CA: Folic acid and homocysteine metabolic defects and the risk of placental abruption, preeclampsia and spontaneous pregnancy loss: A systematic review. Placenta 1999;20:519–529.
49. Nelen WL, Blom HJ, Steegers EA, et al: Hyperhomocysteinemia and recurrent early pregnancy loss: A meta-analysis. Fertil Steril 2000;74:1196–1199.
50. Conard J, Horellou MH, Van Dreden P, et al: Thrombosis and pregnancy in congenital deficiencies in AT III, protein C or protein S: Study of 78 women. Thromb Haemost 1990;63:319–320.
51. Friedrich PW, Sanson BJ, Simioni P, et al: Frequency of pregnancy related venous thromboembolism in anticoagulant-deficient women. Ann Intern Med 1996;125:955–960.
52. Sanson BJ, Friederich PW, Simioni P, et al: The risk of abortion and stillbirth in antithrombin, protein C, and protein S deficient women. Thromb Haemost 1996;75:387–388.
53. Preston FE, Rosendaal FR, Walker ID, et al: Increased fetal loss in women with heritable thrombophilia. Lancet 1996;348: 913–916.

54. Kohler HP, Grant PJ: Plasminogen activator inhibitor type 1 and coronary heart disease. N Engl J Med 2000;342:1792–1801.
55. Glueck CJ, Phillips H, Cameron D, et al: The 4G/4G polymorphism of the hypofibrinolytic plasminogen activator inhibitor type 1 gene: An independent risk factor for serious pregnancy complications. Metabolism 2000;49:845–852.
56. Meijers JC, Tekelenburg WL, Bouma BN, et al: High levels of coagulation factor Xi as a risk factor for venous thrombosis. N Engl J Med 2000;342:696.
57. Kyrle PA, Minar E, Hirschl M, et al: High plasma levels of factor VIII and the risk of recurrent venous thromboembolism. N Engl J Med 2000;343:457.
58. Rosendaal FR: Risk factors for venous thrombotic disease. Thromb Haemost 1999;82:610.
59. van Hylckama Vlieg A, van der Linden IK, Bertina RM, Rosendaal FR: High levels of factor IX increase the risk of venous thrombosis. Blood 2000;95:3678.
60. Cavenagh JD, Colvin BT: Guidelines for the management of thrombophilia. Postgrad Med J 1996;72:87.
61. Clark P, Twaddle S, Walker ID, et al: Cost effectiveness of screening for the factor V Leiden mutation in pregnant women. Lancet 2002;359:1919.
62. Younis JS, Ohel G, Brenner B, et al: The effect of thrombophylaxis on pregnancy outcome in patients with recurrent pregnancy loss associated with factor V Leiden mutation. BJOG 2000; 107:415.
63. Brenner B, Hoffman R, Blumenfeld Z, et al: Gestational outcome in thrombophilic women with recurrent pregnancy loss treated by enoxaparin. Thromb Haemost 2000;83:693.
64. Gris JC, Mercier E, Quere I, et al.: Low molecular weight heparin versus low-dose aspirin in women with one fetal loss and a constitutional thrombophilic disorder. Blood 2004; 103: 3695–3699.
65. Brill-Edwards P, Ginsberg JS, Gent M, et al: Safety of withholding heparin in pregnant women with a history of venous thromboembolism. N Engl J Med 2000;343:1439–1444.
66. Lockwood CJ: Inherited thrombophilias in pregnant patients: Detection and treatment paradigm. Obstet Gynecol 2002;99:333.
67. Eldor A: Thrombophilia, thrombosis and pregnancy. Thromb Haemost 2001;86:104.
68. Roque H, Paidas M, Funai EF, et al: Maternal thrombophilias are not associated with early pregnancy loss. Thromb Haemost 2004; 91: 290–295.
69. Kupferminc MJ, Fait G, Many A, et al: Low molecular weight heparin for the prevention of obstetric complications in women with thrombophilia. Hypertens Pregn 2001;3:35–44.
70. Riyazi N, Leeda M, de Vries JL, et al: Low molecular weight heparin combined with aspirin in pregnant women with thrombophilia and a history of preeclampsia or fetal growth restriction: A preliminary study. Eur J Obstet Gynecol Reprod Biol 1998; 80:49.
71. Ginsberg JS, Hirsh J: Use of antithrombotic agents during pregnancy. Chest 1998;114:524S.
72. American College of Obstetricians and Gynecologists: Anticoagulation with low-molecular-weight heparin during pregnancy: ACOG Committee Opinion 211. Washington, DC, ACOG 1998.
73. Hirsh J: Heparin. N Engl J Med 1991;324:1565–1574.
74. Wessler S, Gitel SN: Heparin: New concepts relevant to clinical use. Blood 1979;53:525–544.
75. Ginsberg J, Hirsh J, Turner DC, et al: Risks to the fetus of anticoagulant therapy during preganancy. Thromb Haemost 1989;61:197–203.
76. Ginsberg J, Kowalchuck G, Hirsh J, et al: Heparin therapy during pregnancy: Risks to the fetus and mother. Arch Intern Med 1989;149:2233–2236.
77. Griffith GC, Nichols G Jr, Asher JD, Flanagan B: Heparin osteoporosis. JAMA 1965:193:85–88.
78. Barbour LA: Current concepts of anticoagulation therapy in pregnancy. Obstet Gynecol Clin North Am 1997;24:499.
79. Hirsh J, Levin MN: Low molecular weight heparin. Blood 1992;79:1–17.
80. Pettila V, Leinonen P, Markkola A, et al: Postpartum bone mineral density in women treated for thromboprophylaxis with unfractionated heparin or LMW heparin. Thromb Haemost 2002;87:182–186.
81. Hull RD, Raskob GE, Rosenbloom D, et al: Heparin for 5 days compared with 10 days in the initial treatment of proximal venous thrombosis. N Engl J Med 1990;332:1260–1264.
82. Hull A, Delmore T, Carter C, et al: Adjusted subcutaneous heparin versus warfarin sodium in long term treatment of venous thrombosis. N Engl J Med 1982;306:189–194.
83. Fejgin MD, Lourwood DL: Low molecular weight heparins and their use in obstetrics and gynecology. Obstet Gynecol Surv 1994;49:424–431.
84. Hirsh J: Oral anticoagulant drugs. N Engl J Med 1991;324: 1865–1875.
85. Elkayam UR: Anticoagulation in pregnant women with prosthetic heart valves: A double jeopardy. J Am Coll Cardiol 1996;27:1704.
86. Turpie AG, Gent M, Laupacis A, et al: Comparison of aspirin with placebo in patients treated with warfarin after heart valve replacement. N Engl J Med 1993;329:524–529.
87. Fialkow PJ, Faguet GB, Jacobson RJ, et al: Evidence that essential thrombocythemia is a clonal disorder in a multipotent cell. Blood 1981;58:916–919.
88. Mesa RA, Silverstein MN, Jacobsen SJ: Population-based incidence and survival figures in essential thrombocythemia and angogenic myeloid metaplasia: An Olmsted County Study, 1976–1995. Am J Hematol 1999;61:10–15.
89. Kobayashi S, Teramura M, Hoshino S: Circulating megakaryocyte progenitors in myeloproliferative disorders are hypersensitive to interleukin-3. Br J Haematol 1993;83:539–544.
90. Murphy S: Therapeutic dilemmas: Balancing the risk of bleeding, thrombosis, and leukemic transformation in myeloproliferative disorders. Thromb Haemost 1997;78:622–626.
91. Koudstaal PJ, Koudstaal A: Neurologic and visual symptoms in essential thrombocythemia: Efficacy of low-dose aspirin. Semin Thromb Haemost 1997;23:365–370.
92. Van Genderen PJ, Michiels J: Erythromelalgia: A pathognomonic microvascular thrombotic complication in essential thrombocythemia and polycythemia vera. Semin Thromb Haemost 1997;23:357–364.
93. Fenaux P, Simon M, Caulier M, et al: Clinical course of essential thrombocythemia in 147 cases. Cancer 1990;66:549–556.
94. Colombi M, Radaelli F, Zocchi L, et al: Thrombotic and hemorrhagic complications in essential thrombocythemia. Cancer 1991;67:2926–2930.
95. Budde U, Scharf RE, Franke P, et al: Elevated platelet count as a cause of abnormal von Willebrand factor multimer distribution in plasma. Blood 1993;82:1749–1757.
96. Van Genderen PJ, Michiels J, van der Poel-van de Luytgaarde SC, et al: Acquired von Willebrand disease as a cause of recurrent mucocutaneous bleeding in primary thrombocythemia: Relationship with platelet count. Ann Hematol 1994;69:81–84.
97. Tefferi A, Ho TC, Ahmann GJ, et al: Plasma interleukin-6 and C-reactive protein levels in reactive versus clonal thrombocytosis. Am J Med 1994;97:374–378.
98. Thiele J, Zankovich R, Steinberg T, et al: Primary (essential) thrombocythemia versus initial (hyperplastic) stages of agnogenic myeloid metaplasia with thrombocytosis: A critical evaluation of clinical and histomorphological data. Acta Haematol 1989;81:192–202.

99. Tiziano B: What is the standard treatment in essential thrombocytopenia. Int J Hematol 2002;76 (Suppl II):311–317.
100. Barbui T, Finazzi G, Dupuy E, et al: Treatment strategies in essential thrombocythemia. Leuk Lymphoma 1996;22 (Supp 1): 149–160.
101. Pearson TC: Primary thrombocythaemia: Diagnosis and management. Br J Haematol 1991;78:145–148.
102. Finazzi G, Budde U, Michiels J: Bleeding time and platelet function in essential thrombocythemia and other myeloproliferative syndromes. Leuk Lymphoma 1996;22 (Suppl 1):71–78.
103. van de Pette J, Prochazka A, Pearson T, et al: Primary thrombocythemia treated with busulfan. Br J Haematol 1986;62: 229–237.
104. Berk P, Goldberg J, Donovan P, et al: Therapeutic recommendations in polycythemia vera study group protocols. Semin Hematol 1986;223:132–143.
105. Lengfelder E, Griesshammer M, Hehlmann R: Interferon-alpha in the treatment of essential thrombocythemia. Leuk Lymphoma 1996;22 (Suppl 1):135–142.
106. Tefferi A, Elliot M, Solberg L Jr, et al: New drugs in essential thrombocythemia and polycythemia vera. Blood Rev 1997; 11:1–7.
107. Murphy S, Iland H: Thrombocytosis. In Loscalzo J, Schafer AL (eds): Thrombosis and Hemorrhage. Baltimore, Williams & Wilkins, 1994, pp 597–612.
108. Pagliaro P, Arrigioni L, Muggiasca M, et al: Primary thrombocythemia and pregnancy: Treatment and outcome in fifteen cases. Am J Hematol 1996;53:6 10.
109. Beressi A, Tefferi A, Silverstein M, et al: Outcome analysis of 34 pregnancies in women with essential thrombocythemia. Arch Intern Med 1995;155:1217–1222.
110. Shpilberg O, Shimon I, Sofer O, et al: Transient normal platelet count and decreased requirement for interferon during pregnancy in essential thrombocythemia. Br J Haematol 1996;92: 491–493.
111. Mercer B, Drouin J, Jolly E, et al: Primary thrombocythemia in pregnancy: A report of two cases. Am J Obstetr Gynecol 1988; 159:127–128.
112. Beard J, Hillmen P, Anderson CC, et al: Primary thrombocythaemia in pregnancy. Br J Haematol 1990;77:371–374.
113. Williams JM, Schlesinger PE, Gray AG: Successful treatment of essential thrombocythaemia and recurrent abortion with alpha interferon. Br J Haematol 1994;88:647–648.
114. Delage R, Demers C, Cantin G, et al: Treatment of essential thrombocythemia during pregnancy with interferon-alpha. Obstet Gynecol 1996;87:814–817.
115. Laszik Z, Silva F: Hemolytic-uremic syndrome, thrombotic thrombocytopaenia purpura, and systemic sclerosis (systemic scloeroderma). In Jennett JC, Olson JL, Schwartz MM, Silva FG (eds): Heptinstall's Pathology of the Kidney, 5th ed. Philadelphia, Lippincott-Raven, 1998, pp 1003–1057.
116. George JN, Gilcher RD, Smith JN, et al.: Thrombotic thrombocytopenic purpura-hemolytic uremic syndrome: diagnosis and management. J Clin Apheresis 1998; 13:120–125.
117. George JN: How I treat patients with thrombotic thrombocytopenic purpura-hemolytic uremic syndrome. Blood 2000;96: 1223–1229.
118. Dang CT, Magid MS, Weksler B, et al: Enhanced endothelial cell apoptosis in splenic tissues of patients with thrombotic thrombocytopenic purpura. Blood 1999;93:1264–1270.
119. Mitra D, Jaffe EA, Weksler B, et al: Thrombotic thrombocytopenic purpura and sporadic hemolytic-uremic syndrome plasmas induce apoptosis in restricted lineages of human microvascular endothelial cells. Blood 1997;89:1224–1234.
120. Moake J, Pudy C, Troll J: Unusually large plasma factor VIII: Von Willebrand factor multimers in chronic relapsing thrombotic thrombocytopenic purpura. N Engl J Med 1982;307: 1432–1435.
121. Furlan M, Robles R, Galbusera M, et al: Von Willebrand factor-cleaving protease in thrombotic thrombocytopenic purpura and the hemolytic uremic syndrome. N Engl J Med 1998;339: 1578–1584.
122. Tsai HM, Lian ECY: Antibodies to von Willebrand factor-cleaving protease in acute thrombotic thrombocytopenic purpura. N Engl J Med 1998;339:1585–1594.
123. Oleksowicz L, Bhagwati N, DeLeon-Fernandez M: Deficient activity of von Willebrand's factor-cleaving protease in patients with disseminated malignancies. Cancer Res 1999;59: 2244–2250.
124. Hayward CPM, Sutton DMC, Carter WH Jr, et al: Treatment outcomes in patients with adult thrombotic thrombocytopenic purpura-hemolytic uremic syndrome. Arch Intern Med 1994;154:982–987.
125. George J, Vesely S: Thrombotic thrombocytopenic purpura-hemolytic uremic syndrome: Diagnosis and treatment. Cleve Clin J Med 2001;68:857–878.
126. Pritchard JA, Cunningham FG, Mason RA: Coagulation changes in eclampsia: Their frequency and pathogenesis. Am J Obstet Gynecol 1976;124:855–864.
127. Martin JN, Blake PG, Perry KG, et al: The natural history of HELLP syndrome: Patterns of disease progression and regression. Am J Obstet Gynecol 1991;164:1500–1513.
128. Sibai BM, Ramadan MK, Usta I, et al: Maternal morbidity and mortality in 442 pregnancies with hemolysis, elevated live enzymes and low platelets (HELLP syndrome). Am J Obstet Gynecol 1993;169:1000–1006.
129. Rock GA, Shumak KH, Buskard NA, et al: Comparison of plasma exchange with plasma infusion in the treatment of thrombotic thrombocytopenic purpura. N Engl J Med 1991;325:393–397.
130. Mokrzycki MH, Rickles FR, Kaplan AA, Kohn OF: Thrombotic thrombocytopenic purpura in pregnancy: Successful treatment with plasma exchange. Blood Purif 1995;13:271–282.
131. Dashe JS, Ramin S III, Cunningham FG: The long-term consequences of thrombotic microangiopathy (thrombotic thrombocytopenic purpura and hemolytic uremic syndrome) in pregnancy. Obstet Gynecol 1998;91:662–668.
132. British Society for Haematology: Investigation and management of heritable thrombophilia. Br J Haematol 2001;114:512–528.
133. Lindquist P, Dahlback B, Marsal K: Thrombotic risk during pregnancy: a population study. Obstet Gynecol 1999;94:595–599.
134. Royal College of Obstetricians and Gynecologists: Thromboprophylaxis during pregnancy, labour, and after vaginal delivery. Guideline #37, January 2004.
135. Cark SL, Porter TF, West FG: Coumarin derivatives and breast-feeding. Obstet Gynecol 2000;95:938–940.

CHAPTER 43

Thromboembolic Disease

Roy G. Farquharson / Michael Greaves

INTRODUCTION

Venous thromboembolism (VTE) is the most common cause of maternal death in the United Kingdom. From 1997 to 1999, 31 women died during pregnancy or soon after delivery.[1] This figure equates to a rate of 1.45 deaths per 100,000 pregnancies. Pulmonary embolism remains the leading direct cause of maternal mortality, and the total number is still disappointingly similar to numbers reported in previous 3-year periods, with the exception of 1994 to 1996, when the total peaked at 46 deaths. The encouraging news is that after cesarean delivery, the number of fatal VTE events decreased dramatically for the first time, from a total of 15 to 4, after the introduction of the Royal College of Obstetricians and Gynaecologists (RCOG) guidelines on thromboprophylaxis, which were published in 1995.[2] Even early pregnancy is a significant risk period for VTE; eight cases (25%) occurred at 8 weeks' gestation. Fatal VTE may occur before the first prenatal visit. Even if the risk of VTE could be predicted accurately, it would not be possible to prevent all fatalities caused by pulmonary embolism in pregnancy.

An accurate measure of the total incidence of VTE in the United Kingdom is difficult to determine because there is no national registry. The Swedish national register suggests an overall incidence of 1.3 events per 1000 deliveries[3] for all types of VTE, including deep venous thrombosis and fatal and nonfatal pulmonary embolism. This rate corresponds closely to the incidence reported in a large, unselected cohort of pregnant women in Glasgow, Scotland.[4]

MATERNAL RISKS

Pregnancy introduces a significant risk of VTE events. Many important changes in the coagulation and vascular systems occur during pregnancy, and these changes support the accepted orthodoxy that pregnancy is a state of hypercoagulation. Each element of Virchow's triad is present: venous stasis, hypercoagulability, and vascular damage. Table 43–1 summarizes additional features in pregnancy that add to the risk of VTE, based on individual case analysis reporting.[1]

Inherited thrombophilia carries an increased risk of thrombosis for both the nonpregnant (Table 43–2) and pregnant populations. In patients with a strong family history of VTE in a first-degree relative, screening for thrombophilia has been suggested as part of the first prenatal visit. Unfortunately, this approach identifies few susceptible carriers of thrombophilia.[5] Further, screening for the most common heritable thrombophilia, heterozygosity for factor V Leiden, is not considered a cost-effective method for the prevention of pregnancy-related VTE.[6] The clinical value of testing for heritable thrombophilia is questioned in most clinical situations.[7] Testing in this context represents screening for what is usually a late-onset, nonfatal clinical disorder of low penetrance. Pretest counseling is mandatory, and non-evidence-based interventions determined by the results of testing must be avoided.[8]

The maternal risks of a VTE event are considerable (discussed earlier). An untreated pulmonary embolism has an estimated mortality rate of 13%. Although recovery from a nonfatal pulmonary embolism is considered complete, subtle residual effects may be detected by pulmonary function testing. The recurrence risk is difficult to quantify, particularly with modern-day aggressive recognition and treatment, but may be as high as 26% in untreated cases. Deep venous thrombosis is associated with valvular damage. Despite recanalization, many patients have postphlebitic syndrome (swelling, pain, skin ulceration) as a long-term consequence. The risks of treatment with anticoagulants include bleeding, thrombocytopenia, and osteoporosis (discussed later).

TABLE 43–1

Risk Factors Identified from Individual Case Analysis of 31 Maternal Deaths as a Result of Venous Thromboembolism (1997–1999)

RISK FACTOR	NUMBER OF CASES	COMMENT
Age	31	The rate of death is doubled in women older than 30 years.
Obesity	13	Body mass index >30. All patients diagnosed in the third trimester were overweight. Increased dosage of low-molecular-weight heparin is recommended for the treatment of venous thromboembolism (VTE).
Immobility	5	All patients had prolonged bed rest.
Family history of VTE	4	Strong history of VTE. All deaths occurred in the antenatal period.
Cesarean delivery	4	The number of events decreased dramatically from the previous report after the 1995 Royal College of Obstetricians and Gynaecologists guideline.
History of VTE	3	Two patients were obese.
Air travel	2	Both cases occurred antenatally.

From Why Mothers Die 1997–1999: The confidential enquiries into maternal deaths in the United Kingdom. London, RCOG Press, 2001, pp 49–71.

FETAL RISKS

Most fetal risk relates to maternal decompensation as a result of the acute VTE event and therapeutic interventions. Hypoxia and cardiovascular collapse are not uncommon in pulmonary embolus. These systemic injuries may directly affect placental and fetal homeostasis. Although heparin does not cross the placenta, its use to treat VTE can precipitate adverse pregnancy outcomes by causing maternal hemorrhage. Warfarin crosses the placenta and is associated with specific teratogenic effects. Except under unusual circumstances, or when given inadvertently when early pregnancy is not suspected, warfarin is not used in pregnancy (discussed later).

Underlying causes of VTE, such as inherited and acquired thrombophilias, are being actively explored for their relationship to poor pregnancy outcomes, such as early and late fetal loss, growth restriction, and early-onset preeclampsia.[9,10] These conditions are discussed in the chapters on clotting disorders and autoimmune disease in pregnancy (Chapters 42 and 44).

TABLE 43–2

Type and Prevalence of Inherited Thrombophilia with the Relative Risk of Venous Thromboembolic Disease

TYPE	PREVALENCE	RELATIVE RISK
Homozygous factor V Leiden	0.1%	×80
Heterozygous factor V Leiden	4%	×5
Protein C deficiency	0.2%	×12
Heterozygous prothrombin gene mutation	2%	×3
Hyperhomocysteinemia	>10%	×2
Increased factor VIII level	Low	×6

THROMBOEMBOLISM IN PREGNANCY

General

The key elements of the management of VTE in pregnancy are a high index of clinical suspicion, objective confirmation by imaging, and administration of heparin for the rest of the pregnancy followed by heparin or warfarin for at least 6 weeks postpartum and 6 months in total.

Diagnosis

The typical clinical features of deep vein thrombosis in pregnancy differ somewhat from those in the nonpregnant patient in relation to lateralization and extent. In up to 90% of cases, thrombosis affects the left leg, and in most patients, the proximal veins are affected. Deep venous thrombosis restricted to the calf veins is uncommon during pregnancy, although it may complicate the postpartum period.

The differential diagnosis of a painful, swollen leg in this situation is narrow. Alternative causes, such as ruptured Baker's cyst and hematoma, are rare in this age group, and cellulitis is uncommon. Symptoms may be subtle and may be confused with common benign changes in pregnancy, such as lower extremity edema or muscle cramping. The unilateral nature of VTE is a useful distinguishing characteristic. Generalized and point tenderness are common features. Dorsiflexion of the calf causes pain (Homan's sign) if the clot is in that region. Tender, indurated veins may be palpable on careful inspection of the popliteal fossa. Asymmetry of the legs is usually seen below the level of the venous obstruction. Localized erythema suggests concomitant superficial thrombosis.

The clinical features of pulmonary embolism are no different from those in the nonpregnant patient, but may be masked by the physiologic dyspnea seen in pregnancy. In most cases, the features are those of pulmonary infarction, with pleuritic chest pain of acute or subacute onset, with or without dyspnea. Patients may have hemoptysis and low-grade fever. The differential diagnosis includes chest infection with pleurisy and pneumothorax, but in the face of the symptoms described earlier, pulmonary infarction should be considered the most likely cause until it has been excluded or an alternative diagnosis is identified. Atypical patients have increasing dyspnea only and present a diagnostic challenge. Less commonly, patients may have a submassive or massive pulmonary embolism. Patients with a submassive pulmonary embolism have increasing severe dyspnea that develops over a few days, with evidence of arterial oxygen desaturation. They may also have increased jugular venous pressure and other evidence of right heart strain. In massive pulmonary embolism, patients have acute severe dyspnea, cyanosis, and collapse, often with hypotension. They may have no chest pain or central chest pain as a result of myocardial ischemia from increased right ventricular work in the face of low arterial oxygen tension. Clinical and electrocardiographic evidence of increased right heart pressure and right ventricular strain are often evident.

Clinical risk factors in addition to pregnancy should be considered because they support the clinical suspicion of the diagnosis. Approximately two thirds of patients have a recognizable risk factor, for example, increased parity, age older than 35 years, obesity, recent immobilization, and operative delivery.[4]

Confirmation of the Diagnosis

A diagnosis of VTE means a commitment to full anticoagulant therapy for several months, with its attendant risks of iatrogenic injury and its effect on the management of delivery. VTE also affects the management of future pregnancies, contraceptive choices, and the use of hormone replacement therapy as well as the perceived level of risk of VTE in first-degree relatives. Objective confirmation is essential to establish the diagnosis.

In lower limb deep venous thrombosis, compression ultrasonography is the test of choice because it is noninvasive and sensitive to thrombi in the proximal veins. The typical criteria for diagnosis are lack of vessel compressibility, absence of blood flow, and vessel dilation or visualization of the thrombus. The principal limitation is reduced sensitivity for thrombi confined to the distal calf veins. Other sources of diagnostic error relate to diminished flow in a patent femoral or iliac vein as a result of extrinsic compression from the gravid uterus and persistent flow in the face of a nonocclusive thrombus in the iliac vein. When the diagnosis is in doubt, additional imaging is needed. Contrast venography with shielding of the uterus is most commonly used. Although it is invasive, causes some discomfort, and inevitably involves radiation exposure, the diagnostic sensitivity is high. An alternative that is under development is direct thrombus magnetic resonance imaging, although this technique is not readily accessible in many centers.

When there is clinical suspicion of a venous thrombosis restricted to the calf veins (most commonly postpartum), an alternative strategy to contrast venography is to withhold anticoagulant therapy after a first negative ultrasound examination and then to repeat the study in 3 to 5 days to exclude progression to the popliteal vein. However, this is an extrapolation from nonpregnant subjects with deep vein thrombosis. Anticoagulant therapy is introduced only if progression is seen. This approach is based on the observations that progression occurs in only approximately 30% of cases and that pulmonary embolism is uncommon in deep venous thrombosis restricted to the calf veins.

When pulmonary embolism is suspected based on the clinical features, imaging is essential to confirm the diagnosis or establish an alternative. Although it is usually performed, electrocardiography is insensitive and insufficiently specific. Arterial blood gas analysis is useful to indicate the degree of hypoxia, but does not exclude other causes. A chest x-ray should be obtained with lead apron shielding of the fetus. Although the findings are often normal at presentation with pulmonary embolism and are rarely diagnostic in isolation, they may indicate an alternative cause of the symptoms (e.g., pneumothorax, pneumonia). A chest x-ray is also required for interpretation of the results of a ventilation-perfusion scan. Concomitant ultrasonography examination of the lower extremities is of value because anticoagulation therapy is indicated for an asymptomatic thrombus in this setting. However, a negative finding on ultrasound study of the legs does not exclude pulmonary embolism because the clot already may have embolized or an alternative source of the thrombus (e.g., pelvic veins) may be present. Isotopic scanning is indicated when a pulmonary embolism is suspected. The unavoidable radiation exposure has been calculated to be acceptable in pregnancy and can be minimized by performing the perfusion scan first and proceeding to the ventilation scan only if perfusion is abnormal. The principal limitation of this technique is a lack of specificity. Although a normal scan reasonably excludes pulmonary embolism and a scan showing unmatched perfusion defects at the segmental level or greater can be considered diagnostic, many scans are interpreted as intermediate probability. Because the level of diagnostic precision is inadequate in this category, additional imaging is indicated. Until recently, pulmonary angiography was required. Spiral computed axial tomography is the preferred approach, and in some centers, it is the first-line study. Radiation scatter to the abdomen is sufficiently low for this method to be considered for use in pregnancy. Magnetic resonance imaging techniques are also being developed to confirm the presence of pulmonary embolism.

There has been increasing interest in the use of D-dimer assay alongside a clinical algorithm to assess patients with suspected deep venous thrombosis. D-dimer is a product of the fibrinolytic digestion of cross-linked fibrin. An increased concentration in plasma is a marker for thrombus formation. Although this test is sensitive, it is not specific and is insufficient to confirm the diagnosis. Further, diagnostic algorithms that use a

D-dimer assay were validated only in previously healthy, nonpregnant, nonhospitalized subjects.[11] The use of this laboratory parameter in pregnancy requires the establishment of gestation-specific laboratory ranges. Plasma products of fibrin dissolution increase in concentration from approximately 10 weeks' gestation in healthy pregnancy and increase further and abruptly immediately postpartum. This diagnostic strategy is impractical and is not recommended.

Pharmacologic and Nonpharmacologic Approaches

Interventions to prevent and treat VTE are pharmacologic antithrombotics, thrombolytics, and mechanical measures (Table 43–3). Among the pharmacologic agents, heparins and warfarin are the principal drugs. The efficacy of aspirin in preventing VTE is debated. A meta-analysis[12] and a randomized study of thromboprophylaxis in lower limb orthopedic surgery[13] showed evidence of an antithrombotic effect, but the use of aspirin for this purpose in pregnancy cannot be supported. Novel oral anticoagulants are under investigation, including an oral direct thrombin inhibitor, ximelagatran. The role of these agents has not been established, and there are no data on their use in pregnancy. In VTE, thrombolytic therapy is restricted to emergency management of massive pulmonary embolism and limb salvage in rare cases of massive lower limb deep venous thrombosis with venous gangrene. Thrombolytic agents are associated with miscarriage or fetal death and maternal bleeding. Their use is relatively contraindicated in pregnancy. Similarly, these agents would likely induce massive uterine hemorrhage soon after delivery and therefore empirically should not be used. Under these circumstances, massive pulmonary embolism has been treated with heparin anticoagulation and emergency pulmonary embolectomy. A recent review of anecdotal reports of thrombolytic therapy in pregnancy implied that the risks to the mother and fetus may be lower than previously suggested.[14]

TABLE 43–3

Pharmacologic and Nonpharmacologic Interventions

ANTITHROMBOTIC AND THROMBOLYTIC AGENTS	MECHANICAL MEASURES
Heparins Unfractionated heparin Low-molecular-weight heparin Synthetic pentasaccharide	Graduated compression stockings Mechanical calf compression
Oral anticoagulants Warfarins Direct thrombin inhibitors	Filters
Aspirin	
Thrombolytics Streptokinase Urokinase Recombinant tissue plasminogen activator	

Heparins

Unfractionated heparin (UH) is manufactured from mammalian intestinal mucosa. It consists of a heterogeneous mixture of highly sulfated polysaccharide chains. The molecular weight ranges from 5000 to 35,000 daltons. Its anticoagulant action is principally the result of binding, through a specific pentasaccharide sequence, to antithrombin III, with a resultant profound acceleration in the rate of inhibition of coagulation enzymes, particularly thrombin and factor Xa.

Although UH is an effective antithrombotic agent, laboratory monitoring of the anticoagulant effect is necessary when it is used to treat established thrombosis. Activated partial thromboplastin time (aPTT) is typically used, but there is marked variation in reagent sensitivity to heparin, and laboratory standardization of heparin dosage control has not been achieved.

Low-molecular-weight heparin (LMWH) is prepared from UH. These products, with an average molecular weight of approximately 5000 daltons, contain a high concentration of molecules with fewer than 18 saccharides. These molecules cannot bind to antithrombin III and thrombin simultaneously, a feature necessary for thrombin inhibition. However, the anti-Xa effect is preserved because there is no requirement for direct binding to factor Xa for the acceleration of inhibition by the heparin–antithrombin III complex. The anti-Xa effect, in relation to the antithrombin effect, is greater in LMWH compared with UH. In addition, the bioavailability from subcutaneous tissues is greater and the plasma half-life is longer than that of UH, permitting effective anticoagulation by once- or twice-daily subcutaneous administration without a requirement for laboratory monitoring. The attributes of LMWH have led to the replacement of UH for many clinical indications. This development is supported by clinical trials in nonpregnant subjects that show at least equivalence to UH in safety and efficacy in the prevention and treatment of VTE. Deep venous thrombosis can be treated safely in the community setting with LMWH,[15] although data on pregnant patients are limited. The efficacy, ease of administration, and possible greater safety of LMWH suggest that these agents are preferable to UH in pregnancy. However, the pharmacokinetics of LMWH may be altered in pregnancy. This consideration is important because the dosing of LMWH has been extrapolated from data on nonpregnant subjects. Some early observational studies of LMWH in pregnancy have design flaws, including nonstandardized gestation intervals, a nonhomogenous case mix, and small numbers of patients with few serial observation points.[16] A systematic review reported 40 citations of LMWH use in 728 pregnant and postpartum women. However, only 2 articles were categorized as level I with regard to the quality of evidence,[17] and 19 of the articles were less than level III. Variations in dosage regimens were marked and ranged from 2500 to 22,000 units daily, which included fixed dosages, increasing dosages as pregnancy progressed, dosages based on body weight, and dosages titrated according to anti-Xa levels. The wide variation in dosage regimens highlights the uncertainty about the pharmacokinetics of heparin in pregnancy.

However, useful data are emerging. In a longitudinal study of LMWH prophylaxis in pregnancy the group mean peak anti-Xa level occurred later, at 4 hours, compared with 2 hours in the nonpregnant state.[18] Group mean peak values showed significant differences at 12 and 36 weeks' gestation, compared with the nonpregnant state, at the 2-hour time point. The threshold for thromboprophylaxis was reached at the 4-hour peak assessment (Fig. 43–1).[18] A previous study in a smaller cohort with nonstandardized gestation intervals supports this trend.[19] Compared with the nonpregnant state, the area under the anti-Xa curve (AUC) is less in pregnancy, with the lowest median reading occurring at 36 weeks' gestation (Fig. 43–2).[18] The AUC reflects LMWH activity and therefore reduced plasma activity with advancing gestation. Renal excretion is the principal route of clearance of LMWH. In contrast, UH is cleared in part by the reticuloendothelial system. Pregnancy-related physiologic adaptations in renal function probably account for the altered pharmacokinetics of LMWH. Renal clearance for LMWH may increase, accounting for the lower AUC of anti-Xa in pregnancy. This observation is supported by higher AUC values in 12 healthy, nonpregnant volunteers who were given LMWH.[20] Conversely, in renal failure, the biologic half-life of LMWH is increased.[21] These issues highlight the unresolved question as to whether dosing regimens based on trials in nonpregnant individuals can be used in pregnancy. Hunt et al.[22] recommended dose escalation after 20 weeks' gestation to

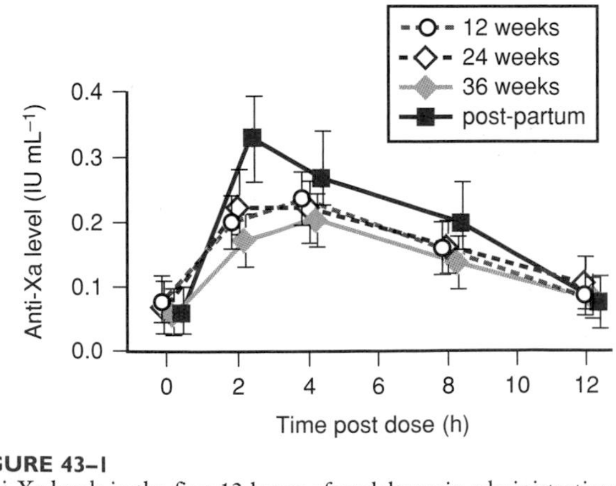

FIGURE 43–1
Anti-Xa levels in the first 12 hours after dalteparin administration, expressed as mean and 95% confidence intervals (12 weeks, n = 29; 24 weeks, n = 26; 36 weeks, n = 24; postpartum, n = 24).

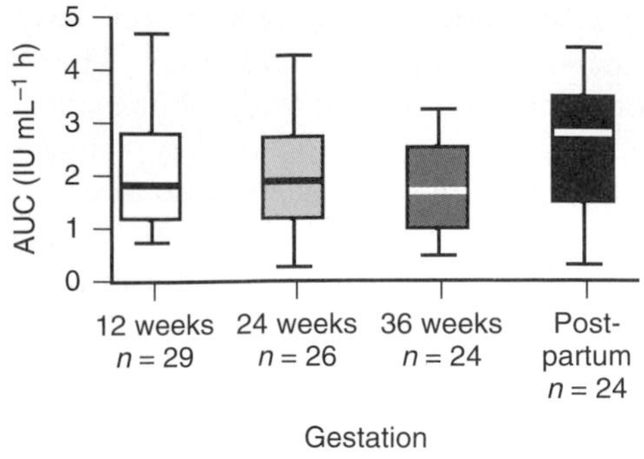

FIGURE 43–2
Area under the curve (AUC) of anti-Xa activity, subclassified by gestational age. Central bar, median; box area, interquartile range; whiskers, range.

overcome these altered heparin pharmacokinetics in pregnancy.

The principal side effect of heparin therapy is bleeding. Heparin-induced thrombocytopenia with paradoxical thrombosis is a less common, but potentially lethal side effect. It is caused by platelet consumption and activation by a heparin-induced antibody. Typically, the platelet count begins to decrease 5 to 10 days after exposure to heparin, even at a low dose, and in many cases, new or worsening thrombosis is noted. This decrease is 10-fold more likely to occur with UH than with LMWH,[23] and fortunately, it has been reported only rarely in pregnant patients treated with heparin.

Clinically significant osteoporosis is a rare consequence of pregnancy and also of long-term (>3 months) exposure to heparin. Evidence is accumulating that it is less likely to occur with LMWH than with UH. The potential threat of osteoporosis was addressed by several prospective studies that showed that the physiologic effect of pregnancy-induced bone loss is probably greater than that seen with long-term heparin use (Table 43–4). During pregnancy, bone remodeling is uncoupled, with a marked increase in early bone resorption followed by late bone formation[24] and alteration of bone architecture.[25] Osteoporotic fracture in pregnancy is an alarming condition. Fortunately, it is rare and sporadic.

A novel synthetic pentasaccharide factor Xa inhibitor (fondaparinux) is undergoing clinical investigation.[26] Early results suggest that it may be even less likely to cause thrombocytopenia and osteoporosis than currently available antithrombotics. No data on pregnancy are available.

Warfarin (Coumarins)

Warfarins, prescribed by oral tablet, are vitamin K antagonists. They inhibit the complete synthesis of the vitamin K-dependent procoagulants (prothrombin, factors VII, IX, and X) as well as the anticoagulant proteins C and S. Because a degree of inhibition of coagulation is required for efficacy, but excessive warfarin use causes bleeding, close laboratory monitoring is critical. The adoption of

TABLE 43–4

Effect of Pregnancy on Bone Mineral Density in the Lumbar Spine (L1–L4) Compared with Heparin Expressed as Percentage Loss (Number of Patients)

STUDY	CONTROL (%)	LOW-MOLECULAR-WEIGHT HEPARIN (%)	UNFRACTIONATED HEPARIN (%)
Shefras and Farquharson 1996[50]	3.13 (8)	5.1 (17)	
Backos et al. 1999[51]		3.7 (77)	3.7 (46)
Black et al. 2000[24]	3.5 (10)		
Carlin et al. 2004[52]	3.56 (20)	4.17 (55)	

the international normalized ratio (INR) system to express prothrombin time has ensured uniformity between laboratories. Prospective clinical trials established the appropriate target INR in a variety of clinical situations. However, there is a substantial risk of hemorrhage. In unselected series, the prevalence of life-threatening bleeding in subjects treated with warfarin was approximately 1 event per 100 treatment-years.[27] The risk is greatest in subjects with peripheral or cerebrovascular disease and in older patients. The risk may be lower in women of childbearing age. Bleeding is most likely to occur during the first weeks of warfarin therapy. The bleeding risk increases markedly when the INR is greater than 4.5, but approximately 25% of bleeds occur when the INR is less than 3.0. The principal cause of unexpected fluctuation in the INR is drug interaction.

Warfarin is teratogenic. Up to 30% of fetuses exposed between 6 and 10 weeks' gestation are affected. The developing skeleton is the principal target, with abnormalities ranging from subclinical stippling of the epiphyses on x-ray, to nasal deformity, to severe phocomelia. Because heparin is a safer alternative, warfarin is never used to manage VTE during the first trimester. Further, because of reports of intracranial abnormalities and developmental problems attributed to maternally derived inadvertent anticoagulation, warfarin is rarely the anticoagulant of choice to treat or prevent VTE in pregnancy. Commonly, anticoagulation with heparin that was instituted during pregnancy is switched to warfarin postpartum because of the ease of administration.

Mechanical Measures

Well-fitted graduated compression hosiery is widely used to prevent VTE. Although there are few data in pregnancy, there is evidence of efficacy perioperatively in nonpregnant patients. There is also evidence that symptoms of postphlebitic syndrome are less likely to develop if compression stockings are worn regularly for 2 years after an episode of lower limb deep vein thrombosis.[28] Whether below-the-knee stockings are as effective as full-length hosiery is the subject of debate.

Mechanical devices that stimulate calf muscle contraction have been used perioperatively to prevent deep vein thrombosis. They may be indicated in subjects who are not candidates for pharmacologic thromboprophylaxis because of a high risk of bleeding.

Filters that can be located in the inferior vena cava, either temporarily or permanently, have been used in subjects with proximal lower limb deep vein thrombosis who are considered to be at high risk for pulmonary embolism. The frequency of their use varies substantially between nations and is low in the United Kingdom. Risks include inferior vena cava thrombosis and migration of the filter. Their principal use is in patients in whom anticoagulant therapy is contraindicated (e.g., those with recent cerebral hemorrhage). Specific difficulties are associated with their use in pregnancy, in particular, the need to use radiologic screening to ensure safe placement and the possibility of compression of the inferior vena cava by the gravid uterus. Successful use has been reported,[14] however, and these devices may be helpful in some postpartum patients.

Management Options: Established VTE in Pregnancy

Treatment protocols with heparin have been based largely on those used in nonpregnant individuals and seem safe and effective. Treatment with heparin should be initiated when there is clinical suspicion of deep vein thrombosis and continued after the diagnosis is confirmed. Because of the advantages of LMWH (described earlier), most clinicians consider LMWH the anticoagulant of choice. LMWH should be administered by subcutaneous injection at the recommended dose for the particular product, based on prepregnancy body weight. Although there is evidence of more rapid clearance of LMWH in later pregnancy, once-daily administration appears to be satisfactory. Laboratory monitoring for the anticoagulant effect is not essential, although many clinicians prefer to ascertain that the plasma concentration of LMWH is within the therapeutic range on at least one occasion once treatment is established. Coagulation times, such as aPTT, are not of value for this purpose. The aPTT may remain within the nontherapeutic range, even in patients who are given full doses of LMWH. The anti-Xa assay gives an indication of the pharmacologic response, but is a poor predictor of further thrombosis and provides limited information on bleeding risk.[29] A peak (3–4 hours after injection) plasma anti-Xa concentration of 0.4 to 1.0 anti-Xa units appears to be acceptable. A level greater than 1.0 suggests that the daily dose could be reduced.

Treatment with UH is initiated by intravenous bolus injection of at least 5000 units, followed by continuous intravenous infusion at an initial rate of 1000 units hourly, with adjustment to maintain the aPTT ratio to control of 1.5 to 2.5. This value is often difficult to achieve, especially in late pregnancy. Once the patient's condition is stabilized, the dose of heparin can be delivered in 12-hourly divided doses by subcutaneous injection.

Whether UH or LMWH is administered, the platelet count should be monitored from day 5 until at least day 20. A progressive, unexplained decrease in the platelet count suggests heparin-induced thrombocytopenia, although this complication is rare in this patient group. Heparin should be discontinued and alternative strategies considered until the diagnosis can be reasonably excluded. Although lepirudin is the alternative anticoagulant of choice in the nonpregnant patient with heparin-induced thrombocytopenia, there is no information on its use in pregnancy. The heparin-like preparation danaparoid may be a better choice.

The anticoagulant effect of UH can be reversed rapidly with protamine. However, protamine is of limited efficacy in reversing the effect of LMWH. If bleeding occurs, treatment is supportive, with red cell transfusion if indicated. Plasma infusion is of no value.

The initial management of most cases of pulmonary embolism is comparable to that of deep vein thrombosis. The exception is life-threatening massive pulmonary embolism, in which the relative risks of surgical embolectomy and thrombolytic therapy must be considered urgently.

Additional management issues should be considered. Elevating the affected limb helps to relieve symptoms, but analgesia is frequently necessary because of the considerable swelling and discomfort caused by proximal venous occlusion or pulmonary infarction. Bed rest is not indicated. Compression stockings should be used as soon as resolution of swelling allows them to be worn without discomfort.

Full-dose heparin treatment should be maintained to term. Once labor has begun, the patient should be advised to withhold the next dose of heparin. A recent concern has arisen about the safety of spinal or epidural anesthesia in laboring women who are receiving anticoagulants.[30] For this reason, some clinicians opt to switch from LMWH to UH at approximately 36 weeks' gestation, taking advantage of the shorter half-life of UH. Insertion and withdrawal of a spinal catheter should be avoided within 12 hours of a therapeutic dose. Whether risk is increased after this period is unclear, but the potential risk must be balanced against the needs for analgesia and anesthesia during labor.

If no abnormal bleeding occurs during delivery, heparin is reintroduced 12 to 24 hours postpartum. Alternatively, warfarin may be introduced (along with heparin) and continued postpartum. In this case, heparin is discontinued only when an INR of 2.0 or greater is achieved with warfarin therapy. Treatment is continued with a target INR of 2.5 for 6 weeks postpartum or a total of 6 months from the initial diagnosis of VTE, whichever is longer. Although warfarin is secreted in breast milk, the breast-fed neonate of a treated mother is not adversely affected. However, warfarin is best avoided when the mother is expressing milk to feed to a severely premature neonate.

SUMMARY OF MANAGEMENT OPTIONS

Established Thromboembolism in Pregnancy

Management Options	Quality of Evidence	Strength of Recommendation	References
Initial Management	Ia/Ib	A	32–36
Give unfractionated heparin (UH) 5000–10,000 units IV loading dose then continuous IV 1000–2000 U/hr or low-molecular-weight heparin (LMWH) [for example, dalteparin 5000 units three times daily SC].			
Monitor activated partial thromboplastin time (UH) or peak heparin level (anti-Xa) [LMWH]; obtain serial platelet counts.			
Maintenance	Ia	A	36–38
Give UH (10,000 units SC twice daily) or LMWH (dalteparin 5000 three times daily).			
Monitor activated partial thromboplastin time (1.5–2.5 times control) [UH] or peak anti-Xa(>0.2 Us/mL) [LMWH]; obtain platelet counts.			

SUMMARY OF MANAGEMENT OPTIONS

Established Thromboembolism in Pregnancy *(Continued)*

Management Option	Quality of Evidence	Strength of Recommendation	References
Intrapartum	IIa	B	39,40
Temporarily discontinue therapy with onset of labor.			
Epidural block and operative delivery are not contraindicated if clotting is normal.			
Reinitiate treatment with UH or LMWH approximately 12 hours after delivery if no active bleeding occurs.			
Postpartum	IIa	B	34,39,41,42
Continue LMWH, UH, or warfarin (with monitoring) for 6 weeks or at least 6 months after an acute event.			
Measure bone density of the maternal spine and hip if long-term therapy is anticipated.			
Graduated elastic compression stockings should be worn for 2 years.	III	B	43
Breast-feeding is not contraindicated.			

Management Options: Thromboprophylaxis in Pregnancy

Thromboprophylaxis should not be offered to all pregnant women. Routine population screening for hereditary thrombophilias is not justified. In assessing thrombotic risk, acquired factors are at least as important as genetic predisposition. A history of VTE is an important consideration for thromboprophylaxis in pregnancy. In addition, patient age, parity, and weight are associated with venous thrombotic risk during pregnancy and in the puerperium. Immobilization and serious medical disorders are other important risk factors. In the postpartum period, the risk of venous thrombosis is increased in women who have had cesarean delivery, especially as an emergency procedure.

The risk of VTE in women with a history of thrombosis may be lower than previously considered. In a persuasive prospective study of 125 women who had a history of venous thrombosis and in whom antenatal thromboprophylaxis was withheld, the overall rate of recurrence was only 2.4%. No recurrence was reported in the subgroup of women who had a temporary risk factor at the time of the first event.[31] This study also suggested that the recurrence rate may be higher in heritable thrombophilia, but was too small to allow firm conclusions to be drawn. The risk of pregnancy-associated first occurrence of VTE in women with heritable thrombophilia has been overstated. The best available data show a substantial risk of approximately 1 in 3 in women with antithrombin deficiency. The risk is probably approximately 1 in 100 in asymptomatic patients with protein C deficiency and lower still in asymptomatic women with factor V Leiden.[4] Based on these observations, an attempt to stratify risk has been made, with recommendations for thromboprophylaxis of graded intensity, depending on these factors. Table 43–5 is modified from the recommendations of the British Committee for Standards in Haematology.[8] In deciding on the use of pharmacologic thromboprophylaxis based on the diagnosis of asymptomatic heritable thrombophilia (slightly increased risk), it must be borne in mind that this therapy is invasive, that approximately 5% of the healthy female population will be so classified, and that most do not have pregnancy-related VTE. The recommendations are pragmatic because there are no randomized controlled trials.

The use of compression stockings antenatally and postpartum is a reasonable precaution at all levels of increased risk. In general, for the reasons discussed earlier, LMWH is preferable to UH for pharmacologic thromboprophylaxis. The use of preloaded syringes is convenient and increases safety. The platelet count must be monitored. If anti-Xa levels are used to guide dosing of LMWH, the factors discussed earlier should be considered in the interpretation of the results. Warfarin can be used for postpartum prophylaxis, with a target INR of 2.5. Recently updated thromboprophylaxis recommendations have been published by the Royal College of Obstetricians and Gynaecologists.[53]

TABLE 43-5

Recommendations for Thromboprophylaxis in Pregnancy

RISK CATEGORY	MANAGEMENT
Slight	
Women who have no personal history of venous thrombosis, but a positive family history and who are heterozygous for protein S deficiency, heterozygous for factor V Leiden, or heterozygous for prothrombin G20210A Women with a history of venous thrombosis in association with a temporary risk factor that is no longer present	In general, pharmacologic thromboprophylaxis is not required antenatally, but anticoagulant prophylaxis may be considered after delivery in those with previous venous thromboembolism and others who have an additional risk factor.
Intermediate	
Women who have a personal history of apparently spontaneous venous thromboembolism who are no longer receiving anticoagulant prophylaxis Women who have no personal history of venous thrombosis, but a positive family history of venous thrombosis and who are heterozygous for protein C deficiency, are homozygous for factor V Leiden or the prothrombin G20210A mutation, or have combinations of defects	Postpartum thromboprophylaxis with heparin or warfarin should be given. Antenatal thromboprophylaxis should be considered, such as fixed prophylactic doses of unfractionated or low-molecular-weight heparin (e.g., 4000–5000 units dalteparin once daily SC or unfractionated heparin 7500 IU every 8–12 hours SC).
High	
Women who are receiving long-term anticoagulant therapy for venous thromboembolism Women who have type I antithrombin deficiency or a type II reactive site antithrombin defect (regardless of whether they have had a thrombotic episode)	Adjusted doses of low-molecular-weight or unfractionated heparin, higher than those usually used to prevent venous thrombosis, should be administered (e.g., low-molecular-weight heparin introduced at approximately dalteparin 75 units/kg early pregnancy weight every 12 hours SC; the dose may be adjusted to give a peak anti-Xa level of 0.35 to 0.5 units 3–4 hours after injection). The use of fixed prophylactic doses of unfractionated or low-molecular-weight heparin (e.g., heparin 7500 IU every 12 hours SC or dalteparin 4000–5000 units once daily SC, respectively) is an alternative strategy.

From Walker ID, Greaves M, Preston PE: Investigation and management of inherited thrombophilia. Br J Haematol 2001;114:512–528.

SUMMARY OF MANAGEMENT OPTIONS

Thromboprophylaxis in Pregnancy

Management Options	Quality of Evidence	Strength of Recommendation	References
Low Risk Patients	Ia	A	38,44,45,53
Initiate low-molecular-weight heparin (LMWH) (dalteparin 5000 units daily SC) or unfractionated heparin (UH) 7500 units twice daily SC after delivery.			
Continue LMWH or UH for 6 weeks postpartum or convert to oral warfarin after 1 week of heparin treatment.			
Breastfeeding is not contraindicated.			
High Risk Patients	III	B	38,46–48,53
Initiate LMWH (dalteparin enoxaprim, tinzaparin—see reference for dosage), increasing to twice daily after 20 weeks' gestation, or UH 10,000 units twice daily SC on diagnosis.			
Give UH or LMWH for 1 week postpartum, then continue heparin, LMWH, or warfarin for 5 weeks.			
Breastfeeding is not contraindicated.			

SUMMARY OF MANAGEMENT OPTIONS
Thromboprophylaxis in Pregnancy *(Continued)*

Management Options	Quality of Evidence	Strength of Recommendation	References
Cesarean Section			
Low Risk Patients			
Early mobilization and hydration	Ia	A	49
Medium Risk Patients			
SC heparin or stockings	Ia	A	38,44,46–49
High Risk Patients			
Heparin and stockings	Ia	A	38,44,46–49

CONCLUSIONS

- Thromboembolism is an important cause of maternal death, and effective preventative measures are available.
- Pregnancy increases the risk of thromboembolism. Additional risk factors include maternal age, obesity, a family history of thromboembolism, a previous thromboembolic event, immobility, cesarean delivery, and air travel.
- Women with a personal or family history of recurrent thromboembolism may be tested for an inherited thrombophilia.
- Key management strategies for a woman with a thromboembolic event are as follows:
  - Induction of intravenous or subcutaneous heparin, followed by maintenance therapy, with brief suspension of therapy for labor and delivery
  - Continuation of treatment for at least 6 weeks after delivery
- Thromboprophylaxis is the key management strategy for a woman with a previous thromboembolic event. The extent and type of thromboprophylaxis are determined by the nature of the risk.
- Anticoagulation is not a contraindication to breastfeeding.

REFERENCES

1. Why Mothers Die 1997–1999: The confidential enquiries into maternal deaths in the United Kingdom. London, RCOG Press, 2001, pp 49–71.
2. Royal College of Obstetricians and Gynaecologists: Report of a working party on prophylaxis against thromboembolism in gynaecology and obstetrics. London, RCOG Press, 1995.
3. Lindqvist P, Dahlback B, Marsal K: Thrombotic risk during pregnancy: A population study. Obstet Gynecol 1999;94: 595–599.
4. McColl MD, Ramsay JE, Tait RC, et al: Risk factors for pregnancy associated venous thromboembolism. Thromb Haemost 1997;78:1183–1188.
5. Cosmi B, Legnani C, Bernardi F, et al: Value of family history in identifying women at risk of venous thromboembolism during oral contraception: Observational study. BMJ 2001;322: 1024–1025.
6. Nelson-Piercy C: Inherited thrombophilia and adverse pregnancy outcome: Has the time come for screening? BJOG 1999;106:513–515.
7. Greaves M, Baglin T: Laboratory testing for heritable thrombophilia: Impact on clinical management of thrombotic disease Br J Haematol 2000;109:699–703.
8. Walker ID, Greaves M, Preston PE: Investigation and management of inherited thrombophilia. Br J Haematol 2001;114: 512–528.
9. Preston FE, Rosendaal FR, Walker ID, et al: Increased fetal loss in women with heritable thrombophilia. Lancet 1996;348: 913–916.
10. Branch WD, Khamashta MA: Antiphospholipid syndrome: Obstetric diagnosis, management and controversies. Obstet Gynecol 2003;101:1333–1344.
11. Wells PS, Anderson DR, Ginsberg J: Assessment of deep vein thrombosis or pulmonary embolism by the combined use of clinical model and noninvasive diagnostic tests. Semin Thromb Hemost 2000;26:643–656.
12. Collins R, Baigent C, Sandercock P, Peto RO: Antiplatelet therapy for thromboprophylaxis: The need for careful consideration of the evidence from randomised trials. BMJ 1994;309: 1215–1217.
13. Pulmonary Embolism Prevention (PEP) Trial Collaborative Group: Prevention of pulmonary embolism and deep vein thrombosis with low dose aspirin. Lancet 2000;355: 1295–1302.

14. Ahearn GS, Hadjiliadis D, Govert JA, Tapson VF: Massive pulmonary embolism during pregnancy successfully treated with recombinant tissue plasminogen activator: case report and review of treatment options. Arch Intern Med 2002;162:1221–1227.
15. Levine M, Gent M, Hirsch J, et al: A comparison of low molecular weight heparin administered primarily at home with unfractionated heparin administered in hospital for proximal deep vein thrombosis. N Engl J Med 1996;334:677–688.
16. Sanson BJ, Lensing AW, Prins MH, et al: Safety of low molecular weight heparins in pregnancy: A systematic review. Thromb Haemost 1999;81:668–672.
17. Ensom MH, Stephenson MD: Low molecular weight heparins in pregnancy. Pharmacotherapy 1999;19:1013–1025.
18. Sephton V, Farquharson RG, Topping J, et al: A longitudinal study of maternal dose response to low molecular weight heparin in pregnancy. Obstet Gynecol 2003;101:1307–1311.
19. Blomback M, Bremme K, Hellgren M, Lindberg H: A pharmacokinetic study of dalteparin during late pregnancy. Blood Coagul Fibrinolysis 1998;9:343–350.
20. Eriksson BI, Soderberg K, Widlund L, et al: A comparative study of three low molecular weight heparins and unfractionated heparin in healthy volunteers. Thromb Haemost 1995;73: 398–401.
21. Hirsh J, Levine M: Low molecular weight heparin. J Am Soc Hematol 1992;79:1–17.
22. Hunt BJ, Doughty HA, Majmdar G, et al: Thromboprophylaxis with low molecular weight heparin in high-risk pregnancies. Thromb Haemost 1997;77:39–43.
23. Warkentin TE, Levine MN, Hirsh J, et al: Heparin-induced thrombocytopenia in patients treated with low molecular heparin or unfractionated heparin. N Engl J Med 1995;332: 1330–1335.
24. Black AJ, Topping J, Durham B, et al: A detailed assessment of alterations in bone turnover, calcium homeostasis, and bone density in normal pregnancy. J Bone Miner Res 2000;15:557–563.
25. Shahtaheri SM, Aaron JE, Johnson DR, Purdie DW: Changes in trabecular bone architecture in women during pregnancy. BJOG 1999;106:432–438.
26. Bounameaux H, Perneger T: Fondaparinux: A new synthetic pentasaccharide for thrombosis prevention. Lancet 2002;359: 1710–1711.
27. Palareti G, Leali N, Coccheri S, et al: Bleeding complications of oral anticoagulant treatment: An inception cohort, prospective collaborative study (ISCOAT). Italian Study on Complications of Oral Anticoagulant Therapy. Lancet 1996;348:423–428.
28. Brandjes DP, Buller HR, Heijboer H, et al: Randomised trial of effect of compression stockings in patients with symptomatic proximal-vein thrombosis. Lancet 1997;349:759–762.
29. Greaves M: Limitations of the laboratory monitoring of heparin therapy: Scientific and Standardization Committee Communications. On behalf of the Control of Anticoagulation Subcommittee of the Scientific and Standardization Committee of the International Society of Thrombosis and Haemostasis. Thromb Haemost 2002;87:163–164.
30. Wysowski DK, Talarico L, Bacsanyi J, Botstein P: Spinal and epidural hematoma and low-molecular-weight heparin. N Engl J Med 1998;338:1774–1775.
31. Brill-Edwards P, Ginsberg JS: Safety of withholding antepartum heparin in women with a previous episode of venous thromboembolism. N Engl J Med 2000;343:1439–1444.
32. Barritt DV, Jordan SC: Anticoagulant drugs in the treatment of pulmonary embolism: A controlled trial. Lancet 1960;1: 1309–1312.
33. Brandjes DP, Heijboer H, Buller HR, et al: Acenocoumarol and heparin compared with acenocoumarol alone in the initial treatment of proximal vein thrombosis. N Engl J Med 1992;327: 1485–1489.
34. Hyers TM, Hull RD, Weg JG: Antithrombotic therapy for venous thromboembolic disease. Chest 1995;108:335.
35. Levine M, Gent M, Hirsch J, et al: A comparison of low molecular weight heparin administered primarily at home with unfractionated heparin administered in hospital for proximal deep vein thrombosis. N Engl J Med 1996;334:677–688.
36. Gould MK, Dembitzer AD, Doyle RL, et al: Low molecular weight heparins compared with unfractionated heparin for treatment of acute DVT. Ann Intern Med 1999;130:800–809.
37. Monreal M: Long-term treatment of venous thromboembolism with low molecular weight heparin. Curr Opin Pulm Med 2000;6:326–329.
38. van den Belt AGM, Prins MH, Lensing AWA, et al: Fixed dose subcutaneous low molecular heparins versus adjusted dose unfractionated heparin for venous thromboembolism. Cochrane Database of Systematic Reviews, Issue 4, 2000.
39. Toglia MR, Weg JG: Venous thromboembolism during pregnancy. N Engl J Med 1996;335:108–114.
40. Checketts MR, Wildsmith JA: Central nerve block and thromboprophylaxis: Is there a problem? Br J Anaesth 1999;82: 164–167.
41. Ginsburg JS, Greer IA, Hirsh J: Use of antithrombotic agents during pregnancy. Chest 2001;119:1315.
42. Brandjes DP, Buller HR, Heijboer H, et al: Randomised trial of effect of compression stockings in patients with proximal venous thrombosis. Lancet 1997;349:759–762.
43. Orme ML-E, Lewis PJ, de Swiet M, et al: May mothers given warfarin breast-feed their infants? BMJ 1977;1:1564–1565.
44. Antiplatelet Trialists Collaboration: Collaborative overview of randomised trials of antiplatelet therapy. BMJ 1994;308: 235–246.
45. Derry S, Loke YK: Risk of gastrointestinal haemorrhage with long term use of aspirin: Meta-analysis. BMJ 2000;321: 1183–1188.
46. Nelson-Piercy C, Letsky EA, de Swiet M: Low molecular weight heparin for obstetric thromboprpohylaxis: Experience of sixty nine pregnancies in sixty one women at risk. Am J Obstet Gynecol 1997;176:1062–1068.
47. Hunt BJ, Doughty H, Majumdar G, et al: Thromboprophylaxis with low molecular weight heparin in high risk pregnancies. Thromb Haemost 1997;1:39–43.
48. Chan WS, Ray JG: Low molecular weight heparin during pregnancy: Safety and practicality. Obstet Gynecol Surv 1999;54: 649–654.
49. Amigiri SV, Lees TA: Elastic compression stockings for prevention of deep venous thrombosis. Cochrane Database of Systematic Reviews, Issue 4, 2000.
50. Shefras J, Farquharson RG: Bone density studies in pregnant women receiving heparin. Eur J Obstet Gynaecol 1996;65: 171–174.
51. Backos M, Rai R, Thomas E, et al: Bone density changes in pregnant women treated with heparin: A prospective longitudinal study. Hum Reprod 1999;14:2876–2880.
52. Carlin A, Farquharson RG, Quenby S, et al: Prospective observational study of bone mineral density during pregnancy: Low molecular weight heparin versus control. Hum Reprod 2004;19: 1211–1214.
53. Royal College of Obstetricians and Gynaecologists: Thromboprophylaxis during pregnancy, labour and after normal vaginal delivery. Guideline No.37. London, RCOG Press, 2004. Available at www.rcog.org.uk.

CHAPTER 44

Autoimmune Diseases

T. Flint Porter / D. Ware Branch

INTRODUCTION

The immune system's remarkable ability to protect the body from invasion by foreign pathogens stems from its capacity to distinguish biologic "self" from "nonself." An aberration in this normally well-regulated process leads to a state of so-called *autoimmunity*, in which immune effector cells are directed against "self" tissues. Persistent immunologic activation results in an *autoimmune disease*, characterized by a typical pattern of clinical signs and symptoms of disease and confirmed by the serologic presence of immune effector cells, usually autoantibodies. For many autoimmune conditions, serologically detected autoantibodies play an active role in tissue damage. In others, their presence may serve only to confirm the existence of an autoimmune process.

The pathophysiologic mechanisms that lead to autoimmune diseases have been studied extensively. The earliest theory held that autoimmunity resulted from a failure in the normal deletion of lymphocytes that recognized self-antigens. More recently, investigators have suggested that autoimmunity results from a failure of the normal regulation of the immune system (which contains many immune cells that recognize self-antigens but are normally suppressed). Regardless of what fundamental immunologic disturbance allows autoimmunity, it appears that a combination of environmental, genetic, and host factors must be present for the full expression of an autoimmune disease.

Autoimmune diseases have a predilection for reproductive-age women and are frequently encountered during pregnancy. Indeed, more than 70% of patients with autoimmune disease are women of reproductive age.[1] Studies in both animal models and humans support the role that sex hormones play in the development of autoimmunity; estrogens accelerate disease while androgens are protective.[2–6] It should come as no surprise that pregnancy-associated fluctuations in sex hormones substantially influence disease severity. Interestingly, the effect of pregnancy depends on whether the autoimmune disease is innate (cellular) or adaptive (humoral) in nature. Diseases with strong cellular pathophysiology, such as rheumatoid arthritis (RA) and multiple sclerosis, are associated with remission during pregnancy, whereas diseases characterized by autoantibody production, such as systemic lupus erythematosus (SLE) and Graves' disease, tend toward increased severity in pregnancy. Still others are unique to pregnancy or have unique features associated with pregnancy. Thus, the obstetrician should be familiar with the more common autoimmune diseases, how they influence and are influenced by pregnancy, and what special medical risks may be in store for mother or the conceptus.

SYSTEMIC LUPUS ERYTHEMATOSUS

General

Systemic lupus erythematosus is an idiopathic chronic inflammatory disease that affects skin, joints, kidneys, lungs, serous membranes, nervous system, liver, and other organs of the body. Like other autoimmune diseases its course is characterized by periods of remission and relapse. The most common complaint among patients with SLE is extreme fatigue (Table 44–1). Fever, weight loss, myalgia, and arthralgia are also particularly common symptoms.

The prevalence of SLE is 5 to 100 per 100,000 individuals, depending on the population studied. The disease is at least 5, and probably closer to 10 times, more common among adult women than adult men.[1] The lifetime risk of developing SLE for a white woman is 1 in

TABLE 44–1

Approximate Frequency of Clinical Symptoms in SLE

SYMPTOMS	PATIENTS (%)
Fatigue	80–100
Fever	80–100
Arthralgia, arthritis	95
Myalgia	70
Weight loss	>60
Skin	
Butterfly rash	50
Photosensitivity	60
Mucous membrane lesions	35
Renal involvement	50
Pulmonary	
Pleurisy	50
Effusion	25
Pneumonitis	5–10
Cardiac (pericarditis)	10–50
Lymphadenopathy	50
CNS	
Seizures	15–20
Psychosis	<25

700,[7] with an overall incidence of 1 in 2000 in the United States. The incidence varies among populations and is approximately two to four times higher in African Americans and Hispanic Americans.[7] A genetic predisposition to SLE is likely, given that approximately 10% of patients with SLE also have an affected relative[8]; concordance between twins is reportedly greater than 50%.[9] Several alterations in the human leukocyte antigen (HLA) system have been linked to the development of SLE, and homozygous carriers of mutations responsible for complement deficiency disorders also appear to be predisposed to development of the disease.

Diagnosis

Serologic Markers

The diagnosis of SLE, suspected by the clinical presentation, is confirmed by demonstrating the presence of circulating autoantibodies. Patients are initially screened for nonspecific antibodies directed against nuclear antigens. Cumbersome biologic assays of antibodies directed against nucleoprotein (nucleohistone) commonly referred to as the *LE phenomenon*, have been replaced by immunofluorescent assays for nonspecific antinuclear antibodies (ANA). Findings are interpreted according to antibody titer and to some degree on the pattern of antibody binding. The *homogeneous* pattern is found most commonly in patients with SLE (65%), though its specificity is low. A peripheral pattern is the most specific for SLE, even if it is not very sensitive. The speckled and nucleolar patterns are more specific for other autoimmune diseases.

Immunofluorescent assays that identify specific nuclear antigen-antibody reactions are better for confirming the diagnosis of SLE, monitoring disease activity, and guiding immunotherapy. Particularly useful are anti-double-stranded DNA (anti-dsDNA) antibodies, present in 80% to 90% of patients with newly diagnosed SLE, elevations of which precede symptomatic flare in 80% of SLE patients followed prospectively.[10,11] In one randomized, placebo-controlled trial, glucocorticoid treatment in patients with elevated anti-dsDNA titers resulted in fewer relapses of disease. In pregnancy, anti-dsDNA antibodies correlate with flare and preterm delivery.[11,12]

Antibodies to single-stranded DNA (anti-ssDNA) are also found in a large number of untreated SLE patients, but are less specific for SLE than anti-dsDNA. Patients with SLE may also have antibodies to RNA-protein conjugates, often referred to as *soluble or extractable antigens*, since they can be separated from tissue extracts. These antigens include the Sm antigen, nuclear ribonucleoprotein (nRNP), the Ro/SS-A antigen, and the La/SS-B antigen. The Sm and nRNP antigens are nuclear in origin, and the presence of anti-Sm, found in about 30% to 40% of patients with SLE, is highly specific for the disease. Anti-Ro/SS-A and anti-La/SS-B, found in the sera of both SLE patients and patients with Sjögren's syndrome, are of particular importance to obstetricians, because they are associated with neonatal lupus.

Diagnostic Criteria

In 1971, the American Rheumatism Association devised criteria for SLE as a framework for comparing studies of patients with SLE. These were revised in 1982[13] and again in 1997[14] (Table 44–2). To be classified as having SLE, an individual must have at least 4 of 11 clinical and laboratory criteria at one time or serially. These criteria are very sensitive and specific for SLE, but were never intended to form the *sine qua non* for the diagnosis of SLE. Many patients have less than four clinical or laboratory features of SLE and do not meet strict diagnostic criteria. Exclusion of patients with an autoimmune diathesis from the diagnosis of SLE by the dogmatic use of strict diagnostic criteria can result in patients being confused and frustrated. Although these patients should not be considered to have SLE, they are often referred to as having lupus-like disease. Such individuals may benefit from therapies for SLE and often require special care during pregnancy. A subset of these patients will ultimately develop the clinical syndrome.

Lupus Nephritis

Clinically obvious renal disease is a relatively common complication of SLE, eventually occurring in about 50% of patients with SLE. Lupus nephropathy probably results from immune complex deposition leading to complement activation and inflammatory tissue damage in

TABLE 44–2

Revised American College of Rheumatology Classification Criteria for SLE

CRITERION	DEFINITION
1. Malar rash	Fixed erythema, flat or raised, over the malar eminences, tending to spare the nasolabial folds
2. Discoid rash	Erythematous raised patches with adherent keratotic scaling and follicular plugging; atrophic scarring possible in older lesions
3. Photosensitivity	Skin rash as a result of unusual reaction to sunlight, by patient history or physician observation
4. Oral ulcers	Oral or nasopharyngeal ulceration, usually painless
5. Arthritis	Nonerosive arthritis involving two or more peripheral joints, characterized by tenderness, swelling, or effusion
6. Serositis	a) Pleuritis—convincing history of pleuritic pain or rubbing heard by a physician, or evidence of pleural effusion b) Pericarditis—documented by ECG or rub or evidence of effusion
7. Renal	a) Persistent proteinuria >0.5 g/day or >3+ if quantitation not performed b) Cellular casts—red cell, hemoglobin, granular, tubular, or mixed
8. Neurologic	a) Seizures—in the absence of offending drugs or known metabolic derangements (e.g., uremia, ketoacidosis, or electrolyte imbalance) b) Psychosis—in the absence of drugs or metabolic derangements
9. Hematologic	a) Hemolytic anemia—with reticulocytosis b) Leukopenia—<4,000/μL on 2 or more occasions c) Lymphopenia—<1,500/μL on 2 or more occasions d) Thrombocytopenia—<100,000/μL in absence of drugs
10. Immunologic	a) Anti-DNA—antibody to native DNA in abnormal titer b) Anti-Sm—presence of antibody to Sm nuclear antigen c) Positive finding of antiphospholipid antibodies based on (1) an abnormal serum level of IgG or IgM anticardiolipin antibodies, (2) a positive test result for lupus anticoagulant using a standard method, or (3) a false-positive serologic test for syphilis for 6 months
11. Antinuclear antibody	An abnormal ANA titer by immunofluorescence or an equivalent assay at any time and in the absence of drugs known to be associated with "drug-induced lupus" syndrome

From Tan EM, Cohen AS, Fries JF, et al: The 1982 revised criteria for the classification of systemic lupus erythematosus. Arthritis Rheum 1982;25:1271–1277 and Hochberg MC: Updating the American College of Rheumatology revised criteria for the classification of systemic lupus erythematosus. Arthritis Rheum 1997;40:1725.

the kidney. The most common presentation is proteinuria, which occurs at some time in up to 75% of patients. About 40% of patients will have hematuria or pyuria, and about a third will have urinary casts.

Renal biopsy is necessary to confirm the diagnosis of lupus nephropathy and is important for determining the prognosis and providing appropriate treatment. Renal biopsy findings are used to group lupus nephropathy into four basic histologic and clinical categories. Of these, *diffuse proliferative glomerulonephritis* (DPGN) is the most common (40%) and most severe, with 10-year survival around 60%. Patients with DPGN typically present with hypertension, moderate to heavy proteinuria and nephrotic syndrome, hematuria, pyuria, casts, hypocomplementemia, and circulating immune complexes. *Focal proliferative glomerulonephritis* is usually associated with mild hypertension and proteinuria; serious renal insufficiency is uncommon. *Membranous glomerulonephritis* typically presents with moderate to heavy proteinuria but lacks the active urinary sediment and does not cause renal insufficiency. *Mesangial glomerulonephritis* appears to be the least clinically severe lesion and carries the best long-term prognosis.

The first line of therapy in patients with active lupus nephropathy has traditionally been glucocorticoids, usually given as oral prednisone, 40 to 50 mg/day for several weeks to several months. Thereafter, the dose is tapered while carefully watching the patient for evidence of signs and symptoms of worsening disease. Severe proliferative lesions, such as seen in moderate to severe DPGN, have been shown to respond best to cytotoxic agents. Cyclophosphamide, in a divided monthly dose of 0.5 to 1.0 g/m^2, is now generally used.

Lupus Cerebritis

Up to 20% of patients with SLE develop CNS manifestations of their disease, also referred to as lupus cerebritis. Patients most often present with new onset seizures, although peripheral neuropathy, headaches, chorea, stroke, mood disorders, transverse myelitis, and psychosis are also reported. The severity of lupus cerebritis may also be influenced by other problems commonly encountered in patients with SLE, including metabolic abnormalities, infection, and chronic steroid use. An evaluation for lupus cerebritis should include an assessment for the presence of infection, including lumber puncture if necessary, radiologic imaging, and electroencephalogram. Patients with lupus cerebritis who present with chorea, transverse myelitis, or stroke should be tested for antiphospholipid antibodies. Empiric therapy for lupus cerebritis typically includes glucocorticoids as a first-line therapy, with cyclophosphamide and intravenous immune globulin (IVIG) reserved for refractory cases.

Risks of SLE and Pregnancy

The Risk of SLE Exacerbation (Flare)

Whether pregnancy is associated with a higher rate of SLE exacerbation is a matter of considerable debate.

Early studies on the subject were hampered by poor study design, not to mention the difficulty differentiating between normal manifestations of pregnancy and the signs and symptoms typically associated with SLE. At the same time, common complications of pregnancy such as preeclampsia may mimic exacerbations of SLE.

Between the early 1950s and the early 1970s, the findings of several small retrospective series suggested that women with SLE were placing themselves at substantial risk for severe morbidity and even mortality during pregnancy.[15] Many also reported relatively high rates of pregnancy wastage among women with SLE.[16] These concerns led many practitioners to the opinion that SLE patients should not become pregnant. However, these early studies were plagued by several problems, and their conclusions should not be the basis of clinical decision making today. All were retrospective, relatively small, and, because of the lack of generally agreed-upon criteria for the classification of SLE, were predisposed to include a disproportionate number of more severe cases. In addition, without standardized diagnostic criteria for SLE exacerbation, early investigators may have incorrectly diagnosed preeclampsia and other obstetric complications as SLE exacerbations.

Studies done since 1980 have done much to clarify the relationship of pregnancy to the rate and nature of SLE exacerbations. Overall, the rate of flare during pregnancy or the postpartum period varies between 15% to 60% of women.[8,17–29] Several prospective studies deserve special consideration. Lockshin and colleagues[17] matched nonpregnant SLE patients with 28 SLE patients undertaking 33 pregnancies and used a previously published scoring system to define SLE exacerbations. There was no difference in the flare score between the cases and controls, and a similar number in both groups required a change in their medication. The same investigators have now followed 80 consecutive pregnancies in women with SLE and conclude that exacerbations occur in less than 25% of cases and that most are mild in nature. If only signs or symptoms specific for SLE are included, exacerbations occurred in only 13% of cases.

Mintz and colleagues[19] prospectively studied 92 pregnancies in women with SLE and used a similar group of nonpregnant SLE patients on oral contraceptives derived from a previous study as controls. Exacerbations were defined by criteria different from those used by Lockshin and colleagues. As a matter of policy, all pregnant women were started on 10 mg prednisone daily, even if there was no evidence of SLE activity. The rate of SLE flares per month at risk was similar in both groups. As in Lockshin's studies, most of the exacerbations tended to be easily controlled with low to moderate doses of glucocorticoids, but seven patients (8%) had severe exacerbations requiring more aggressive therapies. Interestingly, the majority (54%) of the exacerbations occurred in the first trimester.

Using criteria for SLE flare that differed from either of the other two studies, Petri and colleagues[8] found SLE flares (flares per person-years) to be more common among pregnant women than among controls. Fortunately, over three quarters of the flares were mild to moderate in nature.

Urowitz and colleagues[21] reported their experience comparing 79 pregnancies in patients with active SLE to a matched control group of 59 nonpregnant women with active SLE. They also compared these women to 216 women with inactive disease. Using a previously defined SLE exacerbation score, they found no significant differences in disease activity between the three groups. Only inactive patients at the onset of pregnancy showed a significant reduction in SLE activity (41%).

Ruiz-Irastorza and colleagues[22] analyzed the course of SLE in 78 pregnancies in 68 patients and a matched control group of 50 nonpregnant women. Sixty-five percent of the patients experienced an exacerbation of SLE during pregnancy, for a flare rate of 0.082 per patient-month. In the control group, 42% of the patients experienced a flare, with a flare rate of 0.039 per patient-month, representing a statistically significant difference.

Georgiou and colleagues[27] prospectively evaluated the frequency of SLE exacerbation during 59 pregnancies in 47 women with SLE and 59 nonpregnant women matched for parameters other than disease activity and duration. Using accepted clinical criteria, they reported SLE exacerbation in 8 (13.5%) of pregnant patients compared to 13 (22%) of nonpregnant women. More than half of the exacerbations in the pregnant group occurred during the first trimester. As in the previous studies, all exacerbations were mild and easily treated with glucocorticoids.

Preexisting disease activity undoubtedly plays a large role in risk of SLE flare during pregnancy. Derksen and colleagues[25] reported that SLE exacerbation occurred in fewer than 20% of women with sustained remission prior to pregnancy. More recently, Cortez-Hernandez and colleagues[28] studied 60 women with 103 pregnancies and found that SLE exacerbations during pregnancy were more likely in women who discontinued maintenance therapy before pregnancy and/or had a history of more than three severe flares prior to pregnancy. The findings of several other studies support the notion that women with active disease should postpone pregnancy until sustained remission can be achieved.[26,27,29]

In summary, the question of whether pregnancy predisposes to SLE exacerbation is not yet settled. At most, the predisposition to SLE flare during pregnancy is modest. Importantly, in a majority of studies of pregnant women with SLE, flares have been mild to moderate in nature and easily treated with glucocorticoids.[17,19,21,22,26,27,29] Moreover, the routine use of glucocorticoids or antimalarial agents in all pregnant SLE patients, as suggested by some investigators, seems unwarranted in view of the excellent results achieved by others without routine prophylactic immunosuppression.

The Risk of Lupus Nephritis Exacerbation

Women with lupus nephropathy face several challenges during pregnancy. Not only is there some evidence suggesting that pregnancy may worsen renal function. In turn, underlying renal disease presages increased risks of maternal and fetal complications. In addition, those with chronic renal disease are likely to have worsening proteinuria during gestation as renal perfusion increases. In turn, this inevitably poses the question of whether the increased proteinuria represents an exacerbation of underlying renal disease, preeclampsia, or both.

Whether renal flares are more common in pregnancy in all women with SLE remains controversial. Two studies reported high frequencies of renal flares (43% to 46%) during pregnancy,[30,31] whereas others have reported lower figures (9% to 28%).[19,22,32,33] Three studies describe the patients' status during pregnancy in terms of whether the SLE was active or in remission prior to conception.[34–36] In all three, the rate of SLE exacerbation was lower among pregnancies in which the patient was in remission prior to conception.

Studies on pregnancy outcome in women with past or current SLE nephritis are scarce. This may be explained, in part, by (1) the reduced fertility associated with long-term cyclophosphamide or impaired renal function, or both, and (2) the classical assumption that pregnancy should be discouraged in women with a history of lupus nephritis. The earliest reports suggested that lupus nephropathy was a major contributor to serious maternal morbidity or death.[15,16,37] However, larger, more recent series suggest that the outlook for pregnancy in women with lupus nephropathy is usually favorable if the disease is well-controlled and renal function preserved.[38] Oviasu and colleagues[39] reviewed eight studies (151 pregnancies) published between 1973 and 1991 on the effect of completed pregnancy on maternal renal function in established lupus nephritis, and reported that transient deterioration of renal function occurred in only 17% of pregnancies and permanent deterioration in 8%.

Even better outcomes were reported in three studies published in the 1990s.[39–41] Out of 143 patients with lupus nephropathy, only 1 developed irreversible loss of renal function after pregnancy. Importantly, the majority of women in these studies had normal renal function, mild proteinuria, and well-controlled hypertension *before* conception. Petri and colleagues at the Hopkins Lupus Pregnancy Center reported that only women who began pregnancy with nephrotic syndrome went on to renal failure after delivery.[32] Hayslett and Lynn[34] and Bobrie and colleagues[36] also found that the rate of renal deterioration was somewhat lower among pregnancies in which the patient was in remission prior to conception. Most recently, Moroni and colleagues[42] reported that renal flare occurred in 5% (1/20) of pregnancies in women with inactive lupus nephropathy prior to conception compared to 39% (12/31) in women with active lupus nephropathy prior to conception ($P < 0.01$). The sole predictors for renal flare were a plasma creatinine greater than 1.2 mg/dL or proteinuria ≥500 mg in 24-hour collection. Permanent deterioration occurred in two women with active lupus nephropathy prior to conception, one of whom eventually died.

Based on the published data summarized in Table 44-3, approximately one third of women with lupus nephropathy experience SLE exacerbation during pregnancy and 21% experience some form of renal deterioration. The median rate for permanent deterioration is 7%. Women with inactive lupus nephropathy prior to conception rarely suffer permanent deterioration during pregnancy.

Medical prudence would strongly suggest that pregnancy is contraindicated in patients with active lupus nephropathy (especially DPGN), nephrotic syndrome, and severe hypertension. Pregnancy should only be attempted if immunosuppressive therapy is effective in reducing disease activity, and antihypertensive therapy reduces blood pressure to acceptable levels. Moderate renal failure (creatinine 1.5 to 2.0 mg/dL) is a relative contraindication to pregnancy, and advanced renal failure (creatinine >2.0 mg/dL) should be considered an absolute contraindication to pregnancy.

Problems of Detection of SLE Exacerbation (Flare) in Pregnancy

Thorough and frequent clinical assessment remains essential for the timely and accurate detection of SLE exacerbation. However, detection of flare during pregnancy is hampered by the fact that many of the typical signs and symptoms associated with flare are considered normal manifestations of pregnancy. In addition, common complications of pregnancy such as preeclampsia may be mistaken for SLE exacerbation. Nevertheless, criteria for measuring SLE flare during pregnancy have been recently tested and have been found valid.[46] As in all patients with SLE, the most common presenting symptom of flare during pregnancy is extreme fatigue (see Table 44–1). In addition, skin lesions occur in >90% and arthritis/arthralgias >80% SLE exacerbations during pregnancy.[27,31]

Serologic evaluation of SLE disease activity may be beneficial in confirming flare in confusing cases. Most specific are elevations in anti-dsDNA titers that precede lupus flare in more than 80% of patients.[10,11] In pregnancy, elevated anti-dsDNA titers have also been shown to correlate with the need for preterm delivery.[12] In combination with anticardiolipin antibodies, elevated levels of anti-dsDNA are associated with an increased risk of fetal loss.

Early reports suggested that serial serologic evaluation of complement components and activation products were

TABLE 44-3

Renal Deterioration during Pregnancy in Patients with Lupus Nephritis

AUTHOR	PATIENTS	PREGNANCIES	EXACERBATIONS NO	EXACERBATIONS YES	DETERIORATION NO	DETERIORATION YES	PERMANENT
Hayslett[34]							
inactive PTC	23	31	21/31 (68%)	10/31 (32%)	24/31 (77%)	7/31 (23%)	2/31 (6%)
active PTC	24	25	13/25 (52%)	12/25 (48%)	16/25 (64%)	9/25 (36%)	5/25 (20%)
Fine[43]	13	14	NA	NA	10/14 (71%)	4/14 (29%)	2/14 (14%)
Jungers[35]							
inactive PTC	8	11	9/11 (82%)	2/11 (18%)	9/11 (82%)	2/11 (18%)	1/11 (9%)
active PTC	8	15	4/15 (27%)	11/15 (73%)	13/15 (87%)	2/15 (13%)	1/15 (7%)
Imbasciati[44]	6	18	8/18 (44%)	10/18 (56%)	14/18 (78%)	4/18 (22%)	2/18 (11%)
Devoe[45]	14	17	13/17 (76%)	4/17 (24%)	12/17 (71%)	5/17 (29%)	2/17 (12%)
Bobrie[36]	35	53	35/53 (66%)	18/53 (34%)	NA	NA	4/53 (8%)
Julkunen[40]	16	26	24/26 (92%)	2/26 (8%)	25/26 (96%)	1/26 (4%)	0/26
Packham[41]	41	64	NA	NA	52/64 (81%)	12/64 (19%)	1/64 (2%)
Oviasu[39]	25	53	NA	NA	22/28 (79%)	6/28 (21%)	0/28
Moroni[42]							
inactive PTC	19	20	19/20 (95%)	1/20 (5%)	NA	NA	0/20
active PTC	20	31	19/31 (61%)	12/31 (39%)	NA	NA	2/31 (6%)
Total	252	378					
Median Rates of Exacerbation/Deterioration				**33%**		**21%**	**7%**

PTC, prior to conception.

beneficial in predicting SLE flare during pregnancy. In two studies, Devoe and colleagues[45,47] found that SLE exacerbation was signaled by a decline of C3 and C4 into the subnormal range. More recently, Buyon and colleagues[48] found that SLE exacerbation was associated with an absence of the usual increase in C3 and C4 levels during normal pregnancies. However, the practical utility of serial determinations of complement components or their activation products during pregnancy remains unproven. Lockshin and colleagues[49] reported that low-grade activation of the classical pathway may be attributed to pregnancy alone. Wong and colleagues[30] prospectively studied 19 continuing SLE pregnancies and found that neither ANA, C3 nor C4 levels predicted which patients were going to have a flare; Nossent and Swaak[50] observed that fewer than half of the pregnancies with decreased serum C3 levels were associated with a clinical SLE flare. Finally, although some have found that hypocomplementemia has been reported to correlate with poor pregnancy outcomes,[51-53] there is also evidence that hypocomplementemia may occur in pregnant patients without SLE and no adverse pregnancy outcomes.[54]

Laboratory confirmation of SLE flare is probably most helpful in women with active lupus nephropathy in whom proteinuria, hypertension, and evidence of multiorgan dysfunction may easily be confused with preeclampsia. Table 44-4 outlines features that may prove helpful in distinguishing between the two conditions. Preeclampsia is more likely in women with decreased levels of antithrombin III.[55,56] Complement concentrations are not always helpful because activation may also occur in women with preeclampsia.[57] In the most severe and confusing cases, the correct diagnosis is possible only by renal biopsy. However, in reality, concerns about maternal and fetal well-being often prompt delivery, rendering the distinction between SLE flare and preeclampsia clinically moot.

TABLE 44-4

Distinguishing between Preeclampsia and SLE/Lupus Nephropathy Flare

TEST	PREECLAMPSIA	SLE
Serologic		
Decreased complement	++	+++
Elevated Ba or Bb fragments with low CH50	±	++
Elevated anti-dsDNA	−−	+++
Antithrombin III deficiency	++	±
Hematologic	++	−−
Microangiopathic hemolytic anemia	−−	++
Coombs' positive hemolytic anemia	++	++
Thrombocytopenia	−−	++
Leukopenia		
Renal	+	+++
Hematuria	−−	+++
Cellular casts	±	++
Elevated serum creatinine	++	±
Elevated ratio of serum blood urea nitrogen/creatinine	++	±
Hypocalciuria		
Liver transaminases	++	±

Risks of Immunosuppressive Agents in Pregnancy

GLUCOCORTICOIDS

The group of drugs most commonly given to pregnant women with SLE is the glucocorticoid preparations, both as maintenance therapy and in "bursts" to treat suspected SLE flares. The doses used in pregnancy are the same as those used in nonpregnant patients. Pregnancy per se is not an indication to reduce the dose of glucocorticoids, though a carefully monitored reduction in dosage may be reasonable in appropriately selected women whose disease appears to be in remission.

Some groups have recommended prophylactic glucocorticoid therapy during pregnancy,[19,29,33] but there are no controlled studies to show this practice to be prudent or necessary in the face of inactive SLE. Moreover, good maternal and fetal outcomes are achieved without prophylactic treatment of women with stable disease.[25] In contrast, glucocorticoid treatment of women with active disease and/or elevated anti-dsDNA titers has been shown to result in fewer relapses and better pregnancy outcomes.[11,27]

Although glucocorticoids have a low potential for teratogenesis, they are not without risk during pregnancy. Patients requiring chronic maintenance therapy are best treated with prednisolone or methylprednisolone because of their conversion to relatively inactive forms by the abundance of 11-β-ol dehydrogenase found in the human placenta. Glucocorticoids with fluorine at the 9-α position (dexamethasone, betamethasone) are considerably less well metabolized by the placenta, and chronic use during pregnancy should be avoided. Both have been associated with untoward fetal effects. Maternal side effects of chronic glucocorticoid therapy are the same as in nonpregnant patients and include weight gain, striae, acne, hirsutism, immunosuppression, osteonecrosis, and gastrointestinal ulceration. During pregnancy, chronic glucocorticoid therapy has also been associated with an increased risk of preeclampsia,[58–60] uteroplacental insufficiency and intrauterine growth restriction (IUGR),[61] and glucose intolerance.[59,60] Women undergoing chronic treatment with glucocorticoids should be screened for gestational diabetes at 22 to 24 weeks', 28 to 30 weeks', and 32 to 34 weeks' gestation.

ANTIMALARIALS

An accumulating body of evidence suggests that antimalarial drugs, such as hydroxychloroquine, may be used safely for the treatment of SLE during pregnancy.[52–66] In the past, many patients and their physicians have discontinued antimalarials during pregnancy because of concerns about teratogenicity, including ototoxicity[67] and eye damage.[68] The latter was of particular concern because of the affinity of antimalarials for melanin containing tissues found in the eye. However, hydroxychloroquine has been used in women considered at risk for malaria for years without any reported adverse fetal effects. This experience has been confirmed in recent large series showing hydroxychloroquine to be relatively safe during pregnancy.[62–65] Furthermore, they may be more beneficial than glucocorticoids for women who need maintenance therapy during pregnancy. In a recent randomized controlled trial, women who continued hydroxychloroquine during pregnancy experienced a significant reduction in SLE disease activity compared to women who changed to glucocorticoid therapy.[69] The findings of a recent case-control trial, which compared the effects of in utero exposure to hydroxychloroquine, were very reassuring.[66] There were no differences between 122 infants with in utero exposure to hydroxychloroquine and 70 control infants in the number and type of defects identified at birth or in the proportion of infants with visual, hearing, growth, or developmental abnormalities at follow-up (median, 24 months).

CYTOTOXIC AGENTS

Cytotoxic agents, including azathioprine, methotrexate, and cyclophosphamide, are used to treat only the most severely affected patients with SLE. Limited data suggest that azathioprine, a derivative of 6-mercaptopurine, is not a teratogen in humans but has been associated with IUGR[70,71] and evidence of impaired neonatal immunity.[72] Women who require azathioprine to control SLE disease activity should not necessarily be discouraged from becoming pregnant, though potential fetal risks should be carefully weighed against the benefits of the medication. Cyclophosphamide has been reported to be teratogenic in both animal[73] and human studies[74,75] and should be avoided during the first trimester. Thereafter, cyclophosphamide should be used only in unusual circumstances such as in women with severe, progressive proliferative glomerulonephritis.[76] Methotrexate is known to kill chorionic villi and cause fetal death, and its use should be scrupulously avoided.

NONSTEROIDAL ANTI-INFLAMMATORY DRUGS

The most common types of analgesics used in the treatment of SLE outside of pregnancy are nonsteroidal anti-inflammatory drugs (NSAIDs). Unfortunately, they readily cross the placenta and block prostaglandin synthesis in a wide variety of fetal tissues. Maternal ingestion of normal adult doses of aspirin in the week before delivery has been associated with intracranial hemorrhage in preterm neonates.[77] Although short-term tocolytic therapy with indomethacin appears to be safe,[78,79] chronic use has been associated with a number of untoward fetal effects; when used after 32 weeks' gestation, chronic indomethacin therapy may result in constriction or closure of the fetal ductus arteriosus.[80] Long-term use of all NSAIDs has been associated with decreased fetal urine output and oligohydramnios as well as neonatal renal insufficiency.[81] Given these risks, chronic use of adult dosages of aspirin and other NSAIDs should be avoided during pregnancy, especially after the first trimester. Acetaminophen and narcotic-containing preparations are acceptable alternatives if analgesia is needed during pregnancy.

OTHER IMMUNOSUPPRESSIVE AGENTS

Several new treatment regimens including cyclosporine, high-dose IVIG, mycophenolate mofetil, and thalidomide, have been studied in the treatment of nonpregnant patients with SLE.[76] Only IVIG has been used during pregnancy without reports of adverse fetal effects. Obviously, thalidomide is strictly contraindicated during pregnancy because of its known potent teratogenicity. Complete immunoablative therapy followed by bone marrow stem cell transplantation has also been studied in patients with the most severe, unresponsive SLE.[76]

TREATMENT OF SLE EXACERBATION IN PREGNANCY

Mild to moderate symptomatic exacerbations of SLE without CNS or renal involvement may be treated with initiation of glucocorticoids or an increase in the dose of glucocorticoids. Relatively small doses of prednisone (e.g., 15 to 30 mg/day) will result in improvement in most cases. For severe exacerbations without CNS or renal involvement, doses of 1.0 to 1.5 mg/kg/day of prednisone in divided doses should be used, and a good clinical response can be expected in 5 to 10 days. Thereafter, glucocorticoids may be tapered by several different approaches (Table 44–5).

Severe exacerbations, especially those involving the CNS or kidneys, are treated more aggressively. In recent years, an intravenous pulse glucocorticoid approach has become popular. The initial regimen involves a daily intravenous dose of methylprednisolone at 10 to 30 mg/kg (about 500 to 1000 mg) for 3 to 6 days. Thereafter, the patient is treated with 1.0 to 1.5 mg/kg/day of prednisone in divided doses and rapidly tapered over the course of 1 month. One can expect that 75% of patients will respond favorably to this approach.[82] This regimen may be repeated every 1 to 3 months in severe cases as an alternative to cytotoxic drugs.

In nonpregnant patients, both azathioprine and cyclophosphamide may be used in severe SLE exacerbations to control disease, reduce irreversible tissue damage, and reduce glucocorticoid doses.[83–85] In particular, severe proliferative lupus nephritis may be treated more effectively with cyclophosphamide, usually in combination with glucocorticoids.[85] The drug may be given either orally or intravenously, but the most effective cyclophosphamide regimen is uncertain. Cyclophosphamide appears to be useful in the treatment of severe cerebral lupus as well.

TABLE 44–5

Suggested Methods for Tapering Prednisone

1. Consolidate to a single morning dose of prednisone. Reduce the daily dose by 10% per week, as tolerated. When a dose of 20 to 30 mg/day is reached, reduce by 2.5-mg increments per week. If the patient remains asymptomatic at a dose of 15 mg/day, reduce the dose by 1-mg increments per week to a dose of 5 to 10 mg/day.
2. Consolidate to a single morning dose of prednisone. Taper to 50 to 60 mg/day by reducing the dose 10% per week. Thereafter eliminate the alternate-day dose by tapering it 10% per week, as tolerated. Thereafter, taper the remaining every other day dose by 10% per week, as tolerated.

Plasmapheresis and IVIG have been used to treat severe cases of SLE flare unresponsive to standard treatments. Plasmapheresis should be considered in life-threatening disease that is unresponsive to other treatments. A cytotoxic agent should also be administered soon after plasmapheresis is initiated (days 5 through 10 of therapy) if the patient is no longer pregnant. IVIG has been used for salvage treatment of recalcitrant SLE flare with neuropsychiatric or renal involvement.[86]

Obstetric Complications in Women with SLE

GESTATIONAL HYPERTENSION AND PREECLAMPSIA

The exact incidence of pregnancy-related hypertension associated with SLE is difficult to estimate due to inconsistencies in the definition and classification of these disorders, as well as the inclusion of patients with lupus nephropathy in the various studies. Nevertheless, it appears that between 20% and 30% of women with SLE develop either gestational hypertension or preeclampsia (gestational hypertension with proteinuria) sometime during pregnancy.[23,34,58,87–89] Women with lupus nephropathy are undoubtedly most vulnerable given the known association between preeclampsia and underlying renal disease of any origin.[90] In one prospective series, preeclampsia occurred in 7 of 19 (37%) women with lupus nephritis, compared with 15 of 106 (14%) without.[17] Other important predisposing factors include chronic hypertension, secondary antiphospholipid syndrome, and chronic steroid use.[23,34,40,41,43,91,92]

PREGNANCY LOSS

Women with SLE are probably more likely to have an unsuccessful pregnancy than women in the general obstetric population. The exact physiologic mechanisms responsible for pregnancy loss in women with SLE and other immunologic diseases remain uncertain, though a clear relationship between pregnancy failure and histologic evidence of inflammation has been well documented. Recent experimental observations suggest that altered complement regulation causes and may perpetuate pregnancy loss.[54]

In most retrospective studies, the rate of pregnancy loss appears to be higher in women with SLE than in the general obstetric population, ranging between 8% and 41%, with a median of 22%.[15,18,34,43,89,93–98] In one case-control trial comparing obstetric outcomes between 481 pregnancies in 203 lupus patients and 566 pregnancies in 177 healthy relatives and 356 pregnancies in 166 healthy unrelated women, investigators found that pregnancy loss occurred significantly more often in women with SLE (21%) than in either their healthy relatives (8%) or unrelated healthy controls (14%).[99] In the group of women with SLE and prior pregnancy, those whose diagnosis was made with SLE onset *after* their first pregnancy had a higher rate of loss once the diagnosis was made

(27% vs. 19%). The pregnancy loss rates observed in most prospective trials of lupus pregnancies have been better than those found in retrospective trials, possibly because of careful monitoring of SLE activity and routine antenatal surveillance. Still, from the data summarized in Table 44–6, between 11% and 34% of women with SLE experienced pregnancy loss, with a median of 24%. A disproportionate number of these occur in the second or third trimester. In the most recent, well-detailed prospective trials, fetal deaths in the second or third trimester accounted for between 10% and 40% of the total number of losses.[27,28]

Control of disease activity appears to have a salutary effect on the rate of pregnancy loss,[24] with one early study reporting live births in 64% of women with active disease within 6 months of conception, compared to 88% in women with quiescent disease.[34] In a more recent prospective study of pregnancy in SLE patients, pregnancy loss occurred in 75% of women with active disease compared to 14% of women with inactive disease.[27] Not surprisingly, pregnancy loss is more likely if SLE is diagnosed during the index pregnancy.[44,96,97]

Preexisting renal disease increases the rate of pregnancy loss in women with SLE. Table 44–7 summarizes obstetric outcomes in 411 pregnancies in 261 women with a diagnosis of lupus nephropathy prior to conception. Excluding therapeutic abortions, the median rates of miscarriage, fetal and neonatal death, and live birth were 13%, 7%, and 75%, respectively, figures not remarkably different from those for all patients with SLE shown in Table 44–6. Pregnancy loss rates in individual studies vary widely, probably because of variations in the degree of renal impairment of included patients, as well as definitions of pregnancy loss.

The degree of renal impairment no doubt influences the likelihood of pregnancy loss in women with lupus nephropathy. In a recent study of lupus nephropathy in pregnancy that included only women with inactive disease and normal renal function (serum creatinine <0.8 mg/dL), the overall fetal survival rate was >90%, after exclusion of embryonic losses (losses <10 weeks' gestation).[102] These results contrast markedly to those of another study in which the rate of fetal loss was 50% in pregnant women with lupus nephropathy and moderate to severe renal insufficiency (serum creatinine ≥1.5 mg/dL).[34] In a study comparing obstetric outcomes according to the degree of renal impairment in women with lupus nephropathy, spontaneous abortion occurred in 26% of women with minimally impaired renal function (serum creatinine <1 mg/dL, creatinine clearance >80 mL/min, and proteinuria <1 g/day) and 36% in women with mild impairment (creatinine clearance 50–80 mL/min, proteinuria 1–3 g/day).[43]

Among SLE patients, fetal deaths are associated with the presence of antiphospholipid antibodies (see Antiphospholipid Syndrome). In several studies, the presence of antiphospholipid (aPL) antibodies has been the single most sensitive predictor of fetal death.[103] The positive predictive value of aPL antibodies for fetal death is over 50%[58]; for women with SLE and a prior fetal death, the predictive value is over 85%.[104] In the most recent prospective trial, the presence of any aPL was the single strongest predictor of subsequent pregnancy loss, even in women with active disease and underlying renal impairment.[105]

PRETERM BIRTH

Preterm birth has been reported in as few as 3% and as many as 73% of pregnancies complicated by SLE.[19,30,34,35,43,44,97,103–107] Not surprisingly, the presence of aPL antibodies, chronic hypertension, and disease activity have all been reported to increase the likelihood of preterm birth in women with SLE.[27,105] Only a handful of studies have compared preterm birth rates in

TABLE 44–6

Fetal Outcome in Prospective Cohort Studies of Women after the Diagnosis of SLE

AUTHOR	PREGNANCIES	LIVE BIRTHS	THERAPEUTIC ABORTIONS*	PREGNANCY LOSSES: MISCARRIAGE	PREGNANCY LOSSES: FETAL DEATHS	PREGNANCY LOSSES: TOTAL
Devoe[47]	11	8 (73%)	1 (9%)	2 (18%)	0	3 (27%)
Mintz[19]	102	80 (78%)	0	17 (17%)	5 (5%)	22 (22%)
Lockshin[17]	80	61 (76%)	NA	NA	NA	19 (24%)
Nossent[50]	39	33 (85%)	0	4 (10%)	2 (5%)	6 (15%)
Wong[30]	24	17 (71%)	5 (21%)	2 (8%)	0	7 (29%)
Derksen[25]	35	25 (71%)	1 (3%)	8 (23%)	1 (3%)	10 (29%)
Huong[29]	99	76 (77%)	5 (5%)	13 (13%)	5 (5%)	23 (23%)
Lima[101]	108	89 (82%)	2 (2%)	7 (7%)	10 (9%)	19 (18%)
Georgiou[27]	59	36 (61%)	3 (5%)	9 (15%)	1 (2%)	13 (22%)
Cortes-Hernandez[28]	103	68 (66%)	8 (8%)	15 (15%)	12 (12%)	35 (34%)
Total	**660**					
Median Rates		**75%**	**5%**	**14%**	**5%**	**24%**

*Elective terminations were excluded.

TABLE 44–7

Pregnancy Outcomes among Women with SLE Nephropathy

				PREGNANCY LOSSES		LIVE BIRTHS		
AUTHOR	PATIENTS	PREGNANCIES	THERAPEUTIC ABORTIONS	MISCARRIAGE	FETAL DEATHS	PRETERM	TERM	TOTAL
Hayslett[34]								
remission PTC	23	31	7	1 (4%)	2 (8%)	1 (4%)	20 (84%)	21 (88%)
active PTC	24	25	3	3 (14%)	5 (23%)	0	14 (64%)	14 (64%)
Jungers[35]								
remission PTC	8	11	0	0	0	1 (9%)	10 (91%)	11 (100%)
active PTC	8	15	3	3 (25%)	0	2 (17%)	7 (58%)	9 (75%)
Imbasciati[44]	6	18	2	0	4 (25%)	10 (62%)	2 (12%)	12 (75%)
Gimovsky	19	46	6	16 (40%)	5 (12%)	9 (23%)	10 (25%)	19 (48%)
Devoe[45]	14	17	2	2 (13%)	1 (7%)	3 (20%)	9 (60%)	12 (80%)
Bobrie[36]	35	53	15	5 (13%)	0	5 (13%)	28 (74%)	33 (87%)
Julkunen[38]	16	26	2	1 (4%)	1 (4%)	6 (25%)	16 (67%)	22 (92%)
Packham[41]	41	64	5	5 (9%)	10 (17%)	19 (32%)	24 (41%)	43 (73%)
Oviasu[39]	25	53	6	8 (17%)	1 (2%)	10 (21%)	28 (60%)	38 (81%)
Huong	22	32	0	7 (22%)	2 (6%)	17 (53%)	6 (19%)	23 (72%)
Cortes-Hernandez[28]	20	20	1	5 (26%)	6 (32%)	3 (16%)	5 (26%)	8 (42%)
Total	**261**	**411**						
Median Rates				**13%**	**7%**	**19%**	**58%**	**75%**

PTC, prior to conception.

women with SLE and healthy controls. In one retrospective case-control study, preterm birth occurred more commonly in a group of women with SLE than in a group of matched controls (12% vs. 4%).[100] This was not the case in a more recent prospective trial, in which the rates of preterm birth in women with SLE and healthy controls were statistically similar (8% vs. 15%).[27] Interestingly, preterm birth was more common among women with active SLE compared to those with inactive disease (12.5% vs. 4%).

A substantial proportion of preterm birth associated with SLE is undoubtedly a result of iatrogenic delivery for obstetric and medical indications, rather than idiopathic preterm labor. From the few studies that provide sufficient detail, between 28% and 66% of preterm deliveries are indicated because of preeclampsia and another 12% to 33% because of suspected or confirmed fetal compromise.[8,97,100,104–106] An association between SLE and preterm premature rupture of membranes (PPROM) has also been reported, occurring in 39% of pregnancies delivered at 24 to 36 weeks' gestation.[104]

INTRAUTERINE FETAL GROWTH RESTRICTION

Uteroplacental insufficiency resulting in IUGR or small-for-gestational-age neonates has been reported in between 12% and 40% of pregnancies complicated by SLE.[22,24,26,41,89,105] Mintz and colleagues[19] reported higher rates of IUGR in pregnancies complicated by SLE than in pregnancies in normal controls (23% vs. 4%). However, the higher rate of IUGR associated with SLE may have been due to all the women with SLE receiving prophylactic glucocorticoid therapy during pregnancy. In a more recent prospective trial during which glucocorticoids were given only for symptomatic SLE flare, Georgiou and colleagues[27] reported no significant differences in the rate of IUGR between SLE pregnancies and healthy controls. Factors that have been associated with a higher rate of IUGR in SLE pregnancies include renal insufficiency and/or hypertension.[61,89]

NEONATAL LUPUS ERYTHEMATOSUS

Neonatal lupus erythematosus is a rare condition of the fetus and neonate, occurring in 1 in 20,000 of all live births and in fewer than 5% of all women with SLE.[105] Dermatologic manifestations are the most common manifestation of neonatal lupus and are described as erythematous, scaling annular or elliptical plaques occurring on the face or scalp, analogous to the subacute cutaneous lesions in adults. Lesions appear in the first weeks of life, probably induced by exposure of the skin to ultraviolet light, and may last for up to 6 months.[110] Hypopigmentation may persist for up to 2 years. A small percentage of affected infants will go on to have other autoimmune diseases later in life.[110] Hematologic neonatal lupus is rare and may be manifest as autoimmune hemolytic anemia, leukopenia, thrombocytopenia, and hepatosplenomegaly.

Cardiac neonatal lupus lesions include congenital complete heart block and the less frequently reported endocardial fibroelastosis. Congenital complete heart block is due to disruption of the cardiac conduction system, especially in the area of the atrioventricular node. The diagnosis of congenital complete heart block is typically made around 23 weeks' gestation,[111] when a fixed bradycardia, in the range of 60 to 80 beats/minute, is detected during a routine prenatal visit. Fetal echocardiography reveals complete atrioventricular dissociation with a structurally normal heart. Confirmation of neonatal lupus is based on the presence of autoantibodies in maternal circulation. Endomyocardial damage is irreversible; in the most severely affected cases, cardiac failure leads to hydrops fetalis and fetal death. In less severely affected neonates, pacemaker placement is not uncommonly necessary to ensure survival. In the largest series of prenatally diagnosed congenital complete heart block, the 3-year survival was only 79%; the majority of deaths occurred before 90 days of life.[111] Cutaneous manifestations of neonatal lupus have also been reported in infants with congenital complete heart block.[110]

Not all women who give birth to babies with neonatal lupus have been previously diagnosed with an autoimmune disorder.[106,108] However, in one study, 7 of 13 previously asymptomatic mothers who delivered infants with dermatologic neonatal lupus were later diagnosed with one of several autoimmune disorders.[110] Surprisingly, asymptomatic women who deliver infants with congenital complete heart block were less likely to develop an autoimmune disorder than those who delivered infants with dermatologic manifestations.[112]

A model of passively acquired autoimmunity, neonatal lupus manifestations are presumed to arise from the transplacental passage of autoantibodies directed against Ro/SS-A and La/SS-B ribonucleoprotein antigens.[111,113–116] Anti-Ro/SS-A antibodies are found in 75% to 95% of mothers who deliver babies with neonatal lupus.[111,117,118] A smaller percentage have anti-La/SS-B, and some have both.[118] Dermatologic neonatal lupus has also been associated with anti-U1RNP without anti-Ro/SS-A or anti-La/SS-B.[118] Among all mothers with SLE, the risk of neonatal lupus is less than 5%.[109] Of mothers with SLE who are serologically positive for anti-Ro/SS-A antibodies, 15% will have infants affected with dermatologic neonatal lupus; the proportion that delivers infants with congenital complete heart block is much smaller. However, once a women with SLE and anti-Ro/SS-A antibodies delivers one infant with congenital complete heart block, her risk for recurrence is at least two to threefold higher than women with anti-Ro/SS-A or anti-La/SS-B antibodies who have never had an affected child.[111] Recurrence of dermatologic neonatal lupus is approximately 25%.[89,119]

There is no known in utero therapy that completely reverses fetal congenital complete heart block secondary to SLE. However, some evidence suggests that glucocorticoids, plasmapheresis, and IVIG, or some combination thereof, may slow the progression of prenatally diagnosed congenital complete heart block or prevent recurrence in a future pregnancy.[120,121] In utero treatment with dexamethasone was felt to slow disease progression in one case report of hydrops secondary to congenital complete heart block.[122] In one retrospective study, maternally administered dexamethasone appeared to prevent progression from second-degree block to third-degree block.[123] In a large series of 87 pregnancies at risk for neonatal lupus, mothers who received corticosteroids before 16 weeks' gestation were less likely to deliver infants with congenital complete heart block compared to mothers who received no therapy.[124] However, there was no benefit to treatment when congenital complete heart block was diagnosed in utero. In utero treatment with digoxin is not beneficial for prenatally diagnosed congenital complete heart block.[125]

Taken together, the currently available data indicate that newly discovered cases of congenital complete heart block in utero should be evaluated by sonographic examination of the fetal heart and determination of maternal anti-Ro/SS-A and anti-La/SS-B status. If the diagnosis of congenital complete heart block due to neonatal lupus is made, experts currently recommend administration of a glucocorticoid that crosses the placenta (e.g., dexamethasone, 4 mg/day) to limit further immunologic damage to the fetal heart. The efficacy of this approach is being examined in a registry of cases collected by Dr. J.P. Buyon at the Hospital for Joint Diseases, in New York City (212-598-6283).

Management Options

Prepregnancy

Women with SLE who are contemplating pregnancy should be counseled before conception about potential obstetric problems, including pregnancy loss, preterm birth, gestational hypertension/preeclampsia, and IUGR. They should also be informed of the risk of SLE flare as well as special concerns related to antiphospholipid syndrome and neonatal lupus. Preconceptional laboratory evaluation should include an assessment for anemia and thrombocytopenia, underlying renal disease (urinalysis, serum creatinine, and 24-hour urine for creatinine clearance and total protein), and aPL antibodies (lupus anticoagulant and anticardiolipin). It is also common practice to obtain anti-Ro/SS-A and anti-La/SS-B antibodies on all patients with SLE, but the cost-effectiveness of these tests is not proven.

Women with active SLE should be discouraged from embarking on pregnancy until remission can be attained. Cytotoxic drugs and NSAIDs should be stopped before pregnancy. However, maintenance therapy with hydroxychloroquine or glucocorticoids need not be discontinued.

Prenatal

The obstetric management of the patient with SLE is guided by the potential risks to the mother and fetus. As mentioned, prenatal visits should occur every 1 to 2 weeks in the first and second trimesters and every week thereafter. A primary goal of the antenatal visits after 20 weeks gestation is the detection of hypertension and/or proteinuria. Because of the risk of uteroplacental insufficiency, fetal ultrasonography should be performed every 4 to 6 weeks starting at 18 to 20 weeks' gestation. In the usual case, fetal surveillance (daily fetal movement counts and once weekly nonstress tests and amniotic fluid volume measurements) should be instituted at 30 to 32 weeks' gestation. More frequent ultrasonography and fetal testing is indicated in patients with SLE flare, hypertension, proteinuria, clinical evidence of IUGR, or antiphospholipid syndrome. In the patients with antiphospholipid syndrome, fetal surveillance as early as 24 to 25 weeks' gestation may be justified.[126]

Labor and Delivery

The management of the gravida with SLE during labor and delivery represents a continuation of her antenatal care. Exacerbations of SLE can occur during labor and may require the acute administration of steroids. Regardless, stress doses of glucocorticoids should be given during labor or at the time of cesarean delivery to all patients who have been treated with chronic steroids within the previous year. This compensates for the anticipated endogenous adrenal insufficiency in these patients. Intravenous hydrocortisone, given in three doses of 100 mg every 8 hours is an acceptable regimen. Complications such as preeclampsia and IUGR should be dealt with based on obstetric concerns; their management is not specifically altered by the presence of SLE. Neonatology support may be needed at delivery for problems associated with congenital complete heart block and other manifestations of neonatal lupus.

Postnatal

The true predisposition for SLE exacerbation following delivery is uncertain. Regardless, care should be taken to examine for these flares in the symptomatic parturient. If gestational hypertension complicates the intrapartum process, it should be anticipated that the patient will clear these acute effects in a manner similar to otherwise normal women with this condition. Maintenance medications should be restarted immediately after delivery, at similar doses as during the pregnancy. Further dose adjustments can be handled in the outpatient setting.

SUMMARY OF MANAGEMENT OPTIONS

Systemic Lupus Erythematosus

Management Options	Quality of Evidence	Strength of Recommendation	References
Prepregnancy			
Establish good control of SLE; adjust maintenance medications.	–	GPP	–
Discontinue azathioprine, methotrexate, and cyclophosphamide if possible and only under careful supervision.	IIb	B	72,74,75,78, 79,82,84
It is not necessary to discontinue hydroxychloroquine.	IIa	B	62–66
Perform laboratory assessment for anemia, thrombocytopenia, renal disease, antibodies (anti-phospholipid, anti-Ro/SS-A, anti-La/SS-B).	–	GPP	–
Counsel patient regarding risks (exacerbations, preeclampsia, fetal/neonatal).	–	GPP	–
Prenatal			
Provide multidisciplinary care.	–	GPP	–
Encourage early prenatal care.	–	GPP	–
Perform dating scan.	–	GPP	–
Perform frequent antenatal checks: every 2 weeks in the 1st and 2nd trimesters, weekly in 3rd.	–	GPP	–
Maintain vigilance for SLE flare, preeclampsia, IUGR.	–	GPP	–
For SLE patients with renal involvement, perform monthly 24-hr urine collections for creatinine clearance and total protein.	–	GPP	–
Possible drugs:			
• Antimalarials	IIa	B	62–66
• Glucocorticoids	IIb	B	72,82

SUMMARY OF MANAGEMENT OPTIONS

Systemic Lupus Erythematosus *(Continued)*

Management Options	Quality of Evidence	Strength of Recommendation	References
Prenatal *(Continued)*			
• Azathioprine (if steroids are ineffective)	III	B	72,84
• Methotrexate/cyclophosphamide as third choice	III	B	74,75
• Avoid full-dose NSAIDs	III	B	78,79
Perform serial biometry, Doppler studies, and amniotic fluid volume every 3–4 wks.	–	GPP	–
Begin prenatal testing at 30–32 weeks' gestation (earlier in patients with worsening disease, evidence of fetal compromise, or history of poor pregnancy outcome).	III	B	118
Consider low-dose aspirin, especially if history of recurrent miscarriages or early-onset severe preeclampsia.	Ib	A	59,60
Labor and Delivery			
Deliver at term. Avoid postdates.	–	GPP	–
Maintain continuous fetal heart rate monitoring.	–	GPP	–
Intravenous glucocorticoids for delivery in patients who have received maintenance or steroid bursts during pregnancy.	IIb	B	82
Postnatal			
Monitor for SLE exacerbation.	–	GPP	–
Restart maintenance therapy.	–	GPP	–
Check neonate for SLE manifestations.	–	GPP	–

ANTIPHOSPHOLIPID SYNDROME

Antiphospholipid antibodies are a family of autoantibodies that bind to negatively charged phospholipids, phospholipid-binding proteins, or a combination of the two. The association between aPL antibodies and hypercoagulability was first reported 50 years ago; a link with pregnancy loss was not established until the mid-1970s. Since then, collaboration between international laboratory researchers and clinicians from various specialties has led to the development of definitive diagnostic criteria for so-called *antiphospholipid syndrome* (APS).[127] However, the obstetric aspects of APS continue to generate considerable controversy, and refining the diagnostic criteria for APS is an ongoing process.

The first aPL detected was the false-positive Wassermann test. The key antigenic component was later found to be cardiolipin, a phospholipid found in mitochondrial membranes. Lupus anticoagulant was first described in the early 1950s and was later found to be associated with false-positive tests for syphilis and (paradoxically) with thrombosis. Anticardiolipin antibodies eventually were found to be strongly associated with lupus anticoagulant and thrombosis. Most recently, investigators reported that anticardiolipin binding sometimes requires the presence of a phospholipid-binding protein known as β_2-glycoprotein I (GPI).[128] As a result, APS research has become more focused on phospholipid-binding proteins, rather than the phospholipids themselves.

The association between aPL antibodies and thrombosis and pregnancy loss is now well established. Correctly identifying patients with APS is important given the efficacy of heparin treatment in reducing the recurrence risk of thromboembolism and improvement in pregnancy outcomes.[101,129,130] Nevertheless, aPL antibodies are found in up to 5% of apparently healthy controls and up to 35% of patients with SLE.[131] The prospective risks of a positive test for aPL antibodies in otherwise healthy subjects are unknown.

The Pathogenesis of Antiphospholipid Syndrome

The mechanism(s) by which aPL antibodies cause thrombosis most likely involves interference with normal hemostasis by interaction with phospholipids or phospholipid-binding protein components such as β_2-GPI (which has anticoagulant properties), prostacyclin, prothrombin, protein C, annexin V, and tissue factor.[127]

Antiphospholipid antibodies also appear to activate endothelial cells, indicated by increased expression of adhesion molecules, secretion of cytokines, and production of arachidonic acid metabolites.[132] The findings that some anticardiolipin antibodies cross-react with oxidized low-density lipoprotein[133] and that human anticardiolipin antibodies bind to oxidized, but not reduced, cardiolipin[134] imply that aPL may participate in oxidant-mediated injury of the vascular endothelium. However, aPL do bind perturbed cells, such as activated platelets[135] or apoptotic cells,[136] which typically lose normal membrane symmetry and express anionic phospholipids on their surface.

Whether aPL per se are the cause of adverse obstetric outcomes is also a matter of debate. Investigators working with murine models have found that passive transfer of aPL results in clinical manifestations of APS, including fetal loss and thrombocytopenia.[137,138] One group has used a murine pinch-induced venous thrombosis model to demonstrate that human polyclonal and murine monoclonal aPL are associated with larger and more persistent thrombi than in mice treated with control antibodies.[139] Recent work points to the complement system as having a major role in APS-related pregnancy loss, showing that C3 activation is required for fetal loss in a murine model.[140] In humans, APS-related pregnancy complications are probably related to abnormal placental function. Some authorities have focused on abnormalities in the decidual spiral arteries as the immediate cause of fetal loss in APS pregnancies. Some investigators have found narrowing of the spiral arterioles, intimal thickening, acute athetosis, and fibrinoid necrosis.[141–143] In addition, placental histopathology demonstrates extensive necrosis, infarction, and thrombosis.[141] These abnormalities might result from thrombosis during the development of normal maternoplacental circulation via interference with trophoblastic annexin V[143] or by impairing trophoblastic hormone production or invasion.[144]

Diagnostic Evaluation of Antiphospholipid Syndrome

Diagnostic Criteria

The 1999 International Consensus Statement provides simplified criteria for the diagnosis of APS.[127] Patients with bona fide APS must manifest at least one of two clinical criteria (vascular thrombosis or pregnancy morbidity) and at least one of two laboratory criteria (positive lupus anticoagulant or medium to high titers of β_2-GPI-dependent IgG or IgM isotype anticardiolipin antibodies), confirmed on two separate occasions, at least 6 weeks apart. Thrombosis may be either arterial or venous and must be confirmed by an imaging or Doppler study or by histopathology. Pregnancy morbidity is divided into three categories: (1) otherwise unexplained fetal death (10 weeks' gestation), (2) preterm birth (34 weeks' gestation) for severe preeclampsia or placental insufficiency, or (3) otherwise unexplained recurrent preembryonic or embryonic pregnancy loss. Autoimmune thrombocytopenia and amaurosis fugax are often associated with APS but are not considered sufficient diagnostic criteria. Antiphospholipid syndrome may exist as an isolated immunologic derangement (primary APS) or in combination with other autoimmune diseases (secondary APS), most commonly SLE.

Laboratory Testing

Patients suspected of having APS should be tested using at least two aPL assays for several reasons. First, there is no definitive association between any of the clinical manifestations of APS and a particular aPL antibody. Second, there is substantial interlaboratory variation in assay performance and interpretation. Currently, the most commonly performed aPL antibody assays are for lupus anticoagulant and anticardiolipin antibodies (IgG and IgM isotypes). These are also the most commonly detected aPL antibodies and the only two currently recognized by the 1999 International Consensus Statement. Testing for lupus anticoagulant utilizes an in vitro coagulation assay in which the antibodies prolong clotting times, and the test for anticardiolipin antibodies is a standardized enzyme-linked immunosorbent assay. Lupus anticoagulant tests are reported as being positive or negative, whereas anticardiolipin antibodies are reported in terms of international units (designated GPL for IgG binding and MPL for IgM binding). Approximately 70% of patients with bona fide APS have both LAC and anticardiolipin antibodies.

The assay for anticardiolipin antibodies is a more sensitive test for detection of APS; the assay for lupus anticoagulant is more specific. Low titers of anticardiolipin antibodies are present in up to 5% of normal individuals and should not be used to make the diagnosis of APS. Medium to high titers of anticardiolipin antibodies are more specific for the diagnosis of APS, as is the specificity of the IgG isotype compared to the IgM isotype.

Several areas of controversy surround laboratory testing for aPL. First, relevance of low positive IgG anticardiolipin antibodies is questionable. Many of the studies reporting a relationship between aPL antibodies and recurrent pregnancy loss have included patients who test positive solely for low levels of IgG anticardiolipin antibodies.[145–147] Yet, marked differences have been reported in low levels of IgG anticardiolipin antibodies in women with recurrent first-trimester miscarriage and the much higher levels found in women with APS characterized by fetal death or thrombosis.[148] In addition, women with low levels of IgG anticardiolipin antibodies have been found to have no greater risk for aPL antibody-related events than women who tested negative.[149]

The presence of isolated IgM or IgA aPL antibody levels is also of questionable clinical significance. Women with isolated IgM aCL antibodies are no more likely to suffer aPL-related morbidity than women who tested negative for all aPL antibodies.[149] Although the 1999 International Consensus Statement considers medium to high titers of IgM anticardiolipin antibodies as diagnostic criteria for APS, clinicians should exercise caution when the diagnosis is based on their presence alone. Several treatment trials have included women with isolated IgM anticardiolipin antibodies, but have failed to analyze their outcomes separately.[145–147,150] Isolated IgA anticardiolipin antibodies should also be viewed with suspicion. Testing for IgA anticardiolipin antibodies appears to add little diagnostic benefit compared with IgG and IgM anticardiolipin antibodies; IgA anticardiolipin antibodies are not considered criteria in the 1999 International Consensus Statement.

Some investigators have attempted to link poor obstetric outcomes to aPL antibodies other than lupus anticoagulant and anticardiolipin antibodies. These include antibodies to phosphatidylserine, phosphatidylethanolamine, phosphatidylinositol, phosphatidylglycerol, phosphatidylcholine, and phosphatidic acid.[151,152] However, such antibodies do appear to be associated with poor obstetric outcomes once women who are positive for lupus anticoagulant and anticardiolipin antibodies are excluded.[153] In addition, multiple aPL antibody tests do not increase the diagnostic yield for APS.[154] Indeed, substituting negatively charged phospholipids, such as phosphatidylserine or phosphatidylinositol, for cardiolipin in the immunoassay system yields comparable results. The most persuasive argument against using alternative phospholipid assays for the diagnosis of APS is undoubtedly the fact that none of them have been standardized in the same fashion as the assay for anticardiolipin antibodies.

The demonstration that antibodies to cardiolipin are directed against β_2-GPI or an epitope formed by the interaction of phospholipids and β_2-GPI, has led to the development of anti-β_2-GPI antibody assays. Although they are not considered criteria in the 1999 International Consensus Statement, their presence is strongly associated with clinical features of APS and they are sometimes the only aPL antibody detected in patients who are suspected of having the syndrome.[155] Some authorities predict that internationally standardized anti-β_2-GPI assays will replace lupus anticoagulant and anticardiolipin antibody assays for the diagnosis of APS. Current recommendations are to reserve the use of anti-β_2-GPI assays for patients who are strongly suspected of having APS but in whom standard aPL antibody assays are negative.[131,155]

As a final note, the 1999 International Consensus Statement criteria were developed primarily for research purposes to ensure more uniform patient characterization as well as disease subcategorization in APS studies. Not unlike the situation with autoimmune conditions such as SLE, some patients will present with one or more clinical or laboratory features suggestive but not diagnostic of APS. In such cases, the decision to proceed with therapies generally reserved for patients with APS should be based on experienced clinical judgment.

Risks of APS and Pregnancy

Thrombotic Complications of APS in Pregnancy

Numerous retrospective studies confirm a link between aPL and venous or arterial thrombosis.[156,157] Approximately 70% of thrombotic events occur in the venous system, although arterial thromboses and cerebrovascular accidents are also common.[158] Transient CNS manifestations of ischemia also are common in APS patients.[148] Antiphospholipid antibodies are present in approximately 2% of individuals with unexplained thrombosis[159] and are the only identifiable predisposing factor in 4% to 28% of cases of stroke in otherwise healthy patients younger than age 50.[160–162]

In the only prospective study of untreated APS patients (who also had SLE), 50% of those with lupus anticoagulant had a thrombotic episode during the study period; the annual risk of venous thrombosis and arterial thrombosis was 13.7% and 6.7%, respectively.[163] The lifetime risk of thromboembolism in women with APS is unknown. However, over half occur in relation to pregnancy or the use of combination oral contraceptives.[164] In the two largest series of prospectively followed APS pregnancies, the rates of thrombosis and stroke were 5% and 12%, respectively.[101,130]

Obstetric Complications of APS in Pregnancy

GESTATIONAL HYPERTENSION/PREECLAMPSIA

The median rate of gestational hypertension/preeclampsia in pregnancies complicated by APS is 32%, with a range up to 50%.[101,130,165,166] Preeclampsia may develop as early as 15 to 17 weeks' gestation.[101] The rate of gestational hypertension/preeclampsia does not appear to be markedly diminished by treatment with either glucocorticoids and low-dose aspirin or heparin and low-dose aspirin. In contrast to the high rate of preeclampsia observed in some case series of women previously diagnosed with APS, aPL antibodies are not found in a statistically significant proportion of a general obstetric population presenting with preeclampsia[167] or in women at moderate risk to develop preeclampsia because of conditions such as underlying chronic hypertension or preeclampsia in a prior pregnancy.[168] However, two groups of investigators have reported that women with early-onset, severe preeclampsia are more likely to test positive for aPL antibodies compared to healthy controls.[169,170] Based on these findings, testing for aPL antibodies should only be considered in early-onset, severe preeclampsia.

UTEROPLACENTAL INSUFFICIENCY AND PRETERM BIRTH

Several investigators have found relatively high rates of IUGR in association with aPL antibodies.[101,130,169,171,172]

Even with currently used treatment protocols, the rate of IUGR approaches 30%.[101,130] Pregnancies complicated by APS are also more likely to exhibit nonreassuring fetal heart rate patterns during antenatal tests of fetal well-being and intrapartum monitoring.[101,103,130] Not surprisingly, the rate of preterm birth in these series ranges from 32% to 65%.[101,130,166]

PREGNANCY LOSS

In the original description of APS, the sole obstetric criterion for diagnosis was fetal loss (>10 menstrual weeks of gestation).[156] At least 40% of pregnancy losses reported by women with lupus anticoagulant or medium to high positive IgG anticardiolipin antibodies occur in the fetal period.[130,146,173,174,176] More recently, APS-related pregnancy loss has been extended to include women with early recurrent pregnancy loss, recurrent pregnancy loss including those occurring in the preembryonic (<6 menstrual weeks of gestation) and embryonic periods (6 through 9 menstrual weeks of gestation).[127] In serologic evaluation of women with recurrent pregnancy loss, 10% to 20% have detectable aPL antibodies.[145,150–152,170,177]

Fetal death and early recurrent pregnancy loss are seen by some as two points along the same continuum of APS-related pregnancy loss. However, women with APS identified because of a prior fetal death and/or thromboembolism seem to have more serious complications in subsequent pregnancies than those with early recurrent pregnancy loss.[176] Recent prospective treatment trials of APS during pregnancy have been comprised mainly of women with early recurrent pregnancy loss and no other APS-related medical problems.[145,151,177–180] Accordingly, the rates of obstetric complications were relatively low, with fetal death, preeclampsia, and preterm birth occurring in 4.5% (0% to 15%), 10.5% (0% to 15%), and 10.5% (5% to 40%), respectively. Only 1 of 300 women suffered a thrombotic event, and no neonatal deaths due to complications of prematurity were reported. Based on these data, it seems unlikely that early recurrent pregnancy loss, fetal death, and preterm birth resulting from severe preeclampsia or placental insufficiency result from the same pathophysiologic mechanism. Certainly, hypercoagulability causing defective uteroplacental circulation that results in diminished intervillous blood flow might be responsible for later pregnancy complications. Women with early recurrent pregnancy loss probably represent a different patient population with pregnancy losses due to different mechanisms, perhaps relating to different aPL specificities or aPL operating on a fundamentally different pathophysiologic background.

Postpartum and Catastrophic Antiphospholipid Syndrome

Catastrophic APS is a rare but devastating syndrome characterized by multiple simultaneous vascular occlusions throughout the body, often resulting in death. The diagnosis should be suspected if at least three organ systems are affected and confirmed if there is histopathologic evidence of acute thrombotic microangiopathy affecting small vessels. Renal involvement occurs in 78% of patients. Most have hypertension; 25% eventually require dialysis. Other common manifestations described by Asherson[181] include adult respiratory distress syndrome (66%), cerebral microthrombi and microinfarctions (56%), myocardial microthrombi (50%), dermatologic abnormalities (50%), and disseminated intravascular coagulation (25%). Death from multiorgan failure occurs in 50% of patients.[181] The pathophysiology of catastrophic APS is poorly understood. However, the onset may be presaged by several factors, including infection, surgical procedures, discontinuation of anticoagulant therapy, and the use of drugs such as oral contraceptives.[181–183]

Early and aggressive treatment of catastrophic APS appears prudent. Patients should be transferred to an intensive care unit where supportive care can be provided. Hypertension should be aggressively treated with appropriate antihypertensive medication. Although no treatment has been shown to be superior to another, a combination of anticoagulants (usually heparin) and steroids plus either plasmapheresis or IVIG has been successful in some patients.[181,182] Streptokinase and urokinase have also been used to treat acute vascular thrombosis.[181] Women suspected of catastrophic APS during pregnancy should probably be delivered.

Management Options (General Considerations)

Treatment for Antiphospholipid Syndrome during Pregnancy

The ideal treatment for APS during pregnancy should include: (1) improvement in maternal and fetal-neonatal outcome by preventing pregnancy loss, preeclampsia, placental insufficiency, and preterm birth, and (2) reduction or elimination of the risk of thromboembolism. Early enthusiasm for treatment with glucocorticoids to reduce the risk of pregnancy loss waned after publication of a small, randomized trial found maternally administered heparin to be as effective as prednisone.[179] At present, maternally administered heparin is considered the treatment of choice (Table 44–8); it is usually initiated in the early first trimester after ultrasonographic demonstration of a live embryo. In most case series and trials, daily low-dose aspirin is included in the treatment regimen.[145,150,177–180,184] In a recent meta-analysis of treatment trials, the live-birth rate was improved by 54%.[184]

The decision to use one of the currently recommended anticoagulation regimens should be based on individual clinical and laboratory characteristics (see Table 44–8). Women with APS and a history of thromboembolism should probably receive full anticoagulation with heparin during pregnancy because of their substantial risk of recurrent thromboembolism.[129,185,186] Most authorities recommend full, adjusted-dose anticoagulation.[187,201]

TABLE 44–8

Subcutaneous Heparin Regimens Used for Antiphospholipid Syndrome during Pregnancy

Prophylactic Regimens

Recommended in women with no history of thrombotic events—diagnosis of recurrent preembryonic and embryonic loss or prior fetal death or early delivery because of severe preeclampsia or severe placental insufficiency

Standard Heparin

7,500-10,000 U q12h in the first trimester, 10,000 U q12h in the second and third trimesters

Low Molecular Weight Heparin

1) Enoxaparin 40 mg once daily or dalteparin 5000 U once daily
2) Enoxaparin 30 mg q12h or dalteparin 5000 U q12h

Anticoagulation Regimens

Recommended in women with a history of thrombotic events

Standard Heparin

Every 8-12 hours, adjusted to maintain the midinterval heparin levels* in the therapeutic range

Low Molecular Weight Heparin

1) Weight-adjusted (enoxaparin 1/mg/kg q12h or dalteparin 200 U/kg q12h)
2) Intermediate dose (enoxaparin 40 mg once daily or dalteparin 5000 U once daily until 16 weeks of gestation and q12h from 16 weeks on

*Heparin levels, anti-factor Xa levels. Women without a lupus anticoagulant in whom the activated partial thromboplastin time (aPTT) is normal can be observed using the aPTT.

In contrast, women diagnosed with APS *without* a history of thromboembolic disease may have less risk of thromboembolism during pregnancy. Women with early recurrent pregnancy loss alone, without a history of thromboembolism, have been treated with both low-dose prophylaxis and adjusted-dose anticoagulation regimens.[186] Live-birth rates have exceeded 70% using either strategy.[145,151,179] In one trial of nearly 100 women, two thirds of whom had recurrent preembryonic and embryonic pregnancy loss and none of whom had a history of thromboembolic disease, an unfractionated heparin dose of 5000 U twice daily was associated with a 71% live-birth rate.[145] Another study of women with aPL antibodies and predominantly preembryonic and embryonic pregnancy loss, none of whom had a history of thromboembolic disease, with heparin administered in a twice-daily regimen and adjusted to keep the midinterval activated partial thromboplastin time (aPTT) approximately 1.5 times the control mean, was associated with an 80% live-birth rate.[151] In most case series and trials, daily low-dose aspirin is included in the treatment regimen.

Women with a history of fetal death or neonatal death after delivery at less than 34 weeks' gestation for severe preeclampsia or placental insufficiency, without prior thromboembolism, may be at higher risk for thromboembolism during pregnancy.[188] It is our practice to treat such women with generous thromboprophylaxis (e.g., 15,000 to 20,000 units of standard unfractionated heparin or 60 mg of enoxaparin [low molecular weight heparin, or LMWH] in divided doses daily).[130,179,189]

Women with APS should be counseled about the potential risks of heparin therapy during pregnancy, including heparin-induced osteoporosis and heparin-induced thrombocytopenia (HIT). Osteoporosis resulting in fracture occurs in 1% to 2% of women treated during pregnancy.[190] Women treated with heparin should be encouraged to take daily supplemental calcium and vitamin D (e.g., prenatal vitamins). It also seems prudent to encourage daily axial skeleton weight-bearing exercise (e.g., walking). Immune-mediated HIT is much less common but potentially more serious. Most cases have their onset 3 to 21 days after heparin initiation and are relatively mild in nature.[191] A more severe form of HIT paradoxically involves venous and arterial thromboses, resulting in limb ischemia, cerebrovascular accidents, and myocardial infarctions, as well as venous thromboses.[192] It may occur in up to 0.5% of patients treated with unfractionated sodium heparin.[191] LMWH is much less likely to be associated with HIT, compared with unfractionated sodium heparin.[193]

Other pregnancy complications associated with APS occur in spite of appropriate treatment.[130,194] In a recent observational study of 107 pregnancies complicated by APS, preeclampsia occurred in 20%, preterm birth in 24%, and IUGR in 15% of treated women.[194]

Pregnancy losses continue to occur in 20% to 30% of cases, even when heparin prophylaxis is given.[131,179,184] Several alternative therapies have been tried in so-called refractory cases. Glucocorticoids, often in high doses, have sometimes been added to regimens of heparin and low-dose aspirin. Although there are anecdotal reports of success, this practice has never been studied in appropriately designed trials; the combination of glucocorticoids and heparin may increase the risk of osteoporotic fracture.[195] IVIG has also been used in pregnancies complicated by APS, especially in women with particularly poor past histories or recurrent pregnancy loss during heparin treatment.[196] However, a small randomized, controlled, pilot study of IVIG treatment found no benefit to this expensive therapy compared to heparin and low-dose aspirin.[197] Hydroxychloroquine has been shown to diminish the thrombogenic properties of aPL antibodies in a murine thrombosis model.[198] There are few case reports and no trials of APS patients being treated during pregnancy with hydroxychloroquine. Finally, women with particularly egregious thrombotic histories, such as recurrent thrombotic events or cerebral thrombotic events, are understandably viewed as being at very high risk for thrombosis during pregnancy. In selected such cases, some authorities recommend the judicious use of warfarin anticoagulation rather than heparin.

Healthy women with recurrent embryonic and preembyronic loss and low titers of aPL do not require treatment.[199] The controlled trial of Pattison and colleagues included a majority of such women and found no difference in live-birth rates using either low-dose aspirin or placebo.[177]

Prepregnancy

Women with APS will preferably seek preconception counseling. At that time, the presence of clinically significant levels of aPL antibody should be confirmed and potential maternal and obstetric complications discussed, including thrombosis, pregnancy loss, preterm delivery, gestational hypertension/preeclampsia, and uteroplacental insufficiency. Primary APS patients, like patients with SLE, should be assessed for evidence of anemia, thrombocytopenia, and underlying renal disease (urinalysis, serum creatinine, 24-hour urine for creatinine clearance, and total protein).

The various anticoagulation prophylaxis regimens should be discussed, along with their risks and limitations. Patients should also be informed about the risks of heparin-induced osteoporosis and HIT, and recommendations for appropriate protective measures should be provided. Some authorities recommend instituting daily low-dose aspirin (81 mg) prior to conception.

Prenatal

Women with APS who suspect they are pregnant should be evaluated immediately. An early transvaginal ultrasound is useful to confirm an intrauterine pregnancy as well as provide accurate dating of the pregnancy. One of the anticoagulation prophylaxis regimens discussed previously (see Table 44–8) should be instituted, and appropriate precautions against heparin-induced osteoporosis and HIT should be taken. Calcium supplementation is encouraged, as well as the performance of daily weight-bearing exercise.

Prenatal visits should occur every 2 to 4 weeks until 20 to 24 weeks' gestation and every 1 to 2 weeks thereafter. Patient visits should be specifically designed to monitor for the development of preeclampsia and thrombosis and to monitor fetal well-being. Because of the risk of IUGR and oligohydramnios secondary to uteroplacental insufficiency, serial ultrasound examinations should be performed every 3 to 4 weeks after 17 to 18 weeks' gestation. Antenatal surveillance (daily fetal movement counts and at least once-weekly nonstress tests with amniotic fluid volume measurements) should be initiated at 30 to 32 weeks' gestation (or earlier if uteroplacental insufficiency is suspected). More frequent ultrasound examinations and more frequent or earlier fetal testing may be indicated in selected cases.

Labor and Delivery

Labor and delivery in women with APS should be managed in the same way as in any patient who is considered at high risk for preeclampsia and uteroplacental insufficiency. Most authorities recommend continuous electronic fetal monitoring throughout labor, given the increased risk of nonreassuring fetal heart rate tracings noted in women with APS.

The most common management dilemma in women with APS probably involves the need to alter anticoagulation regimens in a way that minimizes the risk of bleeding at the time of delivery without placing the patient at a prohibitively high risk of thromboembolism. Treatment approaches vary and there is no evidence that one method is better than another. Patients receiving prophylactic anticoagulation with heparin can be instructed to withhold their injections at the onset of labor. Alternatively, injections can be discontinued 12 hours before a planned induction. The most common practice in women with APS on full-dose anticoagulation (unfractionated heparin or LMWH) is to hold the last injection 24 hours prior to a planned induction of labor or cesarean delivery. As an alternative for women deemed at extremely high risk for thromboembolism, including those with an event within 2 weeks of delivery, intravenous heparin can be started in labor and discontinued 2 to 4 hours prior to anticipated delivery. Intravenous heparin can be resumed 4 to 6 hours after vaginal delivery and 12 hours after cesarean.

Spontaneous labor is problematic for women who are fully anticoagulated, particularly those receiving LMWH preparations. Anti-factor Xa levels might be helpful but have been found to underestimate the risk of bleeding in some patients. Protamine sulfate may be necessary in the event of surgical intervention. For those on adjusted-dose unfractionated heparin, careful monitoring of the aPTT (or heparin level) is required. If the aPTT is prolonged near delivery, protamine sulfate may be necessary to reduce the risk of bleeding.

Many anesthesiologists are particularly concerned that anticoagulation in any form increases the risk of spinal hematoma formation in women receiving regional anesthesia in labor or for cesarean delivery. The American Society of Regional Anesthesia (ASRA) recommends that neuraxial blockade should be withheld until 24 hours after the last injection in women on full anticoagulation with LMWH.[200] The same recommendation has been made for women receiving adjusted-dose anticoagulation with unfractionated heparin.[201] For women receiving low-dose thromboprophylaxis (low-dose twice-daily unfractionated heparin or once-daily LMWH), ASRA has recommended that needle placement be delayed until 10 to 12 hours after the last dose.

Postpartum

Anticoagulant coverage of the postpartum period in women with APS and prior thrombosis is critical.[201] We prefer initiating warfarin thromboprophylaxis as soon as possible after delivery, with doses adjusted to achieve an

International Normalized Ratio of 3.0. There is no consensus regarding the postpartum management of APS patients without prior thrombosis, although most is diagnosed because of prior fetal loss or neonatal death after delivery at or before 34 weeks' gestation for severe preeclampsia or placental insufficiency, though experts agree that there is an increased risk of thrombosis. The recommendation in the United States is to treat with anticoagulant therapy for 6 weeks after delivery. The need for postpartum anticoagulation in women with APS diagnosed solely on the basis of recurrent preembryonic or embryonic losses is uncertain. Both heparin and warfarin are safe for breast-feeding mothers. Finally, oral contraceptives containing estrogen are absolutely contraindicated.

SUMMARY OF MANAGEMENT OPTIONS

Antiphospholipid Syndrome

Management Options	Quality of Evidence	Strength of Recommendation	References
Prepregnancy			
Counsel regarding risks of thromboembolism, pregnancy loss, and pregnancy complications.	–	GPP	–
Check for anemia, thrombocytopenia, and renal compromise.	III	B	130
Discuss anticoagulation prophylaxis options and risk of heparin therapy.	III	B	130
Prenatal			
Institute joint obstetrician and physician surveillance.	–	GPP	–
Start anticoagulation prophylaxis (usually low-dose aspirin and subcutaneous LMWH), and take the appropriate precautions against heparin-induced osteoporosis and HIT.	III Ib	B A	130 145,150,179
Encourage calcium supplementation and weight-bearing exercise.	–	GPP	–
Monitor platelet counts for the first 2 to 3 weeks of heparin therapy.	–	GPP	–
Prenatal visits should occur every 2 to 4 weeks until 20 to 24 weeks' gestation and every 1 to 2 weeks thereafter.	III	B	134
Monitor fetal growth (every 3 to 4 weeks after 17 to 18 weeks' gestation) and health.	III	B	134
Screen for preeclampsia.	III	B	134
Antenatal surveillance should be initiated at 30 to 32 weeks of gestation or earlier if uteroplacental insufficiency is suspected	–	GPP	–
Labor and Delivery			
Deliver near term. Avoid postdates.	–	GPP	–
Adjust anticoagulation prophylaxis to minimize the risk of thromboembolism.	III	B	134
Consider sequential compression devices.	–	GPP	–
Maintain continuous fetal heart rate monitoring through labor.	–	GPP	–
Postpartum			
Resume anticoagulation 4 to 6 hours after vaginal delivery and 8 to 12 hours after cesarean delivery.	III	B	134
Warfarin may be substituted.	III	B	134
Continue anticoagulation prophylaxis for at least 6 weeks after delivery. Consider consultation with subspecialist in thrombophilic disorders.	III	B	134

RHEUMATOID ARTHRITIS

Rheumatoid arthritis (RA) is a debilitating disease, the hallmark feature of which is chronic symmetrical inflammatory arthritis of the synovial joints. RA is more common than SLE, with an incidence of from 2.5 to 7 per 10,000 per year and a prevalence of approximately 1% in the adult U.S. population. Although found in virtually all populations, it is more common in some populations (Native American) and less common in others (Native African). Although it is often said to peak in the 40s or 50s, RA can appear at any age of life (including in children), and the prevalence increases with age into the 60s or 70s in both females and males. As with virtually all autoimmune conditions, RA is more common in women than men with a ratio of 2:1 to 3:1 women to men.[202]

Pathogenesis of Rheumatoid Arthritis

Histologic features of RA are described as symmetrical inflammatory synovitis marked by cellular hyperplasia, accumulation of inflammatory leukocytes, and angiogenesis with membrane thickening, edema, and fibrin deposition as common early findings. Inflammatory damage at the synovium eventually leads to typical joint erosion involving a locally invasive synovial tissue called *pannus*.

The characteristic autoantibody in patients with RA is rheumatoid factor (RF), an autoantibody made by oligoclonal activated B cells in the peripheral circulation and synovium of RA patients. This group of autoantibodies, which reacts with antigens on the Fc portion of IgG, is composed of a heterogeneous group of antibodies containing light and heavy chains distributed among all the variable region subgroups. It is unknown whether RF autoantibodies are simply markers for RA or whether they are directly responsible for tissue damage. There is some evidence that RF autoantibodies form IgG aggregates in synovial fluid, resulting in complement activation and local inflammation and eventual joint erosion.

Concordance for RA is found in approximately 15% of monozygotic twins and 5% of dizygotic twins. It is estimated that heritable factors account for approximately 60% of the predisposition to RA.[203] The human leukocyte antigen (HLA) region (HLA class II gene locus DRB1, encoding HLA-DR), is of primary importance in RA susceptibility. Variant forms of DRB1 have been identified in association with RA, including DRB1*0401, *0404, *0405, *0101, *1402 and *1001. These alleles encode for similar amino acid sequences *(shared epitopes)* that are suspected of bestowing susceptibility to RA. Other suspect HLA complex genes are located on chromosomes 1p and 1q, 9, 12p, 16cen, and 18q.[204,205]

Juvenile rheumatoid arthritis (JRA) is a somewhat different, but related arthritis. It is probably a heterogeneous group of diseases. By definition, JRA has its onset in individuals younger than age 16 years; males and females are equally represented. One prominent subgroup is comprised of individuals with Still's disease. This condition is initially systemic in nature and includes fever, skin rash, serositis, and lymphadenopathy. Arthritis occurs late in the course of disease and tends not to be as destructive or chronic as classic RA. Nearly three quarters of children with JRA have spontaneous, permanent remission by the time they reach adulthood.

Diagnostic Evaluation of Rheumatoid Arthritis

Clinical Presentation

The symptoms of RA develop insidiously over several months; the clinical course is variable. Less commonly, disease onset is acute and somewhat rapid. Twice as many patients present during winter months compared to summer months, and trauma (including surgery) is a frequent precursor. Morning stiffness, pain, and swelling of peripheral joints are the most common initial features. The disease tends to involve primarily the joints of the wrists, knees, shoulders, and metacarpophalangeal joints in an erosive arthritis that typically follows a slowly progressive course marked by exacerbations and remissions. Eventually, joint deformities may occur; these are especially obvious at the metacarpophalangeal joint and proximal and distal interphalangeal joints of the hands. Fatigue, weakness, weight loss, and malaise are also common.

Rheumatoid nodules, present in 20% to 30% of affected patients, are made up of a local proliferation of small vessels, histiocytes, fibroblasts, and other cells, and are usually located in the subcutaneous tissues of the extensor surfaces of the forearm. Uncommonly, extra-articular tissues may also be affected, including the lung (pleuritis, pleural effusions, interstitial fibrosis, pulmonary nodules, pneumonitis, and airway disease) and heart (pericarditis, effusion, myocarditis, endocardial inflammation, conduction defects, and arteritis leading to myocardial infarction).

Diagnostic Criteria

The classification criteria published by the American College of Rheumatology are shown in Table 44-9. Physical examination should reveal evidence of joint inflammation, including joint tenderness, synovial thickening, joint effusion, erythema, and decreased range of motion. Symmetric involvement should be noted. Radiographic evidence of RA includes joint space narrowing and erosion; although too expensive for routine use, magnetic resonance imaging may detect synovial hypertrophy, edema, and early erosive changes.

TABLE 44–9

Classification Criteria for the Diagnosis of Rheumatoid Arthritis

CRITERIA*	DEFINITION
Morning stiffness	Morning stiffness in and around the joints, lasting at least 1 hour before maximal improvement
Arthritis of ≥3 joint areas	At least 3 joint areas simultaneously have had soft tissue swelling or fluid (not bony overgrowth alone) observed by a physician. The 14 possible areas are right or left proximal interphalangeal, metacarpophalangeal, wrist, elbow, knee, ankle, and metatarsophalangeal joints
Arthritis of hand joints	At least 1 area swollen (as defined above) in a wrist, metacarpophalangeal, a proximal interphalangeal joint
Symmetric arthritis	Simultaneous involvement of the same joint areas (as defined above) on both sides of the body (bilateral involvement of proximal interphalangeals, metacarpophalangeals, and metatarsophalangeals is acceptable without absolute symmetry)
Rheumatoid nodules	Subcutaneous nodules, over bony prominences or extensor surfaces, or in juxta-articular regions, observed by a physician
Serum rheumatoid	Demonstration of abnormal amounts of serum rheumatoid factor by any method for which the result has been positive in <5% of normal control subjects
Radiographic changes	Radiographic changes typical of rheumatoid arthritis on posteroanterior hand and wrist radiographs, which must include erosions or unequivocal bony decalcification localized in or most marked adjacent to the involved joints (osteoarthritis changes alone do not qualify)

*For classification purposes, a patient shall be said to have rheumatoid arthritis if he/she has satisfied at least 4 of these 7 criteria. Criteria 1 through 4 must have been present for at least 6 weeks. Patients with 2 clinical diagnoses are not excluded. Designation as classic, definite, or probable rheumatoid arthritis is *not* to be made.

Laboratory Criteria

More than 70% of patients with clinical features of RA are also seropositive for RF. In addition, some of those who are initially seronegative will eventually convert, leaving only 10% of RA patients without a positive RF. Approximately 5% of the general population also test positive for RF, as do many patients with other autoimmune conditions (e.g., SLE, scleroderma, and mixed connective tissue disease), viral infections, parasitic infections, chronic bacterial infections, and after irradiation or chemotherapy.

Rheumatoid Arthritis in Pregnancy

The relationship between RA and pregnancy is fascinating even if the basic scientific understanding of the relationship remains elusive. The observation that in many patients RA dramatically improves during pregnancy[199] eventually led Philip Hench to discover cortisone. Numerous studies (Table 44-10) show that at least 50% of patients with RA demonstrate improvement in their disease in at least 50% of their pregnancies.[206–212] In addition, Hazes and colleagues[213] reported a protective effect of pregnancy in development of RA.

For a majority of patients, the improvement in RA starts in the first trimester heralded by a reduction in joint stiffness and pain.[208] The peak improvement in symptoms generally occurs in the second or third trimester. Other aspects of the disease may also improve during pregnancy, with studies indicating that the subcutaneous nodules associated with RA may disappear during pregnancy.[210] Even with the overall improvement in symptoms, the clinical course of RA during pregnancy is characterized by short-term fluctuations in symptoms, as in the nonpregnant state. Most patients who experience an improvement in RA during pregnancy will have a similar improvement in subsequent pregnancies. However, this is not a given, and some patients will have relatively less improvement in a second or third pregnancy. There are no laboratory or clinical features that predict improvement of RA in pregnancy.

A quarter of RA patients have no improvement in their disease during pregnancy, and in a small number of cases the disease may actually worsen. Unfortunately, nearly

TABLE 44–10

Improvement of Rheumatoid Arthritis in Pregnancy

AUTHOR	PATIENTS	PATIENTS WITH IMPROVEMENT	PREGNANCIES	PREGNANCIES WITH IMPROVEMENT
Hench[206]	22	20 (91%)	37	33 (89%)
Oka[212]	93	73 (78%)	114	88 (77%)
Betson[209]	21	13 (62%)	21	13 (62%)
Ostensen[210]	10	8 (80%)	10	9 (90%)
Ostensen*,[214]	51	NA	76	35 (46%)

*Study of patients with juvenile rheumatoid arthritis.

three quarters of patients whose disease has improved during pregnancy will suffer a relapse in the first several postnatal months.[208,210] The level of disease during the first postnatal year generally returns to that of a year before conception, but may be worse.[212]

In contrast to SLE, there are no data to suggest that RA in remission is likely to have a better course during pregnancy than active RA. The long-term prognosis for RA patients undertaking pregnancy appears to be similar to those that avoid pregnancy. Oka and Vainio[212] compared 100 consecutive pregnant RA patients with age- and disease-matched controls and found no significant differences between the groups in terms of the severity of their disease. There are few studies of JRA, but one study found that only 1 case in 20 had a worsening or reactivation of their disease associated with pregnancy.[214]

The mechanism(s) by which pregnancy favorably affects RA is unknown. Plasma cortisol, which rises during pregnancy to peak at term, was initially thought to be important to the amelioration of RA.[206] However, there is no correlation between cortisol concentrations and disease state.[215] Some studies suggest that estrogens or estrogens and progestagens favorably affect arthritis,[216] but there are conflicting studies,[217] and a double-blind crossover trial found that estrogen did not benefit RA.[218] Sex hormones may interfere with immunoregulation and interactions with the cytokine system.[219] Promising data suggest that certain proteins circulating in higher concentrations during pregnancy or unique to pregnancy are associated with improvement of RA. These include pregnancy-associated α_2-glycoprotein[220] and gamma globulins eluted from the placenta.[221] Other investigators feel that the placenta may modify RA by clearing immune complexes[222] or that modification of immune globulins during pregnancy alters their inflammatory activity.[223] Nelson and coworkers suggested that amelioration of disease was associated with a disparity in HLA class II antigens between mother and fetus. Thus, the maternal immune response to paternal HLA antigens may have a role in pregnancy-induced remission of arthritis.[224]

Risks of Rheumatoid Arthritis in Pregnancy

Obstetric Complications and Rheumatoid Arthritis

About 15% to 25% of pregnancies in women with RA end in miscarriage,[225,226] a figure that may or may not be slightly higher than in normal women. One controlled study found that women with RA have a significantly higher frequency of miscarriage than normal women, even before the onset of their disease (25% vs. 17% before disease, 27% vs. 17% after disease).[225] Another controlled study did not find that women with RA have a higher proportion of miscarriage prior to the onset of disease.[211] Interestingly, this same study found that the frequency of fetal death was higher in patients who later develop RA than in nonaffected relatives. There are scant data available, but women with RA do not appear to be at significant risk for preterm birth, preeclampsia, or IUGR.

Management Options

Prepregnancy

The prepregnancy management of RA is similar to that of any of the other autoimmune disorders. This includes stabilization of the underlying disease process, reducing maintenance medications to minimize early fetal risks, and avoidance of known teratogenic agents.

Prenatal

As with SLE, a physician should see a woman with RA every 2 to 4 weeks throughout the pregnancy, especially if the patient is having trouble with her disease. Rest is an important part of the management of RA, and the patient should be counseled to plan adequately for this. Physical therapy can be helpful in patients whose disease does not improve with pregnancy.

ANTIRHEUMATIC DRUGS AND PREGNANCY

It is best to use acetaminophen for simple analgesia. If possible, the patient should avoid NSAIDs and aspirin (see discussion in SLE). Glucocorticoids should be considered for patients whose RA does not improve during pregnancy. Relatively low doses of prednisone are usually adequate for RA during pregnancy and are not often necessary for maintenance therapy. Intra-articular steroids can also be used if necessary in pregnancy. If NSAIDs prove necessary, the minimum dose necessary to control inflammation should be used. Methotrexate is absolutely contraindicated during the first trimester and relatively contraindicated thereafter. The anti-tumor necrosis factor-α (TNF-α) agents are of unknown safety in pregnancy and probably should avoided. Leflunomide is teratogenic in animals.

Labor and Delivery

Because RA has little, if any, adverse effect on pregnancy outcome, there are no special prenatal obstetric concerns. In a rare case, severe deforming RA can pose a problem to the mechanics of vaginal delivery; such cases are obvious and require individualized care.

Postnatal

Postpartum management of the RA parturient is similar to that of patients with other autoimmune disorders (see SLE).

SUMMARY OF MANAGEMENT OPTIONS

Rheumatoid Arthritis

Management Options	Quality of Evidence	Strength of Recommendation	References
Prepregnancy			
Counsel regarding risk of exacerbation during pregnancy and risk of medication exposure.	III	B	207–215
Establish good control of RA and adjust maintenance medications.	–	GPP	–
If possible, discontinue cytotoxic medications before conception. This should be done only under careful supervision.	III	B	207–215
Reduce dosage to lowest levels achieving therapeutic effect.	–	GPP	–
Avoid known teratogens.	–	GPP	–
Prenatal			
Review regularly (joint obstetrician and physician surveillance).	–	GPP	–
Prescribe rest (general and local).	–	GPP	–
Physiotherapy/Physical therapy recommended in some patients.	–	GPP	–
Possible drugs:	III	B	207–215
• Avoid full-dose aspirin and NSAIDs if possible (or use minimum doses to control inflammation).			
• Prescribe steroids for worsening disease (RCT not in pregnancy).			
• Avoid methotrexate in the first trimester.			
• D-Penicillamine is contraindicated.			
• Use glucocorticoids judiciously for exacerbations of disease. Use lowest dosage possible.			
• Avoid teratogenic medications.			
Prenatal visits should occur every 2 to 4 weeks throughout pregnancy.	–	GPP	–
Labor and Delivery			
Individualize care according to physical abilities.	–	GPP	–
Postpartum			
Monitor for RA exacerbations.	–	GPP	–
Consult with rheumatology subspecialist.	–	GPP	–

SYSTEMIC SCLEROSIS

The term *scleroderma* is derived from words referring to hardening *(scleros)* and skin *(derma)*, the hallmark feature of this disease. Systemic sclerosis (SSc) refers to internal organ involvement, characterized histologically by a marked increase in collagen, mostly in the dermis with hyalinization and often obliteration of small blood vessels. Early in the disease process, the dermis contains mononuclear cell infiltrates and sometimes calcium, due to the deposition of calcium hydroxyapatite. Pathologic changes also include thinning of the epidermis and loss of normal dermal appendages. Most patients with SSc report Raynaud's phenomenon, and vascular features are evident in biopsies from SSc patients. Small arteries and arterioles exhibit characteristic endothelial cell proliferation and intimal thickening as well as increased amounts of fibrinogen and fibrin, with lumina often occluded by fibrosis. Remaining vessels become dilated, visible through the skin as telangiectases.

Internal organs have similar histologic changes. Fibromucoid intimal thickening in the kidney results in narrowing and thinning of the lumen. Cortical glomerular involvement is usually focal and includes endothelial cell proliferation and thickening of the basement membrane. In the lung, the most common finding is interstitial fibrosis with increased numbers of fibroblasts, capillary congestion, and thickening and occlusion of alveolar walls and arteriolar intima. Densely hyalinized fibrosis is found in the gastrointestinal tract and random focal fibrosis in the myocardium.

The disease is uncommon, occurring in no more than 10 to 15 individuals per million per year. The ratio of females to males is 10:1 in the 15- to 44-year age-group. The mean age of onset is in the early 40s, when many affected women may potentially become pregnant.[227]

Pathogenesis of Systemic Sclerosis

The pathophysiologic changes of SSc include vascular abnormalities, immunologic abnormalities, and disordered collagen synthesis. The initial event most likely occurs in small blood vessels with early proliferation of intimal layer endothelial cells that produce cytokines, growth factors, adhesion proteins, vasoactive proteins, coagulation factors, and extracellular matrix. Aberrant production of factors such as von Willebrand factor also occurs. A hallmark feature of SSc is clearly increased fibroblast activity with an accelerated rate of fibroblast collagen synthesis.

An association between an increase of HLA-DR11 (whites) and HLA-DR15 (Asians) in patients with diffuse SSc has been described. Associations have also been described with the SSc-associated autoantibodies topoisomerase I and anticentromere antibody although results have varied in different ethnic and racial groups.[228]

A number of different non-HLA genes have most recently been identified in association with SSc. Genes encoding for extracellular matrix proteins have been identified, notably C0L1A1 and C0L1A2, genes encoding type I collagen. Other interesting studies have identified a candidate gene near the fibrillin 1 gene on chromosome 15q in studies of a Native American population with a particularly high prevalence of SSc. Polymorphisms in transforming growth factor-β 1, 2, and 3 genes have also been identified in association with SSc, as have polymorphisms in TNF-α, TNF-β, CXCR2, tissue inhibitor of metalloproteinase-1, and interleukin-4 receptor-α.[229]

Diagnostic Evaluation of Systemic Sclerosis

Clinically, the expression of SSc varies considerably; the morbidity depends on the extent of skin or internal organ involvement. Raynaud's phenomenon is common, especially in patients with CREST syndrome (calcinosis of involved skin, Raynaud's phenomenon, esophageal dysmotility, sclerodactyly, and telangiectasias), a more limited form of scleroderma. Patients who eventually develop diffuse disease involving the internal organs are more likely to present with arthritis, finger and hand swelling, and skin thickening. The skin thickening, which usually starts on the fingers and hands, eventually involves the neck and face. In severe, progressive disease, much of the skin may be involved and marked deformities of the hands and fingers may occur. Raynaud's phenomenon and internal organ damage are attributed to fibrosis of arterioles and small arteries. In these circumstances, the normal vasoconstrictor response to various stimuli, including cold, causes near-complete obliteration of the vessel. As a result, digital ischemia may occur. A similar vasculopathy is probably responsible for internal organ involvement. Lower esophageal dysfunction is most common. Other portions of the gastrointestinal tract may be involved, producing malabsorption, diarrhea, and/or constipation.

A variety of pulmonary lesions may occur, with the most common being progressive interstitial fibrosis. Pulmonary hypertension, a problem of special interest to the obstetrician, may also occur in longstanding disease. Nearly half of the patients with well-established SSc have evidence of myocardial involvement. Arrhythmias are probably the most common sign encountered. Renal disease occurs to some extent in many patients and is a major cause of mortality among patients with SSc. Severely involved cases may present with proteinuria and renal insufficiency, hypertension, or both. Sudden onset of severe hypertension and progressive renal insufficiency with microangiopathic hemolysis is known as *scleroderma renal crisis*. These crises usually occur in cold weather, suggesting that the pathophysiology is similar to that of Raynaud's phenomenon.

Antinuclear antibodies are present in most patients with SSc, but anti-DNA antibodies are not. About half of patients have serum cryoglobulins. Antibodies to centromere detected by indirect immunofluorescence are common among patients with limited scleroderma (CREST syndrome), but not among those with diffuse disease. Up to 40% of patients have antibody to an extractable nuclear antigen designated ScI. The biologic significance of these autoantibodies is unclear.

Risks of Systemic Sclerosis in Pregnancy

Complications of Systemic Sclerosis in Pregnancy

Pregnancy in women with SSc is uncommon, with fewer than 200 reports in the published literature. Early reports suggested that fertility was impaired in women with SSc, although this has not been confirmed in more recent studies.[230] Rather, women in the SSc group were older and had either waited to have children or had not desired pregnancy.[227] The effect that pregnancy might have on the course of SSc depends to some extent on the degree of preexisting disease involvement. Published data regarding the risks of pregnancy in women with SSc are scarce, and the findings of case reports and small series that suggest pregnancy should be avoided in women with SSc should be regarded with caution. The findings of the largest and most complete studies suggest that overall maternal outcomes are more salubrious, with worsening of disease in pregnancy in no more than 20% of cases.[227,230,231] Postpartum, approximately one third of women with SSc have exacerbations of Raynaud's phenomenon, arthritis, and skin thickening.[231]

Pregnancy is probably safest in SSc patients without obvious renal, cardiac, or pulmonary disease. Although data are scant, women with SSc with moderate to severe cardiac or pulmonary involvement likely face increased risks of substantial morbidity or mortality and should not undertake pregnancy. In addition, SSc patients with moderate to severe renal disease and hypertension probably face a substantial risk for preeclampsia and perhaps mortality due to renal crisis. Pregnancy should be discouraged in these women as well. Finally, there may be an increased risk of renal crisis in patients with early diffuse SSc[231]; therefore, some authorities suggest that these patients delay pregnancy.

Obstetric Complications in Women with Systemic Sclerosis

PREGNANCY LOSS

Fetal outcomes in SSc pregnancies are mixed, with half or more ending in term live births and another quarter ending in liveborn premature infants.[230,232–238] Preterm birth is particularly prominent in women with early, diffuse disease. Women with late, diffuse scleroderma may be at increased risk for miscarriage, reported at 65% in one case series. There has been some suggestion that a predisposition to pregnancy loss predates the onset of SSc in some women. Of 154 patients who eventually developed SSc and 115 matched controls, a significantly greater number of women with SSc had a history of miscarriage (29% vs. 17%).[238] However, only 3 met the definition for recurrent miscarriage (three or more consecutive losses). The most recent large case-control trial failed to find any association between a history of pregnancy loss and the subsequent development of SSc.[231]

GESTATIONAL HYPERTENSION/PREECLAMPSIA AND IUGR

Given the microvascular nature of the condition and the relative frequency of renal involvement in SSc, one might speculate that preeclampsia and IUGR would occur significantly more often in SSc pregnancies. This is supported by high rates of preeclampsia in case reports but not by case series. In one case series, 10% of pregnancies were complicated by IUGR.[230] Neonatal involvement with skin sclerosis possibly attributable to SSc have been reported in a few cases. The risks of this condition, as well as its relationship to SSc itself, remain unclear. Among the 29 pregnancies accumulated in case reports, there were 2 miscarriages (7%), 2 fetal deaths (7%), and 1 neonatal death attributable to prematurity. Two other infants died because of multiple anomalies. Among the 103 pregnancies in the small series,[233–236] there were 24 miscarriages (23%), 3 fetal deaths (3%), and 2 neonatal deaths due to prematurity. Thus, noncontrolled reports suggest that 72% to 83% of pregnancies among women with SSc are successful (excluding perinatal deaths due to anomalies). In the case-control study by Giordano and colleagues,[237] 80 SSc patients had 299 pregnancies. Of these, 50 ended in miscarriage (17%), significantly higher than the rate of miscarriage in the matched controls (10%). There was no difference in the miscarriage rate between patients with diffuse versus limited SSc. The retrospective study of Steen and colleagues[232] included 86 pregnancies after the onset of SSc. Of these, 15% ended in miscarriage and 2% ended in midtrimester fetal deaths. These percentages were not significantly different from those in RA controls or neighborhood controls. The later prospective study by this same group found that 18% of 67 SSc pregnancies ended in miscarriage, compared to 158 control pregnancies. Taken together, the available data suggest that the rate of miscarriages and fetal deaths in patients with SSc might be slightly increased compared with controls.

Management Options

Prepregnancy

Before pregnancy, management of SSc follows the basic guidelines set out for the other autoimmune disorders. Patients with early diffuse scleroderma and with significant cardiopulmonary involvement or severe renal disease should be counseled against getting pregnant.

Prenatal

Systemic sclerosis patients considering pregnancy and any patient with SSc who presents for medical care already pregnant should have her clinical situation thoroughly investigated. Special attention should be given to the evaluation of possible renal or cardiopulmonary involvement. It is prudent to recommend pregnancy termination in patients with diffuse SSc and cardiopulmonary involvement or moderate to severe renal involvement.

Even in the nonpregnant state, there is no satisfactory therapy for SSc. Patients with limited disease are usually managed with vasodilators and anti-inflammatory agents. As discussed previously, NSAIDs should be avoided if at all possible during pregnancy. Oral vasodilators for the prevention and treatment of Raynaud's phenomenon may be continued, although substantial data to prove fetal safety are not available. Patients with diffuse SSc may be taking glucocorticoids; see Systemic Lupus Erythematosus in this chapter. Other immunosuppressive or cytotoxic agents should be avoided.

Angiotensin-converting enzyme inhibitors appear to be particularly efficacious in treating SSc-related hypertension and renal crises. These drugs have been associated with fetal/neonatal renal insufficiency in a small number of cases. However, in SSc-related hypertension, the benefits of these medications probably outweigh the risks of discontinuing them.[239]

Patients with continuing pregnancies should be seen by a physician every 1 to 2 weeks in the first half of pregnancy and once weekly thereafter. Although serial laboratory testing is not necessary, laboratory assessment of unusual or suspicious symptoms or signs may be helpful. The possible risk of IUGR and fetal death requires serial examination of the fetus by sonography. Fetal surveillance should be instituted by 30 to 32 weeks' gestation, or sooner if the clinical situation demands.

Labor and Delivery

In patients with mild to moderate disease, few additional precautions are needed during the labor and delivery process. Again, signs of preeclampsia should be sought, since this complication may be more likely with scleroderma.[224] Wound healing may be a problem in patients with advanced disease or those on steroids. Therefore, operative interventions require meticulous attention to this issue. In patients with significant pulmonary, cardiac, or renal impairment, intensive care management may be needed.

Postnatal

Postpartum care represents a continuation of the intrapartum management plan. Most often, reinstitution of maintenance medication is all that is required. Complications of scleroderma, as previously outlined, require individualization of care.

SUMMARY OF MANAGEMENT OPTIONS

Systemic Sclerosis

Management Options	Quality of Evidence	Strength of Recommendation	References
Prepregnancy			
Counsel regarding risk of exacerbation during pregnancy and risk of medication exposure.	IIa	B	230
Establish good control of SSc and adjust maintenance medications.	III	B	231
If possible, discontinue cytotoxic medications before conception. This should be done only under careful supervision.	–	GPP	–
Assess cardiopulmonary and renal function (advise against conception if significantly compromised?).	III	B	231
Prenatal			
Institute joint obstetrician and physician surveillance.	III	B	231
Prenatal visits should occur every 2 to 4 weeks until 20 to 24 weeks' gestation and every 1 to 2 weeks thereafter.	III IV	B C	227 231
Monitor cardiopulmonary and renal function (consider termination of pregnancy if severe compromise).	IV	C	227
Possible drugs:			
• Anti-inflammatory for moderate joint problems	–	GPP	–
• Vasodilators for pulmonary problems	–	GPP	–
• Steroids for worsening disease	–	GPP	–
Be vigilant for preeclampsia.	IV	C	227
Use of ACE inhibitors a dilemma if hypertension is present; avoid if possible.	III	B	231
Check fetal growth (every 3 to 4 weeks after 17 to 18 weeks) and health.	IIa	B	230
Initiate antenatal surveillance initiated at 30 to 32 weeks' gestation or earlier if uteroplacental insufficiency is suspected.	–	GPP	–
Labor and Delivery			
Deliver near term. Avoid postdates.	–	GPP	–
Intensive/high dependency care may be necessary.	–	GPP	–
Take special precautions to ensure would healing if cesarean section delivery.	–	GPP	–
Postnatal			
Provide initial care in intensive/high dependency care setting.	–	GPP	–
Review dosage of drugs and resume maintenance medications.	–	GPP	–

MYASTHENIA GRAVIS

Myasthenia gravis (MG) is an autoimmune disorder affecting neuromuscular transmission, resulting in variable weakness and fatigability of skeletal muscle. Increasing weakness with repetitive use of the muscle(s) is the characteristic feature. Occurring in only 2 to 10 per 100,000 individuals, MG affects twice as many women as men, with an onset usually in the second or third decade in women.[240,241] The immediate cause of the disease is probably an autoimmune attack on the acetylcholine receptor complex of the neuromuscular junction. Serum autoantibodies against acetylcholine receptors (anti-AChR) are found in the serum of 85% of patients with MG.[242] The disease can be transferred passively to laboratory animals by the injection of IgG from affected individuals.[243] Accordingly, 10% to 20% of infants born to women with MG show signs of neonatal MG, thought to be caused by the transplacental passive transfer of antibodies from mother to child.[244,245]

Ocular muscle weakness resulting in diplopia or eyelid ptosis is the usual presenting problem. Some patients have difficulty with chewing or talking. In a large majority of patients, MG progresses from ocular to generalized skeletal muscle involvement over a 1- to 2-year period. Any trunk or limb muscle may be involved, but the neck flexors, deltoids, and wrist extensors are notable. Death results from severe respiratory muscle fatigue. Muscle weakness varies throughout the day but is usually worse toward the end of the day. The long-term course of disease is likewise variable and is characterized by periodic fluctuations in severity. For unclear reasons, MG tends to be worsened by emotional distress, systemic illness, and increased temperature (fever, hot weather).

Pathogenesis of Myasthenia Gravis

It is apparent that the pathophysiology of disease is not simply the blockade of AChR by antibody. The muscle endplate, wherein the AChR resides, is misshapen and bears a reduced number of AChR.[246] This is presumed to be due to autoimmune damage, perhaps mediated through complement destruction. The net result is a diminished depolarization response to a normal amount of released acetylcholine at the postsynaptic membrane.

Abnormalities of the thymus are found in most patients with MG. In total, 75% have lymph follicle hyperplasia and 10% to 15% have lymphoblastic or epithelial thymic tumors. Thymectomy results in remission in 35% and improvement in 50% of patients.[247] These observations suggest that MG may be due to (1) an autoimmune attack on the antigens common to the thymus and motor endplate, or (2) abnormal clone(s) of immune cells in the thymus.

Treatment of Myasthenia Gravis

Myasthenia gravis is treatable but not curable. The use of anticholinesterase drugs is reportedly safe during pregnancy. Pyridostigmine, an analogue of neostigmine, is the most commonly used anticholinesterase medication. These medications impede degradation of acetylcholine and bring about improvement in muscle function. Some patients with MG may only respond to immunosuppressive therapy with corticosteroids, azathioprine, and cyclosporine.[247] In the occasional patient with refractory MG, IVIG and plasmapheresis have been used with some success.[240]

Diagnostic Evaluation of Myasthenia Gravis

The diagnosis of MG rests on the clinical presentation, physical examination, and confirmatory diagnostic procedures. Repetitive use of the muscle under study results in apparent exhaustion. The muscle vigor can be dramatically restored with short-acting anticholinesterase drugs, such as edrophonium in doses of 210 mg given by intravenous injection. More sophisticated tests are now available, including single-fiber electromyography and repetitive nerve stimulation studies.

Risks of Myasthenia Gravis in Pregnancy

Complications of Myasthenia Gravis in Pregnancy

Several pregnancy-related physiologic changes may have detrimental effects on MG. Nausea, vomiting, altered gastrointestinal absorption, expanded plasma volume, and increased renal clearance require adjustment of anticholinesterase throughout pregnancy. Elevation of the maternal diaphragm by the gravid uterus causes hypoventilation of the lower portions of the lungs, which exacerbates respiratory compromise in some women with MG. Maternal predisposition to infections such as pyelonephritis can precipitate an exacerbation of MG. Increased physical exertion in the second and third trimesters and the emotional stress of pregnancy itself may also result in MG exacerbation.

The course of MG during pregnancy is highly variable. Cartlidge[248] recommends postponement of pregnancy in women recently diagnosed with MG because this period represents the time of greatest risk. In an extensive review, approximately 40% of women with MG had exacerbation of their disease during pregnancy; approximately 30% had no change and 30% had postpartum exacerbations that were frequently sudden and serious in nature.[249] Moreover, of the approximately 30% of MG patients whose disease remained unchanged during pregnancy, several had significant postpartum exacerbations. In the most recent review that included both patients who were in remission prior to pregnancy and patients who were taking therapy, exacerbations occurred in 10 of 54 pregnancies (19%), improvement in

12 (22%), and no change in 32 (59%).[242] Plauche found an overall maternal mortality of 4% (9 of 225 reported cases).[249] The majority of these (7 of 9) were due to refractory MG.

Obstetric Complications in Myasthenia Gravis

The rates of miscarriage and fetal death in pregnancies complicated by MG do not appear to be significantly different from those of the normal population.[240,250] However, early series suggested preterm birth in up to two thirds of patients with MG,[250–253] and anticholinesterase drugs are thought to have an oxytocic action.[254] However, in the most recent and largest series to date, there was a difference in the prevalence of preterm birth and low birth weight in 54 MG patients compared to the general population.[240]

The transplacental passage of anti-AChR antibodies can lead to fetal or neonatal MG. Only about 10% to 15% of infants born to mothers with MG show signs of MG.[255] The relative infrequency of fetal involvement was due to alpha-fetoprotein, which has been shown to inhibit the binding of anti-AChR to AchR.[256,257] Most infants with neonatal MG have high concentrations of anti-AChR in their circulation.

The diagnosis of neonatal MG is made by observation of poor sucking, feeble cry, and respiratory difficulties that respond to edrophonium. Neonatal MG is transient, usually abating over a period of 1 to 4 weeks. The symptoms usually develop within the first several days of life, but are often absent initially, perhaps because of the presence of alpha-fetoprotein.[257] When properly recognized, the disease is easily managed with supportive care and anticholinesterase drugs. There does not appear to be any correlation between the risk of neonatal MG and severity of maternal MG manifestations[242] or the level of maternal anti-AChR antibodies.[258,259] However, there does appear to be a relationship between neonatal levels and the severity of neonatal MG.[242] Arthrogryposis multiplex congenita (AMC), a nonprogressive congenital contraction disorder thought to result from poor fetal movement, has rarely been reported in infants born to women with MG.[255,260,261] There is some evidence that plasmapheresis and immunosuppressive therapy may reduce the recurrence of AMC in MG patients with a prior neonatal death presumably due to AMC.

Management Options

Prepregnancy

Adjustment of medication to establish quiescence/control of the disease process is vital before pregnancy. Patients should be appropriately educated regarding the need for close supervision, the expected increase in fatigue, and the potential for respiratory compromise (especially late in pregnancy); the fetal risks of preterm delivery, the potential for associated anomalies, and the transient nature of neonatal MG should be discussed.

Prenatal

Treatment is frequently necessary before, during, and after pregnancy to ensure maternal and fetal well-being. Pregnancy-related changes in drug absorption, increased renal clearance, and expanded plasma volume may require alterations in medication in order to maintain adequate drug levels. The first line of therapy is quaternary ammonium compounds with anticholinesterase activity. Although neostigmine (Prostigmin) was the first such drug to be used, its short half-life was a major drawback. Pyridostigmine (Mestinon), which has a longer half-life, is the most popular long-acting medication currently used for maintenance therapy of MG. There is now a sustained-release form of the drug (Mestinon Timespan, 180 mg), but its popularity is limited by concerns about irregular absorption and drug preparation. Oral pyridostigmine is typically given in doses of 240 to 1500 mg/day in divided doses at 3- to 8-hour intervals. When used, the sustained-release preparation is typically given as a single bedtime dose of 180 to 540 mg. If the patient requires more drug, as is often the case with advancing pregnancy, it is best to first shorten the interval between doses. If this fails to control symptoms, the dose of pyridostigmine should be increased by increments of 15 to 30 mg. Such maneuvers usually lead to adequate control of MG during pregnancy. The most common side effects of these medications are due to the accumulation of acetylcholine (muscarinic effects). These include gastrointestinal symptoms (nausea, vomiting, cramping, diarrhea) and increased oral and bronchial secretions. Overdose of anticholinesterase drugs results in the rare so-called *cholinergic crisis*, which paradoxically includes muscle weakness and respiratory failure.

Glucocorticoids are effective in most patients with MG. Most authorities prefer high doses (prednisone 60 to 80 mg/day) to start; the dose is tapered over many months after improvement is noted. The disease may transiently worsen soon after the steroids are started; for this reason, patients should be hospitalized for steroid therapy. Unfortunately, remission appears to be maintained only if the patient continues on steroids, and withdrawal of steroids may cause myasthenic exacerbations. For these reasons, pregnant MG patients should maintain glucocorticoid therapy through pregnancy and the postpartum period. Some authors believe that glucocorticoid-induced remission is a particularly good time for pregnancy in patients with MG.

Plasmapheresis has been used with success in severe MG. Most patients were also taking glucocorticoids. There is one case report of using plasmapheresis to successfully treat MG in pregnancy.[262] It may be that maternal plasmapheresis might be the treatment of choice in MG pregnancies in which the fetus has markedly reduced or absent fetal movement predisposing it to AMC.

Thymectomy may result in improvement in many patients with MG by mechanisms that are unknown. However, resorting to thymectomy during pregnancy would seem imprudent because of frequent long delays before improvement and perioperative maternal and fetal concerns.

Patients with MG should be seen relatively frequently throughout pregnancy, every 2 weeks in the first and second trimester, and every week in the third trimester. Undue emotional and physical stress are to be avoided, since they may result in exacerbation of MG. The patient and physician should be alert to the possibility of preterm labor, and appropriate preventive steps instituted. Although care must be individualized, limiting exercise and work is probably in order for many patients. Infections may also result in exacerbation of MG. Respiratory and urinary tract infections must be identified and treated promptly.

Fetal involvement with MG is suspected by poor fetal movement and hydramnios. This is not treatable in utero. Differentiating poor fetal movement due to MG from that due to fetal hypoxemia may be difficult, but normal fetal heart rate tests, especially a negative contraction stress test, and a normal biophysical profile score, are reassuring.

Labor and Delivery

The management of labor and delivery in patients with MG requires limitation of emotional and physical stress and the appropriate use of parenteral anticholinesterase drugs. Neostigmine can be given subcutaneously, intramuscularly, or intravenously. As a rough guide, 60 mg oral pyridostigmine is equivalent to 0.5 mg IV neostigmine and 1.5 mg subcutaneous neostigmine. The usual dose of parenteral neostigmine is 0.5 to 2.5 mg. Maximal effects on skeletal muscle may occur 2 to 30 minutes after intramuscular injection; the effects last for about 2.5 hours. Pyridostigmine can be given intramuscularly or very slowly intravenously. The usual dose is 2 mg (approximately 1/30 of the usual oral dose) every 2 to 3 hours. The course of the first stage of labor in patients with MG is not altered because MG does not affect smooth muscle.[245] The second stage of labor could be affected by the weakened material expulsive efforts, although the average duration of labor in MG patients is normal.

It is important to recognize that certain medications that may be used in the management of obstetric concerns are contraindicated in patients with MG. These are listed in Table 44–11. Magnesium sulfate is absolutely contraindicated because it further interferes with the neuromuscular blockade of MG. Preterm labor can probably be treated with beta-sympathomimetics,[260] but the associated hypokalemia should be carefully avoided. A small number of patients with MG have an associated cardiomyopathy, which could increase the risks of beta-sympathomimetics.

Because the patient with MG is particularly sensitive to neuromuscular drugs, analgesic and anesthetic considerations are important before the onset of labor. All patients with MG should be seen in consultation with an anesthesiologist early in the course of pregnancy. Epidural anesthesia is probably best because it limits the need for analgesia, may help prevent anxiety and fatigue, and is excellent for forceps procedures. Amide-type local anesthesia agents are used.[263] Some authors recommend general endotracheal anesthesia for cesarean section in patients with respiratory involvement. Myasthenic crises requiring ventilatory support may be precipitated by the stress of labor and delivery, an inadvertent change in medication, or surgery. Rarely, cholinergic crises may result from overdosage with anticholinesterase drugs. These patients have prominent muscarinic symptoms in addition to respiratory weakness. In all patients with MG, labor and delivery management should include the immediate availability of personnel and equipment for ventilatory support and airway maintenance. Postoperative care may be best accomplished in an intensive care setting.

Postnatal

It would be difficult to find a patient, following delivery, who is not fatigued and weakened. Differentiating this normal state of affairs from exacerbation of MG may be difficult without objective testing. Drug dosages may need to be rapidly adjusted, in particular downward, as the effects of the volume expansion of pregnancy clear.

TABLE 44–11

Medications that May Exacerbate or Cause Muscle Weakness in Patients with Myasthenia Gravis

Magnesium salts	Cholistin
Aminoglycosides	Polymyxin B
Halothane	Quinine
Propranolol	Lincomycin
Tetracycline	Procainamide
Barbiturates	Ether
Lithium salts	Penicillamine
Trichlorethylene	

SUMMARY OF MANAGEMENT OPTIONS
Myasthenia Gravis

Management Options	Quality of Evidence	Strength of Recommendation	References
Prepregnancy			
Counsel regarding risk of exacerbation during pregnancy and risk of medication exposure.	III	B	240
Review therapy; establish good control of MG; adjust maintenance medications.	III	B	249–255
If possible, discontinue cytotoxic medications before conception. This should be done only under careful supervision.	III	B	–
Consider thymectomy in symptomatic women who are refractory to therapy.	III	B	–
Prenatal			
Institute joint obstetrician and physician surveillance.	III	B	252
Continue pre-existing drugs:			
• Anticholinesterase	III	B	240
• Steroids			
• Azathioprine			
Consider plasmapheresis and IVIG in refractory cases.	III	B	240
Maintain fetal surveillance, especially activity (?biophysical profile score).	–	GPP	–
Initiate antenatal surveillance at 30 to 32 weeks' gestation.	–	GPP	–
Avoid/minimize physical/emotional stress.	III	B	249–255
Labor and Delivery			
Minimize stress.	III	B	–
Continue anticholinesterase drugs (parenteral).	III	B	–
Prescribe intravenous glucocorticoids for delivery in patients who have received maintenance or steroid bursts during pregnancy.	–	GPP	–
Regional analgesia preferable to narcotics for pain relief and general anesthesia.	III	B	249–255
Consult with experienced anesthetists if general anesthesia (advisable to consult in prenatal period).	III	B	249–255
Assisted second stage more likely.	III	B	249–255
Avoid magnesium sulfate (and other contraindicated drugs) in patients with preeclampsia.	IV	C	254
Postnatal			
Provide special care and surveillance of newborn; may need short-term anticholinesterases.	III	B	240, 259
Review dosage of drugs.	III	B	240

CONCLUSIONS

- Autoimmune disorders in pregnancy carry risks to mother (especially miscarriage, preeclampsia, and thromboembolism) and fetus (especially IUGR and fetal death); the newborn can show residual effects of transplacental maternal antibody passage.
- Prepregnancy care should cover explaining the risks of the condition and optimizing medical control, ideally using drugs that are safe in pregnancy.

CONCLUSIONS (Continued)

- Prenatal care largely focuses on maintenance of disease control, anticoagulation where indicated, and surveillance for preeclampsia in the mother and uteroplacental disease in the fetus.
- Labor and delivery are usually determined by the development of complications; anticoagulation will need to be reduced in the short term.
- After delivery the priority is to maintain vigilance for maternal exacerbation.
- Maternal therapy should be adjusted as indicated.
- Neonatal surveillance and management is required if maternal antibodies persist.

REFERENCES

1. Beeson PB: Age and sex associations of 40 autoimmune diseases. Am J Med 1994;96:457–462.
2. Ahmed SA, Dauphinee MJ, Talal N: Effects of short term administration of sex hormones on normal and autoimmune mice. J Immunol 1985;134:204–210.
3. Blank M, Mendlovic S, Fricke H, et al: Sex hormone involvement in the induction of experimental systemic lupus erythematosus by a pathogenic anti-DNA idiotype in naive mice. J Rheumatol 1990;17:311–317.
4. Block SR, Winfield JB, Lockshin MD, et al: Studies of twins with systemic lupus erythematosus: A review of the literature and presentation of 12 additional sets. Am J Med 1975;59:533–552.
5. Jungers P, Dougados M, Pellissier C, et al: Influence of oral contraceptive therapy on the activity of systemic lupus erythematosus. Arthritis Rheum 1982;25:618–623.
6. Mackworth-Young CG, Parke AL, Morley KD, et al: Sex hormones in male patients with systemic lupus erythematosus: A comparison with other disease groups. Eur J Rheumatol Inflamm 1983;6:228–232.
7. Kotzin BL: Systemic lupus erythematosus. Cell 1996;85:303–306.
8. Petri M, Howard D, Repke J: Frequency of lupus flare in pregnancy: The Hopkins lupus pregnancy center experience. Arthritis Rheum 1991;34:1538–1545.
9. Hayslett JP: The effect of systemic lupus erythematosus on pregnancy and pregnancy outcome. Am J Reprod Immunol 1992;28:199–204.
10. Ter Borg EJ, Hurst G, Hummel EJ, et al: Measurements of increases in anti-double-stranded DNA antibody levels as a predictor of disease exacerbation in SLE: A long term, prospective study. Arthritis Rheum 1990;33:634–643.
11. Bootsma H, Spronk PE, Derksen R, et al: Prevention of relapses in systemic lupus erythematosus. Lancet 1995;345:1595–1599.
12. Tomer Y, Viegas OAC, Swissa M, et al: Levels of lupus autoantibodies in pregnant SLE patients: Correlations with disease activity and pregnancy outcome. Clin Exper Rheumatol 1996;14:275–280.
13. Tan EM, Cohen AS, Fries JF, et al: The 1982 revised criteria for the classification of systemic lupus erythematosus. Arthritis Rheum 1982;25:1271–1277.
14. Hochberg MC: Updating the American College of Rheumatology revised criteria for the classification of systemic lupus erythematosus. Arthritis Rheum 1997;40:1725.
15. Garenstein M, Pollach VE, Kark RM: Systemic lupus erythematosus and pregnancy. N Engl J Med 1962;267:165–169.
16. Estes D, Larson DL: Systemic lupus erythematosus and pregnancy. Clin Obstet Gynecol 1965;8:307–321.
17. Lockshin MD, Reinits E, Druzin ML, et al: Case-control prospective study demonstrating absence of lupus exacerbation during or after pregnancy. Am J Med 1984;77:893–898.
18. Meehan RT, Dorsey JK: Pregnancy among patients with systemic lupus erythematosus receiving immunosuppressive therapy. J Rheumatol 1987;14:252–258.
19. Mintz R, Niz J, Gutierrez G, et al: Prospective study of pregnancy in systemic lupus erythematosus: Results of a multidisciplinary approach. J Rheumatol 1986;13:732–739.
20. Lockshin MD: Pregnancy does not cause systemic lupus erythematosus to worsen. Arthritis Rheum 1989;32:665–670.
21. Urowitz MB, Gladman DD, Farewell VT, et al: Lupus and pregnancy studies. Arthritis Rheum 1993;36:1392–1397.
22. Ruiz-Irastorza G, Lima F, Alves J, et al: Increased rate of lupus flare during pregnancy and the puerperium: A prospective study of 78 pregnancies. Br J Rheumatol 1996;35:133–138.
23. Kleinman D, Katz VL, Kuller JA: Perinatal outcomes in women with systemic lupus erythematosus. J Perinatol 1998;18:178–182.
24. Johns KR, Morand EF, Littlejohn GO: Pregnancy outcome in systemic lupus erythematosus (SLE): A review of 54 cases. Aust N Z J Med 1998;28:18–22.
25. Derksen RH, Bruinse HW, de Groot PG, Kater L: Pregnancy in systemic lupus erythematosus: A prospective study. Lupus 1994;3:149–155.
26. Aggarwal N, Sawhney H, Vasishta K, et al: Pregnancy in patients with systemic lupus erythematosus. Aust N Z J Obstet Gynaecol 1999;39:28–30.
27. Georgiou PE, Politi EN, Katsimbri P, et al: Outcome of lupus pregnancy: A controlled study. Rheumatol (Oxford) 2000;39:1014–1019.
28. Cortes-Hernandez J, Ordi-Ros J, Labrador M, et al: Predictors of poor renal outcome in patients with lupus nephritis treated with combined pulses of cyclophosphamide and methylprednisolone. Lupus 2003;12(4):287–296.
29. Huong DL, Wechsler B, Vauthier-Brouzes D, et al: Outcome of planned pregnancies in systemic lupus erythematosus: A prospective study on 62 pregnancies. Br J Rheumatol 1997;36:772–777.
30. Wong KL, Chan FY, Lee CP: Outcome of pregnancy in patients with systemic lupus erythematosus. A prospective study. Arch Intern Med 1991;151:269–273.
31. Petri M: Hopkins Lupus Pregnancy Center: 1987 to 1996. Rheum Dis Clin North Am 1997;23:1–13.
32. Nossent HC, Koldingsnes W: Long-term efficacy of azathioprine treatment for proliferative lupus nephritis. Rheumatol (Oxford) 2000;39:969–974.
33. Tincani A, Faden D, Tarantini M, et al: Systemic lupus erythematosus and pregnancy: A prospective study. Clin Exp Rheumatol 1992;10:439–446.
34. Hayslett JP, Lynn RI: Effect of pregnancy in patients with lupus nephropathy. Kidney Int 1980;18:207–220.
35. Jungers P, Dougados M, Pelissier C, et al: Lupus nephropathy and pregnancy. Arch Intern Med 1982;142:771–776.

36. Bobrie G, Liote F, Houillier P, et al: Pregnancy in lupus nephritis and related disorders. Am J Kidney Dis 1987;9:339–343.
37. Bear R: Pregnancy and lupus nephritis: A detailed report of six cases with a review of the literature. Obstet Gynecol 1976;47: 715–718.
38. Julkunen H: Pregnancy and lupus nephritis. Scand J Urol Nephrol 2001;35:319–327.
39. Oviasu E, Hicks J, Cameron JS: The outcome of pregnancy in women with lupus nephritis. Lupus 1999;1:19–25.
40. Julkunen H, Kaaja R, Palosuo T, et al: Pregnancy in lupus nephropathy. Acta Obstet Gynecol Scand 1993;72:258–263.
41. Packham DK, Lam SS, Nichols K, et al: Lupus nephritis and pregnancy. Quart J Med 1992;83:315–324.
42. Moroni G, Quaglini S, Banfi G, et al: Pregnancy in lupus nephritis. Am J Kidney Dis 2002;40:713–720.
43. Fine LG, Barnett EV, Danovitch GM, et al: Systemic lupus erythematosus in pregnancy. Arch Intern Med 1981;94:667–677.
44. Imbasciati E, Surian M, Bottino W, et al: Lupus nephropathy and pregnancy. Nephron 1984;36:46–51.
45. Devoe LD, Taylor RL: Systemic lupus erythematosus in pregnancy. Am J Obstet Gynecol 1979;135:473–479.
46. Ruiz-Irastorza G, Khamashta MA, Gordon C, et al: Measuring systemic lupus erythematosus activity during pregnancy: Validation of the lupus activity index in pregnancy scale. Arthritis Rheum 2004;51:78–82.
47. Devoe LD, Loy GL: Serum complement levels and perinatal outcome in pregnancies complicated by systemic lupus erythematosus. Obstet Gynecol 1984;63:796–800.
48. Buyon JP, Cronstein BN, Morris M, et al: Serum complement values (C3 and C4) to differentiate between systemic lupus activity and preeclampsia. Am J Med 1986;81:194–200.
49. Lockshin MD, Qamar T, Redecha P, Harpel PC: Hypocomplementemia with low C1s-C1 inhibitor complex in systemic lupus erythematosus. Arthritis Rheum 1986;29:1467–1472.
50. Nossent HC, Swaak TJ: Systemic lupus erythematosus. VI. Analysis of the interrelationship with pregnancy. J Rheumatol 1990;17:771–776.
51. Shibata S, Sasaki T, Hirabayashi Y, et al: Risk factors in the pregnancy of patients with systemic lupus erythematosus: Association of hypocomplementaemia with poor prognosis. Ann Rheum Dis 1992;51:619–623.
52. Rubbert A, Pirner K, Wildt L, et al: Pregnancy course and complications in patients with systemic lupus erythematosus. Am J Reprod Immunol 1992;28:205–207.
53. Girardi G, Salmon JB: The role of complement in pregnancy and fetal loss. Autoimmunity 2003;36:19–26.
54. Adelsberg BR: The complement system in pregnancy. Am J Reprod Immunol 1983;4:38–44.
55. Weiner CP, Brandt J: Plasma antithrombin III activity: An aid in the diagnosis of preeclampsia-eclampsia. Am J Obstet Gynecol 1982;142:275–281.
56. Weiner CP, Kwaan HC, Xu C, et al: Antithrombin III activity in women with hypertension during pregnancy. Obstet Gynecol 1985;65:301–306.
57. Mellembakken JR, Hogasen K, Mollnes TE, et al: Increased systemic activation of neutrophils but not complement in preeclampsia. Obstet Gynecol 2001;97:371–374.
58. Lockshin MD, Qamar T, Druzin ML: Hazards of lupus pregnancy. J Rheumatol 1987;14:214.
59. Laskin CA, Bombardier C, Hannah ME, et al: Prednisone and aspirin in women with autoantibodies and unexplained recurrent fetal loss. N Engl J Med 1997;337:148–153.
60. Vaquero E, Lazzarin N, Valensise H, et al: Pregnancy outcome in recurrent spontaneous abortion associated with antiphospholipid antibodies: A comparative study of intravenous immunoglobulin versus prednisone plus low-dose aspirin. Am J Reprod Immunol 2001;45:174–179.
61. Rahman P, Gladman DD, Urowitz MB: Clinical predictors of fetal outcome in systemic lupus erythematosus. J Rheumatol 1998;25:1526–1530.
62. Buchanan NM, Toubi E, Khamashta MA, et al: Hydroxychloroquine and lupus pregnancy: Review of a series of 36 cases. Ann Rheum Dis 1996;55:486–488.
63. Khamashta MA, Buchanan NM, Hughes GR: The use of hydroxychloroquine in lupus pregnancy: The British experience. Lupus 1996;5(Suppl 1):S65–S66.
64. Klinger G, Morad Y, Westall CA, et al: Ocular toxicity and antenatal exposure to chloroquine or hydroxychloroquine for rheumatic diseases. Lancet 2001;358:813–814.
65. Motta M, Tincani A, Faden D, et al: Antimalarial agents in pregnancy. Lancet 2002;359:524–525.
66. Costedoat-Chalumeau N, Amoura Z, Duhaut P, et al: Safety of hydroxychloroquine in pregnant patients with connective tissue diseases: A study of 133 cases compared with a control group. Arthritis Rheum 2003;48:3207–3211.
67. Hart C, Naughton RF: The ototoxicity of chloroquine phosphate. Arch Otolaryngol 1964;80:407.
68. Nylander U: Ocular damage in chloroquine therapy. Acta Ophthalmol 1967;45(Suppl 92):5.
69. Levy RA, Vilela VS, Cataldo MJ, et al: Hydroxychloroquine (HCQ) in lupus pregnancy: Double-blind and placebo-controlled study. Lupus 2001;10:401–404.
70. Armenti VT, Ahlswede KM, Ahlswede BA, et al: National transplantation pregnancy registry: Outcomes of 154 pregnancies in cyclosporine-treated female kidney transplant recipients. Transplantation 1994;57:502.
71. Armenti VT, Moritz MJ, Davison JM: Drug safety issues in pregnancy following transplantation and immunosuppression: Effects and outcomes. Drug Saf 1998;19:219–232.
72. Cote CJ, Meuwissen HJ, Pickering RJ: Effects on the neonate of prednisone and azathioprine administered to the mother during pregnancy. J Pediatr 1974;85:324.
73. Ujhazy E, Balonova T, Durisova M, et al: Teratogenicity of cyclophosphamide in New Zealand white rabbits. Neoplasma 1993;40:45.
74. Kirshon B, Wasserstrum N, Willis R, et al: Teratogenic effects of first-trimester cyclophosphamide therapy. Obstet Gynecol 1988;72:462–464.
75. Enns GM, Roeder E, Chan RT, et al: Apparent cyclophosphamide (Cytoxan) embryopathy: A distinct phenotype? Am J Med Genet 1999;86:237–241.
76. Ruiz-Irastorza G, Khamashta MA, Castellino G, Hughes GR: Systemic lupus erythematosus. Lancet 2001;357:1027–1032.
77. Stuart JJ, Gross SJ, Elrad H, et al: Effects of acetylsalicylic acid ingestion on maternal and neonatal hemostasis. N Engl J Med 1982;307:909.
78. Macones GA, Robinson CA: Is there justification for using indomethacin in preterm labor? An analysis of neonatal risks and benefits. Am J Obstet Gynecol 1997;177:819–824.
79. Vermillion ST, Newman RB: Recent indomethacin tocolysis is not associated with neonatal complications in preterm infants. Am J Obstet Gynecol 1999;181:1083–1086.
80. Pryde PG, Besinger RE, Gianopoulos JG, Mittendorf R: Adverse and beneficial effects of tocolytic therapy. Semin Perinatol 2001;25:316–340.
81. Ostensen M, Villiger PM: Nonsteroidal anti-inflammatory drugs in systemic lupus erythematosus. Lupus 2001;10: 135–139.
82. Isenberg DA, Morrow WJ, Snaith ML: Methylprednisolone pulse therapy in the treatment of systemic lupus erythematosus. Ann Rheum Dis 1982;41:347–351.
83. Sesso R, Monteiro M, Sato E, et al: A controlled trial of pulse cyclophosphamide versus pulse methylprednisolone in severe lupus nephritis. Lupus 1994;3:107–112.

84. Nossent HC, Koldingsnes W: Long-term efficacy of azathioprine treatment for proliferative lupus nephritis. Rheumatol (Oxford) 2000;39:969–974.
85. Austin HA, Balow JE: Treatment of lupus nephritis. Semin Nephrol 2000;20:265–276.
86. Rauova L, Lukac J, Levy Y, et al: High-dose intravenous immunoglobulins for lupus nephritis—a salvage immunomodulation. Lupus 2001;10:209–213.
87. Nicklin JL: Systemic lupus erythematosus and pregnancy at the Royal Women's Hospital, Brisbane 1979–1989. Aust N Z J Obstet Gynaecol 1991;31:128–133.
88. Yasmeen S, Wilkins EE, Field NT, et al:. Pregnancy outcomes in women with systemic lupus erythematosus. J Matern Fetal Med 2001;10:91–96.
89. Julkunen H, Jouhikainen T, Kaaja R, et al: Fetal outcome in lupus pregnancy: A retrospective case-control study of 242 pregnancies in 112 patients. Lupus 1993;2:125.
90. Fisher KA, Luger A, Spargo BH, et al: Hypertension in pregnancy: Clinical-pathologic correlations and remote prognosis. Medicine 1981;60:267–276.
91. Oviasu E, Hicks J, Cameron JS: The outcome of pregnancy in women with lupus nephritis. Lupus 1991;1:19–25.
92. Ramsey-Goldman R, Kutzer JE, Kuller LH, et al: Pregnancy outcome and anti-cardiolipin antibody in women with systemic lupus erythematosus. Am J Epidemiol 1993;138:1057–1069.
93. Fraga A, Mintz G, Orozco J, et al: Sterility and fertility rates, fetal wastage and maternal morbidity in systemic lupus erythematosus. J Rheumatol 1974;1:293–298.
94. McHugh NJ, Reilly PA, McHugh LA: Pregnancy outcome and autoantibodies in connective tissue disease. J Rheumatol 1989;16:42–46.
95. Zulman Jl, Talal N, Hoffman GS, et al: Problems associated with the management of pregnancies in patients with systemic lupus erythematosus. J Rheumatol 1979;7:37–49.
96. Jungers P, Dougados M, Pellissier C, et al: Influence of oral contraceptive therapy on the activity of systemic lupus erythematosus. Arthritis Rheum 1982;25:618–623.
97. Gimovsky ML, Montoro M, Paul RH: Pregnancy outcome in women with systemic lupus erythematosus. Obstet Gynecol 1984;63: 686–692.
98. Siampoulou-Marridou A, Manoussakis MN, Mavrıdıs AK, et al: Outcome of pregnancy in patients with autoimmune rheumatic disease before the disease onset. Ann Rheum Dis 1988; 47:982–987.
99. Huong DL, Wechsler B, Vauthier-Brouzes D, et al: Pregnancy in past or present lupus nephritis: A study of 32 pregnancies from a single centre. Ann Rheum Dis 2001;60(6):599–604.
100. Petri M, Allbritton J: Fetal outcome of lupus pregnancy: A retrospective case-control study of the Hopkins Lupus Cohort. J Rheumatol 1993;20:650–656.
101. Lima F, Khamashta MA, Buchanan NM, et al: A study of sixty pregnancies in patients with the antiphospholipid syndrome. Clin Exper Rheumatol 1996;14:131–136.
102. Huong DL, Wechsler B, Vauthier-Brouzes D, et al: Pregnancy in past or present lupus nephritis: A study of 32 pregnancies from a single centre. Ann Rheum Dis 2001;60:599–604.
103. Lockshin MD, Druzin ML, Goei S, et al: Antibody to cardiolipin as a predictor of fetal distress or death in pregnant patients with systemic lupus erythematosus. N Engl J Med 1985;313:152–156.
104. Englert HJ, Derue GM, Loizou S, et al: Pregnancy and lupus: Prognostic indicators and response to treatment. Quart J Med 1988;66:125–136.
105. Cortes-Hernandez J, Ordi-Ros J, Povedes F, et al: Clinical predictors of fetal and maternal outcome in systemic lupus erythematosus: A prospective study of 103 pregnancies. Rheumatology 2002;41(6):643–650.
106. Varner MW, Meehan RT, Syrop CH, et al: Pregnancy in patients with systemic lupus erythematosus. Am J Obstet Gynecol 1983;145:1025–1037.
107. Houser MT, Fish AJ, Tagatz GE, et al: Pregnancy and systemic lupus erythematosus. Am J Obstet Gynecol 1980;138:409–413.
108. Johnson MJ, Petri M, Witter FR, et al: Evaluation of preterm delivery in a systemic lupus erythematosus pregnancy clinic. Obstet Gynecol 1995;86:396–399.
109. Lockshin MD, Bonfa E, Elkon D, Druzin ML: Neonatal lupus risk to newborns of mothers with systemic lupus erythematosus. Arthritis Rheum 1988;31:697–701.
110. Neiman AR, Lee LA, Weston WL, Buyon JP: Cutaneous manifestations of neonatal lupus without heart block: Characteristics of mothers and children enrolled in a national registry. J Pediatr 2000;137:674–680.
111. Buyon JP, Hiebert R, Copel J, et al: Autoimmune-associated congenital heart block: Demographics, mortality, morbidity and recurrence rates obtained from a national neonatal lupus registry. J Am Coll Cardiol 1998;31:1658–1666.
112. Lawrence S, Luy L, Laxer R, et al: The health of mothers of children with cutaneous neonatal lupus erythematosus differs from that of mothers of children with congenital heart block. Am J Med 2000;108:705–709.
113. Scott JS, Maddison PJ, Taylor MV, et al: Connective tissue disease, antibodies to ribonucleoprotein and congenital heart disease. N Engl J Med 1983;309:209–212.
114. Lee LA: Neonatal lupus erythematosus. J Invest Dermatol 1993; 100:9S–13S.
115. Reed BR, Lee LA, Harmon C, et al: Autoantibodies to SS-A/Ro in infants with congenital heart block. Pediatr 1983;103:889–891.
116. Buyon JP, Clancy RM: Neonatal lupus syndromes. Curr Opin Rheumatol 2003;15:535–541.
117. Buyon JP, Winchester RJ, Slade SG, et al: Identification of mothers at risk for congenital heart block and other neonatal lupus syndromes in their children: Comparison of enzyme-linked immunosorbent assay and immunoblot for measurement of anti-SS-A/Ro and anti-SS-B/La antibodies. Arthritis Rheum 1993;36:1263–1273.
118. Lee LA, Frank MB, McCubbin VR, Reichlin M: Autoantibodies of neonatal lupus erythematosus. Invest Dermatol 1994; 102:963–966.
119. Waltuck J, Buyon JP: Autoantibody associated complete heart block: Outcome in mothers and children. Ann Intern Med 1994;120:544–551.
120. Barclay CS, French MAH, Ross LD, Sokol RJ. Successful pregnancy following steroid therapy and plasma exchange in women with anti-Ro (SS-A) antibodies: Case report. BJOG 1987;94: 369–371.
121. Kaaja R, Julkunen H, Ammala P, et al: Congenital heart block: Successful prophylactic treatment with intravenous gamma globulin and corticosteroid therapy. Am J Obstet Gynecol 1991;165:1333–1334.
122. Carreira PE, Gutierrez-Larraya F, Gomez-Reino JJ: Successful intrauterine therapy with dexamethasone for fetal myocarditis and heart block in a woman with systemic lupus erythematosus. J Rheumatol 1993;20:1204–1207.
123. Saleeb S, Copel J, Friedman D, Buyon JP: Comparison of treatment with fluorinated glucocorticoids to the natural history of autoantibody-associated congenital heart block: Retrospective review of the research registry for neonatal lupus. Arthritis Rheum 1999;42:2335–2345.
124. Shinohara K, Miyagawa S, Fujita T, et al: Neonatal lupus erythematosus: Results of maternal corticosteroid therapy. Obstet Gynecol 1999;93:952–957.
125. Eronen M, Heikkila P, Teramo K: Congenital complete heart block in the fetus: Hemodynamic features, antenatal treatment, and outcome in six cases. Pediatr Cardiol 2001;22:385–392.

126. Druzin ML, Locksrun M, Edersheim TG, et al: Second trimester fetal monitoring and preterm delivery in pregnancies with systemic lupus erythematosus and/or circulating anticoagulant Am J Obstet Gynecol 1987;157:1503–1510.
127. Wilson WA, Gharavi AE, Koike T, et al: International consensus statement on preliminary classification criteria for definite antiphospholipid syndrome: Report of an international workshop. Arthritis Rheum 1999;42:1309–1311.
128. Roubey RA, Eisenberg RA, Harper MF, Winfield JB: "Anticardiolipin" autoantibodies recognize β2-glycoprotein I in the absence of phospholipid. Importance of Ag density and bivalent binding. Immunol 1995;154:954–960.
129. Khamashta MA, Cuadrado MJ, Mujic F, et al: The management of thrombosis in the antiphospholipid-antibody syndrome. N Engl J Med 1995;332:993–997.
130. Branch DW, Silver RM, Blackwell JL, et al: Outcome of treated pregnancies in women with antiphospholipid syndrome: An update of the Utah experience. Obstet Gynecol 1992; 80:614–620.
131. Levine J, Branch DW, Rauch J: The antiphospholipid syndrome. N Engl J Med 2002;346:752–763.
132. Meroni PL, Raschi E, Camera M, et al: Endothelial activation by aPL: A potential pathogenetic mechanism for the clinical manifestations of the syndrome. J Autoimmun 2000;15:237–240.
133. Vaarala O, Alfthan G, Jauhiainen M, et al: Crossreaction between antibodies to oxidised low-density lipoprotein and to cardiolipin in systemic lupus erythematosus. Lancet 1993;341: 923–925.
134. Hörkkö S, Miller E, Dudl E, et al: Antiphospholipid antibodies are directed against epitopes of oxidized phospholipids: recognition of cardiolipin by monoclonal antibodies to epitopes of oxidized low density lipoprotein. J Clin Invest 1996;98:815–825.
135. Shi W, Chong BH, Chesterman CN: β2-Glycoprotein I is a requirement for anticardiolipin antibodies binding to activated platelets: Differences with lupus anticoagulants. Blood 1993;81:1255–1262.
136. Price BE, Rauch J, Shia MA, et al: Antiphospholipid autoantibodies manner. J Immunol 1996;157:2201–2208.
137. Blank M, Cohen J, Toder V, et al: Induction of antiphospholipid syndrome in naive mice with mouse lupus monoclonal and human polyclonal anticardiolipin antibodies. Proc Natl Acad Sci USA 1991;88:3069–3073.
138. Chamley LW, Pattison NS, McKay EJ, et al: The effect of human anticardiolipin antibodies on murine pregnancy. J Reprod Immunol 1994;27:123–134.
139. Pierangeli SS, Harris EN: In vivo models of thrombosis for the antiphospholipid syndrome. Lupus 1996;5:451–455.
140. Holers VM, Girardi G, et al: Complement C3 activation is required for antiphospholipid antibody-induced fetal loss. J Exp Med 2002;195:211–220.
141. De Wolf F, Carreras LO, Moerman P, et al: Decidual vasculopathy and extensive placental infarction in a patient with repeated thromboembolic accidents, recurrent fetal loss, and a lupus anticoagulant. Am J Obstet Gynecol 1982;142:829–834.
142. Erlendsson K, Steinsson K, Johannsson JH, et al: Relation of antiphospholipid antibody and placental bed inflammatory vascular changes to the outcome of pregnancy in successive pregnancies of 2 women with systemic lupus erythematosus. J Rheumatol 1993;20:1779–1785.
143. Rand JH, Wu X-X, Andree HAM, et al: Pregnancy loss in the antiphospholipid-antibody syndrome—a possible thrombogenic mechanism. N Engl J Med 1997;337:154–160.
144. di Somone N, Meroni PL, del Papa N, et al: Antiphospholipid antibodies affect trophoblast gonadotropin secretion and invasiveness by binding directly and through adhered β2-glycoprotein I. Arthritis Rheum 2000;43:140–150.
145. Rai R, Cohen H, Dave M, Regan L: Randomised controlled trial of aspirin and aspirin plus heparin in pregnant women with recurrent miscarriage associated with phospholipid antibodies (or antiphospholipid antibodies). BMJ 1997;314:253–257.
146. Pattison NS, Chamley LW, McKay EJ, et al: Antiphospholipid antibodies in pregnancy: Prevalence and clinical associations. BJOG 1993;100:909–913.
147. Farquharson RG, Quenby S, Greaves M: Antiphospholipid syndrome in pregnancy: A randomized, controlled trial of treatment. Obstet Gynecol 2002;100:408–413.
148. Silver RM, Draper ML, Scott JR, et al: Clinical consequences of antiphospholipid antibodies: An historic cohort study. Obstet Gynecol 1994;83:372–377.
149. Silver RM, Porter TF, van Leeuwen I, et al: Anticardiolipin antibodies: Clinical consequences of "low titers." Obstet Gynecol 1996;87:494–500.
150. Kutteh WH: Antiphospholipid antibody-associated recurrent pregnancy loss: Treatment with heparin and low-dose aspirin is superior to low-dose aspirin alone. Am J Obstet Gynecol 1996;174:1584–1589.
151. Aoki K, Dudkiewicz AB, Matsuura E, et al: Clinical significance of β_2-glycoprotein I-dependent anticardiolipin antibodies in the reproductive autoimmune failure syndrome: Correlation with conventional antiphospholipid antibody detection systems. Am J Obstet Gynecol 1995;172:926–931.
152. Yetman DL, Kutteh WH: Antiphospholipid antibody panels and recurrent pregnancy loss: Prevalence of anticardiolipin antibodies compared with other antiphospholipid antibodies. Fertil Steril 1996;66:540–546.
153. Branch DW, Silver R, Pierangeli S, et al: Antiphospholipid antibodies other than lupus anticoagulant and anticardiolipin antibodies in women with recurrent pregnancy loss, fertile controls, and antiphospholipid syndrome. Obstet Gynecol 1997; 89:549–555.
154. Bertolaccini ML, Roch B, Amengual O, et al: Multiple antiphospholipid tests do not increase the diagnostic yield in antiphospholipid syndrome. Br J Rheumatol 1998;37: 1229–1232.
155. Carreras LO, Forastiero RR, Martinuzzo ME: Which are the best biological markers of the antiphospholipid syndrome? J Autoimmun 2000;15:163–172.
156. Harris EN: Syndrome of the black swan. Br J Rheumatol 1987;26:324–326.
157. Hughes GRV, Harris EN, Gharavi AE: The anticardiolipin syndrome. J Rheumatol 1986;13:486–489.
158. Khamashta MA, Harris EN, Gharavi AE, et al: Immune mediated mechanism for thrombosis: Antiphospholipid antibody binding to platelet membranes. Ann Rheum Dis 1988;47: 849–854.
159. Maim J, Laurell M, Nilsson IM, et al: Thromboembolic disease—critical evaluation of laboratory investigation. Thromb Haemost 1992;68:7–13.
160. Brey RL, Hart RG, Sherman DG, et al: Antiphospholipid antibodies and cerebral ischemia in young people. Neurology 1990;40:1190–1196.
161. Ferro D, Quintarelli C, Rasura M, et al: Lupus anticoagulant and the fibrinolytic system in young patients with stroke. Stroke 1993;24:368–370.
162. Hart RG, Miller VT, Coull BM, et al: Cerebral infarctions associated with lupus anticoagulant. Stroke 1987;18:257–263.
163. Glueck HI, Kant KS, Weiss MA, et al: Thrombosis in systemic lupus erythematosus: Relation to the presence of circulating anticoagulant. Arch Intern Med 1985;145:1389–1395.
164. Branch DW: Antiphospholipid antibodies and pregnancy: Maternal implications. Semin Perinatol 1990;14:139–146.
165. Pauzner R, Dulitzki M, Langevitz P, et al: Low molecular weight heparin and warfarin the treatment of patients with antiphospholipid syndrome during pregnancy. Thromb Haemost 2001;86:1379–1384.
166. Huong DLT, Wechsler B, Bletry O, et al: A study of 75 pregnancies in patients with antiphospholipid syndrome. J Rheumatol 2001;28:2025–2030.

167. Dreyfus M, Hedelin G, Kutnahorsky R, et al: Antiphospholipid antibodies and preeclampsia: A case-control study. Obstet Gynecol 2001;97:29–34.
168. Branch DW, Porter TF, Rittenhouse L, et al: Antiphospholipid antibodies in women at risk for preeclampsia. Am J Obstet Gynecol 2001;184:825–832.
169. Branch DW, Dudley DJ, Mitchell MD, et al: Immunoglobulin G fractions from patients with antiphospholipid antibodies cause fetal death in BALB/c mice: A model for autoimmune fetal loss. Am J Obstet Gynecol 1990;163:210–216.
170. Moodiey J, Bhoola V, Duursma J, et al: The association of antiphospholipid antibodies with severe early onset preeclampsia. S Afr Med J 1995;85:105–107.
171. Lockshin MD, Druzin ML, Qamar T: Prednisone does not prevent recurrent fetal death in women with antiphospholipid antibody. Am J Obstet Gynecol 1989;160:439–443.
172. Polzin WJ, Kopelman IN, Robinson RD, et al: The association of antiphospholipid antibodies with pregnancy complicated by fetal growth restriction. Obstet Gynecol 1991;78: 1108–1111.
173. Oshiro BT, Silver RM, Scott JR, et al: Antiphospholipid antibodies and fetal death. Obstet Gynecol 1996;87:489–493.
174. Lockwood CJ, Romero R, Feinberg RF, et al: The prevalence and biologic significance of lupus anticoagulant and anticardiolipin antibodies in a general obstetric population. Am J Obstet Gynecol 1989;161:369–373.
175. Clifford K, Rai R, Watson H, Regan L: An informative protocol for the investigation of recurrent miscarriage: Preliminary experience of 500 consecutive cases. Hum Reprod 1994; 9:1328–1332.
176. Branch DW: Antiphospholipid antibodies and reproductive outcome: The current state of affairs. J Reprod Immunol 1998; 38(1):75–87.
177. Pattison NS, Chamley LW, Birdsall M, et al: Does aspirin have a role in improving pregnancy outcome for women with the antiphospholipid syndrome? A randomized controlled trial. Am J Obstet Gynecol 2000;183(4):1008–1112.
178. Silver RK, MacGregor SN, Sholl JS, et al: Comparative trial of prednisone plus aspirin versus aspirin alone in the treatment of anticardiolipin antibody-positive obstetric patients. Am J Obstet Gynecol 1993;169:1411–1417.
179. Cowchock FS, Reece EA, Balaban D, et al: Repeated fetal losses associated with antiphospholipid antibodies: A collaborative randomized trial comparing prednisone with low-dose heparin treatment. Am J Obstet Gynecol 1992;166:1318–1323.
180. Granger KA, Farquharson RG: Obstetric outcome in antiphospholipid syndrome. Lupus 1997;6:509–513.
181. Asherson RA, Cervera R, de Groot PG, et al: Catastrophic Antiphospholipid Syndrome Registry Project Group. Catastrophic antiphospholipid syndrome: International consensus statement on classification criteria and treatment guidelines. Lupus 2003;12:530–534.
182. Schaar CG, Ronday KH, Boets EP, et al: Catastrophic manifestation of the antiphospholipid syndrome. J Rheumatol 1999;26:2261–2264.
183. Camera A, Rocco S, De Lucia D, et al: Reversible adult respiratory distress in primary antiphospholipid syndrome. Haematologica 2000;85:208–210.
184. Empson M, Lassere M, Craig JC, Scott JR: Recurrent pregnancy loss with antiphospholipid antibody: A systematic review of therapeutic trials. Obstet Gynecol 2002;99:135–144.
185. Rosove MH, Brewer PM: Antiphospholipid thrombosis: Clinical course after the first thrombotic event in 70 patients. Ann Intern Med 1992;117:303–308.
186. Rivier G, Herranz MT, Khamashta MA, Hughes GR: Thrombosis and antiphospholipid syndrome: A preliminary assessment of three antithrombotic treatments. Lupus 1994;3: 85–90.
187. American College of Obstetricians and Gynecologists: Thromboembolism in pregnancy. ACOG Practice Bulletin 19. Washington, DC, ACOG, 2000.
188. Erkan D, Merrill JT, Yazici Y, et al: High thrombosis rate after fetal loss in antiphospholipid syndrome: Effective prophylaxis with aspirin. Arthritis Rheum 2001;44:1466–1467.
189. Branch DW, Kamashta MA: Antiphospholipid syndrome: Obstetric diagnosis, management, and controversies. Obstet Gynecol 2003;101:1333–1344.
190. Dahlman TC: Osteoporotic fractures and the recurrence of thromboembolism during pregnancy and the puerperium in 184 women undergoing thromboprophylaxis with heparin. Am J Obstet Gynecol 1993;168:1265–1270.
191. Kelton JG: Heparin-induced thrombocytopenia: An overview. Blood Rev 2002;16:77–80.
192. Warkentin TE, Kelton JG: Delayed-onset heparin-induced thrombocytopenia and thrombosis. Ann Intern Med 2001;135(7):502–506.
193. Warkentin TE, Levine MN, Hirsh J, et al: Heparin-induced thrombocytopenia in patients treated with low-molecular-weight heparin or unfractionated heparin. N Engl J Med 1995;332: 1330–1335.
194. Backos M, Rai R, Baxter N, et al: Pregnancy complications in women with recurrent miscarriage associated with antiphospholipid antibodies treated with low dose aspirin and heparin. BJOG 1999;106:102–107.
195. Cowchock S: Treatment of antiphospholipid syndrome in pregnancy. Lupus 1998;7(Suppl 2):S95–S97.
196. Wapner RJ, Cowchock FS, Shapiro SS: Successful treatment in two women with antiphospholipid antibodies and refractory pregnancy losses with intravenous immunoglobulin infusions. Am J Obstet Gynecol 1989;161:1271–1272.
197. Clark AL, Branch DW, Silver RM, et al: Pregnancy complicated by the antiphospholipid syndrome: Outcomes with intravenous immunoglobulin therapy. Obstet Gynecol 1999;93:437–441.
198. Edwards MH, Pierangeli S, Liu X, et al: Hydroxychloroquine reverses thrombogenic properties of antiphospholipid antibodies in mice. Circulation 1997;96:4380–4384.
199. Cowchock S, Reece EA: Do low-risk pregnant women with antiphospholipid antibodies need to be treated? Organizing Group of the Antiphospholipid Antibody Treatment Trial. Am J Obstet Gynecol 1997;176:1099–1100.
200. American Society of Regional Anesthesia (ASRA): Recommendations for neuraxial anesthesia and anticoagulation. Richmond, VA, ASRA, 1998.
201. Ginsberg JS, Greer I, Hirsh J: Use of antithrombotic agents during pregnancy. Chest 2001;119(Suppl 1):122S–131S.
202. Silman AJ, Hochberg MC (eds): Epidemiology of the Rheumatic Diseases, 2nd ed. London, Oxford University Press, 2001.
203. MacGregor AJ, Snieder H, Rigby AS, et al: Characterizing the quantitative genetic contribution to rheumatoid arthritis using data from twins. Arthritis Rheum 2000;43:30–37.
204. Jawaheer D, Seldin JM, Anoms CI, et al: Screening the genome for rheumatoid arthritis susceptibility genes. Arthritis Rheum 2003;48:906–916.
205. Fisher SA, Lanchbury JS, Lewis CM: Meta-analysis of four rheumatoid arthritis genome-wide linkage studies: Confirmation of a susceptibility locus on chromosome 16. Arthritis Rheum 2003;48:1200–1206.
206. Hench PS: The ameliorating effect of pregnancy on chronic atrophic (infectious) rheumatoid arthritis, fibrositis, and intermittent hydrarthritis. Proc Mayo Clinic 1938;13:161–167.
207. Oka M: Effect of pregnancy on onset and course of rheumatoid arthritis. Ann Rheum Dis 1953;12:227–229.
208. Persellin RH: The effect of pregnancy on rheumatoid arthritis. Bull Rheum Dis 1977;27:922–927.
209. Betson JR, Dorn RV: Forty cases of arthritis and pregnancy. J Int Coll Surg 1964;42:521–526.

210. Ostensen M, Husby G: A prospective clinical study of the effect of pregnancy on rheumatoid arthritis and ankylosing spondylitis. Arthritis Rheum 1983;26:1155–1159.
211. Silman AJ, Roman E, Beral V, Brown A: Adverse reproductive outcomes in women who subsequently develop rheumatoid arthritis. Ann Rheum Dis 1988;47:979–981.
212. Oka M, Vainio V: Effect of pregnancy on the prognosis and serology of rheumatoid arthritis. Acta Rheumatologica Scandinavica 1966;12:47–52.
213. Hazes JM, Dijkmans BAC, Vandenbroucke JP, et al: Pregnancy and the risk of developing rheumaoid arthritis. Arthritis Rheum 1990;33:1770–1775.
214. Ostensen M: Pregnancy in patients with a history of juvenile rheumatoid arthritis. Arthritis Rheum 1991;34:881–887.
215. Ostensen M: Glucocorticosteroids in pregnant patients with rheumatoid arthritis. Z Rheumatol 2000;59(Suppl 2): II70–II74.
216. Royal College of General Practitioners: Oral contraceptives and health: Interim report. London, Pitman, 1974.
217. Gilbert M, Rotstein J, Cunningham C: Norethynodrel with mestranol in the treatment of rheumatoid arthritis. JAMA 1964;190:235.
218. Bijlsma WJ, Huger-Bruning O, Thijssen JHH: Effect of estrogen treatment on clinical and laboratory manifestations of rheumatoid arthritis. Ann Rheum Dis 1987;46:777–779.
219. DaSilva JA, Hall GM: The effects of gender and sex hormones on outcome in rheumatoid arthritis. Bailliers Clin Rheumatol 1992;6:196.
220. Kasukawa R, Ohara M, Yoshida H, Yoshida T: Pregnancy-associated α_2-glycoprotein in rheumatoid arthritis. Int Arch Allergy Appl Immunol 1979;58:67–74.
221. Sany J, Clot J, Borneau M, Ardary M: Immunomodulating effect of human placenta-eluted gamma globulins in rheumatoid arthritis. Arthritis Rheum 1982;25:17–24.
222. Klippel GL, Cerere FA: Rheumatoid arthritis and pregnancy. Rheum Dis Clin North Am 1989;15:213–239.
223. Mannik M, Nardella FA: IgG rheumatoid factor and self-association of these antibodies. Clin Rheum Dis 1985;11:551–572.
224. Nelson JL, Voigt LF, Koepsell TD, et al: Pregnancy outcome in women with rheumatoid arthritis before disease onset. J Rheumatol 1993;19:18.
225. Kaplan D: Fetal wastage in patients with rheumatoid arthritis. J Rheumatol 1986;13:857–877.
226. Morris WIC: Pregnancy in rheumatoid arthritis and systemic lupus erythematosus. Aust N Z J Obstet Gynaecol 1969;9: 136–144.
227. Steen VD: Scleroderma and pregnancy. Rheum Dis Clin North Am 1997;23:133–147.
228. Morrow J, Nelson JL, Watts R, Isenberg DA (eds): Autoimmune Rheumatic Diseases, 2nd ed. Oxford, UK, Oxford University Press, 1999.
229. Johnson RW, Tew MB, Arnett FC: The genetics of systemic sclerosis. Curr Rheumatol Rep 2002;4:99–107.
230. Steen VD, Conte C, Day N, et al: Pregnancy in women with systemic sclerosis. Arthritis Rheum 1989;32:151–157.
231. Steen VD: Pregnancy in women with systemic sclerosis. Obstet Gynecol 1999;94:15–20.
232. Englert H, Brennan P, McNeil D, et al: Reproductive function prior to disease onset in women with scleroderma. J Rheumatol 1992;19:1575–1579.
233. Black CM: Systemic sclerosis and pregnancy. Bailliere Clin Rheumatol 1990;4:105–124.
234. Johnson TR, Banner EA, Winkelmann RK: Scleroderma and pregnancy. Obstet Gynecol 1964;23:467–469.
235. Slate WG, Graham AR: Scleroderma and pregnancy. Am J Obstet Gynecol 1968;101:335–341.
236. Weiner RS, Brinkman CR, Paulus HE: Scleroderma, CREST syndrome and pregnancy. Arthritis Rheum 1986;29:51(suppl).
237. Giordano M, Valentini G, Lupoli S: Pregnancy and systemic sclerosis. Arthritis Rheum 1985;28:237–238.
238. Silman AJ, Black C: Increased incidence of spontaneous abortion and infertility in women with scleroderma before disease onset: A controlled study. Ann Rheum Dis 1988;47:441–444.
239. Baethge BA, Wolf RE: Successful pregnancy with scleroderma renal disease and pulmonary hypertension in a patient using angiotensin converting enzyme inhibitors. Ann Rheum Dis 1989;48:776–778.
240. Batocchi AP, Majolini L, Evoli A, et al: Course and treatment of myasthenia gravis during pregnancy. Neurol 1999;52:447–452.
241. Oosterhuis HJGH: Myasthenia Gravis. Groningen, Groningen Neurological Press, 1997, pp 39–40.
242. Vincent A, Newsom-Davis J: Acetylcholine receptor antibody as a diagnostic test for myasthenia gravis: Results in 153 validated cases and 2967 diagnostic assays. J Neurol Neurosurg Psychiatry 1985;48:1246–1252.
243. Lindstrom J: An assay for antibodies to human AChR in serum from patients with myasthenia gravis. Clin Immunol Immunopathol 1977;7:36–43.
244. Donaldson JO, Penn AS, Lisak RP, et al: Anti-acetylcholine receptor antibody in neonatal myasthenia gravis. Am J Dis Child 1981;135:222–226.
245. Plauche WC: Myasthenia gravis. Clin Obstet Gynecol 1983;26:592.
246. Engle AG, Santa T: Histometric analysis of ultrastructure of the neuromuscular junction in myasthenia gravis and in the myasthenic syndrome. Ann NY Acad Sciences 1971;183:46–63.
247. Drachman DB: Myasthenia gravis. N Engl J Med 1994;330: 1797.
248. Cartlidge NEF: Neurologic disorders. In Barron WM, Lindheimer MD (eds): Medical Disorders During Pregnancy, 2nd ed. St Louis, Mosby, 1995, p 430.
249. Plauche WC: Myasthenia gravis in mothers and their newborns. Clin Obstet Gynecol 1991;34:82–99.
250. Plauche WC: Myasthenia gravis in pregnancy: An update. Am J Obstet Gynecol 1979;135:691–697.
251. McNall PG, Jafarnia MR: Management of myasthenia gravis in the obstetrical patient. J Obstet Gynecol 1965;92:518–525.
252. Chambers DC, Hall JE, Boyce J: Myasthenia gravis and pregnancy. Obstet Gynecol 1967;76:323–324.
253. Hay DM: Myasthenia gravis in pregnancy. BJOG 1967;76: 323–324.
254. Catanzarite VA, McHargue AM, Sandberg EC, et al: Respiratory arrest during therapy for premature labor in a patient with myasthenia gravis. Obstet Gynecol 1984;64:819–822.
255. Polizzi A, Husson SM, Vincent A: Teratogen update: Maternal myasthenia gravis as a cause of congenital arthrogryposis. Tetratol 2000;62:332–341.
256. Brenner T, Beyth Y, Abramsky O: Inhibitory effect of α-fetoprotein on the binding of myasthenia gravis antibody to acetylcholine receptor. Proc Natl Acad Sciences USA 1980;77: 3635–3639.
257. Donaldson JO, Penn AS, Lisak RP, et al: Anti-acetylcholine receptor antibody in neonatal myasthenia gravis. Am J Dis Child 1981;135:222–226.
258. Lefvert AK, Osterman PO: Newborn infants to myasthenic mothers: A clinical study and an investigation of acetylcholine receptor antibodies in 17 children. Neurology 1983;33:133–138.
259. Bartoccioni E, Evoli A, Casali C, et al: Neonatal myasthenia gravis: Clinical and immunological study of seven mothers and their newborn infants. J Neuroimmunol 1986;12: 155–161.
260. Shepard MK: Arthrogryposis multiplex congenita in sibs. Birth Defects 1971;7:127.

261. Holmes LB, Driscoll SG, Bradley WG: Multiple contractures in newborn of mother with myasthenia gravis. Pediatr Res 1979;13:486.
262. Levine SE, Keesey JC: Successful plasmapheresis for fulminant myasthenia gravis during pregnancy. Arch Neurol 1986; 42:197–198.
263. Bader AM: Neurological and neuro muscular disease. In Chestnut DH (ed): Obstetric Anesthesia: Principles and Practice. St Louis, Mosby, 1994.

CHAPTER 45

Diabetes

Christine Ang / David Howe / Mary Lumsden

INTRODUCTION

Diabetes mellitus is a group of metabolic diseases characterized by hyperglycemia resulting from defects in insulin secretion, insulin action, or both. Approximately 150 million are affected worldwide. The World Health Organization (WHO) has predicted that between 1995 and 2025 there will be a 35% increase in the worldwide prevalence of diabetes. In the United Kingdom, it was estimated in the year 2000 that 1.4 million people suffer from diabetes and another million remain undiagnosed. It is variously estimated that 3% to 5% of pregnancies are complicated by diabetes. Approximately 0.2% to 0.5% of all pregnancies occur in women with a preexisting diagnosis of type 1 diabetes mellitus,[1] and a similar number have preexisting type 2 diabetes mellitus.[2] An additional 1% to 6% of women will develop sufficient hyperglycemia during pregnancy to meet the criteria for a diagnosis of diabetes (termed *gestational diabetes*, or GDM).[3] Of those women with gestational diabetes, between 20% and 50% subsequently develop type 2 diabetes mellitus.[3]

Chronic hyperglycemia is associated with long-term damage, dysfunction, and failure of various organs, especially the eyes, kidneys, nerves, heart, and blood vessels.[4] Women entering pregnancy with a preexisting diagnosis of diabetes historically had a poor prognosis for successful pregnancy. Numerous studies have shown that with careful attention to control of blood sugar near-normal outcomes can be achieved and the risk of progression of diabetic complications during pregnancy is minimal. Sadly, many diabetic women are unable to achieve ideal glucose control for whatever reason, and diabetic pregnancy remains associated with increased rates of congenital abnormality, miscarriage, hypertension, late stillbirth, fetal macrosomia, and obstructed labor.[1,5,6] Additionally, the physiologic changes that occur in pregnancy can accelerate the progression of diabetic complications, such as retinopathy and nephropathy, particularly if the diabetes is poorly controlled. These issues are considered in more detail in the section on established diabetes.

More controversial is the diagnosis of gestational diabetes, in which hyperglycemia develops in pregnancy. Undoubtedly, many of the obstetric complications of diabetes occur to some degree across a continuum of glucose concentrations. The difficulty lies in deciding at which level of glucose to intervene. Setting the threshold too low will result in overinvestigation and treatment of many women who can be expected to have a good pregnancy outcome. Furthermore, it is not entirely clear that rigorous glucose control instituted in late pregnancy successfully reduces the risks of these complications.[3,7–9] The evidence for screening for gestational diabetes is considered in the Gestational Diabetes section.

Several bodies, including the Scottish Intercollegiate Guidelines Network (SIGN), Diabetes UK, The American Diabetes Association, and the American College of Obstetricians and Gynecologists, have produced guidelines and position statements on the management of pregnant women with diabetes and on screening for gestational diabetes and fetal macrosomia.[10–15]

CLASSIFICATION AND DIAGNOSIS OF DIABETES

Traditionally, diabetes mellitus has been divided into insulin dependent (type 1) and noninsulin dependent (type 2) forms. More recently, a classification into five groups (see Table 45–1) has been advanced, based on patterns of inheritance and clinical presentation. Pregnancy itself is a state of physiologic insulin resistance. In a number of women the physiologic increase in insulin resistance during pregnancy on a background of inherited insulin resistance or obesity is enough to make them overtly diabetic. GDM refers to women who are shown to be diabetic for the first time during pregnancy, regardless of whether the diabetes persists after pregnancy.[9]

TABLE 45–1

Classification of Diabetes Mellitus

Type 1 diabetes mellitus	Immune-mediated DM (cell-mediated immune destruction of beta cells of pancreas) Idiopathic DM (forms of the disease with no known etiology)
Type 2 diabetes mellitus	Relative rather than absolute insulin deficiency
Impaired glucose homeostasis	Impaired fasting glucose (fasting glucose higher than normal, but less than diagnostic) Impaired glucose tolerance (plasma glucose following a 75 g challenge higher than normal, but less than diagnostic)
Gestational diabetes mellitus	Glucose intolerance in pregnancy
Other specific types	DM due to specific etiologies: • Genetic defects of beta cell function (MODY 1, 2, 3) • Genetic defects of insulin action • Disease of exocrine pancreas (pancreatitis, cystic fibrosis) • Endocrine (Cushing's) • Drug or chemical induced • Infection (rubella, coxsackie, cytomegalovirus) • Uncommon forms of immune-related diabetes • Other genetic syndromes

From Abbertini K, Zimmet P: Definition, diagnosis and classification of diabetes mellitus and its complications. Part 1: Diagnosis and classification of diabetes mellitus. Provisional report of a WHO consultation. Diabetes Med 1998;15:539–553.

The diagnosis of diabetes in nonpregnant subjects is made on the finding of elevated fasting blood glucose and/or elevated blood glucose following an oral glucose challenge. Multiple genetic and epigenetic factors modify fasting glucose concentrations and the response to an oral glucose challenge, so that there is not a clear bimodal separation of "normal" glucose tolerance and "diabetic" states. Instead there is a continuum of fasting blood glucose concentrations and of the response to an oral glucose challenge. The accepted criteria used to diagnose diabetes are shown in Table 45–2.[16,17] In addition, for glucose values falling between "normal" and "diabetic," the terms *impaired glucose tolerance* and *impaired fasting glycemia* have been coined. Impaired glucose homeostasis and impaired fasting glycemia are not recognized as diseases, but their presence does indicate an increased likelihood of developing diabetes.

TABLE 45–2

World Health Organization Criteria for the Diagnosis of Diabetes

	FASTING PLASMA GLUCOSE		120 MIN GLUCOSE
Impaired fasting glucose	6.1–6.9 mmol/L		
Impaired glucose tolerance	≤7.0 mmol/L	and	7.8–11.0 mmol/L
Diabetes	≥7.0 mmol/L	or	≥11.1 mmol/L

Key:
Blood glucose levels are plasma levels in venous blood following a 75-g oral glucose challenge in fasted subjects. *Values in mg/dL: 6.1 mmol/L = 110 mg/dL, 7.0 mmol/L = 126 mg/dL, 7.8 mmol/L = 140 mg/dL, 11.1 mmol/L = 200 mg/dL.*

From Abbertini K, Zimmet P: Definition, diagnosis and classification of diabetes mellitus and its complications. Part 1: Diagnosis and classification of diabetes mellitus. Provisional report of a WHO consultation. Diabetes Med 1998;15:539–553.

MATERNAL AND FETAL GLUCOSE HOMEOSTASIS IN PREGNANCY

During pregnancy there is a physiologic increase in insulin resistance in maternal tissues, presumably to satisfy the nutritional demands of the fetus.[18] Placental glucose transport is noninsulin sensitive. Instead glucose is moved across the placenta by facilitated diffusion down a concentration gradient. High levels of maternal glucose result in high levels of fetal glucose. The fetal pancreas is stimulated by hyperglycemia, and there is an early increase in beta cell mass of the pancreatic islets, so that the pancreas of fetuses exposed to repeated hyperglycemia secretes relatively more insulin than that of normoglycemic fetuses.[19] Insulin appears to promote fetal growth, either directly through insulin receptors or by increasing the bioactivity of insulin-like growth factor-1 (IGF-1). The mechanism of fetal macrosomia in diabetes is likely due to accelerated pancreatic maturation and higher fetal insulin levels, and this has come to be known as the *Pedersen hypothesis*.[20] Other factors besides glucose stimulate fetal insulin release, and this may be one reason why maternal glucose levels explain only a limited amount of birth weight variation.

Impact of Maternal Diabetic Vascular Disease

Diabetes is associated with both microvascular and macrovascular disease. Microvascular disease leads to retinopathy, nephropathy, and neuropathy, whereas accelerated atherosclerosis of large vessels predisposes to myocardial infarction, stroke, and limb ischemia. Microvascular disease seems to be a result of sustained episodes of hyperglycemia with increased production of metabolites that lead to vascular damage.[21] The endothelial lining of blood vessels plays a pivotal role in the regulation of tissue blood flow, and hyperglycemia-induced endothelial dysfunction of small-resistance arteries leads ultimately to tissue hypoperfusion. There are probably several phases to vascular damage mediated by hyperglycemia. In animal models endothelial-dependent vasodilation is sequentially increased, unaltered, and impaired by hyperglycemia.[22] Studies in pregnant humans have found either normal or impaired function.[23,24]

The fetal placental circulation by definition develops during pregnancy, and numerous researchers have sought evidence for abnormal development of the placental circulation in diabetic pregnancies. Any structural changes are relatively subtle.[25] The regulation of fetal placental blood flow is poorly understood, but in the absence of autonomic or cholinergic innervation is entirely dependent on circulating hormonal and autocrine factors. There is evidence for disturbances in the activity of endothelial-derived nitric oxide in the diabetic placenta.[26]

ESTABLISHED/PREEXISTING DIABETES

Maternal Risks

Prior to the discovery of insulin in 1921 by Frederic Banting and Charles Best, women with diabetes rarely became pregnant, and those who did experienced a high incidence of maternal and fetal morbidity. Nowadays, most women starting pregnancy with a preexisting diagnosis of diabetes have their diabetes relatively well controlled. Nonetheless pregnancy is associated with a physiologic worsening of tissue insulin resistance and with renal and cardiovascular adaptations that might be expected to accelerate the progression of diabetic complications such as retinopathy and nephropathy. Diabetic women are more prone to developing hypertension in pregnancy, and the increased susceptibility to infection means that diabetic women are more likely to suffer from pyelonephritis and perhaps from other infection-mediated adverse obstetric events. Several large studies in nonpregnant subjects have convincingly shown that intensive glucose control reduces the development and progression of diabetic complications.[27–30] The same is true during pregnancy; women can be encouraged that improvement in glycemic control during pregnancy has long-term health benefits. At the same time, intensive glycemic control increases the risk of hypoglycemia and may be one reason why some women choose not to comply with suggested treatment.

Hypoglycemia

For many women, the degree of glycemic control encouraged during pregnancy is much tighter than normal. Concerns about hypoglycemia may be a reason for poor compliance with diet and insulin regimens. Most hypoglycemic episodes occur in the first 20 weeks and in women who have experienced hypoglycemic episodes before pregnancy.[31] It has been estimated that for every 1% fall in glycosylated hemoglobin (HbA_{1c}) levels, there is approximately a 33% increase in hypoglycemic attacks. It is important that family members are educated about the use of glucagon injection for emergency treatment of profound hypoglycemia.

Diabetic Ketoacidosis

In established diabetics ketoacidosis is rare, affecting less than 1% of pregnancies, due to the increased level of supervision and tighter glycemic control generally seen during pregnancy.[1] Occasionally the first presentation of type 1 diabetes mellitus may be with ketoacidosis in pregnancy. The 1994–1996 Report on Confidential Enquiries into Maternal deaths in the United Kingdom reported two indirect maternal deaths from diabetes mellitus and two late deaths from diabetic ketoacidosis. The risk of ketoacidosis increases in the presence of obvious precipitants such as hyperemesis and infection. Obstetricians should be aware that tocolytic therapy with beta-sympathomimetics and corticosteroid therapy results in increased insulin requirements. The metabolic effects of antenatal corticosteroids, are prolonged, and it may be appropriate to use a sliding scale of intravenous insulin to maintain normoglycemia.

Retinopathy

Diabetic retinopathy complicates both type 1 and type 2 diabetes mellitus. In patients who developed diabetes before age 30 and who have had diabetes for more than 20 years, almost all will have retinopathy, and about half of these will have proliferative retinopathy.[32] In women with minimal or early retinopathy, there is a 10% chance of progression during pregnancy; in those with proliferative retinopathy, there is a 50% chance of progression.[33] Hypertension and preeclampsia further increase the risk of progressive retinopathy.[34] Instituting a regimen of intensive glycemic control in patients with moderate to severe nonproliferative retinopathy may result in progression of retinopathy; it is usual to increase the frequency of funduscopic examination.[32]

Nephropathy

End-stage renal disease is one of the major complications of diabetes and accounts for 40% of all patients on dialysis.[35] The incidence of diabetic nephropathy increases with duration of disease and is present in around 25% of diabetics after 15 years.[36] It is estimated that about 6% of pregnant type 1 diabetics will have clinically significant renal impairment.[37]

The impact of pregnancy on diabetic nephropathy depends on prepregnancy renal function. Most case series are small, but in general in women with good renal function (creatinine <150 micromol/L; <1.70mg/dL), there is little evidence of worsening of renal function.[38,39]

In women with markedly decreased glomerular filtration rates prior to pregnancy there is a significant risk of permanent decline in renal function.[39,40] Renal disease is a risk factor for the development of hypertension in pregnancy, and hypertension further accelerates the decline in renal function. Microalbuminuria in early pregnancy is a sensitive predictor of those women likely to develop hypertension.[41] Women with nephropathy are more likely to suffer from pregnancy complications. The incidences of low birth weight, preeclampsia, and preterm delivery are increased in women with nephropathy.[39,42,43]

Hypertension

In diabetic women with chronic hypertension, the normal physiologic changes in blood pressure occur during pregnancy but start from a higher baseline.[44] Chronic hypertension is a risk factor for the development of preeclampsia, and worsening proteinuria and hypertension in later pregnancy may indicate the development of superimposed preeclampsia.[44] Clinically, however, it can be difficult to distinguish between preeclampsia and worsening nephropathy. The development of proteinuric hypertension is reported to complicate 12% to 40% of diabetic pregnancies.[45–48] The presence of microvascular disease (as indicated by the presence of retinopathy) increases the risk of developing hypertension.[49,50]

Atherosclerosis

Macrovascular disease is also a feature of diabetes; the exaggerated lipid changes in pregnancy, along with rheologic and prothrombotic changes, might be expected to accelerate atherosclerosis. Myocardial infarction, however, remains a rare event in pregnant diabetics[51]; equally, there is little evidence of progression of peripheral arterial disease during pregnancy.[52]

Neuropathy

Peripheral neuropathy has usually developed to some degree in most diabetics after 10 to 15 years. Autonomic neuropathy may delay gastric emptying and blunt cardiovascular reflexes, but there are few case reports in the literature suggesting that these considerations are not common.[53] Autonomic neuropathy also results in lack of hypoglycemic awareness. Painful *insulin neuritis*, often described as an ache or burning sensation, sometimes complicates a rapid tightening of glycemic control.[54]

Infection

Maternal infections are more common in diabetics. It has been estimated that about 80% of pregnancies in women with type 1 diabetes mellitus will have at least one episode of infection, compared with 25% of pregnancies in nondiabetic women.[55] Infection is a risk factor for preterm labor and for ketoacidosis. Chronic urinary tract infection, besides being a risk factor for preterm labor, contributes to nephropathy. Pyelonephritis complicates about 4% of diabetic pregnancies and only 1% of nondiabetic pregnancies.[56] Postpartum endometritis and wound infections are also more common in diabetics.

Other Associated Endocrine Diseases

Type 1 diabetes mellitus is an autoimmune condition, and women with type 1 diabetes are at risk of other autoimmune endocrine diseases, notably those affecting the thyroid. The incidence of thyroid dysfunction during pregnancy and the first year postpartum in type 1 diabetics is about 3 times higher than that of the normal population.[57]

Operative Delivery

Maternal diabetes is a risk factor for cesarean delivery. Reported rates of cesarean section in diabetic women range from 25% to 80% and reflect wide divergences in obstetric practice.[39,43,58–61] Many factors account for the high cesarean section rate, including prematurity, macrosomia, and the presence of diabetic complications such as nephropathy. The diagnosis of diabetes, or the knowledge that women are being treated with insulin, triggers an increase in intervention among obstetricians.[62]

Pelvic Floor Trauma

Macrosomia, nulliparity, episiotomy, and instrumental delivery are established risk factors for third- and fourth-degree tears. Approximately 20% of diabetic women who deliver vaginally suffer second-, third-, or fourth-degree tears.[59] Shoulder dystocia is also a risk factor for perineal trauma. Langer reported that when the birth weight was less than 4000 g, the incidence of shoulder dystocia was 0.3%, which rose to 4.9% when the birth weight was above 4000 g. Furthermore, as a group, nondiabetic women had shoulder dystocia rate of 0.5% compared to 3.2% in women who were diabetic.[63]

Fetal Risks

Maternal diabetes mellitus increases the risks of congenital abnormalities, miscarriage, unexplained stillbirth, premature delivery, macrosomia, and traumatic delivery, and also of a number of neonatal complications. In the pre-insulin era, fetal and neonatal losses were in the order of 65%. Improvements in insulin therapy and obstetric approaches to the pregnant diabetic have progressively improved outcomes. The perinatal mortality rate of infants of diabetic mothers has declined from 250 per 1000 live births in the 1960s to 20 per 1000 live births in the 1980s. Furthermore, it has been established that tight glycemic control before conception and during pregnancy can reduce the rate of congenital malformations, miscarriage, and fetal macrosomia. Fatal congenital abnormalities now appear to be the leading cause of perinatal death, but unexplained late stillbirth remains a problem.

Congenital Anomalies

Many centers around the world continue to report that approximately 3% to 8% of infants of diabetic mothers suffer from major congenital abnormalities.[64–67] The reduction in the incidence of congenital anomalies remains a major goal, especially when it is considered that congenital anomalies account for between 20% and 50% of the perinatal deaths to diabetic women.[64,68] The increased risk of congenital anomaly is found in type 1 and type 2 diabetics who had hyperglycemia during early pregnancy. Women with gestational diabetes diagnosed later in pregnancy do not seem to be at risk.

The congenital abnormalities found in the infants of diabetic women do not form a clear syndrome. Neural tube defects and cardiac malformations are more common than in the nondiabetic population, and caudal regression (or sacral agenesis) is reported to be 200 to 400 times more common in infants of women with diabetes.[69–71] There is good evidence that the abnormalities arise as a consequence of poor glycemic control periconceptually and during embryogenesis.[70] When the HbA_{1c} is less than 6 standard deviations above the mean, the congenital anomaly rate is about 3%, but when the HbA_{1c} is more than 12 standard deviations above the mean, the anomaly rises to rate 35%. Figure 45–1 shows the relationship between first-trimester HbA_{1c} and congenital abnormalities. Small studies have reported low rates of congenital abnormality where preconceptual input has optimized glycemic control.[72,73] In the larger Diabetes In Early Pregnancy Study, where women were enrolled within 21 days of conception, infants of diabetic mothers had higher rates of congenital abnormality than those of nondiabetic mothers, but the investigators were unable to relate the risk of abnormality to mean glucose or to glycosylated HbA_{1c}.[74] The randomized prospective Diabetes Control and Complications Trial showed that the timely institution of intensive therapy for blood glucose control is associated with rates of spontaneous abortion and congenital malformations that are similar to those in the nondiabetic population.[75]

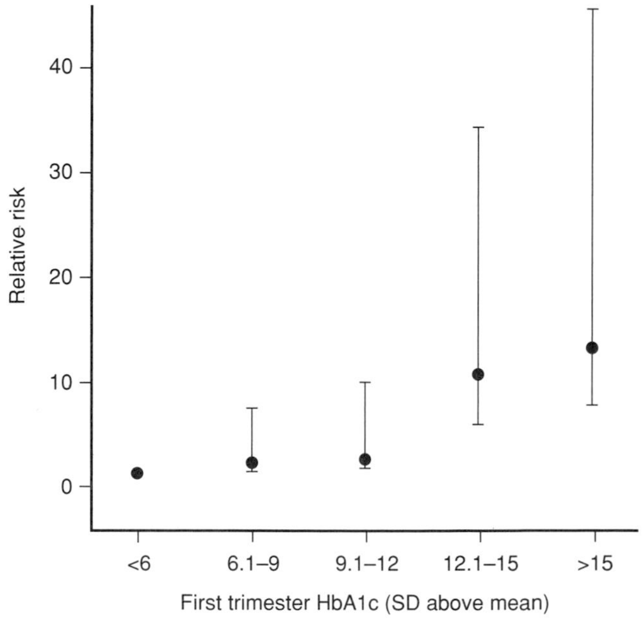

FIGURE 45–1
Relative risk of major congenital malformations (and 95% confidence intervals) for given HbA_{1c} values (expressed as SD above mean).
Adapted from Greene MF: Prevention and diagnosis of congenital anomalies in diabetic pregnancies. Clin Perinatol 1993;20:533–47.

Both hyperglycemia and hypoglycemia have been suggested as possible causes of congenital anomaly. Studies with nonhuman embryos in culture identified that hypoglycemia is teratogenic.[71] In clinical practice, however, increased frequency of hypoglycemic episodes does not increase the incidence of congenital anomaly, suggesting that human embryos in utero can tolerate short-lived periods of hypoglycemia.[73] More likely, hyperglycemia or some metabolic derangement consequent on hyperglycemia is responsible for damage to the developing embryo. Intensive control of glucose concentrations around the time of conception and embryogenesis can reduce the incidence of congenital abnormalities in infants of diabetic women to that seen in nondiabetic women.[72,73,75] The higher incidence of neural tube defects in diabetic pregnancies does not seem to be associated with deranged folate metabolism, though this is not to argue against the importance of folate supplementation.[76]

Early Pregnancy Losses

The incidence of miscarriage is increased in diabetic pregnancies and, as with all complications, is related to the degree of glycemic control since it increases with greater HbA_{1c} levels.[77,78] Figure 45–2 shows the relationship between first-trimester HbA_{1c} and miscarriage. The Diabetes Control and Complications Trial showed that intensive therapy for blood glucose control reduces the rate of spontaneous abortion to that in the nondiabetic population.[75]

Preterm Labor

The frequency of spontaneous preterm labor is reported to be higher in diabetics (in one series complicating about 20% of pregnancies).[79,80] The mechanism of preterm labor is not known. Polyhydramnios and increased susceptibility to infection in poorly controlled diabetics may both be contributory factors.

Fetal Growth

The birth weight of infants of diabetic mothers is greater than those of nondiabetic mothers, and the incidences of obstructed labor and shoulder dystocia are correspondingly increased. The distribution of standardized birth weight in infants of diabetic women is unimodal and

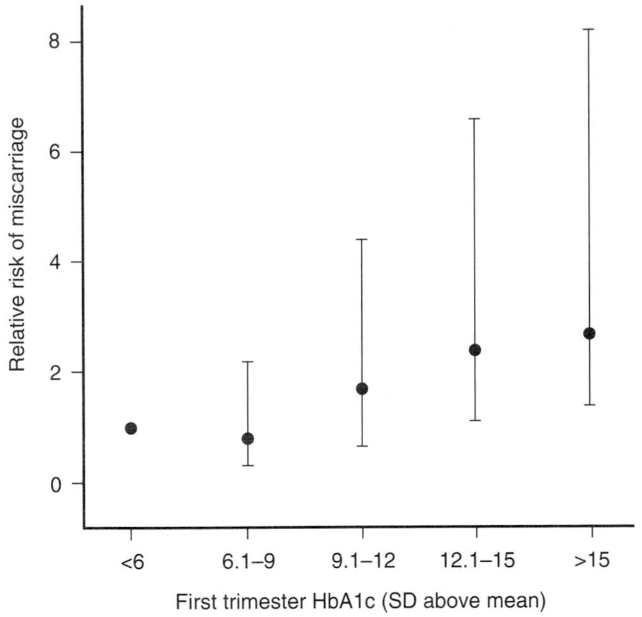

FIGURE 45–2
Relative risk of miscarriage (and 95% confidence intervals) for given HbA_{1c} values (expressed as SD above mean). Adapted from Greene MF: Prevention and diagnosis of congenital anomalies in diabetic pregnancies. Clin Perinatol 1993;20:533–547.

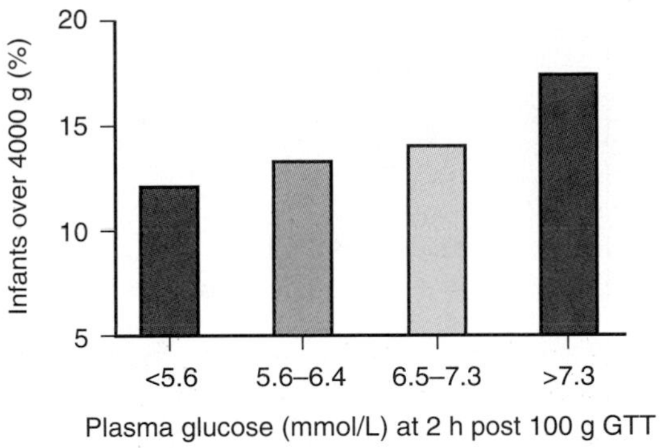

FIGURE 45–3
Birth weight related to the 2-hour glucose level in 3637 pregnancies with a normal 100 g glucose tolerance test between 24 and 28 weeks' gestation in the Toronto Tri-Hospitals study. From Sermer M, Naylor CD, Gare DJ, et al: Impact of increasing carbohydrate intolerance on maternal-fetal outcomes in 3637 women without gestational diabetes: The Toronto Tri-Hospital Gestational Diabetes Project. Am J Obstet Gynecol 1995;173:146–156.

shifted about 1.2 to 1.5 standard deviations to the right.[81,82] Between 20% and 40% of infants of diabetic mothers have a birth weight over the 90th percentile for gestation.[19] Fetal macrosomia develops from about 20 weeks' gestation on.[83] At birth, diabetic infants have significantly more adipose tissue, larger shoulders, and decreased head-to-shoulder ratio compared to nondiabetic infants of similar birth weight and length.[84] The widely accepted Pederson model suggests that maternal hyperglycemia leads to fetal hyperglycemia, and this in turn leads to hyperplasia of fetal pancreatic beta cells and increased fetal insulin concentrations. Insulin can be detected in increased amounts in the cord blood and amniotic fluid of diabetic women from 20 weeks' gestation onward.[85,86]

Much effort has been devoted to identifying which parameter of glycemic control best predicts the development of macrosomia. Mean daily glucose, preprandial glucose, and postprandial glucose concentrations have all been advocated. At the center of the debate is the concept that the peak excursions of hyperglycemia associated with meals may be relatively more important in determining macrosomia than the average background glucose. In both diabetic and nondiabetic women, postprandial glucose concentrations in the third trimester rather than fasting glucose levels are correlated with fetal size and birth weight.[87,88] Figure 45–3 shows the relationship between birth weight and the 2-hour plasma glucose following a 100-g oral glucose tolerance test (GTT) in women with a normal glucose tolerance. In diabetic women, mean postprandial whole blood glucose above 6.7 mmol/L (120 mg/dL) was associated with a 30% chance of macrosomia.[87]

Polyhydramnios is considered a complication of diabetes. The precise mechanism of polyhydramnios is not known, but it may relate to the higher incidence of congenital anomalies, to increased osmotic pressure in amniotic fluid (due to high glucose concentrations), or to fetal polyuria.[89,90] Polyhydramnios does not necessarily indicate that the pregnancy is at risk. A review of all cases of polydramnios, regardless of diabetic status from a database of over 40,000 women concluded that the overall incidence of polyhydramnios was about 1% and that the diagnosis of polyhydramnios was associated with an increase in perinatal mortality and congenital anomalies.[91]

Perinatal Mortality

The perinatal mortality rate in diabetic pregnancies remains consistently higher than the background perinatal mortality rate.[64,92–98] It is estimated that between 10% and 50% of perinatal mortality in women with diabetes is due to congenital abnormalities.[64,68,97] There is also a significantly higher rate of stillbirth unrelated to congenital anomaly in diabetic pregnancies in most case series.[64,92–94,97] It is likely that some of the stillbirths seen in diabetic pregnancies are due to intrauterine growth restriction (IUGR) produced by the usual mechanisms that affect nondiabetic pregnancies. The rightward shift in the birth weight distribution of diabetic infants can mask the diagnosis of significant IUGR.

Stillbirths are more common in diabetic pregnancies across all infant birth weights, suggesting that factors other than placental insufficiency are involved (Figure 45–4).[99] It is generally stated that "poor glycemic control" is associated with stillbirth. In animal models, fetal hyperglycemia results in increased oxygen consumption and ultimately hypoxia and acidosis.[100,101] Fetal cord

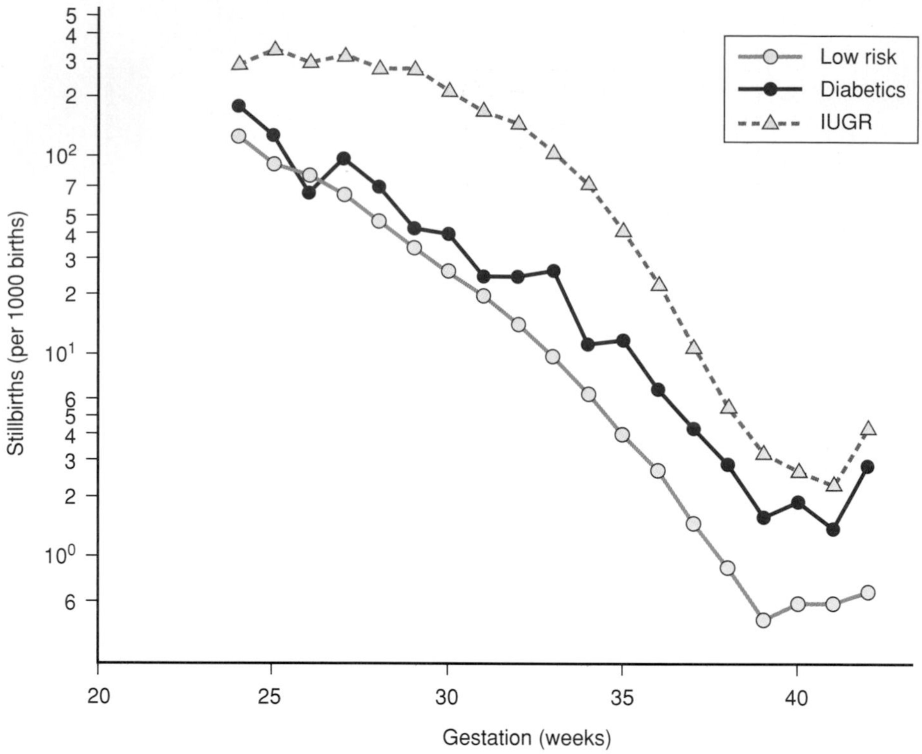

FIGURE 45–4
Fetal death rates by gestational age for low risk pregnancies (*open circles*) compared with diabetes pregnancies (*filled circles*) and pregnancies complicated by intrauterine growth restriction (*open triangles*).
Key: Note rates are displayed on a logarithmic scale. Adapted from Smulian JC, Ananth CV, Vintzileos AM, et al: Fetal deaths in the United States: Influence of high-risk conditions and implications for management. Obstet Gynecol 2002;100:1183–1189.

blood sampling in human diabetic pregnancies has confirmed that fetal acidemia is significantly associated with both the maternal and fetal blood glucose concentrations.[102] Furthermore, chronic fetal hypoxia may be exacerbated in poorly controlled patients in whom a shift to the left in the maternal oxyhemoglobin dissociation curve results in reduced red cell oxygen delivery at tissue level.[103] Although uncommon, maternal ketoacidosis is also associated with a high (20% to 50%) fetal mortality rate.[104] Interestingly, reversible fetal hydrops, presumably due to fetal tachyarrhythmia, has been reported in a case of maternal ketoacidotic coma.[105] It is suggested that tachycardia, particularly in the context of fetal hypertrophic obstructive cardiomyopathy, may further contribute to unexplained stillbirth in diabetic women. Whatever the mechanism, unexplained stillbirth remains difficult to predict or prevent: There are reports of stillbirth within 72 hours of seemingly normal fetal monitoring.[106]

Shoulder Dystocia and Birth Trauma

The macrosomic fetus is at an increased risk of traumatic delivery, particularly shoulder dystocia. Diabetic women were six times as likely as nondiabetic women to suffer shoulder dystocia (see also Figure 45–5).[63] A 13-year retrospective review of 231 infants weighing over 4500 g born vaginally found that around 8% had serious trauma (brachial plexus injuries or clavicular fracture).[107]

Neonatal Complications of Diabetic Infant

A number of neonatal complications have been well characterized in the infants of diabetic pregnancies.[108] These are summarized in Table 45–3. Hypoglycemia is relatively common but usually of little consequence and results from a rapid drop in plasma glucose concentrations following clamping of the umbilical cord. Even in well-controlled diabetic mothers, the incidence of early hypoglycemia in infants is still high, particularly in those mothers who had a longer duration of diabetes. Hypocalcemia and hypomagnesemia are also more common in infants of diabetic mothers. The etiology is unknown, but adult diabetics seem to have a lower set point for parathyroid hormone regulation of calcium.[109] More strict control of glucose during pregnancy is associated with a reduction in the incidence of hypocalcemia.

Infants of diabetic mothers typically have elevated cord blood erythropoeitin levels and are polycythemic.[102] The increased red cell mass contributes to a higher incidence of postnatal hyperbilirubinemia and the need for phototherapy.

Classically, the incidence of respiratory distress syndrome in infants of diabetic mothers was reported to be higher than that of nondiabetics. More recent data (from women with better glycemic control) indicate that this statement is no longer true.[110] Routine fetal lung maturity testing in well-controlled diabetics at term is not required, because less than 1% of infants will develop respiratory distress.[111] Furthermore, not all cases of respiratory distress in term infants of diabetic mothers are due to pulmonary surfactant deficiency; transient tachypnea, polycythemia, and hypertrophic obstructive cardiomyopathy also contribute.[112] Nonetheless, hyperglycemia and hyperinsulinemia do seem to delay lung maturation and the production of surfactant in experimental models.[113]

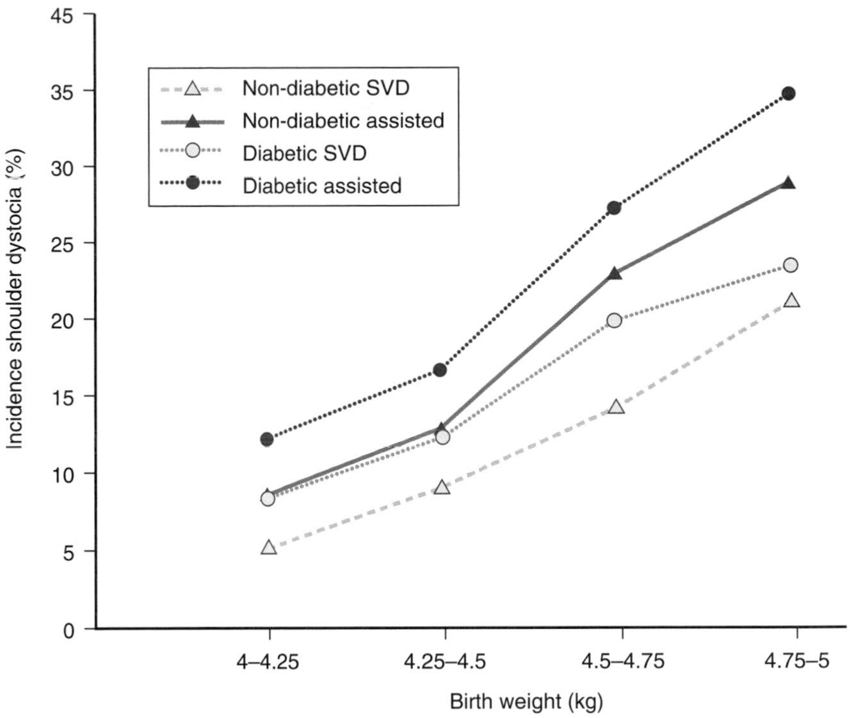

FIGURE 45–5
Incidence of shoulder dystocia in diabetic (*circles*) and nondiabetic pregnancies (*triangles*) for increasing birth weight. Key: Spontaneous vaginal deliveries are shown as open symbols, and assisted deliveries (forceps and vacuum) are shown as filled symbols.
Adapted from Nesbitt TS, Gilbert WM, Herrchen B, et al: Shoulder dystocia and associated risk factors with macrosomic infants born in California. Am J Obstet Gynecol 1998;179:476–480.

Fetal hyperinsulinemia is also believed to cause hypertrophy of the myocardium and particularly of the ventricular septum.[114] The ventricular hypertrophy in infants of diabetic pregnancies may be asymptomatic and only picked up on echocardiographic screening.[108,115] It is estimated that as many as 30% of fetuses may have cardiac hypertrophy. Intensive glycemic control during pregnancy reduces the incidence of hypertrophic myopathy.[116] Importantly, the prognosis is good: hypertrophy seems reversible in the neonatal period.[115,116]

Management Options

Prepregnancy and Prenatal Care—Diabetes Management

TARGET PLASMA GLUCOSE CONCENTRATION

In nondiabetic subjects, glucose remains between about 4 mmol/L (70mg/dL) in the fasting state and 7 mmol/L (126 mg/dL) in the immediate aftermath of a meal.[117] Diabetic subjects tend to have higher postprandial peaks and sustained minor elevations of glucose between meals. The goal of intensive treatment must be to try to reproduce near physiologic levels of glucose throughout the day. Diabetic women are routinely asked to measure their own blood glucose several times a day to aid adjustment of insulin doses. A thorough daily profile requires patients to check blood glucose early morning (fasting) and before meals, at 2 hours after meals, and during the night, but it is probably unrealistic to expect patients to comply with this sort of monitoring every day. Physicians should be aware that self-recorded log books may not always be accurate.[118] Table 45–4 shows typical target figures for blood glucose recommended in UK and North American guidelines.[13–15]

TABLE 45–3

Neonatal Complications of Maternal Diabetes

COMPLICATION	INCIDENCE (%)
Hypoglycemia	25–40
Hypocalcemia	50
Hypomagnesemia	10
Polycythemia	33
Hyperbilirubinemia	20–25
Cardiomyopathy	10
RDS	<2

From Reece EA, Homko CJ: Infant of the diabetic mother. Semin Perinatal 1994;18:459–469.

GLYCOSYLATED HEMOGLOBIN

Proteins react spontaneously with glucose to form glycosylated derivatives. HbA_{1c} serves as a retrospective indicator of the average glucose concentration over the previous 8 to 10 weeks.[119,120] The HbA_{1c} level is more strongly correlated to preprandial than postprandial glucose concentrations. In the third trimester, however, HbA_{1c} levels may only reflect mean glucose values over the previous 2 weeks, presumably because of increased rates of erythropoiesis.[121] HbA_{1c} is expressed as a percentage of the normal hemoglobin, and the normal range is approximately 4% to 6%.[122]

DIETARY REGULATION

For some women, alteration in diet alone is enough to ensure a more normal level of blood glucose. Dietary advice should include a redistribution of meals to ensure a

TABLE 45–4

Target Blood Glucose Concentrations in Pregnancy

	BEFORE MEALS	2 H POSTPRANDIAL
Whole blood glucose	3.9–5.6 mmol/L (70-100 mg/dL)	<7.8 mmol/L (140 mg/dL)
Plasma glucose	4.4–6.1 mmol/L (80-110 mg/dL)	<8.6 mmol/L (155 mg/dL)

From American Diabetes Association guidelines: Preconception care of women with diabetes. Diabetes Care 2003;26:591–593. The Scottish Intercollegiate Guidelines Network[13] and Diabetes UK[15] give similar values.

regular intake of low glycemic index carbohydrates, low in fat and sugar. Recommended caloric intake is tailored to prepregnancy weight.[69] Women with a normal body mass index (BMI) prepregnancy are advised to consume about 30 kcal/kg/day and are expected to gain 28 to 40 pounds during pregnancy. Women with a BMI more than 120% of ideal are advised to cut back caloric intake to 24 kcal/kg/day and aim to gain 25 to 35 pounds during pregnancy. Women significantly underweight prior to pregnancy are advised to consume 36 to 40 kcal/kg/day and to aim to gain 15 to 25 pounds during pregnancy. It is suggested that carbohydrate make up about 40% to 50% of the diet, which is less than is usually advised for nonpregnant patients, in an attempt to limit postprandial peaks of glucose.

INSULIN REGIMENS

Women with type 1 diabetes mellitus require increasing doses of insulin as their pregnancies advance due to changes in carbohydrate metabolism. Those with type 2 diabetes mellitus controlled either by diet or with oral hypoglycemic drugs prepregnancy usually require treatment with insulin once pregnant. In women with established type 2 diabetes controlled by diet alone, persistent postprandial hyperglycemia (>7.5 to 8.0 mmol/L; 120 mg/dL) or fasting hyperglycemia (>6.0 mmol/L; 105 mg/dL) are indications for the introduction of insulin therapy.[15]

Women requiring insulin during pregnancy are managed on a regimen requiring multiple daily dosing. Once-daily or twice-daily subcutaneous doses of intermediate or long-acting insulin are combined with doses of regular insulin before meals. The pharmocodynamics of regular insulin absorption from subcutaneous injections dictates that injections need to be given at least 1/2 hour before meals and that the effects may last for several hours afterward.[123] The insulin analogue Lispro offers a better pharmacodynamic profile than insulin[123] and appears to be safe in pregnancy.[124]

ORAL HYPOGLYCEMIC AGENTS

Oral hypoglycemic drugs (both sulfonylureas and biguanides) are usually avoided in pregnancy because they cross the placenta, potentially resulting in fetal hypoglycemia. However, they have been used in all trimesters and are reportedly safe.[125] Hypoglycemic agents might therefore provide an alternative to insulin for the management of women with type 2 diabetes and with gestational diabetes,[126] especially where self-administration of insulin is difficult for educational or linguistic reasons.

Prepregnancy—Other Issues

Prepregnancy clinics were first introduced in the 1970s in the hope that preconceptual improvements in glycemic control would reduce the number of congenital abnormalities and spontaneous miscarriages in diabetic pregnancies. Several studies have demonstrated the value of this approach.[73,127] A significant number of diabetic women, however, do not plan their pregnancies or choose not to attend such clinics.[128]

Points to be considered during counseling might include the risks of progression of diabetic retinopathy and nephropathy, risks of obstetric outcomes, and risks of diabetes in the offspring. The risk of diabetes in the child is 2% to 3% if the mother has type 1 diabetes mellitus and 4% to 5% if the father is affected. The need for folate supplementation should also be stressed. Women with established diabetes are at an increased risk of having babies with neural tube defects and are therefore recommended to take up to 5 mg of folic acid daily.

A small number of women with complications of diabetes may be on medical treatment that is contraindicated in pregnancy, such as angiotensin-converting enzyme inhibitors to reduce the progression of diabetic nephropathy, and these should be changed to a more appropriate antihypertensive. Lipid-lowering agents that inhibit HMG CoA reductase are also contraindicated in pregnancy because they have been shown to be teratogenic at higher doses in animal studies.

Prenatal—Other Issues

Prenatal care of the diabetic woman is directed at detecting and, if possible, reducing the complications of diabetes.

GLUCOSE CONTROL

Ideally, this will have been optimized before conception, but if not, the prompt confirmation of a viable pregnancy by early scan allows for adjustment of insulin regimens to achieve good glucose control. This requires close liaison between the supervising physician or diabetes nurse and the patient.

BASELINE INVESTIGATIONS

Routine baseline investigations in early pregnancy might be supplemented by an electrocardiogram and by measurement of urea and electrolytes and/or 24-hour urine protein excretion to detect undiagnosed nephropathy if diabetes has been of long duration. A thyroid autoantibody screen and thyroid function test should be done.

CLINICAL REVIEW

If a funduscopic examination has not been done recently, this should be arranged; it should usually be repeated at a later date in pregnancy to exclude proliferative retinopathy. Hypertension should be treated to reduce the risks of progression of retinopathy and nephropathy. A target diastolic blood pressure of 80 mm Hg is advised for nonpregnant hypertensive diabetics, and it is probably wise to aim for similar levels during pregnancy.[129] Meta-analysis suggests that women with risk factors for hypertension and preeclampsia, such as diabetes, might benefit from low-dose aspirin.[130]

SCREENING FOR ABNORMALITY

Early studies of biochemical screening for neural tube defects, trisomy 21, and Edwards syndrome suggested that different reference ranges might be required for diabetics. However, this work has not been supported by later studies.[131] Nuchal translucency measurements in diabetics without congenital anomalies lie in the normal range for the background population.[132] Given the higher incidence of congenital anomalies in diabetic pregnancies, most centers plan to offer a detailed fetal survey around 18 to 20 weeks' gestation. Reported antenatal detection rates for cardiac, CNS, and skeletal abnormalities in insulin-dependent diabetics are around 70%.[133] Approximately 60% to 80% of non-cardiac lesions and 33% to 50% of cardiac lesions are identified antenatally. These rates are not different from routine detailed ultrasonography of low risk populations. Fetal echocardiography can help to identify fetuses with obstructive cardiomyopathy.

FETAL GROWTH

Serial ultrasound estimation of fetal weight is routinely used to identify fetuses showing accelerated growth. Although currently the best tool available, sonographic estimation of fetal weight is often inaccurate, with errors of around 7% of birth weight.[134] It is also worth pointing out that the charts used to calculate fetal weight are not specifically validated for diabetic fetuses, where there are disturbances of body proportions. The positive predictive value of ultrasound measurements for birth weight over 4500 g is only 35%.[135] Magnetic resonance imaging may ultimately offer a more accurate estimate of fetal volume or weight.[136] There has been little published work on the role of more intense insulin therapy in reducing fetal growth in established diabetics once macrosomia has been identified, although most obstetricians use the presence of macrosomia as an indicator of poor control.

FETAL HEALTH SURVEILLANCE

Most obstetricians support a policy of increased fetal assessment in the third trimester to identify impending stillbirth. Paradigms used for monitoring growth-retarded fetuses have been adopted, but these may not be suitable for detecting the acute metabolic decompensation (possibly involving a combination of fetal hypoxia, acidemia, and hypoxia) thought to be involved in late stillbirth in diabetes.[137] Cardiotocography and the biophysical profile (BPP) are acute tests of fetal well-being. There is a correlation between BPP score or fetal heart rate variability and cord pH measured at cordocentesis in diabetic women.[137] In this study, however, 9 of 12 acidotic fetuses had a normal BPP score, and 6 of 12 had normal heart rate variability.[137] It has been suggested that fetal neurobehavioral development in diabetic pregnancies may be different from that of nondiabetic pregnancies, with differences in the baseline breathing and heart rate, frequency of breathing movements, and gross body movements.[138]

Assessment of umbilical blood flow velocity waveform by Doppler is useful in identifying those pregnancies with significant placental vascular resistance. One of the most quoted studies of Doppler ultrasonography in diabetic pregnancy measured the flow velocity waveform every 2 weeks from 28 weeks' gestation in 128 diabetic women and 170 controls.[139] There were 9 abnormal umbilical flow velocity waveforms in the diabetic group, and most of these infants were growth retarded. It was also apparent that significant fetal compromise can occur in the presence of a normal flow waveform. As with nondiabetic pregnancies, abnormal results on Doppler ultrasonography indicate the need for more intense surveillance with cardiotocography or BPP scoring. In women with significant complications of diabetes, where there is an increased risk of IUGR and/or preeclampsia, there is merit in starting fetal surveillance early (from 26 weeks' gestation on), but in those without complications, monitoring could be delayed to after 32 weeks' gestation.[140] There is little evidence to guide the decision about frequency of monitoring, except that twice-weekly nonstress testing in the third trimester is associated with a low perinatal mortality rate.[141] Falling insulin requirements in the third trimester reflect the fact that the fetus is hyperinsulinemic and functioning as a "glucose-sink," draining maternal glucose. It is not clear if such a change indicates the need for increased surveillance.

Labor and Delivery

TIMING AND MODE OF DELIVERY

Decisions regarding the timing and mode of delivery must balance the risks of prematurity with the risks of late intrauterine death and macrosomia. Gestation-specific risks of stillbirth in diabetics continue to fall up to around 38 weeks' gestation and then increase slightly in postdate pregnancies.[142] Most obstetricians and their patients are comfortable with delivery around 38 to 39 weeks. Invasive testing of the lecithin-to-sphingomyelin (L/S) ratio in amniotic fluid to predict fetal lung maturity is difficult to justify in well-controlled term diabetics.[111] The mode of delivery is probably also largely a matter of personal choice, given the increasing cesarean section rate in general. Cost-benefit analysis suggests that in diabetic women, 489 cesarean sections are needed to prevent 1 case of permanent brachial plexus injury where the estimated fetal weight is >4000 g, and 443 cesareans are needed where the estimated fetal weight is >4500 g.[143] Current guidelines issued by the American College of Obstetricians and Gynecologists are to strongly consider elective cesarean where the estimated fetal weight is above 4500 g.[12] Shoulder dystocia remains difficult to predict; in fact the incidence of shoulder dystocia with infants weighing less than 4000 g ranges from 26% to 58% in various reports. There are no conclusive data that early induction of labor prevents dystocia.[12]

GLUCOSE CONTROL

Labor is a time of unpredictable glucose and insulin demands.[69] Unless a rapid labor and delivery is predicted, blood glucose is probably best controlled by a sliding scale of insulin and glucose infusion, adjusted according to regular capillary blood glucose monitoring. Maternal plasma glucose levels during labor and delivery should be maintained at approximately 4 to 8 mmol/L (72 to 144 mg/dL) to avoid maternal hypoglycemia and the associated adverse fetal response.[69]

Postnatal

Following the third stage of labor, the insulin infusion rate is halved; once the woman is eating normally, subcutaneous insulin can be recommenced at the prepregnancy dose.[69] The abrupt decline in pregnancy hormones postpartum results in improved insulin sensitivity, which is further improved by breastfeeding. Insulin doses may need frequent adjustment in the early postpartum period. For breastfeeding women with preexisting type 2 diabetes mellitus, oral hypoglycemic agents should be restarted cautiously because of a risk of hypoglycemia in the infant.

GESTATIONAL DIABETES MELLITUS

Gestational diabetes mellitus (GDM) is defined as "carbohydrate intolerance resulting in hyperglycemia of variable severity with onset or first recognition during pregnancy, whether or not insulin is used and regardless of whether diabetes persists after pregnancy."[17] The original work by O'Sullivan studied women who had been given a 100 g oral glucose challenge test in pregnancy.[144] Diagnostic criteria were developed based on the number of women who subsequently became diabetic. This is not an obstetrically useful outcome, and attention has since focused on defining the relationship between glucose intolerance in pregnancy and outcomes such as macrosomia, operative delivery, and perinatal mortality. Coustan succinctly summarized the issues surrounding the diagnosis of gestational diabetes by posing four key questions[145]:

- What level of maternal hyperglycemia measurably worsens pregnancy outcome?
- Does intervention improve outcome?
- Is such intervention cost effective?
- What is the optimum screening and/or diagnostic test?

Screening for Diabetes in Pregnancy

RATIONALE FOR SCREENING

Successful screening tests require that the condition should be prevalent in the target population, that treatment improves the prognosis, and that treatment is cost effective. Debate continues about the advantages of screening for GDM because not all studies have confirmed a higher incidence of pregnancy complications in women with GDM. A major flaw has been a failure to stratify the degree of hyperglycemia. Some women diagnosed with GDM have severe hyperglycemia and in fact probably have undiagnosed existing diabetes. Others have mild hyperglycemia just above the upper end of the normal range. It is estimated that 70% of women diagnosed with GDM have modest hyperglycemia and require only dietary intervention.[3]

MATERNAL AND FETAL RISKS

The risk of complications is related to the degree of hyperglycemia. In the Toronto Tri-Hospitals study, a cohort of 3637 women who tested negative for GDM at 28 weeks' gestation were followed through pregnancy. Even in these women without GDM, increasing carbohydrate intolerance was associated with a significantly increased incidence of cesarean section, preeclampsia, macrosomia, and need for neonatal phototherapy.[146] In women who have been diagnosed with GDM the incidence of fetal macrosomia is increased. Recent studies suggest 20% to 30% of women with untreated GDM give birth to infants heavier than 4000 g.[62,147] It has been estimated that about 4% of women with GDM will give birth to an infant weighing over 4500 g; the figure for the general obstetric population is about 2% of women.[148] Not surprisingly, most studies of GDM report a cesarean section rate of up to 30%.[62,149–151] It is important, however, to ask if diagnosing and treating GDM significantly changes outcomes. Certainly birth weight can be reduced by insulin treatment in GDM,[151–153] but in the randomized controlled trials reported so far, this does not appear to translate into a reduction in the cesarean section rate or in brachial plexus injury.[3] It should be noted that the trials are small, often the difference in glycemic control between the treated and control groups is minimal, and reductions in birth weight are similarly small.

The evidence for a significant increase in the incidence of preeclampsia and nonproteinuric hypertension in GDM is conflicting. In one case-control study comparing 197 women with GDM to nondiabetic pregnancies, there was a statistically significant but clinically insignificant rise in blood pressure in the third trimester in the diabetic group.[154] Others report an increased incidence of preeclampsia and nonproteinuric hypertension affecting 6% to 20% of pregnancies complicated by GDM, as opposed to 6% to 11% of control pregnancies.[149,153,155,156] Insulin treatment may not reduce the incidence of hypertension, since, even in women with mild glucose intolerance not diagnostic of GDM, preeclampsia and nonproteinuric hypertension were diagnosed in about 20% of cases.[62]

The diagnosis of GDM does not in general indicate increased risk to the fetus and neonate. The perinatal mortality rate for women with GDM or impaired glucose tolerance who are not requiring insulin is low.[157,158]

It has been argued that the principal benefit of screening for GDM is the ability to identify a group of women at risk of subsequently developing diabetes. The cumulative incidence of type 2 diabetes mellitus increases markedly in the first 5 years after delivery and appears to plateau after 10 years.[159] For this to be a justification for screening, however, it would need to be established that such women could successfully be targeted in programs to modify lifestyle (to decrease obesity) and comply with regular follow-up to aid the early identification of diabetes.

SCREENING OPTIONS

The diagnostic test for GDM is the oral GTT. Unfortunately, several bodies have advocated different tests and diagnostic criteria, as shown in Table 45–5.[3] The World Health Association (WHO) definition is based on a 75-g oral test, whereas in North America, a 100-g oral test is used, and two different professional bodies in the United States have even recommended different criteria. Most centers in the United Kingdom use the 75-g oral GTT recommended by the WHO as a single-step screening and diagnostic test. The diagnosis of GDM is made when the fasting and 2-hour glucose values are sufficient for a diagnosis of either impaired glucose tolerance or diabetes. In North America, the American Diabetes Association[160] and National Diabetes Data Group[161] recommend a 100-g oral glucose challenge as the diagnostic test, and a randomly administered 50-g oral glucose challenge as the screening test.[3] The WHO criteria label twice as many women with GDM as do the National Diabetes Data Group criteria.[3] Screening is carried out between 24 and 28 weeks' gestation when insulin resistance tends to be at its maximum.

Several strategies are used for selecting women to undergo diagnostic testing. An inclusive strategy, in which every woman is tested, is expensive and may overdiagnose GDM. A more targeted approach selects women on the basis of risk factors (such as previous GDM, family history, and obesity). It has been estimated that, applying a strategy of universal screening to a population with an average risk of GDM, 8900 women need to be screened to prevent one case of brachial plexus injury using North American criteria.[3] As the prevalence of diabetes increases, the number needed to screen reduces (and this is the advantage of using risk factors to select women for screening). In the Toronto Tri-Hospital study, maternal BMI, age, and race were risk factors for a positive 100-g oral glucose challenge; and using such risk factors meant that about 35% of the general population could be excluded from screening.[162] The American College of Obstetricians and Gynecologists has suggested that women fulfilling the criteria listed in Table 45–6 could be exempted from universal screening.[11]

Another strategy is to take a simple, cheap screening test such as random or fasting blood glucose from all women in pregnancy and to perform formal diagnostic testing on a subgroup identified on the basis of values

TABLE 45–5

Diagnosis of Gestational Diabetes by WHO Criteria (75 g Oral Glucose Tolerance Test) and by National Diabetes Data Group and American Diabetes Association Criteria (100 g Oral Glucose Tolerance Test)

	WHO CRITERIA	NATIONAL DIABETES DATA GROUP CRITERIA	AMERICAN DIABETES ASSOCIATION CRITERIA
Test	75 g oral GTT	100 g oral GTT	100 g oral GTT
Fasting	7.0 mmol/L	5.8 mmol/L	5.3 mmol/L
One hour		10.6 mmol/L	10.0 mmol/L
Two hour	7.8 mmol/L	9.2 mmol/L	8.6 mmol/L
Three hour		8.0 mmol/L	7.8 mmol/L

Key:
Glucose levels are plasma levels in venous blood.
Values in mg/dl: 5.3 mmol/L = 95 mg/dL, 5.8 mmol/L = 105 mg/dL, 7.0 mmol/L = 126 mg/dL, 7.8 mmol/L = 140 mg/dL, 8 mmol/L = 145 mg/dL, 8.6 mmol/L = 155 mg/dL, 9.2 mmol/L = 165 mg/dL, 10 mmol/L = 180 mg/dL, 10.6 mmol/L = 190 mg/dL.

Adapted from Brody SC, Harris R, Lohr K: Screening for gestational diabetes: A summary of the evidence from the US Preventive Service Task Force. Obstet Gynecol 2003;101:380–392.

TABLE 45–6

Criteria Identifying Women at "Low Risk" of GDM

Age <25 years
Low-risk racial or ethnic group (not Hispanic, African, Native American, South or East Asian, or Pacific Islander)
BMI <25
No history of abnormal glucose tolerance
No previous adverse pregnancy outcome associated with GDM
No known first-degree relative with diabetes

From ACOG Practice Bulletin Number 30: Gestational Diabetes. Obstet Gynecol 2001;98:525–538.

from the screening test. Measurements of random blood glucose or glycated proteins such as fructosamine or HbA_{1c}, however, perform poorly as screening tools.[8,163–165] Assessment of fasting blood glucose provides better sensitivity, but even so fasting levels that identify women with GDM on formal testing with either the 75-g or 100-g GTT result in 30% to 50% of women with normal glucose tolerance also requiring testing.[166] In North America, the American Diabetes Association and the National Diabetes Data Group recommend a randomly administered 50-g oral glucose challenge as the screening test.[160,161] Plasma glucose greater than 130 mg/dL or 140 mg/dL 1 hour after a 50-g load indicates the need for a full diagnostic glucose challenge. Screening with a 50-g challenge compared with simple measurement of fasting glucose reduces the number of women requiring a diagnostic GTT from around 30% to 15%.[167]

Management Options

The diagnosis of GDM encompasses a wide range of glucose intolerance; many women can be managed without the need for insulin. A reasonable goal of medical therapy might be to reduce the incidence of macrosomia, because this should impact on the cesarean section rate, shoulder dystocia, and brachial plexus injury. Women with GDM can be taught to monitor blood glucose at home, although the optimum frequency of glucose assessment has not been established. Similarly, women with GDM should be given the same advice about diet as women with established diabetes. About 45% of women with GDM diagnosed by 100-g oral challenge can be managed by diet alone.[150] As the number of abnormal glucose values on the GTT increases, so do the chances of the woman requiring insulin therapy

Several different strategies have been employed when deciding when to start insulin treatment. Fasting plasma glucose above 6.0 mmol/L (108 mg/dL) or a 2-hour postprandial value of 7.0 mmol/L (126 mg/dL) have been incorporated into guidelines as an indication to commence insulin therapy.[10,13] Others have suggested using the presence of fetal macrosomia as the trigger for starting insulin.[168,169] A more invasive, physiologically driven approach involves amniocentesis to measure amniotic fluid insulin and starting insulin treatment where there is evidence of fetal hyperinsulinemia. None of these approaches has been subjected to a sufficiently powered randomized study.[3,19]

The perinatal mortality rate in GDM is generally lower than that in established diabetes, and it is likely to be difficult to establish whether antenatal monitoring reduces the perinatal mortality rate. Pragmatically, however, it may be best to use an approach similar to that used in established diabetes, especially in women with GDM requiring insulin.[170]

Delivery can be planned at 40 weeks' gestation if the GDM is well-controlled, because the incidence of intrauterine death near term is lower than in preexisting diabetes, at least for women not requiring insulin.[157,158] In a randomized controlled trial comparing routine induction of labor between 38 and 39 weeks' gestation to expectant management, there did not appear to be any difference in the incidence of cesarean delivery; however, there were proportionally more babies that were large for gestational age in the group of women that were managed expectantly, compared to those that were induced.[171] Lurie and colleagues showed that there were more cases of shoulder dystocia in women who were managed expectantly compared to those who were induced at 38 to 39 weeks' gestation (10% versus 1.4%), with no difference in the cesarean section rate.[172]

A diagnosis of GDM carries the implication that diabetes may subsequently develop with pregnancy. A formal oral GTT should be carried out some 2 to 3 months after pregnancy, when approximately 3% of women will be found to have diabetes.[159] It would seem prudent to offer advice about lifestyle modifications that might reduce the likelihood of developing diabetes. Follow-up studies of women with GDM indicate that up to 70% will develop diabetes within 28 years.[159] The American Diabetes Association has recommended a 3-yearly oral GTT to screen for the development of diabetes in these women.

CONCLUSIONS

- In most centers the pregnancy outcome goals in women with diabetes is still approximate to that of the nondiabetic woman.
- Some women with long-standing diabetes enter pregnancy with impaired renal function, retinopathy, or chronic hypertension and are predictably at increased risk of a poor outcome.

CONCLUSIONS (Continued)

- All of the recognized pregnancy complications of diabetes (congenital abnormalities, miscarriage, preterm delivery, late stillbirth, macrosomia, and preeclampsia) are exacerbated by hyperglycemia and can be largely negated by strict attention to glycemic control periconceptually and throughout pregnancy.
- Current regimens of insulin do not restore the blood glucose profile throughout the day to normal.
- Women diagnosed with GDM or impaired glucose tolerance are a heterogeneous group:
  - Some have glucose tolerance just above the normal range and are at low risk for pregnancy complications.
  - Others almost certainly have undiagnosed diabetes and require insulin treatment and pregnancy surveillance in the same way as established diabetics.
  - Because of the heterogeneous nature of the group and pregnancy outcomes, the cost-effectiveness of screening for GDM is low; such screening may not be justified.

SUMMARY OF MANAGEMENT OPTIONS

Diabetes in Pregnancy

Management Options	Quality of Evidence	Strength of Recommendation	References
Prepregnancy			
Explain general risks and management of diabetes in pregnancy.	IV	C	175
Evaluate any additional risks with appropriate specialist referral (e.g., renal, ophthalmologic).	III Ib	B A	176 177
Optimize blood glucose control with the same target range as for pregnancy (see Table 45–4) (main aim is to reduce congenital abnormalities).	Ib III	A B	73 127
Discuss effective contraception until good glucose control (avoid estrogen-containing preparations with vascular disease).	–	GPP	–
Provide folate supplementation (4–5 mg daily) for at least 2 months before and during first trimester.	Ib	A	178
Prenatal			
Screen for gestational diabetes ideally in all pregnancies at ~28 weeks; WHO recommends 75-g oral GTT for diagnosis (see Table 45–2).	IV	C	16,179
Perform regular capillary glucose series; start/adjust insulin regimen to keep capillary glucose values within Table 45–4 target range.	IV	C	13,14,15
Insulin pump does not confer advantage over conventional insulin treatment.	Ib	A	180
Data limited but probably best to avoid oral hypoglycemic agents.	III	B	125,126
Suggest appropriate diet in accordance with prepregnancy weight.	IV	C	69
Instruct partners/relatives in glucagon use for hypoglycemic attacks.	–	GPP	–
Monitor baseline renal and possibly cardiac function.	–	GPP	–
Ensure regular ophthalmologic review.	Ib	A	177
Monitor for hypertensive disease; aim to keep diastolic at ~80 mm Hg.	III IV	B C	176 129
Avoid/change from ACE inhibitors.	III	B	181
Low-dose aspirin is safe and may be beneficial; possibly reserve use only to those with vascular disease.	Ia	A	130
Initiate fetal surveillance (limited evidence to determine the value of these tests in diabetic pregnancies):			
• Normality (serum screening, NT, 20-week ultrasound)	III	B	131,132,133
• Growth (Note: limitations and overestimation of fetal weight)	III	B	134,135
• Well-being (Note: NST, BPS, and AFV may not be as predictive of fetal risk as in IUGR)	III	B	137,138,173

Continued

SUMMARY OF MANAGEMENT OPTIONS

Diabetes in Pregnancy *(Continued)*

Management Options	Quality of Evidence	Strength of Recommendation	References
Prenatal—(Continued)			
• Umbilical artery blood flow (Note: predictive of fetal risk in pregnancies complicated by placental vascular disease; uncertain value in other diabetic pregnancies)	III	B	139,173
• Timing and frequency of testing uncertain; possibly from 26 weeks' with vascular disease and 32 weeks' otherwise	III	B	140
Gestational Diabetes			
Initially try to control with diet before insulin.	IV	C	10,13
	III	B	150
• Criteria for starting insulin vary (high glucose values vs macrosomia).	Ib	A	168
	III	B	169
• Otherwise manage as for established diabetics. (Evidence supporting this approach is limited.)	–	GPP	–
• Timing of delivery: conflicting evidence for the value of 38 vs 40 weeks.	Ib	A	171
	III	B	172
• GTT after pregnancy:	Ia	A	159
• at 2-3 months (to confirm resolution)			
• every 3 years (to identify development of type 2 diabetes).			
Labor and Delivery			
Can be delayed until term (38-39 weeks) if diabetes is well controlled and pregnancy uncomplicated.	Ib	A	142,171
Use of tests of lung maturity not considered necessary at that gestation.	IIb	B	111
Method of delivery will depend on complications in mother and/or fetus.	–	GPP	–
No evidence that induction of labor reduces risk of shoulder dystocia.	IV	C	12
ACOG recommends consider elective cesarean section if estimated fetal weight >4.5 kg.	IV	C	12
Maintain good perinatal glucose control.	IV	C	69
Postnatal			
Insulin requirements usually reduced to prepregnancy requirements (often lower if breastfeeding).	IV	C	69
Continue capillary glucose monitoring.	IV	C	69
Encourage breastfeeding.	–	GPP	–
Give contraceptive advice.	–	GPP	–

REFERENCES

1. Garner P: Type 1 diabetes mellitus and pregnancy. Lancet 1995; 346:157–161.
2. Feig DS, Palda VA: Type 2 diabetes in pregnancy: A growing concern. Lancet 2002;359:1690–1692.
3. Brody SC, Harris R, Lohr K: Screening for gestational diabetes: A summary of the evidence from the US Preventive Services Task Force. Obstet Gynecol 2003; 101:380–392.
4. Clark CM, Lee DA: Prevention and treatment of the complications of diabetes mellitus. N Engl J Med 1995;332:1210–1217.
5. Dunne FP: Pregestational diabetes mellitus and pregnancy. Trends Endocrinol Metab 1999;10:179–182.
6. Schwartz R , Teramo KA: Effects of diabetic pregnancy on the fetus and newborn. Semin Perinatol 2000;24:120–135.
7. Greene MF: Screening for gestational diabetes mellitus. N Engl J Med 1997;337:1625–1626.
8. Jarrett RJ: Should we screen for gestational diabetes? The concept of gestational diabetes was popularised before considerations of evidence-based medicine came on the scene. BMJ 1997; 315:736–737.

9. Kjos SL, Buchanan TA: Gestational diabetes mellitus. N Engl J Med 1999;341:1749–1756.
10. American Diabetes Association: Gestational diabetes mellitus. Diabetes Care 2003;26:S103–S105.
11. Gestational diabetes: ACOG Practice Bulletin Number 30. Obstet Gynecol 2001;98:525–538.
12. Fetal macrosomia: ACOG Practice Bulletin Number 22. Obstet Gynecol 2000;96(5).
13. Scottish Intercollegiate Guidelines Network Edinburgh: Management of diabetes. Section 8 Management of diabetes in pregnancy. 2001.
14. American Diabetic Association guidelines: Preconception care of women with diabetes. Diabetes Care 2003;26:S91–S93.
15. Diabetes UK: Recommendations for the management of pregnant women with diabetes (including gestational diabetes). 2002.
16. Albertini K, Zimmet P: Definition, diagnosis and classification of diabetes mellitus and its complications. Part 1: Diagnosis and classification of diabetes mellitus. Provisional report of a WHO consultation. Diabetes Med 1998;15:539–553.
17. Report of the Expert Committee on the Diagnosis and Classification of Diabetes Mellitus. Diabetes Care 2003;26:S5–S20.
18. Buchanan TA, Metzeger BE, Freinkel N, Bergman RN: Insulin sensitivity and beta-cell responsiveness to glucose during late pregnancy in lean and moderately obese women with normal glucose tolerance or mild gestational diabetes. Am J Obstet Gynecol 1990;162:1008–1114.
19. Fraser R: Diabetic control in pregnancy and intrauterine growth of the fetus. BJOG 1995;102:275–277.
20. Pedersen JF: Weight and length at birth of infants of diabetic mothers. Acta Endocrinol (Copenh) 1954;16:330-342.
21. Brownlee M: Biochemistry and molecular cell biology of diabetic complications. Nature 2001;414:813–820.
22. Pieper GM: Enhanced, unaltered and impaired nitric oxide-mediated endothelium-dependent relaxation in experimental diabetes mellitus: importance of disease duration. Diabetologia 1999;42:203–213.
23. Ang C, Hillier C, Johnston F, et al: Endothelial function is preserved in pregnant women with well-controlled type 1 diabetes. BJOG 2002;109:699–707.
24. Ramsay JE, Simms RJ, Ferrell WR, et al: Enhancement of endothelial function by pregnancy: Inadequate response in women with type 1 diabetes. Diabetes Care 2003;26:475–479.
25. Mayhew TM, Jairam IC: Stereological comparison of 3D spatial relationships involving villi and intervillous pores in human placentas from control and diabetic pregnancies. J Anat 2000;197: 263–274.
26. Stanek J, Eis AL, Myatt L: Nitrotyrosine immunostaining correlates with increased extracellular matrix: evidence of postplacental hypoxia. Placenta 2001;22(Suppl):S56–S62.
27. The effect of intensive treatment of diabetes on the development and progression of long-term complications in insulin-dependent diabetes mellitus. N Engl J Med 1993;329:977–986.
28. UK Prospective Diabetes Study (UKPDS) Group: Effect of intensive blood-glucose control with metformin on complications in overweight patients with type 2 diabetes (UKPDS 34). Lancet 1998;352:854–865.
29. UK Prospective Diabetes Study (UKPDS) Group: Intensive blood-glucose control with sulphonylureas or insulin compared with conventional treatment and risk of complications in patients with type 2 diabetes (UKPDS 33). Lancet 1998;352:837–853.
30. Reichard P, Berglund B, Britz A, et al: Intensified conventional insulin treatment retards the microvascular complications of insulin-dependent diabetes mellitus (IDDM): The Stockholm Diabetes Intervention Study (SDIS). J Intern Med 1991;230: 101–108.
31. Kimmerlee R, Heinemann L, Delecki A, Berger M: Severe hypoglycaemia incidence and predisposing factors in 85 pregnancies of type 1 diabetic women. Diabetes Care 1992;15: 1034–1037.
32. Ferris FL, Davis MD, Aiello LM: Treatment of diabetic retinopathy. N Engl J Med 1999;341:667–668.
33. Chew EY, Mills JL, Metzger BE, et al: Metabolic control and progression of retinopathy: the diabetes in early pregnancy study. Diabetes Care 1995;18:631–637.
34. Lovestram-Adrian M, Agardh CD, Aberg A, Agardh E: Pre-eclampsia is a potent risk factor for deterioration of retinopathy in type 1 diabetic patients. Diabetic Medicine 1997; 14:1059–1065.
35. Remuzzi G, Schieppati A, Ruggenenti P: Nephropathy in patients with type 2 diabetes. N Engl J Med 2002;346:1145–1151.
36. Ritz E, Reinhold SR: Nephropathy in patients with type 2 diabetes mellitus. N Engl J Med 1999;341:1127–1133.
37. How HY, Sibai BM: Use of angiotensin-converting enzyme inhibitors in patients with diabetic nephropathy. J Matern Fetal Neonat Med 2002;12:402–407.
38. Rossing K, Jacobsen P, Hommel E, et al: Pregnancy and progression of diabetic nephropathy. Diabetologia 2002;45: 36–41.
39. Biesenbach G, Grafinger P, Stoger H, Zarzgornik J: How pregnancy influences renal function in nephropathic type 1 diabetic women depends on their pre-conceptual creatinine clearance. J Nephrol 1999;12:41–46.
40. Purdy LP, Hantsch CE, Molitch ME, et al: Effect of pregnancy on renal function in patients with moderate-to-severe diabetic renal insufficiency. Diabetes Care 1996;19:1067–1074.
41. Schroder W, Heyl W, Hill-Grasshoff B, Rath W: Clinical value of detecting microalbuminuria as a risk factor for pregnancy-induced hypertension in insulin-treated diabetic pregnancies. Eur J Obstet Gynaecol Reprod Biol 2000;91:155–158.
42. Khoury JC, Miodovnik M, LeMasters G, Sibai BM: Pregnancy outcome and progression of diabetic nephropathy. J Matern Fetal Neonat Med 2002;11:238–244.
43. Dunne FP, Chowdhury A, Hartland A, et al: Pregnancy outcome in women with insulin-dependent diabetes mellitus complicated by nephropathy. Quart J Med 1999;92:451–454.
44. Sibai B: Chronic hypertension in pregnancy. Obstet Gynecol 2002;100:369–377.
45. Hiilesmaa V, Suhonen L, Teramo K: Glycaemic control is associated with pre-eclampsia but not with pregnancy-induced hypertension in women with type 1 diabetes mellitus. Diabetologica 2000;43:1534–1539.
46. Garner PR, D'Alton ME, Dudley DK, et al: Pre-eclampsia in diabetic pregnancies. Am J Obstet Gynecol 1990;163:505–508.
47. Sibai BM, Caritis S, Hauth J, et al: Risks of preeclampsia and adverse neonatal outcomes among women with pregestational diabetes mellitus. National Institute of Child Health and Human Development Network of Maternal-Fetal Medicine Units. Am J Obstet Gynecol 2000;182:364–369.
48. Cundy T, Slee F, Gamble G, Neale L: Hypertensive disorders of pregnancy in women with type 1 and type 2 diabetes. Diabetes Med 2002;19:482–489.
49. Reece EA, Sivan E, Francis G, Homko CJ: Pregnancy outcomes among women with and without diabetic microvascular disease (White's classes B to FR) versus non-diabetic controls. Am J Perinatol 1998;15:549–555.
50. Siddiqi T, Rosenn B, Mimouni F, et al: Hypertension during pregnancy in insulin-dependent diabetic women. Obstet Gynecol 1991;77:514–519.
51. Gordon MC, Landon MB, Boyle J, et al: Coronary artery disease in insulin-dependent diabetes mellitus of pregnancy (class H): A review of the literature. Obstet Gynecol Surv 1996;51:437–444.
52. Hemachandra A, Ellis D, Lloyd CE, Orchard TJ: The influence of pregnancy on IDDM complications. Diabetes Care 1995;18: 950–954.
53. MacLeod AF, Smith SA, Sonksen PH, Lowy C: The problem of autonomic neuropathy in diabetic pregnancy. Diabetes Med 1990;7:80–82.

54. Zachary T, Bloomgarden MD: Neuropathy, womens' health, and socioeconomic aspects of diabetes. Diabetes Care 2002;25: 1085–1094.
55. Stamler EF, Cruz ML, Mimouni F, et al: High infectious morbidity in pregnant women with insulin dependent diabetes: An understated complication. Am J Obstet Gynecol 1990;163: 1217–1221.
56. Cousins L: Pregnancy complications among diabetic women. Obstet Gynecol Surv 1987;42:140–149.
57. Gallas PR, Stolk RP, Bakker K, et al: Thyroid dysfunction during pregnancy and in the first postpartum year in women with diabetes mellitus type 1. Eur J Endocrinol 2002;147:443–451.
58. Howorka K, Pumprla J, Gabriel M, et al: Normalization of pregnancy outcome in pregestational diabetes through functional insulin treatment and modular out-patient education adapted for pregnancy. Diabetes Med 2001;18:965–972.
59. Ray JG, Vermeulen MJ, Shapiro JL, Kenshole AB: Maternal and neonatal outcomes in pregestational and gestational diabetes mellitus, and the influence of maternal obesity and weight gain: The DEPOSIT study. Diabetes Endocrine Pregnancy Outcome Study in Toronto. Quart J Med 2001;94:347–356.
60. Gunton JE, Morris J, Boyce S, et al: Outcome of pregnancy complicated by pregestational diabetes—improvement in outcomes. Austr NZ J Obstet Gynaecol 2002;42:478–481.
61. Dunne FP, Brydon PA, Proffitt M, et al: Fetal and maternal outcomes in Indo-Asian compared to Caucasian women with diabetes in pregnancy. Quar J Med 2000;93:813–818.
62. Naylor CD, Sermer M, Chen E, Sykora RH: Cesarean delivery in relation to birthweight and gestational glucose tolerance: Pathophysiology or practice style? JAMA 1996;275:1165–1170.
63. Langer O, Berkus MD, Huff RW, Samueloff A: Shoulder dystocia: Should the fetus weighing >4000 g be delivered by caesarean section? Am J Obstet Gynecol 1991;165:831–837.
64. Vaarasmaki MS, Hartikainen AL, Anttila M, et al: Factors predicting peri- and neonatal outcome in diabetic pregnancy. Early Hum Devel 2000;59:61–70.
65. Farrell T, Neale L, Cundy T: Congenital anomalies in the offspring of women with type 1, type 2 and gestational diabetes. Diabetes Med 2002;19:322–326.
66. Temple R, Aldridge V, Greenwood R, et al: Association between outcome of pregnancy and glycaemic control in early pregnancy in type 1 diabetes: Population-based study. BMJ 2002;325: 1275–1276.
67. Sheffield JS, Butler-Koster EL, Casey BM, et al: Maternal diabetes mellitus and infant malformations. Obstet Gynecol 2002;100:925–930.
68. Weintrob N, Karp M, Hod M: Short and long-range complications in offspring of diabetic mothers. J Diabetic Complica 1996;10:294–301.
69. Miller EH: Metabolic management of diabetes in pregnancy. Semin Perinatol 1994;18:414-31.
70. Greene MF: Prevention and diagnosis of congenital anomalies in diabetic pregnancies. Clin Perinaol 1993;20:533–547.
71. Reece EA, Homko CJ: Metabolic fuel mixes and diabetic embryopathy. Clin Perinatol 1993;20:517–532.
72. Mills JL, Baker L, Goldman AS: Malformations in infants of diabetic mothers occur before the seventh gestational week: Implications for treatment. Diabetes 1979;28:292–293.
73. Steel JM, Johnstone FD, Hepburn DA, Smith AF: Can prepregnancy care of diabetic women reduce the risk of abnormal babies? BMJ 1990;301:1070–1074.
74. Mills JL, Knopp RH, Simpson JL, et al: Lack of relation of increased malformation rates in infants of diabetic mothers to glycaemic control during organogenesis. N Engl J Med 1988;318:671–676.
75. Pregnancy outcomes in the Diabetes Control and Complications Trial. Am J Obstet Gynecol 1996;174:1343–1353.
76. Kaplan JS, Iqbal S, England BG, et al: Is pregnancy in diabetic women associated with folate deficiency? Diabetes Care 1999;22:1017–1021.
77. Mills JL, Simpson JL, Driscoll SG, et al: Incidence of spontaneous abortion among normal women and insulin-dependent diabetic women whose pregnancies were identified within 21 days of conception. N Engl J Med 1988;319:1617–1623.
78. Rosenn B, Miodovnik M, Combs CA, et al: Glycaemic thresholds for spontaneous abortion and congenital malformations in insulin-dependent diabetes mellitus. Obstet Gynecol 1994;84: 515–520.
79. Kovilam O, Khoury J, Miodovnik M, et al: Spontaneous preterm delivery in the type 1 diabetic pregnancy: the role of glycaemic control. J Matern Fetal Neonat Med 2002;11:245–248.
80. Berkowitz GS, Blackmore-Prince C, Lapinski RH, Savitz DA: Risk factors for preterm birth subtypes. Epidemiol 1998;9: 279–285.
81. Johnstone FD, Mao JH, Steel JM, et al: Factors affecting fetal weight distribution in women with type 1 diabetes. BJOG 2000;107:1001–1006.
82. Bradley RJ, Nicolaides KH, Brudenell MJ: Are all infants of diabetic mothers "macrosomic"? BMJ 1988;297:1583–1584.
83. Raychaudhuri K, Maresh MJ: Glycaemic control throughout pregnancy and fetal growth in insulin dependent diabetics. Obstet Gynecol 2000;95:190–194.
84. McFarland MB, Trylovich CG, Langer O: Anthropometric differences in macrosomic infants of diabetic and nondiabetic mothers. J Matern Fetal Neonat Med 1998;7:292–295.
85. Fallucca F, Sciullo E, Napoli A, et al: Amniotic fluid insulin and C peptide levels in diabetic and nondiabetic women during early pregnancy. J Clin Endocrinol Metab 1996;81:137–139.
86. Weiss PA, Kainer F, Haas J: Cord blood insulin to assess the quality of treatment in diabetic pregnancies. Early Hum Devel 1998;51:187–195.
87. Jovanovic-Peterson L, Peterson CM, Reed GF, et al: Maternal postprandial glucose levels and infant birth weight: The Diabetes in Early Pregnancy Study. Am J Obstet Gynecol 1991; 164:103–111.
88. Parretti E, Mecacci F, Papini M, et al: Third-trimester maternal glucose levels from diurnal profiles in nondiabetic pregnancies: Correlation with sonographic parameters of fetal growth. Diabetes Care 2001;24:1319–1323.
89. Weiss PA, Hofmann H, Winter R, et al: Amniotic fluid glucose values in normal and abnormal pregnancies. Obstet Gynecol 1985;65:333–339.
90. Yasuhi I, Ishimaru T, Hirai M, Yamabe T: Hourly fetal urine production rate in the fasting and the postprandial state of normal and diabetic women. Obstet Gynecol 1994;84:64–68.
91. Biggio JR, Wenstrom KD, Dubard MB, Cliver SP: Hydramnios prediction of adverse perinatal outcome. Obstet Gynecol 1999;94:773–777.
92. Penney GC, Mair G, Pearson DW: Outcomes of pregnancies in women with type 1 diabetes in Scotland: A national population-based study. BJOG 2003;110:315–318.
93. Casson IF, Clarke CA, Howard CV, et al: Outcomes of pregnancy in insulin dependent diabetic women: Results of a five year population cohort study. BMJ 1997;315:275–278.
94. Platt MJ, Stanisstreet M, Casson IF, et al: St Vincent's Declaration 10 years on: Outcomes of diabetic pregnancies. Diabetes Med 2002;19:216–220.
95. Neilsen GL , Neilsen PH: Outcome of 328 pregnancies in 205 women with insulin-dependent diabetes mellitus in the county of Northern Jutland from 1976-1990. Eur J Obstet Gynaecol Reprod Biol 1993;50:33–38.
96. Hawthorne G, Robson S, Ryall EA, et al: Prospective population based survey of outcome of pregnancy in diabetic women: Results of the Northern Diabetic Pregnancy Audit, 1994. BMJ 1997;315:279–281.
97. Cundy T, Gamble G, Townend K, et al: Perinatal mortality in type 2 diabetes mellitus. Diabetes Med 2000;17:33–39.
98. Hadden DR, Alexander A, McCance DR, Traub AI: Obstetric and diabetic care for pregnancy in diabetic women: 10 years outcome analysis, 1985-1995. Diabetes Med 2001;18:546–553.

99. Mondestin MA, Ananth CV, Smulian JC, Vintzileos AM: Birth weight and fetal death in the United States: The effect of maternal diabetes during pregnancy. Am J Obstet Gynecol 2002;187: 922–926.
100. Philipps AF, Dublin JW, Matty PS, Raye JR: Arterial hypoxaemia and hyperinsulinaemia in the chronically hyperglycaemic fetal lamb. Paediatr Res 1982;16:653–658.
101. Miodovnik M, Lavin JP, Barden T, et al: Effect of maternal ketoacidaemia on the pregnant ewe and the fetus. Am J Obstet Gynecol 1982;144:585–583.
102. Salvesen DR, Brudenell MJ, Nicolaides KH: Fetal polythemia and thrombocytopenia in pregnancies complicated by maternal diabetes. Am J Obstet Gynecol 1992;166:1287–1292.
103. Landon MB: Obstetric Management of Pregnancies Complicated by Diabetes Mellitus. Clin in Obstet Gynecol, 2000;43:65–74.
104. Nelson-Piercy C: Diabetes. In Handbook of Obstetric Medicine, 2nd ed. Oxford, Martin Dunitz, 2002, pp 82–99.
105. Greco P, Vimercati A, Giorgino F, et al: Reversal of foetal hydrops and foetal tachyarrhythmia associated with maternal diabetic coma. Eur J Obste Gynaecol Reprod Biol 2000;93:33–35.
106. Girz BA, Divon MY, Merkatz IR: Sudden fetal death in women with well-controlled, intensively monitored gestational diabetes. J Perinatol 1992;12:229–233.
107. Nassar AH, Usta IM, Khalil AM, et al: Fetal macrosomia (≥4500 g): Perinatal outcome of 231 cases according to the mode of delivery. J Perinatol 2003;23:136–141.
108. Reece EA, Homko CJ: Infant of the diabetic mother. Semin Perinatol 1994;18:459–469.
109. Schwarz P, Sorensen HA, Momsen G, et al: Hypocalcaemia and parathyroid hormone responsiveness in diabetes mellitus: A trisodium-citrate clamp study. Acta Endocrinol (Copenh), 1992;126:260–263.
110. Piper JM: Lung maturation in diabetes in pregnancy: If and when to test. Semin Perinatol 2002;26:206–209.
111. Kjos SL, Berkowitz KM, Kung B: Prospective delivery of reliably dated term infants of diabetic mothers without determination of fetal lung maturity: Comparison to historical control. J Matern Fetal Neonat Med 2002;12:433–437.
112. Kjos SL, Walther FJ, Montoro M, et al: Prevalence and etiology of respiratory distress in infants of diabetic mothers: predictive value of fetal lung maturation tests. Am J Obstet Gynecol 1990; 163:898–903.
113. Dekowski SA , Snyder JM: Insulin regulation of messenger ribonucleic acid for the surfactant-associated proteins in human fetal lung in vitro. Endocrinol 1992;131:669–676.
114. Susa JB, McCormick KL, Widness JA, et al: Chronic hyperinsulinaemia in the fetal rhesus monkey. Effects of fetal growth and composition. Diabetes 1979;28:1058–1063.
115. Pedra SRFF, Smallhorn JF, Ryan G, et al: Fetal cardiomyopathies. Pathologenic mechanisms, hemodynamic findings, and clinical outcome. Circulation 2002;106:585–591.
116. Reller MD, Kapla S: Hypertrophic cardiomyopathy in infants of diabetic mothers: An update. Am J Perinatol 1988;5:353–358.
117. Saltiel AR , Kahn CR: Insulin signalling and the regulation of glucose and lipid metabolism. Nature 2001;414:799–806.
118. Langer O, Mazze RS: Diabetes in pregnancy: evaluating self-monitoring performance and glycaemic control with memory-based reflectance meter. Am J Obstet Gynecol 1986;155: 635–637.
119. Rohfling CL, Wiedmeyer HM, Little RR, et al: Defining the relationship between plasma glucose and HbA(1c): Analysis of glucose profiles and HbA(1c) in the Diabetes Control and Complications Trial. Diabetes Care 2002;25:275–278.
120. Hillman N, Herranz L, Grande C, et al: Is HbA_{1c} influenced more strongly by preprandial or postprandial glycemia in type 1 diabetes? Diabetes Care 2002;25:1100–1101.
121. Parfitt VJ, Clark JD, Turner GM, Hartog M: Use of fructosamine and glycated haemoglobin to verify self blood glucose monitoring data in diabetic pregnancy. Diabetes Med 1993;10: 162–166.
122. O'Kane MJ, Lynch PL, Moles KW, Magee SE: Determination of a diabetes control and complications trial-aligned HbA(1c) reference range in pregnancy. Clin Chimica Acta 2001;311: 157–159.
123. Holleman F, Hoekstra JBL: Insulin lispro. N Engl J Med 1997;337:176–183.
124. Bhattacharyya A, Brown S, Hughes S, Vice PA: Insulin lispro and regular insulin in pregnancy. Quart J Med 2001;94:255–260.
125. Coetzee EJ, Jackson WP: Oral hypoglycaemics in the first trimester and fetal outcome. So Afr Med J 1984;65:635–637.
126. Langer O, Oral hypoglycaemic agents in pregnancy: their time has come. J Matern Fetal Neonat Med, 2002;12:376–383.
127. McElvy SS, Miodovnik M, Rosenn B, et al: A focused preconceptual and early pregnancy program in women with type 1 diabetes reduces perinatal mortality and malformation rates to general population levels. J Matern Fetal Med 2000;9:14–20.
128. Holing EV, Beyer CS, Brown ZA, Connell FA: Why don't women with diabetes plan their pregnancies? Diabetes Care 1998;21:889–895.
129. Ramsay LE, Williams B, Johnston GD, et al: British Hypertension Society guidelines for hypertension management 1999: Summary. BMJ 1999; 319:630–635.
130. Coomarasamy A, Honest H, Papaioannou S, et al: Aspirin for prevention of preeclampsia in women with historical risk factors: A systematic review. Obstet Gynecol 2003;101:1319–1332.
131. Evans MI, Harrison HH, O'Brien JE, et al: Correction for insulin-dependent diabetes in maternal serum alpha-fetoprotein testing has outlived its usefulness. Am J Obstet Gynecol 2002;187:1084–1086.
132. Bartha JL, Wood J, Kyle PM, Soothill PW: The effect of metabolic control on fetal nuchal translucency in women with insulin-dependent diabetes: A preliminary study. Ultrasound in Obstet Gynecol 2003;21:451–454.
133. Albert TJ, Landon MB, Wheller JJ, et al: Prenatal detection of fetal anomalies in pregnancies complicated by insulin-dependent diabetes mellitus. Am J Obstet Gynecol 1996;174:1424–1428.
134. Best G, Pressman EK: Ultrasonographic prediction of birth weight in diabetic pregnancies. Obstet Gynecol 2002;99: 740–744.
135. Smith GC, Smith MF, McNay MB, Fleming JE: The relation between fetal abdominal circumference and birth weight: findings in 3512 pregnancies. BJOG 1997;104:186–190.
136. Uotila J, Dastidar P, Heinonen T, et al: Magnetic resonance imaging compared to ultrasonography in fetal weight and volume estimation in diabetic and normal pregnancy. Acta Obstet Gynecol Scand 2000;79:255–259.
137. Salvesen DR, Freeman J, Brudenell MJ, Nicolaides KH: Prediction of fetal acidaemia in pregnancies complicated by maternal diabetes mellitus by biophysical profile scoring and fetal heart rate monitoring. BJOG 1993;100:227–233.
138. Devoe LD, Youssef AA, Castillo RA, Croom CS: Fetal biophysical activities in third trimester pregnancies complicated by diabetes mellitus. Am J Obstet Gynecol 1994;171:298–303.
139. Johnstone FD, Steel JM, Haddad NG, et al: Doppler umbilical artery flow velocity waveforms in diabetic pregnancy. BJOG 1992;99:135–140.
140. Lagrew DC, Pircon RA, Towers CV, et al: Antepartum fetal surveillance in patients with diabetes: When to start? Am J Obstet Gynecol 1993;168:1820–1825.
141. Kjos SL, Leung A, Henry OA, et al: Antepartum surveillance in diabetic pregnancies: predictors of fetal distress in labor. Am J Obstet Gynecol 1995;173:1532–1539.
142. Smulian JC, Ananth CV, Vintzileos AM, et al: Fetal deaths in the United States: Influence of high-risk conditions and implications for management. Obstet Gynecol 2002;100:1183–1189.

143. Rouse DJ, Owen J, Goldenberg RL, Cliver SP: The effectiveness and costs of elective cesarean delivery for fetal macrosomia diagnosed by ultrasound. JAMA 1996;276:1480–1486.
144. O'Sullivan JB, Mahan CM: Criteria for the oral glucose tolerance test in pregnancy. Diabetes 1964;13:278–285.
145. Coustan DR: Management of gestational diabetes mellitus: A self-fulfilling prophecy? JAMA 1996;275:1199–1200.
146. Sermer M, Naylor CD, Gare DJ, et al: Impact of increasing carbohydrate intolerance on maternal-fetal outcomes in 3637 women without gestational diabetes: The Toronto Tri-Hospital Gestational Diabetes Project. Am J Obstet Gynecol 1995;173: 146–156.
147. Garner P, Okun N, Keely E, et al: A randomized controlled trial of strict glycemic control and tertiary level obstetric care versus routine obstetric care in the management of gestational diabetes. Am J Obstet Gynecol 1997;177:190–195.
148. Ales KL, Santini DL: Should all pregnant women be screened for gestational glucose intolerance? Lancet 1989;i:1187–1191.
149. Jensen DM, Sorensen B, Feilberg-Jorgensen N, et al: Maternal and perinatal outcomes in 143 Danish women with gestational diabetes mellitus and 143 controls with a similar risk profile. Diabetes Med 2000;17:281–286.
150. Gruendhammer M, Brezinka C, Lechleitner M: The number of abnormal plasma glucose values in the oral glucose tolerance test and the feto-maternal outcome of pregnancy. Eur J Obstet Gynecol Reprod Biol 2003;108:131–136.
151. Nachum Z, Ben-Shlomo I, Weiner E, Shalev E: Twice daily versus four times daily insulin dose regimens for diabetes in pregnancy: Randomised controlled trial. BMJ 1999;319:1223–1227.
152. Langer O, Levy J, Brustman L, et al: Glycaemic control in gestational diabetes mellitus—how tight is tight enough: Small for gestational age versus large for gestational age? Am J Obstet Gynecol 1989;161:646–653.
153. de Veciana M, Major CA, Morgan MA, et al: Postprandial versus preprandial blood glucose monitoring in women with gestational diabetes mellitus requiring insulin therapy. N Engl J Med 1995;333:1237–1241.
154. Schaffir JA, Lockwood CJ, Lapinski R, et al: Incidence of pregnancy-induced hypertension among gestational diabetics. Am J Perinatol 1995;12:252–254.
155. Casey BM, Lucas MJ, McIntire DD, Leveno KJ: Pregnancy outcomes in women with gestational diabetes compared with the general obstetric population. Obstet Gynecol 1997;90:869–873.
156. Suhonen L, Teramo K: Hypertension and pre-eclampsia in women with gestational glucose intolerance. Acta Obstet Gynecol Scand 1993;72:269–272.
157. Johnstone FD, Nasrat AA, Prescott RJ: The effect of established and gestational diabetes on pregnancy outcome. BJOG 1990;97:1009–1015.
158. Gabbe SG, Mestman JH, Freeman RK, et al: Management and outcome of class A diabetes mellitus. Am J Obstet Gynecol 1977; 127:465–469.
159. Kim C, Newton KM, Knopp RH: Gestational diabetes and the incidence of type 1 diabetes: a systematic review. Diabetes Care 2002;25:1862–1868.
160. Gestational diabetes mellitus. Diabetes Care 2002;25:S94–S96.
161. Classification and diagnosis of diabetes mellitus and other categories of glucose intolerance. Diabetes 1979;28:1039–1057.
162. Naylor CD, Sermer M, Chen E, Farine D: Selective screening for gestational diabetes mellitus. Toronto Tri-Hospital Gestational Diabetes Project Investigators. N Engl J Med 1997;337:1591–1596.
163. Nasrat A, Johnstone FD, Hasan F: Is random plasma glucose an efficient screening test for abnormal glucose tolerance in pregnancy? BJOG 1988;95:855–860.
164. Cousins L, Dattel BJ, Hollingsworth DR, Zettner A: Glycosylated haemoglobin as a screening test for carbohydrate intolerance in pregnancy. Am J Obstet Gynecol 1984;150:455–460.
165. Cefalu WT, Prather KL, Chester DL, et al: Total serum glycosylated proteins in detection and monitoring of gestational diabetes. Diabetes Care 1990;13:872–875.
166. Sacks DA, Chen W, Wolde-Tsadik G, Buchanan TA: Fasting plasma glucose test at the first prenatal visit as a screen for gestational diabetes. Obstet Gynecol, 2003;101:1197–1203.
167. Perucchini D, Fischer U, Spinas GA, et al: Using fasting plasma glucose concentrations to screen for gestational diabetes mellitus: Prospective population based study. BMJ 1999;319:812–815.
168. Kjos SL, Schaefer-Graf U, Sardesi S, et al: A randomised controlled trial using glycemic plus fetal ultrasound parameters versus glycemic parameters to determine insulin therapy in gestational diabetes with fasting hyperglycemia. Diabetes Care 2001;24:1904–1910.
169. Buchanan TA, Kjos SL, Montoro NM, et al: Use of fetal ultrasound to select metabolic therapy for pregnancies complicated by mild gestational diabetes. Diabetes Care 1994;17:275–283.
170. Rosenn BM: Antenatal fetal testing in pregnancies complicated by gestational diabetes mellitus. Semin Perinatol, 2002;26:210–214.
171. Kjos SL, Henry OA, Montoro M, et al: Insulin-requiring diabetes in pregnancy: A randomised controlled trial of active induction of labour and expectant management. Am J Obstet Gynecol 1993;169:611–615.
172. Lurie S, Insler V, Hagay ZJ: Induction of labour at 38-39 weeks of gestation reduces the incidence of gestational diabetic patients class A2. Am J Perinatol 1996;13:293–296.
173. Siddiqui F, James D: Fetal monitoring in type 1 diabetic pregnancies. Early Hum Devel 2003;72:1–13.
174. Nesbitt TS, Gilbert WM, Herrchen B, et al: Shoulder dystocia and associated risk factors with macrosomic infants born in California. Am J Obstet Gynecol 1998;179:476–480.
175. Elixhauser A, Weschler JM, Kitzmiller JL, et al: Cost benefit analysis of pre-conception care for women with established diabetes mellitus. Diabetes Care 1993;16:1146-1157.
176. Gordon M, Landon MB, Samuels P, et al: Perinatal outcome and long term follow-up associated with modern management of diabetic nephropathy. Obstet Gynecol 1996;87:401–409.
177. Laatikainen L, Teramo K, Hieta-Heikurainen H, et al: A controlled study of the influence of CSII treatment of diabetic retinopathy in pregnancy. Acta Medica Scand 1987;221:367–376.
178. MRC Vitamin Research Group: Prevention of neural tube defects: Results of the Medical Research Council Vitamin Study. Lancet 1991;338:131.
179. Carpenter MW, Coustan DR: Criteria for screening tests of gestational diabetes. Am J Obstet Gynecol 1982;144:768.
180. Coustan DR, Reece EA, Sherwin RS, et al: A randomized clinical trial of the insulin pump vs intensive conventional therapy in diabetic pregnancies. JAMA 1986;255:631.
181. Schaefer C: Angiotensin II-receptor-antagonists: Further evidence of fetotoxicity but not teratogenicity. Birth Defects Res 2003;67:591–594.

CHAPTER 46

Thyroid Disease

Anna P. Kenyon / Catherine Nelson-Piercy

INTRODUCTION

Thyroid disease is the second most common cause of endocrine dysfunction in women of childbearing age (diabetes is the first). Thyroid disease can be challenging to diagnose and manage because many of its symptoms are common in pregnancy. Physiologic changes in serum levels of pituitary and thyroid hormones may hamper diagnosis, and a clear understanding of these changes is needed when managing patients with suspected or known thyroid disease.

The thyroid gland is a bilobed gland composed of spherical follicles. Each follicle has a colloid center surrounded by a single layer of follicle cells. Intimately involved with the follicle cells are parafollicular C cells, lymphatic drainage channels, and capillary networks.

Iodide ions are actively transported from the blood onto the apical surface of the follicle cells and are oxidized to iodine through the action of thyroid peroxidase. The thyroid gland regulates the amount of iodide it actively traps and can withstand fluctuations in dietary supply. In the lumen, colloid iodide is incorporated into the tyrosine residues of thyroglobulin (also made in the follicle cells) to produce inactive mono-iodotyrosine and di-iodotyrosine. This process is known as organification of iodide. Combinations of these products lead to the formation of the active thyroid compounds thyroxine (T_4) and tri-iodothyronine (T_3), which are released into the capillary network at the apical surface of follicle cells having re-entered from the colloid at their basal surface (endocytosis).

Production is controlled by the hypothalamus-pituitary-thyroid axis. Thyroid-releasing hormone is released from the hypothalamus, and thyroid-stimulating hormone (TSH) is released from the anterior pituitary. TSH is a glycoprotein with alpha and beta subunits. Many anterior pituitary hormones share the alpha subunits, but the beta subunit is unique. TSH has many actions, including increasing the release of T_4 and T_3 through increased iodide transport into follicular cells, organification and release of thyroglobulin into the follicular lumen, and endocytosis of colloid.

More T_4 than T_3 is produced by the thyroid gland, but T_4 is converted in some peripheral tissues (liver, kidney, and muscle) to the more potent T_3.

In plasma, more than 99% of T_3 and T_4 is bound by carrier proteins to thyroid-binding globulin, albumin, and transthyretin (previously known as thyroid-binding prealbumin). Thyroid-binding globulin has the highest affinity for T_3 and T_4, so although it is present in the lowest concentration, 75% of all thyroid hormones are bound to it. Only the free hormones (free T_4 and free T_3) are biologically active (0.04% of total T_4 and 0.5% of total T_3).

Pregnancy is a state of relative iodine deficiency because of increased renal loss (increased glomerular filtration rate in the early first trimester) and transfer of iodine to the developing fetus. To compensate, the thyroid gland increases its uptake of iodine from the blood. If the supply is insufficient, cellular hyperplasia and goiter result. Although a physiologic goiter may be seen on ultrasound examination by a change in gland size of 10% to 20%, this change is not clinically detectable. A clinically apparent goiter suggests iodine deficiency or pathology.[1]

The fetal thyroid gland begins to form at 5 weeks' gestation and has some function at 10 weeks, but it is only autonomous at 12 weeks, when T_4, T_3, and TSH levels can be measured in fetal serum.[2] Levels continue to increase until 35 to 37 weeks' gestation, when they reach adult levels. The gland is relatively immature, however, with high TSH levels relative to the amount of T_4 produced. The fetal thyroid concentrates iodine at a significantly higher rate than the maternal thyroid. Diagnostic scanning or uptake with radioactive tracers, such as iodine-131 or technetium-99, or radioactive iodine therapy should be avoided because of the risks of exposure to the developing fetus.[3]

TSH and hCG and share a common alpha subunit, and their beta subunits share some similarities, as do their receptors. The increase in hCG that occurs in early pregnancy "spills over" and stimulates the TSH receptor, suppressing TSH and increasing T_4. The reason for this increase may be to provide the fetus with T_4 before it becomes autonomous. These changes must be considered when a diagnosis of hyperthyroidism is contemplated in early pregnancy, especially in the context of hyperemesis gravidarum, where hCG secretion may be exaggerated, or in trophoblastic disease, where it is grossly elevated. Two thirds of women with hyperemesis have abnormal thyroid function test results in the absence of thyroid disease, with 30% having undetectable TSH, 60% having suppressed TSH, and 59% having an elevated free T_4 level.[4]

Little T_4 crosses the placenta after the first trimester, and the placenta is relatively impermeable to TSH and T_3.

Thyroid-releasing hormone, antithyroid medications (propylthiouracil, carbimazole, and methimazole), and iodine cross the placenta and may alter the fetal physiology.

Pregnancy causes an increase in thyroid-binding globulin (and transthyretin) through the effects of estrogen, which increases synthesis and decreases clearance. The elevation is present at 2 weeks' gestation and peaks at 20 weeks' gestation.[1] This elevation necessitates a small increase in the production of T_4 (1%–3%) and T_3 until this plateau is reached. Thus, total T_4 and T_3 are elevated.[5] Because only the free hormone is biologically active, only free hormone measurements are used in pregnancy.

Further physiologic changes in thyroid function occur with advancing gestation, but there is controversy about the precise nature of these changes. As described earlier, TSH decreases in early pregnancy, but may increase in the third trimester,[6,7] although some authors have not shown this finding.[8] Concentrations of free T_4 decrease in the second half of pregnancy (below the range seen outside pregnancy). Peripheral conversion of free T_4 to free T_3 is enhanced, and this increased efficiency may be in preparation for the exertions of labor and delivery.[9]

Table 46–1 shows normal values for thyroid function test results throughout pregnancy.

TABLE 46–1

Normal Values for Thyroid Function Tests during Pregnancy

TEST	NON PREGNANT	FIRST TRIMESTER	SECOND TRIMESTER	THIRD TRIMESTER
Free T_4 (pmol/L)	11–23	10–24	9–19	7–17
Free T_3 (pmol/L)	4–9	4–8	4–7	3–5
TSH (mu/L)	<4	0–1.6	1–1.8	7–7.3

Adapted from Chan BY, Swaminathan R: Serum thyrotropin concentration measured by sensitive assays in normal pregnancy. BJOG 1988;95:1332–1334; Parker JH: Amerlex free triiodothyronine and free-thyroxine levels in normal pregnancy. BJOG 1985;92:1234–1238; Girling JC: Thyroid disorders in pregnancy. Curr Obstet Gynaecol 2003;13:45–51.

Serum autoantibodies to the thyroid are common and may be destructive or stimulating. Occasionally, both coexist in the same patient. TSH receptor-stimulating antibodies (immunoglobulin G) are found in Graves' disease (hyperthyroid), and antimicrosomal (thyroid peroxidase) antibodies are seen in Hashimoto's thyroiditis (hypothyroid). Antithyroglobulin antibodies can cause destruction of thyroid tissue. All of these antibodies freely cross the placenta, with varying possible fetal effects.

HYPERTHYROIDISM

General

Hyperthyroidism affects 0.2% of pregnant women[10,11]; 95% of these have a diagnosis of Graves' disease, an autoimmune disorder associated with circulating immunoglobulin G antibodies to the thyroid TSH receptor that stimulate thyroid hormone production.

Possible causes of hyperthyroidism include the following:

- Graves' disease
- Toxic multinodular goiter
- Toxic nodule or adenoma
- Subacute thyroiditis
- Acute thyroiditis (de Quervain's [viral] or postpartum)
- Iodine treatment
- Amiodarone therapy
- Lithium therapy
- Hyperfunctioning ovarian teratoma (struma ovarii)
- TSH-producing adenoma
- hCG-producing tumor
- Thyroid carcinoma

Diagnosis

Thyrotoxicosis usually occurs in the late first or early second trimester. Symptoms are the same as in thyrotoxicosis outside pregnancy, but they may be unhelpful in establishing a diagnosis and are commonly reported by many euthyroid pregnant women (e.g., palmar erythema, emotional lability, vomiting, goiter, heat intolerance). Discriminatory symptoms include weight loss, tremor, lid lag, lid retraction, and persistent tachycardia greater than 100 beats/minute.

Diagnosing hyperthyroidism in early pregnancy may be difficult. When interpreting the results of thyroid function tests suggesting biochemical thyrotoxicosis in early pregnancy, hyperemesis gravidarum and trophoblastic disease must be excluded.

Symptoms that persist beyond 10 to 20 weeks' gestation, symptoms that antedate the pregnancy, and the presence of thyroid-stimulating antibodies suggest true hyperthyroidism. The diagnosis of hyperthyroidism is confirmed by an elevated free T_4 or free T_3 level with suppressed TSH levels.

Carbimazole (methimazole is similar and available in the United States) and propylthiouracil are used to treat hyperthyroidism in and throughout pregnancy. Both agents are thionamides and act by competitively inhibiting the peroxidase-catalyzed reactions that are necessary for iodine organification. They also block the coupling of iodotyrosine, especially the formation of di-iodothyronine. Their onset of action is delayed until the preformed hormones are depleted, a process that can take 3 to 4 weeks. Thionamides may suppress the immune system, but this effect is controversial (discussed later).[12]

Maternal and Fetal Risks

Important maternal side effects of thionamides are agranulocytosis and hepatitis that is idiosyncratic with propylthiouracil, but dose-related with carbimazole. Monitoring of liver function may be necessary. In women with sore throat or fever, a white blood cell count must be obtained to exclude agranulocytosis. If neutropenia occurs, therapy is discontinued, and thionamides should not be given again. Drug rash or urticaria is reported in 1% to 5% of cases and necessitates a switch to an alternative preparation. Additional symptoms may include nausea, vomiting, and diarrhea.

The two most serious maternal complications of untreated hyperthyroidism are heart failure and thyroid storm. Thyroid storm is a medical emergency with a maternal mortality rate of 25%, even with appropriate management (discussed later).[13] Heart failure, the more common of the two serious maternal complications, is caused by the long-term myocardial effects of T_4 and is intensified by other pregnancy-related conditions, such as preeclampsia, infection, or anemia.[14]

When diagnosed in pregnancy, thyrotoxicosis is associated with adverse outcomes, including miscarriage, growth restriction, premature labor, placental abruption, pregnancy-induced hypertension, preeclampsia, infection, and increased perinatal mortality. One study suggested an increased risk of chromosomal abnormalities.[15] The relative risk of low birth weight was 0.74 in one euthyroid (controlled hyperthyroidism) population, 2.36 in the same population with uncontrolled hyperthyroidism in the first half of pregnancy, and 9.24 in patients with hyperthyroidism throughout pregnancy. The same study showed an odds ratio for preeclampsia of 4.74 in patients with uncontrolled hyperthyroidism at term.[16] This study suggests that treatment improves outcome and is supported by another study showing stillbirth in 24% of women with untreated hyperthyroidism and in 5% to 7% of women receiving treatment. The incidence of prematurity was 53%, decreasing to 9% to 11% with treatment.[17]

There is a risk of fetal or neonatal thyrotoxicosis because of the passive transplacental passage of immunoglobulins that is associated with Graves' disease. These antibodies exert an effect on the fetal thyroid at 20 weeks' gestation.[18] Infants born to mothers with high titers of antibodies or poorly controlled disease[10,18] are particularly at risk. Studies report prevalences of 1% to 17%.[18,19] Fewer cases are diagnosed in utero than in the neonatal period. Fetal thyrotoxicosis may be suspected in a fetus with persistent tachycardia (>160 beats/min), goiter, or growth restriction.[18] The diagnosis may be made on the basis of antenatal ultrasound.[20,21]

Fetal thyrotoxicosis may lead to premature delivery (90%),[18] fetal craniosynostosis, exophthalmos, heart failure (hydrops fetalis), hepatosplenomegaly, thrombocytopenia, goiter (with neck obstruction and polyhydramnios), and growth restriction. Additional neonatal features include jaundice, poor feeding, poor weight gain, and irritability.[18] The mortality rate may be as high as 25%.[11]

Thyrotoxicosis in the neonatal period is usually transient, lasting only 2 to 3 months after delivery. Symptoms may be delayed up to 2 weeks postnatally if the mother was taking medication at the time of delivery. The effects of maternal antithyroid medication are eventually cleared from the neonatal circulation, but thyroid-stimulating antibodies are cleared more slowly.

To predict fetal thyrotoxicosis, maternal TSH receptor autoantibodies are tested in early pregnancy. To predict neonatal disease, they are tested again in late pregnancy.[22] One suggested protocol is to test in the first trimester and again at 6 months' gestation.[23] If high titers of antibodies are detected in early pregnancy or if levels have not decreased with advancing gestation, fetal thyrotoxicosis should be anticipated. Obstetric ultrasound may be recommended to assess fetal growth, heart rate, and goiter. If antibodies are detected in late pregnancy, then cord blood and neonatal (days 3–4 and 7–10)[11,24] thyroid function tests (TSH and free T_4) should be performed.[22]

Fetal thyrotoxicosis can be treated in utero by giving the mother increased doses of antithyroid medication. Subsequent maternal hypothyroidism can be treated with thyroxine, which does not cross the placenta in significant amounts. Percutaneous fetal blood sampling to measure thyroid function (for which normal ranges are available) is technically possible and may play a role in management.[2,25]

Fetal effects of maternal antithyroid medication have been reported, particularly the association of carbimazole or methimazole with aplasia cutis.[26] This condition results in patches of absent skin at birth, 70% to 85% of which occur on the scalp. However, the condition is rare. The natural incidence is 0.03%.[27] However, in one study, in a population of 49,000 infants, none of the mothers who took antithyroid medication had an affected infant and no cases occurred in 643 women with Graves' disease.[28]

High doses of antithyroid medication may cause fetal hypothyroidism, but rarely cause goiter. In one study, 43 women treated with thionamides until delivery were compared with 27 women in whom treatment was discontinued in pregnancy. Free T_4 levels were slightly lower in fetuses compared with mothers in the first group. Levels in fetuses were higher in the second group, and some maternal and cord T_4 levels were in the thyrotoxic range at delivery.[29] If maternal disease is controlled too tightly, some infants may become hypothyroid. Neonatal hypothyroidism usually resolves spontaneously by day 5 of life[30] and occurs in 10% to 20% of patients treated with thionamides.[31]

Management Options

Prepregnancy

Menstrual abnormalities are less common now than reported in previous series. The most common manifestations are hypomenorrhea and oligomenorrhea. However, most thyrotoxic women are believed to remain ovulatory.[32]

Therapy for hyperthyroidism is best begun before pregnancy to allow for the use of radioactive iodine studies for diagnosis, higher initial doses of pharmacologic agents without concern about fetal effects, and surgery, when needed, for patients who do not respond to therapy. Patients who have had radioactive iodine are advised not to conceive until 4 months after the last treatment.[33] Some argue for establishing a euthyroid state 3 months before conception. Counseling should be supportive and reassuring. Treated thyrotoxicosis has a low risk of adverse obstetric outcome. Women should be counseled against discontinuing medication either prepregnancy or antenatally.

Prenatal

The goal of treatment is to maintain a euthyroid clinical state and a free T_4 level at the upper limit of normal for pregnancy-specific ranges. This approach allows use of the lowest possible dose and minimizes the risk of fetal hypothyroidism. Women with newly diagnosed hyperthyroidism should undergo examination and thyroid function tests monthly. Less frequent testing is needed in those with stable disease.

Patients with Graves' disease often have temporary worsening of control in early pregnancy as a result of increasing hCG levels and perhaps reduced absorption of medication as a result of vomiting. Improvement may then occur, with women often requiring less medication as the relative immune suppression of pregnancy results in a decrease in antibody levels. In 30% of patients, all medication can be discontinued in the last weeks of pregnancy.[34]

Block-and-replace regimens that are sometimes used outside pregnancy are not suitable for pregnant women. Antithyroid medications cross the placenta freely, whereas thyroxine does not. Therefore, this regimen places the fetus at risk for hypothyroidism. Fetal abnormalities are more common in the offspring of women receiving thyroxine and carbimazole (9.5%) than in those receiving carbimazole alone (4.1%).[20,28] These regimens may be of use in the treatment of fetal thyrotoxicosis (discussed earlier).

Therapeutic modalities for hyperthyroidism are divided into the following five categories:

- Thionamides (propylthiouracil and carbimazole)
- β-blockers
- Iodides
- Radioactive iodine
- Surgery

Propylthiouracil and carbimazole are the mainstays of treatment for hyperthyroidism in pregnancy. Propylthiouracil crosses the placenta less readily than carbimazole and is usually the first choice; however, women whose disease is well controlled with carbimazole need not change.[35] The disadvantage of propylthiouracil is that more frequent dosing is often necessary compared with carbimazole. Newly diagnosed cases should be treated aggressively initially, with high doses (e.g., carbimazole 40 mg, propylthiouracil 400 mg daily) for 4 to 6 weeks. The doses can be reduced gradually by up to 25%.

In patients with troublesome autonomic (sympathetic) symptoms of palpitations, tachycardia, and tremor, propranolol 20 to 40 mg three times daily may be used for up to 1 month until longer-term treatment with thionamides becomes effective. Longer treatment courses should be avoided because of the risk of growth restriction.[36] β-blockers have the additional benefit of reducing peripheral conversion of T_4 to T_3.

Iodide treatment is an older mode of therapy and is now limited to preoperative use. Long-term use of this therapy results in a high incidence of fetal goiter and hypothyroidism and does not result in adequate control of thyrotoxicosis.[37]

Radioactive iodine (iodine-131) is used widely outside pregnancy to treat Graves' disease and is used in high doses to treat carcinoma. However, it is absolutely contraindicated in pregnancy because it ablates the fetal thyroid, causing fetal and neonatal hypothyroidism. There is additional concern about possible effects on the parental gonads, and pregnancy should be delayed until after treatment. Radioactive iodine also frequently results in maternal hypothyroidism.[17,28]

Surgery is reserved for patients who do not respond to medication or who cannot tolerate the medication. Thyroid surgery is associated with a high incidence of hypothyroidism postoperatively. Other postoperative complications include hypoparathyroidism (1%–2%) and recurrent laryngeal nerve palsy (1%–2%). Surgical and anesthetic morbidity and mortality rates are also increased in pregnancy. The reported pregnancy loss rate associated with general anesthesia and surgery of all types in the first trimester is approximately 8%. The rate decreases to 6.5% in the second trimester. Before surgery, patients should be prepared medically with 7 to 10 days of iodide treatment to decrease gland vascularity and prevent thyroid storm. Overall, surgery is reserved for patients in whom standard medical therapy is unsuccessful and women with a significant goiter that causes stridor, respiratory distress, dysphagia, or carcinoma.

Labor and Delivery

In women with adequately treated thyrotoxicosis, labor and delivery are not associated with increased risks. However, labor and delivery may precipitate thyroid storm in pregnant women with poorly treated or untreated thyrotoxicosis. The patient may have extreme symptoms of hyperthyroidism, particularly cardiovascular symptoms (palpitations, tachycardia, and atrial fibrillation with rapid ventricular response). If the symptoms are severe, high-output cardiac failure may occur. Blood pressure is usually normal, although pulse pressure may be increased. With prolonged duration of symptoms, shock may ensue.[38]

Fever is invariably present, is progressive, begins a few hours after a stressful event, and may exceed 40°C. Mental status is commonly altered, ranging from restlessness and confusion to psychosis, seizures, and coma. Severe diarrhea, nausea, vomiting, and nonspecific abdominal pain may also be present.[39] If the patient has a large goiter, exophthalmos, or a history of hyperthyroidism, the diagnosis of thyroid storm usually is not difficult to establish. However, without the obvious findings or history, the diagnosis may be difficult to establish because the results of biochemical tests may not differ from those in patients who have thyrotoxicosis without thyroid storm. Treatment should not be delayed if the condition is suspected.

The goals of treatment in thyroid storm are to decrease the production of thyroid hormones, to decrease the effect of circulating hormones, to provide supportive therapy, and to treat the underlying cause. Methimazole and carbimazole may be used, although propylthiouracil (300–400 mg every 8 hours orally, by nasogastric tube, or rectally) is preferred because it decreases peripheral conversion of T_4 to T_3 and decreases thyroid hormone production. Potassium iodide (2–5 drops orally) or sodium iodide (0.5–1.0 g IV) every 8 hours should be initiated approximately 1 to 2 hours after the initiation of therapy with thionamides. This treatment is provided in an attempt to block the release of preformed thyroid hormones from the colloid space.[40]

Supportive therapy involves maintaining blood volume, glycemic control, and temperature control, and restoring the electrolyte balance.[40]

Propranolol (40–80 mg orally or 1 mg/min intravenously) is given to reduce adrenergic overactivity.[40]

Postnatal

To exclude hyperthyroidism as a result of passive antibody transfer and hypothyroidism as a result of transfer of antithyroid medications (discussed earlier), thyroid function tests should be performed on umbilical cord blood and in the neonate in women who are breastfeeding. For propylthiouracil, only 0.07% of the maternal dose is excreted in breast milk, with a slightly higher dose excreted for carbimazole (0.5%) and methimazole (10%).[20] Breastfeeding is generally considered safe in patients who take propylthiouracil (<150 mg daily) and carbimazole (<15 mg daily).[20,41]

Graves' disease can flare postnatally as maternal antibody levels increase. In patients who stopped taking medication, it is often necessary to reintroduce it 2 to 3 months postpartum. These changes must be distinguished from true postpartum thyroiditis (discussed later).

SUMMARY OF MANAGEMENT OPTIONS

Hyperthyroidism

Management Options	Quality of Evidence	Strength of Recommendation	References
Prepregnancy			
Establish the diagnosis of hyperthyroidism (elevated free T_4 or free T_3 level with suppressed thyroid-stimulating hormone [TSH] levels) before pregnancy so that a complete diagnostic workup (including radioactive iodine studies) can be performed and therapy instituted.	–	GPP	–
Avoid conception until 4 months after the completion of radioiodine therapy. The patient should be euthyroid for 3 months before conception.	IV	C	32
Prenatal			
Use pregnancy-specific reference ranges when interpreting the results of thyroid function tests.	III	B	6,7

Continued

SUMMARY OF MANAGEMENT OPTIONS

Hyperthyroidism *(Continued)*

Management Options	Quality of Evidence	Strength of Recommendation	References
Prenatal *(Continued)*			
Use caution when interpreting the results of thyroid function tests in early pregnancy: TSH levels decrease as result of increasing levels of hCG.	IIa	B	4
If the cause is autoimmune, disease may improve as pregnancy advances and antibody levels decrease.	–	GPP	–
Continue therapy to maintain the free T_4 level at the upper limit of normal.	–	GPP	–
Test thyroid function every 3 months, more frequently if dosage adjustments are made.	–	GPP	–
Screen for agranulocytosis and hepatitis in patients who are taking thionamides.	–	GPP	–
Measure the TSH receptor antibody titer early in pregnancy (1 month). If it is high, there is a risk of fetal thyrotoxicosis.	III	B	22,23
Perform fetal ultrasound for fetal growth, tachycardia, or goiter.	III	B	11,24
Measure the TSH receptor antibody titer late in pregnancy (at about 28 weeks). If it is high, there is a risk of neonatal thyrotoxicosis.	III	B	22,23
Labor and Delivery			
Labor and delivery may precipitate thyroid storm	–	GPP	–
Postnatal			
Symptoms may worsen in the postpartum period, especially if the medication dosage was reduced. If medication was discontinued, it may need to be reintroduced 2–3 months postpartum.	–	GPP	–
If the TSH receptor antibody titer is high late in pregnancy, screen for neonatal thyrotoxicosis by testing the infant on days 3–4 and 7–10 of life.	III	B	22,23
Observe the neonate for signs of hypothyroidism if the mother is taking high doses of antithyroid medication. Test the cord blood and neonatal blood if the mother is breastfeeding.	III	B	11,22,24
Perform a complete diagnostic evaluation.	–	GPP	–

HYPOTHYROIDISM

General

Hypothyroidism affects 1% of pregnant women, and as with hyperthyroidism, many of the symptoms occur in normal pregnancy. Discriminatory symptoms are cold intolerance, slow heart rate, and delayed relaxation of deep tendon reflexes, particularly those of the ankle.

The most common cause of hypothyroidism is autoimmune associated with thyroid peroxidase autoantibodies, leading to destruction of the gland, lymphoid infiltration, and eventual atrophy and fibrosis. This type is known as atrophic (autoimmune) hypothyroidism. In some cases, antibodies blocking the TSH receptor have been implicated. Hashimoto's thyroiditis is a different form of autoimmune thyroiditis, also with thyroid peroxidase (microsomal) autoantibodies, often at high titers. However, atrophic changes occur with regeneration and result in goiter formation. When the origin is autoimmune, other autoimmune diseases (e.g., pernicious anemia, insulin-dependent [type I] diabetes mellitus, and vitiligo) may be present.

Hypothyroidism may be iatrogenic after treatment with lithium, amiodarone, or antithyroid drugs. Alternatively, it may be transient, occurring as part of the disease course in subacute de Quervain's thyroiditis or postpartum thyroiditis.

Any woman who is taking thyroxine for iatrogenic hypothyroidism should have a careful history taken to determine the original cause of disease. Particular care should be taken in women who are using thyroxine after thyroidectomy or after radioactive iodine treatment when the original diagnosis was hyperthyroidism. Thyrotoxic symptoms in these women should not be attributed to treatment excess until a flare of residual disease has been excluded.[42]

Diagnosis

Hypothyroidism may be diagnosed in patients with a reduced free T_4 concentration in association with an elevated TSH level. Outside pregnancy, an elevated TSH level is a sensitive indicator of the degree of thyroid hormone deficiency. Results must be interpreted with pregnancy-specific reference ranges. Identifying thyroid peroxidase autoantibodies can confirm the diagnosis, but these are nonspecific and are present in 20% to 30% of the normal population.[43]

Maternal and Fetal Risks

The most serious consequence of hypothyroidism is myxoedema coma. This event is extremely rare in pregnancy, but is a true medical emergency, with a 20% mortality rate. The clinical picture includes hypothermia, bradycardia, decreased deep tendon reflexes, and altered consciousness. Hyponatremia, hypoglycemia, hypoxia, and hypercapnia may be present as well. Once the diagnosis is made, therapy should begin immediately with supportive care and thyroid hormone replacement. Symptoms usually improve after 12 to 24 hours of therapy.[44]

Recent studies of subclinical hypothyroidism showed no association with miscarriage. Therefore, screening of thyroid function in asymptomatic women with miscarriage is not recommended.[45]

One study of outcome in hypothyroidism showed that gestational hypertension, (eclampsia, preeclampsia, and pregnancy-induced hypertension) occurred more commonly in patients with overt and subclinical hypothyroidism than in the general population, with rates of 22%, 15%, and 7.6%, respectively. In addition, 36% of patients with overt hypothyroidism and 25% of those with subclinical hypothyroidism who remained hypothyroid at delivery had gestational hypertension. Low birth weight in both groups of patients was secondary to premature delivery for gestational hypertension. Older studies suggested a link with congenital malformations, but more recent studies showed no association.[46]

T_4 is important in the early development of the fetal brain, and some studies[47–49] suggest that neuropsychiatric development is impaired in the offspring of mothers with hypothyroidism. As discussed earlier, the fetus is reliant on maternal T_4 before 12 weeks' gestation. Correction of maternal hypothyroxinemia in the first 12 weeks of pregnancy might be expected to improve neurodevelopmental outcome.[49] A study of intelligence quotient scores in offspring born to mothers with hypothyroidism in early pregnancy who were subsequently treated showed no adverse effect compared with siblings born when the same mothers were euthyroid.[50]

Cretinism (deaf mutism, spastic motor disorder, and hypothyroidism) is a distinct and severe form of brain damage caused by severe maternal iodine deficiency.

Neonatal or fetal hypothyroidism as a result of transplacental transfer of maternal autoantibodies is extremely rare (1 in 180,000 neonates, or approximately 2% of infants with congenital hypothyroidism),[51] if it occurs at all.[52]

Congenital absence of the thyroid gland is exceptionally rare. In these cases, the fetus is reliant on transfer of maternal T_3 and T_4 across the placenta[53] throughout gestation.

All infants are screened for hypothyroidism with the blood spot Guthrie card. Blood is collected with a heel prick on day 6 of life. Those with an abnormality are recalled for further testing (0.2%–0.3% of the general population).

The fetus is not believed to be at risk for hyperthyroidism as a result of maternal T_4 therapy because placental transfer is poor.

Management Options

Prepregnancy

In hypothyroidism, the frequency of menstrual irregularities has been reported at 56% to 80%. Oligomennorhea, amennorhea, polymenorrhea, and menorrhagia have been reported. Most cases are likely to be attributed to anovulatory cycles. However, a recent study reported far fewer menstrual irregularities, only 23.4% in 171 hypothyroid patients studied (three times more frequent than in 124 control subjects). The most common manifestation was oligomenorrhea (42.5%), followed by menorrhagia (30%). Reduced libido may be an associated feature.

Ovulation and conception can occur in patients with mild hypothyroidism.[32] Severe hypothyroidism is likely associated with failure of ovulation; therefore, tests of thyroid function are appropriate in the evaluation of an infertile couple. The Royal College of Obstetricians and Gynaecologists guidelines suggest that testing should be done only when the woman reports menstrual irregularities or other symptoms.[54]

Given the association of hypothyroidism and other autoimmune disease, performing thyroid function tests in women with insulin-dependent (type I) diabetes mellitus before pregnancy may be a useful screening tool.

Patients with hypothyroidism should be counseled to delay pregnancy until maintenance levels of T_4 have been achieved. Reassurance should be given about the safety of T_4 use during pregnancy. It is useful to perform baseline TSH and free T_4 measurements in those contemplating pregnancy in the near future, or testing may be performed as early as possible after conception.

Prenatal

Antithyroid peroxidase and antithyroglobulin antibodies may be found more commonly in women with recurrent miscarriage (three or more),[55] the risk of which may be associated with antibody titer and avidity.[23,55,56] It is not clear whether this increased risk is a manifestation of an altered humoral response to pregnancy or whether the thyroid autoantibodies are implicated in the pathophysiology. These studies tested women because of their history of recurrent miscarriage (they were therefore at risk for subsequent miscarriage) rather than clinical or biochemical features of hypothyroidism. This selection may explain the observation (discussed earlier) that there does not seem to be an increased frequency of miscarriage in patients with mild hypothyroidism.

A new diagnosis of hypothyroidism in pregnancy is uncommon, given the association with infertility. A more common problem is pregnancy in a woman with inadequately treated hypothyroidism or the diagnosis of hypothyroidism after an episode of postpartum thyroiditis that resolved.

Those who enter pregnancy euthyroid can expect a good outcome. Hypothyroidism requires treatment with thyroxine. If there is no coexisting heart disease, an initial dose of thyroxine 100 μg is usually required. In women who are stable while receiving treatment, checking thyroid function in each trimester is sufficient. However, if dosage changes are implemented, thyroid function (TSH and free T_4) should be measured after 4 to 6 weeks. More frequent testing (every 2 weeks) may be needed in patients with very poor control in early pregnancy. When dosage adjustments are made, free T_4 should be used rather than TSH, which may decrease slowly. However, poor compliance may also result in an increased TSH level with a normal free T_4 level. Kaplan (1992),[57] Glinoer (1998),[23] and Mandel and colleagues (1990)[58] variously advocated increasing the dose of thyroxine with advancing gestation. They suggested a dose of 200 μg and an 80% increase in dosage in all patients. They also suggested that patients with a TSH level less than 10 should have a dose increase of 41 plus or minus 24 μg daily. If the TSH level is 10 to 20, a dose increase of 65 plus or minus 19 μg daily is recommended, and if the TSH level is greater than 20, a dose increase of 105 plus or minus 32 μg daily is required. Suggested mechanisms for this increased requirement include an elevated extrathyroidal pool of T_4; the need to saturate large quantities of thyroid-binding globulin; increased degradation of T_4; reduced absorption of T_4, especially if taken with iron supplements; and increased transfer of T_4 from mother to fetus.[59] However, Girling and DeSwiet (1992)[5] and, more recently, Chopra and Baber (2003)[60] suggested that there is no need to adjust the dose of T_4 replacement if replacement was adequate before pregnancy. However, in the Girling and DeSwiet[5] study, in 20% of women, hypothyroidism was not adequately treated on entering the pregnancy.[5] The Chopra and Baber[60] study emphasized that taking T_4 at the same time as iron supplements may reduce its absorption and therefore its effectiveness.[5]

Labor and Delivery

When adequate control is achieved, no specific measures are needed for labor or delivery. However, when a large goiter causes respiratory compromise, anesthetic or surgical advice may be required.

Postnatal

Thyroid peroxidase autoantibodies are significantly associated with postpartum thyroiditis (discussed later) and postpartum depression.[61]

SUMMARY OF MANAGEMENT OPTIONS

Hypothyroidism

Management Options	Quality of Evidence	Strength of Recommendation	References
Prepregnancy			
Consider this diagnosis in patients with fertility or menstrual disorders.	IIa	B	31,53
Optimize medical therapy and delay pregnancy until good control is achieved.	IIa	B	46,48
Prenatal			
Perform baseline thyroid function tests as soon as possible.	–	GPP	–
Use pregnancy-specific reference ranges when interpreting the results of thyroid function tests.	III	B	6,7

SUMMARY OF MANAGEMENT OPTIONS

Hypothyroidism *(Continued)*

Management Options	Quality of Evidence	Strength of Recommendation	References
Perform thyroid function tests every 3 months, more frequently if dosage adjustments are made.	–	GPP	–
Routine increases in thyroxine dosage are not required. Make dosage adjustments based on the results of thyroid function tests.	III	B	5,59
Patients should avoid taking iron supplements at the same time as oral thyroxine therapy. Check compliance in patients with vomiting.	III	B	58,59
Labor and Delivery			
A larger maternal goiter may cause anesthetic complications (difficulties with intubation).	–	GPP	–
Postnatal			
Observe the patient for signs of postpartum thyroiditis.	–	GPP	–
Screen for postpartum depression.	III	B	60

THYROID NODULES AND THYROID CANCER

General

Thyroid nodules, solitary toxic nodules, or adenomas are found in 2% of pregnant women,[62] and they usually cause hyperthyroidism. Although they are rare overall,[14] 90% of thyroid cancers are thyroid nodules. Carcinomas derived from the thyroid epithelium may be papillary, follicular (differentiated), or undifferentiated. They are rarely active hormonally, but 90% secrete thyroglobulin, which is used outside pregnancy as a tumor marker. There may be an increased incidence of malignancy in pregnancy (40%).[20] Enlargement of the thyroid gland in pregnancy[63] and recent pregnancy (within 5 years) have been associated with thyroid cancer.[64,65] However, because these malignancies are most common in women of childbearing age, additional risk in pregnancy may be difficult to determine. Only nodules that are believed to be malignant need further evaluation or treatment, usually with surgery, with or without radioactive iodine. After treatment, T_4 may be used to suppress the production of TSH and prevent stimulation of residual thyroid tissue or tumor.

Diagnosis

Outside pregnancy, radioactive iodine is used to distinguish "cold" (more likely to be malignant) from "hot" (functioning) nodules. However, these studies cannot be performed in pregnancy. Therefore, ultrasound is the main investigative tool. Fine-needle aspiration is reserved for rapidly enlarging nodules, cystic nodules larger than 4 cm, and solid nodules larger than 2 cm.[20] Cystic nodules are usually benign (multinodular goiter or solitary toxic adenoma). Those with retrosternal extension or tracheal deviation and respiratory compromise may require further imaging. Biopsy results are usually of four types: First, the sample may be insufficient (<5%); biopsy should be repeated. Second, the nodule may be definitely benign (75%); these patients should be reassured. Third, the nodule may be definitely malignant (5%); these patients should undergo surgery. Finally, the finding may be indeterminate (20%). This finding usually occurs when follicular cells are seen; patients often require surgery. The prognosis is similar for patients diagnosed during or outside of pregnancy.[62]

Management Options

Prepregnancy

Thyroid nodules should be evaluated and treated before the patient becomes pregnant. Pregnancy should be delayed for 1 year after thyroid cancer has been treated with high-dose radioactive iodine because congenital abnormalities have been reported.[33]

Prenatal

Because of the risk of malignancy, testing should proceed as outlined earlier and should not be delayed because of pregnancy. Antithyroid drugs should be used as described earlier to treat hyperthyroidism, but nodules do not usually remit after this treatment. Only if a nodule is found beyond 20 weeks' gestation should aspiration wait until the postnatal period. If biopsy confirms malignancy, the pregnant patient should undergo surgery unless she is only a few weeks from term. Those with indeterminate pathology may delay surgery until after delivery. Surgery is safest when carried out in the second trimester, and with these exceptions, should not be delayed because of pregnancy.[66,67] Radioactive iodine should not be used in pregnancy. Suppressive doses of T_4 should be safe in pregnancy, but care should be taken to avoid maternal thyrotoxicosis.

Labor and Delivery

In patients with a large goiter with retrosternal extension, careful consideration must be given to possible respiratory compromise and complications of intubation if a general anesthetic agent is used. Retrosternal extension should be suspected in patients with respiratory symptoms or dysphagia and in the rare patient with vocal cord paralysis, Horner's syndrome, and vascular or lymphatic compromise.

Postnatal

Radioactive iodine may be administered after delivery, but not while the patient is breastfeeding. Contact with the infant may need to be limited temporarily to reduce exposure.[68]

SUMMARY OF MANAGEMENT OPTIONS

Thyroid Nodules and Cancer

Management Options	Quality of Evidence	Strength of Recommendation	References
Prepregnancy			
Delay pregnancy for 1 year after thyroid cancer has been treated with high-dose radioactive iodine.	IV	C	32
Prenatal			
If a nodule is identified beyond 20 weeks, perform a biopsy after delivery.	III	C	65,66
If a biopsy confirms malignancy, proceed to surgery.	III	C	65,66
Surgery is safest after the second trimester.	III	C	65,66
If a biopsy shows intermediate pathology, delay surgery until after delivery.	III	C	65,66
Labor and Delivery			
Watch for anesthetic complications in patients with a large goiter or retrosternal extension.	–	GPP	–
Postnatal			
Radioactive iodine may be used, but not while breastfeeding. Contact with the infant may need to be limited temporarily.	IV	C	67

POSTPARTUM THYROIDITIS

General

Postpartum thyroiditis is believed to occur in 5% to 10% of pregnancies.[69] The frequency of diagnosis depends largely on the extent to which it is sought. Women may not report symptoms and may attribute them to normal postpartum physiology. The condition occurs 3 to 4 months postpartum, but has been reported up to 6 months after delivery.[70] It is an autoimmune disorder, and women with thyroid antibodies in the first trimester have a 33% to 50% chance of having postpartum thyroiditis.[69] The disease is more common (threefold higher) in those with insulin-dependent (type I) diabetes mellitus,[71] a family history of the disease, or thyroid peroxidase antibodies (75% of affected individuals).

The differential diagnosis of postpartum hyperthyroidism includes the following:

- Postpartum painless thyroiditis
- Postpartum Graves' disease
- Postpartum Hashimoto's thyroiditis
- Postpartum toxic multinodular goiter

The most common diagnosis is postpartum painless thyroiditis, which is characterized by an initial destructive phase in the first 2 months, with release of preformed thyroid hormone that causes hyperthyroidism. Three months later, hypothyroidism occurs as stores of preformed thyroid hormone are depleted and the gland is destroyed. However, any combination of clinical states is possible at any time. Most cases resolve spontaneously.

Diagnosis

Radioactive iodine uptake studies can be used in women who choose not to breast-feed. Low uptake is seen in postpartum painless thyroiditis, where only preformed T_4 is released. In contrast, in Graves' disease, new T_4 is generated. In women who are breast-feeding, repeat thyroid function tests 1 month later may show a transition from hyperthyroidism to hypothyroidism, confirming the diagnosis.

Management Options

Most cases resolve spontaneously. However, in a recent study of 86 women, only 51% of those who were not treated were biochemically euthyroid at 9 months. Early institution of permanent T_4 replacement is recommended in women with postpartum thyroid dysfunction, elevated TSH levels, and thyroid antibodies.[72] Later, hypothyroidism (23%–39%) may occur in those who recover, particularly when antibodies are found. For this reason, some advocate yearly thyroid function tests. Thyroxine may be discontinued in some patients. Close observation in the puerperium of any future pregnancies should be undertaken in view of the risk of recurrence.

SUMMARY OF MANAGEMENT OPTIONS
Postpartum Thyroiditis

Management Options	Quality of Evidence	Strength of Recommendation	References
Most cases progress through phases: • hyperthyroidism • hypothyroidism • full recovery	IV	C	69,70
In a few cases hypothyroidism persists or develops.	IV	C	69,70
Treat symptomatic hyperthyroidism with thionamides.	IIa	B	71
	III	B	72
Give thyroxine supplementation if hypothyroidism develops.	IIa	B	71
	III	B	72
Annual thyroid function tests	IV	C	69,70

CONCLUSIONS

HYPOTHYROIDISM

- Thyroxine is important in the early development of the fetal brain, and ensuring adequate replacement in the first trimester is important.
- Little T4 crosses the placenta after the first trimester.
- Adequately treated women with hypothyroidism can expect a good pregnancy outcome.

HYPERTHYROIDISM

- Hyperthyroidism can be difficult to diagnose before 20 weeks' gestation. At earlier gestations consider the differential diagnosis carefully.
- Untreated or poorly controlled hyperthyroidism in pregnancy is associated with adverse outcome.
- Antithyroid medications cross the placenta. Using the lowest possible dose will minimize the risk of fetal hypothyroidism: Thyroid function tests in cord blood and from breastfed neonates may be necessary.
- Passive transfer of antibody may cause fetal or neonatal hyperthyroidism: Thyroid function tests in cord blood and from breastfed neonates may be necessary.
- Thionamides can cause maternal agranulocytosis and hepatitis.
- Adequately treated women with hyperthyroidism can expect a good pregnancy outcome.

REFERENCES

1. Glinoer D: Pregnancy and iodine. Thyroid 2001;11:471–481.
2. Thorpebeeston JG, Nicolaides KH, Felton CV, et al: Maturation of the secretion of thyroid-hormone and thyroid-stimulating hormone in the fetus. N Engl J Med 1991;324:532–536.
3. Fisher DA, Klein AH: Thyroid development and disorders of thyroid-function in the newborn. N Engl J Med 1981;304: 702–712.
4. Goodwin TM, Montoro M, Mestman JH: Transient hyperthyroidism and hyperemesis gravidarum: Clinical aspects. Am J Obstet Gynecol 1992;167:648–652.
5. Girling JC, DeSwiet M: Thyroxine dosage during pregnancy in women with primary hypothyroidism. BJOG 1992;99:368–370.
6. Chan BY, Swaminathan R: Serum thyrotropin concentration measured by sensitive assays in normal-pregnancy. BJOG 1988;95:1332–1334.
7. Parker JH: Amerlex free triiodothyronine and free-thyroxine levels in normal-pregnancy. BJOG 1985;92: 1234–1238.
8. Rodin A, Rodin A: Thyroid-disease in pregnancy. Br J Hosp Med 1989;41:238–242.
9. Girling JC: Thyroid disorders in pregnancy. Curr Obstet Gynaecol 2003;13:45–51.
10. Burrow GN: Thyroid-function and hyperfunction during gestation. Endocr Rev 1993;14:194–202.
11. Smith C, Thomsett M, Choong C, et al: Congenital thyrotoxicosis in premature infants. Clin Endocrinol 2001;54:371–376.
12. Neal MJ: Thyroid and Anti Thyroid Drugs: Medical Pharmacology at a Glance. Oxford, Blackwell, 1987, pp 68–69.
13. Mestman JH, Goodwin TM, Montoro MM: Thyroid-disorders of pregnancy. Endocrinol Metab Clin North Am 1995;24:41–71.
14. Glinoer D, Soto MF, Bourdoux P, et al: Pregnancy in patients with mild thyroid abnormalities: Maternal and neonatal repercussions. J Clin Endocrinol Metab 1991;73:421–427.
15. Momotani N, Ito K, Hamada N, et al: Maternal hyperthyroidism and congenital-malformation in the offspring. Clin Endocrinol 1984;20:695–700.
16. Millar LK, Wing DA, Leung AS, et al: Low birth weight and preeclampsia in pregnancies complicated by hyperthyroidism. Int J Gynecol Obstet 1995;50:223.
17. Davis LE, Lucas MJ, Hankins GDV, et al: Thyrotoxicosis complicating pregnancy. Am J Obstet Gynecol 1989;160:63–70.
18. Peleg D, Cada S, Peleg A, Ben Ami M: The relationship between maternal serum thyroid-stimulating immunoglobulin and fetal and neonatal thyrotoxicosis. Obstet Gynecol 2002;99:1040–1043.
19. Burrow GN: Current concepts: The management of thyrotoxicosis in pregnancy. N Engl J Med 1985;313:562–565.
20. O'Doherty MJ, McElhatton PR, Thomas SHL: Treating thyrotoxicosis in pregnant or potentially pregnant women: The risk to the fetus is very low. BMJ 1999;318:5–6.
21. Wallace C, Couch R, Ginsberg J: Fetal thyrotoxicosis: A case-report and recommendations for prediction, diagnosis, and treatment. Thyroid 1995;5:125–128.
22. Laurberg P, Nygaard B, Glinoer D, et al: Guidelines for TSH-receptor antibody measurements in pregnancy: Results of an evidence-based symposium organized by the European Thyroid Association. Eur J Endocrinol 1998;139:584–586.
23. Glinoer D: The systematic screening and management of hypothyroidism and hyperthyroidism during pregnancy. Trends Endocrinol Metab 1998;9:403–411.
24. Polak M: Hyperthyroidism in early infancy: Pathogenesis, clinical features and diagnosis with a focus on neonatal hyperthyroidism. Thyroid 1998;8:1171–1177.
25. Kilpatrick S: Umbilical blood sampling in women with thyroid disease: Is it necessary? Am J Obstet Gynecol 2003;189:1–2.
26. Mandel SJ, Brent GA, Larsen PR: Review of antithyroid drug-use during pregnancy and report of a case of aplasia cutis. Thyroid 1994;4:129–133.
27. Vandijke CP, Heydendael RJ, Dekleine MJ: Methimazole, carbimazole, and congenital skin defects. Ann Intern Med 1987;106:60–61.
28. Ramsay I, Kaur S, Krassas G: Thyrotoxicosis in pregnancy: Results of treatment by anti-thyroid drugs combined with T-4. Clin Endocrinol 1983;18:73–85.
29. Momotani N, Noh J, Oyanagi H, et al: Antithyroid drug-therapy for Graves-disease during pregnancy: Optimal regimen for fetal thyroid status. N Engl J Med 1986;315:24–28.
30. Cheron RG, Kaplan MM, Larsen PR, et al: Neonatal thyroid-function after propylthiouracil therapy for maternal Graves-disease. N Engl J Med 1981;304:525–528.
31. Momotani N, Noh JY, Ishikawa N, Ito K: Effects of propylthiouracil and methimazole on fetal thyroid status in mothers with Graves' hyperthyroidism. J Clin Endocrinol Metab 1997;82: 3633–3636.
32. Krassas GE: Thyroid disease and female reproduction. Fertil Steril 2000;74:1063–1070.
33. Ayala C, Navarro E, Rodriguez JR, et al: Conception after iodine-131 therapy for differentiated thyroid cancer. Thyroid 1998;8:1009–1011.
34. Mestman JH: Thyroid-disease in pregnancy. Clin Perinatol 1985;12:651–667.
35. Drug and therapeutics bulletin: The practical management of thyroid disease in pregnancy. 1995;33:47–48.
36. Pruyn SC, Phelan JP, Buchanan GC: Long term propranolol therapy in pregnancy. Am J Obstet Gynecol 1979;135:485–489.
37. Senior B, Chernoff HL: Iodide goiter in the newborn. Pediatrics 2003;47:510–515.
38. Hoffenberg R: Thyroid emergencies. Clin Endocrinol Metab 1980;9:503–512.
39. Lowy C: Endocrine emergencies in pregnancy. Clin Endocrinol Metab 1980;9:569–581.
40. Kaufman L, Zimmerman L: Thyrotoxicosis and thyroid storm: A review of evaluation and management. Prim Care Update Obstet Gynecol 2003;10:29–32.
41. Lamberg BA, Ikonen E, Osterlund K, et al: Antithyroid treatment of maternal hyperthyroidism during lactation. Clin Endocrinol 1984;21:81–87.
42. Smith CM, Gavranich J, Cotterill A, Rodda CP: Congenital neonatal thyrotoxicosis and previous maternal radioiodine therapy. BMJ 2000;320:1260–1261.
43. Hall R, Richards CJ, Lazarus JH: The thyroid and pregnancy. BJOG 1993;100:942.
44. Cardoso CG, Graca LM, Dias T, et al: Spontaneous ovarian hyperstimulation and primary hypothyroidism with a naturally conceived pregnancy. Obstet Gynecol 1999;93:809–811.
45. Clifford K, Rai R, Watson H, Regan L: An informative protocol for the investigation of recurrent miscarriage: Preliminary experience of 500 consecutive cases. Hum Reprod 1994;9: 1328–1332.
46. Leung AS, Millar LK, Koonings PP, et al: Perinatal outcome in hypothyroid pregnancies. Obstet Gynecol 1993;81:349–353.
47. Pop V, Verkerk G, Kuipens H, et al: Maternal thyroid peroxidase antibodies during pregnancy: A marker of impaired child development? Infant Behav Dev 1996;19:681.
48. Mirabella G, Lobaugh NJ, Newton SC, et al: Thyroid hormone deficiency in pregnancy and early life: Effects on attention, learning, and memory in infancy. Infant Behav Dev 1998;21:580.
49. Haddow JE, Palomaki GE, Allan WC, et al: Maternal thyroid deficiency during pregnancy and subsequent neuropsychological development of the child. N Engl J Med 1999;341: 549–555.
50. Liu H, Momotani N, Noh JY, et al: Maternal hypothyroidism during early-pregnancy and intellectual-development of the progeny. Arch Intern Med 1994;154:785–787.

51. Brown RS, Bellisario RL, Botero D, et al: Incidence of transient congenital hypothyroidism due to maternal thyrotropin receptor-blocking antibodies in over one million babies. J Clin Endocrinol Metab 1996;81:1147–1151.
52. Fisher DA: Fetal thyroid function: Diagnosis and management of fetal thyroid disorders. Clin Obstet Gynecol 1997;40:16–31.
53. Burrow GN: Neonatal goiter after maternal propylthiouracil therapy. J Clin Endocrinol Metab 1965;25:403–408.
54. Royal College of Obstetricians & Gynaecologists: The Initial Investigation and Management of the Infertile Couple: National Evidence Based Clinical Guidelines. London, RCOG, 1998.
55. Muller AF, Mantel MJ, Verhoeff A, et al: Thyroid autoimmunity and abortion: A prospective study in an IVF population. Neth J Med 1996;48:A75.
56. Wilson R, Ling H, MacLean MA, et al: Thyroid antibody titer and avidity in patients with recurrent miscarriage. Fertil Steril 1999;71:558–561.
57. Kaplan MM: Monitoring thyroxine treatment during pregnancy. Thyroid 1992;2:147–152.
58. Mandel SJ, Larsen PR, Seely EW, Brent GA: Increased need for thyroxine during pregnancy in women with primary hypothyroidism. N Engl J Med 1990;323:91–96.
59. Yang K, Burrow GN: Endocrine Problems Section 4 Thyroid Disease. In Lee RV, Rossene-Montella K, Barbor L-A, et al. (eds.) Medical Care of the Pregnant Patient. Philadelphia, American College of Physicians, 2000, pp. 272–286.
60. Chopra IJ, Baber K: Treatment of primary hypothyroidism during pregnancy: Is there an increase in thyroxine dose requirement in pregnancy? Metab Clin Exp 2003;52:122–128.
61. Kuijpens JL, Vader HL, Drexhage HA, et al: Thyroid peroxidase antibodies during gestation are a marker for subsequent depression postpartum. Eur J Endocrinol 2001;145:579–584.
62. Mazzaferri EL: Evaluation and management of common thyroid disorders in women. Am J Obstet Gynecol 1997;176:507–514.
63. Zivaljevic V, Vlajinac H, Jankovic R, et al: Case-control study of female thyroid cancer: Menstrual, reproductive and hormonal factors. Eur J Cancer Prev 2003;12:63–66.
64. Sakoda LC, Horn-Ross PL: Reproductive and menstrual history and papillary thyroid cancer risk: The San Francisco Bay Area thyroid cancer study. Cancer Epidemiol Biomarkers Prev 2002;11:51–57.
65. Memon A, Darif M, Al Saleh K, Suresh A: Epidemiology of reproductive and hormonal factors in thyroid cancer: Evidence from a case-control study in the Middle East. Int J Cancer 2002;97:82–89.
66. Driggers RW, Kopelman JN, Satin AJ: Delaying surgery for thyroid cancer in pregnancy: A case report. J Reprod Med 1998;43:909–912.
67. Wemeau JL, Cao CD: Thyroid nodule, cancer and pregnancy. Ann Endocrinol 2002;63:438–442.
68. Mountford PJ: Risk assessment of the nuclear medicine patient. Br J Radiol 1997;70:671–684.
69. Stagnaro-Green A: Recognizing, understanding, and treating postpartum thyroiditis. Endocrinol Metab Clin North Am 2000;29(2):417–430.
70. Browne Martin K, Emerson CH: Postpartum thyroid dysfunction. Clin Obstet Gynecol 1997;40:90–101.
71. Gallas PRJ, Stolk RP, Bakker K, et al: Thyroid dysfunction during pregnancy and in the first postpartum year in women with diabetes mellitus type I. Eur J Endocrinol 2002;147:443–451.
72. Stuckey BGA, Kent GN, Allen JR: The biochemical and clinical course of postpartum thyroid dysfunction: The treatment decision. Clin Endocrinol 2001;54:377–383.

CHAPTER 47

Pituitary and Adrenal Disease

Mark B. Landon

PITUITARY DISEASE

Normal Changes in Pregnancy

The anterior lobe of the pituitary gland may enlarge significantly during pregnancy as a result of lactotroph proliferation. Magnetic resonance imaging (MRI) scans confirm that the gland more than doubles in size by the end of gestation.[1] Accordingly, prolactin levels increase approximately 10-fold in preparation for lactation.[2]

Pregnancy also affects the levels of other pituitary hormones. Gonadotropin concentrations decrease and show a diminished response to gonadotropin-releasing hormone. The response of growth hormone (GH) to insulin or arginine stimulation is similarly blunted. Plasma levels of adrenocorticotropic hormone (ACTH) increase throughout pregnancy, but absolute levels remain lower in the pregnant than in the nonpregnant state.[3] Curiously, the increase in ACTH levels occurs despite an increase in free and bound cortisol, suggesting an alternate mechanism to the normal negative feedback loop between cortisol and ACTH. The diurnal variation of cortisol, although blunted, is maintained during pregnancy. Thyrotropin levels are unaffected by pregnancy. Free levels of thyroxine and triiodothyronine are unchanged, whereas total levels increase as a result of estrogen-induced synthesis of thyroxine-binding globulin.

Posterior pituitary function is also altered during normal pregnancy. A significant preterm increase in oxytocin is observed, whereas plasma levels of vasopressin remain similar to those obtained in the nonpregnant state. However, plasma osmolality decreases 5 to 10 mOsm/kg in pregnant women, indicating a decreased threshold for vasopressin secretion in pregnancy. During gestation, patients also experience thirst at a lower plasma osmolality.[4]

Prolactin-Producing Adenomas

Maternal and Fetal Risks

Widely available radioimmunoassays for serum prolactin and improved techniques for radiologic diagnosis have led to the detection of an increasing number of prolactin-secreting pituitary adenomas in women. Spontaneous ovulation is uncommon in patients with a pituitary tumor. Therefore, most patients with this disorder have amenorrhea-galactorrhea or anovulatory cycles and infertility. With ovulation induction and suppression of prolactin synthesis by dopaminergic agents, such as bromocriptine, pregnancy can often be achieved in patients with prolactinomas.

Much of the normal pituitary gland enlargement that occurs in pregnancy is secondary to hyperplasia of the anterior pituitary lactotrophic cells, which are stimulated by estrogen. Although this stimulus may cause enlargement of adenomas during pregnancy,[5] most patients with a microadenoma, a pituitary tumor of less than 1 cm, have an uneventful pregnancy.[6–8] In the few patients who have symptoms, regression usually occurs after delivery.

Management Options

PREPREGNANCY

Most women with prolactin-secreting adenomas require ovulation induction to conceive. Nonpregnant patients who have amenorrhea-galactorrhea and hyperprolactinemia (prolactin level >20 ng/mL) should be evaluated for pituitary adenoma. Although serum prolactin levels are correlated with pituitary adenomas, when a patient with hyperprolactinemia is considering pregnancy, a thorough radiologic examination is warranted. MRI has replaced both computed axial tomography and coned down sella turcica radiographs as the procedure of choice to evaluate the size of the pituitary gland.

Once a pituitary tumor is diagnosed, it may be prudent to re-evaluate the gland for growth after several months before attempting ovulation induction. Bromocriptine therapy is often all that is required for patients with microadenomas. Macroadenomas, which are tumors that measure 1 cm or more, should be treated definitively with surgery. These patients are more likely to have symptoms during pregnancy when treated with medical therapy alone.[5,8] Continued bromocriptine therapy after surgery is indicated if symptomatic residual tumor enlargement occurs.

PRENATAL

Evaluation for possible prolactin-secreting tumors is difficult during pregnancy because of the physiologic increase in serum prolactin that occurs in normal gestation. At term, serum prolactin levels may reach values that are 20 times normal. Further, prolactin levels do not always increase during pregnancy in women with prolactinomas, nor do they always increase with pregnancy-induced tumor enlargement (Fig. 47–1).[9] Enlargement usually produces a headache as the first clinical feature, before visual disturbance. Therefore, radiologic diagnosis is necessary for the pregnant patient who has severe headaches or a visual field defect.

Management of the pregnant patient with a previously diagnosed prolactinoma requires careful attention by a team of physicians, including an obstetrician, an endocrinologist, and an ophthalmologist. Women with symptomatic macroadenomas should be seen monthly. Prompt self-referral in patients with headache or visual symptoms should be encouraged. Visual field testing should be performed monthly in women with macroadenomas. Headaches may reflect tumor enlargement and impingement on the diaphragmatic sella or adjacent dura. Visual disturbances are caused by compression of the optic nerve. If the optic chiasm is compressed by superior extension, bitemporal hemianopsia may develop. Although the limitations of serum prolactin levels have been discussed, marked elevations outside the normal range for pregnancy at a given gestational age may signal rapid tumor enlargement.

Gemzell and Wang[5] reviewed the course of 85 women during 91 pregnancies affected by previously untreated microadenomas. Only 5% had complications. Four of the five patients with headache and visual disturbances showed resolution after delivery. One patient who had a visual field defect noted early in pregnancy subsequently underwent transsphenoidal hypophysectomy after cesarean delivery for a triplet gestation at 36 weeks. Similarly, Albrecht and Betz[10] reported a low rate of complications in women with untreated microadenomas during gestation. Of 352 patients, 8 (2.3%) had visual disturbances and 17 (4.8%) had headaches.

Maygar and Marshall[6] reported that symptoms are more common in the first trimester than in the second or third, with a median time at onset of 10 weeks' gestation. However, the likelihood of visual symptoms did not differ among trimesters (Fig. 47–2). In this series, symptoms requiring therapy occurred in more than 20% of the 91 patients with untreated tumors, but in only 1% of women with previously treated adenomas.

Molitch[8] reviewed 16 series that included 246 cases of prolactin-secreting pituitary microadenomas in pregnancy. Only 4 of the 246 women (1.6%) had symptoms of tumor enlargement, and 11 (4.5%) had asymptomatic enlargement on radiologic examination (Table 47–1). In

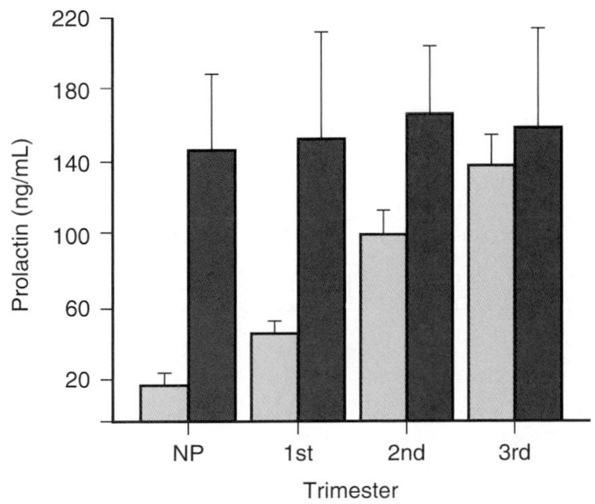

FIGURE 47–1
Maternal serum prolactin concentration in patients with microadenoma (*shaded bars*, *n* = 237) and control subjects (open bars, n = 215) in the nonpregnant state (NP) and during each trimester. (From Divers W, Yen SSC: Prolactin producing microadenomas in pregnancy. Obstet Gynecol 1983;62:425.)

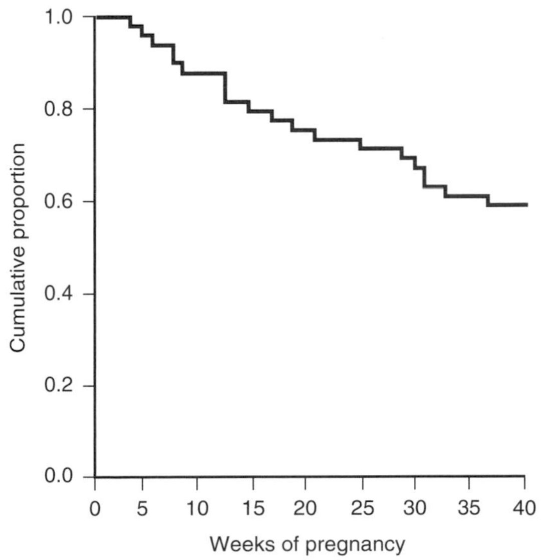

FIGURE 47–2
Time from the beginning of pregnancy to the onset of symptoms (headache or visual disturbances) in 91 pregnancies in women with previously untreated pituitary tumors. (From Maygar DM, Marshall JR: Pituitary tumors and pregnancy. Am J Obstet Gynecol 1978;132:739.)

no case was surgical intervention necessary. Molitch[8] also reviewed 45 patients with macroadenomas, 7 of whom (15.5%) had symptomatic tumor enlargement. Four of these women required surgery during pregnancy. Cabergoline, a dopamine agonist, has been used to treat refractory cases of tumor enlargement during pregnancy.[11] Although data on cabergoline are less extensive, preliminary evidence does not suggest an increase in adverse perinatal outcomes.[12] The risk of symptoms is probably related to the size of the tumor at the onset of pregnancy. Further data are needed to define which group of patients with a microadenoma should be treated with bromocriptine for a prolonged period before conception.

Treatment of complications during pregnancy is influenced by both gestational age and the severity of symptoms. If the fetus is mature, induction of labor or cesarean delivery should be accomplished. Cesarean section is generally performed for obstetric indications. Earlier in gestation, therapy should not be delayed if radiologic evidence suggests tumor enlargement. Medical treatment with bromocriptine or cabergoline is successful in most symptomatic patients and has become the preferred primary approach during pregnancy.[9] Bromocriptine has an established safety profile in early pregnancy, as evidenced by its use to induce ovulation in large groups of women with hyperprolactinemia without an increased incidence of congenital malformations.[13,14] Other treatment modalities used during pregnancy include transsphenoidal surgery,[6–8] and in one case, hydrocortisone therapy.[14] Complications of transsphenoidal surgery include infection, hypopituitarism, hemorrhage, and transient diabetes insipidus. The risk of these complications is probably not increased during pregnancy.

LABOR AND DELIVERY

Intrapartum care of the patient with a prolactin-producing adenoma does not differ from that of the general obstetric population. Some undiagnosed patients may have sudden visual impairment, and prolactinoma must be differentiated from more common conditions, such as preeclampsia and migraine, which may cause the same symptoms.

TABLE 47–1

Effect of Pregnancy on Prolactinomas

TUMOR TYPE	PREVIOUS THERAPY	NO. OF PATIENTS	SYMPTOMATIC ENLARGEMENT
Microadenoma	No	246	4
Macroadenoma	No	45	7
Macroadenoma	Yes	46	2

Adapted from Molitch ME: Pregnancy and the hyperprolactinemic woman. N Engl J Med 1985;312:1364.

POSTNATAL

After delivery, radiologic assessment of tumor size and a serum prolactin assay should be performed at the first postpartum visit. Breast-feeding is not contraindicated in patients with a prolactin-secreting microadenoma.[7] Because serum prolactin levels may remain elevated during breast-feeding, caution must be used in interpreting these results. However, serum prolactin levels do not appear to be significantly higher than prepregnancy levels in women with microadenomas who choose to breastfeed.[15] Counseling patients about future pregnancies requires establishing that progression of tumor growth has not occurred. Some suggest continuing bromocriptine therapy for 12 months before conception to reduce the risk of tumor enlargement during gestation.[12] Gemzell and Wang[5] concluded that in 16 patients with untreated pituitary adenomas, symptoms did not seem to occur with increasing frequency in subsequent pregnancies.

SUMMARY OF MANAGEMENT OPTIONS

Prolactin-Producing Adenomas

Management Options	Quality of Evidence	Strength of Recommendation	References
Prepregnancy			
Treatment (bromocriptine, cabergoline, surgery, or radiation therapy, depending on tumor size)	III	B	15, 52
Advise against pregnancy until cure is achieved.	III	B	7
Prenatal			
Bromocriptine is safe for the fetus.	III	B	7,13,15
Cabergoline is probably also safe, but there is less experience in pregnancy.	III	B	11,12

SUMMARY OF MANAGEMENT OPTIONS

Prolactin-Producing Adenomas *(Continued)*

Management Options	Quality of Evidence	Strength of Recommendation	References
Prenatal—Continued			
Screening or monitoring for recurrence or exacerbation is best undertaken by vigilance for clinical features (headaches, visual disturbance) and prompt testing. Some recommend visual field testing every month.	III	B	7,9,15,50
Interdisciplinary management	III	B	7,9,15,50
If enlargement or recurrence is seen:			
• Bromocriptine if the fetus is not mature; delivery and definitive management if the fetus is mature	III	B	13–15
• Cabergoline for resistant cases (less experience)	III	B	11,12
• Limited experience with hydrocortisone	IV	C	14
• Surgery in extreme cases that do not respond to medical measures	III	B	7,8
Postnatal			
Can breastfeed	III	B	7,15
Monitor symptoms, the prolactin level (may be difficult to interpret in breastfeeding mothers), and tumor size by imaging.	III	B	15

Acromegaly

Maternal and Fetal Risks

Acromegaly is caused by excessive secretion of GH, most often because of an acidophilic or chromophobic pituitary adenoma. Although amenorrhea is common in women with acromegaly, pregnancy occasionally occurs.[16] Pregnancy may be accompanied by tumor expansion that necessitates medical treatment and surgical resection.[17] Patients with acromegaly are at increased risk for diabetes, hypertension, and cardiomyopathy.

Management Options

Documenting elevation of GH levels during pregnancy may be difficult because of placental expression of a GH variant.[18] Few laboratories offer specific radioimmunoassays to differentiate GH from the placental variant. Lack of suppression of GH levels below 5 mg/mL during a glucose tolerance test can help to establish the diagnosis. Measurement of the level of somatomedin C, which mediates the effects of GH, is more useful in establishing the diagnosis of acromegaly in nonpregnant women. Levels of this insulin-like growth factor may increase in normal pregnancy. Definitive surgical treatment or radiation therapy is often undertaken before conception. Dopaminergic agents may paradoxically decrease GH levels in patients with acromegaly. Case reports confirm the lack of tumor expansion during pregnancy in women receiving bromocriptine therapy.[19] More recently, octreotide (Sandostatin) was used to reduce GH levels in women with acromegaly who were pregnant or were attempting pregnancy.[20] Maternal–fetal transfer of octreotide has been shown to occur without side effects. However, few cases have been reported, and the potential benefits of octreotide treatment should be weighed carefully against the potential risks.[21]

SUMMARY OF MANAGEMENT OPTIONS

Acromegaly

Management Options	Quality of Evidence	Strength of Recommendation	References
Prepregnancy			
Definitive surgical management before conception	–	GPP	–

Continued

SUMMARY OF MANAGEMENT OPTIONS

Acromegaly *(Continued)*

Management Options	Quality of Evidence	Strength of Recommendation	References
Prenatal			
Normal elevation of growth hormone levels in pregnancy makes the diagnosis difficult. Lack of suppression of growth hormone levels during a glucose tolerance test is suggestive of the diagnosis. Elevation of somatomedin C levels is a more precise indicator of the diagnosis.	III	B	18
Screen for diabetes, hypertension, and cardiomyopathy.	–	GPP	–
Vigilance for tumor expansion (headaches, visual disturbance)	–	GPP	–
Bromocriptine is an effective and safe treatment in pregnancy.	IV	C	19
Octreotide has been used in pregnancy, but only in a small number of cases, so probably is best avoided.	IV	C	20,21

Diabetes Insipidus

Maternal and Fetal Risks

Diabetes insipidus is rare, with fewer than 100 cases complicating pregnancy reported in the literature. The disease results from inadequate or absent antidiuretic hormone (vasopressin) production by the posterior pituitary gland. The etiology of diabetes insipidus is often unknown, although in most cases, it follows pituitary surgery or destruction of the normal pituitary architecture by tumor. It is a primary idiopathic disorder in up to 50% of cases. Many cases are likely autoimmune, with lymphocytic infiltration of the posterior pituitary gland. Massive polyuria, caused by failure of the renal tubular concentrating mechanism, and dilute urine, with a specific gravity less than 1.005, are characteristic of diabetes insipidus. To combat dehydration and the intense thirst produced by this syndrome, patients consume large quantities of fluid. The diagnosis of diabetes insipidus relies on the finding of continued polyuria and relative urinary hyposmolarity when water is restricted. Administration of intramuscular vasopressin causes water retention and an appropriate increase in urine osmolality. This response is not seen in patients with nephrogenic diabetes insipidus, in which free water clearance is increased because of insensitivity of the renal tubules to antidiuretic hormone. In patients with primary polydipsia or psychogenic diabetes insipidus, urine osmolality increases in response to vasopressin or desmopressin (DDAVP). However, the increase is not as marked as in individuals with central diabetes insipidus. Other conditions that cause polyuria, such as diabetes mellitus, hyperparathyroidism with hypercalcemia, and chronic renal tubular disease, must be considered in the differential diagnosis. However, these conditions usually can be distinguished from central diabetes insipidus by appropriate laboratory testing.

Hime and Richardson[22] reviewed 67 cases of diabetes insipidus complicating pregnancy and noted that 58% of patients showed deterioration during gestation, whereas 20% of patients showed improvement. To explain this phenomenon, it has been suggested that the increased glomerular filtration rate seen in pregnancy may increase the requirement for antidiuretic hormone.[23] Mild disease may worsen during pregnancy because antidiuretic hormone clearance is increased by increased placental vasopressinase activity.[24] Impaired liver function, including fatty liver of pregnancy, is seen with diabetes insipidus during pregnancy, suggesting that several factors may explain the observed worsening of this condition.

Transient diabetes insipidus of pregnancy has been reported during the last trimester.[25] It is associated with acute fatty liver and HELLP syndrome as well as twin gestation. Increased placental vasopressinase activity, along with insufficient liver degradation in HELLP syndrome and acute fatty liver, may unmask this condition.

Management Options

Synthetic vasopressin, in the form of l-deamino-8-D-arginine vasopressin (DDAVP), is the treatment of choice. This drug is given intranasally in doses of approximately 0.1 to 0.25 mg twice daily. Plasma electrolytes and fluid status should be monitored carefully with initiation of therapy. A stable dose is usually easy to achieve. Oxytocic activity is rarely observed. The successful use of DDAVP in pregnancy and the puerperium suggests that this drug is safe for both mother and fetus as well as during lactation.[26]

Spontaneous labor and lactation seem to occur in most patients with diabetes insipidus. Although older reports suggest an increased incidence of dysfunctional labor in affected patients, oxytocin release appears to be independent of vasopressin secretion.[27]

SUMMARY OF MANAGEMENT OPTIONS

Diabetes Insipidus

Management Options	Quality of Evidence	Strength of Recommendation	References
Prepregnancy			
Vigilance for tumor expansion (headaches, visual disturbance)	–	GPP	–
Prenatal			
Continue supplementation with synthetic vasopressin (DDAVP), which is effective and safe in pregnancy. The dose may need to be increased during pregnancy.	IV	C	25,26
Monitor disease control with clinical features and the specific gravity or osmolarity of urine.	IV	C	26
Labor and Delivery			
Vigilance for dysfunctional labor (seen in only a few cases)	IV	C	26,27
Postnatal			
Vigilance for poor lactation (seen in only a few cases)	IV	C	26

Pituitary Insufficiency

Maternal and Fetal Risks

Approximately 65 years ago, Sheehan described postpartum ischemic necrosis of the anterior pituitary.[28] This form of hypopituitarism is usually observed in patients with severe postpartum hemorrhage and hypotensive shock. Because pituitary necrosis is uncommon in patients with other conditions associated with hypovolemic shock, the hyperplastic pituitary gland of pregnancy may be more susceptible to hypoperfusion. Lymphocytic hypophysitis, an autoimmune form of hypopituitarism, is also more common in pregnant women and during the puerperium. It should be considered when hypopituitarism is suspected in patients without preceding postpartum hemorrhage. Slow clinical progression suggests that factors other than ischemia may be involved in the pathogenesis of pituitary insufficiency after pregnancy. Tissue necrosis may release sequestered antigens, triggering autoimmunity of the pituitary and delayed hypopituitarism in Sheehan's syndrome.[29] Destruction of the gland as a result of tumor invasion, surgery, or radiation therapy may accompany pregnancy, although fertility is often compromised. Antepartum pituitary infarction is a rare complication of insulin-dependent diabetes mellitus.[30] In these cases, insulin requirements may decrease dramatically.

Patients with Sheehan's syndrome may have varying degrees of hypopituitarism, and specific assays of tropic hormones as well as stimulation and suppression tests may be necessary to establish the diagnosis. During pregnancy, because of normal physiologic changes, adjustments must be made in interpreting both hormone levels and responses to various stimuli. An average delay of 7 years is observed between onset and diagnosis. Hypovolemic shock from postpartum hemorrhage is a precipitating event in up to 79% of cases.[31] There is no apparent correlation between the degree of hemorrhage and the occurrence of Sheehan's syndrome. The characteristic clinical picture begins with failure to lactate. However, this does not occur in all cases. Some patients have late-onset disease and progress to loss of axillary and pubic hair, oligomenorrhea, or amenorrhea with senile vaginal atrophic changes as well as signs and symptoms of hypothyroidism. Patients with these findings are usually infertile, although the frequency of pregnancy is difficult to ascertain. In a review of 19 patients with Sheehan's syndrome documented by endocrinology studies or postmortem examination, 39 pregnancies occurred after the onset of hypopituitarism.[31] Eleven of these women required hormonal therapy to establish a pregnancy, and replacement therapy was used during 15 (38%) of the 39 pregnancies. The treated group had a live birth rate of 87%, compared with 54% in untreated patients, suggesting that early diagnosis and proper therapy improve outcome.

Because pregnancy may occur in women with Sheehan's syndrome, this diagnosis should be considered in all patients with a history of postpartum hemorrhage. Measuring gonadotropin levels is of little value because levels decrease with normal pregnancy. However, the finding of a low or low-normal level of thyroid-stimulating hormone in conjunction with a low serum thyroxine level is consistent with secondary hypothyroidism. Similarly, low cortisol levels that do not increase with stress and decreased ACTH levels support the diagnosis.

Management Options

The treatment of pituitary insufficiency involves replacement of hormones that are necessary to maintain normal metabolism and respond to stress. Thyroid hormone may be provided as L-thyroxine in doses of 0.1 to 0.2 mg daily. Corticosteroids are essential for patients who have adrenal insufficiency. Maintenance dosage is cortisone acetate 25 mg every morning and 12.5 mg every evening or prednisone 5 mg every morning and 2.5 mg every evening. Mineralocorticoid replacement is rarely necessary because adrenal production of aldosterone is not solely dependent on ACTH stimulation. The dose of glucocorticoids should be increased during the stress of labor and delivery.

SUMMARY OF MANAGEMENT OPTIONS

Pituitary Insufficiency

Management Options	Quality of Evidence	Strength of Recommendation	References
Prepregnancy and Prenatal			
Give appropriate replacement hormones (usually thyroxine and corticosteroids).	–	GPP	–
Monitor clinical features and thyroid-stimulating hormone levels.	–	GPP	–
Labor and Delivery			
Increase the dose of glucocorticoids.	–	GPP	–
Postnatal			
Readjust glucocorticoid and thyroxine dosage if necessary.	–	GPP	–

ADRENAL DISEASE

Normal Changes in Pregnancy

A twofold to threefold increase in cortisol levels is observed by the end of normal pregnancy.[32] Most of this increase is caused by an estrogen-induced increase in cortisol-binding globulin levels; however, biologically active free cortisol levels are also elevated.[33] An increase in free, or unbound, cortisol is apparent by the end of the first trimester. The urinary free cortisol concentration is also elevated during gestation.

Increased cortisol-binding globulin levels prolong the half-life of cortisol in plasma, and cortisol production is also increased. Urinary 17-hydroxycorticosteroid levels are actually lower in pregnancy because excretion of cortisol tetrahedron metabolites is decreased.[34] ACTH levels increase throughout pregnancy, but absolute levels remain lower in the pregnant than in the nonpregnant state.[35] Both ACTH and cortisol surge during labor. Unlike cortisol, ACTH does not cross the placenta. ACTH is manufactured by the placenta, as is corticotropin-releasing hormone. The relationship between these placental hormones and maternal adrenal function is unknown. Aldosterone secretion, which is controlled by the renin-angiotensin system, increases in early pregnancy. Finally, the production of dehydroepiandrosterone in the adrenal cortex is elevated in normal pregnancy. This hormone is aromatized to estradiol and estrone by the placenta.

Cushing's Syndrome

Maternal and Fetal Risks

Cushing's syndrome, which is characterized by excess glucocorticoid production, arises from ACTH-dependent or independent inappropriate hypersecretion of ACTH by a pituitary adenoma or from ectopic production of ACTH. Cushing's syndrome as a result of primary adrenal disease, usually an adrenal adenoma, is more common during pregnancy than in the nonpregnant state. It accounts for approximately 50% of Cushing's syndrome cases during pregnancy.[36] Patients with pituitary disease and secondary adrenal hyperplasia are more likely to have excess androgen secretion, which can inhibit pituitary gonadotropin release. Amenorrhea is common in this setting. In contrast, adrenal adenomas are more likely to be pure cortisol producers and less likely to impair fertility.[32] Other causes of Cushing's syndrome include neoplastic ectopic ACTH production, nodular adrenal hyperplasia, and excessive doses of exogenous corticosteroids.

Because women with Cushing's syndrome are usually infertile, de novo cases are rare in pregnancy. Most cases occur in patients who were previously or partially treated. The clinical features may be difficult to distinguish from many signs and symptoms that accompany normal pregnancy. Weakness, weight gain, edema, striae, hypertension, and impaired glucose tolerance may be observed, both during gestation and in Cushing's syndrome. Early onset of hypertension, with easy bruising and proximal myopathy, strongly suggests the diagnosis and requires further evaluation.

Laboratory diagnosis includes elevated serum cortisol levels without diurnal variation and failure to suppress cortisol secretion with the administration of dexamethasone. Assays for ACTH are of variable accuracy and may confuse the diagnosis. However, an elevated early-morning ACTH value in the presence of high urinary levels of cortisol suggests ACTH-dependent Cushing's syndrome. During gestation, total and free cortisol levels normally increase. Therefore, laboratory results must be compared with established norms for pregnancy. Diurnal variation in cortisol production is maintained in normal pregnancy, although free plasma cortisol levels at term may be two to three times higher than those in nonpregnant women. Further, even in normal pregnant patients, cortisol secretion may not be suppressed with low doses of dexamethasone (1 mg).[35] The preferred screening test for Cushing's syndrome is a 24-hour urine free cortisol measurement. If two collections show elevated levels, then Cushing's syndrome is diagnosed and the cause of excess cortisol production must be determined. A high-dose dexamethasone test may be helpful. Most patients with adrenocortical hyperplasia show a reduction in plasma and urinary corticosteroid levels with an 8-mg dose (2 mg every 6 hours for 2 days). If suppression is unsuccessful, an adrenal tumor, an autonomous adrenal nodule, or ectopic ACTH production must be considered. After testing, pituitary or adrenal gland imaging should be undertaken. MRI is the optimal imaging modality during pregnancy because no radiation is used.

Several reports suggest that Cushing's syndrome may be exacerbated by pregnancy, with improvement of symptoms after delivery.[32,36] In most cases, Cushing's syndrome is associated with an adrenal adenoma.[32] Keegan and colleagues[37] speculated that placental ACTH may stimulate a latent adrenal tumor, with adrenal cortisol secretion decreasing after parturition. The idea that pregnancy may stimulate the development of Cushing's syndrome is supported by the fact that in virtually all reports of Cushing's syndrome in pregnancy, the diagnosis was not established until pregnancy occurred.[32] Several cases of recurrent Cushing's syndrome during pregnancy have been described. These may represent hyperresponsiveness of adrenocortical cells to a non-ACTH or non-corticotropin-releasing hormone substance that is produced during pregnancy.[38]

Pregnancy outcome in Cushing's syndrome is marked by a high rate of preterm delivery (67%) and stillbirth (7%) when elective termination is not performed.[32,33,35,37] Maternal hyperglycemia may be a contributing factor to the intrauterine deaths observed (Table 47–2). Hypertension has been reported in 65% of cases, and preeclampsia in 9%.[32]

Koerten and colleagues[39] reviewed 33 cases of Cushing's syndrome in pregnancy and concluded that maternal complications are more common with adrenal adenomas than with hyperplasia. In this review, every patient with an adenoma had hypertension if the pregnancy progressed beyond the first trimester. Seven of 16 (47%) patients had pulmonary edema, and 1 died. In contrast, only 1 of the 12 patients with adrenal hyperplasia had hypertensive disease. The overall prematurity rate (delivery after 20 weeks' gestation) was 20 of 33 cases (61%); stillbirth occurred in 4 cases.

Management Options

Management of the pregnant patient with cortisol excess includes identifying the source of hormone production and instituting proper therapy. Patients with pituitary disease are most often treated surgically if a tumor can be well defined. Surgical removal of adrenal adenomas can be accomplished through a posterior incision. Bevan and associates[40] examined maternal and fetal outcomes based on the timing of surgery. Fetal loss occurred in 1 of 11 (9%) patients treated during gestation versus 8 of 26 (31%) in whom definitive therapy was delayed. In Buescher's review of 105 cases in which 32 women underwent therapy to relieve hypercortisolism, treatment reduced the perinatal mortality rate from 15% to 6.3%.[32] Again, because the incidence of adrenal adenoma and carcinoma appears to be increased in pregnant patients with Cushing's syndrome, prompt evaluation with MRI is warranted, particularly if high levels of dexamethasone do not suppress excess cortisol production. Surgery is indicated if an adrenal tumor is discovered. Treatment may be delayed in the third trimester if an expedited delivery is planned.

TABLE 47–2

Cushing's Syndrome and Perinatal Complications in 65 Pregnancies

COMPLICATION	N	(%)
Miscarriage	2	(3.1)
Perinatal death		
Neonatal death	5	(7.7)
Stillbirth	5	(7.7)
Premature birth	42	(64.6)
Intrauterine growth retardation	17	(26.2)

Adapted from Buescher MA, McClamrock HD, Adashi EY: Cushing syndrome in pregnancy. Obstet Gynecol 1992;79:130.

SUMMARY OF MANAGEMENT OPTIONS
Cushing's Syndrome

Management Options	Quality of Evidence	Strength of Recommendation	References
Prepregnancy			
Complete testing and treatment (usually surgical) before conception.	–	GPP	–
Prenatal			
If the diagnosis is made during pregnancy, identify and treat the cause or source of hormone production (usually by surgery). The only exception is diagnosis in the third trimester. In this case, delivery and subsequent definitive management may be an option.	III	B	32,36,40
Testing includes magnetic resonance imaging, especially because of the risk of carcinoma.	–	GPP	–

Primary Aldosteronism

Maternal and Fetal Risks

Few cases of primary aldosteronism during pregnancy have been reported. The diagnosis is suggested in a patient with hypertension, hypokalemia, and metabolic alkalosis. Adrenal adenoma is the most common etiology, present in nearly 75% of cases. Glucocorticoid-remediable aldosteronism is a hereditary form of primary aldosterone excess that causes hypokalemia and hypertension in childhood. This diagnosis is established before pregnancy and is amenable to medical treatment. The clinical course of these pregnancies has been described, including a high rate of preeclampsia in patients with underlying chronic hypertension.[41] Because aldosterone secretion is increased during pregnancy, the diagnosis of new-onset hyperaldosteronism can be difficult to establish. However, elevated aldosterone levels accompanied by suppressed renin levels support the diagnosis of primary hyperaldosteronism. High levels of urinary potassium with serum hypokalemia also help to establish the diagnosis. Failure to replace serum potassium may also suppress aldosterone secretion, obscuring the diagnosis.[42] Inappropriately high aldosterone levels are present after suppression testing. The potassium level should be normalized before the administration of suppression tests, such as 9-α-fludrocortisone. Amelioration of hypertension and hypokalemia during gestation is attributed to high levels of progesterone, which may block the action of aldosterone. Even so, patients often have severe hypertension and superimposed preeclampsia.

Management Options

The management of patients without toxemia complicating primary aldosteronism is controversial. Although early case reports suggested prompt surgical excision of underlying adrenal adenomas, Lotgerring and associates[43] described successful medical therapy from midgestation with spironolactone, an aldosterone antagonist, and other antihypertensive medications. This therapy should be used cautiously because spironolactone is an antiandrogen that may cause feminization of a male fetus. Laparoscopic adrenalectomy has been used to treat primary hyperaldosteronism during pregnancy.[44]

SUMMARY OF MANAGEMENT OPTIONS
Primary Aldosteronism

Management Options	Quality of Evidence	Strength of Recommendation	References
Prenatal			
If the diagnosis is made during pregnancy, options are:			
• Medical treatment (antihypertensives and spironolactone), although spironolactone is an antiandrogen, with an associated risk of feminization	IV	C	43
• Laparoscopic adrenalectomy	IV	C	44
• Open surgery	IV	C	42

Adrenal Insufficiency

Maternal and Fetal Risks

Adrenal insufficiency is usually primary (Addison's disease) and caused by autoimmune destruction. Granulomatous diseases, such as tuberculosis, bilateral adrenalectomy, fungal infection, and AIDS, are other rare etiologies. Pituitary failure or adrenal suppression as a result of steroid replacement may also lead to adrenal insufficiency. In these cases, mineralocorticoid production is preserved. Adrenal crisis, an acute, life-threatening condition, may accompany stressful conditions, such as labor, the puerperium, or surgery. Unfortunately, the diagnosis of hypoadrenalism is often difficult, particularly in patients who have enough adrenal reserve to sustain normal daily activity. Postpartum adrenal crisis may lead to the diagnosis of adrenal insufficiency for the first time.[45]

The clinical presentation of Addison's disease during gestation is similar to that in the nonpregnant state. Fatigue, weakness, anorexia, nausea, hypotension, nonspecific abdominal pain, hypoglycemia, and increased skin pigmentation are hallmarks of this endocrinopathy. Mineralocorticoid deficiency leads to renal sodium loss, with resultant depletion of intravascular volume. A small cardiac silhouette on chest radiography is often associated with reduced cardiac output and eventual circulatory collapse. Hypoglycemia, which is common in early pregnancy, may be exacerbated by glucocorticoid deficiency.

Management Options

The diagnosis of adrenal insufficiency is based on specific laboratory findings. Plasma cortisol levels are decreased. However, because the level of cortisol-binding globulin is elevated in pregnancy, even low-normal cortisol values may reflect adrenal insufficiency.[45]

Stimulation of the adrenal gland by synthetic ACTH may help to establish a diagnosis.[46] After intravenous administration of 0.25 mg cosyntropin (Cortrosyn), the plasma cortisol level should be increased at least twofold over baseline values. Failure to respond to this stimulus suggests primary adrenal insufficiency. This test may be used in pregnancy because little ACTH crosses the placenta. A longer ACTH stimulation test is used if the short test does not confirm the diagnosis. Measurement of serum ACTH may also help to distinguish primary adrenal insufficiency from hypopituitarism. Low baseline serum cortisol levels, coupled with ACTH levels greater than 250 pg/mL, confirm the diagnosis of primary adrenal insufficiency.

Pregnancy usually proceeds normally in treated patients. Maintenance replacement of adrenocortical hormones is provided by cortisone acetate 25 mg orally each morning and 12.5 mg in the evening. As an alternative, prednisone may be substituted at doses of 5 mg and 2.5 mg, respectively. Mineralocorticoid deficiency is treated with fludrocortisone acetate (Florinef) 0.05 to 0.1 mg daily. Stress doses of glucocorticoids should be administered during labor and delivery. With doses of glucocorticoids exceeding 300 mg in 24 hours, supplemental mineralocorticoid therapy is unnecessary. The use of a mineralocorticoid requires careful observation for symptoms of fluid overload. Patients with edema, excess weight gain, and electrolyte imbalance require dose adjustment.

Adrenal crisis is a rare, life-threatening condition that requires immediate medical attention. Treatment in an intensive care setting is recommended. Women with undiagnosed Addison's disease may have a crisis during the puerperium. Symptoms include nausea, vomiting, and profound epigastric pain accompanied by hypothermia and hypotension. Treatment initially consists of glucocorticoid and fluid replacement. Intravenous hydrocortisone is given at a dose of 100 mg, followed by repeat doses every 6 hours for up to several days. Mineralocorticoid replacement is indicated in cases of refractory hypotension or hyperkalemia.

Patients with adrenal insufficiency should wear an identifying bracelet. Emergency medical kits are available to help these patients when they travel. Women with Addison's disease require an increase in steroid replacement during periods of infection or stress and during labor and delivery. Cortisol is administered at a dose of 100 mg intravenously every 8 hours for the first 24 hours. The dose of steroids is reduced by 50% the next day.

SUMMARY OF MANAGEMENT OPTIONS

Adrenal Insufficiency

Management Options	Quality of Evidence	Strength of Recommendation	References
Prenatal			
Continue glucocorticoid and mineralocorticoid supplementation.	IV	C	45,46
Vigilance for fluid overload and electrolyte disturbance	IV	C	45,46

Continued

SUMMARY OF MANAGEMENT OPTIONS

Adrenal Insufficiency *(Continued)*

Management Options	Quality of Evidence	Strength of Recommendation	References
Prenatal—Continued			
Vigilance for adrenal crisis: • IV hydrocortisone • IV fluids • Supportive medical therapy • Critical care setting	IV	C	45,46
Labor and Delivery			
Increase glucocorticoid supplementation.	IV	C	45,46

Pheochromocytoma

Maternal and Fetal Risks

Pheochromocytoma is a rare, catecholamine-producing tumor that is uncommon in pregnancy. The tumors arise from the chromaffin cells of the adrenal medulla or sympathetic nervous tissue, including remnants of the organs of Zuckerkandl, neural crest tissue that lies along the abdominal aorta. In pregnancy, as in the nonpregnant state, the tumor is located in the adrenal gland in 90% of cases.[47] The incidence of malignancy, which can be diagnosed only when metastases are present, is approximately 10%. In patients with a family history of pheochromocytoma, multiple endocrine neoplasia syndrome (MEN types IIa and IIb) should be suspected. Pheochromocytoma is more common in patients with neurofibromatosis. Schenker and colleagues[47,48] reported mortality rates of 55% with postpartum diagnosis versus 11% with diagnosis during pregnancy. Fetal loss rates can exceed 50%.

In pregnancy, pheochromocytoma may cause a hypertensive crisis, with cerebral hemorrhage or severe congestive heart failure. Pheochromocytoma is easily confused with other medical diseases. The signs and symptoms may mimic those of severe pregnancy-induced hypertension (Table 47–3). Hypertension, headache, abdominal pain, and blurring of vision are common to both entities. Although not uniformly present, paroxysmal hypertension (particularly before 20 weeks' gestation), orthostasis, and absence of significant proteinuria and edema may be helpful in the differential diagnosis. Severe thyrotoxicosis may also resemble this disease. However, significant diastolic hypertension is rarely seen with hyperthyroidism. Aggravation of hypertension with administration of β-blockers suggests pheochromocytoma. An unexplained hypertensive response to anesthesia or circulatory collapse after delivery should prompt consideration of this diagnosis.

Management Options

PREPREGNANCY

If this condition is suspected, a complete diagnostic evaluation is indicated before pregnancy is attempted. Definitive therapy should be undertaken (discussed later).

PRENATAL

The definitive diagnosis depends on laboratory measurement of catecholamines and their metabolites in a 24-hour urine collection. Elevated metanephrine excretion appears to be the most sensitive and specific finding, although isolated elevated vanillylmandelic acid excretion may be present.[47] Because episodic secretion of catecholamines occurs with some tumors, plasma assay of epinephrine or norepinephrine may be helpful during symptomatic episodes.[48] Levels of catecholamines are unaffected by normal pregnancy. Levels may be elevated after eclamptic seizures. Extra-adrenal tumors have characteristic elevations of norepinephrine, but not epinephrine.

Pharmacologic testing may establish the diagnosis in the nonpregnant patient. The phentolamine (Regitine) test is based on the observation that marked α-adrenergic

TABLE 47–3

Symptoms and Signs in 89 Cases of Pheochromocytoma in Pregnancy

SYMPTOM OR SIGN	%
Paroxysmal or sustained hypertension	82
Headaches	66
Palpitation	36
Sweating	30
Blurred vision	17
Anxiety	15
Convulsion and dyspnea	10

Adapted from Schenker JG, Chowers I: Pheochromocytoma and pregnancy: Review of 89 cases. Obstet Gynecol Surv 1971;26:739.

blockade causes a decrease in blood pressure in many patients with pheochromocytoma. This test is not advised during pregnancy because it is associated with maternal and fetal deaths.[49] Nonetheless, it is of extreme importance that the diagnosis be established. Approximately 90% of maternal deaths as a result of pheochromocytoma occur in patients who are undiagnosed before delivery.[50] When symptoms suggest pheochromocytoma and laboratory findings support the diagnosis, the tumor should be localized with radiologic techniques. MRI is the procedure of choice in pregnancy. In the nonpregnant state, selective venous catheterization of the adrenals may be performed. The tumor is bilateral in approximately 10% of cases, including those that occur during gestation.

Before surgery, the patient's condition should be stabilized with oral doses of phenoxybenzamine and α-adrenergic receptor blockers. Careful evaluation of fluid status with central monitoring is essential when using these preparations. β-Blockade with propranolol or similar selective agents is reserved for the treatment of tachyarrhythmias and should not be instituted before α-blockade because hypertensive crisis may ensue. Labetalol is not recommended because it is a combined adrenergic blocking agent. Hypertensive crisis requires intravenous phentolamine administration in an intensive care setting.

Schenker and Granat[48] recommend prompt surgical removal of pheochromocytomas detected before 24 weeks' gestation. Laparoscopic removal has been achieved during pregnancy.[51] When the diagnosis is made during the early third trimester, maternal stabilization with medical therapy has been successful, allowing further fetal maturation.

LABOR, DELIVERY, AND POSTNATAL

Cesarean delivery is preferred because it minimizes the potential catecholamine surges associated with labor and vaginal delivery. Adrenal exploration is performed at the time of cesarean delivery. Careful follow-up is needed because tumors may recur and are potentially malignant.

SUMMARY OF MANAGEMENT OPTIONS
Pheochromocytoma

Management Options	Quality of Evidence	Strength of Recommendation	References
Prepregnancy			
Avoid pregnancy until definitive treatment is implemented and cure is achieved.	–	GPP	–
Prenatal			
If the diagnosis is suspected clinically, establish the diagnosis with 24-hour catecholamine testing. Establish the location of the tumor (10% are bilateral) with magnetic resonance imaging.	III	B	47–49
Establish medical stabilization and control of blood pressure before and during surgery.	III	B	47–49
Some give medical treatment and defer surgery until after delivery.	IV	C	50
Laparoscopic surgery has been undertaken.	IV	C	51
Labor and Delivery			
Cesarean delivery is preferable once medical stablization is established.	III	B	47–49
Concomitant surgery at the time of cesarean delivery is debatable.	III	B	47–49
Postnatal			
Monitor for recurrence.	III	B	47–49

CONCLUSIONS

- Pituitary and adrenal problems are very rare in pregnancy.
- The evidence underlying management is limited.
- An interdisciplinary approach is needed.
- Ideally, patients should be evaluated and treated before pregnancy.
- Insufficiency requires continuation with supplements in pregnancy.
- Patients taking glucocorticoids need increased doses to cover labor and delivery.
- Although surgery has been performed during pregnancy, most cases can be managed medically and surgery deferred until the pregnancy is complete.

REFERENCES

1. Gonzalez JG, Elizondo G, Saldwar D, et al: Pituitary gland growth during normal pregnancy: An in vivo study using magnetic resonance imaging. Am J Med 1988;85:217.
2. Tyson JE, Hwang P, Guyden H, et al: Studies of prolactin secretion in human pregnancy. Am J Obstet Gynecol 1972;113:14.
3. Rees LH, Burke SW, Chard T, et al: Possible placental origin of ACTH in normal human pregnancy. Nature 1975;254:620.
4. Davison JM, Gilmore EA, Durr J, et al: Altered osmotic thresholds for vasopressin secretion and thirst in human pregnancy. Am J Physiol 1983;246:105.
5. Gemzell C, Wang CF: Outcome of pregnancy in women with pituitary adenoma. Fertil Steril 1979;31:363.
6. Maygar DM, Marshall JR: Pituitary tumors and pregnancy. Am J Obstet Gynecol 1978;132:739.
7. Jewelewicz R, VanDeWiele RL: Clinical course and outcomes of pregnancy in twenty-five patients with pituitary microadenomas. Am J Obstet Gynecol 1980;136:339.
8. Molitch ME: Pregnancy and the hyperprolactinemic women. N Engl J Med 1984;315:21.
9. Divers W, Yen SSC: Prolactin producing microadenomas in pregnancy. Obstet Gynecol 1983;62:425.
10. Albrecht BH, Betz G: Prolactin-secreting pituitary tumors and pregnancy. In Olefsky JM, Robbins RJ (eds): Contemporary Issues in Endocrinology and Metabolism: Prolactinomas, Vol 2. New York, Churchill Livingstone, 1986, pp 195–218.
11. Liu C, Tyrrell JB: Successful treatment of a large macroprolactinoma with cabergoline during pregnancy. Pituitary 2001;4:85.
12. Molitch ME: Pituitary disease in pregnancy. Semin Perinatol 1998;22:157–170.
13. Turkalj I, Braun P, Krup P: Surveillance of bromocriptine in pregnancy. JAMA 1982;247:1589.
14. Jewelewicz R, Zimmerman EA, Carmel PW: Conservative management of a pituitary tumor during pregnancy following induction of ovulation with gonadotropins. Fertil Steril 1977;28:35.
15. Zarate A, Canales ES, Alger M: The effect of pregnancy and lactation on pituitary prolactin secreting tumors. Acta Endocrinol 1979;92:407.
16. Abelove WA, Rupp JJ, Paschkis KE: Acromegaly and pregnancy. J Clin Endocrinol Metab 1954;14:32.
17. Bigazzi M, Ronga R, Lancranjan I, et al: A pregnancy in an acromegalic woman during bromocriptine treatment: Effects of growth hormone and prolactin in maternal, fetal, and amniotic compartments. J Clin Endocrinol Metab 1979;48:9.
18. Frankenne F, Closset J, Gomez F, et al: The physiology of growth hormones in pregnant women and partial characterization of the placental GH variant. J Clin Endocrinol Metab 1988;66:1171.
19. Luboshitzky R, Dickstein G, Barzilai D: Bromocriptine induced pregnancy in an acromegalic patient. JAMA 1989;244:584.
20. Fassnacht M, Capeller B, Arlt W, et al: Octreotide LAR treatment throughout pregnancy in an acromegalic woman. Clin Endocrinol 2001;55:411–415.
21. Neal JM: Successful pregnancy in a woman with acromegaly treated with octreotide. Endocr Pract 2000;6:148–150.
22. Hime MC, Richardson JA: Diabetes insipidus and pregnancy: Case report, incidence and review of the literature. Obstet Gynecol Surv 1978;33:375.
23. Durr JA: Diabetes insipidus in pregnancy. Am J Kidney Dis 1978;9:276.
24. Davidson JM, Shiells EA, Barron WM, et al: Changes in the metabolic clearance of vasopressin and of plasma vasopressinase throughout human pregnancy. J Clin Invest 1989;83:1313.
25. Jin-no Y, Kamiya Y,Okada M, et al: Pregnant woman with transient diabetes insipidus resistant to 1-desamino-8-D-arginine vasopressin. Endocr J 1998;45:693–696.
26. Burrow GN, Wassenaar W, Robertson GL, Sehl H: DDAVP treatment of diabetes insipidus during pregnancy and the postpartum period. Acta Endocrinol 1981;97:23.
27. Shangold MM, Freeman R, Kumaresan P, et al: Plasma oxytocin concentrations in a pregnant woman with total vasopressin deficiency. Obstet Gynecol 1983;61:662.
28. Sheehan HL: Postpartum necrosis and the anterior pituitary. J Pathol Bacteriol 1937;45:189.
29. Goswami R, Kochupillai N, Crock PA, et al: Pituitary autoimmunity in patients with Sheehan's syndrome. J Clin Endocrinol Metab 2002;87:4137–4141.
30. Dorfman SG, Dillaphlain RP, Gambrell RD: Antepartum pituitary infarction. Obstet Gynecol 1979;53:215.
31. Grimes HG, Brooks MH: Pregnancy in Sheehan's syndrome: Report of a case and review. Obstet Gynecol Surv 1980;35:481.
32. Buescher MA, McClamrock HD, Adashi EY: Cushing syndrome in pregnancy. Obstet Gynecol 1992;79:130.
33. Nolten W, Lindheimer M, Rueckert P, et al: Diurnal patterns and regulation of cortisol secretion of pregnancy. J Clin Endocrinol Metab 1980;51:466.
34. Migeon CJ, Kenny FM, Taylor FH: Cortisol production rate: VIII. Pregnancy. J Clin Endocrinol 1968;28:661.
35. Carr BR, Parker CR, Madden JD, et al: Maternal plasma adrenocorticotropin and cortisol relationships throughout human pregnancy. Am J Obstet Gynecol 1982;139:416.
36. Aron DC, Schnall AM, Sheeler LR: Cushing's syndrome and pregnancy. Am J Obstet Gynecol 1990;162:244.
37. Keegan GT, Gravartis F, Roland AS: Pregnancy complicated by Cushing's syndrome. South Med J 1976;69:1207.
38. Hana V, Dokoupilova M, Marek J, Plavka R: Recurrent ACHT-independent Cushing's syndrome in multiple pregnancies and its treatment with metyrapone. Clin Endocrinol (Oxf) 2001; 54:277–281.

39. Koerten JM, Morales WJ, Washington SR, Castaldo TW: Cushing's syndrome in pregnancy: A case report and literature review. Am J Obstet Gynecol 1986;154:626.
40. Bevan JS, Gough MH, Gillmer MDG, et al: Cushing's syndrome in pregnancy: The timing of definitive treatment. Clin Endocrinol 1987;27:225.
41. Wyckoff JA, Seely EW, Hurwitz S, et al: Glucocorticoid-remediable aldosteronism and pregnancy. Hypertension 2000;35: 668–672.
42. Merrill RH, Dombroski RA, MacKenna JM: Primary hyperaldosteronism during pregnancy. Am J Obstet Gynecol 1984; 160:785.
43. Lotgerring FK, Derkx FMH, Wallenburg HCS: Primary hyperaldosteronism in pregnancy. Am J Obstet Gynecol 1986;155:986.
44. Shalhav AL, Landman J, Afane J, et al: Laparoscopic adrenalectomy for primary hyperaldosteronism during pregnancy. Laparoendosc Adv Surg Tech A 2000;10:169–171.
45. Brent F: Addison's disease and pregnancy. Am J Surg 1950; 79:645.
46. O'Shaughnessy RW, Hackett KJ: Maternal Addison's disease and fetal growth retardation. J Reprod Med 1984;29:752.
47. Schenker JG, Chowers I: Pheochromocytoma and pregnancy: Review of 89 cases. Obstet Gynecol Surv 1971;26:739.
48. Schenker JG, Granat M: Pheochromocytoma and pregnancy: An update and appraisal. Aust N Z J Obstet Gynaecol; 1982;22:1.
49. Shapiro B, Fig LM: Management of pheochromocytoma. Endocrinol Metab Clin North Am 1989;18(2):443.
50. Venuto R, Burstein P, Schmeider R: Pheochromocytoma: Antepartum diagnosis and management with tumor resection in the puerperium. Am J Obstet Gynecol 1984;150:431.
51. Finkenstedt G, Gasser RW, Hofle G, et al: Pheochromocytoma and sub-clinical Cushing's syndrome during pregnancy: Diagnosis, medical pre-treatment and cure by laparoscopic unilateral adrenalectomy. J Endocrinol Invest 1999;22:551–557.
52. Wallace EA, Holdaway IM: Treatment of macroprolactinomas at Auckland Hospital 1975-91. N Z Med J 1995;108:50–52.

CHAPTER 48

Hepatic and Gastrointestinal Disease

Catherine Williamson / Joanna Girling

INTRODUCTION

Anatomy and Physiology of the Liver

An understanding of the physiologic changes of normal pregnancy is vital if pathologic conditions are to be correctly defined. False-positive and false-negative interpretations can result if the normal changes due to pregnancy are not fully appreciated.

The liver moves superiorly and posteriorly in pregnancy, such that a palpable liver edge is likely to be pathologic. Absolute blood flow to the liver is unchanged, although the proportion of cardiac output perfusing the liver falls from 35% to 25%. Venous pressure increases in the esophagus due to increased circulating volume, increased portal pressure, and increased pressure from the gravid uterus, thereby diverting a greater proportion of venous return from the inferior vena cava via the azygos system. This results in transient esophageal varices in up to 60% of healthy pregnant women.[1,2] Spider nevi, palmar erythema, and edema are common findings in normal pregnancy, reflecting, in part, peripheral vasodilatation; they should not be assumed to be due to chronic liver disease unless they clearly antedate the pregnancy.

The liver has several important functions, including protein synthesis, metabolism, excretion, and inactivation of a number of substances. Changes in each of these should be considered both in relation to the effect of normal pregnancy and potential overlap with the changes of liver disease outside pregnancy:

- Protein synthesis increases in pregnancy, with rises in coagulation factors VII, VIII, X, and fibrinogen: The last of which has usually doubled by the end of pregnancy, so an apparently normal result may reflect a significant abnormality in, for example, disseminated intravascular coagulopathy (DIC).[3] This increase is probably the main cause of the increase in erythrocyte sedimentation rate that occurs in pregnancy; the 95th percentile for the second trimester in a nonanemic woman being 70 mm/hour.[4] In acute liver failure, prolongation of the prothrombin time may be the first sign of coagulopathy, because prothrombin has the shortest half-life of those coagulation factors manufactured in the liver. Production of albumin is not changed during uncomplicated pregnancy, and hemodilution results in a fall in concentration, so that levels of 28 g/L are commonly seen: these do not reflect failure of hepatic synthesis as might be the case outside pregnancy. The concentration of many hormone-binding proteins is increased, largely due to reduced metabolism rather than increased hepatic synthesis. For example, the higher concentration of estrogen stimulates greater sialylation of the carbohydrate moieties of thyroxine-binding globulin, which extends its half-life from 15 minutes to 3 days[5] and so greatly increases the total T_4.
- Amino acids undergo oxidative deamination in the liver to produce ammonia, which is converted to urea in the Krebs cycle. Failure of this process in severe liver disease can contribute to hepatic encephalopathy. It may also be associated with low urea concentrations, which must not be confused with the fall in urea that occurs as a consequence of the increased glomerular filtration rate of normal pregnancy.[6]
- Hypercholesterolemia occurs in some forms of chronic liver disease due to impaired excretion. Hypertriglyceridemia can occur in chronic alcohol abuse. In normal pregnancy their concentrations increase by 50% and 300%, respectively,[7] and take several months to return to normal after delivery.
- The liver is responsible for postprandial glucose storage and subsequent release during fasting. Hypoglycemia

may occur, despite these large glucose reserves, in patients with massive liver necrosis, for example, in acute fatty liver of pregnancy and is an important cause of liver coma. Serial measurements of blood glucose and subsequently intravenous infusion of 50% dextrose are important in preventing hypoglycemic coma in patients with severe liver failure.

Anatomy and Physiology of the Gastrointestinal Tract

The gastrointestinal tract also undergoes extensive physiological changes in pregnancy. These changes contribute to the common findings of nausea and vomiting, gastroesophageal reflux, constipation, and hemorrhoids, although the exact basis for these changes is not clearly understood. Nausea and vomiting seem to be due to the combined actions of estrogen and progesterone, although this is not certain; human chorionic gonadotrophin may also make a contribution (see hyperemesis gravidarum). Gastroesophageal reflux occurs in up to 80% of pregnancies,[8] and is thought to be due to a combination of reduced lower esophageal sphincter pressure, raised intragastric pressure, reduced pyloric sphincter competence with backwash of alkaline bile and failure of clearance of acid gastric contents. Constipation is traditionally attributed to progesterone-driven smooth muscle relaxation, and increasing transit times allowing more fluid to be absorbed. However, in pregnancy only small bowel transit times have been reported,[9] colonic times have not been studied directly. Iron supplements, dietary changes and altered exercise levels may also contribute, as may mechanical problems in the lower gastrointestinal tract especially the anal sphincter.[10]

Liver Function Tests

So-called "liver function tests" (LFT) are really nonspecific tests of liver cell damage: In essence they reflect the extent of hepatocyte damage, although if damage is extensive and sustained, values may plummet. In pregnancy, significant changes occur in the commonly measured tests of liver function, which must be borne in mind when interpreting blood results. Aspartate transaminase, alanine transaminase, γ-glutamyl transferase, and total bilirubin each fall during pregnancy, the upper limit of normal being about 25% lower than outside pregnancy. This is mainly as a result of haemodilution[11] (Table 48–1). Alkaline phosphatase rises steadily through pregnancy, reaching a peak in the third trimester up to 300% above the nonpregnant range, due to the production of a heat-stable placental isoenzyme: If there is a clinical indication to differentiate the hepatic from the placental form, then the sample can be heat-treated to 60°C for 10 minutes and then reanalyzed, the fall representing the liver isoenzyme.

In the postnatal period, alkaline phosphatase falls steadily, reaching nonpregnant values by day 13 in most women. The transaminases may rise considerably, especially during the first 5 days of the puerperium and can exceed both the pregnant and nonpregnant reference ranges[12] (Table 48–2). This is because they are not specific to liver, occurring also in breast, smooth and striated muscle, and red blood cells. The exercise of labor, the trauma of delivery, and breast-feeding may all contribute to this phenomenon. It is essential to bear this in mind when managing liver disease in the puerperium.

The Fetus and Maternal Liver Disease

In many cases, the fetus is only affected by the maternal liver condition if the pregnant woman is systemically unwell, for example, febrile, dehydrated, hypoglycemic, or profoundly malnourished. Specific issues relating to transmission of infection, the genetic input of the fetus to the maternal condition (e.g., acute fatty liver of pregnancy), the role of the placenta (e.g., preeclampsia and HELLP syndrome), and fetal "poisoning" (e.g., obstetric cholestasis) are covered in the relevant sections. It does not seem that fetal exposure to raised bilirubin, even if prolonged, or toxic metabolites of maternal liver failure

TABLE 48–1

Liver Function Tests in Normal Pregnancy[11]

	NONPREGNANT	FIRST TRIMESTER	SECOND TRIMESTER	THIRD TRIMESTER
AST u/L	7–40	10–28	11–29	11–30
ALT u/L	0–40	6–32	6–32	6–32
Bili μmol/L	0–17	4–16	3–13	3–14
GGT u/L	11–50	5–37	5–43	5–41
Alk phos u/L	30–130	32–100	43–135	130–418

ALT, alanine aminotransaminase; AST, aspartate aminotransaminase; Bili, bilirubin; GGT, γ - glutamyl transferase; Alk phos, alkaline phosphatase.

TABLE 48–2

Liver Function Tests Following Delivery in Normal Pregnancy[12]

	POSTPARTUM PEAK (DAYS)	MEAN RISE (%)	RANGE RISE (%)
AST	2–5	88	0–500
ALT	5	147	0–1140
GGT	5–10	62	0–450
Alk phos	Predelivery	–	–

ALT, alanine aminotransaminase; AST, aspartate aminotransaminase; GGT, γ - glutamyl transferase; Alk phos, alkaline phosphatase.

influence development.[13] Unconjugated bilirubin crosses the placenta bidirectionally, and this is the main route of fetal clearance. There is not a simple link between maternal and fetal levels of bilirubin.

JAUNDICE IN PREGNANCY

Jaundice may be coincidental to the pregnancy or due to a condition that is specific to the pregnancy. Worldwide the most common cause of jaundice in pregnancy is viral hepatitis, usually hepatitis A. In some parts of the world hepatitis B, C, or E are most prevalent. Hepatitis secondary to infection with cytomegalovirus, Epstein-Barr virus, toxoplasmosis, or herpes simplex should also be considered as causes of jaundice in pregnancy, not least because of the other important implications that these infections have for the fetus. Other common causes of jaundice not related to the pregnancy are the complications of gallstones, drug reactions (in the United Kingdom co-amoxiclav is the commonest cause of cholestatic jaundice) and drug abuse, including alcohol.

The pregnancy-specific causes of jaundice are acute fatty liver of pregnancy, HELLP (*h*emolysis, *e*levated *l*iver enzymes, *l*ow *p*latelets) syndrome, obstetric cholestasis, and hyperemesis gravidarum. Only in the first of these, which is also the rarest, is jaundice a common feature.

Physiology

When faced with the challenge of a jaundiced pregnant patient, it is easier to reach a diagnosis if a simple logical pathway is followed. Initially the jaundice should be classified according to its type. Then its cause can usually be determined. An understanding of the physiology of bilirubin handling makes this much easier.

Following the destruction of a red blood cell, the released hemoglobin is broken down into globin and heme; other heme-containing proteins, such as myoglobin, cytochromes, and catalase, contribute up to 15% of the total heme. The heme is broken down to biliverdin, which is reduced to form bilirubin, usually amounting to 250 to 300 mg daily: This is not changed by pregnancy. This bilirubin is unconjugated and water-insoluble, and usually carried to the liver bound to albumin. In this state it is unable to pass through the kidney or the blood-brain barrier. However, unbound unconjugated bilirubin is lipid-soluble and can cross the blood-brain barrier. This is most likely in neonates with immature conjugating mechanisms or in the presence of either profound hypoalbuminemia or displacement of bilirubin from albumin by, for example, fatty acids, salicylates, or sulfonamides.

At the hepatocyte membrane, unconjugated bilirubin is actively taken up and conjugated to two molecules of glucuronide, by the action of uridine diphosphoglucurosyl (UDP) transferase. This conjugated bilirubin is water-soluble and usually remains in the liver. Hepatocyte (or canalicular) damage allows it to enter the blood, and the part that remains unbound passes into urine and causes the dark urine of cholestatic jaundice; it is always abnormal to find bilirubinuria. The protein-bound conjugated bilirubin contributes to the yellow discoloration of skin and mucus membranes and the hyperbilirubinemia of liver disease.

From the hepatocyte, bilirubin is actively taken up by the bile canaliculus. It is these energy-dependent steps that are most likely to be impaired by either liver damage or by increased pressure in the biliary tract. From the canaliculus, conjugated bilirubin drains into the extrahepatic bile ducts, the common bile duct, and finally the small intestine. The conjugated bilirubin is too large to be absorbed from this location. It passes to the terminal ileum where bacterial action hydrolyses it to free bilirubin, which is then reduced to urobilinogen. Some of this undergoes further bacterial action in the stool, changing it to stercobilinogen, which contributes to the dark color of feces—reduced entry of bilirubin into the gut accounts for the pale stool of cholestatic jaundice. The rest of the urobilinogen is absorbed and returns to the liver via the enterohepatic circulation; from there it is re-excreted into the bile. This urobilinogen is water-soluble, and in normal circumstances a small amount passes into the urine. Urinary urobilinogen is increased either if there is an increased load of bilirubin, in which case the hepatic capacity to re-excrete the urobilinogen may be overwhelmed, or if hepatic damage impairs re-excretion.

Classification

In Figure 48–1, the potential points for pathological processes resulting in jaundice are highlighted. Three pathologic processes lead to jaundice:

- Hemolysis
- Congenital hyperbilirubinemia
  - unconjugated
  - conjugated

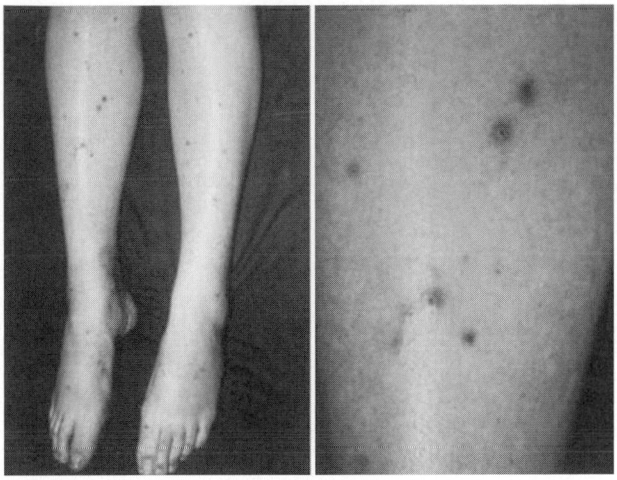

FIGURE 48–1
Dermatologic features observed in obstetric cholestasis cases: Dermatitis artefacta (See Color Plate 41).

- Cholestasis
  - intrahepatic
  - extrahepatic

Hemolytic Jaundice

Hemolytic jaundice occurs when there is excess breakdown of red blood cells and is characterized by increased unconjugated bilirubinemia. There are no abnormalities in transaminases unless liver disease is present as well. Investigations are centered on causes of hemolytic anemia, including hereditary spherocytosis or elliptocytosis, thalassemia, sickle cell disease, glucose-6-phosphate dehydrogenase, blood group incompatibility, or drug reaction. In HELLP syndrome, the main cause of jaundice may be hemolysis.

Congenital Hyperbilirubinemia

In this group of disorders raised bilirubin is the only biochemical abnormality. It occurs when there is either defective conjugation or abnormal handling of bilirubin. The most common condition in this category is Gilbert's syndrome. This benign, familial cause of unconjugated hyperbilirubinemia affects up to 7% of the general population. Most patients have a reduced level of UDP transferase, to around 30% of normal. A number of gene mutations have been described, although phenotypic expression of carriers varies widely, with some individuals being asymptomatic and others experiencing intermittent jaundice. Fasting, intercurrent illness, and pregnancy have been reported to increase the level of unconjugated bilirubinemia, with up to half of pregnant women developing worsening of jaundice.[14] Apart from the raised bilirubin, the other LFTs are normal, and there are no stigmata of chronic liver disease. The reticulocyte count is not raised, thus excluding hemolysis.

Crigler-Najjar syndrome is a very rare and much more serious cause of unconjugated hyperbilirubinemia, which is due to either absence of (autosomal recessive) or marked reduction of (autosomal dominant) UDP transferase. This usually presents at birth, with jaundice and sometimes kernicterus.

Conjugated hyperbilirubinemia is due to defective handling of bilirubin within the liver. Dubin-Johnson syndrome is autosomal recessive and results from a mutation in the *MRP2* (multidrug-resistance protein 2) gene, which is responsible for transporting a wide range of compounds out of the hepatocyte across the canalicular border, including bilirubin and bile salts. It is benign, with a good prognosis, most affected individuals experiencing only mild and fluctuating jaundice. Rotor syndrome is a similar condition, which is often autosomal dominant. In both conditions bilirubinuria is present.

Benign recurrent intrahepatic cholestasis (BRIC) and progressive familial intrahepatic cholestasis (PFIC) are rare causes of conjugated congenital hyperbilirubinemia, which in pregnancy may account for a small proportion of cases of obstetric cholestasis (see following sections).

Cholestatic Jaundice

The broad term *cholestasis* refers to failure to excrete bile from the hepatocyte, the canaliculus (intrahepatic), or the common bile duct (extrahepatic) due to acquired damage or obstruction. Consequently, some or all of the substances usually excreted by this route, including bilirubin, bile salts, cholesterol, and phospholipids, accumulate in the blood. Alkaline phosphatase levels may rise, due to either increased synthesis at the sinusoidal surface of the hepatocyte or to re-entry from the sinusoids into the systemic circulation in response to raised intraductal pressure. Cholestasis may occur without jaundice if excretion of bilirubin is maintained or only part of the liver is affected. Jaundice occurs when the failure of excretion of bilirubin results in its accumulation in the circulation.

Intrahepatic cholestatic jaundice is due to any of a wide range of abnormalities at a cellular level and has a diverse number of clinical causes. Within this category fall viral hepatitis, drug reactions, alcohol abuse, cirrhosis of any cause, obstetric cholestasis, acute fatty liver of pregnancy, and hyperemesis gravidarum. Extrahepatic cholestasis is due to obstruction to the flow of bile at any point beyond the canaliculus; causes include gallstones, biliary stricture, pancreatitis, and malignancy.

In both forms of cholestatic jaundice there may be pale stool, dark urine, and conjugated bilirubinemia. They must be clearly differentiated from each other by careful history, examination, and investigation because they require different management strategies.

In practical terms, an important step in assessing a patient with jaundice is to establish the type of jaundice (see section on Classification and Table 48–3). This is very simply and quickly done by asking the laboratory to report the bilirubin both as the total amount and divided into conjugated and unconjugated forms (also referred to as direct and indirect bilirubin). Commercial urine dipsticks

TABLE 48–3

Serum and Urine Findings in a Jaundiced Patient, Allowing Characterization of the Cause of the Jaundice

	SERUM BILIRUBIN		URINE BILIRUBIN			
CAUSE OF JAUNDICE	UNCONJUGATED	CONJUGATED	BILIRUBIN	UROBILINOGEN	RETICULOCYTE COUNT	ALT
Hemolysis	↑	N	–	↑	↑	N
Gilbert's syndrome	↑↑	N	–	↑	N	N
Crigler-Najjar syndrome	↑↑↑	N	–	↑	N	N
Dubin-Johnson	N/↑	↑	✓	↑	N	N
Hepatocellular	N/↑	↑	✓	↑/N	N	↑
Hepatocanalicular	N/↑	↑	✓	↑/N	N	↑
Extrahepatic	N/↑	↑	✓	↑/N	N	↑

✓, present; –, absent; ↑, increased; ↓, decreased; ALT, alanine transaminase; N, normal.

should be used to test for bilirubinuria (which is always abnormal) and urinary urobilinogen. Table 48–3 can then be used to establish the most likely type of jaundice.

Management Options

Prepregnancy

Some causes of jaundice have long-term implications for maternal health and should be discussed prior to pregnancy.

Prenatal

It is important to determine the type of jaundice and its cause. Management depends on the cause and involves interdisciplinary approaches with health professionals from other specialties according to differential diagnosis.

Labor and Delivery

Planned early delivery may be required as "treatment" for some pregnancy-specific causes of jaundice, but is not inevitable. An epidural should not be sited if a coagulopathy or profound thrombocytopenia is present.

Postnatal

Resolution of jaundice should be confirmed. Care should be taken with the use of the oral contraceptive pill. Implications for future pregnancy depend on the cause and should be discussed with the patient.

SUMMARY OF MANAGEMENT OPTIONS

Jaundice in Pregnancy

Management Options	Quality of Evidence	Strength of Recommendation	References
Prepregnancy			
Jaundice due to conditions with implications for pregnancy should be discussed.	–	GPP	–
Prenatal			
Identify the type of jaundice and its cause.	–	GPP	–
Interdisciplinary management depends on cause.	–	GPP	–
Labor and Delivery			
Plan early delivery if this will improve outcome.	–	GPP	–
Avoid regional analgesia if coagulopathy is present.	–	GPP	–
Postnatal			
Confirm resolution of jaundice	–	GPP	–
Long-term management depends on cause.	–	GPP	–

OBSTETRIC CHOLESTASIS

General

Obstetric cholestasis (OC) affects 0.7% of pregnancies in Caucasians in the United Kingdom and approximately double this proportion of women of South Asian origin.[15,16] It is associated with maternal hepatic impairment and with fetal morbidity and mortality. OC has a complex etiology, with genetic, environmental, and endocrinologic factors playing a role. Evidence for a genetic cause includes the high prevalence in specific ethnic groups; for example, it affects 5.5% of pregnancies in Chilean Araucanians,[17] and the fact that sisters have a relative risk of 17%.[18] Recent genetic studies of cholestasis in nonpregnant cases have also added to our understanding of the etiology of OC. Mutations in genes that influence hepatic bile acid transport (i.e., *MDR3*, *FIC1*, and *BSEP*) have been demonstrated in two conditions: PFIC and BRIC.[19–21] A small proportion of the heterozygous mothers of children with PFIC have been shown to have mutations in at least one of these genes and to have a higher incidence of OC than expected.[21–23]

Women who develop OC are thought to have an increased sensitivity to the cholestatic effect of raised serum estrogens in pregnancy; the condition occurs most commonly in the third trimester when estrogen levels are highest and some women with a previous history of OC develop similar symptoms when taking the oral contraceptive pill[24] or when challenged with exogenous estrogens.[25] It has also been suggested that progesterone may play a role in the etiology of the condition as 34 (68%) of 50 women in a French prospective series of OC cases had been treated with oral micronized natural progesterone for risk of premature delivery.[26]

Diagnosis

The classical maternal symptom of OC is generalized pruritus without a rash. Dark urine, pale stool, or jaundice may also be present, but these are uncommon. If pruritus is associated with abnormal liver transaminases or raised bile acids, a diagnosis of OC should be considered. A recent UK study demonstrated that pruritus without hepatic impairment occurs in approximately 50% of pregnancies, but this is most commonly transient, localized to the abdomen and limited to the first trimester.[27] Amongst women with pruritus, 3% had OC (using a diagnosis of pruritus plus raised serum transaminases or bile acids), and in this group the itch was more commonly described as "all over," "on the legs," or "on the palms and soles." However, OC did also occur in women who only complained of pruritus on the abdomen, so we recommend that the LFTs and serum bile acids should be checked in all pregnant women who complain of pruritus without rash.

Measurement of bile acids is the most useful test for the diagnosis of OC. In unaffected pregnancies the levels of serum bile acids change little.[28] The extent of the rise in OC pregnancies is variable and can be marked. However, more moderate rises in serum bile acids may still be associated with an adverse fetal outcome, so it is important to consider the diagnosis in all women with levels above the normal range. Serum transaminases [alanine aminotransferase (ALT) and aspartate aminotransferase (AST)] also rise in the majority of cases, but the extent of the rise may not be marked (i.e., two- to threefold). The relative value of serum bile acids, ALT and AST for the diagnosis of OC is a matter of debate as it is not yet certain which is the best prognostic indicator: The diagnosis can be entertained if one or more of these are abnormal. Studies have shown that serum bile acids and transaminases are both raised in more than 90%,[29] or all cases,[30,31] although the timing of the changes may be different. In a subgroup of women the rise in serum bile acids and transaminases can occur up to 15 weeks after the onset of pruritus, so it is advisable to repeat the tests in women with persistent symptoms of OC even if the initial results are normal.[32]

Raised bilirubin can occur in OC, but it is not commonly seen and should not be used alone to make the diagnosis. Alkaline phosphatase rises in the third trimester of normal pregnancies, mainly as a consequence of the placental isoenzyme, and is therefore not of value in the diagnosis of OC. Gamma-glutamyltransferase is elevated in approximately 33% of cases.[28]

A new marker of hepatocellular damage, glutathione-*S*-transferase alpha (GSTα), seems to be a better early discriminator between pruritus gravidarum and OC, because in the latter condition it becomes raised 9 weeks before transaminases or bile salts.[33]

Women with pruritus and abnormal LFTs should have viral hepatitis (hepatitis A, B, C, CMV, and EBV) and autoimmune hepatitis excluded: Blood needs to be taken for the appropriate serologic tests, antimitochondrial antibodies to exclude primary biliary cirrhosis and anti-smooth muscle antibodies to exclude autoimmune chronic active hepatitis. An ultrasound scan of the liver and biliary tree should be performed to exclude other causes of biliary obstruction. In a study of 227 UK cases of OC, gallstones were present in 13%, and of these cases 70% had a history of symptoms of cholelithiasis prior to pregnancy.[34] Asymptomatic gallstones are unlikely to cause OC and are more likely to be present because mutations in at least one gene predispose affected women to both OC and gallstones.[35]

The diagnosis of OC should be one of exclusion and be finally confirmed by resolution of symptoms and biochemical abnormalities postpartum. Antenatally, once the diagnosis of OC has been made, the LFTs, including a prothrombin time, should be checked once per week: The purpose of this is not to assess disease severity, because the risk to the fetus is not clearly linked at present to levels of any biochemical markers, but to ensure continued cholestasis.

It is particularly important to establish whether a woman with OC has hepatitis C, because pregnancies in seropositive women are more likely to be complicated by spontaneous prematurity.[36] Also women with hepatitis C infection have a higher prevalence of OC.[36] If a woman is found to be seropositive, it is important to discuss the risk of vertical transmission, although this is currently thought to be low and not markedly influenced by the mode of delivery or breast-feeding. An additional argument for screening for hepatitis C in women with OC is that treatment with interferon and ribavirin postnatally can be curative.

Maternal and Fetal Risks

Maternal Risks

Pruritus can be a very distressing symptom, and some women may have such marked dermatitis artefacta that they develop permanent scars (Fig. 48–1). We are aware of one woman who was so disturbed by pruritus that she put her feet in ice water and developed frostbite.

The main maternal risk in pregnancy is postpartum hemorrhage as a consequence of the prolonged prothrombin time that can occur in association with hepatic impairment.[37]

The pruritus and hepatic impairment resolve rapidly after delivery in the majority of cases, although epidural opiates seem to be associated with a transient deterioration of itch in a few women. If symptoms or biochemical abnormalities persist more than 3 months postpartum, women should be referred to a hepatologist.

There was a 90% risk of recurrence of OC in UK cases. Twenty-seven percent of women complained of either cyclical or oral contraceptive-induced pruritus when they were not pregnant,[34] but the condition did not influence their health in the long term. Therefore, women with OC should be advised to avoid estrogen-containing contraceptives. If no alternatives are suitable, the oral contraceptive pill should only be introduced with serial monitoring of LFTs, surveillance for pruritus, and discontinuation if changes develop.

Fetal Risks

OC has been reported to be associated with increased rates of spontaneous prematurity, fetal distress (defined as meconium-stained amniotic fluid or CTG abnormalities), and intrauterine death (IUD). In the 1995 CESDI report[38] 5% of all full-term stillbirths were attributed to OC. Table 48–4 summarizes the frequency of these complications in each of the studies that has been performed in all successive cases within specific hospitals. Although the rates of IUD have decreased following a policy of delivery by 38 weeks' gestation (see Table 48–4), women are still referred to the obstetric medicine clinic at Queen Charlotte's Hospital having had OC pregnancies complicated by IUD. We suspect that this complication still occurs in approximately 0.5% of affected pregnancies, even with early delivery. The data in Table 48–4 and the results of a study of OC pregnancies complicated by IUD in the UK[34] suggest that delivery by 37 weeks' gestation reduces the risks of IUD. Some data from *in vitro* animal studies suggest that ursodeoxycholic acid (UDCA) and dexamethasone treatment may also be protective.[39] It may be of relevance that these therapeutic agents were given to 40% of women in a recent series of 70 cases in which no IUDs were reported.[16]

Iatrogenic prematurity is also commoner in OC pregnancies,[34] and it is important not to underestimate the fetal risks of elective delivery at 37 weeks' gestation. A study of neonatal respiratory morbidity following elective cesarean section for all indications reported a higher incidence of respiratory distress syndrome and transient tachypnea of the newborn in those that were delivered during the week 37 + 0 to 37 + 6 compared with 38 + 0 to 38 + 6, and a similar difference was seen when this was compared with deliveries the following week of gestation.[40] Another study demonstrated that a markedly

TABLE 48–4

Summary of the Major Studies of Fetal Outcome in Obstetric Cholestasis

YEAR	NO. OF CASES	IUD AND/OR NND (%)	MECONIUM STAINING (%)	PRETERM LABOR (%)	PLANNED DELIVERY <37–38/40*	REFERENCE
1964–1969	87	9	–	54	No	43
1965–1979	56	11	27	36	No	42
post-1969	91	3	–	–	Yes	43
1988	83	4	45	44	Yes	52
1994	320	2	25	12	Yes	161
1990–1996	91	0	15	14	Yes	162
1999–2001	70	0	14	6	Yes	16

IUD, intrauterine death rate as a percentage of all births; NND, neonatal death.
* That is, in the majority of cases in the study.

higher proportion of babies required ventilation for respiratory distress syndrome when delivered at an earlier gestation; that is, 1:73 (1.4%) at 35 weeks, compared with 1:557 (0.2%) at 37 weeks (and 1:1692 at 38 weeks).[41] In our study of 70 women with OC, 58 were delivered at or beyond 37 weeks' gestation, and of these, nine babies were admitted to the special care baby unit and two needed ventilation.[16] However, most women consider these risks to be more acceptable than the risk of IUD in OC pregnancies not delivered by 38 weeks.[42,43]

Management Options

Once the diagnosis of OC has been made, we recommend that affected women are delivered between 37 to 38 weeks' gestation to reduce the risk of IUD. Fetal surveillance can be performed with regular cardiotocography, although there is no evidence that this predicts which pregnancies are at risk of fetal distress or IUD. It is, however, often reassuring for affected women and for the team caring for them. We recommend that vitamin K 10 mg orally should be taken daily to reduce the risk of hemorrhage. Two drugs, UDCA and dexamethasone, have been shown to improve maternal symptoms and biochemical abnormalities in OC. We recommend UDCA treatment for women with distressing symptoms of pruritus. Dexamethasone, and other therapeutic agents discussed in the following sections, can be considered in women who do not respond to UDCA treatment.

Vitamin K

The active vitamin-K-dependent clotting factors (II, VII, IX, and X) are formed from precursors in the liver, and patients with liver disease are at risk of hemorrhage due to deficiency of these clotting factors. In OC, impaired intestinal absorption secondary to steatorrhea is the most likely cause of vitamin K deficiency, although hepatic impairment may also contribute in some cases. It is thought that the increased prevalence of postpartum hemorrhage in OC is related to vitamin K deficiency, although it is feasible that prematurity, induction of labor, instrumental delivery, or other factors are also relevant. There has been one report of reduction in the prothrombin level in a woman with OC[37] and a case report of severe fetal intracranial hemorrhage in a woman treated with cholestyramine that was thought to be due to vitamin K deficiency.[44] Once OC is diagnosed, we recommend that all women are treated with water-soluble oral vitamin K 10 mg daily.

Ursodeoxycholic Acid

There have been more studies of UDCA than any other drug for the treatment of OC. In the Cochrane Database of Systematic reviews, three trials totaling 56 women are identified in which UDCA is compared with placebo: In two there is no difference in relief of symptoms; in one trial, greater reduction in bile salts and liver enzymes was noted with UDCA.[45] When the results of ten studies with a total of 85 affected women who have been treated with UDCA are combined, 74 (87%) showed clinical or biochemical improvement or both.[16] In addition, UDCA has been shown to reduce the levels of bile acids in the cord blood and amniotic fluid at the time of delivery.[47] UDCA is commonly started at a dose of 500 mg twice a day, but doses of up to 2000 mg/day were given in several studies, and some women will only respond to higher doses. All babies born to mothers given UDCA were delivered safely, and no problems attributable to treatment have been reported, although there has been no follow-up of these babies.

Dexamethasone

One Finnish study demonstrated improvement in clinical symptoms and biochemical abnormalities in ten women with OC who were treated with oral dexamethasone 12 mg daily for 7 days, with a gradual reduction in dose over the subsequent 3 days.[48] The results of this study are encouraging, but this is the only series of cases treated with dexamethasone in the literature to date. There has been one case report of worsening of maternal pruritus and ALT following dexamethasone treatment.[49] Our experience of 12 women suggests that approximately 40% of those whose symptoms and biochemical abnormalities do not respond to initial treatment with UDCA will respond to dexamethasone treatment.

There have been no long-term studies of the subsequent effects on the child of antenatal exposure to high doses of dexamethasone in the 7- to 10-day regimen used in obstetric cholestasis, but there is some uncertainty about the fetal risks of such high doses of corticosteroids. It is thought that treatment with two doses of dexamethasone (12 mg IM) for fetal lung maturity is safe, but some animal and human data suggest a possible association between repeated courses of steroids and decreased birth weight[50] and abnormal neuronal development.[51] Widespread use of dexamethasone cannot yet be recommended. Its use should be carefully considered in women with severe resistant symptoms who are remote from delivery.

Other Drugs that Can Be Used to Treat Obstetric Cholestasis

Several other drugs have been used to treat OC, including cholestyramine, *S*-adenosylmethionine, and guar gum (reviewed in reference[46]). Although all resulted in clinical improvement in some studies, none of these agents consistently resulted in a biochemical improvement and no studies were powered to show improvement in fetal outcome.

Aqueous cream with menthol often relieves the pruritus for a short time, and some women find this helps them to fall to sleep.

Amniocentesis and Amnioscopy

Meconium staining of the amniotic fluid is reported in almost all cases of IUD that complicate OC in the current literature. Amniocentesis for the presence of meconium has been proposed as the best way to predict the at-risk fetus.[52] No IUDs were reported in a series of 206 women in whom amnioscopy and amniocentesis were used to test for meconium before 37 weeks' gestation as part of a management protocol for OC.[53] However, such an approach may be considered too intrusive to be used routinely by most obstetricians. Also, amnioscopy or amniocentesis may give misleading results because the passage of maternal bile acids to the fetus may stimulate passage of meconium into the amniotic fluid regardless of whether there is fetal distress. Also the absence of meconium does not guarantee either its ongoing absence or fetal well-being.

SUMMARY OF MANAGEMENT OPTIONS

Obstetric Cholestasis

Management Options	Quality of Evidence	Strength of Recommendation	References
Prepregnancy			
If previous history of OC, advise of recurrence risk of 90%.	III	B	53
Biliary tract ultrasonography to exclude other pathology	III	B	34
Prenatal			
Confirm the diagnosis with serum bile acid, ALT, or AST measurement.	IIa	B	28–32
Exclude viral infection, including hepatitis C, autoimmune hepatitis, and other causes of biliary obstruction.	III	B	34–36
Treatment of maternal symptoms initially is with oral vitamin K and simple topical measures (e.g., aqueous cream with menthol).	IV	C	37, 44
Consider UDCA 500 mg bid for women with severe symptoms.	IIa	B	47
Dexamethasone (problem of possible fetal adverse neurological effects of repeated doses)	IIb	B	48, 49
Cholestyramine, guar gum	IV	C	46
Monitor fetal well-being, though does not predict at-risk fetus.	III	B	16,161,162
Labor and Delivery			
Consider elective delivery at 37–38 weeks.	III	B	16,161,162
Vigilance for postpartum hemorrhage	IV	C	37
Postnatal			
Monitor biochemical resolution; generally long-term maternal and baby health are good.	–	GPP	–
Vitamin K supplement for baby	–	GPP	–
Use oral contraceptives only with close clinical and biochemical monitoring; 27% of cases have cyclical or oral contraceptive-induced pruritus.	III	B	34
Consider referral to hepatologist if symptoms and biochemical abnormalities persist.	–	GPP	–

ALT, alanine aminotransaminase; AST, aspartate aminotransaminase; OC, obstetric cholestasis; UDCA, ursodeoxycholic acid.

ACUTE FATTY LIVER OF PREGNANCY

Acute fatty liver of pregnancy (AFLP) is a rare but dangerous disorder. The clinical symptoms and signs are not specific, the definition is one of exclusion (rather than inclusion), and so the diagnosis can be difficult to reach. However, failure to do so may jeopardize the life of the pregnant woman or her fetus.

General

Definition

AFLP may be defined as acute liver failure with reduced hepatic metabolic capacity in the absence of other causes. Histologically there is panlobular microvesicular steatosis, with sparing of periportal areas and intrahepatic cholestasis: These appearances are not unique to AFLP, and can be difficult to detect with conventional fixing and staining techniques. The very nature of the illness means that a liver biopsy is often not appropriate. In reviewing the literature it is clear that subjective diagnoses are often used, and this, in conjunction with the rarity of the condition, makes evidence-based care of women with AFLP challenging.

Incidence

AFLP has been reported to occur in between 1 in 7000 (clinical diagnosis alone in 27 of 28 cases)[54] and 1 in 13,000 pregnancies (10 cases, all biopsy-proven).[55] Most cases are reported in the third trimester, although it is described as early as 20 weeks and in the puerperium. Age, parity, and race do not seem to influence the risk; multiple pregnancies and male fetuses are reported more commonly than expected, although there is not a clear explanation for the pathophysiology behind this.

Diagnosis

The symptoms and signs of AFLP are vague and nonspecific. It is likely that many women experience a prodromal phase in which there is only a gradual deterioration in their condition and when jaundice may not be apparent: in one study this lasted on average for 9 days, although the range was 1 to 21 days[54] prior to the rapid and sometimes catastrophic decline that can occur with AFLP. There should be a low threshold for performing LFTs on pregnant women who present in the third trimester with prodromal symptoms including new-onset nausea, vomiting, epigastric or right upper quadrant pain, and malaise.

Other features in the condition include pruritus, headache, fever, preeclampsia (hypertension and proteinuria), and, in severe cases, impaired conscious level or coma. Abnormalities in laboratory investigations may include:

- raised transaminases: typically three to ten times the upper limit of normal; transaminase levels above 1000 iμ/L may occur with hepatic ischemia or hypoglycemia
- hyperbilirubinemia
- hypoglycemia
- neutrophil leukocytosis often reaching 20,000-30,000
- hyperuricemia
- prolonged prothrombin time

One of the keys to the diagnosis of AFLP is the rapidity with which LFT can deteriorate in the aggressive phase of the disease. This typically is combined with features of hepatic synthetic failure, including hypoglycemia, deranged clotting, and confusion secondary to hepatic encephalopathy. Other pregnancy-specific liver conditions do not impair liver function in this way. Other causes of fulminating liver failure must be excluded: Paracetamol (acetaminophen) overdose and acute viral hepatitis are the commonest causes, and rarer causes include Wilson's disease, poisoning with carbon tetrachloride, and drug reactions (e.g., to halothane or isoniazid).

Imaging of the liver has not been successful in accurately detecting fatty infiltration nor, if it is present, determining its cause. Techniques that have been used include ultrasound, computed tomography (CT), and magnetic resonance imaging (MRI). Apart from ultrasound, it is unlikely that imaging will be either portable or easily accessible to the delivery suite; abdominal CT is better avoided when possible prior to delivery because of radiation exposure to the fetus, and many pregnant women will be too large to fit inside a standard MRI even if they are well enough to be moved there. False-positive and false-negative diagnoses are equally common with all modalities.[56] If the diagnosis remains in doubt and, in particular, if there is not a rapid improvement after delivery, the place for imaging the liver should be reconsidered.

Liver biopsy is another possibly helpful diagnostic tool. Bearing in mind the histopathologic caveats outlined earlier and the potential complexities of performing a biopsy in the presence of deranged clotting, the need for a tissue diagnosis should be carefully assessed on an individual basis.

Maternal and Fetal Risks

Significant risks, including maternal and fetal mortality, are undoubtedly associated with AFLP. Several case series seem to demonstrate improved outcome for mother and baby in recent years. In the 1960s, 16 cases of AFLP associated with the use of tetracycline were reported, with a 70% maternal mortality.[57] Among 33 pregnancies with biopsy-proven AFLP reported in the 1980s, maternal mortality was 21% and fetal mortality was 27%.[58] More recently, Castro and associates reported 28 clinically diagnosed cases with no maternal mortality and a 7% neonatal mortality.[54]

The Report on Confidential Enquiries into Maternal Deaths in the United Kingdom continues to report maternal death from AFLP, with three women dying in the triennium 2000 to 2002.[59] There is an ongoing need for all obstetricians to be aware of AFLP, not just those in large tertiary referral centers. In 2005 the UK Obstetrics Surveillance System (UKOSS) was launched. AFLP is the subject of their initial surveillance and the results are eagerly awaited.

Etiology

The cause of AFLP is uncertain, but is likely to be multifactorial, with a genetic component in a number of cases. In some women, AFLP may occur because of an autosomal recessive abnormality in fetal long-chain fatty acid beta oxidation. This is an interesting concept, as it demonstrates that the fetus may determine maternal complications of pregnancy. In addition, for these families, the risk of recurrence is significant.

Long-chain hydroxyacyl coenzyme A dehydrogenase (LCHAD) deficiency is a recently described disorder of mitochondrial fatty acid oxidation that is usually asymptomatic in heterozygous carriers. Affected individuals often die in early childhood or sooner from complications of hypoglycemia, cardiomyopathy, or fatty liver failure; those who live longer develop chorioretinopathy, rhabdomyolysis, and peripheral neuropathy, although these can be ameliorated by a high-carbohydrate, low-fat diet, in which the fat component is medium-chain triglycerides. Several mutations of the alpha subunit of the mitochondrial trifunctional protein cause deficiency of LCHAD. In Finland a guanine cytosine transposition, G1528C, and in America a glutamic acid to glutamine change, E474Q, have been identified.[60,61] The latter group estimates that 1 in 175 of their population is heterozygous for E474Q, and therefore that 1 in 62,000 pregnancies results in LCHAD deficiency. Affected fetuses do not metabolize long-chain fatty acids completely, resulting in accumulation of abnormal and highly toxic intermediates in the mother's liver, and the acute clinical picture we recognize as AFLP. It is also hypothesized that fat accumulation may occur in the placenta, and that this may induce the clinical picture of preeclampsia. Preeclampsia has been described in pregnancies with fetuses affected by homozygous LCHAD deficiency more commonly than would be expected, and more than in pregnancies in the same women with unaffected fetuses.[62]

It is not certain what proportion of cases of AFLP may be due to LCHAD deficiency. It is likely that this will vary between countries, depending in part on the prevalence of the known (and unknown) genetic mutations in the local populations. Mansouri and colleagues[63] reported no carriers of the G1528C mutation in 14 histologically proven cases of AFLP, but Treem and associates found that 75% of 12 women with AFLP had LCHAD levels compatible with carrier status.[64] A recent larger study identified LCHAD mutations in 5 of 27 women with AFLP, all of whom had a fetus with LCHAD deficiency.[65] All five affected fetuses had at least one copy of the E474Q mutation, and the authors therefore recommended screening for this mutation in the children of women who have had pregnancies complicated by AFLP. In contrast, the same study demonstrated that only 1 of 81 women with HELLP had an LCHAD mutation and this was not inherited by the fetus, indicating that it is not justified to screen the offspring from all pregnancies affected by HELLP.

Conversely, not all pregnancies where the baby has LCHAD deficiency will result in AFLP or other serious maternal liver disease. Ibdah and colleagues[66] found that in 15 of 24 pregnancies in which the baby had LCHAD deficiency either AFLP (n = 12) or HELLP (n = 3) syndrome developed, and in the other 9 pregnancies there were no complications. These women had 11 other pregnancies with unaffected babies in which maternal liver disease did not occur. Similarly, Tyni and associates[62] found some form of liver disease of pregnancy and or preeclampsia in 15 of 29 pregnancies in which the fetus was homozygous for LCHAD deficiency and described 7 of the remaining 14 pregnancies as completely normal; none of the other 34 pregnancies from these women (when the fetus did not have homozygous LCHAD deficiency) were complicated by significant liver disease.

Management Options

The ultimate management option is to deliver the baby, because this seems to be the optimal way to improve the maternal condition and to protect the fetus. The decision to deliver brings with it a not uncommon conundrum for obstetricians: A vaginal delivery minimizes the risk of maternal hemorrhage in the face of a coagulopathy, but may take several hours or longer to achieve, and this could be significantly detrimental to the mother or fetus; a cesarean section allows delivery to be achieved more quickly but may be complicated by bleeding. An individual decision regarding the severity of the maternal and fetal conditions needs to be made. Often, induction of labor can be started while the maternal condition is stabilized and blood products made available, and then the ongoing management can be reviewed according to the current balance of concerns.

From the maternal perspective, she should have one to one nursing on the delivery suite, preferably in a high-dependency area. All vital signs should be measured and recorded clearly on a 24-hour spread sheet; it is usually advisable to insert a central line early in the course of the disease before coagulopathy ensues. Glucose assessments should be made at least every two hours, and hypoglycemia treated with large doses of high-concentration intravenous glucose via a long line. Prothrombin time should also be measured every six hours along with LFTs, renal function tests and electrolytes, and full blood count. Formal assessment of level of consciousness must be made hourly, as hepatic coma is a potential complication of AFLP.

One of the keys to successful management is a multidisciplinary approach. Senior obstetric, anesthesiology, hematology, and hepatology colleagues should be involved at an early stage. If no hepatologists are in-house, the obstetrician should liaise directly with the nearest liver transplant unit. This serves several purposes: firstly it provides expert advise on both the investigations and the management; secondly it alerts the transplant team who are usually able to accept transfer after delivery if recovery does not commence. Most women will be transferred from the delivery suite to the intensive care unit after delivery.

Follow-up and Recurrence

Once they have recovered, all women affected by AFLP should have the opportunity with their partners to be debriefed about the complications of their pregnancy. In those women who survive, complete recovery of the liver is expected.

Pediatricians should consider screening all babies of women with AFLP for LCHAD deficiency, either by measuring LCHAD activity in cultured skin fibroblasts or liver, or by doing DNA studies looking for the common mutations. Affected babies should be placed on the appropriate dietary restrictions. Not only does this screening minimize the complications for the index baby, but also it allows the couple to make an informed choice about the risks to the mother and fetus in a future pregnancy.

The risk of recurrence of AFLP depends largely on whether the baby has LCHAD deficiency. If he or she does, the rate is between 15% and 25% for future pregnancies from the same partnership; if the baby does not, then the recurrence risk is very much lower, although it is difficult to give a precise figure since so many women decide against a further pregnancy.

When a woman has had an affected baby previously, prenatal diagnosis (of LCHAD) is possible in subsequent

SUMMARY OF MANAGEMENT OPTIONS

Acute Fatty Liver of Pregnancy

Management Options	Quality of Evidence	Strength of Recommendation	References
Prepregnancy			
None, unless previous pregnancy is affected, in which case confirm previous diagnosis, check LFTs, advise risk of recurrence.	IV	C	57, 58
Consider screening for LCHAD deficiency.	III	B	62, 66
Prenatal			
If previous AFLP, check baseline LFT; advise to report any new symptoms; start home testing for urinary protein after 24 weeks; monitor BP every 2 weeks.	–	GPP	–
Establish diagnosis, resuscitate.	–	GPP	–
Intensive care/high dependency setting	–	GPP	–
Supportive therapy (see *Labor/Delivery* below)	–	GPP	–
Plan delivery/end pregnancy	–	GPP	–
Labor and Delivery			
Maternal resuscitation by correction of			
Hypoglycemia	–	GPP	–
Fluid balance			
Coagulopathy			
Multidisciplinary approach ideally in liaison with liver unit to manage liver failure	–	GPP	–
Intensive fetal monitoring	–	GPP	–
Urgent delivery when maternal condition is stabilized, vaginal delivery preferable for mother.	–	GPP	–
Meticulous hemostasis	–	GPP	–
Postnatal			
Continue intensive care management	–	GPP	–
Watch for postpartum wound hematoma formation and sepsis, postpartum hemorrhage.	–	GPP	–
Recurrence risk is difficult to estimate, perhaps as high as 10–20%.	–	GPP	–
Support contraceptive measures.	–	GPP	–
Full hepatic recovery expected without further sequelae; occasionally emergency liver transplant needed.	–	GPP	–

Continued

SUMMARY OF MANAGEMENT OPTIONS
Acute Fatty Liver of Pregnancy *(Continued)*

Management Options	Quality of Evidence	Strength of Recommendation	References
Postnatal			
Pediatricians to consider screening baby for LCHAD deficiency	–	GPP	–
Prenatal diagnosis of LCHAD possible by amniocentesis/CVS if previous baby affected	III	B	66, 67

AFLP, acute fatty liver of pregnancy; CVS, chorionic villus sampling; LCHAD, long-chain hydroxyacyl coenzyme A dehydrogenase; LFT, liver function test.

pregnancies, by enzyme assay in amniocytes[67] or DNA analysis from chorionic villus sampling (CVS).[66]

LIVER HEMATOMA AND NONTRAUMATIC LIVER RUPTURE

General

Liver hematoma is an uncommon and potentially dangerous problem in pregnancy, its most hazardous complication being hepatic rupture. Rupture of the liver capsule occurs in between 1 in 45,000 and 1 in 225,000 deliveries.[68,69]

The vast majority of cases are reported in association with preeclampsia, and a very high proportion are in multiparous women older than 30 years of age. Only two cases have been described in the puerperium following a normal pregnancy.[70] In over 85% of cases, the right lobe of the liver is affected. Rinehart and associates[71] reviewed the literature and presented figures for the common symptoms and signs of hepatic rupture. Not surprisingly, they found that almost 70% of patients had epigastric pain, 65% had hypertension, and over 50% were shocked. However, there was a wide range of other presentations, including some women with mild symptoms prior to massive circulatory collapse. HELLP syndrome seems to be particularly associated with intrahepatic hemorrhage, subcapsular hematoma, and capsular rupture.

The pathogenesis is debated. One attractive theory suggests that preeclampsia causes hepatic ischemia via intravascular volume depletion, which results in local necrosis and hemorrhage. Subsequently, neovascularization occurs, and these vessels are especially susceptible to rupture and further hemorrhage, particularly during hypertensive episodes. Subcapsular hematoma may then expand sufficiently to result in hepatic rupture.[71]

Maternal and Fetal Risks

Hepatic rupture is dangerous for mother and baby. Maternal mortality is between 16% and 60%, and perinatal mortality is between 40% and 60%.[72,73] Current management options have contributed greatly to lowering the mortality rates.

Management Options

The management will obviously be determined by the seriousness of the situation. There should be a low threshold for imaging the liver in older, multiparous women with preeclampsia and epigastric pain. Ultrasound will usually be readily available and is helpful in diagnosing subcapsular hematomas. CT (Fig. 48–2) and MRI hepatic digital subtraction angiography may have greater sensitivity for identifying small amounts of intraperitoneal blood and small hematomas but have the disadvantage of being less readily available and less portable if the patient is unwell.

Treatment of hepatic rupture is based on resuscitating the patient and stopping the hemorrhage. If the diagnosis is suspected, a midline laparotomy with the involvement of an experienced surgeon should be considered: This allows the diagnosis to be confirmed, the baby to be delivered (which will improve the maternal circulation and remove the baby to a place of safety), and treatment to be instituted. If unexplained hemoperitoneum is found at a Pfannenstiel laparotomy for presumed abruption or

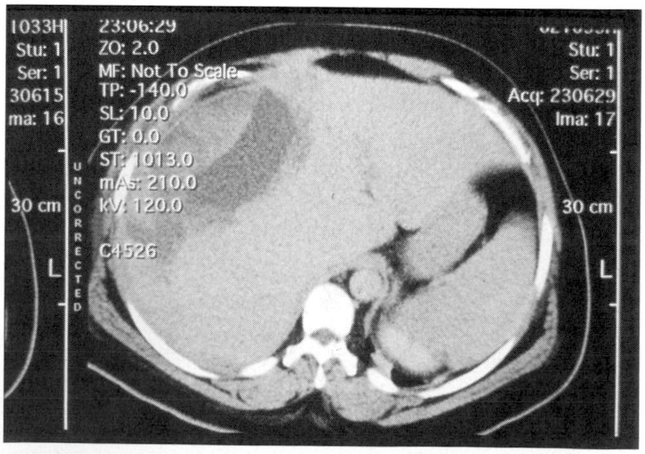

FIGURE 48–2
Liver hematoma.

uterine rupture, careful exploration of the upper abdomen, preferably by an experienced general or hepatic surgeon and possibly with an upper midline incision to improve access, must be strongly considered.

A wide variety of therapeutic maneuvers for liver rupture have been described. Currently the most successful seem to involve digital compression of the hepatic artery and portal vein to temporarily arrest the hemorrhage (Pringle maneuver),[72] evacuation of the residual hematoma, and temporary packing with large dry gauze swabs.[74] Packs are removed at a further laparotomy 24 to 36 hours later, once correction of hypovolemia, coagulopathy, acidosis, and hypothermia is complete. Liver resection and transplantation have also been described, but not surprisingly their mortality rate is very high.

Unruptured small hematomas have been managed conservatively, following delivery of the baby, with serial imaging of their size to exclude expansion[72]: Delayed rupture 6 weeks after initial diagnosis has been reported,[75] so care must be taken if this option is adopted. Tense, large, or expanding hematomas should probably be evacuated surgically to obviate the impending rupture. Hepatic embolization has been described in these circumstances (and in others) but seems to carry a high risk of ischemic necrosis of the liver, liver failure, and sepsis,[76] and may not be accessible to many units; others have described this technique as a "gold standard."[70]

SUMMARY OF MANAGEMENT OPTIONS

Liver Hematoma and Rupture

Management Options	Quality of Evidence	Strength of Recommendation	References
Prepregnancy			
None	–	GPP	–
Prenatal			
Treat upper abdominal discomfort seriously especially in parous women with PET or HELLP; consider imaging the liver.	–	GPP	–
Labor and Delivery			
Liver rupture should be considered in a woman with unexplained shock or if unexpected hemoperitoneum is found at cesarean section.	–	GPP	–
Management:			
Resuscitation	–	GPP	–
Laparotomy and stop hemorrhage (by liver surgeon preferably) with temporary occlusion of portal vein and packing	IV	C	72, 74
Embolization has varied success	III	B	70, 76
Unruptured hematomas can be managed conservatively (though danger of delayed rupture).	IV	C	72
Postnatal			
Patients who survive do not have permanent liver damage.	–	GPP	–
Recurrence has been recorded but very rarely.	–	GPP	–

HELLP, hemolysis, elevated liver enzymes, low platelets; PET, preclampsia toxemia.

HYPEREMESIS GRAVIDARUM

General

Nausea and vomiting affect up to 50% of pregnant women. Most women are able to maintain fluid and nutrient intake by dietary modification, and the symptoms will resolve by the end of the first trimester. Hyperemesis gravidarum affects 0.5% to 1% of pregnancies and causes severe and protracted vomiting that results in ketosis, dehydration, and weight loss. The cause of hyperemesis gravidarum remains unidentified, but it is thought to result from a combination of endocrine, biochemical, and psychological factors. Seropositivity for *Helicobacter pylori* is commoner in women with hyperemesis than in controls,[77,78] and one study of endoscopic biopsy findings demonstrated that the severity of gastric symptoms may be associated with the density of infection.[79]

Diagnosis

The onset of hyperemesis gravidarum is always in the first trimester. In addition to nausea, vomiting, and weight loss, women often report ptyalism (excessive salivation), and there may be signs of dehydration, including postural hypotension and tachycardia. Hyperemesis gravidarum is a diagnosis of exclusion (Table 48–5), and it is important to make a thorough clinical assessment and to ensure that investigations are performed for common and serious causes of vomiting.

An ultrasound of the uterus should be performed to confirm that a woman is pregnant, to establish the number of fetuses, and to exclude hydatidiform mole.

Laboratory investigations commonly reveal hyponatremia, hypokalemia, and raised hematocrit. A biochemical hyperthyroidism and abnormal LFTs may also be present. These are both markers of the severity of the disease and resolve with successful treatment. Women with biochemical hyperthyroidism should be examined for signs of hyperthyroidism, but these are rarely present.

Maternal and Fetal Risks

Maternal Risks

Serious maternal morbidity and mortality may result if hyperemesis gravidarum is not managed correctly. Wernicke's encephalopathy can develop as a result of thiamine (vitamin B_1) deficiency. This is associated with diplopia, sixth nerve palsy, nystagmus, ataxia, and confusion. If untreated, Wernicke's encephalopathy may lead to Korsakoff's psychosis (amnesia, impaired ability to learn) or death. Other vitamin deficiencies may occur, for example, peripheral neuropathy and anemia may result from deficiency of vitamins B_{12} and B_6.

Hyponatremia (plasma sodium <120 mmol/L) can cause confusion, seizures, and respiratory arrest. If hyponatremia is severe, or if it is treated too rapidly, women may develop central pontine myelinolysis. This is caused by symmetrical destruction of myelin at the centre of the basal pons and can result in pyramidal tract signs, spastic quadraparesis, pseudobulbar palsy, and impaired consciousness.

Other risks include deep venous thrombosis that may result from dehydration and reduced mobility, Mallory-Weiss tear due to prolonged vomiting, and muscle wasting with weakness.

Fetal Risks

Infants of mothers with severe hyperemesis, abnormal biochemistry, and weight loss have been reported to have lower birth weights in some studies[80,81] but not others.[82,83]

There are few known fetal risks from the therapeutic agents used to treat hyperemesis.

Management Options

Rehydration and Vitamin Supplementation

Fluid replacement therapy should be with either normal saline (NaCl 0.9%; 150 mmol/L Na^+) or Hartmann's solution (NaCl 0.6%; 131 mmol/L Na^+). Dextrose-containing fluids should not be used because they do not contain sufficient sodium to correct hyponatremia, and Wernicke's encephalopathy can be precipitated by intravenous dextrose and carbohydrate-rich foods. Double-strength saline should not be used to correct hyponatremia in hyperemesis gravidarum, because central pontine myelinolysis can occur if the serum sodium level is corrected too rapidly. Potassium supplements should be added to the intravenous fluid replacement therapy as required. Thiamine supplements should be given, as a daily dose of either 50 to 150 mg orally, or 100 mg diluted in 100 mL normal saline as an intravenous infusion.

TABLE 48–5

Differential Diagnosis of Hyperemesis Gravidarum

SYSTEM	DIAGNOSIS	INVESTIGATION/INITIAL ASSESSMENT
Genitourinary	Urinary tract infection	Mid-stream urine specimen
	Uremia	Urea and electrolytes
	Molar pregnancy	Ultrasound of the uterus
Gastrointestinal	Gastritis/peptic ulceration	*Helicobacter pylori* antibodies
	Pancreatitis	Amylase, blood glucose, calcium
	Bowel obstruction	Plain supine abdominal radiograph
Endocrine	Addison's disease	Urea and electrolytes, early morning cortisol, short synacthen test with ACTH
	Hyperthyroidism	Surveillance for symptoms and signs of hyperthyroidism, TFTs, thyroid autoantibodies
	Diabetic ketoacidosis	Blood glucose, urinary dipstick for ketones, glucose tolerance test
CNS	Intracranial tumor	CNS examination, brain imaging
	Vestibular disease	CNS examination
Drug-induced	–	Discontinue agent

ACTH, adrenocorticotrophic hormone; CNS, central nervous system; TFT, thyroid function test.

Urine output should be monitored and dipsticks used to assess ketonuria. Women should be weighed on admission and regularly thereafter if their symptoms do not resolve. Serial assessments of electrolytes should be carried out.

Antiemetics

There is no evidence for teratogenicity following treatment with dopamine antagonists (metoclopramide, domperidone),[84,85] phenothiazines (chlorpromazine, prochlorperazine),[86,87] anticholinergics (dicyclomine),[88] or antihistamine H_1-receptor antagonists (promethazine, cyclizine), and one of these should be tried in the first instance. Women with hyperemesis often find nonoral preparations, such as rectal domperidone or subcutaneous metoclopramide, preferable.

In women with severe hyperemesis who have not responded to these antiemetic therapies, promising results have been reported with both corticosteroids and 5-hydroxytryptamine$_3$ (5-HT_3) receptor antagonists (ondansetron, cisapride).

Corticosteroids

Corticosteroids have been reported to be an effective treatment for hyperemesis gravidarum in several case reports.[89–91] In an American double-blind study of 40 women with hyperemesis who were randomized to receive either oral methylprednisolone 16 mg or oral promethazine 25 mg (three times daily for both) the response to both drugs was similar after 2 days, but no women who received methylprednisolone were readmitted within 1 week of discharge. In contrast, five (25%) women who received promethazine were readmitted with hyperemesis.[92] A British double-blind study of 25 women who were randomized to receive either 40 mg prednisolone or placebo daily demonstrated a trend toward improved nausea and vomiting and reduced dependence on intravenous fluids, but this did not reach statistical significance. However, steroid therapy did result in an improved sense of well-being, improved appetite, and weight gain compared with placebo.[93] Overall, the studies of corticosteroid treatment for hyperemesis suggest that the treatment is effective for some patients. We recommend starting intravenous hydrocortisone 100 mg three times a day in women with severe and resistant symptoms who are unable to tolerate fluids, followed by prednisolone 40 mg once daily. This should be reduced by approximately 5 mg every 5 days, provided symptoms are controlled.

5-Hydroxytryptamine Receptor Antagonists

Ondansetron is a 5-HT_3 receptor antagonist and is a potent antiemetic drug for the treatment of chemotherapy-associated and postoperative nausea. It has been used to treat hyperemesis successfully in several case reports, in which it was given for between 2 and 19 weeks and was commenced at 11, 14, or 30 weeks' gestation.[94–96] In all cases there were no known adverse fetal events. One double-blind controlled trial in which 30 patients were randomized to receive either 10 mg intravenous ondansetron or 50 mg intravenous promethazine failed to demonstrate any significant difference in the degree of nausea, weight gain, or days of hospitalization between the two groups.[97] However, the entry criteria for this study were less stringent than for the randomized, double-blind studies of corticosteroid treatment for hyperemesis gravidarum.[92,93] Therefore it remains likely that ondansetron may be an effective treatment for women with more severe disease. Experience of its use in the first trimester is limited, and we would recommend reserving ondansetron treatment for the second trimester except in very severe cases.

Other Treatment Options

There has been one double-blind randomized cross-over trial of the efficacy of powdered root ginger and placebo in which women reported a reduced severity and greater relief of symptoms in the period in which ginger was given and no side effects were observed.[98] Several authors have reported success in managing severe hyperemesis gravidarum using enteral and parenteral nutrition.[99–101] However, as the complications can be serious, such treatment is usually reserved for women whose symptoms are sufficiently severe as to be life threatening to the mother. In one series of 16 cases with good pregnancy outcomes, there were 3 cases of line sepsis, and pneumothorax, thrombosis, and dislodgement of the line.[101]

It is advisable to give thromboembolic deterrent stockings and thromboprophylaxis such as enoxaparine 40 mg daily to women with hyperemesis while they are inpatients.

SUMMARY OF MANAGEMENT OPTIONS

Hyperemesis Gravidarum

Management Options	Quality of Evidence	Strength of Recommendation	References
Prepregnancy			
Discuss recurrence risk	–	GPP	–

Continued

SUMMARY OF MANAGEMENT OPTIONS
Hyperemesis Gravidarum *(Continued)*

Management Options	Quality of Evidence	Strength of Recommendation	References
Prepregnancy*(Continued)*			
Advice can be given on treatment options and psychological support provided at an early stage.	–	GPP	–
Give folate supplements.	–	GPP	–
Prenatal			
Remember alternative diagnoses.	–	GPP	–
Rehydration with intravenous fluid and electrolyte therapy	–	GPP	–
Nutrient and vitamin (especially thiamine) supplementation	–	GPP	–
Dietician, parenteral nutrition in extreme cases	III	B	99–101
Psychological and social support	–	GPP	–
Thromboprophylaxis	–	GPP	–
Treatment:			
First line = Conventional antiemetics	III	B	84–87
Alternative agent = Corticosteroids	Ib	A	92,93
Alternative agent = 5-HT_3 antagonist if no response	Ib	A	97
Antigastroesophagal reflux measures may help some.	–	GPP	–
Fetal growth surveillance	–	GPP	–
Labor and Delivery			
Women on corticosteroids prenatally should have IV hydrocortisone to cover labor/delivery.	–	GPP	–
Postnatal			
Review nutritional status.	–	GPP	–
Wean off steroids; most will not need short synacthen test to exclude adrenal suppression.	–	GPP	–
Discuss contraception.	–	GPP	–

PEPTIC ULCERATION IN PREGNANCY

General

Dyspepsia is common, affecting up to 50% of pregnant women.[102] It usually worsens as pregnancy progresses, and it is more prevalent in women who are older, multiparous, or have a prepregnancy history of heartburn.[103]

Peptic ulceration, however, is uncommon in pregnancy.[104] In addition, women with established peptic ulcer disease can report symptomatic improvement. This is thought to be secondary to reduced gastric acid output and increased protective mucus production associated with raised progesterone levels, in addition to a healthier diet and increased medical supervision.

Diagnosis

It is important to have a high index of suspicion for peptic ulcer disease because the classical symptoms (e.g., severe regular dyspepsia) may be absent. Also, symptoms may not correlate with severity of disease. Patients who are smokers and have a previous history of peptic ulcer disease or previous nonsteroidal anti-inflammatory drug use are at highest risk for peptic ulceration in pregnancy.

Investigations should include blood tests for hemoglobin, electrolytes, and serum amylase, as well as LFTs. An abdominal ultrasound is useful to exclude cholelithiasis and pancreatitis secondary to gallstones. However, if peptic ulcer disease is suspected from the history and examination, *Helicobacter pylori* antibodies should be checked for, and if a woman has positive serology, treatment should be considered (Table 48–6). Although endoscopy is the investigation of choice outside pregnancy and is safe in pregnancy,[105] too few cases have been reported for the frequency of complications to be assessed. However, endoscopy does allow direct visualization of upper gastrointestinal tract pathology, permits biopsies to be taken for histopathology, and provides a therapeutic option (e.g., injection of adrenaline for acute bleeding ulcers).

Zollinger-Ellison Syndrome

This syndrome is caused by pancreatic gastrin-secreting tumors that result in a marked increase in gastric acid secretion. If untreated the condition causes severe gastroesophageal reflux, peptic ulceration, and malabsorption, and therefore the acid secretion usually requires treatment. There have been recent reports of the successful management of Zollinger-Ellison syndrome in pregnancy.

Maternal and Fetal Risks

Maternal Risks

Complications of peptic ulcer disease in the general, nonpregnant population include bleeding and perforation. These are rarely reported in pregnancy.

Acute gastrointestinal bleeding presents with hematemesis, melena, or the passage of fresh blood from the rectum. It can be associated with hypotension and tachycardia and may result in anemia. It is important to insert a nasogastric tube if gastrointestinal bleeding is suspected. This will allow upper and lower gastrointestinal bleeding to be distinguished and will help to ensure a clear view for endoscopy. When endoscopy is performed, pregnant women should be placed in the left lateral position to reduce inferior vena caval obstruction and reduced venous return. A large-bore cannula should be sited, the woman should be fasting, and a transfusion should be commenced if acute bleeding is confirmed.

Ulcer perforation is rare in pregnancy. Clinical features include abdominal pain with abdominal guarding and rebound tenderness, nausea, vomiting, pyrexia, dehydration, hypotension, and a leukocytosis. If suspected, an abdominal radiograph should be performed to investigate for the presence of pneumoperitoneum or free gas in the abdomen.

Fetal Risks

The fetus may be compromised if there is major maternal hemorrhage or perforation of a peptic ulcer. Otherwise few fetal risks arise from the drugs that can be used to treat peptic ulcer disease, with the exception of sodium bicarbonate-containing preparations and misoprostol (see subsequent section on Misoprostol).

Management Options

Antacids, H_2-antagonists, or proton pump inhibitors can be used to treat established peptic ulcer disease in pregnancy, including Zollinger-Ellison syndrome. If gastrointestinal bleeding is present, therapeutic endoscopy or surgery is indicated, and perforation requires surgical management.

Antacids

Aluminum and magnesium-containing antacids are generally considered to be safe in pregnancy and breastfeeding,[108,109] as are the nonabsorbed alginate-containing drugs such as Gaviscon[110] and the mucosal protective agent sucralfate.[111] Magnesium-based antacids may be preferred to aluminum-based ones, because the latter can be associated with constipation. Sodium bicarbonate-containing antacids should be avoided because they may cause respiratory alkalosis and fluid overload in the mother and fetus.[112]

Acid-Suppressing Drugs

Several recent studies have indicated that H_2-receptor antagonists[113–116] and proton pump inhibitors[114–117] are safe in pregnancy. Three studies have compared the rate of congenital malformations in pregnancies in which there was first-trimester exposure to either H_2-receptor antagonists or omeprazole. A Swedish cohort study in which H_2-receptor antagonists had been taken in 255 pregnancies, proton pump inhibitors in 275, and both in

TABLE 48–6

Therapeutic Options for *Helicobacter Pylori* in Pregnancy.*

	ANTIBIOTIC		
ACID SUPPRESSANT	AMOXYCILLIN	CLARITHROMYCIN	METRONIDAZOLE
Omeprazole 20 mg bid	1 g bid	500 mg bid	–
Omeprazole 20 mg bid	500 mg tid	–	400 mg tid
Omeprazole 20 mg bid	–	500 mg bid	400 mg bid

bid, twice a day; tid, three time a day.
*Modified from the British National Formulary.

20 pregnancies did not demonstrate an increased rate of congenital malformation compared with all births at that time.[114] Similar results were found in a study of 447 British and 108 Italian pregnancies with first-trimester exposure to ranitidine, cimetidine, or omeprazole.[116] Similarly, there was no evidence of increased risk of major malformations in a prospective, multicenter, controlled study in which two groups of 113 women were treated with either omeprazole or with H_2-receptor antagonists and compared with the same number of controls.[115]

Less is known about lansoprazole than omeprazole, but there has recently been a reassuring report of good fetal outcomes with lansoprazole treatment in six cases where there was first-trimester exposure.[118]

One prospective, controlled, multicenter study of the use of cisapride, a 5-HT_3 receptor antagonist for the treatment of gastroesophageal reflux, gastrointestinal pain, and duodenal ulcer in pregnancy, showed no increase in the rate of major or minor malformations nor fetal distress.[119]

Triple Therapy for Helicobacter Pylori

If peptic ulcer disease is suspected, serology should be sent for *Helicobacter pylori* antibodies. If a woman has distressing symptoms, appropriate therapy will eradicate the infection and may improve the symptoms. Of the recommended therapeutic regimens at the time of writing, only three include the use of omeprazole (see Table 48–6). The others advise the use of alternative acid-suppressant drugs, about which there is little experience in pregnancy. We therefore recommend that one of the three regimens outlined in Table 48–6 should be used, for 7 days. The regimens containing amoxycillin are recommended for community-based use. Studies of the incidence of congenital abnormalities and adverse pregnancy outcomes in women who have taken these antibiotics indicate that there is no increased risk for amoxycillin,[120] clarithromycin,[121] or metronidazole.[122,123]

Misoprostol

Misoprostol is a synthetic prostaglandin E_1 analogue that has antisecretory and protective properties believed to promote healing of peptic ulcers. However its use is contraindicated in pregnancy because it is a potent stimulant of uterine contractions and can induce spontaneous abortion or uterine bleeding. It is also teratogenic.[124–126]

Therapeutic Endoscopy and Surgery

There is very little experience of therapeutic endoscopy in pregnancy. Of four cases in the literature, thermocoagulation was performed in one for bleeding duodenal ulcer,[105] sclerotherapy for bleeding duodenal ulcer was performed in two,[105,127] and sclerotherapy for a bleeding Mallory-Weiss tear in the fourth.[128] The fetal outcome in three cases was good and was not specifically reported in the fourth.[128]

The indications for surgery are the same as in the nonpregnant patient. A perforated ulcer requires emergency surgery, and the patient should receive broad-spectrum antibiotics. Surgery should also be performed in patients with hemorrhage from peptic ulcers if they have not responded to a transfusion of six units of blood.

SUMMARY OF MANAGEMENT OPTIONS
Peptic Ulceration in Pregnancy

Management Options	Quality of Evidence	Strength of Recommendation	References
Prepregnancy			
Advise against agents that may exacerbate peptic ulcer disease (e.g., alcohol, smoking).	–	GPP	–
If taking bicarbonate-containing antacids or misoprostol, advise cessation of treatment.	III	B	112,124–126
Perform investigations to establish the cause of peptic ulceration.	–	GPP	–
Anticipate improvement in clinical symptoms with pregnancy.	–	GPP	–
Aluminum- and magnesium-containing antacids, mucosal protective agents, and histamine receptor blockers are safe in pregnancy.	IIb	B	108–111
Avoid bicarbonate-containing antacids (danger of respiratory alkalosis and fluid overload).	IV	C	112
Consider anti-*Helicobacter* treatment with positive immunological diagnosis and if other therapy has been ineffective.	–	GPP	–

SUMMARY OF MANAGEMENT OPTIONS
Peptic Ulceration in Pregnancy *(Continued)*

Management Options	Quality of Evidence	Strength of Recommendation	References
Prepregnancy*(Continued)*			
Endoscopy is also safe with an experienced operator if no response to medical management; surgery rarely required and mainly needed for those with severe bleeding/perforation.	–	GPP	–
Postnatal			
Symptoms of dyspepsia are likely to improve postnatally.	–	GPP	–
Repeat endoscopy if indicated by initial findings.	–	GPP	–

CELIAC DISEASE

General

Definition and Incidence

Celiac disease, or gluten-sensitive enteropathy, is a common disorder in which gluten-containing foods trigger inflammation of the jejunal mucosa, which improves when a gluten-free diet is taken. In England it occurs in 1 in 1000, and in Ireland 1 in 300 individuals,[129] although more may have silent or undiagnosed celiac disease; it seems to be rare in black Africans, although this may reflect reporting bias. The cause is multifactorial. There is a genetic component, with 10% to 15% of first-degree relatives being affected.[130] However, 30% of identical twins are discordant,[131] suggesting additional factors are involved, such as viral infection.

Etiology

Gluten is present in the cereals wheat, barley, and rye, but not oats. There are four main gluten fractions, but α-gliadin is the most damaging to small intestine mucosa. The enzyme tissue transglutaminase, the main antigen of the endomysial antibody, modifies gliadin and enhances gliadin-specific T-cell responses in genetically predisposed individuals. This is one of several immunologic abnormalities that revert to normal when a gluten-free diet is assumed. Histologically the small bowel shows partial villus atrophy, with crypt hypertrophy and chronic inflammatory changes, the extent of the damage decreasing toward the ileum as gluten is progressively digested into smaller and less damaging moieties.

Diagnosis

Clinically celiac disease presents at any age and is more common in females than males. The symptoms are variable and may include tiredness and malaise (often in conjunction with anemia), diarrhea, steatorrhea, abdominal pain or bloating, weight loss, mouth ulcers, osteoporosis, and neurological symptoms from folate, B_6, or B_{12} deficiency. In pregnancy the most common presentation is with nonspecific symptoms without overt malabsorption, or with anemia.

A new diagnosis of celiac disease should be considered in pregnant women with iron-deficiency anemia or in the presence of otherwise unexplained folate or B_{12}-deficiency anemia. There should be a low threshold for investigating unexplained iron-deficiency anemia, diarrhea, or weight loss in pregnancy, especially if the anemia responds poorly to iron supplementation or folate or B_{12} deficiency is also present. In a study of premenopausal nonpregnant women, 1 in 16 asymptomatic but anemic volunteer blood donors were found to have celiac disease.[132] Among anemic pregnant women, 1 in 43 were found to have antiendomysial antibodies, although apparently none were investigated further for celiac disease.[133] The diagnosis of celiac disease is confirmed by finding endomysial, gliadin, or tissue transglutaminase antibodies, which have high specificity and sensitivity. Outside pregnancy, a jejunal biopsy is usually obtained; within pregnancy most experts feel that this is best avoided, although duodenoscopy can be performed if clinically indicated.

It is important not to miss the diagnosis of celiac disease, because left untreated the condition causes significant morbidity for both the pregnant woman and her fetus and carries with it an increased lifetime increase in mortality mostly from small bowel carcinomas and lymphomas. All of these risks can be ameliorated by assuming a gluten-free diet.

Maternal and Fetal Risks

Maternal Risks

Untreated celiac disease is associated with later menarche, earlier menopause, and a greater risk of secondary amenorrhea compared with control groups of either unaffected women or women with treated celiac disease.[134] Women with treated celiac disease who adhere to a gluten-free diet have no more gynecologic problems than a group of women without celiac disease. Infertility itself is more common in women with celiac disease than in the general population and has been reported to affect 4% to 8% of cases.[135,136] The pathophysiology of these problems remains uncertain.

Male subfertility is also reported in celiac disease. Abnormal sperm forms, which resolve once dietary gluten is withdrawn, have been observed in nearly half of men with untreated disease. Another group found that male fertility improved after treatment.[137–139]

Anemia is common in women with celiac disease. They should take iron and folate supplements throughout pregnancy; they may also need B^{12} supplementation, and so should be monitored appropriately. Women with celiac disease who are not anemic before pregnancy should be tested for anemia and iron, folate and B^{12} deficiency regularly throughout the pregnancy. Hypocalcemia is less common but must be considered.

Ideally women with celiac disease should take 5 mg, not 400 μg of folate preconceptually, in order to optimize their levels of folic acid. There is insufficient evidence to support, or refute, the claim that celiac disease increases the risk of neural tube defect. This may be because most series of women are too small to make meaningful conclusions.

Fetal Risks

Several reports show first-trimester pregnancy loss to be up to nine times more common in women with untreated celiac disease than in those who have received treatment and to be much more common in pregnancies in the same woman before compared with after treatment with a gluten-free diet.[140] Low-birth-weight babies are nearly six times more common in women with untreated compared with treated celiac disease, and in a cohort of 12 women, once they assumed a gluten-free diet, the number of low-birth-weight babies born fell from nearly 30% to 0%.[140] Similarly, a gluten-free diet increased the duration of breast-feeding more than twofold.

Gasbarrini and colleagues investigated a group of 83 women with either two or more consecutive miscarriages or an unexplained growth-restricted baby (<tenth percentile) and 50 controls. In the poor-outcome groups, 8% and 15%, respectively, had immunologic and histologic features of celiac disease, compared with none of 50 controls.[141] They hypothesize that treatment with a gluten-free diet might improve pregnancy outcome. Martinelli and associates found similar results in an Italian population: among 845 pregnant women screened for celiac disease, 12 cases were discovered and these women had more small-for-gestational-age infants than the other women.[142]

More recently an intriguing hypothesis suggests that men with celiac disease may father more pregnancies complicated by low birth weight than other men do. In a prospective, population-based cohort of 10,000 pregnancies in Sweden, babies of the 27 fathers with celiac disease were delivered at the same gestational age as the rest of the population, but weighed on average 266 g less and were five times more likely to weigh less than 2.5 kg; babies of fathers with a wide range of autoimmune conditions were not similarly affected. The babies of the 53 mothers with celiac disease had similar outcomes to those of the babies born to fathers with celiac disease. No difference was noted for babies with siblings or other relatives with celiac disease (n = 512). The exact mechanism for this is uncertain but indicates the importance of non-nutritional factors for neonatal outcome in parents with celiac disease. Genetic factors must be implicated.[143]

Management Options

Women with celiac disease should have a strict gluten-free diet prior to conception to minimize the risk of miscarriage. They should persist with this throughout pregnancy to minimize the risks of growth restriction, prematurity, and anemia. In order to achieve this they should ideally have prepregnancy advice. Once they are pregnant, a management plan should include growth scans, testing for anemia, and iron and possibly folate and B_{12} supplementation. Some women with celiac disease malabsorb calcium: A baseline measurement should be taken, and a calcium-rich diet recommended; supplementation may be necessary for some women.

SUMMARY OF MANAGEMENT OPTIONS

Celiac Disease in Pregnancy

Management Options	Quality of Evidence	Strength of Recommendation	References
Prepregnancy			
Preconception counseling and gluten-free dietary control	IIa	B	140,141
Folic acid supplementation	–	GPP	–

SUMMARY OF MANAGEMENT OPTIONS

Celiac Disease in Pregnancy *(Continued)*

Management Options	Quality of Evidence	Strength of Recommendation	References
Prenatal			
Careful gluten-free dietary surveillance by dietician	IIa	B	140,141
Folic acid supplementation	–	GPP	–
Monitor nutritional status.	–	GPP	–
Replace vitamins, minerals as indicated.	–	GPP	–
Give iron; check for anemia.	–	GPP	–
Screen for fetal abnormality, especially neural tube defect.	–	GPP	–
Monitor fetal growth and well-being.	III	B	141,142
Postnatal			
Monitor nutritional and vitamin adequacy, particularly with lactation.	–	GPP	–
Contraceptive advice and caution with oral preparations if disease active	–	GPP	–

INFLAMMATORY BOWEL DISEASE IN PREGNANCY

General

The term *inflammatory bowel disease* describes Crohn's disease and ulcerative colitis, as well as other less common forms of colitis. Crohn's disease is a chronic, granulomatous inflammatory disease of the intestine in which affected segments of bowel are often separated by normal bowel (skip lesions). It most commonly involves the terminal ileum. Common symptoms are abdominal pain and diarrhea, and there may also be anemia and weight loss, fresh blood or melena per rectum, fistulae, or perianal sepsis. Nonintestinal tract manifestations of the disease include aphthous ulcers, sacroiliitis, sclerosing cholangitis, and uveitis.

Ulcerative colitis is a chronic inflammatory disease of the colon and rectum. It commonly presents with diarrhea and rectal passage of mucus and blood. Typically the disease starts in the rectum and spreads proximally, without skip lesions. Severe attacks are characterized by passage of a large number of bowel movements a day and can be complicated by fever and abdominal distension (toxic megacolon), which can be fatal. Other complications include anemia, weight loss, hypoalbuminemia, electrolyte imbalances, and carcinoma of the colon (with long-standing disease). Nonintestinal features are similar to those seen in Crohn's.

Although Crohn's disease and ulcerative colitis are both chronic inflammatory disorders of the gastrointestinal tract, the cause of the inflammation does not appear to be the same in each condition. Both are thought to be caused by immune dysregulation in response to constituents of normal gut flora in genetically predisposed individuals. The inflammatory response in Crohn's disease is driven by interleukin-12 (IL-12) and interferon-γ (IF-γ),[144] whereas in ulcerative colitis it is caused by IL-13 release by natural killer T (NKT) cells in a murine model.[145]

There is evidence for a genetic origin in both Crohn's disease and ulcerative colitis. A recent study reported that in siblings with similar genetic susceptibility for inflammatory bowel disease, smoking was associated with an increased risk of Crohn's disease and nonsmoking was associated with the development of ulcerative colitis.[146] Laboratory studies have also demonstrated mutations in *NOD2*, a gene that encodes an intracellular receptor for bacterial lipopolysaccharide, in a subgroup of patients with Crohn's ileitis, but not in patients with colitis or anorectal disease.[147]

Diagnosis

If a woman has known inflammatory bowel disease and is complaining of symptoms consistent with an exacerbation, stool culture should be performed to exclude infection. Blood specimens should be taken to establish whether she has anemia, electrolyte imbalance, or hepatic impairment, and inflammatory markers should be checked. The erythrocyte sedimentation rate is raised in normal pregnancy, but the C-reactive protein is not and is of value in the assessment of patients with Crohn's disease and ulcerative colitis. If a flare-up of inflammatory bowel disease is confirmed, care should be shared between obstetricians and gastroenterologists. If there is severe disease or if toxic megacolon is suspected, an abdominal radiograph should be performed, and the woman should be referred for a surgical opinion.

In a woman who does not have a history of inflammatory bowel disease, the diagnosis is based on imaging of the upper and lower gastrointestinal tract, colonoscopy, and biopsy. Most women will have had the diagnosis made before they conceive, but if a new presentation of inflammatory bowel disease occurs in pregnancy, endoscopy and biopsy are preferable to barium studies.

Maternal and Fetal Risks

Maternal Risks

Fertility is reduced in women with active Crohn's disease and possibly in those with ulcerative colitis, but there is no evidence of reduced fertility with quiescent inflammatory bowel disease. The frequency of exacerbations of both Crohn's disease and ulcerative colitis is the same as outside pregnancy (30%–40% women per annum).[148] Flares may occur at any stage of pregnancy although they occur most commonly in the first trimester.

Women who have had an ileostomy or colostomy usually tolerate pregnancy well, providing at least 50% of the small intestine remains. Complications that can occur in patients who have had gut resection include malabsorption of fat, fat-soluble vitamins, vitamin B_{12}, water, and electrolyte imbalance. Also, women can have obstruction of ileostomy as pregnancy progresses.

The mode of delivery is not usually influenced by inflammatory bowel disease, even in those with an ileal pouch-anal anastomosis. There are few reports of the management of labor in such cases, but two studies have reported normal vaginal deliveries in the majority of women.[149,150] However, cesarean section should be considered in women with impaired anal continence, in those who have had extensive perineal surgery due to scarring causing skin inelasticity, or in women with active perianal disease, as episiotomy may result in fistula formation. These cesarean procedures may be complicated, and an experienced obstetrician should be present.

Postpartum flare is not a feature of ulcerative colitis but can occur in Crohn's disease.

Fetal Risks

For the majority of cases, if the maternal inflammatory bowel disease is quiescent at the time of conception, the fetal outcome is no different to that in unaffected pregnancies. However, active disease at the time of conception is associated with an increased rate of miscarriage, and flares during pregnancy result in low birth weight and prematurity.[151–153]

Because the etiology of inflammatory bowel disease has both hereditary and immune components, breastfeeding should be encouraged in an effort to reduce the risks to the children of affected women.

Management Options

Acute exacerbations of inflammatory bowel disease can be treated with 5-aminosalicylic acid (5-ASA)-containing compounds and corticosteroids taken rectally, and then orally if local therapy is not sufficient to control symptoms. In severe attacks intravenous corticosteroids may be required. Loperamide can be used for the treatment of diarrhea. Metronidazole is used to treat anal disease and fistulae, particularly in active Crohn's disease. 5-ASA-containing compounds, corticosteroids, and the immunosuppressives azathioprine and 6-mercaptopurine can be used during remission to prevent relapse rates. Long-term management for recurrent Crohn's disease also includes attention to diet and vitamin supplementation. Pregnant women with inflammatory bowel disease should be advised to take high-dose folate (5 mg daily).

5-Aminosalicylic Acid Derivatives

Many women are now treated with 5-ASA derivatives. Salazopyrin, or Azulfidine (sulfasalazine), is a prodrug that is converted by colonic bacteria into sulphapyridine and 5-ASA. The efficacy of Salazopyrin in the treatment of inflammatory bowel disease resides in the 5-ASA component. Many of the side effects of the drug have been attributed to sulphapyridine, and therefore newer preparations that do not have this component are now used more commonly than Salazopyrin. These include mesalazine (5-ASA), balsalazine (a prodrug of 5-ASA), and olsalazine (a dimer of 5-ASA that is cleaved in the lower bowel). Both oral and topical preparations of 5-ASA and Salazopyrin are safe in pregnancy. In a U.S. study that included 186 cases in which the mother was treated with Salazopyrin, the fetal complication rate was lower than the reported rates in the general population.[154] A prospective Canadian study of 165 women who were exposed to oral mesalazine in pregnancy, 146 of whom had first-trimester exposure, demonstrated no increase in major congenital malformations when compared with matched controls who had not been exposed to teratogenic drugs.[155] In a French study designed to address whether treatment with high doses of mesalazine in pregnancy were associated with an adverse fetal outcome, 86 women who received less than 3 g mesalazine daily were compared with 37 who received more than 3 g daily. The results revealed no difference in the rates of congenital malformations, prematurity, nor fetal death between the groups, and the prevalence of these complications was not different from the quoted rates from the general population.[156] Only very small amounts of 5-ASA pass into breast milk, and the drug is therefore also thought to be safe in lactating women.[157]

Corticosteroids

Corticosteroids taken orally in low doses may reduce recurrence rates, and in higher doses are used for acute intestinal symptoms, orally or intravenously. Distal disease can respond to steroid enemas.

Azathioprine

Azathioprine is an immunosuppressant that is metabolized to 6-mercaptopurine. There are many reports of renal transplant recipients who have conceived while taking azathioprine and who have had normal children. Thus the drug is thought to not be teratogenic in humans. Azathioprine crosses the placenta, but the fetal liver lacks the enzyme that converts it to its active metabolite, and this is thought to explain the fetal protection from teratogenic effects. There is no reason to suspect that the risks in women with inflammatory bowel disease should be different from those who have had renal transplants. One case series reported the outcome of 16 pregnancies in 14 women with inflammatory bowel disease who were treated with azathioprine. There were no congenital abnormalities, and the children's growth and development were normal.[158]

6-Mercaptopurine

There have been very few reports of 6-mercaptopurine use in pregnancy. In one large case series of patients with inflammatory bowel disease treated with the drug, two women had ongoing pregnancies after having stopped the drug at 3 and 4 weeks' gestation, respectively, and no congenital abnormalities were found in their children.[159]

Metronidazole

Because metronidazole is used to treat *Trichomonas vaginalis*, there have been several studies of its use in the first trimester. A Canadian meta-analysis of all studies that contained at least ten women exposed to metronidazole in the first trimester and untreated controls did not find evidence that the drug is teratogenic.[122] A Spanish meta-analysis that included five cohort and case-control studies reported similar results.[123] This study included three series that were also included in the Canadian study.

Antidiarrheal agents

Loperamide is a synthetic piperidine derivative that is used for the treatment of diarrhea. In a prospective, controlled, multicenter study of loperamide in pregnancy in which 105 women were studied and 89 were exposed to loperamide in the first trimester, there were no significant differences in the rate of major or minor congenital malformations when compared with matched controls.[160]

SUMMARY OF MANAGEMENT OPTIONS

Inflammatory Bowel Disease in Pregnancy

Management Options	Quality of Evidence	Strength of Recommendation	References
Prepregnancy			
Preconception counseling and control and encourage conception when disease is quiescent	IIa	B	151–153
Consider modification of drug therapy to those with a good safety record in pregnancy (see below); steroids do not reduce the risk of relapse.	–	GPP	–
Ensure folate supplementation (5 mg/day).	–	GPP	–
Prenatal			
Continue appropriate drug therapy prenatally:			
Salicylates	IIa	B	154–157
Corticosteroids (oral or rectal)	III	B	154
Azathioprine	III	B	158
6-Mercaptopurine – limited experience in pregnancy	III	B	159
Metronidazole	III	B	122,123
Loperamide	IIa	B	160
Flares should be treated in the same way as outside pregnancy.	–	GPP	–
Attention to nutrition, iron, and folate supplementation	–	GPP	–
Monitor fetal growth.	IIa	B	151–153

Continued

SUMMARY OF MANAGEMENT OPTIONS
Inflammatory Bowel Disease in Pregnancy *(Continued)*

Management Options	Quality of Evidence	Strength of Recommendation	References
Labor and Delivery			
Cesarean section is rarely indicated.	–	GPP	–
Exceptions are women with severe perianal disease, postoperative perineal scarring, or impaired anal continence with an ileal pouch-anal anastamosis.	–	GPP	–
Scrupulous attention to wound repair (abdominal and perineal) with Crohn's disease	–	GPP	–
Postnatal			
If severe diarrhea and malabsorption is present, consider alternatives to oral contraceptives.	–	GPP	–
Breast-feeding is safe for women taking sulphasalazine, mesalazine, corticosteroids, and metronidazole.	IIa	B	154–157, 122,123
There are currently insufficient data about azathioprine and breastfeeding to give evidence-based guidance, although most experts in the field feel that the benefits of maintaining remission and achieving lactation outweigh the risks of discontinuing therapy.	III	B	158
An increased frequency of flares in the postpartum period is reported in Crohn's disease but not in ulcerative colitis.	–	GPP	–

CONCLUSIONS

- Jaundice is uncommon in pregnancy and should prompt extensive investigation to find the cause.
- Obstetric cholestasis is common in pregnancy with significant fetal risks; predicting that risk is not reliable; ursodeoxycholic acid is effective against maternal symptoms but its value in improving fetal outcome is not known.
- Acute fatty liver is a rare but dangerous disorder; intensive/high-dependency supportive multidisciplinary care is needed, followed by urgent delivery.
- Liver hematoma and rupture are very rare events; delay in diagnosis is a risk; multidisciplinary care with hepatic surgeon is required.
- Hyperemesis gravidarum affects about 1% of women; if untreated it can lead to dehydration, ketosis, and weight loss; parenteral fluid and vitamin support are often needed together with pharmacologic control of the vomiting; parenteral nutrition is only rarely necessary.
- Peptic ulceration often improves in pregnancy; it can be managed medically in most cases.
- Celiac disease should not result in any serious problems provided the woman religiously adheres to a gluten-free diet prior to and during pregnancy.
- Inflammatory bowel disease often improves in pregnancy; medical management should be used as in the nonpregnant patient, with the only caveat being that the drugs used should be those with a proven safety record in pregnancy.

REFERENCES

1. Kerr MG, Scott DB: Studies of the inferior vena cava in late pregnancy. Br Med J 1964;I:532–533.
2. Schreyer P, Caspi E, El-Hindi JM, et al: Cirrhosis pregnancy and delivery: A review. Obst Gynecol Sur 1982;37:304–312.
3. Bonnar J: Haemostasis and coagulation disorders in pregnancy. In Bloom Al, Thomas DP (eds): Haemostasis and Thrombosis, Edinburgh, Churchill Livingstone, 1987, 570–584.
4. van den Broek, Letsky EA, et al: Pregnancy and the erythrocyte sedimentation rate. BJOG 2001;108:1164–1167.
5. Brent GA: Maternal thyroid function: Interpretation of thyroid function tests in pregnancy. Clin Obstet Gynecol 1997;40:3–15.
6. Dunlop W, Davison JM: Renal haemodynamics and tubular function in normal pregnancy. Clin Obstet Gynaecol 1987;1:769–788.

7. Darmady JM, Postle AD: Lipid metabolism in pregnancy. BJOG 1982;89:211–215.
8. Broussard CN, Richter JE: Treating gastro-oesophageal reflux disease during pregnancy and lactation: What are the safest therapy options? Drug Safety 1998;19:325–337.
9. Parry E, Shields R, Turnbull AC: Transit time in the small intestine in pregnancy. J Obstet Gynaecol Br Commonw 1970;77: 900–901.
10. Marshall K, Thompson KA, Walsh DM, et al: Incidence of urinary incontinence and constipation during pregnancy and postpartum: A survey of current findings at the Rotunda Lying-In Hospital. BJOG 1998;105:400–402.
11. Girling JC, Dow, E, Smith JH: Liver function tests in pre eclampsia: Importance of comparison with a reference range derived for normal pregnancy. BJOG 1997;104:246–250.
12. David AL, Kotecha M, Girling JC: Factors influencing postnatal liver function tests. BJOG 2000;107:1421–1426.
13. Waffarn F, Charles S, Pena I, et al: Fetal exposure to maternal hyperbilirubinaemia. Am J Dis Child 1982;136:416–417.
14. Arias IM: Inheritable and congenital hyperbilirubinaemia. N Engl J Med 1971;285:1416–1421.
15. Abedin P, Weaver JB, Egginton E: Intrahepatic cholestasis of pregnancy: Prevalence and ethnic distribution. Ethn Health 1999;4:35–37.
16. Kenyon AP, Nelson-Piercy C, Girling J, et al: Obstetric cholestasis, outcome with active management: A series of 70 cases. BJOG 2002;109:282–288.
17. Reyes H, Gonzalez MC, Ribalta J, et al: Prevalence of intrahepatic cholestasis of pregnancy in Chile. Ann Intern Med 1978;88:487–493.
18. Eloranta ML, Heinonen S, Mononen T, Saarikoski S: Risk of obstetric cholestasis in sisters of index patients. Clin Genet 2001;60:42–45.
19. Bull LN, van Eijk MJ, Pawlikowska L, et al: A gene encoding a P-type ATPase mutated in two forms of hereditary cholestasis. Nat Genet 1998;18:219–224.
20. Strautnieks SS, Bull LN, Knisely AS, et al: A gene encoding a liver-specific ABC transporter is mutated in progressive familial intrahepatic cholestasis. Nat Genet 1998;20:233–238.
21. Jacquemin E, De Vree JM, Cresteil D, et al: The wide spectrum of multidrug resistance 3 deficiency: From neonatal cholestasis to cirrhosis of adulthood. Gastroenterology 2001;120: 1448–1458.
22. Dixon PH, Weerasekera N, Linton KJ, et al: Heterozygous MDR3 missense mutation associated with intrahepatic cholestasis of pregnancy: Evidence for a defect in protein trafficking. Hum Mol Genet 2000;9:1209–1217.
23. Mullenbach R, Linton KJ, Wiltshire S, et al: ABCB4 gene sequence variation in women with intrahepatic cholestasis of pregnancy. J Med Genet 2003;40:E70.
24. Larsson-Cohn U, Stenram U: Jaundice during treatment with oral contraceptive agents. JAMA 1965;193:422–426.
25. Kreek MJ, Weser E, Sleisenger MH, Jeffries GH: Idiopathic cholestasis of pregnancy. The response to challenge with the synthetic estrogen ethinyl estradiol. N Engl J Med 1967;277: 1391–1395.
26. Bacq Y, Sapey T, Brechot MC, et al: Intrahepatic cholestasis of pregnancy: A French prospective study. Hepatology 1997;26: 358–364.
27. Kenyon AP, Girling J, Nelson-Piercy C, et al: Pruritus in pregnancy and the identification of obstetric cholestasis risk: A prospective prevalence study of 6531 women. J Obstet Gynaecol 2002;22(Suppl 1):S15.
28. Heikkinen J: Serum bile acids in the early diagnosis of intrahepatic cholestasis of pregnancy. Obstet Gynecol 1983;61:581–587.
29. Laatikainen T, Ikonen E: Serum bile acids in cholestasis of pregnancy. Obstet Gynecol 1977;50:313–318.
30. Heikkinen J, Maentausta O, Ylostalo P, Janne O: Changes in serum bile acid concentrations during normal pregnancy, in patients with intrahepatic cholestasis of pregnancy and in pregnant women with itching. BJOG 1981;88: 240–245.
31. Lunzer M, Barnes P, Byth K, O'Halloran M: Serum bile acid concentrations during pregnancy and their relationship to obstetric cholestasis. Gastroenterology 1986;91:825–829.
32. Kenyon AP, Nelson-Piercy C, Girling J, et al: Pruritus may precede abnormal liver function tests in women with obstetric cholestasis: A longitudinal analysis. BJOG 2001;108:1190–1192.
33. Dann AT, Kenyon AP, Girling JC, et al: Serum glutathione *S*-transferase alpha 1-1, An index of hepatocellular damage is raised at 24 weeks' gestation in women who develop obstetric cholestasis. Hepatology 2004;40:1406–1414.
34. Williamson C, Hems LM, Goulis DG, et al: Clinical outcome in a series of cases of obstetric cholestasis identified via a patient support group. BJOG 2004;111:676–681.
35. Rosmorduc O, Hermelin B, Poupon R: MDR3 gene defect in adults with symptomatic intrahepatic and gallbladder cholesterol cholelithiasis. Gastroenterology 2001;120:1459–1467.
36. Locatelli A, Roncaglia N, Arreghini A, et al: Hepatitis C virus infection is associated with a higher incidence of cholestasis of pregnancy. BJOG 1999;106:498–500.
37. Herre HD, Engelmann C, Wiken HP: Diagnosis and therapy of blood coagulation disorders in intrahepatic cholestasis. Zentralbl Gynakol 1976;98:217–219.
38. CESDI Consortium: Confidential enquiry into stillbirths and deaths in infancy. Fifth annual report, 1995. Maternal and Child Health Research Consortium.
39. Gorelik J, Shevchuk A, Diakonov I, et al: Dexamethasone and ursodeoxycholic acid protect against the arrhythmogenic effect of taurocholate in an in vitro study of rat cardiomyocytes. BJOG 2003;110:467–474.
40. Morrison JJ, Rennie JM, Milton PJ: Neonatal respiratory morbidity and mode of delivery at term: Influence of timing of elective cesarean section. BJOG 1995;102:101–106.
41. Madar J, Richmond S, Hey E: Surfactant-deficient respiratory distress after elective delivery at 'term.' Acta Paediatr 1999;88:1244–1248.
42. Reid R, Ivey KJ, Rencoret RH, Storey B: Fetal complications of obstetric cholestasis. Br Med J 1976;1:870–872.
43. Reyes H: The enigma of intrahepatic cholestasis of pregnancy: Lessons from Chile. Hepatology 1982;2:87–96.
44. Sadler LC, Lane M, North R: Severe fetal intracranial haemorrhage during treatment with cholestyramine for intrahepatic cholestasis of pregnancy. BJOG 1995;102:169–170.
45. Burrows RF, Clavisi O, Burrows E for the Cochrane Pregnancy and Childbirth Group: Interventions for treating cholestasis in pregnancy. Cochrane Database Syst Rev 2003;3:1–10.
46. Williamson C: Gastrointestinal disease. Baillieres Best Pract Res Clin Obstet Gynaecol 2001;15:937–952.
47. Mazzella G, Nicola R, Francesco A, et al: Ursodeoxycholic acid administration in patients with cholestasis of pregnancy: Effects on primary bile acids in babies and mothers. Hepatology 2001;33:504–508.
48. Hirvioja ML, Tuimala R, Vuori J: The treatment of intrahepatic cholestasis of pregnancy by dexamethasone. BJOG 1992;99:109–111.
49. Kretowicz E, McIntyre HD: Intrahepatic cholestasis of pregnancy, worsening after dexamethasone. Aust N Z J Obstet Gynaecol 1994;34:211–213.
50. Bloom SL, Sheffield JS, McIntire DD, Leveno KJ: Antenatal dexamethasone and decreased birth weight. Obstet Gynaecol 2001;97:485–490.
51. Modi N, Lewis H, Al-Naqeeb N, et al: The effects of repeated antenatal corticosteroid therapy on the developing brain. Pediatric Research 2001;50:581–585.

52. Fisk NM, Storey GN: Fetal outcome in obstetric cholestasis. BJOG 1988;95:1137–1143.
53. Roncaglia N, Arreghini A, Locatelli A, et al: Obstetric cholestasis: Outcome with active management. Eur J Obstet Gynecol Reprod Biol 2002;100:167–170.
54. Castro MA, Fassett MJ, Reynolds TB, et al: Reversible peripartum liver failure: A new perspective on the diagnosis, treatment and cause of acute fatty liver of pregnancy, based on 28 consecutive cases. Am J Obstet Gynecol 1999;181:389–395.
55. Pockros PJ, Peters RL, Reynolds TB: Idiopathic fatty liver of pregnancy: Findings in 10 cases. Medicine (Baltimore) 1984;63:1–11.
56. Castro MA, Ouzounian JG, Colletti PM: Radiologic studies in acute fatty liver of pregnancy. A review of the literature and 19 new cases. J Reprod Med 1996;41:839–843.
57. Kunelis CT, Peters JL, Edmondson HA: Fatty liver of pregnancy and its relationship to tetracycline therapy. Am J Med 1965;33:359–377.
58. Fagan EA: Disorders of the liver. In de Swiet M(ed): Medical Disorders in Obstetric Practice, 4th ed. London, Blackwell Science, 2002, pp 282–345.
59. RCOG publications: The Report on Confidential Enquiries into Maternal Deaths in the United Kingdom 2000–2002. London, 2004.
60. Ijist L, Ruiter JPN, Hoovers JMN, et al: Common missense mutation G1528C in long chain 3-hydroxyacyl CoA dehydrogenase deficiency—Characterisation and expression of the mutant protein, mutation analysis on genomic DNA and chromosomal localisation of the mitochondrial trifunctional protein alpha subunit gene. J Clin Invest 1996;98:1028–1033.
61. Sims HF, Brackett JC, Powell CK, et al: The molecular basis of pediatric long chain 3-hydroxyacyl CoA dehydrogenase deficiency associated with maternal acute fatty liver of pregnancy. Proc Natl Acad Sci USA 1995;92:841–845.
62. Tyni T, Ekholm E, Pikho H: Pregnancy complications are frequent in long chain 3 hydroxyacyl coenzyme A dehydrogenase deficiency. Am J Obstet Gynecol 1998;178:603–608.
63. Mansouri I, Fromenty B, Durand F, et al: Assessment of the prevalence of genetic metabolic defects in acute fatty liver of pregnancy. J Hepatol 1996;25:781.
64. Treem W, Shoup M, Hale D, et al: Acute fatty liver of pregnancy, haemolysis, elevated liver enzymes and low platelets syndrome and long chain 3-hydroxyacyl coenzyme A dehydrogenase deficiency. Am J Gastroenterol 1996;91:2293–2300.
65. Yang Z, Yamada J, Zhao Y, et al: Prospective screening for pediatric mitochondrial trifunctional protein defects in pregnancies complicated by liver disease. JAMA 2002;288:2163–2166.
66. Ibdah JA, Bennett MJ, Rinaldo P, et al: A fetal fatty-acid oxidation disorder as a cause of liver disease in pregnant women. Engl J Med 1999;340:1723–1731.
67. Perez-Cerda C, Merinero B, Jimenez A, et al: First report of prenatal diagnosis of long-chain 3-hydroxyacyl-CoA dehydrogenase deficiency in a pregnancy at risk. Prenat Diagn 1993;13:529–533.
68. Sherbahn R: Spontaneous ruptured subcapsular liver haemaotma associated with pregnancy: A case report. J Reprod Med 1996;41:125–128.
69. Ibrahim N, Payne E, Owen A: Spontaneous rupture of the liver in association with pregnancy: Case report. BJOG 1985;92:539–540.
70. Abdi S, Cameron IC, Nakielny RA, Majeed AW: Spontaneous hepatic rupture and maternal death following an uncomplicated pregnancy and delivery. BJOG 2001;108:431–433.
71. Rinehart B, Terrone D, Magann E, et al: Pre-eclampsia associated hepatic haemorrhage and rupture: A mode of management related to maternal and perinatal outcome. Obstet Gynaecol Surv 1999;54:196–202.
72. Schwartz M, Lien J: Spontaneous liver haematoma in pregnancy not clearly associated with preeclampsia: A case presentation and literature review. Am J Obstet Gynecol 1997;176:1328–1333.
73. Bis KA, Waxman B: Rupture of the liver associated with pregnancy: A review of the literature and a review of 2 cases. Obstet Gynaecol Survey 1976;31:792–794.
74. Marsh FA, Kaufmann SJ, Bhahra K: Surviving hepatic rupture in pregnancy—A literature review with an illustrative case report. J Obstet Gynaecol 2003;23:109–113.
75. Sheikh R, Yasmeen S, Pauly MP, Riegler JL: Spontaneous intrahepatic haemorrhage and hepatic rupture in the HELLP syndrome. J Clin Gastro 1999;128:323–328.
76. Quinn MF, Lundell CJ, Finck EJ, Pentecost MJ: Spontaneous hepatic hemorrhage in preeclampsia: Treatment with hepatic arterial embolisation. Radiology 1990;174:1039–1041.
77. Kazerooni T, Taallom M, Ghaderi AA: Helicobacter pylori seropositivity in patients with hyperemesis gravidarum. Int J Gynaecol Obstet 2002;79:217–220.
78. Salimi-Khayati A, Sharami H, Mansour-Ghanaei F, et al: Helicobacter pylori seropositivity and the incidence of hyperemesis gravidarum. Med Sci Monit 2003;9:CR12–CR15.
79. Bagis T, Gumurdulu Y, Kayaselcuk F, et al: Endoscopy in hyperemesis gravidarum and helicobacter pylori infection. Int J Gynecol Obstet 2002;79:105–109.
80. Gross S, Librach C, Cecutti A: Maternal weight loss associated with hyperemesis gravidarum. Am J Obstet Gynecol 1989;160:906–909.
81. Godsey RK, Newman RB: Hyperemesis gravidarum: A comparison of single and multiple admissions. J Reprod Med 1991;36:287–290.
82. Tsang IS, Katz VL, Wells SD: Maternal and fetal outcomes in hyperemesis gravidarum. Int J Gynaecol Obstet 1996;55: 231–235.
83. Weigel MM, Weigel RM: Nausea and vomiting of early pregnancy and pregnancy outcome. An epidemiological study. BJOG 1989;96:1304–1311.
84. Buttino L, Gambon C: Home subcutaneous metoclopramide therapy for hyperemesis gravidarum. Prim Care Update Ob Gyns 1998;5:189.
85. Buttino L, Coleman SK, Bergauer NK, et al: Home subcutaneous metoclopramide therapy for hyperemesis gravidarum. J Perinatol 2000;20:359–362.
86. Milkovich L, Van Den Berg BJ: An evaluation of the teratogenicity of certain antinauseant drugs. Am J Obstet Gynecol 1975;125:245.
87. Morelock S, Hingson R, Kayne H, et al: Bendectin and fetal development. A study of Boston City Hospital. Am J Obstet Gynecol 1982;142:209–213.
88. Mazzotta P, Magee LA: A risk-benefit assessment of pharmacological and nonpharmacological treatments for nausea and vomiting of pregnancy. Drugs 2000;59:781–800.
89. Nelson-Piercy C, de Swiet M: Corticosteroids for the treatment of hyperemesis gravidarum. BJOG 1994;101:1013–1015.
90. Taylor R: Successful management of hyperemesis gravidarum using steroid therapy. QJM 1996;89:103–107.
91. Safari HR, Alsulyman OM, Gherman RB, Goodwin TM: Experience with oral methylprednisolone in the treatment of refractory hyperemesis gravidarum. Am J Obstet Gynecol 1998a; 178:1054–1058.
92. Safari HR, Fassett MJ, Souter IC, et al: The efficacy of methylprednisolone in the treatment of hyperemesis gravidarum: A randomized, double-blind, controlled study. Am J Obstet Gynecol 1998b;179:921–924.
93. Nelson-Piercy C, Fayers P, de Swiet M: Randomised, double-blind, placebo-controlled trial of corticosteroids for the treatment of hyperemesis gravidarum. BJOG 2001; 108:9–15.
94. Tincello DG, Johnstone MJ: Treatment of hyperemesis gravidarum with the 5-HT3 antagonist ondansetron (Zofran). Postgrad Med J 1996;72:688–689.
95. Guikontes E, Spantideas A, Diakakis J: Ondansetron and hyperemesis gravidarum. Lancet 1992;340:1223.

96. World MJ: Ondansetron and hyperemesis gravidarum. Lancet 1993;341:185.
97. Sullivan CA, Johnson CA, Roach H, et al: A pilot study of intravenous ondansetron for hyperemesis gravidarum. Am J Obstet Gynecol 1996;174:1565–1568.
98. Fischer-Rasmussen W, Kjaer SK, Dahl C, Asping U: Ginger treatment of hyperemesis gravidarum. Eur J Obstet Gynecol Reprod Biol 1991;38:19–24.
99. Hsu JJ, Clark-Glena R, Nelson DK, Kim CH: Nasogastric enteral feeding in the management of hyperemesis gravidarum. Obstet Gynecol 1996;88:343–346.
100. Charlin V, Borghesi L, Hasbun J, et al:. Parenteral nutrition in hyperemesis gravidarum. Nutrition 1993;9:29–32.
101. Russo-Stieglitz KE, Levine AB, Wagner BA, Armenti VT: Pregnancy outcome in patients requiring parenteral nutrition. J Matern Fetal Med 1999;8:164–167.
102. Bassey OO: Pregnancy heartburn in Nigerians and Caucasians with theories about aetiology based on manometric recordings from the oesophagus and stomach. BJOG 1977;84:439–443.
103. Marrero JM, Goggin PM, de Caestecker JS, et al: Determinants of pregnancy heartburn. BJOG 1992;99:731–734.
104. Baird RM: Peptic ulceration in pregnancy: Report of a case with perforation. Can Med Assoc J 1996;94:861–862.
105. Cappell MS, Colon V, Sidhom OA: A study of eight medical centers of the safety and clinical efficacy of esophagogastroduodenoscopy in 83 pregnant females with follow-up of fetal outcome and comparison to control groups. Am J Gastroenterol 1996;91:348–354.
106. Harper MA, McVeigh JE, Thompson W, et al: Successful pregnancy in association with Zollinger-Ellison syndrome. Am J Obstet Gynecol 1995;173:863–864.
107. Stewart CA, Termanini B, Sutliff VE, et al: Management of the Zollinger-Ellison syndrome in pregnancy. Am J Obstet Gynecol 1997;176:224–233.
108. Lewis JH, Weingold AB: The use of gastrointestinal drugs during pregnancy and lactation. Am J Gastroenterol 1985;80: 912–923.
109. Nelson MM, Forfar JO: Associations between drugs administered during pregnancy and congenital abnormalities of the fetus. Br Med J 1971;1:523–527.
110. Uzan M, Uzan S, Sureau C, Richard-Berthe C: Heartburn and regurgitation in pregnancy. Efficacy and innocuousness of treatment with Gaviscon suspension. Rev Fr Gynecol Obstet 1988;83:569–572.
111. Avery AJ, Carr S: Treatment of common minor and self-limiting conditions. In Rubin P(ed): Prescribing in Pregnancy, 3rd ed. London, BMJ Publishing Group, 2000, pp 15–28.
112. Fagan EA: Disorders of the gastrointestinal tract. In de Swiet M (ed): Medical Disorders in Obstetric Practice, 4th ed. Oxford, Blackwell Science, 2002, pp 346–385.
113. Magee LA, Inocencion G, Kamboj L, et al: Safety of first trimester exposure to histamine H_2 blockers. A prospective cohort study. Dig Dis Sci 1996;41:1145–1149.
114. Kallen B: Delivery outcome after the use of acid-suppressing drugs in early pregnancy with special reference to omeprazole. BJOG 1998;105:877–881.
115. Lalkin A, Loebstein R, Addis A, et al: The safety of omeprazole during pregnancy: A multicenter prospective controlled study. Am J Obstet Gynecol 1998;179:727–730.
116. Ruigomez A, Garcia Rodriguez LA, et al: Use of cimetidine, omeprazole, and ranitidine in pregnant women and pregnancy outcomes. Am J Epidemiol 1999;150:476–481.
117. Kallen BA: Use of omeprazole during pregnancy—No hazard demonstrated in 955 infants exposed during pregnancy. Eur J Obstet Gynecol Reprod Biol 2001;96:63–68.
118. Wilton LV, Pearce GL, Martin RM, et al: The outcomes of pregnancy in women exposed to newly marketed drugs in general practice in England. BJOG 1998;105:882–889.
119. Bailey B, Addis A, Lee A, et al: Cisapride use during human pregnancy: A prospective, controlled multicenter study. Dig Dis Sci 1997;42:1848–1852.
120. Jepsen P, Skriver MV, Floyd A, et al: A population-based study of maternal use of amoxicillin and pregnancy outcome in Denmark. Br J Clin Pharmacol 2003;55:216–221.
121. Einarson A, Phillips E, Mawji F, et al: A prospective controlled multicentre study of clarithromycin in pregnancy. Am J Perinatol 1998;15:523–525.
122. Burtin P, Taddio A, Ariburnu O, et al: Safety of metronidazole in pregnancy: A meta-analysis. Am J Obstet Gynecol 1995;172:525–529.
123. Caro-Paton T, Carvajal A, Martin de Diego I, et al: Is metronidazole teratogenic? A meta-analysis. Br J Clin Pharmacol 1997;44:179–182.
124. Orioli IM, Castilla EE: Epidemiological assessment of misoprostol teratogenicity. BJOG 2000;107:519–523.
125. Gonzalez CH, Vargas FR, Perez AB, et al: Limb deficiency with or without Mobius sequence in seven Brazilian children associated with misoprostol use in the first trimester of pregnancy. Am J Med Genet 1993;47:59–64.
126. Fonseca W, Alencar AJ, Pereira RM, Misago C: Congenital malformation of the scalp and cranium after failed first trimester abortion attempt with misoprostol. Clin Dysmorphol 1993;2:76–80.
127. Potzi R, Ferenci P, Gangl A: Endoscopic sclerotherapy of esophageal varices during pregnancy: A case report. Z Gastroenterol 1991;29:246–247.
128. Macedo G, Carvalho L, Ribeiro T: Endoscopic sclerotherapy for upper gastrointestinal bleeding due to Mallory-Weiss syndrome. Am J Gastroenterol 1995;90:1364–1365.
129. McCarthy CF, Mylotte M: Family studies on coeliac disease in Ireland. In Proceedings of 2nd International Coeliac symposium, Coeliac disease. Stenfert Kroese, Leiden, 1974.
130. Bevan S, Popat S, Braegger CP, et al: Contribution of the MHC region to the familial risk of coeliac disease. J Med Genet 1999;36:687–690.
131. Greco L, Romino R, Coto I, et al: The first large population based twin study of coeliac disease. Gut 2002;50:624–628.
132. Unsworth DJ, Lock RJ, Harvey RF: Iron deficiency anaemia in premenopausal women. Lancet 1999;353:1100.
133. Unsworth DJ; Lock RJ, Haslam N: Coeliac disease and unfavourable pregnancy outcome. Gut 2000;47:598–599.
134. Smeucol E, Maurino E, Vasquez H, et al: Gynaecological and obstetric disorders in coeliac disease: Frequent clinical onset during pregnancy and the puerperium. Eur J Gastroenterol Hepatol 1996;8:63–89.
135. Collin P, Vilska S, Heinonen PK, et al: Infertility and coeliac disease. Gut 1996;39:382–384.
136. Meloni GF, Dessole S, Vargiu N, et al: The prevalence of coeliac disease in infertility. Human Reprod 1999;14:2759–2761.
137. Farthing MC, Rees LH, Edwards CR, et al: Male gonadal function in coeliac disease: 11 Sex hormones. Gut 1983;24:127–135.
138. Baker PG, Read AE: Reversible fertility in male coeliac patients. Br Med J 1975;ii:316–317.
139. Farthing MJ, Edwards CR, Rees LH, et al: Male gonadal function in coeliac disease: 1 Sexual dysfunction, infertility and semen quality. Gut 1982;23:608–614.
140. Ciacci C, Cirillo M, Auriemma G, et al: Celiac disease and pregnancy outcome. Am J Gastroenterol 1996;91:718–722.
141. Gasbarrini A, Torre ES, Trivellini C, et al: Recurrent spontaneous abortion and intrauterine fetal growth retardation as symptoms of coeliac disease. Lancet 2000;356:399–400.
142. Martinelli P, Troncone R, Paparo F, et al: Coeliac disease and unfavourable outcome of pregnancy. Gut 2000;46:332–335.
143. Ludvigsson JF, Ludvigsson J: Coeliac disease in the father affects the newborn. Gut 2001;49:169–175.
144. Okazawa A, Kanai T, Watanabe M, et al: Th1-mediated intestinal inflammation in Crohn's disease may be induced by acti-

vation of lamina propria lymphocytes through synergistic stimulation of interleukin-12 and interleukin-18 without T cell receptor engagement. Am J Gastroenterol 2002;97:3108–3117.
145. Heller F, Fuss IJ, Nieuwenhuis EE, et al: Oxazolone colitis, a Th2 colitis model resembling ulcerative colitis, is mediated by IL-13-producing NK-T cells. Immunity 2002;17:629–638.
146. Bridger S, Lee JC, Bjarnason I, et al: In siblings with similar genetic susceptibility for inflammatory bowel disease, smokers tend to develop Crohn's disease and non-smokers develop ulcerative colitis. Gut 2002;51:21–25.
147. Ogura Y, Bonen DK, Inohara N, et al: A frameshift mutation in NOD2 associated with susceptibility to Crohn's disease. Nature 2001;411:603–606.
148. Hudson M, Flett G, Sinclair TS, et al: Fertility and pregnancy in inflammatory bowel disease. Int J Gynaecol Obstet 1997;58:229–237.
149. Scott HJ, McLeod RS, Blair J, et al: Ileal pouch-anal anastomosis: Pregnancy, delivery and pouch function. Int J Colorectal Dis 1996;11:84–87.
150. Metcalf A, Dozois RR, Beart RW Jr, Wolff BG: Pregnancy following ileal pouch-anal anastomosis. Dis Colon Rectum 1985;28:859–861.
151. Mogadam M, Korelitz BI, Ahmed SW, et al: The course of inflammatory bowel disease during pregnancy and postpartum. Am J Gastroenterol 1981b;75:265–269.
152. Baiocco PJ, Korelitz BI: The influence of inflammatory bowel disease and its treatment on pregnancy and fetal outcome. J Clin Gastroenterol 1984;6:211–216.
153. Morales M, Berney T, Jenny A, et al: Crohn's disease as a risk factor for the outcome of pregnancy. Hepatogastroenterology 2000;47:1595–1598.
154. Mogadam M, Dobbins WO 3rd, Korelitz BI, Ahmed SW: Pregnancy in inflammatory bowel disease: Effect of sulfasalazine and corticosteroids on fetal outcome. Gastroenterology 1981;80:72–76.
155. Diav-Citrin O, Park YH, Veerasuntharam G, et al: The safety of mesalamine in human pregnancy: A prospective controlled cohort study. Gastroenterology 1998;114:23–28.
156. Marteau P, Tennenbaum R, Elefant E, et al: Fetal outcome in women with inflammatory bowel disease treated during pregnancy with oral mesalazine microgranules. Aliment Pharmacol Ther 1998;12:1101–1108.
157. Christensen LA, Rasmussen SN, Hansen SH: Disposition of 5-aminosalicylic acid and *N*-acetyl-5-aminosalicylic acid in fetal and maternal body fluids during treatment with different 5-aminosalicylic acid preparations. Acta Obstet Gynecol Scand 1994;73:399–402.
158. Alstead EM, Ritchie JK, Lennard-Jones JE, et al: Safety of azathioprine in pregnancy in inflammatory bowel disease. Gastroenterology 1990;99:443–446.
159. Present DH, Meltzer SJ, Krumholz MP, et al: 6-Mercaptopurine in the management of inflammatory bowel disease: Short and long-term toxicity. Ann Int Med 1989;111:641–649.
160. Einarson A, Mastroiacovo P, Arnon J, et al: Prospective, controlled, multicentre study of loperamide in pregnancy. Can J Gastroenterol 2000;14:185–187.
161. Rioseco AJ, Ivankovic MB, Manzur A, et al: Intrahepatic cholestasis of pregnancy: A retrospective case-control study of perinatal outcome. Am J Obstet Gynecol 1994;170:890–895.
162. Heinonen S, Kirkinen P: Pregnancy outcome with intrahepatic cholestasis. Obstet Gynecol 1999;94:189–193.

CHAPTER 49

Neurologic Disorders

J. Ricardo Carhuapoma / Mark W. Tomlinson / Steven R. Levine

INTRODUCTION

Neurologic conditions seen in reproductive-age women will be encountered during pregnancy. Table 49–1 shows the incidence of several such neurologic diseases. The relative rarity of many of these conditions limits the actual clinical experience of both the managing obstetrician and neurologist. In addition, the individual practitioner is further hampered by the limited amount of pregnancy-specific information available. The frequent overlap of symptoms associated with common pregnancy complaints, the sometimes disabling and lethal consequences of the disease, and fetal effects of maternal treatment make the diagnosis and management of neurologic disease during pregnancy an often daunting task.

Optimal and effective management commonly requires the expertise of several disciplines. This obviously includes the obstetrician or maternal-fetal medicine specialist and the neurologist. Involvement of an anesthesiologist is essential at the time of labor and delivery to provide appropriate analgesia or anesthesia. Early involvement of the pediatrician or neonatologist is important to anticipating neonatal needs and adequately caring for the newborn. Drugs discussed are listed with a risk factor category used by the Food and Drug Administration (FDA). The categories and definitions are shown in Table 49–2.[1] There are very few randomized clinical trials to guide evidence-based medicine in the field of neurologic complications of pregnancy.

TABLE 49–1

Incidence of Neurologic Disease in Childbearing Population

Migraine	1:5
Epilepsy	1:150
Multiple sclerosis	1:1000
Cerebral venous thrombosis	1:2500–10,000 deliveries
Ruptured cerebral aneurysm	1:10,000 pregnancies
Bleed from cerebral AVM	1:10,000 pregnancies
Myasthenia gravis	1:25,000
Malignant brain tumor	1:50,000
Guillain–Barré syndrome	1.5:100,000

AVM, arteriovenous malformation.

SEIZURES

Neurologic Complications of Preeclampsia and Eclampsia

Maternal and Fetal Risks

Preeclampsia and eclampsia are also discussed in Chapters 37 and 74. The reported incidence of eclampsia in both the United Kingdom and the United States is approximately 0.05% of births.[2] As with preeclampsia, the specific cause and pathophysiology leading to eclampsia is unknown. Postulated contributing factors include cerebral edema, vasospasm, ischemia, hemorrhage, or hypertensive encephalopathy.[3]

Hypertension is an important factor associated with convulsions. Increasing systolic and diastolic blood pressures in a previously normotensive patient challenge the autoregulatory properties of cerebral blood vessels. In normotensive patients, autoregulation is preserved between mean arterial pressure (MAP) values from 50 mm Hg to 150 mm Hg. Beyond this range, cerebral blood vessels lose their tone and an angiographic pattern of vasodilation with segments of vasoconstriction develops. The blood-brain barrier and its "tight junctions" are

TABLE 49–2

Classification System for Fetal Risk Associated with Medications Used during Pregnancy

Category A	Controlled studies in women fail to demonstrate a risk to the fetus in the first trimester (and there is no evidence of a risk in later trimesters), and the possibility of fetal harm appears remote.
Category B	Either animal-reproduction studies have not demonstrated a fetal risk but there are no controlled studies in pregnant women, or animal-reproduction studies have shown an adverse effect (other than a decrease in fertility) that was not confirmed in controlled studies in women in the first trimester (and there is no evidence of a risk in later trimesters).
Category C	Either studies in animals have revealed adverse effects on the fetus (teratogenic or embryocidal, or other) and there are no controlled studies in women, or studies in women and animals are not available. Drugs should be given only if the potential benefit justifies the potential risk to the fetus.
Category D	There is positive evidence of human fetal risk, but the benefits from use in pregnant women may be acceptable despite the risk (e.g., if the drug is needed in a life-threatening situation or for a serious disease for which safer drugs cannot be used or are ineffective).
Category X	Studies in animals or human beings have demonstrated fetal abnormalities, or there is evidence of fetal risk based on human experience, or both, and the risk of the use of the drug in pregnant women clearly outweighs any possible benefit. The drug is contraindicated in women who are or may become pregnant.

disrupted, and vasogenic edema ensues.[4–9] This process occurs preferentially in the occipital lobes and in "watershed" areas of the brain.[10] The neuropathologic changes are widespread throughout the neuraxis.[11] Cerebral edema is evident, and the presence of petechial hemorrhages surrounding arterioles is conspicuous, conceivably rendering certain neuronal populations hyperexcitable. Although hypertension through this cascade of events can initiate the pathogenic process of convulsions in many instances, it does not explain all cases. Eclampsia can be seen in patients without significant blood pressure elevations.[3] As many as 38% of all eclamptics have been reported to have no hypertension or proteinuria identified before the initial seizure.[12]

In addition to convulsions, a variety of visual symptoms may be seen. These may be nonspecific but can include retinal detachments and cortical blindness secondary to hypertension-induced retinal arteriolar dilatation, papilledema,[13] central retinal artery occlusion,[14] and vasospasm.[15] Visual changes generally improve with delivery and hypertension control. Headache is also common and may involve increased intracranial pressure (ICP) resulting from vasogenic edema.[16] More severe findings such as lethargy, stupor, and coma in a preeclamptic patient should always raise the suspicion of an intracerebral hemorrhage or of worsening brain edema with the subsequent risk of brain herniation.[17]

Although maternal mortality rates have decreased over the past several decades, eclampsia continues to be a significant contributor, particularly in underdeveloped countries. During the early 1980s in the Unites States pregnancy-induced hypertension (PIH) was the third leading cause of maternal deaths, accounting for 22.5%. Eclampsia and other central nervous system (CNS) complications were a factor in more than 60% of the PIH deaths.[18] In a more recent series, approximately 1% of pregnancies complicated by eclampsia still resulted in maternal death.[12,19] In developing countries, maternal mortality is reported in 8% to 14% of patients with eclampsia.[20] Fetal and neonatal complication rates also tend to be high and are attributed to prematurity, placental insufficiency, and placental abruption.[21]

Management Options (See also Chapters 36 and 80)

PRENATAL, LABOR, DELIVERY, AND POSTNATAL

Eclampsia most frequently occurs during the antepartum and intrapartum periods, but approximately one third of cases are seen postpartum. Between 28% and 56% of postpartum convulsions occur more than 48 hours after delivery.[22,23] The diagnosis is clinical, and additional diagnostic evaluation is not always necessary when typical preeclampsia precedes the seizure. When the presentation is not classic, however, imaging studies such as brain computed tomography (CT) and magnetic resonance imaging (MRI), including diffusion-weighted imaging (DWI), can be helpful in identifying complications or other causes of seizure, such as hemorrhage, cerebral infarction, or cerebral venous thrombosis (Fig. 49–1).

Magnesium sulfate has been the mainstay of both seizure prophylaxis and abortive therapy in the United States.[24] The precise mechanism of action remains poorly understood. Current hypotheses include reduction in cerebral vasospasm through calcium antagonism, and *N*-methyl-D-aspartate (NMDA) receptor channel blockade providing "neuroprotection" from ischemic injury resulting from vasospasm.[25–28]

The efficacy of magnesium has been established.[29] Recent larger trials provide compelling evidence that magnesium sulfate is superior to phenytoin and diazepam in both treatment and prophylaxis of eclamptic seizures.[30] A multicenter worldwide trial including more than 1600 eclamptic patients reported that magne-

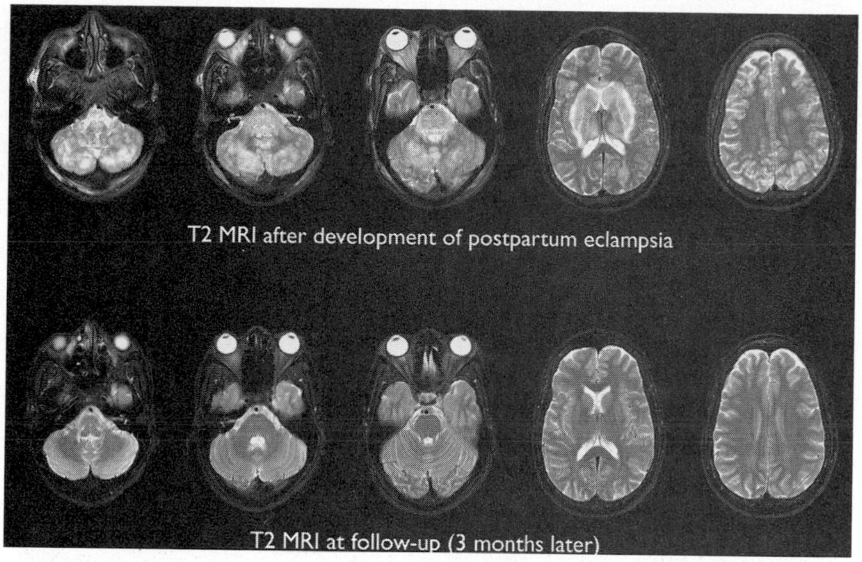

T2 MRI after development of postpartum eclampsia
T2 MRI at follow-up (3 months later)

FIGURE 49–1
Axial head T_2-weighted MRI of a woman with headaches, proteinuria, and postpartum seizures. There are multiple regions of T_2 hyperintensity in the cerebellum, pons, basal ganglia, and the hemispheric white matter consistent with changes seen in eclampsia. These radiologic abnormalities reversed on subsequent MR evaluation that followed the complete clinical resolution of this patient's initial neurologic presentation.

sium sulfate was associated with a 52% lower risk of recurrent seizures than diazepam, and a 67% lower risk than phenytoin. Furthermore, maternal and neonatal morbidity rates were lower in the magnesium group than for those receiving phenytoin. Magnesium sulfate has also been shown to be superior to placebo and phenytoin when used prophylacticly to prevent seizures. A large North American study comparing the efficacy of magnesium and phenytoin for seizure prophylaxis was stopped early when interim analysis showed that phenytoin provided ineffective seizure prophylaxis.[30] Management differences between eclampsia and epilepsy should not be surprising because the pathophysiology of the two conditions is likely to be different. A recent Cochrane Review shows that magnesium sulfate more than halves the risk of eclampsia and probably reduces the risk of maternal death (RR 0.41: 95% CI, 0.29–0.58). Magnesium sulfate does not improve outcome of the newborn. The risk of placental abruption was also reduced.[29]

Specific dosing recommendations have varied, but generally consist of a 4 to 6 g intravenous load given over 5 to 30 min. This is followed by a maintenance dose of 1 to 3 g/hr intravenously. Therapeutic serum levels are in the range of 4 to 8 mEq/L. The magnesium infusion is usually continued for approximately 24 hours into the postpartum period. The duration of therapy is empiric and based on the distribution of postpartum seizure risk. Complications associated with the use of magnesium center on its calcium antagonism at the neuromuscular junction, which can result in neuromuscular blockade. At levels above 10 mEq/L deep tendon reflexes are lost. Lethargy and respiratory depression are also seen. Levels of 12 to 15 mEq/L result in respiratory paralysis. Higher levels can result in cardiac standstill. Management of overdose includes respiratory support, calcium gluconate (1 g), and cardiac monitoring. A recent randomized controlled trial failed to prevent preeclampsia with low-dose aspirin in women with abnormal uterine artery Doppler.[31]

Blood pressure control is also important in both preventing and managing neurologic complications associated with preeclampsia/eclampsia. Some investigators have suggested that a greater emphasis should be placed on blood pressure control with the potential elimination of seizure prophylaxis.[32,33] Hydralazine and labetalol are frequently used as first-line agents, with continuous IV infusions of nicardipine, sodium nitroprusside, and nitroglycerin being used in refractory cases. The NHLBI recently convened a working group on research of hypertension in pregnancy.[34]

Simple first-aid measures (avoiding injury, nursing semiprone, maintaining airway, and giving oxygen) should not be forgotten. Maternal renal, liver, and coagulation status should be monitored, together with the fetal condition if the eclampsia is prenatal. Fluid overload should be avoided. Most obstetricians deliver the fetus once the mother is stable if the eclampsia occurs during pregnancy (see Chapters 36 and 80).

SUMMARY OF MANAGEMENT OPTIONS

Neurologic Complications of Preeclampsia/Eclampsia

Management Options (See also Chapters 36 and 80)	Quality of Evidence	Strength of Recommendation	References
Prenatal, Labor and Delivery, Postnatal			
First-Aid Measures	Ia	A	240
Avoid injury			
Semiprone position			
Maintain airway			
Administer oxygen			
Monitor maternal and fetal condition			
Control and prevent recurrence of seizures; magnesium sulfate is the drug of choice	Ia	A	30
Treat hypertension	Ia	A	240
Avoid fluid overload	–	GPP	–
Check renal, liver, and coagulation status	–	GPP	–
Deliver when stable	–	GPP	–

Epilepsy

Maternal and Fetal Risks

Epilepsy is probably the most common serious neurologic problem faced by obstetricians. Approximately 1 million American women of childbearing age have epilepsy, delivering roughly 20,000 babies annually. Seizures during pregnancy have an incidence of 0.15% to 10%.[35,36] The interrelationship of maternal epilepsy, antiepileptic drug metabolism and pharmacodynamics, genetics, drug-induced embryopathies, and maternal behavior is complex and has led to considerable controversy concerning epilepsy in pregnancy.

One area of unresolved controversy involves the effect of pregnancy on seizure frequency.[37–39] Approximately one third of patient's will have an increase in frequency, whereas the remainder will experience no change or a decrease.[38] Some of the change can be attributed to physiologic changes and psychological stress associated with pregnancy.[40] These factors include increased steroid hormone levels, sleep deprivation, and metabolic changes. More commonly when seizure frequency increases, deliberate patient noncompliance secondary to fear of fetal drug effects is likely to blame.[41] The effect of pregnancy on epilepsy may be inferred from the women's seizure frequency before pregnancy. As a rule, the fewer the number of seizures occurring in the 9 months before conception, the less the risk of worsening epilepsy during pregnancy.[38,41] If the seizure frequency is at least one seizure monthly before pregnancy, then the probability of increased seizure frequency during pregnancy is high. This is in contrast to women having only one seizure during the 9 months before pregnancy. These patients have only a 25% risk of seizing during pregnancy.

Decreases in most antiepileptic drug (AED) levels occur during pregnancy and can affect seizure frequency.[42] Gastrointestinal absorption decreases, whereas hepatic and renal clearance increase for most AEDs. Albumin levels decrease, leading to lower total drug levels.[43] Pregnancy-associated changes in specific agents are described in Table 49–3. Postpartum these changes reverse, with a resultant increase in drug levels. In reality, the availability of serum drug level testing allows women to maintain prepregnancy therapeutic levels. When this is accomplished only 10% of patients will experience increased seizure frequency during pregnancy.[38]

The effects of AEDs on the fetus are complex and controversial.[44,45] The four most commonly used agents (carbamazepine, phenobarbital, phenytoin, and valproic acid) are known to cross the placenta and all are believed to

TABLE 49–3

Antiepileptic Drug Level Changes in Pregnancy Compared with Nonpregnant Baseline

DRUG	TOTAL DRUG LEVEL (%)	FREE DRUG LEVEL (%)
Phenytoin	–56*	–31
Phenobarbital	–55*	–50*
Carbamazepine	–42*	–28
Valproic acid	–39*	+25

*Significantly different from baseline ($P < 0.005$).
Adapted from Yerby MS et al. Antiepileptic drug disposition during pregnancy, Neurology 1992; 42 (Suppl 5): 12–16, in Degado-Escueta AV, Janz D, Beck-Mannagetta G (eds): *Pregnancy and Teratogenesis in Epilepsy*.

have teratogenic effects. The rate of congenital malformations in patients using these drugs is approximately two to three times that of infants of nonepileptic mothers (i.e., 6%–8% in epileptic pregnancies).[41] Thus, more than 90% of mothers taking AEDs during pregnancy will deliver normal children.

Additional factors have been linked to the increased rate of anomalies seen in patients using AEDs. Multiagent therapy appears to enhance malformation rates.[46] In addition, phenytoin,[47] primidone,[48] and carbamazepine[49] have been associated with patterns of malformation that are quite similar. Common anomalies include a mildly dysmorphic face and fingers with stubby distal phalanges and hypoplastic fingernails, suggesting a "fetal AED syndrome."[41] A genetic predisposition may play a role in development of these malformations. Such a link has been reported for the enzyme epoxide hydrolase. A reduction in the enzyme's activity was seen in amniocytes of fetuses who had findings of fetal hydantoin syndrome, but not in those lacking findings.[50] Further confusing the issue is evidence that some anomalies associated with AEDs are found in mothers with epilepsy who have not been exposed to these medications.[51]

Despite the etiologic uncertainty, individual drugs have been associated with specific anomalies. Cleft lip and palate, as well as cardiac and urogenital defects are reported with phenytoin. Spina bifida is found in 1% to 2% of patients taking valproic acid.[52] The malformation pattern associated with phenobarbital is similar to that seen with phenytoin. Carbamazepine was felt to be the safest of the AEDs, but recently it was associated with spina bifida at a rate of approximately 1%.[46] Developmentally, most children have normal motor function but may have some degree of cognitive dysfunction. The latter-observed abnormalities appear more likely to relate to seizures during pregnancy and lower levels of paternal education rather than AEDs.[53]

Coagulopathies have been reported in approximately half of all babies born to mothers taking phenobarbital, primidone, or phenytoin. A deficiency of vitamin K-dependent clotting factors is responsible. Few infants have clinical symptoms.[54]

Management Options

PREPREGNANCY

Ideally patients are seen prior to conception to optimize antiepileptic therapy. The patient should be evaluated for withdrawal of antiepileptic medications in conjunction with a neurologist. Some patients who have been seizure-free for longer than 2 years are potential candidates. However, other factors must also be considered before a decision is made. Age of onset, seizure type, electroencephalographic findings, and number of seizures occurring before control was achieved all affect the risk of recurrence.[55,56] If complete withdrawal is not possible or practical, monotherapy should be attempted to reduce the risk of fetal malformations. The drug chosen should be that which is most effective for a given seizure type.[41]

Those who will be continuing on AEDs should be counseled about the importance of seizure control and the current understanding of fetal risks for malformations. Such counseling may decrease the number of patients who inappropriately discontinue their medication. Initiation of folic acid supplementation should also be considered preconceptionally. Although there is no direct evidence of benefit in epileptic patients, the recommendation is based on findings demonstrating a decrease in recurrence of neural tube defects in women with a previously affected child. The goal of therapy is to maintain normal serum and red cell folate levels.[41]

PRENATAL

Patients on AEDs should have drug levels monitored. They should be maintained on the lowest effective dose. With valproic acid, multiple doses at intervals during the day are preferred. A fall in drug level is common and does not necessarily require an increase in dose. Decisions to change the drug dose should be based on the clinical status, with drug levels used to guide such changes. Free drug levels change to a lesser degree than the total levels and may be used to serially monitor the patient.[41] A targeted ultrasound examination should be performed in the second trimester to search for fetal anomalies. In addition, maternal serum alpha-fetoprotein screening or amniocentesis for alpha fetoprotein and acetylcholinesterase should be considered to screen for neural tube defects in patients taking valproate or carbamazepine. Vitamin K can be given to the mother during the final 4 weeks of gestation to decrease the risk of fetal coagulopathy.[41] Should seizures recur, short-acting benzodiazepines may be used acutely. Free serum levels should be rechecked and drug dosage optimized.

In recent years, the use of new AEDs has become widespread in patients with epilepsy. However, the alterations in the pharmacokinetics of these agents during pregnancy have not been adequately studied. Data are lacking for drugs such as gabapentin (GBP), topiramate (TPM), tiagabine (TGB), oxcarbazepine (OXC), levetiracetam (LEV), and zonisamide (ZNS), but no definitive adverse effects have been demonstrated in humans. All these drugs are classified as category C. Their use during pregnancy should be based on an evaluation of the benefits of the drug in a given patient versus the unknown potential for adverse outcome.

The majority of AEDs are characterized by significant increases in clearance during pregnancy.[57] Limited studies of the newer AEDs indicate similar extensive transplacental transfer (lamotrigine, OXC, TPM, and ZNS). Current recommendations are that ideal AED concentration should be established for each patient before conception and that monitoring of AED levels should be performed during each trimester and the last month of pregnancy.[57]

LABOR AND DELIVERY

Most patients with epilepsy are able to labor normally and achieve a vaginal delivery. Elective cesarean section may be considered in patients refractory to treatment during the third trimester or in those who exhibit status epilepticus with significant stress. During labor, repeated seizures that cannot be controlled or status epilepticus may require an operative delivery. Fetal asphyxia can occur with prolonged or repeated seizures. Cesarean delivery may also be considered when repeated absence or psychomotor seizures limit maternal awareness and ability to cooperate. Tonic-clonic seizures are seen in approximately 1% to 2% of women during labor. Lorazepam, a short-acting benzodiazepine, is the drug of choice for treating seizures acutely.[41] The drug is administered in 2 mg boluses every 5 minutes as necessary. Some use 5 to 10 mg boluses of diazepam as an alternative.

POSTNATAL

Antiepileptic drug levels must be monitored after delivery because reversal of the physiologic alterations causing a decline in levels during gestation leads to a rise postpartum. If the medication dose was increased during pregnancy, the regimen should be returned to that used prior to pregnancy to avoid toxicity. During the first postpartum day an additional 1% to 2% of women will have tonic-clonic convulsions. Again lorazepam is the agent of choice for acute control. New-onset seizures in the postpartum period require complete evaluation to rule out intracerebral hemorrhage, cortical vein thrombosis, infection, or eclampsia.

Neonates should be given vitamin K 1 mg IM after birth to prevent a coagulopathy. All AEDs can cross into the breast milk but breastfeeding is not contraindicated for most agents. The effects of diazepam on nursing infants are unknown, and it should be used with caution. Phenobarbital should only be used when no alternatives exist because neonatal sedation can occur along with neonatal withdrawal on weaning.[58]

Status Epilepticus

Maternal and Fetal Risks

Status epilepticus (SE) is defined as ongoing seizure activity lasting longer than 30 minutes or recurrent seizures without full recovery of consciousness between episodes. The actual incidence during pregnancy is unknown. The important causes are listed in Table 49–4. Predisposing factors include poor compliance with AEDs, CNS infections, trauma, and illicit drug use.[38] Status epilepticus represents a medical emergency. Most seizures are generalized tonic-clonic. During the tonic phase, contractions of the respiratory muscles impair adequate maternal oxygenation, leading to fetal hypoxia and asphyxia. During the convulsive phase, metabolic acidosis ensues. Rhabdomyolysis occurs and can lead to acute renal failure. After 30 minutes of continuous brain electrical activity, even in the absence of the metabolic derangements, irreversible neuronal injury can occur. The hippocampus and amygdala of the temporal lobe are particularly sensitive to permanent damage.[59] Trauma from recurrent seizure activity can result in preterm labor, rupture of membranes, abruptio placenta, and fetal death.[38]

TABLE 49–4

Causes of Prolonged Convulsions
Uncontrolled epilepsy
Eclampsia
Encephalitis
Meningitis
Cerebral tumor
Cerebral trauma
Drug withdrawal
Toxicity (e.g., heavy metals)
Metabolic disturbance
Cerebrovascular disease

Management Options

PRENATAL, LABOR AND DELIVERY, AND POSTNATAL

Diagnostic and therapeutic interventions should be performed simultaneously. A patent airway must be secured and supplemental oxygenation given. Hypotension should be avoided to prevent decreased cerebral perfusion pressure. Complete blood count with differential, electrolyte profile, blood urea nitrogen, creatinine, urine toxicology screen, and AED levels should be obtained. Cerebrospinal fluid (CSF) analysis is performed if meningoencephalitis is suspected.

Intravenous benzodiazepines are used acutely. Again lorazepam is the drug of choice. It is given in 2-mg boluses every 5 minutes. Simultaneously, the patient is loaded with phenytoin 18 mg/kg administered at a rate not exceeding 50 mg/min. The administration of intravenous valproic acid (20 mg/kg loading dose) is an alternative if phenytoin is otherwise contraindicated. The combination of phenytoin and benzodiazepines is effective in controlling 75% to 85% cases of status epilepticus. In those patients with persistent seizures, higher levels of phenytoin can be achieved with an additional 5 mg/kg. In refractory cases where barbiturates or a continuous infusion of benzodiazepines are needed, elective intubation is required to protect the airway. Continuous electroencephalographic monitoring should also be initiated. Once identified, the underlying cause should be treated.

SUMMARY OF MANAGEMENT OPTIONS

Epilepsy

Management Options	Quality of Evidence	Strength of Recommendation	References
Prepregnancy			
Regular check of clinical control and serum anticonvulsant levels	Ia	A	41,241
Adjust anticonvulsant dose to control seizures with serum levels as a guide; avoid toxic doses.	Ia	A	41,241
Folate supplementation	Ia	A	241
Status Epilepticus			
First-aid measures (see "Preeclampsia/Eclampsia")	–	GPP	–
Investigate and treat simultaneously.	Ia	A	241
Control convulsions:			
-Anticonvulsant drugs (IV benzodiazepine as boluses plus either IV phenytoin or IV magnesium if eclampsia is the cause).	Ia	A	41,241
-Ventilate while maintaining anticonvulsants if anticonvulsants alone fail to control seizures.	–	GPP	–
Avoid hypertension.	–	GPP	–
Prenatal			
Regular check of clinical control and serum anticonvulsant levels	Ia	A	41,57,241
Adjust anticonvulsant dose to control seizures with serum levels as a guide; avoid toxic doses.	Ia	A	41,241
Detailed fetal anomaly scan at 20 weeks	Ia	A	41,241
Short-acting benzodiazepine acutely if seizures recur	Ia	A	41,241
Information about safety of more recent anticonvulsants is lacking	IV	C	57
Labor and Delivery			
Continue anticonvulsant medication.	–	GPP	
Short-acting benzodiazepine acutely if seizures recur	Ia	A	41,241
Postnatal			
Examine newborn to confirm normality.	–	GPP	–
Vitamin K to newborn	–	GPP	–
Monitor seizure control and serum levels; dose adjustment may be necessary.	Ia	A	41,241

CEREBROVASCULAR DISEASE

Ischemic Stroke and Transient Ischemic Attacks

Maternal and Fetal Risks

For many years it was believed that the incidence of cerebral ischemia is significantly higher during pregnancy. Currently, controversy exists because the evidence is inconclusive.[60] What seems clear from a recent epidemiologic study is that the relative risk of stroke rises to 8.7 during the postpartum period. In that same population-based report the relative risk of stroke during gestation was found to be 0.7.[61] The incidence of pregnancy-associated ischemic stroke is approximately 3 to 4 cases/100,000/yr.[62] For reasons that are unclear, middle cerebral artery occlusions may be overrepresented during pregnancy and internal carotid artery occlusions during the postpartum period.

Most of the conditions associated with "stroke in the young" are shared by pregnant women suffering cerebral ischemia and therefore demand an extensive diagnostic evaluation to identify the cause and provide optimal treatment. The causes can be divided into processes that involve the "ABCs" of stroke: arteries, blood components, and cardiac sources of emboli. A detailed list of specific causes is given in Table 49–5.

Premature or accelerated atherosclerosis accounts for almost 25% of ischemic strokes in pregnant women.

TABLE 49–5

Causes of Stroke in Pregnancy

Arteriopathies
Atherosclerosis
Arterial dissection
Moyamoya disease
Takayasu's arteritis
Fibromuscular dysplasia
Syphilis
Chronic meningitis
Systemic lupus erythematosus
Pregnancy-related intimal hyperplasia
Hematologic Disorders
Sickle hemoglobinopathies
Antiphospholipid antibody syndrome
Thrombtic thrombocytopenic purpura
Protein C, S, or antithrombin III deficiency
Activated protein C resistance
Paroxysmal nocturnal hemoglobinuria
Polycythemia vera
Thrombocytosis
Leukemia
Systemic malignancy
Disseminated intravascular coagulation
Cardioembolism
Valvular disease
Mitral valve prolapse
Atrial septal defect with paradoxical embolism
Atrial fibrillation
Subacute bacterial endocarditis
Nonbacterial thrombotic endocarditis
Peripartum cardiomyopathy

Women with hypertension, diabetes mellitus, tobacco use, hyperlipidemia, and family history of premature atherosclerotic disease are especially at risk for this stroke mechanism. Identification and treatment of these factors may have contributed to the decline in cerebrovascular events noted in pregnant women.

Less common vascular causes include arterial dissection during labor and delivery,[63] inflammatory arteritis such as Takayasu's arteritis,[64] and fibromuscular dysplasia. The last of these has been associated with cerebral ischemia as well as intracranial aneurysms, carotid artery dissection, and carotid-cavernous fistula.[62,63] Fibromuscular dysplasia appears to occur more commonly in young women and may also affect the renal arteries.[65]

Physiologic alterations seen in pregnancy may theoretically predispose the pregnant woman to develop cerebral ischemia. Increases in clotting factors, including fibrinogen, increased platelet aggregability, decreased antithrombin III concentration,[66,67] and impaired fibrinolytic activity, all occur during normal pregnancy.[68,69] These changes persist through the first several postpartum weeks and may be the only identifiable predisposing risk factors during pregnancy. The risk of thrombosis due to congenital deficiencies in antithrombin III, protein C, or protein S is compounded by pregnancy (see also Chapter 42). Activated protein C resistance is a recently identified cause of thrombosis resulting from a point mutation in factor V, rendering it resistant to inactivation by activated protein C. The abnormal factor V is called factor V Leiden and is the most common hereditary cause of thrombosis.[70] The Leiden mutation may be a risk factor for stroke during pregnancy.[71] It has also been identified in neonates with cerebral ischemic or hemorrhagic infarct and placental infarcts.[72] Thrombotic thrombocytopenic purpura may initially present during pregnancy and is often mistaken for eclampsia.[73]

Substance abuse is an under-recognized cause of stroke, especially in poor, urban woman (see also Chapter 35). Cocaine (Fig. 49–2), amphetamines, heroin, and other sympathomimetics are associated with both ischemic and hemorrhagic stroke.[74–76] Mechanisms of injury include vasospasm (Fig. 49–3), vasculitis, endocarditis, drug-induced cardiomyopathy with cerebral embolism, foreign material embolism, rupture of preexisting arteriovenous malformations (AVMs) and aneurysms, and acute hypertensive hemorrhage.

Antiphospholipid antibody syndrome is also associated with cerebral arterial occlusive disease (Fig. 49–4) (See also Chapter 44).[77] The syndrome consists of venous or arterial thrombosis, recurrent pregnancy loss, or thrombocytopenia in the presence of antiphospholipid antibodies (lupus anticoagulant or anticardiolipin).[78–82] Some of these patients have coexistent systemic lupus erythematosus. Patients with higher titers of IgG anticardiolipin antibodies may be at higher risk for recurrent thrombo-occlusive events.[83,84]

Sickle cell disease and sickle cell trait are associated with an increased risk of stroke. Vessel wall injury may

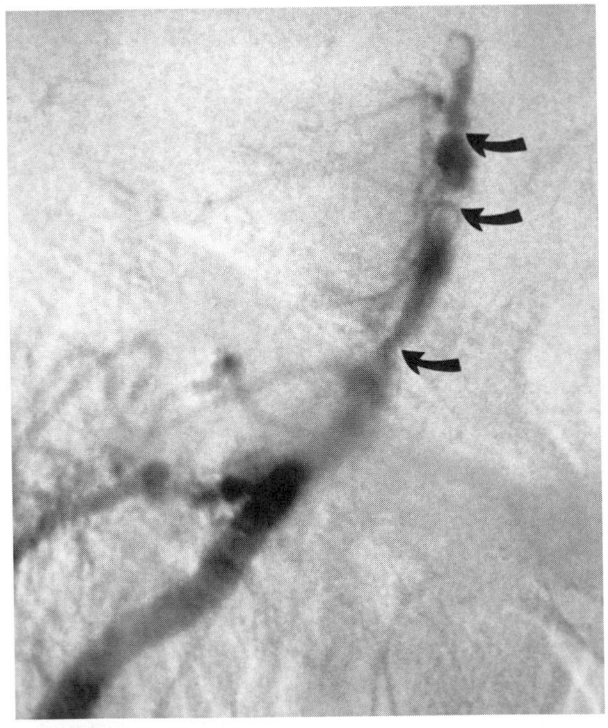

FIGURE 49–2
Conventional cerebral angiography in a young cocaine user showing severe basilar artery irregularities, stenosis, and filling defects (*arrows*).

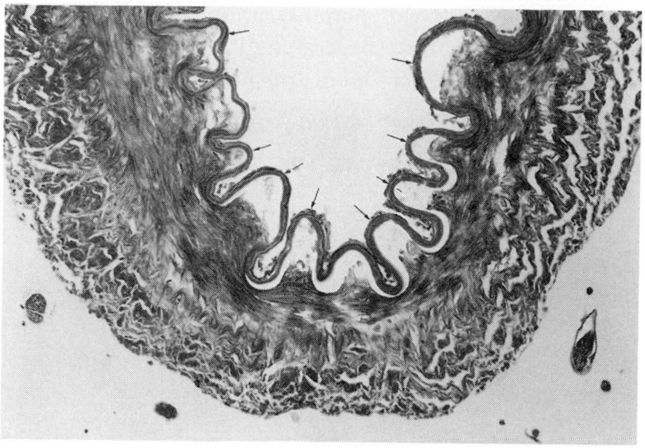

FIGURE 49–3
Histopathology of a cerebral vessel showing an excessively corrugated internal elastic lamina (*arrows*) separated from the media seen after presumably prolonged vasospasm in a young mother with a massive stroke from crack cocaine use.

occur during periods of crises. The recurrent vascular damage can lead to endothelial proliferation and subsequent vessel occlusion.[85] Frequent blood transfusions can dramatically reduce the vessel damage.

Congestive heart failure during pregnancy or the postpartum period is associated with significant maternal morbidity and mortality (see also Chapter 39). Pulmonary or systemic emboli occur in as many as 50% of these patients. Peripartum cardiomyopathy and rheumatic heart disease are causes of congestive heart failure in pregnancy. Emboli result from ventricular wall thrombosis secondary to a low cardiac output or atrial thrombosis from atrial fibrillation.[86] Watershed infarction in the brain has also been reported secondary to low cardiac output.[87]

Cerebral embolism has been associated with mitral valve prolapse (MVP) in case reports.[88] MVP is a common condition with a prevalence of 2% to 4% in the general population and as high as 20% in reproductive age women.[89] The rarity of stroke in pregnancy makes it unlikely to be a significant complication for pregnant women with MVP. Complications associated with atrial septal defects (ASD) are uncommon in reproductive-age women. However, ASD been found in up to 50% of young patients with unexplained ischemic stroke.[90] Paradoxic emboli from the venous to systemic circulation are responsible. Mechanical heart valves may also cause stroke in pregnant women, secondary to emboli from valve thrombosis.[91,92] Bacterial endocarditis can also result in ischemic or hemorrhagic stroke.[93] Cardiac disease associated with systemic lupus erythematosus and antiphospholipid syndrome represents another potential cause.[94]

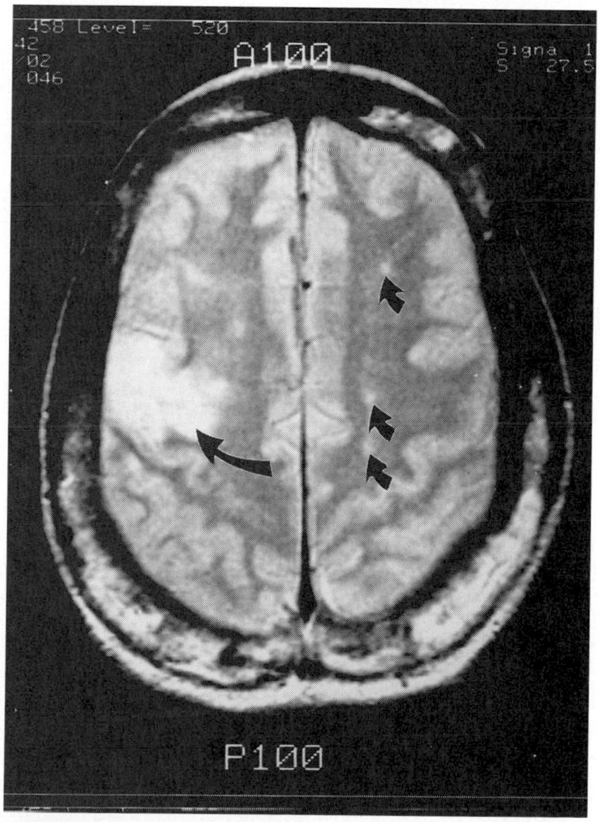

FIGURE 49–4
Axial head MRI (proton-weighted) of a young woman with the antiphospholipid syndrome including recurrent miscarriages, a right middle cerebral artery infarct (*long arrow*), and multiple smaller ischemic lesions in the left cerebral hemisphere (*short arrows*) can be seen.

Management Options

PRENATAL, LABOR, DELIVERY, AND POSTNATAL

Any focal neurologic deficit in the pregnant woman, transient (<24 hr) or persistent, should raise the suspicion of cerebral ischemia. A careful history and physical examination often give enough information to narrow the diagnostic evaluation. An early imaging study of the brain is essential to exclude hemorrhage or a mass lesion. CT is not contraindicated in pregnancy under these circumstances. Abdominal shielding limits the minimal fetal radiation exposure. MRI can also be used during pregnancy. Although it is more sensitive than a CT scan, it is tolerated less well by critically ill patients and is often less available.

Initial blood work should include a complete blood count with differential and platelet counts, electrolytes, serum glucose, blood urea nitrogen, creatinine, prothrombin time/activated partial thromboplastin time (aPTT). Antinuclear antibody, lupus anticoagulant and anticardiolipin antibody, rheumatoid factor, VDRL, and HIV testing should be obtained. Other blood studies include protein C and S and antithrombin III assays, activated protein C resistance and polymerase chain reaction for factor V Leiden, along with serum protein and hemoglobin electrophoresis. Blood and urine toxicology evaluation should be obtained. Carotid and transcranial Doppler should be considered. If cardiac origin is suspected, an electrocardiograph, echocardiogram, Holter monitor, and possibly evaluation for deep venous thrombosis can be performed. A lumbar puncture may also be indicated. In the absence of identified cause, cerebral angiography is recommended. Despite a thorough evaluation, the cause of ischemic stroke is elusive in 20% to 40% of nonpregnant patients. Although no specific data are currently available, this probably holds true for pregnant patients as well.

Many of the thrombotic and embolic conditions leading to stroke require either prophylactic or therapeutic anticoagulation. When anticoagulation is deemed necessary, heparin is the agent of choice in most instances. Warfarin is an option, but first-trimester embryopathy and the potential for fetal hemorrhage limit its usefulness. Heparin does not cross the placenta and is shorter acting than warfarin. This decreases fetal risk while making peripartum management easier and more predictable. Complications associated with heparin include thrombocytopenia and osteopenia, in addition to bleeding.[95,96]

Prophylactic doses of heparin tend to need to be higher in pregnancy and increase with increasing gestational age.[97] Typical doses are 7500 to 10,000 IU/mL, given subcutaneously every 12 hours. As in the nonpregnant patient, full anticoagulation aims to maintain the aPTT 1.5 times control. Therapy is individualized with subcutaneous heparin two to three times daily.

Low-molecular-weight heparin is now commonly used in pregnancy. Advantages over unfractionated heparin include longer duration of action, more reliable antithrombotic effect, and a suggestion of decreased risk of thrombocytopenia and osteopenia.[98,99] Increasing data on use during pregnancy suggest it is safe and effective in preventing noncerebral thrombotic complications.[100,101] Treatment of acute ischemic stroke with low-molecular-weight heparin is of uncertain benefit. Patients with inherited thrombophilias requiring full anticoagulation before pregnancy should be placed on therapeutic doses of heparin preconceptually or once pregnancy is discovered. The optimal therapy for activated protein C resistance during pregnancy is unknown, but likely should at least utilize prophylactic doses of heparin. Optimal treatment for the antiphospholipid antibody syndrome is a matter of current investigation. Some authors recommend the use of low-dose aspirin (60–80 mg/day) and heparin during the pregnancy.[78,79] The role of corticosteroids, immunosuppression or plasma exchange, and intravenous gamma globulin is not well defined.[102] In patients with cardiomyopathy or atrial fibrillation, heparin has been used in both prophylactic and therapeutic doses.[103]

Thrombolytic therapy for acute ischemic stroke is indicated in carefully selected patients within 180 minutes of symptom onset using a defined protocol.[104] Its use in pregnancy is uncertain, however, because pregnant or lactating women were excluded from the trial that demonstrated efficacy. Recent case reports have documented the relative safety of intravenous and intra-arterial thrombolysis used for neurologic and medical indications during early pregnancy.[105] Nevertheless, the widespread use of thrombolytics during pregnancy cannot be recommended, and they should only be used after a careful discussion of the risks and benefits of this form of treatment with the patient or surrogates. Plasmapheresis has been used successfully in some patients with thrombotic thrombocytopenic purpura.[106]

Cerebrovenous Thrombosis

Maternal and Fetal Risks

Cerebrovenous thrombosis has been traditionally associated with pregnancy, especially the puerperium. The condition is seen throughout gestation[107–109] but most commonly is identified during the second to third week postpartum.[107] The incidence is highest in developing countries where it is the most common cause of stroke associated with pregnancy. The original description of severe headache, papilledema, and seizures has evolved through the years. Additional findings at presentation include focal neurologic deficits, bilateral long tract signs, aphasia, visual disturbances, headache, focal seizures and the syndrome of idiopathic intracranial hypertension. When the deep cerebral venous system is involved, lethargy and coma are common. The superficial venous sinuses, particularly the superior sagittal sinus, are commonly involved.

Cerebrovenous thrombosis has classically been associated with infection and dehydration. Other underlying conditions such as hemoglobinopathies, hyperviscosity syndromes, anemia, leukemia, collagen vascular diseases, malignancy, AVM, and paroxysmal nocturnal hemoglobinuria should be sought.[110] In addition, hypercoagulable states such as protein C and S deficiencies have been implicated.[69,111] More recently, activated protein C resistance,[112,113] lupus anticoagulants, and anticardiolipin antibodies have been identified in patients with cerebrovenous thrombosis.[114–116]

Management Options

PRENATAL, LABOR, DELIVERY, AND POSTNATAL

Timely diagnosis of cerebrovenous thrombosis requires a high index of suspicion. During pregnancy the initial evaluation begins with a brain CT without contrast. A partially filled posterior segment of the superior sagittal sinus is seen (empty delta sign) (Fig. 49–5). MRI with MR venography can identify the thrombus. It provides greater sensitivity and is currently the test of choice within the limitations previously described.

The only prospective, randomized, case-controlled study evaluating acute treatment found systemic anticoagulation to be the treatment of choice, even in the presence of intracerebral hemorrhage.[117] Thrombolytic therapy is an emergent therapeutic approach; however, due to the lack of experience in pregnant patients, caution should be exercised.[118] The overall prognosis is generally good in the absence of coma, recurrent seizures, or rapid decline in neurologic function. Long-term outcome is generally better than for arterial stroke. Prolonged anticoagulation with warfarin is required postpartum.

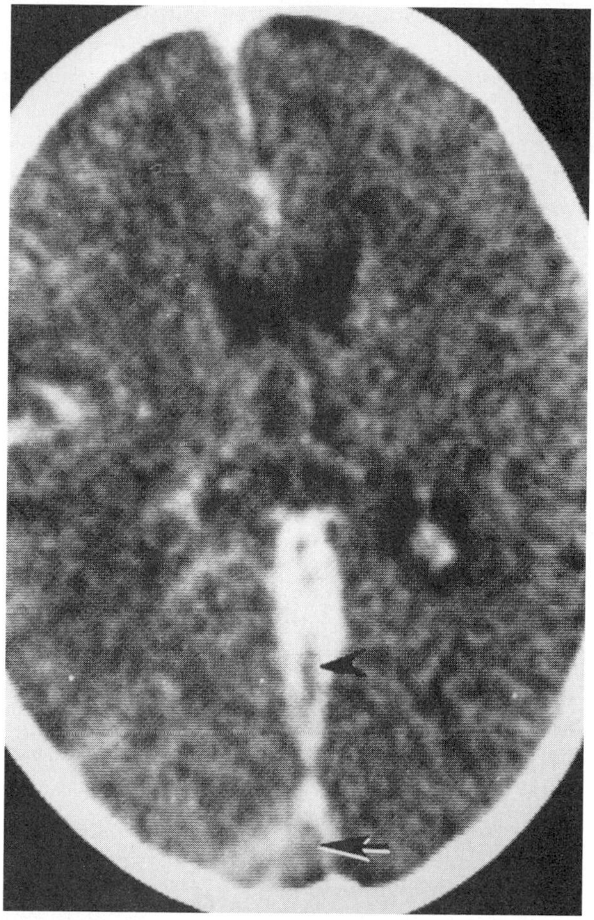

FIGURE 49–5
Axial head CT scan demonstrating cerebrovenous thrombosis of the straight sinus (*arrowhead*) and the empty delta sign (*arrow*).

Subarachnoid Hemorrhage in Pregnancy

Maternal and Fetal Risks

Subarachnoid hemorrhage (SAH) is a rare but often catastrophic event that can occur during pregnancy. The incidence of SAH is 1 to 5/10 000 pregnancies. Maternal mortality is 30% to 40%, but rates as high as 80% have been reported.[119] Fetal outcome parallels that of the mother and reflects the maternal condition and gestational age at delivery.[119] The primary cause during gestation is ruptured cerebral aneurysms or AVMs. Less common causes include moyamoya disease,[120] dural venous sinus thrombosis, mycotic aneurysm, choriocarcinoma, vasculitides, brain tumors,[121] and coagulopathies. Drugs such as cocaine and phenylpropanolamine have been linked with SAH in pregnant patients.[122–124]

Aneurysms and AVMs are believed to develop secondary to congenital defects in cerebral vasculature formation. Aneurysms are generally located at an angle of vessel bifurcation in or near the circle of Willis. AVMs, on the other hand, can be located anywhere between the frontal region and the brainstem, but occur with a higher frequency in the frontoparietal and temporal regions (Fig. 49–6). The anatomic distribution of both lesions is similar to that in the nongravid population.[119]

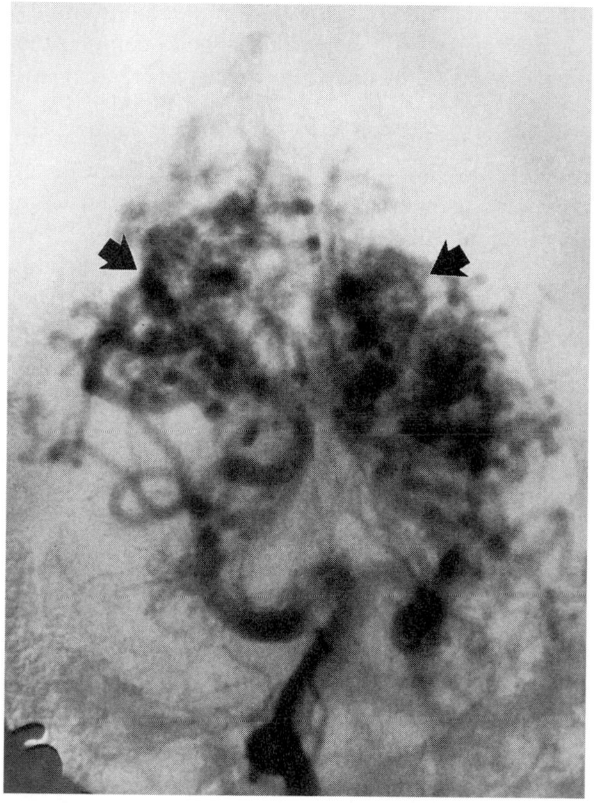

FIGURE 49–6
Conventional cerebral angiography documenting large, bilateral cerebral AVMs (*arrows*).

Information describing the natural history of intracranial aneurysms during pregnancy is scarce. In the nonpregnant patient asymptomatic lesions account for 95% of intracranial aneurysms and are typically identified incidentally. They rupture at a rate of 1% to 2% per year.[125] Activities reported to precede aneurysmal rupture include emotional strain, heavy lifting, coughing, coitus, urination, and defecation. Outcomes of patients with AVMs are influenced by the presenting symptoms and subsequent treatment. Most present with spontaneous bleeding, and these patients have the worst prognosis. Other presenting symptoms in order of frequency include seizures, headache, and neurologic deficit. If left untreated there is an annual hemorrhage rate of 4%.[125]

Rarely, unruptured aneurysms are first identified during pregnancy. Because SAH is uncommon during gestation, the effect of pregnancy on cerebral aneurysms or AVMs is controversial. More than 85% of SAH cases occur during the second or third trimester.[126] Several physiologic changes occur during pregnancy, which may theoretically predispose these cerebrovascular abnormalities to bleed. These factors include increases in blood volume, stroke volume, and cardiac output. Estrogen levels are also increased and may result in vasodilation of already abnormal vessels.[127] The many dynamic events occurring during labor and delivery would seem to make this a time of particularly high risk.

Despite the associated physiologic changes, pregnancy does not appear to increase the incidence of SAH, and, surprisingly, bleeding during the time of labor and delivery is infrequent.[119,128] Most pregnancies complicated by SAH are preceded by unaffected gestations. In a review of 154 patients prepared by Dias and Sekhar only 25% were nulliparous, and the mean parity of patients with aneurysmal and AVM ruptures were 2.0 and 1.4, respectively.[119] Barno and Freeman reviewed 24 years of maternal mortality in Minnesota resulting from SAH. The mean parity among the 37 deaths was 2.9.[129] Forster and colleagues reported their experience with AVMs in reproductive-age women. Although the annual hemorrhage rate was higher when these women were pregnant than when not (9.3% vs. 4.5%), it was no different from the 9.6% annual rate in reproductive age women who never became pregnant.[128] Although Horton and associates identified a lower annual rate of hemorrhage in both pregnant and nonpregnant patients with AVMs (3.5% vs. 3.1%), they too concluded that pregnancy was not a risk factor for bleeding.[130]

Once bleeding has occurred, the patient's course is significantly modified by her neurologic condition at presentation. The Hunt and Hess classification system has prognostic implications and is shown in Table 49–6. Left untreated, half of all nonpregnant patients will die as a result of the initial event, with another 25% to 35% succumbing to a subsequent bleed. Other factors affecting the patient's ultimate outcome are neurologic status, presence of vasospasm, and blood pressure. Maternal mortality rates associated with aneurysmal bleeding do not increase due to pregnancy.[119] Conversely, AVM-associated mortality appears to be increased in gravid compared with nongravid patients. This is likely related to the poor neurologic condition of these patients at presentation.[119]

Pregnancy does not significantly alter the clinical presentation of SAH. Signs and symptoms of aneurysmal or AVM bleeding are indistinguishable. A sudden-onset, "bursting" headache is generally the initial symptom. Frequently other signs and symptoms accompany the headache, which may include nausea and vomiting, meningeal signs, decreased level of consciousness, hypertension, focal neurologic signs, and seizures. Specific findings depend on the size, location, and rapidity of the bleed. When the hemorrhage is massive, the patient may be moribund at presentation.

TABLE 49–6

Hunt and Hess Scale for Grading the Clinical Severity of Subarachnoid Hemorrhage

GRADE	EXAMINATION FINDINGS
I	Normal neurologic examination, mild headache, and slightly stiff neck
II	Moderate-to-severe headache and stiff neck; no confusion or neurologic deficit except for cranial nerve palsy
III	Persistent confusion and/or focal deficit
IV	Persistent stupor; moderate to severe neurologic deficit
V	Coma with moribund appearance

Major complications associated with SAH include vasospasm and recurrent hemorrhage. Vasospasm is a serious problem seen in 30% to 40% of aneurysm patients, but much less commonly in those with AVMs. The resultant ischemia is a major cause of permanent disability and death. Recurrent hemorrhage is a particularly morbid complication. In the untreated nonpregnant patient the risk of rebleeding is 6% during the first 48 hours. Rebleeding continues to occur at a rate of 1.5% per day for the remainder of the first 2 weeks.[125] Mortality increases with each successive bleed with a rate of 64% and 80% after the first and second rebleed, respectively. Although considerably fewer data are available for the pregnant patient, the risk of recurrent bleeding appears to be similar in this population.[126]

Management Options

PRENATAL

Due to the rare and life-threatening nature of the condition, it is important to maintain a high index of suspicion. Occasionally SAH is confused with eclampsia, resulting in diagnostic delays and often a worse outcome. All abnormal neurologic signs and symptoms in the gravid patient should be thoroughly evaluated. CT scan of the brain, lumbar puncture (if necessary), and cerebral angiography is the common sequence of testing. The CT scan can predict, with a high degree of accuracy, the type of hemorrhage and its site of origin. If the CT scan is normal, the CSF should be examined for blood or xanthochromia. Nonclearing bloody CSF found at lumbar puncture supports the diagnosis of SAH, but it may also be seen with other conditions such as preeclampsia. Cerebral angiography remains the best diagnostic tool for identifying any vascular abnormality. Angiography may fail to visualize the cause of SAH in 20% of patients, however. In these cases, a repeat angiogram may be necessary to rule out false-negative results secondary to vasospasm or clot filling of the aneurysm. MRI scan may also be helpful when the initial angiogram fails to identify the lesion. Abdominal shielding should be considered during any radiologic examination of the gravid patient.

Management of SAH is based on standard neurosurgical principles with only slight alterations during pregnancy. The clinical goals remain prevention and treatment of neurologic complications. Early aneurysm clipping (<4 d) is now commonly recommended in the post-SAH period for conscious patients. Early operation also allows for therapies such as induced hypertension and volume expansion to be instituted to combat vasospasm without increasing the risk of rebleeding. Improved outcomes for both the mother and the fetus have been realized with early surgical intervention in pregnant patients.[119] Patients with significant neurologic deficits are less likely to undergo early aneurysm clipping due to an extremely high likelihood of operative mortality. Recent advances with endovascular procedures in the treatment of cerebral aneurysms (e.g., Guglielmi coiling) allow the early securing of these vascular lesions in high risk patients.[131] Medical therapy alone and careful monitoring of these high risk patients remain an alternative to any intervention if the patient is too unstable to leave the ICU.

The proper timing for resection of AVMs is more controversial due to the smaller number of cases. No clear benefit to surgery in these patients has been found,[119] with some surgeons advocating operative intervention in AVMs only to remove clinically significant hematomas.[132] One alternative is embolization of the AVM under angiographic control prior to surgical excision.[133]

A complete discussion of the neurosurgical and anesthetic principles of craniotomy for aneurysm clipping is beyond the scope of this chapter. However, two intraoperative therapies—hypotension and hypothermia—are commonly instituted to reduce complications, which raise special concerns in the pregnant patient. Hypotension is sometimes instituted to reduce the risk of rupture of the aneurysm during surgical dissection. Although maternal hypotension may pose a threat to fetal well-being, it has been successfully induced with sodium nitroprusside or isoflurane in a number of cases.[134,135] Based on experimental evidence, administration of sodium nitroprusside in pregnant patients has raised concerns regarding potential fetal cyanide toxicity. Thus, if surgery is to be performed during pregnancy it is recommended that infusion rates not exceed 10 mg/kg/min.[135] The fetal effects of maternal hypotension should be evaluated throughout the perianesthetic period with electronic fetal heart rate monitoring. Adverse changes in fetal cardiac activity suggest the need for elevation in maternal blood pressure if safe and feasible from the maternal standpoint. Many of the drugs used in anesthesia may decrease fetal heart rate variability, thereby complicating interpretation of the fetal heart rate monitor data. Excessive hyperventilation further decreases uterine blood flow during sodium nitroprusside administration and should be avoided.[136] Because of the potential fetal risks of maternal hypotension, some authors recommend cesarean delivery immediately prior to intracranial surgery if the fetus is mature enough.[137]

Hypothermia is instituted during cerebral aneurysm clipping as a means of cerebral protection from potential ischemia due to aneurysm rupture, retraction injury, or hypotension. Stange and Halldin suggested that hypothermia is well tolerated by the mother and fetus, provided that other confounding variables (e.g., respiratory exchange, acidosis, and electrolyte balance) are controlled.[138] However, most experience with hypothermia and hypotension in pregnancy is anecdotal. Regardless of the neurosurgical technique used, maternal outcome is the most important predictor of eventual fetal outcome.

Adjunctive medical therapy for SAH is directed toward reducing the risks of rebleeding and cerebral ischemia due to vasospasm. Patients are generally confined to bed rest in a dark, quiet room. They are administered stool softeners and analgesics. Because of the presumed benefits of volume expansion, colloid solutions are frequently administered. Nimodipine, a dihydropyridine calcium channel blocker, is often given because it has been shown to improve neurologic outcome following SAH. Caution is advised in using this drug in pregnancy because the fetal effects have not been completely defined. In a small number of preeclamptic patients taking nimodipine for seizure prophylaxis no apparent adverse fetal outcomes were reported.[139] However, in an animal model, nicardipine (another dihydropyridine calcium channel blocker) led to the development of fetal acidosis and hypoxemia.[140]

ε-Aminocaproic acid (EACA) and tranexamic acid have been used to block the activation of plasminogen, a precursor of plasmin, a major fibrinolytic protein, and decrease the incidence of rebleeding. Initial clinical trials did find a reduction in the incidence of rebleeding with these agents; however, later work failed to demonstrate significant improvement in outcome.[141] EACA, because of the lack of proven benefit and potential interference with fetal fibrinolysis, which may be linked to the development of hyaline membrane disease, is not used in current clinical practice.[142]

Cerebral edema can result in elevated ICP. Intracranial invasive monitoring may be necessary. If the ICP elevation is secondary to cerebral edema, mannitol, an osmotic diuretic, may be used. Typically, 1 g/kg of mannitol is administered intravenously, as frequently as needed to keep the ICP below 20 mm Hg. The development of hyperosmolality due to dehydration is a potential hazard of mannitol therapy and can be monitored by frequent determinations of the patient's intravascular volume status. Normal values are 280 to 300 mOsm/L; the drug should be withheld when a level of 315 to 320 mOsm/L is reached. Care must be taken to prevent hypovolemia resulting from the accompanying diuresis, which could aggravate both cerebral and placental hypoperfusion. The use of hypertonic saline solutions (2% and 3% sodium chloride/acetate) is becoming a popular alternative to mannitol due to their efficacy and hemodynamic profile. Nevertheless, their safety during pregnancy is not defined, and the use of these solutions should be limited to only extreme cases of refractory ICP elevation.

LABOR AND DELIVERY

After a successful repair of an aneurysm or AVM, the most frequent obstetric concern relates to mode of delivery. Earlier authors routinely recommended elective cesarean section for these patients. This was particularly true along with consideration of sterilization if an AVM was responsible for the SAH.[143] More recent data and reanalysis of some older studies suggest that labor and vaginal delivery pose no additional risk to mother or fetus.[119,128,130,144] These recommendations probably also hold true for the patient who begins labor before surgical correction is attempted or when the intracranial lesion is inaccessible to surgical intervention, but the data are limited. Young and colleagues have suggested that the rise in physiologic blood pressure known to occur in labor are counterbalanced by a parallel increase in CSF pressure, offering a potential explanation for the foregoing clinical observations.[145] Most authorities still advocate minimizing the hemodynamic stresses of labor, however, by using epidural anesthesia and shortening the second stage of labor with outlet forceps.[146,147] Ultimate management decisions should be individualized based primarily on the maternal condition with modifications for fetal intervention based on gestational age.

SUMMARY OF MANAGEMENT OPTIONS

Cerebrovascular Disease

Management Options	Quality of Evidence	Strength of Recommendation	References
Ischemic Stroke (arterial) and Transient Ischemic Attacks (TIAs)			
General supportive measures (see Chapter 80)	–	GPP	–
Search for cause/associated factors:	III	B	61,62
Investigate CBC, clotting and thrombophilia screen, renal and liver function routinely; other investigations determined by possible cause:			
Treat thrombolic/embolic conditions (see Chapters 41, 42 and 80):			
Cause unknown in 20–40%			
Consider anticoagulation with heparin if no evidence of hemorrhage on MRI or CT	III	B	61,62
Indications for surgery are as for nonpregnant patients.	III	B	61,62
Cerebral Venous Thrombosis			
Control seizures.	III	B	107,111
Ensure adequate hydration.	III	B	107
One randomized case-controlled study suggests anticoagulation beneficial.	Ib	A	117
No experience in pregnancy with thrombolytic therapy.	III	B	118
Subarachnoid Hemorrhage			
Diagnosis			
(following high index of clinical suspicion) by, in order,	IV	C	147
CT scan			
Lumbar puncture			
Cerebral angiography (or MRI)			
Management—Prenatal			
Interdisciplinary care with neurosurgeons	–	GPP	–
In general, normal neurosurgical principles of management apply in pregnancy, though care needed intraoperatively with:			
Hypotension	IV	C	133–135
Hypothermia	IV	C	138
Anticonvulsants, high dose steroids, mannitol and nimodipine (safe in limited pregnancy experience) are used depending on clinical picture/problems.	IIb	B	139
Caution with EACA	Ia	A	141
Trend for early surgery	III	B	119,131
Embolization prior to or without surgery is a new development	IV	C	133

SUMMARY OF MANAGEMENT OPTIONS

Cerebrovascular Disease *(Continued)*

Management Options	Quality of Evidence	Strength of Recommendations	References
Management—Labor and Delivery			
Regional analgesics preferable to narcotics and general anesthetics	–	GPP	–
No evidence to support blanket policy of elective cesarean section, but most advocate:	III	B	119,128,130, 144,146,147
Minimize pushing in second stage.			
Cesarean section for normal obstetric reasons			
Consider life-support machine and care in patient with brain death to gain fetal maturity			

CBC, complete blood count; CT computed tomography; MRI, magnetic resonance imaging.

HEADACHE

Maternal Risks

Headaches during pregnancy are extremely common. The most common categories are migraine and tension-type. Although a new-onset headache during pregnancy is most likely either a migraine or tension-type, it may be the first manifestation of an intracranial process that needs immediate attention.[148–150] Such conditions include aneurysm rupture, AVM, intracranial hypertension, cerebral ischemia, cerebrovenous thrombosis, meningitis, sinusitis, and intracranial masses. In addition, benign intracranial hypertension or pseudotumor cerebri may be seen with pregnancy, but it is uncommon. Patients receiving spinal or epidural analgesia or anesthesia may experience a spinal headache during the postpartum period.

Evaluation of the pregnant patient with headache represents a clinical challenge. The ailment's prevalence and typically benign nature make it desirable to minimize costs by limiting diagnostic testing while being certain to promptly diagnose uncommon but more serious conditions. The medical history is usually very helpful. Migraines are often associated with a history of similar previous episodes. With a history suggestive of migraine headaches, a normal neurologic examination, and resolution with simple measures, the patient may be followed clinically. If a new-onset headache severe enough to justify an emergency room visit or a preexisting condition becomes progressively worse, an "aura" is present, or a neurologic deficit is identified, diagnostic evaluation is indicated.

Migraine

Maternal and Fetal Risk

Migraines can be subdivided into those with or without an aura. The aura is described as the presence of transient neurologic signs or symptoms before, during ,or even after the headache. The pain is often associated with nausea, vomiting, and photophobia. Sleep often provides relief. As with headaches in general during gestation, the course of migraines is variable. A decrease in frequency is seen in 50% to 80% of women, particularly in the third trimester.[151] Those patients experiencing migraines associated with menstruation are especially likely to show improvement. The headaches tend to worsen postpartum, with as many as 40% of patients complaining of pain during this time. Migraine recurred during the first week after childbirth in about one third of women.[152] Migraines may present for the first time during the puerperium in 4.5% of patients, however, and an aura may initially appear during this time period.[153] No demonstrated adverse fetal outcome is associated with migraines.[154]

Management Options

PRENATAL, LABOR, DELIVERY, AND POSTNATAL

A carefully obtained history and physical exam are essential. With a prior personal or family history of migraine and a typical presentation, no further investigation is needed. New-onset migraines represent a diagnosis of exclusion. In the absence of a past history or with focal neurologic findings, neuroimaging studies such as brain CT or MRI are indicated.[151] It is desirable to minimize abdominal and pelvic exposure to x-rays and avoid contrast agents if possible. Radiologic studies should not be avoided on the basis of pregnancy alone, however. Prothrombin time, aPTT, fibrinogen, and complete blood count with platelets should be obtained. Additional investigations should include anticardiolipin antibodies, antithrombin III, protein C, protein S, and activated protein C resistance to exclude thrombophilias. Lumbar puncture is indicated once the absence of an intracranial mass effect has been ruled out by imaging studies. A normal opening pressure (range 5–15 mm Hg) excludes pseudotumor cerebri.

Migraine treatment during pregnancy is complicated by the fact that most drugs cross the placenta and many have potentially adverse fetal effects. As a result, physicians often avoid indicated drug therapy, despite relatively safe and effective options.[151] Therapy can be divided into abortive and prophylactic measures. The latter approach is reserved for patients with debilitating headaches or those with a frequency, for example, exceeding three migraine episodes per month. Beta-blockers (category B and C) are often helpful in this situation. Tricyclic antidepressants (most category D) are a useful second-line approach.

A variety of interventions are available once a headache has begun. When normal daily function is not significantly compromised, nonpharmacologic measures are advised. Such strategies include coping mechanisms such as ice, massage, sleep, and biofeedback. Reassurance is also of value, as many migraine sufferers experience improvement during gestation. When drug therapy is needed, acetaminophen and low-dose caffeine (both category B) can be used as first-line agents. During the first two trimesters, a short course of nonsteroidal anti-inflammatory drugs (NSAIDs) can be tried (many are category B in early pregnancy). Extended use of NSAIDs should be avoided, however, because of potential constriction of the fetal ductus arteriosus and oligohydramnios, particularly late in gestation (category D in the third trimester). Narcotics such as meperidine, morphine, and hydromorphone (category B) can be used if severity warrants.[155] Glucocorticoids (category B) are safe when used for short periods and may help in migraines refractory to standard treatment.[156] Magnesium sulfate can be used for prophylactic or abortive therapy. Benzodiazepines (category D), ergot derivatives (category D), and sumatriptan as well as the newer triptans (category C) should be avoided.[157] Although the association of benzodiazepines with birth defects is not clear, neonatal depression and withdrawal may occur with use during the latter part of pregnancy. Vasoconstriction caused by ergot derivatives may lead to fetal vascular disruption. In addition, these agents may increase uterine activity by an oxytocin-like action. In the most extreme cases, intravenous hydration, prochlorperazine 10 mg IV, and intravenous narcotics or corticosteroids may be necessary.[151]

Nausea is a common accompanying complaint. Mild symptoms can usually be successfully treated with phosphorylated carbohydrate solution (Emetrol) or doxylamine succinate (category B) and pyridoxine (vitamin B_6). In more severe cases, trimethobenzamide (category C) and some phenothiazine compounds including chlorpromazine, prochlorperazine, and promethazine (all category C) can be used parenterally or as suppositories. Most of the medications described above enter the breast milk. Those that can be used in pregnancy can continue to be utilized during breastfeeding. Chlorpromazine is an exception, because it can cause neonatal lethargy.

Tension-Type Headaches

Maternal and Fetal Risks

Tension-type headaches are characterized by daily headaches of mild to moderate severity with a global distribution. They typically worsen throughout the day, and nausea and vomiting are seldom reported. Patients may exhibit symptoms such as depressed mood, anorexia, and insomnia. In contrast with migraine, tension-type headache symptoms do not improve during pregnancy and may actually worsen. The pathogenesis is unclear. Contracture of the neck muscles and stretching of aponeurotic connections may be the result rather than the cause of the headache. Characteristically, the neurologic exam is normal and no neuroimaging studies are required.

Treatment is aimed at behavioral aspects of the condition. Mild analgesics are indicated only when there is considerable pain. Acetaminophen is preferable to aspirin. If depression is a cardinal component, antidepressant agents can be used. Despite their classification, tricyclic antidepressants (most category D) appear to be relatively safe during pregnancy and can be used when clinically indicated. There is considerably less experience with the serotonin reuptake inhibitors (most category B). Available information suggests that these agents may also be used relatively safely when indicated.[158,159]

Spinal Headache

Maternal Risks and Management Options

Spinal headaches are commonly seen after accidental dural puncture during epidural placement. The typical history is that of a severe headache, which is exacerbated with sitting or standing and palliated with lying flat. The frequency of symptoms is related to the large-bore needle used. Such headaches less commonly follow the use of spinal anesthesia. The symptoms are believed to be due to leakage of CSF and subsequent CSF hypotension. Initial management consists of intravenous hydration and bed rest lying flat. If the patient fails to show improvement within 24 hours of conservative management, then a blood patch is indicated. About 2 to 3 mL of autologous blood are injected near the area of the dural puncture. Dramatic resolution of symptoms is typically observed.[160]

TABLE 49–7

Causes of Raised Intracranial Pressure

Benign intracranial hypertension
Cerebral edema
Hypertensive encephalopathy
Lead poisoning
Viral encephalitis
Impaired reabsorption CSF
Venous sinus thrombosis
High CSF protein
Guillain–Barré syndrome
Spinal cord tumor
Postmeningitis
Drugs
Hypervitaminosis A
Tetracycline
Indomethacin
Nitrofurantoin
Space-occupying lesion

CSF, cerebrospinal fluid.

Benign Intracranial Hypertension (Pseudotumor Cerebri)

Maternal Risks

Benign intracranial hypertension is characterized by diffuse global headache, nausea, vomiting, papilledema, and, at times, horizontal diplopia. It is typically worse during early morning hours. The cause of increased ICP is either increased production or decreased reabsorption of CSF.[161] This condition is more common in young, obese, reproductive-age women. There is no evidence that the incidence is higher during pregnancy. Although benign intracranial hypertension can develop throughout pregnancy, it is most often seen during the first half of gestation. Other causes of increased ICP are listed in Table 49–7.

Management Options

PRENATAL, LABOR, AND DELIVERY

The diagnosis is one of exclusion. It is confirmed by demonstrating a high opening pressure at the time of lumbar puncture in the presence of a normal CT scan. Although weight reduction is a part of treatment in nonpregnant individuals, it is not encouraged during pregnancy. However, excess weight gain should be avoided. Treatment is aimed at avoiding visual complications. Acetazolamide, a carbonic anhydrase inhibitor (category C), is used along with repeated lumbar puncture and CSF drainage. Refractory cases may be treated with a lumbar subarachnoid-peritoneal shunt. When vision is threatened, optic nerve sheath fenestration can be performed to relieve pressure on the optic nerve.

Cesarean section is reserved for obstetric indications. As lumbar puncture is a mainstay of treatment, regional anesthesia with either spinal or epidural is not contraindicated.

SUMMARY OF MANAGEMENT OPTIONS

Headache

Management Options	Quality of Evidence	Strength of Recommendation	References
General			
Indications for Further Investigation:	–	GPP	–
Focal/abnormal neurologic signs			
Impaired intellect			
Worsening and/or intractable pain			
Pain that disturbs sleep			
Migraine			
Avoid Precipitating Factors; Nonpharmacologic Measures:	IV	C	151,155
Bed rest			
Avoidance of light			
Coping mechanisms			
Ice			
Massage			
Sleep			

Continued

SUMMARY OF MANAGEMENT OPTIONS

Headache *(Continued)*

Management Options	Quality of Evidence	Strength of Recommendation	References
Migraine			
Analgesics			
Simple agents (e.g., acetaminophen)	IV	C	151,155
Short course of NSAIDs in first two trimesters but not third	IV	C	151,155
Narcotics (e.g., meperidine, morphine) for severe cases	IV	C	155
Short course adjuvant glucocorticoids for refractory cases. (AVOID: benzodiazepines, ergot preparations & sumatriptan)	IV	C	156,157
Prophylaxis	IV	C	151,155
Propranolol (Trial excluded pregnant women.)			
Tricyclic antidepressants			
Antiemetics	IV	C	151,155
Phenothiazines (Trial excluded pregnant women.)			
Tension Headaches			
Reassurance, bed rest	–	GPP	–
Simple analgesia			
Tricyclic antidepressants in extreme			
Spinal Headache			
No evidence that injection of physiologic saline at time of dural tap/puncture is of benefit	–	GPP	–
Analgesia	–	GPP	–
Lying flat	Ib	A	8
Autologous blood patch if analgesia and lying flat fail to work after 24 hr	Ib	A	8
Benign Intracranial Hypertension			
Exclude other causes of raised intracranial pressure.	–	GPP	–
Monitor visual function.	–	GPP	–
Avoid excess weight gain.	III	B	242
If evidence of visual function deterioration, consider			
Acetazolamide	III	B	242
Serial lumbar puncture	III	B	242
If these conservative measures fail: (Extrapolated from management in nonpregnant subjects)			
Shunting	–	GPP	–
Optic nerve sheath fenestration if vision is still threatened	–	GPP	–

VENTRICULOPERITONEAL SHUNTS

Maternal Risks

Advances in extracranial shunt technology during the 1960s improved the prognosis for patients with hydrocephalus. As a result, an increasing number of women with ventriculoperitoneal shunts in place are reaching reproductive age and becoming pregnant.[162] Pregnancy is associated with signs and symptoms of elevated ICP in as many as 58% of patients with previously well-functioning shunts.[163] Several case reports suggest that shunt malfunction is more common in the third trimester. The causes of the malfunctions have been postulated to be functional rather than mechanical, due to increased intraperitoneal pressure associated with advancing gestational age.[164]

Management Options

Prepregnancy

A baseline CT scan or MRI preconceptually may be of value. Further investigation is indicated if there is any suggestion of shunt malfunction.[163] The baseline study can also be of benefit for comparison purposes in the diagnostic evaluation of symptoms suggestive of increased ICP. Patients using AEDs should have their therapy reevaluated. Genetic counseling and preconceptual folic acid should be provided when a maternal neural tube defect is present.[165]

Prenatal

Patients should be monitored for evidence of increased ICP, including headaches, nausea, vomiting, visual changes, and altered sensorium. In the presence of these symptoms a CT scan or MRI should be obtained. With radiologic evidence of elevated ICP, conservative management with bed rest and fluid restriction may be tried. More rapid relief and direct measurement of the ICP can be obtained during aspiration of the shunt reservoir.[166] Pumping of the shunt may also provide symptomatic relief.[167] This method is less invasive and theoretically can decrease the risk of shunt infection. Shunt replacement is reserved for those patients who fail conservative treatment.

Labor and Delivery

Intrapartum treatment of women with ventriculoperitoneal shunts centers on the optimal mode of delivery and the need for prophylactic antibiotics. Most reported cases were allowed to labor and deliver vaginally. No complications were noted.[162] Concern with the potential for intra-abdominal scarring associated with surgery and the favorable outcomes seen with vaginal delivery would suggest that cesarean section should be reserved for routine obstetric indications. Shortening of the second stage with forceps or vacuum can be considered, but it does not appear to be universally necessary.[162] Analgesia and anesthesia choices during labor and delivery are limited. Narcotic use should be minimized because of the potential further increase in ICP and alteration of sensorium. Epidural anesthesia can be used with caution. In patients with elevated ICP or a neural tube defect regional anesthesia should be avoided and general anesthesia used.

The use of prophylactic antibiotics during the intrapartum period is controversial, but the presence of a foreign body with a direct connection to the brain makes prophylaxis theoretically sensible.[163] No adverse outcomes were reported in several patients treated without the routine use of prophylaxis.[162] However, the number of involved patients was small, and increased experience will be required before a true lack of benefit is determined.

SUMMARY OF MANAGEMENT OPTIONS

Ventriculoperitoneal Shunts

Management Options	Quality of Evidence	Strength of Recommendation	References
Prepregnancy			
Check clinically for symptoms suggestive of shunt malfunction; MRI/CT if suspected (? useful as baseline for pregnancy even if asymptomatic).	Ib	A	163,165
Review and rationalize anticonvulsant medication (see above under "Epilepsy").	–	GPP	–
Folate for all and specific genetic counseling if neural tube defect	Ib	A	163,165
Prenatal			
Vigilance for raised intracranial pressure (and shunt malfunction)	–	GPP	–
MRI/CT if suspected	–	GPP	–
If confirmed	IV	C	166,167
Bed rest			
Fluid restriction			
Reservoir aspiration or pumping			
Shunt replacement for those who fail conservative measures	–	GPP	–

Continued

SUMMARY OF MANAGEMENT OPTIONS

Ventriculoperitoneal Shunts *(Continued)*

Management Options	Quality of Evidence	Strength of Recommendation	References
Labor and Delivery			
Vaginal delivery is acceptable; assisted procedure only for normal obstetric indications	III	B	162
Epidural with care; avoid narcotic analgesia (raises intracranial pressure)		GPP	
No evidence of need for prophylactic antibiotics	III	B	162,163

CT, computed tomography; MRI, magnetic resonance imaging.

SPINAL CORD INJURY

Maternal Risks

Modern rehabilitation practices allow many patients with spinal cord injuries to lead increasingly independent lives. Often included is the desire to develop a family. Many of the medical problems common to patients with spinal cord problems may be exacerbated during pregnancy. Urinary tract infections (UTI) often with resistant organisms are common in all patients with spinal cord injury due to incomplete bladder emptying and indwelling or intermittent catheterization. During gestation, 75% or more women will develop a UTI. This increases the risk of pyelonephritis.[168] Anemia is present in 60% to 100% of patients.[168] Chronic constipation, another problem seen in nearly all patients with spinal cord injury, is compounded both by pregnancy itself and iron supplementation used in anemia treatment.[169] Immobility associated with many spinal lesions places patients at risk for pressure ulceration. One quarter to half of gravid patients have pressure sores, which with gestational weight gain is a potential aggravating factor. Patients with lesions above T10 may not feel contractions, resulting in failure to appreciate the onset of term or preterm labor, increasing the risk of precipitous or preterm delivery.

Autonomic dysreflexia is a potential life-threatening complication, which can occur in patients with spinal cord lesions at or above T5. The condition results from stimulation of pelvic or abdominal organs, with resultant sympathetic activation uncontrolled by higher centers. Clinical manifestations can include headache, flushing, sweating, cardiac arrhythmias, and hypertension. Several activities common to pregnancy, including bowel or bladder distension, bladder catheterization, labor, and even vaginal examination, may precipitate autonomic dysreflexia, making this a time of particular concern.

Management Options

Prenatal

Management is aimed at minimizing the risk of the common complications. Urine should be screened for bacteria, with appropriate treatment when significant bacteriuria is identified.[168] Prophylactic antibiotics for suppression may be considered. If bladder catheterization is necessary, intermittent is preferred over an indwelling catheter. Dietary changes, stool softeners, or enemas may be necessary to control constipation, with manual disimpaction used in extreme cases. Attention to padding and position changes is important to avoid skin breakdown. Patients should be monitored for preterm labor. Uterine palpation and serial cervical exams can be applied.

Labor and Delivery

Unnecessary stimuli that may lead to autonomic dysreflexia should be avoided. Since uterine contractions are often associated with the condition, epidural anesthesia may be placed early in labor to eliminate sympathetic tone. This should be done even if the patient does not feel the pain of contractions.

SUMMARY OF MANAGEMENT OPTIONS

Spinal Cord Injury

Management Options	Quality of Evidence	Strength of Recommendation	References
Prenatal			
Prophylactic antibiotics	–	GPP	–
Screen for bacteriuria.	III	B	168
Dietary adjustment and bowel softener	–	GPP	–
Nursing care including attention to pressure areas	–	GPP	–
Vigilance for preterm labor	–	GPP	–
Labor and Delivery			
Avoid unnecessary stimuli; epidural even if no sensation.	–	GPP	–

NEUROMUSCULAR DISEASE

Mononeuropathies

Facial Nerve Palsy (Bell's Palsy)

MATERNAL RISKS

Peripheral facial nerve palsy is characterized by acute-onset facial weakness, occasionally preceded by ipsilateral retroauricular pain. The sense of taste may be diminished over the anterior two thirds of the tongue in lesions proximal to the origin of the corda tympani. Viral infection may play an etiologic role. Bell's palsy appears to be more prevalent during pregnancy, with an increased frequency during the third trimester and postpartum. More than three quarters of the pregnancy-related cases occur during this period. The reported incidence is approximately 50 per 100,000 pregnancies, but only 17 per 100,000 in nonpregnant women of childbearing age.[170]

MANAGEMENT OPTIONS

Although the benefit of prednisone (category B) is uncertain, it is frequently used at a dose of 1 mg/kg/d for 5 to 7 days. Success rates are higher if therapy is started within 7 days of the onset of symptoms. The eye should be protected with drops and glasses or a patch. The outcome is quite favorable, with most women recovering completely within 3 to 6 weeks.

Carpal Tunnel Syndrome

MATERNAL RISKS

Carpal tunnel syndrome results from entrapment of the median nerve in the carpal tunnel of the wrist. It is one of the most common mononeuropathies encountered during pregnancy, with a prevalence of approximately 20%.[171] The syndrome is manifested by wrist pain and numbness in the first three digits (and occasionally part of the fourth) of the affected hand. The symptoms may often be severe enough to interfere with sleep; however, significant weakness and muscle wasting is uncommon. Excessive weight gain and fluid retention are predisposing factors. Symptoms typically begin in the second half of pregnancy; however, carpal tunnel syndrome may initially present in the puerperium.[172,173]

MANAGEMENT OPTIONS

The diagnosis is typically made clinically. Electrophysiologic studies may be used if necessary, which show a decreased conduction velocity in the median nerve across the wrist. Initial therapy is conservative and consists of rest and wrist splinting. Resolution of symptoms usually occurs within a few weeks after delivery. In those cases that first present postpartum, resolution is seen 2 to 3 weeks after breastfeeding is stopped. Very few patients will require surgical nerve decompression.

Lateral Femoral Cutaneous Neuropathy (Meralgia Paresthetica)

MATERNAL RISKS

Meralgia paresthetica is a minor but bothersome sensory disturbance caused by stretching or compression of the lateral femoral cutaneous nerve under the inguinal ligament.[174] Numbness, tingling, burning, or pain in the lateral aspect of the thigh and no other neurologic deficits characterizes it. Standing or walking aggravates the symptoms. Symptoms usually begin during the third trimester and are often associated with obesity and exaggerated lumbar lordosis. Prolonged labor may cause or precipitate this neuropathy due to straining with hips flexed.

MANAGEMENT OPTIONS

During pregnancy pain relief can usually be achieved with sitting. Resolution occurs postpartum without treatment in most instances. Occasionally antiepileptic or antidepressant drugs such as carbamazepine or amitriptyline, respectively, may be required. Local steroid or lidocaine injections may be useful.

Lumbar Disc Disease

MATERNAL RISKS AND MANAGEMENT OPTIONS

Lower back pain is one of the most common complaints during pregnancy affecting more than 50% of pregnancies from the mid-second trimester onward.[175] Significant lumbar disc disease is relatively uncommon, however. Clear clinicoradiologic evidence of herniated disc was found in only 5 of nearly 49,000 consecutive deliveries.[176] Fifty-six of 6048 (0.92%) interviewed women had a confirmed new nerve injury of the lower extremities.[177] Factors associated with nerve injury were nulliparity and prolonged second stage of labor. Median duration of symptoms was 2 months. Diagnostic studies include nerve conduction velocities and electromyography. MRI studies should be used cautiously because there is a significant prevalence of disc bulges and frank disc herniations in asymptomatic individuals.[178] Patients who are refractory to medical therapy after delivery may benefit from lumbar laminectomy. Intraoperative positioning during cesarean section may cause sciatica neuropathy.[179]

SUMMARY OF MANAGEMENT OPTIONS

Mononeuropathies

Management Options	Quality of Evidence	Strength of Recommendation	References
Facial Nerve Palsy (Bell's Palsy)			
High-dose steroids, especially if severe and early presentation, though it may not, be as effective in pregnancy.	III	B	170
Protect eye on affected side.	–	GPP	–
Carpal Tunnel Syndrome			
Explanation and reassurance	III	B	171,172
Wrist exercises in day, elevation at night	III	B	171–173
Wrist splinting	III	B	171–173
Diuretics have been used in severe cases.	III	B	173
Local steroid injection for relief of symptoms	III	B	173
Surgical decompression is not usually necessary in pregnancy.	III	B	173
Lateral Femoral Cutaneous Neuropathy (Meralgia Paresthetica)			
Explanation and reassurance	IV	C	174
Relief with certain positions, especially when sitting	IV	C	174
Rarely anticonvulsants (carbamazepine) or antidepressants (amitriptyline) required	–	GPP	–
Lumbar Disc Disease			
Conservative approach (bed rest, firm supporting mattress)	III	B	175,176
Surgery reserved for cases refractory to conservative measures persisting after pregnancy	III	B	175

Polyneuropathies

Acute Inflammatory Demyelinating Polyneuropathy (Guillain-Barré Syndrome)

MATERNAL RISKS

Acute inflammatory demyelinating polyneuropathy is an acquired condition characterized by demyelination of the motor roots and the proximal segments of the peripheral nerves.[180] Pregnancy appears to have no effect on the incidence or course of the disease, although cases have been reported in the first trimester and 28th week of gestation. Guillain-Barré syndrome also does not adversely affect pregnancy.[181,182] Presentation usually consists of ascending paralysis associated with lower back pain and radicular symptoms. Deep tendon reflexes are typically very depressed or lost. In the most severe cases respiratory muscle paralysis is seen and mechanical ventilation is required. Viral infections such as cytomegalovirus (CMV), Epstein-Barr virus (EBV), HIV-1, and hepatitis virus may play a causative role. Flu-like symptoms often precede the onset of weakness by 2 to 3 weeks. In addition, *Campylobacter jejuni* has been implicated as a causal agent.

MANAGEMENT OPTIONS

The diagnosis is made based on the history and physical examination. Confirmation is obtained with electrophysiologic studies. Abnormal findings become evident more than 7 days after the onset of symptoms. Plasmapheresis has been used in the treatment during pregnancy since 1980.[183] Volume status and fetal well-being should be monitored during therapy because significant hypovolemia can result from fluid shifts occurring during therapy. Intravenous immunoglobulins have been used as an alternative to plasmapheresis.[184] Intubation and mechanical ventilation along with appropriate supportive care should be utilized as indicated. Spontaneous labor and vaginal delivery can be allowed. There is no contraindication to epidural anesthesia.

Chronic Inflammatory Demyelinating Polyneuropathy

MATERNAL RISKS AND MANAGEMENT OPTIONS

Chronic inflammatory demyelinating polyneuropathy is a condition with clinical features similar to Guillain-Barré syndrome. A protracted course extending beyond 6 months and a tendency to relapse differentiates the two conditions. During pregnancy, recurrence is seen more often in the last half of gestation.[185] There are no known adverse fetal effects.

Corticosteroids, plasmapheresis, and immunoglobulins have been used therapeutically, individually or in combination. Treatment response is variable, and sometimes poor outcomes result. Data during pregnancy are limited, but labor and delivery are usually uneventful.

Multifocal motor neuropathy has been reported to worsen during pregnancy and to improve with intravenous immunoglobulin.[186]

SUMMARY OF MANAGEMENT OPTIONS

Polyneuropathies

Management Options	Quality of Evidence	Strength of Recommendation	References
Acute Inflammatory Demyelinating Polyneuropathy			
Monitor respiratory function; ventilatory support may be necessary.	–	GPP	–
Nursing and physiotherapy care	–	GPP	–
Prophylactic heparin	–	GPP	–
Therapy options			
Plasmapheresis	IV	C	183
IV immunoglobulin	Ib	A	184
Chronic Inflammatory Demyelinating Polyneuropathy			
Management similar to Guillain-Barré syndrome	IV	C	185
Treatment with	IV	C	185
Corticosteroids			
Plasmapheresis			
IV immunoglobulin			
Interferon			

Noninflammatory Myopathies (Myasthenia Gravis Is Discussed in Chapter 44)

Myotonic Dystrophy

MATERNAL AND FETAL RISKS

Myotonic dystrophy is an autosomal dominant genetic condition characterized by a progressive distal muscle weakness and wasting. There is an associated delay in relaxation in affected muscles. The effect of pregnancy on myotonic dystrophy is variable. Symptoms may first present during pregnancy,[187] exacerbations may occur particularly in the third trimester,[188] or the patient may remain asymptomatic.[189] Cardiac disease can occur in association with myotonic dystrophy, presenting as conduction defects, arrhythmias, or congestive heart failure.[190,191]

An elevated risk of poor fetal outcome is associated with myotonic dystrophy. There is an increased incidence of spontaneous abortion, preterm labor and delivery, and neonatal death.[187] Polyhydramnios is frequently present and may be associated with an affected fetus.[192] Preterm labor is likely a result of the increased amniotic fluid volume and myotonic involvement of the uterus.[193] Congenital myotonic dystrophy presents as generalized hypotonia and weakness. The respiratory muscles may be involved, resulting in inadequate ventilation at birth. Neonatal death is frequent, but if the affected infant is able to survive the first few weeks, some improvement may be seen.[194] The overall long-term prognosis remains generally poor, however. Developmental milestones are delayed and the incidence of mental retardation is increased.[195] Congenital myotonic dystrophy is usually only found in neonates born to mothers with the disease and differs from the adult form.[196]

MANAGEMENT OPTIONS

Prepregnancy and Prenatal. Any maternal cardiac or pulmonary compromise should be determined. A baseline electrocardiograph and pulmonary function tests should be obtained and the patient informed of the signs and symptoms of arrhythmias. Physical activity should be encouraged to slow clinical progression. Genetic counseling and prenatal diagnosis using DNA linkage analysis should be offered. Serial ultrasonography should be used to assess the amniotic fluid volume. In the presence of polyhydramnios, patients need to be followed for evidence of preterm labor. In the third trimester, fetal surveillance may be indicated.

Labor, Delivery, and Postnatal. Despite the risk of preterm labor, myotonic involvement of the uterine smooth muscle can result in dysfunctional labor. Augmentation with oxytocin is often effective.[197] Shortening of the second stage of labor may be helpful in women with significant weakness. Postpartum hemorrhage is a common complication and should be anticipated.

Respiratory muscle weakness may be present and must be considered when offering analgesia and anesthesia. Local or regional anesthesia is preferred. The risk of apnea with narcotics may be increased, and these agents should be used with caution. Nondepolarizing neuromuscular blocking agents should be avoided because of generalized muscle contracture resulting in difficulty with airway management.[198] Prenatal consultation with an anesthesiologist may be prudent.

A pediatrician should be present in the delivery room to aid in neonatal resuscitation and ventilation. There are no newborn tests for myotonic dystrophy. When the mother is asymptomatic and neonatal myotonia is suspected, electromyographic studies on the mother can confirm the neonatal diagnosis.

SUMMARY OF MANAGEMENT OPTIONS
Myotonic Dystrophy

Management Options	Quality of Evidence	Strength of Recommendation	References
Prepregnancy			
Assess cardiorespiratory status; optimize treatment.	III	B	188
Genetic counseling	III	B	188
Prenatal			
Monitor cardiorespiratory status	III	B	188
Discuss prenatal diagnosis	III	B	188
Vigilance for hydramnios	III	B	188
If hydramnios, vigilance for preterm labor	III	B	188
Inform and arrange consultation with anesthiologist; inform pediatricians if fetus affected.	–	GPP	–
Labor and Delivery			
Augmentation with oxytocin if dystocia in first stage	IV	C	197
May need assisted second stage if significant weakness.	III	B	188
Active management of third stage; vigilance for PPH	–	GPP	–
Regional analgesic preferable to narcotics and/or general anaesthetic; avoid nondepolarising neuromuscular blocking drugs.	III	B	188,198
Pediatrician to be present for delivery	–	GPP	–
Postnatal			
Careful neuromuscular examination and follow-up of newborn	III	B	188

PPH, postpartum hemorrhage.

Demyelinating Diseases

Multiple Sclerosis

MATERNAL AND FETAL RISKS

Multiple sclerosis (MS) is a demyelinating disease that affects the central nervous system at different levels and at varying times.[199] It is a relatively common neurologic disease among young adults, peaking at age 30. The prevalence in the United States is 1/1000. Women are affected twice as often as men.

Common symptoms include acute onset of diplopia, vertigo, gait instability, bladder incontinence, loss of vision, and fatigue. Any CNS symptom can be a manifestation of MS, however. The disease course in an individual patient is unpredictable. Different general disease patterns are recognized. One type is characterized as relapsing and remitting with an identified onset and resolution of symptoms. The chronic progressive pattern follows a protracted course, with worsening of symptoms over a prolonged period. Finally a relapsing progressing course displays identifiable exacerbations with no clear return to baseline neurologic function. Poor prognostic factors include prominent weakness, poor response to steroids, and older age at onset. The common pathologic lesion called a plaque demonstrates myelin loss and gliosis associated with inflammatory infiltrates.

Previous research on the effects of pregnancy on MS has generally been flawed, and well-controlled studies are needed.[200] Pregnancy itself may exert a short-term beneficial effect on the course of MS, including fewer, less severe relapses especially in the third trimester. However, this protection is lost in the postpartum period. The incidence of new cases of MS is decreased during pregnancy, as is the risk of exacerbation and progression of existing disease. Postpartum, the incidence of new-onset disease is not different from that in the nonpregnant population.[201] Exacerbation is reported to increase 20% to 40% during the first 6 months after delivery.[202,203] Despite the increase in disease activity postpartum, there does not appear to be any increase in long-term disability related to pregnancy.[204–206] Objective evidence of decreased MS activity during the latter half of gestation with a return to baseline postpartum has been seen using serial MRI scans in two patients.[207] The relative immunosuppression associated with pregnancy may play a role in pregnancy-related changes seen in MS. Children of MS mothers have a 3% risk of developing MS compared with a 0.1% risk seen in the general population.[208]

MANAGEMENT OPTIONS

Prepregnancy. The diagnosis of MS is made clinically. Brain imaging and CSF studies are used to support the clinical impression. High-intensity signal lesions are found in the CNS white matter on MRI scanning, and oligoclonal banding is seen in the CSF. Few data are available during pregnancy on the three FDA-approved treatments for MS patients with relapsing-remitting disease. The therapies include: copolymer 1 or glatiramer acetate (category B), interferon b1b, and interferon b1a (both category C). Corticosteroid therapy is also used.

Preconceptual evaluation and counseling is desirable. Disease activity should be assessed. In times of remission, with the lack of information regarding MS therapies during gestation and the fact that most patients show improvement during pregnancy, consideration should be given to stopping the drugs or minimizing the dose. Patients should also be informed of the increased risk of their offspring developing the disease.

Prenatal. Patients should be monitored for evidence of increased disease activity and the risks of therapy weighed against the potential concerns associated with lack of information. In those patients with urinary tract involvement, regular screening for asymptomatic bacteriuria should take place. Physical therapy and stretching exercises required prior to conception should be continued.

Labor and Delivery and Postnatal. Labor and delivery should not be significantly affected in patients with MS. Prolonged antepartum corticosteroid use requires stress dose steroids during labor. Hydrocortisone 25 mg parenterally every 8 hours in addition to the usual daily dose is an acceptable regimen.[209] Maternal exhaustion seen in the second stage can be managed with operative vaginal delivery. The use of spinal anesthesia has traditionally been avoided due to fear of increasing the risk of exacerbation. There are no data to support this concern, however, and spinal, epidural, and general anesthesia can all be used safely.[210] Breastfeeding may be encouraged, because there does not appear to be an increase in the frequency or severity of postpartum relapse.[211]

SUMMARY OF MANAGEMENT OPTIONS

Multiple Sclerosis

Management Options	Quality of Evidence	Strength of Recommendation	References
Prepregnancy			
Counsel about risks to mother and baby.	IV	C	200, 208
Consider reducing therapy if disease in remission.	–	GPP	–

Continued

SUMMARY OF MANAGEMENT OPTIONS
Multiple Sclerosis *(Continued)*

Management Options	Quality of Evidence	Strength of Recommendation	References
Prepregnancy			
Counsel about risks to mother and baby.	IV	C	200, 208
Consider reducing therapy if disease in remission.	–	GPP	–
Prenatal			
Monitor for relapse or worsening of disease activity (including use of MRI).	IV	C	207
If necessary increase therapy (lack of information on some drugs in pregnancy)	–	GPP	–
Maintain physical exercises, etc.	–	GPP	–
Labor and Delivery			
"Stress dose" steroids for labor/delivery if patient on corticosteroids prenatally	III	B	209
Assisted second stage may be necessary.	–	GPP	–
No data to suggest spinal, epidural, and general anaesthetics contraindicated.	IV	C	210
Postnatal			
Breastfeeding is acceptable.	III	B	211
Vigilance for relapse	III	B	201–203

MRI, magnetic resonance imaging.

CEREBRAL TUMORS

Primary Brain Tumors

Maternal and Fetal Risks

All types of brain tumors have been described in pregnant women, but the overall incidence of primary brain tumors in pregnancy is small and not different from that seen in nonpregnant women of childbearing age. Nevertheless, normal physiologic changes such as increased fluid volumes and increased sex hormone levels occurring during gestation may have a profound effect on tumor growth and neurologic symptoms. Growth of some tumors with estrogen and progesterone receptors can be altered.[212,213] Although tumor growth may lead to initial diagnosis during pregnancy, signs and symptoms at presentation are the same as those in nongravid individuals.

Presenting symptoms relate to increased ICP or local mass effect. Common complaints or neurologic findings include headache, nausea, vomiting, visual changes, hemiparesis, cranial nerve deficits, and seizures. Most of these findings are nonspecific and commonly associated with normal pregnancy, potentially leading to a delay in diagnosis.

Management Options

PREPREGNANCY AND PRENATAL

Management of primary brain tumors in pregnancy depends on the type of tumor and whether it is benign or malignant. Maternal outcome will depend on these factors as well as histologic grade of malignant lesions.[214] Gestational age will also be an important consideration in determining timing and mode of therapy as well as maternal and fetal risks and benefits.

The diagnosis is made with neuroimaging studies. MRI is preferred because low-grade tumors may present as nonenhancing lesions on brain CT, making their classification difficult. Surgical therapy is the treatment of choice for most lesions. Resection is best performed prior to conception when a diagnosis is made before pregnancy. In benign tumors, such as most meningiomas or in low-grade malignant gliomas diagnosed during pregnancy, resection can often be delayed until after delivery providing the patient is neurologically stable. Malignant tumors should be resected promptly. Adjuvant chemotherapy can be given after the first trimester when maternal benefit outweighs fetal risk.

In tumors where radiation therapy is indicated as a primary treatment modality or an adjuvant, this should be delayed until after delivery if possible. Preterm delivery may be undertaken in the presence of fetal pulmonary maturity to expedite therapy. If gestational age prohibits timely delivery, localized brain radiation may be used with careful abdominal shielding to minimize fetal exposure.

Vasogenic cerebral edema is seen with some tumor types and may require glucocorticoid therapy. Dexamethasone is the drug of choice. This agent readily crosses the placenta, so if prolonged high-dose treatment is required, prednisone may be considered as a substitute to decrease fetal exposure. Seizure prophylaxis with appropriate AEDs is indicated when there is a significant risk of convulsions.

LABOR AND DELIVERY

Little information exists to guide labor and delivery management. Vaginal delivery may be allowed with cesarean section reserved for obstetric indications. The second stage may be shortened with forceps or vacuum to avoid increased ICP with pushing.

Metastatic Brain Tumors (See also Chapter 53)

Maternal Risks and Management Options

The brain is a common site of metastatic cancer. Lung, breast, and gastrointestinal cancers are the most frequent site of the primary tumors. Rarely do maternal cancers spread to the fetoplacental unit.

Choriocarcinoma is a trophoblastic tumor that is rarely found associated with a normal pregnancy. The tumor spreads rapidly by the hematogenous route, with brain metastasis discovered at the time of diagnosis in as many as 20% of patients.[215–217] Brain involvement presenting as an ischemic stroke,[218] intracerebral hemorrhage,[219] or subdural hematoma resulting from metastatic infiltration and proliferation in vascular spaces may actually lead to the diagnosis. Chemotherapy is considered the treatment of choice in choriocarcinoma. Alternatives in special circumstances include surgical resection of single brain metastasis and cranial irradiation. The presence of brain lesions is associated with an overall worse prognosis.

SUMMARY OF MANAGEMENT OPTIONS

Cerebral Tumors

Management Options	Quality of Evidence	Strength of Recommendation	References
Primary Tumors			
Prepregnancy			
Tumors are best treated before commencing pregnancy	III	B	214
Prenatal			
Management depends on:	III	B	214
Tumor type and whether benign or malignant			
Its natural history			
Gestation			
Patient's wishes			
Most tumors are treated by surgery.	III	B	214
Adjuvant chemotherapy can be given after the first trimester.	III	B	214
Radiation is best delayed until after delivery.	III	B	214
High-dose steroids may be necessary with cerebral edema.	III	B	214
Labor and Delivery			
Insufficient data to determine whether assisted second stage is of benefit.	–	GPP	–
Management Options—Secondary/Metastatic Tumors			
Management depends on:	III	B	215–217
Primary			
Site			
Its effects			

Prolactinoma (See also Chapter 47)

Maternal Risks

Prolactinomas are the most common type of pituitary tumor. Most are microadenomas found during an evaluation for amenorrhea, galactorrhea, or infertility. In addition, macroadenomas (>10 mm diameter) may present with headache or bitemporal hemianopia. The use of bromocriptine to treat infertility has allowed women with prolactinomas to become pregnant. Pregnancy can stimulate tumor growth. Although this is rarely a problem with microadenomas, symptoms may develop or worsen in the presence of a macroadenoma.[220]

Management Options

If adenoma size has not previously been determined, neuroimaging studies are indicated to define the extent of the tumor. MRI is able to identify small adenomas and their relation to the optic nerve, whereas CT scan provides better definition of any bony erosion resulting from the tumor expansion.[221] With microadenomas, bromocriptine can be stopped once pregnancy is diagnosed with less than a 5% chance of the lesion becoming symptomatic.[222] Visual fields are periodically tested to detect evidence of tumor growth. Headaches are a useful early symptom of tumor enlargement. Bromocriptine may be started during pregnancy if symptoms develop. Macroadenomas have a 15% to 35% chance of enlargement. Bromocriptine may be continued throughout gestation, or patients must be followed closely for symptoms. Hypophysectomy or radiotherapy are reserved for cases that fail medical management. Adenomas generally decrease in size after delivery.

SUMMARY OF MANAGEMENT OPTIONS

Prolactinoma

Management Options (See also Chapter 47)	Quality of Evidence	Strength of Recommendation	References
Prenatal			
Clinical surveillance (headaches and visual disturbance) for recurrence or expansion in pregnancy	III	B	243
Some screen visual fields through pregnancy	–	GPP	–
Bromocriptine with tumor enlargement (confirmed with CT or MRI)	III	B	221,243,244
Bromocriptine appears to be safe during pregnancy.	III	B	243,244
Hypophysectomy (radiotherapy rarely needed for failed medical management).	III	B	244

CT, computed tomography; MRI, magnetic resonance imaging.

MOVEMENT DISORDERS

Maternal and Fetal Risks

Life-threatening, new-onset movement disorders are extremely rare during pregnancy.[223,224] Movement disorders are classified based on either excessive (hyperkinetic or dyskinetic) or slowed (hypokinetic) motor activity. The findings can be persistent or intermittent. In reproductive-age women, the hyperkinetic or dyskinetic disorders predominate. Several of the movement disorders are associated with abnormalities of tone, but most are not associated with actual weakness.

Most movement disorders are the result of disease involving the basal ganglion (caudate nucleus, globus pallidus, putamen, substantia nigra) and its connections. However, abnormalities of the thalamus, cerebellum, spinal cord, and peripheral nerves can cause abnormal movements. A wide spectrum of pathologic processes, including degenerative conditions, toxins, metabolic aberrations, cerebrovascular disease, neoplasms, autoimmune conditions, infections, and trauma, can lead to movement disorders.[224] In addition, dopamine receptor antagonists commonly used to treat nausea and vomiting in early pregnancy may rarely induce new-onset dystonia, chorea, tremors, and parkinsonism.

Chorea Gravidarum

Maternal and Fetal Risks

Chorea gravidarum, a hyperkinetic disorder, is an uncommon condition that encompasses any cause of chorea occurring during pregnancy.[225–227] In the preantibiotic era, it was commonly due to group A streptococcal infection and rheumatic fever. Clinical manifestations of chorea include abrupt, rapid, unsustained, involuntary, purposeless, irregular, and nonrhythmic movement of a limb or axial structure. The movements may be isolated and of brief duration or they may be more flowing and sustained. Patients are often unable to persist with voluntary motor activity. This is illustrated by difficulty in maintaining protrusion of their tongue or closure of their eyes. There are multiple causes of chorea gravidarum. Most cases are due to medications, toxins, infections (e.g., HIV or cerebral toxoplasmosis), autoimmune disorders, cerebrovascular disease, or an endocrinopathy. Specific causes are shown in Table 49–8.

Management Options

Management of chorea depends on the underlying origin and its severity. The diagnostic evaluation is complex and aimed at excluding the conditions listed in Table 49–8. Therapeutic intervention is aimed primarily at the underlying cause. The actual chorea is usually benign and of secondary concern. Treatments typically offer only symptomatic relief and have the potential for adverse effects. Expectant management is preferred except when movements may lead to dehydration, malnutrition, or insomnia or when they are exceedingly violent and pose a risk of maternal injury. Short-term use of low-dose haloperidol (category C) can reduce chorea movements.

Wilson's Disease

Maternal and Fetal Risks

Wilson's disease is an autosomal recessive disorder of copper metabolism associated with a deficiency of the copper-binding and carrier protein, ceruloplasmin. Disease manifestations include chorea, tremors, hypersalivation, dystonia, myoclonus, or slurred speech. Copper deposition in the brain is responsible for the clinical findings. Kayser-Fleischer rings describe copper deposition in the cornea and are one of the classic physical findings. Other organ systems are also affected. The defective gene is located on chromosome 13 (p14).[223,224] The carrier frequency in the population is between 1/90 and 1/200.

TABLE 49–8

Causes of Chorea Gravidarum

Sydenham's (rheumatic)
Systemic lupus erythematosus
Antiphospholipid syndrome
Wilson's disease
Cerebrovascular disease
Meningovascular syphilis
Hyperthyroidism
Neuroacanthocytosis
Huntington's disease
Adult-onset Tay–Sachs disease
Medications/drugs
Antepileptic drugs
Neuroleptics
Theophylline derivatives
Lithium
Tricyclic antidepressants
Lead toxicity
Amphetamines
Cocaine
Metaclopramide

Management Options

Typically the diagnosis is made when serum ceruloplasmin levels are less than 20 mg/dL. Half of patients with Wilson's disease will have levels less than 5 mg/dL. The diagnosis may be complicated in pregnancy because increased estrogen levels increase ceruloplasmin levels, leading to false-negative assays. Prior to penicillamine therapy pregnancy was uncommon because of the development of infertility, and when conception did occur the rate of spontaneous abortions was increased.[228,229]

Penicillamine (category D) therapy is the first-line treatment of Wilson's disease.[230] Five consecutive successful pregnancies in the same woman with Wilson's disease have been reported.[231] Therapy has been associated with adverse fetal effects. Fetal connective tissue anomalies secondary to an inhibition of collagen synthesis can result.[230,232] Also neonatal inguinal hernia, reversible cutis laxa,[223,224] hyperflexible joints, vascular fragility, and poor wound healing have all been reported.[233,234] Many infants born to mothers taking penicillamine during pregnancy are free of defects, however.

With proper therapy the course of Wilson's disease does not appear to be affected by pregnancy. Penicillamine therapy should be continued during pregnancy. Halting therapy could lead to irreversible damage to the maternal brain, liver, and other organs. To minimize the risk of poor wound healing following delivery, the daily penicillamine dose should be decreased from 1 g to 250 mg during the third trimester. An alternative therapy uses zinc and trientine. Collagen synthesis is not adversely affected, but experience with this regimen in pregnancy is limited.[228]

Restless Leg Syndrome

Maternal Risks

Restless leg syndrome is a common condition with 11% to 19% of pregnant women affected.[235] It consists of an unpleasant sensation of the legs often associated with periodic movements during or just before sleep, or in the late evening when fatigue is present. Clinically there is flexion of the hip and knee with dorsiflexion of the ankle and extension of the great toe. The cause is unclear; however, in nonpregnant patients there has been an association with iron deficiency. Treatment aimed at iron replacement has been associated with an improvement in symptoms.[236] Symptoms often disappear with walking.

Management Options

Treatment is supportive and includes reassurance, massage, flexion and extension leg exercises, and walking. With the high incidence of iron deficiency in pregnancy, iron supplementation may be a prudent early intervention. Severe cases can be managed with opiates.

Parkinson's Disease

Maternal and Fetal Risks

Parkinson's disease is an idiopathic hypokinetic disorder typically seen after the age of 40, but approximately 5% of cases may present earlier.[223] Thus Parkinson's disease may be seen in women of childbearing age. The condition is a degenerative disorder of unknown origin related to a deficiency of dopamine-secreting neurons in the substantia nigra of the brainstem mesencephalon (midbrain). Manifestations include slowed movements (bradykinesia), increased tone (rigidity), resting tremor, loss of postural reflexes, masked facies, and transient akinesia. Patients often have difficulty initiating movements, and automatic movements are reduced. This constellation of findings is termed parkinsonism and represents a common clinical presentation for a variety of conditions in addition to Parkinson's disease. The differential diagnosis includes intracranial processes such as hydrocephalus, head trauma, subdural hematomas, cerebrovascular disease, and encephalitis. Carbon monoxide poisoning, metabolic abnormalities, and cyanide and manganese toxicity have also been implicated. Also several medications, including alpha methyldopa, disulfiram, dopamine receptor antagonists, lithium, methanol, reserpine, and tetrabenazine, may lead to parkinsonism. Discontinuation of the offending drug if clinically feasible may lead to varying degrees of symptomatic improvement.

Information describing the course of Parkinson's disease in pregnancy is limited. There are reports of worsening during pregnancy with improvement postpartum.[223,224] Symptoms may be exacerbated by several factors, including hormonal changes, medications, weight gain, increased fatigue, and dehydration.

Management Options

Initial evaluation of a patient suspected of having Parkinson's disease should exclude other conditions associated with parkinsonism. As with the condition itself, information regarding the safety of antiparkinsonism medications during pregnancy is limited. Use of the combination of levodopa/carbidopa (not categorized), a mainstay in the treatment of Parkinson's disease, has been associated with malformations in animals, but adequate human data are not available. These medications should be used with caution. Amantidine (category C) has also been associated with malformations in animals. In humans, the overall malformation rate is reported to be higher, but there is no specific pattern. Again, data are limited, and caution should precede its use.[1]

Bromocriptine (category C) is a second-line agent for the treatment of Parkinson's disease. Although it is not as efficacious as the levodopa/carbidopa combination, there is considerably more experience during pregnancy. The information is based on lower doses used to treat prolactinomas.[237] It is considered safe without excess risk of complications based on 1335 women receiving it during pregnancy for a prolactinoma. Bromocriptine may be added to the levodopa/carbidopa combination when disabling symptomatology appears such as dopa-induced dyskinesias. Selegiline (Category C) and pergolide (category B) are newer treatments that lack adequate pregnancy data.[238]

SUMMARY OF MANAGEMENT OPTIONS

Movement Disorders

Management Options	Quality of Evidence	Strength of Recommendation	References
Chorea Gravidarum			
Management depends on cause	IV	C	224
Treatment only given if:	IV	C	224
Dehydration			
Malnutrition			
Insomnia			
Violence			
Risk of maternal injury			
Short-term low-dose haloperidol commonly used.	IV	C	224

SUMMARY OF MANAGEMENT OPTIONS
Movement Disorders (Continued)

Management Options	Quality of Evidence	Strength of Recommendation	References
Wilson's Disease			
Penicillamine is the treatment of choice, but lowest dose that gives disease control should be used (risk of fetal defects).	III IV	B C	228–230,232
Restless Leg Syndrome			
Supportive treatment:	III	B	235
Reassurance			
Massage, exercises, and physiotherapy			
Walking			
Iron supplementation if deficient	IV	C	236
Opiates for severe cases	III	B	235
Parkinson's Disease			
Levodopa/cardidopa is probably safe for the fetus (limited human data).	–	GPP	–
Bromocriptine is often added to this with severe cases.	III	B	237
Amantadine, selegiline, and pergolide have limited published data.	–	GPP	

CEREBRAL ABSCESS

Maternal Risks

Pregnancy and puerperium-associated cerebral abscesses are exceedingly rare, with fewer than 15 cases reported.[239] Although most abscesses are supratentorial and solitary (Fig. 49 7), focal neurologic deficits are not always present despite headache, fever, seizures, or depressed level of consciousness. Sources of infection include otitis media, venous sinus thrombosis, and hemorrhage into the basal ganglia. In most cases a source is not found. Cerebral abscesses have been reported in immunocompetent hosts. Approximately half the cases have been associated with eclampsia. Overall mortality is 35%, and when the abscess is associated with eclampsia, mortality reaches 50%.

Management Options

Although rare, a cerebral abscess should be a part of the differential diagnosis when a mass lesion is seen on brain imaging. As a rule, aggressive medical management of the abscess is often adequate, and surgical evacuation may not be necessary. Medical therapy includes the appropriate use of intravenous antibiotic(s) to cover a broad spectrum of potential organisms. A source for the infection should be promptly and thoroughly sought and treated and when found may give information about the responsible organism(s). Surgical drainage may be indicated if there is an initial poor response to the antibiotics.

ACKNOWLEDGEMENTS

We thank Sabrina Hinton and Srinath R. Geetla for their expert technical assistance in manuscript/reference list preparation.

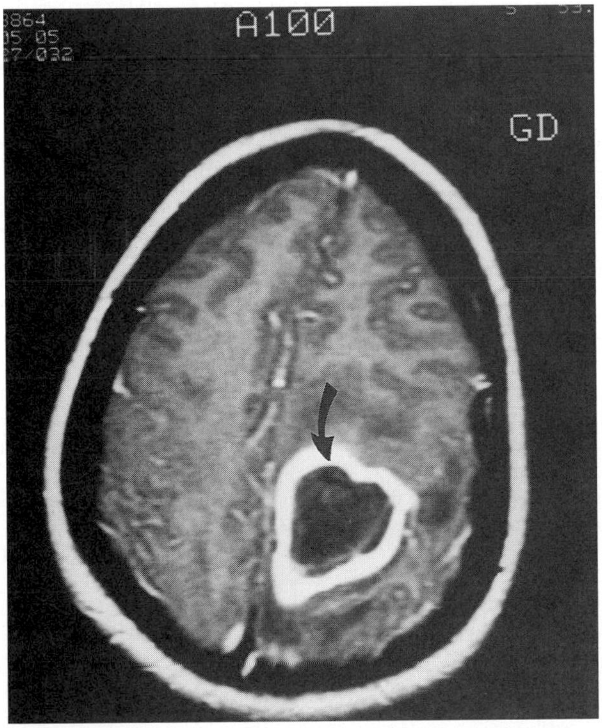

FIGURE 49–7
Axial head MRI revealing a ring-enhancing lesion, proven to be a puerperal cerebral abscess (*curved arrow*) at surgery.

SUMMARY OF MANAGEMENT OPTIONS
Cerebral Abscess

Management Options	Quality of Evidence	Strength of Recommendation	References
Aggressive IV antibiotics (broad spectrum)	III	B	239
Find and treat source of infection.	III	B	239
Surgical drainage for the few cases that fail to respond to antibiotics	III	B	239

CONCLUSIONS

- The optimal and effective management of neurologic complications of pregnancy include the early involvement of the obstetrician, anesthesiologist, and neurologist. The early participation of the pediatrician/neonatologist is also important to anticipating and treating neonatal needs.
- Eclampsia most frequently occurs during the antepartum and intrapartum periods, but approximately one-third of cases are seen postpartum.
- Magnesium sulfate and blood pressure control have been mainstay of both seizure prophylaxis and abortive therapy in patients with preeclampsia and eclampsia.
- Although it was believed that the incidence of stroke is higher during pregnancy, the most recent evidence is less conclusive. Nevertheless, the relative risk of stroke rises to 8.7 during the postpartum period.
- Despite the associated physiologic changes associated with pregnancy and delivery, the risk of subarachnoid hemorrhage does not appear to increase during these physiologic states and bleeding during the time of labor and delivery is infrequent.
- Although previous research on the effects of pregnancy on multiple sclerosis (MS) has been flawed, it is now thought that pregnancy itself may exert a short-term beneficial effect on the course of MS.
- Carpal tunnel syndrome is one of the most common mononeuropathies encountered during pregnancy, with a prevalence of about 20%. Resolution of symptoms usually occurs within the first few weeks after delivery.
- In cases of benign tumors, such as most meningiomas or in low-grade malignant gliomas diagnosed during pregnancy, resection often can be delayed until after delivery, providing the patient is neurologically stable. Malignant tumors should be resected promptly.
- Aggressive medical management of brain abscesses during pregnancy is often adequate, and surgical evacuation is not necessary unless there is poor response to appropriate antibiotic therapy.

REFERENCES

1. Briggs GG, Freeman RK, Yaffe SJ: Drugs in pregnancy and Lactation: a Reference Guide to Fetal and Neonatal Risk, 4th ed. Baltimore, Williams & Williams; 1994.
2. Saftlas AF, Oslon DR, Franks AL, et al: Epidemiology of preeclampsia and eclampsia in the United States. Am J Obstet Gynecol 1990;163:460–465.
3. Barton JR, Sinbai BM: Cerebral pathology in eclampsia. Clin Perinatol 1991;18:891–910.
4. Sheehan HL, Lynch JB: Pathology of Toxemia of Pregnancy. Baltimore, Williams & Wilkins; 1973.
5. Colosimo C, Fineli A, Moschini M, et al: CT findings in eclampsia. Neuroradiology 1985;27:313–317.
6. Crawford S, Varner MW, Digre KB, et al: Cranial magnetic resonance imaging in eclampsia. Obstet Gynecol 1985;70: 474–477.
7. Lewis LK, Hinshaw DB, Will AD, et al: CT and angiographic correlation of severe neurological disease in toxemia of pregnancy. Neuroradiology 1988;30:59–64.
8. Raroque JG, Orrison WW, Rosenberg GA: Neurologic involvement in toxemia of pregnancy: Reversible MRI lesions. Neurology 1990;40:167–169.
9. Schwaighofer BW, Jesselink JR, Jealy ME: MR demonstration of reversible brain abnormalities in eclampsia. J Comput Assist Tomogr 1989;13:310–312.
10. Cunningham FG, Fernandez CO, Hernandez C: Blindness associated with preeclampsia and eclampsia. Am J Obstet Gynecol 1995;172:1291–1298.
11. Richards A, Graham D, Bullock R: Clinicopathological study of neurological complications due to hypertensive disorders of pregnancy. J Neurol Neurosurg Psychiatr 1988;51:416–421.
12. Douglas KA, Redman CWG: Eclampsia in the United Kingdom. Br Med J 1994;309:1395–1400.
13. Hallum AV: Eye changes in hypertensive toxemia of pregnancy. JAMA 1936;106:1649–1651.
14. Carpenter F, Kava HL, Plotkin D: The development of total blindness as a complication of pregnancy. Am J Obstet Gynecol 1953;66:641–647.
15. Will AD, Lewis KL, Hinshaw DB, et al: Cerebral vasoconstriction in toxemia. Neurology 1987;37:1555–1557.
16. Schaefer PW, Buonanno FS, Gonzalez RG, et al: Diffusion-weighted imaging discriminates between cytotoxic and vasogenic edema in a patient with eclampsia. Stroke 1997;28:1082–1085.

17. Beck DW, Menezes AH: Intracerebral hemorrhage in a patient with eclampsia. JAMA 1981;246:1442–1443.
18. Atrash HK, Koonin LM, Lawson HW, et al: Maternal mortality in the United States 1979–1986. Obstet Gynecol 1990;76:1055–1060.
19. Mattar F, Sibai BM: Eclampsia: VIII. Risk factors for maternal morbidity. Am J Obstet Gynecol 2000;182:307–312.
20. Duley L: Maternal mortality associated with hypertensive disorders of pregnancy in Africa, Asia, Latin America and the Caribbean. BJOG 1992;99:547–553.
21. Sibai BM: Eclampsia: VI. Maternal-perinatal outcome in 254 consecutive cases. Am J Obstet Gynecol 1990;163:1049–1055.
22. Miles Jr JF, Martin Jr JN, Blake PG, et al: Postpartum eclampsia: A recurring perinatal dilemma. Obstet Gynecol 1990;76:328–331.
23. Lubarsky SL, Barton JR, Friedman SA, et al: Late postpartum eclampsia revisited. Obstet Gynecol 1994;83:502–505.
24. Sibai BM: Magnesium sulfate is the ideal anticonvulsant in preeclampsia-eclampsia. Am J Obstet Gynecol 1990;162: 1141–1145.
25. Coan EJ, Collinridge GL: Magnesium ions block an *N*-methyl-D-aspartate receptor-mediated component of synaptic transmission on rat hippocampus. Neuroscience Letters 1985;53:21–26.
26. Stasheff SF, Anderson WW, Clark S, et al: NMDA antagonists differentiate epileptogenesis from seizure expression in an in vitro model. Science 1989;245:648–651.
27. Standley CA, Irtenkauf SM, Stewart L, et al: Magnesium sulfate versus phenytoin for seizure prevention in amygdala kindled rats. Am J Obstet Gynecol 1994;171:948–951.
28. Mason BA, Standley CA, Irtenkauf SM, et al: Magnesium is more efficacious than phenytoin in reducing *N*-methyl-D-aspartate seizures in rats. Am J Obstet Gynecol 1994;171:999–1002.
29. Duley L, Gulmezoglu AM, Henderson-Smart DJ: Magnesium sulfate and other anticonvulsants for women with pre-eclampsia. Cochrane Database Syst Rev 2003:CD000025.
30. Lucas MJ, Leveno KJ, Cunningham FG: A comparison of magnesium sulfate with phenytoin for the prevention of eclampsia. N Engl J Med 1995;333:201–205.
31. Yu CK, Papageorghiou AT, Parra M, et al: Randomized controlled trial using low-dose aspirin in the prevention of preeclampsia in women with abnormal uterine artery Doppler at 23 weeks' gestation. Ultrasound Obstet Gynecol 2003;22:233–239.
32. Chua S, Redman CWG: Are prophylactic anticonvulsants required in severe preeclampsia? 1991;337:250–251.
33. Burrows RF, Burrows EA: The feasibility of a control population for a randomized control trial of seizure prophylaxis in the hypertensive disorders of pregnancy. Am J Obstet Gynecol 1995;173:929–935.
34. Roberts JM, Pearson G, Cutler J, Lindheimer M: Summary of the NHLBI working group on research on hypertension during pregnancy. Hypertension 2003;41:437–445.
35. O'Brien MD, Gilmour-White S: Epilepsy and pregnancy. Br Med J 1993:492–495.
36. Brodie MJ: Management of epilepsy during pregnancy and lactation. Lancet 1990:426–427.
37. Devinsky O, Yerby MS: Women with epilepsy, reproduction and effects of pregnancy on epilepsy. Neurol Clin 1994;12:479–495.
38. Yerby MS, Devinsky O: Epilepsy and pregnancy. Adv Neurol 1994;64:45–63.
39. Schmidt D: The effect of pregnancy on the natural history of epilepsy: A review of literature. In Janz D, Bossi L, Dam M, et al, eds: Epilepsy, Pregnancy and the Child. New York, Raven Press, 1982, pp 3–14.
40. Schmidt D, Conyen R, Avanzini GM, et al: Change of seizure frequency in pregnancy epileptic women. J Neurol Neurosurg Psychiatr 1983;46:751–755.
41. Delgado-Escueta AV, Jantz D: Consensus guidelines: Preconception counseling, management, and care of the pregnant women with epilepsy. Neurology 1992;42:149–160.
42. Yerby M, Freil PN, McCormick KB, et al: Pharmacokinetics of anticonvulsants in pregnancy: Alteration in plasma protein binding. Epilepsy Res 1990;5:223–228.
43. Perruca E, Crema A: Plasma protein binding of drugs in pregnancy. Clin Pharmacokinet 1982;7:336–352.
44. Nelson KB, Ellenberg JH: Maternal seizure disorder, outcome of pregnancy, and neurologic abnormalities in the children. Neurology 1982;32:1247–1254.
45. Samren EB, van Duijn CM, Koch S, et al: Maternal use of antiepileptic drugs and the risk of major congenital malformations: A joint European prospective study of human teratogenesis associated with maternal epilepsy. Epilepsia 1997;38:981–990.
46. Lindhout D, Rene JE, Hoppener A, et al: Teratogenicity of antiepileptic drug combinations with special emphasis on epoxidation of carbamazepine. Epilepsia 1984;25:77–83.
47. Hanson JW, Smith DW: The fetal hydantoin syndrome. J Pediatr 1975;87:285–290.
48. Rudd NL, Freedom RM: A possible primidone embryopathy. J Pediatr 1979;94:835–837.
49. Jones KL, Lacro RV, Johnson KA, et al:. Pattern of malformations in the children of women treated with carbamazepine during pregnancy. N Engl J Med 1989;320:1661–1666.
50. Buehler BA, Delimont D, van Waes M, et al: Prenatal prediction of risk of the fetal hydantoin syndrome. N Engl J Med 1990;322:1567–1572.
51. Gaily E, Granstorm ML, Hiilesmaa V, et al: Minor anomalies in offspring of epileptic mothers. J Pediatr 1988;112:520–529.
52. Lindhout D, Omzigt JGC, Cornel MC: Spectrum of neural tube defects in 34 infants prenatally exposed to antiepileptic drugs. Neurology 1992;42(Suppl 5):111–118.
53. Gaily E, Kantola-Sorsa E, Granstorm ML: Specific cognitive dysfunction in children with epileptic mothers. Dev Med Child Neurol 1990;32:403–414.
54. Vert P, Deblay MF: Hemorrhagic disorders in infants of epileptic mothers. In Janz D Bossi L, Dam M, et al, eds: Epilepsy, Pregnancy and the Child. New York, Raven Press; 1982.
55. Callaghan N, Garrett A, Goggin T: Withdrawal of anticonvulsant drugs in patients free of seizures for two years. N Engl J Med 1988;318:942–946.
56. Shinnar S, Vining EPG, Mellits ED, et al: Discontinuing antiepileptic medication in children with epilepsy after two years without seizures. N Engl J Med 1985;313:976–980.
57. Pennell PB: Antiepileptic drug pharmacokinetics during pregnancy and lactation. Neurology 2003;61:S35–S42.
58. Committee on Drugs: The transfer of drugs and other chemicals into human milk. Pediatrics 1994;93:137–150.
59. Donaldson JO: Neurologic emergencies in pregnancy. Obstet Gynecol Clin North Am 1991;18:199–211.
60. Sloan MA, Stern BJ: Cerebrovascular disease in pregnancy. Curr Treat Options Neurol 2003;5:391–407.
61. Kittner SJ, Stern BJ, Feeser BR, et al: Pregnancy and the risk of stroke. N Engl J Med 1996;335:768–774.
62. Wiebers D: Ischemic cerebrovascular complications of pregnancy. Arch Neurol 1985;42:1106–1113.
63. Wiebers D, Mokri B: Internal carotid artery dissection after childbirth. Stroke 1985;16:956–959.
64. Wong V, Wang R, Tse T: Pregnancy and Takayasu's arteritis. Am J Med 1983;75:597–601.
65. Ezra Y, Kidron D, Beyth Y: Fibromuscular dysplasia of the carotid arteries complicating pregnancy. Obstet Gynecol 1989;73:840–843.
66. Fletcher A, Alkjaersig N, Burstein R: The influence of pregnancy upon blood coagulation and plasma fibrinolytic enzyme function. Am J Obstet Gynecol 1979;134:743–751.
67. Crowley J: Coagulopathy and bleeding in the parturient patient. Rhode Island Med 1989;72:135–143.
68. Donaldson JO: Thrombophilic coagulopathies and pregnancy-associated cerebrovascular disease. Curr Obstet Gynaecol 1991;1:186–190.
69. Roos KL, Pascuzzi RM, Kuharik MA, et al: Postpartum intracranial venous thrombosis associated with dysfunctional protein c and deficiency of protein S. Obstet Gynecol 1990;76:492–494.

70. Koster T, Rosendaal FR, de Rhonda H, et al: Venous thrombosis due to poor anticoagulant response to activated protein c: Leiden thrombophilia study. Lancet 1993;342:1503–1506.
71. Boketwa MI, Bremme K, Blomback M: Arg 506-gln mutation in factor V and risk of thrombosis during pregnancy. Br J Haematol 1996;92:473–478.
72. Thorarensen O, Ryan S, Hunter J, et al: Factor v Leiden mutation: An unrecognized cause of hemiplegic cerebral palsy, neonatal stroke, and placental thrombosis. Ann Neurol 1997;42:372–375.
73. Weiner CP: Thrombotic microangiopathy in pregnancy and the postpartum period. Semin Hemtol 1987;24:119–129.
74. Kaku DA, Lowenstein DH: Emergence of recreational drug abuse as a major risk factor for stroke in young adults. Ann Intern Med 1990;113:821–827.
75. Levine SR, Brust JCM, Futrel N, et al: Cerebrovascular complication of the use of the "crack" forms of alkaloidal cocaine. N Engl J Med 1990;323:699–704.
76. Mercado A, Johnson G, Calver D, et al: Cocaine, pregnancy, and post partum intracerebral hemorrhage. Obstet Gynecol 1989;73:467–468.
77. Galli M, Barbui T: Antiphospholipid antibodies and thrombosis: Strength of association. Hematol J 2003;4:180–186.
78. Levine SR, Welch KMA: Antiphospholipid antibodies. Ann Neurol 1989;26:386–389.
79. Branch DW: Antiphospholipid antibodies and pregnancy: Maternal implications. Semin Perinatol 1990;14:139–146.
80. Triplett DA: Antiphospholipid protein antibodies: Laboratory detection and clinical relevance. Thrombosis Res 1995;78:1–31.
81. Wilson JJ, Zahn CA, Ross SD, et al: Association of embolic stroke in pregnancy with lupus anticoagulant. J Reprod Med 1986;31:725–728.
82. Shapiro SS: The lupus anticoagulant/antiphospholipid syndrome. Ann Rev Med 1995;47:533–553.
83. Levine SR, Brey RL, Sawaya KL, et al: Recurrent stroke and thrombo-occlusive events in the antiphospholipid syndrome. Ann Neurol 1995;38:119–124.
84. Levine SR, Salowich-Palm L, Sawaya KL, et al: IgG anticardiolipin antibody titer > 40 gpl and the risk of subsequent thrombo-occlusive events and death: A prospective cohort study. Stroke 1997;28:1660–1664.
85. Grotta J, Manner C, Pettigrew L, et al: Red blood cell disorders and stroke. Stroke 1986;17:811–817.
86. Hodgman MT, Pessin MS, Homans DC, et al: Cerebral embolism as the initial manifestation of peripartum cardiomyopathy. Neurology 1982;32:668–671.
87. Connor RCR, Adams JH: Importance of cardiomyopathy and cerebral ischemia in the diagnosis of fatal coma in pregnancy. J Clin Pathol 1996;19:244–249.
88. Bergh PA, Hollander D, Gregori CA, et al: Mitral valve prolapse and thromboembolic disease in pregnancy; a case report. Int J Gynecol Obstet 1988;27:133–137.
89. Levy D, Savage D: Prevalence and clinical features of mitral valve prolapse. Am Heart J 1987;113:1281–1290.
90. Webster MWI, Chancellor AM, Smith HJ, et al: Patent foramen ovale in young stroke patients. Lancet 1988;2(8601):11–12.
91. Salazar E, Zajarias A, Gutierrez N, Iturbe E: The problem of cardiac valve prostheses, anticoagulants and pregnancy. Circulation 1984;70(Suppl I):169–177.
92. Sareli E, England M, Berk M, et al: Maternal and fetal sequelae of anticoagulation during pregnancy in patients with mechanical heart valve prostheses. Am J Cardiol 1989;63:1462–1465.
93. Cox S, Hankins G, Leveno K, et al: Bacterial endocarditis: A serious pregnancy complication. J Reprod Med 1988;33: 671–674.
94. Hojnik M, George J, Ziporen L, et al: Heart valve involvement (Libman-Sacks endocarditis) in the antiphospholipid syndrome. Circulation 1996;93:1579–1587.
95. Dahlman T, Lindvall N, Hellgren M: Osteopenia in pregnancy during long term heparin treatment: A radiological study postpartum. BJOG 1990;97:221–228.
96. Ginsberg J, Hirsh J: Anticoagulants during pregnancy. Ann Rev Med 1989;40:79–86.
97. Brancazio L, Ropertik K, Stierer R, et al: Pharmacokinetics and pharmacodynamics of subcutaneous heparin during the early third trimester of pregnancy. Am J Obstet Gynecol 1995;173:1240–1245.
98. Hirsh J, Levine M: Low molecular weight heparin. Blood 1992;79:1–17.
99. Melissari E, Parker CJ, Wilson NV, et al: Use of low molecular weight heparin in pregnancy. Thromb Haemost 1992;68: 652–656.
100. Dultizki MD, Pauzner R, Langevitz P, et al: Low molecular weight heparin during pregnancy and delivery: Preliminary experience with 41 pregnancies. Obstet Gynecol 1996;87:380–383.
101. Fejgin MD, Lourwood DL: Low molecular weight heparins and their use in obstetrics and gynecology. Obstet Gynecol Surv 1994;49:424–431.
102. Brey RL, Levine SR: Treatment of neurologic complications of antiphospholipid antibody syndrome. Lupus 1996;5:473–476.
103. Witlin AG, Mabie WC, Sibai BM: Peripartum cardiomyopathy: An ominous diagnosis. Am J Obstet Gynecol 1997;176:182–188.
104. The National Institute of Neurological Disorders and Stroke: The rt-PA Stroke Study Group. Tissue plasminogen activator for acute ischemic stroke. N Engl J Med 1995;33:1581–1587.
105. Elford K, Leader A, Wee R, Stys PK: Stroke in ovarian hyperstimulation syndrome in early pregnancy treated with intraarterial rt-pa. Neurology 2002;59:1270–1272.
106. Upshaw J, Reidy T, Groshart K: Thrombotic thrombyocytopenic purpura in pregnancy: Response to plasma manipulations. South Med J 1985;78:677–680.
107. Srinivasan K: Cerebral venous and arterial thrombosis in pregnancy and puerperium: A study of 135 patients. Angiology 1983;34:731–774.
108. Chopra JS, Banerjee AK: Primary intracranial sinovenous occlusions in youth and pregnancy. In Vinken PJ BG, Klawans HL, eds: Handbook of Clinical Neurology. Amsterdam, Elsevier Science Publishers, 1989, pp 425–452.
109. Fehr PR: Sagittal sinus thrombosis in early pregnancy. Obstet Gynecol 1982;59:7–9.
110. Wozniak AJ, Kitchens CS: Prospective hemostatic studies in patient with paroxysmal nocturnal hemoglobinuria, pregnancy and cerebral venous thrombosis. Am J Obstet Gynecol 1982;142:591–593.
111. Bousser MG, Chiras J, Bories J, et al: Cerebral venous thrombosis—A review of 38 cases. Stroke 1985;16:199–213.
112. Deschiens MA, Conard J, Horellou MH, et al: Coagulation studies, factor V Leiden, and anticardiolipin antibodies in 40 cases of cerebral venous thrombosis. Stroke 1996;27:1724–1730.
113. Zuber M, Toulon P, Marnet L, et al: Factor V Leiden mutation in cerebral venous thrombosis. Stroke 1996;27:1721–1723.
114. Carhuapoma JR, Mitsias P, Levine SR: Cerebral venous thrombosis and anticardiolipin antibodies. Stroke 1997;28:2363–2369.
115. Levine SR, Kieran S, Puzio K, et al: Cerebral venous thrombosis with lupus anticoagulants. Report of two cases. Stroke 1987;18:801–804.
116. Provenzale JM, Loganbill HA: Dual sinus thrombosis and venous infarction associated with antiphospholipid antibodies: MR findings. J Comput Assist Tomogr 1994;18:719–723.
117. Einhaupl KM, Villringer A, Meister W, et al: Heparin treatment in sinus venous thrombosis. Lancet 1991;338:597–600.
118. Horowitz M, Purdy P, Unwin H, et al: Treatment of dural sinus thrombosis using selective catherization and urokinase. Ann Neurol 1995;38:58–67.
119. Dias M, Sekhar L: Intracranial hemorrhage from aneurysms and arteriovenous malformations during pregnancy and puerperium. Neurology 1990;27:855–866.

120. Enomoto H, Got H: Moyamoya disease presenting as intracerebral hemorrhage during pregnancy: Case report and review of the literature. Neurosurgery 1987;20:33–35.
121. Isla A, Alvarez F, Gonzalez A, et al: Brain tumor and pregnancy. Obstet Gynecol 1997;89:19–23.
122. Henderson CE, Torbey M: Rupture of intracranial aneurysm associated with cocaine use during pregnancy. Am J Perinatol 1988;5:142–143.
123. Iriye BK, Asrat T, Adashek JA, et al: Intraventricular haemorrhage and maternal brain death associated with antepartum cocaine abuse. BJOG 1995;102:68–69.
124. Maher LM: Postpartum intracranial hemorrhage and phenylpropanolamine use. Neurology 1987;37:1686.
125. Barrow DL, Reisner A: Natural history of intracranial aneurysms and vascular malformations. Clin Neurosurg 1993;40:3–39.
126. Wilterdink JL, Feldman E: Cerebral hemorrhage. In Devinsky O, Feldman E, Hairlire B, eds: Neurological Complications of Pregnancy New York, Raven Press, 1994, pp 12–23.
127. Pritchard J, MacDonald P, Grant N: Maternal adaptation to pregnancy. In Eastman NJ ed: Williams Obstetrics, 11th ed. New York, Appleton-Century-Crofts, 1985.
128. Forster DMC, Kunkler IH, Hartland P: Risk of cerebral bleeding from arteriovenous malformations in pregnancy: The Sheffield experience. Stereotact Funct Neurosurg 1993;61 (Suppl 1):20–22.
129. Barno A, Freeman DW: Maternal deaths due to spontaneous subarachnoid hemorrhage. Am J Obstet Gynecol 1976;125: 384–392.
130. Horton JC, Chambers WA, Lynos SL, et al: Pregnancy and the risk of hemorrhage from cerebral arteriovenous malformations. Neurosurgery 1990;27:867–871.
131. Piotin M, de Souza Filho CB, Kothimbakam R, Moret J: Endovascular treatment of acutely ruptured intracranial aneurysms in pregnancy. Am J Obstet Gynecol 2001;185: 1261–1262.
132. Aminoff MJ: Maternal neurologic disorders. In Creasy RK, Resnik R, eds: Maternal-Fetal Medicine Principles and Practice. Philadelphia, WB Saunders, 1994.
133. Rigg D, McDonogh A: Use of sodium nitroprusside in deliberate hypotension during pregnancy. Br J Anaesth 1981;53:985–987.
134. Willoughby JS: Sodium nitroprusside, pregnancy and multiple intracranial aneurysms. Anaesth Intensive Care 1984; 12:358–360.
135. Newman B, Lam AM: Induced hypotension for clipping of a cerebral aneurysm during pregnancy: A case report and brief review. Anesth Analg 1986;65:675–678.
136. Kassel NF, Sasaki T, Colohan ART, et al: Cerebral vasospasm following aneurysmal subarachnoid hemorrhage. Stroke 1985;16:562–572.
137. Grenvik A, Safar P: Brain Failure and Resuscitation. New York, Churchill Livingstone, 1981.
138. Strange K, Halldin M: Hypothermia in pregnancy. Anesthesiology 1983;58:460–461.
139. Belfort MA, Saade GR, Moise Jr KJ, et al: Nimodipine in the management of preeclampsia: Maternal and fetal effects. Am J Obstet Gynecol 1994;171:417–424.
140. Ducsay CA, Thompson JS, Wu AT, et al: The effects of calcium entry blocker (nicardipine) tocolysis in rhesus macaques: Fetal plasma concentrations and cardiorespiratory changes. Am J Obstet Gynecol 1987;157:1482–1486.
141. Van Rossum J, Wintzen AR, Endtz LJ, et al: Effect of tranexamic acid on rebleeding after subarachnoid hemorrhage: A double blind control trial. Ann Neurol 1977;2:238–242.
142. Beller FK: Treatment of coagulation disorders in pregnancy. Zentralbl Gynakol 1973;95(32):1089–1100.
143. Robinson JL, Hall CS, Sedzimir CB: Av malformations, aneurysms and pregnancy. J Neurosurg 1974;41:63–70.
144. Parkinson D, Bachers G: Arteriovenous malformations: Summary of 100 consecutive supratentorial cases. J Neurosurg 1980;53:285.
145. Young DC, Leveno KJ, Whalley PS: Induced delivery prior to surgery for ruptured cerebral aneurysm. Obstet Gynecol 1983;61:749–752.
146. Hunt HB, Schifrin BS, Suzuki K: Ruptured berry aneurysms and pregnancy. Obstet Gynecol 1974;43:827–837.
147. Tuttleman RM, Gleicher N: Central nervous system hemorrhage complicating pregnancy. Obstet Gynecol 1981;58:651–657.
148. Silberstein SD: Evaluation and emergency treatment of headache. Neurol Clin 1997;15(1):209–231.
149. Fox MW, Harms RW, Davis DH: Selected neurologic complications of pregnancy. Mayo Clin Proc 1990;65:1595–1618.
150. Hainline B: Headache. Headache 1994;12(3):443–460.
151. Silberstein SD: Migraine and pregnancy. Neurol Clin 1997;15:209.
152. Sances G, Granella F, Nappi RE, et al: Course of migraine during pregnancy and postpartum: A prospective study. Cephalalgia 2003;23:197–205.
153. Stein GS: Headaches in the first postpartum week and their relationship to migraine. Headache 1981;21:201–205.
154. Wainscott G, Sullivan FM, Volans GN: The outcome of pregnancy in women suffering from migraine. Postgrad Med J 1978; 54:98–102.
155. Silberstein SD: Headaches and women. Treatment of the pregnant and lactating migraineur. Headache 1993;33:533–540.
156. Schulman EA, Silberstein SD: Symptomatic and prophylactic treatment of migraine and tension type headache. Neurology 1992;42(Suppl):16–21.
157. Loder E: Safety of sumatriptan in pregnancy: A review of the data so far. CNS Drugs 2003;17:1–7.
158. Nulman I, Rover J, Stewart DE, et al: Neurodevelopment of children exposed in utero to antidepressant drugs. N Engl J Med 1997;336:258–262.
159. Chambers CD, Johnson KA, Dick LM, et al: Birth outcomes in pregnant women taking fluoxetine. N Engl J Med 1996;335: 1010–1015.
160. Seebacher J, Ribeiro V, LeGillou JL, et al: Epidural blood patch in the treatment of post dural puncture headache: A double blind study. Headache 1989;29:630–632.
161. Rottenberg DA, Foley KM, Posner JB: Hypothesis: The pathogenesis of pseudotumor cerebri. Medical Hypothesis 1980;6: 913–918.
162. Landwehr Jr JB, Isada NB, Pryde PG, et al: Maternal neurosurgical shunts and pregnancy outcome. Obstet Gynecol 1994; 83:134–137.
163. Wisoff JH, Kartzert KJ, Handwerker SM: Pregnancy in patients with cerebrospinal fluid shunts: Report of a series and review of the literature. Neurosurgery 1991;29:827–831.
164. Hanakita J, Suzuki T, Yamamoto Y, et al: Ventriculoperitoneal shunt malfunction during pregnancy. J Neurosurg 1985;63: 459–460.
165. MRC Vitamin Study Research Group: Prevention of neural tube defects: Results of the medical research council vitamin study. Lancet 1991;338:131–137.
166. Houston CS, Clein LJ: Ventriculoperitoneal shunt malfunction in a pregnant patient with meningomyelocele. CMAJ 1989;141: 701–702.
167. Kleinman G, Sutherling W, Martinez M, et al: Malfunction of ventriculoperitoneal shunts during pregnancy. Obstet Gynecol 1983;61:753–754.
168. Baker ER, Cardenas DD, Benedetti TJ: Risks associated with pregnancy in spinal cord injured women. Obstet Gynecol 1992;80:425–428.
169. Feyi-Waboso PA: An audit of five years experience of pregnancy in spinal cord damaged women. A regional units experience and a review of literature. Paraplegia 1992;30:631–635.
170. Falco NA, Eriksson E: Idiopathic facial palsy in pregnancy and puerperium. Surg Gynecol Obstet 1989;169:337–340.

171. Viotk AJ, Mueller JC, Farlinger DE, et al. Carpal tunnel syndrome in pregnancy. Canadian Medical Association. 1983; 128:277.
172. Wand JS: Carpal tunnel syndrome in pregnancy and lactation. J Hand Surg [Br] 1990;15:93–95.
173. Snell NJC, Coysh HL, Snell BJ: Carpal tunnel syndrome presenting in the puerperium. Practitioner 1980;224:191–193.
174. Peterson PH: Meralgia paresthetica related to pregnancy. Am J Obstet Gynecol 1952;64:690–691.
175. Fast A, Shapiro D, Ducommun EJ, et al: Low-back pain in pregnancy. Spine 1987;12(4):368–371.
176. LaBan MM, Perrin JCS, Latimer FR: Pregnancy and the herniated lumbar disc. Arch Phys Med Rehab 1983;64:319.
177. Wong CA, Scavone BM, Dugan S, et al: Incidence of postpartum lumbosacral spine and lower extremity nerve injuries. Obstet Gynecol 2003;101:279–288.
178. Weinreb JC, Wolbarsht LB, Cohen JM, et al: Prevalence of lumbosacral intervertebral disc abnormalities on MR images in pregnant and asymptomatic women. Radiology 1989; 170:125–128.
179. Roy S, Levine AB, Herbison GJ, Jacobs SR: Intraoperative positioning during cesarean as a cause of sciatic neuropathy. Obstet Gynecol 2002;99:652–653.
180. Rodin A, Ferner R, Russell R: Guillain-Barré syndrome in pregnancy and puerperium. J Obstet Gynaecol 1988;9:39–42.
181. Zeeman GG: A case of acute inflammatory demyelinating polyradiculoneuropathy in early pregnancy. Am J Perinatol 2001; 18:213–215.
182. Yamada H, Noro N, Kato EH, et al: Massive intravenous immunoglobulin treatment in pregnancy complicated by Guillain-Barré syndrome. Eur J Obstet Gynecol Reprod Biol 2001;97: 101–104.
183. Watson WJ, Katz VL, Bowes WA: Plasmapheresis during pregnancy. Obstet Gynecol 1990;76:451–457.
184. van der Merche FGA, Schmitz PIM, Group DG-BS: A randomized trial comparing intravenous immune globulin and plasma exchange in Guillain-Barré syndrome. N Engl J Med 1992; 326:1123–1129.
185. Dyck PJ, Prneas J, Pollard J: Chronic inflammatory demyelinating polyradiculoneuropathy. In Dyck PJ TP, Griffin JW, Low PA, Poduslo JF, eds: Peripheral Neuropathy. Philadelphia, WB Saunders, 1993, pp 1498–1517.
186. Chaudhry V, Escolar DM, Cornblath DR: Worsening of multifocal motor neuropathy during pregnancy. Neurology 2002;59: 139–141.
187. Sarnat HGB, O'Connor T, Byrne PA: Clinical effects of myotonic dystrophy on pregnancy and the neonate. Arch Neurol 1976;33:459–465.
188. Jaffe R, Mock M, Abramowitz J, et al: Myotonic dystrophy and pregnancy: A review. Obstet Gynecol Surv 1986;41:272–278.
189. Hughes RG, Lyall EGH, Liston WA: Obstetric and neonatal complications of myotonic dystrophy. J Obstet Gynaecol 1991;11:191–193.
190. Fall LH, Young WW, Power JA, et al: Severe congestive heart failure and cardiomyopathy as a complication of myotonic dystrophy in pregnancy. Obstet Gynecol 1990;76:481–485.
191. Moorman J, Coleman R, Packer D, et al: Cardiac involvement in myotonic dystrophy. Medicine 1985;64:371–387.
192. Webb D, Muir I, Faulker J, et al: Myotonia dystrophica: Obstetric complications. Am J Obstet Gynecol 1978;132:265–270.
193. Broekhuizen FF, Elejalde M, Elejalde R, et al: Neonatal myotonic dystrophy as a cause of hydramnios and neonatal death. J Reprod Med 1983;28:595–599.
194. Rutherford MA, Heckmatt JZ, Dubowitz V: Congenital myotonic dystrophy: Respiratory function at birth determines survival. Arch Dis Child 1989;64:191–195.
195. Dyken PR, Harper PS: Congenital dystrophia myotonica. Neurology 1973;23:465–473.
196. Harper PS: Congenital myotonic dystrophy in Britain: Genetic basis. Arch Dis Child 1975;50:514–521.
197. Hilliard GD, Harris RE, Gilstrap LC, et al: Myotonic muscular dystrophy in pregnancy. South J Med 1977;70:446–447.
198. Mudge BJ, Taylor PB, Vanderspeck AFL: Perioperative hazards in myotonic dystrophy. Anaesthesia 1980;35:492–495.
199. Poser CM, Paty DW, Scheinberg L, et al: New diagnostic criteria for multiple sclerosis: Guidelines for research protocols. Ann Neurol 1983;13:227–231.
200. Dwosh E, Guimond C, Duquette P, Sadovnick AD: The interaction of ms and pregnancy: A critical review. Int MS J 2003; 10:38–42.
201. Runmarker B, Anderson O: Pregnancy is associated with a lower risk of onset and a better prognosis in multiple sclerosis. Brain 1995;118:253–261.
202. Cook SD, Troiano R, Bansil S, et al: Multiple sclerosis and pregnancy. In Devinsky O, Feldman E, Hainline B, eds: Neurologic Complications of Pregnancy. New York, Raven Press, 1993, pp 83–95.
203. Korn-Lubetzki I, Kahan E, Cooper G, et al: Activity of multiple sclerosis during pregnancy and puerperium. Ann Neurol 1984;16:229–231.
204. Birk K, Ford C, Smeltzer S, et al: The clinical course of multiple sclerosis during pregnancy and the puerperium. Arch Neurol 1990;47:738.
205. Worthington J, Jones R, Crawford M, et al: Pregnancy and multiple sclerosis: A 3 year prospective study. J Neurol 1994;241: 228–233.
206. Bernardi S, Grasso MG, Bertollini R, et al: The influence of pregnancy on relapses in multiple sclerosis: A cohort study. Acta Neurol Scand 1991;84:403–406.
207. Van Walderveen MAA, Tas MW, Barkhof F, et al: Magnetic resonance evaluation of disease activity during pregnancy in multiple sclerosis. Neurology 1994;44:327–329.
208. Sadovnick AD: Empiric recurrence risks for use in the genetic counseling of multiple sclerosis patients. Am J Med Genet 1984;17:713–714.
209. Salem M, Tainsh RE Jr, Bromberg J, et al: Perioperative glucocorticoid coverage. A reassessment 42 years after emergence of a problem. Ann Surg 1994;219:416–425.
210. Warren TM, Datta S, Ostheimer GW: Lumbar epidural anesthesia in a patient with multiple sclerosis. Anesth Analg 1982;61:1022.
211. Nelson LM, Franklin GM, Jones MC, et al: Risks of multiple sclerosis exacerbation during pregnancy and breast feeding. JAMA 1988;259:3441.
212. Moguilewsky M, Pertuiseet BF, Versat C, et al: Cytosolic and nuclear sex steroid receptors in meningioma. Clin Neuropharmacol 1984;7:375.
213. Poisson M, Pertuiseet BF, Hauw JJ, et al: Steroid hormone receptors in human meningiomas, gliomas and brain metastases. J Neurooncol 1983;1:179.
214. Burger PC, Green SB: Patient age, histologic features, and length of survival in patients with glioblastoma multiforme. Cancer 1987;59:1617.
215. Athanassiou A, Begent RHJ, Newlands ES, et al: Central nervous system metastases of choriocarcinoma. Cancer 1983;52:1728.
216. Weed JC, Hunter VJ: Diagnosis and management of brain metastasis from gestational trophoblastic disease. Oncology 1991;5:48.
217. Weed JC, Wood KT, Hammond CB: Choriocarcinoma metastatic to the brain: Therapy and prognosis. Semin Oncol 1982; 9:208.
218. Nakagawa Y, Tashiro K, Isu T, et al: Occlusion of cerebral artery due to metastasis of chorioepithelioma. J Neurosurg 1979; 51:247.
219. Aguilar MM, Rabinovitch R: Metastic chorioepithelioma simulating multiple strokes. Neurology 1964;14:933.

220. Scheithauer BW, Sano T, Kovacs KT, et al: The pituitary gland in pregnancy: A clinico-pathologic and immunohistochemical study of 69 cases. Mayo Clin Proc 1990;65:461.
221. Kulkarni MV, Lee KF, McArdle CB, et al: 1.5 t MR imaging of pituitary microadenomas: Technical consideration and ct correlation. Am J Neuroradiol 1988;9:5.
222. Tindall G, Reisner A: Prolactinomas. In Wilkins RH, Rengachary SS, eds: Neurosurgery, 2nd ed. New York, McGraw-Hill, 1996, pp 1299–1307.
223. Golbe LI: Pregnancy and movement disorders. Neurol Clin 1994;12:497–508.
224. Rogers JD, Fahn S: Movement disorders and pregnancy. Adv Neurol 1994;64:163–178.
225. Donaldson IM, Espiner EA: Disseminated lupus erythematosus presenting as chorea gravidarum. Arch Neurol 1971;25:240–244.
226. Jones S, Spagnuolo M, Kloth HH: Chorea gravidarum and streptococcal infection. Obstet Gynecol 1972;39:77–79.
227. Caviness JN, Muenter M: An unusual cause of recurrent chorea. Mov Disord 1991;6:355–357.
228. Walshe JM: The management of pregnancy in Wilson's disease treated with trientine. Quart J Med 1986;58:81–87.
229. Dreifuss FE, McKinney WM: Wilson's disease (hepatolenticular degeneration) and pregnancy. JAMA 1966;195:960–962.
230. Scheinberg IH, Sternlieb I: Pregnancy in penicillamine treated patients with Wilson's disease. N Engl J Med 1975;293: 1300–1302.
231. Furman B, Bashiri A, Wiznitzer A, et al: Wilson's disease in pregnancy: Five successful consecutive pregnancies of the same woman. Eur J Obstet Gynecol Reprod Biol 2001;96:232–234.
232. Biller J, Swiontoniowski M, Brazis PW: Successful pregnancy in Wilson's disease: A case report and review of the literature. Eur Neurol 1985;24:306–309.
233. Rasmussen BK, Rigmor J, Schroll M, et al: Epidemiology of headache in a general population: A prevalence study. J Clin Epidemiol 1991;44:1147–1157.
234. Geever EF, Youseff S, Seifter E, et al: Penicillamine and wound healing in young guinea pigs. J Surg Res 1967;7:160–167.
235. Goodman JDS, Brodie C, Ayida GA: Restless leg syndrome in pregnancy. BMJ 1988;297:1101–1102.
236. Allen RP, Earley CJ: Restless legs syndrome: A review of clinical and pathophysiologic features. J Clin Neurophysiol 2001;18: 128–147.
237. Turkalj I, Braun P, Krupp P: Surveillance of bromocriptine in pregnancy. JAMA 1982;247:1589–1591.
238. Olin ER: Antiarrhythmic agents. In Olin ER, ed: Facts and Comparisons. St Louis, JB Lippincott; 1992.
239. Aboukasm AG, Levine SR, Donaldson JO: Pregnancy related cerebral abscess. Neurologist 1996;2:73–76.
240. Magee LA, Ornstein MP, von Dadelszen P: Management of hypertension in pregnancy. BMJ 1999;318:1332–1336.
241. Crawford P, Appleton R, Betts T, et al: Best practice guidelines for the management of women with epilepsy. The Women with Epilepsy Guidelines Development Group 1999. Seizure 8 (4):201–217.
242. Kassam SH, Hadi HA, Fadel HE, et al: Benign intracranial hypertension in pregnancy: Current diagnostic and therapeutic approach. Obstet Gynecol Surv 1983;38(6):314–321.
243. Hammond CB, Haney AF, Land MR, et al: The outcome of pregnancy in patients with treated and untreated prolactin-secreting pituitary tumors. Am J Obstet Gynecol 1983;147:148–157.
244. Samaan NA, Schultz PN, Leavens TA, et al: Pregnancy after treatment in patients with prolactinoma: Operation versus bromocriptine. Am J Obstet Gynecol 1986;155:1300–1305.

CHAPTER 50

Renal Disorders

David Williams

INTRODUCTION

The kidneys undergo marked hemodynamic, renal tubular, and endocrine changes during pregnancy. A failure of these adaptations in women with renal disease creates a suboptimal environment for fetal development and increases the risk of obstetric complications such as preeclampsia, preterm labor, and intrauterine growth restriction (IUGR). In turn, during pregnancy the diseased maternal kidneys are exposed to the damaging consequences of a prothrombotic state, ascending urinary infections, gestational hypertension, and altered hemodynamics that exacerbate proteinuria. Women with a preconception glomerular filtration rate (GFR) of less than 25 mL/min, (serum creatinine >177 μmol/L; 2.0 mg/dL) have a 1:3 chance of a pregnancy-related decline to end-stage renal failure (ESRF) and are likely to have preterm, growth-restricted babies. Preexisting hypertension, proteinuria, recurrent urinary tract infections (UTIs), and in women with diabetic nephropathy—poor glycemic control, are all independently, but cumulatively detrimental to maternal and fetal outcome. Women with ESRF are far more likely to have a successful pregnancy following a kidney transplant compared with those on dialysis. Pregnancy itself can cause acute renal disease or uncover a previously subclinical renal condition. This chapter describes gestational changes to the kidney during healthy pregnancy, the influence of pregnancy on chronic renal disease, and, conversely, the effect of chronic renal disease on pregnancy outcome. The management of specific acute and chronic renal diseases during pregnancy is also discussed.

RENAL CHANGES DURING NORMAL PREGNANCY

Renal Glomerular Function during Pregnancy

Renal adaptation to pregnancy is anticipated prior to conception, during the luteal phase of each menstrual cycle. Renal blood flow and GFR increase by 10% to 20% before menstruation.[1,2] If pregnancy is established, the corpus luteum persists and these hemodynamic changes continue.[2,3] By 16 weeks' gestation GFR is 55% above nonpregnant levels.[3,4] This increment is mediated through an increase in renal blood flow that reaches a maximum of 70% to 80% above nonpregnant levels by the second trimester, before falling to around 45% above nonpregnant levels at term.[5] Elegant human studies have confirmed that unlike the hyperfiltration that precedes diabetic nephropathy, gestational hyperfiltration is not associated with a damaging rise in glomerular capillary blood pressure (BP).[4]

The changes to renal physiology in healthy pregnancy can both hide and mimic renal disease (Table 50–1). The increased GFR of pregnancy leads to a fall in serum creatinine concentration (SCr), so that values considered normal in the nonpregnant state may be abnormal during pregnancy. SCr levels fall from a nonpregnant mean value of 73 μmol/L (0.82 mg/dL) to 60 μmol/L (0.68 mg/dL), 54 μmol/L (0.61 mg/dL) and 64 μmol/L (0.72 mg/dL) in successive trimesters.[6] SCr is not, however, linearly correlated with creatinine clearance and is influenced by muscle mass, physical exercise, racial differences, and dietary intake of meat. As SCr roughly doubles for every 50% reduction in GFR, a more useful parameter by which to monitor serial changes in renal function is the reciprocal of SCr (1/SCr). Estimates of GFR can be further refined using the Cockcroft-Gault equation, which calculates GFR using SCr, maternal age, and prepregnancy weight.[7] For women, the Cockcroft-Gault equation is

$$\text{GFR (mL/min)} = 0.8 \times [140 - \text{age (years)} \times \text{weight (kg)}] / \text{SCr } (\mu\text{mol/L})$$

$$(1 \text{ mg/dL creatinine} = 88.4\ \mu\text{mol/L creatinine})$$

The gestational rise in renal blood flow also causes the kidneys to swell so that bipolar renal length increases by approximately 1 cm. During the third trimester renal blood flow falls, leading to a fall in creatinine clearance

TABLE 50–1

Physiologic Changes of Pregnancy Can Both Mask and Mimic Renal Disease in Pregnancy

Pregnancy Mimics Renal Disease
Increased proteinuria (should not exceed 200 mg/24h)
Decreased serum albumin (reduced by 5–10 g/L)
Increased cholesterol by 50% in third trimester[16]
Salt and water retention (dependent edema)
Dilatation of the renal tracts (mimics renal obstruction, especially on right side)
Glycosuria (present in 10% of nondiabetic mothers)
Hypercalciuria
Physiologic reduction in hemoglobin concentration
Symptoms mimicking cystitis
Metabolic acidosis (bicarbonaturia to compensate for respiratory alkalosis)
Pregnancy Masks Renal Disease
Physiologic vasodilatation reducing systemic BP
Increased GFR reducing SCr and serum urea

BP, blood pressure; GFR, glomerular filtration rate; SCr, serum creatinine.

and a rise in reciprocal SCr. Serum urea levels, however, continue to fall in the third trimester due to reduced maternal hepatic urea synthesis.[8] This metabolic adaptation ensures that more nitrogen is available for fetal protein synthesis.[8]

The renal pelvicaliceal system and ureters, particularly on the right side, dilate and can appear obstructed to those unaware of these changes.[9] The right pelvicaliceal system dilates by a maximum of 0.5 mm each week from 6 to 32 weeks, reaching a maximum diameter of approximately 20 mm (90th percentile), which is maintained until term.[10] The left pelvicaliceal system reaches a maximum diameter of 8 mm (90th percentile) at 20 weeks' gestation.[10]

Proteinuria increases as pregnancy progresses, but levels over 200 mg/24 hours during the third trimester are above the 95% confidence limit for the normal population.[11] A random urine protein:creatinine ratio is a useful guide to 24-hour urinary protein excretion, but is not a substitute for either a 12-hour[12] or 24-hour urine collection, due to the high incidence of both false-positive and false-negative results.[13,14] A random urine sample that gives a protein (mg): creatinine (mmol) ratio of more than 0.19 is a good predictor of significant proteinuria[13] and is an indication for more accurate assessment of proteinuria with a 12- or 24-hour urine collection.

Serum albumin levels fall by 5 to 10 g/L,[15] serum cholesterol and triglyceride concentrations increase significantly,[16] and dependent edema affects most pregnancies at term. Normal pregnancy therefore simulates the classic features of nephrotic syndrome (see Table 50–1).

Renal Tubular Function During Pregnancy

Increased alveolar ventilation causes a respiratory alkalosis to which the kidney responds by increased bicarbonaturia and a compensatory metabolic acidosis.[17] Other renal tubular changes include reduced tubular glucose reabsorption, which leads to glycosuria in approximately 10% of healthy pregnant women,[18] a 250% to 300% increase in urinary calcium excretion,[19] and a first-trimester increase in urate excretion that decreases toward term, at which time plasma urate levels rise again to nonpregnancy levels.[20]

During healthy pregnancy a mother gains 6 to 8 kg of fluid, of which approximately 1.2 L is due to an increase in plasma volume.[3] Plasma osmolality falls by 10 mOsm/kg by 5 to 8 weeks' gestation due to a fall in both the threshold for thirst and for the release of antidiuretic hormone (vasopressin).[21] During pregnancy, vasopressin is metabolized by placental vasopressinase, and at term the maternal posterior pituitary produces four times as much vasopressin to maintain physiologic concentrations.[22] Failure of the maternal pituitary to keep up with the increased metabolic clearance of vasopressin leads to a transient polyuric state in the third trimester, which is known as transient diabetes insipidus of pregnancy.[23]

Renal Endocrine Function During Pregnancy

The kidney also acts as an endocrine organ that produces erythropoietin,[24] active vitamin D,[25] and renin.[3] The production of all three hormones increases during healthy pregnancy, but their effects are masked by other changes.[3,24,25] In early pregnancy, peripheral vasodilatation exceeds renin/aldosterone-mediated plasma volume expansion, so diastolic BP falls by 12 weeks.[26] Conversely, plasma volume expansion exceeds the erythropoietin-mediated increase in red cell mass, causing a "physiologic anemia," which should not normally lead to a hemoglobin (Hb) concentration of less than 9.5 g/dL.[27] Similarly, extra active vitamin D produced by the placenta circulates at twice nongravid levels, but concomitant halving of parathyroid hormone levels, hypercalciuria, and increased fetal requirements keep maternal plasma ionized calcium levels unchanged.[19,28]

LOWER URINARY TRACT INFECTION

General

The incidence of asymptomatic bacteriuria (significant growth of a uropathogen in the absence of symptoms) is 2% to 10%, which is the same during pregnancy as it is in sexually active nonpregnant women.[29] However, the structural and immune changes to the urothelium of the renal tracts during pregnancy[30] make it more likely that a lower UTI will ascend to cause acute pyelonephritis.[29,31] During pregnancy, 12.5% to 30% of women with untreated asymptomatic bacteriuria will develop acute pyelonephritis,[29–33] a serious infection with significant morbidity to mother and fetus.

Diagnosis of a Urinary Tract Infection

During pregnancy symptoms suggestive of a UTI are dysuria and offensive-smelling urine. Other symptoms, usually associated with a UTI are urinary frequency, nocturia, urge-incontinence, and strangury (the urge to pass urine having just done so), but these symptoms are also found in healthy pregnant women.

Microscopy and culture of a freshly voided midstream urine sample will allow quantification of pyuria (leukocytes in the urine) and growth of a urinary pathogen. Bacterial UTI is the most common cause of pyuria and is considered significant if microscopy of a sample of unspun midstream urine reveals more than 10 leukocytes per microliter. Urine culture is conventionally recognized as significant if there is growth of more than 10^5 colony forming units per milliliter (CFU/mL) of a single recognized uropathogen in association with pyuria.[34] Low counts of bacteriuria (10^2–10^4 CFU/mL) may still be significant if symptomatic women have a high fluid intake or are infected with a slow-growing organism. If left untreated, most symptomatic women with "low-count bacteriuria" will have 10^5 CFU/mL 2 days later.[34] During pregnancy, the most common uropathogens are bowel commensals, *Escherichia coli* (70%–80%), *Klebsiella*, *Proteus*, *Enterobacter*, and *Staphylococcus saprophyticus*.

If urine from a symptomatic pregnant woman is cloudy and positive on dipstick testing for nitrite (produced by most uropathogens) and leukocyte esterase (produced by white blood cells), then a UTI is likely, and empirical treatment can be started.[34] These urine sticks are not sensitive enough to be used for screening for asymptomatic bacteriuria in early pregnancy;[35] therefore, microscopy and culture of a clean catch midstream urine sample is necessary. Hematuria and proteinuria are unreliable indicators of a UTI, but are important signs of renal disease (see later discussion).

Asymptomatic Bacteriuria

Maternal and Fetal Risks

During pregnancy, untreated asymptomatic bacteriuria will develop into acute pyelonephritis in 12.5% to 30% of women, but if treated less than 1% of pregnant women develop pyelonephritis.[29–33] A systematic review of 14 studies confirmed that antibiotic treatment of asymptomatic bacteriuria, compared with placebo or no treatment, significantly reduced the incidence of pyelonephritis (odds ratio 0.24; 95% CI 0.19–0.32).[36] Following successful treatment of asymptomatic bacteriuria, monthly screening of midstream urine is necessary, because approximately 30% of women will have a relapse of bacteriuria, making them vulnerable to acute pyelonephritis again.[29]

Asymptomatic bacteriuria has also been associated with an increased risk of preterm delivery and low birth weight.[37] Treatment of asymptomatic bacteriuria has been shown to reduce the incidence of preterm delivery and low-birth-weight babies (odds ratio 0.60; 95% CI 0.45–0.80).[36] Others have not, however, found the same association between preterm labor and bacteriuria.[31] It has been suggested that the underlying renal pathology, which is commonly associated with bacteriuria, is responsible for poor pregnancy outcomes.[31] Further good quality studies are needed to settle this issue.

Management Options

Contrary to much published advice, not all pregnant women need to be screened for asymptomatic bacteriuria. There are two main reasons. Firstly, the prevalence of asymptomatic bacteriuria varies among populations, and where it is low (<2.5%) it is hard to justify the cost-effectiveness of screening. In populations where the prevalence of asymptomatic bacteriuria is greater than 5%, the case for screening is much stronger.[32] Secondly, approximately 1% to 2% of the 90% to 98% of asymptomatic women who test negative for bacteriuria in the first trimester will develop a symptomatic UTI.[33,38] Therefore a third of all women who develop a UTI in late pregnancy would have been missed on first-trimester screening.[33,38] Women at increased risk of pyelonephritis or renal impairment should be screened for asymptomatic bacteriuria every 4 to 6 weeks throughout pregnancy (Table 50–2).

Treatment of Urinary Tract Infections

There is no consensus about the optimal treatment of asymptomatic bacteriuria[47] nor the empirical treatment of symptomatic UTIs in pregnancy.[48] Most UTIs during pregnancy (approximately 75%) are caused by *E. coli*, which is usually sensitive to nitrofurantoin (89%), trimethoprim (with or without sulfamethoxazole) (87%), ampicillin (72%), or cephalosporins.[49,50] Therefore until well-structured trials are done, the most cost-effective treatment regimen for treating asymptomatic bacteriuria or a first episode of cystitis is either nitrofurantoin monohydrate macrocrystals (100 mg bid for 3 days) or

TABLE 50–2

Screening for Asymptomatic Bacteriuria (every 4–6 weeks) Is Recommended for the Following Groups of Pregnant Women

History of asymptomatic bacteriuria[39]
Previous recurrent UTIs[39]
Preexisting renal disease, especially scarred kidneys due to reflux nephropathy[36,40–42]
Structural and neuropathic abnormalities of the renal tracts[31,43]
Renal calculi[44]
Preexisting diabetes mellitus[45] but not gestational diabetes[46]
Sickle cell disease and trait[39]
Low socioeconomic group and less than 12 years higher education[33,39]

UTI, urinary tract infection.

trimethoprim (200 mg bid for 3 days).[50] Nitrofurantoin should be avoided after the onset of labor in patients with glucose-6-phosphate dehydrogenase deficiency, although no well-documented cases of hemolysis in neonates have ever been recorded,[51] and trimethoprim should be avoided in the first trimester because it is a folic acid antagonist associated with an increased risk of neural tube defect.[52]

Screening for recurrent infections should begin one week after completion of initial treatment and then every 4 to 6 weeks for the rest of pregnancy. Recurrent infections or a first infection in a pregnant woman at high risk of pyelonephritis (see Table 50–2) should be treated with a 7- to 10-day course of an antibiotic that reflects antibacterial sensitivities.[50] Women who have had two episodes of asymptomatic bacteriuria or cystitis should be considered for low-dose antibiotic prophylaxis—guided by the sensitivities of the most recent infective organism, for the remainder of pregnancy and until 4 to 6 weeks postpartum.[53] Suitable regimes for long-term antibiotic prophylaxis include nitrofurantoin 50 to 100 mg at night, amoxicillin 250 mg at night, cephalexin 125 to 250 mg at night, or trimethoprim 100 to 150 mg at night.[53] These women should also be investigated for structural abnormalities of the renal tracts or renal calculus, using ultrasonography.

SUMMARY OF MANAGEMENT OPTIONS

Lower Urinary Tract Infections

Management Options	Quality of Evidence	Strength of Recommendation	References
Prepregnancy			
Identify women at high risk of UTI to screen for asymptomatic bacteriuria (see Table 50–2).	III	B	39,40,43, 44,45
Prenatal Screening			
All women at high risk for pyelonephritis or renal impairment should be screened (see Table 50–2).	III	B	39,40,43,44, 45
Screening in a low risk population is more controversial; possibly base the screening policy on the prevalence of asymptomatic bacteriuria.	Ib	A	32
Prenatal Treatment			
If asymptomatic or symptomatic UTI, treat with nitrofurantoin or trimethoprim or according to antibiotic sensitivities.	III	B	49,50
Repeat MSU 7–10 days after antibiotic course.	IV	C	53
Repeat MSU every 4–6 wk.	IV	C	53
If recurrent UTI:	IV	C	53
1. Treat with antibiotics for 7–10 days.			
2. Ultrasound renal tracts for calculus or renal tract anomaly.			
3. Consider low-dose antibiotics for remainder of pregnancy (see text for possible regimens).			
Postnatal			
Repeat MSU 6 wk postpartum.	IV	C	53

MSU, midstream urinalysis; UTI, urinary tract infection.

ACUTE PYELONEPHRITIS

General

The same uropathogens that cause asymptomatic bacteriuria and cystitis are responsible for acute pyelonephritis.[54] Therefore the prevalence of asymptomatic bacteriuria in a pregnant population (see previous section), dictates the incidence of acute pyelonephritis. Screening and treating a high risk population for asymptomatic bacteriuria (see Table 50–2) reduces the incidence of acute pyelonephritis to less than 1%.[33,36] Unless acute pyelonephritis is treated promptly there is considerable maternal and fetal morbidity.[54]

Maternal Symptoms and Signs

Most women with acute pyelonephritis present in the second and third trimester.[54] Over 80% of women present with backache, fever, rigors, and costovertebral angle tenderness, and about half have lower urinary tract symptoms, nausea, and vomiting.[54] Bacteremia is present in 15% to 20% of pregnant women with acute pyelonephritis,[54] and a small proportion of these women will develop septic shock and increased capillary leak, leading to pulmonary edema.[55] It is important, therefore, to differentiate the hypotension due to reduced intravascular volume (fever, nausea and vomiting) from that due to septic shock. Women with pyelonephritis at risk of serious complications are those who present with the highest fever (>39.4°C), tachycardia (>110 bpm), at more than 20 weeks' gestation and who have received tocolytic agents and injudicious fluid replacement.[56]

Fetal Risks

Acute pyelonephritis can trigger uterine contractions and preterm labour.[57] Antibiotic treatment of pyelonephritis will reduce uterine activity, but those with recurrent infection or marked uterine activity are at increased risk of preterm labour.[57] Because uterine activity often occurs in the absence of cervical change and because tocolysis using β-adrenergics aggravates the cardiovascular response to endotoxaemia,[56] tocolytic therapy should be used with care and only in those with cervical changes.[58]

Management Options

Women suspected of having acute pyelonephritis from their history, symptoms, and signs should be admitted to the hospital. Laboratory tests should include full blood count, SCr, urea, electrolytes, and urine culture. If systemic symptoms or septic shock are present, a blood culture may be useful. Pregnant women with pyelonephritis and septic shock need intensive care. In these women, assessment of the state of hydration is critical and often requires invasive hemodynamic monitoring with a central venous pressure line. This will optimize fluid balance, aiming for a urine output greater than 30 mL/hour to minimize renal impairment and reduce the risk of pulmonary edema. Intravenous antibiotics should be started empirically (see following section) until sensitivities of blood and urine cultures are known. These women often have transient renal impairment, thrombocytopenia, and hemolysis, suggesting that the alveolar capillary endothelium is damaged by endotoxin.[55] A blood film and lactate dehydrogenase concentration will diagnose hemolysis.

Trials investigating the outpatient management of pyelonephritis in pregnancy have identified a group of women who can be treated at home.[58] These women should be at less than 24 weeks' gestation, be relatively healthy, and understand the importance of compliance. They should have an initial period of observation in the hospital to demonstrate their ability to take oral fluids and receive intramuscular cefuroxime/ceftriaxone, and following satisfactory laboratory tests can go home to be seen again within 24 hours for a second intramuscular dose of a cephalosporin. They then start a 10-day course of oral cephalexin 500 mg four times daily or appropriate antibiotic with regular outpatient follow-up.[57] Following this regimen 90% of women will improve as outpatients and 10% will require hospital admission due to sepsis or recurrent pyelonephritis. Women with acute pyelonephritis who are over 24 weeks' gestation should be admitted for at least 24 hours to observe the maternal condition as described earlier and to monitor uterine activity and fetal condition including heart rate.[58]

Choice of Antibiotic

Gram-negative bacteria causing pyelonephritis in pregnancy are often resistant to ampicillin,[59] therefore, intravenous cefuroxime 750 mg to 1.5 g (depending on severity of condition) every 8 hours is an effective first choice until sensitivities are known.[48] Women allergic to β-lactam antibiotics can be given IV gentamicin (1.5 mg/kg /8h) for the initial treatment of acute pyelonephritis. A single-dose regimen (7 mg/kg/24h) should be avoided during pregnancy to reduce the very small risk of eighth nerve damage to the fetus.[50] Serum concentrations of gentamicin should be measured and dose adjustments made according to levels. Intravenous antibiotics should be continued until the patient has been afebrile for 24 hours. Oral antibiotics should then be given for 7 to 10 days, according to bacterial sensitivities, or, if not available, as if for symptomatic lower UTI (see previous section).[50]

Failure of these measures to improve the maternal clinical condition within 48 to 72 hours suggests an underlying structural abnormality. Ultrasonography is an easy but inconclusive way of excluding stones. If clinical suspicion is high, a plain abdominal radiograph will identify 90% of renal stones, and a one-shot intravenous urogram (IVU) at 20 to 30 minutes will identify the rest.[58] The risk to the fetus from radiation of one or two radiographs is minimal, especially when compared with the clinical benefit of identifying an obstructed, nonfunctioning kidney. Urinary tract obstruction can also be detected using magnetic resonance urography, especially during the second and third trimesters.[60]

Following one episode of pyelonephritis, pregnant women should have monthly urine cultures to screen for a recurrence.[58] The risk of recurrent pyelonephritis can be reduced with antimicrobial prophylaxis, according to the sensitivities of initial bacterial infection[53,61] or with nitrofurantoin 100 mg at night continued until 4 to 6 weeks postpartum.[58]

SUMMARY OF MANAGEMENT OPTIONS
Acute Pyelonephritis

Management Options	Quality of Evidence	Strength of Recommendation	References
Prepregnancy			
Identify women at high risk of UTI to screen for asymptomatic bacteriuria (see Table 50–2).	III	B	39,40,43, 44,45
Prenatal Screening			
All women at high risk for pyelonephritis or renal impairment should be screened (see Table 50–2).	III	B	39,40,43, 44,45
Prenatal Treatment			
Initial diagnosis of acute pyelonephritis is clinical (symptoms: back/loin ache, fever, rigors, nausea, and vomiting; signs: pyrexia, tachycardia, costovertebral angle tenderness).	–	GPP	–
If acute pyelonephritis is suspected, admit to hospital (if septic shock, admit to HDU/ITU).	–	GPP	–
Investigate: CBC (thrombocytopenia, hemolysis), serum creatinine, BUN, LDH (hemolysis), urine culture, blood culture, ultrasound renal tracts	–	GPP	–
Intravenous fluid if vomiting and/or shocked.		GPP	–
Monitor with CVP/PAWP if renal impairment and/or shocked.	–	GPP	–
IV antibiotic; cefuroxime 750 mg–1.5 g q8h or gentamicin 1.5 mg/kg/q8h.	Ia	A	48,50
Switch to oral antibiotic for 7–10 days when apyrexial for 24 h and bacterial sensitivities are known.	–	GPP	–
Repeat MSU 7–10 days after antibiotic course completed.	IV	C	58
Repeat MSU every 4 wk.	IV	C	58
If recurrent UTI: 1. Treat with antibiotics for 7–10 days. 2. Ultrasound renal tracts for calculus or renal tract anomaly. 3. Consider low-dose antibiotics for remainder of pregnancy (see text for possible regimens).	III	B	53,58,60
Postnatal			
Repeat MSU 6 wk postpartum; possible referral for renal team follow-up.	IV	C	53,58

BUN, blood urea nitrogen; CBC, complete blood count; CVP/PAWP, central venous pressure/pulmonary artery wedge pressure; HDU/ITU, hemodialysis unit/intensive therapy (care) unit; LDH, lactate dehydrogenase; MSU, midstream urinalysis; UTI, urinary tract infection.

ACUTE RENAL FAILURE IN PREGNANCY

General

Acute renal failure (ARF) is now a rare, but serious complication of pregnancy. In early pregnancy ARF is associated with septic abortion (a complication now largely confined to the developing world) and dehydration related to hyperemesis gravidarum. Around the time of delivery, ARF is most commonly caused by gestational syndromes such as preeclampsia/hemolysis, elevated liver enzymes, and low platelets (HELLP) syndrome and abruptio placentae (Table 50–3). Pregnancy is, however, a prothrombotic state, associated with heightened inflammation[62] and major changes to the vascular endothelium,[63] in particular the glomerular capillary endothelium.[64] These physiologic changes predispose pregnant women to acute glomerular capillary thrombosis. Whereas nonpregnant patients who suffer an acute prerenal insult, such as hemorrhage, dehydration, or septic shock, may develop transient acute tubular necrosis (ATN) if inadequately treated, the same prerenal insult in pregnancy is more likely to develop into renal cortical necrosis with permanent renal impairment. This is even more likely to occur if a prerenal insult coexists with a pregnancy-related condition that induces a consumptive coagulopathy or endothelial damage (e.g., preeclampsia/HELLP syndrome).

TABLE 50–3

Causes of Acute Renal Failure in Pregnancy

Most common causes	Placental abruption Severe preeclampsia/HELLP syndrome
Early pregnancy	Septic abortion Hyperemesis gravidarum Ovarian hyperstimulation syndrome
Rare causes	Amniotic fluid embolus HUS/TTP Acute fatty liver of pregnancy. Acute obstruction of renal tracts

HELLP, hemolysis, elevated liver enzymes, low platelets; HUS, hemolytic uremic syndrome; TTP, thrombotic thrombocytopenic purpura.

The principles of management are aimed at identification and correction of the precipitating insult and optimal fluid resuscitation, which is best guided by monitoring the central venous pressure (CVP) and ideally pulmonary artery wedge pressure. If oliguria persists despite euvolemia, with deteriorating renal function or fluid overload, then fluid restriction followed by renal replacement therapy is indicated (Table 50–4).

Acute Renal Failure Associated with Preeclampsia (See also Chapters 36 and 80)

General

Preeclampsia rarely causes ARF severe enough to require dialysis.[65] In a cohort of South African women with severe preeclampsia and renal impairment, 7 of 72 (10%) required temporary dialysis and none developed chronic renal failure.[65] All women who needed dialysis either had hemorrhage due to abruptio placentae or HELLP syndrome.[65] Preeclampsia causing mild transient renal impairment (SCr up to 125 μmol/L; 1.41 mg/dL) is common, but with appropriate management, recovery of renal function should be complete (see next section).

Women with preexisting renal disease are more vulnerable to preeclampsia, especially when it is associated with chronic hypertension.[66] A meta-analysis of trials investigating the effectiveness of low-dose aspirin (50–150 mg/day) in pregnant women with moderate to severe renal disease revealed a significant reduction in the risk of preeclampsia and perinatal death.[67]

TABLE 50–4

Indications for Renal Replacement Therapy (RRT), (Dialysis)

Hyperkalemia (K >7.0 mmol/L), refractory to medical treatment
Pulmonary edema, refractory to diuretics
Acidosis producing circulatory problems
Uremia (there is no absolute level of uremia above which dialysis is mandatory for new-onset acute renal failure, but a serum urea over 25–30 mmol/L or SCr >500–700 mmol/L (5.65–7.91 mg/dL) usually indicates a need for dialysis).

Conversely, 2% to 5% of women with preeclampsia have been found to have underlying renal disease when assessed more than 3 months postpartum.[68] Women who have had preeclampsia should therefore be checked for persistent postpartum hypertension and proteinuria. Gestational hypertension usually resolves within 3 months of delivery, but heavy proteinuria due to preeclampsia can take up to 12 months to disappear. Women who have had preeclampsia are more likely to have persistent microalbuminuria compatible with microvascular disease and an increased risk of cardiovascular disease in later life.[69,70]

Women who develop high levels of proteinuria (>10 g/24h) tend to have earlier onset preeclampsia and deliver at an earlier gestational age as compared with preeclamptic women who have less marked proteinuria (<5 g/24h).[71] It is of note, that after correction for prematurity, however, massive proteinuria (>10 g/24h) has no significant effect on neonatal outcome.[71] Increasing proteinuria per se is not therefore an indication for delivery. Pregnant women who develop proteinuria greater than 1 to 3 g/24h (the threshold influenced by other maternal risk factors for thrombosis) should be started on thromboprophylaxis with enoxaparin 40 mg SC (optimal dose) or fragmin 5000 units SC (optimal dose).

The diagnosis of preeclampsia is difficult if there is chronic hypertension and preexisting proteinuria, especially as these two parameters become more marked in late pregnancy. Furthermore, hyperuricemia and IUGR are common features of both preeclampsia and chronic renal impairment, but the presence of raised hepatic transaminases and thrombocytopenia support a diagnosis of preeclampsia.[72]

Management Options for Acute Renal Failure with Preeclampsia

The cure for severe preeclampsia is delivery of the baby and placenta. Delivery may halt the general progression of preeclampsia, but postpartum maternal renal function usually deteriorates before improving.[65] Dialysis is very rarely necessary, but is most common in preeclamptic women who have HELLP syndrome or placental abruption and who double their SCr in the first 24 to 48 hours after admission.[65] Women with preeclampsia who have a rise in SCr from approximately 70 μmol/L (0.79 mg/dL) to greater than 120 μmol/L (1.36 mg/dL) should be delivered to prevent ongoing renal impairment.

Fluid balance is critical to the management of ARF during pregnancy. Too little intravascular fluid leads to prerenal failure, which is especially damaging to chronically impaired kidneys, whereas too much fluid risks pulmonary edema, adult respiratory distress syndrome, and maternal death.[73] Furthermore, transient oliguria (<100 mL over 4 hr) is a common observation in the first 24 hours immediately after a healthy pregnancy. If a preeclamptic woman is not obviously hypovolemic and has a serum urea less than or equal to 5 mmol/L (14 mg/dL) and SCr less than or equal to 90 µmol/L (1.02 mg/dL) repeated fluid challenges to increase urine output are unnecessary and will only increase the maternal risk of pulmonary edema. Women with severe preeclampsia and renal impairment (SCr >120 µmol/L; 1.36 mg/dL) should have their fluid balance guided by either a CVP catheter or, when available, a pulmonary artery flotation catheter on a intensive care unit familiar with this equipment.[74] The rate of fluid replacement should take account of central venous filling pressure, pulmonary wedge pressure, hourly urine output, and insensible losses. Once euvolemic, the rate of IV fluid replacement should equal the previous hours' urine output plus insensible losses—usually 30 mL/hour, if afebrile. The amount of IV fluid replacement can be reduced, once the mother can take oral fluid and her renal impairment starts to improve. IV fluid regimens that stick to a fixed hourly replacement can lead to fluid overload in oliguric woman and to reduced intravascular volume in those undergoing diuresis. Fluid replacement should include blood to replace blood loses, then isotonic sodium chloride or compound sodium lactate (Hartmann's solution). Dextrose solutions are hypotonic and lead to maternal hyponatremia (5% dextrose contains only 30 mmol/L NaCl, compared with 150 mmol/L NaCl in 0.9% NaCl solution).

Low dose "renal" dopamine infusion (3 µg/kg/min) was previously used to increase renal blood flow in people with ARF. However, a group of 60 South African women with severe preeclampsia and ARF had a similar improvement in urine output and renal function following furosemide infusion (5 mg/hr) as compared with dopamine infusion.[100] Because furosemide has fewer side-effects than dopamine, it is recommended that once hypovolemia has been corrected, as judged by the CVP or pulmonary wedge pressure, preeclamptic women with oliguria (<200 mL/12 hr) and a serum urea greater than 14 mmol/L (39.2 mg/dL) and SCr greater than 500 µmol/L (5.65 mg/dL) may benefit from a furosemide infusion in an effort to avoid hemodialysis.[75] Despite a combination of furosemide followed by low-dose dopamine infusion and vice versa, 13/60 preeclamptic women with oliguric renal failure required temporary dialysis.[75]

Once ATN is established, with oliguria and a rising SCr, despite adequate intravascular volume and BP, fluid intake should then be restricted to avoid fluid overload. Under these circumstances, renal replacement therapy is indicated (see Table 50–4). No good studies have followed women with ARF related to preeclampsia, but those with the most severe renal impairment will undoubtedly be left with a degree of permanent renal impairment that might not manifest until later in life.[65]

Hypertension due to preeclampsia is caused by vasoconstriction around a reduced plasma volume.[72] For this reason and despite the lack of evidence from randomized trials,[76] women with severe preeclampsia often receive plasma volume expansion prior to therapeutic vasodilatation.[77] Unless signs of pulmonary edema are present, (basal crackles and Po_2 <95% on air), 500 mL of colloid or crystalloid given over 30 to 60 minutes, or 250 mL/hour until the pulmonary wedge pressure is 10 to 12 mm Hg, can improve both maternal and fetal well-being in severe preeclampsia.[78,79] A vasodilator given alone can cause profound hypotension that may threaten maternal renal, cerebral, and uteroplacental blood flow.

Acute Renal Failure Associated with the Hemolytic Uremic Syndrome/Thrombotic Thrombocytopenic Purpura

Hemolytic uremic syndrome (HUS) and thrombotic thrombocytopenic purpura (TTP) are very similar syndromes (from here on designated HUS/TTP). They are characterized by microangiopathic hemolytic anemia and thrombocytopenia. Both congenital and acquired forms of HUS/TTP are more common in late pregnancy.[80] Women with HUS/TTP develop platelet thrombi attached to von Willebrand factor multimers in end-organ microvessels. This typically results in a multiorgan disorder with gastrointestinal ischemia and renal or neurologic impairment.[81] A recently discovered plasma metalloproteinase (ADAMTS13), which normally cleaves von Willebrand factor multimers to prevent microthrombi, is deficient in some women with congenital HUS/TTP,[82] and antibodies that neutralize ADAMTS13 have been found in women with acquired HUS/TTP.[83]

HUS/TTP is more common in women (approximately 70% of all cases) and more common in association with pregnancy (approximately 13% of all cases).[80] During pregnancy, the levels of ADAMTS13 progressively fall.[84] This may explain why women with a congenital deficiency of ADAMTS13 or with other risk factors for thrombosis (e.g., obesity or a thrombophilia) are predisposed to peripartum HUS/TTP.

Hemolytic Uremic Syndrome/Thrombotic Thrombocytopenic Purpura and Preeclampsia

Preeclampsia shares many similarities with HUS/TTP, not least that both syndromes occur most frequently in the third trimester or immediately postpartum. It is, however, most important to differentiate between them, because their management is different. Women with HUS/TTP often present with gastrointestinal or neurologic abnormalities,[80] and they are more likely to have severe renal impairment, hemolysis, and thrombocytopenia compared with women who have preeclampsia. Disseminated intravascular coagulation (DIC) is rare in HUS/TTP, so prothrombin time and kaolin clotting time are usually normal.[81] Women with preeclampsia are more likely to have elevated hepatic transaminases, heavy proteinuria, and abnormal clotting compared with women with HUS/TTP.[72] However, in many women the distinction between preeclampsia and HUS/TTP can only be determined by the course of the illness following delivery,[85] but here again ARF due to preeclampsia usually gets transiently worse before improving.[65]

Management Options for Acute Renal Failure with Hemolytic Uremic Syndrome/Thrombotic Thrombocytopenic Purpura (See also Chapters 42 and 80)

Maternal survival from HUS/TTP has greatly improved since treatment with plasmapheresis—infusion of fresh plasma and removal of old plasma.[86] Until recently it was unclear why plasmapheresis worked, but the recent discovery of antibodies to ADAMTS13 (removed with old plasma) and a congenital deficiency of ADAMTS13 (replenished with infusion of fresh plasma), gives reason to this process. However, a severe deficiency in ADAMTS13, which is not currently a routine laboratory measurement, is not present in all cases of HUS/TTP, and plasmapheresis is effective in pregnant women who have milder deficiencies of ADAMTS13.[87]

Steroids are often added to the plasma exchange regime and are a rationale choice for acquired HUS/TTP with an autoimmune pathology, but there are no randomized controlled trials of their use. Antiplatelet regimes with aspirin and dipyridamole may also be beneficial in conjunction with plasma exchange.[88] Conversely, administration of platelets to thrombocytopenic patients with HUS/TTP can result in a precipitous decline in clinical status.

Acute Renal Failure due to Acute Renal Cortical Necrosis

Risks and Management Options

In the developed world, acute renal cortical necrosis (ARCN) has become a rare complication of pregnancy. The reduced incidence of septic abortion and improved management of peripartum obstetric emergencies has prevented prerenal impairment developing into ATN and then renal ARCN. In the developing world, however, obstetric emergencies are still responsible for the majority of cases of ARCN.[89] ARF following septic abortion or peripartum obstetric emergencies developed into ARCN in 20% of women following a prolonged period of ATN.[90]

ARCN is most commonly caused by abruption of the placenta with hemorrhage, amniotic fluid embolus, and sepsis associated with DIC.[91] Following hemorrhage or sepsis with hypotension, prerenal failure will, without adequate resuscitation, lead to ATN. If anuria persists for longer than a week, then ARCN should be suspected. A definitive diagnosis can be made with renal biopsy, but is often missed due to the patchy nature of cortical necrosis. Selective renal angiography will also confirm the diagnosis, but introduces another nephrotoxic agent and is usually unnecessary. Due to the serious nature of the precipitating illness and the limited availability of renal replacement therapy in the developing world, maternal mortality is still high.[90] However, for those women who survive the acute illness, renal function usually returns slowly over the next 6 to 24 months. Long-term renal function depends on the extent of cortical necrosis, which is often incomplete. Hyperfiltration through remnant glomeruli usually leads to a subsequent progressive decline in renal function.

Acute Renal Failure Due to Acute Fatty Liver of Pregnancy (See also Chapters 48 and 80)

Risks and Management Options

Acute fatty liver of pregnancy (AFLP) causes reversible peripartum liver and renal impairment in 1:5000 to 1:10,000 pregnancies.[92] The diagnosis is made on clinical and laboratory findings of impaired liver and on renal and clotting function, rather than on histologic or radiologic evidence of a fatty liver.[92] Women with AFLP usually present with nausea, vomiting, and abdominal cramps. Impaired renal function and reduced plasma antithrombin levels are early findings of AFLP that may precede liver dysfunction.[92] In established cases of AFLP, depressed function of the liver with prolonged prothrombin time, hypoglycemia, and DIC are more markedly abnormal than liver transaminases, which may only be moderately elevated.[92] In a series of 28 women with AFLP, other ubiquitous laboratory findings at the time of delivery were elevated serum total bilirubin (mean 128 μmol/L; 7.5 mg/dL), creatinine (mean 205 μmol/L; 2.32 mg/dL), and uric acid levels (mean 654 μmol/L; 11mg/dL).[92]

A recessively inherited fetal inborn error of mitochondrial fatty acid oxidation may explain up to 20% of AFLP.[93] Mitochondrial fatty acid oxidation is important for both normal renal and liver function and may therefore explain the dual vulnerability of these organs in women with AFLP.

In women with AFLP, maternal renal impairment is aggravated by hypotension secondary to hemorrhage, which is itself most likely to follow an emergency operative delivery.[92,94] The combination of renal dysfunction, hemorrhage, and DIC secondary to liver failure during pregnancy or postpartum requires intensive care with a multidisciplinary team of hepatologists, nephrologists, intensivists, and obstetricians. Management is supportive, aimed at maintaining adequate fluid balance for renal perfusion, replacing blood, correcting the coagulopathy with fresh frozen plasma and possibly with antithrombin concentrate and fresh platelets. Hypoglycemia should be corrected with 10% dextrose solutions. Temporary dialysis may be necessary, but with good supportive care, recovery of normal renal and liver function is usual.[92] Perinatal survival in association with AFLP is improving, but depends on the early recognition of the maternal condition, close fetal surveillance, timely delivery, and excellent neonatal care.

Acute Renal Failure due to Nephrotoxic Drugs During Pregnancy

Risks and Management Options

Nonsteroidal anti-inflammatory drugs (NSAIDs), including the more selective COX-2 inhibitors, when given to the mother peripartum, reduce renal blood flow and can cause acute renal impairment to both mother and fetus.[95,96] Women with reduced intravascular volume, especially with preexisting renal impairment, are particularly vulnerable and should be prescribed NSAIDs with caution. Aminoglycosides are also nephrotoxic and should be prescribed with care and attention to drug plasma levels in women with mild renal impairment.

Acute Renal Failure due to Renal Obstruction in Pregnancy

Risks and Management Options

Obstruction of the renal tracts during pregnancy may be due to renal calculi (see later discussion), congenital renal tract abnormalities or a gestational overdistension syndrome. Women born with congenital obstructive uropathies at the pelvo- or vesico-ureteric junction (PUJ or VUJ) are at increased risk for urine outflow obstruction in the second half of pregnancy, even if they have had surgical correction in childhood[97] (Fig. 50–1). Congenital abnormalities of the lower urinary tracts including the bladder and urethra are varied and usually require extensive surgical correction in childhood. During pregnancy, these women are at increased risk of recurrent urine infections and, less commonly, of outflow obstruction requiring either temporary nephrostomy or ureteric stent.[98]

Women with a single kidney and urologic abnormalities are particularly vulnerable to developing postrenal failure in relation to gestational obstruction of their solitary kidney (see Fig. 50–1). An incomplete obstruction can cause renal impairment with an apparently good urine output. High back-pressures compress and damage the renal medulla, leading to a loss of renal concentrating ability and production of dilute urine that is passed through an incomplete obstruction. It is also important for the obstetrician to remember that a congenitally single kidney is often associated with other abnormalities of the genital tracts, such as a unicornuate uterus.[99]

During pregnancy the renal tracts can rarely and spontaneously become grossly overdistended. If untreated this overdistension can very rarely lead to rupture of the kidney or renal tracts.[100] Women with overdistension of the renal tracts initially present with severe loin pain, most commonly on the right side and radiating to the lower abdomen. The pain is positional and inconstant; it is characteristically relieved by lying on the opposite side and tucking the knees up to the chest. A palpable tender flank mass may suggest renal tract rupture.[100] Rupture of the kidney almost always occurs in a previously diseased kidney, usually in association with a benign hamartoma or renal abscess.[100] Urinalysis will reveal either gross or microscopic hematuria. A renal ultrasound will detect a hydronephrotic kidney with a grossly dilated pelvicaliceal system (see previous discussion for physiologic pelvicaliceal dimensions). Occasionally a urinoma will be evident around the kidney, indicating rupture of the renal pelvis that can sometimes seal spontaneously.

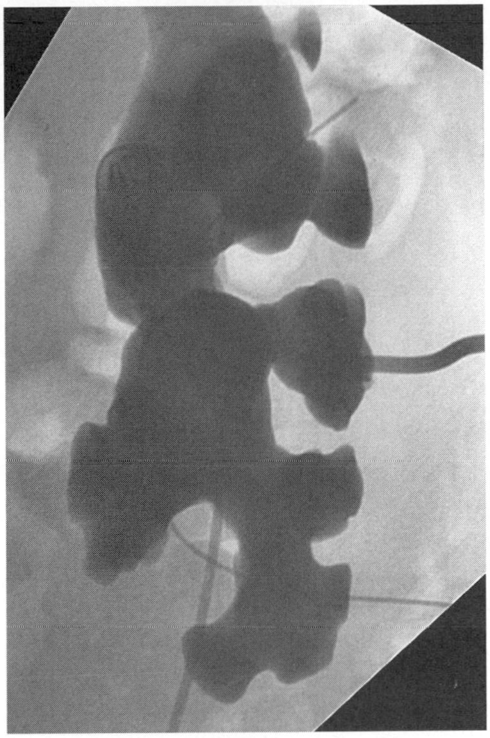

FIGURE 50–1
A postpartum nephrostogram of a dilated collecting system in a solitary cross-fused left kidney that obstructed at 22 weeks' gestation. This 28-year-old primigravida presented with nausea and mild left loin pain and was admitted with severe hypertension 180/110 mm Hg. Her SCr rose from 162 μmol/L (1.83 mg/dL) to 298 μmol/L (3.37 mg/dL) in 3 days, despite a urine output of 4 L/24 hr. Pelvicaliceal dilatation (36-mm diameter) was noted on renal ultrasound, indicating partial urinary outflow obstruction. Within days of a nephrostomy, her symptoms dissipated and the hypertension and SCr had returned to normal; the pregnancy went to 37 weeks. Labor failed to progress and a caesarean section was complicated by an abnormal unicornuate uterus. The nephrostomy remained in situ until 6 weeks postpartum, at which time a ureteric stent was inserted. (Figure shows stent and nephrostomy tube.)

The pain from the overdistension syndrome varies from mild to very severe. Women with mild symptoms can usually be treated with advice on positional relief and regular analgesia. Women with severe unremitting pain, hematuria, and grossly distended renal tracts on ultrasound, in the absence of structural or infected masses, usually have immediate pain relief following decompression of the system with either a ureteric stent or nephrostomy. Rupture of the kidney necessitates immediate surgery and almost invariably an emergency nephrectomy.[100]

SUMMARY OF MANAGEMENT OPTIONS
Acute Renal Failure

Management Options	Quality of Evidence	Strength of Recommendation	References
Identify and Treat Precipitating Cause			
Severe Preeclampsia			
Delivery	III	B	65
Fluid balance	III	B	74
Furosimde if necessary	Ib	A	75
Dialysis in rare cases	Ib	A	75
Hemorrhage			
Blood and clotting factor replacement	–	GPP	–
Medical/surgical methods to stop bleeding			
Sepsis	–	GPP	–
Antibiotics			
Surgical drainage if appropriate			
HUS/TTP			
Plasmapheresis	Ib	A	86
Steroids	III	B	88
Antiplatelet therapy (e.g., aspirin)	III	B	88
FFP	III	B	88
ARCN	III	B	90
Supportive management			
Often with RRT until renal function returns			
Acute Fatty Liver of Pregnancy	III	B	92,94
Delivery			
Supportive management			
Correct clotting, hypoglycemia, and fluid balance			
Urinary Tract Obstruction	III	B	98,100
Correction of obstruction			
Nephrotoxic Drugs	III	B	95,96
Stop			
Monitoring and Optimising Fluid Balance			
Clinical assessment; thirst, urine output (catheter), skin turgor, JVP (difficult in pregnancy).	III	B	150–152
Biochemical SCr, BUN, urine chemistry (but rarely useful).			
If SCr >120 μmol/L (1.36 mg/dL) and clinical uncertainty of fluid balance, use invasive monitoring (CVP/PAWP).			
In severe preeclampsia/HELLP in the absence of pulmonary edema (Po_2 > 95% on air), give fluid to expand plasma volume prior to vasodilator.			
Treatment			
Recognize deteriorating renal function despite euvolemia and need for RRT (see Table 50–4).	III	B	150–152
If new onset proteinuria (>10 g/24h and SCr >120 μmol/L) remote from term (i.e., < 30–32 wk), consider diagnostic renal biopsy.			
Proteinuria >1–3 g/24h, give thromboprophylaxis with LMW heparin until 6 wk postpartum or until proteinuria resolves.			

ARCN, acute renal cortical necrosis; BUN, blood urea nitrogen; CVP/PAWP, central venous pressure/pulmonary artery wedge pressure; FFP, fresh frozen plasma; HELLP, hemolysis, elevated liver enzymes, low platelets (syndrome); HUS/TTP, hemolytic uremic syndrome/thrombotic thrombocytopenic purpura; JVP, jugular venous pressure; LMW, low molecular weight; RRT, renal replacement therapy; SCr, serum creatinine.

CHRONIC RENAL DISEASE IN PREGNANCY

General

The effect of pregnancy-related changes on women with preexisting renal disease depends on the type of renal disease; the level of renal impairment; and complications such as hypertension, proteinuria, and infection (Table 50–5). Advice to women with renal impairment regarding pregnancy must take into account all these parameters in an effort to answer the two most important questions:

- What effect will the pregnancy have on the mother's kidney disease?
- What effect will the mother's kidney disease have on the pregnancy?

The Effect of Pregnancy on the Mother's Kidney Disease—Risks and Management Options

The gestational increment in GFR is attenuated in women with moderate renal impairment and absent in those with a SCr greater than 200 μmol/L (2.26 mg/dL).[101–104] Similarly, the gestational increase in blood volume and erythropoiesis is inversely related to the preconception SCr.[103] However, the anemia of renal impairment can be safely corrected during pregnancy with human recombinant erythropoeitin.[105] At all levels of preconception renal impairment, the likelihood of renal damage as a consequence of pregnancy is increased by the coexistence of other factors, in particular, hypertension, proteinuria, and infection.[101-108]

TABLE 50–5

Features Detrimental to Long-term Maternal Renal Function and Pregnancy Outcome

Impaired Renal Function	Preconception SCr >177 μmol/L (2.00 mg/dL) or GFR <25 mL/min. Two thirds of mothers have an accelerated decline in renal function and one third develop ESRF in association with pregnancy. Increased risk of preterm labor, IUGR, and preeclampsia.
Hypertension	Increased risk of preeclampsia, IUGR, and preterm labor and an accelerated decline in maternal renal function
Proteinuria	Nephrotic levels associated with maternal thromboembolism. Variable reports of IUGR, preterm labor, and poorer long-term maternal renal prognosis
Urinary Tract Infections	Increased maternal and fetal morbidity with acute pyelonephritis and preeclampsia and probable increased risk of preterm labor
Reduced Plasma Volume	IUGR
Hyperglycemia	Large-for-gestational-age babies, but with microvascular disease there is an increased risk of IUGR

ESRF, end-stage renal failure; GFR, glomerular filtration rate; IUGR, intrauterine growth restriction; SCr, serum creatinine.

Effect of Pregnancy on Maternal Kidney Disease in Women with Preexisting Mild to Moderate Renal Impairment

Women who become pregnant with renal disease, but with normal or near normal renal function at conception and a SCr <120 μmol/L (1.36 mg/dL) carry only a slightly increased risk of long-term damage to their kidneys from pregnancy compared with women with mild renal disease who had never become pregnant.[102,109] However, more accurate data using creatinine clearance instead of SCr is still needed.

In a large multicenter series, 40% of women with moderate renal impairment (SCr 124–168 μmol/L; 1.49–1.90 mg/dL) had a pregnancy-related deterioration in renal function, which persisted after delivery in about half of the cases.[110,111] In one series, only 1 of 49 (2%) pregnancies in women with an initial SCr below 177 μmol/L (2.00 mg/dL) rapidly declined to ESRF.[110]

Effect of Pregnancy on Maternal Kidney Disease in Women with Preexisting Severe Renal Impairment

Two-thirds of women with a SCr greater than 177 μmol/L (2.00 mg/dL) have a gestational deterioration in renal function that nearly always persists postpartum.[110] Unlike women who have mild to moderate renal impairment, those with severely impaired renal function do not tend to recover their renal function postpartum. One-third of women with a SCr above 177μmol/L (2.00 mg/dL) (creatinine clearance <25 mL/min) will develop ESRF during or following pregnancy.[110]

There is no guarantee that aborting the pregnancy will reverse a decline in renal function. Indeed, women with severe renal impairment who have a gestational decline in renal function requiring dialysis, might consider continuing the pregnancy, (in the absence of other complications), as there is an 80% chance of a live birth outcome when dialysis is started after conception.[112] Women who are established on dialysis with ESRF have no further renal function to lose, but they put themselves at high risk of morbidity from pregnancy complications such as preeclampsia (see following section).

Effect of Pregnancy on Maternal Kidney Disease in Women with Preexisting Proteinuria and Hypertension

Asymptomatic proteinuria (>500 mg/day) detected in early pregnancy, usually indicates underlying renal impairment.[113] These women have an increased risk of preeclampsia (30%), which increases further in those who also have chronic hypertension.[113] Limited postpartum follow-up of women with proteinuria identified in early pregnancy has shown that they have an increased risk of progressive renal impairment.[113] It is therefore most important that women with proteinuria recognized during early pregnancy are investigated for previously occult renal disease and monitored serially throughout pregnancy for changes in renal function, level of proteinuria, BP, and occult urinary infection. Chronic hypertension and preconception proteinuria usually worsen in the third trimester[110] and in most series provoke an accelerated decline in renal function postpartum.[101–108]

Effect of the Mother's Kidney Disease on the Pregnancy—Risks and Management Options

Improved neonatal and obstetric care over the last few decades are responsible for the impressive improvement in neonatal outcome from women with impaired renal function.[101,104,110] However, women with the most severe renal impairment still have the worst fetal outcome.[101,103,110] Furthermore, early pregnancy losses are often ignored in analyses of pregnancy outcome, but are also more common in women with severe renal impairment.[101,114,115]

Effect of Preexisting Mild to Moderate Renal Impairment on Pregnancy Outcome

Women with normal or near-normal renal function have a higher incidence of preterm delivery and IUGR.[102] In a retrospective study of 240 pregnancies in 166 Japanese women who delivered between 1970 and 1988, the perinatal mortality rate was significantly higher if the GFR was less than 70 mL/minute (22%; versus 4% if GFR > 70 mL/min).[116]

Effect of Preexisting Severe Renal Impairment on Pregnancy Outcome

A ubiquitous observation is that a SCr greater than 220 μmol/L is associated with more preterm deliveries and lower birth weights than a lower SCr.[110] In one series, 73% of women with a preconception SCr greater than 221 μmol/L were delivered before 37 weeks and 57% had IUGR, compared with 55% and 31%, respectively, for women who had a SCr less than 221 μmol/L.[110] Neonatal survival was an impressive 100% in the group with severe renal insufficiency.[110]

A cesarean section rate of around 60% is a consistent finding in most series with women who have markedly impaired renal function, but relatively good perinatal outcome.[101,106,110] Therefore, when the fetus is put at risk by maternal disease, it seems inadvisable to prolong pregnancy beyond a point when intact neonatal survival is expected. Although it is difficult to dissect apart the independent contribution to poor fetal outcome of maternal hypertension, proteinuria, and renal impairment, the balance of evidence suggests that each parameter is individually and cumulatively detrimental to fetal outcome.[101-103,114]

Effect of Hypertension on Pregnancy Outcome

In one study, women with moderate to severe renal impairment (SCr 110–490 μmol/L; 1.24–5.54 mg/dL) who were hypertensive at conception or in early pregnancy had a 10.6 times higher relative risk of fetal loss than normotensive women with the same level of renal function.[101] Another study found that if the preconception BP was greater than 140/90 mm Hg, perinatal mortality was 23% versus 4% for normotensives with renal disease.[116] Furthermore, treatment of chronic hypertension before conception reduces the incidence of fetal and maternal complications toward that of normotensive women.[114]

Outside of pregnancy, hypertension related to chronic renal disease is often treated with angiotensin-converting enzyme (ACE) inhibitors or angiotensin II antagonists. These drugs are particularly useful for women with diabetic nephropathy and can be taken up to the sixth week of pregnancy, but due to their effect on fetal renal development and other teratogenic effects, they should be stopped as soon as pregnancy is diagnosed. Some women have continued these drugs throughout the first trimester, without apparent harm to the neonate, but without any detailed assessment of neonatal renal function.

Antihypertensive medications that can be safely used to control hypertension in pregnant women with renal impairment include methyldopa, labetolol, nifedipine SR, or alpha antagonists. Thiazide diuretics mildly attenuate gestational plasma volume expansion and show a trend toward mild fetal IUGR.

Effect of Preexisting Proteinuria on Pregnancy Outcome

One series of women with primary glomerulonephrosis demonstrated a linear relationship between increasing proteinuria and decreasing infant weight,[117] and in another that included 398 pregnancies, there were 34 stillbirths (9%), all associated with significant proteinuria.[114] In another series, women with asymptomatic proteinuria (>500 mg/24 hr) in early pregnancy had 53/57 live births, but 45% were preterm, 23% were complicated by IUGR, and 62% had superimposed preeclampsia.[113] However, in a further series of 82 pregnancies affected by moderate to severe renal impairment, high-grade proteinuria had no effect on pregnancy outcome.[110]

Patients with nephrotic syndrome are at increased risk of thromboembolism, but outside of pregnancy this risk is not usually considered high enough to warrant thromboprophylaxis with heparin. Pregnant women, however, are already in a prothrombotic state, and thromboembolism is a major cause of maternal death.[73] Thromboprophylaxis with low-molecular-weight (LMW) heparin (e.g., enoxaparin 40 mg SC once daily) is therefore essential for all pregnant women with more than 3 g proteinuria per 24 hours, including those with proteinuria due to preeclampsia. In women with 1 to 3g proteinuria per 24 hours, heparin thromboprophylaxis should be considered, especially if additional risk factors exist, such as obesity (BMI >30), maternal age older than 35 years, cigarette smoking, and immobility. Thromboprophylaxis with LMW heparin should continue for at least 6 weeks postpartum if the proteinuria persists.

Women with heavy proteinuria will often have a low plasma albumin concentration and massive systemic edema. This is particularly seen in some pregnant women with diabetic nephropathy. In order for them to tolerate the pregnancy, small doses of a loop diuretic, furosemide, may be necessary to reduce edema. Thromboprophylaxis with LMW heparin is essential for this group of women.

Prophylactic Low-Dose Aspirin and Pregnancies Complicated by Renal Disease

Women with renal disease often hyperfilter through remaining glomeruli and have microalbuminuria. During healthy pregnancy women develop a prothrombotic and proinflammatory state, which, even if preeclampsia does not occur, is often associated with a degree of glomerular endothelial swelling.[64] If preeclampsia does emerge, the glomerular capillary endothelial cells swell and the narrowed lumen is filled with thrombus.[64] Thrombosis and infarction within a glomerular capillary lead to the loss of a functioning nephron and loss of renal function. Subclinical cortical necrosis due to glomerular capillary thrombosis is a possible explanation for the gestational loss of renal function associated with pregnancies complicated by moderate to severe renal impairment, especially in relation to sepsis due to recurrent UTIs.[104] In an attempt to prevent glomerular capillary thrombi, preserve maternal renal function, and reduce the risk of preeclampsia,[67] the author prescribes prophylactic low-dose aspirin (75 mg/day) throughout pregnancy to all women with a history of renal disease, especially those who have recurrent UTIs and who are immunosuppressed with renal transplants.

SUMMARY OF MANAGEMENT OPTIONS

Chronic Renal Failure

Management Options	Quality of Evidence	Strength of Recommendation	References
Prepregnancy			
Counsel about increased risk of Pregnancy complications (IUGR, preeclampsia, preterm labor)	–	GPP	–
Deteriorating maternal renal function			
Prenatal			
Low-dose aspirin (50–150 mg/day to reduce risk of preeclampsia and perinatal death)	Ia	A	67
Monitor maternal:	III	B	101,102,103
-urine for infection every 4–6 wk			
-proteinuria			
-hematuria			
-blood pressure			
-serum creatinine, BUN, CBC			
-baseline renal ultrasound (pelvicaliceal dimensions)			
Monitor fetal			
-growth and health	III	B	102,110,116
Urine infection screening–(keep urine sterile with antibiotics)	–	GPP	–
Proteinuria and hypoalbuminemia—thromboprophylaxis with LMW heparin/aspirin	III	B	73
Hematuria—red cell casts suggest renal parenchymal disease, normal red cell morphology suggests urological pathology and need for nephro-urologic advice	–	GPP	–

Continued

SUMMARY OF MANAGEMENT OPTIONS

Chronic Renal Failure *(Continued)*

Management Options	Quality of Evidence	Strength of Recommendation	References
Blood pressure—keep BP less than or equal to 140/90 mm Hg with antihypertensive treatment (methyldopa, nifedine, labetol; not beta blockers, ACE inhibitors, or thiazide diuretics)	–	GPP	–
Serum creatinine, BUN, CBC. Recognize acute on chronic renal impairment and need for RRT; erythropoietin can be used for severe anemia	III	B	105,112
Baseline renal ultrasound (pelvicaliceal dimensions)	–	GPP	–
Cesarean section commoner	III	B	101,106,110

ACE, angiotensin-converting enzyme; BP, blood pressure; BUN, blood urea nitrogen; CBC, complete blood count; IUGR, intrauterine growth restriction; LMW, low molecular weight; RRT, renal replacement therapy.

SPECIFIC RENAL DISEASES IN PREGNANCY

Risks and Management Options

Primary Glomerulonephritis

The histologic type of primary glomerulonephritis does not affect pregnancy outcome as much as the clinical parameters, hypertension, proteinuria, level of renal impairment, and incidence of UTIs.[116] Suggestions that certain histopathologic diagnoses have a worse fetal or maternal outcome probably reflect the increased incidence of these clinical complications in certain histopathologic diagnoses.[108,116] However, the presence of severe vessel lesions on renal biopsy has been associated with increased perinatal mortality, but had no significant effect on maternal complications during pregnancy.[114] On the rare occasion that sudden renal impairment (SCr >120 µmol/L; 1.36 mg/dL) or new-onset heavy proteinuria (>5 g proteinuria per 24 hr) occurs before 30 to 32 weeks' gestation in the absence of preeclampsia, a renal biopsy is indicated to exclude a steroid-responsive glomerular disease.

IgA Disease

IgA nephropathy is the most common type of chronic primary glomerulonephritis in young people and is consequently highly represented in pregnant women. Most women with IgA nephropathy who are normotensive and have a GFR above 70 mL/minute have a good obstetric and renal outcome following pregnancy.[108,116] Those women who have a preconception SCr greater than 120 µmol/L (1.36 mg/dL; GFR <50 mL/min), hypertension, heavy proteinuria, and the most severe histologic lesions on renal biopsy are more likely to have an accelerated deterioration in renal function.[108,116]

Women who had Henoch-Schönlein purpura (HSP) with IgA glomerulonephritis as children are at an increased risk of recurrent proteinuric hypertension during their pregnancies (70% in one series).[118] There are also reports of pregnancy triggering recurrent HSP.[119]

Autosomal Dominant Polycystic Kidney Disease

Women with autosomal dominant polycystic kidney disease (ADPKD) who have normal renal function and BP, usually have a successful, uncomplicated pregnancy.[120] However, preexisting hypertension is a significant risk factor for preeclampsia and fetal prematurity.[120] In one study of 468 live births from women with ADPKD there were no more fetal complications compared with 200 live births from family members who did not have ADPKD.[120] As this is an autosomal dominant condition, the parents must be aware before pregnancy that there is a 50% chance of their offspring being affected.

Reflux Nephropathy

Reflux nephropathy is one of the most common renal conditions in women of childbearing age. Women who had vesicoureteric reflux (VUR) in childhood are at risk of reflux nephropathy in later life. Reflux nephropathy is characterized by renal scarring, reduced GFR, recurrent UTIs, proteinuria, and hypertension. This combination of clinical features makes pregnancy in women with reflux nephropathy particularly high risk. Pregnancy complications include superimposed preeclampsia (≤75%), recurrent UTIs (28%–65%), deterioration of renal function (≤13% have an irreversible decline in renal function), gestational ureteric obstruction requiring drainage (2/47), and increased fetal morbidity and mortality influenced by maternal hypertension and SCr at conception.[104,121,122] Women with reflux nephropathy who have impaired renal function (SCr >110 µmol/L; 1.24 mg/dL) at conception are at particularly high risk of poor pregnancy outcome.[104]

All women with reflux nephropathy, even those who have had VUR successfully treated by ureteric reimplantation during childhood, should be screened for asymptomatic bacteriuria every 4 to 6 weeks throughout pregnancy (see Table 50–2). Acute pyelonephritis is twice as common in women with persistent VUR than in those who have had spontaneous or surgical resolution of VUR.[104] Following one UTI, low-dose prophylactic antibiotics, chosen according to the sensitivity of the most recent UTI, would reduce the risk of further UTIs and may therefore preserve renal function. Women with persistent VUR, especially those with a history of upper UTI and those who are contemplating pregnancy, should consider prepregnancy correction of VUR to reduce maternal and fetal morbidity.

Women with congenital urologic defects, including reflux nephropathy or PUJ obstruction, are at increased risk of upper renal tract obstruction requiring nephrostomy or stenting, even if they have had urologic correction as children.[121] Throughout pregnancy they should be monitored regularly with serial assessment of renal function (blood urea nitrogen, BUN), midstream urine, and BP. Ultrasonography of the renal pelvis at the end of the first trimester will provide a useful baseline measurement with which to compare future measurements. A repeat ultrasound scan is indicated if there is renal pain suggestive of obstruction, persistent infection, or a rise in SCr in a woman with a single kidney.

VUR is a familial disorder, which affects 20% of infants who have a parent with a family history of VUR, compared with a 1% to 2% frequency of VUR in the general population.[123] Prevention of damaging reflux nephropathy requires diagnosis and treatment before the neonate develops a UTI.[124] Fetal VUR can be detected antenatally by obstetric ultrasound[124] or in newborn babies soon after delivery using cystography, not renal ultrasonography.[123] Evidence for renal scarring can safely be sought in those positive for VUR using a dimercaptosuccinic acid (DMSA) radioisotope scan at 3 months of age.[123]

SUMMARY OF MANAGEMENT OPTIONS

Primary Glomerulonephritis, Autosomal Dominant Polycystic Kidney Disease, Reflux Nephropathy

Management Options	Quality of Evidence	Strength of Recommendation	References
Primary Glomerulonephritis			
Prenatal			
Control BP	–	GPP	–
Low-dose aspirin throughout pregnancy	Ia	A	67
Screen for preeclampsia	III	B	118
Fetal surveillance	III	B	114
Steroids if worsening disease with known steroid-responsive disease *not* due to preeclampsia	–	GPP	–
Autosomal Dominant Polycystic Kidney Disease			
Prenatal and Postnatal			
Fetal surveillance, screen for preeclampsia especially coexisting hypertension	III	B	120
Screen baby/infant for disease	–	GPP	–
Reflux Nephropathy			
Prepregnancy			
Baseline assessment of GFR and proteinuria	III	B	104
Optimal control of BP (<140/90 mm Hg)	III	B	104
Advise of risks of complicated pregnancy	–	GPP	–
Prenatal			
Baseline renal US at 12 wk	III	B	104,120,121

Continued

SUMMARY OF MANAGEMENT OPTIONS

Primary Glomerulonephritis, Autosomal Dominant Polycystic Kidney Disease, Reflux Nephropathy *(Continued)*

Management Options	Quality of Evidence	Strength of Recommendation	References
Reflux Nephropathy			
Repeat US if renal angle pain or increase in SCr.	–	GPP	–
Low-dose aspirin through pregnancy	Ia	A	67
Screen for preeclampsia; fetal surveillance	III	B	104,120,121
MSU every 4–6 wk until 6 wk postpartum	III	B	104
Prophylactic antibiotics if recurrent UTIs	III	B	104
Screen fetus for VUR	III	B	123
Postnatal			
Screen infant shortly after delivery for VUR with cystography.	III	B	123

BP, blood pressure; GFR, glomerular filtration rate; MSU, midstream urinalysis; SCr, serum creatinine; US, ultrasound; UTI, urinary tract infection; VUR, vesicoureteric reflux.

Nephrolithiasis

The incidence of symptomatic renal stone disease during pregnancy is similar to that in the nongravid state.[125] One large series has shown that symptomatic nephrolithiasis affects 1 in 244 pregnancies,[126] despite an apparently ideal environment for renal stone formation that includes gestational renal tract dilatation, urinary stasis, and hypercalciuria. However, during pregnancy there is also increased excretion of inhibitors of stone formation, such as magnesium, citrate, and nephrocalcin, an acidic glycoprotein. Symptomatic renal calculi are, however, more common in whites than African Americans and in multigravidas than primigravidas.[125,126] Renal colic is also more common in the second and third trimester.[125,126]

One large series including 90 pregnancies in 78 women with renal stones, found an increased frequency of UTIs.[127] UTIs associated with renal stones should be treated for longer than isolated UTIs and followed up with antibiotic prophylaxis. Another large series found that women with symptomatic renal stones had an increased risk of preterm rupture of membranes,[126] possibly related to the increased frequency of urinary infection.

Acute Renal Colic

Pregnant women in the process of passing a renal calculus usually develop severe colicky lumbar pain, associated with fever, lower UTI, and hematuria. An ultrasound of the renal tracts will identify a renal calculus in about half of these women.[128] In those women with a normal ultrasound, but symptoms still suggestive of a renal calculus, a kidneys, ureters, bladder (KUB) and single-shot IVU radiocontrast study can identify most other renal calculi.[129] However, in an effort to avoid even a small dose of radiation to the fetus, magnetic resonance urography has recently been used to differentiate between physiologic urinary tract dilatation and obstruction due to calculi.[60]

Initial conservative management of renal colic during pregnancy will result in up to 75% of women passing their stones spontaneously.[128,129] Women must be well hydrated, given pain relief with meperidine (pethidine) and antibiotics. Continued symptoms may necessitate passage of a ureteric stent, but this is difficult to do without radiologic guidance. A percutaneous nephrostomy is another option, especially for an obstructed single kidney, but the nephrostomy is likely to have to remain in place for the rest of the pregnancy.

Recent advances in fiberoptics have allowed the development of holmium laser lithotripsy. This technique allows a ureteroscope to be passed into the upper renal tracts, facilitating direct stone crushing energy to within 0.5 mm of the laser fiber tip. This technique has been successfully and safely used in all stages of pregnancy.[130]

Women who are recurrent stone formers with persistent gross hypercalciuria, despite increased fluid intake, can use thiazide diuretics in pregnancy to increase distal tubular reabsorption of calcium. Uric acid and cystine stones rarely form in pregnancy owing to the physiologic alkalinization of the urine. If problematic, both conditions may be controlled by increasing urine output and further alkalinizing the urine to a pH above 6. During pregnancy, xanthine oxidase inhibitors for uric acid stones and D-penicillamine for cystine stones should probably be avoided, especially during the first trimester.

SUMMARY OF MANAGEMENT OPTIONS

Nephrolithiasis, Renal Colic

Management Options	Quality of Evidence	Strength of Recommendation	References
Prepregnancy			
Identify women with renal calculi; for 4–6 weekly MSU during pregnancy; consider definitive treatment to remove calculus.	III	B	60,127–129
Prenatal			
If UTI with renal calculi, treat for 10 days then give prophylactic antibiotics.	IV	C	127
If renal colic: • Give IV NS and pain relief (pethidine rather than NSAID even in first or second trimester). • Identify renal calculus with KUB, or single-shot IV urography, or MRU, if available. • Most (75%) renal calculi will pass spontaneously.	III	B	128,129
Renal calculi causing obstruction, especially in a single kidney, need treatment with a uretric stent or nephrostomy, or ureteroscopic holium laser lithotripsy, if available.	III	B	128–130
Postnatal			
Definitive removal of obstructing calculus	III	B	128–130

IV, intravenous; KUB, kidneys, ureter, bladder; MRU, magnetic resonance urography; NS, normal saline; NSAID, nonsteroidal anti-inflammatory drug; UTI, urinary tract infection.

Diabetic Nephropathy (See also Chapter 45)

Diabetic nephropathy eventually affects about 30% of all patients with type 1 (insulin-dependent diabetes mellitus, IDDM). Before the onset of renal impairment and proteinuria, there is glomerular hyperfiltration and increased urinary albumin excretion—microalbuminuria. The hyperfiltration of early diabetic nephropathy is damaging to the glomerulus, as it is mediated by an increase in glomerular capillary pressure. The increase in renal blood flow due to pregnancy further augments the hyperfiltration of early diabetic nephropathy, but this only partly explains the transient rise in microalbuminuria (30–300 mg albuminuria) and preexisting proteinuria during the third trimester.[131]

Microalbuminuria in early pregnancy is, however, associated with an increased prevalence of preeclampsia and as a consequence preterm delivery.[132] An elevated glycosylated hemoglobin (HbA_{1c}) in the first trimester,[132] prepregnancy duration of diabetes,[132] and maternal blood pressure[133] are all independently associated with an increased risk of preeclampsia. However, improved perinatal care is allowing approximately 95% perinatal survival.[133]

Pregnancy in women with type 1 diabetes does not precipitate the onset of diabetic nephropathy, and those who have established diabetic nephropathy with well-preserved renal function do not progress more rapidly to ESRF as a consequence of pregnancy.[134] Conversely, the majority of women with diabetic nephropathy and moderate to severe renal impairment (SCr >124 μmol/L; 1.4 mg/dL) have more than a 40% chance of an accelerated decline in renal function associated with an exacerbation of hypertension or preeclampsia.[135]

Due to the risk of an accelerated decline in maternal renal function, pregnancy should be discouraged in women with diabetic nephropathy who have a GFR lower than 70 mL/minute, (SCr >124 μmol/L; 1.4 mg/dL), especially in association with uncontrolled hypertension. If pregnancy occurs in this group of women, they must understand the risks to their own renal function and the importance of regular antenatal care. Good control of maternal blood glucose levels and hypertension before conception and during pregnancy will improve both perinatal and maternal outcome.[133] If maternal BP remains persistently over 130/90 mm Hg, a calcium-channel blocker can be safely used throughout pregnancy to lower systemic pressures to protect maternal kidneys and reduce the risk of preeclampsia. Low-dose aspirin (50–150 mg/day) also has a role in reducing the risk of preeclampsia in women with diabetic nephropathy.[67]

Women with diabetic nephropathy who develop nephrotic syndrome are at increased risk of thromboembolism during pregnancy and for 6 weeks postpartum. These women should receive thromboprophylaxis with LMW heparin if proteinuria exceeds 1 to 3 g/24 hours, depending on the presence of other risk factors, such as obesity, smoking, age older than 35 years, history of thrombosis, and immobility. Diuretics used with caution may have a role in the symptomatic relief of gross edema.

SUMMARY OF MANAGEMENT OPTIONS

Diabetic Nephropathy (See also Chapter 45)

Management Options	Quality of Evidence	Strength of Recommendation	References
Prepregancy			
Advise that pregnancy with diabetic nephropathy and SCr >124 μmol/L; 1.4 mg/dL at conception is associated with a 40% risk of gestational decline in renal function	III	B	134,135
Advise that increased risk of adverse pregnancy outcome	III	B	132
Try and achieve euglycemia	III	B	133
Prenatal			
Every 4–6 wk monitor BP, BUN, Glucose, MSU until 24 wk, then every 2 wk until 32 wk, then weekly	III	B	132,134,135
Try and achieve euglycemia	III	B	133
Give aspirin 75 mg once daily to reduce risk of preeclampsia	Ia	A	67
Control hypertension to <140/90 mm Hg	III	B	133
Screen for preeclampsia; fetal surveillance	III	B	132,134,135
Give LMW heparin when >1–3 g proteinuria/24h and hypoalbuminemia	–	GPP	–
A diuretic may be necessary for symptomatic relief of gross edema with nephrotic syndrome	–	GPP	–
Postnatal			
Reassess renal function (GFR) postpartum	III	B	134,135

BP, blood pressure; BUN, blood urea nitrogen; GFR, glomerular filtration rate; LMW, low molecular weight; MSU, midstream urinalysis; SCr, serum creatinine.

Lupus Nephritis (See also Chapter 44)

Systemic lupus erythematosus (SLE) is a multisystem autoimmune disorder that predominantly affects young women and is characterized by a relapsing and remitting course. Renal involvement (lupus nephritis) is recognized by proteinuria, elevated SCr, hypertension, and often thrombocytopenia and hyperuricemia. Consequently, a relapse of SLE during the second half of pregnancy is difficult to distinguish from preeclampsia. Clinical features that may be discriminatory are the presence of hematuria and red cell casts in active lupus nephritis, as well as extrarenal manifestations affecting the skin and joints. The laboratory findings of active SLE include consumption of complement (C3 and C4), which is not consumed during preeclampsia,[136] and a rising titer of double-stranded DNA antibody. The erythrocyte sedimentation rate (ESR) can reach as high as 70 in healthy pregnancy and is therefore not useful in identifying a flare of lupus nephritis during pregnancy. The C-reactive protein (CRP) level is unchanged in active lupus. If there is clinical doubt remote from term (before 32 weeks' gestation), a renal biopsy may help to differentiate between active lupus nephritis and preeclampsia.

Women with quiescent lupus nephritis, absent antiphospholipid antibodies (APL ab), normal or near normal renal function (SCr <120 μmol/L), limited proteinuria (< 500 mg/24 hr), and controlled hypertension for at least 6 months before conception can expect a good fetal and maternal outcome.[137,138] Relapses of SLE are more common in pregnant women who have had more than three flares before pregnancy, who have APL ab, C3 hypocomplementemia, and hypertension. Women with active lupus nephritis at conception, especially in association with proteinuria, hypertension, and APL ab, have an increased risk of early pregnancy loss, IUGR, preterm delivery, preeclampsia, and perinatal and maternal mortality.[138] The presence of maternal APL ab is specifically associated with an increased risk of early pregnancy loss and extractable nuclear antibodies (ENA: anti-Ro and anti-La) are associated with an increased risk of congenital fetal heart block.

Prednisolone, azathioprine, and hydroxychloroquine have all been safely used to control SLE during pregnancy for many years. A flare of lupus nephritis during pregnancy is usually treated with IV methylprednisolone 500 mg daily, for 3 days, and an increase of oral prednisolone to around 40 mg daily. Steroid-resistant and progressive lupus nephritis has been successfully treated during pregnancy with IV cyclophosphamide. However, when a severe flare of lupus nephritis occurs during pregnancy, the effects of this life-threatening condition on the mother need to be balanced against the likelihood of a successful fetal outcome. Difficult decisions regarding continuation of the pregnancy sometimes need to be made. Additional treatment includes antihypertensive medication to control BP to ≤140/90 mm Hg and thromboprophylaxis with low-dose aspirin and LMW heparin, especially in the presence of APL ab and proteinuria greater than 1 g/24 hours. Lupus nephritis is slightly more likely to flare postpartum, but the consensus is not to use prophylactic steroids peripartum, unless there are signs of disease activity.[137]

SUMMARY OF MANAGEMENT OPTIONS

Lupus Nephropathy (See also Chapter 44)

Management Options	Quality of Evidence	Strength of Recommendation	References
Prepregnancy			
Advise to postpone pregnancy until at least 6 months in remission	III	B	138
Advise increased risk of adverse pregnancy outcome, if previous frequent relapses, (SCr >120 μmol/L; 1.36 mg/dL), BP >140/90 mm Hg	III	B	137,138
Advise of significance of ENA to fetus	III	B	138
Prenatal			
Prednisolone, azathioprine, hydroxychloroquine to be used to treat lupus nephritis as necessary	III	B	137
Recognize lupus nephritis flare—rise in dsDNA antibodies and consumption of complement	III	B	136
Treat lupus flare with prednisolone/methylprednisolone	III	B	137
Surveillance for • Preeclampsia • Poor placental function • Fetal congenital heart block if ENA positive	III	B	138
Thromboprophylaxis with LMW heparin if >1 g proteinuria	–	GPP	–
Postnatal			
Advise increased risk of postpartum lupus flare, but no need for prophylactic increase in immunosuppression	III	B	137
Some advise limited breast-feeding if on azathioprine but no strong evidence to support this	–	GPP	–

dsDNA, double-stranded DNA; ENA, extractable nuclear antibodies; LMW, low molecular weight; SCr, serum creatinine.

CHRONIC DIALYSIS AND PREGNANCY

Women with ESRF have reduced fertility, but improvements in hemodialysis and the use of erythropoietin to treat chronic renal failure-induced anemia have increased the likelihood of women conceiving and of producing a surviving infant.[139] The incidence of pregnancy in women on hemodialysis is variably reported between 0.44% and 7%, depending on the criteria that define the female dialysis population.[140] Up to 60% of reported pregnancies now result in a live infant,[105,140] but 80% of pregnancies are preterm at around 32 weeks.[105,140] High fetal urinary urea causes an osmotic diuresis, which probably explains why polyhydramnios affects more than 50%

of such pregnancies. Premature rupture of membranes and maternal hypertension are other causes for preterm delivery.

Women on peritoneal dialysis (PD) are less likely to conceive than women on hemodialysis.[140] Furthermore, as pregnancy progresses the physiologic demands of pregnancy are increasingly difficult to meet by increasing the number of PD exchanges. There are, however, many case reports of successful pregnancies in women on PD.[141] Complications include peritonitis that should be treated in the same way as for nonpregnant patients with intraperitoneal antibiotics and awareness of drug levels.

The key to a successful pregnancy for women with ESRF is that their renal replacement therapy should match as closely as possible the healthy gestational changes to kidney function. This requires knowledge of the timing and extent of these pregnancy-related changes and a willingness by the woman to eventually have almost daily hemodialysis and monitoring. Frequent dialysis should aim to keep the predialysis serum urea at less than 17 mmol/L (BUN <50 mg/dL). This strategy will also reduce the need for large volumes of fluid to be removed at any one time and is therefore less likely to compromise uteroplacental blood flow. In those women who have some residual renal function or who can still produce urine, fluid balance is easier to manage, which increases the likelihood of a successful pregnancy outcome.

Women who increase their dialysis regimen to more than 20 hours per week are also more likely to have a successful pregnancy outcome.[141] Further improvements are likely with more than 24 hours per week.[139] Fluid balance and weight gain should recognize an average gestational weight gain of 1 pound (0.5 kg) per week during the second and third trimesters.[142] Maternal BP should be kept just under 140/90 mm Hg. Rises in BP might initially respond to extra fluid removal, but resistant hypertension in a euvolemic woman may herald gestational hypertension requiring antihypertensive medication.

Increased dialysis will, however, lead to hypokalemia and a higher concentration of potassium in the dialysate, or potassium supplements may be necessary. Furthermore, a gestational reduction in serum sodium concentration necessitates a concomitant reduction in dialysate sodium concentration to around 135 mmol/L, and the gestational reduction in serum bicarbonate concentration (18–22 mmol/L) should be matched with a low bicarbonate dialysate.[143] Increased dialysis frequency will also allow for a greater protein intake, which is variably recommended to be between 1.2 and 1.8 g/kg/day.[140]

Anemia and hemorrhage are common in the dialysis population. Serum iron and Hb levels need to be monitored monthly, and iron supplements with erythropoietin given to maintain a Hb between 10 and 11 g/dL. The dose of erythropoietin needs to increase by 50% to 100% in pregnancy. It does not cross the placenta, to consequently there have been no reports of teratogenicity or polycythemia in the infant.[141,144] The dialysis circuit should be heparinized as usual. Folate supplementation (2–5 mg/day) is recommended throughout pregnancy, and low-dose aspirin (75 mg/day) taken from shortly after conception may reduce the risk of preeclampsia.[67] The requirement for calcium and vitamin D supplements is also likely to change as pregnancy progresses, and therefore plasma levels of calcium and phosphate need to be monitored and doses of phosphate binders adjusted or stopped accordingly.

Cesarean section is necessary in approximately 50% of pregnancies in women on dialysis. After cesarean section women on peritoneal dialysis will need to have a temporary rest from PD for up to 72 hours, after which time, small 1-L volumes can be used, gradually building back up to 2 L.

SUMMARY OF MANAGEMENT OPTIONS
Chronic Dialysis

Management Options	Quality of Evidence	Strength of Recommendation	References
Prepregnancy			
Women on dialysis have reduced fertility, but pregnancy is more likely if optimal Hb and iron status and if hemodialysis rather than PD	III	B	114,140
Advise increased risk of adverse pregnancy outcome (preterm labor, IUGR, hydramnios, and preeclampsia)	III	B	105,140
Prenatal			
Hemodialysis regime to mimic physiological renal changes of pregnancy	III	B	139–141
After Ist trimester, increase the dialysis regime to almost daily (20–24 h/wk) to keep predialysis BUN <50 mg/dL (17 mmol/L).	III	B	139–141
Increase erythropoietin and iron (may need IV iron) to keep Hb 10–11 g/dL	III	B	141,144

SUMMARY OF MANAGEMENT OPTIONS
Chronic Dialysis *(Continued)*

Management Options	Quality of Evidence	Strength of Recommendation	References
Prenatal—*Continued*			
Recognize gestational weight gain, approximately 0.5 kg/wk in 2nd and 3rd trimester	IV	C	142
Recognize hypertension may be caused by fluid overload before using antihypertensive medicines	–	GPP	–
Give aspirin 75 mg and folic acid 5 mg/day throughout pregnancy	Ia	A	67
Adjust calcium and phosphate binders according to serum chemistry	–	GPP	–
Screen for complications (preterm labor, IUGR, hydramnios, and preeclampsia)	III	B	105,140
Labor and Delivery			
Cesarean section most likely	–	GPP	–
Women on PD will need temporary hemodialysis	–	GPP	–
Fetal monitoring for last 30 min of hemodialysis	–	GPP	–
Postnatal			
Keep close monitoring of BP and fluid balance	–	GPP	–
Gradually return to nonpregnant dialysis regime over 2 wk	–	GPP	–

BP, blood pressure; BUN, blood urea nitrogen; Hb, hemoglobin; IUGR, intrauterine growth restriction; IV, intravenous; PD, peritoneal dialysis.

RENAL TRANSPLANT PATIENTS AND PREGNANCY (See also Chapter 54)

After renal transplantation a women's fertility usually returns toward normal.[145] Pregnancy should, however, be delayed for around 2 years after transplantation or until renal function and immunosuppressive therapy is stabilised.[145] About 1 in 20 women of childbearing age who have a functioning kidney transplant will become pregnant, and of those that go beyond the first trimester, 90% will end successfully.[146] These pregnancies are, however, more likely to be complicated by preterm labor (50%), preeclampsia (30%), and IUGR (20%).[146] Despite these complications the majority of controlled studies have shown that pregnancy has no influence on long-term maternal renal function if SCr is less than 133 μmol/L (1.5 mg/dL).[145] However, as for all renal disease, obstetric and maternal outcome is worse if there is hypertension, recurrent UTIs, proteinuria, and renal impairment (SCr >133 μmol/L).

Pregnancy does not appear to affect the rate of rejection.[145] However, the plasma levels of cyclosporine usually decrease in pregnancy, and controversy has arisen as to whether the dose of cyclosporine should be adjusted according to plasma levels. Small studies suggest that it is unnecessary to increase the dose of cyclosporine to prevent rejection,[147] and it is the author's practice to keep the level of immunosuppression the same as prepregnancy levels. Women taking cyclosporine appear to have small-for-gestational-age babies compared with women who take prednisolone and azathioprine.[148] However, cyclosporine is otherwise well tolerated in pregnancy with no increased risk of teratogenesis.

Prednisolone (5–10 mg) rarely causes problems for the neonate, as only small amounts cross the placenta as judged by maternal-to-cord blood ratios of approximately 10:1. Azathioprine passes easily across the placenta, but it is not converted to its active metabolite, 6-mercaptopurine, by the immature fetal liver. It has been taken by thousands of pregnant women over 3 decades and appears to be safe. A series of 100 pregnancies in which the mother took tacrolimus revealed a similar side effect profile to cyclosporine.[149] At present very few women have been treated with mycophenolate mofetil, but successful pregnancies and healthy offspring have been reported. Too few women have received ornithine ketoacid transaminase 3 (OKT3) or antithymocyte globulin (ATG) to recommend their use in pregnancy, but sometimes difficult decisions need to be made between treating steroid-resistant rejection and continuing the pregnancy.

Pregnant women on immunosuppression should receive prophylactic antibiotics for all surgical interventions, including delivery. Furthermore, monthly urine cultures should be taken to screen for asymptomatic bacteriuria, which should be treated when isolated. Just one UTI during pregnancy in a transplant patient would be an indication for long-term low-dose antibiotic prophylaxis.[150] During labor, the pelvic kidney does not obstruct labor; therefore, a spontaneous vaginal delivery should be the aim if the maternal and fetal condition remain satisfactory. Cesarean section is, however, necessary in 50% of women with renal transplants.[145] Furthermore, the dose of steroids should be temporarily increased at this physically stressful time. The presence of azathioprine and cyclosporine in breast milk suggests that breastfeeding should be limited, although additional exposure for a few weeks postpartum is unlikely to be harmful compared with in utero exposure over the previous 9 months.

SUMMARY OF MANAGEMENT OPTIONS
Renal Transplant (See also Chapter 54)

Management Options	Quality of Evidence	Strength of Recommendation	References
Prepregnancy			
Advise to delay pregnancy until 2 yr post-transplantation	III	B	145
Advise increased risk of adverse pregnancy outcome, though pregnancy does not increase likelihood of rejection	III	B	145,146
Prenatal			
Advise aspirin 75 mg once daily throughout pregnancy	Ia	A	67
Keep maintenance immunosuppression the same as before pregnancy, despite dilutional fall in cyclosporine level	III	B	147,149
Monitor BP, BUN, MSU, proteinuria 4–6 weekly throughout pregnancy	–	GPP	–
Screen for preeclampsia and fetal compromise	III	B	146,148
Labor and Delivery			
Peripartum prophylactic antibiotics	–	GPP	–
Spontaneous vaginal delivery usually possible, despite pelvic kidney	III	B	145
Temporary increase in steroid dose to cover stress of delivery	–	GPP	–
Postnatal			
No good evidence that limited breastfeeding while taking azathioprine and cyclosporine is harmful (≤ 4 weeks)	–	GPP	–

BP, blood pressure; BUN, blood urea nitrogen; MSU, midstream urinalysis.

CONCLUSIONS

Women with chronic renal disease who continue with their pregnancy need extra prenatal screening for and management of:

- Urine infections—The aim is to keep the urine sterile.
- Hypertension—The aim is to keep the BP below 140/90 mm Hg.
- Proteinuria—If it is above 1 g–3 g/24 hour (depending on presence of other risk factors for thrombosis e.g. BMI >30, age >35years), the aim is to implement thromboprophylaxis with LMW heparin or low-dose aspirin.
- Deteriorating renal function—The aim is to remove or treat the cause of acute renal impairment, effect a timely delivery, and implement dialysis in specific cases.
- Preterm labor—If this is a risk, the aim is to implement tocolytic therapy and management in a center with appropriate neonatal facilities.
- Fetal well-being—The aim is to try and achieve maximum fetal maturity while avoiding irreversible maternal injury or acute fetal compromise.
- Severe acute gestational syndromes need removal or treatment of the nephrotoxic insult, intensive monitoring of fluid balance, and awareness of the need for dialysis.
- Women with ESRF are far more likely to have a successful pregnancy outcome if they have a renal transplant compared with those on dialysis.

REFERENCES

1. Van Beek E, Houben AJHM, van Es PN, et al: Peripheral haemodynamics and renal function in relation to the menstrual cycle. Clin Sci 1996;91:163–168.
2. Chapman AB, Zamudio S, Woodmansee W, et al: Systemic and renal hemodynamic changes in the luteal phase of the menstrual cycle mimic early pregnancy. Am J Physiol (Renal Physiol) 1997;273:F777–782.
3. Chapman AB, Abraham WT, Zamudio S, et al: Temporal relationships between hormonal and hemodynamic changes in early human pregnancy. Kidney Int 1998;54:2056–2063.
4. Roberts M, Lindheimer MD, Davison JM: Altered glomerular permselectivity to neutral dextrans and heteroporous membrane modeling in human pregnancy. Am J Physiol 1996;270: F338–343.
5. Sturgiss SN, Dunlop W, Davison JM: Renal haemodynamics and tubular function in human pregnancy. Bailliere's Clin Obstet Gynaecol 1994;8:2:209–234.
6. Davison J, Baylis C: Renal disease. In de Swiet M (ed): Medical Disorders in Obstetric Practice, 3rd ed. Oxford, UK, Blackwell Science, 1995, pp 226–305.
7. Quadri KH, Bernardini J, Greenberg A, et al: Assessment of renal function during pregnancy using a random urine protein to creatinine ratio and Cockcroft-Gault formula. Am J Kidney Dis 1994;24:416–420.
8. Kalhan SC: Protein metabolism in pregnancy. Am J Clin Nutr 2000;71(Suppl):1249S–1255S.
9. Hertzberg BS, Carroll BA, Bowie JD, et al: Doppler US assessment of maternal kidneys: Analysis of intrarenal resistivity indexes in normal pregnancy and physiological pelvicaliectasis. Radiology 1993;186:689–692.
10. Faundes A, Bricola-Filho M, Pinto e Silva LC: Dilatation of the urinary tract during pregnancy: Proposal of a curve of maximal caliceal diameter by gestational age. Am J Obstet Gynecol 1998;178:1082–1086.
11. Kuo VS, Koumantakis G, Gallery ED: Proteinuria and its assessment in normal and hypertensive pregnancy. Am J Obstet Gynecol 1992;167:723–728.
12. Rinehart BK, Terrone DA, Larmon JE, et al: A 12-hour urine collection accurately assesses proteinuria in the hospitalized hypertensive gravida. J Perinatol 1999;19:556–558.
13. Rodriguez-Thompson D, Lieberman ES: Use of random urinary protein-to-creatinine ratio for the diagnosis of significant proteinuria during pregnancy. Am J Obstet Gynecol 2001;185:808–811.
14. Durnwald C, Mercer B: A prospective comparison of total protein/creatinine ratio versus 24-hour urine protein in women with suspected preeclampsia. Am J Obstet Gynecol 2003;189: 848–852.
15. Kametas N, Krampl E, McAuliffe F, et al: Haemorheological adaptation during pregnancy in a Latin American population. Eur J Haematol 2001;66:305–311.
16. Okazaki M, Usui S, Tokunaga K, et al: Hypertriglyceridemia in pregnancy does not contribute to the enhanced formation of remnant lipoprotein particles. Clin Chim Acta 2004;339:169–181.
17. Lim VS, Katz AI, Lindheimer MD: Acid-base regulation in pregnancy. Am J Physiol 1976;231:1764–1769.
18. Davison JM, Hytten FE: The effect of pregnancy on the renal handling of glucose. Br J Obstet Gynaecol 1975;82:374–381.
19. Seely EW, Brown EM, DeMaggio DM, et al: A prospective study of calcitropic hormones in pregnancy and postpartum: Reciprocal changes in serum intact parathyroid hormone and 1,25-dihydroxyvitamin D. Am J Obstet Gynecol 1997;176:214–217.
20. Dunlop W, Davison JM: The effect of normal pregnancy upon the renal handling of uric acid. Br J Obstet Gynaecol 1977;84:13–21.
21. Davison JM, Shiells EA, Philips PR, Lindheimer MD: Serial evaluation of vasopressin release and thirst in human pregnancy. Role of human chorionic gonadotrophin in the osmoregulatory changes of gestation. J Clin Invest 1988;81:798–806.
22. Davison JM, Sheills EA, Barron WM, et al: Changes in the metabolic clearance of vasopressin and in plasma vasopressinase throughout human pregnancy. J Clin Invest 1989;83:1313–1318.
23. Williams DJ, Metcalfe KA, Skingle L, et al: Pathophysiology of transient cranial diabetes insipidus during pregnancy. Clin Endocrinol 1993;38:595–600.
24. McMullin MF, White R, Lappin T, et al: Haemoglobin during pregnancy: Relationship to erythropoietin and haematinic status. Eur J Haematol 2003;71:44–50.
25. Verhaeghe J, Bouillon R: Calcitropic hormones during reproduction. J Steroid Biochem Mol Biol 1992;41:469–477.
26. Halligan A, O'Brien E, O'Malley K, et al: Twenty-four hour ambulatory blood pressure measurement in a primigravid population. J Hypertens 1993;11:869–873.
27. Steer PJ: Maternal haemoglobin concentration and birth weight. Am J Clin Nutr 2000;71 (Suppl):1285S–1287S.
28. Prentice A: Calcium in pregnancy and lactation. Annu Rev Nutr 2000;20:249–272.
29. Little PJ: The incidence of urinary infection in 5000 pregnant women. Lancet 1966;2:925–928.
30. Nowicki B: Urinary tract infection in pregnant women: Old dogmas and current concepts regarding pathogenesis. Cur Infect Dis Rep 2000;4:529–535.
31. Kincaid Smith P, Bullen M: Bacteriuria in pregnancy. Lancet 1965;191:359–399.
32. Campbell-Brown M, McFadyen IR, Seal DV, Stephenson ML: Is screening for bacteriuria in pregnancy worthwhile? BMJ 1987;294:1579–1582.
33. Cunningham FG, Lucas MJ: Urinary tract infections complicating pregnancy. Baillieres Clin Obstet Gynaecol 1994;8:353–373.
34. Tomson C: Urinary tract infection. In Warrell DA, Cox TM, Firth J, Benz EJ (eds): Oxford Textbook of Medicine, 4th ed. Oxford, Oxford University Press, 2003, pp 420–433.
35. Tincello DG, Richmond DH: Evaluation of reagent strips in detecting asymptomatic bacteriuria in early pregnancy: prospective case series. BMJ 1998;316:435–437.
36. Smaill F: Antibiotics for asymptomatic bacteriuria in pregnancy. Cochrane Database Syst Rev 2001;2;CD000490.
37. Romero R, Oyarzun E, Mazor M, et al: Meta-analysis of the relationship between asymptomatic bacteriuria and preterm delivery/low birth weight. Obstet Gynecol 1989;73:576–582.
38. Whalley PJ: Bacteriuria of pregnancy. Am J Obstet Gynecol 1967;97:723–738.
39. Pastore LM, Savitz DA, Thorp JM Jr: Predictors of urinary tract infection at the first prenatal visit. Epidemiology 1999;10: 282–287.
40. McGladdery SL, Aparicio S, Verrier-Jones K, et al: Outcome of pregnancy in an Oxford-Cardiff cohort of women with previous bacteriuria. Quart J Med 1992;303:533–539.
41. Smellie JM, Prescod NP, Shaw PJ, et al: Childhood reflux and urinary infection: A follow up of 10–41 years in 226 adults. Pediatr Nephrol 1998;12:727–736.
42. Bukowski TP, Betrus GG, Aquilina JW, Perlmutter AD: Urinary tract infections and pregnancy in women who underwent antireflux surgery in childhood. J Urol 1998;159:1286–1289.
43. Natarajan V, Kapur D, Sharma S, Singh G: Pregnancy in patients with spina bifida and urinary diversion. Int Urogynecol J Pelvic Floor Dysfunct 2002;13:383–385.
44. Abrahams HM, Stoller ML: Infection and urinary stones. Curr Opin Urol 2003;13:63–67.
45. Golan A, Wexler S, Amit A, et al: Asymptomatic bacteriuria in normal and high-risk pregnancy. Eur J Obstet Gynecol Reprod Biol 1989;33:101–108.
46. Rizk DE, Mustafa N, Thomas L: The prevalence of urinary tract infections in patients with gestational diabetes mellitus. Int Urogynecol J Pelvic Floor Dysfunct 2001;12:317–321.

47. Villar J, Lydon-Rochelle MT, Gulmezoglu AM, Roganti A: Duration of treatment for asymptomatic bacteriuria during pregnancy. Cochrane Database Syst Rev 2000;2:CD000491.
48. Vazquez JC, Villar J: Treatments for symptomatic urinary tract infections during pregnancy. Cochrane Database Syst Rev 2003;4:CD002256.
49. Jamie WE, Edwards RK, Duff P: Antimicrobial susceptibility of gram-negative uropathogens isolated from obstetric patients. Infect Dis Obstet Gynecol 2002;10:123–126.
50. Duff P: Antibiotic selection in obstetrics: Making cost-effective choices. Clin Obstet Gynaecol 2002;45:59–72.
51. Gait JE: Hemolytic reactions to nitrofurantoin in patients with glucose-6-phosphate dehydrogenase deficiency: Theory and practice. DICP 1990;24:1210–1213.
52. Hernandez-Diaz S, Werler MM, Walker AM, Mitchell AA: Neural tube defects in relation to use of folic acid antagonists during pregnancy. Am J Epidemiol 2001;153:961–968.
53. Dwyer PL, O'Reilly M: Recurrent urinary tract infection in the female. Curr Opin Obstet Gynaecol 2002;14:537–543.
54. Gilstrap LC, Cunningham FG, Whalley PJ: Acute pyelonephritis in pregnancy: An anterospective study. Obstet Gynecol 1981;57:409–413.
55. Cunningham FG, Lucas MJ, Hankins GD: Pulmonary injury complicating antepartum pyelonephritis. Am J Obstet Gynecol 1987;156:797–807.
56. Towers CV, Kaminskas CM, Garite TJ, et al: Pulmonary injury associated with antepartum pyelonephritis: Can patients at risk be identified? Am J Obstet Gynecol 1991;164:974–978.
57. Millar LK, DeBuque L, Wing DA: Uterine contraction frequency during treatment of pyelonephritis in pregnancy and subsequent risk of preterm birth. J Perinat Med 2003;31:41–46.
58. Wing DA: Pyelonephritis in pregnancy. Treatment options for optimal outcomes. Drugs 2001;61:2087–2096.
59. Dunlow SG, Duff P: Prevalence of antibiotic-resistant uropathogens in obstetric patients with acute pyelonephritis. Obstet Gynecol 1990;76:241–245.
60. Spencer JA, Chahal R, Kelly A, et al: Evaluation of painful hydronephrosis in pregnancy: Magnetic resonance urographic patterns in physiological dilatation versus calculous obstruction. J Urol 2004;171:256–260.
61. Sandberg T, Brorson JE: Efficacy of long-term antimicrobial prophylaxis after acute pyelonephritis in pregnancy. Scand J Infect Dis 1991;23:221–223.
62. Redman CW, Sacks GP, Sargent IL: Preeclampsia: An excessive maternal inflammatory response to pregnancy. Am J Obstet Gynecol 1999;180:499–506.
63. Poston L, Williams DJ: Vascular function in normal pregnancy and preeclampsia. In BJ Hunt, L Poston, M Schachter, A Halliday (eds): An Introduction to Vascular Biology. Cambridge, UK, Cambridge University Press, 2002, pp 398–425.
64. Spargo B, McCartney CP, Winemiller R: Glomerular capillary endotheliosis in toxaemia of pregnancy. Arch Pathol 1959;63: 593–599.
65. Drakely AJ, Le Roux PA, Anthony J, Penny J: Acute renal failure complicating severe preeclampsia requiring admission to an obstetric intensive care unit. Am J Obstet Gynecol 2002;186:253–256.
66. Fink JC, Schwartz SM, Benedetti TJ, Stehman-Breen CO: Increased risk of adverse maternal and infant outcomes among women with renal disease. Paediatr Perinat Epidemiol 1998;12: 277–287.
67. Coomarasamy A, Honest H, Papaioannou S, et al: Aspirin for prevention of preeclampsia in women with historical risk factors: A systematic review. Obstet Gynecol 2003;101:1319–1332.
68. Reiter L, Brown MA, Whitworth JA: Hypertension in pregnancy: The incidence of underlying renal disease and essential hypertension. Am J Kidney Dis 1994;24:883–887.
69. Bar J, Kaplan B, Wittenberg C, et al: Microalbuminuria after pregnancy complicated by preeclampsia. Nephrol Dial Transplant 1999;14:1129–1132.
70. Williams DJ: Pregnancy—A stress test for life. Curr Opin Obstet Gynaecol 2003;15:465–471.
71. Newman MG, Robichaux AG, Stedham CM, et al: Perinatal outcomes in preeclampsia that is complicated by massive proteinuria. Am J Obstet Gynecol 2003;188:264–268.
72. Williams DJ, de Swiet M: Pathophysiology of preeclampsia. Intensive Care Med 1997;23:620–629.
73. Why Mothers Die 1997–1999. The Confidential enquiries into maternal deaths in the United Kingdom. London, The Stationary Office Ltd., 2001.
74. Gilbert WM, Towner DR, Field NT, Anthony J: The safety and utility of pulmonary artery catheterization in severe preeclampsia and eclampsia. Am J Obstet Gynecol 2000;182:1397–1403.
75. Keiseb J, Moodley J, Connolly CA: Comparison of the efficacy of continuous furosemide and low-dose dopamine infusion in preeclampsia/eclampsia related oliguria in the immediate postpartum period. Hypertens Pregnancy 2002;21:225–234.
76. Duley L, Williams J, Henderson-Smart DJ: Plasma volume expansion for treatment of women with preeclampsia. Cochrane Database Syst Rev 2000;CD001805.
77. Young PF, Leighton NA, Jones PW, et al: Fluid management in severe preeclampsia (VESPA): Survey of members of ISSHP. Hypertens Pregnancy. 2000;19:249–259.
78. Boito SME, Struijk PC, Pop GAM, et al: The impact of maternal plasma volume expansion and antihypertensive treatment with intravenous dihydralazine on fetal and maternal haemodynamics during preeclampsia: A clinical, echo-Doppler and viscometric study. Ultrasound Obstet Gynecol 2004;23:327–332.
79. Visser W, Wallenberg HCS: Maternal and perinatal outcome of temporizing management in 254 consecutive patients with severe preeclampsia remote from term. Eur J Obstet Gynecol Reprod Biol 1995;63:147–154.
80. George JN: The association of pregnancy with thrombotic thrombocytopenic purpura-hemolytic uremic syndrome. Current Opin Hematol 2003;10:339–344.
81. Yarranton H, Machin SJ: An update on the pathogenesis and management of acquired thrombotic thrombocytopenic purpura. Curr Opin Neurol 2003;16:367–373.
82. Bianchi V, Robles R, Alberio L, et al: Von Willebrand factor-cleaving protease (ADAMTS13) in thrombocytopenic disorders: A severely deficient activity is specific for thrombotic thrombocytopenic purpura. Blood 2002;100:710–713.
83. Tsai HM, Lian EC: Antibodies to von Willebrand factor-cleaving protease in acute thrombotic thrombopurpura. N Engl J Med 1998;339:1585–1594.
84. Mannucci PM, Canciani MT, Forza I, et al: Changes in health and disease of the metalloprotease that cleaves von Willebrand factor. Blood 2001;98:2730–2735.
85. McMinn JR, George JN: Evaluation of women with clinically suspected thrombotic thrombocytopenic purpura-hemolytic uremic syndrome during pregnancy. J Clin Apheresis 2001;16: 202–209.
86. Rock GA, Shumak KH, Buskard NA, et al: Comparison of plasma exchange with plasma infusion in the treatment of thrombotic thrombocytopenic purpura. Canadian Apheresis Study Group. N Engl J Med 1991;325:393–397.
87. Vesely SK, George JN, Lammle B, et al: ADAMTS13 activity in thrombotic thrombocytopenic purpura-hemolytic uremic syndrome: Relation to presenting features and clinical outcomes in a prospective cohort of 142 patients. Blood 2003;102:60–68.
88. Bobbio-Pallavicini E, Gugliotta L, Centurioni R, et al: Antiplatelet agents in thrombotic thrombocytopenic purpura (TTP): Results of a randomised multicenter trial by the Italian Cooperative group for TTP. Haematologica 1997;82:429–435.
89. Chugh KS, Jha V, Sakhuja V, Joshi K: Acute renal cortical necrosis—A study of 113 patients. Ren Fail 1994;16:37–47.
90. Prakash J, Triathi K, Pandey LK, et al: Renal cortical necrosis in pregnancy-related acute renal failure. J Indian Med Assoc 1996;94:227–229.

91. Pertuiset N, Grunfeld JP: Acute renal failure in pregnancy. Baillieres Clin Obstet Gynaecol 1994;8:333–351.
92. Castro MA, Fassett MJ, Reynolds TB, et al: Reversible peripartum liver failure: A new perspective on the diagnosis, treatment, and cause of acute fatty liver of pregnancy, based on 29 consecutive cases. Am J Obstet Gynecol 1999;181:389–395.
93. Yang Z, Yamada J, Zhao Y, Set al: Prospective screening for pediatric mitochondrial trifunctional protein defects in pregnancies complicated by liver disease. JAMA 2002;288: 2163–2166.
94. Pereira SP, O'Donohue J, Wendon J, Williams R: Maternal and perinatal outcome in severe pregnancy-related liver disease. Hepatology 1997;26:1258–1262.
95. Landau D, Shelef I, Polacheck H, et al: Perinatal vasoconstrictive renal insufficiency associated with maternal nimesulide use. Am J Perinataol 1999;16:441–444.
96. Steiger RM, Boyd EL, Powers DR, et al: Acute maternal renal insufficiency in premature labor treated with indomethacin. Am J Perinatol 1993;10:381–383.
97. Mor Y, Leibovitch I, Fridmans A, et al: Late post-reimplantation ureteral obstruction during pregnancy: A transient phenomenon. J Urol 2003;170:845–848.
98. Greenwell TJ, Venn SN, Creighton S, et al: Pregnancy after lower urinary tract reconstruction for congenital abnormalities. BJU Int 2003;92:773–777.
99. Bingham C, Ellard S, Cole TR, et al: Solitary functioning kidney and diverse genital tract malformations associated with hepatocyte nuclear factor-1beta mutations. Kidney Int 2002;61: 1243–1251.
100. Meyers SJ, Lee RV, Munschauer RW: Dilatation and nontraumatic rupture of the urinary tract during pregnancy: A review. Obstet Gynecol 1985;66:809–815.
101. Jungers P, Chauveau G, Choukroun G, et al: Pregnancy in women with impaired renal function. Clin Nephrol 1997;47:281–288.
102. Katz AI, Davison JM, Hayslett JP, et al: Pregnancy in women with kidney disease. Kidney Int 1980;18:192–206.
103. Cunningham FG, Cox SM, Harstad TW, et al: Chronic renal disease and pregnancy outcome. Am J Obstet Gynecol 1990;163: 453–459.
104. Jungers P, Houillier P, Chauveau D, et al. Pregnancy in women with reflux nephropathy. Kidney Int 1996;50:593–599.
105. Chao A, Huang J, Lien R, et al: Pregnancy in women who undergo long-term hemodialysis. Am J Obstet Gynecol 2002; 187:152–156.
106. Imbasciati E, Pardi G, Capetta P, et al: Pregnancy in women with chronic renal failure. Am J Nephrol 1986;6:193–198.
107. Hemmelder MH, de Zeeuw D, Fidler V, de Jong PE: Proteinuria: A risk factor for pregnancy-related renal function decline in primary glomerular disease? Am J Kidney Dis 1995;26:187–192.
108. Jungers P, Houillier P, Forget D, Henry-Amar M: Specific controversies concerning the natural history of renal disease in pregnancy. Am J Kidney Dis 1991;17:116–122.
109. Jungers P, Houillier P, Forget D, et al: Influence of pregnancy on the course of primary glomerulonephritis. Lancet 1995;346: 1122–1124.
110. Jones DC, Hayslett JP: Outcome of pregnancy in women with moderate or severe renal insufficiency. N Engl J Med 1996;335:226–232.
111. Epstein FH: Pregnancy and renal disease. N Engl J Med 1996;335:277–278.
112. Hou S: Frequency and outcome of pregnancy in women on dialysis. Am J Obstet Gynecol 1994;23:60–63.
113. Stettler RW, Cunningham FG: Natural history of chronic proteinuria complicating pregnancy. Am J Obstet Gynecol 1992;167:1219–1224.
114. Packham DK, North RA, Fairley KF, et al: Primary glomerulonephritis and pregnancy. Quart J Med 1989;266:537–553.
115. Holley JL, Bernardini J, Quadri KHM, et al: Pregnancy outcomes in a prospective matched control study of pregnancy and renal disease. Clin Nephrol 1996;45:77–82.
116. Abe S: An overview of pregnancy in women with underlying renal disease. Am J Kidney Dis 1991;17:112–115.
117. Barcelo P, Lopez-Lillo J, Cabero L, Del Rio G: Successful pregnancy in primary glomerular disease. Kidney Int 1986;30: 914–919.
118. Ronkainen J, Nuutinen M, Koskimies O: The adult kidney 24 years after childhood Henoch-Schönlein purpura: A retrospective cohort study. Lancet 2002;360:666–679.
119. Cummins DL, Mimouni D, Renic A, et al: Henoch-Schönlein purpura in pregnancy. Br J Dermatol 2003;149:1282–1285.
120. Chapman AB, Johnson AM, Gabow PA: Pregnancy outcome and its relationship to progression of renal failure in autosomal dominant polycystic kidney disease. J Am Soc Nephrol 1994;5: 1178–1185.
121. Mansfield JT, Snow BW, Cartwright PC, Wadsworth K: Complications of pregnancy in women after childhood reimplantation for vesicoureteral reflux: An update with 25 years of follow-up. J Urol 1995;154:787–790.
122. Mor Y, Leibovitch I, Zalts R, et al: Analysis of the long term outcome of surgically corrected vesico-ureteric reflux. BJU Int 2003;92:97–100.
123. Scott JE, Swallow V, Coulthard MG, et al: Screening of newborn babies for familial ureteric reflux. Lancet 1997;350: 396–400.
124. Ylinen E, Ala-Houhala M, Wikstrom S: Risk of renal scarring in vesicoureteral reflux detected either antenatally or during the neonatal period. Urology 2003;61:1238–1242.
125. Lattanzi DR, Cook WA: Urinary calculi in pregnancy. Obstet Gynecol 1980;56:462–466.
126. Lewis DF, Robichaux AG 3rd, Jaekle RK, et al: Urolithiasis in pregnancy. Diagnosis, management and pregnancy outcome. J Reprod Med 2003;48:28–32.
127. Coe FL, Parks JH, Lindheimer MD: Nephrolithiasis during pregnancy. N Engl J Med 1978;298:324–326.
128. Hendricks SK, Ross SO, Krieger JN: An algorithm for diagnosis and therapy of management and complications of urolithiasis during pregnancy. Surg Gynecol Obstet 1991;172:49–54.
129. Butler EL, Cox SM, Eberts EG, Cunningham FG: Symptomatic nephrolithiasis complicating pregnancy. Obstet Gynecol 2000;96:753–756.
130. Watterson JD, Girvan AR, Beiko DT, et al: Ureteroscopy and holmium:yag laser lithotripsy: An emerging definitive management strategy for symptomatic ureteral calculi in pregnancy. Urology 2002;60:383–387.
131. Biesenbach G, Zazgornik J, Stoger H, et al: Abnormal increases in urinary albumin excretion during pregnancy in IDDM women with pre-existing microalbuminuria. Diabetologia 1994;37: 905–910.
132. Ekbom P, Damm P, Feldt-Rasmussen B, et al: Pregnancy outcome in type 1 diabetic women with microalbuminuria. Diabetes Care 2001;24:1739–1744.
133. Reece EA, Leguizamon G, Homko C: Pregnancy performance and outcomes associated with diabetic nephropathy. Am J Perinatol 1998;15:413–421.
134. Rossing K, Jacobsen P, Hommel E: Pregnancy and progression of diabetic nephropathy. Diabetologia 2002;45:36–41.
135. Purdy LP, Hantsch CE, Molitch ME, et al: Effect of pregnancy on renal function in patients with moderate to severe diabetic renal insufficiency. Diabetes Care 1996;19:1067–1074.
136. Buyon JP, Cronstein BN, Morris M, et al: Serum complement values (C3 and C4) to differentiate between systemic lupus activity and preeclampsia. Am J Med 1986;81:194–200.
137. Moroni G, Quaglini S, Banfi G, et al: Pregnancy in lupus nephritis. Am J Kidney Dis 2002;40:713–720.
138. Rahman FZ, Rahman J, Al-Suleiman SA, Rahman MS: Pregnancy outcome in lupus nephropathy. Arch Gynaecol Obstet 2004;
139. Hou SH: Modifications of dialysis regimens for pregnancy. Int J Artif Organs 2002;25:823–826.

140. Holley JL, Reddy SS: Pregnancy in dialysis patients: A review of outcomes, complications and management. Semin Dial 2003;16:384–387.
141. Okundaye I, Abrinko P, Hou S: Registry of pregnancy in dialysis patients. Am J Kidney Dis 1998;31:766–773.
142. Giatras I, Levy DP, Malone FD, et al: Pregnancy during dialysis: Case report and management guidelines. Nephrol Dial Transplant 1998;13:3266–3272.
143. Hou S, Firanek C: Management of the pregnant dialysis patient. Adv Ren Replace Ther 1998;5:24–30.
144. Schneider H, Malek A: Lack of permeability of the human placenta for erythropoietin. J Perinatal Med 1995;23:71–76.
145. EBPG Expert Group on Renal Transplantation: European best practice guidelines for renal transplantation. Section IV: Long-term management of the transplant recipient. IV 10. Pregnancy in renal transplant recipients. Nephrol Dial Transplant 2002;17 (Suppl) 4:50–55.
146. Davison JM: Towards long-term graft survival in renal transplantation: Pregnancy. Nephrol Dial Transplant 1995;10:85–89.
147. Thomas AG, Burrows L, Knight R, et al: The effect of pregnancy on cyclosporine levels in renal allograft patients. Obstet Gynecol 1997;90:916–919.
148. Armenti VT, Wilson GA, Radomski JS, et al: Report from the National Transplantation Pregnancy Registry (NTPR): Outcomes of pregnancy after transplantation. Clin Transplant 1999;111–116.
149. Kainz A, Harabacz I, Cowlrick IS, et al: Analysis of 100 pregnancy outcomes in women treated systemically with tacrolimus. Transplant Int 2000;13(Suppl):S299–S300.
150. Davison JM, Milne JEC: Pregnancy and renal transplantation. Br J Urol 1997;80(Suppl 1):29–32.
151. Sibai BM, Villar MA, Mabie BC: Acute renal failure in hypertensive disorders in pregnancy. Pregnancy outcome and remote prognosis in thirty-one consecutive cases. Am J Obstet Gynecol 1990;162:777–783.
152. Nzerue CM, Hewan-Lowe K, Nwawka C: Acute renal failure in pregnancy: A review of clinical outcomes at an inner-city hospital from 1986–1996. J Natl Med Assoc 1998;90:486–490.

CHAPTER 51

Spine and Joint Disorders

Ralph B. Blasier / Michael J. Mendelow

INTRODUCTION

During pregnancy, maternal anatomic changes present mechanical challenges to the musculoskeletal system. Hormonal changes occur that modify the connective tissues and their response to mechanical stress. Complaints of musculoskeletal discomfort during pregnancy are common[1–5] and may be temporarily disabling.[6] These problems usually do resolve spontaneously with completion of pregnancy, but occasionally they may remain as chronic disorders. Some musculoskeletal conditions that exist prior to pregnancy may affect the course of the pregnancy.

LOW BACK AND PELVIC PAIN

General Considerations

Back and pelvic pain has been reported to occur in 48% to 90% of pregnancies.[1–12] Of 855 women followed prospectively throughout pregnancy by Ostgaard, 49% complained of back pain. Of these, 22% noted ongoing back pain at the time they became pregnant, leaving a true incidence rate of 27%. In this series, the back and posterior pelvic pain prevalence rate was 22% to 28% throughout pregnancy, and pain was often present before the 12th week. Kristiansson and colleagues followed 200 women prospectively through pregnancy. They noted prevalence rates of pain of 19% at week 12, gradually increasing to 47% at week 24, with a peak prevalence of 49% at week 36. If mechanical factors were predominant in causing pain, a greater increase in prevalence would be expected with advancing gestation.[1,8] Overall prevalence of back pain with onset before or during pregnancy was 81.5%, but prevalence rates during pregnancy were two to three times greater than those before. Studies of nonpregnant women of similar demographics report prevalence rates of back pain of 20% to 25%. Lumbar pain may be more common during pregnancy in women who noted back pain before pregnancy, whereas onset during pregnancy is more commonly described as sacral pain.[1,8] The findings of Berg, in a study of the pregnancies of 862 women, are similar, with pain in the sacroiliac area being most common (67% of women with pain).[9] The pain has been noted to be so severe that patients are unable to continue to work in 9% to 10% of women and work function and daily routine are compromised in 30% to 36% of pregnant women.[1,8]

The many terms used in the literature such as *sacroiliac joint dysfunction*, *pelvic girdle relaxation*, *pelvic insufficiency*, and even *sacroiliac joint pain* allude to an unjustified knowledge of pain mechanisms and describe a mixed group of patients.[13] More recent prospective studies incorporating pain diagrams, serial interviews, and provocative physical examination[1,10,12,13] have been helpful in our understanding and progress toward rational management. Berg and associates differentiate a *muscular insufficiency*, usually noted by patients having *mild back pain*, from a diagnosis of *sacroiliac dysfunction* made in two thirds of women with severe back pain.[9] The former diagnosis was made in patients with tender paravertebral muscles who had normal range of motion and no neurologic signs. The latter term was applied to patients with evidence of sacroiliac pain or decreased sacroiliac motion on provocative or functional testing (or both). Ostgaard and colleagues suggest the terms *low back pain* and *posterior pelvic pain*.[13]

Hormonal Considerations

Relaxin is a polypeptide hormone. In the human female, production sites for relaxin are the corpus luteum, deciduas, and chorion. Postulated receptor sites and target organs are the pubic symphysis, myometrium, cervix, placenta, breasts, and skin fibroblasts.[14] Relaxin is thought to relax connective tissue and relax myometrium. The association of estrogen and relaxin with separation of the pubic symphysis has been demonstrated in three orders of mammals, including Rodentia, Primatia, and Chiroptera, presumably those with narrow pelves relative to the size of their offspring.[15] Relaxin values in humans peak in the first trimester.[7,16] The effect of relaxin is remodeling of connective tissue, a side effect of which may be pelvic pain.[7]

MacLennan found relaxin levels to be higher in the first half of pregnancy and decreasing toward the end of gestation. In early labor, levels increase again, but by the third day postpartum, relaxin is almost undetectable.[16] Relaxin levels are higher in the patients with symptoms, and the highest levels were found in women most affected clinically. Moreover, patients with the highest levels took longer to recover after the pregnancy, and some had recurrent high levels and symptoms with subsequent pregnancies. The relationship between hormone levels and joint pain in pregnancy is unclear. Marnach and associates found pain to be associated with elevated levels of estradiol and progesterone, but not relaxin, cortisol, or measured joint laxity.[17]

Mechanical Explanations for Back and Pelvic Pain in Pregnancy

Load on the spine is increased by general weight gain and the weight of the uterus, fetus, and breasts.[11] Theories of increasing lumbar lordosis occurring in response to the more anterior center of mass, and producing increased shear stresses across the motion segments of the lumbar spine have long been entertained.[2,11] The contribution of abdominal musculature to support of the spine may be diminished, and postural adjustments and response to increased loads are required.[18,19] General changes in laxity of supporting soft tissues occur under hormonal influences, and, because of higher receptor concentration, may be concentrated in the pelvic area. A generalized systemic effect on ligaments may cause lower back and posterior pelvic pain, because muscle forces are concentrated in the lumbar and lumbosacral region.[8,11]

Radicular symptoms are commonly noted in pregnancy.[20] This may be caused by direct pressure of the uterus on nerve roots and lumbar and sacral plexi. Bushnell is credited with describing the "parietal neuralgia of pregnancy" as mechanical pressure on nerve roots by ligamentous structures of an increasingly lordotic spine.[21] With descent of the fetus into the pelvis in late pregnancy, radicular symptoms attributed to pressure on the lumbosacral plexus may be experienced.

Ostgaard and colleagues[11] provided a biomechanical analysis, which demonstrates that the flexion moment caused by the more anterior center of increasing mass of the fetus and uterus can be accommodated with large increases in extensor muscle forces and consequential lumbar spine compression forces. Extension of the upper trunk, head, and neck can offset the increase in flexion moment by maintaining a new center of gravity closer to the spine. Ostgaard and colleagues analyzed biomechanical factors and low back pain in 855 pregnant women and found that lumbar lordosis did not increase during gestation. In two separate prospective studies, no correlation was found between spinal configuration and complaints of back pain.[11,22] Hip joint extension, rather than lumbar spine extension, must be a major mechanism used by pregnant women to cope with the increased flexion moment produced by pregnancy.[11] Whether a population of women with back pain has intrinsic limitation of hip extension, or whether women with hip flexion contractures have a greater tendency toward back pain with pregnancy, remains to be studied.

A correlation has been identified between back pain and prepartum lumbar lordosis, suggesting that women with increased lumbar lordosis for any reason prior to pregnancy may be at higher risk for back pain when pregnant.[11] Fast and associates found that, despite expectedly significant differences in abdominal length and in the ability to perform a sit-up, there was no correlation with apparent decrease in abdominal strength and back pain.[18] Ostgaard found that no biomechanical parameter correlated with sick leave for back pain during pregnancy. Sick leave taken correlated with pain intensity and with pain in the sacroiliac joint areas, as opposed to other areas of back pain, suggesting that posterior pelvic pain is more disabling than back pain.[1,23]

Peripheral laxity, followed throughout pregnancy in the prospective back pain study by Ostgaard of biomechanical factors, was measured by presence of *striae distensae*, by serial measurement of ulnar deviation angle of the fourth finger to a defined force, and by Bishop score (a 1–10 scale of cervix "ripeness"). Peripheral laxity was seen to significantly increase from weeks 12 through 20 in primiparous women. Laxity in multiparous women was the same at 12 weeks as that in primigravidas at 36 weeks and did not change during pregnancy. The correlation between increased peripheral laxity and increased abdominal sagittal diameter was strong. These data suggest that an increase in laxity after an initial pregnancy does not necessarily return to normal. All persons lose stature (total height) with physical exertion. Control individuals and pregnant women without back pain regain stature after exertion faster than pregnant women with symptoms of back pain.[24]

A presumed common inheritable disorder called benign joint hypermobility syndrome has been recognized in the medical literature since 1967. At times linked to entities such as fibromyalgia, osteogenesis imperfecta, and Ehlers-Danlos and Marfan syndromes, recent investigation has suggested the underlying pathophysiology for this ill-defined condition may relate to altered collagen synthesis. Grahame and colleagues[25] have attempted to establish specific clinical diagnostic criteria for this constellation of joint-related symptoms. Their revised Brighton criteria for diagnosis include major and minor articular and extra-articular symptoms or physical examination findings. Several lines of investigation have noted an increased incidence of genitourinary relaxation and pelvic prolapse in women with this condition. Relative to spine and joint disorders in pregnancy, this underlying syndrome may add risk to those affected individuals and requires further study.

Lumbar Disc Disease

The association of lumbar disc disease and pregnancy has been suggested by several authors. Relaxin may weaken the annulus of the intervertebral discs.[2,19] LaBan found five patients in a very large series of deliveries to have clinical, electromyographic, and surgically proven findings of herniated lumbar discs, a rare event.[26] Magnetic resonance imaging (MRI) evaluation of pregnant and nonpregnant women revealed the same prevalence of disc abnormalities in both groups. No prospective, controlled studies have related lumbar disc disease to pregnancy. However, the potential for disc herniation and lumbar nerve root compression, with radicular pain and definite neurologic loss, should be considered in the evaluation of the pregnant patient with back pain. Electromyographic studies may be helpful in diagnosis and management. Progressive paralysis or loss of bowel and bladder control require urgent imaging studies, usually with MRI, and urgent surgical decompression.

Vascular Congestion and Night Backache

Back pain in pregnancy has been shown to be common in the evening.[5,12] It has been proposed that this pain is due to increased venous flow through lumbar veins, the vertebral plexus, and paraspinal and azygous veins occurs at night in response to redistribution of an already-large extracellular and venous fluid volume, and that this may be worsened due to mechanical vena caval compression in the supine patient. Edema and increased pressure occur with subsequent pain.

Pain during menstruation, which may be associated with pelvic venous congestion, has been relieved by dihydroergotamine, which causes venous constriction. Patients with symptomatic lumbar stenosis and congestive heart failure have increased symptoms at night, which are relieved with management of heart failure. Venous congestion may be relieved by positional changes, and beyond a search for other musculoskeletal causes, pain that persists should be investigated as a sign of venous pathology, such as proximal venous thrombosis.[2,12]

Sacroiliac Pain, Osteitis Condensans Illii, and an Association with the Inflammatory Processes

Inflammatory changes in the sacroiliac joints are suggested as a cause for sacroiliac pain.[27] "Osteitis condensans illii," as described by Wells, is a "fairly uniform area of increased density in the lower iliac bone, adjacent to the sacroiliac joint, unilateral or bilateral."[28] This finding is most common in women, particularly those who have been pregnant. Of the 67 patients reported by Wells, all were females, 80% had been pregnant, and 30 patients had had low back pain.[28] Shipp and Haggart, in 1950, suggested that the motion or strain associated with pregnancy on the sacroiliac ligaments may explain the finding of osteitis condensans illii most commonly in postpartum women.[29] Wells concluded that there is likely little relationship between back pain and oteitis condensans illii and that the association with pregnancy is due to some unknown mechanism.[28]

Risk Factors

Risk factors for back pain during pregnancy include increasing parity, younger age, back pain before pregnancy, increased lordosis before pregnancy, smoking, and physically strenuous work.[1,8,11,23] Specifically, perceived physical heaviness of work, frequency of twisting and forward bending, and sitting work posture are important risk factors. Housewives had the same prevalence of back pain as working women. Women without previous back pain and women who believed they had a "normal or strong back" were less likely to experience back pain. Pain intensity tends to increase more and to be more severe in younger women.[8]

Risk factors for postpartum pain include twin pregnancy, first pregnancy, higher age at first pregnancy, increased weight of the baby, forceps or vacuum extraction, fundus expression, and a flexed position of the women at childbirth. Cesarean section is negatively associated with persistent postpartum pain.[30]

GENERAL LOW BACK AND PELVIC PAIN

Management Options

Evaluation

History and physical examination can give some insight into pain mechanisms and direct the management of back and pelvic pain. Extraskeletal causes for backache must be considered. Obstetric complications and urologic disorders may present with symptoms ranging from vaginal discharge, flank pain, nausea, vomiting, and dysuria.[31] Atypical presentations of refractory pain may indicate more significant and rare pathology such as disc herniation, infection, or tumor. Spinal cord tumors, including schwannomas, presenting during pregnancy have been reported. Sacroiliac joint infection has been diagnosed using MRI.[32] Although complaints of back pain are common, vigilance must be maintained if serious diagnoses are not to be missed.

For example, a history of pain at night, a radicular pain distribution, paresthesias, and bowel or bladder dysfunction may herald radiculopathy from nerve root irritation by lumbar disc disease. Differentiation from similar symptoms related to direct fetal pressure on nerve roots, such as paresthesias in the distribution of the ilioinguinal and iliofemoral nerves and even of quadriceps weakness and "giving-way" episodes is necessary.[31] The patient with sacroiliac pain will complain of pain, either unilaterally, or bilaterally. Unilateral pain is more commonly sacroiliac pain than pain from other causes.

Straight-leg raise testing (Lasègue's sign) is performed with the "patient supine, noting the presence and distribution of pain and the angle of lower limb elevation at which it occurs as the examiner raises the straight leg from the examining table by flexion at the hip only." In the normal patient, the angle between the leg and the examining table should reach 70 degrees or more without pain, and the maneuver should not cause any pain beyond hamstring discomfort with stretching. A positive test reproduces the patient's radicular pain and suggests nerve root compression.

Specific provocative tests for assessment of lumbosacral or sacroiliac pain have been described that correlate with, and discriminate more effectively between, specific sources of pain. Being more reproducible, such provocative tests may have greater clinical value.[10,13,27] Posterior superior iliac spine pressure in the standing patient may provoke pain in the sacroiliac region. Sacrospinous and sacrotuberous ligament tenderness by direct pressure during vaginal examination suggests a pelvic contribution to the patient's pain. Symphyseal pain is provoked by direct pressure over the pubic symphysis.

The femoral compression test, or posterior shear or "thigh thrust" test,[10,27] is performed with the patient supine and the hip in 90 degrees of flexion. Axial pressure is applied to the femur. The test is positive if pain is produced in the sacral area or ipsilateral buttock.

The iliac or ventral gapping test involves lateral opening pressure against the medial aspect of the anterosuperior iliac spine, that is, the pelvis of the supine patient is pressed apart.

The iliac compression or dorsal gapping test involves compressive or closing pressure against the lateral iliac wings of the patient in a lateral decubitus or supine position. Pain provoked in either right or left sacral and or buttock area denotes a positive test.

The Patrick test is performed on the supine patient by flexing, abducting, externally rotating, then extending the hip, placing the ankle of the side being tested across the thigh of the opposite leg. The examiner places one hand on the contralateral pelvis to stabilize it. The test is positive if pain is provoked in the sacroiliac area with the pelvis stabilized. Pain with the pelvis free to roll may be of lumbar origin.

Pelvic torsion, or the Gaenslen test, performed on the supine patient positioned near the edge of the examining table, involves maximum flexion of one hip and simultaneous maximal extension of the other hip held over the edge of the table.[27]

The "Fortin finger test"[33] is considered positive if the patient can localize pain with one finger immediately inferomedial to, and within 1 cm from, the posterior superior iliac spine and if the patient consistently points to this area.

Pain provoked in the groin with rotation suggests the hip itself as a source of the pain, whereas posterior pelvic or symphyseal pain indicates sacral or symphyseal causes. Limitation of extension (flexion contracture) may be associated with increased lumbar lordosis, likely of long duration (before pregnancy) and predisposing to low back pain with pregnancy.[11]

Radiographic evaluation, undesirable during pregnancy, may be warranted if pain cannot be explained by the hormonal, mechanical, and vascular mechanisms, especially if neoplasm or infection is being considered. No harm to the fetus has been demonstrated with fetal exposure of less than 10 rads, a dose much greater than that incurred in a routine spine radiography series or bone scan.[31] MRI may be helpful in diagnosis of tumor and infection, although safety in pregnancy has not been established by long-term follow-up. Mass lesions impinging on nerve roots, such as disc herniations, can be evaluated with electromyographic and nerve conduction studies.[31,32]

Treatment

Most complaints regarding back and pelvic pain during pregnancy require only symptomatic care. Lumbar disc disease, urologic disorders, venous thrombosis, or other vascular or visceral causes for back pain must be considered in refractory or atypical cases.

SUMMARY OF MANAGEMENT OPTIONS

Back and Pelvic Pain—General

Management Options	Quality of Evidence	Strength of Recommendation	References
Evaluation			
Consider extraskeletal causes for backache (e.g., obstetric complications and urologic disorders).	IV	C	1,2
Atypical presentations or pain refractory to the usual care may indicate more significant, although rare, pathology (e.g., disc herniation, infection, tumor).	IV	C	3,63
Differentiation from similar symptoms from direct fetal pressure on nerve roots (e.g., paresthesias in the distribution of the ilioinguinal and iliofemoral nerves and even of quadriceps weakness and "giving-way") is necessary.	–	GPP	–
Routine examination includes inspection of the patient while she is standing, then while bending forward, followed by palpation about the spine, paraspinal area, and sacrum.	–	GPP	–
Radiographic evaluation, although undesirable during pregnancy, may be warranted if insidious causes for pain are suspected.	IV	C	3
MRI may be particularly helpful in the diagnosis of tumor and infection.	–	GPP	–
Mass lesions compressing nerve roots, such as disc herniations, can be initially evaluated with electromyographic and nerve conduction studies without exposure to radiation.	–	GPP	–
Treatment			
Daily low back exercises help develop abdominal tone with standing, lateral bending, and rotational trunk exercises.	IV III	C B	1,2 76
The pelvic tilt exercise, anecdotally provides marked relief of low back pain.	IV III	C B	1,2 76
Simple measures taught in back care programs, such as placing one foot on a foot stool when standing for a prolonged period, can give some relief.	IV III	C B	1,2 76
For mild to moderate pain, general comfort measures including rest, activity modification, and physical therapy, including massage and pelvic and low back exercises, as well as general back care are helpful.	IV III	C B	1,2 76
For night pain, the use of a "maternity cushion" may give relief.	Ib	A	77
Elastic compression stockings worn throughout the day may, by limiting lower extremity edema, diminish the fluid shifts and venous engorgement that occur at night.	–	GPP	–
Analgesic options are limited, and nonsteroidal anti-inflammatory drugs (NSAIDs) should be specifically avoided because of concern for potential adverse fetal effects.	–	GPP	–
Persistent pain, including discogenic pain, not responsive to rest, may benefit from lumbar epidural steroids.	–	GPP	–
Transcutaneous electrical nerve stimulation (TENS) may be helpful.	–	GPP	–
Muscle weakness is a concern, but only acute loss of bowel and bladder function or acute paralysis would indicate a need for decompressive surgery during pregnancy.	IV	C	63
Mobilization techniques applied to the sacroiliac area have been reported to provide relief, commonly permanent, in some women.	IV III	C B	1,2 8,76
Treatment with a trochanteric belt provides relief, particularly for women with posterior pelvic pain.	IV III	C B	1,2,13 8
Sacroiliac injection with corticosteroids and local anesthetic may be indicated in severe cases.	–	GPP	–

SPONDYLOLYSIS AND SPONDYLOLISTHESIS

Spondylolysis is a bony insufficiency at the pars interarticularis of the spine. The condition can cause instability and pain. Spondylolisthesis is the slipping forward of one vertebra on another. This can result from a spondylolytic defect, or from degenerative change in the facet joints.[19,34] Depending on the cause and the nature of the defect, the disorder is classified into five different types. Dysplastic and isthmic spondylolisthesis represent congenital and developmental disorders, which have a high familial incidence. These slips are more common in males than females (2:1), although females have a higher chance of progression. These slips most commonly occur at the L5–S1 level. The condition probably develops or presents in the first two decades of life with the diagnosis most often being made in adolescence.[18,29,30]

Risks

The influence of pregnancy on spondylolisthesis is an interesting issue, but little has been written on the subject. Saraste[35,36] provided a long-term review of 255 patients with isthmic and dysplastic spondylolysis, diagnosed at between 9 and 40 years old, with average age at diagnosis of 24 years. The length of follow-up ranged from 20 to 44 years. A comparison of the 171 men, 21 nulliparous women, and 63 parous women, showed no significant differences in symptomatology, impairment, degree of slip, or progression of slip. Moreover, spondylolysis, with or without spondylolisthesis, was not a risk factor for pregnancy complications.

Degenerative spondylolisthesis usually occurs at the L4–L5 level and presents later in life and more commonly in women than in men (4:1). Sanderson and Fraser found, in a review of radiographs of 949 women, that those who had borne children had a significantly higher incidence of degenerative spondylolisthesis than those who had not. Nulliparous women had twice the incidence of degenerative slips as men. Proposed explanations for their findings include the generalized increase in laxity of pregnancy and residual relative joint relaxation, and the effects of relaxin on the collagen of the facet joint capsules and of the annulus of the intervertebral disc.[19]

Women have generally greater joint laxity than men. Possibly, compromised abdominal musculature in parous women may allow perpetually increased sheer and rotatory stresses at the L4–L5 joints.[19]

Management Options

The management of spondylolysis and spondylolisthesis during pregnancy differs little from that in the nonpregnant patient. Symptomatic relief can be obtained by rest and immobilization. The choice of analgesic is limited in pregnancy and should not include aspirin or nonsteroidal anti-inflammatory agents. In the event that significant neurologic impairment is suspected, consultation should be obtained emergently.

SCOLIOSIS

Scoliosis is a three-dimensional deformity of the spine, most prominently manifested by curvature in the coronal plane. The disorder is usually idiopathic, commonly familial, and presents and progresses most dramatically during the adolescent growth spurt. Spinal curvature may also be due to congenital defects in the vertebral bodies, to spinal cord disorders, to intracranial pathology, or to muscle spasm and back pain. Scoliosis is more common in females than in males.

Risks

The influence of pregnancy on preexisting scoliosis, particularly with regard to curve progression, has been controversial. An increase in curve progression during pregnancy has been demonstrated in scoliosis patients in small series. In particular, those treated with bracing who have multiple pregnancies before age 23, those with curves greater than 25 degrees, and patients who already had ongoing curve progression at the time of the pregnancy, have been found to have increases in their curves during pregnancy. Subsequent reviews have not found the same associations.[37–39]

Betz and colleagues[32] retrospectively reviewed 355 women with idiopathic scoliosis who had reached skeletal maturity. Two groups, 175 who had had at least one pregnancy and 180 who had never been pregnant, were compared. No effects on curve progression during pregnancy were demonstrated with regard to age of the patient at the time of pregnancy, ongoing progression of the curve at the time of pregnancy, the number of pregnancies, or the presence of a spinal pseudarthrosis (incidence 77%). Those having severe back pain during pregnancy (12%) may be slightly higher in unfused patients with scoliosis than in nonscoliotic patients. In patients who had undergone posterior spinal fusion, no progression of the unfused portion of the curve was demonstrated. In these patients, no problems during the pregnancy were attributed to the scoliosis.

In 159 deliveries of women who had scoliosis without a spinal fusion, spinal anesthesia could not be administered in two because of the scoliosis, and cesarean section was necessary in 12 (7.4%) for reasons unrelated to the scoliosis. In patients who had undergone posterior fusion, two patients had minor problems during delivery related to the fusion. In one, spinal anesthesia could not be administered, and in the other, proper positioning was difficult. The incidence of complications or deformity in the newborn was not increased.

In the series by Betz and colleagues,[37] postpartum back pain in scoliotic women or women with scoliosis who had not been pregnant was no greater than in the general population. As in other series, potential for progression of curves greater than 30 degrees during adulthood at a general rate of 1 degree per year was seen. However, increased progression, especially of the 6 to 8 degrees per pregnancy previously reported, was not found. They recommend that, for women of childbearing age with curves greater than 30 degrees, radiographs should be done soon after each delivery to minimize the potential for fetal exposure.[37,39]

Management Options

Prepregnancy and Prenatal

The influence of pregnancy on preexisting scoliosis, particularly with regard to curve progression, has been controversial. The affected patient should be counseled that no significant increase in the rate or incidence of curve progression during pregnancy has been demonstrated in large series of pregnant scoliosis patients compared with nonpregnant ones. In patients who had undergone posterior spinal fusion, no progression of the unfused portion of the curve is seen in the majority.

Labor and Delivery

In patients who had undergone posterior fusion, 1.5% have minor problems during delivery related to the fusion. In one report, spinal anesthesia could not be administered, and in another, proper positioning for delivery was difficult. Overall, less than 3% of deliveries in women who had undergone posterior spinal fusion for scoliosis had problems requiring cesarean section. The indications for section were unrelated to the fusion or the scoliosis. The incidence of complications or deformity in the newborn was not increased in patients who had undergone posterior fusion for scoliosis.

Postpartum

Scoliotic women show no increase in postpartum back pain compared with women with scoliosis who had not been pregnant. Therefore, no specific postpartum recommendations are offered. In general, for women with curves greater than 30 degrees, radiographs should be done every 2 years up to age 25, and every 5 years thereafter. Appropriate radiographic and clinical evaluation by a surgeon who manages scoliosis should be considered in the months following delivery, taking the opportunity to have a radiograph when pregnancy is unlikely.

PELVIC ARTHROPATHY AND RUPTURE OF THE PUBIC SYMPHYSIS

Pelvic arthropathy usually occurs in two recognizable syndromes, though there may be overlap between them:

- Abnormal mobility of the pelvic joints may lead to pain and a waddling gait; or
- After a difficult delivery, there may be a rupture of the symphysis.

PELVIC ARTHROPATHY

The increased lumbar lordosis caused by the weight and position of the developing fetus increases the stress on the lumbosacral junction and the sacroiliac joints. In patients with a more sagittal than oblique orientation of these joints, there is less inherent stability, and there may be a predisposition to pelvic laxity. Under hormonal influence, the ligaments of the pubic symphysis and the sacroiliac joints relax during the first half of pregnancy, returning to normal in the typical patient at 6 months postpartum. Excessive relaxation of the ligaments of the pelvis may cause symptoms at about the sixth or seventh month, consisting of pain with walking, turning in bed, or other exertion. There may be a unilateral limp or even a bilateral waddling gait. The pain may rarely be so severe that standing or walking is precluded. Asymmetrical sacroiliac laxity (right different from left) is much more strongly associated with pelvic pain than is the absolute amount of laxity.[40–42]

In some cases, symptoms appear only during labor, due to excessive loosening of the symphysis and sacroiliac joints. Separation of the pubic symphysis during pregnancy is common, varying between 0 and 35 mm (average 7–8 mm). Separation over 8 to 9 mm is considered pathologic. Rupture of the ligaments of the pubic symphysis may occur during labor as a result of forceps delivery, especially in case of fetal/pelvic disproportion. Patients often complain of prelabor pain in the pubis and sacroiliac joints. During and after labor, the patient may complain of pain over the symphysis and sacroiliac joints, radiating down the thighs. The lower limbs are externally rotated, and she may be unable to walk normally for weeks or months. The diagnosis is made with a history of pregnancy, pain at the pubic symphysis or the sacroiliac joints, tenderness at the pubic symphysis or the sacroiliac joints, and excessive laxity of the ligaments. A gap may be felt at the symphysis externally or by vaginal examination. Relaxation of the symphysis can be ascertained by placing the examiner's fingers on the superior edges of the pubic bones and noting vertical translation during walking. A pre-vaginal examination of the symphysis can be made while an assistant pulls down on one of the patient's ankles while pushing up on the other.

Ultrasonography has been used to confirm the diagnosis, with symptomatic patients having a symphyseal gap of 20 mm (range 10–35 mm) and asymptomatic controls 4.8 mm (range 4.3–5.1 mm).[43,44] MRI has been used to diagnose postpartum pubic and pelvic pin, but its clinical benefit has not been established.[45,46]

Management Options

Treatment is generally by rest, with or without a pelvic band or girdle. Some investigators report treatment with early injection of steroid or local anesthetic or use of oral anti-inflammatories. A limited number of reports mention pelvic arthropathy with onset 1 to 2 days after delivery, characterized by pain and tenderness at the symphysis, but without swelling or bruising and without widening or abnormal mobility of the symphysis. Symptoms abate within a week or two with rest and analgesics. It has been speculated that this is caused by swelling and pressure within the fibrous confines of a relatively normal pubic symphysis.[47]

RUPTURE OF THE PUBIC SYMPHYSIS

Separation of the pubic symphysis in association with labor and delivery is rare and is sometimes unrecognized when it does occur. Some widening of the pubic symphysis has been noted as being necessary for normal delivery, and some widening normally does occur. Rarely, the separation is greater than 10 mm, and this is usually symptomatic.[48] The pubic symphysis comprises a thick fibrocartilagenous disc between two thin layers of hyaline cartilage covering the articular surfaces of the bone. It is held together by four ligaments: the anterior pubic (strong), the superior and inferior arcuate, and the posterior pubic (weak). Progesterone and relaxin are known to increase the elasticity of the pubic ligaments. A slight widening of the symphysis occurs during a normal pregnancy, but not normally more than 8 to 9 mm. Occasionally, actual rupture of the pubic symphysis may occur.[48] Occasionally, the onset of pain may be abrupt and may even be accompanied by an audible "crack."[49] Associated factors may include hard labor, precipitous labor, difficult forceps delivery, cephalopelvic disproportion, abnormal presentation, multiparity, forceful abduction of the thighs, or previous pelvic trauma.[30,48,50–54] Estimates of incidence range between 1/500 and 1/30,000.[48,49] The incidence appears to be decreasing over time, as many difficult vaginal deliveries are being replaced by cesarean section.[48] Separations of as much as 120 mm have been reported, and the sacroiliac joints become affected with more than 40-mm separation.[48]

Management Options

Treatment may begin with tight pelvic binding and rest in the lateral decubitus position. Symptoms may last as little as 2 days, typically 8 weeks, or (reportedly) up to 8 months.[48] For inadequate reduction, recurrent diastasis, or persistent symptoms, external skeletal fixation is the treatment of choice to maintain stability while the ligaments heal.[55,56] Pin tract infections in association with the external fixation pins are common and are usually readily manageable.[55,56] Internal fixation by plate and screws or cerclage wire have also been reported.[56,57] One case has been reported of anterior plate fixation of the pubis with simultaneous posterior fixation by sacroiliac screws.[58]

Complications of separation of the pubic symphysis include nonunion (failure to heal with reduction), pubic degenerative joint disease, osteitis pubis, and hemorrhage. The separation may occur in association with a connecting vaginal laceration, and there have been reports of these being complicated by suppurative arthritis, abscess of the vulva, and abscess of the space of Retzius.[48] Some investigators report irrigation and immediate closure of such a connecting vaginal laceration, under the belief that lack of a cortical fracture, unexposed bone ends, and coverage of the bone by articular cartilage may decrease the chance of wound infection.[59]

POSTPARTUM OSTEITIS PUBIS

Osteitis pubis is a self-limited, apparently noninfective, osteonecrosis that begins at the pubic symphysis and extends into the pubic bones. It is rarely associated with pregnancy, either antepartum or postpartum. It is similar to pelvic arthropathy in its presentation, with accompanying pubic tenderness and pain that may prevent ambulation. It is differentiated from pelvic arthropathy and symphyseal disruption by radiographic rarefaction of the pubic bones, without symphyseal widening. It is differentiated from septic symphysitis by its lack of fever, leukocytosis, and radiographic bony sequestrum. Steroids and nonsteroidal anti-inflammatories have been recommended for treatment.[60] Treatment of symptomatic osteitis pubis with intravenous pamidronate has been reported.[61]

SEPTIC PUBIC SYMPHYSITIS AND SACROILITIS

Osteomyelitis in or adjacent to the pubic symphysis has rarely been reported in association with pregnancy. Fever is not universal, though leukocyte count, erythrocyte sedimentation rate, and C-reactive protein levels are usually elevated. Surgical drainage and antibiotics should be curative.[62,63]

STRESS FRACTURES OF THE PUBIC BONE

Stress fracture of the body of the pubic bone have rarely been reported during pregnancy, unrelated to athletics or physical training. In the few cases reported, no underlying pathologic process has been found. The cause is thought to be due to ligament laxity, muscle imbalance, and increased load. Pain is usually insidious in onset. There is tenderness at the fracture. Radiography is diagnostic, but not usually until some healing has occurred. MRI has been suggested to diagnose pelvic stress fractures immediately.[64,65] Management is usually directed toward symptomatic relief.

PELVIC TRAUMA AND PREGNANCY

In a study of 34 women who had had a displaced pelvic ring fracture, all of whom had at least one full-term pregnancy after healing, only two required elective cesarean section, and the need for the cesarean section was determined at the first presentation by pelvimetry. Of these 34 women, 17 had healed with displacement of the fracture involving the birth canal. Of eight who had had previous traumatic pubic symphyseal disruption, two had recurrence of pain during pregnancy.

In a case of trauma very shortly after delivery, there is a report of a very wide traumatic diastasis of the pubic symphysis, which was "surprisingly easy" to reduce, with apparently no lasting injury to the sacroiliac ligaments. It was reasoned that the physiologic relaxation of the pelvis during pregnancy protected the ligaments from gross disruption during the injury.[66] Successful surgical fixation of a severely displaced acetabular fracture has been reported in a patient 20 weeks pregnant, without affecting the pregnancy.[67]

TRANSIENT OSTEOPOROSIS OF THE HIP

Transient osteoporosis of the hip is a rare condition. It has been defined by multiple case reports over the last 41 years.[68] It is characterized by a gradually developing pain in the hip with weight bearing.[69] Symptoms begin in the third (or late second) trimester. The pain is predominantly in the anterior thigh and the groin. For unknown reasons, the left hip is affected more often than the right, though both may be affected.[68] The pain is relieved by rest. There is no associated history of trauma or illness. Musculoskeletal examination is normal, except for discomfort at the extremes of hip motion and a slight decrease in total range of hip motion.[69] Joints other than the hip may become involved, and the process may regress at one joint and progress at another.[70] Other areas affected may include knee, ankle, foot, ribs, shoulders, and spine.[68,71]

Radiographic osteopenia can occur, beginning 2 to 4 weeks after onset of symptoms. Radiographically, the joint space is preserved.[68,69] The indistinctness of the subchondral cortical bone is "striking."[70] MRI of the involved joint reveals a joint effusion and diffuse signal abnormalities in the marrow, suggestive of marrow edema (decreased signal on T_1-weighted images and increased signal on T_2-weighted images).[68,72] The differential diagnosis includes joint infection, rheumatoid arthritis, pigmented villinodular synovitis, and osteonecrosis.[70] Radionucleide bone scanning shows an increased uptake in the affected femoral head and often the acetabulum.[70,73] One report of a case followed by serial dual-photon x-ray absorptiometry (DXA) over a period of 4 years showed a loss of 20% of bone mineral density (compared with age-matched controls), which resolved rapidly in the first year and returned to the normal range after cessation of lactation.[68]

Management Options

The condition is self-limiting. Treatment is conservative, including protection from weight bearing, maintenance of joint motion, and analgesic medications.[69] Bone and synovial biopsies are not necessary.[69] In cases in which joint aspiration has been performed, the effusion is sterile, and the joint fluid is normal.[68–70] Some cases report associated pathologic fracture of the pubic rami or the femoral neck.[55]

Various treatments have been used, including limitation of weight bearing by wheelchairs, crutches, or canes. Corticosteroids, phenylbutazone, and calcitonin have been tried without beneficial effect.[69,71] After delivery, symptoms completely resolve over 3 to 9 months.[69]

The cause of transient osteoporosis of the hip is unknown.[70] Some hypothesize that the cause may be neurovascular and perhaps related to reflex sympathetic dystrophy. However, lack of trauma; lack of the characteristic burning, pulsing pain; lack of changes in skin color, temperature, and moisture; and failure to respond to sympathetic blockade all mitigate against this explanation.[65] Some authors have speculated about other causes, including abnormalities in local blood flow, viral infection, rheumatic and other inflammatory conditions, and metabolic abnormalities, but none of these explanations has been convincingly upheld.[73] Other investigators have speculated that mechanical compression of the obturator nerve in pregnancy may be a causative factor, but animal experimentation has failed to produce hip osteoporosis by this mechanism.[71] It appears that by an unknown stimulus, intense bone resorption is initiated in the femoral head. Later, during resolution, osteoid is laid down and mineralized. Between resorption and remineralization, the bone is weak and susceptible to microtrauma, thus explaining the pain with weight bearing. If the microtrauma accumulates faster than it can be repaired, a pathologic fracture may ensue. For this reason, weight bearing should be limited until resolution of osteopenia.[71]

AVASCULAR NECROSIS OF THE HIP

It is not entirely clear that there is any difference between pregnancy-related transient osteoporosis of the hip and pregnancy-related avascular necrosis of the hip. Some authors have defined aseptic necrosis of the femoral head during pregnancy as an entity separate from transient osteoporosis of the hip in pregnancy, but the clinical presentation is very similar to transient osteoporosis.[74] Symptoms begin in the third trimester; the hip is painful with weight bearing; the pain is relieved by rest; there is no associated history of trauma or illness; and the musculoskeletal examination is normal, except for discomfort at the extremes of hip motion and a slight decrease in total range of hip motion. Radiographs show osteoporotic changes, and radionucleide bone scanning shows an increased uptake in the affected femoral head.[74] Unlike nonpregnancy-related aseptic necrosis of the hip, which often mandates operative treatment and often leads to predictable degenerative joint disease, it has been observed that aseptic necrosis of the hip in pregnancy gives good results with conservative treatment, consisting of reduction in weight bearing.

One radiographic finding that may differentiate aseptic necrosis of the femoral head during pregnancy from transient osteoporosis of the hip has been a "crescent sign," with subchondral lucency or subchondral collapse of the weight-bearing dome of the femoral head. Actual bone necrosis, dead osteocytes, or empty osteocyte lacunae have not been well documented. The crescent sign of the femoral head radiographically resembles other proven cases of aseptic necrosis that occur without pregnancy, and this has been the basis for calling the osteoporotic hip with a crescent sign in pregnancy, "aseptic necrosis during pregnancy." However, the crescent sign might as well be a pathologic fracture in osteoporotic bone, making the distinction between these two entities questionable. MRI should be able to differentiate between these two entities if they actually differ; however, this has not been studied to date.

HIP ARTHROPLASTY

Generally, hip joint replacement should not occur in a woman of childbearing age, as this operation is typically reserved for patients with limited physical activities and relatively short expected life span. However, there are a few rare indications for hip joint replacement in the young, such as avascular necrosis of the hip, severe rheumatoid disease, or certain aggressive tumorous conditions. Reckling has reported a completely normal impregnation, labor, and delivery in a 19-year-old girl who had had a prior total hip replacement.[75]

A prosthetic hip does not have as much inherent joint stability as a biologic hip. Dislocation during positioning is a theoretical concern. However, hip flexion with abduction or external rotation ought to be relatively safe. The dangerous positions are hip flexion with internal rotation and, to a lesser extent, hip extension with external rotation. Neither of these positions would be likely to occur during delivery, with or without stirrups, or squatting with a birthing chair. Other preexisting hip conditions, such as severe slipped capital femoral epiphysis, especially bilateral, or hip fusion, may make positioning for delivery challenging. They do not otherwise preclude vaginal delivery.

SUMMARY OF MANAGEMENT OPTIONS
Back and Pelvic Pain—Specific Conditions

Management Options	Quality of Evidence	Strength of Recommendation	References
Scoliosis			
Prepregnancy and Prenatal	–	GPP	–
Curvature does not usually worsen.			
Compromise of respiratory function may occur in some (see Chapter 38).			
Labor and Delivery	–	GPP	–
Regional analgesia may not be possible.			
Positioning for delivery may have to be individualized.			
For respiratory compromise, see Chapter 38.			
Pelvic Arthropathy			
Rest, with or without a pelvic band or girdle.	–	GPP	–
Analgesia and anti-inflammatory drugs.	III	B	54
If this fails, consider injection of steroids and local anesthetic.	III	B	54

SUMMARY OF MANAGEMENT OPTIONS

Back and Pelvic Pain—Specific Conditions *(Continued)*

Management Options	Quality of Evidence	Strength of Recommendation	References
Rupture of the Pubic Symphysis			
Treatment is generally nonsurgical, and complete recovery is to be expected.	–	GPP	–
Steroids and anti-inflammatory drugs.	IV	C	60
Treatment may begin with tight pelvic binding and rest in the lateral decubitus position.	–	GPP	–
Symptoms may last as little as 2 days, typically 8 weeks, or reportedly up to 8 months.	–	GPP	–
For inadequate reduction, recurrent diastasis, or persistent symptoms, external skeletal fixation is the treatment of choice to maintain stability while the ligaments heal.	–	GPP	–
Internal fixation by plate and screws or metallic cerclage wire only considered in extreme cases.	–	GPP	–
Hip Problems			
Transient Osteoporosis—Conservative Approach	IV	C	69
Limit weight bearing.			
Encourage movement.			
Analgesia.			
Avascular Necrosis	–	GPP	–
Manage as for transient osteoporosis.			
Hip Arthroplasty	–	GPP	–
Usually no significant problem encountered nor special management required.			
Normal birthing position can be used.			
Avoid flexion to more than 90 degrees and internal rotation or adduction of the hips, which can provoke dislocation.			

CONCLUSIONS

- Back and pelvic pain are common complaints in pregnancy.
- Risk factors for back pain during pregnancy include increasing age, increasing parity, younger age, back pain before pregnancy, increased lumbar lordosis before pregnancy, smoking, physically strenuous work.
- Risk factors for persistent pain postpartum include twin pregnancy, first pregnancy, higher age at first pregnancy, increased weight of the baby, forceps or vacuum extraction, fundus expression, a flexed position of the women at childbirth.
- Cesarean section is negatively associated with persistent postpartum pain.
- Extraskeletal causes should always be remembered in the initial evaluation.
- Atypical presentations, or pain refractory to the usual care, may indicate more significant, although rare, pathology.
- Radiographic evaluation, although undesirable during pregnancy, may be warranted if insidious causes for pain are suspected.
- MRI may be helpful in the diagnosis of tumor and infection.
- Lesions compressing nerve roots, such as disc herniations, can be initially evaluated with electromyographic and nerve conduction studies, without exposure to radiation.

REFERENCES

1. Ostgaard HC, Andersson G, Karlsson K: Prevalence of back pain in pregnancy. Spine 1991;16:549–552.
2. Hainline B: Low-back pain in pregnancy. Adv Neurol 1994;64:65–76.
3. Turgut F, Turgut M, Cetinsahin M: A prospective study of persistent back pain after pregnancy. Eur J Obstet Gynecol Reprod Biol 1998;80:45–48.
4. Stapleton DB, MacLennan AH, Kristiansson P: The prevalence of recalled low back pain during and after pregnancy: A South Australian population survey. Aust N Z J Obstet Gynaecol 2002;42:482–485.
5. Fast A, Weiss L, Parikh S, et al: Night backache in pregnancy. Am J Phys Med Rehabil 1989;68(5):227–229.
6. Heckman JD, Sassard R: Current concept review musculoskeletal considerations in pregnancy. J Bone Joint Surg 1994; 76-A,11:1720–1730.
7. Kristiansson P, Svardsudd K, von Schoultz B: Serum relaxin, symphyseal pain, and back pain during pregnancy. Am J Obstet Gynecol 1996;175:1342–1347.
8. Kristiansson P, Svardsudd K, von Schoultz B: Back pain during pregnancy: A prospective study. Spine 1996;21:702–709.
9. Berg G, Hammer M, Müller-Nielson J, et al: Low back pain during pregnancy. Obstet Gynecol 1988;71:71–75.
10. Kristiansson P, Svardsudd K: Discriminatory power of tests applied in back pain during pregnancy. Spine 1996;21: 2337–2344.
11. Ostgaard HC, Anderson GBJ, Schultz AB, et al: Influence of some biomechanical factors on low-back pain in pregnancy. Spine 1993;18:61–65.
12. Fast A, Shapiro D, Ducommun EJ, et al: Low-back pain in pregnancy. Spine 1987;12:368–371.
13. Ostgaard HC, Zetherstorm G, Roos-Hansson E, Svanberg B, Reduction of back and posterior pelvic pain in pregnancy. Spine 1994;19:894–900.
14. MacLennan AH: The role of the hormone relaxin in human reproduction and pelvic girdle relaxation. Scand J Rheumatol Suppl 1991;88:7–15.
15. Samuel C, Butkas A, Coghlan JP, et al: The effect of relaxin on collagen metabolism in the nonpregnant rat pubic symphysis: The influence of estrogen and progesterone in regulating relaxin activity. Endocrinology 1996;137:3884–3890.
16. MacLennan AH, Nicolson R, Green RC, et al: Serum relaxin and pelvic pain of pregnancy. Lancet 1986;ii:243–245.
17. Marnach ML, Ramin KD, Ramsey PS, et al: Characterization of the relationship between joint laxity and maternal hormones in pregnancy. Obstet Gynecol 2003;101:331–335.
18. Fast A, Weiss L, Ducommun EJ, et al: Low-back pain in pregnancy: Abdominal muscles, sit-up performance, and back pain. Spine 1990;15:28–30.
19. Sanderson PL, Fraser RD: The influence of pregnancy on the development of degenerative spondylolisthesis. J Bone Joint Surg 1996;78-B,6:951–954.
20. Wong CA, Scavone BM, Dugan S, et al: Incidence of postpartum lumbosacral spine and lower extremity nerve injuries. Obstet Gynecol 2003;101:279–288.
21. Bushnell LF: Postural backache of the gynecic patient. Clin Orthop 1955;5:164–168.
22. Bullock JE, Jull GA, Bullock M: The relationship of low back pain to postural changes during pregnancy. Aust J Physiother 1987;33:10–17.
23. Ostgaard HC, Andersson GB: Previous back pain and risk of developing back pain in a future pregnancy. Spine 1991;16: 432–436.
24. Rodacki CL, Fowler NE, Rodacki AL, et al: Stature loss and recovery in pregnant women with and without low back pain. Arch Phys Med Rehabil 2003;84:507–512.
25. Grahame R, Bird HA, Child A: The revised (Brighton 1998) criteria for the diagnosis of Benign Joint Hypermobility Syndrome (BJHS). J Rhematol 2000;27:1777–1779.
26. LaBan MM, Perrin JC, Latimer FR: Pregnancy and the herniated lumbar disc. Arch Phys Med Rehabil 1983; 64(7):319–321.
27. Laslett M, Williams M: The reliability of selected pain provocation tests for sacroiliac joint pathology. Spine 1994;19:1243–1249.
28. Wells J: Osteitis condensans ilii. Am J Roentgenol Radium Ther Nucl Med 1956;76(6):1141–1143.
29. Shipp FL, Haggart GE: Further experience in the management of osteitis condensans ilii. J Bone Joint Surg (Am): 1950;32(4):841–847.
30. Mens JM, Vleeming A, Stoeckart R, et al: Understanding peripartum pelvic pain—Implications of a patient survey. Spine 1996;21:1363–1370.
31. Rungee JL: Low back pain during pregnancy. Orthopedics 1993;6:1339–1344.
32. Wilbur A, Langer B, Spigos D: Diagnosis of sacroiliac joint infection in pregnancy by magnetic resonance imaging. Magn Reson Imaging 1988;6:341–343.
33. Fortin JD, Falco FJ: The Fortin finger test: An indicator of sacroiliac pain. Am J Orthop 1997;26:477–480.
34. Bradford DS, Hu SS: Spondylolysis and spondylolisthesis. In Weinstein SL (ed): The Pediatric Spine: Principles and Practice. New York, Raven Press, 1994, pp 585–601.
35. Saraste H: Long-term clinical and radiological follow-up of spondylolysis and spondylolisthesis. J Pediatr Orthop 1987;7:631–638.
36. Saraste H: Spondylolysis and pregnancy—A risk analysis. Acta Obstet Gynecol Scand 1986;65:727–729.
37. Betz RR, Bunnell WP, Lombrecht-Mulier E, et al: Scoliosis and pregnancy. J Bone Joint Surg 1987;69-A,1:90–96.
38. Ascani E, Bartolozzi P, Logroscino CA, et al: Natural history of untreated idiopathic scoliosis after skeletal maturity. Spine 1986;11:784–789.
39. Weinstein SL: Adolescent idiopathic scoliosis: Prevalence and natural history. In Weinstein SL (ed): The Pediatric Spine: Principles and Practice. New York, Raven Press, 1994, pp 463–478.
40. Damen L, Buyruk HM, Guler-Uysal F, et al: Pelvic pain during pregnancy is associated with asymmetrical laxity of the sacroiliac joints. Acta Obstet Gynecol Scand 2001;80:1019–1024.
41. Damen L, Buyruk HM, Guler-Uysal F, et al: The prognostic value of asymmetrical laxity of the sacroiliac joints in pregnancy-related pelvic pain. Spine 2002;27:2820–2824.
42. Van Dongen PW, De Boer M, Lemmens WA, et al: Hypermobility and peripartum pelvic pain syndrome in pregnant South African women. Eur J Obstet Gynecol Reprod Biol 1999;84:77–82.
43. Scriven MW, Jones DA, McKnight L: The importance of pubic pain following childbirth: A clinical and ultrasonographic study of diastasis of the pubic symphysis. J R Soc Med 1995;88:28–30.
44. Bjorklund K, Nordstrom ML, Bergstrom S: Sonographic assessment of symphyseal joint distention during pregnancy and post partum with special reference to pelvic pain. Acta Obstet Gynecol Scand 1999;78:125–130.
45. Wurdinger S, Humbsch K, Reichenbach JR, et al: MRI of the pelvic ring joints postpartum: Normal and pathologic findings. J Magn Reson Imaging 2002;15:324–329.
46. Kurzel RB, Au AH, Rooholamini SA, et al: Magnetic resonance imaging of peripartum rupture of the symphysis pubis. Obstet Gynecol 1996;87:826–829.
47. Driessen F: Postpartum pelvic arthropathy with unusual features. Br J Obstet Gynaecol 1987;94:870–872.
48. Lindsey RW, Leggon RE, Wright DG, et al: Separation of the symphysis pubis in association with childbearing: A case report. J Bone Joint Surg 1988;70-A,2:289–292.

49. Dhar S, Anderton J: Rupture of the symphysis pubis during labor. Clin Orthop Relat Res 1992;283:252–257.
50. Davidson MR: Examining separated symphysis pubis. J Nurse-Midwifery 1996;41:259–262.
51. Cappiello GA, Oliver BC: Rupture of symphysis pubis caused by forceful and excessive abduction of the thighs with labor epidural anesthesia. JFMA 1995;82:261–263.
52. Dunbar RP, Ries AM: Puerperal diastasis of the pubic symphysis: A case report. J Reprod Med 2002;47:581–583.
53. Heath T, Gherman RB: Symphyseal separation, sacroiliac joint dislocation and transient lateral femoral cutaneous neuropathy associated with McRobert's manoeuvre: A case report. J Reprod Med 1999;44:902–904.
54. Kharrazi FD, Rodgers WB, Kennedy JG, et al: Parturition-induced pelvic dislocation: A report of four cases. J Orthop Trauma 1997;11:277–281.
55. Petersen AC, Rasmussen KL: External skeletal fixation as treatment for total puerperal rupture of the pubic symphysis. Acta Obstet Gynecol Scand 1992;71:308–310.
56. Kotwal PP, Mittal R: Disruption of symphysis pubis during labor. Int J Gynecol Obstet 1996;54:51–53.
57. Rommens PM: Internal fixation in postpartum symphysis rupture: Report of three cases. J Orthop Trauma 1997;11: 273–276.
58. Shuler TE, Gruen GS: Chronic postpartum pelvic pain treated by surgical stabilization. Orthopedics 1996;19:687–689.
59. Kowalk DL, Perdue PS, Bourgeois FJ, et al: Disruption of the symphysis pubis during vaginal delivery: A case report. J Bone Joint Surg 1996;78-A:1746–1748.
60. Gonik B, Stringer A: Postpartum osteitis pubis. South Med J 1985;78:213–214.
61. Maksymowych WP, Aaron SL, Rusel AS: Treatment of refractory symphysitis pubis with intravenous pamidronate. J Rheumatol 2001;28:2754–2757.
62. Magnusdottir R, Franklin J, Gestsson J: Septic symphysial disruption presenting as severe symphysiolysis in pregnancy. Acta Obstet Gynecol Scand 1996;75:681–682.
63. Lovisetti G, Sala F, Battaini A, et al: Osteomyelitis of the pubic symphysis, abscess and late disjunction after delivery: A case report. Chir Organi Mov 2000;85:85–88.
64. Moran JJ: Stress fractures in pregnancy. Am J Obstet Gynecol 1988;158:1274–1277.
65. Mikawa Y, Watanabe R, Yamano Y, et al: Stress fracture of the body of pubis in a pregnant woman. Arch Orthop Trauma Surg 1988;107:193–194.
66. Baijal E: Multiple fractures of the pelvis with an unusually wide disruption of the symphysis pubis sustained in an accident shortly after childbirth: A case report. Injury 1974;6:57–59.
67. Yosipovitch Z, Goldberg I, Ventura E, et al: Open reduction of acetabular fracture in pregnancy: A case report. Clin Orthop Relat Res 1992;282:229–232.
68. Funk JL, Shoback DM, Genant HK: Transient osteoporosis of the hip in pregnancy: Natural history of changes in bone mineral density. Clin Endocrinol 1995;43:373–382.
69. Bruinsma BJ, LaBan MM: The ghost joint: Transient osteoporosis of the hip. Arch Phys Med Rehabil 1990;71:295–298.
70. Bramlett KW, Killian JT, Nasca RJ, et al: Transient osteoporosis. Clinl Orthop Relat Res 1987;222:197–202.
71. Shifrin L, Reis ND, Zinman H, et al: Idiopathic transient osteoporosis of the hip. J Bone Joint Surg 1987;69-B:769–773.
72. Takatori Y, Kokubo T, Ninomiya S, et al: Transient osteoporosis of the hip: Magnetic resonance imaging. Clin Orthop Relat Res 1991;271:190–194.
73. Brodell JD, Burns Jr JE, Heiple KG: Transient osteoporosis of the hip of pregnancy. J Bone Joint Surg 1989;71-A:1252–1257.
74. Myllynen P, Makela A, Kontula K: Aseptic necrosis of the femoral head during pregnancy. Obstet Gynecol 1988;71:495–498.
75. Reckling FW: Normal pregnancy and delivery following total hip joint replacement. Clin Orthop Relat Res 1976;115:169–171.
76. McIntyre IN, Broadhurst NA: Effective treatment of low back pain in pregnancy. Aust Fam Physician 1996;25:S65–S67.
77. Young G, Jewell D: Interventions for preventing and treating backache in pregnancy. Cochrane Database Syst Rev 2000;2: CD001139.

CHAPTER 52

Skin Disease

George Kroumpouzos / Lisa M. Cohen

INTRODUCTION

Skin problems in pregnancy can be categorized as follows[1]:

- physiologic skin changes of pregnancy
- preexisting skin diseases and tumors affected by pregnancy
- pruritus in pregnancy
- specific dermatoses of pregnancy.

Prompt recognition and correct classification of the skin problem are essential for treatment, when necessary. The pregnant woman should be counseled about the nature of her skin condition, possible maternal or fetal risks associated with it, and management options.

PHYSIOLOGIC SKIN CHANGES OF PREGNANCY

The skin undergoes changes during pregnancy that are caused by the profound endocrine and metabolic alterations during the gestational period. The physiologic skin changes of pregnancy include pigmentary changes such as hyperpigmentation and melasma, vascular changes such as spider angiomas (Fig. 52–1), palmar erythema, nonpitting edema and varicosities, stretchmarks (*striae gravidarum*) (Fig. 52–2), as well as mucosal, hair (Fig. 52–3), nail, and glandular changes.[1–3] These changes are not associated with any risks for the mother or fetus and are expected to resolve postpartum.

The types of pigmentation seen in pregnancy are summarized in Table 52–1. The most common pigmentary changes of pregnancy are hyperpigmentation and melasma (Fig. 52–4). Uncommon pigmentary patterns, such as pseudoacanthosis nigricans (Fig. 52–5) and dermal melanocytosis (Fig. 52–6), can also be seen.[4–8] Furthermore, postinflammatory hyperpigmentation secondary to specific dermatoses of pregnancy (Fig. 52–7) is particularly common in skin of color. A mild form of localized or generalized hyperpigmentation occurs to some extent in up to 90% of pregnant women[1,3] and shows accentuation of the areolae, nipples, genital skin, axillae, and inner thighs. The most familiar examples are darkening of the linea alba (*linea nigra*) (see Fig. 52–2) and periareolar skin (*secondary areolae*).

Melasma (*chloasma*, or *mask of pregnancy*) is a type of facial melanosis reported in up to 70% of pregnant women[2] and one third of nonpregnant women taking an oral contraceptive.[9] Although the malar pattern is common, the entire central face is affected in most patients *(centrofacial pattern)* (see Fig. 52–4) and less often the ramus of the mandible *(mandibular pattern)*.[10] Melasma results from melanin deposition in the epidermis (70%, accentuated by Wood's lamp examination), dermal macrophages (10% to 15%) or both (20%). This type of melanosis is thought to be associated with the hormonal changes of gestation and worsens with exposure to ultraviolet and visible light.[10–11] Melasma usually resolves postpartum but may recur in subsequent pregnancies or with the use of oral contraceptives. The dermal type of melasma is less responsive to treatment than the epidermal. Mild gestational melasma can be treated with azelaic acid, which is safe during pregnancy. Persistent melasma can be treated postpartum with topical hydroquinone 2% to 4% and a broad-spectrum sunscreen, with[12] or without a topical retinoid and mild topical steroid. Melasma, whether caused by pregnancy or oral contraceptives,[3] is resistant to treatment in 30% of patients. Combination therapies, including laser treatment[13,14] and chemical peels,[15] may be effective to some extent in resistant cases.

The physiologic vascular, connective tissue, mucosal, glandular, hair, and nail changes of pregnancy are summarized in the Summary of Management Options box. The oral pyogenic granuloma of pregnancy (*granuloma gravidarum*, or *pregnancy epulis*) is discussed under Skin Tumors.

SUMMARY OF MANAGEMENT OPTIONS

Physiologic Skin Changes of Pregnancy

Management Options	Quality of Evidence	Strength of Recommendation	References
Pigmentation			
Follow-up for spontaneous resolution in postpartum period.	–	GPP	–
Sun protection mandatory in all cases.	–	GPP	–
For persistent cases postpartum, consider:			
• Hydroquinone 2%-4% cream with or without tretinoin and mild topical steroids	IV	C	12
• Combination therapies including laser treatment (erbium: YAG, Q-switched ruby, or Q-switched Nd:YAG)	IIa	B	13,14
• Combination therapies, including chemical peels (glycolic acid and Jessner's solution)	IIb	B	15
Spider Nevus (see Fig. 52–1)			
Reassure (occurs in 67% of white women, in the second to fifth months; resolves within 3 months' postpartum); persistent lesions can be treated with fine-needle electrocautery, cryotherapy, or laser.	–	GPP	–
Palmar Erythema			
Reassure (occurs in 70% of white and 30% of African American women).	–	GPP	–
Varicosities			
Explain (occurs in 40% of women; thrombosis in <10%); recommend leg elevation, compression stockings.	–	GPP	–
To treat symptomatic hemorrhoids, recommend stool softeners, hot sitz baths, topical anesthetics, suppositories, laxatives.			
Nonpitting Edema			
Reassure; exclude preeclampsia. Recommend leg elevation; compression stockings, diuretics if severe.	–	GPP	–
Striae Gravidarum (see Fig. 52–2)			
Reassure (occurs in 90% of white women; less common in other groups; less apparent postpartum but may never disappear); prescribe antipruritics, topical steroids if itchy; laser can improve the color changes.	–	GPP	–
Pyogenic Granuloma (*Granuloma Gravidarum*)			
Reassure (occurs in 2% of pregnant women at second to fifth months; typically on the gingivae; postpartum shrinkage).	–	GPP	–
Recommend good dental hygiene; excision if excessive discomfort or bleeding.			
Gum Hyperemia/Gingivitis			
Seen in most pregnant women in the third trimester; resolves postpartum.	–	GPP	–
Reassure; recommend good dental hygiene.			

Continued

SUMMARY OF MANAGEMENT OPTIONS

Physiological Skin Changes of Pregnancy *(Continued)*

Management Options	Quality of Evidence	Strength of Recommendations	References
Hair Changes (see Fig. 52–3)			
Mild hursutism regresses within 6 months' postpartum. Postpartum hair shedding (*telogen effluvium*) lasts 1 to 5 months. Frontoparietal hair recession and diffuse thinning also reported. Exclude pathologic androgen production if hirsutism. Follow-up postpartum hair changes.	–	GPP	–
Glandular Changes			
Reassure (enlargement of sebaceous glands of the areolae); axillary sweating can be controlled with aluminum chloride solution (20%).	–	GPP	–
Nail Changes			
Reassure (start in the first trimester; onycholysis, subungual hyperkeratosis, transverse grooving, brittleness).	–	GPP	–

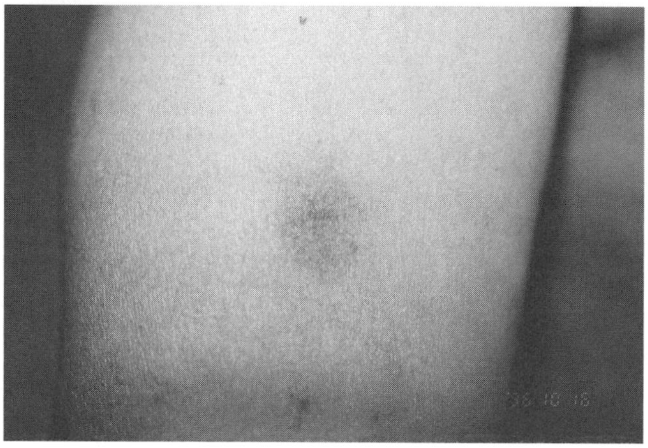

FIGURE 52–1
Spider angioma (telangiectasia) on the arm (see Color Plate 42).

PREEXISTING SKIN DISEASES AND TUMORS AFFECTED BY PREGNANCY

The pregnant woman is susceptible to aggravation or less often to improvement of skin diseases and tumors.[16] The conditions that may improve during pregnancy are listed in Table 52–2.

Inflammatory Skin Diseases

Risks and Management Options

ATOPIC DERMATITIS (ECZEMA)

Eczema is the most common pregnancy dermatosis, accounting for 36% of total cases.[17] Atopic dermatitis

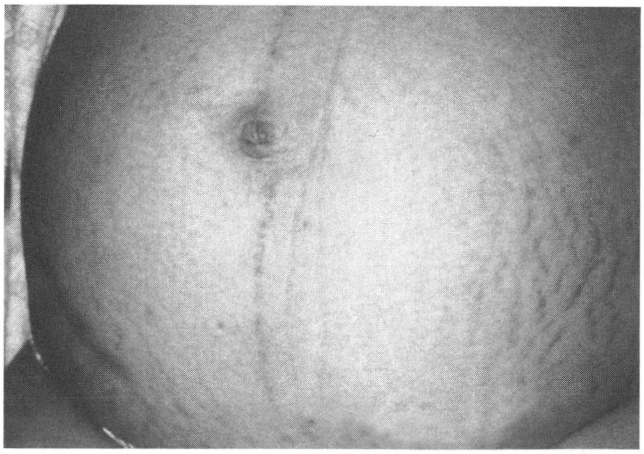

FIGURE 52–2
Stretchmarks (striae gravidarum) on the lateral aspects of the abdomen and hyperpigmentation of the linea alba, causing development of the *linea nigra* (see Color Plate 43).

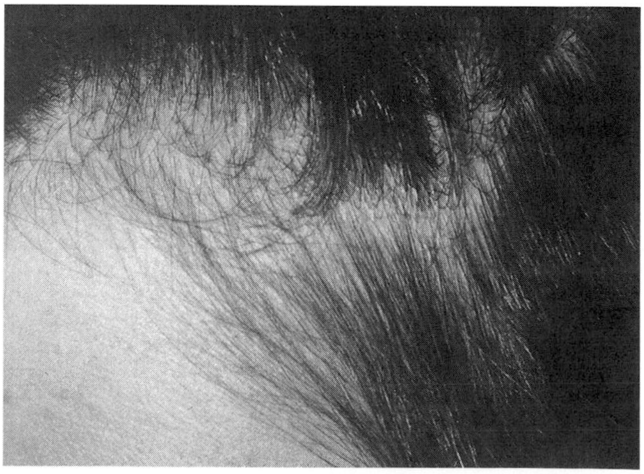

FIGURE 52–3
Telogen effluvium, which developed in the immediate postpartum period, with typical temporal recession and thinning (see Color Plate 44).

TABLE 52–1

Patterns of Pigmentation in Pregnancy

PATTERNS

- **Common hypermelanoses**
  - Hyperpigmentation
  - Melasma
- **Uncommon hypermelanoses**
  - Pseudoacanthosis nigricans
  - Dermal melanocytosis
  - Vulvar melanosis
  - Verrucous areolar pigmentation
  - Localized reticulate pigmentation
- **Darkening of preexisting pigmentation**
  - Acanthosis nigricans
  - Pigmentary demarcation lines
- **Darkening of benign skin lesions**
  - Scars
  - Melanocytic nevi
  - Skin tags; seborrheic keratoses
- **Postinflammatory hyperpigmentation**
  - Secondary to specific dermatoses of pregnancy (see specific section in text)
- **Jaundice** (see specific section in text)

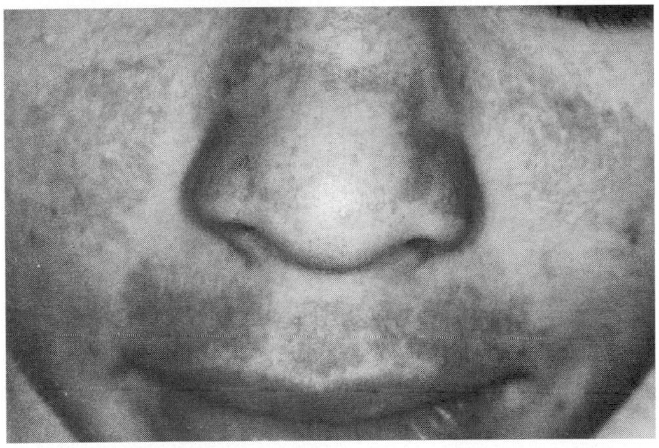

FIGURE 52–4
Melasma of the entire central face (see Color Plate 45).

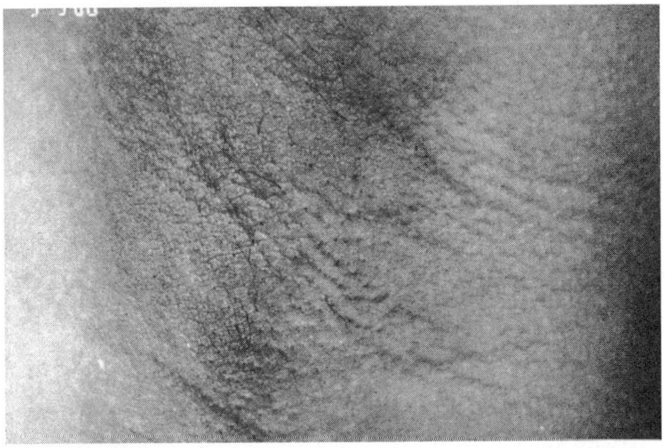

FIGURE 52–5
Pseudoacanthosis nigricans may develop in skin of color during pregnancy and manifests itself as hyperpigmented velvety plaques on the axillae (as shown) and neck (see Color Plate 46).

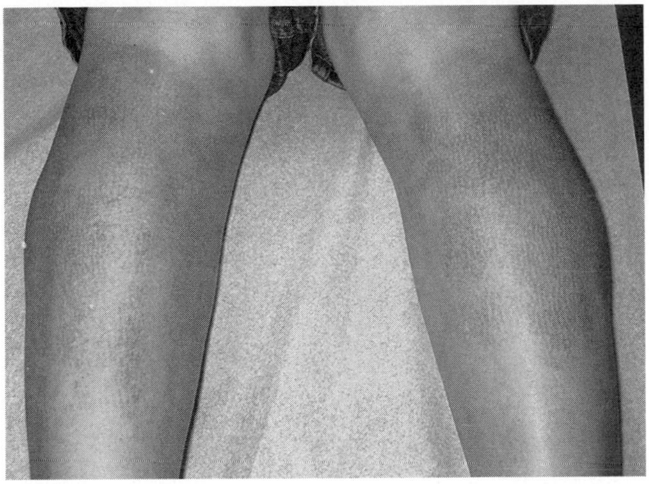

FIGURE 52–6
Grayish-brown ill-defined patches of dermal melanocytosis may develop in pregnancy and persist in the postpartum period (see Color Plate 47).

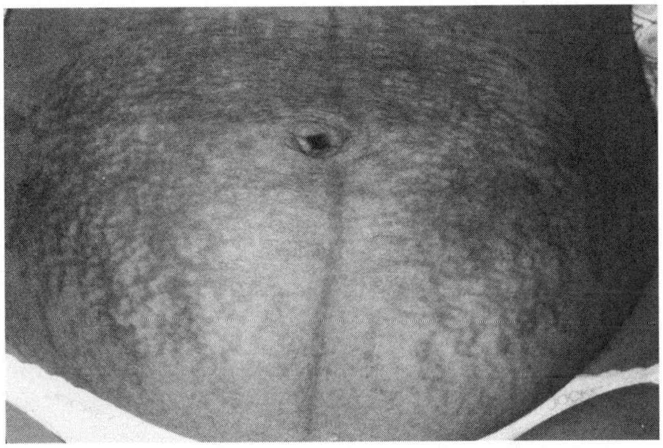

FIGURE 52–7
Extensive postinflammatory hyperpigmentation secondary to pruritic urticarial papules and plaques of pregnancy in an Asian female (see Color Plate 48).

TABLE 52–2

Preexisting Disorders That May Improve in Pregnancy

- Atopic dermatitis
- Acne vulgaris
- Chronic plaque psoriasis
- Fox-Fordyce disease
- Hidradenitis suppurativa
- Linear IgA disease
- Rheumatoid arthritis
- Sarcoidosis

is more likely to worsen than remit in pregnancy, although remission has been reported in up to 24% of cases. There is a personal history of atopy in 27% of pregnant females with atopic dermatitis, a family history of atopy in 50% of cases, and infantile eczema in 19% of offspring. There have been no adverse effects on the fetal outcome. Maternal smoking may be implicated in the development of atopic eczema during pregnancy and lactation.[18] The effect of breast-feeding on atopic eczema has been debated. Gestational atopic eczema is treated with moisturizers and low- to mid-potency topical steroids. A short course of oral steroid may be required for severe eczema. Systemic antibiotics, such as erythromycin base or penicillin, are necessary in superinfected eczema. Systemic antihistamines, such as diphenhydramine, are often required for severe pruritus. Ultraviolet B light (UVB) is a safe adjunct in treating chronic eczema. Irritant hand dermatitis and nipple eczema are often seen postpartum.[1] Nipple eczema can show painful fissures and be complicated with bacterial infection, most commonly from *Staphylococcus aureus*.

ACNE VULGARIS

The effect of pregnancy on acne vulgaris is unpredictable. Some patients may develop acne for the first time during pregnancy, and acne conglobata may worsen during pregnancy. Comedonal acne can be treated with topical keratolytic agents, such as benzoyl peroxide, whereas inflammatory acne can be treated with azelaic acid, topical erythromycin, topical clindamycin phosphate, or oral erythromycin base. All these medications are safe to use during gestation.[19]

Urticaria may worsen in pregnancy, whereas hidradenitis suppurativa and Fox-Fordyce disease may remit during gestation as a result of reduced apocrine gland activity.[1]

CHRONIC PLAQUE PSORIASIS

Chronic plaque psoriasis is the most common type of psoriasis to develop or exacerbate during pregnancy.[20] It is more likely to improve (40% to 63%) than worsen (14%) during gestation; it commonly flares, however, within 4 months of delivery. Psoriatic arthritis may develop or worsen during pregnancy, and often starts postpartum or perimenopausally (30% to 45%).[21] Topical steroids and topical calcipotriene as well as topical anthralin and topical tacrolimus appear to be safe treatment options for localized psoriasis in pregnancy.[22] UVB is the safest treatment for severe psoriasis that has not responded to topical medications. A short course of cyclosporine can be administered for psoriasis that has not responded to UVB.

GENERALIZED PUSTULAR PSORIASIS/IMPETIGO HERPETIFORMIS

A very rare variant of generalized pustular psoriasis develops in pregnancy, often associated with hypocalcemia[23] or low serum levels of vitamin D.[24] When compared with nonpregnant women with various forms of psoriasis, pregnant women with impetigo herpetiformis rarely have a personal or family history of psoriasis, develop the eruption strictly during pregnancy, and improve postpartum. The eruption usually starts in the third trimester. It often persists until delivery and occasionally runs a protracted course postpartum. It can exacerbate with the use of oral contraceptives.[25] Impetigo herpetiformis is manifested as grouped discrete sterile pustules at the periphery of erythematous patches (Fig. 52–8*A*). The lesions start in the major flexures and extend centrifugally onto the trunk and around the umbilicus, usually sparing the face, hands, and feet. The lesions may become crusted (Fig. 52–8*B*) or vegetative, and the mucous membranes may show erosive or circinate lesions. Postinflammatory hyperpigmentation commonly develops; nail changes secondary to subungual pustules are exceptionally seen.

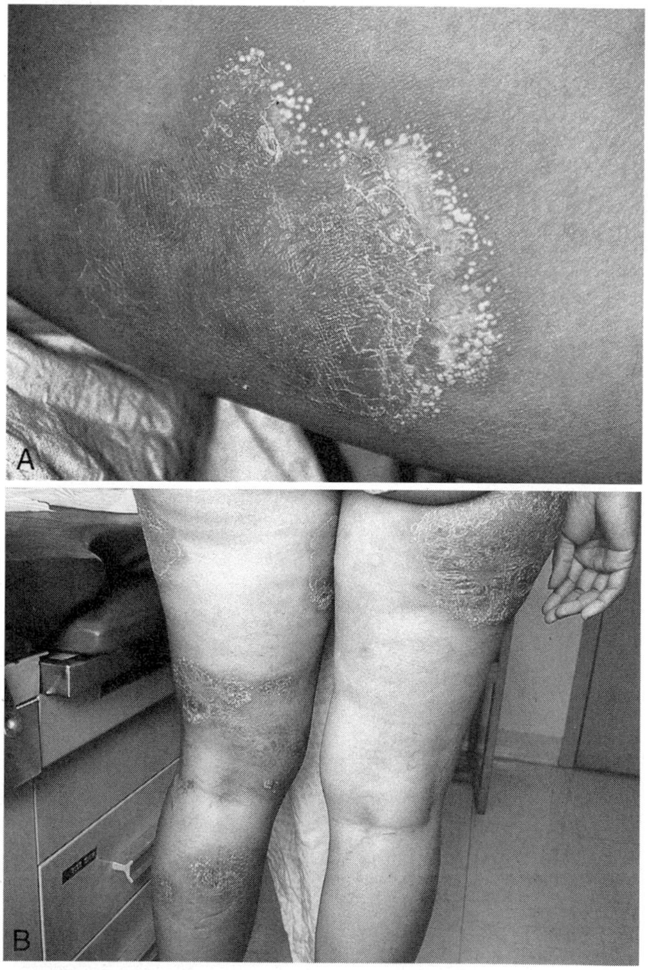

FIGURE 52–8
A, Early impetigo herpetiformis: discrete group sterile papules at the periphery of erythematous patch. *B*, Generalized advanced lesions of impetigo herpetiformis show crusting or vegetations.(see Color Plate 49.) (Photographs courtesy of Aleksandr Itkin, MD.)

Skin histopathology shows features of pustular psoriasis, and direct immunofluorescence is negative. The laboratory workup reveals leukocytosis, elevated erythrocyte sedimentation rate, and occasionally hypocalcemia or decreased serum vitamin D levels. Impetigo herpetiformis is thought to be an outbreak of psoriasis probably triggered by a metabolic milieu, such as pregnancy or hypocalcemia.[1] The latter is known to exacerbate generalized pustular psoriasis and can develop secondary to hypoalbuminemia in pregnancy. A report[26] that showed reduced levels of an inhibitor of skin elastase in a patient with impetigo herpetiformis warrants further investigation. Furthermore, a recent report[27] raised speculation that infections during pregnancy may trigger a flare of pustular psoriasis in an individual with psoriatic tendency.

Impetigo herpetiformis can be treated with systemic steroids at daily doses up to 60 mg/day of prednisone. Calcium and vitamin D replacement therapy should be undertaken if necessary and can lead to remission of the eruption.[23] A severe case was treated with cyclosporine.[28] Impetigo herpetiformis has been treated postpartum with oral retinoids[29] or PUVA[30] (psoralens with ultraviolet A light). Systemic antibiotics should be administered in superinfected cases. The eruption commonly resolves postpartum but recurs in each successive pregnancy with earlier onset and increased morbidity.[25,31] There are serious risks for the mother and fetus. Maternal risks include tetany, seizures, delirium, and exceptionally death from cardiac or renal failure. Fetal risks[25] such as stillbirth, neonatal birth, and fetal abnormalities may result from placental insufficiency, which often complicates impetigo herpetiformis, and have been reported even when the skin disease was well controlled.[31] Maternal and fetal monitoring is of utmost importance. In severe cases termination of pregnancy is warranted, the timing of which depends on the maternal and fetal status. The eruption resolves promptly afterwards.

Infections

Risks and Management Options

Pregnancy can affect the vast majority of common infections, causing an increase in the prevalence or exacerbation of candida vaginitis, *Trichomonas*, *Pityrosporum* folliculitis, and papillomavirus infections.[1,16] Other infections, such as recurrent genital herpes simplex virus infection, are not exacerbated in pregnancy but are of critical interest because they significantly increase fetal morbidity and mortality[32] (see Chapter 31). Disseminated infections are more likely to occur during gestation and may have devastating effects for the fetus. Viral exanthems can have significant maternal and/or fetal complications; their management options are summarized in Table 52–3. The consequences for the mother and fetus are also reviewed in Chapters 30 to 33.

The prevalence of candida vaginitis increases during pregnancy. The infection has been reported in 17% to 50% of pregnant women[33]; of those, 10% to 40% are asymptomatic.[34] *Candida albicans* has been associated with intra-amniotic infection.[35] The organism can be cultured from up to 50% of neonates born to infected mothers.[16] Neonatal candidiasis can result from passage of the infant through an infected birth canal and congenital candidiasis from an ascending infection in utero. The latter is characterized by generalized skin lesions that appear within 12 hours of delivery.[16] *Trichomonas* infection is seen in 12% to 27% of pregnant women.[36] An association with preterm delivery and low birth weight[37] has been debated.[38] *Pityrosporum* folliculitis and tinea versicolor (Fig. 52–9), both caused by yeasts of the *Malassezia* species, occur with greater frequency in pregnant women.[39] Papillomavirus infections may worsen during gestation, and condylomata acuminata can show accelerated growth, blocking the birth canal.[16]

Early studies showed exacerbation of leprosy during pregnancy or within the first 6 months of lactation,[40] a finding that was debated by a recent study.[41] Leprosy reactions are triggered by pregnancy: type 1 (reversal) reaction occurs maximally postpartum,[42] when the cell-mediated immunity returns to prepregnancy levels, and type 2 reaction (*erythema nodosum leprosum*) throughout pregnancy and lactation.[43] The increased incidence of erythema nodosum leprosum in pregnant women has been associated with early loss of nerve function secondary to "silent neuritis."[44] Multidrug therapy of rifampin, dapsone, and clofazimine is the treatment of choice during pregnancy. Leprosy reactions should be treated with oral steroids and not thalidomide which is contraindicated in pregnancy. Patients with leprosy should be counseled about the effects of pregnancy on the disease before they become pregnant, and pregnancies should be planned when the disease is well controlled. Leprosy has been associated with increased fetal mortality and low birth weight.[40] Approximately 20% of children born to mothers with leprosy will develop the disease by puberty.

Autoimmune Disorders

Risks and Management Options

SYSTEMIC LUPUS ERYTHEMATOSUS

Chronic discoid lupus is not affected by pregnancy. The data[45–47] as to whether flares of systemic lupus erythematosus (SLE) are more common during pregnancy are conflicting. The discrepancy among previous studies is due to methodologic differences,[48] including the definition of lupus flare, and the fact that several typical manifestations of active SLE, such as facial erythema (Fig. 52–10), alopecia, fatigue, edema, anemia, musculoskeletal pain, mild proteinuria, and elevated ESR, are common findings in pregnancy. In most studies the frequency of flare during pregnancy was higher than 57%.[48]

TABLE 52-3

Viral Exanthems: Maternal and Fetal Risks and Management Options

VIRUS	MATERNAL RISKS	FETAL RISKS	MANAGEMENT OPTIONS	LEVEL OF EVIDENCE	GRADE OF RECOMMENDATION
Varicella-Zoster	Pneumonitis (14%) Death (3%)	0–20 weeks: congenital varicella syndrome → skin lesions or limb hypoplasia to severe multisystem involvement	Give VZIG to seronegative mother within 72 hours postexposure; treat confirmed maternal varicella early with acyclovir for pneumonitis or other complications.	Ib	A
		13–40 weeks: herpes zoster in infancy (1–2%)			
		−1 to +1 week from delivery: neonatal varicella	Provide VZIG prophylaxis if mother has varicella or infant of seronegative mother has maternal or other VZV contact before 28 days; treat neonatal varicella with intravenous acyclovir.	Ib	A
Rubella	None	0–8 weeks: spontaneous abortion (20%)	HNIG may be offered to seronegative pregnant contacts of rubella for whom termination is unacceptable.	III	B
		0–12 weeks: congenital rubella syndrome (85%) → sensorineural deafness, congenital heart defects, retinopathy, cataract, microphthalmia, psychomotor retardation	Recommend therapeutic abortion.	III	B
		13–16 weeks: congenital rubella → sensorineural deafness, retinopathy			
Erythema Infectiosum (Parvovirus B19)	Aplastic crisis in patients with hemoglobinopathy	0–20 weeks: midtrimester abortion 4–6 weeks later (↑ by 9%)			
		9–20 weeks: hydrops fetalis after 12 weeks (3%)	Monitor for hydrops fetalis; consider intrauterine transfusion.	IIa	B
		Congenital red cell aplasia?			
Enteroviruses (Echo Virus, Coxsackie Virus)	None	Perinatal maternal infection: neonatal infection of variable severity symptomatic → fulminant multisystem disease: pneumonitis, hepatitis, meningoencephalitis, myocarditis, pancreatitis, disseminated intravascular coagulation	Give HNIG to neonates born within 5 days of maternal infection (efficacy unproven).	III	B
			Provide infection control measures to prevent nosocomial spread from index case.	IIb	B
Measles	Increased mortality from pneumonia (3%), encephalitis, hepatitis, myocarditis, nephritis, appendicitis, mesenteric adenitis, thrombotic thrombocytopenic purpura	Preterm labor; ↓ birth weight within 2 weeks of rash; fetal death in utero uncommon	Provide prophylactic IG within 6 days postexposure.	IIb	B
		Congenital infection to the neonate ranges from mild disease to death	Offer symptomatic treatment.	GPP	GPP
			Give MMR postpartum to susceptible women.	Ib	A

HNIG, human normal immunoglobulin; VZIG, varicella zoster immune globulin.
Table modified from Mahon E, Ruiter A, Lockwood D: Infectious diseases in pregnancy. In Black M, McKay M, Braude P, et al (eds): Obstetric and Gynecologic Dermatology, 2nd ed. London, Mosby, 2002, pp 80–81.

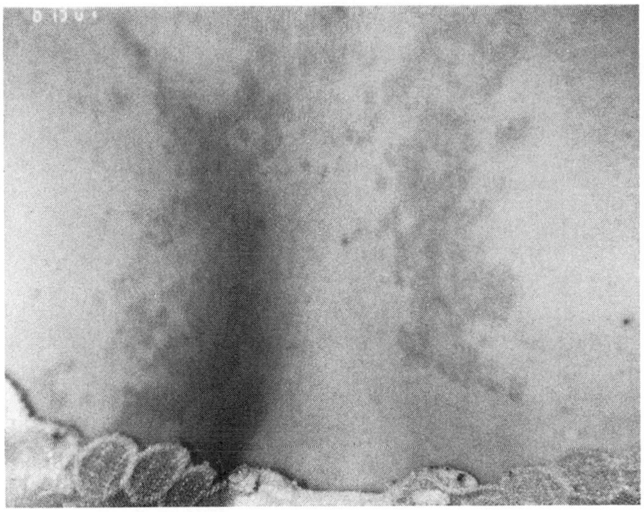

FIGURE 52–9
Hyperpigmented minimally scaly patches on the chest in a pregnant female with tinea versicolor (see Color Plate 50).

Pregnancy is well tolerated by mothers in remission for at least 3 months before conception, but if conception occurs during the active stage of disease 50% of gravidas will worsen during pregnancy and may experience life-threatening progression of the renal disease.[45] When SLE first appears during pregnancy it may show severe manifestations but usually remits postpartum. Cutaneous flares and arthralgias are the most common manifestations of SLE in pregnancy. Flares are not more severe during than outside of pregnancy and can be treated with

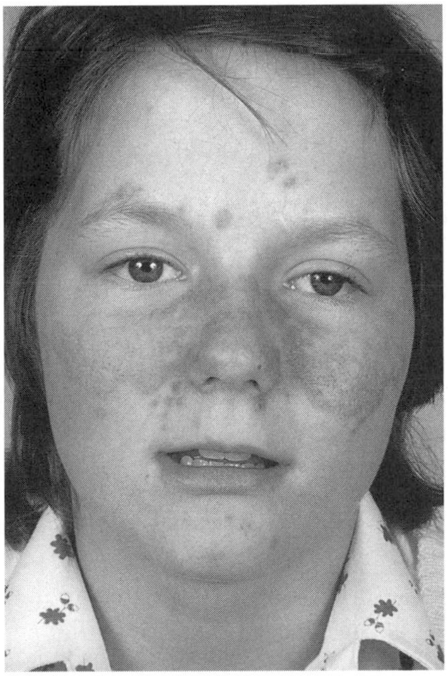

FIGURE 52–10
Malar erythema in a butterfly distribution in a pregnant woman with systemic lupus erythematosus. (see Color Plate 51). (Photograph courtesy of Cameron Thomas, Campbell Kennedy, and Phillipa Kyle from second edition.)

oral steroids. Yet, steroids do not prevent flares and should not be prescribed prophylactically.

The effects of lupus on fetal outcome correlate with the severity of maternal lupus, active disease at the time of conception or first presentation of SLE during pregnancy, and presence of anticardiolipin antibody or lupus anticoagulant. Preterm delivery occurs in 16% to 37% of pregnancies, and spontaneous abortion rates are two to four times normal; other risks include fetal death, intrauterine growth restriction (IUGR), and preeclampsia.[48] These obstetric complications have been associated with uteroplacental hypoperfusion, defective placentation, and chronic inflammation. The antiphospholipid syndrome[49] may complicate SLE, but many patients have primary antiphospholipid syndrome without lupus. It presents with manifestations that can worsen or lead to its initial diagnosis during gestation, such as recurrent miscarriage, thrombosis, livedo reticularis, migraine, stroke, and thrombocytopenia. Treatment with low-molecular-weight heparin or aspirin and close antenatal surveillance for maternal and fetal complications is warranted.

NEONATAL LUPUS

Neonatal lupus[50] can develop due to transplacental passage of maternal anti-Ro (SS-A), and less commonly anti-La (SS-B) or anti-U1-RNP antibody. The risk is 5% if anti-Ro positive, and the incidence is 1.6% of all lupus pregnancies. An association with HLA DR2 and DR3 positivity in the mother has been reported. The female-to-male ratio is 3:1. Neonatal lupus is characterized by a transient skin eruption and systemic manifestations, including congenital heart block (15% to 30%), cytopenias, hepatosplenomegaly, and pericarditis/myocarditis. The eruption become manifest several weeks into postnatal life and resolves by 6 to 8 months of age, coincident with the clearance of maternal autoantibody from the infant's circulation. The skin lesions frequently affect the face and scalp, with a predilection for the eyelids. Other sun-exposed areas may be also affected; occasionally the eruption becomes generalized. The lesions are papulosquamous or annular/polycyclic, indistinguishable from subacute cutaneous lupus of the adult. Skin histopathology shows interface dermatitis and superficial dermal mononuclear cell infiltrate. Immunofluorescence shows a particulate pattern of IgG in the epidermis.

Congenital heart block carries a substantial neonatal morbidity and mortality, and can be detected in utero at 18 to 20 weeks' gestation. Twenty-two percent of affected infants die in the perinatal period, and 62% of the infants require a pacemaker. The risk of bearing a second child with heart block is 25%, rising to 50% after two or more affected infants. The maternal and fetal anti-Ro, anti-La, and anti-U1-RNP status should be determined, and the newborn should be screened for heart block. Survivors of neonatal lupus may be at increased risk of developing connective tissue disease in adulthood.

DERMATOMYOSITIS/POLYMYOSITIS

Dermatomyositis/polymyositis may show a flare of the heliotrope rash, worsening of proximal muscle weakness, or subcutaneous calcification in approximately half of the affected individuals.[51] When the disease is in remission during pregnancy there are no maternal or fetal risks involved. Nevertheless, when the disease starts or relapses during gestation, it can be detrimental to the mother and/or fetus. High doses of oral steroids may be required to control the disease. Fetal demise due to abortion, stillbirth, or neonatal death has been reported in over half of the cases of active disease, and prenatal surveillance is crucial. An assisted vaginal delivery may be required in case of active myositis during labor. If the disease is diagnosed in the first trimester, the option of therapeutic abortion should be offered to the mother because of the high risk of maternal and/or fetal complications.

SYSTEMIC SCLEROSIS

The course of scleroderma is not significantly altered by pregnancy. Gravidas with limited scleroderma without systemic disease do better than those with diffuse scleroderma.[52] Women with early (less than 4 years) diffuse scleroderma are at high risk for hypertension, renal failure, premature delivery, and small full-term infants. The risk of hypertension and renal failure is greatest during the third trimester and postpartum period. Nevertheless, renal crisis during gestation is less common than previously thought. Successful pregnancy is now reported in 70% to 80% of patients. The skin disease usually does not progress during pregnancy, whereas reflux esophagitis and articular disease worsen. Raynaud's phenomenon usually improves secondary to gestational vasodilation and increased blood flow.

BULLOUS DISORDERS

Pemphigus vulgaris, vegetans, or foliaceus may present or worsen during gestation.[53] Linear immunoglobulin A (IgA) disease may improve in pregnancy and relapse postpartum.[54] Pemphigus vulgaris is rare during pregnancy; it usually worsens in the first or second trimester. Skin immunofluorescence studies are required to differentiate pemphigus from herpes gestationis (see Herpes Gestationis in this chapter). Neonatal pemphigus can develop from transplacental transfer of IgG antibodies. Most neonates require no therapy as the blisters heal spontaneously within 2 to 3 weeks. Eight out of 26 documented pregnancies in 22 women with pemphigus resulted in stillbirth or abortion. Stillborn infants have been found to have skin lesions and immunofluorescence findings consistent with pemphigus. Pemphigus during pregnancy can be controlled with high doses of oral steroids.

Metabolic Disorders

Risks and Management Options

PORPHYRIA

Porphyria cutanea tarda, acute intermittent porphyria, and variegate porphyria can present problems in pregnancy because they are adversely affected by estrogen. Patients with porphyria cutanea tarda demonstrate bullous lesions, skin fragility, and milia on sun-exposed areas, such as the dorsa of the hands and forearms; other skin changes include facial hypertrichosis, periorbital hyperpigmentation, scarring alopecia, and dystrophic calcification with ulceration. Reports of porphyria cutanea tarda and pregnancy have been scarce in the literature; these reports have provided conflicting results.[55] Symptomatic exacerbation of the disease has been often reported during the first trimester followed by improvement later in pregnancy. These changes parallel a rise in serum estrogen and porphyrin excretion in the first trimester and a fall in serum iron levels and urinary porphyrins later in gestation. Nevertheless, some authors reported exacerbation of the disease with oral contraceptives and not in pregnancy. The fetal prognosis is not usually affected by this disorder. Lists of drugs that are safe and unsafe for porphyria patients have been published.[56] Management of porphyria cutanea tarda during pregnancy includes sun protection, avoidance of alcohol and iron, and repeated phlebotomies in retractable cases. Chloroquine is contraindicated in pregnancy because of its teratogenicity. The newborn should be assessed and screened for porphyria cutanea tarda in the immediate postpartum period, both for genetic counseling and avoidance of inducing factors in the child.

ACRODERMATITIS ENTEROPATHICA

Acrodermatitis enteropathica is a rare autosomal disorder of zinc deficiency characterized by dermatitis, diarrhea, and alopecia. The skin lesions are vesiculobullous and eczematous and are distributed on the extremities and periorificial sites, such as the mouth, anus, and genital areas. The disease usually flares during gestation, because serum levels decrease early in pregnancy.[57] This decline is not attributed to fetal demands only, because acrodermatitis enteropathica can also flare with oral contraceptive use. The skin lesions in pregnancy need to be differentiated from pemphigoid gestationis and impetigo herpetiformis. Most often, having first appeared in childhood, the skin disease reappears during pregnancy, worsens until delivery, and clears postpartum.[57] The disorder usually has no effect on fetal outcome. Fetal malformations and neonatal death have been reported in a few cases of untreated maternal disease.

Connective Tissue Disorders

Risks and Management Options

EHLERS-DANLOS SYNDROMES I TO X

Ehlers-Danlos syndromes I to X are a group of inherited disorders of collagen metabolism that manifest with skin fragility, easy bruising, joint hypermobility, and skin hyperelasticity. Women with Ehlers-Danlos syndromes type I (classic, or gravis) and IV (ecchymotic, or arterial) are particularly likely to develop complications during pregnancy. The risks include premature rupture of the membranes; postpartum bleeding; rupture of major vessels (especially in type IV), including the aorta and pulmonary artery; poor wound healing and dehiscence; uterine lacerations; bladder and uterine prolapse; and abdominal hernias.[58] The reported maternal mortality in type IV disease is 20% to 25%. The risks are such that women with Ehlers-Danlos syndromes types I or IV should be counseled against pregnancy. A favorable outcome of pregnancy, however, has been reported for types II (mitis) and X (fibronectin abnormality).

PSEUDOXANTHOMA ELASTICUM

Gestation may worsen the vascular complications of pseudoxanthoma elasticum. The main complication is massive hematemesis from gastrointestinal (particularly gastric) bleeding, but repeated epistaxis and congestive heart failure with ventricular arrhythmia have been also reported.[59] Hypertension is frequent and should be treated aggressively. An increased risk of first-trimester miscarriage and IUGR secondary to placental insufficiency has been reported.

Skin Tumors

Risks and Management Options

MISCELLANEOUS LESIONS

Most benign skin tumors can appear for the first time, increase in number, or enlarge during gestation as a result of the effects of high estrogen levels on vascular and soft tissues. The most common lesions that change during pregnancy are melanocytic nevi, seborrheic keratoses, and skin tags. Melanocytic nevi may develop, enlarge, or darken during pregnancy (Fig. 52–11). The pigmentary changes observed in melanocytic nevi during pregnancy are thought to be due to the melanogenic effects of high estrogen levels and increased levels of melanocyte-stimulating hormone. An increase in estrogen and progesterone receptors in melanocytic nevi in pregnancy has been demonstrated. A mild degree of histopathologic atypia has been reported in a few studies but there is no evidence that pregnancy induces malignant transformation of preexisting nevi. Seborrheic keratoses may also enlarge or darken during gestation. Skin tags (*molluscum fibrosum gravidarum*) usually appear during the later months of pregnancy and may partially or completely disappear postpartum. In all these cases, the pregnant woman needs to be reassured that these skin lesions are common during pregnancy and may improve postpartum.

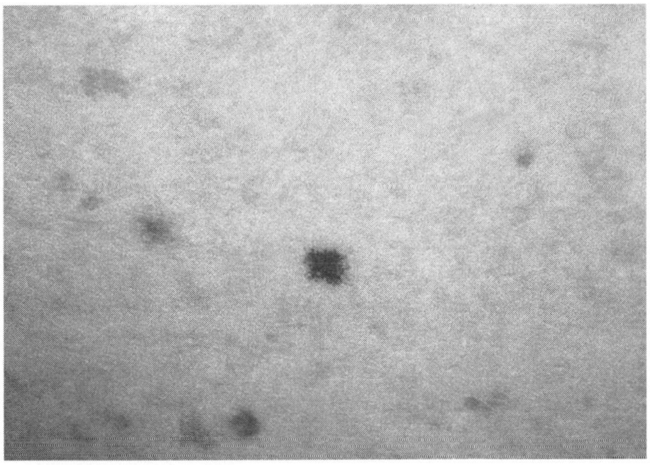

FIGURE 52–11
Melanocytic nevus that became darker and developed a mild border irregularity during gestation (see Color Plate 52).

Vascular tumors may also be affected or present during pregnancy. The pyogenic granuloma of pregnancy (*granuloma gravidarum*, pregnancy tumor, or pregnancy epulis) is a benign proliferation of capillaries within the gingivae that appears between the second and fifth months of pregnancy. The prevalence of *granuloma gravidarum* is estimated to approach 2% of all pregnancies. It may be caused by trauma to inflamed mucosa and presents as a vascular deep-red or purple nodule between the teeth or on the buccal or lingual surface of the marginal gingiva. Occasionally, pyogenic granulomas can develop on the lip or extramucosal sites (Fig. 52–12). Typical histopathologic features of a pyogenic granuloma are seen in all cases. Spontaneous shrinkage of the tumor usually occurs postpartum, and most cases do not require

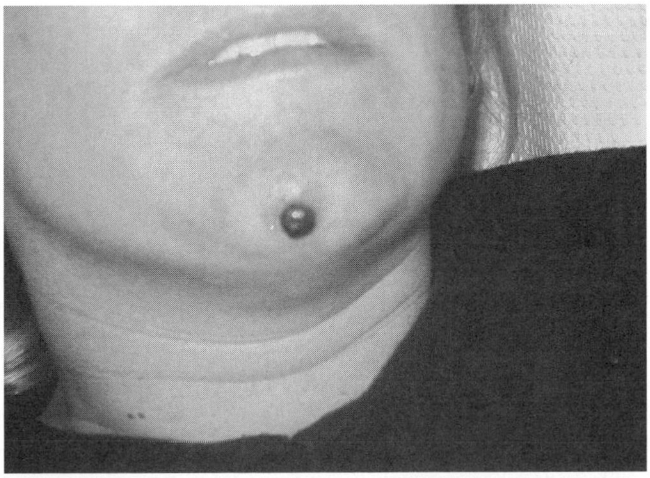

FIGURE 52–12
Pyogenic granuloma of pregnancy (*granuloma gravidarum*), typically seen on the gingivae, can also develop on extramucosal sites (see Color Plate 53).

treatment. Surgical excision, however, is necessary in cases of excessive bleeding. An increased frequency of other vascular tumors, such as hemangioma, hemangioendothelioma, glomus tumor, and glomangioma, has been reported in pregnancy. Large hemangiomas that exceptionally cause arteriovenous shunt and high-output cardiac failure in pregnancy partially regress postpartum, tending to enlarge again in subsequent pregnancies.

Dermatofibromata, dermatofibrosarcomata protuberans, leiomyomata, and keloids may develop or enlarge during pregnancy (Fig. 52–13). Desmoid tumors often develop in the rectus abdominis muscle. Neurofibromas may enlarge or arise *de novo* during gestation, often complicated with massive hemorrhage within the tumor; these lesions may partially resolve postpartum.

NEUROFIBROMATOSIS

Women with neurofibromatosis are at high risk for vascular complications during pregnancy such as hypertension and renal artery rupture.[60] A higher prevalence of maternal and fetal risks, such as first-trimester spontaneous abortion, stillbirth, IUGR, and perinatal complications, has been reported in neurofibromatosis.

MALIGNANT MELANOMA

Malignant melanoma accounts for 8% of malignant neoplasms during pregnancy. Most studies[61-63] have showed that melanomas that develop during pregnancy are thicker than melanomas in nonpregnant women and show a trend toward shorter disease-free survival. These findings are thought to be due to a delay in the diagnosis of melanoma during gestation, but the data to support this speculation is insufficient. Grin and colleagues[64] reviewed controlled clinical trials in pregnant women with melanoma and indicated that pregnancy does not influence the 5-year survival rate. These results were confirmed by a recent study[65] in pregnant women with stage I to II melanoma, which did not reveal any difference in the 10-year disease-free survival and overall survival between pregnant and nonpregnant women. Moreover, no differences were found in the histologic subtype, tumor location, ulceration, and vascular invasion between the two groups. There was a trend toward shorter disease-free survival in pregnant women that did not reach statistical significance. The authors concluded that the overall survival for women with melanoma during pregnancy is dependent only on the tumor thickness and ulceration.

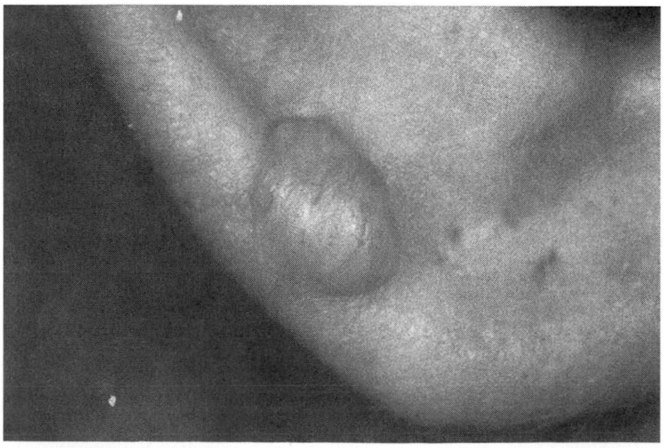

FIGURE 52–13
Keloid that developed during pregnancy without previous trauma (see Color Plate 54).

Surgery is the treatment of choice in patients with early melanoma. Correct staging is crucial, and sentinel lymph node biopsy using preoperative intradermal injection of technetium-99m-sulfur colloid is considered safe during pregnancy.[66] For pregnant women with advanced disease the prognosis, risks, and benefits from systemic therapy should be discussed. Systemic chemotherapy during the second and third trimesters does not usually cause fetal abnormalities, except in the case of alkylating agents.[67] Nevertheless, given that the effectiveness of chemotherapy in advanced melanoma is at present limited, systemic chemotherapy should not be given in pregnancy in other than exceptional circumstances. In some cases, termination of pregnancy may be the least damaging course of action to allow systemic therapy to be offered.

There are currently no standard guidelines for patients who desire a pregnancy after the diagnosis and treatment of melanoma. Based on the fact that 50% of recurrences develop by 3 years in patients with thick lesions, MacKie[67] suggested that women who have melanoma should not become pregnant not should they take oral contraceptive or postmenopausal hormonal replacement therapy for 2 years after initial treatment unless there are exceptional circumstances. The recommendation of other authors[66] about how long to wait before becoming pregnant after a diagnosis of melanoma is on case-by-case basis, depending on tumor thickness and stage, age of the patient, and desire to become pregnant. Although placental and/or fetal metastasis is extraordinarily rare (19 cases),[66] melanoma is the most common type of malignancy to metastasize to the placenta and fetus, representing 30% of placental metastases and 58% of fetal metastases. Maternal and fetal death invariably occurs; 80% of maternal deaths occur within 3 months of delivery. When a gravida is diagnosed with melanoma the placenta should be sent for histologic examination. Some authors[67] suggested that blood from both the mother and umbilical cord be examined cytologically.

Miscellaneous Skin Disorders

Risks and Management Options

A variety of skin disorders have been reported to start or flare during pregnancy, but large series are missing for most of them. Sarcoidosis of the skin is one of the most studied and has been shown to improve in pregnancy. Figure 52–14 demonstrates minimal residual skin lesions of sarcoidosis in a pregnant female who demonstrated generalized skin sarcoidosis before gestation. Exacerbation or new onset of erythema nodosum (adversely affected by

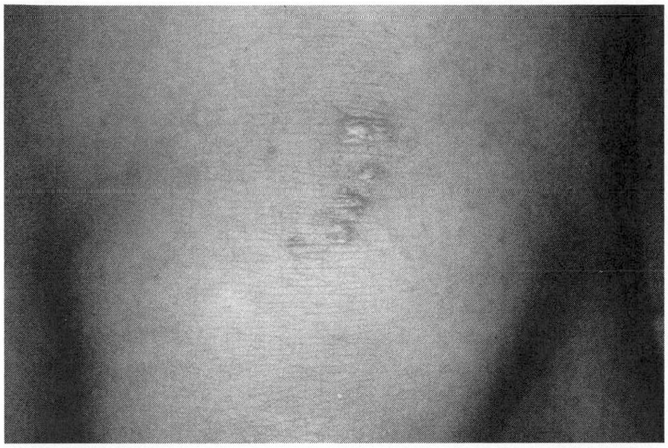

FIGURE 52–14
Minimal residual skin lesions of sarcoidosis on the knee in a pregnant female who showed severe generalized skin sarcoidosis before gestation (see Color Plate 55).

estrogen), keratosis pilaris, erythema multiforme, bowenoid papulosis, mycosis fungoides, Langerhans cell histiocytosis, mastocytosis, erythrokeratodermia variabilis, hereditary angioedema, tuberous sclerosis, Marfan syndrome, and hereditary hemorrhagic telangiectasia during pregnancy have been reported. The serious maternal risks related to vascular complications of tuberous sclerosis, Marfan syndrome, and hereditary hemorrhagic telangiectasia should be promptly assessed. The management of the rest of the aforementioned conditions should be individualized.

SUMMARY OF MANAGEMENT OPTIONS

Preexisting Skin Disorders

Management Options	Quality of Evidence	Strength of Recommendation	References
Atopic Dermatitis (Eczema)			
• Emollients	–	GPP	–
• Low- or mid-potency topical steroids			
• Oral antihistamines			
• UVB phototherapy			
• Short-course oral steroid for severe disease			
Acne Vulgaris			
Comedonal Acne	–	GPP	–
Treat with benzoyl peroxide.			
Inflammatory Acne	–	GPP	–
Treat with:			
• Azelaic acid			
• Topical erythromycin or clindamycin			
• Oral erythromycin			
Psoriasis			
Chronic Plaque Psoriasis			
Treat with:			
• Topical steroids, calcipotriene, anthralin, tacrolimus	IV	C	22
• UVB	–	GPP	–
• Short-course cyclosporine	–	GPP	–
Generalized Postular Psoriasis			
• Monitor maternal BP, cardiac and renal function.	–	GPP	–
• Institute fetal monitoring, vigilance for IUGR.	IV	C	25
• Prescribe high-dose oral steroids as first-line therapy.	–	GPP	–
• UVB and cyclosporine are second-line therapies.	IV	C	28

Continued

SUMMARY OF MANAGEMENT OPTIONS

Preexisting Skin Disorders *(Continued)*

Management Options	Quality of Evidence	Strength of Recommendation	References
Psoriasis—Continued			
• Give calcium and vitamin D if necessary.	IV	C	23
• Prescribe systemic antibiotics if superinfection.	–	GPP	–
Infections (See Chapters 30–32 and Table 52–3)			
Autoimmune Disorders			
• **SLE**			
Give oral steroids for skin and joint exacerbation.	IV	C	48
Neonatal Lupus	IV	C	50
• Skin biopsy if diagnosis uncertain.			
• Screen fetus/newborn for heart block.			
• Assess maternal/fetal anti-Ro, anti-La, anti-RNP.			
• Test ECG, liver function, platelets in newborn.			
• Give topical steroids, UV protection for skin rash.			
• See Chapter 37 for discussion congenital heart block.			
Dermatomyositis/Polymyositis	III	B	51
• Prescribe oral steroids; second line: methotrexate.			
• Be vigilant for IUGR and preterm labor.			
• Consider assisted vaginal delivery.			
Systemic Sclerosis	IV	C	52
• Monitor for hypertension and renal failure.			
• Be vigilant for preterm delivery and small-for-dates infants.			
Bullous Disorders—Pemphigus	III	B	53,54
• Prescribe oral steroids.			
• Institute vigilance for miscarriage/fetal death.			
• Institute vigilance for neonatal lesions.			
Metabolic and Connective Tissue Disorders			
Porphyria Cutanea Tarda			
• Be vigilant for exacerbation. Avoid sun, iron, and alcohol. Consider venesection.	IV	C	55
• Avoid chloroquine in first trimester. Avoid drugs that cause exacerbation.	IV	C	56
Acrodermatitis Enteropathica	IV	C	57
• Offer zinc supplementation.			
• Screen carefully for fetal malformations.			
Ehlers-Danlos Syndromes I and IV	III	B	58
• Prepregnancy counsel against conception.			
• Maintain vigilance for rupture of major vessels, postpartum hemorrhage, wound dehiscence.			
• Maintain vigilance for uterine or bladder prolapse.			
• Be vigilant for preterm delivery.			
• Provide IV access and crossmatch blood for delivery.			
• Avoid excessive trauma at operative delivery.			

SUMMARY OF MANAGEMENT OPTIONS

Preexisting Skin Disorders *(Continued)*

Management Options	Quality of Evidence	Strength of Recommendation	References
Metabolic and Connective Tissue Disorders—*Continued*			
• Use nonabsorbable sutures for cesarean section.			
• Consider termination of pregnancy if no response to therapy.			
Pseudoxanthoma Elasticum	IV	C	59
• Institute vigilance for GI bleeding, hypertension.			
• Institute vigilance for first-trimester miscarriage, IUGR.			
Skin Tumors			
Malignant Melanoma			
• If before pregnancy, avoid conception for up to 2 years.	IV	C	66
• Perform prompt excision and staging for definitive management.	III	B	64,65
• Chemotherapy may be used after first trimester with low risk of fetal anomaly.	IV	C	67
• Perform biopsy of placenta for metastasis (very rare).	IV	C	66,67
Neurofibromatosis			
• Monitor for hypertension and vascular complications.	IV	C	60
• Monitor fetal growth and health.	IV	C	60

BP, blood pressure; EKG, electrocardiogram; GI, gastrointestinal; IUGR, intrauterine growth restriction; UVB, ultraviolet light B.

PRURITUS IN PREGNANCY

Pruritus has been reported in 17% of pregnancies. As shown in Table 52–4, a broad differential diagnosis needs to be considered, and the constellation of clinical and laboratory findings is the most helpful approach to establishing a diagnosis and reaching management decisions. In summary, a patient with pruritus in pregnancy should be evaluated as follows:

- A detailed history, past medical history, obstetric history, and physical examination are imperative for determining the cause of pruritus. The laboratory workup should be directed by the clinical findings. The constellation of clinical and laboratory data will help identify pruritic skin diseases that are not specifically related to pregnancy, such as scabies, or systemic disorders with skin manifestations (see previous section).
- In the patient with pruritus and no eruption, one should consider systemic causes of pruritus such as lymphoma and liver, renal, and thyroid disease.
- In the patient with pruritus, jaundice, and no eruption, one should consider hepatitides, obstetric cholestasis, hyperbilirubinemic states, and other liver diseases.
- In the patient with pruritus and eruption, one should consider specific dermatoses of pregnancy (see following section), allergic reactions, drug eruptions, and urticarial lesions of hepatitis B.
- In the patient with pruritus, no jaundice, no eruption, no systemic disease, and no specific pregnancy dermatosis, one should consider intrahepatic cholestasis of pregnancy, pruritus associated with striae gravidarum and hyperemesis gravidarum complicated with cholestasis.

TABLE 52–4

Etiology of Pruritus in Pregnancy

COMMON CAUSES
• Intrahepatic cholestasis of pregnancy • Preexisting skin diseases • Specific dermatoses of pregnancy • Systemic diseases with skin involvement • Allergic reactions • Drug eruptions • Pruritus associated with striae gravidarum
UNCOMMON CAUSES
• Systemic causes of pruritus (lymphoma; liver, thyroid, or renal disease) • Viral hepatitis • Hyperbilirubinemic states • Hyperemesis gravidarum

Obstetric Cholestasis (See also Chapter 48)

Risks and Management Options

Generalized pruritus without a skin rash often results from obstetric cholestasis, the most common pregnancy-induced liver disorder. The condition manifests itself with jaundice (*intrahepatic jaundice of pregnancy*) or without (*pruritus gravidarum*). Viral hepatitis is the most common cause of jaundice in pregnancy with obstetric cholestasis second. Obstetric cholestasis is very common in Chile, Bolivia, and Scandinavia.[68] The incidence of obstetric cholestasis is lower in Europe (0.1% to 1.5%), the United States, Canada, and Australia. This geographic variation is thought to be due to environmental and/or dietary factors. Obstetric cholestasis recurs in 60% to 70% of subsequent pregnancies.[69] Oral contraceptives can cause a recurrence of pruritus and cholestasis. In half of the cases there is a family history of this condition or an association with multiple-gestation pregnancy.[68] Some authors suggested that obstetric cholestasis occurs more frequently and at an earlier gestational age in pregnant women who are positive for hepatitis C virus.[70]

Obstetric cholestasis manifests itself in 80% of cases after the 30th week of pregnancy,[68] although initial presentation as early as 6 weeks' gestation has been reported. The pruritus, which may precede the liver function abnormalities of the condition, affects the palms and soles and extends to the legs and abdomen. Excoriations due to scratching are invariably seen. Obstetric cholestasis is occasionally preceded by a urinary tract infection. Mild nausea and discomfort in the upper right quadrant may accompany the pruritus. Mild jaundice (20%) usually develops 2 to 4 weeks after the onset of itching and may be associated with subclinical steatorrhea and increased risk of hemorrhage.[69] Up to 50% of patients develop darker urine and light-colored stools. The symptoms and biochemical abnormalities of obstetric cholestasis usually resolve within 2 to 4 weeks postpartum. An increased risk of cholelithiasis has been debated.

Elevated serum bile acids, especially postprandial elevations, are the most sensitive marker of obstetric cholestasis[69] and correlate with the severity of the pruritus. Mild abnormalities on liver function tests are commonly found, namely elevated cholesterol, transaminases, alkaline phosphatase, and lipids. The conjugated bilirubin is mildly to moderately elevated (2 to 5 mg/dL) in jaundiced patients. Malabsorption of fat may cause vitamin K deficiency, resulting in a prolonged prothrombin time. Skin biopsy is unnecessary because there are no primary skin lesions. Liver biopsy is not indicated, but if performed shows centrilobular cholestasis, bile thrombi within dilated canaliculi, and minimal inflammatory changes.

Hormonal, immunologic, genetic, environmental, and probably alimentary factors may play a role in the etiology of obstetric cholestasis.[68] It has been suggested that the relative decrease in hepatic blood flow during gestation causes decreased elimination of toxins and estrogens. Estrogens interfere with bile acid secretion and increase biliary cholesterol secretion. Progestins inhibit hepatic glucuronyltransferase, thus reducing the clearance of estrogens and amplifying their effects. Monosulfated or disulfated progesterone metabolites, in particular the 3α, 5α-isomers, are substantially increased in obstetric cholestasis secondary to decreased biliary and fecal excretion. The increased serum levels of sulfated progesterone metabolites may saturate the maximal transport capacity of membrane transport proteins of the hepatocyte. Recent immunologic studies[71] showed a predominance of Th1 cytokines (cell-mediated immune reaction) and decreased maternal-fetal lymphocyte reaction in obstetric cholestasis. These findings show that immunologic mechanisms may be implicated in the pathogenesis of obstetric cholestasis.

Genetic factors have been suggested by the existence of familial cases and geographic variation of obstetric cholestasis. A high prevalence of the HLA haplotype Aw31B8 has been reported. A higher incidence of obstetric cholestasis has been observed in mothers of patients with progressive familial intrahepatic cholestasis (PFIC) or benign recurrent intrahepatic cholestasis. Patients with PFIC type 3 show mutations of the multidrug resistance 3 (MDR3) gene, which encodes the canalicular phosphatidylcholine translocase, a biliary transport protein. Recently, in a family of PFIC type 3 patients, 6 women with a history of obstetric cholestasis were heterozygous for the familial mutation in the MDR3 gene.[72] Environmental factors, as indicated by the geographic variation of obstetric cholestasis and its higher incidence during the winter, and alimentary factors have been implicated in the pathogenesis of obstetric cholestasis; the importance of these factors, however, has been debated.

Fetal risks in obstetric cholestasis include fetal distress, stillbirth, and preterm delivery. Malabsorption of vitamin K increases the risk of intracranial hemorrhage. The pathogenesis of fetal complications is associated with decreased fetal elimination of toxic bile acids, which can cause vasoconstriction of human placental chorionic veins. Furthermore, a higher incidence of meconium passage has been reported in stillbirths in obstetric cholestasis. Meconium can cause acute umbilical vein obstruction. The incidence of meconium passage was increased with the infusion of cholic acid in animal studies. The risk of serious fetal complications in obstetric cholestasis makes intensive fetal surveillance mandatory. Obstetric management should weigh the risk of preterm delivery against the risk of sudden death in utero.

Mild cholestasis can be treated symptomatically with topical antipruritics and emollients; oral antihistamines are rarely effective. Epomediol and silymarin have been helpful in mild cases.[68] The effectiveness of intravenous S-adenosylmethionine was not confirmed by a randomized, placebo-controlled study.[73] Treatment with activated charcoal has met limited success. Phenobarbital has shown minimal effect on the pruritus of obstetric cholestasis and variable effects on the biochemical abnormalities of the condition.[74] UVB has been variably effective and can be safely used when pharmacologic treatments fail. Dexamethasone suppression of fetoplacental estrogen production was effective (uncontrolled) and deserves further evaluation.[75]

Cholestyramine decreases the enterohepatic circulation of bile acids. It needs to be administered (up to 18 g/day) for several days before a clear benefit for pruritus can be obtained and does not improve the biochemical abnormalities of obstetric cholestasis.[74] Furthermore, it has the disadvantage of precipitating vitamin K and should be administered in conjunction with weekly vitamin K supplementation.[68] A case of severe fetal intracranial hemorrhage during treatment with cholestyramine for obstetric cholestasis has been reported. Vitamin K and cholestyramine should be given at different times of the day so that cholestyramine does not interfere with vitamin K absorption. A decrease in pruritus has been reported in approximately half of the patients studied (uncontrolled), but recurrence of itching was common after the first week of treatment. Patients with high serum bile acids may not respond to cholestyramine,[74] and several patients who did not respond to cholestyramine subsequently responded to other agents, such as ursodeoxycholic acid and dexamethasone. It may be concluded that cholestyramine can be effective only in mild to moderate obstetric cholestasis.

Ursodeoxycholic acid, a naturally occurring hydrophilic bile acid, protects against injury to bile ducts by hydrophobic bile acids and stimulates the excretion of these and other hepatotoxic compounds as well as sulfated progesterone metabolites. The medication has been shown to reduce bile acid levels in colostrum, cord blood, and amniotic fluid. A meta-analysis[69] of randomized controlled trials indicated that ursodeoxycholic acid, when administered in doses between 450 and 1200 mg daily, was highly effective in controlling the pruritus and liver dysfunction associated with obstetric cholestasis.[70,76,77] Ursodeoxycholic acid may have a synergistic effect with S-adenosylmethionine.[76] Ursodeoxycholic acid has been safe for both mother and fetus, and may decrease the fetal mortality associated with obstetric cholestasis.[78] Compared to cholestyramine, ursodeoxycholic acid is safer, works faster, has a more sustained effect on pruritus, and shows higher efficacy in improving the biochemical abnormalities of obstetric cholestasis.[68] Data that are available support the use of ursodeoxycholic acid as a first-line agent and cholestyramine as a second-line agent in the treatment of moderate to severe obstetric cholestasis.

SUMMARY OF MANAGEMENT OPTIONS

Pruritus in Pregnancy

Management Options	Quality of Evidence	Strength of Recommendation	References
Establish the Diagnosis			
Consider:	–	GPP	–
• **Specific systemic diseases** with skin involvement (see previous sections)			
• **No eruption:** other systemic diseases with pruritus (lymphoma; liver, renal, thyroid disease)			
• **No eruption and jaundice:** hepatitides, obstetric cholestasis, hyperbilirubinemic states, and other liver diseases			
• **Eruption:** specific dermatoses of pregnancy (see following section), allergic reactions, drug eruptions, and urticarial lesions of hepatitis B			
• **No eruption/jaundice/systemic disease or dermatosis:** obstetric cholestasis, pruritus associated with striae gravidarum, and hyperemesis gravidarum complicated with cholestasis			
Management depends on cause—see below for Obstetric Cholestasis			
Obstetric Cholestasis			
Maternal Treatment			
• Symptomatic in mild cases	–	GPP	–
• First line: ursodeoxycholic acid	III	B	70
• Second line: cholestyramine and vitamin K	IIa	B	68,74
• Dexamethasone?	IIb	B	75
• UVB?	–	GPP	–

Continued

SUMMARY OF MANAGEMENT OPTIONS

Pruritus in Pregnancy *(Continued)*

Management Options	Quality of Evidence	Strength of Recommendation	References
Obstetric Cholestasis—*Continued*			
Management of Fetal Risks			
Institute fetal surveillance in last trimester (possibly from as late	III	B	101,102
as 34 weeks' gestation?).	IIa	B	103
Options for Overall Management	–	GPP	–
• Initiate fetal surveillance.			
• Perform elective delivery at 37–38 weeks.			
• Perform elective delivery at 36–37 weeks if fetal lung maturity and favorable cervix.			
• Consider maternal treatment with URSO.			
• Monitor LFTs and bile acids every 2–4 weeks.			

LFTs, liver function tests; URSO, ursodeoxycholic acid; UVB, ultraviolet light B.

SPECIFIC DERMATOSES OF PREGNANCY

Specific dermatoses of pregnancy are encountered predominantly during gestation or in the puerperium and include only those skin diseases that result directly from the state of gestation or the products of conception.[17] The classification of specific dermatoses of pregnancy into herpes gestationis, pruritic urticarial papules and plaques of pregnancy (PUPPP), prurigo gestationis, and pruritic folliculitis of pregnancy that was proposed by Holmes and Black[79] is now accepted by most authors.

Herpes (Pemphigoid) Gestationis

Risks and Management Options

Herpes gestationis is a rare autoimmune bullous disease of pregnancy and the puerperium. It has been rarely associated with choriocarcinoma and molar pregnancy.[80] The disease is more prevalent in white females, and its incidence is estimated between 1 in 10,000 and 1 in 50,000 pregnancies.[80] Herpes gestationis usually starts in the second or third trimester, with an average onset at 21 weeks' gestation, although initial onset in the immediate postpartum period occurs in about 20% of cases.[80,81] Herpes gestationis starts with severely pruritic urticarial abdominal lesions in half of the cases (Fig. 52–15*A*). The lesions do not spare the umbilicus. A generalized bullous eruption rapidly ensues (Fig. 52–15*B*), which may affect the palms and soles; facial and mucosal involvement is rare. Bullous lesions arise in both inflamed and clinically normal skin and, unless superinfected, heal without scarring.

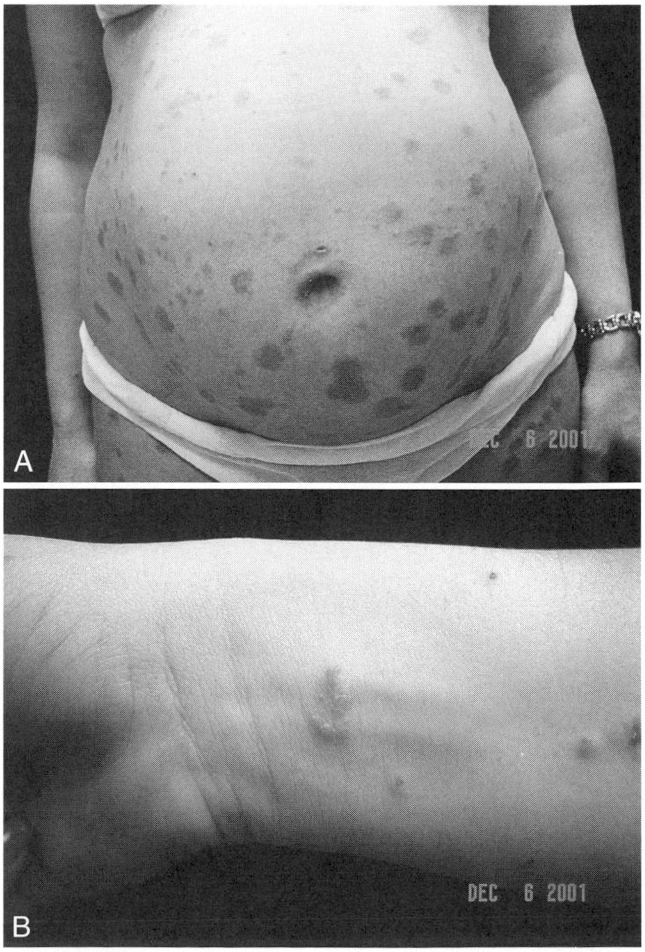

FIGURE 52–15
A, Pruritic abdominal urticarial lesions usually develop in the early phase of herpes gestationis. *B*, Characteristic tense vesicles on an erythematous base on the forearm in a patient with herpes gestationis (see Color Plate 56.). (Photographs courtesy of Jeffrey Callen, MD.)

A flare at the time of delivery, preceded by a period of quiescence in late pregnancy, is typically seen (75%).[80] The disease spontaneously resolves in the postpartum period, although a protracted course and "conversion" to bullous pemphigoid have been reported. Cases with overlapping features of herpes gestationis and bullous pemphigoid have been described. Herpes gestationis often recurs in subsequent pregnancies, usually appearing at an earlier gestational age and more severely. Nevertheless, skip pregnancies occur (8%).[81,82] The postpartum duration of herpes gestationis may increase with the number of involved pregnancies. Recurrence with menses or ovulation or subsequent use of oral contraceptives has been reported.[82] The effects of breast-feeding and prolactin on prolonging the duration of herpes gestationis deserve further clarification. The above data underscore the importance of hormonal factors in the pathogenesis of the disease.

Histopathology of early urticarial lesions shows a spongiotic epidermis, marked papillary dermal edema, and a mild perivascular infiltrate of lymphocytes, histiocytes, and characteristically many eosinophils. Focal necrosis of the basal keratinocytes leads to subepidermal blister formation. Direct immunofluorescence of perilesional skin shows linear C3 along the basement membrane zone.[1] In salt-split skin specimens, the antibody binds to the roof of the vesicle. Concomitant IgG deposition is detected in about 25% to 30% of patients. However, IgG is always positive when indirect complement-added immunofluorescence is used.[1] Deposition of IgG1 has been found in virtually all patients studied with monoclonal antibodies. Linear deposition of C3 and IgG1 has also been seen in the skin of neonates of affected mothers and in the basement membrane zone of amniotic epithelium.[80]

The antibody in herpes gestationis belongs to the IgG1 subclass and is believed to activate complement through the classical pathway. The major pathogenic antigen is the bullous pemphigoid 180 kd hemidesmosomal glycoprotein.[83] Reactivity against both the 180 kd and 240 kd bullous pemphigoid antigens is detected in 10% of cases—the reactivity against the 240 kd antigen is thought to develop later during the disease process as a secondary response to basal keratinocyte injury[80] *(epitope spreading)*. Serum antibody levels and eosinophilia do not correlate with the severity of disease. Antibody titers and immunofluorescence for C3 may remain positive even after clearance of the skin lesions or in subsequent disease-free pregnancies. The major antigenic epitopes (A1, A2, A.25, and A3)[84] are located in the noncollagenous domain (NC16A) of the transmembrane 180 kd antigen. Autoantibodies and autoimmune T lymphocytes from herpes gestationis patients recognize the NC16A2 (MCW-1) epitope[84]; these T cells express a Th1 cytokine profile. Several authors postulate that an immunologic insult occurs against class II placental antigens of paternal haplotype, and the antibody then cross-reacts with a maternal skin basement membrane epitope.[85]

The association of herpes gestationis with alleles of the human leukocyte antigens HLA-DR3 (61% to 80%), HLA-DR4 (52%), or both (43% to 50%)[86] and with the C4 null allele indicates that genetic factors may play an important role in the pathogenesis of the disease. Nonetheless, the finding of anti-HLA antibodies in all patients with herpes gestationis is considered an epiphenomenon in the disease process.[80] A change in partner has been occasionally associated with the onset of the disease,[82] and an increased prevalence of HLA-DR2 among husbands has been associated with herpes gestationis among their wives, particularly females positive for HLA-DR3/DR4. Yet, an association between change in consort and development of herpes gestationis has not been consistently found,[81] and skip pregnancies despite having the same partner[81,82] would argue against this association. The role of paternal factors is intriguing but not yet entirely understood.

The differential diagnosis of herpes gestationis includes drug eruptions, erythema multiforme, allergic contact dermatitis, PUPPP, and preexisting bullous disease with exacerbation during gestation, such as bullous pemphigoid. A careful history and clinical examination are usually sufficient to rule out allergic contact dermatitis, drug eruptions, and preexisting bullous disease with flare during pregnancy. Of note, bullous pemphigoid has not been reported during gestation, usually affects the elderly, and is equally common among males and females. The lesions in bullous pemphigoid are more prominent on the lower abdomen and thighs, and do not cluster around the umbilicus. Erythema multiforme can be differentiated by histopathologic and immunofluorescence studies. PUPPP is the most common specific dermatosis of pregnancy that needs to be differentiated from herpes gestationis. Interestingly, PUPPP can manifest with urticarial and/or vesicular lesions almost indistinguishable from those of herpes gestationis. The two diseases, however, can be distinguished by direct immunofluorescence, which is negative in PUPPP.

Herpes gestationis is associated with no maternal risks other than an increased risk of Graves' disease. Neonatal vesiculobullous lesions occur in 10% of cases[87] secondary to passive transplacental transfer of herpes gestationis antibody. The eruption is usually mild and resolves spontaneously in a few weeks as the maternal antibodies disappear from the infant's blood. Superinfection of bullous lesions warrants prompt treatment with systemic antibiotics. Monitoring for evidence of adrenal insufficiency is necessary for infants of mothers treated with oral steroids. Although an association with small for gestational age infants and preterm delivery has been reported,[88] no increase in fetal morbidity or mortality has been documented, with the exception of one case of fetal cerebral hemorrhage. The fetal complications may not be altered by the use of systemic steroids and are thought to be due to low-grade placental insufficiency.[80]

Early urticarial lesions may respond to topical steroids with or without an oral antihistamine, but most cases require oral steroids. Even though doses of prednisone up to 180 mg daily have been reported, most patients respond to lower doses (20 to 40 mg daily). The dose should be tapered 7 to 10 days after control is achieved. Most patients can be maintained on 5 to 10 mg of prednisone daily. The dosage should be increased at the time of delivery to control postpartum exacerbation. Plasmapheresis or chemical oophorectomy with goserelin have been used in recalcitrant herpes gestationis with some success.[80] Plasmapheresis can be considered for patients who do not respond to high doses of oral steroids or when oral steroids are contraindicated. High-dose intravenous immune globulin combined with cyclosporine has been used to treat herpes gestationis with some success.[89] Early delivery may be warranted in refractory cases. A case report indicated some benefit from minocycline in postpartum herpes gestationis. Intractable cases may respond to postpartum administration of cyclophosphamide, pyridoxine, gold, methotrexate, or dapsone.[1,80] Nevertheless, these agents have not been consistently effective, and their use is limited to patients who are not breastfeeding.

Pruritic Urticarial Papules and Plaques of Pregnancy

Risks and Management Options

Pruritic urticarial papules and plaques of pregnancy is the most common specific dermatosis of pregnancy, affecting between 1 in 130 and 1 in 300 gravidas.[79] The term *PUPPP* was coined by Lawley and colleagues,[90] who reported a specific pruritic urticarial eruption in 7 pregnant women. *Polymorphic eruption of pregnancy* is the term used in the British literature. PUPPP occurs predominantly in primigravidas in the third trimester, with a mean onset at 35 weeks' gestation, and occasionally postpartum.[79,91] Familial occurrence and recurrence in subsequent pregnancies, with menses, or with oral contraceptive use are uncommon. The lesions start in the abdominal striae in two thirds of the cases (Fig. 52–16*A*), and characteristically show periumbilical sparing.[1] The eruption is polymorphous, showing urticarial and at times vesicular, purpuric, polycyclic, or targetoid lesions[91] (Fig. 52–16*B*). Lesions can spread over the trunk and extremities, usually sparing the palms and soles. Involvement of the face is rare (G. Kroumpouzos, unpublished observation); dyshidrosis-like lesions on the extremities are unusual. When generalized, PUPPP may resemble a toxic erythema (Fig. 52–16*C*) or resolving atopic eczema. On resolution of PUPPP, extensive postinflammatory hyperpigmentation can be seen, especially in skin of color (see Fig. 52–7).

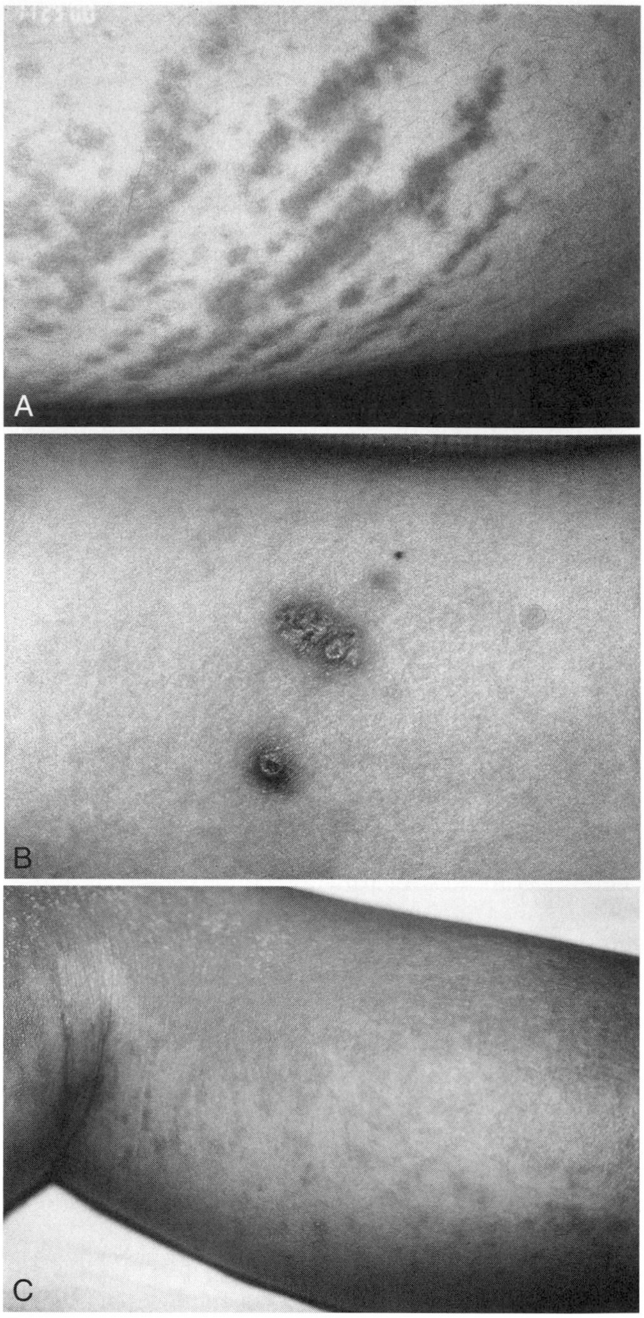

FIGURE 52–16
A, Early PUPPP showing typical urticarial lesions in the abdominal striae. *B*, Lesions with microvesiculated appearance on the forearm in PUPPP. *C*, Widespread PUPPP may resemble a toxic erythema (see Color Plate 57.). (Photograph courtesy of Helen Raynham, MD.)

Pruritic urticarial papules and plaques of pregnancy is a clinical diagnosis because it lacks pathognomonic histopathologic features and laboratory abnormalities. The histopathology shows spongiotic dermatitis, a perivascular or upper dermal inflammatory cell infiltrate with variable numbers of eosinophils, and occasionally mild epidermal changes such as parakeratosis, acanthosis, and exocytosis.[1] Results from immunofluorescence and serology studies are negative. Differentiation from the urticarial prebullous phase of herpes gestationis requires immunofluorescence studies (positive in herpes gestationis). Mild PUPPP requires symptomatic treatment with antipruritic topical medications, topical steroids, and oral antihistamines. Rarely, a short course of oral prednisone may be necessary. UVB can be effective.[79] The maternal and fetal prognosis is not affected. Early delivery in refractory cases is not indicated because there are no maternal or fetal risks.

The pathogenesis of PUPPP has not been fully clarified. The clinical presentation and immunohistologic profile suggest a delayed hypersensitivity reaction. No immunologic or hormonal abnormalities have been found, with the exception of a decrease in serum cortisol in one study.[17] A role for estrogen and/or progesterone has been suggested by clinical observations. It has been postulated that rapid abdominal wall distention in primigravidas may trigger an inflammatory process. This hypothesis was proposed by Cohen and colleagues,[92] who first reported an association with twin pregnancy and abnormal weight gains in the mother and fetus. Our recent meta-analysis[92] of 282 PUPPP cases revealed 29 multiple gestation pregnancies (11.7%). This prevalence is at least 10-fold higher than the prevalence of multiple gestation in the USA (1%). The association of PUPPP with multiple gestation is also supported by the recent study of Elling and colleagues.[93] Furthermore, multiple gestation is characterized by higher estrogen and progesterone levels, and progesterone has been shown to aggravate the inflammatory process at the tissue level. Interestingly, increased progesterone receptor immunoreactivity has been detected in skin lesions of PUPPP.[94]

Immunohistochemical studies[95] showed an infiltrate composed predominantly of T-helper lymphocytes. Activated T cells (HLA-DR+, CD25+, LFA-1+) were found in the dermis associated with increased numbers of CD1a+, CD54+ (ICAM+-1+) dendritic cells, and CD1a+ epidermal Langerhans cells in skin lesions, as compared to unaffected skin. This immunohistologic profile may imply a delayed hypersensitivity reaction to an unknown antigen. Fetal DNA was recently detected in skin lesions of PUPPP by Aractingi and colleagues.[96] The authors suggested that fetal cells can migrate to maternal skin and cause PUPPP because pregnancy is associated with peripheral blood chimerism, particularly during the third trimester. The importance of microchimerism in the pathogenesis of PUPPP awaits further clarification.

Prurigo Gestationis

Risks and Management Options

Prurigo gestationis affects between 1 in 300 and 1 in 450 pregnant females.[79] The condition usually begins at about 25 to 30 weeks' gestation and manifests itself with grouped excoriated or crusted pruritic papules over the extensor surfaces of the extremities (Fig. 52–17) and occasionally on the abdomen and elsewhere.[1] Prurigo gestationis commonly resolves in the immediate postpartum period but may occasionally persist for up to 3 months. On resolution of the lesions, postinflammatory hyperpigmentation develops. Recurrence in subsequent pregnancies has not been adequately studied. Serology may show an elevated IgE.[17] Results of immunofluorescence studies are negative; the histopathology is nonspecific. Although Spangler and colleagues[97] reported a dismal fetal outcome in their series, fetal or maternal risks have not been confirmed by any other studies. The differential diagnosis includes other specific dermatoses of pregnancy, pruritic dermatoses unrelated to pregnancy, drug eruptions, arthropod bites, and infestations such as scabies. The treatment is symptomatic with moderately potent topical steroids, if necessary intralesional or under occlusion, and oral antihistamines.[1]

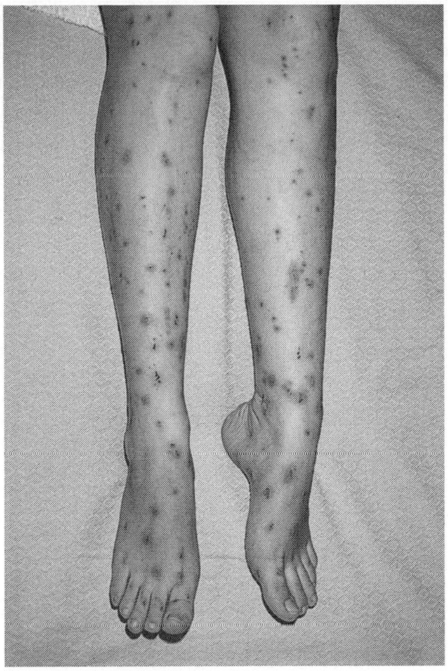

FIGURE 52–17
Prurigo gestationis: excoriated papules and nodules on the extensor surfaces of the extremities (see Color Plate 58.). (Photograph courtesy of Cameron Thomas, Campbell Kennedy, and Phillipa Kyle from second edition.)

Prurigo gestationis is the least studied of the specific dermatoses of pregnancy. Although its clinical presentation is indistinguishable from that of prurigo nodularis in nonpregnant women, a flare of prurigo nodularis during pregnancy has not been reported. Prurigo gestationis has been associated with a family history of obstetric cholestasis. Vaughan Jones and colleagues[17] postulated that prurigo gestationis and obstetric cholestasis are closely related conditions, being distinguished only by the absence of primary lesions in obstetric cholestasis. The authors reported an association with personal or family history of atopic dermatitis and elevation of serum IgE, and suggested that prurigo gestationis may be the result of obstetric cholestasis in women with an atopic predisposition. The strong association of prurigo nodularis in nonpregnant women with atopy and psychosomatic factors supports the hypothesis of Vaughan Jones and colleagues. Yet, the association with atopy was not confirmed by other studies. The role of atopy and psychosomatic factors in prurigo gestationis definitely warrants further study.

Pruritic Folliculitis of Pregnancy

Risks and Management Options

Pruritic folliculitis of pregnancy is a rare specific dermatosis of pregnancy first described by Zoberman and Farmer.[98] In 2 of the original 6 cases, pruritic folliculitis of pregnancy had occurred in previous pregnancies. Since the original description, 24 cases have been reported.[79] Decreased awareness of the condition and the fact that many cases may be misdiagnosed as infectious folliculitis or PUPPP may have contributed to an underestimate of its true prevalence. The lesions are pruritic follicular erythematous papules (Fig. 52–18*A*) and pustules (Fig. 52–18*B*) that predominate on the trunk.[99] The eruption develops during the second or third trimester and clears spontaneously at delivery or in the postpartum period. The histopathology is that of a sterile folliculitis. Results of immunofluorescence and serology tests are negative. The differential diagnosis includes infectious folliculitis and specific dermatoses of pregnancy. An infectious folliculitis can be ruled out with special stains and cultures from the pustules. The largest series[17] of pruritic folliculitis of pregnancy patients showed a decreased birth weight and a male-to-female ratio of 2:1. Preterm delivery was reported in one case. No other maternal or fetal risks have been documented.

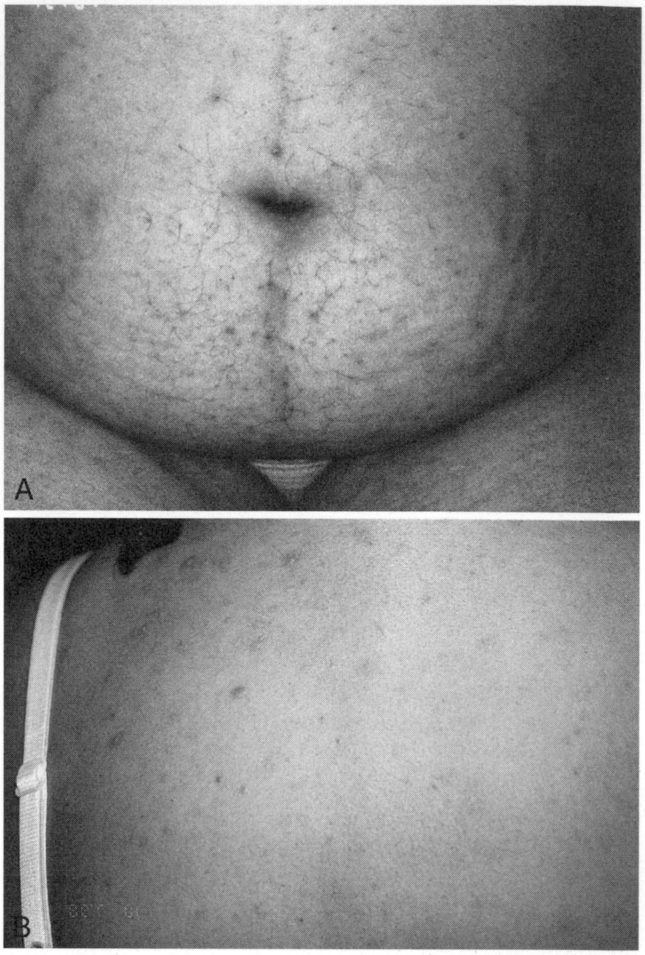

FIGURE 52–18
A, Pruritic folliculitis of pregnancy: typical follicular erythematous or pigmented papules on the abdomen. *B*, Follicular acneform pustules and papules on the upper back in pruritic folliculitis of pregnancy (see Color Plate 59).

The patient should be reassured that the eruption resolves after delivery and has not been associated with substantial fetal risks. Symptomatic pruritic folliculitis of pregnancy can be treated with low- or mid-potency topical steroids, benzoyl peroxide, and UVB therapy.[1] The pathogenesis of pruritic folliculitis of pregnancy has not been determined. No immunologic or hormonal abnormalities have been found. Associations with increased serum levels of androgens or obstetric cholestasis have been reported but were not confirmed in the majority of published cases. It has been suggested[79] that pruritic folliculitis of pregnancy may be a form of hormonally induced acne, similar to the monomorphic type of acne that develops after the administration of systemic steroids or progestogens. This intriguing hypothesis has not been supported by any data. Other authors[100] have considered pruritic folliculitis of pregnancy to be a variant of PUPPP. Although follicular lesions have been reported in PUPPP, the clinical presentation and histopathology of pruritic folliculitis of pregnancy differ from that of PUPPP. For the time being, pruritic folliculitis of pregnancy can be considered a specific dermatosis of pregnancy until further data about the condition becomes available.

SUMMARY OF MANAGEMENT OPTIONS
Rashes in Pregnancy

Management Options	Quality of Evidence	Strength of Recommendation	References
Establish the Cause—Two Possibilities:			
• Preexisting skin conditions	–	GPP	–
• Dermatoses of pregnancy	–	GPP	–
Herpes (Pemphigoid) Gestationis			
• Perform skin immunofluorescence to confirm the diagnosis.	IV	C	80
• Give topical steroids with or without an oral antihistamine (e.g., diphenhydramine) for early urticarial lesions.	IV	C	80
• Give oral steroids in most cases.	IV	C	80
• Perform plasmapheresis if oral steroids fail.	IV	C	80
• Cyclosporine with IVIG may be beneficial.	IV	C	89
• Immunosuppressants postpartum in non–breastfeeding mothers can be considered.	IV	C	80
• Maintain fetal surveillance (growth and health).	III	C	88
• Maintain vigilance for neonatal herpes gestations.	IV	C	87
PUPPP (Polymorphic Eruption of Pregnancy)			
• Perform skin biopsy if herpes gestation is a consideration.	III	B	91
• Reassure that there are no fetal risks.	III	B	91
• Prescribe topical steroids and/or antipruritic medications with or without an oral antihistamine.	III	B	91
• Give oral steroids in severe cases.	III	B	91
• UVB can be tried.	IV	C	90
Prurigo of Pregnancy			
• Reassure that there are no fetal risks.	IV	C	1
• Give topical steroids with or without an oral antihistamine.	IV	C	1
• Give oral steroids in severe cases.	–	GPP	–
Pruritic Folliculitis of Pregnancy			
• Perform cultures and special stains to rule out infectious folliculitides.	IV	C	1
• Reassure that there are no fetal risks.	–	GPP	–
• Topical benzoyl peroxide, low- or mid-potency topical steroids, and UVB can be tried.	IV	C	1

UVB, ultraviolet light B.

CONCLUSIONS

- **Physiologic skin changes of pregnancy:** no risks for the mother or fetus
- **Preexisting skin disorders:** more likely to worsen than improve during pregnancy
- **Melanoma:** prognosis not adversely affected by pregnancy
- **Impetigo herpetiformis:** form of pustular psoriasis associated with decreased calcium or vitamin D and serious maternal and fetal risks
- **Obstetric cholestasis:** check serum bile acids; ursodeoxycholic acid effective; fetal risks: distress, stillbirth, preterm delivery

CONCLUSIONS

- **Herpes gestationis:** flare at delivery; treatment with oral steroids; fetal risks: small for gestational age infants, preterm delivery, neonatal herpes gestationis
- **PUPPP:** starts in the abdominal striae and shows periumbilical sparing; associated with multiple gestation pregnancy; no maternal or fetal risks
- **Prurigo gestationis** and **pruritic folliculitis of pregnancy:** no maternal or fetal risks

REFERENCES

1. Kroumpouzos G, Cohen LM: Dermatoses of pregnancy. J Am Acad Dermatol 2001;45:1–19.
2. Winton GB, Lewis CW: Dermatoses of pregnancy. J Am Acad Dermatol 1982;6:977–998.
3. McKay M: Physiologic skin changes of pregnancy. In Black M, McKay M, Braude P, et al (eds): Obstetric and Gynecologic Dermatology, 2nd ed. London, Mosby, 2002, pp 17–22.
4. Kroumpouzos G, Avgerinou G: Acanthosis nigricans without diabetes during pregnancy (letter). Br J Dermatol 2002;146:925–928.
5. Rubin AI, Laborde SV, Stiller MJ:Aquired dermal melanocytosis: Appearance during pregnancy. J Am Acad Dermatol 2001;45: 609–613.
6. Garcia RL: Verrucose areolar hyperpigmentation of pregnancy (letter). Arch Dermatol 1973;107:774.
7. Schiller M, Kütting B, Luger T, Metze D: [Localized reticulate hyperpigmentation]. Hautarzt 1999;50:580–585.
8. Galasso F, Sbano E, Altamura V, Della Corte G: [Acanthosis nigricans in pregnancy]. G Ital Dermatol Venereol 1989;124: 511–515.
9. McKenzie AW: Skin disorders in pregnancy. Practitioner 1971;206:773–780.
10. Sanchez NP, Pathak MA, Sato S, et al: Melasma: A clinical, light microscopic, ultrastructural, and immunofluorescence study. J Am Acad Dermatol 1981;4:698–710.
11. Snell RS, Bischitz PG: The effects of large doses of estrogen and progesterone on melanin pigmentation. J Invest Dermatol 1960; 35:73–82.
12. Kligman AM, Willis I: A new formula for depigmenting human skin. Arch Dermatol 1975;111:40–48.
13. Angsuwarangsee S, Polnikorn N. Combined ultrapulse CO2 laser and Q-switched alexandrite laser compared with Q-switched alexandrite laser alone for refractory melasma: Split-face design. Dermatol Surg 2003;29:59–64.
14. Tse Y, Levine VJ, McClain SA, Ashinoff R: The removal of cutaneous pigmented lesions with the Q-switched ruby laser and the Q-switched neodymium:yttritium-aluminum-garnet laser. A comparative study. J Dermatol Surg Oncol 1994; 20:795–800.
15. Lee GY, Kim HJ, Whang KK: The effect of combination treatment of the recalcitrant pigmentary disorders with pigmented laser and chemical peeling. Dermatol Surg 2002; 28:1120–1123.
16. Winton GB: Skin diseases aggravated by pregnancy. J Am Acad Dermatol 1989;20:1–13.
17. Vaughan Jones SA, Hern S, Nelson-Piercy C, et al: A prospective study of 200 women with dermatoses of pregnancy correlating the clinical findings with hormonal and immunopathological profiles. Br J Dermatol 1999;141:71–81.
18. Schafer T, Dirschedl P, Kunz B: Maternal smoking during pregnancy and lactation increases the risk for atopic eczema in the offspring. J Am Acad Dermatol 1997;36:550–556.
19. Hale EK, Pomeranz MK: Dermatologic agents during pregnancy and lactation: An update and clinical review. Int J Dermatol 2002;41:197–203.
20. Boyd AS, Morris LF, Phillips CM, Menter MA: Psoriasis and pregnancy: Hormone and immune system interaction. Int J Dermatol 1996;35:169–172.
21. McHugh NJ, Laurent MR: The effect of pregnancy on the onset of psoriatic arthritis. Br J Rheumatol 1989;28:50–52.
22. Tauscher AE, Fleischer AB Jr, Phelps KC, Feldman SR: Psoriasis and pregnancy. J Cutan Med Surg 2002;6:561–570.
23. Bajaj AK, Swarup V, Gupta OP, Gupta SC: Impetigo herpetiformis. Dermatologica 1977;155:292–295.
24. Ott F, Krakowski A, Tur E, et al: Impetigo herpetiformis with lowered serum level of vitamin D and its diminished intestinal absorption. Dermatologica 1982;164:360–365.
25. Oumeish OY, Farraj SE, Bataineh AS: Some aspects of impetigo herpetiformis. Arch Dermatol 1982;118:103–105.
26. Kuijpers ALA, Schalkwijk J, Rulo HFC, et al: Extremely low levels of epidermal skin derived antileucoproteinase/elafin in a patient with impetigo herpetiformis. Br J Dermatol 1997;137: 123–129.
27. Rackett SC, Baughman RD: Impetigo herpetiformis and *Staphylococcus aureus* lymphadenitis in a pregnant adolescent. Pediatr Dermatol 1997;14:387–390.
28. Finch TM, Tan CY: Pustular psoriasis exacerbated by pregnancy and controlled by cyclosporin A (letter). Br J Dermatol 2000; 142:582–584.
29. Gimenez-Garcia R, Gimenez Garcia MC, Llorente de la Fuente A: Impetigo herpetiformis: Response to steroids and etretinate. Int J Dermatol 1989;28:551–552.
30. Breier-Maly J, Ortel B, Breier F, et al: Generalized pustular psoriasis of pregnancy (Impetigo herpetiformis). Dermatol 1999; 198:61–64.
31. Beveridge GW, Harkness RA, Livingston JRB: Impetigo herpetiformis in two successive pregnancies. Br J Dermatol 1966;78:106–112.
32. Spence MR: Genital infections in pregnancy. Med Clin North Am 1977;61:139–151.
33. Hopsu-Havu VK, Grönroos M, Punnonen R: Vaginal yeasts in parturients and infestation of the newborns. Acta Obstet Gynecol Scand 1980;59:73–77.
34. Sobel JD: Epidemiology and pathogenesis of recurrent vulvovaginal candidiasis. Am J Obstet Gynecol 1985;152:924–935.
35. Gravett MG, Hummel D, Eschenbach DA, Holmes KK: Preterm labor associated with subclinical amniotic fluid infection and with bacterial vaginosis. Obstet Gynecol 1986; 67:229–237.
36. Cotch MF, Pastorek JG II, Nugent RP, et al: Demographic and behavioral predictors of *Trichomonas vaginalis* infection among pregnant women. Obstet Gynecol 1991;78:1087–1092.
37. Cotch MF, Pastorek JG II, Nugent RP, et al: *Trichomonas vaginalis* associated with low birth weight and preterm delivery. The vaginal infections and prematurity study group. Sex Transm Dis 1997;24:353–360.
38. Association of *Chlamydia trachomatis* and *Mycoplasma hominis* with intrauterine growth retardation and preterm delivery. The Johns Hopkins study of cervicitis and adverse pregnancy outcome. Am J Epidemiol 1989;129:1247–1257.

39. Heymann WR, Wolf DJ: *Malassezia (pityrosporum)* folliculitis occurring during pregnancy. Int J Dermatol 1986;25:49–51.
40. Lockwood DN, Sinha HH: Pregnancy and leprosy: A comprehensive literature review. Int J Lep Mycobact Dis 1999;67:6–12.
41. Ulrich M, Zulueta AM, Caceres-Dittmat G, et al: Leprosy in women: Characteristics and repercussions. Soc Sci Med 1993; 37:445–456.
42. Duncan ME, Pearson JMH, Ridley DS, et al: Pregnancy and leprosy: The consequences of alterations of cell-mediated and humoral immunity during pregnancy and lactation. Int J Lepr 1982;50:425–435.
43. Duncan ME, Pearson JMH: The association of pregnancy and leprosy. III. Erythema nodosum leprosum in pregnancy and lactation. Lepr Rev 1984;55:129–142.
44. Duncan ME, Pearson JMH: Neuritis in pregnancy and lactation. Int J Lepr Mycobact Dis 1982;50:31–38.
45. Lockshin MD: Pregnancy does not cause systemic lupus erythematosus to worsen. Arthritis Rheum 1989;32:665–670.
46. Petri M, Howard D, Repke J: Frequency of lupus flares in pregnancy. Arthritis Rheum 1991;34:1538–1545.
47. Ruiz-Irastorza G, Lima F, Alves J, et al: Increased rate of lupus flare during pregnancy and the puerperium: A prospective study of 78 pregnancies. Br J Rheumatol 1996;35:133–138.
48. Khamashta MA, Ruiz-Irastorza G, Hughes GRV: Systemic lupus flares during pregnancy. Rheum Dis Clin North Am 1997;23: 15–30.
49. Frances C, Piette JC: Cutaneous manifestations of Hughes syndrome occurring in the context of lupus erythematosus. Lupus 1997;6:139–144.
50. Tseng C-E, Buyon JP: Neonatal lupus syndromes. Rheum Dis Clin North Am 1997;23:31–54.
51. Gutierrez G, Dagnino R, Mintz G: Polymyositis/dermatomyositis and pregnancy. Arthritis Rheum 1984;27:291–294.
52. Steen VD: Scleroderma and pregnancy. Rheum Dis Clin North Am 1997;23:133–147.
53. Daniel Y, Shenhav M, Botchan A, et al: Pregnancy associated with pemphigus. BJOG 1995;102:667–669.
54. Collier PM, Kelly SE, Wojnarowska FW: Linear IgA disease and pregnancy. J Am Acad Dermatol 1994;30:407–411.
55. Loret de Mola JR, Muise KL, Duchon MA: Porphyria cutanea tarda and pregnancy. Obstet Gynecol Surv 1996;15:493–497.
56. Moore MR: Porphyria—A Patient's Guide (web publication). The Porphyria Charitable Trust, Porphyria Research Unit, The University of Queensland, Brisbane, Australia, 1996.
57. Bronson DM, Barsky R, Barsky S: Acrodermatitis enteropathica: Recognition at long last during a recurrence in pregnancy. J Am Acad Dermatol 1983;9:140–144.
58. Rudd NL, Nimrod C, Holbrook KA, et al: Pregnancy complications in type IV Ehlers-Danlos syndrome. Lancet 1983;I:50–53.
59. Berde C, Willis DC, Sandberg EC: Pregnancy in women with pseudoxanthoma elasticum. Obstet Gynecol Surv 1983;38: 339–344.
60. Swapp GH: Neurofibromatosis in pregnancy. Br J Dermatol 1973;80:431–435.
61. Slingluff CL Jr, Reintgen DS, Vollmer RT, Seigler HF: Malignant melanoma arising during pregnancy. A study of 100 patients. Ann Surg 1990;211:552–557.
62. Mackie RM, Bufalino R, Morabito A, et al: Lack of effect of pregnancy on outcome of melanoma. For the World Health Organization Melanoma Programme. Lancet 1991;337:653–655.
63. Travers RL, Sober AJ, Berwick M, et al: Increased thickness of pregnancy-associated melanoma. Br J Dermatol 1995;132: 876–883.
64. Grin CM, Driscoll MS, Grant-Kels JM: The relationship of pregnancy, hormones and melanoma. Semin Cutan Med Surg 1998;17:167–171.
65. Daryanani D, Plukker JT, De Hullu JA, et al: Pregnancy and early-stage melanoma. Cancer 2003;97:2248–2253.
66. Schwartz JL, Mozurkewich EL, Johnson TM: Current management of patients with melanoma who are pregnant, want to get pregnant, or do not want to get pregnant (editorial). Cancer 2003;97:2130–2133.
67. Mackie RM: Pregnancy and exogenous female sex hormones in melanoma patients. In Balch CM, Houghton AN, Sober AJ, Soong S-J (eds): Cutaneous Melanoma, 3rd ed. St Louis, Mo., QMP Publishing, 1998, pp. 187–193.
68. Kroumpouzos G: Intrahepatic cholestasis of pregnancy: What's new (editorial). J Eur Acad Dermatol Venereol 2002;16:316–318.
69. Kroumpouzos G, Cohen LM: Specific dermatoses of pregnancy: An evidence-based systematic review. Am J Obstet Gynecol 2003;188:1083–1092.
70. Laifer SA, Stiller RJ, Siddiqui DS, et al: Ursodeoxycholic acid for the treatment of intrahepatic cholestasis of pregnancy. J Matern Fetal Med 2001;10:131–135.
71. Peng B, Liu S: [Study of relationship between T helper cell type-1 and type-2 cytokines and intrahepatic cholestasis of pregnancy]. Chung-Hua Fu Chan Ko Tsa Chih. Chin J Obstet Gynecol 2002; 37:516–518.
72. Dixon PH, Weerasekera N, Linton KJ, et al: Heterozygous MDR3 missense mutation associated with intrahepatic cholestasis of pregnancy: Evidence for a defect in protein trafficking. Hum Mol Genet 2000;9:1209–1217.
73. Ribalta J, Reyes H, Gonzales M, et al: S-adenosyl-L-methionine in the treatment of patients with intrahepatic cholestasis of pregnancy: A randomized, double-blind, placebo-controlled study with negative results. Hepatol 1991;13:1084–1089.
74. Laatikainen T: Effect of cholestyramine and phenobarbital on pruritus and serum bile acid levels in cholestasis of pregnancy. Am J Obstet Gynecol 1978;132:501–506.
75. Hirvioja M-L, Tuimala R: The treatment of intrahepatic cholestasis of pregnancy by dexamethasone. BJOG 1992;99:109–111.
76. Nicastri PL, Diaferia A, Tartagni M, et al: A randomized placebo-controlled trial of ursodeoxycholic acid and S-adenosylmethionine in the treatment of intrahepatic cholestasis of pregnancy. BJOG 1998;105:1205–1207.
77. Palma J, Reyes H, Ribalta J, et al: Ursodeoxycholic acid in the treatment of cholestasis of pregnancy: A randomized, double-blind study controlled with placebo. J Hepatol 1997;27:1022–1028.
78. Davies MH, da Silva RCMA, Jones SR, et al: Fetal mortality associated with cholestasis of pregnancy and the potential benefit of therapy with ursodeoxycholic acid. Gut 1995;37: 580–584.
79. Holmes RC, Black MM: The specific dermatoses of pregnancy. J Am Acad Dermatol 1983;8:405–412.
80. Engineer L, Bhol K, Ahmed AR: Pemphigoid gestationis: A review. Am J Obstet Gynecol 2000;183:483–491.
81. Jenkins RE, Hern S, Black MM:. Clinical features and management of 87 patients with pemphigoid gestationis. Clin Exp Dermatol 1999;24:255–259.
82. Holmes RC, Black MM, Jurecka W, et al: Clues to the etiology and pathogenesis of herpes gestationis. Br J Dermatol 1983;109: 131–139.
83. Morrison LH, Labib RS, Zone JJ, et al: Herpes gestationis autoantibodies recognize a 180-kd human epidermal antigen. J Clin Invest 1988;81:2023–2026.
84. Lin M-S, Gharia M, Fu C-L, et al: Molecular mapping of the major epitopes of BP180 recognized by herpes gestationis autoantibodies. Clin Immunol 1999;92:285–292.
85. Kelly SE, Black MM: Pemphigoid gestationis: Placental interactions. Semin Dermatol 1989;8:12–17.
86. Shornick JK, Stastny P, Gilliam JN: High frequency of histocompatibility antigens HLA-DR3 and DR4 in herpes gestationis. J Clin Invest 1981;68:553–555.
87. Karna P, Broecker AH: Neonatal herpes gestationis. J Pediatr 1991;119:299–301.
88. Shornick JK, Black MM: Fetal risks in herpes gestationis. J Am Acad Dermatol 1992;26:63–68.

89. Hern S, Harman K, Bhogal BS, Black MM: A severe persistent case of pemphigoid gestationis treated with intravenous immunoglobulins and cyclosporine. Clin Exp Dermatol 1998; 23:185–188.
90. Lawley TJ, Hertz KC, Wade TR, et al: Pruritic urticarial papules and plaques of pregnancy. JAMA 1979;241:1696–1699.
91. Aronson IK, Bond S, Fiedler VC, et al: Pruritic urticarial papules and plaques of pregnancy: Clinical and immunopathologic observations in 57 patients. J Am Acad Dermatol 1998;39:933–939.
92. Cohen LM, Capeless EL, Krusinski PA, Maloney ME: Pruritic urticarial papules and plaques of pregnancy and its relationship to maternal-fetal weight gain and twin pregnancy. Arch Dermatol 1989;125:1534–1536.
93. Elling SV, McKenna P, Powell FC: Pruritic urticarial papules and plaques of pregnancy in twin and triplet pregnancies. J Eur Acad Dermatol Venereol 2000;14:378–381.
94. Im S, Lee E-S, Kim W, et al: Expression of progesterone receptor in human keratinocytes. J Korean Med Sci 2000;15: 647–654.
95. Carli P, Tarocchi S, Mello G, Fabbri P: Skin immune system activation in pruritic urticarial papules and plaques of pregnancy. Int J Dermatol 1994;33:884–885.
96. Aractingi S, Bertheau P, Le Goue C, et al: Fetal DNA in skin of polymorphic eruptions of pregnancy. Lancet 1998;352: 1898–1901.
97. Spangler AS, Reddy W, Bardawil WA, et al: Papular dermatitis of pregnancy. A new clinical entity? JAMA 1962;181:577–581.
98. Zoberman E, Farmer ER: Pruritic folliculitis of pregnancy. Arch Dermatol 1981;117:20–22.
99. Kroumpouzos G, Cohen LM: Pruritic folliculitis of pregnancy. J Am Acad Dermatol 2000;43:132–134.
100. Roger D, Vaillant L, Fignon A, et al: Specific pruritic dermatoses of pregnancy. A prospective study of 3192 women. Arch Dermatol 1994;130:734–739.
101. Mahon E, de Ruiter A, Lockwood D: Infectious diseases in pregnancy. In Black M, McKay M, Braude P, et al (eds): Obstetric and Gynecologic Dermatology, 2nd ed. London, Mosby, 2002, pp 80–81.
102. Alsulyman OM, Ouzounian JG, Ames-Castro M, Goodwin TM: Intrahepatic cholestasis of pregnancy: Perinatal outcome associated with expectant management. Am J Obstet Gynecol 1996; 175:957–960.
103. Fisk NM, Storey GNB: Fetal outcome in obstetric cholestasis. BJOG 1988;95:1137–1143.
104. Rioseco AJ, Ivankovic MB, Manzur A, et al: Intrahepatic cholestasis of pregnancy: A respective case control study of perinatal outcome. Am J Obstet Gynecol 1994; 170:890–895.

CHAPTER 53

Malignant Disease

Adnan R. Munkarah / Robert T. Morris / Veronica L. Schimp

INTRODUCTION

Cancer is the second leading cause of death in women of reproductive age, and fortunately, a rare cause of maternal mortality.[1,2] Between birth and 39 years of age, 1 in 52 females has invasive cancer, and approximately 3500 women between the ages of 15 and 34 years die annually of cancer in the United States.[2] It is estimated between 1 in 1000 and 1 in 1500 women will be affected by cancer while pregnant each year. The predominant malignancies associated with pregnancy are cervical cancer, breast cancer, melanoma (see Chapter 52), hematologic cancer (See Chapter 50), thyroid cancer (see Chapter 46), and colorectal cancer (Table 53–1).[3] No convincing data show that pregnancy adversely influences the biology, natural history, prognosis, or treatment of maternal cancer.[4,5]

The evaluation and treatment of pregnant women with cancer is similar to that of nonpregnant women, with a few exceptions, and both maternal and fetal outcomes should be considered when planning therapy during pregnancy. One major dilemma encountered in the treatment of pregnant women with cancer is the timing of therapeutic intervention with regard to fetal growth, development, and viability. For most malignancies, the presence of the cancer does not adversely affect the fetus; the major risk to fetal survival and normal development is the toxic effect of the various treatment modalities. Conversely, continuation of pregnancy has not been associated with accelerated tumor growth for most malignancies; therefore, elective abortion offers no therapeutic advantage to the mother. Intuitively, however, any cancer left untreated is being given an optimal opportunity to grow and metastasize. It is a therapeutic challenge for the medical team to weigh the need for immediate intervention for maternal indications against the need to delay therapy for fetal indications.

RADIATION

Radiation therapy is an effective treatment modality for a variety of cancers encountered during pregnancy. In addition, many diagnostic procedures, such as regular x-rays, radioisotope scans, and computed tomography, used in the pretreatment evaluation of malignancies are associated with radiation exposure to the mother and potentially to the fetus (Table 53–2).[6] The effects of radiation on tissues are the result of multiple cellular events that include mitotic delay, cytogenetic abnormalities, and mutagenesis and apoptotic cell death.

The effects of radiation on the fetus depend on the dose of radiation delivered as well as the stage of gestation during which exposure occurred. The dose to the embryo or fetus depends on several factors. These include the teletherapy machine used and its leakage, the target dose, the size of the radiation fields, the distance from the edge of the field to the embryo or fetus, and the use of wedges, lead blocks, compensators, and other scattering objects. Factors that decrease the radiation dose to the embryo or fetus include less leakage, a lower target dose, smaller irradiation fields, greater distance between the edges of the radiation fields and the embryo or fetus, and avoidance of wedges and other scattering objects. A distance of more than 30 cm between the edges of the radiation fields and the embryo or fetus yields a fetal exposure of only 4 to 20 cGy. Lead shielding can further reduce exposure.[7]

Before implantation, the embryo is a multicellular organism that is mostly sensitive to the lethal effects of radiation.[8,9] Exposure to high-energy radiation at that stage may induce cytogenetic abnormalities that will result in an abortion.[10–12]

The teratogenic effects of radiation are a significant risk if the fetus is exposed during organogenesis, which usually lasts for 10 days to 7 weeks after conception. The congenital malformations that are most frequently described with exposure to high-dose radiation involve the central nervous system, skeleton, and genitals. Microcephaly is the most common malformation reported.[13] Other malformations include eye abnormalities, such as microphthalmia, retinal changes, and cataracts. Growth retardation and abortion can also occur during this period.

TABLE 53-1

Incidence of Cancer in Pregnancy

SITE OR TYPE	ESTIMATED INCIDENCE PER 1000 PREGNANCIES
Cervix uteri	
Noninvasive	1.3
Invasive	1.0
Breast cancer	0.33
Melanoma	0.14
Ovary	0.10
Thyroid	Unknown
Leukemia	0.01
Lymphoma	0.01
Colorectal	0.02

From Allen H, Nisker J (eds): Cancer in Pregnancy: Therapeutic Guidelines. New York, Futura, 1986.

Later in gestation, except for the central nervous system, the fetal organs become more resistant to the teratogenic effects of radiation. Exposure to high-dose radiation at that stage mainly results in growth retardation and neurophysiologic and behavioral changes that may become obvious in infancy or childhood. Data show that central nervous system malformations and growth retardation have occurred after acute exposure to more than 50 rad.[13] Fetal exposure to less than 5 rad has not been associated with such effects. In utero exposure to radiation may result in an increased risk of leukemia in childhood.[13–16] This effect, however, is the subject of debate among investigators. Ample evidence shows that radiation therapy delivered to the abdomen and pelvis results in fetal exposure to dangerous radiation doses.

TABLE 53-2

Estimated Average Fetal Dose

ROENTGENOGRAM OF MOTHER	DOSE TO FETUS (RAD)
Barium enema	0.800
Upper gastrointestinal series	0.560
Intravenous pyelogram	0.400
Hip	0.300
Abdomen	0.290
Lumbar spine	0.275
Cholecystography	0.200
Pelvis	0.040
Chest	0.008
Skull	0.004
Cervical spine	0.002
Shoulder	0.001
Extremity (upper or lower)	0.001
Computed tomography scan of the abdomen and pelvis	3.000

From Deppe G, Munkarah A, Malone JM Jr: Neoplasia. In Gleicher N (ed): Principles and Practice of Medical Therapy in Pregnancy, 2nd ed. Norwalk, Conn, Appleton & Lange, 1998, pp 1231–1234.

CHEMOTHERAPY

Chemotherapy is an essential part of the treatment of many malignancies that can occur during pregnancy, such as breast and ovarian cancers, lymphomas, and leukemias.[17–22] Before the initiation of treatment with an antineoplastic agent in a pregnant woman, the potential benefits to the mother should be weighed against the potential risks to the mother and fetus. When cure is a realistic goal, appropriate treatment should be initiated as needed, without modifications that may adversely affect maternal outcome.

The physiologic changes that accompany pregnancy may alter the pharmacokinetics of various drugs, including many chemotherapeutic agents.[23] For water-soluble drugs, the increase in plasma volume and decrease in albumin concentration may lead to a decreased concentration of the drug after bolus administration; however, its half-life will be longer. On the other hand, an increase in the activity of the hepatic oxidases and an increase in glomerular filtration may lead to an increase in the hepatic or renal clearance of some agents. Like other substances, the transfer of antineoplastic agents to the fetus through the placenta is controlled by the molecular weight, lipid solubility, and protein binding of the agents. For example, the highly protein-bound nature of vinca alkaloids makes transplacental passage to the fetus inefficient.

The timing of fetal exposure to the chemotherapeutic agents is one of the most important determinants of pregnancy outcome. In the first trimester, exposure to chemotherapy can result in congenital malformations or abortion.[22–24] The risk of congenital malformations has been reported to be as high as 17%. The folic acid antagonists aminopterin and methotrexate, when used in the first trimester, seem to be more teratogenic than other antineoplastic agents. Syndromes of congenital anomalies that include cranial anomalies, cleft palate, anencephaly, and micrognathia have been associated with the use of aminopterin. Similarly, the use of methotrexate has led to skull abnormalities known as cloverleaf skull, or oxycephaly.[25–30] First-trimester use of alkylating agents and procarbazine is also associated with an increased risk of fetal malformations.[31]

Second- and third-trimester exposure to chemotherapy does not seem to result in an increased risk of congenital malformations. This exposure has been associated with low birth weight, intrauterine growth retardation, spontaneous abortion, premature birth, microcephaly, and mental retardation and impaired learning behavior.

Myelosuppression is a side effect common to many chemotherapeutic agents. Maternal thrombocytopenia or leukopenia at the time of the delivery can result in significant complications, including massive hemorrhage and serious infections. Therefore, the timing of delivery should be well planned in a woman who is receiving chemotherapy.

SUMMARY OF MANAGEMENT OPTIONS
Cancer Treatment

Management Options	Quality of Evidence	Strength of Recommendation	References
Radiation			
Fetal exposure from imaging doses are given in Table 53-2	III	B	6
Lead screening reduces embryo/fetal exposure and risk	III	B	7
Main risk to early embryo is miscarriage	III	B	10–12
Main risks between 10d and 7w is teratogenesis (? only if >50 rads)	III	B	13
After embryogenesis main risks are	III	B	13–16
growth restriction			
impaired neurobehavioral development (? only if >50 rads)			
Chemotherapy			
Physiological changes of pregnancy may alter the pharmacokinetics of chemotherapeutic agents	III	B	23
In first trimester the main risks are	III	B	22–30
miscarriage			
fetal abnormality (?17%) especially with the folate antagonists			
In second and third trimester the main risks are	III	B	29
growth restriction			
preterm delivery			
impaired neurobehavioral development			

CERVICAL CANCER

Cervical cancer is the most common malignancy diagnosed in pregnancy, with a frequency of 1.6 to 10.6 cases per 10,000 pregnancies.[32] The wide variability in the incidence reported in the literature seems to be caused by the inclusion of patients with postpartum cancer and carcinoma in situ. It is estimated that between 1% and 3% of patients with cervical cancer are pregnant at the time of diagnosis.[33] The mean age of pregnant patients at the time of diagnosis of cervical cancer is 31.6 years (range, 31–36.5 years).[34] As in nonpregnant patients, the most common histologic type is squamous cell carcinoma, which accounts for more than 80% of all cervical cancers.[35] More than 70% of patients have early-stage disease, which includes FIGO (International Federation of Gynecology and Obstetrics) stage I and IIA lesions.[35–38] Diagnosis may be made at an earlier stage in pregnancy because pregnant women are seen frequently by health care providers and undergo routine examinations and Papanicolaou (Pap) smears. One third of pregnant patients who are diagnosed with cervical cancer are asymptomatic, with diagnosis made at the time of an abnormal Pap smear result.

The interpretation of Pap smears obtained during pregnancy can be problematic, because several common physiologic changes associated with the gravid state can lead to false-positive results. For example, eversion of the transformation zone and exposure of columnar cells to the acid pH of the vagina cause squamous metaplasia that may be falsely interpreted as dysplasia. The Arias-Stella reaction can resemble an adenocarcinoma.[39,40] In one study of gravid hysterectomy specimens, Arias-Stella reaction was reported in 9% of specimens examined.[41] Another false-positive cause of low-grade dysplasia on Pap smear is retrieval of trophoblastic cells. It is essential to inform the cytopathologist interpreting the Pap smear that the patient is pregnant.

Historically, it was believed that pregnancy had an adverse effect on the natural history of cervical cancer. Recent studies, however, showed no difference in survival between pregnant and nonpregnant women with cervical cancer when matched by age, stage, and year of diagnosis.[33–35,38,39,42–44] In addition, several studies show that, contrary to a common misconception, the mode of delivery does not seem to affect outcome.[32,44,45]

Management Options

Colposcopy is a safe and reliable method for evaluating pregnant patients with abnormal cervical cytologic findings.[46–50] Colposcopy-directed biopsy can be performed during any trimester, although most colposcopists suggest delaying biopsy until the second trimester. The main complication associated with cervical biopsy during pregnancy is bleeding; however, this usually can be controlled with the application of Monsel's solution and pressure. Endocervical biopsy must be avoided during pregnancy because of the risk of premature rupture of the membranes, preterm labor, and uncontrollable bleeding.[51]

During pregnancy, diagnostic cervical conization is reserved for selected indications that include the finding of minimal stromal invasion on a colposcopically directed biopsy and persistent cytologic suggestion of invasive carcinoma on Pap smear.[52,53] Fortunately, eversion of the squamocolumnar junction during pregnancy improves access to the endocervix and decreases the necessary volume of tissue to be removed. The risks of immediate and delayed bleeding after conization are 8.9% and 3.7%, respectively.[43] Other infrequent complications include premature labor, chorioamnionitis, and fetal loss.

Pregnant women who are diagnosed with invasive cervical cancer should be counseled extensively about treatment options as well as the effect of the treatment on the mother and fetus. Many factors should be considered in treatment planning, including gestational age, tumor size and stage, and the patient's desire to preserve the pregnancy. Few recent studies have evaluated the effect of delaying definitive therapy until fetal maturity is reached.[36–38,45,54–56] In these reports, treatment delays ranged from 53 to 212 days and did not result in decreased maternal survival. However, the number of patients in these series is too small to allow definite conclusions to be drawn. Treatment delay seems to be a reasonable option in a patient who is more than 20 weeks' pregnant when diagnosed with early-stage disease (FIGO IA1–IB1). In patients who elect to continue with the pregnancy and delay treatment, cervical cancer does not seem to adversely affect the fetus; the incidence of intrauterine growth restriction and stillbirth is not increased in these cases.[42] Repeat examination every 6 to 8 weeks (including colposcopy) is recommended until surgery. For patients with more advanced disease, such as International Federation of Gynecology and Obstetrics (FIGO) stages IB2 and IIA, early treatment is suggested.[33,57]

The choice of treatment modality for pregnant patients with cervical cancer is based on the same principles that are used in the nonpregnant state. Patients with early-stage disease can be treated surgically with radical hysterectomy and bilateral pelvic lymphadenectomy.[54,55,58,59] Depending on the time of diagnosis, surgery can be done early in gestation, with termination of the pregnancy, or at cesarean delivery. Except for increased blood loss, there is no significant increase in other perioperative complications compared with nonpregnant patients, and the cure rates are comparable.[55]

Radiation therapy is used to treat advanced disease that is not amenable to surgical management. When radiation is administered in the first trimester, spontaneous abortion usually occurs at a cumulative dose of 30 to 50 Gy. Treatment in the second trimester results in abortion at a higher cumulative dose and less reliably. If abortion did not occur by the end of the external radiation therapy, surgical evacuation can be performed before brachytherapy.[60] For patients who are treated after delivery, most radiotherapists wait a few weeks for the uterus to involute before starting treatment.

Tumor stage is an important predictor of survival in cervical cancer. The outcome of patients with early-stage disease is excellent, with 5-year survival rates exceeding 90%.[35] However, in a recent report, the survival rate was worse in women who were diagnosed postpartum than in those diagnosed during pregnancy, and women diagnosed postpartum were at significant risk for recurrent disease, particularly if delivery was vaginal.[45] One site of tumor recurrence when cervical cancer occurs in pregnancy is in the episiotomy site.[61–63] It is believed that tumor cells can implant at the site of episiotomy incision after vaginal delivery. Treatment usually includes local excision and radiation.

SUMMARY OF MANAGEMENT OPTIONS
Cervical Cancer

Management Options	Quality of Evidence	Strength of Recommendation	References
Diagnosis			
Physical examination and cervical smear at first prenatal visit in high risk and those without smear in previous 3 years	III	B	46–50
Colposcopy and directed biopsies for suspicious lesions though measures needed to deal with increased bleeding risk	III	B	43,51
Cone biopsy when microinvasion suspected on directed biopsies; loop excision may be associated with increased preterm births	III	B	52,53

SUMMARY OF MANAGEMENT OPTIONS
Cervical Cancer *(Continued)*

Management Options	Quality of Evidence	Strength of Recommendation	References
Treatment			
Cervical Intraepithelial Neoplasia:			
follow-up with colposcopy during pregnancy	III	B	51
Micro-Invasive Cancer:			
after careful maternal counseling consider delaying definitive therapy until fetal maturity reached (enhance with steroids) and delivery completed	III	B	36–38
Invasive Cancer:			
Use same therapy guidelines as for non-pregnant patient:			
before 20 weeks: Consider termination and immediate therapy	III	B	54, 55, 58, 59
after 20 weeks: consider awaiting fetal maturity (enhance with steroids), then deliver and implement therapy postnatally	III	B	54, 55, 58, 59
Elective cesarean hysterectomy can be considered with early stage disease	III	B	9
Careful patient counseling required with either presentation	III	B	54, 55, 58, 59
Prognosis			
Recent studies suggesting worse prognosis when diagnosed after pregnancy	III	B	45
Reports of recurrences in episiotomy sites after vaginal birth	III	B	63

OVARIAN CANCER

Ovarian cancer occurs in between 1 in 12,000 and 1 in 20,000 pregnancies.[64–66] It is the second most common malignancy diagnosed in pregnancy.[67] During pregnancy, most ovarian masses are diagnosed incidentally at the time of obstetric ultrasound. Most adnexal masses are nonmalignant and usually are functional cysts (17%), dermoid cysts (36%), or cystadenomas (27%).[57] The risk that an ovarian neoplasm in pregnancy is malignant ranges from 2% to 5%, compared with 20% outside of pregnancy.[68–70]

The histologic distribution of ovarian cancers in pregnancy is different from that seen in the general population, partly because pregnant women are relatively young and have a higher incidence of germ cell tumors. Germ cell tumors account for 33% to 40% of malignant neoplasms complicating pregnancy, epithelial malignancies account for 33% to 53%, and gonadal stromal tumors account for 9% to 20%.[71–74] The distribution of subtypes of germ cell tumors diagnosed during pregnancy is a matter of debate. Whereas some series indicate that dysgerminomas are the most common subtype,[69,73,74] others indicate that malignant teratomas[71,72] and endodermal sinus tumors[75] are more common. Most ovarian malignancies diagnosed in pregnancy are stage I, as would be expected with germ cell tumors.

Management Options

Management of an adnexal mass during pregnancy depends on the ultrasonographic characteristics of the mass and the gestational age. Current recommendations are to proceed with surgical exploration with a midline incision at 16 to 18 weeks for masses that are larger than 6 cm, have a significant solid component, are bilateral, or persist after 14 weeks' gestation.[76,77] The serum cancer antigen 125 level can be elevated in normal pregnancies, especially in the first trimester, and should not be used to decide on surgical intervention.[78] Ovarian neoplasms, even when benign, are associated with increased risk of complications during pregnancy. Adnexal torsion is reported in up to 25% of patients[79,80]; other complications include rupture and hemorrhage. The risk of pregnancy loss or preterm labor is increased if surgery is performed for one of these acute complications.

Unilateral salpingo-oophorectomy with staging biopsy is the recommended surgery for stage I germ cell tumors. Patients with dysgerminomas and stage IA, grade 1 immature teratomas do not require further adjuvant therapy. The remaining germ cell tumors behave more aggressively and should be treated with adjuvant chemotherapy. Treatment of advanced germ cell tumors of any histologic subtype includes chemotherapy. In anecdotal reports of pregnant patients treated with combination chemotherapy regimens (bleomycin, etoposide, cisplatin, and vinblastine), good maternal and fetal outcomes were achieved.[81,82]

In epithelial carcinomas, patients with early-stage disease can be treated successfully with conservative surgery, including salpingo-oophorectomy and staging biopsy. Advanced disease presents a management problem. Tumor debulking surgery is often extensive and may result in adverse pregnancy outcome. Cisplatin-based chemotherapy is usually used postoperatively. Few case reports describe successful treatment of advanced ovarian cancer in pregnancy with surgery and chemotherapy.[16,20,77]

Gonadal stromal tumors are uncommon in pregnancy. They are often confined to the ovary and have an indolent course. Treatment involves unilateral salpingo-oophorectomy.

SUMMARY OF MANAGEMENT OPTIONS

Ovarian Cancer

Management Options	Quality of Evidence	Strength of Recommendation	References
Diagnosis			
Often diagnosed as chance finding during an obstetric ultrasound examination	III	B	76, 77
CA-125 levels are unhelpful as can be raised in normal pregnancy	III	B	78
MRI helpful	IV	C	67
Treatment			
Surgical exploration ideally performed in second trimester	III	B	71–73
Pregnancy preservation and conservative surgery with unilateral salpingo-oophorectomy and staging biopsies are possible in most early stage ovarian cancers (uncommon)	III	B	71–73
Chemotherapy, if needed, has risks (see above and Chapter 50)	III	B	16, 20, 23–30
Salvage of the pregnancy may not be possible with advanced disease	III	B	71–73

OTHER GYNECOLOGIC MALIGNANCIES

Vulvar carcinoma in pregnancy is extremely rare. The most common histologic varieties are invasive squamous cell carcinoma and melanoma.[83] Radical excision of the primary lesion with inguinofemoral node dissection is the treatment of choice for stage I and II tumors. The timing of treatment and mode of delivery are usually dependent on the time of diagnosis during pregnancy. The current recommendation is to proceed with definitive surgical treatment at any time during pregnancy, up to 36 weeks' gestation.[83–85] Patients can be allowed to deliver vaginally if the wounds have healed.

Twelve cases of endometrial carcinoma have been reported during pregnancy.[86–88] Surprisingly, five cases were associated with a viable fetus.[71,72] The remaining cases were diagnosed at the time of dilation and curettage performed for abnormal bleeding.

SUMMARY OF MANAGEMENT OPTIONS

Other Gynecological Malignant Disease In Pregnancy

Management Options	Quality of Evidence	Strength of Recommendation	References
Vulval Carcinoma			
Rare; histological varieties most commonly encountered are invasive squamous cell carcinomas and melanomas	III	B	83, 85
Radical excision of the primary lesion and inguinal femoral node dissection is the treatment of choice for stage I and II squamous cell cancer	III	B	84, 85
Timing of treatment and mode of delivery are usually dependent on the time of diagnosis during pregnancy. It has been recommended to proceed with	III	B	83, 85

SUMMARY OF MANAGEMENT OPTIONS

Other Gynecological Malignant Disease In Pregnancy *(Continued)*

Management Options	Quality of Evidence	Strength of Recommendation	References
Vulval Carcinoma—*Continued*			
definitive surgical treatment at any time during pregnancy up to 36 weeks of gestation. Patients can be allowed to deliver vaginally provided the wounds have healed			
Endometrial Carcinoma			
There have been twelve cases of **endometrial carcinomas** reported during pregnancy. Surprisingly five cases were associated with a viable fetus. The remaining cases were diagnosed at the time of dilatation and curettage performed for irregular bleeding	III	B	86–88

BREAST CANCER

Pregnancy-associated breast cancer is usually defined as carcinoma that is diagnosed during pregnancy or within 1 year postpartum.[89,90] It is the most common tumor in women of reproductive age. Approximately 3% of breast cancers occur in pregnancy, for a rate of 10 to 40 cases per 100,000 deliveries. The incidence is approximately 3 in 10,000 pregnancies.[4,91,92] Approximately 15% of breast cancers occur in women of childbearing age, and there is evidence that the incidence of premenopausal breast cancer is on the rise. Traditionally, it was believed that pregnancy adversely affected the outcome of patients with breast cancer. Many older reports showed poor survival in women with pregnancy-associated breast cancer.[93–95] In contrast, more recent data show identical survival rates in pregnant women and nonpregnant cohorts, when matched for disease stage.[57,90] The 5-year survival rate is reported to be 90% for patients with stage I disease, 37% for those with stage II disease, 15% for those with stage III disease, and 0% for those with stage IV disease.[96] One explanation for the lower survival rates in earlier reports is that pregnant women are more likely to be diagnosed at advanced stages.[90,97–99] Between 53% and 74% of pregnant women who are diagnosed with breast cancer have evidence of lymph node metastases. Physiologic changes that affect the breast during gestation make clinical examination difficult and inaccurate. In addition, physicians may be reluctant to perform breast biopsy during pregnancy and lactation because of the increased risk of bleeding, infection, and milk fistulas. Delays of several months between the diagnosis of breast mass and biopsy are common.[90] Delay in the diagnosis contributes to the advanced disease and poor prognosis associated with gestational breast cancer.

Management Options

Pregnant women should have a baseline breast examination at the first prenatal visit. Mammography can be performed safely during pregnancy; however, it may not be done routinely because of concern about fetal irradiation. A bilateral mammogram performed with modern equipment yields less than 500 μGy to the human embryo, which is well below the 100-mGy toxic level.[7] The mammogram may have limited diagnostic utility because of the hyperemia and edema that affect the mammary tissues and contribute to the generalized radiographic density of the breasts. Ultrasound is accurate in differentiating between cystic and solid masses. The detection of a mass necessitates prompt evaluation with fine-needle aspiration or surgical biopsy. An experienced cytologist should evaluate the cells obtained from aspirates because hyperproliferative physiologic changes in the mammary tissue may be mistaken for malignancy. The increased risk of complications associated with breast biopsy during pregnancy should not deter the surgeon from performing these procedures when clinically indicated.[90]

As in the nonpregnant patient, staging of breast cancer during pregnancy involves a complete physical examination, blood testing, and chest x-ray with abdominal shielding. Ultrasonographic evaluation of the liver should be performed only if the patient has localizing symptoms or abnormal liver chemistry findings.[100] A radionuclide bone scan can cause significant fetal exposure to radiation. Because of their low yield in early-stage disease, bone scans should be limited to patients with more advanced disease. Magnetic resonance imaging during pregnancy is safe for the mother and fetus; it is being used with increasing frequency to diagnose bone, liver, and brain metastases.

Stage I and II breast cancers are best treated with surgery. Modified radical mastectomy is the standard treatment.[90,101–103] It can be performed safely during pregnancy under general anesthesia. Treatment modalities that include breast preservation with radiation therapy should be avoided in pregnant women because of the risk of fetal exposure to a potentially mutagenic and lethal radiation dose. The standard breast radiation therapy course of approximately 5000 cGy exposes the fetus to a radiation dose that varies according to gestational age and the associated anatomic changes. Early in pregnancy, when the uterus is still in the pelvis, fetal exposure may be as low as 10 cGy. However, in late pregnancy, when the fetus moves up into the mother's abdomen, fetal exposure can reach 200 cGy. Conversely, for some women diagnosed with early breast cancer in the third trimester, delaying treatment until after parturition is an acceptable option with minimal maternal risks and obvious fetal benefit.[104,105]

Adjuvant chemotherapy is indicated in patients with lymph node metastases and in some with large tumors and negative lymph nodes. During organogenesis in the first trimester, the risks of teratogenicity and fetal malformations should be weighed carefully against the potential benefits. Later in pregnancy, regimens that include cyclophosphamide and doxorubicin can be given relatively safely.[57] Methotrexate should be avoided, when possible, because of its associated teratogenicity. In addition to fetal effects, a course of chemotherapy during pregnancy may result in possible maternal complications, including sepsis and hemorrhage, with unplanned labor and delivery.

Advanced-stage disease requires both chemotherapy and radiation therapy. The prognosis is poor, and maternal survival is limited. Management of these patients during pregnancy presents ethical and medical dilemmas and should be planned on an individual basis.

Recent literature does not support the role of routine therapeutic abortion in pregnant patients with breast cancer.[90] Many authors showed that survival is not improved by pregnancy termination for maternal indications.[97,101,106] In some cases, therapeutic abortion may be strongly recommended because of potential fetal damage from the proposed chemotherapy or radiation treatments. In early pregnancy, treatment is greatly simplified with therapeutic abortion.[90]

Subsequent pregnancy in women who have been treated for breast cancer does not seem to confer a worse prognosis than that in patients who did not get pregnant.[107] Population-based studies show that a subsequent pregnancy results in an improvement in survival, with favorable relative risks of 0.2 (range, 0.1–0.5)[89] to 0.8 (range, 0.3–2.3).[104,105] However, it is difficult to draw definite conclusions from available studies because of the small number of patients reported and the associated selection bias. Because recurrence is most likely in the first 2 years, most investigators recommend delaying conception for 2 to 3 years after treatment.

SUMMARY OF MANAGEMENT OPTIONS
Breast Cancer and Pregnancy

Management Options	Quality of Evidence	Strength of Recommendation	References
Diagnosis			
Physiologic changes of pregnancy reduce the sensitivity of physical examination and mammography	IV	C	90
Fine needle aspiration of any suspicious lesion	IV	C	90
Open biopsy if the results of needle biopsy are equivocal	IV	C	90
Treatment			
Radical mastectomy is the preferred treatment for early cancers	III	B	91
Adjuvant chemotherapy may be indicated for some patients with high risk cancers. Both maternal benefits and potential risks to the fetus should be weighed carefully	III IV	B C	91 90
If diagnosis is made late in pregnancy and chemotherapy or radiation treatment are indicated, consider delaying therapy until after delivery	IIb	B	102
Routine therapeutic abortions are not indicated	III	B	91,96
Termination of pregnancy may be considered in patients with advanced disease if chemotherapy and/or radiation treatment are indicated in early pregnancy	IIb	B	102
Recommend delaying conception for 2–3 years after treatment	IIa	B	97

PLACENTAL METASTASES

Metastasis of maternal malignancy into the placenta is rare. Malignant melanoma is the most common maternal malignancy associated with placental metastasis; it accounts for nearly one third of reported cases.[106] Next in frequency are hematopoietic malignancies and breast carcinoma.[106,107] Fetal metastasis is extremely rare, even when the maternal surface of the placenta contains evidence of metastatic tumor. The low incidence of fetal metastasis has been attributed to two factors: inherent resistance of the trophoblast to tumor invasion and possible immune rejection by the fetal immune system.[107] Interestingly, after delivery, some infants with metastatic melanoma have complete tumor regression and long-term survival.

CONCLUSIONS

- Between 1 in 1000 and 1 in 1500 gravidas will be affected by cancer each year.
- Cervical cancer is the most common malignancy diagnosed in pregnancy, followed by ovarian cancer.
- Abnormal Pap smears should be thoroughly evaluated in pregnant women; colposcopy is a safe and reliable method for evaluating cytologic abnormalities in pregnancy.
- Treatment of cervical cancer in pregnancy is based on disease stage and gestational age; the same principles should be applied as in the nonpregnant state.
- The histologic distribution of ovarian cancers in pregnancy is different from that seen in the general population, partly because of the younger age group and the higher incidence of germ cell tumors.
- Management of the asymptomatic adnexal mass in pregnancy is dependent on size, ultrasonographic characteristics, and gestational age at diagnosis.
- Surgical exploration (optimally in the early second trimester) for ovarian cancer diagnosis and staging are established recommendations; early-stage disease can be treated successfully with conservative surgery. Extensive surgical debulking can be problematic in pregnancy.
- Adjuvant chemotherapy has been used during pregnancy with good maternal and fetal outcomes.
- Routine breast examination is recommended in pregnancy. Breast masses can be further studied by mammography, ultrasonography, and fine needle aspiration or biopsy.
- Stage I and II breast cancers are best treated by a surgical approach.
- The recommendation for routine therapeutic abortion in breast cancer patients in the interest of maternal survival is not supported by current literature.
- Malignant melanoma is the most common maternal malignancy associated with placental metastases.

REFERENCES

1. Centers for Disease Control and Prevention: Maternal mortality: United States, 1982–1996. JAMA 1998;280:1042.
2. Lundig S, Murray T, Bolden S, Wingo PA: Cancer statistics, 1999. CA Cancer J Clin 1999;48:6.
3. Allen H, Nisker J (eds): Cancer in Pregnancy: Therapeutic Guidelines. New York, Futura, 1986.
4. Gallenberg MM, Lopinzi CI: Breast cancer and pregnancy. Semin Oncol 1989;16:369–376.
5. Colbourn DS, Nathanson L, Belilos E: Pregnancy and malignant melanoma. Semin Oncol 1989;16:377–387.
6. Deppe G, Munkarah A, Malone JM Jr: Neoplasia. In Gleicher N (ed): Principles and Practice of Medical Therapy in Pregnancy, 2nd ed. Norwalk, Conn, Appleton & Lange, 1998, pp 1231–1234.
7. Wagner LK, Lester RG, Saldana LR: Exposure of the pregnant patient to diagnostic radiation: A guide to medical management. Madison, WI, Medical Physics Publishing, 1997.
8. Brent RL, Bolden BT: The indirect effect of irradiation on embryonic development: III. The contribution of ovarian irradiation, oviduct irradiation and zygote irradiation to fetal mortality and growth retardation in the rat. Radiat Res 1967;30:759–773.
9. Russell LB: X-ray-induced developmental abnormalities in the mouse and their use in analysis of embryological patterns: I. External gross visceral changes. J Exp Zool 1950;114:545–547.
10. Russell LB, Saylors CL: The relative sensitivity of various germ-cell stages of the mouse to radiation-induced nondisjunction, chromosome losses and deficiencies. In Sobel's Repair from Genetic Radiation. New York, Pergamon, 1963, pp 313–336.
11. Rugh R: Effect of ionizing radiation, including radioisotopes on the placenta and embryo. Birth Defects 1964;1:64–72.
12. Hall EJ: Effects of radiation on the embryo and fetus. In Hall EJ (ed): Radiobiology for the Radiologist, 4th ed. Philadelphia, Lippincott, 1994, pp 363–392.
13. Dekaban AS: Abnormalities in children exposed to x-irradiation during various stages of gestation: Tentative timetable of radiation injury to the human fetus. J Nucl Med 1968;9:471–477.
14. Stewart A, Kneale GW: Radiation dose effects in relation to obstetric x-rays and childhood cancers. Lancet 1970;1:1185–1188.
15. Mole RH: Antenatal irradiation and childhood cancer: Causation or coincidence. Br J Cancer 1974;30:199–208.
16. Wong PJ, Rosemark PJ, Wexler MR, et al: Doses to organs at risk from mantle field radiation therapy using 10 MV x-rays. Mt Sinai J Med 1985;52:216–220.
17. Henderson CE, Elia G, Garfinkel D, et al: Platinum chemotherapy during pregnancy for serous cystadenocarcinoma of the ovary. Gynecol Oncol 1993;49:92–94.
18. Turchi JJ, Villases C: Anthracyclines in the treatment of malignancy in pregnancy. Cancer 1988;61:435–440.
19. Zuazu J, Julia A, Sierra J, et al: Pregnancy outcome in hematologic malignancies. Cancer 1991;67:703–709.

20. Reynoso E, Shepherd F, Messner HA, et al: Acute leukemia during pregnancy: The Toronto Leukemia Study Group experience with long-term follow-up of children exposed in utero to chemotherapeutic agents. J Clin Oncol 1987;5:1098–1106.
21. Malfetano JH, Goldkrand JW: Cisplatinum combination chemotherapy during pregnancy for advanced epithelial ovarian carcinoma. Obstet Gynecol 1990;75:545–547.
22. Doll DC, Ringenberg QS, Yarbro JW: Antineoplastic agents in pregnancy. Semin Oncol 1989;16:337–346.
23. Wieve VJ, Sipila PEH: Pharmacology of antineoplastic agents in pregnancy. Crit Rev Oncol Hematol 1994;16:75–81.
24. Beeley L: Adverse effects of drugs in the first trimester of pregnancy. Clin Obstet Gynecol 1986;13:177–195.
25. DeAlvarez RR: An evaluation of aminopterin as an abortifacient. Am J Obstet Gynecol 1962;83:1467–1477.
26. Emerson JK: Congenital malformation due to attempted abortion with aminopterin. Am J Obstet Gynecol 1962;84: 356–357.
27. Goetsch C: An evaluation of aminopterin as an abortifacient. Am J Obstet Gynecol 1962;83:1474–1477.
28. Panchalingham S: Post-methotrexate babies. Ceylon Med J 1973;18:93–97.
29. Schein PS, Winokur SH: Immunosuppressive and cytotoxic chemotherapy: Long-term complications. Ann Intern Med 1975;82:84–96.
30. Warkany J: Aminopterin and methotrexate: Folic acid deficiency. Teratology 1978;17:353–357.
31. Glantz JC: Reproductive toxicology of alkylating agents. Obstet Gynecol Surv 1994;49:709–715.
32. Hacker NF, Berek JS, Lagase LD, et al: Cervical carcinoma associated with pregnancy. Obstet Gynecol 1995;59:735–746.
33. Sood AK, Sorosky JI: Invasive cervical cancer complicating pregnancy. Obstet Gynecol Clin North Am 1998;25:343–383.
34. Nevin J, Soeters R, Dehaeck K, et al: Cervical carcinoma associated with pregnancy. Obstet Gynecol Surv 1995;50:228–239.
35. Jones WB, Shingleton HM, Russell A, et al: Cervical carcinoma and pregnancy: A national patterns of care study of the American College of Surgeons. Cancer 1996;77:1479–1488.
36. Duggan B, Muderspach LI, Roman LD, et al: Cervical cancer in pregnancy: Reporting on planned delay in therapy. Obstet Gynecol 1993;82:598–602.
37. Greer BE, Easterling TR, McLennan DA, et al: Fetal and maternal consideration in the management of stage IB cervical cancer during pregnancy. Gynecol Oncol 1989;34:61–65.
38. Hopkins MP, Morley GW: The prognosis and management of cervical cancer associated with pregnancy. Obstet Gynecol 1992;80:9–13.
39. Rhatigan RM: Endocervical gland atypia secondary to Arias-Stella change. Arch Pathol Lab Med 1992;116:943.
40. Pisharodi L, Jovanoska S: Spectrum of cytologic changes in pregnancy. Acta Cytol 1995;39:905.
41. Schneider V: Arias-Stella reaction of the endocervix: Frequency and location. Acta Cytol 1981;25:224.
42. Baltzer J, Regenbrecht ME, Kopcke W, et al: Carcinoma of the cervix and pregnancy. Int J Gynecol Obstet 1990;31: 317–323.
43. Hannigan EV: Cervical cancer in pregnancy. Clin Obstet Gynecol 1990;33:837–845.
44. Zemlickis D, Lishner M, Degendorfer P, et al: Maternal and fetal outcome after invasive cervical cancer in pregnancy. J Clin Oncol 1991;9:1956–1961.
45. Sood AK, Sorosky JI, Mayr N, et al: Cervical cancer diagnosed shortly after pregnancy: Prognostic variables and delivery routes. Obstet Gynecol 2000;95:832–838.
46. Benedet JL, Selke PA, Nickerson KG: Colposcopic evaluation of abnormal Papanicolaou smears in pregnancy. Am J Obstet Gynecol 1987;157:932–937.
47. Hellberg D, Axelson D, Gad A, et al: Conservative management of the abnormal smear during pregnancy: A long-term follow-up. Acta Obstet Gynecol Scand 1987;66:195–199.
48. Madej JG Jr: Colposcopy monitoring in pregnancy complicated by CIN and early cervical cancer. Eur J Gynaecol Oncol 1996;17:59–65.
49. Campion MJ, Sedlacek TV: Colposcopy in pregnancy. Obstet Gynecol Clin North Am 1993;20:153–163.
50. Harper DM, Roach MSI: Cervical intraepithelial neoplasia in pregnancy. J Fam Pract 1995;42:79–83.
51. Ostergard DR, Nieberg RK: Evaluation of abnormal cervical cytology during pregnancy with colposcopy. Am J Obstet Gynecol 1979;34:756–761.
52. Choo YC, Chan OLY, Ma HK: Colposcopy in microinvasive carcinoma of the cervix: An enigma of diagnosis. BJOG 1984;92:1156–1160.
53. Hannigan EV, Whitehouse HH, Atkinson WD, et al: Cone biopsy during pregnancy. Obstet Gynecol 1992;60:450–459.
54. Monk BJ, Montz FJ: Invasive cervical cancer complicating intrauterine pregnancy: Treatment with radical hysterectomy. Obstet Gynecol 1992;80:199–203.
55. Sood AK, Sorosky JI, Krogman S, et al: Surgical management of cervical cancer complicating pregnancy: A case-control study. Gynecol Oncol 1996;63:294–298.
56. Sorosky JI, Squatrito R, Ndubisis BU, et al: Stage I squamous cell cervical carcinoma in pregnancy: Planned delay in therapy awaiting fetal maturity. Gynecol Oncol 1995;59:207–210.
57. Greer BE, Goff BA, Koh W-J, et al: Cancer in the pregnant patient. In Hoskins WJ, Perez CA, Young RC (eds): Principles and Practice of Gynecologic Oncology, 3rd ed. Philadelphia, Lippincott-Raven, 2000, pp 501–528.
58. Nisker JA, Shubat M: Stage IB cervical carcinoma and pregnancy: Report of 49 cases. Am J Obstet Gynecol 1983;145: 203–206.
59. Sivanesaratnam V, Jayalakshmi P, Loo C: Surgical management of early invasive cancer of the cervix associated with pregnancy. Gynecol Oncol 1993;48:68–75.
60. Sood AK, Sorosky JI, Mayr N, et al: Radiotherapeutic management of cervical carcinoma that complicates pregnancy. Cancer 1997;80:1073–1078.
61. Cliby WA, Dodson MK, Podratz KC: Cervical cancer complicated by pregnancy: Episiotomy site recurrences following vaginal delivery. Obstet Gynecol 1994;84:179–182.
62. Copeland LJ, Saul PB, Sneige N: Cervical adenocarcinoma: Tumor implantation in the episiotomy sites of two patients. Gynecol Oncol 1987;28:230–235.
63. Gordon AN, Jensen R, Jones HW III: Squamous carcinoma of the cervix complicating pregnancy: Recurrence in episiotomy after vaginal delivery. Obstet Gynecol 1989;73:850–852.
64. Chung A, Birnbaum SJ: Ovarian cancer associated with pregnancy. Obstet Gynecol 1973;41:211–214.
65. Munnell EW: Primary ovarian cancer associated with pregnancy. Clin Obstet Gynecol 1963;6:983–993.
66. White KC: Ovarian tumors in pregnancy: A private hospital 10-year survey. Am J Obstet Gynecol 1973;116:544–550.
67. Boulay R, Podczaski E: Ovarian cancer complicating pregnancy. Obstet Gynecol Clin North Am 1998;25:385–399.
68. Beischer NA, Buttery BW, Fortune DW, et al: Growth and malignancy of ovarian tumors in pregnancy. Aust N Z J Obstet Gynecol 1971;11:208–220.
69. Dgani R, Shoham Z, Atat E, et al: Ovarian carcinoma during pregnancy: A study of 23 cases in Israel between the years 1960 and 1984. Gynecol Oncol 1989;33:326–331.
70. Young RH, Dudley AG, Scully RE: Granulosa cell, Sertoli-Leydig, and unclassified sex cord-stromal tumors associated with pregnancy: A clinicopathological analysis of 36 cases. Gynecol Oncol 1984;18:181–205.

71. Antonelli NM, Dotters DJ, Katz VL, et al: Cancer in pregnancy: A review of the literature. Part I. Obstet Gynecol Surv 1996;51:125–134.
72. Antonelli NM, Dotters DJ, Katz VL, et al: Cancer in pregnancy: A review of the literature. Part II. Obstet Gynecol Surv 1996;51:135–142.
73. Creasman WT, Rutledge F, Smith JP: Carcinoma of the ovary associated with pregnancy. Obstet Gynecol 1971;38:111–116.
74. Novak ER, Lambrou CD, Woodruff DJ: Ovarian tumors in pregnancy. Obstet Gynecol 1975;46:401–406.
75. Talerman A: Letter. Ovarian endometrial sinus tumor associated with pregnancy: review of the literature. Gynecol Oncol 1992;44:291–292.
76. Katz VL, Watson WJ, Hansen WF, et al: Massive ovarian tumor complicating pregnancy: A case report. J Reprod Med 1993;38:907–910.
77. King LA, Nevin PC, Williams PP, et al: Treatment of advanced epithelial ovarian carcinoma in pregnancy with cisplatin-based chemotherapy. Gynecol Oncol 1991;41:78–80.
78. Kobayashi F, Sagawa N, Nakamura K, et al: Mechanism and clinical significance of elevated CA-125 levels in the sera of pregnant women. Am J Obstet Gynecol 1989;160:563–566.
79. El Yahia AR, Rahman J, Rahman MS, et al: Ovarian tumors in pregnancy. Aust N Z J Obstet Gynecol 1991;31:327–330.
80. Struyk AP, Treffers PE: Ovarian tumors in pregnancy. Acta Obstet Gynecol Scand 1984;63:421–424.
81. Christman JE, Teng NN, Lebovic GS, et al: Delivery of a normal infant following cisplatin, vinblastine and bleomycin (PVB) chemotherapy for malignant teratoma of the ovary during pregnancy. Gynecol Oncol 1990;37:292–295.
82. Malone JM, Gershenson DM, Creasy RK: Endodermal sinus tumor of the ovary associated with pregnancy. Obstet Gynecol 1986;68:865–889.
83. Regan MA, Rosenzweig BA: Vulvar carcinoma in pregnancy: A case report and literature review. Am J Perinatol 1993;10:334–335.
84. Barclay DL: Surgery of the vulva, perineum and vagina in pregnancy. In Barber HR, Graber EA (eds): Surgical Disease in Pregnancy. Philadelphia, Saunders, 1974, pp 320–348.
85. Monaghan JM, Lindegue G: Vulvar carcinoma in pregnancy: Commentary. BJOG 1986;93:7785–7786.
86. Carinelli SG, Cefis F, Merol D: Epithelial neoplasia of the endometrium in pregnancy: A case report. Tumori 1987;73:175–180.
87. Fine BA, Baker TR, Hempling RE, et al: Pregnancy coexisting with serous papillary adenocarcinoma involving both uterus and ovary. Gynecol Oncol 1994;53:369–372.
88. Ojomo EO, Ezimokhai M, Raele FR, et al: Recurrent postpartum hemorrhage caused by endometrial carcinoma coexisting with endometrioid carcinoma of the ovary in a full-term pregnancy. BJOG 1993;100:489–491.
89. Sankila R, Heinavaara S, Hakulinen T: Survival of breast cancer patients after subsequent term pregnancy: 'Healthy mother effect.' Am J Obstet Gynecol 1994;170:818–823.
90. Petrek JA: Breast cancer and pregnancy. Monogr Natl Cancer Inst 1994;16:113–121.
91. King RM, Welch JS, Martin JK Jr, et al: Carcinoma of the breast associated with pregnancy. Surg Gynecol Obstet 1985;160:228–232.
92. Petrek JA: Breast cancer and pregnancy. In Harris JR, Hellman S, Henderson IC, Kinne DW (eds): Breast Diseases, 2nd ed. Philadelphia, Lippincott, 1991, p 809.
93. Haagensen CD, Stout AP: Carcinoma of the breast: Criteria of operability. Ann Surg 1943;118:859–870.
94. Kilgore AR, Bloodgood JC: Tumors and tumor-like lesions of the breast in association with pregnancy. Arch Surg 1929;18:2079–2098.
95. White TT: Carcinoma of the breast and pregnancy. Ann Surg 1954;139:9–18.
96. Clark RM, Chua T: Breast cancer and pregnancy: The ultimate challenge. Clin Oncol 1989;1:11–18.
97. Petrek JA, Dukoff R, Rogatko A: Prognosis of pregnancy-associated breast cancer. Cancer 1991;67:869–872.
98. Zemlickis D, Lishner M, Degendorfer P, et al: Maternal and fetal outcome after breast cancer in pregnancy. Am J Obstet Gynecol 1992;166:781–787.
99. Fiorica JV: Special problems: Breast cancer and pregnancy. Obstet Gynecol Clin North Am 1994;21:721–732.
100. Difronzo LA, O'Connel TX: Breast cancer in pregnancy and lactation. Surg Clin North Am 1996;76:267–278.
101. Shousha L: Breast carcinoma presenting during or shortly after pregnancy and lactation. Arch Pathol Lab Med 2000;124:1053–1060.
102. Nettleton J, Long J, Kuban D, et al: Breast cancer during pregnancy: Quantifying the risk of treatment delay. Obstet Gynecol 1996;87:414–418.
103. Antypas C, Sandilos P, Kouvavis J, et al: Fetal dose evaluation during breast cancer radiotherapy. Int J Radiat Oncol Biol Phys 1998;40:995–999.
104. Velentgas P, Daling JR, Malone KE, et al: Pregnancy after breast carcinoma: Outcomes and influence on mortality. Cancer 1999;85:2424–2432.
105. Upponi SS, Ahmad F, Whitaker IS, Purushotham AD: Pregnancy after breast cancer. Eur J Cancer 2003;39:736–741.
106. Shanklin DR: Tumors of the Placental and Umbilical Cord. Philadelphia, Marcel Decker, 1990, pp 154–159.
107. Eltorky M, Khare VK, Osborne P, et al: Placental metastasis from maternal carcinoma. J Reprod Med 1995;40:499–503.

CHAPTER 54

Pregnancy After Transplantation

Vincent T. Armenti / Michael J. Moritz / John M. Davison

INTRODUCTION

Transplantation is now an accepted therapeutic option for patients with end-stage organ failure. The first successful human kidney transplant took place in 1954.[1] However, it was not until the 1960s that immunosuppression became available and not until the 1980s, with the introduction of cyclosporine, that consistently acceptable graft and patient survival was achieved. With the restoration of organ function, patients experience an overall improvement in their health, increased libido, and return of fertility.

The first post-transplant pregnancy occurred in March 1958 and was reported in 1963. It occurred in a patient who had received a kidney from her identical twin.[2] This pregnancy resulted in cesarean delivery of a healthy boy. As transplantation has progressed, with improvements in surgical techniques and medical therapy and advances in immunosuppression, pregnancies have been reported in recipients of each organ type. Most outcomes reported are in kidney transplant recipients. Issues that must be considered include maternal graft function and maternal health, the effect of pregnancy on graft function, and the effect of the medications and graft function on the developing fetus. There is also concern about the long-term effects of pregnancy on graft function. Finally, there is the question of whether more subtle and long-term effects, although not apparent at birth, may affect the growth and development of the offspring of these recipients or future generations. These issues are discussed in this chapter.

ORGAN TRANSPLANTATION

Patients with end-stage renal disease who are receiving or will soon need dialysis are candidates for renal transplantation. Common indications for renal transplantation are glomerulonephritis, diabetes, polycystic kidney disease, and hypertension. In 2002 in the United States, 14,710 kidney transplants were performed. The 1-year graft survival rate was 90% for deceased donor kidneys and 95% for donor kidneys.[3] Recent technical advances that allow laparoscopic removal of living donor kidneys have helped to make living donation more acceptable, removing disincentives.[4] In 2001, the number of kidney transplants from living donors exceeded the number from deceased donors.[5] Standard requirements for donor–recipient pairs for kidney transplantation are ABO compatibility and a negative pretransplant cross-match (i.e., absence of preformed anti-donor antibodies). Efforts to increase the number of kidney transplants include the use of methods to use ABO-incompatible donors as well as treatment protocols to reduce antibody levels in patients with antidonor antibodies, making transplantation possible.

Patients with both type I diabetes and end-stage renal disease are candidates for simultaneous kidney–pancreas transplantation. These patients may opt for a kidney transplant first, especially if they have a living donor, and later undergo a pancreas transplant. Patients who do not have diabetic nephropathy, but have other severe complications of diabetes, such as hypoglycemic unawareness, may be candidates for pancreas transplantation alone. In 2002, there were 771 pancreas–kidney transplants performed in the United States, with a 1-year graft survival rate of 76%.[3]

Patients with end-stage liver disease are candidates for liver transplantation. The first successful human liver transplant was performed in 1967.[1] Of candidates for liver transplantation, 95% have chronic liver disease (i.e., cirrhosis) and 5% have fulminant hepatic failure, a disorder that progresses rapidly. Chronic diseases that require transplantation include cirrhosis as a result of hepatitis C, hepatitis B, alcohol use, biliary cirrhosis, or primary sclerosing cholangitis. In children, the most common cause of liver failure is biliary atresia. Complications of end-stage liver disease that suggest the need for transplantation include ascites, encephalopathy, and bleeding as a result of esophageal varices. In 2002, in the United States, 5040 liver transplants were performed, with a 1-year graft survival rate of 80% to 85%.[3] Living donation, in which part of an adult liver is donated, is now an option for both adult and pediatric recipients.

Although most pregnancies reported in the literature and to the registries have been in kidney or liver recipients, numbers are starting to accrue in the other groups as well, except for small bowel recipients. Candidates for heart transplantation have end-stage heart disease. Cardiomyopathy and coronary artery disease are the most common indications. On average, these adults are older than patients in other organ groups, which is likely part of the reason why fewer pregnancies have been reported. In the United States, 1975 heart transplants were performed in 2002, with a 1-year graft survival rate of 85%.[3] Fewer heart–lung and liver–kidney transplants are performed, and few pregnancies have been reported in these recipients.

Patients with end-stage lung disease and an anticipated survival of less than 2 years without transplantation are candidates for lung transplantation. Three common indications are emphysema or chronic obstructive pulmonary disease, including α_1-antitrypsin deficiency, primary pulmonary hypertension, and cystic fibrosis. The 1-year graft survival rate is the lowest of all of the groups discussed, at 76%, with 957 transplants performed in the United States in 2002.[3] Living donation is an option.

SUCCESS OF TRANSPLANTATION

Medication regimens to maintain graft survival and prevent rejection have been evolving since the 1960s. In general, these can be divided into the following three categories:

- Induction regimens are used in the first week after transplantation. These include agents such as antilymphocyte sera and interleukin-2-receptor blockade antibodies.
- Antirejection regimens are used to treat episodes of rejection. They typically include high-dose, short-term treatments with either corticosteroids or antilymphocyte sera.
- Maintenance regimens are initiated soon after transplantation to prevent acute rejection episodes and provide long-term immunosuppression. The goal of this treatment is to minimize acute rejection episodes and toxicity. Combination therapies are used to balance benefits against side effects and toxicities.

A major goal of therapy is to avoid acute rejection episodes, which affect graft survival. Different organs show different effects of acute rejection, but the result can be chronic rejection, which has no effective treatment and ultimately leads to graft demise.

Maintenance regimens in the early 1960s included azathioprine and prednisone. In the 1980s, the mainstay of immunosuppression was cyclosporine, either in combination with azathioprine and prednisone or with prednisone alone. Tacrolimus, introduced in the 1990s, is another calcineurin inhibitor that is similar to cyclosporine, but more potent and with different side effects. Mycophenolate mofetil was introduced in the mid-1990s, and like azathioprine, belongs to the antimetabolite class. This agent essentially replaced azathioprine, and in most cases, is used with a calcineurin inhibitor. A newly introduced agent is sirolimus, which has a different mechanism of action and the added advantage of not being nephrotoxic. Two drugs of the same class are not used in combination (e.g., cyclosporine and tacrolimus). Table 54–1 summarizes the current agents and their mechanisms of action and side effects, including agents used for induction and rejection.[6] The U.S. Food and Drug Administration (FDA) categories for these drugs are shown in Table 54–2, including information on published reproductive or clinical outcome data.[7]

RISKS OF TRANSPLANTATION

Immunosuppressive Agents and Teratology

Corticosteroids

In animal studies, corticosteroids have caused cleft palate.[8] Clinically, these agents are associated with an increased risk of premature rupture of the membranes and adrenal insufficiency in newborns.[9] Prednisone has been used for more than 40 years for maintenance therapy, and intravenous methylprednisolone is used for induction and treatment of rejection. At current doses, it is considered an adjunctive drug. More recently, given the many side effects, steroid withdrawal and steroid avoidance have been attempted.

Azathioprine

Azathioprine (1.5–3 mg/kg/day), a primary drug used for immunosuppression before the introduction of cyclosporine, is now an adjunctive agent at doses of 0.5 to 1.5 mg/kg/day. Clinical data do not support early concerns about teratogenicity in animal studies, nor has a predominant structural malformation pattern been identified. It is listed as a category D agent, and reviews show attributable newborn problems, including thymic atrophy, transient leukopenia, anemia, thrombocytopenia, chromosomal aberrations, sepsis, and reduced immunoglobulin levels.[10,11]

Cyclosporine

As the first calcineurin inhibitor, cyclosporine became the mainstay of immunosuppression and remains a commonly

TABLE 54–1

Immunosuppressive Drugs

DRUG	USES	EFFECTS	SIDE EFFECTS	COMMENTS
Cyclosporine	Maintenance	Profound inhibitor of helper T cell function	Nephrotoxicity, hypertension, tremor, hirsutism	Relatively selective for alloimmune responses; cannot be used with tacrolimus because of synergistic nephrotoxicity
Tacrolimus	Maintenance, antirejection	Profound inhibitor of helper T cell function	Nephrotoxicity, neurotoxicity, diabetes	
Corticosteroids (oral prednisone, IV methylprednisolone)	Maintenance, antirejection	Inhibits all leukocytes; high doses cause lymphocytosis	Cushingoid fascies, diabetes, excessive weight gain, aseptic necrosis of the hip	Many troublesome side effects; nonspecific immunosuppressant
Azathioprine	Maintenance	Inhibits clonal proliferation of T cells	Leukopenia	Nonspecific
Muromonab-CD3 (OKT3)	Antirejection, induction	Disables or depletes all T cells	First dose can cause fever, chills, or bronchospasm as a result of cytokine release	Low frequency of development of anti-OKT3 antibodies; maximum duration of therapy 2–3 weeks
Antithymocyte globulin	Antirejection, induction	Depletes T cells	Fevers, chills	Maximum duration of therapy 2–3 weeks
Mycophenolate mofetil (CellCept)	Maintenance	Akin to azathioprine	Diarrhea, leukopenia	More lymphocyte-selective than azathioprine
Sirdimus (Rapamune)	Maintenance	Inhibits helper T cells	Potential thrombocytopenia and hyperlipidemia	Some similarities to cyclosporine and tacrolimus; synergistic only with cyclosporine
Basiliximab (Simulect)	Antirejection prophylaxis	Inhibits interleukin-2-mediated activation of lymphocytes	Possible anaphylactoid reaction	Immunosuppressive chimeric monoclonal antibody
Daclizumab (Zenapax)	Antirejection prophylaxis	Inhibits interleukin-2-mediated activation of lymphocytes	Possible anaphylactoid reaction	Immunosuppressive chimeric humanized antibody

Adapted from Moritz MJ, Armenti VT: Organ transplantation. In Jarrell BE, Carabasi RA (eds): National Medical Series for Independent Study: Surgery. Philadelphia, Lippincott Williams & Wilkins, 2000, pp 461–477.

TABLE 54–2

Immunosuppressive Drugs Commonly Used in Transplantation

DRUG	USUSAL ORAL DOSAGE	ANIMAL REPRODUCTIVE DATA	PUBLISHED PREGNANCY CLINICAL OUTCOMES?	FDA PREGNANCY CATEGORY
Corticosteroids (prednisone, prednisolone, methylprednisolone)	5–20 mg/day 500–1000 mg/day (antirejection)	Yes Yes	Yes* Yes*	B B
Azathioprine	0.5–1.5 mg/kg/day	Yes	Yes*	D
Cyclosporine (Sandimmune, Neoral)	3–10 mg/kg/day	Yes	Yes*	C
Cyclosporine (Gengraf)	3–10 mg/kg/day	Yes	No*	C
Tacrolimus	0.05–0.2 mg/kg/day	Yes	Yes*	C
Mycophenolate mofetil	2–3 g/day	Yes	Yes*†	C
Muromonab-CD3 (OKT3)	2.5–10 mg/day IV	No	Yes*†	C
Antithymocyte globulin (Atgam, ATG)	15–30 mg/kg/day IV	No	Yes†	C
Antithymocyte globulin (Thymoglobulin)	1.0–1.5 mg/kg/day IV	No	No*	C
Sirolimus	2–5 mg/day	Yes	No*	C
Basiliximab	20 mg/day IV	Yes	No	B
Daclizumab	1 mg/kg/day IV	No	No	C

*Registry data.
†Case reports only.
B, no evidence of risk in humans; C, risk cannot be excluded; D, positive evidence of risk; FDA, U.S. Food and Drug Administration.
Adapted from Armenti VT, Moritz MJ, Davison JM: Drug safety issues in pregnancy following transplantation and immunosuppression. Drug Saf 1998; 19:219–232.

used agent. Cyclosporine was originally available as Sandimmune, which was later reformulated as Neoral. Generic versions are available. It is usually used with one or two adjunctive agents. Maternal problems include hypertension and nephrotoxicity. Although fetal toxicity and abnormality have been reported in animal studies, these occurred at dosages higher than those used clinically.[12,13] Some early clinical reports suggested a greater risk of fetal growth restriction,[14] but the magnitude of teratogenic risk appears minimal and no predominant pattern of newborn malformations is evident.

Tacrolimus

Tacrolimus, which was approved for use in the United States in 1995, is more potent than cyclosporine. In animal studies, fetal resorption occurred at doses higher than those used clinically.[15] Transient neonatal hyperkalemia has been reported,[16] as has a higher incidence of diabetes. Tacrolimus can be used alone or with an adjunctive agent.

Mycophenolate Mofetil

Mycophenolate mofetil, which was approved for use in 1995, is typically used in combination with a calcineurin inhibitor. In contrast to the calcineurin inhibitors, there is greater concern about the potential risk of teratogenicity, based on reproductive toxicity studies in animals. Developmental toxicity in rats and rabbits included malformations and intrauterine growth restriction. Death occurred at dosages that appeared to be within the recommended clinical dosages based on body surface area.[17] Limited clinical data show no particular pattern of malformation.[18,19] Given these concerns, when a patient who is taking mycophenolate mofetil becomes pregnant or is considering pregnancy, the dosage may be decreased or mycophenolate mofetil is discontinued and another agent substituted.

Sirolimus

Sirolimus, which was approved for use in the United States in 1999, is an antiproliferative agent of its own class. It is used in combination with cyclosporine or tacrolimus, or with prednisone alone (European and U.S. labeling). There are concerns about its use in pregnancy, but teratogenicity has not been noted in animal studies, although decreased fetal weight and delayed ossification have been reported.[20] When it was used with cyclosporine in pregnant animals, resorption and fetal mortality rates were increased, suggesting increased toxicity; however, insufficient data on clinical outcome are available.[19]

Other agents used for short-term induction or rejection have a minor role in pregnancy. In a small series of patients, muromonab-CD3 (OKT3)[7] and corticosteroids were used for rejection in pregnancy (discussed later).

Maternal Risks

Transplant recipients have varying degrees of post-transplant recovery. One difficulty in assessing pregnancy risk in this population overall is that many of the conclusions have been derived from experience in kidney transplant recipients. In 1976, a management plan was suggested in a detailed case report of a renal transplant recipient during pregnancy.[21] Based on this information and a survey of literature at the time, the following criteria were derived for counseling renal recipients who are contemplating pregnancy:

- Good general health for at least 2 years after the transplant
- Stature compatible with good obstetric outcome
- No proteinuria
- No significant hypertension
- No evidence of renal rejection
- No evidence of renal obstruction on excretory urogram or ultrasound
- Stable renal function
- Stable immunosuppressive therapy

Most of these guidelines still apply, although recipients can safely become pregnant sooner than 2 years post-transplant and hypertension is now much more prevalent. It has been more difficult to identify criteria for recipients of other organs, but good, stable graft function is essential for pregnancy to be well tolerated. The appropriate interval after transplant and the features of good, stable graft function for each group of organ recipients are harder to define. For renal recipients, graft function can be assessed by measuring the serum creatinine level or creatinine clearance. Extensive studies in both clinical and animal models in the non-transplant population have evaluated the effect of pregnancy on renal function. Renal function is unaffected if the kidney is stable.[22] In the transplant population, this finding is supported by well-designed case–control studies showing that pregnancy does not cause deterioration of graft function when prepregnancy graft function is stable.[23–25] Factors that must be considered in nonrenal recipients are the nephrotoxic effect of calcineurin inhibitors on native kidney function and the increased likelihood of hypertension. Thus, nonrenal recipients who receive calcineurin inhibitor therapy often have renal impairment.

Literature surveys from the azathioprine era of the 1970s and 1980s attest to thousands of successful post-transplant pregnancies in renal transplant recipients. The spontaneous abortion rate was approximately 14%, and the therapeutic abortion rate was approximately 20%. Of pregnancies that continued beyond the first trimester, more than 90% were successful. Renal impairment occurred in approximately 15% of women, and hypertension complicated approximately 30% of pregnancies. Preterm delivery was common, affecting 45% to 60%

of pregnancies, with fetal growth restriction occurring in approximately 20%.[26,27]

Initial reports of cyclosporine exposure during pregnancy raised concern because a higher rate of fetal growth restriction, which may have been related to higher doses, was noted.[14] Also apparent was a higher incidence of hypertension than was previously noted in the azathioprine era.[28] With the advent of cyclosporine, it was suggested that this drug might not be optimal for use in pre gnancy and that patients be switched back to azathioprine-based regimens because of the longer experience with these drugs. Given the need to provide more consistent and effective surveillance for the transplant community, the National Transplantation Pregnancy Registry (NTPR) was established in 1991, with the goal of maintaining an ongoing database to assess the safety of pregnancy in transplant recipients as well as pregnancies fathered by male transplant recipients. A National Transplant Pregnancy Register was established in the United Kingdom in 1997, but discontinued in 2002.[29] After the introduction of cyclosporine, case and individual transplant center reports and registry data reported successful pregnancies in female transplant recipients while highlighting consistent risks to mothers and newborns. Most conclusions came from data on renal recipients, but information is accruing from other organ recipients with differences evident among the groups.

Overall, compared with the general population, female transplant recipients are at greater risk for preeclampsia and hypertension during pregnancy. A higher percentage of cesarean deliveries is reported as well. The balance between graft function and management of immunosuppression during pregnancy is crucial. Fortunately, in organ recipients, the incidence of rejection during pregnancy is no higher than that in the nonpregnant population, and graft loss within 2 years of delivery does not appear to be affected by pregnancy. When irreversible, unpredictable graft events occur, they more often happen in patients with impaired prepregnancy graft function. Many recipients have had successful successive pregnancies, and some have had successful outcomes with multiple gestations and in vitro fertilization.[30–32]

Current data for each organ recipient group reported to the NTPR are summarized in Tables 54–3 to 54–7.[19] High incidences of prematurity and low birth weight are reported and are more apparent among pancreas–kidney recipients and less apparent in liver and heart recipients. Pancreas–kidney recipients usually tolerate pregnancy without gestational diabetes. Most infectious complications involve the urinary tract. Rejection during pregnancy is associated with poorer outcomes for the newborn and for graft survival (Tables 54–8 and 54–9). Rejection should be biopsy-proven, if possible; treatment is with steroids, antilymphocyte sera or adjustment of baseline immunosuppression.

TABLE 54–3

Pregnancies in Female Transplant Recipients

ORGAN	RECIPIENTS	PREGNANCIES	OUTCOME*
Kidney	677	1030	1060
Liver	102	173	174
Liver–kidney	3	5	6
Pancreas–kidney	34	47	49
Heart	31	52	52
Heart–lung	3	3	3
Lung	13	14	14
Total	863	1324	1358

*Includes twins and triplets.
From Armenti VT, Radomski JS, Moritz MJ, et al: Report from the National Transplantation Pregnancy Registry (NTPR): Outcomes of Pregnancy after Transplantation. In Cecka JM, Terasaki PI (eds): Clinical Transplants 2002. Los Angeles, UCLA Immunogenetics Center, 2003, pp 121–130.

Fetal Risks

Two large reports on the two primary calcineurin inhibitors, cyclosporine and tacrolimus, examined the overall prevalence of malformations in newborns. In the offspring of cyclosporine-treated recipients, the malformation rate was 4.1% (14 of 339 births), based on a meta-analysis.[33] NTPR data on the offspring of cyclosporine-treated liver or kidney recipients showed malformations in 3% to 5% of a total of 425 liveborn infants.[34] The types of malformations varied among different systems, with no predominant type noted. No structural malformations were noted in newborns of pancreas–kidney (21 liveborn infants), heart (27 liveborn infants), or lung recipients (3 liveborn infants). In a report of patients treated with tacrolimus during pregnancy (84 women, 100 pregnancies), 4 of 71 liveborn infants analyzed (5.6%) had evidence of structural malformations, but no specific pattern was evident.[35] Transplant recipients, on average, delivered 1 month early, with birth weights of 2200 to 2800 g reported. Differences were seen among organ recipient groups. Genetic considerations must be taken into account. They may contribute to organ failure in the mother and must be considered in the assessment of risk to the newborn. Table 54–10 summarizes the incidence of malformations reported to the NTPR in transplant recipients receiving the newer immunosuppressants. Of concern is the potential for more subtle effects that may not be apparent at birth, but may affect long-term growth and development as well as the next generation.[36] Clinical reports noted that children of recipients are developing well, although there is concern that alterations in T cell subpopulations may affect vaccinations or long-term immunity.[37,38] A large series of 175 newborns of cyclosporine-treated kidney recipients reported to the NTPR showed no evidence of an increased incidence of developmental delays over that expected, given the high percentage of premature offspring in this group.[39]

TABLE 54–4

Female Kidney Recipients

	CYCLOSPORINE (SANDIMMUNE) [321 RECIPIENTS, 485 PREGNANCIES]	CYCLOSPORINE (NEORAL) [100 RECIPIENTS, 133 PREGNANCIES]	TACROLIMUS (38 RECIPIENTS, 47 PREGNANCIES)
Maternal Factors			
Transplant-to-conception interval	3.3 yr	5.2 yr	2.8 yr
Hypertension during pregnancy	63%	72%	53%
Diabetes during pregnancy	12%	5%	15%
Infection during pregnancy	23%	23%	33%
Rejection episode during pregnancy*	4%	2%	5%
Preeclampsia	29%	30%	32%
Mean serum creatinine level (mg/dL)			
Before pregnancy	1.4	1.3	1.3
During pregnancy	1.4	1.4	1.7
After pregnancy	1.6	1.5	1.6
Graft loss within 2 yr of delivery	9%	2%	17%
Outcome (*n*)†	494	141	48
Therapeutic abortion	8%	1%	2%
Spontaneous abortion	12%	18%	25%
Ectopic pregnancy	1	0	0
Stillbirth	3%	1%	4%
Live birth	76%	79%	69%
Live Births (*n*)	374	111	33
Mean gestational age	36 wk	36 wk	35 wk
Mean birth weight	2499 g	2460 g	2260 g
Premature birth (<37 wk)	52%	54%	56%
Low birth weight (<2500 g)	45%	51%	58%
Cesarean delivery	51%	43%	53%
Newborn complications	40%	48%	55%
Neonatal death (*n*) [%] (within 30 days of birth)	3 (1%)	0	1 (3%)

*Rejection for Sandimmune, including chronic rejection, Neoral, and tacrolimus biopsy-proven acute rejection.
†Includes twins and triplets.
From Armenti VT, Radomski JS, Moritz MJ, et al: Report from the National Transplantation Pregnancy Registry (NTPR): Outcomes of Pregnancy after Transplantation. In Cecka JM, Terasaki PI (eds): Clinical Transplants 2002. Los Angeles, UCLA Immunogenetics Center, 2003, pp 121–130.

Childhood transplant recipients who subsequently become pregnant in adulthood are of increasing relevance (Table 54–11).[40] The risk of malformations in newborns of these patients is not increased, but a small percentage of recipients have graft rejection, dysfunction, or even loss within 2 years of delivery. Consistent features of obstetric outcome are higher incidences of prematurity and low birth weight, depending on the type of organ transplant. These rates are always much higher than in the general population.

MANAGEMENT OPTIONS

Prepregnancy and Prenatal

Recommendations for the management of pregnancy after transplantation have been published.[41–56] Transplantation restores fertility, and patients must be advised about appropriate birth control. For all organ recipients, an interval from transplant to conception is advisable to allow establishment of stable graft function and reduction of immunosuppression to maintenance levels, with concomitant reduction of the risk of more serious post-transplant infections. NTPR data showed a higher incidence of pregnancy termination and peripartum rejection with transplant-to-conception intervals of less than 6 months compared with longer intervals in cyclosporine-treated kidney recipients. Waiting at least 6 months, and preferably, 1 year from transplant seems advisable.[57] It is important to note whether the recipient has been rejection-free (and for how long) as well as the level and stability of graft function.

No specific combination of immunosuppressive agents is known to be teratogenic, although there is concern about the newer agents mycophenolate mofetil and sirolimus, given their mechanisms of action. Clinical data are sparse, and there are no definitive recommendations for switching a recipient from one regimen to another prepregnancy or for a specific regimen for women of reproductive age. Pregnancy should be considered high risk, and there should be close communication among the transplant surgeons, transplant physicians, and obstetricians.

A significant percentage of recipients have hypertension and may be receiving a combination of antihypertensive medications. Angiotensin-converting enzyme

TABLE 54-5

Pregnancy Outcomes in Female Liver Recipients*

	CYCLOSPORINE (SANDIMMUNE) [59 RECIPIENTS, 94 PREGNANCIES]	CYCLOSPORINE (NEORAL) [21 RECIPIENTS, 29 PREGNANCIES]	TACROLIMUS (28 RECIPIENTS, 41 PREGNANCIES)
Maternal Factors			
Transplant-to-conception interval	3.4 yr	6.1 yr	2.8 yr
Hypertension during pregnancy	40%	39%	25%
Diabetes during pregnancy	2%	0	15%
Infection during pregnancy	32%	36%	17%
Rejection episode during pregnancy	13%	3%	8%
Preeclampsia	25%	32%	14%
Graft loss within 2 yr of delivery	8%	10%	4%
Outcome (*n*)†	95	29	41
Therapeutic abortion	11%	0	0
Spontaneous abortion	14%	24%	27%
Ectopic pregnancy	0	0	0
Stillbirth	3%	0	2%
Live birth	73%	76%	71%
Live Births (*n*)	69	22	29
Mean gestational age	37 wk	38 wk	37 wk
Premature birth (<37 wk)	38%	27%	38%
Mean birth weight	2635 g	2768 g	2828 g
Low birth weight (<2500 g)	35%	35%	28%
Cesarean delivery	42%	18%	30%
Newborn complications	26%	32%	31%
Neonatal death (within 30 days of birth)	0	0	0

*Some recipients had a subsequent pregnancy while receiving a different regimen; two recipients with five pregnancies that occured while they were receiving no immunosuppression are not included in this table.

†Includes twins.

From Armenti VT, Radomski JS, Moritz MJ, et al: Report from the National Transplantation Pregnancy Registry (NTPR): Outcomes of Pregnancy after Transplantation. In Cecka JM, Terasaki PI (eds): Clinical Transplants 2002. Los Angeles, UCLA Immunogenetics Center, 2003, pp 121–130.

inhibitors and angiotensin II receptor antagonists are contraindicated during pregnancy, but their adverse effects have been noted from midpregnancy onward, so it can be argued that they may be continued until conception.[45,58] If dosage adjustments or changes to hypertensive agents are needed, these changes can be made in anticipation of pregnancy. In addition to hypertension and preeclampsia, attention should be focused on other comorbid conditions that are likely to occur, including infections and gestational diabetes.

Rejection, although not common, must be considered in the face of graft dysfunction. The etiology of graft dysfunction in any solid organ recipient must be investigated. There are special clinical considerations for each organ group. In the renal transplant group, the group with the most data, the usual pattern for the serum creatinine level is a slight decrease in early pregnancy, with a return to baseline postpartum. Increases during pregnancy and postpartum should be evaluated. Pancreas–kidney recipients usually can tolerate pregnancy without problems with glucose control, but additional comorbid conditions caused by cardiovascular disease must be considered. Lung recipients appear to have a higher incidence of peripartum problems in terms of both graft function and patient survival.

Infectious complications during pregnancy are most often urinary tract infections. Therefore, monthly urine culture should be performed. Occasionally, more serious yeast infections, pneumonia, sepsis, or unspecified viral infections complicate pregnancy. Cytomegalovirus is usually asymptomatic and is detected by serologic, antigen, or viral monitoring. If a primary infection occurs during pregnancy, there is a risk of transmission with fetal sequelae, but the effectiveness of treating the mother's infection in preventing or ameliorating fetal sequelae is uncertain.

The rate of hepatitis C transmission from mother to child in the nontransplant population is 5%,[59] with one case reported to the NTPR. Recipients with acute hepatitis B infection may transmit it to their offspring. Administration of hepatitis B immune globulin and hepatitis B virus vaccine to the newborn within a few hours of birth usually prevents transmission. Estimates of the incidence of acute infection with toxoplasmosis are 0.2% to 1%, with most cases undiagnosed and asymptomatic. Congenital toxoplasmosis can have severe consequences, and the diagnosis is dependent on culture, direct antigen detection, or serologic tests.[60]

Scrutiny for hypertensive changes and preeclampsia is essential, although the diagnosis of preeclampsia may be difficult because serum uric acid levels and urinary

TABLE 54–6

Pregnancy Outcomes in 31 Female Pancreas–Kidney Recipients with 47 Pregnancies

MATERNAL FACTORS	
Transplant-to-conception interval	3.8 yr
Hypertension during pregnancy	78%
Diabetes during pregnancy	0
Infection during pregnancy	50%
Rejection episode during pregnancy	7%
Preeclampsia	36%
Graft loss within 2 yr of delivery	18%
Outcome (*n*)*	49
Therapeutic abortion	6%
Spontaneous abortion	12%
Ectopic pregnancy	2%
Stillbirth	0
Live birth	80%
Live Births (*n*)	39
Mean gestational age	35 wk
Premature birth (<37 wk)	74%
Mean birth weight	2159 g
Low birth weight (<2500 g)	59%
Cesarean delivery	54%
Newborn complications	56%
Neonatal death† (within 30 days of birth)	1 (3%)
Immunosuppression by pregnancy *n* (%)	
Cyclosporine, azathioprine, and prednisone	19 (40)
Cyclosporine and prednisone	6 (13)
Cyclosporine (Neoral), azathioprine, and prednisone	12 (26)
Neoral and prednisone	3 (6)
Tacrolimus, azathioprine, and prednisone	4 (9)
Tacrolimus and azathioprine	2 (4)
Tacrolimus and prednisone	1 (2)

*Includes twins.
†One neonatal death as a result of sepsis (26 wk, 624 g).
From Armenti VT, Radomski JS, Moritz MJ, et al: Report from the National Transplantation Pregnancy Registry (NTPR): Outcomes of Pregnancy after Transplantation. In Cecka JM, Terasaki PI (eds): Clinical Transplants 2002. Los Angeles, UCLA Immunogenetics Center, 2003, pp 121–130.

TABLE 54–7

Pregnancy Outcomes in 31 Female Heart and 13 Female Heart-Lung Transplant Recipients

	ORGAN (*N*)	
MATERNAL FACTORS	HEART (31)	LUNG (13)
Transplant-to-conception interval	4.0 yr	2.7 yr
Hypertension during pregnancy	48%	50%
Diabetes during pregnancy	4%	21%
Infection during pregnancy	12%	15%
Rejection episode during pregnancy	22%	31%
Preeclampsia	11%	13%
Graft loss within 2 yr of delivery	0	23%
Outcome (*n*)	52	14
Therapeutic abortion	10%	36%
Spontaneous abortion	17%	7%
Ectopic pregnancy	2%	0
Stillbirth	2%	0
Live births	69%	57%
Live Births (*n*)	36	8
Mean gestational age	37 wk	35 wk
Premature birth (<37 wk)	43%	63%
Mean birth weight	2711 g	2285 g
Low birth weight (<2500 g)	36%	63%
Cesarean delivery	30%	38%
Newborn complications	23%	75%
Neonatal death (within 30 days of birth)	0	0

From Armenti VT, Radomski JS, Moritz MJ, et al: Report from the National Transplantation Pregnancy Registry (NTPR): Outcomes of Pregnancy after Transplantation. In Cecka JM, Terasaki PI (eds): Clinical Transplants 2002. Los Angeles, UCLA Immunogenetics Center, 2003, pp 121–130.

TABLE 54–8

Outcomes of Cyclosporine (Neoral) or Tacrolimus Treatment in Female Kidney Recipients with Biopsy-Proven Acute Rejection Episodes during Pregnancy

CASE	REGIMEN	PREPREGNANCY LEVEL CREATININE (mg/dL)	REJECTION TREATMENT	GRAFT LOSS <2 YR POSTPARTUM	OUTCOME	GESTATIONAL AGE (WK)	BIRTH WEIGHT (G)
1	Cyclosporine (Neoral) switched to tacrolimus during pregnancy*	1.3	OKT3 and radiation	Yes	Spontaneous abortion	6	N/A
2	Tacrolimus	2.8	Muromonab-CD3 (OKT3) and methylprednisolone	No	Spontaneous abortion	7	N/A
3	Neoral	1.2	Methylprednisolone	No	Live birth	32	1378
4	Neoral	3.0	Methylprednisolone	No	Live birth	29	1247
5	Neoral	2.6	Reinitiate immuno-suppression†	No	Live birth	32	1417
6	Tacrolimus	1.0	Antithymocyte globulin (Thymoglobulin) and sirolimus	Yes	Live birth	32	1531

*Both recipients stopped taking their medications during pregnancy.
†The recipient was being treated for cancer.
From Armenti VT, Radomski JS, Moritz MJ, et al: Report from the National Transplantation Pregnancy Registry (NTPR): Outcomes of Pregnancy after Transplantation. In Cecka JM, Terasaki PI (eds): Clinical Transplants 2002. Los Angeles, UCLA Immunogenetics Center, 2003, pp 121–130.

TABLE 54-9

National Transplantation Pregnancy Registry: Live Birth Outcomes of Liver Recipients with Biopsy-Proven Acute Rejection during Pregnancy

CASE	MATERNAL IMMUNOSUPPRESSION	GESTATIONAL AGE (WK)	BIRTH WEIGHT (G)	NEWBORN COMPLICATIONS
1	Cyclosporine	35	1673	Jaundice
2	Cyclosporine	34	1474	
3	Cyclosporine	37	2693	
4	Cyclosporine	39	2920	
5	Cyclosporine	27	964	Bronchopulmonary dysplasia requiring oxygen for 3 yr and pyloric stenosis repair at 3 mo
6	Tacrolimus	38	2892	
7	Tacrolimus	34	2268	
8	Cyclosporine	27	680	Death at 3.5 mo as a result of complications of prematurity
Mean		33.8	1946	

From Armenti VT, Herrine SK, Radomski JS, et al: Pregnancy after liver transplantation. Liver Transplant 2000;6:671–685.

protein excretion may be well above expected normal ranges without preeclampsia, as a result of drug nephrotoxicity or the renal allograft. Other complications include HELLP syndrome, ureteral obstruction, and complications of cesarean delivery. Peripartum ultrasound assessment to exclude urinary obstruction is warranted if the serum creatinine level increases.

Unless obvious immunosuppressive toxicity or rejection occurs, it is best to maintain baseline immunosuppressive dosing. Blood concentrations are likely to decrease during pregnancy, given the increased maternal volume of distribution as well as fetal metabolism of drugs. Some recipients are noncompliant, choosing to stop taking medications during pregnancy for fear that the medication will harm the fetus. Reports to the registry show that, in most pregnancies, immunosuppressive doses have been kept the same or increased during pregnancy. Regardless of dosing during pregnancy, many changes that occur peripartum mandate that postpartum immunosuppressive dosing should be directed by blood level, when possible.

Significant unexplained deterioration in graft function should be assessed with biopsy. For heart recipients to avoid x-ray exposure, biopsy can be done with echocardiographic guidance.[49] If the diagnosis of acute rejection is made, then appropriate antirejection regimens are necessary. Given the risk of rejection and preeclampsia, more frequent monitoring is warranted from midpregnancy onward, including blood pressure measurements, assessment of graft function, and measurement of immunosuppressive drug levels.

In liver recipients, worsening liver function with chronic rejection or hepatitis C has been noted, with further deterioration in subsequent pregnancies.[61] Whether such deterioration is time-linked or pregnancy-induced requires further study. Recipients with stable graft function have tolerated subsequent pregnancies. Data to support this observation have been noted in each recipient group but are more easily quantified among kidney recipients.

Labor and Delivery

A high incidence of cesarean delivery is reported in all organ recipient groups. Cesarean delivery is performed for obstetric indications only. Immunosuppression must not be interrupted during labor and delivery.

TABLE 54-10

Reported Birth Defects in Offspring of Female Kidney Recipients Taking Cyclosporine (Neoral) or Tacrolimus during Pregnancy

DEFECT	*N*	REGIMEN
Cleft lip and palate and ear deformity	1	Tacrolimus, mycophenolate mofetil, then sirolimus and prednisone
Hypoplastic nails and shortened fifth fingers	1	Tacrolimus, mycophenolate mofetil, and prednisone
Renal cystic dysplasia	1	Tacrolimus, alone
Submucosal cleft palate	1	Neoral, azathioprine, and prednisone
Tongue-tied	1	Neoral, azathioprine, and prednisone
Pyloric stenosis	1	Neoral, azathioprine, and prednisone
Imperforate anus, clubbed feet, hypospadias	1	Neoral, azathioprine, and prednisone
Total number of live-born infants with birth defects	7/140 (5%)	

From Armenti VT, Radomski JS, Moritz MJ, et al: Report from the National Transplantation Pregnancy Registry (NTPR): Outcomes of Pregnancy after Transplantation. In Cecka JM, Terasaki PI (eds): Clinical Transplants 2002. Los Angeles, UCLA Immunogenetics Center, 2003, pp 121–130.

TABLE 54–11

National Transplantation Pregnancy Registry: Outcomes in Pediatric Female Kidney Recipients (Younger Than 21 Years at Transplant)

	CYCLOSPORINE (SANDIMMUNE) [86 RECIPIENTS, 142 PREGNANCIES; 1 OUTCOME UNKNOWN]	CYCLOSPORINE (NEORAL) [25 RECIPIENTS, 31 PREGNANCIES]	TACROLIMUS-PROGRAF (11 RECIPIENTS, 13 PREGNANCIES)
Maternal Factors			
Transplant-to-conception interval*	3.9 yr	7.2 yr	3.3 yr
Hypertension during pregnancy	56%	68%	54%
Diabetes during pregnancy	2%	3%	0
Infection during pregnancy	26%	26%	67%
Rejection episode during pregnancy	1%	0	15%
Preeclampsia	26%	45%	8%
Mean serum creatinine level (mg/dL)			
Before pregnancy	1.4	1.3	1.2
During pregnancy	1.4	1.3	2.9
After pregnancy	1.7	1.4	1.9
Graft loss within 2 yr of delivery	12%	0	36%
Outcome (*n*)†	145	33	13
Therapeutic abortion	9%	0	0
Spontaneous abortion	10%	9%	15%
Ectopic pregnancy	0	0	0
Stillbirth	5%	3%	15%
Live birth	76%	88%	69%
Live Births (*n*)	110	29	9
Mean gestational age	36 wk	37 wk	35 wk
Mean birth weight	2512 g	2547 g	2422g
Premature birth (<37 wk)	49%	52%	44%
Low birth weight (<2500 g)	46%	48%	56%
Cesarean delivery	52%	46%	67%
Newborn complications	38%	24%	56%
Neonatal death (within 30 days of birth) [*n* (%)]	1 (1)	0	0

*Calculated from the most recent transplant before the estimated date of conception.
†Includes twins and triplets.
From Armenti VT, Moritz MJ, Davison JM: Pregnancy in female pediatric solid organ transplant recipients. Pediatr Clin North Am 2003;50:1543–1560.

Postnatal

Most oral maintenance agents are easily absorbed, and treatment can usually be resumed shortly after cesarean delivery. When oral treatment cannot be resumed, intravenous formulations are available for most, but not all, agents. Immunosuppressive drug levels should be monitored and dosage adjusted appropriately, which may affect blood pressure, renal function, and other toxicities.

One must be aware of postpartum depression among transplant recipients, as medications may be missed or not taken. Therefore, close monitoring is required for several months postpartum.

Breastfeeding is controversial.[61–64] Although exposure of the newborn to an immunosuppressive drug may be detrimental, a newly emerging view is that the benefits of breastfeeding outweigh the minimal risk. Further study of potential long-term effects is needed.

CONCLUSIONS

- Successful pregnancy is possible after transplantation.
- Before becoming pregnant, recipients should have stable graft function and optimal control of comorbid conditions.
- Although the shortest safe interval between transplant and conception has not been established, 1 year is a reasonable milestone, given the prerequisites of stable, adequate graft function and maintenance-level immunosuppression.
- Stable medical regimens should be changed as little as possible, and close maternal and fetal surveillance is required during pregnancy.
- These pregnancies are high risk and require coordinated care by perinatal specialists and transplant personnel.

SUMMARY OF MANAGEMENT OPTIONS

Pregnancy after Transplantation

Management Options	Quality of Evidence	Strength of Recommendation	References
Prepregnancy			
Patients should defer conception for at least 1 year after transplantation, with adequate contraception.	IIb	B	26,55,57,65
Assessment of graft function:	III	B	26,46,65
• Recent biopsy	III	B	66
• Proteinuria	III	B	66
• Hepatitis B and C status	IV	C	44
• Cytomegalovirus, toxoplasmosis, and herpes simplex status	IV	C	44, 46
Maintenance immunosuppression options: • Azathioprine • Cyclosporine • Tacrolimus • Corticosteroids • Mycophenolate mofetil • Sirolimus	IV	C	7,19,28,33, 35,41,42,44, 49,54,67,68
The effect of comorbid conditions (e.g., diabetes, hypertension) should be considered and their management optimized; nonrenal recipients should have their baseline kidney function assessed.	III	B	22,26,45,69
Vaccinations should be given, if needed (e.g., rubella).	IV	C	26,44
Explore the etiology of the original disease; discuss genetic issues, if relevant.	IV	C	26,70
Discuss the effect of pregnancy on renal allograft function.	IIa	B	23–26
Discuss the risks of intrauterine growth restriction, prematurity, and low birth weight.	III	B	19,26–28,56
Prenatal			
Accurate early diagnosis and dating of pregnancy	IV	C	26
Clinical and laboratory monitoring of the functional status of transplanted organs and immunosuppressive drug levels: • Every 4 weeks until 32 weeks • Every 2 weeks until 36 weeks • Then weekly, until delivery	III	B	26,44,46, 49,71,72
Monthly urine culture	IV	C	26,44,47
Surveillance for rejection, with biopsy considered if it is suspected	III	B	19,26,44,61
Surveillance for bacterial or viral infection (e.g., cytomegalovirus, toxoplasmosis, hepatitis)	IV	C	26,44,46
Fetal surveillance	IV	C	26,46,55
Monitoring for hypertension and nephropathy	IV	C	26,28,44,48,69
Surveillance for preeclampsia	IV	C	26,46
Screening for gestational diabetes	IV	C	26
Labor and Delivery			
Vaginal delivery is optimal; cesarean delivery is used for obstetric reasons.	IV	C	26,47
For kidney recipients, episiotomy is performed on the side opposite the allograft.		GPP	
For heart, lung, or heart–lung recipients: • Vigilance for poor or absent cough reflex and the need for airway protection • Unpredictable response to vasoactive medications • Judicious use of intravenous fluids		GPP	

SUMMARY OF MANAGEMENT OPTIONS
Pregnancy after Transplantation *(Continued)*

Management Options	Quality of Evidence	Strength of Recommendation	References
Postnatal			
Monitor immunosuppressive drug levels for at least 1 month postpartum, especially if dosages were adjusted during pregnancy.	III	B	44,49,67,71
Surveillance for rejection, with biopsy considered if it is suspected	III	B	19,26,61
Breastfeeding	III	B	61–64
Contraception counseling	IV	C	26

REFERENCES

1. United Network for Organ Sharing: Time line of key events in U.S. transplantation and UNOS history. Retrieved November 5, 2003, from UNOS Web site: http://www.unos.org/inthenews/factsheets.asp.
2. Murray JE, Reid DE, Harrison JH, et al: Successful pregnancies after human renal transplantation. N Engl J Med 1963;269:341–343.
3. Worldwide Transplant Center Directory. In Cecka JM, Terasaki PI: Clinical Transplants 2002. Los Angeles, UCLA Immunogenetics Center, 2003, pp 428–537.
4. Bartlett ST: Laproscopic donor nephrectomy after seven years. Am J Transplant 2002;2:896–897.
5. Stuart FP: Annual literature review: Clinical transplants 2001–2002. In Cecka JM, Terasaki PI (eds): Clinical Transplants 2002. Los Angeles, UCLA Immunogenetics Center, 2003, pp 273–298.
6. Moritz MJ, Armenti VT: Organ transplantation. In Jarrell BE, Carabasi RA (eds): National Medical Series for Independent Study: Surgery. Philadelphia, Lippincott Williams & Wilkins, 2000, pp 461–477.
7. Armenti VT, Moritz MJ, Davison JM: Drug safety issues in pregnancy following transplantation and immunosuppression. Drug Saf 1998;19:219–232.
8. Fraser FC, Fainstat TD: The production of congenital defects in the offspring of pregnant mice treated with cortisone: A progress report. Pediatrics 1951;8:527–533.
9. Hou S: Pregnancy in transplant recipients. Med Clin North Am 1989;73:667–683.
10. Davison, JM: Dialysis, transplantation, and pregnancy. Am J Kidney Dis 1991;17:127–132.
11. Leb DE, Weisskopf B, Kanovitz BS: Chromosome aberrations in the child of a kidney transplant recipient. Arch Intern Med 1971;128:441–444.
12. Mason RJ, Thomson AW, Whiting PH, et al: Cyclosporine-induced feto-toxicity in the rat. Transplantation 1985;39:9–12.
13. Fein A, Vechoropoulos M, Nebel L: Cyclosporin-induced embryotoxicity in mice. Biol Neonate 1989;56:165–173.
14. Pickrell MD, Sawers R, Michael J: Pregnancy after renal transplantation: Severe intra-uterine growth retardation during treatment with cyclosporin A. BMJ 1988;296:825.
15. Farley DE, Shelby J, Alexander D, Scott JR: The effect of two new immunosuppressive agents, FK506 and didemnin B, in murine pregnancy. Transplantation 1991;52:106–110.
16. Jain A, Venkataramanan R, Fung JJ, et al: Pregnancy after liver transplantation under tacrolimus. Transplantation 1997;64:559–565.
17. Roche Laboratories: Mycophenolate mofetil package insert. Nutley, NJ, Roche Laboratories, 2000.
18. Pérgola PE, Kancharla A, Riley DJ: Kidney transplantation during the first trimester of pregnancy: Immunosuppression with mycophenolate mofetil, tacrolimus and prednisone. Transplantation 2000;71:94–97.
19. Armenti VT, Radomski JS, Moritz MJ, et al: Report from the National Transplantation Pregnancy Registry (NTPR): Outcomes of Pregnancy after Transplantation. In Cecka JM, Terasaki PI (eds): Clinical Transplants 2002. Los Angeles, UCLA Immunogenetics Center, 2003, pp 121–130.
20. Wyeth-Ayerst Pharmaceuticals: Sirolimus package insert. Philadelphia, Wyeth Laboratories, 2001.
21. Davison JM, Lind T, Uldall PR: Planned pregnancy in a renal transplant recipient. BJOG 1976;83:518–527.
22. Baylis C: Glomerular filtration and volume regulation in gravid animal models. In Lindheimer MD, Davison JM (eds): Ballieres Clin Obstet Gynaecol 1994;8(2):235–264.
23. First MR, Combs CA, Weiskittel P, et al: Lack of effect of pregnancy on renal allograft survival or function. Transplantation 1995;59:472–476.
24. Sturgiss SN, Davison JM: Effect of pregnancy on long-term function renal allografts. Am J Kidney Dis 1992;19:167–172.
25. Sturgiss SN, Davison JM: Effect of pregnancy on the long-term function of renal allografts: An update. Am J Kidney Dis 1995;26:54–56.
26. Davison JM: Pregnancy in renal allograft recipients: Problems, prognosis and practicalities. In Lindheimer MD, Davison JM (eds): Ballieres Clin Obstet Gynaecol 1994;8(2):501–525.
27. Davison JM: Renal disorders in pregnancy. Curr Opin Obstet Gynecol 2001;13:109–114.
28. Armenti VT, Ahlswede KM, Ahlswede BA, et al: National Transplantation Pregnancy Registry: Outcomes of 154 pregnancies in cyclosporine-treated female kidney transplant recipients. Transplantation 1994;57:502–506.
29. Davison JM, Redman CWG: Pregnancy post-transplant: The establishment of a UK registry. BJOG 1997; 104:1106–1107.
30. Case AM, Weissman A, Sermer M, Greenblatt EM: Successful twin pregnancy in a dual-transplant couple resulting from in-vitro fertilization and intracytoplasmic sperm injection. Hum Reprod 2000;15:626.
31. Coscia LA, Cardonick EH, Moritz MJ, Armenti VT: Multiple gestations in female kidney transplant recipients maintained on calcineurin inhibitors. Am J Transplant 2003;5:A1603.
32. Jimenez E, Gonzalea-Carabello Z, Morales-Otero L, Santiago-Delpin EA: Triplets born to a kidney transplant recipient. Transplantation 1995;59:435–436.
33. Oz BB, Hackman R, Einarson T, Koren G: Pregnancy outcome after cyclosporine therapy during pregnancy: A meta-analysis. Transplantation 2001;71:1051–1055.

34. Armenti VT, Radomski JS, Moritz MJ, et al: National Transplantation Pregnancy Registry (NTPR): Outcomes of pregnancy after transplantation. In Cecka JM, Terasaki PI (eds): Clinical Transplants 2001. Los Angeles, UCLA Immunogenetics Center, 2002, pp 97–105.
35. Kainz A, Harabacz I, Cowlrick IS, et al: Review of the course and outcome of 100 pregnancies in 84 women treated with tacrolimus. Transplantation 2000;70:1718–1721.
36. Scott JR, Branch DW, Holman J: Autoimmune and pregnancy complications in the daughter of a kidney transplant patient. Transplantation 2002;73:815–816.
37. Pilarski LM, Yacyshyn BR, Lavarovits AI: Analysis of peripheral blood lymphocyte populations and immune function from children exposed to cyclosporine or azathioprine in utero. Transplantation 1994;57:133–144.
38. Di Paolo S, Schena A, Morrone L, et al: Immunologic evaluation during the first year of life of infants born to cyclosporine-treated kidney transplant recipients: Analysis of lymphocyte subpopulation and immunoglobulin serum levels. Transplantation 2000;69:2049–2054.
39. Stanley CW, Gottlieb R, Zager R, et al: Developmental well-being in offspring of women receiving cyclosporine post-renal transplant. Transplant Proc 1999;31:241–242.
40. Armenti VT, Moritz MJ, Davison JM: Pregnancy in female pediatric solid organ transplant recipients. Pediatr Clin North Am 2003;50:1543–1560.
41. Barrou BM, Gruessner AC, Sutherland DER, et al: Pregnancy after pancreas transplantation in the cyclosporine era. Transplantation 1998;65:524–527.
42. Nagy S, Bush M, Berkowitz R, et al: Pregnancy outcome in liver transplant recipients. Obstet Gynecol 2003;102:121–128.
43. Scantlebury V, Gordon R, Tzakis A, et al: Childbearing after liver transplantation. Transplantation 1990;49:317–321.
44. Hou S: Pregnancy in chronic renal insufficiency and end-stage renal disease. Am J Kidney Dis 1999;33:235–252.
45. EBPG Expert Group on Renal Transplantation: European best practice guidelines for renal transplantation. Nephrol Dial Transplant 2002;17:50–55.
46. Armenti VT, Moritz MJ, Davison JM: Medical management of the pregnant transplant recipient. Adv Renal Replace Ther 1998;5:14–23.
47. McGrory CH, Groshek MA, Sollinger HW, et al: Pregnancy outcomes in female pancreas-kidney recipients. Transplant Proc 1999;31:652–653.
48. Carr DB, Larson AM, Schmucker BC, et al: Maternal hemodynamics and pregnancy outcome in women with prior orthotopic liver transplantation. Liver Transplant 2000;6:213–221.
49. Wagoner LE, Taylor DO, Olsen SL, et al: Immunosuppressive therapy, management, and outcome of heart transplant recipients during pregnancy. J Heart Lung Transplant 1993;12:993–999.
50. Branch KR, Wagoner LE, McGrory CH, et al: Risks of subsequent pregnancies on mother and newborn in female heart transplant recipients. J Heart Lung Transplant 1998;17:698–702.
51. Gertner G, Coscia L, McGrory C, et al: Pregnancy in lung transplant recipients. Prog Transplant 2000;10:109–112.
52. Donaldson S, Novotny D, Paradowski L, Aris R: Acute and chronic lung allograft rejection during pregnancy. Chest 1996;110:293–296.
53. Armenti VT, Herrine SK, Moritz MJ: Reproductive function after liver transplantation. Clin Liver Dis 1997;1:471–485.
54. Molmenti EP, Jain AB, Marino N, et al: Liver transplantation and pregnancy. Clin Liver Dis 1999;3:163–174.
55. Laifer SA, Guido RS: Reproductive function and outcome of pregnancy after liver transplantation in women. Mayo Clin Proc 1995;70:388–394.
56. Armenti VT, Ahlswede KM, Ahlswede BA, et al: Variables affecting birthweight and graft survival in 197 pregnancies in cyclosporine-treated female kidney transplant recipients. Transplantation 1995;59:476–479.
57. Gaughan WJ, Coscia LA, Dunn, SR, et al: National Transplantation Pregnancy Registry: Relationship of transplant to conception interval to pregnancy outcome in cyclosporine-treated female kidney recipients. Am J Transplant 2001;1:S377.
58. Hanssens M, Keirse MJNC, Vankelecom F, Van Assche FA: Fetal and neonatal effects of treatment with angiotensin-converting enzyme inhibitors in pregnancy. Obstet Gynecol 1991;78:128–135.
59. Conte D, Fraquell M, Prati D, et al: Prevalence and clinical course of chronic hepatitis C virus (HCV) infection and rate of vertical transmission in a cohort of 15,250 pregnant women. Hepatology 2000;31:751–755.
60. Wong SY, Remington JS: Toxoplasmosis in pregnancy. Clin Infect Dis 1994;18:853–862.
61. Armenti VT, Herrine SK, Radomski JS, et al: Pregnancy after liver transplantation. Liver Transplant 2000;6:671–685.
62. Nyberg G, Haljamäe U, Frisenette-Fich C, et al: Breast-feeding during treatment with cyclosporine. Transplantation 1998;65: 253–255.
63. Thiagarajan KD, Easterling T, Davis C, et al: Breast-feeding by a cyclosporine treated mother. Obstet Gynecol 2001;97:816–817.
64. French AE, Soldin SJ, Soldin OP, Koren G: Milk transfer and neonatal safety of tacrolimus. Ann Pharmacother 2003;37: 815–818.
65. Rudolph J, Schweizer RT, Bartus SA: Pregnancy in renal transplant patients. Transplantation 1979;27:26–29.
66. Kozlowska-Boszko B, Lao M, Gaciong Z, et al: Chronic rejection as a risk factor for deterioration of renal allograft function following pregnancy. Transplant Proc 1997;29:1522–1523.
67. Armenti VT, Moritz MJ, Cardonick EH, Davison JM: Immunosuppression in pregnancy: Choices for infant and maternal health. Drugs 2002;62:2361–2375.
68. Toma H, Kazunari T, Tokumoto T, et al: Pregnancy in women receiving renal dialysis or transplantation in Japan: A nationwide survey. Nephrol Dial Transplant 1999;14:1511–1516.
69. Lindheimer MD, Katz AI: Gestation in women with kidney disease: Prognosis and management. In Lindheimer MD, Davison JM (eds): Ballieres Clin Obstet Gynaecol 1994;8(2):387–404.
70. Cowan SW, Coscia LA, Philips LZ, et al: Pregnancy outcomes in female heart and heart-lung transplant recipients. Transplant Proc 2002;34:1855–1856.
71. Armenti VT, Jarrell BE, Radomski JS, et al: National Transplantation Pregnancy Registry (NTPR): Cyclosporine dosing and pregnancy outcome in female renal transplant recipients. Transplant Proc 1996;28:2111–2112.
72. Bumgardner GL, Matas AJ: Transplantation and pregnancy. Transplant Rev 1992;6:139–162.

CHAPTER 55

Trauma

Renee A. Bobrowski

INCIDENCE AND RISKS

General

Trauma occurs in 6% to 7% of all pregnancies and is the leading cause of nonobstetric maternal death.[1,2] Motor vehicle accidents (MVAs) are the most frequent cause of injury, followed by falls, direct assault to the abdomen, and penetrating trauma. Although most injuries during pregnancy are minor, 2% to 8% of victims have a life-threatening injury and require admission to an intensive care unit.[3] Maternal mortality from trauma approximates 10%, but is the same as for nonpregnant patients, when matched for injury severity.[4]

Trauma places the mother and fetus at increased risk, and fetal loss occurs in at least 40% of critically injured gravidas. Injury severity score, increasing fluid requirement during resuscitation, Glasgow coma score, and maternal acidosis and hypoxia appear to predict an increase in fetal loss.[3–7] The rate of adverse pregnancy outcome, however, is approximately 4%, even when maternal injuries are minor.[8] Because 90% of all trauma in pregnant women is minor, more fetuses die as a result of lesser injuries than as a result of catastrophic trauma.

The obstetrician must be prepared to work in concert with the trauma team to evaluate and treat an injured pregnant woman. It is imperative to understand the physiologic changes of pregnancy and the implications for managing gravid trauma patients. The presence of a fetus may be extremely unnerving to even the most experienced emergency team, and obstetric consultation can be invaluable. The basic principles of trauma management apply to injured pregnant women, and maternal resuscitation is the first priority under all circumstances. Once the maternal condition is stable, diagnostic evaluation, fetal assessment, and treatment can proceed.

Physiologic Changes of Pregnancy and Trauma

Among the many physiologic changes that occur during pregnancy, some assume greater importance in trauma. Understanding a pregnant woman's response to injury will facilitate her care from the moment of arrival in the emergency department. Table 55–1 outlines changes that are pertinent to the care of gravid trauma victims and their clinical implications.

The fetal response to trauma depends on the severity of maternal injury and the adequacy of placental perfusion. Uterine perfusion depends on maternal blood pressure because the uterine arteries lack autoregulation and are maximally dilated during pregnancy. Maternal hypotension and hypoxia increase the secretion of catecholamines, which are potent vasoconstrictors of the uterine artery. Normal maternal heart rate and blood pressure do not ensure adequate placental perfusion and fetal oxygenation. Therefore, these vital signs are poor indicators of fetal well-being.[4]

MANAGEMENT OPTIONS—GENERAL

Basic Principles of Trauma Resuscitation During Pregnancy

Emergency department evaluation and treatment of the injured gravida should proceed in a timely and organized fashion. Ideally, each member of the trauma team is assigned specific tasks to avoid confusion and duplication of services. Patients with minor injuries should receive routine medical treatment and appropriate fetal assessment. The management of gravidas with moderate to severe injuries can be divided into the following steps:

- Primary survey
- Resuscitation

TABLE 55–1

Clinical Implications of the Physiologic Changes of Pregnancy in the Patient with Traumatic Injury

PHYSIOLOGIC CHANGE	CLINICAL IMPLICATION
Blood volume increases 50%	Blood loss may exceed 30% before clinical signs of hypovolemia occur Aggressive volume replacement is needed
Systemic vascular resistance decreases	Misinterpreted as hemodynamic instability
Heart rate increases	Misinterpreted as early decompensation
Respiratory rate and tidal volume increase	Normal P_{CO_2} = 30 mm Hg
Minute ventilation and oxygen consumption increase	More susceptible to hypoxemia with apnea
Diaphragm is elevated	Perform thoracostomy 1–2 interspaces higher than normal
Gastrointestinal motility decreases	Aspiration risk increases
Distended abdomen occurs with advancing gestation	Sensitivity of peritoneal signs decreases
Uterine enlargement occurs	Protects bowel with lower abdominal penetrating trauma
Uterine blood flow increases	Risk of hemorrhage and retroperitoneal bleeding increases
Bladder is displaced into the abdomen	More susceptible to injury
Renal blood flow increases	Normal serum blood urea nitrogen and creatinine levels = 12 and 0.8 mg/dL, respectively
Hypomotility of the renal collecting system occurs	Ureteral dilation and mild hydronephrosis (right > left)
White blood cell count increases	Nonspecific for injury
Levels of fibrinogen and factors VII, VIII, IX, and X increase	Hypercoaguable state; risk of thrombosis increases

- Secondary survey
- Laboratory and diagnostic studies
- Definitive treatment (Table 55–2)[9,10]

The steps in this algorithm may occur simultaneously in the emergency department.

Primary Survey

The primary survey focuses on identifying life-threatening injuries and initiating resuscitative measures. Details of the event, the mechanism of injury, resuscitation attempts in the field, and the patient's medical history should be obtained from the transporting paramedics. The components of the primary survey include the ABCs of resuscitation (airway, breathing, and circulation), an initial physical examination with adequate exposure to identify injuries, and a brief neurologic assessment.

The highest priority is to establish that the patient has an adequate airway. This can be accomplished in many cases by talking to the patient. A patient who can speak in complete sentences, in a normal voice, and can respond appropriately has a patent airway as well as adequate oxygenation and brain perfusion. If there is evidence of airway compromise, endotracheal intubation should be performed without delay.

Once the airway is deemed adequate, breathing must be assessed. The chest should be examined for expansion, breath sounds, crepitus, subcutaneous emphysema, and open wounds. Supplemental oxygen, 100% by mask, is administered until respiratory assessment is completed. Pulse oximetry can objectively confirm normal oxygen saturation unless the patient has hypotension, peripheral

TABLE 55–2

Summary of General Principles of Trauma Resuscitation

Primary Survey

Identify and treat life-threatening conditions
- Airway
- Breathing
- Circulation
  - Venous access
  - Fluid and blood component therapy
  - Left lateral positioning
- Initial neurologic assessment
- Appropriate exposure for initial physical examination

Resuscitation

Response to initial treatment
- Pulse rate and blood pressure
- Urinary output
- Continue resuscitative measures

Secondary Survey

Initiate once patient is stabilized
- Complete physical examination
- Obstetric evaluation
  - Fundal height
  - Uterine tone, contractions, and tenderness
  - Fetal assessment: fetal heart rate, nonstress test, ultrasonographic examination
  - Pelvic examination
- Laboratory studies (See Table 55–3)
- Diagnostic studies
  - Focused assessment with sonography for trauma
  - Computed tomography
  - Diagnostic peritoneal lavage

Definitive Treatment

Consult with appropriate specialists for treatment of specific injuries
Assess the need for transport
Provide deep vein thrombosis prophylaxis
Give tetanus immunization as needed
Administer Rh-immune globulin if the patient is Rh-negative

vasoconstriction, or severe anemia. If there is evidence of maternal hypoxia, arterial blood gas analysis should be obtained while the patient breathes room air (when possible). Oxygen can be weaned based on the clinical assessment and the patient's condition. When a nasogastric tube is required for gastric decompression, it should be placed after adequate ventilation is established.

Endotracheal intubation and mechanical ventilation may be required when a patient cannot maintain adequate ventilation or oxygenation. Intubation should not be delayed with the expectation that a patient's respiratory status will quickly and spontaneously improve. Blood gas analysis can be helpful in the decision-making process, but clinical judgment is equally important. Indications for intubation and mechanical ventilation include airway obstruction, inability to protect the airway, hypoxia, coma, shock, flail chest, open chest wounds, and ineffective ventilation. Adequate preoxygenation before intubation and prompt reoxygenation afterward are important because oxygen consumption increases during pregnancy. Because lower esophageal sphincter tone is decreased during pregnancy, rapid-sequence induction with cricoid pressure should be performed. Postintubation chest radiography is mandatory to confirm proper tube placement.

Circulation is the third component of the ABCs that requires immediate assessment. The hemodynamic changes of pregnancy can result in a misleading impression of maternal stability. Blood volume increases 50% during pregnancy, and gravid women tolerate a greater degree of acute blood loss before hemodynamic compromise occurs. Pulse rate and blood pressure may not change until 30% to 35% of blood volume has been lost.[11] Tachycardia and hypotension therefore are absent in a pregnant woman during the early phase of shock. Conversely, a gravida who has tachycardia and hypotension has lost a significant proportion of her blood volume and will need aggressive resuscitation with fluids and blood products.

A pregnant patient who is lying supine should have a left lateral tilt, particularly during the second and third trimesters. Left lateral positioning maximizes cardiac output by reducing uterine pressure on the inferior vena cava and allowing adequate venous return. If a spine injury is suspected or documented, a rolled towel or blanket can be placed beneath the spine board at the level of the hips without risking neurologic compromise.

The physical examination during the primary survey should be thorough and efficient. In patients with moderate to severe injuries, all clothing must be removed to allow adequate visualization and assessment of injuries. Obvious hemorrhage should be controlled with direct pressure to the wound. A rapid neurologic assessment is included, and the initial examination includes determination of orientation and responsiveness, pupillary reaction, motor response, and the Glasgow Coma Scale.

Concurrent with the initial evaluation of a moderately to severely injured patient, intravenous access must be established. A large-bore (14–16-gauge) peripheral catheter is preferred because it allows the quickest infusion of fluids and blood products. The number of peripheral catheters placed should increase as injury severity increases; patients with moderate injuries should have two secure catheters in place. Central venous access is required when peripheral access cannot be established because of absent veins, hypotension, or large surface area burns. Subclavian line placement in hypotensive trauma patients, however, carries a 12% complication rate, including pneumothorax, hemothorax, thrombosis, and infection.[12] Additionally, the infusion ports of a double- or triple-lumen central venous catheter are generally 18-gauge, and the maximum flow rate is slower than with a large-bore peripheral intravenous line. Another option for central access is placement of a large-bore (8.5 Fc) central catheter; if needed, this line can be converted over a guidewire to a triple-lumen catheter after resuscitation.

Crystalloid (lactated Ringer's solution) is the fluid of choice for initial resuscitation for many physicians. Replacement should be at a rate of 3:1 crystalloid to blood lost. Others use colloid or plasma expanders. If the patient remains hypotensive despite infusion of 2 to 3 L crystalloid, transfusion of packed red blood cells should begin. In the emergency setting, type O negative blood is administered until blood type and crossmatch are obtained. When possible, a warming device helps to prevent hypothermia as a result of infusion of crystalloid and blood products. Coagulation products should be administered based on abnormal laboratory parameters.

Military antishock trousers are controversial in the management of traumatic shock. They have not been well studied nor widely used in pregnant women. In the injured gravida, the lower extremity compartments can be inflated, but this may increase bleeding from injured pelvic structures. Generally, the abdominal compartment should not be inflated in the second and third trimesters, because it can compromise venous return and precipitate or exacerbate respiratory compromise from increased intra-abdominal pressure. Military antishock trousers are recommended for an injured pregnant woman only when major pelvic fractures are accompanied by uncontrollable hemorrhage.[9,10]

Resuscitation

The goal of the resuscitation phase is to monitor the patient's response to initial treatment and optimize intravascular volume and oxygen delivery. Adequate maternal resuscitation is of paramount importance to fetal survival. Blood pressure and pulse rate are frequently monitored, although these parameters are not reliable in detecting early shock in the gravida.[4]

Measurement of central venous pressure has been used in the acute setting, but absolute values should be viewed with great caution because central venous pressure is lowered by pregnancy. A pulmonary artery catheter is rarely indicated during initial resuscitation attempts. Vasopressors are contraindicated in hemorrhagic shock unless the patient has cardiogenic shock as a result of cardiac contusion or neurogenic shock associated with spinal cord injury.[10]

A urinary catheter is diagnostic and therapeutic; it allows accurate measurement of urine output and assessment of the urine for hematuria, and provides adequate drainage. The kidney is sensitive to the effects of hypotension, and urine output decreases as the kidney attempts to conserve fluid and maintain intravascular volume. An output of 30 mL/hr or more indicates adequate renal perfusion. Evidence of blood at the urethral meatus or difficulty in passing a catheter suggests bladder or urethral injury. If no urine is obtained through the catheter, bladder rupture must be considered. This condition is most commonly associated with a pelvic fracture. Gross or microscopic hematuria mandates evaluation to exclude urinary tract injury.

If an injured patient in shock is unresponsive to aggressive resuscitative measures, immediate operative intervention must be considered. A number of causes of refractory shock should be eliminated, however, before proceeding to the operating room. In the pregnant woman who is seriously injured, volume replacement may be inadequate, particularly in the third trimester, when blood volume is at its peak. Concealed hemorrhage associated with abruptio placentae can result in maternal shock, and amniotic fluid embolism is a rare but potential cause of cardiovascular collapse. Additional causes of persistent shock include tension pneumothorax, cardiac tamponade, neurogenic shock, uncorrected hypothermia, significant electrolyte and acid–base disturbances, and hypoxia.[11]

Secondary Survey

The secondary survey is performed once the maternal condition is stabilized. A complete physical examination should be conducted in an ordered fashion. Particular attention must be given to sites of bleeding, injured limbs, and entrance and exit wounds in cases of penetrating trauma. Head injuries account for nearly 50% of deaths in trauma patients. A complete neurologic assessment should be performed and compared with the initial examination.[13] The most common underlying etiologies of central nervous system impairment in a trauma patient include alcohol intoxication, diabetic ketoacidosis, narcotic and barbiturate overdose, hypovolemic shock, and cerebrovascular accidents. All neck injuries should be presumed to be life-threatening until excluded by appropriate evaluation. Tension and open pneumothorax, flail chest, and massive hemothorax are thoracic injuries that require rapid diagnosis and treatment. A chest tube should be placed one to two interspaces higher in pregnant patients to compensate for diaphragm elevation.[14] Although an abdominal examination should be conducted on all injured patients, the absence of findings does not exclude an acute intra-abdominal process. A rectal examination should be performed in patients with moderate to severe injuries to exclude gastrointestinal bleeding and document normal sphincter tone.

A complete obstetric examination is included in the secondary survey. Fundal height should be measured and fetal heart tones auscultated. Uterine tone and the presence of contractions and tenderness are assessed. Pelvic examination should be performed on all gravidas unless contraindicated. A sterile speculum examination assists in identifying membrane rupture or genitourinary bleeding. Contraindications to the pelvic examination include unstable spine, pelvic, and femur fractures because positioning may risk additional injury. Examination may be possible after orthopedic consultation. Digital examination can be performed if there is no vaginal bleeding or, in the presence of bleeding, once placenta previa has been excluded by ultrasonographic examination.

Fetal assessment begins with estimating gestational age by last menstrual period, fundal height, and ultrasonography. If the gestational age is uncertain, ultrasonographic measurements can quickly approximate dating of the pregnancy. When the potential for fetal survival must be determined urgently, a biparietal diameter of 54 mm or greater measured by ultrasonography has been suggested as more predictive than estimated fetal weight.[15] Fetal heart tones can be auscultated intermittently by Doppler in a previable fetus.

Continuous fetal heart rate monitoring of a viable fetus should be instituted in the emergency room as soon as possible, once initial resuscitation of the mother has begun. Changes in the fetal heart rate pattern may be the first sign of compromise and may occur despite normal maternal vital signs. Fetal tachycardia, bradycardia, late decelerations, and decreased beat-to-beat variability can indicate deterioration in fetal status. The tocodynameter can be helpful in detecting contractions that may not be perceived by an injured patient. Obstetric staff must be immediately available to interpret the fetal heart rate tracing before the patient is transferred to the obstetrics unit.

A variety of laboratory studies and diagnostic modalities are available to assist in evaluating and managing an injured gravida. Diagnostic peritoneal lavage (DPL), abdominal–pelvic computed tomography (CT) scan, and focused abdominal sonography of trauma (FAST) can be helpful in determining whether a patient requires operative intervention for intra-abdominal injuries. The study or combination of studies performed should be tailored to the clinical situation (discussed later).

Laboratory Studies in the Gravid Trauma Victim

Complete laboratory evaluation must be initiated quickly for patients with moderate to severe injuries. Suggested studies are listed in Table 55–3. Additional tests should be ordered as dictated by the patient's condition and the clinical situation.

Pregnant women have a physiologic anemia because plasma volume increases to a greater degree than red cell volume. Nevertheless, the hemoglobin level during pregnancy is normally 10 g/dL or higher. An initial hemoglobin level of less than 8 g/dL has been associated with ongoing hemorrhage and an increased mortality rate in nonpregnant trauma patients.[16] A normal hemoglobin level, however, does not exclude excessive bleeding because several hours may be required for equilibration to occur. Activated partial thromboplastin time (aPTT) and prothrombin time (PT) are unaffected by pregnancy. Fibrinogen increases during pregnancy, and a low-normal fibrinogen level (200–250 mg/dL) suggests a consumptive coagulopathy.[17]

Serum chemistry values provide additional information. Although electrolyte levels are usually normal in young, healthy gravidas, a decreased bicarbonate level is correlated with fetal demise in pregnant trauma patients. Determining a baseline creatinine level is helpful in case renal complications develop. Elevation of the aspartate aminotransferase (AST) or alanine aminotransferase (ALT) level above 130 IU/L is associated with a sixfold increase in the risk of intra-abdominal injury and is an indication to pursue diagnostic imaging in the stable nonpregnant patient.[18]

The Kleihauer-Betke stain determines the presence of fetal blood cells in the maternal circulation as well as the degree of fetomaternal hemorrhage (FMH). Determining the amount of FMH is important to ensure that Rh-negative gravidas receive an adequate dose of anti-D immunoglobulin to prevent isoimmunization. Fetal cells and ghost maternal cells are counted after acid elution and staining of the maternal blood sample. A normal maternal blood volume of 5 L (5000 mL) is commonly assumed. The laboratory reports the ratio of fetal to maternal cells, and the volume of FMH is calculated:

$$\frac{\text{Fetal cells}}{\text{Maternal cells}} \times \text{Maternal blood volume}$$

Unfortunately, alcohol and illicit substance use is common in trauma patients, and urine and blood toxicology screens should be performed. The results of testing provide information that is important for both medical and legal reasons. The physiologic effects of illicit substances can alter a patient's response to the stress of trauma. Alcohol lowers sympathetic response, whereas cocaine can cause sympathetic stimulation or paradoxical depression. Cocaine use has been associated with placental abruption and should be considered in the gravid trauma patient with an adverse fetal outcome. Organic pathology should be excluded in patients with neurologic compromise, but their condition may reflect the effects of an illicit substance.

TABLE 55–3

Suggested Laboratory Studies for Patients with Moderate to Severe Traumatic Injury

Complete blood count and platelet count
Coagulation profile
Type and crossmatch
Serum electrolytes, blood urea nitrogen, and creatinine
Serum glucose
Aspartate aminotransferase and alamine aminotransferase
Amylase
Lipase
Arterial blood gas analysis
Urinalysis
Urine and blood toxicology screens
Kleihauer-Betke stain

Diagnostic Studies in the Gravid Trauma Victim

Diagnostic procedures can be pursued once initial resuscitation is completed and the mother and fetus are stable. Radiographic screening of patients with moderate to severe injuries consists of cervical spine, chest, and pelvis films. Cervical spine films exclude cervical spine injury in most patients with blunt trauma. Chest x-ray evaluates the presence of hemothorax, pneumothorax, or ruptured diaphragm. A plain film of the abdomen should be obtained if abdominal injury or a foreign body is suspected.

Radiation exposure should be considered when caring for the pregnant patient. Examinations that assist management should be performed, and necessary tests should not be omitted because the patient is pregnant. Fetal risk is negligible if maternal exposure is limited to less than 5 to 10 rad (5000–10,000 mrad).[19] Abdominal shielding and avoiding duplication of films (e.g., intravenous pyelogram scout film and pelvic film) minimize fetal exposure. The radiation dose to the fetus from common radiologic studies has been estimated at 0.02 to 0.07 mrad per chest radiograph, 100 mrad per abdominal film, 200 mrad per hip film, and 3 to 5 rad per CT scan of the abdomen and pelvis.[19] Studies with the highest radiation dose include pelvic CT, pelvic angiography, and pelvic fluoroscopy.

Intra-abdominal injury must be excluded, as in the nonpregnant patient. Clinical examination of the abdomen in nonpregnant patients with blunt trauma detects only 60% of intra-abdominal injuries. During pregnancy, signs and symptoms of an acute intra-abdominal process are often further obscured as the uterus stretches the anterior abdominal wall. Three diagnostic modalities are available to exclude abdominal injury when the patient does not require emergent laparotomy: DPL, CT scan, and FAST. Each has its advantages, disadvantages, and limitations.

DPL is highly sensitive and accurately detects 94% to 98% of intra-abdominal injuries.[20,21] Traditional indications for DPL include equivocal findings on physical examination, unexplained hypotension, an unresponsive patient, and spinal cord injury. DPL can be performed in a pregnant patient without compromising safety and accuracy.[22,23] Although CT scan and FAST are becoming more common, DPL is still useful for evaluation of unstable blunt trauma or an indeterminate FAST study. DPL is more accurate than CT for early diagnosis of hollow visceral and mesenteric injury, but does not reliably exclude retroperitoneal injury. DPL also cannot assess the specific site of bleeding or the extent of injury. Previous laparotomy, massive obesity, and advanced third-trimester pregnancy are relative contraindications to DPL, although no gestational age cutoff has been defined.[24] The complication rate for DPL is 1% in nonpregnant patients and does not appear to be increased during pregnancy.[22–24]

The standard technique for DPL is modified somewhat for the pregnant patient. As for any DPL, the bladder and stomach must be emptied before the procedure. Location of the incision is dependent on the stage of gestation. During the first trimester, a standard infraumbilical incision may be used. As pregnancy advances, however, the incision must be supraumbilical and above the uterine fundus. Once the peritoneum has been entered under direct visualization, the catheter is placed into the abdominal cavity and aspirated to detect gross blood. One liter Ringer's lactate is infused into the peritoneal cavity, and the fluid is allowed to drain into a sterile bag by gravity. An aliquot of returned fluid is then sent for red blood cell count, white blood cell count, and amylase measurement. A minimum of 200 mL fluid must be recovered to allow accurate interpretation. Standard criteria for a positive DPL finding include aspiration of at least 10 mL gross blood, bloody lavage effluent, red blood cell count greater than $100{,}000/mm^3$, white blood cell count greater than $500/mm^3$, amylase level greater than 175 IU/dL, and detection of bile, bacteria, or food particles.[9]

CT scanning is recommended when a patient with blunt trauma is hemodynamically stable but has unreliable or equivocal findings on physical examination or findings suggestive of significant trauma. It is the diagnostic modality of choice for nonoperative management of solid viscus injuries and has the advantage of detecting clinically unsuspected injuries. Its negative predictive value is excellent. Experience with abdominopelvic CT in pregnant trauma victims is limited, but a case series of 42 patients undergoing helical CT for trauma has been published. The radiation exposure of 0.87 to 1.75 mrad calculated in this study was less than the traditional amount and was determined by the scan pitch.[25] Disadvantages of CT include a lower sensitivity for hollow viscus injury, possible dye reactions, and lack of portability, which requires patients to be moved from the resuscitation area of the emergency department.

FAST is a relatively new modality, but it is rapidly becoming the diagnostic study of choice for hemodynamically stable patients.[26,27] It is noninvasive, can be performed at the bedside in the emergency room, and can be repeated easily if the results are equivocal. The examination focuses on identifying fluid in the pericardium, pleural cavity, pararenal retroperitoneum, and peritoneal cavity. The sensitivity of FAST is 73% to 88%, and its accuracy is 96% to 99%.[21] FAST appears to decrease the need for both DPL and CT scan, allowing more selective and cost-effective use of these modalities.[26] A review of FAST in pregnant blunt trauma victims showed sensitivity and specificity similar to nonpregnant patients, suggesting that it can be useful in assessing the need for additional evaluation or emergent laparotomy.[28]

An evidence-based algorithm incorporating hemodynamic status and the findings on physical examination was developed by the EAST Practice Management Guidelines Work Group.[21] FAST is considered the diagnostic examination of choice for patients who are hemodynamically unstable, with DPL as an alternative to exclude hemoperitoneum. Patients who are hemodynamically stable, with a reliable physical examination, undergo serial examinations or diagnostic testing, depending on the findings on initial clinical examination. Patients with an unreliable physical examination should undergo FAST or CT scan, depending on institution and physician preference, with subsequent management determined by results.

Definitive Treatment

Definitive treatment is instituted according to the type and severity of injuries as well as the clinical condition. A patient with hemorrhagic shock and obvious intra-abdominal injury is unlikely to remain in the emergency department longer than necessary and will have undergone minimal diagnostic evaluation before operative intervention. In a patient who is hemodynamically stable, adequate time is available to assess the full extent of injuries. Once diagnostic studies have been completed and interpreted, a treatment plan can be devised in consultation with appropriate specialty services.

Trauma victims are frequently transported to the nearest hospital. However, not all institutions are equipped to care for a patient with major injuries, and transfer to a tertiary care center may be necessary for definitive therapy. Maternal stability and fetal well-being must be ensured before land or air transport. Copies of medical notes and the results of laboratory and radiologic studies should accompany the patient to avoid duplication and unnecessary delays. A patient should not be transferred if there is any sign of hemodynamic compromise, ongoing hemorrhage, severe uncorrected anemia, nonreassuring fetal status, or danger of delivery en route. Personnel equipped to handle emergencies should always accompany a pregnant patient during transport.

Tetanus immunization is the first of two treatment issues that should be addressed before a patient leaves the emergency department. Tetanus occurs almost exclusively in patients who have been inadequately immunized. Preventing tetanus after injury entails ensuring adequate immunity and local wound care, with elimination of necrotic tissue and foreign bodies. Tetanus toxoid (0.5 mL IM) is administered when a patient has been appropriately immunized, but the most recent booster was longer than 5 years ago. Previously unimmunized patients require both tetanus immune globulin (500 U IM) and the first of three doses of tetanus toxoid. The immune globulin and toxoid must be injected into different sites to ensure adequate protection.

The second issue is the extremely high risk of deep venous thrombosis (DVT) in patients with moderate to severe injuries. Blood transfusion, surgery, femur or tibia fracture, and spinal cord injury are associated with an increased risk of DVT.[29] However, only a small percentage of patients have clinical signs of DVT in the days after the traumatic event. Young patients with injuries are at high risk, and DVT has been reported to occur in 46% of trauma victims younger than 30 years of age.[29] The American College of Chest Physicians[30] recommends DVT prophylaxis for trauma patients with an identifiable risk factor. Low-molecular-weight heparin (LMWH) should be administered if the patient has no contraindications to heparin therapy. If LMWH prophylaxis is contraindicated, mechanical prophylaxis (elastic stockings or intermittent pneumatic compression) should be instituted. An inferior vena caval filter is not recommended for prophylaxis.[30] LMWH has been used successfully during pregnancy, but studies showing its efficacy in gravid trauma victims are lacking. The hypercoaguable state of pregnancy is an additional risk factor for thrombosis, and DVT prophylaxis should be initiated once the injured gravida is stable.

SUMMARY OF MANAGEMENT OPTIONS

Trauma in Pregnancy—General Management

Management Options (See Table 55–2)	Quality of Evidence	Strength of Recommendation	References
Overall Primary Survey			
Multidisciplinary team approach	–	GPP	–
Airway	IV	C	11
Breathing	IV	C	11
Circulation	IV	C	11
-venous access	Ia	A	12
-fluid/blood/blood product replacement			
-left lateral position			
Initial neurological assessment	IV	C	10
Initial physical examination	IV	C	10
Resuscitation			
Response to initial treatment	IV	C	4,11
-pulse and blood pressure			
-urine output			
-continued resuscitation			
Secondary Survey			
Initiate after stabilization	IV	C	11,24
-complete physical examination	III	B	23
-obstetric assessment			
-laboratory investigations (see Table 55–3)			
-diagnostic studies			

Continued

SUMMARY OF MANAGEMENT OPTIONS

Trauma in Pregnancy—General Management *(Continued)*

Management Options (See Table 55–2)	Quality of Evidence	Strength of Recommendation	References
Definitive Treatment			
See specific sections (below)	–	–	–
Assess need for transfer to tertiary center	–	GPP	–
Thromboprophylaxis	IV	C	19,30
	III	B	29
Tetanus immunization if needed	–	GPP	–
Rh-immunoglobulin if Rh negative	IIa	B	8

BLUNT TRAUMA

Incidence

MVAs are responsible for 60% to 75% of cases of blunt trauma, making it the most common mechanism of injury and the leading cause of fetal death related to maternal trauma.[4,31] The severity of the crash appears to be the most significant factor in prediciting fetal outcome.[32] Although most injuries are minor, each year in the United States, an estimated 1300 to 3900 women experience a fetal loss as a result of an MVA.[33] Obstetric complications associated with blunt trauma include abruptio placentae, preterm labor, uterine rupture, fetomaternal hemorrhage, direct fetal injury, and fetal demise. The incidence of abruptio placentae, direct fetal injury, and fetal death in non-life-threatening blunt abdominal trauma is fortunately low (1.6%, 0.8%, and 1.6%, respectively), but the fetus is nevertheless at risk, even when maternal injuries are minor.[34] The incidence of preterm delivery associated with noncatastrophic blunt trauma is also infrequent, at 0.86%.[35]

Falls are the second most common form of blunt trauma, but direct abdominal assault is occurring with increasing frequency in pregnant women. The prevalence of physical abuse of pregnant women is 6% to 31%. Morbidity and adverse outcomes of pregnancy appear to be more common with direct assaults than with MVAs.[36,37] Physical abuse is often a repetitive event that may prompt multiple emergency room visits. It is important to ask specific questions about abusive relationships because women frequently do not volunteer such information. As the only health care provider many patients sees regularly during pregnancy, the obstetrician has the best opportunity to offer assistance to victims of abuse.

General Management

The initial management of a pregnant woman who has blunt trauma was discussed earlier (see Table 55–2). The trauma team may have performed a primary survey and begun resuscitation efforts before an obstetrician is summoned. This approach is appropriate because maternal stabilization is always the priority. The obstetric consultant should assume comanagement responsibilities for the mother and fetus once notified of the patient's admission to the emergency department.

Injury patterns associated with MVAs vary depending on whether the victim was restrained, the type of safety belt system in use, and the patient's place in the vehicle. Unbelted individuals usually sustain injuries to the head, face, chest, abdomen, and pelvis when they hit the interior of the car or are ejected. A lap belt prevents ejection from the vehicle, but hollow viscus and lumbar spine injuries are common. Those wearing a shoulder harness without the lap component often have cervical spine, clavicular, chest, liver, and spleen injuries. A three-point lap–shoulder system offers optimal protection, but injuries do occur, and include rib, sternum, and clavicular fractures. Air bag deployment may cause face, arm, and chest abrasions, and chemical keratitis has been reported.

Abdominal injuries are common in victims of blunt trauma. Specific injuries sustained during pregnancy change with advancing gestation. By 12 weeks, the bladder has become an intra-abdominal organ and thus is more susceptible to injury. As the uterus enlarges and rises out of the pelvis, the risk of injury increases. Life-threatening retroperitoneal hemorrhage occurs more frequently during pregnancy, when pelvic blood flow is markedly increased.[38] Bowel injuries, however, tend to occur less often because the small intestine is compressed into the upper abdomen.

Accurate and timely diagnosis of intra-abdominal injury requiring surgical intervention is one of the challenges in blunt trauma. Findings on physical examination of the abdomen may be normal initially despite visceral injury. Serial examinations are therefore important to detect deterioration in the patient's condition. Intra-abdominal hemorrhage should be suspected in patients with rib and pelvic fractures. Rib fractures are frequently associated with liver and spleen injuries, and pelvic fractures are associated with genitourinary injuries and retroperitoneal hemorrhage. FAST, DPL, and abdominal–pelvic CT scan should be used, as previously discussed, to determine the need for operative intervention.

Information on pelvic fracture during pregnancy is limited to a literature review of 101 cases of pelvic and acetabular fracture during pregnancy.[39] Mechanisms of injury included automobile–pedestrian accidents, MVAs, and falls. The overall maternal mortality rate was 9%, and the fetal mortality rate was 35%. Fractures in the third trimester were associated with an 18% incidence of fetal skull fracture. As reported by other authors, increasing severity of maternal injury increased both maternal and fetal mortality rates. The trimester of pregnancy during which the injury occurred did not influence fetal death. Repair of the fracture usually is not performed during pregnancy, and the mode of delivery depends on the type of fracture and the interval between injury and delivery.

Abruptio Placentae

Abruptio placentae occurs in 1% to 5% of gravidas with minor injuries and 6% to 37% of those with major injuries.[34–36,38,40–42] It is the most common cause of fetal death when the mother survives blunt trauma. Placental abruption cannot be predicted based on placental location, severity of maternal injury, or vehicle damage (in the case of an MVA), and it can occur without obvious injury to the mother.[6,8,43,44] A small series reported an increased incidence of abruption in patients involved in MVAs at speeds of 30 mph and greater and those with a higher injury severity score.[7]

When a gravida is involved in an MVA, intrauterine pressure at the time of impact is estimated to be 10 times greater than the forces generated with labor.[45] Although the uterus is considered more elastic than the placenta, recent models indicate that their mechanical properties are similar and there is overlap. The uteroplacental interface appears to fail at a lower strain than either the uterus or the placenta.[32] The increase in intrauterine pressure generated on impact may propagate placental separation, with subsequent formation of a retroplacental hematoma.[45]

Placental abruption usually occurs soon after the traumatic event. Classic signs and symptoms include vaginal bleeding, abdominal pain, and fundal tenderness as well as uterine irritability, high-frequency contractions, and increased tone. Back pain and vaginal bleeding may be the most prominent symptoms in women with separation of a posterior placenta.[46] The absence of vaginal bleeding, however, does not exclude the diagnosis. Bleeding can be concealed within the uterus and may be detected only by increasing fundal height, fetal heart rate abnormalities, or maternal hypovolemia. A hypertonic uterus and evidence of fetal compromise are highly suggestive of abruptio placentae. Cardiotocographic monitoring is the most sensitive method of surveillance after a traumatic event (discussed later).[8,35,36]

Management of a patient with abruptio placentae after traumatic injury is similar to that of an uninjured gravida with this complication. As soon as abruption is suspected, intravenous access must be established. A urinary catheter allows accurate measurement of output. Complete blood and platelet counts, fibrinogen level, aPTT, and PT should be obtained and repeated every 4 to 6 hours to detect disseminated intravascular coagulation. A minimum of two units of packed red blood cells must be crossmatched and immediately available in the blood bank. Fresh frozen plasma and packed red blood cells should be administered based on abnormal laboratory findings and estimates of ongoing hemorrhage. Obstetric management depends on the maternal condition, fetal status, and severity of abruption. If there are signs of maternal hypovolemia or shock, fluid resuscitation and administration of blood products should begin promptly. Disseminated intravascular coagulation is not an indication to proceed with cesarean section, and abdominal delivery only increases the risk of bleeding complications.

Fetal status and the severity of abruption direct the clinical course once the mother is stable. When the fetus is alive, gestational age and plans for intervention must be established quickly. Hysterotomy offers no benefit to either mother or fetus if a previable fetus shows signs of compromise. Continuous fetal monitoring and close observation are reasonable approaches for a preterm gestation when the heart rate pattern is reassuring. Corticosteroids should be administered to minimize the complications of prematurity if the gestational age is 24 to 34 weeks. As always, the risks of prematurity must be weighed against the risks of continuing the pregnancy. Delivery is generally indicated in a term pregnancy with abruptio placentae, but cesarean delivery is unnecessary if the fetal status is reassuring. If the fetus has died, induction of labor and vaginal delivery can be anticipated because this is the safest method of delivery for the mother.

Preterm Labor

Preterm labor requiring tocolysis occurs in 11% to 28% of gravidas who have blunt trauma.[35,37,47] Delivery before 34 weeks' gestation, however, is uncommon and experienced by only 0.86% of gravidas with blunt trauma.[35] Extravasation of blood into the myometrium appears to be a stimulus for uterine contractions associated with traumatic events. Uterine muscle injury can also cause release of lysosomal enzymes, generation of prostaglandins, and subsequent uterine activity.

When uterine contractions occur after blunt trauma, it may be difficult to determine whether they represent placental abruption or isolated preterm labor. Tocolysis is discouraged by those who believe that uterine activity is an indication of the former. Uterine contractions developing after blunt trauma abate without treatment in 90% of gravidas.[40] On the other hand, successful tocolysis has been reported after blunt trauma.[47] Regardless of whether pharmacologic inhibition of labor is used, fetal heart rate and uterine contractions should be monitored continuously during observation of the patient.

If a tocolytic is administered, the agent should be selected with an awareness of its potential complications. β-Mimetic preparations (ritodrine, terbutaline) are relatively contraindicated in patients at risk for hemorrhage because drug-induced tachycardia may mask early signs of hypovolemia. Magnesium sulfate has fewer cardiac side effects than the β-mimetics. However, patients with renal dysfunction are at increased risk for toxicity because magnesium is excreted through the kidneys. Indomethacin may be used to inhibit preterm labor, although it can cause transient or premature closure of the fetal ductus arteriosus and oligohydramnios. Additionally, nonsteroidal anti-inflammatory agents, such as indomethacin, may be contraindicated in severely injured patients because the drug can adversely affect platelet and renal function. Calcium channel blockers (e.g., nifedipine) have also been used successfully as an oral tocolytic. This class of drugs may cause maternal hypotension, however, and may imitate early shock in a gravid trauma patient.

Uterine Rupture

Uterine rupture occurs in 0.6% to 1% of gravidas who have blunt trauma and is most frequently associated with maternal pelvic fracture.[48–50] It is an uncommon complication of trauma because uterine muscle retains its elasticity and resistance to rupture, even at advanced gestation. When the uterus ruptures, however, the site is often fundal.[51] A scarred uterus has a greater propensity to rupture than an unscarred uterus. Uterine rupture usually occurs as a result of direct abdominal trauma during the late second and third trimesters. It is much more devastating for the fetus than for the mother, with a 10% maternal mortality rate, but a fetal mortality rate of nearly 100%.[47]

The diagnosis of uterine rupture can be difficult. Signs and symptoms may be limited to vague abdominal pain. Uterine tenderness, a nonreassuring fetal heart rate pattern, absence of the presenting part, palpable fetal parts outside the uterus, fetal demise, and maternal shock are more dramatic presentations. When fetal death occurs after a serious accident, uterine rupture must be considered. Rupture of the uterus may first be suspected when induction of labor is unsuccessful. DPL results are generally positive when the uterus has ruptured and major vessels have been damaged.

If rupture of the uterus is suspected, exploratory laparotomy should be performed to control maternal hemorrhage. Ideally, a trauma surgeon will be in attendance to explore the abdomen for additional injuries. A vertical abdominal incision allows maximum exposure, particularly if surgical repair of intra-abdominal injuries is required. Conservation of fertility is always a consideration because a patient's wishes may be unknown or uncertain at the time of the accident. However, uterine repair should be undertaken only if the patient is hemodynamically stable and hemorrhage can be controlled. When the uterus is extensively damaged and repair is impossible or the patient is in hemorrhagic shock, hysterectomy is indicated.

If the uterus is to be repaired, the site of rupture should be assessed after delivery of the fetus and once hemostasis is achieved. Necrotic tissue along the rupture site may be excised to allow reapproximation of well vascularized tissue. The uterine defect can then be repaired in layers. The risk of uterine rupture in future pregnancies is certainly present, but not prohibitive. It would seem prudent to offer elective cesarean delivery in subsequent pregnancies, especially if the rupture site was fundal or damage was extensive.

Fetal Injury

The exact incidence of fetal injury as a result of maternal trauma is unknown. An incidence of 0.49% has been noted in gravidas with noncatastrophic trauma.[35] Fetal skull fractures, long bone fractures, intracranial hemorrhage, and soft tissue injury have been reported. Skull fracture or head injury is most commonly described and is associated with maternal pelvic fracture late in gestation, when the fetal head is engaged.[39]

The management of fetal injuries must be individualized, and experience is limited. If the fetus is alive and without signs of distress, delivery may be delayed in very premature gestation. Serial ultrasonography and frequent assessment of fetal well-being may be beneficial until maturity is reached. If pregnancy is advanced or delivery is indicated for fetal compromise, a pediatrician should be consulted and in attendance for the delivery. Accurate and unbiased documentation is always important, given the medicolegal ramifications of fetal injury.

Fetal Assessment

The prediction of adverse fetal outcome after a traumatic event has been a controversial subject. Cardiotocographic monitoring is currently the most sensitive method of immediate fetal surveillance.[40] Clinical risk factors for fetal death include injury severity score, severe abdominal injury, hypotension, hemorrhagic shock, DIC with or without abruption, and gestational age less than 23 weeks.[52–56] Because almost all patients who have placental abruption after trauma manifest signs soon after the event, it is important to institute fetal heart rate and uterine activity monitoring once the mother is stable. Delayed abruption several days after an accident is described, but has been questioned. The few patients reported were not monitored immediately after the event, and early signs of abruption may have been overlooked.[57,58]

Uterine activity appears to be the most sensitive indicator of abruption after blunt trauma.[35,36,59,60] The presence of six to eight or more contractions per hour identifies a patient who is at risk for adverse pregnancy outcome.[8,35,36] Approximately 14% of women who had contractions every 2 to 5 minutes immediately after blunt trauma subsequently had abruption. No patient with fever than eight contractions per hour had abruption.[8] Similarly, a second study showed that when uterine contractions, tenderness, or vaginal bleeding were present, 19% of patients had obstetric complications compared with 0.9% who did not have these symptoms.[36]

Although obstetric ultrasonographic examination can be helpful in fetal assessment, normal findings do not exclude or reduce the risk of abruption. The sensitivity of ultrasonography in predicting abruption in blunt trauma patients is only 40%.[8,40] Cardiotocographic monitoring appears to be more sensitive than ultrasonography in detecting acute abruption.[48,61] Ultrasonography is useful to exclude placenta previa, document fetal viability, establish gestational age, estimate fetal weight, measure amniotic fluid volume, and assess fetal well-being.

Guidelines for monitoring pregnant trauma victims have been suggested. If a patient does not have uterine tenderness, contractions, or vaginal bleeding on presentation, 2 to 6 hours of cardiotocographic monitoring is sufficient.[35–37,47,48] Patients may be released home if they do not have symptoms, the fetal heart rate pattern is reassuring, and maternal injuries have been appropriately evaluated and treated. These patients are not at increased risk for adverse pregnancy outcome compared with uninjured control subjects.[8] They should be instructed about the symptoms and signs of preterm labor and abruption as well as indications to return to the hospital.

Approximately 52% of gravidas have uterine tenderness, irritability or contractions, or vaginal bleeding after blunt trauma.[37] These patients require additional observation and continuous fetal monitoring; a minimum of 24 hours has been recommended, even if symptoms resolve.[35] A more recent study recommends at least 24 hours of fetal monitoring if the maternal heart rate is greater than 110 beats/min, the injury severity score is greater than 9, the fetal heart rate is less than 120 beats/min or greater than 160 beats/min, or there is evidence of placental abruption, and for victims of ejections or motorcycle or pedestrian collisions.[62] The hospital stay should be extended as maternal and fetal conditions dictate. Seriously injured patients who require surgery or transfer to the intensive care unit present a challenge to the obstetrician. If the fetus is viable, continuous monitoring should be used; obstetrics personnel must be readily available to evaluate the fetal heart rate tracing.

Fetomaternal Hemorrhage

Fetomaternal hemorrhage (FMH) occurs in a significant number of gravidas who are victims of blunt trauma. The incidence is 8.7% to 30% in gravid trauma patients compared with 1.8% to 8% in pregnant control subjects.[8,36,37,60,63] The mean volume of transfusion was reported in two studies as 12 mL and 16 mL, with a range of 5 to 69 mL.[8,63] Although no clinical signs reliably predict FMH, an increased incidence is noted in women who have an anterior placenta or uterine tenderness.[8,36] Most fetuses with FMH have a normal outcome, but anemia, supraventricular tachycardia, and fetal demise are recognized complications.[8,63]

The most important role of Kleihauer-Betke (KB) testing in trauma patients is to identify a large volume of fetomaternal transfusion in the Rh-negative gravida. Massive FMH occasionally occurs, even with relatively minor maternal injuries, so all Rh-negative gravidas should undergo KB testing after any trauma. Although routine testing of all gravid blunt trauma victims has been suggested, the clinical utility of this approach is uncertain.[37] Unfortunately, the KB result does not correlate with the occurrence of placental abruption or fetal distress.[35,60] The KB test predicted obstetric complications in only 27% of pregnant trauma patients in one study, and the sensitivity for adverse outcome was only 18% in a second series.[37,60] Testing may, however, identify FMH as the cause of an otherwise unexplained fetal death.

Isoimmunization can occur very early in pregnancy because the Rh antigen is present on fetal red blood cells 34 days after conception. The amount of fetal blood required to stimulate maternal antibody formation may be as little as 0.01 mL. The KB test, however, is not sensitive enough to detect such a small amount of fetal blood in the maternal circulation. Because an undetectable amount of fetal blood can lead to sensitization in early pregnancy, all unsensitized Rh-negative women who have trauma should be considered candidates for Rh immune globulin.[35,48]

The amount of immune globulin administered depends on the volume of FMH as calculated from the KB stain results. Anti-D immunoglobulin (300 μg or 1500 IM) IU administered within 72 hours of the event protects against maternal antibody formation for transfusion of up to 15 mL fetal red blood cells (30 mL whole blood). If KB testing is unavailable, 300 μg is adequate in most women and can be administered empirically.[36,40] The precise doses used should be in accordance with local guidelines.

Seat Belt Use

Passenger restraint systems have saved thousands of lives. The use of lap–shoulder belts reduces the likelihood of fatal injury by 45% and the likelihood of moderate to critical injury by 50%.[64] Safety belts minimize injuries by limiting passenger contact with the interior of the vehicle, preventing ejection, and spreading the force of deceleration over a larger area. Although air bags have augmented the reduction in rates of injury and death, they do not offer protection in lateral collisions and do not prevent ejection. Combined lap–shoulder restraint systems must continue to be worn for optimal crash protection. Air bags should not be disconnected during pregnancy.

MVAs are the most common mechanism of fetal death associated with maternal trauma.[31] The leading cause of fetal death in MVAs is maternal death, and the most common cause of maternal death is ejection from the vehicle.[65] The maternal mortality rate is 33% when the woman is ejected from the vehicle versus only 5% when she is not. When the mother is ejected, the fetal mortality rate is 47% compared with 11% when the mother remains in the vehicle. The rate of fetal death is decreased by seat belt use because seat belts prevent ejection and decrease the maternal mortality rate.[65]

The addition of a shoulder harness to the lap belt reduces the risk of maternal head injury and fetal death. The shoulder component decreases the maternal morbidity rate by preventing jack-knifing of the mother's torso over the lap belt and increasing the area over which deceleration forces dissipate. Decreasing force over the abdomen reduced the fetal mortality rate in animal studies from 50% with a lap belt alone to 12% with the three-point restraint system.[66] Crash simulation with a pregnant crash dummy also provides evidence that the three-point restraint system decreases the likelihood of injury.[67]

Despite the benefits of safety belts, pregnant women often hesitate to use them; 30% of gravidas either do not wear a safety belt or wear it incorrectly.[33] The perception of increased risk of fetal injury with seat belt use is a major factor contributing to the reluctance of pregnant women to use restraint systems. During the first antenatal visit, all pregnant women should be counseled on the importance and proper use of safety belts. Unfortunately, only 42% to 55% of gravidas receive information on the use of restraint systems during pregnancy.[33,68,69] It is equally important to give patients correct information.[68] Women should be instructed to place the lap portion of the belt under the abdomen and across both the anterior and superior iliac spines. The belt should be snug, but comfortable. The shoulder restraint should cross the shoulder without rubbing the neck and should be positioned between the breasts.[70] Lap and shoulder belts should be worn together because neither is as effective as the combination.[66,71] It is helpful to remind women during the course of pregnancy that safety belts should be worn and that they save the lives of both mother and fetus.

SUMMARY OF MANAGEMENT OPTIONS
Blunt Trauma in Pregnancy

Management Options	Quality of Evidence	Strength of Recommendation	References
General Management			
See above	–	–	–
Kleihauer-Betke (KB) test, fetal heart rate monitoring (FHR), and fetal ultrasound are advisable for all	III	B	35
Abruptio Placentae			
Assess maternal condition	III	B	46
Assess fetal condition with FHR	IIa	B	8,36
	III	B	35
See Chapter 59 for detailed discussion of management	–	–	–
Preterm Labor			
Be alert for evolving abruption	–	GPP	–
Consider tocolysis	III	B	35,37
See Chapters 61 and 62 for detailed discussion of management	–	–	–
Uterine Rupture			
Exploratory laparotomy when suspected	III	B	23

SUMMARY OF MANAGEMENT OPTIONS

Blunt Trauma in Pregnancy

Management Options	Quality of Evidence	Strength of Recommendation	References
Uterine Rupture ***(Continued)***			
Midline incision for adequate exposure			
Uterine repair if the patient is hemodynamically stable			
Cesarean hysterectomy if the patient has uncontrollable hemorrhage or excessive uterine damage			
Fetal Injury			
Individualize management, as experience is limited; gestation and fetal condition will influence the management; ultrasound evaluation may help	–	GPP	–
Fetomaternal Hemorrhage			
KB test: if positive confirms significant fetomaternal hemorrhage; if negative does not exclude a small bleed	III	B	35
Give Rh immune globulin to all Rh-negative women in accordance with local guidelines; increased doses required with positive KB test	III IV	B C	35 48
Fetal Assessment			
FHR monitoring is the most sensitive assessment of immediate fetal condition	III IV	B C	40 48
Normal obstetric ultrasound does not exclude fetal risk (e.g. abruption); confirms viability, approximate weight, and presentation; excludes placenta previa	IIa III	B B	8 40
Clinical risk factors for adverse fetal outcome are severity of injury, shock, disseminated intravascular coagulation, and gestation <23 weeks	III	B	52,53
Guidelines for fetal monitoring:	III	B	35–37
-no uterine tenderness, contractions or bleeding: 2–6h continuous FHR monitoring	III IV	B C	47 48
-uterine tenderness, contractions or bleeding: 24-h continuous FHR monitoring			

PENETRATING TRAUMA

Incidence

Pregnant women are the victims of penetrating trauma with increasing frequency. Gunshot and stab wounds are the most common, but injury occurs by other mechanisms as well, and may be self-inflicted.[72] Firearm injuries are the second most common mechanism of fetal death associated with maternal trauma.[31] The exact incidence of these injuries in pregnancy, however, is uncertain because some cases may not be reported. The mortality rate associated with penetrating injury in nonpregnant victims increases with the number of organs injured, but the rate of visceral injury and the mortality rate are lower during pregnancy.

The mother usually fares much better than the fetus when the injury is caused by a gunshot or stab wound.[10,73] The maternal mortality rate is 0% to 9% for gunshot wounds during pregnancy, whereas the perinatal mortality rate is 41% to 71%.[73] When the mother is stabbed, fetal injury and fetal death occur in 93% and 50% of cases, respectively.[74] Although direct fetal injury is responsible for most perinatal deaths, some deaths results from premature delivery, with it attendant complications.[75] Fetal survival is affected by several factors, including the severity of fetal and maternal injury, the presence and extent of placental hemorrhage, and gestational age at delivery.

General Management Options

Maternal injury patterns change with advancing gestation. Penetrating trauma in the first trimester causes wounds similar to those in nonpregnant victims. As the uterus enlarges and occupies more space in the abdominal cavity, it is more likely to be injured than any other intra-abdominal organ. The uterus offers relative protection to other abdominal organs by the third trimester. Hence, bowel injury is uncommon when a pregnant woman has a penetrating injury to the lower abdomen, but the small bowel is at high risk for injury when entry is in the upper abdomen. Multiple bowel wounds are more common in pregnant victims than in their nonpregnant counterparts because the intestine is compressed in the upper abdomen with advancing gestation.

As with other forms of trauma, the emergency team, trauma surgeon, and obstetrician must coordinate the care of a pregnant woman. Maternal resuscitation and hemodynamic stability are a priority, and the leading cause of early death from gunshot wounds is hypovolemia as a result of major vessel injury. The injured woman must be thoroughly examined and each entrance and exit wound noted. If exploratory laparotomy is indicated, a midline vertical incision offers optimal exposure to the abdomen.

An indication for exploratory laparotomy, however, is not an indication to empty the uterus. Abdominal delivery concurrent with exploratory laparotomy increases operative time and blood loss. A patient may undergo induction of labor and vaginal delivery postoperatively without increased risk of morbidity.[76] The only indication for hysterotomy is to provide adequate surgical exposure for repair of maternal injuries. Cesarean hysterectomy is indicated when damage to the uterus is extensive or uterine injury is associated with uncontrollable hemorrhage. Specific guidelines for treating pregnant women with gunshot and stab wounds are discussed later, but these guidelines should be individualized based on obstetric and surgical needs.

Gunshot Wounds

The size of the entrance wound does not predict the internal damage caused by a bullet. If no exit wound is found, radiographic studies are performed to localize the bullet. A flat plate and lateral film usually suffice. Intra-abdominal bullet wounds may be managed in one of the following ways:

- Observation
- Exploratory laparotomy with cesarean delivery
- Exploratory laparotomy without delivery

Surgical exploration has been considered standard practice for managing bullet wounds of the abdomen and flank. However, careful observation of a wounded gravida has been suggested as an alternative in the following situation:

- The mother is hemodynamically stable
- The bullet has entered below the uterine fundus
- The bullet can be localized to within the uterus
- There is no evidence of maternal genitourinary or gastrointestinal injury[77]

Additionally, the fetus should be free of injury or compromise, or dead, if the mother is managed conservatively.[78,79] Broad-spectrum antibiotic coverage is prudent, at least initially. This conservative approach should be considered only in trauma centers in which experienced surgeons manage trauma care. With this approach, it has been suggested that fewer than 20% of gravidas require surgical intervention for visceral wounds.[77]

Although this type of nonoperative management has been reported, this approach has not been prospectively tested in gravidas with penetrating injuries. Radiologic studies may give a false impression of the location of the bullet in the uterus when significant maternal injury has occurred.[80] DPL can be performed to exclude intra-abdominal hemorrhage. Exploratory laparotomy, however, is the most reliable means for detecting intra-abdominal injury should doubt exist. The ultimate decision about the need for operative intervention rests with the surgical team.

The decision to deliver the fetus is based on gestational age, fetal status, and exposure required for surgical exploration and repair of maternal injuries. If the fetus is alive and, near term and the uterus is injured, cesarean delivery with uterine repair is reasonable. When a viable fetus is alive but remote from term, suggested indications for delivery include evidence of fetal hemorrhage, uteroplacental insufficiency, and infection.[73]

Although fetal injury can occur when a bullet enters the mother's lower abdomen, the risks of prematurity may outweigh the risk of delaying repair of fetal injuries. Although obstetric ultrasonography and radiography may be helpful, the diagnosis of in utero injuries can be difficult. Neonatal and pediatric surgical consultation is invaluable in planning care.

If the fetus has died, vaginal delivery is preferred if there is no evidence of uterine hemorrhage. Options include awaiting spontaneous labor and induction of labor with prostaglandins or oxytocin. If laparotomy is required and the uterus prevents exposure for repair of maternal injuries, evacuation of the dead fetus is indicated.

Stab Wounds

When a patient has a stab wound, attempts should be made to determine the object used and its length. The longer the object, the more likely it is that the peritoneum has been penetrated when the abdomen is wounded. The risk of intestinal injury in nonpregnant stabbing victims is less than that with gunshot injuries because bowel tends to move away from a penetrating object (sliding effect). This effect explains, in part, the lower mortality rate with stab wounds than with gunshot wounds. The sliding effect may be less during pregnancy because bowel is compressed into the upper abdomen with advancing gestation.

Traditionally, all abdominal stab wounds have been regarded as an indication for exploratory laparotomy. More recently, nonoperative management has been considered for some patients.[72] Two of the most important factors in assessing the need for laparotomy in injured gravidas are peritoneal penetration and location of the entrance wound. A wound can be probed, and a fistulogram may assist in determining whether the peritoneal cavity has been entered. If a conservative approach is chosen, the patient must be closely monitored and exploration undertaken without delay if the mother has signs of hemorrhage or evidence of sepsis. Contraindications to observation include the following:

- Penetration of the peritoneal cavity
- Entry above the fundus
- Hemodynamic instability of the mother
- Fetal compromise at a viable gestational age

As with gunshot wounds to the abdomen, the surgical consultant should make the final decision about the need for operative intervention.

DPL may be used to identify intra-abdominal injury requiring laparotomy, but it has several limitations in patients with penetrating injuries.[4] First, the findings may be negative in nonpregnant victims, despite hollow viscus injury, because bleeding is usually minimal. Second, the leukocyte response to bowel injury may be delayed, causing a false-negative finding. Finally, the accuracy of DPL in pregnant women with stab wounds is unknown. Although a positive finding would be expected when uterine vessels are injured, the size of a uterine wound and the depth of penetration cannot be ascertained.

FAST was prospectively evaluated in 75 patients with penetrating abdominal trauma and was shown to be useful as the initial diagnostic test.[81] It is not, however, as reliable as in blunt trauma, and a negative result requires additional testing. Additionally, it has not been studied in pregnant victims of penetrating trauma, and its accuracy is unknown in this setting.

A lower abdominal stab wound with adequate force is likely to damage the uterus as well as the fetus. Management options include the following:

- Observation
- Uterine repair with delivery of the fetus
- Uterine repair with the fetus left in utero[82]

No outcome data are available comparing repair of a uterine wound with no repair. The risks of infection and uterine rupture associated with each approach are unknown, given the limited number of patients with these injuries. Indications for delivery are the same as those for gravidas with a gunshot wound.

Based on reported cases of stab wounds to the pregnant uterus, Sakala and Kort[74] proposed the following management plan. A nonperforating injury of the uterus may be repaired without disturbing the pregnancy. Perforating injuries, however, carry a much higher rate of fetal injury. A fetus at or near term should be considered for cesarean delivery and uterine repair. If the fetus is premature, alive, and not compromised, the uterus may be repaired, with vaginal delivery anticipated. When the fetus has died, both perforating and nonperforating injuries should be repaired and the fetus delivered vaginally. The injured uterus maintains its ability to labor and deliver an infant.[83] Antibiotic prophylaxis seems reasonable in these cases, although no data are available to support this recommendation.

Stab wounds to the upper abdomen are three times more frequent than lower abdominal wounds. Upper abdominal wounds that penetrate the peritoneum require surgical exploration because of the high likelihood of small bowel injury. If doubt exists, exploratory laparotomy is the safest approach to exclude intra-abdominal injury. When the peritoneum of the upper abdomen has been penetrated, laceration of the diaphragm must be excluded because it can result in bowel herniation, strangulation, and sepsis. After diaphragm repair, labor and second-stage Valsalva efforts should be avoided and cesarean delivery should be performed, presumably to avoid increasing intra-abdominal pressure.[74]

SUMMARY OF MANAGEMENT OPTIONS
Penetrating Trauma in Pregnancy

Management Options	Quality of Evidence	Strength of Recommendation	References
General Management			
See above	–	–	–
Examine patient for entrance and exit wounds	IV	C	10
	III	B	73
Exploratory Laparotomy			
Midline vertical incision	IV	C	10
	III	B	73

Continued

SUMMARY OF MANAGEMENT OPTIONS
Penetrating Trauma in Pregnancy *(Continued)*

Management Options	Quality of Evidence	Strength of Recommendation	References
Exploratory Laparotomy *(Continued)*			
Uterine evacuation is not mandatory	IV	C	10
	III	B	73
Cesarean hysterectomy may be necessary if the patient has uncontrollable hemorrhage or excessive uterine damage	IV III	C B	10 73
Gunshot Wounds			
Obtain flat plate and lateral radiograph if no exit wound visible	IV	C	78
Surgical exploration if:			
-signs of intra-abdominal injury	III	B	76
-positive peritoneal lavage	III	B	4
-persistent unexplained shock	–	GPP	–
Consider conservative management if:			
-the mother is hemodynamically stable	IV	C	77,78
-the bullet entered below the uterine fundus	III	B	76
-the bullet can be localized to the uterus	III	B	76
-the fetus is without injury or dead	III	B	76
-the mother has no genitourinary or gastrointestinal injury	III	B	76
Deliver fetus if:			
-evidence of fetal hemorrhage	IV	C	77
-uteroplacental insufficiency	IV	C	77
-infection	–	GPP	–
Stab Wounds			
Determine peritoneal penetration; options:			
-probe wound	–	GPP	–
-fistulogram	IV	C	74
-diagnostic peritoneal lavage	III	B	4
Surgical exploration if:			
-peritoneal penetration	IV	C	74
-entry above the uterine fundus	–	GPP	–
-hemodynamically unstable mother	IV	C	82
-fetal compromise at viable gestation	IV	C	74
Consider conservative management if:			
-no peritoneal penetration	IV	C	74
-entry below the uterine fundus	IV	C	74
-guidelines for delivery of the fetus are the same as for gunshot wounds (above)	IV	C	74
Uterine injury with lower abdominal stab wound; options			
-observation	IV	C	74
-uterine repair with delivery	IV	C	74
-uterine repair and fetus remains in utero	IV	C	74

BURNS

Incidence

Fortunately, most burns sustained during pregnancy are minor, and more severe burns are uncommon. Most burns occur in the home and are the result of a house fire, hot water or flammable liquids, and gases. Pregnant women account for 0.4% to 7% of all patients who are hospitalized with major burns.[84–88]

Maternal survival is dependent on the percentage of total body surface area (TBSA) burned.[87,89–91] When 20% to 39% of TBSA has been burned, 97% to 100% of gravidas survive. The mortality rate increases when 40% to 59% of TBSA is burned, and ranges from 27% to 50%. Burns exceeding 60% of TBSA are associated with an increasing maternal death rate.[86,87,90–93] Survival in pregnant women with burn injuries is comparable to that in their nonpregnant counterparts, when matched for burn severity.[89] Concurrent inhalation injury, however, is associated with an increased mortality rate in nonpregnant patients.

Fetal survival is also affected by the percentage of maternal TBSA involved. The fetal mortality rate is negligible when the burn affects less than 20% of maternal TBSA. When 20% to 39% of the mother's TBSA is involved, the fetal loss rate ranges from 11% to 27%. The fetal mortality rate increases to 45% to 53% with burns that affect 40% to 59% of maternal TBSA. When a pregnant woman has a burn that involves greater than 60% of TBSA, fetal loss approaches 100%.[86,87,90–93] The largest reported burn survived by both mother and fetus is 58% of TBSA.[94]

Classification of Burns

The depth of a burn is classified by degree. A first-degree burn is confined to the epidermis. Second-degree burns are superficial and deep partial-thickness burns. Adequate epithelial cells remain and allow skin to regenerate. Clinically, blistering, erythema, and pain characterize superficial partial-thickness burns. Deep partial-thickness lesions are characterized by blisters; a pale, white appearance; and no pain sensation. Full-thickness burns, previously known as third-degree burns, destroy all epithelial elements. Regeneration is not possible without grafting. The burned area appears charred and leathery, without blisters; thrombosed superficial vessels may be visible; and pain sensation is absent. Fourth-degree burns involve structures beneath the skin.

Burn size estimates the extent of injury. The "rule of nines" is a method used to estimate the percentage of body surface area involved. Each upper extremity and the head and neck are 9% of TBSA. The lower extremities and the anterior and posterior surface's of the trunk are 18% each. This system was devised for nonpregnant patients, however, and does not account for the presumed increase in abdominal surface area with advancing gestation.

Burns severity is defined as minor, moderate, or major. A minor burn is a superficial, or partial-thickness, burn that covers less than 15% of TBSA or a full-thickness burn that covers more than 2% of TBSA. Major burns include partial-thickness burns covering more than 25% of TBSA, full-thickness burns covering more than 10% of TBSA, and burns meeting the criteria for admission to a burn unit (discussed later). Major burns are classified according to the TBSA involved: moderate (10% to 19% of TBSA), severe (20%–39% of TBSA), and critical (>40% of TBSA).[92]

Management of Minor Burns

Minor burns may be treated on an outpatient basis if the burn does not affect an area of critical function (i.e., hand, across a joint) or an area in which cosmesis is a concern (i.e., face). Superficial (first-degree) burns do not require specific treatment beyond keeping the area clean and protected. A mild analgesic may be prescribed. A narcotic, such as oxycodone, may be required for pain control in patients with partial-thickness burns. The burned area should be cleansed with sterile saline and devitalized tissue removed. Large blisters may be incised and debrided. Blisters should not be aspirated because this practice can introduce bacteria into a closed space. A nonadherent sterile dressing can be used to protect the burned area. Patients with partial-thickness burns should be re-evaluated in 24 hours. At this time, the wound is evaluated and the dressing changed. Complete healing can be expected in 2 to 3 weeks, with no adverse effects on the pregnancy.

Management of Major Burns

The basic principles of resuscitation also apply to the patient with a major burn injury. Fluid administration is the most important initial treatment. Venous access should be established with a 14- to 16-gauge catheter placed through unburned skin, when possible. Immediate removal of clothing prevents continued burning by smoldering synthetic fabric. All skin surfaces must be examined, burned areas assessed for depth and surface area involved, and additional injuries excluded. Inhalation injury should be suspected and 100% oxygen given by face mask. Arterial blood gas analysis and carbon monoxide level measurement are standard features of laboratory evaluation. A burn specialist should be consulted. Admission to a burn unit is considered for patients with any of the following injuries[95]:

- Partial-thickness burn affecting greater than 10% of TBSA
- Burns of the face, hands, feet, genitalia, perineum, or skin over major joints

- Third-degree burns
- Electrical injury, including lightning injury
- Chemical burns
- Inhalation injury
- Burn injury in patients with preexisting medical disorders that could complicate management or affect the risk of death
- Burns and associated trauma
- Burn injury in a patient who requires special social, emotional, or long-term rehabilitation

The systemic response to a major burn is a massive release of vasoactive mediators that cause a decrease in plasma and blood volumes, shifting intravascular fluid to intracellular and interstitial compartments. Thus, the goal of fluid resuscitation is to correct hypovolemia during the initial 24 to 48 hours. Hypovolemic shock develops in a patient with burns covering more than 15% to 20% of TBSA if fluid resuscitation is not instituted promptly.[96] Hypovolemia in the pregnant patient can also lead to decreased placental perfusion and fetal compromise. Therefore, proper resuscitation is critical for both mother and fetus.

The essential component of fluid resuscitation is crystalloid (normal saline or lactated Ringer's solution). The amount of fluid that a patient requires during the first 24 hours after a burn injury can be estimated with one of several formulas. The Parkland formula estimates fluid requirements during the first 24 hours as 4 mL/kg/% TBSA burned. Edema formation at the burn site is most rapid during the initial 6 to 8 hours after the a burn, and fluid is administered at a rate to compensate for the intravascular loss. One half of the total fluid required is administered during the first 8 hours after the burn (not after admission), and the remaining half is administered over the next 16 hours. The Brooke and Evans formulas are also used to estimate fluid requirements, but differ from the Parkland protocol in their administration of colloid and free water in addition to crystalloid. Additional fluid may be required for adequate resuscitation in pregnant women with major burns because blood volume increases with advancing gestation. Inhalation injury also increases the amount of fluid required during initial resuscitation. Fluid administration is adjusted to maintain urinary output of 0.5 mL/kg/hr. Most patients remain tachycardic despite adequate fluid resuscitation; therefore, heart rate is not a good clinical measure. Pregnant patients also have a baseline increase in heart rate. Electrolyte balance must be closely monitored during and after resuscitation, with imbalances corrected on an ongoing basis.

Diligent wound care is critical to preventing infectious complications. In the emergency department, personnel should wear sterile gloves and gowns while caring for the patient. Once clothing has been removed, burned areas are covered with sterile dry dressings or sterile sheets. An intravenous narcotic should be administered, as needed, for pain control. Debridement and application of antibiotic ointment should not be performed in the trauma room, but under proper conditions in a burn unit. Topical antimicrobial agents delay colonization of the wounded area. Three have established efficacy in the treatment of major burns: 11.1% mafenide acetate, 1% silver sulfadiazine, and 0.5% silver nitrate. Silver sulfadiazine must be used with caution, and long-term use is relatively contraindicated in pregnant women because of the theoretical risk of kernicterus in the newborn. Iodine-containing solutions are frequently used for wound care, but their use must be limited during pregnancy because of the absorption of the iodine and the risk of fetal thyroid dysfunction.[91] All patients with a burn affecting greater than 10% of TBSA should receive tetanus toxoid with immunoglobulin if their previous immunization status is uncertain.

Carbon monoxide (CO) poisoning can occur whenever carbonaceous material is released as a result of incomplete combustion. The affinity of CO for hemoglobin is more than 200 times that of oxygen, and it readily displaces oxygen from hemoglobin.[97] Carbon monoxide causes a left shift of the oxyhemoglobin dissociation curve and increases the affinity of hemoglobin for the remaining bound oxygen. Tissue oxygenation decreases as less oxygen is released from hemoglobin in the periphery. Signs and symptoms of CO poisoning correlate with the blood level. A CO level of less than 10% is unlikely to cause symptoms, whereas levels of 10% to 20% cause a mild headache and palpitations. Once the level reaches 20% to 40%, dizziness, agitation, confusion, and incoordination become apparent. Patients with a CO level of greater than 40% are at risk for progressive dyspnea, lethargy, coma, and death.

CO readily crosses the placenta and may cause fetal malformations, hypoxia, neurologic dysfunction, low birth weight, and death in utero. CO levels rise more slowly in the fetus than in the mother, and continue to increase for up to 24 hours after the maternal level has reached a steady state. Once fetal CO reaches a steady state, the concentration is 10% to 15% higher than the mother's concentration. Likewise, the fetus requires a much longer time for elimination than the mother does. The maternal half-life of CO in a sheep model was 2.5 hours compared with 7 hours in the fetus.[97]

The blood level determines the urgency of treatment for CO poisoning. Observation is sufficient if the CO level is less than 10%. When the level is 10% to 20%, treatment with 100% inspired oxygen is indicated. High-concentration oxygen administered with a tight-fitting face mask decreases the half-life of carboxyhemoglobin in adults from 2 to 3 hours in room air to 45 minutes.[97] Similarly, 100% oxygen decreases the half-life of carboxyhemoglobin in the fetus from 7 hours to 2 to 3 hours, but it is still longer than that in the mother. Based on mathematical calculations, a pregnant woman with CO poisoning should receive 100% oxygen for up to five times longer than needed to reduce her own level to normal (<5%).[97,98] This extended period of treatment allows for the longer elimination time required by the fetus.

Hyperbaric oxygen therapy is used for nonpregnant patients with a CO level greater than 25% or with neurologic changes, regardless of the blood level. It has been used to treat pregnant women with CO poisoning, with no adverse fetal effect. Therapy has been recommended for pregnant women with a maternal CO level of more than 20%; neurologic changes, regardless of the CO level; or signs of fetal compromise.[99] However, hyperbaric oxygen therapy in patients with a major burn presents a number of logistic problems, and care must be individualized.

Inhalation injury occurs as a result of exposure to smoke particles and chemicals. Patients who are burned in a closed space are at increased risk, and the incidence increases with burn severity. Two thirds of patients with burns affecting more than 70% of TBSA have concurrent inhalation injury.[96] Singed nasal hair, facial burns, inflamed oropharyngeal mucosa, carbonaceous sputum, and a CO level greater than 15% suggest injury. Laryngeal edema should be suspected in a patient with hoarseness, stridor, or cough. Intubation may be required to maintain a patent airway. The initial chest radiograph, however, may not show the severity of injury. If the diagnosis of inhalation injury is in doubt, laryngobronchoscopy can be performed. Treatment includes warm humidified oxygen, bronchodilators, pulmonary toilet, nebulized heparin, and therapeutic bronchoscopy. Mechanical ventilation is required if respiratory failure occurs.

Patients with major burns are at risk for many complications, including pulmonary edema, pneumonia, wound infections, septic shock, electrolyte disturbances, nutritional deficiencies, and scar formation. Sepsis is the major cause of death in patients with burns, emphasizing the importance of sterile technique.[91] A circumferential burn of the thorax or abdomen may cause respiratory compromise or vena caval compression in pregnant victims. Early escharotomy improves respiratory excursion and relieves increased intra-abdominal pressure. Scar formation can be physically limiting, but successful pregnancies have been reported in patients with significant abdominal scarring after burn injuries. Surgical release and grafting can be performed in a scar that becomes restrictive with advancing pregnancy, and uninvolved expanded abdominal skin has been used as a flap to reconstruct a scar after delivery.[100,101] Clinically significant thromboembolism is an infrequent complication in patients with a major burn. Nevertheless, prophylaxis has been suggested for patients with additional risk factors, including lower extremity trauma, extensive burns, morbid obesity, prolonged bed rest, and central venous lines.[30] Although data on the risk of thromboembolism in pregnant burn victims are not available, pregnancy is an additional risk factor and prophylaxis seems reasonable if no other contraindications exist.

Obstetric complications associated with major burns include spontaneous abortion, premature labor, and fetal death in utero. The first week after injury seems to be the period of highest risk, and medical complications often precede obstetric complications. The physiologic response to burns includes hypovolemia, hypoxia, acidosis, electrolyte imbalance, and sepsis. Each of these, alone or in combination, can lead to uterine activity or fetal compromise.[94] Septicemia is the most common cause of spontaneous abortion in women with burns.[84]

An increased incidence of premature labor has been associated with burns affecting more than 30% to 35% of TBSA.[94] In addition to the mechanisms that can stimulate the uterus (discussed earlier), prostaglandins and leukotrienes are released from macrophages, neutrophils, and platelets at the burn site. Prostaglandin E_2, a uterine stimulant, is produced by scalded skin. Because prostaglandins are associated with uterine activity, pregnant women who have a burn injury should be monitored for uterine contractions. Tocolytic agents, particularly β-mimetics, must be used cautiously, and only after the mother is clinically stable and the fetal heart rate tracing is reassuring.

Intervention on behalf of a viable fetus may be required in a gravida with a major burn. The following recommendations are based on combined experiences of various authors caring for pregnant burn victims. Delivery is suggested when a significant medical complication develops in a woman with moderate burns, because fetal survival in this group appears to be influenced by maternal complications. Likewise, early obstetric intervention has been advocated for a gravely ill woman who has complications that jeopardize the fetus and any woman with extensive burns who is beyond 32 weeks' gestation.[85,89] Fetal death occurs most commonly during the first week after a major burn and is a likely event when a gravida has severe to critical burns.[94,102] Delivery after maternal stabilization is recommended for women at 26 weeks' gestation and beyond with burns affecting greater than 40% to 50% of TBSA.[87,92,93,102] This recommendation is based on older literature, and the gestational age for intervention should be adjusted based on institutional neonatal survival at the limits of viability and on patient and family wishes. Cesarean delivery is reserved for obstetric indications, and vaginal delivery has been accomplished, even in women with perineal burns. If abdominal delivery is indicated, the incision may be performed through burned skin without increasing morbidity.

SUMMARY OF MANAGEMENT OPTIONS

Burns in Pregnancy

Management Options	Quality of Evidence	Strength of Recommendation	References
Minor Burns			
Out-patient treatment if burn does not cover area of critical function or cosmetic importance	–	GPP	–
Superficial burn:			
-analgesia	–	GPP	–
-keep burned area clean and protected	–	GPP	–
Partial full-thickness burn:			
-clean, debride and irrigate	–	GPP	–
-bacitracin ointment	–	GPP	–
-nonadherent dressing	–	GPP	–
-adequate analgesia	–	GPP	–
-re-evaluate in 24h	–	GPP	–
Major Burns			
Resuscitation			
See General Management (above)	–	–	–
Fluid balance management:	IV	C	96
-adequate fluid administration (Parkland, Brooke, or Evans formula)			
-monitor urinary output to maintain 0.5 mL/kg/h			
Examine entire body surface: assess depth of burn and surface area involved	IIa	B	87,90
Arterial blood gas analysis and carbon monoxide level	IV	C	97
Wound care:			
-sterile technique	–	GPP	–
-topical antimicrobial agent	–	GPP	–
-silver sulfadiazine relatively contraindicated in late pregnancy	–	GPP	–
-surgery for debridement, prevention of cicatrization	–	GPP	–
-cicatrized abdominal wounds may require release in pregnancy	IV	C	100
-minimal use of iodine-containing topical cleansing solutions	IV	C	91
Carbon monoxide poisoning:			
-100% inspired oxygen by face mask if CO level ≥10%	IV	C	97
-treat five times longer than required to lower maternal level below 5%	IV	C	97
-hyperbaric oxygen therapy if	IV	C	99
• maternal CO level is >20%			
• neurologic changes occur (regardless of CO level)			
• signs of fetal compromise are noted			
Inhalation injury:	IV	C	96
-intubation if laryngeal edema develops			
-warm humidified oxygen			
-pulmonary toilet			
-mechanical ventilation as indicated			
-therapeutic bronchoscopy			
Preterm labor:	III	B	94
-cautious use of tocolysis if preterm labor			
-steroids if preterm delivery likely			

SUMMARY OF MANAGEMENT OPTIONS

Burns in Pregnancy *(Continued)*

Management Options	Quality of Evidence	Strength of Recommendation	References
Major Burns *(Continued)*			
Consider delivery of the fetus if:	IIa	B	87,90
-significant medical complications in a gravida with a moderate -to severe burn injury			
-complications occur in a gravely ill woman			
-gravely ill woman who develops complications			
-extensive burns at >32 weeks' gestation			
->40%–50% of the total body surface area is burned			

ELECTRICAL INJURY

Incidence

Reports of electrical injuries in pregnant women are exceedingly uncommon. A total of 21 pregnant women with electrical injury and 11 gravidas struck by lightning have been reported.[103,104] Although one study reported no maternal deaths from conductive and lightning injuries, the fetal mortality rate was 73% and 45%, respectively.[103] The fetal death rate was only 6%, however, in 31 women who were followed prospectively after predominantly household electrical injuries.[104] Minor injuries are less likely to be reported than catastrophic events, however, and the true incidence of electrical injury in pregnancy is likely to be underestimated. Most victims of electrical injury have multisystem trauma, and should be transferred to an experienced center for optimal care.

Management

The direct effects of the current and the heat it generates cause physical damage, as does trauma as a result of electrical injury. Electrical injury can be thermal, conductive, or caused by lightning; conductive injuries are the most common. The type of current, its path through the body, and its voltage also affect the type of injury. Cardiac and respiratory arrest are the main causes of death after injury from domestic alternating current and lightning. The current passing through the body can cause cardiac dysrhythmia, asystole, respiratory arrest, muscle contraction, tetany, skeletal fractures, and neurologic injury. Continuous cardiac monitoring is recommended for patients who have loss of consciousness, cardiac dysrhythmia, abnormal findings on 12-lead electrocardiogram, abnormal mental status or physical examination findings, or burns or tissue damage expected to cause hemodynamic instability or electrolyte abnormalities.[105] Fractures may be caused by a fall occurring with the shock, and cervical spine injury as a result of muscular contraction must be excluded. Rhabdomyolysis can cause renal failure if adequate intravenous hydration is not maintained until myoglobinuria resolves. Tissue necrosis may be extensive, and antibiotic prophylaxis with penicillin decreases the risk of muscle and fascial infection. Surgical consultation may be required for wound care, debridement, and fasciotomy. Most victims of electrical injury have multisystem trauma and require transfer to an experienced center for optimal care.

Resistance to current varies among tissues of the body. Blood offers little resistance compared with muscle, skin, tendon, fat, and bone. Amniotic fluid, the uteroplacental circulation, and fetal skin offer low resistance to electrical current flow.[103,106] As a result, the fetus is very vulnerable to electrical injury. When the current takes a hand-to-foot path through the mother, it presumably passes through the uterus.[104,106] The current path may therefore be an important factor in fetal outcome, and may account for the difference in mortality rates among reported cases.[103,104]

The severity of maternal injury is not predictive of fetal outcome, and minor exposure can have a profound fetal effect. Significantly less current is required to produce injury in the fetus than in the mother.[103] In cases of fetal demise, cardiac arrest appears to have been the cause of death. This observation is consistent with maternal reports of sudden cessation of fetal movement after the injury. Intrauterine growth restriction and oligohydramnios have been reported in fetuses surviving maternal electrical injury.[103,106] An animal model also showed growth restriction in 71% of rabbit fetuses subjected to electrically induced thermal injury of the placenta.[107]

The paucity of data makes it difficult to offer management recommendations for a gravida who has an electrical injury. Care of the mother should follow established guidelines. Fetal cardiac activity should be confirmed after electrical injury. If the fetus is alive and viable, continuous cardiotocographic monitoring should be started at the time of initial maternal evaluation. Monitoring for 4 hours is suggested when minor mechanical trauma (i.e., fall to the floor) is associated with electrical injury. Twenty-four hours of maternal and fetal monitoring has been recommended if the results of maternal electrocardiogram are abnormal, maternal loss of consciousness occurred, or there is a history of cardiovascular disease.[105] Monitoring for oligohydramnios and fetal growth restriction throughout the rest of the pregnancy is also recommended for the surviving fetus.[106]

SUMMARY OF MANAGEMENT OPTIONS

Electrical Injury in Pregnancy

Management Options	Quality of Evidence	Strength of Recommendation	References
Maternal Resuscitation (See Table 54–2)			
Management of multisystem trauma in cooperation with subspecialists (see above)	–	–	–
Continuous cardiac monitoring with:	III	B	105
• Loss of consciousness			
• Cardiac dysrhythmia			
• Abnormal 12-lead electrocardiogram reading			
• Abnormal mental status or physical examination findings			
• Burn or tissue damage is expected to cause hemodynamic instability or electrolyte abnormalities			
Adequate intravenous hydration if rhabdomyolysis develops	III	B	103,104
Antibiotic prophylaxis	III	B	103,104
Wound and burn care	III	B	103,104
Obstetric Management			
Confirm the presence of a fetal heart rate.	–	GPP	–
Maternal injury does not correlate with fetal injury.	III	B	103
Continuous cardiotocographic monitoring for 4 hours:	III	B	106
• Minor mechanical trauma			
Continuous cardiotocographic monitoring for 24 hours:	III	B	106
• Abnormal maternal electrocardiogram reading			
• Maternal loss of consciousness			
• History of maternal cardiac disease			
Consider surveillance for oligohydramnios and fetal growth restriction if the fetus survives the event.	III	B	103,106

PERIMORTEM CESAREAN SECTION

Incidence

The concept of perimortem and postmortem cesarean delivery dates back thousands of years. Fortunately, it is an uncommon occurrence, and the exact incidence is difficult to calculate.

Management Options

Injuries in a pregnant trauma patient occasionally are so severe that the mother dies, despite maximal resuscitation efforts. The decision to perform perimortem cesarean delivery in an attempt to save the fetus is based on gestational age and the duration of cardiac arrest. The operation should not be performed in anticipation of a cardiopulmonary arrest, but only once cardiovascular collapse has occurred.

One of the most important questions is the effect of cesarean delivery on the efficiency of cardiopulmonary resuscitation (CPR). Even under optimal conditions, CPR generates a cardiac output that is only 30% of normal.[108] Shunting of 10% of the cardiac output to the uterus and the left lateral tilt recommended to decrease vena caval compression by the uterus further reduce the effectiveness of chest compressions. Oxygen consumption increases during pregnancy as well and predisposes pregnant women to rapid desaturation with hypoventilation. It is presumed that delivery of the fetus allows more efficient CPR by relieving vena caval obstruction and increasing blood volume by autotransfusion.

The sooner the infant is delivered after a maternal arrest, the better the chance of intact neurologic survival. Optimal neonatal outcome is achieved when delivery occurs less than 5 minutes from the arrest. There are no documented cases of intact fetal survival beyond 35 minutes from the onset of cardiac arrest in the mother.[108] Therefore, it seems reasonable to proceed with delivery up to 35 minutes after maternal collapse. If the duration of arrest is unknown, proceeding with delivery is also reasonable.

Once maternal cardiopulmonary arrest has occurred and the decision is made to intervene on behalf of the fetus, the following steps are suggested. Initiate delivery 4 minutes after maternal arrest, with the intention to deliver the fetus 5 minutes after the arrest.[108] Continue CPR throughout the procedure to offer every chance for maternal survival. Do not waste precious time preparing a sterile field or instrument tray or attempting to perform an ultrasound examination. Each surgeon should approach the abdominal incision in the most efficient fashion. Consider a low transverse uterine incision because less blood loss occurs and closure can be achieved more quickly than with a classical incision. If more than 4 minutes have passed, but signs of fetal life are present, proceed with delivery.

SUMMARY OF MANAGEMENT OPTIONS
Perimortem Cesarean Section

Management Options	Quality of Evidence	Strength of Recommendation	References
Perform when maternal cardiopulmonary arrest occurs, not in anticipation of it.	IV	C	108
Initiate delivery 4 minutes after arrest if maternal resuscitation is unsuccessful: The goal is delivery 5 minutes after arrest.	IV	C	108
Continue cardiopulmonary resuscitation during delivery.	IV	C	108
Use time efficiently:	IV	C	108
• Do not prepare a sterile field or a full instrument table.			
• Use the quickest incision possible.			
• Consider a low transverse uterine incision.			
Proceed with delivery if >4 minutes have passed since maternal arrest but signs of fetal life are still present.	IV	C	108

CONCLUSIONS

- Trauma occurs in 6% to 7% of all pregnancies and is the leading cause of non-obstetric maternal mortality.
- Physiologic changes associated with pregnancy can significantly influence the clinical presentation after trauma as well as the response to initial resuscitative attempts.
- The management of gravidas with moderate to severe injuries should follow an organized plan, including a primary survey, an initial resuscitation attempt, a secondary survey, laboratory and diagnostic testing and definitive treatment. With few exceptions, both the diagnostic and therapeutic approach to trauma in pregnancy should differ minimally from that of a non-pregnant patient.
- Gestational age assessment should be determined quickly, and monitoring of the potentially viable fetus should be a component of the initial evaluation.
- Blunt trauma can lead to pregnancy-specific injuries including abruptio placenta, preterm labor, uterine rupture, and fetomaternal hemorrhage.

Continued

CONCLUSIONS *(Continued)*

- With penetrating trauma, exploratory laparotomy is not necessarily an indication for operative delivery of the fetus. This latter decision should be based on gestational age, fetal and maternal stability, and the ability to gain adequate surgical exposure for the repair of maternal injuries.
- Maternal and fetal survival in burn victims are dependent on the percentage of total body surface area burned in the mother.
- With electrical injuries, the severity of maternal injury is not predicitive of fetal outcome. Significantly less current is required to produce injury in the fetus than in the mother.
- A perimortem cesarean delivery should be initiated within 4 minutes after arrest with continuation of the CPR process throughout the surgical procedure.

REFERENCES

1. Fildes J, Reed L, Jones N, et al: Trauma: The leading cause of maternal death. J Trauma 1992;32:643–645.
2. Van Hook JW: Trauma in pregnancy. Clin Obstet Gynecol 2002;45:414–424.
3. Drost TF, Rosemurgy AS, Sherman HF, et al: Major trauma in pregnant women: Maternal/fetal outcome. J Trauma 1990; 30:574–578.
4. Esposito TJ, Gens DR, Smith LG, et al: Trauma during pregnancy: A review of 79 cases. Arch Surg 1991;126:1073–1078.
5. Scorpio RJ, Esposito TJ, Smith LG, Gens DR: Blunt trauma during pregnancy: Factors affecting fetal outcome. J Trauma 1992;32:213–216.
6. Schiff MA, Holt VL: The injury severity score in pregnant trauma patients: Predicting placental abruption and fetal death. J Trauma 2002;53:946–949.
7. Reis PM, Sander CM, Pearlman MD: Abruptio placentae after auto accidents: A case control study. J Reprod Med 2000; 45:6–10.
8. Pearlman MD, Tintinalli JE, Lorenz RP: A prospective controlled study of outcome after trauma during pregnancy. Am J Obst Gynecol 1990;162:1502–1510.
9. Macho JR, Lewis FR, Krupski WC: Management of the injured patient. In Way LW (ed): Current Surgical Diagnosis & Treatment, 10th ed. Norwalk, Conn, Appleton & Lange, 1994, pp 213–240.
10. Esposito TJ: Trauma during pregnancy. Emerg Med Clin North Am 1994;12:167–199.
11. Esposito TJ: Pitfalls in resuscitation and early management of the pregnant trauma patient. Trauma 1988;5:1–22.
12. Arrighi DA, Farnell MB, Mucha P Jr, et al: Prospective, randomized trial of rapid venous access for patients in hypovolemic shock. Ann Emerg Med 1989;18:927–930.
13. Jordan BD: Maternal head trauma during pregnancy. In Devinsky O, Feldmann E, Hainline B (eds): Neurological Complications of Pregnancy. New York, Raven Press, 1994, pp 131–138.
14. Morkovin V: Trauma in pregnancy. In Farrell RG (ed): Ob/Gyn Emergencies: The First 60 Minutes. Rockville, Md, Aspen, 1986, p 81.
15. Smith RS, Bottoms SF: Ultrasonographic prediction of neonatal survival in extremely low-birth-weight infants. Am J Obstet Gynecol 1993;169:490–493.
16. Knottenbelt JD: Low initial hemoglobin levels in trauma patients: An important indicator of ongoing hemorrhage. J Trauma 1991;31:1396–1399.
17. Neufeld JDG: Trauma in pregnancy: What if . . . . ? Emerg Med Clin North Am 1993;11:207–224.
18. Sahdev P, Garramone RR, Schwartz RJ, et al: Evaluation of liver function tests in screening for intra-abdominal injuries. Ann Emerg Med 1991;20:838–841.
19. American College of Obstetricians and Gynecologists: Guidelines for diagnostic imaging during pregnancy. ACOG Committee Opinion No. 158. Washington, DC, September, 1995.
20. Fischer RP, Beverlin BC, Engrav LH, et al: Diagnostic peritoneal lavage: Fourteen years and 2,586 patients later. Am J Surg 1978;136:701–704.
21. Hoff WS, Holevar M, Nagy KK, et al: Practice management guidelines for the evaluation of blunt abdominal trauma: The EAST Practice Management Guidelines Work Group. J Trauma 2002;53:602–615.
22. Rothenberger DA, Quattlebaum FW, Zabel J, Fischer RP: Diagnostic peritoneal lavage for blunt trauma in pregnant women. Am J Obstet Gynecol 1977;129:479–481.
23. Esposito TJ, Gens DR, Smith LG, Scorpio R: Evaluation of blunt abdominal trauma occurring during pregnancy. J Trauma 1989;29:1628–1632.
24. McAnena OJ, Moore EE, Marx JA: Initial evaluation of the patient with blunt abdominal trauma. Surg Clin North Am 1990;70:495–513.
25. Lowdermilk C, Gavant ML, West OC, Goldman SM: Screening helical CT for evaluation of blunt traumatic injury in the pregnant patient. Radiographics 1999;19:S243–S258.
26. Dolich MO, McKenny MG, Varela E, et al: 2,576 ultrasounds for blunt abdominal trauma. J Trauma 2001;50:108–112.
27. Boulanger BR, McLellan BA, Brenneman FD, et al: Prospective evidence of the superiority of a sonography-based algorithm in the assessment of blunt abdominal trauma. J Trauma Injury Infect Crit Care 1999;47:632–637.
28. Goodwin H, Holmes JF, Wisner DH: Abdominal ultrasound examination in pregnant blunt trauma patients. J Trauma 2001;50:689–694.
29. Geerts WH, Code KI, Jay RM, et al: A prospective study of venous thromboembolism after major trauma. N Engl J Med 1994;331:1601–1606.
30. Sixth ACCP Consensus Conference on Antithrombotic Therapy: Prevention of venous thromboembolism. Chest 2001;119:132S–175S.
31. Weiss HB, Songer TJ, Fabio A: Fetal deaths related to maternal injury. JAMA 2001;286:1863–1868.
32. Pearlman MD, Klinich KD, Schneider LW: A comprehensive program to improve safety for pregnant women and fetuses in motor vehicle crashes: A preliminary report. Am J Obstet Gynecol 2000;182:1554–1564.

33. Pearlman MD, Phillips ME: Safety belt use during pregnancy. Obstet Gynecol 1996;88:1026–1029.
34. Pearlman MD: Motor vehicle crashes, pregnancy loss and preterm labor. Int J Gynecol Obstet 1997;57:127–132.
35. Dahmus MA, Sibai BM: Blunt abdominal trauma: Are there any predictive factors for abruptio placentae or maternal-fetal distress? Am J Obstet Gynecol 1993;169:1054–1059.
36. Goodwin TM, Breen MT: Pregnancy outcome and fetomaternal hemorrhage after noncatastrophic trauma. Am J Obstet Gynecol 1990;162:665–671.
37. Connolly A, Katz VL, Bash KL, et al: Trauma and pregnancy. Am J Perinatol 1997;14:331–336.
38. Elliott M: Vehicular accidents and pregnancy. Aust N Z J Obstet Gynaecol 1996;6:279–286.
39. Leggon RE, Wood C, Indeck MC: Pelvic fractures in pregnancy: Influencing maternal and fetal outcomes. J Trauma 2002; 3:796–804.
40. Pearlman MD, Tintinalli JE, Lorenz RP: Blunt trauma during pregnancy. N Engl J Med 1991;323:1609–1613.
41. Rothenberger D, Quattlebaum FW, Perry JF Jr, et al: Blunt maternal trauma: A review of 103 cases. J Trauma 1978; 18:173–179.
42. Crosby WM: Automobile trauma in pregnancy: Prevention and treatment. Prim Care Update Obstet Gynecol 1996;3:6–12.
43. Stafford PA, Biddinger PW, Zumwalt RE: Lethal intrauterine fetal trauma. Am J Obstet Gynecol 1988;159:485–489.
44. Farmer DL, Adzick NS, Crombleholme WR, et al: Fetal trauma: Relation to maternal injury. J Pediatr Surg 1990;25:711–714.
45. Crosby WM, Snyder RG, Snow CC, Hanson PG: Impact injuries in pregnancy. Am J Obstet Gynecol 1968;101:100–110.
46. Notelovitz M, Bottoms SF, Dase DF, Leichter PJ: Painless abruptio placentae. Obstet Gynecol 1979;53:270–272.
47. Williams JK, McClain L, Rosemurgy AS, Colorado NM: Evaluation of blunt abdominal trauma in the third trimester of pregnancy: Maternal and fetal considerations. Obstet Gynecol 1990;75:33–37.
48. American College of Obstetricians and Gynecologists: Obstetric aspects of trauma management. ACOG Educational Bulletin No. 251. Washington, DC, September, 1998.
49. Mighty H: Trauma in pregnancy. Crit Care Clin 1994;10:623–634.
50. Lavin JP, Polsky SS: Abdominal trauma during pregnancy. Clin Perinatol 1983;10:423–438.
51. Pepperell RJ, Rubinstein E, MacIsaac IA: Motor-car accidents during pregnancy. Med J Aust 1977;1:203–205.
52. Shah KH, Simons RK, Holbrood T, et al: Trauma in pregnancy: Maternal and fetal outcomes. J Trauma Injury Infect Crit Care 1998;45:83–86.
53. Ali J, Yeo A, Gana TJ, McLellan BA: Predictors of fetal mortality in pregnant trauma patients. J Trauma Injury Infect Crit Care 1997;42:782–785.
54. Theodorou DA, Velmahos GC, Souter I, et al: Fetal death after trauma in pregnancy. Am Surg 2000;66:809–812.
55. George ER, Vanderwaak T, Scholten DJ: Factors influencing pregnancy outcome after trauma. Am Surg 1992;58:594–598.
56. Baerga-Varela Y, Zietlow SP, Bannon MP, et al: Trauma in pregnancy. Mayo Clin Proc 2000;75:1243–1248.
57. Higgins SD, Garite TJ: Late abruptio placentae in trauma patients: Implications for monitoring. Obstet Gynecol 1984;63:10S–12S.
58. Lavin JP, Miodovnik M: Delayed abruption after maternal trauma as a result of an automobile accident. J Reprod Med 1981;26:621–624.
59. Pearlman MD, Tintinalli JF: Evaluation and treatment of the gravida and fetus following trauma during pregnancy. Obstet Gynecol Clin North Am 1991;18:371–381.
60. Towery R, English P, Wisner D: Evaluation of pregnant women after blunt injury. J Trauma 1993;35:731–736.
61. Hurd WW, Miodovnik M, Hertzberg V, Lavin JP: Selective management of aburptio placentae: A prospective study. Obstet Gynecol 1983;61:467–473.
62. Curet MJ, Schermer CR, Demarest GB, et al: Predictors of outcome in trauma during pregnancy: Identification of patients who can be monitored for less than 6 hours. J Trauma 2000;49:18–25.
63. Rose PG, Strohm PL, Zuspan FP: Fetomaternal hemorrhage following trauma. Am J Obstet Gynecol 1985;153:844–847.
64. US Department of Transportation, National Highway Traffic Safety Administration: 1991 Occupant protection facts. Washington, DC, NHTSA, 1992.
65. Crosby WM, Costiloe JP: Safety of lap-belt restraint for pregnant victims of automobile collisions. N Engl J Med 1971;284:632–636.
66. Crosby WM, King AI, Stout LC: Fetal survival following impact: Improvement with shoulder harness restaint. Am J Obstet Gynecol 1972;112:1101–1106.
67. Pearlman MD, Viano D: Automobile crash stimulation with the first pregnant crash test dummy. Am J Obstet Gynecol 1996;175: 977–981.
68. Hammond TL, Mickens-Powers BF, Stickland K, Hankins GDV: The use of automobile safety restraint systems during pregnancy. J Obstet Gynecol Neonatal Nurs 1990;19:339–343.
69. Griffiths M, Hillman G, Usherwood MM: Seat belt injury in pregnancy resulting in fetal death: A need for education? Case reports. BJOG 1991;98:320–321.
70. American College of Obstetricians and Gynecologists: Automobile passenger restraints for children and pregnant women. Technical Bulletin no. 151. Washington, DC, ACOG, 1995.
71. Schoenfeld A, Ziv E, Stein L, et al: Seat belts in pregnancy and the obstetrician. Obstet Gynecol Surv 1987;42:275–282.
72. Sandy EA, Koerner M: Self-inflicted gunshot wound to the pregnant abdomen: Report of a case and review of the literature. Am J Perinatol 1989;6:30–31.
73. Kuhlmann RS, Cruikshank DP: Maternal trauma during pregnancy. Clin Obstet Gynecol 1994;37:274–293.
74. Sakala EP, Kort DD: Management of stab wounds to the pregnant uterus: A case report and a review of the literature. Obstet Gynecol Surv 1988;43:319–324.
75. Buchsbaum HJ: Diagnosis and management of abdominal gunshot wounds during pregnancy. J Trauma 1975;15:425–430.
76. Awwad JT, Azar GB, Seoud MA, et al: High-velocity penetrating wounds of the gravid uterus: Review of 16 years of civil war. Obstet Gynecol 1994;83:259–264.
77. Franger AL, Buchsbaum HJ, Peaceman AM: Abdominal gunshot wounds in pregnancy. Am J Obstet Gynecol 1989;160: 1124–1128.
78. Iliya FA, Hajj SN, Buchsbaum HJ: Gunshot wounds of the pregnant uterus. J Trauma 1980;20:90–92.
79. Pimentel L: Mother and child: Trauma in pregnancy. Emerg Med Clin North Am 1991;9:549–563.
80. Kirshon B, Young R, Gordon AN: Conservative management of abdominal gunshot wound in a pregnant woman. Am J Perinatol 1988;5:232–233.
81. Udobi KF, Rodriguez A, Chiu WC, Scalea TM: Role of ultrasonography in penetrating abdominal trauma: A prospective clinical study. J Trauma 2001;50:475–479.
82. Grubb DK: Nonsurgical management of penetrating uterine trauma in pregnancy: A case report. Am J Obstet Gynecol 1992; 166:583–584.
83. Pierson R, Thomas L, Beatty R: Penetrating abdominal wounds in pregnancy. Ann Emerg Med 1986;15:1232–1234.
84. Jain ML, Garg AK: Burns in pregnancy: A review of 25 cases. Burns 1993;19:166–167.
85. Unsur V, Oztopeu C, Atalay C, et al: A retrospective study of 11 pregnant women with thermal injury. Eur J Obstet Gynecol Reprod Biol 1996;64:55–58.
86. Amy BW, McManus WF, Goodwin CW, et al: Thermal injury in the pregnant patient. Surg Obstet Gynecol 1985;161:209–212.

87. Taylor JW, Plunkett GD, McManus WF, Pruitt BA: Thermal injury during pregnancy. Obstet Gynecol 1976;47:434–438.
88. Cheah SH, Sivanesaratnam V: Burns in pregnancy: Maternal and fetal prognosis. Aust N Z J Obstet Gynaecol 1989;29:143–145.
89. Rode H, Millar AJ, Cywes S, et al: Thermal injury in pregnancy: The neglected tragedy. S Afr Med J 1990;77:346–348.
90. Akhtar MA, Mulawkar PM, Kulkarni HR: Burns in pregnancy: Effect on maternal and fetal outcomes. Burns 1994;20:351–355.
91. Polko LE, McMahon MJ: Burns in pregnancy. Obstet Gynecol Surv 1998;53:50–56.
92. Smith BK, Rayburn WF, Feller I: Burns and pregnancy. Clin Perinatol 1983;10:383–398.
93. Matthews RN: Obstetric implications of burns in pregnancy. BJOG 1982;89:603–609.
94. Rayburn W, Smith B, Feller I, et al: Major burns during pregnancy: Effects on fetal well-being. Obstet Gynecol 1984;63:392–395.
95. Guidelines for the operation of burn units: Resources for optimal care of the injured patient. Committee on Trauma, American College of Surgeons, 1999.
96. Monafo WW: Initial management of burns. N Engl J Med 1996;335:1581–1586.
97. Longo LD: The biological effects of carbon monoxide on the pregnant woman, fetus, and newborn infant. Am J Obstet Gynecol 1977;129:69–97.
98. Hill EP, Hill JR, Power GG, et al: Carbon monoxide exchange between the human fetus and mother: A mathematical model. Am J Phys 1977;232:H311–H323.
99. Van Hoesen KB, Camporesi EM, Moon RE, et al: Should hyperbaric oxygen be used to treat the pregnant patient for acute carbon monoxide poisoning? A case report and literature review. JAMA 1989;261:1039–1043.
100. Widgerow AD, Ford TD, Botha M: Burn contracture preventing uterine expansion. Ann Plast Surg 1991;27:269–271.
101. Webb JC, Baack BR, Osler TM, et al: A pregnancy complicated by mature abdominal burns scarring and its surgical solution: A case report. J Burn Care Rehab 1995;16:276–279.
102. Chama CM, Na'Aya HU: Severe burn injury in pregnancy in Northern Nigeria. J Obstet Gynaecol 2002;22:20–22.
103. Fatovich DM: Electric shock in pregnancy. J Emerg Med 1993; 11:175–177.
104. Einarson A, Bailey B, Inocencion G, et al: Accidental electric shock in pregnancy: A prospective cohort study. Am J Obstet Gynecol 1997;176:678–681.
105. Fish RM: Electric injury: Part III. Cardiac monitoring indications, the pregnant patient and lightning. J Emerg Med 2000;18:181–187.
106. Leiberman JR, Mazor M, Molcho J, et al: Electrical accidents during pregnancy. Obstet Gynecol 1986;67:861–863.
107. Rosati P, Exacoustos C, Puggioni GF, Mancuso S: Growth retardation in pregnancy: Experimental model in the rabbit employing electrically induced thermal placental injury. Int J Expr Pathol 1995;76:174–181.
108. Whitty JE: Maternal cardiac arrest in pregnancy. Clin Obstet Gynecol 2002;45:379–392.

CHAPTER 56

Psychiatric Illness

Roger F. Haskett

INTRODUCTION

Recognition of psychiatric illness during pregnancy and the postnatal period is vitally important for the health of the mother and infant. Psychiatric disorders, such as depression, are commonly associated with impaired functioning that can significantly interfere with a pregnant woman's ability to care for herself, including participating in optimal prenatal care and maintaining an appropriate diet, as well as increasing the risk of using substances such as tobacco and alcohol. Women with psychiatric and substance use disorders during pregnancy are reported to have at least twice the risk of inadequate prenatal care compared to women without these diagnoses.[1] This association with inadequate prenatal care persists after controlling for other known risk factors and is associated with more adverse pregnancy outcomes and decreased use of pediatric care after birth. These findings are consistent with studies of patients in other primary care settings, noting that depressed individuals are much less likely to comply with treatment recommendations. In addition the presence of mood or anxiety disorders during pregnancy is a strong predictor of psychiatric illness and disability in the postpartum period.

In obstetrics and gynecology practices, the prevalence of psychiatric disorders, including substance abuse disorders, is reported to range from 20% to 48%; this number is even higher in clinics serving low-income women. In particular, the prevalence of major depression in these settings is reported to be as high as 22%. This high prevalence should not be unexpected, considering that adult women suffer from depression and anxiety disorders at rates two to three times higher than men, and that the increased prevalence tends to be most prominent following puberty and throughout the reproductive years.[2] When detected it will be noted that the onset of these psychiatric disorders may predate pregnancy, occur during pregnancy, or most commonly appear during the postpartum period.

In addition to appropriately administering specific treatments,[3] successful management of psychiatric illness in pregnancy and the postpartum period requires effective collaboration between the obstetrician, pediatrician, psychiatrist, and other mental health professionals as well as the participation of relatives and other key social supports.

PREVALENCE OF PSYCHIATRIC ILLNESSES IN PREGNANCY

Recognition of the high frequency of psychiatric symptoms in obstetric and gynecology practices has followed the recent development of screening tools for use in these settings. One study in a university-based obstetric clinic providing prenatal care for low-income minority women reported that 38% of women screened positive for psychiatric disorders including substance abuse.[4] One in five pregnant women screened positive for alcohol or other substance abuse, and more than half of the women who screened positive for a psychiatric disorder (21%) met criteria for a depressive disorder, including 4% with major depression. Other identified diagnoses were anxiety disorder (5%) and eating disorder (5%). Women with psychiatric disorders were more likely to have public insurance, an unexpected pregnancy, and a previous history of psychiatric treatment. More significantly, they tended to be more likely to have received inadequate prenatal care and to be referred to child protective services. Another study of 766 women attending gynecologic practices in Sweden[5] found that 30% met criteria for a psychiatric disorder, although these investigators deleted the screening questions for alcohol abuse. Overall 27% of women screened positive for a depressive disorder, including 10% for major depression, and 12% were positive for an anxiety disorder. Of more concern was the finding that only one out of five women with a psychiatric diagnosis was receiving any treatment, either medication or psychotherapy.

The PRIME-MD Patient Health Questionnaire (PHQ) was the screening instrument used in these studies to assess current psychiatric disorders. The PHQ is a four-page self-report measure that assesses eight common psychiatric diagnoses, including mood, anxiety, eating, alcohol, and somatoform disorders. Although developed in other primary care settings,[6] the validity and utility of the PHQ has been assessed in a multisite sample of 3000 patients attending obstetric/gynecology outpatient clinics or office practices.[7] In addition to assessing the eight psychiatric diagnoses, the PHQ screens for disorders that are more common among or restricted to women, such as premenstrual syndrome, postpartum and menopausal mood disorders, and posttraumatic stress disorder. Information about reproductive history, psychosocial stressors, and severity of impairment is also included. In the validation study, 20% of women met criteria for a psychiatric diagnosis; the majority were unrecognized prior to reviewing the questionnaire. Most physicians and nurse practitioners (89%) reported that the diagnostic information provided by the PHQ was "very" or "somewhat" useful in management or treatment planning.

MAJOR DEPRESSION

General

In 1992 the Global Burden of Disease study reported that unipolar major depression was the most common cause of disease burden in women aged 15 to 44.[8] This heavy burden of depression-related disability in women results not only from the high prevalence of depression, but also from a clinical course that is characterized by early onset, recurrence, chronicity, and comorbidity.[9] Typically major depression is found to be one and a half to three times more prevalent in women than men. This higher prevalence of depression among women has been detected throughout the world using a variety of epidemiologic study designs.[2] Similar gender differences have been found for chronic minor depression or dysthymia and recurrent minor depression. The gender difference in prevalence appears at age 11 to 14 and is consistently found through midlife.[10,11] The literature is inconsistent about the presence of a gender difference in prevalence following menopause, and some reports suggest that the prevalence in men and women converges after age 55 due to an absolute fall in the female prevalence.[12] There does not appear to be a gender difference in the course of depression. The higher prevalence of depression among women is due to a higher risk of first onset, not to a differential risk of recurrence, speed of episode recovery or chronicity of depression.[13] In addition, although limited, research has not found an effect of pregnancy on the onset or recurrence of major depression. Pregnancy does not protect against depression, as was once believed, nor does it appear to increase the risk of depression compared to nonpregnant controls. An emerging consensus holds that significant distress and impairment is also associated with the presence of "minor depression," or depressive symptoms that do not reach a level of severity to meet criteria for major depression. In a recent systematic review of depression in pregnancy, the prevalence rates were reported as 7.4%, 12.8%, and 12.0% for each trimester of pregnancy, respectively.[14]

Diagnosis

Depression during pregnancy may be difficult to detect because many symptoms characteristic of depression, such as sleep and appetite disturbance, low energy, and diminished libido, are common in pregnant women who are not depressed. Although five of nine symptoms (Table 56–1) must be present over the same 2-week period to meet criteria for major depression, one of the symptoms must be either (1) depressed mood most of the day and nearly every day or (2) markedly diminished interest or pleasure in activities, often referred to as *anhedonia.* Using these symptoms in a two-question case-finding instrument is an effective means for identifying major depression. A positive response to either of the questions (1) "During the past month, have you often been bothered by feeling down, depressed, or hopeless?" or (2) "During the past month, have you often been bothered by little interest or pleasure in doing things?" had a sensitivity of 96% and a specificity of 57%; a negative response made a diagnosis of major depression very unlikely.[15] In women who give a positive response to either question, additional inquiry should be made about the presence of the other seven features of depression—such as change in sleep or appetite, physical agitation, fatigue, worthlessness or guilt, poor concentration, and suicidal thinking. In pregnant women, the most useful confirming symptoms are anhedonia, guilt, hopelessness, and suicidal thinking.

Many pregnant women do not seek treatment; identification of their depression is dependent on adequate screening by their obstetrician during antenatal visits. Risk factors for depression in pregnancy include a

TABLE 56–1

Diagnostic Criteria for Major Depression

1. Depressed mood most of the day, nearly every day*
2. Markedly diminished interest or pleasure in activities*
3. Major change in appetite or weight
4. Decrease or increase in sleep
5. Psychomotor agitation or retardation
6. Fatigue or loss of energy
7. Feelings of worthlessness or excessive or inappropriate guilt
8. Diminished ability to think or concentrate; indecisiveness
9. Recurrent thoughts of death or suicide

American Psychiatric Association: Diagnostic and Statistical Manual of Mental Disorders, Fourth Edition, Text Revision. Washington DC, American Psychiatric Association, 2000.
*Must be present to establish diagnosis

personal and family history of mood disorder, marital conflict, younger age, and limited social support with greater numbers of children. In a recent study of 3472 women at 10 obstetric clinics, who were screened for depression during a prenatal visit,[16] 20% were found to have elevated depressive symptom scores (CES-D ≥16) but less than 1 in 7 of these women was receiving treatment for depression. Among the 28% of women who were positive on the lifetime depression screen items ("you had 2 weeks or more when nearly every day you felt sad, blue, or depressed or in which you lost interest in things like work"), nearly one half (42.6%) reported increased depressive symptoms during pregnancy. Women having a prior history of depression were nearly five times more likely to have elevated depressive symptoms during pregnancy than women without this history. Other factors predicting elevated depression scores were a self-rating of poor overall health, greater alcohol use problems, smoking, being unmarried, being unemployed, and lower educational attainment. Other studies have reported low levels of spousal support predicting depression during pregnancy.[17]

Maternal and Fetal Risks

Recent literature reviews summarize the reported association between depressive symptoms during pregnancy and poor neonatal outcomes, such as low birth weight, increased risk of premature delivery, and maternal preeclampsia.[18–21] In a study of African-American women, who have twice the risk of spontaneous preterm birth relative to white women, an association was found between elevated maternal depressive symptoms and spontaneous preterm birth.[22] In addition there have been reports linking developmental delays, antisocial behavior, and criminality in individuals whose mothers were depressed during pregnancy.[23,24] Pregnant women with depression may have decreased appetite and inadequate weight gain during pregnancy and are more likely to use tobacco, alcohol, or illicit drugs.[25] In addition, depression during pregnancy is a strong predictor of postpartum depression.

Management Options

Screening for depression is feasible and when using self-report instruments does not require clinical staff. In the Marcus study 90% of women approached were willing to be screened[16]; in the study by Scholle, 82% of screened women agreed to a clinical research review of their results.[26] Identification of risk factors for depression in pregnancy can increase the efficiency of screening, for example, women with a past history of depressive illness should be specifically targeted for appropriate screening.

Standard treatments for depression with demonstrated efficacy include psychotherapy, antidepressant medications, and electroconvulsive therapy (ECT).[27] Selection of a specific intervention will be influenced by the severity of depression and level of impairment, specific information related to use of the intervention in pregnancy, and the woman's preferences.[28–30] Nonpharmacologic treatments such as interpersonal psychotherapy have been adapted successfully for use during pregnancy[31] and are sometimes preferred by women concerned about exposing the fetus to antidepressant medications.

When considering pharmacologic treatments for depression in pregnancy, the risks to the developing fetus can be divided into risks of physical malformations (*teratogenesis*), risks of neonatal toxicity or withdrawal syndromes following delivery, and risks of long-term behavioral effects (*behavioral teratogenesis*). Although the Food and Drug Administration established a system to advise physicians about the safety of medications in pregnancy, these categories should be used with caution. The majority of psychotropic medications are categorized as Category C, which indicates "human studies are lacking . . . risk cannot be ruled out." No psychotropic medications are in Category A, indicating that they are safe for use in pregnancy, because ethical concerns do not permit the randomized studies needed to generate the data for this classification. Clinicians should note that medications in Category B should not be assumed to be safer than those in Category C because, although the former indicates that there is no evidence of risk in humans, this may be the result of an absence of human studies.

On review of the literature there is no evidence that tricyclic or selective serotonin reuptake inhibitor/serotonin and norepinephrine reuptake inhibitor (SSRI/SNRI) antidepressants are associated with an increased risk of major malformations.[32] Reports have linked exposure to tricyclic antidepressants during the third trimester with neonatal toxicity manifesting as lethargy, hypotonia, and anticholinergic symptoms as well as withdrawal syndromes comprising irritability, tachypnea, tachycardia, and feeding difficulties.[33] Although reports have been inconsistent and generated from small numbers of women, fluoxetine, paroxetine, and sertraline have been linked to transient neonatal difficulties for some women taking these medications in late pregnancy. There is limited data assessing behavioral teratogenesis or neurologic and behavioral developmental outcomes following prenatal exposure of the developing brain to tricyclic and SSRI antidepressants.[34,35] Fortunately the studies that have been published were unable to detect any differences between children exposed to antidepressants in utero and unexposed children at ages varying from 4 months to 7 years.[36]

The treatment of depression during pregnancy raises the following issues, which must be addressed by the treating physician and the patient:

- Risk of exposing the fetus to antidepressant medication
- Risk of untreated depression in the mother
- Risk of relapse of depression in the mother following antidepressant withdrawal.[21]

Obstetricians may encounter these issues in two possible circumstances: a pregnant woman who is recently diagnosed with depression or a woman who is not currently depressed or pregnant and who seeks consultation before conception. In women who present with a new onset or recurrence of depression during pregnancy, the choice of antidepressant treatment will be influenced by the severity of the current episode and any prior episodes of depression. In milder forms of depression, interpersonal or cognitive behavioral psychotherapy alone may be an appropriate treatment. Alternatively, in women who have failed psychotherapy alone or who have severe symptoms, such as weight loss or suicidality, or marked functional impairment, antidepressant medication is likely to be strongly recommended. In these latter women, the risks to the pregnancy associated with their depressive illness will usually exceed the known risks of exposure to an antidepressant medication.[37] Many of the women who seek consultation about antidepressant treatment prior to conception will have suffered prior episodes of depression and may be taking maintenance treatment. In these circumstances, the decision to continue or withdraw antidepressant medications prior to conception will be influenced by the risk for relapse of depression, including the severity and frequency of prior episodes of depression. Up to 75% of women who discontinue an antidepressant during pregnancy will suffer a depressive relapse,[38] although assessing a specific woman's prognosis should focus on the number of prior episodes and the time to relapse after previous attempts at antidepressant discontinuation. Women with a history of rapid and severe relapses following antidepressant discontinuation are likely to be most appropriately treated by continuing medication throughout pregnancy. These risk-benefit discussions with the mother should be documented in the medical record and if possible should occur with the father present.

SUMMARY OF MANAGEMENT OPTIONS

Major Depression

Management Options	Quality of Evidence	Strength of Recommendation	References
Prepregnancy/Prenatal			
Women with previous depressive illness are at risk of relapse during or after pregnancy.	–	GPP	–
Institute specialist team management with access to Mother and Baby Units if available.	–	GPP	–
Psychotherapy (interpersonal and/or cognitive behavioral) has been effective for milder disease.	IV	C	31
Tricyclics and SSRIs have been effective in pregnancy.	Ib	A	32
	IIb	B	33,36
Counsel about fetal risks from medication; withdrawal syndrome reported but no evidence of teratogenic or long-term risks.	Ib	A	32
	IIb	B	33,36
Counsel about danger of relapse with reduction in medication.	IIb	B	38
Check for drug/alcohol abuse.	IIb	B	24
Institute surveillance for fetal growth, preeclampsia, and preterm labor.	III	B	18,19
	IV	C	20
Postnatal			
Be vigilant for maternal relapse in postnatal period.	–	GPP	–
Be vigilant for neonatal withdrawal.	IIb	B	33,34

ANXIETY DISORDERS

General

Studies of women in the general population[39] have reported that the 12-month prevalence of anxiety disorders is 4.3% for generalized anxiety disorder (GAD), 3.2% for panic disorder, and 1.8% for obsessive-compulsive disorder (OCD). Prevalence of posttraumatic stress disorder (PTSD) in a recently reported cohort of economically disadvantaged pregnant women was 7.7%, with these women being five times more likely to have a major depressive disorder and three times more likely to have a generalized anxiety disorder.[40] Unfortunately, in contrast to depression, the systematic data on the frequency and course of anxiety disorders during pregnancy are limited. Some of the difficulty in characterizing anxiety disorders in pregnancy results from the frequent overlap of depressive and anxiety symptoms and from the past convention of subsuming all combined presentations under a depressive diagnosis. Surveys that distinguish between anxiety and depressive disorders, however, find a prevalence of anxiety disorders in obstetrics and gynecology practices that ranges from 5% to 12%.[41] Little is known about the influence of pregnancy on the course of anxiety disorders, although a small number of retrospective accounts and case reports have suggested that symptoms of anxiety and panic disorder decrease and symptoms of OCD increase during pregnancy.[42]

Diagnosis

Anxiety is frequently free-floating, although it may focus on specific pregnancy fears, and is accompanied by symptoms of autonomic arousal. In women with panic disorder, chronic feelings of elevated anxiety are interspersed by the abrupt onset of episodes of pronounced fear, sometimes described as a fear of dying, going crazy, or losing control, which is associated with prominent physical symptoms of distress. These include shortness of breath, dizziness, unsteady feelings or faintness, palpitations or tachycardia, chest pain or discomfort, trembling or shaking, sweating, hot flashes or chills, choking, nausea or abdominal distress, numbness or paresthesias, as well as depersonalization (feeling separated from their body) or derealization (familiar surroundings feel unfamiliar). Episodes of panic usually begin to ease within 30 minutes but may be followed by a lingering period of increased anxiety and impaired function. Women with OCD describe recurrent thoughts that are unpleasant and out of character, often involving personally unacceptable aspects of aggression or sexuality, or repetitive compulsive behavioral rituals that are experienced as unreasonable; attempts to resist are followed by increased and incapacitating anxiety.

Maternal and Fetal Risks

There is some evidence for a deleterious effect of increased maternal stress and anxiety on birth weight and premature delivery.[43,44] Other obstetric complications associated with increased maternal anxiety include preeclampsia,[45] increased analgesic use,[46] and increased rate of cesarean sections.[47] Adverse effects on the fetus include increased uterine artery resistance, as well as changes in fetal hemodynamics and autonomic reactivity.[48,49]

Management Options

Nonpharmacologic treatments are often effective in decreasing anxiety symptoms and include cognitive behavioral therapy and relaxation techniques. Pharmacologic treatment of anxiety disorders during pregnancy is indicated in women who have severe symptoms and are unresponsive to psychotherapy. Use of SSRI antidepressants is favored, due to their demonstrated effectiveness in anxiety disorders and accumulating evidence for their safety in pregnancy. Because of persistent concerns about an increased frequency of oral clefts as well as signs of toxicity in neonates born to women taking high doses of benzodiazepines in late pregnancy, these medications should be used cautiously and at the lowest effective dose. Abrupt withdrawal of benzodiazepines during pregnancy, however, is not recommended. There are insufficient data to determine the safety of buspirone during pregnancy.

SUMMARY OF MANAGEMENT OPTIONS

Anxiety Disorders

Management Options	Quality of Evidence	Strength of Recommendation	References
Prepregnancy and Prenatal			
Recommend psychotherapy (cognitive behavioral or relaxation techniques).	–	GPP	–
Prescribe SSRIs if medication is required.	–	GPP	–
Avoid benzodiazepines.	–	GPP	–
Institute surveillance for fetal growth, preeclampsia, and preterm labor.	III	B	44–46

BIPOLAR DISORDER

General

The prevalence of mania and bipolar disorder is about 1%; in contrast to depression, there is no significant gender difference. Despite this, there appears to be a relationship between childbirth and the first episode of mania in women with bipolar illness, as noted by reports that childbirth predated the first episode of mania in one of four women with this illness.[50,51] In addition, Hunt and Silverstone[52] reported from a study of patients with severe bipolar illness that 39% of the mothers but none of the fathers had their first episode after childbirth. Epidemiologic studies also note a marked excess of postpartum psychosis after the first child compared to subsequent pregnancies, suggesting that there is a particular change occurring at the first delivery that is less evident at other births. Overall the risk of relapse of mania after delivery is estimated to be between 1 in 3 and 1 in 4.[52] Diagnostic and management issues associated with depressive episodes occurring during the course of a bipolar disorder are similar to those for unipolar depressive episodes described previously.

Diagnosis

The essential criterion for the diagnosis of mania is the presence of abnormally and persistently elevated, expansive, or irritable mood for at least 1 week. This must be accompanied by at least three of the following clinical features: inflated self-esteem or grandiosity, decreased need for sleep, increased talkativeness or pressure to keep talking, flight of ideas or subjective experience of racing thoughts, distractibility, increase in goal-directed activity (socially, at work or school, or sexually) or psychomotor agitation, disinhibited behavior, excessive involvement in pleasurable activities with high potential for painful consequences (engaging in unrestrained buying sprees, sexual indiscretions, or foolish business investments). The overall severity must lead to marked functional impairment or need for hospitalization. Women with bipolar illness may also present with less severe forms of mania, diagnosed as *hypomania*, which are of shorter duration and are usually associated with less functional impairment. Although the euphoric or irritable mood changes are usually evident in a patient being followed longitudinally, the most informative diagnostic feature of mania, especially during the assessment of current and past episodes in a new patient, is persistently decreased need for sleep without daytime fatigue or lowered energy.

Maternal and Fetal Risks

Risks to the mother and fetus result from the impulsive, disinhibited, or high risk behavior that is seen in mania, as well as from the commonly associated substance abuse and dependence. In addition, women with untreated mania or hypomania are unlikely to participate in appropriate prenatal care or maintain an adequate diet.

Management Options

Treatment considerations should address two separate groups of women:

- those presenting with mania during pregnancy
- women with an established diagnosis of bipolar disorder requesting advice about a planned or recently confirmed pregnancy.

In the former, the risks to the mother and fetus from untreated mania are prominent, and the risks of failure to treat must be balanced against the risks of effective pharmacologic treatment.[53,54] Admission to a psychiatric facility is necessary if there is a high risk of imminent harm to the mother or fetus and the woman has reduced insight and is unwilling to cooperate with appropriate outpatient treatment. Medication choices for mania in pregnancy should include lithium carbonate, despite early reports about the risk of Ebstein's anomaly and other cardiovascular abnormalities in infants exposed to lithium during the first trimester.[55] Subsequent studies of lithium in pregnancy suggest a more modest teratogenic relationship, with a risk of cardiovascular abnormalities that is 10 to 20 times higher in exposed children than the normal population, but with an actual occurrence rate that is low (0.05% to 0.1%).[56,57] It is recommended that fetuses who have first-trimester exposure to lithium should be screened for cardiovascular abnormalities by ultrasound in the mid-trimester. Despite these concerns, the risk of lithium for mania must be balanced against the increased teratogenic potential of the anticonvulsants that are the other established pharmacologic treatment for this disorder.[58] Valproate and carbamazepine have been linked to neural tube defects in 2% to 5% of exposed babies; there is insufficient data to assess the risks with the newer, more novel anticonvulsants. It does appear, however, that teratogenic risk is increased by the use of combinations of anticonvulsants and high plasma levels. In addition, a third class of medications is now under consideration for the treatment of mania, the atypical antipsychotics. Olanzapine was the first approved for this indication and is likely to be followed by others in the class. Although currently there is limited safety data available, which limits use of these drugs in pregnancy, studies of small numbers of women taking olanzapine during pregnancy have not revealed any teratogenicity. Finally, ECT should also be considered as an alternative to psychotropic medication exposure. It has demonstrated effectiveness for treatment of mania and depression, and reviews support the relative safety of ECT during pregnancy provided that specific modifications are made to the anesthetic procedure.[59]

Ideally, a woman with well-controlled bipolar illness will address the specific management of pregnancy prior to conception. Unfortunately the rate of unplanned pregnancy in women with bipolar illness is even higher than the 50% seen in the general population.[60] In these women pregnancy will commonly be at an advanced gestational age when diagnosed. As neural tube closure usually occurs by the end of the fourth week and development of the heart by the end of the eighth week, the period of risk for major organ malformation may have passed by the time many women taking maintenance psychotropic medication have confirmed pregnancy. This is particularly important information for women considering a rapid discontinuation of medications once pregnancy is detected. Studies have shown a 50% recurrence rate within 2 to 10 weeks of discontinuation of lithium in patients with bipolar illness, and this is increased if medication is discontinued abruptly. Considering the lack of data of a clear safety advantage for a specific mood stabilizer and the risks of relapse following a change in treatment, there is little support for switching a woman from one mood stabilizer to another once pregnancy is detected. If the decision is made to continue medication during pregnancy, the minimum effective dose should be used. In women who are planning pregnancy and report only occasional episodes of moderately severe mania or hypomania, medication discontinuation before conception may be a supportable option, provided that the taper occurs over 2 to 4 weeks' minimum and there is close collaboration between the obstetrician and psychiatrist.

SUMMARY OF MANAGEMENT OPTIONS

Bipolar Disorder

Management Options	Quality of Evidence	Strength of Recommendation	References
Prepregnancy and Prenatal			
Lithium is effective; increased risk of fetal cardiovascular abnormalities though low prevalence.	Ia IV III	A C B	55 56 57
Anticonvulsants are effective; increased risk of fetal neural tube defects.	IV	C	58
Atypical antipsychotics (e.g., olanzapine) have no reported risks in pregnancy.	–	GPP	–
For severe episodes, ECT has been used effectively in pregnancy (with appropriate anesthetic precautions).	III	B	59
Perform careful detailed fetal anomaly scan at 20 weeks, especially if on medication.	Ia IV III	A C B	55 56,58 57
Hospitalize in a psychiatric facility if safety concerns present (Mother and Baby Unit if postnatal).	–	GPP	–
Screen for substance abuse.	–	GPP	–
Postnatal			
Be vigilant for recurrence after delivery.	III	B	52
Perform careful neonatal examination to exclude abnormality.	Ia IV III	A C B	55 56,58 57

SCHIZOPHRENIA

General

Pregnancy in women with schizophrenia occurs under very different circumstances today compared to a few decades ago.[61] The first and most influential change resulted from the release of patients to the community, instead of confining them to institutions, providing them with increased opportunities to meet partners. Despite this, although the fertility rates for women with schizophrenia have increased, its occurrence remains between 30% and 80% of the general population.[62] Because effective utilization of birth control practices is limited in women with schizophrenia, one important contributing factor for this decrease in fertility is the high prevalence of hyperprolactinemia in patients taking the older class of antipsychotic medications. More recently, the treatment of schizophrenia has seen an increased utilization of a new generation of atypical antipsychotics that are much less likely to produce elevated prolactin levels. As a result, it is very likely that the frequency of pregnancy in women with schizophrenia will increase.

Diagnosis

The diagnostic criteria for schizophrenia require the presence of at least two of the following over a 1-month period: delusions, hallucinations, disorganized speech, grossly disorganized or catatonic behavior, and affective flattening or markedly decreased volition. These features should be associated with prominent social and occupational dysfunction of at least 6 months' duration. The diagnostic evaluation should focus on the chronic and persistent features of the illness because the clinician may have difficulty during a cross-sectional assessment in differentiating psychosis in schizophrenia from psychotic symptoms in a patient with mood disorder. Particular presentations that may have diagnostic challenges are the delusional denial of the pregnancy or the incorporation of the pregnancy into established delusional systems.

Maternal and Fetal Risks

Prenatal care may not be appropriately sought or maintained by these women, especially in cases in which the pregnancy was not planned and in women with prominent volitional deficits. Individuals with this illness are also noted to have great difficulty maintaining healthy lifestyle choices for diet, exercise, and avoidance of alcohol and tobacco. All of these factors are associated with worse outcomes from pregnancy. The use of older antipsychotic medications conveys some increased risk of teratogenicity, although further examination of this data linked the low-potency phenothiazines, such as chlorpromazine, with an increased risk of malformations. The depot antipsychotics are not recommended during pregnancy because they have been associated with an increased risk of extrapyramidal side effects in the neonate.

Management Options

Although it may be desired by the patient, discontinuation of psychotropic medication during pregnancy in women with schizophrenia is associated with a markedly increased risk of relapse. Considering that treatment of relapse is likely to require higher doses of medication than maintenance treatment, one alternative is to attempt reduction to the lowest effective dosage of medication, especially during the first trimester. Although low doses of the more potent older antipsychotics, such as haloperidol, are preferred for the treatment of schizophrenia in pregnancy, the new atypical antipsychotics are commonly being continued in pregnancy, despite the limited amount of safety data currently available. Any indication of psychotic relapse should be managed by prompt admission to a psychiatric facility for restabilization. A key aspect of management during pregnancy is to evaluate the options for the mother and child after delivery. Assessment of the woman's capacity to provide appropriate care for the infant should begin during the pregnancy; this should include review of the stability of the illness, the woman's adherence to outpatient care, and the quality of psychosocial supports.

SUMMARY OF MANAGEMENT OPTIONS
Schizophrenia

Management Options	Quality of Evidence	Strength of Recommendation	References
Prepregnancy, Prenatal, and Postnatal			
Decrease oral medication to lowest level consistent with a therapeutic effect.	–	GPP	–
Avoid depot preparations.	–	GPP	–
Check for substance abuse.	–	GPP	–
Offer psychosocial support and encouragement to take up prenatal care.	–	GPP	–
Hospitalization in a psychiatric facility may be necessary with acute relapses (Mother and Baby Unit preferable).	–	GPP	–
Assess ability of patient to care for baby and need for additional psychosocial support.	–	GPP	–

SUBSTANCE ABUSE AND DEPENDENCY (See also Chapter 34)

General

Considering that substance abuse and dependence are chronic relapsing disorders, women with these diagnoses are at particular risk when they become pregnant. Identification of prenatal substance use, including alcohol and nicotine, is a critical public health issue in the care of pregnant women.[63] In 1992 the National Pregnancy and Health Survey reported an estimated prevalence among U.S. women during pregnancy of alcohol (18.8%) and illicit drug use (5.5%). Another report of prospectively screened newborns in an urban population noted that 44% of infants tested positive for opiates, cocaine, or cannabis. Although many women report spontaneously quitting substance use on learning of the pregnancy, maintenance of abstinence is problematic without participation in treatment programs.[64] A key strategy in the accurate identification of affected women is the use of self-report screening instruments. These tend to identify much higher rates of substance use than detected by maternal interview alone. For example, one report contrasted the 65% to 70% correct identification of prenatal drinkers using a questionnaire with the 20% having documentation of alcohol use in the obstetric record.

Diagnosis

One of the strongest risk factors for substance abuse is the presence of other psychiatric disorders. Depression, mania, and schizophrenia are all associated with an increased prevalence of substance use and abuse. Other risk factors identified for frequent drinking in pregnancy were being unmarried, smoking, age ≥25 years, and having a college education, although the applicability of these findings to other populations requires further study.[65] Interviewing individuals who are aware of the mother's behavior, such as the spouse/partner and other relatives, can be informative, although the presence of substance abuse in these individuals may decrease the reliability of their responses. Urine screening of the mother has been controversial, although with the mother's consent it may be a useful strategy for identifying mothers who should be referred for treatment.

Maternal and Fetal Risks

The legality of substances does not lessen their serious implications for the health of the fetus; legal substances are probably associated with more widespread use.[66] The fetal consequences of maternal smoking are well established. These include intrauterine growth restriction, low birth weight, and developmental delays. Fetal alcohol syndrome (FAS) is associated with alcohol consumption during pregnancy. The three critical features are growth deficiency, facial phenotype, and brain damage dysfunction. A recent preclinical study showed that alcohol blocked N-methyl-D-aspartate receptors and excessively activated GABA receptors, leading to extensive neuron degeneration. The damage was dependent on the rapidity of dose administration and the duration of blood alcohol level elevation.[67] This suggests that peak levels during a drinking episode are most critical to developing FAS. Maternal use of benzodiazepines and barbiturates is known to be associated with neonatal withdrawal syndromes, but of more concern is the recent report suggesting that these substances may delete neurons from the developing brain through a mechanism similar to that proposed for alcohol. Considering their relatively common use in pregnant women and infants, there is an urgent need for more systematic examination of these risks.

Maternal use of illicit substances is associated with significant risk of adverse effects on the fetus.[68] Cannabis use during pregnancy has been associated with effects on the exposed infant's cognitive development and behavior, with at least one report linking hyperactivity, inattentiveness, and impulsivity at age 10 with first- and third-trimester exposure to cannabis.[69] Prenatal cocaine use is reported to be associated with a dose-dependent decrease in head circumference and head weight.[70] There has been a report of increased frequency of cardiovascular and musculoskeletal anomalies in infants exposed to methylenedioxymethamphetamine (Ecstasy) during pregnancy,[71] but further study is needed. Opiate withdrawal is the primary risk for infants born to opiate-dependent mothers and is characterized by autonomic dysfunction, as well as gastrointestinal and respiratory symptoms.

Management Options

The key to management of substance abuse is detection. The use of screening instruments is valuable; a questionnaires such as CAGE or T-ACE (Table 56–2) are commonly used for the detection of alcohol misuse.[72] Although the literature suggests that six drinks daily can cause overt FAS, the safe level has not been identified and the comparative risks for binge drinking and daily drinking are not clear. Risk-drinking (enough to *potentially* damage the offspring) has been defined as an average of more than one drink (0.5 oz) per day, or less if massed (binges of >5 drinks per episode.[73] In the United States, a conservative position has been adopted that essentially recommends total abstinence during pregnancy.

Unfortunately there are few screening tools for detection of the use of other substances. When diagnosed, a comprehensive treatment program is indicated, with individual and group therapy, behavioral incentives, and in some situations, pharmacologic agents such as methadone. These interventions have demonstrated positive effects on both maternal and neonatal outcomes.

The Summary of Management Options for this section is found in Chapter 34.

POSTPARTUM DEPRESSION CONDITIONS

General

The psychiatric diagnostic system (i.e., *DSM-IV*) does not recognize postpartum disorders as discrete diagnoses but permits "postpartum onset" to be used as a specifier

TABLE 56–2

T-ACE Screening Tool for Pregnancy Risk-Drinking*

Tolerance
"How many drinks can you hold?"
(A positive answer, scored a 2, is at least a 6-pack of beer, a bottle of wine, or 6 mixed drinks. This suggests tolerance of alcohol and very likely a history of at least moderate to heavy alcohol intake.)
Annoyed
"Have people annoyed you by criticizing your drinking?"
Cut Down
"Have you felt you ought to cut down on your drinking?"
Eye Opener
"Have you ever had a drink first thing in the morning to steady your nerves or get rid of a hangover?"

* From Sokol RJ, Delaney-Black V, Nordstrom B: Fetal alcohol spectrum disorder. JAMA 2003;290:2996–2999. The first question is scored 0 or 2 points. The last 3 questions are scored 1 point if answered affirmatively. A total score of 2 or more is considered positive for risk-drinking.

for episodes of illness appearing within 4 weeks of childbirth. There is continued debate about this relatively brief interval for the definition of postpartum illness, most epidemiologic studies use a 3-month period, which captures the peak prevalence of psychiatric illness and hospitalization after childbirth, and other researchers and clinicians are extending their focus to the events occurring during the first postnatal year.[74] Postpartum mood changes include three distinct clinical syndromes: postpartum blues, postpartum depression, and postpartum psychosis, although a single cross-sectional evaluation of all three may be indistinguishable. Fortunately, the prevalence of these three disorders varies inversely to their severity.

Postpartum "Blues"

General

Although not actually listed in *DSM-IV* as a psychiatric disorder, this well-recognized, common disorder occurs in 25% to 80% of women following delivery. Sadness may be prominent, but the syndrome is commonly characterized by emotional lability, bursting into tears without apparent cause, increased anxiety, insomnia, and negative thinking. Symptoms usually appear within the first postpartum week and, in the majority of women, peak around day 5 postpartum and resolve within 2 weeks. Given the timing and self-limiting nature of this syndrome, there have been many reports and hypotheses linking its pathophysiology to the rapid and profound changes occurring at parturition, but so far none have achieved wide support.

Diagnosis

The key to the diagnosis of this state is its time course.[75] Distinguishing between postpartum blues and postpartum depression has great clinical significance. Persistence of depressive symptoms past the second week postpartum should result in a careful reassessment of the original diagnosis. In addition, prominent insomnia and mood lability in a woman with risk factors for postpartum psychosis, even if it occurs in the first 2 weeks after childbirth, should prompt an urgent psychiatric consultation.

Maternal and Fetal Risks

Generally this syndrome is not associated with significant functional impairment of the mother and does not significantly increase risks to the infant.

Management Options

Provide support and education about the typically self-limiting nature of this condition, but monitor for progression and development of postpartum depression.

SUMMARY OF MANAGEMENT OPTIONS

Postpartum "Blues"

Management Options	Quality of Evidence	Strength of Recommendation	References
Postnatal			
Confirm that this is not postnatal depression and that it resolves within 2 weeks.	–	GPP	–
Offer explanation and support.	–	GPP	–

Postpartum Depression

General

The prevalence of postpartum depression is 10% to 15%; it occurs in 1 of every 7 to 10 women after delivery, making it the most common complication of childbirth. Women with a past history of depression have an elevated risk of postpartum depression, estimated to range from 25% to 50%. Although the psychiatric diagnostic system focuses on depression appearing up to 4 weeks after delivery, a significant body of data emphasizes the importance of depression having an onset up to 1 year after childbirth. Due to its temporal association, the cause of postpartum depression is commonly attributed to the rapid and profound hormonal changes occurring after delivery. Other factors that increase the risk of postpartum depression are also seen in women suffering from depression unrelated to childbirth, such as past and family history of depressive episodes, poor marital relationship, low social support, stressful life events, and low socioeconomic status.[17,76]

Diagnosis

The clinical features and diagnostic process for postpartum depression are similar to those for women suffering from depression at other times. The first step is to identify a period of persistent depressed mood or anhedonia lasting at least 2 weeks. Several screening instruments have been utilized for this purpose. The most commonly reported instrument in the literature is the Edinburgh Postnatal Depression Scale (EPDS), a 10-item self-report instrument designed to assess the presence of depressive symptoms in women after childbirth.[77] Each symptom item is scored from 0 to 3 according to severity. A score >9 on the EPDS should be followed by a brief focused interview to determine the presence of a depressive diagnosis. Other instruments include a two-question case-finding instrument assessing the presence of depressed mood or anhedonia.[15] A positive response to either of the two items suggests that a diagnosis of depression should be explored.

In women who were screened during the second trimester of pregnancy and again during the postpartum year, the two independently predictive risk factors for postpartum depression were high depressive symptoms during pregnancy and a past personal history of depressive disorder.[78] Another study of first-time otherwise healthy mothers found that women reporting high levels of depressive symptomatology at 2 months' postpartum had an increased risk of high levels of depressive symptoms continuing through the first year postpartum.[79] This emphasizes the persistence of depressive symptoms with associated impairment of function and reinforces the importance of identifying depressed mothers soon after childbirth, preferably with routine use of screening instruments, and referring for appropriate interventions.[80]

Considering that bipolar illness can present with an episode of depression, it is essential to ask the depressed woman about the features of past hypomania or mania, particularly when psychotic features are present. This can be done by asking about the past occurrence of at least 3 to 4 days of a markedly decreased need for sleep (i.e., feeling rested after 3 to 4 hours sleep per night, without daytime fatigue or decreased energy). A positive response to this question or one about periods of persistently elevated or irritable mood that others thought were abnormal indicates that further evaluation for possible bipolar disorder is indicated and psychiatric referral is recommended.

Maternal and Fetal Risks

Although the overall risk of suicide in postpartum women is low, those who develop a severe psychiatric illness in the first year after childbirth are at a significantly increased risk. In one study, the long-term risk of suicide in women admitted to a psychiatric hospital in the first year after childbirth was increased 17 times.[81] In these women the risk of completed suicide during the first postpartum year was markedly increased to 70 times greater than the age-specific mortality rate. A recent report from the United Kingdom noted that suicide was the leading cause of maternal death during the first year after childbirth.[82]

Adverse effects of maternal depression on infant development have been widely reported,[83–85] including reports of an association between maternal depression and an increased risk of sudden infant death syndrome.[86] Children of depressed parents are at high risk for anxiety and depressive disorder in childhood, depression in adolescence, and alcohol dependence as adults.[87] Children of depressed mothers are also less likely to benefit from appropriate parental prevention practices.[88] Depressed mothers reported a three times greater risk of serious emotional problems in their children and more functional disability.[89]

Homicide is the leading cause of infant deaths due to injury, 9 per 100,000 live births from 1988 to 1991.[90] This study revealed that children born to young unmarried and poorly educated mothers were several times more likely to be killed. In this group of mothers, the most important risk factors were maternal age <17 years and birth of the second or subsequent child before age 19; these accounted for 17% of the infant deaths. Five percent of homicides occurred on the first day of the infant's life; 95% of these infants were not born in a hospital compared to 8% of all infants killed during the first year of life who were not born in a hospital. Infants killed immediately after birth appeared to be the result of unwanted or disguised pregnancies. Identification of adolescents who have hidden their pregnancies and provision of appropriate prenatal care is particularly important. Maternal depression may play a role in the deaths occurring after the first day of life. The combination of depressed mood, low self-esteem, pessimism and hopelessness may reach delusional levels in some mothers, leading them to believe that their babies and themselves are better off dead.[91] In addition, reports suggest that infants of depressed mothers are more irritable, less easily consoled, and have disrupted sleep and wake cycles, all increasing their risks of being abused.

Management Options

Women receiving a diagnosis of depression after childbirth are commonly treated with antidepressant medication.[92] Uncontrolled studies have reported improvement in postpartum depression after treatment with antidepressants such as sertraline, fluvoxamine, and venlafaxine. Unfortunately only one placebo-controlled trial of antidepressants in postpartum depression has been published. This study compared antidepressant medication (fluoxetine) with psychotherapy (cognitive-behavioral therapy; CBT). Results indicated that fluoxetine was more effective than placebo. With regard to the role of psychotherapy, six sessions of CBT were more effective than one session, but the addition of multiple CBT sessions to fluoxetine did not provide any additional benefit.[93]

Women with postpartum depression appear abnormally sensitive to the withdrawal of high levels of gonadal steroids following parturition. A preliminary placebo-controlled study showed that transdermal estrogen was an effective treatment for women with severe postpartum depression, although more research is needed to assess the safety of estrogen in the postpartum period.[94]

Due to the reluctance of some postpartum women to take medication, psychotherapy has been studied as an alternative to antidepressant medication as well as an adjunct to medication. In addition to the study noted previously, several randomized controlled trials have shown that individual psychotherapy is an effective treatment for postpartum depression.[95] There was greater improvement of maternal mood and social functioning in women receiving interpersonal psychotherapy than in women in the waiting list control group.[96] Other studies have shown the benefit of including the partner in the psychotherapy sessions, although the results from group therapy are mixed.[97]

Many women who express reluctance to take medication after childbirth identify concern about the possible adverse effects on breastfeeding infants. Because all antidepressants are excreted in breast milk, many studies have evaluated the serum levels of antidepressant in breastfeeding infants. With few exceptions, these reports have found that the serum levels of antidepressants in infants were either very low or undetectable.[98,99] Reports of adverse effects in breastfed infants of mothers taking antidepressants have included increased crying, colic, and decreased sleep in three infants whose mothers were taking fluoxetine and who were found to have serum levels of fluoxetine and its metabolite that were in the adult therapeutic range. Citalopram, sertraline, and doxepin have been identified in case reports with either adverse effects or elevated serum levels. It should be noted that most reports were of one or two cases, methodologies varied, and with the exception of one study the follow-up was brief.

SUMMARY OF MANAGEMENT OPTIONS

Postpartum Depression

Management Options	Quality of Evidence	Strength of Recommendation	References
Postnatal			
Maintain vigilance for the condition by all health providers in the puerperium.	–	GPP	–
Antidepressants (SSRIs are first choice) are effective.	III	B	91
More information required about estrogen as a therapy.	Ib	A	93
Interpersonal psychotherapy is an effective alternative.	Ib	A	94
Cognitive behavioral psychotherapy does not give additional benefit when used with antidepressants.	Ib	A	92
Suggest Mother and Baby Unit admission in extreme cases.	–	GPP	–
Breastfeeding is safe with antidepressants.	–	GPP	–

Postpartum Psychosis

General

Postpartum psychosis is the most severe postpartum mood disorder; fortunately it is rare, affecting 1 to 2 women per 1000 deliveries. Current literature generally reflects the view that postpartum psychosis, in the majority of cases, is a presentation of bipolar disorder following childbirth.[52,100] Women with a history of bipolar disorder have a 100-fold higher risk of developing postpartum psychosis than women without bipolar disorder.[101] In addition, women with bipolar disorder and a family history of postpartum psychosis have a rate of postpartum episodes twice that seen in women with bipolar disorder and no family history.[102]

Diagnosis

Symptoms of insomnia, prominent mood lability, restlessness, sadness, and irritability appear within 2 weeks of childbirth, followed by the development of psychotic features, such as delusions, hallucinations, and thought disorder. Insomnia is an early and common symptom and is found in 42% to 100% of women with psychosis.[103] The presence of perplexity and confusion are also noted to be common, unlike in nonpuerperal manic episodes. Some researchers have commented on the role of sleep loss in the precipitation of mania generally[104]; this may be of particular importance following childbirth.[105] Studies of sleep in the later stages of pregnancy show prominent sleep disruption, with prolonged sleep latency, more awakenings, decreased total sleep time, and suppression of stage 4 sleep; recovery of stage 4 sleep and reduction in REM sleep occur in the early postpartum period.[106,107] More importantly a prospective study of sleep in pregnancy revealed a differential effect depending on the presence of a past history of mood disorders. In addition sleep disruption during late pregnancy and the early postpartum period appears to be more pronounced in first-time mothers than in mutiparous women. This may be relevant for the observed increase in the risk of postpartum psychosis after the first child compared to later deliveries.

Maternal and Fetal Risks

In almost all instances, women with postpartum psychosis are unable to provide adequate care for themselves or their child and require additional support and supervision. Thoughts of harming the infant are common in women with postpartum psychosis; sometimes they act on their thoughts. Postpartum women who commit infanticide or suicide more commonly present with depressed mood than mania.

Management Options

Early identification of sleep impairment is important in the management of women with a history of bipolar disorder or postpartum psychosis. Prevention of sleep loss in vulnerable women by daytime delivery and reduction of nocturnal stimulation may be appropriate. Prompt treatment of decreased sleep in these women, with a high potency benzodiazepine such as clonazepam or a sedating antipsychotic, is essential. Due to the high risk of recurrence, prophylactic treatment of women with a history of postpartum psychosis or bipolar disorder is often considered, although there is no consensus about the optimal time to begin prophylaxis. Many patients prefer to defer starting prophylactic medication until immediately after delivery.

Established postpartum psychosis requires admission to a psychiatric hospital. Mother and baby units are optimal but are relatively uncommon in the United States. Because there are no adequately controlled studies of psychopharmacologic treatment of postpartum psychosis, the standard treatments for a psychotic manic or depressed episode are used, including new generation antipsychotics, lithium, valproate, and antidepressants. If an antidepressant is used, a mood stabilizer such as lithium or valproate should be given in combination. There are numerous reports that ECT is effective in the treatment of postpartum psychosis, but there are no controlled studies of this strategy. A small open-label pilot study of 17β-estradiol in the treatment of postpartum psychosis found encouraging results but requires further investigation.[108]

SUMMARY OF MANAGEMENT OPTIONS

Postpartum Psychosis

Management Options	Quality of Evidence	Strength of Recommendation	References
Postnatal			
All health providers in the puerperium must maintain vigilance for the condition.	–	GPP	–
Psychiatric admission usually mandatory to protect baby, Mother and Baby Unit preferred if available	–	GPP	–
Medication may include a combination of lithium, valproate, antidepressants; benzodiazepines for sleep problems.	–	GPP	–
Role of ECT and estrogen therapy uncertain.	–	GPP	–

CONCLUSIONS

PSYCHIATRIC AND SUBSTANCE ABUSE DISORDERS

- Relatively common in women during pregnancy and the postnatal period
- Present in up to 50% of women seen in obstetric and gynecology practices
- Commonly not recognized unless standard clinical assessments are supplemented with screening instruments
- Associated with twice the risk of inadequate antenatal care
- Collaborative care with a psychiatrist or other mental health clinician frequently beneficial

DEPRESSION AND ANXIETY DISORDERS

- Most common in women during the reproductive years
- More likely to develop during pregnancy in women with personal and family history of mood disorder, marital conflict, younger age, and limited social support

Continued

CONCLUSIONS (Continued)

DEPRESSION AND ANXIETY DISORDERS (Continued)

- Failure to treat is associated with negative obstetric and neonatal outcomes
- Standard psychotherapeutic and pharmacologic treatments are effective; many can be used in pregnancy
- Withdrawal of treatment is commonly followed by relapse

BIPOLAR DISORDER AND SCHIZOPHRENIA

- Present particular risks during pregnancy
- Untreated mania is associated with impulsive high risk behaviors, often including substance abuse
- Use of effective antimanic treatments during pregnancy requires careful assessment of the risk-benefit relationship
- Psychotic symptoms and volitional deficits in women with schizophrenia may result in major impediments to antenatal care and ability to care for the infant

SUBSTANCE ABUSE

- Associated with adverse effects on the infant
- May be difficult to detect without specific screening and corroborative information
- Responds favorably to comprehensive treatment programs, although they are frequently characterized by a relapsing course before sustained abstinence is achieved

POSTPARTUM MOOD DISORDERS

- Common
- Distinguishing the three forms of disorder is crucial
- Postpartum blues spontaneously remits within 2 weeks of delivery
- Postpartum depression may become apparent at any time during the first year after childbirth; the strongest predictors are a past history of depressive disorder and depression during pregnancy
- Standard antidepressant treatments are indicated for postpartum depression
- Postpartum psychosis is rare but usually appears within 2 weeks of childbirth and requires urgent psychiatric inpatient care
- Postpartum psychosis is most common in women with a history of bipolar illness

REFERENCES

1. Kelly RH, Danielsen BH, Golding JM, et al: Adequacy of prenatal care among women with psychiatric diagnoses giving birth in California in 1994 and 1995. Psychiatr Serv 1999; 50:1584–1590.
2. Kessler RC: Epidemiology of women and depression. J Affect Disord 2003;74:5–13.
3. Miller LJ: Psychiatric medication during pregnancy: Understanding and minimizing risks. Psychiatr Ann 1994; 24:69–75.
4. Kelly RH, Zatzick DF, Anders TF: The detection and treatment of psychiatric disorders and substance use among pregnant women cared for in obstetrics. Am J Psychiatr 2001; 158:213–219.
5. Sundström IME, Bixo M, Björn I, Åström M: Prevalence of psychiatric disorders in gynecologic outpatients. Am J Obstet Gynecol 2001;184:8–13.
6. Spitzer RL, Kroenke K, Williams JBW: Validation and utility of a self-report version of PRIME-MD: The PHQ primary care study. JAMA 1999;282:1737–1744.
7. Spitzer RL, Williams JBW, Kroenke K, et al: Validity and utility of the PRIME-MD Patient Health Questionnaire in assessment of 3000 obstetric-gynecologic patients: The PRIME-MD Patient Health Questionnaire obstetrics-gynecology study. Am J Obstet Gynecol 2000;183:759–769.
8. Lopez AD, Murray CC: The Global Burden of Disease, 1990–2020. Nat Med 1998;4:1241–1243.
9. Steiner M, Dunn E, Born L: Hormones and mood: From menarche to menopause and beyond. J Affect Disord 2003;74:67–83.
10. Angold A, Costello EJ, Worthman CM: Puberty and depression: The roles of age, pubertal status and pubertal timing. Psychol Med 1998;28:51–61.
11. Hankin BL, Abramson LY, Moffitt TE, et al: Development of depression from preadolescence to young adulthood: Emerging gender differences in a 10-year longitudinal study. J Abnorm Psychol 1998;107:128–140.
12. Bebbington PE, Dunn G, Jenkins R, et al: The influence of age and sex on the prevalence of depressive conditions: Report from the National Survey of Psychiatric Morbidity. Psychol Med 1998;28:9–19.
13. Kessler RC, McGonagle KA, Swartz M, et al: Sex and depression in the National Comorbidity Survey I: Lifetime prevalence, chronicity and recurrence. J Affect Disord 1993;39:85–96.
14. Bennett HA, Einarson A, Taddio A, et al: Prevalence of depression during pregnancy. Systematic review. Obstet Gynecol 2004;103:698–709.
15. Whooley MA, Alvins AL, Miranda J, Browner WS: Case-finding instruments for depression. J Gen Intern Med 1997;12:439.

16. Marcus SM, Flynn HA, Blow FC, Barry KL: Depressive symptoms among pregnant women screened in obstetrics settings. J Women's Health 2003;12:373–380.
17. O'Hara MW: Social support, life events, and depression during pregnancy and the puerperium. Arch Gen Psychiatr 1986; 43:569.
18. Steer RA, Scholl TO, Hediger ML, Fischer RL: Self-reported depression and negative pregnancy outcomes. J Clin Epidemiol 1992;45:1093–1099.
19. Orr ST, Miller CA: Maternal depressive symptoms and the risk of poor pregnancy outcome: Review of the literature and preliminary findings. Epidemiol Rev 1995;17:165–171.
20. Hendrick V, Altshuler L: Management of major depression during pregnancy. Am J Psychiatr 2002;159:1667-1673.
21. Kurki T, Hiilesmaa V, Raitasalo R, et al: Depression and anxiety in early pregnancy and risk for preeclampsia. Obstet Gynecol 2000;95:487–90.
22. Orr ST, James SA, Prince CB: Maternal prenatal depressive symptoms and spontaneous preterm births among African-American women in Baltimore, Maryland. Am J Epidemiol 2002;156:797–802.
23. Rutter M, Quinton D: Parental psychiatric disorder: Effect on children. Psychol Med 1984;14:853–880.
24. Mäki P, Veijola J, Räänen P, et al: Criminality in the offspring of antenatally depressed mothers: A 33-year follow-up of the Northern Finland 1966 Birth Cohort. J Affect Disord 2003;74:273–278.
25. Zuckerman B, Amaro H, Bauchner H, Cabral H: Depressive symptoms during pregnancy: Relationship to poor health behaviors. Am J Obstet Gynecol 1989;160:1107–1111.
26. Scholle SH, Haskett RF, Hanusa BH, et al: Addressing depression in obstetrics/gynecology practice. Gen Hosp Psychiatr 2003;25:83–90.
27. Steiner M, Yonkers KA: Evidence-based treatment of mood disorders in women. Mental Fitness 2003;2:34–67.
28. Nonacs R, Cohen LS: Depression during pregnancy: Diagnosis and treatment options. J Clin Psychiatr 2002;63:24–30.
29. Wisner KL, Gelenberg AJ, Leonard H, et al: Pharmacologic treatment of depression during pregnancy. JAMA 1999; 282:1264–1269.
30. Wisner KL, Zarin DA, Holmboe ES, et al: Risk-benefit decision making for treatment of depression during pregnancy. Am J Psychiatr 2000;157:1933–1940.
31. Spinelli MG, Endicott J: Controlled clinical trial of interpersonal psychotherapy versus parenting education program for depressed pregnant women. Am J Psychiatr 2003; 160:555–562.
32. Einarson A, Fatoye B, Sarkar M, et al: Pregnancy outcome following gestational exposure to venlafaxine: A multicenter prospective controlled study. Am J Psychiatr 2001; 158:1728–1730.
33. Laine K, Heikkinen T, Ekblad U, Kero P: Effects of exposure to selective serotonin reuptake inhibitors during pregnancy on serotonergic symptoms in newborns and cord blood monoamine and prolactin concentrations. Arch Gen Psychiatr 2003; 50:720–726.
34. Goldstein DJ: Effects of third trimester fluoxetine exposure on the newborn. J Clin Psychopharmacol 1995;15:417–420.
35. Kulin NA, Pastuszak A, Sage SR, et al: Pregnancy outcome following maternal use of the new selective serotonin reuptake inhibitors: A prospective controlled multicenter study. JAMA 1998;279:609–610.
36. Nulman I, Rovet J, Stewart DE, et al: Neurodevelopment of children exposed in utero to antidepressant drugs. N Engl J Med 1997;336:258–262.
37. Einarson A, Selby P, Koren G: Abrupt discontinuation of psychotropic drugs during pregnancy: Fear of teratogenic risk and impact of counseling. J Psychiatr Neurosci 2001;26:44–48.
38. Cohen LS, Altshuler LL, Stowe ZN: MGH Prospective Study: Depression in pregnancy in women who decrease or discontinue antidepressant medication. Annual Meeting Syllabus and Proceedings Summary. Washington, DC, American Psychiatric Association, 1999.
39. Kessler RD, McGonagle KA, Zhao S, et al: Life-time and 12-month prevalence of DSM-III-R psychiatric disorders in the United States. Arch Gen Psychiatr 1994;51:8–19.
40. Cook CAL, Flick JH, Homan SM, et al: Posttraumatic stress disorder in pregnancy: Prevalence, risk factor and treatment. Obstet Gynecol 2004;103:710–717.
41. Matthey S, Barnett B, Howie P, Kavanagh DJ: Diagnosing postpartum depression in mothers and fathers: Whatever happened to anxiety? J Affect Disord 2003;74:139–147.
42. Cohen LS, Sichel DA, Dimmock JA, Rosenbaum JF: Impact of pregnancy on panic disorder: A case series. J Clin Psychiatr 1994;55:284–288.
43. Berkin MR, Bland JM, Peacock JL, Anderson HR: The effect of anxiety and depression during pregnancy on obstetric complications. BJOG 1993;100:629–634.
44. Paarlberg KM, Vingerhoets JJM, Passchier J, et al: Psychosocial predictors of low birthweight. BJOG 1999;106:834–841.
45. Atiba EO, Adeghe A-H, Murphy PJ, et al: Patient's expectation and cesarean section rate. Lancet 1993;341:246.
46. Sjogren B, Thomassen P: Obstetric outcome in 100 women with severe anxiety over childbirth. Acta Obstet Gynecol Scand 1997;76:948–952.
47. Ryding EL, Wijma B, Wijma K, Rydhstrom H: Fear of childbirth during pregnancy may increase the risk of emergency cesarean section. Acta Obstet Gynecol Scand 1998;77:542–547.
48. McCubbin JA, Lawson EJ, Cox S, et al: Prenatal maternal blood pressure response to stress predicts weight and gestational age: A preliminary study. Am J Obstet Gynecol 1996; 175:706–712.
49. Sjostrom K, Valentin L, Thelin T, Marsal K: Maternal anxiety in late pregnancy and fetal hemodynamics. Eur J Obstet Gynecol Reprod Biol 1997;74:149–155.
50. Ambelas A: Life events and mania: A special relationship? Br J Psychiatry 1987;501:235–240
51. Whalley L, Roberts D, Wentzel J, Wright A: Genetic factors in puerperal affective psychoses. Acta Psychiatr Scand 1982; 65:180–193.
52. Hunt N, Silverstone T: Does puerperal illness distinguish a subgroup of bipolar patients? J Affect Disord 1995;34:101–107.
53. Viguera AC, Cohen LS: The course and management of bipolar disorder during pregnancy. Psychopharmacol Bull 1998; 34:339–346.
54. Altschuler LL, Cohen LS, Szuba MP, et al: Pharmacologic management of psychiatric illness in pregnancy. Am J Psychiatr 1996;153:592–606.
55. Llewellyn A, Stowe ZN, Strader JR: The use of lithium and management of women with bipolar disorder during pregnancy and lactation. J Clin Psychiatr 1998;59(suppl 6):57–64.
56. Jacobson SJ, Jones K, Johnson K, et al: Prospective multicentre study of pregnancy outcome after lithium exposure during first trimester. Lancet 1992;339:530–533.
57. Cohen LS, Friedman JM, Jefferson JW, et al: A reevaluation of risk of in utero exposure to lithium. JAMA 1994;271:146–150.
58. Holmes LB, Harvey EA, Coull BA, et al: The teratogenicity of anticonvulsant drugs. N Engl J Med 2001;244:1132–1138.
59. Miller LJ: Use of electroconvulsive therapy during pregnancy. Hosp Community Psychiatr 1994;45:444–450.
60. Finnerty M, Levin Z, Miller LJ: Acute manic episodes in pregnancy. Am J Psychiatr 1996;153:261–263.
61. Empfield MD: Pregnancy and schizophrenia. Psychiatr Ann 2000;30:61–66.
62. Nanko S, Moridaira J: Reproductive rates in schizophrenic outpatients. Acta Psychiatr Scand 1993;87:400–404.

63. Johnson K, Gerada C, Greenough A: Substance misuse during pregnancy. Br J Psychiatr 2003;183:187–189.
64. Colman GJ, Joyce T: Trends in smoking before, during and after pregnancy in ten states. Am J Med 2003;24:29–35.
65. Floyd RL, Decoufle P, Hungerford DW: Alcohol use prior to pregnancy recognition. Am J Prevent Med 1999; 17:101–107.
66. Mick E, Biederman J, Faraone SV, et al: Case-control study of attention-deficit hyperactivity disorder and maternal smoking, alcohol use and drug use during pregnancy. J Am Acad Child Adolesc Psychiatry 2002;41:378–385.
67. Ikonomiou C, Bittigau P, Ishimaru MJ, et al: Ethanol-induced apoptic neurodegeneration and fetal alcohol syndrome. Science 2000;287:1056–1059.
68. Jones H, Johnson R: Pregnancy and substance abuse. Curr Opin Psychiatr 2001;14:187–193.
69. Goldschmidt L, Day NL, Richardson GA: Effects of prenatal marijuana exposure on child behavior problems at age 10. Neurotoxicol Teratol 2000;22:325–336.
70. Bateman DA, Chiriboga CA: Dose-response effect of cocaine on newborn head circumference. Pediatr 2000;106:33–39.
71. McElhatton PR, Bateman DN, Evans C, et al: Congenital anomalies after prenatal ecstasy exposure. Lancet 1999;354: 1441–1442.
72. Midanik LT, Zahnd EG, Klein D: Alcohol and drug CAGE screeners for pregnant, low-income women: The California Perinatal Needs Assessment. Alcohol Clin Exp Res 1998; 22:121–125.
73. Sokol RJ, Delaney-Black V, Nordstrom B: Fetal alcohol spectrum disorder. JAMA 2003;290:2996–2999.
74. Brockington I: Postpartum psychiatric disorders. Lancet 2004;363:303–310.
75. O'Hara MW, Schlechte JA, Lewis DA, Wright EJ: Prospective study of postpartum blues: Biologic and psychosocial factors. Arch Gen Psychiatr 1991;48:801.
76. Righetti-Veltema M, Conne-Perréard E, Bousquet A, Manzano J: Risk factors and predictive signs of postpartum depression. J Affect Disord 1998;49:167–180.
77. Cox JL, Holden JM, Sagovsky R: Detection of postnatal depression: Development of the 10-item Edinburgh Postnatal Depression Scale. Br J Psychiatry 1987;150:782–786.
78. Verkerk GJM, Pop VJM, Van Son MJM, Van Heck GL: Prediction of depression in the postpartum period: A longitudinal follow-up study in high-risk and low-risk women. J Affect Disord 2003;77:159–166.
79. Beeghly M, Weinberg MK, Olson KL, et al: Stability and change in level of maternal depressive symptomatology during the first postpartum year. J Affect Disord 2002;71:169–180.
80. Philipps LHC, O'Hara MW: Prospective study of postpartum depression: 41/2-year follow-up of women and children. J Abnorm Psychol 1991;100:151–155.
81. Appleby L, Mortensen PB, Faragher EB: Suicide and other causes of mortality after postpartum psychiatric admission. Br J Psychiatr 1998;173:209–211.
82. Oates M: Suicide: The leading cause of maternal death. Br J Psychiatr 2003;183:279–281.
83. Cogill SR, Caplan HL, Alexandra H, et al: Impact of maternal postnatal depression on cognitive development of young children. BMJ 1986;292:1165–1167.
84. McCook A: Postpartum depression linked to later violence in children. Dev Psychol 2003;39:1083–1094.
85. Vidyashankar C: Postnatal depression linked to poor growth of infants. Arch Dis Child 2003;88:34–37.
86. Sanderson CA, Cowden B, Hall DMB, et al: Is postnatal depression a risk factor for sudden infant death? Br J Gen Pract 2002; 52:636–640.
87. Weissman MM, Warner V, Wickramaratne P, et al: Offspring of depressed parents. Arch Gen Psychiatr 1997;54:932–940.
88. McLennan JD, Kotelchuck M: Parental prevention practices for young children in the context of maternal depression. Pediatr 2000;105:1090–1095.
89. Weissman MM, Feder A, Pilowsky DJ, et al: Depressed mothers coming to primary care: Maternal reports of problems with their children. J Affect Disord 2004;78:93–100.
90. Overpeck MD, Brenner RA, Trumble AC, et al: Risk factors for infant homicide in the United States. N Engl J Med 1998; 339:1211–1215.
91. Wissow L: Infanticide. N Engl J Med 1998;339:1239-1241.
92. Hendrick V: Treatment of postnatal depression. BMJ 2003;327:1003–1004.
93. Appleby L, Warner R, Whitton A, Faragher B: A controlled study of fluoxetine and cognitive-behavioral counseling in the treatment of postnatal depression. BMJ 1997;314:932–936.
94. Gregoire AJP, Kumar R, Everitt B, et al: Transdermal oestrogen for treatment of severe postnatal depression. Lancet 1996;347:930–933.
95. Cooper PJ, Murray L, Wilson A, Romaniuk H: Controlled trial of the short- and long-term effect of psychological treatment of post-partum depression. Impact on maternal mood. Br J Psychiatr 2003;182:412–419.
96. O'Hara MW, Stuart S, Gorman LL, Wenzel A: Efficacy of interpersonal psychotherapy for postpartum depression. Arch Gen Psychiatr 2000;57:1039.
97. Dennis CE: Treatment of postpartum depression, Part 2: A critical review of nonbiological interventions. J Clin Psychiatry 2004;65:1252–1265.
98. Gjerdingen D: The effectiveness of various postpartum depression treatments and the impact of antidepressant drugs on nursing infants. J Am Board Fam Pract 2003;16:372–382.
99. Misri S, Kim J, Riggs KW, Kostaras X: Paroxetine levels in postpartum depressed women, breast milk and infant serum. J Clin Psychiatr 2000;61:828–832.
100. Kendell R, Chalmers J, Platz C: Epidemiology of puerperal psychoses. Br J Psychiatr 1987;150:662–673.
101. Pariser SF: Women and mood disorders. Menarche to menopause. Ann Clin Psychiatr 1993;5:249–254.
102. Jones I, Coyle N, Robertson E, et al: Puerperal psychosis: evidence for familiarity of the puerperal trigger. Mol Psychiatr 1999;4:S26.
103. Rhode A, Marneros A: Postpartum psychoses: Onset and long-term course. Psychopathology 1993;26:203–209.
104. Wehr TA, Sack DA, Rosenthal NE: Sleep reduction as a final common pathway in the genesis of mania. Am J Psychiatry 1987; 144:201–204.
105. Sharma V, Mazmanian D: Sleep loss and postpartum psychosis. Bipolar Disord 2003;5:98–105.
106. Hoppenrouwers T, Hodgman JE, Bernsten I, et al: Sleep in women during the last semester of pregnancy. Sleep Res 1979;8:150.
107. Karacan I, Williams RL, Hursch CJ, et al: Some implications of the sleep patterns of pregnancy for postpartum emotional disturbances. Br J Psychiatry 1969; 115:929–935.
108. Ahokas A, Aito M, Rimón R: Positive treatment effect of estradiol in postpartum psychosis: A pilot study. J Clin Psychiatr 2000;61:166–169.

SECTION SIX

Prenatal—General

CHAPTER 57

Abdominal Pain

Kassam Mahomed

INTRODUCTION AND OVERVIEW

Abdominal pain during pregnancy presents unique clinical challenges; the differential diagnosis during pregnancy is extensive. The pain may result from three broad sources:

- Physiologic effects of pregnancy
- Pathologic conditions related to pregnancy
- Pathologic conditions unrelated to pregnancy

The clinical presentation and natural history of many abdominal disorders are altered during pregnancy; the diagnostic evaluation is altered and constrained by pregnancy; and finally, the interests of both the mother and the fetus must be considered in pain management.

The initial step in management of abdominal pain is to establish a diagnosis by a detailed history, a thorough physical examination, and specific investigations (Tables 57–1 to 57–4). Details of this process will be covered in sections devoted to specific conditions.

Abdominal assessment during pregnancy is modified by displacement of abdominal viscera by the enlarging gravid uterus, because of which abdominal masses may also be missed on physical examination.

Physiologic changes in laboratory values during pregnancy which need to be remembered in clinical evaluation include mild leukocytosis, dilutional anemia, increased alkaline phosphatase levels, hyponatremia, hypercoagulability, and fasting hypoglycemia with postprandial hyperglycemia.

DIAGNOSTIC IMAGING IN PREGNANCY

Fetal safety during diagnostic imaging is a concern in pregnancy. Ultrasonography is considered safe during pregnancy, although sensitivity for nonobstetric conditions may be decreased.[1] Magnetic resonance imaging (MRI) is preferable to computed tomography (CT) scanning to avoid ionizing radiation.[2,3] Rapid sequence MRI is preferable to conventional MRI because of briefer exposure.[4] Radiation dosage is the most important risk factor and is worse in earlier gestation. Exposure of more than 15 rads during the second and third trimester, or more than 5 rads in the first trimester, should be of concern because of the associated increased risk of miscarriage, chromosomal and fetal abnormalities, as well as increased likelihood of malignancies in childhood.[5] Diagnostic studies with the most radiation exposure, such as intravenous pyelogram (IVP) and barium enema, typically expose the fetus to less than 1 rad.[2]

Sigmoidoscopy, especially flexible sigmoidoscopy, seems to be relatively safe in pregnancy; it does not induce labor and should be considered in medically stable patients with important indications, as opposed to routine screening.[6] Informed consent, however, should be routine in such cases.

PHYSIOLOGIC CONDITIONS IN PREGNANCY (See Table 57–1)

Round Ligament Pain

Round ligament pain occurs in 10% to 30% of pregnancies and most commonly occurs toward the end of the first trimester and in the second trimester. It is more common in multigravidae than primigravidae and is said to be due to stretching of the round ligaments, but there is no documented evidence for this. The pain, which is usually described as cramplike or stabbing and is made worse by movement, is in the lower quadrant and can radiate to the groin. It is often associated with some tenderness over the area of the round ligaments.

Risks

The main risk is failure or delay in diagnosis of a significant pathologic condition (see later discussion).

TABLE 57–1

Physiologic Conditions in Pregnancy

	ROUND LIGAMENT PAIN	UTERINE TORSION	BRAXTON HICKS CONTRACTIONS	MISCELLANEOUS MILD DISCOMFORT
History				
Pain	Cramplike/stabbing, aggravated by movement	Recurrent attacks, pain can be severe	Irregular tightenings	Mild/varied
Urine	–	± urinary retention		–
Trimester	Late 1st/2nd	3rd	Late 2nd/3rd	3rd
Previous disease	–	Uterine anomaly, pelvic mass, previous surgery		Fibroids
Examination				
Shock	–	+	–	–
Uterus	Soft	Very tender	Irregular contractions	–
Tenderness	Over area of round ligament insertion	Very tender over adnexa	–	–
Others	–	Vagina distorted/ changed	No show, no cervical change	–
Investigations				
All	Negative or normal	Negative or normal	Negative or normal	Negative or normal

+, Present; –, absent; ±, may be present.

Management Options

Management is conservative and includes reassurance, reducing physical activity, avoiding movements or postures that exacerbate the symptoms, and in some cases analgesics. Failure to respond to conservative measures or worsening of symptoms are indications for further investigations.

Severe Uterine Torsion

Mild asymptomatic axial rotation of the uterus (<40 degrees), usually to the right, is observed in the majority of pregnancies.[7] However, of rotations greater than 45 degrees, 6% occur in the first, 26% in the second, and 49% in the third trimester. The features of pain, shock, intestinal complaints, urinary symptoms, bleeding, and obstructed labor are related to the degree of torsion and can be acute, subacute, chronic, or intermittent.[8] In 80% to 90% of cases, there is a predisposing factor such as a fibroid, congenital anomaly, torsion of a gravid horn of a didelphic uterus,[9] adnexal mass, or a history of pelvic surgery.[10]

Risks

Maternal vasovagal shock and possible fetal asphyxia (both acute and chronic) are the main risks of severe uterine torsion.

Management Options

Conservative measures such as bed rest, analgesia, and altering the position of the mother can be used to try to produce a spontaneous correction of the torsion. Often laparotomy is performed for detorsion of the uterus, hoping the pregnancy will continue. If the fetus is viable, cesarean section is performed following detorsion of the uterus[8] (level IV, grade C).

Braxton Hicks Contractions

Many women experience Braxton Hicks contractions in the latter half of pregnancy.[11] They are irregular in frequency and inconsistent in intensity. Although in the majority of women these contractions are painless, some women find them painful.

Risks

The main danger is to mistake the uterine activity of true preterm labor for Braxton Hicks contractions.

Management Options

A careful history and examination should be performed to exclude genuine labor. Absence of a "show" or membrane rupture together with a high presenting part would be reassuring. Value of absent fetal breathing movements with true labor is yet to be established. Vaginal examination, perhaps repeated in 4 hours, may be the only satisfactory way to assess the significance of these uterine contractions. Once the diagnosis is made, reassurance is all that is necessary.

Miscellaneous Nonpathologic Causes of Discomfort

Heartburn, excessive vomiting, and constipation are common causes of mild discomfort or pain, especially during early pregnancy. A full discussion of the risks and management of hyperemesis gravidarum is given in Chapter 48.

During the third trimester, most pregnant women will experience varying degrees of these symptoms, which some will describe as "discomfort" and others as "pain."[11] Normal events causing such symptoms include abdominal wall distention, vigorous fetal activity, engagement of the fetal head, and pressure effect of the fetal head with breech presentation.

Risks

The main risk is to miss a pathologic cause for the pain.

Management Options

Heartburn may be helped by reassurance, avoidance of bending, and lying flat in bed. Antacids[12,13] and H_2 receptor antagonists[14] are of proven benefit if simple measures do not help. If vomiting is excessive and not relieved by reassurance and dietary adjustments, hospital admission may be required, especially if there is dehydration (level Ib, grade A).

Constipation may be relieved by increasing dietary fiber[15] and avoiding iron unless absolutely necessary. In severe cases laxatives may be tried[16] (level III, grade B).

SUMMARY OF MANAGEMENT OPTIONS

Round Ligament Pain

Management Options	Quality of Evidence	Grade of Recommendation	References
Exclude pathologic causes of pain	–	GPP	–
Reassure	–	GPP	–
Reduce physical activity	–	GPP	–
Provide local heat	–	GPP	–

SUMMARY OF MANAGEMENT OPTIONS

Severe Uterine Torsion

Management Options	Quality of Evidence	Grade of Recommendation	References
Exclude pathologic cause of pain	–	GPP	–
Conservative measures	–	GPP	–
Bed rest			
Analgesia			
Alter maternal position			
Screen for acute and chronic fetal hypoxia.			
Surgical measures (diagnosed at laparotomy)	IV	C	8
Correct the torsion			
Deliver by cesarean section during laparotomy or later (either vaginal or by cesarean) if preterm			

SUMMARY OF MANAGEMENT OPTIONS

Heartburn, Excess Vomiting and Constipation

Management Options	Quality of Evidence	Grade of Recommendation	References
Heartburn			
Reassure	–	GPP	–
Avoid bending	–	GPP	–
Avoid lying flat in bed (more pillows/raise head of bed)	–	GPP	–
Antacids	Ib	A	12,13
H_2 antagonists if severe	Ia	A	14
Excess Vomiting			
Exclude pathologic cause	–	GPP	–
Reassure	–	GPP	–
Dietary adjustment	–	GPP	–
Rectal antiemetics (? avoid first trimester)	–	GPP	–
Consider hospital admission (especially if dehydration/ketosis):	–	GPP	–
Nothing else as first measure			
Consider IV fluids and IV antiemetics if continued problem			
See Chapter 48 for discussion of hyperemesis gravidarum			
Give steroids in extreme cases			
Constipation			
Dietary adjustment, increase fiber	IIb	B	15
Stop iron therapy unless absolutely indicated	–	GPP	–
Consider laxatives	III	B	16
Consider suppositories/enema only if severe	–	GPP	–

PATHOLOGIC CONDITIONS RELATED TO PREGNANCY (See Tables 57–2 and 57–3)

Spontaneous Miscarriage

Chapter 4 provides a detailed discussion of risks and management options.

Uterine Leiomyoma

Chapter 58 provides a detailed discussion of risks and management options.

Placental Abruption

Chapter 59 provides a detailed discussion of risks and management options.

Chorioamnionitis

Chapters 27 and 63 provide detailed discussions of risks and management options.

Preterm Labor

Chapter 62 provides a detailed discussion of risks and management options.

Uterine Rupture

Chapter 77 provides a detailed discussion of risks and management options, and Chapters 68 and 75 contain discussions of specific issues.

Ectopic Pregnancy

Chapter 4 provides a detailed discussion of risks and management options.

TABLE 57–2

Pathologic Conditions Related to Pregnancy: Uterine

	ABORTION/ MISCARRIAGE	FIBROIDS	PLACENTAL ABRUPTION	CHORIOAMNIONITIS	PRETERM LABOR	UTERINE RUPTURE
History						
Pain	+	Localized ± severe	Mild to very severe	±	+	+
Vaginal bleeding	++	±	Mild to severe	–	± Show	+
Urinary	–	–	–	–	–	± Hematuria
Alimentary	–	± Vomiting	–	–	–	–
Trimester	1st/early 2nd	Late 2nd/3rd	Late 2nd/ early 3rd	3rd	Late 2nd/3rd	3rd
Previous disease	±	+	Hypertension, fibroids	Draining liquor	–	Uterine scar
Others	–	–	Multiple pregnancy	–	Multiple pregnancy, PROM, ± Polyhydramnios	Oxytocin
Examination						
Shock	±	–	±	–	–	±
Pyrexia	±	Low-grade	–	±	±	–
Hypertension	±	–	±	–	±	–
Uterus	± Tender	Tender fibroid	± Tender	± Tender	Contractions	++ Tender
Fetal heart	–	–	±	Fetal tachycardia	–	FHR abnormality/ fetal death
Proteinuria	–	–	±	–	±	±
Others	Open cervical os	–	± Oliguria ± Coagulopathy	–	Cervical dilatation	–
Investigations						
Hemoglobin	± Low	± Low	± Low	± Low	–	± Low
Leukocytes	± Raised	± Raised	± Low	Raised	± Raised	–
Platelet	–	–	± Low	–	–	–
Ultrasound scan	+	+	± Retroplacental clot	–	Absent fetal breathing movement	–
Others	–	Low-grade fever Malpresentation	± Positive Kleihauer sign	–	–	–

+, Present; –, absent; ±, may be present.
FHR, fetal heart rate; PROM, prelabor rupture of membranes.

Ovarian Pathology

Chapter 58 provides a detailed discussion of risks and management options.

Abdominal Pregnancy

General

Advanced abdominal pregnancy is a rare event. In the United States it has been estimated that there are 10.9 abdominal pregnancies per 100,000 births, and 9.2 abdominal pregnancies per 1000 ectopic gestations.[17]

It is more commonly seen in patients of low socioeconomic status and in developing countries and in those with a history of infertility or a previous history of pelvic infection.

Advanced abdominal pregnancy has been divided into primary and secondary forms:

- In primary abdominal pregnancy, the tubes and ovaries are normal, and there is no evidence of uteroplacental fistula. The pregnancy is related exclusively to the peritoneal surface very early in pregnancy.
- Secondary abdominal pregnancy occurs after tubal abortion or rupture, with subsequent implantation of the conceptus on a nearby peritoneal surface.

Diagnosis

Early diagnosis requires a high index of suspicion. Abdominal pain is present in 80% of cases, often noticed in early pregnancy, and varies from mild discomfort to severe and unbearable pain. Fetal movements may be painful or absent with fetal death. In 30% of cases vaginal bleeding occurred in early pregnancy. Examination reveals abdominal tenderness, with easily palpable fetal parts.

TABLE 57-3

Pathologic Conditions Related to Pregnancy: Extrauterine

	ECTOPIC PREGNANCY	CORPUS LUTEUM CYST	HEMORRHAGE INTO CYST/TORSION
History			
Pain	± Severe ± Shoulder tip	+ Aching unilateral	Intermittent lower quadrant
Vaginal bleeding	+	±	±
Trimester	1st	1st	1st/2nd
Previous disease	±	–	±
Others	±	–	Nausea/vomiting
Examination			
Shock	±	–	±
Pyrexia	±	–	± Low grade
Extrauterine	Tenderness ± Mass	Mild tenderness ± Mass	± Tenderness + Mass
Others	Cervical excitation tenderness Os closed		
Investigations			
Hemoglobin	± Low	–	–
White blood cell count	–	–	± Raised
Ultrasound scan	+	+	+
Others	Beta hCG positive	–	–

+, Present; –, absent; ±, may be present
hCG, human chorionic/gonadotropin.

Abnormal lie occurs in 15% to 20% of cases. Vaginal examination often reveals a closed, uneffaced cervix occasionally displaced anteriorly. Absence of palpable uterine contractions to oxytocin stimulation or to induction of labor by prostaglandins is one of the most helpful clinical clues to the diagnosis.[18] Even with a high index of suspicion, confirmation of the diagnosis is not always easy.

Ultrasound scan should reveal one or more of the following features: the fetal head is located outside the uterus; the fetal body is outside the uterus, as is the ectopic placenta; failure to demonstrate a uterine wall between the fetus and the urinary bladder; and there is recognition of a close approximation of fetal parts and the maternal abdominal wall.

Radiography should reveal one or more of the following features: absence of a definite uterine shadow around the fetus; maternal intestine shadows intermingling with fetal parts in the anteroposterior view; overlapping of the maternal spine by fetal small parts in the lateral film.

MRI can safely produce images in different planes without the use of ionizing radiation. This method seems to be a very sensitive diagnostic tool where facilities exist.

Risks

Perinatal mortality rate is reported to be greater than 50%.[19] If there is reduced liquor volume there is an increased incidence of fetal malformation, pressure deformities, and pulmonary hypoplasia. Maternal mortality rate depends on availability and accessibility of services but has been reported as 5 per 1000 cases.[17]

Management Options

Management is based on an empiric approach derived from a review of cases[20] rather than evidence from controlled trials (level III, grade B).

Timing and the nature of the intervention will depend on the gestation and viability of the fetus at the time of diagnosis. If the fetus is dead, then surgery is indicated. Some advocate waiting 3 to 8 weeks to allow atrophy of the placental vessels with a possible decrease in intraoperative complications. If the fetus is alive but nonviable (before 24 weeks), immediate surgery is thought to be indicated by many authors. If the pregnancy is 24 or more weeks, a conservative approach may be contemplated to allow time for further development of the fetus. This approach requires thorough and careful counseling of the parents. There are no data that define the risks for the conservative versus surgical options at either gestation.

NATURE OF INTERVENTION

Preoperative preparations should include having several units of blood available and, if possible, carrying out the delivery with a general, vascular, or genitourinary surgeon. A midline vertical incision is always advisable to improve access. The amniotic sac should be carefully incised in an avascular area free of placenta. Removal of the fetus should be done in a way to minimize manipulation of the placenta and surrounding membranes and the likelihood of bleeding.

MANAGEMENT OF THE PLACENTA

If the blood supply to the placenta can be safely secured, complete removal of the placenta usually results in an uncomplicated postoperative recovery, and most authors now agree that removal of the placenta, if straightforward, should be the optimal approach.

If the placenta cannot be removed safely, other options include ligating the cord close to the placenta and leaving it in situ or ligating the placental blood supply and removing the pelvic organ upon which implantation has occurred (e.g., hysterectomy or salpingo-oophorectomy).

Partial removal of the placenta when its whole blood supply cannot be ligated may result in massive hemorrhage, shock, and death. This is not recommended. In such situations it is best that the placenta be left in situ. However, this option is often accompanied by ileus, peritonitis, abscess formation, and prolonged hospital stay.

Some advocate leaving the placenta in situ with later use of methotrexate to increase the rate of absorption/destruction of the retained placental tissue. However, this leads to rapid destruction of the placenta with accelerated accumulation of necrotic placental tissue, which often becomes infected. This is therefore not a recommended method of treatment.

SUMMARY OF MANAGEMENT OPTIONS COVERED IN OTHER CHAPTERS
Pathologic Conditions Related to Pregnancy

Topics	Summary of Management Options Found in Chapter
Spontaneous miscarriage	4
Uterine leiomyoma	58
Placental abruption	59
Chorioamnionitis	27 and 63
Preterm labor	62
Uterine rupture	77 plus 68 and 75
Ectopic pregnancy	4
Ovarian pathology	58

SUMMARY OF MANAGEMENT OPTIONS
Abdominal Pregnancy

Management Options	Quality of Evidence	Grade of Recommendation	References
Dead Fetus			
Delivery by laparotomy, possibly with a delay to reduce complication rates.	IV	C	19
Live Fetus Before 24 Weeks			
Delivery by laparotomy.	–	GPP	–
Live Fetus After 24 Weeks			
Consider a conservative approach after careful counseling. Possibly undertaken as inpatient.	–	GPP	–
Laparotomy and delivery if oligohydramnios and/or compressional deformities.	–	GPP	–
Guidelines for laparotomy and delivery:	IV	C	19
Ideally perform jointly with general/vascular surgeon.			
Have several units of blood available.			

Continued

SUMMARY OF MANAGEMENT OPTIONS
Abdominal Pregnancy *(Continued)*

Management Options	Quality of Evidence	Grade of Recommendation	References
Live Fetus After 24 Weeks—*Continued*			
Make midline vertical incision in abdomen.			
Incise sac away from placenta.			
Avoid placental manipulation during delivery.			
If blood supply to placenta can be secured, remove placenta completely.			
If blood supply to placenta cannot be secured, ligate cord only (greater postoperative morbidity).			

PATHOLOGIC CONDITIONS UNRELATED TO PREGNANCY (See Table 57–4)

Gastrointestinal Tract

Acute Appendicitis

GENERAL

Acute appendicitis is the most common nonobstetric surgical emergency during pregnancy complicating about 1 in 1000 pregnancies,[21] the same as in nonpregnant women.[22] The incidences are approximately 30%, 45%, and 25% in the first, second, and third trimesters, respectively.[23] The incidence among teenagers is higher than in older age groups.[24]

DIAGNOSIS

The diagnosis is challenging as the typical symptoms, anorexia, nausea, and vomiting mimic normal pregnancy, and the anatomic location of the appendix during pregnancy can be different from that in the nonpregnant patient. Conventional teaching maintains that appendicitis pain "migrates" upward with the growing uterus. However, a recent review of cases over a 10-year period[23] showed that pain in the right lower quadrant of the abdomen is the most common presenting symptom in pregnancy, regardless of gestational age. Appendicitis should always be considered when a pregnant woman presents with persistent abdominal pain and tenderness, nausea, vomiting, and fever. Rebound tenderness and muscle guarding are valuable signs in the diagnosis of appendicitis, but because of the laxity of the abdominal wall, these signs are found less frequently in pregnant women.[25]

Normal pregnant women may have mild leukocytosis, but serial white blood cell counts can prove helpful when evaluating patients over several hours when a shift to the left may be very valuable.[26]

Pyelonephritis is the most common differential diagnosis of abdminal pain that mimics acute appendicitis in pregnancy.[27] Interestingly, a review of 50 women presenting with right lower abdominal pain clinically diagnosed and operated upon for acute appendicitis revealed that 80% of the appendices were histologically normal.[28]

Use of high resolution ultrasound with graded compression technique allows direct visualization of an acutely inflamed appendix[29] with reported 100% sensitivity and 96% specificity.

RISKS

Similarity with normal symptoms in pregnancy can lead to a delay in the diagnosis. Reluctance to operate in a pregnant woman causes further delay and thus increases the risk of perforation, peritonitis, and septicemia as well as a substantial risk of miscarriage, preterm labor, and fetal demise. A review[22] of 56 women who underwent appendectomy during pregnancy showed that 33% aborted after surgery in the first trimester. Second-trimester surgery resulted in preterm delivery in 14%. This is more likely when the inflamed appendix has perforated. Maternal mortality rates have declined from 40% in 1908 to 0.5% in 1977.

MANAGEMENT OPTIONS

Despite the difficulty in making the diagnosis, surgery should not be delayed when the clinical suspicion is high. Laparoscopy can be performed safely in pregnancy especially before 20 weeks (see later discussion)[26] and may be considered during the first two trimesters for nonperforated appendicitis or when the diagnosis is uncertain. Use of ultrasound[30] to guide first trocar insertion to prevent

TABLE 57–4

Pathologic Conditions Unrelated to Pregnancy

	ACUTE APPENDICITIS	INTESTINAL OBSTRUCTION	CHOLECYSTITIS	INFLAMMATORY BOWEL DISEASE	PEPTIC ULCER	ACUTE PANCREATITIS
History						
Pain	Right lower quadrant, lumbar, loin	Colicky	Right upper quadrant, epigastric-colicky/stabbing	+	Epigastric pain	Central upper abdomen, radiating into back
Urinary	± Frequency	–	–	–	–	–
Alimentary	Nausea/vomiting	Nausea/vomiting, constipation	Nausea/vomiting	Diarrhea	Nausea/vomiting	
Trimester	–	Late 2nd/3rd postnatal	–	–	–	3rd/postnatal
Previous disease	–	±	–	+	+	Alcohol gallstones
Others	–	–	Jaundice	Weight loss	–	–
Examination						
Shock	±	±	±	–	If perforation	±
Pyrexia	+	±	±	–	–	–
Extrauterine	Tender	Distention/tenderness	Tenderness	±	Tender epigastrium	Tender
Others	–	Bowel sounds high pitched	–	–	–	–
Investigations						
Leukocytes	Raised	Raised	Raised	Raised	–	± Raised
Urine	± Pyuria	–	–	–	–	–
Ultrasound scan	–	–	Gallstones	–	–	–
Radiographic abnormality	–	+	–	–	If perforation	–
Others	–	–	–	Endoscopy/biopsy	Endoscopy	Amylase +

+, present; –, absent; ±, may be present.

injury to the uterus may be a useful adjunct to improve safety (level III, grade B).

Because the location of the appendix is variable in pregnancy, the incision used with laparotomy needs to be individualized. In the first trimester, as the appendix remains in its usual location and the uterus does not obstruct access to it, a low transverse or McBurney incision can be used. In the second and third trimesters, a right paramedian incision over the area of maximal tenderness allows better access to the appendix and the option of extending the incision if needed. It is thought preferable to extend the incision to gain adequate exposure rather than to extensively compress or manipulate the pregnant uterus. There are, though, no studies that address this issue.

During the postoperative period one must be alert for signs of preterm labor, monitoring for contractions and cervical dilation. Peri- or postoperative use of tocolysis is debatable. Those who are against using tocolysis[31] fear the risk of potential fluid overload and adult respiratory distress syndrome. Others[32] have used prophylactic tocolysis successfully. There are no reported trials to resolve this issue[32,33] (level III, grade B). Postoperative antibiotics are normally recommended. Clindamycin and gentamicin in combination are thought to be effective and safe even though they are both category B drugs in pregnancy (see Chapter 35).

Intestinal Obstruction

Acute intestinal obstruction is the second most common nonobstetric abdominal emergency complicating pregnancy. It occurs in 1 in 1500 pregnancies and is increasingly being reported as a cause of acute abdominal pain requiring surgery in pregnancy.[34] This trend is attributed to a number of factors, including an increase in the number of surgical procedures performed in young women[35] and an increased number of pregnancies occurring in older women.[36,37] Obstruction most likely occurs in the third trimester because of the added mechanical effects of the enlarged gravid uterus.[38]

Clinical presentation is similar to that in the nonpregnant state, with colicky abdominal pain, vomiting, and constipation. Abdominal distention and high-pitched bowel sounds are found. If the diagnosis is suspected, there should be no delay in requesting an erect abdominal x-ray to demonstrate dilated loops of bowel with fluid levels.

RISKS

Like appendicitis, delay in diagnosis is common and is often the explanation for the morbidity and fatality that accompany intestinal obstruction in pregnancy. High maternal and fetal mortality rates of 10% to 20% and 30% to 50%, respectively, are reported, especially if the obstruction is complicated by strangulation or perforation, or by fluid and electrolyte imbalance.[34,36]

MANAGEMENT OPTIONS

If there are no signs of strangulation, conservative management with intravenous fluids and nasogastric aspiration may be tried for a few hours. Where there is any doubt, however, early surgery after correcting fluid and electrolyte imbalance would be the safest option in view of the high complication rate. A vertical midline incision is usually necessary, and occasionally the definitive surgical procedure may have to be preceded by cesarean section if access becomes a problem and fetal maturity is assured. Use of perioperative tocolysis to prevent preterm labor in a continuing pregnancy is debatable, as discussed earlier[34] (level IV, grade C).

Acute Cholecystitis and Cholelithiasis

Physiologic changes of the biliary system in pregnancy including decreased gallbladder motility and delayed emptying results in an increase in gallbladder disease in pregnancy. In a large ultrasound study in Chile, 12% of pregnant women versus 1.3% of nonpregnant control subjects had gallstones.[39] Most gallstones are asymptomatic in pregnancy, but when symptoms occur they are the same as in nonpregnant women. Acute cholecystitis as a result of cystic duct obstruction complicates about 1 in 1000 pregnancies, and many women will get their first attack during pregnancy.

DIAGNOSIS

Pain is located in the epigastrium and right upper quadrant and can vary in severity. It may be sudden in onset and become intermittent. Colicky pain is often a result of a stone obstructing the common bile duct. There may be nausea, vomiting, pyrexia, tachycardia, and right subcostal tenderness. The tenderness on deep palpation under the right costal margin on deep exhalation is known as positive Murphy's sign. Leukocytosis is common. Serum liver function tests and amylase may be mildly abnormal. The differential diagnosis includes viral hepatitis, pneumonia, appendicitis, acute fatty liver of pregnancy, and shingles. Ultrasound scan of the gallbladder and the common bile duct will demonstrate gallstones in more than 90% of cases.[40] Cholangiography is contraindicated in pregnancy.

It is important to differentiate cholecystitis from the hemolysis, elevated liver enzymes, and low platelets (HELLP) syndrome and severe preeclampsia, which are associated with great risk to the mother and fetus. Abnormal renal function, raised serum uric acid levels, and low platelet counts will help to make the correct diagnosis of HELLP syndrome.

RISKS

Spontaneous rupture of the gallbladder may occur. There is a possible risk of miscarriage and preterm delivery when surgery is required during pregnancy.

MANAGEMENT OPTIONS

Management is similar to that in the nonpregnant woman. Initially, and particularly in the first and third trimesters, conservative treatment should be advocated.[41] This approach includes analgesia with meperidine but not morphine, intravenous fluids, and nasogastric suction. Antibiotics may be used. Recurrent attacks, failure to respond to conservative treatment, suspected perforation, empyema of the gallbladder, peritonitis, and doubt about the diagnosis are indications for surgery.

Cholecystectomy is not indicated when asymptomatic gallstones are present. If symptomatic, it is preferable to operate in the second trimester, although more aggressive surgical options have now become more acceptable during all trimesters because of advances in maternal and fetal monitoring and advances in laparoscopic surgery.[42,43] Fever and pulmonary complications can occur postoperatively.[44] Tocolysis prior to surgery has not been generally recommended[45] (level III, grade B).

Inflammatory Bowel Disease

Chapter 48 provides a detailed discussion of risks and management options.

Gastroesophageal Reflux and Peptic Ulcer Disease

Chapter 48 provides a detailed discussion of risks and management options.

Acute Pancreatitis

Although acute pancreatitis is rare in pregnancy (1 in 4000), it is said to be more common in pregnancy because of the higher risk of gallstones. It tends to present in late pregnancy or soon after delivery.[40] Gallstones cause more than 70% of cases by obstructing the sphincter of Oddi. Typical symptoms include fever and often sudden midepigastric pain, which may localize to the left upper quadrant and often radiates into the left flank. Anorexia, nausea, and vomiting are common. There may be mild pyrexia with varying degree of abdominal tenderness. Ultrasonography will demonstrate gallstones in more than 70% of cases. Raised serum amylase and lipase concentrations will confirm the diagnosis.[40] False-negative results may occasionally occur with hemorrhagic pancreatitis with massive necrosis or when the blood is taken 24 to 72 hours after the attack. A CT scan may be used for severe cases to delineate areas of pancreatic necrosis.[40]

RISKS

Dehydration and shock may contribute to a high maternal mortality rate particularly in the third trimester. An acute episode may be associated with preterm labor.[46]

MANAGEMENT OPTIONS

The recommended treatment is similar to that for the nonpregnant patient and includes taking nothing by mouth, intravenous fluids, gastric acid suppression, analgesia, and possibly nasogastric suction. Meperidine is the traditional choice for analgesia and seems to be relatively safe in pregnancy. In most cases pancreatitis subsides in 3 to 7 days after such treatment. In patients with gallstones and pancreatitis, surgery may be performed as noted earlier after inflammation subsides. Some, however, recommend aggressive surgical intervention[46,47] (level III, grade B).

Urinary Tract Pathology

Chapter 50 provides detailed discussions of risks and management options.

Liver Disease

Acute Fatty Liver of Pregnancy

Chapter 48 provides a detailed discussion of risks and management options.

Severe Preeclampsia and Eclampsia

Chapters 36 and 80 provide detailed discussions of risks and management options.

SUMMARY OF MANAGEMENT OPTIONS

Appendicitis

Management Options	Quality of Evidence	Grade of Recommendation	References
Diagnosis is not easy; risk to mother and fetus greatly increased with perforation.	III	B	**32**
Laparoscopy can be performed safely especially before 20 weeks.	–	GPP	–
Use of ultrasound scan to guide trocar is a useful adjunct for safety.	III	C	**30**
Laparotomy performed with right paramedian incision at site of maximal tenderness.	–	GPP	–
There is conflicting evidence for the use of prophylactic tocolysis postoperatively for 2–3 days.	III	B	**32,33**
Administer postoperative antibiotics.	–	GPP	–

SUMMARY OF MANAGEMENT OPTIONS

Intestinal Obstruction

Management Options	Quality of Evidence	Grade of Recommendation	References
Once diagnosis is made, conservative vs. surgical approach is cause for debate:	IV	C	34
Conservative (nasogastric suction and IV fluids) may be considered for a few hours if no strangulation/perforation is present.			

Continued

SUMMARY OF MANAGEMENT OPTIONS

Intestinal Obstruction *(Continued)*

Management Options	Quality of Evidence	Grade of Recommendation	References
Surgical approach (laparotomy and surgical correction of obstruction) always indicated if strangulation/perforation, though some would advocate early surgery for all cases.			
If surgical option chosen:	IV	C	34
Obstetrician and surgeon should operate together.			
Make adequate vertical incision.			
Cesarean section may be necessary for adequate surgical field in late pregnancy.			
Give careful attention to fluid and electrolyte balance.	–	GPP	–
Tocolysis for 2–3 days after surgery is common practice.	–	GPP	–
Administer perioperative antibiotics.	–	GPP	–

SUMMARY OF MANAGEMENT OPTIONS

Cholecystitis

Management Options	Quality of Evidence	Grade of Recommendation	References
Prepregnancy			
Consider cholecystectomy prior to conception with symptomatic gallstones.	–	GPP	–
Prenatal			
Conservative approach first:	III	B	42
Bed rest			
Analgesia/sedation			
IV fluids			
Nasogastric suction			
Antibiotics (e.g., amoxicillin, cefradine, or co-amoxiclav) (chenodeoxycholic acid is contraindicated because of possible teratogenic effects)			
Dietary adjustment after attack has subsided (avoiding fatty foods, etc.)			
Indications for cholecystectomy	III	B	43
(preferably in second trimester):	IV	C	41
Recurrent cholecystitis attacks			
Jaundice			
Abnormal liver function			
Empyema of gallbladder			
Bile duct dilatation suggestive of obstruction			
Pancreatitis			
Laparotomy is also indicated if appendicitis cannot be excluded			

SUMMARY OF MANAGEMENT OPTIONS
Acute Pancreatitis

Management Options	Quality of Evidence	Grade of Recommendation	References
Prepregnancy			
Discuss specific measures in women with risk factors:	–	GPP	–
Cholecystectomy in women with known gallstones and previous attacks of cholecystitis or pancreatitis			
Various strategies in women with alcohol abuse (see Chapter 34)			
Change treatment in women taking thiazide diuretics			
Prenatal			
Prevent and treat shock with IV fluids and monitoring of electrolyte, calcium, and glucose concentrations.	III	B	46
Analgesia	–	GPP	–
Administer prophylactic antibiotics (such as amoxicillin, cefradine or co-amoxiclav).	III	B	46
Suppression of pancreatic activity (no Randomized Controlled Trials):	–	GPP	–
Anticholinergic drugs			
Steroids			
Prostaglandins			
Glucagon			
Cimetidine			
Trypsin inhibitors			
Use of nasogastric suction is questioned	–	GPP	–
Prompt recognition and treatment of surgical complications:	–	GPP	–
Laparotomy usually performed with cholecystectomy if conservative measures fail.			
Cholecystectomy can be an early option when pancreatitis occurs with gallstones in first or second trimester.			
Postnatal			
Cholecystectomy possible if pancreatitis with gallstones successfully treated conservatively in pregnancy.	–	GPP	–

MISCELLANEOUS CAUSES (See Table 57–5)

Rectus Hematoma

Bleeding into the rectus muscle and subsequent hematoma formation following rupture of a branch of the inferior epigastric vessels may occur following a bout of coughing or direct trauma, usually in late pregnancy. A large unilateral painful swelling may be confused with an ovarian cyst, degenerating fibroid, uterine rupture, or placental abruption. However, its superficial location in the abdominal wall should enable accurate diagnosis.

Management Options

If diagnosed early, treatment consists of analgesia and bed rest. If, however, diagnosis is only made at the time of surgery, the hematoma can be evacuated and hemostasis secured.

Sickle Cell Crisis

Chapter 39 provides a detailed discussion of risks and management options.

Porphyria (See also Chapter 52)

Porphyrias are rare diseases caused by deficiency of various heme biosynthetic enzymes that result in accumulation of toxic prophyrin precursors. Acute intermittent porphyria is the most common of these diseases, and women present with diffuse abdominal pain, gastrointestinal symptoms, and autonomic nervous system disturbances.[48] Exacerbations

TABLE 57–5

Miscellaneous Conditions

	RECTUS HEMATOMA	SICKLE CRISIS	PORPHYRIA	MALARIA	ARTERIO VENOUS HEMORRHAGE
History					
Pain	+	+	+	+	+
Alimentary	–	±	±	±	±
Urinary	–	–	±	±	–
Previous disease	–	+	Precipitating factor	–	±
Others	Trauma/cough	Precipitating factor	Psychological, autonomic	Travel to malaria area	–
Examination					
Shock	±	+	–	±	++
Pyrexia	±	±	–	+	–
Uterine	–	–	–	–	Tender if uterine vein rupture
Extrauterine	Tender	–	–	–	–
Others	± Mass	–	–	Spleen enlarged	–
Investigations					
Hemoglobin	–	Low	–	Low	Low
Ultrasound scan	± Mass				±
Radiologically abnormal	–	±	–	–	–
Others	–	HbS, sickling	Urinary porphyrins	Positive malaria slide	–

+, presence –, absent; ±, may be present.

first presenting during pregnancy can mimic various neuropsychiatric disorders and present a challenging diagnosis.[49] Pregnancy itself can precipitate an attack, and so porphyria may present for the first time in pregnancy.

Increased urinary levels of porphobilinogen and delta-aminolevulinic acid are diagnostic. Management includes avoidance of precipitating drugs, avoidance of fasting, and possible administration of parenteral glucose.[49] Genetic counseling would be recommended.

Malaria

Chapter 33 provides a detailed discussion of risks and management options

Arteriovenous Hemorrhage

Miscellaneous, very rare conditions resulting in intra-abdominal hemorrhage can cause abdominal pain in pregnancy. These conditions include rupture of the utero-ovarian veins, rupture of aneurysms (splenic, hepatic, renal, aortic), and spontaneous rupture of the uterine vein.[50] In addition to the abdominal pain, rapidly progressing shock is a feature.

Risks

The main risks of these conditions are maternal and fetal demise.

Management Options

Speed of action is imperative in these cases, and even then, death may not be avoided. In all conditions, the principles of management are the same: namely, surgical control of the hemorrhage, correction of shock, and specific measures for specific problems (such as splenectomy with splenic rupture or insertion of a graft with aortic rupture). If the patient survives long enough for such definitive measures to be considered, practical assistance from a general or vascular surgeon is mandatory.

Tuberculosis

Chapter 33 provides a detailed discussion of risks and management options.

Psychological Causes

About 1% of laparoscopies performed for abdominal pain in pregnancy reveal no cause for the pain.[51] Many of these patients have psychological stress that affects the irritable bowel syndrome. Pregnant women with idiopathic abdominal pain are often single, are smokers, and have financial problems.[52] However, this diagnosis is made by exclusion and requires comprehensive diagnostic evaluation to exclude organic disease and to avoid surgical intervention. Reporting a high number of ailments during antenatal care may be an indication for psychosocial support.[53] Domestic volence should also be considered in these cases (see Chapter 81).

PROCEDURE: LAPAROSCOPY IN PREGNANCY

INDICATIONS

Laparoscopy has become an increasingly popular option for many conditions. The most common indication has been laparoscopic cholecystectomy, which though initially reserved for the second trimester, is now being more widely and safely performed in any of the three trimesters as surgeons become more aggressive in their management approach. Other indications include appendicitis and ovarian cyst complications in early pregnancy.

PROCEDURE

In pregnancy patients should be counseled adequately regarding the risks from the procedure. In late pregnancy ultrasound-guided Verres needle insertion has been shown to reduce injury to the uterus.[30] An experienced anesthetist would be recommended to ensure that respiration is not compromised by the pneumoperitoneum.

COMPLICATIONS

Lachman and associates[51] recently reviewed the literature on the subject and cautioned on the lack of adequate data on the possible harmful effect of intra-abdominal pressure as a result of the pneumoperitoneum as well as any possible effect of carbon dioxide absorption on the fetus. The long-term consequences have also been questioned in another review article.[54] Use of ultrasound scan to guide the Verres needle has been suggested to avoid needle injury to the uterus.[30] In terms of short-term risks of miscarriage and preterm labor, the numbers studied to date are too small to be reassured and caution would still need to be exercised.

PROCEDURE: LAPAROTOMY IN PREGNANCY

INDICATIONS

The indications for laparotomy in pregnancy are discussed in the different sections of this chapter. In general, they are the same as in the nonpregnant patient. Obstetricians arguably are more comfortable with the idea of operating on a pregnant woman than are general surgeons. They are also often more familiar with the alterations in disease presentation and differential diagnosis in pregnancy than general surgeons. For these reasons, it is advisable that obstetricians do not simply turn the care of their patients over to surgical specialists for diagnosis and treatment, but rather remain actively involved in their patients' management throughout the period of evaluation, treatment, and postoperative care.[55]

PROCEDURE

Anesthetic Considerations

The choice of the anesthesia for surgery during pregnancy depends on the operation proposed, the skill of the anesthesiologist, and the preference of the surgeon and the patient. Although it has been suggested that chronic exposure of operating room personnel to anesthetic agents leads to an increased rate of miscarriage, the hazard associated with acute general anesthetic administration to the patient is not well characterized. It seems that the risk is very small. It is probably more important that meticulous attention is paid to maintenance of maternal homeostasis. The fetus is totally dependent on adequate maternal oxygenation and uterine perfusion. Any compromise of maternal oxygenation will potentially affect the fetus. Both conduction or regional anesthesia and general anesthesia can be used in pregnancy with safety for both the mother and fetus.

Operation

Abdominal incisions in pregnancy are the same as those used in nonpregnant patients. McBurney and low transverse incisions are best limited to the first trimester. Later in pregnancy, the enlarged uterus so completely fills the lower abdomen that access to organs other than the anterior, lower uterine segment (as for cesarean section) is extremely difficult. It is generally advisable to make an incision that can be extended if necessary, rather than attempting to use a small and poorly placed incision and being forced to manipulate the uterus in an attempt to accomplish the operation. Midline or paramedian incisions work well. Healing in pregnancy is generally without complications, though there may be some skin scar spreading as the abdomen enlarges through pregnancy and keloid formation in some women. If labor occurs shortly after surgery, the fresh incision may inhibit maternal expulsive efforts during the second stage necessitating an assisted delivery.

COMPLICATIONS

There is an increased risk of miscarriage in association with laparotomy performed during early pregnancy.[55] This risk exists especially in the first trimester and is considerably reduced on planned procedures carried out in the second trimester. Preterm delivery and technical difficulty are problems encountered when laparotomy is carried out during the third trimester. However, although the risks of laparotomy in pregnancy should not be underestimated, the risks to the mother and baby of the condition for which the surgery is required are usually greater than the risks of the operation itself.

CONCLUSIONS

- Abdominal pain in pregnancy is a common complaint.
- There are diverse obstetric, gynecologic, surgical, medical, and psychiatric causes of abdominal pain.
- A careful history and methodical physical examination aided by selective investigations will usually reveal the cause of the pain in most cases.
- Physiologic changes that occur in pregnancy may make diagnosis more difficult.
- Diagnosis of some conditions (e.g., appendicitis) can be delayed or missed during pregnancy; a high index of suspicion together with a knowledge of the ways in which different pathologic conditions present in pregnancy is needed.

REFERENCES

1. Derchi LE, Serafini G, Gandolfo N, et al: Ultrasound in gynecology. Eur Radiol 2001;11:2137–2155.
2. Karam PA: Determining and reporting fatal radiation exposure from diagnostic radiation. Health Phys 2000;79(Suppl 5):585–590.
3. Timins JK: Radiation during pregnancy. NJ Med 2001;98:29–33.
4. Kennedy A: Assessment of acute abdominal pain in the pregnant patient. Semin Ultrasound CT MR 2000;21:64–77.
5. Streffer C, Shore R, Konermann G, et al: Biological effects after prenatal irradiation (embryo and fetus). A report of the International Commission on Radiological Protection. Ann ICRP 2003;33:5–206.
6. Cappell MS, Colon VJ, Sidhom OA: A study of 10 medical centres of the safety and efficacy of 48 flexible sigmoidoscopies and 8 colonoscopies during pregnancy with follow-up of fetal outcome and with comparison to control groups. Dig Dis Sci 1996;41:2353–2361.
7. Smith CA: Pathological uterine torsion: A catastrophic event in late pregnancy. Am J Obstet Gynecol 1975;123:32–33.
8. Gronkjaer Jensen J: Uterine tortion in pregnancy. Acta Obstet Gynecol Scand 1992;71:260–265.
9. Achanna S, Monga D, Hassan MS: Case report: Tortion of a gravid horn of a didelphic uterus. J Obstet Gynecol Res 1996;22(2):107–109.
10. Taylor ES: Editorial comment. Obstet Gynecol Surv 1985;40:81.
11. Setchell M: Abdominal pain in pregnancy. In Studd J (ed): Progress in Obstetrics and Gynaecology, Vol. 6. London, Churchill Livingstone, 1987, pp 89–99.
12. Shaw RW: Randomized controlled trail of Syn-Ergel and an active placebo in the treatment of heartburn of pregnancy. J Int Med Res 1978;6:147–151.
13. Atley RD, Weekes AR, Parkinson DJ: Treating heartburn in pregnancy: Comparison of acid and alkali mixtures. Br Med J 1978;2:919–920.
14. Redstone HA, Barrowman N, Veldhuyzen SJ: H_2-receptor antagonists in the treatment of functional (non-ulcer) dyspepsia: A meta-analysis of randomized controlled clinical trails. Aliment Pharmacol Therapeut 2001;15:1291–1299.
15. Anderson AS, Whichelow MJ: Constipation during pregnancy: Dietary fibre intake and the effect of fibre supplementation. Hum Nutr Appl Nutr 1985;39:202–207.
16. Signorelli P, Croce P, Dede A: A Clinical study of the use of a combination of glucomannan with lactulose in the constipation of pregnancy. Minerva Ginecol 1996;48(12):577–582.
17. Atrash HK, Friede A, Hogue CJR: Abdominal pregnancy in the United States. Frequency and maternal mortality. Obstet Gynecol 1987;69:333.
18. Delke I, Veridiano NP, Tancer ML: Abdominal pregnancy: Review of current management and addition of 10 cases. Obstet Gynecol 1982;60:200.
19. Opare-Addo HS, Deganus S: Advanced abdominal pregnancy: A study of 13 consecutive cases seen in 1993 and 1994 at Komfo Anoyke Teaching Hospital, Kumasi Ghana. Afr J Reprod Health 2000;4(1):28–39.
20. Costa SD, Presley J, Bastert G: Advanced abdominal pregnancy. Obstet Gynecol Surv 1991;46:515–525.
21. Tracey M, Fletcher HS: Appendicitis in pregnancy. Am Surg 2000;66:555–559.
22. Anderson B, Nielson TF: Appendicitis in pregnancy: Diagnosis, management and complications. Acta Obstet Gynecol Scand 1998;78:758–762.
23. Mourad J, Elliot JP, Erickson L, Lisboa L: Appendicitis in pregnancy: New information that contradicts long-held clinical beliefs. Am J Obstet Gynecol 2000;182:1027–1029.
24. Mazze R, Kallen B: Appendicectomy during pregnancy: Swedish registry study of 728 cases. Obstet Gynecol 1991;77:835–840.
25. Cunningham FG, McGubbin JH: Appendicitis complicating pregnancy. Obstet Gynecol 1975;45:415–420.
26. Angelini DJ: Obstetric triage: Management of acute nonobstetric abdominal pain in pregnancy. J Nurse Midwifery 1999;44:572–585.
27. Sharp H: Gastrointestinal surgical conditions during pregnancy. Clin Obstet Gynecol 1994;37:306–315.
28. Archibong EA, Eskandar M, Sobande AA, Ajao OG: Right lower quadrant pain in females. Is it appendicitis or gynaecological? Saudi Med J 2002;23(1):30–33.
29. Chang T, Lepanto L: Ultrasonography in the emergency setting. Emerg Med Clin North Am 1992;210:1–25.
30. Wang CJ, Yen CF, Lee CL, Soong YK: Minilaparoscopic cystectomy and appendicectomy in late second trimester. Journal of the Society of Laproscopic Surgeons 2002;6(4):373–375.
31. Kort B, Katz V, Watsor W: The effect of nonobstetric operation during pregnancy. Surg Gynecol Obstet 1993;177:371–376.
32. Al Mulhim AA: Acute appendicitis in pregnancy. Int Surg 1996;81:295–297.
33. To WWK, Ngai CS, Ma HK: Pregnancies complicated by acute appendicitis. Aust NZ J Surg 1995;65:799–803.
34. Connoly MM, Unti JA, Nora PF: Bowel obstruction in pregnancy Surg Clin North Am 1995;75:101–113.
35. Gleicher N (ed): Principles and Practice of Medical Therapy in Pregnancy, 2nd ed. Norwalk, CT, Appleton & Lange, 1992, p 950.
36. Meyerson S, Holtz T, Ehringreis M, et al: Small bowel obstruction in pregnancy. Am J Gastroenterol 1995;90:299–302.
37. Hill LM, Symmonds RE: Small bowel obstruction in pregnancy: A review and report of four cases. Obstet Gynecol 1977;49:170–173.

38. Davis MR, Bohon CJ: Intestinal obstruction in pregnancy. Clin Obstet Gynecol 1983;26:832–842.
39. Valdivieso V, Covarrubias C, Siegel F, et al: Pregnancy and cholelithiasis: Pathogenesis and natural course of gallstones diagnosed in early puerperium. Hepatology 1993;17:1–4.
40. Sharp HT: Gastrointestinal surgical conditions during pregnancy. Clin Obstet Gynecol 1994;37:306.
41. Ghumman E, Barry M, Grace PA: Management of gallstones in pregnancy. Br J Surg 1997;84:1646–1650.
42. Landers D, Carmona R, Crombleholme W, et al: Acute cholecystitis in pregnancy. Obstet Gynecol 1987;69:131–133.
43. Dixon NP, Faddis DM, Silberman H: Aggressive management of cholecystitis during pregnancy. Am J Surg 1987;154: 292–294.
44. Davis A, Katz V, Cox R: Gallbladder disease in pregnancy. J Reprod Med 1995;40:759–762.
45. Schucker J, Mercer B: Surgical disease of the gallbladder. In Gleicher N (ed): Principles and Practice of Medical Therapy in Pregnancy, 3rd ed. Stamford, CT, Appelton & Lange, 1998, pp 1516–1518.
46. Ramin KD, Ramin SM, Richey SD, Cunningham FG: Acute pancreatitis in pregnancy. Am J Obstet Gynecol 1995;173: 187–191.
47. Howden C: Small and large bowel disease In Gleicher N (ed): Principles and Practice of Medical Therapy in Pregnancy, 3rd ed. Stamford, CT, Appelton & Lange, 1998, pp 1102–1108.
48. Grandchamp B: Acute intermittent porphyria. Semin Liv Dis 1998;18:7–24.
49. Soriano D, Seidman DS, Mashiach S, et al: Acute intermittent porphyria first diagnosed in the third trimester of pregnancy: A case report. J Perinatal Med 1996;24(2):185–189.
50. Kuppuvelumani P, Rachagan SP, Khin MS: Spontaneous intrapartum rupture of uterine vein—An uncommon cause of intraabdominal hemorrhage. Med J Malaysia 1994;49:185–186.
51. Lachman E, Schienfield A, Voss E, et al: Pregnancy and laparoscopic surgery. J Am Assoc Gynecol Laparosc 1999;6: 347–351.
52. Baker PN, Madeley RJ, Symonds EM: Abdominal pain of unknown aetiology in pregnancy. Br J Obstet Gynaecol 1989;96: 688–691.
53. Forde R: Pregnant women's ailments and psychosocial conditions. Fam Pract 1992;9:270–273.
54. Fatum M, Rojanshy N: Laparoscopic surgery during pregnancy. Obstet Gynecol Surv 2001;56:50–59.
55. Kammerer WS: Non-obstetric surgery during pregnancy. Med Clin North Am 1979;6:1157–1163.

CHAPTER 58

Nonmalignant Gynecology

Kassam Mahomed

INTRODUCTION

This chapter discusses the significance of a number of gynecologic problems in association with pregnancy that are not covered elsewhere in the book. For malignant gynecologic problems, see Chapter 53. Nonmalignant topics discussed elsewhere include infection (see Chapter 32), female circumcision (see Chapter 73), previous pelvic floor surgery, and previous third-degree tear (see Chapter 73).

OVARIAN CYSTS IN PREGNANCY (See Chapters 53 and 55)

Introduction

With routine ultrasonographic examination during the first trimester, the discovery of an ovarian cyst has become relatively common early in pregnancy. Ovarian cysts that are 6 cm or larger are estimated to occur in 0.5 to 2 per thousand pregnancies.[1] Most unilocular and anechoic ovarian cysts with thin borders that are seen during the first trimester are corpus luteum cysts. These cysts are not usually present after the end of the first trimester. Three fourths of these cysts are asymptomatic, and most resolve without treatment.[2] Further evaluation or management of cysts in early pregnancy is usually left until the second trimester.[3]

After 16 weeks of amenorrhea, organic cysts are the most common, mainly dermoid cysts. A review of series noted three stage Ia borderline tumors, accounting for 3.6% of cysts and 10% of persisting masses.[4] No prospective studies are available to assess the risk of cancer or the complications associated with a cyst larger than 6 cm in diameter and without malignant criteria.

Risks

The major risk of ovarian cysts in pregnancy is to the mother. Between 10% and 15% of ovarian cysts undergo torsion and cause pain.[4] If the cyst is large enough, it may cause malpresentation or may obstruct labor and increase the risk of cesarean delivery.[5] The most important fetal risk is miscarriage (4.7% risk after elective surgery) or premature delivery (9%), which may be induced by surgical removal.[6]

Management Options

Prepregnancy

Surgical treatment is indicated for cysts that are detected before pregnancy, are larger than 5 cm or contain echogenic material, and persist for longer than 4 weeks or are symptomatic.[7] Aspiration of cysts, either laparoscopically or ultrasonically, with cytologic examination of the fluid, is no longer favored because cystadenomas or cystadenocarcinomas may be misdiagnosed.[8]

Prenatal

More than 90% of cysts that occur in pregnancy are nonneoplastic.[9] Corpus luteum cysts usually begin to regress after 12 weeks.[10] Asymptomatic ovarian cysts with benign sonographic features may be followed closely by serial scanning into the second trimester, when surgery can be planned, if necessary.[11,12] However, if the cyst is not enlarging, conservative management may be preferred. Surgery, even in the second trimester, may result in premature delivery in approximately 9% of cases.[6]

If ultrasound examination of an ovarian cyst larger than 5 cm shows echogenic features, surgery may be indicated.[11] Although laparotomy is the preferred management option, experienced gynecologists remove persistent smaller cysts laparoscopically without increased risk to the pregnancy.[13]

Torsion of ovarian cysts is treated by surgery.[14] Progestogen support, such as with medroxyprogesterone acetate 20 mg twice daily, may be advised.[15] There is no evidence that untwisting of an ovary that has undergone torsion increases the risk of venous embolism.[14] The use of tocolysis to reduce the risk of preterm delivery is controversial, and there are no reported trials to help to resolve this issue.[16]

Evacuation by puncture is not well evaluated and is not recommended during pregnancy.[8] If intervention is necessary, laparoscopy is the preferred method.

Labor and Delivery

If an ovarian cyst causes obstruction in labor, delivery is by cesarean section.[3] The ovarian mass is managed in the usual manner at the same time. Aspiration is not advisable because the chance of malignancy is approximately 2%.[8]

PROCEDURE

OVARIAN CYSTECTOMY IN PREGNANCY

Indications

Cystectomy is performed in patients with a symptomatic cyst (e.g., torsion, hemorrhage, rupture) and in those with an asymptomatic cyst that is recognized ultrasonically, but does not regress by 16 weeks. Other indications include echogenic material that suggests a dermoid or has a septate or multilocular appearance.

Gestation

The procedure should be performed ideally at 18 to 20 weeks' gestation. A cyst noted earlier in gestation may be corpus luteum.

Description

Preoperative and perioperative measures include antithromboembolic stockings and the use of subcutaneous heparin postoperatively.

Anesthesia

A general anesthetic agent is used.

Incision

A longitudinal midline incision is used. The incision extends from below the umbilicus to just above the pubic bone. The actual size of the incision depends on the size of the cyst.

Method

The uterus is retracted gently to one side. The ovary with the cyst is usually very mobile, unless the cyst is associated with infection, endometriosis, or malignancy. The ovary and cyst are gently drawn through the incision. The mesenteric border is identified. Two Allis forceps are placed on the antimesenteric border near each pole of the ovary (Fig. 58–1*A*).

The ovarian capsule only (not the cyst) is incised along the antimesenteric border, between the two forceps (taking care not to puncture the cysts) [Fig. 58–1*B*].

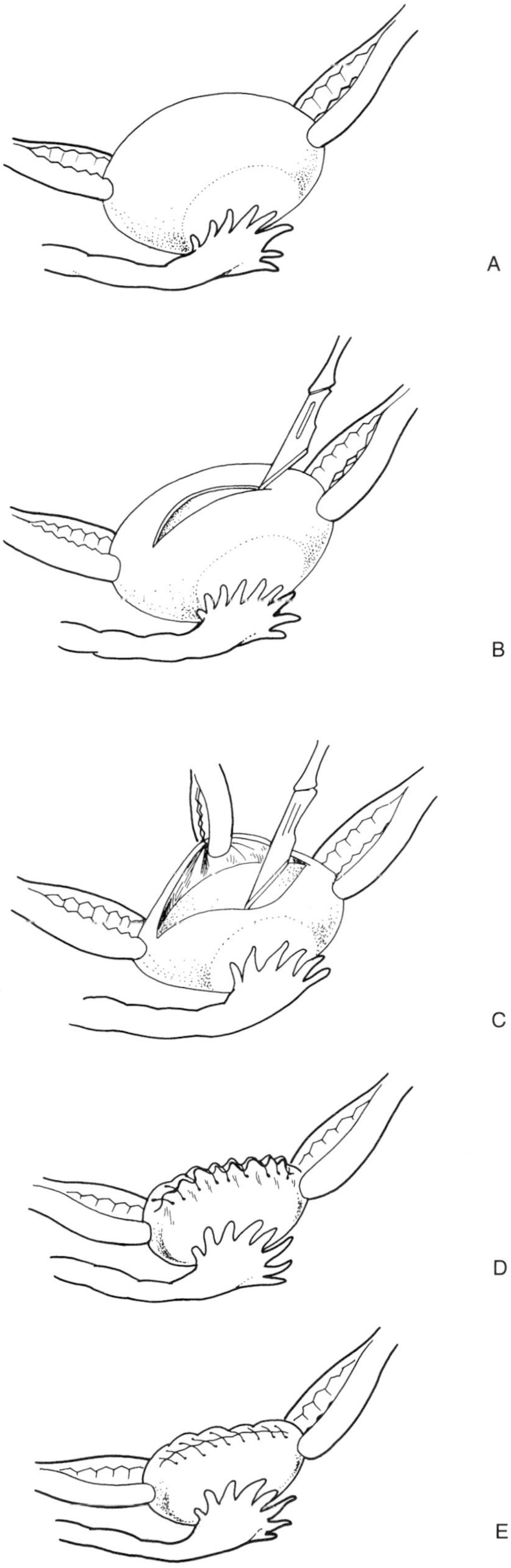

FIGURE 58–1
Ovarian cystectomy.

The handle of the scalpel or closed scissor blades is used to bluntly dissect the capsule away from the cyst, using tissue forceps on the margin of the capsule as counteraction (Fig. 58–1*C*). The blunt dissection is continued close to the cyst, including along the mesenteric aspect. The cyst can then be removed and sent for histologic evaluation.

Hemostasis

Spot diathermy is applied to bleeding points arising from the mesenteric aspect of the ovary.

Repair of the Ovary

Usually the cut edges of the ovary are everted, and repair is advised because of the risk of adhesions from bowel. However, the goal of repair is to minimize damage to the vascular supply within the ovary and to the capsule. If repair is necessary, it is done with polyglactic (Vicryl) or polyglycolic (Dexon) acid sutures rather than catgut sutures to minimize the inflammatory reaction. Sutures (3–0) should be placed carefully and without causing tension (Fig. 58–1*D*). Careful tissue handling is required, and microsurgical technique (i.e., forceps) is preferred to gross handling (Fig. 58–1*E*). The abdominal wall is closed as usual.

Postoperative Management

Narcotic analgesia is used. The use of prophylactic tocolysis is debatable. The fetal heart rate is monitored, and histologic studies are performed.

Complications

The major complication of ovarian cystectomy in pregnancy is miscarriage or premature labor; the risk probably depends on the amount of inflammation caused by the operation.

Tubal adhesions of the fimbria to the incision in the ovarian capsule may occur and impair future fertility. This complication is not usually recognized until subsequent laparoscopic examination.

If the lesion does not appear to be a dermoid and could be a mucinous or serous cystadenoma, ovarian cystectomy rather than oophorectomy is probably the treatment of choice, because malignancy is rare. In young women, it is probably better to repeat the laparotomy to remove the ovary later rather than remove an ovary for what may be a benign condition.

Rarely, ileus may occur, but because there is usually no need to handle bowel, the risk is low.

SUMMARY OF MANAGEMENT OPTIONS
Ovarian Cysts

Management Options	Quality of Evidence	Strength of Recommendation	References
Prepregnancy			
Treat symptomatic cysts, sonolucent cysts, and echogenic cysts 8 cm or more in diameter.	III	B	7
Prenatal			
Treat ovarian hyperstimulation symptomatically. Do not aspirate cysts, but thoracentesis or paracentesis for effusions or ascites may be necessary.	–	GPP	–
Functional corpus luteum cysts regress by 16 weeks.	III	B	10,16
Remove symptomatic cysts.	–	GPP	–
Perform laparoscopy (laparotomy) for cysts 8 cm or more in diameter and those with echogenic features. Leave cysts caused by endometriosis and tuberculosis; remove others. The ideal time for surgery is 18 to 20 weeks' gestation.	III	B	13,17
If cysts are asymptomatic, with benign sonographic features, conservative management is acceptable.	III	B	11
Provide progesterone support if a corpus luteum cyst is removed before 10 weeks.	III	B	15
Untwisting a torsioned ovary does not increase the risk of embolism.	III	B	14
Provide tocolysis to cover surgery and the postoperative period.	III	B	16
Avoid cyst aspiration because of the risk of missing a malignancy.	III	B	8
Labor and Delivery			
For cysts impacted in the pouch of Douglas, perform LSCS and ovarian cystectomy rather than cyst aspiration.	III	B	3

LSCS, lower segment cesarean section.

FIBROIDS (See Chapter 57)

Introduction

Fibroids are more common in primiparous women than in multiparous women.[17] Fibroids are usually asymptomatic and may be seen in up to 80% of women of reproductive age, although only approximately 4% of pregnant women have ultrasonographically visible uterine fibroids.[18] They may interfere with conception and maintenance of pregnancy.[19]

Risks

Although it was believed that fibroids increase in size during pregnancy, those that are initially less than 5 cm in diameter usually involute completely during pregnancy. Larger fibroids may undergo hemorrhagic infarction and can cause pain of varying severity associated with nausea, vomiting, and mild pyrexia.[20] Classically, this complication occurs at approximately 20 to 22 weeks' gestation.

Other risks of fibroids in pregnancy relate to their size and position. These risks include recurrent pregnancy loss, preterm labor, fetal malposition, obstructed labor, retained placenta, and postpartum hemorrhage.[18,21–23] The need for cesarean delivery is at least doubled in patients with fibroids in the lower uterine segment and those larger than 5 cm.[18]

Management Options

Prepregnancy

Because most complications of pregnancy are associated with submucosal fibroids, their removal is advised before pregnancy,[23] usually hysteroscopically, with or without the use of goserelin.[24] The appropriate interval from surgery to conception is not known.

Intramural or subserosal fibroids should be removed only if they are large, distorting the uterine cavity, or are symptomatic, and then only after careful patient counseling,[25] because hysterectomy may become necessary if excessive bleeding occurs. Preoperative gonadotropin-releasing hormone analogue therapy may reduce the risk of hemorrhage.[24]

Prenatal

Most fibroids are asymptomatic during pregnancy and are diagnosed on routine ultrasound examination. If degeneration occurs and causes pain, then analgesia is necessary. Application of local heat or ice packs to the abdomen may provide relief.[26] Prostaglandin inhibitors may also be useful, but should be prescribed for only a few days because of their possible adverse fetal effects.[27] Rarely, the degree of maternal discomfort indicates the need to remove a large subserosal pedunculated fibroid during pregnancy. A subserosal fibroid that becomes impacted in the pouch of Douglas and interferes with micturition may be managed conservatively by catheterization. The patient should be encouraged to spend time resting prone in the head-down position.[28]

If a fibroid (usually a lower-segment fibroid) causes an abnormal lie of the fetus after 36 weeks' gestation, elective abdominal delivery at 38 to 39 weeks' gestation is advised.[29]

Labor and Delivery

Management during labor of a patient with a fibroid depends on whether the fibroid is obstructing delivery. If a lower-segment fibroid causes obstruction, cesarean delivery is indicated.[30] If it is not, then problems associated with poor uterine contractility, particularly postpartum hemorrhage, should be anticipated. Adequate oxytocic therapy should be prescribed and blood transfusion anticipated. Blood should be typed and held in case urgent crossmatch is required.[21–23] A wide-bore intravenous cannula should be in situ.

PROCEDURE

CESAREAN DELIVERY WITH A LOWER-SEGMENT FIBROID

Indication

Cesarean delivery is indicated when a lower-segment fibroid causes an abnormal lie at 38 weeks' gestation or is larger than 6 cm at 38 weeks' gestation and is palpable below the fetal head, either abdominally or vaginally. Smaller fibroids are usually soft and "drawn" or "pressed" out of the way during labor.

The ultrasonographic dimensions may not accurately reflect the true size of the fibroid, so clinical evaluation is more important than ultrasonographic assessment.

Preoperative Preparation

In preparation for cesarean delivery, crossmatched blood should be available. In addition, the patient is given antibiotics. Antithromboembolic stockings are used as well.

Anesthetic

Spinal or epidural anesthesia is used.

Skin Incision

A midline subumbilical incision is advisable if the fibroid is large or if a classic procedure is anticipated. However, if the fibroid is small or posterior, a routine lower transverse incision may be performed.

Uterine Incision

The type of incision used depends on the observed site of the fibroid. If the lower segment is well formed around the fibroid and a transverse lower-segment incision can be made, allowing a 2- to 3-cm margin with the fibroid, then a lower-segment approach is used. If access through the lower segment with a 2- to 3-cm margin is not possible, then a classic cesarean section should be performed, again ensuring a 2- to 3-cm safety margin with the fibroid. Concurrent myomectomy should be avoided because of the high risk of hemorrhage.

Complications and Postnatal Care

There are no complications, other than the usual complications of cesarean delivery. As a result of the hypoestrogenic state that occurs in the puerperium, the fibroid normally regresses and degenerates, possibly causing pain. Occasionally, this involution does not occur in the puerperium, and medical therapy, such as gonadotropin-releasing hormone analogues or embolization, can be used to induce regression. If myomectomy is indicated, bleeding may be reduced.

Previous Myomectomy

If the patient had a previous myomectomy in which the endometrial cavity was opened, then the standard advice is to perform elective cesarean delivery, especially if the implantation site is likely to be over the previous myomectomy incision scar. However, if myomectomy was performed for subserosal fibroids only, there is less risk of uterine rupture during labor. In this case, conservative management is usually advised, although labor should be managed as in a patient with a previous cesarean delivery.

SUMMARY OF MANAGEMENT OPTIONS
Fibroids

Management Options	Quality of Evidence	Strength of Recommendation	References
Prepregnancy			
Remove endometrial or submucosal fibroids hysteroscopically, with or without the use of a gonadotropin-releasing hormone analogue, if the patient has a history of subfertility.	III	B	24
Most women with fibroids have no problem conceiving or with pregnancy.	Ia	A	19
Consider myomectomy for other fibroids if they are symptomatic, and only after careful counseling.	Ia	A	19
Prenatal			
Red degeneration is treated with bed rest, analgesics, local heat, ice	III	B	26
Prostaglandin synthetase inhibitors may be used with caution.	IIb	B	27
Removal of a pedunculated serosal fibroid producing severe symptoms is rare.	–	GPP	–
Ligate and avulse cervical fibroid polyps.	–	GPP	–
Consider elective LSCS if: • Lower segment or cervical fibroids cause unstable lie or failure of engagement of the fetal head • The patient had a previous myomectomy for intramural fibroids	III	B	29
Labor and Delivery			
LSCS if a fibroid leads to obstructed labor	III	B	30
Vigilance for postpartum hemorrhage	III	B	21–23
Do not remove fibroids at LSCS	–	GPP	–
For cesarean delivery, consider a classic or upper-segment approach if access through the lower segment with 2 to 3 cm normal tissue is not possible.	III	B	29
Postnatal			
Analgesia for excessive pain (GnRH analogue in extreme cases)	–	GPP	–

LSCS, lower segment cesarean section.

SUBFERTILITY

Introduction

One in six couples of reproductive age needs specialist help because of inability to conceive (primary infertility) or inability to conceive the number of children they wanted (secondary infertility).[30] This figure may increase in the future as more women delay having children until an age when natural fertility is in decline because of increased aneuploidy of oocytes.[31,32] The problem is compounded by the fact that most couples who seek treatment are not sterile, but have decreased fertility, and many eventually conceive spontaneously.

A male factor is the dominant cause of subfertility in 20% to 25% of couples.[33,34] Female causes of subfertility include problems with ovulation, defects in sperm–mucus interaction, and tubo-peritoneal disorders. In 25% to 30% of couples who undergo evaluation, inability to conceive is unexplained.[33] Endometriosis causes subfertility in approximately 5% of women through any of these mechanisms.

Treatments to assist conception include ovulatory drugs, tubal or ovarian microsurgery, and assisted reproductive technology. This technology may include intrauterine insemination; in vitro fertilization, with or without intracytoplasmic sperm injection; or donor insemination.

Risks Associated with Pregnancies Conceived Using Fertility Treatments

Ovarian stimulation is associated with a risk of theca lutein cysts in the ovary; these cysts are more common with gonadotropin (6%) than with clomiphene therapy (3%).[35] When cysts are associated with ascites, pleural effusions, hemoconcentration, or hypoalbuminemia, the syndrome is called ovarian hyperstimulation syndrome.

Clomiphene or gonadotropin therapy is associated with spontaneous miscarriage rates of approximately 25%.[36]

Women with polycystic ovary syndrome who conceive spontaneously or with the use of drugs also have an increased risk of impaired glucose tolerance and pregnancy-induced hypertension. This risk is independent of body mass index, although women with polycystic ovary disease generally have a higher body mass index than other women.[37] In a case–control study, pregnant women with polycystic ovary syndrome had a much higher incidence of pregnancy-induced hypertension, 31.8%, versus women without polycystic ovary syndrome, who had a pregnancy-induced hypertension incidence of 3.7%.[38]

Multiple pregnancy is a major risk factor associated with ovulation induction, intrauterine insemination, and assisted reproductive technology, including in vitro fertilization, gamete intrafallopian transfer, and zygote intrafallopian transfer. The maternal morbidity rate is sevenfold greater in multiple pregnancy than in singleton pregnancy. In addition, perinatal mortality rates are fourfold higher for twins and sixfold higher for triplets, and cerebral palsy rates are 1% to 1.5% in twin and 7% to 8% in triplet pregnancies.[39] Restricting the number of embryos transferred to one or two[40] can reduce this risk.

Compound heterozygosity for the cystic fibrosis transmembrane regulator (CFTR) mutation for cystic fibrosis is increased in patients with infertility associated with azoospermia and congenital bilateral absence of the vas deferens.[41] The frequency of mutations differs significantly from that in the general population (2% vs. 40%, respectively).[42]

Management Options

Prepregnancy

When a couple seeks treatment for infertility, the woman must undergo an assessment that includes a thorough history and examination to ensure that she does not have a medical problem that must be treated or controlled before conception to minimize subsequent risks during pregnancy. All women with infertility should be tested for rubella. Those who are not immune should be vaccinated at least 3 months before pregnancy.[43]

More than half of patients who undergo in vitro fertilization are of advanced reproductive age and at risk for producing offspring with age-related aneuploidies, which contribute significantly to the risk of spontaneous abortion and implantation failure. Aneuploidy rates of greater than 50% are reported. These patients must be informed about the availability of preimplantation genetic diagnosis. They can use this option to improve their relatively poor chances of becoming pregnant, especially with the current tendency to limit the number of transferred embryos to avoid the complications of multiple pregnancy.[44]

For all women contemplating pregnancy, folic acid supplementation should be initiated.[45]

Preventive strategies for ovarian hyperstimulation attempt to identify women who are at increased risk (using ultrasound and serum estradiol measurements). The lowest possible dose of gonadotropin is used to reduce the granulosa and luteal mass. In patients with a large number of follicles (>20) and an increasing serum estradiol level, the most widely used and most cost-effective approach is to withhold gonadotropin stimulation (coasting) while continuing down-regulation.[46] Other methods include early unilateral ovarian follicular aspiration; administration of glucocorticoids, macromolecules, and progesterone; cryopreservation of all embryos; and electrocautery or laser vaporization of one or both ovaries.[47]

Identification of the CFTR gene mutation in couples with subfertility associated with oligospermia would assist in the selection of the most suitable method of assisted reproduction.[41]

Prenatal

The first, and probably most important, management step is to confirm that the missed period is associated with at least one viable intrauterine pregnancy and to identify multiple pregnancy, if present.

All caregivers should recognize the likelihood of anxiety and the need for supportive counseling in patients who conceive after in vitro fertilization.[48]

Vigilance for ectopic pregnancy should be maintained in women with a history of tubal disease.[49]

If pregnancy is associated with the use of hyperstimulatory drugs, corpus luteum cysts are commonly seen until 12 weeks.[10,16] Surgical therapy or aspiration should be avoided. Sometimes the need for stimulation of ovulation is associated with an endocrine dysfunction, such as a progesterone defect, in early pregnancy. High-dose progestogen therapy has been advocated, but should be initiated only in women whose progesterone levels are lower than the fifth percentile for their gestation.[14] Interestingly, only half of women with low serum progesterone levels miscarry, suggesting that the endometrial and myometrial roles of progesterone are uncertain.

Prenatal screening should be discussed, especially with older women. As the value of first-trimester screening becomes more evident and practical, and if the risk of chorionic villus sampling becomes an acceptable norm, a select patient population will reach the second trimester of pregnancy, and few patients will need second-trimester screening and invasive testing.[50]

Women with polycystic ovary disease should be screened for gestational diabetes during pregnancy, with frequent surveillance of blood pressure.[37]

Ultrasound is frequently performed to evaluate fetal growth and well-being, especially to allay the anxiety of the couple and the physician.[48]

The prenatal management of multiple pregnancy is discussed in Chapter 60. However, if there are three or more fetuses, the risk of prematurity is high and selective reduction may need to be considered.

Ideally, the number of people caring for these patients should be restricted, especially so that consistent information and advice can be given to the couple, who may be anxious. The couple may believe that their only difficulty was in conceiving and that once this goal has been achieved, the pregnancy is not at additional risk. Counseling may be necessary.[48]

Labor and Delivery

The "preciousness" of these pregnancies, with the associated anxiety and stress, results in an increased rate of operative deliveries. In addition, catecholamines released as a result of anxiety may theoretically inhibit labor or affect the fetus, leading to increased numbers of cesarean deliveries because of failure to progress or fetal distress. Continuous fetal heart monitoring is advisable and may be demanded by the patient. Immediate measurement of fetal scalp pH is important when fetal heart irregularities occur. Otherwise, physician or midwife anxiety may lead to unnecessary cesarean delivery.

Postnatal

Contraception is not usually an issue in these couples, but must be discussed. The usual contraindications to the use of intrauterine devices in women with a recent history of tubal disease apply. Contraceptives that may delay the return of ovulation (progesterone-only preparations) should be avoided in couples who may want another pregnancy soon.

SUMMARY OF MANAGEMENT OPTIONS
Subfertility

Management Options	Quality of Evidence	Strength of Recommendation	References
Prepregnancy			
Check for underlying medical disease (e.g., hypertension, diabetes, renal disease, chlamydial infection).	–	GPP	–
Counsel women undergoing assisted reproduction about the rates of multiple pregnancy.	III	B	39,40
Use preconceptual and periconceptual folate supplementation.	Ia	A	45
Discuss the preimplantation genetic diagnosis.	III	B	44
Ensure that the patient is immune to rubella.	III	B	43
Follow protocols to avoid hyperstimulation and multiple pregnancy.	III	B	46,47
If the male partner has obstructive azoospermia, the couple should be screened for cystic fibrosis carrier status. Males should also be screened for Y chromosome deletions.	III	B	41

SUMMARY OF MANAGEMENT OPTIONS

Subfertility *(Continued)*

Management Options	Quality of Evidence	Strength of Recommendation	References
Prenatal			
Check the viability and number of intrauterine pregnancies.	III	B	39
Diagnose ectopic pregnancy early.	–	GPP	–
Check progesterone levels until 12 weeks in patients who undergo clomiphene (Clomid) or gonadotropin therapy	–	GPP	–
Screen for hypertension and gestational diabetes in women with polycystic ovary syndrome.	III	B	37
Check fetal growth and development in pregnancies achieved through in vitro fertilization.	–	GPP	–
For multiple pregnancies, see Chapter 60.			
Provide reassurance.	IIb	B	48
Labor and Delivery			
Provide continuous fetal heart rate monitoring for psychological reasons.	IIb	B	48
Postnatal			
Contraception is not usually an issue.	–	GPP	–
Avoid IUCD use in patients with a history of tubal disease.	–	GPP	–
Avoid progestogens in patients with a history of ovulatory disorders.	–	GPP	–

IUCD, intra-uterine contraceptive device.

OTHER GYNECOLOGIC DISEASES AND PROBLEMS

Congenital Disorders

Some women have congenital abnormalities of the genital tract that affect pregnancy or labor and delivery. Most uterine abnormalities are diagnosed by hysterosalpingogram. Bicornuate uterus, uterus didelphys, and septate uterus constitute 80% of cases.[51] These conditions are associated with preterm delivery (29%), spontaneous first-trimester miscarriage (24%), ectopic pregnancy (3%), fetal malpresentation (23%), and a high cesarean delivery rate (27.5%). Cervical cerclage improved obstetric outcomes in patients with cervical incompetence.[52] In patients with other abnormalities, fetal survival rates improved from 13% to 91% after hysteroscopic metroplasty and from 3% to 86% after an abdominal procedure.[52] The other disorder of the lower tract is a vaginal septum. A septum that is fenestrated superiorly may obstruct labor. This complication can usually be managed acutely simply by dividing the septum in the second stage under epidural or pudendal anesthesia. Hemostatic measures are not usually required.

CERVICAL STENOSIS OR INCOMPETENCE AS A RESULT OF PREVIOUS CONE BIOPSY

Cone biopsy may affect conception because the destruction of mucus-producing glands may cause cervical stenosis or incompetence. The overall rate of normal term vaginal delivery is reported as 46.6% and is inversely proportional to cone size. The incidence of both spontaneous midtrimester abortion and prematurity is increased in direct proportion to cone size. Cervical stenosis necessitating cesarean delivery is associated with small rather than large cones.[53] The role of cervical cerclage is uncertain.[54]

PREGNANCY AFTER PREVIOUS ENDOMETRIAL ABLATIVE THERAPY

Endometrial ablation by numerous methods is used in women with dysfunctional menstrual bleeding and usually is performed only in women who do not wish to retain reproductive capacity. Pregnancy is rare, presumably because of incomplete endometrial resection or regrowth of the endometrium. The risks of pregnancy may be comparable to those in women with Asherman's syndrome.[55] In one series, only 17 of 43 pregnancies had progressed beyond 20 weeks.[56]

VULVAL VARICOSITY

Vulval varicosities are common during pregnancy, especially in multipara. This familial condition is slight during a first pregnancy, but varicosities develop earlier and are larger as the number of pregnancies increases. They cause discomfort, heaviness in the pubic region, and sometimes pruritus or even pain, which is most often relieved by lying flat. They usually disappear completely postpartum. Bed rest and support may provide symptomatic relief. They are also significantly relieved by sclerosing agents.[57]

SUMMARY OF MANAGEMENT OPTIONS
Other Gynecologic Diseases and Problems

Management Options	Quality of Evidence	Strength of Recommendation	References
Congenital Anatomic Defects			
Evaluate and treat prepregnancy.	III	B	51
Evaluate prenatally and plan delivery.	III	B	51,52
Divide vaginal septa.	III	B	51
Cervical Stenosis or Incompetence			
Evaluate prenatally and plan delivery.	III	B	53
Cervical suture	Ia	A	54
Vigilance for dystocia in labor and the need for LSCS	–	GPP	–
Endometrial Resection			
Counseling and vigilance for a higher risk of miscarriage, preterm delivery, intrauterine growth restriction, and fetal death	IV III	C B	55 56
Vulval Varicosity			
Provide symptomatic treatment prenatally (bed rest, support).	–	GPP	–
Sclerosing therapy may be used.	IV	C	56
Avoid trauma during delivery.	–	GPP	–

LSCS, lower segment cesarean section.

CONCLUSIONS

OVARIAN CYSTS

- Ovarian cysts are common in pregnancy. Most are benign and regress spontaneously.
- An ultrasound scan is useful in assessing the nature of the cyst.
- When surgical treatment is required, laparoscopy is the preferred method, but the risk of preterm labor should be discussed.

FIBROIDS

- Fibroids are common in pregnancy. Small fibroids usually cause no problems.
- Fibroids that distort the uterine cavity should be resected, preferably hysteroscopically, before conception. Gonadotropin-releasing hormone analogues have been used to reduce their size preoperatively.
- Pain during pregnancy can usually be managed conservatively, but care is required during labor for delay and postpartum hemorrhage.

SUBFERTILITY

- Assisted reproduction is being used with increasing frequency, and techniques to avoid ovarian hyperstimulation are becoming more refined.
- The risk of multiple pregnancy, with its associated risks, is still high. Even after conception, these pregnancies should be considered high risk. Counseling is essential.

REFERENCES

1. Sergent F, Verspyck E, Marpeau L: Management of an ovarian cyst during pregnancy. Presse Med 2003;32:1039–1045.
2. Zanetta G, Mariani E, Lissoni A, et al: A prospective study of the role of ultrasound in the management of adnexal masses in pregnancy. BJOG 2003;110:578–583.
3. Perkins KY, Johnson JL, Kay HH: Simple ovarian cysts: Clinical features on a first trimester ultrasound scan. J Reprod Med 1997;42:440–444.
4. Struyk AP, Treffers BE: Ovarian tumours in pregnancy. Acta Obstet Gynecol Scand 1984;63:421–424.
5. Goffinet F: Ovarian cysts and pregnancy J Gyncol Obstet Biol Reprod (Paris) 2001;30(Suppl 1):S100–S108.
6. Sherard GB III, Hodson CA, Williams HJ, et al: Adnexal masses and pregnancy: A 12-year experience. Am J Obstet Gynecol 2003;189:358–362.
7. Kobayashi H, Yoshida A, Kobayashi M, et al: Changes in size of the functional cyst on ultrasonography during early pregnancy. Am J Perinatol 1997;14:1–4.
8. Caspi B, Ben-Arie A, Appleman Z, et al: Aspiration of simple pelvic cysts during pregnancy. Gynecol Obstet Invest 2000; 49:102–105.
9. Hess LW, Peaceman A, O'Brien WF, et al: Adnexal mass occurring with intrauterine pregnancy: Report of fifty-four patients requiring laparotomy for definitive management. Am J Obstet Gynecol 1988;158(5):1029–1034.
10. Derchi LE, Serafini G, Gandolfo N, et al: Ultrasound in gynecology. Eur Radiol 2001;11:2137–2155.
11. Usui R, Miri Kami H, Kosuge S, et al: Retrospective survey of clinical, pathologic, and prognostic features of adnexal masses operated on during pregnancy. J Obstet Gynaecol Res 2000;26:89–93.
12. Hill LM, Conners-Beauty DJ, Nowak A, et al: The role of ultrasonography in the detection and management of adnexal masses during the second and third trimesters of pregnancy. Am J Obstet Gynecol 1998;179:703–707.
13. Toen PM, Chang AM: Laparoscopic management of adnexal mass during pregnancy. Acta Obstet Gynecol Scand 1997;76:173–176.
14. Cohen SB, Oelsner G, Seidman DS, et al: Laparoscopic detorsion allows sparing of the twisted ischemic adnexa. J Am Assoc Gynecol Laparosc 1999;6:139–143.
15. Perkins KY, Johnson JL, Kay HH: Simple ovarian cysts: Clinical features on a first-trimester ultrasound scan. J Reprod Med 1997;42:440–444.
16. To WWK, Ngai CS, Ma HK: Pregnancies complicated by acute appendicitis. Aust N Z J Surg 1995;65:799–803.
17. Parazzini F, La Vecchia C, Negri E, et al: Epidemiologic characteristics of women with uterine fibroids: A case-control study. Obstet Gynecol 1988;72:853–857.
18. Exacoustos C, Rosati P: Ultrasound diagnosis of uterine myomas and complications in pregnancy. Obstet Gynecol 1993;82:97–101.
19. Pritts EA: Fibroids and infertility: A systematic review of the evidence. Obstet Gynecol Surv 2001;56:483–491.
20. Strobelt N, Ghidini A, Cavallone M, et al: Natural history of uterine leiomyomas in pregnancy. J Ultrasound Med 1994;13: 399–401.
21. Vergani P, Ghidini A, Strobelt N, et al: Do uterine leiomyomas influence pregnancy outcome? Am J Perinatol 1994; 11:356–358.
22. Phelan JP: Myomas and pregnancy. Obstet Gynecol Clin North Am 1995;22:801–805.
23. Lanouette JM, Diamond MP: Pregnancy in women with uterine myoma. Infertil Reprod Med North Am 1996;7:19–32.
24. Narayan R, Rajat K, Gesurmy K, et al: Treatment of submucus fibroids, and outcome of assisted conception. J Am Assoc Gynecol Laparosc 1994;1: 307–311.
25. Roberts WE, Fulp KS, Morrisson JC, et al: The impact of leiomyomas on pregnancy. Aust N Z J Obstet Gynaecol 1999;39:43–47.
26. Koike T, Minakami H, Kosuge S, et al: Uterine leiomyoma in pregnancy: Its influence on obstetric performance. J Obstet Gynaecol Res 1999;25:309–313.
27. Higby K, Suiter CR: A risk-benefit assessment of therapies for premature labour. Drug Saf 1999;21:35–56.
28. Yang JM, Huang WC: Sonographic findings of acute urinary retention secondary to an impacted pelvic mass. J Ultrasound Med 2002;21:1165–1169.
29. Coronado GD, Marshall LM, Schwartz SM: Complications in pregnancy, labour, and delivery with uterine leiomyomas: A population-based study. Obstet Gynecol 2000;95:764–769.
30. Sherer DM, Schwartz SM, Mahon TR: Intrapartum ultrasonographic depiction of fetal malpositioning and mild parietal bone compression in association with large lower segment uterine leiomyoma. J Maternal Fetal Med 1999;8:28–31.
31. Hull MG, Glazener CM, Kelly NJ, et al: Population study of causes, treatment and outcome of infertility. BMJ 1985;291: 1693–1697.
32. Delhanty JD: Preimplantation genetics: An explanation for poor human fertility? Ann Hum Genet 2001;65:331–338.
33. Snick HK, Snick TS, Evers JL, Collins JA: The spontaneous pregnancy prognosis in untreated sub fertile couples: The Walcheren primary care study. Hum Reprod 1997;12:1582–1588.
34. Evers LH: Female sub fertility. Lancet 2002; 360 (9327):151–160.
35. Ziadeh SM, Zakaria MR, Abu-Hieja A: Pregnancy rates using CC/hMG or hMG alone. J Obstet Gynaecol Res 1997;23:97–101.
36. Costello MF, Hughes GJ, Garrett DK, et al: A spontaneous luteinising surge is beneficial in women with unexplained infertility undergoing controlled ovarian hyper stimulation without in vitro fertilisation. Int J Fertil Womens Med 1997;43:28–33.
37. Urman B, Sarac E, Dogan L, Gurgan T: Pregnancy in infertile PCOD patients: Complications and outcome. J Reprod Med 1997;42:501–505.
38. Kashyap S, Claman P: Polycystic ovary disease and the risk of pregnancy-induced hypertension. J Reprod Med 2000;45:991–994.
39. Wimalasundera RC, Trew G, Fisk NM: Reducing the incidence of twins and triplets. Best Pract Res Clin Obstet Gynaecol 2003;17:309–329.
40. Bergh C, Bryman I, Nilsson L, Janson PO: Results of gonadotrophin stimulation with the option to convert cycles to in vitro fertilisation in cases of multifollicular development. Acta Obstet Gynecol Scand 1998;77:68–73.
41. Cruger DG, Agerholm I, Byriel L, et al: Genetic analysis of males from intracytoplasmic sperm injection couples. Clin Genet 2003;64:198–203.
42. Leonardi S, Bombace V, Rotolo N, et al: Congenital absence of vas deferens and cystic fibrosis. Minn Pediatr 2003;55:43–50.
43. McElhaney RD Jr, Ringer M, DeHart DJ, Vasillenko P: Rubella immunity in a cohort of pregnant women. Infect Control Hosp Epidemiol 1999;20:64–66.
44. Kuliev A, Verlinsky Y: The role of preimplantation genetic diagnosis in women of advanced reproductive age. Curr Opin Obstet Gynecol 2003;15:233–238.
45. Lumley J, Watson L, Watson M, et al: Periconceptual supplementation with folate and/or multivitamin for prevention of neural tube defects: Cochrane review. In Cochrane library, issue 3. Oxford, UK, Update Software, 2003.
46. Al-Shawaf T, Grudzinskas JG: Prevention and treatment of ovarian hyperstimulation syndrome. Best Pract Res Clin Obstet Gynaecol 2003;17:249–261.

47. Delvigne A, Rozenberg S: Epidemiology and prevention of ovarian hyperstimulation syndrome (OHSS): A review. Hum Reprod Update 2002;8:559–577.
48. McMahon CA, Ungerer JA, Beaurepaire J, et al: Anxiety during pregnancy and fetal attachment after in-vitro fertilisation. Hum Reprod 1997;12:176–182.
49. Ankum WM, Mol BW, Van der Veen F, Bossuyt PM: Risk factors for ectopic pregnancy: A meta-analysis. Fertil Steril 1996;65:1093–1099.
50. Budorick NE, O'Boyle MK: Prenatal diagnosis for detection of aneuploidy: The options. Radiol Clin North Am 2003;41: 695–708.
51. Golan A, Langer R, Neuman M, et al: Obstetric outcome in women with congenital uterine malformations. J Reprod Med 1992;37:233–236.
52. Heinonen PK: Reproductive performance of women with uterine anomalies after abdominal or hysteroscopic metroplasty or no surgical treatment. J Am Assoc Gynecol Laparosc 1997;4:311–317.
53. Leiman G, Harrison NA, Rubin A: Pregnancy following conization of the cervix: Complications related to cone size. Am J Obstet Gynecol 1980;136:14–18.
54. Drakeley AJ, Roberts D, Alfirevic Z: Cervical stitch (cerclage) for preventing pregnancy loss in women: Cochrane review. In Cochrane library, issue 4. Chester, UK, John Wiley, 2003.
55. Wood C, Rogers P: A pregnancy after planned partial endometrial resection. Aust N Z J Obstet Gynaecol 1993;33:316–318.
56. Cook JR, Seman EI: Pregnancy following endometrial ablation: Case history and literature review. Obstet Gynecol Surv 2003;58:551–556.
57. Marhic C: Vulvar varicosity and pregnancy. Rev Fr Gynecol Obstet 1991;25(2 Pt 2):184–186.

CHAPTER 59

Bleeding in Late Pregnancy

Justin C. Konje / David J. Taylor

INTRODUCTION

Bleeding in late pregnancy, or antepartum hemorrhage, is defined as bleeding from the genital tract after 20 weeks' gestation. This type of bleeding complicates 2% to 5% of all pregnancies[1] and has various causes (Table 59–1).

MANAGEMENT OF BLEEDING IN LATE PREGNANCY (See Chapter 79)

Antepartum hemorrhage is unpredictable, and the patient's condition may deteriorate rapidly before, during, or after presentation. Management starts with general measures to treat or prevent deterioration, followed by specific treatment measures. The general measures discussed in this chapter apply to all cases of antepartum hemorrhage, but they may be modified, depending on the severity of bleeding. The specific measures depend on the diagnosis and are discussed under the various causes of bleeding.

TABLE 59–1

Causes of Bleeding in Late Pregnancy

CAUSE	INCIDENCE
Placenta previa	31.0
Abruptio placentae	22.0
Unclassified	47.0
Marginal	60.0
Show	20.0
Cervicitis	8.0
Trauma	5.0
Vulvovaginal varicosity	2.0
Genital tumor	0.5
Genital infection	0.5
Hematuria	0.5
Vasa praevia	0.5
Other	0.5

INITIAL ASSESSMENT (Fig. 59–1)

Management of the patient with antepartum hemorrhage must be in a hospital with adequate facilities for transfusion, cesarean delivery, and neonatal resuscitation and intensive care. In the patient with significant vaginal bleeding, immediate transfer to a hospital by ambulance is recommended.

Initial management includes a history, evaluation of the patient's general condition, and initiation of testing and treatment.

History

The history should identify initiating factors, such as trauma or coitus, the amount and character of bleeding, associated abdominal pain or regular uterine contractions, a history of ruptured membranes or previous vaginal bleeding, gestational age as determined by early ultrasound scan or the last menstrual period, information about the site of the placenta from previous scans, and information about fetal movements.

Physical Examination

Physical examination should assess both the maternal and the fetal condition, including the following features:

- Maternal pulse, blood pressure, and respiratory rate
- Clinical evidence of shock (restlessness; cold, clammy extremities; poor skin perfusion; piloerection response)
- Abdominal examination to determine whether the uterine fundus is compatible with the estimated gestational age and to assess the presence of tenderness, the number and viability of fetuses, the presence of uterine contractions, and the lie and presentation of the fetus or fetuses
- Vaginal examination. Traditionally, digital or speculum examination is considered inadvisable unless placenta previa has been excluded. However, despite this

conventional guidance, in practice, careful vaginal examinations are undertaken by experienced clinicians when they are certain that the fetal head is engaged, making the diagnosis of placenta previa unlikely. In most cases, only an inspection of the vulva to quickly assess the amount of blood loss and to determine whether bleeding has stopped or is continuing is necessary. When placenta previa has been excluded, speculum examination may be performed.

Testing and Immediate Management

Initially, the patient with antepartum hemorrhage should be evaluated and managed as discussed later, but subsequent management is determined by gestational age and the severity and type of bleeding. Initial management includes the following:

- Insertion of an intravenous line with a wide-bore cannula (preferably size 14–16 French)
- Obtaining blood for immediate hemoglobin or hematocrit estimation, complete blood count and typing, and holding of serum for potential crossmatching. If bleeding is continuing or is heavy, then at least four units of blood must be crossmatched. When placental abruption is suspected, a coagulation profile and measurement of urea and electrolytes should be performed. Other tests that may be performed are the Kleihauer-Betke test on maternal blood and the Apt test on vaginal blood.
- Administration of intravenous fluids if bleeding is continuing or severe while crossmatched blood is awaited. Colloids are the most suitable fluids. Consideration should be given to transfusing type O, Rhesus-negative blood if crossmatching is delayed.
- Performing an ultrasound scan to exclude placenta previa if a scan has not been done previously or to exclude a major abruption with placental separation. However, a scan should be performed only if maternal and fetal conditions are stable.

After initial management, one of the following conditions is likely to be present:

- Bleeding has stopped.
- Bleeding is continuing, and is mild to moderate and non-life-threatening.
- Bleeding is continuing and is severe and life-threatening.
- The fetus is in distress, regardless of the bleeding pattern.
- The fetus is dead, regardless of the bleeding pattern.

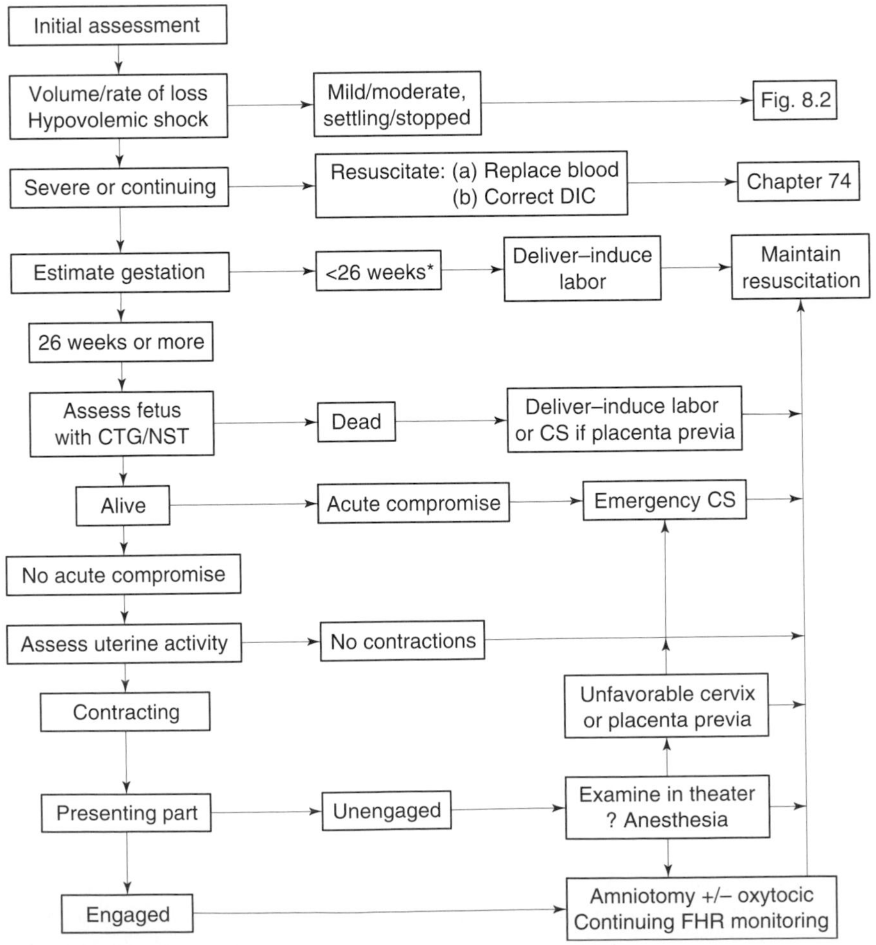

FIGURE 59–1
Management of bleeding in late pregnancy. Initial assessment and management of severe bleeding. (*The gestation after which survival rates are considered high enough to influence the mode of delivery of the preterm fetus varies in different centers from 24 to 28 weeks.)

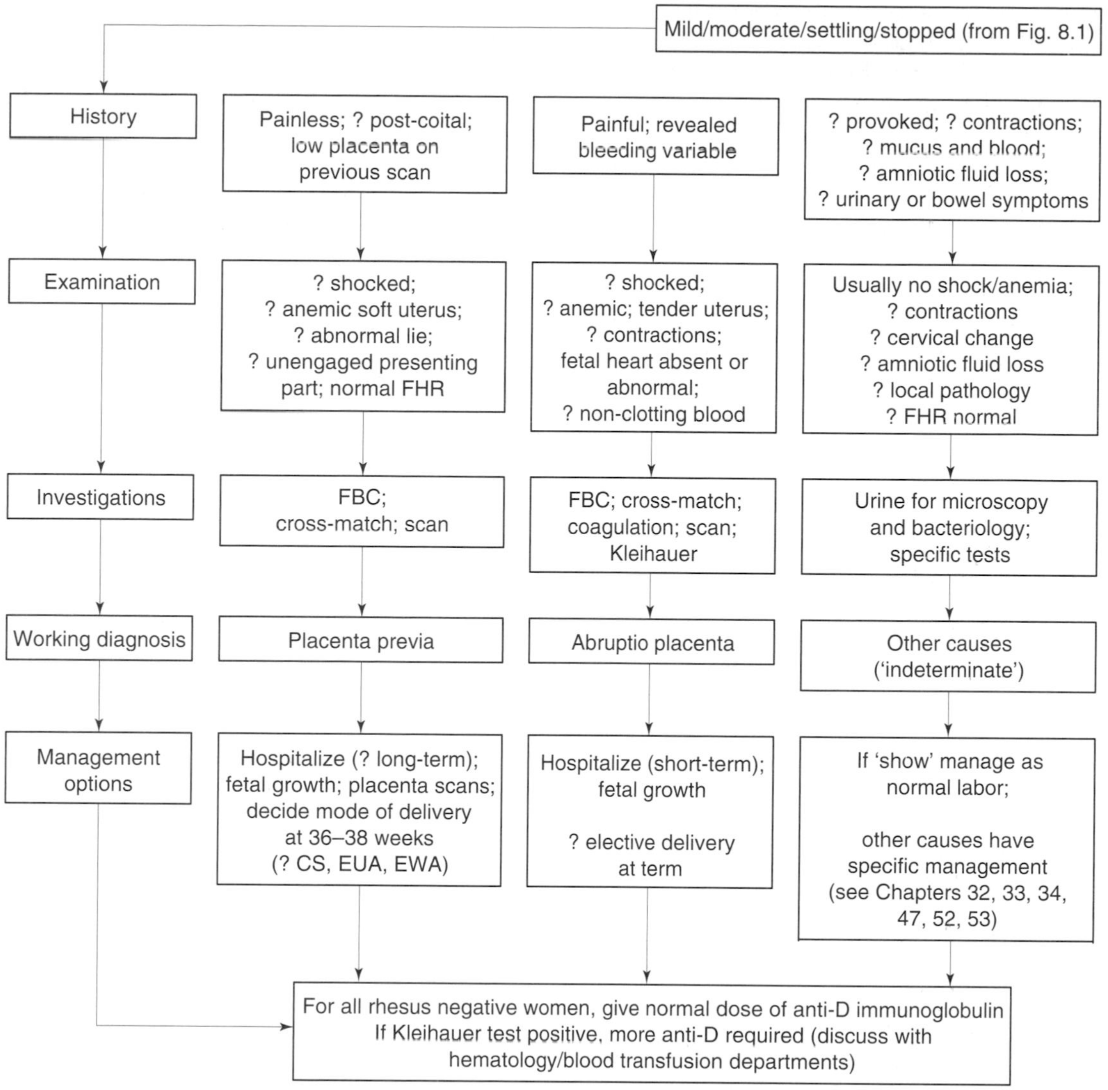

FIGURE 59–2
Management of bleeding in late pregnancy. Subsequent assessment and specific management of mild bleeding. (EUA, EWA, examination in the theater with and without anesthesia, respectively.)

Subsequent management is determined by these circumstances. Options include immediate delivery and expectant management. These are discussed under the various types of antepartum hemorrhage. The flow charts in Figures 59–1 and 59–2 outline the steps in management.

PLACENTA PREVIA

In placenta previa, the placenta is inserted partially or entirely into the lower uterine segment. Four grades have been defined (Table 59–2 and Fig. 59–3). Figures 59–4 and 59–5 show two of these grades. This condition occurs in 0.4% to 0.8% of pregnancies,[2] although an incidence of 0.16% was recently reported in an unselected population in Finland.[3]

The etiology of placenta previa is unknown, but various associations have been identified. These include age, parity, and previous cesarean delivery.[4–7] A single cesarean delivery increases the risk by 0.65%, two increase the risk 1.5%, three increase the risk by 2.2%, and four or more increase the risk by 10%.[7] Other risk

TABLE 59–2

Grading of Placenta Previa

GRADE	DESCRIPTION
I	The placenta is in the lower segment, but the lower edge does not reach the internal os
II	The lower edge of the low-lying placenta reaches, but does not cover, the internal os
III	The placenta covers the internal os asymmetrically
IV	The placenta covers the internal os symmetrically

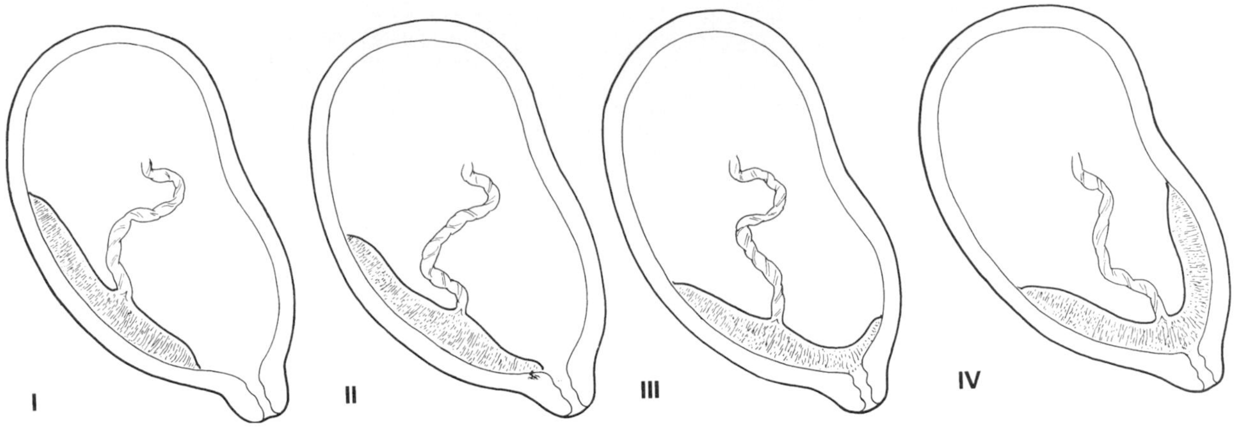

FIGURE 59–3
Grades of placenta previa. I, Encroaching on the lower segment; II, reaching the internal OS; III, asymmetrically covering the internal os; IV, symmetrically covering the internal os.

factors include cigarette smoking,[8] drug abuse (especially cocaine), a history of abortion, and previous placenta previa. A recurrence risk of 4% to 8% after one pregnancy affected by placenta previa has been reported.[9] The association with abortion (spontaneous or induced) is greater with an increasing number of previous abortions.[10,11]

Placenta accreta and placenta percreta are discussed in Chapter 77.

Maternal Risks

Maternal mortality as a result of hemorrhage decreased from 29 cases in 1952–1954 to none in 1985–1987, but increased to 5 in 1988–1990, 4 in 1991–1993, 3 in 1994–1996, and 4 in 2000–2002.[12] Postpartum hemorrhage is believed to be caused by inadequate occlusion of the sinuses in the lower segment after delivery. Anesthetic and surgical complications may occur, especially in women with major placenta previa who have emergency cesarean delivery with suboptimal preparation for surgery. Air embolism occurs when the sinuses in the placental bed are torn. Postpartum sepsis is caused by ascending infection of the raw placental bed. Placenta accreta occurs in up to 15% of women with placenta previa. The risk of recurrence is approximately 4% to 8% after one previous placenta previa.

Fetal Risks

The fetal risks of placenta previa include the following:

- Preterm birth. Cotton and colleagues[13] reported a perinatal mortality rate of 100% at less than 27 weeks,

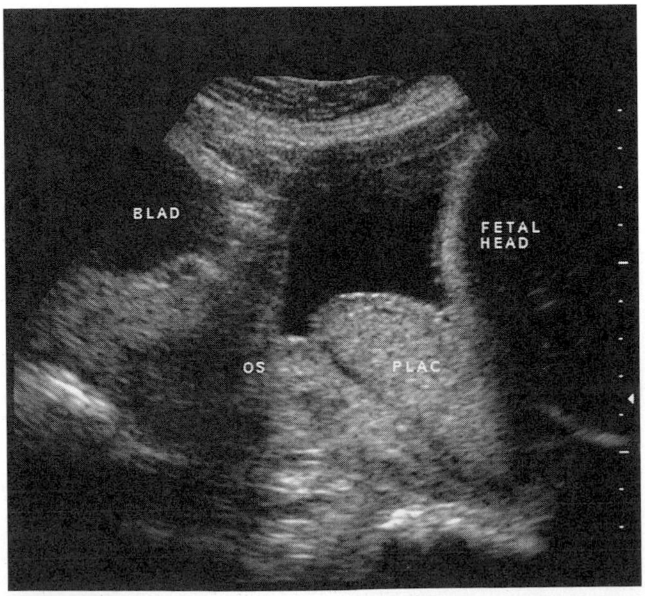

FIGURE 59–4
Grade II posterior placenta previa. The placenta extends to the cervical os, but does not cover it.

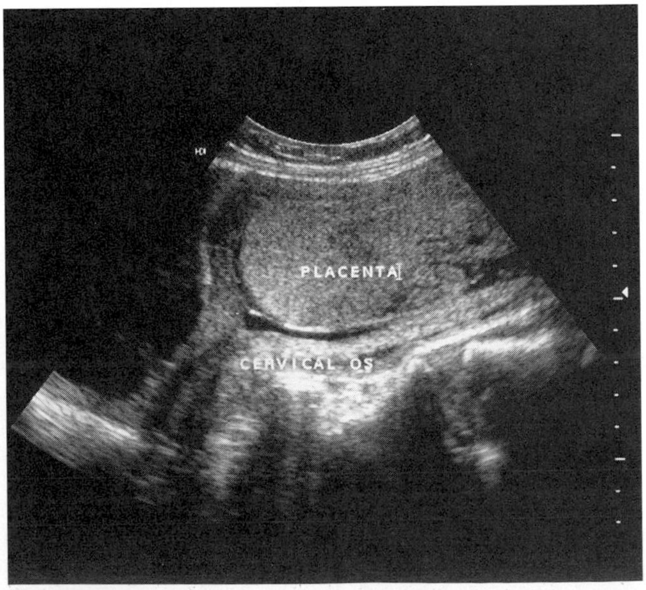

FIGURE 59–5
Grade IV placenta previa. The placenta covers the os symmetrically.

19.7% at 27 to 32 weeks, 6.4% at 33 to 36 weeks, and 2.6% after 36 weeks. These figures, however, represent the outcome nearly 23 years ago. In recent years, the overall perinatal mortality rate has dropped from 126 per 1000[12] to 42 to 81 per 1000[4] as a result of conservative management and improved neonatal care.
- Fetal growth restriction, which may occur in up to 16% of cases. The incidence is higher in patients with multiple episodes of antepartum hemorrhage.[14]
- Placenta previa. The incidence of serious malformations is doubled in women with placenta previa. The most common malformations are those of the central nervous system and the cardiovascular, respiratory, and gastrointestinal systems.[3]
- Other risks. Additional fetal risks include umbilical cord complications, such as prolapse and compression,[10] malpresentation, fetal anemia, and unexpected intrauterine death (e.g., rupture of vasa previa, severe maternal hypovolemic shock).

Presentation

Placenta previa characteristically causes unprovoked painless vaginal bleeding. Occasionally, it is caused by sexual intercourse. Threatened second-trimester miscarriage may precede placenta previa,[15] although bleeding may be minor and in some cases unreported. The initial episode of bleeding has a modal incidence at approximately 34 weeks and occurs before 36 weeks in more than 50% of cases. It occurs after 40 weeks in only 2% of cases.[4]

The absence of pain is often considered a significant distinguishing factor between placenta previa and placental abruption, but 10% of women with placenta previa have coexisting abruption.[10] These patients and those who seek care for the first time while in labor and are therefore experiencing painful uterine contractions (25% of women with placenta previa[16]) may present a diagnostic problem.

Because ultrasound scanning is performed in early pregnancy in most centers, some patients with a low-lying placenta may be identified before 20 weeks' gestation, but the diagnosis of placenta previa cannot be made because the lower segment has not formed at this time.

Abdominal findings in placenta previa include malpresentation, which is either breech or transverse in 35% of cases[13]; slight, but consistent deviation of the presenting part from the midline; and difficulty with palpating the presenting part.

Diagnosis

Various approaches have been used to diagnose placenta previa.

Vaginal Examination

Digital vaginal examination may cause hemorrhage. Because local causes are likely to be benign, speculum examination is probably best deferred until ultrasonography has excluded the diagnosis. If digital vaginal examination is necessary because of excessive bleeding, it should be performed only in an operating room, with full preparation for cesarean delivery (discussed later).

Placental Localization

Diagnostic ultrasound scanning is safe, accurate, and noninvasive, and is the diagnostic method of choice. Although routine placental localization is considered part of the anomaly scan at 20 to 22 weeks' gestation, several questions arise from this practice. For example, is a low-lying placenta at this stage predictive of placenta previa at delivery, and does this screening reduce the likelihood of adverse outcome? More important, should the scan be repeated at 32 to 34 weeks' gestation? Must the asymptomatic patient be admitted, and if so, when?

Unfortunately, the earlier the scan is performed, the more likely the placenta is to be found in the lower pole of the uterus. For example, approximately 28% of placentas in women who undergo transabdominal scanning before 24 weeks are "low," but by 24 weeks, this number drops to 18%, and only 3% are low-lying by term.[17] Conversely, a false-negative scan for a low placenta is found in as many as 7% of patients at 20 weeks.[18] These results are more common when the placenta is posterior, the bladder is overfilled, the fetal head obscures the margin of the placenta, or the operator does not scan the lateral uterine wall.[19] A low-lying placenta is more common in early pregnancy because the lower segment does not exist. The apparent placental migration is caused by enlargement of the upper segment and formation of the lower segment. Many apparently low placentas are found above the lower segment. Comeau and associates[20] and Ruparelia and Chapman[21] showed that the more advanced the pregnancy, the more accurate the diagnosis of placenta previa based on scanning findings.

When a transvaginal ultrasound scan is performed for placental localization and the distance between the lower edge of the placenta and the internal cervical os is measured, the persistence of a low-lying placenta at a later gestation is higher. Taipale and colleagues[22] observed that if a placenta overlapped the internal os by at least 25 mm at 18 to 23 weeks, the positive predictive value for placenta previa at delivery was 40%, with a sensitivity of 80%. Becker and associates[23] found that when the lower edge overlapped the os by at least 25 mm at 20 to 23 weeks, vaginal delivery was not possible at term (i.e., 100% positive predictive value).

Although no randomized controlled trials have been conducted, case studies advocate localization of the placenta at the routine anomaly scan. Practitioners must recognize the limitations of this practice, and whenever possible, offer transvaginal ultrasound scans to improve the accuracy of localization and measure the distance from the os to the placental edge to help define the extent to which the placenta is low-lying.

Because there are no randomized controlled trials of the maternal and fetal effects of routine localization versus no localization, current practice must be governed by large cohort case studies. It is assumed that when there is a low-lying placenta, education of patients and careers enhances the chance of better maternal and fetal outcome but this is not always the case. Whether these patients should be admitted routinely at a later gestation is debatable. Most units do not routinely admit these patients, but repeat the scans at 32 to 34 weeks' gestation. Dasche and colleagues[24] observed that in 34% of cases, placenta previa that was diagnosed at 20 to 23 weeks was still present at delivery, whereas 73% of those present at 32 to 35 weeks persisted at delivery. A policy of routine scanning will reduce the false-positive rate, but at the expense of increasing workload and patient anxiety. Unfortunately, none of the studies reported the proportion of patients with low-lying placenta diagnosed at 32 to 34 weeks who had bleeding later in gestation. For units that do not routinely scan for placental site at 20 weeks, this 32 to 34 week scanning is indicated only in patients with an indication such as abnormal presentation, vaginal bleeding, or a chance finding when ultrasound was undertaken in late pregnancy for other reasons. In these cases, a transvaginal approach is recommended because it has better diagnostic accuracy, especially with posterior placenta previa.[25,26] This approach is safe and well tolerated. Placenta previa is diagnosed on transvaginal ultrasound scan when the placental edge is less than 3 cm from the internal os.

The findings on placenta previa can be summarized as follows:

- Routine location of the placental site at the 20-week transabdominal ultrasound has a low positive predictive value for placenta previa later in pregnancy.
- Transvaginal ultrasound is more accurate than transabdominal in diagnosing placenta previa.
- There is no evidence that either of these interventions or rescanning "at-risk" patients in the third trimester reduces adverse maternal or fetal outcomes from placenta previa, and randomized trials addressing these issues are needed.

Magnetic resonance imaging may be a diagnostic technique of the future, but its high cost limits its availability.[27,28]

Management Options (See Fig. 59–2)

General management options were discussed earlier (see Fig. 59–1). Specific measures include immediate delivery and expectant management.

Immediate Delivery

If bleeding continues, but is neither profuse nor life-threatening and the gestation is more than 34 weeks, delivery is preferred after resuscitation is initiated. The mode of delivery depends on the grade of placenta previa and the state of the cervix. Occasionally, placental localization leads to inaccurate grading of placenta previa. In addition, some units do not have facilities for emergency placental localization. Options include immediate cesarean section and examination in an operating room, with or without anesthesia ("double setup"). Cesarean section is the only option in patients with profuse, life-threatening bleeding.

PROCEDURE

EXAMINATION IN AN OPERATING ROOM (DOUBLE SETUP)

Indications

Examination in an operating room provides the most accurate assessment of the relationship between the lower edge of the placenta and the cervical os. It should be done only when delivery will be undertaken. This approach is contraindicated by active, profuse hemorrhage mandating immediate delivery; fetal malposition or malpresentation precluding vaginal delivery; fetal heart rate abnormality; and clear ultrasonographic evidence of major placenta previa. It may be considered when ultrasonographic evidence of placenta previa is inconclusive or when grade I or II anterior previa is suspected in patients with ongoing, but not life-threatening, uterine bleeding in active labor.

Preparation

Before this procedure is undertaken, crossmatched blood must be available. An anesthetist must be present, a midwife or operating room nurse must be scrubbed and gowned, and a cesarean section tray prepared. A second obstetrician should be scrubbed and ready to operate. The procedure must be performed by an experienced obstetrician, and a pediatrician must be present. Opinions vary as to whether the procedure should be carried out under general anesthesia. A survey of anesthetic management of cesarean section for placenta previa in the United Kingdom showed that 86% of anesthetists were willing to use regional anesthesia for a minor degree of placenta previa, but only 15% were prepared to offer these techniques for all degrees of placenta previa.[29] One advantage of general anesthesia is proper relaxation of the patient, which makes examination easier and allows rapid progression to cesarean section, if necessary. The main disadvantage is the need to wake the patient from anesthesia before inducing labor if vaginal delivery is possible. In addition, if cesarean section becomes necessary, a second anesthetic increases the risks. Performing the procedure under epidural anesthesia is an alternative, but this approach causes peripheral vasodilation and may worsen the effects of hypovolemia if hemorrhage is severe. A compromise appears to be drawing the drugs for induction of general anesthesia and preparing the anesthetic machine and instruments before the procedure. With such precautions, and in experienced hands, the interval between examination and delivery can be short.

Procedure

The patient is placed in the lithotomy position and draped with sterile towels after the vulva, but not the vagina, is cleaned. The bladder is catheterized, and two fingers are gently introduced into the vagina, with care taken to avoid the cervical os. Each vaginal fornix is palpated in turn to feel whether there is placenta between the presenting part and the finger. If placental tissue is present, a sensation of "bogginess" is felt. If the four fornices are empty, the index finger is gently introduced into the cervical os and the surroundings felt for the placental edge. If the cervix is closed, it should not be forced open and cesarean section should be performed. If the cervix admits a finger and no placental tissue is felt, the fetal membranes should be ruptured. An organized blood clot in the cervix may be mistaken for placental tissue. Persistent bright red bleeding after membrane rupture is an indication for cesarean delivery. If the placental edge is felt anteriorly but does not extend to the os and no bleeding is provoked, the decision may be made to rupture the membranes in preparation for vaginal delivery. If brisk vaginal bleeding occurs at any stage during the procedure, the procedure should be abandoned immediately and cesarean section performed.

Expectant Management

The perinatal mortality rate in placenta previa is directly related to gestational age at delivery.[13,30–32] Macafee and associates[30] and Johnson and colleagues[32] introduced expectant management of placenta previa to achieve the maximum fetal maturity possible while minimizing maternal and fetal risks. The overall objective is to reduce perinatal and maternal mortality. The basis of this approach is that most episodes of bleeding are small and self-limited and are not fatal to the fetus or mother in the absence of provoking trauma (e.g., intercourse, vaginal examination) or labor. A major advantage of expectant management is that in some patients, particularly those presenting early with lesser degrees of previa, the condition may resolve to permit vaginal delivery. More recently, several groups reported an improvement in perinatal mortality rates that was attributed mainly to prolongation of pregnancy.[33,34]

Macafee and associates[30] recommended treating the patient as an inpatient in a fully equipped, fully staffed maternity hospital from initial diagnosis to delivery. Permitting some women to return home is advocated[35] as part of expectant management. This practice is controversial because reports from some units have been conflicting. Cotton and colleagues[13] reported no difference in perinatal and maternal mortality rates in those sent home and those managed in hospitals, whereas D'Angelo and Irwin[36] suggested that keeping the mother in the hospital until delivery was justified because neonatal mortality and morbidity rates and treatment costs were reduced. Kaunitz and colleagues,[37] in a review of 355 patients who were managed at home, however, reported one intrapartum death as a result of placenta previa. This controversy is more evident when asymptomatic placenta previa is diagnosed on ultrasonography. It is becoming increasingly acceptable to manage these patients at home.[38,39] Love and Wallace,[40] in a review of 15,930 deliveries in Edinburgh, concluded that although clinical outcomes were variable and could not be predicted from antenatal events, most patients with or without bleeding, regardless of the degree of previa, could be managed on an outpatient basis. Randomized controlled trials are needed to justify the merits of this conservative approach.

Severe hemorrhage (heavy vaginal bleeding that causes maternal hypovolemia) was originally considered a contraindication to expectant management.[40] However, in one study in which approximately 20% of the women lost more than 500 mL blood, half were managed expectantly, with a mean gain in gestation of 16.8 days.[11] Crenshaw and colleagues[31] managed only 43% to 46% of patients successfully with an aggressive expectant approach, whereas Cotton and associates[13] successfully managed 66% of women expectantly with an aggressive approach.

During expectant management, preterm labor is a problem. Brenner and associates[41] found that 40% of women with placenta previa had rupture of the membranes, spontaneous labor, or other problems that resulted in delivery before 37 weeks' gestation. Inhibiting contractions in those with preterm labor seems logical, but some consider antepartum hemorrhage a contraindication to the use of tocolytics.[42] With vaginal bleeding and uterine contractions, placental abruption, which is widely considered a contraindication to tocolysis, cannot be excluded. In addition, placental abruption may coexist with placenta previa in 10% of cases. Further, tocolytics cause maternal tachycardia and palpitations, features that may be confused with hypovolemia. Sampson and associates[43] advocate the use of tocolytics in cases of placenta previa and uterine contractions after 21 weeks and reported a reduction in the perinatal mortality rate from 126 to 41 per 1000.

The perinatal mortality rate is also directly related to the total amount of blood lost antepartum. Liberal use of blood transfusions may nullify this effect.[13] There is no limit to the number of blood transfusions a patient can have. To optimize the oxygen supply to the fetus and protect the mother against anticipated blood loss, the aim of transfusion is to maintain hemoglobin of at least 10 g/dL or hematocrit of 30%.

Despite expectant management, 20% of women with placenta previa are delivered earlier than 32 weeks.

These cases account for 73% of perinatal deaths.[13] These premature deliveries are a major problem, and although cervical cerclage has been advocated, it is not normally used. Neonatal mortality and morbidity rates are reduced in this group by maternal corticosteroid administration. The use of thyroid-releasing hormones[44] should be limited to randomized controlled trials until more evidence is available.

The main disadvantages of continuous hospitalization are the cost and the psychological effect of separation on families. For many families, hospitalization means prolonged separation, and in some extreme cases, the breakup of marriages. Advantages include easy access to resuscitation and prompt delivery and ensuring bed rest (which may decrease the occurrence of hemorrhage) and limitation of activities. With improvement in transportation facilities and ambulance services, highly motivated women who clearly understand the need for restriction of activity and are within approximately 15 to 30 minutes of the hospital may be monitored at home. This approach applies only to women with grade I to III placenta previa or asymptomatic grade IV placenta previa. In all cases of expectant management, two units of crossmatched blood must be available at all times.

Method of Delivery

In general, the diagnosis of placenta previa means cesarean delivery. When the degree of placenta previa is minor (grade I or II anterior) and the fetal head is engaged, pregnancy may be allowed to continue beyond 37 to 38 weeks and vaginal delivery anticipated. In these patients, amniotomy followed by oxytocin (Syntocinon) administration can be considered. In those with more severe placenta previa, emergency or elective cesarean delivery is commonly used. Elective delivery is ideal because emergency delivery has a negative effect on perinatal mortality and morbidity rates, independent of gestational age. Cotton and associates[13] found that 27.7% of infants delivered emergently had anemia compared with 2.9% delivered electively. Cesarean section for placenta previa poses several problems. It should never be left to an inexperienced obstetrician. The Royal College of Obstetricians and Gynaecologists in the United Kingdom recommends that such cesarean sections be performed by senior obstetricians (consultants in the U.K). Although general anesthesia was preferred to regional anesthesia in the past, there is an increasing tendency to use the latter, and Frederiksen and colleagues[45] showed its safety and a reduction in intrapartum blood loss compared with general anesthesia.

PROCEDURE

Although epidural anesthetic is increasingly advocated for cesarean delivery, Moir[46] described placenta previa as an absolute contraindication to epidural anesthesia. Epidural anesthesia, by lowering blood pressure, may critically reduce uterine and placental perfusion. Crawford,[47] however, believes that in experienced hands, an epidural is safe. An increasing number of anesthetists offer regional anesthesia to these patients.[28] When the patient's condition is stable and there is no active bleeding, epidural or spinal anesthesia should not be regarded as contraindicated, provided an experienced anesthetist is available. Because patients and their partners may experience severe anxiety in the presence of profuse bleeding during cesarean delivery, careful consideration should be given to the decision to allow partners in the operating room.

A transverse incision of the lower segment of the uterus is commonly used, provided there is a lower segment. When the lower segment is nonexistent or is very vascular, some obstetricians advocate a classical or De Lee's incision. Scott,[48] however, believes that such incisions are rarely justified because of their consequences and long-term disadvantages. When difficulties occur with transverse incisions of the lower segment, the incision may be converted to an inverted T-, J-, or U-shaped incision.

If the incision in the uterus is transverse and the placenta is anterior, two approaches are available: going through the placenta or defining its edge and going through the membranes above or below the placenta. The former approach requires speed and may cause significant fetal blood loss.[49] The latter approach, however, may be associated with undue delay in the delivery of the fetus, more troublesome bleeding from a partially separated placenta, and resultant fetal blood loss and anoxia. Myerscough[49] advises against cutting or tearing through the placenta because of the inevitable fetal blood loss that occurs as fetal vessels are torn. Because the lower segment is less muscular, contraction and retraction cause inadequate occlusion of the sinuses of the placental bed, and intraoperative hemorrhage is not uncommon.[50] When hemostasis is difficult, bleeding sinuses can be oversewn with atraumatic sutures.[48] If this approach is unsuccessful, the uterus can be packed, but if the pack is left in situ during closure of the uterus, bleeding may continue but remain concealed for some time. Intramyometrial injection of prostaglandin $F_{2\alpha}$ is useful in these cases.[49] When bleeding is uncontrollable, ligation of the internal iliac artery or even hysterectomy may be necessary as a last resort.

PLACENTAL ABRUPTION

Placental abruption is bleeding after premature separation of a normally situated placenta. The reported incidence varies from 0.49% to 1.8%.[51] The wide variation in reported incidence is believed to be caused by variations in diagnosis. Fox[52] found evidence of abruption in 4.5% of placentas examined routinely, suggesting that small episodes of placental abruption are more common than those diagnosed clinically. Placental abruption is concealed in 20% to 35% of cases and revealed in 65%

to 80% of cases.[26,28] The concealed type is more dangerous, with more severe complications. Four grades of placental abruption have been described (Table 59–3). The most severe type (grade 3) occurs in approximately 0.2% of pregnancies.[26]

The etiology of placental abruption is unknown in most cases. In a few, however, the cause is obvious, such as in direct trauma to the uterus. Various risk factors are associated with placental abruption. The risk of recurrence in subsequent pregnancies is significant, varying from 6%[51] to 16.7%[53–55] It is more common in older women, but this increase has been attributed to parity and is independent of age.[54] Cigarette smoking increases the incidence of placental abruption.[56] Naeye[4] reported an incidence of 1.69% in nonsmokers, 2.46% in smokers, and 1.87% in smokers who had quit. In the smokers, evidence of decidual necrosis at the edge of the placenta was found. This finding may represent the effect of smoking on uteroplacental blood flow[57,58] and decidual integrity.

Other etiologic factors include sudden decompression of the uterus after membrane rupture in patients with polyhydramnios and multiple pregnancy, external cephalic version,[59] placental abnormalities (especially circumvallate placenta),[60,61] abdominal trauma,[62] and increased levels of α-fetoprotein.[63,64] Although maternal hypertension is considered a risk factor, there is no consensus on whether hypertension precedes abruption or vice versa. Naeye and colleagues[65] found no evidence of placental abruption in patients with hypertension, but Abdella and associates[66] observed that the incidence of placental abruption in patients with preeclampsia was twice that in those without preeclampsia. In a meta-analysis, Ananth and associates[67] concluded that chronic hypertension was associated with a threefold increased risk of abruption compared with normotensive patients, whereas the odds ratio for patients with preeclampsia was 1.73. The suggestion that folic acid deficiency may have an etiologic role in placental abruption has not been confirmed. Large prospective studies[68,69] have not shown an association between placental abruption and folate supplementation. More recently, hyperhomocysteinemia and protein C deficiency[70] and other thrombophilias were reported to be more common in women with placental abruption.[71] Although inferior vena caval compression and the use of lupus anticoagulant have been suggested as possible etiologic factors, there is no convincing evidence.

TABLE 59–3

Grading of Placental Abruption

GRADE	DESCRIPTION
0	Asymptomatic patient with a small retroplacental clot
1	Vaginal bleeding; uterine tetany and tenderness may be present; no signs of maternal shock or fetal distress
2	External vaginal bleeding possible; no signs of maternal shock; signs of fetal distress
3	External bleeding possible; marked uterine tetany, yielding a boardlike consistency on palpation; persistent abdominal pain, with maternal shock and fetal demise; coagulopathy may be evident in 30% of cases

Maternal Risks

- The maternal mortality rate is approximately 1%. In the last confidential enquiry into maternal deaths in the United Kingdom (2000–2002),[12] four maternal deaths were caused by placental abruption. The maternal mortality rate decreased from 8% in 1919 to less than 1% in 1995.[72] Although severe hemorrhage is usually the major cause of other complications that lead to mortality, disseminated intravascular coagulation may cause severe hemorrhage, renal failure, and death.
- The recurrence rate is generally reported as 6% to 17% after one episode and increases to 25% after two episodes. Approximately 7% of women with abruption severe enough to kill the fetus have the same outcome in subsequent pregnancies, and 30% of all future pregnancies of women who have a placental abruption do not produce a living child.[1]
- Hypovolemic shock. Blood loss may be underestimated in placental abruption because concealed bleeding into the myometrium may be difficult to quantify.
- Acute renal failure can result from hypovolemia or disseminated intravascular coagulation.
- Disseminated intravascular coagulation
- Postpartum hemorrhage can result from coagulation failure or from a Couvelaire uterus, in which severe bleeding occurs into the myometrium and impairs the ability to contract.
- Fetomaternal hemorrhage can lead to severe Rhesus sensitization in Rhesus-negative patients. All Rhesus-negative patients must undergo a Kleihauer-Betke test and have anti-D immunoglobulin administered to prevent immunization.

Fetal Risks

Fetal risks include the following:

- The perinatal mortality rate varies from 4.4% to 67.3%, depending on neonatal facilities.[73] More than 50% of the perinatal deaths are stillbirths.[9] Of the infants delivered alive, Abdella and associates[66] reported a 16% mortality rate within 4 weeks, with most infants weighing less than 2500 g. The perinatal mortality rate is closely related to gestational age. Paterson[54] reported survival rates varying from 23% at 28 to 32 weeks to 87.6% at 37 to 40 weeks. However, survival rates today are probably higher than these figures suggest because they were reported before the advances that have occurred in modern neonatal care. For example, in Norway, the rate decreased from 2.5 per 1000 to 0.9 per 1000 between 1967 and 1991.[51] The higher incidence of fetal malformations[72] and intrauterine growth restriction[1] contributes to the high perinatal mortality rate. For babies weighing more than 2500 g, the reported survival rate is 98%.[74] In the presence of associated complications, such as hypertension, the fetal mortality rate increases threefold.[66]

- Fetal growth restriction is reported in up to 80% of infants born before 36 weeks' gestation.
- The rate of congenital malformations may be as high as 4.4% (twice that in the general population[75]). The rate of major malformations is increased threefold. Most involve the central nervous system, and these can occur at five times the normal incidence.[72]
- The neonatal hematologic findings may be abnormal. Anemia results from significant fetal bleeding.[68]

Diagnosis

The diagnosis is usually made on clinical grounds, but ultrasonography is helpful in some cases (e.g., when there is a large retroplacental hematoma, although this is uncommon, even in severe cases). The symptoms and signs are diagnostic in moderate to severe cases. In mild forms, the diagnosis may not be obvious until after delivery, when a retroplacental clot is identified.

Placental abruption causes vaginal bleeding, abdominal pain, uterine contractions, and tenderness. Vaginal bleeding occurs in no more than 70% to 80% of cases.[26] This bleeding is characteristically dark and nonclotting. It occurs after 36 weeks' gestation in approximately 50% of cases.[26] In a study of 193 cases, Paterson[54] found that 18% occurred before 32 weeks, 40% occurred between 34 and 37 weeks, and 42% occurred after 37 weeks. Because labor is the most common factor precipitating placental separation,[9] nearly 50% of patients with placental abruption are in established labor. Uterine contractions may be difficult to distinguish from the abdominal pain of abruption. When this distinction is possible, the contractions are characteristically very frequent, often with more than five occurring in 10 minutes.[76]

Although abdominal pain is common, it is not invariable and is less common in posteriorly sited placentas. This is evidenced by unsuspected, or silent, abruption described by Notelovitz and colleagues[77] and the higher pathologic incidence of placental abruption reported by Fox.[52] Pain probably indicates extravasation of blood into the myometrium. In severe cases (grade 3), the pain is sharp, severe, and sudden in onset. In addition, some patients may have nausea, anxiety, thirst, restlessness, and a feeling of faintness, whereas others report absent or reduced fetal movements.

If blood loss is significant, the patient may have signs of shock (tachycardia predominates; blood pressure is poorly correlated with blood volume in this condition). Hypertension may mask true hypovolemia, but increasing abdominal girth or fundal height suggests significant concealed hemorrhage. The uterus is typically described as "woody hard" in severe placental abruption. In such cases, the fetus is difficult to palpate, and a continuous fetal heart rate monitor or real-time ultrasonography must be used to identify the fetal heartbeat. The fetus may be "distressed," with fetal heart rate abnormalities, or may be dead. Fetal distress occurs in grade 1 to 2 abruption, but in grade 3 abruption, fetal death is inevitable, by definition.[78] In severe cases complicated by disseminated intravascular coagulation, there may be no clotting in the vaginal blood, which is dark. The incidence of coagulopathy is 35% to 38%,[53,79] and it occurs mainly in the severe forms.

Typically, blood clots are found in the vagina, except if the blood is nonclotting. Serous fluid from a retroplacental clot may be confused with liquor. The cervix may be dilating because 50% of patients are in labor. If the membranes are ruptured, blood-stained liquor is seen.

Ultrasonography is not a sensitive method of diagnosing placental abruption, but it is useful in excluding coincident placenta previa, which is present in 10% of cases. When the retroplacental clot is large, ultrasonography identifies it as hyperechogenic or isoechogenic compared with the placenta. This echogenicity may be misinterpreted as a thick placenta.[80] Resolving retroplacental clots appear hyperechogenic within 1 week and sonolucent within 2 weeks. Although ultrasonography is not an accurate diagnostic tool, it is useful in monitoring cases managed expectantly, and Rivera-Alxima and colleagues[81] used it to determine the time of delivery. The size of the hematoma, its location and change in size over time, and fetal growth are monitored by ultrasound scan. The Kleihauer-Betke test may be useful in making the diagnosis when a patient has abdominal pain without vaginal bleeding and in cases of unsuspected (silent) abruption.

The differential diagnosis of placental abruption includes conditions that can be broadly classified into two groups. These are other causes of vaginal bleeding and causes of abdominal pain. The former groups are discussed elsewhere in this chapter. The latter groups are discussed in Chapter 57.

Management Options (See Fig. 59–2)

Once the diagnosis of placental abruption has been made, management depends on its severity, associated complications, the condition of the mother and the fetus, and gestational age. Management is divided into general and specific measures. For management, Sher and Statland[82] divided placental abruption into three degrees of severity. These are summarized in Table 59–3.

The general management options were discussed earlier (see Fig. 59–1). Specific measures to be considered are the following:

- Immediate delivery
- Expectant management
- Management of complications

Immediate Delivery

The need for immediate delivery depends on the severity of abruption and whether the fetus is alive or dead. If the fetus is dead, vaginal delivery is the goal. Maternal resuscitation is emphasized because fetal death is common in severe placental abruption, often with coagulopathy. Once resuscitation has been initiated, the fetal membranes should be ruptured to hasten the onset of labor. This approach is effective in most cases, but in a few, augmentation with oxytocin is needed. This drug must be administered cautiously because uterine rupture may be caused by an overstimulated uterus. Barron[83] reported that membrane rupture should be reserved for dead fetuses and patients who are in advanced labor.

If the fetus is alive, the decision as to how best to achieve delivery is not always easy. In addition, the outlook for the fetus is poor not only in terms of immediate survival but also because studies show that as many as 15.4% of liveborn infants do not survive.[66] However, when the mortality rate associated with vaginal delivery is compared with that of cesarean section in nonrandomized controlled trials (52% vs. 16%, Okonofua and Olatubosun[73]; 20% vs. 15%, Hurd and associates[76]), cesarean delivery has advantages. Hibbard[9] stated that many of the poor results associated with cesarean section are largely the result of indecision and delay in the last quarter of pregnancy. He stated that cesarean delivery must be considered when the fetus is alive, particularly if there is evidence of fetal distress. However, coagulopathy adds considerable maternal risk, and the likelihood of injury or death may be increased by surgery.

If the decision is made to deliver and the fetus is alive, the degree of abruption and the state of the fetus are important determining factors. When abruption is severe, cesarean section must be performed once resuscitation has started. Delivery should be performed promptly, especially because most postadmission fetal deaths occur in fetuses delivered more than 2 hours after admission.

In mild to moderate cases of abruption, the mode of delivery is determined by the condition of the fetus, its presentation, and the state of the cervix. Abnormal fetal heart rate patterns are an indication for immediate cesarean delivery. However, if the decision is made to deliver vaginally, continuous fetal monitoring must be available to identify early abnormal fetal heart rate patterns. Golditch and Boyce,[68] Lunan,[74] and Okonofua and Olatubosun[73] showed that the perinatal mortality rate is higher with vaginal delivery in the absence of electronic fetal monitoring. Prostaglandins are used to ripen the cervix in women with mild abruption, but the danger of inducing tetanic contractions must be remembered. When feasible, amniotomy often hastens delivery, but when it is not possible, oxytocin can be used. However, vigilance must be maintained for the development of hyperstimulation.

Expectant Management

The goal of expectant management is to prolong pregnancy, with the hope of improving fetal maturity and survival. Expectant management is usually considered in cases of mild placental abruption occurring before 37 weeks' gestation. Vaginal bleeding is slight, abdominal pain is mild and usually localized, and the patient is cardiovascularly stable. Once conservative management has been chosen, the fetal condition must be monitored closely. No evidence supports the routine admission of patients who are being managed expectantly, especially when there is no evidence of maternal or fetal compromise or uterine contractions. Fetal growth restriction is a common finding in association with placental abruption. The timing of delivery depends on the finding of further vaginal bleeding, the fetal condition, gestational age, and the availability of neonatal care facilities. If bleeding episodes are recurrent, induction at 37 to 38 weeks is usually undertaken if fetal indices of health (e.g., biophysical parameters and growth; see Chapters 11 and 12) are satisfactory. When the initial episode is small and self-limiting and there is no acute (abnormal cardiotocographic findings or biophysical profile score) or chronic (growth restriction, oligohydramnios, or abnormal umbilical artery Doppler recording) fetal compromise, no evidence supports the induction of labor. Despite this lack of evidence, induction of labor at term is often advocated in such patients using the speculative argument that undetected damage might have occurred to the integrity and function of the placenta, and in the face of uncertainty, delivery at term confers more advantages.

If the initial ultrasound scan showed a retroplacental clot, the clot may be monitored by serial ultrasound scans. If the fetal condition deteriorates, delivery is expedited, with the speed and urgency determined by whether fetal compromise is acute or chronic.

Some cases of mild abruption may be complicated by labor. In such cases, it is difficult to establish which came first. Many consider tocolytics contraindicated in the presence of placental abruption because they may worsen abruption.[42] Sholl[84] stated that a trial of tocolytics in mild abruptio placentae and labor may successfully prolong pregnancy without jeopardizing the mother and fetus. There have been no large trials to confirm this statement.

Management of Complications

The major complications of placental abruption are hemorrhagic shock, disseminated intravascular coagulation, ischemic necrosis of the distal organs (especially the kidneys and brain), and postpartum hemorrhage. These are discussed in Chapters 50, 77, 79, and 80.

Rhesus Isoimmunization

Fetomaternal hemorrhage during abruption can be significant.[85] All Rhesus-negative women with abruption must undergo a Kleihauer-Betke test and receive an appropriate dose of anti-D immunoglobulin to prevent immunization. Repeated doses depend on the amount of fetomaternal hemorrhage, as determined by the Kleihauer-Betke test. This treatment must be given within 72 hours of the onset of abruption. When management is expectant in a patient with intermittent recurrent bleeding, regular Kleihauer-Betke testing and assays of therapeutic anti-D immunoglobulin levels can be performed to guide further anti-D administration. Collaboration with the hematologist and blood bank is advisable to determine the correct dose when the Kleihauer-Betke test result is positive.

UNCLASSIFIED BLEEDING

The exact cause of bleeding in late pregnancy is unknown in 47% of patients. The reported incidence varies from 38% to 74%.[86–90] The cause of bleeding may become apparent later, but in most cases, no cause is seen.[28] When causes are identified, they include marginal sinus rupture (60%), "show" (20%), cervicitis (18%), trauma (5%), vulvovaricosities (2%), genital tumors, hematuria, genital infections, and vasa previa (0.5% each). Although this group of causes is referred to as unclassified bleeding, it invariably includes unrecognized cases of minor abruption or placenta previa. Marginal sinus rupture is the most common source of bleeding in antepartum hemorrhage of unknown cause.[60]

Risks

The risks of unclassified bleeding depend on the cause. More serious causes are discussed in the relevant chapters. This type of bleeding is associated with a higher perinatal mortality rate, which varies from 3.5% to 15.7%.[86–88] This rate is higher than that associated with placenta previa (4.2%–8.1%), suggesting some degree of placental dysfunction. Preterm labor is more common in these patients and is a contributor to the higher perinatal mortality rate.

In vasa previa, fetal exsanguination after rupture or compromise of placental circulation as a result of compression of the abnormal vessels may cause fetal death. Seventy-five percent of deaths in vasa previa are caused by exsanguination. Other fetal risks include increased incidence of intrauterine growth restriction and congenital malformations. The main risk to the mother is bleeding, but often, maternal blood loss is mild and therefore not life-threatening.

Diagnosis

There are usually no signs and symptoms diagnostic of either placenta previa or placental abruption. In most cases, bleeding is mild and resolves spontaneously. Approximately 60% of cases occur after 37 weeks, and of these, 15% of patients are delivered within 10 days of the initial hemorrhage.[88] When marginal bleeding occurs with clot formation, serum separated from the clot may be confused with liquor after spontaneous rupture of fetal membranes.[91]

The diagnosis of unclassified bleeding is often made after placental abruption and placenta previa are excluded. An ultrasound scan is necessary to exclude placenta previa because minor grades may present in a similar manner.

Speculum examination should be performed in patients with unclassified bleeding. Opinions differ about the timing of this examination. Some believe that it should be delayed until bleeding has stopped, whereas others advocate immediate examination once placenta previa has been excluded. Some advocate immediate examination because they want to exclude advanced labor and local causes of bleeding. Others advocate delayed examination because they believe that a delay does not affect management and that other local causes of bleeding are usually benign and need no immediate action. No controlled trials have compared these different types of management.

Management Options

If placenta previa and abruption have been excluded, further management depends on gestational age, the nature of the bleeding (severity and persistence or recurrence), the state of the fetus (abnormal fetal heart rate patterns), and the presumed cause of bleeding.

Options for further management include delivery and an expectant approach. At or beyond 37 weeks' gestation, when bleeding is recurrent or significant or associated fetal factors (e.g., growth restriction, abnormal heart rate patterns) are present, delivery is the management option of choice. Vaginal delivery is not contraindicated if there is no fetal compromise. Before 37 weeks' gestation, if bleeding is recurrent and significant, immediate delivery may be needed. The mode of delivery is determined by the state of the fetus, its lie, and other associated factors, such as the state of the cervix.

If expectant management is chosen, the patient may be monitored at home or in the hospital. Most units monitor patients in the hospital until bleeding has stopped for at least 24 hours. Watson,[88] in a retrospective review, showed no significant advantage in admitting patients to the hospital. A randomized controlled trial comparing inpatient versus outpatient care in these cases is needed, especially with the current emphasis on community-based care for pregnancy. Regardless of where the patient is managed, fetal surveillance should be implemented because of the increased risk of perinatal death (discussed earlier). Where awaiting the spontaneous onset of labor is the practice,[87] the perinatal mortality rate is not increased. Some advocate induction at 38 weeks[87,90] because any bleeding carries a theoretical risk of disrupting placental function and should be considered an indication for delivery at 38 weeks' gestation.[92] We recommend awaiting the spontaneous onset of labor if fetal growth and welfare are satisfactory (because no evidence supports the proposition of placental disruption) and use induction only when there is evidence of fetal compromise.

One potential hazard of vaginal bleeding in late pregnancy is fetal exsanguination as a result of vasa previa. This complication usually occurs at amniotomy or when fetal membranes rupture spontaneously. Classically, profuse vaginal bleeding follows amniotomy, with subsequent fetal bradycardia. The diagnosis of this condition before these events occur is difficult, but an experienced observer may be able to feel vessels coursing over the membranes. Speculum examination may also show the vessels. In some cases, when mild bleeding occurs after amniotomy but the fetal heart rate is normal, this diagnosis cannot be excluded. An Apt[93] test (discussed earlier) must be performed. If fetal blood is found, the infant should be delivered immediately by cesarean section.

CONCLUSIONS

GENERAL

- Bleeding in late pregnancy is an important cause of fetal and maternal morbidity and mortality.
- The etiology of the various types of bleeding is poorly understood.
- The principles are initial assessment of the patient's condition and subsequent planned management aimed at resuscitation and prolongation of pregnancy, if possible, or immediate delivery for either fetal or maternal indications.

PLACENTA PREVIA

- Previous cesarean delivery increases the risk of occurrence from 0.65% after one cesarean delivery to 10% after four or more.
- Transvaginal ultrasound provides the most reliable diagnosis and poses no maternal risk.
- Routine anomaly scans at 20 to 22 weeks' gestation have a high false-positive rate of 40% to 70% and a 7% false-negative rate for diagnosis, depending on whether transabdominal or transvaginal scanning is performed.
- Management depends on presentation, gestational age, and the degree of previa. When the mother's life is not at risk, expectant management (with or without blood transfusion) will improve neonatal outcome.
- When major placenta previa is present, delivery is by cesarean section, preferably under regional anesthesia (provided by an experienced anesthetist) and performed by an experienced obstetrician.

PLACENTAL ABRUPTION

- Risk factors include age, parity, smoking, thrombophilia, hyperhomocysteinemia, and increased maternal serum levels of α-fetoprotein.
- The diagnosis is made clinically rather than radiologically.
- Major risks include intrauterine fetal death, maternal disseminated intravascular coagulation, and renal failure.
- Management depends on the grade. If the fetus is alive and is not distressed or is dead, vaginal delivery should be offered; otherwise, cesarean delivery should be performed. Correction of a coagulopathy is essential before embarking on delivery; however, when correction is not possible, adequate blood products must be available.
- The recurrence risk is 6% to 17% after one episode and 25% after two episodes.

UNCLASSIFIED BLEEDING

- The diagnosis is one of exclusion.
- Vasa previa must be considered as part of the differential diagnosis.
- Unclassified bleeding increases the risk of an adverse perinatal outcome and is an indication for ongoing fetal monitoring.

SUMMARY OF MANAGEMENT OPTIONS

Bleeding in Late Pregnancy

Management Options	Quality of Evidence	Strength of Recommendation	References
Prenatal			
Identification of at-risk women, with delivery in units with facilities for blood transfusion and cesarean delivery:	III	B	94,95
• Previous cesarean delivery (risk of placenta previa)	IIb	B	96
• Proven placenta previa (on ultrasound)	III	B	17,18
• Clinical diagnosis of abruption	IV	C	53
• Clinical diagnosis of unclassified bleeding	IV	C	88
Initial assessment of severity of bleeding	III	B	97,98
Severe and continuing bleeding:			
• Resuscitate (IV access, blood and clotting factors) and correct coagulopathy (if possible).	III	B	97,99
• A major obstetric hemorrhage protocol should be available.	IV	C	12
• Deliver the infant or empty the uterus (the route depends on gestation, fetal condition, maternal condition, amount of blood loss, fetal presentation, and whether the patient is in labor)	–	GPP	–
• In most cases of placenta previa, cesarean delivery is used.	IV	C	47
Mild to moderate bleeding or bleeding that is resolving:			
Establish the cause and manage bleeding appropriately:			
Placenta previa			
• Expectant management	III	B	37,40
Controversy about whether to admit an asymptomatic patient to the hospital			
Hospital admission (and readiness for blood transfusion and cesarean delivery) if the patient is symptomatic (considerable variation in practice)			
• Elective or planned delivery	IV	C	13
Anesthesia for cesarean delivery in patients with placenta previa cesarean			
Emergency delivery: Regional or general anesthesia	III	B	82
Elective delivery: Regional anesthesia	III	B	43,82
Placental abruption or unclassified bleeding:	III	B	100–103
• Serial fetal assessment			
• Elective delivery at term			
Anti-D for Rhesus-negative women	IV	C	104
Labor and Delivery			
Crossmatch in patients with severe or active bleeding or placenta previa	III	B	97,99
Postnatal			
Vigilance for postpartum hemorrhage	IV	C	105
Anti-D for Rhesus-negative women (if not already given)	IV	C	104
Treatment of anemia	–	GPP	–

REFERENCES

1. McShane PM, Heye PS, Epstein MF: Maternal and perinatal mortality resulting from placenta praevia. Obstet Gynecol 1985;65:176–182.
2. MacGillivray I, Campbell DM: Management of twin pregnancies. In MacGillivray I, Campbell DM, Thompson B (eds): Twinning and Twins. Chichester, John Wiley, 1988, p 324.
3. Taipale P, Hiilesmaa V, Ylostalo P: Diagnosis of placenta previa by transvaginal sonographic screening at 12–16 weeks in a non-selected population. Obstet Gynecol 1997;89:364–367.
4. Naeye ER: Placenta praevia: Predisposing factors and effects on the fetus and the surviving infants. Obstet Gynecol 1978;52:521–525.
5. Newton ER, Barss V, Cetrulo CL: The epidemiology and clinical history of asymptomatic mid-trimester placenta praevia. Am J Obstet Gynecol 1984;148:743–748.
6. Clark SL, Koonings PP, Phelan JP: Placenta praevia, accrete and prior caesarean section. Obstet Gynecol 1985;66:89–92.
7. Naeye RL: Abruptio placenta and placenta praevia: Frequent, perinatal mortality and cigarette smoking. Obstet Gynecol 1980;55:701–704.
8. Kelly JV, Iffy L: Placenta praevia. In Iffy L, Kaminetzky HA (eds): Principles and Practice of Obstetrics and Perinatology, Vol. 2. New York, John Wiley, 1981.
9. Hibbard BM: Bleeding in late pregnancy. In Hibbard BM (ed): Principles of Obstetrics. London, Butterworths, 1988.
10. Hershkowitz R, Fraser D, Mazor M, Leiberman JR: One or more multiple previous caesarean sections are associated with similar increased frequency of placenta previa. Eur J Obstet Gynecol Reprod Biol 1995;62:185–188.
11. Ananth CV, Smulian JC, Vinsileos AM: The association of placenta previa with history of cesarean section and abortion: A metaanalysis. Am J Obstet Gynecol 1997;177:1071–1078.
12. Department of Health: Why Mothers Die: A report on confidential enquiries into maternal deaths in the United Kingdom 2000–2002. London, The Stationary Office, 2004.
13. Cotton DB, Read JA, Paul RH, Quilligan EJ: The conservative aggressive management of placenta praevia. Am J Obstet Gynecol 1980;137:687–695.
14. Varma TR: Fetal growth and placental function in patients with placenta praevia. J Obstet Gynaecol Br Commonw 1971;80:311–315.
15. Konje JC, Ewings PD, Adewunmi OA, et al: The effect of threatened abortion on pregnancy outcome. J Obstet Gynecol 1992;12:150–155.
16. Hibbard LT: Placenta praevia. In Sciarra JJ (ed): Gynecology and Obstetrics, Vol. 2. New York, Harper & Row, 1981.
17. Chapman MG, Furness ET, Jones WR, Sheat JH: Significance of the location of placenta site in early pregnancy. BJOG 1989;86:846–848.
18. McClure N, Dornan JC: Early identification of placenta praevia. BJOG 1990;97:959–961.
19. Laing FC: Placenta praevia: Avoiding false-negative diagnosis. J Clin Ultrasound 1981;9:109–113.
20. Comeau J, Shaw L, Marcell CC, Lavery JP: Early placenta praevia and delivery outcome. Obstet Gynecol 1983;61:577–580.
21. Ruparelia BA, Chapman MG: Early low-lying placenta ultrasonic assessment, progress and outcome. Eur J Obstet Gynecol Reprod Biol 1985;20:209–213.
22. Taipale P, Hiiesmaa V, Ylostalo P: Transvaginal ultrasonography at 18–23 weeks in predicting placenta previa at delivery. Ultrasound Obstet Gynecol 1998;12:422–425.
23. Becker RH, Vonk R, Mende BC, et al: The prevalence of placental localisation at 20–23 gestational weeks for prediction of placenta previa at delivery: Evaluation of 8650 cases. Ultrasound Obstet Gynecol 2001;17:496–501.
24. Dasche JS, McIntire DD, Ramus RM, et al: Persistence of placenta previa according to gestational age at ultrasound detection. Obstet Gynecol 2002;99:692–697.
25. Tan NH, Abu M, Woo JLS, Tahir HM: The role of transvaginal sonography in the diagnosis of placental praevia. Aust N Z J Obstet Gynaecol 1995;35:42–45.
26. Knuppel AR, Drukker JE: Bleeding in late pregnancy: Antepartum bleeding. In Hayashi RH, Castillo MS (eds): High Risk Pregnancy: A Team Approach. Philadelphia, Saunders, 1986.
27. Powell MC, Buckley J, Price H, et al: Magnetic resonance imaging and placenta praevia. Am J Obstet Gynecol 1986;154:565–569.
28. Fraser R, Watson R: Bleeding during the latter half of pregnancy. In Chalmers I (ed): Effective Care in Pregnancy and Childbirth. London, Oxford University Press, 1989.
29. Bonner SM, Haynes SR, Ryall D: The anaesthetic management of caesarean section for placenta praevia: A questionnaire survey. Anaethesia 1995;50:992–994.
30. Macafee CHG, Millar WG, Harley G: Maternal and fetal mortality in placenta praevia. J Obstet Gynaecol Br Emp 1962;52: 313–324.
31. Crenshaw C, Jones DED, Parker RT: Placenta praevia: A survey of 20 years experience with improved perinatal survival by expectant therapy and caesarean delivery. Obstet Gynecol Surv 1973;28:461–470.
32. Johnson HW, Williamson JC, Greeley AV: The conservative management of some varieties of placenta praevia. Am J Obstet Gynecol 1945;49:398–406.
33. Besinger RE, Moniak CW, Paskiewicz LS, et al: The effect of tocolytic use in the management of placenta previa. Am J Obstet Gynecol 1995;172:1770–1778.
34. Towers CV, Pircon RA, Heppard M: Is tocolysis safe in the management of third trimester bleeding? Am J Obstet Gynecol 1999;180:1572–1578.
35. Silver R, Depp R, Sabbagha RE, et al: Placenta praevia: Aggressive expectant management. Am J Obstet Gynecol 1984; 150:15–22.
36. D'Angelo LJ, Irwin LF: Conservative management of placenta praevia: A cost benefit analysis. Am J Obstet Gynecol 1984;149: 320–323.
37. Kaunitz AM, Spence C, Danielson TS, et al: Perinatal and maternal mortality in a religious group avoiding obstetric care. Am J Obstet Gynecol 1984;150:826–831.
38. Rosen DMB, Peek MJ: Do women with placental praevia without antepartum haemorrhage require hospitalisation? Aust N Z J Obstet Gynaecol 1994;34:130–134.
39. Anon: Editorial comment. Aust NZ J Obstet Gynaecol 1994; 34:130–131.
40. Love CDB, Wallace EM: Pregnancies complicated by placenta previa: What is appropriate management? BJOG 1996; 103:864–867.
41. Brenner WE, Edelman DA, Hendricks CH: Characteristics of patients with placenta praevia and results of 'expectant management.' Am J Obstet Gynecol 1978;132:180–189.
42. Besinger RE, Niebyl JR: The safety and efficacy of tocolytics agents for the treatment of preterm labour. Obstet Gynecol Surv 1990;45:415–440.
43. Sampson MB, Lastres O, Thomasi AM, et al: Tocolysis with terbutaline sulphate in patients with placenta praevia complicated by premature labour. J Reprod Med 1984;29:248–250.
44. Ballard BR, Ballard PL, Creasy RK, et al: Respiratory disease in very-low-birthweight infants after prenatal thyrotropin releasing hormone and glucocorticoid. Lancet 1992;339:510–515.
45. Frederiksen MC, Glassenberg R, Stika CS: Placenta previa: A 22-year analysis. Am J Obstet Gynecol 1999;180:1432–1437.
46. Moir DD: Obstetric and Anaethesia and Analgesia, 2nd ed. London, Bailliere Tindall, 1980.

47. Crawford JS: Principles and Practice of Obstetrics Anaesthesia, 15th ed. Oxford, Blackwell, 1985.
48. Scott JS: Antepartum haemorrhage. In Whitefield CR (ed): Dewhurst's Textbook of Obstetrics and Gynaecology for Postgraduates, 4th ed. Oxford, Blackwell, 1986.
49. Myerscough PR: Munro Kerr's Operative Obstetrics, 10th ed. London, Bailliere Tindall, 1982.
50. Williamson HC, Greeley AV: Management of placenta praevia: 12 year study. Am J Obstet Gynecol 1945;50:987–991.
51. Rasmussen S, Irgrens KM, Dalaker K: The occurrence of placental abruption in Norway 1967–1991. Acta Obstet Gynecol Scand 1996;75:222–228.
52. Fox H: Pathology of the Placenta. London, Saunders, 1978.
53. Pritchard JA, Brekken AL: Clinical and laboratory studies on severe abruption placentae. Am J Obstet Gynecol 1967;97: 681–700.
54. Paterson MEL: The aetiology and outcome of abruption placentae. Acta Obstet Gynecol Scand 1979;58:31–35.
55. Rasmussen S, Irgrens KM, Dalaker K: The effect on the likelihood of further pregnancy of placental abruption and the rate of its recurrence. BJOG 1997;104:1292–1295.
56. Kramer MS, Usher RH, Pollack R, et al: Etiologic determinants of abruptio placentae. Obstet Gynecol 1997;89:221–226.
57. Ananth CV, Smulian JC, Vintzileos AM: Incidence of placental abruption in relation to cigarette smoking and hypertensive disorders during pregnancy: A meta-analysis of observational studies. Obstet Gynecol 1999;93:622–628.
58. Lehtovirta P, Forss M: The acute effect of smoking on intervillous blood flow of the placenta. BJOG 1978;85: 729–737.
59. Savona-Ventura C: The role of external cephalic version in modern obstetrics. Obstet Gynecol Surv 1986;41:393–400.
60. Scott JS: Placenta extrachoralis (placenta marginata and placenta circumvallata). J Obstet Gynaecol Br Emp 1960;67:904–918.
61. Wilson D, Paalman RJ: Clinical significance of circumvallate placenta. Obstet Gynecol 1967;29:774–778.
62. Crosby WM, Costila JP: Safety of lap-belt restraint for pregnant victims of automobile collisions. N Engl J Med 1971;284: 632–635.
63. Egley C, Cefalo R: Abruptio placenta. In Studd J (ed): Progress in Obstetrics and Gynaecology, Vol. 5. London, Churchill Livingstone, 1985, pp 108–120.
64. Yaron Y, Cherry M, Kramer RL, et al: Second trimester maternal serum marker screening: Maternal serum alpha-fetoprotein, beta-human chorionic gonadotrophin, estriol, and their various combinations as predictors of pregnancy outcome. Am J Obstet Gynecol 1999;181:968–974.
65. Naeye RL, Harknes WL, Utts J: Abruptio placenta and perinatal death: A prospective study. Am J Obstet Gynecol 1977;128: 710–714.
66. Abdella TN, Sibai BM, Hays JM, Anderson GD: Relationship of hypertensive diseases to abruption placentae. Obstet Gynecol 1984;63:365–370.
67. Ananth CV, Savitz DA, Williams MA: Placental abruption and its association with hypertension and prolonged rupture of membranes: A methodologic review and meta-analysis. Obstet Gynecol 1996;88:309–318.
68. Golditch IA, Boyce NE: Management of abruptio placenta. JAMA 1970;212:288–293.
69. de Valera E: Abruptio placentae. Am J Obstet Gynecol 1968;100: 599–606.
70. De Vries JIP, Dekker GA, Huijgens PC, et al: Hyperhomocysteinemia and protein S deficiency in complicated pregnancies. BJOG 1997;104:1248–1254.
71. Kupferminc MJ, Eldor A, Steinman N, et al: Increased frequency of genetic thrombophilia in women with complications of pregnancy. N Engl J Med 1999;340:9–13.
72. Egley C, Cefalo RC: Abruptio placenta. In Studd J (ed): Progress in Obstetrics and Gynaecology, Vol. 5. Edinburgh, Churchill Livingstone, 1985.
73. Okonofua FE, Olatubosun OA: Caesarean versus vaginal delivery in abruptio placentae associated with live fetuses. Int J Gynecol Obstet 1985;23:471–474.
74. Lunan CB: The management of abruptio placentae. J Obstet Gynecol Br Commonw 1973;80:120–124.
75. Niswander KR, Friedman EA, Hoover DB, et al: Fetal morbidity following potentially atoxigenic obstetric conditions: I. Abruptio placentae. Am J Obstet Gynecol 1996;95:838–845.
76. Hurd WW, Miodovnik M, Lavin JP: Selective management of abruptio placentae: A prospective study. Obstet Gynecol 1983;61:467–473.
77. Notelovitz M, Bottoms SF, Dase DF, Leichter PJ: Painless abruptio placentae. Obstet Gynecol 1979;53:270–272.
78. Page EW, King EB, Merril JA: Abruptio placentae: Dangers of delayed delivery. Obstet Gynecol 1954;3:385–393.
79. Green-Thompson RW: Antepartum haemorrhage. Clin Obstet Gynaecol 1982;9:479–515.
80. Nyberg DA, Cyr DR, Mack LA, et al: Sonographic spectrum of placental abruption. Am J Radiol 1987;148:161–167.
81. Rivera-Alxima ME, Saldana LR, Maklad N, Korp S: The use of ultrasound in the expectant management of abruptio placentae. Am J Obstet Gynecol 1983;146:924–927.
82. Sher G, Statland BE: Abruptio placentae with coagulopathy: A rational basis for management. Clin Obstet Gynaecol 1985;28:15–23.
83. Barron SL: Antepartum haemorrhage. In Chaimberlain G, Turnbull A (eds): Obstetrics. London, Churchill Livingstone, 1989.
84. Sholl JS: Abruptio placentae: Clinical management in nonacute cases. Am J Obstet Gynecol 1987;156:40–51.
85. Pritchard JA, MacDonald PC, Gant NF: Obstetric hemorrhage. In Williams' Obstetrics. New York, Appleton-Century-Crofts, 1985, pp 389–423.
86. Macafee CHG, Harley JMG: Antepartum haemorrhage. In Claye A (ed): British Obstetric Practice: Obstetrics, 3rd ed. London, Heinemann, 1963.
87. Willcocks J: Antepartum haemorrhage of uncertain origin. J Obstet Gynaecol Br Commonw 1971;78:987–991.
88. Watson R: Antepartum haemorrhage of uncertain origin. Br J Clin Pract 1982;36:222–226.
89. Butler NR, Bromham DG: The first report of the 1958 British Perinatal Mortality Survey. Edinburgh, Livingstone, 1963.
90. Roberts G: Unclassified antepartum haemorrhage: Incidence and perinatal mortality in a community. J Obstet Gynaecol Br Commonw 1970;77:492–495.
91. Naftolin F, Khudr G, Benirschke K, Hutchinson DL: The syndrome of chronic abruptio placentae, hydorrhoea and circumvallate placenta Am J Obstet Gynecol 1973;116:347–350.
92. Walker J, MacGillivary I, MacNaughton MC: Combined Textbook of Obstetrics and Gynaecology, 9th ed. Edinburgh, Churchill Livingstone, 1976.
93. Apt L, Downey WS: Melena neonatorum: The swallowed blood syndrome. J Pediatr 1955;47:6–16.
94. Silver R, Depp R, Sabbagha RE, et al: Placenta praevia: Aggressive expectant management. Am J Obstet Gynecol 1984;150:15–22.
95. Abdella TN, Sibai BM, Hays JM Jr, et al: Relationship of hypertensive disease to abruptio placentae. Obstet Gynecol 1984;63:365–370.
96. Lydon-Rochelle M, Holt VL, Easterling TR, et al: First-birth cesarean and placental abruption or previa at second birth. Obstet Gynecol 2001;97:765–769.
97. Golditch IA, Boyce NE: Management of abruptio placentae. JAMA 1970;212:288–293.
98. Lunan CB: The management of abruptio placentae. BJOG 1973;80:120–124.
99. Hurd WW, Miodovnik M, Hertzberg V,et al: Selective management of abruptio placentae: A prospective study. Obstet Gynecol 1983;61:467–473.

100. Brenner WE, Edelmann DA, Hendricks CH, et al: Characteristics of patients with placenta praevia and results of 'expectant management.' Am J Obstet Gynecol 1978;132:180–189.
101. Sampson MB, Lastres O, Tomasi AM, et al: Tocolysis with terbutaline sulphate in patients with placenta praevia complicated by premature labour. J Reprod Med 1984;29:248–250.
102. Rivera-Alxima ME, Saldana LR, Maklad N, et al: The use of ultrasound in the expectant management of abruptio placentae. Am J Obstet Gynecol 1983;146:924–927.
103. Willocks J: Antepartum haemorrhage of uncertain origin. J Obstet Gynaecol Br Commonw 1971;78:987–991.
104. Consensus Conference on Anti-D Prophylaxis: Papers and abstracts. Edinburgh, April 8–9, 1997. BJOG 1998;105(Suppl 18):1–44.
105. Jouppila P: Postpartum haemorrhage. Curr Opin Obstet Gynecol 1995;7:446–450.

CHAPTER 60

Multiple Pregnancy

Caroline Anne Crowther / Jodie Michele Dodd

INTRODUCTION

Multiple pregnancy rates vary worldwide. The lowest prevalence for twin births is reported in Japan (6.7 per 1000 deliveries), with intermediate prevalence reported in North America and Europe (11 per 1000 deliveries), and the highest prevalence reported in Africa, particularly Nigeria (40 per 1000 deliveries). The frequency of twin births in tertiary centers ranges from 1 in 25 to 1 in 100, with the highest rate reflecting the hospital referral population rather than the true rate for the population. The incidence of monozygous twinning is relatively constant worldwide, at 3.5 per 1000 births.[1] Dizygous twinning rates and higher-order birth rates vary widely and are affected by age, parity, racial background, and the use of assisted reproductive techniques. This chapter discusses the general and obstetric risks and problems associated with multiple pregnancy. Specific fetal problems (e.g., poor fetal growth, single fetal death in twins, congenital anomaly in one twin, twin reversed arterial perfusion sequence, monoamniotic twins, twin–twin transfusion syndrome [TTTS]) in multiple pregnancy are discussed in Chapter 24.

RISKS

Multiple pregnancy is associated with greater maternal and fetal risks than singleton pregnancy.

Maternal Risks (Table 60–1)

Increased Symptoms of Early Pregnancy

Nausea and vomiting are common and may arouse the suspicion of a multiple pregnancy. Higher levels of pregnancy hormones are implicated.[2]

Increased Risk of Miscarriage

Miscarriage is more common in multiple pregnancy than in singleton pregnancy. The rate of missed abortion is approximately twice as high as the 2% rate seen in singletons at 10 to 14 weeks' gestation. The risk of miscarriage with one missed abortion is ten times that of a normal twin pregnancy.[3]

Vanishing Twin Syndrome

Twins and higher-order multiple gestations are more often conceived than born. During the first trimester, arrest of development and subsequent reabsorption of one or more of the fetuses may occur. This event can be seen ultrasonographically and is known as the "vanishing twin" phenomenon.[4] First-trimester vaginal bleeding may be related to this syndrome. The prognosis for the

TABLE 60–1

Maternal Risks Associated with Multiple Pregnancy
Increased symptoms of early pregnancy
Increased risk of miscarriage
Vanishing twin syndrome
Minor disorders of pregnancy
Anemia
Preterm labor and delivery
Hypertension
Antepartum hemorrhage
Hydramnios
Possible need for prenatal hospitalization
Single fetal death in twins
Increased risk of an operative vaginal birth
Increased likelihood of cesarean birth
Postpartum hemorrhage
Postnatal problems
Maternal mortality

remaining fetus after loss of a cotwin at this early stage of pregnancy is good.[4]

Minor Disorders of Pregnancy

The extra weight carried with a multiple pregnancy exaggerates the minor symptoms of pregnancy. Backache, breathlessness, difficulty walking (especially toward the end of pregnancy), and pressure problems (e.g., varicose veins) are more common in multiple pregnancy.

Anemia

Anemia is more frequent in multiple than in singleton pregnancy. The greater increase in blood volume compared with the red cell mass decreases the hemoglobin concentration, producing a more pronounced decrease in hemoglobin compared with singleton pregnancy.[5] However, mean corpuscular hemoglobin concentration, used as a measure of anemia, does not differ in multiple versus singleton pregnancy. In a retrospective case–control study comparing hemoglobin concentration in twin and singleton gestations matched for parity, no statistically significant differences in third-trimester hemoglobin levels were identified between the two groups.[6] The lower levels identified in the first and second trimesters of pregnancy in twins compared with singletons reflected lower values in multiparous women with a twin pregnancy. Fetal demands in a multiple pregnancy are greater, particularly for folate, and megaloblastic anemia has been reported.

Preterm Labor and Delivery

Preterm birth (birth <37 weeks) occurred in 43.6% of all twin pregnancies compared with 5.6% of singleton pregnancies in the Scottish Twin Study.[7] In the United States, there has been an increase in the preterm birth rate for twins, from 40.9% in 1981 to 55.0% in 1996.[8] Very preterm birth (birth <32 weeks) occurred in 6% of women with a twin pregnancy in South Australia in 1995.[9] The mean duration of pregnancy decreases as the number of fetuses in utero increases. The risks to the mother of a preterm birth relate to the need for hospitalization and the possible use of tocolytic therapy, with potential side effects. Premature rupture of the membranes occurs more frequently in multiple gestations, and preterm labor and birth are frequent sequelae.

Hypertension

The incidence of pregnancy-induced hypertension, preeclampsia, and eclampsia is increased in multiple pregnancy.[10–12] A primigravida with a twin pregnancy has a five times greater risk of severe preeclampsia than a primigravida with a singleton pregnancy, and for a multigravida, the risk is 10 times greater.[13] Some report a higher risk of hypertension with monozygotic twins,[10,14] but others do not.[15,16]

Antepartum Hemorrhage

Antepartum hemorrhage as a result of placenta previa[17] and placental abruption[18] is increased in multiple gestations.

Hydramnios

Hydramnios is suspected clinically in up to 12% of multiple pregnancies[19] and is associated with an increased risk of preterm labor. Acute polyhydramnios may occur, particularly with monoamniotic twins, and may cause significant abdominal discomfort for the mother. Hydramnios may be associated with TTTS (see Chapter 24).

Possible Need for Prenatal Hospitalization

With the increased risk of threatened preterm labor, hypertension, fetal growth restriction, and minor disorders of pregnancy, women with a multiple pregnancy often require hospital admission, sometimes for prolonged periods, during the prenatal period. For the mother, prolonged separation from her family is often a disruptive and stressful experience. Specific complications of twinning, such as TTTS or single fetal death, may require hospitalization.

Single Fetal Death in Twins

The risk of single fetal death in a multiple pregnancy is 2% to 6%. Psychological trauma may be considerable and is enhanced by concerns about the health of the surviving fetus or fetuses. The mother who experiences fetal death of one twin during the antepartum period must adjust to a future without one of the twins while developing a bond with the surviving twin. The mother also must adjust to the additional risk of death and morbidity from cerebral and renal lesions for the surviving twin (see Chapter 24).

Risk of Operative Vaginal Birth

Compared with a vaginal singleton birth, there is an increased likelihood of operative delivery for one or both twins, with the associated maternal risks of trauma, infection, and hemorrhage.

Increased Likelihood of Cesarean Birth

Twins are more frequently born by cesarean section than singletons, either as an elective procedure or as an emergency procedure before or after the birth of the first twin. Presentation and gestational age influence this likelihood.[20] The higher the order of multiple birth, the higher the likelihood of cesarean birth.[21]

Postpartum Hemorrhage

The risk of postpartum hemorrhage is greater in multiple pregnancy because of the increased placental site, uterine overdistention, and a greater tendency to uterine atony.[11]

Postnatal Problems

Learning to cope with the demands of two or more infants can be stressful. A higher percentage of depression is reported in mothers of twins.[22] Given the increased perinatal mortality rate among higher-order multiple pregnancies, the problems of coping with the loss of one or more infants may be an added burden in the postnatal period.

Maternal Mortality

Women with a multiple pregnancy have a twofold increase in the risk of death compared with women with a singleton gestation.[11]

Fetal Risks (Table 60–2)

Stillbirth and Neonatal Death

In reports from Australia, the United Kingdom, the United States, Scandinavia, and Zimbabwe, multiple pregnancy contributed up to 10% of perinatal mortality.[7,23–27] The perinatal mortality rate in twins is up to 10 times that in singletons,[7,19,23,28,29] and if a broader concept of loss is used to include late abortion, late neonatal death, and infant death related to perinatal causes, the mortality risk is further doubled. Cause-specific mortality among twins is considerably higher for every major cause of death.[30] At all weeks of gestation, the risk of stillbirth and neonatal death is increased compared with singletons.[31] Same-sex twins have a poorer prognosis than opposite-sex twins.[29,32]

Higher mortality rates are reported for monochorionic compared with dichorionic twins,[33] although not by all.[34] For dichorionic twins, the risk of death increased throughout gestation, whereas the risk for monochorionic twins reached a maximum at 28 weeks' gestation and then remained constant.[34] In a review of 1051 twin pairs, factors associated with one or both twins dying in utero related to monochorionicity (odds ratio [OR], 2.0; 95% confidence interval [CI], 1.2–3.4) and discordant birth weight (OR, 4.3; 95% CI, 2.5–7.3), after correcting for gestational age at birth.[35]

TABLE 60–2

Fetal Risks Associated with Multiple Pregnancy

Stillbirth or neonatal death
Single fetal death in twins
Preterm labor and delivery
Intrauterine growth restriction
Congenital anomalies
Congenital anomaly in one twin
Twin reversed arterial perfusion sequence
Conjoined twins
Cord accident
Zygosity
Monoamniotic twins
Hydramnios
Twin–twin transfusion syndrome
Risk of asphyxia
Operative vaginal birth, especially for the second twin
Twin entrapment
Cerebral palsy

Single Fetal Death in Twins (See Chapter 24)

Preterm Labor and Birth

Preterm birth (<37 completed weeks) is the main reason for the poor perinatal outcome in multiple pregnancy. All studies of perinatal mortality in multiple pregnancy agree that preterm birth is the greatest single threat to infants. The preterm birth rate in twin pregnancy varies among populations from 30%[36] to 50%.[37] Triplets have a higher risk of preterm birth than twins, up to 80%.[38,39]

The median gestational age at birth for monochorionic twins is 36 weeks compared with 37 weeks for dichorionic twins. However, 9.2% of monochorionic twins are born before 32 weeks' gestation compared with 5.5% of dichorionic twins (Fig. 60–1).[3]

Intrauterine Growth Restriction

The incidence of small-for-gestational-age infants (birthweight <10th percentile for gestational age standards in pregnancy) is common in multiple pregnancy. Rates vary between populations from 25%[37] to 33%.[40] These infants are at increased risk for perinatal mortality and morbidity. The risk of low birth weight is increased in monochorionic twin pregnancies.[41–43]

Fetal Problems Specific to Multiple Pregnancy

Major congenital abnormalities are more common in multiple pregnancies compared with singletons, with rates reported as 4.9%.[44] Several fetal problems are specific to multiple pregnancy, including conjoined twins (discussed later), twin reversed arterial perfusion sequence, monoamniotic twins, and TTTS (see Chapter 24).

Conjoined Twins

Conjoined twins is a congenital abnormality that occurs only in multiple pregnancy and affects 1 in 200 monozygotic twins.[45]

Cord Accident

Preterm birth, preterm prelabor rupture of the membranes, hydramnios, malposition, and malpresentation are more likely to increase the risk of a cord accident in multiple pregnancies than in singleton pregnancies.

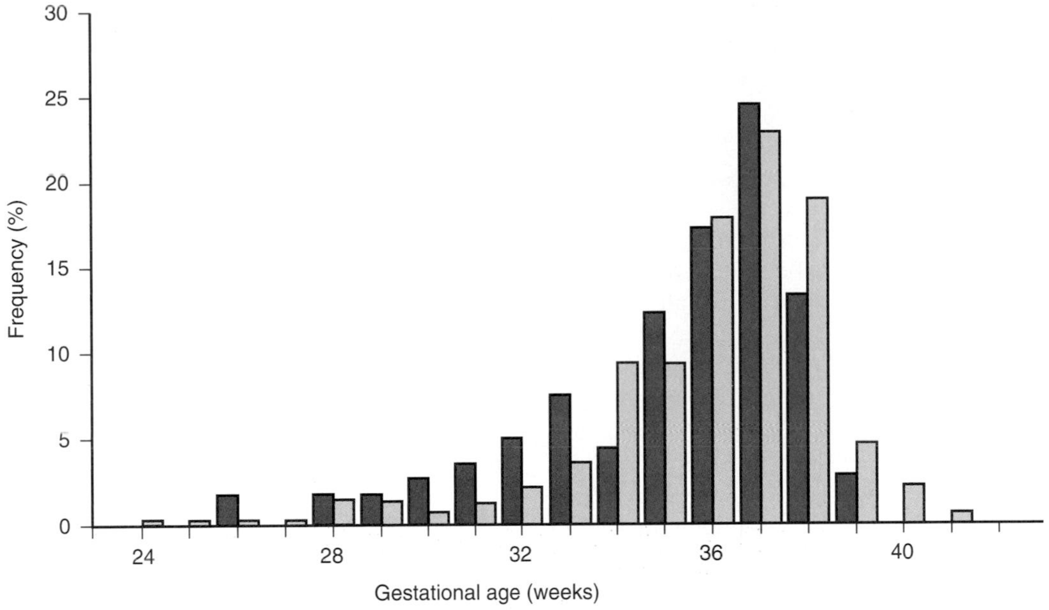

FIGURE 60–1
Gestational age at birth for monochorionic and dichorionic twin pregnancies. (From Sebire N, Thornton S, Hughes K, et al: The prevalence and consequence of missed abortion in twin pregnancies at 10–14 weeks of gestation. BJOG 1997;104:847–848.)

Chorionicity

Chorionicity has an important effect on pregnancy outcome. Two thirds of monozygous twins are monochorionic and are at increased risk for mortality and morbidity compared with dichorionic twins. Risk factors include increased risk of TTTS, congenital anomalies, single fetal death in utero, and acute hydramnios (see Chapter 24).

Hydramnios

Hydramnios may occur in one gestational sac in both TTTS and the "stuck twin" phenomenon (see Chapter 24). It may be caused by fetal anomalies such as upper gastrointestinal tract atresias and hydrops fetalis, possibly as a result of congenital heart anomalies. In some cases of gross hydramnios in both sacs, no causal factor is evident. Hydramnios is a major cause of preterm birth because of increased intrauterine volume. The associated perinatal mortality rate is high.[46]

Risk of Asphyxia

The risk of mortality as a result of asphyxia in a twin is four to five times that in a singleton.[30] Important risk factors include the increased occurrence of intrauterine growth restriction, cord prolapse, and hydramnios.

Operative Vaginal Birth, Especially for the Second Twin

The likelihood of operative birth is increased, especially for the second twin, who may require internal podalic version. Operative birth is associated with an increased risk of birth trauma, low Apgar scores, and hyperbilirubinemia compared with a normal vaginal birth.

Twin Entrapment

Twin entrapment is rare and is reported to occur in 1 in 817 twin pregnancies.[47] The risk of fetal death of the first twin is high, as is the risk of fetal hypoxia in both twins. Twin entrapment is associated with monoamniotic twins.

Cerebral Palsy

The prevalence of cerebral palsy in triplets is 47 times that in singletons. The risk in twins is eight times that in singletons.[48] Lower gestational age at birth is associated with a greater risk of cerebral palsy.[49]

MANAGEMENT OPTIONS

Prepregnancy

The risk of multiple pregnancy for women undergoing ovulation induction is increased to 20% to 40%. After the use of clomiphene, the twinning rate is 5% to 10%.[50] Appropriate counseling about this increased risk should be provided to women who are offered this treatment. The risk of multiple pregnancy as a result of the use of assisted reproductive techniques correlates directly with the number of embryos or zygotes transferred, increasing from 1.4% when a single embryo is transferred with in vitro fertilization, to 17.9% after transfer of two embryos, and

24.1% after transfer of four embryos.[51] Similarly, the risk of multiple pregnancy after gamete intrafallopian transfer correlates with the number of oocytes transferred, with a risk of 18.7% after transfer of two oocytes and 25.8% after transfer of three oocytes.[51] The rate of multiple pregnancy at 20 weeks' gestation after zygote intrafallopian transfer with three zygotes is 27%.[52]

When deciding how many embryos, zygotes, or oocytes to transfer, a compromise between a wanted high conception rate and an acceptable risk of multiple pregnancy is necessary. The best way to reduce the risk of multiple pregnancy is to reduce the number of embryos, zygotes, or oocytes transferred after full discussion of the risks and benefits with the couple. Two randomized controlled trials compared single versus double embryo transfer,[53,54] and another compared double embryo transfer with transfer of four embryos.[55] In a meta-analysis of these trials, when single embryo transfer was compared with double embryo transfer, fewer women became pregnant (relative risk [RR], 0.69; 95% CI, 0.51–0.93), but the risks of twin pregnancy (RR, 0.12; 95% CI, 0.03–0.48) and low birth weight (RR, 0.17; 95% CI, 0.04–0.79) were markedly reduced.[56] No statistically significant differences were identified for outcomes relating to singleton pregnancy, pregnancy loss at less than 20 weeks' gestation, extrauterine pregnancy, or preterm birth at less than 37 weeks.[56] When the transfer of two embryos was compared with the transfer of four embryos, no statistically significant differences were seen in the number of women who became pregnant with a multiple or singleton pregnancy or the risk of pregnancy loss.[55] However, these trials were significantly underpowered to be able to detect all but large differences, and they did not report other important clinical outcomes.

Periconceptual folate supplementation is recommended as a general measure for all women to reduce the risk of neural tube defects.[57]

Prenatal

Overall Care

Regular antenatal attendance for pregnancy care is accepted practice. Most clinicians increase the number of times women with a multiple pregnancy are seen during the prenatal period. Many forms of care are practiced, ranging from modified shared care, with a general practitioner seeing the woman at the hospital for alternate prenatal visits, to seeing her weekly at the hospital prenatal clinic from 20 weeks' gestation. Specialized multidisciplinary twin clinics have been advocated, and some nonrandomized cohort data suggest that perinatal outcome can be improved by intensive preterm birth education, continuity of care providers, and individualized care.[58–60] Prospective randomized data are lacking.

Frequent prenatal visits permit extra vigilance in the early detection of pregnancy-induced hypertension.[61] Routine screening for gestational diabetes is often performed, although evidence to support this practice is conflicting, with some reports suggesting an increased risk in twins and others suggesting no increased risk.[62,63]

Antepartum hemorrhage can be neither predicted nor prevented by additional prenatal visits or any other strategy. In addition, iron and folate supplementation is frequently advised from the beginning of the second trimester for women with multiple pregnancy, although the evidence to support this practice is limited.[5,6]

Diagnosis of Chorionicity by Early Ultrasound

Amnionicity and chorionicity can be determined by ultrasound.[64] Hazards for monochorionic twins include TTTS, and for monoamniotic twins, cord entanglement. Knowledge of amnionicity and chorionicity may be useful in predicting which pregnancies are at greater risk for TTTS or to differentiate TTTS from a twin pregnancy complicated by growth restriction. Similarly, this knowledge may be useful in the management of twin pregnancy when one twin has a major congenital malformation and selective termination is considered, or in the management of pregnancy after a single fetal death.[65] Screening for amnionicity and chorionicity is best performed in the first trimester, although it is not always easy, even for a skilled ultrasonographer.[66]

Monochorionic twins are the same sex and have one placental mass, with a thin dividing membrane (two amnions, no chorions) and a T insertion.[35,67] Because the dividing membrane is so thin, it is often difficult to identify, and the pregnancy may be misidentified as monoamniotic. Visualization of the dividing membrane is facilitated by searching over the fetal chin or away from the fetal body and around the limbs. A dichorionic placenta essentially eliminates the diagnosis of TTTS.

The dividing membrane is thicker in dichorionic twins than in monochorionic twins (contains two layers of amnion and two layers of chorion). Measuring the membrane thickness by ultrasound, using a cutoff of 2 mm to characterize a dichorionic or monochorionic placenta,[68] has been described as a good, but suboptimal, test for determining chorionicity.[66] High interobserver and intraobserver variation, together with differences related to gestational age and sampling site, lead to suboptimal accuracy of the determination of chorionicity.[67] Ultrasonic detection of the lambda sign[69] (an echogenic V-shaped chorionic projection of tissue between the dividing membranes in dichorionic placentation) is reported as more reliable, especially if the scan is performed at 10 to 14 weeks' gestation (Fig. 60–2).[70] As gestational age increases, the lambda sign is more difficult to see, and after 20 weeks, it may disappear. The lambda sign is also known as the twin peak sign.[71] Given the prognostic value for later risks of pregnancy, attempting to establish the chorionicity of the placenta between 10 and 14 weeks' gestation may be appropriate.

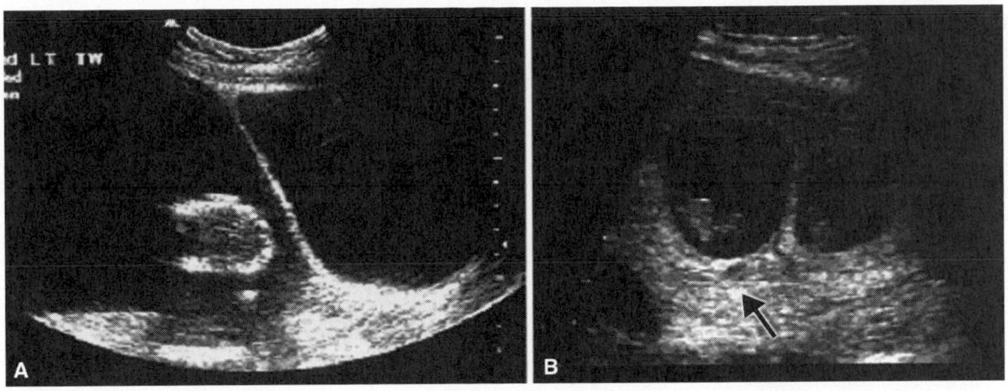

FIGURE 60–2
Ultrasonography to establish chorionicity. *A*, Monochorionic twin pregnancy. *B*, Dichorionic twin pregnancy showing the lambda sign (*arrow*).

Accuracy rates for determining chorionicity with first-trimester ultrasound, determined by subsequent pathologic examination, are reported as up to 96% with transabdominal sonography[72] and up to 100% with transvaginal sonography.[73]

No prospective clinical studies show that knowledge of chorionicity should alter subsequent clinical management or whether pregnancy outcome can be improved by changes in clinical care.

Nuchal Translucency Screening

The use of nuchal translucency screening for trisomy 21 and aneuploidy in singleton gestation is widespread, and it has been used to screen women with twin pregnancy. In a study of 448 women with twin pregnancy, nuchal translucency was measured for each fetus and combined with maternal age to derive a risk estimate. The detected nuchal translucency was greater than the 95th percentile for gestational age (using crown–rump length derived from singletons) in 7.3% of fetuses, including 88% of those with trisomy 21. These findings suggest that in dichorionic twin pregnancies, the sensitivity and false-positive rate of fetal nuchal translucency as a screening tool for trisomy 21 are similar to those reported for singleton pregnancies.[74] In monochorionic twin pregnancies, the false-positive rate of screening is higher than that reported in singleton pregnancies, and discordance in nuchal translucency measurements raise the possibility of early-onset TTTS.[75]

Pregnancy Reduction

Couples who are faced with the dilemma of a triplet or higher-order multiple pregnancy have several options. Termination of the entire pregnancy generally is not acceptable to women, particularly those with a history of infertility. Attempting to continue the pregnancy with all of the fetuses is associated with inherent problems related to preterm birth, survival, and long-term morbidity. Reduction in the number of fetuses by selective termination has been advocated in an attempt to reduce the risk of adverse obstetric and perinatal outcomes.[76] This practice involves intracardiac injection of potassium chloride (see Chapter 24). Many prospective nonrandomized studies have compared pregnancy outcome after multifetal pregnancy reduction in twins conceived spontaneously or after assisted reproduction[77–79] with multifetal pregnancy reduction in expectantly managed triplet pregnancies.[79–82] A systematic review assessed the effects of multifetal pregnancy reduction on fetal loss, preterm birth, and perinatal and infant mortality and morbidity rates in women with triplet and higher-order multiple pregnancies. This review included prospective nonrandomized studies, but excluded[83,84] case series, retrospective studies, and prospective studies that used historical controls as well as those in which selective fetal reduction was performed because of fetal anomaly. The overall quality of the included studies was poor, with inconsistent allocation of patients to treatment groups. However, when pregnancy was reduced to twins, the reported outcomes appeared comparable to those in twins conceived spontaneously or those conceived with assisted reproductive techniques (Table 60–3). Counseling these patients is further complicated by the varying preterm delivery rates and their consequences (Table 60–4). No randomized controlled trials have assessed multifetal reduction. The available nonrandomized studies provide limited insight into the benefits and risks associated with fetal reduction procedures.[84] Although a randomized controlled trial would provide the most reliable evidence, selective termination may not be acceptable to couples, particularly those with a history of infertility, and consequently, recruitment to such a trial may be exceptionally difficult.

Fetal Anomaly Scanning

A complete abdominal ultrasound scan performed by an operator with expertise in obstetric anomaly scanning is essential. The goals of midtrimester sonographic examination are to document fetal biometric discordance, seek evidence of discordant fetal anomalies or infection, and localize the placenta. The likelihood of a chromosomal

TABLE 60–3

Pregnancy Outcomes in Multifetal Pregnancy Reduction

OUTCOME (% OF PREGNANCIES)	TRIPLETS UNREDUCED	TRIPLETS REDUCED TO TWINS	TWINS UNREDUCED	TWINS REDUCED TO SINGLETONS
Miscarriage Rate	20.2%	8.6%	7.8%	5.6%
Very Preterm Birth	22.1%*	9.3%*	13.8%†	13.3†

*<32 weeks.
†<34 weeks.
From Dodd J, Crowther C: Reduction of the number of fetuses for women with triplet and higher order multiple pregnancies (Cochrane Review). In Cochrane Library, Issue 4, 2003. Chichester, UK, John Wiley & Sons.

abnormality is increased greatly in the presence of a structural malformation.

Given the increased risk of congenital abnormalities, an anomaly scan of each fetus is suggested, usually between 18 and 20 weeks' gestation. In centers offering routine ultrasound scanning at this stage of pregnancy, undetected multiple pregnancy should be diagnosed. Early diagnosis allows appropriate counseling and planning for future care and has been reported to reduce perinatal loss related to twin pregnancy.[85] Conjoined twins can be diagnosed if an ultrasound scan is performed at this stage.

In one series, prenatal ultrasonography, including cardiac screening limited to the four-chamber view, resulted in the detection of up to 39% of all major congenital anomalies in twins.[86] However, none of the cardiac lesions were detected. Of major noncardiac anomalies, 55% were detected, as were 69% of major anomalies that could alter prenatal management.[86] In a retrospective study of 245 women with twin pregnancy, ultrasound screening for fetal anomalies identified a 4.9% prevalence of congenital malformations. For the detection of each individual anomaly, sensitivity was 82%, specificity was 100%, positive predictive value was 100%, and negative predictive value was 98%.[44]

Conjoined Twins

Conjoined twins are usually diagnosed antenatally.[87] Determination of the conjoined site permits multidisciplinary discussion before birth as to the prognosis and the possibility of surgical correction and allows full involvement of the parents. Unless birth is necessary for other reasons, preterm cesarean section is recommended. The use of steroids to stimulate fetal lung maturity is advisable. Some test for fetal lung maturity before birth. Many obstetricians recommend elective cesarean delivery at 38 weeks; however, this procedure can be difficult technically. Some recommend a classic incision, but this approach seems to offer little fetal benefit over a lower-segment incision and increases the maternal risks, particularly of uterine scar rupture in subsequent pregnancy. At delivery, two neonatal teams should be available, with the neonatal surgical team and operating room on standby.

Preterm Labor

Preterm labor and subsequent birth presents the greatest risk for fetal morbidity and mortality. Patient counseling as to the signs and symptoms of preterm labor may be of value, and parents should be given a written information

TABLE 60–4

Likelihood of Preterm Delivery and Subsequent Preterm Mortality and Neurodevelopmental Morbidity (NDM) Rates in Unreduced Triplets (URT) and Triplets Reduced to Twins (TWN)

OUTCOME	24 WK		26 WK		28 WK		30 WK		32 WK		REFERENCE
	URT	TWN	URT	TWN	URT	TWN	URT	TWN	URT	TWN	
Percentage of pregnancies undelivered at a given gestation	80	90	75	87	70	87	65	87	55	82	149
Percentage survival if delivered at a given gestation (95% CI)	21 (16–25)		62 (58–65)		88 (68–90)		96 (95–97)		99 (97–99)		150
Percentage with no NDM ("no disability") if delivered at a given gestation (95% CI)	30* (8–58)		55* (35–75)		70* (62–88)		Proportion of survivors with "no disability" continues to rise with gestation at delivery, but no accurate current data available for each gestational period >28 wk*				151*, 152*

*Mortality and neurodevelopmental morbidity assessed at 4 years in survivors.
CI, confidence interval.

sheet. If uterine activity is noted, the woman should go to the hospital promptly.

It is difficult to predict which patients will have preterm labor. Cervical assessment by either digital[88–90] or ultrasound examination[91–94] has been suggested as a useful way to evaluate the risk of preterm delivery. How frequently such an assessment should be made (e.g., weekly, every 2 weeks, monthly) is uncertain, and whether such assessment is more beneficial than harmful is not known. Cervical assessment allows calculation of the cervical score (cervical length [in centimeters]—cervical dilation [in centimeters]). A cervical score of 2 or less at or before 34 weeks' gestation has a positive predictive value of 75% for preterm birth,[89] with other authors reporting that a cervical score of 0 or less has a positive predictive value of 75% for preterm birth.[90] As part of a study of the prediction of preterm delivery, cervical length was prospectively assessed by ultrasound in 147 women with a twin pregnancy. A short cervix (<25 mm) was consistently associated with spontaneous preterm birth at less than 32 weeks' gestation (OR, 6.9; 95% CI, 2.0–24.2), less than 35 weeks' gestation (OR, 3.2; 95% CI, 1.3–7.9), and less than 37 weeks' gestation (OR, 2.8; 95% CI, 1.1–7.7).[91]

The presence of fetal fibronectin in cervical secretions has been used to predict preterm birth.[91,92] In multiple pregnancy, a positive fetal fibronectin test result at 28 to 30 weeks was associated with preterm birth before 32 weeks' gestation.[91] A positive fetal fibronectin test result at 28 weeks' gestation predicted birth before 35 weeks, with sensitivity, specificity, positive predictive value, and negative predictive value of 50.0%, 92.0%, 62.5%, and 87.3%, respectively.[92] The ability of fetal fibronectin to predict very preterm birth requires ongoing prospective evaluation to determine whether such prediction can lead to effective interventions that would reduce the risk of preterm birth.

If cervical change is noted, hospital admission is the most generally accepted management. Routine hospital admission and subsequent rest, however, seem to offer little benefit in delaying labor.[95,96] It is unknown whether prophylactic tocolysis is of value in this identifiable group at high risk for preterm birth.

Several prenatal interventions have been tried to reduce the risk of preterm birth in multiple pregnancies and have been evaluated by randomized clinical trials. These include prophylactic cervical cerclage,[97,98] prophylactic β-mimetic agents,[99,100] bed rest in the hospital,[95] and home uterine activity monitoring.[101,102] However, none of these have proven to be of value in reducing the incidence of preterm birth and the associated high perinatal mortality rate in multiple pregnancy.

Prophylactic cervical cerclage in twin pregnancy does not show benefit when the results of randomized trials are reviewed.[103] It seems prudent to reserve the insertion of a cervical suture for women with evidence of cervical incompetence. Prophylactic tocolytic agents are occasionally used in multiple pregnancy. Systematic review of randomized trials of prophylactic β-mimetics does not show a benefit in the incidence of preterm labor,[104] and their use cannot be recommended.

Admission of women with an uncomplicated twin pregnancy to the hospital for rest does not reduce the risk of preterm birth. The Cochrane systematic review of randomized trials of routine hospitalization for rest shows an increased likelihood of preterm birth in women who were admitted, compared with control subjects who continued normal activity at home.[105] Hospital admission for rest in an uncomplicated twin pregnancy should be considered only if the woman requests admission. Women may request hospital admission for several reasons, including discomfort, difficulty coping at home, or living a significant distance from the hospital.

The value of hospital admission for rest in triplet or higher-order multiple pregnancy is uncertain. Only one small randomized study has been done. In this study, hospitalization for rest showed a beneficial trend in reducing the incidence of preterm delivery in 19 triplet pregnancies. In addition, the hospitalized group had infants with higher birth weight.[106] All of these benefits are also compatible with chance variation. A multicenter trial is needed to evaluate further the effects of hospital admission for rest in triplet pregnancy.

Home uterine activity monitoring (HUAM) has been suggested to permit the diagnosis of preterm labor at an early stage, allowing successful tocolysis and fewer preterm births. A small randomized trial of 45 women reported these benefits.[101] However, in subgroup analysis of the 844 twin gestations in a multicenter trial comparing HUAM with weekly or daily nursing contact, HUAM did not reduce the risk of preterm birth.[102] HUAM, when combined with daily nursing contact, resulted in more unscheduled visits and increased use of tocolytics.

A course of prenatal corticosteroids should be given to improve fetal outcome in women with multiple pregnancy who are considered at risk for preterm birth at less than 34 weeks, if birth is planned or if there is a high risk of birth within the next 48 hours.[107] Whether a larger dose of corticosteroids than that given in singleton pregnancies would be more beneficial in twin gestations has been suggested but not adequately assessed.[107] The efficacy of repeat doses of steroids is uncertain in women with multiple pregnancy who have not been delivered 7 or more days after a first course of steroids but are still at high risk for preterm birth. This issue is being addressed by ongoing randomized trials in Australia, New Zealand, Canada, the United States, and Scandinavia.

Fetal Assessment

Fetal assessment during pregnancy includes regular ultrasound to determine fetal growth and well-being. The recommended frequency of scanning varies (e.g., from every 2 weeks from 24 weeks' gestation to every 3 to 4 weeks from 20 weeks' gestation). Umbilical artery Doppler improves pregnancy outcome in high risk pregnancy, and is often included as part of routine fetal assessment.[108] Some centers suggest obtaining biophysical profiles from 30 weeks' gestation, although the evidence to support this strategy is not strong.

The use of umbilical artery Doppler studies in the assessment of twin pregnancy was evaluated in three randomized controlled trials.[109–111] Giles and colleagues[111] randomly allocated 526 women with a twin pregnancy at 25 weeks' gestation to biometry only or to biometry and umbilical artery Doppler waveform at 25, 30, and 35 weeks' gestation. This study of close antenatal surveillance identified a lower than expected fetal mortality rate from 25 weeks' gestation in both the biometry alone and combined biometry and Doppler groups.

Maternal Education and Support

During the prenatal period, the couple will need specific information and support to help prepare for the birth and care of their infants.[25] The most likely mode of birth, care in labor, and the use of analgesia, especially epidural, should be discussed.[112] Many countries have multiple pregnancy support groups. The opportunity to contact a local group during the prenatal period, attend meetings, and make personal contact with other families who have had a multiple birth is recommended.

Labor and Delivery

Birth in a hospital is accepted practice,[113] with many advising birth in a tertiary unit, when possible. Induction of labor may be indicated for complications such as preeclampsia or growth restriction. The benefit of elective birth at 37 weeks' gestation to reduce the risk of antepartum stillbirth as a result of intrauterine growth restriction is controversial.

Retrospective data suggest that the lowest rate of perinatal mortality and morbidity in twin pregnancies occurs at 36 to 38 weeks' gestation, with the risk of adverse outcome increasing as gestation advances.[31,114–118] A recent Cochrane systematic review of the role of elective birth in twin pregnancy from 37 weeks' gestation[119] identified a single small randomized controlled trial from Japan[120] assessing elective birth with continued expectant management. This study identified no statistically significant differences. However, the sample size was underpowered to detect meaningful differences, and insufficient data are available to support the practice of elective birth from 37 weeks' gestation in women with an otherwise uncomplicated twin pregnancy. A multicenter randomized controlled trial is in progress, coordinated by the Maternal Perinatal Clinical Trials Unit at the University of Adelaide, to assess the optimal timing of birth in women with twin pregnancy at term.

Intrapartum blood loss is greater in multiple pregnancy, as is the risk of postpartum hemorrhage. An intravenous access line should be inserted early in labor and blood obtained to estimate maternal hemoglobin or hematocrit and to hold serum for crossmatching, if needed later.

For a vaginal birth, both twins should be monitored continuously.[113] Initially, only external fetal monitoring will be possible. When feasible, a scalp electrode should be placed on the first twin, with continuation of external monitoring of the second twin. The use of a twin fetal heart rate monitor allows simultaneous recording of the two fetal heart rate tracings. If continuous monitoring of the second twin is impossible, some recommend cesarean section because of the higher risk of fetal asphyxia in twins, which may go undetected without adequate monitoring.

Epidural analgesia is widely used, providing the mother with adequate pain relief, and minimizes the risk that she will push before full dilation occurs.[113] In addition, adequate analgesia is provided in the event that operative birth, internal podalic version of the second twin, or cesarean delivery is needed. The widespread use of epidural anesthesia often negates the need for emergency general anesthesia with the complications discussed earlier, although it may still be needed for emergency cesarean section for fetal distress.

The optimal mode of birth in multiple pregnancy is controversial.[121] For triplets and higher-order multiple gestations, the most frequent mode of delivery is cesarean section,[122–124] although no randomized studies are available to support this mode of birth over vaginal birth. Reports suggest that the risk of lower Apgar scores in higher-order multiple gestations is reduced with cesarean delivery[38,125]; in addition, there are fewer perinatal deaths.[38]

Neonatal respiratory disease was more common in twins born by cesarean section at 36 to 38 weeks than in those born vaginally at 38 to 40 weeks.[126] A more recent report suggested higher perinatal mortality rates with cesarean delivery, primarily as a result of respiratory distress syndrome.[127]

The Cochrane systematic review of the mode of birth for the second twin[128] identified a single randomized trial[129] comparing planned vaginal birth with planned cesarean birth for the second, nonvertex twin. This study highlighted the need for further evidence from randomized controlled trials to inform practice. To provide more reliable information about the optimal mode of birth for women with twin pregnancy, a randomized controlled trial (Twin Birth Study) is in progress, coordinated by the University of Toronto, Maternal, Infant and Reproductive Health Research Unit, at the Centre for Research in Women's Health.

Based on the literature on twin pregnancy, some recommendations can be made. The mode of birth is often affected by the presentation of the twins, which may be divided into the following three groups:

- First twin vertex, second twin vertex
- First twin vertex, second twin nonvertex
- First twin nonvertex

First Twin Vertex, Second Twin Vertex

The most common presentation of twins is vertex–vertex. In this case, most obstetricians recommend vaginal birth,[130–133] and the literature supports vaginal birth, even of very low-birth-weight infants (<1500 g).[131,134,135]

First Twin Vertex, Second Twin Nonvertex

For twins presenting as first twin vertex, second twin nonvertex, opinion is divided as to the optimal mode of birth. Some recommend elective cesarean delivery,[132,136] reporting reduced neonatal mortality and morbidity rates for the second twin. Others suggest that there is no increase in neonatal risk associated with vaginal birth of the second twin weighing 1500 g or more, either as breech presentation after internal podalic version if the fetus does not have a longitudinal lie, or as cephalic presentation after external cephalic version.[137–142] The only randomized study found no difference in neonatal outcome in 60 nonvertex second twins at 35 weeks' gestation or more. Study subjects were randomly allocated to either vaginal delivery or cesarean section.[129,143] Assessment of whether vaginal breech delivery is appropriate is necessary using the standard criteria for singleton birth. These include exclusion of cephalopelvic disproportion, estimated fetal weight of less than approximately 3500 g, and the finding of a flexed fetal head on ultrasound.

For a nonvertex second twin of very low birth weight (<1500 g), the mode of birth is controversial. Some recent reports recommend cesarean delivery to minimize birth trauma to the preterm infant,[131,137,139,140,144] whereas others show no neonatal benefit and emphasize that vaginal delivery has reduced risks for the mother.[134] No randomized studies have compared vaginal and cesarean birth in these infants.

First Twin Nonvertex

When the first twin is nonvertex, cesarean delivery is often preferred[121,133] and advised,[131] although no series suggests that vaginal birth is inappropriate. It is likely that this approach is influenced by the data on the optimum mode of delivery in singleton breech presentations (see Chapter 64). By following such a policy, the risk of twin entrapment by interlocking chins or heads can be avoided.

PROCEDURE

TWIN BIRTH

For a vaginal twin birth, at least one experienced obstetrician, anesthetist, pediatrician, and neonatal nurse should be in attendance. Depending on gestational age (e.g., if preterm) and circumstances (e.g., operative birth, abnormal CTG findings), a double pediatric team (two pediatricians and two neonatal nurses) may be appropriate. For higher-order multiple births, one pediatric team should be present for each infant. Some recommend having a nurse scrubbed and the operating room prepared for emergency cesarean section.

For a vaginal birth, delivery of the first twin should be as for a singleton. After the birth of the first twin, an experienced obstetrician assesses the lie and presentation of the second twin. This assessment can be done by vaginal examination, abdominal palpation, or transabdominal ultrasound examination. The lie should be corrected to longitudinal by external version or internal podalic version.[145] External version (Fig. 60–3) gently turns the fetus so that the vertex lies above the pelvic brim. Amniotomy can be performed if there are uterine contractions (discussed later), and then delivery is completed. Version is more likely to be successful with epidural anesthesia and when the twins are of similar weight (difference of <500 g).[138]

In two series, external version was less likely than breech extraction to result in a vaginal birth.[140,146] Emergency cesarean section and complications such as cord prolapse and fetal distress were more frequent in the external version group. Although these were not randomized studies, in view of these findings, internal podalic version, if necessary, and breech delivery are recommended by some obstetricians if the lie is nonlongitudinal or the breech is presenting. However, others prefer to use external cephalic version and perform amniotomy once the lie is longitudinal and there are regular uterine contractions. They advocate cesarean delivery if the lie remains nonlongitudinal. Oxytocin (Syntocinon) infusion is mandatory if there is uterine inertia, and it is normal practice in many units to

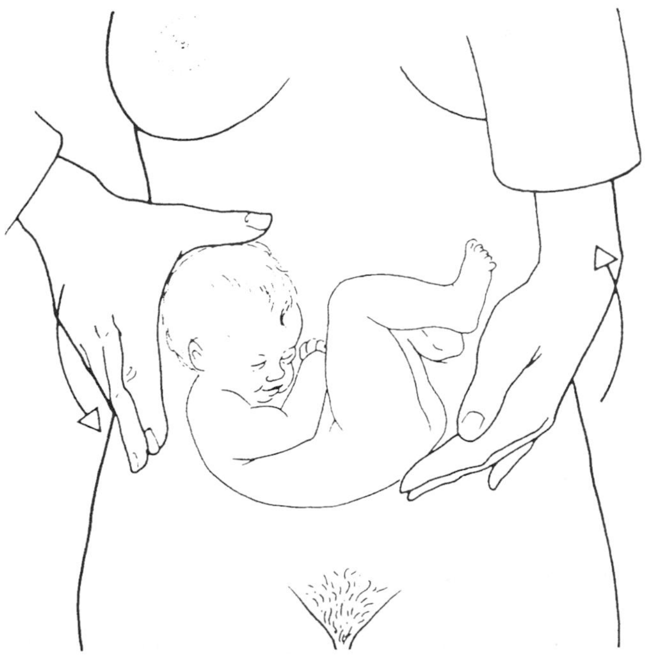

FIGURE 60–3
Modified external version for delivery of the second twin.

have an infusion ready at the onset of the second stage of labor. Once there are contractions and the lie is longitudinal, amniotomy is performed and birth proceeds with maternal effort during contractions. A scalp electrode can be applied after amniotomy to permit continuous fetal heart rate monitoring, or an external monitor can be used. Most authors advise continuous monitoring of the second twin throughout the second stage of labor, given the increased risk of intrapartum asphyxia. The risk of fetal distress and acidosis is increased if the twin–twin delivery interval exceeds 30 minutes.[147] If fetal distress develops and birth cannot be achieved safely, or if the second twin does not descend into the pelvis, emergency cesarean delivery is necessary.

After birth of the second infant, active management of the third stage of labor is recommended with an oxytocic agent.[148] To prevent uterine atony, in many units, infusion of oxytocin is continued for 3 to 4 hours.

Internal podalic version with vaginal breech delivery remains an option for birth of the second twin when a non-longitudinal lie persists and the membranes are intact (Fig. 60–4). This approach involves the following steps:

- Use adequate analgesia, usually epidural, but possibly a general anesthetic.
- Place the patient in the lithotomy position.
- Provide continuous fetal heart rate monitoring.
- Use aseptic technique, and catheterize the patient.
- Ensure that a pediatrician is present.
- Determine the lie of the second twin by abdominal palpation, internal examination, or transabdominal ultrasound examination.
- Locate a fetal foot. Confirm that the structure is a foot rather than a wrist by palpating the heel.
- Perform an amniotomy.
- Grasp the foot, and pull down into the vagina. Grasp both feet, if possible.
- With maternal effort during contractions, deliver the fetus as an assisted breech.

Complications

Complications include the following:

- Fetal anoxia
- Difficulty with delivery of the head with breech presentation
- Fetal trauma as a result of breech delivery (e.g., dislocated hips)
- Inadvertent delivery of a hand with shoulder presentation
- Placental abruption
- Cord accident
- Endometritis
- Maternal trauma (e.g., ruptured uterus)

Twin Entrapment

Twin entrapment may occur if the first twin is delivered as a breech and the second twin is cephalic and the head of the second twin enters the pelvis before the head of the leading

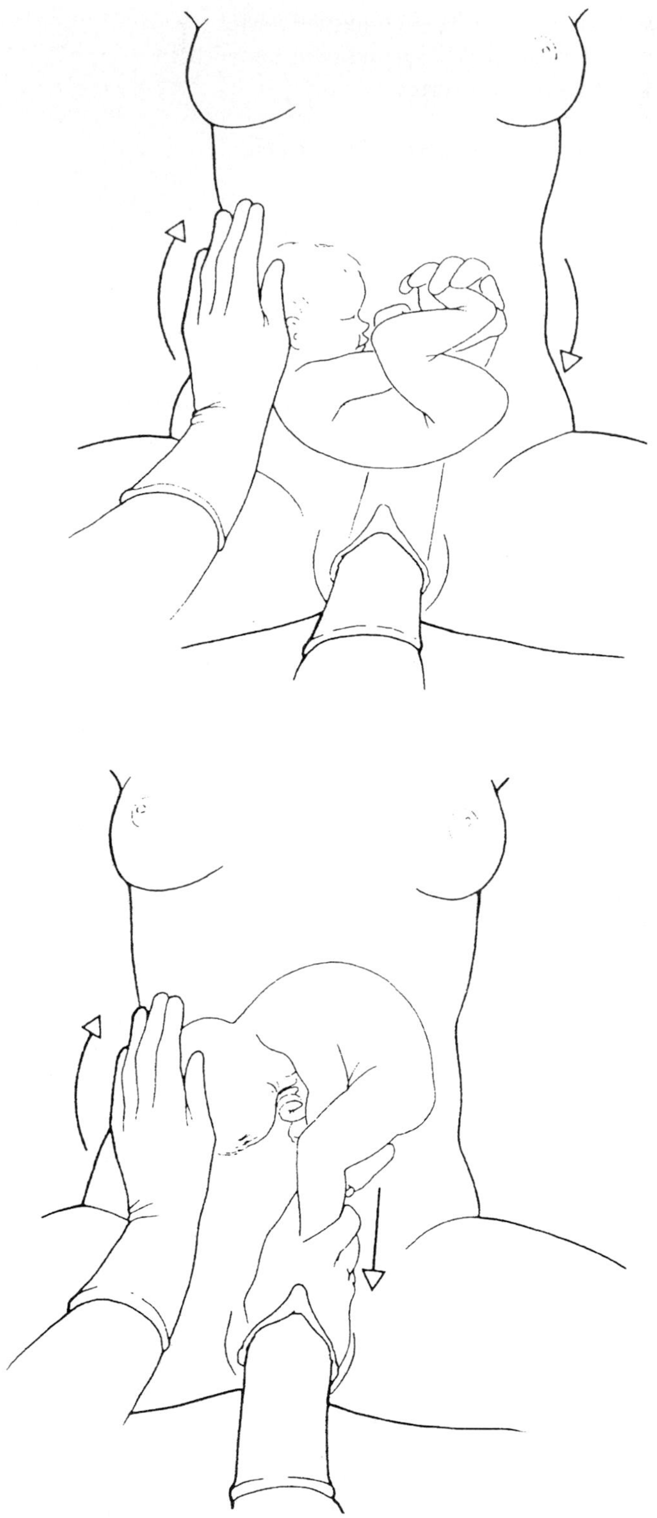

FIGURE 60–4
Internal podalic version.

twin. Some maintain that the risk of twin entrapment can be avoided by performing elective cesarean section if the first twin is breech and the second twin is cephalic. In an emergency, an attempt may be made to separate the locked twins by passing a hand vaginally between the chins of the fetuses and pushing the second twin upward. If this attempt fails, emergency cesarean section is necessary. Alternatively, an attempt may be made to push back the first twin, presenting as a breech, and allow the "second" twin, presenting cephalically, to deliver first. Again, if this attempt fails, emergency cesarean delivery is necessary.

During cesarean section, the head of the first twin is maneuvered upward, enabling birth of the second twin's head and body. The "first" twin may then be delivered. Some recommend having a second obstetrician available to manipulate the infants vaginally, if necessary.

If the first twin is already dead, rather than cesarean birth, there is the option of decapitation of the first twin, vaginal delivery of the second twin, and delivery of the head of the first twin. Such a destructive procedure should be performed under general anesthesia to protect the mother from seeing it. Many believe that this option should not be used in modern obstetrics, and some would argue that abdominal delivery may be associated with a lower incidence of perinatal asphyxia for the second twin.

Complications

In twin entrapment, the risk of fetal death of the first twin is high, as is the risk of fetal hypoxia for both twins. Maternal risks relate to the need for emergency cesarean section, endometritis, and the possible need for general anesthesia.

Postnatal

After the birth of twins, the mother may require a prolonged hospital stay. Breastfeeding should be encouraged, and additional support is important. The provision of adequate contraception is necessary and should be discussed. Coordinated support to help the parents care for their infants should be available.[25]

Before discharge, if extra help is not available at home, additional community support may need to be arranged. Maintaining contact with the local multiple birth support group during the puerperium is important.

CONCLUSIONS

- Multiple pregnancy is associated with maternal and fetal risks.
- Prepregnancy care centers on avoiding multiple conceptions in women who undergo assisted reproductive techniques.
- Early prenatal care focuses on determining chorionicity and diagnosing fetal anomalies.
- Later prenatal care is directed toward the prevention, prediction, and detection of preterm birth and intrauterine growth restriction.
- The optimal timing and mode of delivery in twins are not clear, and the results of ongoing multicenter randomized trials are awaited.

SUMMARY OF MANAGEMENT OPTIONS
Multiple Pregnancy

Management Options	Quality of Evidence	Strength of Recommendation	References
Prepregnancy			
Counsel women who are undergoing assisted conception techniques about the risks of multiple pregnancy.	III	B	32, 52
No data are available to guide the "ideal" number of embryos or oocytes to replace.	Ia	A	56
Preconceptual and periconceptual folate supplementation	Ia	A	57
Prenatal			
Specialized twin clinics may lessen adverse outcomes. Little evidence supports other forms of prenatal care.	III	B	58–60
Documentation of zygosity or chorionicity at 10 to 14 weeks	III	B	70

Continued

SUMMARY OF MANAGEMENT OPTIONS

Multiple Pregnancy *(Continued)*

Management Options	Quality of Evidence	Strength of Recommendation	References
No prospective data on whether this documentation improves outcome			
Increased surveillance if twins are monozygous or monochorionic	IIb	B	41
Monochorionic twins are at increased risk for adverse outcome.			
No prosospective data on whether increased surveillance improves outcome			
Iron and folate supplementation from the second trimester	IIb	B	6
Screening for hypertension	IIa	B	61
Conflicting evidence of the value of screening for gestational diabetes	IIa	B	62, 63
Nuchal translucency measurement of each fetus identifies fetuses at risk for trisomy 21, cardiothoracic abnormalities, and twin–twin transfusion syndrome	III	B	74
Routine anomaly ultrasound scan at 18 to 20 weeks	III	B	44
Conjoined twins:	III	B	87
• Careful ultrasonographic evaluation of anatomy			
• Interdisciplinary discussion of therapeutic options			
Vigilance for early symptoms of preterm labor; prompt self-referral if it is suspected	Ib	A	101
Possible ultrasound assessment of cervical changes and fetal fibronectin as part of preterm delivery screening	IIa	B	91
Prenatal corticosteroids preterm birth before 34 weeks is possible	Ia	A	107
No evidence that hospitalization to prevent preterm labor and delivery is effective	Ia	A	105
No evidence that prophylactic cervical cerclage is effective to prevent preterm labor and delivery	Ia	A	103
Regular fetal ultrasound assessment of growth and umbilical artery Doppler	Ib	A	111
Hospitalization at the woman's request or if complications are detected	Ia	A	105
Consider therapeutic amniocentesis (repeated if necessary) for extreme hydramnios and maternal distress.	IIb	B	46
Prenatal education about the possible modes of delivery, analgesia, and care in labor	IV	C	112
Labor and Delivery			
Hospital delivery	III	B	113
Experienced obstetrician and other health professionals	III	B	113
Await spontaneous labor if no complications occur.	Ia	A	119
Pediatrician neonatal nurse, and anesthetist available at delivery, with one pediatrician per infant present if preterm or operative delivery or fetal problems are anticipated	–	GPP	–
Continuous monitoring of all fetuses during labor	III	B	113
IV access	–	GPP	–
Epidural analgesia recommended	III	B	113
Aim for vaginal delivery unless the leading twin has a nonlongitudinal lie.	III	B	126,134
Some advocate elective cesarean delivery if the first twin is not cephalic.	III	B	126,134
Vaginal delivery of the first twin, if appropriate	III	B	134
Synthetic oxytocin infusion for uterine inertia, especially after the first twin is delivered	–	GPP	–

SUMMARY OF MANAGEMENT OPTIONS
Multiple Pregnancy *(Continued)*

Management Options	Quality of Evidence	Strength of Recommendation	References
If the second twin has a longitudinal lie, amniotomy and delivery	III	B	145
If an infant has a nonlongitudinal lie, convert to a longitudinal lie by external version or internal podalic version.	III	B	145
Prophylactic oxytocin infusion after delivery to reduce the risk of postpartum hemorrhage	Ia	A	147
Some advocate elective cesarean delivery for triplets and higher-order births	IIb	B	127
Postnatal			
Extra support while in the hospital to assist with infant care	–	GPP	–
Offer longer in-patient stay.	–	GPP	–
Arrange support at home.	–	GPP	–
Provide adequate contraceptive advice.	–	GPP	–

REFERENCES

1. Little J, Thompson B: Descriptive epidemiology. In MacGillivray I, Campbell D, Thomson B (eds): Twinning & Twins. Chichester, Wiley, 1988, pp 37–66.
2. Vandekerckhove F, Dhont M, Thiery M, Derom R: Screening for multiple pregnancy. Acta Genet Med Gemellol 1984;33: 571–574.
3. Sebire N, Thornton S, Hughes K, et al: The prevalence and consequence of missed abortion in twin pregnancies at 10–14 weeks of gestation. BJOG 1997;104:847–848.
4. Landy HJ, Weiner S, Corson SL, et al: The 'vanishing twin': Ultrasonographic assessment of fetal disappearance in the first trimester. Am J Obstet Gynecol 1986;155:14–19.
5. Krafft A, Breymann C, Streich J, et al: Hemoglobin concentration in multiple versus singleton pregnancies: Retrospective evidence for physiology not pathology. Eur J Obstet Reprod Biol 2001;99:184–187.
6. Blickstein I, Goldschmit R, Lurie S: Hemoglobin levels during twin vs singleton pregnancies: Parity makes a difference. J Reprod Med 1995;40:47–50.
7. Patel N, Barrie W, Campbell D, et al: Scottish twin study 1983: Preliminary report. Glasgow, University of Glasgow, Departments of Child Health and Obstetrics, Social Paediatric and Obstetric Research Unit, 1983.
8. Kogan M, Alexander G, Kotelchuck M, et al: Trends in twin birth outcomes and prenatal care utilization in the United States, 1981–1997. JAMA 2000;284:335–341.
9. Chan A, Scott J, McCaul K, Keane R: Pregnancy Outcomes in South Australia in 1995. Adelaide, Pregnancy Outcome Unit, South Australian Health Commission, 1996.
10. Campbell D, MacGillivray L: Pre-eclampsia in twin pregnancies: Incidence and outcome. Hypertens Pregnancy 1999;18:197–207.
11. Monde-Agudelo A, Belizan J, Lindmark G: Maternal morbidity and mortality associated with multiple gestations. Obstet Gynecol 2000;95(6 Pt 1):899–904.
12. Macfarlane AJ, Price, FV, Daw EG: Antenatal care. In Botting BJ, Macfarlane AJ, Price FV (eds): Three, Four and More: A Study of Triplet and Higher Order Births. London, HMSO, 1990.
13. MacGillivray I, Campbell D: Management of twin pregnancies. In MacGillivray I, Campbell D (eds): Twinning and Twins. Chichester, John Wiley, 1988, pp 111–139.
14. McMullan P, Norman R, Marivate M: Pregnancy-induced hypertension in twin pregnancy. BJOG 1984;91:240–243.
15. Maxwell C, Liebermann E, Norton M, et al: Relationship of twin zygosity and risk of pre-eclampsia. Am J Obstet Gynecol 2001;185:819–821.
16. Savvidou M, Kartanastasi E, Skentou C, et al: Twin chorionicity and pre eclampsia. Ultrasound Obstet Gynecol 1996;18: 228–231.
17. Ananth C, Demissie K, Smulian J, Vintzileos A: Placental previa in singleton and twin births in the United States, 1989 through 1998: A comparison of risk factor profiles and associated conditions. Am J Obstet Gynecol 2003;188:275–281.
18. Ananth C, Smulian J, Vintzileos A, Knuppel R: Placental abruption among singleton and twin births in the United States: Risk factor profiles. Am J Epidemiol 2001;153:771–778.
19. Keith L, Ellis R, Berger G, et al: The Northwestern University multihospital twin study: A description of 588 twin pregnancies and associated pregnancy loss, 1971 to 1975. Am J Obstet Gynecol 1980;138:781–789.
20. Roberts C, Phipps H, Nassar N, Raynes-Greenow C: The management of twin births in Australia and New Zealand. Aust N Z J Obstet Gynaecol 2003;43(5):397.
21. Lipitz S, Frenkel Y, Watts C, et al: High-order multifetal gestation: Management and Outcome. Obstet Gynecol 1990;76: 215–218.
22. Thorpe K, Golding J, MacGillivray I, Greenwood R: Comparison of prevalence of depression in mothers of twins and mothers of singletons. BMJ 1991;302:875–878.
23. Hawrylyshyn PA, Barkin M, Bernstein A, et al: Twin pregnancies: A continuing perinatal challenge. Obstet Gynecol 1982;59:463–466.
24. Hartikainen-Sorri A, Kauppila A, Tuimala R, Koivisto M: Factors related to an improved outcome for twins. Acta Obstet Gynecol Scand 1983;62:23–25.
25. Bryan E: Educating families, before, during and after multiple birth. Semin Neonatol 2002;7:241–246.

26. Crowther C: Perinatal mortality in twin pregnancy: A review of 799 twin pregnancies. S Afr Med J 1987;71:73–74.
27. Doherty J: Perinatal mortality in twins, Australia, 1973–1980: 1. Acta Genet Med Gemellol 1988;37:313–319.
28. Fowler M, Kleinman J, Kiely J, Kessel S: Double jeopardy: Twin infant mortality in the United States, 1983 and 1984. Am J Obstet Gynecol 1991;165:15–22.
29. Rydhstroem H, Heraib F: Gestational duration, and fetal and infant mortality for twins vs singletons. Twins Res 2001;4:227–231.
30. Kleinman J, Fowler M, Kessel S: Comparison of infant mortality among twins and singletons: United States 1960–1983. Am J Epidemiol 1991;133:133–143.
31. Dodd J, Robinson J, Crowther C, Chan A: Stillbirth and neonatal outcomes in South Australia, 1991–2000. Am J Obstet Gynecol 2003;189(6):1731–1736.
32. Northern Regional Perinatal Mortality Survey Steering Group. Twin Res 1998;1:189–195.
33. Dube J, Dodds L, Armston B: Does chorionicity or zygosity predict adverse perinatal outcomes in twins? Am J Obstet Gynecol 2002;186:579–583.
34. Baghdadi S, Gee H, Whittle M, Khan K: Twin pregnancy outcome and chorionicity. Acta Obstet Gynecol Scand 2003;82:18–21.
35. Barrs V, Benacerraf B, Firgoletto F: Ultrasonographic determination of chorion type in twi gestation. Obstet Gynecol 1985;66:779–783.
36. Kauppila A, Jouppila A, Koivisto M, et al: Twin pregnancy: A clinical study of 335 cases. Acta Obstet Gynecol Scand 1975;44 (suppl):5–8.
37. Houlton M, Marivate M, Philpott R: The prediction of fetal growth retardation in twin pregnancy. BJOG 1981;88:264–273.
38. Crowther C, Hamilton R: Triplet pregnancy: A 10 year review of 105 cases at Harare Maternity Hospital, Zimbabwe. Acta Genet Med Gemellol 1989;38:271–278.
39. Sassoon D, Castro L, Davis J, Hobel C: Perinatal outcome in triplet versus twin gestations. Obstet Gynecol 1990;75:817–820.
40. Jeffrey RL, Bowes WA, Delaney JJ: Role of bed rest in twin gestation. Obstet Gynecol 1974;43:822–826.
41. Minakami H, Honma Y, Matsubara S, et al: Effects of placental chorionicity on outcome in twin pregnancies: A cohort study. J Reprod Med 1999;44:595–600.
42. Beeby P, Vaughan H: Twin pregnancy outcome and choronicity. Paper presented at the Perinatal Society of Australia and New Zealand 7th Annual Congress, Hobart, Australia, March 2003.
43. Lynch A, McDuffie RC, Murphy J, et al: The contribution of assisted conception, chorionicity and other risk factors to very low birthweight in a twin cohort. BJOG 2003;110:405–410.
44. Edwards M, Ellings J, Newman R, Menard M: Predictive value of antepartum ultrasound examination for anomalies in twin gestations. Ultrasound Obstet Gynecol 1995;6:43–49.
45. Hanson J: Incidence of conjoining twinning. Lancet 1975;ii: 1257.
46. Hecher K, Plath H, Bregenzer T, et al: Endoscopic laser surgery versus serial amniocenteses in the treatment of severe twin-twin transfusion syndrome. Am J Obstet Gynecol 1999;180:717–724.
47. Cohen M, Kohl S, Rosenthal A: Fetal interlocking complicating twin gestation. Am J Obstet Gynecol 1965;91:407–411.
48. Petterson B, Nelson KB, Watson L, Stanley F: Twins, triplets, and cerebral palsy in births in Western Australia in the 1980s. BMJ 1993;307:1239–1243.
49. Yokoyama Y, Shimizu T, Hayakawa K: Prevalence of cerebral palsy in twins, triplets and quadruplets. Int J Epidemiol 1995;24: 943–948.
50. Pritchard J, MacDonald P, Grant N: Multi-fetal pregnancy. In Williams J, Pritchard J, MacDonald P (eds): Williams' Obstetrics, 17th ed. New York, Appleton-Century-Crofts, 1985, p 503.
51. Hurst T, Lancaster P: Assisted conception Australian and New Zealand 1999 and 2000. Sydney, Australian Institute of Health and Welfare, National Perinatal Statistic, 2001.
52. Bollen N, Camus M, Staessen C, et al: The incidence of multiple pregnancy after in vitro fertilization and embryo transfer, gamete or zygote intra fallopian transfer. Fertil Steril 1991;55:314–318.
53. Gerris J, Neuberg D, Mangelschots K, et al: Prevention of twin pregnancy after in-vitro fertilization or intracytoplasmic sperm injection based on strict embryo criteria: A prospective randomized clinical trial. Hum Reprod 1999;14:2581–2587.
54. Martikainen H, Tiitinen A, Tomas C, et al: One versus two embryo transfer after IVF and ICSI: A randomised study. Hum Reprod 2001;16:1900–1903.
55. Vauthier-Brouzes D, Lefebvre G, Lesourd S, et al: How many embryos should be transferred in invitro fertilization? A prospective randomized study. Fertil Steril 1994;62:339–342.
56. Dare M, Crowther C, Dodd J, Norman RJ: Single or multiple embryo transfer following in vitro fertilization (IVF) for improved pregnancy outcome: A systematic review of the literature. Aust N Z J Obstet Gynaecol 2004;44(4):283–291.
57. Lumley J, Watson L, Watson M, Bower C: Periconceptional supplementation with folate and/or multivitamins for preventing neural tube defects (Cochrane Review). In Cochrane Library, Issue 4, 2003. Chichester, UK, John Wiley & Sons.
58. Ellings J, Newman J, Hulsey T, et al: Reduction in very low birth weight deliveries and perinatal mortality in a specialized, multidisciplinary twin clinic. Obstet Gynecol 1993;81:387–388.
59. Newman R, Ellings J: Antepartum management of the multiple gestation: The case for specialized care. Semin Perinatol 1995;19:387–403.
60. Ruiz R, Brown C, Peters M, Johnston A: Specialized care for twin gestations: Improving newborn outcomes and reducing costs. J Ostet Gynecol Neonatal Nurs 2001;30:52–60.
61. Santema J, Koppelaar I, Wallenburg H: Hypertensive disorders in twin pregnancy. Eur J Obstet Gynecol Reprod Biol 1995;58:9–13.
62. Henderson C, Scarpelli S, LaRosa D, Divon M: Assessing the risk of gestational diabetes in twin gestation. J Natl Med Assoc 1995;87:757–758.
63. Schwartz D, Daoud Y, Zazula P, et al: Gestational diabetes mellitus: Metabolic and blood glucose parameters in singleton versus twin pregnancies. Am J Obstet Gynecol 1999;181:912–914.
64. Mahony BS, Filly RA, Callen PW: Amnionicity and chorionicity in twin pregnancies: Prediction using ultrasound. Radiology 1985;155:205–209.
65. D'Alton M, Mercer B: Antepartum management of twin gestation: Ultrasound. Clin Obstet Gynecol 1990;33:42–51.
66. Sepulveda W: Chorionicity determination in twin pregnancies: Double trouble? Ultrasound Obstet Gynecol 1997;10:79–81.
67. Stagiannis KD, Sepulveda W, Southwell D, et al: Ultrasonographic measurement of the dividing membrane in twin pregnancy during the second and third trimesters: A reproducibility study. Am J Obstet Gynecol 1995;173:1546–1550.
68. Winn HN, Gabrielli S, Reece EA, et al: Ultrasonographic criteria for the prenatal diagnosis of placental chorionicity in twin gestations. Am J Obstet Gynecol 1989;161(6 Pt 1):1540–1542.
69. Bessies R, Papiernik E: Echographic imagery of amniotic membranes in twin pregnancies. In Gedda L, Parisi L (eds): Twin Research 3: Twin Biology and Multiple Pregnancy. New York, Alan R Liss, 1981, pp 183–187.
70. Sepulveda W, Sebire N, Hughes K, et al: The Lambda sign at 10–14 weeks of pregnancy as a predictor of chorionicity in twin pregnancies. Ultrasound Obstet Gynecol 1996;7:421–423.
71. Finberg HJ: The 'twin peak' sign: Reliable evidence of dichorionic twinning. J Ultrasound Med 1992;11:571–577.
72. Kurtz AB, Wapner RJ, Mata J, et al: Twin pregnancies: Accuracy of first-trimester abdominal US in predicting chorionicity and amnionicity. Radiology 1992;185:759–762.
73. Monteagudo A, Timor Tritsch IE, Sharma S: Early and simple determination of chorionic and amniotic type in multifetal-

gestations in the first fourteen weeks by high-frequency transvaginal ultrasonography. Am J Obstet Gynecol 1994;170:824–829.
74. Sebire N, Snijders R, Abraha H, et al: Screening trisomy 21 in twin pregnancies by maternal age and fetal nuchal translucency thickness at 10–14 weeks of gestation. BJOG 1996;103:999–1003.
75. Nicolaides K, Sebire N, Snijders R: The 11–14 week scan: The diagnosis of fetal abnormalities. New York, Parthenon, 1999.
76. Evans MI, Dommergues M, Timor Tritsch I, et al: Transabdominal versus transcervical and transvaginal multifetal pregnancy reduction: International collaborative experience of more than one thousand cases. Am J Obstet Gynecol 1994;170:902–909.
77. Donner C, de Maertelaer V, Rodesch F: Multifetal pregnancy reduction: Comparison of obstetrical results with spontaneous twin gestation. Eur J Obstet Gynecol Reprod Biol 1992;44:181–184.
78. Groutz A, Yovel I, Yaron Y, et al: Pregnancy outcome after multifetal pregnancy reduction to twins compared with spontaneously conceived twins. Hum Reprod 1996;11:1334–1336.
79. Mansour R, Aboulghar M, Serour G, et al: Multifetal pregnancy reduction: Modification of the technique and analysis of the outcome. Fertil Steril 1999;71:380–384.
80. Porreco RP, Burke S, Hendrix ML: Multifetal reduction of triplets and pregnancy outcome. Obstet Gynecol 1991;78(No. 3, Part 1):335–339.
81. Boulot P, Hedon B, Pelliccia G, et al: Multifetal pregnancy reduction: A consecutive series of 61 cases. BJOG 1993;100:63–68.
82. Lipitz S, Reichman B, Uval J, et al: A prospective comparison of the outcome of triplet pregnancies managed expectantly or by multifetal reduction to twins. Am J Obstet Gynecol 1994;170:874–879.
83. Dodd J, Crowther C: Multifetal pregnancy reduction: Systematic review. Fertil Steril 2003 (in press).
84. Dodd J, Crowther C: Reduction of the number of fetuses for women with triplet and higher order multiple pregnancies (Cochrane Review). In Cochrane Library, Issue 4, 2003. Chichester, UK, John Wiley & Sons.
85. Persson P-H, Grennert L, Gennser G, Kullander S: On improved outcome of twin pregnancies. Acta Obstet Gynecol Scand 1979;58:3–7.
86. Allen S, Gray L, Frentzen B, Cruz A: Ultrasonographic diagnosis of congenital anomalies in twins. Am J Obstet Gynecol 1991;165:1056–1060.
87. Barth R, Filly R, Goldberg J, et al: Conjoined twins: Prenatal diagnosis and assessment of associated malformations. Radiology 1990;177:201–207.
88. Houlton M, Marivate M, Philpott R: Factors associated with preterm labour and changes in the cervix before labour in twin pregnancy. BJOG 1982;89:190–194.
89. Neilson J, Verkuyl D, Crowther C, Bannerman C: Preterm labor in twin pregnancies: Prediction by cervical assessment. Obstet Gynecol 1988;72:719–723.
90. Newman R, Godsy R, Ellings J, et al: Quantification of cervical change: Relationship to preterm delivery in the multifetal gestation. Am J Obstet Gynecol 1991;165:264–271.
91. Goldenberg R, Iams J, Miodovnik M, et al: The preterm prediction study: Risk factors in twin gestations. Am J Obstet Gynecol 1996;175:1047–1053.
92. Wennerholm U, Holm BN, Mattsby-Baltzer I, et al: Fetal fibronectin, endotoxin, bacterial vaginosis and cervical length as predictors of preterm birth and neonatal morbidity in twin pregnancies. BJOG 1997;104:1398–1404.
93. Maymon R, Merman A, Jauniauz E, et al: Transvaginal sonographic assessment of cervical length changes during triplet gestation. Hum Reprod 2001;16:956–960.
94. Skentou C, Souka A, To M, et al: Prediction of preterm delivery in twins by cervical assessment at 23 weeks. Ultrasound Obstet Gynecol 2001;B17:7–10.
95. Crowther C, Chalmers I: Bed rest and hospitalization during pregnancy. In Chalmers I, Enkin M, Keirse M (eds): Effective care in pregnancy and childbirth. Oxford, Oxford University Press, 1989:624–632.
96. Crowther C, Neilson J, Verkuyl D, et al: Preterm labour in twin pregnancies: Can it be prevented by hospital admission? BJOG 1989;96:850–853.
97. Weekes A, Menzies D, de Boer C: The relative efficacy of bed rest, cervical suture, and no treatment in the management of twin pregnancies. BJOG 1977;84:161–164.
98. Sinha D, Nandakumar V, Brough A, Beebeejaun M: Relative cervical incompetence in twin pregnancy: Assessment and efficacy of cervical suture. Acta Genet Med Gemellol 1979;78:322–331.
99. Tambi Raja R, Atputharajah V, Salmon Y: Prevention of prematurity in twins. Aust N Z J Obstet Gynaecol 1978;18:179.
100. Ashworth M, Spooner S, Verkuyl D, et al: Failure to prevent preterm labour and delivery in twin pregnancy using prophylactic oral salbutamol. BJOG 1990;97:878–882.
101. Knuppel R, Lake M, Watson D, et al: Preventing preterm birth in twin gestation: Home uterine activity monitoring and perinatal nursing support. Obstet Gynecol 1990;76:24S–27S.
102. Dyson D, Danbe K, Bamber J, et al: A multicentre randomised trial of three levels of surveillance in patients at risk for preterm labor: Twin gestation subgroup analysis. Am J Obstet Gynecol 1997;176(SPO Abstract S18, A399):S118.
103. Grant A: Cervical cerclage to prolong pregnancy. In Chalmers I, Enkin MW, Keirse M (eds): Effective Care in Pregnancy and Childbirth. Oxford, Oxford University Press, 1989, pp 633–645.
104. Keirse M, Grant A, King J: Preterm labour. In Chalmers I, Enkin MW, Keirse M (eds): Effective Care in Pregnancy and Childbirth. Oxford, Oxford University Press, 1989, pp 694–749.
105. Crowther C: Hospitalization for bed rest in multiple pregnancy (Cochrane Review). In Cochrane Library, Issue 4, 2003. Chichester, UK, John Wiley & Sons.
106. Crowther C, Verkuyl D, Ashworth M, et al: The effects of hospitalization for bed rest on duration of gestation, fetal growth and neonatal morbidity in triplet pregnancy. Acta Genet Med Gemellol 1991;40:63–68.
107. Crowley P: Antenatal corticosteriods prior to preterm birth (Cochrane Review). In Cochrane Library, Issue 4, 2003. Chichester, UK, John Wiley & Sons.
108. Neilson J, Alfirevic Z: Doppler ultrasound for fetal assessment in high risk pregnancies (Cochrane Review). In Cochrane Library, Issue 4, 2003. Chichester, UK, John Wiley & Sons.
109. Omtzigt A: Clinical value of umbilical Doppler velocimetry: A randomised controlled trial. Utrecht, University of Utrecht, 1990.
110. Johnstone F, Prescott R, Hoskins P, et al: The effect of introduction of umbilical Doppler recordings to obstetric practice. BJOG 1993;100:733–741.
111. Giles W, Bisits A, O'Callaghan S, et al: The Doppler assessment in multiple pregnancy: Randomised controlled trial of ultrasound biometry versus umbilical artery Doppler ultrasound and biometry in twin pregnancy. BJOG 2003;110: 593–597.
112. Hofmeyr G, Drakely A: Delivery of twins. Baillieres Clin Ostet Gynaecol 1998;12:91–108.
113. Osbourne G, Patel N: An assessment of perinatal mortality in twin pregnancies in Dundee. Acta Genet Med Gemellol 1985;34:193–199.
114. Luke B, Minogue J, Witter F, et al: The ideal twin pregnancy: Patterns of weight gain, discordance, and length of gestation. Am J Obstet Gynecol 1993;169:588–597.
115. Cincotta R, Flenady V, Hockey R, King J: Mortality of twins and singletons by gestational age: A varying coefficient approach. In 5th Annual Congress, Perinatal Society of Australia and New Zealand, Canberra, March 13–16, 2001, p 22.

116. Minakami H, Sato I: Reestimating date of delivery in multifetal pregnancies. JAMA 1996;275:1432–1434.
117. Cheung YB, Yip P, Karlberg J: Mortality of twins and singletons by gestational age: A varying-coefficient approach. Am J Epidemiol 2000;152:1107–1116.
118. Hartley R, Emanuel I, Hitti J: Perinatal mortality and neonatal morbidity rates among twin pairs at different gestational ages: Optimal delivery timing at 37–38 weeks' gestation. Am J Obstet Gynecol 2001;184:451–458.
119. Dodd J, Crowther C: Elective delivery from 37 weeks gestation in women with a twin pregnancy (Cochrane Review). In Cochrane Library, Issue 4, 2003. Chichester, UK, John Wiley & Sons.
120. Suzuki S, Otsubo Y, Sawa R, et al: Clinical trial of induction of labor versus expectant management in twin pregnancy. Gynecol Obstet Invest 2000;49(1): 24–27.
121. Hogle K, Hutton E, McBrien K, et al: Cesarean delivery for twins: A systematic review and meta-analysis. Am J Obstet Gynecol 2003;188:220–227.
122. Newman R, Hamer C, Miller C: Outpatient triplet management: A contemporary review. Am J Obstet Gynecol 1989;161: 547–555.
123. Lipitz S, Reichman B, Paret G, et al: The improving outcome of triplet pregnancies. Am J Obstet Gynecol 1989;161:1279–1284.
124. Collins M, Bleyl J: Seventy-one quadruplet pregnancies: Management and outcome. Am J Obst Gynecol 1990;162: 1384–1392.
125. Petrikovsy B, Vintzilees A: Management and outcome of multiple pregnancy of high fetal order: Literature review. Obstet Gynecol Surv 1989;44:578–584.
126. Chasen S, Madden A, Chervenak F: Caesarean delivery of twins and neonatal respiratory disorders. Am J Obstet Gynecol 1999;181:1052–1056.
127. Wildschut H, van Roosmalen J, van Leeuwen E, Keirse M: Planned abdominal compared with planned vaginal birth in triplet pregnancies. BJOG 1995;102:292–296.
128. Crowther C: Caesarean delivery for the second twin (Cochrane Review). In Cochrane Library, Issue 4, 2003. Chichester, UK, John Wiley & Sons.
129. Rabinovici J, Barkai G, Reichman.B, et al: Randomised management of the second non-vortex twin: Vaginal or caesarean. Am J Obstet Gynecol 1987;156:52–56.
130. Rayburn W, Lavin J, Miodovnik M, Varner M: Multiple gestation: Time interval between delivery of the first and second twins. Obstet Gynecol 1984;63:502–506.
131. Chervenak F, Johnson R, Youcha S, et al: Intrapartun Management of twin gestation. Obstet Gynecol 1985;65:119–124.
132. Cetrulo C: The controversy of mode of delivery in twins: The intrapartum management of twin gestation. Semin Perinatol 1986;10:39–40.
133. Hutton E, Hannah M, Barrett J: Use of external cephalic version for breech pregnancy and mode of delivery for breech and twin pregnancy: A survey of Canadian practitioners. J Obstet Gynaecol Can 2002;24:804–810.
134. Morales WJ, O'Brien WF, Knuppel RA, et al: The effect of mode of delivery on the risk of intraventricular hemorrhage in nondiscordant twin gestations under 1500g. Obstet Gynecol 1989;73:107–110.
135. Hays P, Smeltzer J: Multiple gestation. Clin Obstet Gynecol 1986;29:264–285.
136. Barrett JM, Staggs SM, van Hooydonk JE, et al: The effect of type of delivery upon neonatal outcome in premature twins. Am J Obstet Gynecol 1982;143:360–365.
137. Acker D, Lieberman M, Holbrook H, et al: Delivery of the second twin. Obstet Gynecol 1982;59:710–711.
138. Chervenak F, Youcha S, Johnson R, et al: Intrapartum external version of the second twin. Obstet Gynecol 1983;62:160–164.
139. Blickstein I, Swarts-Shoran Z, Lautz M, Borenstein R: Vaginal delivery of the second twin in breech presentation. Obstet Gynecol 1987;69:774–776.
140. Gocke SE, Nageotte MP, Garite T, et al: Management of the nonvertex second twin: Primary caesarean section, external version, or primary breech extraction. Am J Obstet Gynecol 1989;161:111–114.
141. Adam C, Allen AC, Baskett TF: Twin delivery: Influence of the presentation and method of delivery on the second twin. Am J Obstet Gynecol 1991;165:23–27.
142. Fishman A, Grubb DK, Kovacs BW: Vaginal delivery of the nonvertex second twin. Am J Obstet Gynecol 1993;168:861–864.
143. Rabinovici J, Barkai G, Reichman.B, et al: Internal poldalic version with unruptured membranes for the second twin in transverse lie. Obstet Gynecol 1988;71:428–430.
144. Doyle LW, Hughes CD, Guaran RL, et al: Mode of delivery of preterm twins. Aust N Z J Obstet Gynaecol 1988;28:25–28.
145. Kaplan B, Peled Y, Rabinerson D, et al: A successful external version of B-twin after birth of A-twin for vortex: Non vortex twins. Eur J Obstet Gynecol Reprod Biol 1995;58:157–160.
146. Wells SR, Thorp JM, Bowes WA: Management of the nonvertex second twin. Surgery 1991;172:383–385.
147. Leung T, Tam W, Leung T, et al: Effects of twin-to-twin delivery interval on umbilical cord blood gas in the second twins. BJOG 2002;109:1424–1425.
148. Prendiville W, Elbourne D, McDonald S: Active versus expectant management in the third stage of labour (Cochrane Review). In Cochrane Library, Issue 4, 2003. Chichester, UK, John Wiley & Sons.
149. Lipitz S, Reichman, B, Uval J, et al: A prospective comparison of the outcome of triplet pregnancies managed expectantly or by multifetal reduction to twins. Am J Obstet Gynecol 1994;170: 974–990.
150. Draper E, Maktelow B, Field D, James D: Prediction of survival for preterm births by weight and gestational age: Retrospective population based study. BMJ 1999;319:1093–1097.
151. Johnson A, Townshend P, Yudkin P, et al: Functional abilities at age 4 years of children born before 29 weeks gestation. BMJ 1993;306:1715–1718.
152. Bhutta A, Cleves M, Casey P, et al: Cognitive and behavioural outcomes of school-aged children who were born preterm: a meta-analysis. JAMA 2002;288:728–737.

CHAPTER 61

Screening for Spontaneous Preterm Labor and Delivery

Robert Ogle / Jonathan Hyett

INTRODUCTION

Preterm birth is associated with significant perinatal morbidity and mortality rates. Adverse outcomes from preterm birth include cerebral palsy, developmental delay, chronic lung disease, and visual and hearing loss. About 40% of preterm births follow idiopathic preterm labor, 35% follow preterm prelabor rupture of membranes, and the remainder are iatrogenic because of obstetric or medical indications.[1] The early detection of preterm labor or preterm rupture of membranes in traditional antenatal care is often problematic because symptoms or signs may vary only a little from the normal physiologic symptoms and signs of pregnancy. The criteria for diagnosis of preterm labor, defined by the onset of increasingly frequent and painful uterine contractions with progressive effacement and dilation of the cervix, can be assessed most accurately once contractions occur at least once every 10 minutes, there is 80% cervical effacement, and the cervix is at least 3 cm dilated.[2,3] However, the patient may frequently present with relatively mild symptoms and signs suggestive of labor, which may be features of normal pregnancy.[4] Using lower thresholds for contraction frequency and cervical change will therefore affect the sensitivity and positive predictive value of clinical assessment for detection of preterm labor.

Prediction of preterm birth would ideally involve a screening test with high sensitivity and high negative predictive value. It should also enable effective intervention if the test gives a positive result. The screening tools and interventions that are currently available have not enabled obstetricians to decrease the incidence of preterm birth and do not satisfy the requirements of an optimal screening test. However, they may allow time for transfer of a pregnancy at risk to an appropriate tertiary referral center, as well as the administration of glucocorticoids to enhance fetal lung maturity and antibiotic prophylaxis to reduce the risk of neonatal sepsis.

A wide variety of screening tools have been evaluated in research, and those most extensively evaluated fall into four groups:

- Monitoring of uterine activity
- Assessment of cervical length
- Measurement of cervical fetal fibronectin
- Presence of bacterial vaginosis in early pregnancy

Other forms of screening have been looked at in small series and include estimation of estriol, interleukins, ferritin, and corticotropin-releasing hormone, but findings in relation to these measures have not been consistently associated with preterm labor. This chapter will review the four major areas of screening and evaluate their effectiveness in screening for preterm labor and preterm rupture of membranes.

MONITORING UTERINE ACTIVITY

If the onset of increasingly frequent and painful uterine contractions precedes effacement and dilation of the cervix, then assessment of uterine activity may identify pregnancies at risk of preterm delivery at an early stage of preterm labor, allowing effective intervention.

The simplest method for assessing uterine activity relies on teaching the patient to palpate and record her own contractions. Increased uterine activity appears to precede a clinical diagnosis of preterm labor by less than 24 hours.[5] Most obstetricians using this technique would therefore advise the patient to monitor her own contractions for an hour twice a day. Although this technique has the advantage that it does not involve any expensive equipment, it is completely subjective and has been shown to have poor sensitivity, with 89% of women palpating less than 50% of their contractions.[6] In addition, the process of monitoring is time-consuming, is generally limited to high risk groups, and potentially increases patient anxiety, which is itself associated with an increased risk of preterm delivery. This issue applies equally to other forms of uterine activity monitoring; indeed, these techniques require intense patient support through a process of education, analysis of results, and encouragement to continue monitoring on a regular basis, and it has frequently been suggested that it is this support that leads to an improvement in outcome more often than the process of monitoring itself.[7]

A more objective approach to uterine activity monitoring involves tocography, monitoring activity indirectly via a pressure transducer attached to a recording device and placed against the maternal abdominal wall. Early studies with this technique demonstrated that normal uterine activity increases with advancing gestation and is more pronounced at night. Uterine activity was monitored in a series of 109 low risk pregnancies that delivered at term; the 95th percentile was 1.3 contractions per hour at 21 to 24 weeks, 2.9 contractions per hour at 28 to 32 weeks, and 4.9 contractions per hour at 38 to 40 weeks.[8] It was found that 96% of recordings had less than 4 contractions per hour, and this threshold is often used to define a risk of preterm labor. An early case control study recruited 76 women at high risk of preterm labor to assess whether daily ambulatory home uterine monitoring could facilitate an early diagnosis of preterm labor and compared them to 76 matched control subjects.[9] The rates of threatened preterm labor were similar in the study and control groups (51% vs. 45%), but the cervix was significantly less effaced and dilated and there were no cases of ruptured membranes at the time of diagnosis in the monitored group. Consequently, all cases were considered suitable for long-term tocolytic therapy, and the preterm delivery rate was lower in the monitored group (22%) than in the control group (41%).

Although this initial series appeared to give encouraging results, there are several problems with this technique. Few studies have validated the instrumentation used in home monitoring. Those that have been performed suggest that patients are readily able to use the machines, that home machines appear to be of similar sensitivity as hospital machines, and that they detect more than 90% of contractions recorded by an intrauterine pressure catheter during normal term labor.[10–12] However, the sensitivity and specificity of the tocometer vary according to its position, the tension on the belt, and the thickness of the maternal abdominal wall, so the amplitude of the waveform seen on a tocogram cannot be related to the strength of uterine activity. Data interpretation is also subject to observational error, with one study finding that the results were interpreted reliably in only 70% of cases by a single observer.[13]

Perhaps more important, monitoring uterine activity does not lend itself to screening a low risk population; the equipment is relatively expensive, monitoring is time-consuming, studies need to be repeated regularly for many weeks of pregnancy, and data analysis requires a skilled health care professional. The technique is, therefore, suitable only for pregnancies deemed to be at high risk for preterm labor. Many randomized controlled trials have evaluated the use of home uterine activity monitoring in such high risk pregnancies. The first six series were reviewed in a meta-analysis that accessed previously unpublished data from the study groups and defined four outcome measures: incidence of preterm birth, incidence of preterm labor with a cervical dilation of over 2 cm at diagnosis, neonatal admission to intensive care, and mean birth weight.[7,14–19] The meta-analysis, presenting data from six studies on a total of only 697 pregnancies, concluded that home uterine monitoring in singleton pregnancies was associated with a 24% reduction in preterm birth, a 52% reduction in "late presentation" with cervical dilation greater than 2 cm, and a significant mean increase in birth weight of 126 g. There was, however, no difference in the admission rate to neonatal intensive care.[20] This analysis was controversial, however, as a previous analysis had suggested serious methodologic deficiencies in some of the studies, had found no significant benefit of monitoring, and concluded that it should not be used clinically without further validation.[21]

One of the criticisms of early trials of home uterine monitoring was that the increased level of support that the monitored patients received may have been responsible for any improvement seen in the outcome. Three trials addressed this possibility, one using a sham monitor but offering all patients nursing support, the second offering monitoring without any nursing support, and the third randomly assigning patients to both nursing support and home monitoring.[22–24] The first of these studies randomized 1992 women, 1165 of whom used home monitoring devices, but only 842 (72.3%) of them completed the study, suggesting that there may be difficulties with compliance when home monitoring devices are used for wider indications. The study concluded that there was no evidence that either home uterine activity monitoring or daily nursing contact improved early diagnosis of preterm labor or reduced the rates of preterm birth or neonatal morbidity.[22] In contrast, the second, smaller study (n = 218), which also had a significant dropout rate in monitoring (15% did not complete the monitoring), found that the diagnosis of preterm labor could be made significantly earlier and that this affected the outcome, measured in terms of the interval between the diagnosis of labor and delivery, and was independent of nursing support.[23] However, the third study, which randomly assigned 2422 women to combinations of nurse contact and home monitoring concluded that neither daily contact nor home monitoring improved pregnancy outcome beyond that seen with weekly nurse contact.[24]

Because little evidence indicates that home uterine monitoring is a useful screening tool for preterm labor, the number of studies examining its role has dropped significantly over the last few years. During this time, interest in other markers for preterm delivery, such as sonographic assessment of the cervix and measurement of fetal fibronectin has grown. Consequently, the recent data sets that review home uterine monitoring are often acquired in trials primarily designed to assess other screening tests or a combination of screening tools.

Although most of the original trials defined preterm delivery before 37 weeks as their end point, most recent data sets are concerned with delivery before 34 weeks' gestation. Morrison and associates assessed 85 asymptomatic women at high risk of preterm labor with both serial fetal fibronectin measurement and home uterine monitoring.[25] They reported that 14 (16.5%) of the 85 women delivered before 34 weeks and the sensitivity and specificity of fetal fibronectin and home uterine monitoring alone were 43% and 89% (fetal fibronectin) and 64% and 85% (home uterine monitoring alone). When the two tests were combined, the specificity improved substantially but the sensitivity of a double positive result was poor (3 of 14 cases: 21%), so they are not usefully combined in this manner.

Most recently, home uterine monitoring was used to assess the risk of preterm labor in 306 high risk singleton pregnancies.[26] These patients were also seen regularly at the hospital for serial assessment of fetal fibronectin and for sonographic assessment of the cervix. All three investigations had a low sensitivity and poor positive predictive value for preterm delivery. The authors concluded that although the likelihood of preterm delivery is associated with an increased frequency of uterine contractions, assessment is not clinically useful for predicting preterm delivery.

CERVICAL SCREENING

Ultrasound assessment of the cervix in normal pregnancy shows that cervical effacement starts around 32 weeks. In pregnancies affected by preterm labor, the process may begin between 16 and 24 weeks. Effacement begins at the internal os and can be visualized as cervical shortening and funneling, a process that occurs before dilation of the external cervical os. Ultrasound assessment potentially allows changes other than cervical dilation to be assessed with a higher degree of accuracy, and using a transvaginal route, assessment is possible in virtually all cases.[27,28]

Ultrasound assessment of the cervix has been used in a variety of situations to improve the accuracy of a diagnosis of preterm labor and to predict the likelihood of a woman going into preterm labor. Screening has been studied in both high and low risk populations, and because the prevalence of preterm labor varies in these groups, these data sets are considered separately. A variety of techniques have been used to assess the cervix with ultrasound, and the multitude of studies describing the use of this test are heterogeneous in design, assessing the cervix at different stages of pregnancy, using either single or serial examinations, and choosing varying gestational ages at delivery to report the sensitivity and specificity of the test. A recent meta-analysis of antenatal transvaginal ultrasound assessment of the cervix identified 46 studies involving 31,577 pregnancies describing the effectiveness of this screening technique.[29] The review concluded that assessment of both cervical length and funneling, either alone or in combination, appeared to be useful in predicting spontaneous preterm birth in asymptomatic women, although there was less data available to assess the usefulness of this technique in symptomatic patients.

Ultrasound Measurement of the Cervix

One of the problems with comparison of studies measuring cervical change is a lack of standardization of the investigational technique. Most sonographers assess the cervix using a transvaginal scan, but transabdominal and transperineal routes can also be used. The cervix may be curved, and there may evidence of funneling; it is important to establish a method that allows for these differences in a consistent manner. The cervix is a dynamic structure, and measurements are affected by factors such as bladder filling and abdominal pressure.

A standardized technique for transvaginal cervical assessment has been described.[30] After the patient has emptied her bladder, a transvaginal probe (5–7 MHz) is introduced into the anterior fornix of the vagina, taking care to optimize image quality while avoiding undue pressure on the cervix that will distort anatomy. The whole length of the sonolucent endocervical mucosa is identified in a sagittal section, and the image is magnified so that this occupies 75% of the screen. Calipers are placed from the triangular echodense area marking the external os to the V-shaped indentation marking the internal os, and this distance is measured in a straight line. Three measurements are made over a period of 3 minutes to allow for any change in the state of the cervix, and the shortest measurement is reported. This technique allows clear views of the cervix and lower uterine segment and is acceptable to the majority of patients.

For women who do not find transvaginal sonography acceptable, or in circumstances in which vaginal examination ideally would be avoided (such as preterm prelabor rupture of membranes), alternative techniques such as transabdominal or transperineal/translabial assessment may be used. The limitations of these techniques, however, must be recognized. Transabdominal cervical assessment in 149 low risk singleton pregnancies at 23 weeks' gestation demonstrated that it was harder to visualize the cervix as it became shorter: a cervical length of less than 20 mm could be identified only 13% of the time, while a cervical length greater than 40 mm could be identified 51% of the time. In addition, the cervix was significantly easier to visualize when the bladder was fuller, but this state is associated with an artificial increase in the length of the cervix.[31] Visualization can also be difficult using a transperineal/translabial approach, and there is some evidence that the "operator learning curve" with this technique is substantial, making it a less appropriate test for screening.[32] Many authors have reported a poor correlation between transvaginal and transperineal/translabial techniques, making interpretation of data more difficult.[32–34] Cervical length in a low risk population is normally distributed, with a mean length at 23 weeks' gestation of 35 to 38 mm; the 10th and 90th percentiles are approximately 25 mm and 45 mm, respectively.

Other cervical parameters have also been investigated. In many circumstances, a sagittal section of the entire length of the endocervical canal shows that it is in fact curved, and direct measurement from the internal to external os does not take this curvature into account. In these circumstances, cervical length would be undermeasured, and there would be a potential for false-positive screening results. To and associates investigated this in a prospective series of 300 singleton pregnancies undergoing transvaginal cervical assessment at 23 weeks' gestation.[35] A curved cervix was seen in 48% of patients: in 51% of those with cervical length of 26 mm or more, 25% of those with cervical length of 16 to 25 mm, but 0% in those with cervical length of 15 mm or less. This group had previously defined that pregnancies with cervical length less than 15 mm should be considered to have a positive test result, and in these circumstances, the effect of cervical curvature would not be important.

Early studies of transvaginal cervical screening suggested that cervical funneling could also be reported, and that this finding had an independent predictive role for preterm delivery.[36] Funneling can be assessed in a number of ways; subjectively, describing presence or absence, by measuring dilation at the internal os and the length of the endocervical canal that is involved, or by combining these features to give a cervical index.[37] In a series of 469 high risk pregnancies assessed longitudinally, funneling, determined in terms of width and length and the percentage of the cervix involved, was not found to give any additional information about risk if the cervical length was less than a screen-positive cutoff of 25 mm.[38] This was also the case in a series of 6819 low risk pregnancies screened at 23 weeks' gestation, in which funneling was defined as being present if the width at the internal cervical os was greater than 5 mm.[39] In this series, funneling appeared to be almost universally associated with a short cervix, and there was no apparent advantage to its inclusion as a screening criterion.

Cervical Assessment in Asymptomatic Patients at High Risk of Preterm Labor

Women with a previous history of preterm labor or preterm prelabor rupture of membranes together with women who have previously had cervical surgery or have a known uterine anomaly are considered to be at high risk of preterm labor. Other inclusion criteria have included extreme maternal age, in utero exposure to diethylstilbestrol, and maternal genetic anomalies such as Elhers-Danlos syndrome. The rationale for screening in this group is to allow early intervention that would prevent the onset of preterm delivery of preterm prelabor rupture of membranes.[40–42] It is not currently clear what the optimum gestation for screening is, what cervical cutoff should be used to define a screen-positive group, or whether serial scans would be more appropriate than a single scan.

There is a strong association between a short cervix and preterm delivery in high risk pregnancies. Cook and associates showed that cervical length less than 21 mm at less than 20 weeks' gestation was associated with 95% delivery by 34 weeks' gestation.[43] Guzman and associates examined 469 women at high risk of preterm delivery with singleton pregnancies serially (mean of three occasions) between 15 and 24 weeks' gestation.[37] The cervix was 25 mm or less in length in 23.4% of women, including 76% of those delivering before 34 weeks' gestation. The negative predictive value of this cutoff was 96%. Similarly, Owen and associates demonstrated that a single examination at 16 to 19 weeks' gestation with a cervix 25 mm or less in length increased the risk of preterm delivery by 35 weeks' gestation 3.3 times (95% confidence interval [CI]: 2.1–5.0) and found that if serial examinations up to 24 weeks' gestation were performed, a single cervical length of less than 25 mm increased the risk of preterm labor 4.5 times (95% CI: 2.7–7.6).[33] Only limited data are available about the value of serial screening beyond 24 weeks' gestation, but in one small study (n = 69) of high risk pregnancies examined every fortnight from 16 to 30 weeks' gestation, cervical length and funneling were found to be significant at evaluations performed at 20 to 24 weeks as well as 25 to 29 weeks.[44]

Cervical Assessment in Asymptomatic Patients at Low Risk of Preterm Labor

The rationale for screening in a general, low risk population is that a significant proportion of preterm deliveries occur in pregnancies with no historical risk factors. The apparent effectiveness of screening high risk populations has lead many groups to examine screening in a low risk group, and evaluation of cervical length seems to be of similar predictive value in this setting.[45–49] Iams and associates reported a multicenter study of 2915 pregnancies recruited through 10 university perinatal centers in the United States.[45] Investigators used a clearly described method to assess cervical length; the process involved initial training, a period of standardization of technique, and continuing audit of the quality of examinations. Both cervical length and funneling were examined, but although funneling seemed to be equally predictive of outcome, the authors noted that determination of this sign was less consistent, with a prevalence of 0% to 12.7% across centers. The predictive value of cervical assessment was reported in terms of the proportion of spontaneous preterm deliveries that occurred before 35 weeks of gestation; this occurred in 126 (4.3%) of the pregnancies enrolled. A cervical length less than 20 mm was found in less than 5% of women, and this group included 23% of preterm births. The relative risk of preterm labor associated with various cervical lengths was also reported. These data were calculated relative to the risk of preterm delivery in the top quartile rather than relative to the background population as a whole. This approach demonstrated that there is a significant association between the risk of preterm labor and a short cervix. It also demonstrated that there was a continuum of risk and the authors suggested that this challenged the traditional concept that the cervix is either competent or incompetent and provided evidence that cervical competence should be considered as a continuous variable.

There are four other studies that have examined large (>500 pregnancies) groups of low risk singleton pregnancies.[46–49] Although they are not directly comparable with the study of Iams described earlier, a review of their results demonstrates similar findings, i.e., the risk of spontaneous preterm birth is inversely related to cervical length (Table 61-1).

Unfortunately, there is little evidence to suggest that screening a low risk population is useful, as an effective intervention to improve pregnancy outcome has not yet been demonstrated. Therefore, it could be argued that such a screening policy is not appropriate or that such a policy is relevant only in units with an active interest in interventions for preterm labor where screen-positive patients would be recruited for further research.

Cervical Assessment in Patients Symptomatic of Preterm Labor

Early diagnosis of preterm labor potentially allows early intervention to reduce the risk of preterm delivery or to optimize conditions for the premature neonate. The clinical diagnosis of labor is dependent on the presence of uterine activity with cervical effacement and dilation, and accurate cervical assessment is therefore important. Traditional, digital examination tends to be imprecise, with large margins of inter- and intraoperator error. The rationale for using ultrasound to assess the cervix in women presenting with symptoms of preterm labor is that cervical assessment will be more precise, allowing earlier treatment of women with evidence of cervical change, but reducing the proportion of women who are not in preterm labor and have unnecessary treatment.

Cervical effacement has many potential causes. This process may be biologic or may represent a mechanical weakness that is revealed as the uterus becomes distended. Alternatively, it may be secondary to the onset of uterine contraction or to inflammation and the release of local hormones—frequently a response to infection or hemorrhage. It is unlikely that a single form of therapy will resolve all the etiologies underlying cervical effacement and dilation, and this may explain why most randomized controlled trials of cervical cerclage have not shown this to be an effective method of preventing preterm birth.

Cervical Screening in Twin Pregnancies

The incidence of preterm delivery is significantly higher in multiple pregnancies, with a consequent effect on perinatal mortality and morbidity rates in these infants. From 5% to 10% of twins deliver before 33 weeks' gestation, a sixfold increase over the rate of preterm delivery in singleton pregnancies by this gestation.[50] Despite this, fewer studies have assessed the use of cervical screening in twin pregnancies, and it is less clear whether ultrasound assessment is useful or at what week of gestation ultrasound should be performed.

A prospective cohort of 177 pregnancies was used to evaluate cervical length in normal twin pregnancies.[51] Of these 177, 28 (16.3%) pregnancies delivered before 34 weeks' gestation and were excluded from further analysis. In the remainder, the mean cervical length decreased from 47 mm at 13 weeks' gestation to 32 mm at 32 weeks' gestation in a linear fashion. The rate of cervical shortening was 0.8 mm per week.

Ong and associates suggested that, from a clinical perspective, it is not the estimation of risk per se that is important, but the prediction of preterm labor within a limited time frame, allowing admission, preparative treatment (such as steroid therapy), and transfer to a unit with appropriate neonatal facilities.[52] Cervical length was assessed every 2 weeks in 46 twin pregnancies between 24 weeks' gestation and delivery. Only data from pregnancies that labored spontaneously were subsequently included in the analysis. There was no difference in the rate of shortening between pregnancies delivering before and after 37 weeks' gestation. An absolute threshold for cervical length was, however, more useful: cervical lengths of less than 20 mm and less than 25 mm had relative risks of delivery within 1 week of 11.67 (95th CI: 4.23–32.17) and 4.12 (95th CI: 1.10–15.47), respectively. A similar longitudinal study of only 20 twin pregnancies suggested a difference in the rate of cervical shortening between women delivering preterm (<36 weeks' gestation) and those delivering at term. After excluding one preterm delivery that had a short cervix at the time of the first scan (10 mm at 24 weeks' gestation), the rate of shortening was found to be 2.9 mm/week and 1.8 mm/week in preterm and term pregnancies, respectively. This difference was not statistically significant, but this may have been due to the relatively low numbers enrolled.[53]

Skentou and associates also examined various thresholds for cervical length to predict the risk of preterm delivery.[54] This prospective study of 464 twin pregnancies involved a single transvaginal ultrasound assessment at 23 (22–24) weeks' gestation. This study included 313 (67.5%) dichorionic and 151 (32.5%) monochorionic twin pregnancies and found no significant difference in the rate of preterm delivery (defined as before 34 weeks' gestation) in these two groups. A significant inverse relationship was found between cervical length and the risk of preterm birth (risk = 26.48 × cervical length − 1.688)

TABLE 61-1

Comparison of Studies Reporting the Predictive Value of Transvaginal Ultrasound Assessment of Cervical Length for Preterm Labor.*

FIRST AUTHOR	HASSAN[47]				HEATH[46]			
CENTER	US, SINGLE CENTER				UK, SINGLE CENTER			
N GESTATION AT TEST	6877				2567			
GESTATION OF OUTCOME†	19 (14–24) WK				23 (22–24) WK			
	32 WK (2.9%)				32 WK			
	CX	PREV	OR	SENS	CX	PREV	OR	SENS
					5		51.5	
	10	0.3%	29.3		10			
	15	0.6%	24.3	8.2%	15	1.7%	2.7	58%
	20	0.9%	18.3	10.6%	20	3.4%		
	25	1.7%	13.4	14.7%	25	8.0%	0.71	
	30	9.1%	3.2		30	18.0%		
	40	71.6%			40		0.45	
					50		0.24	

*The studies are heterogeneous in nature, reflected in the tabulated data.
†The prevalence of preterm delivery in the study population is given in parentheses.
Cx, cervical length (mm); Prev, prevalence of preterm delivery; OR, odds ratio for preterm delivery; Sens, sensitivity of cutoff for prediction of preterm labor.

such that thresholds of 15 mm, 20 mm, and 25 mm detected 17.6%, 39.1%, and 46.4% of twin pregnancies delivering before 34 weeks, respectively. The corresponding screen-positive rates were higher than those seen in singleton pregnancies: 2.1%, 4.7%, and 9.6%.

In addition to assessing cervical length, Guzman and associates looked at cervical funneling and the effect of transfundal pressure during the examination.[55] A series of 131 pregnancies were examined serially between 15 and 28 weeks' gestation. The effectiveness of assessments at 15 to 20, 21 to 24, and 25 to 28 weeks' gestation for the prediction of preterm delivery by 28, 30, 32, and 34 weeks' gestation were evaluated. Although the cervix was significantly shorter with transfundal pressure, this application did not improve the investigators' ability to predict preterm labor. A cervical length of less than 20 mm was found to be at least as good as any other characteristic at predicting spontaneous preterm delivery.

These data differ slightly from the findings of another group, who investigated the associations between preterm delivery and a short cervix and cervical funneling in a series of 251 twin pregnancies, examined at 22 and 27 weeks' gestation.[56] A receiver operating characteristic curve showed no clear best cutoff point for cervical length at 22 weeks' gestation, although a cutoff of 25 mm appeared best at 27 weeks' gestation. Using this cutoff at 22 weeks (for comparison to other data sets) gave a sensitivity of 38% and specificity of 97% for preterm delivery before 32 weeks' gestation. Cervical funneling, considered to be present when the lateral border of the funnel was more than 3 mm in length, was present in 12.4% of pregnancies at 22 weeks' gestation, and this finding had a sensitivity of 54% and a specificity of 89% as an indicator of preterm birth by 32 weeks' gestation. The authors concluded that cervical length and funneling both predict very preterm birth and that although cervical length is the method of choice at 27 weeks' gestation, at 22 weeks the diagnostic characteristics of both parameters are close.

CERVICOVAGINAL FETAL FIBRONECTIN

Fetal fibronectin is a glycoprotein found in amniotic fluid, placental tissue, and the decidua basalis.[57] It is normally found in cervicovaginal secretions before 16 to 18 weeks' gestation, before fusion of the fetal membranes and the decidua is complete. Similarly, it is found at the end of pregnancy, prior to the onset of labor, but it is not normally present in cervicovaginal secretions between 22 and 37 weeks. It has been suggested that the presence of fetal fibronectin in cervicovaginal secretions in the later part of the second trimester and in the third trimester of pregnancy is due to disruption of the chorionic-decidual interface and is often secondary to infection.[58]

Initial studies establishing the presence of fetal fibronectin in cervicovaginal secretions involved extensive laboratory analysis that delayed the availability of results. More recently, an enzyme-linked immunosorbant assay containing the FDC-6 monoclonal antibody has been developed that can be used at the bedside, potentially making this test a much stronger clinical tool.[59]

A large systematic review of 64 primary articles reporting the effectiveness of screening for preterm delivery by the detection of cervicovaginal fetal fibronectin in a total of 26,876 women has recently been published.[60] There were two large subsets of women, asymptomatic and symptomatic of preterm labor. Among asymptomatic women, the likelihood ratio for predicting preterm delivery before 34 weeks was 4.01 (95% CI 2.93–5.49) with a likelihood ratio for negative results of 0.78 (95% CI 0.72–0.84). Among those women who were symptomatic, the likelihood ratio for positive results was 5.42 (95% CI

HIBBARD[48] US, SINGLE CENTER 760 20 (16–22) WK 32 WK (3.6%)				IAMS[45] US, MULTICENTER 2915 24 WK 35 WK (4.3%)				TAIPALE[49] FINLAND, SINGLE CENTER 3694 (18–22) WK 35 WK (0.8%)			
CX	PREV	RR	SENS	CX	PREV	RR	SENS	CX	PREV	RR	SENS
				13		13.99					
22	2.5%	8.4	18.5%	22		9.46	23%				
27	5.0%	9.7	29.6%	26		6.19	37%	25	0.3%	20	100%
30	10.0%	5.2	44.4%	30		3.79	54%	29	3.0%	8	97%
38.5	50.0%			35		2.35		35	27.0%	2.2	73%
				40		1.98		40	52.0%	1.7	38%

4.36–6.74) for predicting birth between 7 and 10 days of testing, with a corresponding negative likelihood ratio of 0.25 (95% CI 0.20–0.31).

Another meta-analysis, confined to reports in the English language, found that fetal fibronectin was useful in the prediction of delivery before 34 weeks, with an overall sensitivity of 53% and specificity of 89%.[61] The sensitivities for prediction of delivery within 7, 14, and 21 days were 71%, 67%, and 59%, respectively. The corresponding specificities were 89%, 89%, and 92%. Further analysis of studies in asymptomatic women who could be divided into low risk and high risk showed that for a single sampling of fibronectin, sensitivity for detection of delivery prior to 34 weeks was 41% (21%–59%) for low risk women with a specificity of 94% (91%–96%). For high risk women the sensitivity was considerably lower at 23% (14%–32%) but with a comparable specificity of 94% (93%–96%). The studies of serial sampling of cervical fibronectin showed a higher sensitivity of prediction of delivery prior to 34 weeks with low risk and high risk groups showing a sensitivity of 68% (52%–83%) and 92% (62%–100%), respectively. Predictably the specificities in each group of serial sampling were significantly reduced (there is an independent chance of a false-positive result every time the test is done, so the specificity falls as the number of samples, and hence false positives, increases). The few studies looking at multiple pregnancies have small numbers and result in sensitivities and specificities with such broad confidence intervals that a meaningful conclusion cannot be drawn.

Subgroup analysis of symptomatic and asymptomatic pregnancies demonstrated that this test was most sensitive in women with symptoms of preterm labor, but its usefulness as a screening test for decisions about hospital admission and the administration of glucocorticoids is reduced by the fact that the specificity is significantly lower than in asymptomatic women. The authors concluded that fetal fibronectin is a reasonably effective marker in predicting preterm delivery in the short term, particularly if there are symptoms of preterm labor.

Combined Cervical Screening and Fibronectin

The combined use of ultrasound and fibronectin has been evaluated in only a few studies, and in symptomatic women. Rizzo and associates found that combining cervical sonography with fibronectin screening improved diagnostic accuracy and allowed better prediction of the admission to delivery time.[62] Other investigators have found that fibronectin and cervical length had comparable ability to distinguish those at high and low risk of preterm delivery, but that their combination provides little added benefit.[63] Hincz and associates proposed a two-step test only when the cervical length was in an immediate range of 21 to 31 mm. This form of testing had an overall sensitivity of 86% with a specificity of 90% for predicting delivery within 28 days.[64]

SCREENING FOR BACTERIAL VAGINOSIS IN EARLY PREGNANCY

Bacterial vaginosis (BV) is characterized by an overgrowth of a mixture of organisms (*Gardnerella vaginalis*, *Mobiluncus*, *Bacteroides* spp., and *Mycoplasma hominis*), is often asymptomatic, and may resolve spontaneously. Although the role of BV in preterm labor is poorly understood, several reports[65,66] found that the relative risk of preterm labor is doubled if the mother has BV. The hypothesis is that the organisms found in BV ascend into and colonize the chorionic-decidual space, resulting in preterm labor or preterm rupture of membranes. This increase in invasion of the genital tract may be due to the rise in pH, which is a key feature of BV, allowing vaginal bacteria to proliferate relatively unchecked. Two studies[67,68] suggest that infection in early pregnancy may be a greater risk factor than BV infection in the late second trimester and early third trimester of pregnancy.

Leitich and associates[69] performed a meta-analysis to evaluate the risk of preterm delivery associated with BV; 20,232 patients in 18 studies were included. They found that BV increased the risk of early delivery (less than 37 weeks' gestation) with an odds ratio of 2.19 (95% CI 1.54–3.12). A subgroup analysis showed that if BV was identified prior to 16 weeks, then the risk of preterm birth was further increased with an odds ratio of 7.55 (95% CI 1.80–31.65). Even at less than 20 weeks, a finding of BV was associated with an odds ratio of 4.20 (95% CI 2.11–8.39) for preterm birth. This analysis found no particular association of BV with delivery prior to 34 weeks; however, few studies used that gestation time as an outcome and the studies that used early screening used less than 37 weeks as their criteria for preterm delivery. There is little evidence that screening for BV in specific subgroups, particularly in women with a prior preterm delivery and in multiple gestations, improves its sensitivity or specificity.

Despite this reasonably convincing evidence of a link between early infection with BV and preterm delivery, screening and subsequently treatment of BV remain controversial. The recent review of the Cochrane Collaboration[70] of 10 trials of 4249 women showed that antibiotic therapy successfully treated BV but failed to reduce the risk of preterm birth before 37 weeks, with odds ratio 0.95 (95% CI 0.82–1.10); at 34 weeks, with odds ratio 1.20 (95% CI 0.69–2.07); or 32 weeks, with odds ratio 1.08 (95% CI 0.70–1.68). In those women who had a previous preterm birth, treatment of BV did not decrease the risk of a subsequent preterm birth, odds ratio 0.83 (95% CI 0.59–1.17), but did decrease the risk of preterm premature rupture of membranes, odds ratio 0.14 (95% CI 0.05–0.38). Similarly, Carey and associates[71] failed to show oral metronidazole therapy to be useful in prevention of preterm labor in a mixed population.

At present the role of screening for BV and then treating it is not clear in a low risk population. It possibly has benefit in a high risk population, but further controlled studies are required.

CONCLUSIONS

- The successful prediction of preterm labor potentially allows interventions to reduce preterm delivery rates and improve perinatal outcome.
- Four screening methods have been extensively evaluated.
- Uterine contraction monitoring has poor sensitivity as a screening tool and is of limited clinical value.
- Assessment of cervical length and cervical fibronectin may have a role in screening for preterm labor, particularly in high risk populations.
- Although there is limited evidence of successful intervention to prevent preterm labor, it is possible to improve perinatal outcome by arranging delivery in an appropriate setting and by giving steroids.
- An additional use of fetal fibronectin and cervical length assessment is the value of a negative result. The prediction that delivery is not imminent has practical applications, such as a reduction in inpatient admission, a reduction in unnecessary interventions such as cervical cerclage, and a reduction in the number of courses of steroids given to promote fetal maturity.[72]
- It remains unclear whether the presence of bacterial vaginosis is predictive of preterm labor, and further studies are needed to assess the effectiveness of antibiotic treatment in early pregnancy in reducing of rate of preterm labor and preterm rupture of membranes.
- To take full advantage of these screening tests, clinicians should aim to use the findings to focus interventions in those truly at high risk and to reduce interventions in other pregnancies.

SUMMARY OF MANAGEMENT OPTIONS

Screening for Spontaneous Preterm Labor and Delivery

Management Options	Quality of Evidence	Strength of Recommendation	References
Uterine Activity Monitoring			
Self-monitoring applies to whole population but has a poor sensitivity.	IIb	B	6
Any improved outcome reported in monitored pregnancies may represent the benefits of increased education and support inherent in the studies.	Ib	A	7

SUMMARY OF MANAGEMENT OPTIONS

Screening for Spontaneous Preterm Labor and Delivery

Management Options	Quality of Evidence	Strength of Recommendation	References
Uterine Activity Monitoring—Continued			
Tocography is only practically applicable to high risk groups rather than whole populations.	–	GPP	–
Two meta-analyses of the same 6 studies in 697 high risk pregnancies have reached opposite conflicting conclusions; further studies are needed.	Ia	A	20,21
The addition of fetal fibronectin testing to uterine activity monitoring does not confer any benefit in practice.	IIb	B	25
Cervical Ultrasound			
It is important to use a standardized technique.	IV	C	30
Transvaginal route is significantly better than translabial/transperineal or transabdominal approaches.	IIa	B	31–34
Most studies have been performed at ≤ 24 weeks.	III	B	33,44
Assessment of cervical length or funneling is predictive of preterm labor and delivery in:	Ia	A	29
Asymptomatic high risk patients	III	B	33,37,43,45
Asymptomatic low risk women	III	B	44–49
Twins	III	B	51–54,56
More data needed about value in patients with symptoms suggestive of preterm labor.	Ia	A	29
No evidence yet shows that incidence of preterm delivery is reduced with use of cervical ultrasound though allow rational approach to Maternal steroids Use of tocolysis Transfer to a tertiary center	Ia	A	29
Main advantage could be in negative predictive value to avoid unnecessary interventions.	Ia	A	29
Fetal Fibronectin (FFN)			
Positive test significantly increases the likelihood of preterm labor and delivery before 34 weeks.	Ia	A	60,61
Negative test significantly reduces the likelihood of preterm labor and delivery within 10 days.	Ia	A	60,61
Serial sampling improves positive predictive accuracy but with a lower specificity.	Ia	A	60,61
FFN gives better predictive performance in symptomatic women than in asymptomatic.	Ia	A	60,61
Insufficient data about twin pregnancies.	Ia	A	60,61
Conflicting data about whether combination of FFN and cervical ultrasound improves predictive accuracy.	III	B	62,63
Screening for Bacterial Vaginosis (BV)			
Role of BV screening in practice is uncertain.	Ia	A	69,70
Positive screening for BV in early pregnancy is associated with an increased risk of delivery <37 weeks; but no evidence of increased risk of preterm delivery <34 weeks.	Ia	A	69
Antibiotic therapy in BV positive women reduces incidence of BV colonization but not the incidence of preterm delivery.	Ia	A	70
More studies needed of BV screening and antibiotic use in high risk pregnancies.	Ia	A	69,70

REFERENCES

1. Iams JD: Preterm birth. Gabbe SG, Niebyl JR, Simpson JL (eds): Obstetrics: Normal and Problem Pregnancies, 4th ed. Philadelphia, Churchill Livingstone, 2002, pp 755–826.
2. Hueston WJ: Preterm contractions in community settings: II. Predicting preterm birth in women with preterm contractions. Obstet Gynecol 1998;92:43–46.
3. Macones GA, Segel SY, Stamilio DM, Morgan MA: Predicting delivery within 48 hours in women treated with parenteral tocolysis. Obstet Gynecol 1999;93:432–436.
4. King JF, Grant A, Keirse MJ, Chalmers I: Beta-mimetics in preterm labour: An overview of the randomized clinical trials. Br J Obstet Gynaecol 1988;95:211–222.
5. Iams JD, Johnson FF, Parker M: A prospective evaluation of the signs and symptoms of preterm labor. Obstet Gynecol 1994;84:227–230.
6. Newman RB, Gill RJ, Wittreich P, Katz M: Maternal perception of prelabor uterine activity. Obstet Gynecol 1986;160:1172–1178.
7. Iams JD, Johnson FF, O'Shaughnessy RW: A prospective random trial of home uterine activity monitoring in pregnancies at increased risk of preterm labor: Part II. Am J Obstet Gynecol 1988;159:595–603.
8. Moore TR, Iams JD, Creasy RK, et al: Diurnal and gestational patterns of uterine activity in normal human pregnancy. Obstet Gynecol 1994;83:517–523.
9. Katz M, Gill PJ, Newman RB: Detection of preterm labor by ambulatory monitoring of uterine activity: A preliminary report. Obstet Gynecol 1986;68:773–778.
10. Katz M, Gill PJ: Initial evaluation of an ambulatory system for home monitoring and transmission of uterine activity data. Obstet Gynecol 1985;66:273–277.
11. Paul MJ, Smeltzer JS: Relationship of external tocodynamometry with measured internal uterine activity. Am J Perinatol 1991;8:417–420.
12. Dickenson JE, Godfrey M, Legge M, Evans SF: A validation study of home uterine activity monitoring technology in Western Australia. Aust NZ J Obstet Gynaecol 1997;37:39–44.
13. Scheerer LJ, Campion S, Katz M: Ambulatory tocodynamometry data interpretation: Evaluating variability and reliability. Obstet Gynecol 1990;76(Suppl 1):67S–69S.
14. Morrison JC, Martin JN, Martin RW, et al: Prevention of preterm birth by ambulatory assessment of uterine activity: A randomised study. Am J Obstet Gynecol 1987;156:536–543.
15. Iams JD, Johnson FF, O'Shaughnessy RW, West LC: A prospective random trial of home uterine activity monitoring in pregnancies at increased risk of preterm labor. Am J Obstet Gynecol 1987;157:638–643.
16. Hill WC, Fleming AD, Martin RW, et al: Home uterine activity monitoring is associated with a reduction in preterm birth. Obstet Gynecol 1990;76(Suppl 1):13S–18S.
17. Dyson DC, Crites YM, Ray DA, Armstrong MA: Prevention of preterm birth in high-risk patients: The role of education and provider contact versus home uterine monitoring. Am J Obstet Gynecol 1991;164:756–762.
18. Mou SM, Sunderji SG, Gall S, et al: Multicenter randomised clinical trial of home uterine activity monitoring for detection of preterm labour. Am J Obstet Gynecol 1991;165:858–866.
19. Blondel B, Breart G, Berthoux Y, et al: Home uterine activity monitoring in France: A randomised controlled trial. Am J Obstet Gynecol 1992;167:424–429.
20. Colton T, Kayne HL, Zhang Y, Heeren T: A meta-analysis of home uterine activity monitoring. Am J Obstet Gynecol 1995;173:1499–1505.
21. Grimes DA, Schulz KF: Randomized controlled trials of home uterine activity monitoring: A review and critique. Obstet Gynecol 1992;79:137–142.
22. The Collaborative Home Uterine Monitoring Group: A multicentre randomized controlled trial of home uterine monitoring: Active versus sham device. Am J Obstet Gynecol 1995;173: 1120–1127.
23. Wapner RJ, Cotton DB, Artal R, et al: A randomized multicentre trial assessing a home uterine activity monitoring device used in the absence of daily nursing contact. Am J Obstet Gynecol 1995;172:1026–1034.
24. Dyson DC, Danbe KH, Bamber JA, et al: Monitoring women at risk for preterm labor. N Engl J Med 1998;338:15–19.
25. Morrison JC, Naef RW, Botti JJ, et al: Prediction of spontaneous preterm birth by fetal fibronectin and uterine activity. Obstet Gynecol 1996;87:649–655.
26. Iams JD, Newman RB, Thom EA, et al: Frequency of uterine contractions and the risk of spontaneous preterm delivery. N Engl J Med 2002;346:250–255.
27. Sonek J, Iams JD, Blumenfeld M, et al: Measurement of cervical length in pregnancy: Comparison between vaginal ultrasonography and digital examination. Obstet Gynecol 1990;76:172.
28. Zilianti M, Azuaga A, Calderon F, et al: Monitoring the effacement of the uterine cervix by transperineal sonography: A new perspective. J Ultrasound Med 1995;14:719–724.
29. Honest H, Bachmann LM, Coomarasamy A, et al: Accuracy of cervical transvaginal sonography in predicting preterm birth: A systematic review. Ultrasound Obstet Gynecol 2003; 22:305–322.
30. Colombo DF, Iams JD: Cervical length and preterm labor. Clin Obstet Gynecol 2000;43:735–745.
31. To MS, Skentou C, Cicero S, Nicolaides KH: Cervical assessment at the routine 23-weeks' scan: Problems with transabdominal sonography. Ultrasound Obstet Gynecol 2000;15: 292–296.
32. Cicero S, Skentou C, Souka A, et al: Cervical length at 22–24 weeks of gestation: Comparison of transvaginal and transperineal-translabial ultrasonography. Ultrasound Obstet Gynecol 2001;17:335–340.
33. Owen J, Yost N, Berghella V, et al: Mid-trimester endovaginal sonography in women at high risk for spontaneous preterm birth. JAMA 2001;286:1340–1348.
34. Carr DB, Smith K, Parson L, et al: Ultrasonography for cervical length measurements: Agreement between transvaginal and translabial techniques. Obstet Gynecol 2000;96:554–558.
35. To MS, Skentou C, Chan C, et al: Cervical assessment at the routine 23 week anomaly scan: Standardising techniques. Ultrasound Obstet Gynecol 2001;17:217–219.
36. Berghella V, Kuhlonon K, Weiner S, et al: Cervical funneling: Sonographic criteria predictive of preterm delivery. Ultrasound Obstet Gynecol 1997;10:161–166.
37. Guzman ER, Walters C, Ananth CV, et al: A comparison of sonographic cervical parameters in predicting spontaneous preterm birth in high-risk singleton pregnancies. Ultrasound Obstet Gynecol 2001;18:204–210.
38. To MS, Skentou C, Liao AW, et al: Cervical length and funneling at 23 weeks of gestation in the prediction of spontaneous preterm birth in high-risk singleton pregnancies. Ultrasound Obstet Gynecol 2001;18:200–203.
39. Hassan SS, Romero R, Berry SM, et al: Patients with an ultrasonographic cervical length <15 mm have nearly a 50% risk of early spontaneous preterm delivery. Am J Obstet Gynecol 2000;182:1458–1467.
40. Varma TR, Patel RH, Pillai U: Ultrasonic assessment of the cervix in at risk patients. Int J Obstet Gynecol 1987;25: 25–34.

41. Podobnik M, Bulnic M, Smiljanic N, Bistricki J: Ultrasonography in the detection of cervical incompetency. J Clin Ultrasound 1988;13:383–391.
42. Michaels WH, Schreiber FR, Padgett RJ, et al: Ultrasound surveillance of the cervix in twin gestations: Management of cervical incompetence. Obstet Gynecol 1991;78:739–744.
43. Cook CM, Ellwood DA: The cervix as a predictor of preterm delivery in "at risk" women. Ultrasound Obstet Gynecol 2000;15:109–113.
44. Andrews WW, Copper R, Hauth JC, et al: Second trimester cervical ultrasound: associated with increased risk for recurrent early spontaneous delivery. Obstet Gynecol 2000;95: 222–226.
45. Iams JD, Goldenberg RL, Meis PJ, et al: The length of the cervix and the risk of spontaneous preterm delivery. N Engl J Med 1996;334:567–572.
46. Heath VC, Southall TR, Souka AP, et al: Cervical length at 23 weeks of gestation: Prediction of spontaneous preterm delivery. Ultrasound Obstet Gynecol 1998;12:312–317.
47. Hassan SS, Romero R, Berry SM, et al: Patients with an ultrasonographic cervical length <15 mm have nearly a 50% risk of early spontaneous preterm delivery. Am J Obstet Gynecol 2000;182:1458–1467.
48. Hibbard JU, Tart M, Moawad AH: Cervical length at 16–22 weeks' gestation and risk for preterm delivery. Obstet Gynecol 2000;96:972–978.
49. Taipale P, Hiilesmaa V: Sonographic measurement of uterine cervix at 18–22 weeks' gestation and the risk for preterm delivery. Obstet Gynecol 1998;92:902–907.
50. Sebire NJ, Snijders RJ, Hughes K, et al: The hidden mortality of monochorionic twin pregnancies. Br J Obstet Gynaecol 1997;104:1203–1207.
51. Fujita MM, Brizot Mde L, Liao AW, et al: Reference range for cervical length in twin pregnancies. Acta Obstet Gynecol Scand 2002;81:856–859.
52. Ong S, Smith A, Smith N, et al: Cervical length assessment in twin pregnancies using transvaginal ultrasound. Acta Obstet Gynecol Scand 2000;79:851–853.
53. Bergelin I, Valentin L: Cervical changes in twin pregnancies observed by transvaginal ultrasound examination during the latter half of pregnancy: A longitudinal, observational study. Ultrasound Obstet Gynecol 2003;21:556–563.
54. Skentou C, Souka AP, To MS, et al: Prediction of preterm delivery in twins by cervical assessment at 23 weeks. Ultrasound Obstet Gynecol 2001;17:7–10.
55. Guzman ER, Walters C, O'Reilly-Green C, et al: Use of cervical ultrasonography in prediction of spontaneous preterm birth in twin gestations. Am J Obstet Gynecol 2000; 183(5):1103–1107.
56. Vayssiere C, Favre R, Audibert F, et al: Cervical length and funnelling at 22 and 27 weeks to predict spontaneous birth before 32 weeks in twin pregnancies: A French prospective multicentre study. Am J Obstet Gynecol 2002;187:1596–1604.
57. Feinberg RF, Kleiman HJ, Lockwood CJ: Is oncofetal fibronectin a trophoblast glue for human implantation? Am J Pathol 1991;138:537–543.
58. Lockwood CJ: Recent advances in elucidating the pathogenesis of preterm delivery, the detection of patients at risk and preventative therapies. Curr Opin Obstet Gynecol 1994;6:7–18.
59. Erikesen NL, Parisi VM, Daoust S, et al: Fetal fibronectin: A method for detecting the presence of amniotic fluid. Obstet Gynecol 1992;80:451–454.
60. Honest H, Bachmann LM, Gupta JK, et al: Accuracy of cervical fetal fibronectin test in predicting risk of spontaneous preterm birth: Systematic review. Br Med J 2002;325:301–310.
61. Leitich H, Kaider A: Fetal fibronectin—How useful is it in the prediction of preterm birth? Br J Obstet Gynaecol 2003;110(suppl 20):66–70.
62. Rizzo G, Capponi A, Arduini A, et al: The value of fetal fibronectin in cervical and vaginal secretions and of ultrasonographic examination of the uterine cervix in predicting premature delivery for patients with preterm labour and intact membranes. Am J Obstet Gynecol 1996;175:1446–1451.
63. Rozenberg P, Goffinet F, Malagrida L, et al: Evaluating the risk of preterm delivery: A comparison of fetal fibronectin and transvaginal ultrasonographic measurement of cervical length. Am J Obstet Gynecol 1997;176:196–199.
64. Hincz P, Wilczynski J, Kozarzewski M, Szaflik K: Two-step test: The combined use of fetal fibronectin and sonographic examination of the uterine cervix for prediction of preterm delivery in symptomatic patients. Acta Obstet Gynecol Scand 2002;81:58–63.
65. Goldenberg RL, Iams JD, Mercer BM, et al: The preterm prediction study: The value of new vs. standard risk factors in predicting early and all spontaneous preterm births. Am J Publ Health 1998;88:233–238.
66. Flynn CA, Helwig AL, Meurer LN: Bacterial vaginosis in pregnancy and the risk of prematurity: Meta-analysis. J Fam Pract 1999;48:885–892.
67. Hay PE, Lamont RF, Taylor-Robinson D, et al: Abnormal bacterial colonization of the genital tract and subsequent preterm delivery and late miscarriage. BMJ 194;308:295–298.
68. Kurki T, Sivonen A, Renkonen O-V, et al: Bacterial vaginosis in early pregnancy and pregnancy outcome. Obstet Gynecol 1992;80:173–177.
69. Leitich H, Bodner-Adler B, Brunbauer M, et al: Bacterial vaginosis as a risk factor for preterm delivery: A meta-analysis. Am J Obstet Gynecol 2003;189:139–147.
70. McDonald H, Brocklehurst P, Parsons J, Vigneswaran R: Antiobiotics for treating bacterial vaginosis in pregnancy (Cochrane Review). In The Cochrane Library. Issue 3. Oxford, Update Software, 2003.
71. Carey JC, Klebanoff MA, Hauth JC, et al: Metronidazole to prevent preterm delivery in pregnant women with asymptomatic bacterial vaginosis. N Engl J Med 2000;342:534–540.
72. Iams JD: Prediction and early detection of preterm labour. Obstet Gynecol 2003;101:402–412.

Threatened and Actual Preterm Labor Including Mode of Delivery

John M. Svigos / Jeffrey S. Robinson / Rasniah Vigneswaran

INTRODUCTION, DEFINITION, AND INCIDENCE

Preterm labor refers to the onset of labor after the gestation of viability (20–28 weeks, depending on definition) and before 37 completed weeks or 259 days of pregnancy. The onset of labor may be determined by documented uterine contractions (at least one every 10 minutes) and ruptured fetal membranes or documented cervical change with an estimated length of less than 1 cm or cervical dilation of more than 2 cm. Threatened preterm labor may be diagnosed when there are documented uterine contractions but no evidence of cervical change.

Despite these apparently clearly defined entities, and because of the need for early management of suspected preterm labor, it is common for clinicians to make the diagnosis before the foregoing criteria are met. Hence, the reported incidence of threatened preterm labor is likely to be considerably greater than the incidence of actual preterm labor. For example, O'Driscoll[1] suggested that the pregnant woman's own diagnosis of preterm labor, based on her perception of uterine contractions, may be incorrect in as up to 80% of instances. Kragt and Keirse[2] demonstrated that 33% of women presenting with contractions could safely be discharged home in 48 hours without needing treatment.

Amon and Petrie[3] suggest that 50% of women presenting with uterine contractions do not need tocolytics, and Gonik and Creasy[4] in their review found that only 18% to 20% of women presenting with possible preterm labor were candidates for long-term tocolytic agents. Even more sobering was Gonik and Creasy's assessment of a 20% to 45% efficacy rate of placebo treatment for suspected preterm labor.

In South Australia in 2001,[5] the overall preterm delivery (PTD) rate was 8.1%. Since 1981, the percentage of babies born preterm has increased from 5.5% to 8.1%; however, in recent years this rate has remained stable. If we assume that about 50% of women who present in threatened preterm labor eventually deliver at term, then the proportion of the obstetric population presenting for diagnosis will be approximately 16.2%. As in previous years, two thirds of cases were associated with preterm premature rupture of the membranes (PPROM) and only one third (or 2.7% overall) were due to preterm labor (PTL) without PPROM.

The incidence of preterm delivery in most developed countries has remained frustratingly constant over the past 3 decades at about 5% to 10%, with some regions, including our own, noticing a small increase above the usual incidence over the last 5 years. In institutions serving as referral centers the rate, as would be expected, is much higher. In South Australia, the major tertiary center, the Women's and Children's Hospital, Adelaide, had a 14.3% rate of PTD in 2002.[6] There are a number of explanations to account for this lack of success.

First, doubts have been expressed about the comparability of current estimates of the incidence of preterm delivery with previous years, as they increasingly reflect the increased survival of the extremely preterm, very low birth weight infants, who would previously have been regarded as "nonviable." Registration practices can alter so that some babies are registered as births when previously they would have been regarded as midtrimester miscarriages. Change in requirements for registrations and increased ascertainment may account for some of the increase in preterm births in South Australia since 1981.[5]

Additionally, there is only a relatively limited window of opportunity during which the presently available tocolytic agents can be used, and because of their poor efficacy they prolong pregnancy only marginally. Thus, they should not be expected to impact substantially on the actual preterm delivery rate.

Tucker and associates' study[7] (1991) of 13,119 consecutive singleton births demonstrated this problem. There were 1445 (11%) preterm births in the study group, but 630 (44%) of them were at more than 34 weeks' gestation, and consequently treatment to prevent labor was not attempted. Another 241 (16.6%) of women had PPROM, and hence, tocolysis was withheld. A total of 238 women (16.5%) had medical or obstetric indications for delivery (vaginal bleeding, hypertension, intrauterine fetal death, intrauterine fetal growth restriction), and 189 (13%) were too far advanced in labor (cervical dilation >3 cm) to be considered for tocolytic therapy. Thus, in only 147 women (10.2% of the subgroup; 5% of women presenting at <35 weeks' gestation, and only 1% of the total obstetric population studied) was it appropriate to use a tocolytic agent. Therefore, the opportunity to make a significant impact on the incidence of PTD was limited.

In Project 27/28 in the United Kingdom, 3522 babies born between 27^0 and 28^6 weeks of gestation were reported to The Confidential Enquiry into Stillbirths and Deaths in Infancy (CESDI) in 1 year. A 2-year follow-up of 761 babies showed that major placental bleeding (18%), pregnancy-induced hypertension (21%), prelabor rupture of the membranes (31%), clinical chorioamnionitis (11%), preterm labor (55%), cervical incompetence (5%), bacteriuria (7%), and maternal smoking remain important antecedents of preterm birth. Thus, the strategies that would be required to prevent them are many and varied. In the CESDI report, emphasis was given to reduction of smoking as being the cause of preterm delivery most amenable to intervention.[8]

MATERNAL RISKS

General Risks

Consideration of preterm birth makes it clear that many of its causes have their origins in maternal pathology, which carries a risk for the mother as well as the fetus. Excluding PPROM and "idiopathic" PTL,[9] which together constitute approximately 66% of cases, the two most common maternal conditions associated with preterm birth are pregnancy-induced hypertension and antepartum hemorrhage.[4] These two conditions may either precipitate PTL spontaneously or prompt the deliberate induction of PTL as a way to resolve the problem or to deliver the fetus from an adverse environment. Induction of labor may of itself carry risks for the mother (see Chapter 68). Additionally, if "idiopathic" PTL is studied in detail, the following associations have been recognized: intrauterine infection (47%), placental abruption or previa (40%), uterine factors (anomalies, polyhydramnios 20%), cervical incompetence (17%), immunologic factors (33%), maternal factors (systemic infection, preeclampsia 10%), fetal anomalies (7%), trauma (surgical, others 3%), and true "idiopathic" PTL (1%). Often more than one factor may be present and will contribute to the maternal risks associated with PTL.

Risks of Tocolytic Agents

Beta-Sympathomimetics

Another area of significant risk to the pregnant woman with threatened or actual PTL is the risk from the treatment regimens currently employed. Although beta-sympathomimetic agents, mainly ritodrine, have been studied in randomized controlled trials to determine their efficacy in the treatment of PTL, unfortunately the total number of women studied is not able to provide meaningful information regarding the incidence of serious maternal hazards associated with such therapy. However, a systematic review by Gyetvai and associates[10] demonstrated the following adverse maternal effects when compared to no treatment or placebo: palpitations (48% with beta-sympathomimetic vs. 5% with no treatement or placebo), tremor (39% vs. 4%), nausea (20% vs. 12%), headache (23% vs. 6%), and chest pain (10% vs. 1%). Rare but serious and potentially life-threatening adverse effects have been reported following beta-sympathomimetic use. Pulmonary edema has become increasingly recognized as a serious maternal hazard, with many but not all cases being due to fluid overload. The actual incidence of this problem is difficult to estimate from the literature but varies from 5% of treated women[11] to "a few cases." Women receiving associated corticosteroid therapy for fetal lung maturity enhancement, women receiving combinations of tocolytic agents (e.g., beta-sympathomimetics and magnesium sulfate), those with unrecognized chorioamnionitis, and women with multiple pregnancies are reported to be at increased risk of pulmonary edema.[10] Myocardial ischemia, possibly as a result of diffuse myocardial micronecrosis, has been reported in women receiving beta-sympathomimetic tocolytic therapy and constitutes an infrequent but serious maternal hazard.[10,11] A number of maternal biochemical effects occur with these agents, but they rarely cause serious problems unless there are underlying maternal diseases such as diabetes, thyrotoxicosis, or cardiac disease. Blood sugar levels increase in approximately 40% of women receiving beta-sympathomimetic agents, particularly if combined with corticosteroid administration, and may occasionally result in severe ketoacidosis in pregnant diabetic women.[9,11] Serum potassium levels generally fall, owing to a net influx of potassium from the maternal extracellular fluid into the intracellular fluid compartments as a result of the changes in carbohydrate metabolism. The resulting hypokalemia, however, is usually transient and unlikely to be of serious concern.[10,12]

Although beta-sympathomimetic tocolytic agents have been the mainstay of regimens for the treatment of PTL, other agents are now being used increasingly, as they appear to have fewer adverse effects with comparable effectiveness. However, none of these agents are without risk for the mother.

Nonsteroidal Anti-inflammatory Agents

Nonsteroidal anti-inflammatory drugs (NSAIDs) are inhibitors of the cyclooxygenase enzyme (prostaglandin synthetase), which plays an integral role in the initiation and maintenance of labor. Indomethacin has been the most commonly used NSAID for tocolysis over the past 20 years. The most likely maternal side effects of treatment include peptic ulceration, gastrointestinal bleeding, thrombocytopenia, and allergic reactions that can occur irrespective of the mode of administration. Less common complications include the risk of postpartum hemorrhage, renal function impairment, particularly if aminoglycoside antibiotics are used, and severe hypertension if beta-blocking agents are used. Long-term use has been associated with depression, dizziness, psychosis, and frequent headaches. It is believed that some of these unwanted side effects may be mediated through the constitutive type 1 isoform of cyclooxygenase (COX-1), as this enzyme is responsible for the unwanted renal and gastric side effects in nonpregnant subjects.[13] It has been shown that labor is associated with up-regulation of the expression of COX-2 and not COX-1 within the uterus,[14] and therefore, there is increasing interest in the newer COX-2 selective NSAIDs. Trials evaluating the safety of these drugs is awaited.

Magnesium Sulfate

A recent systematic review of more than 2000 women in 23 trials failed to find support for use of magnesium sulfate because it did not delay birth or prevent preterm birth.[15]

However, surprisingly, despite this apparently complete lack of effectiveness, magnesium sulfate has been the most popular parenteral drug used for tocolysis in North America. Elliott's study[16] of maternal side effects found that side effects occurred in 7% of patients and necessitated stopping treatment in 2%. Cutaneous vasodilation, flushing, nausea, vomiting, palpitations, and headaches are common side effects. Less frequent but troublesome problems are maternal hypothermia, bone demineralization, and paralytic ileus. The most significant maternal side effect is the development of pulmonary edema and an adult respiratory distress–like syndrome in approximately 1% of patients. This appears to be less frequent than that seen with the use of beta-sympathomimetic tocolytic agents. Hypermagnesemia may lead to maternal respiratory depression, cardiac arrest, and even death on rare occasions. Because of these significant side effects, and the complete lack of efficacy of this medication, it is difficult to see how its use for tocolysis can continue to be justified.

Calcium-Channel Blockers

Following the early favorable report of Read and Wellby[17] regarding the use of calcium-channel blockers for tocolysis, nifedipine has been increasingly used in the management of preterm labor. Analysis of adverse maternal effects is limited due to inconsistent reporting in individual trials. One review[18] reported fewer interruptions of treatment due to adverse effects with nifedipine compared to beta-sympathomimetics (0% vs. 7%). Fewer adverse effects were reported among women allocated nifedipine rather than ritodrine. However, there have been reports of pulmonary edema, maternal hypotension, and hepatotoxicity, which justify caution with their use.

Oxytocin Receptor Antagonist (Atosiban)

The oxytocin receptor antagonist atosiban has been compared with three different beta-sympathomimetics (ritodrine, salbutamol, and terbulaline) in a large multicenter study.[19] When compared with beta-sympathomimetics, atosiban was associated with fewer maternal adverse effects such as chest pain (1% vs. 5%), palpitations (2% vs. 16%), tachycardia (6% vs. 76%), hypertension (3% vs. 6%), (dyspnea (0.3% vs. 7%), nausea (12% vs. 16%), vomiting (7% vs. 22%), and headache (10% vs. 19%). There was one case of pulmonary edema in the atosiban group and two in the beta-sympathomimetic group. Atosiban has recently been licensed in Europe and the United Kingdom for use as a tocolytic, and evaluation of its more widespread use is awaited, although its high cost may prove to be a significant factor limiting its use.

Nitric Oxide Donors

There have been reports of some small observational studies of the use of nitric oxide donors (e.g., glyceryl trinitrate) for tocolysis.[20] The reported side effects have been few, but clearly, randomized evaluation in studies of sufficient size and with sufficient power to test efficacy and to note rare adverse effects is necessary before any meaningful comments can be made with regard to maternal safety.[21]

Risks Associated with the Mode of Delivery in Preterm Labor

Cesarean section as the preferred mode of delivery for the very preterm infant is a practice that did not receive adequate scrutiny before it came into common use. With it came significant maternal morbidity related to a poorly formed lower uterine segment, increased operative hemorrhage, infection, and compromised future uterine function—all this without documented improvement in perinatal mortality or morbidity rates.[22–24]

A survey of members of the Society of Perinatal Obstetricians (SPO)[22] demonstrated a doubling over a 5-year period of the elective cesarean section rate for infants born between 24 and 28 weeks' gestation. However, Sanchez-Ramos and associates[23] were able to demonstrate that a significant decrease in the cesarean section rate over the same 5-year period for very low birth weight infants did not alter the neonatal mortality rate, the incidence of low Apgar scores, or cord blood gas values, intraventricular hemorrhage, or the median length of stay in the neonatal intensive care unit. Grant and associates'[24] systematic review of six trials of elective versus selective cesarean delivery for infants less than 37 weeks' gestation not only demonstrated the difficulty of randomization of mode of delivery in this clinical situation, with only 122 women recruited, but concluded that decision making on an individual case-by-case basis, taking into account parental preference, was all that could be recommended from the available data.

The use of classical cesarean section for gestations less than 30 weeks, although often suggested, carries more risk of morbidity than the lower segment procedure and has very little data to recommend it. Unpublished data from Stacey and Steer[25] suggest that it confers no particular benefit, with 8 of 17 babies dying when delivered by the classic route before 30 weeks' gestation, compared to none of 21 babies of similar gestation delivered by lower segment cesarean section.

Assessing the psychosocial trauma experienced by the patient, her partner, and her family in relation to the management of threatened or actual PTL is difficult, and this short paragraph cannot do justice to the importance and magnitude of the problem. The physical restrictions imposed by the use of intravenous tocolytics, the impersonality of the multidisciplinary approach, the geographic dislocation that is commonly necessary, the uncertainty of the perinatal outcome, and delayed maternal-infant bonding are probably the major conflicts experienced. These factors need to be kept in mind as we attempt to further reduce the maternal risk associated with threatened and actual preterm labor.

FETAL AND NEONATAL RISKS

Risks of Associated Pathology

Compromised fetal health is often the precipitating factor in threatened or actual PTL. Hence, intrauterine fetal death, intrauterine growth restriction, major congenital anomalies, unrecognized intrauterine infection, and complicated multiple pregnancy will all contribute to the perinatal mortality and morbidity rates associated with PTL.

Risks of Prematurity

The gestational age at which threatened or actual PTL presents, together with the birth weight, influences both the management and the outcome (Fig. 62–1). In women presenting between 20 and 24 weeks' gestation, the management decision after discussion with the parents may be to allow delivery to occur because of the maternal risks from treatment and the likely poor prognosis for the baby if, as is often the case, delivery can be postponed only for a few hours or days.

Fetal intrapartum hypoxia and birth trauma associated with PTL involving the very low birth weight infant, whether birth is by the vaginal or abdominal route, will contribute to the perinatal risk. The risks in the neonatal period are those of congenital malformation, the sequelae of intrauterine growth restriction, respiratory distress syndrome, necrotizing enterocolitis, intracranial hemorrhage, convulsions, and septicemia. The fetal and neonatal risks associated with the medical management of PTL have not been accurately quantified, but certainly they require consideration in the overall management.

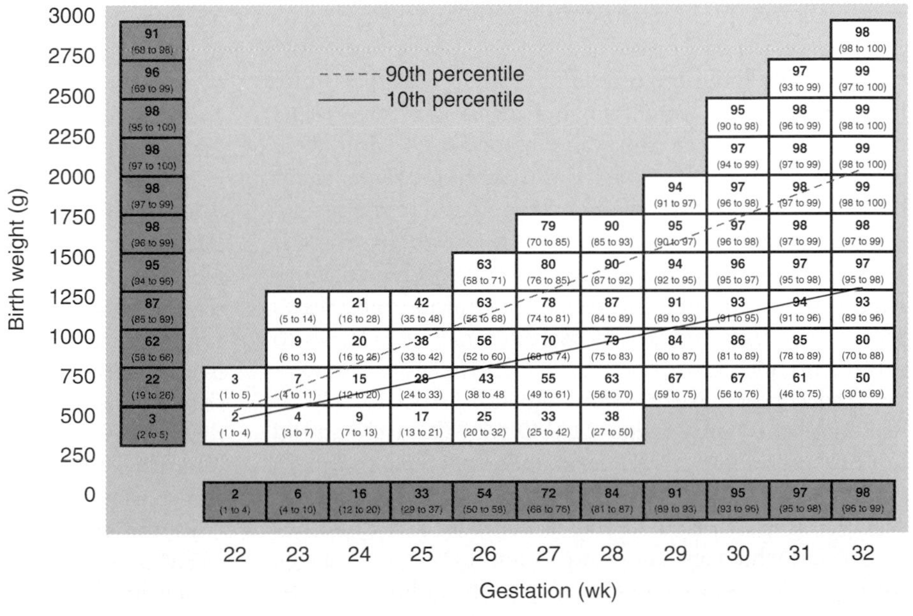

Figure 62–1
Median (95% confidence interval) predicted survival rates for European infants known to be alive at onset of labor. Values above 90th percentile represent infants large for gestational age; values below 10th percentile represent infants small for gestational age (see reference source for other ethnic groups). (From Draper ES, Manktelow B, Field DJ, James D: Prediction of survival for preterm births by weight and gestational age: Retrospective population based study. BMJ 1999;319:1093–1097.)

Risks of Tocolytic Agents

Beta-sympathomimetic tocolytic agents cross the placenta and may cause fetal tachycardia and occasionally other adverse fetal cardiac effects, which may be significant in an already compromised fetus.[10,26] The maternal hyperglycemia commonly associated with the use of these agents may result in neonatal hypoglycemia. There is a suggestion that neonatal intraventricular hemorrhage may be associated with the use of oral beta-sympathomimetic drugs, although the data are preliminary.[27] There have been only a few small studies of possible long-term ill effects for the neonate, and currently it appears there is no difference in developmental outcome if all confounding factors are taken into account.

Prostaglandin synthetase inhibitors (NSAIDs) cross from the mother to the fetus, potentially resulting in prolonged bleeding time, cardiopulmonary effects (predominantly premature closure or constriction of the ductus arteriosus and persistent fetal circulation), renal dysfunction, and reduced urinary output. Necrotizing enterocolitis and neonatal intraventricular hemorrhage have also been recorded in association with the use of these agents.[28–30] Most studies have limited the use of prostaglandin synthetase inhibitors to short-term therapy (48–72 hours) before 32 to 34 weeks' gestation. Newer and possibly more specific prostaglandin synthetase inhibitors such as sulindac,[31] ketorolac,[32] and the COX-2 selective agents (e.g., nimesulide) are currently being evaluated, as there is some evidence that they have fewer fetal side effects.

Magnesium sulfate also readily crosses the placenta and may compromise fetal cardiac activity, with reduced baseline variability of the fetal heart rate demonstrated by cardiotocography being a common association, which in turn may lead to unnecessary intervention. The neonate may exhibit hypotonia and hypocalcemia as a consequence of the hypermagnesemia.[33] The more controversial aspects of magnesium sulfate are related to its possible fetal neuroprotective role, as several observational studies indicated a reduction in cerebral palsy rate in very low birth weight infants in association with its use. However, Mitterdorf and associates,[34] who were originally enthusiasts for its use as a tocolytic agent because of this presumed effect, have found in their small randomized controlled trial (MagNET trial) that there is a highly significant association between tocolytic magnesium sulfate exposure and total neonatal mortality rates as well as a trend toward worse outcomes in relation to intraventricular hemorrhage, periventricular leukomalacia, and cerebral palsy. Crowther and associates (2003) presented the much larger ACTO $MgSO_4$ trial and did not observe an increase in perinatal or neonatal mortality rate.[35] A nonsignificant reduction of adverse neurologic sequelae was reported. If this is confirmed in the other large trials which are under way, then there may be a role for magnesium sulfate before very preterm birth.

Calcium-channel blockers[18] have not been adequately evaluated with regard to fetal or neonatal effects, and the Cochrane reviewers recommended the assessment of different dose and formulations on maternal and neonatal outcomes. Some animal studies have demonstrated profound metabolic alterations in the fetus, but to date these changes have not been confirmed in the fetuses of pregnant women.[4]

Newer tocolytic agents such as nitric oxide donors and oxytocin receptor antagonists have not been sufficiently assessed for us to be able to make meaningful comments at this stage.[19,21]

The maternal administration of thyrotropin-releasing hormone (TRH) in association with corticosteroids was thought, from preliminary studies, to enhance the development of fetal lung maturity, but the ACTOBAT Study[36] demonstrated results to the contrary (see later discussion), and hence, its use is now discouraged.[37]

Maternal corticosteroid administration to enhance fetal lung maturity is beneficial for the preterm neonate but may carry a number of risks, including infection, although the latest available data do not confirm this potential complication.[38,39] These potential risks must be balanced against the proven beneficial effect on neonatal pulmonary function and the possible reduction in intraventricular hemorrhage and necrotizing enterocolitis.[34] The Dutch trial,[40] which studied the effects of maternal prenatal corticosteroid administration, suggested a long-term increase in the incidence of pharyngeal and ear infections in infants of treated mothers but reported no clear evidence of significant fetal or neonatal infection in PTL associated with intact membranes.

The former practice of repeated maternal corticosteroid administration encouraged by the NIH Consensus Statement (1994)[38] for pregnancies at risk for preterm delivery between 24 and 34 weeks' gestation raised the question of whether long-term studies were advisable to detect any adverse effects on the fetus and neonate. Crowley and associates,[39] in an early overview of three studies, suggested that there was little evidence of adverse long-term outcomes with repeated maternal corticosteroid administration and questioned the need for further long-term studies. Walfisch and colleagues[41] reviewed 280 articles on this topic and concluded that there are no well-designed randomized controlled trials (RCTs) in humans that support the advantages of multiple courses over a single course of antenatal corticosteroids. They also commented that an increasing body of evidence raises the concern of adverse consequences from the use of repeated courses. This conclusion is consistent with the current Cochrane systematic review of three trials, which included 551 women. However, fewer infants required surfactant and there were fewer cases of severe respiratory distress syndrome (RDS).[42]

In the randomized trial conducted by the NICHD MFMU Network it was planned to recruit 2200 women, which has been reported in abstract form).[43] However, the trial was stopped after an interim analysis when only 495 women had been entered. There was no difference in the primary outcome, the respiratory distress syndrome, but infants delivered before 32 weeks may benefit with less use of surfactant, mechanical ventilation, and hypotension. There was a reduction in birth weight, particularly if four or more courses of steroids had been given.[43]

While awaiting full publication of the NICHD MFMU trial and results from RCTs in progress (such as the Australasian Collaborative Trial of Repeat Doses of Corticosteroids for the Prevention of Neonatal Respiratory Disease Study [ACTORDS] coordinated by Crowther and associates at the Women's and Children's Hospital, South Australia), it is recommended that only a single course of antenatal corticosteroids be given to all women at risk for preterm birth at 24 to 34 weeks' gestation.[41] (For a more detailed discussion of this topic, see Chapter 67.)

MANAGEMENT OPTIONS

Prepregnancy

The prevention and treatment of preterm birth has been the subject of extensive study. Risk-scoring strategies have been used to assess individual potential for preterm birth based on socioeconomic status, clinical history, lifestyle, and past obstetric and current prenatal complications. Unfortunately, there is little evidence from randomized trials of preterm preventive programs based on prospective risk scoring, whether they be hospital-based or require local social intervention, to suggest that there has been an overall reduction in the incidence of preterm delivery.[44] This failure is due both to a low sensitivity (generally below 50%) and a poor predictive value (17%–34%), particularly in primigravid women (previous pregnancy history is consistently reported to be one of the most important predictors). In addition, the value of prediction is limited when there are few, if any, effective treatments to alter the outcome.[45]

Hewitt and Newnham's study[46] of very low birth weight infants (weighing less than 1500 g) illustrates the limitations of preterm preventive programs. For infants born without major congenital anomalies, only 24% of the mothers had a history of a previous preterm birth. A total of 48% of the women were in their first pregnancy, and therefore, by definition they had no risk factors related to past obstetric history; of the multiparous women, 38% had no factors in their previous pregnancies indicating high risk. Another important feature revealed by this study was that idiopathic PTL was once again shown not to be the major factor in delivery at early gestations, occurring in only 17% of women studied, with PPROM in 30%, hypertension in 19%, antenatal hemorrhage in 17%, major anomalies in 8%, and fetal death in utero in 5%.

Thus, blanket preventive programs aimed indiscriminately at preterm delivery would not appear to be logical, other than as part of a scientific trial. With the assistance of the perinatal pathologist,[47] a significant proportion of women with "idiopathic" PTL can be demonstrated to have specific etiologic factors, and knowledge of these factors may be of assistance in the counseling and management of individual women with a previous preterm birth. In the situation of preterm birth without known causation, it is useful in prepregnancy counseling to estimate the likely recurrence risk. In their prospective study of preterm deliveries without uterine anomalies or medical problems, Ashmead and associates[48] determined that women with one previous preterm delivery had a 15% chance and those with two previous preterm births a 41% chance of another preterm delivery. These statistics may be useful in counseling patients who live in an area remote from a perinatal center, as it can be suggested that they move to a more convenient location during the critical period of a subsequent pregnancy in order to enhance the outcome.

More general advice with regard to daily work activity (avoidance of heavy manual labor or mental stress when family economics permit) and specific habits such as alcohol, smoking, and chemical dependency should be given, as there is some evidence that these factors may play a role in preterm birth.[49–51]

Hence, at the present time specific prepregnancy preventive measures for PTL might be considered for multiparous patients, but for nulliparous patients, apart from those with a known genital tract anomaly for which surgical correction might be possible, there do not appear to be any proven strategies to prevent PTL.

Prenatal

Assessment of Risk

At the first prenatal visit, assessing the risk of preterm delivery based on the history and examination may be useful as an initial screen to identify women at particularly high risk. The risk can be updated during the pregnancy if complications develop. An adaptation of the score devised by Creasy and associates[52] combines socioeconomic factors, previous medical history, daily habits, and aspects of the current pregnancy and is probably the most acceptable system, but its predictive value overall is only 17% to 34% owing to the multifactorial nature of PTL. In all women, but particularly those at risk of PTL, it is preferable that gestational age be confirmed by an early ultrasound scan.

Women with Previous Preterm Labor and Delivery: Cervical Problems

If cervical incompetence is suspected on the basis of a previous midtrimester miscarriage or known physical damage to the cervix (e.g., following surgery), then cervical cerclage (ideally as a planned procedure) can be performed at 12 to 14 weeks' gestation. It has been calculated, from the evidence of randomized trials, that 1 woman in 30 will benefit from a cervical suture.[53] Systematic review of randomized trials does not support use of cervical cerclage in women at low or medium risk of midtrimester loss, and its use for a short cervix remains uncertain.[54] Placement of a cervical stitch is usually a vaginal procedure, but on rare occasions it may have to be performed by the abdominal route (see Chapters 6 and 7). Late cervical cerclage in the face of cervical dilation is a less successful procedure and should only be considered under certain circumstances, preferably using a scoring system as an aid to prognosis.[55]

The Role of Infection

In acknowledgment of the increasing emphasis of the role of subclinical infection in PTL, particularly if an infective etiology is suspected from a previous preterm birth, it seems reasonable to take vaginal and cervical microbiologic swabs electively in high risk women at 20 to 24 weeks' gestation.[56] Even if the patient is not subjected to prophylactic antibiotic therapy (see later discussion), knowledge of the potential microbiologic milieu at the time of PTL will assist both the obstetrician in the management of maternal pyrexia and the neonatologist in the management of suspected infection in the preterm infant. Identification of group B streptococcus carriers is of particular value, as it enables appropriate intrapartum treatment with intravenous penicillin in nonallergic women.

Patient Education

Education of the patient with a previous preterm birth about the signs and symptoms of PTL is a useful option to consider. The perception of contractions, menstrual-like cramps, pelvic pressure sensations, low, dull backache, abdominal cramping with or without diarrhea, an increase or change in vaginal discharge, and a "show" may all prove to be significant, but are, individually, not particularly predictive.[57] Nonetheless, if they occur in any women at risk of PTL, then a thorough cervical assessment should be performed, whether this be by digital examination or by ultrasonography.

Antenatal Care

In those women suspected of being at increased risk of PTL, more frequent antenatal assessment, particularly in the latter half of pregnancy, is a common option employed. The rationale for this form of management is based on indirect evidence that absent or delayed onset of prenatal care is associated with an increased rate of preterm birth and low birth weight infants. Of course, it is possible that those patients who are sufficiently motivated to seek early and regular prenatal care are intrinsically healthier and better motivated than those who do not. However, prenatal care does provide the opportunity to detect (and possibly treat) some of the maternal and fetal conditions (for example, anemia, hypertension, and bacteriuria) that can lead to preterm birth. Although multiple pregnancy and fetal anomalies cannot be treated, early warning may allow for decisions to be made regarding the place, the timing, and the route of delivery, which in turn may enhance the outcome.[58] Bowes[59] perhaps best summarized the contributions of prenatal care in preterm birth management by suggesting that success is related to the continuity of care, time available for patients to talk about their problems, ready access to ancillary services when needed, and a prenatal record that provides fail-safe reminders of critical procedures and screening tests.[59] Enhanced prenatal care may have the potential to become more effective as better predictive tests for PTL and more selective prophylactic agents are developed to deal with women at risk of preterm birth. This must be balanced by current evidence from the Cochrane overview that social support does not appear to reduce the risk of preterm birth.

Prediction of Preterm Labor

Prediction of PTL (see Chapter 61) has dominated research efforts for the past decade or more. Outpatient and home monitoring of uterine contractions, regular cervical assessment both clinically and ultrasonographically, the use of biochemical markers such as placental corticotropin-releasing hormone (CRH) and its binding protein, salivary estriol, the inflammatory cytokines and prostaglandins, fetal fibronectin (FFN), cervical ferritin, and most recently noninvasive cutaneous cardiovascular dynamics (CVD) have either come and gone or are being evaluated or reevaluated in the hope that we might obtain a reliable predictor with high sensitivity and specificity in order to judiciously manage patients at increased risk of preterm delivery.

Strategies for Prevention

A number of strategies involving the prophylactic use of oral tocolytics, antibiotics, and corticosteroids have been used in the prenatal management of women at high risk of PTL and are worthy of further discussion.

TOCOLYTICS

Several controlled trials of the prophylactic administration of beta-sympathomimetic drugs for the prevention of PTL have been reported in the literature.[10] Detailed analysis gives no indication that these agents decrease the incidence of PTD or low birth weight in multiple or singleton pregnancies, with odds ratios for both being 1.17 and 1.02, respectively. Hence, their use in the preventive management of PTL cannot be recommended.

ANTIBIOTICS

In some obstetric populations 40% to 50% of preterm labors have an infective basis that, through the inflammatory process, triggers the cytokine cascade, which is responsible for PTL and membrane rupture. Vaginal colonization with *Bacteroides*, *Trichomonas vaginalis*, *Ureaplasma urealyticum*, *Mycoplasma hominis*, *Gardnerella vaginalis*, *Neisseria gonorrhoeae*, or hemolytic streptococcus group B or asymptomatic bacteriuria appears to increase the risk of PTL, PPROM, and PTD.[60] Once labor has begun under these circumstances, then it is almost certainly too late for antibiotics to have any effect in delaying birth (see later discussion), and it would seem more logical to treat biologically relevant microorganisms early in pregnancy in order to prevent activation of the cytokine cascade. The current data suggest that bacterial vaginosis (BV) is the most closely associated with the foregoing outcomes, and Morales and associates[61] were able to demonstrate a significant reduction in the incidence of PTL, PTD, low birth weight (<2500 g), and PPROM using oral metronidazole compared to placebo. Subsequently, McGregor and associates[62] performed a randomized placebo-controlled trial using 2% clindamycin vaginal cream, but were unable to demonstrate a significant change in pregnancy outcome with locally administered antibiotics, and this was confirmed by a similar multicenter trial.[63] This led to the conclusion that systemic therapy may be required to reduce the incidence of PTD through the eradication of upper genital tract organisms. Hauth and associates[64] helped to clarify this question in a randomized study, from which they concluded that treatment with systemic therapy (specifically metronidazole and erythromycin) reduced the rate of preterm delivery in a high risk group with known BV. More recently, work by McDonald and associates[65] has shown in a subgroup analysis that in women with a history of PTD, treatment of BV-positive women with oral metronidazole during the second trimester reduces the incidence of preterm birth, but this benefit of treatment did not extend to all women with heavy growth of *Gardnerella vaginalis*. Further study of broad-based screening and treatment of asymptomatic carriers of BV, both at high risk and low risk for PTL, is necessary in order to evaluate the efficacy of this potential form of prophylaxis for PTL.

Fetal fibronectin (FFN) may offer some assistance in this regard, as preliminary studies have demonstrated that a positive FFN test at 24 weeks' gestation is associated with a twofold risk of BV, which in turn is predictive (20-fold increased risk) of subsequent chorioamnionitis and neonatal sepsis (6-fold increased risk) 6 to 8 weeks later.[66] Gibbs[67] did not support the prenatal treatment of BV as being effective in the prevention of intrauterine infection and PTD, and this view was supported by the large study of Carey and associates.[68] However, their conclusions continue to be challenged by the NICHD MFMU Network Study[69] and the previously mentioned authors Morales and associates, McDonald and associates, Hauth and associates, and McGregor and associates and by the separate appraisals of Lamont[70] and Vigneswaran.[71] With regard to asymptomatic bacteriuria, Romero and associates[72] in their meta-analysis demonstrated that antibiotic therapy led to a significant reduction in low birth weight, although a similar effect on the rate of PTD was not seen.

The ORACLE trials,[73–75] although not directly answering the question of the use of prophylactic antibiotics for the prevention of PTL in women with intact membranes, nevertheless gave some important insights into the use of antibiotics in the management of PTL and PPROM. ORACLE II[75] confirmed the generally held view that antibiotics should not be prescribed routinely for women in spontaneous preterm labor without evidence of clinical infection, and ORACLE I considered the issue of antibiotic prophylaxis for PPROM (see Chapter 63). The explanation of a lack of beneficial effect may be that the population studied had a much lower incidence of asymptomatic vaginal infection and colonization than anticipated, and hence the sample size would be inadequate to show a positive effect. Additionally it is possible that once labor is established, then the cascade effect of cytokine/prostaglandin release would render antibiotics useless, and antibiotics might well aggravate the situation and contribute to neonatal morbidity by increasing the release of inflammatory cytokines.

CORTICOSTEROIDS

The use of "prophylactic" maternal corticosteroids to enhance fetal lung maturity in women at risk for PTD has currently been restricted to situations of threatened PTL and established PPROM during the immediate episode if it occurs before 34 weeks' gestation. A repeat course of corticosteroids may be given at 32 weeks' gestation should delivery be imminent more than 4 weeks since the last dose of corticosteroids. As mentioned previously, the results of the NICHD MFMU Network and ACTORDS trials are awaited with interest in view of experimental studies[76] and retrospective human studies, which have suggested caution with regard to the former practice of repeated maternal corticosteroid administration in high risk women because of possible fetal intrauterine growth restriction and neonatal neurodevelopmental impairment.[77]

PROGESTERONE

Supplemental progesterone to prevent PTD has been revisited with studies by da Fonseca and associates[78] and Meis[79] showing encouraging results with improvements in intermediate endpoints for prematurity reduction but with the sample size being insufficient to demonstrate a reduction in perinatal morbidity rate.

Management of Women Presenting with Threatened or Acute Preterm Labor

Once the diagnosis of threatened or actual PTL is established, then parenteral tocolytic therapy should be considered. After a careful clinical appraisal of the maternal and fetal condition, preliminary investigations should be performed. Ultrasonography can be used to ascertain fetal number, estimate fetal weight, check fetal morphology and presentation, measure the volume of amniotic fluid, and identify the placental site. It can also be used to assess fetal well-being. Fetal breathing movements may also be visualized during this evaluation, and although suppression of fetal breathing movements was found in preliminary studies to predict the likelihood of PTL,[80] it has never been incorporated into routine management.

Testing for an infective etiology is important in the initial assessment and includes culture of vaginal and cervical secretions and a midstream specimen of urine, a complete blood count (including a white blood cell count), and C reactive protein estimation. Amniocentesis with Gram stain and culture and, more recently, interleukin 6 (IL-6) estimation, may be considered if infection is suspected. At the same time fetal lung maturity can be assessed by lecithin/sphingomyelin ratio or phosphotidyl glycerol measurement. If indicated by an abnormal fetal morphology, fetal karyotype determination, possibly using fluorescent labeled in situ hybridization (FISH) or rapid techniques for diagnosis of aneuploidy, should be considered. Not all obstetricians would perform amniocentesis routinely in this situation both because of the possibility of inducing further uterine activity and because of the lack of randomized data to guide management decisions based on the findings.

Determination of the presence or absence of PPROM by clinical and, if necessary, additional investigations is essential to the management.

Although acknowledging that positive FFN tests in symptomatic women have only a 29.3% predictability of delivery before 34 weeks' gestation, a large body of evidence now exists of a greater than 95% accuracy of a negative FFN test predicting that preterm delivery will not occur before 34 weeks[81] and should probably be utilized to stop unnecessary and potentially dangerous intervention in women presenting with threatened preterm labor, particularly in remote areas where unnecessary and costly maternal-fetal transfer may also be avoided. A number of noninterventional studies have confirmed the usefulness of fetal fibronectin testing in this situation, and its use merits consideration in regionalized perinatal networks.

Once gestational age is established, the universally poor immediate and longer-term fetal outcomes of infants born between 20 and 24 weeks' gestation require considerable discussion between the parents, the obstetrician, and the neonatologist either before or shortly after the initiation of tocolytic therapy.[22,82] In cases of extreme fetal immaturity the parents may well choose to allow delivery to occur rather than to invoke risky, uncomfortable, and expensive delaying tactics of poor efficacy, but caution must be exercized because fetal weight and gestational estimates are subject to significant variation between 20 and 24 weeks. Perhaps a more pragmatic method of dealing with this dilemma is to transfer the patient to a tertiary center and allow her to deliver vaginally without intervention but with a neonatologist present at delivery to assess the delivered neonate with regard to the potential need for further neonatal support.

Whether continuous electronic fetal monitoring should be carried out during such a labor is a matter of dispute. Some argue that recording a potentially abnormal fetal heart rate while prescribing nonintervention is distressing for parents and staff, whereas others argue that the normality or otherwise of the fetal heart rate may be important for the neonatologist in deciding whether or not to resuscitate or support the neonate.

The use of tocolytic therapy between 24 and 34 weeks' gestation is not only to facilitate the in utero transfer of the fetus to a tertiary referral center[83] but also to enable sufficient time to enhance fetal lung maturity by the concomitant use of maternal corticosteroid therapy. The systematic review of 17 trials[10] with a total of 2284 women comparing tocolytics with no treatment or placebo and including some women with ruptured membranes found that ritodrine was the most frequently evaluated drug, but other agents were also used including isoxsuprine, terbutaline, magnesium sulfate, indomethacin, and atosiban. Overall, tocolytics were associated with a significant reduction in the odds of delivery within 24 hours (OR [odds ratio] 0.47; 95% CI [confidence interval] 0.29–0.77), 48 hours (OR 0.57, CI 0.38–0.83), and 7 days (OR 0.60; CI 0.38–0.95). For beta-sympathomimetics, indomethacin, and atosiban these effects were statistically significant, but for magnesium sulfate they were not. However, there was no statistically significant reduction in births before 30 weeks (OR 1.33; CI 0.53–3.33) or before 32 weeks (OR 0.81, CI 0.61–1.07) or before 37 weeks (OR 0.17; CI 0.02–1.62). Tocolysis was not associated with any clear effects on perinatal death (OR 1.22, CI 0.84–1.78) or on any measure of neonatal morbidity such as respiratory distress (OR 0.82; CI 0.61–1.07) or intraventricular hemorrhage (OR 0.73; CI 0.46–1.15). Trials for glyceryl trinitrate[21,84] have been too small to make any firm conclusions, and there are no placebo-controlled trials of calcium-channel blockers despite their increasing popularity as tocolytic agents. However, the latest Cochrane review did report on 11 randomized trials involving 870 women, comparing nifedipine with other tocolytics, and concluded that nifedipine was more effective than beta-mimetics and had fewer side effects.[18]

There are a number of explanations for the apparent negative (although not significantly so) effect of tocolysis on the perinatal mortality rate. Perhaps too many women in the trials were at an advanced gestation when prolongation of the pregnancy would have had little potential benefit for their babies; the time gained by tocolysis may not have been used productively (i.e., administration of corticosteroids, transfer to a tertiary unit), and there may have been direct or indirect adverse effects of the tocolytic agents used which outweighed the benefits of pregnancy prolongation (e.g., their use in the presence of abruptio, severe hypertension, and intrauterine growth restriction).

Currently there appears to be a trend away from the use of beta-sympathomimetics as first-line tocolytics, with a swing toward nifedipine or, particularly in the United Kingdom, atosiban, because of their fewer side effects. Nifedipine does have the advantages of cheapness, ease of administration, and availability. However, there continues to be a lack of consensus in administration regimens. The lack of any trials that show an advantage against placebo means that we should continue to be intolerant of any harmful short- or long-term side effects.

Tocolytic therapy should be continued if possible for 48 hours to try to maximize the enhancement of fetal lung maturity by maternally administered corticosteroids. Data from the 12 controlled trials reviewed by Crowley and associates,[85] and later by the NIH Consensus group,[38] demonstrate that corticosteroids not only reduce the occurrence of neonatal respiratory distress, but are also associated with reductions in the risk of neonatal intraventricular hemorrhage, necrotizing enterocolitis, and neonatal death, particularly in extremely preterm infants (less than 28 weeks' gestation).

The place of other maternally administered agents to enhance fetal outcome requires further discussion in the light of completed studies. The Australian collaborative trial of antenatal thyrotropin-releasing hormone (TRH) for the prevention of neonatal respiratory disease in women at high risk of preterm delivery who also received corticosteroids (the ACTOBAT study)[36] concluded that the increased maternal side effects and the increased ventilatory requirements of the treated neonates could not justify the widespread use of TRH. This finding is supported in a systematic review of 11 trials that included more than 4500 women. The subsequent 12-month follow-up study of ACTOBAT,[86] which suggests the additional possibility of abnormal neurodevelopment, should alert clinicians to be cautious in their use of TRH unless it is under the strict conditions of a clinical trial.

The prophylactic use of maternally administered vitamin K and phenobarbitone to reduce the incidence of neonatal intracerebral hemorrhage has not been validated scientifically in clinical trials[87] and, similarly, cannot be recommended as part of the routine management of PTL.[88]

If the initially selected tocolytic agent is unsuccessful, or is not tolerated in the suppression of PTL, then an alternative agent may be considered. This agent can be given alone or in combination with the initial tocolytic agent. Any such strategy should only be instituted after a careful reappraisal of maternal and fetal well-being. In particular, intrauterine infection should be excluded as far as possible, because it is notorious for producing a "failure" of tocolysis and is potentially dangerous not only to the fetus but also to the mother. The results of the ORACLE trial[74] should discourage the routine use of antibiotic therapy as an adjunct to tocolysis unless there is clinical evidence of maternal infection or when the mother is known to be a group B streptococcus carrier.

After an initial 48 hours of labor suppression by intravenous tocolysis, some workers have continued oral tocolytic agents until 34 to 37 weeks' gestation in an effort to prolong gestation. Although a trial[89] using a sustained-release oral tocolytic agent suggested benefit, continuing oral tocolysis has not been commonly employed by many perinatal centers, nor is it currently widely used.

More recently the role of cervical cerclage has been expanded to include women with nonreassuring sonographic cervical findings in the midtrimester.[90] Results of both retrospective cohort series and randomized trials of cerclage in women with shortened cervical length are inconclusive at this time. So-called rescue cerclage should therefore only be performed under the conditions of a randomized trial.[54,91,92]

Treatment of PTL after 34 weeks' gestation has little to recommend it because the additional expense and the maternal risks of tocolysis are not justified in view of the minimal neonatal morbidity potentially avoided between 34 and 37 weeks' gestation.[93]

Labor and Delivery

Once preterm delivery seems inevitable, the mode of delivery and the neonatal outcome should be discussed with the parents. The parents should discuss the further management with an obstetrician and a neonatologist as well as with an experienced obstetric anesthetist.[94] They play an essential part in establishing management guidelines that will be acceptable to all parties. The other central person in the management team in some countries is the midwife, who should also be included in discussions concerning the management of labor and the delivery.

In general, before 24 completed gestational weeks, vaginal delivery should be the accepted route, with expert neonatal evaluation at delivery to determine if further neonatal supportive care is warranted. Between 24 and 34 weeks the management of labor should not differ significantly from that beyond 34 weeks.[22] Continuous electronic fetal monitoring and a preference for regional analgesia are of unproven benefit but are commonly used in the contemporary management of established PTL.

Once labor is established, maternal antibiotic therapy should be commenced if signs of intrauterine infection are present. Earlier reservations regarding the possibility of inducing superinfection with resistant bacteria and complicating the diagnosis of infection in the neonate have not been borne out in clinical practice.[95,96] A reduction in maternal infectious morbidity rate has been shown in most studies, and although the authors currently favor the use of intravenous ampicillin 2 g every 8 hours and gentamicin 80 g every 8 hours during labor, this combination of antibiotics is currently under review in the light of new evidence suggesting that beta-lactam antibiotics may have deleterious effects on the neonate as a result of the sudden release of cytokines and aggravation of the fetal inflammatory response syndrome (FIRS).[97]

Evaluation of the available randomized trials would suggest that "prophylactic" outlet forceps or "elective" episiotomy does not contribute significantly to the neonatal outcome and hence should only be performed for standard obstetric indications.[98] Early cord clamping has not been proved to confer an advantage to the neonate and so cannot be recommended in the routine management of a preterm birth.[98] Standard management of the third stage is recommended in PTL.

From the neonatal aspect, the significantly higher risk of morbidity and fatality of infants born outside a tertiary perinatal center makes a compelling argument for maternal-fetal transport (preferably with the baby in utero) to a tertiary perinatal center with neonatal intensive care facilities, providing such transport does not jeopardize the safety of the mother.[99,100] When transport is not possible (in some series up to 50% of cases), then specifically trained and equipped obstetric and neonatal retrieval teams with appropriate nursing and medical personnel should attend the birth. They can supervise or perform the delivery of the neonate and then stabilize the mother and her premature infant prior to their respective transfers to the tertiary perinatal center if this is deemed necessary.[99,100]

Postnatal

Maternal Considerations

Encouragement of parent-infant bonding is a major consideration in postnatal management. Continuous access by the parents to the neonatal nursery should be encouraged to facilitate the bonding process. Breastfeeding should be encouraged in a compassionate and pragmatic manner.

Continuing psychosocial support is important, utilizing the services of a domiciliary midwife, a social worker, and if indicated, a psychiatrist. This staff support is likely to be essential if there is significant neonatal morbidity or a perinatal death.

An early postnatal evaluation of possible etiologic factors related to the PTL should be considered by the perinatal team, which should include an obstetrician, neonatologist, perinatal pathologist, and where indicated, input from an obstetric physician, pediatric surgeon, geneticist, and ultrasonologist in order to construct a rational plan of management for further pregnancies.

Neonatal Considerations

Premature birth requires adaptation to extrauterine life while the different organ systems undergo continued structural and functional development and maturation. Thus, premature infants can be expected to have a variety of problems in the neonatal period with the risk of complications being proportional to the degree of prematurity.

Premature infants are likely to have difficulties in maintaining body temperature and in oral feeding, as well as having a greater risk of infection. Lung maturity of premature infants is proportional to their gestation and is the major cause of respiratory distress syndrome in these infants. Poorly developed respiratory control may lead to recurrent apnea in premature infants.[101]

Congestive cardiac failure may occur as a result of a patent ductus arteriosus associated with prematurity. Liver immaturity is likely to be associated with severe neonatal jaundice, and the baby is more vulnerable to the neurotoxic effects of unconjugated bilirubin. There is also an increased risk of intracranial hemorrhage and necrotizing enterocolitis in these infants, and in the extremely premature infant, chronic lung disease, retinopathy, cerebral palsy, and developmental delay are more likely in the longer term.[101]

Maturity of organ systems, particularly the lung, is the key factor determining the ultimate prognosis of the premature infant. Minimizing the incidence and severity of respiratory distress has been the major factor in the substantial improvement in neonatal morbidity and mortality rates over the past 2 decades. Previously mentioned strategies of regionalization of perinatal care, selective use of tocolytic agents, and the antenatal administration of corticosteroids to enhance fetal lung maturity have all been positive contributing factors.

Evaluation of the "prophylactic use" of exogenous surfactant has demonstrated a favorable outcome with a significant reduction in the incidence of respiratory distress syndrome.[102–104] Additionally, the course of established respiratory distress can be significantly modified by the administration of surfactant "rescue" therapy in association with mechanical respiratory support.[105] It cannot be emphasized too strongly that the antenatal administration of corticosteroids to the mother is equally as important as exogenous surfactant in minimizing respiratory morbidity.

Although there has been a significant increase in neonatal survival rates at 24 to 27 weeks' gestation over the past decade,[106] it appears that prematurity per se has a deleterious effect on neonatal growth and development, which contributes to a poorer outcome. This must be taken into account, particularly when assessing survival rates in premature infants in the less than 24 weeks' gestational ("previable") age group.[107]

Despite the very substantial medical advances in neonatal intensive care, it must be emphasized that not every premature newborn infant can be salvaged, and on some occasions survival will be accompanied by severe handicap, either physical or mental. Prolonging life in these circumstances may not be beneficial to the infant and may be unacceptably burdensome to the parents. Consideration of withdrawing life support in such tragic circumstances should be undertaken after detailed and extensive consultation and counseling of the parents.[108,109]

In addition to these medical and ethical challenges confronting the neonatologist are the immediate and delayed financial costs of neonatal intensive care. Economic constraint applies a brake to the tendency of the specialist to attempt to overcome all these medical and ethical challenges, as neonatologists are increasingly being required to apply evidence-based medical practice in an environment of cost containment.

The final measure of the quality of a tertiary neonatal service is the dedication and commitment of its long-term follow-up program. All perinatal centers must be prepared continuously to maintain and even upgrade this essential service in order to practice early intervention so as to reduce to the minimum possible the physical and mental handicaps inevitable in very premature infants, and provide crucial information to obstetricians and subspecialists in maternal-fetal medicine of the potential outcome of infants of all gestational ages and birth weight groups. They must promulgate appropriate and relevant advice and support, reassure, and counsel the parents who will continue to bear the brunt of the care for the infant who is born prematurely.

CONCLUSIONS

- Since the last edition of this text in 1999 there have been numerous efforts made on many fronts not only to try to reduce the incidence of preterm delivery and the neonatal mortality rate associated with such an event but also to reduce the neonatal morbidity rate.
- Sadly, we have not reduced the incidence of preterm delivery, and indeed, in some centers there has been a small but significant increase in the incidence of preterm delivery. This rise may be due to expanding indications for obstetric intervention before term (in consultation with our neonatology colleagues) rather than a true increase in spontaneous preterm labor.
- Much effort continues in the quest to find accurate markers of preterm labor (see Chapter 61) to allow the use of interventions such as prophylactic progesterone therapy and cerclage after sonographic cervical evaluation. These possible interventions require further evaluation in large, well-conducted clinical trials.
- Our attempts to reduce neonatal morbidity rate may come to fruition with our rapidly increasing knowledge of the role of cytokines in the fetal inflammatory response syndrome, leading to the development of nonantibiotic anti-inflammatory agents that may play a significant role in the future management of preterm labor.

SUMMARY OF MANAGEMENT OPTIONS
Threatened and Actual Preterm Labor

Management Options	Quality of Evidence	Grade of Recommendation	References
Prepregnancy (Previous Preterm Delivery)			
Establish cause/precipitating factors; estimate risk of recurrence; be honest about the value of preventive measures.	III	B	44,47,48
Give advice about lifestyle, work, place of residence at critical phase of pregnancy, diet, smoking, alcohol and drug abuse.	III	B	49–51
Prenatal—Assessment of Risk			
Careful history taking for presence of specific risks (e.g., previous preterm birth), but value of formal risk scoring systems uncertain.	III	B	44,47,48, 52
Establish gestational age early and accurately.	–	GPP	–
Prenatal—Previous Preterm Labor and Delivery			
General advice about lifestyle, work, place of residence at critical phase of pregnancy, diet, smoking, alcohol and drug abuse.	III	B	49–51
If cervical incompetence, suture at 12–14 weeks.	Ib	A	53
Patient education about clinical features may alert clinician but overall has poor predictive value and no evidence of improved outcome.	Ia	A	109

Continued

SUMMARY OF MANAGEMENT OPTIONS

Threatened and Actual Preterm Labor *(Continued)*

Management Options	Quality of Evidence	Grade of Recommendation	References
Prenatal—Previous Preterm Labor and Delivery—*Continued*			
Increased attendance and discussion for women at increased risk helpful to allow decision on place, timing, and mode of delivery.	III	B	58
Prenatal—Strategies Needing Further Evaluation			
Screening	See Chapter 61		
Monitoring uterine contractility			
Regular cervical assessment (clinical and ultrasound)			
Infection screening			
Biochemical screening			
Prophylaxis			
Tocolytics offer no value.	Ia	A	10
Antiobiotics (general) offer no value.	Ib	A	74
Treatment of bacterial vaginosis with systemic metronidazole and erythromycin reduces preterm delivery.	Ib	A	64
Steroids should be used in women in genuine preterm labor; concerns over repeated courses.	Ia	A	39,77
Presenting with Threatened or Actual Preterm Labor			
Initial assessment to determine whether genuine preterm labor	–	GPP	–
Uterine activity			
Bleeding			
Membrane rupture			
Presentation			
Engagement of head			
Cervical status (clinical and ultrasound)			
Gestational age			
Biochemical tests (e.g., fetal fibronectin) may be of more value in excluding diagnosis	III	B	81
Search for a cause/precipitating factor (e.g., fetal abnormality, placental bleeding, infection, multiple pregnancy, membrane rupture)	–	GPP	–
Discuss prognosis with parents (see text)	III	B	22,82
Transfer to tertiary center preferably in utero	III	B	83,99,100
Liaison with pediatricians	–	GPP	–
Tocolysis (influenced by factors including gestation, cause, contraindications)	Ia	A	10,18,21,84
Beta-sympathomimetics most widely used; nifedipine and atosiban use increasing (alternatives: atosiban, nifedipine, indomethacin before 24 weeks).			
Justified for at least 48 h to administer steroids; probably not justified beyond 34 weeks.			
BEWARE PULMONARY EDEMA AND HYPERGLYCEMIA ESPECIALLY WHEN USED WITH MATERNAL STEROIDS.			
Consider oral maintenance tocolytic therapy after successful abolition of contractions.	Ib	A	89
Maternal steroids	Ia	A	38,85
Thyroid releasing hormone, vitamin K, and phenobarbitone are not justified.	Ib	A	36,86,87

SUMMARY OF MANAGEMENT OPTIONS

Threatened and Actual Preterm Labor *(Continued)*

Management Options	Quality of Evidence	Grade of Recommendation	References
Presenting with Threatened or Actual Preterm Labor—*Continued*			
Rescue cerclage only in the context of RCT.	Ia	A	54
Antibiotic therapy cannot be recommended at present as an adjunct to tocolysis (except in labor with group B streptococcus carrier and use of erythromycin for preterm premature rupture of membranes; see Chapter 63).	Ia	A	74
Labor and Delivery			
Interdisciplinary approach (obstetric, nursing, pediatric, anesthetic)	–	GPP	–
Before 24 Weeks			
Careful discussion with parents about prognosis (see text)	–	GPP	–
Aim for vaginal delivery; experienced pediatrician in attendance			
From 24 Weeks			
Careful discussion with parents about prognosis (see text)	–	GPP	–
If cephalic presentation, aim for vaginal delivery with cesarean for normal obstetric indications. Some would not perform cesarean sections at 24 or 25 weeks.	–	GPP	–
If breech presentation, see Chapter 64.			
Continuous fetal heart rate monitoring	IV	C	110
Many use regional analgesia.	IV	C	94
Instrumental vaginal delivery only for standard obstetric indications.	IV	C	98
Antibiotics if features of infection (may reduce maternal/fetal infective risk)	–	GPP	–
Experienced pediatrician in attendance	See Chapter 82		
Postnatal			
Maternal	–	GPP	–
Encourage breast-feeding			
Psychological support			
Give adequate information about baby			
Allow continuous access to neonatal care unit			
Look for causes/precipitating factors and establish plan for future pregnancies			
Appropriate neonatal care	–	GPP	–

REFERENCES

1. O'Driscoll MK: Preterm labour. In Anderson A, Beard R, Brudenall JM, Dunn PM (eds): Proceedings of the Fifth Study Group of the Royal College of Obstetricians and Gynaecologists. London, Royal College of Obstetricians and Gynaecologists, 1977, pp 369–370.
2. Kragt H, Keirse MJNC: How accurate is a woman's diagnosis of threatened preterm delivery. In Chalmers I, Enkin M, Keirse MJNC (eds): Pre-term Labour: Effective Care in Pregnancy and Childbirth, Vol. 1. Oxford, Oxford University Press, 1989, pp 694–745.
3. Amon E, Petrie RH: Tocolytic agents. In Charles D, Glover DD (eds): Current Therapy in Obstetrics. Toronto, BC Decker, 1988, pp 267–270.
4. Gonik B, Creasy RK: Preterm labor: Its diagnosis and management. Am J Obstet Gynaecol 1986;154:3–9.
5. Chan AM, Scott J, Nguyen AM, Keen R: Pregnancy outcome in South Australia 2001. Annual report of the Pregnancy Outcome Unit, Epidemiology Branch, South Australian Health Commision, 2002.
6. Clinical Information Services Annual Report, Adelaide Women's and Children's Hospital, 2002.
7. Tucker JM, Goldenberg RL, Davis RO, et al: Etiologies of preterm birth in an indigent population: Is prevention a logical expectation? Obstet Gynecol 1991;77:343–347.
8. Cemach Project 27/28: An enquiry into quality of care and its effects on the survival of babies born at 27–28 weeks. London, UK, CESDI, CEMACH, 2003. Available at www.cemach.org.uk.
9. Lettieri L, Vintzileos AM, Rodis JF, et al: Does "idiopathic" preterm labor resulting in preterm birth exist? Am J Obstet Gynecol 1993;168:1480–1485.

10. Gyetvai K, Hannah ME, Modnett ED, Ohlsson A: Tocolytics for preterm labor: A systematic review. Obstet Gynecol 1999;94: 869–877.
11. Katz M, Robertson PA, Creasy RK: Cardiovascular complications associated with terbutaline treatment for preterm labor. Am J Obstet Gynecol 1981;139:605–608.
12. Ingemarsson L, Arulkumaran S, Kottegoda SR: Complications of betamimetic therapy in preterm labor. Aust NZ J Obstet Gynaecol 1985;25:182–189.
13. Zuckerman H, Shalev F, Gilad G, Katzuni E: Further study of the inhibition of premature labor by indomethacin. Part II: Double-blind study. J Perinatal Med 1984;12:25–29.
14. Slater DM, Berger LC, Newton R, et al: Expression of cyclo-oxygenases types 1 and 2 in human fetal membranes at term. Am J Obstet Gynecol 1995;172:77–82.
15. Crowther CA, Moore VM, Hiller JE, Doyle LW: Magnesium sulphate for preventing preterm birth in threatened preterm labour. In The Cochrane Library, Issue 2. Oxford, Update Software, 2003.
16. Elliott JP: Magnesium sulfate as a tocolytic agent. Am J Obstet Gynecol 1983;147:277–284.
17. Read MD, Wellby DE: The use of a calcium antagonist (nifedipine) to suppress preterm labour. Br J Obstet Gynaecol 1986;93: 933–937.
18. King JF, Flenady VJ, Papatsonis DN, et al: Calcium channel blockers for inhibiting preterm labor. Cochrane review. In The Cochrane Library, Issue 2. Oxford, Update Software, 2003.
19. Worldwide Atosiban versus Beta-agonists Study Group (2001): Effectiveness and safety of the oxytocin antagonist versus beta-adrenergic agonists in the treatment of preterm labor. Br J Obstet Gynaecol 2001;108:133–142.
20. Rowlands S, Trudinger B, Visva-Lingam S: Treatment of preterm cervical dilatation with glyceryl trinitrate, a nitric oxide donor. Aust NZ J Obstet Gynaecol 1996;36:377–381.
21. Duckitt K, Thornton S: Nitric oxide donors for the treatment of preterm labor (Cochrane Review). In The Cochrane Library, Issue 2. Oxford, Update Software, 2003.
22. Amon F, Moyn S: Caesarean section for fetal indications at the limits of fetal viability (1986–1991). 12th Annual SPO Meeting No. 4. Am J Obstet Gynecol 1992;166:274.
23. Sanchez-Ramos L, Walker C, Briones D, Cullen MT: Decreasing caesarean section rates in very low birthweight infants: Effective on perinatal outcome. Am J Obstet Gynecol 1992;166:444.
24. Grant A, Penn ZJ, Steer PJ: Elective or selection caesarean delivery of the small baby? A systematic review of the controlled trials. Br J Obstet Gynaecol 1996;103:1197–1200.
25. Stacey L, Steer PJ: Personal communication, 1997.
26. Friedman DM, Blackstone J, Young BK, Hoskins IA: Fetal cardiac effects of oral ritodrine tocolysis. Am J Perinatol 1994;11:109–112.
27. Groome LJ, Goldenberg RL, Cliver SP, et al: Neonatal periventricular-intraventricular hemorrhage after maternal beta-sympathomimetic tocolysis. The March of Dimes Multicenter Study Group. Am J Obstet Gynecol 1992;167:873–879.
28. Gersony WM, Peckham GJ, Ellison RC, et al: Effects of indomethacin in premature infants with patent ductus arteriosus: Results of a national collaborative study. J Pediatr 1982;102: 895–896.
29. Gleason CA: Prostaglandins and the developing kidney. Semin Perinatol 1987;11:12–21.
30. Hennessy MD, Livinston EC, Papagianos J, Killam AP: The incidence of ductal constriction and oligohydramnios during tocolytic therapy with ibuprofen. 12th Annual SPO Meeting No. 163. Am J Obstet Gynecol 1992;166:324.
31. Carlan SJ, O'Brien WF, O'Leary TD, Mastrogiannis D: Randomized comparative trial of indomethacin and sulindac for the treatment of refractory preterm labor. Obstet Gynecol 1992;79:223–228.
32. Schorr SJ, Ascarelli MH, Rust OA, et al: A comparative study of ketorolac (Toradol) and magnesium sulfate for arrest of preterm labor. South Med J 1998;91:1028–1032.
33. Wright JW, Ridgeway LE, Wright BD, et al: Effects of $MgSO_4$ on heart rate monitoring in the preterm fetus. J Reprod Med 1996;41:605–608.
34. Mittendorf R, Dambrosia J, Pryole PG, et al: Association between the use of antenatal magnesium sulphate in preterm labor and adverse health outcomes in infants. Am J Obstet Gynecol 2002;186:1111–1118.
35. Crowther CM, Hiller J, Doyle L, Coordinating Committee ACTO $MgSO_4$: Australasian Collaborative Trial of Magnesium Sulphate Use in Pregnancy (ongoing trial). Women's and Children's Hospital, Adelaide, South Australia.
36. ACTOBAT Study Group: Australian collaborative trial of antenatal thyrotropin-releasing hormone (ACTOBAT) for prevention of neonatal respiratory disease. Lancet 1995;345:877–881.
37. Crowther CA, Alfirevic Z, Haslam RR: Prenatal thyrotropin-releasing hormone for preterm birth. In The Cochrane Library, Issue 2. Oxford, Update Software, 2003.
38. NIH Consensus Statement: Effect of Corticosteroids for Fetal Maturation on Perinatal Outcomes, Vol. 12, No. 2. Bethesda, National Institutes of Health, 1994.
39. Crowley P, Chalmers I, Keirse MJNC: The effects of corticosteroid administration before preterm delivery: An overview of the evidence from controlled trials. Br J Obstet Gynaecol 1990;97:11–25.
40. Smolders de Haas H, Neuvel J, Schmand B, et al: Physical development and medical history of children who were treated antenatally with corticosteroids to prevent respiratory distress syndrome: A 10- to 12-year follow-up. Pediatrics 1990;86:65–70.
41. Walfisch A, Hallak M, Mazor M: Multiple courses of antenatal steroids: Risks and benefits. Obstet Gynecol 2001;98(3):491–497.
42. Crowther CA, Harding J: Repeat doses of prenatal corticosteroids for women at risk of preterm birth for preventing neonatal respiratory disease (Cochrane Review). In the Cochrane Library, Issue 1. Chichester, UK, John Wiley & Sons, 2004.
43. Wapner RJ for the NICHD MFMU Network: A randomised trial of single vs weekly courses of corticosteroids. Am J Obstet Gynecol 2003;189:S56.
44. Connon AF: An assessment of key aetiological factors associated with preterm birth and perinatal mortality. Aust NZ J Obstet Gynaecol 1992;32:200–203.
45. McLean M, Walters WAW, Smith R: Prediction and early diagnosis of preterm labor: A critical review. Obstet Gynecol Surv 1993;48:209–225.
46. Hewitt BG, Newnham JP: A review of the obstetric and medical complications leading to the delivery of infants of very low birthweight. Med J Aust 1988;149:234–238.
47. Chambers H: The perinatal autopsy. Med J Aust 1990;153: 578–579.
48. Ashmead G, Burrows W, Krew M, et al: Predicting preterm labour and birth. 12th Annual SPO Meeting No. 486. Am J Obstet Gynecol 1990;164:379.
49. Fox SH, Brown C, Koontz AM, Kessel SS: NHIS findings. Publ Health Rep 1990;102:73–75.
50. Mozurkewich F, Luke B, Papiernik E: The association between working conditions and preterm birth: A meta-analysis. Society of Perinatal Obstetricians Abstract No. 86. Am J Obstet Gynecol 1997;176:36.
51. Newman R: Occupational fatigue and preterm premature rupture of membranes. Society of Perinatal Obstetricians Abstract No. 84. Am J Obstet Gynecol 1977;176:35.
52. Creasy RK, Gummer BA, Liggins GC: A system for predicting spontaneous preterm birth. Obstet Gynecol 1980;55:692–698.
53. MCR/RCOG Working Party on Cervical Cerclage: Final report on the multicentre randomized trial of cervical cerclage. Br J Obstet Gynaecol 1993;100:516–523.
54. Drakeley AJ, Roberts D, Alfirevic Z: Cervical stitch (cerclage) for preventing pregnancy loss in women (Cochrane Review). In The Cochrane Library, Issue 2. Oxford, Update Software, 2003.

55. Balucci I, Drews M, Rawlinson K, Fenton AN: Cervical cerclage. Risks versus benefits. Am J Obstet Gynecol 1991;165:380.
56. Gibbs RS, Romero R, Hillier SL, et al: A review of premature birth and subclinical infection. Am J Obstet Gynecol 1992;166: 1515–1528.
57. Iams JD, Parker M, Johnson FF: A prospective evaluation of the signs and symptoms of preterm labor. Obstet Gynecol 1992;84: 227–230.
58. Buescher PA, Ward NI: A comparison of low birth weight among Medicaid patients of public health departments and other providers of prenatal care in North Carolina and Kentucky. Publ Health Rep 1992;107:54–59.
59. Bowes WA: Enhanced prenatal care in the prevention of preterm labor. Editorial. Obstet Gynecol Surv 1992;47: 474–475.
60. McDonald HM, O'Loughlin JA, Jolly P, et al: Vaginal infection and preterm labour. Br J Obstet Gynaecol 1991;98:427–435.
61. Morales WJ, Schorr S, Albritton J: Effect of metronidazole in patients with preterm birth in preceding pregnancy and bacterial vaginosis: A placebo-controlled, double blind study. Am J Obstet Gynecol 1994;171:345–347.
62. McGregor JA, French JL, Jones W, et al: Bacterial vaginosis is associated with prematurity and vaginal fluid mucinase and sialidase: Results of a controlled trial of clindamycin cream. Am J Obstet Gynecol 1994;170:1048–1060.
63. Joesoef MR, Hillier SL, Wiknjosastro U, et al: Intravaginal clindamycin treatment for bacterial vaginosis: Effects on preterm delivery and low birth weight. Am J Obstet Gynecol 1995;173: 1527–1531.
64. Hauth JC, Goldenberg RL, Andrews W, et al: Reduced incidence of preterm delivery with metronidazole and erythromycin in women with bacterial vaginosis. N Engl J Med 1995;333: 1732–1736.
65. McDonald HM, O'Loughlin JA, Vigneswaran R, et al: Impact of metronidazole therapy on preterm birth in women with bacterial vaginosis flora (Gardnerella vaginalis): A randomised, placebo controlled trial. Br J Obstet Gynaecol 1997;104: 1391–1397.
66. Goldenberg RL, Thom E, Moawad AH, et al: The preterm prediction study: Fetal fibronectin, bacterial vaginosis and peripartum infection. Obstet Gynecol 1996;87:656–660.
67. Gibbs RS: Chorioamnionitis and bacterial vaginosis. Am J Obstet Gynecol 1993;169:460–462
68. Carey JC, Klebanoff MA, Harth JC, et al: Metronidozale to prevent preterm delivery in pregnant women with asymptomatic bacterial vaginosis. National Institute of Child Health and Human Development Network of Maternal-Fetal Med Units. N Engl J Med 2000;342:534–540.
69. Meis PJ, Goldenberg RL, Mercer B, et al: The preterm prediction study: Significance of vaginal infections. National Institute of Child Health and Human Development Maternal-Fetal Medicine Units Network. Am J Obstet Gynecol 1995;173: 1231–1235.
70. Lamont RF: Antiobiotics for the prevention of preterm birth. N Engl J Med 2000;342:581–583.
71. Vigneswaran R: Infection and preterm birth: Evidence of a common causal relationship with bronchopulmonary dysplasia and cerebral palsy. J. Paediatr Child Health 2000;36:293–296.
72. Romero R, Oyarzun F, Mazor M, et al: Meta-analysis of the relationship between asymptomatic bacteriuria and pre-term delivery/low birth weight. Obstet Gynecol 1989;73:576–582.
73. Kenyon SL, Taylor DJ, Tarnow-Mordi W, Oracle Collaborative Group: Broad spectrum antibiotics for preterm, prelabour rupture of fetal membranes: The ORACLE I randomized trial. Lancet 2001;357:979–988.
74. Kenyon SL, Taylor DJ, Tarnow-Mordi W, Oracle Collaborative Group: Broad spectrum antibiotics for spontaneous preterm labor: The ORACLE II randomized trial. Lancet 2001;357: 989–994.
75. Kenyon SL, Taylor DJ, Tarnow-Mordi W: Broad-spectrum antibiotics for preterm, prelabour rupture of the membranes: The ORACLE I randomised trial. ORACLE Collaborative Group. Lancet 2001;357:979–988.
76. Ikegami M, Jobe AH, Newnham J, et al: Repetitive prenatal glucocorticoids improve lung function and decrease growth of preterm lambs. Am J Respir Crit Care Med 1997;156:178–184.
77. Seckl JR, Miller WL: How safe is long term prenatal glucocorticoid treatment? JAMA 1997;277:1077–1079.
78. da Fonseca EB, Bittar RE, Carvalho MHB, Zugaib M: Prophylactic administration of progesterone by vaginal suppository to reduce the incidence of spontaneous preterm birth in women at increased risk: A randomized placebo-controlled double-blind study. Am J Obstet Gynecol 2003;188:419–424.
79. Meis PJ, Klebanoff AA, Thom E, et al, NICHD and MFMU Network: Prevention of recurrent preterm delivery by 17 alphahydroxyprogesterone caproate. N Engl J Med 2003;348: 2379–2385.
80. Castle BM, Turnbull AC: The presence or absence of fetal breathing movements predicts outcome of preterm labour. Lancet 1983;2:471–473.
81. Morrison JC, Allbert JR, McLaughlin BN, et al: Oncofetal fibronectin in patients with false labor as a predictor of preterm delivery. Am J Obstet Gynecol 1993;168:538–542.
82. Robertson PA, Sniderman SH, Laros RK, et al: Neonatal morbidity according to gestational age and birthweight from five tertiary care centres in the United States 1983 through 1986. Am J Obstet Gynecol 1992;166:1629–1635.
83. Tsokos N, Newnham J, Langford SA: Intravenous tocolytic therapy for long distance aeromedical transport of women in preterm labour in Western Australia. Asia Oceania J Obstet Gynaecol 1988;14:21 25.
84. Smith GN, Walker MC, McGrath MJ: Randomised, double-blind, placebo controlled pilot study assessing nitroglycerin as a tocolytic (1999). Am J Obstet Gynaecol 1999;106:736–739.
85. Crowley P, Chalmers I, Keirse MJNC: The effects of corticosteroid administration before preterm delivery. An overview of the evidence from controlled trials. Br J Obstet Gynaecol 1990;97:11–25.
86. Crowther CA, Hiller JE, Haslam RR, Robinson JS: Australian Collaboration Trial of Antenatal Thyrotropin-Releasing Hormone: Adverse effects at 12 month follow-up ACTOBAT Study Group. Pediatrics 1997;99:311–317.
87. Thorp JA, Poskin MF, McKenzie DR, Heimes B: Perinatal factors predicting severe intracranial haemorrhage. Am J Perinatol 1997;14:631–636.
88. Doyle L: Antenatal phenobarbitone and neonatal outcome. Lancet 1996;348:975–976.
89. Holleboom CAG, Merkus JMWM, van Elferen LWM, Keirse MJNC: Double-blind evaluation of ritodrine sustained release for oral maintenance of tocolysis after active preterm labour. Br J Obstet Gynaecol 1996;103:702–705.
90. Owen J, Iams JD, Havth JC: Vaginal sonography and cervical incompetence. Am J Obstet Gynecol 2003;188:586–596.
91. Althuisius SM, Dekker GA, Hummel P, et al: Final results of the Cervical Incompetence Prevention Randomized Cerclage Trial (CIPRACT): Therapeutic cerclage with bed rest versus bed rest alone. Am J Obstet Gynecol 2001;185:1106–1112.
92. Rust OA, Atlas RO, Reed J, et al: Revisiting the short cervix defected by transvaginal ultrasound in the secnd trimester: Why cerclage may not help. Am J Obstet Gynecol 2001;185: 1095–1105.
93. Fox JF, McCaul RW, Martin WE, et al: Neonatal morbidity between 34–37 weeks gestation. Am J Obstet Gynecol 1992; 166:360.
94. Crowhurst JA: Epidural blockade in obstetrics—How safe? Med J Aust 1992;157:220–222.
95. Isaacs D, Barfield CP, Grimwood K, et al: Systemic bacterial and fungal infections in infants in Australian neonatal units. Australian Study Group for Neonatal Infections. Med J Aust 1995;162:198–201.
96. Katz V: Management of group B streptococcal disease in pregnancy. Clin Obstet Gynecol 1993;36:832–842.

97. Svigos JM: The fetal inflammatory response syndrome and cerebral palsy: Yet another challenge and dilemma for the obstetrician. Aust NZ J Obstet Gynaecol 2001;41(2):170–176.
98. Keirse MJNC: Preterm labour. In Chalmers I, Enkin M, Keirse MJNC (eds): Effective Care in Pregnancy and Childbirth, Vol. 2. Oxford, Oxford University Press, 1989, pp 695–745.
99. Paneth N: The choice of place of delivery. Effect of hospital level on mortality in all singleton births in New York City. Am J Dis Child 1987;141:60–64.
100. Towers CV, Bonebrake R, Padilla G, Rumney P: The effect of transport on the rate of severe intraventricular haemorrhage in very low birth weight infants. Obstet Gynecol 200;95:291–295.
101. Kitchen W, Yu VYH, Orgill AA, et al: Infants born before 29 weeks gestation: Survival and morbidity at 2 years of age. Br J Obstet Gynaecol 1982;89:887–889.
102. Corbett A, Bucciarelli R, Goldman S, et al: Decreased mortality rate in small premature infants treated at birth with a single dose of synthetic surfactant: A multicentre controlled trial. J Pediatr 1991;118:277–284.
103. Long W, Stevenson D, Pauly T: Effects of a single prophylactic dose of Exosurf Neonatal in 215 500–700 gram infants. Pediatr Res 1991;29:223A.
104. Stevenson D, Walther F, Long W, et al: Controlled trial of a single dose of synthetic surfactant at birth in premature infants weighing 500 to 699 grams. The American Exosurf Neonatal Study Group I. J Pediatr 1992;120:S3–S12.
105. Gitlin JD, Soll RF, Parad RB, et al: Randomised controlled trial of exogenous surfactant for the treatment of hyaline membrane disease. Pediatrics 1987;79:31–37.
106. Creasy RD: Assessment and care of the fetus. In Eden RD, Buehin FK (eds): Preterm Labor. New York, Oxford University Press, 1990, pp 617–633.
107. Nwaesi CG, Young DC, Byrne JM, et al: Preterm birth at 23 to 26 weeks gestation: Is active management justified? Am J Obstet Gynecol 1987;157:890–897.
108. Young ENT, Stevenson DK: Limiting treatment for extremely premature, low-birth-weight infants (500–700 grams). Am J Dis Child 1990;144:549–552.
109. Hueston WJ, Know MA, Eilers G, et al: The effectiveness of preterm-birth prevention educational programmes for high-risk women: A meta-analysis. Obstet Gynecol 1995;86:705–712.
110. NICE. Electronic fetal monitoring guideline. May 2001. http://www.nice.org.uk/

CHAPTER 63

Prelabor Rupture of the Membranes

John Michael Svigos / Jeffrey S. Robinson / Rasniah Vigneswaran

DEFINITIONS AND INCIDENCE

Prelabor rupture of the membranes (PROM) is an obstetric conundrum; it has been poorly defined with an obscure etiology, difficult to diagnose, and associated with significant maternal, fetal, and neonatal risks and management strategies that are often diverse and controversial. It may be defined as rupture of the fetal membranes with a latent period before the onset of spontaneous uterine activity. The length of this latent period varies in different definitions from not being specified to up to 8 hours.

It is generally accepted that PROM occurs in 10% of all pregnancies,[1] with the majority of cases occurring after 37 completed weeks of gestation. If PROM occurs before 37 completed weeks of gestation, then the condition is referred to as preterm prelabor rupture of the membranes (PPROM). PPROM occurs in approximately 2% of all pregnancies.[2–4] These statistics refer to the general obstetric population, but clearly, the incidence of PPROM recorded for any particular hospital will be determined by the level of perinatal care provided, and hence in a hospital accepting fetal-maternal transfers the incidence of PPROM may be recorded as 5% of all pregnancies delivering there.[5]

RISKS

Maternal Risks

Significant maternal risks are associated with PROM, especially PPROM, and these problems can occur antepartum, intrapartum, and postpartum. Although the incidence of subclinical chorioamnionitis may be as high as 30% with PPROM,[6,7] serious maternal systemic infection is rare if treatment is initiated promptly.

The use of a number of therapeutic agents such as corticosteroids, antibiotics, and tocolytic agents, particularly with PPROM, may pose some additional maternal risk, which must be considered in the overall management. Abruptio placentae is evident in 4% to 7% of women with PPROM, and hence vaginal bleeding in the presence of PROM must be regarded seriously and managed accordingly.[8–11]

The undoubted psychosocial sequelae, particularly related to PPROM, with the disruption created by maternal hospitalization and continued observation associated with the uncertain fetal/neonatal prognosis, should never be underestimated and should be addressed on an individual basis within the overall management strategy.

The maternal intrapartum consequences of PROM are predominantly related to the induction of labor. The latent phase of labor under these circumstances may be as long as 16 to 20 hours, and thus unrealistic limits must not be set regarding the duration of labor when counseling the patient and attendant staff. The increased likelihood of operative delivery associated with induction of labor will increase the chance of maternal complications.[12]

Pathologic examination of placentas associated with PROM demonstrates an increased incidence of marginal cord insertion and battledore placentae, which may account for the increased incidence of retained placenta in this condition.[13] This in turn may be associated with the known increase in the incidence of primary and secondary postpartum hemorrhage. The latter complication is also probably associated with the 10% incidence of endometritis and myometritis that occur with PROM.

The complications described here account for a significant proportion of puerperal maternal morbidity, and the impaired maternal-infant bonding, particularly seen with PPROM, and which results in maternal psychological and lactation problems, will contribute to the remainder.

Fetal and Neonatal Risks

Prematurity is the most significant factor in the increased perinatal morbidity and mortality associated with preterm rupture of the membranes, because delivery occurs within 7 days of PPROM in over 80% of cases.[14,15]

Although the incidence of chorioamnionitis is 30%, the reported incidence of neonatal sepsis is only 2% to 4%.[16–18] Gestational age at the time of rupture of the membranes will have some influence on the incidence of neonatal sepsis (the earlier the gestation, the greater the chance of infection), as will the length of the latent period (the longer the latent period, the smaller the chance of infection). A growing body of epidemiologic data has demonstrated a relationship between intrauterine infection and the development of neonatal intraventricular hemorrhage, periventricular leukomalacia, and the subsequent occurrence of cerebral palsy.[19] Recent evidence suggests this damage is the result of the fetal inflammatory response syndrome (FIRS)[20] initiated by placental inflammation rather than infection with the local generation of arachidonic acid and the proinflammatory cytokines (i.e., interleukin 1 [IL-1], interleukin 6 [IL-6], and tumour necrosis factor-α [TNF-α]) thought to be responsible.

Oligohydramnios, particularly if there is prolonged PPROM, may result in the neonatal "oligohydramnios tetrad" of facial anomalies, limb position defects, pulmonary hypoplasia, and impaired fetal growth, all of which will add to neonatal morbidity.[13]

Fetal hypoxia is also more likely, due to the greater possibility of cord prolapse, cord compression, and abruptio placentae associated with PROM, particularly with PPROM. Neonatal morbidity will also be increased because of the mechanical difficulties encountered with delivery, either by the vaginal or abdominal route, as a result of the increased incidence of malpresentations and reduced volume of amniotic fluid.

MANAGEMENT OPTIONS

Prepregnancy

Prepregnancy counseling has only a limited role in the management of PROM, particularly PPROM, because in the vast majority of cases the cause is unknown.

The recurrence risk for PPROM has not been extensively studied, but Naeye's original observations[21] of a recurrence rate of 21% to 32% were subsequently confirmed by Asrat and associates.[22] More recently, a somewhat lower recurrence rate of 16.7% has been reported by Lee and associates,[23] but in this study, after one pregnancy complicated by PPROM, the subsequent overall preterm delivery rate in the next pregnancy was 34.2%.

A detailed examination of etiologic associations of PPROM by Harger and associates[24] suggested that the only independent risk factor that might be amenable to prepregnancy intervention was cigarette smoking, and the risk appeared to be dose-related.

Other less constant associations that might be amenable to intervention include cocaine abuse, intrauterine diethylstilbestrol (DES) exposed women, and possibly nutritional deficiencies of ascorbic acid, copper, zinc, and iron.[25–28] However, evidence that implementing intervention strategies improves outcomes is lacking.

There is substantial direct and indirect evidence that reproductive tract infections and associated inflammatory changes are responsible for many instances of PPROM.[27] Group B streptococci, chlamydia, gonorrhea, syphilis, *Mycoplasma hominis*, and *Ureaplasma urealyticum* have all been variously incriminated, but good evidence that prophylactic treatment is effective at reducing the incidence of PPROM is lacking. The prophylactic antimicrobial treatment of bacterial vaginosis during pregnancy in high risk women was reported in three studies to show a 66% to 70% reduction in the expected incidence of PPROM.[28] However, the study by Gibbs[29] did not support the value of such prophylactic treatment, and the much larger study by Carey and associates[30] would tend to confirm his view. Despite the lack of consistent evidence, two recent separate appraisals by Lamont[31] and Vigneswaran[32] were supportive of the treatment of bacterial vaginosis as an effective preventive measure for PPROM. The Cochrane Systematic Review concludes that antibiotics are associated with delay in delivery and reduction in markers of neonatal morbidity,[33] but largely on the basis of the large multinational ORACLE trial, which showed a benefit only for the use of erythromycin in the presence of ruptured membranes (see later discussion).

In light of the foregoing information, prepregnancy vaginal cultures would appear to be a useful investigation in women with a past history of PPROM, especially in relation to the detection of group B streptococcus and bacterial vaginosis.

Antimicrobial treatment of the sexual partner is more controversial, but the avoidance of coital activity during the course of further pregnancies appears to be unnecessarily restrictive given the available evidence. If there is concern on the part of the woman that infection might be introduced by the male partner, then this risk might be reduced by the use of condoms.

Prenatal

Diagnosis and Further Assessment

The diagnosis of PROM requires a judicious assessment of the history, clinical findings, and specialized testing. Whenever the history is suggestive of PROM, a sterile vaginal speculum examination should be performed. Visualization of amniotic fluid draining through the cervix provides the most reliable diagnosis. In cases of doubt, demonstration that vaginal fluid has an alkaline pH on nitrazine yellow testing (the pH indicator turning black) is suggestive, but not conclusive evidence of PROM. The normal vaginal pH is acid, and becomes neutral or alkaline due to the presence of amniotic fluid; however, such loss of acidity can also be due to vaginal infections, urine, or even bathwater. Ferning on microscopy is also a useful sign that the fluid is of amniotic origin and this simple test, which is easy to perform, should be more widely used in the diagnosis of PROM. However, both pH tests and ferning are less reliable with increasing prematurity.

When the diagnosis is in doubt, then further investigations, including the use of a modified vaginal pouch to collect the amniotic fluid,[34] ultrasound evaluation of amniotic fluid volume, and intra-amniotic dye injections, may be required. However, ultrasonographic diagnosis of oligohydramnios is often possible only with a large fluid loss that is clinically obvious. Furthermore, intra-amniotic injection of dyes is not without risk and is not widely practiced.[35,36] Alternatively, if conservative management is deemed appropriate, a "wait and see" policy may be adopted. Repeatedly dry pads and a normal amniotic fluid volume on scan make the diagnosis less likely, and the converse is also true.

Fetal fibronectin immunoenzyme testing has been utilized in the more precise diagnosis of PROM and may become a useful confirmatory test when the diagnosis is in doubt.[37]

The initial clinical assessment of the patient with PROM will determine the further management. All efforts must be directed initially at the exclusion of overt chorioamnionitis with attention to the detection of maternal tachycardia, pyrexia, uterine tenderness, purulent vaginal discharge, and fetal tachycardia (see also Chapter 27). Thereafter, there should be an evaluation of the fetal gestational age (from the history, clinical examination, and ultrasonographic assessment), immediate assessment of fetal well-being (clinical examination and fetal cardiotocography), and the exclusion of abruptio placentae and preterm labor.

The subsequent management of the patient will depend very heavily on the particular combination of the abovementioned features. The management alternatives that can be considered are discussed in the following sections.

Expectant Management

Expectant management consists of hospitalization and continued clinical observation of the mother and fetus. The role of bed rest is controversial but may aid diagnosis by allowing a pool of amniotic fluid to collect in the posterior fornix. Maternal activity also seems sometimes to increase the rate of fluid leakage, perhaps by dislodging the presenting part. Specialized assessments of continued fetal well-being using cardiotocography (nonstressed testing, NST) and biophysical profiles have been advocated,[38] and obstetric ultrasonographic evaluation of fetal growth is usually performed every 2 weeks.

The detection of covert chorioamnionitis using serial white blood cell differential counts and C-reactive protein estimates, in association with an initial and then weekly vaginal microbiologic cultures, has been advocated. The use of amniocentesis in clarifying the possibility of covert chorioamnionitis is more controversial and has yet to be tested adequately.[39] A number of small clinical trials have studied the relationship of proinflammatory cytokines (IL-6, IL-8, LL-18) and microbial invasion of the amniotic cavity in PPROM, but these have yet to be validated as markers for obstetric intervention[40] and may not be better than clinical findings or fetal fibronectin.[41]

Of recent interest are the observations that early intrauterine infection appears to be associated with disturbances in neurobehavioral physiology.[40] Abnormalities of the fetal heart rate (NST) and the biophysical profile score (BPS) correlate closely with proven intrauterine sepsis. These noninvasive tests have obvious advantages over amniocentesis. However, at present, it is not known whether the use of these tests will be helpful in determining the appropriate management and improving fetal outcome.

Active Management

Active management may be defined as the expectant management plus the use of one or more of the following pharmacologic agents:

- Maternal corticosteroids
- Tocolytics
- Prophylactic antibiotic administration.

In the contemporary management of PPROM, there is good evidence to recommend corticosteroids before 34 weeks' gestation to enhance fetal lung maturity.[42] However, the repeated use of corticosteroids in women with a prolonged latent phase after PPROM is currently in question, awaiting the results of large multicenter trials (including NICHD MFMU trial[43] and ACTORDS[44]) to determine neonatal safety, particularly in relation to intrauterine growth, pulmonary structural development, and neurodevelopment despite the reassuring original work by Liggins and Howie[45] (see Chapters 62 and 67).

With regard to tocolytic agents, it would seem logical that if maternal corticosteroids are advocated, then tocolysis for at least 48 hours should be acceptable (again, provided there is no overt evidence of infection). However, there is no good evidence available to support this view, and a high index of suspicion of intrauterine infection must be maintained if tocolytic therapy is to be instituted under these circumstances. The use of tocolytics to facilitate maternal-fetal transfer to an appropriate tertiary center has been supported, but on the basis of limited evidence.[46,47]

It is believed that membrane rupture is preceded by structural weakness associated with extracellular matrix degradation and cellular apoptosis[46–48] with a considerable number being associated with covert chorioamnionitis. Microorganisms appear to degrade the fetal membranes either directly with proteases or phospholipases or indirectly by the activation of collagenases such as the matrix metalloproteinases (MMPs).[49]

Administration of antibiotics to the mother should improve neonatal outcome by preventing infectious morbidity in the fetus and perhaps by prolonging the latency period. The latest Cochrane review of antibiotics for PPROM[50] demonstrated a reduction in maternal infection, delay in delivery, reduction in neonatal infection, and a reduction in the number of neonates requiring surfactant or oxygen therapy at 28 days. However, there did not appear to be a reduction in necrotizing enterocolitis, major cerebral abnormality, respiratory distress syndrome, stillbirth, or neonatal death rates. Co-amoxiclav (ampicillin and clavulanic acid) should be avoided as it was associated with an increased risk of necrotizing enterocolitis.

The ORACLE II[51] randomized trial attempted to answer the question of the value of prophylactic antibiotics by randomly assigning women with PPROM to the following groups: oral erythromycin (n = 1197), oral augmentin (n = 1212), both (n = 1192), or placebo (n = 1225). The primary outcome measure was a composite of neonatal death, chronic lung disease, or major cerebral abnormality on ultrasound before discharge from the hospital. Analysis was by intention to treat. Among the 2415 infants born to women allocated erythromycin only or placebo, fewer in the erythromycin only group had the primary composite outcome. Co-amoxiclav alone and co-amoxiclav plus erythromycin groups had no benefit over the placebo group. Use of erythromycin was also associated with prolongation of pregnancy, reductions in the need for neonatal treatment with surfactant, decreases in oxygen dependence at 28 days of age and older, fewer major cerebral abnormalities on ultrasound, and fewer positive blood cultures. Although the co-amoxiclav alone group and the co-amoxiclav plus erythromycin group were associated with a greater chance of prolongation of the pregnancy, they were also associated with a significantly higher rate of neonatal necrotizing enterocolitis. The authors concluded that treatment with erythromycin was associated with the best range of health benefits for the neonate and suggested that there might be a reduction in childhood disability. This view was challenged in an accompanying leading article.[52]

With our increased understanding of the role of proinflammatory cytokines and their undesirable intestinal, pulmonary, and neurologic effects on the fetus, the choice of antibiotics used in PPROM may well be critical.[19] Macrolide antibiotics such as erythromycin, clindamycin, aminoglycosides, and metronidazole tend to shut down bacterial virulence factor production, exert antiprotease activity, and stabilize activated inflammatory cells. Beta-lactam antibiotics such as penicillins and cephalosporins act primarily by impairing cell wall synthesis with the release of endotoxins, which promote proinflammatory cytokine release and increase the potential for deleterious effects on the neonate. These views would appear to be supported by the ORACLE I trial, but much longer neonatal follow-up is required before definite conclusions can be drawn.

The ORACLE I trial utilized oral antibiotic therapy four times daily for 10 days or until delivery, but earlier evidence suggested that initial aggressive broad-spectrum intravenous antibiotic therapy was desirable,[51] even though it was not clear if extended antibiotic therapy was necessary. More recent trials suggest that 72 hours of antibiotic therapy after PPROM is sufficient to gain benefit.

Currently the authors favor the use of intravenous ampicillin 2 g every 8 hours and gentamicin 80 mg every 8 hours for 48 hours followed by oral therapy with amoxicillin every 8 hours for 5 days, as suggested by Mercer and Arheart,[53] but this regimen is under review in light of the ORACLE trial.

Aggressive Management

Aggressive management is employed when delivery is deemed necessary as a result of obstetric indications, such as fetal distress, maternal sepsis, or abruptio placentae, or is requested by the parents in the face of marked fetal immaturity (<24 weeks) or of demonstrated fetal maturity (after 34 weeks). This form of management implies an increased incidence of induction and augmentation of labor, operative delivery, and associated maternal and neonatal morbidity. We are presently fortunate to have the results of a prospective randomized trial to aid us in the management of PROM at term[54] (see following discussion). Unfortunately, prospective, randomized trials have yet to be done for PPROM at different gestational age groups, and this remains a challenge for contemporary perinatology.

Management Strategies

Generally, the recommended management of PROM has shifted from an expectant mode to a more active mode, with accurate assessment of fetal gestational age being crucial to the decision-making process. It is useful to consider prenatal management strategies in relation to five gestational periods.

PPROM AT LESS THAN 24 COMPLETED GESTATIONAL WEEKS

The most appropriate management at this gestation is not clear and must be individualized, the wishes of the parents being paramount. Aggressive management is almost always indicated if active labor, abruptio placentae, or clinical evidence of maternal-fetal infection are present. It may also be requested by the parents if they fear delivery at a subsequent gestation (e.g., 25–26 weeks) when there is the possibility of survival, but also a high likelihood of serious neonatal complications and long-term handicap.

Expectant management is being increasingly considered, but with reported neonatal survival rates of less than 50% at gestations less than 24 weeks, even in the very latest and most optimistic studies[55–58] and with "normal" neonatal development in less than 40% after a 12-month follow-up period, care must be taken to ensure that parental counseling is thorough and cautious when there is PPROM at less than 24 weeks' gestation. The parents must be helped to understand that the neonatal prognosis is at best guarded and the likelihood of neonatal death and morbidity is significant. The prognosis for delivery at preterm gestations is also discussed in Chapter 62.

In view of the uncertainty of the outcome, an alternative management strategy has evolved for women who experience PPROM at less than 24 weeks' gestation. After initial hospitalization for 72 hours, the patient can be managed at home, restricting her physical activity, taking her own temperature, and reporting weekly for prenatal evaluation and microbiologic/hematologic surveillance. This management alternative has yet to be tested in randomized trials but would clearly have merit with regard to economic and psychosocial considerations.

PPROM AT 24 TO 31 COMPLETED GESTATIONAL WEEKS

At this gestation, the greatest risk to the fetus is still prematurity, and this risk currently outweighs any potential advantage in delivering a patient with occult intrauterine infection. Consequently, expectant management is the most favored option at this gestation.

The use of amniocentesis to detect the possibility of occult amniotic infection remains controversial at this gestation, particularly as fetal lung maturity is unlikely. It may be specifically indicated in certain circumstances, particularly if there are potential signs of chorioamnionitis, such as mild pyrexia, raised white blood cell count, and an elevated C-reactive protein.

A randomized study,[59] which assessed hospital versus home management after 72 hours of PPROM at 26 to 31 weeks' gestation, suggested that home management was a safe protocol to adopt, in terms of neonatal and maternal outcome, with significant savings in maternal hospital bed days. Hoffmann and associates[60] suggested that this form of management may be more appropriate for a subset of patients with PPROM characterized by the absence of labor or evidence of infection for 1 week, with adequate amniotic fluid volume demonstrated by ultrasonographic assessment. We await the outcome of similar larger randomized studies to determine the appropriate management of PPROM at this gestation.

Included in the prenatal management of PPROM at 24 to 31 weeks' gestation must be a discussion with the parents regarding the likely mode of delivery, should expectant management not be appropriate. In this regard, some interesting trends in clinical practice have evolved. A survey of members of the Society of Perinatal Obstetricians conducted by Amon and associates (1992)[61] regarding the use of cesarean section for fetal indications, particularly at the limits of fetal viability, in women delivering between the years 1986 and 1992, showed a doubling of the cesarean section rate for infants delivered between 24 and 28 weeks' gestation. Sanchez-Ramos and associates,[62] however, were able to demonstrate that a significant decrease in the cesarean section rate from 55% to 40% ($P < 0.05$) for very low birth weight infants delivering between the years 1986 and 1990 did not alter the neonatal mortality rate, the incidence of low Apgar scores, cord blood gas values, the incidence of intraventricular hemorrhage, or the median length of stay in the neonatal intensive care unit. Weiner[63] specifically studied breech presentation before 32 weeks' gestation and concluded that cesarean section reduced the perinatal mortality rate by a reduction in the incidence of intraventricular hemorrhage, confirming the study by Olofsson and associates.[64]

On balance, it would appear that aiming for vaginal delivery of the very low birth weight infant would be a reasonable management option to put before the parents during counseling, with resort to cesarean section for standard obstetric indications, save perhaps for those infants presenting by the breech before 32 weeks' gestation (for a fuller description of the mode of delivery of the preterm breech, see Chapter 64).

PPROM AT 31 TO 33 COMPLETED GESTATIONAL WEEKS

At our institution, neonatal survival at this gestation exceeds 95%, and thus, the risk from prematurity is similar to the risk to the neonate from sepsis. Although the use of amniocentesis would appear to be an attractive refinement in the management of patients with PPROM at this gestation,[64–66] its value has never been adequately evaluated. Success rates in obtaining amniotic fluid at amniocentesis in women with PPROM have varied from 45% to 97%. If fluid is obtained successfully, then the lack of a "gold standard" for the diagnosis of occult intrauterine infection versus colonization makes interpretation of the results of Gram stain, fluid microbiologic culture, leukocyte esterase testing, and gas liquid chromatography studies particularly difficult.[67] Fisk's review[68] of six studies using culture or Gram staining to diagnose infection of the amniotic fluid revealed sensitivities of 55% to 100%, and specificities of 76% to 100%. The outcome studied is important in interpreting the sensitivity and specificity of tests designed to diagnose occult infection; for example, if the presence of pathogenic organisms is regarded as diagnostic of infection, then the sensitivity of demonstrating such organisms on Gram staining and culture of the amniotic fluid is by definition 100%, whereas if neonatal death from sepsis is used as the end-point, sensitivity will be much lower and significant morbidity will be ignored. Fisk used histopathologic evidence of chorioamnionitis as definitive evidence of infection, but this has been disputed as an end-point by Ohlsson and Wang,[69] who accepted clinical chorioamnionitis and all its shortcomings; Dudley and associates,[39] who used neonatal sepsis (proven or suspected); and Vintzileos and associates,[38] who used both clinical chorioamnionitis and neonatal sepsis (proved or possible).

With regard to fetal lung maturity, Dudley and associates[39] demonstrated its presence in 58% of specimens obtained at amniocentesis at this gestation. This result was consistent with other studies,[64,66] which showed a 50% to 60% incidence of fetal lung maturity. With regard to neonatal respiratory distress with PPROM, pulmonary maturity testing (L/S ratio) had a positive predictive value of 68% and a negative predictive value of 79%. The specific situations of occult amniotic fluid infection but fetal lung immaturity, and fetal lung maturity but absent fluid infection, have not been adequately evaluated to determine the correct management option.

If amniocentesis is unsuccessful in obtaining an adequate amniotic fluid sample, then the management must be on a clinical basis with its inherent limitations, in association with the less precise hematologic parameters of serial C-reactive protein estimation and complete blood pictures to assess the presence of infection.[67–71] Although Yeast and associates[72] found no evidence that amniocentesis induces labor, the procedure is not entirely free of complications, and this must be considered when counseling the parents. It would appear that further evaluation of the role of amniocentesis in the management of PPROM, particularly at this gestation, requires a large prospective randomized trial before it can take its place as a legitimate management option.

PPROM AT 34 TO 36 COMPLETED GESTATIONAL WEEKS

Although an expectant management policy is commonly employed at this gestation, this is by no means the standard approach, with many favoring induction of labor as outlined by Olofsson and associates[64] in their review of the practice of Swedish obstetricians with regard to PPROM. The possibility of failed induction is more likely at this gestation than at term, but this has not been adequately evaluated to date.

Clearly, aggressive management is indicated if there is evidence of intrauterine infection, abruptio placentae, or fetal distress.

PPROM AFTER 36 COMPLETED GESTATIONAL WEEKS

In women with PROM after 36 completed gestational weeks, an expectant management policy may be justified initially because it can be anticipated that 75% to 85% of these women will enter labor within 24 hours. The controversial aspects of management at this gestation center around the risks of maternal and neonatal infection as the latency period lengthens, set against the risks of induction of labor and a possible increase in cesarean section rate. The study by Hannah and associates[54] in which 5041 women with PROM at term were randomly assigned to expectant management for up to 4 days or to induction of labor with intravenous oxytocin or vaginal prostaglandin E_2 gel has helped clarify this controversy. These authors found that the rates of neonatal infection and cesarean section were not significantly different among the study groups. The rates of neonatal infection were 2.0% for the induction with oxytocin group, 3.0% for the induction with prostaglandin group, 2.8% for the expectant management (with subsequent oxytocin) group, and 2.7% for the expectant management (with subsequent prostaglandin) group. Clinical chorioamnionitis and maternal colonization with group B streptococcus were important predictors of neonatal infection.[55] The rates of cesarean section ranged from 9.6% to 10.9% in the four groups. Hence, in PROM after 36 completed gestational weeks, induction of labor with oxytocin or prostaglandin E_2 and expectant management result in similar rates of neonatal infection and cesarean section. However, clinical chorioamnionitis was less likely to develop in the women in the induction with oxytocin group than in those in the expectant management (oxytocin) group (4.0% versus 8.6%, $P < 0.001$), as was postpartum fever (1.9% versus 3.6%, $P = 0.008$). Induction of labor with intravenous oxytocin therefore results in a lower risk of maternal infection than does expectant management. Hannah and associates[54] also found that the women viewed induction of labor more positively than expectant management and, although it is important to give women choices in their management, if the cost implications are also taken into account, then induction of labor with intravenous oxytocin would appear to be the most appropriate management in this clinical situation.

Special Circumstances

THE "HINDWATER" LEAK

This poorly defined clinical entity is of unknown frequency and is often a diagnosis of exclusion. The natural history of this phenomenon is unknown and awaits further evaluation.

RESEALED PROM

Once again this is a poorly defined clinical entity that may encompass a number of women with "hindwater" leak.[72,73] Mercer and associates,[53] in a study of 220 conservatively managed women with PPROM between 20 and 34 weeks' gestation, identified eight women (3.6%) in whom there was cessation of leakage. At approximately the same time Carlan and associates[74] reported on 349 women with PPROM of whom 14 (4%) apparently resealed after initial confirmation of PPROM. In both studies those women who resealed were of a younger age group, had PPROM at an earlier gestation, and had larger pockets of residual amniotic fluid at the initial ultrasonographic examination than the women with PPROM who did not reseal. After resealing, the pregnancies proceeded normally without any increased likelihood of rerupture.

MULTIPLE PREGNANCY AND PROM

Currently there is little information regarding the latency period and perinatal outcome after PPROM in multiple gestations. Additionally, the relative risks of morbidity and mortality between presenting and nonpresenting infants have not been addressed. The study by Mercer and associates[75] showed only a brief latency period, regardless of gestational age, with no difference in infant survival between twins, but with a significant increase in respiratory morbidity in the nonpresenting infant. In their case-controlled study, Montgomery and associates[76] suggested that the natural history of PPROM in the twin gestation parallels that in the singleton pregnancy and that similar antepartum management strategies are appropriate for both groups.

Labor and Delivery

If labor occurs in the presence of PROM, then it should be monitored closely and augmented promptly if there is any delay, because of the increased risk of infection. The only exception to this rule is to allow transfer to a tertiary care center if labor is preterm and begins in a hospital without appropriate neonatal care facilities. Vaginal delivery should generally be the objective, with decisions regarding the mode of delivery and the need for cesarean section not differing substantially from other preterm deliveries with intact membranes.

Once labor is established, maternal antibiotic therapy is often commenced, particularly if signs of intrauterine infection are present. Although this policy has not been addressed specifically by controlled studies, earlier reservations regarding the possibility of inducing superinfection with resistant bacteria and complicating the diagnosis of infection in the neonate have not been borne out in clinical practice.

This has been demonstrated in particular by the controlled trials of antibiotic use in maternal group B hemolytic streptococcal colonization.[45] A documented reduction in anticipated maternal puerperal infectious complications has been confirmed in most studies advocating this approach.[72] The authors would favor the use of intravenous ampicillin 2 g, every 8 hour and gentamicin 80 mg, every 8 hour during labor. An alternative regimen to prevent neonatal group B sepsis is recommended particularly when two or more of the following are present: previous baby affected by group B streptococcus (GBS), GBS bacteriuria in the current pregnancy, preterm labor, prolonged rupture of the membranes, or fever in labor. Penicillin, initially 3 g is given intravenously, followed by 1.5 g (2.5 million units) intravenously at 4-hour intervals until delivery. If the woman is allergic to penicillin, then clindamycin 900 mg every 8 hours until delivery should be used instead. These regimens are currently recommended in the United Kingdom and most of Europe, where it is argued that it reduces GBS infection by more than 90%.[77] This regimen avoids use of ampicillin because of concerns about its association with an increase in the rate of gram-negative sepsis.

Labors following PROM carry an increased risk of fetal distress, often as a result of umbilical cord compression due to the associated oligohydramnios. The use of amnioinfusion to counter this complication has shown some promise in the controlled trial by Nageotte and associates[78] and in the prospective randomized study conducted by Schrimmer and associates[79] and can be used before 26 weeks' gestation with potential benefit.[80]

At the time of delivery, the presence of a neonatologist, with the backup of an appropriate neonatal support team, is essential to the optimization of perinatal outcome.

Postnatal

With regard to the woman delivering after PROM, an awareness of the risks associated with endometritis, not only postpartum genital sepsis/septicemia but also postpartum hemorrhage and venous thrombosis, is essential for effective management. Active promotion of maternal-infant bonding, particularly with PPROM, deserves special consideration.

All infants born after PROM should be thoroughly screened for sepsis, irrespective of the antepartum or intrapartum use of maternal antibiotic therapy. Screening investigations usually include neonatal blood culture, endotracheal aspirate culture, urinary latex particle agglutination testing, and a complete blood picture. Lumbar puncture and cerebrospinal fluid examination should be reserved for clinically septic neonates and for those with positive blood cultures. Initial antibiotic therapy using a combination of intravenous penicillin and gentamicin may be employed while awaiting the results of the screening investigations. Often the results are inconclusive or equivocal, and discontinuation of the antibiotic therapy may then have to be based on clinical judgment.

Prematurity remains the greatest hazard encountered with PROM, and hence, hyaline membrane disease requiring mechanical ventilation is common. This can be aggravated by pulmonary hypoplasia, which is usually only significant if PPROM occurs before 25 weeks' gestation, with a latent period of more than 5 weeks before delivery.[81] The outcome of PPROM at later gestations is more optimistic than is reported for other causes of oligohydramnios.

The other complications associated with prematurity and its management, including intracranial hemorrhage, jaundice, and feeding difficulties, must be attended to in the usual fashion, and there should be provision made for long-term neonatal follow-up, particularly in view of preliminary data suggesting a higher risk of neurodevelopment impairment in preterm infants delivered after prolonged PPROM, compared to those born after spontaneous preterm labor (PTL) with intact membranes.[81] For example, placentas of infants that develop cerebral palsy are more likely to be infected with *Escherichia coli* and perhaps GBS than placentas from control cases.[82]

CONCLUSIONS

- A recent survey of perinatologists in the United States[83] has demonstrated national consensus in the use of steroids, antibiotics, and fetal monitoring, which represents a major change from 15 years ago, but beyond this, there continues to be little consensus regarding the optimal management of PPROM.
- Part of the problem continues to be our lack of progress in determining the etiology of PPROM and our inability to offer appropriate management options based on an understanding of the pathophysiology.
- The current interest in proinflammatory cytokines has shown that both PTL and PROM are associated with their overproduction, and increasing evidence suggests that TNF-α may represent the switch[84] between the PTL and PROM pathways because of its ability to engender MMP-9 activity and activate apoptosis in the fetal membranes. Nitric oxide synthetase inhibitors and *N*-methyl-D-aspartate receptor antagonists, which counter the effects of TNF-α, may represent a future sphere of activity for preventive therapy.[19]
- The ORACLE I trial,[50] which consolidated the place of antibiotic therapy in PPROM, has also opened up further areas for investigation. Not only has this study resulted in a reconsideration of the choice of antibiotic therapy, but it also has drawn attention to the potential deleterious effects of PPROM on fetal brain development. Murphy and associates[85] and Spinillo and associates[86] have suggested that the risk of neonatal neurologic handicap is related to the duration of membrane rupture. This in turn would suggest that FIRS with the elaboration of proinflammatory cytokines and the associated complications of intraventricular hemorrhage, periventricular leukomalacia, and cerebral palsy may not be prevented by antibiotic therapy alone. Animal experiments using anti-inflammatory agents and chemical agents to counteract the effects of IL-1 and IL-6 represent new areas, which may see them incorporated in a combined fashion with the current regimens employed to prevent or treat the fetal morbidity associated with intrauterine infection/inflammation related to PPROM.[19]

SUMMARY OF MANAGEMENT OPTIONS

Prelabor Rupture of the Membranes

Management Options	Quality of Evidence	Strength of Recommendation	References
Prepregnancy (Especially Previous Preterm PROM)			
Counsel about recurrence risks (21–32% for PROM; up to 34% for preterm delivery).	III	B	22, 23
Search for causes/precipitating factors has limited overall value.	–	GPP	–
Stress value of preventive measures, such as patient education and smoking cessation.	III	B	24
Note conflicting data on the value of vaginal bacteriologic screening and antimicrobial treatment of woman and partner.	Ib	A	28–32
Prenatal: Prevention			
There are conflicting data on the value of vaginal bacteriologic screening and antimicrobial treatment of woman and partner.	Ib	A	28–32
Cervical ultrasound assessment with fetal fibronectin (and similar biochemical screening tests) in women with previous history of PROM may be of benefit.	III	B	37

SUMMARY OF MANAGEMENT OPTIONS

Prelabor Rupture of the Membranes *(Continued)*

Management Options	Quality of Evidence	Strength of Recommendation	References
Prenatal: Confirm Diagnosis			
Perform history and physical examination (especially sterile speculum) and collection of amniotic fluid; make repeated pad checks to confirm diagnosis.	–	GPP	–
Additional tests ("ferning," alkaline pH turning nitrazine blue/black, presence of vernix or meconium) all have limitations, especially being unreliable/inappropriate at preterm gestations.	–	GPP	–
Presence of fetal fibronectin (and other biochemical markers) may be useful confirmatory test indicating the likelihood of ensuing preterm labor—may allow intervention to reduce the likelihood of both complications.	III	B	37
Intraamniotic injection of dyes is not without risk and is not widely practiced.	IV	C	35, 36
Ultrasound diagnosis of oligohydramnios associated only with substantial fluid loss, which is usually clinically obvious.	–	GPP	–
Prenatal Management: General			
Maintain vigilance for chorioamnionitis (CA) (see also Chapter 27):	IIb	B	67–70
• Clinical: maternal fever, tachycardia, uterine pain/tenderness, purulent vaginal discharge, fetal tachycardia			
• Laboratory investigations (unreliable):			
– White blood cell count (and differential count)	–	GPP	–
– C-reactive protein	–	GPP	–
– Amniotic fluid Gram stain, white cells and culture (role of amniocentesis is uncertain).	IIa	B	38,39,64–66
– Gas chromatography	–	GPP	–
– Biophysical testing (NST and/or BPS)	III	B	38, 40
– Value of pro-cytokine testing is uncertain	IIb	B	40, 41
Delivery is indicated if chorioamnionitis is diagnosed or fetal "distress" occurs (NST/BPS)	–	GPP	–
Prenatal Management: <24 Weeks with No Evidence of CA or Fetal Distress			
Individualized management including: parental input.	–	GPP	–
Careful counseling of parents needed (see also Chapter 62).	–	GPP	–
If decision is to continue with pregnancy, then implement surveillance for sepsis (see above) (possibly at home).	IIb	B	67–70
Mode of delivery is usually vaginal.	IV	C	61, 62
Prenatal Management: 24–31 Weeks with No Evidence of CA or Fetal Distress			
The upper gestational age chosen will vary depending on local neonatal survival rates.	–	GPP	–
Expectant/conservative management (possibly at home after initial hospital assessment and exclusion of sepsis) is recommended.	Ib	A	59, 60
Counsel parents regarding prognosis (see Chapter 62).	–	GPP	–
Look for clinical evidence of chorioamnionitis (CA) (see above).	IIb	B	67–70

Continued

SUMMARY OF MANAGEMENT OPTIONS
Prelabor Rupture of the Membranes *(Continued)*

Management Options	Quality of Evidence	Strength of Recommendation	References
Prenatal Management: 24–31 Weeks with No Evidence of CA or Fetal Distress—*Continued*			
Treatments:			
Steroid use is variable.	Ia	A	42–44
Many only use tocolysis for transfer to tertiary unit.	IV	C	46,47
Many give antibiotics (erythromycin common; *not* Co-amoxyclav).	Ia	A	50–52
Assessment of fetal pulmonary maturity is a variable practice and of uncertain value.	IIa	B	39,64,66
Aim for vaginal delivery if cephalic; most undertake cesarean section for breech (see also Chapter 64).	IV	C	61–64
Prenatal Management: 31–36 Weeks with No Evidence of CA or Fetal Distress			
Options used in practice:	–	GPP	–
Expectant/conservative (wait for 24–72 hours and if then not in labor, opt for induction)			
Aggressive (induce labor at presentation)			
Prenatal Management: After 36 Completed Weeks with No Evidence of CA or Fetal Distress			
Discuss options with patient:	Ib	A	54
Expectant/conservative (wait for 24–72 h and if not in labor, opt for induction)			
Aggressive (induce labor at presentation) (waiting up to 4 days increases maternal septic morbidity but no other outcome measures)			
Special Circumstances			
"Hindwater leak"—poorly defined, difficult to diagnose; if definite proof of PROM (irrespective of whether cervical membranes intact), then manage as any other PROM case.	–	GPP	–
Cessation of PROM—manage normally.	Ia	A	53, 74
Multiple pregnancy—manage as for singleton.	IIa	B	75, 76
Labor and Delivery			
Continue observing for evidence of infection.	–	GPP	–
Use of maternal antibiotics prophylactically during labor remains controversial (except with group B streptococcal colonization when antibiotics reduce maternal septic morbidity).	IIa	B	45
Consider amnioinfusion for fetal distress.	Ib	A	78, 79
Cesarean section for normal obstetric indications.	–	GPP	–
Pediatrician should attend delivery.	–	GPP	–
Postnatal			
Maintain vigilance and screening for infection.	–	GPP	–
Neonatal screen for sepsis and appropriate care.	–	GPP	–
Long-term pediatric follow-up, especially neurodevelopmental.	–	GPP	–

REFERENCES

1. Mead PB: Management of the patient with premature rupture of the membranes: A review. Clin Perinatol 1980;7:243–255.
2. Gibbs RS, Blanco JD: Premature rupture of the membranes. Obstet Gynecol 1982;60:671–679.
3. Graham RL, Gilstrap LC, Hauth JC, et al: Conservative management of patients with premature rupture of fetal membranes. Obstet Gynecol 1982;59:607–610.
4. Cox SM, Williams ML, Leveno KJ: The natural history of preterm ruptured membranes: What to expect of expectant management. Obstet Gynecol 1988;71:558–562.
5. Clinical Information Services Report. Adelaide, South Australia, Women's and Children's Hospital, 1995.
6. Levy DL, Arquembourg PC: Maternal and cord blood complement activity: Relationship to premature rupture of the membranes. Am J Obstet Gynecol 1981;139:38–40.
7. Garite TJ, Freeman RK: Chorioamnionitis in the preterm gestation. Obstet Gynecol 1982;59:539–545.
8. Breese MW: Spontaneous premature rupture of the membranes. Am J Obstet Gynecol 1961;81:1086–1088.
9. Nelson DM, Stempel LE, Zuspan FP: Association of prolonged preterm premature rupture of the membranes and abruptio placentae. J Reprod Med 1986;31:249–253.
10. Vintzileos AM, Campbell WA, Nochimson DJ, Weinbaum PJ: Premature rupture of the membranes: A risk factor for the development of abruptio placentae. Am J Obstet Gynecol 1987;156: 1235–1238.
11. Major CA, de Veciana M, Lewis DF, Morgan MA: Preterm premature rupture of the membranes and abruptio placentae: Is there an association between these pregnancy complications? Am J Obstet Gynecol 1995;172:672–676.
12. Asrat T, Garite TJ: Management of preterm rupture of membranes. Clin Obstet Gynecol 1991;34:730–741.
13. Allen SR: Epidemiology of premature rupture of the fetal membranes. Clin Obstet Gynecol 1991;34:685–693.
14. Taylor J, Garite TJ: Premature rupture of the membranes before fetal viability. Obstet Gynecol 1984;64:615–620.
15. Beydoun SN, Yasin SY: Premature rupture of the membranes before 28 weeks: Conservative management. Am J Obstet Gynecol 1986;155:471–479.
16. Knudsen FU, Steinrud J: Septicaemia of the newborn associated with ruptured foetal membranes, discoloured amniotic fluid or maternal fever. Acta Paediatr Scand 1976;65:725–731.
17. Cederqvist LL, Zervoudakis IA, Ewool LC, Litwin SD: The relationship between prematurely ruptured membranes and fetal immunoglobulin production. Am J Obstet Gynecol 1979;134: 784–788.
18. Siegel JD, McCracken GH Jr: Sepsis neonatorum. N Engl J Med 1981;304:642–647.
19. Svigos JM: The feta inflammatory response syndrome and cerebral palsy: Yet another challenge and dilemma for the obstetrician. Aust N Z J Obstet Gynaecol 2001;41:170–176.
20. Gomez R, Romero R, Ghezzi F, et al: The fetal inflammatory response syndrome. Am J Obstet Gynecol 1998;179:194–202.
21. Naeye RL: Factors that predispose to premature rupture of the fetal membranes. Obstet Gynecol 1982;60:93–98.
22. Asrat T, Lewis DF, Garite TJ, et al: Rate of recurrence of preterm premature rupture of membranes in consecutive pregnancies. Am J Obstet Gynecol 1991;165:1111–1115.
23. Lee T, Carpenter MW, Heber WW, Silver HM: Preterm premature rupture of membranes: Risks of recurrent complications in the next pregnancy among a population-based sample of gravid women. Am J Obstet Gynecol 2003;188:209–213.
24. Harger JH, Hsing AW, Tuomala RE, et al: Risk factors for preterm premature rupture of fetal membranes: A multicenter case-control study. Am J Obstet Gynecol 1990;165:130–137.
25. Cherukuri R, Minkoff H, Feldman J, et al: A cohort study of alkaloidal cocaine ("crack") in pregnancy. Obstet Gynecol 1988;72:147–151.
26. Ludmir J, Landon MB, Gabbe SC, et al: Management of the diethylstilboestrol-exposed pregnant patient: A prospective study. Am J Obstet Gynecol 1987;157:665–669.
27. Artal R, Burgeson R, Fernandez FJ, Hobel CJ: Fetal and maternal copper levels at term with and without premature rupture of membranes. Obstet Gynecol 1979;53:608–610.
28. Kiilholma P, Gronroos M, Erkkola R, et al: The role of calcium, copper, iron and zinc in preterm delivery and premature rupture of the fetal membranes. Gynecol Obstet Invest 1984;17: 194–201.
29. Gibbs RS: Chorioamnionitis and bacterial vaginosis. Am J Obstet Gynecol 1993;169:460–462.
30. Carey JC, Klebanoff MA, Harth JC, et al: Metronidazole to prevent preterm delivery in pregnant women with asymptomatic bacterial vaginosis. National Institute of Child Health and Human Development Network of Maternal-Fetal Medicine Units. N Engl J Med 2000;342:534–540.
31. Lamont RF: Antibiotics for the prevention of preterm birth. N Engl J Med 2000;342:581–583.
32. Vigneswaran R: Infection and preterm birth: Evidence of a common causal relationship with bronchopulmonary dysplasia and cerebral palsy. J Paediatr Child Health 2000;36:293–296.
33. Kenyon S, Boulvain M, Neilson J: Antibiotics for preterm rupture of membranes (Cochrane Review). In The Cochrane Library, Issue 2. Oxford, Update Software, 2003.
34. O'Brien JM, Mercer BM, Sibai BM: The use of a modified vaginal pouch for the diagnosis and management of premature rupture of the membranes. Am J Obstet Gynecol 1995;172: 1565–1566.
35. Nicolini U, Monni G: Intestinal obstruction in babies exposed in utero to methylene blue. Lancet 1990;336:1258–1259.
36. Fish WH, Chazen EM: Toxic effects of methylene blue on the fetus. Am J Dis Child 1992;146:1412–1413.
37. Mercer BM, Goldenberg RL, Meis PJ, et al: The preterm prediction study: Prediction of preterm premature rupture of membranes through clinical findings and ancillary testing. The National Institute of Child Health and Human Development Maternal-Fetal Medicine Units Network. Am J Obstet Gynecol 2000;183:738–745.
38. Vintzileos AM, Campbell WA, Rodis JF: Antepartum surveillance in patients with preterm premature rupture of the membranes. Clin Obstet Gynecol 1991;34:779–793.
39. Dudley J, Malcolm G, Ellwood D: Amniocentesis in the management of preterm premature rupture of the membranes. Aust N Z J Obstet Gynaecol 1991;31:331–336.
40. Spinillo A, Capuzzo E, Stronati M, et al: Effect of preterm premature rupture of membranes on neurodevelopment outcome: Follow-up at two years of age. BJOG 1995;102: 882–887.
41. Coleman MA, Keelan JA, McCowan LM, et al: Predicting preterm delivery: Comparison of cervicovaginal interleukin (IL)-1beta, IL-6 and IL-8 with fetal fibronectin and cervical dilatation. Eur J Obstet Gynaecol Reprod Biol 2001;95:154–158.
42. Crowley P: Prophylactic corticosteroids for preterm birth (Cochrane Review). In The Cochrane Library, Issue 2. Oxford, Update Software, 2003.
43. Wapner RJ, for the NICHD MFMU Network: A randomised trial of single vs weekly courses of corticosteroids. Am J Obstet Gynecol 2003;198:S56.
44. Crowther CM, ACTORDS – Australasian Collaborative Trial of Repeat Doses of Corticosteroids for the Prevention of Neonatal Respiratory Disease (ongoing trial). Women's and Children's Hospital, Adelaide, South Australia.

45. Liggins GC, Howie RN: A controlled trial of antepartum glucocorticoid treatment for prevention of the respiratory distress syndrome in premature infants. Pediatrics 1972;50:515–525.
46. Keirse MJNC, Ohlsson A, Treffers PE, Kanhai HHH: Pre-labor rupture of the membranes preterm. In Chalmers I, Enkin M. Keirse MJNC (eds): Effective Care in Pregnancy and Childbirth, Vol. 1. Oxford, Oxford University Press, 1989, pp 666–692.
47. Harlass FE: The use of tocolytics in patients with preterm premature rupture of the membranes. Clin Obstet Gynecol 1991;34:751–758.
48. McLaren J, Malak TM, Bell SC: Structural characteristics of term human fetal membranes prior to labor: Identification of an area of altered morphology overlying the cervix. Hum Reprod 1999;14:237–241.
49. Bell SC: Mechanisms underlying prelabor rupture of the fetal membranes. In Kingdom J, Javniaux E, O'Brien S (eds): The Placenta: Basic Science and Clinical Practice. London, RCOG Press, 2000, pp 187–204.
50. Kenyon S, Neilson J: Antibiotics for preterm rupture of membranes (Cochrane Review). In The Cochrane Library, Issue 2. Oxford, Update Software, 2003.
51. Kenyon S, Taylor DJ, Tarnow-Mordi W, for the ORACLE Collaborative Group: Broad spectrum antibiotics for preterm, prelabor rupture of fetal membranes: The ORACLE II randomized trial. Lancet 2001;357:979–988.
52. Hannah ME: Antibiotics for preterm premature rupture of the membranes and preterm labour? Lancet 2001;357:973–974.
53. Mercer BM, Arheart KL: Antimicrobial therapy in expectant management of preterm premature rupture of the membranes. Lancet 1995;346:1271–1279.
54. Hannah ME, Ohlsson A, Farine D, et al: Induction of labor compared with expectant management for prelabor rupture of the membranes at term. TERMPROM Study Group. N Engl J Med 1996;334:1005–1010.
55. Seaward PG, Hannah ME, Myhr TL, et al: International multicenter term PROM study: Evaluation of predictors of neonatal infection in infants born to patients with premature rupture of membranes at term. Am J Obstet Gynecol 1998;179:635–639.
56. Helewa M, Menticoglu S, Heaman M, Dancombe L: Spontaneous preterm premature rupture of membranes (SPPROM): Experience with community based care vs traditional in hospital care at two Canadian tertiary centers. Society for Perinatal Obstetrics abstract no. 510. Am J Obstet Gynecol 1997;176:147.
57. Majors CA, Kitzmiller JL: The healthy neonate – Expectant management of midtrimester rupture of membranes. Society for Perinatal Obstetrics abstract no. 104. Am J Obstet Gynecol 1990;163:14.
58. Morales W, Talley T: Premature rupture of membranes at < 25 weeks – A management dilemma. Am J Obstet Gynecol 1991;168:503–507.
59. Carlan SJ, O'Brien WF, Parsons M, Lense JJ: Preterm premature rupture of the membranes: A randomised study of home versus hospital management. Obstet Gynecol 1991;81:61–64.
60. Hoffmann D, Hansen G, Ingardia C, Philipson E: Preterm premature rupture of membranes: Is outpatient management appropriate? Society for Perinatal Obstetrics abstract no. 467. Am J Obstet Gynecol 1992;166:403.
61. Amon E, Shyken JM, Sibai BM: How small is too small and how early is too early? A survey of American obstetricians specializing in high-risk pregnancies. Am J Perinatol 1992;9:17–21.
62. Sanchez-Raimos L, Walker C, Briones D, Cullen MT: Decreasing caesarean section rates in very low-birthweight infants: Effect on perinatal outcome. Society for Perinatal Obstetrics abstract no. 655. Am J Obstet Gynecol 1992;166:444.
63. Weiner CP: Vaginal breech delivery in the 1990s. Clin Obstet Gynecol 1992;35:559–569.
64. Olofsson P, Rydhstrom H, Sjoberg NO: How Swedish obstetricians manage premature rupture of the membranes in preterm gestations. Am J Obstet Gynecol 1988;159:1028–1034.
65. Broekhuizen FF, Gilman M, Hamilton PR: Amniocentesis for gram stain and culture in preterm premature rupture of the membranes. Obstet Gynecol 1985;66:316–321.
66. Burke MS, Porreco RP: Use of amniotic fluid analysis in the management of preterm premature rupture of the membranes. J Reprod Med 1986;31:31–38.
67. Garite TJ, Freeman RK, Linzey EM, Braly P: The use of amniocentesis in patients with premature rupture of the membranes. Obstet Gynecol 1979;54:1226–1230.
68. Fisk NM: Modifications to selective conservative management in preterm premature rupture of the membranes. Obstet Gynecol Surv 1988;43:328–334.
69. Ohlsson A, Wang E: An analysis of antenatal tests to detect infection in preterm premature rupture of the membranes. J Obstet Gynecol 1990;162:809–818.
70. Cotton DB, Hill LM, Strassner HT, et al: Use of amniocentesis in preterm gestation with ruptured membranes. Obstet Gynecol 1984;63:38–43.
71. Norman K, Louw JP: C-Reactive protein in premature rupture of membranes. Contemp Rev Obstet Gynecol 1991;3:148–151.
72. Yeast JD, Garite TJ, Dorchester W: The risks of amniocentesis in the management of premature rupture of the membranes. Am J Obstet Gynecol 1984;149:505–508.
73. Johnson JW, Egerman RS, Moorhead J: Cases with ruptured membranes that 'reseal.' Am J Obstet Gynecol 1990;163: 1024–1032.
74. Carlan SJ, O'Brien WF, Olock JL: Clinical characteristics and outcome of patients with resealed, preterm premature rupture of membranes. Society for Perinatal Obstetrics abstract no. 657. Am J Obstet Gynecol 1992;166:445.
75. Mercer B, Crocker L, Dahmus M, et al: Clinical characteristics and outcome of twin pregnancies complicated by preterm premature rupture of the membranes. Am J Obstet Gynecol 1993;168:1467–1473.
76. Montgomery DM, Perlow JH, Asrat T, et al: Preterm premature ruptured membranes in the twin gestation: A controlled study. Society for Perinatal Obstetrics abstract no. 301. Am J Obstet Gynecol 1992;166:360.
77. RCOG Guideline No 36: Prevention of early onset neonatal group B streptococcal disease. London, RCOG, 2003. Accessed at Web site http://rcog.org.uk/guidelines.asp?PageID106&GuidelineID=56.
78. Nageotte MP, Feeman RK, Garite TJ, Dorchester W: Prophylactic intrapartum amnioinfusion in patients with preterm premature rupture of the membranes. Am J Obstet Gynecol 1985;153:557–562.
79. Schrimmer DB, Macri CJ, Paul RH: Prophylactic amnioinfusion as a treatment for oligohydramnios in laboring patients: A prospective randomised trial. Am J Obstet Gynecol 1991;165: 972–975.
80. Locatelli A, Vergani P, Di Pirro G, et al: Role of amnioinfusion in the management of premature rupture of the membranes at < 26 weeks' gestation. Am J Obstet Gynecol 2000;183:878–882.
81. Nimrod C, Varela-Gittings F, Machin G, et al: The effect of very prolonged membrane rupture on fetal development. Am J Obstet Gynecol 1984;148:540–543.
82. Vigneswaran R, Aitchison SJ, McDonald HM, et al: Cerebral palsy and placental infection: A case-cohort study. BMC Pregnancy Childbirth 2004;4:1–12.
83. Bonebrake R, Simigiannis H, Rust M, Repke J: Is there a national consensus of treatment of PPROM? SMFM abstract no. 262. Am J Obstet Gynecol 2002;187:6.
84. Fortunato SJ, Menon R, Lombardi SJ: Role of tumor necrosis factor-alpha in the premature rupture of membranes and

preterm labor pathways. Am J Obstet Gynecol 2002;187: 1159–1162.

85. Murphy DJ, Sellers S, MacKenzie IZ, et al: Case-control study of antenatal and intrapartum risk factors for cerebral palsy in very preterm singleton babies. Lancet 1995;346:1449–1454.

86. Spinillo A, Capuzza E, Stronati M, et al: Effect of preterm premature rupture of membranes on neurodevelopmental outcome: Follow-up at two years of age. Am J Obstet Gynecol 1995;102: 882–887.

CHAPTER 64

Breech Presentation

Zoë Penn

INTRODUCTION

The intense obstetric controversy that breech presentation has generated is drawing to an end. The place of external cephalic version for the preterm and term fetus (unnecessary and beneficial, respectively) has been largely resolved, as has the optimum mode of delivery. Vaginal delivery of the breech was the norm (and an essential manipulative skill to be acquired by all obstetricians) until the late 1950s, when cesarean section was first recommended on a routine basis. This opinion gained ground steadily, but it was not until the third millennium that a trial was published that finally convinced most of the world's obstetricians that it was evidence based.

However, another fundamental shift in opinion over the last 10 to 15 years has been the realization that breech presentation may well be a bad prognostic variable in itself.[1] Any studies, clinical trials, or proposed clinical management must take this into account.

INCIDENCE

The incidence of breech presentation varies with gestational age, being approximately 14% at 29 to 32 weeks and 2.2 to 3.7% at term (depending on the use of external cephalic version), giving an overall figure of 3% to 4%.[2,3]

ETIOLOGY

Although in many cases no specific underlying cause of breech presentation is apparent, in some cases a cause can be identified (Table 64–1).

Preterm Labor

A major reason for breech presentation is the preterm onset of labor (probably the chance lie of a highly mobile fetus in relatively copious liquor); most of these babies are structurally normal. It remains unclear whether breech presentation per se predisposes to preterm labor.

Fetal Abnormality

Lamont and associates[4] found that 18% of preterm breech infants were congenitally abnormal. Collea and associates[5] quoted a 5% incidence of congenital abnormality in term breech fetuses, two and a half times higher than in their vertex counterparts (2.1%). Central nervous system abnormalities are the most commonly noted; approximately 50% of all babies with hydrocephalus and myelomeningocele present by the breech, as do 50% of those with Prader-Willi syndrome and trisomy. Despite the association of breech presentation with preterm labor, labor at term is still most common and 90% of abnormal breech babies weigh more than 2000 g.

Breech presentation is also associated with fetal growth restriction and with abnormalities of amniotic fluid volume (either oligo- or polyhydramnios). The association between fetal growth restriction and breech presentation is particularly marked in the preterm fetus. Breech fetuses tend to have reduced fetal-placental ratios, to be small for gestational age, and to have an increased head circumference regardless of the mode of delivery. This difference in weight persists at 18 months of age but disappears by 4 years.[6] Breech presentation has also been linked with relatively short umbilical cords.

Maternal Abnormality

Uterine size or shape may also influence presentation. The narrower cephalic pole of the fetus usually fits better than the breech into the narrower lower segment, and the breech and legs into the wider upper segment, especially if the legs of the fetus are flexed at the knee. However, if the knees are extended, the hips flexed, and the uterine space limited, the head and feet may lie alongside each other, making the cephalic pole of the fetus larger and thus encouraging a breech presentation.

TABLE 64–1

Etiology of Breech Presentation

Preterm labor
Fetal abnormality (especially central nervous system)
Oligo- or polyhydramnios
Fetal growth restriction
Short umbilical cord
Extended legs in the fetus
Uterine abnormality (e.g., bicornuate uterus)
Placenta previa
Cornual placenta
Contracted pelvis
Multiple pregnancy
Maternal anticonvulsants
Maternal substance abuse

Uterine tone is greatest in nullipara, limiting the available space, and breech presentation is reported to be more common in nulliparous women. On the other hand, the relaxed uterus of the grand multipara encourages an unstable lie, so that the fetus enters labor by chance in a breech presentation.

Other less benign conditions may alter the uterine capacity or the intrauterine shape. Uterine anomaly, such as bicornuate uterus, is associated with breech presentation. Placenta previa is well recognized in association with breech presentation, as this changes the intrauterine shape and prevents engagement of the head. Cornual implantation of the placenta, an otherwise benign condition, is also strongly associated with breech presentation; only 5% of vertex-presenting fetuses have a cornual placenta in comparison to 73% of those presenting by the breech.

A contracted pelvis is also associated with breech presentation, probably by limiting uterine space in the lower segment.

Other Reasons for Breech Presentation

Women who have had a breech presentation at term are significantly more likely to have another in a subsequent pregnancy. This is usually associated with extended fetal legs and may indicate a genetic predisposition to this posture in the fetus.

Multiple pregnancy is strongly associated with breech presentation. The reader is referred to Chapter 60 for further discussion of management.

Medication with anticonvulsants in pregnancy also seems to be associated with breech presentation,[7] as does maternal alcohol abuse[8]; both substances have a profound influence on intrauterine fetal neurologic function. Fetal behavior in utero in fetuses with persistent breech presentation is also subtly different. They demonstrate more state transitions in fetal activity and heart rate patterns in utero than their cephalic presenting counterparts.[9]

RISKS AND SIGNIFICANCE

Although fetuses presenting by the breech have an increased perinatal mortality rate, it has proved difficult to separate and quantify the independent risks of the breech position itself and to distinguish the problems of the delivery from the problems of the fetus being abnormal. The perinatal mortality rate remains increased even when delivery is by cesarean section, and this is true even after correction for gestational age, congenital defects, and birth weight.

Many retrospective reviews of breech presentation and trials of antepartum and intrapartum management compare the breech-presenting infant with the vertex-presenting infant, and because of its associated problems, the breech-presenting infant is more likely to perform unfavorably, regardless of the mode of delivery. Nelson and Ellenberg[10] looked at all the obstetric factors that could be associated with the development of cerebral palsy using a multiple regression technique and found that breech presentation was an independent predictor for cerebral palsy. There were a number of small randomized controlled trials and meta-analyses studying the role of the mode of delivery of the term breech in relation to neonatal performance and long-term outcome, but they produced conflicting results.[5,11–15] (It should be noted that functional and behavioral outcomes by mode of delivery need to be considered independently of perinatal mortality; see the later section on mode of delivery.)

Some of the association of breech presentation with cerebral palsy can be accounted for by the excess of low birth weight in breech presentation, and this factor is independent of the mode of delivery.[16]

More subtle aspects of neuromotor development may also be manifest in breech-presenting fetuses. These may represent a continuum, with subtle differences in in utero fetal behavioral states being evident.[16] Bartlett and coworkers compared 90 morphologically normal term breech-presenting singletons having birth weights greater than 2500 g and delivered by cesarean section with similar cephalically presenting infants, matched for gender and mode of delivery. They prospectively collected data on neurologic status and motor performance over the first 18 months of life. They found that not only did breech-presenting infants have more open popliteal angles at birth (an unsurprising observation) but also they had significantly lower motor scores at 6 weeks and an excess of neurologic problems diagnosed at 18 months.[17]

The risks to the mother are easier to quantify. Breech presentation confers an increased likelihood of cesarean section with its attendant risks of morbidity and death.[5] It has been calculated by some that the risk of maternal fatality in cesarean section is up to 38 times that of a vaginal delivery.[18] However, others have suggested a relative risk as low as 7, decreasing to 5 after exclusion of women with medical or life-threatening complications.[19]

In the latter study, most of the surplus risk occurred in emergency cesarean sections, when the relative risk was 11, compared with elective cesarean sections when the risk was only 4. There is some evidence that breech presentation and cesarean section may reduce the subsequent pregnancy rate, probably because of the woman's decision not to reproduce again.[20]

DIAGNOSIS

Three clinical types of breech presentation are recognized. This classification is useful in that it may indicate the cause of the presentation and the complications to be anticipated. As with most clinical classifications, there is overlap of the associated factors between the groups:

- The frank (or extended) breech indicates that the legs of the fetus are flexed at the hip and extended at the knee. This type accounts for 60% to 70% of all breech presentations at term. The risks of fetal-pelvic disproportion and of cord prolapse are lowest in this group.
- The complete (or flexed) breech indicates that the hips and knees are flexed so that the feet are presenting in the pelvis.
- The incomplete (or footling) breech indicates that one leg is flexed and the other extended.

The woman with a breech presentation, especially towards term, may complain of subcostal discomfort and of feeling the baby kick in the lower part of the uterus. On palpation the hard round ballotable head is found at the fundus, and the softer breech is at the lower pole. The fetal heart sounds are more commonly heard above the umbilicus. One diagnostic pitfall is the confusion of a deeply engaged head and a breech presentation. The examiner thinks that the shoulders are above the pelvic brim when in fact the breech is over the pelvis.

At vaginal examination, if the cervix is sufficiently dilated, the fetal ischial tuberosities and the sacrum provide the bony landmarks. The anus and the genitalia may also be felt but are less useful in diagnosis due to their softness and compressibility. If the membranes are ruptured, the examining finger in the anus may produce meconium staining. The main diagnostic confusion is face presentation. Face presentation produces the characteristic bony landmarks of the malar eminences, mouth, and mentum that produce a bony triangle, whereas the ischial tuberosities and the sacrum are in line. The mouth, in contrast to the anus, has a firm unyielding margin of bone. Engagement of the breech implies that the bitrochanteric diameter has passed through the pelvic brim.

Because of the difficulties described earlier, approximately 45% of breech presentations are not diagnosed until after 38 weeks, and 30% remain undiagnosed until labor.[21] If there is any doubt about presentation, an ultrasound scan is mandatory if mistakes are to be avoided. Some clinicians even advocate routine late third trimester ultrasonography to determine presentation and ensure time for external cephalic version (ECV) (thus decreasing the need for cesarean section).[21]

THE PRETERM BREECH PRESENTATION

The search for methods of preventing or suppressing preterm labor has proved disappointing, and obstetricians have been forced to look at other techniques for optimizing the condition of preterm infants at birth so as to minimize neonatal complications. This has focused predominantly on the mode of delivery and has led to an increase in the cesarean section rate. For breech-presenting fetuses at 23 weeks the cesarean section rate has risen approximately threefold between 1995 and 2002, reflecting the increasingly aggressive management policies for extremely preterm infants.

Risks

General

The proportion of babies delivered before 37 weeks' gestation in the United Kingdom has been remarkably constant over the years at about 7%. However, the mortality and morbidity rates of babies delivered between 33 and 36 weeks inclusive is now very low and not significantly influenced by mode of delivery, provided that cesarean section is undertaken for the usual clinical indications. Discussion is focused here on the gestation range of 26 to 32 weeks, when approximately 2% of all pregnant women with viable fetuses will deliver. About 25% of all babies delivered at these gestations are in breech presentation, probably due to the chance lie of a very mobile fetus in the relatively copious amniotic fluid. Thus, the overall incidence of very preterm (<33 weeks) breech presentation at delivery is 0.5%.

The premature baby in breech presentation shares many of the characteristics of the mature breech. The premature breech baby also has a higher rate of congenital abnormality than its vertex presenting counterpart, up to 18%.[22,23] The preterm breech has a higher antepartum stillbirth and neonatal death rate than babies presenting by the head, regardless of mode of delivery.[2] It is probably even more true of the preterm breech than the term infant that poor outcome in survivors, such as mild neurologic dysfunction, cannot safely be attributed solely to the fact of vaginal breech delivery but is often due to the abnormalities associated with breech presentation. The premature breech shows other differences from the premature cephalic-presenting infant; it is more commonly small for gestational age and has a lower fetal-placental ratio. It also tends to have a larger head circumference for a given birth weight than babies delivered in vertex presentation, probably due to the lack of the compressive effect of the lower segment. It seems likely that in many cases of breech presentation at delivery, prematurity and poor fetal outcome are both determined by the same prenatal influences.

At Delivery

OCCIPITAL DIASTASIS AND CEREBELLAR INJURY

Experienced obstetricians have recognized that cesarean section is not always an atraumatic option for the fetus, and the preterm breech infant faces some formidable difficulties whichever route of delivery is employed. Wigglesworth and Husemeyer[24] have emphasized the vulnerability of the occipital bone to damage during vaginal breech delivery, due to its impact on the maternal pubis during descent of the fetal head into the pelvis during the second stage. These forces tend to separate the squamous part of the occipital bone from the lateral part (occipital diastasis). This produces a ridge in the posterior fossa and hence bruising or laceration of the cerebellum. The squamous part of the occipital bone is forced anteriorly to distort the foramen magnum and produce pressure on the spinal cord. Cerebellar bruising can be present in the absence of occipital diastasis, and although the fracture may be easily diagnosable after delivery with a lateral skull x-ray, the cerebellar bruising alone will not be diagnosable unless the cerebellum is scanned routinely by the neonatologist using ultrasound. The injury is commonly not discovered at postmortem examination if traditional dissection techniques have been used. The damage to the brain may not be clinically apparent until the age of approximately 2 years, when the child will manifest signs of clumsiness and poor coordination consequent upon its cerebellar damage (ataxic cerebral palsy).

INTRAVENTRICULAR AND PERIVENTRICULAR DAMAGE

In addition, the preterm infant is vulnerable to intraventricular and periventricular damage secondary to hemorrhage or ischemia, which can be due to hypoxic or acidotic insults in the antepartum, intrapartum, and neonatal periods. The premature breech may be still more susceptible to these as a consequence of the peculiar circumstances surrounding delivery. However, avoiding vaginal delivery will not necessarily prevent intracranial bleeding. Tejani and associates (1984) have shown that premature labor of itself can produce intracranial hemorrhage even if delivery is delayed or by cesarean section.[25]

GENERALIZED TRAUMA AND NERVE INJURIES

A traumatic breech delivery in which there is widespread limb and body bruising can produce gross skeletal muscle damage that results in large quantities of hemoglobin and myoglobin being liberated. This can lead to severe jaundice and damage to the kidneys in a premature infant whose hepatic capacity to deal with bilirubin is limited and whose renal excretory capacity is poor. This can produce a form of "shock lung" in the neonate manifesting as severe respiratory distress syndrome.

The premature breech infant is also susceptible to damage to internal organs, transection of the spinal cord, and other nerve palsies consequent on traction, especially the brachial plexus and fractures of long bones similar to its more mature counterpart. Because the widest diameter of the fetus is the biparietal diameter and the discrepancy between the diameters of the head and the body is most pronounced in the premature fetus, it is possible for the body and limbs of the premature breech to slip through a cervix that is still incompletely dilated and the head will be unable to follow. This "entrapment" of the after-coming head is more likely in the mother who commences active pushing prior to second stage, with a footling presentation, especially with the preterm fetus in whom the subcutaneous fat has not yet been laid down and the liver is not of the large size reached in the mature fetus; hence, the abdominal circumference is relatively smaller. Recommended management is usually to incise the cervix with scissors at 4 and 8 o'clock, but inevitably there is delay in delivery and therefore an increase in the hypoxic stress to the fetus, together with a likely increase in traumatic morbidity to both mother and child. However, Robertson and associates,[26] after studying 132 consecutive preterm singleton breech deliveries, demonstrated that there did not seem to be a difference in the incidence of head entrapment by mode of delivery for breech infants at 28 to 36 weeks' gestation, and nor did there appear to be a difference in adverse neonatal outcomes after entrapment.

Injuries are not confined to babies delivered vaginally in breech presentation. Any very low birth weight baby is susceptible to trauma from a difficult delivery through a poorly formed lower segment. If the presentation is breech, a limited uterine incision can impede the delivery of the head to the same degree as a difficult vaginal delivery and is analogous in every way to the entrapment of the after-coming head that is such a feared complication of the premature breech delivered vaginally. To some extent this can be avoided by performing an anterior vertical uterine incision (ideally De Lee's incision, but often in a very small uterus it becomes a classical incision). However, this carries increased risks for the mother, particularly in respect to uterine rupture in a future pregnancy or labor, but occasionally also in terms of poor healing and postpartum hemorrhage. The incidence of intraventricular hemorrhage in the fetus and neonate is also closely related to the occurrence of preterm labor of itself, independent of the mode of delivery.[25]

Management Options for the Preterm Breech in Labor

Most elective deliveries of the preterm breech when the woman is not in labor are for fetal or maternal indications when the preferred route of delivery is cesarean section. The controversy about management mainly centers on the preterm breech presentation in labor, in which the initial priorities are (1) the accurate diagnosis of premature labor, (2) the confirmation of presentation, and (3) the exclusion of fetal abnormality.

It is evident that in up to 80% of cases in which the mother thinks she is in premature labor, contractions cease spontaneously and the pregnancy continues. The definitive diagnosis of labor therefore rests on demonstrating progressive dilation of the cervix. Careful cervical assessment of all women in suspected premature labor is imperative to confirm or refute the diagnosis. In the presence of ruptured membranes this should be done using full aseptic technique and the number of examinations limited to minimize the risk of introducing infection, causing chorioamnionitis. Vaginal examination can confirm the presentation and can even reveal the presence of fetal abnormality (for example, imperforate anus!). In view of the recognized association of fetal abnormality with premature breech presentation, all previous ultrasound examinations should be carefully reviewed. A further detailed ultrasound scan should be performed if possible to confirm the normality of the fetus and check on placental position at the same time. An estimate of fetal weight may allow a more rational decision to be made about the optimum place and mode of delivery. Ultrasound fetal weight estimation is possible to ± 15% in skilled hands, although when performed by junior residents outside of normal hours, errors greater than 15% have been reported in over 40% of cases.[27] This has led some workers to suggest that the outcome for the infant is best predicted by accurate knowledge of gestational age.[21]

Administration of tocolytics may be appropriate in an effort to delay delivery long enough to administer steroids to promote surfactant production in the fetal lung prior to preterm delivery or to arrange delivery in a site with appropriate neonatal intensive care facilities. It is now clear that tocolytic therapy is ineffective in preventing premature delivery in the longer term and that its use beyond 48 to 72 hours is probably inappropriate.

The Optimum Mode of Delivery of the Preterm Breech

The preterm breech on the labor ward presents the obstetrician with a heterogeneous group of clinical problems. Some will present not in labor but with spontaneous rupture of the membranes only; others will present at 7 cm dilation in strong labor and deliver after only a short interval. As with all premature deliveries, premature vaginal breech delivery is sometimes precipitate and may therefore occur in the absence of skilled medical attendants. It is important to realize that, in common with all preterm labors, the antecedents are often pathologic, and therefore, a decision about the mode of delivery is uncontentious. If there has been a placental abruption or cord prolapse, then clearly cesarean section is indicated.

However, if the clinical situation is of "the uncomplicated preterm breech in labor," that is, if fetal and maternal condition are good, and labor is progressing at a normal rate, it is necessary to decide whether a vaginal delivery is to be allowed or a cesarean section should be undertaken.

One of the first suggestions that cesarean section should be undertaken routinely for the delivery of the preterm breech was in 1977 when Goldenberg and Nelson reviewed the outcome of 224 babies less than 1500 g delivered between 1965 and 1969.[28] They compared babies delivered vaginally in breech presentation with babies delivered vaginally in vertex presentation, and all those delivered by cesarean section. For reasons enumerated earlier (in particular, the differing incidence of congenital anomaly) their comparisons were not valid. The other problem highlighted by these authors was the noncomparability of the study groups in other respects. The authors reported that many fetuses below 1000 g were not monitored during labor as they were thought to be nonviable, or if they were monitored, when signs of fetal distress supervened surgical intervention was often not performed as the fetus was thought to be "too small to live." This approach resulted in infants being delivered vaginally who happened to survive despite nonintervention being compared with infants who were thought to be viable and not "too small to live" and who were therefore delivered electively by cesarean section, attended by senior and experienced members of staff. Such a comparison is inherently likely to show a better outcome for the latter group and therefore lead to the (potentially) erroneous conclusion that cesarean section improves the outcome for the preterm breech infant.

Further retrospective reviews of clinical practice were published over the next few years, some comparing the vertex with the breech,[29] some correctly comparing the vaginally delivered breech with the breech delivered by cesarean section, but then only stratifying by birth weight below and above 2500 g or in other similarly wide weight bands.[30] Some advocated cesarean section,[30] and some advised that selected preterm breeches should be allowed to deliver vaginally.[31] Most of these latter authors felt that outcome was more related to obstetric variables other than the mode of delivery. Other authors advised that all premature infants are best delivered by classical cesarean section.[32] Wolf and associates[33] observed the natural experiment of two adjacent maternity units both with different policies for the delivery of the preterm breech (26–31 weeks). One unit chose to deliver vaginally (17% cesarean section rate) and the other by cesarean section (85% cesarean section rate), but they did not observe any differences in survival rates.

Further evidence of the noncomparability of the vaginally delivered and cesarean delivered breeches is reported in a paper by Jain and associates.[34] He noted that even within the weight range of 1000 to 1499 g there was a marked difference in the average weight, with the babies delivering vaginally being significantly lighter and at a lower gestation than those delivered by cesarean section, a difference likely to account for any differences in survival. A further series of retrospective and uncontrolled studies were then reported to show a better outcome after cesarean section for babies weighing 1000 to 1500 g, but no advantage to babies weighing less than this.[22,35,36]

In order to overcome the noncomparability of groups in these retrospective reviews of practice, there has been a series of attempts at using statistical techniques to determine the contribution that mode of delivery makes to outcome for the preterm breech.[37,38] Kitchen and associates[38] found that the mode of delivery was a significant factor in the likelihood of survival for the preterm breech. Rosen and associates,[37] on the other hand, found that variables such as gestational age or administration of steroids antenatally were more significantly associated with outcome.

Thus, all currently existing evidence has major methodologic flaws that make it unreliable as a guide to clinical decision making and have led to a number of calls for a randomized controlled trial to settle the question of optimum mode of delivery. Despite this, there has only been one such randomized trial which has actually been completed. Viegas and associates randomized 23 women, but unfortunately their analysis was fundamentally flawed by inappropriate withdrawals and no conclusions can be drawn from their results.[39] Two other randomized trials of the optimum mode of delivery of the preterm infant (both vertex and breech presenting) have been initiated, but both were terminated prematurely and produced no interpretable results.[40,41] Lumley and associates[40] randomized only 4 subjects out of a possible 33 who were eligible over a 5-month period and terminated the trial after drawing the conclusion that clinicians were unwilling to randomize their management. Wallace, Schifrin, and Paul[41] aborted their randomized trial of the optimum mode of delivery of the preterm infant because they found that an unacceptably high number of the babies (63%) were above the 1500-g upper weight limit for the trial. They concluded that a more accurate way of estimating fetal weight prior to delivery was needed before a further attempt was feasible. The subjects they did randomize were analyzed according to the eventual mode of delivery, not according to the randomized mode of delivery, thereby invalidating the randomizing process.

A prospective randomized multicenter trial to determine the best mode of delivery for the preterm breech (26–32 weeks) recruiting subjects in the United Kingdom was also abandoned.[42] The recruitment rate was disappointing, with only 10% of eligible subjects being randomized, despite large numbers of women consenting to take part in the trial antenatally and sufficient numbers of premature breeches presenting for randomization. No definitive conclusion was reached. The authors concluded that the failure of the trial did not mean obstetricians were insisting on cesarean delivery; 30% of preterm breeches not entered in the trial were allowed to deliver vaginally. Instead, they concluded that obstetricians were reluctant to abandon individualized decisions about management even in the presence of a high degree of scientific uncertainty about the basis on which their decisions were being made. Also, some evidence suggested that if the clinician was unsure of the optimum mode of delivery, then women wished to make a choice for themselves and withdrew from randomization. It therefore appears likely that the optimal mode of delivery of the preterm breech will remain uncertain for the foreseeable future. At gestations above 32 weeks but below 37 weeks and when the fetus weighs 1500 to 2500 g, current evidence does not suggest any advantage to routine cesarean section. Under this gestation and weight but at more than 26 weeks' gestation, the optimal mode of delivery remains uncertain in the absence of any clinical feature specifically indicating cesarean section. The advantage, if any, that routine section confers on the fetus is likely to be small, otherwise it would already be obvious in the multiplicity of published data already available. What is certain is that if a policy of routine cesarean section for the preterm breech fetus is followed, a number of cesarean sections will be performed unnecessarily for the fetus that is congenitally abnormal, for the fetus that is over 1500 g and therefore unlikely to benefit, for babies mistakenly thought to be in breech presentation (of which there were two in the U.K. study), and for some that will not actually be in established premature labor and were destined to deliver at a later gestation. A policy of routine cesarean section will also expose the mother to a definite risk of maternal mortality and morbidity.

PROCEDURE: CONDUCT OF DELIVERY

Vaginal delivery of the preterm breech should be supervised by an experienced obstetrician. An effective epidural anesthetic is preferable to prevent the woman from pushing prior to full dilation, to allow manipulation of the breech, or painless operative intervention either with forceps or rapid recourse to cesarean section. The anesthetist and pediatrician should be in attendance for the second stage. There is no clear evidence to favor the use of obstetric forceps to the after-coming head; the pelvis will be relatively capacious for the premature neonate, and it will not be subject to the rapid compression-decompression forces applied to the head of the mature infant in breech presentation. There is some evidence that delivery with intact membranes is an advantage.[29] Should the cervix clamp down over the head or the body be delivered through an incompletely dilated cervix, the head should be flexed abdominally and the finger of the vaginal hand should be inserted into the mouth of the fetus to flex the head and facilitate delivery. If this is not possible, then scissors with the intracervical blade guarded by a finger should be introduced at 4 and 8 o'clock, and the cervix should be incised. The carefully flexed head should then deliver easily. The cervix is usually repaired easily provided analgesia is adequate.

If cesarean section is indicated, the abdominal incision used should be considered carefully. Although a Pfannenstiel will give good access for a lower segment uterine incision, if this needs to be extended in an emergency (for example, if the after-coming head becomes entrapped), then a vertical midline incision will be an advantage (it can be extended upward as far as is necessary). The advent of mass closure with nylon has reduced the morbidity of the midline approach so that it is now on a par with the Pfannenstiel, apart from the obvious cosmetic drawback of the midline scar. As well as providing improved access, it is also quicker. If a transverse uterine incision needs extending, then a J shape is to be preferred to an inverted T, as the latter leaves a point of marked scar weakness at its center, which may rupture in a future pregnancy. The De Lee or classical uterine incision appears to confer little benefit on the fetus in terms of reduced trauma, from 28 weeks onward (Patterson, Stacey, and Steer, unpublished data). On the other hand, neonatal mortality rates below 28 weeks can be high.[43] Because of the maternal morbidity involved, it is probably unwise to use the classical approach to try to salvage the preterm baby if its viability seems doubtful.

THE BREECH PRESENTATION AT TERM

Management Options

Version of the Breech

SPONTANEOUS VERSION

The fact that breech presentation is so uncommon at term implies that spontaneous version usually occurs in the weeks before term and so breech presentation becomes less common as the third trimester progresses. The incidence of spontaneous version after 32 weeks maybe as high as 57% and after 36 weeks' gestation may still be as high as 25%.[44] Spontaneous version is more likely in multiparas without a previous breech birth and is less likely in nulliparous women and in the breech with extended legs. Prior to cesarean section solely for breech presentation at term, the presentation should be checked immediately before surgery by ultrasound scanning, as the chances of spontaneous version even at this late stage are not insignificant.[44]

PROMOTION OF SPONTANEOUS VERSION

Techniques to promote spontaneous version have been investigated following Hofmeyr's observation that in some cases version from breech to cephalic occurred between the preliminary scan and the planned external cephalic version (ECV).[45] He postulated that the combination of disengagement of the breech and postural change might have promoted spontaneous version. A variety of other techniques have been described including the knee chest position, with the buttocks higher than the torso and the chest lying on a flat surface for 10 minutes every day, and another technique describes elevation of the pelvis, and abduction of the thighs. The Cochrane review of five studies, including 392 women, of randomized or quasi-randomized controlled trials compared postural management of the breech with control subjects. There was no effect on the rate of noncephalic births, the rate of cesarean section, or the incidence of low Apgar scores.[46] Therefore, although there is likely to be no significant adverse effects from postural management, there is currently no evidence to support its efficacy.

EXTERNAL CEPHALIC VERSION

External cephalic version fell from favor in the mid-1970s. Prior to this time it was performed without medication (except occasionally sedation), without tocolysis, and usually prior to 36 weeks' gestation. It was thought that because ECV was easier to perform prior to 36 weeks, it must therefore be safer. Without tocolysis it was often unsuccessful after 36 weeks. Bradley-Watson in 1975 reported a 1% fetal mortality rate for ECV done prior to 36 weeks without tocolysis, which was considered unacceptably high.[47] As a result, the use of ECV declined and was almost abandoned in most institutions as cesarean section was seen as a safer alternative. Another significant disadvantage of preterm ECV is that fetal bradycardia may precipitate immediate delivery by cesarean section, with the risk of ensuing respiratory distress syndrome. To avoid this, it was traditional to manage acute bradycardia by reversion of the fetus to breech, which did not always work and in any case defeated the objective of the ECV. In addition, spontaneous reversion to breech occurred quite often prior to delivery. Thus, the effectiveness of ECV was controversial, especially as the fetal mortality rate was reported to be higher in the preterm than the term breech.

The Cochrane review included three randomized controlled trials of the use of ECV before term involving 899 women and showed no significant effect on noncephalic presentation, cesarean section, low Apgar scores, or perinatal mortality rate, and the practice cannot currently be recommended.[48] There are no published data on the use of ECV in the management of the preterm breech in labor. The antecedents of the preterm breech in labor are often abnormal, and ECV is therefore less relevant as a management strategy.

Any consideration of the efficacy and safety of the technique of external cephalic version should include a likelihood of spontaneous version, the effectiveness of ECV of producing a cephalic presentation at the time of birth, the risks to the mother and the baby, and the utility of cephalic presentation at birth to the mother and the baby (i.e., if some preexisting abnormality or fetal compromise determines the mode of delivery rather than the presentation itself and also if the prognosis of the baby is determined by its condition rather than the mode of delivery, correction of the breech presentation will then not alter the outcome for the fetus).

The advantage of performing ECV at term is that it allows time for spontaneous version to occur and the clarification of conditions that of themselves may require delivery by cesarean section. This will result in fewer uneccessary attempts being made. Also, should complications of ECV occur, then prompt recourse to cesarean section will result in the birth of a mature infant. It also appears that ECV at term results in fewer complications.

The Cochrane review[48] looked at six trials of a randomized or quasi-randomized nature and concluded that ECV at term was associated with a significant reduction in noncephalic births (relative risk 0.42) and a reduction in cesarean section (relative risk 0.52), although there was no significant effect on perinatal mortality rate. This review also concluded that there was insufficient evidence to assess any risks associated with ECV at term.

The implications of these data are that every 100 ECV attempts should prevent 34 breech births and 14 cesarean sections. A conservative estimate of the impact of performing ECV on 2% of the 750,000 pregnancies in the United Kingdom every year would be a reduction in the number of breech births by 5100 and a reduction in the number of cesarean sections by 2100.[48]

However, the impact of ECV on the rate of cesarean sections for this indication will depend on the success rate of ECV. There seems to be a wide variation in the reported success rate. Trials performed in Africa on black African women have much higher success rates. This success is probably due to the tendency of late engagement of the presenting part in the pelvis in black African women.[49] Success rates as high as 77% have been reported,[50] but in general, success rates of 50% or even less are acceptable.

Various methods of predicting the success of an attempted ECV have been devised. Most studies have found that nulliparity, increased uterine tone, a posterior fetal spine, the breech engaged in the pelvis, a frank breech, and gestations above 38 weeks are bad prognostic indicators for success.[51] One study found that if the presenting part in a nullipara was engaged and there was difficulty in palpating the fetal head, then no attempt at ECV was successful. On the other hand, if the presenting part was not engaged in a multipara and the fetal head was easily palpable, then 94% of attempts were successful.[52] ECV in the preterm breech tends to be more successful but does not promote more cephalic deliveries at term.[53]

Because of the observation that increased uterine tone decreases the chances of success of ECV, the use of tocolytics has been investigated. A variety of tocolytics have been used. The Cochrane database reviewed six trials of routine tocolysis and showed that its use was associated with fewer failures. Use of fetal acoustic stimulation (FAS) was also associated with fewer failures of ECV.

In a randomized controlled trial of the use of tocolysis in ECV, Marquette and associates[54] confirmed the efficacy of ritodrine in promoting success of ECV in nulliparous patients but not in parous patients. They found that ritodrine increased the success rate of ECV from 25% to 43% in nulliparous women. Fernandez and coworkers also assessed the efficacy of terbutaline (0.25 mg subcutaneously) in comparison with placebo for ECV and found a significant decrease in noncephalic presentations and cesarean sections because of increased chances of success with ECV.[55] There has been an evaluation of glyceryl trinitrate in a placebo-controlled randomized trial for women whose first attempt at ECV without tocolysis had failed, but no significant differences between groups were observed.[56]

Because one of the main reasons for the failure or abandonment of ECV is maternal discomfort, the use of epidural analgesia for the procedure has been suggested. There has been only one randomized controlled trial of the use of epidural anesthesia to improve the success of ECV. This trial had approximately 35 women randomized to epidural anesthesia versus no epidural and found that the success rate was significantly increased (risk ratio 2:12), and that the chances of success were not affected by an anterior placenta or oligohydramnios.[57] As reported earlier, observational studies suggest a doubling of the success rate for ECV using tocolysis. Two studies have examined the use of epidural anesthesia if initial attempts performed using tocolysis have failed. Both these studies reported fetal complications of the procedure and, although they reported favorable success rates, commented that the "safety of the procedure remains in question."

BENEFITS TO THE FETUS OF ECV

It is clear that ECV reduces the incidence of breech presentation at term and of breech delivery, whether vaginal or by cesarean section. It will therefore decrease the incidence of cord prolapse and unattended precipitate breech birth. Unattended or precipitate breech birth has been shown to be associated with an eightfold increase in the risk of poor condition at birth in comparison to women expertly attended and assessed for vaginal delivery ante partum.[58] It may be that the rate of cesarean section is higher than the average for cephalic presentations even after successful version, although not all studies have found this.[59,60] However, it would be a mistake to suppose that elective cesarean section eliminates all risks for the fetus: cesarean delivery of the preterm breech may still be traumatic, and the risk of pulmonary hypertension of the newborn may be increased.[61,62]

RISKS TO THE FETUS OF ECV

The risk to the fetus is difficult to quantify because there is at present no randomized controlled trial large enough to clarify the issue, and the authors of the Cochrane review were unable to draw any overall conclusions regarding risks. However, in a review of 979 reported cases of ECV at term with neither inhalational analgesia nor general anesthesia, there were no fetal losses.[37] ECV has been associated with demonstrable changes in the fetal circulation.[63] An 8% incidence of fetal bradycardia has been reported in association with ECV.[64] If an ECV (whether successful or not) produces a fetal bradycardia, it is possible that subsequent labor is more likely to be complicated by fetal heart rate abnormality and result in cesarean section.[64] Lau and associates demonstrated changes in the fetal circulation, but not placental circulation, associated with attempted ECV. The pulsatility index was reduced in the middle cerebral artery, and these authors postulated that this was merely a physiologic response to manipulation of the fetal head.[63] Isolated cases of cord presentation and even fetal demise have also been reported. Kouam[65] followed up 116 children born after ECV. Developmental screening at 2 to 5 years of age showed no developmental delay. Although the short-term neonatal outcomes reported in the randomized controlled trials are essentially normal and compare favorably with control subjects, they are only surrogates for definitive follow-up studies of the effects of this procedure.

Fetal-maternal hemorrhage has been reported in association with ECV. The risk has been quoted at approximately 5% using tocolysis, whereas the risk without tocolysis has been reported to be as high as 28%. The experience of ECV prior to 36 to 37 weeks demonstrates that the risks to the fetus are related to gestational age and the use of general anesthesia. It may be that an anterior placenta also represents a risk. However, the risks of ECV set in the overall context of the risks of breech presentation in itself or of the risks of breech delivery vaginally or abdominally are small.

BENEFITS TO THE MOTHER OF ECV

There will be a decrease in the number of cesarean sections performed and possibly in the number of vaginal breech deliveries, which often entails episiotomy and forceps delivery. The maternal morbidity rate is usually higher after cesarean section than after vaginal delivery. Cesarean section may compromise future reproductive function,[66,20] and there may be adverse emotional sequelae for the mother and the maternal-infant pair.[67] All these aspects are aside from the higher maternal death rate associated with cesarean section.

Interestingly, although ECV has become much more widely used over the last decade and more pregnant women (and their clinicians) have become aware of the procedure, pregnant women may be less inclined to take up the option of ECV and opt for planned cesarean section instead.[68]

The contraindications for the performance of ECV are outlined in Table 64–2. The absolute contraindications are uncontroversial. However, the relative contraindications are more debatable. It may be that uterine anomalies and excessive maternal body weight should be regarded as relative contraindications. An amniotic fluid volume of less than 2 cm in depth in any pocket, the fetal back lying anteriorly, a tense uterus, difficulty palpating the fetal head, an engaged breech, and nulliparity will decrease the chance of success.[51] Chances of success are increased with increasing parity and a breech lying more in the iliac fossae than in the midline. Fetal abdominal circumference is related to the chances of success, whereas the biparietal diameter is not. Gestational age and estimated fetal weight, provided the attempt was after 37 weeks, had no relationship with the chances of success, as success rates were found to be the same at 37, 38, and 40 weeks.

Although previous cesarean section is a relative contraindication to ECV, there is a small series of 36 women who had one previous cesarean section and underwent an ECV, of which 66% were successful, and of these, 76% had a vaginal birth. There were no maternal or neonatal complications.[69] Maternal Rh negativity is a relative contradiction. If ECV is used, a Kleihauer test should be done and anti-D (Rhogam) administered.

TABLE 64–2

Indications and Contraindications for External Cephalic Version (ECV)

Indications for ECV
Any breech presentation after 36/37 weeks' gestation
Suspected fetopelvic disproportion
Unengaged breech
Absolute Contraindications to ECV
Multiple pregnancy*
Antepartum hemorrhage
Placenta previa
Ruptured membranes
Significant fetal abnormality
Need for cesarean section for other indications
Relative Contraindications to ECV
Previous cesarean section
Intrauterine growth restriction
Severe proteinuric hypertension
Obesity
Rhesus isoimmunization
Evidence of macrosomia
(Grand multiparity)
(Anterior placenta)
("precious baby")
(previous antepartum hemorrhage)
Any suspected fetal compromise: unreactive cardiotocogram

*Apart from the second twin after the vaginal delivery of the first.
Note: If tocolysis is to be used, women with congenital or acquired heart disease, diabetes, or thyroid disease should be excluded because of possible adverse reactions.

PROCEDURE – EXTERNAL CEPHALIC VERSION

PREREQUISITES

1. Recent ultrasound to confirm a normal fetus and an adequate liquor volume
2. Reassuring fetal heart rate pattern

3. Informed consent-in which the mother is specifically advised of the risks of provoking labor, ruptured membranes, and cord and placental accidents
4. Facilities for the performance of a cesarean section

PROCEDURE

ECV may be performed in the labor room or the clinic room, if there is rapid access to delivery facilities. The woman is positioned either in steep or slight lateral tilt or in Trendelenburg position. It is sometimes recommended that a Kleihauer test be performed before and after the procedure. Some also recommend placing an intravenous line and cross matching blood for a possible cesarean section. If tocolysis is to be used, some practitioners perform an electrolyte and glucose estimation as well. A clinical pelvimetry should be judged as adequate. An ultrasound scan should be performed in order to assess the liquor volume, fetal attitude, and position of the fetal legs. The fetal heart rate pattern should be normal and reassuring prior to commencement. Some authorities recommend that a contraction stress test be performed prior to version. It has even been suggested that the maternal blood pressure be taken every 5 minutes throughout the procedure[53] and that the maternal heart rate be monitored electronically. This is probably unnecessary if the mother appears well throughout but could be important if tocolysis is used.

If tocolysis is employed, this can be given in a variety of ways: 10 μg of hexaprenaline given intravenously over 1 minute, terbutaline 0.25 mg subcutaneously or in 5 mL of normal saline over 5 minutes intravenously; terbutaline 0.5 μg/minute intravenously or terbutaline 0.5 μg/minute intravenously over 15 to 20 minutes; or ritodrine 0.2 mg/minute intravenously for 20 minutes. Some authors give the chosen tocolytic as a stat dose and commence the ECV almost immediately. Others increase the dose steadily or wait until adequate uterine relaxation is achieved, all contractions have ceased, or there is softening of the uterus and easy palpation of fetal parts.

The ECV should be performed as one episode by one operator, and continuous pressure on the uterus should be limited to 5 minutes. Many recommend that uterine manipulation should continue for only 10 minutes, although waiting for the fetus to be active spontaneously (helping to dislodge it from the pelvis) and then applying pressure may be advantageous. Others have recommended stimulating the fetus to move using a vibroacoustic stimulator.[70] Mohamed and associates[50] reported that 55% are successful after 1 minute and only 15% require up to 5 minutes continuous pressure on the abdomen. The increased incidence of fetal heart rate abnormalities with failed ECV suggests that persistence in an attempt beyond these suggested times may be counterproductive. The incidence of fetal heart rate abnormalities may be higher when the procedure is unsuccessful. Mohamed and associates[50] also report that 73% were deemed by the obstetricians to be easy versions with 90% of women reporting little or no discomfort.

A variety of techniques of ECV are also employed. A forward or backward somersault can be performed: the forward somersault is the classically described maneuver. A technique is described which involves placing the woman in a steep lateral tilt with her back against the wall behind the examination couch. A forward somersault is recommended if the fetal back is downward and a backward somersault if the fetal back is upward. If the breech is engaged, the breech must first be pushed out of the pelvis with the operator's right hand prior to correction of the presentation. There is a general consensus that vaginal disengagement should not be performed if the breech will not easily come out of the pelvis with abdominal pressure. Occasionally the fetal head is caught under the costal margin and this prevents the disengagement of the breech. In such a case the fetal head should be manipulated down and sideways prior to the disengagement of the breech and forward somersault. The actual version is accomplished using flexion of the fetal head and encouragement of a forward somersault by pressure on the uterus. Some practitioners pause as the breech is about to negotiate the transverse diameter of the uterus and apply acoustic stimulation. This may causes fetal kicking, which assists the version.[70]

If the fetal back is anterior, version is often impossible to achieve, either with a backward or forward somersault. Johnson and associates[70] suggest that fetal acoustic stimulation will convert the anterior to a lateral position in 90% of cases and thus make version possible.

After successful version, the attitude of the fetus should be maintained manually for a few minutes.

The fetal heart can be monitored continuously through the procedure or every 2 minutes. A repeat fetal heart rate tracing should be performed immediately after the ECV. If this is normal, the woman may go home. She should return within a few days so that the position of the fetus can be rechecked. Some practitioners perform a cesarean section if the breech presentation recurs, while others follow their protocol for selection for vaginal breech delivery. Others continue to correct the presentation repeatedly. There is some evidence that the latter approach does result in more vertex presentations at delivery.

Current evidence indicates that ECV performed at term, and particularly with tocolysis, is a safe procedure for carefully selected women. The short-term complications are negligible, and although the long-term complications are harder to determine, overall it seems likely that the benefits will outweigh the risks.

Assessment of the Fetus

The presentation of the fetus should be checked using ultrasound scanning. This should be possible in most cases even if the woman presents in labor. The fallibility of conventional abdominal palpation as a screening test for malpresentation has been demonstrated many times, including personally by the author! Thorp and associates[71] showed that palpation only had a sensitivity of 28% and a specificity of 94% in the detection of breech presentation, using ultrasound scanning as the "gold standard."

X-ray erect lateral pelvimetry (see later discussion) to investigate pelvic capacity has been traditional but has been increasingly abandoned because of a possible long-term increased incidence of myelodysplasia.[72] If used, CT scanning is preferred because it reduces the radiation dosage. The presentation of the fetus can be confirmed at the same time. Radiologic exclusion of a nuchal arm, with an estimated incidence of 4%, has been suggested as a possible advantage, because this complication can produce delay and trauma during the second stage of labor. Magnetic resonance imaging is being used in some centers, but the same caveats about the value of the measurements apply.

As x-ray pelvimetry is abandoned, assessment of the fetus using ultrasound has become mandatory. If ECV is contemplated, then placental site, adequacy of fetal growth, and liquor volume are the minimum information required from ultrasound examination. More detailed information about the fetus should be obtained if vaginal delivery is being contemplated. Ultrasound examination will provide an estimate of fetal weight, which is crucial to the management of breech delivery. However, it should always be remembered that estimation of fetal weight has, at best, an error of ± 15%, which is ± 600 g in the 4-kg fetus. Chauhan and associates[73] have also demonstrated that fetal weight is less accurately estimated in the breech- than in the vertex-presenting infant. Placenta previa should also be excluded, as far as possible, prior to any decision about ECV or the mode of delivery. It has been suggested that, prior to attempts at ECV or vaginal breech delivery, a nuchal cord should be excluded on ultrasound examination. Successful detection of a nuchal cord has been reported but is unlikely to be practicable on a routine basis.

The validity of ultrasound measurement of fetal size measurements, especially the biparietal diameter, has long been debated. Bader and associates[74] performed ultrasound measurements in 450 fetuses in breech presentation and compared them with 1880 fetuses in cephalic presentation between 15 and 40 weeks' gestation. They found no difference between the biparietal diameter, head circumference, and the cephalic index (CI = BPD/occipital frontal distance × 100) in the two groups in uncomplicated pregnancy. However, in complicated pregnancies the CI was found to be lower in breech-presenting fetuses, indicating the dolichocephalic head shape that is commonly noted (the complications included premature rupture of the membranes, premature labor, intrauterine growth restriction, fetal anomaly, polyhydramnios or oligohydramnios, drug and alcohol abuse, maternal diabetes, and hypertension.) Neck hyperextension (the stargazing fetus) is an important condition that can cause spinal cord and brain injuries at delivery. Proposed etiologies are cord around the neck, fundal placenta, spasm of the fetal musculature, and fetal and uterine anomalies. It is of interest that most mammals other than the human deliver their young with the neck of the fetus in a hyperextended position. Flexion of the neck in the human fetus is probably an adaptation to the necessity of delivering a large brain in a large fetal skull through a relatively small pelvis. Although the incidence of neck extension in the fetus has been quoted as 7.4%,[44] its significance is hard to ascertain. It is regarded as an unfavorable prognostic sign with regard to successful vaginal breech delivery, but few authors indicate how it is to be diagnosed ante partum. Rojansky and associates[75] have validated the ultrasound determination of fetal neck extension comparing ultrasound scans with the "gold standard" of x-rays and found a high correlation. They measured the craniospinal angle by obtaining a sagittal view of the fetus visualizing the orbital ridge and the occipital eminence along with the spine in the same plane. A line is drawn between the orbital ridge and occipital eminence and the angle formed with the second line, which passes through the cervical and thoracic vertebrae, is measured. Other adverse features if ECV or vaginal breech delivery are contemplated include intrauterine growth restriction and rhesus isoimmunization.

Choice of Mode of Delivery – Vaginal Breech Delivery

It was not until the late 1950s that the increasing safety of cesarean section led to it becoming the preferred mode of delivery, and elective cesarean section began to be recommended on a routine basis to minimize perinatal morbidity and mortality. In the 50 years that followed, the controversy continued until the frequent calls for a randomized controlled trial were finally answered.[76] Clinicians now have robust data on which to base their recommendations. These data strongly supports the view that elective cesarean section is the safest option for the baby, at a marginally increased risk to the mother.[77,78]

Risks of Vaginal Breech Delivery for the Fetus

The risks and benefits of vaginal breech delivery are shown in Table 64–3.

TABLE 64–3

Risks and Benefits of Vaginal Breech Delivery for the Fetus

Risks
Poor condition at birth
Intracranial hemorrhage
Medullary coning
Severance of the spinal cord
Brachial plexus injury
Occipital diastasis
Fracture of the long bones
Epiphyseal separation
Rupture of internal organs
Long-term neurologic damage
Genital damage in the male
Hypopituitarism
Damage to the mouth and pharynx
Benefits
Reduction in idiopathic pulmonary hypertension

SHORT-TERM NEONATAL/PERINATAL OUTCOME AND FOLLOW-UP

Many of the studies performed to assess the mortality and morbidity rates for fetuses undergoing vaginal breech delivery have been poor. They were mostly retrospective reviews of practice and often simply compared babies delivered vaginally by the breech and by the head. This approach does not compare like with like and is therefore invalid for our purposes. However, because of the rise in the popularity of elective cesarean section for breech presentation, increasingly vaginal breech delivery was being performed only when the woman presented in advanced labor with an unexpected breech presentation. This situation increased the risk of a breech birth being attended by inadequately trained or experienced personnel. Moreover, there was no opportunity for prior assessment for suitability for vaginal breech delivery. These women were a high risk group. Many of the long-term and short-term follow-up studies of vaginally delivered breech babies were performed on populations born in the 1950s and 1960s and reflected the standards of care being offered at that time. More recent studies have reported careful selection criteria for vaginal breech delivery and a cesarean section rate of 20% to 60%. Most of these have shown no difference in short-term outcomes for the fetus.[14,58,79–82] However, this was not accompanied by any reported overall decrease in the rate of birth asphyxia. Moreover, the evidence based on these retrospective reviews of practice remained contradictory. Mecke and associates[80] demonstrated a higher 1-minute Apgar score in breech neonates delivered by cesarean section compared to those delivered vaginally. Babies delivered by cesarean section also had higher pH values at delivery. Similar differences were observed when babies in cephalic presentation were compared by mode of delivery. That the breech delivered vaginally has a lower pH than the cephalic infant or the breech infant delivered vaginally is not in doubt; it is what this difference means clinically that is difficult to ascertain. Despite this continuing uncertainty, the cesarean section rate for breech presentation increased steadily, in some centers during the 1970s from 22% to 94%.

Some specific conditions associated with breech presentation probably increase the chances of trauma during delivery. Fetal neck hyperextension, which can cause damage to the cervical spine, is a contraindication to vaginal birth. Flexed legs appears to increase the risk of cord prolapse to as much as 15% compared with 1.4% to 6% if the legs are extended (the risk of cord prolapse with a cephalic presentation is only 0.24%–0.5%). If the arms are caught across the back of the neck at delivery (nuchal arm), the risk of brachial plexus injury is about 8.5% at term, although 70% of these injuries have resolved fully by 3 months of age.

Until the Hannah trial, there had been only two small randomized controlled trials of the mode of delivery of the term breech. Collea and associates[14] randomized 208 women at term in labor to receive a cesarean section or a vaginal delivery. Despite this intention, 45% of the latter group were delivered by cesarean section. Although there are some caveats about their methodology, they showed no statistically significant differences in short-term neonatal outcome between babies delivered vaginally and babies delivered by cesarean section, either by intention to treat or actual mode of delivery. By contrast, they showed "striking and concerning differences in maternal outcome," with higher maternal morbidity rates associated with cesarean section. Gimovsky and associates[15] recruited 105 women with non-frank breech presentation into another randomized controlled trial. They also showed no statistically significant differences in short-term neonatal outcome. The two meta-analyses of the mode of delivery of the term breech did not significantly challenge these findings.[12,13]

Eventually, the uncertainty about the best management, and the need for reliable information became so great that pressure built up for someone to organize a properly planned randomized trial. Hannah and coworkers accepted the challenge, and in 2000 they published the results of a multicenter randomized controlled trial of the optimum mode of delivery of the term breech.[76] From 121 centers in 26 countries, 2088 women with a frank or complete breech were recruited. By the time the trial ended, 1041 women had been assigned to planned cesarean section, of whom 941 (90.4%) were actually delivered by cesarean section, and 1041 women had been assigned to planned vaginal delivery of whom 591 (56.7%) were actually delivered vaginally. The trial was halted before the planned total had been recruited, on the advice of the data monitoring group because a highly significant difference had already emerged. Perinatal mortality, neonatal morbidity, and serious neonatal morbidity rates were significantly lower for the planned cesarean section group (1.6%) than for the planned vaginal birth group (5.0%) (relative risk 0.33), and there were no significant differences between groups in terms of maternal mortality or serious maternal morbidity rates (3.9% versus 3.2%).[75] These relative differences in outcome between planned cesarean section and vaginal breech delivery persist even when a variety of clinical differences between groups are taken into account: parity, type of breech, whether the fetus was larger or smaller than 3000 g, whether the pelvis had been assessed clinically or radiologically, whether labor was induced or augmented, the use of epidural anesthesia, presentation, the degree of experience of the clinician, and a variety of other clinical parameters that are usually held to be important predictors of the success and safety of attempted vaginal delivery. The only significant interaction was between the treatment group and the countries' reported perinatal mortality/morbidity rate (PNMMR) for the combined outcome of perinatal mortality, neonatal mortality, or serious neonatal morbidity rates. In countries with a low PNMMR (≤ 20 in 1000 births) the risk from planned cesarean section compared with planned vaginal birth was 0.4% versus 5.7%, whereas the rates in countries with a high PNMMR (>20 in 1000 births) were 2.9% versus 4.4%. This difference in the developed countries disappeared when just the outcome of perinatal or neonatal death was considered. Neonatal morbidity showed the greatest differences according to geography, with reductions in morbidity being much greater for countries with low PNMMRs than for those with high PNMMRs. It is not clear why this might be the case. Possible explanations include incomplete ascertainment of poor neonatal condition in the first week of life or death before morbidity can be recognized. The observation might even be real, possibly because of high levels of experience with vaginal breech birth in countries with low cesarean section rates and high perinatal mortality rates—certainly fewer women allocated to vaginal breech delivery in those countries ended up with a cesarean birth.[83] Overall, this study indicated that, with a policy of planned cesarean section, for every additional 14 cesarean sections done, one baby will avoid death or serious morbidity. In countries with high PNMMR as many as 39 additional cesarean sections would need to be done to avoid one dead or compromised baby, whereas in countries with low PNMMR the number of additional cesarean sections required may be as low as seven.

Vaginal delivery still carries the risk of cord prolapse and extended arms at delivery as well as difficult delivery of the head. This risk may be approximately 1% to 2%.[14] Therefore, obstetric expertise should be maintained for dealing with unexpected breech presentations and for the late presenting (usually previously undiagnosed) breech in labor in whom cesarean section is logistically impossible; this may amount to 11% or more of all breech deliveries.[58] How to achieve this maintenance of competence in an era of few vaginal breech deliveries and many trainees with restricted hours for teaching has not yet been fully established; training on sophisticated mannequins is probably the best approach.

LONG-TERM INFANT FOLLOW-UP

Long-term follow-up studies fall into two main groups: those that review infants born prior to 1970 and those born after 1970. The standards of obstetric and neonatal care have changed so dramatically since 1970 that studies prior to this time demonstrate more about factors other than mode of delivery.

Those studies reviewing later born (1970–1980) children reflect the impact of rising cesarean section rates and more modern obstetric care. They are still mostly retrospective reviews of practice.

In one case-controlled study, breech-delivered infants were compared with cephalic-delivered infants (matched for sex, birth weight, gestational age, maternal age, parity, and year of delivery) at 4 to 10 years of age. A slight excess of minor neurologic dysfunction was found in the breech group but was not statistically significant.[84]

In a population-based study, Danielian and associates[82] compared the long-term outcome of infants delivered in breech presentation at term by intended mode of delivery. They identified 1645 infants from the Grampian region in Scotland during the years 1981 to 1990 who had been delivered alive at term after breech presentation. Elective cesarean section was performed in 35.9% of cases, and 64.1% were intended vaginal deliveries. There were no significant differences in terms of severe handicap, developmental delay, or neurologic deficit up to school age.

A variety of other prospective evaluations of long-term outcome have shown no difference in neurologic outcome, psychomotor problems, or cerebral palsy.[6,85]

Another long-term follow-up of infants born by the breech either spontaneously or using the Bracht maneuver for delivery of the head showed that psychometric and intellectual development were superior in those infants delivered spontaneously.[86]

Despite the fact that many of the studies are of dubious quality, they are remarkably consistent in reporting minimal risk of long-term neurologic damage after careful selection for vaginal delivery: Handicap rates are not demonstrably higher than for babies delivered by cesarean section (after correction for congenital anomalies).

Risk of Breech Delivery for the Mother

The risks of breech delivery to the mother are shown in Table 64–4.

Assessment for Vaginal Breech Delivery (Table 64–5)

All the available literature stresses the importance of adhering to an appropriate protocol when assessing women for vaginal breech delivery. These protocols have produced elective cesarean section rates from 25% to 65%.

Close consultation with the mother and partner and counseling about the implications of the choice of vaginal breech delivery versus elective cesarean section is important. It is the responsibility of the obstetrician to explain the options and the evidence to the woman and her family in the clearest possible terms. Although

TABLE 64–4

Comparison of Risks to the Mother of Vaginal Breech Delivery and Cesarean Section

Risks of vaginal breech delivery for the mother
Perineal discomfort and morbidity
Difficult birth experience
Risks of cesarean section for the mother
Short-term morbidity: increased postpartum pyrexia, increased need for blood transfusion
Increased maternal mortality rate
Reduction in future fertility[20]
Difficult birth experience
Entering a subsequent pregnancy with a scar on the uterus

TABLE 64–5

Assessment for Vaginal Breech Delivery

Assessment of the cause of breech presentation
Exclude:
Placenta previa
Multiple pregnancy
Fibroids/pelvic tumors
Oligohydramnios/polyhydramnios
Hydrocephalus/anencephaly
Other congenital abnormality
Assessment of fetal condition
Exclude:
Intrauterine growth restriction
Rhesus disease
Fetal abnormality
Other
Assessment of fetal weight and attitude
Assessment of the maternal pelvis
Clinical pelvimetry (important for medicolegal reasons) (x-ray erect lateral pelvimetry no longer advocated)
Computed tomography scanning pelvimetry and magnetic resonance imaging may be unnecessary and unreliable
Assessment of maternal condition
Exclude significant maternal disease: diabetes, proteinuric hypertension, cardiac or renal disease
Assessment of maternal and parental wishes

cesarean section will be the recommended option for the vast majority of women, especially in the developed world, some women when informed of the options will still wish to attempt a vaginal delivery, and their wishes should be respected.

ASSESSMENT OF PELVIC CAPACITY – CLINICAL

Clinical pelvimetry is a low technology screening investigation that is probably of benefit only if there is gross contraction of the pelvis. A subjective assessment of the bony features of the pelvic cavity is made, including the sacral promontory, the curvature of the sacrum, whether the side walls are convergent or the ischial spines prominent, whether the sacrospinous ligaments will accommodate two fingers, whether the intertuberous diameter will accommodate the clenched fist, and whether the pubic arch is greater than 90 degrees. The success or otherwise of clinical pelvimetry is hard to assess, and most discussions about the assessment of pelvic capacity center on x-ray pelvimetry. With regard to a clinical assessment of the size of the pelvis, a consideration of the woman's height alone is probably useful.[87]

ASSESSMENT OF PELVIC CAPACITY

No prospective randomized trials have ever been performed to assess the value of x-ray pelvimetry. There is no absolute level of pelvic contraction as assessed by x-ray below which vaginal delivery is impossible, and antenatal assessment of fetal weight is probably a more important determinant of the success of attempted vaginal delivery.[87,88] One report, comparing three different protocols for the assessment for vaginal breech delivery, concluded that the one that did not include x-ray pelvimetry produced a lower elective cesarean section rate and similar emergency cesarean section rates to protocols that included x-ray measurements. The authors concluded that progress in labor is the best indicator of pelvic adequacy.[89]

There is one reported study of the comparison of ultrasound with x-ray for determining the obstetric conjugate.[73] They found a highly significant correlation between the two measurements, but ultrasound measurements were consistently found to be 1 cm smaller than the x-ray values.

The advantage of computed tomography (CT) scanning for pelvimetry is clear: it will reduce the radiation dosage and is more accurate.[77] However, there is no evidence that it will predict the outcome of a trial of vaginal breech delivery any better than standard pelvimetry. Normal measurements do not guarantee vaginal delivery, and the Royal College of Obstetricians and Gynaecologists has concluded that no data support the routine use of radiologic pelvimetry before term breech delivery.[72]

One randomized controlled trial of magnetic resonance (MR) pelvimetry has been performed. Two hundred thirty-five women had MR pelvimetry and were then randomly assigned to two groups. In the study group, the results of the pelvimetry were disclosed to the clinicians who used them to decide on the optimal route of delivery. In the control group the clinicians assigned the route of delivery after consideration of other clinical factors alone. The authors found that the overall cesarean section rate was the same, although the emergency cesarean section rates were lower in the MR group. There were no significant differences in the baby's condition at birth or in the early neonatal period between the two groups.[90]

CRITERIA FOR SELECTION FOR VAGINAL BREECH DELIVERY

Various criteria have been proposed. In summary, the fetus should be neither too small nor too big and should have a well-flexed head; the mother should have at least an average capacity pelvis, judged clinically; and the mother and the baby should be in "good" condition.

An estimated fetal weight of 1500 to 3900 g is probably appropriate (for discussion of the delivery of the preterm breech, see previous section); however, the limits of fetal weight and gestation are contentious, with many different limits being suggested. In addition, clinical estimation of fetal weight is unreliable, and even when ultrasound is used, there is a margin of error of ± 15%. The error of the estimation of weight is greater in the breech than the vertex fetus.

It is probably wise to perform a clinical pelvimetry to exclude the obviously contracted pelvis, but x-ray pelvimetry should not be done because there is no clear evidence of its value and there is inevitably some very small risk from the radiation involved in its use. It is good practice and probably wise from the medicolegal point of view to explain this to the mother before labor.

Some authors would exclude the nulliparous woman with a breech from consideration of vaginal delivery, yet others consider the grand multiparous patient also at high risk.[10] The evidence for either proposition is not compelling. The fetus should ideally be in frank or complete breech presentation (not a footling), and absence of detectable congenital abnormality should be confirmed using ultrasound.

It is commonly assumed that the undiagnosed breech in labor is at higher risk of complications than those that have been diagnosed prelabor and adequately assessed for suitability for trial of vaginal delivery. However, the experience of some authors[91,92] is that these women do well and are more likely to deliver vaginally with no greater mortality or morbidity rates than those diagnosed and assessed prior to labor. They suggest that there are no grounds for delivering all undiagnosed breeches in labor by cesarean section.

PROCEDURE – VAGINAL BREECH DELIVERY

PRACTICAL CONSIDERATIONS IN THE CONDUCT OF ASSISTED VAGINAL BREECH DELIVERY

The essence of the assisted vaginal breech delivery is allowing as much spontaneous delivery by uterine action and maternal effort as possible. Operator intervention should be limited to the maneuvers described here, which are designed to correct any deviation from the normal mechanism of spontaneous delivery. The operator may make the delivery more complicated by injudicious traction that encourages displacement of the fetal limbs from their normal flexed position across the fetal body or by promoting hyperextension of the fetal head. Traction can also cause injury of itself. The fetal body should, at all times, be treated with the utmost care and grasped, if at all, by the bony parts. Some authors recommend using a towel to cover the baby to prevent friction injury, to improve grip without the need for too much squeezing, and to keep the baby warm. Within these limits, there are many described procedures for the vaginal delivery of the breech.

First Stage

Many authors suggest that spontaneous labor increases the chance of successful vaginal delivery, and that if delivery is required before the onset of spontaneous labor, elective cesarean section is preferable to induction of labor.

Labor should be conducted in a labor ward with all the facilities needed to perform a cesarean section, with a full anesthetic service and senior obstetric staff available. The woman should be instructed to arrive early in labor so that her progress and the condition of the fetus may be monitored. Similarly, if the membranes rupture, she should attend the hospital because of the risks of cord prolapse. Rupture of the membranes at any point during the labor should prompt immediate vaginal examination.

On presentation in labor an intravenous line should be sited and blood taken for typing and to save serum. Because of the relatively high risk of cesarean section, oral intake should be avoided for the duration of the labor. After the usual assessment of the woman in labor she should be told that continuous electronic fetal monitoring is advisable and that an epidural anesthetic may be preferable. The latter will make any manipulation in the second stage more comfortable and make any urge to push prior to full dilation easier to resist. Bearing down prior to full dilation may push the relatively smaller breech through the incompletely dilated cervix and entrap the after-coming head behind the cervix. Epidural anesthesia is not essential, and some obstetricians suggest that there is a higher chance of spontaneous vaginal delivery without one. Chadha and associates[93] reported that epidural analgesia was associated with a longer duration of the second stage, an increased need for augmentation of labor with oxytocin infusion, and a significantly higher cesarean section rate in the second stage of labor. There is little doubt that epidural anesthesia obtunds the urge to bear down. However, the counter argument is that if a baby does not deliver easily with an epidural in situ, then it is better delivered by cesarean as there is likely to be mild relative disproportion. Because there is no clear scientific evidence to resolve this issue, it seems appropriate at the present time to allow the woman a major degree of personal choice in this respect. Whatever she chooses, however, an anesthetist should be in attendance during the second stage of labor in case rapid anesthesia should be required for an unexpectedly difficult delivery. Although on first principles the use of oxytocics should be avoided because of the risk of uterine hyperstimulation and consequent fetal hypoxia, in practice if the labor progress is slow, there is no evidence that the careful use of oxytocin is dangerous. Oxytocin is particularly appropriate if there is a primary dysfunctional labor (slow progress in the active phase, less than 1 cm cervical dilation every 2 hours). The use of an intrauterine pressure transducer may reassure the obstetrician that excessive uterine activity is not being generated. The other fear with oxytocin is that its use will produce descent of the breech in the presence of fetal-pelvic disproportion; hence, the disproportion will be detected only when the head is entrapped above the pelvic brim and the body is already delivered. The bitrochanteric diameter is usually smaller than the biparietal, and if the former does not easily traverse the pelvis, neither will the latter. However, Collea and associates[14] demonstrated that the use of oxytocin in selected patients does not produce an excess rate of maternal or neonatal complications.

Failure to make expected progress in cervical dilation or for the breech to descend appropriately in the first 4 hours of labor, or the appearance of cardiotocographic abnormalities, should prompt careful consideration of whether cesarean section is advisable. Total labor duration should be similar to that in cephalic presentation, although descent of the breech may be slow. The progress of the labor should therefore be plotted on a partogram in the usual way. There is evidence that the use of the World Health Organization partogram in breech labor reduces the incidence of prolonged labor, reduces the incidence of cesarean section (at least in multigravidae), and improves the condition of the neonate at birth.[94] This probably reflects the importance of good progress in labor as a favorable prognostic variable for successful vaginal breech delivery.

Meconium staining of the liquor is common in breech labor, and its predictive value for asphyxia is poor. In early labor it is often found on the glove at the end of a vaginal examination. Its passage when the breech is still high in the birth canal in first stage may indicate "fetal distress," and careful evaluation of the fetal heart rate pattern at this stage will be necessary. However, the passage of meconium in the second stage is almost universal and is of no prognostic value. Cardiotocographic fetal heart rate abnormalities should be investigated using fetal blood sampling, preferably obtaining the blood from the region around the ischial tuberosity and avoiding the genitalia. The blade may have to be pressed firmly onto the buttock in order to ensure a good flow of capillary blood. There is no evidence that an adequate sample of blood obtained in this way has a different pH than blood obtained from the fetal scalp, and so the usual criteria of acidosis can be applied.

Second Stage (See Fig.64–1)

The second stage should be supervised by an experienced obstetrician (Fig. 64–1). The active second stage with vaginal breech delivery does not start until the cervix is fully dilated and the fetal anus is seen on the perineum without having to part the mother's labia. The woman should then be placed in the lithotomy position with her buttocks just over the end of the delivery couch. She should be cleaned and draped as for ventouse or forceps delivery. Care should be taken to avoid the completely supine position in case this causes hypotension secondary to caval compression, and lateral tilt using a wedge is probably advisable. It is best if the bladder and lower bowel are empty, and elective bladder catheterization is probably advisable, with an "in and out" catheter. Routine enemas are not, however, usually recommended. If effective regional anesthesia is not in place, a pudendal block with perineal infiltration should be used. An episiotomy is generally advised and should be performed at this point. An episiotomy will always be required if forceps are to be used to achieve delivery of the after-coming head, if extensive manipulation of the fetus is anticipated, and in all nulliparas. The breech, legs and abdomen should be allowed to deliver spontaneously to the level of the umbilicus; the only intervention recommended up to this stage is to correct the position to sacroanterior if it is not this already. At this point the obstetrician should deliver the legs, if they are extended, by abduction of the thigh and flexion of the fetal knee (using finger pressure in the popliteal fossa), allowing the fetal thigh to pass lateral to the fetal body. A loop of umbilical cord should then be brought down to minimize traction and possible tearing with consequent loss of fetal blood. The prognostic significance of the absence of cord

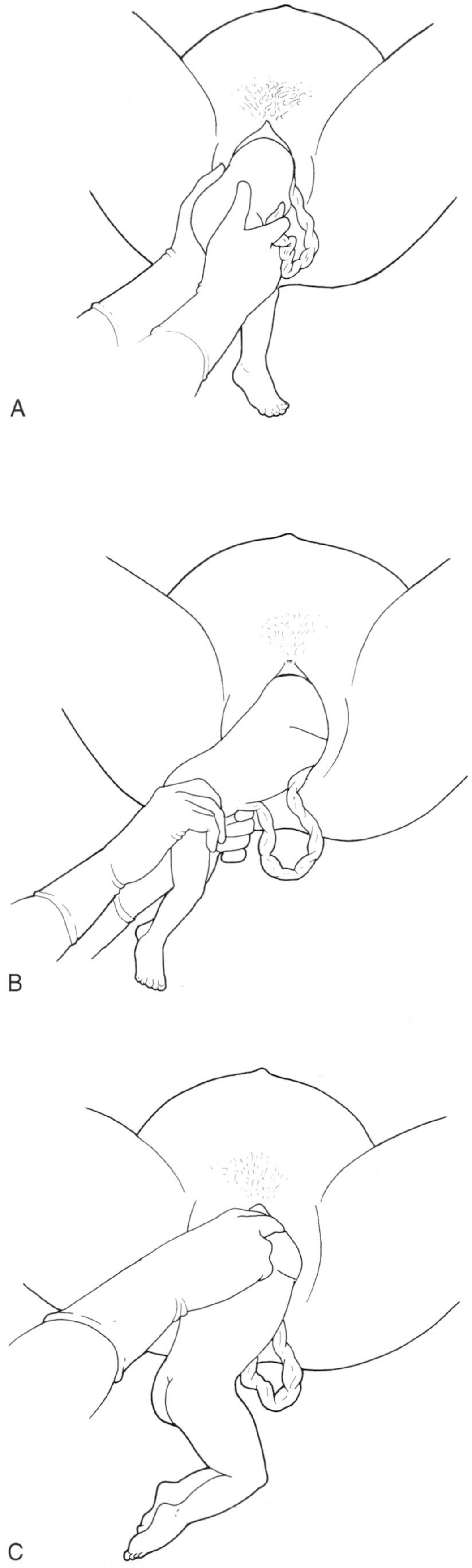

FIGURE 64–1
The second stage of vaginal breech delivery. Delivering the shoulder by Lövsett's maneuver.

pulsation is controversial. Fetal condition is probably better assessed by noting fetal tone and color.

Delivery to this point should ideally have been achieved with one contraction and one maternal expulsive effort. Delivery of the rest of the body, to delivery of the mouth, should be achieved over the next one or two contractions. The duration of time that should be allowed to elapse between delivery just below the umbilicus to delivery of the mouth is 5 to 10 minutes. Arulkumaran and associates[95] examined two different ways of delivering the breech. They allowed spontaneous delivery to the hip with one contraction, and maternal effort followed by an assisted delivery of the rest of the body and head in the next contraction in one group of women, and in another group they assisted delivery to the shoulders with one contraction and then an assisted delivery of the head was performed with the next contraction. The former method produced babies with a smaller fall in fetal blood pH and in better condition at delivery, judged by the Apgar score and need for ventilation. They hypothesized that this was due to exposure, stretching, and compression of the umbilical cord over a longer period of time during the delivery of the latter group, or possibly due to premature separation of the placenta. It should be noted, however, that the pH and the Apgar scores are anyway usually lower in vaginally delivered breeches than in babies delivered head first.[84]

Once the legs and abdomen have emerged, the fetus should be allowed to hang from the vulva until the wing of the scapula is seen. The arms are often found folded over the fetal chest, flexed at the shoulder and elbow, and in this case no particular maneuver is required to effect their delivery. If injudicious traction is exerted in order to deliver the breech, the arms may become extended over the fetal head. In this case the Lovsett's maneuver may be used to free the arm. This involves wrapping the fetus in a warm dry towel and grasping the body over the bony pelvis with the thumbs along the sacrum. The fetal back should then be turned through 180 degrees until the posterior arm comes to lie anteriorly. The elbow will appear below the symphysis pubis, and that arm and hand can be delivered by sweeping it across the fetal body. This maneuver is repeated in reverse to deliver the other arm. If these maneuvers fail, the traditional last resort is to induce deep anesthesia and push the body of the fetus well up, pass the hand along its ventral aspect and bring down the most accessible arm. This may then allow completion of vaginal birth. However, having pushed the fetus up successfully, it may well be safer to proceed with cesarean section.[95] The nuchal arm, where the arm is flexed at the elbow and extended at the shoulder coming to lie behind the fetal head, may be dealt with by a modified Lovsett's maneuver: rotating the fetal back through 180 degrees in the direction of the trapped arm may draw the elbow forward toward the face and over the fetal head by friction on the birth canal and render it amenable to a traditional Lovsett's maneuver to deliver the arm. If this technique does not suffice to release the nuchal arm, it may be forcibly extracted by hooking the finger over it, in which case it is almost always fractured.

The fetus should be allowed to hang from the vulva for a few seconds again until the nape of the neck is visible at the anterior vulva. This allows descent of the head into the pelvis and at this point the head may be delivered. Downward traction before spontaneous descent may result in hyperextension of the fetal head rather than flexion and descent, so again, operator interference can cause complications in the delivery. If the head negotiates the inlet of the pelvis easily, there is little danger that the progress of the head will be arrested in midcavity. If there is difficulty with the head in the midcavity, or the outlet, a properly performed Mauriceau-Smellie-Veit maneuver will overcome this (see later full description). Should the head fail to descend into the pelvis after the shoulders have delivered, the body of the fetus should be turned sideways and suprapubic pressure used to flex the head and push it into the pelvis in the occipitotransverse position. A vaginal finger in the mouth of the fetus may also tend to flex the head and help it to descend into the pelvis prior to delivery. A McRoberts maneuver can be used to facilitate delivery of the head if it is arrested at the inlet and suprapubic pressure and the Mauriceau-Smellie-Veit maneuver have failed. This involves a sharp flexion of the maternal thighs toward the maternal abdomen, and abduction of the legs, in a way directly analogous to the management of shoulder dystocia in the vertex delivery.[96] Continued failure of the head to descend into the pelvis may be due to hydrocephalus, in which case the head can be perforated through the foramen magnum (an epidural needle is a suitable instrument) and the cerebrospinal fluid drained. Such a maneuver should be performed only if the diagnosis has been confirmed by ultrasound and the fetus is already dead. Alternatively, the cervix may not be fully dilated, in which case the cervix must be incised. This is done with round-ended scissors, and the incisions made at 4 and 8 o'clock to avoid the bladder and rectum and the main blood vessels (which supply the cervix at 3 and 9 o'clock). If there are locked twins, there is no choice but to do a cesarean section; the traditional technique of decapitating the first twin is no longer acceptable. If none of these causes is present, then the operator must assume that cephalopelvic disproportion is present and there is then a strong case for the performance of a symphysiotomy.[97] With proper predelivery assessment and conduct of labor this situation should only arise very rarely.

PERFORMING A SYMPHYSIOTOMY (Fig. 64–2)

The episiotomy should be enlarged. If the mother does not have epidural analgesia, the anterior, superior, and inferior aspects of the symphysis should be infiltrated with lidocaine 0.5%. The usual precautions to prevent intravenous injection should be taken. While waiting for the analgesia to take effect, an indwelling urinary catheter should be inserted. The suprapubic skin should then be cleaned with antiseptic solution. Following this, the index finger should be placed in the vagina and lateral pressure applied to the catheter to move the urethra away from the midline. A thick, firm-bladed

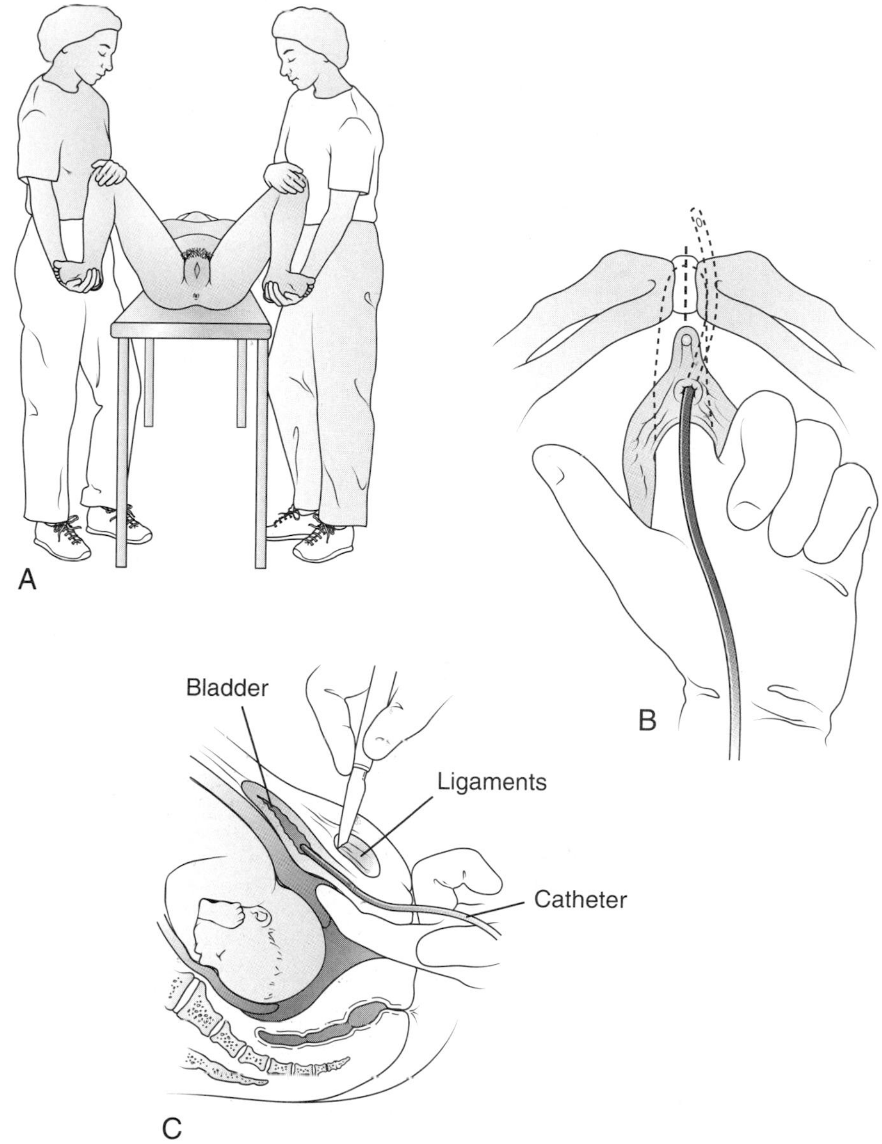

FIGURE 64–2
Performance of a symphysiotomy. *A*, Position of the woman for symphysiotomy. *B*, Pushing the urethra to one side using a finger to press on the urinary catheter. *C*, Incising the symphysis, with the finger pushing the urethra to one side, to avoid damaging it with the knife. (From WHO: Managing complications in pregnancy and childbirth: A guide for midwives and doctors. Accessed at www.who.int/reproductive-health/impac/procedures/symphysiotomy_P53_P56.html)

scalpel should then be used to make a vertical stab incision over the symphysis. Keeping to the midline, the knife should be pressed down through the cartilage joining the two pubic bones until the pressure of the scalpel blade can be felt on the finger in the vagina. If the cartilage is not fully divided, the blade can be rotated and the cutting movement can be made back toward the top of the symphysis to finish the process. Following the delivery, there is no need to close the incision unless there is bleeding. It is, however, wise to give prophylactic antibiotics, e.g. ampicillin, gentamicin, and metronidazole. Elastic strapping from one iliac crest to the other will reduce postoperative pain, but analgesia will be necessary. The urinary catheter should be left in situ for a minimum of 5 days.

Techniques for Delivering the Head (See Fig.64–3)

It should be remembered that entrapment of the after-coming head can also occur with cesarean section, especially if an inadequate-size abdominal incision has been made. Robertson and associates[26] found no significant difference in the incidence of head entrapment by mode of delivery from 28 to 36 weeks' gestation, nor any association with adverse outcome following head entrapment. The techniques for delivery of the after-coming head are various (Fig. 64–3). Some authorities advise that the body should be supported on the right forearm of the operator and not be raised above the horizontal in order to minimize the chance of hyperextension of the fetal head. Others advise that the operator's assistant should grasp the ankles of the fetus and raise the body vertically above the mother's abdomen prior to any attempt to deliver the fetal head, as this will promote rotation of the fetal head and place it in the anteroposterior diameter of the pelvis. This is called the Burns-Marshall technique and may rotate the head and deliver it over the perineum without further intervention. It is therefore advisable to cover the perineum with the hand to prevent precipitate delivery of the head as the body is swung upward. The operator's hand can then be opened slowly in order to

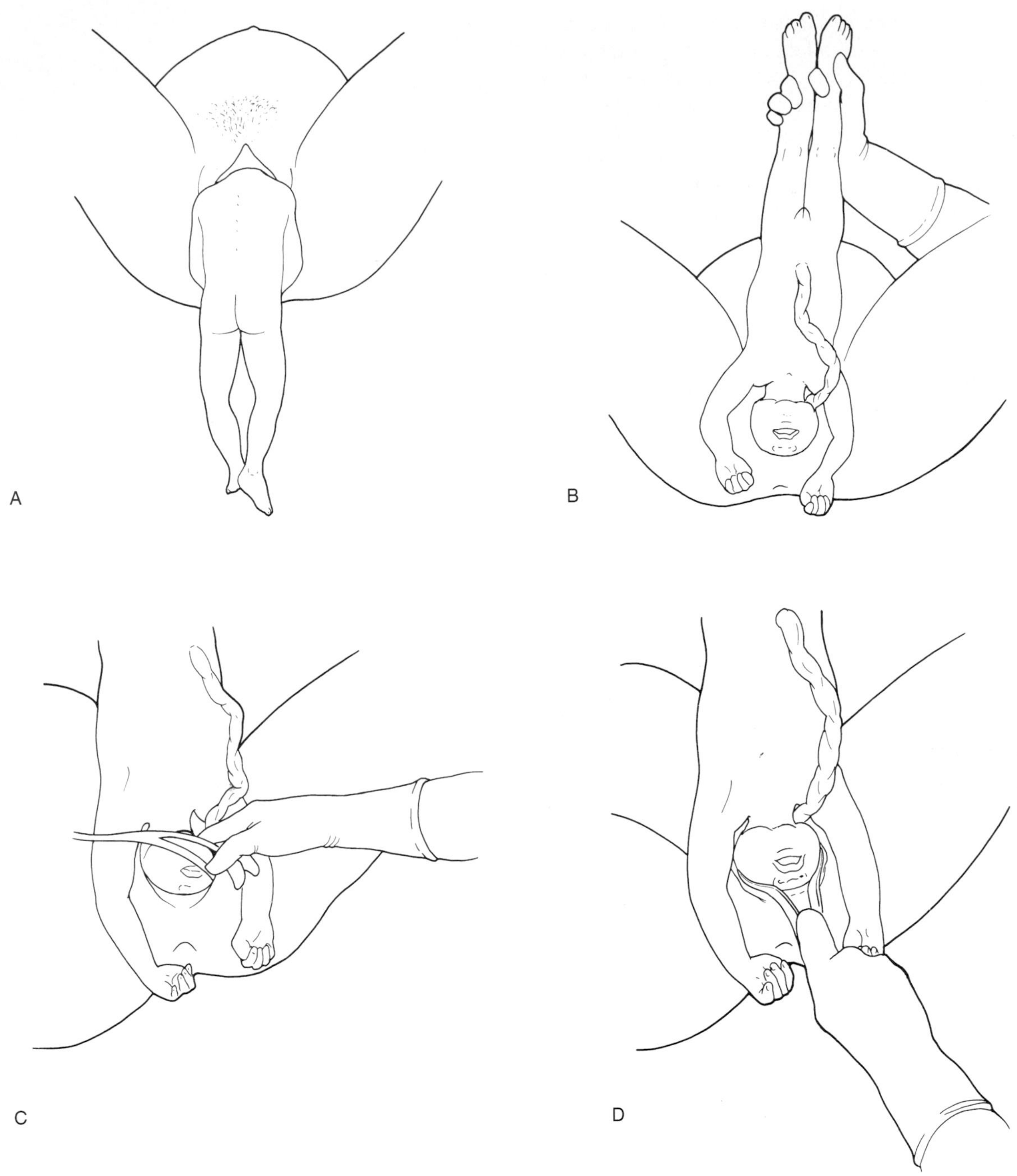

FIGURE 64–3
Forceps delivery of the aftercoming head. *A*, Allowing the trunk to hang flexes the head and encourages descent. *B*, Once the head is in the pelvis, rotating the trunk over the mother's abdomen delivers the face. *C*, Applying forceps to the aftercoming head. *D*, Forceps used to control the rate of delivery of the head.

allow the rest of the head to deliver. Often, however, further assistance is required to deliver the head. The head may be delivered from this position using forceps applied below the fetal body. The operator should remember that the smallest part of the head is lowest in the vagina and that the tip of the forceps blade must accommodate the occiput; therefore, premature straightening of the forceps blade during application will cause undue pressure on the side of the fetal head. Forceps should be of a type with a long enough shank to permit the operator to visualize the maneuver, as often the fetal arms obstruct the view, and if the fetal body is in the horizontal position, access is further reduced. The head should be delivered slowly (over about 1 minute) to reduce the compression-decompression forces on the fetal skull that may cause tentorial tears and intracranial bleeding.

The other frequently described technique of delivering the fetal head is the so-called "Mauriceau-Smellie-Veit" maneuver. This is actually a variety of techniques. The principle is that of traction down the axis of the birth canal while encouraging flexion of the fetal head to present the most favorable diameters to the pelvis. With the fetus supported on the right forearm, the middle finger of the right hand is passed into the fetal throat and the forefinger and the ring finger are placed either on the fetal shoulders or the malar eminences. Pressure is applied on the tongue to flex and deliver the head. The middle finger should not be just inside the fetal mouth, as traction can produce dislocation or fracture of the mandible. If the finger is inserted too far down the throat, creation of a pseudodiverticulum of the pharynx has been described. The left hand is used to exert pressure upward and posteriorly on the fetal occiput to encourage flexion. Alternatively, suprapubic pressure can be applied to encourage head flexion and descent. All these maneuvers can be performed with the operator's assistant elevating the fetal body above the horizontal. Downward traction on the fetal shoulders tends to stretch the cervical spine and in combination with flexion of the fetal head will draw the base of the skull away from the vault, thus causing a tentorial tear. Therefore, traction on the trunk should not be used. All these permutations have been described by various authors as the Mauriceau-Smellie-Veit maneuver.

A pediatrician should always be present at the delivery, and ideally the mouth and pharynx should be sucked out on the perineum prior to complete delivery of the head, although often the head delivers too quickly for this to be done.

The Zavanelli maneuver has also been described for the delivery of the breech with an entrapped after-coming head. Tocolysis is used to facilitate replacement of the fetal body into the uterus, and cesarean section completes the delivery.[98] As experience with this maneuver is very limited, its use in this desperate situation remains controversial.

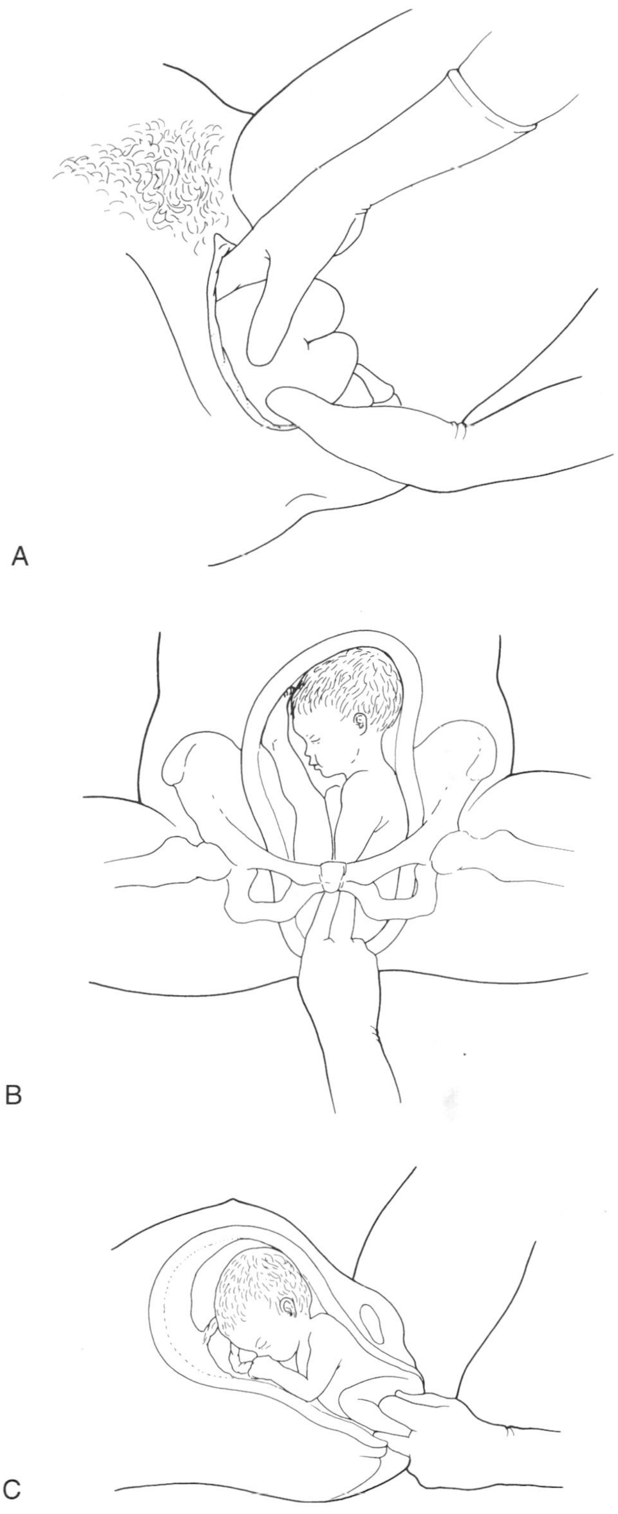

FIGURE 64–4
Active breech delivery (Breech extraction).

Considerations in the Performance of Breech Extraction (Fig. 64–4)

Currently, breech extraction is rarely performed because of the risks of fetal and maternal trauma and because of the effects of excessive traction on the fetal body. Its main current indication is for the delivery of a second twin after internal podalic version, or if cord prolapse complicates the late second stage. It may also be appropriate if the fetus is dead. Groin traction is performed to draw the breech over the perineum, Lovsett's maneuver is employed routinely, and downward traction is exerted to bring the head into the pelvis. In effect, all the stages of assisted breech delivery are achieved actively by the obstetrician.

Choice of Mode of Delivery

CESAREAN SECTION

Practical considerations in the performance of cesarean section for the delivery of the term breech. The orthodox obstetric practice of considering any woman with a breech presentation and any other medical or obstetric complication for delivery by elective cesarean section has much to recommend it. Elective and even emergency cesarean section for the term breech should present few technical problems. It should be remembered that the performance of a cesarean section does not prevent the possibility of birth injury and many of the foregoing considerations about the careful delivery of the after-coming head and the dangers of traction on the fetal spine still apply. The lower segment will be the site of choice for the incision with a term breech presentation. Schutterman and Grimes[99] reviewed 416 breeches of all gestations allocated randomly to transverse or low vertical incisions in the uterus and found no advantages for low vertical incisions. An elective cesarean section when adequate liquor is still present and the uterus is less likely to contract rapidly before completion of delivery of the breech will present few problems to the experienced operator. Forceps may be employed for delivery of the after-coming head. Cesarean delivery at full dilation in the absence of liquor may be difficult because an arm may prolapse through the uterine incision; it should immediately be pushed back. Instead, a leg should be grasped and brought through the incision. Traction will then effect the rest of the delivery. The head can be trapped by a well-contracted lower segment, and the incision will then need to be enlarged in a J-shaped fashion to increase access. In general the mode of effecting delivery through the uterine incision is the same as for vaginal breech delivery, and many of the same complications may arise.

The fetal head may become entrapped in the uterine incision at the point of delivery, as the lower uterine segment contracts rapidly down. For this reason, even at an elective cesarean section it is prudent to have a pediatrician present for delivery. Because of this complication, uterine tocolysis has been evaluated to see if its use improved the ease of delivery or the condition of the fetus at birth. Ritodrine was compared with nitroglycerin and no therapy. No effect was found for the fetus or the mother, and the incision-delivery interval was not significantly different. Tocolytics cannot be recommended for routine deliveries but might be useful when delivery is expected to be difficult or traumatic.[100]

Deficiencies in the conduct of vaginal breech deliveries, resulting in perinatal death, have been systematically evaluated in a blinded case-controlled audit. The authors concluded that infant death at term was to a large extent potentially avoidable but that in control breech infants who survived, suboptimal care was not uncommon.[84]

ACTIVE BREECH DELIVERY

With increasing consumer pressure over the last few years toward less interventionist obstetrics, a demand for an active method of delivering the breech has appeared. This demand has been satisfied in the United Kingdom by a group of mainly midwife practitioners who perform the so-called "active breech delivery." This encourages women to be active during labor, and although encouraging the woman to adopt the most comfortable position during labor, they favor a standing position for the delivery itself. They emphasize nonpharmacologic analgesia, and encourage maternal participation in the birth. The breech is usually allowed to deliver spontaneously without any interference from the birth attendants. The author's experience of 21 of such deliveries being conducted in her own maternity unit is that one baby died during the final stages of birth, one definitely has persisting neurologic damage, and another may have. In the light of these poor outcomes, the technique cannot be recommended.

CONCLUSIONS

For the Preterm Breech in Labor:

- Exclude, as far as possible, congenital abnormality and placenta previa.
- Accurately determine and confirm presentation (preferably with ultrasound).
- Accurately diagnose and confirm preterm labor by careful vaginal examination, cervical ultrasound, and biochemical markers (see Chapter 61).
- Carefully observe fetal and maternal condition.
- Use epidural anesthesia (with maternal agreement).
- Involve an experienced obstetrician.
- Clear-cut recommendations about the optimal mode of delivery will have to await the performance of a properly conducted trial, which in the light of previous experience, seems unlikely ever to be performed. In the absence of such evidence, the decision about the mode of delivery should be reached after close consultation with the laboring woman and her partner.

For the Term Breech (37 weeks and over):

- The presence of breech presentation in both the term and the preterm pregnancy confers an increased risk on the fetus regardless of the mode of delivery. This increased risk is only partly due to an increased rate of congenital malformations.
- The use of external cephalic version in the appropriately assessed woman after 37 weeks' gestation shows a clear benefit in the reduced numbers of cesarean sections and an increased rate of vaginal delivery in the cephalic position and has a good safety record.

CONCLUSIONS *(Continued)*

For the Term Breech (37 weeks and over): (Continued)

- There is now convincing evidence that women with a term breech should be advised that planned elective cesarean section reduces the risk of death or serious morbidity for the fetus with no evidence of increased morbidity in the mother.
- Despite this, some women (particularly in less developed countries) may still choose to try to deliver vaginally.
- Consideration for vaginal delivery:
  - Fetal morphology
  - Estimated fetal weight
  - Fetal attitude
  - Fetal well-being
  - Placental location
  - An assessment of the maternal pelvis
  - Assessment of any maternal conditions that would preclude vaginal delivery
- Approximately 50% of women who go into labor with a breech fetus at term will require an emergency cesarean section.
- Approximately 10% of breech presentations at term will be undetected until presentation in labor; because of this, vaginal breech deliveries will continue to occur, and thus, the skills to accomplish vaginal breech delivery as safely as possible should not be forgotten.

SUMMARY OF MANAGEMENT OPTIONS
Breech Presentation

Management Options	Quality of Evidence	Strength of Recommendation	References
Term Breech Presentation			
Fetal Assessment			
Confirm diagnosis and determine placental site.	–	GPP	–
Confirm normality as association of breech presentation with congenital anomalies.	III	B	10
Version in Prenatal Period			
There is insufficient evidence to advocate postural methods to promote spontaneous version.	Ia	A	46
External cephalic version (ECV) at 36+ weeks' gestation should be recommended.	Ia	A	48
Tocolysis increases the success of ECV.	Ib	A	54,55,56
There is insufficient evidence that epidural anesthesia increases the effectiveness of ECV.	Ib	A	57
Need for fetal heart rate monitoring before and after ECV.	III	B	45
If the Woman Chooses to Attempt a Vaginal Delivery			
The health of the mother and baby should be assessed.	IV	C	72
Ultrasound should be performed to confirm the diagnosis, check for fetal abnormalities, and assess placental site, fetal attitude, and estimated fetal weight.	IV	C	72,75
A written protocol is advisable, and a skilled birth attendant for labor and delivery is mandatory.	IIb	B	76
Pelvimetry need not be used routinely.	III	B	72,87,89

SUMMARY OF MANAGEMENT OPTIONS
Breech Presentation *(Continued)*

Management Options	Quality of Evidence	Strength of Recommendation	References
Labor and Delivery			
Evidence is that planned cesarean section for breech at term is the preferred method of delivery because it significantly reduces perinatal mortality and morbidity rates.	Ia Ib	A	12,13 76
Preterm Breech Presentation			
Prenatal			
There is insufficient evidence that ECV before term offers any benefit.	Ia	A	42, 53
Labor and Delivery			
There is insufficient evidence to recommend cesarean section for the preterm breech.	Ib	B	41
For the preterm breech in labor an ultrasound scan should be performed to confirm the presentation and normality; the mode of delivery should be determined in close consultation with the woman and her family.	IV	C	72

REFERENCES

1. Hytten F: Breech presentation: Is it a bad omen? Br J Obstet Gynaecol 1982;60:417–420.
2. Haughey MJ: Fetal position during pregnancy. Am J Obstet Gynecol 1985;153:885–886.
3. Coltart T, Edmonds DK, Al-Mufti R: External cephalic version at term: A survey of consultant obstetric practice in the United Kingdom and Republic of Ireland. Br J Obstet Gynaecol 1997; 104:544–547.
4. Lamont RF, Dunlop PDM, Crowley P, et al: Spontaneous preterm labor and delivery at under 34 weeks gestation. Br Med J 1983;286:454–457.
5. Collea JV, Rabin SC, Weghorst GR, et al: The randomised management of term frank breech presentation: Vaginal delivery versus cesarean section. Am J Obstet Gynecol 1978;134:186.
6. Luterkort M, Polberger S, Persson PH, Bjerre I: Role of asphyxia and slow intrauterine growth among breech delivered infants. Early Hum Dev 1987;14:19–31.
7. Robertson IS: Breech presentation associated with anticonvulsant drugs. J Obstet Gynecol 1984;4:174–177.
8. Manzke H: Morbidity among infants born in breech presentation. J Perinat Med 1987;6:127–138.
9. Kean LH, Suwanrath C, Gargari SS, et al: A comparison of fetal behaviours in breech and cephalic presentations at term. Br J Obstet Gynaecol 1999;106:1209–1213.
10. Nelson KB, Ellenberg JH: Antecedents of cerebral palsy. Multivariate analysis of risk. N Engl J Med 1990;315:81.
11. Rovinsky JJ, Miller JA, Kaplan S: Management of breech presentation at term. Am J Obstet Gynecol 1973;115:497–513.
12. Cheng M, Hannah M: Breech delivery at term: A critical review of the literature. Obstet Gynecol 1993;82:605–618.
13. Gifford DS, Morton SC, Kahn K: A meta-analysis of infant outcomes after breech delivery. Obstet Gynecol 1995;88: 1047–1054.
14. Collea JV, Chien C, Quilligan EJ: The randomised management of term frank breech presentation: A study of 208 cases. Am J Obstet Gynecol 1980;137:253–239.
15. Gimovsky ML, Petrie RH, Todd WD: Randomised management of the non-frank breech presentation at term: A preliminary report. Am J Obstet Gynecol 1983;146:34–40.
16. Krebs L, Topp M, Langhoff-Roos J: The relation of breech presentation at term to cerebral palsy. Br J Obstet Gynaecol 1999;106:943–947.
17. Bartlett DJ, Okun NB, Byrne PJ, et al: Early motor development of breech- and cephalic presenting infants. Obstet Gynecol 2000;95:425–432.
18. Hofmeyr GJ: Breech presentation and abnormal lie in late pregnancy. In Chalmers I, Enkin M, Kierse MJNC (eds): Effective Care in Pregnancy and Childbirth. Oxford, Oxford University Press, 1989, pp 653–665.
19. Lilford RJ, Van Coeverden De Groot HA, Moore PJ, Bingham P: The relative risks of caesarean section (intrapartum and elective) and vaginal delivery: A detailed analysis to exclude the effects of medical disorders and other acute pre-existing physiological disturbances. Br J Obstet Gynaecol 1990;97:883–892.
20. Albrechtsen S, Rasmussen S, Dalaker K, Irgens LM: Reproductive career after breech presentataion: Subsequent pregnancy rates, interpregnancy interval and recurrence. Obstet Gynecol 1998;92:345–350.
21. Flamm BL, Ruffini RM: Undetected breech presentation: Impact on external version and caesarean rates. Am J Perinatol 1998;15:287–289.
22. Kierse MJNC: Preterm delivery. In Chalmers I, Enkin M, Kierse MJNC (eds): Effective Care in Pregnancy and Childbirth. Oxford, Oxford University Press, 1995, Chap. 74, pp 666–693.
23. Karp LE, Doney JR, McCarthy T, et al: The premature breech: Trial of labor or cesarean section? Obstet Gynecol 1979;53: 88–92.

24. Wigglesworth JS, Husesmeyer RP: Intracranial birth trauma in vaginal breech delivery. Br J Obstet Gynaecol 1977;84:684–691.
25. Tejani N, Rebold B, Tuck S, et al: Obstetric factors in the causation of early periventricular-intraventricular haemorrhage. Obstet Gynecol 1984;64:510–515.
26. Robertson PA, Foran CM, Croughane-Minihane MS, Kilpatrick SJ: Head entrapment and neonatal outcome by mode of delivery in breech deliveries from 28 to 36 weeks of gestation. Am J Obstet Gynecol 1996;174:1742–1747.
27. Tahilrameny MP, Platt LD, Sze-Ya YEH, et al: Ultrasonic examination of weight in the very low birth weight fetus: A resident versus staff physician comparison. Am J Obstet Gynecol 1985; 151:90–91.
28. Goldenberg RL, Nelson KG: The premature breech. Am J Obstet Gynecol 1977;27:240–244.
29. Miller EC, Kouam S, Schweintek S: The problem of the increased perinatal mortality rate in premature breech deliveries, compared to premature vertex deliveries. Geburts Fraunheilk 1980;40:1013–1021.
30. Demol S, Bashiri A, Furman B, et al: Breech presentation is a risk factor for intrapartum and neonatal death in preterm delivery. Eur J Obstet Gynecol Reprod Biol 2000;93:47–51.
31. Paul RH, Koh KS, Monfared AH: Obstetric factors influencing outcome in infants weighing from 1001 to 1500 grams. Am J Obstet Gynecol 1979;133:503–508.
32. Haesslin HC, Goodlin RC: Delivery of the tiny newborn. Am J Obstet Gynecol 1979;134:192–200.
33. Wolf H, Schaap AH, Bruinse HW, et al: Vaginal delvery compared with caesarean section in early preterm breech delivery: A comparison of long term outcome. Br J Obstet Gynaecol 1999;106:486–491.
34. Jain L, Ferre C, Vidyasagar D: Cesarean delivery of the breech very-low-birth-weight: Does it make a difference? J Matern Fetal Med 1998;7:28–31.
35. Yu VYH, Bajuk B, Cutting D, et al: Effect of mode of delivery on the outcome of very low birth weight infants. Br J Obstet Gynaecol 1984;91:633–639.
36. Feige A, Douros A: Mortality and morbidity of small premature infants (<1500 g) in relation to presentation and delivery mode. Z Geburtsh Neonatol 2002;2:50–55.
37. Kitchen W, Ford GW, Doyle LW, et al: Cesarean section or vaginal delivery at 24–28 weeks gestation: Comparison of survival and neonatal and two year morbidity. Obstet Gynecol 1985; 66(2):149–157.
38. Rosen MG, Chik L: The effect of route of delivery on outcome in breech presentation. Am J Obstet Gynecol 1984;148:909–914.
39. Viegas OAC, Ingemarsson I, Low PS, et al: Collaborative Study on Preterm Breeches: Vaginal delivery versus cesarean section. Asia Oceania J Obstet Gynecol 1985;11(3):359–365.
40. Lumley J, Lester A, Renon P, Wood C: A failed RCT to determine the best mode of delivery for the very low birth weight infant. Con Clin Trials 1985;6:120–127.
41. Wallace RL, Schifrin BS, Paul RH: The delivery route for very-low-birth-weight infants. J Reprod Med 1984;29:736–740.
42. Penn ZJ, Steer PJ, Grant A: A randomised controlled trial of the optimum mode of delivery of the preterm fetus in breech presentation. Br J Obstet Gynaecol 1996;103:684–689.
43. Haddad NG, Irvine DS: Classical versus lower segment caesarean section in very preterm deliveries (Letter). Lancet 1988; i:762.
44. Westgren M, Edvall H, Nordstrom E, Svalenius E: Spontaneous cephalic version of breech presentation in the last trimester. Br J Obstet Gynaecol 1985;92:19–22.
45. Hofmeyr GJ: Effect of external cephalic version in late pregnancy on breech presentation and caesarean section rate: A controlled trial. Br J Obstet Gynaecol 1983;90:392–399.
46. Hofmeyer GJ, Kulier R: Cephalic version by postural management for breech presentation. Cochrane Database Syst Rev 2000;2:CD000051.
47. Bradley-Watson PJ: The decreasing value of external cephalic version in modern obstetrics. Am J Obstet Gynecol 1975;13:237–241.
48. Hofmeyr GJ: External cephalic version facilitation for breech presentation at term. Cochrane Database Syst Rev. 2000;2:CD000184 (update: 2001;4:CD000184).
49. Hofmeyr GJ: ECV at term: How high the stakes? Br J Obstet Gynaecol 1991;98:1–3.
50. Mahomed K, Seeras R, Coulson R: External cephalic version at term: A randomised controlled trial using tocolysis. Br J Obstet Gynaecol 1991;98:8–13.
51. Aisenbrey GA, Catanzarite VA, Nelson C: External cephalic version: Predictors of success. Obstet Gynecol 1999;94:783–786.
52. Norchi S, Tenore AC, Lovotti M, et al: Efficacy of external cephalic version performed at term. Eur J Obstet Gynecol Reprod Biol 1998;76(2):161–163.
53. Hofmeyr GJ: External cephalic version for breech presentation before term. Cochrane Database of Syst Rev 2000;2:CD000084.
54. Marquette GP, Boucher M, Theriault D, Rinfret D: Does the use of a tocolytic agent affect the success rate of external cephalic version. Am J Obstet Gynecol 1996;174:859–864.
55. Fernandez CO, Bloom SL, Smulian JC, et al: A randomised placebo controlled evaluation of terbutaline for external cephalic version. Obstet Gynecol 1997;90:775–779.
56. Yanny H, Johanson R, Balwin KJ, et al: Double-blind randomised controlled trial of glyceryl trinitrate spray for external cephalic version. BJOG: Int J Obstet Gynaecol 2000;107: 562–564.
57. Schorr SJ, Speights SE, Ross EL, et al: A randomised trial of epidural anesthsia to improve external cephalic version success. Am J Obstet Gynecol 1997;177:1133–1137.
58. Gimovsky ML, Petrie RH: The intrapartum management of the breech presentation. Clin Perinatol 1989;16:976–986.
59. Lau TK, Kit KW, Rogers M: Pregnancy outcome after successful external cephalic version for breech presentation at term. Am J Obstet Gynecol 1997;176:218–223.
60. Egge T, Schauberger C, Schaper A: Dysfunctional labor after external cephalic version. Obstet Gynecol 1994;83:771–773.
61. Ilagan NB, Key-Chyang Liang, Piligan J, Poland R: Thoracic spinal cord transection in a breech presenting cesarean section delivered preterm infant. Am J Perinatol 1987;4:232–233.
62. Heritage CK, Cunningham MD: Association of elective repeat cesarean section and persistent pulmonary hypertension of the newborn. Am J Obstet Gynecol 1985;152:627–629.
63. Lau TK, Leung TY, Lo KW, et al: Effect of external cephalic version at term on fetal circulation. Am J Obstet Gynecol 2000;182:1239–1242.
64. Lau TK, Lo KW, Leung TY, et al: Outcome of labour after successful external cephalic version at term complicated by isolated transient fetal bradycardia. Br J Obstet Gynaecol 2000;107: 410–415.
65. Kouam L: Child development after abdominal version of the fetus from breech presentation near term (English Abstract). Geburtsh Frauenheilk 1985;45:83–90.
66. Hemminki E: Pregnancy and birth after cesarean section: A survey based on the Swedish Birth Register. Birth 1987;14:12–17.
67. Garel M, Lelong N, Marchand A, Kaminski M: Psychological consequences of cesarean childbirth: A 4 year follow-up study. Early Hum Dev 1990;21:105–114.
68. Yogev Y, Horowitz E, Ben-Haroush A, et al: Changing attitudes toward mode of delivery and external cephalic version in breech presentations. Int J Gynaecol Obstet 2002;79:221–224.
69. De Meeus JB, Ellia F, Magnin G: External cephalic version after previous caesarean section: A series of 38 cases. Eur J Obstet Gynecol Reprod Biol 1998;81:65–68.
70. Johnson RL, Elliott JP: Fetal acoustic stimulation, an adjunct to external cephalic version: A blinded, randomized crossover study. Am J Obstet Gynecol 1995;173:1369–1372.

71. Thorp JM, Jenkins T, Watson W: Utility of Leopold maneuvers in screening for malpresentation. Obstet Gynecol 1991;78: 394–396.
72. Royal College of Obstetricians and Gynaecologists: The management of breech presentation at term. London, RCOG Press, 2001, Guideline No 20.
73. Chauhan SP, Mangann EF, Naef RW, et al: Sonographic assessment of birth weight among breech presentations. Ultrasound Obstet Gynecol 1995;6:54–57.
74. Bader B, Graham D, Stinson S: Significance of ultrasound measurements of the head of the breech fetus. J Ultrasound Med 1987;6:437–439.
75. Rojansky N, Tanos V, Lewin A, Weinstein D: Sonographic evaluation of fetal head extension and maternal pelvis in cases of breech presentation. Acta Obstet Gynecol Scand 1994;73:607–611.
76. Hannah ME, Hannah WJ, Hewson SA, et al: Planned caesarean section versus planned vaginal birth for breech presentation at term: A randomised multicenter trial. Term Breech Trial Collaborative Group. Lancet 2000;356:1375–1383.
77. Committee on Obstetric Practise: ACOG Committee opinion. Mode of term singleton breech delivery. Number 265, December 2001, American College of Obstetricians and Gynecologists. Int J Obstet Gynaecol 2002;77:65–66.
78. Hofmeyr GJ, Hannah ME: Planned caesarean section for term breech delivery. Cochrane Database of Systematic Rev 2001;1:CD000166.
79. Croughan-Minihane MS, Pettiti DB, Gordis L, Golditch I: Morbidity amongst breech infants according to method of delivery. Obstet Gynecol 1990;75:821–825.
80. Mecke H, Weisner D, Freys I, Semm K: Delivery of breech presentation infants at term. An analysis of 304 breech deliveries. J Perinat Med 1989;17:121–126.
81. Otamiri G, Berg G, Ledin T, et al: Influence of elective caesarean section and breech delivery on neonatal neurological condition. Early Hum Dev 1990;23:53–66.
82. Danielian PJ, Wang J, Hall MH: Longterm outcome by method of delivery of fetuses in breech presentation at term: Population based follow-up. Br J Med 1996;312:1451–1453.
83. Lumley J: Any room left for disagreement about assisting breech births at term? Lancet 2000;356:1368–1369.
84. Krebs L, Langhoff-Roos J, Bodker B: Are intrapartum and neonatal deaths in breech delivery at term potentially avoidable? A blinded controlled audit. J Perinat Med 2002;30:220–224.
85. Hutchcroft SA, Wearing MP, Buck CW: Late results of cesarean section and vaginal delivery in cases of breech presentation. Can Med Assoc 1981;125:726–730.
86. Krause W, Voigt C, Donzik J, et al: Assisted spontaneous delivery versus Bracht manual aid within the scope of vaginal delivery in breech presentation. Late morbidity in children 5–7 years of age. Z Geburtsh Perinatol 1991;195:76–81.
87. Mahamood TA: The influence of maternal height, obstetrical conjugate and fetal birth weight in the management of patients with breech presentation. Aust NZ J Obstet Gynaecol 1990;30:10–14.
88. Beischer NA: Pelvic contraction in breech presentation. J Obstet Gynaecol Br Commonw 1966;73:421–427.
89. Biswas A, Johnstone MJ: Term breech delivery: Does X-ray pelvimtetry help? Aust NZ J Obstet Gynaecol 1993;33:150–154.
90. van Loon AJ, Manting A, Surlier EK, et al: Randomised controlled trial of magnetic resonance pelvimetry in breech presentation at term. Lancet 1999;350:1799–1804.
91. Leung WC, Pun TC, Wong WM: Undiagnosed breech revisited. Br J Obstet Gynaecol 1999;106:638–641.
92. Nowsu EC, Walkinshaw S, Chia P, et al: Undiagnosed breech. Br J Obstet Gynaecol 1993;100:531–535.
93. Chadha YC, Mahmood TA, Dick MJ, et al: Breech delivery and epidural analgesia. Br J Obstet Gynaecol 1992;99:96–100.
94. Lennox CE, Kwast BE, Farley TM: Breech labour on WHO partograph. Int J Obstet Gynaecol 1998;62:117–127.
95. Arulkumaran S, Thavarasah AS, Ingemarsson I, Ratnam SS: An alternative approach to assisted vaginal breech delivery. Asia Oceania J Obstet Gynecol 1989;15:47–51.
96. Shushan A, Younis JS: McRoberts maneuver for the management of the after-coming head in breech delivery. Gynecol Obstet Invest 1992;32:188–189.
97. Menticoglou SM: Symphysiotomy for the trapped aftercoming parts of the breech: A review of the literature and a plea for its use. Aust NZ J Obstet Gynaecol 1990;30:1–9.
98. Sandberg EC: The Zavanelli maneuver extended: Progression of a revolutionary concept. Am J Obstet Gynecol 1988;158: 1347–1353.
99. Schutterman EB, Grimes DA: Comparative safety of the low transverse versus the low vertical uterine incision for the delivery of breech infants. Obstet Gynecol 1985;61:593–597.
100. Ezra Y, Wade C, Rolbin SH, Farine D: Uterine tocolysis at caesarean breech delivery with epidural anaesthesia. J Reprod Med 2002;47:555–558.

CHAPTER 65

Unstable Lie, Malpresentations, and Malpositions

I. Z. MacKenzie

INTRODUCTION

Near term and during labor, the fetus normally assumes a longitudinal lie and presents with the cephalic pole to the maternal pelvis with the neck flexed and the vertex in the lowermost part of the uterus. In approximately 5% of labors, the lie is not longitudinal. This is usually associated with dangers to both mother and fetus and demands intervention. As with much of medicine, the prior identification of the pregnancy at particular risk of an unstable lie, malpresentation, or malposition can allow intervention in advance of a complication developing and improve the outcome for mother and baby. This chapter will not consider issues relating to fetal breech presentation as these are dealt with elsewhere (see Chapter 64).

DEFINITIONS

Unstable Lie

This is a description generally used beyond 37 weeks' gestation when the fetal lie and presentation repeatedly change, the lie varying from longitudinal, to transverse, and oblique, and the presentation from cephalic, to back, limbs, breech, or a combination. By 37 weeks the fetus usually adopts a "stable" lie and a presentation that will be unchanging until labor and delivery; the fetal position, describing the relationship of the fetal back to the maternal side may, however, change.

Malpresentation Including Compound Presentation

This refers to the fetus that does not present to the maternal pelvis by the vertex alone. The presenting part is defined as that part of the fetus that is lowermost in the uterus. Alternatives include face, brow, breech, and shoulder, as well as compound presentations that involve more than one fetal part, including a combination of the head or breech with a limb or limbs or umbilical cord or a combination of limbs with or without the umbilical cord.

Malposition

A fetal malposition refers to when the fetal vertex presents to the maternal pelvis in a position other than flexed in an occipitoanterior position. Malpositions include occipitotransverse and occipitoposterior positions and may involve some degree of asynclitism (sideways tilt of the head).

Figure 65–1 is an illustration of the various positions that the vertex and brow or face may adopt during labor.

ETIOLOGY

Unstable Lie

Unstable lie is much more common in parous than nulliparous women, but may be caused by or associated with a number of factors. Any situation that discourages or prevents the fetal head or breech from entering the maternal pelvis will predispose to an abnormal and unstable fetal lie. Figure 65–2 illustrates some of the factors associated with an unstable fetal lie.

Maternal Factors

HIGH PARITY

Increasing muscle laxity in the maternal anterior abdominal wall so that it fails to act as a brace and encourage

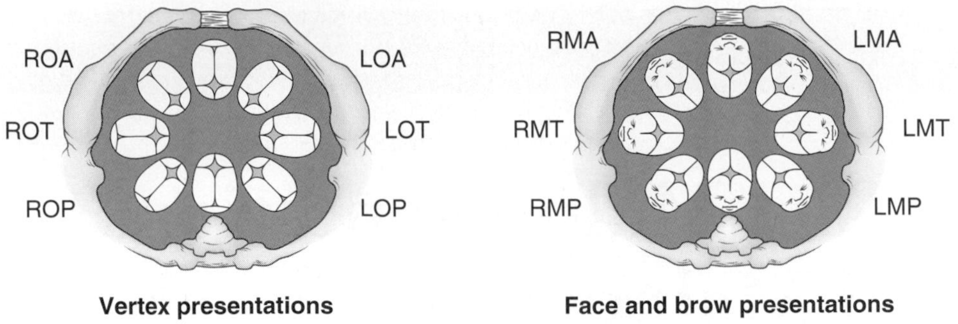

FIGURE 65–1
Diagrammatic representation of the positions for vertex and face presentations. A, anterior; L, left; m, mento; O, occipito; R, right; T, transverse.

and maintain a longitudinal fetal lie is probably the most frequent associated factor. In addition, there is a commonly held view that the highly parous uterus has reduced myometrial tone, thereby encouraging an unstable lie; this has not been proven and is of doubtful relevance.

PLACENTA PREVIA

A persistently changing fetal lie may be the only clinical feature leading to the diagnosis of placenta previa. In addition, a placenta situated in the fundus may also predispose to an unstable lie.[1]

PELVIC TUMORS

Ovarian cysts and low-lying fibroids can obstruct the fetal head or breech entering the pelvis and may result in a high head or breech and transverse or oblique lie.

UTERINE MALFORMATION

Uterus cordiformis, subseptus, or septus may be causative. More severe forms of uterine anomaly, including uterus bicornis and uterus didelphys, are less likely to lead to an unstable lie due to the restricted uterine capacity; a predisposition to fetal breech presentation, however, results.

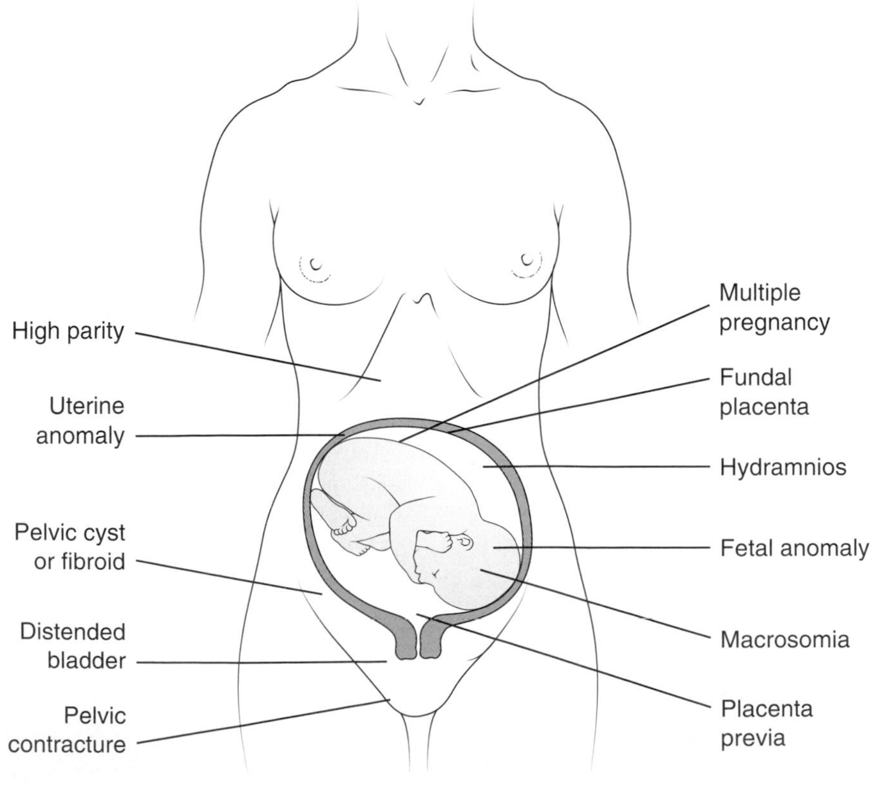

FIGURE 65–2
Etiologic factors and conditions associated with unstable fetal lie.

DISTENDED MATERNAL URINARY BLADDER

Maternal urinary retention with a distended bladder can cause a changing fetal lie, usually only temporarily, with resolution occurring with urinary voiding or bladder catheterization.

Fetal Factors

POLYHYDRAMNIOS

Polyhydramnios, excessive volumes of amniotic fluid, may produce marked uterine distension, enabling the fetus to move around more freely. This probably represents the most common "pathologic" cause for an unstable lie and is also potentially the most hazardous for mother and fetus (see Chapter 13).

OLIGOHYDRAMNIOS

By restricting fetal movement, oligohydramnios can prevent the breech fetus from undergoing spontaneous version to cephalic.

MULTIPLE PREGNANCY

The discovery of an abnormal lie during the last three weeks of pregnancy may arouse suspicion of a multiple pregnancy and lead to investigations that result in the diagnosis being reached; nowadays such a diagnosis is unlikely to have been missed until this stage of pregnancy because of the widespread use of routine ultrasonography during the early weeks of gestation. When the lie of one or both fetuses repeatedly changes, there is usually polyhydramnios.

FETAL MACROSOMIA

Fetal macrosomia produces the same effect as pelvic contracture and must also be considered in such cases.

FETAL ABNORMALITIES

Significant hydrocephaly, tumors of the fetal neck or sacrum, fetal abdominal distension as occurs with hydrops fetalis, and fetal neuromuscular dysfunction (including extended legs) may impede or discourage engagement of a fetal pole in the maternal pelvis. In cases of intrauterine death, the fetus is more likely to present abnormally due to loss of tone, sometimes even requiring delivery by cesarean section because vaginal delivery is impossible.

Compound Presentation

Compound presentations are most usually associated with polyhydramnios and high parity and are more common during the early weeks of the third trimester. Multiple pregnancies, especially those that are monoamniotic, represent a particular risk. Pelvic tumors, including uterine fibroids low in the uterine body or an ovarian cyst situated in the pouch of Douglas, also predispose to compound presentations.

Presentations that involve the umbilical cord are similarly associated with the features previously mentioned. Fetal breech presentation, notably the nonextended breech presentation, is the most common malpresentation associated with cord presentation and prolapse.[2–5]

Brow and Face Presentations

The majority of cases of brow and face presentation are thought to arise when there is a minor degree of deflexion of the presenting vertex that then undergoes further extension; with a more exaggerated extension, a brow presentation will become a face presentation. This may occur during the antepartum period, resulting in a primary face presentation, or develop during the course of labor, resulting in a secondary face presentation.

Primary face presentations are generally associated with fetal malformations, such as anencephaly, meningocele, dolichocephaly, congenital branchiocele, goiter or other anterior neck tumors, and tense extensor neck muscles. Polyhydramnios with the increased space within the uterus and a tight nuchal cord have also been implicated as predisposing factors.

Secondary face presentations are thought to be associated with a contracted or abnormally shaped pelvis. This was considered responsible for 40% of face presentations in a series reported from the Johns Hopkins Hospital early in the last century.[6] It is also much commoner in preterm labor, probably due to the more capacious pelvis accommodating the relatively small fetus.[7]

Malpositions

Recent data derived from ultrasound examinations at the start of labor have suggested that the majority (68%) of posterior positions confirmed toward the end of labor were in an occipitoanterior position at the beginning of labor. The other 32% began labor as an occipitoposterior position, and these labors are more likely to result in an assisted delivery.[8]

Maternal pelvic shape is thought probably to be the major determinant of fetal position prior to labor. When the anteroposterior pelvic dimension of the brim equals or exceeds that of the transverse dimension, occipitoposterior positions are favored. Thus women with an android pelvis are more likely to have an occipitoposterior position in late pregnancy and at the start of labor since the larger dimensions toward the back of the pelvis encourage the broader occiput to be accommodated there rather than in the anterior compartment. In addition, when there is a high assimilation pelvis, with an extra vertebra included in the formation of the sacrum, the inclination of the brim increases, which favors an occipitoposterior position. The much less common anthropoid-shaped pelvis, with the lessening of the posterosagittal diameter (the distance between the midpoint of the widest transverse diameter and the sacrum), affects not only the brim but commonly extends to the lower levels of the pelvis and to the outlet. In particular, the concavity of the sacrum from promontory to tip is often reduced or abolished (flat sacrum), leaving a reduced space in which the sinciput can turn should internal rotation commence. This leads to the head impacting in the pelvic cavity, resulting in a "deep transverse arrest." It has been suggested that increased muscle tone in the extensor muscles of the fetus might also predispose to an occipitoposterior position, but there is little evidence to support this theory.

Most important is the observation that a high proportion of patients with a malposition making poor progress through labor respond to augmentation of uterine contractions with oxytocin and deliver spontaneously vaginally.[9] This suggests that the quality of uterine contractions plays a significant part in determining the position and attitude of the fetal head. As well as uterine contraction strength being important, there is now good evidence that the tone of the pelvic floor is also relevant. Use of regional anesthesia for the management of pain relief during labor has been implicated as a mechanism for the increased rates of malposition in late labor[10,11] although this is disputed. Regional anesthesia provides an extremely effective method of reducing the distress of labor, distress that is more common with a preexisting occipitoposterior position. The issue of cause and effect thus comes into play. The experience reported from Dublin provides some evidence to suggest that regional blockade is not causal in the evolution of fetal malposition. It was noted that despite a 30-fold increase in intrapartum epidural usage between 1975 and 1998, occipitoposterior position at the end of a first labor decreased from 3.8% to 2.4%.[12]

INCIDENCE

Unstable Lie

Figures are not generally available for the incidence with which unstable lie is encountered in a population. The incidence will be influenced mainly by the proportion of multiparae and particularly the numbers of grand-multiparae. Similarly, in societies where malnutrition is prominent and maternal or fetal skeletal deformities are relatively common, the incidence will be higher. In a well-nourished and developed population where high parity (greater than four) is uncommon, the incidence will be in the range of 0.1% to 1.0%, and the occurrence rate of transverse lie in labor is in the region of 0.4%.[13]

Compound Presentations

There is a relatively sparse literature on the incidence of compound presentations that involve one or more limbs and the fetal head or breech. Overall the incidence has been quoted to be between 1:377 and 1:1213 deliveries;[14–16] personal experience suggests that the lower incidence is more usual in the developed world. Combinations involving the upper limbs and head are the most common. Diagnosis in late labor is the usual situation, with as many as 50% of compound presentations being diagnosed during the second stage of labor.

The incidence of cord presentation has not been widely reported although cord prolapse occurs in around 1:300 to 1:700 total births[3,5,17,18]: 1:900 cephalic presentation labors, 1:56 breech labors, 1:23 twin labors,[5] and 1:5 to 1:10 compound presentations that involve a limb.[14,15,19] Thus cord prolapse in a singleton pregnancy with a cephalic presentation at term has an incidence of around 1:1400 labors. These rates are almost certainly lower than the incidence of cord presentation, since recognized cord presentation is likely to be managed by cesarean section before a prolapse can occur.

Brow and Face Presentation

Brow presentation in labor has an incidence of between 1:200 and 1:500 labors.[20–22] Face presentations are generally quoted to occur in around 1:1000 to 1:1500 deliveries.[23] The incidences during pregnancy are less well documented, especially for brow presentation, since it is probable that this presentation is usually only transient, with reversion to vertex with flexion of the neck or face presentation with further deflexion.

Malpositions

During the antepartum period, prior to the onset of labor, the occipitoposterior position exists in around 11% of singleton pregnancies.[24,25] Once labor starts, the incidence is in the region of 20% to 25%; if the fetal back is on the maternal left, the occipitoposterior position is much less common than when the back is on the maternal right.[20] It is said to be more common in cases of membrane rupture before the onset of labor with an incidence of 27%.[26] Between 20% and 35% of those that start labor in an occipitoposterior position remain in that position to the end of labor, indicating that 65% to 80% undergo spontaneous rotation during labor. As few as 1% to 5% are delivered in an occipitoposterior position.[27,28]

DIAGNOSIS

Unstable Lie

This diagnosis is usually suspected when repeated clinical examinations show a variable fetal lie during the last month of gestation. Occasionally, in those women in whom clinical examination is not easy (including those with a raised body mass index), the diagnosis may fortuitously be made by an ultrasound examination performed for other reasons. An unstable lie would appear to be more common than is presently thought, from the evidence of the frequency with which fetal breech presentation is missed prior to the onset of labor, despite frequent and recent antenatal clinical examinations. Further, the observation of spontaneous and unexpected version of the fetus from a cephalic to breech presentation during the last weeks before delivery adds weight to this observation.[29,30]

Compound Presentations

A compound presentation involving a fetal arm with the head, or an arm with a leg is only likely to be diagnosed during the antepartum period as a coincidental finding at an ultrasound examination or in rare circumstances on radiographic or magnetic resonance imaging examination. The high nonengaged head that cannot be encouraged into the maternal pelvis might prompt an ultrasound examination, leading to the diagnosis.

Diagnosis during labor may be suspected because of a delay in the presenting part entering the pelvis and is confirmed on vaginal examination by identifying an errant limb or limbs. Occasionally, the diagnosis is made unexpectedly at a vaginal examination when the maternal pelvis is large and the interloping limb with the head or breech does not delay engagement of the presenting part.

Compound presentations involving the umbilical cord are usually classified according to Naegele, who distinguished between "presentation" before membrane rupture and "prolapse" after membrane rupture. A diagnosis of cord presentation will not usually be made prior to the onset of labor except in those cases of an unstable lie when a vaginal examination is performed as part of the assessment of the strategy for continued management. Although some have documented reaching the diagnosis with ultrasound, this is not a widely reported observation.[31]

Face Presentation

Older texts report that abdominal palpation allows the diagnosis of a fetal face presentation to be made by the recognition of a much broader lower pole presenting to the pelvis than usual and the palpation of a marked depression between the fetal back and the occiput (Fig. 65–3). This is more easily demonstrated if the fetus is lying in a dorsoanterior, or mentoposterior presentation; this is less common than a mentoanterior presentation.[20] It is also said that the fetal heart sounds are very easily heard when listened to over the fetal chest, especially with a mentoanterior position; this potentially valuable clinical sign is lost if hand-held Doppler machines are routinely used to detect fetal heart pulsations in preference to a Pinnard stethoscope. Despite this, it is the author's experience that these clinical signs are difficult to elicit, even in those cases of face presentation already confirmed by radiology or ultrasonography.

Confirmation of the presentation should be made by vaginal examination during the intrapartum period. The obstetrician, however, should be wary of confusion between a face and a breech presentation, due to the inevitable facial edema that readily forms during labor, and the added difficulty associated with a high presenting part and a poorly dilated cervix. Identification of the supraorbital ridges, the ridge of the nose, and the alveolar processes within the mouth should lead to the diagnosis. If the technology is available, an ultrasound examination can be used to confirm the clinical suspicion.[32]

Brow Presentation

Although occasionally a brow presentation may be recognized during the antenatal period, usually coinciden-

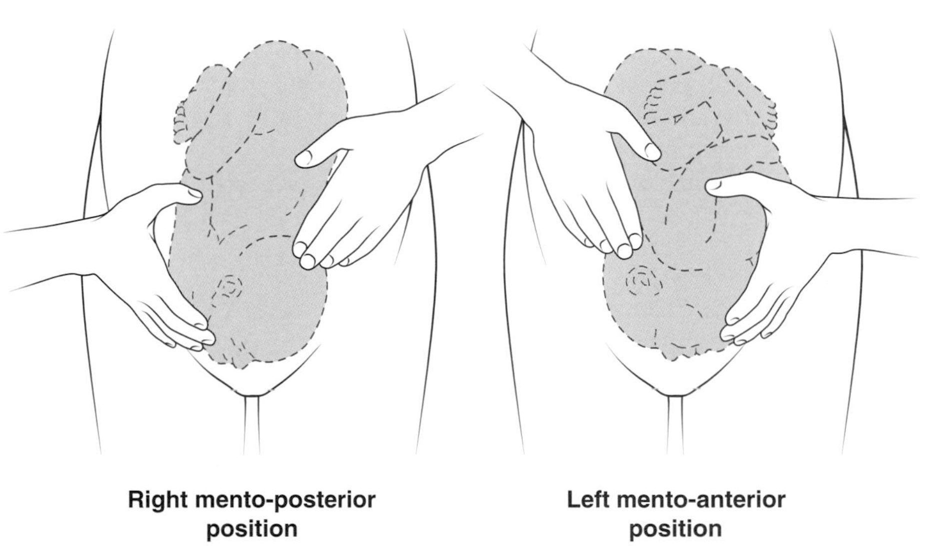

FIGURE 65–3
Palpation of the fetus and the landmarks associated with a face presentation.

tally at an ultrasound examination, in most instances this is not a permanent position. The suspicion of a broader head than expected for the overall size of the fetal body resting above the pelvic brim may (rarely) lead the astute clinician to suspect this possible diagnosis. Diagnosis during the intrapartum period is only likely to be made during advanced labor when the cervix is moderately well dilated and the brow palpable to the examining fingers. Identification of the anterior fontanelle and the supraorbital ridges confirms the diagnosis, but any significant caput succedaneum can mask these landmarks. As with face presentations, ultrasound examination is the most practical way to confirm or refute the diagnosis.

Malpositions

It is often written that the outline of the distended uterus occasionally suggests an occipitoposterior position; a flatness with a dip between the head and the trunk may be evident. Certainly fetal movements may be readily observed over much of the anterior surface of the abdomen if the baby is active at the time of the examination. However, the fetal back may be difficult to identify on palpation although the shoulder is felt toward the flank with the limbs often obvious to palpation over the abdomen. With Pawlik's grip, the sinciput is said to be prominent, but personal experience would not suggest this to be a reliable feature. Importantly, the fetal heart is heard maximally in the flank to which the back is directed; the Pinard stethoscope allows this clinical sign to be elicited while the small Doppler fetal heart detectors generally do not. An ultrasound examination should confirm or refute the clinical findings.

During labor, the anterior fontanelle is easier to reach when the position is occipitoposterior than occipitoanterior, although caput succedaneum may make this more difficult, especially late in labor. Palpation of the more anterior of the two ears can be helpful, but this may be misleading if the pinna has been turned forward. At this examination, not only should the degree of flexion be noted but also any asynclitism. Diagnosis of a deep transverse arrest should not present difficulties unless caput succedaneum or anterior or posterior asynclitism is marked. Once again, palpation of the fetal ear could be helpful, or if available, ultrasound will confirm the position.[33,34]

RISKS

Unstable Lie and Compound Presentation

There are no hazards to mother or fetus during the antenatal period from an unstable lie per se. It is possible that cord entanglement is a greater risk, although this has not been positively shown. During the latter weeks of pregnancy, spontaneous resolution to a longitudinal lie before labor starts occurs in the region of 85%.[35–37]

There are, however, very serious risks to mother and fetus with the onset of labor if the lie is not longitudinal. Once the membranes rupture, with or without accompanying uterine contractions, there is a risk of cord prolapse if the fetal lie is oblique or transverse, or the presenting part is high above the pelvic inlet. Cord prolapse may result in damaging hypoxia or even stillbirth. Perinatal death has variously been reported to occur as frequently as 5% to 10% of cases[5,38,39] or even as often as 43%.[40] The risk of hypoxic damage is less well documented and it may be as little as 1% in survivors.[5] Keeping the interval between cord prolapse and delivery as brief as possible is likely to be important.[39,41]

If labor starts when the lie is not longitudinal, a compound presentation may result, or the pelvis may remain empty. If left unattended, fetal distress will eventually supervene, ultimately resulting in fetal death. A Bandl's ring or retraction ring (Fig. 65–4) may form, making delivery even by cesarean section potentially hazardous.[42] In addition uterine rupture is a real possibility, especially in multiparae, with potentially serious consequences for mother and fetus (see Chapter 77).

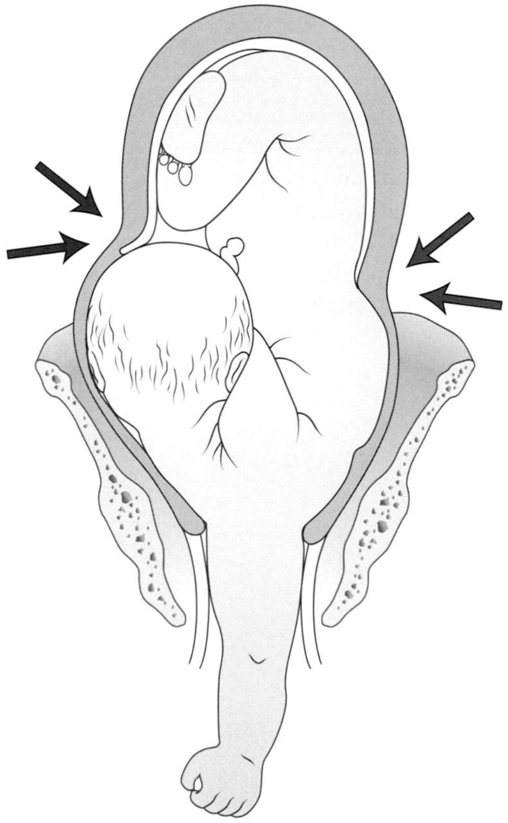

FIGURE 65–4
Fetal shoulder presentation, illustrating the site of Bandl's, or retraction, ring forming at the junction of the upper and lower uterine segments with an obstructed labor.

Malpresentation

Face

Cord prolapse may be marginally increased over a vertex presentation, but once established in labor with the head engaged in the pelvis, this is unlikely. Progress should be as for a vertex presentation without any additional risk to the fetus since the presenting head diameters are similar (Fig. 65–5). However, with the largest presenting diameter (biparietal) displaced toward the back of the pelvis, a generous episiotomy should be performed, to reduce the risk of a third-degree tear. Providing the face is mentoanterior, vaginal delivery is likely. If there is any delay in delivery, forceps rather than a ventouse should be used, as the ventouse cannot be applied effectively or safely with the face presenting. The parents should be advised in advance of the delivery that their baby will appear very unattractive initially due to the inevitable bruising and marked edema, both of which disappear within a few hours of birth.

Brow

There are no added risks to the mother with a fetal brow presentation during the antenatal period. As with a face presentation, the risk of cord presentation and prolapse is increased.

Except with very preterm labor, the fetus cannot be delivered as a persistent brow unless there is a very capacious pelvis, because of the large mentovertical diameter that presents to the pelvis (see Fig. 65–5). If continued extension of the neck to a face presentation does not occur and the brow presentation persists, the chance of fetal distress and even uterine rupture is high if labor in a parous woman is not progressing and is left to continue for too long.

Malpositions

Few risks are associated with a fetal malposition prior to labor. As already stated, there is a belief that prelabor rupture of the membranes is more common with an occipitoposterior position. Since the head is usually not engaged and may not be well settled into the pelvis, the risk of cord prolapse is increased.

Once in labor, progress may be slower than with an anterior position, and maternal distress is often increased, with discomfort felt particularly in the back. As well as a protracted first stage of labor, there is often a delay during the second stage with the need for augmentation of contractions with oxytocin, or assistance with manual rotation, forceps delivery with or without rotation, or assistance with the ventouse. With a current reluctance to engage in rotational procedures, especially if fetal distress is suspected, there is an increased risk of cesarean section.

It has recently been shown by one group that the occipitoposterior position that persists to the time of vaginal delivery presents a significant risk of anal sphincter damage for both nulliparae and multiparae.[12]

MANAGEMENT

Unstable Lie and Compound Presentation

Antenatal

During the antenatal period management can be expectant or active, while delivery can either await spontaneous onset of labor or be arranged as a planned event. An algorithm of the various options is illustrated in Figure 65–6.

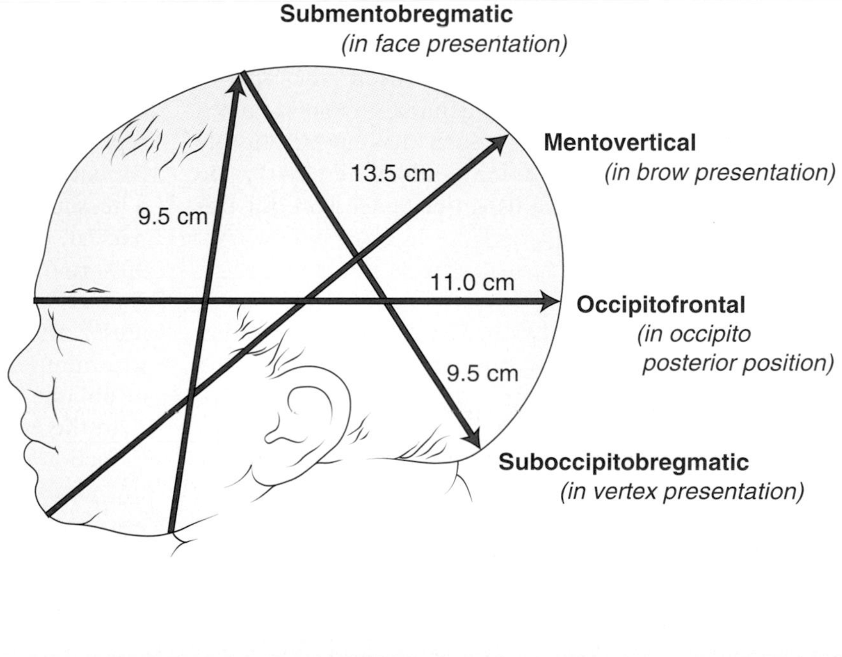

FIGURE 65–5
The sagittal dimensions of the fetal head according to the presentation.

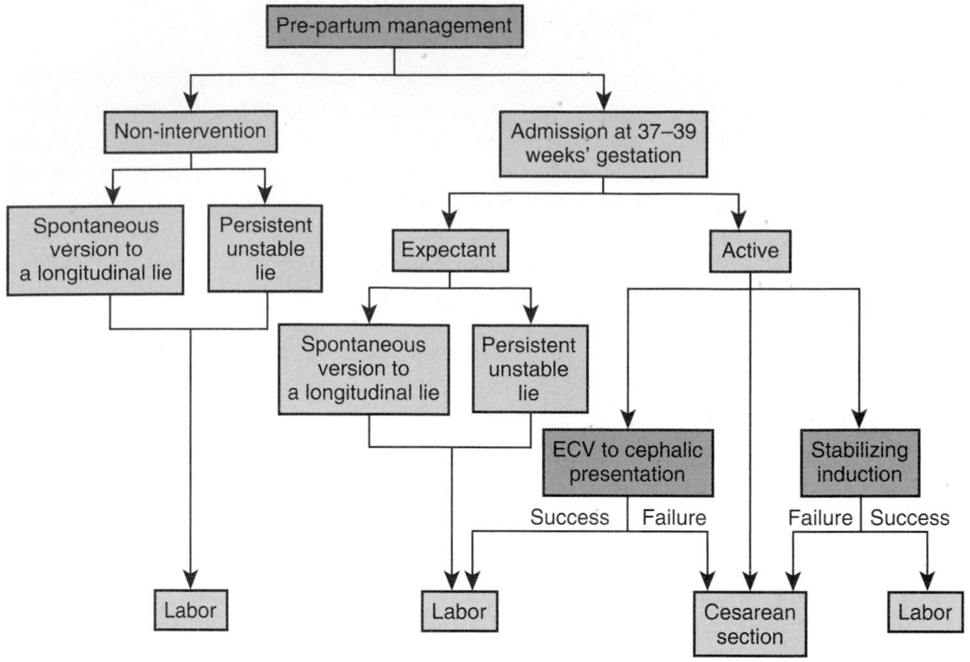

FIGURE 65–6
Algorithm for the prenatal management of unstable lie in late pregnancy. ECV, external cephalic version.

NONINTERVENTION

Once an unstable lie is identified, no specific action is taken in anticipation that the lie will become longitudinal before the membranes rupture or labor starts: this is likely to occur in more than 80% of cases.[35–37] Manipulation to a longitudinal lie at an antenatal examination can sometimes be performed. Every attempt should be made to identify any obvious mechanical cause for the unstable lie, especially if it is likely to result in obstructed labor, thus requiring elective cesarean section. The patient should be advised of the risks associated with an unstable lie and the need for urgent attention should labor start or the membranes rupture. If the woman lives very far from the delivery unit, it may be necessary to admit her from about 37 weeks to await the onset of labor to ensure prompt attention at the onset of labor.

A number of physical exercises, such as the woman adopting the knee-elbow position for short periods on a number of occasions each day, have been advocated to promote spontaneous version, generally from a breech to cephalic presentation.[43–46] Such maneuvers possibly improve the chances of a longitudinal lie by 5% to 10%, but there is no established evidence base for this proposition.

INTERVENTION

Admission may be advised from 37 to 39 weeks' gestation onward. This enables daily observations of fetal lie and presentation to be made; provides the opportunity for active treatment to correct the lie if necessary; allows for immediate clinical assistance upon membrane rupture or the onset of labor; and facilitates urgent management if the lie is not longitudinal, fetal distress occurs, or the cord is presenting or prolapsed.

If spontaneous resolution to a longitudinal lie occurs and is established as cephalic or breech presentation and maintained for 48 hours, the patient may be discharged home to await labor; some currently discourage labor with a breech presentation and reference should be made to the relevant chapter on this topic.

If spontaneous resolution of an abnormal lie does not occur, an active approach to management may be adopted. External cephalic version can be attempted if facilities permit immediate delivery in the event of placental abruption, membrane rupture, cord prolapse, or acute fetal distress for any reason[41,47] (see also Chapter 64 on breech presentation). If a longitudinal lie is established and maintained, the patient may be released home to await spontaneous onset of labor; rhesus immunoprophylaxis should be given to at-risk women either before or soon after the version attempt, and a Kleihauer-Betke test is ideally checked about 20 minutes after the attempt to determine whether additional prophylaxis is necessary. If a longitudinal lie is not maintained, the version can be repeated as often as necessary, and if not successful the patient can be kept in the hospital until labor supervenes. The success of version antenatally for unstable lie is unclear, but in cases of breech presentation it is around 40% to 65%.[39,40,48] Tocolysis can be used, such as intravenous infusions of ritodrine 50 μg/minute for 15 minutes[39] or terbutaline sulfate 250 μg intravenously over 1 to 2 minutes,[24] but is often unnecessary with a transverse or oblique lie (see Chapter 64).

In the event of a continuing unstable lie, a stabilizing induction may be performed, either immediately following admission or when an appropriate gestation (usually 38–39 weeks) has been reached during the following days or weeks. Following transfer to the labor suite an external cephalic version is performed converting the fetal lie to longitudinal. Once in position, regular abdominal palpations are performed to confirm the longitudinal lie is maintained and a titrated intravenous infusion of oxytocin is commenced to stimulate uterine contractility.[38] As soon as contractions are occurring at 10-minute intervals or more frequently, a low amniotomy is performed, having ensured the lie is still longitudinal and the presentation is not compound and in particular that the cord is not presenting. If the cord presents, an emergency cesarean section is necessary. Once low amniotomy is performed, a reasonable volume of amniotic fluid should be released, followed by confirmation that the cord is not presenting and the presenting part is fixed in the pelvic brim. Thereafter, once labor is established, management continues as for an uncomplicated labor. A hindwater amniotomy using a Drew-Smythe catheter[49] can be performed. This catheter is passed through the cervix, behind the presenting part between the uterine wall and the fetal membranes, taking every possible care to avoid trauma to the fetus and the placenta, especially if it is posterior. The stylet within the catheter is advanced to puncture the membranes and allow a controlled release of amniotic fluid. This procedure aims to reduce the chances of cord prolapse occurring, but is rarely done in modern practice because of a fear that the rigid catheter will damage the fetus or placenta or perforate the uterus. A more modern approach to hindwater rupture is to use an intrauterine catheter (preferably a solid-state blunt-ended transducer) passed up alongside the fetal head. This has the advantage that the catheter can then be used to measure uterine activity as an aid to appropriately controlling it. Uterine contractility can also be stimulated with local (vaginal) or oral prostaglandins, but this is probably less advisable since the response to prostaglandins is unpredictable and occasionally hyperstimulation can occur, requiring either acute tocolysis or emergency cesarean section, especially if the lie reverts to oblique or transverse.

Finally, a decision to deliver by elective antepartum cesarean section can be made at a convenient time, often at 38 to 40 weeks' gestation,[37] ideally converting the lie to longitudinal at laparotomy and using a lower segment incision rather than a classical (vertical midline). This approach is particularly appropriate if there is a contraindication to external version, external version fails, or there is a mechanical obstruction to vaginal delivery.

Intrapartum

When the fetal lie is transverse or oblique and the membranes rupture or labor starts, the options for management illustrated in the algorithm in Figure 65–7 indicate that a cord presentation or prolapse will prompt different immediate decisions on management depending on the stage of labor and whether the membranes are intact or ruptured.

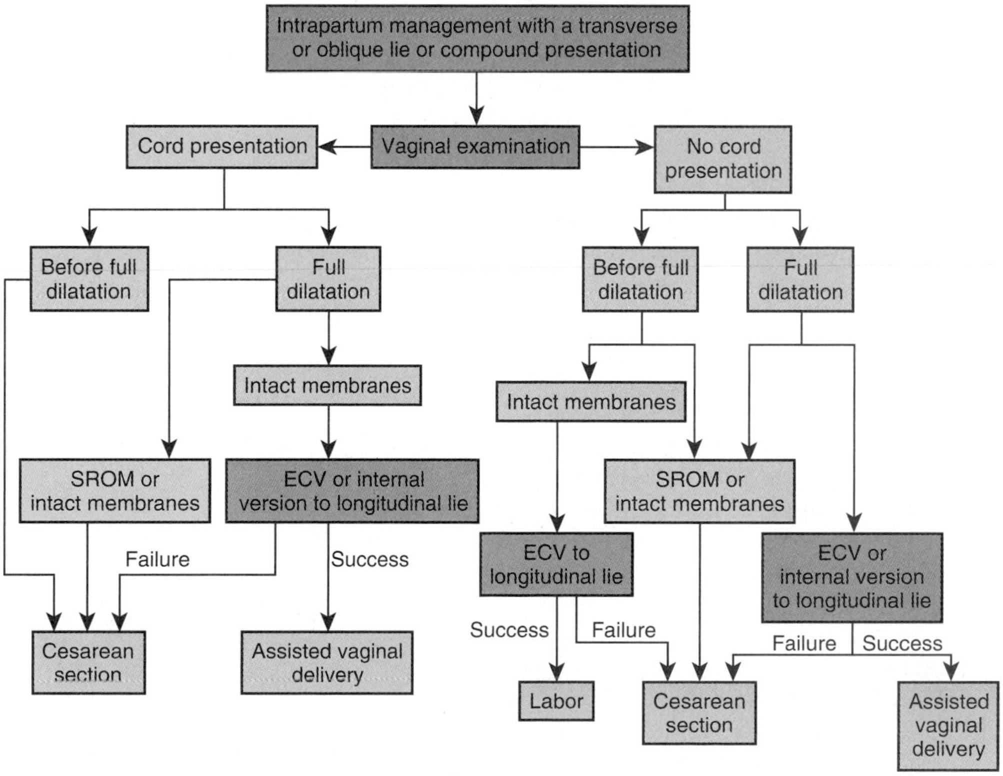

FIGURE 65–7
Algorithm for the intrapartum management of unstable lie. ECV, external cephalic version; SROM, spontaneous rupture of membranes.

CORD PRESENTATION BEFORE FULL CERVICAL DILATATION

Delivery by cesarean section should be organized in this case; an ultrasound examination at this stage has been used to demonstrate the umbilical cord in the lower pole of the uterus.[31] If there is evidence suggesting fetal distress, the arrangements should be made with urgency. If there is a cord prolapse before full dilatation of the cervix, a "crash" procedure to deliver by cesarean section is required. An attempt is made to reduce pressure on the umbilical cord with digital counterpressure within the vagina or use of the Trendelenberg or knee-chest positions; an attempt to replace the cord may be successful[18] (see Chapter 71 on fetal distress). Cord presentation at full dilatation may be managed by external cephalic or internal cephalic version; delivery by cesarean section should be arranged urgently if the expertise for version is not immediately available or the attempt is unsuccessful. If a cord prolapse is present and the lie is not longitudinal, urgent crash cesarean section is required. Immediate vaginal delivery with forceps for a cephalic presentation, or a breech extraction, should be considered if the necessary skills are available and the presenting part is low enough in the pelvis; the ventouse is a slower option in the hands of many clinicians compared with forceps.[50]

NO CORD PRESENTATION AND THE CERVIX NOT FULLY DILATED

Management of this circumstance will depend on whether the fetal membranes are intact or ruptured. With intact fetal membranes an external version can be performed, and, if successful, labor can continue, with close observation to ensure the lie remains longitudinal until the presenting part engages in the maternal pelvis. Either the attempt at external version is made between contractions, or a tocolytic agent can be infused to relax the uterus. Tocolytic agents that can be used in this situation include β-agonists such as terbutaline infused at 5 to 20 μg/minute, salbutamol (albuterol) 2.5 to 4.5 μg/minute, ritodrine 100 to 350 μg/minute,[51] or the oxytocin antagonist, atosiban, given as a single IV bolus dose of 6.75 mg.[42] If the version is successful, a repeat vaginal examination should be performed to exclude cord presentation or prolapse. Once this has been done, labor can be allowed to establish and progress augmented with oxytocin if necessary. If the version has been unsuccessful, delivery by cesarean section should be performed (see later discussion). With ruptured membranes, delivery by cesarean section is generally the only option unless the patient is in very early labor and an attempt at external cephalic version is successful. If the compound presentation involves the fetal head and a hand or arm is also present, attempts should be made to push the arm up or nip one of the fetal fingers to try to encourage its withdrawal out of the pelvis. It is also reasonable to allow the labor to continue with close supervision in anticipation that spontaneous withdrawal will occur with continuing uterine contractions, causing discomfort to the arm and hand. If it is still present at full dilatation with the head engaged in the pelvis, a decision will need to be reached to determine whether vaginal manipulation can encourage the hand out of the pelvis so that vaginal delivery can continue or whether cesarean section should be performed. A shoulder presentation, sometimes with a prolapsed arm into the vagina, is a serious situation (see Fig. 65–5). Clamping of the uterine wall around the fetus by a retraction or Bandl's ring may have contributed. Delivery must be by cesarean section. Administration of a uterine relaxant such as halothane administered by the anesthetist can facilitate the delivery, which is most safely achieved through a classical uterine incision. This incision allows the fetus to be withdrawn through the fundus of the uterus, whereas a lower segment incision makes it nearly impossible to manipulate the fetus into a position that will allow delivery without damage to the fetus. This management is indicated even if the fetus has already died, to avoid uterine rupture and other serious uterine trauma at the time of the delivery.

A TRANSVERSE LIE AT FULL DILATATION WITH INTACT MEMBRANES

This condition can be managed by external cephalic version with an assisted vaginal cephalic or breech delivery following. If an internal podalic version is attempted, a conclusion should have been reached that there is no anticipated fetopelvic disproportion. With adequate anesthesia (either a general or fully effective regional block) using an appropriate aseptic technique, the obstetrician introduces a hand into the uterus, identifies the foot of the anteriorly positioned leg and applies traction on the leg, withdrawing the foot and leg and subsequently the breech through the vagina (Fig. 65–8). It is even better if both feet can be grasped and pulled down, as this avoids the "splits," with one leg down and one leg

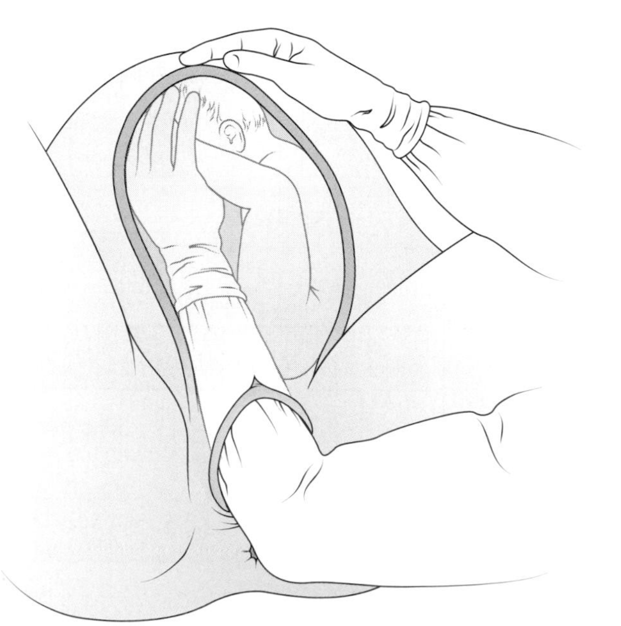

FIGURE 65–8
Principle of securing the foot of the anterior leg at internal podalic version.

up, which can splint the baby and make it difficult to deliver. The delivery is as described for a breech extraction (see Chapter 64). Great care must be taken to avoid both fetal bony injury and laceration of the uterus. Tocolysis may be helpful for this procedure. If version is not successful, delivery should be achieved by cesarean section; attempts at version should only be performed when immediate resort to section is available.

ALREADY RUPTURED MEMBRANES AT FULL DILATATION

If the fetus is in a transverse or oblique lie or there is a compound presentation, delivery should be performed as urgently as possible, using the classical cesarean section incision unless an attempt at external version can be successfully made on opening the abdominal wall and immediately before the uterine is incised. A transverse incision in the lower uterine segment is likely to be inadequate for fetal extraction because the loss of amniotic fluid reduces the surgeon's ability to manipulate the fetus within the uterus. Struggling to deliver the fetus through a lower segment incision can cause serious trauma to the fetus, uterus, or both; or the uterine incision will need to be extended as an inverted T or as a U-shape incision. Such incision extensions may result in compromised healing and a vulnerable area of scar integrity, which may predispose to uterine rupture in future labors.

SUMMARY OF MANAGEMENT OPTIONS
Unstable, Transverse, and Oblique Lie

Management Options	Quality of Evidence	Strength of Recommendation	References
Prenatal See Figure 65–6			
Confirm diagnosis with ultrasound if necessary.	–	GPP	–
Investigate for possible causes including history and ultrasound examination.	–	GPP	–
Discuss options and risks.	–	GPP	–
Expectant Management			
If noncephalic after 36 weeks— "wait and see" policy—danger of cord prolapse or admission in advanced labor with a malpresentation		GPP	–
Advice to adopt knee–chest maneuver to promote cephalic version has not been shown to be of value and is not recommended.	Ia	A	52
Active Management			
Admit to hospital at 37–39 weeks; assess daily; if spontaneous conversion to cephalic presentation occurs, subsequent options are:	–	GPP	–
- Allow patient to return home to await spontaneous labor			
- Induce labor			
If noncephalic after 36 weeks, offer ECV if no contraindications; if successful conversion to cephalic is achieved:	Ia	A	54
- Allow patient to return home to await spontaneous labor.	–	GPP	–
- Stabilizing induction between 38–39 weeks	III	B	38
If ECV fails or version contraindicated, cesarean section is necessary	Ia	A	55
Labor and Delivery See Figure 65–7			
Confirm diagnosis by examination ± ultrasound examination.	–	GPP	–
First Stage of Labor			
If cord presentation or prolapse, cesarean section is necessary	–	GPP	–
If no cord presentation,	–	GPP	–
- For ECV if membranes intact and allow to labor if successful			
- Otherwise for cesarean section			

SUMMARY OF MANAGEMENT OPTIONS

Unstable, Transverse, and Oblique Lie

Management Options	Quality of Evidence	Strength of Recommendation	References
Second Stage of Labor			
Confirm diagnosis by examination ± ultrasound examination	–	GPP	–
If membranes ruptured, for cesarean section	–	GPP	–
If membranes not ruptured	–	GPP	–
- For ECV or internal version* and vaginal delivery if successful			
- If version is unsuccessful, cesarean section is necessary			

ECV, external cephalic version.
*The use of internal podalic version should be limited to the obstetrician with experience of the technique and when fetopelvic disproportion is not suspected.

Malpresentation

Antenatal

Once an identifiable specific cause for the malpresentation has been diagnosed, treatment of the precipitating condition may be indicated (see relevant chapters). For those cases without identifiable cause, there are no recognized and universally accepted managements to adopt for correcting a fetal brow or face presentation. In view of the increased risk of cord presentation and thus cord prolapse, the patient should be advised of early admission when labor starts or membrane rupture occurs.

As with an unstable lie, admission from 39 weeks' gestation should be considered for this reason. If delivery is indicated for other reasons, planned cesarean section without recourse to labor may be a safer option than inducing labor if there is a high presenting fetal part. The alternative is labor induction with either local prostaglandins or intravenous oxytocin and low amniotomy once contractions are established and the fetal head fixed or engaged in the pelvic brim. Preparation should have been made to allow for rapid cesarean section should cord presentation or prolapse be diagnosed, with the patient forewarned of this possibility.

Intrapartum

Labor management should be the same as for a vertex presentation, assuming routine maternal and fetal observations are satisfactory and good progress is maintained; many brow presentations convert to a face or vertex and the majority of face presentations present as mentoanterior. Oxytocin augmentation is acceptable if uterine contractions are inadequate, but caution should always be shown since labor may become obstructed with dire consequences if left unattended. If progress in labor is slow, resort to cesarean section may be a wiser option. Figure 65–9 illustrates the management options.

Once full dilatation is reached with a brow presentation, spontaneous delivery will not follow unless the fetus is very small or the pelvis is unusually capacious. Providing the assessment of the pelvis indicates that there is no evidence of absolute disproportion, the presentation can be converted with rotational forceps to face or vertex, whichever proves to be the easier, and then delivered. Some have advised the use of the ventouse in this situation but this requires the cup to be applied behind the bregma and this is unlikely to be possible in the majority of cases (see Chapter 74). The current majority view is that unless the head is engaged in the pelvis at the start of vaginal manipulations, delivery by cesarean section is recommended.

With a face presentation, vaginal delivery should be anticipated if the head is engaged, with the delivery occurring spontaneously or assisted with forceps. The head should be a mentoanterior position at the delivery, achieved by forceps rotation if necessary (see Chapter 74). The ventouse has no place in the management of a face presentation. Thus cesarean section to complete the delivery may be necessary if the obstetrician does not have the necessary skills to conduct a rotational forceps procedure.

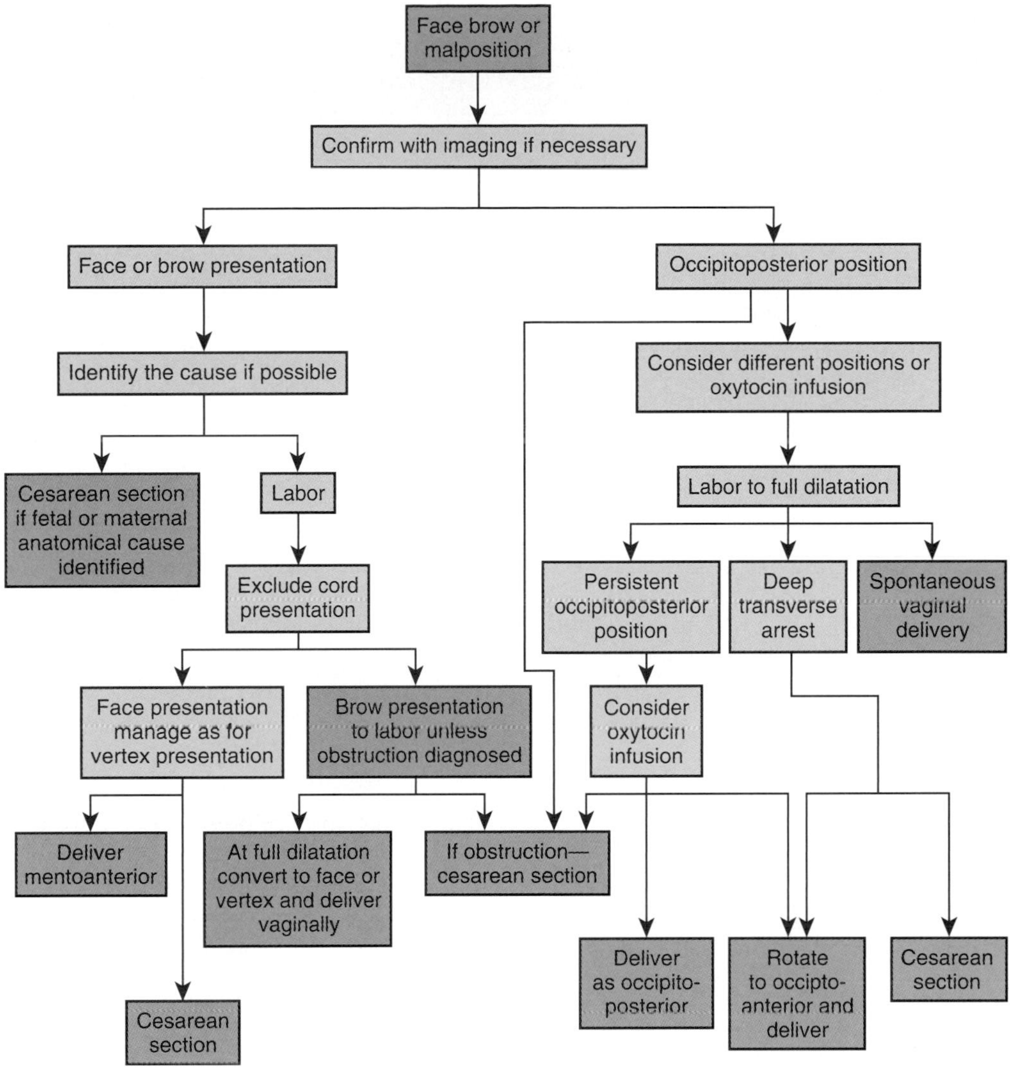

FIGURE 65–9
Algorithm for the intrapartum management of malpresentation and malposition of the fetal head.

SUMMARY OF MANAGEMENT OPTIONS
Face and Brow Presentation

Management Options	Quality of Evidence	Strength of Recommendation	References
	Prenatal		
Confirm diagnosis—examination; ultrasound	–	GPP	–
Assess for causal factors	–	GPP	–
Interventions			
Perform cesarean section if arrested progress in labor.	–	GPP	–
Offer cesarean section as an alternative to labor.	–	GPP	–
Labor and Delivery See Figure 65–9			
First Stage of Labor			
Establish diagnosis by vaginal examination ± ultrasound	–	GPP	–

Continued

SUMMARY OF MANAGEMENT OPTIONS
Face and Brow Presentation *(Continued)*

Management Options	Quality of Evidence	Strength of Recommendation	References
Prenatal			
Brow Presentation	–	GPP	–
Allow labor to progress with careful monitoring of progress.			
If spontaneous conversion to face or vertex, anticipate spontaneous vaginal delivery			
Assisted vaginal delivery			
Cesarean section if arrested progress in labor			
Offer cesarean section if pelvic disproportion suspected.			
Face Presentation	–	GPP	–
If mento-anterior, allow labor to proceed anticipating vaginal delivery.			
Offer cesarean section If mento-posterior or if pelvic disproportion suspected.			
Second Stage of Labor			
Persistent Brow Presentation	–	GPP	–
Rotate and convert to vertex or face and deliver.			
Recommend cesarean section if pelvic disproportion suspected.			
Face Presentation	–	GPP	–
Spontaneous delivery as mentoanterior with adequate episiotomy.			
Rotate to mentoanterior and deliver.			
Recommend cesarean section if pelvic disproportion suspected.			

Malposition

Antenatal

There is probably little benefit from trying to alter an occipitoposterior position diagnosed during the antenatal period because the majority of cases correct themselves once labor starts. There may be some virtue in advising the patient that her membranes may rupture prior to the onset of contractions, that labor may be more uncomfortable and possibly more prolonged, and that there is a greater chance of requiring assistance with a vaginal delivery and need for delivery by cesarean section, when compared with a more optimal position. Some women say that they find difficult labor easier to cope with if forewarned, and they may be more inclined to choose an epidural early in labor. On the other hand, many occipitoposterior positions will correct spontaneously to occipitoanterior during labor, in which case anxiety will have been generated to no purpose, and it may increase the likelihood of maternal request for delivery by elective cesarean section. Some have suggested the patient adopts a variety of positions to encourage rotation of the fetus. An analysis of the literature, concentrating on the use of the maternal hands/knees position during the antenatal and intrapartum periods, concluded that this position compared with others resulted in a short-term reversion to an anterior position. There was no indication that this maneuver enhanced labor outcome, however.[52]

Intrapartum

When the diagnosis of malposition is made early in labor, as much information as possible should be gathered at this time about the fetal position, including the amount of head palpable per abdomen, the degree of deflexion and asynclitism, the amount of molding and caput formation, the level of the presenting part in relation to the ischial spines, and maternal pelvis size and shape. Issues relating to fetal well-being including fetal heart rate pattern and the color of the liquor should also be taken into account as with any labor.

Options at this point are as illustrated in the algorithm (see Fig. 65–9) and include

- no specific action if acceptable progress is being made.
- provide oxytocin augmentation if uterine contractions are incoordinate, infrequent, or of poor quality.
- abandoning labor in favor of cesarean section.
- encouraging the patient to lie on the same side as the fetal back.[53]

Once the second stage of labor has been reached, spontaneous delivery in the occipitoposterior position may occur, or spontaneous rotation may still occur with spontaneous delivery as occipitoanterior. Alternatively, delivery may be delayed by a persistence of the occipitoposterior position or the evolution of a deep transverse arrest. It has been suggested that vaginal manipulation to rotate the fetus to an occipitoanterior position should be avoided if fetal distress is suspected at that time, with resort instead to delivery by cesarean section. The decision on management at this stage should be determined by assessing which method of delivery is most likely to result in earlier delivery.

SUMMARY OF MANAGEMENT OPTIONS
Malposition

Management Options	Quality of Evidence	Strength of Recommendation	References
Prenatal			
No specific managements of proven benefit	Ib	A	52
Labor and Delivery See Figure 65–9			
First Stage of Labor			
Anticipate possible protracted uncomfortable labor.			
Offer regional analgesia if appropriate.	–	GPP	–
Augment with oxytocin infusion.	Ib	A	56
Consider cesarean section if secondary arrest.	–	GPP	–
Second Stage of Labor			
Spontaneous rotation and delivery in occipitoanterior position	–	GPP	–
Spontaneous delivery in occipitoposterior position:	–	GPP	–
Partial resolution to deep transverse arrest	–	GPP	–
-Rotation and delivery in occipitoanterior position			
-Cesarean section			
Persistent occipitoposterior position:	–	GPP	–
-Oxytocin augmentation to achieve a spontaneous delivery			
-Assisted delivery in occipitoposterior position			
-Rotation to occipitoanterior position and delivery			
-Cesarean section			

CONCLUSIONS

UNSTABLE LIE AND COMPOUND PRESENTATIONS

- A fetal or uterine abnormality can be responsible for the changing lie and compound presentation.
- The risk of complications such as cord prolapse and uterine rupture exists when the membranes rupture or once contractions begin.
- Some of the risks can be reduced by antenatal admission with action to correct the lie or deliver by cesarean section before labor.
- The most significant risk when the membranes rupture or labor starts is umbilical cord prolapse. This usually mandates delivery by cesarean section, but replacement of the cord is sometimes possible and should be considered.
- External or internal version at full dilatation should be considered if the lie is transverse or oblique and the membranes are intact.
- If there is a compound presentation with ruptured membranes, cesarean section is usually necessary, and a classical incision may be needed.

MALPRESENTATION AND MALPOSITION

- A primary face presentation may indicate a fetal abnormality and warrants appropriate investigation.
- During labor with a malpresentation, there is an increased risk of cord prolapse.
- In general, a fetus with a persistent brow presentation cannot be delivered vaginally, but conversion to vertex or face at full dilatation should be considered unless pelvic disproportion is anticipated.
- Fetuses with a face presentation can deliver vaginally in a mentoanterior position.
- Fetuses in an occipitoposterior position at full dilatation may deliver spontaneously occipitoanterior or posterior, require an assisted delivery occipitoposterior, or be rotated and delivered occipitoanterior, or may need to be delivered by cesarean section.
- A deep transverse arrest can usually be delivered vaginally by rotation and assisted delivery.

REFERENCES

1. Stevenson CS: Transverse or oblique presentation of the fetus in the last ten weeks of pregnancy: Its causes, general nature and treatment. Am J Obstet Gynecol 1994;58:432–446.
2. Savage E, Kohl SG, Wynn RM: Prolapse of the umbilical cord. Obstet Gynecol 1970;36:502–509.
3. Levy H, Meier PR, Makowski EL: Umbilical cord prolapse. Obstet Gynecol 1984;64:499–502.
4. Mesleh R, Sultan M, Sabagh T, Algwiser A: Umbilical cord prolapse. J Obstet Gynaecol 1993;13:24–28.
5. Murphy DJ, MacKenzie IZ: The mortality and morbidity associated with umbilical cord prolapse. BJOG 1995; 102:826–830.
6. Hellman LM, Epperson JWW, Connally F, Baltimore MD: Face and brow presentation. The experience of the Johns Hopkins Hospital 1896–1948. Am J Obstet Gynecol 1950; 59:831–842.
7. Vago T: Prolapse of the umbilical cord: A method of management. Am J Obstet Gynecol 1970;107:967–969.
8. Gardberg M, Laakkonen E, Salevaara M: Intrapartum sonography and persistent occiput posterior position: A study of 408 deliveries. Obstet Gynecol 1998;91:746–749.
9. O'Driscoll K, Jackson RJA, Gallagher JT: Active management of labour and cephalopelvic disproportion. J Obstet Gynaecol Br Commonw 1970;77:385–389.
10. Hoult IJ, MacLennan AH, Carrie LE: Lumbar epidural analgesia in labour: Relation to fetal malposition and instrumental delivery. Br Med J 1977;i:14–16.
11. Robinson CA, Macones GA, Roth NW, Morgan MA: Does station of the fetal head at epidural placement affect the position of the fetal vertex at delivery. Am J Obstet Gynecol 1996; 175:991–994.
12. Fitzpatrick M, McQuillan K, O'Herlihy C: Influence of persistent occiput posterior position on delivery outcome. Obstet Gynecol 2001;98:1027–1031.
13. Pritchard JA, MacDonald PC: Williams' Obstetrics, 16th ed. New York, Appleton-Century-Croft, 1980.
14. Breen JL, Wiesmeien E: Compound presentation—A survey of 131 patients. Obstet Gynecol 1968;32:419–422.
15. Cruikshank DP, White CA: Obstetric malpresentations—Twenty years experience. Am J Obstet Gynecol 1973; 116:1097–1104.
16. Weissberg SM, O'Leary JA: Compound presentation of the fetus. Obstet Gynecol 1973;41:60–64.
17. Yla-Outinen A, Heinonen PK, Tuimala R: Predisposing and risk factors of umbilical cord prolapse. Acta Obstet Gynecol Scand 1985;64:567–569.
18. Barrett JM: Fundic reduction for the management of umbilical cord prolapse. Am J Obstet Gynecol 1991;165:654–657.
19. Goplerud J, Eastman NJ: Compound presentation: Survey of 65 cases. Obstet Gynecol 1953;1:59–66.
20. Moir JC: Munro Kerr's Operative Obstetrics, 6th ed. London, Bailliere Tindall and Cox, 1956.
21. Posner LB, Rubin EJ, Posner AC: Face and brow presentations: A continuing study. Obstet Gynecol 1963;21:745–749.
22. Mostar S, Akaltin E, Babunca C: Deflexion attitudes: Median vertex, persistent brow and face presentations. Obstet Gynecol 1966;28:49–56.
23. Cruikshank DP, Cruikshank JE: Face and brow presentation: A review. Clin Obstet Gynecol 1981;24:333–351.
24. Dyson DC, Ferguson JE, Hensleigh P: Antepartum external cephalic version under tocolysis. Obstet Gynecol 1986;67:63–68.

25. Dawson JB: Occipito posterior position: Review of 415 cases. Br Med J 1940;i:612–613.
26. Miller D: The occipito posterior case: Its diagnosis and management. Br Med J 1930;i:1036–1039.
27. Gardberg M, Tuppurainen M: Persistent occipito posterior presentation—A clinical problem. Acta Obstet Gynecol Scand 1994;73:45–47.
28. Neri A, Kaplan B, Rabinson D, et al: The management of persistent occipito-posterior position. Clin Exp Obstet Gynecol 1995;22:126–131.
29. Westgren M, Edvall H, Nordstrom L, et al: Spontaneous cephalic version of breech presentation in the last trimester. BJOG 1985;92:19–22.
30. Nwosu EC, Walkinshaw S, Chia P, et al: Undiagnosed breech. BJOG 1993;100:531–535.
31. Lange IR, Manning FA, Morrison I, et al: Cord prolapse: Is antenatal diagnosis possible? Am J Obstet Gynecol 1985; 151:1083–1085.
32. Sherer DM, Onyeije CI, Bernstein PS, et al: Utilization of real-time ultrasound in labor and delivery in an active academic teaching hospital. Am J Perinatol 1999;16:303–307.
33. Kreiser D, Schiff E, Lipitz S, et al: Determination of fetal occiput position by ultrasound during the second stage of labor. J Matern Fetal Med 2001;10:283–286.
34. Akmal S, Tsoi E, Kametas N, et al: Intrapartum sonography to determine fetal head position. J Matern Fetal Med 2002;12:172–177.
35. Fried AW, Cloutier M, Woodring JH, et al. Sonography on the transverse fetal lie. AJR 1984;142:421–423.
36. Hughey MJ: Fetal position during pregnancy. Am J Obstet Gynecol 1985;153:885–886.
37. Phelan JP, Boucher M, Mueller E, et al: The nonlaboring transverse lie: A management dilemma. J Reprod Med 1986;1:184–186.
38. Edwards RL, Nicholson HO: The management of the unstable lie in late pregnancy. J Obstet Gynaecol Br Commonw 1969;76:713–718.
39. Brocks V, Philipsen T, Secher NJ: A randomised trial of external cephalic version with tocolysis in late pregnancy. BJOG 1984;91:653–656.
40. Fall O, Nilsson BA: External cephalic version in breech presentation under tocolysis. Obstet Gynecol 1979;53:712–715.
41. Hibbard LT, Schumann WR: Prophylactic external cephalic version in an obstetric practice. Am J Obstet Gynecol 1973;116:511–516.
42. Atosiban Study Group: Effectiveness and safety of the oxytocin antagonist atosiban versus beta-adrenergic agonists in the treatment of preterm labour. BJOG 2001;108:133–142.
43. Elkins V: In Enkin M, Chalmers I (eds): Effectiveness and Satisfaction in Antenatal Care. London, Spastics International Medical Publishers, 1982, p 216.
44. Hofmeyr GJ: Effect of external cephalic version in late pregnancy on breech presentation and caesarean section rate: A controlled trial. Br Med J 1983;90:392–399.
45. Bung P, Huch R, Huch A: Ist die indische wendung eine erfolgreiche methode zur senking der beckenendlage-frequenz? Geburtshilfe Frauenheilkd 1987;47:202–205.
46. Chenia F, Crowther C: Does advice to assume the knee-chest position reduce the incidence of breech presentation at delivery? Birth 1987;14:75–78.
47. Ranney B: The gentle art of external cephalic version. Am J Obstet Gynecol 1973;116:239–245.
48. Saling E, Muller-Holve W: External cephalic version under tocolysis. J Perinat Med 1975;3:115–122.
49. Drew-Smythe HG: Indications for the induction of premature labour. Br Med J 1931;1:1018–1020.
50. Okunwobi-Smith Y, Cooke IE, MacKenzie IZ: Decision to delivery intervals for assisted vaginal vertex delivery. BJOG 2000;107:467–471.
51. Phelan JP, Stine LE, Edwards NB: The role of external version in the intrapartum management of the transverse lie presentation. Am J Obstet Gynecol 1985;151:724–726.
52. Hofmeyr GJ, Kulier R: Hands/knees posture in late pregnancy or labour for fetal malposition (lateral or posterior). Cochrane Database Syst Rev 2000;(2):CD001063.
53. Wu X, Fan L, Wang Q: Correction of occipito-posterior by maternal postures during the process of labor. Zhonghua Fu Chan Ke Za Zhi 2001;36:468–469.
54. Hofmeyr GJ, Kulier R: External cephalic version for breech presentation at term. Cochrane Database Syst Rev 2002; (2):CD000083.
55. Hofmeyr GJ, Hannah ME: Planned caesarean section for term breech delivery. Cochrane Database Syst Rev 2001; (2):CD000166.
56. Cammu H, Van Eeckhout E: A randomised controlled trial of early versus delayed use of amniotomy and oxytocin infusion in nulliparous labour. BJOG 1996;103:313–318.

CHAPTER 66

Prolonged Pregnancy

John M. Grant

INTRODUCTION

Induction of labor for prolonged pregnancy is one of the commonest interventions in pregnancy, with up to one quarter of pregnant women undergoing this procedure. Obstetricians may fear prolonged pregnancy, for if the infant is stillborn at 43 weeks' gestation, they will be criticized by the parents and by their peers, and can be subject to litigation. Pregnant women may ask for induction of labor to relieve themselves of the discomforts of pregnancy in the later weeks. Midwives may comfortably undertake induction of labor, bearing in mind the ease of administration of vaginal prostaglandin. It is not surprising, therefore, that induction of labor for prolonged pregnancy is so common. So secure seems the practice of induction of labor for prolonged pregnancy that authoritative organizations recommend that "women should be offered induction of labor after 41 weeks gestation."[1,2] Yet this recommendation is founded on uncertain clinical science.

DEFINITION

This is the first uncertainty. Even the name of the condition is uncertain, and may be called "prolonged pregnancy," "postmaturity," "post-dates pregnancy," and "post-term pregnancy." The International Federation of Gynecologists and Obstetricians defines prolonged pregnancy as one that is longer than 294 days after the last menstrual period.[3] The Cochrane Collaboration has identified 13 randomized trials of induction of labor after 41 weeks' gestation.[4–17] In 10 of the trials, prolonged pregnancy was defined: prolonged pregnancy was considered to be 287 days after the last menstrual period in two trials,[9,15] 290 to 297 days in one,[10] 292 to 294 days in one,[8] 293 days in one,[5] 294 days in four,[6,9,11,14] and 287 to 301 days in one.[16] The largest trial, which contributed 59% of women to the systematic review, used 287 days as the definition of prolonged pregnancy.[15] This variation in the definition of prolonged pregnancy is important, for a pregnancy at 287 days' gestation is biologically different from a pregnancy at 301 days, both from the risk of uteroplacental insufficiency and from the ease of induction of labor. This variation in definition contributes much to the confusion surrounding prolonged pregnancy.

INCIDENCE

Why are we so exercised by the concept of prolonged pregnancy? It is because of the risk of intrauterine death of the infant, birth asphyxia in labor, and shoulder dystocia at delivery. Induction of labor for prolonged pregnancy is intended to be a prophylactic measure to prevent these serious complications. These risks increase with increasing gestational age after term, but are still small. After 42 weeks' gestation the risk of stillbirth is about 1 in 1000 pregnancies, and after 43 weeks' gestation it is about 1 in 500 pregnancies.[18] There are similar risks of neonatal death at these gestational ages. Thus, even after 43 weeks' gestation the risk of perinatal death is small, about 1 in 250 pregnancies. Observational studies show that the frequency of birth asphyxia is also small, the estimate being 1 in 350 pregnancies at 42 weeks' gestation in one study[19] and 1 in 490 pregnancies in another.[20] Shoulder dystocia in prolonged pregnancy is due to increasing birth weight in the infant beyond term. It may be more frequent than fetal death in pregnancy and birth asphyxia in labor. The estimates for shoulder dystocia are 1 in 75 pregnancies at 42 weeks' gestation in one study,[21] 1 in 28 pregnancies in a second,[22] and 1 in 77 pregnancies in a third.[23] Shoulder dystocia also has a variable definition, according to the perception of the obstetrician. Probably, shoulder dystocia that matters requires procedures beyond the McRobert's maneuver for its resolution. These procedures are not commonly stated in the literature, and so the frequency of important shoulder dystocia in prolonged pregnancy is unknown.

Many more women are considered to have prolonged pregnancy than are at risk of these serious complications. After the due date, spontaneous labor will occur every day in 10% of women who have not yet delivered. This means that the proportions of women who have not yet delivered will be about 24% at 41 weeks', 11% at 42 weeks', and 5% at 43 weeks' gestation. Many women are delivered before the due date by elective cesarean section, many women undergo induction of labor before the due date for preeclampsia and other medical indications, and many women undergo induction of labor before the due date for social reasons or because of the discomforts of late pregnancy. The variation in the definition of prolonged pregnancy, and the variation in the frequency of elective delivery before the due date partly account for the variation in the incidence of prolonged pregnancy in different populations.[18–23] Measurement of gestational age by ultrasound in early pregnancy reduces the incidence of mistaken prolonged pregnancy.[24–27] Another consideration is the definition of the due date. This may be defined as 280 days or 40 weeks after the date of the first day of the last menstrual period, which is the mean value if gestational age is assumed to adopt a statistical normal distribution. However, the distribution is not normal, for it is skewed toward lower gestational ages on account of prematurity, and also toward higher gestational ages, perhaps on account of some pregnancies that are genuinely pathologically prolonged. It is statistically more correct to consider the due date as the median or the mode. The median is 282 days, and the mode is 283 days.[28] If the due date is counted as 283 days after the last menstrual period, then a definition of prolonged pregnancy of an arbitrarily chosen number of days after this date would reduce the number of women who would be considered eligible for induction of labor by about 27%.

RISKS

Maternal Risks

The main risk to the pregnant woman is not from prolonged pregnancy itself, but from the consequences of induction of labor to prevent prolonged pregnancy.

The Cochrane Collaboration has carried out a meta-analysis of the effect of induction of labor at 41+ weeks' gestation on the likelihood of cesarean section. The meta-analysis suggests that the risk of cesarean section is reduced by 13% (typical odds ratio 0.87; 95% confidence interval [CI] 0.76–0.99; $P = 0.02$).[5,6,8–17] This information has been used by authoritative organizations to support their recommendation for the routine offer of induction of labor after 41 weeks' gestation.

However, analysis of these trials shows that clinically they were quite different. We have already noted the variation in the definition of prolonged pregnancy. There were also variations in the physical characteristics of the cervix at induction of labor. In five randomized trials, women with both favorable and unfavorable cervices were included[5,8,10,11,13]; in four trials women with unfavorable cervices only were included[6,9,16,17]; and in the trial by Hannah and colleagues the cervix had to be less than 3 cm dilated.[12] In the other three trials the state of the cervix was not mentioned. There was variation in the methods of induction of labor. In five randomized trials, labor was induced by low amniotomy and simultaneous oxytocin infusion[5,6,10,11,13]; in one trial by 3 mg of vaginal prostaglandin[8]; in one trial initially by 3 mg of vaginal prostaglandin followed by 0.5 mg intracervical prostaglandin[9]; in one trial by 3 mg intracervical prostaglandin[15]; and in two trials by 0.5 mg intracervical prostaglandin.[16,17] But the greatest variation was in the methods of fetal monitoring in the control subjects: amnioscopy[5]; urinary estriols[11,13]; nonstressed cardiotocography[8–10,15–17]; fetal movement charts[6,8,15,16]; oxytocin challenge test[6,11]; fetal biometry[8]; amniotic fluid volume[6,8,9,16,17]; and the "atropine test."[13]

These randomized trials show such clinical variation that they should never have been combined in a meta-analysis. Variations in the definitions of prolonged pregnancy, the state of the cervix at induction of labor, the methods of induction of labor, and the methods of fetal monitoring in the control group have a much greater influence on cesarean section than induction of labor overall. We cannot be confident that randomization would have smoothed out all the variation in prognostic factors between the experimental and the control groups, for many of the trials were small, and differences in prognostic factors in each trial may have occurred by chance. Many of the trials are old and used methods of induction of labor and fetal monitoring that are not used today. We cannot be confident even of the largest, most recent randomized trial.[16] This trial used a method of induction of labor that is not common in the United Kingdom, intracervical prostaglandins; women in the control group did not have intracervical prostaglandins if uteroplacental insufficiency was suspected; and obstetricians may have been more likely to perform a cesarean section in the control group if they suspected fetal hypoxia in labor.

This misleading meta-analysis shows the dangers of a systematic review performed by statisticians, and not by obstetricians. In this systematic review far too much attention was paid to the mathematics of meta-analysis than to the clinical characteristics of the trials contributing to the systematic review. Obstetricians should not accept the results of a systematic review unless they themselves have analyzed the content of the randomized trials contributing to the review. If there is clinical variation in the trials, the statistical results of any meta-analysis arising from the systematic review should be rejected.

Almost certainly, in primigravidas at least, in most maternity units induction of labor increases the risk of cesarean section. I carried a systematic review in MEDLINE of observational studies carried out from 1995 to 2001, of induction of labor in primiparas, using the keywords *primipara, induction of labor* and *cesarean section*. In each study women who underwent induction of labor were compared with women who did not undergo induction of labor. The overwhelming indication for induction of labor was "post dates," genuine medical indications such as preeclampsia being very much in the minority. Fourteen such studies were found.[29–42] Because the frequency of uteroplacental insufficiency in prolonged pregnancy is rare, it is likely that uteroplacental function in the women who underwent induction of labor was no different from uteroplacental function in the women who did not undergo induction of labor. If induction of labor did not increase the likelihood of cesarean section, we would expect, by chance, that in these 14 studies induction of labor would be associated with a decrease in the rate of cesarean section just as often as an increase in the rate of cesarean section. Two of the 14 studies showed a decrease, and 12 showed an increase in the rate of cesarean section with induction of labor. By the sign test this difference is statistically significant, the probability that this difference is due to chance being 0.008. Thus, in general, induction of labor in primiparas results in an increase in the risk of cesarean section.

Why should the results of the randomized trials be so different from the observational studies? Almost certainly the interpretation of the randomized trials has been too naïve, for induction of labor, and labor itself, are very complex processes. We know that in spontaneous labor the risk of cesarean section strongly depends upon organizational factors governing the management of labor in maternity hospitals. These factors include policies concerning active management of labor; a dedicated midwife; a member of the family or other companion during labor; the timing of routine vaginal examinations; the training of obstetricians and midwives in electronic fetal monitoring; and the number and seniority of the midwives and obstetricians attending the labor ward. In most maternity units it is likely that induction of labor will act adversely, in conjunction with one or more of these factors, to increase the likelihood of cesarean section. Induction of labor is a complex procedure that involves much work and supervision by midwives and obstetricians—administration of vaginal prostaglandins, amniotomy, electronic fetal monitoring, and intravenous oxytocin infusion. There is an increased chance of slow labor, epidural analgesia, and abnormalities of the fetal heart rate. Thus, in an understaffed maternity unit induction of labor is an unwelcome burden and will result an increased likelihood of cesarean section in order to clear the decks for women who actually have an important medical complication of pregnancy, such as preeclampsia.

Less commonly, induction of labor will act beneficially, in conjunction with one or more of these factors, to decrease the likelihood of cesarean section. Thus, in a well-staffed maternity unit with a midwife dedicated to the care of each woman in labor and who is well trained in the interpretation of fetal heart rate traces, induction of labor may increase the chance of a vaginal delivery.

The important lesson is that maternity units should not turn to meta-analyses of randomized trials to guide their policies concerning induction of labor, but that each maternity unit should make its own comparison of primiparas who have their labor induced and primiparas who do not have their labor induced. If the rate of cesarean section in women who undergo induction of labor is significantly higher than in women who do not undergo induction of labor, as in 12 of the maternity hospitals in this survey, then induction of labor for "post-dates" pregnancy should be restricted. If the rate of cesarean section in women who undergo induction of labor is lower than in women who do not undergo induction of labor, as in two of the maternity hospitals in this survey, then induction of labor for "post-dates" pregnancy should be liberal.

Fetal and Neonatal Risks

The risk of stillbirth from 37 weeks onward is 1 in 3000 pregnancies, from 42 weeks onward it is 1 in 1000 pregnancies, and from 43 weeks onward it is 1 in 500 pregnancies.[18] The risk of neonatal death from birth asphyxia and from trauma in prolonged pregnancy is not certain. The systematic review in the Cochrane Collaboration involved 6073 women, 3071 allocated to induction of labor and 3002 allocated to fetal surveillance.[4–12] There was one perinatal death in the women who underwent induction of labor and seven perinatal deaths in the control group (odds ratio 0.22; 95% CI 0.05–0.87; $P = 0.03$). The odds ratio is impressive, suggesting that the risk of perinatal death is reduced by a factor of 4 with a policy of induction of labor. The 95% CI does not cross unity, suggesting that even allowing for statistical sampling error, the risk of perinatal death is reduced by a policy of induction of labor.

This information has been used to justify a policy of induction of labor at 41 weeks' gestation and beyond, but is this policy justifiable? The 13 randomized trials in the Cochrane Collaboration resulted in only eight perinatal deaths in more than 6000 women. This is surely a tiny number of perinatal deaths with which to justify such an invasive intervention in so many women in pregnancy. By 41 weeks' gestation, one quarter of all pregnant women would be considered eligible for induction of labor. According to the results of this systematic review 498 women would have to undergo induction of labor at 41 weeks' gestation and beyond in order to prevent one perinatal death. This would not matter if induction of labor were a trivial procedure, but as we have seen, it is a very complex procedure. If in this systematic review there had been two perinatal deaths in the women who were allocated to induction of labor, the difference in perinatal mortality between induction of labor and fetal surveillance would no longer be statistically significant (odds ratio 0.32; 95% CI 0.09–1.19; $P = 0.09$). Thus, we would be less secure in advocating a policy of induction of labor from 41 weeks onward. This illustrates the marginal nature of the evidence underlying current recommendations.

Almost certainly, the combined size of the 13 randomized trials in the Cochrane Collaboration is too small to be able to show reliably a reduction in perinatal mortality rate with induction of labor. The results of the systematic review in the Cochrane Collaboration show that perinatal death occurred in about 1 of 500 pregnancies in the women allocated to fetal surveillance. In order to test the hypothesis that induction of labor will reduce this rate of perinatal mortality by one half, 47,000 women at 41 weeks' gestation would be required to participate in the trial ($\alpha = 0.05$; $1 - \beta = 0.80$). The power of the 13 trials in this systematic review is 0.17. In this systematic review, therefore, with 6073 participants, there was only a 17% chance of being able to show a reduction in perinatal mortality rate with induction of labor. The apparent significant reduction in perinatal mortality rate found in this systematic review could easily be a type I statistical error. The justification for supposing that a policy of induction of labor from 41 weeks onward will reduce perinatal mortality rate is therefore very shaky.

MANAGEMENT OPTIONS

Prepregnancy

Nothing can be done before pregnancy to influence the problems of post-term pregnancy.

Prenatal

Estimation of gestational age by ultrasound examination in early pregnancy will reduce the number of women who are subjected to induction of labor.[24–27] In the Western world estimation of gestational age by ultrasound has become routine, for reasons that are not connected with prolonged pregnancy, such as the timing of prenatal diagnosis. In maternity units with a high rate of induction of labor for prolonged pregnancy, assessment of gestational age in early pregnancy should be performed.

Fetal Surveillance

The focus of randomized trials in prolonged pregnancy has been the comparison of a surgical intervention, induction of labor, and "fetal surveillance," in its broadest sense. Little attention has been paid to a comparison of various forms of fetal surveillance and no surveillance, or various forms of fetal surveillance with one another. Observational studies suggest that cardiotocography, measurement of the volume of amniotic fluid by ultrasound, and Doppler assessment of fetal and uteroplacental arteries are unlikely to predict fetal outcome reliably. A randomized trial of cardiotocography and measurement of the amniotic fluid index compared with induction of labor suggested that the rates of cesarean section and meconium below the vocal cords were increased in pregnancies beyond 42 weeks' gestation.[43] Another trial compared amniotic fluid index with maximum depth of the amniotic fluid in prolonged pregnancy, and found that use of the amniotic fluid index increased the likelihood of induction of labor with no apparent benefit to the infant.[44] A third randomized trial compared a modified biophysical profile score with cardiotocography combined with maximum depth of the amniotic fluid, and found that there were more abnormal results in the women randomized to measurement of the biophysical profile score with no apparent benefit to the infant.[45] Counting of fetal movements by the pregnant woman in prolonged pregnancy does not decrease the risk of stillbirth.[46]

Prolonged pregnancy is the commonest indication for induction of labor and involves an enormous expenditure of effort by obstetricians and midwives, yet its pathophysiology is poorly understood. In some respects the effect of prolonged pregnancy is similar to idiopathic intrauterine growth restriction, but whereas the pathophysiology of the latter condition is well understood, the pathophysiology of the former has been scarcely researched. In intrauterine growth restriction biopsies of the decidua at the site of attachment of the placenta show failure of trophoblastic invasion of the spiral arteries, resulting in reduced uteroplacental blood flow, reduction of growth of the infant, and progressive fetal hypoxia and metabolic acidosis.[47] Because uteroplacental insufficiency is a progressive phenomenon in pregnancy, some cases of fetal death in prolonged pregnancy may be due to the syndrome of idiopathic growth restriction continuing beyond term. Certainly we know that when fetal death occurs in prolonged pregnancy the birth weight is lower than when fetal death does not occur, yet other parameters of uteroplacental compromise, such as umbilical blood flow and amniotic fluid volume, are not abnormal in prolonged pregnancies (see earlier discussion). Could the problem with prolonged pregnancy lie with cellular function in the trophoblast? Does apoptosis occur to a greater degree when fetal death occurs in prolonged pregnancy?[48] The controversies surrounding prolonged pregnancy will not be resolved until these and similar questions are answered by research into the basic science of the problem.

Other Interventions

Certainly it defies common sense to subject so many women to such an invasive procedure as induction of labor in the face of so little understanding of the scientific nature of prolonged pregnancy. Above all, there should be an embargo on randomized trials of induction of labor in prolonged pregnancy, and maternity units should seek ways of reducing the number of women subjected to induction of labor.

The very existence of "prolonged pregnancy" has even been questioned. It probably does exist, because perinatal mortality rate increases progressively from term onward, but even at 43 weeks' gestation this risk is still very small. Even at this gestational age fetal hypoxia and metabolic acidosis are rare.

The obstetrician is therefore faced with a dilemma when attempting to give advice to a woman about prolonged pregnancy. Induction of labor has entered the culture of obstetrics in the Western world, and women may wish to have labor induced, even long before 41 weeks' gestation. Refusal to induce labor risks losing the trust of the pregnant woman, especially given the current widespread practice of recommending induction at 41 weeks; and if the tragedy of a stillbirth occurs, the obstetrician may become involved in unpleasant litigation.[49] The obstetrician will find it difficult to defend the concept that prolonged pregnancy does not exist. It is probably wise to recommend induction of labor after 42 completed weeks' gestation, this being the definition of prolonged pregnancy by an authoritative body, the International Federation of Gynecologists and Obstetricians.[3] If before that time the woman is anxious about prolonged pregnancy, then sweeping of the membranes may be performed[50]; this simple procedure will result in natural labor occurring in three quarters of the women. If the woman prefers induction of labor before 42 weeks' gestation, she must be made to understand the risks of failed induction of labor, cesarean section, fetal distress due to hypertonic uterine action, greater need for epidural analgesia, and a greater chance of vacuum extraction or forceps delivery.

CONCLUSIONS

- Prolonged pregnancy has an uncertain definition and uncertain pathophysiology; more basic research into the pathophysiology of prolonged pregnancy is required.
- If a definition of 41 weeks is used, about one quarter of all women will be considered to have prolonged pregnancy; using 42 weeks as the definition will reduce this figure to 11%.
- Meta-analysis of randomized trials of induction of labor in prolonged pregnancy suggests a reduction in perinatal mortality rate and a reduction in the rate of cesarean section; but the randomized trials are so variable clinically that these conclusions are not justified.
- Observational data suggest that routine induction of labor for prolonged pregnancy increases the risks of cesarean section (especially in primigravidas), fetal distress, greater need for epidural analgesia, and a greater chance of an assisted vaginal delivery.

SUMMARY OF MANAGEMENT OPTIONS
Prolonged Pregnancy

Management Options	Quality of Evidence	Strength of Recommendation	References
Prenatal—General			
Establish accurate gestational age as early as possible.	Ia	A	4, 24–27
Menstrual dates overestimate gestation. Routine early scan of value in preventing induction for "post dates."	Ia	A	4, 24–27
Sweeping membranes at term reduces chances of pregnancy going beyond 41 weeks.	Ia	A	50
Prenatal—At 41 Weeks			
Re-evaluate for possible risk factors.	–	GPP	–
Active Management Option (induction of labor): Controversy continues over this issue			
a) RCT evidence supports this approach: Routine induction of labor for prolonged pregnancy reduces perinatal mortality.	Ia	A	4
Labor induction does not increase cesarean section rate or operative vaginal delivery rate if cervix made favorable first.			

SUMMARY OF MANAGEMENT OPTIONS
Prolonged Pregnancy *(Continued)*

Management Options	Quality of Evidence	Strength of Recommendation	References
Prenatal—At 41 Weeks			
The author believes that the interpretation of the RCT data is flawed because			
Randomization does not preclude an effect from the varied clinical practice between the trials.			
Although a difference in perinatal mortality was observed, this was on the basis of very small differences.			
b) Observational data do not support this approach	IIa–III	B	29–42
Routine induction of labor for prolonged pregnancy increases the risks of cesarean section (especially in primigravidae), fetal distress, greater need for epidural analgesia, and a greater chance of an assisted vaginal delivery.			
Expectant Management Option (fetal surveillance): *Overall very little evidence to suggest that monitoring identifies at-risk fetuses or improves outcome though most studies underpowered.*			
Routine fetal movement counts alone not shown to reducing perinatal deaths—no specific data in prolonged pregnancies.	Ib	A	46
NST and measurement of the amniotic fluid index in pregnancies beyond 42 weeks have higher rates of cesarean section and meconium below the vocal cords compared to induction of labor.	Ib	A	43
Modified biophysical profile score testing in prolonged pregnancy results in more abnormal results and interventions compared to NST combined with maximum depth of the amniotic fluid with no apparent benefit to the infant.	Ib	A	45
Assessment of amniotic fluid index versus vertical pockets of amniotic fluid increase obstetric intervention.	Ib	A	44
Labor and Delivery			
Vigilance for fetal hypoxia and shoulder dystocia	–	GPP	–

AFV, amniotic fluid volume; NST, non-stress test.

REFERENCES

1. Royal College of Obstetricians and Gynaecologists: Induction of Labour. Evidence-based Clinical Guideline. London, RCOG Press, 2001, pp 24–26.
2. Maternal-Fetal Medicine Committee of the Society of Obstetricians and Gynaecologists of Canada: Postterm Pregnancy (Committee Opinion). SOGC Clinical Practice Guidelines, No. 15. 1997.
3. International Federation of Gynecologists and Obstetricians: International classification of diseases: Update. Int J Obstet Gynecol 1980;17:634–640.
4. Crowley P: Interventions for preventing or improving the outcome of delivery at or beyond term. Cochrane Database Syst Rev 2001;issue 2.
5. Henry GR: A controlled trial of surgical induction of labour and amnioscopy in the management of ptolonged pregnancy. J Obstet Gynaecol Br Commonw 1969;76:795–798.
6. Katz Z, Yemini M, Lancet M, et al: Non-aggressive management of post-dates pregnancies. Eur J Obstet Gynecol Reprod Biol 1983;15:71–79.
7. Suikkari AM, Jalkanen M, Heiskala H, Koskela O: Prolonged pregnancy: Induction or observation. Acta Obstet Gynecol Scand Suppl 1983;116:58.
8. Cardozo L, Fysh J, Pearce M: Prolonged pregnancy: The management debate. BMJ 1986;293:1059–1063.
9. Dyson DC, Miller PD, Armstrong MA: Management of prolonged pregnancy: Induction of labour versus antepartum fetal testing. Am J Obstet Gynecol 1987;156:928–934.
10. Augensen K, Bergsjo P, Eikeland T, et al: Randomised comparison of early versus late induction of labor in post-term pregnancy. BMJ 1987;294:1192–1195.
11. Witter FR, Weitz CM: A randomized trial of induction of labour at 42 weeks gestation versus expectant management for postdates pregnancies. Am J Perinatol 1987;4:206–211.
12. Martin JN, Sessums JK, Howard P, et al: Alternative approaches to the management of gravidas with prolonged post-term postdate pregnancies. J Miss State Med Assoc 1989;30:105–111.
13. Bergsjo P, Huang GD, Yu SQ, et al: Comparison of induced versus non-induced labor in post-term pregnancy. A random-

ized prospective study. Acta Obstet Gynecol Scand 1989; 68:683–687.
14. Heden L, Ingemarsson I, Ahlstrom H, Solum T: Induction of labour vs conservative management in prolonged pregnancy: Controlled study. Int J Feto-matern Med 1991;4:148–152.
15. Herabutya Y, Prasertsawat PO, Tongyai T, et al: Prolonged pregnancy: The management dilemma. Int J Gynaecol Obstet 1992;37:253–258.
16. Hannah ME, Hannah WJ, Hellmann J, et al: Induction of labor as compared with serial antenatal monitoring in post-term pregnancy. A randomized controlled trial. The Canadian Multicenter Post-term Pregnancy Trial Group. N Engl J Med 1992; 326:1628–1629.
17. National Institute of Child Health and Human Development of Maternal-Fetal Units: A clinical trial of induction of labour versus expectant management in postterm pregnancy. Am J Obstet Gynecol 1994;170:716–723.
18. Hilder L, Costeloe K, Thilaganathan B: Prolonged pregnancy: Evaluating gestation-specific risks of fetal and infant mortality. BJOG 1998;105:169–173.
19. Usher RH, Boyd ME, McLean FH, Kramer MS: Assessment of fetal risk in postdates pregnancies. Am J Obstet Gynecol 1988;158:259–264.
20. Alexander JM, McIntyre DD, Leveno KJ: Forty weeks and beyond: Pregnancy outcomes by week of gestation. Obstet Gynecol 2000;96:291–294.
21. Baskett TF, Allen AC: Perinatal complications of shoulder dystocia. Obstet Gynecol 1995;86:14–17.
22. Acker DB, Sachs BP, Friedman EA: Risk factors for shoulder dystocia. Obstet Gynecol 1985;66:762–768.
23. Eden RD, Seifert LS, Winegar A, Spellacy WN: Perinatal characteristic of uncomplicated postdate pregnancies. Obstet Gynecol 1987;69:296–299.
24. Bakketeig LS, Jacobsen G, Brodtkorb CJ, et al: Randomised controlled trial of ultrasonographic screening in pregnancy. Lancet 1984;ii:207–210.
25. Waldenstrom U, Axelsson O, Nilsson S, et al: Effects of routine one-stage ultrasound screening in pregnancy: A randomised controlled trial. Lancet 1988;ii:585–588.
26. Ewigman B, Lefevre M, Hesser J: A randomised trial of routine prenatal ultrasound. Obstet Gynecol 1990;76:189–194.
27. Ewigman BG, Crane JP, Frigoletto FD, et al and the RADIUS study group: Effect of prenatal ultrasound screening on perinatal outcome. N Engl J Med 1993;329:821–827.
28. Bergsjo P, Denman DW, Hoffman HJ, Meirik O: Duration of human singleton pregnancy. A population-based study. Acta Obstet Gynecol Scand 1990;69:197–207.
29. Weeks JW, Pitman T, Spinnato JA: Fetal macrosomia: Does prediction affect delivery route and birth outcome? Am J Obstet Gynecol 1995;173:1215–1219.
30. Prysak M, Castronova FC: Elective induction versus spontaneous labor: A case-control analysis of safety and efficacy. Obstet Gynecol 1998;92:1056–1057.
31. Parry E, Parry D, Pattison N: Induction of labour for post-term pregnancy: An observational study. Aust N Z J Obstet Gynaecol 1998;38:275–280.
32. Yeast JD, Jones A, Poskin M: Induction of labor and the relationship to cesarean delivery: A review of 7001 consecutive inductions. Am J Obstet Gynecol 1999;180:628–633.
33. Seyb ST, Berka RJ, Socol ML, Dooley SL: Risk of cesarean delivery with elective induction of labor at term in nulliparous women. Obstet Gynecol 1999;94:600–607.
34. Nuutila M, Halmesmaki E, Hiilesmaa V, Ylikorkala O: Women's anticipations of and experiences with induction of labor. Acta Obstet Gynecol Scand 1999;78:704–709.
35. Buist R: Induction of labour: Indications and obstetric outcomes in a tertiary referral hospital. N Z Med J 1999;112: 251–253.
36. Dublin S, Lydon-Rochelle M, Kaplan RC, et al: Maternal and neonatal outcomes after induction of labor without an identified indication. Am J Obstet Gynecol 2000;183:986–994.
37. Maslow AS, Sweeny AL: Elective induction of labor as a risk factor for cesarean delivery among low-risk women at term. Obstet Gynecol 2000;95:917–922.
38. Duff C, Sinclair M: Exploring the risks associated with induction of labour: A retrospective study using the NIMATS database. Northern Ireland Maternity System. J Adv Nurs 2000;31: 310–417.
39. Coonrod DV, Bay RC, Kishi GY: The epidemiology of labor induction: Arizona, 1997. Am J Obstet Gynecol 2000;182: 1355–1362.
40. Yawn BP, Wollan P, McKeon K, Field CS: Temporal changes in rates and reasons for medical induction of term labor. Am J Obstet Gynecol 2001;184:611–619.
41. Sue-Quan AK, Hannah ME, Cohen MM, et al: Effect of labour induction on rates of stillbirth and cesarean section in post-term pregnancies. Can Med Assoc J 1999;160:1145–1149.
42. Beebe LA, Rayburn WF, Beaty CM, et al: Indications for labor induction. Differences between university and community hospitals. J Reprod Med 2000;45:469–475.
43. Roach VJ, Rogers MS: Pregnancy outcomes beyond 41 weeks gestation. Int J Gynaecol Obstet 1997;59:19–24.
44. Alfiveric Z, Luckas M, Walkinshaw SA, et al: A randomised comparison between amniotic fluid index and maximum pool depth in the monitoring of post-term pregnancies. BJOG 1997;104: 207–211.
45. Alfiveric Z, Walkinshaw SA: A randomised controlled trial of simple compared with complex antenatal monitoring after 42 weeks of gestation. BJOG 1995;102:638–643.
46. Grant A, Elbourne D, Valentin L, Alexander S: Routine formal movement counting and risk of antepartum late death in normally formed singletons. Lancet 1989;ii:345–349.
47. Gerretsen G, Huisjes HJ, Hardonk MJ, Elema JD: Trophoblast alterations in the placental bed in relation to physiological changes in spiral arteries. BJOG 1983;90:34–39.
48. Smith SC, Baker PN: Placental apoptosis in post-term pregnancies. BJOG 1999;106:861–862.
49. Dimond B: Legal aspects of consent 3: Duty of care to inform. Br J Nurs 2001;10:466–468.
50. Boulvain M, Stan C, Irion O: Membrane sweeping for induction of labour. Cochrane Database Syst Rev 2005;issue2

CHAPTER 67

Labor—An Overview

Philip J. Steer

WHY HUMAN LABOR IS DIFFICULT

Recent years have seen an explosion of knowledge about early human origins (see, for example, www.modernhumanorigins.com and www.talkorigins.org); it is now thought that bipedal apes were living in Africa as long ago as 6.5 million years (MY) ago.[1,2] By about 3 MY ago, it is likely that at as many as six separate species of hominid coexisted in Africa.[3–5] These Australopithecines ("southern apes") had an almost human-shaped pelvis and walked erect efficiently, but still had a brain capacity equivalent to that of a chimpanzee—about 400 cm.[3] Among the many theories for the evolution of erect posture are that it provided an expanded visual horizon from standing upright on the savannah, which by then covered much of Africa, exposed less body area to the direct rays of the noonday sun, conferred the ability to go fishing in shallow water, and freed the hands for tool holding. Whatever the selectional advantages of the upright posture, the narrow pelvis that resulted (aiding the efficient transfer of forces from the legs to the spine while running) severely limits the cranial capacity of any infant that can be born successfully. However, the development of rotational birth enabled larger fetal heads to pass through the maternal pelvis,[6] and about 1.5 MY *Homo erectus* appeared with an adult cranial capacity of 900 cm^3.[7] It was probably the demands of socialization in troupes (or tribes) that selected for higher brain capacity, with the development of a language instinct being particularly advantageous.[8] The mechanism may well have been neoteny, the persistence of the fetal form into adult life, producing in this case a larger brain/body ratio. Species such as *Homo neanderthalensis* and *Homo sapiens* emerged, both with cranial capacities ranging from 1000 to 1800 cm^3.[3] It may have been *Homo sapiens*' superior language skills that allowed it to succeed by developing a culture, which could be passed down the generations, whereas *Homo neanderthalensis* showed no such progress and died out about 30,000 years ago.[8]

Although being able to run fast and think quickly are both advantageous, they produce an obvious conflict at the time of birth. Babies with large heads can (and do) wreak havoc on their mother's pelvis, causing urinary[9] and fecal[10] incontinence, and even vesicovaginal fistulae.[11] Neglected, prolonged, obstructed labor can in addition lead to renal failure, pelvic inflammatory disease, osteitis pubis, foot drop, and secondary infertility. In rural Africa, the lifetime risk of maternal mortality from childbirth may be as high as 1 in 15.[11] One study has shown that even in Sweden, where birth injury is relatively uncommon, 1 in 40 women will experience some degree of anal sphincter rupture during childbirth.[12]

The growing appreciation of the risk of normal childbirth to pelvic function in women[13–15] as well as the increasing safety of cesarean section[16,17] have led more women (especially doctors!) to request elective cesarean section,[18] to which obstetricians are increasingly likely to accede.[19–21] Many women see the predictability and control of an elective procedure as important advantages.[22]

It may appear paradoxical that the increase in cesarean section rates seen in most developed countries[23–29] and the widespread uptake of epidural anesthesia[30] has occurred against the background of a rising tide of pressure by women's groups to be allowed "natural labor."[31] Such pressure may be due to "female machismo" the desire of some women to "do it by themselves" without assistance (especially from male obstetricians). It can be speculated that such a philosophy has resulted in part at least from the century-long tradition of female emancipation, and feminism, sometimes referred to as "women's lib(eration)." Whatever the root cause of the natural childbirth movement, it has given rise to increasing numbers of "alternative birth centers,"[32,33] and in some countries, even to increases in home birth.[34,35] Most studies show such "low tech" births to be safe, provided careful selection is practised.[34–38] Some women will persist in their aim to achieve a vaginal birth even when it is not safe, and this may lead to the death of her fetus, or even herself. The obstetrician must accept even this extreme view, and, provided the woman is mentally competent, the law in the United Kingdom prevents compulsory cesarean section,[39] a stance that is supported in the United Kingdom by the Royal College of Obstetricians and Gynaecologists.[40] Women have autonomy in childbirth.[41]

FEAR OF CHILDBIRTH

An underappreciated reason why women request cesarean section is a natural fear of childbirth. Historically, childbirth has been dangerous, and in many parts of the world, it still is, with maternal mortality rates per pregnancy approaching 1%,[40,42–50] giving a lifetime risk of 5% or more. Each year, about half a million women die in childbirth.[42] Many of these deaths are a direct consequence of prolonged labor (associated with hemorrhage and sepsis, for example), which, as explained earlier, is a particularly human problem. Prolonged labor also produces a huge toll of maternal morbidity, as detailed previously. In African cities such as Kano and Lagos in Nigeria and Addis Ababa in Ethiopia some hospitals specialize entirely in the repair of vesicovaginal fistula. In the developing world, even where cesarean section is available, mortality is still significant. In a recent study of over 8000 cesarean sections in Malawi, two thirds were performed because of obstructed labor, and 1% of mothers died.[51] Two thirds of the surgeons were not medically qualified.

We often forget that it is less than 100 years since the maternal mortality rate in the developed world was similar to that in India today, about one maternal death in every 250 pregnancies. British history is littered with disastrous labors such as that of Princess Charlotte in 1817. Her labor lasted over 2 days, and resulted in a stillborn male infant; the mother herself died the following day, and the obstetrician committed suicide some time later. Even at the famous Queen Charlotte's Hospital (London, United Kingdom) in the 1940s, mothers were dying after being in labor for 5 or 6 days.[52] There were also high perinatal mortality rates; 1 baby in 15 did not survive birth in the 1930s.

In more modern practice, obstetricians and midwives can be lulled into believing that labor is no longer a painful experience. I became aware of the error of this view in the early 1990s, when I analyzed a national survey of pain relief in labor for the National Birthday Trust (set up in the 1930s to campaign for better pain relief for women in labor). Even with the ready availability of analgesics and epidural anesthesia, only 6.5% of women said that pain in labor was mild. Overall 37.5% said that they had experienced severe pain, and 56% said that pain had been "unbearable."[53] Even in the last few years, the media in the United Kingdom have carried articles from women reporting terrifying experiences. Jane Dewar, in *You* magazine, April 1999, wrote "it took me two years to recover from the trauma of giving birth. I didn't feel joyful after the birth of my son—I felt violated, angry and betrayed." Cristina Odone, writing in the *Daily Telegraph* on the 15th of August 2003, wrote about the "pointless suffering inflicted by some dogmatic midwives" who encouraged her to persevere with a "natural" approach to labor against her wishes. She went on to describe how 48 hours of latent labor left her cervix "stubbornly undilated," and she castigated the "self-righteous mantras about bravery and perseverance." She was petrified and indignant about her experience. There is now a UK website devoted to fear of childbirth (www.tokophobia.com). In Finland, Sweden, and the United Kingdom, fear of childbirth is the reason that many women request cesarean section, accounting for up to a fifth of all cesarean births.[54] Previous complicated childbirth or inadequate pain relief are the most common reasons for requesting a cesarean section among women who have previously given birth..[55] Even counseling by specially trained midwives does not appear to be sufficient to dispel the fear of childbirth. In a prospective trial, women who had been treated for the fear of childbirth reported a rather more frightening experience of delivery, and more frequent symptoms of posttraumatic stress related to delivery than women in a comparison group.[56]

In contrast to the fear of natural childbirth, cesarean sections are often perceived as relatively straightforward and a guarantee that senior staff will be involved in the delivery. This perception has been enhanced by adverse publicity regarding the shortage of midwives in the United Kingdom;[57] mothers fear that they will not be adequately supported if they attempt a normal labor and vaginal birth. In Brazil, similar maternal concerns have resulted in cesarean section rates exceeding 80% in some areas.[27] It has also been shown in South America that as disposable income increases, there is a parallel rise in the demand for elective cesarean section.[29]

Perhaps a lesson to be drawn is the importance of women's choice, and the role of technology as a facilitator, allowing choice to be exercised safely. In this context, technology includes the diagnostic tests that enable the identification of those women who will be safest in hospital delivered by cesarean section (e.g., those with placenta previa) and those who can deliver at home with relative safety (e.g., the multipara with a previous normal birth). The availability and the cost of technologic interventions must also be taken into account. It should be with these considerations in mind that we consider the purpose of intrapartum care and even whether, given modern technology, it is necessary for women to labor at all.

SHOULD WOMEN BE ALLOWED AN ELECTIVE CESAREAN ON REQUEST? (See also Chapters 75 and 76)

Although some have argued that to carry out a cesarean section without a medical indication is unethical,[58–60] in most countries, obstetricians are willing to give women the choice.[61–63] Recently, the American College of Obstetricians and Gynecologists has reaffirmed the need to allow women the choice to elect an epidural anesthetic before 5 cm dilatation, even if this results in an increased cesarean section rate.[64] An ACOG bulletin in November 2003 advocated that elective cesarean section was an option that should be considered under the principle of patient autonomy.[65] The National Institute for Clinical Excellence in the United Kingdom recently (April 2004) published guidelines on cesarean section (www.nice.org.uk). Section 4.8 of the guidelines specifically addresses the issue of cesarean section for maternal request. The recommendations are:

- Maternal request is not on its own an indication for cesarean section and specific reasons for the request should be explored, discussed and recorded.
- When a woman requests a cesarean section in the absence of an identifiable reason, the overall benefits and risks of cesarean section compared with vaginal birth should be discussed and recorded.
- When a woman requests a cesarean section because she has a fear of childbirth, she should be offered counselling (such as cognitive behavioural therapy) to help her to address her fears in a supported manner, because this results in reduced fear of pain in labor and shorter labor. *(Although it should be noted that in the single prospective randomized study on which this recommendation was based there was no significant difference in the proportion of women in the counseled or noncounseled groups who eventually went ahead with their planned cesarean section.[66])*
- An individual clinician has the right to decline a request for cesarean section in the absence of an identifiable reason. However, the woman's decision should be respected and she should be offered referral for a second opinion.

It is quite clear from recommendation four that "the woman's decision (for cesarean section) should be respected," and thus maternal choice should be accommodated. Despite this clarity, however, the media in the United Kingdom widely portrayed this guideline as an attempt to restrict cesarean section for maternal choice. For example, a national newspaper, the *Daily Mail*, reported on the 28th of April 2004 that "a major clampdown on Caesarean births has been ordered by Health Chiefs. Doctors have been told that they must have a valid reason to perform (a cesarean section), not just because the mother is 'too posh to push.' Women will instead be encouraged to endure (sic) natural labor—and could face private medical bills of up to £5,000 if they insist on the surgical birth." I support John Queenan, deputy editor of *Obstetrics and Gynecology*, in his recent call to work toward a consensus on this issue.[67] As cesarean section becomes progressively safer year after year (e.g., with reductions in mortality and morbidity rates secondary to the use of prophylactic antibiotics and anticoagulants, and the improvement in surgical techniques, especially those for controlling hemorrhage), the demand for elective cesarean section is likely to grow rather than diminish. We may arrive at a situation in which elective cesarean section is actually safer than spontaneous labor, particularly as successful vaginal delivery cannot be guaranteed, and spontaneous labor therefore always carries an unavoidable risk of a more dangerous emergency section. If this happens, then arguments in favor of universal elective cesarean section become stronger, and we will need to consider the question of whether all women should be offered this alternative.[68] Probably, such a question could only be answered by a prospective randomized controlled trial, which would need to include indicators of long-term outcome, both for the mother and baby.

INTRAPARTUM CARE

What Is its Purpose?

When asked to state the purpose of intrapartum care, contributors to the first edition of this book gave an interesting variety of answers. One considered that it was to ensure the delivery of the fetus in optimal condition for gestation while minimizing the potential hazards of childbirth and any underlying pathology to the mother; a very medical approach. Another also mentioned easing the physical and emotional burden on the parturient and her partner and the creation of a healthy family. A third said providing reassurance and guidance to the woman and her partner was its primary purpose and put identification of abnormalities in labor second. When considering the place of birth, the first contributor said the hospital was the predominant venue, the second said home intrapartum care and delivery was discouraged, while the third said that 40% of births in his area took place at home and that 60% of births were supervised by midwives and family doctors. These answers illustrate the current tension between the medical and midwifery models of care. The former declares that labor is only ever normal in retrospect (i.e., all labors should be considered a complication waiting to happen until proved otherwise), whereas the latter says that most labors are normal and should be treated as such, lest negative thoughts impair the natural process. Doctors tend to intervene surgically in labor because they are trained to do so, because they are afraid of litigation, because they have a heavy workload with conflicting demands, and because they have a perverse financial incentive to do so. Obstetricians are often paid more for surgical intervention than for normal delivery, and even if they are not, an operative delivery taking at the most an hour is much more cost-effective for the physician (although not for the patient or hospital) than the often protracted process of natural birth taking up to a whole day. Midwives, on the other hand, sometimes overlook abnormalities in their ardent desire that things will be normal and are sometimes reluctant to recommend intervention because they will lose control of the case. Despite a wish to do so, they are often unable to provide continuity of care because of limited hours in shifts, and they commonly work in large teams (often because of their own family commitments). Perhaps the only sensible compromise in this situation is to expect a positive outcome to labor, while retaining an awareness that the negative can sometimes happen. A positive, reassuring but constantly vigilant attitude is surely even more important in maternity care than in any other branch of medicine.

Who Should Provide Care in Labor?

There is currently no evidence to suggest that any particular pattern of care is associated with a better perinatal outcome than any other. The first contributor quoted earlier works in a country that spends much more on maternity care than the third, but which has substantially higher perinatal mortality rates. In particular, there is no documented evidence that home birth in low risk cases (probably at least 70% of the population in most developed countries) is associated with higher perinatal mortality rates. Indeed, some have argued that morbidity is lower with home birth because of lower rates of surgical intervention and cross-infection. What therefore must take priority is delivering care that is appropriate to the individual mother. Even in the United States, probably home to the archetypal medical model, demand for birthing centers with all the comforts of home has grown over the last 20 years, and the practice of midwifery is gradually increasing. In Holland, the midwifery model is still preeminent, although there has been a shift to more hospital births over the last 30 years. In the United Kingdom, midwifery reached a low point in the mid-1970s, when medical intervention peaked (e.g., with a national induction rate of 45%), but with the widespread introduction of midwifery teams with improved continuity, and a named caseload with full responsibility for total care in normal cases, the practice has developed renewed confidence. Unfortunately, with a return to a successful national economy and almost full employment, many midwives have left practice for easier, and better remunerated, occupations with no antisocial hours. Moreover, the tendency for maternity services to rely on resident junior medical staff to provide out of hours cover is being challenged in Europe by the "European Working Time Directive," which already limits weekly working hours for junior staff to 56 and plans to reduce them to 48 by the end of the decade. The recent limitation of resident working hours to 80 per week in the United States may presage a similar trend.[69] Perhaps equally important has been the consumer revolution, with women wanting and demanding a greater participation in decisions affecting their care. Increasing moves to patient-held records in the United Kingdom has facilitated this, and it is now the official government policy for maternity records. It is spreading to include a parent-held pediatric record and may become universal with the electronic patient record being developed by the National Health Service (with an investment currently planned of £6 billion). Another current issue is cost-effectiveness; the employment of expensively trained medical staff to perform normal deliveries is hard to defend and even harder to pay for. Although this may be a common pattern in a free-market system, such as that in the United States, there are increasing moves to "managed competition," in which audit and cost considerations play an important part. The widespread publication of birth statistics, including cesarean section rates, will result in a better informed and increasingly vocal public.

THE NEED FOR WOMEN TO HAVE CHOICE

The first aim in intrapartum care should therefore be to select women without obvious risk factors and offer them choice. They should be able to choose their birth attendant, the place of birth, and their mode of birth. There can be no justification for arbitrary rules, and if normal women wish to deliver on a bean bag on the floor surrounded by their family or in a birthing pool with their partner, they should be allowed to do so. There is no evidence that they are exposing themselves or their baby to undue risk, and there is good evidence that a supportive emotional atmosphere is beneficial to progress in labor. In the past, many women have been subjected to demeaning procedures such as pubic shaving and routine enemas, without a shred of evidence that they were beneficial; such practices have fortunately been discontinued in most institutions. On the other hand, many women wish to avail themselves of effective pain relief. The provision of safe epidural anesthesia requires a hospital setting with full staffing and equipment for maternal resuscitation, in case of a rare complication. For this reason alone, hospital maternity units are likely to remain popular. Even apparently normal nulliparas who choose to have their babies at home have a 25% chance of needing to be transferred to the hospital for specialized help, and therefore adequately trained paramedical staff need to be available for such emergencies (and for high risk women who have some sudden complication at home).

ELECTRONIC FETAL MONITORING: YES OR NO? (See Chapter 71)

Electronic fetal monitoring (EFM) remains a conundrum. Despite its many advocates, it has proved impossible to demonstrate its effectiveness conclusively. In addition, the contribution of perinatal events to long-term disability is now believed to be much less than was at one time thought. There is some optimism that this realization might help to reduce the tide of litigation that is engulfing obstetric practice in many western countries, but it also reduces the apparent need for detailed and continuous monitoring in low risk cases. Again, it is important that the parents be involved in the decision about the way that their baby will be monitored in labor. Many obstetricians will have experienced the trauma of parents who decline EFM and who then have an unexpected stillbirth. On the other hand, there can be little doubt that EFM is responsible for many unnecessary cesarean sections, especially in those units where fetal blood sampling and pH estimation is not routinely practiced. The indications for EFM are clearly spelled out in Chapter 71, but the principle of autonomy means that the woman's choice must be paramount. In UK law, for example, the fetus is not a legal "person" until it is born and thus safeguarding the fetus cannot be used as an argument for over riding the mother's wishes. For the professionals' sake, however, clear records of her choice, and the reasons for it, should be kept. If the woman has risk factors but declines monitoring, explanation of the need for EFM should be clearly given and its use firmly advised. However, her choice must be respected, and there is no place for compromising other aspects of her care if she refuses advice on any particular issue. Choice should also be extended to women with complications. As explained in Chapter 64, there is little evidence that cesarean section for a preterm infant in breech presentation results in a better outcome for the child, although most obstetricians practice operative delivery in this situation. It may be difficult to share this uncertainty with a couple at a time of great stress; but not to do so removes from them the option of choosing a vaginal birth should they prefer it. This is particularly important at 24 to 26 weeks' gestation, when the prognosis for the child is very poor and the morbidity from a vertical incision in the uterus very considerable. The physician's first duty is to his or her patient, not to his or her self-esteem.

ACTIVE OR EXPECTANT MANAGEMENT OF LABOR (See Chapter 69)

The active management of labor, like EFM, has its passionate devotees. However, like EFM, the scientific evidence for its superiority is lacking. Although there is little doubt that use of oxytocin in labors progressing more slowly than average shortens labor, the evidence that the mode of delivery is affected is conflicting. Certainly, the risks of inadvertent uterine hyperstimulation are considerable, and inappropriate use of oxytocics is a common cause of litigation in obstetrics. A study from my own unit[70] showed that even if the cervix was dilating at less than 1 cm every 2 hours, 50% of women still achieved a vaginal delivery without the use of oxytocics. An editorial in the *Lancet* in 1988[71] commented: "since 50% of the untreated control group achieved a vaginal delivery, the conservative approach remains a valid clinical option. At present, low dose oxytocin infusion with careful assessment of uterine activity is the best policy in most cases." Almost 20 years later, we have hardly advanced at all in our understanding of slow labor (dystocia). Indeed, the guidelines on dystocia recently published by the American College of Obstetricians and Gynecologists emphasizes that there is a very wide range of acceptable practice.[72] No particular maternal position (or posture) in labor has been shown consistently to enhance the rate of cervical dilatation (although for a variety of reasons, the supine position should be avoided), amniotomy may enhance progress but also increases the incidence of fetal heart rate decelerations and (possibly) chorioamnionitis, high-dose oxytocin infusion speeds labor but increases the rate of uterine hyperstimulation, and there is no clear evidence that continuous EFM is necessary. Minimally effective uterine activity has been defined in the ACOG guidelines as three contractions every 10 minutes averaging more than 25 mm Hg active pressure above baseline. However, although active pressure has been shown to be more important than the frequency of contractions in determining the rate of cervical dilatation[73] and although several studies have shown that manual palpation is often highly inaccurate for the assessment of the pressure of uterine contractions,[74,75] there it is equally no evidence that measuring intrauterine pressure improves outcome. This may be because there have been very few trials of any size assessing the value of intrauterine pressure measurement. Clinical experience suggests that it may be useful in certain circumstances, such as when the mother is very obese or there is a uterine scar. Perhaps the only firm conclusion that one can draw is that women should not be sold active management on the basis that it has proven medical benefit for themselves if the real reason for using it is to speed labor and thus economize on staff time. On the other hand, many women in desultory labor, or with spontaneous prelabor rupture of the membranes, wish to "get on with it," and there is no reason why their views should not be the deciding factor.

INDUCTION OF LABOR (See Chapter 68)

The major factors influencing the outcome of induced labor are parity and the state of the cervix. Failed induction should be a rarity in parous women and is uncommon in nulliparas provided the cervix is favorable (a Bishop score >6). In such women, induction of labor can be undertaken with confidence if there are medical indications (which probably do not exist in more than about 5% of pregnancies). Induction of labor for social reasons remains controversial but widely practiced. Following an era in which in some institutions so-called medical indications were said to exist in more than half of all pregnancies, it would seem perverse if the expertise in induction of labor thus gained should be denied to women who wish to take advantage of it for personal reasons that to them are compelling. In nulliparous women with an unfavorable cervix, two (small) doses of vaginal prostaglandin E_2 24 hours apart can be tried; if this does not precipitate labor or improve the ripeness of the cervix, the indications for induction should be critically reviewed.

THE MANAGEMENT OF PRETERM LABOR (See Chapters 61 and 62)

In many ways, despite continuing improvements in neonatal care, the obstetric management of preterm labor has become more controversial over the last 10 years. Two particular issues are of concern.

Tocolysis

Firstly, following an era in which the use of tocolytics to suppress preterm contractions became de rigueur, the systematic reviews have cast steadily increasing doubt on their efficacy.[76] Early use of alcohol was rapidly supplanted by the use of β-sympathomimetics, and for many years ritodrine was widely used and presumably very profitable for the drug company producing it. However, although they have been shown to delay delivery, β-sympathomimetics have not been shown to improve perinatal outcome, and they have a high frequency of unpleasant and even fatal maternal side effects. In the United States, the use of magnesium sulfate to suppress preterm uterine activity persisted for many years despite the lack of any evidence for its efficacy. The latest *Cochrane Review* has stated that "Magnesium sulphate is ineffective at delaying birth or preventing preterm birth, and its use is associated with an increased mortality for the infant."[77] Therefore, there seems to be no justification for its continuing use for this indication. Nitric oxide donors such as glycerin trinitrate were fashionable briefly, but have been abandoned because they are no more effective than alternatives and give many women in whom they are used a severe headache.[78] In the *Cochrane Systematic Review*, when compared with any other tocolytic agent (mainly β-sympathomimetics), calcium channel blockers reduced the number of women giving birth within 7 days of receiving treatment (RR 0.76; 95% CI 0.60–0.97) and prior to 34 weeks' gestation (RR 0.83; 95% CI 0.69–0.99), "When tocolysis is indicated for women in preterm labour, calcium channel blockers are preferable to other tocolytic agents."[76] However, calcium channel blockers are currently unlicensed for this use. On the other hand, a licensed drug (atosiban) is available in Europe, and in multinational multicenter trials has been shown to be as effective as β-sympathomimetics in suppressing uterine contractions, but with far fewer side effects.[79] Thus, it would probably be the treatment of choice, but unfortunately it is very expensive, and in a cash-limited National Health Service, this presents a problem. The cost of a day's treatment with atosiban is approximately £200 ($300), whereas nifedipine costs about 50p (£0.5, $0.75) per dose. The controversy regarding which drug to use was highlighted by the editor of the *British Journal of Obstetrics and Gynaecology* (BJOG) when he wrote "the economic arguments do not make much sense. Nifedipine is cheaper predominantly because it has not undergone the expensive pregnancy licensing process. There may also be unseen late costs. In the short run, hospital trusts [governing boards] risk being sued for using an unlicensed drug when the licensed one is available, and in the long run refusal to prescribe an effective licensed drug will discourage future drug development in pregnancy. If pharmaceutical companies make a good new drug, we should use it." His editorial raised concerns because the editor declared that he had been paid to advise the drug company that produces atosiban on their drug development program. In a subsequent letter to the BJOG it was noted that at a recent senior staff conference of the Royal College of Obstetricians and Gynaecologists, the majority of the obstetricians present indicated that their first-choice tocolytic agent was nifedipine.[80] The authors also pointed out that atosiban had been refused a license both in the United States and in Australia. Where does this leave us? Perhaps we should end with a comment from the current Royal College of Obstetricians and Gynaecologists guidelines* that "in the absence of clear evidence that tocolytic drugs improve outcome following preterm labor, it is reasonable not to use them."[81]

Antenatal Steroids for Fetal Lung Maturation

Since their introduction in the 1980s,[82] antenatal steroids have been used widely and have been shown to reduce both neonatal respiratory distress syndrome and mortality at or before 34 weeks' gestation.[83] Following a period during which major efforts were made to make sure that the mothers of all babies that could potentially benefit had received an appropriate course of steroids, the use of this powerful medication began to increase to include, for example, routine administration before elective cesarean section at 38 weeks' gestation and multiple courses in women considered to be at increased risk of preterm delivery. In the last 5 years, questions have been raised about the wisdom of such an approach. There is particular concern about potential long-term side effects. Animal studies have shown that maternal corticosteroid administration delays myelination in the fetal brain and reduces the growth of all fetal brain areas, particularly the hippocampus.[84] There may also be long-

---

*www.rcog.org.uk/guidelines.asp?pageID=106&guidelineID=44

term effects on the setting of the hypothalamopituitary axis and glucose homeostasis.[84–86] These latter changes are consistent with the Barker hypothesis of intrauterine fetal programming.[87,88] Some studies have already suggested that antenatal corticosteroid therapy is associated with higher systolic and diastolic blood pressures in adolescence and might lead to clinical hypertension in survivors well beyond birth.[89] Moreover, studies are now suggesting that repeated courses of antenatal steroids may result in a decreased neonatal head circumference[90] and decreased birth weight.[91] Multivariate analyses of the behavior of children in the Western Australian Preterm Infant Follow-up Study have shown that increasing the number of glucocorticoid exposures, for the purpose of enhancing lung maturation prior to preterm birth, is associated with both reduced birth weight and an increase in behavioral disorders at 3 years of age.[85] In 2000, the NIH (http://odp.od.nih.gov/consensus/cons/112/112_intro.htm) issued the following consensus statement: "The current benefit and risk data are insufficient to support routine use of repeat or rescue courses of antenatal corticosteroids in clinical practice. Clinical trials are in progress to assess potential benefits and risks of various regimens of repeat courses. Until data establish a favorable benefit-to-risk ratio, repeat courses of antenatal corticosteroids, including rescue therapy, should be reserved for patients enrolled in clinical trials." This conclusion has subsequently been supported by the American College of Obstetricians and Gynecologists[92] and a *Cochrane Review*.[93] A leading article in the *Journal of the American Medical Association* drew attention to the rapidly increasing number of papers reporting adverse long-term effects of antenatal steroids.[94] It should not be forgotten that before the adverse effects of the antenatal use of diethylstilbestrol were recognized, it had been given in over 4.5 million pregnancies, and more than 2 million men and women exposed in utero had their reproductive function adversely affected[95,96]; and that thalidomide resulted in the birth of over 10,000 babies with phocomelia before its dangers were appreciated.[97,98]

In summary, with systematic review and meta-analysis we are becoming better at understanding what we know, and defining what we know we do not know. However, it is those things that we do not know that we do not know which sometimes give us the most serious cause for concern when eventually the facts emerge. It is always best to remember "First do no harm."

CONCLUSIONS

- Human birth is difficult because of an evolutionary conflict between a small pelvis adapted for walking upright and an enlarged brain adapted to toolmaking and interpersonal communication.
- Fear of childbirth is therefore justified
- Caesarean section is increasingly requested by choice and most obstetricians will accede to this provided the woman is fully informed of the risks and benefits
- The most important component of intrapartum care is the presence of an experienced and competent birth attendant
- Electronic fetal monitoring makes labor safer for the fetus but increases the likelihood of operative intervention
- Active management does not affect the outcome of labor but may shorten it and this can have logistic advantages for both parturient and accoucheur
- Tocolytics are largely ineffective and not to use them is an acceptable option
- Steroids administered to the mother reduce neonatal mortality and morbidity if the baby delivers before 34 weeks, but have long term adverse consequences for babies that deliver at term because their mother was not really in labor.

REFERENCES

1. Gee H: Palaeontology. Return to the planet of the apes. *Nature* 2001;412:131–132.
2. Haile-Selassie Y: Late Miocene hominids from the Middle Awash, Ethiopia. Nature 2001;412:178–181.
3. Johanson DC, Edey MA: Lucy—The Beginnings of Humankind. London, Penguin Books, 1990.
4. Kingdon J: Lowly Origin. Princeton, New Jersey, Princeton University Press, 2003.
5. Bryson B: A Short History of Everything. London, Black Swan Books, 2003.
6. Ruff CB: Biomechanics of the hip and birth in early Homo. Am J Phys Anthropol 1995;98:527–574.
7. Rightmire GP: Brain size and encephalization in early to Mid-Pleistocene Homo. Am J Phys Anthropol 2004;124:109–123.
8. Pinker S: The Language Instinct. London, Penguin Books, 1994.
9. Viktrup L, Lose G, Rolff M, Barfoed K: The symptom of stress incontinence caused by pregnancy or delivery in primiparas. Obstet Gynecol 1992;79:945–949.
10. MacArthur C, Bick DE, Keighley MR: Faecal incontinence after childbirth. BJOG 1997;104:46–50.
11. Arrowsmith S, Hamlin EC, Wall LL: Obstructed labor injury complex: Obstetric fistula formation and the multifaceted morbidity of maternal birth trauma in the developing world. Obstet Gynecol Surv 1996;51:568–574.

12. Fornell EK, Berg G, Hallbook O, et al: Clinical consequences of anal sphincter rupture during vaginal delivery. J Am Coll Surg 1996;183:553–558.
13. Peschers UM, Sultan AH, Jundt K, et al: Urinary and anal incontinence after vacuum delivery. Eur J Obstet Gynecol Reprod Biol 2003;110:39–42.
14. Chaliha C, Sultan AH, Bland JM, et al: Anal function: Effect of pregnancy and delivery. Am J Obstet Gynecol 2001;185:427–432.
15. Sultan AH: Anal incontinence after childbirth. Curr Opin Obstet Gynecol 1997;9:320–324.
16. Sachs BP, Yeh J, Acker D, et al: Cesarean section-related maternal mortality in Massachusetts, 1954–1985. Obstet Gynecol 1988;71:385–388.
17. Lilford RJ, van Coeverden de Groot HA, Moore PJ, Bingham P: The relative risks of caesarean section (intrapartum and elective) and vaginal delivery: A detailed analysis to exclude the effects of medical disorders and other acute pre-existing physiological disturbances. BJOG 1990;97:883–892.
18. Al-Mufti R, McCarthy A, Fisk NM: Survey of obstetricians' personal preference and discretionary practice. Europ J Obstet Gynecol Reprod Biol 1997;73:1–4.
19. Paterson-Brown S, Fisk NM: Caesarean section: Every woman's right to choose? Curr Opin Obstet Gynecol 1997;9:351–355.
20. Cotzias CS, Paterson-Brown S, Fisk NM: Obstetricians say yes to maternal request for elective caesarean section: A survey of current opinion. Eur J Obstet Gynecol Reprod Biol 2001;97:15–16.
21. Paterson-Brown S: Should doctors perform an elective caesarean section on request? Yes, as long as the woman is fully informed. BMJ 1998;317:462–463.
22. Ryding EL: Investigation of 33 women who demanded a cesarean section for personal reasons. Acta Obstet Gynecol Scand 1993;72:280–285.
23. Kabir AA, Steinmann WC, Myers L, et al: Unnecessary cesarean delivery in Louisiana: An analysis of birth certificate data. Am J Obstet Gynecol 2004;190:10–19.
24. Khawaja M, Jurdi R, Kabakian-Khasholian T: Rising trends in cesarean section rates in Egypt. Birth 2004;31:12–16.
25. Lee SI, Khang YH, Lee MS: Women's attitudes toward mode of delivery in South Korea—A society with high cesarean section rates. Birth 2004;31:108–116.
26. Walker R, Turnbull D, Wilkinson C: Increasing cesarean section rates: Exploring the role of culture in an Australian community. Birth 2004;31:117–124.
27. Behague DP, Victora CG, Barros FC: Consumer demand for caesarean sections in Brazil: Informed decision making, patient choice, or social inequality? A population based birth cohort study linking ethnographic and epidemiological methods. BMJ 2002;324:942–945.
28. Roberts CL, Tracy S, Peat B: Rates for obstetric intervention among private and public patients in Australia: Population based descriptive study. BMJ 2000;321:137–141.
29. Belizan JM, Althabe F, Barros FC, Alexander S: Rates and implications of caesarean sections in Latin America: Ecological study. BMJ 1999;319:1397–1400.
30. Zhang J, Yancey MK, Klebanoff MA, et al: Does epidural analgesia prolong labor and increase risk of cesarean delivery? A natural experiment. Am J Obstet Gynecol 2001;185:128–134.
31. Changing Childbirth. Part 1: Report of the Expert Maternity Group (Chairman, J Cumberlege). London, HMSO, 1993.
32. Garite TJ, Snell BJ, Walker DL, Darrow VC: Development and experience of a university-based, freestanding birthing center. Obstet Gynecol 1995;86:411–416.
33. Gottvall K, Grunewald C, Waldenstrom U: Safety of birth centre care: Perinatal mortality over a 10-year period. BJOG 2004;111:71–78.
34. Gulbransen G, Hilton J, McKay L, Cox A: Home birth in New Zealand 1973–1993: Incidence and mortality. N Z Med J 1997;110:87–99.
35. Davies J, Hey E, Reid W, Young G: Prospective regional study of planned home births. Home Birth Study Steering Group. BMJ 1996;313:1302–1306.
36. Bastian H, Keirse MJ, Lancaster PA: Perinatal death associated with planned home birth in Australia: Population based study. BMJ 1998;317:384–388.
37. Wiegers TA, Keirse MJ, van der ZJ, Berghs GA: Outcome of planned home and planned hospital births in low risk pregnancies: Prospective study in midwifery practices in the Netherlands. BMJ 1996;313:1309–1313.
38. Blais R: Are home births safe? CMAJ 2002;166:335–336.
39. Dyer C: Appeal court rules against compulsory caesarean sections. BMJ 1997;314:993.
40. Dyer C: Colleges say no to forced caesarean sections. BMJ 1994;308:224.
41. Goldbeck-Wood S: Women's autonomy in childbirth. BMJ 1997;314:1143–1144.
42. Harrison KA: Maternal mortality in developing countries. BJOG 1989;96:1–3.
43. Rosenfield A: Maternal mortality in developing countries. An ongoing but neglected "epidemic." JAMA 1989;262:376–379.
44. Etard JF, Kodio B, Traore S: Assessment of maternal mortality and late maternal mortality among a cohort of pregnant women in Bamako, Mali. BJOG 1999;106:60–65.
45. Mungra A, Vanaja K: Kanhai HH, Van Kanten RW. Nationwide maternal mortality in Surinam. BJOG 1999;106:55–59.
46. de Bernis L, Dumont A, Bouillin D, et al: Maternal morbidity and mortality in two different populations of Senegal: A prospective study (MOMA survey). BJOG 2000;107:68–74.
47. Geelhoed DW, Visser LE, Asare K, et al: Trends in maternal mortality: A 13-year hospital-based study in rural Ghana. Eur J Obstet Gynecol Reprod Biol 2003;107:135–139.
48. Etard JF, Kodio B, Traore S: Assessment of maternal mortality and late maternal mortality among a cohort of pregnant women in Bamako, Mali. BJOG 1999;106:60–65.
49. Vork FC, Kyanamina S, van Roosmalen J: Maternal mortality in rural Zambia. Acta Obstet Gynecol Scand 1997;76:646–650.
50. Nkata M: Maternal mortality due to obstructed labor. Int J Gynaecol Obstet 1997;57:65–66.
51. Fenton PM, Whitty CJ, Reynolds F: Caesarean section in Malawi: Prospective study of early maternal and perinatal mortality. BMJ 2003;327:587.
52. MacRae DJ: Primary uterine inertia. J Obstet Gynaecol Br Emp 1952;59:785–798.
53. Steer PJ: The availability of pain relief. In Chamberlain G, Wraight A, Steer PJ (eds): Pain and Its Relief in Childbirth. Edinburgh, Churchill Livingstone, 1993.
54. Saisto T, Halmesmaki E: Fear of childbirth: A neglected dilemma. Acta Obstet Gynecol Scand 2003;82:201–208.
55. Saisto T, Ylikorkala O, Halmesmaki E: Factors associated with fear of delivery in second pregnancies. Obstet Gynecol 1999;94:679–682.
56. Ryding EL, Persson A, Onell C, Kvist L: An evaluation of midwives' counseling of pregnant women in fear of childbirth. Acta Obstet Gynecol Scand 2003;82:10–17.
57. Ashcroft B, Elstein M, Boreham N, Holm S: Prospective semi-structured observational study to identify risk attributable to staff deployment, training, and updating opportunities for midwives. BMJ 2003;327:584.
58. Bewley S, Cockburn J II: The unfacts of 'request' caesarean section. BJOG 2002;109:597–605.
59. Bewley S, Cockburn J: Responding to fear of childbirth. Lancet 2002;359:2128–2129.
60. Bewley S, Cockburn J: I. The unethics of 'request' caesarean section. BJOG 2002;109:593–596.
61. Kwee A, Cohlen BJ, Kanhai HH, et al: Caesarean section on request: A survey in the Netherlands. Eur J Obstet Gynecol Reprod Biol 2004;113:186–190.

62. Bergholt T, Ostberg B, Legarth J, Weber T: Danish obstetricians' personal preference and general attitude to elective cesarean section on maternal request: A nation-wide postal survey. Acta Obstet Gynecol Scand 2004;83:262–266.
63. Penna L, Arulkumaran S: Cesarean section for non-medical reasons. Int J Gynaecol Obstet 2003;82:399–409.
64. ACOG Committee Opinion number 269 February 2002: Analgesia and cesarean delivery rates. American College of Obstetricians and Gynecologists. Obstet Gynecol 2002;99: 369–370.
65. ACOG committee opinion. Surgery and patient choice: The ethics of decision making. Number 289, November 2003. Int J Gynaecol Obstet 2004;84:188–193.
66. Saisto T, Salmela-Aro K, Nurmi JE, et al: A randomized controlled trial of intervention in fear of childbirth. Obstet Gynecol 2001;98:820–826.
67. Queenan JT: Elective cesarean delivery. Obstet Gynecol 2004;103:1135–1136.
68. Nygaard I, Cruikshank DP: Should all women be offered elective cesarean delivery? Obstet Gynecol 2003;102:217–219.
69. Queenan JT: Work-hour limitations: Let's solve our own problems. Obstet Gynecol 2004;103:611–612.
70. Bidgood KA, Steer PJ: A randomized control study of oxytocin augmentation of labor. 1. Obstetric outcome. BJOG 1987;94: 512–517.
71. Anonymous: How actively should dystocia be treated? Lancet 1988;i:160.
72. ACOG Practice Bulletin Number 49, December 2003: Dystocia and augmentation of labor. Obstet Gynecol 2003;102: 1445–1454.
73. Woolfson J, Steer PJ, Bashford CC, Randall NJ: The measurement of uterine activity in induced labor. BJOG 1976;83: 934–937.
74. Arrabal PP, Nagey DA: Is manual palpation of uterine contractions accurate? Am J Obstet Gynecol 1996;174:217–219.
75. Miles AM, Monga M, Richeson KS: Correlation of external and internal monitoring of uterine activity in a cohort of term patients. Am J Perinatol 2001;18:137–140.
76. King JF, Flenady VJ, Papatsonis DN, Dekker GA, Carbonne B. Calcium channel blockers for inhibiting preterm labor. Cochrane Database Syst Rev 2003;CD002255.
77. Crowther CA, Hiller JE, Doyle LW: Magnesium sulphate for preventing preterm birth in threatened preterm labor. Cochrane Database Syst Rev 2002;CD001060.
78. Duckitt K, Thornton S: Nitric oxide donors for the treatment of preterm labor. Cochrane Database Syst Rev 2002;CD002860.
79. Effectiveness and safety of the oxytocin antagonist atosiban versus beta-adrenergic agonists in the treatment of preterm labor. The Worldwide Atosiban versus Beta-agonists Study Group. BJOG 2001;108:133–142.
80. Jones B, Mohan A, Bennett P: The drugs we deserve. BJOG 2004;111:392–393.
81. Hannah ME: Search for best tocolytic for preterm labor. Lancet 2000;356:699–700.
82. Liggins GC: Can the benefits of antepartum corticosteroid treatment be improved? Eur J Obstet Gynecol Reprod Biol 1989;33:25–30.
83. Crowley P: Prophylactic corticosteroids for preterm birth. Cochrane Database Syst Rev 2000;CD000065.
84. Whitelaw A, Thoresen M: Antenatal steroids and the developing brain. Arch Dis Child Fetal Neonatal Ed 2000;83:F154–F157.
85. Newnham JP, Moss TJ, Nitsos I, Sloboda DM: Antenatal corticosteroids: The good, the bad and the unknown. Curr Opin Obstet Gynecol 2002;14:607–612.
86. Welberg LA, Seckl JR, Holmes MC:. Prenatal glucocorticoid programming of brain corticosteroid receptors and corticotrophin-releasing hormone: Possible implications for behavior. Neuroscience 2001;104:71–79.
87. Newnham JP: Is prenatal glucocorticoid administration another origin of adult disease? Clin Exp Pharmacol Physiol 2001;28:957–961.
88. Seckl JR, Cleasby M, Nyirenda MJ: Glucocorticoids, 11-beta-hydroxysteroid dehydrogenase, and fetal programming. Kidney Int 2000;57:1412–1417.
89. Doyle LW, Ford GW, Davis NM, Callanan C: Antenatal corticosteroid therapy and blood pressure at 14 years of age in preterm children. Clin Sci (Lond) 2000;98:137–142.
90. Walfisch A, Hallak M, Mazor M: Multiple courses of antenatal steroids: Risks and benefits. Obstet Gynecol 2001;98:491–497.
91. Bloom SL, Sheffield JS, McIntire DD, Leveno KJ: Antenatal dexamethasone and decreased birth weight. Obstet Gynecol 2001;97:485–490.
92. Committee on Obstetric Practice. ACOG committee opinion: Antenatal corticosteroid therapy for fetal maturation. Obstet Gynecol 2002;99:871–873.
93. Crowther CA, Harding J: Repeat doses of prenatal corticosteroids for women at risk of preterm birth for preventing neonatal respiratory disease. Cochrane Database Syst Rev. 2003;CD003935.
94. Lawson EE: Antenatal corticosteroids—too much of a good thing? JAMA 2001;286:1628–1630.
95. Goldstein DP: Incompetent cervix in offspring exposed to diethylstilbestrol in utero. Obstet Gynecol 1978;52:73S–75S.
96. Kaufman RH, Adam E, Hatch EE, et al: Continued follow-up of pregnancy outcomes in diethylstilbestrol-exposed offspring. Obstet Gynecol 2000;96:483–489.
97. Newman CG: The thalidomide syndrome: Risks of exposure and spectrum of malformations. Clin Perinatol 1986;13:555–573.
98. Smithells D: Was the thalidomide tragedy preventable? Lancet 1998;351:1591.

CHAPTER 68

Induction of Labor and Pregnancy Termination for Fetal Abnormality

Luis Sanchez-Ramos / Isaac Delke

INDUCTION OF LABOR

Definition

Labor induction is the stimulation of regular uterine contractions before the spontaneous onset of labor, using mechanical or pharmacologic methods in order to generate progressive cervical dilation and subsequent delivery. Although the term generally refers to patients who are at term, it is also employed for women who are at least 20 weeks' gestation. It is important to distinguish labor induction from augmentation, which refers to stimulation of uterine contractions when spontaneous contractions during labor have been considered inadequate.

Introduction

Induction of labor is an important and common clinical procedure in obstetrics. The rate of labor induction in the United States continues to rise significantly for all gestational ages. Preliminary data for the year 2002 from the National Center for Health Statistics indicate that the rate was 20.5% for the year 2001, more than twice the 1989 level of 9%.[1] The reason for this increase is unclear, although it may partly reflect a growing use of labor induction for post-date pregnancies and an increasing trend toward elective induction of labor for other indications (including maternal request).

Indications and Contraindications

Generally, labor induction is indicated when the benefits of delivery to the mother or fetus outweigh the potential risks of continuing the pregnancy. The most appropriate timing for labor induction is the point at which the maternal or perinatal benefits are greater if the pregnancy is interrupted than if the pregnancy is continued. Ideally, most pregnancies should be allowed to reach term, with the onset of spontaneous labor being the sign of physiologic termination of pregnancy. However, occasionally a woman is best delivered before the spontaneous onset of labor. Commonly accepted indications for labor induction are listed in Table 68–1. Of the standard indications for labor induction, pregnancy-induced hypertension and post-date pregnancies are among the most common, accounting for more than 80% of reported inductions. Given that there is an indication for induction, the risks to mother and fetus must then be considered, to make sure that the benefit outweighs these risks. The risks to the mother are mainly related to an increased chance that she will need operative delivery, compared with labor following the spontaneous onset of labor. The risks to the fetus are those of prematurity. Whenever there is evidence of fetal lung maturity, or the pregnancy has reached at least 39 weeks (confirmed by an early ultrasound) the decision to induce labor is not difficult. Maternal consent to any increased risk of operative delivery can be obtained, and the fetus is not likely to be at risk for complications that cannot be dealt with in a modern neonatal unit. However, the decision to induce labor prior to fetal maturity having been achieved is far more difficult. In such cases, premature delivery should offer the fetus clear benefits that outweigh the potential problems associated with preterm birth. Although elective induction of labor (without medical or obstetric indications) is generally not recommended, logistic factors such as distance from the hospital or a history of rapid labor and delivery may be reasonable indications for elective induction. The issue of induction of labor from 39 weeks at maternal request (usually due to intolerance of the discomforts of pregnancy, but sometimes for social reasons, e.g., the limited availability of the father to attend the birth) remains controversial.

Generally recognized relative and absolute contraindications to labor induction are listed in Table 68–2. There

TABLE 68–1

Commonly Accepted Indications for Labor Induction

Pregnancy-induced hypertension
Prelabor rupture of membranes
Chorioamnionitis
Severe intrauterine growth restriction
Isoimmunization
Maternal medical problems (diabetes mellitus, renal disease, lupus)
Fetal demise
Postdates pregnancy
Oligohydramnios
Logistic factors (risk of rapid labor, distance from hospital)

TABLE 68–3

Criteria for Fetal Maturity

Fetal heart tones have been documented for 20 weeks by nonelectronic fetoscope or for 30 weeks by Doppler.
It has been 36 weeks since a positive serum or urine human chorionic gonadotropin pregnancy test was performed by a reliable method.
An ultrasound measurement of the crown-rump length, obtained at 6–11 weeks, supports a gestational age of 39 weeks or more.
An ultrasound scan, obtained at 12–20 weeks, confirms the gestational age of 39 weeks or more determined by clinical history and physical examination.

are few absolute contraindications to labor induction, and there can be certain clinical situations in which induction is usually contraindicated but exceptional circumstances make induction appropriate (i.e., prolapsed umbilical cord in the presence of fetal demise). A number of clinical situations that are not generally considered contraindications to labor induction but require caution include breech presentation, borderline clinical pelvimetry, grand multiparity, nonreassuring fetal testing not requiring emergency delivery, polyhydramnios, and multifetal gestation.

Requirements for Labor Induction

Prior to inducing labor, the obstetrician should carefully review the indication(s) for ending the pregnancy and obtain informed consent. In addition, the mother and fetus should be carefully examined and, if indicated, fetal pulmonary maturity should be documented. In order to avoid iatrogenic prematurity, an amniocentesis to assess fetal lung maturity may be required. Table 68–3 lists criteria, which if met, allow fetal maturity to be assumed, so that amniocentesis need not be performed.[2]

Preinduction Status of the Cervix

Successful labor induction is clearly related to the state of the cervix. Women with an unfavorable cervix, who have not experienced a cervical ripening phase prior to labor, present the greatest challenge with regard to labor induction. In addition, the duration of labor induction is affected by parity and to a minor degree by baseline uterine activity and sensitivity to oxytocic drugs. Many investigators have identified the importance of assessing cervical status prior to induction of labor. Calkins and colleagues were the first to carry out systematic studies of the factors influencing the duration of the first stage of labor.[3] The authors concluded that the length, thickness, and particularly the consistency of the cervix were important parameters. In 1955, Bishop devised a cervical scoring system for multiparous patients with planned elective induction of labor in which 0 to 3 points are given for each of five factors.[1] He determined that when the total score was at least 9, the likelihood of vaginal delivery following labor induction was similar to that observed in patients with spontaneous onset of labor. Although several modifications have been suggested, the Bishop score has become a classical parameter in obstetrics and has since been applied to a much wider group of patients. Nulliparous women with a Bishop score no greater than 3 have a 23-fold increased risk of induction failure and a two- to fourfold increased risk of cesarean delivery compared with nulliparous women with a Bishop score of at least 4.[5] Similarly, multiparous women with a Bishop score of no greater than 3 have a sixfold increased risk of failed induction and twofold increased risk of cesarean birth compared with those women with higher Bishop scores.[5,6]

The Bishop score has become the most commonly employed preinduction scoring system. Several recent studies have assessed the predictive accuracy of ultrasound for successful labor induction.[7–9] However, there is a lack of convincing evidence that this technique provides significant additional information when compared to digital examination.

TABLE 68–2

Contraindications to Labor Induction

Placenta or vasa previa
Transverse fetal lie
Prolapsed umbilical cord
Prior classical uterine incision
Active genital herpes infection
Pelvic structural deformities

Preinduction Cervical Ripening

Cervical ripening is the process that culminates in the softening and distensibility of the cervix, thus facilitating labor and delivery. There is an inverse relationship between the Bishop score and the failure of labor induction, with low scores being associated with a high rate of failed induction. Moreover, not only is inducing uterine contractions in the presence of an unripe cervix more likely to lead to delivery by cesarean section, but even if vaginal delivery is eventually achieved, the labor will often have been prolonged. This is a particular problem if the induction is for fetal indications, as then prolonged fetal monitoring is also required. In addition, an extended exposure to uterine contractions and the resulting reduction in intervillous blood flow can result in fetal hypoxia and acidosis. Thus, it is useful to employ cervical ripening agents to prepare the unripe cervix for labor induction. Ideally, a ripening agent would act upon the cervix to make it more favorable without inducing uterine activity; the length of the active phase of labor would thereby be minimized, limiting the stress on the fetus to the minimum. Unfortunately, it has proved difficult to separate methods of cervical ripening and labor induction. Patients with an unripe cervix may undergo cervical ripening without initiating labor contractions when a pharmacologic agent such as dinoprostone (PGE_2) is employed, but sometimes contractions ensue before the cervix has ripened. A considerable amount of research has been directed toward various methods to prepare or ripen the cervix prior to the induction of labor. Although many of these methods also initiate uterine activity, it should be appreciated that the principal role of these agents is to soften the unripe cervix independently of uterine activity. The various methods for cervical ripening can be divided into two categories (Table 68–4):

- Mechanical
- Pharmacologic

Mechanical Methods

FOLEY CATHETER

Mechanical methods have been employed for many years to ripen the cervix prior to labor induction.[10] Barnes, in the mid-19th century, was one of the first to describe the use of a balloon catheter to ripen the uterine cervix.[11] Since that time several variations of this method have been popularized. The balloon catheter currently most frequently used is a Foley catheter with a 25- to 50-mL balloon, which can be passed through an undilated cervix before inflation of the balloon above the internal os. It is thought that the mechanical separation of the fetal membranes from the cervix and lower segment stimulates local cytokine and prostaglandin release, and these act upon the ground substance of the cervix to break down the cross-links between the glycosaminoglycans. More recently, extra-amniotic saline infusion has been a successful modification to the use of balloon catheters for cervical ripening, presumably by enhancing this effect.[12–14] A recent review of 13 trials in which balloon catheters were used for cervical ripening concluded that with or without extra-amniotic saline infusion, the method resulted in improved Bishop scores and decreased induction-to-delivery intervals.[15] Simultaneous use of balloon-tipped catheters and pharmacologic agents has been shown to be even more effective for cervical ripening than for labor induction; however, the cost of such combination therapy is substantial.

TABLE 68–4

Cervical Ripening Methods

Mechanical methods
Foley catheter
Laminaria tents
Hygroscopic dilators
Acupuncture
Membrane stripping
Pharmacologic methods
Dinoprostone (PGE_2)
Misoprostol (PGE_1)
Cytokines
Nitric oxide
Relaxin

LAMINARIA TENTS

Laminaria tents, natural and synthetic, have been used as a mechanical method for cervical ripening for many years. Although their safety and efficacy in the second trimester have been established, use of laminaria during the third trimester of pregnancy is associated with a high incidence of infection.[16] Synthetic hygroscopic cervical dilators have also been used for many years as agents to prepare the cervix for pregnancy termination. Several studies have shown that these osmotic dilators can also be successfully employed for cervical ripening in viable pregnancies with an unripe cervix.[17–19] Advantages to the use of osmotic dilators are their low cost and ease of placement and removal.

MEMBRANE STRIPPING

Membrane stripping (sometimes known as "membrane sweep") is a simple technique not infrequently used to ripen the cervix, in which a finger is inserted through the cervix and "swept" around the lower segment above the internal os in a circular motion. As with the Foley catheter, it appears to work by release of prostaglandin (especially prostaglandin $F_{2\alpha}$) from the decidua and the adjacent membranes. However, presumably because it is more vigorous, it often stimulates uterine contractions as well as causing ripening. A recent systematic review showed no evidence of an increase in the risk of maternal or perinatal infection when "sweeping" is used.[20] However, there are adverse effects such as discomfort during the necessarily vigorous vaginal examination and occasionally bleeding from the cervix or placental margins if the placenta is low lying. Moreover, if the induction is for fetal compromise, the ensuing contractions mandate fetal monitoring even if labor does not become established.

ACUPUNCTURE

Although much more common in Asia, acupuncture for cervical ripening and labor induction is also becoming more available in the Western world. A recent study concluded that acupuncture at points LI 4 (large intestine 4) and SP 6 (spleen 6) induces cervical ripening at term, and in postdated pregnancies it shortens the time interval between the estimated date of confinement and the actual time of delivery.[21]

Pharmacologic Methods

PROSTAGLANDINS

The use of prostaglandins for cervical ripening has been reported extensively, involving a variety of prostaglandin classes, doses, and routes of administration.[22–24] The distinction between cervical ripening and labor induction is blurred in patients receiving prostaglandins because many women will go into labor even when prostaglandins are being used primarily for ripening. Dinoprostone, or PGE_2, is the prostaglandin most commonly employed. The local application of PGE_2 results in direct softening of the cervix by at least three mechanisms: (1) It softens the cervix by altering the extracellular ground substance of the cervix, (2) it increases the activity of the smooth muscle of the cervix and uterus, and (3) it leads to gap junction formation that is necessary for the coordinated uterine contractions of labor.[25,26]

Meta-analyses have shown that prostaglandins are superior to placebo and oxytocin alone in ripening the cervix.[27,28] A systematic review including at least 5000 pregnancies from more than 70 prospective trials suggests that PGE_2 is superior to placebo or no therapy in enhancing cervical effacement and dilation.[27]

Two forms of PGE_2 (dinoprostone) are available commercially in the United States, although even more forms are available in other Western countries. In randomized trials, the two forms are similar in efficacy.[29–31] The first is formulated as a gel and is placed endocervically, but not above the internal os. The application, 0.5 mg, can be repeated in 6 hours, not to exceed three doses in 24 hours. The second form is a 10-mg vaginal insert that is placed in the posterior fornix of the vagina. This formulation allows for controlled release of dinoprostone over 12 hours, after which it is removed.

Misoprostol (synthetic analogue of PGE_1) has been the subject of numerous recent articles describing its use as a cervical ripening agent.[32–50] Doses of 25 to 50 μg administered vaginally or orally have been shown in several studies to be effective in inducing cervical ripening and labor. However, because the majority of patients experience regular uterine contractions soon after the initial dose, misoprostol should be considered primarily a labor induction agent, which occasionally ripens the cervix without uterine activity.

The role of cytokines in cervical ripening has been the subject of several recent studies.[51] Interleukin 8 (IL-8) can lead to neutrophil chemotaxis, which is associated with collagenase activity and cervical ripening.[52] These inflammatory agents may be particularly important as mediators of cervical ripening associated with preterm labor. Nitric oxide synthase (NOS) and nitric oxide (NO) have been postulated to have a regulatory role in the myometrium and cervix during pregnancy and parturition.[53–55] In the human cervix, ripening is associated with an increase in inducible NOS (iNOS) and neural NOS expression in the cervix.

Resident and migrating inflammatory cells can cause an increase in iNOS activity. In the primate, cervical ripening has many aspects of an inflammatory process: tissue remodeling and breakage of chemical bridges between collagen fibers. Inflammatory agents such as IL-1, tumor necrosis factor-alpha, and IL-8 all seem to be involved in cervical ripening.[56–58] Currently, however, there is no commercial product available that exploits these properties directly.

Relaxin is a polypeptide hormone, similar to insulin, produced by the ovaries, decidua, and chorion. Because of its effect on connective tissue remodeling, it has been studied as a cervical ripening agent.[59,60] Based on data from animal studies, relaxin was predicted to have a cervical ripening effect in humans. The findings that porcine relaxin induces cervical ripening in humans supported this prediction. However, because studies showed that in fact administered human relaxin has no effect on the human cervix, the usual role played by relaxin in human pregnancy and parturition is unclear. At the present time, relaxin, either purified porcine or recombinant human, is not produced commercially as a cervical ripening agent, and its future potential in this context remains unclear.

Pharmacologic Methods for Labor Induction

Oxytocin

Oxytocin, a neurohormone originating in the hypothalamus and secreted by the posterior lobe of the pituitary gland, is the most commonly used drug for the purpose of labor induction in viable pregnancies. This octapeptide is secreted in a pulsatile manner, a fact that is reflected in the marked variability observed in minute-to-minute measurements of maternal plasma oxytocin concentration.[61] The half-life of oxytocin is 10 to 12 minutes.[62] The metabolic clearance rate is similar for men, pregnant women, and nonpregnant women: 20 to 27 mL/kg/minute.[63] The similarity of the metabolic clearance rate between men and pregnant women is striking in view of the large increase that occurs during pregnancy in the plasma concentration of leucine-aminopeptidase, an enzyme capable of hydrolyzing oxytocin. This suggests that factors other than this enzyme are responsible for the degradation of oxytocin.

There is considerable confusion regarding the pharmacokinetics of oxytocin; much of the original pharmacokinetic work was done prior to the availability of a reliable radioimmunoassay for oxytocin.[64] Indeed, the potency of oxytocin is still based on a bioassay of avian vasopressive activity with 1 United States Pharmacopeia (USP) unit being equivalent to 2 μg of oxytocin.

Traditionally, it has been held that oxytocin levels reached a steady-state level within 15 to 20 minutes of beginning an infusion or increasing the dosage. Recent work using a sensitive oxytocin radioimmunoassay has shown that approximately 40 minutes are required for any particular dose of oxytocin to reach a steady-state plasma concentration.[65]

It is well established that there is a marked variability in the response of the uterus to oxytocin, but in general, the sensitivity of the uterus to oxytocin increases dramatically as pregnancy progresses.[66] This increase in responsiveness is likely due to the increasing concentrations of oxytocin receptors in the myometrium and decidua with increasing gestational age.[67] It appears that oxytocin has direct stimulatory effects on the myometrium in addition to stimulating decidual prostaglandin production.[68] An increased level of prostaglandin $F_{2\alpha}$ ($PGF_{2\alpha}$) metabolite was demonstrated in women undergoing successful oxytocin induction of labor, whereas this increase was not present in failed inductions.[69] The direct effect of oxytocin on the myometrium is believed to be mediated by polyphosphoinositide hydrolysis with production of inositol phosphates that act as a second messenger and lead to the mobilization of intracellular calcium ion.[70]

Other organs that show a response to oxytocin include breast, vascular smooth muscle, and kidney. Oxytocin stimulates contraction of the myoepithelium surrounding the alveoli of the mammary gland, leading to the milk ejection reflex. At dosages typically used for the induction of labor, there is no demonstrable effect on vascular smooth muscle tone. However, intravenous boluses of as little as 0.5 IU transiently decrease peripheral vascular tone, leading to hypotension.[71] Similarly, at low dosages, oxytocin exerts negligible effect on renal function; however, at high infusion rates, it exhibits a marked antidiuretic effect (which is not surprising, given its similarity in structure to antidiuretic hormone, also produced in the posterior pituitary). Excessively high infusion rates, coupled with infusion of crystalloid, have led to deaths from water intoxication.

Oxytocin can be administered by any parenteral route. It is also absorbed by the buccal and nasal mucosa. When administered orally and swallowed, oxytocin is rapidly inactivated by trypsin. The intravenous route is now used almost exclusively to stimulate the pregnant uterus because it allows precise measurement of the amount of medication being administered and a relatively rapid discontinuation of the effects of the drug when infusion is discontinued.

TECHNIQUES FOR THE ADMINISTRATION OF OXYTOCIN

Oxytocin is administered as a dilute solution with the flow rate into the intravenous line precisely regulated by an infusion pump. The health care professionals who attend the patient during an induced labor must be familiar with the use and potential complications of oxytocin. Likewise, a qualified physician who is able to manage any complications that may arise with the use of oxytocin should be readily available. Fetal monitoring is indicated prior to beginning the infusion to assess the baseline level of uterine activity and fetal status, and should then be continued during the infusion. Either external or internal monitoring is acceptable as long as uterine activity and fetal heart rate are adequately documented. Consideration should be given to the use of internal monitoring when high doses of oxytocin are required or when satisfactory progress in labor is not being made (see also Chapter 69 on the augmentation of labor). The tracing should be inspected frequently and carefully for any evidence of hyperstimulation as manifested by increased baseline tonus, tachysystole, or the onset of late decelerations; and the infusion of oxytocin must be stopped immediately should they occur.

Significant difference of opinion exists regarding the initial dose of oxytocin and the interval and frequency of dosage increase. A controlled intravenous oxytocin infusion remains the preferred method of induction of labor. Several trials have compared various regimens of oxytocin dosage increase and time intervals between dose increases.[72–76] Starting doses have ranged from 0.5 to 2.0 mU/minute, with some as high as 6 mU/minute. Increments of dose increase have ranged from a low of 1 to 2 mU/minute up to 6 mU/minute, with adjustments for increased uterine activity. Time intervals between increases have ranged from 15 to 40 minutes. Although low-dose regimens (initial dose 0.5–2.0 mU/minute, with incremental increases of 1–2 mU/minute every 15–40 minutes) are commonly utilized in the United States, high-dose regimens (initial dose 6–8 mU/minute, with incremental increases of 6 mU/minutes every 15–40 minutes) have been reported to be safe and effective for labor induction in patients with viable pregnancies, provided there was close fetal monitoring and early recourse to cesarean delivery in the event of fetal distress.[77] A meta-analysis of 11 trials comparing low-dose with high-dose oxytocin for labor induction found that larger dose increases and shorter intervals between increases were associated with shorter labors and lower rates of intra-amniotic infections and cesarean delivery for dystocia, but more hyperstimulation was noted.[78] Based on recent pharmacokinetic data,[79,80] many obstetricians have moved to a regimen whereby the dose of oxytocin is increased by 1 to 2 mU/minute every 40 minutes. Advantages of this regimen derive from not increasing the oxytocin dose before steady-state levels of oxytocin have been reached. This leads to a lower total dosage of oxytocin being used, in addition to a lower incidence of the hyperstimulation that can result from increasing the oxytocin dose before a steady state is reached. A potential disadvantage is that women who are relatively insensitive to oxytocin may have a very prolonged course before adequate labor is established. Nearly 90% of patients will respond to 16 mU/minute or less, and it is most unusual for a patient to require more than 20 to 40 mU/minute.[81]

The recognition that endogenous oxytocin is secreted in spurts during pregnancy and spontaneous labor has prompted exploration of a more physiologic manner of inducing labor with this agent. In 1978, Pavlou and associates were the first to describe a protocol of pulsatile infusion.[82] More recently, several randomized trials have compared the safety and efficacy of pulsatile oxytocin administration with continuous infusion.[83–85] Most authors conclude that although there does not appear to be a shortening of the induction-to-delivery interval, pulsatile administration of oxytocin reduces the amount of oxytocin required for successful labor induction.

SIDE EFFECTS AND COMPLICATIONS OF OXYTOCIN INFUSION

Although oxytocin is a safe medication with appropriate administration and monitoring, there is always the potential for adverse occurrences. The most common complication related to oxytocin induction of labor is uterine hyperstimulation. Uterine hyperstimulation may present as tachysystole with more than five contractions in 10 minutes, contractions of greater than 90 seconds' duration, or an increase in the baseline uterine tonus. The decreased intervillous blood flow associated with hyperstimulation ultimately leads to decreased oxygen transfer to the fetus, as indicated by the appearance of late decelerations. Oxytocin infusion should be discontinued immediately in the presence of hyperstimulation. If there is evidence of fetal distress, standard intrauterine resuscitation measures should be instituted, including oxygen administration and positioning the patient in the left lateral decubitus position.

Uterine rupture is a very uncommon complication when oxytocin is used appropriately. There are no prospective data in the literature describing the incidence of uterine rupture in oxytocin-induced labor. Retrospective series of uterine rupture have implicated oxytocin in 4.3%[86] to 12.5%[87] of occurrences. Factors that may reduce the risk of uterine rupture include avoidance of oxytocin in the grand multipara, use of internal uterine pressure monitoring for patients with previous cesarean delivery and when high doses of oxytocin are required, and avoidance of oxytocin in obstructed labors.

Water intoxication, an infrequent complication of oxytocin administration, may be avoided with appropriate management. The minimum effective dose of oxytocin should be used to avoid the antidiuretic effects of high-dose oxytocin. The risk of water intoxication increases in women who have received large volumes of free water; therefore, 5% dextrose solutions without electrolytes should generally not be used during labor induction. Symptoms occur as the plasma sodium concentration falls below 120 to 125 mEq/L and may include nausea and vomiting, mental status changes, and ultimately seizures and coma. Mild instances of water intoxication can be treated by discontinuing the hypotonic fluid and restricting fluid intake. With severe symptoms, correction of hyponatremia by saline infusion may be necessary.

Concern has been raised regarding a possible association between oxytocin-induced labor and an increased incidence of neonatal jaundice. Many of the older studies claiming that oxytocin leads to neonatal jaundice failed to control for confounding variables such as gestational age and the infusion of large volumes of free water. The more recent literature has not identified any correlation between oxytocin induction and neonatal hyperbilirubinemia.[88,89]

Prostaglandins

Exogenous prostaglandins, particularly dinoprostone (PGE_2), are frequently used as cervical ripening agents.[90–97] Because the prostaglandin-induced cervical ripening process often includes initiation of labor, approximately half of treated women with dinoprostone enter labor and deliver within 24 hours. Prostaglandins have the dual capability to ripen the cervix and initiate uterine contractility. As a consequence, induced labor with prostaglandins appears to be similar to that of spontaneous labor. The use of prostaglandins (PGs) as labor induction agents has been reported extensively in a variety of PG classes, doses, and routes of administration.[27] Prior to 1992 most trials assessing the impact of prostaglandins as cervical ripening and labor induction agents included various dosages of intracervical (0.3–0.5 mg) or intravaginal (3–5 mg) dinoprostone (PGE_2). In 1992, the Food and Drug Administration (FDA) approved PGE_2 (0.5 mg intracervically) for cervical ripening and labor induction. In 1995, a slow-release 10-mg dinoprostone vaginal insert also was approved for the same indications. Because most trials have compared these prostaglandin preparations with placebo, the relative efficacy of these two prostaglandin preparations has been difficult to assess. Additionally, once cervical ripening was completed and uterine activity initiated, most patients studied required further augmentation with oxytocin.

The optimal route for PGE_2 administration has not yet been determined. The intracervical route has been used in the majority of trials, especially those comparing the effectiveness of the FDA-approved formulations (Prepidil and Cervidil). Although intracervical administration of gel is more difficult than intravaginal administration, the former route appears to cause more significant cervical ripening. The intracervical method also appears to be associated with a lower risk of hyperstimulation. However, the easiest and most practical way to apply PGE_2 in routine clinical practice is via the vaginal route. The most commonly used doses are 3 to 5 mg. It has been suggested that the dose of PGE_2 should be varied according to the patient's cervical score, permitting a lower dose of PGE_2 to be used in many cases. Just as there is no consensus about the optimal dose and route of administration of PGE_2, the optimal frequency of administration is still a matter of debate. A commonly used approach to cervical ripening and labor induction with PGE_2 is to administer approximately 3 mg at 4- to 6-hour intervals for two doses, followed by oxytocin induction or augmentation in 12 to 18 hours if necessary. Irrespective of the route and dose of PGE_2 employed, for the majority of patients, dinoprostone preparations should be regarded mainly as cervical ripening agents, and are not reliable as labor induction agents.

MISOPROSTOL FOR LABOR INDUCTION

Misoprostol is a synthetic prostaglandin E_1 (PGE_1) analogue that has been marketed in the United States since 1988 as a gastric protective agent for the prevention and treatment of peptic ulcers. It was licensed in a tablet form designed for oral absorption. Early studies performed in the late 1980s and early 1990s demonstrated that oral administration of misoprostol caused uterine contractions in early pregnancy.[98–100] Subsequent studies, performed abroad and in the United States, showed that intravaginal administration of misoprostol tablets can terminate first-trimester and second-trimester pregnancies.[101–105] A large number of published controlled trials have shown that misoprostol, administered either vaginally or via the oral route, is an effective agent for cervical ripening and labor induction in patients with viable pregnancies.[32–50,106–114] An initial meta-analysis suggested a significantly reduced cesarean delivery rate for patients induced with misoprostol.[115] Follow-up meta-analysis has shown that 84% of patients receiving misoprostol go into active labor, with only 29.4% requiring oxytocin augmentation. A significantly higher proportion of patients receiving misoprostol achieved a vaginal delivery within 12 hours (37.6% versus 23.9%). Similarly, 68.1% of patients receiving misoprostol achieved a vaginal delivery within 24 hours. Use of misoprostol for cervical ripening and labor induction is associated with an approximate 5-hour reduction of the interval from the first dose to delivery when compared with dinoprostone. The reduced induction-to-delivery interval seen with misoprostol compared with dinoprostone implies that either it produces higher levels of uterine activity, or that it is a more efficient cervical ripening agent. Consistent with the former hypothesis, compared with women receiving dinoprostone, Foley catheter, or placebo, women receiving misoprostol are twice as likely to experience tachysystole and uterine hyperstimulation, with the incidence of these conditions closely related to the dose of misoprostol administered.[115]

In relation to cervical ripening, most of the individual studies in meta-analyses assessing the efficacy and safety of misoprostol and dinoprostone have not shown a significant reduction in the overall cesarean delivery rate. However, the lack of a positive finding was probably because the sample sizes of the trials were small. The 44 trials included in the recent meta-analysis[115] provide data for 5735 subjects participating in trials assessing the impact of misoprostol treatment on the cesarean delivery rate. When all the trials were pooled, subjects receiving misoprostol had a significantly lower cesarean rate than subjects in the comparison groups (17.3% versus 22.9%). The most common indications for cesarean delivery were arrest of dilation or descent, failed induction, and abnormal fetal heart rate tracings. The rate of cesarean deliveries performed because of fetal heart rate abnormalities was similar for misoprostol-induced patients and those in the comparison group. Similarly, no difference was noted for the rate of cesarean deliveries because of dystocia. Patients receiving misoprostol had a significantly lower rate of cesarean deliveries because of failed induction. This suggests that it may be better at ripening the cervix than dinoprostone.

No evidence of adverse perinatal or maternal effects has been noted.[116] The statistical power resulting from the aggregation of 44 studies included in the meta-analysis increases confidence in our ability to assess safety. The number of subjects studied affords a power of at least 90% to detect a difference in neonatal intensive care unit admission rates of at least 4 percentage points (from 14% to 18%). Sufficient power was also noted for the detection of at least a doubling in the rate of abnormal 5-minute Apgar scores (from 1.4% to 2.8%).

Accordingly, these data provide strong support for the conclusion that misoprostol safely decreases the cesarean delivery rate among women undergoing labor induction compared with women receiving alternate induction agents.

ORAL VERSUS VAGINAL ADMINISTRATION

Initial pharmacokinetic studies compared the pharmacokinetics of vaginal and oral administration of misoprostol.[117–120] These studies showed that the peak plasma concentration of misoprostolic acid was higher and achieved earlier after oral administration, but the detectable plasma concentration lasted longer after vaginal administration. Systemic bioavailability of vaginally administered misoprostol was noted to be three times higher than that of orally administered misoprostol.[117] In all patients studied, independent of the dose or route of administration, the first effect of misoprostol treatment was an increase in uterine tonus. After oral administration, the effect was more rapid and the initial increase was more pronounced than after vaginal treatment. However, after vaginal treatment, tonus remained at a higher level for a longer time.

A significant proportion of the published randomized studies have evaluated the safety and efficacy of vaginally administered misoprostol for cervical ripening and labor induction. During the past few years, seven randomized trials have compared oral versus vaginal administration of misoprostol for labor induction.[109–114,121] In aggregate, 1191 patients were randomized to receive misoprostol orally ($n = 602$) or by the vaginal route ($n = 589$). The oral doses employed ranged from 50 μg to 200 μg every 4 to 6 hours. Vaginal misoprostol was administered in doses ranging from 25 μg to 100 μg every 3 to 4 hours. No difference was noted in the proportion of patients who delivered vaginally within 12 and 24 hours in each group. Similarly, the intervals from start of induction to vaginal delivery were not different. The proportion of patients experiencing increased uterine activity (tachysystole or hyperstimulation) was similar for both groups. Additionally, no difference was noted for the incidence of abnormal 5-minute Apgar scores and rates of NICU (neonatal intensive care unit) admissions. Interestingly, the rate of cesarean delivery was significantly lower among those induced with oral misoprostol. Although both routes of misoprostol administration seem to be efficacious, the evidence documenting the safety of vaginally administered misoprostol is much more extensive.

DOSES OF MISOPROSTOL FOR LABOR INDUCTION

Owing to the small number of studies employing oral misoprostol, and the lack of uniformity in dosage, the most appropriate dose of misoprostol for labor induction has not been determined. At the present time, oral doses of 100 μg administered every 3 to 4 hours appear to be safe and effective. Further studies are needed to determine whether higher doses can improve efficacy without increasing the rate of adverse maternal and perinatal outcomes.

Since the majority of studies have assessed the safety and efficacy of vaginal administration, more data are available to determine the most appropriate dose. Although dosing regimens as high as 200 μg have been reported in the literature, most authors have used vaginal misoprostol doses of 25 or 50 μg. Because of the increased incidence of uteronic effects, some authors have advised against the use of doses greater than 25 μg. However, the data that form the basis for this recommendation are limited. Six randomized clinical trials have been specifically designed to compare the safety and effectiveness of 25 or 50 μg of misoprostol administered intravaginally.[122–127] These trials, although generally well designed, are hampered by small sample size and thus prone to type II errors. A systematic review with meta-analysis of five randomized trials concluded that intravaginal misoprostol at doses of 50 μg for cervical ripening and labor induction is more efficacious, but it is unclear whether it is as safe as the 25-μg dose.[128]

In addition to the six randomized trials and the systematic review, two separate studies have compared the two doses (25 versus 50 μg). These two studies compared intravaginal misoprostol with intracervical dinoprostone gel (Prepidil).[37,38] The misoprostol dosage for the first study was 50 μg every 3 hours for a maximum of six doses, whereas the second study used 25 μg every 3 hours for a maximum of eight doses. Taken together, these two studies indirectly compared two doses of misoprostol: 25 μg and 50 μg. Subjects allocated to receive 50 μg experienced shorter intervals to vaginal delivery and no differences in overall cesarean or operative delivery rates, cesarean deliveries for fetal heart rate (FHR) abnormalities, or NICU admission rates. Although subjects receiving 50 μg of misoprostol experienced a greater incidence of tachysystole, no significant increases in adverse maternal or perinatal outcomes were noted. Meconium-stained fluid was noted more frequently for those receiving 50 μg of misoprostol. Given the reassuring perinatal findings noted previously, this latter finding, however, is of questionable importance. Because these two separate studies by Wing and associates[37,38] indirectly compare two doses of misoprostol, 25 μg and 50 μg, they were incorporated into the present analysis. Altogether, 906 patients were compared: 479 received doses of 25 μg and 427 received doses of 50 μg (Table 68–5). Patients who received the 25-μg dose had a lower incidence of tachysystole and hyperstimulation; however, they also had a longer interval to vaginal delivery, and a lower proportion of these patients delivered vaginally within 12 and 24 hours. No differences were noted in the cesarean delivery rate, cesareans performed for FHR abnormalities, operative delivery rates, or NICU admissions.

A recent ACOG (American College of Obstetricians and Gynecologists) Committee Opinion states that if misoprostol is used for cervical ripening and labor induction, 25 μg should be considered for the initial dose.[129] This opinion is based on the greater incidence of tachysystole noted with larger doses of misoprostol. Despite increased uterine activity with greater doses, however, greater rates of adverse maternal or perinatal outcomes have not been reported. Although existing evidence suggests that both the 25- and 50-μg doses of misoprostol are currently appropriate for intravaginal administration, we agree that further large prospective trials are required to define an optimal dosing regimen.

Cervical Ripening and Labor Induction in Special Circumstances

Previous Cesarean Delivery

Among patients with a previous cesarean section, the incidence of uterine disruption is greater with induced labor than with spontaneous labor (0.65% versus 0.40%).[130] Patients in this group undergoing cervical ripening and labor induction with PGE_2 (dinoprostone) experience a rupture rate of 0.9%.[131]

In women with unscarred uteri, vaginal or oral administration of misoprostol has been found safe and effective for patients with unfavorable cervices who require labor induction. There are indirect data, however, from which to assess the risks and benefits of using misoprostol to ripen the cervix and induce labor in women with a previous lower uterine segment scar. Recent publications have suggested that the use of misoprostol in patients with

TABLE 68–5

Second-Trimester Termination of Pregnancy (TOP) by Misoprostol-only Regimen

MISOPROSTOL REGIMEN	NUMBER OF SUBJECTS	GESTATIONAL AGE (WEEKS)	TOP RATE IN 24 h (%)	MEAN INDUCTION-TOP INTERVAL (h)	REFERENCES
1. Misoprostol 200 µg vaginal q12h × 2	28	12–22	89	12.0	Jain & Mishell[100]
2. PGE_2 20 mg vaginal q3h	27		81	10.6	
1. Misoprostol 100 µg vaginal q6h for 36 h max	27	12–24	74 (48 h)	23.1	Nuutila et al[223]
2. Misoprostol 200 µg vaginal q12h for 36 h max	26		92	27.8	
3. Gemeprost 1 mg vaginal q3h for 36 h max	27		89	14.5	
1. Misoprostol 200 µg vaginal q12h × 2	50	16–22	70.6 (48 h)	45	Herabutya et al[224]
2. Misoprostol 400 µg vaginal q12h × 2	50		82	33.4	
3. Misoprostol 600 µg vaginal q12h × 2	50		96	22.3	
1. Misoprostol 200 µg vaginal q6h × 8	51	12–22	87.2 (48 h)	13.8	Jain et al[225]
2. Misoprostol 200 µg vaginal q12h × 4	49		89.2	14.0	
1. Misoprostol 400 µg vaginal q3h	74	14–20	73.0	15.2 (median)	Wong et al[226]
2. Misoprostol 400 µg vaginal q6h	74		60.8	19.0	
1. Misoprostol 200 µg vaginal q6h	50	14–30	59	18.2 (median)	Dickinson & Evans[227]
2. Misoprostol 400 µg vaginal q6h	50		76	15.1	
3. Misoprostol 600 µg vaginal; then 200 µg q6h	50		80	13.2	
1. Misoprostol 200 µg oral q1h × 3; then misoprostol 400 µg oral q4h	65	12–20	39.5	34.5	Bebbington et al[228]
2. Misoprostol 400 µg vaginal q4h × 6	49		85.1	19.6	
1. Misoprostol 800 µg vaginal; then 400 µg oral q8h × 5	21	14–23		15.9	Feldman et al[229]
2. Misoprostol 800 µg vaginal; then 400 µg vaginal q8h × 5	23			21.1	
3. Misoprostol 400 µg vaginal q12h	60			26.0	
1. Misoprostol 400 µg vaginal q6h	28	14–26	86	14.5 (median)	Dickinson & Evans[231]
2. Misoprostol 400 µg oral q3h	29		45	25.5	
3. Misoprostol 600 µg vaginal; then 200 µg oral q3h	27		74	16.4	
1. Sublingual misoprostol 400 µg q3h × 5	18	14-20	100	11.6	Tang & Ho[232]

previous cesarean delivery is associated with a high frequency of uterine disruption (dehiscence or frank rupture).[132–138] Most of these publications consist of a few case reports or are based on retrospective uncontrolled studies. A randomized trial designed to compare the safety and efficacy of vaginally administered misoprostol in women with previous cesarean deliveries was prematurely terminated.[133] At the time this study was halted, however, the study had not met specific criteria for early termination.[139]

We used several sources to identify all publications that have reported the use of misoprostol for cervical ripening and labor induction in women with previous cesarean delivery. Eleven studies have been published indicating the use of misoprostol for cervical ripening and labor induction in women with scarred uteri.[132–138,140–143] Uterine disruptions, dehiscence, or rupture were reported in six of the studies.[132–137] Of 355 patients included in these 11 studies, 16 (4.5%) experienced uterine disruption. Because several confounding factors were present, however, it is important to analyze these data in detail. Data are available for 10 of 16 patients reported to have experienced uterine disruptions. The mean age of the patients was 29.6 ± 4.7 years with a mean gestational age of 39.5 ± 2.1 weeks. Three patients had two previous cesarean deliveries and, in two other patients, the type of scar was unknown. Although the information is not precise, it appears that in at least in three cases, the patients had a dehiscence of the previous incision. Most patients were induced with single or multiple vaginal doses of 25 μg of misoprostol. Two patients received four doses, and two others received at least three doses of misoprostol. The median interval from the last dose of misoprostol until the diagnosis of uterine disruption was 10 hours (interquartile range 8.5–17.2 hours). Seven patients received oxytocin infusion after misoprostol was administered and before the diagnosis of uterine disruption. Only two experienced tachysystole, and all patients were delivered by cesarean. The mean birth weight was 3438 ± 572 g. Four cases of neonatal acidemia and one neonatal death were reported.

Because of the paucity of data, there is a lack of sufficient evidence from which to assess the risks and benefits of using misoprostol or other prostaglandins to induce labor in women with a scar from a previous lower segment cesarean delivery. Randomized controlled trials are needed to assess outcomes including vaginal delivery rates, interval to delivery, and number of failed inductions. We are currently completing a trial comparing intravaginal misoprostol with oxytocin infusion in patients with previous cesarean delivery. Because uterine disruption is such an uncommon event, however, only a large multicenter randomized controlled trial will yield adequate statistical power to assess safety in this population of patients. To detect a difference in uterine rupture from 1% to 3.7%, such a trial would have to include 565 patients in each group ($\alpha = 0.05$, $\beta = 0.80$). Until such a trial is performed, an alternative approach would be to perform a case-control study. In the meantime, the use of misoprostol for cervical ripening and labor induction in women with a previously scarred uterus should occur only in the setting of a research protocol.

Twin Pregnancies

Twin pregnancies frequently involve maternal and fetal complications, which require early delivery. Additionally, the optimal timing of birth for women with an otherwise uncomplicated twin pregnancy at term is uncertain, with clinical support for both elective delivery at 37 weeks as well as expectant management. Elective delivery at term may be performed via an elective cesarean or vaginally with the use of mechanical or pharmacologic agents for cervical ripening and labor induction. At present, there are insufficient data to support a practice of elective cesarean delivery for women with an otherwise uncomplicated twin pregnancy at term.

The safety and efficacy of uterotonic agents, particularly oxytocin, for labor induction in women with twins are not as clear as in those with singleton pregnancies. Some clinicians believe that the overdistended uterus encountered with twins is resistant to oxytocin and may require high doses to obtain adequate uterine contractions. Additionally, some clinicians suspect that a gravida with twins is prone to hyperstimulation or even uterine rupture with relatively low doses of oxytocin. Although there are no large randomized trials attesting to the safety and efficacy of cervical ripening and labor induction in patients with twin pregnancies, several retrospective studies have suggested that labor induction, with a variety of induction agents, is acceptably safe. A recent case-matched control study compared the safety and efficacy of labor induction with oxytocin versus spontaneous labor in 62 women with twin pregnancies.[144] Twin pregnancy had no adverse impact on the effectiveness or efficiency of oxytocin labor stimulation; indeed it appeared to be associated with fewer side effects. Additional case series of labor induction in twin pregnancies have included the use of intrauterine balloon catheters,[145] oral dinoprostone or PGE_2,[146] and oxytocin.[147]

Although misoprostol has been shown to be a safe and effective agent for labor induction in singleton pregnancies, there are no published studies in women with twin pregnancies. If misoprostol is chosen for labor induction in twins, continuous monitoring of the fetal heart rate and uterine contractions should be performed. Repeated doses should only be used if there is definitely no evidence of regular uterine activity.

According to the American College of Obstetricians and Gynecologists, twin pregnancies do not necessarily constitute a contraindication to labor induction.[148] However, as with misoprostol, patients with twin pregnancies who undergo labor induction with oxytocin, or with any other agent, need to be monitored very closely.

Fetal Death

The ideal method for termination of pregnancy in cases of intrauterine fetal demise should be effective and safe and should have minimal side effects. In the past, oxytocin infusion and PGE_2 vaginal suppositories (referred to as pessaries in the United Kingdom) were the most commonly used methods for labor induction in patients with fetal death.

INTRAVENOUS OXYTOCIN

Intravenous oxytocin is a time-honored, effective, and safe method for inducing labor in cases of intrauterine fetal demise. However, oxytocin infusion is less effective when used in patients with a very unripe cervix and in those remote from term. Large doses and prolonged administration may be required, circumstances that increase the risk of water intoxication and attendant central nervous system complications. For patients who are remote from term, some authors have reported the use of high-dose oxytocin.[149] One regimen describes the use of approximately 300 mU/minute (200 units of oxytocin in 500 mL of 5% dextrose lactated Ringer solution or 5% dextrose and half normal saline at 50 mL/hour). In this setting, 5% dextrose and water has been associated with hyponatremia. Electrolytes should be checked before beginning oxytocin and should be repeated every 24 hours or if signs and symptoms of water intoxication occur. Attention should be paid to fluid intake and urinary output. For patients at or near term, lower doses of oxytocin are usually required. Laminaria, or other mechanical means of cervical ripening, may be beneficial before the use of oxytocin for induction.

PROSTAGLANDINS

Many cases of fetal death can be managed simply and effective by PGE_2 vaginal suppositories. The customary dose is one 20-mg suppository inserted vaginally every 4 hours until contractions are sufficient to promote progressive cervical change. Generally, this dose is used only for patients who are at no more than 28 weeks' gestation. However, some authors have reported safe use in the third trimester.[150] Reported side effects with higher doses (20 mg) of PGE_2 vaginal suppositories include fever, nausea, vomiting, and diarrhea. These annoying side effects may be ameliorated with appropriate and specific pretreatment medications. Although PGE_2 vaginal suppositories have been used safely in the third trimester, the risk of uterine rupture is increased.

More recently, misoprostol (synthetic analogue of PGE_1) has been used safely and effectively for cervical ripening and labor induction in patients with fetal death. Mariani-Neto and associates first reported the use of oral misoprostol (400 μg every 4 hours) for induction of labor following fetal death.[151] The authors reported their experience with 20 patients with fetal demise at 19 to 41 weeks' gestation. All patients delivered successfully with a mean interval to delivery of 552 minutes. The mean dose of misoprostol required was 1000 μg (400 to 2800 μg). Additional studies have assessed the safety and efficacy of misoprostol in the management of fetal death.[152–153] The doses and routes of administration have varied significantly among the studies. Oral doses of 200 μg and vaginal doses ranging from 50 to 200 μg every 4 to 6 hours have been employed. Some authors have combined misoprostol with mifepristone; patients receive a single dose of 200 mg mifepristone orally, following which a 24- to 48-hour interval is recommended prior to administering 100 to 200 μg of misoprostol in the vagina every 3 hours.[152,153]

Wagaarachchi and associates first reported a combination of vaginal and oral misoprostol after priming with mifepristone.[154] Women received a single dose of 200 mg mifepristone followed by a 24- to 48-hour interval before administration of misoprostol. For gestations of 24 to 34 weeks, 200 μg of intravaginal misoprostol was administered, followed by four oral doses of 200 μg at three 1-hour intervals. Gestations over 34 weeks were given a similar regimen but a reduced dose of 100 μg misoprostol. The average induction-to-delivery interval was 8.5 hours, which was the shortest among the previous regimens. Improved patient acceptability and reduced risk of introducing intrauterine infection are potential advantages of oral over vaginal route.

High doses of misoprostol (vaginal or oral administration) may be associated with fever, chills, and diarrhea. Pretreatment with antidiarrheal and antiemetic agents may reduce adverse effects.

EXTRA-AMNIOTIC SALINE INFUSION

Extra-amniotic saline infusion has been shown to be successful in inducing labor in antepartum deaths after 20 weeks' gestation.[155] A size 18 Foley catheter is inserted through the cervix under direct vision. The balloon is inflated with 30 mL of sterile water, and the catheter is usually strapped to the thigh under slight traction. Normal saline (0.9%) infusion is started to run at 30 drops per minute, and a maximum volume of 2 L should be infused into the extra-amniotic space.

CONCLUSIONS

INDUCTION OF LABOR

- Labor induction is indicated when the benefits of delivery to the mother and/or fetus outweigh the risks of continuing the pregnancy.
- More than 80% of inductions are for post-dates and hypertension.
- Social inductions are controversial and should not be performed before 39 weeks because of the risks to the neonate of pulmonary immaturity.
- The success of induction is higher in parous than nulliparous women, and is also strongly dependent on the ripeness of the cervix.
- The most widely used index of cervical ripeness is the Bishop score.
- If the Bishop score is 6 or less, induction is best done with an agent that ripens the cervix as well as producing uterine activity; this is usually a form of prostaglandin.
- Mechanical methods, such as laminaria tents and balloons, are also effective at ripening the cervix.
- Dinoprostone (prostaglandin E_2) is widely used for ripening and induction but misoprostol has the advantages of easier storage (because it is stable at room temperature and does not need to be stored in a refrigerator) and cheapness. Appropriate doses (for parous/nulliparous women) are 1-2mg of dinoprostone and 25–50 μg of misoprostol.
- Parenteral administration of oxytocin is effective at inducing labor, especially when combined with artificial rupture of the membranes. It has no direct effect on ripening of the cervix.
- The safest and most widely used regimens for induction with intravenous oxytocin commence at 1-2 mU/min and increase the dose by 1–2 mU/min every 40 minutes until contractions are effective (with a contraction frequency of no more than five in ten minutes). Less than 10% of women will require more than 16 mU/min to establish satisfactory uterine activity.
- All oxytocics carry a small risk of causing uterine rupture; the risk is higher in parous women and even higher in women with a scarred uterus. The risk is higher with prostaglandins (including misoprostol) than with oxytocin because the oxytocic effect is less controllable.

SUMMARY OF MANAGEMENT OPTIONS
Induction of Labor

Management Options	Quality of Evidence	Strength of Recommendation	References
Prenatal—General			
Bishop score is still the most reliable indicator of success of induction.	III	B	4
Prenatal—Indications			
Women should have a valid indication for IOL and no contraindications (see Tables 68–1 and 68–2).	III	B	81
Indications should be such that mother or fetus will benefit from a higher probability of a healthy outcome than if birth is delayed.	III	B	81
For a consideration of the validity of specific indication for induction of labor, see specific chapters.	–	–	–
Preinduction Cervical Ripening:			
Mechanical Methods			
Foley catheter	Ia	A	15
Laminaria tents	Ib	A	17,18
Membrane sweep	Ia	A	8
Acupuncture	IIb	B	21
Pharmacologic Methods			
Prostaglandins	Ia	A	27,28

Continued

SUMMARY OF MANAGEMENT OPTIONS

Induction of Labor *(Continued)*

Management Options	Quality of Evidence	Strength of Recommendation	References
Labor Induction			
Oxytocin is effective.	Ib	A	73,74,76
Prostaglandins are effective.	Ia	A	267
In women with intact membranes, vaginal prostaglandin E_2 is superior to oxytocin.	Ia	A	27,28
Although both routes are equally effective, intravaginal PGE_2 is preferable to intracervical as it is less invasive.	Ia	A	267
PG tablets (3 mg) are equally effective as PG gel (1–2 mg) every 6 hours, but tablets offer financial savings.	Ia	A	267
Oxytocin use in women with intact membranes should be combined with amniotomy.	III	B	81
Oxytocin should not be started for 6 hours following prostaglandin administration.	III	B	81
Oxytocin starting dose is 1–2 mU/minute, increased at intervals of 30–40 min.	III	B	81
Misoprostol appears to be a cheap, effective induction agent. Safety issues are probably related to dose or route and are being assessed.	Ia	A	115
Other methods such as mechanical methods, estrogens, relaxin, hyaluronidase, castor oil, bath, enema, and breast stimulation have varying efficacy.	III	B	81
Labor-Monitoring			
Fetal well-being should be established prior to induction of labor.	III	B	81
Following insertion of prostaglandin, fetal well-being should be established once contractions begin.	III	B	81
When oxytocin is being used for induction, continuous electronic monitoring should be used.	III	B	81
If there is uterine hypercontractility, tocolysis should be considered.	Ia	A	37,38,128

TERMINATION OF PREGNANCY FOR FETAL ANOMALY

Introduction

In 2001, 12% of all legal terminations of pregnancy (TOP) reported to the U.S. Centers for Disease Control and Prevention (CDC) occurred after 12 weeks' gestation. Only 5.6% were performed after 15 weeks' gestation: 4.2% at 16 to 20 weeks and 1.4% at 21 to 24 weeks. Dilation and evacuation (D&E) accounted for 96% of these procedures. From 1974 through 2001, the percentage of second-trimester TOP performed by D&E increased from 31% to 96%; and the percentage of second-trimester TOP performed by intrauterine instillation (intra-amniotic, extra-amniotic) using hypertonic saline, urea, or prostaglandin $F_{2\alpha}$ ($PGF_{2\alpha}$) decreased from 57% to 1.3%.[156] D&E, preceded by cervical preparation, is safe and effective when undertaken with appropriate instruments by practitioners who have a sufficient workload to maintain their skills.[157,158] Compared with intra-amniotic instillation methods, dilation and evacuation has lower complication rates.[158–161] However, almost all the comparative data relate to obsolete abortifacients (such as saline and urea solutions) that are rarely used today.

The introduction of PG analogues in the late 1970s changed the management of TOP in the second trimester; they were initially instilled into the amniotic cavity, and later used for cervical ripening. The subsequent introduction of the antiprogestin, mifepristone, shortened the induction-to-TOP interval still further, and the dosage of PG analogues required was reduced. Today, medical TOP is the method of choice in many centers that perform second-trimester TOP.[162–164]

Both D&E and medical induction are relatively safe, with low complication rates.[159,165] The method chosen is largely dependent on physician preference and level of technical expertise, coupled with the patient's informed decision.

Definition

Termination of pregnancy is the medical or surgical removal of a pregnancy before the time of fetal viability while preserving the life and health of the mother. Patients in need of TOP can be identified at any gestational age; however, the great majority are performed at 24 weeks' gestation or less.

Indications

The most commonly accepted indications for TOP are as follows:

- A pregnancy that would result in the birth of a child with anomalies incompatible with life or associated with significant physical or mental morbidity
- Fetal death
- To save the life of the mother or preserve the health of the mother

Fetal Conditions

Significant structural and chromosomal conditions affect at least 3% to 5% of all births, and an increasing number of women will be faced with the decision to end a pregnancy based on fetal health concerns.[166,167] Unfortunately, because fetal assessment (e.g., using biochemical screening, ultrasound, chorionic villus sampling, or amniocentesis) is not available until the second trimester, TOP for this indication is usually later in gestation than TOP for social indications. The number of fetal conditions that can be identified during pregnancy continues to expand because of the steady improvement of the technology available for prenatal diagnosis. Conditions that can be identified include the following:

1. Chromosomal disorders (e.g., trisomy 21, 18, 13)
2. X-linked disorders (e.g., hemophilia)
3. Metabolic disorders (e.g., Tay-Sachs)
4. Neural tube defects (e.g., anencephaly, spina bifida)
5. Structural anomalies associated with exposure to teratogens
6. Infections (e.g., rubella, cytomegalovirus, toxoplasmosis)
7. Structural anomalies of multifactorial or unknown etiology
8. Other fetal indications, including preterm prelabor rupture of membranes prior to 24 weeks and fetal death at 24 weeks or less

Maternal Conditions

Terminations of pregnancy to save the life or preserve the health of the mother are rare events. Some women with chronic medical conditions choose pregnancy termination only after discovering for the first time during pregnancy that continuing the pregnancy poses significant health risks for themselves. This failure of preconception counseling is unfortunately more common than it should be. For most chronic medical conditions, sufficient data exist to permit accurate decisions as to the likelihood and magnitude of risks associated with a continuing pregnancy, although it is often impossible to say precisely who will be affected. For example, although one can quote 30% to 50% mortality rate for pregnancy in association with Eisenmenger syndrome or pulmonary hypertension, half the women counseled will survive, and it is usually impossible to say which half. In the case of other medical indications for TOP, such as severe hypertensive vascular disease and certain malignancies, the prognosis can be given with more certainty.[168–170] Decision for TOP in this context should be based on the collaborative agreement of a multidisciplinary team. At minimum, the team should consist of the patient, the obstetrician, a medical specialist, and an expert in genetic counseling. Additional members may include family members, spiritual counselors, nurses, intensive care specialists, and ethicists. The decision must be individualized for each patient.

Legal Termination of Pregnancy Services

In the United States, only a few states provide public funding for TOP, and one third of private insurance plans provide limited or no coverage.[171] Women with federally funded medical care are covered for TOP services only if the woman's life is threatened, or in cases of rape or incest (32 states), when medically necessary (16 states), and in cases of life endangerment (2 states). Hence, cost considerations pose formidable barriers to women seeking TOP, even when there is gross fetal malformation.

Clinicians performing D&E procedures need training from an experienced mentor and the opportunity to maintain proficiency through ongoing experience. In the United States only 44% of all facilities providing TOP offer services at 14 weeks' gestation; the proportion declines dramatically as gestation advances, to 22% at 20 weeks and 7% at 24 weeks.[172] Moreover, only 7% of obstetrics and gynecology residency programs currently provide routine training in second-trimester TOP.[173] Labor induction is an integral part of obstetrics and gynecology training; training in D&E for second-trimester TOP is not. Among graduating obstetrics and gynecology residents in U.S. programs, 43% had never performed a D&E, and 81% had performed 10 or fewer procedures.[173] Therefore, despite the safety advantages of D&E, women requesting second-trimester TOP may be limited to labor induction methods simply because practitioners trained and willing to perform D&E are unavailable. Thus, the future availability of D&E, especially beyond 15 weeks of gestation, is uncertain. As the availability of D&E procedures decreases, the need for safe, efficacious methods of medical TOP will increase.

Patient Assessment and Counseling (See also Chapter 9)

Patient assessment should include history, physical examination, appropriate laboratory studies, and counseling.

History

The complete medical history should focus on the timing and reliability of the last normal menstrual period. If there is the slightest doubt about gestational age (for example, a discrepancy between the history and examination findings), assessment of fetal size with ultrasound is crucial. Knowledge of past reproductive history, sexual history, current medications, allergies, prior pelvic surgery, and any known uterine anomalies is important. Women with medical conditions severe enough to warrant TOP may require additional evaluation and stabilization prior to the procedure.

Physical Examination

Physical examination must include vital signs, weight, uterine size, and cardiopulmonary assessment. A sterile speculum examination should be done, seeking cervical pathologic problems, such as active cervicitis, deformities, and past trauma. A small, stenotic, or scarred cervical os may impair the cervical dilation necessary for safe surgical TOP.

Laboratory Studies

Few laboratory studies are required in young healthy women, but hematocrit, Rh status, indirect Coombs, and urinalysis results should be obtained.

- A complete blood count (CBC) and blood typing are the minimum laboratory studies required for surgical TOP.
    - A CBC is required to identify patients with significant anemia, who are at risk if excessive blood loss occurs. Transfusion may be needed, particularly in second-trimester TOPs. Patients with severe anemia are best treated in a setting where transfusion is available.
    - Blood typing is required so that Rh-negative women can be identified and given anti-D immunoglobulin (RhoGAM) to prevent Rh sensitization in subsequent pregnancies.
    - Screening for common sexually transmitted infections (STIs) should be addressed in geographic areas of high prevalence, in age groups at high risk (i.e., <25 years), and in at-risk groups (e.g., those with histories of STIs, multiple sex partners, substance abuse).
- Additional laboratory testing is dictated by the medical history and physical examination findings.

Coagulation studies are indicated for patients with conditions such as a history of coagulopathy, hematologic malignancies, hemorrhage with previous surgical procedures, petechiae, bruising, and hepatosplenomegaly.

Liver function tests are indicated for patients with conditions such as hepatitis, alcohol abuse, cancer, hepatomegaly, and jaundice. Renal function tests are indicated for patients with conditions such as renal disease, recurrent urinary tract infections, oliguria, hematuria, and proteinuria.

Electrolyte assays are necessary in patients who develop significant vomiting associated with the use of medical TOP techniques.

Ultrasound, in addition to its value for prenatal diagnosis, is used for determination of gestational age, placental location, and detection of uterine fibroids or the presence of uterine anomalies (e.g., uterus didelphys, unicornuate uterus, septate uterus).

Counseling

When a congenital fetal anomaly is diagnosed, the clinician should meet with the patient for the following reasons:

- To explain to the patient the nature and severity of the anomaly
- To discuss the treatment options available for the management of the anomaly
- To explain the implication(s) of the anomaly for the child and on the family
- To refer the patient for expert opinion if the clinician is uncertain about the congenital anomaly or its implication(s), treatment, and so on

The purpose of counseling is to help the patient understand her options regarding the pregnancy. In cases with severe anomaly, TOP may be offered as an option when there is a substantial risk that if the child were born, it would suffer from such physical or mental abnormality as to be seriously handicapped. If the clinician, based on his or her professional opinion, disagrees with the patient on her decision regarding TOP, the patient should be reminded that she can seek a second opinion.

At the minimum, the patient should know the diagnosis, purpose of the procedure, risks and possible complications, alternative treatments, and the likelihood of successful treatment.

Therefore, the woman should be given appropriate information related to the choice between TOP and continuing her pregnancy to viability, regardless of the physician's personal views about rearing a child with such an anomaly or about TOP. However, although physicians have a duty to give full and accurate information, they have no obligation to be involved in the procedure itself if they have ethical objections. For this reason, training in carrying out TOP should not be mandatory, although it is mandatory for physicians to be knowledgeable about the procedure and its complications so that they can give accurate advice and make an appropriate referral to someone who is willing to perform it.[174]

Choice of Methods

Termination of pregnancy can be achieved by surgical means or with pharmacologic agents alone, in combination, or as an adjunct to a surgical method. The methods described refer to pregnancy termination at 13 to 24 weeks' gestation. The decision over which method to use is primarily determined by the following factors:

- The gestational age
- The expertise of the available medical staff
- Patient preference
- The clinical importance of obtaining an intact fetus
- Presence of other complicating clinical conditions

Generally, dilation and suction evacuation can be used up to 14 weeks' gestation, but thereafter, specific techniques of cervical preparation and special instruments for D&E need to be used. Modern methods of aggressive cervical preparation coupled with extensive clinical experience of the procedure have resulted in improved safety for D&E.[175] Moreover, there are limited data on the new labor induction agents compared to D&E.[166]

From a provider perspective, D&E allows predictable scheduling and avoids the prolonged period of medical observation typical of labor induction. Patients having a TOP for fetal anomaly may find that the prospect of a prolonged induction and delivery compounds the anguish of their decision and loss. A surgical TOP, possibly under general anesthesia, may be less traumatic emotionally. Shulman and colleagues observed recently that patients in their institution recovered more quickly after D&E and required fewer referrals for postoperative counseling than patients having a medical TOP.[176] However, D&E places a greater emotional burden on the surgeon and support staff.[177]

Although some women elect to have a medical TOP out of a desire to avoid surgery, the rate for the use of surgical aspiration or curettage to treat incomplete TOP is 15% to 30% or higher.[165–167]

On the other hand, grieving is important for many parents of a fetus with congenital abnormality, and seeing and holding the fetus are important components of healing.[178] In addition, medical TOP results in the delivery of an intact fetus and therefore allows optimal evaluation and confirmation of suspected genetic or structural abnormalities. This information is vital in counseling couples about the likelihood of recurrence.

Currently, medical TOP with misoprostol is a safe alternative to surgical TOP in patients with acute medical conditions and chronic debilitating illnesses. In our experience, misoprostol combined with mechanical cervical dilators such as a Foley catheter or laminaria tents can be used safely in patients with severe hypertensive disorders, cardiac disease, or asthma.[179]

In difficult or challenging cases, especially at or beyond 16 weeks, the physician, in consultation with the patient, must choose the most appropriate method based upon the patient's individual circumstances.[180,181]

Clincal Setting

Surgical D&E can be performed safely in a variety of outpatient settings, including a physician's office, provided there is an efficient system for emergency transfer.[182–184] In contrast, medical TOP services are usually provided in hospital settings.

Surgical Methods

Surgical methods include dilation and evacuation (D&E), dilation and intact extraction (D&X), hysterotomy, and hysterectomy. The use of real-time ultrasound scanning during D&E can reduce perforation rates.[185] Hysterotomy or hysterectomy is seldom used owing to higher rates of morbidity and mortality.[186] Prerequisites for surgical TOP include cervical preparation, adequate cervical dilation to use a 16-mm suction cannula, special grasping forceps, adequate anesthesia, oxytocic agents, antibiotic prophylaxis, and appropriate postoperative care.

Dilation and Evacuation

Anesthesia

The choice of anesthesia must be based on the medical, psychiatric, and emotional condition of the patient. Consultation with anesthetists, medical specialists, and psychiatric specialists may be necessary to determine the best choice for the individual patient. In general, paracervical block with light sedation provides sufficient anesthesia for many patients; however, the full range of anesthesia options must be available. Use of short-acting barbiturates by intravenous bolus infusion is a simple, effective form of general anesthesia that obviates the need for muscle relaxants, intubation, and halogenated gases.[187]

Cervical Preparation

A variety of mechanical and pharmacologic methods have been utilized (see –4).

Use of Osmotic Dilators

There are four types of osmotic dilators—laminaria japonica, two synthetic dilators (Lamicel, Dilapan) (Fig. 68–1),[188] and isaptent. Laminaria, derived from the seaweed genus *Laminaria* (*L. japonica*, *L. digitata*), are one of the oldest devices used for cervical ripening. Tents prepared from *L. japonica* are commercially available and are packaged in a variety of sizes. Although tents prepared from *L. digitata* are available, they are less

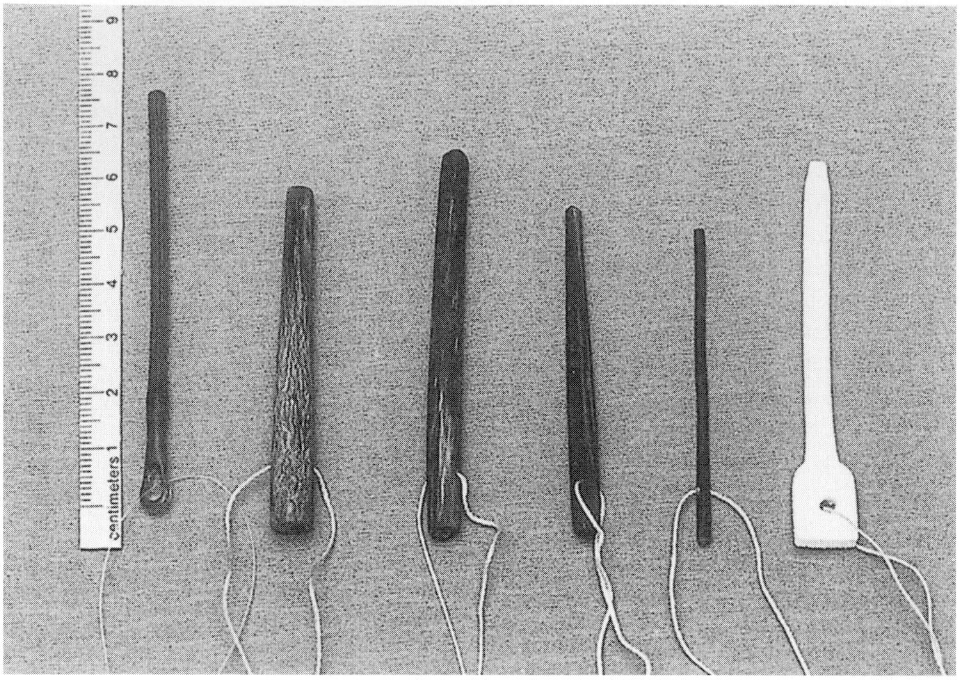

Figure 68–1
Osmotic dilators. Left to right: Dilapan, a single-sized synthetic polyacrylonitrile rod (hypan) currently available outside the United States; *Laminaria japonicum*, dried and compressed stalks of seaweed, four sizes (available in sizes ranging from 2 to 10 mm); Lamicel, a magnesium sulfate-impregnated polyvinyl alcohol sponge (available as 3 and 5 mm). (From Williamson DW: Resources for abortion providers. In Paul M, Lichtenberg ES, Borgatta L, et al [eds]: A Clinician's Guide to Medical and Surgical Abortion. New York, Churchill Livingstone, 1999, p 292, Fig. 20–13.)

useful clinically; they become gelatinous with expansion and are prone to fragment or become trapped in the cervix. The tents absorb water, swell, and ultimately dilate and soften the cervix. The tents expand most rapidly in the first 4 to 6 hours but continue to swell for up to 24 hours. In general, laminaria will expand up to four times their original diameter, resulting in concomitant dilation of the cervix. Placement of several smaller tents rather than one large tent may result in improved dilation and facilitate their later removal.

Compared to laminaria, Dilapan swells more rapidly and to a greater diameter, therefore, fewer Dilapan on average are needed for similar efficacy.[189] However, Dilapan is more likely to disintegrate, or retract, and it is no longer available in the United States.[190] Lamicel was found to be inferior to laminaria for midtrimester cervical ripening prior to D&E.[191] Lamicel is seldom used alone, as the sponges are difficult to insert in aggregate and become too soft on expansion to achieve the dilation needed.

Isaptent, although not used widely in the United States, is an alternative osmotic dilator that is effective for midtrimester cervical ripening. These commercially available tents (Dilex C.; Central Drug Research Institute, Lucknow, India) are prepared from granulated seed husk powder, derived from the isopgol plant (*Plantago ovata*), which is compressed and sealed into a cylindrical polythene sheath. The tents expand to a maximum diameter of 9 to 11 mm within 8 to 12 hours.[192] Comparison of isaptent to laminaria for cervical ripening demonstrates similar efficacy.[193]

Strategies may range from use of a single osmotic dilator with same-day surgery during the early second trimester to serial insertion of a variety of types and size of dilators for more advanced gestations. For procedures at up to 16 weeks' gestation, placing the dilators 4 to 8 hours prior to surgery may suffice. Beyond 16 weeks it is common practice to allow overnight dilation, and some mid to late second-trimester procedures call for a second insertion in 12 to 24 hours. Repeated laminaria applications significantly increase cervical dilation as compared to a single application, and therefore, treatment must be individualized.[190,194]

Adequate dilation is required in order to pass the 16-mm suction cannula and grasping forceps and to remove all the fetal parts. The minimum dilation required to insert grasping forceps depends on the type and size of the instrument used (13 mm for small Sopher, 14 to 15 mm for large Sopher, 16 mm for small Bierer, and 17 mm for large Bierer).[158] Prior to starting the procedure, sufficient cervical dilation must be confirmed. If cervical dilation is inadequate, additional osmotic dilators can be placed and the procedure delayed for at least 4 to 6 hours (or rescheduled to the next day).

Adequate pretreatment with laminaria may effect enough dilation prior to D&E to avoid the need for additional forced dilation in the operating room. Laminaria is the current mainstay in the United States for achieving cervical dilation for second-trimester TOP. Dilapan is still used widely in countries where it is available.

Methods of Insertion

After placing the speculum in the vagina and exposing the cervix, the cervix should be cleaned with antiseptic solution. Some women require no anesthesia or analgesia, but local anesthesia is helpful in women who are anxious or when the procedure is technically difficult. Use of a 50:50 mixture of lidocaine (1% or 0.5%) and bupivacaine (0.25%) provides rapid onset and a longer duration of action than does lidocaine alone.

The anterior lip of the cervix is grasped with a long Allis clamp. The cervical canal is carefully sounded, without rupturing the membranes, to identify its length. If desired, the cervix can be dilated mechanically using finely tapered dilators (such as Pratt and Denniston), and this allows insertion of more or larger osmotic dilators.

The large end of each osmotic dilator is grasped with a ring, packing, or ovum forceps and inserted into the cervical canal, laying successive dilators on top or next to the previous ones. Coating the dilators with lubricating jelly may ease insertion. Laminaria should be inserted leaving a 2- to 4-mm length protruding from the external os to facilitate its removal. The surgeon should ensure that the tips of the osmotic dilators pass through the internal os (Fig. 68–2).[158] If not, the result is a funnel-shaped canal and an inadequately dilated internal os (Fig. 68–3).[180] After inserting the dilators, they can be kept in place while the speculum is removed by placing a gauze sponge in a sponge holder over the cervix. The number and type of osmotic dilators inserted should be recorded.

In the event of inadvertent or spontaneous membrane rupture, the osmotic dilators should still be placed, but left in place for only 12 hours rather than 24 hours. The patient may resume normal activities, depending on how she feels.

Cervical Priming with Prostaglandins Prior to D&E

Lauersen and colleagues found a superior dilating effect with four to six laminaria tents placed 12 hours prior to D&E than with either PGE_2 vaginal suppositories (30 or 60 mg) or 15(S)-methyl $PGF_{2\alpha}$ (0.5 or 1.0 mg).[195] Vaginal and oral misoprostol have also been found useful in this setting.[196,197] More recently, buccal administration of misoprostol (600 μg given 2 to 4 hours prior to the procedure) was found to be as effective as laminaria tent for cervical preparation.[198]

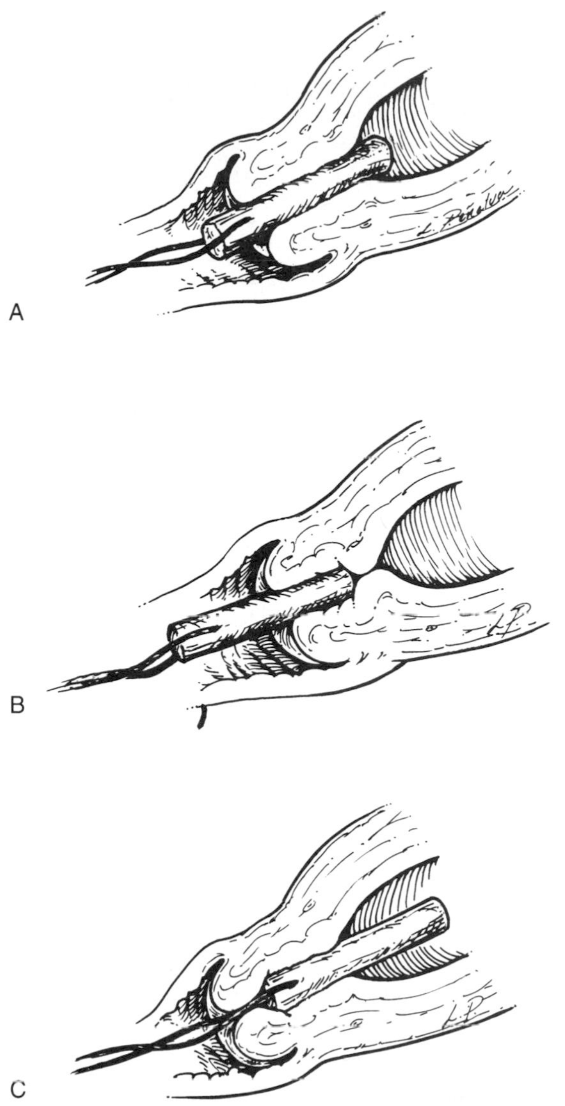

Figure 68–2
Osmotic dilator insertion. *A*, Laminaria placed appropriately through the internal os. *B*, Laminaria does not pass through the internal os. Swelling results in funneling of the endocervical canal and inadequate dilation of the internal os. *C*, Laminaria inserted too far into the endocervical canal. This placement may result in rupture of the membranes and difficult removal. (From Haskell WM, Easterling TR, Lichtenberg ES: Surgical abortion after the first trimester. In Paul M, Lichtenberg ES, Borgatta L, et al [eds]: A Clinician's Guide to Medical and Surgical Abortion. New York, Churchill Livingstone, 1999, p 130, Fig. 10–2.)

PROCEDURE: DILATION AND EVACUATION

This procedure consists of removal of the osmotic dilators, assessment of cervical dilation, and insertion of a 16-mm suction cannula to rupture the membranes and evacuate the amniotic fluid and fetal elements, followed by mechanical destruction and evacuation of fetal parts using special grasping forceps (preferably under ultrasound guidance).

The osmotic dilators are removed digitally or with packing forceps. The number of dilators should be counted to ensure they are all removed. Following this, a gentle digital examination will establish the extent of cervical dilation (particularly at the internal os). If sufficient dilation cannot be accomplished, the procedure should be delayed to repeat the osmotic dilation, or consideration should be given to admitting the patient for a medical TOP.

Once dilation is deemed adequate, the bladder should be emptied with a rubber catheter before D&E is started. The cervix is grasped with a long Allis clamp and a cannula is passed into the uterine cavity to rupture the membranes and evacuate as much amniotic fluid as possible with vacuum suction. The suction cannula should always be advanced fully into the uterine cavity before suction is applied. Up to 15 weeks' gestation, a 14-mm cannula should suffice, but gestations of 16 weeks and more require a 16-mm cannula. During removal of the amniotic fluid it is common for some membranes and placental tissue to be evacuated. However, complete placental extraction is generally delayed until the fetal parts have been removed.

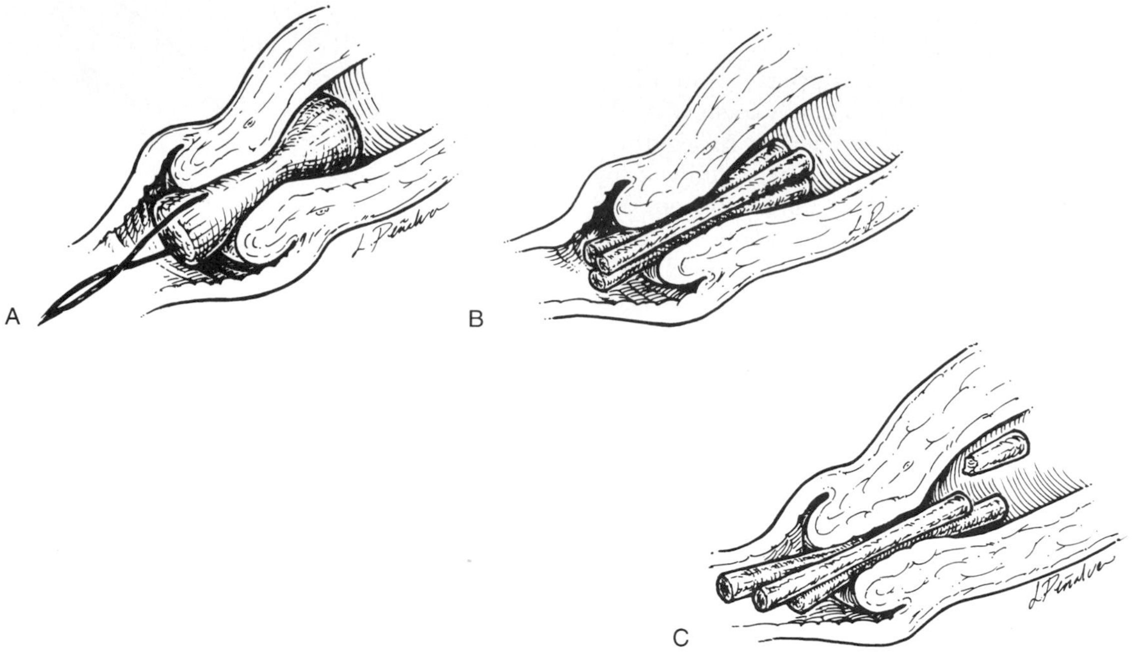

Figure 68–3
Dumbbelled osmotic dilator. *A*, A single large osmotic dilator is "dumbbelled" by the stiff internal os. Removal of this dilator may be difficult. *B*, Several small dilators are dumbelled. Because they are smaller, it may be possible to remove one. The others are then looser. *C*, When there are several dilators that cannot be removed, an alternative is to fracture one deliberately. The other dilators are then loosened and easier to remove. One fragment here has entered the uterine cavity and must be removed by suction or other means. (From Borgatta L, Burnhill MS, Karlin E: The challenging abortion. In Paul M, Lichtenberg ES, Borgatta L, et al [eds]: A Clinician's Guide to Medical and Surgical Abortion. New York, Churchill Livingstone, 1999, p 177, Fig. 13–5.)

With a 14-mm cannula, suction alone is usually adequate to remove 13- to 16-week pregnancies. Beyond 16 weeks some fetal parts remain in the uterus after suctioning and require extraction by forceps; most commonly these remnants include the spinal cord and calvarium. To extract the remaining fetal parts, a grasping forceps appropriate for the amount of cervical dilation should be used. In cases past 16 weeks, the fetus is extracted, usually in parts, using Sopher or similar forceps and other destructive instruments.

The choice of forceps (Fig. 68–4)[199] depends on operator preference and the extent of cervical dilation. We prefer Sopher forceps with its long shafts and bulkier grasping surfaces with sheltered serrations.

Once inserted, the forceps should be opened widely and one blade inserted along the anterior uterine wall in order to grasp the fetal parts. When fetal parts are felt between the blades on closing the handles, they are removed with a gentle twisting motion. The calvarium is the part most likely to be left behind. If fetal parts remain in the uterus, gentle probing with a small sharp curette may locate and retrieve them, although use of a sharp curette always carries the risk of perforating the uterine wall. Alternatively, sonography can be used to locate any remaining fetal parts and aid in their evacuation. In one study, use of intraoperative ultrasonography reduced the incidence of uterine perforation at D&E from 1.4% to 0.2%.[185]

Complete removal of the placenta generally requires one or more passes with the 14- to 16-mm suction curette. Before concluding the procedure, the fetal parts should be assembled to determine whether TOP was complete. Similarly, the quantity of placental tissue should be visually assessed to ensure that it is commensurate with the gestation.

USE OF OXYTOCIC AGENTS

The use of uterotonic agents during surgical TOP is a matter of preference. We use an intravenous infusion of oxytocin 20 to 40 units in 500 mL crystalloids given intraoperatively after rupture of membranes and continued postoperatively for 30 minutes. If the full 40 units is given, care should be taken to avoid excessive further infusion of crystalloid, because of the risk of water intoxication due to the antidiuretic effect of oxytocin.

ANTIBIOTIC PROPHYLAXIS

Routine oral antibiotic prophylaxis reduces the risk of infection after surgical TOP.[200–202] It is commonly started on the first day of osmotic dilator placement. Antibiotics such as tetracycline, clindamycin, and metronidazole have all been used to good effect.

POSTOPERATIVE CARE

Minimum observation periods for recovering D&E patients are 1 hour for early and mid second-trimester cases and 2 hours for late D&E, usually defined as more than 19 to 20 weeks' gestation.

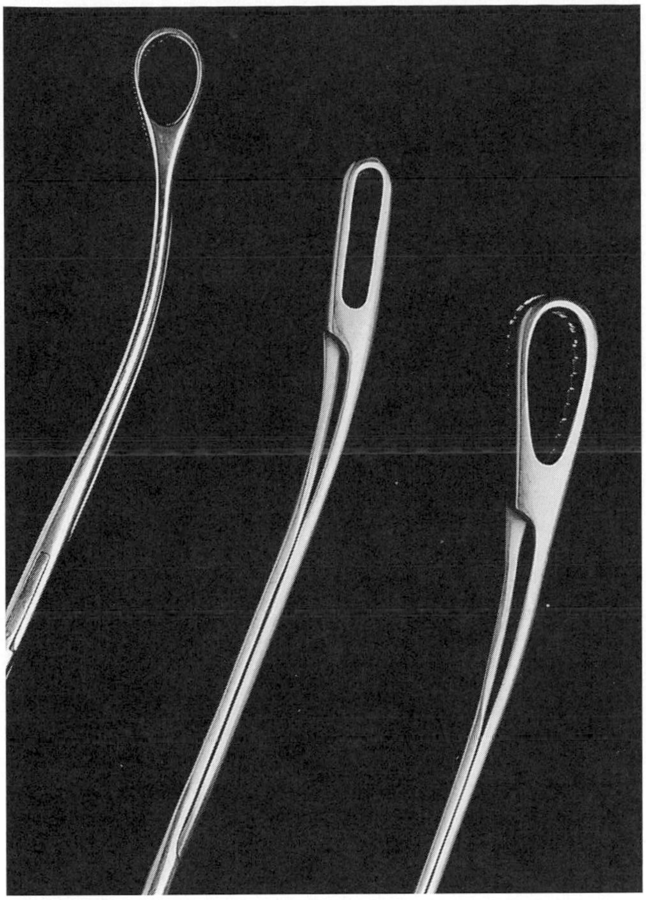

Figure 68–4
Instruments for D&E. Kelly placental forceps, Sopher forceps, and Bierer forceps (left to right). (From Ludmir J, Stubblefield PG: Surgical procedures in pregnancy. In Gabbe SG, Niebyl JR, Simpson JL [eds]: Obstetrics: Normal and Problem Pregnancies. New York, Churchill Livingstone, 2002, p 639, Fig. 19–25.)

Intact Dilation and Extraction

The American College of Obstetricians and Gynecologists in its general policy statement related to TOP described "intact dilation and extraction" (intact D&X) as containing all the following four elements.[203]

- Deliberate dilation of the cervix, generally accomplished with multiple, serial osmotic dilators over 2 days or more
- Instrumental conversion of the fetus to a footling breech
- Breech extraction of the body excepting the head
- Partial evacuation of the intracranial contents of a living fetus to effect vaginal delivery of a dead but otherwise intact fetus

According to the Centers for Disease Control, only 5.6% of TOP performed in the United States in 2001 (the most recent data available) were performed after the 16th week of pregnancy.[156] It is unknown how many of these were performed using intact D&X.

Intact D&X is a very controversial procedure in the United States. A select panel convened by the American College of Obstetricians and Gynecologists could identify no circumstances under which this procedure, as defined here, would be the only option to save the life or preserve the health of the woman.[203] In the authors' institution, medical TOP, with concurrent use of a 30-mL balloon Foley catheter or laminaria tents and misoprostol, is the method of choice after 18 weeks' gestation. The physician, in consultation with the patient, must choose the most appropriate method based upon the patient's individual circumstances.

Hysterotomy and Hysterectomy

In rare circumstances, hysterotomy or hysterectomy for TOP is preferable to either D&E or medical TOP. The possible indications include failed medical TOP if D&E cannot be safely performed, myomas in the lower uterine segment obstructing extraction, prior placement of an abdominal cerclage, which it is desired to leave in place, uterine anomalies (e.g., uterus didelphys, unicornuate or septate uterus), and some cases of cervical cancer.[180]

Another clinical challenge is the patient with complete placenta previa presenting for second trimester TOP.[204] In ultrasound studies, the reported prevalence of second-trimester placenta previa ranges from 2% to 6%. Thomas and colleagues reported on 131 patients with and without placenta previa who underwent second-trimester D&E. The 23 patients (17.6%) with ultrasound-documented placenta previa averaged only 21 mL more blood loss and had no other complications.[205]

On the other hand, placenta accreta occurs in 1 to 2 per 10,000 second-trimester TOP and usually results in heavy bleeding during the procedure. Placenta accreta is frequently associated with previous uterine surgery, suggesting a preexisting defect in the basal layer of the endometrium (decidua basalis).[206] Occasionally, patients with placenta accreta or placenta percreta require laparotomy with hysterotomy or hysterectomy despite the increased morbidity and mortality risks associated with these procedures.[207] These patients may benefit from preoperative placement of embolization balloon catheters using interventional radiology techniques.[208,209]

Medical Termination of Pregnancy

The introduction of prostaglandin analogues and mifepristone has revolutionized the management of second-trimester TOP and fetal death in the last 2 decades. Gemeprost and misoprostol are the two most extensively studied prostaglandin analogues that are used in this period. Gemeprost is the only licensed synthetic prostaglandin analogue for second-trimester TOP in the United Kingdom. However, it is expensive and needs to be stored in a refrigerator. Misoprostol is inexpensive and can be stored at room temperature. It has been widely used for induction of labor in cases of fetal death and second-trimester TOP for fetal anomaly. The combination of either gemeprost or misoprostol with mifepristone is most effective. With these regimens, over 90% of women abort within 24 hours and the mean induction-to-delivery interval is about 6 hours. Mifepristone is expensive and is not available in many countries. Therefore, prostaglandin analogue-only regimens can be the only option. These regimens are still effective, with TOP rate above 90% in 48 hours; however, the induction to TOP interval (15 hours) is much longer. Intracervical tents can be used to shorten the induction-to-delivery interval.[163,164]

Instillation into the uterine cavity through the intra-amniotic or extra-amniotic routes of substances designed to kill the fetus and promote delivery (such as hypertonic saline, hyperosmolar urea, $PGF_{2\alpha}$, ethacride lactate) is obsolete.[162–164] A recent review by Ramsey and coworkers detailed the limited role of vaginal PGE_2 and intramuscular $PGF_{2\alpha}$ as well as high-dose oxytocin infusion for second-trimester TOP.[210]

Fetocidal Procedures

Use of medical TOP has been associated with live birth rates from 4% to 10%.[167,211] In borderline viable gestations, patients, physicians, and nurses express concern about the dilemma of resuscitation in the event of a live birth after a PG-induced TOP. Moreover, such live birth is beset with ethical, medical, and legal implications. Because of concern among patients, practitioners, and hospitals, many TOP services perform a fetocidal procedure prior to or concomitantly with PG-induced TOP at 20 weeks' gestation or more.

The most common fetocidal agents used in developed countries are potassium chloride (KCl) and digoxin.[212,213] The procedure involves transabdominal insertion of a 20-gauge spinal needle into the fetal cardiac chambers by ultrasound guidance and instillation of 2 to 3 mL of potassium chloride in a concentration of 2 mEq/mL. Cardiac standstill is usually observed within 1 to 3 minutes. An alternative is the instillation of digoxin in doses varying from 0.25 to 2 mg, by the intracardiac, intrathoracic, intrafetal, and intra-amniotic routes.

Cervical Preparation

PHYSICAL METHODS

Osmotic dilators can be useful before induction of labor (see earlier discussion). There has been a resurgence of interest in catheter-based techniques, specifically in relation to the concurrent use of extra-amniotic saline infusion and misoprostol. A variety of balloon-catheter devices have been shown to be effective for cervical ripening.[210] Foley catheters with a 30-mL balloon are more commonly used in the United States. Extra-amniotic saline infusion (EASI) is an effective adjuvant to both midtrimester and term labor inductions.[214] Using aseptic technique and countertraction, a lubricated 26F Foley catheter with a 30- to 50-mL balloon is grasped with ring forceps and inserted through the internal os, after which the catheter balloon is inflated in the lower uterine segment. For the tightly closed, nulliparous cervix, a smaller diameter catheter (e.g., 18F) can also be used. Normal saline is infused through the catheter lumen at a nominal rate of 30 to 60 mL/hour, and traction is not used. Overall, EASI appears to be a safe and effective alternative to laminaria for midtrimester cervical priming. Advantages of EASI include low cost, reversibility, and lack of systemic side effects. Although EASI and laminaria appear to be equally efficacious, EASI offers the potential advantage of easier placement and less patient discomfort.

PHARMACOLOGIC CERVICAL RIPENING

Mifepristone (RU-486; Mifeprex) received Food and Drug Administration (FDA) approval in the United States in September 2000. Mifepristone was found to be more effective than laminaria tents in shortening the induction-to-delivery interval in a study using gemeprost.[215,216] The value of intracervical tents in regimens using misoprostol is less clear.[217] The World Health Organization (WHO) recommended that cervical preparation should precede all TOPs induced after 14 weeks.[218] Whenever possible, mifepristone should be used as the cervical priming agent before second-trimester TOP. If mifepristone is not available, an intra-cervical tent should be used.

Prostaglandins and Their Analogues

Prostaglandin receptors are present throughout all stages of pregnancy, and thus, PGs and their analogues are effective in terminating both first- and second-trimester pregnancy. The natural PGs, $PGF_{2\alpha}$ and PGE_2, were the first to be tested clinically for medical TOP but they were soon replaced by synthetic PG analogues because of the high incidence of gastrointestinal side effects when given parenterally or vaginally.[162–165]

The PGE and PGF analogues have been used clinically for second-trimester TOP. The PGE analogue is preferable as it has a more selective action on the myometrium and causes less gastrointestinal side effects. The most extensively studied PGE and PGF analogues for second-trimester TOP are carboprost, meteneprost, sulprostone, gemeprost, and misoprostol.

PROSTAGLANDIN E_2 (PGE_2) ANALOGUES

Two PGE_2 analogues, dinoprostone (Prostin) and meteneprost (9-methylene PGE_2), are commercially available and have been investigated for midtrimester TOP. Of these, only Prostin is FDA approved in the United States as an abortifacient in the midtrimester and for fetal death up to 28 weeks' gestation. The recommended dosage regimen of Prostin for second-trimester termination is 20 mg administered as a vaginal suppository every 3 to 4 hours (maximal exposure: 24 hours). In a series of midtrimester TOPs with vaginal PGE_2, 20 mg every 4 hours with osmotic dilators, the mean induction-to-delivery interval was 17 hours.[163,164] PGE_2 is not thermally stable and must be kept refrigerated. It has been widely investigated and has been proved effective for second-trimester TOP. However, intravaginal misoprostol was at least as effective as PGE_2 and without the cost and side effects associated with PGE_2 use.[100]

PROSTAGLANDIN $F_{2\alpha}$ ($PGF_{2\alpha}$) ANALOGUE

A synthetic $PGF_{2\alpha}$ analogue, carboprost tromethamine (15S)-15-methyl-$PGF_{2\alpha}$ tromethamine (Hemabate), is the only other commercially available PG that is FDA-approved and marketed in the United States as a midtrimester abortifacient at 13 to 20 weeks of gestation. The recommended dosage regimen of carboprost for second-trimester TOP is 250 µg, administered by intramuscular injection every 1.5 to 3.5 hours (maximal exposure: 12 mg or 48 hours). A test dose of 100 µg may be administered to confirm patient tolerance before administration of the full 250 µg dose. The successful TOP rate with intramuscular carboprost reached 80% to 90% in 36 hours, but it was associated with a high rate of gastrointestinal side effects.[163,164]

PROSTAGLANDIN E_1 (PGE_1) ANALOGUES

The three most extensively studied PGE analogues are sulprostone, gemeprost, and misoprostol. Sulprostone (16-phenoxy-(ω)-17-18,19,20-tetranor PGE_2 methyl sulphonylamide) was studied in the early 1980s for medical termination of second-trimester pregnancies. However, intramuscular sulprostone is no longer used clinically for medical TOP because of its association with myocardial infarction.[219] Therefore, gemeprost and misoprostol are the principal drugs used for second-trimester medical TOP today.

GEMEPROST

Gemeprost (16,16-dimethyl trans-Δ^2 PGE_1 methyl ester) is a PGE_1 analogue. It is the only prostaglandin licensed in the United Kingdom for medical TOP. It is administered as a vaginal pessary. Studies using a vaginal gemeprost-only regimen gave a complete TOP rate of 80% to 96.5% in 48 hours.[220–223] The commonest regimen is 1 mg every 3 to 6 hours for five doses in 24 hours. It is repeated if delivery does not occur in this time. The mean induction-to-delivery interval ranged from 14 to 18 hours. The commonest side effects were vomiting, diarrhea, and fever. Cost and the need for refrigeration are the drawbacks with gemeprost; these factors make its use practical only in developed countries.

MISOPROSTOL

Misoprostol (15-deoxy-16-hydroxy-16-methyl PGE_1) is a synthetic PGE_1 analogue. It was discovered that it could be used "off-label" as an abortifacient. It is cheap, stable at room temperature, and readily available in many developing countries. Vaginal misoprostol is as effective as gemeprost.[221–223]

Recent studies mainly focus on the optimization of misoprostol dosing regimens by comparing various dosages, dosing intervals, and routes of administration.[224–229] The dosage of misoprostol used ranged from 100 to 800 µg with dosing intervals of 3 to 12 hours. The efficacy of misoprostol is improved when a higher dose (400 to 800 µg) is given at a shorter intervals (3 to 4 hours) (Table 68–5). The vaginal route is more effective than the oral route.[228,230] The greater bioavailability of vaginal misoprostol probably explains the clinical results. Zieman and colleagues compared the absorption kinetics of misoprostol with oral versus vaginal (400 µg) administration in pregnant women.[120] It was shown that the systemic bioavailability of vaginally administered misoprostol is three times higher than that of the oral route. The plasma level was sustained up to 4 hours after vaginal administration. However, women preferred the oral route because it was less painful, gave more privacy, and was more convenient.[230]

A randomized study demonstrated that misoprostol 600 µg given vaginally, then 200 µg orally every 3 hours was probably the optimal regimen for second-trimester TOP.[231] A regimen that involves the administration of the first dose of misoprostol vaginally and subsequent doses orally might have a number of beneficial effects. It will minimize the number of vaginal examinations required to insert subsequent doses while preserving the possible direct cervical priming effect of the first dose.

Recently, sublingual administration of misoprostol has been developed. The sublingual route was chosen because it was considered as the most vascular area of the buccal cavity. It also avoids the first-pass effect through the liver in oral administration and the uncomfortable vaginal administration. One pilot study using 400 µg misoprostol every 3 hours for a maximum of five doses achieved a 100% second-trimester abortion rate with a median induction-to-abortion interval of 11.6 hours.[232] It was shorter than a similar dose regimen of vaginal misoprostol alone (15.2 hours), as shown in Table 68–5.[226]

MIFEPRISTONE AND SYNTHETIC PROSTAGLANDIN ANALOGUES

Mifepristone is the anti-progestin that is approved for use clinically for induction of TOP. It increases the sensitivity of the uterus to PGs. The use of oral mifepristone 36 to 48 hours before PG administration can increase the successful TOP rate, shorten the induction-to-delivery interval, and reduce the total dose of PGs required (see Table 68–6).[233–242] The first recommended dose of mifepristone was 600 mg, but it has been shown in a randomized trial that the successful TOP rate and induction-to-delivery interval were the same even if the dose was reduced to 200 mg.[239]

If mifepristone pretreatment is used before gemeprost (1 mg every 6 hours), the induction-to-delivery interval can be decreased from 15.7 hours to 6.6 hours and the successful TOP rate in 24 hours is increased from 72% to 95% (see Table 68–6).[237]

TABLE 68–6

Second-Trimester Termination of Pregnancy (TOP) by using Mifepristone Prior to Misoprostol

TREATMENT WITH ORAL MIFEPRISTONE 36–48 HOURS BEFORE MISOPROSTOL/GEMEPROST REGIMEN	NO. OF SUBJECTS	GESTATIONAL AGE (WEEKS)	TOP RATE IN 24 h (%)	INDUCTION-TOP INTERVAL (h)	REFERENCES
1. Mifepristone 600 mg + misoprostol 800 μg vaginal; then 400 μg vaginal q3h	35	13–20	97	6.0	El-Refaey & Templeton[238]
2. Mifepristone 600 mg + misoprostol 800 μg vaginal; then 400 μg oral q3h	34		97	6.7	
1. Mifepristone 600 mg + misoprostol 800 μg vaginal; then 400 μg oral q3h × 4	35	13–20	94	6.9	Webster et al[239]
2. Mifepristone 200 mg + misoprostol 800 μg vaginal; then 400 μg oral q3h × 4	35		97	6.9	
1. Mifepristone 200 mg + misoprostol 200 μg vaginal q3h × 5	49	14–20	90	9.0 (median)	Ho et al[240]
2. Mifepristone 200 mg + misoprostol 200 μg oral q3h × 5	49		69	13.0	
1. Mifepristone 200 mg + misoprostol 400 μg oral q3h × 5	70	14–20	81.4	10.4 (median)	Ngai et al[242]
2. Mifepristone 200 mg + misoprostol 200 μg vaginal q3h × 5	69		84.0	10.0	
Mifepristone 200 mg + misoprostol 800μg vaginal; then misoprostol 400 μg oral q3h × 4	500	13–21		6.5 (median)	Ashok & Templeton[241]
1. Mifepristone 200 mg + 1 mg gemeprost q6h × 3	50	12–20		6.6 (median)	Bartley et al[237]
2. Mifepristone 200 mg + misoprostol 800 μg vaginal; then misoprostol 400 μg oral q3h × 4	50			6.1	

To improve patient acceptability and to maintain the efficacy, a combination regimen including both the oral and vaginal routes has been developed. El-Refaey and Templeton (1995) compared two misoprostol regimens in women pretreated with 600 mg mifepristone for 36 to 48 hours.[238] The first group received 800 μg vaginal misoprostol as the first dose and 400 μg vaginal misoprostol every 3 hours. The second group received 800 μg vaginal misoprostol as the first dose and 400 μg oral misoprostol every 3 hours. The mean induction-to-TOP interval was 6.0 and 6.7 hours, respectively. The 24-hour TOP rate was 97% in both groups (see Table 68–6). Ashok and associates (1999) used mifepristone 200 mg followed by 800 μg vaginal misoprostol as the first dose and 400 μg oral misoprostol every 3 hours. They achieved 97% abortion rate; the median induction-to-abortion interval was 6.5 hours.[241] Pretreatment with mifepristone significantly reduced the induction-to-TOP interval when compared with a misoprostol-only regimen. It was thought that vaginal misoprostol as the first dose could have a cervical priming effect.

Current evidence shows that the combination of oral mifepristone and vaginal misoprostol is an effective method for termination of second-trimester pregnancy. If mifepristone is not available, vaginal misoprostol alone can be used but the induction-to-TOP interval will be slightly longer.

USE OF PROSTAGLANDIN WITH A SCARRED UTERUS

With the rising cesarean delivery rate, an increasing number of women undergoing second-trimester TOP will have a previous uterine scar. No matter what method is used, the risk of uterine rupture is higher than for those without a scar. The reported risk of scar rupture at the time of medical termination in the presence of a previous uterine scar varies from 3.8%[243] to 4.3%.[244] This rate compares with a uterine rupture rate of 0.2% in patients with an intact uterus.[245,246] Uterine scar rupture has been reported with both gemeprost and misoprostol regimens with or without priming by mifepristone.[247–255] No well-controlled study has shown any method as being better than the others. All oxytocic agents should be used with caution in patients with previous cesarean deliveries. Women should be appropriately counseled about the risks and consequences, and practitioners should be prepared to deal with a rupture if and when it occurs. The optimum chance for successful outcome is provided by an informed and alert clinician who appreciates the potential risks of the procedure and who is prepared to deal with those risks.

Side Effects and Complications

Second-trimester TOP is a relatively safe procedure in countries where it is legal, accessible, and performed under modern medical conditions. However, both the patient and practitioner must be aware of procedure- and medication-related side effects and complications, including acute medical events and potential long-term reproductive risks.

SIDE EFFECTS OF PROSTAGLANDIN-INDUCED TOP

The use of PGs gemeprost and misoprostol, with or without mifepristone, is a safe and effective method of second-trimester TOP. Side effects including nausea, vomiting, and diarrhea are characteristics of prostaglandin administration and are due to prostaglandin's stimulatory effect on the gastrointestinal tract. Diarrhea is more common in women using gemeprost, whereas fever is more common with misoprostol.[163,164] The advantages of using misoprostol for second-trimester TOP compared with other PG agents are the relatively low incidence of reported side effects (Table 68–7). Side effects reported from the use of high-dose oxytocin regimens include nausea and vomiting. Prolonged usage may cause water intoxication. The suggested high-dose oxytocin regimen includes an alternating period of oxytocin infusion and a drug-free interval to allow for clearance of the oxytocin to avoid water intoxication.

COMPLICATIONS ASSOCIATED WITH MEDICAL TOP

Complications common to most medical TOP include retained placenta and associated hemorrhage or infection, failed TOP, live birth, and serious complications such as uterine rupture.

Retained Placenta (incomplete abortion). Patients who underwent medical TOP compared to those who had D&E were more likely to have retained products of conception that required operative intervention (21% versus 0.7%). Although patients who underwent medical TOP with misoprostol were less likely to have complications than patients who underwent medical TOP by other methods (22% versus 55%), these patients still had more complications than surgical patients (22% versus 4%). Patients who elect to undergo second-trimester medical abortion should be advised that they have a significant risk (21%) of requiring surgery for retained products of conception because this knowledge may assist them in making an informed decision.[166]

Sixty percent of subjects passed the placenta spontaneously within 2 hours, with approximately two-thirds of the expulsions occurring within the first 30 minutes. The rate of complications (hemorrhage and febrile morbidity) increased over time, reaching 4% at 30 minutes and 9% at 2 hours.[256] Retained tissues can lead to hemorrhage, infection, or both and usually manifests itself within several days of the TOP. Cramping and bleeding can be accompanied by fever. If complete placental expulsion did not occur within 2 hours of fetal delivery, the placenta was removed manually or by forceps or curettage.[256]

Infection. During the second trimester infection rates for both medical and surgical TOP methods have remained within the narrow range of 0.4% to 2.0% in North America and Great Britain.[165,166] Infection is usually associated with retained products of conception, but there are no data to analyze the incidence of infection separately in cases with or without retained tissue. Typically, signs and symptoms of post-TOP infection arise within the first 48 to 96 hours. The patient may present with pain, fever, and pelvic tenderness. The cervix should be cultured for sexually transmitted pathogens—*Neisseria* (gonorrhea) and *Chlamydia*. Established risk factors for post-TOP infection

TABLE 68–7

Induction Agents and Reported Adverse Effect (% occurrence)

AGENT	INDUCTION-ABORTION INTERVAL (h)	ADVERSE EFFECTS (%)	COMMENTS
Hypertonic saline	20–46	Fever, vomiting (5–12%) Hemorrhage	Intraamnotic injection; used with oxytocin augmentation
Oxytocin	8–13	Water intoxication (rare) Nausea and vomiting (less than with PGs)	Inexpensive Significantly fewer gastrointestinal side effects than prostaglandins (PGs) Requires intravenous infusion
$PGF_{2\alpha}$	14–37 (dose-dependent)	Incomplete abortion Hemorrhage Live-born fetus (rates higher than with saline) Nausea, vomiting, diarrhea (30%)	Intraamniotic instillation; most patients require oxytocin augmentation No longer available in United States in form used for induction Potent bronchoconstrictor
15-Methyl $PGF_{2\alpha}$	8–16	Vomiting, diarrhea, fever (2–3 episodes per patient)	Intramuscular (has also been used via intra-amniotic, extra-amniotic, vaginal routes)
Dinoprostone (PGE_2)	11–14 (6–7 h with cervical ripening)	Fever, nausea, vomiting, diarrhea (most patients experience at least one side effect)	Vaginal suppositories Must be refrigerated
Sulprostone (PGE_2)	11	Vomiting (12–46%) Diarrhea (6–17%)	Given intramuscular or intravenously Not available in United States
Gemeprost (PGE_1) + mifepristone	15 6–8	Vomiting (1–14%) Diarrhea (2–20%)	Vaginal pessary Not available in United States
Misoprostol (PGE_1) + mifepristone + laminaria	9–14 6–10 10–22	Vomiting (4–10%) Diarrhea (4–15%)	Oral or vaginal routes Inexpensive; no refrigeration required

include age younger than 20 years, nulliparity, previous pelvic inflammatory disease, and presence of pathogens in the cervix at the time of TOP. The latter association has been reported with documented *Chlamydia* infection, gonorrhea, and bacterial vaginosis.[201] Most post-TOP infections, however, occur in women without these risk factors. Routine antibiotic prophylaxis may prevent up to half of all post-TOP infections in the United States and is highly cost-effective. Tetracyclines or nitroimidazoles (metronidazole or tinidazole) were equally efficacious for preventing infection.[200] Ascending genital tract infections are typically polymicrobial. Patients who present with post-TOP metritis should receive a full course of broad-spectrum antibiotic therapy. When retained tissue is evident or suspected, prompt evacuation is indicated.

Failure of Medical TOP. Failed induction has been defined as a failure to achieve TOP within 24 to 48 hours and is a significant clinical problem. Management options include deferring TOP when membranes are intact for a predetermined time, aggressive cervical dilation with sequential laminaria application and another trial of induction, changing the induction agent used, or recommending D&E.

Uterine Rupture. Serious complications including uterine rupture, major hemorrhage, and cervical tear are rare.[163,164] Cases of uterine rupture were reported to occur with both gemeprost and misoprostol, and the use of mifepristone did not exclude the possibility.[243–255] The incidence of uterine rupture was estimated to be 0.2% in the second trimester. Risk factors for uterine rupture include previous cesarean delivery, grand multipara, advanced gestation, prolonged PG therapy, and use of oxytocin in addition to PGs.[252]

Live Birth. Second-trimester medical TOP with PG analogues has been associated with live birth rates of 4% to 10%.[167,211] Physicians should have a protocol to induce fetal death (e.g., fetal intracardiac potassium chloride or digoxin) before induction, and patients should be apprised of the risk for live birth and should understand the plan in advance.

COMPLICATIONS ASSOCIATED WITH D&E (Table 68–8)

Based on the data from the 1970s and 1980s, D&E is clearly safer than intra-amniotic instillation methods and hysterotomy or hysterectomy for second-trimester TOP through 16 weeks' gestation.[159,165,182–184] In these investigations most of the specific complications associated with D&E occurred at rates well below 1%. A recent report by Autry and colleagues confirmed both the low complication rate that is associated with D&E and its superiority over medical TOP.[166] When skilled operators are available, D&E after cervical preparation with laminaria should be considered the preferred method for second-trimester TOP. Hence, the choice of TOP method at this later stage usually hinges on nonmedical considerations: cost, convenience, comfort, and compassion.

In challenging or difficult cases, careful assessment and choice of TOP method should be made to minimize complications. Intraoperative ultrasonography may be helpful in difficult cases.[185] Previous cesarean delivery scar does not seem to increase the perioperative risk of late termination (14 to 22 weeks) by the laminaria and evacuation technique.[207]

Hemorrhage. Reported rates of hemorrhage vary widely, reflecting both diverse definitions and imprecise estimation of blood loss. Hemorrhage associated with TOP is not common and the RCOG guideline group reported this complication as 1.5 per 1000 TOPs overall.[161] Factors associated with increased risk of uterine hemorrhage were operator inexperience, advanced gestational age, advanced maternal age and parity, prior cesarean delivery, uterine fibroids, and past history of post-TOP or postpartum bleeding.[159,162] Hemorrhage associated with D&E may indicate cervical laceration, perforation, retained tissue, uterine atony, placental abnormalities, or coagulopathy. Advances in operative technique and use of uterotonic agents have resulted in reduction of both mean and median blood loss in North America.

Intraoperative use of oxytocin, ergots, and PGs reduces blood loss from uterine atony during D&E.

TABLE 68–8

Comparison of Complication Rates among Medical and Surgical TOP Study Subjects

COMPLICATION	MEDICAL (n = 158)	SURGICAL (n = 139)	*P* VALUE
Patients with any complication	45 ± 28.5	5 ± 3.6	<.001
Failed initial method	11 ± 7.0	0 ± 0	<.01
Hemorrhage with transfusion	1 ± 0.6	1 ± 0.7	NS
Infection with intravenous antibiotics	2 ± 1.3	0 ± 0	NS
Retained products of conception	33 ± 20.9	1 ± 0.7	<.001
Cervical laceration with repair	2 ± 1.3	3 ± 2.2	NS
Organ damage	2 ± 1.3	0 ± 0	NS
Hospital readmission	1 ± 0.6	1 ± 0.7	NS

Modified from Autry AM, Hayes EC, Jacobson GF, Kirby RS: A comparison of medical induction and dilation and evacuation for second-trimester abortion. Am J Obstet Gynecol 2002;187:393–397.

Treatment of uterine atony includes manual uterine compression, oxytocin infusion, ergot derivatives, and PGs (15-methyl $PGF_{2\alpha}$, PGE_1).

Second-trimester TOP by D&E in the presence of placenta previa appears to be safe and apparently does not increase maternal morbidity as compared with the outcome in patients without placenta previa undergoing the same procedure.[204] All placenta accreta patients had at least one cesarean delivery (mean 1.7), and prior to a preoperative sonogram demonstrating some form of placenta previa. The prevalence of clinical placenta accreta encountered during D&Es in the second trimester was 0.04%, the same as that reported for placenta accreta diagnosed clinically in the third trimester. Placenta accreta can be a potential complicating factor in the patient undergoing D&E in the second trimester.

Cervical Injury. The most common type of cervical injury is a superficial laceration caused by the tenaculum or Allis forceps tearing off during dilation. At the other extreme are the cervicovaginal fistula and the longitudinal laceration ascending to the level of the uterine vessels. Rates of cervical injury range from 0.01 to 1.6 per 100 suction curettage TOP.[157,158]

Several risk factors of cervical injury during suction curettage have emerged. Among factors within the control of the physician, use of laminaria and performance of the TOP by an attending physician (rather than a resident) lower the risk significantly. Among factors beyond the control of the physician, a history of prior abortion lowers the risk, and age of 17 years or under increases the risk. Use of laminaria and performance of the TOP under local anesthesia by an attending physician together yield a 27-fold protective effect.[159] Cervical preparation with misoprostol may confer similar benefits as laminaria, although more extensive experience will be needed to confirm this.

Perforation. Perforation is a potentially serious, but infrequent, complication of D&E. According to most reports, the incidence of perforation is about 0.2 per 100 suction curettage TOP.[157]

Several risk factors for perforation exist. Performance of a curettage TOP by a resident rather than an attending physician increases the risk more than fivefold; on the other hand, cervical dilation by laminaria decreases the risk about fivefold. The risk of perforation increases significantly with advancing gestational age. Previous gynecologic surgery including TOP, cesarean delivery, and large loop excision of the transformation zone of the cervix (LLETZ) procedure is a risk factor for tearing of the internal os leading to perforation of the uterus during subsequent D&E procedures.[257] Dilation of the cervix particularly for these “at-risk” procedures should be predominantly passive by the use of oral prostaglandins such as misoprostol and osmotic dilators. The overall perforation rate was 0.029%.[258]

The use of real-time ultrasound scanning during D&E can reduce perforation rates. The routine intraoperative use of ultrasonographic imaging to guide intrauterine forceps during uterine evacuation for second-trimester TOP resulted in a significant reduction in uterine perforation, the rate declining from 1.4% to 0.2%.[185] These findings support the routine use of intraoperative ultrasonography for second-trimester TOP to reduce the incidence of uterine perforation and make the procedure a safer one.

The two principal dangers of perforation are hemorrhage and damage to the abdominal contents. Lateral perforations in the cervico-isthmic region are particularly hazardous because of the proximity of the uterine vessels. Perforations of the fundus are more likely to be innocuous. Many suspected or documented perforations require only observation. Perforation with a dilator or sound is unlikely to damage abdominal contents. On the other hand, a suction cannula or forceps in the abdominal cavity can be devastating.

If the physician suspects a perforation, the procedure should stop immediately. If unmanageable hemorrhage, expanding hematoma, or injury to abdominal content occurs, prompt laparotomy is necessary. Laparoscopy can be useful in documenting perforation and assessing damage; if necessary, the physician can complete the abortion under laparoscopic visualization. Any woman with severe pain within hours after D&E should be evaluated for possible perforation with bowel injury.

Acute Medical Events

Acute medical events, such as vasovagal reaction, asthmatic reactions, amniotic fluid embolism, anaphylaxis, and seizures to anesthetic agents or laminaria can occur at the time of TOP.[259–261] The safety of PG agents used for TOP has been established. Side effects are usually of a minor nature, although life-threatening complications can occur and include cardiac arrest.[262] This severity emphasizes the importance of medical supervision when the procedure is carried out.[238]

Long-Term Reproductive Risks

The bulk of evidence would suggest that D&E is a very safe procedure with few long-term problems. There is no proven association between D&E and subsequent fertility difficulty.[263] Second-trimester D&E is not a risk factor for midtrimester pregnancy loss or spontaneous preterm birth. Preterm delivery in future gestations appears less likely when greater preoperative cervical dilation is achieved with laminaria, possibly because of a decrease in cervical trauma.[264–266] Published studies have not been prospective and have not been able to control for competing risk factors, such as smoking or exposure to sexually transmitted infections that might overestimate the impact of induced TOP on poor reproductive outcome. Long-term complications associated with medical TOP in the second trimester using gemeprost and misoprostol with or without mifepristone are rarely reported.

CONCLUSIONS

GENERAL

- The introduction of prostaglandin analogues and mifepristone has revolutionized the management of second-trimester TOP and fetal death in the last 2 decades.
- Prostaglandin analogues provide a safe and effective method for induction of second-trimester TOP and intrauterine death.
- Gemeprost is the drug licensed for this purpose but misoprostol is a cheaper alternative and can be stored and transferred at room temperature. It provides a suitable alternative of particular relevance to resource-poor areas of the world.

GENERAL

- Prostaglandin analogues can also be used as cervical priming agents prior to D&E. D&E is safe and effective. TOP services can be difficult to organize; the skill and expertise to provide a safe D&E may not always be available.
- The choice of TOP methods continues to extend with new developments in medical termination across all gestations. There is no comparative trial evidence of late D&E against modern methods of midtrimester medical termination.
- Debate continues regarding appropriate techniques for terminating more advanced pregnancies.
- Practitioners should be specifically trained, competent, and comfortable with the procedure they provide.
- Clinical preassessment, counseling, and informed choice form the basis of good practice.
- Ultrasound is useful, but there is no randomized trial evidence of its value.
- Health care professionals should be aware of choices for TOP methods, and women should receive information that helps them to choose a method that is right for them.

DILATION AND EVACUATION

- Cervical ripening facilitates cervical dilation and reduces risk for certain complications.
- Antibiotic prophylaxis reduces short-term infective morbidity rate and should be offered as a minimum, but a screen-and-treat policy for infection is an alternative; both together might confer even greater health advantage.
- Aseptic technique should be observed for D&E with careful and gentle instrumentation to avoid injury to cervix or uterus.
- D&E needs specific training and requires special cervical preparation and instruments.
- Patients must have access to services for post-TOP advice and management of complications.

MEDICAL TOP

- Gemeprost and misoprostol are the two most extensively studied prostaglandin analogues that are used for mid-trimester TOP.
- The combination of either gemeprost or misoprostol with mifepristone is most effective. With these regimens, TOP rate within 24 hours is over 90% and the mean induction-to-TOP interval is about 6 hours. Mifepristone is expensive and is not available in many countries.
- Therefore, prostaglandin analogue-only regimens might be the only option. These regimens are still effective with a TOP rate of over 90% in 48 hours. However, the induction-to-TOP interval (15 hours) is much longer.
- Intracervical tents can be used to shorten the induction-to-TOP intervals.

FUTURE RESEARCH AGENDA

- Comparison of late D&E and modern midtrimester medical TOP with mifepristone and prostaglandin
- Prospective studies on the influence of medical and surgical TOP on future reproductive health (fertility and obstetric outcome)

SUMMARY OF MANAGEMENT OPTIONS
Second-Trimester Termination of Pregnancy

Management Options	Quality of Evidence	Strength of Recommendation	References
Prenatal—General			
Accurate estimation of gestational age	III	C	160,161
Accurate diagnosis	–	GPP	–
Patient assessment and counseling	–	GPP	–
Dilation and Evacuation (D&E)			
Cervical preparation			
Laminaria	IIa	B	190,191,194
Misoprostol	IIb	B	195,196,197
Use of prophylactic antibiotics	–	GPP	–
Use of intraoperative ultrasound	–	GPP	–
Use of intraoperative oxytocin	–	GPP	–
Medical Abortion			
Fetocidal agent – KCl or digoxin	III	B	212,213
Mifepristone 36–48 h, then vaginal misoprostol followed by oral misoprostol	Ia	A	238,241
Laminaria/Foley + vaginal misoprostol, then oral misoprostol concurrently	IIb	B	217
Failed Medical Abortion	III	B	180
D&E or			
Hysterotomy or hysterectomy			

REFERENCES

1. Hamilton BE, Martin JA, Sutton PD: Births: Preliminary data for 2002. Nation Center for Health Statistics. National Vital Stat Rep 2003;51:1–20.
2. American College of Obstetrics and Gynecologists: Assessment of Fetal Lung Maturity. ACOG Educational Bulletin No. 230. Washington, DC, ACOG, 1996.
3. Calkins LA, Irvine JH, Horsley GW: Variation in the length of labor. Am J Obstet Gynecol 1930;19:294–297.
4. Bishop EH: Elective induction of labor. Obstet Gynecol 1955;5:519–527.
5. Poma PA: Cervical ripening—A review and recommendations for clinical practice. J Reprod Med 1999;44:657–668.
6. Xenakis EMJ, Piper JM, Conway DL, et al: Induction of labor in the nineties: Conquering the unfavorable cervix. Obstet Gynecol 1997;90:235–239.
7. Gonen R, Degani S, Ron A: Prediction of successful induction of labor: Comparison of transvaginal ultrasonography and the Bishop score. Eur J Ultrasound 1998;3:183–187.
8. Ware V, Raynor BD: Transvaginal ultrasonographic cervical measurement as a predictor of successful labor induction. Am J Obstet Gynecol 2000;182:1030–1032.
9. Gabriel R, Darnaud T, Chalot F, et al: Transvaginal sonography of the uterine cervix prior to labor induction. Ultrasound Obstet Gynecol 2002;3:254–257.
10. Krammer J, O'Brien WF: Mechanical methods of cervical ripening. Clin Obstet Gynecol 1995;38:280–286.
11. Woodman WB: Induction of labor at eight month, and delivery of a living child in less than four hours by Dr. Barnes's method. Lancet 1863;I:10.
12. Vengalil SR, Guinn DA, Olabi NF, et al: A randomized trial of misoprostol and extra-amniotic saline infusion for cervical ripening and labor induction. Obstet Gynecol 1998;91:774–779.
13. Sherman DJ, Frenkel E, Pansky M, et al: Balloon cervical ripening with extra-amniotic infusion of saline or prostaglandin E2: A double-blind, randomized controlled study. Obstet Gynecol 2001;97:375–380.
14. Lin A, Kupferminc M, Dooley SL: A randomized trial of extra-amniotic saline infusion versus laminaria for cervical ripening. Obstet Gynecol 1995;86:545–549.
15. Sherman DJ, Frenkel E, Tovbin J, et al: Ripening of the unfavorable cervix with extra-amniotic catheter balloon: Clinical experience and review. Obstet Gynecol Surv 1996;51:621.
16. Kazzi GM, Bottoms SF, Rosen MG: Efficacy and safety of Laminaria digitata for preinduction ripening of the cervix. Obstet Gynecol 1982;60:440–443.
17. Gilson GJ, Russell DJ, Izquierdo LA, et al: A prospective randomized evaluation of a hygroscopic cervical dilator, Dilapan, in the preinduction ripening of patients undergoing induction of labor. Am J Obstet Gynecol 1996;175:145–149.
18. Krammer J, Williams MC, Sawai SK, O'Brien WF: Preinduction cervical ripening: A randomized comparison of two methods. Obstet Gynecol 1995;85:614–618.
19. Guinn DA, Goepfert AR, Christine M, et al: Extra-amniotic saline infusion, laminaria, or prostaglandin E2 gel for labor induction with unfavorable cervix: A randomized trial. Obstet Gynecol 2000;96:106–112.
20. Boulvain M, Irion O, Marcoux S, Fraser W: Sweeping of the membranes to prevent post-term pregnancy and to induce

labour: A systematic review. Br J Obstet Gynaecol 1999;106: 481–485.
21. Tsuei JJ, Yiu-Fun L, Sharma S: The influence of acupuncture stimulation during pregnancy: The induction and inhibition of labor. Obstet Gynecol 1977;50:479–488.
22. Macer J, Buchanan D, Yonekura ML: Induction of labor with prostaglandin E2 vaginal suppositories. Obstet Gynecol 1984;63:664–668.
23. Gordon-Wright AP, Elder MG: Prostaglandin E2 tablets used intravaginally for the induction of labor. Br J Obstet Gynaecol 1979;86:32–36.
24. Craft I: Amniotomy and oral prostaglandin E2 titration for induction of labor. BMJ 1972;2:191–194.
25. Uldbjerg N, Ekman G, Malmstrom A, et al: Biochemical and morphological changes of human cervix after local application of prostaglandins. Lancet 1981;1:267–268.
26. Rath W, Adelman-Girill BC, Pieper U, Kuhn W: The role of collagenases and proteases in prostaglandin induced cervical ripening. Prostaglandins 1987;34:119–127.
27. Keirse MJ: Prostaglandins in preinduction cervical ripening. Meta-analysis of worldwide clinical experience. J Reprod Med 1993;38:89–100.
28. Owen J, Winkler CL, Harris BA Jr, et al: A randomized, double-blind trial of prostaglandin E2 gel for cervical ripening and meta-analysis. Am J Obstet Gynecol 1991;165:991–996.
29. Vollebregt A, van't Hof DB, Exalto N: Prepidil compared to Propess for cervical ripening. Eur J Obstet Gynecol Reprod Biol 2002;104:116–119.
30. Stewart JD, Rayburn WF, Farmer KC, et al: Effectiveness of prostaglandin E2 intracervical gel (Prepidil), with immediate oxytocin, versus vaginal insert (Cervidil) for induction of labor. Am J Obstet Gynecol 1998;179:1175–1180.
31. Hennessey MH, Rayburn WF, Stewart JD, Liles EC: Pre-eclampsia and induction of labor: a randomized comparison of prostaglandin E2 as an intracervical gel, with oxytocin immediately, or as a sustained-release vaginal insert. Am J Obstet Gynecol 1998;179:1204–1209.
32. Sanchez-Ramos L, Kaunitz AM, Del Valle GO, et al: Labor induction with the prostaglandin E1 methyl analogue misoprostol versus oxytocin: A randomized trial. Obstet Gynecol 1993;81:332–336.
33. Fletcher HM, Mitchell S, Simeon D, et al: Intravaginal misoprostol as a cervical ripening agent. Br J Obstet Gynaecol 1993;100:641–644.
34. Fletcher H, Mitchell S, Simeon D, et al: Intravaginal misoprostol versus dinoprostone as cervical ripening and labor-inducing agents. Obstet Gynecol 1994;83:244–247.
35. Campos GA, Guzman S, Rodriguez JG, et al: Misoprostol-Un analogo de la PGE1-para la induccion de parto a termino: Estudio comparativo y randomizado con oxitocina. Rev Chil Obstet Ginecol 1994;59:190–196.
36. Tabor B, Anderson J, Stettler B, Wetwiska T: Misoprostol versus prostaglandin E2 gel for cervical ripening. Am J Obstet Gynecol 1995;172:425 (Abstract no. 605).
37. Wing DA, Jones MM, Rahall A, et al: A comparison of misoprostol and prostaglandin E2 gel for preinduction cervical ripening and labor induction. Am J Obstet Gynecol 1995;172: 1804–1810.
38. Wing DA, Rahall A, Jones MM, et al: Misoprostol: An effective agent for cervical ripening and labor induction. Am J Obstet Gynecol 1995;172:1811–1816.
39. Varaklis K, Gumina R, Stubblefield PG: Randomized controlled trial of vaginal misoprostol and intracervical prostaglandin E2 gel for induction of labor at term. Obstet Gynecol 1995;86:541–544.
40. Chuck FJ, Huffaker BJ: Labor induction with intravaginal misoprostol versus intracervical prostaglandin E2 gel (Prepidil Gel): Randomized comparison. Am J Obstet Gynecol 1995;173: 1137–1142.
41. Echeverria E, Rocha M: Estudio comparativo randomizado de induccion de parto con ocitocina y misoprostol en embarazos en vias de prolongacion. Rev Chil Obstet Ginecol 1995;60:108–111.
42. Ngai SW, To WK, Lao T, Ho PC: Cervical priming with oral misoprostol in prelabor rupture of membranes at term. Obstet Gynecol 1996;87:923–926.
43. Mundle WR, Young DC: Vaginal misoprostol for induction of labor: A randomized controlled trial. Obstet Gynecol 1996;88: 521–525.
44. Kadanali S, Kucukozkan T, Zor N, Kumtepe Y: Comparison of labor induction with misoprostol vs. oxytocin/prostaglandin E2 in term pregnancy. Int J Gynecol Obstet 1996;55:99–104.
45. Rust OA, Greybush M, Singleton C, et al: A comparison of preinduction cervical ripening techniques. Am J Obstet Gynecol 1999;180:S126.
46. Kolderup L, McLean L, Grullon K, et al: Misoprostol is more efficacious for labor induction than prostaglandin F2, but is it associated with more risk? Am J Obstet Gynecol 1999;180: 1543–1550.
47. Danielian P, Porter B, Ferri N, et al: Misoprostol for induction of labor at term: A more effective agent than dinoprostone vaginal gel. Br J Obstet Gynaecol 1999;106:793–797.
48. Nunes F, Rodrigues R, Meirinho M: Randomized comparison between intravaginal misoprostol and dinoprostone for cervical ripening and induction of labor. Am J Obstet Gynecol 1999;181:626–629.
49. Abramovici D, Goldwasser S, Mabie BC, et al: A randomized comparison of oral misoprostol versus Foley catheter and oxytocin for induction of labor at term. Am J Obstet Gynecol 1999;181:1108–1112.
50. Butt KD, Bennett KA, Crane JMG, et al: Randomized comparison of oral misoprostol and oxytocin for labor induction in term prelabor membrane rupture. Obstet Gynecol 1999;94: 994–999.
51. Sennstrom MB, Ekman G, Westergren-Thorsson G, et al: Human cervical ripening and inflammatory process mediated by cytokines. Mol Hum Reprod 2000;6:375–381.
52. Sennstrom MK, Brauner A, Lu Y, et al: Interleukin-8 is a mediator of the final cervical ripening in humans. Eur J Obstet Gynecol Reprod Biol 1997;74:89–92.
53. Vaisanen-Tommiska M, Nuutila M, Aittomaki K, et al: Nitric oxide metabolites in cervical fluid during pregnancy: Further evidence for the role of cervical nitric oxide in cervical ripening. Am J Obstet Gynecol 2003;188:779–785.
54. Ekerhovd E, Weijdegard B, Brannstrom M, et al: Nitric oxide induced cervical ripening in the human: Involvement of cyclic guanosine monophosphate, prostaglandin F(2 alpha), and prostaglandin E2. Am J Obstet Gynecol 2002;186:745–750.
55. Maul H, Longo M, Saade GR, Garfield RE: Nitric oxide and its role during pregnancy: From ovulation to delivery. Curr Pharm Des 2003;9:359–380 (review).
56. Bao S, Rai J, Screiber J: Brain nitric oxide synthase expression is enhanced in the human cervix in labor. J Soc Gynecol Investig 2001;8:158–164.
57. Nicoll AE, Mackenzie F, Greer IA, Norman JE: Vaginal application of the nitric oxide donor isosorbide mononitrate for preinduction cervical ripening: A randomized controlled trial to determine effects on maternal and fetal hemodynamics. Am J Obstet Gynecol 2001;184:958–964.
58. Chanrachakul B, Herabutya Y, Punyavachira P: Potential efficacy of nitric oxide for cervical ripening in pregnancy at term. Int J Gynaecol Obstet 2000;71:217–219.
59. Riskin-Mashiah S, Wilkins I: Cervical ripening. Obstet Gynecol Clin North Am 1999;26:243–257.
60. Brennand JE, Calder AA, Leitch CR, et al: Recombinant human relaxin as a cervical ripening agent. Br J Obstet Gynaecol 1997;104:775–780.
61. Dawood MY, Ylikorkala O, Trivedi D, Fuchs F: Oxytocin in maternal circulation and amniotic fluid during pregnancy. J Clin Endocrinol Metab 1979;49:429–434.

62. Seitchik J, Amico J, Robinson AG, Castillo M: Oxytocin augmentation of dysfunctional labor. IV. Oxytocin pharmacokinetics. Am J Obstet Gynecol 1984;150:225–228.
63. Leake RD, Weitzman RE, Fisher DA: Pharmacokinetics of oxytocin in the human subject. Obstet Gynecol 1980;56:701–704.
64. Seitchik J: The management of functional dystocia in the first stage of labor. Clin Obstet Gynecol 1987;30:42–49.
65. Seitchik J, Amico J, Robinson AG, Castillo M: Oxytocin augmentation of dysfunctional labor. IV. Oxytocin pharmacokinetics. Am J Obstet Gynecol 1984;150:225–228.
66. Caldeyro-Barcia R, Sereno JA: The response of the human uterus to oxytocin throughout pregnancy. In Caldeyro-Barcia R, Heller H (eds): Oxytocin. New York, Pergamon Press, 1961, pp 177–200.
67. Fuchs A, Fuchs F, Husslein P, et al: Oxytocin receptors in the human uterus during pregnancy and parturition. Am J Obstet Gynecol 1984;150:734–741.
68. Fuchs A, Fuchs F, Husslein P, et al: Oxytocin receptors and human parturition: A dual role for oxytocin in the initiation of labor. Science 1982;215:1396–1398.
69. Husslein P, Fuchs A, Fuchs F: Oxytocin and the initiation of human parturition. I. Prostaglandin release during induction of labor by oxytocin. Am J Obstet Gynecol 1981;141:688–693.
70. Tomasi A, Bangalore S, Phillippe M: Myometrial contractile and inositol-phosphate response to oxytocin. Abstract 357, Society for Gynecologic Investigation, 34th Annual Meeting, Atlanta, 1987.
71. Hendricks CH, Brenner WE: Cardiovascular effects of oxytocic drugs used post partum. Am J Obstet Gynecol 1970;108: 751–760.
72. Blakemore KJ, Qin N-G, Petrie RH, Paine LL: A prospective comparison of hourly and quarter-hourly oxytocin dose increase intervals for the induction of labor at term. Obstet Gynecol 1990;75:757–761.
73. Mercer B, Pilgrim P, Sibai B: Labor induction with continuous low-dose oxytocin infusion: A randomized trial. Obstet Gynecol 1991;77:659–663.
74. Chua S, Arulkumaran S, Kurup A, et al: Oxytocin titration for induction of labour: A prospective randomized study of 15 versus 30 minute dose increment schedules. Aust N Z J Obstet Gynaecol 1991;31:134–137.
75. Satin AJ, Leveno KJ, Sherman ML, McIntire D: High-dose oxytocin: 20-versus 40-minute dosage interval. Obstet Gynecol 1994;83:234–238.
76. Muller PR, Stubbs TM, Laurent SL: A prospective randomized clinical trial comparing two oxytocin induction protocols. Am J Obstet Gynecol 1992;167:373–381.
77. Merrill DC, Zlatnik FJ: Randomized, double-masked comparison of oxytocin dosage in induction and augmentation of labor. Obstet Gynecol 1999;94:455–463.
78. Crane JM, Young DC: Meta-analysis of low-dose versus high-dose oxytocin for labour induction. J Soc Obstet Gynaecol Can 1998;20:1215–1223.
79. Seitchik J: The management of functional dystocia in the first stage of labor. Clin Obstet Gynecol 1987;30:42–49.
80. Seitchik J, Amico J, Robinson A, Castillo M: Oxytocin augmentation of dysfunctional labor. IV. Oxytocin pharmacokinetics. Am J Obstet Gynecol 1984;150:225–228.
81. American College of Obstetricians and Gynecologists: Induction and augmentation of labor. ACOG Technical Bulletin No. 110. Washington, DC, ACOG, 1987.
82. Cummiskey KC, Dawood MY: Induction of labor with pulsatile oxytocin. Am J Obstet Gynecol 1990;163:1868–1874.
83. Salamalekis E, Vitoratos N, Kassanos D, et al: A randomized trial of pulsatile vs. continuous oxytocin infusion for labor induction. Clin Exp Obstet Gynecol 2000;27:21–23.
84. Reid GJ, Helewa ME: A trial of pulsatile versus continuous oxytocin administration for the induction of labor. J Perinatol 1995;15:364–366.
85. Willcourt RJ, Pager D, Wendel J, Hale RW: Induction of labor with pulsatile oxytocin by a computer-controlled pump. Am J Obstet Gynecol 1994;170:603–608.
86. Schrinsky DC, Benson RC: Rupture of the pregnant uterus: A review. Obstet Gynecol Surv 1978;33:217–232.
87. Eden RD, Parker RT, Gall SA: Rupture of the pregnant uterus: A 53-year review. Obstet Gynecol 1986;68:671–674.
88. Johnson JD, Aldrich M, Angelus P, et al: Oxytocin and neonatal hyperbilirubinemia: Studies of bilirubin production. Am J Dis Child 1984;138:1047–1050.
89. Linn S, Schoenbaum SC, Monson RR, et al: Epidemiology of neonatal hyperbilirubinemia. Pediatrics 1985;75:770–774.
90. Macer J, Buchanan D, Yonekura ML: Induction of labor with prostaglandin E2 vaginal suppositories. Obstet Gynecol 1984;63: 644–648.
91. Gordon-Wright AP, Elder MG: Prostaglandin E2 tablets used intravaginally for the induction of labor. Br J Obstet Gynaecol 1979;86:32–36.
92. Craft I: Amniotomy and oral prostaglandin E2 titration for induction of labor. BMJ 1972;2:191–194.
93. Ulmsten U, Ekman G, Belfrage P, et al: Intracervical versus intravaginal PGE_2 for induction of labor at term patients with an unfavorable cervix. Arch Gynecol 1985;236:243–248.
94. Darroca RJ, Buttino L Jr, Miller J, Khamis HJ: Prostaglandin E2 gel for cervical ripening in patients with an indication for delivery. Obstet Gynecol 1996;87:228–230.
95. Rayburn WF, Wapner RJ, Barss VA: An intravaginal controlled-release prostaglandin E2 pessary for cervical ripening and induction of labor at term. Obstet Gynecol 1992;79:374–379.
96. Sanchez-Ramos L, Farah LA, Kaunitz AM, et al: Preinduction cervical ripening with commercially available prostaglandin E2 gel: A randomized, double-blind comparison with a hospital-compounded preparation. Am J Obstet Gynecol 1995;173: 1079–1084.
97. Stempel JE, Prins RP, Dean S: Preinduction cervical ripening: A randomized prospective comparison of the efficacy and safety of intravaginal and intracervical prostaglandin E2 gel. Am J Obstet Gynecol 1997;176:1305–1309.
98. Rabe T, Basse H, Thuro H, et al: Effect of PGE_1 methyl analog misoprostol on the pregnant uterus in the first trimester. Geburtsh Frauenheilk 1987;47:324–331.
99. Normal JE, Thong KJ, Baird DT: Uterine contractility and induction of abortion in early pregnancy by misoprostol and mifepristone. Lancet 1991;338:1233–1236.
100. Jain JK, Mishell DR Jr: A comparison of intravaginal misoprostol with prostaglandin E2 for termination of second-trimester pregnancy. N Engl J Med 1994;331:290–293.
101. Bugalho A, Faundes A, Jamisse L, et al: Evaluation of the effectiveness of vaginal misoprostol to induce first trimester abortion. Contraception 1996;53:244–246.
102. Koopersmith TB, Mischell DR Jr: The use of misoprostol for termination of early pregnancy. Contraception 1996;53:238–242.
103. Wiebe ER: Abortion induced with methotrexate and misoprostol. Can Med Assoc J 1996;154:165–170.
104. Creinin MD, Vittinghoff E, Galbraith S, Klaisle C: A randomized trial comparing misoprostol three and seven days after methotrexate for early abortion. Am J Obstet Gynecol 1995;173: 1578–1584.
105. Baird DT, Sukcharoen N, Thong KJ: Randomized trial of misoprostol and cervagem in combination with a reduced dose of mifepristone for induction of abortion. Hum Reprod 1995;10:1521–1527.
106. Lemancewicz A, Urban R, Skotnicki MZ, et al: Uterine and fetal Doppler flow changes after misoprostol and oxytocin therapy for induction of labor in post-term pregnancies. Int J Gynecol Obstet 1999;67:139–145.
107. Thomas N, Longo SA, Rumney PJ, et al: Intravaginal misoprostol in prelabor rupture of membranes. Am J Obstet Gynecol 2000;182:S136.

108. Ngai SW, Chan YM, Lam SW, Lao TT: Labour characteristics and uterine activity: misoprostol compared with oxytocin in women at term with prelabor rupture of membranes. Br J Obstet Gynaecol 2000;107:222–227.
109. Bennett KA, Butt K, Crane JMG, et al: A masked randomized comparison of oral and vaginal administration of misoprostol for labor induction. Obstet Gynecol 1998;92:481–486.
110. Adair CD, Weeks JW, Barrilleaux S, et al: Oral or vaginal misoprostol administration for induction of labor: A randomized, double-blind trial. Obstet Gynecol 1998;92:810–813.
111. Wing DA, Ham D, Paul RH: A comparison of orally administered misoprostol with vaginally administered misoprostol for cervical ripening and labor induction. Am J Obstet Gynecol 1999;180:1155–1160.
112. Kwon JS, Mackenzie VP, Davies GAL: A comparison of oral and vaginal misoprostol for induction of labour at term: A randomized trial. Am J Obstet Gynecol 1999;180:S128.
113. Wing DA, Park MR, Paul RH: Oral administration of 100 microgram tablets of misoprostol for cervical ripening and labor induction. Am J Obstet Gynecol 2000;95:905–908.
114. Dyar TR, Greig P, Cummings R, Nichols K: The efficacy and safety of oral versus vaginal misoprostol for the induction of term labor. Am J Obstet Gynecol 2000;182:S135.
115. Sanchez-Ramos L, Kaunitz AM, Wears RL, et al: Misoprostol for cervical ripening and labor induction: A meta-analysis. Obstet Gynecol 1997;89:633–642.
116. Sanchez-Ramos L, Kaunitz AM: Misoprostol for cervical ripening and labor induction: A systematic review of the literature. Clin Obstet Gynecol 2000;43:475–488.
117. Khan R-U, El-Refaey H: Pharmacokinetics and adverse-effect profile of rectally administered misoprostol in the third stage of labor. Obstet Gynecol 2003;101:968–974.
118. Tang OS, Schweer H, Seyberth HW, et al: Pharmacokinetics of different routes of administration of misoprostol. Hum Reprod 2002;17:332–336.
119. Gemzell Danielsson K, Marions L, Rodriguez A, et al: Comparison between oral and vaginal administration of misoprostol on uterine contractility. Obstet Gynecol 1999;93:275–280.
120. Zieman M, Fong SK, Benowitz NL, et al: Absorption kinetics of misoprostol with oral or vaginal administration. Obstet Gynecol 1997;90:88–92.
121. Toppozada MK, Answar MYM, Hassan HA, El-Gazaerly WS: Oral or vaginal misoprostol for induction of labor. Int J Gynecol Obstet 1997;56:135–139.
122. Farah LA, Sanchez-Ramos L, Rosa C, et al: Randomized trial of two doses of the prostaglandin E1 analog misoprostol for labor induction. Am J Obstet Gynecol 1997;177:364–371.
123. Srisomboon J, Singchai S: A comparison between 25 micrograms and 50 micrograms of intravaginal misoprostol for labor induction. J Med Assoc Thai 1998;81:779–784.
124. Diro M, Adra A, Gilles JM, et al: A double-blind randomized trial of two dose regimens of misoprostol for cervical ripening and labor induction. J Matern Fetal Med 1999;8:114–118.
125. Wang H, Li L, Pu L: The effect of 25 μg misoprostol on induction of labor in late pregnancy. Chin J Obstet Gynecol 1998;33:469–471.
126. El-Sherbiny MT, El-Gharieb IH, Gewely HA: Vaginal misoprostol for induction of labor: 25 μg vs. 50 μg dose regimen. Int J Gynaecol Obstet 2001;72:25–30.
127. Meydanli MM, Caliskan E, Burak F, et al: Labor induction post-term with 25 micrograms vs. 50 micrograms of intravaginal misoprostol. Int J Gynaecol Obstet 2003;81:249–255.
128. Sanchez-Ramos L, Kaunitz AM, Delke I: Labor induction with 25 μg versus 50 μg intravaginal misoprostol: A systematic review. Obstet Gynecol 2002;99:145–151.
129. American College of Obstetricians and Gynecologists: Induction of Labor with Misoprostol. ACOG Committee Opinion No. 228. Washington, DC, ACOG, 1999.
130. Rageth JC, Juzi C, Grossenbacher H: Delivery after previous cesarean: A risk evaluation. Obstet Gynecol 1999;93:332–337.
131. Vause S, Macintosh M: Use of prostaglandins to induce labour in women with a cesarean section scar. BMJ 1999;318:1056–1058.
132. Sciscione AC, Nguyen L, Manley JS, et al Uterine rupture during preinduction cervical ripening with misoprostol in a patient with previous cesarean delivery. Aust NZ Obstet Gynaecol 1998;38:96–97.
133. Wing DA, Lovett K, Paul RH: Disruption of prior uterine incision following misoprostol for labor induction in women with previous cesarean delivery. Obstet Gynecol 1998;91:828–830.
134. Blanchette H, Nayak S, Erasmus S: Comparison of the safety and efficacy of intravaginal misoprostol (prostaglandin E1) with those of dinoprostone (prostaglandin E2) for cervical ripening and induction of labor in a community hospital. Am J Obstet Gynecol 1999;180:1551–1559.
135. Plaut MM, Schwartz ML, Lubarsky SL: Uterine rupture associated with the use of misoprostol in the gravid patient with a previous cesarean section. Am J Obstet Gynecol 1999;180: 1535–1542.
136. Cunha M, Bugalho A, Bique C, Bergstrom S: Induction of labor by vaginal misoprostol in patients with previous cesarean delivery. Acta Obstet Gynecol Scand 1999;78:653–654.
137. Choy-Hee I, Raynor BD: Misoprostol induction in women with prior cesarean. Am J Obstet Gynecol 2000;182:S159.
138. Bennett KA, Elmore L, Fleischman S, et al: Prostaglandin induction in women with prior cesarean delivery increases induction time and risk of uterine rupture. Am J Obstet Gynecol 2000;182:S130.
139. Pocock SJ: When to stop a clinical trial. BMJ 1992;305:235–240.
140. Chuck FJ, Huffaker BJ: Labor induction with intravaginal misoprostol versus intracervical prostaglandin E2 gel (Prepidil Gel): Randomized comparison. Am J Obstet Gynecol 1995;173: 1137–1142.
141. Vengalil SR, Guinn DA, Olabi NF, et al: A randomized trial of misoprostol and extra-amniotic saline infusion for cervical ripening and labor induction. Obstet Gynecol 1998;91:774–779.
142. Perry KG, Larmon JE, May WL, et al: Cervical ripening: A randomized comparison between intravaginal misoprostol and an intracervical balloon catheter combined with intravaginal dinoprostone. Am J Obstet Gynecol 1998;178:1333–1340.
143. Carlan SJ, Bouldin S, O'Brien WF: Extemporaneous preparation of misoprostol gel for cervical ripening: A randomized trial. Obstet Gynecol 1997;90:911–915.
144. Fausett MB, Barth WH Jr, Yoder BA, Satin AJ: Oxytocin labor stimulation of twin gestations: Effective and efficient. Obstet Gynecol 1997;90:202–204.
145. Manor M, Blickstein I, Ben-Arie A, et al: Case series of labor induction in twin gestations with an intrauterine balloon catheter. Gynecol Obstet Invest 1999;47:244–246.
146. Suzuki S, Otsubo Y, Sawa R, et al: Clinical trial of induction of labor versus expectant management in twin pregnancy. Gynecol Obstet Invest 2000;49:24–27.
147. Neimand KM, Gibstein A, Rosenthal AH: Oxytocin in twin gestation. Am J Obstet Gynecol 1967;99:533–538.
148. American College of Obstetricians and Gynecologists: Induction of labor. ACOG Practice Bulletin No. 10. Washington, DC, ACOG, 1999.
149. Toaff R, Ayalon D, Gogol G: Clinical use of high concentration oxytocin drip. Obstet Gynecol 1971;37:112–120.
150. Kent DR, Goldstein AI, Linzey EM: Safety and efficacy of vaginal prostaglandin E2 suppositories in the management of third-trimester fetal demise. J Reprod Med 1984;29:101–102.
151. Mariani-Neto C, Leao EJ, Barreto EM, et al: Use of misoprostol for labor induction in stillbirth. Rev Paul Med 1987;105: 325–328.
152. Bugalho A, Bique C, Machungo F, Bergstrom S: Vaginal misoprostol as an alternative to oxytocin for induction of labor in women with late fetal death. Acta Obstet Gynecol Scand 1995; 74:194–198.

153. Nakintu N: A comparative study of vaginal misoprostol and intravenous oxytocin for induction of labour in women with intrauterine fetal death in Mulago Hospital, Uganda. Afr Health Sci 2001;1:55–59.
154. Wagaarachchi PT, Ashok PW, Narvekar NN, et al: Medical management of late intrauterine death using a combination of mifepristone and misoprostol. Br J Obstet Gynaecol 2002;109: 443–447.
155. Mohomed K, Jayaguru AS: Extra-amniotic saline infusion for induction of labour in antepartum fetal death: A cost effective method worthy of wider use. Br J Obstet Gynaecol 1997;104: 1058–1061.
156. Strauss LT, Herndon J, Chang J, et al: Abortion surveillance – United States, 2001. MMWR 2004;53(SS09):1–32.
157. Flett GM, Templeton A: Surgical abortion. Best Pract Res Clin Obstet Gynaecol 2002;16:247–261.
158. Haskell WM, Easterling TR, Lichtenberg ET: Surgical abortion after the first trimester. In Paul M, Lichtenberg ES, Borgatta L, et al (eds): A Clinician's Guide to Medical and Surgical Abortion. New York, Churchill Livingstone, 1999, pp 123–138.
159. Grimes DA, Schulz KF, Cates W Jr, Tyler CW: Mid-trimester abortion by dilatation and evacuation: A safe and practical alternative. N Engl J Med 1977;296:1141.
160. American College of Obstetricians and Gynecologists: Methods of midtrimester abortion. ACOG Tech Bull 1987;109:602–605.
161. Royal College of Obstetricians and Gynaecologists: The Care of Women Requesting Induced Abortion. London, RCOG Press, 2004.
162. Blumenthal PD, Castleman LD, Jain JK: Abortion by labor induction. In Paul M, Lichtenberg ES, Borgatta L, et al (eds): A Clinician's Guide to Medical and Surgical Abortion. New York, Churchill Livingstone, 1999, pp 139–154.
163. Tang OS, Ho PC: Medical abortion in the second trimester. Best Pract Res Clin Obstet Gynaecol 2002;16:237–246.
164. Ngai SW, Tang OS, Ho PC: Prostaglandins for induction of second-trimester termination and intrauterine death. Best Pract Res Clin Obstet Gynaecol 2003;17:765–775.
165. Lichtenberg ES, Grimes DA, Paul M: Abortion complications: Prevention and management. In Paul M, Lichtenberg ES, Borgatta L, et al (eds): A Clinician's Guide to Medical and Surgical Abortion. New York, Churchill Livingstone, 1999, pp 197–216.
166. Autry AM, Hayes EC, Jacobson GF, Kirby RS: A comparison of medical induction and dilation and evacuation for second-trimester abortion. Am J Obstet Gynecol 2002;187:393–397.
167. Owen J, Hauth JC: Concentrated oxytocin plus low-dose prostaglandin E2 compared with prostaglandin E2 vaginal suppositories for second-trimester pregnancy termination. Obstet Gynecol 1996;88:110.
168. Yentis SM, Steer PJ, Plaat F: Eisenmenger's syndrome in pregnancy: Maternal and fetal mortality in the 1990s. Br J Obstet Gynaecol 1998;105:921–922.
169. Weiss Bm, Zemp L, Seifert B, Hess OM: Outcome of pulmonary vascular disease in pregnancy: A systematic overview from 1978 through 1996. J Am Coll Cardiol 1998;31:1650–1657.
170. Gleicher N, Midwall J, Hochberger D, Jaffin H: Eisenmenger's syndrome and pregnancy. Obstet Gynecol Surv 1979;34: 721–741.
171. Henshaw SK, Finer LB: The accessibility of abortion services in the United States, 2001. Perspect Sex Reprod Health 2003;35: 16–24.
172. Henshaw SK: Factors hindering access to abortion services. Fam Plann Perspect 1995;27:54–87.
173. Westhoff C, Marks F, Rosenfield A: Residency training in contraception, sterilization and abortion. Obstet Gynecol 1993;81: 311–314.
174. Chervenak FA, McCullough LB, Skupski D, Chasen ST: Ethical issues in the management of pregnancies complicated by fetal anomalies. Obstet Gynecol Surv 2003;58:473–483.
175. Cates W Jr, Schulz KF, Grimes DA, et al: Dilatation and evacuation procedures and second-trimester abortions: The role of physician skill and hospital setting. JAMA 1982;248:559–563.
176. Shulman LP, Grimes DA, Stubblefield PG: ACOG Update: Abortion. Washington, DC, American College of Obstetricians and Gynecologists, 1997 (no. 7), p 22.
177. Kaltreider NB, Goldsmith S, Margolis AJ: The impact of midtrimester abortion techniques on patients and staff. Am J Obstet Gynecol 1979;135:235.
178. Geerinck-Vercammen CR, Kanhal HH: Coping with termination of pregnancy for fetal abnormality in a supportive environment. Prenat Diagn 2003;23:543–548.
179. Del Valle GO, Sanchez-Ramos L, Jordan CW, et al: Use of misoprostol (prostaglandin E1 methyl analogue) to expedite delivery in severe preeclampsia remote from term. J Matern Fetal Med 1996;5:39–40.
180. Borgatta L, Burnhill MS, Karlin E: The challenging abortion. In Paul M, Lichtenberg ES, Borgatta L, et al (eds): A Clinician's Guide to Medical and Surgical Abortion. New York, Churchill Livingstone, 1999, pp 169–182.
181. Dark AC, Miller L, Kothenbeutel RL, Mandel L: Obesity and second-trimester abortion by dilation and evacuation. J Reprod Med 2002;47:226–230.
182. Hern WM, Ferguson KA, Hart V, et al: Outpatient abortion for fetal anomaly and fetal death from 15–34 menstrual weeks' gestation: Techniques and clinical management. Obstet Gynecol 1993;81:301.
183. Peterson WF, Berry N, Grace MR, et al: Second trimester abortion by dilatation and evacuation: An analysis of 11,747 cases. Obstet Gynecol 1983;62:185–190.
184. Jacot FRM, Poulin C, Bilodeau AP, et al: A five-year experience with second-trimester induced abortions: No increase in complication rate as compared to the first trimester. Am J Obstet Gynecol 1993;168:633–637.
185. Darney PD, Sweet RL: Routine intraoperative sonography for second trimester abortion reduces incidence of uterine perforation. J Ultrasound Med 1989;8:71–75.
186. Lawson HW, Frye EA, Atrash HK: Abortion mortality, United States, 1972 through 1987. Am J Obstet Gynecol 1994;171: 1365–1372.
187. MacKay HT, Schulz KF, Grimes DA: Safety of local versus general anesthesia for second-trimester dilatation and evacuation abortion. Obstet Gynecol 1985;66:661–665.
188. Williams DW: Resources for abortion providers. In Paul M, Lichtenberg ES, Borgatta L, et al (eds): A Clinician's Guide to Medical and Surgical Abortion. New York, Churchill Livingstone, 1999, p 292.
189. Blumenthal PD: Prospective comparison of Dilapan and laminaria for pretreatment of the cervix in second-trimester induction abortion. Obstet Gynecol 1988;72:243–246.
190. Hern WM: Laminaria versus Dilapan osmotic cervical dilators for outpatient dilation and evacuation abortion: Randomized cohort comparison of 1001 patients. Am J Obstet Gynecol 1994;171:1324–1328.
191. Grimes DA, Ray IG, Middleton CJ: Lamicel versus laminaria for cervical dilation before early second-trimester abortion: A randomized clinical trial. Obstet Gynecol 1987;69:887–890.
192. Khanna NM, Sarin JPS, Nandi RC, et al: Isaptent: A new cervical dilator. Contraception 1980;21:29–40.
193. Sema S, Hingorani V, Kumar S, Kinra G: Three methods for gradual cervical dilatation prior to vacuum aspiration in late first trimester pregnancy. Contraception 1983;28:223–231.
194. Stubblefield PG, Altman AM, Goldstein SP: Randomized trial of one versus two days of laminaria treatment prior to late midtrimester abortion by uterine evacuation: A pilot study. Am J Obstet Gynecol 1982;143:481–482.
195. Lauersen NH, Den T, Iliescu C, et al: Cervical priming prior to dilatation and evacuation: A comparison of methods. Am J Obstet Gynecol 1982;144:890–894.

196. MacIsaac L, Grossman D, Balistreri E, Darney P: A randomized controlled trial of laminaria, oral misoprostol, and vaginal misoprostol before abortion. Obstet Gynecol 1999;93:766–770.
197. Gottlieb C, Lundstrom-Lindstedt V, Swahn ML, Bygdeman M: Vacuum aspiration for termination of early second trimester pregnancy after treatment with vaginal prostaglandin. Acta Obstet Gynecol Scand 1991;70:41–45.
198. Todd CS, Soler M, Castleman L, et al: Buccal misoprostol as cervical preparation for second trimester pregnancy termination. Contraception 2002;65:415–418.
199. Ludmir J, Stubblefield PG: Surgical procedures in pregnancy. In Gabbe SG, Niebyl JR, Simpson JL (eds): Obstetrics: Normal and Problem Pregnancies. New York, Churchill Livingstone, 2002, p 639.
200. Sawaya GF, Grady D, Kerlikowske K, et al: Antibiotics at the time of induced abortion: The case for universal prophylaxis based on a meta-analysis. Obstet Gynecol 1996;87:884–890.
201. Blackwell AL, Thomas PD, Wareham K, Emery SJ: Health gains from screening for infection of the lower genital tract in women attending for termination of pregnancy. Lancet 1993;342:206–210.
202. Penney GC, Thomson M, Norman J: A randomized comparison of strategies for reducing infective complications of induced abortion. Br J Obstet Gynaecol 1998;105:599–604.
203. American College of Obstetricians and Gynecologists: Abortion Policy. ACOG Statements of Policy. Washington, DC, ACOG, 2000.
204. Halperin R, Vaknin Z, Langer R, et al: Late midtrimester pregnancy termination in the presence of placenta previa. J Reprod Med 2003;48:175–178.
205. Thomas AG, Alvarez M, Friedman F, et al: The effect of placenta previa on blood loss in second-trimester pregnancy termination. Obstet Gynecol 1994;84:58–60.
206. Clark SL, Koonings PP, Phelan JP: Placenta previa/accreta and prior cesarean section. Obstet Gynecol 1985;66:89–92.
207. Schneider D, Bukovsky I, Caspi E: Safety of midtrimester pregnancy termination by laminaria and evacuation in patients with previous cesarean section. Am J Obstet Gynecol 1994;171: 554–557.
208. Rashbaum WK, Gates EJ, Jones J, et al: Placenta accreta encountered during dilation and evacuation in the second trimester. Obstet Gynecol 1995;85:701–703.
209. Kerr A, Karlin D, Mikhail M, et al: Intraoperative embolization for pelvic hemorrhage following termination of pregnancy. Am J Perinatol 1996;13:151–153.
210. Ramsey PS, Owen J: Midtrimester cervical ripening and labor induction. Clin Obstet Gynecol 2000;43:495–512.
211. Stroh G, Hinman AR: Reported live births following induced abortion: Two and one-half years' experience in upstate New York. Am J Obstet Gynecol 1976;126:83–90.
212. Elimian A, Verma U, Tejani N: Effect of causing fetal cardiac asystole on second-trimester abortion. Obstet Gynecol 1999;94:139–141.
213. Jackson RA, Teplin VL, Drey EA, et al: Digoxin to facilitate late second-trimester abortion: A randomized, masked, placebo-controlled trial. Obstet Gynecol 2001;97:471–476.
214. Sherman DJ, Frenkel E, Tovbin J, et al: Ripening of the unfavorable cervix with extra-amniotic catheter balloon: Clinical experience and review. Obstet Gynecol Surv 1996;51:621–627.
215. Thong K J, Baird DT: A study of gemeprost alone, dilapan or mifepristone in combination with gemeprost for the termination of second trimester pregnancy. Contraception 1992;46:11–17.
216. Ho PC, Tsang SSK, Ma HK: Reducing the induction to abortion interval in termination of second trimester pregnancies: A comparison of mifepristone with laminaria tent. Br J Obstet Gynaecol 1995;102:648–651.
217. Jain JK, Mishell DR Jr: A comparison of misoprostol with and without laminaria tents for induction of second trimester abortion. Am J Obstet Gynecol 1996;175:173–177.
218. WHO Scientific Group on Medical Methods for Termination of Pregnancy: Method of abortion after 14 weeks of gestation. In WHO Technical Report Series on medical method for termination of pregnancy. Geneva, WHO, 1997, pp 42–54.
219. Ulmann A, Silvestre L, Chemama L, et al: Medical termination of early pregnancy with mifepristone (RU486) followed by a prostaglandin analogue. Study in 16,369 women. Acta Obstet Gynecol Scand 1992;71:278–283.
220. Thong KJ, Baird DT: An open study comparing two regimens of gemeprost for the termination of pregnancy in the second trimester. Acta Obstet Gynecol Scand 1992;71:191–196.
221. Wong KS, Ngai CSW, Chan KS, et al: Termination of second trimester pregnancy with gemeprost and misoprostol: A randomized double-blind placebo-controlled trial. Contraception 1996;54:23–25.
222. Wong KS, Ngai CSW, Wong AYK, et al: Vaginal misoprostol compared with vaginal gemeprost in termination of second trimester pregnancy. Contraception 1998;58:207–210.
223. Nuutila M, Toivonen J, Ylikorkala O, Halmesmäki E: A comparison between two doses of intravaginal misoprostol and gemeprost for induction of second-trimester abortion. Obstet Gynecol 1997;90:896–900.
224. Herabutya Y, O-Prasertsawat P: Second trimester abortion using intravaginal misoprostol. Int J Gynecol Obstet 1998;60: 161–165.
225. Jain JK, Kuo J, Mishell DR Jr: A comparison of two dosing regimens of intravaginal misoprostol for second-trimester pregnancy termination. Obstet Gynecol 1999;93:571–575.
226. Wong KS, Ngai CSW, Yeo ELK: A comparison of two regimens of intravaginal misoprostol for termination of second trimester pregnancy: A randomized comparative trial. Hum Reprod 2000;15:709–712.
227. Dickinson JE, Evans SF: The optimization of intravaginal misoprostol dosing schedules in second-trimester pregnancy termination. Am J Obstet Gynecol 2002;186:470–474.
228. Bebbington MW, Dent N, Lim K, et al: A randomized controlled trial comparing two protocols for the use of misoprostol in midtrimester pregnancy termination. Am Obstet Gynecol 2002;187:853–857.
229. Feldman DM, Borgida AF, Rodis JF, et al: A randomized comparison of two regimens of misoprostol for second-trimester pregnancy termination. Am J Obstet Gynecol 2003;189: 710–713.
230. Ho PC, Ngai SW, Liu KL, et al: Vaginal misoprostol compared with oral misoprostol in termination of second-trimester pregnancy. Obstet Gynecol 1997;90:735–738.
231. Dickinson JE, Evans SF: A comparison of oral misoprostol with vaginal misoprostol administration in second-trimester pregnancy termination for fetal abnormality. Obstet Gynecol 2003;101:1294–1299.
232. Tang OS, Ho PC: Pilot study on the use of sublingual misoprostol for medical abortion. Contraception 2001;64:315–317.
233. Thong KJ, Baird DT: Induction of second trimester abortion with mifepristone and gemeprost. Br J Obstet Gynaecol 1993;100:758–761.
234. El-Refaey H, Hinshaw K, Templeton A: The abortifacient effect of misoprostol in the second trimester. A randomized comparison with gemeprost in patients pre-treated with mifepristone (RU486). Hum Reprod 1993;8:1744–1746.
235. Thong KJ, Lynch P, Baird DT: A randomised study of two doses of gemeprost in combination with mifepristone for induction of abortion in the second trimester of pregnancy. Contraception 1996;54:97–100.
236. Ho PC, Chan YF, Lau W: Misoprostol is as effective as gemeprost in termination of second trimester pregnancy when combined with mifepristone: A randomised comparative trial. Contraception 1996;53:281–283.
237. Bartley J, Baird DT: A randomized study of misoprostol and gemeprost in combination with mifepristone for induction of

abortion in the second trimester of pregnancy. Br J Obstet Gynaecol 2002;109:1290–1294.
238. El-Refaey H, Templeton A: Induction of abortion in the second trimester by a combination of misoprostol and mifepristone: A randomized comparison between two misoprostol regimens. Hum Reprod 1995;10:475–478.
239. Webster D, Penny GC, Templeton A: A comparison of 600 mg and 200 mg mifepristone prior to second trimester abortion with the prostaglandin misoprostol. Br J Obstet Gynaecol 1996;103: 706–709.
240. Ho PC, Ngai SW, Liu KL: Vaginal misoprostol compared with oral misoprostol in termination of second-trimester pregnancy. Obstet Gynecol 1997;90:735–738.
241. Ashok PW, Templeton A: Nonsurgical mid-trimester termination of pregnancy: A review of 500 consecutive cases. Br J Obstet Gynaecol 1999;106:706–710.
242. Ngai SW, Tang OS, Ho PC: Randomized comparison of vaginal (200 every 3 h) and oral (400 every 3 h) misoprostol when combined with mifepristone in termination of second trimester pregnancy. Hum Reprod 2000;15:2205–2208.
243. Chapman SJ, Crispens M, Owen J, Savage K: Complications of midtrimester pregnancy terminations: The effect of prior cesarean delivery. Am J Obstet Gynecol 1996;175:889–892.
244. Boulot P, Hoffet M, Bachelard G, et al: Late vaginal induced abortion after a previous caesarean birth: Potential for uterine rupture. Gynecol Obstet Invest 1993;36:87–90.
245. Letourneur B, Parant O, Tofani V, Berrebi AJ: Uterine rupture on unscarred uterus following labor induction for 2(nd) trimester termination of pregnancy with oral misoprostol: Conservative management. Gynecol Obstet Biol Reprod 2002;31:371–373.
246. Al-Hussaini TK: Uterine rupture in second trimester abortion in a grand multiparous woman. A complication of misoprostol and oxytocin. Eur J Obstet Gynecol Reprod Biol 2001;96:218–219.
247. Jwarah E, Greenhalf JO: Rupture of the uterus after 800 micrograms misoprostol given vaginally for termination of pregnancy. Br J Obstet Gynaecol 2000;107:807.
248. Berghahn L, Christensen D, Droste S: Uterine rupture during second-trimester abortion associated with misoprostol. Obstet Gynecol 2001;98:976–977.
249. Herabutya Y, Chanarachakul B, Punyavachira P: Induction of labor with vaginal misoprostol for second trimester termination of pregnancy in the scarred uterus. Int J Gynaecol Obstet 2003;83:293–297.
250. Rouzi AA: Second-trimester pregnancy termination with misoprostol in women with previous cesarean sections. Int J Gynaecol Obstet 2003;80:317–318.
251. Pongsatha S, Tongsong T: Misoprostol for second trimester termination of pregnancies with prior low transverse cesarean section. Int J Gynaecol Obstet 2003;80:61–62.
252. Norman JE: Uterine rupture during therapeutic abortion in the second trimester using mifepristone and prostaglandin. Br J Obstet Gynaecol 1995;102:332–333.
253. Phillips K, Berry C, Mathers AM: Uterine rupture during second trimester of pregnancy using mifepristone and a prostaglandin. Eur J Obstet Gynaecol 1996;65:175–176.
254. Chen M, Shih JC, Chiu WT, Hsieh FJ: Separation of cesarean scar during second-trimester intravaginal misoprostol abortion. Obstet Gynecol 1999;94:840.
255. Xu J, Chen H, Ma T, Wu X: Termination of early pregnancy in the scarred uterus with mifepristone and misoprostol. Int J Gynaecol Obstet 2001;72:245–251.
256. Kirz DS, Haag MK: Management of the third stage of labor in pregnancies terminated by prostaglandin E2. Am J Obstet Gynecol 1989;160:412–414.
257. Pridmore BR, Chambers DG: Uterine perforation during surgical abortion: A review of diagnosis, management and prevention. Aust NZ J Obstet Gynaecol 1999;39:349–353.
258. Grimes DA, Schulz KF, Cates W Jr: Prevention of uterine perforation during curettage abortion. JAMA 1984;251:2108–2111.
259. Chanda M, MacKenzie P, Day JH: Hypersensitivity reactions following laminaria placement. Contraception 2000;62:105–106.
260. Sutkin G, Capelle SD, Schlievert PM, Creinin MD: Laminaria cervical dilation might be associated with toxic shock syndrome. Obstet Gynecol 2001;98:959–961.
261. Cole DS, Bruck LR: Anaphylaxis after laminaria insertion. Obstet Gynecol 2000;95:1025.
262. Kallra PA, Litherland D, Sallomi DF, et al: Cardiac standstill induced by prostaglandin pessaries. Lancet 1989;1:1460.
263. Lurie S, Levy R, Katz Z, et al: The influence of midtrimester termination of pregnancy on subsequent fertility: Four to five years follow-up. Contraception 1994;50:239–241.
264. Schneider D, Halperin R, Langer R, et al: Abortion at 18–22 weeks by laminaria dilation and evacuation. Obstet Gynecol 1996;88:412–414.
265. Halperin R, Zimmerman A, Langer R, et al: Laminaria dilatation and evacuation for pregnancies with mid-trimester premature rupture of membranes: A retrospective cohort study. Eur J Obstet Gynecol Reprod Biol 2002;100:181–184.
266. Kalish RB, Chasen ST, Rosenzweig LB, et al: Impact of midtrimester dilation and evacuation on subsequent pregnancy outcome. Am J Obstet Gynecol 2002;187:882–885.

CHAPTER 69

Poor Progress in Labor

Harry Gee

INTRODUCTION

Parturition is a physiologic process; therefore, it might be expected that the great majority of cases would progress normally and should not require medical intervention. However, the relatively high incidence of abnormal outcomes in the absence of intervention indicates that the physiology is not robust. The possible evolutionary reasons why this might be so are covered in Chapter 67.

Poor progress in labor is associated with increased morbidity and mortality rates for both the fetus and mother.[1] Poor progress, however, is rarely causative of itself, but is a sign of underlying pathology. Ideally, the recognition of poor progress in labor would result in the diagnosis of the specific underlying cause, and cause-specific treatment would follow, but with our current knowledge and diagnostic ability this is often not possible. Under these circumstances it has become a pragmatic necessity to use interventions on a trial-and-error basis. Such interventions should be validated by properly controlled clinical trials. Unfortunately, such trials have rarely been performed, and even when they have been, many popular and widely adopted interventions have failed to meet expectations. A common response to this failure has all too often been to question whether the intervention had been correctly applied rather than to review the value of the intervention itself or its indication. This failure to acknowledge our ignorance has severely limited our ability to improve the management of labor.

This chapter aims to provide a critical analysis of the following:

- The physiology of labor
- The methods of monitoring progress of labor
- Our ability to define the boundaries between normal and abnormal progress of labor
- The pathology underlying poor progress of labor, and its consequences
- The effectiveness of interventions

THE ONSET AND DIAGNOSIS OF LABOR

Onset of Labor

In the human, no single trigger for the onset of labor has been identified. Figure 69–1 represents a possible mechanism. Within the fetoplacental unit lies the placental corticotropin model[2,3] that generates the appropriate endocrine environment for the onset of labor via the pituitary-adrenal axis and the placenta. Within the mother, the hormonal environment precipitating labor is created by changes in placental function resulting in the generation of a number of proinflammatory agents (cytokines and interleukins), while the synthesis of prostaglandins and oxytocin integrate myometrial and cervical response.

These positive feedback systems promote change, not homeostasis. The steady-state pregnancy mode is changed to active labor, which is terminated ultimately by delivery. Stimulating or obstructing such a system carries risk: hyperstimulation from uterotonics and uterine rupture from obstruction (in this respect nulliparous women behave differently from multiparous ones, although the reasons for this are not fully understood). When labor is obstructed in nulliparas the uterus tends to become inert, but in multiparas it continues to contract, resulting in an increased risk of rupture.

Efficient labor requires the coordination of myometrium and cervix. The overt nature of myometrial activity has attracted the attention—perhaps to an inordinate degree. Cervical function is much more subtle but no less important. The function of the cervix in pregnancy is to prevent delivery and its collagenous composition with fibers wound tightly in a tubular configuration are ideally suited to retaining the fetus in utero. It is reasonable to propose that some instances of poor progress in the first stage of labor may be due to asynchrony in the coordination between cervical ripening and myometrial contaction,[4] in particular, a cervix that remains

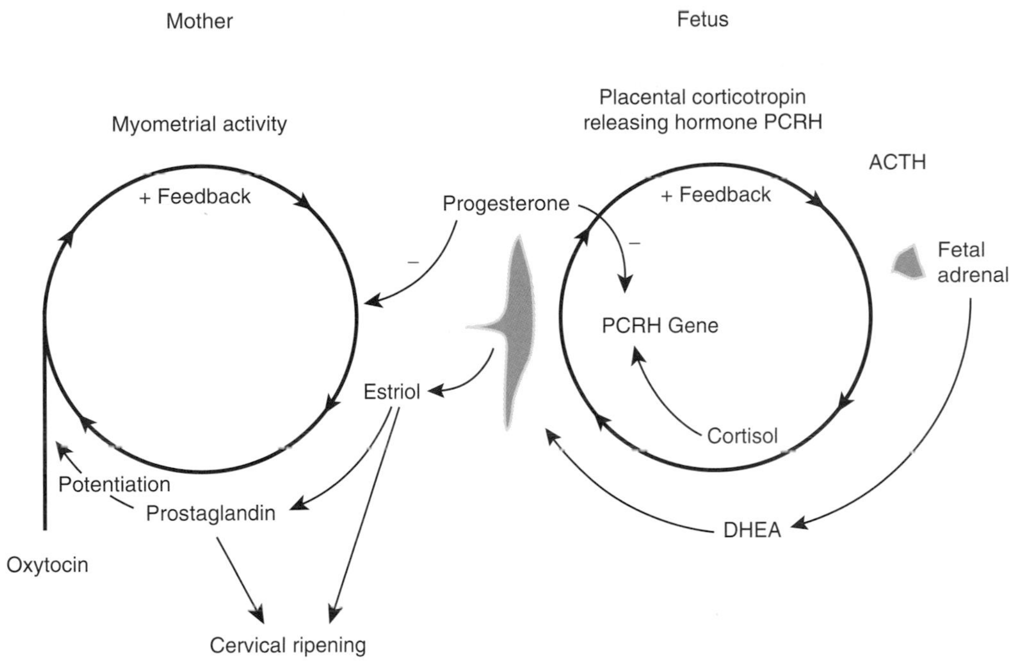

FIGURE 69–1
A model for the initiation of labor.

unripe despite the onset of regular coordinated uterine contractions.

The move from pregnancy to labor mode in the cervix is characterized by "ripening." The resultant increase in tissue compliance permits deformation. Effacement and formation of the lower segment are the initial manifestations of this, followed by dilation. In nulliparous women, these processes are usually sequential, but in parous women dilation may take place before effacement is complete. Either way, effacement redistributes tissue from the cervix to the lower segment and decreases cervical resistance.

Throughout pregnancy, the myometrium is spontaneously active, but before the onset of labor, contractions originating in any particular muscle cell or group of muscle cells are not propagated throughout the myometrium. Under the influence of estrogens and prostaglandins, spontaneous activity rises throughout gestation; in addition, gap junctions (*nexuses*) form between muscle cells.[5] These junctions provide preferential pathways for electrical activity to pass from cell to cell, producing a coordinated response from the myometrium. As coordination increases, contractility becomes sufficient to raise the intrauterine pressure and Braxton Hicks contractions can be perceived by both the mother and an observer palpating the uterus. However, until they are strong enough, and the cervix ripe enough, for cervical dilation to accompany these contractions, they are usually relatively painless.

By the time of the onset of labor, oxytocin is already in high concentrations in the maternal circulation, and oxytocin receptors have developed on the membranes of smooth muscle cells. Thus, oxytocin is thought to facilitate labor rather than initiate it.[6]

Prostaglandins *potentiate* the action of oxytocin. This potentiation results in a greater tonic effect from the combination of prostaglandin and oxytocin than would be achieved from the additive effect of either on its own. Estrogens promote the production of prostaglandins in the decidua, between the fetal membranes and the myometrium.[7] These and other agents, such as interleukins and cytokines, that are involved in the inflammatory cascade[8] characterizing labor have paracrine effects,[7,9] meaning that they act over short distances, stimulating the maternal positive feedback loop, with the result that uterine activity rises exponentially at the beginning of labor and continues to rise thereafter.

Many of the agents involved in the initiation of labor affect both myometrium and cervix in different ways, but all these changes have the net effect of creating the right local environment for labor to occur. Oxytocin is a very unusual hormone in that it is almost entirely specific in its effect on myometrial contractility. There are oxytocin receptors and a small amount of smooth muscle in the cervix that are active in labor,[10] but the effect of oxytocin on the cervix is minimal compared to its effect on the myometrium.

Diagnosis of Labor

Diagnosis of labor is crucial because incorrect diagnosis leads to unwarranted and potentially dangerous interventions. Precise identification of the onset of labor is problematic. Two essential characteristics must be considered:

- The onset of regular uterine contractions
- Progressive change in the cervix

A subsidiary characteristic is spontaneous rupture of the amniotic membranes. Friedman's graphic analysis of labor laid the foundations for current practice.[11–13] Relying for the diagnosis of labor upon recognizing the onset of regular uterine contractions is problematic, because labor is an exponential escalation of uterine activity that can take place over several days, occasionally even weeks. Precise delineation of a transition point from Braxton Hicks contractions to contractions leading to progressive dilation of the cervix is not possible without examining the cervix, as up to the time of writing it has not proved possible to identify any substantial change in the characteristics of the uterine contractions themselves between pregnancy and labor. Measurements assessing the onset, peak, and offset of contractions and the propagation of contractions across the myometrium using electromyography do not show any important differences that would clearly delineate contractions associated with cervical dilation. Thus, fundamentally, the diagnosis of progressive labor relies upon identifying changes in the cervix. Friedman used assessment of the cervix to divide the first stage of labor into latent and active phases (Fig. 69–2).

During the latent phase the cervix is changing (primarily by effacement, and to a lesser extent by softening) but showing little dilation. The active phase is characterized by progressive cervical dilation.

Other definitions of the onset of labor have been used for research purposes and will be found in the literature, including, for example, the time of admission to delivery suite.[14] This is temporally precise but of little physiologic importance. Clinically, it makes good sense to restrict the

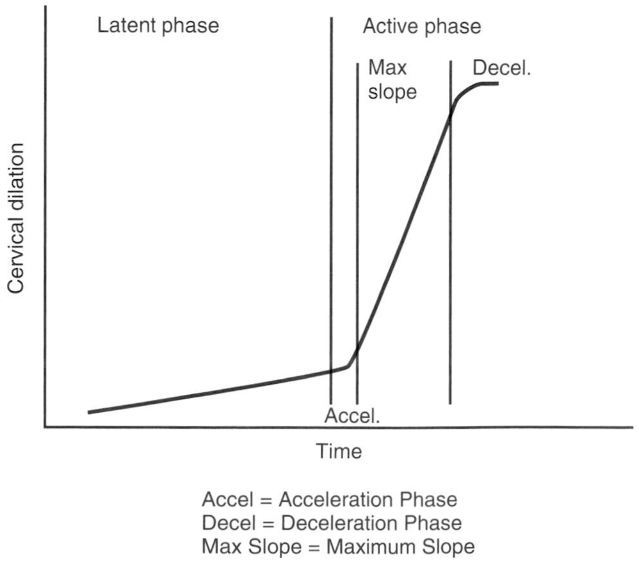

FIGURE 69–2
Friedman's representation of cervical dilation in labor.

diagnosis to evidence of cervical dilation[15] because of the following points:

- Dilation is relatively easy to recognize and record (on a cervicogram).
- Available techniques and limits for monitoring labor apply primarily to the active phase of labor.

A good practice point is that for clinical purposes, all else being normal, only diagnose labor and thereby commence the monitoring of labor when progressive cervical dilation is demonstrable (usually beyond 3 cm dilation).

It should be noted that although regular uterine contractions with intact membranes and without evidence of progressive cervical dilation should probably not be classified as labor, they are still associated with interruptions of the maternal intervillous blood supply and therefore represent a hypoxic challenge to the fetus. Thus, fetuses with poor reserve, such as those suffering from intrauterine growth restriction, should always be monitored carefully when there are contractions, even when there is no progressive cervical dilation.

LABOR MECHANISMS AND PROCESSES

Progress in labor results from the interaction of three factors:

- Powers
- Passages
- Passenger

Powers

Efficient uterine activity is crucial to promote the formation of the birth canal and impart flexion and rotation to the passenger so that it can pass through the complex geometry of the canal.

In the first stage of labor, there is little change in uterine volume. Thus, myometrial contractions are, to all intents and purpose, isometric (i.e., there is minimal shortening of the muscle fibers as they develop tension). Wall tension is required to dilate the cervix. However, it is important that the muscle fibers do not shorten significantly, as this would carry the risk of continuously compressing the blood vessels traversing the myometrium. This in turn would reduce placental perfusion continuously rather than the intermittent reduction associated with the contractions themselves.

Progress is determined by the equilibrium between force (myometrial contractions, especially at the fundus) and resistance (cervix and lower segment). This is almost self-evident, but there is a more subtle effect. The "give" from a compliant cervix attenuates the tension generated by the myometrium.[16,17] Thus, a compliant cervix not only dilates quickly but does so with less uterine activity (as measured by the rise in pressure in the amniotic fluid). The converse is also true.

One apparent paradox is that multiparous women demonstrate faster rates of cervical dilation than nulliparous women but do so with lower uterine activity.[18] This is becuase of their lower resistance.

Assessment of uterine Activity

Uterine activity can be quantified by measurement of intrauterine pressure (IUP), which is directly proportional to wall tension and indirectly proportional to uterine size. Four variables must be taken into account to assess uterine activity, the first three being associated with the contractions themselves: amplitude, duration, repetition frequency, and basal pressure or *tone* (the last one is associated with the elastic recoil and muscular tone of the uterus itself). Measurement of basal tone in absolute terms is sensitive to hydrostatic pressure. Hydrostatic pressure in turn is related to the position of the transducer in relation to the upper fluid level within the uterus. This relationship is affected by posture, and therefore, correct measurement of the baseline tone over and above the hydrostatic pressure requires knowledge of the position of the transducer in relation to the uterus. In current practice, transducers placed at the tip of an intrauterine catheter are often used, and their precise location within the uterus is unknown. Changes in baseline tone can be assessed if the recorded pressure is "zeroed" at the beginning of a recording, but this means that the absolute level always remains uncertain. For this reason, the assessment of uterine activity usually relies upon measuring changes in pressure above baseline tone, ignoring the effect of baseline tone itself. In fact, in the absence of placental abruption or the use of oxytocics (the two most common causes of abnormally elevated baseline tone) most workers have found that the level of baseline tone does not contribute significantly to the rate of cervical dilation and can therefore reasonably be ignored when assessing whether any particular level of uterine activity is likely to be associated with progressive cervical dilation.

IUP monitoring is invasive, requiring insertion of either a fluid-filled catheter connected to an external transducer, or a transducer-tipped catheter, into the amniotic sac. This carries a small risk, from incorrect placement, of abruption, uterine perforation, entanglement, and infection, although these risks are minimal with the modern designs of soft-tipped catheters. IUP monitoring has never been shown in prospective randomized trials to improve the management of labor, but it has been shown repeatedly that under some circumstances, clinical assessment of uterine activity by palpation is unreliable. For this reason, IUP monitoring may be useful in the following circumstances:

- Contractions are difficult to palpate, such occurs in obese patients.
- There is uncertainty as to whether augmentation of labor (for example, with an oxytocin infusion) is producing appropriate increases in uterine activity.
- The data from this labor will be used for research purposes.

Also, in some circumstances it may be of medicolegal value to be able to demonstrate close and accurate monitoring of uterine activity, for example, with induction or augmentation of labor in the presence of a uterine scar, or the use of Syntocinon in grand multiparas, or when the fetus is particularly at risk from uterine hyperstimulation (e.g., when there is evidence of intrauterine growth restriction). The argument is made that if one is prepared to allow spontaneous uterine activity in such cases, then logically one should be prepared to correct low levels of uterine activity up to a physiologic level, provided this can be assessed objectively. However, no studies clearly demonstrate any advantages to IUP monitoring in these circumstances, and some would counsel against such use in case they provide a false sense of security. An equally valid management option at the present time is not to use an oxytocic at all in such cases, resorting instead to cesarean section if there is poor progress.

Because amplitude of contractions correlates with the palpable duration of contractions (most contractions only become palpable when the IUP exceeds baseline tone by more than 15 mm Hg) and overall activity is dependent on repetition frequency, palpation of contractions with timing of duration, and particularly frequency, can give an adequate, semiquantitative assessment of uterine activity for most clinical purposes, including oxytocin augmentation.[19] For these reasons palpation remains the standard method of monitoring uterine activity for clinical purposes.

Normal Range

If progressive cervical dilation is taking place, there is no need for a lower limit to be placed on acceptable uterine activity. Only when there is perceived delay in labor should the adequacy of uterine activity be questioned.

- A contraction frequency of three to four contractions every 10 minutes is optimal.
- Palpable contractions should last for minimum of 40 seconds.

Contractions occurring more frequently than five every 10 minutes with little or no relaxation between them constitute tachysystole (Fig. 69–3).

Uterine activity increases as labor progresses due to prostaglandin release from the decidua and secretion of oxytocin from the maternal posterior pituitary. Spontaneous uterine activity at the end of the first stage can be in excess of levels considered safe for induced or augmented labor.[20,21] The well-being of the fetus in labor is finely balanced. The stronger the contractions, the better the progress but the greater the effect on placental perfusion. The stress of high levels of uterine activity and rapid progress is usually self-limited by early delivery before there is any adverse cumulative effect on the fetus. Poor progress, on the other hand, may result in the

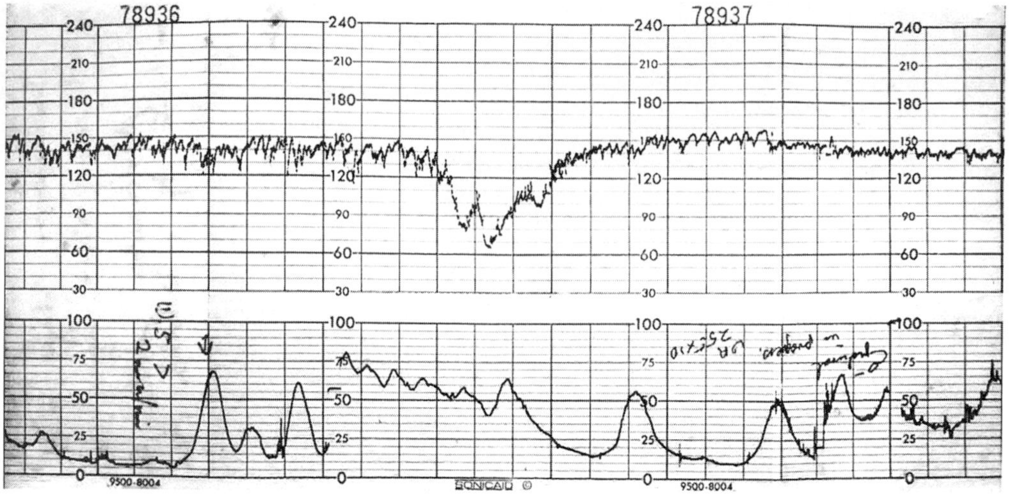

FIGURE 69–3
Hyperstimulation due to oxytocin showing effect on fetal heart rate. Note the frequent small-amplitude contractions and rise in basal tone.

cumulative effects of uterine contractions exceeding the tolerance of the fetus. A compromized fetus will have lower tolerances, and augmented uterine activity will then have a greater and more rapid impact.

Passages

The passages have often been equated solely with the bony pelvis, but the soft tissues are also important, including the cervix and lower segment in the first stage and the pelvic floor in the second stage.

Assessment of the Pelvis

Absolute cephalopelvic disproportion is today rare in well-nourished populations. Childhood rickets used to be a relatively common cause of brim dystocia, hence the importance obstetricians have traditionally given to "engagement," because in previous generations passage of the largest part of the fetus through the narrowest part of the bony pelvis usually guaranteed delivery.

In today's practice, however, clinical and x-ray pelvimetry have poor predictive values[22] and should not be used. More sophisticated imaging techniques, such as magnetic resonance imaging and computed tomography, coupled with ultrasound fetal biometry, have been used to improve diagnosis, and this approach is logical but further clinical research is required to establish their value.[23]

The shortcomings of pelvimetry, and the complex mechanism of labor that relies on flexion, rotation, molding, and even pelvic compliance, means that clinicians have to fall back on "try it and see."

It should be noted that two out of three women who require a cesarean section for failure to progress go on to deliver normally the next time despite birth weight rising with parity. This suggests that cephalopelvic disproportion is not a common cause for failure to progress.

Assessment of the Soft Tissues

The function of the cervix in pregnancy is to obstruct delivery. Failure of the cervix to undergo its correct biophysical preparation may carry its pregnancy function through to labor. Abnormal connective tissue biochemistry has been demonstrated in association with poor progress in labor.[24]

In the second stage of labor the soft tissues of the pelvic floor help to induce the rotational forces necessary for the complex mechanism of labor in the human, while, at the same time, they offer resistance to progress. It is perhaps paradoxical that the resistance necessary to impart rotation also offers resistance to descent.

Measurement of the forces between the cervix and the fetal head has shown differences between progressive and delayed labor.[25–27] These data do not fit simple mechanical relationships, emphasizing that cervical dilation is a more complex process than mere stretching. More work needs to be done to permit clinical application of these experimental techniques.

Clinical monitoring relies on the aggregate response of the cervix during labor. Digital estimation of cervical dilation is plotted against time (cervicography). This is simple and screens for deviation from a normal pattern, but because of the many variables that may be at play, it does not offer a diagnosis. For example, the complex interaction of the head to cervix forces with the stretching of the cervix cannot be assessed clinically at the present time.

Passengers

Birth weight within the normal range has poor predictive value for delivery complications. Figure 69–4 shows that there is some correlation of the duration of labor with birth weight, but the maximum variation over the

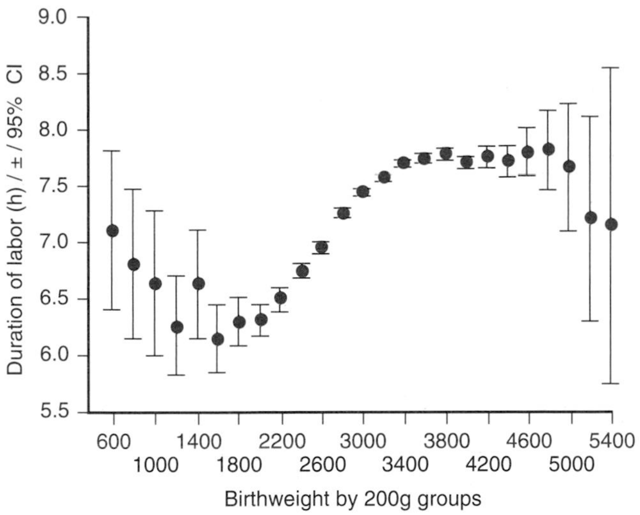

FIGURE 69–4
The duration of labor by birth weight. Data taken from 425,855 births with birth weight and duration of labor recorded in the North West region of London from 1988 to 2000.

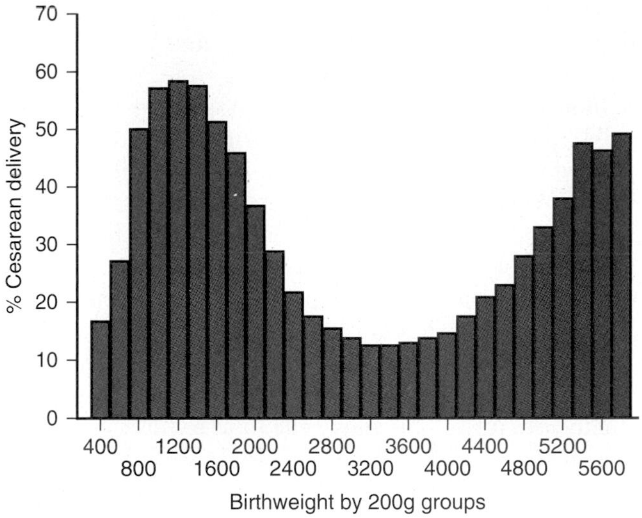

FIGURE 69–5
Percentage of babies delivered by cesarean section, according to birth weight. Data taken from 513,381 births with birth weight and mode of delivery recorded in the North West region of London from 1988 to 2000.

extremes of birth weight is only 1.5 hours. The effects of flexion and rotation on the efficiency of the labor mechanisms are likely to be at least as important. The ability of the fetal head to mold is another important variable. Moreover, in terms of cephalopelvic disproportion, head size is not closely correlated with birth weight. For macrosomic fetuses the main risk is shoulder dystocia. Unlike cephalopelvic disproportion, shoulder dystocia is not reliably predicted by cervical dilation rates in the first stage, and even the descent of the presenting part in the second stage can be normal.[28]

Only the extremes of birth weight have much significance in relation to mode of delivery. In recent U.K. practice, cesarean section was used in up to 60% of pregnancies when the birth weight was less than 2.5 kg, and from 40% to 50% when the birth weight exceeded 5 kg (see Fig. 69–5). However, there was relatively little variation in the use of cesarean section when the birth weight lay between 2.5 kg and 4 kg (Fig. 69–5), and in 513,381 births in the North West region of London between 1988 and 2000, this range accounted for 83.2% of all births. Thus, for the majority of babies, birth weight contributes little to the mode of delivery.

Some evidence suggests that birth weight is rising[29]; even more important than the increasing mean birth weight is the increase in the proportion of babies weighing more than 4 kg, which in some European countries has now reached 30%. However, this increase in birth weight has to be viewed in the context of improved maternal nutrition and the general increase in maternal stature.

Assessment

Even if birth weight was of crucial importance in determining progress in labor, birth weight can only be predicted to an accuracy of ±10% to 15% by ultrasound fetal biometry. The poor predictive value of these estimates means that they have to be factored in very cautiously when planning delivery. They should be taken into consideration, however, when delay is apparent. Other clinical features of cephalopelvic disproportion that should be sought include excessive molding, and failure of the presenting part to engage and descend. Generally speaking, it is reasonable to assume that pelvic capacity is adequate if a woman has delivered vaginally before, but birth weight increases with parity, and the increase may be substantial if the woman has developed gestational diabetes due to advancing maternal age. Therefore, it is wise to check previous birth weights and any features of the current pregnancy (such as glucose intolerance) that may indicate borderline disproportion. This baby may be just that bit too big.

Presentation: Flexion/Deflexion

Flexion and deflexion of the head determines the part that will present. Flexion results in a vertex presentation, that part of the head bounded by the occiput, the posterior part of the anterior fontanel, and the biparietal eminences. This results in the smallest dimensions of the head presenting themselves to the birth canal (9.5 cm × 9.5 cm). Flexion is promoted by efficient powers—uterine contractions in the first stage and the addition of maternal pushing in the second.

Deflexion of the head produces first a brow presentation and then, in complete deflexion, a face presentation. The dimensions of a brow in a term fetus are such (13.5 cm anteroposterior) that they cannot be accommodated by a normal pelvis. Thus, the head remains high, progress of labor may become obstructed with a secondary arrest pattern, or if full dilation is reached, there may be failure of descent. Brow presentation should be considered when a multiparous patient, who has delivered normal-sized babies without a problem before, develops abnormalities of progress. Resort to oxytocin augmentation without this consideration risks uterine rupture.

Judicious prevarication can be adopted to see if there will be spontaneous conversion to either a vertex or a face presentation. If not, cesarean section is usually the only option. Very occasionally, with an occipitoposterior position of the fetal head and a roomy pelvis, deflexion will result in a brow presentation that can be corrected by forceps rotation to occipitoanterior. Such maneuvers are, however, rarely contemplated in modern practice.

Babies with a face presentation can deliver vaginally but only under favorable circumstances. The mentum must rotate anteriorly. This allows the head to flex as it negotiates the curve in the birth canal. To do so with a mentum posterior would require even further deflexion, which is anatomically impossible. A good-sized pelvis and efficient powers are necessary to deliver a face presentation spontaneously. Forceps can be used to add traction.

Assessment is undertaken by digital vaginal examination.

Position: Rotation

The vertex normally engages with the occiput in a lateral position. This allows congruence between the long axis of the head and the widest diameter of the brim of the pelvis from side to side. With descent, the lowest part (occiput) is forced forward by the levator ani muscles that form an inclined plane running from back to front. This occurs in the midpelvis, which when cut across presents a circular shape that is conducive to rotation. With the occiput anterior and the head flexed, the head is now able to fit the diamond-shaped pelvic outlet with matching of the long axes of the head and the outlet. Deflexion of the head is possible as it negotiates the curve of the birth canal.

If the head rotates and maintains a posterior position (OP), there is a tendency to deflex and present a larger dimension to the birth canal. To follow the curve of the birth canal the head has flex further. This is anatomically difficult and unlikely to occur. In the first stage, an OP position may present with any pattern of delay. The options are to wait and hope for spontaneous resolution, augment the powers with a view to encouraging flexion and rotation, or cesarean section if neither produces the desired result. If augmentation is undertaken, the side effects have to be recognized and safeguards employed, meaning continuous electronic fetal monitoring and timely reviews, particularly in a multiparous woman if progress is arrested.

Delay in the second stage can be addressed by instrumentation. For persistent OP, an OP ventouse cup can be used, not only to apply traction, but also to encourage rotation and flexion. Some skill is required to achieve this. Forceps (Kielland's) can be used for simple traction or rotation. These are not maneuvers for the inexperienced.

The head may stay in an occipitolateral position such that it cannot negotiate the diamond-shaped pelvic outlet whose longest dimension lies anteroposterior. This is sometimes termed "deep transverse arrest." It may be due to pelvic abnormality or poor powers failing to impart rotation. Resistance from the pelvic floor is also required for rotation. Epidural analgesia may interfere with this by paralyzing the levator muscles, allowing the head to descend below the midcavity without rotation. Rotation to occipitoanterior is required, using either ventouse or rotational forceps. The latter is more effective but requires skill and practice if maternal and fetal trauma is to be avoided.

Assessment is undertaken by digital vaginal examination. This examination can prove difficult, especially if there is scalp edema (caput). Ultrasound imaging can be helpful by identifying midline structures and the orbits.

CLINICAL ASPECTS OF MANAGEMENT OF LABOR

If a woman delivers vaginally the first time, she is much more likely to do so in the future. Thus, good management of the first labor is crucial and has a bearing on the rest of her reproductive potential.

Active Management

This term carries a number of connotations. In its broadest sense it marked a change in philosophy from reacting to prolonged labor after the event, to prospective monitoring of labor to detect delay early, diagnose its cause, and instigate management.[30] This ideal is often not possible because a precise diagnosis is lacking. A more pragmatic approach emerged whereby prospective detection of departure from normal progress was automatically managed by augmenting the powers to accelerate progress because this was the only variable open to manipulation by the clinician.[15,31]

Whatever the clinician's view of active management, most agree that good management of labor[32] depends upon the following:

- Correct diagnosis of labor
- Use of a partogram
- Adherence to agreed policies of management based on best evidence regarding fetal and uterine contraction monitoring
- Appropriate intervention
- Auditing of outcomes

The Partogram

Figure 69–6 is a chart that represents the essential variables for monitoring both mother and fetus during labor. Graphic representation of data is used whenever possible because trends are important. The three sets of data concern maternal signs, fetal signs, and progress of labor.

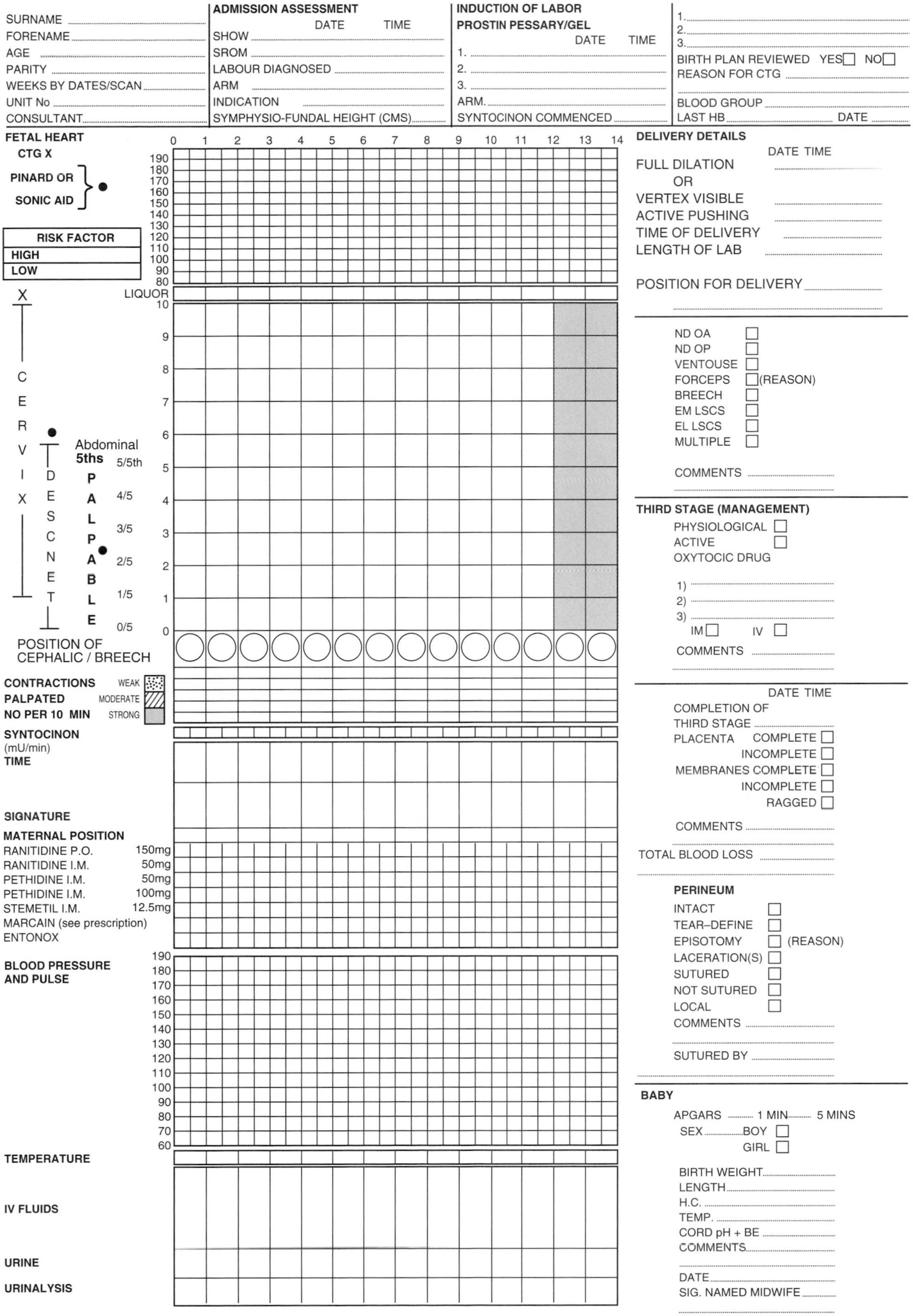

SURNAME
FORENAME
AGE
PARITY
WEEKS BY DATES/SCAN
UNIT No
CONSULTANT

ADMISSION ASSESSMENT
DATE TIME
SHOW
SROM
LABOUR DIAGNOSED
ARM
INDICATION
SYMPHYSIO-FUNDAL HEIGHT (CMS)

INDUCTION OF LABOR
PROSTIN PESSARY/GEL
DATE TIME
1.
2.
3.
ARM.
SYNTOCINON COMMENCED

1.
2.
3.
BIRTH PLAN REVIEWED YES☐ NO☐
REASON FOR CTG
BLOOD GROUP
LAST HB DATE

FETAL HEART
CTG X
PINARD OR SONIC AID }●
0 1 2 3 4 5 6 7 8 9 10 11 12 13 14
190 180 170 160 150 140 130 120 110 100 90 80

RISK FACTOR
HIGH
LOW

LIQUOR
X
C E R V I X
● D E S C E N T
Abdominal **5ths** **PALPABLE**
5/5th 4/5 3/5 2/5 1/5 0/5
10 9 8 7 6 5 4 3 2 1 0
POSITION OF CEPHALIC / BREECH

CONTRACTIONS WEAK
PALPATED MODERATE
NO PER 10 MIN STRONG
SYNTOCINON
(mU/min)
TIME
SIGNATURE
MATERNAL POSITION
RANITIDINE P.O. 150mg
RANITIDINE I.M. 50mg
PETHIDINE I.M. 50mg
PETHIDINE I.M. 100mg
STEMETIL I.M. 12.5mg
MARCAIN (see prescription)
ENTONOX
BLOOD PRESSURE AND PULSE
190 180 170 160 150 140 130 120 110 100 90 80 70 60
TEMPERATURE
IV FLUIDS
URINE
URINALYSIS

DELIVERY DETAILS
DATE TIME
FULL DILATION
OR
VERTEX VISIBLE
ACTIVE PUSHING
TIME OF DELIVERY
LENGTH OF LAB
POSITION FOR DELIVERY

ND OA ☐
ND OP ☐
VENTOUSE ☐
FORCEPS ☐(REASON)
BREECH ☐
EM LSCS ☐
EL LSCS ☐
MULTIPLE ☐
COMMENTS

THIRD STAGE (MANAGEMENT)
PHYSIOLOGICAL ☐
ACTIVE ☐
OXYTOCIC DRUG
1)
2)
3)
IM☐ IV ☐
COMMENTS

DATE TIME
COMPLETION OF THIRD STAGE
PLACENTA COMPLETE ☐
INCOMPLETE ☐
MEMBRANES COMPLETE ☐
INCOMPLETE ☐
RAGGED ☐
COMMENTS
TOTAL BLOOD LOSS

PERINEUM
INTACT ☐
TEAR–DEFINE ☐
EPISOTOMY ☐ (REASON)
LACERATION(S) ☐
SUTURED ☐
NOT SUTURED ☐
LOCAL ☐
COMMENTS
SUTURED BY

BABY
APGARS 1 MIN 5 MINS
SEX BOY ☐
GIRL ☐
BIRTH WEIGHT
LENGTH
H.C.
TEMP.
CORD pH + BE
COMMENTS
DATE
SIG. NAMED MIDWIFE

FIGURE 69–6
Partogram.

Graphic representation of data is used whenever possible becasue trends are important. The three sets of data concern maternal signs, fetal signs, and progress of labor.

Maternal Signs

Maternal data comprise vital signs (pulse, blood pressure, temperature), urinalysis, and medical treatment (analgesia, uterotonics).

Fetal Signs

Fetal data comprise fetal heart rate, state of the membranes, color of the liquor, and descent and position of the presenting part.

Progress of Labor

The cervicogram is a component part of the partogram and, by definition, relates to the first stage. It represents, graphically, cervical dilation over time from the diagnosis of established labor. In practice this applies only to the active phase of dilation (although monitoring the change in the Bishop's score of the cervix may be of value in the latent phase). Because the usual concern is detection of delay, the lower limit of progress has received much attention, with little attention on setting upper limits. Precipitate labor has been associated with risk but this comes mainly from unexpected delivery rather than from the brevity of the process per se (although there is a reported increase in the incidence of Erb's palsy with precipitate labor – see Chapter 70).

MANAGEMENT OF THE FIRST STAGE OF LABOR

Diagnosis of Delay or Aberrance

Friedman selected 200 nulliparous women retrospectively from a larger heterogeneous group of patients[12] and a similar cohort of parous women[13] to identify "ideal" labor, namely, no iatrogenic interventions (apart from "prophylactic low forceps"), vaginal deliveries, and average-sized, healthy neonates. These patients' labor curves were analyzed to identify statistical limits as means and standard deviations.

From these data a lower limit of maximum slope dilation was produced (Fig. 69–7).

The value of 1 cm/hour has now become almost universally accepted for clinical practice. However, this rate may be an overestimate for the following reasons:

- The data are not normally distributed, but have a tail skewed toward higher rates of dilation, bringing into question the validity of the statistical analysis.
- Most clinicians use an average of 1 cm/hour for the whole of the active phase, including the slower phases of acceleration and deceleration and not just the phase of maximum slope.

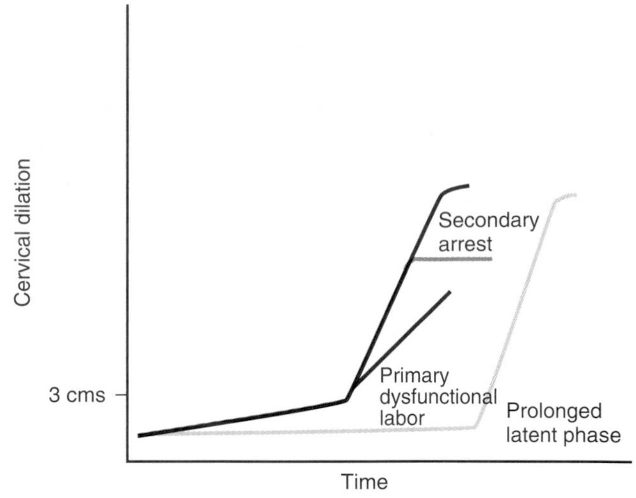

FIGURE 69–7
Patterns of delay. (Data from Friedman.)

Better statistical analysis of progress in normal labor has confirmed these doubts (Fig. 69–8).[33] These data show lower rates of dilation in the early part of the active phase and no inflection points at the end of the phase of maximum slope. This pattern of progress may reflect physiology better, but more clinical evaluation is required.

Several cervicograms have been produced for clinical use. Hendricks[34] produced similar patterns of dilation but chose the slowest 20% as the statistical divide. Philpott and Castle,[35] in a southern African population, demonstrated a marked difference in the rate of maximum slope compared with Friedman's data (median 1.25 cm/hour versus 2.75 cm/hour, respectively) based on data from an unspecified number of cases, representing the slowest 10% of primigravidas, suggesting that there may be significant popula-

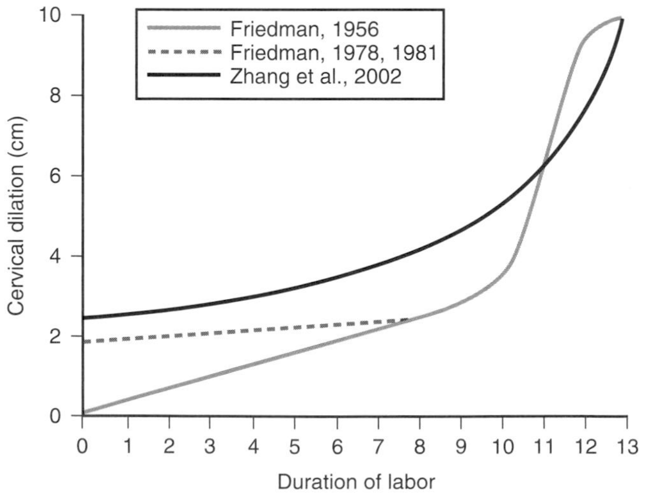

FIGURE 69–8
Reanalysis of progress in nulliparous labor. (Data from Friedman EA: Cervimetry—an objective method for the study of cervical dilation in labor. Am J Obstet Gynecol 1956;71(16):1189–1193; Friedman EA: A cervimeter for continuous measurement of cervical dilatation in labour—preliminary results. BJOG 1978;85(8):638 (letter); Friedman A: The labor curve. Clin Perinatol 1981;8(1):15–25; Zhang J, Troendle JF, Yoncey MK: Reassessing the labor curve in nulliparous women. Am J Obset Gynecol 2002;3(2):288–290.)

tion differences. They introduced the concept of an alert line followed 4 hours later by an action line.[36] This interval has been changed by other researchers, often without clear reason or benefit. Despite the earlier observation that there was a lower maximum slope gradient in their population, the lines were set with gradients of 1 cm/hour. Beazley and Kurjak[37] used a "low risk" population to produce a cervicogram whose limits differentiate progress above the line, resulting in an 80% chance of a favorable outcome, compared with only a 20% chance below it. This cervicogram acknowledges differing limits for nulliparous and parous women. Studd[38] devised a cervicogram from a multiracial population in the United Kingdom having "normal" labor. An S-shaped dilation curve was produced, with the steepest gradient between 4 cm and full dilation. The statistical methodology used to produce these curves was not specified, nor were the biologic limits.

All these cervicograms, in their various ways, attempt to define a boundary that can be used to define slow progress. However, they have been devised using data from specific populations with individual characteristics, and therefore, they may not be generalizable to different populations. Indeed, as they all differ, it is likely that they cannot be used without their clinical value being tested prospectively to determine their predictive value for any particular group. For example, it seems unlikely that the same cervicogram would be applicable to a black African population with their high assimilation pelves and high obstructed labor rates, compared with white Scandinavians with their wide pelves and low cesarean section rates. Prospective evaluation of these various cervicograms in different populations from those in which they were derived has not been done, and the available data does not allow their generalizability to be assessed from the original studies. Using data from later papers, the positive predictive value for operative delivery from an alert line set at 1 cm/hour gradient and an action line 2 hours later (values that are widely used today in the developed world) is only 43%. Use of standard cervicogram limits for the multiethnic populations of many of today's major cities seems unlikely to be adequate.

Thus, cervicography is only an aid to the management of labor and should not be used as a substitute for appropriate diagnosis. Transgression of a lower limit of progress should simply raise awareness of increasing risk, indicating the need to look for an explanation (diagnosis) of the slow progress.

Poor Progress

Friedman described three patterns of aberrance from normal labor[39] (see Fig. 69–7):

- Prolonged latent phase (PLP)
- Primary dysfunctional labor (PDL)
- Secondary arrest (SA)

None of these patterns is pathognomonic of a particular pathology. They are signs of pathology not diagnoses.

Prolonged Latent Phase

Friedman described the latent phase, from the onset of contractions to entry to the active phase of dilation, as lasting up to 20 hours in nulliparas (mean 8.6 hours, SD 6 hours) and 14 hours in parous women (mean 5.3 hours, SD 4.1 hours). The difficulties with defining the start and end of this phase have already been discussed. Thus, the true incidence of prolonged latent phase is difficult to determine, but 3.5 % has been proposed in nulliparas. It is less common in parous women.

The causes of this pattern of delay are uncertain but probably relate to delayed cervical ripening (absent or slow changes in cervical connective tissue biochemistry during the second half of pregnancy).

Augmentation of the powers with oxytocin to accelerate progress in the latent phase is not beneficial.[14,40,41] Such augmented labors still exhibit a 10-fold increase in cesarean section rates compared to normal labors, with a threefold increase in low Apgar scores in the neonates.

From a practical point of view, all else being equal, reassurance for the mother, analgesia, and time are often all that is necessary to allow cervical preparation to synchronize with that of the myometrium.

Primary Dysfunctional Labor

Primary dysfunctional labor is defined as progress slower than 1 cm/hour during the active phase slope with an incidence of 26% in nulliparas and 8% in parous women.[40] About 80% of nulliparas and 90% of parous women will respond to oxytocin, suggesting that poor uterine activity is a significant factor. Unfortunately, response in terms of improvement in cervical dilation rate does not always translate into uncomplicated vaginal delivery. Fetal distress may result from augmentation of the forces, and an increased incidence in instrumental delivery and perinatal morbidity suggest that mechanical factors may also operate. Five percent of augmented labors do not respond in terms of increasing their uterine activity or rates of progress, and these nonresponsive labors are associated with cesarean section rates of 77%. On the other hand, 23% still achieved a vaginal delivery,[14] so even failure of response cannot be seen as an automatic indication for cesarean section. Mechanical abnormalities can be postulated (particularly malposition, malrotation and deflexion, and slow molding of the fetal head) which correct themselves in time, but sound evidence for a single causal effect is hard to find. Other possibilities have not been extensively studied. Abnormalities of cervical mechanics and biochemical preparation have been documented and merit further study.

Secondary Arrest

Secondary arrest can be identified by cessation of progress after normal active phase dilation.[42] The incidence is 6% in nulliparas and 2% in parous women.

A subtle variant of secondary arrest is delay between 7 and 10 cm. Even though full dilation may be achieved, there is an increased risk of difficult instrumental delivery.[43]

Of the three patterns of arrest, secondary arrest has the most convincing link with etiology, namely disproportion and malposition. Although in one series 60% nulliparas and 70% of parous women showed improved progress with augmentation of contractions, cesarean section rates were over 10-fold greater than in normal labor. The effect of uterine stimulation may have been to encourage flexion and rotation of the head, promoting descent and progress along the birth canal.

Practice Point

Whatever the pattern of delay, identification of a clear, single etiologic factor is unlikely. This may be due to complex interactions between multiple factors, an inability detect the contributory factor because the diagnostic tools are imprecise, lack of knowledge of other factors, or finally a combination of all three. Treatment is more likely to be successful when a diagnosis of a single pathologic process is possible. Augmentation of the powers may be the only intervention available, and the "do nothing" arm of clinical trials has been woefully absent, leaving this option surrounded with uncertainty.

Thus, the obstetrician faced with evidence of delay should be conversant with the options available and be prepared to balance the risks and benefits of any intervention to be employed.

Interventions

Amniotomy

It is commonly stated that amniotomy increases uterine activity, although the evidence for this is weak, and there are good reasons to keep the membranes intact. For example, more fetal heart rate decelerations have been noted following amniotomy. Randomized clinical trials of routine amniotomy show that there is no improvement in clinical outcome, though labor may be shortened. Surgical intervention is not reduced, and there are no major benefits for the neonate.[44–46] However, if there is poor progress with intact membranes and uterine activity is thought to be suboptimal, a case for amniotomy can be made. Occasionally, it may also allow the presenting part to descend and press more effectively on the cervix. Perhaps more important than the physical forces induced by amniotomy are its pharmacologic effects. Rupture of the membranes provokes prostaglandin release from the decidua. Prostaglandins may stimulate the positive feedback loop to increase uterine activity and ripen the cervix. Amniotomy has also been advocated to allow early detection of meconium as an aid to the assessment of fetal well-being, and therefore may sometimes be useful if the fetal heart rate pattern is nonreassuring. In summary, all other features of labor being normal, there is no clinical benefit from routine amniotomy.

Oxytocin Augmentation

When oxytocin became readily available for clinical use in the 1960s, obstetricians were given some degree of control over one of the three variables that determine progress, namely the powers. As already stated, the powers also indirectly influence flexion and rotation of the passenger.

Oxytocin is a polypeptide hormone secreted from the posterior pituitary of both mother and fetus. The half-life of oxytocin is only 5 to 7 minutes. Therefore, its effect can be removed rapidly merely by stopping the infusion (Fig. 69–9).

Binding of oxytocin to its receptor[47] opens calcium-activated channels and results in membrane depolarization.[6] This, in turn, opens voltage-dependent channels, producing a rise in intracellular calcium that generates tension in the contractile filaments. The prime effect is to increase the frequency of contractions with a second effect of slowing conduction and recruiting more cells per contraction, thereby increasing duration and amplitude. Thus, palpation of frequency and duration is a logical, simple means of monitoring oxytocin's effect.[17]

Both of these effects are beneficial when the myometrium is hypotonic, but addition of oxytocin to an already optimally acting myometrium frequently induces hypertonus, with resulting fetal hypoxia. Careful monitoring of uterine activity is essential and infusion rates may have to be reduced as labor proceeds. Titration of dosage against uterine activity should be performed using

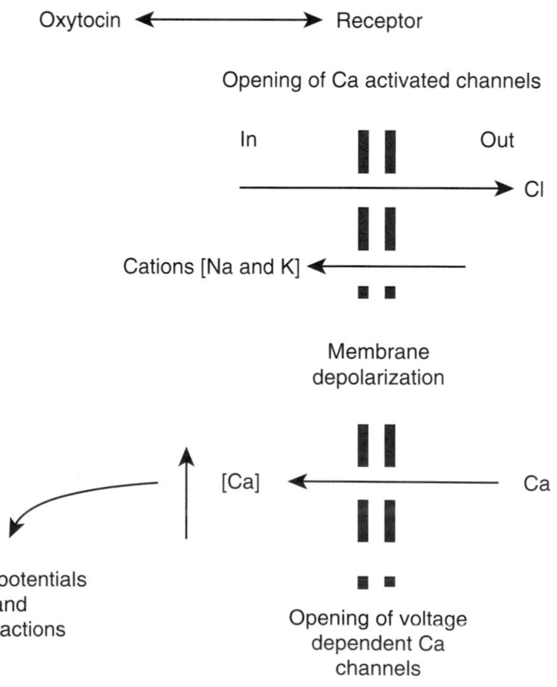

FIGURE 69–9
Action of oxytocin.

regimens that allow time for activity to become stabilized between increments. An interval of 30 minutes between increments is recommended. Published protocols generally recommend a starting dose of 1 to 6 mU/minute; in current practice 1 to 2 mU/minute are usually used. Geometrically increasing regimens (e.g., 1, 2, 4, 8, 16, 32 mU/minute) reach effective doses more quickly but are more prone to cause hyperstimulation, and have therefore generally been replaced by predominantly arithmetic increases (e.g., 1, 2, 4, 6, 8, 10, 12 mU/minute). The majority of women will respond to dose rates of 8 mU/minute, and few will need more than 16 mU/minute.

When oxytocin is used in labor, it must be maintained for the third stage and for an hour thereafter to reduce the risk of uterine atony and postpartum hemorrhage. Postpartum hemorrhage is also associated with prolonged labor.

Meta-analysis[48] of clinical trials of oxytocin augmentation show an increase in the parturient's subjective experience of pain and some increase in the rate of cervical dilation but no reduction in cesarean section and instrumental delivery rates.

Cesarean Section

When interventions for poor progress fail, cesarean section is necessary.

The Active Management of Labor

The widespread availability of oxytocin was followed by the similarly widespread adoption of the use of cervicography to detect slow progress. It was argued by some[15] that the only variable the clinician could influence in the first stage of labor was the powers and that malposition or deflexion of the fetus could only be influenced indirectly via the powers. Hypotonic uterine activity, leading to these abnormalities, should be treated by augmentation. A package of care was proposed for nulliparous women that emphasized the importance of the correct diagnosis of labor (active phase), routine amniotomy, hourly cervical assessment per rectum to determine progress, and augmentation of the powers with intravenous oxytocin if slow active phase progress was detected (the lower limit of normal adopted was 1 cm/hour). This regimen permitted one-to-one midwifery care because within a short measure of time patients progressed normally, responded to augmentation, or underwent cesarean section if they did not progress. The results from uncontrolled cohort studies indicated low cesarean section rates associated with this policy. The simplicity of this approach appealed to many clinicians, and still does.

However, the same results could not be replicated elsewhere and concerns grew over rising cesarean section rates[49] for failure to progress despite the apparent adoption of this philosophy. Moreover, 25 years later, meta-analysis of the individual components of this approach has revealed that the medical interventions proposed are not effective in reducing operative intervention.[48] Randomized controlled clinical trials have now been performed. The first of these[50] showed a decrease in cesarean section associated with the adoption of "active management" from the rate prior to the study, but there was also a decreased rate in the control arm of the study. This was almost certainly a Hawthorne effect (simply by doing the trial and focusing participants' minds on the management issues produced an effect). The end result was not statistically significant. The largest study[51] did not show any improvement in surgical delivery rates, though there was a reduction in maternal postnatal pyrexia. These two studies started with relatively high cesarean section rates, in the region of 20%. Early studies reported the use of oxytocin in up to 50% of nulliparas,[15,53] not a particularly surprising figure if a threshold of 1cm/hour of cervical dilation is chosen as a threshold for augmentation, as this is their average rate of cervical dilation. A third study[52] aimed to test if relaxation of the indications to augment uterine activity that had been adopted as part of a regimen of active management, thereby using less oxytocin, would risk raising a low cesarean section rate. This study reported cesarean section rates of 3.9% in the active management arm compared with 2.6% in the "selective use" arm and spontaneous vaginal delivery rates of 78% and 79%, respectively. Meta-analysis has been performed on clinical studies of active mangement.[54] This analysis combines controlled and uncontrolled trials and concludes that there is reduced operative intervention. Care must be exercized when combining such heterogeneous data. Meta-analysis of only the randomized trials fails to show any benefit. There does not appear to an increase in neonatal problems, probably due to the high degree of intrapartum surveillance that is employed. A study of the promptness with which oxytocin is used (crossing an action line set at 2 or 4 hours after the alert line) did indicate that there was a reduction in cesarean section (RR 0.68) using the more aggressive approach.[53] This trial, though showing benefit, had to be curtailed, and there were protocol violations in the aggressive arm of the study. Confirmation of these findings by similar studies would be helpful.

One-to-One Midwifery Care

This benefit was almost a side effect of the package of active management, but clinical benefit from such intensive care has been demonstrated.[48] Patient confidence and her feeling of control is improved in association with a reduction in the the need for pain relief and a lower incidence of cesarean section and operative vaginal delivery. Who provides the support appears to be less important. Some studies have employed nonclinical but trained lay supporters (doulas).

Interventions demonstrated to be effective are preparation of the mother and personal support during labor and correct diagnosis of labor (active phase) to permit appropriate application of limits of progress.

MANAGEMENT OF THE SECOND STAGE OF LABOR

The second stage of labor starts at full dilation of the cervix and ends with delivery of the fetus. Descent and rotation of the passenger are the main features. Before the advent of epidural analgesia, full dilation of the cervix was apparent because of an urge to push due to the descent of the presenting part onto the pelvic floor. Epidural analgesia may abolish this sensation completely. Thus, there may be no outward signs of entry to the second stage, and diagnosis will only follow vaginal examination. The duration of second stage has thereby become controversial.

Physiology of the Second Stage

Maternal Changes

At full dilation of the cervix, the uterus ceases to be a "closed vessel," cervical resistance is lost, and descent through the birth canal begins. Cervical resistance is necessary for the isometric generation of wall tension. After full dilation, myometrial activity progressively changes toward isotonic activity as the uterus empties. Reduction in uterine volume permits shortening of the myometrial fibers that becomes maximal during the third stage. This form of myometrial activity is crucial for effective hemostasis in the third stage but is potentially dangerous in the second stage.

The myometrium is "inserted" into the pelvis via the connective tissues that surround the cervix, with the round ligaments helping to tether and direct the uterine fundus. These connective tissue supports are elastic. If the force required to stretch them is greater than the resistance offered by the birth canal, there will be progress. The rate of progress will be determined by the equilibrium established between the elasticity of the supports and the resistance offered by the birth canal. Frank obstruction to progress from the bony pelvis will merely direct all force to stretching the cervical supports against this resistance. Descent can occur without pushing, but there is little evidence (other than anecdotal, for example, spontaneous delivery in paraplegic women) to show that delivery can be achieved without the voluntary use of the abdominal muscles to raise intra-abdominal pressure to increase the expulsive forces. Pushing increases maternal effort and interferes with breathing, inducing both respiratory and metabolic acidosis.

Fetal Changes

Studies on the acid-base balance in the fetus in the second stage show a decline in pH and a rise in lactate as pushing and descent progress.[55–57] To a degree, this is physiologic, and the metabolic changes will stimulate the neonate to breathe spontaneously. Too much, however, results in respiratory depression.

Divisions of the Second Stage

It is useful to split the second stage into passive and active sections, depending on whether pushing has commenced.[55]

Passive Section

In the passive section, prior to pushing, there is likely to be little descent to alter the character of myometrial activity, and the mother is not affecting her metabolic state by pushing. Thus, there is minimal effect on the fetus.[55] There does not appear to be a significant risk from waiting at this point prior to pushing, all else being equal. However, there does not appear to be any benefit, either.[58] Thus, whether to commence pushing or wait and the duration of this wait continues to be debated but is probably irrelevant to outcome.[59]

Active Section

The active section commences with pushing. From this point onward, the metabolic changes in the fetus described earlier begin and progress. Descent and rotation of the presenting part should be progressive, irrespective of the presence or not of an epidural anesthetic.

Monitoring Progress

Descent

Descent is monitored and represented on the partogram in two ways: abdominally by the amount of head palpable, usually in fifths, and vaginally as the station, estimated in terms of the level of the lowest point of the presenting part in relation to the ischial spines.

Friedman[60] described progress in terms of the number of expulsive efforts the mother makes; more commonly, time alone is used as the criterion. The former is more physiologic, the latter is easier. If contractions are occurring with the usual frequency of three to four every 10 minutes, the two are the same. No robust clinical trials have been conducted concerning the optimal time for pushing, but traditional limits of 30 minutes for parous and 45 minutes for nulliparous women are reasonable. These times may seem a little short, but it should be remembered that if the woman has not delivered by this time, it can take a further 20 to 30 minutes to prepare for, and carry out, instrumental delivery. There is unlikely to be a problem if delivery occurs within this time but if longer limits are allowed, the extra time may be critical. Progress can be recorded on the partogram, and a second stage nomogram has been produced.[61]

Rotation

Rotation is determined by vaginal examination and palpation of the sutures and fontanels on the fetal head in relation to the maternal pelvis. Scalp edema (caput), which often develops with delay, may make this difficult.

Interventions

Augmentation of the Powers

As with the first stage, efficient powers are paramount. Uterine inertia is not uncommon at full dilation when epidural analgesia is used, due to the abolition of the reflex release of maternal oxytocin produced by the sensation of stretching of the introitus and perineum (Ferguson reflex). Intravenous oxytocin may be required to restore uterine activity.

Use of the mother's abdominal muscles to raise intra-abdominal pressure (Valsalva maneuver) is important. Efficient pushing requires education and encouragement, particularly when epidural analgesia has removed sensation.

Maternal Posture

An upright posture of the mother reduces both the duration of the second stage and the incidence of operative delivery.[62] There are also reductions in the use of episiotomy, perception of pain, and fetal heart rate abnormalities. Maternal posture does not appear to affect malposition. Avoidance of the supine position is beneficial for the acid-base status of the fetus in the second stage.[63]

Manual Rotation

Manual manipulation is an effective way to correct malrotation for those adept at its practice.

Instrumental Delivery

Instrumentation is used to shorten the second stage, either when prolonged or to avoid fetal or maternal complications. The ventouse and variations on its design permit primarily traction on the fetal head from a vacuum applied via a cup. The design of the cup usually produces scalp edema within the lip of the cup that adds to the effect of the vacuum alone. By directing the traction, flexion and rotation can be imparted to the head.

There is less perineal trauma compared with forceps and, therefore, ventouse has been recommended as the instrument of choice for delivery of the head when in an OA position. Cephalhematoma and intraocular hemorrhages have been associated with this instrument, but birth trauma, overall, is no higher than with other instruments.

Forceps are used for traction or rotation according to their design. Correct identification of the position of the fetal head is crucial to avoid trauma. Rotational forceps (Kielland's) can produce spiral tears of the vagina during rotation, an injury that is almost specific to the instrument.

Episiotomy

Episiotomy is surgical reduction of resistance offered by the pelvic floor. There is no benefit from routine episiotomy.[64] Mediolateral episiotomies direct any tearing away from the rectum and anus, resulting in fewer third-degree tears, but cause more bleeding than those in the midline. They also cause more discomfort in the puerperium.

CONCLUSIONS

Principles of good management of labor are summarized as follows:

- Prepare women for labor both physically and mentally and give support.
- Make the correct diagnosis of labor:
  - Only apply cervicogram limits to the active phase.
  - If in doubt, do *not* diagnose labor.
- Understand fetal monitoring.
- Understand interventions and their consequences.
- Agree on a policy:
  - Set policy according to best evidence.
  - Consistently apply policy.
  - Audit the results.

SUMMARY OF MANAGEMENT OPTIONS
Conduct of Normal Labor

Management Options	Quality of Evidence	Strength of Recommendation	References
Use of partogram helps to detect abnormality of labor and poor progress early and thus allow timely intervention.	III	B	36

Continued

SUMMARY OF MANAGEMENT OPTIONS
Conduct of Normal Labor *(Continued)*

Management Options	Quality of Evidence	Strength of Recommendation	References
Use of partogram with an agreed protocol for management reduces maternal morbidity and fetal morbidity and mortality rates.	IIb	B	65
The package of precise diagnosis of labor (active phase), early amniotomy, regular monitoring of cervical dilation rate, and correction with the empirical augmentation of uterine activity reduces the incidence of prolonged labor.	III	B	15
Compared to active management, a policy of no routine amniotomy and selective use of oxytocin does not adversely affect cesarean section rate or neonatal outcome.	Ia, Ib	A	46, 51, 52
Support in labor reduces operative delivery rate.	Ia	A	66

SUMMARY OF MANAGEMENT OPTIONS
Poor Progress in Labor

Management Options	Quality of Evidence	Strength of Recommendation	References
Poor progress in latent phase of first stage:			
Expectant management with careful watch of the fetal heart rate.	III	B	14, 40, 41
Augmentation may increase cesarean section rate.	III	B	14, 40, 41
Poor progress in active phase of first stage:			
Allowing 4 hours of grace after crossing alert line reduces need for augmentation and cesarean section.	Ib	A	53
Judicious augmentation with Syntocinon will reduce labor duration.	Ib	A	51
Studies favor 30-minute incremental intervals with oxytocin infusion.	Ib	A	48
Obstetric outcome is no better by use of intrauterine pressure catheters, compared with use of external tocography, for most cases.	Ib	A	19
Epidural analgesia is associated with prolongation of the first and second stages of labor, malposition, and increased operative vaginal delivery.	Ia	A	67
Poor progress in the second stage of labor:			
Flexibility in the duration of the second stage is permissible.	–	GPP	–
Upright posture of the mother reduces the duration of the second stage and need for operative delivery. It also reduces the need for episiotomy, perception of pain, and fetal heart rate abnormalities.	Ia	A	62
Use of episiotomy should be limited and selective.	Ia	A	64

REFERENCES

1. Rosen MG, Debanne SM, Thompson K: Arrest disorders and infant brain damage. Obstet Gynecol 1989;74(3 Pt 1):321–324.
2. Campbell EA: Plasma corticotrophin-releasing hormone concentrations during pregnancy and parturition. J Clin Endocrinol Metab 1987;64:1054–1059.
3. Schafer WR, Zahradnik HP: Programmed escalation: Models for the control of parturition. Geburtsh Frauenheilk 2001;61(4): 157–166.
4. Gee H: The cervix in labour. Contemp Rev Obstet Gynaecol 1994;6:84–88.

5. Garfield RE, Hayashi RH: Appearance of gap junctions in the myometrium of women during labor. Am J Obstet Gynecol 1981;140(3):254–260.
6. Arias F: Pharmacology of oxytocin and prostaglandins. Clin Obstet Gynecol 2000;43(3):455–468.
7. Nathanielsz PW, Jenkins SL, Tame JD, et al: Local paracrine effects of estradiol are central to parturition in the rhesus monkey. Nat Med 1998;4(4):456–459.
8. Challis JRG, Hooper S (eds): Birth: Outcome of a Positive Cascade. Baillier, 1989.
9. Myers DA, Nathanielsz PW: Biologic basis of term and preterm labor. Clin Perinatol 1993;20(1):9–28.
10. Pajntar M, Verdenik I, Pusenjak S, et al: Activity of smooth muscles in human cervix and uterus. Eur J Obstet Gynecol Reprod Biol 1998;79(2):199–204.
11. Friedman EA: The graphic analysis of labor. Am J Obstet Gynecol 1954;68:1568–1575.
12. Friedman EA: Primigravid labor. Obstet Gynecol 1955;6: 567–589.
13. Friedman EA: Labor in multiparas. Obstet Gynecol 1956;8(6): 691–703.
14. Cardozo LD, Gibb DM, Studd JW, et al: Predictive value of cervimetric labour patterns in primigravidae. BJOG 1982;89(1): 33–38.
15. O'Driscoll K, Jackson JA, Gallagher JT: Prevention of prolonged labour. BMJ 1969;2:447–480.
16. Gee H: The interaction between cervix and corpus uteri in the generation of intra-amniotic pressure in labour. Eur J Obstet Gynecol Reprod Biol 1983;16(4):243–252.
17. Gee H, Olah KS: Failure to progress in labour. In Studd J (ed): Progress in Obstetrics & Gynaecology. London, Blackwell, 1993, p 159–181.
18. Al-Shawaf T, Al-Moghvaby S, Akiel A: Normal levels of uterine activity in primigravidae and mothers of high parity in spontaneous labour. J Obstet Gynecol 1987;8:18–23.
19. Chua S, Kurup A, Arulkumaran S, Ratman SS: Augmentation of labour: Does internal tocography result in better obstetric outcome? Obstet Gynaecol 1990;76:164–167.
20. Gibb DMF, Arulkumaran S, Lun KC, Ratman SS: Characteristics of uterine activity in nulliparous labour. BJOG 1984;89:220–227.
21. Steer PJ, Little DJ, Lewis NL, Kelly MC, Beard RW: Uterine activity in induced labour. Br J Obstet Gynaecol 1975;82:433–441.
22. Krishnamurthy S, Fairlie F, Cameron AD, et al: The role of postnatal x-ray pelvimetry after caesarean section in the management of subsequent delivery. BJOG 1991;98(7): 716–718.
23. Ferguson JE 2nd, Newberry YG, De Angelis GA, et al: The fetal-pelvic index has minimal utility in predicting fetal-pelvic disproportion. Am J Obstet Gynecol 1998;179(5):1186–1192.
24. Granstrom L, Ekman G, Malmstrom A: Insufficient remodelling of the uterine conective tissue in women with protracted labour. BJOG 1991;98:1212–1216.
25. Gough GW, Randall NJ, Genevier ES, et al: Head-to-cervix forces and their relationship to the outcome of labor. Obstet Gynecol 1990;75(4):613–618.
26. Allman AC, Genevier ES, Johnson MR, Steer PJ: Head-to-cervix force: An important physiological variable in labour. 1. The temporal relation between head-to-cervix force and intrauterine pressure during labour. BJOG 1996;103(8):763–768.
27. Allman AC, Genevier ES, Johnson MR, Steer PJ: Head-to-cervix force: An important physiological variable in labour. 2. Peak active force, peak active pressure and mode of delivery. BJOG 1996;103(8):769–775.
28. Lurie S, Levy R, Ben-Arie A, Hagay Z: Shoulder dystocia: Could it be deduced from the labor? Am J Perinatol 1995;12(1):61–62.
29. Rooth G: Increase in birthweight: A unique biological event and an obstetrical problem. Eur J Obstet Gynecol Reprod Biol 2003;106(1):86–87.
30. Beazley JM: The active management of labor. Am J Obstet Gynecol 1975;122(2):161–168.
31. Duignan N: Active management of labour. In Studd J (ed): Active Management of Labour. Oxford, Blackwell, 1985, p 99.
32. World Health Organization partograph in management of labor. Lancet 1994;343(8910):1399–1404.
33. Zhang J, Troendle JF, Yancey MK: Reassessing the labor curve in nulliparous women. Am J Obstet Gynecol 2002;187:824–828.
34. Hendricks CH, Brenner WE, Kraus G: Normal cervical dilatation pattern in late pregnancy and labor. Am J Obstet Gynecol 1970;106:1065–1082.
35. Philpott RH, Castle WM: Cervicographs in the management of labour in primigravidae. I. The alert line for detecting abnormal labour. J Obstet Gynaecol Br Commonw 1972;79:592–598.
36. Philpott RH, Castle WM: Cervicographs in the management of labour in primigravidae. II. The action line and treatment of abnormal labour. J Obstet Gynaecol Br Commonw 1972;79: 599–602.
37. Beazley JM, Kurjak A: Influence of a partograph on the active management of labour. Lancet 1972;2(773):348–351.
38. Studd J: Partograms and nomograms of cervical dilatation in management of primigravid labour. BMJ 1973;4:451–455.
39. Friedman EA, Sachtleben MR: Dysfunctional labor. Obstet Gynecol 1961;17(2):135–148.
40. Friedman EA, Niswander KR, Sachtleben MR, Ashworth M: Dysfunctional labor. IX. Delivery outcome. Am J Obstet Gynecol 1970;106(2):219–226.
41. Chelmow D, Kilpatrick SJ, Laros RK: Maternal and neonatal outcomes after prolonged latent phase. Obstet Gynecol 1993;81: 486–491.
42. Friedman EA, Kroll BH: Computer analysis of labor progression. IV. Diagnosis of secondary arrest of dilatation. J Reprod Med 1971;7(4):176–178.
43. Davidson AC, Weaver JB, Davies P, Pearson JF: The relationship between ease of forceps delivery and speed of cervical dilatation. BJOG 1976;83:279–283.
44. Fraser WD, Marcoux S, Moutquin JM, Christen A: Effect of early amniotomy on the risk of dystocia in nulliparous women. The Canadian Early Amniotomy Study Group. N Engl J Med 1993;328(16):1145–1149.
45. Group UA: A multicentre randomised trial of amniotomy in spontaneous first labour at term. BJOG 1994;101: 307–309.
46. Fraser WD, Turcot L, Krauss I, Brisson-Carrol G: Amniotomy for shortening spontaneous labor. Cochrane Database Syst Rev 2000;(2):CD000015(4).
47. Kimura T, Takemura M, Nomura S, et al : Expression of oxytocin receptor in human pregnant myometrium. Endocrinology 1996;137:780–785.
48 Thornton JG, Lilford RJ: Active management of labour: Current knowledge and research issues. BMJ 1994;309:366–369.
49. Kiwanuka AI, Moore WMO: The changing incidence of caesarean section in the Health District of Central Manchester. BJOG 1987;94:440–444.
50. Lopez-Zeno JA, Peaceman AM, Adashek JA, Socol ML: A controlled trial of a program for the active management of labor. N Engl J Med 1992;326:450–454.
51. Frigoletto FDJ, Lieberman E, JML, et al : A clinical trial of active management of labor. N Engl J Med 1995;333:745–750.
52. Cammu H, Van Eeckhout E: A randomised controlled trial of early versus delayed use of amniotomy and oxytocin infusion in nulliparous labour. BJOG 1996;103:313–318.
53. Pattinson RC, Howarth GR, Mdluli W, et al: Aggressive or expectant management of labour: a randomised clinical trial. BJOG 2003;110:457–461.
54. Glantz JC, McNanley TJ: Active management of labor: A meta-analysis of cesarean delivery rates for dystocia in nulliparas. Obstet Gynecol Surv 1997;52:497–505.

55. Piquard F, Schaefer A, Hsiung R, et al: Are there two biological parts in the second stage of labor? Acta Obstet Gynecol Scand 1989;68(8):713–718.
56. Hagelin A, Leyon J: The effect of labor on the acid-base status of the newborn. Acta Obstet Gynecol Scand 1998;77(8): 841–844.
57. Nordstrom L, Achanna S, Naka K, Arulkumaran S: Fetal and maternal lactate increase during active second stage of labour. BJOG 2001;108:263–268.
58. Fitzpatrick M, Harkin R, McQuillan K, et al: A randomised clinical trial comparing the effects of delayed versus immediate pushing with epidural analgesia on mode of delivery and faecal continence. BJOG 2002;109:1359–1365.
59. Hansen SL, Clark SL, Foster JC: Active pushing versus passive fetal descent in the second stage of labor: A randomized controlled trial. Obstet Gynecol 2002;99:29–34.
60. Friedman EA, Sachtleben MR: Station of the fetal presenting part. V. Protracted descent patterns. Obstet Gynecol 1970;36(4): 558–567.
61. Sizer AR, Evans J, Bailey SM, Wiener J: A second-stage partogram. Obstet Gynecol 2000;96(5):678–683.
62. Gupta JK, Nikodem VC: Woman's position during second stage of labour. Cochrane Database Syst Rev 2000(4).
63. Johnstone FD, Aboelmagd MS, Harouny AK: Maternal posture in second stage and fetal acid base status. BJOG 1987;94(8): 753–757.
64. Carroli G, Belizan J: Episiotomy for vaginal birth. Cochrane Database Syst Rev 2000(4).
65 World Health Organization partograph in management of labour. Lancet 1994;343:1399–1404.
66. Hodnett ED: Caregiver support for women during childbirth. Cochrane Database Syst Rev 2001;(3)(update software).
67. Howell CJ: Cochrane Library, Issue 3. Oxford, Update Software, 2001.

CHAPTER 70

Shoulder Dystocia

Robert B. Gherman

INTRODUCTION

Despite its infrequent occurrence (0.2% – 3% of all deliveries[1]), all health care providers attending vaginal deliveries must be prepared to handle this unpredictable obstetric emergency. Shoulder dystocia represents the failure of delivery of the fetal shoulder(s), whether it be the anterior, posterior, or both fetal shoulders.[2] Shoulder dystocia results from a size discrepancy between the fetal shoulders and the pelvic inlet, which may be absolute or relative (due to malposition). A persistent anterior-posterior location of the fetal shoulders at the pelvic brim occurs when there is increased resistance between the fetal skin and vaginal walls (e.g., with macrosomia), with a large fetal chest relative to the biparietal diameter, and when truncal rotation does not occur (e.g., precipitous labor.)[3] Shoulder dystocia can also occur from impaction of the posterior fetal shoulder on the maternal sacral promontory.

DEFINITION

Most authors have defined this obstetric emergency to include those deliveries requiring maneuvers in addition to gentle downward traction on the fetal head to effect delivery. Several studies have proposed defining shoulder dystocia as a prolonged head-to-body delivery interval (60 sec) or the use of ancillary obstetric maneuvers, as this time represented the mean plus two standard deviations.[4,5]

MATERNAL AND FETAL RISKS

Postpartum hemorrhage and the unintentional extension of the episiotomy or laceration into the rectum (fourth-degree laceration) are the most common maternal complications associated with shoulder dystocia (Table 70–1). In Gherman's study, these occurred in 11% and 3.8%, respectively, of the described shoulder dystocias.[6] Other reported complications have included vaginal lacerations, cervical tears, bladder atony, and uterine rupture. Maternal symphyseal separation and lateral femoral cutaneous neuropathy have also been associated with overly aggressive hyperflexion of the maternal legs.[7] Risks to the physician mainly involve litigation, as brachial plexus palsy, central neurologic dysfunction, and perinatal death account for most of the shoulder dystocia-related lawsuits. A clearly documented medical record may prove to be helpful in the medicolegal arena.[8]

A large retrospective study that evaluated 285 cases of shoulder dystocia found that the fetal injury rate was 24.9%, including 48 (16.8%) brachial plexus palsies, 27 (9.5%) clavicular fractures, and 12 (4.2%) humeral fractures.[9] Unilateral brachial plexus injuries are probably the most common neurologic injury sustained by the neonate. The right arm is more commonly affected (64.6%) due to the fact that the left occiput anterior presentation leaves the right shoulder impinged against the symphysis pubis.[9] Brachial plexus injury has been found to complicate up to 21% of all shoulder dystocia cases.[10] Most (80%) of these nerve injuries have been located within the C5–C6 nerve roots (Erb-Duchenne palsy). Other types of brachial plexus injuries that have been described include Klumpke's palsy (C8–T1), an intermediate palsy, and complete palsy of the entire brachial plexus. Diaphragmatic paralysis, Horner's syndrome, and facial nerve injuries have been reported occasionally to accompany brachial plexus palsy.[3] Approximately one third of brachial plexus palsies will be associated with a concomitant bone fracture, most commonly the clavicle (94%).[8] Neonatal radial fracture can also be associated with the shoulder dystocia or the maneuvers employed to alleviate it.[11]

Gherman's study compared shoulder dystocia cases based on the absence or presence of direct fetal manipulative maneuvers (Woods', posterior arm extraction, or Zavanelli maneuvers). He found that the overall incidence of fetal bone fracture (16.5% vs. 11.4%, $p = 0.21$) and brachial plexus palsy (21.3% vs. 13.3%, $p = 0.1$) were

TABLE 70–1

Common Complications Associated with Shoulder Dystocia

MATERNAL	ACCOUCHEUR	NEONATAL
Third- or fourth-degree lacerations	Terror	Erb-Duchenne palsy
Postpartum hemorrhage	Medical liabilty	Klumpke's palsy Clavicular fracture Humeral fracture Hypoxia Permanent brain injury Death

not significantly different between the two groups.[9] Similar findings had previously been reported by Nocon, who grouped the techniques used to disimpact the shoulder into major treatment categories. None of the major categories revealed a statistically significant difference when compared with respect to fetal injury. In this study, the authors found incidences of injury of 14.9%, 14.3%, 37.9%, and 20%, respectively, associated with the McRoberts' maneuver, rotations, posterior arm delivery, and suprapubic pressure.[12]

PRENATAL: IDENTIFYING THE PREGNANCY AT RISK

It has been clearly shown that risk of shoulder dystocia increases significantly as birth weight increases. The percentages of births complicated by shoulder dystocia for unassisted births not complicated by diabetes were 5.2% for infants weighing 4000 to 4250 g, 9.1% for those 4250 to 4500 g, 14.3% for those 4500 to 4750 g, and 21.1% for those 4750 to 5000 g.[13] It must be remembered, however, that approximately 50% to 60% of shoulder dystocias occur in infants weighing less than 4000 g. Moreover, even if the birth weight of the infant is over 4000 g, shoulder dystocia will only complicate 3.3% of the deliveries.[14,15]

From a prospective point of view, prepregnancy and antepartum risk factors such as previous delivery of a macrosomic infant, preexisting or pregnancy-induced diabetes mellitus, multiparity, excessive maternal weight gain, and postdate gestation have exceedingly poor predictive value for the prediction of shoulder dystocia. For example, one study found that only 32% of patients were obese (>90 kg), 25% had excessive weight gain (>20 kg), 8% had short stature (<60 inches), 6% were more than 42 weeks' gestation, 3% were of advanced maternal age, and 2% had a personal history of diabetes mellitus.[16] In a case-control study from the Northern and Central Alberta Perinatal Outreach Program, maternal obesity (defined as >91 kg) was not associated with shoulder dystocia when multivariable logistic regression analysis was used to control for confounding effects.[17]

Ultrasonographic estimation of fetal weight, performed during either the late third trimester or the intrapartum period, has been commonly employed in order to estimate the risk of shoulder dystocia via prediction of birth weight. To date, however, no studies have specifically evaluated this relationship in a patient population where routine ultrasounds are performed. Late pregnancy ultrasound likewise displays low sensitivity (22% – 44%), poor positive predictive value (30% – 44%), decreasing accuracy with increasing birth weight, and an overall tendency to overestimate the birth weight. For this reason, the American College of Obstetricians and Gynecologists has recently noted that attempted vaginal delivery is not contraindicated for women with estimated fetal weights up to 5000 g in the absence of maternal diabetes.[18,19]

Patients with insulin-requiring diabetes mellitus appear to warrant special evaluation for shoulder dystocia. The risk of shoulder dystocia for unassisted births to diabetic mothers has been found to be 8.4%, 12.3%, 19.9%, and 23.5% when the birth weight is 4000 to 4250 g, 4250 to 4500 g, 4500 to 4750 g, or more than 4750 g, respectively.[13] These values are somewhat higher than for nondiabetics of similar build. Changes in fetal body configuration brought about by increased fat deposition in the fetuses of diabetic mothers, such as larger trunk and chest circumferences, increased bisacromial diameters, and chest-to-head disproportion, impede the rotation of the fetal shoulders into the oblique diameter.

In a similar fashion, patients with a history of shoulder dystocia complicating a prior vaginal delivery have a risk of recurrence, ranging between 11.9% and 16.7%. Maternal and fetal factors that have been shown to be significantly associated with recurrent shoulder dystocia include birth weight greater than the index pregnancy, duration of the second stage of labor, and birth weight more than 4000 g.[1] However, a policy of universal elective cesarean delivery has not been recommended for this cohort of patients because the risks outweigh the benefits.[19] Nonetheless, antepartum counseling and discussion of recurrence risks should be undertaken with consideration of the present estimate of fetal weight, the presence of maternal glucose intolerance, and whether the prior shoulder dystocia resulted in transient or permanent neurologic injury.

PRACTICAL MANAGEMENT OF SHOULDER DYSTOCIA (See Table 70–2)

The patient should be instructed to stop pushing after the shoulder dystocia is initially recognized. Maternal expulsive efforts, however, will need to be reinstituted after the fetal shoulders have been converted to the oblique diameter, in order to achieve delivery. If the provider is alone, additional assistance may be obtained by summoning other obstetricians, an anesthetist or anesthesiologist, additional nursing support, and a pediatrician.

Umbilical cord compression, most commonly between the fetal body and maternal pelvis, leads to a decrease in the fetal pH at a rate of 0.04 units per minute. If a nuchal cord is present and cannot be reduced easily over the fetal head, clamping and cutting of the cord should be avoided until the shoulder dystocia has been alleviated (Table 70–2).[20] Most, if not all, of the commonly encountered shoulder dystocia episodes can be relieved within several minutes. Although research studies have been unable to predict an exact time limit at which irreversible brain injury occurs, it is reasonable to assume that the risk of permanent central neurologic dysfunction is associated with prolongation of the head/shoulder interval thresholds. The length of delay that results in permanent brain injury will depend on the condition of the baby at the point at which the delivery is arrested. It may be as short as 4 to 5 minutes, or as long as 15 minutes.

At the time of delivery, if shoulder dystocia is a concern, some clinicians have empirically advocated proceeding immediately to delivery of the fetal shoulders, in order to maintain the forward momentum of the fetus. Others support a short delay in delivery of the shoulders, arguing that the endogenous rotational mechanics of the second stage may spontaneously alleviate the obstruction. Obstetricians may also employ the McRoberts' maneuver "prophylactically" in order to decrease the risk of shoulder dystocia or shorten the second stage of labor. One clinical trial randomized patients with estimated fetal weights over 3800 g to undergo either prophylactic maneuvers (McRoberts' maneuver and suprapubic pressure or to undergo maneuvers only after delivery of the fetal head, if shoulder dystocia was identified. This study, found that head-to-body delivery times, an indirect proxy for shoulder dystocia, did not differ between the prophylactic and control patients.[21]

Although many maneuvers have been described for the successful alleviation of shoulder dystocia, no randomized controlled trials or laboratory experiments have been conducted that directly compared these techniques. Most obstetricians currently employ the McRoberts' maneuver as their initial step for the disimpaction of the shoulder. In a retrospective review of 236 shoulder dystocia cases occurring between 1991 and 1994 at Los Angeles County/University of Southern California Medical Center, this maneuver alone alleviated 42% of cases. Moreover, trends toward lower rates of maternal and neonatal morbidity were associated with the McRoberts' maneuver.[6]

TABLE 70–2

Maneuvers for the Alleviation of Shoulder Dystocia

- Maternal hip hyperflexion (McRoberts' maneuver)
- Suprapubic pressure
- Rotational maneuvers:
  - Wood's maneuver
  - Rubin's maneuver
- Delivery of the posterior arm (Barnum maneuver)
- "All fours" (Gaskin maneuver)
- Cephalic replacement
  - Zavanelli
  - Modified Zavanelli
- Symphysiotomy
- Abdominal rescue through hysterotomy

The McRoberts' maneuver, performed by sharply flexing the maternal thighs onto the abdomen, results in a straightening of the maternal sacrum relative to the lumbar spine with consequent cephalic rotation of the symphysis pubis.[22] Care should be taken to avoid prolonged or overly aggressive application of the McRoberts' maneuver as the fibrocartilaginous articular surfaces of the symphysis pubis and surrounding ligaments may be unduly stretched.

The overwhelming majority of patients can assume the proper position for the McRoberts' maneuver with little difficulty. Women may be instructed to grasp the posterior aspect of their thighs and pull themselves into position, with family members or health care professionals providing any assistance necessary. The obstetrician may also choose to flex both of the patient's legs. Problems may occur when moving an obese patient or a woman who has undergone a dense epidural motor blockade.

Because shoulder dystocia is considered to be a "bony dystocia," episiotomy alone will not release the impacted shoulder. The need for cutting a generous episiotomy or proctoepisiotomy must be based on clinical circumstances, such as a narrow vaginal fourchette in a nulliparous patient. This may allow the fetal rotational maneuvers to be performed with ease, as well as creating more room for attempted delivery of the posterior arm. Attendants should refrain from applying fundal pressure as a maneuver for the alleviation of the shoulder dystocia. Pushing on the fundus simply duplicates a maternal directional expulsive force that has already failed to deliver the fetal shoulder(s) and serves only to further impact the anterior shoulder behind the symphysis pubis. In addition, the use of fundal pressure has been associated with an increased risk of Erb-Duchenne palsy and thoracic spinal cord injury in the neonate.[23]

Suprapubic pressure, commonly administered by nursing personnel, is typically used immediately prior to or in direct conjunction with the McRoberts' maneuver. This pressure is usually directed posteriorly, in an attempt to force the anterior shoulder under the symphysis pubis. Other described techniques for suprapubic pressure have included lateral application from either side of the maternal abdomen or alternating between sides using a rocking pressure.[24]

Many cases of shoulder dystocia require the performance of several maneuvers to alleviate the impaction. Stallings has found that slightly more than a third of patients required more than two maneuvers.[25] When more complex maneuvers are required, either fetal rotational maneuvers or posterior arm extraction may be employed. In the Woods' corkscrew maneuver, the practioner attempts to abduct the posterior shoulder by exerting pressure onto the anterior surface of the posterior shoulder. In the Rubin's (reverse Woods') maneuver, pressure is applied to the posterior surface of the most accessible part of the fetal shoulder (i.e., either the anterior or posterior shoulder) to effect shoulder adduction. These rotational maneuvers, however, may be difficult to perform when the anterior shoulder is tightly wedged underneath the symphysis pubis. It may therefore be necessary to push the fetus slightly upwards in order to facilitate the rotation.

By replacing the bisacromial diameter with the axilloacromial diameter, posterior arm delivery creates a 20% reduction in shoulder diameter.[26] To perform delivery of the posterior fetal arm, pressure should be applied by the accoucheur at the antecubital fossa in order to flex the fetal forearm. The arm is subsequently swept out over the infant's chest and delivered over the perineum. Rotation of the fetal trunk to bring the posterior arm anteriorly is sometimes required. Grasping and pulling directly on the fetal arm, as well as application of pressure onto the midhumeral shaft, should be avoided as bone fracture may occur.

The previously mentioned maneuvers are typically able to be attempted within 4 to 5 minutes after identification of the shoulder dystocia. If the shoulder dystocia remains uncorrected, a bilateral shoulder dystocia or posterior arm shoulder dystocia may be present. The latter is suggested by the presence of the posterior arm being maintained at the level of the pelvic inlet and an inability to perform posterior arm extraction. These intractable shoulder dystocias warrant the use of heroic techniques, such as the Zavanelli maneuver, symphysiotomy, or hysterotomy.

Performance of these will be complicated by the provider's lack of clinical experience with these maneuvers, performance under emergent conditions, and the significant maternal and neonatal complications inherent in the procedures. In the Zavanelli maneuver, the head is rotated back to a prerestitution position and then gently flexed. Constant firm pressure is used to push the head back into the vagina and cesarean delivery is subsequently performed. Halothane or other general anesthetics, in conjunction with tocolytic agents, may be administered in preparation for and during the Zavanelli maneuver. Oral or intravenous nitroglycerin may be used as well. A modification of the original Zavanelli maneuver may be employed in order potentially to reduce maternal morbidity. As described by Zelig, maternal expulsive efforts were reinitiated after the obstetrician had observed that the biparietal diameter had passed back through the introitus and the shoulders were felt to disimpact.[27] This modification should only be attempted as long as there is no evidence of fetal compromise.

To perform a symphysiotomy, the patient should be placed in an exaggerated lithotomy position. Although its placement may be very difficult secondary to obstruction, a Foley catheter can help to identify the urethra. With the physician's index and middle finger displacing the urethra laterally, the cephalad portion of the symphysis is incised with a scalpel blade or Kelly clamp. The reader is also referred to Chapter 64 (Breech) for further description and discussion of symphysiotomy. Hysterotomy may also be performed to either resolve the shoulder dystocia primarily or assist with vaginal techniques. The abdominal surgeon can apply pressure on the anterior fetal shoulder to allow rotation to the oblique diameter. The posterior fetal arm may be manipulated through the transverse uterine incision with passage of the hand to a vaginal assistant.

Prior to performing these techniques, one may consider using the "all-fours" technique, in which the patient is rolled from her existing position onto her hands and knees.[28] The downward force of gravity or a favorable change in pelvic diameters produced by this maneuver may allow disimpaction of the fetal shoulder. Older textbooks have described deliberate clavicular fracture as a maneuver of last resort, performed by exerting direct upward pressure on the midportion of the fetal clavicle. However, this has not been reported in the recent literature because it is technically difficult to perform and risks serious injury to the underlying vascular and pulmonary structures in the fetus.

SHOULDER DYSTOCIA AND BRACHIAL PLEXUS INJURY

Brachial plexus palsy is currently a major cause of litigation, constituting 11% of the 370 obstetric claims closed by the Norwegian patient insurance system from 1988 to 1997.[29] In the past, textbooks have stated without evidence that brachial plexus palsy is caused by the accoucheur's application of excessive lateral traction on the fetal head and neck during attempts at alleviating the shoulder dystocia. Over the past several

TABLE 70–3

Suggested Medicolegal Documentation for Shoulder Dystocia

When and how dystocia was diagnosed
Progress of labor (active phase and second stage)
Position and rotation of the infant's head
Presence of episiotomy, if performed
Anesthesia required
Estimation of force of traction applied
Order, duration, and results of maneuvers employed
Duration of shoulder dystocia
Documentation of adequate pelvimetry prior to initiating labor induction or augmentation
Neonatal and obstetric impressions of the infant after delivery
Inform gravida that shoulder dystocia had occurred

From Acker DB: A shoulder dystocia intervention form. Obstet Gynecol 1991;78:150–151.

years, multiple lines of evidence have supported the concept that most brachial plexus palsies are not caused by the accoucheur.[3,30–31] This opinion is based on several findings:

- More than 50% of cases of brachial plexus injuries are associated with uncomplicated vaginal deliveries[32,33]
- Brachial plexus palsy can occur in the posterior arm of infants whose anterior arm was impacted behind the symphysis pubis and can also occur with a traumatic cesarean delivery
- There is no statistical correlation with the experience of the obstetric provider nor the number or type of maneuvers used
- Rapid second-stage and disproportionate descent of the head and body of the fetus have been implicated in the pathogenesis of the injury
- Mathematical and computer-simulated models have shown that maternal endogenous forces are far greater than clinician-applied exogenous delivery loads during a shoulder dystocia episode.[34,35]

Despite these observations it is good and prudent practice for obstetricians to make a detailed and accurate account of the procedure when they have managed a case of shoulder dystocia. This should be undertaken as close to the event as possible. Table 70–3 gives a suggested list of items that may be covered in such a report.

CONCLUSIONS

- Knowledge of the maneuvers employed for the alleviation of shoulder dystocia is relevant not only for obstetric residents and attending house staff, but also for family practitioners, nurses, and nurse midwives.
- The performance of shoulder dystocia "drills" can be helpful not only to coordinate a teamwork approach to this obstetric emergency but also to provide an opportunity to practice the maneuvers.
- Shoulder dystocia continues to represent an immense area of clinical interest, due to the fact that it typically occurs unexpectedly.
- All patients in labor should therefore be considered at risk for the development of shoulder dystocia.
- Brachial plexus palsy results from the significant endogenous forces associated with shoulder dystocia; it is not caused by iatrogenic excessive traction, but by an asymmetrical distribution of traction or propulsion forces acting on the fetus.[1,30,36]

SUMMARY OF MANAGEMENT OPTIONS
Shoulder Dystocia

Management Options	Quality of Evidence	Strength of Recommendation	References
Prenatal Identification of At-Risk Pregnancy			
Estimation of fetal weight and risk of SD is of limited value.	III	B	13,14
May be of more use in diabetic pregnancies or those with previous SD.	IIb	B	15
Limited accuracy of ultrasound in estimating fetal weight	III	B	39
ACOG Guidelines:	IV	C	18,19
Vaginal delivery is reasonable with estimated fetal weights up to 5 kg in the absence of diabetes because risks of elective cesarean section			
Despite this guideline women with previous delivery complicated by SD may prefer to have elective cesarean section, especially if estimated fetal weight similar or greater than previously	–	GPP	–
The following are poor predictors of SD: Previous macrosomia/large-for-dates Diabetes (preexisting or gestational) Multiparity Excessive weight gain in pregnancy Postdates pregnancy	IIa	B	16,17
If vaginal delivery is to be attempted following a discussion with an at-risk patient, make a clear record in the patient's notes	–	GPP	–

Continued

SUMMARY OF MANAGEMENT OPTIONS

Shoulder Dystocia *(Continued)*

Management Options	Quality of Evidence	Strength of Recommendation	References
Practical Management of Shoulder Dystocia (See Table 70–2)			
No RCT data covering any aspect of SD management	–	–	–
No evidence that "prophylactic" McRoberts' and suprapubic pressure prevents SD in at-risk cases (i.e., before SD has developed/been recognized)	Ib	A	21
Stop maternal efforts temporarily until SD overcome.	–	GPP	–
Summon help (obstetric, anesthetic, nursing/midwifery, pediatric).	–	GPP	–
Avoid clamping and cutting a nuchal cord until SD overcome.	IV	C	20
McRoberts' maneuver	III	B	6
Suprapubic pressure	IV	C	24
No evidence that episiotomy makes a difference though often advised.	–	GPP	–
Avoid fundal pressure as it increases risk of Erb's palsy and thoracic spine injury.	IV	C	23
Rotational maneuver (Wood or Rubin)	III	B	9
Delivery of posterior arm (Barnum)	III	B	9
Put woman into "all fours" position.	III	B	28
Zavanelli maneuver	III	B	9
Symphysiotomy	IV	C	38
Hysterotomy and abdominal correction	IV	C	37
Make a detailed record as soon as possible after the event (see Table 70–3).	–	GPP	–

ACOG, American College of Obstetricians and Gynecologists; RCT, randomized clinical trial; SD, shoulder dystocia.

REFERENCES

1. Gherman RB: Shoulder dystocia: An evidence-based evaluation of the obstetric nightmare. Clin Obstet Gynecol 2002;45:345–362.
2. Collins JH, Collins CL: What is shoulder dystocia? J Reprod Med 2001;46:148–149.
3. Gherman RB, Ouzounian JG, Goodwin TM: Brachial plexus palsy: An in utero injury? Am J Obstet Gynecol 1999;180: 1303–1307.
4. Spong CY, Beall M, Rodrigues D, et al: An objective definition of shoulder dystocia: Prolonged head-to-body delivery intervals and/or the use of ancillary obstetric maneuvers. Obstet Gynecol 1995;86:433–436.
5. Beall MH, Spong C, McKay J, et al: Objective definition of shoulder dystocia: A prospective evaluation. Am J Obstet Gynecol 1998;179:934–937.
6. Gherman RB, Goodwin TM, Souter I, et al: The McRoberts' maneuver for the alleviation of shoulder dystocia: How successful is it? Am J Obstet Gynecol 1997;176:656–661.
7. Gherman RB, Ouzounian JG, Incerpi MH, et al: Symphyseal separation and transient femoral neuropathy associated with the McRoberts' maneuver. Am J Obstet Gynecol 1998;178:609–610.
8. Acker DB: A shoulder dystocia intervention form. Obstet Gynecol 1991;78:150–151.
9. Gherman RB, Ouzounian JG, Goodwin TM: Obstetrical maneuvers for shoulder dystocia and associated fetal morbidity. Am J Obstet Gynecol 1998;178:1126–1130.
10. Gherman RB, Ouzounian JG, Satin AJ, et al: A comparison of shoulder dystocia-associated transient and permanent brachial plexus palsies. Obstet Gynecol 2003;102:544–548.
11. Thompson KA, Satin AJ, Gherman RB: Spiral fracture of the radius: An unusual case of shoulder dystocia-associated morbidity. Obstet Gynecol 2003;102:36–38.
12. Nocon JJ, McKenzie DK, Thomas LJ, et al: Shoulder dystocia: An analysis of risks and obstetric maneuvers. Am J Obstet Gynecol 1993;168:1732–1739.
13. Nesbitt TS, Gilbert WM, Herrchen B: Shoulder dystocia and associated risk factors with macrosomic infants born in California. Am J Obstet Gynecol 1998;179:476–480.
14. Acker DB, Sachs BP, Friedman EA: Risk factors for shoulder dystocia. Obstet Gynecol 1985;66:762–768.
15. Geary M, McParland P, Johnson H, et al: Shoulder dystocia: Is it predictable? Eur J Obstet Gynecol Reprod Biol 1995;62:15–18.
16. Lewis DF, Edwards MS, Asrat T, et al: Can shoulder dystocia be predicted? Preconceptive and prenatal factors. J Reprod Med 1998;43:654–658.
17. Robinson H, Tkatch S, Mayes DC, et al: Is maternal obesity a predictor of shoulder dystocia? Obstet Gynecol 2003;101; 24–27.
18. American College of Obstetricians and Gynecologists: Fetal Macrosomia. Washington, DC: ACOG, 2000 Practice Bulletin No. 22.
19. American College of Obstetricians and Gynecologists: Shoulder Dystocia. Washington, DC: ACOG, 2002 Practice Bulletin No. 40.
20. Flamm BL: Tight nuchal cord and shoulder dystocia: A potentially catastrophic combination. Obstet Gyncol 1999;94:853.

21. Beall MH, Spong CY, Ross MG: A randomized controlled trial of prophylactic maneuvers to reduce head-to-body time in patients at risk for shoulder dystocia. Obstet Gynecol 2003;102:31–35.
22. Gherman RB, Tramont J, Muffley P, et al: Analysis of McRoberts' maneuver by X-ray pelvimetry. Obstet Gynecol 2000;95:43–47.
23. Hankins GDV: Lower thoracic spinal cord injury: A severe complication of shoulder dystocia. Am J Perinatol 1998;15:443–444.
24. Penney DS, Perlis DW: Shoulder dystocia: When to use suprapubic or fundal pressure. MCN 1992;17:34–36.
25. Stallings SP, Edwards RK, Johnson JWC: Correlation of head-to-body delivery intervals in shoulder dystocia and umbilical artery acidosis. Am J Obstet Gynecol 2001;185:268–274.
26. Poggi SH, Spong CY, Allen RH: Prioritizing posterior arm delivery during severe shoulder dystocia. Obstet Gynecol 2003;101:1068–1072.
27. Zelig CM, Gherman RB: Modified Zavanelli maneuver for the alleviation of shoulder dystocia. Obstet Gynecol 2002;100: 1112–1114.
28. Bruner JP, Drummond SB, Meenan AL, et al: All-fours maneuver for reducing shoulder dystocia during labor. J Reprod Med 1998;43:439–443.
29. Skolbekken JA: Shoulder dystocia: Malpractice or acceptable risk? Acta Obstet Gynecol Scand 2000;79:750–756.
30. Sandmire HF, DeMott RK: Erb's palsy: Concepts of causation. Obstet Gynecol 2000;95:941–942.
31. Sandmire HF, DeMott RK: Erb's palsy causation: A historical perspective. Birth 2002;29:152–154.
32. Gherman RB, Ouzounian JG, Miller DA, et al: Spontaneous vaginal delivery: A risk factor for Erb's palsy? Am J Obstet Gynecol 1998;178:423–427.
33. Sandmire HF, DeMott RK: Erb's palsy without shoulder dystocia. Int J Gynaecol Obstet 2002;78:253–256.
34. Gonik B, Zhang N, Grimm MJ: Defining forces that are associated with shoulder dystocia: The use of a mathematic dynamic computer model. Am J Obstet Gynecol 203;188:1068–1072.
35. Gonik B, Walker A, Grimm M: Mathematic modeling of forces associated with shoulder dystocia: A comparison of endogenous and exogenous sources. Am J Obstet Gynecol 200;182:689–691.
36. Gonik B, Zhang N, Grimm MJ: Prediction of brachial plexus stretching during shoulder dystocia using a computer simulation model. Am J Obstet Gynecol 2003;189:1168–1172.
37. O'Leary JA, Cuva A: Abdominal rescue after failed cephalic replacement. Obstet Gynecol 1992;80:514–516.
38. Goodwin TM, Banks E, Millar LK, Phelan JP: Catastrophic shoulder dystocia and emergency symphysiotomy. Am J Obstet Gynecol 1997;177:463–464.
39. Ben-Haroush A, Yogev Y, Bar J, et al: Accuracy of sonographically estimated fetal weight in 840 women with different pregnancy complications prior to induction of labor. Obstet Gynecol 2004;23:172–176.

CHAPTER 71

Fetal Distress in Labor

Philip J. Steer / Peter Danielian

WHAT IS FETAL DISTRESS?

Fetal distress is a term that is commonly used, but difficult to define. It is probably best taken to mean "an absence of fetal well-being," in a similar way that the expression "a flat baby" means a neonate in need of resuscitation and "an ill person" means someone who is unwell. Thus, its use encompasses many different pathologies affecting the fetus, such as chronic hypoxia leading to a metabolic acidosis, mechanical trauma (e.g., excessive head compression), hyperthermia, meconium aspiration, and sepsis. Hypoxia with acidosis (often referred to as "asphyxia," although originally the term simply meant born without an evident pulse, from the Greek *a-sphyxos*) is widely perceived to be the most important cause, but does not have a simple relationship with the condition of the baby at birth. Beard[1] pointed out as early as 1967 that the Apgar score (a clinical measure of condition at birth) "does not differentiate between asphyxial and non-asphyxial depression of the newborn." In 1982 Sykes and colleagues[2] reported that only 27% of babies with a severe acidosis (umbilical artery pH <7.1 and a base deficit > 12 mmol/L) had a 1-minute Apgar score <7. Similarly, only 21% with a 1-minute Apgar score <7 had a severe acidosis. Lissauer and Steer[3] subsequently noted that more than half of babies born at 32 weeks' gestation or later, and needing resuscitation by intubation and positive pressure ventilation, had either entirely normal fetal heart rate (FHR) patterns throughout labor or normal values for umbilical cord blood pH measurement. In their study, the nonasphyxial associations with depression at birth included operative delivery, anesthetic agents given to the mother, meconium-stained liquor, and tight nuchal cord. Steer and associates[4] subsequently reported that acidosis in the fetus (as measured by cord umbilical artery pH) only accounted for 7.5% of the variation in the 1-minute Apgar score, and 1.8% of the variation in the 5-minute Apgar score. Thorp and colleagues[5] reported that umbilical artery cord pH was normal in 80% of clinically depressed newborns. Chorioamnionitis has in recent years been recognized as an important antecedent of cerebral palsy,[6] but it is not directly associated with asphyxia. Maberry and associates[7] reported that chorioamnionitis does not increase the likelihood of metabolic acidosis at birth; there were no babies with a significant metabolic acidosis or pH <7.0 in 123 cases of confirmed intra-amniotic infection during labor. Instead, the brain damage that later manifests as cerebral palsy may be caused by cytokine release. Nonetheless, chorioamnionitis, or even noninfective fever during labor (see Chapter 72) may potentiate the damaging effects of hypoxia-ischemia on the brain by increasing its metabolic requirements for oxygen.[8]

What Constitutes "Birth Asphyxia"?

Saling's initial publication[9] reported on 306 babies born in vigorous condition and reported their mean capillary fetal blood sample (FBS) pH to be 7.33 with a range (± two standard deviations) of 7.2 to 7.5. An FBS pH of 7.2 subsequently became a widely accepted lower limit of normal, below which values were taken to indicate the need for urgent delivery. However, it has become appreciated over the last 15 years that acidosis has to be very severe (values well below 2 standard deviations from the mean) before it is associated with long-term sequelae. For example, Winkler and colleagues[10] reported that none of 335 infants born with an umbilical artery pH <7.2 but >7.0 had any neonatal complications, and only two of 23 born with a pH <7.0 had any complications attributable to asphyxia. Goodwin and associates[11] reviewed 129 full-term, normally formed, singleton infants born with an umbilical artery pH <7.0 and found that 78% were entirely normal at follow-up, with only 8% having a major neurologic defect. Nagel and colleagues[12] reported 30 newborns with an umbilical artery pH <7.0. All but three had an Apgar score of 6 or more at 5 minutes. In the neonatal period, two babies died, five had mild and two severe encephalopathy. Using the Denver Developmental Screening Test at ages ranging from 14 to 33 months, 23 surviving babies were normal, 2 questionable, and none had major abnormalities (31 lost to follow-up). However, these reports should not be taken as meaning that acidosis is always benign. Severe acidosis (pH <7.0) is still likely to be associated with a much higher incidence of depression at birth than a pH >7.2. Van den Berg and colleagues[13] reviewed the neonatal complications of 84 nonanomalous babies with an umbilical artery pH <7.0 and compared them with a nonacidotic (pH >7.24) matched control group. They found highly significant differences in the proportions of babies requiring intubation (29% cf. 2.4%), and having pulmonary (31% cf. 11%), cardiovascular (15% cf. 8%), and neurologic (23% cf. 7%) complications. Low and associates[14] studied the effect of metabolic acidosis on newborn complications at 10 days of life. Fifty-nine babies had a severe metabolic acidosis (umbilical artery buffer base <30 mmol/L) and were six times more likely to have complications than a control group without acidosis (85% cf. 14%). Neonatal encephalopathy was observed in 61% of the acidotic group cf. 17% of the control group. Socol and colleagues[15] studied 28 newborns with an Apgar score of ≤3 at 5 minutes. They found that 11 of 17 neonates with an umbilical cord arterial pH >7.0 had an uncomplicated neonatal course compared with only 1 of 11 with a pH <7.0. Low's group have subsequently studied the threshold of fetal metabolic acidosis at delivery above which moderate or severe newborn complications may be expected; they found this to be an umbilical artery base deficit of 12 mmol/L.[16] Thereafter, increasing metabolic acidosis is associated with a progression of severity of newborn complications.

On the basis of these findings, it seems reasonable to categorize asphyxia as a cord artery pH <7.0 and a base deficit >12 mMol/L. However, because the large majority of babies with asphyxia by this definition have a normal long-term outcome, it has been suggested that the term *birth asphyxia* should be used to indicate an even more severe situation in which, in addition to acidosis, generalized neonatal dysfunction is evident. Thus, Thorp[17] suggested the inclusion of neonatal depression as measured by the Apgar score, as well as evidence of hypoxic end organ damage such as early neonatal seizures and renal or cardiac dysfunction. Subsequently, the American College of Obstetricians and Gynecologists recommended that birth asphyxia be regarded as resulting from "intrapartum hypoxia sufficient to cause neurological damage," defined by an umbilical artery pH <7.0, a 5-minute Apgar score ≤3, moderate or severe neonatal encephalopathy, and evidence of multiorgan dysfunction (affecting the cardiovascular, renal, and/or pulmonary systems)[18] (Table 71–1). Few depressed neonates fulfill these stringent conditions.[19]

Do Intrapartum Events Lead to Cerebral Palsy?

It is clear that the majority of mental handicap is not caused by intrapartum events. In 1985, the U.S. National Institutes of Health reported that "the causes of severe mental retardation are primarily genetic, biochemical, viral and developmental, and not related to birth events. Associated factors include maternal lifestyle, such as poor nutrition, cigarette smoking, and alcohol and drug abuse."[20] For example, the single most prevalent cause of mental retardation is Down syndrome. However, some forms of mental handicap are likely to be the consequence of birth asphyxia and other adverse intrapartum events. The International Cerebral Palsy Task Force suggested that birth asphyxia was a significant cause of cerebral palsy characterized by nonprogressive abnormal control of movement or posture.[21] The percentage of such cases caused by birth asphyxia remains controversial. It is widely accepted that at least some acute intrapartum events (e.g., placental abruption, cord prolapse) can cause brain injury in previously normal fetuses. In a recent review of 351 babies investigated by MRI or at postmortem, Cowan and colleagues showed that more than 90% of full-term infants with neonatal encephalopathy, seizures, or both, but without specific syndromes or major congenital defects, had evidence of perinatally acquired insults, and in only a few babies was there any evidence of established brain injury acquired before birth.[22] Their data do not exclude the possibility that antenatal factors could initiate a causal pathway for perinatal brain injury and that they might, possibly together with genetic predispositions to hypoxic-ischemic injury, make some infants more susceptible than others to the stresses of labor and delivery. However, although their study was not population-based, it strongly suggests that the potential for avoiding intrapartum brain damage by improved management is substantial. The Western Australia case–control study of neonatal encephalopathy[23] (which was population-based) clearly showed a protective effect of elective cesarean section (adjusted odds ratio [OR] 0.17, 95% confidence

TABLE 71–1

ACOG Definition of Birth Asphyxia, 1991

Intrapartum hypoxia sufficient to cause neurologic damage
Umbilical artery pH <7.00
5-minute Apgar score ≤3
Moderate or severe neonatal encephalopathy
Multiorgan dysfunction (e.g., CVS, renal, pulmonary)

CVS, cardiovascular system.
From ACOG: Utility of umbilical cord blood acid-base measurement. ACOG Committee Opinion 1991;91:33–34.

interval [CI] 0.05–0.56). This demonstrates that intrapartum events play a role in the etiology of neonatal encephalopathy. The question of the proportion of babies with brain injury but no evidence of chromosomal anomaly or congenital anomaly that are due to intrapartum events has been addressed recently by Johnston,[24] who concluded that it was between 30% and 60%, depending on the setting and the efficiency of intrapartum surveillance and the risk status of the population. When addressing the likelihood of perinatal events as a cause of cerebral palsy, the criteria of Nelson can be recommended (Table 71–2).

MANAGEMENT ISSUES

Diagnosis of Fetal Distress

Diagnosis is difficult because of the problems of accessing the fetus in utero. Before the introduction of the Pinard stethoscope, the condition of the fetus remained unknown until the moment of birth. However, once the FHR could be detected with some reliability, it was discovered that both persistent fetal tachycardia and bradycardia were associated with an increased likelihood of poor condition at birth, and that meconium staining of the amniotic fluid could also be an adverse sign. Once continuous electronic fetal monitoring (EFM) was introduced in the 1960s, it was possible to detect reduced FHR variability, which is also associated with an increased risk of depression at birth. The introduction of fetal blood sampling and pH estimation by Saling[9] allowed further assessment of fetal condition. Unfortunately, fetal blood sampling is a complicated and time-consuming technique, which is uncomfortable for the mother. As a result, the approach that developed was to use EFM as a screening tool for asphyxia, and then use fetal blood sampling to confirm or reject the diagnosis. Beard and associates, in their landmark paper of 1971,[25] showed that a normal FHR pattern is associated with a very low risk of acidosis (<2% of fetuses with a normal FHR pattern will have a pH <7.2). However, although increasing abnormality of the FHR is associated with an increasing chance that the fetus is acidotic, even with the most abnormal pattern (a complicated baseline tachycardia), the risk of acidosis is only about 60% (Fig. 71–1). This explains the increased intervention rates for the diagnosis of fetal distress if FHR monitoring is used without the backup of FBS and pH estimation.[26,27] Reviews indicate that the use of FBS and pH measurement not only limits the increase in operative delivery rate seen with EFM, but also improves its ability to reduce the neonatal seizure rate.[28]

Most studies of EFM have examined the relationship between the heart rate pattern and asphyxia. Cardiotocogram (CTG) interpretation can, however, also indicate other pathologies, such as pyrexia (and therefore indirectly, sepsis), which is associated with a fetal tachycardia.[29] Recurrent variable decelerations with a maintained normal FBS pH suggest intermittent cord compression. Repeated umbilical cord compression may cause brain damage without asphyxia because of the major swings in blood pressure induced by repeated occlusion and release.[30] The damage may be exacerbated by nuchal entanglement (cord around the neck) because occlusion of the venous return from the brain increases intracranial pressure. Damage to the hippocampus from intermittent occlusion of the cord has been seen in fetal sheep.[31]

Does Electronic Fetal Monitoring Improve Outcome?

The widespread introduction of EFM in the 1970s was associated with substantial falls in perinatal mortality as reported by a number of retrospective observational

TABLE 71–2

Criteria To Be Fulfilled before Long-term Outcome Can Be Linked with Intrapartum Events

1. Was there evidence of severe, prolonged intrapartum dysfunction?
2. Was the child severely ill as a newborn? Were there disturbances of feeding, tone, and consciousness, and evidence of involvement of other organ systems, of which renal involvement may be especially significant?
3. Is cerebral palsy present?
4. Have other potential explanations been excluded, such as the following:
   - Congenital malformation
   - Infection
   - Metabolic abnormality
   - Familial disease
   - Microcephaly in the neonatal period
   - Abnormal CT or MRI scan suggesting discrete lesions
   - Maternal substance abuse (especially cocaine)
   - Thyroid disease

CT- computed tomography; MRI- magnetic resonance imaging.
From Nelson K: Perspective on the role of perinatal asphyxia in neurologic outcome. CMAJ 1998 (suppl).

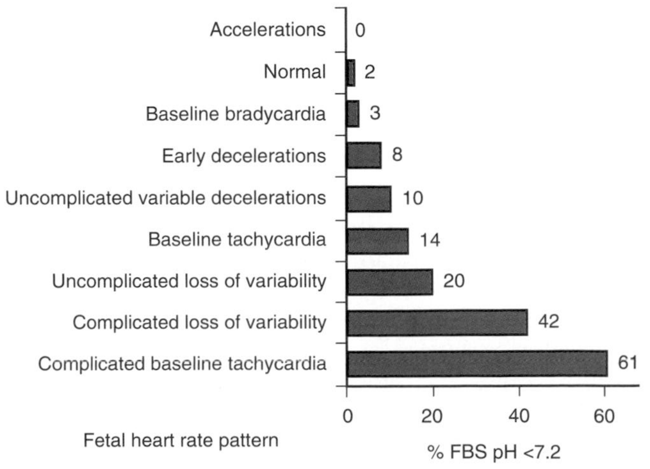

FIGURE 71–1
Fetal heart rate pattern and the associated risk of acidosis.

studies.[32,33] However, during the same period, major advances were being made in neonatal intensive care, and the cesarean section rate also rose substantially. It has proved impossible to establish which of these changes, if any, were responsible for the improvement in outcome. This uncertainty led to calls for prospective randomized controlled trials. None of these trials were, on their own, large enough to have sufficient power to address the long-term outcome of most interest, namely cerebral palsy. Accordingly, there have been a series of meta-analyses, although these are dominated by the effect of the single largest trial, carried out in Dublin in the early 1980s.[34] Vintzileos and associates[26] reviewed nine, including in total 18,561 patients (of which 12,964 were in the Dublin trial). This confirmed a substantial increase in the cesarean section rate associated with EFM (OR 1.53, 95% CI 1.17–2.01) but disappointingly for the advocates of EFM, the reduction in the overall perinatal mortality rate was not significant (4.2/1000 in the EFM group cf. 4.9/1000 in the intermittent auscultation (IA) group). However, in a post hoc analysis, Vintzileos and associates commented that there was a significant reduction in the deaths attributed to hypoxia in the EFM groups, being 0.7/1000 compared with 1.8/1000 in the auscultation group (OR 0.41, 95% CI 0.17–0.98). A similar meta-analysis was performed by Thacker and colleageus[27] with the inclusion of three further studies but with similar conclusions, except that they reported a significant reduction in the incidence of neonatal seizures in the group where EFM had been used (relative risk [RR] 0.5, 95% CI 0.30–0.82). Thus, the studies suggest some improvement in short-term outcome at the expense of an increased operative delivery rate, but were unable to address the issue of long-term outcome (a follow-up study of the Dublin trial showed that three babies in each group developed cerebral palsy[35]; however, even if the number had been doubled in the auscultation group, this would still not have been statistically significant). It should be noted that many authorities, including the National Institute for Clinical Excellence (NICE) in the United Kingdom, state in relation to the meta-analyses that "there was no apparent difference in perinatal death rates between the two groups."[36] This is not actually correct, as most studies show a difference in favor of EFM, which is not, however, statistically significant. As already pointed out, even the meta-analyses are underpowered to address the question of perinatal mortality, let alone long-term outcome. It should always be remembered that absence of evidence is not evidence of absence, and one needs to be aware of the possibility of a type II error (i.e., there is a difference which by chance has not been found to be significant).

Fetal Heart Rate Monitoring and Fetal Blood Sampling

It will be appreciated from the previous discussion that monitoring the heart rate of the fetus should not be expected to detect all pathologies affecting the fetus during labor. For example, maternal intrapartum cardiac arrest, fetal skull fracture with brain infarct, intrapartum fetal stroke, and uterine rupture have been reported as causes of subsequent childhood handicap,[37] but none of these can be predicted reliably beforehand by FHR monitoring (in a recent study of 36 cases of intrapartum rupture of a previous cesarean section scar,[38] no significant differences were noted in rates of mild or severe variable decelerations, late decelerations, prolonged decelerations, fetal tachycardia, or loss of uterine tone. Fetal bradycardia in the first and second stage was the only finding consistently associated with uterine rupture). Equally, although intrapartum infection and meconium aspiration may be associated with fetal tachycardia, neither are consistently associated with acidosis[4,39]; therefore a normal FBS pH may be actively misleading in their management if a normal value is taken as reassurance about fetal condition. Nevertheless, hypoxia and acidosis pose a significant threat to the fetus during labor (accounting for perhaps 20–40% of poor condition at birth), and FHR monitoring remains the best available screening tool for its detection. The best way to detect developing acidosis in the fetus is to measure its pH on an FBS. Clues about other pathologies (e.g., variable decelerations with nuchal cord, FHR tachycardia with infection, sinusoidal variability with fetal anemia) can be obtained from EFM, but its use in these conditions should not be regarded as sensitive or specific.

Human Factors in the Use of Cardiotocography

A human element may factor into our inability to demonstrate that the use of EFM produces an improved outcome to the degree anticipated by the pioneers of the technique. For example, in the Dublin trial, the fetal monitors used were of a relatively primitive design, staff were previously unfamiliar with their use, and during the trial a marked Hawthorne effect was evident, which would have reduced its apparent efficacy. In a later case–control study, the intrapartum treatment of 38 babies severely asphyxiated at birth was compared with 120 controls.[40] In the control group, 29% of babies had an abnormal intrapartum FHR tracing, but in only 9% was the abnormality severe. In contrast, in the babies asphyxiated at birth, 87% had an abnormal FHR tracing, and in 61% of cases the abnormality was severe. The most striking finding, however, was the length of time required for the staff to recognize the FHR abnormality. With moderate abnormalities, the mean time to recognition was 71 minutes, and paradoxically, with severe abnormalities it was 118 minutes. The authors could give no plausible reason why the standard of FHR tracing interpretation was so poor. However, it was clear from this study that if the quality of interpretation of the intrapartum FHR pattern had been higher, the benefits from

EFM would almost certainly have been significantly and substantially enhanced.

In 1990, Ennis and Vincent published the results of their study of 64 cases of poor perinatal outcome from the archives of the Medical Protection Society.[41] In 11 cases, although indicated, continuous EFM was not performed. In six cases, the technical quality of the tracing was inadequate. In 14 cases, a significant abnormality in the FHR pattern was present, but this was either not noticed, or no action was taken upon it. In only 14 cases was appropriate monitoring and action performed (the CTG was missing in 19 cases). In only 16 cases was a consultant involved in the interpretation of the tracing. In a further study from Oxford published in 1994,[19] intrapartum care was assessed in 141 cases of cerebral palsy and 62 perinatal deaths with a potential intrapartum cause. They found that abnormal FHR patterns were 2.3 times as common in babies who went on to develop cerebral palsy compared with controls, and 6.7 times as common in perinatal deaths. They found that failure to respond to these clear signs of abnormality occurred in 26% of cerebral palsy cases and 50% of perinatal deaths, compared with 7% of controls. On the basis of these figures, it can be calculated that there will be approximately one case of potentially preventable cerebral palsy and one potentially preventable perinatal death in every 4000 deliveries. If one assumes 700,000 births per annum in the United Kingdom, 174 cases of cerebral palsy and 158 cases of perinatal death would be preventable.

More recently, Stewart and associates have reported that perinatal mortality in Wales is twice as high at night as during the day, and twice as high in July/August as in the rest of the year.[42] They suggested that the excess of deaths may represent overreliance on inexperienced staff at night and a shortage of staff during the peak summer holiday months, and also that it might be related to physical and mental fatigue of the caregivers. The Confidential Inquiry into Stillbirths and Deaths in Infancy (CESDI) was a U.K. national survey of perinatal deaths, now subsumed into the Confidential Inquiry into Maternal and Child Health (CEMACH, www.cemach.org.uk). The fourth annual report[43] showed that failures in the use and interpretation of CTG were present in more than half of intrapartum-related deaths. The fifth report[44] studied the proportion of 567 cases where there was evidence of suboptimal care in labor, and then classified this by whether improved care could possibly or probably have prevented the adverse outcome. Suboptimal care was identified in 71% of cases, and a better outcome could possibly or probably have been anticipated in 28% and 22% of cases, respectively, if care had been adequate. The report commented that "fetal surveillance problems were the commonest cause (of problems in labor), with CTG interpretation . . . the most frequent criticism."

Maternity care accounts for some 60% of the U.K. National Health Service (NHS) medical litigation bill, with individual settlements reaching £4.6 million and even successful defense costing up to £0.5 million.

Possible Interventions to Improve the Quality of Care

Young and associates[45] have studied the efficacy of intrapartum intervention and found that in cases of low Apgar scores, there was evidence of substandard care in labor in 74%. Following the introduction of regular audit of low Apgar scores, with feedback to clinical staff, this proportion fell to 23%, but crept back up to 32% over the following year. However, following the introduction of compulsory training in FHR pattern interpretation for all staff, the proportion of low Apgar score cases associated with substandard care fell back once again to only 9%.

Indications for Electronic Fetal Monitoring

Intrapartum EFM was intended to be a screening tool for fetal hypoxia, with FBS used as the confirmatory test. Accordingly, many authorities have advocated universal continuous EFM. However, with the growth of the "natural childbirth" movement, and the difficulty in establishing the efficacy of EFM in randomized trials, most guidelines now suggest that intermittent auscultation is an adequate form of FHR monitoring for "low risk" labors and that continuous EFM should be reserved for "high risk" labors. Unfortunately, it is difficult to define "low risk" labor. The guidelines of the NICE in the United Kingdom[36] approach this problem by listing high risk factors that they consider indicate the need for continuous EFM (Table 71–3). I have analyzed 29,443 births at the Chelsea and Westminster Hospital (London, UK) from 1988 thru 1998 inclusive and coded them as low risk if: the mother's age was <40; there was no diabetes, cardiac disease, renal disease, or antepartum hemorrhage; the highest blood pressure at any time during pregnancy was <90 mm Hg diastolic; presentation was cephalic; gestation was 37 to 42 weeks; labor onset was spontaneous; the labor duration was <12 hours; epidural anesthesia was not used; and there was no oxytocin augmentation, meconium staining of the amniotic fluid, or pyrexia. Using these criteria, labors were low risk throughout labor in only 26%. Therefore, according to the NICE guidelines, intermittent auscultation throughout labor was only applicable in about a quarter of labors. In fact, only 11% had no EFM during labor, and the incidence of abnormal FHR pattern was 7.8%. In contrast, in the "high risk" 74%, 4.3% had no EFM during labor, and the incidence of abnormal FHR pattern was 22.8%. A similar analysis of the data from 15 other maternity units in the North West Thames region of London showed a median value for "low risk" labors of 25%, with the highest proportion of low risk labor being 34%, and the lowest 16%. In only one of these units did the proportion of low risk labor where EFM was not used exceed 50%.

TABLE 71-3

Indications for Continuous Electronic Fetal Monitoring

Labor Abnormalities
Induced labor
Augmented labor
Prolonged labor
Prolonged membrane rupture
Regional analgesia
Previous cesarean delivery
Abnormal uterine activity
Suspected Fetal Distress in Labor
Meconium staining of the amniotic fluid
Suspicious fetal heart rate on auscultation
Abnormal fetal heart rate on admission cardiotocography
Vaginal bleeding during labor
Intrauterine infection
Fetal Problems
Multiple pregnancies (all fetuses)
Small fetus
Preterm fetus
Breech presentation
Oligohydramnios
Post-term pregnancy
Rhesus isoimmunization
Maternal Medical Disease
Hypertension
Diabetes
Cardiac disease (especially cyanotic)
Hemoglobinopathy
Severe anemia
Hyperthyroidism
Collagen disease
Renal disease

Mires and colleagues recently reported on a randomized controlled trial of CTG versus Doppler auscultation of the fetal heart at admission in labor in low risk obstetric population.[46] They commented that "as the trial progressed, it became clear that . . . more women had complications that required continuous monitoring than had been predicted"; the overall proportion was 63% and was similar in both groups. In an even more recent study of low risk labors in Dublin, Impey and associates[47] reported that if an admission CTG was performed, 58% of women had continuous EFM during labor, but that even if intermittent auscultation was used from the outset, 42% of women had continuous EFM. Accordingly, using current guidelines, continuous EFM is likely to be used in most settings in over 80% of labors.

Fetal Monitoring by Intermittent Auscultation

Evidence regarding the value of EFM is limited, but the evidence regarding the use of intermittent auscultation is even worse. Recommendations therefore have to depend entirely on custom and practice, and "expert" opinion. These have been summarized in the NICE guidelines.[36] They have followed the American College of Obstetricians and Gynecologists, and the Society of Obstetricians and Gynaecologists of Canada in recommending that (1) during the active phase of the first stage of labor, the FHR should be auscultated and recorded every 15 minutes and (2) during the second stage of labor, the FHR should be auscultated and recorded every 5 minutes. Ideally, the heart rate should be counted over 30 to 60 seconds, in the minute after a contraction (to detect late decelerations).

The "Admission" Cardiotocogram

The incidence of emergency cesarean section for fetal distress is higher in the first hour of labor than in any subsequent single hour. This is because the onset of contractions reveals the fetus that is unable to cope with the relative hypoxia of labor. For this reason, performing EFM for the first hour of labor even in low risk pregnancies ("admission test") has become popular in some maternity units. Unfortunately, no studies of sufficient size have been conducted to enable an evaluation of the usefulness of this approach.[36]

Technical Aspects of Electronic Fetal Monitoring

A cardiotocograph machine is used to produce a continuous recording of FHR and uterine contractions, known as a CTG. It reveals information about aspects of FHR such as baseline variability, which cannot be measured using intermittent auscultation. It also produces recordings of FHR decelerations in relation to contractions, which are easier to detect and analyze, and an automatic paper recording is produced for archival purposes (optical discs are increasingly being used for convenient storage). This record is available for subsequent independent review, which is valuable for audit and teaching, although it may be a mixed blessing in medico-legal terms if it reveals abnormalities previously overlooked.

EFMs can measure the FHR and uterine contractions via external transducers using Doppler ultrasound and a tocodynamometer (strain gauge attached to a belt) or via internal sensors such as a fetal electrode and an intrauterine catheter. Despite the fact that the latter methods are more reliable and accurate, and probably more comfortable for the average woman in labor than the belts necessary to attach the external transducers, they are more invasive and thus most EFM is performed using external devices. This mode of EFM has a number of problems. First, modern machines generally use a form of autocorrelation or cross-correlation analysis to produce the FHR from ultrasound signals, but the systems are now so sensitive that if the fetus is dead they sometimes produce a recording of the maternal rate, which can be mistaken for that of the fetus. This is particularly likely if the mother is anxious and has a tachycardia so that her heart rate is similar to that expected of her fetus and can even lead to the erroneous emergency delivery of a dead baby.[48] To avoid this problem, it is good practice always to ensure that rate calculation is derived from the characteristic signals of the fetal heart (sharp and distinct, sometimes sounding like the hooves of a galloping horse), rather than to rely on the "whooshing" sound produced by reflections from fetal blood vessels.

Second, good recording of the FHR depends greatly on correct placement of the transducers on the abdomen. This is not always achieved, and constant readjustment is often necessary if the mother is very active. Unfortunately, it is often the mothers who wish to have an active birth and who are very mobile who decline the use of internal monitoring. This commonly results in loss of adequate signal and FHR information at a most critical time in the labor, the second stage.

Third, the information obtained about uterine contractions using an external transducer is essentially limited to timing them. The external contraction transducer (tocodynamometer) gives only a relative indication of contraction strength, and the recording is attenuated if, for example, the mother is obese or the transducer is poorly placed. This may mislead the birth attendant into underestimating the strength of contractions, particularly in a stoical woman, and thus lead to overdosage with uterine stimulants such as oxytocin. By comparison, the recordings obtained from a directly applied fetal electrode and an intrauterine catheter are much more accurate and less susceptible to recording failure.

One factor that militates against the use of scalp electrodes is the increasing prevalence of the HIV virus. The Royal College of Obstetricians (UK) advise that women who carry the HIV virus should not have their fetuses monitored using an electrode that breaches its skin, for fear of increasing the risk of transmission of the virus to the fetus. Although women with a detectable viral load are now advised to have their babies delivered by cesarean section, and HIV-infected women only normally choose vaginal delivery if their viral load is undetectable, anonymous testing reveals that in about 25% of cases, women positive for HIV choose not to have antenatal testing and therefore go through labor unaware they are at risk.

Interpretation of Fetal Heart Rate Recordings

The key to reliable and consistent interpretation of FHR tracings from CTG machines is a systematic approach. Four main aspects of the FHR should be assessed: the baseline rate, baseline variability, the presence or absence of accelerations, and the presence and classification of decelerations (slowings of the FHR, or "dips"). Many errors of interpretation occur because of an excessive concern with decelerations and a consequent failure to appreciate the significance of the other three aspects of the FHR. A detailed account of how the FHR can be assessed using CTG is given in Table 71–4.

A normal CTG pattern is highly reassuring that the fetus is not acidotic; the significance of an abnormal pattern is much more difficult to judge. In general, the more of the four basic aspects of the FHR (baseline rate, baseline variability, accelerations, decelerations) that are abnormal, the more likely the fetus is to be acidotic. However, other factors should modulate the response to such a pattern.

The Time Factor

The fetus does not become acidotic as soon as the FHR becomes abnormal; Fleischer and associates[49] showed that a well-grown fetus can cope with hypoxic stress for as long as 90 minutes before the pH of fetal blood starts to fall. Thus, a normal fetal scalp blood pH 60 minutes after the CTG has become abnormal does not indicate that the abnormality is a "false-positive." The pH of the fetus may begin to fall at any subsequent time; accordingly the only safe plan is to repeat the FBS at hourly intervals (more often if the pattern is severely abnormal) or deliver the baby.

In contrast, a low pH may be an acute response to temporary interference with maternal placental blood flow and gas exchange. This can occur, for example, after an epidural top-up (with or without maternal hypotension) or because of uterine hyperstimulation with oxytocics. Action should be taken to correct the problem. This can include turning the mother to the left lateral position to correct supine hypotension, stopping any infusions of oxytocic drugs, and giving the mother oxygen by face mask; persisting hypotension from epidural anesthesia can usually be corrected by intravenous injection of a vasoconstrictor such as ephedrine, and excessive uterine activity may be corrected by an infusion of a tocolytic drug such as ritodrine or salbutamol. If the FHR pattern returns to normal, then a low pH is often corrected, and immediate delivery of the fetus would be inappropriate. Therefore, it is probably unnecessary to take an FBS in response to an acute FHR abnormality unless the resuscitative measures described earlier do not correct the abnormality of the FHR within 15 to 20 minutes.

Intrauterine Growth Restriction

Any baby thought to be seriously small for gestational age on antenatal assessment or with intrauterine growth restriction seen on serial ultrasound scanning should be treated as particularly at risk during labor.[50] There is an increased likelihood of abnormal FHR patterns and acidosis, so FBSs should be taken more readily and more often than with well-grown babies, and the threshold for operative delivery should be reduced.

Early Gestational Age

Preterm babies are more susceptible to the effects of intrauterine hypoxia than full-term babies; in particular

TABLE 71–4

Interpretation of Fetal Heart Rate Pattern (Cardiotocogram)

Admission Test

Normal, reassuring, or reactive
- Two or more accelerations (>15 beats/min for 15 sec) in 20 min
- Baseline FHR 110–150 beats/min
- Baseline variability 5–25 beats/min
- Absence of decelerations
- Moderate tachycardia/bradycardia and accelerations

Interpretation/action: Risk of fetal hypoxia in next 2–3 hr in spontaneous labor, is low other than following acute events

Suspicious, equivocal, or nonreactive
- Absence of accelerations, reduced baseline variability (5–10 beats/min), or silent pattern (5 beats/min), for >40 min, although baseline rate normal (110–150 beats/min)
- Baseline FHR <100 beats/min or >150 beats/min
- Variable decelerations (depth <60 beats/min, duration <60 sec)

Interpretation/action: Continue CTG, consider vibroacoustic stimulation/fetal scalp pH estimation if CTG not normal in 1 hr

Pathologic/ominous
- Silent pattern and baseline FHR >150 beats/min or <110 beats/min with no acceleration
- Repetitive late decelerations and/or complicated variable decelerations
- Baseline FHR <100 beats/min or prolonged bradycardia (>10 min)

Interpretation/action: Exclude cord prolapse, placental abruption and scar dehiscence. If small fetus, or thick meconium, or previously abnormal trace, consider immediate delivery. In other situations, consider fetal scalp pH estimation (and, for example, tocolysis if uterine hyperstimulation, IV fluids if related to epidural 'top-up')

First-Stage Intrapartum CTG

Normal, reassuring, or reactive
- Two or more accelerations (>15 beats/min for >15 sec) in 20 min
- Baseline FHR 110–150 beats/min
- Baseline variability 5–25 beats/min
- Early decelerations (in late first stage)

Suspicious, equivocal, or nonreactive
- Absence of accelerations for >40 min
- Baseline FHR 150–170 beats/min or 100–110 beats/min (normal baseline variability, no decelerations)
- Silent pattern >40 min (normal baseline rate, no decelerations)
- Baseline variability >25 beats/min in the absence of accelerations
- Variable decelerations (depth <60 beats/min, duration <60 sec)
- Occasional transient prolonged bradycardia (FHR drops to <80 beats/min for >2 min or <100 beats/min for >3 min)

Interpretation/action: Continue CTG, vibroacoustic stimulation or fetal scalp pH estimation if CTG not normal in 1 hr

Pathologic/ominous
- Baseline FHR >150 beats/min and silent pattern and/or repetitive late or variable decelerations
- Silent pattern for >90 min
- Complicated variable decelerations (depth ≥60 beats/min, duration ≥60 sec) and changes in shape (overshoot, decreased or increased baseline heart rate following the deceleration, absence of baseline variability, slow recovery)
- Combined/biphasic decelerations (variable followed by late)
- Prolonged bradycardia (FHR drops to <80 beats/min for >2 min or <100 beats/min for >3 min) in a suspicious trace
- Prolonged bradycardia (FHR drops to <80 beats/min for >2 min or <100 beats/min for >3 min) >10 min
- Repetitive late decelerations
- Pronounced loss of baseline variability
- Sinusoidal pattern with no accelerations

Interpretation/action: Consider fetal scalp pH estimation

Second-Stage Intrapartum CTG

Normal, reassuring, or reactive
- Normal baseline heart rate, normal baseline variability and no decelerations, frequent accelerations, both periodic and scattered
- Baseline heart rate 110–150 beats/min and baseline variability 5–25 beats/min or >25 beats/min, with or without early and/or variable decelerations

Suspicious, equivocal, or nonreactive
- Baseline heart rate >150 beats/min, persisting or compensatory following each deceleration
- Reduced baseline variability or silent pattern decelerations of >60 sec duration
- Mild bradycardia, heart rate catches up between contractions and may reach above 100 beats/min, especially when baseline variability is normal

Interpretation/action: Observe trace for increasing baseline heart rate or bradycardia

Pathologic/ominous
- Baseline heart rate <100 beats/min of different patterns
  - Progressive bradycardia: baseline heart rate gradually decreases between contractions; absence of baseline variability can be seen especially when heart rate is <80 beats/min
  - Persisting bradycardia, baseline <80 beats/min. The additional absence of baseline variability represents a more ominous feature
- Baseline tachycardia (>150 beats/min) with reduced variability and severe variable and late decelerations

Interpretation/action: Expedite delivery if not imminent

CTG, Cardiotocography; FHR, Fetal heart rate. Courtesy of Hewlett Packard Asia-Pacific Medical Products Group.

hypoxia has a damaging effect on the type 2 pneumocytes that produce surfactant in the lungs, increasing the incidence and severity of the neonatal respiratory distress syndrome (hyaline membrane disease).[51] However, the incidence of hypoxia and acidosis in fetuses in preterm labor is not increased compared with fetuses in full-term labor.[52] Preterm babies are more likely to have low Apgar scores than full-term babies, but this is due to functional immaturity and not to the effects of hypoxia.[53] A baby born at 28 weeks' gestation is likely to have poor respiratory effort, to have reduced tone, and to have less reflex irritability, and thus a lower Apgar score than its full-term counterpart; however, given a normal FHR pattern, it is no more likely to be hypoxic or acidotic.[52] The interpretation of the FHR pattern of the preterm fetus in labor is similar to that of its full-term counterpart.[54] However, some subtle differences may be seen in the FHR pattern.[55] Short-term baseline variability is often rather less, and FHR accelerations less frequent (the differentiation between quiet and active sleep patterns sometimes does not develop until 28 to 32 weeks' gestation). Small, brief (<20 seconds) decelerations are often seen and are insignificant (cause unknown).

Presentation of the Fetus

Although current recommendations favor elective cesarean delivery for babies in breech position,[56] there is still a place for vaginal delivery if this is what the mother requests (see Chapter 64). The second stage of labor is prolonged when the fetus is in breech presentation, and therefore it is probably wise not to embark on a vaginal breech delivery if there is any suggestion of fetal compromise at the onset of the second stage. Thus, if the FHR pattern is entirely normal, vaginal delivery can proceed, but if the FHR is abnormal, fetal condition should be checked by an FBS pH measurement. This can readily be taken from the buttock, and pH values are the same as for babies in cephalic presentation.[57] If the FBS pH is normal, then the delivery can be allowed to proceed, but if the FHR abnormality persists the FBS should probably be repeated if delivery has not occurred within 30 minutes. The passage of meconium is common with a breech presentation and unless it occurs very early in labor is not a useful monitoring variable.

Twins or Higher Order Pregnancy

Because of the increased risk of perinatal mortality associated with being a second twin, there is an increasing trend for elective cesarean delivery. However, vaginal delivery is a reasonable option if that is the parents' preference.[58] The use of ultrasound allows the heart rate of the second twin to be recorded accurately, and in view of the higher mortality rates for the second twins, such monitoring is recommended. The second twin may have heart rate changes suggestive of hypoxia while that of the first twin remains normal.[59] In this case, since FBS is impossible until the first twin has been delivered, cesarean section is probably appropriate.

Instrumental Delivery

Fetal distress is commonly cited as an indication for urgent instrumental vaginal delivery. However, great caution should be applied if the fetal head needs to be rotated. Hypoxia and acidosis can cause cerebral edema, and an edematous brain is stiffer and less flexible than normal. Twisting forces applied in this situation may cause tentorial tears, which would otherwise not occur. Thus, rotational deliveries when the FHR pattern is abnormal should probably only be undertaken after an FBS pH has been measured and found to be normal.[60]

Maternal Preference

A scientific basis for deciding when labor should be terminated operatively for fetal indications remains elusive. Such decisions cannot therefore be taken in isolation from the social context, and the wishes and anxieties of the parents should always be taken into account. Some parents have particular anxieties about labor; for example they may have a sibling with residual damage attributed to birth asphyxia or trauma. In such cases, they may request delivery by cesarean section if there is any sign of fetal dysfunction or delay in labor. In view of the very low mortality and morbidity rates associated with cesarean section in modern practice, especially in the absence of any acute emergency, it is probably wise to accede to such requests unless delivery is imminent and the obstetrician very confident of a successful outcome.

PROCEDURE

FETAL BLOOD SAMPLING

Position

The use of the lithotomy position should be avoided because of the risk of supine hypotension. This can produce iatrogenic hypoxia and acidosis in the fetus, leading to unnecessary operative delivery. The sampling is most comfortably performed with the woman in the left (or right) lateral position.

Procedure

Under aseptic conditions, an amnioscope is passed up the vagina to rest on the presenting part of the fetus. Sufficient pressure must be used to exclude amniotic fluid, which will otherwise contaminate the sample. The fetal skin is then dried with a dental swab in a holder, and sprayed with ethyl chloride. The evaporation of the ethyl chloride cools the skin, and as it warms up again, a reactive hyperemia is produced, which aids bleeding. The skin is smeared with a water-repellent gel (often silicone) so that when the skin is stabbed with a guarded 2-mm blade a droplet of blood forms. This droplet is allowed to flow into a preheparinized thin glass tube by capillary action (it helps to tilt the tube slightly downward at the operator's end). Mouth operated suction should not be used because of the risk of the operator ingesting potentially infected blood.

Analysis

The sample is then transferred to a blood gas analyzer for measurement. It is preferable to measure Po_2, Pco_2, pH, and calculate the base deficit. If the values are normal, but the FHR pattern remains abnormal, it will usually be necessary to repeat the sampling within 15 to 30 minutes.

Use of Intravenous Fluids during Labor and Its Effect on Fetal Acid–Base Balance

Women in labor are commonly advised not to eat, because of the risk of Mendelson's syndrome (aspiration of stomach contents) should they unexpectedly need general anesthesia. As a result, they often develop ketonemia. For this reason, it is common practice to give parenteral fluid containing glucose and electrolytes, particularly if labor lasts more than a few hours. However, Ames and colleagues reported in 1975 that infusion of glucose-containing solutions could give rise to maternal lactic acidosis.[61] This is because the rise in maternal blood glucose concentration increases the production rate of lactate, according to Michaelis-Menton kinetics. Subsequently, it was confirmed that maternal infusion of glucose at 100 g/hour (1 L of 10% glucose over 1 hr) produced a significant fall in average pH and rise in lactate in fetal as well as maternal blood.[62] However, lactic acidosis does not occur if the glucose infusion rate is restricted to 30 g/hour,[63,64] and there is some evidence to suggest that physiologic amounts of glucose in infused fluids (i.e., 5%) may be associated with less fetal acidosis than glucose-free solutions.[65] These studies indicate that in labor, as at other times, care must be taken to monitor the volume and content of intravenous infusions to ensure they are compatible with the maintenance of normal physiology.

IATROGENIC CAUSES OF FETAL DISTRESS

Excessive Oxytocin Augmentation of Labor

Every uterine contraction above 4 to 6 kPa causes a cessation of maternal intervillous placental blood flow.[66] This produces a period of relative hypoxia for the fetus, such that the fetal Po_2 falls by about 0.5 to 0.75 kPa during each contraction, reaching its lowest level at the end of the contraction, after which the flow is restored and the Po_2 recovers. Because it takes some time for the oxygen-depleted maternal pool of blood to be replaced, recovery takes about 60 to 90 seconds. The total period of reduced oxygenation is therefore 120 to 150 seconds, emphasizing the importance of an adequate intercontraction interval to ensure fetal oxygenation. Poorly controlled oxytocin infusions, which produce excessively frequent contractions, can cause iatrogenic fetal hypoxia and acidosis (see Chapter 69). In practical terms, this means that if the FHR becomes abnormal, oxytocin infusions should be stopped immediately.

Epidural Anesthesia

Before preloading of the circulation with colloid came into practice, abnormalities of the FHR occurred in approximately one third of cases following insertion of an epidural anesthetic. With preloading, this can be reduced by two thirds.[67]

Epidural anesthetics may also cause a fetal tachycardia by inducing hyperthermia in the mother (see Chapter 72). Such tachycardia is not likely to be associated with significant fetal hypoxia, and fetal pH is not affected, but it can give rise to an erroneous diagnosis of fetal distress. It may also lead to a false diagnosis of intrauterine infection, greatly increasing the proportion of newborns investigated with cultures and treated with antibiotics.[68] Probably, the correct response is to cool the mother with tepid sponging.

Drugs

Drugs given to the mother may cross the placenta and affect the fetus. Beta-blockers such as propranolol, and α- and β-blockers such as labetalol may interfere with the reflex responsiveness of the fetal circulation and impair its response to hypoxia. Other hypotensives such as hydralazine can cause hypoxia by producing maternal hypotension. Sedatives such as pethidine (meperidine) and diazepam (Valium) may depress the fetal central nervous system, reducing the variability of the FHR and producing neonatal depression. Care must be taken to give the minimum of any necessary drug in labor, and the effects on the fetus must always be considered.

OTHER METHODS OF MONITORING FOR FETAL DISTRESS

Transcutaneous Gas Measurements

In the late 1970s, transcutaneous Po_2 measurements using a modified Clark electrode became possible. However, the technique was difficult; the scalp had to be shaved, dried, and readily accessible to a fairly large probe, which then had to be glued to the skin or held on by suction. The probe had to be heated to arterialize the circulation and allow oxygen to diffuse out of the fetal arterioles. There were problems with trauma and heat injury. In addition, the measurement of Po_2 is a measure of hypoxic stress but does not quantify response (acid–base buffer reserve) in the way that measuring pH does; it is very susceptible to local and acute changes.

Further attempts to improve acceptability have been made by using pulse oximetry, which does not require the probe to be heated; instead, it uses infrared light to detect changes in oxygenated hemoglobin concentration in the tissues during the arterial pulsation cycle. However, this system also has problems; it cannot work through hair (which leads to practical difficulties with placement) or meconium, it is susceptible to maternal and fetal movement, and sometimes produces inconsistent results. Results suggest that 30% to 60% saturations are the normal range in the human fetus, indicating that prolonged desaturation is physiologic in the human fetus.[69] This makes the significance of the readings difficult to assess clinically. If a cutoff of 30% saturation is used, then values below this have a sensitivity of 94% in detecting pH <7.13, but the specificity is only 38%.[69] This means that the technique is similar to, but not better than, continuous FHR monitoring as a screening test for acidosis.

Near-infrared spectroscopy is a related technique that uses infrared light at two frequencies to assess the difference in concentrations between oxygenated and deoxygenated hemoglobin concentrations and, hence, the oxygen saturation of the blood. However, the method is expensive and presents many technical difficulties, including frequent probe detachment. No published trials have examined the ability of near-infrared spectroscopy in assessing fetal condition during labor.[70]

Fetal Scalp Lactate Measurement

In theory, lactate measurement assesses hypoxic and anaerobic metabolism leading to a metabolic acidosis, which is very similar to that obtained by measuring base deficit. In practice, a randomized controlled trial using lactate compared with pH to assess metabolic acidosis showed no significant differences in clinical performance.[71] The practical advantages in measuring lactate are that very small sample volumes are needed (5 μL compared with 25 μL for pH estimation), and the values are not significantly altered by contamination of the sample with air bubbles.[72]

Electrocardiographic Waveform Analysis

Since the fetal electrocardiogram (ECG) was first demonstrated by Cremer in 1904, attempts have been made to assess fetal well-being by assessing changes in ECG waveform.[73] One approach has been to analyze changes in the PR/RR interval ratio but this has not been found to be of value in a prospective, randomized, controlled trial.[74] Another approach used the T/QRS ratio as a measure of acidosis (based on the hypothesis that it is altered by the production of lactate in the fetal heart secondary to hypoxia) and can reduce the need for FBS.[75,76] Two prospective, randomized, controlled trials[77,78] suggested that it can reduce the need for operative delivery for fetal distress, as well as the incidence of both of metabolic acidosis at delivery and neonatal encephalopathy. However, a recent study of its introduction into routine clinical practice did not show the expected benefits.[79] A particular problem with the use of the ECG waveform analysis is that it requires the application of a fetal scalp electrode.

Expert Systems

Studies of the efficacy of EFM have consistently found the human component to be the weakest link. Computerized analysis is now commonplace in the evaluation of the adult ECG waveform. Keith and associates reported a study in which the ability of an "expert" computer system (Fig. 71–2) designed for the interpretation of FHR and FBS data was compared with the opinions of 17 clinicians experienced in fetal monitoring from 16 centers in the United Kingdom.[80] Fifty cases with

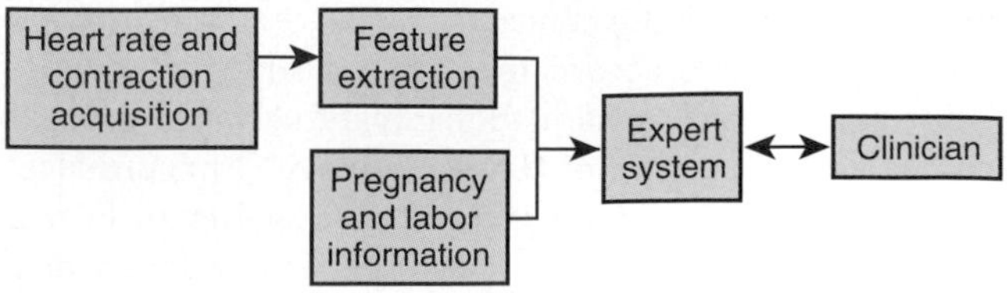

FIGURE 71–2
Principles of expert system cardiotocogram interpretation. (From Keith RDF, Beckley S, Garibaldi JM, et al: A multicentre comparative study of 17 experts and an intelligent computer system for managing labor using the cardiotocogram BJOG 1995;102:688–700.)

complete intrapartum CTGs and clinical data were reviewed by the system and each expert independently on two occasions, at least 1 month apart. The system agreed with the experts well and significantly better than chance (67.3%, $\kappa = 0.31$, $P \ll 0.001$). It was highly consistent (99.16%, $\kappa = 0.98$, $P \ll 0.001$) when used by two operators independently. It recommended no unnecessary intervention in cases that ended with a normal delivery of a baby in good condition (cord artery pH >7.15, vein pH >7.20, 5 min Apgar ≥9, and no resuscitation). This was better than all but two of the experts. It recommended delivery by cesarean section in 11 cases; at least 15 of the 17 experts in each review also recommended cesarean section delivery in these cases. Most did so within 15 minutes of the system, and two thirds did so within 30 minutes. It identified as many of the birth-asphyxiated cases (cord arterial pH <7.05 and base deficit ≥12, and Apgar score at 5 minutes ≤7 with neonatal morbidity) as the majority of the experts, and one more than was acted upon clinically. The experts were found to be consistent and to agree; with the exception of expert "Q." This expert was the only one who declined all information from FBS and attempted to make all decisions on the basis of the FHR alone. In fact, (s)he was the second most inconsistent expert in scoring and obtained the lowest agreement with the other experts (58%, $\kappa = 0.12$). (S)he was also the most inconsistent in recommending cesarean section; in nine cases cesarean section was recommended in the first review and not the second or vice versa. "Q" also recommended two cesarean sections and one second-stage intervention unnecessarily in cases with a normal delivery and a good outcome. Keith and associates commented "in the hands of the experts, this additional information (FBS) clearly adds to the accuracy of decision-making. This information supports the current RCOG (Royal College of Obstetricians and Gynaecologists, 1993) recommendations for using FBS appropriately." This system is currently being prepared for its first clinical trials and shows considerable promise. The outcome of the trials are awaited with interest.

SUMMARY OF MANAGEMENT OPTIONS

Screening for Fetal Distress in Labor

Management Options	Quality of Evidence	Strength of Recommendation	References
Prevention of Fetal Hypoxia			
Avoid unnecessary induction of labor and excessive use of oxtocic agents.	III	B	36
Preload with IV fluids in women who are having epidural analgesia in labor to reduce the risk of maternal hypotension.	Ib	A	67
Remember the effect of maternal drugs on fetal heart rate patterns.	–	GPP	–
Indications for Continuous Electronic Fetal Heart Rate Monitoring (EFM)			
See Table 71–3 for conditions associated with an increased risk of intrapartum fetal hypoxia. These indications may classify up to 80% of women as at-risk.	III	B	36
Fetal Monitoring in "Low risk" Labor			
The advice from the American, Canadian, and British Colleges is that intermittent auscultation can be used in such labors; however, there are no studies of sufficient size to evaluate this approach.	III	B	36
Use of EFM in "High risk" Labor			
Meta-analysis of randomized controlled trials shows significant reductions in the short-term neonatal morbidity rate and a significant reduction in perinatal deaths due to hypoxia, but a significant increase in cesarean delivery rates. However, studies are under powered to show an effect on overall perinatal mortality or cerebral palsy rates.	Ia	A	26,27
Concomitant use of fetal blood sampling (FBS) to estimate pH significantly reduces rates of cesarean delivery.	Ia	A	26–28
Admission EFM Recording ("Admission Test")			
Common practice, but no studies of sufficient size to evaluate this approach.	Ib	A	36, 46, 47
Interpretation of EFM Findings			
Human factors that adversely affect the outcome of EFM are delays in response times and failure to interpret the findings accurately. Education improves human responses, but this benefit is lost with time.	III	B	19,40–43,45
Because of the rate of decline in fetal pH after fetal hypoxia, FBS should be performed at least hourly if EFM abnormality is detected. Shorter intervals are advisable with intrauterine growth restriction.	III	B	49,50
If EFM abnormality is detected: • Correct caval compression. • Give maternal facial oxygen. • Correct hyperstimulation (stop oxytocics, use tocolytics). • Give IV fluids if the patient has epidural-induced hypotension.	III	B	36
EFM in a preterm fetus requires the use of slightly different criteria.	IV	C	55
The maternal pulse may be mistakenly recorded as fetal. The maternal pulse should be regularly recorded clinically by palpation to reduce this risk.	IV	C	48
FBS can be used in breech presentations.	IV	C	57
EFM in twins requires careful confirmation of separate fetal recordings.	IV	C	59
The use of rotational forceps with abnormal EFM is controversial and they should not be used if the fetal scalp pH is <7.15.	IV	C	60

Continued

SUMMARY OF MANAGEMENT OPTIONS

Screening for Fetal Distress in Labor *(Continued)*

Management Options	Quality of Evidence	Strength of Recommendation	References
Technical Aspects			
EFM recordings should be retained.	–	GPP	–
External tocometry can lead to difficulty in interpreting the timing of EFM abnormalities (e.g., with movement, maternal obesity).	–	GPP	–
The conventional advice is that fetal scalp electrodes should not be used in women with HIV.	III	B	36
Other Methods of Fetal Monitoring			
Evidence suggests that pulse oximetry is no better than EFM.	III	B	69
No data are available on the value of near-infrared spectroscopy.	Ia	A	70
Fetal scalp lactate measurement offers practical advantages over pH measurement (less volume of blood and less affected by air bubbles), but no evidence of clinical advantage over pH.	Ib	A	71,72
Electrocardiogram shows no evidence of improved outcome in practice.	Ib	A	73–79
Expert systems should give better interpretative accuracy. Randomized controlled trials are awaited.	III	B	80

CORD PROLAPSE

Prolapse of the umbilical cord in labor is an uncommon event; reported incidences vary from 1 in 265 to 426 labors. The occurrence of cord prolapse is most commonly associated with breech and other malpresentations, a high head at the onset of labor, multiple gestation, grand multiparity, abnormal placentation, preterm labor, polyhydramnios, and obstetric manipulations such as forceps delivery.[81] The diagnosis is commonly made during a vaginal examination, the examiner feeling a soft, usually pulsatile structure. In one series,[82] in 4% the cord was presenting, in 11% it was alongside the presenting part, in 45% it was in the vagina, and in 39% the cord appeared at the introitus. The last mentioned is more likely to occur after artificial, or sudden spontaneous rupture of the forewaters, than in association with a hindwater leak. Occasionally, the diagnosis may be suggested by the sudden appearance of large variable decelerations on the CTG. The mode of delivery remains controversial. As neonatal care has improved, so has the perinatal mortality associated with cord prolapse steadily declined, irrespective of the mode of delivery. For example, in one series reported in 1977, the perinatal mortality rate was 430 per 1000 births,[82] in 1985 162 per 1000 births, and in 1988 55 per 1000 births[83]; although a recent report from Israel found a perinatal mortality of 83 per 1000.[81] Some studies emphasized the danger of prolonged prolapse to delivery interval and urged prompt cesarean section unless the cervix is fully dilated and the presenting part is at or below the ischial spines so that the fetus is immediately deliverable by forceps (which is the case in about 20%–30%). While the woman is being prepared for the operation, it is usually recommended that she be nursed in the traditional knee-chest position facing downward, or alternatively (and often more practically) in steep Trendelenburg's position. It may be necessary for a birth attendant to keep a gloved hand in the vagina to elevate the presenting part and relieve pressure on the cord. One technique first suggested by Vago in 1970 and since commended by others[84] is to fill the urinary bladder with 500 to 700 mL of saline, elevating the presenting part and relieving pressure on the cord. However, more recently one paper championed manual replacement of the cord[83] (termed funic reduction), describing a successful vaginal delivery in seven of eight cases so treated (one was too far advanced in labor for this to be feasible and a cesarean section was performed). The interval between replacement of the cord and final delivery ranged from 14 to 512 minutes (8.5 hours!).

SUMMARY OF MANAGEMENT OPTIONS

Cord Prolapse

Management Options	Quality of Evidence	Strength of Recommendation	References
Cesarean section while pressure on the cord is relieved until delivery.	III	B	84
Manual elevation of the head away from the cord.			
Knee-chest position.			
Steep Trendelenburg position.			
Filling of the bladder with up to 700 mL normal saline.			
Instrumental delivery if the patient is in the second stage of labor, the presenting part is below the level of the ischial spines, and easy, prompt vaginal delivery is anticipated.	III	B	84
The value of funic reduction (manual replacement) is uncertain because few patients have been studied.	III	B	83

INTRAPARTUM FETAL RESUSCITATION

In general, if acute fetal hypoxia is evident and acidosis is rapidly developing, the best management is emergency cesarean section, preferably within 15 minutes. If the presentation is occipitoanterior, the presenting part is at or below the spine, and there is no obvious evidence of disproportion, then a nonrotational forceps delivery is an appropriate alternative. Various studies have reported attempts at intrauterine resuscitation of the fetus, and maneuvers recommended include turning the mother to the left side, giving her oxygen by face mask, stopping any oxytocic infusion, uterine tocolysis, and correction of any hypotension. While there is anecdotal evidence that these maneuvers may be effective in appropriate circumstances, no randomized studies attest to their efficacy.

MECONIUM STAINING OF THE AMNIOTIC FLUID

Aspiration of meconium by the fetus remains a relatively common cause of perinatal mortality and morbidity because it is difficult to prevent. The fetus passes meconium into the amniotic fluid in approximately 10% of all pregnancies; in up to 5% of these (i.e., in 1:200 of all pregnancies) the meconium is aspirated and can then lead to meconium aspiration syndrome (MAS). MAS can cause, or contribute to, neonatal death in up to 0.05% (i.e., 1:2000 of all pregnancies).[85,86] In addition, up to one third of all cases in which aspiration occurs develop long-term respiratory compromise.[87,88] The incidence of MAS may be falling in developed countries: fewer pregnancies are proceeding beyond 42 weeks because of increased use of ultrasound dating of pregnancy and induction between 41 and 42 weeks.[89]

It seems likely that the causes of meconium passage by the fetus are not necessarily the same as those that cause aspiration, and so in the account that follows, the two aspects will be addressed separately.

Passage of Meconium

Mechanism

Meconium is passed into the amniotic fluid by peristalsis of the fetal gut accompanied by relaxation of the internal and external anal sphincters. In the adult this process is a complex interaction of hormonal, myogenic, and neurogenic factors. Peristalsis is principally controlled by local reflexes acting via the neural complexes in the gut wall, but is usually modified by extrinsic innervation. Sympathetic activity inhibits rectal activity and causes constriction of the internal anal sphincter, whereas parasympathetic activity has the opposite effects. In the resting state the internal and external sphincters are constricted. In the adult, involuntary defecation can occur in response to stress ("flight-or-fight reaction"). This is mediated centrally by the hypothalamus (and possibly the amygdala), which in turn causes stimulation of the visceral parasympathetics.[90,91] In contrast, pathophysiologic stresses such as pain, heat, cold, injury, exercise, and nonintestinal infections all produce gut stasis and constipation.[90] It is attractive to suggest that the fetus may exhibit a similar response to the "emotional" stress of labor, but this concept is likely to remain an untested theory. The fetus is stressed pathophysiologically in labor by hypoxia, pyrexia, or compression, which by extrapolation from adult physiology would be more likely to produce gut stasis than increased motility. However, fetal physiology differs in many ways from that of the adult, and our knowledge of the mechanisms of gut motility and meconium passage in the fetus is poor.

The Effect of Maturity and Gestation on Passage of Meconium

Meconium is found in the fetal gut from 10 weeks' gestation,[92] but passage of meconium is rare before 34 weeks.[93] The incidence of meconium passage increases with gestational age and reaches approximately 30% at 40 weeks' gestation and 50% at 42 weeks.[93,94] The presence of meconium in the amniotic fluid may reflect fetal gastrointestinal maturity.[95] Fetal gut transit time does decrease with gestational age, and gut motility increases.[96] The low gut motility in the preterm fetus has been attributed to a lack of gut wall musculature, but this is unlikely because peristalsis has been reported before 12 weeks' gestation, and muscle development must have occurred before this.[97]

Immature innervation of the fetal gut is more likely, with preterm fetuses having fewer myelinated axons and ganglion cells in the colon than full-term infants. Meconium passage in the preterm fetus can occur if it becomes infected with organisms that can cause a fetal enteritis (e.g., *Listeria monocytogenes*, *Ureaplasma urealyticum*, rotaviruses).[98] The fetal gut must be sufficiently developed for peristalsis to occur and meconium to be passed even in the preterm fetus.

Hormonal Control of the Passage of Meconium

The intestinal hormone motilin has been implicated in the passage of meconium in utero; it causes contraction of smooth muscle in the gut wall. Motilin levels in umbilical venous blood increase with gestation, and if they reflect levels in the fetal gut, could be a factor in explaining the tendency for the mature fetus to pass meconium.[99] Cord levels are also higher in infants that have passed meconium prenatally,[99,100] and one study found that they were also higher if an FHR abnormality had occurred in labor.[99] This latter finding was not confirmed in a later study,[100] but different definitions of FHR abnormality were used. It is possible that stress on the fetus could cause release of motilin and thus passage of meconium, but this remains conjectural. The hormonal and other factors that control gut motility are largely unknown, even in the adult.

Infection and the Passage of Meconium

Meconium-stained amniotic fluid is associated with increased peripartum infection rates, independent of other risk factors for infection. Thick meconium, in particular, is associated with a marked increase in peripartum infectious morbidity.[101-103] It is not yet clear whether the presence of meconium encourages infection, or whether infection promotes the passage of meconium by the fetus. In favor of the former, prophylactic intravenous ampicillin-sulbactam significantly reduces intra-amniotic infection in patients with meconium-stained amniotic fluid,[104] although the possibility remains that the presence of the infection antedated the appearance of the meconium and was unrecognized. In addition meconium is a chemoattractant and activator of polymorphonuclear leukocytes in vitro, and for cytokines such as TNF-α, IL-1, and IL-8.[105] It may be that meconium increases the damaging effects of infection by increasing the presence of these inflammatory mediators.

Obstetric Cholestasis

The risk of meconium passage increases in association with cholestasis of pregnancy.[106] This may be secondary to elevated levels of bile acids in the maternal circulation, which cross the placenta and affect the fetus. Cholestasis of pregnancy also increases the bile acid content of meconium.[107] The same study also found that although maternal ursodeoxycholic acid (UDCA) therapy caused a reduction in serum bile acid levels in the mother, there was no associated reduction in the levels of meconium passage in the fetus. The implications of this are unclear, but it is possible that if UDCA does not affect fetal bile acid levels significantly, perinatal loss rates associated with cholestasis of pregnancy will not improve.

Risks

Fetal Hypoxia

An association between meconium passage in utero and poor condition of the neonate has been suggested since ancient times. Aristotle reported opium-like effects in neonates born through meconium-stained fluid, and there have been references to meconium in association with perinatal death from as early as 1676 (quoted in Schulze).[108] Subsequently many authors have suggested that fetal hypoxia causes intestinal peristalsis, relaxation of the anal sphincter, and thus passage of meconium. This view has largely been assumption, with little or no direct evidence to support such a hypothesis. Stander[109] claimed that meconium was a sign of impending fetal "asphyxia" due to "relaxation of the sphincter ani muscle induced by faulty aeration of the blood" and proposed prompt delivery whenever meconium was seen. Desmond and colleagues[110] claimed that meconium staining of the amniotic fluid was a marker of fetal hypoxia, but no blood gas analysis of either fetal or neonatal blood was performed; the diagnosis of hypoxia being made on clinical grounds alone. These observations were made despite the report of Schulze,[108] who had concluded from a study of a series of more than 5500 births in California, that passage of meconium during labor "is in the large majority of cases independent of fetal asphyxia" and that the presence of old meconium in the amniotic fluid was of no prognostic significance for the later development of asphyxia (asphyxia here was not defined but appears to mean lack of respiratory effort at birth). She also observed that in cases associated with asphyxia there were always changes of the FHR during labor, and that these changes should be the sole guide to the necessity for delivery. However in a later study, meconium passage was associated with low umbilical vein oxygen saturation, and thick meconium with lower levels of Po_2 than thin meconium.[111] This remained the principal experimental evidence linking fetal hypoxia with meconium passage and was widely quoted, often as the sole evidence, for at least the subsequent 20 years.

Fenton and Steer[112] made one of the first attempts to separate meconium passage from other markers of fetal compromise such as abnormality of heart rate, but again had only presumptive evidence of hypoxia in the fetus. They stated that there were other, benign causes of meconium passage and suggested that the passage of meconium was not significant if the FHR was greater than 110 beats/minute. The introduction of FBS began to clarify the situation. Miller and associates[113] found no difference in scalp blood pH, umbilical cord artery and vein pH, and neonatal arterial pH up to 64 minutes of life, between meconium and nonmeconium groups, if the FHR during labor had been normal. They concluded that meconium in the absence of other signs was not a sign of fetal distress (defined as late decelerations on the CTG and umbilical artery acidosis). More recent studies confirmed that infants who have normal FHR patterns have similar outcomes whether or not meconium is present, at least as far as acid–base status is concerned.[114]

If the FHR pattern is abnormal, however, the presence of meconium is associated with an increased chance of a baby being acidotic, born in poor condition, and needing resuscitation at birth.[93,113] In the data presented by Steer and colleagues,[93] 140 babies had an abnormal CTG pattern in the first stage of labor. The mean cord artery pH was 7.22 (SD = 0.10) in the 108 cases with clear amniotic fluid, compared with 7.17 (SD = 0.12) in the 32 cases with meconium-stained amniotic fluid (t = 2.37, P = 0.0096, one-tailed). The incidence of 1-minute Apgar scores <7 was 19% (3% at 5 minutes) if the amniotic fluid was clear, compared with 56% (9% at 5 minutes) if the amniotic fluid was meconium-stained. The difference was significant at 1 minute (P = 0.0001; Fisher's exact test). However, they commented that the reduction in the 1-minute Apgar score may have been due at least in part to the use of pharyngeal suction or endotracheal intubation by the attending pediatrician suppressing spontaneous respiration and thus iatrogenically reducing the Apgar score.

Despite the lack of a clear relationship between meconium staining of the amniotic fluid and fetal acidosis in the absence of FHR changes, we cannot conclude that the presence of meconium is not a threat to the fetus or neonate even if the FHR is normal. Yeomans and associates[115] studied 323 pregnancies with meconium-stained amniotic fluid at 36 to 42 weeks' gestation. Although there was a significantly higher incidence of meconium below the vocal cords if an umbilical artery pH was <7.20 compared with when the umbilical artery pH was ≥7.20 (34% compared with 23%), the difference in the incidence of clinical meconium aspiration syndrome according to pH was not significant. Moreover, 69% of babies with meconium below the cords had cord arterial pH of ≥7.2. Thus a normal pH does not exclude the possibility of meconium aspiration, and most babies with meconium aspiration do not have acidosis. These data do not support the hypothesis that fetal hypoxia is a major cause of meconium passage in labor, and indeed Naeye and colleagues[116] reported that meconium staining of the amniotic fluid was not more common, even when the neonate was hypoxic.

Evidence that hypoxia per se does not lead to passage of meconium has been available for many years. Becker and associates[95] showed reduced peristalsis in the fetal guinea pig after induction of maternal hypoxemia, and a similar result was seen in the monkey fetus. In the adult with spinal shock, although the external sphincter relaxes, constipation occurs due to the loss of the other defecation reflexes. If meconium passage does occur in response to reduced intestinal blood flow, it must be an early event for the neurogenic reflexes still to be present. Meconium passage may occur as a result of vagal stimulation, and this could account for coexisting reduction in the FHR.[112] Parasympathetic stimulation is known to occur with cord compression, and this is supported by meconium passage being more common with increasing gestational age. Emmanouilides and colleagues[64] found that in the sheep fetus, if one umbilical artery was ligated, passage of meconium only occurred as a very late phenomenon, after chronic fetal wasting had developed. Although it is widely stated that fetal hypoxia leads to meconium passage in laboratory animals, the studies usually cited were concerned with the investigation of fetal breathing movements and do not state that meconium was passed in response to hypoxia.[66,117]

Meconium Aspiration

The passage of meconium is not a risk to the fetus, but aspiration of the meconium into the fetal or neonatal lung is associated with clinical disease ranging from mild transitory respiratory distress to severe respiratory compromise and occurs in up to one third of cases. Meconium aspiration is commonly defined as the presence of meconium below the vocal cords and occurs in up to 35% of live births with meconium-stained liquor.

Aspiration of meconium was thought by many authors to occur at delivery as the newborn infant took its first breath. Oropharyngeal suction, and endotracheal intubation of the infant before the first breath were widely promoted, to prevent meconium aspiration. However it now seems likely that meconium aspiration is largely an intrauterine event. This change of view has occurred because of compelling evidence that severe meconium aspiration syndrome still occurs despite adequate suction at delivery.[115,118,119]

The current view is that meconium aspiration occurs due to fetal breathing movements, causing inhalation of amniotic fluid, with meconium if present. Two types of breathing movements cause inhalation of amniotic fluid: gasping and deep breathing. Gasping is a normal response to hypoxemia and can be induced experimentally by occluding the umbilical cord or by occluding the maternal aorta.[66,117]

The fetus may also inhale meconium by deep irregular breathing in utero, not initiated by hypoxia. These breaths become more frequent as gestation advances and comprise 10% of all fetal breathing movements.[117] The passage of amniotic fluid deep into the lung has been demonstrated by radiolabeling experiments that also showed that the human fetus inhales 200 mL/kg/24 hours of amniotic fluid.[120] Fetal hypercapnia and acidemia also increase these breathing movements, but they still occur in most, if not all, normal fetuses.[117,121] Although some infants with meconium aspiration are severely compromised at birth, there is little or no difference in umbilical cord acid–base status between infants with meconium below the cords and those without.[115] Meconium aspiration is more common if the meconium is thick rather than thin. This may be a reflection of the fact that oligohydramnios (and therefore thick undiluted meconium) is more likely to lead to fetal hypoxia due to cord compression and, consequently, increased fetal breathing.

Meconium Aspiration Syndrome

GENERAL

MAS represents a wide spectrum of disease ranging from transient respiratory distress with little therapy required, to severe respiratory compromise requiring prolonged mechanical ventilation and high levels of oxygen administration. Neonatal death occurs in up to 40% of cases.[118]

Severe MAS is associated with profound hypoxia, which is secondary to right-to-left shunting, a persistent fetal circulation, resistant pulmonary hypertension, pulmonary hemorrhage, necrosis of pulmonary vessels, and muscularization of distal pulmonary arterioles.[86,122,123] These changes may be due to intrauterine hypoxia, rather than to the meconium itself, although the inhalation of meconium exacerbates the problem in several ways in the neonatal period.

Meconium inhaled in an infant who has not been subjected to hypoxia usually causes mild disease only, and is asymptomatic in 90% of cases. Exposure to intrauterine hypoxia causes pulmonary vasoreactivity that persists after birth. Large increases in pulmonary artery pressure in response to very small falls in oxygen tension then result. The severity of this pulmonary vasospasm seems to depend on the severity of the fetal hypoxia and may be fixed (completely unresponsive) in the most severe cases. These changes have been demonstrated experimentally and observed clinically. A vicious cycle of hypoxia, pulmonary vasospasm, shunting, and therefore worsening hypoxia can develop. Jovanovic and Nguyen[124] showed in the guinea pig that meconium or amniotic fluid aspiration in the absence of hypoxia caused minimal damage, whereas lung damage (necrosis of alveoli and diffuse hemorrhage) in the hypoxic cases was severe whether the amniotic fluid contained meconium or not. The degree of lung destruction seems to depend primarily on the length and degree of hypoxia, not simply the aspiration of meconium. Hypoxic damage also reduces the clearance of aspirated meconium or amniotic fluid.[125] Meconium does, however, exacerbate the problems faced by the neonate. It displaces surfactant, causing atelectasis and hyaline membrane formation[126–128] and causes a chemical pneumonitis possibly due to cytotoxicity to the type II pneumocytes caused by bile salt-induced accumulation of calcium.[129] In addition it enhances bacterial growth and is associated with intrauterine infections. Aspiration may lead to infectious pneumonitis.

Some bacterial toxins cause pulmonary vascular spasm, exacerbating the effects of hypoxia.[98,130,131] Meconium has been demonstrated to cause vascular necrosis and vasoconstriction in the umbilical cord and may cause similar damage in the lung.[132] The umbilical vasoconstriction may cause hypoxia in utero, leading to aspiration. Inhaled thick meconium may cause a physical obstruction to the airways, leading to distal lung collapse, with hyperinflation in other areas of the lung. In total, 95% of severe cases of MAS occur when the meconium is thick, which is more common in post-term pregnancies when a relative oligohydramnios develops. Oligohydramnios may also be due to hypoxia, causing reduced fetal urine output[133] or may be a sign of uteroplacental insufficiency.

METHODS OF PREVENTING MAS

During the 1950s and 1960s, it was thought that meconium-stained amniotic fluid was a marker of fetal compromise, and efforts were made to detect meconium in the amniotic fluid in late pregnancy and to deliver the fetus either before, or as soon as, meconium appeared. Amnioscopy was introduced for pregnancies more than 10 days past the expected date of confinement. It was stated that the finding of meconium indicated "impending danger," and that immediate amniotomy and fetal blood sampling should be performed; the ensuing uterine contractions were thought to be therapeutic for the fetus. A threefold reduction in perinatal mortality was claimed, but other investigators have been unable to reproduce these results.[134,135] Saldana and associates[136] showed no benefit from amnioscopy and delivery. Amnioscopy has not been shown to be beneficial, is uncomfortable for the mother, may result in accidental rupture of the membranes or induce labor, can cause infection, and has to be repeated at regular arbitrary intervals until delivery.

Benacerraf and colleagues[137] reported the detection of thick meconium by ultrasonography, but further studies showed that vernix can produce an ultrasonically indistinguishable image in the absence of meconium.[138,139]

Because meconium passage is more common with advanced gestational age, many studies have investigated the effect of inducing labor at an earlier gestation. In a controlled trial Cole and associates[140] significantly reduced the incidence of meconium-stained liquor by inducing at 39 to 40 weeks' gestation, but no effect on perinatal mortality or respiratory disease was seen. Other studies of induction of labor have not shown a decrease in meconium aspiration, even if the incidence of meconium staining of the liquor was reduced.[141-143] There is thus no evident benefit from induction of labor before meconium appears, or from the routine use of amnioscopy, and disadvantages to both procedures exist.

In the 1970s it was widely believed that meconium aspiration developed by inhalation of the meconium at delivery when the infant took its first breath. To prevent this, aggressive policies of oropharyngeal suction, endotracheal intubation, and splinting of the thorax to prevent aspiration were proposed. Despite these interventions, cases of meconium aspiration still occurred, and further studies showed little or no reduction in MAS. A decline in the mortality from meconium aspiration is probably due to concurrent advances in perinatal medicine, rather than to the introduction of suction protocols. Suction and intubation are not free of risk. Cordero and Hon[144] reported apnea and bradycardia in infants having nasopharyngeal suction, and Linder and colleagues[145] found no benefit from the intubation at birth of meconium-stained but otherwise normal infants. All cases of meconium aspiration in this study occurred in the intubated group, and two cases of laryngeal stridor also required repeated hospitalization with residual hoarseness at 6 months of age. Cunningham and associates[119] recommended routine oropharyngeal suction but not intubation. There is now widespread acceptance that routine suctioning and intubation of neonates that have passed meconium have little if any effect on aspiration and may have deleterious side effects.

Amnioinfusion, the instillation of normal saline into the uterus during labor, has been proposed as a method to reduce meconium concentration and therefore the effects of aspiration. It may reduce cord compression in cases of oligohydramnios and therefore fetal gasping. Recent meta-analysis of the randomized studies investigating amnioinfusion has shown a significant reduction in overall cesarean section rate and in the rate specifically for fetal distress.[146] The incidence of meconium aspiration, MAS, and umbilical artery pH <7.20 appear to be reduced. The beneficial effect of amnioinfusion may be due to a reduction in cord compression during uterine contractions and therefore possible fetal hypoxia, or directly to a reduction in the concentration of meconium. However, because thick meconium is often associated with oligohydramnios, the benefits of amnioinfusion may be due solely to correction of amniotic fluid volume. Although amnioinfusion is a promising technique for reducing the incidence and severity of MAS, one study found that amnioinfusion is not clinically feasible in 53% of cases, and no benefit was seen.[147]

Attempts have been made to classify meconium in labor according to its concentration, because thick meconium has been associated with increased incidence and severity of the aspiration syndrome. However, any grading system is subjective because amniotic fluid draining during labor may not be representative of the fluid in utero, and no fluid may drain at all in cases of oligohydramnios, masking the presence of meconium. Quantifying the meconium concentration by centrifuging samples of amniotic fluid and measuring the amount of solid matter in the sample has been attempted,[148,149] but the same problems of obtaining amniotic fluid representative of the intrauterine milieu exist. In addition, neither author addressed the problem of vernix, and solid matter other than meconium in the liquor, producing false-positive results.

Two reports suggested that social support during labor reduces the incidence of meconium staining,[150,151] but in both cases more oxytocin was used in the group with no support, which could have lead to unphysiologic contractions and fetal hypoxia.

Evidence linking fetal distress and meconium should be viewed with caution because the events during labor and delivery do not represent the intrauterine environment at the time of meconium passage. In addition it is unlikely that prevention of meconium passage or aspiration will be successful until there is some elucidation of the underlying causes. Intrauterine probes to measure meconium concentration in the amniotic fluid continuously during labor, using a light-reflectance method have been developed.[152] Although this enabled observation of the events at the time of meconium passage (e.g., FHR changes, epidural top-ups) and was able to detect meconium not otherwise visible to the birth attendants, it is unlikely to be clinically useful in the foreseeable future.

Management Options with Meconium Staining of the Amniotic Fluid

When amniotic fluid is seen to drain, it should always be inspected carefully for the presence of meconium. If meconium is detected, continuous electronic FHR monitoring is recommended. If the FHR pattern remains normal, no specific action is necessary, except to avoid actions that might precipitate acute fetal hypoxia (supine hypotension, epidural hypotension, uterine hyperstimulation with oxytocics). In particular, there is no indication for routine FBS and pH estimation as long as the FHR pattern is normal. At delivery, a pediatrician should be present. If the baby is vigorous and cries promptly, there is no need for further action. Although there is no proof of efficacy, some pediatricians prefer to suction the pharynx as soon as possible after delivery of the head, and this is acceptable as long as care is taken not to traumatize the pharynx or larynx, as this may precipitate meconium aspiration.

If the FHR pattern is abnormal during labor, the likelihood of acidosis is substantially increased. Consideration should be given to immediate delivery, if necessary by cesarean section. If rapid progress in cervical dilation is occurring, it may be appropriate to take an FBS and allow the labor to continue if the pH is above 7.20, but this decision must take into account other factors such as the wishes of the mother, and whether there are other risk factors, such as intrauterine growth restriction. Amnioinfusion should be considered if it is decided to allow the labor to continue. Amnioinfusion can also be considered even if the FHR pattern is normal, as a preventive measure.

SUMMARY OF MANAGEMENT OPTIONS

Meconium Staining of the Amniotic Fluid

Management Options	Quality of Evidence	Strength of Recommendation	References
Incidence			
Meconium aspiration syndrome contributes to neonatal death in approximately 1 in 2000 births.	III	B	85–87
The main influence on the passage of meconium is gestational age.	III	B	94–96
Meconium aspiration is associated with infection, particularly in the lungs.	III	B	101–104
Fetal passage of meconium is more common in cholestasis of pregnancy.	III	B	106,107
Hypoxia and acidosis do not per se lead to the passage of meconium.	III	B	114,115
The combination of severe hypoxia and meconium aspiration causes lung damage.	III	B	125–127
Prevention			
A pediatrician should be present for delivery, but should not perform routine oropharyngeal suction in the absence of evidence of fetal hypoxia because suction does not reduce the incidence of meconium aspiration syndrome.	IIa	B	144,145
Meconium aspiration and acidosis are reduced by amnioinfusion of normal saline.	Ia	A	146

CONCLUSIONS

FETAL HEART RATE MONITORING

- Intermittent fetal heart rate auscultation is advocated as adequate screening for intrapartum fetal hypoxia in low risk women; however, the trials are of insufficient size.
- Electronic fetal heart rate monitoring in high risk labors produces significant reductions in short-term neonatal morbidity and a significant reduction in perinatal deaths due to hypoxia but a significant increase in cesarean section rates; but all studies were insufficiently robust to be able to demonstrate any effect on perinatal mortality or cerebral palsy rates.
- Concomitant use of fetal blood sampling to estimate pH significantly reduces cesarean section rates.
- An “admission test” is commonly used in practice, but there are no studies of sufficient size to evaluate this approach.
- Human error (especially delays in response times and misinterpretation) contributes to poor outcome in monitored labors.
- Corrective actions to consider with an abnormality in electronic fetal monitoring are
    - Correcting caval compression
    - Maternal facial oxygen
    - Correct hyperstimulation (stop oxytocics, use tocolytics)
    - Intravenous fluids if epidural induced hypotension

CONCLUSIONS (Continued)

CORD PROLAPSE

- Conventional approaches to this problem are
  - If diagnosed in first stage—relief of pressure on cord while performing an emergency cesarean section
  - If diagnosed in the second stage—expedite vaginal delivery

MECONIUM STAINING OF THE AMNIOTIC FLUID

- Most cases are a reflection of fetal gestational maturity.
- Hypoxia is the cause in a minority and thus this is an indication for continuous electronic fetal monitoring.
- Hypoxia and aspiration of meconium can lead to lung damage.
- The incidence of meconium aspiration and acidosis are reduced by amnioinfusion of normal saline.
- A pediatrician should be present for delivery, but routine oropharyngeal suction in the absence of evidence of fetal hypoxia should not be performed as it does not reduce the incidence of meconium aspiration syndrome.

REFERENCES

1. Beard RW, Morris ED, Clayton SG: pH of foetal capillary blood as an indicator of the condition of the foetus. J Obstet Gynaecol Br Commonw 1967;74:812–822.
2. Sykes GS, Molloy PM, Johnson P, et al: Do Apgar scores indicate asphyxia? Lancet 1982;i:494–495.
3. Lissauer TJ, Steer PJ: The relation between the need for intubation at birth, abnormal cardiotocograms in labor and cord artery blood gas and pH values. BJOG 1986;93:1060–1066.
4. Steer PJ, Eigbe F, Lissauer TJ, Beard RW: Interrelationships among abnormal cardiotocograms in labor, meconium staining of the amniotic fluid, arterial cord blood pH and Apgar scores. Obstet Gynecol 1989;74:715–721.
5. Thorp JA, Dildy GA, Yeomans ER, et al: Umbilical cord blood gas analysis at delivery. Am J Obstet Gynecol 1996;175:517–522.
6. Wu YW, Escobar GJ, Grether JK, et al: Chorioamnionitis and cerebral palsy in term and near-term infants. JAMA 2003;290:2677–2684.
7. Maberry MC, Ramin SM, Gilstrap LC III, et al: Intrapartum asphyxia in pregnancies complicated by intra-amniotic infection. Obstet Gynecol 1990;76:351–354.
8. Banerjee S, Steer PJ: The rise in maternal temperature associated with epidural analgesia is harmful and should be treated. Int J Obstet Anaesth 2003;12:280–286.
9. Saling E: Neues Vorgehen zur Untersuchung des Kindes unter der Geburt: Ein Fuhrung, Technick und Grundlagen. Arch Gynakol 1962;197:108–122.
10. Winkler CL, Hauth JC, Tucker JM, et al: Neonatal complications at term as related to the degree of umbilical artery acidaemia. Am J Obstet Gynecol 1991;164:637–641.
11. Goodwin TM, Belai I, Hernandez P, et al: Asphyxial complications in the term newborn with severe umbilical acidemia. Am J Obstet Gynecol 1992;167:1506–1512.
12. Nagel HT, Vandenbussche FP, Oepkes D, et al: Follow-up of children born with an umbilical arterial blood pH < 7. Am J Obstet Gynecol 1995;173:1758–1764.
13. van den Berg PP, Nelen WL, Jongsma HW, et al: Neonatal complications in newborns with an umbilical artery pH < 7.00. Am J Obstet Gynecol 1996;175:1152–1157.
14. Low JA, Panagiotopoulos C, Derrick EJ: Newborn complications after intrapartum asphyxia with metabolic acidosis in the term fetus. Am J Obstet Gynecol 1994;170:1081–1087.
15. Socol ML, Garcia PM, Riter S: Depressed Apgar scores, acid-base status, and neurologic outcome. Am J Obstet Gynecol 1994;170:991–998; discussion 998–999.
16. Low JA, Lindsay BG, Derrick EJ: Threshold of metabolic acidosis associated with newborn complications. Am J Obstet Gynecol 1997;177:1391–1394.
17. Thorp JA: What is birth asphyxia: Reply. Am J Obstet Gynecol 1990;163:1368.
18. ACOG: Utility of umbilical cord blood acid-base measurement. ACOG Committee Opinion 1991;91:33–34.
19. Gaffney G, Sellers S, Flavell V, et al: Case-control study of intrapartum care, cerebral palsy, and perinatal death. BMJ 1994;308:743–750.
20. The task force on joint assessment of prenatal and perinatal factors associated with brain disorders: National Institutes of Health report on cause of mental retardation and cerebral palsy. Pediatrics 1985;76:457–458.
21. MacLennan A: A template for defining a causal relation between acute intrapartum events and cerebral palsy: International consensus statement. BMJ 1999;319:1054–1059.
22. Cowan F, Rutherford M, Groenendaal F, et al: Origin and timing of brain lesions in term infants with neonatal encephalopathy. Lancet 2003;361:736–742.
23. Badawi N, Kurinczuk JJ, Keogh JM, et al: Intrapartum risk factors for newborn encephalopathy: The Western Australian case-control study. BMJ 1998;317:1554–1558.
24. Johnston MV: MRI for neonatal encephalopathy in full-term infants. Lancet 2003;361:713–714.
25. Beard RW, Filshie GM, Knight CA, Roberts GM: The significance of the changes in the continuous foetal heart rate in the first stage of labor. J Obstet Gynaecol Br Commonw 1971;78:865–881.
26. Vintzileos AM, Nochimson DJ, Guzman ER, et al: Intrapartum electronic fetal heart rate monitoring versus intermittent auscultation: A meta-analysis. Obstet Gynecol 1995;85:149–155.
27. Thacker SB, Stroup DF, Peterson HB: Efficacy and safety of intrapartum electronic fetal monitoring: An update. Obstet Gynecol 1995;86:613–620.
28. Thacker SB, Stroup DF: Continuous electronic heart rate monitoring for fetal assessment during labor. Cochrane Database Syst Rev 2000;CD000063.
29. Fusi L, Steer PJ, Maresh MJA, Beard RW: Maternal pyrexia associated with the use of epidural anaesthesia in labour. Lancet 1989;i:1250–1252.
30. Ozden S, Demirci F: Significance for fetal outcome of poor prognostic features in fetal heart rate traces with variable decelerations. Arch Gynecol Obstet 1999;262:141–149.

31. Keunen H, Deutz NE, Van RJ, Hasaart TH: Transient umbilical cord occlusion in late-gestation fetal sheep results in hippocampal damage but not in cerebral arteriovenous difference for nitrite, a stable end product of nitric oxide. J Soc Gynecol Invest 1999;6:120–126.
32. Sibanda J, Beard RW: Influence on clinical practice of routine intra-partum fetal monitoring. BMJ 1975;3:341–343.
33. Beard RW, Edington PT, Sibanda J: The effects of routine intrapartum monitoring on clinical practice. Contrib Gynecol Obstet 1977;3:14–21.
34. MacDonald D, Grant A, Sheridan-Pereira M, et al: The Dublin randomized controlled trial of intrapartum fetal heart rate monitoring. Am J Obstet Gynecol 1985;152:524–539.
35. Grant A, O'Brien N, Joy MT, et al: Cerebral palsy among children born during the Dublin randomised trial of intrapartum monitoring. Lancet 1989;2:1233–1236.
36. NICE fetal monitoring guidelines, May 2001. http://www.nice.org.uk/page.aspx?o=20257.200.
37. Goodlin RC: Do concepts of causes and prevention of cerebral palsy require revision? Am J Obstet Gynecol 1995;172:1830–1834; discussion 1834–1836.
38. Ridgeway JJ, Weyrich DL, Benedetti TJ: Fetal heart rate changes associated with uterine rupture. Obstet Gynecol 2004;103:506–512.
39. Yeomans ER, Gilstrap LC, Leveno KJ, Burris JS: Meconium in the amniotic fluid and fetal acid-base status. Obstet Gynecol 1989;73:175–178.
40. Murphy KW, Johnson P, Moorcraft P, et al: Birth asphyxia and the intrapartum cardiotocograph. BJOG 1990;97:470–479.
41. Ennis M, Vincent CA: Obstetric accidents: A review of 64 cases. BMJ 1990;300:1365–1367.
42. Stewart JH, Andrews J, Cartlidge PH: Numbers of deaths related to intrapartum asphyxia and timing of birth in all Wales perinatal survey, 1993–5. BMJ 1998;316:657–660.
43. Confidential inquiry into stillbirths and deaths in infancy: Fourth annual report, 1st January to 31st December 1995. London, Maternal and Child Health Research Consortium, 1997.
44. Confidential inquiry into stillbirths and deaths in infancy: Fifth annual report, 1st January to 31st December 1996. London, Maternal and Child Health Research Consortium, 1998.
45. Young P, Hamilton R, Hodgett S, et al: Reducing risk by improving standards of intrapartum fetal care. J R Soc Med 2001;94:226–231.
46. Mires G, Williams F, Howie P: Randomised controlled trial of cardiotocography versus Doppler auscultation of fetal heart at admission in labor in low risk obstetric population. BMJ 2001;322:1457–1460.
47. Impey L, Reynolds M, MacQuillan K, et al: Admission cardiotocography: A randomised controlled trial. Lancet 2003;361:465–470.
48. Amato JC: Fetal heart rate monitoring. Am J Obstet Gynecol 1983;147:967–969.
49. Fleischer A, Schulman H, Jagani N, et al: The development of fetal acidosis in the presence of an abnormal fetal heart rate tracing. Am J Obstet Gynecol 1982;144:55–60.
50. Steer P: The management of large and small for gestational age fetuses. Semin Perinatol 2004;28:59–66.
51. Hobel CJ, Hyvarinen MA, Oh W: Abnormal fetal heart rate patterns and fetal acid-base balance in low birth weight infants in relation to the respiratory distress syndrome. Obstet Gynecol 1972;39:83–88.
52. Dickinson JE, Eriksen NL, Meyer BA, Parisis VM: The effect of preterm birth on umbilical cord blood gases. Obstet Gynecol 1992;79:575–578.
53. Catlin EA, Carpenter MW, Brann BS, et al: The Apgar score revisited: Influence of gestational age. J Pediatr 1986;109: 865–868.
54. Zanini B, Paul RH, Huey JR: Intrapartum fetal heart rate: Correlation with scalp pH in the preterm fetus. Am J Obstet Gynecol 1980;136:43–47.
55. Wheeler T, Murrills A: Patterns of fetal heart rate during normal pregnancy. BJOG 1978;85:18–27.
56. Hannah ME, Hannah WJ, Hewson SA, et al: Planned caesarean section versus planned vaginal birth for breech presentation at term: A randomised multicentre trial. Term Breech Trial Collaborative Group. Lancet 2000;356:1375–1383.
57. Wheeler T, Greene KR: Breech management with fetal blood sampling. BMJ 1973;1:802–803.
58. Winn HN, Cimino J, Powers J, et al: Intrapartum management of nonvertex second-born twins: A critical analysis. Am J Obstet Gynecol 2001;185:1204–1208.
59. Steer PJ, Beard RW: Two cases of continuous fetal heart rate monitoring in twins. BMJ 1973;3:263–265.
60. Paintin DB: Midcavity forceps delivery. BJOG 1982;89:495–500.
61. Ames AC, Cobbold S, Maddock J: Lactic acidosis complicating treatment of ketosis of labor. BMJ 1975;4:611–613.
62. Philipson EH, Kalhan SC, Riha MM, Pimentel R: Effects of maternal glucose infusion on fetal acid-base status in human pregnancy. Am J Obstet Gynecol 1987;157:866–873.
63. Piquard F, Hsiung R, Haberey P, Dellenbach P: Does fetal acidosis develop with maternal glucose infusions during normal labor? Obstet Gynecol 1989;74:909–914.
64. Emmanouilides GC, Townsend DE, Bauer RA: Effects of single umbilical artery ligation in the lamb fetus. Pediatrics 1968;42:919.
65. Fisher AJ, Huddleston JF: Intrapartum maternal glucose infusion reduces umbilical cord acidemia. Am J Obstet Gynecol 1997;177:765–769.
66. Duenhoelter JH, Pritchard JA: Fetal respiration: A review. Am J Obstet Gynecol 1977;129:326–338.
67. Collins KM, Bevan DR, Beard RW: Fluid loading to reduce abnormalities of fetal heart rate and maternal hypotension during epidural analgesia in labor. BMJ 1978;2:1460–1461.
68. Lieberman E, Lang JM, Frigoletto F Jr, et al: Epidural analgesia, intrapartum fever, and neonatal sepsis evaluation. Pediatrics 1997;99:415–419.
69. Dildy GA, Thorp JA, Yeast JD, Clark SL: The relationship between oxygen saturation and pH in umbilical blood: Implications for intrapartum fetal oxygen saturation monitoring. Am J Obstet Gynecol 1996;175:682–687.
70. Mozurkewich E, Wolf FM: Near-infrared spectroscopy for fetal assessment during labor (Cochrane Review). Issue 2, 2004. Chichester, UK, John Wiley & Sons.
71. Westgren M, Kruger K, Ek S, et al: Lactate compared with pH analysis at fetal scalp blood sampling: A prospective randomised study. BJOG 1998;105:29–33.
72. Westgren M, Kublickas M, Kruger K: Role of lactate measurements during labor. Obstet Gynecol Surv 1999;54:43–48.
73. Deans AC, Steer PJ: The use of the fetal electrocardiogram in labor. BJOG 1994;101:9–17.
74. Strachan BK, van Wijngaarden WJ, Sahota D, et al: Cardiotocography only versus cardiotocography plus PR-interval analysis in intrapartum surveillance: A randomised, multicentre trial. FECG Study Group. Lancet 2000;355:456–459.
75. Westgate J, Greene KR: Comparison of the T/QRS ratio of the fetal electrocardiogram and the fetal heart rate during labor and the relation of these variables to condition at delivery. BJOG 1991;98:1057–1059.
76. Westgate J, Harris M, Curnow JS, Greene KR: Plymouth randomized trial of cardiotocogram only versus ST waveform plus cardiotocogram for intrapartum monitoring in 2400 cases. Am J Obstet Gynecol 1993;169:1151–1160.
77. Noren H, Amer-Wahlin I, Hagberg H, et al: Fetal electrocardiography in labor and neonatal outcome: Data from the Swedish randomized controlled trial on intrapartum fetal monitoring. Am J Obstet Gynecol 2003;188:183–192.
78. Amer-Wahlin I, Hellsten C, Noren H, et al: Cardiotocography only versus cardiotocography plus ST analysis of fetal electrocardiogram for intrapartum fetal monitoring: A Swedish randomised controlled trial. Lancet 2001;358:534–538.

79. Haberstich R, Vayssiere C, David E, et al: Routine use of ST-segment of fetal electrocardiogram for monitoring labor: A year's experience (preliminary results). Gynecol Obstet Fertil 2003;31:820–826.
80. Keith RDF, Beckley S, Garibaldi JM, et al: A multicentre comparative study of 17 experts and an intelligent computer system for managing labour using the cardiotocogram. BJOG 1995;102:688–700.
81. Kahana B, Sheiner E, Levy A, et al: Umbilical cord prolapse and perinatal outcomes. Int J Gynaecol Obstet 2004;84:127–132.
82. Yla-Outinen A, Heinonen PK, Tuimala R: Predisposing and risk factors of umbilical cord prolapse. Acta Obstet Gynecol Scand 1985;64:567–570.
83. Barrett JM: Funic reduction for the management of umbilical cord prolapse. Am J Obstet Gynecol 1991;165:654–657.
84. Katz Z, Shoham Z, Lancet M, et al: Management of labor with umbilical cord prolapse: A 5-year study. Obstet Gynecol 1988;72:27.
85. Coltart TM, Byrne DL, Bates SA: Meconium aspiration syndrome: A 6-year retrospective study. BJOG 1989;96:411–414.
86. Wiswell TE, Tuggle JM, Turner BS: Meconium aspiration syndrome: Have we made a difference? Pediatrics 1990;85:715–721.
87. Macfarlane PI, Heaf DP: Pulmonary function in children after neonatal meconium aspiration syndrome. Arch Dis Child 1988;63:368–372.
88. Lung function in children after neonatal meconium aspiration. Lancet 1988;i:317–318.
89. Yoder BA, Kirsch EA, Barth WH, Gordon MC: Changing obstetric practices associated with decreasing incidence of meconium aspiration syndrome. Obstet Gynecol 2002;99(5 Pt 1):731–739.
90. Thomas JE: Organ systems in adaptation: The digestive system. In Dill D, Adolp EF, Wilber CG (eds): Handbook of Physiology: Section 4. Adaptation to the environment. Washington, DC, American Physiological Society, 1964, pp 207–214.
91. Guyton AC: In Textbook of Physiology, 8th ed. Philadelphia, WB Saunders, 1991, pp 651–656.
92. Smith CA: In The Physiology of the Newborn Infant. Springfield Ill, Charles C Thomas, 1976.
93. Steer PJ, Eigbe F, Lissauer TJ, Beard RW: Interrelationships among abnormal cardiotocograms in labor, meconium staining of the amniotic fluid, arterial cord blood pH and Apgar scores. Obstet Gynecol 1989;74:715–721.
94. Miller FC, Read JA: Intrapartum assessment of the postdate fetus. Am J Obstet Gynecol 1981;141:516–520.
95. Becker RF, Windle WF, Barth EE, Schulz MD: Fetal swallowing, gastro-intestinal activity and defecation in amnio. Surg Gynecol Obstet 1940;70:603–614.
96. McLain CR: Amniography studies of the gastrointestinal motility of the human fetus. Am J Obstet Gynecol 1963;86:1079–1087.
97. Woods JR, Dolkart LA: Significance of amniotic fluid meconium. In Creasy RK, Resnik R (eds): Maternal-Fetal Medicine: Principles and Practice, 2nd ed. Philadelphia, WB Saunders, 1989, pp 404–413.
98. Romero R, Hanaoka S, Mazor M, et al: Meconium-stained amniotic fluid: A risk factor for microbial invasion of the amniotic cavity. Am J Obstet Gynecol 1991;164:859–862.
99. Lucas A, Christofides ND, Adrian TE, et al: Fetal distress, meconium, and motilin. Lancet 1979;i:718.
100. Mahmoud EL, Benirschke K, Vaucher YE, Poitras P: Motilin levels in term neonates who have passed meconium prior to birth. J Pediatr Gastroenterol Nutr 1988;7:95–99.
101. Seaward PG, Hannah ME, Myhr TL, et al: International Multicentre Prelabor Rupture of Membranes Study: Evaluation of predictors of clinical chorioamnionitis and postpartum fever in patients with prelabor rupture of membranes at term. Am J Obstet Gynecol 1997;177:1024–1029.
102. Jazayeri A, Jazayeri MK, Sahinler M, Sincich T: Is meconium passage a risk factor for maternal infection in term pregnancies? Obstet Gynecol 2002;99:548–552.
103. Tran SH, Caughey AB, Musci TJ: Meconium-stained amniotic fluid is associated with puerperal infections. Am J Obstet Gynecol 2003;189:746–750.
104. Adair CD, Ernest JM, Sanchez-Ramos L, et al: Meconium stained amniotic fluid-associated infectious morbidity: A randomized, double blind trial of ampicillin sulbactam prophylaxis. Obstet Gynecol 1996;188:216–220.
105. Yamada T, Minakami H, Matsubara S, et al: Meconium-stained amniotic fluid exhibits chemotactic activity for polymorphonuclear leukocytes in vitro. J Reprod Immunol 2000;46:21–30.
106. Roncaglia N, Arreghini A, Locatelli A, et al: Obstetric cholestasis: Outcome with active management. Eur J Obstet Gynecol Reprod Biol 2002;100:167–170.
107. Rodrigues CM, Marin JJ, Brites D: Bile acid patterns in meconium are influenced by cholestasis of pregnancy and not altered by ursodeoxycholic acid treatment. Gut 1999;45:446–452.
108. Schulze M: The significance of the passage of meconium during labor. Am J Obstet Gynecol 1925;10:83–88.
109. Stander HJ: Prolapse of the cord: Asphyxia. In Williams' Obstetrics, 8th ed. New York, D. Appleton Century, 1941, p 1104.
110. Desmond MM, Moore J, Lindley JE, Brown CA: Meconium staining of the amniotic fluid. Obstet Gynecol 1957;9:91–103.
111. Walker J: Foetal anoxia. J Obstet Gynaecol Br Emp 1954;61:162–180.
112. Fenton AN, Steer CM: Fetal distress. Am J Obstet Gynecol 1962;83:354–362.
113. Miller FC, Sacks DA, Yeh S-Y, et al: Significance of meconium during labor. Am J Obstet Gynecol 1975;122:573–580.
114. Baker N, Kilby MD, Murray H: An assessment of the use of meconium alone as an indication for fetal blood sampling. Obstet Gynecol 1992;80:792–796.
115. Yeomans ER, Gilstrap LC, Leveno KJ, Burris JS: Meconium in the amniotic fluid and fetal acid-base status. Obstet Gynecol 1989;73:175–178.
116. Naeye RL, Peters EC, Bartholomew M, Landis JR: Origins of cerebral palsy. Am J Dis Child 1989;143:1154–1161.
117. Dawes GS, Fox HE, Leduc BM, et al: Respiratory movements and rapid eye movement sleep in the foetal lamb. J Physiol 1972;220:119–143.
118. Davis RO, Philips JB, Harris BA, et al: Fatal meconium aspiration syndrome occurring despite airway management considered appropriate. Am J Obstet Gynecol 1985;151:731–736.
119. Cunningham AS, Lawson EE, Martin RJ, Pildes RS: Tracheal suction and meconium: A proposed standard of care. J Pediatr 1990;116:153–154.
120. Duenholter JH, Pritchard JA: Fetal respiration: Quantitative measurements of amnionic fluid inspired near term by human and rhesus fetuses. Am J Obstet Gynecol 1976;25:306–309.
121. Harding R: Fetal breathing. In Beard RW, Nathanielsz PW (eds): Fetal Physiology and Medicine, 2nd ed. New York, Marcel Dekker, Inc., Butterworths, 1984, pp 255–286.
122. Murphy JD, Vawter GF, Reid LM: Pulmonary vascular disease in fatal meconium aspiration. J Pediatr 1984;104:758–762.
123. Brown BL, Gleicher N: Intrauterine meconium aspiration. Obstet Gynecol 1981;57:26–29.
124. Jovanovic R, Nguyen HT: Experimental meconium aspiration in guinea pigs. Obstet Gynecol 1989;73:652–656.
125. Tyler DC, Murphy J, Cheney FW: Mechanical and chemical damage to lung tissue caused by meconium aspiration. Pediatrics 1978;62:454–459.
126. Clark DA, Nieman GF, Thompson JE, et al: Surfactant displacement by meconium free fatty acids: An alternative explanation for atelectasis in meconium aspiration syndrome. J Pediatr 1987;110:765–770.

127. Auten RL, Notter RH, Kendig JW, et al: Surfactant treatment of full-term newborns with respiratory failure. Pediatrics 1991;87:101–107.
128. Moses D, Holm BA, Spitale P, et al: Inhibition of pulmonary surfactant function by meconium. Am J Obstet Gynecol 1991;164:477–481.
129. Oelberg DG, Downey SA, Flynn MM: Bile salt-induced intracellular Ca^{++} accumulation in type II pneumocytes. Lung 1990;168:297–308.
130. Hammerman C, Komar K, Abu-Khudair H: Hypoxic vs septic pulmonary hypertension. Am J Dis Child 1988;142:319–325.
131. Florman AL, Teubner D: Enhancement of bacterial growth in amniotic fluid by meconium. J Pediatr 1969;74:111–114.
132. Alsthuler G, Arizawa M, Molnar-Nadasy G: Meconium-induced umbilical cord vascular necrosis and ulceration: A potential link between the placenta and poor pregnancy outcome. Obstet Gynecol 1992;79:760–766.
133. Drummond WH, Bissonnette JM: Persistent pulmonary hypertension in the neonate: Development of an animal model. Am J Obstet Gynecol 1978;131:761–763.
134. Browne ADH, Bernan RK: The application, value, and limitations of amnioscopy. J Obstet Gynaecol Br Commonw 1968;75:616.
135. Huntingford PJ, Brunello LP, Dunstan M, et al: The technique and significance of amnioscopy. J Obstet Gynaecol Br Commonw 1968;75:610–615.
136. Saldana LR, Schulman H, Chin-Chu L: Routine amnioscopy at term. Obstet Gynecol 1976;47:521–524.
137. Benacerraf BR, Gatter MA, Ginsburgh F: Ultrasound diagnosis of meconium-stained amniotic fluid. Am J Obstet Gynecol 1984;149:570–572.
138. Sepulveda WH, Quiroz VH: Sonographic detection of echogenic amniotic fluid and its clinical significance. J Perinat Med 1989;17:333–335.
139. Sherer DM, Abramowicz JS, Smith SA, Woods JR: Sonographically homogeneous echogenic amniotic fluid in detecting meconium-stained amniotic fluid. Obstet Gynecol 1991;78:819–822.
140. Cole RA, Howie PW, Macnaughton MC: Elective induction of labor: A randomised prospective trial. Lancet 1975;ii:767–770.
141. Martin DH, Thompson W, Pinkerton JHM, Watson JD: A randomized controlled trial of selective planned delivery. BJOG 1978;85:109–113.
142. Cardozo L, Fysh J, Pearce JM: Prolonged pregnancy: The management debate. BMJ 1986;293:1059–1063.
143. Witter FR, Weitz CM: A randomized trial of induction at 42 weeks gestation versus expectant management for postdates pregnancies. Am J Perinatol 1987;4:206–211.
144. Cordero L, Hon EH: Neonatal bradycardia following nasopharyngeal suction. J Pediatr 1971;78:441–447.
145. Linder N, Aranda JV, Tsur M, et al: Need for endotracheal intubation and suction in meconium-stained neonates. J Pediatr 1988;112:613–615.
146. Hofmeyr GJ: Amnioinfusion for meconium-stained liquor in labor. Cochrane Database Syst Rev 2002;1:CD000014.
147. Usta IM, Mercer BM, Aswad NK, Sibai BM: The impact of a policy of amnioinfusion for meconium-stained amniotic fluid. Obstet Gynecol 1995;85:237–241.
148. Weitzner JS, Strassner HT, Rawlins RG, et al: Objective assessment of meconium content of amniotic fluid. Obstet Gynecol 1990;76:1143–1144.
149. Trimmer KJ, Gilstrap LC: "Meconiumcrit" and birth asphyxia. Am J Obstet Gynecol 1991;165:1010–1013.
150. Sosa R, Kennell J, Klaus M, et al: The effect of a supportive companion on perinatal problems, length of labor, and mother-infant interaction. N Engl J Med 1980;303:597–600.
151. Klaus MH, Kennell JH, Robertson SS, Sosa R: Effects of social support during parturition on maternal and infant morbidity. BMJ 1986;293:585–587.
152. Genevier ES, Danielian PJ, Randall NJ, et al: A method for the continuous monitoring of meconium concentration in the amniotic fluid during labour. J Biomed Eng 1993;15:229–234.

CHAPTER 72

Central Neuraxial, Analgesia, and Anesthesia in Obstetrics

Lawrence C. Tsen

INTRODUCTION

With the application of diethyl ether to aid in a vaginal delivery in 1847, James Young Simpson, an obstetrician, ushered in the use of anesthetic agents for obstetrics. Over the next half-century, inhaled agents would enable the use and evolution of other agents and techniques in the setting of labor and delivery. Regional anesthetic techniques, which deliver pain relief to a discrete region of the body, were introduced to obstetrics in 1900, when Oskar Kreis described the use of spinal anesthesia. Since that time, central neuraxial techniques, which comprise regional techniques that reversibly interrupt the central neuraxial system, have evolved from single, limited duration injections into the intrathecal sac (spinal) to titratable, controlled infusions through flexible catheters most commonly placed into the epidural space. The combined spinal-epidural (CSE) technique, first introduced to obstetrics in the 1980s, consists of a spinal blockade and an epidural catheter placement during the same procedure (Fig. 72–1).[1] Now rivaling the popularity of the epidural technique, the CSE technique provides rapid and profound initial pain relief with virtually no motor blockade when opioids, sometimes with small amounts of local anesthetics, are used for the spinal injection. Together, the use of the epidural, spinal, and CSE techniques has increased dramatically; in major part, this success has been driven by the quality and safety of the analgesia and anesthesia produced, the ability to titrate the degree and duration of pain relief as required by the circumstances, and an expanding number of situations in which their use is appropriate. Currently, in developed countries, central neuraxial techniques provide labor analgesia for 30% to 50% of all parturients, and the anesthesia for the majority of instrumental and operative deliveries.[2–4]

In this chapter, the indications and implications of central neuraxial techniques to provide obstetric analgesia and anesthesia will be discussed. Emphasis will be placed on the novel indications for these techniques as well as the association of these techniques with two outcomes of common obstetric and anesthetic concern: progress and outcome of labor and maternal temperature alterations.

INDICATIONS

The use of epidural, spinal, and CSE techniques for vaginal, instrumental, and operative deliveries has been well described in numerous texts and articles.[5–7] The use of these techniques, as well as nonpharmacologic modalities, systemic medications, and peripheral nerve blocks, will be discussed in the obstetric setting. The philosophical shift favoring the use of regional versus general anesthesia will be further elucidated, and two novel obstetric applications of these techniques will be discussed in greater detail: external cephalic version and postoperative pain management.

Although the quality, titratability, and patient satisfaction associated with the use of neuraxial analgesia and anesthesia have increased the use of such techniques, perhaps an even more important reason is the reduction in maternal mortality. In relation to anesthetic interventions, maternal death is overwhelmingly the result of airway management difficulties during the provision of sedative or general anesthetic agents.[8–10] Although in the United States the number of deaths involving general anesthesia has remained stable, the estimated rate of maternal deaths from complications of general anesthesia increased from

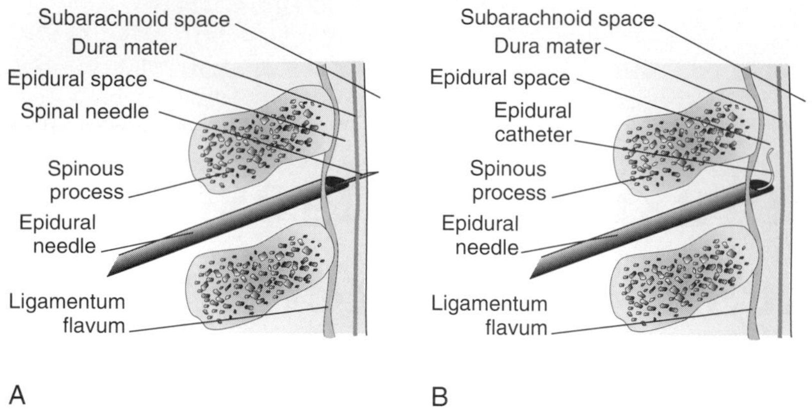

FIGURE 72–1
Combined spinal-epidural (CSE) technique. *A*, The spinal needle is introduced through the epidural needle and punctures the dura matter. The initial medication is dosed into the subarachnoid (spinal) space. *B*, After the withdrawal of the spinal needle, a catheter is introduced into the epidural space and secured in place. (From Rawal N, Holmström B, Zundert A, et al: The combined spinal-epidural technique. In Birnbach DJ, Gatt SP, Datta S [eds]: Textbook of Obstetric Anesthesia. Philadelphia, Churchill Livingstone, 2000, p 159.)

20.0 to 32.3 deaths per million in the time periods of 1979–1984 to 1985–1990, respectively (Fig. 72–2).[11] In addition, the case fatality ratio for general versus regional anesthesia over the same periods increased from 2.3:1 to 16.7:1. These changes have occurred primarily through an increase in the use of central neuraxial anesthesia and a decrease in its associated maternal mortality rate, and the fact that general anesthesia is now used mainly for high risk emergent cases in which regional anesthesia is avoided owing to the urgency of the case, the failure of neuraxial techniques, or the presence of comorbid conditions.

Despite these trends, central neuraxial techniques may still be underutilized in patients who would benefit from the avoidance of systemic sedation or general anesthesia. This group includes parturients with a high likelihood of having a difficult airway and an operative delivery (e.g., obesity, placenta previa, vaginal births after cesarean [VBACs]). In such parturients, consultation optimally should occur early in the third trimester and shortly following their arrival on the labor and delivery ward. If they are admitted in labor, evaluation should be made regarding the suitability of a neuraxial technique (Table 72–1) and early placement of an epidural catheter should be considered, even if the birth attendants or the woman herself are not sure that a regional block will definitely be required. The catheter need not be dosed immediately; such dosing can occur at a later time when an analgesic or anesthetic is required. This approach will decrease the incidence of "perceived lack of time" as a reason for administering a sedative (such as meperidine) or general anesthetic.[4]

The antenatal consultation should focus on the physiologic changes of pregnancy that can make airway management more difficult. As early as the fourth week of gestation, and particularly with preeclampsia/eclampsia,[12]

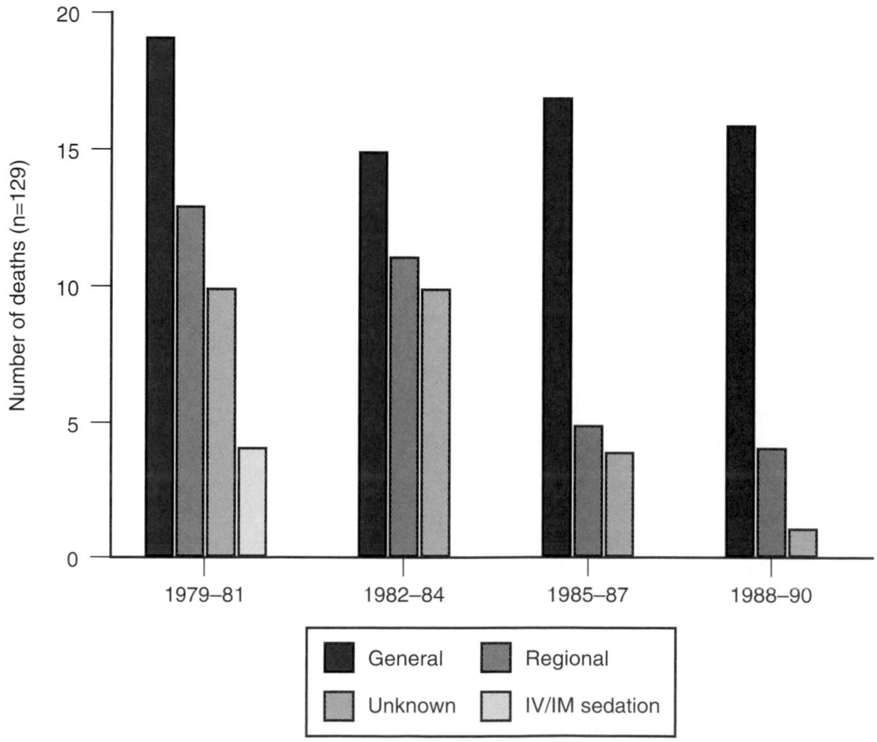

FIGURE 72–2
Anesthesia-related maternal deaths by types of anesthesia, United States, 1979–1990. (From Hawkins JL, Koonin LM, Palmer SK, et al: Anesthesia-related deaths during obstetric delivery in the United States, 1979–1990. Anesthesiology 1997;86:277–284.)

TABLE 72–1

Contraindications to Central Neuraxial Anesthesia

Absolute Contraindications
Patient refusal or inability to cooperate
Localized infection at the insertion site
Sepsis
Severe coagulopathy
Uncorrected hypovolemia
Relative Contraindications
Mild coagulopathy
Severe maternal cardiac disease (including congenital and acquired disorders)
Neurologic disease (including intracranial and spinal cord disorders)
Severe fetal depression

capillary engorgement of the oropharyngeal and respiratory mucosa makes these structures more friable, vascular, and edematous.[13] With labor, the airway structures become further engorged, making the oropharyngeal area even smaller.[14] In addition, the anteroposterior and transverse diameters of the thorax increase during pregnancy, resulting in a substernal angle that, in combination with increases in breast tissue, serve to make laryngoscopy more challenging. Finally, arterial oxygen desaturation occurs more quickly in apneic parturients due to a smaller functional residual capacity and increased oxygen consumption. These alterations make the provision of general anesthesia more challenging; difficult intubations with the need for special airway management devices and techniques were observed in up to 16% of the cases in a 6-year report of general anesthesia performed for cesarean delivery in a tertiary care hospital.[4] Complications such as these have promoted the use of central neuraxial techniques for labor and delivery.

MANAGEMENT OPTIONS FOR PAIN DURING PARTURITION

Nonpharmacologic Techniques

Psychological support and sensory stimulation are two basic classifications of nonpharmacologic modalities for the reduction of pain during labor. The most popular forms of psychological support are "natural childbirth" and "psychoprophylaxis," which were popularized by Dick-Read and Fernand Lamaze, respectively. These methods, which utilize a series of preparative classes to explain the process of labor and teach methods for relaxation and allaying pain, have been observed to reduce the amount of analgesia used,[15] but the degree of pain relief experienced appears limited.[16,17] Potential problems with these techniques include hyperventilation[18] and postpartum depression if analgesic techniques are eventually utilized.[19] Hypnosis, a temporary alteration in consciousness characterized by increased suggestibility, focuses on producing physical and mental relaxation and changing the interpretation of physical stimuli. Although few randomized controlled trials have evaluated the modality, a recent meta-analysis[20] reports that hypnosis can be successful in the management of labor pain. Trained individuals called doulas can also be a source of emotional and physical support during labor. When doulas provide continuous, rather than intermittent, support during labor and delivery, a decrease in analgesia, labor duration, and instrumented deliveries has been observed.[21]

Sensory stimulation, including massage, superficial application of heat and cold, hydrotherapy, acupuncture and acupressure, transcutaneous electrical nerve stimulation (TENS), intradermal sterile water blocks, and music and audio analgesia are all methods of sensory stimulation and have been used with some success during labor. These methods are hypothesized to use innocuous stimuli, such as touch, vibration, and pressure, to compete with painful stimuli at the site of their convergence in the substantia gelatinosa of the dorsal horn of the spinal cord. This competitive inhibition, accompanied by descending messages from the brain cortex and brainstem, is believed to modulate the transmission of pain information. To date, few randomized controlled trials have been performed with these modalities, and thus, only limited conclusions can be drawn. Reviews of trials with labor analgesia produced by acupuncture and TENS demonstrate a high degree of patient acceptability and satisfaction, despite a weak analgesic-sparing effect.[20,22] The novel use of TENS as an adjuvant to other modalities has been investigated. Tsen and associates found that TENS was ineffective in augmenting the duration or quality of analgesia produced by small amounts of spinal or epidural local anesthetics and opiates during labor.[23,24] Overall, despite the limited scientific evidence supporting the analgesic value of these psychological and sensory stimulation modalities, many patients consider them to be an integral and helpful part of their labor experience.

Systemic Medications

Medications given by injection were among the first agents routinely utilized for childbirth pain relief. The combination of scopolamine, an anticholinergic, and morphine to induce a combination of analgesia, sedation, and amnesia termed "twilight sleep" was utilized routinely in the 1950s and 1960s for labor and delivery.[25] Scopolamine, now more commonly utilized as an antiemetic, eventually lost favor to other more effective forms of analgesia with fewer side effects such as delirium, agitation, and excitement.

Oral, subcutaneous, intramuscular, and intravenous injection techniques have all been utilized for administration of systemic labor analgesia. Owing to their more rapid onset and ease of administration, intramuscular

(IM) and intravenous (IV) routes have emerged as the most popular forms. Time to onset, duration, and degree of analgesia with IM analgesic agents can be affected by the habitus of the patient and the site of the injection. Injection into the deltoid muscle, for instance, will result in better absorption than injection into the less perfused gluteus muscle. Patient-controlled analgesia (PCA), which utilizes a pump programmed to give a dose of an IV analgesic on demand outside a defined lock-out period, has created interest, especially when neuraxial analgesia is not available or is contraindicated.[26]

Opioids, despite their side effects of nausea, emesis, drowsiness, dysphoria, hypoventilation, and neonatal respiratory depression, are the most widely used medications for labor analgesia because of their availability and the degree of analgesia produced. Although frequently substituted with meperidine, an agent which results in less neonatal depression at equianalgesic doses,[27] morphine is given in doses of 5 to 10 mg IM or 2 to 3 mg IV for a peak effect in 2 hours and 20 minutes, respectively. Meperidine (trade name Demerol; known as pethidine in Europe), the most commonly used narcotic for labor analgesia, is given in dosages of 50 to 100 mg IM or 10 to 50 mg IV to produce 2 to 4 hours of pain relief. To minimize neonatal respiratory depression, IM administration of meperidine should be avoided within a window of 1 to 3 hours before delivery.[28] (Of course, that is easier said than done; many women thought to be hours away from giving birth deliver suddenly and unexpectedly. In practice, provided that bag and mask ventilation of the neonate and IM naloxone are given, the risk to the baby from IM meperidine is minimal.) Fentanyl, alfentanil, and sufentanil are potent synthetic morphine analogues that are generally not used intramuscularly due to their short duration of action and narrow therapeutic index; with the advent of PCA, however, these agents are being used more frequently.[26] Opioids with agonist/antagonist properties have the advantage of a "ceiling effect" for maternal respiratory depression, and include pentazocine, nalbuphine and butorphanol. Pentazocine is utilized less commonly because of its potential for the psychomimetic effects of dysphoria and a perception of impending death.[29] Nalbuphine and butorphanol are given in IM or IV doses of 3 to 5 mg or 1 to 2 mg, respectively, and are equianalgesic to meperidine with less nausea and emesis.[30]

Tranquilizers such as benzodiazepines and phenothiazines are occasionally used to reduce anxiety during labor and delivery. Diazepam can be used in doses up to 10 mg,[31] but lorazepam and midazolam should be avoided owing to their pronounced neonatal depressant and maternal amnesic effects, respectively. Phenothiazines can be used synergistically to reduce the dose of opioids, thereby increasing sedation and reducing side effects. Hydroxyzine given in doses of 50 to 100 mg IM and promethazine given in doses of 24 to 50 mg IM or 15 to 25 mg IV have been observed to improve maternal analgesia without significant neonatal effects.[32] Promazine, chloropromazine, and prochlorperazine are avoided because of their strong alpha-adrenergic blocking activity, which can produce hypotension.[33]

Barbiturates, such as secobarbital and pentobarbital, can allay anxiety. However, as a class, the efficacy of these agents during labor is limited owing to their lack of analgesic properties, their potential to increase the sensation of pain, and the presence of protracted effects on the newborn.[34] In low doses of 0.2 to 0.5 mg/kg IV, ketamine can produce intense analgesia with limited neonatal effects; however, maternal dysphoric reactions may result.[35] Midazolam 2 to 4 mg IV can decrease these effects. In higher doses of 1 to 2 mg/kg, ketamine can be used as induction agent for general anesthesia; however, when the dose exceeds 2 mg/kg, increases in uterine tone may occur and be associated with lower Apgar scores or abnormally increased neonatal muscle tone.[35]

Inhalational Analgesia

The first form of analgesia used for labor in modern medicine, inhalational analgesia remains popular in many institutions, particularly in Europe. Inhalation of subanesthetic doses of nitrous oxide, trichloroethylene, methoxyflurane, enflurane, isoflurane, and recently, sevoflurane has been used to provide safe and effective analgesia during labor and delivery. Most effective during the early stages of labor, inhaled analgesics are administered either intermittently (i.e., during contractions only) or continuously with the dose regulated according to the patient's response. The most common formulation in current use, a mixture of 50% nitrous oxide and 50% oxygen (Entonox),[36] has been demonstrated to bring relief to approximately 50% of parturients and can be used as an adjuvant, but not a complete analgesic, to a pudendal nerve block for forceps delivery, perineal suturing, or manual removal of the placenta.[37] Advocates who embrace the inhalational technique suggest that it safely provides amnesia and analgesia; those who do not use the technique, cite the possible loss of consciousness, diminished airway reflexes with the associated risk for aspiration and hypoxia, and unscavenged gas pollution of the labor suite. The risk for loss of consciousness and airway reflexes are more commonly witnessed with halogenated agents.

In rare instances, general anesthesia is induced with inhalational halogenated agents (e.g., isoflurane) for vaginal delivery. Two of the more common scenarios include a need for greater anesthesia without time to administer a regional anesthetic (i.e., fetal distress requiring forceps delivery) or a need for maximum uterine relaxation (i.e., need for intrauterine manipulation). In contrast to regional anesthetics, halogenated agents cause uterine relaxation in a dose-dependent manner,[38] with the administration of greater than 0.5% minimum alveolar concentration (MAC) potentially decreasing uterine smooth muscle responses to oxytocin.[39]

Regional Analgesia and Anesthesia

A variety of regional techniques can provide pain relief for labor and delivery. As both expected and unexpected physiologic sequelae may occur following these techniques, intravenous access should be established and resuscitation equipment should be readily available.

Paracervical Block

A technique that relies on blocking the nerve ganglion located immediately lateral and posterior to the cervicouterine junction, the paracervical block is primarily effective for the first stage of labor. Owing to the frequent occurrence of fetal bradycardia, which may result from local anesthetic-induced uteroplacental vasoconstriction or direct fetal myocardial depression, this technique is now used infrequently.[40]

Lumbar Sympathetic Block

By blocking the visceral afferent sensory fibers that accompany the lumbar sympathetic chain, lumbar sympathetic block provides analgesia limited primarily to the first stage of labor. Although seldom used due to the need for multiple injections, this technique has been advocated for labor analgesia due to the near absence of motor blockade.[26,41]

Pudendal Block

Effective for the second stage of labor, the use of outlet forceps, and episiotomy repairs, this block interrupts the terminal nerve transmissions of the pudendal nerve. Owing to the distal nature of the nerve blockade, this form of anesthesia is not effective for midforceps delivery, postpartum examination or repair of the upper vagina or cervix, or exploration of the uterine cavity.[42] Maternal and neonatal blood levels of local anesthetic following a pudendal block are comparable to those seen following an epidural technique.[43]

Perineal Infiltration

Perhaps the most commonly performed local anesthetic technique for labor and delivery, perineal infiltration interrupts pain transmissions from the terminal nerves in the posterior fourchette. Because direct injection into the fetal scalp can occur, the quickly metabolized agent 2-chloroprocaine may be preferable to lidocaine or longer-acting local anesthetics.[44]

Caudal Block

A technique that uses the lowermost segment of the epidural space, the caudal block has lost favor to the higher, more approachable lumbar block. The change to the lumbar approach was also motivated by the association of the caudal block with inadvertent injections of anesthetic into the fetal head, the theoretical increased risks of infection due to a closer proximity to the rectum, and difficulty in extending the cephalad level of the blockade for cesarean delivery.

Antenatal Use of Regional Techniques: External Cephalic Version

Epidural, spinal, and combined spinal-epidural (CSE) techniques have all been used to promote external cephalic version (ECV) and have all been reported to improve success rates compared with control subjects. Schorr and associates[45] randomized 69 patients (all of whom received tocolytics to relax the uterus) to undergo an ECV attempt either with or without epidural anesthesia. In demographically and obstetrically similar groups, the success on the first attempt as well as the overall success rate of ECV was higher in the epidural group (69% versus 32%). No cases of fetal distress or abruptio placentae were observed in either group, and ultimately, vaginal delivery occurred in 66% of the epidural group versus 21% in the control group. In comparison to tocolytics, a preliminary report by Samuels and associates[46] noted greater success with an epidural anesthetic versus ritodrine (29 of 38, 76.3% versus 23 of 38, 60.1%).

Spinal techniques have also been used for ECV attempts, with varying analgesic doses resulting in contrasting results. Dugoff and associates[47] noted no improvement with the spinal administration of bupivacaine 2.5 mg with sufentanil 10 μg (44% versus 42%), whereas Birnbach and associates[48] noted a significant improvement (80% versus 33%) with the use of sufentanil 10 μg alone. Reasons for these contrasting outcomes may reflect differences in obstetric or patient factors, including the amount of force applied or the degree of maternal discomfort tolerated for a given level of analgesia. As a consequence, the ability of spinal analgesia to improve ECV version success requires further investigation. By contrast, when spinal anesthesia (lidocaine 45 mg with fentanyl 10 μg) was used, even in the more difficult setting of previously failed ECV attempts, a high success rate (83%) has been reported.[49]

Whether utilized for primary or failed ECV attempts, a CSE technique with a short duration spinal anesthetic may represent the optimal technique.[49] The short anesthetic duration allows for a timely discharge from hospital in the event of a successful version, and if success or failure results in either a trial of labor or an operative delivery on the same day, the epidural catheter can be left in place to allow additional analgesia or anesthesia to be administered.

Central neuraxial analgesic and anesthetic techniques most likely improve ECV success by relaxing the abdominal wall muscles, improving patient comfort during the ECV attempt, and allowing the obstetrician to make a more concerted attempt.[48,50] The use of anesthetic techniques for ECV attempts has been associated with an improved maternal and fetal outcome, a reduced need for emergent operative deliveries, and a favorable cost-benefit analysis.[50,51]

Anesthesia for Vaginal Delivery

Spinal Anesthesia

The finite duration of action of a single injection, and an increased risk of a postdural puncture headache with multiple injections, limit the utility of spinal anesthesia for the management of labor. Spinal techniques, however, can be used successfully during delivery, especially in the event of an assisted vaginal breech delivery, the need to use outlet forceps or vacuum extraction, or the repair of extensive tears or lacerations. For these procedures, a low level spinal anesthetic block can be used; in the event of a "trial of forceps," consideration should be given to providing a dose appropriate for a cesarean delivery. Clear communication between the obstetrician and anesthetist on their expectations regarding delivery is essential if the optimal technique is to be chosen. Applications of the spinal technique that offer more flexibility include its use as part of a CSE technique (discussed later) or the placement of a catheter into the spinal space, called a "spinal catheter" or "continuous spinal anesthesia" technique. The benefits of these techniques have been observed particularly in patients with conditions such as morbid obesity and cardiac disorders, or following an unintentional dural puncture with an attempted epidural catheter placement as a method for providing a reliable, precisely titratable blockade.[52] For most patients, however, the spinal catheter option is less attractive, as it most often accompanies the use of epidural equipment (17-gauge Touhy needle to place a 20-gauge catheter), which results in a large dural puncture and a significant risk of a postdural puncture headache. Current trials with smaller needles and catheters for labor and delivery are currently being conducted in the United States and Europe, with the hope that a better understanding of the technique and the medications utilized will avoid the complications observed with earlier trials of microcatheters.[53,54]

COMPLICATIONS

A number of complications may occur following a spinal technique. Hypotension, defined as a 20% to 30% decrease in systolic blood pressure from baseline, can be observed in 20% to 100% of pregnant women and is due to the sympathetic vasomotor blockade produced.[55] If left uncorrected for even a brief period of time, hypotension may result in decreased uteroplacental perfusion with resulting hypoxia and fall in pH of the fetus.[56] Preventive measures include maternal intravascular volume expansion (preloading with IV fluid, usually 500 to 1000 mL of crystalloid such as Hartmann's solution) and avoidance of aortocaval compression, and treatment includes titrated doses of vasopressors such as ephedrine (5–10 mg) and phenylephrine (40–100 μg) given intravenously. The nausea and vomiting following a spinal technique may be associated with reductions in sympathetic tone, blood pressure, and cerebral blood flow and can be reduced significantly with vasopressor use.[57] Postdural puncture headache (PDPH) occurs in approximately 1% to 3% of the obstetric population following a spinal technique and is most likely related to the needle size and tip design, with larger, cutting needles associated with a greater incidence.[58] Typically, a PDPH presents as a positional headache that worsens in the upright position and improves in the recumbent position. The differential diagnosis should include other types of headache, hypertensive disorders, infectious diseases, dural venous sinus thromboses, and other intracranial pathologies. If the diagnosis is a PDPH, bed rest may aid in pain relief,[59] and conservative measures of hydration and oral intake of caffeinated and analgesic products (including Fioricet or Fiorinal) may be used for 24 to 48 hours. An epidural blood patch, whereby 10 to 20 mL of autologous blood is placed in the epidural space, has been associated with a greater than 80% incidence of success in most trials.[58,60] Although the incidence of neurologic complications as a result of spinal anesthesia in the obstetric population is extremely rare,[60] consultation with a neurologist may assist in diagnosis and treatment. Finally, an unexpected high level of anesthesia can result in hypotension, dyspnea, the inability to speak, and a loss of consciousness; ventilatory and circulatory support should always be readily available when this technique is provided.

Epidural Analgesia and Anesthesia

One of the most effective methods of pain relief for labor and delivery,[5] the epidural technique with an indwelling catheter provides a reliable form of analgesia that can be titrated as the situation evolves. Should the need arise for surgical anesthesia for an instrumental or operative delivery, laceration repair, or postpartum tubal ligation, this can be provided with a change in the local anesthetics used through the catheter.

The choice of agents for use in the epidural space depends on the degree of pain relief required. During labor and delivery, adequate sensory analgesia with minimal motor blockade is the goal. Optimally, this would allow the pregnant woman to appreciate a sense of pressure, without pain, during each contraction. Almost every local anesthetic developed has been tested for its value in obstetric analgesia. Of the shorter-acting agents, mepivacaine has been reported as having a prolonged half-life and causing neonatal depression. Chloroprocaine 3% and lidocaine 2% produce surgical anesthesia, and the dense sensory and motor block they produce make them less appropriate for vaginal delivery. The longer-acting agents are best suited for labor analgesia when used in low concentrations. Bupivacaine, with a high degree of sensory to motor block, is the most commonly used agent for labor epidural analgesia worldwide. Concentrations of 0.0625% to 0.125% are commonly used to initiate and maintain the block. Ropivacaine and levo-bupivacaine are two newer longer-acting agents that, when given in equipotent concentrations to bupivacaine, may result in slightly less motor blockade and cardiotoxic effects.[61,62] The dose, onset, and duration of various local anesthetics for epidural labor analgesia are well characterized (Table 72–2). Although sufficient for many parturients in the first stage of labor, epidural narcotics alone routinely fail during the second and third stages of labor.[63,64] The combination of narcotics with local anesthetics in the epidural space, however, enhances the quality of analgesia and allows a decrease in the total dose of local anesthetic required. Epidural administration of small doses of sufentanil (0.2–0.3 μg/mL) or fentanyl (0.2 μg/mL) combined with the low doses of bupivacaine 0.0625% or 0.125% result in excellent analgesia for vaginal delivery. In addition, an epidural fentanyl bolus of 50 μg, with or without local anesthetic, can be of assistance during the second stage of labor when patchy analgesia or perineal sparing cannot be remedied with local anesthetics alone.[65]

Once the initial sensory blockade has been established, epidural analgesia can be maintained by intermittent bolus injections, a continuous infusion, or both techniques simultaneously. The development of inexpensive infusion pumps has offered perhaps the optimal method: a continuous infusion coupled with patient-controlled intermittent bolus top-up injections through the epidural catheter. This combined method reduces the total amount of medication used, decreases the amount of motor blockade, and increases patient satisfaction when compared to continuous infusions or intermittent bolus methodologies alone.[66,67]

Combined Spinal-Epidural Analgesia

Introduced in the early 1980s for surgical procedures, the CSE technique, with a few modifications, has become one of the most popular techniques for labor analgesia. The technique consists of epidural needle placement, intraspinal medication administered via a spinal needle placed through the shaft of the epidural needle into the subarachnoid space, and then placement of an epidural catheter. In comparison to the epidural or spinal techniques alone, the CSE technique has a number of advantages (Table 72–3). A mixture of local anesthetics with narcotics appears to be the optimal combination for initial labor analgesia with this technique, and its application, even early in labor, may have beneficial effects on the progress of labor.[68] Used later in labor, the CSE technique can provide quick onset of analgesia and the ability to extend the duration or level of the blockade should delivery methods mandate such augmentation.

COMPLICATIONS

Relatively few complications are inherent to the CSE technique. The risks of a dural puncture with the epidural needle may actually be reduced, as the spinal needle, when placed in through the shaft of the epidural needle, emerges 10 to 15 mm beyond the tip of the epidural needle.[69] The emergence of cerebrospinal fluid through the spinal needle indicates that the dura has been traversed and thus serves to locate the relative position of the tip of the larger epidural needle. The likelihood of the epidural catheter passing through the spinal needle dural puncture site is low, based on laboratory-based and clinical studies.[70] Drugs placed in the epidural space can pass through the dural hole created by the spinal needle and there is a theoretical possibility of producing a dense or high spinal blockade. In the majority of cases, however, the amount of medication is very

TABLE 72–2

Local Anesthetics for Epidural Analgesia and Anesthesia

ANESTHETIC	USUAL CONCENTRATION (%)	ONSET	DURATION
Analgesia			
Lidocaine	1–1.5	Moderate	Intermediate
Bupivacaine	0.0625–0.25	Slow	Long
L-Bupivacaine	0.0625–0.25	Slow	Long
Ropivacaine	0.1–0.2	Slow	Long
Anesthesia			
2-Chloroprocaine	2–3	Fast	Short
Lidocaine	2–5	Moderate	Intermediate
Mepivacaine	2	Moderate	Intermediate
Bupivacaine	0.5	Slow	Long
L-Bupivacaine	0.5	Slow	Long
Ropivacaine	0.5–1	Slow	Long
Tetracaine	1	Slow	Long

TABLE 72–3

Advantages of the Combined Spinal-Epidural Technique for Labor Analgesia

Advantages over an Epidural Technique
More rapid onset
Lower maternal, fetal, and neonatal blood concentrations of local anesthetic than with epidural techniques alone.
Better sacral analgesia
Assists in identification of the epidural space in technically difficult placements
Advantages over a Spinal Technique
Allows ability to titrate the level, density, and duration of the blockade
Catheter can be used for postoperative pain management

limited and may actually improve sacral or perineal analgesia[71]; the risk of a high spinal blockade appears in practice to be negligible.

The failure of subsequent medication given through the epidural catheter to produce adequate analgesia/anesthesia is of greater concern. Because the spinal portion of a CSE technique gives an initial period of analgesia, the epidural catheter that has been placed is "untested" and may not be reliable as a route for further injection of anesthetic should an emergency arise. Although epidemiologic evidence suggests that the epidural catheter following a CSE technique has a lower failure rate than a solely epidural technique,[72] in those parturients with a difficult airway or a high probability of an instrumental or operative delivery, a standard epidural technique, which tests the function of the catheter at the time of placement, may be safer.

MANAGEMENT OPTIONS FOR ANESTHESIA FOR CESAREAN DELIVERY

Despite repeated calls to reduce the rate of cesarean deliveries from both lay and professional organizations in the United States and Europe, the incidence of surgical delivery continues to increase. Although there is now a long history of safety improvements for general anesthesia for cesarean delivery, the majority of maternal deaths due to anesthesia still occur during the actual or attempted provision of general anesthesia. However, in deciding between regional and general anesthetic techniques, the urgency of the procedure, the health and comorbidities of the mother and fetus, and the desires of the mother and health care providers all need to be considered.

Spinal Anesthesia

A simple and reliable technique with rapid onset, spinal anesthesia optimally provides an awake and comfortable patient with minimal risks for aspiration. Despite the lower abdominal incision, a T4 dermatome level is required to prevent referred pain from traction on the peritoneum and uterus. The type and dose of local anesthetic medications used to provide the spinal anesthetic must include consideration of the level of medication desired, the duration of the surgery, the postoperative analgesia plan, and the preference of the anesthesiologist. Hyperbaric bupivacaine is the agent most commonly used because it provides a blockade of long duration while avoiding the extensive motor block produced by tetracaine. The potential toxicity advantages of ropivacaine and levo-bupivacaine are limited given the extremely small doses of agent used. The use of adjuvant spinal medications, such as narcotics and epinephrine, may augment the quality and duration of the anesthesia and analgesia.[73,74]

Following the administration of a spinal technique, the patient may complain of dyspnea. Dyspnea can be due to several factors, including the blunting of thoracic proprioception, the partial blockade of abdominal and intercostal muscles, and the recumbent position increasing the pressure of the abdominal contents against the diaphragm. Despite these changes, significant respiratory compromise is unlikely as the blockade rarely affects the cervical nerves that control the diaphragm. Should the patient lose the ability to vocalize, give a strong hand grip, or demonstrate normal oxygen saturation by pulse oximetry, a rapid sequence induction with cricoid pressure and placement of an endotracheal tube can be performed to maintain ventilation and prevent pulmonary soiling with gastrointestinal contents.

The most common complications of spinal anesthesia have been described earlier and include hypotension, nausea and vomiting, and the risk of a postdural puncture headache. Hypotension presents the greatest risk to maternal and fetal comfort and health[55]; prevention and prompt treatment with infusion of IV fluid and administration of vasopressors have been noted to be beneficial but, on occasion, not completely successful.[75,76] In terms of volume expansion, spinal anesthesia in the urgent setting should not be delayed until a fixed, arbitrary volume has been infused. In addition, aggressive hydration with large fluid volumes (greater than 20 mL/kg crystalloid) may increase the risk of edema with only limited reductions in hypotension.[75] Colloid solutions appear more effective than crystalloids in preventing the hemodynamic consequences of spinal anesthesia[77] but have allergic, cost, and coagulation implications. Current investigations in vasopressors for prevention and treatment of hypotension in this setting include the use of phenylephrine, sometimes in combination with ephedrine, and the use of infusion pumps.[78]

Epidural Anesthesia

Epidural anesthesia for cesarean delivery has increased since the 1980s, primarily due to the widespread use of the epidural technique for labor analgesia; the use of epidural anesthesia for cesarean section has also increased. Although medications used in the spinal and epidural space are identical, epidural doses are 5 to 10 times greater and of much larger volumes to encourage adequate blockade and spread. These dose alterations can be explained primarily by anatomic differences in nerve exposure and the capacity of the spaces.

Advantages of the epidural technique include a lower incidence and degree of maternal hypotension due to the ability of the compensatory mechanisms to respond to the more slowly developing sympathetic blockade. In addition, if a catheter is used, the level, density, and duration of the anesthesia can be titrated. The greater sensitivity of nerves to local anesthetics during pregnancy has been observed clinically through a decrease in anesthetic requirements for epidural blockade.[79,80] For cesarean delivery, the most common agents used are 2% lidocaine with epinephrine 1:200,000 and 3% 2-chloroprocaine. Chloroprocaine is the agent of choice for emergency cesarean deliveries because of its rapid onset and rapid maternal and fetal metabolism; fetal accumulation, especially when acidosis is present, is therefore minimized.[81] By contrast, chloroprocaine is avoided for routine, nonurgent deliveries as the short duration requires multiple doses, and its use can adversely affect the efficacy of subsequent epidural opioid analgesia.[82] In addition, when used in higher total volumes (>40 mL), chloroprocaine can increase the incidence of back pain.[83] Alkalinization with sodium bicarbonate hastens the onset time of local anesthetics significantly and is recommended for use in urgent cesarean deliveries;[84] caution must be applied in its use, however, as certain local anesthetics (particularly bupivacaine) have a low threshold for precipitation.[85]

The complications of epidural anesthesia have been described previously and include hypotension, risk of postdural puncture headache, systemic toxic reactions, and rarely, neurologic complications. Epidural techniques can provide patchy or inadequate blockade due to anatomic or technical reasons;[86] often, these failures can be identified a priori through observation of the degree of labor epidural analgesia, or quickly after partial augmentation of the blockade. Alternative techniques, such as supplementation with intravenous or inhalational agents, spinal anesthesia, or general anesthesia, must always be considered as options.

Combined Spinal-Epidural Anesthesia

The principal advantage of the CSE technique is the ability to augment the density or duration of the anesthesia through the use of the epidural catheter. This is particularly useful in obstetrics, in which a delay in the timing prior to or during surgery can potentially occur (e.g., possible placenta accreta, history of multiple abdominal surgeries, high index of suspicion for gravid hysterectomy). A guiding principle in the selection of the CSE technique is whether the parturient appears to have an airway that would be difficult to intubate; a patient who presents as an intubation risk would perhaps be better served by avoiding the CSE technique, as the epidural catheter is "untested" and may not provide optimal anesthesia when needed.

Contraindications to Regional Anesthesia

Although regional anesthesia is used whenever possible to avoid the potential airway complications associated with general anesthesia, certain conditions or time constraints may contraindicate its use.[4] Such comorbidities include localized infection or generalized sepsis, coagulations disorders, severe hypovolemia, or cardiac disorders in which hypotension may be detrimental. Severe obstetric hemorrhage in the antepartum period, including uterine rupture and acute, severe fetal distress, may also contraindicate regional anesthesia procedures because of the time necessary to establish a surgical anesthetic.

Patients with severe preeclampsia or hypertension may undergo rapid hemodynamic changes with regional techniques; however, both epidural and spinal techniques can and have been used successfully in this setting.[87,88] In addition, gravid hysterectomies have been performed safely with regional techniques.[89] Overall, however, if questions exist regarding the ability of maternal compensatory mechanisms to react to the regional anesthetic or surgery, general anesthesia should be considered.

General Anesthesia

There are few, if any, absolute contraindications to general anesthesia; however, regional anesthesia remains a preferred method to avoid the risks of airway management and allow the patient the ability to witness the delivery. General anesthesia, however, may offer advantages when uterine relaxation would be beneficial; such cases include difficult breech extractions, retained placenta, uterine inversion, or in utero fetal surgery.

The importance of proper airway evaluation, during the antenatal period or in early labor if possible, cannot be overemphasized, as failed intubation, failed ventilation and oxygenation, and pulmonary aspiration of gastric contents are the leading anesthetic causes of maternal death.[90,91] If the airway evaluation suggests the possibility of a difficult intubation, strong consideration should be given to the establishment of a continuous neuraxial technique early in labor.[92] If a difficult airway is discovered upon an intubation attempt, options include allowing the patient to awaken, using alternate techniques to place an endotracheal tube, or using alternative airway devices. The laryngeal mask airway (LMA), although not able to prevent pulmonary soiling with gastric contents as efficiently as an endotracheal tube, can be a lifesaving measure in failed intubation situations,[93] and has been used safely in elective cesarean deliveries.[94]

Attempts should be made to minimize the risk of maternal aspiration, even when the need for intubation is not anticipated. With an elective cesarean delivery, adherence to a nil per os (NPO, nil by mouth) policy for 8 hours prior to surgery is advised. A nonparticulate antacid is believed to decrease the damage to the respiratory epithelium if aspiration occurs,[95] and H_2 antagonists (cimetidine, ranitidine) and promotility agents (metoclopramide) can reduce gastric acid secretion and facilitate emptying, respectively.[96,97]

Preoxygenation and denitrogenation with 100% oxygen reduces the rapidity of onset of any hypoxemia due to the parturient's decreased functional residual capacity and increased oxygen consumption. In urgent situations, four vital capacity breaths of 100% oxygen will provide adequate preoxygenation.[98] Succinylcholine is given with a defasciculating dose of a nondepolarizing agent and can be continued as an infusion, or a short-acting nondepolarizing agent can be used alone. Although nitrous oxide is often used in concentrations of 50% until delivery, the addition of halogenated volatile anesthetics reduces the response to surgical stimulation, although it also reduces awareness, which may be less desirable.[99] The 25% to 40% increase in sensitivity to halogenated agents during pregnancy allows lower doses to be used;[100] this may be of benefit in attenuating the side effects of volatile agents, which reduce uterine tone and interfere with the action of oxytocin.[101] Comparisons of neonatal outcomes following general versus epidural anesthesia for cesarean delivery suggest small, transient differences;[102] however, with either technique, when the uterine incision to delivery is greater than 180 seconds, lower Apgar scores and greater fetal acidosis have been observed (although this may reflect relative difficulty in delivery of the baby rather than the direct effects of the anesthetic agents).[103] Later redistribution of general anesthetic agents from the fetal fat to the circulation can result in secondary depression of neonatal ventilatory effort; and the presence of a pediatrician in such cases is probably advisable until a normal ventilatory pattern is observed.

MANAGEMENT OPTIONS FOR POSTOPERATIVE PAIN

Since 1979, when Wang and associates[104] published the first report of spinal opioid administration in humans, the analgesic efficacy of epidural and spinal opioids has been demonstrated by numerous investigations.[105] By directly activating spinal and supraspinal opioid receptors, epidural and spinal opioids blunt nociceptive input and produce analgesia of greater intensity than doses administered parenterally or intramuscularly (Fig. 72–3).[106,107] As such, a number of opioids, including meperidine, fentanyl, sufentanil, hydromorphone, diamorphine, methadone, buprenorphine, and butorphanol, have been utilized in the epidural and spinal spaces (Table 72–4). Morphine, however, has emerged as the most common agent used internationally for postcesarean delivery pain management owing to its long duration of action and low cost.

In the epidural space, the low lipid solubility of morphine slows the penetration into the spinal tissues. This results in peak analgesic effects that are delayed 60 to 90 minutes[108] but persist to provide reliable analgesia for up to 24 hours.[108,109] Up to 5 mg of epidural morphine has been used for postcesarean analgesia, although lower amounts have been utilized with similar success.[109–111] In a prospective, randomized manner, Palmer and associates[111] performed a dose ranging study of 1.25 to 5 mg of morphine used epidurally for postcesarean analgesia, and observed that the quality of analgesia increased to a dose of 3.75 mg; increasing the dose further to 5 mg did not further improve analgesia. Of interest, the side effects of pruritus and nausea were not dose-related. The use of an infusion of naloxone, a narcotic antagonist, can reduce the severity but not the incidence of pruritus following epidural morphine.[112]

The choice of local anesthetic for epidural anesthesia may influence the efficacy of epidural morphine. Kotelko

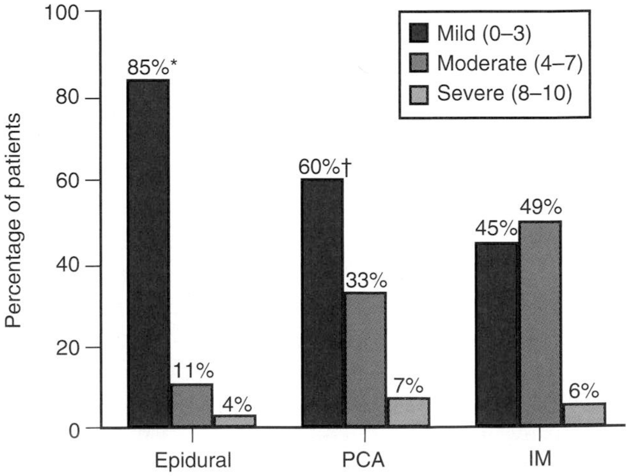

FIGURE 72–3
Percentage of patients recovering from cesarean section and treated with either epidural, patient-controlled intravenous analgesia (PCA), or intramuscular morphine (IM) and reporting mild, moderate, or severe discomfort over a 24-hour period. $^*P < 0.05$ denotes epidural versus PCA and IM. $^†P$ = NS denotes PCA versus IM. (From Harrison DM, Dinatra RS, Morgese L, et al: Epidural narcotic and PCA for postcesarean section pain relief. Anesthesiology 1988;68:454–457.)

TABLE 72-4

Neuraxial Opioids

OPIOID	EPIDURAL DOSE	SPINAL DOSE	DURATION (H)	COMMENTS
Morphine	2.5–5 mg	0.1–0.2 mg	18–24	Gold standard
Fentanyl	50–100 μg	10–20 μg	3–4	Useful as an intraoperative adjuvant
Sufentanil	10–20 μg	5–10 μg	3–4	Useful as an intraoperative adjuvant
Meperidine	25 mg		2–3	
Hydromorphone	1 mg		12	
Methadone	4–5 mg		5–6	
Diamorphine	2.5–5 mg		5–15	Not available in United States

and associates[113] observed that postcesarean analgesia was significantly reduced, usually to less than 3 hours, in patients who received 2-chloroprocaine (a short-acting, rapid-onset local anesthetic used primarily for emergent cesarean deliveries) versus other local anesthetics.

Continuous, low concentration epidural infusions of local anesthetics with opioids may also offer an analgesic option in patients in whom prolonged duration and level of analgesia are desired.[114] The infusion of low doses of bupivacaine combined with either fentanyl or morphine has been noted to provide good postcesarean analgesia and can be operated via patient-controlled infusion pumps.[115]

The delivery of a single spinal dose of opioid has also become an attractive option for postcesarean analgesia. With a duration of action (18 to 24 hours) and side effect profile similar to its use in the epidural space, morphine has also become the leading opioid utilized spinally.[116,117] Owing to the direct access to opioid receptors, such agents are given spinally at approximately one tenth of their epidural dose. Despite this degree of access, morphine still requires 45 to 60 minutes for peak effect. Palmer and associates[73] observed little advantage in utilizing greater than 0.1 mg of morphine for postcesarean analgesia when compared to doses up to 0.5 mg; a greater incidence of pruritus, but not nausea and vomiting, was noted with higher doses.

Postoperative analgesia has been greatly improved through the use of central neuraxial techniques, most commonly provided through a single-dose administration of morphine. Given in the spinal and epidural compartments, opioids provide an enhanced quality and duration with a very acceptable side effect profile when compared to oral or intravenous analgesics.

MANAGEMENT OPTIONS FOR ANALGESIA AND ANESTHESIA IN HIGH RISK PARTURIENTS

Invasive Monitoring (See also Chapter 80)

Although the noninvasive measurement of blood pressure, heart rate, oxygen saturation, urinary output, and fetal cardiotocography is standard practice in most modern labor and delivery facilities, the use of invasive monitors is variable and controversial. Monitoring data, and particularly those from invasive hemodynamic monitors, are best interpreted in relation to all pertinent medical history and physical findings. However, the interpretation of data from cardiovascular monitors remains difficult, despite practice guidelines written by a number of professional organizations, including the joint task force of the American College of Physicians, the American College of Cardiology, and the American Heart Association.[118] A number of studies suggest that the poor collection and incorrect interpretation of hemodynamic data from invasive monitors remain the key problem with their use.[119,120]

In addition to understanding the data produced, knowing when to use invasive monitoring is a vital clinical skill. The indications for invasive arterial blood pressure monitoring during pregnancy are relatively straightforward and include a desire to more carefully manage blood pressure, the lack of reliable noninvasive cuff measurements, the need for vascular access for blood studies, and the planned use of certain hemodynamic agents. By contrast, the indications for invasive central monitoring are not as clear or uniformly accepted. A central venous pressure (CVP) catheter is often placed to yield an approximation of volume status (or to follow a trend in blood loss or replacement therapy) and give a greater understanding of the mechanical phases of the cardiac cycle. Management of oliguria unresponsive to a fluid challenge, pulmonary edema, and refractory hypertension are clinical situations in which some clinicians desire CVP monitoring.

Although a pulmonary artery (PA) catheter can also assist in determining the etiology of pulmonary edema, oliguria with a normal CVP, or cardiovascular failure, its use is the most controversial. Advocates of PA catheter use suggest that it can provide information on left and right ventricular function, systemic vascular resistance, and cardiac output. Detractors question the validity of the data, noting that in the setting of preeclampsia, for example, the correlation between CVP and the pulmonary capillary wedge pressure (PCWP) is unreliable

TABLE 72–5

Pulmonary Artery (PA) Pressures Observed with Different Etiologies of Pulmonary Edema

ETIOLOGY	PA WEDGE PRESSURE	STROKE WORK INDEX
Left ventricular dysfunction	Increased	Decreased
Altered capillary permeability	Normal	Normal or increased
Low hydrostatic-oncotic pressure	Increased	Normal

From Benedetti TJ, Kates R, Williams V: Hemodynamic observations in severe preeclampsia complicated by pulmonary edema. Am J Obstet Gynecol 1985;152:330–334.

when the CVP reading exceeds 6 cm H_2O.[121] In deciding between a PA versus CVP catheter, the clinician should recognize that although the insertion-related complications are similar,[124] the PA catheter is associated with more use-related complications including balloon rupture, pulmonary infarction, valvular damage, and erosion of the pulmonary artery. Thus, the benefits of PA catheter use should clearly outweigh its inherent risks before it can be recommended; the 1999 practice guidelines of the American Society of Anesthesiologists Task Force on Obstetrical Anesthesia state that "the decision to perform invasive hemodynamic monitoring should be individualized and based on clinical indications that include the patient's medical history and cardiovascular risk factors."[125] To date, although PA catheter use has been reported in parturients (primarily with cardiac disease), no controlled trials are available that confirm the benefit of PA catheter monitoring on maternal or fetal outcome. This being noted, the PA pressures observed with different etiologies of pulmonary edema are shown in Table 72–5.[122] Similarly, the PA pressures observed with different etiologies of oliguria are shown in Table 72–6.[123]

Despite being noninvasive (unless a transthoracic probe is placed for echocardiography), future modalities for hemodynamic monitoring may offer greater advantages than currently available. These monitors include Doppler ultrasound and two-dimensional echocardiography, which are able to give detailed, dynamic information on cardiac structures and function.[126]

Hypertensive Disorders of Pregnancy

Whether preexisting, gestational, or a function of preeclampsia or eclampsia, hypertension is a common medical problem in parturients and is associated with higher maternal, fetal, and neonatal mortality and morbidity. Preeclampsia, with its systemic vasoconstriction, intravascular volume and protein depletion, and simultaneous retention of extravascular sodium and water, is of particular concern to anesthesiologists. In addition to individual organ dysfunction, abnormalities in coagulation, and edema of the brain, larynx, and lungs may occur. Medical management of blood pressure should be optimized prior to obstetric or anesthetic interventions if possible, and control with labetalol and hydralazine or infusions of nitroglycerin or nitroprusside should be commenced with arterial and central venous monitoring in severe cases. Prehydration to maintain CVP has been demonstrated to improve urine output, maintain mean arterial pressure, and decrease diastolic pressure.[127] If oliguria persists after normalization of the CVP (usually between 2 and 3 cm H_2O), or the physiologic state is complicated with pulmonary edema or cardiovascular decompensation, a PA catheter may be helpful. A cardiology consultation and an assessment of cardiopulmonary function with a transthoracic echocardiogram may also assist with the diagnosis and management. The course of preeclampsia can be complicated by mild to severe coagulopathy even in the presence of a normal platelet

TABLE 72–6

Pulmonary Artery (PA) Pressures Observed with Different Etiologies of Oliguria

ETIOLOGY	PA WEDGE PRESSURE	LEFT VENTICULAR FUNCTION	SYSTEMIC VASCULAR RESISTANCE	TREATMENT
Low volume	Low	Increased	Increased	Fluid
Renal arteriospasm	Normal	Normal	Normal	Hydralazine
Decreased cardiac output	Increased	Decreased	Increased	Decrease/restrict fluid

From Clark SL, Cotton DB: Clinical indications for pulmonary artery catheterization in the patient with severe preeclampsia. Am J Obstet Gynecol 1988;158:453–458.

count.[128,129] For the benefit of both obstetric and anesthetic management, if the initial platelet count is less than an arbitrary 70 to 75 cells/L^{-9}, the clinical history and the results of additional studies such as a PT/PTT (prothrombin time/partial thromboplastin time) or a thromboelastograph should be reviewed. A risk-benefit analysis will ultimately determine the anesthetic technique of choice and whether the administration of blood products such as fresh frozen plasma or pooled platelets should commence prior to any intervention.

During labor, epidural analgesia offers the advantage of limiting pain or stress, thus reducing catecholamine release, decreasing maternal blood pressure, and indirectly increasing placental perfusion.[127] Epidural anesthesia can also be a preferred technique for cesarean delivery due to the ability to slowly titrate the dose of medications as an aid to the management of blood pressure. The possibility of spinal technique–induced hypotension should not necessarily eliminate this anesthetic option. Although data are limited, one small prospective randomized study of preeclamptic women did not reveal significant blood pressure differences between spinal and epidural anesthesia.[130] A retrospective study of women with severe preeclampsia also observed that the incidence of hypotension was not different between spinal or epidural anesthesia use.[131] As a method of avoiding general anesthesia, spinal anesthesia is a viable option.

Because of the hypovolemia associated with preeclampsia, the use of antihypertensive medications, and the administration of magnesium as seizure prophylaxis, marked hypotension may develop as a result of the sympathectomy produced by neuraxial techniques. Restraint, however, is advocated when responding pharmacologically to hypotension; patients with hypertensive disorders may be exquisitely sensitive to these agents. The induction and emergence from general anesthesia can be associated with reflex hypertension and result in ruptured aneurysms and pulmonary edema.[132] This hypertension can be blunted with a number of agents, including β-blockers, calcium-channel blockers, hydralazine, nitroprusside, nitroglycerine, trimethaphan, and narcotics. Finally, airway changes, including worsening edema, may be encountered in preeclamptic patients and preparations for the management of a potentially difficult airway should be made.

Cardiac Disease

Cardiac disease is becoming increasingly prevalent during pregnancy. Although stable in overall adult prevalence, coronary heart diseases (including those associated with hypertension) and valvular pathologies have become more relevant as the parturient population ages. More significant, however, is the dramatic increase in adult patients who have benefited from improvements in the diagnosis, treatment, and surgical correction of congenital heart disorders (CHDs). In the United States alone, adults with CHDs have grown from an estimated 300,000 in the 1980s to an anticipated 1.4 million in the year 2020.[133] Many of these individuals are women of childbearing age, and with pregnancy, CHD can have profound effects on maternal and fetal outcome.

At one time, general anesthesia was regarded as the method of choice for all cesarean deliveries in patients with both acquired and congenital heart disorders. However, with advances in the understanding of cardiac disorders and the effects of anesthesia, especially in the relation to the anomalous or diseased myocardium, regional techniques have been reconsidered. Regional anesthesia has many beneficial effects, including the ability to provide pain relief, decrease the release and effects of catecholamines, and avoid airway manipulation. General anesthesia can result in moderate, sometimes detrimental inotropic and chronotropic alterations in heart physiology, especially during the induction, intubation, and extubation periods.

The independent and related complexities of cardiac disorders and pregnancy make the sharing of patient data with all interested parties of vital importance. As the cardiac alterations of pregnancy usually plateau from the 20th to 24th gestational weeks until the onset of labor, this represents an ideal time to assess whether adequate compensation is occurring. This is not to say that decompensation cannot occur prior to this period or at any time during the peripartum experience. Although benign arrhythmias occur commonly without symptoms or sequelae during pregnancy,[134] in the setting of corrected congenital cardiac lesions, hemodynamic compromise may result. Communication with the patient's cardiologist is vital, and a full analysis of prior diagnostic studies should be made. Despite the presence of CHD, other causes of arrhythmias or decompensation (electrolyte and thyroid abnormalities, magnesium use, etc.) should be evaluated. Should complete cardiopulmonary arrest occur late (after the 24th week) in pregnancy, an event that occurs in approximately 1 in 30,000 pregnancies,[135] resuscitation must consider both maternal and fetal health. Rapid CPR (cardiopulmonary resuscitation), intubation, prevention of aortocaval compression with uterine displacement, and immediate delivery within 4 to 5 minutes of maternal cardiac arrest may maximize the chances of maternal and fetal survival.[136] In terms of medications, intubation, and defibrillation protocols, there are no alterations to the basic ACLS (advanced cardiorespiratory life support) algorithms.[136]

Acquired Cardiac Disorders

Despite the widespread use of antibiotics, in many parts of the developing world rheumatic heart disease remains the leading cause of cardiac abnormalities in women of childbearing age.[137] Valvular lesions include mitral stenosis (75%–90%), mitral regurgitation (6%–12%), aortic regurgitation (2%–5%), and aortic stenosis (1%).

In general, the primary goal with stenotic lesions is to maintain a normal to slow sinus heart rate with preservation of systemic vascular resistance (SVR). These goals are particularly important when controlling the physiologic responses to central neuraxial blockade, which can often dramatically reduce the SVR (i.e., cause hypotension) and result in compensatory tachycardia. Incremental titration of catheter-based epidural or spinal techniques, or initial use of spinal analgesia with narcotics alone, can limit the sympathetic blockade produced by local anesthetics. Treatment of hypotension with phenylephrine (an α-adrenergic vasopressor) may avoid the tachycardia observed with the use of ephedrine (a combined α- and β-adrenergic vasopressor). In contrast to stenotic lesions, regurgitant valvular disorders, such as mitral and aortic insufficiency, are best managed with normal to slight increases in sinus heart rate and reductions in SVR. Thus, the sympathetic blockade observed with central neuraxial blockade can be beneficial in providing afterload reduction and minimizing the influences of stress catecholamines on SVR. Preserving venous return and intravascular volume are important; however, on occasion, the normally helpful increased intravascular volume of pregnancy or the rapid return of SVR following delivery can result in left ventricular failure and pulmonary edema.[138]

Congenital Cardiac Disorders

Congenital heart disease in the adult is not simply a continuation of the childhood experience. The growth of the cardiac chambers allows arrhythmias to change in character and frequency and ventricular dysfunction and failure to occur. Bioprosthetic replacement valves and conduits can also fail over time, often as a result of adult comorbidities or conditions, including pregnancy. With some congenital disorders, a complete repair is made and cardiovascular function, pressures, and blood flow patterns develop relatively normally. For the most part, these individuals require no special treatment. However, three important differences should be recognized: First, as some cardiac disorders are inherited, fetal echocardiography at 20 to 24 weeks' gestation is desirable. Second, antibiotic prophylaxis may be warranted. Third, arrhythmias are more common as the scar tissue in the heart can act as an arrhythmogenic focus. Other disorders, however, may present as uncorrected or partially corrected lesions in decompensated or poorly compensated states, thereby making the anesthetic management more challenging. The most commonly observed congenital heart disorders during pregnancy include left-to-right shunts, tetralogy of Fallot, Eisenmenger syndrome, and aortic coarctation (see Chapter 37).

The physiologic impact of a small septal defect or a patent ductus arteriosus is usually a trivial to modest left-to-right intracardiac shunt. In general, modest left-to-right shunts are well tolerated during pregnancy, although several alterations in management have been suggested.[139] Because air embolization may occur through intravenous lines, or with the loss-of-resistance-to-air technique of epidural placement, the use of air filters and alternate (loss-of-resistance-to-saline) epidural placement techniques is recommended.[140] In addition, as increases in pulmonary vascular resistance with hypoxia, hypercarbia, and acidosis may allow for reversal of shunt flow, the application of supplemental oxygen appears prudent. Finally, the overall management goal for these defects should focus on limiting maternal catecholamine and systemic vascular resistance (SVR) increases. In this regard, the use of central neuraxial analgesia provides exceptional control; however, the block should be administered slowly, as rapid decreases in SVR may result in a pronounced right-to-left shunt with maternal hypoxemia.[139]

Parturients with uncorrected or partially corrected cyanotic congenital heart disease (i.e., right-to-left shunts) may tolerate pregnancy poorly. Management focuses on maintaining adequate SVR, intravascular volume, and venous return and preventing increases in PVR (often due to pain, hypoxemia, hypercarbia, and acidosis). The use of supplemental oxygen and the use of arterial and central venous catheters may facilitate care and hemodynamic management. The use of pulmonary artery catheters remains controversial owing to difficulties in placement, the risk of pulmonary artery rupture and cardiac arrhythmias, and the limited information obtained in the setting of a severe fixed pulmonary hypertension and a large intracardiac shunt.[141] Neuraxial analgesia produced with intrathecal opioid administration may minimize decreases in SVR, and if provided with a CSE technique, the judicious addition of epidural local anesthetics can be titrated as needed. In the event of a cesarean delivery, regional anesthesia remains preferable to general anesthesia owing to the diminished cardiac output that can occur from halogenated agents and positive pressure ventilation. If regional anesthesia is contraindicated, a controlled versus rapid sequence induction of general anesthesia minimizes critical decreases in SVR and myocardial function. Regardless of the technique employed, hemodynamic alterations must be promptly resolved, and ephedrine and dopamine, rather than phenylephrine, are vasopressors of choice because of their maintenance of both SVR and heart rate.

Diabetes

Analgesic and anesthetic management of diabetic parturients should focus on glucose management and the responses of the physiologic systems most affected: coronary, cerebral and peripheral vascular, gastrointestinal, renal, and autonomic systems. The analgesia and anesthesia produced by neuraxial techniques can increase placental perfusion through reductions in maternal catecholamines and decrease the incidence of fetal acidosis occurring with maternal labor hyperventilation. The cardiovascular, autonomic, and uteroplacental blood flow changes caused by diabetes make the prevention and early treatment of hypotension a significant concern. The frequent and severe maternal hypotension witnessed in diabetics can be associated with spinal and epidural anesthesia for cesarean delivery;[142] however, it is possible that dextrose-containing IV fluids may have played a role. With strict observation and reaction to maternal blood pressure, volume expansion with a non-dextrose-containing solution, and maternal glucose control, spinal anesthesia can be performed without an associated fetal acidosis.[143]

In addition to the improved hemodynamic control seen with the slow initiation of epidural analgesia and anesthesia, this technique may offer other beneficial effects during labor and delivery. Insulin resistance has been demonstrated to occur in a dose-response relationship with the amount of stress following surgery, burns, trauma, and sepsis. More recently, pain per se has been demonstrated to impair insulin sensitivity by affecting nonoxidative glucose metabolism.[144] Although studies have not been performed in laboring diabetic parturients or even in females, this suggests that glucose regulation can be improved by the administration of pain relief in stressful states. Indeed, when epidural anesthesia was compared to general anesthesia as a control group, an attenuation of the hyperglycemic response to abdominal surgery was observed through a modification of glucose production, without affecting glucose utilization.[145] Protein metabolism, by contrast, was not influenced by epidural blockade. These investigations suggest a possible benefit from the use of neuraxial analgesia and anesthesia in parturients with diabetes.

If general anesthesia is required, the possibilities of gastroparesis, limited atlanto-occipital joint extension, and impaired counterregulatory hormone responses to hypoglycemia should be considered and integrated into the management.[146]

EFFECTS OF NEURAXIAL ANALGESIA ON PROGRESS AND OUTCOME OF LABOR

Whether central neuraxial analgesia affects the progress and outcome of labor remains a controversial topic. The myriad of maternal and fetal variables adds complexity to the issue, as well as differing institutional and individual anesthetic and obstetric practices. Moreover, the contemporary pattern and progress of labor appears slower than previously described a half a century earlier by Friedman.[147] Zhang and associates,[148] noting a significant delay in the progress of labor in nulliparous women, pointed to several factors possibly responsible including higher maternal age and weight, increasing fetal size, and higher induction and epidural use rates. Together, these changes make practice patterns and outcomes difficult to compare.

Study Design Issues

The greatest challenge in uncovering an association between neuraxial analgesia and progress of labor is that the ideal prospective, randomized, double-blinded, placebo-controlled study is exceptionally difficult, if not impossible, to perform. Retrospective or nonrandomized studies may underestimate the importance of confounders. For instance, women requesting epidural labor analgesia may be inherently different from those choosing natural childbirth; such differences have included having smaller pelves, more occiput posterior fetal presentations,[149] greater use of oxytocin for induction or augmentation, and more painful labors (which may be associated with slower labor and instrumental delivery).[150] Moreover, in nulliparous parturients with larger fetuses and eventual dystocia, a requirement for larger amounts of epidural local anesthetic for pain relief has been reported.[151–153]

The complexity of assessing prospective studies begins with enrollment procedures, as women open to randomization of the timing and technique of analgesia may not be representative of the majority of parturients. In addition, parturients who deliver either very slowly or very quickly may not remain in their randomized group. Blinding the obstetrician, anesthesiologist, nurse, and patient to central neuraxial versus other analgesic forms is also difficult. Such blinding is necessary to remove any subtle or overt influences on decision-making; for example, instrumental deliveries may be more common in those patients with epidural analgesia because they can more comfortably accept forceps delivery.[154] Finally, women utilizing parenteral opioids, commonly used as a control group, may not progress in a manner representative of the natural progress of labor,[155] thus not giving a true comparison of epidural techniques with the natural birth experience. No study has so far succeeded in meeting all these objectives; however, certain insights can be gained from the literature to date.

Study Results

The American College of Obstetricians and Gynecologists (ACOG) recently issued guidelines on the use of obstetric anesthesia services. Among the recommendations to reduce the incidence of cesarean delivery was delaying epidural analgesia initiation until cervical dilation of 5 cm or greater was achieved.[156] The data cited, primarily observational and nonrandomized, found an association between earlier epidural placement and dystocia. Using a case-control methodology, investigators at the National Maternity Hospital in Dublin (the pioneers of the active management of labor) observed that epidural initiation at greater than 2 cm dilation was a significant risk factor for prolonging labor in nulliparous women.[157] Thorp and associates,[158] in nulliparous women with cervical dilation less than 5 cm and dilation rate less than 1 cm/hour, observed a sixfold increase in cesarean delivery for dystocia in association with the use of regional analgesia. Similarly, Lieberman and associates,[159] using a multivariate regression technique on observational data, noted cervical dilation less than 5 cm and station less than 0 at time of epidural initiation as strong risk factors for cesarean delivery. Such cohort studies, however, have not uniformly supported differences in progress and outcome with epidural analgesia; Ohel and Harats[160] failed to show any difference in labor outcome when epidural analgesia was initiated prior to or after 3 cm cervical dilation. Holt, and associates,[161] in a prospective cohort study, found an association between cesarean delivery and higher station, but not cervical dilation, at the time of epidural placement.

An interesting form of retrospective analysis evaluates those institutions in which epidural analgesia becomes suddenly available. These studies, though nonrandomized, offer an analysis of an entire patient cohort in which a "sentinel event" has occurred but other variables, such as obstetric practice styles, are unlikely to change dramatically. A meta-analysis of such studies found no association between a sudden increase in the utilization of epidural analgesia and higher rates of cesarean delivery.[162]

The majority of randomized controlled trials indicate little overall effect of epidural analgesia on the progress and outcome of labor. Luxman and associates[163] found no difference in length of labor or mode of delivery in 60 nulliparous parturients randomized to receive epidural analgesia prior to or after 4 cm cervical dilation (mean 2.3 cm versus 4.5 cm). Chestnut and associates, in evaluating women closer to 5 cm cervical dilation (mean 4 cm versus 5 cm), demonstrated no differences in labor outcome in either spontaneous[164] or induced[165] labors. A recent meta-analysis of 10 trials comparing parturients of mixed parity randomized to epidural analgesia or parenteral opioids noted a prolongation of the first and second stages of labor by 42 minutes and 14 minutes, respectively, in association with the use of epidurals.[166]

Specific studies, however, do appear to indicate that anesthetic practice differences may influence the progress and outcome of labor. Although the COMET trial found no differences in the incidence of cesarean delivery, a higher proportion of instrumental deliveries was observed in patients with "traditional" epidurals versus CSE or parenteral narcotics. In the "traditional" epidural group, intermittent boluses of 0.25% bupivacaine were administered, a method not commonly used in contemporary practice in which lower concentrations and continuous infusion pumps are usual. Regardless, the findings suggest that differences in neuraxial technique may alter outcomes; this conclusion has been supported by other studies comparing CSE and epidural techniques. In nulliparous parturients at less than 3 cm cervical dilation, Tsen and associates,[68] using 1 mL versus 12 to 15 mL of 0.25% bupivacaine in the spinal and epidural spaces, respectively, observed faster cervical dilation and progress of labor in the spinal group.

Obstetric practice style may also influence the outcome and progress of labor. Meta-analyses of randomized trials have found that although instrumental delivery rates increased in patients receiving epidural analgesia, the resulting incidences were widely divergent, perhaps reflecting substantial practice style differences.[166,167] In terms of cesarean delivery, one study noted that apart from nulliparity, the identity of the individual obstetrician was the variable with the greatest influence on cesarean delivery rates.[168] Moreover, the use of peer review and education have been demonstrated to result in a 50% decrease in cesarean rates despite a simultaneous doubling of epidural analgesia use.[169,170]

In summary, although problems with methodology make an association difficult to evaluate, the use of epidural analgesia appears to affect the progress and outcome of labor remarkably little. Although the risk of cesarean delivery does not appear to be influenced, instrumental vaginal delivery appears to be increased with the use of epidural analgesia. It is possible that these associations may reflect variances in patient demographics or differences in anesthetic and obstetric practice styles.

TEMPERATURE CHANGES IN LABOR

Humans have the ability to maintain body temperature within a narrow range despite changes in environmental temperature. Although the extremities and skin can vary over several degrees, the average core body temperature of healthy adults is 37°C with diurnal variations of ± 0.5°C.[171] Thermoregulation is centered in the hypothalamus and responds to receptors found predominantly in the skin and spinal cord. Established through a balance of heat uptake, production, and loss, temperature equilibrium can be distorted by processes that change the thermoregulatory threshold (set value) or the response to temperatures above or below this value.

Clinically, a temperature greater than 38°C represents a fever. Most commonly, fever is the result of exogenous or endogenous pyrogens that disturb the "thermostat" set value to allow thermoregulatory mechanisms to maintain an elevated temperature. Less commonly, thermoregulatory responses to hyperthermia are prevented (such as a blockade of sympathetically mediated vasodilation or sweating) or overwhelmed (such as immersion in hot water). Of interest, endogenous pyrogens, which act on the thermoregulatory center and are triggered by the release of interleukins 1 and 6 from macrophages, are partially mediated by prostaglandin metabolism;[172] the relationship of this finding to the many pregnancy-induced alterations in the production and distribution of prostaglandins has yet to be elucidated.[173]

Thermoregulation During Pregnancy

During pregnancy, the mother attempts to maintain a normal temperature. The fetus relies on the uteroplacental circulation and the amniotic fluid interface for heat exchange; these limited routes for heat egress result in a normal fetal temperature approximately 0.5°C to

0.75°C higher than maternal body temperature.[174] With extreme hyperthermia, experimental evidence suggests that fetal deterioration may occur. Morishima and associates,[175] utilizing radiant heat to produce maternal hyperthermia of 107°F in anesthetized baboons, observed increased uterine activity and deterioration in fetal condition. Similarly, Cefalo and Hellegers[176] demonstrated fetal deterioration in anesthetized gravid ewes with levels of hyperthermia that produced maternal cardiovascular collapse. Although these extreme degrees of hyperthermia are unlikely to be clinically applicable, lesser increases of temperature may have various effects, including changes in umbilical blood flow.[176]

In terms of neonatal effects, epidemiologic evidence suggests that mild maternal fever may not be as benign as previously assumed based on the animal data. Lieberman and associates,[177] in a retrospective review of 1218 nulliparous women with singleton, term pregnancies in spontaneous labor who were afebrile on admission, noted that 1-minute Apgar scores less than 7, hypotonia, and the need for bag and mask ventilation were more common in parturients with a body temperature greater than 101°F. Although it remains unclear whether temperature per se, independent from underlying infectious or inflammatory processes, can cause neurologic injury, an association between maternal intrapartum fever and neonatal encephalopathy,[178] cerebral palsy,[179]and persistent developmental cognitive deficits[180] has been observed. Moreover, maternal outcome may be directly or indirectly influenced by the presence of even low-grade fever. Lieberman and associates[181] retrospectively observed a twofold higher incidence in operative vaginal and cesarean deliveries in nulliparous women who were afebrile at admission and subsequently developed a fever greater than 99.5°F, compared to those who remained afebrile, even when controlled for birth weight, length of labor, and analgesic choice. More recently, Shipp and associates[182] noted an association between postpartum fever after cesarean delivery and an increased risk of uterine rupture in a subsequent trial of labor.

Epidural Analgesia and Maternal Pyrexia

Study Design Issues

To date, nearly all the clinical studies of maternal fever associated with epidural analgesia have been nonrandomized. Similar to the progress and outcome of labor studies, it is possible that women who request epidural labor analgesia have risk factors that predispose them to fever, including greater rates of nulliparity,[183] prolonged rupture of membranes,[183,184] prolonged labor,[183,185,186] higher temperature on admission,[183] early chorioamnionitis,[183] and frequent cervical examinations.[187] Using a case-control methodology, Vallejo and associates[186] compared women with histologically confirmed chorioamnionitis with two groups of women who received epidural analgesia (with and without chorioamnionitis). Fever was more common in infected women in all groups; however, the incidence of fever in uninfected women with epidurals was only 1%. In a similar study of 149 women who delivered greater than 6 hours following membrane rupture, Dashe and associates[188] noted an increased incidence of fever in 54% of parturients who received epidurals. However, when parturients with evidence of placental inflammation were excluded, the incidence of fever was similar in women with and without epidural analgesia (11% versus 9%).

Study Results

Although an infection is the most common reason for fever during pregnancy, the influence of neuraxial techniques on maternal temperature is of interest. Regional anesthesia administered for surgery, including cesarean delivery, typically results in peripheral vasodilation, redistribution of body heat, and hypothermia.[189] By contrast, in laboring women receiving regional analgesia, a rise in temperature has been noted. Fusi and associates[190] reported an increase in vaginal temperatures of approximately 1°C over 7 hours in 18 parturients receiving epidural analgesia with no evidence of infection; this contrasted to stable temperatures in 15 parturients who received intramuscular meperidine. Using a method perhaps more reflective of core temperature, Camann and associates[185] measured tympanic membrane temperature in 53 laboring parturients divided into three groups. One group received intravenous nalbuphine; the other two groups, composed of women who chose epidural analgesia, were randomized to receive epidural bupivacaine with or without fentanyl. With ambient room temperature maintained at 20°C to 22°C, epidural analgesia did not affect maternal temperature for the first 4 hours. Thereafter, the mean tympanic membrane temperature increased by 0.07°C/hour in both epidural groups, with no differences observed in those receiving epidural fentanyl (Fig. 72–4).

Macaulay and associates[191] evaluated maternal oral and intrauterine and fetal skin temperatures in 33 and 27 parturients undergoing labor with and without epidurals, respectively. With an ambient temperature ranging from 23.3°C to 29°C, 10 fetuses within mothers with epidurals reached a maximum fetal skin temperature of greater than 38°C versus none in the group without epidurals. Of interest, only two women, both in the epidural group, reached an oral temperature greater than 37.5°C. Ultimately, no differences in Apgar scoring or umbilical cord blood gases were found. Overall, a number of investigators have observed an incidence of clinical fever (greater than 38°C) in 1% to 36% of laboring women receiving epidural analgesia, with a temperature elevation rate of approximately 0.1°C/hour of epidural analgesia, usually after a 4- to 5-hour delay.[183,184,192,193]

The mechanisms by which epidural analgesia may produce changes in maternal temperature during labor

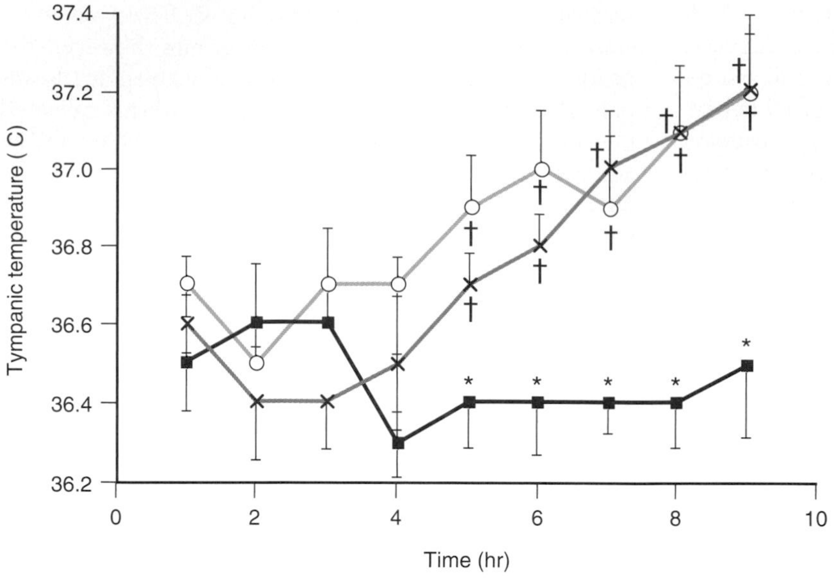

FIGURE 72–4
Mean tympanic temperatures during labor in three groups of patients: Epidural bupivacaine-fentanyl (0), epidural bupivacaine only (X), and parenteral opioids (v) groups. *$P < 0.01$ compared with the epidural group. †$P < 0.01$ compared with the preepidural temperature. (From Camann WR, Hortvet LA, Hughes N, et al: Maternal temperature regulation during extradural analgesia for labour. Br J Anaesth 1991;67:565–568.)

remain unclear. Although high ambient temperatures (24°C to 26°C) have been suggested as a possible etiology,[190] an association between ambient temperature and maternal or fetal temperatures has not been uniformly demonstrated.[184,191] A second possibility could be epidural-induced reductions in heat loss mechanisms, including an increase in sweating thresholds (by 0.55°C in volunteers)[194] and a reduction in hyperventilation during labor.[195,196] A third possibility could be alterations that result in, or are related to, shivering; in those parturients who shivered following the initiation of epidural analgesia versus those who do not, pyrexia developed as early as 1 hour later, in comparison to greater than 4 hours later.[197] In addition, shivering parturients ultimately attained higher maximum temperatures and had a threefold increase in clinical fever. A final possibility could be alterations in the parturients not receiving an epidural technique; the opioids frequently utilized in these groups may suppress temperature elevations.[198] A retrospective study of systemic use[199] and a prospective, randomized study of epidural use[185] of opioids, however, failed to demonstrate temperature curve changes with the addition of opioids.

Impact and Interventions

In addition to the fetal concerns discussed earlier, temperature elevations may alter neonatal exposure to antibiotics and subsequent care. Mayer and associates[200] retrospectively evaluated 300 low risk nulliparous women who received systemic opioids, epidural analgesia, or both ($n = 100$ in each group). The incidence of maternal fever (2%, 16%, and 24% in the preceding groups, respectively) and intrapartum maternal antibiotics (6%, 19%, 22%) was highest in the combined opioid and epidural group. Of note, in the 10 patients who ultimately demonstrated laboratory evidence of chorioamnionitis, maternal fever was not the only presenting symptom; fetal tachycardia and meconium-stained or abnormal amniotic fluid were also found. This suggests that the administration of antibiotics should not be guided by maternal fever alone. In a secondary analysis of 1657 low risk nulliparous women enrolled in a trial of active management of labor, the incidence of maternal fever (15% versus 1%), neonatal sepsis evaluation (34% versus 10%), and antibiotic treatment (15% versus 4%) was increased when epidural analgesia was used.[192] However, the incidence of actual neonatal sepsis was exceedingly low in epidural and nonepidural groups (0.3% versus 0.2%), and of interest, although the indications for sepsis evaluations was not provided, was the finding that two thirds of the evaluations occurred in infants of mothers who did not have intrapartum fevers. Moreover, the mothers who received epidural analgesia had larger infants, longer labors, and a twofold increase in the labor induction rate. Although it is possible that the active management protocol of frequent cervical examinations and early amniotomy may have influenced the risk of fever, a subsequent study evaluated nonrandomized parturients whose temperature remained below 100.4°C throughout labor.[201] Neonatal sepsis evaluations were more common in parturients who had epidural analgesia (20.4% versus 8.9%) even after controlling for gestational age, birth weight, maternal smoking history, active labor management, premature rupture of membranes, and admission cervical dilation. Epidural analgesia was associated with both major (rupture of membranes >24 hours, fetal heart rate >160) and minor criteria (maternal temperature >99.5°F, rupture of membranes 12 to 24 hours) for sepsis evaluation. These data suggest that multiple factors should be present prior to initiating a sepsis evaluation; moreover, of those babies investigated for sepsis because of risk factors, few will ultimately prove to have been infected.

The rate of neonatal sepsis evaluation and treatment can be modified by neonatology admission criteria and practice style. Yancey and associates,[202] reviewing the effects of an on-demand epidural analgesia service where epidural use increased overnight (because of a change in policy in the unit) from 1% to 83%, observed that maternal temperatures greater than 99.5°F and 100.4°F increased threefold and 18-fold, respectively. Despite this increase in maternal temperatures, neonatal blood counts and cultures increased modestly (RR 1.5–1.7), and no changes in the proportion of infants who received antibiotic treatment for presumed sepsis were observed. Similarly, Kaul and associates[203] noted in a retrospective review of the delivery records of 1177 nulliparous women that the incidence of neonatal sepsis evaluations was no different (7.5% versus 9.4%) despite women with epidural analgesia having more fever. Both investigators cited more stringent neonatal sepsis treatment guidelines, which did not include the treatment for maternal fever in the absence of chorioamnionitis, as being responsible for their results.

Attempts to diminish maternal temperature increases during labor have thus far been limited. Goetzl and associates[204] randomized 42 nulliparous women to receive acetaminophen 650 mg every 4 hours versus placebo in women receiving epidural analgesia. The incidence of fever did not differ between groups (23.8%). Of note, despite all neonatal blood cultures being negative, maternal serum and cord blood markers of inflammation (IL-6) were higher in mothers who had fever. This suggests that inflammatory markers can be elevated in the absence of neonatal infection.

In conclusion, epidural analgesia does appear associated with increases in temperature, although most of these increases are mild. This being said, maternal fever has been linked with adverse neonatal outcomes. Further studies of the mechanism of these temperature elevations with epidural use and a reanalysis of maternal and neonatal evaluation and treatment policies are warranted.

CONCLUSIONS

- Central neuraxial techniques, including spinal, epidural, and combined spinal-epidural techniques, are commonly used in modern obstetric care for the provision of labor analgesia and anesthesia for instrumental and operative deliveries.
- Philosophical and clinical shifts in practice have expanded the indications for the use of these techniques. Most recently, these techniques have been applied to the following:
    - External cephalic version: Success has been improved significantly with all central neuraxial techniques for both primary attempts and reattempts.
    - Postoperative pain management: The use of long-acting opioids such as morphine via spinal and epidural techniques has dramatically improved the postoperative analgesia and recovery following cesarean delivery.
- The basic properties of epidural, spinal, and CSE techniques may indicate advantages for specific situations.
- All three techniques can utilize a catheter to allow flexibility in titrating the onset and duration of the blockade; however, this is less commonly done with the spinal technique because of the size of the dural puncture and the resulting high incidence of headache.
- A number of analgesic and anesthetic options exist for labor and delivery, including nonpharmacologic modalities, systemic agents, and peripheral nerve blocks.
- A number of disease processes are being seen more commonly during pregnancy. Hypertensive disorders, cardiac diseases including acquired and congenital heart disorders, and diabetes are comorbid conditions that have implications for obstetric and anesthetic care. On occasion, invasive monitoring may be required for the optimal care of the parturient with these significant disease states, and a risk-benefit analysis for their use should be considered in advance.
- Whether central neuraxial analgesia affects the progress and outcome of labor remains controversial, in part due to the complexity in study design. However, the following should be noted:
    - The majority of studies appear to indicate little overall effect of epidural analgesia on progress and outcome of labor.
    - Anesthetic and obstetric practice styles may influence who ultimately receives an instrumental or operative delivery.
- Although the etiology remains unclear, epidural labor analgesia appears to increase maternal temperature; however, the following should be noted:
    - Study design issues also exist.
    - A delay of 4 to 5 hours is observed prior to a mean increase of approximately 0.1°C/hour following epidural initiation.
    - The impact of these changes remains controversial, and the direct and indirect implications of these changes on neonatal sepsis evaluations deserve further investigation.
- Awareness and communication of the indications and implications of central neuraxial techniques among the entire obstetric care team, including obstetric, anesthetic, neonatal, and nursing care providers, remain of paramount importance to the continued welfare of the expectant mother and fetus.

SUMMARY OF MANAGEMENT OPTIONS
Central Neuraxial Analgesia and Anesthesia

Management Options	Quality of Evidence	Strength of Recommendation	References
External Cephalic Version			
Epidural use is associated with higher success rates compared to no epidural; it is not clear whether spinal or combined-spinal epidural (CSE) has the same effect.	Ib	A	45–49
Pain Relief during Parturition			
Nonpharmacologic methods:			
All nonpharmacologic methods have limited analgesic action.	Ib	A	15–17
Psychological support is of benefit and reduces the need for pain relief.	Ia	A	20
Hypnosis can be beneficial.	Ia	A	21
The presence of a doula or other nonprofessional support in labor reduces need for pain relief.	Ia	A	20,22
Sensory stimulation (e.g., acupuncture, TENS) is claimed to be of some benefit in early labor.	III	B	26–28
Pharmacological methods:			
Systemic medications shown to be effective include opioids and patient-controlled anesthesia.	III	B	36,37
Inhalational analgesia: Entonox—50% NO/50% oxygen—is widely used, but evidence mainly observational.	Ib	A	42
Regional analgesia/anesthesia:			
Most often used are pudendal block and perineal block.	IIb	B	44
Paracervical, caudal, and lumbar sympathetic blocks are infrequently used.	Ib	A	40,41
Pain Relief during Parturition			
Neuraxial analgesia:			
Spinal block is effective for assisted vaginal delivery and cesarean section (CS) but not labor.	IV	C	52
Epidural block is effective for assisted vaginal delivery, and CS; addition of fentanyl and local anesthetic improves short-term effectiveness (especially for an assisted vaginal delivery).	IIa	B	65
CSE technique is effective for assisted vaginal delivery and CS; possibly it has a lower complication rate than epidural alone.	Ib	A	68
Dural puncture managed by:			
analgesia	Ib	A	75
IV fluids	Ia	A	76
blood patch	IV	C	58
Cesarean Section			
Spinal, epidural, and CSE are preferred to general anesthesia; addition of narcotics and ephedrine may result in increased effectiveness.	Ib	A	56,73,74, 79,80
With general anesthesia (GA):			
Use laryngeal mask if intubation is difficult.	IIb	B	94
Use nonparticulate antacid and/or H_2 antagonist in advance of all CS in case GA necessary.	Ib	A	95–97
Use pre- and perioperative oxygenation.	III	B	98

SUMMARY OF MANAGEMENT OPTIONS

Central Neuraxial Analgesia and Anesthesia *(Continued)*

Management Options	Quality of Evidence	Strength of Recommendation	References
Postoperative Pain Relief			
Diclofenac is effective in reducing postpartum pain.	Ia	A	205
Epidural is more effective than parenteral opioids.	Ib	A	105–107
High Risk Pregnancies—Special Considerations			
Invasive monitoring (see also Chapter 80) is valuable but requires skill and experience.	IV	C	118–120
Hypertension:	III	B	127–129
Fluid overload may occur, especially with fluid preloading for epidural analgesia.			
Neuraxial analgesia is difficult with a coagulopathy.			
Induction of general anesthesia is associated with significant rise in blood pressure.			
Cardiac disease:			
Use caution with epidural anesthetic in stenotic lesions where reduced systemic vascular resistance (SVR) may precipitate reduced cardiac output and failure.	IV	C	138
There is a danger of left-to-right shunts reversing with use of epidural anesthesia and fall in SVR resulting in maternal hypoxemia.	IV	C	139
Adverse Effects of Epidural Analgesia			
Prolonged labor and maternal hyperpyrexia both more common, but best management strategy is uncertain.	–	GPP	–

REFERENCES

1. Cook TM: Combined spinal-epidural techniques. Anaesthesia 2000;55:42–64.
2. Palot M, Chale JJ, Colladon B, et al: Anesthesia and analgesia practice patterns in French obstetrical patients. Ann Fr Anesth Reanim 1998;17:210–219.
3. O'Connell MP, Tetsis AV, Lindow SW: The management of the second stage of labor. Int J Gynaecol Obstet 2001;74:51–56.
4. Tsen LC, Pitner R, Camann WR: General anesthesia at a tertiary care hospital 1990–1995: Indications and implications. Int J Obstet Anesth 1998;7:147–152.
5. Eltzschig HK, Lieberman ES, Camann WR: Regional anesthesia and analgesia for labor and delivery. N Engl J Med 2003; 348:319–332.
6. Birnbach DJ, Ojea LS: Combined spinal-epidural (CSE) for labor and delivery. Int Anesthesiol Clin 2002;40:27–48.
7. Rawal N, Holmstrom B, Crowhurst JA, Van Zundert A: The combined spinal-epidural technique. Anesthesiol Clin North Am 2000;18:267–295.
8. Chadwick HS, Posner K, Caplan RA, et al: A comparison of obstetric and nonobstetric anesthesia malpractice claims. Anesthesiology 1991;74:242–249.
9. Turnbull AC, Tindall VR, Robson G, et al: Report on confidential enquiries into maternal deaths in England and Wales 1979–1981. Rep Health Soc Subj (Lond) 1986;29:1–147.
10. Turnbull A, Tindall VR, Beard RW, et al: Report on confidential enquiries into maternal deaths in England and Wales 1982–1984. Rep Health Soc Subj (Lond) 1989;34:1–166.
11. Hawkins JL, Koonin LM, Palmer SK, Gibbs CP: Anesthesia-related deaths during obstetric delivery in the United States, 1979–1990. Anesthesiology 1997;86:277–284.
12. Heller PJ, Scheider EP, Marx GF: Pharyngolaryngeal edema as a presenting symptom in preeclampsia. Obstet Gynecol 1983; 62:523–525.
13. Leontic EA: Respiratory disease in pregnancy. Med Clin North Am 1977;61:111–128.
14. Chandrasekhar S, Topulos G, Bhavani-Shankar K: Upper airway study in pregnancy using acoustic reflectometry. Anesthesiology 2001;94(4)Suppl:A-1035.
15. Hetherington SE: A controlled study of the effect of prepared childbirth classes on obstetric outcomes. Birth 1990;17:86–90.
16. Stone CI, Demchik-Stome DA, Horan JJ: Coping with pain: A component analysis of Lamaze and cognitive-behavioral procedures. J Psychosom Res 1977;21:451–456.
17. Scott JR, Rose NB: Effect of psychoprophylaxis (Lamaze preparation) on labor and delivery in primiparas. N Engl J Med 1976; 294:1205–1207.
18. Motoyama EK, Rivard G, Acheson F, Cook CD: Adverse effect of maternal hyperventilation on the foetus. Lancet 1966; 1:286–288.

19. Stewart DE: Psychiatric symptoms following attempted natural childbirth. Can Med Assoc J 1982;127:713–716.
20. Smith CA, Collins CT, Cyna AM, Crowther CA: Complementary and alternative therapies for pain management in labour. Cochrane Database Syst Rev 2003;CD003521.
21. Scott KD, Berkowitz G, Klaus M: A comparison of intermittent and continuous support during labor: A meta-analysis. Am J Obstet Gynecol 1999;180:1054–1059.
22. Carroll D, Tramer M, McQuay H, et al: Transcutaneous electrical nerve stimulation in labour pain: A systematic review. BJOG 1997;104:169–175.
23. Tsen LC, Thomas J, Segal S, et al: Transcutaneous electrical nerve stimulation does not augment combined spinal epidural labour analgesia. Can J Anaesth 2000;47:38–42.
24. Tsen LC, Thomas J, Segal S, et al: Transcutaneous electrical nerve stimulation does not augment epidural labor analgesia. J Clin Anesth 2001;13:571–575.
25. Eger EI 2nd: Atropine, scopolamine, and related compounds. Anesthesiology 1962;23:365–383.
26. Paech M: Newer techniques of labor analgesia. Anesthesiol Clin North Am 2003;21:1–17.
27. Way WL, Costley EC, Leongway E: Respiratory sensitivity of the newborn infant to meperidine and morphine. Clin Pharmacol Ther 1965;11:454–461.
28. Shnider SM, Moya F: Effects of meperidine on the newborn infant. Am J Obstet Gynecol 1964;89:1009.
29. Coalson DW, Glosten B: Alternatives to epidural analgesia. Semin Perinatol 1991;15:375–385.
30. Hodgkinson R, Huff RW, Hayashi RH, Husain FJ: Double-blind comparison of maternal analgesia and neonatal neurobehaviour following intravenous butorphanol and meperidine. J Int Med Res 1979;7:224–230.
31. Whitelaw AG, Cummings AJ, McFadyen IR: Effect of maternal lorazepam on the neonate. BMJ (Clin Res Ed) 1981;282:1106–1108.
32. Busacca M, Gementi P, Gambini E, et al: Neonatal effects of the administration of meperidine and promethazine to the mother in labor. Double blind study. J Perinat Med 1982;10:48–53.
33. Clark RB, Seifen AB: Systemic medication during labor and delivery. Obstet Gynecol Annu 1983;12:165–197.
34. Brazelton TB: Effect of prenatal drugs on the behavior of the neonate. Am J Psychiatry 1970;126:1261–1266.
35. Akamatsu TJ, Bonica JJ, Rehmet R, et al: Experiences with the use of ketamine for parturition. I. Primary anesthetic for vaginal delivery. Anesth Analg 1974;53:284–287.
36. Holdcroft A, Morgan M: An assessment of the analgesic effect in labour of pethidine and 50 per cent nitrous oxide in oxygen (Entonox). J Obstet Gynaecol Br Commonw 1974;81:603–607.
37. Rosen M: Recent advances in pain relief in childbirth. I. Inhalation and systemic analgesia. Br J Anaesth 1971;43:837–848.
38. Munson ES, Embro WJ: Enflurane, isoflurane, and halothane and isolated human uterine muscle. Anesthesiology 1977;46:11–14.
39. Marx GF, Kim YI, Lin CC, et al: Postpartum uterine pressures under halothane or enflurance anesthesia. Obstet Gynecol 1978;51:695–698.
40. Asling JH, Shnider SM, Margolis AJ, et al: Paracervical block anesthesia in obstetrics. II. Etiology of fetal bradycardia following paracervical block anesthesia. Am J Obstet Gynecol 1970;107:626–634.
41. Leighton BL, Halpern SH, Wilson DB: Lumbar sympathetic blocks speed early and second stage induced labor in nulliparous women. Anesthesiology 1999;90:1039–1046.
42. Hutchins CJ: Spinal analgesia for instrumental delivery. A comparison with pudendal nerve block. Anaesthesia 1980;35:376–377.
43. Merkow AJ, McGuinness GA, Erenberg A, Kennedy RL: The neonatal neurobehavioral effects of bupivacaine, mepivacaine, and 2-chloroprocaine used for pudendal block. Anesthesiology 1980;52:309–312.
44. Philipson EH, Kuhnert BR, Syracuse CD: 2-Chloroprocaine for local perineal infiltration. Am J Obstet Gynecol 1987;157:1275–1278.
45. Schorr SJ, Speights SE, Ross EL, et al: A randomized trial of epidural anesthesia to improve external cephalic version success. Am J Obstet Gynecol 1997;177:1133–1137.
46. Samuels P, Cheek TG, Ludmir J: Epidural anesthesia for external version. SOAP 23rd Annual Meeting Abstracts. Boston, MA, 1991.
47. Dugoff L, Stamm CA, Jones OW 3rd, et al: The effect of spinal anesthesia on the success rate of external cephalic version: A randomized trial. Obstet Gynecol 1999;93:345–349.
48. Birnbach DJ, Matut J, Stein DJ, et al: The effect of intrathecal analgesia on the success of external cephalic version. Anesth Analg 2001;93:410–413.
49. Cherayil G, Feinberg B, Robinson J, Tsen LC: Central neuraxial blockade promotes external cephalic version success after a failed attempt. Anesth Analg 2002;94:1589–1592.
50. Carlan SJ, Dent JM, Huckaby T, et al: The effect of epidural anesthesia on safety and success of external cephalic version at term. Anesth Analg 1994;79:525–528.
51. Hoffmeyr GJ, Kulier R: Cephalic version by postural management for breech presentation. Cochrane Dtabase Syst Rev 2000;CD000051.
52. Arkoosh VA: Continuous spinal analgesia and anesthesia in obstetrics. Reg Anesth 1993;18:402–405.
53. Huckaby T, Skerman JH, Hurley RJ, Lambert DH: Sensory analgesia for vaginal deliveries: A preliminary report of continuous spinal anesthesia with a 32-gauge catheter. Reg Anesth 1991;16:150–153.
54. Lambert DH, Hurley RJ: Cauda equina syndrome and continuous spinal anesthesia. Anesth Analg 1991;72:817–819.
55. Tsen LC, Boosalis P, Segal S, et al: Hemodynamic effects of simultaneous administration of intravenous ephedrine and spinal anesthesia for cesarean delivery. J Clin Anesth 2000;12:378–382.
56. Corke BC, Datta S, Ostheimer GW, et al: Spinal anaesthesia for caesarean section. The influence of hypotension on neonatal outcome. Anaesthesia 1982;37:658–662.
57. Datta S, Alper MH, Ostheimer GW, Weiss JB: Method of ephedrine administration and nausea and hypotension during spinal anesthesia for cesarean section. Anesthesiology 1982;56:68–70.
58. Turnbull DK, Shepherd DB: Post-dural puncture headache: Pathogenesis, prevention and treatment. Br J Anaesth 2003;91:718–729.
59. Jones RJ: The role of recumbency in the prevention and treatment of postspinal headache. Anesth Analg 1974;53:788–796.
60. Abouleish E, Vega S, Blendinger I, Tio TO: Long-term follow-up of epidural blood patch. Anesth Analg 1975;54:459–463.
61. Santos AC, DeArmas PI: Systemic toxicity of levobupivacaine, bupivacaine, and ropivacaine during continuous intravenous infusion to nonpregnant and pregnant ewes. Anesthesiology 2001;95:1256–1264.
62. Ohmura S, Kawada M, Ohta T, et al: Systemic toxicity and resuscitation in bupivacaine-, levobupivacaine-, or ropivacaine-infused rats. Anesth Analg 2001;93:743–748.
63. Booker PD, Wilkes RG, Bryson TH, Beddard J: Obstetric pain relief using epidural morphine. Anaesthesia 1980;35:377–379.
64. Camann WR, Denney RA, Holby ED, Datta S: A comparison of intrathecal, epidural, and intravenous sufentanil for labor analgesia. Anesthesiology 1992;77:884–887.
65. Celleno D, Capogna G: Epidural fentanyl plus bupivacaine 0.125 per cent for labour: Analgesic effects. Can J Anaesth 1988;35:375–378.
66. van der Vyver M, Halpern S, Joseph G: Patient-controlled epidural analgesia versus continuous infusion for labour analgesia: A meta-analysis. Br J Anaesth 2002;89:459–465.

67. Paech MJ, Pavy TJ, Sims C, et al: Clinical experience with patient-controlled and staff-administered intermittent bolus epidural analgesia in labour. Anaesth Intensive Care 1995;23:459–463.
68. Tsen LC, Thue B, Datta S, Segal S: Is combined spinal-epidural analgesia associated with more rapid cervical dilation in nulliparous patients when compared with conventional epidural analgesia? Anesthesiology 1999;91:920–925.
69. Castillo D, Tsen LC: Epidural blood patch placed in the presence of an unknown cervical epidural hematoma. Anesth Analg 2003;97:885–887.
70. Holmstrom B, Rawal N, Axelsson K, Nydahl PA: Risk of catheter migration during combined spinal epidural block: Percutaneous epiduroscopy study. Anesth Analg 1995;80:747–753.
71. Suzuki N, Koganemaru M, Onizuka S, Takasaki M: Dural puncture with a 26-gauge spinal needle affects spread of epidural anesthesia. Anesth Analg 1996;82:1040–1042.
72. Albright GA, Forster RM: The safety and efficacy of combined spinal and epidural analgesia/anesthesia (6,002 blocks) in a community hospital. Reg Anesth Pain Med 1999;24:117–125.
73. Palmer CM, Emerson S, Volgoropolous D, Alves D: Dose-response relationship of intrathecal morphine for postcesarean analgesia. Anesthesiology 1999;90:437–444.
74. Abouleish EI: Epinephrine improves the quality of spinal hyperbaric bupivacaine for cesarean section. Anesth Analg 1987;66: 395–400.
75. Park GE, Hauch MA, Curlin F, et al: The effects of varying volumes of crystalloid administration before cesarean delivery on maternal hemodynamics and colloid osmotic pressure. Anesth Analg 1996;83:299–303.
76. Lee A, Ngan Kee WD, Gin T: A quantitative, systematic review of randomized controlled trials of ephedrine versus phenylephrine for the management of hypotension during spinal anesthesia for cesarean delivery. Anesth Analg 2002;94:920–926.
77. Ueyama H, He YL, Tanigami H, et al: Effects of crystalloid and colloid preload on blood volume in the parturient undergoing spinal anesthesia for elective cesarean section. Anesthesiology 1999;91:1571–1576.
78. Mercier FJ, Riley ET, Frederickson WL, et al: Phenylephrine added to prophylactic ephedrine infusion during spinal anesthesia for elective cesarean section. Anesthesiology 2001;95:668–674.
79. Datta S, Lambert DH, Gregus J, et al: Differential sensitivities of mammalian nerve fibers during pregnancy. Anesth Analg 1983;62:1070–1072.
80. Bromage PR: Continuous lumbar epidural analgesia for obstetrics. Can Med Assoc J 1961;85:1136–1140.
81. Philipson EH, Kuhnert BR, Syracuse CD: Fetal acidosis, 2-chloroprocaine, and epidural anesthesia for cesarean section. Am J Obstet Gynecol 1985;151:322–324.
82. Camann WR, Hartigan PM, Gilbertson LI, et al: Chloroprocaine antagonism of epidural opioid analgesia: A receptor-specific phenomenon? Anesthesiology 1990;73:860–863.
83. Stevens RA, Urmey WF, Urquhart BL, Kao TC: Back pain after epidural anesthesia with chloroprocaine. Anesthesiology 1993; 78:492–497.
84. Stevens RA, Chester WL, Schubert A, et al: pH-adjustment of 2-chloroprocaine quickens the onset of epidural anaesthesia. Can J Anaesth 1989;36:515–518.
85. Peterfreund RA, Datta S, Ostheimer GW: pH adjustment of local anesthetic solutions with sodium bicarbonate: Laboratory evaluation of alkalinization and precipitation. Reg Anesth 1989; 14:265–270.
86. Portnoy D, Vadhera RB: Mechanisms and management of an incomplete epidural block for cesarean section. Anesthesiol Clin North Am 2003;21:39–57.
87. Aya AG, Mangin R, Vialles N, et al: Patients with severe preeclampsia experience less hypotension during spinal anesthesia for elective cesarean delivery than healthy parturients: A prospective cohort comparison. Anesth Analg 2003;97:867–872.
88. Santos AC, Birnbach DJ: Spinal anesthesia in the parturient with severe preeclampsia: Time for reconsideration. Anesth Analg 2003;97:621–622.
89. Chestnut DH, Dewan DM, Redick LF, et al: Anesthetic management for obstetric hysterectomy: A multi-institutional study. Anesthesiology 1989;70:607–610.
90. Ross BK: ASA closed claims in obstetrics: Lessons learned. Anesthesiol Clin North Am 2003;21:183–197.
91. Royal College of Obstetricians and Gynaecologists: Why mothers die 1997–1999. The fifth report of the Confidential Enquiries into Maternal Deaths in the United Kingdom. London, RCOG Press, 2001.
92. Malan TP Jr, Johnson MD: The difficult airway in obstetric anesthesia: Techniques for airway management and the role of regional anesthesia. J Clin Anesth 1988;1:104–111.
93. Practice guidelines for management of the difficult airway: An updated report by the American Society of Anesthesiologists Task Force on Management of the Difficult Airway. Anesthesiology 2003;98:1269–1277.
94. Han TH, Brimacombe J, Lee EJ, Yang HS: The laryngeal mask airway is effective (and probably safe) in selected healthy parturients for elective cesarean section: A prospective study of 1067 cases. Can J Anaesth 2001;48:1117–1121.
95. James CF, Modell JH, Gibbs CP, et al: Pulmonary aspiration—Effects of volume and pH in the rat. Anesth Analg 1984;63: 665–668.
96. Johnston JR, Moore J, McCaughey W, et al: Use of cimetidine as an oral antacid in obstetric anesthesia. Anesth Analg 1983; 62:720–726.
97. Murphy DF, Nally B, Gardiner J, Unwin A: Effect of metoclopramide on gastric emptying before elective and emergency caesarean section. Br J Anaesth 1984;56:1113–1116.
98. Norris MC, Dewan DM: Preoxygenation for cesarean section: A comparison of two techniques. Anesthesiology 1985;62:827–829.
99. Chin KJ, Yeo SW: Bispectral index values at sevoflurane concentrations of 1% and 1.5% in lower segment cesarean delivery. Anesth Analg 2004;98:1140–1144.
100. Palahniuk RJ, Shnider SM, Eger EI 2nd: Pregnancy decreases the requirement for inhaled anesthetic agents. Anesthesiology 1974;41:82–83.
101. Dogru K, Yildiz K, Dalgic H, et al: Inhibitory effects of desflurane and sevoflurane on contractions of isolated gravid rat myometrium under oxytocin stimulation. Acta Anaesthesiol Scand 2003;47:472–474.
102. Mattingly JE, D'Alessio J, Ramanathan J: Effects of obstetric analgesics and anesthetics on the neonate: A review. Paediatr Drugs 2003;5:615–627.
103. Datta S, Ostheimer GW, Weiss JB, et al: Neonatal effect of prolonged anesthetic induction for cesarean section. Obstet Gynecol 1981;58:331–335.
104. Wang JK, Nauss LA, Thomas JE: Pain relief by intrathecally applied morphine in man. Anesthesiology 1979;50:149–151.
105. Cousins MJ, Mather LE: Intrathecal and epidural administration of opioids. Anesthesiology 1984;61:276–310.
106. Pan PH, James CF: Anesthetic-postoperative morphine regimens for cesarean section and postoperative oxygen saturation monitored by a telemetric pulse oximetry network for 24 continuous hours. J Clin Anesth 1994;6:124–128.
107. Harrison DM, Sinatra R, Morgese L, Chung JH: Epidural narcotic and patient-controlled analgesia for post-cesarean section pain relief. Anesthesiology 1988;68:454–457.
108. Rosen MA, Hughes SC, Shnider SM, et al: Epidural morphine for the relief of postoperative pain after cesarean delivery. Anesth Analg 1983;62:666–672.
109. Carmichael FJ, Rolbin SH, Hew EM: Epidural morphine for analgesia after caesarean section. Can Anaesth Soc J 1982;29: 359–363.
110. Fuller JG, McMorland GH, Douglas MJ, Palmer L: Epidural morphine for analgesia after caesarean section: A report of 4880 patients. Can J Anaesth 1990;37:636–640.

111. Palmer CM, Nogami WM, Van Maren G, Alves DM: Postcesarean epidural morphine: A dose-response study. Anesth Analg 2000;90:887–891.
112. Thind GS, Wells JC, Wilkes RG: The effects of continuous intravenous naloxone on epidural morphine analgesia. Anaesthesia 1986;41:582–585.
113. Kotelko DM, Dailey PA, Shnider SM, et al: Epidural morphine analgesia after cesarean delivery. Obstet Gynecol 1984;63: 409–413.
114. Sharar SR, Ready LB, Ross BK, et al: A comparison of postcesarean epidural morphine analgesia by single injection and by continuous infusion. Reg Anesth 1991;16:232–235.
115. Fischer RL, Lubenow TR, Liceaga A, et al: Comparison of continuous epidural infusion of fentanyl-bupivacaine and morphine-bupivacaine in management of postoperative pain. Anesth Analg 1988;67:559–563.
116. Zakowski MI, Ramanathan S, Sharnick S, Turndorf H: Uptake and distribution of bupivacaine and morphine after intrathecal administration in parturients: Effects of epinephrine. Anesth Analg 1992;74:664–669.
117. Chadwick HS, Ready LB: Intrathecal and epidural morphine sulfate for post-cesarean analgesia—A clinical comparison. Anesthesiology 1988;68:925–929.
118. Clinical competence in hemodynamic monitoring: A statement for physicians from the ACP/ACC/AHA Task Force on Clinical Privileges in Cardiology. Circulation 1990;81:2036–2040.
119. Sibbald WJ, Keenan SP: Show me the evidence: A critical appraisal of the Pulmonary Artery Catheter Consensus Conference and other musings on how critical care practitioners need to improve the way we conduct business. Crit Care Med 1997;25:2060–2063.
120. Connors AF Jr, Speroff T, Dawson NV, et al: The effectiveness of right heart catheterization in the initial care of critically ill patients. SUPPORT Investigators. JAMA 1996;276:889–897.
121. Newsome LR, Bramwell RS, Curling PE: Severe preeclampsia: Hemodynamic effects of lumbar epidural anesthesia. Anesth Analg 1986;65:31–36.
122. Benedetti TJ, Kates R, Williams V: Hemodynamic observations in severe preeclampsia complicated by pulmonary edema. Am J Obstet Gynecol 1985;152:330–334.
123. Clark SL, Cotton DB: Clinical indications for pulmonary artery catheterization in the patient with severe preeclampsia. Am J Obstet Gynecol 1988;158:453–458.
124. Sise MJ, Hollingsworth P, Brimm JE, et al: Complications of the flow-directed pulmonary artery catheter: A prospective analysis in 219 patients. Crit Care Med 1981;9:315–318.
125. Practice guidelines for obstetrical anesthesia: A report by the American Society of Anesthesiologists Task Force on Obstetrical Anesthesia. Anesthesiology 1999;90:600–611.
126. Belfort MA, Mares A, Saade G, et al: Two-dimensional echocardiography and Doppler ultrasound in managing obstetric patients. Obstet Gynecol 1997;90:326–330.
127. Jouppila P, Jouppila R, Hollmen A, Koivula A: Lumbar epidural analgesia to improve intervillous blood flow during labor in severe preeclampsia. Obstet Gynecol 1982;59:158–161.
128. VanWijk MJ, Boer K, Berckmans RJ, et al: Enhanced coagulation activation in preeclampsia: The role of APC resistance, microparticles and other plasma constituents. Thromb Haemost 2002;88:415–420.
129. Kelton JG, Hunter DJ, Neame PB: A platelet function defect in preeclampsia. Obstet Gynecol 1985;65:107–109.
130. Wallace DH, Leveno KJ, Cunningham FG, et al: Randomized comparison of general and regional anesthesia for cesarean delivery in pregnancies complicated by severe preeclampsia. Obstet Gynecol 1995;86:193–199.
131. Hood DD, Curry R: Spinal versus epidural anesthesia for cesarean section in severely preeclamptic patients: A retrospective survey. Anesthesiology 1999;90:1276–1282.
132. Fox EJ, Sklar GS, Hill CH, et al: Complications related to the pressor response to endotracheal intubation. Anesthesiology 1977;47:524–525.
133. Perloff JK: Congenital heart disease in adults. A new cardiovascular subspecialty. Circulation 1991;84:1881–1890.
134. Rotmensch HH, Rotmensch S, Elkayam U: Management of cardiac arrhythmias during pregnancy. Current concepts. Drugs 1987;33:623–633.
135. Rees GA, Willis BA: Resuscitation in late pregnancy. Anaesthesia 1988;43:347–349.
136. The American Heart Association in collaboration with the International Liaison Committee on Resuscitation: Guidelines 2000 for Cardiopulmonary Resuscitation and Emergency Cardiovascular Care. Part 6: Advanced cardiovascular life support. Section 4: Devices to assist circulation. Circulation 2000;102:I105–111.
137. Lim ST: Rheumatic heart diseases in pregnancy. Ann Acad Med Singapore 2002;31:340–348.
138. Khanlou H, Khanlou N, Eiger G: Relationship between mitral valve regurgitant flow and peripartum change in systemic vascular resistance. South Med J 2003;96:308–309.
139. Tsen LC: Anesthetic management of the parturient with cardiac and diabetic diseases. Clin Obstet Gynecol 2003;46:700–710.
140. Naulty JS, Ostheimer GW, Datta S, et al: Incidence of venous air embolism during epidural catheter insertion. Anesthesiology 1982;57:410–412.
141. Daliento L, Somerville J, Presbitero P, et al: Eisenmenger syndrome. Factors relating to deterioration and death. Eur Heart J 1998;19:1845–1855.
142. Datta S, Brown WU Jr: Acid-base status in diabetic mothers and their infants following general or spinal anesthesia for cesarean section. Anesthesiology 1977;47:272–276.
143. Datta S, Kitzmiller JL, Naulty JS, et al: Acid-base status of diabetic mothers and their infants following spinal anesthesia for cesarean section. Anesth Analg 1982;61:662–665.
144. Greisen J, Juhl CB, Grofte T, et al: Acute pain induces insulin resistance in humans. Anesthesiology 2001;95:578–584.
145. Lattermann R, Carli F, Wykes L, Schricker T: Epidural blockade modifies perioperative glucose production without affecting protein catabolism. Anesthesiology 2002;97:374–381.
146. Jones TW, Porter P, Sherwin RS, et al: Decreased epinephrine responses to hypoglycemia during sleep. N Engl J Med 1998;338:1657–1662.
147. Friedman EA: Primigravid labor: A graphicostatistical analysis. Obstet Gynecol 1955;6:567–589.
148. Zhang J, Troendle JF, Yancey MK: Reassessing the labor curve in nulliparous women. Am J Obstet Gynecol 2002;187:824–828.
149. Floberg J, Belfrage P, Ohlsen H: Influence of the pelvic outlet capacity on fetal head presentation at delivery. Acta Obstet Gynecol Scand 1987;66:127–130.
150. Wuitchik M, Bakal D, Lipshitz J: The clinical significance of pain and cognitive activity in latent labor. Obstet Gynecol 1989;73:35–42.
151. Hess PE, Pratt SD, Lucas TP, et al: Predictors of breakthrough pain during labor epidural analgesia. Anesth Analg 2001;93: 414–418.
152. Hess PE, Pratt SD, Soni AK, et al: An association between severe labor pain and cesarean delivery. Anesth Analg 2000;90:881–886.
153. Panni MK, Segal S: Local anesthetic requirements are greater in dystocia than in normal labor. Anesthesiology 2003;98: 957–963.
154. Bofill JA, Vincent RD, Ross EL, et al: Nulliparous active labor, epidural analgesia, and cesarean delivery for dystocia. Am J Obstet Gynecol 1997;177:1465–1470.
155. Kowalski WB, Parsons MT, Pak SC, Wilson L Jr: Morphine inhibits nocturnal oxytocin secretion and uterine contractions in the pregnant baboon. Biol Reprod 1998;58:971–976.

156. American College of Obstetricians and Gynecologists Task Force on Cesarean Delivery Rates: Evaluation of Cesarean Delivery. Washington, DC: ACOG, 2000.
157. Malone FD, Geary M, Chelmow D, et al: Prolonged labor in nulliparas: Lessons from the active management of labor. Obstet Gynecol 1996;88:211–215.
158. Thorp JA, Eckert LO, Ang MS, et al: Epidural analgesia and cesarean section for dystocia: Risk factors in nulliparas. Am J Perinatol 1991;8:402–410.
159. Lieberman E, Lang JM, Cohen A, et al: Association of epidural analgesia with cesarean delivery in nulliparas. Obstet Gynecol 1996;88:993–1000.
160. Ohel G, Harats H: Epidural anesthesia in early compared with advanced labor. Int J Gynaecol Obstet 1994;45:217–219.
161. Holt RO, Diehl SJ, Wright JW: Station and cervical dilation at epidural placement in predicting cesarean risk. Obstet Gynecol 1999;93:281–284.
162. Segal S, Su M, Gilbert P: The effect of a rapid change in availability of epidural analgesia on the cesarean delivery rate: A meta-analysis. Am J Obstet Gynecol 2000;183:974–978.
163. Luxman D, Wolman I, Groutz A, et al: The effect of early epidural block administration on the progression and outcome of laobr. Int J Obstet Anesth 1998;7:161–164.
164. Chestnut DH, McGrath JM, Vincent RD Jr, et al: Does early administration of epidural analgesia affect obstetric outcome in nulliparous women who are in spontaneous labor? Anesthesiology 1994;80:1201–1208.
165. Chestnut DH, Vincent RD Jr, McGrath JM, et al: Does early administration of epidural analgesia affect obstetric outcome in nulliparous women who are receiving intravenous oxytocin? Anesthesiology 1994;80:1193–1200.
166. Halpern SH, Leighton BL, Ohlsson A, et al: Effect of epidural vs parenteral opioid analgesia on the progress of labor: a meta-analysis. JAMA 1998;280:2105–2110.
167. Leighton BL, Halpern SH: Epidural analgesia: Effects on labor progress and maternal and neonatal outcome. Semin Perinatol 2002;26:122–135.
168. Goyert GL, Bottoms SF, Treadwell MC, Nehra PC: The physician factor in cesarean birth rates. N Engl J Med 1989;320:706–709.
169. Socol ML, Garcia PM, Peaceman AM, Dooley SL: Reducing cesarean births at a primarily private university hospital. Am J Obstet Gynecol 1993;168:1748–1758.
170. Lagrew DC Jr, Morgan MA: Decreasing the cesarean section rate in a private hospital: Success without mandated clinical changes. Am J Obstet Gynecol 1996;174:184–191.
171. Mackowiak PA, Wasserman SS, Levine MM: A critical appraisal of 98.6 degrees F, the upper limit of the normal body temperature, and other legacies of Carl Reinhold August Wunderlich. JAMA 1992;268:1578–1580.
172. Resch GE, Millington WR: Inhibition of interleukin-1beta and prostaglandin E(2) thermogenesis by glycyl-glutamine, a pro-opiomelanocortin-derived peptide. Brain Res 2001;894:316–320.
173. Kelly RW: Inflammatory mediators and cervical ripening. J Reprod Immunol 2002;57:217–224.
174. Walker DW, Wood C: Temperature relationship of the mother and fetus during labor. Am J Obstet Gynecol 1970;107: 83–87.
175. Morishima HO, Glaser B, Niemann WH, James LS: Increased uterine activity and fetal deterioration during maternal hyperthermia. Am J Obstet Gynecol 1975;121:531–538.
176. Cefalo RC, Hellegers AE: The effects of maternal hyperthermia on maternal and fetal cardiovascular and respiratory function. Am J Obstet Gynecol 1978;131:687–694.
177. Lieberman E, Lang J, Richardson DK, et al: Intrapartum maternal fever and neonatal outcome. Pediatrics 2000;105:8–13.
178. Impey L, Greenwood C, MacQuillan K, et al: Fever in labour and neonatal encephalopathy: A prospective cohort study. BJOG 2001;108:594–597.
179. Grether JK, Nelson KB: Maternal infection and cerebral palsy in infants of normal birth weight. JAMA 1997;278:207–211.
180. Dammann O, Drescher J, Veelken N: Maternal fever at birth and non-verbal intelligence at age 9 years in preterm infants. Dev Med Child Neurol 2003;45:148–151.
181. Lieberman E, Cohen A, Lang J, et al: Maternal intrapartum temperature elevation as a risk factor for cesarean delivery and assisted vaginal delivery. Am J Public Health 1999;89: 506–510.
182. Shipp TD, Zelop C, Cohen A, et al: Post-cesarean delivery fever and uterine rupture in a subsequent trial of labor. Obstet Gynecol 2003;101:136–139.
183. Herbst A, Wolner-Hanssen P, Ingemarsson I: Risk factors for fever in labor. Obstet Gynecol 1995;86:790–794.
184. Vinson DC, Thomas R, Kiser T: Association between epidural analgesia during labor and fever. J Fam Pract 1993;36: 617–622.
185. Camann WR, Hortvet LA, Hughes N, et al: Maternal temperature regulation during extradural analgesia for labour. Br J Anaesth 1991;67:565–568.
186. Vallejo MC, Kaul B, Adler LJ, et al: Chorioamnionitis, not epidural analgesia, is associated with maternal fever during labour. Can J Anaesth 2001;48:1122–1126.
187. Dolak JA, Brown RE: Epidural analgesia and neonatal fever. Pediatrics 1998;101:492 (author reply 493–494).
188. Dashe JS, Rogers BB, McIntire DD, Leveno KJ: Epidural analgesia and intrapartum fever: Placental findings. Obstet Gynecol 1999;93:341–344.
189. Glosten B, Sessler DI, Faure EA, et al: Central temperature changes are poorly perceived during epidural anesthesia. Anesthesiology 1992;77:10–16.
190. Fusi L, Steer PJ, Maresh MJ, Beard RW: Maternal pyrexia associated with the use of epidural analgesia in labour. Lancet 1989;1:1250–1252.
191. Macaulay JH, Bond K, Steer PJ: Epidural analgesia in labor and fetal hyperthermia. Obstet Gynecol 1992;80:665–669.
192. Lieberman E, Lang JM, Frigoletto F Jr, et al: Epidural analgesia, intrapartum fever, and neonatal sepsis evaluation. Pediatrics 1997;99:415–419.
193. Ploeckinger B, Ulm MR, Chalubinski K, Gruber W: Epidural anaesthesia in labour: Influence on surgical delivery rates, intrapartum fever and blood loss. Gynecol Obstet Invest 1995;39: 24–27.
194. Glosten B, Savage M, Rooke GA, Brengelmann GL: Epidural anesthesia and the thermoregulatory responses to hyperthermia—Preliminary observations in volunteer subjects. Acta Anaesthesiol Scand 1998;42:442–446.
195. Goodlin RC, Chapin JW: Determinants of maternal temperature during labor. Am J Obstet Gynecol 1982;143:97–103.
196. Hagerdal M, Morgan CW, Sumner AE, Gutsche BB: Minute ventilation and oxygen consumption during labor with epidural analgesia. Anesthesiology 1983;59:425–427.
197. Gleeson NC, Nolan KM, Ford MR: Temperature, labour, and epidural analgesia. Lancet 1989;2:861–862.
198. Oka T: 5-HT and narcotic-induced hypothermia. Gen Pharmacol 1978;9:151–154.
199. Gross JB, Cohen AP, Lang JM, et al: Differences in systemic opioid use do not explain increased fever incidence in parturients receiving epidural analgesia. Anesthesiology 2002;97:157–161.
200. Mayer DC, Chescheir NC, Spielman FJ: Increased intrapartum antibiotic administration associated with epidural analgesia in labor. Am J Perinatol 1997;14:83–86.
201. Goetzl L, Cohen A, Frigoletto F Jr, et al: Maternal epidural use and neonatal sepsis evaluation in afebrile mothers. Pediatrics 2001;108:1099–1102.
202. Yancey MK, Zhang J, Schwarz J, et al: Labor epidural analgesia and intrapartum maternal hyperthermia. Obstet Gynecol 2001;98:763–770.

203. Kaul B, Vallejo M, Ramanathan S, Mandell G: Epidural labor analgesia and neonatal sepsis evaluation rate: A quality improvement study. Anesth Analg 2001;93:986–990.
204. Goetzl L, Evans T, Rivers J, et al: Elevated maternal and fetal serum interleukin-6 levels are associated with epidural fever. Am J Obstet Gynecol 2002;187:834–838.
205. Windle ML, Booker LA, Rayburn WF: Postpartum pain after vaginal delivery. A review of comparative analgesic trials. J Reprod Med 1989;34:891–895.

Author's note: The author would like to thank the gracious mentorship, friendship, and scholarship of Sanjay Datta, MD, FFARCS (Eng.), who richly contributed to the author's appreciation and enthusiasm for the patients and science within the specialty of obstetric anesthesia.

CHAPTER 73

Perineal Repair and Pelvic Floor Injury

Colm O'Herlihy / Rohna Kearney

INTRODUCTION

Pelvic floor injury at the time of vaginal delivery can result in the later development of urinary incontinence, pelvic organ prolapse and fecal incontinence. In the United States the direct annual cost of pelvic organ prolapse surgery alone is estimated to be over $1 billion, with 22 women per 10,000 requiring surgical correction for this indication.[1,2] The annual direct cost of urinary incontinence is even higher, at $12.4 billion.[3] The lifetime risk of a woman in the United States undergoing surgery for incontinence or prolapse by the age of 80 is 11%.[4] With growing awareness of the impact of pelvic floor injury, attention is now increasingly focused on the prevention of these problems. Vaginal delivery is the factor most subject to modification in the etiology of pelvic floor injury.[5–7] In order to prevent injury and minimize the impact of delivery on the pelvic floor, it is necessary to have an understanding of the anatomy and the pathophysiology of injury.

Anatomy

The primary function of the pelvic floor is to prevent the pelvic organs from downward displacement in the upright position, while at the same time allowing parturition and elimination. The levator ani muscles, which are composites of the pubococcygeus, puborectalis, and iliococcygeus on each side, are the most important constituents of the pelvic floor and resemble a horizontal shelf that acts to close like a valve when the female assumes the upright position.[8] The pubococcygeus comprises the puboanalis, pubovaginalis, and puboperineus subdivisions.[9] The pubococcygeus and puborectalis arise from the inner surface of the pubic bone, whereas the iliococcygeus arises from the arcus tendineus levator ani. The pubococcygeus inserts into the vaginal wall (pubovaginalis), perineal body (puboperineus), and intersphincteric groove (puboanalis). The puborectalis forms a sling around the rectum and inserts into the deep external sphincter and the iliococcygeus inserts into the iliococcygeal raphe.

The perineal membrane is a triangular sheet of fibromuscular tissue with the striated urogenital sphincter lying above. It provides support by attaching the vagina, urethra and perineal body to the ischiopubic rami. Above it the striated urogenital sphincter consists of the compressor urethra urethrovaginal sphincter, and the sphincter urethra.

The endopelvic fascia refers to the condensation of the adventitial layers of the pelvic organs. This connective tissue layer attaches the pelvic organs to the lateral pelvic walls and, together with the levator ani, shares the load on the pelvic floor. Support for the vagina has been identified at three levels[10,11] (Fig. 73–1). Level I consists of the uterosacral and cardinal ligaments, which represent a medial and lateral thickening of the endopelvic fascia connecting the cervix and upper vagina to the pelvic sidewalls. These structures are vertical in the standing position and serve to keep the uterus, cervix, and upper vagina tethered in a posterior position over the levator ani muscles.

At level II, the middle third of the vagina is attached by the paracolpium to the arcus tendineus and levator ani muscle fascia. The arcus tendineus fascia pelvis runs from the pubic bone anteriorly to the ischial spines posteriorly. At level III, the lower third of the vagina is attached directly to the perineal membrane, perineal body, and levator ani.

The proximal urethra is supported by the endopelvic fascia and anterior vaginal wall, which act like a hammock and attach it to the arcus tendineus fascia and levator ani, thus resulting in compression and closure of the urethral lumen in response to increases in intra-abdominal pressure.[12]

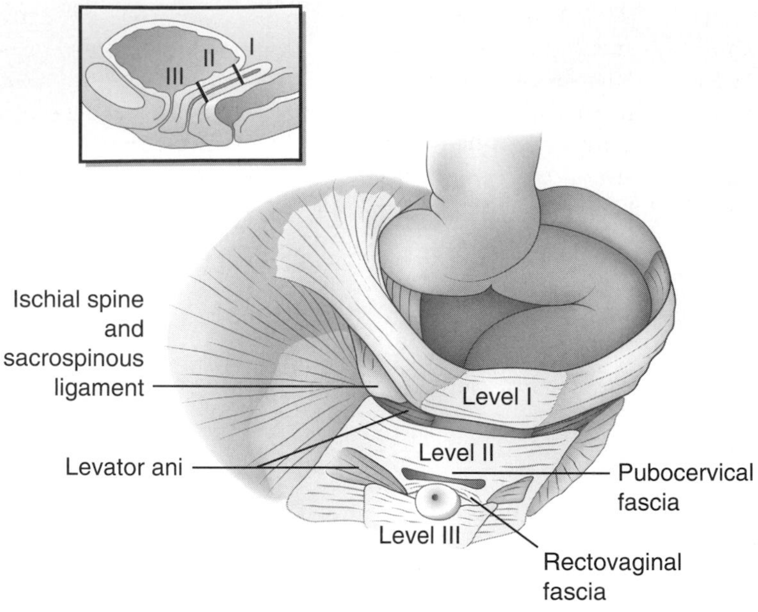

FIGURE 73–1
Illustration of the three levels of vaginal support. (From Delancey JO: Anatomic aspects of vaginal eversion after hysterectomy. Am J Obstet Gynecol 1992;166:1717–1728.)

The perineal body is covered by skin and lies between the lower vagina and the anus. It is attached by the perineal membrane to the inferior pubic rami and ischial tuberosities. The perineal body receives the insertion of the bulbocavernosus muscles and posteriorly is attached to the coccyx by the external anal sphincter.

The anal sphincters are located in the posterior compartment of the pelvic floor. The external anal sphincter is a voluntary muscle consisting of three components, a subcutaneous part, a superficial part connecting the perineal body to the coccyx, and a deep part, which surrounds the rectum. The internal anal sphincter is a downward extension and thickening of the circular smooth muscle of the rectum. The intersphincteric groove runs between the internal and external anal sphincters. The ischiorectal fossas lie between the levator ani and the obturator internus muscles. The external anal sphincter and bulbocavernosus muscles are supplied by the pudendal nerve, which arises from the anterior primary rami of S2, S3, and S4. The nerve leaves the pelvis through the greater sciatic foramen and runs in the pelvic side wall close to the ischial spine and sacrospinous ligament to enter the pudendal (Alcock's) canal through the lesser sciatic foramen. It divides into three terminal branches—the clitoral, perineal, and inferior rectal. Autonomic nerves from the pelvic plexus supply the internal anal sphincter.

Pathophysiology

Pelvic floor injury can result from damage to the nerve supply, muscles, or connective tissue, which together maintain pelvic floor function. There is good evidence that damage to the innervation of the pelvic floor is a causative factor in the development of urinary and fecal incontinence following vaginal delivery.[13,14] Partial denervation of the pelvic floor has been shown in 80% of women following a single vaginal delivery.[15] Fetal macrosomia and a prolonged second stage (either active or passive) are associated with an increased risk of neuropathic damage.[16]

The levator ani and endopelvic fascia act together to maintain urinary continence and pelvic organ support. If the muscle is damaged, the connective tissue has to play a greater compensatory role, and this frequently fails over time, most commonly after the menopause. The arcus tendineus fascia is found to be detached (most commonly from the ischial spines) in women with anterior vaginal wall prolapse,[10] and histologic studies have documented levator ani muscle fibrosis following vaginal delivery.[17] Such changes are also seen in women with stress urinary incontinence and pelvic organ prolapse.[18] Magnetic resonance imaging is providing increasing information about pelvic floor injury following childbirth, demonstrating, for example, abnormalities in the levator ani in women with stress urinary incontinence and prolapse.[19,20] A recent study has shown levator ani muscle abnormality in 20% of women following their first vaginal delivery,[21] although it has not yet been established whether these defects are related to muscle or nerve injury or a combination of insults. As well as a prolonged second stage of labor and fetal macrosomia, instrumental delivery, midline episiotomy, and occipitoposterior fetal position have also been implicated in pelvic floor injury.[15,16,22–24]

UTEROVAGINAL PROLAPSE

Effects of Pregnancy, Childbirth, and Parity

Nulliparous pregnant women have been shown to exhibit altered pelvic floor support when compared with nulliparous nonpregnant women. In the nonpregnant group, 43% had stage 0 prolapse and 57% had stage 1, but in the pregnant group 10% had stage 0, 43% had stage 1, and

48% had stage 2.[25] Interestingly, the greatest changes observed were in the length of the anterior wall and the perineal body, which may explain the common occurrence of urinary incontinence during pregnancy. The increase in perineal body length may represent an adaptation that reduces the occurrence of anal sphincter damage. Another study of nulliparous women delivered at term showed that at 36 weeks' gestation 46% had prolapse, with 26% having a stage 2 prolapse[26]; at 6 weeks postpartum there was a similar incidence of new prolapse in women delivered vaginally and by cesarean section. Thus, regardless of the mode of delivery, being pregnant of itself impairs pelvic floor support.

That the risk of prolapse increases with the number of vaginal deliveries is well documented. Mant and associates have shown that a woman after two vaginal deliveries has an eightfold increased risk of developing pelvic organ prolapse compared with the nulliparous woman and that this risk rises to 12-fold after four vaginal deliveries.[5]

Risks

Uterine prolapse occurring for the first time during pregnancy is rare, occcurring in 1 in 10,000 to 15,000 deliveries.[27] It can occur acutely following a fall or trauma in nulliparous women[27] but is more commonly seen in parous women with prolapse prior to pregnancy. Much of the literature relating to uterine prolapse in pregnancy consists of case reports prior to 1970,[27–31] when the condition was seen more frequently owing to higher average parity.[32] Thus, current data on maternal and fetal risks are lacking. A large review up to 1940 reported a substantial fetal and maternal complication rate,[27] which included a 10% risk of miscarriage[28] and an increased risk of preterm birth.[29] Fetal and maternal death have also been reported.[29] Cervical elongation, hypertrophy, and edema are present in all cases in which the pregnancy progresses to term.[27] Urinary obstruction can occur and may require catheterization. Abnormalities of labor are common. On the one hand, weakness of the pelvic floor can lead to precipitate delivery with resultant cervical lacerations. On the other hand, cervical infection and bleeding during pregnancy are common and can lead to scarring and fibrosis with resultant cervical dystocia. This typically manifests as secondary arrest in cervical dilation, usually between 5 and 7 cm.[30] At one time it would have been managed by Duhrssen's cervical incisions with or without the use of forceps, but presently cesarean section is preferred. Accordingly, although spontaneous vaginal delivery rates of 40% to 80% have been reported,[29,30] cesarean or instrumental deliveries are more common. Primary postpartum hemorrhage, due to uterine atony, may be difficult to control, as manual uterine compression is hindered by the prolapse.

Management Options

Prenatal

Uterine prolapse occurring prenatally requires admission to hospital if it is not possible to reduce the prolapse in the clinic. Treatment consists of bed rest in the Trendelenburg position combined with an indwelling urinary catheter and saline soaks to reduce cervical edema. Once edema has been reduced, the prolapse can usually be manually replaced and a pessary then inserted to prevent reccurrence; a Hodge pessary is the one most commonly used. Antibiotic creams are often prescribed to reduce associated cervicitis. There is no evidence that systemic antibiotics are beneficial. In the past vaginal packing and even surgical closure of the introitus have been described as effective.[32] The introitus is reopened at term to allow vaginal delivery. Pessary treatment is often required only until the fifth month of pregnancy, when the uterus lifts out of the pelvis, thereby alleviating prolapse symptoms.[33]

Labor and Delivery

Careful intrapartum monitoring of the rate of cervical dilation is essential for early detection of both precipitate delivery and cervical dystocia. In the event of the latter, (Duhrssen's) intracervical incisions can be considered, but today cesarean section is usually more appropriate.

Postnatal

If the prolapse is untreated, it will almost certainly recur in future pregnancies. Surgery is the definitive cure, but a vaginal pessary is an appropriate immediate treatment during postnatal genital involution. Longer term use of a pessary should be considered if more pregnancies are desired, as a surgical repair is likely to be undone by another vaginal delivery, and an elective cesarean to avoid recurrent prolapse carries its own risks.

SUMMARY OF MANAGEMENT OPTIONS

Uterovaginal Prolapse

Management Options	Quality of Evidence	Strength of Recommendation	References
Prepregnancy			
Consider deferring formal repair until family is complete.	–	GPP	–

Continued

SUMMARY OF MANAGEMENT OPTIONS
Uterovaginal Prolapse *(Continued)*

Management Options	Quality of Evidence	Strength of Recommendation	References
Prenatal			
Bed rest in Trendelenburg position	–	GPP	–
Saline soaks	–	GPP	–
Antibiotic cream	–	GPP	–
Hodge pessary	–	GPP	–
Labor/Delivery			
Critical review of cervical dilation	–	GPP	–
Active management of third stage and vigilance for postpartum hemorrhage	–	GPP	–
Postnatal			
Formal prolapse management	–	GPP	–

PREVIOUS PELVIC FLOOR REPAIR/ VAGINAL SURGERY

Maternal Risks

Despite a general decline in family size, the combined effects of increasing rates of surgical intervention for pelvic organ prolapse and urinary incontinence and delayed childbearing mean that many women are becoming pregnant having previously undergone reconstructive surgery. This poses a dilemma for the obstetrician. Both pregnancy and especially delivery can pose a threat to the continued efficacy of successful surgical repair. It is important to provide the woman with information on the likelihood of symptoms recurring during pregnancy, persisting following delivery and necessitating further treatment. However, published evidence on which to base management is scanty. The urethra lengthens during pregnancy,[34] and the bladder becomes an abdominal organ. Stress incontinence occurs commonly in pregnancy[35] and is a risk factor for persistent urinary incontinence. Thus, pregnancy of itself poses a risk of prolapse recurring. However, the main obstetric concern following previous successful pelvic floor surgery is mode of delivery. Reported outcomes among women delivered abdominally or vaginally following previous surgery for pelvic organ prolapse and stress urinary incontinence provide conflicting results. In the largest series of 89 women who conceived following colporrhaphy (66 of whom had undergone cervical amputation), 34 miscarried or delivered prior to 32 weeks. Twenty-four had a cesarean section to preserve pelvic floor function. At 6 to 8 weeks post partum, there was recurrence of symptoms in 7% of women, but at 1 year postpartum, 22% had symptoms severe enough to require further surgery.[36] Cesarean section failed to prevent recurrence, with 9 of the 25 (36%) delivered abdominally suffering recurrence at 5 years compared to 7 of the 49 (14%) delivered vaginally. On the other hand, in another series of 78 women who had surgery for prolapse, 31 were followed up after subsequent pregnancy. Twenty-five had vaginal deliveries and four of them had recurrent prolapse,[37] six had cesarean section, and none had any recurrence of prolapse (although this difference is not statistically significant). Another study of five women who delivered vaginally following a previous Burch colposuspension reported that three suffered recurrent incontinence,[38] whereas all the women delivered by cesarean section had maintained continence at 1 year post cesarean (despite a majority having had incontinence in the third trimester). Of six reported vaginal deliveries following uterosacral sacrospinous suspension for prolapse, one patient suffered a recurrence of symptoms requiring further surgery.[39]

Fetal Risks

The Manchester repair (Fothergill) operation performed prior to pregnancy has been associated with greater miscarriage and preterm delivery rates, but this operation is now rarely performed.

Management Options

Prepregnancy

All women planning a pregnancy after previous pelvic floor surgery for urinary incontinence or prolapse should be advised of a possible functional deterioration during pregnancy that may persist, even if an elective cesarean section is performed.

Prenatal

Timely assessment of symptom recurrence and reassurance of probable resolution of symptoms following delivery are important. Intensive pelvic floor physiotherapy may be indicated, but there are inadequate data on its effectiveness in this situation for it to be recommended with confidence.

Labor and Delivery

If symptoms have been largely cured by a prolapse or incontinence repair procedure, current consensus would favor performing an elective cesarean section in order to minimize the risk of recurrent symptoms. There have, however, been many reports of women delivering vaginally with no recurrence of symptoms. If a vaginal delivery is planned, an episiotomy may be beneficial to reduce stretching of rigid or scarred tissues.[36]

Postnatal

Pelvic floor exercises should be continued. A decision regarding further surgical management should ideally be deferred until 6 months following delivery, as recovery of function continues to occur until then.[40] Any plans for further childbearing should be discussed; the woman should be made aware that any subsequent pregnancy risks producing a recurrence of symptoms requiring further surgery once childbearing is complete.

SUMMARY OF MANAGEMENT OPTIONS

Previous Pelvic Floor Repair or Vaginal Surgery

Management Options	Quality of Evidence	Strength of Recommendation	References
Prepregnancy			
Advise that further pregnancy can result in functional deterioration even if cesarean section performed.	–	GPP	–
Prenatal			
Assess current status of pelvic floor function.	–	GPP	–
Advise that pregnancy and delivery may result in deterioration or recurrence of symptoms.	–	GPP	–
Refer for physiotherapy (uncertain benefit).	–	GPP	–
Labor/Delivery			
Consensus favors cesarean section.	–	GPP	–
Episiotomy may be benficial if vaginal delivery is undertaken.	III	B	36
Postnatal			
Arrange postnatal review after 6 months.	III	B	40

PERINEAL INJURY

Trauma to the perineum, of varying degree, constitutes the most common form of obstetric injury. Its severity is generally classified according to the degree of perineal disruption:

- First-degree tear involves only perineal or vaginal skin.
- Second-degree tear occurs when perineal skin and muscles are torn.
- Third-degree tear occurs when, in addition to perineal skin and muscle, the anal sphincter muscle is torn.
- Fourth-degree tear occurs when sphincter muscle disruption is complete with additional extension into the anal mucosa; this implies that both external and internal anal sphincter muscles have been severed.

Further subdivision of third-degree tears, in particular, has been proposed[41] according to the depth of torn sphincter muscle, but such differentiation can be difficult in clinical practice.

First- and Second-Degree Tears

General

First- and second-degree perineal tears are very common. The incidence of intact perineum following delivery after a first vaginal birth is very low, approximately 6%.[42] The maternal position at delivery may be important; one study reported an overall 66% intact perineum rate associated with the lateral position at delivery, compared to 42% in the squatting position.[43] Because of the frequent need for suturing of tears and the limited availability of experienced surgeons, repair is often performed by relatively inexperienced personnel. All staff supervising even the most normal births should therefore receive early and thorough training in perineal repair. The principles of management include immediate assessment to exclude deeper injury involving the anal sphincter, appropriate surgical repair, and effective postpartum analgesia and advice.

Maternal Risks

Second-degree tears can result in significant morbidity. Women who sustain them resume sexual intercourse later and report greater frequency of dyspareunia than women who have intact perineums or first-degree tears.[44] Use of teaching models for instruction of midwifery and medical staff in repair technique is effective in reducing such complications.[45]

Management Options

PRENATAL

Prenatal and intrapartum perineal massage have been advocated as interventions to reduce the incidence of second- and greater-degree tears, but the evidence in its favor is conflicting. In one study of 1340 women, massage and stretching during the second stage of labor did not increase the rate of perineums intact after delivery.[46] However, a second study of 861 nulliparas randomized to antenatal perineal massage demonstrated a reduction in episiotomy, and second- and third-degree lacerations, with the greatest benefit among women over 30 years old.[47] Pelvic floor muscle exercises performed prenatally and postnatally have been shown to reduce self-reported incontinence in late pregnancy and up to 6 months postpartum.[48]

LABOR AND DELIVERY

Several studies have examined the method of perineal repair. Use of polyglactin suture material is associated with less perineal pain lower resuture rates compared to chromic catgut.[49,50] A two-stage continuous repair leaving the skin unsutured also seems to be associated with less pain.[50,51]

THE ROLE OF CESAREAN SECTION

There is no consensus about the role of elective cesarean section in the prevention of obstetric pelvic floor injury. However, some are so convinced of its benefit that they even advocate obtaining "informed consent" regarding the risks of perineal injury before women elect to have a vaginal birth.[52] Although traumatic mechanical injury to the anal sphincter occurs only with vaginal delivery, evidence exists to show that if performed late in labor cesarean section may fail entirely to protect the anal sphincter mechanism, with one study showing neurologic injury in women delivered by cesarean section after 8 cm dilation.[53] Parous women delivered only by cesarean section still have a 3.5-fold increased relative risk of urinary incontinence compared to women who have never been pregnant, although the risk is higher still after vaginal delivery.[54] These data suggest that the pregnant state of itself (regardless of mode of delivery) can influence function and indicate that more research is required into the pathogenesis of obstetric pelvic floor injury before definitive advice on mode of delivery can be offered.

POSTNATAL

Analgesia is the main priority.

SUMMARY OF MANAGEMENT OPTIONS

First- and Secondary-Degree Tear

Management Options	Quality of Evidence	Strength of Recommendation	References
Prenatal			
There is conflicting evidence on the value of perineal massage before and during labor.	Ib	A	46, 47
Pelvic floor exercises before and after labor are associated with a lower incidence of self-reported incontinence up to 6 months.	III	B	48

SUMMARY OF MANAGEMENT OPTIONS

First- and Secondary-Degree Tear *(Continued)*

Management Options	Quality of Evidence	Strength of Recommendation	References
Labor and Delivery			
Polyglactin suture material is associated with a lower incidence of pain and lower resuture rates than chromic catgut.	Ib	A	49, 50
Two-stage continuous suture leaving skin unsutured is associated with less pain.	Ib	A	50, 51
Postnatal			
Analgesia and pelvic floor exercises are recommended.	III	B	48

Third-Degree Anal Sphincter Injury

General

Altered fecal continence is common following primary repair of third- and fourth-degree perineal injury, that is, when anal sphincter muscle disruption is clinically recognized after vaginal delivery. Up to 50% of women experience some incontinence symptoms within the weeks and months after a third-degree tear.[55,56] These symptoms do not correlate with the mode of sphincter repair. Consequently, all women known to have sustained anal sphincter trauma should have their continence routinely assessed at the conclusion of the puerperium.

Postnatal continence assessment should include direct questioning using a standardized bowel function questionnaire (Table 73–1)[57] so that a reliable continence score can be allotted to facilitate monitoring of the progress of symptoms over time. Continence of flatus, liquid, and solid feces should be documented, together with inquiry concerning fecal urgency, a socially debilitating symptom defined as an inability to defer defecation for longer than 5 minutes; the complaint of urgency incontinence may reflect external anal sphincter dysfunction.

Digital examination of the anal canal may provide an approximation of the integrity of the sphincter and perineal body but is not otherwise diagnostically reliable. On the other hand, palpable defects in the levator ani musculature have been shown to correlate with magnetic resonance images of the pelvic floor.[21] Nevertheless, anorectal physiologic testing is necessary to determine objectively the nature and prognosis of any residual anal sphincter damage and routinely consists of the following investigations:

- Anal manometry is performed to evaluate sphincter tone and contractile function.
- Endoanal ultrasound is used to examine the anatomic integrity of the sphincter.
- Neurophysiologic testing of the pelvic floor is done to identify pudendal neuropathy.

These tests should be applied not only to women who have sustained third- and fourth-degree tears but also to other puerperal patients complaining of fecal incontinence. Disturbance of resting tone on anal manometry is indicative of predominant internal anal sphincter dysfunction, whereas a reduction in squeeze incremental pressure on voluntary contraction is consistent with reduced external sphincter muscle power. Manometry is performed using a multichannel, water-perfused catheter in the left lateral position, and reductions in the pressure profile, while diagnostically reliable, do not differentiate traumatic muscular from neurologic injury. High-quality endoanal endosonography provides clear and reproducible images of both internal and external

TABLE 73–1

Standardized Bowel Function Questionnaire: Fecal Continence Scoring System

FEATURE	NEVER	RARELY	SOMETIMES	USUALLY	ALWAYS
Incontinence for solid stool	0	1	2	3	4
Incontinence for liquid stool	0	1	2	3	4
Incontinence for flatus	0	1	2	3	4
Wears pad	0	1	2	3	4
Fecal urgency	0	1	2	3	4

Add one score from each row. A score of 0 implies complete continence. A score of 20 implies complete incontinence.

sphincters [58,59] but may overestimate the significance of muscular defects. Many women are found to have small defects that do not correlate with antecedent obstetric events or fecal incontinence symptoms.[60]

Pudendal nerve assessment should include testing both conduction along the entire length of the nerve, for example, using clitoral-anal reflex assessment, and anal sphincter electromyography (EMG), which assesses motor unit recruitment and action potential morphology. Neuropathy is responsible for at least one third of fecal continence disturbances, and its assessment provides essential information on prognosis and appropriate management.[61]

Risk Factors for Anal Sphincter Injury (Table 73–2)

VAGINAL DELIVERY

Normal vaginal delivery inevitably increases the risk of damage to the sphincter mechanism, compared with prelabor cesarean section. Nonetheless, intrapartum cesarean section can be followed by continence disturbance, consistent with first stage influences on anal sphincter function.[53] Prelabor cesarean section should, therefore, be chosen when any risk to the pelvic floor is to be avoided.

PRIMIPARITY

Because first labors are most often associated with inefficient uterine contractility, dystocia, prolonged labor, use of epidural anesthesia and episiotomy, puerperal fecal incontinence most often follows first vaginal delivery. Risk is increased between two- and fivefold,[62] which reflects the reduced elasticity of the pelvic floor among nulliparas.

INSTRUMENTAL DELIVERY

Both forceps and vacuum extraction significantly increase the risk to the fecal continence mechanism two- to sevenfold.[16,62] Although vacuum extraction is somewhat less commonly traumatic, completion of the delivery with forceps when a vacuum attempt fails, generally due to poor adhesion of the vacuum cup, compounds the incontinence risk.[63]

TABLE 73–2

Obstetric Risk Factors for Anal Sphincter Injury

First vaginal delivery
Instrumental delivery (forceps > vacuum)
Prolonged second stage of labor (>1 hour)
Epidural anesthesia
Persistent occipitoposterior position
Macrosomia (birth weight > 4 kg)
Shoulder dystocia
Previous third-degree perineal tear
Midline episiotomy

PROLONGED SECOND STAGE OF LABOR AND EPIDURAL ANALGESIA

Effective epidural analgesia, now a very widely applied form of intrapartum pain relief, abolishes the maternal bearing down reflex in late labor. As a consequence, the passive phase of the second stage of labor is prolonged, sometimes for several hours, before maternal pushing is encouraged. Such a prolonged passive second stage doubles the risk of subsequent incontinence, apparently secondary to pudendal neuropathy. Randomized evidence does not support an expectant policy in the second stage under epidural blockade, because the instrumental delivery rate is not reduced and the duration of labor is needlessly prolonged.[64]

INTRAPARTUM MECHANICAL FACTORS

Third-degree tears occur three times more frequently when the fetus is macrosomic (birth weight >4 kg) compared with lower birth weights. Shoulder dystocia also predisposes to anal sphincter injury, as does persistent occipitoposterior position of the fetal head in the second stage of labor.[22]

MIDLINE EPISIOTOMY

Episiotomy is performed with the objective of preventing deep perineal lacerations and anal sphincter trauma, and is one of the most frequent surgical interventions. The perineal incision can be made either mediolaterally or in the midline posteriorly. Although there is a widespread assumption that it can do more harm than good,[65–67] recent population data suggest that selective mediolateral episiotomy may be protective of the sphincter mechanism.[68,69] On the other hand, there is little doubt that midline episiotomy, which is particularly favored in North America, greatly increases the risk of third-degree tear[70] to the extent that its use should probably be abandoned. This risk is compounded when midline episiotomy is combined with other interventions, such as epidural analgesia and instrumental delivery.

PREVIOUS ANAL SPHINCTER DISRUPTION

The incidence of third-degree tears of varying severity is about 2.5% of primiparous and 0.5% of multiparous vaginal deliveries, with an overall average rate of about 1.5%.[59] Following satisfactory postnatal repair, at subsequent vaginal delivery the risk of a further tear increases fourfold to about 4%[71] if mediolateral episiotomy is practiced and to over 10% with midline episiotomy.[72]

Management Options

Bearing in mind the inherent anatomic vulnerability of the anal sphincter during childbirth, some risk of trauma exists even when obstetric management is optimal. Avoidance of postpartum fecal incontinence rests partly with measures to avoid occurrence of third-degree tears but even more significantly, in the appropriate management of anal sphincter injury when it occurs at delivery.

PRIMARY PREVENTION

Primary preventive measures include augmentation of myometrial contractions during first labors, using intravenous oxytocin to correct dystocia; in this way the incidences of instrumental delivery, occipitoposterior position, and prolonged first and second stages of labor can be minimized (for a somewhat different view, see Chapter 69). Vacuum extraction should be the first choice for low-cavity instrumental delivery, although the potentially traumatic sequence of failed vacuum followed by forceps delivery should not be ignored. Abbreviation of the passive, nonpushing second stage of labor is advisable, even in the presence of effective epidural anesthesia (again, for a somewhat different view, see Chapter 72). When episiotomy is performed, midline procedures should be eschewed in favor of mediolateral incisions approximating as closely as possible to 45 degrees.

OPTIMIZING PERINEAL REPAIR

A standard classification of the severity of anal sphincter injury has not been generally adopted. It is inevitable that the functional outcome following repair of extensive tears involving the internal anal sphincter and anal mucosa (fourth-degree tears) will be intrinsically more predisposed to continence sequelae than when only partial-thickness external sphincter trauma has occurred. Nevertheless, well-trained obstetric surgeons using appropriate operative techniques will produce the best functional outcomes, regardless of the extent of injury.

MANAGEMENT OF OBSTETRIC SPHINCTER DISRUPTION

Timing of Repair Procedure. It is standard obstetric practice to repair anal sphincter tears immediately or within a few hours of vaginal delivery—the so-called primary repair. Early repair abbreviates the patient's inconvenience and discomfort but should not preclude performance of the repair procedure by an appropriately trained obstetric surgeon. If a skilled operator is not immediately available, then delayed primary repair within 24 hours has much to recommend it, provided that hemostasis and analgesia have been produced. Delayed repair will, however, almost inevitably enhance the patient's anxiety and sense of grievance concerning her injury, with a potential incremental effect on resort to complaint and litigation.

Surgical Technique. Anal sphincter repair should be conducted with full surgical precautions, instrumentation, and lighting in an operating room setting. Slowly absorbed synthetic monofilament suture materials such as polyglyconate (Maxon) or polydioxone (PDS) should be used. Although coloproctologists employ an overlapping "figure-of-eight" approximation of the anal sphincter muscle stumps when performing secondary repairs following an interval of fibrosis and cicatrization, direct approximation of the disrupted sphincter appears to provide equally effective functional results in the well-perfused muscle found immediately after injury at primary repair.[55] Distortion of the normal anal anatomic relationships following deep perineal lacerations means that endoanal ultrasound does not appear to offer useful intraoperative assistance in improving surgical muscle realignment. Ultrasound may have a potential role, however, in the early postnatal screening of women with ostensibly intact anal sphincters so as to facilitate selective monitoring of fecal continence among those who sustain occult forms of anal sphincter injury.

Postnatal Management. Although firm evidence is scanty, it appears likely that prophylactic broad-spectrum antibiotic therapy (e.g., co-amoxyclavulanic acid) enhances the integrity of primary anal sphincter repair during the first 3 to 5 postnatal days. On the other hand, firm randomized, controlled data exist to support the use of a laxative rather than a constipating postoperative regimen during the early puerperium.[73] Use of lactulose or ispaghula to soften the stool is associated with a shorter and less painful recovery period when compared with codeine phosphate treatment as employed by coloproctologists following elective anal surgery.

Routine Postnatal Review of Fecal Continence. Because up to 50% of women who sustain a third- or fourth-degree tear experience some puerperal symptoms of fecal incontinence, routine follow-up assessment of anal sphincter function is advisable once postnatal healing is complete. Such a review is probably best performed at 8 to 12 weeks following delivery and should consist, as delineated previously, of an assessment of fecal continence symptoms, anal manometry, and endoanal ultrasound combined with pudendal nerve evaluation, if indicated. The examination should optimally take place in an obstetric setting because it provides the patient with an opportunity to discuss not only her current continence status but also the antecedent circumstances surrounding her anal injury. The results of the anal physiology investigations facilitate the planning of further treatment and provide invaluable insights into prognosis.

Symptomatic Therapy. Minor postnatal fecal incontinence symptoms such as intermittent fecal urgency or constipation are frequently transient in nature and can often be effectively managed using loperamide or ispaghula, respectively. Perineal pain, secondary to discomfort in the sutured tissues, is amenable to targeted local injection of a combination of 2% bupivicaine, hyaluronidase, and methylprednisolone acetate. More significant tenderness and dyspareunia associated with perineal anatomic distortion can be corrected by minor surgical intervention under local or general anesthesia. Associated psychosexual dysfunction responds to early psychotherapeutic counseling initiated before secondary deterioration in sexual interaction has developed.

Postnatal Physiotherapy. Even without active treatment, fecal incontinence symptoms of minor degree are frequently transient and disappear or attenuate within a few

TABLE 73–3

Proposed Management of Multiparas in Pregnancies after Anal Sphincter Injury

TYPE OF INJURY	INVESTIGATION PROFILE	MANAGEMENT
1. Previous third-degree tear—asymptomatic	Normal manometry and ultrasound	Allow vaginal delivery
2. Previous third-degree tear—symptomatic incontinence	Abnormal manometry and/or ultrasound	Prelabor cesarean section
3. Successful secondary sphincter repair	Normal manometry and ultrasound	Prelabor cesarean section
4. Previous third-degree tear or "occult" injury—asymptomatic	Abnormal manometry and ultrasound	Discuss vaginal or cesarean delivery

months of delivery. Kegel pelvic floor exercises are not effective in alleviating incontinence, but the addition of operant conditioning through biofeedback physiotherapy using an endoanal stimulating probe[74] significantly improves anal sphincter function. Biofeedback therapy is particularly effective in maintaining muscle bulk while healing occurs and neuropathy recovers.

Secondary Anal Sphincter Repair. Persistent symptoms of fecal incontinence lasting for more than 6 months following delivery usually necessitate surgical repair of the damaged anal sphincter muscle. Before considering surgery, it is mandatory to exclude a coexistent neuropathic cause for the symptoms and to confirm pudendal nerve integrity. If severe neuropathy is identified, then colostomy diversion or an artificial sphincter procedure may be necessary.

Counseling during Subsequent Pregnancies. Women who suffer persistent and debilitating fecal incontinence after childbirth are likely to experience deterioration in their symptoms after further vaginal deliveries.[75] Transient symptoms that do not persist but are associated with abnormally low resting and squeeze manometric pressures and a large residual anal sphincter defect may recur following further vaginal deliveries. On the other hand, the continence of asymptomatic women with relatively normal manometric profiles is not likely to deteriorate, even in the presence of documented anal sphincter scarring on endoanal ultrasound examination. Ultrasound tends to overdiagnose functional deficits in continence[60] but should, nonetheless, be performed, together with anal manometry, when planning the mode of next delivery in women with a history of third- or fourth-degree anal sphincter injury.

As a generalization, in the absence of clear evidence of the optimal approach in such women, it is probably best to individualize the management. An empiric approach is suggested in Table 73–3.

In women who have achieved normal continence following primary obstetric anal sphincter injury and repair, further vaginal delivery is a reasonable option. However, elective prelabor cesarean section is advisable to protect the continence mechanism following successful secondary repair of the anal sphincter. The use of prophylactic cesarean delivery in women with asymptomatic ultrasonically identified sphincter defects is not justified by the published evidence.

SUMMARY OF MANAGEMENT OPTIONS

Third-Degree Tear

Management Options	Quality of Evidence	Strength of Recommendation	References
Prevention			
Oxytocin augmentation of first labor	–	GPP	–
Appropriate episiotomy technique (avoid midline)	–	GPP	–
Vacuum extraction as first choice for assisted vaginal delivery	–	GPP	–
Short passive phase of second stage of labor (see Chapters 69 and 72 for contrasting views on these options)	–	GPP	–
Optimal Perineal Repair Technique			
Formal training of obstetric trainees	–	GPP	–
Primary approximation or overlap sphincter repair with slowly absorbed suture material	Ib	A	55
Appropriate suture material (e.g., polyglyconate or polydioxone)	–	GPP	–

SUMMARY OF MANAGEMENT OPTIONS
Third-Degree Tear *(Continued)*

Management Options	Quality of Evidence	Strength of Recommendation	References
Focused Postnatal Management			
Laxative regimen postnatally	Ib	A	73
Prophylactic antibiotic therapy	–	GPP	–
Analgesia and other symptomatic therapy	–	GPP	–
Biofeedback physiotherapy	Ib	A	74
Appropriate assessment of fecal continence following sphincter injury	–	GPP	–
Selected secondary overlap sphincter repair for persistent incontinence	–	GPP	–
Subsequent Pregnancies			
Those at risk:	–	GPP	–
Persistent fecal incontinence symptoms			
Previous third-degree tear			
Poor antenatal manometry profile			
Individualize management (see Table 73–3)	–	GPP	–

FEMALE CIRCUMCISION (FEMALE GENITAL MUTILATION)

The World Health Organization defines female genital mutilation (FGM) as including all procedures involving partial or total removal of the external female genitalia or other injury to the female genital organs for cultural, religious, or nontherapeutic reasons.[76] This practice occurs predominantly in Africa, although affected women and girls may present anywhere in the world as immigrants from these countries. Consequently, FGM is now a global concern with human rights organizations devoted to the elimination of this practice and many countries prohibiting it by law. Medical professionals caring for affected women require knowledge and understanding of FGM.[77] Countries where there is a high prevalence of FGM include Egypt, Sudan, Eritrea, Ethiopa, Djibouti, Somalia, Mali, Senegal, Guinea, and Sierra Leone, and the WHO estimates that currently 100 million to 140 million women live with the consequences of this procedure, with a further 2 million girls at risk each year.

There are several forms of FGM that carry differing health implications:

- Type I: excision of the prepuce with or without excision of the entire clitoris
- Type II: excision of the clitoris with partial or total excision of the labia minora
- Type III: excision of part or all of the external genitalia and stitching or narrowing of the vaginal opening (infibulation)
- Type IV: pricking, piercing, or incising of the clitoris or labia, stretching of the clitoris and labia, or cauterization of the clitoris and surrounding tissue including scraping of the introital skin (angurya cuts) or cutting the vagina (gishiri cuts) and the introduction of corrosive substances or herbs into the vagina to cause bleeding and cicatrization

The greatest health risks are in women who have undergone infibulation, which accounts for about 15% of cases. FGM is usually performed on women between 5 and 8 years of age and has physical, psychological, and sexual consequences.

General Risks

Immediate risks of the FGM procedure itself when performed by a traditional practitioner using crude instruments and no anesthesia include shock, hemorrhage, sepsis, and death. There are few reliable figures of FGM-related mortality rate. Ulceration of the genitalia and acute urinary retention can also follow, as can transmission of HIV and hepatitis.

Delayed complications include urinary and vaginal infections, large epidermal cysts, abscesses, keloid scarring, obstructed menstruation, urinary incontinence, and coital and psychosexual problems which may lead to infertility.[78]

Maternal Risks

The incidence of pregnancy complications or maternal deaths related to FGM is unknown. The risks depend on the type of FGM performed; infibulation in particular can cause tender introital scarring which precludes adequate prenatal examination, investigation, and treatment. Vaginitis is common, as are urinary tract infections. Miscarriage may be complicated by retention of products in the vagina, leading to sepsis. When labor occurs, assessment of cervical dilation may be difficult or impossible. Urinary retention in labor is common. Dystocia, usually due to soft tissue obstruction in the second stage, can have serious consequences for the mother and fetus if undetected or improperly managed. Vaginal delivery is associated with increased risks of perineal damage and hemorrhage.[79] The increased incidence of postpartum hemorrhage is mainly due to the need for anterior episiotomy or lacerations extending to the urethra, bladder, or rectum. Postpartum pain is also more severe due to a greater degree of perineal injury. Postnatal wound infections, dehiscence, and fistulas can occur.

Fetal Risks

Stillbirth and neonatal death have been reported with higher frequency in circumcised women, secondary to fetal asphyxia due to prolonged obstructed labor.[80] This sequence is generally confined to women with severe types of FGM.

Management

Prenatal

Sensitive prenatal care is essential. Women may not volunteer that they are affected by FGM, necessitating an increased awareness when treating women originating from countries where FGM is practiced. Early recognition provides sufficient time for assessment, discussion, and the development of a management plan. The extent of damage, scar tissue, and physical obstruction to vaginal delivery should be clearly documented so that unnecessary repeated examinations can be avoided. Women with a tight introitus, 1 cm or less, have the greatest risk of perineal damage. However, if the urinary meatus can be observed or two fingers can be inserted on digital examination, significant delivery problems are unlikely to ensue. Parous women who have been sutured at a previous delivery are at risk of developing significant scar tissue with subsequent infection and wound problems. Antenatal assessment also provides an opportunity to establish if the woman would wish introital dilation to allow comfortable intercourse, or to undergo a complete reversal of the procedure. Ideally, complete reversal should be avoided during pregnancy or immediately post-partum owing to the greater likelihood of hemorrhage at that time. Optimally, an anterior episiotomy sufficient only to expose the urethra should be performed during the late second stage, but occasionally this procedure must be performed earlier to allow adequate investigation or treatment during pregnancy, for example, in the case of pain and bleeding in early pregnancy. Antenatally, the health care provider can also educate affected women so as to eliminate the practice of FGM in her offspring.

Labor and Delivery

The diagnosis of labor may be difficult in the presence of a small introitus. In this case defibulation may need to be performed to allow adequate assessment. In skilled hands, intrapartum defibulation is a safe and effective procedure.[80] This procedure can be done under local anesthesia. If the opening is large enough to permit digital examination, then the decision on defibulation can be deferred to the second stage. Extra care is essential in the second stage as the delivery of the fetal head may be obstructed by scar tissue. This can result in fetal asphyxia or severe tearing in the mother, leading to hemorrhage and fistula development. If introital obstruction develops, a timely anterior episiotomy should be performed to the urethra but not beyond because of the risk of hemorrhage.

Following delivery of the placenta, a careful examination of the genital tract is necessary. In particular, the presence of high vaginal lacerations and damage to the anal sphincter, rectum, or bladder should be noted. The sides of the midline anterior incision should be oversewn to secure hemostasis, leaving the urethra exposed. Reinfibulation should not be performed, irrespective of the wishes of the woman, as this will result in further scarring and problems; ideally, this issue will have been discussed prenatally.

Postnatal

Good postnatal analgesia is important because anterior divisions are associated with more pain. Affected women may need education in relation to differences in urination, menstruation, and coital function. A specific postnatal visit should be arranged to assess healing and to discuss sexual activity.

DEFIBULATION PROCEDURE

1. Locate opening and paint with antiseptic solution.
2. Administer local anesthetic to the introitus if epidural anesthesia is not present.
3. Raise scar tissue from underlying area and incise in midline to expose urethral meatus. Do not incise beyond this.
4. Suture raw edges for hemostasis.

SUMMARY OF MANAGEMENT OPTIONS
Female Genital Mutilation or Circumcision

Management Options	Quality of Evidence	Strength of Recommendation	References
Prenatal			
Identify women at risk.	–	GPP	–
Sensitive approach: Educate couple and obtain consent for examination and treatment.	–	GPP	–
Establish type of female genital mutilation and determine if defibulation is required.	III	B	80
Discuss timing of defibulation and postnatal result.	III	B	80
Labor/Delivery			
Observe for obstructed second stage.	–	GPP	–
Perform timely defibulation or episiotomy if required.	–	GPP	–
Inspect genital tract after delivery of placenta for extension of lacerations.	–	GPP	–
Repair perineal damage and provide hemostasis.	–	GPP	–
Postnatal			
Provide analgesia and follow-up and education.	–	GPP	–

CONCLUSIONS

UTEROVAGINAL PROLAPSE IN PREGNANCY

- Troublesome prolapse is rare in pregnancy but more common during the puerperium.
- Vaginal pessary treatment is the first, and usually most effective, choice of treatment for pregnancy and postnatal prolapse.
- Persistent prolapse carries an increased risk of preterm birth.
- Delivery by prelabor cesarean section is recommended in pregnancies following previous successful repair of prolapse or urinary or fecal incontinence.

OBSTETRIC ANAL SPHINCTER INJURY

- Anal sphincter disruption follows 1% to 2% of vaginal births, more commonly first deliveries.
- Other obstetric risk factors include instrumental delivery, prolonged second stage of labor, midline episiotomy, and previous sphincter disruption.
- Enquiry about fecal continence should form part of the routine postnatal assessment.

POSTPARTUM FECAL INCONTINENCE

- Damage to the anal sphincter mechanisms can be traumatic/muscular (especially primiparas) or neurologic or a combined injury.
- Fecal incontinence symptoms require appropriate postpartum anal physiologic investigation to define both the type of injury and the most appropriate management.
- Many fecal continence disturbances are transient and can be managed effectively with drugs and biofeedback physiotherapy.
- Secondary surgical repair is necessary for women with fecal incontinence persisting for some months post-partum.

FEMALE GENITAL MUTILATION

- Medical professionals should not be involved in supervising or performing genital mutilation procedures.
- The degree of mutilation is variable and, if extensive, can interfere with management of subsequent pregnancy and delivery.
- Counseling should be provided during pregnancy with a view to postnatal surgical correction of symptomatic genital distortion.

REFERENCES

1. Brown JS, Waetjen LE, Subak LL, et al: Pelvic organ prolapse surgery in the United States, 1997. Am J Obstet Gynecol 2002; 186:712–716.
2. Subak LL, Waetjen LE, Van den Eeden S, et al: Cost of pelvic organ prolapse surgery in the United States. Am J Obstet Gynecol 2001;98:646–651.
3. Wilson L, Brown JS, Shin GP, et al: Annual direct cost of urinary incontinence. Obstet Gynecol 2001;98:398–406.
4. Olsen AL, Smith VJ, Bergstrom JO, et al: Epidemiology of surgically managed pelvic organ prolapse and urinary incontinence. Obstet Gynecol 1997;89:501–506.
5. Mant J, Painter R, Vessey M: Epidemiology of genital prolapse: Observations from the Oxford Family Planning Study. BJOG 1997;104:579–585.
6. Skoner MM, Thompson WD, Caron VA: Factors associated with risk of stress urinary incontinence in women. Nurs Res 1994;43:301–306.
7. Viktrup L, Lose G, Rolff M, Barfoed K: The symptom of stress incontinence caused by pregnancy or delivery in primiparas. Obstet Gynecol 1992;79:945–949.
8. Porges RF, Porges JC, Blinick G: Mechanisms of uterine support and the pathogenesis of uterine prolapse. Obstet Gynecol 1960;15:711–726.
9. Lawson JO: Pelvic anatomy. I. Pelvic floor muscles. Ann R Coll Surg Engl 1974;54:244–252.
10. DeLancey JO: Fascial muscular abnormalities in women with urethral hypermobility and anterior vaginal wall prolapse. Am J Obstet Gynecol 2002;187:93–98.
11. Delancey JO: Anatomic aspects of vaginal eversion after hysterectomy. Am J Obstet Gynecol 1992;166:1717–1728.
12. Delancey JO: Structural support of the urethra as it relates to stress urinary incontinence: The hammock hypothesis. Am J Obstet Gynecol 1994;170:1713–1723.
13. Snooks SJ, Swash M: Innervation of the muscles of continence. Ann R Coll Surg Engl 1986;18:45–49.
14. Neill ME, Swash M: Increased motor unit fibre density in the external anal sphincter muscle in ano-rectal incontinence: A single fibre EMG study. J Neurol Neurosurg Psych 1980;43(4):343–347.
15. Allen RE, Hosker GL, Smith ARB, Warrell DW: Pelvic floor damage and childbirth: A neurophysiological study. BJOG 1990;97:770–779.
16. Sultan AH, Kamm MA, Hudson CN, et al: Anal sphincter disruption during vaginal delivery. N Engl J Med 1993;329: 1905–1911.
17. Dimpfl T, Jaegar C, Mueller-Felber W, et al: Myogenic changes of the levator ani muscle in premenopausal women: The impact of vaginal delivery and age. Neurourol Urodynam 1998;17:197–206.
18. Koebl H, Strassegger H, Riss PA, Gruber H: Morphologic and functional aspects of pelvic floor muscle in patients with pelvic relaxation and genuine stress incontinence. Obstet Gynecol 1989;74:789–795.
19. Tunn R, Paris S, Fischer W, et al: Static magnetic resonance imaging of the pelvic floor muscle morphology in women with stress urinary incontinence and pelvic prolapse. Neurourol Urodynam 1998;17:579–589.
20. Kirschner-Hermanns R, Wein B, Niehaus S, et al: The contribution of magnetic resonance imaging of the pelvic floor to the understanding of urinary incontinence. Br J Urol 1993;72:715–718.
21. Delancey JOL, Kearney R, Chou Q, et al: Levator ani muscle abnormalities seen in MR images after vaginal delivery. Obstet Gynecol 2003;101:46–53.
22. Fitzpatrick M, McQuillan K, O'Herlihy C: Influence of persistent occiput posterior position on delivery outcome. Obstet Gynecol 2001;98:1027–1031.
23. Coats P, Chan K, Wilkins M: A comparison between midline and mediolateral episiotomies. BJOG 1980;87: 408–413.
24. Richter HE, Brumfield CG, Cliver SP, et al: Risk factors associated with anal sphincter tear: A comparison of primiparous patients, vaginal births after cesarean deliveries, and patients with previous vaginal delivery. Am J Obstet Gynecol 2002;187:1194–1198.
25. O'Boyle A, Woodman P, O'Boyle J, et al: Pelvic organ support in nulliparous pregnant and nonpregnant women: A case control study. Am J Obstet Gynecol 2002;187:99–102.
26. Sze E, Sherard G, Dolezal J: Pregnancy, labor, delivery and pelvic organ prolapse. Obstet Gynecol 2002;100:981–986.
27. Keetel W: Prolapse of the uterus during pregnancy. Am J Obstet Gynecol 1941;42:121–126.
28. Suzuki K, Shane J: Uterine prolapse in the pregnant primigravida. Am J Obstet Gynecol 1972;112:303–304.
29. Mufarrij I, Keetel W: Prolapse of the uterus associated with pregnancy. Am J Obstet Gynecol 1957;73:899–903.
30. Schinfeld J: Prolapse of the uterus during pregnancy: A report of two cases and review of management. Am J Obstet Gynecol 1977;129:587–588.
31. Bluett D: Uterine prolapse in pregnancy: Case report and description of pessary. Am J Obstet Gynecol 1968;101:574–575.
32. Myerscough PR: Munro Kerr's Operative Obstetrics, 9th ed. London, Bailliere Tindall, 1977.
33. Piver M, Spezia J: Uterine prolapse during pregnancy. Obstet Gynecol 1968;32:765.
34. Iosif F, Ingemarsson I, Ulmstein U: Urodynamic studies in normal pregnancy and in the puerperium. Am J Obstet Gynecol 1980;137:696.
35. Viktrup L, Lose G, Rolff M, et al: The symptom of stress incontinence caused by pregnancy or delivery in primiparas. Obstet Gynecol 1992;79:945.
36. Taylor R: Pregnancy after pelvic floor repair. Am J Obstet Gynecol 1996;94:35–39.
37. Allahbadia G: Obstetric performance following conservative surgery for pelvic relaxation. Int J Obstet Gynecol 1992;38:293–298.
38. Abu Heija A: Long-term results of colposuspension operation for genuine stress incontinence. Asia Oceania J Obstet Gynaecol 1994;20:179–181.
39. Kovac R, Cruikshank S: Successful pregnancies and vaginal deliveries after sacrospinous uterosacral fixation in five of nineteen patients. Am J Obstet Gynecol 1993;168:1778–1786.
40. Tunn R, DeLancey JOL, Howard D, et al: MR imaging of levator ani muscle recovery following vaginal delivery. Int Urogynecol J Plevic Floor Dysfunct 1999;10:300–307.
41. Sultan AH: Obstetrical perineal injury and anal incontinence. Clin Risk 1999;5:193–196.
42. Samuelsson E, Ladfors L, Lindblom BG, Hagberg H: A prospective observational study on tears during vaginal delivery: Occurrences and risk factors. Acta Obstet Gynecol Scand 2002;81:44–49.
43. Webb D, Culhane J: Hospital variation in episiotomy use and the risk of perineal trauma during childbirth. Birth 2002;29:132–136.
44. Signorello L, Harlow B, Chekos A, Repke J: Postpartum sexual functioning and its relationship to perineal trauma: A retrospective cohort study of primiparous women. Am J Obstet Gynecol 2001;184:881–888.
45. Cain J, Shirar E: A new method for teaching the repair of perineal trauma of birth. Fam Med 1996;28:107–110.
46. Stamp G, Kruzins G, Crowther C: Perineal massage in labour and prevention of perineal trauma: A randomised controlled trial. BMJ 2001;322:1277–1280.
47. Shipman M, Boniface D, Teft M, McCloghry F: Antenatal perineal massage and subsequent perineal outcomes: A randomised controlled trial. BJOG 1997;104:787–791.
48. Sampselle C, Miller J, Mims B, et al: Effect of pelvic muscle exercise on transient incontinence during pregnancy and after birth. Obstet Gynecol 1998;91:406–412.

49. Upton A, Roberts C, Ryan M, et al: A randomised trial, conducted by midwives, of perineal repairs comparing a polyglycolic suture material and chromic catgut. Midwifery 2002;18:223–229.
50. Macrodt C, Gordon B, Fern E, et al: The Ipswich childbirth study: 2. A randomised comparison of polyglactin 910 with chromic catgut for postpartum perineal repair. BJOG 1998;105:441–445.
51. Oboro V, Taboweit D, Loto O, Bosah A: Multicentre evaluation of the two layered repair of postpartum perineal trauma. J Obstet Gynecol 2003;23:5–8.
52. O'Boyle A, Davis GD, Calhoun BC: Informed consent and birth: Protecting the pelvic floor and ourselves. Am J Obstet Gynecol 2002;187:981–983.
53. Fynes M, Donnelly V, O'Connell PR, et al: Cesarean delivery and anal sphincter injury. Obstet Gynecol 1998;92:496–500.
54. Guarisi T, Pinto-Neto AM, Herrmann V, Faundes A: Urodynamics in climacteric women with urinary incontinence: Correlation with route of delivery. Int Urogynecol J Pelvic Floor Dysfunct 2002;13:366–371.
55. Fitzpatrick M, Behan M, O'Connell PR, O'Herlihy C: A randomised clinical trial comparing primary overlap with approximation repair of third-degree obstetric tears. Am J Obstet Gynecol 2000;183:1220–1224.
56. Sultan AH, Monga AK, Kumar D, Stanton S: Primary repair of obstetric anal sphincter rupture using the overlap technique. BJOG 1999;106:318–323.
57. Jorge JM, Wexner SD: Aetiology and management of faecal incontinence. Dis Colon Rectum 1993;36:77–79.
58. Bartram CI, Burnett SJD: Atlas of Anal Endosonography. Oxford, Butterworth-Heinemann, 1997, pp 7–16.
59. Fitzpatrick M, Fynes M, Cassidy M, et al: Prospective study of the influence of parity and operative technique on the outcome of primary anal sphincter repair following obstetrical injury. Eur J Obstet Gynecol 2000;89:159–160.
60. Voyvodic F, Rieger N, Skinner S, et al: Endosonographic imaging of anal sphincter imaging: Does size of tear correlate with degree of dysfunction? Dis Colon Rectum 2003;46:735–741.
61. Fitzpatrick M, O'Brien C, O'Connell PR, O'Herlihy C: Patterns of abnormal pudendal nerve conduction associated with postpartum fecal incontinence. Am J Obstet Gynecol 2003;189: 730–735.
62. Donnelly VS, Fynes M, Campbell DM, et al: Obstetric events leading to anal sphincter damage. Obstet Gynecol 1998;92: 955–961.
63. Fitzpatrick M, Behan M, O'Connell PR, O'Herlihy C: Randomised clinical trial to assess anal sphincter function following forceps or vacuum assisted vaginal delivery. BJOG 2003;110:424–429.
64. Fitzpatrick M, Harkin R, McQuillan K, et al: A randomised clinical trial comparing the effects of delayed versus immediate pushing with epidural analgesia on mode of delivery and faecal continence. BJOG 2002;109:1359–1365.
65. Myers-Helfgott M, Helfgott A: Routine use of episiotomy in modern obstetrics—Should it be performed? Obstet Gynecol Clin North Am 1999;26:305–325.
66. Anthony S, Buitendijk S, Zondervan K: Episiotomies and the occurrence of severe perineal lacerations. BJOG 1994;101: 1064–1067.
67. Henrikson T, Bek K, Hedegaard M: Episiotomy and perineal lacerations in spontaneous vaginal deliveries. BJOG 1992;99:950–954.
68. Carroli G, Belizan J: Episiotomy for vaginal birth. Cochrane Data Syst Rev 2000;2:CD000081
69. de Leeuw JW, Struijk PC, Vierhout ME, et al: Risk factors for third degree perineal ruptures during vaginal delivery. BJOG 2001;108:383–387.
70. Signorello L, Harlow B, Chekos A, et al: Midline episiotomy and anal incontinence: Retrospective cohort study. BMJ 2000;320:86–90.
71. Harkin R, Fitzpatrick M, O'Connell PR, O'Herlihy C: Anal sphincter disruption at vaginal delivery: Is recurrence predictable. Eur J Obstet Gyn Reprod Gynecol 2003;109:149–152.
72. Payne TN, Carey JC, Rayburn WF: Prior third and fourth degree perineal tears and recurrence risks. Int J Gynecol Obstet 1999;64:55–57.
73. Mahony R, Behan M, O'Herlihy C, O'Connell PR: Randomised, clinical trial of bowel confinement vs laxative use after primary repair of a third degree obstetric anal sphincter tear. Dis Colon Rectum 2004;47:12–17.
74. Fynes M, Marshall K, Cassidy M, et al: A randomised control trial on the effect of biofeedback therapy on anorectal physiology and faecal continence. Dis Colon Rectum 1999;42:753–758.
75. Fynes M, Donnelly V, Behan M, et al: Effect of second vaginal delivery on anorectal physiology and faecal continence: A prospective study. Lancet 1999;354:983–988.
76. Management of pregnancy, childbirth and the postpartum period in the presence of female genital mutilation. Report of a WHO Technical Consultation, Geneva, October 15–17, 1997.
77. Rushwan H: Female genital mutilation (FGM) management during pregnancy, childbirth and the postpartum period. Int J Gynaecol Obstet 2000;70:99–104.
78. Hakim LY: Impact of female genital mutilation on maternal and neonatal outcomes during parturition. East Afr Med J 2001;78(5):255.
79. Larsen U, Okonofua FE: Female circumcision and obstetric complications. Int J Gynaecol Obstet 2002;77:255–265.
80. Rouzi AA, Aljhadali EA, Amarin ZO, Abduljabbar HS: The use of intrapartum defibulation in women with female genital mutilation. BJOG 2001;108:949–951.

CHAPTER 74

Assisted Vaginal Delivery*

Robert Hayashi

INTRODUCTION

Assisted vaginal delivery (AVD) offers the option of an operative procedure to safely and quickly remove the infant, mother, and obstetrician from a difficult or even hazardous situation. When spontaneous vaginal delivery does not occur within a reasonable time, a successful assisted or operative vaginal delivery trial avoids cesarean section with its attendant uterine scar and implications for a future pregnancy, and avoids potential birth asphyxia from prolonged fetal and cord compression. Reviews of delivery statistics[1] show considerable variation in the incidence of AVD, but the range is usually between 10% and 20% of all deliveries. Whether the method employed is the ventouse (vacuum extractor) or obstetric forceps, the operator can expect optimal results only when careful attention is given to the indications, prerequisites, and performance of the procedure.

INDICATIONS

Maternal indications are most commonly those of maternal distress, maternal exhaustion, or undue prolongation of the second stage of labor. Prolongation of the second stage of labor is a relative indication. Many have argued that specific time limits are not needed if monitoring of the fetus shows no evidence of distress and progress is not obviously arrested. However, in cases without regional anesthesia and with reassuring fetal monitoring parameters (e.g., a normal fetal heart rate pattern) it is probably appropriate to consider intervention if the second stage in a nullipara lasts longer than 2 hours (1 hour in a multipara). A further hour is often allowed in the presence of regional anesthesia, provided the mother wishes it and fetal condition is satisfactory. The increased need for intervention following epidural anesthesia has been well documented.[2,3] This approach conforms to the ACOG (American College of Obstetricians and Gynecologists) guidelines.[4] Less common but more medically significant indications for AVD include cardiopulmonary or vascular conditions in which the stresses of the second stage should be minimized. With vaginal birth after previous cesarean section, decreasing the stress on the uterine scar may be a relative indication, although dehiscence or rupture is rare if the ACOG guidelines are followed. It has been suggested that if use of the ventouse has failed to deliver the infant but the fetal head has been brought down sufficiently, a cautious low or outlet forceps procedure is safe.[5] Significant bleeding per vaginam is also an indication for terminating labor; the source of the bleeding may be maternal or fetal (for example, placental abruption or vasa previa).

Fetal indications commonly encountered are malpositions of the fetal head, with relative dystocia. The occiput posterior (OP) and occiput transverse (OT) positions occur more frequently with regional anesthesia.[3,6] This may result from disturbance of the tone of the musculature of the pelvic floor impeding spontaneous rotation to the optimal occiput anterior (OA) position. Similarly, the maternal expulsive (bearing down) force may be compromised. Intervention with forceps for protection of the premature infant remains controversial. In the infant weighing below 1500 g, forceps delivery offers no advantage[7] and may in fact be deleterious,[8] owing to an increased incidence of intracranial bleeding. Use of the ventouse carries the same risk; vacuum extraction is probably best avoided at less than 34 weeks. Spontaneous delivery (with a generous episiotomy if delivery is delayed at the perineum, or the outlet appears tight) and manual control of the head appear preferable, with abdominal delivery if operative intervention is needed.[8]

*This chapter is based extensively on the chapter in the previous edition, by Philip Dennen and Robert Hayashi. As Philip Dennen has now retired, the responsibility for the current chapter, and especially the updates, rests with Robert Hayashi. However, the prior contribution of Philip Dennen is gratefully acknowledged.

In the low-birth-weight infant (1500–2500 g) assisted vaginal delivery is more widely accepted but should be managed with caution and minimal force.[9,10]

Fetal distress is a commonly cited indication. This expression is subject to varied interpretation, which may range from a brief bradycardia to prolonged late decelerations with acidosis. "Presumed fetal jeopardy" may be a preferable term, in conjunction with recording of as precise a description of the situation as possible in order to validate the indication.[4]

Vaginal delivery of the breech is considered by some to be an indication for forceps to the aftercoming head.[11,12] When the management decision is made to deliver vaginally (see Chapter 64), forceps to the aftercoming head may be considered routinely. The procedure becomes mandatory if the body has delivered and the Mauriceau-Smellie-Veit maneuver has failed. A putative advantage is the avoidance of traction force on the trunk and cervical spine, together with automatic control of the flexion of the fetal head. This may decrease the risk of hyperextension[13] and cervical plexus injuries.[14]

CONTRAINDICATIONS

Lack of engagement (leading bony point at or above the level of the ischial spines) suggests pelvic inlet dystocia and is usually considered an absolute contraindication to AVD. Conditions in which vaginal delivery per se is contraindicated include known pelvic abnormality with fetopelvic disproportion and fetal anomalies if obstructive or subject to damage from vaginal delivery. Certain fetal malpositions, such as a brow presentation or a face presentation in other than chin anterior position, are not suitable cases, nor is the dead fetus with postmortem changes. Inability to diagnose the position of the fetal head accurately or to apply the instrument properly are major contraindications.[1,15,16]

Several factors are relative contraindications. Fetal macrosomia may be such a factor. In general, the higher the head, the greater the difficulty and the need for performance skill. An increased risk of shoulder dystocia with midcavity procedures with macrosomia and an arrest has been reported.[17] The proficiency and experience of the operator are also factors to be considered. Finally, caution should be used with a ventouse procedure on a fetus who has had fetal scalp blood samplings performed because of the possibility of enhanced fetal scalp bleeding.[11]

DEFINITIONS

Significant comparative statistics have always been difficult to collect owing to differences in the classification, initially of forceps, but now of all assisted vaginal deliveries. ACOG has proposed a more specific classification,[4,18] which has proved to be of clinical value[19,20] and deserves universal adoption. This classification is given in Table 74–1. It applies equally to vacuum extractor and forceps procedures.[4] To the classification of low forceps, a significant clinical addition would be the observation that, on examination, the head must fill the hollow of the sacrum.[21] Station of the head is measured in plus or minus centimeters of distance between the leading bony point of the skull and the ischial spines.

Neonatal results comparable to those of spontaneous delivery can be expected, with procedures categorized as outlet or low with rotation less than 45 degrees.[1,22,23–26] Midpelvic and rotational procedures are generally associated with a higher rate of morbidity than spontaneous delivery.[27] However, when compared more properly with appropriate alternatives of management, namely, manual rotation followed by forceps or ventouse extraction or delivery by cesarean section, results are equivalent.[23,27–31] It is clear that abdominal delivery is associated with a much higher rate of maternal febrile morbidity. The controversy continues; appropriate selection and proficiency in execution of the maneuver remain the unmeasurable variables that often determine the results of trials.

"Failed forceps" and "failed ventouse" are terms that have a pejorative implication. They can carry the stigma of poor judgment, poor obstetrics, and perhaps negligence in that disproportion was unrecognized. Alternatively, a "trial" (psychologically a better term) of forceps or ventouse connotes a cautious attempt at vaginal delivery with the option of altering management if unusual difficulty is met.[13] A trial of forceps or ventouse is appropriately carried out in an operating theater with immediate recourse to cesarean section if vaginal delivery is not achieved. The

TABLE 74–1

Classification of Forceps Deliveries According to Station and Rotation

TYPE OF PROCEDURE	CLASSIFICATION
Outlet forceps	Scalp is visible at the introitus without separating labia Fetal skull has reached pelvic floor Sagittal suture is in anteroposterior diameter or right or left occiput anterior or posterior position Fetal head is at or on perineum Rotation does not exceed 45 degrees
Low forceps	Leading point of fetal skull is at station ≥ + 2 cm, and not on the pelvic floor Rotation ≤45 degrees (left or right occiput anterior to occiput anterior, or left or right occiput posterior to occiput posterior)
Midforceps	Rotation >45 degrees Station above +2 cm but head engaged
High forceps	Not included in classification

From American College of Obstetricians and Gynecologists: Operative vaginal delivery. Technical Bulletin No. 196. Washington, DC, 1994.

procedure deserves greater utilization.[32] A gentle negative trial should not alter outcome.[33,34]

PREREQUISITES

In management of an AVD certain prerequisites must be met.[4] The head must be engaged (as defined by the biparietal diameter having passed through the plane of the inlet of the pelvis (Fig. 74–1)). Generally this will have occurred when the leading bony point has reached the ischial spines. It must be remembered that certain conditions may lead to a higher than anticipated level of the biparietal diameter.[21] This is true with molding, particularly with macrosomia. Asynclitism and occiput posterior positions are associated with a higher level of the biparietal diameter, as is any extension of the fetal vertex away from a well-flexed position. These factors must always be considered when estimating engagement of the head if the assessment is to be accurate.

The position and attitude of the head must also be known if an accurate and effective application of the chosen instrument is to be made. Should the operator be unable to diagnose the position of the fetal head from the fontanels and suture lines, feeling for the location of an ear can be helpful. This can, however, produce a loss of station and backward rotation of the head due to the necessary displacement of the vertex, which may then mitigate against delivery. The use of ultrasound (with the transducer placed just above the symphysis pubis) may also help determine fetal head position.

The maternal pelvis should be evaluated for the adequacy of the fetopelvic relationship. Factors such as maternal overweight or diabetes with related fetal macrosomia should be considered. An obvious disproportion contraindicating vaginal delivery must not be present. Clinical evaluation rather than radiographic pelvimetry should be adequate for estimation of the midpelvis and the pelvic outlet.

The bladder should be empty for procedures at other than outlet level. Membranes must be ruptured and the

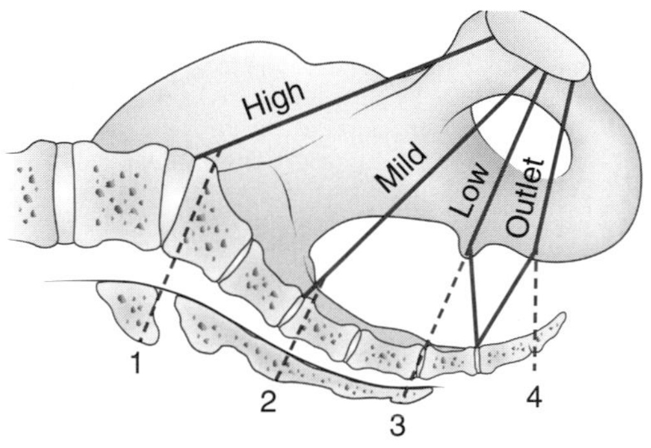

FIGURE 74–1
The obstetric planes of the pelvis and forceps classification: 1, Plane of inlet. 2, Plane of greatest pelvic dimension. 3, Plane of least pelvic dimension. 4, Plane of outlet. (From Dennen PC: Forceps Deliveries, 3rd ed. Philadelphia, F.A. Davis, 1988.)

cervix must be fully dilated and retracted, or marked obstruction to rotation or decent of the head will result. There is no place in modern obstetrics for manual or mechanical dilation of the cervix or for cervical incisions to facilitate an operative procedure.[13] The rare exception may be the trapped head in a breech delivery.[35] Appropriate anesthesia is needed for any AVD, although applying the ventouse usually causes less maternal discomfort and the requirement for anesthesia may therefore be less. Although outlet and possibly some low forceps procedures may be performed with local perineal infiltration, a pudendal block is usually more appropriate. For any rotational procedure a regional block (epidural or spinal) is necessary.[35] In rare circumstances, a general anesthetic may be necessary. In the UK, it has been suggested to be medicolegally advisable to have an anesthesiologist attend and confirm that adequate analgesia has been produced before proceeding with any but the most urgent operative vaginal delivery. This does not happen in the majority of units.

Although the simplest operations may be undertaken in an informal birthing room setting, most procedures deserve a delivery room/operating theater. Facilities, equipment, and personnel should be adequate for support of patient, infant, and operator in case of any adverse development. A negative trial of AVD should result swiftly in abdominal delivery instead.[4]

Because complications tend to increase in inverse ratio to the technical skill and experience of the operator, physician knowledge of the instruments and the physical forces involved in their use is essential. The operator must know his or her limitations and be prepared to abandon the procedure in case of difficulty. The use of greater force is the worst of the available options.

COMPLICATIONS

Most of the complications of AVD have also been reported following spontaneous vaginal and even abdominal delivery, but their incidence is greater with AVD. Assessment of causation is frequently problematic because this type of delivery is so often accompanied by other fetal and labor factors that commonly are associated with birth injury. However, it is obviously difficult for the operator to disclaim responsibility for an injury subsequent to an instrumental delivery. Maternal complications are usually those of soft tissue trauma and tend to be reported more frequently with the use of forceps than with ventouse. They can include uterine, cervical, or vaginal injury, laceration, or hematoma. Bladder or urethral injury may occur, including postpartum urinary retention and late fistula formation. Rectal laceration (with or without episiotomy) and subsequent fistula may occur, as well as later problems in defecation.[1] Increased blood loss is common with more difficult procedures. Maternal injury with use of the ventouse includes inadvertent entrapment of the cervix or vaginal wall between the cup edge and fetal head with consequent laceration of the maternal periurethral and vaginal tissues. Placement of the cup should never be done carelessly or forcefully.

Fetal complications of forceps delivery include transient facial marks, facial palsies, and fracture of facial bones or skull. Severe cervical cord damage following midforceps rotation has been reported,[36] but such serious trauma is extremely rare. Injury from the ventouse includes minor, and occasionally severe, scalp injury, including scalp bruising, abrasion, laceration, cephalhematoma, subgaleal hematoma, and intracranial hemorrhage. Subgaleal hematomas are thought to be due to disruption of the diploic vessels in the loose subaponeurotic scalp tissue that allows a large volume of bleeding to occur over time.[19] The entire scalp can be elevated. Tentorial tears have been associated with mechanical injury to the fetal cranium and are thought to be related to the shearing forces on the tentorium, resulting in rupture of the deep venous system or laceration of the inferior surface of the cerebellum.[20] Although the pathophysiology is not clearly understood, the vacuum extractor may produce stress on the fetal cranium in the occipital frontal diameter, with tension on the tentorium. The tentorium may then rupture, causing intracranial hemorrhage. Because of these uncommon, but serious, sequelae in infants following a ventouse delivery, all such infants should be carefully observed following birth for any neurologic signs of irritability, drowsiness, tachypnea, seizure activity, or an enlarging head size.[37] Any such signs should be carefully investigated.

Cephalhematoma may be associated with an underlying skull fracture.[38] Fortunately, most documented series of vacuum extractions report no such serious complications. However, neonatal jaundice and retinal hemorrhage are found more frequently with the ventouse.[35] Brachial plexus palsy related to shoulder dystocia and facial nerve palsies are slightly more common after AVD than after spontaneous deliveries.[37,39] Opinions vary on the risk of long-term neurologic damage related to AVD. The subject is under continuing investigation.[10] Some studies show a relationship between cerebral palsy and difficult forceps procedures, whereas others fail to confirm such a relationship.[28] It is generally believed that most neurologic deficit is unrelated to incidents occurring at delivery or to substandard intrapartum obstetric care.[40]

RISK MANAGEMENT

In the vast majority of AVDs the normal outcome gives no reason for complaint. However, in our litigious society a bad outcome increases the risk of litigation against the operator or hospital, regardless of the cause.

In lawsuits against physicians who chose the option of AVD, the common allegations[41] are inadequate indication, failure to rule out cephalopelvic disproportion, and faulty performance causing fetal injury (this may include incorrect diagnosis of station or position, improper use of instruments, or the use of excessive force). The lack of informed consent is frequently cited. Although strongly urged by attorneys, obtaining fully informed consent is often not feasible in an emergency situation. In such circumstances, the best defense is to be able to demonstrate the need for and appropriateness of the procedure and its performance (in other words, the indications for intervention should be absolute and not relative, and execution of the intervention must be competent). As an absolute minimum, if prior informed signed consent is not obtained, the chart should note a discussion of the procedure with the woman, her partner, and even (if appropriate and there is time) with her family. Physicians in training may be particularly vulnerable to lawsuits unless adequate supervision is present. The "learning curve" excuse is invalid because all patients are entitled to the same standard of care.

In any suit following a bad outcome, regardless of the delivery mode, the operator is forced into a defensive position, attempting to prove that the outcome was due to factors other than the alleged misdeeds. After the fact verbal explanations of usually poorly remembered events may appear to be merely an effort to escape responsibility. Careful documentation is the keystone in the operator's defense. Notes that outline the clinical circumstances, the cognitive steps in choice of options of delivery, and a detailed operative note of maneuvers used are mandatory. Consideration of a cesarean section option, possibly with simultaneous preparations, should be noted, particularly with a midpelvic procedure. Many institutions routinely measure cord gases in all assisted vaginal deliveries in order to document the infant's condition at birth. Finally, the fear of litigation should not dictate medical practice; AVD remains good medical practice in appropriate circumstances and with appropriate safeguards. Despite this exhortation, however, a survey showed that by 1996 over half of ACOG fellows had already abandoned midcavity AVDs in favor of cesarean section.[42]

INSTRUMENTS AND CHOICE OF PROCEDURE

Ventouse/Vacuum

The principal idea of the vacuum extractor is to use a cup device attached by tubing to a pump to create enough negative pressure to allow traction on the cup. In this way, traction is transferred to the fetal head (scalp) which is thereby pulled along the birth canal axis. Traction is applied during a uterine contraction, resulting in descent of the fetal head by a push-pull effect. Positioning of the cup on the fetal head and the development of a caput succedaneum are important considerations.

Malström devised a metal cup with rounded edges and an outside diameter of 60 mm, with the vacuum tubing and traction chain coming off the center of the back of the cup dome. By gradual increments of negative pressure, the fetal scalp is sucked into the hollow of the shallow cup to create a caput succedaneum called a "chignon." Placement of the chignon is very important and a major determinant of outcome. If properly placed at the "flexing point" of the fetal head, a point located on the sagittal suture 3 cm in front of the posterior fontanel, traction will result in maximal flexion of a synclitic head.[43,44] Incorrect placement may result in deflexed and asynclitic fetal head attitudes and consequent failure of the vacuum extractor technique (Fig. 74–2). Assuming that the length of the sagittal suture is approximately 9 cm at term, when the cup is properly placed on the flexion point, the leading edge of the cup will be about 3 cm away from the anterior fontanel.[44] Proper cup positioning is crucial to move the fetal head from a midpelvic level to the plane of the outlet of the birth canal, and thus, positioning should always be a primary concern when performing a ventouse delivery.

An important modification to the Malström vacuum extractor was designed by Bird.[43] He moved the vacuum hose and traction chain attachment from the dome to the lateral wall or rim of the cup. This modified cup was to be used specifically for posterior and lateral positions of the occiput. This alteration allowed easier placement of the cup over the flexing point, and its utility has been supported by an observational study in Portsmouth.[45]

Traction force studies have suggested that 22.7 kg (50 lb) of traction force may be the upper limit of fetal safety for assisted deliveries.[46–48] Duchon noted that with a vacuum cup having a diameter of 60 mm, a vacuum of 550 to 600 mm Hg (0.8 kg/cm^2) will allow 22 kg of traction force before detachment or "pop off" occurs.[49] This should be considered the end point of safety, and inappropriate increases in vacuum should be avoided to minimize fetal morbidity. Repeated detachments of the cup are often associated with scalp injury.

In 1973, Kobayashi introduced a single unit pliable Silastic cup with a stainless steel valve on the stem that allows for relief of a significant amount of the suction force to the scalp between contractions without loss of application of the cup to the fetal head.[50] The Silastic cup diameter is 65 mm and fits over the fetal occiput like a skull cap. The advantage of this design over the metal cup is that there is less scalp trauma because the cup has no rigid edge and can shape to the fetal head. Also, there is no need to take time to develop a chignon so that traction can be applied shortly after proper application. The disadvantage is that placement of the cup center over the flexing point of the fetal head is not easily done on a nonflexed head in the midpelvic area. Two randomized comparisons of the soft cups with rigid cups have been reported.[51,52] Both found a higher failure rate with the Silastic cup, especially with occiput posterior positions. On this basis, use of the Silastic cup should be restricted to easy or outlet procedures. Nevertheless, because of the perceived increased safety and convenience of the soft cup, this device has almost completely replaced the metal cup for use in vacuum extractor deliveries in the United States.

In 1973, a three-component plastic system vacuum extractor composed of a disposable plastic replica of the Malström cup with a flexible handle stem that can be attached to disposable plastic tubing and reusable hand pump was described by Paul and associates[53] from the University of Southern California. They reported favorably on their experience with the device. The cup was 50 mm in diameter and required the development of a chignon as with the rigid cup. The advantage over the rigid cup was the simplicity of assembly because there were fewer parts to fit together. Also, defective tubing and rough edges on the cup were avoided. In later years, the cup was modified to remove the necessity of forming a chignon before traction. The cup diameter was increased to 60 mm and the cup shaped like a teacup (i.e., the dome was deepened). This device is called a Mityvac.

A new device, called the Kiwi Complete Delivery System, has been introduced that has incorporated several important aspects of past experience and innovative new ideas. The innovative aspect of this completely disposable system is the use of a hand-pump/traction system directly attached to the vacuum cup that allows the obstetrician to develop the negative pressure via an accurate vacuum indication gauge in the traction handle. The two vacuum cups utilize past experience for design. The Kiwi Pro Cup is a soft, flexible, 65-mm diameter cup, similar

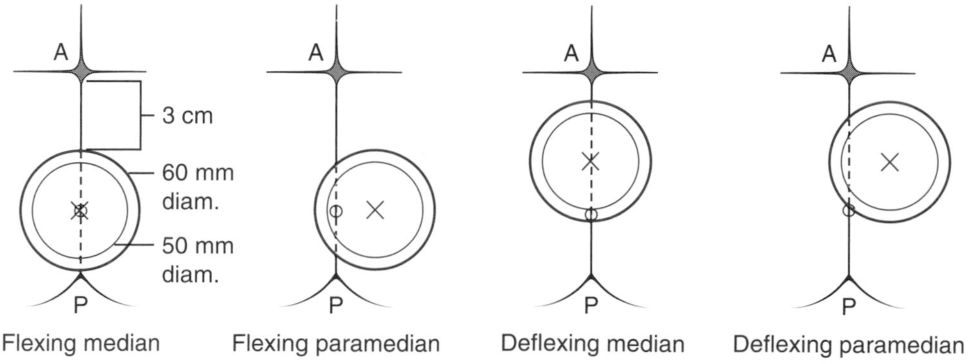

FIGURE 74–2
Applications of a 50-mm vacuum cup: the "flexing median" application should be used in order to avoid deflexion and asynclitism. (From Chalmers I, Enkin M, Keirse MJNC (eds): Effective Care in Pregnancy and Childbirth. Oxford, Oxford University Press, 1989.)

to the Kobayashi cup that expands to mold to the fetal head in the low occiput anterior position. The Kiwi Omni Cup is a rigid, flat plastic cup, 50 mm in diameter, similar to the Malström metal cup. The traction/suction line is anchored in the center of the back of the cup and can flex into a radial recession on the back side of the cup to allow lateral traction like the Bird modification of the Malström cup. This design facilitates rotational function of the device for malpositions such as occiput transverse or posterior. Because of its unique design and convenience for the operator, the Kiwi Complete Delivery System is becoming popular (Fig. 74–3).

Because maintained vacuum or negative pressure is crucial for effective use of the ventouse extractor and "pop off" can result in fetal scalp trauma, properly maintained equipment to provide an airtight seal within the pump and tubing is essential. The equipment should be regularly serviced and defective parts (including smooth-rimmed cups) replaced. The operator should test run the system for air leakage immediately before applying the cup to the fetal head.

PROCEDURE: VENTOUSE DELIVERY

GENERAL

After determining that there is a clear indication for a ventouse delivery, the operator should discuss the following issues with the patient or her partner:

- The alternative methods of delivery available
- The advantages and disadvantages of the vacuum extractor
- The expected outcome
- Any possible complications (both minor and serious)

These issues should be recorded in the notes at some time close to the procedure. Ideally, the operator should have a choice of vacuum extractor type, so that they can choose an appropriate instrument for the situation.

SILASTIC OR PLASTIC CUP

This can be used for a flexed, relatively synclitic fetal head at the pelvic outlet, whereas for a deflexed, asynclitic fetal

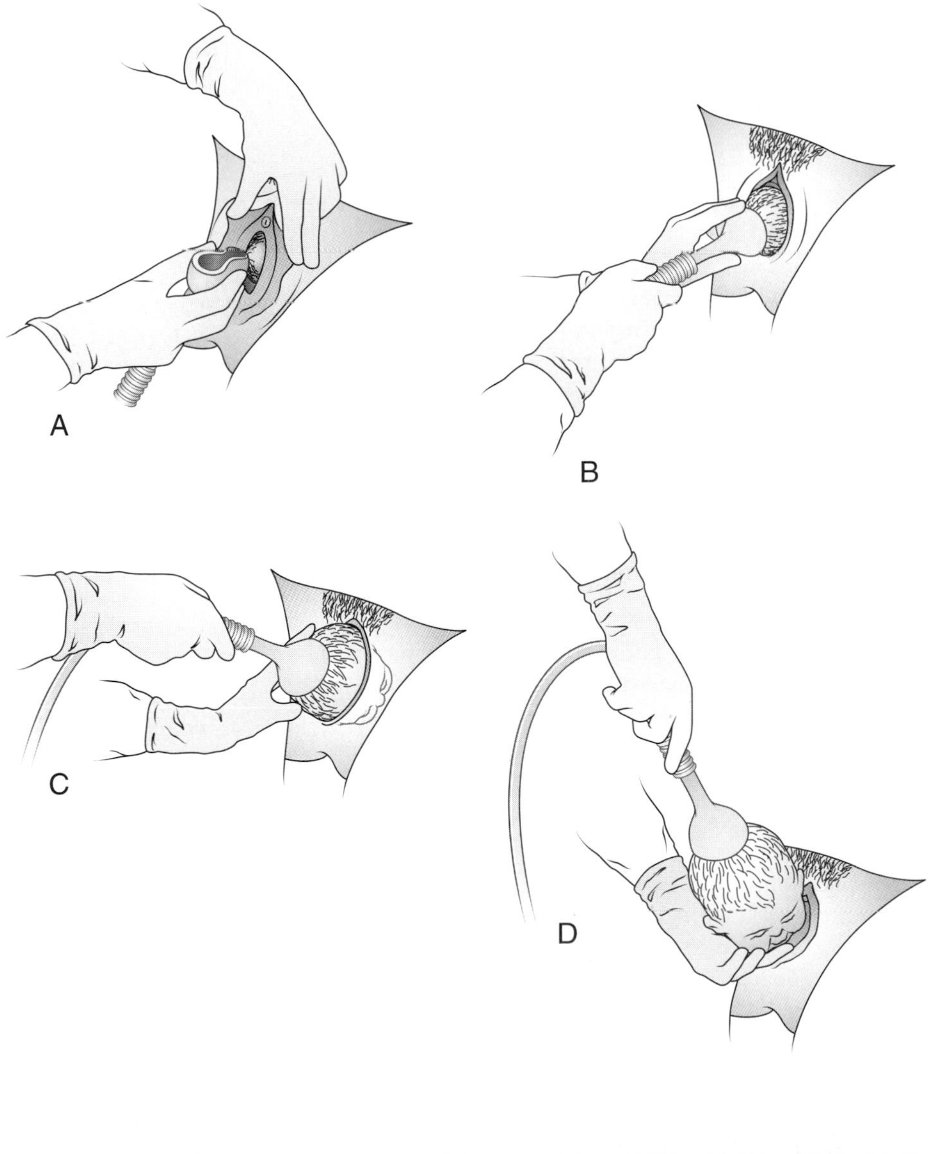

FIGURE 74–3
Delivery with ventouse/vacuum.

head, use of the Kiwi cup carries a higher chance of successful delivery. If fetal head malposition, such as occiput posterior or transverse, causes dystocia, then use of the Bird cup (or Kiwi Omni Cup) would be a good choice. An incorrectly chosen instrument lessens the chance of a successful outcome. Before application of the cup to the fetal head, the operator must check the pump, hose, and cup, fully assembled, for proper and maintained negative pressure when the cup is applied to the palm of a gloved hand.

After the patient has been washed with antiseptic solution and draped in the dorsal lithotomy position for delivery, the operator should empty the urinary bladder and then check the fetal head position and station. Analgesia should preferably be by regional block, placed previously. However, an alternative for deliveries expected to be straightforward is a pudendal block with perineal infiltration of local anesthetic.

The application technique of the cup will differ, depending on whether the cup is metal or soft.

MALSTRÖM METAL CUP

For the Malström metal cup, betadine or an antiseptic soap solution is applied to the rim of the cup and the cup slipped carefully into the vagina. The cup is then positioned over the flexing point of the fetal head with the rim nearest to the anterior fontanel positioned 3 cm from it (see Fig. 74–2). The negative pressure of the system is increased to 0.2 kg/cm^2, and the perimeter of the cup is checked for entrapped cervical or vaginal tissue. Negative pressure is increased by 0.2 kg/cm^2 every 2 minutes to a maximum pressure of 0.8 kg/cm^2 in order to build the chignon. At this point, traction in the axis of the birth canal can be applied during uterine contractions.

By placing a hand in the vagina with the thumb on the cup and index finger on the fetal scalp, traction force can be monitored in the following manner:

- Gradually increase the traction force until the cup begins to slip away from the fetal scalp, diminish the traction somewhat, and then hold for the remainder of the uterine contraction.
- Release traction between uterine contractions.

The expectation is that the presenting part should descend with each push-pull event and that the head will be delivered within approximately five pulls. The fetal heart rate is monitored throughout the procedure with an external fetal heart rate monitor. Once the head is delivered, the suction is disconnected and the cup is removed.

SOFT CUP (See Fig. 74–3)

For application of the soft cup, a flexed synclitic fetal head position is presumed. After application of betadine or antiseptic soap solution to the cup rim, the edges of the cup are carefully folded in to diminish its diameter and it is then inserted into the vagina. Because of the larger overall size of the Silastic cup, periurethral and labial lacerations can occur easily unless extra care is taken. Once on the fetal head, the operator should palpate around the edges of the cup to clear any trapped tissues, move the stem of the cup as close to the flexing point near the occiput as possible, and pump the negative pressure to 0.2 kg/cm^2. A further check should be made for any tissue under the cup rim, then a uterine contraction should be awaited. With the onset of a uterine contraction, the negative pressure is increased to 0.8 kg/cm^2 and traction exerted, placing the intravaginal hand and fingers as noted previously to monitor the traction force (see Fig. 74–3). After the contraction, the partial release valve mechanism is triggered to drop the negative pressure to 0.2 kg/cm^2 between contractions. Expectations for progress are the same as noted previously. The operator using a vacuum extractor must be willing to abandon the technique if obvious progress of descent is not evident with approximately five push-pull events or after several "pop offs." An attempt at forceps delivery at this point is ill-advised.

FORCEPS

Obstetric forceps in current use may be loosely grouped in two major categories—classical and special. Classical instruments are related to those devised by Sir James Y. Simpson (1848) and by George T. Elliot (1858). Simpson type forceps are characterized by a spread shank and somewhat longer cephalic curve. Examples of the type are the long and short Simpson, Simpson-Braun, Luikart-Simpson, DeLee, Hawks-Dennen, Neville Barnes, and Wrigley, as well as the DeWees and many obsolescent axis traction instruments. They are preferred by many for their superior traction ability. The Elliot type forceps are characterized by overlapping shanks and a shorter cephalic curve. Examples of the type include the Elliot, Tucker-MacLane and its Luikart modification, Bailey-Williamson, and others.

Special instruments include the Piper forceps designed for the aftercoming head in breech delivery, the Kielland forceps for rotational delivery at any station, the Barton forceps for transverse arrest in the flat pelvis, the divergent forceps of Laufe and Zeppelin, the Moolgaoker, the Shute, and other cleverly designed instruments. A key feature of instruments such as Kielland or Moolgaoker forceps is their lack of pelvic curve, which facilitates atraumatic rotation but reduces their effectiveness for axis traction.

The choice of instrument is often influenced by regional as well as personal preferences. For example, the Wrigley and Neville Barnes instruments commonly used in the United Kingdom and Canada are almost unknown in the United States. Some operators prefer to approach most clinical situations with the same instrument, thereby losing the unique clinical advantages of the various available forceps. The larger, more molded head is more accurately contacted by the blades with the longer tapering cephalic curve of a Simpson type, whereas the unmolded head is better accommodated by the shorter, full cephalic curve of an Elliot type.[21,35,54]

With the occiput in an anterior quadrant any classical instrument with the appropriate cephalic curve may be chosen. Most commonly used for outlet or low forceps are the Wrigley, the Simpson (short or long), or an Elliot type of instrument. For low forceps with rotation greater than 45 degrees several alternatives are available. Most operators prefer a special instrument for rotation, such as the Kielland, the Moolgaoker, or Shute; however, either an Elliot or Simpson type of classical forceps may also be used. At midforceps level the same choices apply, but the need for axis traction principles becomes more important. In the United Kingdom it is traditional not to use forceps with a cephalic curve because of the supposed increased risk of spiral tears of the vagina. For forceps to the aftercoming head, Piper forceps are generally preferred, although the Kielland forceps and even classical forceps have been used effectively.

PROCEDURE: FORCEPS DELIVERY

POSITION

Numerous texts outline many of the specifics of procedure for forceps delivery. Certain principles given here have universal pertinence to the use of forceps, regardless of the type of instrument chosen. In some areas, the least complicated procedures may be performed with the patient in Sims' lateral recumbent position. For clarity, the use of the lithotomy position (with wedging under the right buttock to produce some lateral tilt and avoid caval compression and maternal hypotension) is assumed in the following discussion. Once the prerequisites for forceps use have been observed (indication explained to the mother and permission obtained, adequate analgesia ensured, maternal bladder emptied, membranes ruptured, position and station of the head determined), the aspects of application and traction must be considered.

APPLICATION (Fig. 74–4)

Application is extremely important to the safe and accurate control of the head as force is transmitted from the operator to the fetal skull via the instrument. To minimize the amount of force required and the potential of trauma, descent of the long axis of the head must be accomplished in the axis of the pelvis. If the landmarks on the head are obscured and the fetal position is unknown, the operator should not use forceps.[15]

In an oblique anterior position of the occiput, the blade of a classical instrument going to the posterior segment of the pelvis should be inserted first.[4] The posterior blade then splints the head, preventing rotation to a less favorable occiput transverse as the anterior blade is wandered into place. With classical instrument applications, the left blade is held in the left hand and is applied to the left side of the mother's pelvis and to the left side of the fetal head. These four points of laterality are reversed for the right blade.

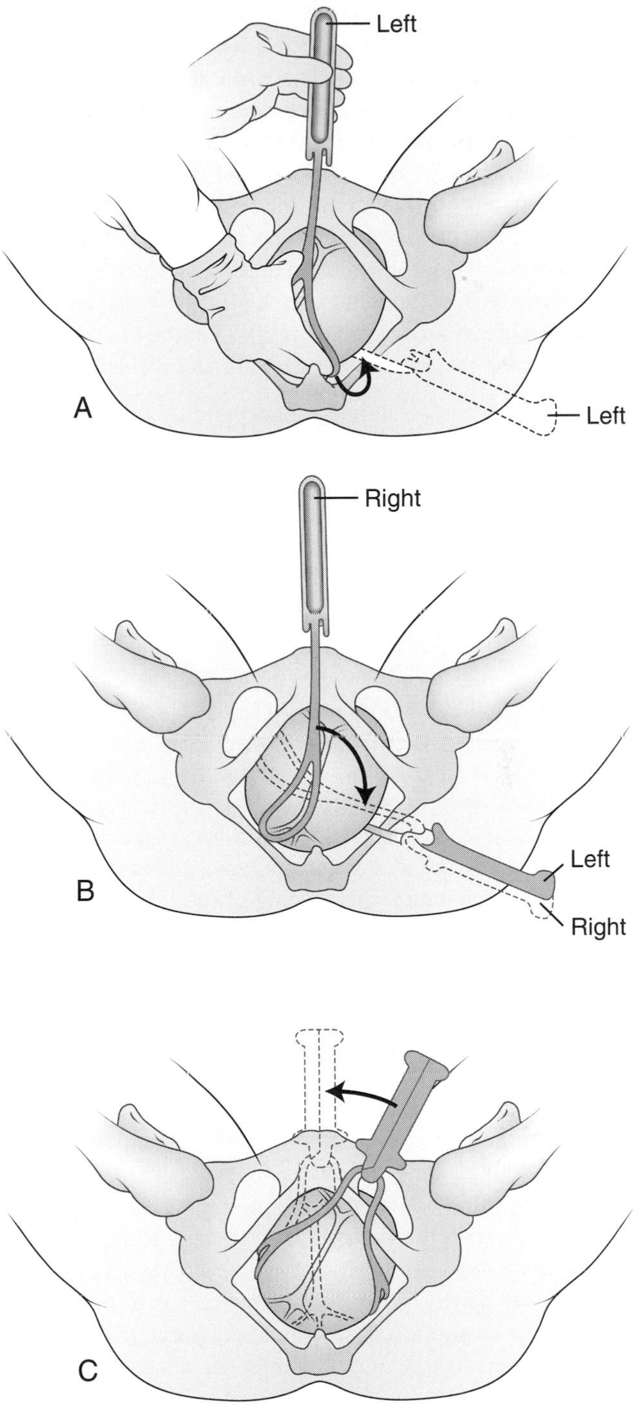

FIGURE 74–4
Forceps application left occiput anterior position.

Exceptions, when a left blade would go to the right side of the head, would include application to an OP position, to an aftercoming head, or with certain special instruments and maneuvers such as the Scanzoni rotation.

To commence insertion, the posterior blade is held vertically, perpendicular to the long axis of the patient. The cephalic curve of the instrument is approximated to the curve of the fetal skull, guided by the fingers of the opposite hand. The handle is gently moved in an arc away from the midline toward the thigh, then downward, then back toward the midline. The toe of the blade slides higher on the head to seat over the malar eminence. This is repeated with the anterior blade. The amount of downward component in the arc traversed by the handles is the same for each blade in the case of an occiput anterior (OA) position. Increasing rotation of the occiput away from OA decreases the downward component of the arc of the posterior blade insertion while increasing the downward arc of the anterior blade insertion. The anterior blade is often more subject to temporary obstruction as it is wandered into the anterior segment of the pelvis. The blades are locked and the application is checked.

Checks for accurate application are as follows[21]:

- The sagittal suture should be perpendicular to the plane of the shanks of the forceps. Any other situation is an asymmetrical application.
- The posterior fontanel should be midway between the blades and one fingerbreadth above the plane of the shanks. Greater distance above the plane of the shanks indicates an extended head, whereas a lesser distance indicates an overflexed attitude. In either case, a less favorable diameter is presented to the pelvic axis and relative resistance to descent results. This applies to all vertex presentations.
- With fenestrated blades, a small but equal amount of fenestration should be felt on each blade. The presence of a large amount of palpable fenestration suggests a short application of the blades on the head, increasing the risk of facial nerve injury and slipping of the blades.

When the checks indicate improper application, readjustment is necessary. Should the sagittal suture be oblique to the plane of the shanks rather than perpendicular, a dangerous brow-mastoid application is present. The blades must be unlocked, then separately wandered to the correct position. The blades are relocked and rechecked. Correction of the flexion attitude is readily accomplished by unlocking and separately shifting the blades to bring the plane of the shanks to one fingerbreadth below the posterior fontanel. The presence of more than a fingertip of fenestration is an indication to unlock the blades and separately adjust them higher in the pelvis. These readjustments are all done without removal of the forceps. If proper application cannot be accomplished, removal of the forceps, reevaluation of the situation, then reapplication are indicated.

TRACTION

The ultimate and dominant function of the obstetric forceps is traction to accomplish descent of the head in the birth canal. The pelvic curve, so carefully designed into the instrument, is mechanically effective with the occiput in the anterior position. Increasing rotation of the occiput away from OA decreases the pelvic curve until it is nonexistent in occiput transverse (OT). Thus, a correctional rotation of the head to OA should be accomplished either before or with the onset of traction. The head is rotated along its long axis by rotating the handles in a wide arc ending with the occiput at OA. The toes of the blades should describe as small an arc as possible in the upper pelvis.

Compression of the fetal head is an undesirable forceps effect and should be minimized by the use of the fingerguards rather than squeezing the handles during traction. Force applied at the fingerguards is so close to the fulcrum at the adjacent lock that negligible compressive force is applied to the head. The natural compression supplied by the pelvic walls and intervening soft tissues serves to maintain the position of the instrument on the head. Assuming that the clinical situation permits, traction should be timed to coincide with uterine contractions and voluntary expulsive effort by the mother. The operator may be seated or standing, well balanced, using principally shoulder and arm muscles. Traction force should be increased gradually rather than rapidly. Jerking the instrument increases the risk of injury to fetus and mother. A steady pull should be maintained and then gradually released as the contraction wanes. The number of pulls and the force required will vary with the case. Delivery should usually be effected by traction with no more than three contractions, employing no more than moderate force. There are two components of traction, both of which must be considered: direction and amount.

The direction of traction must be in the axis of the pelvic curvature, the curve of Carus. This direction alters with the different obstetric planes of the pelvis (see Fig. 74–1). The critical head diameter that must be moved is the biparietal diameter. Effective force must be directed as a perpendicular to the plane of the pelvis at the level of the biparietal diameter (Fig. 74–5) using an axis traction principle. This is done manually with the Pajot-Saxtorph maneuver with traction outward on the fingerguards and downward on the shanks of the instrument (Fig. 74–6). The resultant vector of force ideally is in the proper direction. This vector must be estimated by the operator and is more difficult with the biparietal diameter at higher station. The axis traction

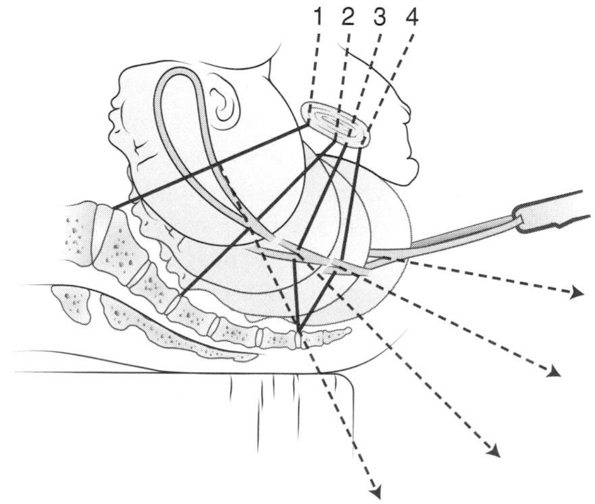

FIGURE 74–5
Line of axis traction (perpendicular to the plane of the pelvis at which the head is stationed) at different planes of the pelvis: 1, High. 2, Mid. 3, Low. 4, Outlet. (From Dennen PC: Forceps Deliveries, 3rd ed. Philadelphia, F.A. Davis, 1988.)

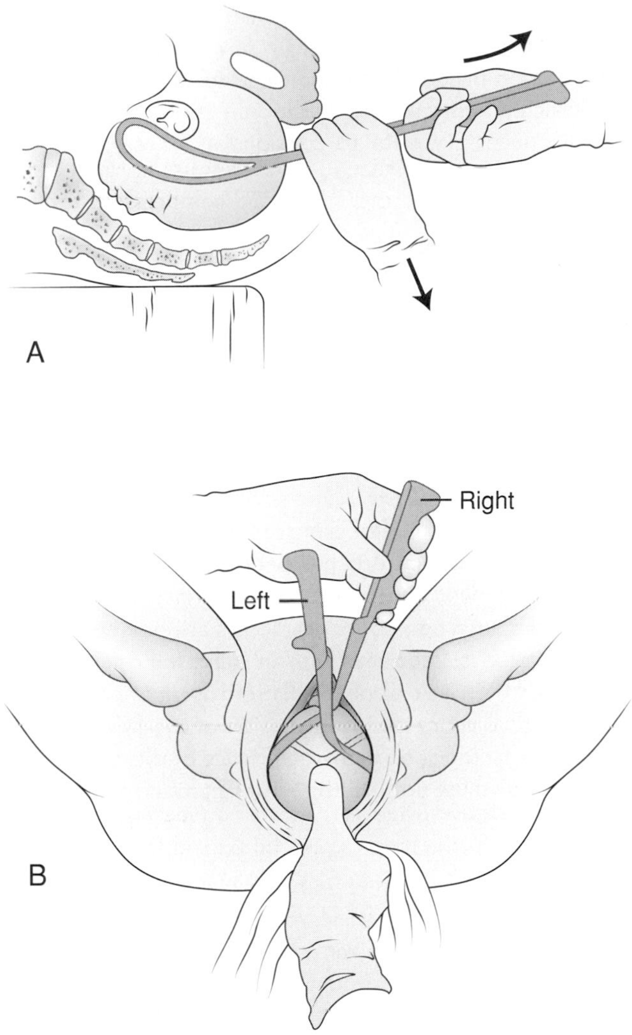

FIGURE 74–6
A, Traction. *B*, Removal of forceps; Ritgen head control.

principle is more easily accomplished instrumentally with an attachment such as the Bill handle which will fit any classical forceps, or with an axis traction instrument.

As the biparietal diameter descends, the direction of traction and the level of the handles rise. The long axis of the head tends to be held in the axis of the pelvis by maternal structure pressure. With traction and elevation of the handles, observation of the edge of the instrument in relation to the adjacent scalp can show the operator the proper direction of pull. If the instrument is elevated too soon, the scalp appears to sink in relation to the upper edge of the blade. Conversely, late elevation of the instrument results in the scalp rising as the head is forced to extend. As the occiput passes under the symphysis pubis, the handle elevation may reach 45 degrees above the horizontal. Higher elevation of the handles increases the risk of vaginal sulcus tears.

The amount of traction force should always be the least possible to accomplish reasonable descent. Maximum permissible force is 45 lb (20 kg) in the nullipara or 30 lb (13 kg) in the multipara.[13] Most deliveries are accomplished with considerably less force. The amount of vectored force may be difficult to estimate when using manual axis traction. With a traction attachment, the vectored force is equal to the total traction force exerted.

Episiotomy, quite popular in North America, is less so in other areas of the world. Regardless of the controversy over routine use of the procedure, episiotomy results in the need for less tractive force. There is continuing controversy about whether the episiotomy should be mediolateral (posterolateral) or midline; this author prefers the median approach as more cosmetic, easier to repair, and much less painful in the puerperium. However, although data from controlled trials are lacking, it seems likely that the median episiotomy is associated with a higher rate of third- or fourth-degree tears than the mediolateral.[15] Thus, either approach appears valid at the present time.

During extension of the head over the perineum, the forceps may be removed and a Ritgen maneuver performed for completion of delivery of the head. The fetus should be monitored between contractions throughout the procedure.

Should reasonable effort not produce descent of the head, the initial management should be to direct traction force to a lower plane, rather than using more force. If this is not helpful, the blades should be removed and the situation completely reevaluated. The same, or another, instrument may be carefully applied. Abdominal delivery is the appropriate alternative for a second negative trial. A ventouse trial is not advised following a failed forceps delivery.

MANAGEMENT OF SPECIAL SITUATIONS

Occiput Transverse Position

Although possible with a flat pelvis, spontaneous delivery as an OT rarely occurs; most will rotate to OA or OP. Should timely delivery become necessary with an OT position, or in cases of the relatively common persistent OT and deep transverse arrest, several options are available, with equivalent results for all methods.[55]

PROCEDURE: OCCIPUT TRANSVERSE POSITION

MANUAL ROTATION

Manual rotation (Fig. 74–7) is a method used successfully by some operators. Used alone and followed by spontaneous delivery there is a significant decrease in the danger of sulcus and vaginal tears.[54] Assuming planned subsequent forceps use, the hand used for rotation depends upon the location of the occiput. Because the left hand would be used to guide the toe of the right forceps blade after manual rotation from an ROT OT to OA, the left hand is used for rotation from ROT. Conversely, the right hand rotates from LOT. The fingers are introduced into the vagina behind the posterior parietal bone with the palm upward and the thumb over the anterior

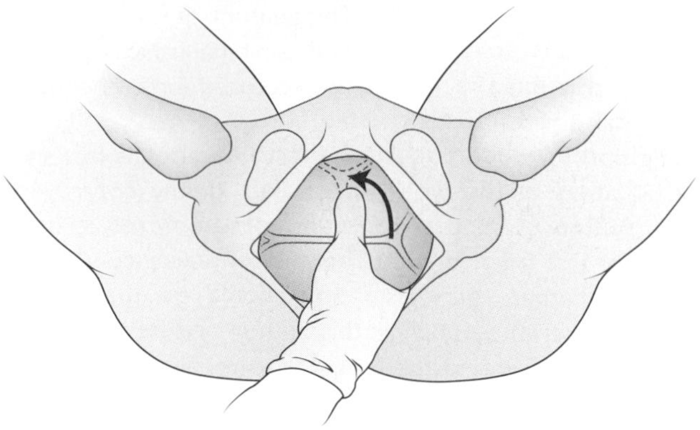

FIGURE 74–7
Manual rotation of the head.

parietal bone. The head is then flexed, if possible, and rotated toward OA. Fundal pressure fixes the head, and the posterior blade of the forceps is applied as the fingers splint the head in its new position. Rotation is usually easiest with the biparietal diameter at the plane of greatest pelvic dimension. Higher displacement of the head, even disengagement, is considered potentially hazardous. Some operators feel that resorting to this alternative is an acceptable risk, with fundal pressure reengaging the rotated head in OA, provided that immediate recourse to abdominal delivery is available.

CLASSICAL FORCEPS

Classical forceps rotation is commonly used, although accurate application to the head in OT is more difficult to accomplish than in anterior positions. More points of obstruction may be met in wandering the anterior blade. Midforceps rotations are particularly difficult because the pelvic curve of the instrument is not available in the transverse position, and in application the perineum may obstruct adequate depression of the handle of the anterior blade. The Simpson type instrument may be used, but the Elliot type overlapping shanks offer less resistance to rotation and application may be slightly easier.[56]

Initial application of the anterior blade has been advocated.[15] Most prefer application of the posterior blade first. The blade (left blade in an LOT) is introduced directly posterior to the head following the plane of least resistance until the handle is below the horizontal. The handle is lower with increasing height of the head. To compensate for the pelvic curve of the instrument, the handle must deviate laterally away from the midline during insertion so that the toe stays in the midline. The anterior blade (the right blade in the case of an LOT) is introduced as high as possible under the pubic ramus with the handle initially almost vertical. The handle descends through an arc of nearly 180 degrees. The heel of the blade is simultaneously wandered upward with pressure from the fingers of the vaginal hand. The blades are locked with the shanks as close as possible to one fingerbreadth medial to the posterior fontanel. Standard checks of application apply. Rotation is then accomplished with rotation of the handles upward through a wide arc consistent with the pelvic curve of the instrument. If obstruction is met, the head may require slight upward displacement so that rotation may be facilitated close to the plane of greatest pelvic dimension. The application is rechecked and readjusted, if necessary, prior to traction for delivery.

KIELLAND FORCEPS

Kielland forceps (Fig. 74–8) are the most popular instrument worldwide for transverse positions of the occiput, although this may be changing.[57] The construction of the instrument offers a single accurate application for correction of asynclitism, rotation, and extraction, with a semiaxis traction pull. Use of the instrument should yield fetal results equivalent to those of cesarean section for the same clinical situation.[28–30,58] Early studies, which suggested a poor outcome, have since been criticized as indicating that inappropriate selection criteria had been used.[58,59]

The instrument should not be used in a flat pelvis or when short anteroposterior diameters are present. In such cases, rotation is associated with an increased risk of maternal injury.[56] The lack of pelvic curve may also increase the risk of vaginal injury during extension of the head at delivery. Owing to the special characteristics of this instrument, the operator must not use the same approach as with conventional forceps.

Before application, the bladder should always be emptied and the patient positioned with the buttocks slightly overhanging the edge of the delivery table. The instrument is oriented in a position of use with the knobs, or buttons, on the shanks toward the occiput. The anterior blade is always inserted first. Four application methods are possible. With a very low station, the blade may be applied directly from below upward. In Kielland's original inversion application (sometimes called the classical application) the blade is inserted in an inverted manner, concavity of the cephalic curve upward, beneath the symphysis and anterior to the head. The toe is carried into the uterus until the "elbow" of the leading edge of the shank is close to the pubis. At this point the blade is rotated 180 degrees on its own axis in the direction of the button. The blade will then drop onto the head with the cephalic curve applied to the anterior parietal bone. If difficulty is encountered, the anterior blade is removed in favor of a wandering application. The third and fourth methods involve wandering over the occiput in case of a flexed head or over the face in case of an extended head. Some operators mistakenly fear the inversion method will tear the lower segment, and routinely use the wandering method. With the anterior blade in place, the posterior blade is introduced posterior to the head, with the cephalic curve upward, following the plane of least resistance. Obstruction is frequently met at the sacral promontory. This is overcome with a lateral shift to avoid the obstruction. When in place, the instrument's sliding lock is engaged with the handles at approximately 45 degrees below the horizontal in a midforceps procedure. The level of the handles depends on the level of the biparietal diameter, being higher with a lower head.

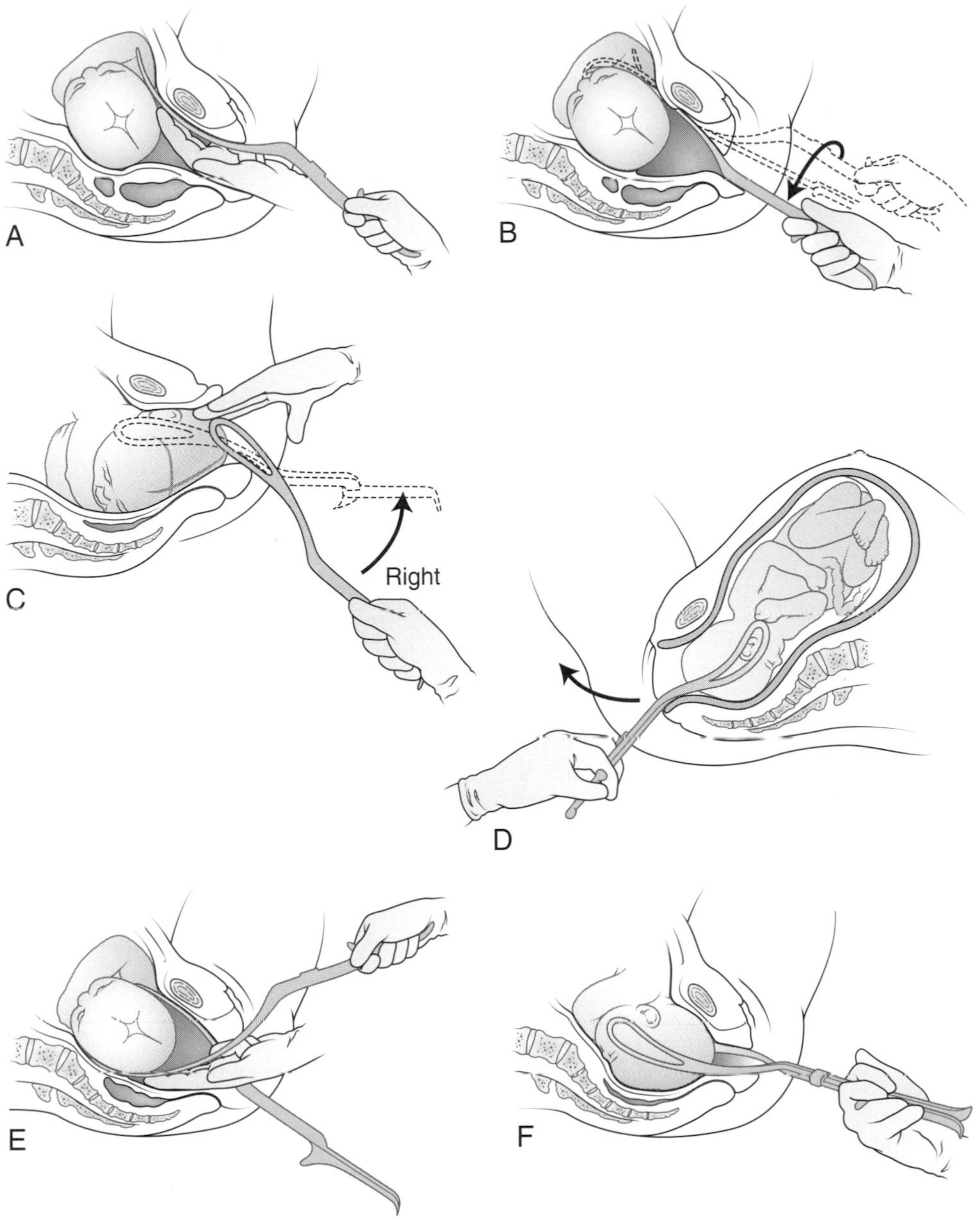

FIGURE 74–8
The use of Kielland's forceps with a left occiput transverse position. *A* and *B*, Classical (inversion) method of application of anterior blade. *C*, Direct application of anterior blade to low head. *D*, Wandering application of anterior blade. *E*, Direct application of posterior blade (anterior blade in place). *F*, Traction after rotation to occiput anterior position.

Any asynclitism is corrected by equalizing the level of the fingerguards. Correction of inadequate flexion is facilitated if the blades are unlocked and separately wandered to one fingerbreadth medial to the posterior fontanel. They are then relocked and moved back toward the midline.

Rotation toward OA position is accomplished, usually with remarkably little effort, by rotating the instrument along its own axis. If resistance is met, lowering the plane of the handles should be tried. Continued resistance may be due to a relative obstruction at that level. The head should first be drawn downward in transverse position for 1 cm and rotation attempted. If unsuccesful, the head should be displaced to 1 cm above the original station and rotated. Following rotation to OA, the application should be rechecked. Extraction may be performed with the Kielland forceps. The operator must remember that the nearly straight instrument must be pulled in a lower plane below the horizontal and should not be raised above the horizontal at delivery. Some operators change to another instrument for better traction.

OTHER FORCEPS

Barton forceps, with its hinged anterior blade, is another alternative for managing transverse arrest. Its main indication is a flat maternal pelvis, which is a contraindication for the Kielland forceps.[21,54,60] With Barton forceps, the head is brought down in the transverse position, then rotated to OA as it traverses the plane of the outlet. The need for this instrument is so infrequent that the reader is referred to a standard text for its use.[13,15]

In the United States and Canada, special instruments (Mann, Laufe, Shute, and other forceps) have been devised for rotation from OT or from OP. These instruments have regional advocates. Similarly, the Moolgaoker[61] has attracted followers in the United Kingdom and on the European continent. The ventouse and, of course, cesarean section are also alternate management options.

Occiput Posterior Position

Heads in OP position may eventually spontaneously rotate to OA and deliver. Similar options to those for the OT are available when delivery is required from an OP. Before any procedure is carried out the operator must know in which direction to rotate the head, if it is not in an oblique posterior position. The recorded position earlier in labor, palpation of the fetal back, or even ultrasonographic location of the back should resolve the question. Obviously the occiput must only be rotated in the direction of the fetal back.

PROCEDURE: OCCIPUT POSTERIOR POSITION

MANUAL ROTATION

Manual rotation either with or without subsequent forceps extraction is an option. The technique is similar to that for an OT with rotation being carried up to 180 degrees rather than 90 degrees.

CLASSICAL FORCEPS

Classical forceps rotation from OP is usually performed with the modified Scanzoni maneuver, a double forceps application method. A single upside-down application from below followed by a 180-degree rotation has been described but is not popular.[54] In the Scanzoni technique an Elliot-type instrument is preferred.[56] It is applied to the OP head as if it were an OA. In an ROP position the blades would be applied as if the position were LOA. When the application is checked, the plane of the shanks should be just above the posterior fontanel. The rotation to OA is accomplished with rotation of the handles through a wide arc, ending with the handles pointing downward. The blades are now upside-down with toes pointing posteriorly. One blade should be left as a splint against backward rotation while the other is removed downward, then inverted and reinserted between the splinting blade and the head. The splinting blade is then removed downward prior to reapplication in standard manner to the vertex, which is now in OA position. An ordinary forceps technique is then used for delivery. Some operators prefer to substitute a better tractor at the reapplication. The use of a solid blade or indented fenestration instrument for rotation prevents insertion of the blade through the fenestration of the vaginal splinting blade.

KIELLAND FORCEPS

Kielland forceps rotation is probably the most popular method of rotation of an OP. The previous comments on the instrument (see OT management, discussed earlier) apply. Application to an OP differs in that the blades, with buttons toward the occiput, are applied directly from below the thighs to the appropriate position on the head. Other aspects of technique are not different from those discussed in rotation from OT.

OCCIPUT POSTERIOR DELIVERY

Delivery from the OP position is an option that is advocated by those who fear that rotational procedures may be traumatic. An indication for delivery without rotation can exist in an anthropoid pelvis with narrow transverse dimensions. Also, with a funnel pelvis, usually android, with the head molded into the outlet under a narrow arch, delivery in OP may be indicated. An OP delivery is relatively traumatic as unfavorable diameters must be brought through the pelvis. The biparietal diameter is usually at a higher station than anticipated. More force is required and the direction of the force is critical. More perineal space is required. An axis traction instrument or at least a Simpson type instrument should be employed. Applied as in the first step of a Scanzoni, the shanks are depressed against the perineum to get close to the posterior fontanel. The blades are then locked and the application is checked. With traction, after the anterior fontanel clears the symphysis, the head is delivered by flexion rather than by extension.

PROCEDURE: 'AFTERCOMING' HEAD OF A BREECH

Following delivery of the arms and body of the infant, the body is wrapped in a towel, care of which is placed in the hands of the necessary assistant. This serves to keep fetal extremities out of the field, and when excessive elevation of the body is avoided, there is less chance of cervical hyperextension injury.[14] In the controlled breech delivery, the back is upward and the head enters the pelvis within a few degrees of mentum posterior. The position is determined by palpation. The Piper forceps are applied upward from a kneeling position. The left blade is applied first, guided by two fingers of the right hand. The handle is started beneath the patient's right thigh, then swept downward and medially as the toe passes upward to the right parietal area of the infant. The handle then rests 45 to 50 degrees below the horizontal. The right blade is similarly applied upward from beneath the left thigh. The application is checked by palpation of the chin between the shanks of the instrument. The infant is then allowed to straddle the instrument, and traction is applied in a direction and manner similar to routine forceps use. Vectoring is not needed because the reverse pelvic curve of the instrument gives the instrument axis traction. The head is routinely delivered with the forceps in place.

PROCEDURE AT CESAREAN SECTION (See also Chapter 76)

Although cesarean section is not within the purview of AVD, it should be noted that the use of instruments to deliver the head from the uterine incision at cesarean section[54] can decrease traumatic extension of that incision. Wrigley or short Simpson forceps are often employed. A single vectis blade, to turn and elevate the occiput through the uterine incision, can have the same effect, as can the curved, unhinged blade of the Barton forceps. The Murless instrument, with a single, hinged, locking blade, is more popular in the United Kingdom. It is introduced laterally and slipped beneath the head. When locked in position, it acts as a vectis and elevator to deliver the head.[54] The ventouse has also been advocated for this purpose, and is an excellent option.

Comparison of Ventouse and Forceps

Operative vaginal delivery trials comparing the obstetric forceps with the vacuum extractor have documented that the vacuum technique offers lower rates of maternal trauma such as genital tract lacerations, but higher rates of newborn scalp trauma and cephalhematoma than forceps. Efficacy of the two techniques are fairly equivalent.[62–77]

In a mid-1990s survey of residency training programs in the United States, 210 of 291 identified programs answered a questionnaire about their practice.[69] Forceps are the primary instrument in most programs (68%), but nearly one third of responding centers prefer vacuum extraction. Nearly all the responding programs (199 of 209, 95%) teach AVD using vaccum, mainly the soft cup vacuum extractor (metallic cups are used in only 14% of centers). Instruction in midpelvic operative vaginal delivery is currently offered in only 64% of the programs. Deep transverse arrest is handled initially by forceps in half the responding centers, whereas 28% and 22% would proceed with cesarean section or attempt a vacuum extraction, respectively.

CONCLUSIONS

- Appropriate use of the ventouse or the obstetric forceps as options in management of the second stage of labor is good medical practice.
- Careful attention to indications, contraindications, prerequisites, and performance should lead to a positive outcome. Mounting evidence attests to the safety of appropriate procedures.
- The instruments are not inherently dangerous. The manner in which they are used may be. In addition to a working knowledge of the instruments, the operator must have the willingness to abandon an unsuccessful procedure.
- Injury is the result of force applied to tissues that resist that force. That resistance can be felt and is obvious. The operator who refuses to apply force of injurious dimension does not injure.
- More important than the leading bony point of the head is the biparietal diameter, the widest and critical diameter, which must be moved. It contains the pivot point of the head.
- All operative procedures in assisted vaginal delivery may be considered a trial, to be performed with care and with adequate facilities for timely abdominal delivery in case of a negative trial.
- Protection is afforded to the operator by recording of the cognitive processes of decision for and execution of the operative procedure. A specific detailed documentation in the patient's record is always indicated.

SUMMARY OF MANAGEMENT OPTIONS
Assisted Vaginal Delivery

Management Options	Quality of Evidence	Strength of Recommendation	References
Indications			
Maternal indications include distress, exhaustion, and certain maternal medical disorders (see text).	IV	C	4, 72, 73
Fetal indications include presumed fetal jeopardy and breech delivery (forceps to aftercoming head).	IV	C	4, 72, 73
Process indications include malposition (OP, OT, asynclitism) and unsuccessful ventouse procedure (forceps trial with caution and facilities for cesarean section standing by).	IV	C	4, 72, 73

Continued

SUMMARY OF MANAGEMENT OPTIONS
Assisted Vaginal Delivery *(Continued)*

Management Options	Quality of Evidence	Strength of Recommendation	References
Indications—*Continued*			
Practitioners should be aware that no indication is absolute and must be able to distinguish "standard" from "special" indications.	IV	C	72
Contraindications			
Unengaged head (two fifths or more palpable abdominally or at or above ischial spines vaginally)	IV Ia IIa	C A B	72 74 68
Inability to define position	IV	C	75, 76
Malposition (face, brow)			
Suspected or actual cephalopelvic disproportion (pelvic anatomy or macrosomia related)			
Certain fetal anomalies			
Prematurity (? <34 weeks for ventouse) or <1500 g			
Repeated scalp pH estimations (ventouse)			
Operator inexperience or lack of training with instrument			
Prerequisites			
Engaged head (but one fifth palpable abdominally or above +2 station is potentially hazardous)	IV	C	72, 73
Fully dilated (some argue for 9+ cm with ventouse), membranes ruptured			
Empty bladder (? not for outlet delivery)			
Known presentation, position, and station			
Adequate analgesia/anesthesia			
Experienced operator and adequate support facilities			
Willingness to abandon procedure if difficult			
Informed and consenting patient			
Working, serviced equipment for ventouse and matching blades for forceps			
OT or OP Options			
Manual rotation/ventouse/rotational forceps	–	GPP	–
Possible delivery as OP position	–	GPP	–
Selection by circumstances, individual experience, and preferences rather than scientific guidelines	IV	C	72
Requires experience and skill	IV	C	72
Choice of Instrument			
Practitioners should use the most acceptable intrument for individual circumstances.	IV	C	72
Deficient knowledge and incorrect technique contribute to increased complications. Practitioners should be aware of the potential risks and necessary safety measures.	IV	C	72
Vacuum versus forceps:	Ia	A	74
Vacuum has higher rates of delivery failure, cephalhematomas, retinal hemorrhages, and jaundice.			

SUMMARY OF MANAGEMENT OPTIONS

Assisted Vaginal Delivery *(Continued)*

Management Options	Quality of Evidence	Strength of Recommendation	References
Choice of Instrument—*Continued*			
Forceps has higher rates of regional/general anesthesia and maternal trauma.			
No differences in rates of cesarean section, Apgar scores, long-term (5 y) maternal and baby follow-up.			
Soft versus metal vacuum cups:	Ia	A	77
Soft cup has higher rates of delivery failure (especially with OP, OT, and difficult OA positions).			
Metal cup has higher rates of neonatal scalp trauma.			

REFERENCES

1. Hankins GDV, Rowe TF: Operative vaginal delivery—Year 2000. Am J Obstet Gynecol 1994;175:275–282.
2. Kaminski HM, Stafl A, Aiman J: The effect of epidural analgesia on the frequency of instrumental obstetric delivery. Obstet Gynecol 1987;69:770.
3. Hoult IJ, MacLennan AH, Carrie LES: Lumbar epidural analgesia in labour: Relation to fetal malposition and instrumental delivery. BMJ 1977;1:14–16.
4. American College of Obstetricians and Gynecologists: Operative Vaginal Delivery. Technical Bulletin No. 196. Washington, DC, ACOG, 1994.
5. Williams MC, Knuppel RA, O'Brien WF, et al: A randomized comparison of assisted vaginal delivery by obstetric forceps and polyethylene vacuum cup. Obstet Gynecol 1991;78:789.
6. Perkins RP: Fetal dystocia. Clin Obstet Gynecol 1987;30:56.
7. Fairweather DVI: Obstetric management and follow-up of the very-low-birthweight infant. J Reprod Med 1981;26:387.
8. O'Driscoll K, Meagher D, MacDonald D, Goeghegan F: Traumatic intracranial hemorrhage in firstborn infants and delivery with obstetric forceps. BJOG 1981;88:577.
9. Schwartz DB, Miodovnik M, Lavin JP: Neonatal outcome among low birth weight infants delivered spontaneously or by low forceps. Obstet Gynecol 1983;62:283.
10. Laube DW: Forceps delivery. Clin Obstet Gynaecol 1986; 29:286.
11. Milner RDG: Neonatal mortality of breech deliveries with and without forceps to the aftercoming head. BJOG 1975;82:783.
12. Myers SA, Gleicher N: Breech delivery: Why the dilemma? Am J Obstet Gynecol 1987;156:6.
13. Dennen PC: Forceps Deliveries, 3rd ed. Philadelphia, F.A. Davis, 1988.
14. Yeomans ER, Gilstrap LC: The role of forceps in modern obstetrics. Clin Obstet Gynecol 1994;37:785–793.
15. O'Grady JP: Modern Instrumental Delivery. Baltimore, Williams & Wilkins, 1988.
16. Bowes WA, Katz VL: Operative vaginal delivery: Forceps and vacuum extractor. Curr Probl Obstet Gynecol Fertil 1994;17(3): 84–109.
17. Benedetti TJ, Gabbe SG: Shoulder dystocia. A complication of fetal macrosomia and prolonged second stage of labor with midpelvic delivery. Obstet Gynecol 1978;52:526.
18. American College of Obstetricians and Gynecologists: Obstetric Forceps. ACOG Committee Opinion No. 71. Washington, DC, ACOG, 1989.
19. Hagadorn-Freathy AS, Yoemans ER, Hankins GDV: Validation of the 1988 ACOG forceps classification system. Obstet Gynecol 1991;77:356.
20. Robertson PA, Laros RK, Zhao RL: Neonatal and maternal outcome in low-pelvic and midpelvic operative deliveries. Am J Obstet Gynecol 1990;162:1436.
21. Dennen EH: Forceps Deliveries, 2nd ed. Philadelphia, F.A. Davis, 1965.
22. Niswander KR, Gordon M: Safety of the low forcep operation. Am J Obstet Gynecol 1973;117:619.
23. Gilstrap LC, Hauth JC, Schiano S, Connor KD: Neonatal acidosis and method of delivery. Obstet Gynecol 1984;63:681.
24. Seidman DS, Laor A, Gale R, et al: Long-term effects of vacuum and forceps deliveries. Lancet 1991;337:1583.
25. Yancey MK, Herpolsheimer A, Jordan GD, et al: Maternal and neonatal effects of outlet forceps delivery compared with spontaneous vaginal delivery in term pregnancies. Obstet Gynecol 1991;78:646.
26. Richardson DA, Evans MI, Cibils LA: Midforceps delivery: A critical review. Am J Obstet Gynecol 1983;145:621.
27. Friedman EA, Sachtleben-Murray MS, Dahrouge D, Neff RK: Long-term effects of labor and delivery on offspring: A matched pair analysis. Am J Obstet Gynecol 1984;150:941.
28. Dierker LJ, Rosen MG, Thompson K, Lynn P: Midforceps deliveries: Long-term outcome of infants. Am J Obstet Gynecol 1986;154:764.
29. Bashore RA, Phillips WH, Brinkman CR: A comparison of the morbidity of midforceps and cesarean delivery. Am J Obstet Gynecol 1990;162:1428.
30. Dierker LJ, Rosen MG, Thompson K, et al: The midforceps: Maternal and neonatal outcomes. Am J Obstet Gynecol 1985;152:176.
31. Hughey MJ, McElin TW, Lusskey R: Forceps operations in perspective. I. Mid forcep rotation operations. J Reprod Med 1978;20:253.
32. Lowe B: Fear of failure: A place for the trial of instrumental delivery. BJOG 1987;94:60.
33. Boyd ME, Usher RH, McLean FH, Norman BE: Failed forceps. Obstet Gynecol 1986;68:779.
34. Revah A, Ezra Y, Farine D, Ritchie K: Failed trial of vacuum or forceps—Maternal and fetal outcome. Am J Obstet Gynecol 1997;176:200–204.
35. Pritchard JA, MacDonald PC, Grant NF(eds): Williams Obstetrics, 19th ed. Norwalk, CT, Appleton & Lange, 1988.

36. Mentiglou SM, Perlman M, Manning FA: High cervical spinal cord injury in neonates delivered with forceps: Report of 15 cases. Obstet Gynecol 1995;86:589–594.
37. Tan KL: Brachial palsy. J Obstet Gynaecol Br Emp 1973;117:51.
38. Zelson C, Lee SJ, Pearl M: The incidence of skull fractures underlying cephalhematomas in newborn infants. J Pediatr 1974;85:371.
39. Levine MG, Holroyde J, Woods JR, et al: Birth trauma: Incidence and predisposing factors. Obstet Gynecol 1984;63:792.
40. Niswander K, Henson G, Elborne D, et al : Adverse outcome of pregnancy and the quality of obstetric care. Lancet 1984;ii:827.
41. Dennen PC: Operative vaginal delivery. In Donn SM, Fisher CW (eds): Risk Management Techniques in Perinatal and Neonatal Practice. Armonk, NY, Futura, 1996.
42. Bofill JA, Rust OA, Perry KG, et al: Operative vaginal delivery: A survey of fellows of ACOG. Obstet Gynecol 1996;88: 1007–1010.
43. Bird GC: The importance of flexion in vaccum extractor delivery. BJOG 1976;83:194–200.
44. Vacca A: The pace of the vacuum exterior in modern obstetric practice. Fetal Med Rev 1990;2:103–122.
45. Vacca A, Grant A, Wyatt G, Chalmers I: Portsmouth operative delivery trial: A comparison of vacuum extraction and forceps delivery. BJOG 1983;90:1107–1112.
46. Wylie B: Traction in forceps deliveries. Am J Obstet Gynecol 1935;29:425.
47. Moolgaoker A, Ahamed O, Payne P: A comparison of different methods of instrumental delivery based on electronic measurments of compression and traction. Obstet Gynecol 1979;54:299–309.
48. Laufe LE: Divergent and crossed obstetric forceps: Comparative study of compression and traction forces. Obstet Gynecol 1971;38:885–887.
49. Duchon M, DeMund M, Brown R: Laboratory comparison of modern vacuum extractors. Obstet Gynecol 1988;71:155–158.
50. Maryniak G, Frank J: Clinical assessment of the Kobayashi vacuum extractor. Obstet Gynecol 1984;64:431–435.
51. Hammarstrom M, Csemiczky G, Belfrage P: Comparison between the conventional Malström extractor and a new extractor with Silastic cup. Acta Obstet Gynecol Scand 1986;65:791–792.
52. Dohn M, Barclay C, Fraser R, et al: A multicentre randomized trial comparing delivery with a silicone rubber cup and rigid metal vacuum extractor cups. BJOG 1989;96:545–551.
53. Paul R, Staisch K, Pine S: The "new" vacuum extractor. Obstet Gynecol 1973;41:800–802.
54. Douglas-Stromme RG: Operative Obstetrics, 5th ed. Norwalk, CT, Appleton & Lange, 1988.
55. Healy DL, Quinn MA, Pepperell RJ: Rotational delivery of the fetus: Kielland's forceps and two other methods compared. BJOG 1982;89:501.
56. Dennen EH: Choice of forceps. Clin Obstet Gynecol 1959;2:367.
57. Jain V, Guleria K, Gopalan S, Narang A: Mode of delivery in deep transverse arrest. Int J Gynaecol Obstet 1993;43:129–135.
58. Traub AI, Morrow RJ, Ritchie JWK, Dorman KJ: A continuing use for Kielland's forceps. BJOG 1984;91:894.
59. Cardozo LD, Gibb DMF, Studd JWW, Cooper DJ: Should we abandon Kielland's forceps? BMJ 1983;287:315–317.
60. Traub AI, Morrow RJ, Ritchie JWK Dornan KJ: A continuing use for Kielland's forceps? BJOG 1984;91:894–898.
61. Moolgaoker A: A new design of obstetric forceps. J Obstet Gynaecol Br Commonw 1962;69:450.
62. Bofill J, Rust O, Schort S, et al: A randomised prospective trial of the obstetric forceps versus the M-cup vacuum extractor. Am J Obstet Gynecol 1996;175:1325–1350.
63. Vacca A, Grant A, Wyatt G, Chalmers I: Portsmouth operative delivery trial: a comparison of vacuum extraction and forceps delivery. BJOG 1983;90:1107–1112.
64. Johanson R, Pusey J, Livera N, Jones P: North Staffordshire/ Wigan assisted delivery trial. BJOG 1989;96: 537–544.
65. Cohn M, Barclay C, Fraser R, et al: A multicentre randomized trial comparing delivery with a silicone rubber cup and rigid metal vacuum extractor cups. BJOG 1989;96:545–551.
66. Chenoy R, Johanson R: A randomized prospective study comparing delivery with metal and silicone rubber vacuum extractor cups. BJOG 1992;99:360–363.
67. Low J, Ng TY, Chew SY: Clinical experience with the Silc Cup Vacuum Extractor. Singapore Med J 1993;34:135–138.
68. Johanson RB, Rice C, Doyle M, et al: A randomised prospective study comparing the new vacuum extractor policy with forceps delivery. BJOG 1993;100:524–530.
69. Bofill JA, Rust OA, Perry KGJ, et al: Forceps and vacuum delivery: A survey of North American residency programs. Obstet Gynecol 1996;88:622–625.
70. Channa S, Monga D: Outcome of forceps delivery versus vacuum extraction—A review of 200 cases. Singapore Med J 1994;35:605–608.
71. Lucas MJ: The role of vacuum extraction in modern obstetrics. Clin Obstet Gynecol 1994;37:794–805.
72. Johanson, RB: Instrumental Vaginal Delivery. RCOG Clinical "Green Top" Guideline. London, RCOG, 2000.
73. Gei AF, Belfort MA: Forceps-assisted vaginal delivery. Obstet Gynecol Clin North Am 1999;26:345–370.
74. Johanson RB, Menon V: Vacuum extraction versus forceps for assisted vaginal delivery. The Cochrane Database of Systematic Reviews 1999, Issue 2. Art. No.: CD000224. DOI: 10.1002/ 14651858.CD000224.
75. Thiery M: Fetal hemorrhage following blood samplings and use of vacuum extractor. Am J Obstet Gynecol 1979;134:231.
76. Roberts IF, Stone M: Fetal hemorrhage: Complication of vacuum extractor after fetal blood sampling. Am J Obstet Gynecol 1978;132:109.
77. Johanson R, Menon V: Soft versus rigid vacuum extractor cups for assisted vaginal delivery. The Cochrane Database of Systematic Reviews 2000, Issue 2. Art No.: CD000446. DOI: 10.1002/ 14651858.CD000446.

CHAPTER 75

Delivery After Previous Cesarean Section

Gordon C. S. Smith

INTRODUCTION

Rates of primary cesarean section have increased over the last 20 years. Consequently, increasing numbers of women present with second pregnancies and face the issue of mode of delivery. The dictum of "once a cesarean always a cesarean" largely applied in the United States until the 1980s (although not in the United Kingdom or Europe). However, a series of studies in the 1980s reported the relative safety of attempting vaginal birth following cesarean delivery (VBAC). Rates of VBAC increased in the United States until 1996[1] and then declined following reports of the risks of uterine rupture.[2] Further studies over the last 2 to 3 years have described risks of VBAC which may well increase the trend toward planned repeat cesarean delivery (PRCD). The choice between PRCD and VBAC, like virtually every other medical choice, involves the balancing of risks and benefits.

Estimating these risks and benefits requires the interpretation of large numbers of studies which are almost exclusively observational in nature. The risks of mode of delivery in women with a previous cesarean delivery can be classified at several different levels. First, risks can be divided into maternal risks and risks to the infant. Each can be further divided into short term and long term. Frequently, the different risks favor different modes of delivery. Furthermore, the research question of how to assess the risks and benefits of VBAC versus PRCD is complex due to an absolute reliance on observational data. Virtually all studies are open to some form of criticism. However, even studies with obvious weaknesses can still yield useful information if assessed in an unbiased manner. Many parties involved in the debate about VBAC start with strongly held prior beliefs about whether it is a "good" or "bad" thing. Consequently, there is a tendency in much of the literature for reviews of VBAC to fall into camps of believers and nonbelievers. The reliance of analyses on frequently flawed but partially informative research studies means that biased parties can interpret the literature in a way that confirms their prior belief. The aim of this chapter is to attempt an unbiased summary of the risks and benefits associated with delivery of pregnant women who have previously been delivered by cesarean section.

METHODOLOGIC ISSUES WHEN COMPARING RATES OF ADVERSE OUTCOMES BETWEEN VAGINAL BIRTH AFTER CESAREAN AND PLANNED REPEAT CESAREAN DELIVERY

Selection Bias and Randomized Controlled Trials

Theoretically, the ideal method for comparing the relative risk of VBAC and PRCD would be a randomized controlled trial (RCT). In practice this is unlikely to occur since most women would not accept the choice being made in a random fashion. Moreover, many of the events of interest are relatively uncommon, such as uterine rupture, hysterectomy, perinatal or maternal death. Consequently, it is unlikely that even if a trial was organized that it would be statistically powered to address the questions of central clinical interest. Although RCTs are clearly the gold standard in evidence-based medicine, it would be wrong to overstate their importance. The main utility of an RCT is to produce a bias-free estimate of relative risk. Two of the major questions relating to VBAC are:

- Does PRCD protect the fetus from severe adverse events in the short term?
- Is PRCD harmful to the mother in the long term?

Because severe adverse events are rare, it would be extremely difficult to organize an adequately powered trial to address the first question. Regarding the second, even if the long-term effects were confined to the outcome of the next pregnancy, follow-up would be required for years after initial recruitment, which is unlikely to be a practical proposition.

The major weakness of observational studies is the issue of selection bias, namely differences might be observed that are not due to the grouping but to factors that determined the grouping. However, observational data have some strengths when comparing outcomes following VBAC and PRCD. The issue of selection bias is less problematic in the context of assessing potentially beneficial effects of PRCD. Women who have PRCD are systematically more likely to have complications such as preexisting maternal disease or gestational diabetes, and they are also older and shorter.[3,4] Selection of women for VBAC is likely to identify a healthy cohort. It follows that if better outcomes are observed in observational studies among women having PRCD, it is very likely that the differences were observed despite rather than because of selection bias. Moreover, it follows that where the outcomes are equivalent between PRCD and VBAC or are better for VBAC, selection bias is likely to have given the VBAC group an advantage. Observational data can allow identification of different pregnancies in the same woman. Analysis of such data may allow assessment of some of the absolute risks of rare adverse events in future pregnancies.

Definition of Vaginal Birth After Cesarean

Another methodologic issue is the question of whether a trial of labor was truly attempted. A proportion of women who elect to have a PRCD will present prior to their scheduled date of cesarean delivery in early labor. Often, these women will be delivered in early labor by emergency cesarean section. Many of the databases that contain sufficient numbers of cases to make adequately powered comparisons of key outcomes will lack the detailed information required to distinguish between these women and women who were genuinely attempting VBAC but required emergency cesarean delivery. This problem can be overcome by comparing the outcomes of apparent VBAC before and at or after 40 weeks' gestation. In the latter group, the majority of women scheduled for PRCD will have been delivered. If similar absolute risks are observed before and after the start of the 40th week, results are likely to be robust. However, even in the most detailed databases, there is likely to be some ambiguity about whether a trial of labor was truly attempted. This uncertainty might sometimes reflect a flexible clinical plan. For example, a woman presenting in early labor might elect for planned repeat cesarean delivery if vaginal examination demonstrated minimal cervical dilation, whereas VBAC would have been attempted if cervical findings were more promising. It is important for the comparison of studies that the definition of VBAC is explicit in all published work.

Ascertainment Bias

The issue of ascertainment bias has also not been properly addressed. Many studies of uterine rupture include both symptomatic uterine rupture and asymptomatic dehiscence. Diagnosis of the latter is most likely to be made at the time of cesarean section since the practice of confirming the integrity of the scar following vaginal birth is no longer recommended. It follows, therefore, that ascertainment of uterine rupture will be increased for any exposure associated with an increased risk of cesarean delivery. Ascertainment bias cannot explain the increased rates of uterine rupture observed among women attempting VBAC following one previous cesarean delivery[3] since the comparison group, PRCD, would have 100% ascertainment of uterine rupture. However, among those attempting VBAC, any factor associated with an increased risk of emergency cesarean section will necessarily be associated with an apparent increased risk of uterine rupture due to ascertainment bias. For example, a study of women who had two previous cesarean deliveries demonstrated an increased risk of uterine rupture among women delivered by planned cesarean section.[5] This finding was almost certainly due to the combined effects of selection bias and ascertainment bias. Ascertainment bias could be overcome by confining analysis to those women who have a symptomatic rupture. However, the data required to discriminate this group are lacking from many of the administrative databases that contain sufficient numbers of women who experience uterine rupture.

Influence of Risk of Emergency Cesarean Delivery

Many of the risks described for PRCD, such as infection and hemorrhage, are more common among women who attempt VBAC but then require emergency cesarean delivery than among women who are delivered by PRCD.[2] It follows, therefore, that among groups who have a high risk of emergency cesarean section, comparison of outcomes of VBAC and PRCD are likely to favor the latter. The greater risk of adverse events following emergency rather than planned cesarean delivery[6] indicate that at certain levels of risk of emergency cesarean delivery, a strategy of delivering all women by a planned procedure may actually carry a lower risk of adverse events directly attributable to surgery. The full-term breech trial, the largest RCT of planned cesarean section, confirmed this proposition, demonstrating similar rates of maternal morbidity comparing those delivered by planned cesarean section with those for whom vaginal birth was attempted.[7] This paradoxical neutral rate of surgical complications despite close to 100% cesarean delivery in the intervention group reflects the 36% emergency cesarean section rate among those attempting vaginal breech birth. It follows, therefore, that comparisons of outcomes between women attempting VBAC and women having PRCD will differ according to the emergency cesarean delivery rate in the former group.

Relative and Absolute Risks

Medical research tends to follow an analytical paradigm inherited from the basic experimental sciences. The approach is to determine a measurable variable, to make a comparison between two groups, and to determine whether the dependent variable differs in a way that exceeds what is consistent with chance. RCTs are the clearest manifestation of the experimental scientific approach in medicine. However, this focus is sometimes inappropriate in medicine, and its shortcomings can be appreciated in the case of VBAC. First, there may be many outcomes that differ between the two groups. By their nature, RCTs tend to concentrate on short-term outcomes due to the expense and practical difficulties of long-term follow-up. For instance, in the case of the full-term breech trial, the analysis was confined to short-term neonatal and maternal outcomes. If the women were followed up to the end of their reproductive careers, detrimental effects of a first cesarean delivery may become evident. However, by the nature of the question, this could never be addressed by an RCT, and inferences can only be drawn from observational data. The focus on the experimental paradigm also leads to emphasis being placed on the relative rather than the absolute risk. This can lead to bizarre misinterpretation of the data. For instance, a meta-analysis of observational studies quoted absolute risks of perinatal death of 5.8 per 1000 for VBAC and 3.4 per 1000 for PRCD with an odds ratio of 1.7 for perinatal death in the VBAC group.[8] However, many of these deaths were not truly related to the chosen mode of delivery. A large scale retrospective cohort study then described more accurate estimates of absolute risks related to the mode of delivery of 1.2 per 1000 and 0.1 per 1000 respectively with an odds ratio of approximately 12 for VBAC.[4] Despite the fact that the true absolute risk of VBAC described in that study was five times lower than previously described, the greater relative risk when compared with PRCD led to it being interpreted by some observers as justification of PRCD because of a much greater true relative risk.

COMPARISON OF OUTCOMES OF VBAC AND PRCD

Maternal Risks

Short Term

Vaginal birth carries some direct risks, such as vaginal and perineal laceration, including trauma to the anal sphincter and mucosa. However, the major sources of significant short-term maternal morbidity in the context of attempted VBAC are emergency cesarean delivery and uterine rupture. The balance of risks comparing VBAC and PRCD depends on the extent to which the excess of cesarean deliveries in the PRCD group is compensated by more severe complications in the VBAC group. The greater severity of complications in the VBAC group is because the cesarean delivery is performed as an emergency[6] and because there is more likely to be a uterine rupture.[3] Since the comparison depends on the excess of cesarean deliveries in the PRCD group, VBAC will compare more favorably when the rate of successful vaginal birth is higher.

A large-scale, population-based study in 2001 demonstrated a significantly increased risk of uterine rupture among women attempting VBAC following spontaneous onset of labor (5.2 per 1000) compared with those having PRCD (1.6 per 1000),[3] which was consistent with an earlier meta-analysis of approximately 40,000 women.[8] The meta-analysis was dominated by a single large-scale study in which uterine rupture was not defined.[9] However, the population-based cohort defined rupture on the basis of International Classification of Diseases (ICD)9 codes, which include antepartum and intrapartum rupture.[3] Since the former is likely to include cases of asymptomatic dehiscence in the PRCD group, the true excess of clinically significant uterine rupture may be higher in the VBAC group.

The net effect on maternal morbidity can be inferred from analysis of outcomes that indicate surgical problems. Overall, women attempting VBAC have decreased rates of febrile morbidity (odds ratio = 0:7), blood transfusion (odds ratio = 0:6), hysterectomy (odds ratio = 0:4), and venous thromboembolism (odds ratio = 0:4) compared with PRCD.[8,9] However, the lower rates of complications in the VBAC group could reflect selection bias. For instance, over 30% of women having PRCD wish to have a tubal ligation.[9] Systematic variation in plans for further pregnancies could lead to a bias toward hysterectomy to manage intraoperative bleeding in women having PRCD. Attempted VBAC has been associated with an increased risk of serious intraoperative injury (vascular, bowel, or urinary tract) affecting 1.3% compared with 0.6% of women having PRCD, which presumably reflects difficulties that arise due to uterine rupture and the greater risk of emergency versus planned cesarean delivery.[2] Current studies are too small to determine the relationship among VBAC, PRCD, and maternal death. There is a nonsignificant trend toward greater maternal mortality in the meta-analysis among women attempting VBAC, with three deaths among 27,504 attempting VBAC and no deaths among 17,740 women having PRCD.[8] Two of the maternal deaths in the VBAC group were due to venous thromboembolism. If any difference is confirmed in this regard with further observational studies, it is unlikely to be explained by selection bias due to the greater likelihood of pre-existing maternal disease and older age of the PRCD mothers.

Long Term

Long-term maternal consequences of the choice between VBAC and PRCD are numerous. If attempted VBAC results in vaginal birth, particularly operative vaginal delivery, recent observational studies suggest that a woman may be at increased risk of urinary incontinence (overall prevalence 15.9% among those delivered by cesarean section versus 21% delivered vaginally).[10] If VBAC is attempted and results in catastrophic uterine rupture, the uterus will be vulnerable to antepartum uterine rupture in future pregnancies. Due to the rarity of these events and the lack of detail in most administrative databases, the absolute risk is difficult to quantify.

Observational studies have suggested that women delivered by cesarean section are more likely to experience difficulty in conceiving (odds ratio = 1.5).[11] The implications of this for the decision between VBAC and PRCD are difficult to define. First, these women have already had a cesarean delivery and it is unclear whether there is a "dose-response" relationship between number of cesarean deliveries and lowered fertility. Second, lowered fertility prior to the first birth is a risk factor for cesarean delivery,[11] and it is questionable, therefore, whether the relationship between cesarean delivery and lowered fertility is causal. This question may be resolved by examining the association according to the indication for the first cesarean delivery.

The major long-term effect of PRCD is on the outcome of future pregnancies. Previous cesarean delivery is associated with an increased risk of placental abruption in future pregnancies (odds ratio = 1.3).[12] Moreover, multiple previous cesarean deliveries are also associated with an increased risk of placenta previa and, in particular, placenta previa associated with morbid adherence of the placenta. The overall incidence of placenta previa is 0.3%.[13] Compared with women who had no previous cesarean deliveries, the odds ratio for placenta previa in relation to number of previous cesarean deliveries is 1.2 for one procedure, 2.6 for two procedures, and 3.6 for three or more previous cesarean deliveries.[14] Combining these data, there appears to be an absolute risk of placenta previa of 0.5% to 1% among women with repeated cesarean deliveries. Morbid adherence of the placenta, placenta accreta, or percreta, is a rarer and still more serious complication of placentation associated with anterior placenta previa among women with a previous cesarean delivery. The overall incidence of severe placenta accreta (defined as resulting in death, hysterectomy, blood transfusion, coagulopathy, or being associated with placenta percreta) was estimated as 0.05%, and the odds ratio for women with repeated cesarean deliveries is 3.3.[15] Although the absolute risk of this event in future pregnancies is low, in the region of 1 in 1000, clearly the consequences can be severe.

Multiple cesarean deliveries could, theoretically, also affect surgical procedures outside pregnancy, for example, by increasing the likelihood of bladder trauma at the time of hysterectomy. A history of multiple previous cesarean deliveries is quoted as a relative contraindication to vaginal hysterectomy. However, recent studies do not suggest either increased rates of complications overall or a trend of increasing risk of complications with the number of previous cesarean deliveries.[16,17]

Fetal/Neonatal Risks

Short Term

Both PRCD and VBAC carry risks for the offspring. The major risk of PRCD for the neonate is the possibility of neonatal respiratory morbidity, specifically, respiratory distress syndrome, transient tachypnea of the newborn, and primary pulmonary hypertension.[18] The incidence of composite respiratory morbidity at term following vaginal delivery is 0.5%, for emergency cesarean delivery 1.2%, and for planned cesarean delivery before labor 3.5%.[19] Persistent pulmonary hypertension is the most serious of these problems. It is estimated to affect 0.4% of neonates delivered by planned cesarean section, an incidence four to five times greater than among infants delivered vaginally.[18]

The potential adverse effects of VBAC on the neonate relate both to specific issues of uterine rupture and emergency cesarean delivery but also to general adverse associations of vaginal birth. An analysis of a cohort of infants born at term to women with a previous cesarean delivery described increased rates of suspected and proven sepsis among infants delivered following attempted VBAC compared with PRCD (1% vs. 0.1%, respectively for proven sepsis), primarily due to increased rates among those who ended up having an emergency cesarean delivery.[20] The net effect of reduced respiratory morbidity and increased sepsis following VBAC compared with PRCD may favor the former since the risk of admission to special care is lower among infants delivered following attempted VBAC than PRCD (4.6% vs. 7%, respectively).[9] However, the caveat must be applied, as in all cases where VBAC is associated with lower risks, that women attempting VBAC are likely to be a "healthy cohort" due to selection bias. For instance, macrosomic offspring of diabetic women with a previous cesarean delivery will almost inevitably have PRCD, and these infants are at very high risk of neonatal complications.

Planned cesarean delivery clearly has some protective effect on the fetus by avoiding the stress of labor and the potential for trauma during vaginal delivery. Planned cesarean delivery is associated with the lowest rates in the offspring of intracranial hemorrhage[21] and hypoxic ischemic encephalopathy (HIE).[22] The overall net effect on serious but rare complications in the offspring is difficult to assess since relatively detailed information is required. Generally, the studies that are large and robust enough to detect differences in rare outcomes lack detailed information for adequate analysis. Death in the neonatal period can be used as a composite measure of severe neonatal complications. A meta-analysis of observational studies demonstrated an increased risk of perinatal death among the offspring of women attempting VBAC compared with PRCD. The absolute risks quoted were 0.6% and 0.3%, respectively, and the odds ratio for death in the VBAC group was 1.7 (1.3–2.3).[8] However, the meta-analysis was dominated by a single study from Switzerland that made up 75% of the patients analyzed. The Swiss study included deaths from 28 weeks onward, and the vast majority of the deaths included in this study would not be causally related to the mode of delivery.[9] A population-based retrospective cohort study in Scotland addressed this issue by linking national databases of perinatal death data and maternity data. Using this approach, it was possible to identify perinatal deaths occurring at term among women with previous cesarean births and compare the absolute and relative risks of these events in relation to mode of delivery. Among women attempting VBAC, the rate of intrapartum stillbirth was 0.05%, and the rate of neonatal death was 0.08%. In comparison, women delivered by PRCD had no risk of intrapartum stillbirth, and the rate of neonatal death was 0.01%, which was significantly lower than among women attempting VBAC.[4] The absolute risks of death were similar when the analysis was confined to births at or after 40 weeks' gestation. The relative risk of perinatal death unrelated to congenital abnormality for attempted VBAC with reference to PRCD was approximately 12. However, the absolute risk of perinatal death among women attempting VBAC was very similar to nulliparous women. The overall rate of delivery-related perinatal death associated with VBAC at term was 0.13%: one third were due to uterine rupture, one third were due to other causes of intrapartum asphyxia, and one third were due to nonasphyxial causes. The single death among over 9000 PRCDs at term was attributed to maternal disease.[4] This analysis suggests that the balance of serious but rare complications favors planned repeat cesarean section. It might be argued that PRCD may have carried additional serious neonatal respiratory morbidity. However, it seems reasonable to speculate that sublethal serious morbidity might also favor PRCD. Although there may have been an excess of severe respiratory problems among the PRCD group that did not result in death, it is equally likely that, as in previous studies,[21,22] serious morbidity such as intracranial hemorrhage and HIE were less common in the PRCD group.

Whereas the analysis of the risks and benefits of cesarean delivery has tended to focus on delivery-related events, the major cause of perinatal death overall is stillbirth prior to the onset of labor. The risk of this event increases with advancing gestational age, and the cumulative risk of unexplained stillbirth is the major determinant of perinatal loss associated with continuing pregnancy beyond the 39th week.[23] Among 15,000 women delivered at term by a means other than PRCD, there were 20 delivery-related perinatal deaths. Among the same group there were 35 stillbirths in which death of the fetus occurred before the onset of labor, and 20 of these occurred at or after the 39th week and could potentially have been prevented by PRCD.[4] Recent analyses indicate that among all women having a second birth, a previous cesarean delivery is associated with a two- to threefold increased risk of unexplained stillbirth compared with women whose first birth was vaginal and that this is independent of the indication for the first cesarean delivery or maternal characteristics.[24] This demonstrates that an additional potential benefit of PRCD may be to reduce the risk of antepartum stillbirth. The absolute risk of this event is, however, relatively low at approximately 1 per 1000.

Long Term

There is some evidence that obstetric complications can affect a number of aspects of health in later life. Recent studies have demonstrated that children delivered by cesarean section have an increased risk of hospital admission for asthma in childhood, with odds ratios in the region of 1.2 to 1.3 compared with vaginal birth.[25,26] It has been hypothesized that this may be explained by effects of mode of delivery on the gut and susceptibility to atopy. However, cesarean delivery is a well-recognized cause of neonatal respiratory morbidity at term, specifically, transient tachypnea of the newborn and respiratory distress syndrome.[19,27] A number of previous studies have demonstrated that neonatal respiratory morbidity secondary to preterm delivery is associated with an increased risk of later asthma.[28–31] It is likely that the association with later asthma is a long-term consequence of neonatal respiratory morbidity.[32]

The reduced risk of HIE among infants delivered by planned cesarean delivery suggests that these children may be at reduced risk of developing cerebral palsy in later life. However, an adequate analysis of this issue has not been published. A meta-analysis of observational studies has demonstrated that "complicated" cesarean delivery is associated with a 10-fold excess risk of early-onset schizophrenia in later life.[33] Although this issue is still unclear and is likely to remain unclear for many years, the possible lifelong effects of both cesarean delivery and traumatic birth should be considered and should be an area of active research.

FACTORS AFFECTING THE BALANCE OF RISKS AND BENEFITS

Likelihood of Success of VBAC

One of the key features in deciding between PRCD and attempted VBAC is the background risk of emergency cesarean section associated with VBAC. The choice is not between PRCD and certain vaginal delivery. Rather, it is the choice between planned cesarean delivery and attempting vaginal birth with the possibility of emergency cesarean delivery.

Large-scale European population-based studies have demonstrated successful VBAC rates of approximately 75%.[4,9] A number of factors associated with increased or decreased chance of success have been identified. The indication for the first cesarean delivery gives some predictive information regarding the probability of successful VBAC. Women whose first cesarean section was for failure to progress had an increased proportion of emergency cesarean deliveries (37%) during attempted VBAC, whereas those delivered for breech presentation in their first pregnancy had a lower rate of emergency cesarean delivery (14%), which was comparable to nulliparous women.[34] Women with no previous successful vaginal birth are at five to seven times greater risk of requiring emergency cesarean delivery compared with those who have had a previous vaginal birth.[35] A history of gestational diabetes is also associated with a significantly higher risk of emergency cesarean section during VBAC compared with controls (36% vs. 23%, respectively).[36]

A number of factors during labor and delivery are also predictive of the risk of emergency cesarean delivery. The risk of cesarean delivery increases with increasing birth weight of the neonate.[37,38] This post hoc knowledge has little practical use at present due to the inherent inaccuracy of ultrasonic prediction of birth weight.[39] Further studies are required that relate the ultrasound estimated fetal weight to the risk of cesarean delivery to determine whether this association might have some clinical application in risk assessment in the future. Slow progress during labor is also associated with increased rates of cesarean delivery as demonstrated by associations with limited cervical dilation on admission (odds ratio 1.9)[35] and the need for augmentation of labor (odds ratio 2.2).[35]

As the previous discussion indicates, a number of factors are associated with an increased risk of emergency cesarean delivery during VBAC. However, counseling about the risk of VBAC is, at best, semiquantitative. An effective statistical method is required to give women individual assessments of risk. Risk scoring is widely used elsewhere in medicine, such as in the intensive care unit and for cardiac surgery. The relevance of this to VBAC would be at several levels. First, PRCD and VBAC are thought to be economically equivalent when the rate of emergency cesarean delivery is 25% to 30%.[40] Second, the benefits of VBAC are related to avoiding cesarean delivery. For women at high risk of emergency cesarean delivery, the main advantage is lost. Moreover, due to the higher directly attributable adverse effects of emergency cesarean delivery, PRCD is likely to be associated with lower rates of maternal complications, such as febrile morbidity and blood transfusion, when the background risk of emergency cesarean delivery is high.

Factors Determining Risk of Uterine Rupture

Clearly one of the major issues when considering VBAC is the probability of uterine rupture. This outcome is significant as it can affect the health of the child and mother and may determine complications in future pregnancies. This has led to a number of studies that have attempted to address the factors predicting uterine rupture.

Previous classical cesarean section is associated with a much greater risk of antepartum and intrapartum uterine rupture and is an indication for planned cesarean delivery at 36 to 37 weeks' gestation. In contrast, previous vertical lower uterine segment cesarean delivery does not appear to be associated with an increased risk of uterine rupture compared with a low transverse incision,[41] although this analysis is based on reported data for fewer than 400 women with such incisions. Single-layer closure of a low transverse incision was associated with a four- to fivefold risk of uterine rupture after adjustment in multivariate analysis for a number of maternal and demographic factors.[42]

A number of studies have demonstrated that the risk of rupture varies inversely with the interval between the previous cesarean delivery and the next pregnancy.[42-45] Increased birth weight is also associated with an increased risk of rupture,[37] but again the clinical utility of this association in risk scoring is limited due to the inaccuracy of antenatal estimation of fetal weight.

Reports of increased risk of uterine rupture associated with prostaglandins (rate 2.4% compared with 0.5–0.7% for other women in labor)[3,46] has led the ACOG (American College of Obstetrics and Gynecology) to discourage the use of prostaglandin when inducing labor among women attempting VBAC.[47] In contrast, the risk of uterine rupture is not increased when labor is induced with oxytocin when compared with women in spontaneous labor.[3] The overall absolute risk of uterine rupture was 0.2% among women with a previous vaginal birth, which was fivefold lower than among women with no previous vaginal birth. The apparent protective effect was observed whether the vaginal births were before or after the cesarean delivery.[48]

Influence of Future Reproductive Intentions

Perhaps one of the key issues when deciding about mode of delivery in women with one previous cesarean section is the individual's intentions regarding further pregnancies. The natural focus when making decisions regarding VBAC and PRCD is the possibility of serious adverse consequences in the current pregnancy. Although VBAC is associated with lower rates of non-life-threatening complications, the potential for catastrophic uterine rupture raises the possibility that PRCD may be associated with lower risks of severe maternal morbidity and mortality. Consistent with this, there is a trend toward lower maternal mortality in the PRCD group, as discussed earlier. This argument would not hold, however, when the mother is planning many future births. Logically, one could not support a decision to have a PRCD after a first cesarean and then attempt vaginal birth after a second cesarean. Women who elect for PRCD and are planning future pregnancies must consider the additional future risks associated with multiple previous cesarean deliveries. In the context of complications likely to lead to severe maternal morbidity or death, the major factor is placenta previa with accreta or percreta. It is currently very difficult to assess the balance of the risk of severe morbidity and mortality of uterine rupture during VBAC and of complications of abnormal placentation in future pregnancies. These questions will only be addressed by high-quality observational studies using detailed and large-scale databases, probably involving record linkage to maternal death inquiry data and obstetric data. However, it seems currently plausible that the balance of risks and benefits of VBAC favors attempted vaginal birth among women who desire to have many future pregnancies. [Editor's note: Although it should also be borne in mind that the techniques for cesarean section have improved steadily in recent years and will presumably continue to improve. In particular, imaging techniques for the detection of placenta accreta are improving rapidly, and surgical techniques are being devised to improve the safety of dealing with such cases (including approaches such as selective embolization and leaving the placenta in situ with the subsequent use of methotrexate—see Chapter 77)].

SUMMARY OF MANGEMENT OPTIONS

Delivery After Cesarean Section Decisions Regarding Mode of Delivery

Management Options	Quality of Evidence	Strength of Recommendation	References
The evidence that forms the basis of informed discussion of VBAC vs PRCD is based on observational studies only with the potential for bias			
Overall, women attempting VBAC have 50% greater morbidity although this depends on the background risk of failure	III	B	58
Absolute risk of maternal morbidity:	III	B	58
Highest with failed VBAC—14.1%			
Intermediate with PRCD—3.6%			
Lowest with successful VBAC—2.4%			
No validated predictive tool for assessing risk of failed VBAC	III	B	59
The major risks of VBAC are:			
Uterine rupture risk is 5.2 per 1000 VBAC compared with 1.6 per 1000 PRCD; can be catastrophic, leading to perinatal death (1 per 2000) and very rarely maternal death (<1 in 10,000)	III	B	3,8,9,60
General risks associated with vaginal birth, such as intrapartum asphyxia and perineal trauma			
Likelihood of perinatal death higher in low throughput obstetric units	III	B	57
Other risks of VBAC are:			
Urinary incontinence in later life (approximately 5% higher incidence)	III	B	10
Neonatal sepsis, intracerebral hemorrhage, HIE	III	B	20–22
The major risks of PRCD are:			
Short-term maternal complications (febrile, blood transfusion, hysterectomy, thromboembolism)	III	B	8,9
Neonatal respiratory morbidity, which can be severe (respiratory distress OR = 7.0; pulmonary hypertension OR = 4–5)	III	B	18
Rare but serious complications in future pregnancies relating to morbid placental implantation (placental abruption OR = 1.3; placenta previa OR ~3.0; morbid adherence OR = 3.3)	III	B	12,14,15
Other risks of PRCD are:			
Childhood asthma (OR = 1.3)	III	B	25

Continued

SUMMARY OF MANGEMENT OPTIONS

Delivery After Cesarean Section
Decisions Regarding Mode of Delivery *(Continued)*

Management Options	Quality of Evidence	Strength of Recommendation	References
Successful VBAC more likely with:			
Breech or fetal distress as indication for original CS (rather than poor progress)	III	B	34
Previous vaginal delivery (5–7 times more successful)	III	B	35
No diabetes	III	B	36
Lower birth weight	III	B	37,38
Normal progress in labor	III	B	35
Uterine rupture more likely with:			
Previous classical CS	III	B	41
No previous vaginal birth	III	B	48
Single layer closure	III	B	42
Shorter interpregnancy interval	III	B	42–45
Higher birth weight	III	B	37
Induction of labor with prostaglandin, relative risk = 4.7	III	B	3,55
Cost effectiveness of VBAC vs. PRCD is equivalent if emergency CS rate = 25–30%	III	B	40
The decision to attempt VBAC is complex, requires careful counseling and should take into consideration:	–	GPP	–
Maternal preferences and priorities including motivation to achieve a vaginal birth			
Importance placed on rare but serious adverse outcomes (see above)			
Presence of factors that influence likelihood of successful VBAC vs uterine rupture (see above)			
Plans for future pregnancies			

CS, cesarean section; HIE, hypoxic ischemic encephalopathy; OR, odds ratio; PRCD, planned repeat cesarean delivery; VBAC, vaginal birth after cesarean.

MANAGEMENT OF WOMEN ATTEMPTING VBAC

The management of labor in a woman attempting VBAC cannot be based on RCT evidence, since the trials have not been conducted (and almost certainly never will be) that are sufficiently robust to determine the effects of management on the risk of rare events, such as perinatal death at term. Management must be guided, therefore, on the basis of understanding the risks of VBAC. Given the small but finite risks involved, a conservative approach is justified. Rejection of caution in this context on the basis that "there is no evidence that demonstrates X is useful" is not justified when the issue is lack of evidence rather than convincing data that indicate no benefit.

Given that the absolute risk of uterine rupture is in the region of 1 in 100 to 1 in 200 and that it can result in rapid fetal demise and life-threatening maternal hemorrhage, it seems self-evident that VBAC should be attempted only in units with immediate access to facilities for the management of uterine rupture. This will usually require resident obstetric, anesthetic, and neonatology services with access to hematology and other support services. Uterine rupture is classically diagnosed by pain, vaginal bleeding, maternal hypotension, or collapse. However, the earliest warning sign may be an abnormal fetal heart rate pattern. Given this, and the risk of intrapartum asphyxia due both to the rupture and other events, a recommendation for continuous electronic fetal monitoring is mandatory. A small proportion of women will be requesting VBAC because they want "natural childbirth," and they may refuse continuous electronic fetal monitoring. In such cases, it is essential on both ethical and medicolegal grounds that appropriate attempts are made to persuade the woman to accept continuous monitoring, and these attempts should be fully documented, together with the names of witnesses to the discussion. It is quite often possible to persuade many of these women to accept almost continuous fetal monitoring using a handheld Doppler ultrasound fetal heart detector, and if fetal heart rate decelerations are clearly audible, most women will then accept continuous monitoring. Concerns that the symptoms of uterine rupture might be masked by epidural anesthesia have not been sustained and use of epidural analgesia is appropriate when attempting VBAC.[49] The use of intrauterine pressure catheters was previously widespread, but this is no longer the case as they do not appear to indicate reliably the event of a uterine rupture and may, therefore, be falsely reassuring.[50] Oxytocin as a means of inducing labor does not appear to be associated with an increased risk of uterine rupture compared with women in spontaneous labor.[3] However, oxytocin should be used extremely cautiously to augment the progress of women in labor. It should only be used when uterine activity is clearly inadequate, and great care should be taken to avoid uterine hyperstimulation. In women who are obese, or very restless, it is often difficult to assess uterine contractions adequately by external palpation and there may be a specific case for the use of intrauterine pressure catheters to measure uterine activity in these circumstances. Regular cervical examinations should be performed in all cases and there should be a low threshold for emergency cesarean delivery when cervical dilation is inadequate in the presence of normal uterine activity. Postpartum examination of the uterine scar at the time of vaginal examination is no longer recommended since cases where surgical repair is required are almost invariably symptomatic.[51]

VBAC in "Special" Situations

The classic determinants of eligibility for VBAC are that a woman has had a single previous cesarean section through a low transverse uterine incision for a nonrecurrent indication and that she has a singleton infant in a longitudinal lie and cephalic presentation in her present pregnancy with no other contraindication for vaginal birth. A number of studies have examined the risks and benefits of VBAC in other situations. For instance, a number of studies have reported that no excess risks are associated with VBAC among women with twins.[52-54] However, none of these included more than 100 pregnancies. In order to exclude a 1% incidence of an adverse event with conventionally accepted levels of statistical certainty, a trial would have to examine the outcome of approximately 350 cases and see no events. Clearly, if a single event was observed, the finding would be consistent with a true incidence of less than 1%, but then even greater numbers would be required to define the limits of the estimated risk.

Other examples of special situations include suspected fetal macrosomia, multiple previous cesarean deliveries, and induction of labor with an unfavorable cervix. These and other indications regarded as "special" are usually referred to in these terms due to an increased risk of uterine rupture and, often, an increased risk of emergency cesarean section. As discussed earlier, there are multiple risk factors for uterine rupture, such as single-layer closure, a short interval between the previous cesarean delivery and the next pregnancy, macrosomia, prostaglandin induction, and no previous vaginal birth. Some combinations of these events have been shown to be associated with high absolute risks of uterine rupture. For example, a short interpregnancy interval and a previous single-layer closure is associated with a 5% to 6% risk of uterine rupture during a future VBAC attempt.[42] This is much higher than the absolute risk associated with prostaglandin induction.[3] Nevertheless, prostaglandin induction is now discouraged by the ACOG.[47] However, statements that VBAC is or is not recommended in the presence of a single risk factor are potentially misleading. For instance, if the fivefold reduction in risk associated with a previous vaginal birth is correct[48] and there is no interaction between parity and use of prostaglandin, then women with a previous vaginal birth being induced with prostaglandin would have a risk of uterine rupture of less than 1%.

It is, therefore, currently impossible to address fully the risks of VBAC in association with different maternal characteristics to provide women with an individualized risk of uterine rupture and probability of successful vaginal birth. Ideally, one could take the prior odds of such outcomes and obtain a best estimate of these risks on the basis of the key maternal and obstetric characteristics. At present the best approach is to assess the presence of single or multiple risk factors for uterine rupture and emergency cesarean delivery and discuss these with each individual woman. When assessing evidence, a clear distinction must be made between lack of adequate evidence and adequately powered studies that find no increase in risk. Attempting VBAC in twin pregnancy falls into the former category.

RECENT STUDIES

A number of areas discussed above have recently been addressed. First, a study has been reported where the outcome studied was uterine rupture leading to death of the infant.[57] This confirmed that prostaglandin induction and no previous vaginal birth were associated with an increased risk of catastrophic rupture and that the previously described associations could not be explained by ascertainment bias. This study did not demonstrate an association between the use of oxytocin to induce labor and the risk of uterine rupture. The study also demonstrated that if a uterine rupture occurred, it was approximately three times more likely to result in death of the infant in a low throughput hospital. This was thought to reflect the fact that high throughput hospitals are more likely to have the facilities available for immediate delivery and resuscitation of the infant (resident experienced obstetric, anaesthetic, and pediatric staff; a dedicated obstetric operating room; and a neonatal intensive care unit). This study provides empirical data to support the proposition that attempted VBAC should only take place in units with these facilities.

Second, a large scale, multi-center prospective cohort study of approximately 18,000 VBAC attempts and 16,000 PRCD was reported at the end of 2004.[58] This is the only large scale prospective study of VBAC to be reported. Significant maternal morbidity was, overall, approximately 50% more common among women attempting VBAC. However, the best outcomes, as previously described, were to women who attempted VBAC and were successful. The absolute risk of one or more serious maternal complications was 14.1% among women attempting VBAC and failing, 3.6% among women having a planned repeat cesarean delivery and 2.4% among women who had a successful attempt at VBAC. There were only two perinatal deaths (both neonatal) attributed to uterine rupture among the offspring of women attempting VBAC and this likely reflects the fact the study was confined to high throughput centers. There was a 1 in 2000 risk of hypoxic ischemic encephalopathy among women attempting VBAC and no such events among women having a PRCD.

The foregoing underlines the importance of the background risk of cesarean delivery on the risks and benefits of attempting VBAC. A meta-analysis of observational studies of scoring systems for predicting the risk of cesarean section demonstrated that there were only two validated methods for predicting the risk of cesarean section and both utilized data that would only be available during the intrapartum period.[59] They stated that "conducting high-quality research on the factors that delineate women who are at higher likelihood of vaginal delivery without complications and developing accurate user-friendly screening tools to integrate these data should be a national research priority."

Finally, a recent large scale retrospective analysis of Canadian data allowed some estimates of the absolute risk of maternal death.[60] They estimated a 1–2 per 100,000 risk of death associated with an attempt at VBAC. The risk of death was 5–6 per 100,000 among women having a PRCD, after excluding complex cases such as placenta previa. However, they did not have information on the number of previous cesarean deliveries and were unable to adjust for key maternal characteristics other than age. Therefore, the apparent increased risk of death among women having PRCD needs to be interpreted with caution.

FUTURE PRIORITIES FOR RESEARCH

A simple and pragmatic method for quantifying the risk of emergency cesarean delivery and uterine rupture during attempted VBAC in relation to combinations of maternal characteristics would help decision-making considerably. Currently, there is no practical method for giving a woman an individualized risk of adverse events during attempted VBAC. Ideally, some of the key issues discussed above would be resolved by a large scale randomized controlled trial. The problems with this ideal are that it would have to be very large and allow long term follow-up and a truly informative trial is unlikely to be a practical proposition.

SUMMARY OF MANAGEMENT OPTIONS
Conduct of Trial of Labor

Management Options	Quality of Evidence	Strength of Recommendation	References
Attempt at VBAC should only be conducted in a setting with resident obstetric/anesthetic/neonatal staff and access to full laboratory support.	III	B	57
The issue of intravenous access and crossmatching of blood are controversial.	–	GPP	–
Conduct critical review of progress of labor.	–	GPP	–
Judicious use of oxytocin is acceptable but should be discontinued if response to uterine stimulation does not occur promptly, and vigilance for uterine hyperstimulation should be maintained.	III	B	57
Continuously monitor fetal heart rate.	III	B	56
Routine insertion of intrauterine pressure catheter is of no proven benefit and may be falsely reassuring.	III	B	50
Regional anesthesia is not contraindicated.	IV	C	49
Digital palpation/examination of scar is not indicated.	III	B	51

VBAC, vaginal birth after cesarean.

CONCLUSIONS

The evidence informing decisions between PRCD and VBAC is based entirely on observational data and, therefore, open to biased interpretation.

The major risks of VBAC are:

- uterine rupture (overall approximately 0.4–0.5%), which can be catastrophic, leading to perinatal death in about 1 per 2000 and very rarely leading to maternal death (<1 in 10,000)
- general risks associated with vaginal birth, such as intrapartum asphyxia and birth trauma
- an increased risk of perioperative morbidity among those women requiring emergency cesarean delivery

The major risks of PRCD are:

- an increased risk of mild to moderate short-term complications in the mother
- an increased risk of respiratory morbidity in the neonate, which can be severe
- an increased risk of rare but serious complications in future pregnancies relating to morbid placental implantation

The balance of risks and benefits depends on the background risk of emergency cesarean delivery if VBAC is attempted, which itself depends on:

- whether the mother has had previous vaginal births
- the indication for the first cesarean delivery
- whether the onset of labor in the current pregnancy will be induced or spontaneous
- progress in early labor

The decision to attempt VBAC is complex, requires careful counseling, and will depend on:

- the mother's motivation to achieve a vaginal birth
- plans for future pregnancies
- the importance placed on rare but serious adverse outcomes

REFERENCE

1. Menacker F, Curtin SC: Trends in caesarean birth and vaginal birth after previous caesarean, 1991–99. Natl Vital Stat Rep 2001;49:1–16.
2. McMahon MJ, Luther ER, Bowes WA Jr, Olshan AF: Comparison of a trial of labor with an elective second caesarean section. N Engl J Med 1996;335:689–695.
3. Lydon-Rochelle M, Holt VL, Easterling TR, Martin DP: Risk of uterine rupture during labor among women with a prior caesarean delivery. N Engl J Med 2001;345:3–8.
4. Smith GCS, Pell JP, Cameron AD, Dobbie R: Risk of perinatal death associated with delivery after previous caesarean section. JAMA 2002;287:2684–2690.
5. Phelan JP, Ahn MO, Diaz F, et al: Twice a caesarean, always a caesarean? Obstet Gynecol 1989;73:161–165.
6. Lilford RJ, van Coeverden de Groot HA, Moore PJ, Bingham P: The relative risks of caesarean section (intrapartum and elective) and vaginal delivery: A detailed analysis to exclude the effects of medical disorders and other acute pre-existing physiological disturbances. BJOG 1990;97:883–892.
7. Hannah ME, Hannah WJ, Hewson SA, et al: Planned caesarean section versus planned vaginal birth for breech presentation at term: A randomised multicentre trial. Term Breech Trial Collaborative Group. Lancet 2000;356:1375–1383.
8. Mozurkewich EL, Hutton EK: Elective repeat caesarean delivery versus trial of labor: A meta-analysis of the literature from 1989 to 1999. Am J Obstet Gynecol 2000;183:1187–1197.
9. Rageth JC, Juzi C, Grossenbacher H: Delivery after previous caesarean: A risk evaluation. Swiss Working Group of Obstetric and Gynecologic Institutions. Obstet Gynecol 1999;93:332–337.
10. Rortveit G, Daltveit AK, Hannestad YS, Hunskaar S: Urinary incontinence after vaginal delivery or caesarean section. N Engl J Med 2003;348:900–907.
11. Murphy DJ, Stirrat GM, Heron J: The relationship between caesarean section and subfertility in a population-based sample of 14, 541 pregnancies. Hum Reprod 2002;17:1914–1917.
12. Lydon-Rochelle M, Holt VL, Easterling TR, Martin DP: First-birth caesarean and placental abruption or previa at second birth. Obstet Gynecol 2001;97:765–769.
13. Clark SL, Koonings PP, Phelan JP: Placenta previa/accreta and prior caesarean section. Obstet Gynecol 1985;66:89–92.
14. Gilliam M, Rosenberg D, Davis F: The likelihood of placenta previa with greater number of caesarean deliveries and higher parity. Obstet Gynecol 2002;99:976–980.
15. Gielchinsky Y, Rojansky N, Fasouliotis SJ, Ezra Y: Placenta accreta—summary of 10 years: A survey of 310 cases. Placenta 2002;23:210–214.
16. Unger JB, Meeks GR: Vaginal hysterectomy in women with history of previous caesarean delivery. Am J Obstet Gynecol 1998;179:1473–1478.
17. Poindexter YM, Sangi-Haghpeykar H, Poindexter AN, et al: Previous caesarean section: A contraindication to vaginal hysterectomy? J Reprod Med 2001;46:840–844.

18. Levine EM, Ghai V, Barton JJ, Strom CM: Mode of delivery and risk of respiratory diseases in newborns. Obstet Gynecol 2001;97:439–442.
19. Morrison JJ, Rennie JM, Milton PJ: Neonatal respiratory morbidity and mode of delivery at term: Influence of timing of elective caesarean section. BJOG 1995;102:101–106.
20. Hook B, Kiwi R, Amini SB, et al: Neonatal morbidity after elective repeat caesarean section and trial of labor. Pediatrics 1997;100:348–353.
21. Towner D, Castro MA, Eby-Wilkens E, Gilbert WM: Effect of mode of delivery in nulliparous women on neonatal intracranial injury. N Engl J Med 1999;341:1709–1714.
22. Badawi N, Kurinczuk JJ, Keogh JM, et al: Intrapartum risk factors for newborn encephalopathy: The Western Australian case-control study. BMJ 1998;317:1554–1558.
23. Smith GC: Life-table analysis of the risk of perinatal death at term and post term in singleton pregnancies. Am J Obstet Gynecol 2001;184:489–496.
24. Smith GCS, Pell JP, Dobbie R: Caesarean section and the risk of unexplained stillbirth in subsequent pregnancy. Lancet 2003;In press.
25. Xu B, Pekkanen J, Jarvelin MR: Obstetric complications and asthma in childhood. J Asthma 2000;37:589–594.
26. Kero J, Gissler M, Gronlund MM, et al: Mode of delivery and asthma—Is there a connection? Pediatr Res 2002;52:6–11.
27. Dani C, Reali MF, Bertini G, et al: Risk factors for the development of respiratory distress syndrome and transient tachypnoea in newborn infants. Italian Group of Neonatal Pneumology. Eur Respir J 1999;14:155–159.
28. Bertrand JM, Riley SP, Popkin J, Coates AL: The long-term pulmonary sequelae of prematurity: The role of familial airway hyperreactivity and the respiratory distress syndrome. N Engl J Med 1985;312:742–745.
29. Pelkonen AS, Hakulinen AL, Turpeinen M: Bronchial lability and responsiveness in school children born very preterm. Am J Respir Crit Care Med 1997;156:1178–1184.
30. Evans M, Palta M, Sadek M, et al: Associations between family history of asthma, bronchopulmonary dysplasia, and childhood asthma in very low birth weight children. Am J Epidemiol 1998;148:460–466.
31. Ng DK, Lau WY, Lee SL: Pulmonary sequelae in long-term survivors of bronchopulmonary dysplasia. Pediatr Int 2000;42:603–607.
32. Smith GCS, Wood AM, White IR, et al: Neonatal respiratory morbidity at term and the risk of childhood asthma. Arch Dis Child 2005;89:956–960.
33. Verdoux H, Geddes JR, Takei N, et al: Obstetric complications and age at onset in schizophrenia: An international collaborative meta-analysis of individual patient data. Am J Psychiatry 1997;154:1220–1227.
34. Shipp TD, Zelop CM, Repke JT, et al: Labor after previous caesarean: Influence of prior indication and parity. Obstet Gynecol 2000;95:913–916.
35. Macones GA, Hausman N, Edelstein R, et al: Predicting outcomes of trials of labor in women attempting vaginal birth after caesarean delivery: A comparison of multivariate methods with neural networks. Am J Obstet Gynecol 2001;184:409–413.
36. Coleman TL, Randall H, Graves W, Lindsay M: Vaginal birth after caesarean among women with gestational diabetes. Am J Obstet Gynecol 2001;184:1104–1107.
37. Elkousy MA, Sammel M, Stevens E, et al: The effect of birth weight on vaginal birth after caesarean delivery success rates. Am J Obstet Gynecol 2003;188:824–830.
38. Zelop CM, Shipp TD, Repke JT, et al: Outcomes of trial of labor following previous caesarean delivery among women with fetuses weighing >4000 g. Am J Obstet Gynecol 2001;185:903–905.
39. Smith GCS, Smith M-FS, McNay MB, Fleming J-EE: The relation between fetal abdominal circumference and birthweight: Findings in 3512 pregnancies. BJOG 1997;104:186–190.
40. Clark SL, Scott JR, Porter TF, et al: Is vaginal birth after caesarean less expensive than repeat caesarean delivery? Am J Obstet Gynecol 2000;182:599–602.
41. Shipp TD, Zelop CM, Repke JT, et al: Intrapartum uterine rupture and dehiscence in patients with prior lower uterine segment vertical and transverse incisions. Obstet Gynecol 1999;94:735–740.
42. Bujold E, Mehta SH, Bujold C, Gauthier RJ: Interdelivery interval and uterine rupture. Am J Obstet Gynecol 2002;187:1199–1202.
43. Huang WH, Nakashima DK, Rumney PJ, et al: Interdelivery interval and the success of vaginal birth after caesarean delivery. Obstet Gynecol 2002;99:41–44.
44. Shipp TD, Zelop CM, Repke JT, et al: Interdelivery interval and risk of symptomatic uterine rupture. Obstet Gynecol 2001;97:175–177.
45. Esposito MA, Menihan CA, Malee MP: Association of interpregnancy interval with uterine scar failure in labor: A case-control study. Am J Obstet Gynecol 2000;183:1180–1183.
46. Taylor DR, Doughty AS, Kaufman H, et al: Uterine rupture with the use of PGE2 vaginal inserts for labor induction in women with previous caesarean sections. J Reprod Med 2002;47: 549–554.
47. ACOG Committee opinion. Induction of labor for vaginal birth after caesarean delivery. Obstet Gynecol 2002;99:679–680.
48. Zelop CM, Shipp TD, Repke JT, et al: Effect of previous vaginal delivery on the risk of uterine rupture during a subsequent trial of labor. Am J Obstet Gynecol 2000;183:1184–1186.
49. Flamm BL: Vaginal birth after caesarean (VBAC). Best Pract Res Clin Obstet Gynaecol 2001;15:81–92.
50. Beckley S, Gee H, Newton JR: Scar rupture in labour after previous lower uterine segment caesarean section: The role of uterine activity measurement. BJOG 1991;98: 265–269.
51. Silberstein T, Wiznitzer A, Katz M, et al: Routine revision of uterine scar after caesarean section: Has it ever been necessary? Eur J Obstet Gynecol Reprod Biol 1998;78:29–32.
52. Sansregret A, Bujold E, Gauthier RJ: Twin delivery after a previous caesarean: A twelve-year experience. J Obstet Gynaecol Can 2003;25:294–298.
53. Odeh M, Tarazova L, Wolfson M, Oettinger M: Evidence that women with a history of caesarean section can deliver twins safely. Acta Obstet Gynecol Scand 1997;76:663–666.
54. Myles T: Vaginal birth of twins after a previous caesarean section. J Matern Fetal Med 2001;10:171–174.
55. RCOG Clinical Effectiveness Support Unit: Induction of labour. Evidence based guideline No 9. London, RCOG Press; 2001.
56. RCOG Clinical Effectiveness Support Unit: The use of electronic fetal monitoring. Evidence based clinical guideline number 8. London, RCOG Press; 2001.
57. Smith GCS, Pell JP, Pasupathy D, Dobbie R: Factors predisposing to perinatal death related to uterine rupture during attempted vaginal birth after caesarean section: Retrospective cohort study. BMJ 2004;329:375.
58. Landon MB, Hauth JC, Leveno KJ, et al: Maternal and perinatal outcomes associated with a trial of labor after prior cesarean delivery. N Engl J Med 2004;351:2581–2589.
59. Guise JM, Hashima JN, Eden KB, Osterweil P: Predicting vaginal birth after cesarean delivery: A review of prognostic factors and screening tools. Am J Obstet Gynecol 2004;190:547–555.
60. Wen SW, Rusen ID, Walker M, et al: Comparison of maternal mortality and morbidity between trial of labor and elective cesarean section among women with previous cesarean delivery. Am J Obstet Gynecol 2004;191:1263–1269.

CHAPTER 76

Cesarean Section

Jan E. Dickinson

INTRODUCTION

Of the profound alterations in the practice of obstetrics over the past century, one of the most apparent has been the progressive increase in the frequency of cesarean delivery. Sporadically reported throughout medical history, cesarean birth has only during the last century been technically refined and rendered safe for both mother and fetus. The safety of the lower uterine segment technique, the evolution of anesthetic proficiency, the availability of blood products and antibiotics, the broadening of indications for the operation, the recognition of the fetus as a patient, the feasibility of vaginal delivery following cesarean section, and the acceptance of this procedure by women have characterized the evolution of cesarean birth in the twentieth century. These factors have all contributed to the rise in the incidence of cesarean birth over the past 50 years. The past decade has seen further evolution of cesarean birth as an issue of choice for women as a preferred mode of delivery, producing intense polarization of both medical and lay opinion.[1–7] Additionally, the secondary rise in repeat cesarean delivery has been associated with an increase in severe complications of cesarean birth, particularly complications of placentation.[8,9] Placenta accreta and its subtypes have been reported with increasing frequency in association with repeat cesarean birth.[10,11] Such abnormalities of placentation clearly have great potential to increase maternal morbidity for repeat cesarean birth.

INCIDENCE OF CESAREAN SECTION

During the 1970s and early 1980s, the cesarean delivery rate progressively increased throughout the world, more dramatically in some countries than in others (Fig. 76–1). By the 1990s and beyond, most countries observed a progressive increase in cesarean birth. Women are now four times more likely to have a cesarean birth than 30 years ago.[12] The reasons for this increase in cesarean birth are multifactorial and include the increasing number of women with a prior cesarean delivery, the increase in multifetal gestations, the use of intrapartum electronic fetal monitoring, changes in obstetric training, medicolegal concerns, alterations in parental and societal expectations of pregnancy outcome, and maternal autonomy in decision-making regarding delivery mode.

In 1984, cesarean delivery became the number one in-hospital operative procedure in the United States[13] and accounted for 21% of all live births. By 1988, this figure climbed to 24.7%.[14] Advocacy for vaginal birth after cesarean (VBAC) in the late 1980s and 1990s was probably associated with a lessening of the incidence in the United States; in 1999 the incidence declined to 22%.[15] However increasing concerns for the potential complications of VBAC[16,17] have reduced some of the early enthusiasm for this technique, and the observed decline has been short lived, with the resumption of a progressive increase in the cesarean birth rate. In 2001 the US cesarean delivery rate was 24.4%, the fifth consecutive annual rise, and the VBAC rate fell 20%.[18]

In Europe and the United Kingdom, an increase in cesarean birth has also been evident, but with wide national variation. A recent review of cesarean birth in Norway showed a sharp increase in the cesarean delivery rate, from 2.5% in 1972 to 12.8% in 1987 with a slight rise to 13.6% in 1999.[19] This relatively low rate of cesarean delivery in Nordic countries has not been manifest in other areas of Europe. In 1980 the cesarean delivery rate in England was 9%, increasing to 13% in 1992[20]; a recent audit of rates demonstrated an abrupt rise to 21.3% in 2000.[21] Similar rates have been reported in Italy (22.5% in 1995),[22] with France midway at 17.5% in 1995.[23]

In Australia, there has been a continual increase in the incidence of cesarean birth. In the author's state of Western Australia, rates of cesarean birth have steadily increased, from 15.7% in 1986, to 20.3% in 1995, and to

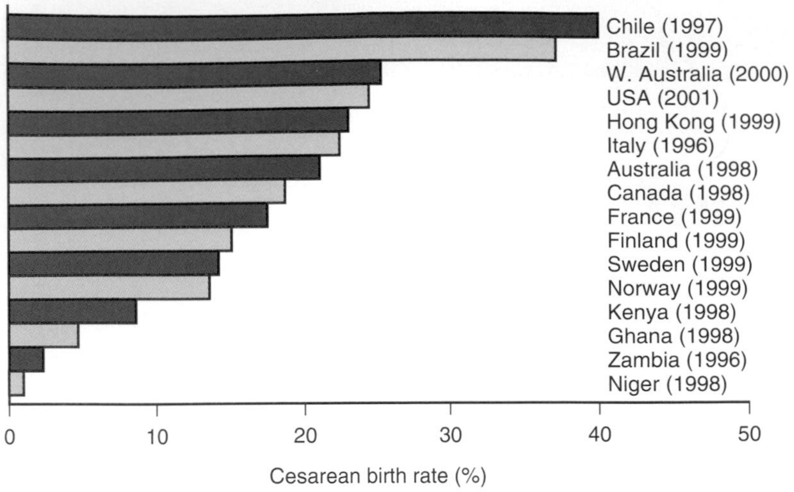

FIGURE 76–1
Contemporary international cesarean delivery rates

25.3% in 2000,[24] with no suggestion of a decline or plateau in the incidence.

Data from South America have consistently demonstrated some of the highest cesarean birth rates internationally.[25] In Chile the incidence of cesarean birth increased from 27.7% in 1986 to 37.2% in 1994.[25] In Brazil a high incidence of cesarean delivery has been present for many years, reaching 50% in some areas.[26] The contrary situation exists in sub-Saharan Africa, where very low cesarean birth rates, generally less than 5%, have been reported for many years. This phenomenon most likely represents inadequate access to medical services in economically depressed countries. High maternal and perinatal mortality rates are typical in many areas of sub-Saharan Africa. In Zambia the cesarean delivery rate was 1.6% in 1996; other countries' rates were similarly low: Ghana, 4.1% (1996); Tanzania, 2.2% (1998); and Kenya, 6.7% (1998).[27]

INDICATIONS FOR CESAREAN SECTION

There are four principal indications for cesarean delivery:

- dystocia (inadequate labor progress)
- suspected fetal compromise
- malpresentation
- prior cesarean birth.

These indications account for more than 70% of cesarean deliveries and are therefore the major determining factors of the cesarean birth rate[28] (Table 76–1). Programs designed to alter cesarean delivery rates have tended to focus on modifying these four primary operative indications (e.g., active management of labor protocols, increasing VBAC rates). Several other issues have been correlated with cesarean birth rates, including hospital type and facilities, individual medical practices, health insurance status, women's childbirth attitudes, and medicolegal influences.

Recently, much attention has been given to maternal requests for cesarean birth in the absence of a traditional obstetric indication. Although there are bipartisan views on this contentious issue, several points need to be addressed. First, it is recognized that women must be involved in the management decisions regarding their pregnancy and birth. Women vary greatly in their birth experience desires, and individualization is central to any delivery mode policy. Second, it is now appreciated that much of the increased mortality previously ascribed to cesarean birth did not discriminate between elective procedures and nonelective procedures. In a low risk woman an elective cesarean section with appropriate perioperative care has an extremely low mortality risk. Third, there is an increasing amount of knowledge and discussion of the long-term effects of vaginal birth on the female pelvic floor and sexual function. Fourth, although the first cesarean delivery may be uncomplicated, subsequent pregnancies are clearly associated with an increased risk of placenta previa and accreta. Finally, within the specialty of obstetrics are several practitioners who believe cesarean birth to be the most appropriate delivery mode and have published their

TABLE 76–1

Indications for Cesarean Section

Previous cesarean section	26.1%
Dystocia	23.0%
Malpresentation	11.7%
Suspected fetal compromise	10.7%
Others	28.5%
Placental disorders	
Multifetal gestations	
Fetal disease	
Maternal medical/physiologic conditions	

Data from Perinatal Statistics in Western Australia, 2000. Eighteenth Annual Report of the Western Australian Midwives' Notification System. Department of Health, Western Australia, July 2002.

views widely, whereas others believe it is a major surgical procedure with attendant risks.[29] The debate will continue; however, it is clear that obstetric paternalism is giving way to patient autonomy. Education and discussion remain the keystones in obstetric care, and continuing audit of outcomes is essential.

ISSUES IN THE OPERATIVE TECHNIQUE OF CESAREAN BIRTH

Cesarean delivery is the most frequent major surgical procedure performed in obstetrics and gynecology. There is, however, wide variation in the surgical techniques used in cesarean birth and the quality of evidence to support the techniques used.[30] Randomized controlled clinical trials are not widely used in the evaluation of surgical procedures, with such therapies usually characterized by observational evidence. The lack of randomized controlled trials of surgical interventions has not gone unnoticed.[31] History, personal prestige, commercial competition, surgical equipoise, inadequate funding and infrastructure, inadequate surgeon education in epi demiology, and the presence of emergency or rare conditions are cited as obstacles to the conduct of randomized clinical trials in surgery.[31] The particular issue of the "learning curve" is problematic in the conduct of the surgical randomized clinical trial, because there will inevitably be a bias in favor of the familiar technique and errors are more likely to occur during the acquisition of skills with a new procedure.

A recent survey of British obstetricians observed a wide range in the techniques for procedures in cesarean delivery.[30] Relative concordance of technique was observed in only a few aspects of cesarean delivery (e.g., double-layer closure of the uterine incision, prophylactic antibiotic use, and Pfannenstiel abdominal entry).[30] There were large variations in the technique of uterine entry, abdominal packing, uterine closure techniques, peritoneal closure, used of subrectus sheath wound drainage, and superficial fat closure. Despite evidence from randomized clinical trials, many obstetricians continued to use practices that have been demonstrated to increase morbidity (e.g., 27.6% performed manual removal of the placenta).

SURGICAL TECHNIQUES IN CESAREAN DELIVERY

The Abdominal Incision for Cesarean Birth

Preparation of the Patient

Preoperative positioning with left lateral tilt will minimize maternal inferior vena caval compression, reducing the risk of hypotension and reductions in placental perfusion. A urinary catheter usually remains in situ perioperatively, draining continuously to a closed system. Suprapubic and abdominal hair should be removed as short a time before the procedure as possible. Skin infections may occur if shaving is performed remote from the surgery, due to the occurrence of grazes during shaving, and may increase the incidence of wound infections. An antiseptic solution, usually povidone-iodine, is applied to the skin. Iodophor-impregnated adhesive films have been assessed in a small clinical trial,[32] and although they did not appear to alter postoperative wound infection rates, they did reduce the skin preparation time, a consideration in emergency situations. Standard plastic adhesive drapes are no more effective than linen drapes in preventing wound infections and may adversely affect healing if dislodged.[33] They have become popular when coupled with integral gutters to collect the blood and amniotic fluid shed during the operation, reducing contamination, a consideration of particular importance in areas of high hepatitis B and HIV prevalence.

The Choice of Skin Incision

The choice of the abdominal incision and its closure should be individualized to the characteristics of the woman and the circumstances demanding operative intervention. The massively obese multigravida will require a different operative technique than that used on the unscarred abdomen of a thin primigravida. The ideal incision provides prompt surgical access, adequate exposure, and a secure wound closure.

The transverse suprapubic skin incision is the most common technique used for cesarean delivery in the developed world. The Joel-Cohen incision has been proposed as the quickest method of delivering the fetus compared, with the Pfannenstiel, or midline vertical abdominal incision.[34–36] The Pfannenstiel incision is a straight horizontal incision about 2 cm above the pubic symphysis with its mid-portion within the shaved area of the pubis. A Joel-Cohen incision is also a straight horizontal incision, but higher, being about 3 cm below the line joining the anterior and superior iliac spines. It can therefore be rather longer than the Pfannenstiel incision, and it is easier to pull aside the rectus muscles at this level. Three randomized controlled trials have examined abdominal entry techniques.[37–39] The first, published in 1987, used a quasi-randomized study design and compared the Maylard transverse muscle-splitting incision with the Pfannenstiel incision in 97 women.[37] In this small study the time to achieve delivery was longer in the Maylard group (10.4 ± 3.1 minutes vs. 7.6 ± 4.1 minutes, Maylard vs. Pfannenstiel, respectively, $P < 0.05$). There was no significant difference in febrile morbidity (OR, 0.72; 95% CI, 0.22–2.39) or blood loss as estimated by hemoglobin alteration (3.1 ± 0.6 g/L vs. 3.0 ± 0.8 g/L). The Maylard incision was significantly larger than the Pfannenstiel (18.3 ± 4.5 cm vs. 14 ± 2.1 cm), which, although providing an increased surgical field, may have some cosmetic disadvantages in contemporary elective cesarean birth. The size of the abdominal incision was a critical factor in the degree of difficulty of delivery, with a significant negative correlation between perceived delivery difficulty and incision size reported. An abdominal incision size of 15 cm or greater was associated with significantly less difficulty in cesarean delivery.

The second study, available only in abstract form,[38] compared the Pfannenstiel and Joel-Cohen incisions in 268 women. A reduction in operating time (35 vs. 26 minutes) and maternal composite morbidity (16.3% vs. 7%, P <0.05) was reported with the Joel-Cohen technique.

The most recent trial also compared the Pfannenstiel and Joel-Cohen incisions in 310 women with pregnancies beyond 32 weeks' gestation.[39] The total operative time was similar (Pfannenstiel 33 minutes (range, 18–70 minutes) vs. Joel-Cohen 32 minutes (range, 12–60 minutes), although the time taken to deliver the fetus was more rapid with the Joel-Cohen incision (Pfannenstiel, 240 seconds [range, 50–600 sec] vs. Joel-Cohen, 90 seconds [range, 60–600 sec] P = 0.05). There was no significant difference in the incidence of perioperative complications nor infant neurodevelopmental outcome at 6 months. The reduction in fetal extraction time did not appear to have a clear maternal-fetal benefit. Additionally, the authors of this study commented that the cosmesis of the Joel-Cohen incision (a component of the technique known in toto as the Misgav Ladach method) was inferior to that for the Pfannenstiel incision.

A vertical skin incision was the original approach to enter the peritoneal cavity, although it now has been usurped by the more cosmetic low transverse incision. The main indications for its use are a previous midline vertical incision, obesity, or uncertain operative diagnosis for example, in trauma to the pregnant abdomen or an intra-abdominal tumor mass. In an observational study in 1976, Haeri[40] reported no significant difference between the two incisions in terms of operating time (53 minutes vs. 45 minutes, transverse vs. vertical incision, respectively), postoperative febrile morbidity (30% vs. 48%), and postcesarean hemoglobin <10 g/dL (28% vs. 36%). There was, however, an increase in the incidence of complete wound breakdown in the vertical skin incision group (0% vs. 7%) and total maternal morbidity (OR, 0.46; 95% CI, 0.25–0.86).

In the massively obese patient, a vertical skin incision with avoidance of the subpanniculus fold may be indicated. The higher wound infection rate in this subpopulation requires modifications of perioperative procedures. Gallup[41] reduced the wound infection rate from 42% to 3% by careful perioperative techniques. If a transverse incision is chosen for the obese patient, it should be away from the subpanniculus fold, and a subcutaneous closure should be used to reduce dead space and subsequent seroma formation.

The Uterine Incision for Cesarean Birth

The clinical situation prompting the need for abdominal delivery determines the uterine incision to deliver the fetus. The low transverse uterine incision is used in over 90% of cesarean deliveries. This high prevalence is due to its ease of repair, reduced adhesion formation, decreased blood loss, and low incidence of dehiscence or rupture in subsequent pregnancies.[42] A previous low transverse uterine incision may render the woman eligible for a trial of labor in a subsequent pregnancy. The disadvantages of the low transverse incision are primarily restricted to situations in which the lower uterine segment is undeveloped. In this circumstance there is a greater chance of lateral extension into the major uterine vessels, resulting in maternal morbidity from hemorrhage. If the initial incision is inadequate to deliver the fetus, extension of the uterine incision to a J or a U or an inverted T incision will be required, creating a more vulnerable scar.

The low vertical incision, also a lower-segment incision, may be used in situations in which the transverse incision is inappropriate, predominantly in patients with an underdeveloped lower uterine segment. When used in these circumstances, there is a lower risk of lateral extension into the uterine vessels. The incision may be extended upward into the body of the uterus if more room is needed. An upper uterine segment extension renders closure more difficult and precludes a subsequent trial of labor. More extensive dissection of the bladder is necessary to keep the vertical incision within the lower uterine segment. If the incision extends downward, it may tear through the cervix into the vagina and possibly the bladder. The low vertical incision may be used if a contraction ring needs to be cut in order to deliver the infant. If the vertical incision is confined to the lower uterine segment there is a lower probability of dehiscence and/or rupture in a subsequent pregnancy.[42]

Infrequently performed in modern obstetrics, the classical uterine incision is a vertical incision into the upper uterine segment. It is required in circumstances where exposure of the lower uterine segment is inadequate, in elective cesarean hysterectomy, or in cases of a noncorrectable back-down transverse lie. The incision permits rapid delivery and reduces the risk of bladder injury, because the bladder is not dissected. When an anterior placenta previa is present, an upper segment incision may be used to avoid incising the placenta. However, dissection around the placenta following a lower-segment incision can eliminate the need for a classical uterine incision. The many disadvantages of the classical uterine incision result in its limited use in obstetrics today. The incision is more complicated and time-consuming to repair, the incidence of infection is higher, and adhesion formation is common. There is a greater risk of incision rupture during subsequent pregnancies[42,43]; if rupture occurs, the resultant bleeding is much greater than with the relatively avascular lower segment. The fetus is also more likely to be expelled from the uterus into the peritoneal cavity. For these reasons, most obstetricians consider a vertical upper uterine incision to be a contraindication to a trial of vaginal delivery, committing women to elective repeat cesarean deliveries.

In a recent review of 19,726 consecutive cesarean deliveries between 1980 and 1998, Patterson and colleagues[44] observed a distribution of uterine incisions of 98.5% low transverse, 1.1% classical, and 0.4% inverted T. Over the period of the study there was an increase in the incidence of inverted T incisions, from 0.2% to 0.9%. Maternal morbidity, expressed as puerperal infection, blood transfusion, hysterectomy, intensive care unit admission, and maternal death, was significantly higher in classical cesarean delivery compared with the low transverse incision. Perinatal morbidity was also increased in classical and inverted T incisions compared with low transverse cesarean, reflecting the preterm birth preponderance with the former incisions.

Considerable variation exists among obstetricians in the surgical technique used in the conduct of a low transverse uterine incision for cesarean birth. In the survey by Tully and colleagues,[30] 54.7% of surgeons used predominantly blunt dissection and 45.7% predominantly sharp dissection to enter the uterine cavity. Manual removal of the placenta was utilized by 24.7%, and 33.7% routinely closed the parietal peritoneum.

Formal investigation of the creation of the uterine incision consists of four randomized controlled trials involving 526 women[45–48] assessing the use of absorbable staples compared with extending the incision manually or with scissors in low transverse uterine cesarean delivery. Stapling techniques have been introduced to decrease blood loss from the incision margins. In a meta-analysis of these trials by the Cochrane Collaboration,[49] the stapling technique did not offer any reduction in total operation time (weighted mean difference = −1.17 minutes; 95% CI, −3.57, 1.22), although there was a significant increase in the incision to fetal delivery time (0.85 minutes; 95% CI, 0.48–1.23). There was a reduction in intraoperative blood loss with stapling techniques (weighted mean difference = − 41.22 mL; 95% CI, −50.63 to −31.8). The evidence currently available does not warrant the routine use of stapling techniques in the creation of the lower uterine segment incision, and the incision-to-delivery interval delay could have adverse consequences in some situations. In addition, the cost of the guns and staples is considerable; this will probably limit their wider use.

The comparison of blunt and sharp extension of the uterine incision has been compared in a small randomized trial involving 286 women.[50] There was no reported difference in the incidence of unintended uterine incision extension, intraoperative duration, or estimated blood loss between the two techniques. The primary correlate of incision extension was the stage of labor, being significantly greater when cesarean section was performed in the second stage of labor regardless of the uterine incision technique employed. The small sample size of this trial does render the conclusion of the study that the techniques are equivalent open to some debate.

Techniques for the delivery of the placenta at cesarean birth have been the subject of three randomized controlled clinical trials[51–53] involving 224 women; these studies were also assessed by the Cochrane Collaboration.[54] Manual removal of the placenta was associated with a significant increase in maternal blood loss and postoperative infectious morbidity. Lasley and coworkers[55] randomized 333 women to manual or spontaneous placental delivery and observed an increase in wound infection rates (OR, 2.33; 95% CI, 0.72 8.73) and a strong trend to an increase in endometritis with manual removal (OR, 1.85; 95% CI, 0.97–3.53). Manual placental removal at cesarean section should therefore be performed only when clinically indicated and not as a routine practice. Disappointingly, in the survey by Tully and colleagues,[30] 25.1% of obstetricians routinely employed manual removal of the placenta at cesarean delivery.

Maternal antibiotics to decrease the incidence of postoperative endomyometritis are administered prophylactically in many centers, although there remain a surprising number who do not use the technique[56] despite compelling evidence of its efficacy in trials involving over 10,000 women.[57] Commonly a single dose of a first- or second-generation cephalosporin is given, although either the addition of metronidazole or the use of ampicillin plus clavulanic acid or sulbactam to cover gram-negative anaerobes is increasing and has been shown to be more effective than ampicillin alone.[58] The Cochrane Collaboration meta-analysis of 47 published randomized controlled trials of antibiotic prophylaxis regimens[59] demonstrated ampicillin and first-generation cephalosporins have a similar efficacy in reducing endometritis (OR, 1.27; 95% CI, 0.84–1.93), with no benefit in using more broad-spectrum agents (ampicillin versus second- or third-generation cephalosporin OR, 0.83; 95% CI, 0.54–1.26; first-generation cephalosporin versus second- or third-generation cephalosporin OR, 1.21; 95% CI, 0.97–1.51). A multiple-dose regimen for prophylaxis was not more effective than a single-dose regimen (OR, 0.92; 95% CI, 0.70–1.23). Antibiotic administration is sometimes on a selective rather than comprehensive basis (e.g., in cases of nonelective cesarean section with prior rupture of the membranes), although the evidence suggests it is of value in all cases.[60]

The uterus may be exteriorized for repair. This procedure is not a necessary routine but does assist visualization and technically facilitates repair of the uterine incision, especially if there have been lateral extensions. The relaxing uterus can be promptly recognized and massage applied, potentially decreasing intraoperative blood loss. Hershey and Quilligan[61] reported lower blood loss in women undergoing exteriorization repair (mean reduction in hematocrit, 6.2 ± 0.35 vs. 7.0 ± 0.43, exteriorization vs. intraperitoneal, respectively, $P < 0.01$), although Magann and coworkers[51] did not confirm this significant reduction in their trial. No increase in febrile morbidity has been reported with uterine exteriorization.[51,61] The main adverse effect is pain and vagal-induced vomiting with traction when the woman is awake and the cesarean is being performed under regional analgesia. The incidence of venous air embolism is increased when uterine exteriorization and manual removal of the placenta are performed at cesarean section.[62]

The Cochrane Collaboration has provided a review including two of the five randomized controlled trials of uterine exteriorization versus intraperitoneal repair at cesarean delivery.[63] These two trials involved 486 women, but neither was felt to be methodologically strong. Uterine exteriorization was associated with a reduction in the duration of postcesarean fever (OR, 0.40; 95% CI, 0.17–0.94), and a nonsignificant trend to less infections and gastrointestinal disturbance. No difference in blood loss was found. This review concluded there was insufficient information to make a recommendation on the routine use of uterine exteriorization. Since that Cochrane review was published a further three trials have been published.[64–67] These three trials have not reported results markedly different from those in the Cochrane review.

Surgical Closure Techniques

The uterine incision can be closed with one or two layers. Use of a single-layer closure technique reduces operating time without any obvious short-term detrimental effects.[67–69] A small follow-up study from Tucker and colleagues[70] involving 292 women did not demonstrate an increase in uterine scar dehiscence in the single-layer closure compared with the conventional two-layer closure group. Jelsema and coworkers,[69] in an observational study of 200 women, compared continuous, nonlocking, single-layer closure with the standard two-layer uterine closure. No differences in the febrile morbidity rates were observed, although there was an increased need for additional hemostatic sutures. The Cochrane review of single-versus two-layer uterine closure concludes, on the basis of two randomized trials involving 1006 women available at the time of review,[67,68] that the only advantage to single-layer closure is a reduction in operating time.[71] In that review, based only on one study, there were fewer uterine scar deformities as assessed by hysterosalpingogram, 3 months after delivery. In the United Kingdom, the vast majority of surgeons (96.3%) use a two-layer uterine closure technique.[30] The number of published trials is small; further information is required before single-layer closure can be recommended as a routine.

It has been traditional surgical procedure to close the peritoneum. The reasons for peritoneal closure have never been scientifically validated, however, they include restoration of surgical anatomy and a potential reduction in infection, wound dehiscence, and adhesion formation. Animal experimentation has suggested that adhesion formation may in fact be greater with peritoneal closure due to foreign body reaction to the suture material.[72,73] No significant short-term differences in postoperative complications have been observed in trials of peritoneal nonclosure in general surgery[74,75] or gynecology.[76,77] The Cochrane review of peritoneal closure includes four trials involving 1194 women.[78] There was no difference in short-term postoperative morbidity in women regardless of peritoneal closure or nonclosure. Operating time was reduced if the peritoneum was not closed. The reviewers concluded that there was insufficient data to warrant a practice alteration; although there were no short-term disadvantages in peritoneal nonclosure, no long-term data were available.

Subsequent to the Cochrane review, a further three trials of peritoneal closure have been published.[79-81] A concern with most published trials is the lack of standardization of other aspects of surgical technique of cesarean delivery. A significant reduction in postoperative febrile morbidity (OR, 0.36; 95% CI, 0.17–0.72) and operating time (7.9 minutes) was reported by Grundsell and colleagues[79] in a trial involving 361 women. Assessment of postoperative pain with peritoneal closure has been assessed. In a small study of 40 women, Højberg and colleagues[80] reported no significant difference in postoperative pain scores based on peritoneal closure, although the nonclosure group required less oral analgesia. Rafique and coworkers[81] observed lower narcotic analgesic requirements and greater patient satisfaction (possibly due to a reduction in the narcotic side effects in addition to a reduction in pain) in women randomized to peritoneal nonclosure. Again, a significant reduction in operating time was reported, and a consistent reduction of 5 to 8 minutes has been observed in all the studies. The available clinical and nonclinical data appear to support the concept of peritoneal nonclosure at cesarean birth. These data have been reflected in clinical practice, with the majority of obstetricians favoring nonclosure of both the pelvic (71.1%) and parietal (66.2%) peritoneum in the survey by Tully and colleagues.[30]

Closure of the subcutaneous tissue has been the subject of two trials.[82,83] Del Valle and colleagues[82] investigated the efficacy of subcutaneous closure in 438 women and concluded that a running closure with absorbable suture such as plain catgut was associated with a lower incidence of superficial wound disruption. A similar randomized controlled trial conducted in women with more than 2 cm of subcutaneous fat also demonstrated a lower incidence of wound disruption (14.5% vs. 26.6%, $P = 0.02$), a lower seroma formation rate (6% vs. 19%, $P = 0.003$), and a trend to lower overt wound infection rate (6.0% vs. 7.8%, NS) in the women allocated to the subcutaneous closure group.[83]

Closure of the skin following a cesarean birth may be achieved with interrupted sutures, staples, or a subcuticular suture, the technique and suture material usually being related predominantly to personal preference. Skin closure with staples is more rapid than other techniques[84] but has been associated with increased wound pain and reduced cosmesis. Skin closure techniques have been the subject of three clinical studies.[85–87] Frishman and coworkers[85] conducted a randomized trial comparing skin closure with subcuticular suture or staples for Pfannenstiel incisions in 66 women. The operating time was less in those women randomized to skin closure with staples. Analgesic use was less in women randomized to the suture group and there was also a suggestion of improved cosmesis; however, this is a small trial with methodologic problems, limiting the validity of the results. The use of blunt and sharp-tipped needles produced no difference in wound infections.[86] The overall incidence of wound infection in this study of 204 women was low and the study underpowered for the conclusion. In a small trial of the cosmesis of intracuticular and subcuticular sutures, satisfaction scores were higher for the intracuticular suturing technique at greater than 4 months' postprocedure.[87] The Cochrane review of skin closure techniques at cesarean delivery reported on the only available randomized controlled trial[88] and commented on the lack of available evidence in this aspect of cesarean delivery. Despite the lack of data, the majority of British obstetricians reported subcuticular skin closure as their routine (73.9%).[30]

Alternative Techniques for Cesarean Birth

Alternative surgical techniques to the traditional surgical approach to cesarean birth have been reported in recent years. The Misgav Ladach, Pelosi, and Stark techniques of cesarean section have been the subject of several reports.[35,36,89–92] The Misgav Ladach technique was developed in Israel and involves the Joel-Cohen abdominal incision, single-layer uterine closure, and nonclosure of the visceral and parietal peritoneum. Björklund and coworkers[89] evaluated this technique in Africa in a randomized controlled trial of 339 women and reported a 20% reduction in blood loss, a 50% reduction in the use of suture material, and a reduction in operating time of 7.3 minutes. There was no difference in overall postoperative infection rates. Similarly, Darj and Nordström[36] observed a reduction in operating time (mean, 13.4 minutes) and blood loss (mean, 160 mL) with the Misgav Ladach compared with the Pfannenstiel technique. The Stark technique, which also involves omission of peritoneal closure and single-layer uterine closure, was associated with a lower febrile morbidity rate (7.7% vs. 19.8%), reduced antibiotic use (33.3% vs. 81.3%), and a lower adhesion incidence in subsequent surgery (6.3% vs. 28.8%) compared with the Pfannenstiel incision, double-layer uterine closure, and peritoneal closure in an observational study of 125 women.[92] The Pelosi technique, in which the formation of the bladder flap is eliminated, has been associated with decreased operating time, postoperative febrile morbidity, and hospital costs when compared with traditional techniques.[90,91]

It is clear that eliminating operative steps in cesarean delivery reduces the total operating time. It is not clear whether this reduction is translated into other benefits or if the infectious morbidity, pain, and blood loss alterations are real or the effect of small trials with inadequate methodology. It is also clear that large, rigorously designed and conducted clinical trials with assessment of both short- and long-term outcomes are required to adequately address the surgical technique issues in cesarean delivery. In the United Kingdom this issue is being addressed by the conduct of the CAESAR Study, a randomized controlled trial to evaluate three alternative cesarean section operative techniques.

COMPLICATIONS OF CESAREAN SECTION

Cesarean delivery is a major abdominal surgical procedure and is thus subject to the standard complications—medical, anesthetic, and surgical—associated with a laparotomy (Table 76–2). It is beyond the scope of this chapter to deal with all the potential complications that may surround a cesarean birth. However, maternal morbidity and mortality associated with cesarean delivery are increased in women with preexisting medical disorders.

Hemorrhage

Hemorrhage at the time of cesarean delivery may be related to the operative procedure, such as damage to the uterine vessels, or be incidental, such as occurs due to uterine atony, placenta previa, or placenta accreta. The origin of the excess blood loss is generally apparent at the time of surgery and is dealt with as is appropriate to the etiology. Management is covered in detail in Chapter 77.

TABLE 76–2

Complications of Cesarean Section

Anesthesia-related
aspiration syndrome
hypotension
spinal headache
Hemorrhage
uterine atony
placenta previa/accreta
lacerations
Urinary tract and gastrointestinal injuries
General postoperative complications
respiratory: atelectasis/pneumonia
gastrointestinal: ileus
urinary tract infections
thromboembolism
Endomyometritis
Wound infection

The incidence of placenta accreta appears to be increasing[10,11] and is second only to uterine atony as an indication for emergency hysterectomy for obstetric hemorrhage. There is an association of placenta accreta with placenta previa and previous cesarean delivery, incidence of which have both increased with the recent trend toward more liberal indications for cesarean delivery. Clark and colleagues[10] reported that 25% of women undergoing cesarean delivery for placenta previa in the presence of one or more uterine scars subsequently underwent cesarean hysterectomy for placenta accreta. This risk appears to increase directly with the number of previous uterine incisions. If the placenta is accreta, effective management usually requires total abdominal hysterectomy, although additional options, including the use of uterine compression sutures or leaving the placenta in situ, have been reported. The uterus, vagina, or broad ligament may be lacerated during a cesarean delivery. Traumatic deliveries or poor delivery technique are associated with an increased frequency of operative lacerations. Lacerations involving uterine tissue are usually sutured without difficulty. Vertical lacerations into the vagina or lateral extensions into the broad ligament may be associated with substantial blood loss and the potential for ureteric damage during their repair. Before beginning repair of lacerations into the broad ligament, identification of the ureter is frequently necessary. The initial suture must be inserted just distal to the apex of the laceration.

Urinary Tract Injuries

Injuries to the urinary bladder occur with variable incidence during the course of cesarean delivery.[93,94] The Pfannenstiel incision, with lower entry into the peritoneal cavity, increases the risk of inadvertent cystotomy, especially after prolonged labor in which the bladder is pulled cephalad. Scarring and secondary obliteration of the vesicouterine space following previous cesarean section increase the incidence of trauma secondary to attempts at dissection. The bladder may also be damaged secondary to a uterine laceration, particularly in association with a low vertical uterine incision.

Various techniques are employed to reduce the incidence of intraoperative bladder injury. Preoperative catheterization of the bladder and peritoneal entry as far cephalad as possible are important. Injuries to the base of the bladder are most frequent during a repeat procedure, in which clear tissue planes do not always exist. Careful sharp rather than blunt dissection of the bladder will reduce the occurrence of inadvertent cystotomy as well as reducing blood loss. If there is concern as to possible bladder injury, the abdomen must not be closed until the issue is resolved by transurethral instillation of methylene blue-colored saline with leakage of fluid identifying the cystotomy site.

Full-thickness bladder lacerations should be repaired with a two-layer closure with continuous or interrupted 2-0 or 3-0 chromic catgut. The site of the bladder laceration is important, because repair of a laceration of the bladder dome is usually straightforward. The bladder base is thinner, receives less blood flow, and appears to heal more slowly, and occlusion of the ureteric orifice is also a possibility. Fistula formation is not usually a problem if accidental cystotomy is promptly recognized and repaired.

Ureteric injury is one of the most dreaded complications of any pelvic operation. It is, however, an uncommon occurrence at cesarean section. Eisenkop and colleagues[94] reported 7 ureteric injuries in 7527 women undergoing cesarean delivery. In 5, the ureteric injury occurred during an attempt to control hemorrhage from extension of the uterine incision. When controlling hemorrhage, it is useful to apply direct pressure while identifying the course of the ureter to permit accurate suture placement and reduce the potential for ureteral injury.

Postoperative Complications

Respiratory complications remain a primary cause of postoperative morbidity following major surgical procedures. Deep breathing exercises, incentive spirometry, chest percussion, and postural drainage all have merit, depending on the clinical circumstance.

Gastrointestinal dysfunction is not uncommon after a cesarean delivery; it is usually restricted to a transient ileus. The Cochrane Review of postoperative feeding assessed six trials to evaluate the effect of early and delayed oral intake after cesarean birth.[95] Although the studies were of variable quality, on the available data the review concluded there was no justification to withholding early oral intake after cesarean birth. Early oral intake was associated with a reduced time to return of bowel sounds, a reduced postoperative stay, and a trend to a reduction in abdominal distension.

Urinary tract infections are a common complication of cesarean section and occur with a variable frequency of 2% to 16%, the rate depending on the duration of catheterization and the preoperative health of the woman.[93,96]

Thromboembolic disease during pregnancy is an uncommon event but remains a major cause of maternal morbidity and mortality. Indeed, pulmonary thromboembolism is a leading cause of maternal death in the United Kingdom.[97] The greatest incidence in the puerperium is among cesarean patients, particularly if the surgery is performed as an emergency procedure during labor. Other factors increasing the risk of venous thromboembolism include advanced maternal age, obesity, and inherited thrombophilia disorders. The risk of a deep venous thrombosis after cesarean delivery is 3 to 5 times greater than after vaginal delivery.[98] The reactive thrombocytosis after cesarean birth, the impact of which is compounded by anemia, infection, and postpartum hemorrhage, further increases the risk. In 1995 the Royal College of

Obstetricians and Gynaecologists[99] published a Working Party Report on prophylaxis against thromboembolism in the United Kingdom. This document has drawn attention to the risks of thromboembolic disorders after cesarean birth and the need to consider prophylaxis for high risk women. Routine prophylaxis against postoperative deep vein thrombosis now includes the use of mechanical calf compression intraoperatively (e.g., Flowtron boots), the use of calf compression stockings (e.g., TED), and subcutaneous heparin, either unfractionated or high-molecular weight heparin.[100] Low-molecular weight heparin is now commonly used peripartum, because it can be administered on a once-daily dosage regimen.[101] These heparins are not secreted in breast milk and therefore can be used in lactating women.

Endomyometritis

In the absence of prophylactic antibiotics, postcesarean endomyometritis occurs with an incidence of 20% to 40%.[102,103] Postoperative infections may be reduced by 50% to 60% with the use of prophylactic antibiotics at the time of cesarean delivery.[104,105] In approximately 10% of cases, concurrent bacteremia will accompany postcesarean endomyometritis.[102,104] Uncommonly, postcesarean endomyometritis may be complicated by pelvic abscess, septic shock, and septic pelvic thrombophlebitis. The major risk factors for the development of postcesarean infection are young age, low socioeconomic status, prolonged labor, prolonged rupture of membranes, and multiple vaginal examinations.

Postcesarean section endomyometritis is a polymicrobial infection with bacteria normally present in the lower genital tract: aerobic streptococci (group B and D streptococci), anaerobic gram-positive cocci (peptococcus and peptostreptococcus), aerobic (*E. coli*, *Klebsiella pneumoniae*, *Proteus* spp.) and anaerobic gram-negative bacilli (*Bacteroides* spp. and *Gardnerella vaginalis*).[102] The symptoms and signs of endomyometritis usually develop 24 to 48 hours after surgery. The main clinical manifestations are fever, tachycardia, lower abdominal pain, uterine and adnexal tenderness, and peritoneal irritation. After appropriate laboratory investigation, including complete blood count, aerobic and anaerobic blood cultures, and aerobic and anaerobic endometrial cultures, antibiotic therapy is instituted. Several effective regimens are available: clindamycin plus an aminoglycoside or aztreonam, penicillin plus aminoglycoside and metronidazole or one of the extended-spectrum penicillins such as ticarcillin/clavulanic acid or ampicillin/sulbactam. If a cephalosporin has been administered for prophylaxis, a penicillin should be used due to the possibility of *Enterococcus*.

Most patients show a clear response to treatment within 72 hours. The two most common causes of apparent treatment failure are concurrent wound infection and resistant microorganisms. If a wound infection develops, incision and drainage is indicated, but a change in antibiotics is not usually necessary. The principal microorganisms likely to be resistant to initial treatment regimens are aerobic gram-negative bacilli, enterococci, and *Bacteroides* spp. If a resistant organism is thought to be present, antibiotic therapy should be modified. Parenteral therapy should be continued for a minimum of 24 hours after the patient becomes afebrile and asymptomatic. At this point, therapy may be discontinued. Patients do not need to be maintained on oral antibiotics after discharge from hospital.[104] Extended therapy of this nature is expensive and increases the risk of side effects without providing any measurable therapeutic benefit.

In patients who fail to improve after a change in antibiotic therapy, another detailed examination should be performed to detect a wound infection or pelvic abscess. Other possible causes of poor treatment response include viral infections, venous thrombophlebitis, and drug fever.

Wound Infection

Adverse outcomes associated with abdominal wounds in the obstetric patient occur more frequently in the presence of anemia, premature rupture of the membranes, prolapsed cord, and meconium staining. Reported wound infection rates associated with cesarean section range from 2.5% to 16.1%.[106–108] Nielson and Hokegard[109] found rates of 4.7% for elective cases and 24.2% for emergency cases. A mixture of anaerobic and aerobic bacteria (*E. coli*, *Proteus mirabilis*, *Bacteroides* spp., beta-hemolytic streptococci) are isolated from postcesarean wound infections, similar to those found in postpartum endomyometritis. *Staphylococcus aureus* is isolated from postcesarean wound infections in 25% of cases and appears to originate from the skin rather than the endometrium.[110] Early diagnosis is important, and frequent inspection of the cesarean wound and temperature review is paramount.

Prevention of wound infections involves careful preoperative preparation. Preoperative hexachlorophene showers,[111] clipping of abdominal hair rather than shaving,[111,112] liberal application of skin antiseptic agents in the operating room, and use of wound drapes are simple but effective measures to decrease the incidence of wound infection. Sterile technique, attention to hemostasis, obliteration of tissue dead space and removal of devitalized tissues are important surgical factors that promote appropriate wound healing and prevent wound infection. The use of closed drainage systems is preferable to Penrose-type drains, because the former remain sterile as long as flow continues.

As with any infective process, prompt recognition and treatment are essential. An infected wound is usually characterized by localized pain, tenderness, erythema, and purulent discharge, typically becoming clinically evident 4 to 7 days after surgery. Systemic evidence may also be present, with fever and leukocytosis. The early development of a wound infection, usually in association with cellulitis and high spiking fever, is characteristic of group A and group B beta-hemolytic streptococci. Initial treatment involves opening the wound along the affected area to the fascia and culturing the exudate (anaerobic and aerobic). Incision and drainage with debridement of necrotic tissue is vital. Applications of hydrogen peroxide to chemically debride the area should follow initial local surgical efforts. Because antiseptic solutions are cytotoxic, saline lavage must follow their application, then wet-to-dry dressings. When all necrotic tissue is removed and granulation tissue forms, cessation of debriding agents and the use of wet-to-wet dressings is important. The wound may be reapproximated once granulation tissue appears or be left to close by secondary intention. Drainage is usually sufficient, and systemic antibiotics are not indicated for simple wound infections. A serious complication of wound infection is necrotizing fasciitis, a synergistic infection that destroys subcutaneous tissues. Repeated, aggressive debridement in association with broad-spectrum antibiotics and hyperbaric oxygen therapy is vital to achieve cure.

CONCLUSIONS

- Obstetric practice has altered markedly over the past 50 years. With a progressive reduction in maternal and perinatal mortality rates, the focus of care centers now on continuing improvements in morbidity.
- Cesarean delivery has emerged as a centerpoint of obstetric care with liberalization of the indications for such delivery.
- It is clear that ongoing research is required into the surgical techniques for cesarean delivery to promote improved outcomes for women, not just in the first cesarean birth, but also in subsequent procedures.

SUMMARY OF MANAGEMENT OPTIONS

Cesarean Section

Management Options	Quality of Evidence	Strength of Recommendation	References
Preparation			
Vaginal preparation with povidone-iodine does not reduce postcesarean infectious morbidity.	Ib	A	113
Left lateral tilt for cesarean section reduces the incidence of low Apgar scores.	Ia	A	114
No evidence that adhesive drapes confer benefit over conventional linen drapes.	Ib III	A B	32 33
Cross-match blood with anticipated above-average blood loss (e.g., placenta previa, multiple cesarean sections).	–	GPP	–
Experienced surgeon for anticipated complicated cases (e.g., fibroid uterus, extreme prematurity, placenta previa, multiple cesarean sections).	–	GPP	–
Skin Incision			
Transverse incisions are associated with lower maternal morbidity, including dehiscence, compared to vertical incisions.	Ib	A	40
Pfannenstiel incisions result in faster operations than Maylard incisions.	IIa	B	37
Joel-Cohen incision is faster than Pfannenstiel incision but cosmetically less acceptable. No other differences.	Ib	A	38,39
Uterine Incision			
Transverse lower uterine incision is associated with less maternal morbidity.	III	B	42,43,115,116
Absorbable staples for uterine wound cannot at present be recommended for routine practice.	Ia	A	49
There is no evidence of benefit of blunt versus sharp dissection/extension of uterine incision.	Ib	A	50

SUMMARY OF MANAGEMENT OPTIONS
Cesarean Section *(Continued)*

Management Options	Quality of Evidence	Strength of Recommendation	References
Delivery of the Placenta			
Manual removal is associated with increased maternal blood loss and infection.	Ia	A	54
Oxytocic Agents			
Active management using oxytocic agent is better than expectant management in vaginal deliveries and one would expect the same with cesarean section.	Ia	A	117
Ergometrine-oxytocin is statistically better in preventing postpartum hemorrhage than oxytocin alone but has more side effects.	Ia	A	118
Bolus oxytocin is as effective as intramyometrial prostaglandin and misoprostol in preventing postpartum hemorrhage, but the latter two were more often associated with retained placenta.	Ib	A	119,120
Carbetocin may be associated with less intraoperative blood loss compared to oxytocin.	Ib	A	121
Exteriorization of Uterus			
No evidence of increased morbidity associated with exteriorization of the uterus.	Ia	A	63
Closure			
Uterus: A single-layer uterine incision closure is not associated with increased maternal morbidity; but trials are small and no justification for changing practice exists.	Ia	A	71
Peritoneum: Closure is not necessary in routine practice.	Ia	A	78
Subcutaneous layer: Closure is associated with less superficial wound dehiscence, especially in obese women.	Ib	A	82,83
Subrectus suction drainage: This reduces the rate of wound infection.	Ib	A	122
Skin closure: No data to guide optimum method.	Ia	A	88
Perioperative Measures			
Prophylactic antibiotics are associated with reduced maternal morbidity in emergency cesarean section and with reduced incidence of endometritis in elective cesarean section.	Ia	A	59
Antibiotic regimens: Ampicillin and first-generation cephalosporins are equally effective in reducing postoperative endometritis. Single-dose regimens are as effective as repeat doses, with the exception of urinary tract infection.	Ia	A	123
Thromboprophylaxis is recommended for all women undergoing cesarean section.	IV	C	99
Oral intake: No justification in withholding early oral intake.	Ia	A	95

REFERENCES

1. Paterson-Brown S, Fisk NM: Caesarean section: Every woman's right to choose? Curr Opin Obstet Gynecol 1997;9:351–355.
2. Paterson-Brown S: Should doctors perform an elective caesarean section on request? Yes, as long as the woman is fully informed. BMJ 1998;317:462–465.
3. Quinlivan JA, Petersen RW, Nichols CN: Patient preference the leading indication for elective caesarean section in public patients–Results of a 2-year prospective audit in a teaching hospital. Aust NZ J Obstet Gynaecol 1999;39:207–14.
4. DeMott RK: A blatant misuse of power? Birth 2000;27(4):264–265.

5. Gamble JA, Creedy DK: Women's request for a cesarean section: A critique of the literature. Birth 2000;27:256–263.
6. Cotzias CS, Paterson-Brown S, Fisk NM: Obstetricians say yes to maternal request for elective caesarean section: A survey of current opinion. Eur J Obstet Gynecol Reprod Biol 2001;97: 15–16.
7. Morrison J, MacKenzie IZ: Cesarean section on demand. Semin Perinatol 2003;27:20–33.
8. McMahon MJ, Li R, Schenck AP, et al: Previous cesarean birth. A risk factor for placenta previa? J Reprod Med 1997;42: 409–412.
9. Ananth CV, Smulian JC, Vintzileos AM: The association of placenta previa with history of cesarean delivery and abortion: A meta-analysis. Am J Obstet Gynecol 1997;177:1071–1078.
10. Clark SL, Koonings PP, Phelan JP: Placenta previa/accreta and prior cesarean section. Obstet Gynecol 1985;66:89–92.
11. Manyonda IT, Varma TR: Massive obstetric hemorrhage due to placenta previa/accreta with prior cesarean section. Int J Gynaecol Obstet 1990;34:183–186.
12. Usha Kiran TS, Jayawickrama NS: Who is responsible for the rising caesarean section rate? J Obstet Gynaecol 2002;22: 363–365.
13. Rutkow IM: Obstetric and gynecologic operations in the United States, 1979 to 1984. Obstet Gynecol 1986;67:755–759.
14. Clarke SC, Taffel S: Changes in cesarean delivery in the United States, 1988 and 1993. Birth 1995;22:63–67.
15. Ventura SJ, Martin JA, Curtin SC, et al: Births: Final data for 1999. Natl Vital Stat Rep 2001;49:1–100.
16. Chazotte C, Cohen WR: Catastrophic complications of previous cesarean section. Am J Obstet Gynecol 1990;163:738–742.
17. McMahon MJ, Luther ER, Bowes WA Jr, Olshan AR: Comparison of a trial of labor with an elective second cesarean section. N Engl J Med 1996;335:689–695.
18. Martin JA, Hamilton BE, Ventura SJ, et al: Births: Final data for 2001. Natl Vital Stat Rep 2002;51:1–102.
19. Kolås T, Hofoss D, Daltveit AK, et al: Indications for cesarean deliveries in Norway. Am J Obstet Gynecol 2003;188:864–870.
20. Treffers PE, Pel M: The rising trend for caesarean birth. BMJ 1993;307:1017–1018.
21. Royal College of Obstetricians and Gynaecologists: The national sentinel caesarean section audit report. RCOG clinical effectiveness support unit. London, RCOG Press, 2001.
22. Evans L: Italy has Europe's highest caesarean section rate. BMJ 1995;310:487.
23. Guihard P, Blondel B: Trends in risk factors for caesarean section in France between 1981 and 1995: Lessons for reducing the rates in the future. BJOG 2001;108:48–55.
24. Perinatal Statistics in Western Australia, 2000. Eighteenth Annual Report of the Western Australian Midwives' Notification System. Department of Health, Western Australia. July 2002.
25. Murray SF, Serani Pradenas F: Cesarean birth trends in Chile, 1986 to 1994. Birth 1997;24:258–263.
26. Belizan JM, Althabe F, Barros FC, Alezander S: Rates and implications of caesarean sections in Latin America: Ecological study. BMJ 1999;319:1397–1400.
27. Buekens P, Curtis S, Alayón S: Demographic and health surveys: Caesarean section rates in sub-Saharan Africa. BMJ 2003;326:136.
28. Anderson GM, Lomas J: Determinants of the increasing cesarean birth rate. Ontario data 1979 to 1982. N Engl J Med 1984;311:887–892.
29. Hussen P: Elective caesarean section versus vaginal delivery. Whither the end of traditional obstetrics? Arch Gynecol Obstet 2001;265:169–174.
30. Tully L, Gates S, Brocklehurst P, et al: Surgical techniques used during caesarean section operations: Results of a national survey of practice in the UK. Eur J Obstet Gynecol Reprod Biol 2002; 102:120–126.
31. McCulloch P, Taylor I, Sasako M, et al: Randomized trials in surgery: Problems and possible solutions. BMJ 2002;324: 1448–1451.
32. Lorenz RP, Botti JJ, Appelbaum PC, Bennett N: Skin preparation methods before cesarean section: A comparative study. J Reprod Med 1988;33:202–204.
33. Alexander JW, Aerni S, Plettner JP: Development of a safe and effective one-minute preoperative skin preparation. Arch Surg 1985;120:1357–1361.
34. Stark M, Finkel AR: Comparison between the Joel-Cohen and Pfannenstiel incisions in cesarean section. Eur J Obstet Gynecol Reprod Biol 1994;53:121–122.
35. Holmgren G, Sjöholm L, Stark M: The Misgav Ladach method for cesarean section: Method description. Acta Obstet Gynecol Scand 1999;78:615–621.
36. Darj E, Nordström ML: The Misgav Ladach method for cesarean section compared to the Pfannenstiel method. Acta Obstet Gynecol Scand 1999;78:37–41.
37. Ayers JW, Morley GW: Surgical incision for cesarean section. Obstet Gynecol 1987;70:706–708.
38. Decavalas G, Papadopoulos V, Tzingounis V: A prospective comparison of surgical procedures in caesarean section. Acta Obstet Gynecol Scand 1997;S167:13.
39. Franchi M, Ghezzi F, Raio L, et al: Joel-Cohen or Pfannenstiel incision at cesarean delivery: Does it make a difference? Acta Obstet Gynecol Scand 2002;81:1040–1046.
40. Haeri AD: Comparison of transverse and vertical skin incisions for caesarean section. S Afr Med J 1976;50:33–34.
41. Gallup DG: Modifications of celiotomy techniques to decrease morbidity in obese gynecologic patients. Am J Obstet Gynecol 1984;150:171–178.
42. Tahilramaney MP, Boucher M, Eglinton GS, et al: Previous cesarean section and trial of labor. Factors related to uterine dehiscence. J Reprod Med 1984;29:17–21.
43. Pedowitz P, Schwartz RM: The true incidence of silent rupture of cesarean section scars: A prospective analysis of 403 cases. Am J Obstet Gynecol 1957;74:1071–1081.
44. Patterson LS, O'Connell CM, Baskett TF: Maternal and perinatal morbidity associated with classic and inverted T cesarean incisions. Obstet Gynecol 2002;100:633–637.
45. Dargent D, Audra G, Noblot G: Utilization de la pince POLY CS 57 pour l'operation cesarienne. Un essai randomize. J Gynecol Obstet Biol Reprod (Paris) 1990;18:961–962.
46. Hoskins IA, Ordorica SA, Frieden FJ, Young BK: Performance of cesarean section using absorbable staples. Surg Gynecol Obstet 1991;172:108–112.
47. van Dongen PW, Nijhuis JG, Jongsma HW: Reduced blood loss during caesarean section due to a controlled stapling technique. Eur J Obstet Gynecol Reprod Biol 1989;32:95–102.
48. Villeneuve MG, Khalife S, Marcoux S, Blanchet P: Surgical staples in cesarean section: A randomized controlled trial. Am J Obstet Gynecol 1990;163:1641–1646.
49. Wilkinson C, Enkin MW: Absorbable staples for uterine incision at caesarean section (Cochrane Review). In The Cochrane Library, Issue 2, 2003. Oxford, Update Software, 2003.
50. Rodriguez AI, Porter KB, O'Brien WF: Blunt versus sharp expansion of the uterine incision in low-segment transverse cesarean section. Am J Obstet Gynecol 1994;171:1022–1025.
51. Magann EF, Dodson MK, Allbert JR, et al: Blood loss at time of cesarean section by method of placental removal and exteriorization vs. in situ repair of the uterine incision. Surg Gynecol Obstet 1993;177:389–392.
52. McCurdy CM Jr, Magann EF, McCurdy CJ, Saltzman AK: The effect of placental management at cesarean delivery on operative blood loss. Am J Obstet Gynecol 1992;167:1363–1367.
53. Notelovitz M, Dalrymple D, Grobbelaar B, Gibson M: Transplacental haemorrhage following caesarean section. S Afr J Obstet Gynaecol 1972;10:28–29.
54. Wilkinson C, Enkin MW: Manual removal of placenta at caesarean section (Cochrane Review). In The Cochrane Library, Issue 2, 2003. Oxford, Update Software, 2003.

55. Lasley DS, Eblen A, Yancey MK, Duff P: The effect of placental removal method on the incidence of postcesarean infections. Am J Obstet Gynecol 1997;176:1250–1254.
56. Pedersen TK, Blaakaer J: Antibiotic prophylaxis in cesarean section. Acta Obstet Gynecol Scand 1996;75:537–539.
57. Smaill F: Antibiotic prophylaxis and caesarean section. BJOG 1992;99:789–790.
58. Rijhsinghani A, Savopoulos SE, Walters JK, et al: Ampicillin/sulbactam versus ampicillin alone for cesarean section prophylaxis: A randomized double-blind trial. Am J Perinatol 1995;12: 322–324.
59. Hopkins L, Smaill F: Antibiotic prophylaxis regimens and drugs for cesarean section (Cochrane Review). In The Cochrane Library, Issue 2, 2003. Oxford, Update Software, 2003.
60. Jakobi P, Weissman A, Sigler E, et al: Post-cesarean section febrile morbidity. Antibiotic prophylaxis in low-risk patients. J Reprod Med 1994;39:707–710.
61. Hershey DW, Quilligan EJ: Extra-abdominal uterine exteriorization at cesarean section. Obstet Gynecol 1978;52:189–192.
62. Lowenwirt IP, Chi DS, Handwerker SM: Nonfatal venous air embolism during cesarean section: A case report and review of the literature. Obstet Gynecol Surv 1994;49:72–76.
63. Wilkinson C, Enkin MW: Uterine exteriorization versus intraperitoneal repair at caesarean section (Cochrane Review). In The Cochrane Library, Issue 2, 2003. Oxford, Update Software, 2003.
64. Edi Osagie EC, Hopkins RE, Ogbo V, et al: Uterine exteriorisation at caesarean section: Influence on maternal morbidity. BJOG 1998;105:1070–1078.
65. Wahab MA, Karantzis P, Eccersley PS, et al: A randomized, controlled study of uterine exteriorisation and repair at caesarean section. BJOG 1999;106:913–916.
66. Magann EF, Washburne JF, Harris RL, et al: Infectious morbidity, operative blood loss, and length of the operative procedure after cesarean delivery by method of placental removal and site of uterine repair. J Am Coll Surg 1995;181:517–520.
67. Lal K, Tsomo P: Comparative study of single layer and conventional closure of uterine incision in cesarean section. Int J Gynaecol Obstet 1988;27:349–352.
68. Hauth JC, Owen J, Davis RO: Transverse uterine incision closure: One versus two layers. Am J Obstet Gynecol 1992;167:1108–1111.
69. Jelsema RD, Wittingen JA, Vander Kolk KJ: Continuous, nonlocking, single-layer repair of the lower transverse uterine incision. J Reprod Med 1993;38:393–396.
70. Tucker JM, Hauth JC, Hodgkins P, et al: Trial of labor after a one- or two-layer closure of a low transverse uterine incision. Am J Obstet Gynecol 1993;168:545–546.
71. Enkin MW, Wilkinson C: Single-versus two-layer closure for closing the uterine incision at caesarean section (Cochrane Review). In The Cochrane Library, Issue 2, 2003. Oxford, Update Software, 2003.
72. Parulkar BG, Supe AN, Vora IM, Mathur SK: Effects of experimental non-closure of peritoneum on development of suture line adhesions and wound strength in dogs. Ind J Gastroenterol 1986;5:251–253.
73. Kyzer S, Bayer I, Turani H, Chaimoff C: The influence of peritoneal closure on formation of intraperitoneal adhesions: An experimental study. Int J Tissue React 1986;8:355–359.
74. Gilbert JM, Ellis H, Foweraker S: Peritoneal closure after lateral paramedian incision. Br J Surg 1987;74:113–115.
75. Hugh TB, Nankivell C, Meagher AP, Li B: Is closure of the peritoneal layer necessary in the repair of midline surgical abdominal wounds? World J Surg 1990;14:231–233.
76. Lipscomb GH, Ling FW, Stovall TG, Summitt RL Jr: Peritoneal closure at vaginal hysterectomy: A reassessment. Obstet Gynecol 1996;87:40–43.
77. Kananali S, Erthen O, Kucikozkan T: Pelvic and peritoneal closure and nonclosure at lymphadenectomy in ovarian cancer: Effects on morbidity and adhesion formation. Eur J Surg Oncol 1996;22:282–285.
78. Wilkinson CS, Enkin MW: Peritoneal non-closure at caesarean section (Cochrane Review). In The Cochrane Library, Issue 2, 2003. Oxford, Update Software, 2003.
79. Grundsell HS, Rizk DE, Kumar RM: Randomized study of non-closure of peritoneum in lower segment cesarean section. Acta Obstet Gynecol Scand 1998;77:110–115.
80. Højberg KE, Aagaard J, Laursen H, et al: Closure versus non-closure of peritoneum at cesarean section—evaluation of pain. A randomized study. Acta Obstet Gynecol Scand 1998;77:741–745.
81. Rafique Z, Shibli KU, Russell IF, Lindow SW: A randomized controlled trial of the closure or non-closure of peritoneum at caesarean section: Effect on post-operative pain. BJOG 2002; 109:694–698.
82. Del Valle GO, Combs P, Qualls C, Curet LB: Does closure of Camper fascia reduce the incidence of post cesarean superficial wound disruption? Obstet Gynecol 1992;80:1013–1016.
83. Naumann RW, Hauth JC, Owen J, et al: Subcutaneous tissue approximation in relation to wound disruption after cesarean delivery in obese women. Obstet Gynecol 1995;85:412–416.
84. Gatt D, Quick CR, Owen-Smith MS: Staples for wound closure: A controlled trial. Ann R Coll Surg Engl 1985:67:318–320.
85. Frishman GN, Schwartz T, Hogan JW: Closure of Pfannenstiel skin incisions. Staples vs. subcuticular suture. J Reprod Med 1997;42:627–630.
86. Stafford MK, Pitman MC, Nanthakumaran N, Smith JR: Blunt-tipped versus sharp-tipped needles: Wound morbidity. J Obstet Gynaecol 1998;18:18–19.
87. Lindholt JS, Moller-Christensen T, Steele RE: The cosmetic outcome of the scar formation after cesarean section: Percutaneous or intracutaneous suture? Acta Obstet Gynaecol Scand 1994;73:832–835.
88. Alderdice F, McKenna D, Dornan J: Techniques and materials for skin closure in caesarean section (Cochrane Review). In The Cochrane Library, Issue 2, 2003. Oxford, Update Software, 2003.
89. Björklund K, Kimaro M, Urassa E, Lindmark G: Introduction of the Misgav Ladach caesarean section at an African tertiary centre: A randomized controlled trial. BJOG 2000;107:209–216.
90. Pelosi MA, Pelosi MA III: Simplified cesarean section. Contemp Obstet Gynecol 1995;40:89–100.
91. Wood RM, Simon H, Oz A-U: Pelosi-type vs. traditional cesarean delivery. A prospective comparison. J Reprod Med 1999;44:788–795.
92. Stark M, Chavkin Y, Kupfersztain C, et al: Evaluation of combinations of procedures in caesarean section. Int J Gynaecol Obstet 1995;48:273–276.
93. Buchholz NP, Daly-Grandeau E, Huber-Buchholz MM: Urological complications associated with caesarean section. Eur J Obstet Gynaecol Reprod Biol 1994;56:161–163.
94. Eisenkop SM, Richman R, Platt LD, Paul RH: Urinary tract injury during cesarean section. Obstet Gynecol 1982;60:591–596.
95. Mangesi L, Hofmetr GJ: Early compared with delayed oral fluids and food after caesarean section (Cochrane Review). In The Cochrane Library, Issue 2, 2003. Oxford, Update Software, 2003.
96. Farrell SJ, Anderson HF, Work BA Jr: Cesarean section: Indications and postoperative morbidity. Obstet Gynecol 1980;56:696–700.
97. Why mothers die 1997–1999. The Confidential Enquiries into Maternal Deaths in the United Kingdom London, RCOG Press, 2001 or free at http://www.cemach.org.uk/publications.htm
98. Macklon NS, Greer IA: The deep venous system in the puerperium: An ultrasound study. BJOG 1997;104:198–200.
99. Royal College of Obstetricians and Gynaecologists: Report of a Working Party on prophylaxis against thromboembolism in gynaecology and obstetrics. London, Royal College of Obstetricians and Gynaecologists, 1995.

100. Nelson-Piercy C: Obstetric thromboprophylaxis. Br J Hosp Med 1996;55:404–408.
101. Hunt BJ, Doughty HA, Majumdar G, et al: Thromboprophylaxis with low molecular weight heparin (Fragmin) in high risk pregnancies. Thromb Haemost. 1997;77:39–43.
102. Duff P: Pathophysiology and management of postcesarean endomyometritis. Obstet Gynecol 1986;67:269–276.
103. Magann EF, Dodson MK, Harris RL: Does method of placental removal or site of uterine incision repair alter endometritis after cesarean delivery? Infect Dis Obstet Gynecol 1993;1:65–70.
104. Swartz WH, Grolle K: The use of prophylactic antibiotics in cesarean section. A review of the literature. J Reprod Med 1981;26:595–609.
105. Cartwright PS, Pittaway DE, Jones HW, Entman SS: The use of prophylactic antibiotics in obstetrics and gynecology. A review. Obstet Gynecol Surv 1984;39:537–554.
106. Ortona L, Federico G, Fantoni M, et al: A study on the incidence of postoperative infections and surgical sepsis in a university hospital. Infect Control 1987;8:320–324.
107. Mugford M, Kingston J, Chalmers I: Reducing the incidence of infection after caesarean section: Implications of prophylaxis with antibiotics for hospital resources. BMJ 1989;229:1003–1006.
108. Webster J: Post-caesarean wound infections: A review of the risk factors. Aust NZ J Obstet Gynaecol 1998;28:201–207.
109. Nielsen TF, Hokegard KH: Postoperative cesarean section morbidity: A prospective study. Am J Obstet Gynecol 1983;146: 911–915.
110. Emmons SL, Krohn M, Jackson M, Eschenbach DA: Development of wound infections among women undergoing cesarean section. Obstet Gynecol 1988;72:559–564.
111. Cruse PJ, Foord R: A five-year prospective study of 23,649 surgical wounds. Arch Surg 1973;107:206–210.
112. Alexander JW, Fischer JE, Boyajian M, et al: The influence of hair-removal methods on wound infections. Arch Surg 1983; 118:347–352.
113. Reid VC, Hartmann KE, McMahon M, Fry EP: Vaginal preparation with povidone iodine and postcesarean infectious morbidity: A randomised controlled trial. Obstet Gynecol 2001;97:147–152.
114. Wilkinson C, Enkin MW: Lateral tilt for caesarean section (Cochrane Review). In The Cochrane Library, Issue 2, 2001. Oxford, Update Software, 2001.
115. Irvine DS, Haddad NG: Classical versus low-segment transverse incision for preterm caesarean section: Maternal complications and outcome of subsequent pregnancies. BJOG 1989;96:371–372.
116. Lao TT, Halpern SH, Crosby ET, Huh C: Uterine incision and maternal blood loss in preterm caesarean section. Arch Gynecol Obstet 1993;252:113–117.
117. Prendiville WJ, Elbourne D, McDonald S:. Active versus expectant management in the third stage of labour (Cochrane review). In The Cochrane Library, Issue 4, 2001. Oxford, Update Software, 2001.
118. McDonald S, Elbourne D, Prendiville WJ: Prophylactic syntometrine versus oxytocin for delivery of the placenta (Cochrane Review). In The Cochrane Library, Issue 2, 2000. Oxford, Update Software, 2000.
119. Acharya G, Al-Sammarai MT, Patel N, et al: A randomized, controlled trial comparing effect of oral misoprostol and intravenous syntocinon on intra-operative blood loss during caesarean section. Acta Obstet Gynecol Scand 2001,80:245–250.
120. Chou MM, MacKenzie IZ: A prospective, double-blind, randomized comparison of prophylactic intramyometrial 15-methyl prostaglandin $F_{2\alpha}$, 125 micrograms, and intravenous oxytocin, 20 units, for the control of blood loss at elective caesarean. Am J Obstet Gynecol 1994;171:1356–1360.
121. Dansereau J, Joshi AK, Helewa ME, et al: Double-blind comparison of carbetocin versus oxytocin in prevention of uterine atony after caesarean section. Am J Obstet Gynecol 1999;180:670–676.
122. Loong RLC, Rogers MS, Chang AM: A controlled trial on wound drainage in Caesarean section. Aust NZ J Obstet Gynaecol 1988;28:266–269.
123. Hofmeyr GJ, Smaill F: Antibiotic prophylaxis regimens and drugs for caesarean section (Cochrane review). In The Cochrane Library, Issue 2, 2001. Oxford, Update Software, 2001.

SECTION SEVEN

Postnatal

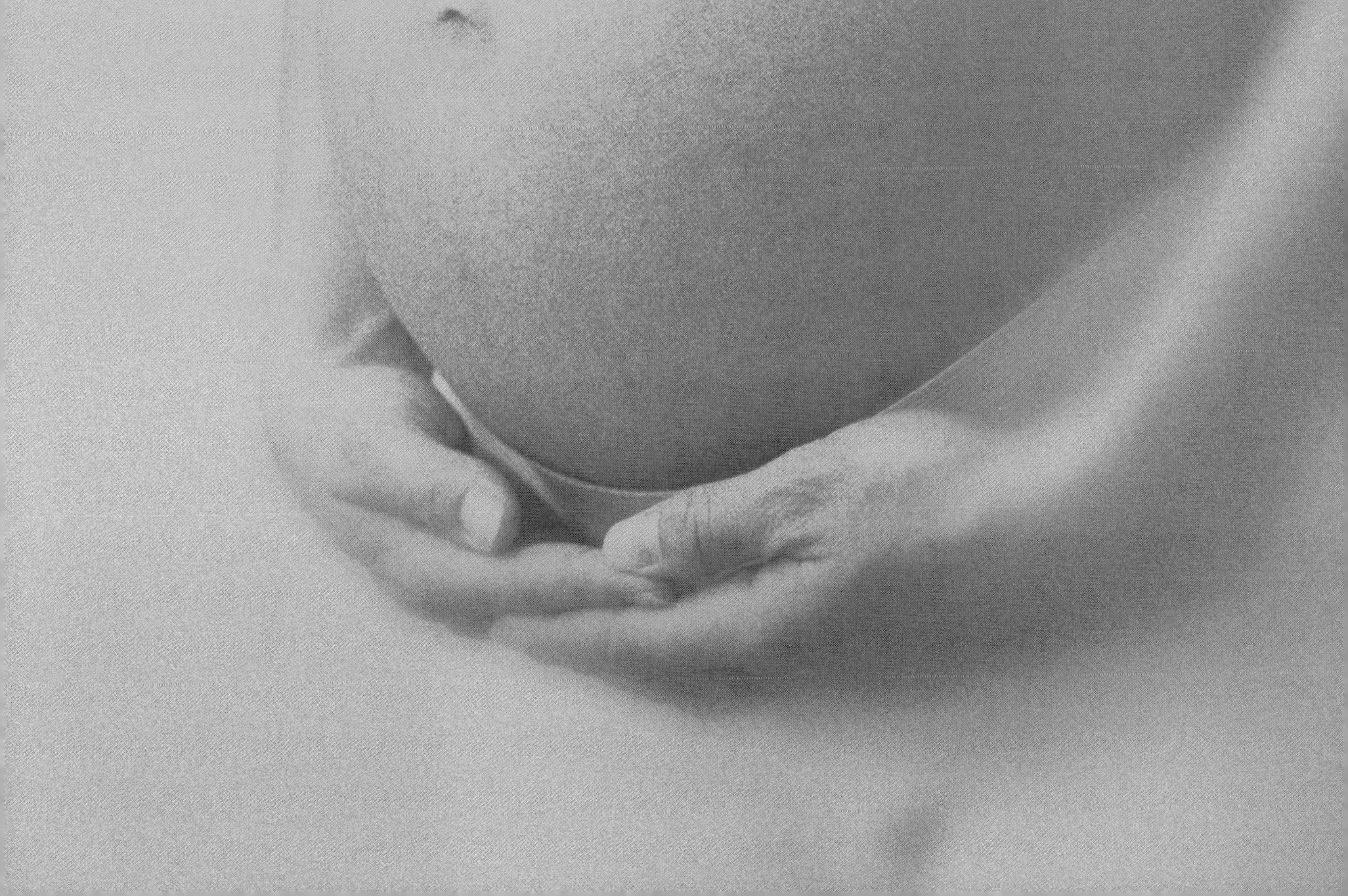

CHAPTER 77

Postpartum Hemorrhage and Other Problems of the Third Stage

Michael S. Rogers / Alan M. Z. Chang

INTRODUCTION

The major cause of maternal death worldwide is hemorrhage. The World Health Organization (WHO) estimated that 25% of 585,000 maternal deaths in 1990 worldwide were due to severe peripartum hemorrhage,[1] with a further 20 million mothers per year suffering significant morbidity from this cause. In developed countries hemorrhage still figures in the top four obstetric causes of maternal mortality, ranking third or fourth after thromboembolism, hypertensive diseases, and amniotic fluid embolism (AFE).

This chapter deals primarily with methods of managing the third stage of labor and the various severe complications that the obstetrician may be faced with, including primary postpartum hemorrhage (PPH), uterine inversion, lower genital tract trauma, uterine rupture, and AFE.

Many complications associated with maternal mortality are preventable and avoidable if rational scientific approaches are taken to management. The 1997–1999 UK Confidential Enquiry[2] concluded that the routine use of national guidelines, developed in part as a result of findings and recommendations from previous reports, had resulted in significant decreases in deaths, and that guidelines had not been followed in the cases in which deaths occurred from these causes. Because most deliveries are rightfully under the control of midwives, it is essential that obstetricians and midwives reach a consensus on the implementation of appropriate management techniques if maternal morbidity and mortality are to be minimized.

THE NORMAL THIRD STAGE OF LABOR

Recognizing the sequence of events in the third stage of labor and understanding the mechanism of placental separation may aid the detection of cases at risk of third-stage complications and the management of pathology.

Prostaglandin F (PGF), $PGF_{2\alpha}$, and oxytocin are the biochemical agents primarily involved in the third stage of labor. During the first and second stages of labor only $PGF_{2\alpha}$ and oxytocin are significantly raised in maternal plasma compared to prelabor concentrations. At 5 minutes after birth, maternal PGF and $PGF_{2\alpha}$ concentrations peak at about twice the levels found at the commencement of the second stage. A rapid increase in prostaglandin concentrations is also found in umbilical cord venous blood, suggesting that this postpartum prostaglandin surge originates in the placenta.[3] After placental separation the concentrations decrease but at rates slower than the metabolic clearance of prostaglandin, indicating that its production continues in the decidua and myometrium. Plasma oxytocin also drops to prelabor levels within 30 minutes of delivery, unless sustained by exogenous infusion.

Continuous real-time ultrasound, performed during the third stage of labor, has revealed that the process of placental separation can be divided into four phases:[4]

1. **Latent**—uterine wall at the placental site remains thin; placenta-free wall contracts
2. **Contraction**—thickening of uterine wall at the placental site
3. **Detachment**—actual separation of the placenta from the adjacent uterine wall
4. **Expulsion**—sliding of the placenta out of the uterine cavity.

Forceful uterine contractions in the latent phase induce shearing forces between the uterine wall and the unyielding placental tissue, initiating the separation of the placenta. A wave of separation begins at one of the placental poles, usually at a point near to the lower segment, and propagates toward the fundus during the contraction and detachment phases.[5] Separation of the fundal placenta begins at more than one of the placental poles, and the central part is last to separate. (This is the reverse of the Schultze and Mathews Duncan mechanisms described in most texts.) In almost half of the cases with a previous cesarean section the separation pattern was reversed, commencing at the fundus, suggesting that myometrial strength in the region of the uterine scar may have been compromised.[5]

Although spontaneous delivery of the placenta usually occurs within 10 minutes of the baby's birth, the third stage is not considered prolonged unless it lasts more than 30 minutes. Combs and Laros,[6] in an 11-year study of 12,979 consecutive, singleton vaginal deliveries, demonstrated that the duration of the third stage followed a log-normal distribution, with a median of 6 minutes (interquartile range, 4 to 10 minutes). The prevalence of a third stage in excess of 30 minutes was 3.3%. Although stating that prophylactic oxytocic agents were not used routinely, their figures for duration are remarkably similar to those from the much larger series (45,869 singleton vaginal deliveries) reported by Dombrowski and colleagues,[7] who estimated that using active management of the third stage, 90% of term placentas will deliver spontaneously by 15 minutes and only 2.2% will be undelivered at 30 minutes. A series of reports from our unit have also confirmed similar third-stage duration, and rates of prolonged third stage associated with different uterotonic agents (oxytocin [Pitocin, Syntocinon]: 1.4% to 1.8%; oxytocin/ergometrine [Syntometrine]: 1.6% to 2.8%; misoprostol [Cytotec]: 1.4%).[8,9,10]

Management Options

There are markedly polarized views between those who believe in active management and those who believe in expectant (natural) management of the third stage.

Active management of the third stage includes:

- Administration of a prophylactic oxytocic agent or prostaglandin within 2 minutes of the baby's birth to induce uterine contraction
- Immediate cutting and clamping of the cord to enhance placental separation
- Placental delivery by controlled cord traction.

In expectant management there is:

- No prophylactic oxytocic
- No cord clamping until pulsations cease
- Delivery of placenta is by maternal effort and gravity rather than cord traction.

Use of Prophylactic Uterotonic Agents

There no longer appears to be any valid argument in favor of the physiologic approach, because two substantive studies comparing active management with expectant management have clearly indicated the advantages of active management. The Bristol trial,[11] where active management had been the norm, and the Hinchingbrooke trial,[12] where expectant management had been the norm, both demonstrated significant reductions in the incidence of PPH with active management compared with expectant management (5.9% versus 17.9% and 6.8% versus 16.5%, respectively). Both studies were terminated after interim analysis because the difference in PPH rate was so great.

Which Uterotonic Agent?

In recent years, considerable attention has been paid to the choice of a uterotonic agent, in particular comparing the cheap and orally administered prostaglandin misoprostol with the combination agent Syntometrine (oxytocin/ergonovine). The findings seem to indicate that rectal misoprostol is a viable alternative to oxytocin in areas where storage and parenteral administration of drugs are problems (oxytocin has to be stored at 4°C to retain its efficacy, whereas tablets of misoprostol kept dry retain their efficacy even at tropical temperatures for several years or more),[13] but its side effects (shivering, nausea, and diarrhea) and slightly lower efficacy make it unsuitable for routine prophylaxis against PPH. Oxytocin (Pitocin) or oxytocin combined with ergometrine (Syntometrine) therefore remain the preferred drugs for routine use in developed countries. Some trials have suggested that oxytocin alone is as efficacious as Syntometrine, whereas others have reported that it is not as effective. Intravenous ergometrine is associated with an increase in the incidence of retained placenta, possibly as a result of myometrial spasm distal to a fundally placed placenta leading to its forced retention, and should not be the agent of choice for routine administration.[14] Ergometrine also causes peripheral vasoconstriction and a rise in blood pressure and should only be given with caution, if at all, to women with hypertension. Oxytocin, on the other hand, when given as an acute bolus, can cause a marked drop in blood pressure. Caution should therefore be exercised when giving oxytocin to women with cardiovascular problems, and a continuous low-dose infusion is probably preferable to bolus injection.

The active and passive management approaches represent the two extremes of the spectrum of common practice. Although the randomized controlled trials performed to date have only compared these two approaches, the benefits of early cord clamping and controlled cord traction in the prevention of PPH have not been established separately from the use of prophylactic uterotonic agents. It is from these two aspects that most criticisms of active management arise.

Timing of Cord Clamping

The umbilical cord can be clamped immediately after birth, clamped after pulsations cease, or left unclamped.

The cord may need to be clamped before birth if there is tight nuchal entanglement. Although early clamping of the cord has been reported to be associated with significant shortening of the third stage, this has only been demonstrated in trials where no prophylactic oxytocin was given.[15,16] The difference in the effects of early versus late cord clamping on the neonate are relatively minor, and opinions differ as to their relative risks and benefits. The deferral of cord clamping until 3 minutes after birth results in a neonatal transfusion of about 80 mL of blood from the placenta.[17] This contributes about 50 mg of iron, which may reduce the frequency of iron-deficiency anemia later in childhood.[18] The theoretical downsides of this blood transfusion are hypervolemia, polycythemia, hyperviscosity, and hyperbilirubinemia. In practice however, these have not been found to produce a clinically relevant increase in neonatal morbidity.[19]

The WHO review of evidence on management of the third stage concludes

> there is no clear evidence to favor one practice over the other. Delaying cord clamping until the pulsations stop is the physiological way of treating the cord and is not associated with adverse effects, at least in normal deliveries. Early cord clamping conflicts with traditional beliefs and is an intervention that needs justification.[20]

In preterm infants, delay in cord clamping has demonstrable benefits and has been shown to decrease the need for blood (P <0.001) and albumin (P <0.03) transfusions during the first 24 hours of life.[21]

Controlled Cord Traction

The use of cord traction has a long history, with the earliest records dating back to Aristotle. Simple cord traction was displaced in the 1800s by the introduction of the Credé maneuver.[22] In this maneuver, the placenta is expelled by downward pressure on the fundus of the uterus in the direction of the birth canal, with the thumb placed on the posterior surface and the flat of the hand on the anterior surface of the fundus. This was proposed as an alternative means to manual removal for expelling the retained placenta and was found to avoid the uterine inversion that was occasionally associated with cord traction. Brandt in 1933 and Andrews in 1940 independently introduced similar methods to improve the use of cord traction to deliver the retained placenta. These involved traction on the cord with countertraction applied to the uterus abdominally. It was not until the 1960s, however, that the modern technique known as *controlled cord traction* was introduced by Spencer,[23] accompanied by the routine administration of ergonovine.

The current consensus is that, when traction is applied to the umbilical cord, it should be done only during a uterine contraction while controlling the uterus by Brandt-Andrews maneuver to prevent uterine inversion. However, it should be noted that the benefits of both early cord clamping and the use of routine controlled cord traction to prevent PPH have not as yet been supported by evidence from randomized controlled trials.

SUMMARY OF MANAGEMENT OPTIONS

Normal Third Stage of Labor

Management Options	Quality of Evidence	Strength of Recommendation	References
Active management of third stage is advised for all women, and includes all the following:	Ia	A	11–13,45
• Administer oxytocic agent (Pitocin (oxytocin) or Syntometrine (oxytocin and ergometrine) more commonly used than misoprostol).	Ib	A	8,13
• Clamp and cut cord.	–	GPP	–
• Use controlled cord traction (no randomized controlled data to show it reduces PPH rates of itself).	III	B	23
Timing of cord clamping			
• No evidence to indicate optimum timing in term delivery.	Ia	A	20
• In preterm infants, delay in clamping may be of benefit.	III	B	21
Ensure intravenous access for women at risk.	–	GPP	–
Save serum for rapid cross-match if needed, or actually cross-match 2 units, for women at risk.	–	GPP	–

RETAINED PLACENTA

Diagnosis and Definition

Using a diagnostic cutoff of 30 minutes for a prolonged third stage, 42% of retained placentas deliver spontaneously within the next 30 minutes,[24] with very few delivering spontaneously after 1 hour.[25] Because the incidence of significant PPH rises after 30 minutes in the third stage,[6] it therefore seems logical to institute some form of active intervention in an attempt to deliver the placenta between 30 and 60 minutes into the third stage. Dombrowski and colleagues[7] noted that, compared with term pregnancies, the frequency of retained placenta (2.0% overall) was markedly increased among very preterm (gestation <27 weeks) and preterm pregnancies (gestation <37 weeks), with odds ratios of 20.8 and 3.0, respectively.

Management Options

Manual removal appears to be the management of choice for retained placenta. However, it is associated with a risk of infection (endometritis) and trauma (perforation of the uterine wall involved with the procedure). Ely and colleagues,[26] in a retrospective study of 1052 manual removals, found that clinical endometritis developed in 6.7% of cases compared with only 1.8% following spontaneous placental delivery.

In some studies, manual removal appears to be aggressively pursued, with rates exceeding 3% and often performed only 15 to 20 minutes into the third stage. The rate generally quoted internationally is 1% to 2%.

In the absence of hemorrhage there is no urgency to resort to manual removal when less invasive alternatives are available.

Patients with a prolonged third stage are often treated as a homogeneous group, although they have different clinical conditions. These include the retention of an already detached placenta (trapped placenta), an adherent placenta, and placenta accreta. Each condition should be distinguished from the others, and each requires a specific clinical approach. Herman[27] notes that each of these conditions is associated with a different sonographic appearance, and concludes that "proper utilization of ultrasound may be crucial for optimal management."

Trapped Placenta

Trapped placenta often follows the intravenous administration of ergometrine when the onset of uterine contraction is very rapid. This tends to close the cervix at the same time as the placental detachment occurs, trapping the placenta. Intramuscular injection of ergometrine results in the onset of uterine contraction in 10 minutes, which is likely to follow rather than precede placental separation, so trapped placenta is less likely to occur. The clinical findings of a trapped placenta include a small, contracted fundus, with some vaginal bleeding and cord lengthening indicative of placental separation, and the placental margin may be palpable through the closed cervical os. On ultrasound examination the entire myometrium is thickened and a clear demarcation may be seen between it and the placenta.[4]

Delivery of a trapped placenta can usually be achieved using controlled cord traction, which encourages cervical dilation. Intravenous glyceryl trinitrate (100 to 200 μg) is useful as a short-term tocolytic agent, appears efficacious and safe, and may obviate the need for general anesthesia for uterine relaxation.[28] Releasing the cord clamp, to allow blood trapped in the placenta to drain, may also help.

Adherent Placenta

With an adherent placenta, the uterine fundus remains broad and high and myometrial contractions may be weak or absent, but there is no bleeding while the placenta remains wholly attached. Adherent placenta is caused by a deficiency in the contractile force exerted by the myometrium underlying the placental site despite normal anatomy (i.e., it is not caused by pathologic invasion of the placenta into the uterine muscle, known as *placenta accreta*). On ultrasound the myometrium appears thick and contracted in all areas, except where the placenta remains attached, and the uterine wall remains less than 2 cm in thickness.[4] If the placenta becomes partly separated the myometrium over the detached area appears thicker, but that underlying the adherent part remains thin (<2 cm).[4] Detachment usually starts in the lower part of the uterus and is associated with bleeding from the placental bed.[5] Treatment options depend on the amount of bleeding:

- In the absence of bleeding, a conservative approach can be adopted and manual removal of the placenta can be postponed while the problem is investigated (by ultrasound).
- Where there is active bleeding, immediate active management is necessary.

Effective treatment of the adherent placenta is based on stimulating a contraction of the underlying myometrium that has sufficient strength to induce separation of the placenta. Oxytocin, ergonovine, and misoprostol are all capable of inducing sustained myometrial contractions. However, there is no evidence that systemic and repeated administration of either oxytocics or prostaglandins is able to assist in the delivery of the adherent placenta.

Recent studies have shown that uterotonic agents administered via umbilical vein injection may be effective in causing the adherent placenta to separate, and this method is currently recommended as the first line of treatment by the WHO.[29]

The Pipingas technique has been shown effective in delivering drugs to the placental bed.[30] A size 10 nasogastric tube is passed along the umbilical vein until resistance is felt, then retracted about 5 cm, and prostaglandin $F_{2\alpha}$ (20 mg diluted in 20 mL of normal saline) or oxytocin (30 IU diluted in 20 mL of normal saline) is injected through the catheter.[31]

SUMMARY OF MANAGEMENT OPTIONS

Retained Placenta

Management Options	Quality of Evidence	Strength of Recommendation	References
Retained placenta should be diagnosed if it is not delivered within 30–60 minutes.	III	B	24, 25
Trapped Placenta			
• Perform ultrasound to confirm separation.	III	B	4
• Use controlled cord traction with a short-acting tocolytic such as glyceryl (rinitrate)	III	B	28
Adherent Placenta			
• If there is active bleeding, manual removal is necessary.	–	GPP	–
• If there is no active bleeding, consider intraumbilical uterotonic agents before resorting to manual removal.	III	B	29–31

ADHERENT PLACENTA (PLACENTA ACCRETA, INCRETA, PERCRETA)

Placenta accreta is a condition in which all or part of the placenta is adherent to the uterine wall because of myometrial invasion by chorionic villi. It may occur when there is either a primary deficiency of, or secondary damage to, the decidua basalis.

Three grades are defined according to the depth of myometrial invasion:

- Accreta—chorionic villi are in contact with the myometrium, rather than being contained within the decidua (80% of cases)
- Increta—extensive villous invasion into the myometrium (15% of cases)
- Percreta—villous invasion extends to (or through) the serosal covering of the uterus (5% of cases).

Placenta accreta was previously reported to be rare (1 in 30,000 deliveries between 1930 and 1950), but the prevalence has risen considerably (1 in 2500 deliveries),[25] a rise attributed to the rise in cesarean section rates. All three grades of placenta accreta are most commonly found in patients with a history of uterine surgery, principally cesarean section, with the probability of placenta previa being accreta rising as high as 67% after four cesarean sections.[32] Placenta accreta is associated both with placenta previa and advanced maternal age. This close association with both previous cesarean section and placenta previa means that placenta accreta rarely complicates vaginal delivery. In fact, in the series reported by Miller and colleagues,[33] 55 of the 62 cases were associated with placenta previa and all were delivered by cesarean section. The rate of placenta accreta was therefore only 1 in 22,000 in the absence of placenta previa. Rarely, abnormal attachment is seen in the absence of prior surgery (e.g., associated with Ascherman syndrome and submucous fibroids). Interestingly, the adherence is not necessarily over the site of the previous scar.

All three grades of placenta accreta can result in profuse postpartum hemorrhage due to incomplete separation of the placenta. Being alert to this possibility is essential in patients who have a combination of placenta previa and a history of previous uterine surgery. If the diagnosis of placenta accreta can be confirmed, plans for delivery by cesarean section by a surgeon experienced in dealing with such cases, and in a facility where resuscitation and intensive care are available, should be made.

Diagnosis

The diagnosis of placenta accreta can be made using color flow Doppler ultrasound as early as the second trimester. Typical features of a placenta accreta include the following:[27]

- The normal hypo-echoic boundary between the placenta and the urinary bladder or serosa is lost.
- The placenta appears to be contiguous with the bladder wall.
- Sonolucent spaces are visible within the placenta, adjacent to the uterine wall.
- Color Doppler reveals persistent blood flow between the basal placenta and the myometrium.[34]

A thickness of myometrial involvement greater than 1 mm, accompanied by the presence of large placental lakes, can predict myometrial invasion with a sensitivity of 100% and specificity of 72%.[35] Magnetic resonance imaging may be useful in the presence of a posterior placenta and for assessing deep myometrial, parametrial, and bladder involvement, or when the ultrasound findings are equivocal.[36]

Management Options

Attempts to physically remove an accretic placenta may lead to severe and uncontrollable hemorrhage. If the diagnosis can be made before delivery, the following options can be considered:

- Scan the uterus intraoperatively using an ultrasound transducer in a sterile sleeve, placing the transducer directly onto the uterus to obtain a detailed view. This enables delineation of the placental attachment. The baby can then be delivered through an incision designed to avoid the placenta (this may need to be fundal or deviated to one side or the other, avoiding the vessels in the broad ligament). The placenta can then be left in situ and its degeneration followed by weekly serum β-human chorionic gonadotropin (β-hCG) measurements and ultrasound evaluation of placental bed vascularity. Remnants can be removed manually or by curettage when β-hCG levels become undetectable and placental blood flow is no longer seen on ultrasound.[37] This is usually successful in avoiding the need for further intervention, but major secondary postpartum hemorrhage can still occur, and occasionally hysterectomy is required.
- If the placenta is left in situ, treatment with methotrexate (50 mg IV on alternate days with folinic acid rescue) may speed degeneration of the placenta and resorption of persisting chorionic villi.[38]
- Elective cesarean hysterectomy may be required as a definitive therapy, and it can be the management of choice if the woman has completed her family.

If a placenta accreta is diagnosed before delivery, the following issues should be considered:

- General anesthesia is probably wise, because it can be difficult to cope with major blood loss while the patient is awake. However, placement of an epidural catheter preoperatively is useful to achieve postoperative pain control.
- It may be useful to pass a nasogastric tube.
- An arterial line for detailed intrapartum blood pressure monitoring should be inserted.
- Insertion of a central venous pressure monitoring line is also wise, and the use of a Swan-Ganz catheter can be considered if facilities are available.
- Calf compressors can be used to minimize the risk of deep vein thrombosis during prolonged surgery, and subcutaneous heparin postsurgery should also be considered.
- Involvement of urologists and vascular surgeons may be necessary. Cystoscopy prelaparotomy can be useful to check for any bladder invasion by the placenta.
- Preparations for major blood transfusion should be made in conjunction with the hematology department.

There are occasions when conservation of the uterus is desired by the patient; in such cases an attempt to avoid hysterectomy can be made. However, only a few cases using this more conservative management have been reported, and hemorrhage and infection are common complications. The cesarean hysterectomy rate is much higher for placenta accreta (>50%) than for placenta previa alone (2%). Although mortality for placenta accreta is now uncommon,[25] morbidity remains high; consequently peripartum hysterectomy remains the current treatment of choice in most cases.

The more usual presentation is discovery of a partially accretic placenta during cesarean section. Hemostasis may be achieved if the accretic area is not too extensive, by placing sutures deep into the myometrial bed using a multiple 3-cm square suturing pattern over the area of maximal bleeding: Cho and colleagues[39] reported successful use of this technique in 23 cases of refractory bleeding with apparently normal uterine cavities on follow-up evaluation.

Other methods have been attempted but hysterectomy is often required, particularly when the bleeding site is from the lower uterine segment.[40]

SUMMARY OF MANAGEMENT OPTIONS
Placenta Accreta

Management Options	Quality of Evidence	Strength of Recommendation	References
Diagnosis of problem is difficult, but real-time ultrasound, color Doppler, and MRI in advance of labor/delivery may help.	III	B	34–36
Ensure intravenous access and resuscitation.	–	GPP	–
Options for treatment:			
• Leave in situ and monitor provided no PPH.	III	B	37
• Administer methotrexate.	III	B	38
• Perform curettage once β-HCG levels become undetectable.	III	B	103
• Removal manually.	III	B	103

SUMMARY OF MANAGEMENT OPTIONS

Placenta Accreta *(Continued)*

Management Options	Quality of Evidence	Strength of Recommendation	References
• Perform hysterectomy.	III	B	103
• Others include oversewing implantation site, resection of implantation site, stepwise uterine devascularization.	III	B	103
Treat any associated uterine atony as described under Primary Postpartum Hemorrhage.	–	GPP	–

CONCLUSIONS

- Prophylactic uterotonics reduce the incidence and severity of PPH, but have limited effects on the actual duration of the third stage of labor; thus, a prophylactic uterotonic agent should be administered to all mothers, with the choice of the agent depending on the clinical situation and on its availability.
- If delivery can be achieved without clamping and cutting of the umbilical cord, this can be delayed until cord pulsation ceases (this will usually occur within 1 to 3 minutes of birth). In the meantime, resuscitation of the newborn can be attended to.
- When clinical signs of separation are present (uterine fundus contracted and palpable above the umbilicus, a show of blood seen vaginally and the umbilical cord lengthens), the placenta is either in the lower uterine segment or in the vagina. Placental expulsion can be achieved by maternal effort or by gentle controlled cord traction, after ensuring the uterus is contracted. In the absence of bleeding, there is no immediate need for active measures, and it is appropriate to wait for up to 30 minutes for the placenta to separate.
- If spontaneous placental separation does not occur within 30 minutes and there is no bleeding, there is no need for immediate active management. However, the uterus should be examined frequently to ensure there is no undetected bleeding, and an ultrasound examination of the placental site may be beneficial in distinguishing the stage of separation and the possible cause of delay, providing a rational basis for further management (Table 77–1). Sublingual glyceryl trinitrate can be given for the "trapped" placenta. In both preterm and term pregnancies with adherent placenta, separation may be achieved by the injection of 20 to 30 mL of oxytocin or prostaglandin solution into the placental bed via an infant nasogastric tube threaded down the umbilical vein. Failure of this technique should alert the clinician that placenta accreta may be present.[41]
- If bleeding is suspected or seen, a systemic uterotonic (oxytocin 10 IU intravenously, Hemabate 250 μg intramuscularly, or misoprostol 1000 μg per rectum) should be given while arrangements are made for manual removal of the placenta (Fig. 77–1) or for transfer of the patient to another facility if appropriate.

PRIMARY POSTPARTUM HEMORRHAGE

Definition

Primary (early) PPH refers to excessive blood loss (>500 mL) during the third stage of labor or in the first 24 hours after delivery; thereafter, significant bleeding is referred to as secondary (late) PPH. Secondary PPH is discussed in detail in Chapter 78.

Significance

In the absence of anemia, blood loss up to 500 mL can be considered physiologic (i.e., within normal limits) and is unlikely to lead to cardiovascular compromise. For those who already have severe anemia (<5 g/dL), this amount of blood loss may induce heart failure or cardiovascular collapse.[42]

Maternal deaths due to obstetric hemorrhage are often associated with substandard care.[2,43] Accurate estimation of blood loss, prompt recognition and treatment of clotting disorders, early involvement of experienced clinicians, availability of anesthetic support, appropriate fluid replacement, and adequate physiologic monitoring are factors that govern maternal survival.

Etiology

Approximately 80% to 90% of cases of primary PPH are associated with uterine atony. However, a combination of

TABLE 77–1

Summary of Clinical and Ultrasound Findings at Different Stages of Placental Separation and Recommendations for Management

	STAGE OF PLACENTAL SEPARATION			
	FULLY ADHERENT	PARTIALLY SEPARATED	FULLY SEPARATED: TRAPPED	FULLY SEPARATED: NORMAL
Clinical Signs				
Duration third stage		>30 minutes		< 30 minutes
Uterine fundus	Above umbilicus			Below umbilicus
Uterus	Broad	Broad	Small, contracted	Small, contracted
Cord lengthening	No	No	Sometimes	Yes
Bleeding	No	Yes	Yes	Yes
Ultrasound Appearance				
Myometrium (placental site)	<2 cm thick across entire placental site	<2 cm thick at fundus >2 cm at lower pole	<2 cm thick at all levels; surrounding placenta	>2 cm thick at all levels; above placenta
Placental position	Upper segment	Upper segment	Upper segment	Lower segment or vagina
Doppler flow (myometrium-placenta)	Present	Absent	Absent	
Management				
Initial: 30–60 minutes	Expectant	Hemabate 250 μg IM; misoprostol 1000 μg PR	Controlled cord traction; glyceryl trinitrate	Maternal effort; gentle controlled cord traction
>60 minutes	Umbilical vein uterotonic	Manual removal	Manual removal	
Failed	Methotrexate/ hysterectomy	Hysterectomy		

improvements in drug therapy for uterine atony and increased cesarean section rates in developed countries have resulted in uterine atony often taking second place to placenta accreta as a cause of morbidity.[44] Less common causes of PPH are upper (uterus, cervix) and lower (vagina, perineum) genital tract trauma, uterine inversion, retained placental tissue, and disseminated intravascular coagulation (DIC).

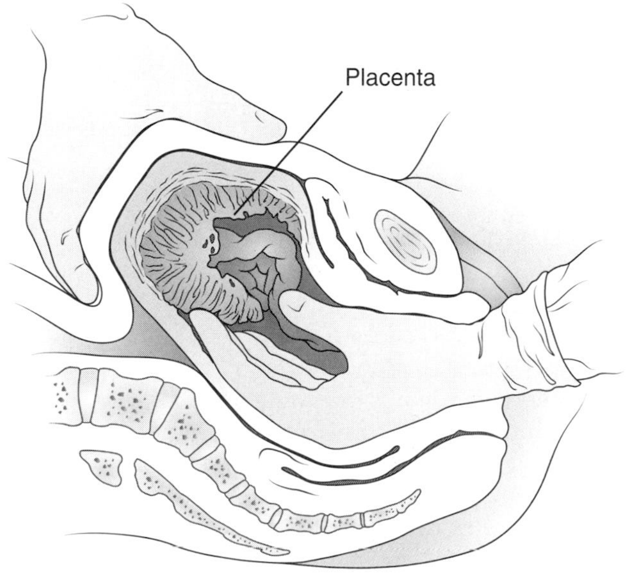

FIGURE 77–1
Manual removal of placenta. The fingers are moved from side to side until the placenta is completely detached. Reproduced with permission from Cunningham FG, MacDonald PC, Gant NF: Williams Obstetrics, 18th ed. Norwalk, Conn, Appleton & Lange, 1989.

Management Options

Prevention

Major reductions in the frequency and severity of PPH have followed the adoption of routine prophylactic administration of oxytocics in the management of the third stage.[45] This consists of injections of synthetic oxytocin, methylergometrine, or a combination of the two (Syntometrine) with crowning of the head, delivery of the baby's anterior shoulder, or immediately after delivery.

In high risk situations (multiple pregnancy, obstructed labor, or manual removal of the placenta), prophylaxis may be extended by the infusion of 40 units oxytocin in 500 mL Hartmann's solution over 4 hours. However, the effectiveness of this has not yet been proven by randomized controlled trial, and many of those delivered by emergency cesarean section show evidence of loss of myometrial oxytocin receptors, reflected by a decrease in binding sites and very low mRNA concentrations.[46]

Treatment

The management of primary PPH will depend on the presence of risk factors and the probable cause. For example (Table 77–2), uterine atony may follow

TABLE 77–2

Summary of Risk Factors, Clinical Findings, and Recommendations for Management for the Major Causes of Primary PPH

RISK FACTORS	CLINICAL FINDINGS	DIAGNOSIS	INITIAL ACTION	SECOND-LINE
Obstructed labor Multiple pregnancy, polyhdramnios Tocolytics	Soft, relaxed uterus	Uterine atony	Massage/compression Repeat oxytocin, either systemic or intramyometrial	Hemabate 250 μg, either systemic or intramyometrial
Obstructed labor Fetal distress Difficult or rotational forceps delivery PROM	Contracted uterus	Uterine rupture	Repair rupture if possible	Hysterectomy
Delayed second stage Ventouse/forceps delivery Precipitate labor	Contracted uterus	Cervical/vaginal tear	Repair tears	Vaginal tamponade
Retained placenta	Fundus not palpable abdominally	Uterine inversion	Reduce inversion by manual or hydrostatic pressure; tocolysis if necessary	Hysterectomy
Retained placenta	Fundus palpable	Retained products	Uterine exploration/ curettage	Hysterectomy
Amniotic fluid embolism	Contracted uterus	Disseminated intravascular coagulation	Fresh frozen plasma, fresh whole blood transfusion	Heparin
Placental abruption	Bleeding from IV site or sutures			
Fulminating preeclampsia				

obstructed labor, multiple pregnancy, or polyhydramnios, in which the myometrium is overexerted or overstretched.

Where primary PPH is caused by failure of the uterus to contract, the condition is easily recognized by the soft relaxed uterus. Bimanual compression and abdominal massage will usually stimulate a contraction and stop the bleeding, although bleeding may resume as soon as such stimulation is stopped (Fig. 77–2). For this reason uterotonic agents such as oxytocin or Syntometrine and prostaglandins such as Hemabate or misoprostol should also be administered to achieve a longer period of myometrial contraction, allowing clotting mechanisms to become fully activated. Because the immediate administration of these agents is essential, it is important that front-line staff, such as midwives or traditional birth attendants, are empowered to do so on their own initiative.

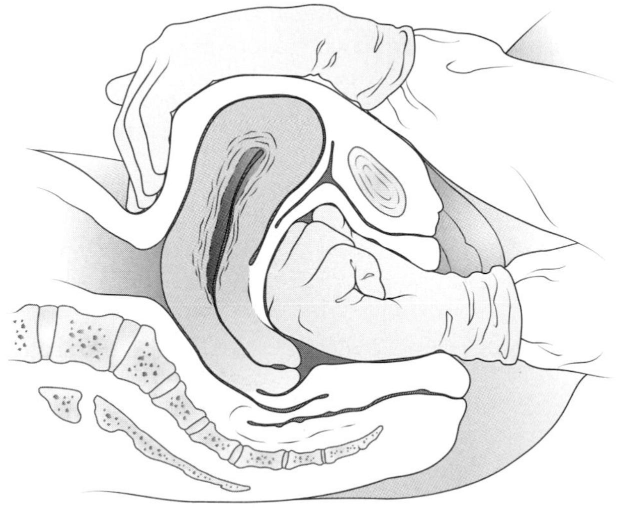

FIGURE 77–2
Bimanual compression of the uterus and massage with abdominal hand will usually effectively control hemorrhage from uterine atony. Reproduced with permission from Cunningham FG, MacDonald PC, Gant NF: Williams Obstetrics, 18th ed. Norwalk, Conn, Appleton & Lange, 1989.

If bleeding continues despite adequate uterine contraction, exploration of the genital tract is necessary to detect other causes such as trauma (uterine, cervical, or vaginal tears) or retained placental tissue, particularly in cases where risk factors were present (i.e., obstructed labor, fetal distress, difficult operative delivery, manual removal of placenta).

In the event that these measures fail to control bleeding, hysterectomy may be resorted to as a life-saving procedure. However, as with placenta accreta, there will be occasions when conservation of the uterus is important to the patient, and alternative therapies may be attempted.

Bilateral internal iliac artery ligation (Fig. 77–3) may reduce the pulse pressure and allow the normal coagulation mechanism to engage,[47] but the procedure is technically difficult during pregnancy and has a poor success rate (less than 50% success).[48] Waters[49] proposed the alternative of bilateral uterine artery ligation (Fig.77–4); reported success rates for this procedure vary between 80% and 96%.[50] AbdRabbo[51] subsequently reported a 100% success rate by also ligating the ovarian vessels where uterine artery ligation alone was unsuccessful (Fig. 77–5).

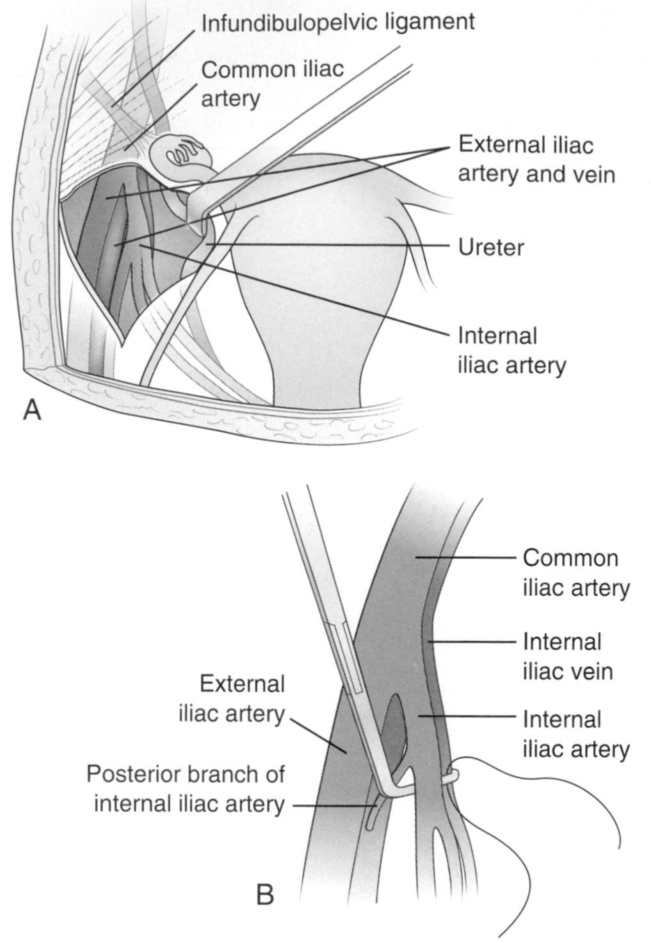

FIGURE 77–3
Operative technique of internal iliac artery ligation. *A*, The retroperitoneal space over the right internal and external iliac vessels has been opened and the ureter retracted medially. *B*, A right-angled clamp is passed between the iliac artery and vein to receive a ligature of number 0 silk. The vessel should be doubly ligated. Reproduced with permission from Pauerstein C: Clinical Obstetrics. New York, Wiley, 1987.

Arterial embolization is highly effective (>95% success)[52] but requires time and specialized facilities to carry out. When the situation is urgent, uterine tamponade can be achieved either by packing the uterine cavity[53] or applying uterine compression sutures such as those described by B-Lynch.[54] In their simplest form, compression sutures are the insertion of absorbable sutures (e.g., Dexon) from the front to the back of the uterus through the lower segment about 1 cm above the cervix and about 2 cm medial to the uterine artery on each side.[55] These are then tied over the top of the uterus, compressing the uterine body (the loose ends can be tied together at the top to prevent the sutures slipping down the side) (Figs. 77–6 to 77–9). Lower segment bleeding from placenta previa or accreta may respond to sutures placed deep into the myometrial bed.

If compression sutures on their own are insufficient or a laparotomy has not yet been performed, another useful technique is to inflate a sterile saline-filled balloon inside the uterine cavity[56-58] (e.g., the Rusch balloon or Cook's

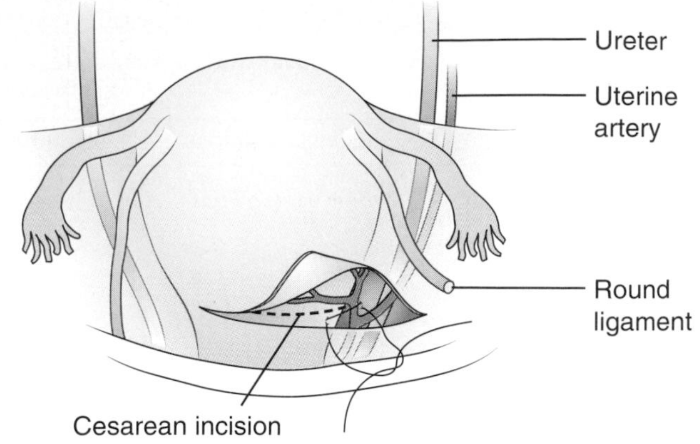

FIGURE 77–4
Operative technique for uterine artery ligation. The vesicouterine fold of peritoneum has been incised transversely and the bladder mobilized inferiorly. A number 1 chromic catgut suture on a large smooth needle has been placed through the avascular space of the broad ligament and through the uterus. The suture includes the uterine vessels and several centimeters of myometrium. Reproduced with permission from Pauerstein C: Clinical Obstetrics. New York, Wiley, 1987.

balloon; see Fig. 77–10). Some types can be inflated with up to 500 mL of sterile saline. This type of tamponade can also be used to arrest bleeding from extensive vaginal lacerations and can even be used to stem bleeding in the pelvis following hysterectomy (the tube used to inflate the balloon is passed through the vagina, and then traction toward the feet is applied to maintain pressure within the pelvic cavity[59]; see Fig. 77–11).

Finally, DIC may complicate any situation in which coagulation factors are exhausted, such as in severe preeclampsia, placental abruption, AFE, or protracted hemorrhage.

While measures are being taken to control obstetric hemorrhage, the patient will require transfusion with adequate volumes of whole blood and/or blood substitutes to maintain blood volume and tissue perfusion. In facilities where cross-matched blood is not readily avail-

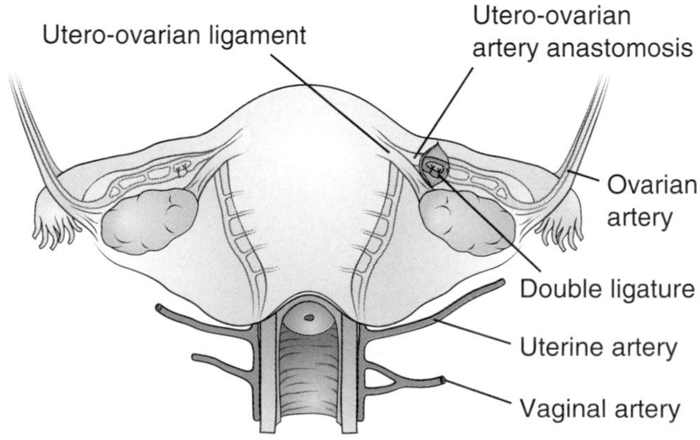

FIGURE 77–5
Area for ovarian artery ligation. Two free ties of 2–0 silk suture are used to ligate the ovarian artery bilaterally near its anastomosis with the uterine artery. An avascular area of mesovarium near the junction of the utero-ovarian ligament with the ovary is the site chosen. Reproduced with permission from Pauerstein C: Clinical Obstetrics. New York, Wiley, 1987.

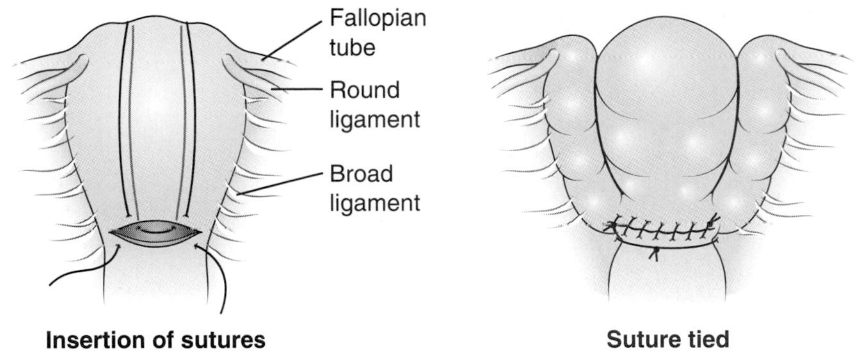

FIGURE 77–6
The B-Lynch suture for the control of massive postpartum hemorrhage. From B-Lynch C, Coker A, Lawal AH, et al: The B-Lynch surgical technique for the control of massive postpartum hemorrhage: An alternative to hysterectomy? Five cases reported. BJOG 1997;104:372–375.

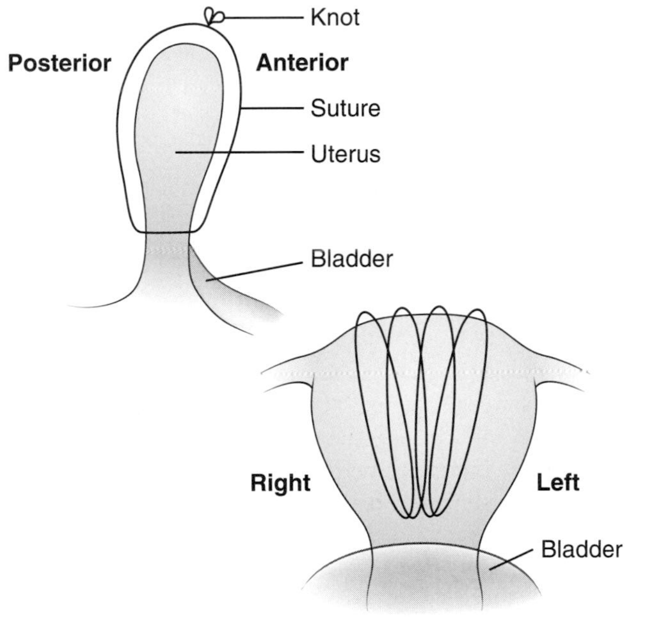

FIGURE 77–7
Simplified uterine compression sutures. From Hayman RG, Arulkumaran S, Steer PJ: Uterine compression sutures: Surgical management of postpartum hemorrhage. Obstet Gynecol 2002;99:502–506.

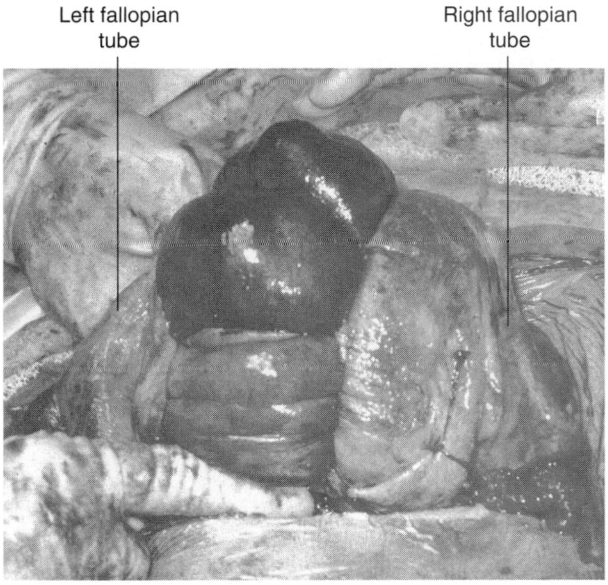

FIGURE 77–9
Posterior view of compression sutures. (see Color Plate 60) From Hayman RG, Arulkumaran S, Steer PJ: Uterine compression sutures: Surgical management of postpartum hemorrhage. Obstet Gynecol 2002;99:502–506.

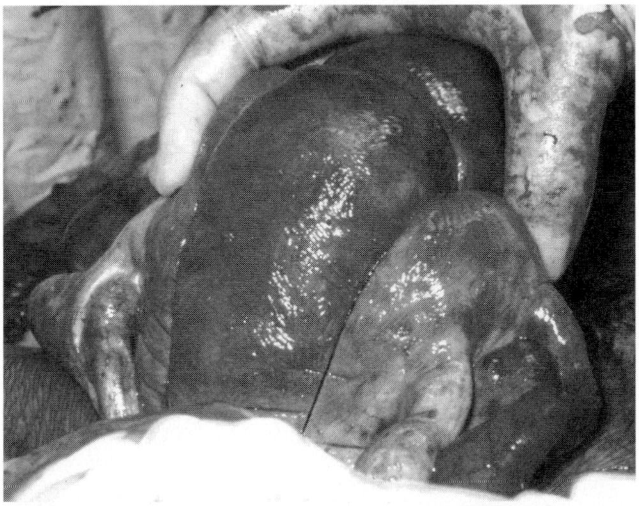

FIGURE 77–8
Anterior view of compression sutures. From Hayman RG, Arulkumaran S, Steer PJ: Uterine compression sutures: Surgical management of postpartum hemorrhage. Obstet Gynecol 2002;99:502–506.

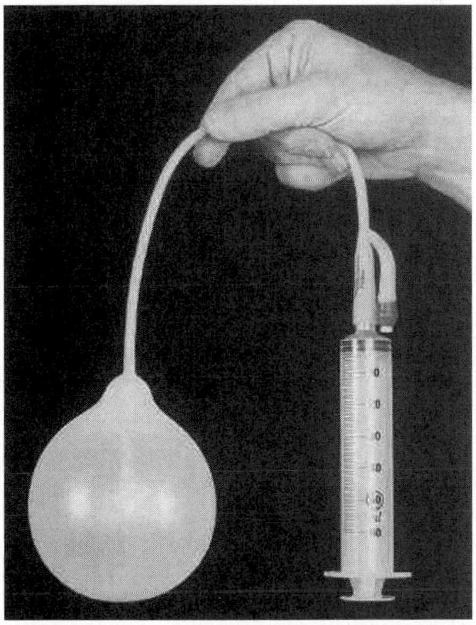

FIGURE 77–10
Example of a balloon used for intrauterine tamponade. From Johanson R, Kumar M, Obhrai M, Young P: Management of massive postpartum haemorrhage: Use of a hydrostatic balloon catheter to avoid caparotomy. BJOG 2001;108:420–422.

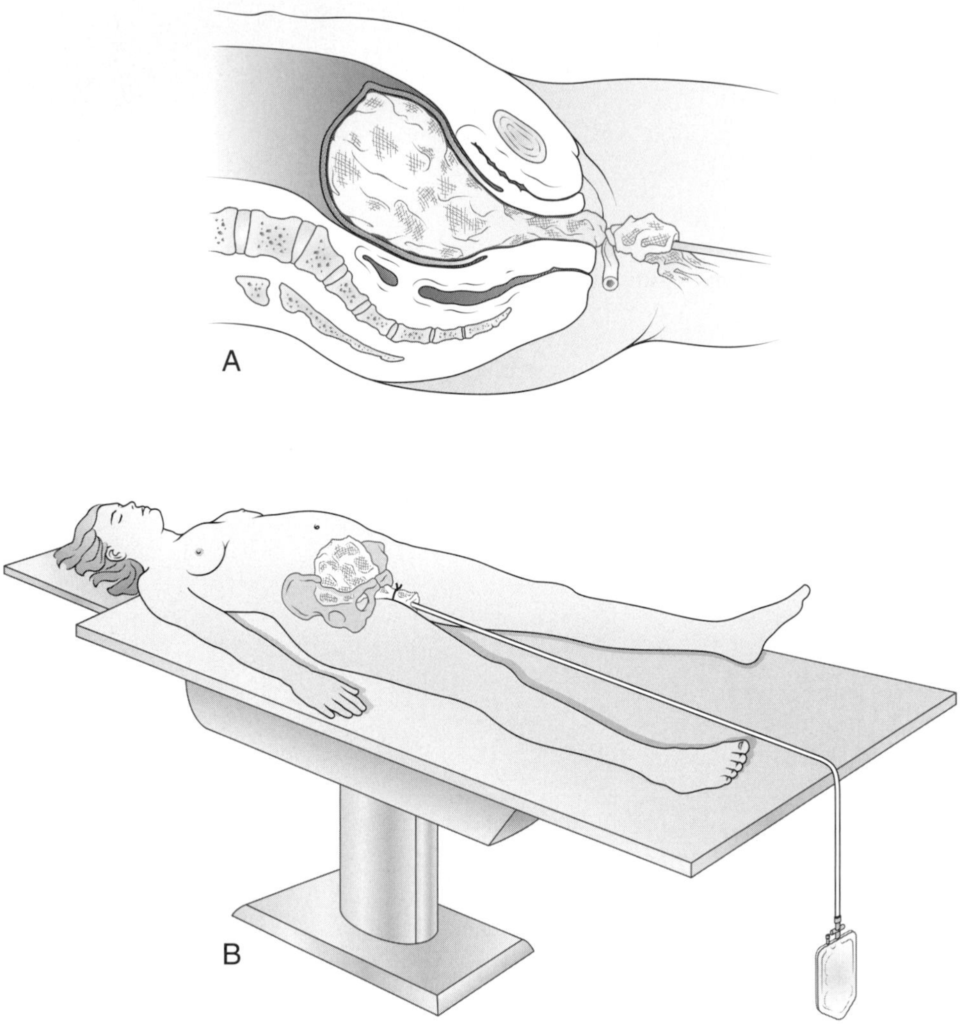

FIGURE 77–11
Use of pelvic tamponade, in this case a Logothetopulos pack. From Robie GF, Morgan MA, Payne GGJ, Wasemiller-Smith L: Logothetopulos pack for the management of uncontrollable postpartum hemorrhage. Am J Perinatol 1990;7:327–328.

able, autologous autotransfusion may be considered. The Cell Saver is an autotransfusion device that collects blood from the operative site using an anticoagulated suction device, separates red blood cells from contaminants by filtration and differential centrifugation, and re-infuses them into the patient. The process appears to be effective in removing fetal and amniotic debris and has not been reported to be complicated by infection, AFE, or DIC.[60]

SUMMARY OF MANAGEMENT OPTIONS

Primary Postpartum Hemorrhage

Management Options	Quality of Evidence	Strength of Recommendation	References
Prevention			
Active management of third stage advised for all women, comprising all the following:	Ia	A	11–13,45
• Administer oxytocic agent (Oxytocin or Syntometrine more commonly used than misoprostol).	Ib	A	8,13
• Clamp and cut cord.	–	GPP	–
• Use controlled cord traction (no randomized controlled data to show that it reduces PPH rates).	III	B	23
No evidence that oxytocin infusion in high risk settings improves outcome.	III	B	104

SUMMARY OF MANAGEMENT OPTIONS

Primary Postpartum Hemorrhage *(Continued)*

Management Options	Quality of Evidence	Strength of Recommendation	References
Treatment			
Initial emergency measures:	–	GPP	–
• Rub-up contraction.			
• Administer intravenous oxytocin (5–10 units) (ergometrine 0.25–0.5 mg i.m. an alternative but should be avoided in hypertensive patients).			
• Establish intravenous access.			
• Cross-match blood.			
General management options for major obstetric hemorrhage	See Chapter 79		
Specific measures:			
• Examine uterus to confirm atony is cause.	–	GPP	–
• Confirm placenta appears intact or perform uterine exploration and removal of placental fragments if suspicion of incomplete third stage.	–	GPP	–
• Bimanual compression is a temporary measure.	–	GPP	–
• Commence i.v. oxytocin infusion.	III	B	104
• Give further i.v. bolus of oxytocin.	III	B	104
• Rule out trauma to vagina, cervix, or uterus.	–	GPP	–
• Use uterine packing or balloon tamponade.	III	B	53,56–58
• Prostaglandin options include:			
• 15-methyl-PGFa (0.25 mg) i.m. or $PGF_{2\alpha}$ (0.5–1.0 mg) into uterine muscle	III	B	105
• Rectal misoprostol 1000μg	III, Ib	B, A	106
• Use B-Lynch sutures or simpler alternatives.	III	B	54,55
• Perform arterial embolization if units have resources and experience.	III	B	52
• Perform bilateral uterine artery ligation.	III	B	50
• Perform bilateral internal iliac artery ligation.	III	B	47
• Perform bilateral ovarian artery ligation.	III	B	51
• Perform hysterectomy.	III	B	107
• Consider Cell Saver.	III	B	60

UTERINE INVERSION

Definition

The uterus is partially (first-degree) or completely (second- and third-degree) turned inside out. Second-degree inversion refers to cases in which the fundus has passed through the cervix but not outside the vagina.

Etiology

Inversion of the uterus is principally a complication of the third stage of labor, and the most common cause is traction applied to the umbilical cord while the uterus is relaxed. The institution of active management of the third stage of labor is associated with a fourfold decrease in the incidence of acute uterine inversion following vaginal delivery.[61] In a case in which the placenta is adherent or accretic, the thin and relaxed myometrium is prone to inversion when traction is applied.[62] This is particularly so if the placenta is fundally situated, because there is direct traction on the central portion of the noncontracted muscle.[50]

Diagnosis

Uterine inversion is often associated with acute lower abdominal pain and profound shock of neurogenic and hemorrhagic origin. The shock is often out of proportion to the degree of blood loss, although if the placenta remains attached following inversion shock is less likely to occur. Bimanual examination will confirm the diagnosis and also reveal the degree of inversion.

Management Options

Once inversion is recognized, oxytocin should be withheld until correction has been established. If puerperal inversion of the uterus is recognized immediately, the uterine corpus can usually be pushed back through the cervical ring, by pressure directed toward the umbilicus, either manually (Johnson maneuver)[63] or by hydrostatic pressure[64] (Fig. 77-12). Tocolysis with beta-mimetics or magnesium sulfate may facilitate the procedure, although glyceryl trinitrate is unlikely to prove effective unless the placenta is still in situ.[65] When reduction under tocolysis fails, general anesthesia with halothane may be induced to provide uterine relaxation and reduction attempted again, although hysterectomy will frequently be indicated. Tews and colleagues have recently reported a new abdominal, uterus-preserving approach for such cases.[66] At laparotomy, the bladder is dissected off the cervix and the vagina entered by a longitudinal incision. Two fingers are advanced through this incision, above the invaginated uterine body and, exerting counterpressure with the other hand, the inversion can be reversed. Uterotonic drugs are then given immediately to maintain uterine contraction and to prevent reinversion.

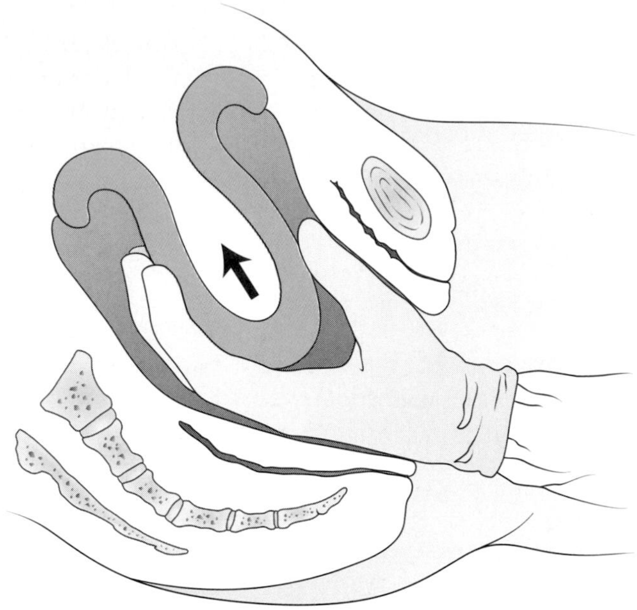

FIGURE 77–12
Manual replacement of uterine inversion. Reproduced with permission from Baskett TF: Essential Management of Obstetric Emergencies. Chichester, UK, Wiley, 1985.

SUMMARY OF MANAGEMENT OPTIONS
Uterine Inversion

Management Options	Quality of Evidence	Strength of Recommendation	References
Prompt recognition and treatment are keys to successful outcome.	III	B	61, 63
Provide intravenous access and resuscitation.	III	B	61, 63
Options for treatment:			
• Manual replacement (with or without a general anesthetic	III	B	62
and/or tocolytics)	III	B	64, 65
• Hydrostatic replacement	III	B	64
• Laparotomy and correction "from above"	III	B	66
Uterotonic drugs may be given after correction.	–	GPP	–

UTERINE RUPTURE

Definition

Uterine rupture (full-thickness tear through myometrium and serosa) is an uncommon obstetric complication, which may occur in a previously intact uterus or in one with a previous cesarean or myomectomy scar. Different terms are sometimes used to describe partial separation (dehiscence) or healing defects (windows) of uterine scars.

Etiology

The approximate incidence of uterine rupture is 0.05%[67] to 0.086%[68] of all pregnancies. Changes in obstetric practice have variable effects on the prevalence. The increasing rates of cesarean section make subsequent rupture more likely, and dehiscence of a cesarean section scar is the most common cause of uterine rupture reported in recent series.[69] However, the tendency to do fewer classical cesarean sections, the more frequent performance of elective repeat cesarean section,[53] and lower overall parity[70] have reduced the overall rate of uterine rupture.

Uterine rupture is rarely encountered in developed countries in the absence of previous surgery, but is more commonly seen when iatrogenically caused by the excessive and prolonged use of oxytocics in the presence of a uterine scar.[54,71] Taylor and colleagues, in a recent multicenter study, showed that the risk of uterine rupture in patients undergoing a trial of labor after previous cesarean section was significantly higher when vaginal PGE_2 was used (6/58 [10.3%] vs. 8/732 [1.1%]).[72]

Uterine rupture is more frequent when women are left for prolonged periods in obstructed labor. This is more likely to occur in developing countries, although the situation has improved greatly in recent years following improvements in medical facilities, transport systems, organization of medical care, and levels of patient education.[73,74] However, unrelieved obstructed labor remains the major cause of uterine rupture, usually occurring in grand multiparous patients when the fetus is macrosomic or abnormal, or when malpresention occurs.

Uterine rupture can occur in nulliparous patients, but the risk is relatively low, accounting for less than 10% of cases, despite the higher incidence of obstructed labor in nulliparous patients compared with multiparae. Maternal and fetal outcomes are usually worse in women with an unscarred uterus than in those with a previous uterine scar whose delivery is planned.[75] If patients with a uterine scar fail to seek medical attention and labor at home, their outcome tends to be worse.[76]

Diagnosis

A nonreassuring fetal heart rate with recurrent variable decelerations may be indicative of imminent uterine rupture. On abdominal palpation a retraction (Bandl's) ring may be palpable at the junction between the upper segment and a grossly distended lower segment. Severe pain is usually elicited by palpation over the rupture site. Vaginal bleeding in a case of obstructed labor is diagnostic but may be hidden above an impacted presenting part.[77] Catheterization of the bladder will almost always reveal blood-stained urine, but fresh arterial blood indicates that the rupture actually involves the bladder.[78]

Once uterine rupture has occurred, the fetus extrudes through the defect and placental separation will begin. Immediate maternal cardiovascular collapse is a rare event unless the tear extends into the broad ligament vessels. Usually maternal condition deteriorates progressively as bleeding continues and eventually leads to collapse only if the situation is left unattended. Examination of the abdomen will reveal generalized tenderness, easily palpable fetal parts, and absent fetal heart activity.[72]

Occasionally the rupture occurs during vaginal delivery of the infant (usually an operative procedure for delay and fetal distress) and presents as a primary PPH.[73] Thus uterine rupture remains a differential diagnosis in PPH, particularly among those with a previous uterine scar.

Management Options

Emergency laparotomy is indicated whenever the diagnosis is suspected:

> It is much better to diagnose rupture of the uterus too readily than to miss it, as any delay gravely impairs the patient's chances of survival.[67]

When confronted with uterine rupture, the clinician should repair the uterus if this is possible. However, in many cases the damage will be too extensive for repair, particularly if spontaneous rupture occurs in an unscarred uterus; for these, hysterectomy may be necessary.

The presence of a repaired ruptured uterus imposes difficult decisions in the management of future pregnancies. If the defect is confined to the lower segment the risk of rupture in a subsequent pregnancy will be similar to that of someone with a previous cesarean section. Extensive tears involving the upper segment will carry a greater risk, and future pregnancy may be contraindicated, particularly in developing countries where access to an adequately staffed and equipped health care facility is absent. In this situation, sterilization may be safer for the woman.

When future pregnancy occurs, the planning of the delivery is essential, and the treatment of choice is an elective cesarean section at term (37 to 38 weeks' gestation).

SUMMARY OF MANAGEMENT OPTIONS
Uterine Rupture

Management Options	Quality of Evidence	Strength of Recommendation	References
Confirm diagnosis by examination under anesthesia or laparotomy.	III	B	67–69
Surgical Options	III	B	67–69
• Hysterectomy			
• Repair			
In subsequent pregnancies, elective cesarean section is advocated by most.	III	B	67–69

AMNIOTIC FLUID EMBOLISM (See also Chapter 80)

Definition

Amniotic fluid embolism is a rare event occurring during labor usually after spontaneous or artificial rupture of membranes (70%), at cesarean section (19%), or during the 48 hours after delivery (11%), although others have also reported it occurring following first-trimester termination of pregnancy[79] and after amniocentesis.[80]

Epidemiology

The reported incidence of AFE ranges from 1 in 8000 births[81] to 1 in 80,000 births.[82] Twenty-five percent of patients die within 1 hour of the onset of symptoms; overall, the reported mortality is 61% to 86%, and the interval from onset of symptoms to death varies between 10 minutes and 32 hours.[83] Even in those that survive, the initial hypoxemia is often so profound that irreversible neurologic injury occurs despite appropriate resuscitation. In Clark's analysis of the American national registry, less than 3 out of 20 survivors had no residual neurologic damage.[82] Because mortality for this condition is so high and the incidence so uncommon, the proportion of maternal deaths attributed to AFE is largely dependent on the prevalence of other causes of maternal death and the efficacy of treatments for these conditions. In the United Kingdom, for example, AFE rates fifth as a cause of direct maternal deaths with thromboembolic disease rated first,[84] whereas in Hong Kong the situation is reversed because of the rarity of deep vein thrombosis among the predominantly Chinese population. In mainland China AFE accounts for 15% of maternal deaths and as a cause rates second after hemorrhage.[85] Similarly, AFE is the most common cause of maternal death in Singapore, accounting for over 30% of all maternal deaths, with thromboembolic disease rated second (20%) due to the more mixed Asian population.[86] In developing countries maternal deaths due to other causes may be so common that AFE is not even considered as a separate category. Preliminary data from the United Kingdom National Register of cases suggest that mortality may not be as high as described above, with only 16% mortality reported to date, although maternal and neonatal morbidity rates are high.[84]

Clinical Manifestations

The onset of symptoms in AFE is sudden and catastrophic: 27% to 51% present with acute respiratory distress (tachypnea, shortness of breath, cyanosis), 13% to 27% with acute hypotension, 17% with fetal distress, 10% to 30% with convulsions,[82,87] and up to 12% with DIC alone (PPH, bleeding from abdominal or perineal sutures or IV sites).[88] Other symptoms include nausea and vomiting, anxiety, shivering, and sweating. These are followed within 1 to 4 hours by evidence of DIC in virtually all cases.[82]

There are no consistent identifiable predisposing factors for AFE apart from the timing of the event.[83]

Etiology

There is no evidence to support the misconception that amniotic fluid enters the maternal circulation at delivery in most women.[89] The presence of squamous cells in the pulmonary circulation is no longer considered diagnostic of AFE, because squamous cells can also be found in nonpregnant patients in blood samples taken from the lungs at pulmonary artery catheterization.[90] In patients with clinical evidence of AFE, blood aspirated from the pulmonary artery contains mucin, vernix, and lanugo and occasionally meconium, as well as squamous cells, which are frequently coated with leukocytes, suggesting a maternal reaction to this fetal debris.[91] The mechanism by which amniotic fluid suddenly enters the maternal circulation is unknown but most likely involves tears in the veins of the lower uterine segment or endocervix.[92]

Pathophysiology

Once AFE has occurred, it induces two potentially fatal processes: cardiopulmonary collapse and DIC. Clark and colleagues noted the similarity between AFE and other shock states, and proposed that the condition resulted from an anaphylactoid response to the presence of amniotic fluid constituents such as meconium or lanugo.[82] In the presence of meconium or a dead fetus, the time from initial presentation to cardiac arrest and death is shorter than following embolization with clear amniotic fluid.[82] Various mediators such as endothelin[93] are released from the maternal tissues in response to AFE, causing myocardial depression, increases in systemic and pulmonary vascular resistance, decreased cardiac output, and DIC.

It is also possible that bioactive chemicals already present in amniotic fluid cause these events directly. Experimental models of AFE using pregnant animals injected with autologous amniotic fluid[94] produce changes consistent with the presence of a potent vasoconstrictor in amniotic fluid. El Maradny and colleagues have shown that the vasoconstrictor is likely to be endothelin, although their study was performed in rabbits using human rather than autologous amniotic fluid.[95] In humans the major haemodynamic abnormality is left ventricular failure, possibly with transient pulmonary hypertension;[96] endothelin causes increases in both systemic and pulmonary vascular resistance. Other factors, including proteolytic enzymes, histamine, serotonin, platelet-activating factor, prostaglandins, and other potent vasoconstrictive arachidonic acid metabolites such as leukotrienes and isoprostanes, have been implicated in the hemodynamic changes and the development of DIC.[83]

Diagnosis

Early diagnosis may be the best way to improve outcome of AFE. At present the diagnosis is made clinically on the basis of the sudden onset of signs and symptoms after excluding the differential diagnoses (Table 77-3).

The diagnosis can be confirmed by retrieval of fetal debris from the pulmonary artery via a Swan-Ganz catheter. Samples may occasionally be contaminated by maternal cells, but large numbers of squamous cells are strongly supportive of the diagnosis, particularly if they are coated with neutrophils.[97] Many patients do not survive long enough for the diagnosis to be confirmed by this method, but postmortem diagnosis can be made by detection of such debris in the pulmonary vessels.

Kobayashi and colleagues have developed a rapid blood test for AFE that shows promise but still requires clinical evaluation. It is based on an immunoassay for Sialyl, a mucin-type glycoprotein originating from the intestinal and respiratory tracts that is present in both meconium and in clear amniotic fluid.[98]

TABLE 77-3

Differential Diagnoses for Amniotic Fluid Embolism

1. Air embolus
2. Pulmonary thromboembolism
3. Septic shock
4. Myocardial infarction
5. Cardiomyopathy
6. Anaphylaxis
7. Aspiration pneumonitis
8. Placental abruption
9. Preeclampsia/eclampsia
10. Uterine atony, rupture, or other cause of major PPH
11. Transfusion reaction
12. Drug toxicity ($MgSO_4$, local anesthetic)
13. Malignant hyperpyrexia

Management Options

Amniotic fluid embolism is managed symptomatically by maintenance of oxygenation, circulatory support, and correction of DIC. If the fetus is undelivered, cesarean section should be performed as soon as possible, because perinatal mortality and morbidity from hypoxia-ischemia is very high in such instances.[99] Oxygen should be given in all cases, with the concentration and mode of delivery adjusted according to the patient's oxygen saturation, which should be maintained as close to 100% as possible.[100] Initial treatment of shock includes rapid blood volume expansion and direct-acting vasopressors such as phenylephrine to optimize perfusion pressure; dopamine can be used later to improve myocardial function.[101] Pulmonary artery wedge pressure should be monitored via a Swan-Ganz catheter to assist in adjusting therapy, and blood aspirated via the catheter can be examined to confirm the diagnosis.[96] Diuretics or systemic vasodilators may be indicated in some cases.

Disseminated intravascular coagulation should be managed initially by transfusion of packed red cells or fresh whole blood to maintain tissue oxygenation, because significant hemorrhage will usually have occurred. Therapy should be guided by the clinical condition of the patient and laboratory evidence of continuing coagulopathy. Fresh frozen plasma and platelet transfusion should also be given to replace clotting factors consumed by the process. Case reports suggest that plasma exchange techniques may be helpful in clearing fibrin degradation products from the circulation. Use of cryoprecipitate, FOY (a serine proteinase inhibitor), cardiopulmonary bypass and pulmonary thromboembolectomy, nitric oxide, and inhaled aerosolized prostacyclin have also been reported.[83] Clark[82] has also suggested the use of corticosteroids and epinephrine, but these have yet to be evaluated in clinical trials.

SUMMARY OF MANAGEMENT OPTIONS

Amniotic Fluid Embolism

Management Options (See also Chapter 80)	**Quality of Evidence**	**Strength of Recommendation**	**References**
If diagnosed before death, management is largely directed toward general, resuscitative, and supportive measures:			
• Oxygen	III	B	100
• Maintain circulation (e.g., dopamine, digoxin)	IV	C	101
• Intensive care unit	–	GPP	–
• Treat any DIC	–	GPP	–

PREECLAMPSIA/ECLAMPSIA (See also Chapters 36 and 80)

A frequently forgotten risk in the third stage of labor is that of preeclampsia or eclampsia. The onset of preeclampsia is extremely variable, and in the Chinese population in Hong Kong up to 50% of cases develop proteinuria and hypertension for the first time during labor or in the immediate puerperium. A similar phenomenon is seen in the black African population, in whom eclamptic convulsions are commonly seen up to 48 hours after delivery. Eclamptic convulsions can occur at any time, before or after the development of proteinuria. Douglas and Redman[102] surveyed 383 cases of eclampsia that were reported in the United Kingdom in 1992 (incidence 4.9/10,000 maternities) and found that 85% of these cases had attended for antenatal care within 1 week prior to the convulsion. Of these cases 11% had no evidence of proteinuria or hypertension, 10% exhibited proteinuria only, and 22% hypertension only, leaving only 57% with the classical picture of proteinuric PPH with both hypertension and proteinuria.

CONCLUSIONS

- Mothers are at their highest risk of death during the third stage of labor, and yet this is the least studied part of obstetric practice.
- Recent ultrasound studies during the third stage have helped define the process of placental separation and development of a more rational approach to management where separation is delayed.
- Prevention of PPH remains a primary concern, and despite the clear-cut advantages of routine oxytocin administration, the practice is not yet ubiquitous.
- Scientific evaluation of both established and new management protocols is also required to minimize morbidity associated with excessive intervention.
- All of the complications considered in this chapter can lead to rapid deterioration of the mother, and how decisions are made is therefore critical to their survival.
- Key to successful outcome is appropriate emergency resuscitation and transfer to a properly equipped facility, with early involvement of experienced obstetricians and anesthetists.

REFERENCES

1. Revised 1990 estimates of maternal mortality: A new approach by WHO and UNICEF. Geneva, World Health Organization, 1996.
2. Confidential Enquiry in the United Kingdom (CEMD): Why mothers die. Report for 1997–1999 and Executive Summary. *http://www.cemach.org.uk*
3. Husslein P, Fuchs AR, Fuchs F: [Oxytocin- and prostaglandin plasma concentrations before and after spontaneous labor: Evidence of involvement of prostaglandins in the mechanism of placental separation]. [German] Wien Klin Wochensch 1983;95:367–371.
4. Herman A, Weinraub Z, Bukovsky I, et al: Dynamic ultrasonographic imaging of the third stage of labor: New perspective into third stage mechanism. Am J Obstet Gynecol 1993;168: 1469–1496.
5. Herman A, Zimerman A, Arieli S, et al: Down-up sequential separation of the placenta. Ultrasound Obstet Gynecol 2002;19:278–281.
6. Combs CA, Laros RK Jr: Prolonged third stage of labor: Morbidity and risk factors. Obstet Gynecol 1991;77:863–867.
7. Dombrowski MP, Bottoms SF, Saleh AAA, et al: Obstetrics: Third stage of labor: Analysis of duration and clinical practice. Am J Obstet Gynecol 1995;172:1279–1284.
8. Yuen PM, Chan NST, Yim SF, Chang AMZ: A randomised double blind comparison of Syntometrine and Syntocinon in the management of the third stage of labor. BJOG 1995;102:377–380.
9. Ng PS, Chan ASM, Sin WK, et al: A multicentre randomized trial of oral misoprostol and i.m. Syntometrine in the management of the third stage of labor. Hum Reprod 2001;16:31–35.
10. Choy CMY, Lau WC, Tam WH, Yuen PM: A randomised controlled trial of intramuscular Syntometrine and intravenous oxytocin in the management of the third stage of labor. BJOG 2002;109:173–177.
11. Prendiville W, Harding JE, Elbourne DR, Stirrat GM: The Bristol third stage trial: Active versus physiological management of the third stage of labor. BMJ 1988;297:1295–1300.
12. Rogers J, Wood J, McCandlish R, et al: Active versus expectant management of third stage of labor: The Hinchingbrooke randomised controlled trial. Lancet 1998;351:693–699.
13. Çaliskan E, Meydanli M, Dilbaz B, et al: Is rectal misoprostol really effective in the treatment of third stage of labor? A randomized controlled trial. Am J Obstet Gynecol 2002;187: 1038–1045.
14. Begley CM: A comparison of "active" and "physiological" management of the third stage of labor. Midwifery 1990;6:3–17.
15. Botha MC: The management of the umbilical cord in labor. S Afr J Obstet Gynaecol 1968;6:30–33.
16. Pau-Chen W, Tsu-Shan K: Early clamping of the umbilical cord. A study of its effect on the infant. Chin Med J 1960;80:351–355.
17. Yao AC, Lind J, Vourenkosky V: Expiratory grunting in the late cord clamped normal infant. Pediatrics 1971;48:865–870.
18. Pisacane A: Neonatal prevention of iron deficiency. Placental transfusion is a cheap and physiological solution. BMJ 1996;312:136–137.
19. Prendiville W, Elbourne D: Care during the third stage of labor. In I Chalmers, M Enkin, M Kierse (eds): Effective Care in Pregnancy and Childbirth. Oxford University Press, 1989, pp. 1145–1169.

20. Care of the umbilical cord: A review the evidence 1998—WHO/RHTMSM/98.4. http://www.who.int/reproductive-health/publications/MSM_98_4
21. Ibrahim HM, Krouskop RW, Lewis DF, Dhanireddy R: Placental transfusion: Umbilical cord clamping and preterm infants. J Perinatol 2000;20:351–354.
22. C. S. F. Credé: Handgriff zur Entfernung der Placenta. Klin Vorträge über Geburtsh Berlin, 1854, pp 927 and 599–603. Who Named It? http://www.whonamedit.com/
23. Spencer PM: Controlled cord traction in management of the third stage of labor. BMJ 1962;5294:1728–1732.
24. Carroli G, Bergel E: Umbilical vein injection for management of retained placenta (Cochrane Review). In The Cochrane Library, Issue 1, 2003. Oxford, Update Software, 2003.
25. Bider D, Dulitzky M, Goldenberg M, et al: Intraumbilical vein injection of prostaglandin $F_{2\alpha}$ in RP. Eur J Obstet Gynecol Reprod Biol 1996;64:59–61.
26. Ely JW, Rijhsinghani A, Bowdler NC, Dawson J: The association between manual removal of the placenta and postpartum endometritis following vaginal delivery. Obstet Gynecol 1995; 86:1002–1006.
27. Herman A: Complicated third stage of labor: Time to switch on the scanner. [Editorial]. Ultrasound Obstet Gynecol 2000;15:89–95.
28. Lowenwirt IP, Zauk RM, Handwerker SM: Safety of intravenous glyceryl trinitrate in management of retained placenta. Aust N Z J Obstet Gynaecol 1997;37:20–24.
29. Purwar MB: Practical recommendations for umbilical vein injection for management of retained placenta. In AM Gulmezoglu, J Villar (eds): The WHO Reproductive Health Library, vol. 4. Geneva, World Health Organization, 2001.
30. Pipingas A, Hofmeyr GJ, Sesel KR: Umbilical vessel oxytocin administration for retained placenta: In vitro study of various infusion techniques. Am J Obstet Gynecol 1993;168:793–795.
31. Bider D, Dulitzky M, Goldenberg M, et al: Intraumbilical vein injection of prostaglandin $F_{2\alpha}$ in retained placenta. Eur J Obstet Gynecol Reprod Biol 1996;64:59–61.
32. Zaki ZMS, Bahar AM, Ali ME, et al: Risk factors and morbidity in patients with placenta previa accreta compared to placenta previa non-accreta. Acta Obstet Gynecol Scand 1998;77: 391–394.
33. Miller DA, Chollet JA, Goodwin TM: Clinical risk factors for placenta previa/placenta accreta. Am J Obstet Gynecol 1997;177:210–214.
34. Krapp M, Baschat A, Hankeln M, Gembruch U: Gray scale and color Doppler sonography in the third stage of labor for early detection of failed placental separation. Ultrasound Obstet Gynecol 2000;15:138–142.
35. Twickler DM, Lucas MJ, Balis AB, et al: Color flow mapping for myometrial invasion in women with a prior cesarean delivery. J Matern Fetal Med 2000;9:330–335.
36. Levine D, Hulka CA, Ludmir J, et al: Placenta accreta: Evaluation with color Doppler US, power Doppler US, and MR imaging. Radiology 1997;205:773–776.
37. Dunstone SJ, Leibowitz CB: Conservative management of placenta previa with a high risk of placenta accreta. Aus N Z J Obstet Gynaecol 1998;38:429–433.
38. Arulkumaran S, Ng CSA, Ingemarsson I, Ratnam SS: Medical treatment of placenta accreta with methotrexate. Acta Obstet Gynecol Scand 1986;65:285–286.
39. Cho JH, Jun HS, Lee CN: Hemostatic suturing technique for uterine bleeding during cesarean delivery. Obstet Gynecol 2000;96:129–131.
40. Strong TH Jr: Obstetric hemorrhage. In MR Foley, TH Strong Jr. (eds): Obstetric Intensive Care: A Practical Manual. Philadelphia, WB Saunders, 1997.
41. Weeks A, Mirembe FM: The retained placenta—new insights into an old problem [Editorial]. Eur J Obstet Gynecol Reprod Biol 2002;102:109–110.
42. Harrison KA: Anemia, malaria and sickle cell disease. Clin Obstet Gynaecol 1982;9:445–477.
43. Bouvier-colle MH, El-Joud DO, Varnoux N: Groupe MOMS-B. [Maternal mortality and severe morbidity in 3 French regions: Results of MOMS, a European multicenter investigation]. J Gynecol Obstet Biol Reprod 2001;30(Suppl): S5–S9.
44. Mousa HA, Walkinshaw S: Major postpartum hemorrhage. Curr Opin Obstet Gynaecol 2001;13:595–603.
45. Prendiville W, Elbourne D, Chalmers I: The effects of routine oxytocic administration in the management of the third stage of labor: An overview of the evidence from controlled trials. BJOG 1988;95:3–16.
46. Phaneuf S, Rodriguez Linares B, TambyRaja RL, et al: Loss of myometrial oxytocin receptors during oxytocin-induced and oxytocin-augmented labor. J Reprod Fertil 2000;120:91–97.
47. Reich WJ, Nechtow MJ: Ligation of the internal iliac arteries: A life-sparing procedure for uncontrollable gynecologic and obstetric hemorrhage. J Int Coll Surg 1961;36:157.
48. Clark SL, Phelan JP, Yeh S-Y, et al: Hypogastric artery ligation for obstetric hemorrhage. Obstet Gynecol 1985;66:353–356.
49. Waters E: Surgical management of postpartum hemorrhage with particular reference to ligation of uterine arteries. Am J Obstet Gynecol 1952;64:1143–1148.
50. O'Leary JA: Uterine artery ligation for control of postpartum hemorrhage. Obstet Gynecol 1974;43:849–853.
51. AbdRabbo SA: Stepwise uterine devascularization: A novel technique for management of uncontrollable postpartum hemorrhage with preservation of the uterus. Am J Obstet Gynecol 1994;171:694–700.
52. Dildy GA III: Postpartum hemorrhage: New management options. Clin Obstet Gynecol 2002;45:330–344.
53. Maier RC: Control of postpartum hemorrhage with uterine packing. Am J Obstet Gynecol 1993;169:317–323.
54. B-Lynch C, Coker A, Lawal AH, et al: The B-Lynch surgical technique for the control of massive postpartum hemorrhage: An alternative to hysterectomy? Five cases reported. BJOG 1997;104:372–375.
55. Hayman RG, Arulkumaran S, Steer PJ: Uterine compression sutures: Surgical management of postpartum hemorrhage. Obstet Gynecol 2002;99:502–506.
56. Marcovici I, Scoccia B: Postpartum hemorrhage and intrauterine balloon tamponade. A report of three cases. J Reprod Med 1999;44:122–126.
57. Bakri YN, Amri A, Abdul JF: Tamponade-balloon for obstetrical bleeding. Int J Gynaecol Obstet 2001;74:139–142.
58. Johanson R, Kumar M, Obhrai M, Young P: Management of massive postpartum haemorrhage: Use of a hydrostatic balloon catheter to avoid laparotomy. BJOG 2001;108:420–422.
59. Robie GF, Morgan MA, Payne GGJ, Wasemiller-Smith L: Logothetopulos pack for the management of uncontrollable postpartum hemorrhage. Am J Perinatol 1990;7:327–328.
60. Rebarber A, Lonser R, Jackson S, et al: The safety of intraoperative autologous blood collection and autotransfusion during cesarean section. Am J Obstet Gynecol 1998;179:715–720.
61. Baskett TF: Acute uterine inversion: A review of 40 cases. J Obstet Gynaecol Canada 2002;24:953–956.
62. Brar HS, Greenspoon JS, Platt LD, Paul RH: Acute puerperal uterine inversion. New approaches to management. J Reprod Med 1989;34:173–177.
63. Hostetler DR, Bosworth MF: Uterine inversion: A life-threatening obstetric emergency. J Am Board Fam Pract 2000;13: 120–123.
64. Ogueh O, Ayida G: Acute uterine inversion: A new technique of hydrostatic replacement. BJOG 1997;104:951–952.
65. Harnett MJ, Segal S: Presence of placental tissue is necessary for TNG to provide uterine relaxation. Anesth Analges 2000;91: 1043–1044.

66. Tews G, Ebner T, Yaman C, et al: Acute puerperal inversion of the uterus—treatment by a new abdominal uterus preserving approach. Acta Obstet Gynecol Scand 2001;80:1039–1040.
67. Eden RD, Parker RT, Gall SA: Rupture of the pregnant uterus: A 53-year review. Obstet Gynecol 1986;68:671–674.
68. Lynch JC, Pardy JP: Uterine rupture and scar dehiscence: A five-year survey. Anaesth Intensive Care 1996;24:699–704.
69. Diaz SD, Jones JE, Seryakov M, Mann WJ: Uterine rupture and dehiscence: Ten-year review and case-control study. South Med J 2002;95:431–435.
70. Fuchs K, Peretz BA, Marcovici R, et al: The "grand multipara"—is it a problem? A review of 5785 cases. Int J Gynaecol Obstet 1985;23:321–326.
71. Chung T, Rogers MS, Gordon H, Chang AMZ: Pre-labor rupture of the membranes at term and unfavourable cervix: A randomised placebo-controlled trial on early intervention with intra-vaginal prostaglandin E_2 gel. Aust N Z J Obstet Gynaecol 1992;32:25–27.
72. Taylor DR, Doughty AS, Kaufman H, et al: Uterine rupture with the use of PGE_2 vaginal inserts for labor induction in women with previous cesarean sections. J Reprod Med 2002;47:549–554.
73. Rashmi, Radhakrisknan G, Vaid NB, Agarwal N: Rupture uterus—changing Indian scenario. J Indian Med Assoc 2001;99:634–637.
74. Nagarkatti RS, Ambiye VR, Vaidya PR: Rupture uterus: Changing trends in etiology and management. J Postgrad Med 1991;37:136–139.
75. Rouzi AA, Hawaswi AA, Aboalazm M, et al: Uterine rupture incidence, risk factors, and outcome. Saudi Med J 2003;24: 37–39.
76. Personal communication.
77. Lawson JB: Sequelae of obstructed labor. In JB Lawson, DB Stewart (eds): Obstetrics and Gynaecology in the Tropics and Developing Countries. London, Edward Arnold, 1967.
78. Webb JC, Gilson G, Gordon L: Late second stage rupture of the uterus and bladder with vaginal birth after cesarean section: A case report and review of the literature. J Matern Fetal Med 2000;9:362–365.
79. Lawson HW, Atrash HK, Franks AL: Fatal pulmonary embolism during legal induced abortion in the United States from 1972 to 1985. Am J Obstet Gynecol 1990;162:986–990.
80. Bell JA, Pearn JH, Wilson BH, Ansford AJ: Prenatal cytogenetic diagnosis—a current audit. A review of 2000 cases of prenatal cytogenetic diagnoses after amniocentesis, and comparisons with early experience. Med J Aust 1987;146:12–15.
81. Steiner PE, Lushbaugh CC: Landmark article, Oct. 1941: Maternal pulmonary embolism by amniotic fluid as a cause of obstetric shock and unexpected deaths in obstetrics. JAMA 1986;255:2187–2203.
82. Clark SL, Hankins GD, Dudley DA, et al: Amniotic fluid embolism: Analysis of the national registry. Am J Obstet Gynecol 1995;172:1158–1167.
83. Davies S: Amniotic fluid embolus: A review of the literature. Can J Anaesth 2001;48:88–98.
84. Tuffnell DJ: Amniotic fluid embolism. Curr Opin Obstet Gynecol 2003;15:119–122.
85. Weiwen Y, Ningyu Z, Lanxiang Z, Yu L: Study of the diagnosis and management of amniotic fluid embolism: 38 cases of analysis. Obstet Gynecol 2000;95(Suppl 1):S38.
86. Lau G: Are maternal deaths on the ascent in Singapore? A review of maternal mortality as reflected by coronial casework from 1990 to 1999. Ann Acad Med Singapore 2002;31:261–275.
87. Morgan M: Amniotic fluid embolism. Anesth 1979;34:20–32.
88. Davies S: Amniotic fluid embolism and isolated disseminated intravascular coagulation. Can J Anaesth 1999;46:456–459.
89. Dolyniuk M, Orfei E, Vania H, et al: Detection and significance of maternal pulmonary amniotic fluid embolism. Obstet Gynecol 1974;43:729–731.
90. Clark SL, Pavlova Z, Greenspoon J, et al: Squamous cells in the maternal pulmonary circulation. Am J Obstet Gynecol 1986;154: 104–106.
91. Lee KR, Catalano PM, Ortiz-Giroux S: Cytologic diagnosis of amniotic fluid embolism. Report of a case with a unique cytologic feature and emphasis on the difficulty of eliminating squamous contamination. Acta Cytol 1986;30:177–182.
92. Bastien JL, Graves JR, Bailey S: Atypical presentation of amniotic fluid embolism. Anesth Analg 1998;87:124–126.
93. Lockwood CJ, Bach R, Guha A, et al: Amniotic fluid contains tissue factor, a potent initiator of coagulation. Am J Obstet Gynecol 1991;165:1335–1341.
94. Hankins GDV, Snyder RR, Clark SL, et al: Acute hemodynamic and respiratory effects of amniotic fluid embolism in the pregnant goat model. Am J Obstet Gynecol 1993;168:1113–1130.
95. El Maradny E, Kanayama N, Halim A, et al: Endothelin has a role in early pathogenesis of amniotic fluid embolism. Gynecol Obstet Invest 1995;40:14–18.
96. Clark SL, Cotton DB, Gonik B, et al: Central hemodynamic alterations in amniotic fluid embolism. Am J Obstet Gynecol 1988;158:1124–1126.
97. Masson RG: Amniotic fluid embolism. Clin Chest Med 1992;13:657–665.
98. Kobayashi H, Ohi H, Terao T: A simple, noninvasive, sensitive method for diagnosis of amniotic fluid embolism by monoclonal antibody TKH-2 that recognizes NeuAc2-6GalNAc. Am J Obstet Gynecol 1993;168:848–853.
99. Davies MG, Harrison JC: Amniotic fluid embolism: Maternal mortality revisited. Br J Hospital Med 1992;47:775–776.
100. Syed SA, Dearden CH: Amniotic fluid embolism: Emergency management. J Accid Emerg Med 1996;13:285–286.
101. Byrick RJ: Comment implantation syndrome: A time limited embolic phenomenon (Editorial). Can J Anaesth 1997;44: 107–111.
102. Douglas KA, Redman CWG: Eclampsia in the United Kingdom—A descriptive study. 1Xth International Congress of the International Society for the Study of Hypertension in Pregnancy, 1994. Sydney, Australia.
103. Read JA, Cotton DB, Miller FC: Placenta accreta: Changing clinical aspects and outcome. Obstet Gynecol 1980;56:31–34.
104. Daro AF, Gollin HA, Lavieri V: A management of postpartum hemorrhage by prolonged administration of oxytocics. Am J Obstet Gynecol 1952;64:1163–1166.
105. Hayashi RH, Castillo MS, Noah ML: Management of severe postpartum hemorrhage with a prostaglandin $F_{2\alpha}$ analogue. Obstet Gynecol 1984;63:806–809.
106. Lokugamage AU, Sullivan KR, Niculesci I, et al: A randomized study comparing rectally administered misoprostol versus Syntometrine combined with an oxytocin infusion for the cessation of primary post partum hemorrhage. Acta Obstet Gynecol Scand 2001;80:835–839.
107. Castaneda S, Karrison T, Ciblis LA: Peripartum hysterectomy. J Perinat Med 2000;28:472–481.
108. Lee CY, Madroazo B, Drukker BH: Ultrasonic evaluation of the postpartum uterus in the management of postpartum bleeding. Obstet Gynecol 1981;58:227–232.
109. King PA, Duthie SJ, Dong ZG, et al: Secondary postpartum haemorrhage. Aust N Z J Obstet Gynaecol 1989;29:394–398.

CHAPTER 78

Puerperal Problems

Anthony Ambrose / John Repke

INTRODUCTION AND GENERAL APPROACH

The puerperium has been referred to as the "fourth trimester" of pregnancy, encompassing the period between delivery and complete physiologic involution and psychological adjustment.[1] Although this component of the human reproductive process does not get the same attention as many other aspects of pregnancy (there is no specific current American College of Obstetrics and Gynecology (ACOG) recommendation or board standard; there is no specific UpToDate* article), its importance remains indisputable. In both developing countries and the United States, more than 60% of maternal deaths occur in the postpartum period. The first 24 hours postpartum and the first postpartum week are both critical periods, with 45% of postpartum deaths occurring within 1 day of delivery, more than 65% within 1 week, and in excess of 80% within 2 weeks.[2] It is a period of cataclysmic change in which the mother returns to her usual physiology after the dramatic but more gradual adaptations of the previous 266 days.

The role of the obstetrician is to conduct the parturient through this period, gradually passing the management of any chronic or lingering problems to her primary care provider.

As patient populations become more ethnically diverse, it is important to realize that postpartum health beliefs and practices, while often similar among cultures, may also differ drastically. Practitioners should make efforts to develop their knowledge regarding the beliefs and traditions of all their patients.[3]

Maternal obesity contributes to postpartum complications, as reported after a retrospective analysis of data from a validated maternity database system in the United Kingdom. Compared with women with a normal body mass index (BMI), women with a BMI greater than 25 were at increased risk for postpartum hemorrhage (odds ratio, OR = 1:1.6), genital tract infection (OR = 1:2.4), urinary tract infection (OR = 1:1.7), and wound infection (OR = 1:2.7).[4]

Bereavement

Unfortunately, not all pregnancy outcomes are happy. As many as one woman in five will suffer a perinatal loss through neonatal death, stillbirth, elective abortion, or miscarriage, and as many as one in five of these will suffer some form of prolonged psychological abnormality.[5,6] The birth of an anomalous[7] or severely ill infant can be almost as difficult to bear. Mothers experiencing an emergency hysterectomy for hemorrhage, or even a planned surgical sterilization, can manifest grief.[8] Postpartum depression may be more common and more severe when a perinatal loss has occurred.[9]

Interestingly, a recent review of the literature for evidence concerning programs of support aimed at encouraging acceptance of loss, specific bereavement counseling, or specialized psychological support or counseling, to include psychotherapy for women and families experiencing perinatal loss, was unable to locate any randomized trials.[5] On the other hand, a number of reports of personal and institutional experiences in providing such services exist and arguably provide reasonable support for such programs.[10–12] Tasteful and good-quality photographs of the deceased child, especially, would seem to be valued by parents and families.[13,14]

It is incumbent for the staff of the birthing facility to recognize patients who are in need of bereavement services, and then to provide what is generally a multidisciplinary approach to assisting the family through the immediate and long-term dilemmas such a loss causes. Many coordinated and formalized programs do this very well. The perceptions of healthcare professionals about

*UpToDate is a medical information resource provider that can be found at www.uptodate.com.

the emotional care needs of families experiencing perinatal loss were significantly increased after attending a formal educational program about bereavement.[15]

In the late 1970s, individuals at Gundersen Lutheran Medical Center in La Crosse, Wisconsin, providing emotional support for families whose babies died during pregnancy or shortly after birth, became increasingly aware of the pain and grief that families experience when a baby dies. This emotional support effort served as the prototype for *Resolve Through Sharing* (RTS), a perinatal bereavement program formally launched there in 1981, which has subsequently spread nationally and even internationally.

Families experiencing the loss of a baby grieve for their baby and the loss of an entire lifetime with that child. RTS recognizes that the support, acceptance, and gentle guidance given by professionals upon learning of a loss are important first steps in the journey of grief. The caregiver's knowledge and guidance validate that grief is a normal response to loss, allowing bereaved families to grieve in their own way, in their own time. Families are involved in the decision-making process. Education, consultation, and evaluation are integral parts of the program. The RTS support person remains in touch with the family for a year or more, referring to other health-care professionals when additional management support is necessary.[16]

Examination of Placenta

Examination of the placenta in the delivery or operating room should be a standard, especially in the case of a less than optimal outcome. The placenta can provide the clinician with much information regarding the roots of various problems of the mother and newborn. After gross examination, the decision can be made whether to enlist the assistance of the pathologist for careful gross and microscopic examination.[17] Pathology reports may be particularly helpful during preconception counseling. Indeed, any patient experiencing a less than optimal outcome should be offered the opportunity for counseling before considering another conception.

Pain Relief

The advent of patient-controlled analgesia/anesthesia utilizing indwelling epidural catheters has revolutionized pain management in the immediate puerperium. For patients not having epidurals, evidence about various methods remains somewhat murky. Prostaglandin synthetase inhibitors, while affording effective control of uterine contractions, may produce excessive bleeding as a side effect. The broad spectrum of perceived pain among women experiencing delivery remains unexplained.

Calvert and Fleming in Glasgow, Scotland, have reviewed the literature concerning approaches to dealing with perineal pain following vaginal delivery. They note the dearth of data to support many traditional and apparently efficacious practices and emphasize the need for careful evaluation of damage, use of nontraumatic suture when repair is necessary, and listening carefully to the patient as she describes her pain.[18]

Education: Assuming the Role of the Mother

Many normal psychological changes take place to prepare the mother for her new responsibilities. Any impediment to these changes may result in a lack of emotional response to the infant at delivery. During the immediate newborn period, prenatal preparation needs to be recalled and developed, in addition to many new and often unanticipated tasks as the maternal role is taken on.[19]

Medications

The administration of appropriate medications such as Rh-immune globulin, vaccinations, and others must not be overlooked prior to discharge. It should be remembered that dosages of many medications for chronic disease states (e.g., thyroid disease, hypertension, seizure disorders) likely were changed (generally increased) during pregnancy because of maternal physiologic adaptations (e.g., the increase in plasma volume, or changes in the rate of drug metabolism). During the puerperium these drug dosages usually need to be restored to prepregnancy levels. The blood levels of antiseizure medications may rise dramatically in the early puerperium if dosages are not adjusted. Coordination with the patient's primary care provider is vital.

General Health Considerations

The puerperium also offers an opportunity for the caregiver to reinforce the healthy lifestyle that many women adopt during pregnancy. This is the time to intervene to prevent recidivism into unhealthy habits, such as the use of tobacco, alcohol, and other unhealthy substances. The nutrition counseling many women undergo during pregnancy, whether or not they have been diagnosed with gestational diabetes, will serve them well in the nonpregnant state and should be reinforced. Even pregestational diabetics often embrace long-overlooked advice for the sake of the babies they carry; this is an opportunity to bolster that resolve.

Length of Stay

At least eight trials have attempted to compare early discharge (with substantial variation in the definition thereof) of healthy mothers with term infants, with standard care in the settings in which the trials were conducted. Investigational problems included high postrandomization exclusions, protocol violations, and failure to use a well-validated standardized instrument to assess postpartum depression. So, although there seems to be no evidence of adverse outcomes associated with policies of early postnatal discharge, methodologic limitations of included studies mean that such complications cannot be ruled out.[20] Indeed, such difficult-to-measure outcomes such as fatigue due to sleep deprivation may be affected by length of stay.

Returning to Exercise

As morphologic and physiologic adaptations to pregnancy recede gradually over many weeks, it seems prudent that mothers return progressively to prepregnancy levels of exercise and physical conditioning. Complications associated with the resumption of physical training, even among elite athletes, seem to be rare.[21] Modest weight reduction during lactation appears to be safe and does not seem to compromise infant weight gain in most cases.[22,23] As a general rule, feeding their babies before exercise helps mothers avoid problems associated with breast engorgement and lactic acid accumulation in breast milk.[24,25]

Returning to Work

This remains a topic replete with opinion but generally unencumbered by data. Although published in the past, ACOG has withdrawn written guidelines. A survey was done by Contemporary OB/GYN in 1983, in which 803 questionnaires were mailed to readers; 392 responses were received (49%). When asked "How many days should patients wait before returning to work after undergoing, [Page no. 5] . . . scheduled repeat caesarean section, . . .?", responses were, on average, 34.7 days (sedentary job), 39.5 days (job that requires standing or walking), and 47.6 days (job that requires heavy physical exertion).[26] Provisions of legislation such as the Family and Medical Leave Act produce a dilemma for the obstetrician, who generally is in no position objectively to assess the capabilities of the patient and has little or no medical evidence on which to rely. The facts that every patient is different and every employment situation is different would seem to demand individualization from the advising provider, but the dearth of evidence-based data to support one's recommendation invites criticism and inappropriate intrusion into the contractual arrangements between employers and employees. In our own practice we tend to deal with this by informing patient and employer that there is little or no data to support a firm recommendation, and advise the patient to return to work, and to do work, according to her comfort level. This allows the patient and her employer to negotiate, compromise, and come to a mutually acceptable arrangement.

SUMMARY OF MANAGEMENT OPTIONS
Overall Care in the Puerperium

Management Options	Quality of Evidence	Strength of Recommendation	References
Bereavement (see also Chapter 26)			
Psychological and general support	III	B	10–12
Photographs and other mementos	IV	C	13,14
Multidisciplinary approach	–	GPP	—
Staff training	III	B	15
Examination of the Placenta			
General macroscopic examination of all placentas, cords, and membranes	–	GPP	–
Formal pathologic examination with identified abnormalities	IV	C	17
Pain Relief (especially with perineal pain) Medications etc			
Local measures and oral analgesia	IV	C	18
Rh immune globulin if indicated	–	GPP	–
Vaccines (e.g., rubella) if indicated	–	GPP	–
Drug therapy to return to prepregnancy doses	–	GPP	–
Most drugs are safe in breast-feeing (see Chapter 35)	–	GPP	–
Advice about smoking, alcohol, etc.	–	GPP	–
General			
No clear data about length of in-hospital stay	Ia	A	20

Continued

SUMMARY OF MANAGEMENT OPTIONS

Overall Care in the Puerperium *(Continued)*

Management Options	Quality of Evidence	Strength of Recommendation	References
Exercise			
Gradual increase to prepregnancy levels	–	GPP	–
Most exercise is safe in the puerperium	IV	C	21
Breast-feeding is better before exercise	Ib	A	24, 25
Work			
Lack of data to give advice about resumption of work; common sense approach and comfort is usual	–	GPP	–

SECONDARY POSTPARTUM HEMORRHAGE (See also Chapter 77)

Excessive vaginal bleeding between 24 hours and 6 weeks following delivery is the traditional definition of secondary or late postpartum hemorrhage (PPH).[27,28] It is a major cause of maternal morbidity and potential maternal mortality.[29,30] Calculating its precise incidence is challenging, as the definition varies; however, it is undoubtedly uncommon, having been reported to complicate fewer than 1% of deliveries.[31]

Secondary PPH is a clinical diagnosis of exclusion, generally presenting as abrupt onset of heavy, sometimes massive (>10% of total blood volume) bleeding 7 to 14 days after delivery.[29] Such bleeding may sometimes represent the initial menstrual period after childbirth, which is often the result of an anovulatory cycle and thus may be heavy, painful, and prolonged.[30]

Differential Diagnosis

The most common causes of late hemorrhage (Table 78–1) include subinvolution of the placental site, retained products of conception, and infection; previously undiagnosed tumors may rarely present in this fashion.[32] It is often attributed to sloughing of the placental eschar.[29] Subinvolution would seem to be the consequence of failure of obliteration of the vessels underlying the placental site; its mechanism is poorly understood.[33]

Women suffering delayed postpartum hemorrhage frequently have retained placental fragments, especially if the bleeding is heavy. This group was noted to have had an increased incidence, in prior pregnancies, of complications, which might reflect aberrant maternal-trophoblastic interaction, such as preeclampsia, intrauterine growth restriction, spontaneous abortion, or retained placenta.[34]

Another possible cause is endometritis, which should be suspected if the history includes uterine tenderness, fever, or foul lochia. This is effectively treated by antibiotics without dilation and curettage (to avoid Asherman's syndrome). If curettage is undertaken, it is probably wise to give antibiotics for at least 6 to 12 hours before the procedure, to guard against bacteremia, unless the bleeding mandates urgent intervention. In such a case, intravenous antibiotics should be given at the time of the procedure. The combination of estrogens and progesterone may allow adequate regeneration of the endometrium and may help prevent formation of synechiae.[28] Therefore, in women with secondary postpartum hemorrhage, prescribing a progesterone-only contraceptive pill would be a mistake, as this would have neither a beneficial effect on the endometrium, nor would it accelerate placental site involution.[30]

Occasionally, relatively earlier secondary PPH (later in the first week) may be related to coagulopathy, especially von Willebrand's disease. As von Willebrand's factor is physiologically increased in pregnancy, a patient may be well during pregnancy, but develop a problem as she returns to the nonpregnant state; unexpected severe bleeding may occur despite only mildly reduced levels of factor VIII. All of these women are at risk for both intrapartum and postpartum bleeding. Mild disease usually requires no therapy, especially if factor VIII levels remain

TABLE 78–1

Causes of Secondary Postpartum Hemorrhage

Abnormalities of placentation
Idiopathic subinvolution of uteroplacental vessels
Retained placental tissue
Placenta accreta
Infection
Endometritis, myometritis, parametritis
Infection/dehiscence of cesarean scar
Preexisting uterine disease
Leiomyomata
Cervical neoplasm
Trauma: rupture of vulvar or vaginal hematoma
Coagulopathy

Modified from Neill A, Thornton S: Secondary postpartum hemorrhage. J Obstet Gynaecol 2002;22:119–122.

within normal limits. In the case of severe disease, (factor VIII levels < 5%), the risk of bleeding is substantial.

Management Options

Management of suspected secondary postpartum hemorrhage consists of stabilization, investigation to establish a cause for the bleeding, and appropriate treatment. Invasive examination in the office setting (e.g., using endometrial sampling devices) may result in a dramatic increase in the volume of bleeding, and uterine perforation is possible, especially if the uterus or its contents are infected. For this reason, investigation should be performed in a more controlled setting.

Crystalloid and blood products should be given as necessary to maintain intravascular volume and coagulability. The initial treatment of late postpartum hemorrhage consists of oxytocic agents plus antibiotics. Pelvic ultrasonography can be helpful in investigating whether there is clot or other debris within the endometrial cavity. However, bear in mind that ultrasound cannot reliably differentiate retained placental fragments from retracted blood clots. Thus, diagnoses of retained placental fragments are not always reliable. If significant bleeding persists despite medical therapy, suction or sharp curettage (or both) should be considered, especially if retained products of conception are suspected after ultrasound examination. The use of sharp curettage probably increases the risk of both uterine perforation and Asherman's syndrome. Ultrasonography may be helpful during curettage, allowing visualization of the location of instruments. Although it is probably wise to send evacuated tissue for histologic examination to rule out trophoblastic disease, degenerating chorionic villi and decidua will be also obtained from all postpartum uteri if samples are taken and do not therefore necessarily warrant a diagnosis of "significant retained products."

Authors in Belgium evaluated color Doppler and the gray-scale sonographic appearance of the uterus after pregnancy. Areas of enhanced vascularity of the uterus, ranging from a focal vascular pedicle to a larger area of the myometrium, were relatively common, predominantly seen in the presence of placental remnants, in the early postpartum period, and after instrumental or manual delivery of the placenta. These investigators felt their results may prove to be of practical value in the management of abnormal uterine bleeding in the puerperium.[35]

In cases of exceptionally heavy bleeding, before hysterectomy or surgical exploration is undertaken, angiographic embolization by skilled interventional radiologists can be considered.[36,37] Hysterectomy is only indicated in the rare patient in whom conservative therapy fails.

SUMMARY OF MANAGEMENT OPTIONS

Secondary Postpartum Hemorrhage

Management Options	Quality of Evidence	Strength of Recommendation	References
Clinical features important in making diagnosis.	III	B	241
Ultrasonography of uterine contents does not distinguish blood clot from placenta; echogenic masses are found in asymptomatic women. Empty uterus on scan may allow a conservative approach.	III	B	241
IV fluids and blood for hemodynamic stabilisation may be necessary in some patients; correct coagulation defects	–	GPP	–
Antibiotics for 12–24 h prior to surgical evacuation	–	GPP	–
Uterotonics and antibiotics may reduce need for curettage	III	B	241
Surgical/suction evacuation of uterus	III	B	242
Embolization may be tried in persistent bleeding after evacuation before resorting to hysterectomy	IIb	B	36, 37
Send surgical products for histologic examination	–	GPP	–

PUERPERAL PYREXIA/INFECTION

Uterine Infection

Approximately 1% to 3% of women having vaginal delivery will develop what is frequently referred to as puerperal endometritis, although these infections may more validly be described as endoparamyometritis, as they often involve more than the innermost tissue layers of the uterus and sometimes surrounding structures as well (Table 78–2). Cesarean deliveries performed prior to the onset of labor and rupture of membranes may be associated with an incidence of 5% to 15% of such infections, and when a cesarean section is performed after lengthy labor or ruptured membranes, the incidence may be in excess of 30%. Rates will vary widely among populations and depending on definitions used.[38]

TABLE 78–2

Differential Diagnosis of Persistent Puerperal Fever

DIAGNOSIS	DIAGNOSTIC TESTS	TREATMENT
Resistant microorganisms	Endometrial and blood culture	Modify antibiotic therapy
Wound infection	Physical examination	Incision, drainage
	Needle aspiration Ultrasound	Antibiotics
Pelvic abscess	Physical examination Ultrasound, CT, MRI	Drainage Antibiotics
Septic pelvic vein thrombophlebitis	Ultrasound, CT, MRI	Anticoagulation Antibiotics
Recrudescence of autoimmune disease	Serology	Corticosteroids
Drug fever	Inspect temperature graph, identify eosinophilia	Discontinue antibiotics
Mastitis	Physical examination	Modify antibiotic coverage to cover staphylococci

CT, computed tomography; MRI, magnetic resonance imaging.
Modified from Duff: Maternal and pernatal infection. In Gable SG, Nielge JR, Simpson JL (eds). *Obstetrics: Normal & Problem Pregnancies*, 4th ed. New York, Churchill Livingstone, 2002.

These infections are generally polymicrobial, caused by organisms present in the normal vaginal flora, now granted access to the upper genital tract, peritoneal cavity, and circulation. The more common pathogenic bacteria include group B, β-hemolytic streptococcus (GBS), anaerobic streptococci, aerobic gram-negative bacilli (usually *E. coli*, *Klebsiella pneumoniae*, and *Proteus*), and anaerobic gram-negative bacilli (generally *Bacteroides* and *Prevotella*).[38] These too may vary among populations.

Although familiar mostly to students of medical history who read the 1843 paper of Oliver Wendell Holmes "The Contagiousness of Puerperal Fever,"[39] or readers of Morton Thompson's historical fiction about Ignaz Semmelweis, "The Cry and the Covenant,"[40] group A streptococci (GAS) are not just of historical interest but can still be an important source of postpartum metritis and sepsis. GAS carrier status may occasionally be identified during routine screening for GBS, and this finding may presage serious postpartum infection.[41] A recently reported 7-month outbreak of 15 cases of postpartum sepsis due to group A hemolytic streptococci was traced to a nurse with atopic dermatitis who carried the organism,[42] raising a chilling memory of similar outbreaks that occurred in Budapest and other locales in the mid-nineteenth century.[43] The Centers for Disease Control and Prevention recently hosted a workshop to formulate recommendations for control of GAS disease among household contacts of persons with invasive GAS infections and for responding to postpartum and postsurgical invasive GAS infections.[44]

Risk factors for metritis include young maternal age, cesarean delivery, low socioeconomic status, extended duration of labor, prolonged rupture of membranes, and multiple vaginal examinations.[38] Puerperal pyrexia due to metritis typically presents with fever and temperatures in excess of 38°C, between 24 and 36 hours of delivery. Controversy exists as to whether temperature elevations within 24 hours of delivery are pathologic because they can be due to overheating of the mother secondary to the efforts of labor, especially if she had an epidural. "Milk fever" can also be a benign cause (see later discussion). Careful evaluation of intrapartum events and observations is necessary to distinguish benign from infectious pyrexia. Other findings and complaints may include tachycardia, pelvic and lower abdominal pain, uterine tenderness, foul lochia, and general malaise.[38]

Patients with such findings or complaints deserve a thorough evaluation, because the differential diagnosis is broad, and metritis should not be assumed. Differential diagnosis includes mastitis, urinary tract infection, atelectasis (especially following cesarean delivery), and bacterial or viral infections virtually anywhere within the respiratory, genitourinary, and gastrointestinal tracts. Examination of the breasts, percussion of the sinuses, inspection of the pharynx, auscultation of the lungs and heart, and other diagnostic techniques may discover a process not related to the uterus. Laboratory tests, with the exception of evaluation of the urine, are not generally helpful initially. Controversy exists as to whether endometrial cultures, white blood counts, chest radiograph, and other diagnostic modalities are helpful prior to starting therapy. If endometrial cultures are attempted, some data support the use of multiple-lumen catheters in order to avoid vaginal contamination.[45] Manual examination, plus or minus visual inspection of the vagina and cervix, should always be done, even thought this may be uncomfortable for the patient. Discovering a hematoma or abscess is important as it directs appropriate therapy; finding and removing an overlooked vaginal sponge benefits the patient and, at the very least, prevents further embarrassment for the provider who left it behind!

Management Options

Once a thorough examination has been done, and the provider has concluded the uterus is the source of the infection, treatment generally consists of broad-spectrum parenteral antibiotics, to include coverage for β-lactamase-producing anaerobes.[46] In most cases the combination of clindamycin (900 mg IV every 8 hr) plus gentamicin (1.5 mg/kg IV every 8 hr), with gentamicin levels followed, will be safe and effective, with cure rates of 90% to 97% reported in several studies.[47–56] Parenteral therapy should continue until the patient is afebrile for 24 to 48 hours, and oral antibiotic therapy thereafter is generally not necessary, barring staphylococcal bacteremia.[57]

If the patient does not respond to the initial antibiotic regimen after 48 to 72 hours, modification in therapy may be necessary. In this case, cultures may prove valuable. Resistant organisms such as enterococci are responsible for many treatment failures. Adding ampicillin (2 g IV every 4 hr) may improve the rate of response.[58]

Should the patient still not improve, evaluation should be repeated and extended. Wound infection, pelvic abscess, septic pelvic thrombophlebitis, and drug fever should be added to the differential diagnosis.[46]

A standardized protocol similar to the aforementioned was evaluated with respect to its efficacy against postcesarean endometritis in Alabama. Twenty percent (322) of 1643 patients delivered by cesarean were diagnosed with endometritis and treated with clindamycin-gentamicin; 129 of these women also received either ampicillin or vancomycin; only 19 of 322 (6%) had persistent fever. Six of these had a wound complication, 1 an infected hematoma, and 12 were suspected as having antimicrobial resistance. Their standardized protocol resulted in a 94% initial cure rate.[59]

A recent prospective, placebo-controlled, double-blinded study in Tennessee investigated whether once-daily dosing of gentamicin and clindamycin (gentamicin 5 mg/kg and clindamycin phosphate 2700 mg) would be as efficacious as administration every 8 hours. There was no difference in the mean time from starting therapy until becoming afebrile between the groups, and success rates were similar (82% in the daily-dose group, and 69% in the thrice-daily dose group).[60]

Septic Pelvic Vein Thrombophlebitis

Septic pelvic vein thrombophlebitis (SPT) is probably a rather infrequent postpartum complication, occurring in only 1:2000 pregnancies. Intrauterine infection may cause seeding of pathogens into the venous circulation, leading to endothelial damage and thrombosis.[61]

Duff[62] has reported that SPT may occur in two rather distinct forms:

- Ovarian vein syndrome/thrombosis
- "Enigmatic fever"

More common is ovarian vein syndrome, which is acute thrombosis of one (usually the right) or both ovarian veins.[63] Common findings are moderate fever, pain, gastrointestinal symptoms, and tachycardia. The abdomen is often tender, and the patient may have guarding and decreased bowel sounds. Differential diagnoses include pyelonephritis, renal stone, appendicitis, broad ligament hematoma, adnexal torsion, and pelvic abscess.[61] Ultrasound, computed tomography, and other imaging modalities have been reported to demonstrate extensive thrombosis of an ovarian vein. Medical treatment consists of thrombolytic agents, heparin, and antibiotics.[64]

Less common is so-called enigmatic fever.[65] Patients initially seem to have metritis and receive systemic antibiotics. Initially, there may be some improvement, but patients frequently have temperature instability. Fever and tachycardia may persist. Differential diagnoses include drug fever, viral syndrome, autoimmune disease, and pelvic abscess.[61]

Management Options

Diagnostic imaging (CT, MRI) may help to detect large thrombi. A group in Winnipeg reported the result of an CT scan of the abdomen and pelvis with infused IV contrast, which demonstrated a massive thrombosis extending from the superior vena cava to the femoral vein, and which responded to a regimen of clindamycin, gentamicin, and unfractionated heparin (Figure 78–1).[66]

Diagnostic imaging may miss thrombi in smaller vessels. In this case, a favorable response to therapeutic-dose heparin supports the diagnosis.[67,68] Patients generally respond within 2 to 3 days. If there is no response and the patient worsens, consultation with a vascular surgeon may be prudent.[62,67]

Although most would recommend the use of heparin in the treatment of SPT, this is not entirely uncontroversial. A study in Dallas used abdominopelvic CT imaging to search for evidence of puerperal SPT in women diagnosed with pelvic infection and fever that persisted after 5 days of adequate antimicrobial therapy with clindamycin, gentamicin, and ampicillin. Sixty-nine women met the criteria for prolonged infection, and 15 (22%) of these were found to have SPT. Four of these women had delivered vaginally; 11 by cesarean section. Of the 15, all

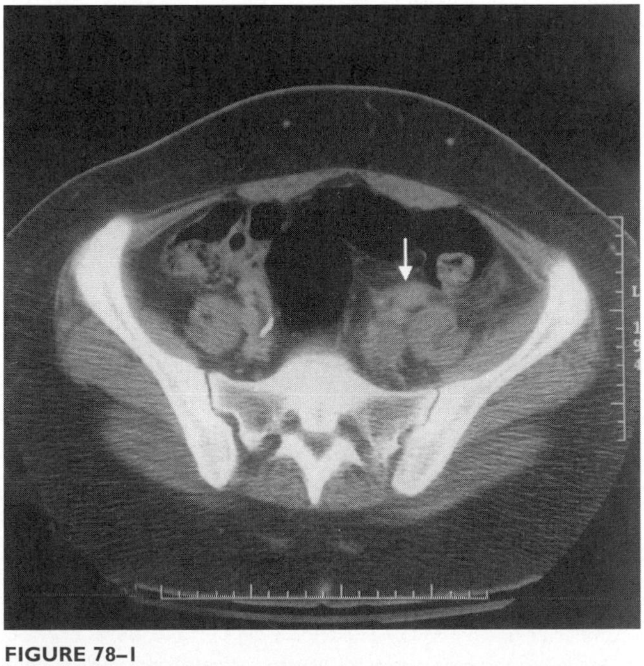

FIGURE 78–1
Infused CT of the abdomen, with the arrow demonstrating left ileofemoral thrombosis. The associated low-density area surrounding the vein represents perivascular inflammation.

were treated with continued antimicrobial therapy, 6 with the addition of heparin and 9 without. There was no significant difference between the responses of women who were and those who were not given heparin. This study, using their criteria for diagnosis of SPT, reported a 1:9000 incidence of SPT after vaginal delivery, and a 1:800 incidence following cesarean section.[69]

Urinary Tract Infections

Factors such as vaginal examinations, urethral catheterization, and the 5% to 10% incidence of asymptomatic bacteruria[61] during pregnancy place the just-delivered mother at risk for infection in any part of her urinary tract. Other risk factors appearing in the literature include being black, native-American, or Hispanic American, unmarried status, cesarean delivery, tocolysis, renal disease, preeclampsia-eclampsia, and abruptio placentae.[70] Urinary tract infections in pregnancy are caused primarily by *Escherichia coli*, *Klebsiella pneumoniae*, and *Proteus* species. Pyelonephritis is a particularly serious infection in pregnancy because it may be complicated by preterm labor, bacteremia, and acute respiratory distress syndrome (ARDS).[61]

SUMMARY OF MANAGEMENT OPTIONS

Puerperal Pyrexia

Management Options	Quality of Evidence	Strength of Recommendation	References
Uterine Infection			
Prevention:			
Limit vaginal examinations, intrauterine monitoring, exteriorizing the uterus at CS and manual removal of placenta at CS	–	GPP	–
Prophylactic antibiotics at the time of CS	Ia	A	243
Management:			
Gentamycin and clindamycin or extended spectrum β-lactam (e.g., imipenem-cilastatin)	Ia	A	244
Continue until afebrile for at least 24 h	–	GPP	–
If patient not responding after 48–72 h seek other causes (e.g. retained products of conception, abscess, hematoma, ovarian vein thrombosis etc), review microbiology and antibiotic regimen	–	GPP	–
Septic Pelvic Vein Thrombophlebitis			
Diagnosis of exclusion; no localizing symptoms	IV	C	62
At least 7 days of therapeutic heparin	Ib	A	70
Broad-spectrum antibiotics	Ib	A	70
Ovarian Vein Thrombosis			
CT/MRI for diagnosis	IV	C	66,68
Heparin and long-term anticoagulation as for thromboembolic disease elsewhere	IV	C	63
Broad-spectrum antibiotics	IV	C	63
Vascular surgery if failed response to medical treatment	–	GPP	–
Urinary Infection			
Culture urine; appropriate antibiotics (oral or parenteral depending on clinical severity)	–	GPP	–
Puerperal Hematomas			
Expectant management and compression if less than 5 cm and not expanding	IV	C	247
Large hematomas require evacuation, hemostasis, restoration of anatomy, closed drainage	IV III	C B	245 246
Large hemotomas above the levators require imaging for detection and surgical correction	IV	C	247

CS, cesarean section; CT, computed tomography; MRI, magnetic resonance imaging.

DISORDERS OF THE BREASTS

For various reasons, approximately half of U.S. women do not breast feed their newborns.[71] Although it is well known that women may experience great discomfort before lactation ceases, precise data about this annoyance is lacking.

Lactation: Suppression and Stimulation

Over the years a number of nonpharmacologic means have been used to suppress lactation and relieve symptoms of engorgement. These include, but are not limited to, strapping or binding the breasts, forcing fluids, restricting fluids and diet, applying various ointments and other products (e.g., cabbage leaves, ice packs) to the breasts and nipples, narcotics, wearing a tightly fitting brassiere, emptying the breasts by massage or pump, and avoiding expression of milk.[72-76] It is evident that a number of these approaches are contradictory.

In the United States, various pharmacologic methods for lactation suppression were used during most of the 20th century.[77] The natural suppression of prolactin secretion results in breast involution; this was approximated pharmacologically with medicines such as bromocriptine. However, since 1988 the U.S. Food and Drug Administration has recommended against the routine use of pharmacologic methods (save analgesics) for lactation suppression and relief of associated symptoms because evidence from randomized controlled studies on the safety and efficacy of those drugs for that purpose is lacking.[78,79] Reports linked bromocriptine with cerebrovascular accident, myocardial infarction, seizure, and other problems in puerperal women. Because of associations with such serious complications, this drug is no longer approved for lactation suppression.[80-85]

Peterson and colleagues at the Centers for Disease Control and Prevention searched the world literature in 1998 to locate data about the postpartum symptoms experienced by women who do not breast feed, and to review data on the efficacy of nonpharmacologic methods of lactation suppression. Their findings were disappointing: extant data suggested that, in spite of current nonpharmacologic treatment for lactation suppression, as many as one woman in three may experience severe breast pain postpartum. Moreover, they found no studies focusing primarily on the symptoms of such women. They did offer directions for future research, suggesting studies that included treatment groups for wearing a breast binder, wearing a tightly fitting brassiere, pumping breast milk mechanically or manually, applying ice packs to the breasts, applying topical analgesics or other substances to the breasts, and taking only oral analgesics. Between 30% and 50% of nonnursing patients will have engorgement and pain that may persist for up to a week.[79]

Unwanted lactation failure is a rare complication that has been associated with retained placenta, via suppression of prolactin.[86] Prolactin may also be suppressed by ergot, pyridoxine, and some diuretics.

It has been reported that metoclopramide[87] and sulpiride[88] may enhance lactation. Use of oxytocin (which has to be taken as snuff, to avoid first-pass inactivation in the liver) has been demonstrated to improve milk let-down and may help with the successful establishment of breast-feeding in some women, especially those with preterm babies.

Mastitis and Abscess

It is not unusual for the breasts to become distended and firm during the first day or two after delivery; this may be accompanied by a transient temperature elevation.[89] It has been reported that 13% of all postpartum women may demonstrate such "breast fever," which seldom lasts more than 24 hours.[90] When fever develops during the puerperium, however, breast fever should be a diagnosis of exclusion, as it is important not to miss more dangerous pathology.

Puerperal mastitis or breast abscess is the most frequent significant complication of nursing. Fever, localized pain, and erythema, often confined to one or more quadrants, are common findings. Onset is generally in the first or second postpartum week, but it may also develop later. It may be related to an obstruction in the milk ducts. When initiating lactation, the nipple and areolar skin often undergo local inflammation and swelling until the nipple is conditioned to frequent suckling. This swelling causes a relative obstruction to milk flow and can be seeded by skin bacteria especially staphylococci or streptococci, leading to bacterial mastitis. There is some evidence that the immediate source of these organisms is the infant's nose and throat. The breast (generally unilaterally and in one quadrant) becomes painful, swollen, warm, and red. An abscess develops in approximately 10% of such women; there may be local fluctuance and pointing.[91,92]

Cultures of the milk are usually unhelpful; infection is almost always with a maternal skin organism. Treatment with antibiotics generally results in prompt resolution of symptoms, and following prompt treatment, the development of abscesses is rare. Dicloxacillin (500 mg PO every 6 hr) may be started empirically.[93] When they do develop, abscesses require surgical incision and drainage[94,95] or aspiration with ultrasound guidance.[96] Continuing to breast feed may be extremely important: the only women who developed abscesses in a series of 65 woman with puerperal mastitis were among the small group who chose to cease nursing.[97] This is probably because continuing to breast feed allows the flow of milk to flush infection from the duct system.

A prospective study done in Turkey assessed contributing factors in puerperal breast abscess. Mastitis patients who were treated with antibiotics did not develop breast abscess. Ultrasonography was helpful, allowing needle aspiration; healing times were similar to those in abscess patients treated with incision and drainage. Needle aspiration patients were reported to have excellent cosmetic results.[98]

SUMMARY OF MANAGEMENT OPTIONS

Breast Problems

Management Options	Quality of Evidence	Strength of Recommendation	References
Lactation Suppression			
Physical support; evidence for value of other topical measures is poor	III	B	72–76
Analgesia should be the only pharmacologic agent used	Ia	A	78,79
Bromocriptine should not be used	IV	C	80–85
Lactation Enhancement			
Metoclopramide	IV	C	87
Sulpiride	IV	C	88
Mastitis and Breast Abscesses			
Oral dicloxacillin (erythromycin if allergic)	IIa	B	93
IV oxacillin for treatment failures	–	GPP	–
Ultrasonography to rule out abscess if there is poor response or fluctuant mass	III	B	96
Open or closed (ultrasound-guided) drainage for abscess	III	B	94–96
Culture milk with complicated mastitis or abscess	–	GPP	–
Continued pumping/expressing and feeding	IIa	B	97

MEDICAL COMPLAINTS IN THE PUERPERIUM

During the "fourth trimester," the recently delivered woman must negotiate the dramatic changes from late pregnancy and delivery and return to her normal non-pregnant physiology.

Cardiovascular Complications

Maternal cardiac output remains elevated for at least 2 days postpartum, primarily because of increased stroke volume from increased venous return. Cardiac output and blood volume drop rapidly thereafter and are almost back to normal by 2 weeks after delivery. Women with stenotic lesions, real or potential left-to-right shunts, or low cardiac output are at particularly high risk for cardiac failure in the immediate postpartum period because of both high stroke volume and cardiac output, and the sudden fluid shifts that occur during the return to nonpregnant physiology. Such women are at higher risk for cardiovascular collapse during the first 10 to 14 days postpartum than they are even during pregnancy.[99]

ARDS may occur during pregnancy or the puerperium. A group in San Diego reported that ARDS occurred approximately 10 times more frequently in or following pregnancy (1 per 6277 deliveries) than the 1.5 cases per 100,000 per year reported for the general population. Leading causes were infection, preeclampsia/eclampsia, and aspiration.[100]

Hypertension

Between 1% and 5% of pregnancies are complicated by chronic hypertension. These women are at risk for superimposition of preeclampsia. Many will have entered pregnancy having been taking antihypertensive medication; some will have had changes made to those regimens because of concerns about possible fetal effects. For example, angiotensin-converting enzyme (ACE) inhibitors, a mainstay of many chronic hypertension treatment regimens, are generally contraindicated during pregnancy because of concerns about harmful fetal effects in the 2nd and 3rd trimester.[101,102] Once the patient has delivered, however, she can usually reinstate them. It is important to coordinate such a change with the baby's pediatrician, however; although the American Academy of Pediatrics considers ACE inhibitors to be compatible with breastfeeding,[103] the ultimate responsibility for the baby's health falls to the pediatrician. It is also prudent to coordinate management of hypertension with the patient's primary care provider upon discharge from hospital.

Cardiomyopathy

Approximately 1000 women in the United States annually suffer from peripartum cardiomyopathy, and some will not survive. Human peripartum cardiomyopathy remains a difficult problem, whose cause and mechanisms of pathogenesis remain a mystery. Recent evidence suggests that this is an autoimmune disease with many contributing factors and effector mechanisms. Investigators from

Emory University have found that sera from these patients contain high titers of autoantibodies against some human cardiac tissue proteins, which were not present in the sera of patients with idiopathic cardiomyopathy. Advances in medical therapy and cardiac transplantation have significantly improved quality of life and survival, but it remains a challenging problem.[104,105]

Diabetes

Women who were diagnosed with gestational diabetes generally do not require treatment following delivery. However, they are at increased risk for developing type II diabetes (approximately 50% will do so within 10 years). Following the traditional postpartum visit at 6 to 8 weeks, they should be directed to follow-up with their primary care providers in 2 to 3 months, at which time they should discuss with their providers the possibility of having provocative testing for diabetes. This may be accomplished by an oral glucose tolerance test, in which a plasma glucose level equal to or more than 200 mg/dL (11 mmol/L) would be sufficient for a diagnosis of diabetes. The test should be performed as described by the World Health Organization, using a glucose load containing the equivalent of 75 g of anhydrous glucose dissolved in water.[106]

In the case of women with pregestational diabetes, their treatment following delivery depends on their glucose levels as they return to their usual diet and activity levels. Upon discharge from the hospital, they can generally return to a management program similar to the one they observed prior to conception. Coordination with the providers furnishing that management is prudent.

Thromboembolic Disease

Due largely to the physiologic changes of pregnancy, as well as relative immobilization during the latter parts of pregnancy, venous thromboembolism is much more common in the puerperium than during a similar period in women who have not recently been pregnant. Maternal deep vein thromboses (DVTs) are more common (80%–90%) in the left leg, occur usually in the iliofemoral veins, and are often associated with pulmonary embolism. Those with prior DVT and with hereditary thrombophilias are at highest risk.[107]

Women with inherited thrombophilias have an increased risk for venous thromboembolism, particularly during the puerperium. The overall prevalence of thrombophilic traits in the general population may be 10% or more; the probability of carrying multiple defects is therefore not that rare. Screening for these traits should be done liberally.[108]

In an ACOG high risk pregnancy monograph, Lockwood recommended that, no matter their past history, asymptomatic pregnant women with antithrombin deficiency and women who are homozygotes or compound heterozygotes for factor V Leiden or prothrombin (G20210A) mutations are at very high risk for thromboembolic episodes and should have anticoagulant therapy throughout pregnancy and in the puerperium.[109,110] Following delivery (6–12 hr), heparin therapy should be resumed and warfarin (Coumadin) therapy begun. Until the internationalized ratio (INR) has been in the therapeutic range for two consecutive days, heparin should be continued. Coumadin should be continued for at least 6 weeks, and longer if there have been prior thromboembolic events.

If a woman developed a venous thromboembolism (VTE) during pregnancy, whether or not she was found to have an inherited or acquired thrombophilia, Lockwood recommends full anticoagulation during pregnancy, resumption of heparin after delivery, and establishment and maintenance of therapeutic levels of oral anticoagulation for 6 to 18 weeks thereafter. He is careful to note that, as there are no randomized clinical trials to assess the efficacy of anticoagulation therapy in preventing maternal or fetal complications, recommendations must rely on expert opinion.[110]

Similar recommendations were published by a group in Australia and New Zealand, recommending 6 months of therapy and treatment for at least 6 weeks postpartum for women who experienced VTE either during pregnancy or postpartum.[72]

For women who had a previous thromboembolism, they recommend therapy postpartum, with the decision whether to treat during pregnancy based upon whether the index event was spontaneous or provoked, the presence or absence of a family history of VTE, the presence of a known thrombophilia, and whether there have been multiple episodes of VTE.[72,111]

Women with a past history of a single provoked thrombotic event with an underlying thrombophilia may be treated by careful observation before delivery and 6 weeks of postpartum prophylaxis.[72,111]

Women with recurrent VTE, previous idiopathic VTE, or a previous VTE and strong family history, but no demonstrated thrombophilia are advised to use thrombophylaxis throughout pregnancy and for 6 weeks thereafter.[72,111]

In our own practice, we liberally solicit input from hematologists on a case-by-case basis, as clinical knowledge about the thrombophilias and their role in VTE during and after pregnancy is increasing rapidly.

Finally, the puerperium offers an opportunity to perform or complete a thrombophilia workup, which may have either been delayed or done only partially during pregnancy, because of physiologic changes elevating a number of clotting factors, including factor VIII, protein S, and protein C.

Postpartum Alopecia

An uncommon complication of pregnancy is a diffuse shedding of scalp hair, often beginning 2 to 5 months after delivery. It is not well described in the medical literature, nor is its cause clearly elucidated. Treatment approaches have severally included topical estrogens and progesterone, as well as thyroid supplementation, all with inconsistent results. It remains a puzzling problem.[112]

SUMMARY OF MANAGEMENT OPTIONS
Medical Problems

Management Options	Quality of Evidence	Strength of Recommendation	References
Cardiovascular			
See Chapter 37 for Management Options			
Main complications of note are heart failure and ARDS	–	GPP	–
Cardiomyopathy			
See Chapter 37 for Management Options			
Hypertension			
See Chapters 36 and 80 for Management Options			
ACE inhibitors can be reintroduced into management	III	B	101–103
Diabetes			
See Chapter 45 for Management Options			
Women with presumed gestational diabetes should stop all medication and perform glucose series to confirm return of glucose homeostasis to normal	–	GPP	–
Thromboembolic Disease			
See Chapters 42, 43, and 44 for Management Options			
Alopecia			
Various treatments have been advocated but without clear evidence of benefit:	IV	C	112
Estrogen creams			
Progesterone creams			
Thyroid supplementation			

ACE, angiotensin-converting enzyme; ARDS, acute respiratory distress syndrome.

CHANGES IN COGNITION AND MOOD: PUERPERAL PSYCHOLOGICAL REACTIONS

Several authors have suggested that women may show specific areas of cognitive changes during and after pregnancy, notably deficits in verbal learning and memory (See also Chapter 56). Mood appears to be affected as well. Steroidal hormones are increasingly recognized as highly relevant in multiple aspects of brain functioning.[113] Although steroid hormones show a pattern of associations with mood during and after pregnancy, no such pattern is evident for cognition.

The postpartum period may represent a time of increased vulnerability to depression for some women.[114] Postpartum "blues" is a transient condition characterized by mild, and often rapid, mood swings, from elation to sadness, irritability, anxiety, decreased concentration, insomnia, tearfulness, and crying spells.[115] Due largely to inconsistencies in diagnostic criteria, the data regarding incidence conflict. Major depressive disorders are thought to afflict 5% to 9% of women at any time, with a lifetime risk of 10% to 25%.[116] New episodes of depression in the first 4 to 6 weeks after delivery occur three times more frequently than in nonpregnant controls.[117] Depression has been described in up to 30% of women in the first postpartum year.[118–120] Other studies have not confirmed this relation, observing rates of postpartum depression similar to depression diagnosed without relation to pregnancy.[121–123]

Hormonal changes following delivery are often presumed to play a role in the development of PPD; however, the relationship between postpartum changes and the development of depression is not well understood.[114] Women may complain of depressive symptoms shortly after delivery, at any time during the following few months, and at cessation of lactation, although it is unclear whether stopping nursing child is cause or effect.[124] Moreover, there is good evidence that, in many cases, PPD may begin well before delivery. One study reported that the prevalence of depression at 32 weeks (13.5%) was higher than postpartum (9.1%).[125] In another study, half of all women diagnosed with PPD had onset of symptoms during or even before their pregnancies.[126]

Wickberg and Hwang investigated the use of the Edinburgh Postnatal Depression Scale (EPDS) on a population-based sample of 1655 women who completed the scale at 2 and 3 months postpartum. They also interviewed 128 using the Montgomery Asberg Depression Rating Scale (MADRS) and assessed them according to DSM-III-R criteria for major depression. A cut-off score of 11.5 on the EPDS identified all but two women with major depression (sensitivity = 96%, specificity 49%, positive predictive value 59%).[127]

Thoppil and others presented at the 2002 Armed Forces District ACOG meeting a report of their institution's multidisciplinary approach to identifying women at risk for depression during pregnancy and postpartum (Table 78–3). Called ISIS (identify, screen, intervene, and support), it was developed and supported by their psychiatry, obstetrics, and social work groups. Social workers educate patients about signs and symptoms of depression at the obstetrics orientation visit. Risk factors for depression are screened for at the first visit with midwife or obstetrician. The EPDS is applied at the 32-week visit. Patients with elevated scores are further evaluated, and consultation and treatment may be initiated by the psychiatry department. Although outcomes data are not yet available, the authors have found that this program thus far has worked smoothly.[128]

Management Options

Psychotherapy is the first-line treatment for depression during pregnancy or after the birth of a child. In some cases, antidepressant treatment may be warranted. The decision to prescribe an antidepressant drug during pregnancy or the postpartum period must be made on an individual basis.[129] Use of pharmacologic therapy in postpartum lactating women must balance the risk of possible deleterious drug effects on the infant via the mother's milk versus the risk of not treating a serious psychiatric condition. All medicines used for this purpose appear in breast milk in varying amounts. The provider must consider such risks to the baby as drug toxicity and the possibility of long-term effects on behavior and neurologic development, which have not as yet been elucidated.[130] Coordination with the baby's pediatrician is essential. Another consideration that must be dealt with before prescribing an antidepressant drug during pregnancy or the postpartum period concerns the matter of who will assume the responsibility for the patient's treatment once the puerperium has passed.

In one study, 25 women met standard diagnostic criteria for postpartum depression. They took 10, 20, or 40 mg/day of paroxetine for at least 4 weeks, and no other mood-altering drugs. Researchers studied fresh breast milk, collected within 6 hours of taking the drug, along with maternal and infant blood samples. Even the lowest dosage of paroxetine improved depression in some of the women. There were no differences among groups in the milk/plasma ratio, no matter what dosage the women took. Only very small amounts were found in breast milk and the infants' serum. These findings imply that one may treat a nursing woman safely with paroxetine,[131,132] as has been shown in similar studies of fluoxetine and sertraline. Prudence may be important, however; Stowe has found that in studying infants exposed to paroxetine via mother's milk, the drug was not found in their blood, similar to studies of sertraline and fluoxetine. However, he warns that one cannot assume it was not in the baby's brain, and it may be premature to base safety conclusions on undetectable concentrations in infant serum.[132]

The reader is referred to Chapter 56 for a more detailed discussion of the management options for postpartum blues, depression, and psychosis.

TABLE 78–3

DSM-IV Criteria for a Major Depressive Episode

A.	Five or more of the following symptoms must be present daily or almost daily for at least 2 consecutive weeks: 1. Depressed mood* 2. Loss of interest or pleasure* 3. Significant increase or decrease in appetite 4. Insomnia or hypersomnia 5. Psychomotor agitation or retardation 6. Fatigue or loss of energy 7. Feelings of worthlessness or guilt 8. Diminished concentration 9. Recurrent thoughts of suicide or death
B.	The symptoms do not meet the criteria for other psychiatric conditions.
C.	The symptoms cause significant impairment in functioning at work, school, and social activities.
D.	The symptoms are not caused directly by a substance or general medical condition.
E.	The symptoms are not caused by bereavement after the loss of a loved one.

*At least one of the five symptoms must be item 1 or 2.
Modified from: American Psychiatric Association: *Diagnostic and Statistical Manual of Mental Disorders*, 4th ed. Washington, D.C., 2000.

SEPARATED SYMPHYSIS PUBIS

Separated symphysis pubis (SSP) is a rare condition involving separation of the symphysis pubis in late pregnancy or during delivery. It usually occurs in otherwise healthy pregnancies and is likely to be the result of hormonal or biomechanical factors (or both). It is also referred to severally as subluxation (an incomplete or partial dislocation[133] of the symphysis pubis), diastasis of the symphysis pubis (probably erroneously),[133] and pelvic girdle relaxation.[134] This entity appears to be more common in the Scandinavian countries, raising the question of a genetic link. Symptoms may range from mild discomfort to total debilitation. Differential diagnosis is broad (osteitis pubis; sports injury; osteomyelitis; postsurgical injury; neoplasm; pubic osteolysis; idiopathic lower back pain; posttraumatic back pain; herniated nucleus pulposus; and various orthopedic, urologic, gynecologic problems) and requires exclusion of more serious medical and orthopedic conditions.

Separation of the symphysis pubis associated with pregnancy has striking clinical similarities to osteitis pubis. However, radiographic findings associated with SSP lack the typical rarefaction and sclerosis seen with osteitis pubis. Often, all that is seen is symphyseal separation, usually of more than 10 mm.[135] Kubitz and Goodlin cited seven cases of symptomatic subluxation in pregnancy or parturition with a prevalence of 1 in 300 births, which is more common than pregnancy complicated by osteitis pubis.[136]

SSP is thought to be caused by hormonal (relaxin and progesterone)[137,138] or biomechanical factors, relaxation, and weakening of the pelvic joints during pregnancy, because the joints of the pelvic girdle are forced to carry the additional weight of the uterus and its contents.[137,139] It is believed the symphysis pubis itself has limited movement, limited to a 3° rotation and a maximum vertical movement of 2 mm.[134] As the movement of the sacroiliac joints is also limited, this would tend to put more pressure on the symphysis.[140] Mechanical precipitating factors include tumultuous labor, difficult assisted vaginal delivery, large baby, excessive abduction of the thighs at the time of delivery, and sudden pressure on the symphysis pubis. In a group of 14 women evaluated by CT scan of the pelvis within 24 hours of delivery, 42% of these asymptomatic women had, on average, a 6.5 mm widening of the symphysis relative to age-matched nonpregnant controls, implying that some degree of asymptomatic separation of the symphysis is normal postpartum.[134,141]

SSP symptoms may present at any time intrapartum or postpartum, with a broad range of symptoms, including pain in the back or pelvic area, difficulty with ambulation, and local manifestation over the symphysis such as tenderness, induration, ecchymoses, and a palpable joint defect.[142]

Management Options

Successful treatment approaches include analgesia, bedrest, binders, limitation of ambulation, walking in a shuffling style when ambulating, avoiding both adduction and abduction of the hips, injections of local anesthetics, steroids, and other medications. Because of ambulation limitations, DVT becomes a risk, and thromboprophylaxis should be considered. Patient education and emotional support is critical, and follow-up with rehabilitative services, orthopedics, home nursing, and social work may be appropriate.[137,142,143]

Apparent paralysis of the lower limbs can sometimes be due to separation of the symphysis pubis or one of the synchondroses of the sacroiliac joint during labor. This may be followed by pain and continuing significant interference with locomotion as recovery occurs.[99]

OBSTETRIC PARALYSIS

The earliest well-documented report of maternal obstetric paralysis, albeit partial, in the English language literature comes from Dublin, around 1838,[145] describing how a young primigravida suffered foot-drop and loss of sensation in the right leg after a normal delivery.

In most cases of maternal obstetric paralysis, symptoms are unilateral, consisting of leg weakness, or, in more severe cases, foot drop. Prognosis for recovery from mild injuries is excellent with physical therapy; however, if fatty degeneration of nerve fibers has occurred, in which the nerves have been functionally severed from their nutritive centers (wallerian degeneration), recovery may take much longer and may never be complete.[133,147]

The incidence of obstetric paralysis is difficult to estimate due to the rapid evolution of obstetric practice during the past several decades. Data from series gathered from the 1930s to the 1970s suggest estimates of intrinsic obstetric maternal paralysis and adverse neurologic outcomes of between 1:2100 and 1:3000.[146,148,149] More contemporary estimates suggest this to be a much more rare complication, probably between 1:7000 and 1:14,000 in patients who do not receive regional anaesthesia/analgesia.[150]

In the industrialized world, obstetric paralysis is an entity seldom reported unless regional anesthesia/analgesia is involved; neurologic complications that follow childbirth are frequently blamed on epidurals and spinals, even when this is not the case.[151] The mechanisms whereby regional/conduction anesthesia/analgesia may be associated with neurologic damage have been well-documented and include neurotoxicity, ischemia, trauma, and compression that may be due to hematomata or abscesses.[151]

Bademasi and colleagues[152] in 1980 presented the results of a prospective study of 34 Nigerian women with puerperal paresis of the lower limbs. These patients tended to be shorter than average. Lumbosacral plexus injury with foot-drop was the most frequent presenting feature (88%); 38% had bilateral involvement; 26% had femoral neuropathy; and 35% absent ankle tendon jerks. Fifteen percent had spastic paraparesis. Electromyographic examination and conduction velocity examination were consistent with proximal neuropraxia of the lumbosacral trunk in 88%. The major predisposing factor was prolonged labor. Further associations with paralysis were hydroureter, vesicovaginal fistula, and rectovaginal fistula (possibly due to pressure necrosis). Recovery was complete in 76%. The authors concluded that direct pressure on the lumbosacral plexus and nerve trunks by the presenting fetal part is the major factor in the pathogenesis of obstetric neuropraxia.

A later paper by Feasby and associates[144] used comprehensive electrophysiologic testing to document two cases of lumbosacral plexus injury, which localized the site of this obstetric paralysis to the lumbosacral trunk (L4-5) and S1 root where they join and pass over the pelvic rim. They noted that paralysis may be mild or severe. Small maternal size, large fetus, midforceps rotation, and fetal malposition were noted to be conditions that might place the mother at risk for nerve injury.

These findings are consistent with earlier reports that the roots of the sciatic nerve may be compressed in the pelvis by the fetal head or obstetric forceps, and the brunt of the resulting motor deficit is then borne by muscles supplied by the common perineal fibers because of their relationship to the bony pelvis. This type of lumbosacral plexus injury seems to be more likely when a short patient with a small pelvis carries a rather large baby, so that labor is complicated by minor disproportion, or when midforceps are used during delivery because of malpresentation.[149] Mothers with a straight sacrum, a flat wide posterior pelvis, posterior displacement of the transverse diameter of the inlet, wide sacroiliac notches, and prominent ischial spines have been thought to have a predisposition to this complication.

Neurotoxicity within the epidural space has been reported to cause paraplegia following the injection of various substances, including a relatively large dose of hypertonic potassium chloride.[153] Several years ago, several cases of neurologic deficit were attributed to the use of 2-chloroprocaine containing the antioxidant 0.2% sodium bisulfite. It would seem that the problem was not the medication but the preservative.[154] In general, however, injections into the epidural space would be expected to be well tolerated[155] as opposed to subarachnoid injections; nerve roots are extremely vulnerable to neurolytic substances.[156] Disastrous consequences of spinal anesthesia/analgesia, albeit rare, have been reported.[157,158]

Ischemia may lead to spinal cord damage; reports have associated this with arterial constriction,[159] vascular malformation,[160] disc herniation,[161,162] vertebral canal stenosis,[163] abscess,[164,165] and hematoma.[166,167] The last condition is of particular concern in this era of prophylactic use of anticoagulants in a growing number of patients. Anesthesiologists especially have expressed a concern about needle or catheter placement in patients who have been using low-molecular-weight heparins. However, to date reports of catastrophic hematoma formation have been lacking.

Management Options

When neurologic damage follows childbirth, it is important to elucidate the mechanism of its occurrence; it is generally advisable to seek the opinion of a neurologist early in the course of the problem.

URINARY RETENTION

Although there would seem to be no universally accepted definition of postpartum urinary retention, this has frequently been classified as either clinically overt postpartum urinary retention, that is, the inability to void spontaneously after delivery, or covert urinary retention, identified through measurements of postvoid bladder residual volumes, measured or calculated by either catheterization or bladder imaging.[168–170]

The cause of postpartum urinary retention has not been clearly elucidated: in normal micturition, afferent input arises from stretch receptors in the bladder that travel through myelinated fibers in the pelvic nerve to the spinal cord and pontine micturition center. Efferent signals mediate relaxation of the urethral and periurethral striated muscles and pelvic floor through the pudendal and sacral nerves; detrusor muscle contraction and relaxation of urethral smooth muscle are mediated by the pelvic nerve and parasympathetic outflow.[171,172]

The capacity of the puerperal bladder is increased over that of the nonpregnant state; it is relatively insensitive to intravesical fluid pressure. Overdistention, incomplete emptying, and excessive residual urine are not unusual. This may be contributed to by anesthetic effects, especially after spinal or epidural analgesia/anesthesia. Conditions are ripe for the development of urinary tract infection because of bladder trauma and dilated renal pelves and ureters, which will not return to their prepregnant state until 2 to 8 weeks after delivery.[88]

The physiologic changes of pregnancy, regional anesthesia, instrumental delivery, cesarean delivery, perineal trauma, protracted labor,[173] and primiparity have variously been associated with postpartum urinary retention, as have rare instances of lumbar disk disease,[174] spinal subdural hematoma,[175] postpartum uterine retroversion,[176] and impacted pelvic masses.[177]

Impaired function of the detrusor can result from overdistention and might account for some cases in which prolonged urinary retention is seen. Postpartum urinary retention observed after regional analgesia/anesthesia may be due to temporary disruption of afferent input. It may be that urinary retention because of instrument-assisted vaginal delivery is related to impaired reflex and voluntary relaxation of the urethral sphincter, periurethral muscles, and pelvic floor. Instrument-assisted vaginal delivery may also result in mechanical outlet obstruction because of the perineal edema that often accompanies such procedures.[178]

Kerr-Wilson and colleagues studied the effect of labor on postpartum bladder function. Urodynamic investigations were performed on 20 patients at 48 hours and at 4 weeks after delivery to assess the effect of modern obstetric practice on the postpartum bladder. Their idea was to assess this by comparing function within 48 hours of delivery with findings at 4 weeks postpartum.

Water cystometry and uroflowmetry were performed. Studies demonstrated a slight but significant decrease in bladder capacity (from 395.5 to 331 mL) and volume at first void (from 277 to 224 mL) in the study interval. All urodynamic values studied were within normal limits on both occasions. Results were not affected by the weight of the infant or by an episiotomy. However, prolonged labor and the use of epidural anesthesia appeared to diminish postpartum bladder function transiently.[179]

In this study, the bladder was not found to be hypotonic postpartum as had been noted by other investigators previously.[180,181] This difference in more contemporary patients was attributed to active management of labor with oxytocin and more frequent cesarean delivery, which allowed for avoidance of prolonged labor, as well as earlier catheterization if the patient was unable to void.

The effects of analgesia and anesthesia are less clear. A study from Geneva suggested that the use of epidural pain relief was associated with postpartum bladder hypotonia and urinary retention, although the cause for this may actually be the fact that their labors were significantly longer.[182] These authors concluded that, as long as prolonged labors were avoided and catheterization done promptly for bladder distention, there was no evidence for any increased risk for bladder hypotonia.

Andolf and coinvestigators[169] used ultrasonography to measure residual bladder volumes 3 days after vaginal delivery in 539 unselected consecutive women. Only 1.5% had abnormal volumes, and only 0.5% needed urinary catheters. Urinary retention was more common after instrumental delivery or epidural analgesia. Despite these reassuring findings, the same women were rescanned 4 years later and by this time one in three was experiencing voiding difficulties. This suggests that such difficulties are not due primarily to postpartum retention.

Viktrup and colleagues[183] followed 305 nulliparous women during pregnancy and the puerperium; 7% developed stress incontinence after delivery. Obstetric factors such as the length of the second stage, infant head circumference, birth weight, and episiotomy were associated with the development of stress incontinence after delivery. Impaired muscle function in or around the urethra during vaginal delivery was proposed as the pathophysiology underlying puerperal incontinence. Most women returned to normal micturition by 3 months postpartum.

A retrospective, case-control study in Minnesota identified 51 cases of clinically overt urinary retention occurring after 11,332 vaginal deliveries (incidence = 0.45%). Individually, statistically significant associations with primiparity, forceps/vacuum use, epidural/spinal anesthesia, and mediolateral episiotomy were identified, but by multivariate analysis, only instrument-assisted vaginal delivery and regional anesthesia were identified as independent risk factors.[178]

A study in Hong Kong based upon telephone interviews of 394 women, 73 of whom had been diagnosed with postpartum urinary retention, concluded that the retention cohort did not suffer statistically significantly higher subsequent rates of stress urinary incontinence, urinary frequency, nocturia, or urgency.[184] This same group reported that covert postpartum urinary retention, while documented in 9.7% of women delivering vaginally, seemed to be self-limited, with postvoid residuals returning to normal within 4 days without specific treatment.[173]

Vasovagal collapse is a dramatic but uncommon sequel to postpartum urinary retention. This can occur especially with lumbar epidural or spinal anesthesia. Even if the patient becomes aware of pain, this might signify return of the sympathetic afferents, while the sacral parasympathetics remain paralyzed. As the sacral parasympathetic supply remains insensate, the patient perceives no subjective sensation of bladder stretching. If untreated (with catheterization), bladder distention can lead to excessive supraspinal parasympathetic outflow resulting in vasovagal syncope.[185]

Evidence to date would suggest that careful attention to all postpartum women, with prompt catheterization for those who cannot void, will prevent most problems related to urinary retention.

SUMMARY OF MANAGEMENT OPTIONS
Other Puerperal Problems

Management Options	Quality of Evidence	Strength of Recommendation	References
Pubic Symphysis Separation			
Most resolve with rest, trochanter belts, analgesics, weight bearing assistance and time	III	B	143
Consider injection of symphysis with mixture of hydrocortisone and lidocaine (chymotrypsin)	III	B	143
Consider thromboprophylaxis with prolonged bedrest	–	GPP	–
Orthopedic treatment reserved for severe cases	–	GPP	–
Obstetric Paralysis—Prevention:			
Avoid prolonged, obstructed labor	–	GPP	–
Proper lithotomy and pushing positions			
Avoid regional anesthesia when coagulopathy or infection is present (systemic or local)			

SUMMARY OF MANAGEMENT OPTIONS
Other Puerperal Problems *(Continued)*

Management Options	Quality of Evidence	Strength of Recommendation	References
Obstetric Paralysis—Management			
Seek neurological opinion and identify the cause	IV	C	157
Splinting, physical therapy, electrical nerve stimulation			
Paraplegia warrants immediate MRI			
Emergency surgery for epidural abscess or hematoma			
Urinary Retention			
12–24 h continuous drainage if > 400 mL residual; majority recover spontaneously	–	GPP	–
Exclude infection	–	GPP	–
Rarely, intermittent self-catheterization required	III	B	184
Investigate if self-catheterization required	–	GPP	–

CONTRACEPTION

It has been demonstrated that ovulation may occur as early as 27 days after delivery (mean: 70–75 days in the absence of lactation).[186,187] Among nursing mothers, the mean time to ovulation is about 6 months.[8] Variables affecting this include frequency of suckling, duration of each suckling period, and amount of supplementation.[188]

Persistently elevated serum prolactin levels appear to be responsible for the suppression of ovulation among lactating women.[189] Levels of prolactin decrease to the normal range by the third week postpartum in nonlactating women, but remain elevated for several more weeks in lactating patients. Immediately after delivery, levels of estrogen fall in all women and remain low in lactating patients. In women not lactating, estrogen levels begin to rise 2 weeks after delivery and are significantly higher than in lactating women by day 17 postpartum. Follicle-stimulating hormone (FSH) levels are identical in women regardless of whether they are lactating. It is therefore assumed that the ovary does not respond to FSH stimulation in the presence of increased prolactin levels.[8]

It is generally advised that vaginal coitus may be resumed when the perineum is comfortable and lochia has slowed. Desire and willingness to resume vaginal coitus after delivery varies greatly among women—this may depend on several factors, including return of libido, presence of vaginal atrophy because of lactation, and presence and state of healing of incisions and lacerations.[190] Most women have resumed intercourse by 3 months, some much earlier.[191] On the other hand, Ryding[192] reported that 20% of women had little desire for sexual activity 3 months after delivery, and an additional 21% had complete loss of desire or aversion to sexual activity.

Abstinence, or, more properly, the intention to abstain from vaginal coitus, is not an effective means of postpartum contraception. Even though it is traditional for obstetricians to advise postponing coitus, sometimes until after the traditional 6- to 8-week postpartum examination, and in spite of lochia, which may persist for 3 to 8 weeks, coitus is likely to occur, and it is prudent to have a contraception plan in effect beforehand.

Management Options

Choice of Contraceptive Method

BARRIER METHODS

In general, barrier methods of contraception have fewer side effects than hormonal methods, and, with the exception of cervical caps and diaphragms, are available without prescription. In addition, under some circumstances they have been shown to provide protection against sexually transmitted diseases. A meta-analysis has shown that regular use of latex condoms decreased the coital transmission of HIV infection by 69%. Epidemiologic studies have shown a decreased risk of genital herpes simplex, gonorrhea, and nongonococcal urethritis in women whose partners faithfully use condoms.[193–195] Unfortunately, the efficacy of barrier methods in preventing both conception and infection depends heavily on the users adhering to manufacturer's recommendations. Most studies have demonstrated a significant difference between method effectiveness and use-effectiveness.

HORMONAL CONTRACEPTION

ACOG has recommended that progestin-only methods are the hormonal method of choice in breastfeeding women and may slightly increase the volume of breast milk (Table 78–4).[196] Manufacturers have recommended that their use be postponed until 6 weeks postpartum in breastfeeding women, because very small amounts of progestin are passed into breast milk, although no adverse effects on infants have been noted when these medications have been started earlier.[197]

The World Health Organization (WHO) has recommended that the breastfeeding woman wait at least 6 months after childbirth to start using estrogen-progestin contraceptives.[198] ACOG has called this and a similar FDA recommendation "a conservative approach" resulting for the most part from experience of earlier combination oral contraceptive studies using higher doses of estrogens. They note "low-dose tablets (35 μg or lower) probably have a lesser effect on quality and quantity of breast milk." If combination oral contraceptives are prescribed, they should not be started before 6 weeks postpartum, and the physician should continue to evaluate the woman's individual breastfeeding experience.[8,193,199]

INTRAUTERINE CONTRACEPTIVE DEVICES

Copper-containing and hormone-releasing intrauterine devices (IUCDs) have been shown to be effective in preventing conception, with failure rates on the order of 2 to 3 pregnancies per 100 women-years.[200,201] Objections that the principal mode of action of IUCDs was, in essence, the abortion of a viable conceptus have been effectively laid to rest.[202] This concept has been supported by both the ACOG and the WHO.[8,203] It is important to inform women that, unlike barrier contraceptives, IUCDs do not provide protection against HIV or other sexually transmitted diseases.

NATURAL FAMILY PLANNING

Natural family planning (NFP) remains a controversial topic. On the basis of mailing a questionnaire to 840 Missouri physicians (obstetrician/gynecologists, family practice physicians, general practice physicians, internal medicine specialists) (65% response rate), authors concluded that most physicians underestimate the effectiveness of NFP and do not give information of modern methods to women.[204] NFP methods are based on the prediction of ovulation using temperature, cervical mucus assessment, and timing. They are not reliable in the absence of relatively regular menstrual cycles, which may take some time to reestablish following delivery.[205] Success rates similar to barrier methods have been reported.[206]

NFP methods vary greatly, but all utilize to some extent selective timing of coitus according to some or all of a variety of methods, to include periodic abstinence, use of menstrual calendars, ovulation prediction, withdrawal, and lactational amenorrhea.

LACTATIONAL AMENORRHEA METHOD

Exclusive breastfeeding helps prevent pregnancy for the first 6 months after delivery but should be relied on only temporarily and when it meets carefully observed criteria of the lactational amenorrhea method (LAM) of contraception.[199] The suckling stimulus provides the only truly physiologic signal that suppresses fertility in normally nourished, healthy women. The variability in the duration of lactational amenorrhea between women is related to the variation in the strength of the suckling stimulus, a unique situation between each mother and baby. Full breastfeeding can provide a reliable contraceptive effect in the first 6 to 9 months. In women, suckling seems to increase the sensitivity of the hypothalamus to the negative feedback effect of estradiol on suppressing the gonadotropin-releasing hormone/luteinizing hormone (GnRH/LH) pulse generator. Practical guidelines for using breast-feeding as a natural contraceptive have been developed, which allows mothers to utilize the only natural suppressor of fertility in women as an effective means of spacing births.[206]

Table 78–5 lists the comparative effectiveness of the different methods of contraception.

TABLE 78–4

ACOG Recommendations for Hormonal Contraception if Used by Breastfeeding Women

Progestin-only oral contraceptives prescribed or dispensed at discharge from hospital to be started 2–3 weeks postpartum (e.g., the first Sunday after the newborn is 2 weeks old)
Depot medroxyprogesterone acetate initiated at 6 weeks postpartum (earlier initiation might be considered in certain clinical situations)
Hormonal implants inserted at 6 weeks postpartum
Combined estrogen-progestin contraceptives, if prescribed, should not be started before 6 weeks postpartum, and only when lactation is well established and the infant's nutritional status well monitored

Modified from American College of Obstetrics and Gynecology. Breastfeeding: Maternal and Infant Aspects. Washington, D.C., 2000. ACOG Educational Bulletin No. 258.

STERILIZATION

Female Sterilization

Tubal sterilization is the most frequently used method of contraception in the United States.[207] More than 600,000 female sterilization procedures, and more than 500,000 male sterilization procedures are performed each year in the United States.[208,209] Preoperative counseling should include a clear discussion about risks of, alternatives to, possibility of failure, and planned irreversibility of permanent surgical sterilization.

Complication rates are low, with an overall mortality rate of 1 to 2 deaths per 100,000 sterilization procedures.[210] Long-term effects of tubal sterilization on pelvic pain, menstrual patterns, and the need for subsequent pelvic surgery are controversial and inconsistent.[211]

The findings of the U.S. Collaborative Review of Sterilization (CREST) were published by the Centers for

TABLE 78-5

Contraceptive Techniques. Comparison of Effectiveness in Terms of Number of Pregnancies per 100 Women during First Year of Use

TECHNIQUE	TYPICAL USE*	PERFECT USE†	RISK REDUCTION FOR SEXUALLY TRANSMITTED INFECTIONS
Continuous abstinence	0.00	0.00	Complete
Nonpenetration	N/A‡	N/A	Some
Hormone implant	0.05	0.05	None
Sterilization			
Male	0.15	0.10	None
Female	0.50	0.50	None
Depot medroxyprogesterone	0.30	0.30	None
Intrauterine device			
Copper	2.0	1.5	None
Hormonal	0.1–0.8	0.1–0.6	None
Oral contraceptives			
Combination	5.0	0.1	None
Progestin-only	5.0	0.5	None
Male condom	14.0	3.0	Good vs. HIV; reduces risk of others
Withdrawal	19.0	4.0	None
Diaphragm	20.0	6.0	Limited
Cervical cap			
Nulliparas	20.0	9.0	Limited
Paras	40.0	30.0	Limited
Female condom	21.0	5.0	Some
Predicting fertility			
periodic abstinence	20.0		None
postovulation method		1.0	None
symptothermal method		2.0	None
cervical mucus method		3.0	none
calendar method		9.0	None
Fertility awareness methods			
with condom	N/A	N/A	None
with diaphragm or cap	N/A	N/A	None
with withdrawal or other methods	N/A	N/A	None
Spermicide	26.0	6.0	Limited
No method	85.0	85.0	None

*Typical use refers to failure rates for women and men whose use is not consistent or always correct.
†Perfect use refers to failure rates for those whose use is consistent and always correct.
‡N/A:Effectiveness rates not available.
Modified from Facts about Birth Control. www.plannedparenthood.org.

Disease Control and Prevention in 1996;[212] these present the only available long-term failure rate data in a very large[10] group of women, with 58% still providing follow-up data at 8 to 14 years after their procedures. CREST showed a 10-year cumulative failure rate of 18.5 per 1000 for all sterilization methods combined. During that interval, postpartum tubal ligation and interval laparoscopic unipolar coagulation were the most effective methods (7.5 failures per 1000).[212] Sterilization failures are frequently manifested as ectopic pregnancies; CREST showed a 10-year cumulative probability of ectopic pregnancy of 7.3 per 1000. The specific ectopic rate following postpartum partial salpingectomy was the lowest among all methods (1.5 per 1000).[213]

In the United States, the strongest indicator of future regret is young age at the time of sterilization, regardless of parity or marital status.[211,214] Women 20 to 24 years of age at sterilization are twice as likely to experience regret as women 10 years older.[215] Approximately 6% of sterilized women report regret or request information about sterilization reversal within 5 years of the procedure;[211] approximately 1% to 2% of men having vas ligation seek information on reversal.[215,216]

The success of surgical reversal of tubal sterilization would seem to be mainly related to the amount of undamaged fallopian tube remaining for reanastomosis.[217] It is difficult to compare studies concerning the success of sterilization, as they generally have small numbers, and because investigators use different preoperative exclusion criteria; length of follow-up also varies significantly.[218] After a Pomeroy-type procedure was reversed, studies report subsequent term pregnancy rates of 41% to 74% in a total of 198 patients, with ectopic rates of 6% to 9%.[219–221] Following bipolar cautery, reversal success as measured by term pregnancy was 42% to 52% in a total of 137 patients, with ectopic pregnancy rates of 3% to 17%.[217,219,220]

Intrapartum or early puerperium procedures are convenient as the patient is already hospitalized. Cesarean delivery gives excellent access to the fallopian tubes. Following vaginal delivery, an epidural catheter may be left in place and then used to provide anesthesia and analgesia for a procedure later in the day or on the following day. On the other hand, waiting another couple of months for an interval procedure allows time to gain confidence in the health of the baby and dispassionately discuss all implications of permanent surgical sterilization.[8]

For years there have been concerns about a syndrome of poststerilization pain and menstrual disturbances. A large review comparing women who had tubal sterilization with controls showed no consistent differences in outcomes such as levels of hormones, and little difference in the characteristics of menses, although there is, understandably, an increase in menstrual flow in women who had been using oral contraceptives.[222] On the other hand, a cohort study with 6 years of follow-up reported that sterilized women were more likely to be hospitalized because of menstrual disorders, usually to have curettage (RR = 2.4).[223] The subgroup of women under 30 years of age studied in CREST who had menstrual dysfunction predating their sterilization procedures had more menstrual changes and, ultimately, were more likely to undergo hysterectomy than controls.[218,223,224]

Transcervical, intrauterine instillation of quinacrine may be a simple, inexpensive, effective, acceptable, and safe method of nonsurgical permanent female sterilization. A study in Bangladesh reported a 1.9% failure rate using 252 mg of quinacrine with or without adjuvant ampicillin or ibuprofen (or both). No serious complications were reported.[225] A larger study in Vietnam, however, reported higher failure rates (13% in women younger than 35, 6.8% in women older than 35). Moreover, these authors noted that toxicology studies of locally applied quinacrine were thought by WHO to be inadequate.[226] It would seem that more study is needed before this method can be recommended in the United States.

Some years ago there was in the United States enthusiasm for scheduled cesarean hysterectomy as a sterilization procedure.[227] It was thought by some that this might prove to be a life-saving measure in some cases, for example, for women with cervical dysplasia who were either noncompliant with follow-up, or had limited access to care. Most studies, however, reported worrisome complication rates, especially regarding the need for blood product replacement. Even though a group in Israel reported an improvement in the need for transfusion from 64% to 17% as their experience increased,[228] the prevailing feeling would seem to be that cesarean hysterectomy without other indications likely has, in most cases, an unfavorable benefit/risk ratio.

Although there is some confidence that tubal ligation protects from recurrent pelvic inflammatory disease, more than 70 cases of salpingitis and almost 40 cases of tubo-ovarian abscess in women who had undergone tubal occlusion have been published. Most cases of salpingitis developed more than a year after either laparoscopic or laparotomy procedures. Tubo-ovarian abscesses developed over a broad interval of time following operation, ranging from weeks to decades.[229]

Male Sterilization

Surgical ligation of the vas deferens is a safe and highly effective means of permanent surgical sterilization. Outpatient ligation of the vas deferens has been a popular procedure since the mid-1960s. As of 1988, at least 5,000,000 U.S. men had undergone this procedure.[230] Most series report subsequent pregnancy rates of less than 1%.[231] In one study, only 20 of 1000 men had a positive semen analysis during a 3-year follow-up period,[232] and the sperm count was less than 10,000/mL in 17 of these men, none of whom reported an unwanted pregnancy.

As with any such procedure, men should be counseled about the risks of, and alternatives to, the procedure, the possibility of failure, and the planned irreversibility of vas ligation. Alternative contraception should be used until at least 90 days have elapsed since the procedure, and semen analyses show either no sperm at all or, at least, no motile sperm. As life circumstances change, however, some men will decide to consider reversal of the procedure, and 50% to 70% of men in whom a reversal operation is undertaken are fertile.[233,234] The reversal success rate depends upon the duration between vasectomy and the reversal procedure; in general, the longer after vasectomy, the less the likelihood of success.[193,235]

Concern that the risk of testicular and prostate cancer may be increased in men after vasectomy would seem to be unfounded. Earlier population-based series showed no increase in risk of testicular cancer among vasectomized men,[236,237] nor any increased risk of prostate cancer.[231,238] However, a recent quantitative review of prostate cancer studies suggested that men with a prior vasectomy may be at an increased risk. However, this increase may not be causal since potential bias cannot be discounted. The overall association was small and therefore could be explained by bias. Interestingly, the relative risk increased over time.[239] Finally, a study of 22,071 U.S. physicians showed that vasectomy did not increase the risk of subsequent cardiovascular disease, even 15 or more years after the procedure.[240]

SUMMARY OF MANAGEMENT OPTIONS
Puerperal Contraception and Sterilization

Management Options	Quality of Evidence	Strength of Recommendation	References
Contraception			
See Table 78–5 for relative effectiveness of different methods	IV	C	248
Barrier:			
Few side effects, some protection against sexually transmitted disease	III	B	193–195
Effectiveness totally dependent on user compliance	–	GPP	–
Hormonal:			
Progestin-only preparations for breast-feeding women	IV	C	196
Relies on user compliance	–	GPP	–
IUCD:			
Main concerns relate to failure to protect against infection	–	GPP	–
Natural family planning:			
Main problem as a method in the puerperium is that the method relies on a regular menstrual cycle, which is uncommon initially	IV	C	205
Lactation amenorrhea method:			
Much debate in the literature over the value of this method/approach	III	B	199,206
Sterilization			
Tubal sterilization (different techniques):			
Patients must be counseled about			
The procedure	–	GPP	–
The irreversibility (varies with method)	III	B	217
Failure rates (varies with method and timing with respect to delivery)	III	B	210
Complications (e.g., regret, ectopics, menstrual disturbance, death)	III	B	211
Cesarean hysterectomy–Should only be considered in a few selected cases	III	B	227,228
Chemical methods—Not currently advocated; further research needed	IIb	B	225,226
Vasectomy:			
Same counseling as with female sterilization:	III	B	231,236–238,240
The procedure			
The irreversibility			
Failure rates			
Complications (generally safe, with no evidence of prostate or testicular cancer or cardiovascular disease)			

CONCLUSIONS

- The puerperium is a neglected phase of pregnancy.
- Surveillance for normal recovery following pregnancy and dealing with minor complaints is all the majority of women require.
- It is an opportunity for health promotion (e.g., smoking cessation, elimination of alcohol, vaccinations, and family planning).
- A few women will develop significant problems that must be recognized and managed promptly especially those with:
    - Puerperal pyrexia
    - Breast infection
    - Medical problems

REFERENCES

1. Jennings B, Edmundson M: The postpartum periods: After confinement: The fourth trimester. Clin Obstet Gynecol 1980;23:1093–1103.
2. Li XF, Fortney JA, Kotelchuck M, Glover LH: Int J Gynaecol Obstet 1996;54:1–10.
3. Kim-Godwin YS: Postpartum beliefs and practices among non-Western cultures. Am J Matern Child Nurs 2003;28:74–78.
4. Sebire NJ, Jolly M, Harris JP, et al: Maternal obesity and pregnancy outcome: A study of 287,213 pregnancies in London. Int J Obesity Related Metabol Disord 2001;25:1175–1178.
5. Chambers HM, Chan FY: Support for women/families after perinatal death. Cochrane Database Syst Rev, 1998, Issue 2, Art. No. CD000452. DOI:10.1002/14651858.CD000452.
6. Forrest G: Effective Care in Pregnancy and Childbirth. Oxford, Oxford University Press, 1989, p. 1423.
7. Drotar D, Baskiewicz A, Irvin N, et al: The adaptation of parents to the birth of an infant with a congenital malformation: A hypothetical model. Pediatrics 1975;6:710–717.
8. Bowes WA Jr., Katz VL: Postpartum Care. In Gabbe SG, Niebyl JR, Simpson JL (eds): Obstetrics: Normal & Problem Pregnancies, 4th ed. New York, Churchill Livingstone, 2002.
9. Rowe J, Clyman R, Green C, et al: Follow-up of families who experience perinatal death. Pediatrics 1978;62:166–170.
10. Brost L, Kenney JW: Pregnancy after perinatal loss: Parental reactions and nursing interventions. J Obstet Gynecol Neonatal Nurs 1992;21:457–463.
11. Chez RA: Acute grief and mourning: One obstetrician's experience. Obstet Gynecol 1995;85:1059–1061.
12. Calhoun LK: Parents' perceptions of nursing support following neonatal loss. J Perinat Neonatal Nurs 1994;8:57–66.
13. Alexander KV: The one thing you can never take away. Am J Matern Child Nurs 2001;26:123–127.
14. Primeau MR, Recht CK: Professional bereavement photographs: One aspect of a perinatal bereavement program. J Obstet Gynecol Neonatal Nurs 1994;23:22–25.
15. DiMarco M, Renker P, Medas J, et al: Effects of an educational bereavement program on health care professionals' perceptions of perinatal loss. J Continuing Educ Nurs 2002;33:180–186.
16. Midland D, Gensch B, Rybarik F: RTS Bereavement Training, 4th ed. La Crosse, WI: Gundersen Lutheran Medical Foundation, 2001.
17. Kaplan CG: Postpartum examination of the placenta. Clin Obstet Gynecol 1996;39:535–548.
18. Calvert S, Fleming V: Minimizing postpartum pain: A review of research pertaining to perineal care in childbearing women. J Advanced Nurs 2000;32:407–415.
19. Attrill B: The assumption of the maternal role: A developmental process. Aust J Midwifery 2002;15:21–25.
20. Brown S, Small R, Faber B, et al: Early postnatal discharge from hospital for healthy mothers and term infants. Cochrane Database Syst Rev CD002958, 2002.
21. Hale RW, Milne L: The elite athlete and exercise in pregnancy. Semin Perinatol 1996;20:277–284.
22. McCrory MA, Nommsen-Rivers LA, Mole PA, et al: Randomized trial of short-term effects of dieting compared with dieting plus aerobic exercise on lactation performance. Am J Clin Nutr 1999;69:959–967.
23. Dewey KG, Lovelady CA, Nommsen-Rivers LA, et al: A randomized study of the effects of aerobic exercise by lactating women on breast-milk volume and composition. N Engl J Med 1994;330:449–453.
24. Kulpa PJ, White BM, Visscher R: Aerobic exercise in pregnancy. Am, J Obstet Gynecol 1987:156:1395–1403.
25. Artal R: Recommendations for exercise during pregnancy and the postpartum period. UpToDate, 2003.
26. Barman MR, Queenan JT: Advising pregnant and postop working patients. Contemporary OB/GYN April 1984.
27. Dewhurst CJ: Secondary postpartum hemorrhage. J Obstet Gynaecol Br Comm 1966;73:53.
28. American College of Obstetricians and Gynecologists: Diagnosis and Management of Postpartum Hemorrhage. ACOG Technical Bulletin No. 143. Washington, D.C., July 1990.
29. King PA, Duthie SJ, Glickman MG, Schwartz PE, Secondary postpartum hemorrhage. Aust N Z J Obstet Gynaecol 1989;29: 394–398.
30. Neill A, Thornton S: Secondary postpartum hemorrhage. J Obstet Gynaecol 2002;22:119–122.
31. Lee CY, Madrazo B, Drukker BH: Ultrasonic evaluation of the postpartum uterus in the management of postpartum bleeding. Obstet Gynecol 1981;58:227–232.
32. Beydoun SN: Postpartum hemorrhage and hypovolemic shock. In Hassam F (ed): Diagnosis and Management of Obstetric Emergency. Manlo Park, CA, Addison-Wesley, 1982, p. 193.
33. Andrew AC, Bulmer JN, Wells M, et al: Subinvolution of the uteroplacental arteries in the human placental bed. Histopathology 1989;15:395–405.
34. Khong TY, Khong TK: Delayed postpartum hemorrhage: A morphologic study of causes and their relation to other pregnancy disorders. Obstet Gynecol 1993;82:17–22.
35. Van den Bosch T, Van Schoubroeck D, et al: Color Doppler and gray-scale ultrasound evaluation of the postpartum uterus. Ultrasound Obstet Gynecol 2002;20:586–591.
36. Pelage J-P, Philippe S, Repiquet D, et al: Secondary postpartum hemorrhage: Treatment with selective arterial embolization. Radiology 1999;212:385–389.
37. Greenwood LH, Dong ZG, Ma HK, et al: Obstetric and nonmalignant gynecologic bleeding: Treatment with angiographic embolization. Radiology 1987;164:155–159.
38. Duff P: Pathophysiology and management of postcesarean endomyometritis. Obstet Gynecol 1986;67:269–276.
39. Putnam CE: Poetry, physiology, and puerperal fever: Understanding the young Oliver Wendell Holmes. Acta Physiol Hungarica 2001;88:155–172.
40. Thompson M: The Cry and the Covenant. New York, Garden City Books, 1949.
41. Stefonek KR, Maerz LL, Nielsen MP, et al: Group A streptococcal puerperal sepsis preceded by positive surveillance cultures. Obstet Gynecol 2001;98:846–848.
42. Ejlertsen T, Prag J, Pettersson E, Holmskov A: A 7-month outbreak of relapsing postpartum Group A streptococcal infections linked to a nurse with atopic dermatitis. Scand J Infect Dis 2001;33:734–737.
43. Adriaanse AH, Pel M, Bleker OP: Semmelweis: The combat against puerperal fever. Eur J Obstet Gynecol Reprod Biol 2000;90:153-158.
44. The Prevention of Invasive Group A Streptococcal Infections Workshop Participants: Prevention of invasive group A streptococcal disease among household contacts of case patients and among postpartum and postsurgical patients: Recommendations from the Centers for Disease Control and Prevention. Clin Infect Dis 2002;35:950–959.
45. Duff P, Gibbs RS, Blanco JD, et al: Endometrial culture techniques in puerperal patients. Obstet Gynecol 1983;61:217–222.
46. Chen KT, Barbieri RL: Acute and chronic endometritis. UpToDate, 2002.
47. diZerega G, Yonekura L, et al: A comparison of clindamycin-gentamicin and penicillin-gentamicin in the treatment of post-cesarean section endomyometritis. Am J Obstet Gynecol 1979;134:238–242.
48. Gibbs RS, Blanco JD, et al: A double-blind, randomized comparison of clindamycin-gentamicin versus cefamandole for treat-

ment of post-cesarean section endomyometritis. Am J Obstet Gynecol 1982;144:261–267.
49. Gibbs RS, Blanco JD, Duff P, et al: A double-blind, randomized comparison of moxalactam versus clindamycin-gentamicin in treatment of endomyometritis after cesarean section delivery. Am J Obstet Gynecol 1983;146:769–772.
50. Gilstrap LC, Maier RC, Gibbs RS, et al: Piperacillin versus clindamycin plus gentamicin for pelvic infections. Obstet Gynecol 1984;64:762–766.
51. Herman G, Cohen AW, Talbot GH, et al: Cefoxitin versus clindamycin and gentamicin in the treatment of postcesarean section infections. Obstet Gynecol 1986;67:371–376.
52. Faro S, Phillips LE, Baker JL, et al: Comparative efficacy and safety of mezlocillin, cefoxitin, and clindamycin plus gentamicin in postpartum endometritis. Obstet Gynecol 1987;69:760–767.
53. Alvarez RD, Kilgore LC, Huddleston JF: A comparison of mezlocillin versus clindamycin/gentamicin for the treatment of postcesarean endomyometritis. Am J Obstet Gynecol 1988;158:425–429.
54. Faro S, Martens M, Hammill H, et al: Ticarcillin/clavulonic acid versus clindamycin and gentamicin in the treatment of post-cesarean endometritis following antibiotic prophylaxis. Obstet Gynecol 1989;73:808–812.
55. Sweet RL, Roy S, Faro S, et al: Piperacillin and tazobactam versus clindamycin and gentamicin in the treatment of hospitalized women with pelvic infection. The Piperacillin/tazobactam Study Group. Obstet Gynecol 1994;83:280–286.
56. French LM, Smaill FM: Antibiotic regimens for endometritis after delivery. Cochrane Database Syst Rev CD001067, 2002.
57. Dinsmoor MJ, Newton ER, Gibbs RS: A randomized, double-blind placebo-controlled trial of oral antibiotic therapy following intravenous antibiotic therapy for postpartum endometritis. Obstet Gynecol 1991;77:60–62.
58. Walmer D, Walmer KR, Gibbs RS: Enterococci in post-cesarean endometritis. Obstet Gynecol 1988;71:159–162.
59. Brumfield CG, Hauth JC, Andrews WW: Puerperal infection after cesarean delivery: Evaluation of a standardized protocol. Am J Obstet Gynecol 2000;182:1147–1151.
60. Livingston JC, Llata E, Rinehart E, et al: Gentamicin and clindamycin therapy in postpartum endometritis: The efficacy of daily dosing versus dosing every 8 hours. Am J Obstet Gynecol 2003;188:149–152.
61. Duff P: Maternal and perinatal infection. In Gabbe SG, Niebyl JR, Simpson JL (eds): Obstetrics: Normal & Problem Pregnancies, 4th ed. New York, Churchill Livingstone, 2002, p.16.
62. Duff P, Gibbs RS: Pelvic vein thrombophlebitis: Diagnostic dilemma and therapeutic challenge. Obstet Gynecol Surv 1983;38:365–373.
63. Brown TK, Munsick RA: Puerperal ovarian vein thrombophlebitis: A syndrome. Am J Obstet Gynecol 1971;109: 263–273.
64. Lee EH, Im CY, Kim JW: Ultrasound diagnosis of postpartum ovarian vein thrombosis. Ultrasound Obstet Gynecol 2001;18:384–386.
65. Dunn LJ, Van Voorhis LW: Enigmatic fever and pelvic thrombophlebitis. N Engl J Med 1967;276:265–268.
66. Jassal DS, Fjeldsted FH, Smith ER, et al: A diagnostic dilemma of fever and back pain postpartum. Chest 2001;120:1023–1024.
67. Duff P: Septic pelvic vein thrombophlebitis. In Charles D (ed): Obstetric and Perinatal Infections. St. Louis, Mosby Year Book, 1993, pp.104–108.
68. Brown CE, Lowe TW, Cunningham FG, Weinreb JC: Puerperal pelvic vein thrombophlebitis: Impact on diagnosis and treatment using x-ray computed tomography and magnetic resonance imaging. Obstet Gynecol 1986;68:789–794.
69. Brown CE, Stettler RW, Twickler D, et al: Puerperal septic pelvic thrombophlebitis: Incidence and response to heparin therapy. Am J Obstet Gynecol 1999;181:143–148.
70. Schwartz MA, Wang CC, Eckert LO, et al: Risk factors for urinary tract infection in the postpartum period. Am J Obstet Gynecol 1999;181:547–548.
71. Ryan AS, Rush D, Krieger FW, et al: Recent declines in breast feeding in the U.S., 1984 through 1989. Pediatrics 1991;88: 719–727.
72. Hague WM, North RA, Gallus AS, et al: A Working Group on Behalf of the Obstetric Medicine Group of Australia. Anticoagulation in pregnancy and the puerperium. Med J Aust 2001;175:258–263.
73. Storrs HJ: Checking the secretion of the lactating breast. Surg Gynecol Obstet 1909;9:401.
74. Duckman S, Hubbard JF: The role of fluids in relieving breast engorgement without the use of hormones. Am J Obstet Gynecol 1950;60:200.
75. Fildes VA: Breasts, Bottles, and Babies. Edinburgh, Edinburgh University Press, 1986.
76. Eaton J: Suppressing lactation. Nurs Times 1991;87:27.
77. Parazzini F, Zanaboni F, Liberati A, Tognoni G: Relief of breast symptoms in women who are not breastfeeding. In Chalmers I, Enkin M, Keirse M (eds): Effective Care in Pregnancy and Childbirth. Oxford, Oxford University Press, 1989, p. 1390–1402.
78. U.S. Food and Drug Administration, Fertility and Maternal Health Drugs Advisory Committee. Summary minutes: Prevention of postpartum breast engorgement with sex hormones and bromocriptine. Washington, U.S. Food and Drug Administration, 1989.
79. Spitz AM, Lee NC, Peterson HB: Treatment for lactation suppression: Little progress in one hundred years. Am J Obstet Gynecol 1998;179:1485–1490.
80. Sandoz Pharmaceuticals: Drug information brochure re. Parlodel (bromocriptine mesylate). East Hanover, NJ, Sandoz Pharmaceuticals, 1987.
81. Willis J (ed): Postpartum hypertension, seizures, and strokes reported from bromocriptine. FDA Drug Bull 1984;14:3.
82. Katz M, Krill I, Pak I: Puerperal hypertension, stroke, and seizures after suppression of lactation with bromocriptine. Obstet Gynecol 1985;66:822–824.
83. Iffy L, TenHove W, Frisoli G: Acute myocardial infarction in the puerperium in patients receiving bromocriptine. Am J Obstet Gynecol 1986;155:371–372.
84. Ruch A, Duhring J: Postpartum myocardial infarction in a patient receiving bromocriptine. Obstet Gynecol 1989;74: 448–451.
85. Morgans D: Bromocriptine and postpartum lactation suppression. BJOG 1995;102:851–853.
86. Neifert MR, McDonough SI, Neville MC: Failure of lactogenesis associated with placental retention. Am J Obstet Gynecol 1981;140:477–478.
87. Sousa PL: Metoclopramide and breast feeding. BMJ 1975;1:512.
88. Aono T, Shioji T, Aki T, et al: Augmentation of puerperal lactation by oral administration of sulpiride. J Clin Endocrinol Metab 1979;48:478–482.
89. The puerperium (Chapter 17): In Cunningham FG, Gant NF et al (eds): Williams Obstetrics, 21st ed. New York, McGraw-Hill, 2001, p. 406–407.
90. Almeida OD, Kitay DZ: Lactation suppression and puerperal fever. Am J Obstet Gynecol 1986;154:940–941.
91. Shirley RL: Breast Pain. UpToDate 2003.
92. Niebyl JR, Spence MR, Parmley TH: Sporadic (nonepidemic) puerperal mastitis. J Reprod Med 1978;20:97–100.
93. Thomsen AC, Espersen T, Maiggard S: Course and treatment of milk stasis, noninfectious inflammation of the breast, and infectious mastitis in nursing women. Am J Obstet Gynecol 1984;149: 492–495.
94. Hindle WH: Other benign breast problems. Clin Obstet Gynecol 1994;37:916–924.

95. Stehman FB: Infections and inflammations of the breast. In Hindle WH (ed): Breast Disease for Gynecologists. Norwalk CT, Appleton & Lange, 1990, p. 151.
96. Karstrup S, Solvin J, Nolsoe CP, et al: Acute puerperal breast abscesses: US-guided drainage. Radiology 1993;188:807–809.
97. Marshall BR, Hepper JK, Zirbel CC: Sporadic puerperal mastitis—An infection that need not interrupt lactation. JAMA 1975;344:1377–1379.
98. Dener C, Inan A: Breast abscesses in lactating women. World J Surg 2003;27:130–133.
99. Varner MW: Medical conditions of the puerperium. Clin Perinatol 1998;25:403–416.
100. Catanzarite V, Willms D, Wong D, et al: Acute respiratory distress syndrome in pregnancy and the puerperium: Causes, courses, and outcomes. Obstet Gynecol 2001;97:760–764.
101. Lindheimer MD, Katz AI: Hypertension in pregnancy. N Engl J Med 1985;313:675–680.
102. Lindheimer MD, Barron WM: Enalapril and pregnancy-induced hypertension. Ann Intern Med 1988;108:911.
103. Committee on Drugs, American Academy of Pediatrics: The transfer of drugs and other chemicals into human milk. Pediatrics 1994;93:137.
104. Ansari AA, Fett JD, Carraway RE, et al: Autoimmune mechanisms as the basis for human peripartum cardiomyopathy. Clin Rev Allergy Immunol 2002;23:301–324.
105. Brown CS, Bertolet BD: Peripartum cardiomyopathy: A comprehensive review. Am J Obstet Gynecol 1998;178:409–414.
106. Jameson LJ: Revised classification and criteria for the diagnosis of diabetes mellitus (Chapter 323). In Harrison's Online. New York, McGraw-Hill, 2003.
107. Ballard JO: Unpublished communication, 2003.
108. DeStefano V, Rossi E, et al: Screening for inherited thrombophilia: Indications and therapeutic implications. Haematologica 2002;87:1095–1118.
109. Lockwood CJ: Inherited thrombophilias in pregnant patients: Detection and treatment paradigm. Obstet Gynecol 2002;99: 333–341.
110. McColl MD, Walker ID, Greer IA: The role of inherited thrombophilia in venous thromboembolism associated with pregnancy. BJOG 1999;106:756–766.
111. Letsky EA: Peripartum prophylaxis of thrombo-embolism. Baillieres Clin Obstet Gynaecol 1997;11:523–543.
112. Eastham JH: Postpartum alopecia. Ann Pharmacotherapy 2001;35:255–258.
113. Buckwalter JG, Buckwalter DK, Bluestein BW, Stanczyk FZ: Pregnancy and postpartum: Changes in cognition and mood. Prog Brain Res 2001;133:303–319.
114. Misri S, Lusskin SI, Lachman A: Postpartum Blues and Depression. UpToDate, 2003.
115. O'Hare MW, Schlechte JA, Lewis DA, et al: Prospective study of postpartum blues. Biological and psychosocial factors. Arch Gen Psychiatry 1991;48:801–806.
116. American Psychiatric Association: Diagnostic and Statistical Manual of Mental Disorders, 4th ed. Washington, D.C., 1994.
117. Cox JL, Murray D, Chapman G: A controlled study of the onset, duration, and prevalence of postnatal depression. Br J Psychiatry 1993;163:27–31.
118. Pop VJM, Essed GG, deGeus CA, et al: Prevalence of postpartum depression or is it postpuerperium depression? Acta Obstet Gynecol Scand 1993;72:354–358.
119. Pederson CA: Postpartum mood and anxiety disorders: A guide for the nonpsychiatric clinician with an aside on thyroid associations with postpartum mood. Thyroid 1999;9:691–697.
120. Stagnaro-Green A: Recognizing, understanding, and treating postpartum thyroiditis. Endocrinol Metab Clin North Am 2000;29:417–430.
121. O'Hara NW, Zekoski EM, Philipps LH, et al: Controlled prospective study of postpartum mood disorders: Comparison of childbearing and non-childbearing women. J Abnorm Psychol 1990;99:3–15.
122. Troutman BR, Cutrona CE: Nonpsychotic postpartum depression among adolescent mothers. J Abnorm Psychol 1990;99: 69–78.
123. Kessler RC, McConagle KA, Zhao S: Lifetime and 12-month prevalence of DSM-III-R psychiatric disorders in the United States. Results from the National Comorbidity Study. Arch Gen Psychiatry 1994;51:8–19.
124. Misri S, Sinclair DA, Kuan AJ: Breast-feeding and postpartum depression: Is there a relationship? Can J Psychiatry 1997;42: 1061–1065.
125. Evans J, Heron J, Francomb H, et al: Cohort study of depressed mood during pregnancy and after childbirth. BMJ 2001;323: 257–260.
126. Yonkers KA, Ramin SM, Rush AJ, et al: Onset and persistence of postpartum depression in an inner-city maternal health clinic system. Am J Psychiatry 2001;158:1856–1863.
127. Wickberg B, Hwang CP: The Edinburgh Postnatal Depression Scale: Validation on a Swedish community sample. Acta Psychiatr Scand 1996;94:181–184.
128. Thoppil CK: ISIS: A New Approach to Postpartum Depression Screening. Poster presented at the 41st Clinical Conference, Armed Forces District, American College of Obstetricians and Gynecologists, October 20, 2002.
129. Gupta S, Masand PS, Rangwani S: Selective serotonin reuptake inhibitors in pregnancy and lactation. Obstet Gynecol Sur 1998;53:733–736.
130. Misri S, Lusskin SI, Lachman A: Use of psychotropic medications in breastfeeding women. UpToDate, 2003.
131. Misri S, Kim J, Riggs KW, et al: Paroxetine levels in postpartum depressed women, breast milk, and infant serum. J Clin Psychiatry 2000;61:828–832.
132. Stowe ZN, Cohen LS, Hostetter A, et al: Paroxetine in human breast milk and nursing mothers. Am J Psychiatry 2000;157: 185–189.
133. Agnew LRC, Aviado DM, Brody JI, et al (eds): Dorland's Illustrated Medical Dictionary, 24th ed. Philadelphia, W.B. Saunders Company, 1965.
134. Davidson MR: Examining separated symphysis pubis. J Nurse Midwifery 1996;41:259–262.
135. Lentz SS: Osteitis pubis: A review. Obstet Gynecol Surv 1995;50:310–315.
136. Kubitz RL, Goodlin RC: Symptomatic separation of the pubic symphysis. South Med J 1986;79:578–580.
137. Fuller JG, Janzen J, Gambling DR: Epidural analgesia in the management of symptomatic symphysis pubis diastasis. Obstet Gynecol 1989;73:855–857.
138. Lindsey RW, Leggon RE, Wright DG, et al: Separation of the symphysis pubis in association with childbearing. J Bone Joint Surg 1988;70:289–292.
139. Musumeci R, Villa E: Symphysis pubis separation during vaginal delivery with epidural anesthesia. Reg Anesth 1994;19:289–291.
140. Dietrichs E: Anatomy of the pelvic joints: A review. Scand J Rheumatol (Suppl) 1991;88:4–6.
141. Garagiola DM, Tarver RD, Gibson L, et al: Anatomic changes in the pelvis after uncomplicated vaginal delivery: A CT study of 14 women. AJR 1989;153:1239–1241.
142. Oxome H: Human Labor and Birth, 5th ed. East Norwalk, CT, Appleton, Century, Croft; 1986, p. 552.
143. Schwartz Z, Katz Z, Lancet M: Management of puerperal separation of the symphysis pubis. Int J Gynecol Obstet 1985;23: 125–128.
144. Feasby TE, Burton SR, Hahn AF: Obstetrical lumbosacral plexus injury. Muscle Nerve 1992;15:937–940.
145. Beatty TE: Second report of the new Lying-in Hospital, Dublin. Dublin J Med Sci 1838;12:273.
146. Bromage PR: Neurologic complications of regional anesthesia for obstetrics. In Shnider SM, Levinson G (eds): Anesthesia

for Obstetrics, 3rd ed. Baltimore, Williams & Wilkins, 1993, p.433–453.

147. Aminoff MJ: Neurologic disorders. In Creasy RK, Resnik R (eds): Maternal-Fetal Medicine, 4th ed. Philadelphia, W.B. Saunders, 1999, p.217
148. Tillman AJB: Traumatic neuritis in the puerperium. Am J Obstet Gynecol 1935;29:660.
149. Hill ED: Maternal obstetric paralysis. Am J Obstet Gynecol 1962;83:1452.
150. Murray RR: Maternal obstetric paralysis. Am J Obstet Gynecol 1964;88:399–403.
151. Scott DB, Hibbard BM: Serious nonfatal complications associated with extradural block in obstetric practice. Br J Anaesth 1990;64:537–541.
152. Bademasi O, Osuntokun BO, van de Werd HH, et al: Obstetric neuropraxia in the Nigerian African. Int J Gynaecol Obstet 1980;17:611–614.
153. Rendell-Baker L: Paraplegia from accidental injection of potassium solution. Anesthesia 1985;40:912–913.
154. Gissen AJ, Datta S, Lambert D: The chloroprocaine controversy, II. Is chloroprocaine neurotoxic? Reg Anesth 1984;9:135–144.
155. Hawkins JL, Chestnut DH, Gibbs CP: Obstetric anesthesia. In Gabbe SG, Niebyl JR, Simpson JL (eds): Obstetrics: Normal and Problem Pregnancies. New York, Churchill Livingstone, 2002, pp. 431–472.
156. Reynolds F: Maternal sequelae of childbirth. Br J Anaesth 1995;75:515–517.
157. Silva M, Mallinson C, Reynolds F: Sciatic nerve palsy following childbirth. Anesthesia 1996;51:1144–1148.
158. Reisner LS, Hochman BN, Plumer MH: Persistent neurologic deficit and adhesive arachnoiditis following intrathecal 2-chloroprocaine injection. Anesth Analg 1980;59:452–454.
159. Drasner K, Rigler ML, Sessler DI, et al: Cauda equina syndrome following intended epidural anesthesia. Anesthesiology 1992;77:582–585.
160. Sghirlanzoni A, Gemma M, Pareyson D, et al: Spinal arteriovenous fistula: A possible cause of paraparesis after epidural anaesthesia. Anaesthesia 1989;44:831–833.
161. Ackerman WE, Andrews PJD, Juneja MM, et al: Cauda equina syndrome: A consequence of lumber disk protrusion or continuous subarachnoid analgesia? Anesth Analg 1993;76:898–901.
162. O'Connell JE: Lumbar disc protrusions in pregnancy. J Neurol Neurosurg Psychiatry 1960;23:138–141.
163. Chaudhari LS, Kop BP, Dhruva AJ: Paraplegia and epidural analgesia. Anaesthesia 1978;33:722–725.
164. Borum SE, McLeskey CH, Williamson JB, et al: Epidural abscess after obstetric epidural analgesia. Anesthesiology 1995; 82:1523–1526.
165. Male CG, Martin R: Puerperal spinal epidural abscess. Lancet 1973;1:608–609.
166. Packer NP, Cummins BH: Spontaneous epidural haemorrhage: A surgical emergency. Lancet 1978;1:356–358.
167. Ackerman WE, Juneja MM, Knapp RK, et al: Maternal paraparesis after anesthesia and cesarean section. South Med J 1990;83: 695–697.
168. Yip SK, Brieger G, Hin LY, Chung T: Urinary retention in the post-partum period: The relationship between obstetric factors and the post-partum post-void residual bladder volume. Acta Obstet Gynecol Scand 1997;76:667–672.
169. Andolf E, Iosif CS, Jergensen C, Rydhstrom H: Insidious urinary retention after vaginal delivery. Prevalence and symptoms at follow-up in a population-based study. Gynecol Obstet Invest 1994;38:51–53.
170. Barrington JW, Edwards G, Ashcroft M, Adekanmi O: Measurement of bladder volume following cesarean section using bladderscan. Int Urogynecol J 2001;12:373–374.
171. Weidner AC, Versi E: Physiology of micturition. In Ostergard DR, Bent AE (eds): Urogynecology and Urodynamics: Theory and Practice, 4th ed. Baltimore, Williams & Wilkins, 1996, p. 33–63.
172. Benson JT, Walters MD: Neurophysiology of the lower urinary tract. In Walters MD, Karram MM (eds): Urogynecology and Reconstructive Pelvic Surgery, 2nd ed. St Louis, Mosby, 1999, p.15–24.
173. Yip SK, Hin LY, Chung TK: Effect of the duration of labor on postpartum postvoid residual bladder volume. Gynecol Obstet Investig 1998;45:177–180.
174. Garmel SH, Guzelian GA, D'Alton JG, D'Alton ME: Lumber disk disease in pregnancy. Obstet Gynecol 1997;89:821–822.
175. Yamada K, Nakahara T, et al: Nontraumatic spinal subdural hematoma occurring in a postpartum period. Acta Neurochirurgica 2003;145:151.
176. Haylen BT, Cerqui AJ: Postpartum uterine retroversion causing bladder outflow obstruction: Cure by laparoscopic ventrosuspension. Int Urogynecol J 1999;10:353–355.
177. Yang JM, Huang WC: Sonographic findings of acute urinary retention secondary to an impacted pelvic mass. J Ultrasound Med 2002;21:1165–1169.
178. Carley ME, Carley JM, Vasdev G, et al: Factors associated with clinically overt postpartum urinary retention after vaginal delivery. Am J Obstet Gynecol 2002;187:430–433.
179. Kerr-Wilson RH, Thompson SW, Orr JW, et al: Effect of labor on the postpartum bladder. Obstet Gynecol 1984;64: 115–118.
180. Bennetts FA, Judd CE: Studies of the post-partum bladder. Am J Obstet Gynecol 1941;42:419.
181. Youssef AF: Cystometric studies in gynecology and obstetrics. Obstet Gynecol 1956;8:181–188.
182. Weil A, Reyes H, Rottenberg RD, et al: Effect of lumbar epidural analgesia on lower urinary tract function in the immediate postpartum period. BJOG 1983;90:428–432.
183. Viktrup L, Lose G, Rolff M, Barfoed K: The symptoms of stress incontinence caused by pregnancy or delivery in primipara. Obstet Gynecol 1992;79:945–949.
184. Yip SK, Sahota D, Chang AM, Chung TK: Four-year follow-up of women who were diagnosed to have postpartum urinary retention. Am J Obstet Gynecol 2002;187:648–652.
185. Coleman MM, Bardwaj A, Chan VV: Back pain and collapse associated with receding subarachnoid blockade. Can J Anaesth 1999;46:464–466.
186. Cronin TJ: Influence of lactation upon ovulation. Lancet 1968;2:422–424.
187. Perez A, Uela P, Masnick GS, Potter RG: First ovulation after childbirth: The effect of breast feeding. Am J Obstet Gynecol 1972;114:1041.
188. Gray RH, Campbell ON, Apelo R, et al: Risk of ovulation during lactation. Lancet 1990;335:25–29.
189. Bonnar J, Franklin M, Nott PN, McNeilly AS: Effect of breast feeding on pituitary-ovarian function after childbirth. BMJ 1975;4:82–84.
190. Reamy K, White SE: Sexuality in pregnancy and the puerperium: A review. Obstet Gynecol Surv 1985;40:1–13.
191. Robson KM, Brant K, Kumar R: Maternal sexuality during first pregnancy after childbirth. BJOG 1981;88:882–889.
192. Ryding E-L: Sexuality during and after pregnancy. Acta Obstet Gynecol Scand 1984;63:679–682.
193. Martin KA, Barbieri RL: Overview of Contraception. UpToDate 2003.
194. Weller SC: A meta-analysis of condom effectiveness in reducing sexually transmitted HIV. Soc Sci Med 1993;36: 1635–1644.
195. Cates W Jr. Stone KM: Family planning, sexually transmitted diseases and contraceptive choice: A literature update. Fam Plann Perspect 1992;24:75–84.
196. Koetsawang S: The effects of contraceptive methods on the quality and quantity of breast milk. Int J Gynaecol Obstet 1987;25(Suppl):115–127.
197. Halderman LD, Nelson AL: Impact of early postpartum administration of progestin-only hormonal contraceptives compared

with nonhormonal contraceptives on short-term breastfeeding patterns. Am J Obstet Gynecol 2002;186:1250–1256.
198. World Health Organization. Division of Family and Reproductive Health: Improving Access to Quality Care in Family Planning: Medical Eligibility Criteria for Contraceptive Use. Geneva, WHO, 1996.
199. American College of Obstetricians and Gynecologists. Breastfeeding: Maternal and Infant Aspects. Washington, D.C., 2000. ACOG Educational Bulletin No. 258.
200. Harlap S, Kost K, Forrest JD: Preventing Pregnancy, Protecting Health: A New Look at Birth Control Choices in the U.S. New York, The Alan Guttmacher Institute, 1991.
201. Dardano KL, Burkman RT: The intrauterine contraceptive device: An often-forgotten and maligned method of contraception. Am J Obstet Gynecol 1999;181:1–5.
202. Alvarez T, Brache V, Fernandez E, et al: New insights on the mode of action of intrauterine contraceptive devices in women. Fertil Steril 1988;49:768.
203. Rivera R, Yacobson I, Grimes D: The mechanism of action of hormonal contraceptives and intrauterine contraceptive devices. Am J Obstet Gynecol 1999;181:1263–1269.
204. Stanford JB, Thurman PB, Lemaire JC: Physician's knowledge and practices regarding natural family planning. Obstet Gynecol 1999;94:672–678.
205. Flynn AM: Natural methods of family planning. Clin Obstet Gynaecol 1984;11:661–678.
206. McNeilly AS: Lactational control of reproduction. Reprod Fertil Dev 2001;13:583–590.
207. Peterson LS: Contraceptive use in the U.S.: 1982–1990. Advanced Data from Vital Health Statistics. No. 260. Hyattsville, MD, National Center for Health Statistics, 1995 (DHHS publication no. PHS 95-1250).
208. Schwartz DB, Wingo PA, et el: Female sterilizations in the United States, 1987. Fam Plann Perspect 1989;21:209–212.
209. Marquette CM, Koonin LM, Antarsh L, et al: Vasectomy in the United States, 1991. Am J Public Health 1995;85:644–649.
210. Escobedo LG, Peterson HB, Grubb GS, et al: Case-fatality rates for tubal sterilization in U.S. hospitals, 1979–1980. Am J Obstet Gynecol 1989;160:147–150.
211. Pollack AE: Sterilization. American College of Obstetricians and Gynecologists. Washington, D.C., 1996. ACOG Technical Bulletin No. 222.
212. Peterson HB, Xia Z, Hughes JM, et al: The risk of pregnancy after tubal sterilization: Findings from the U.S. Collaborative Review of Sterilization. Am J Obstet Gynecol 1996;174:1161–1168.
213. Peterson HB, Xia Z, Hugh JM, et al: The risk of ectopic pregnancy after tubal sterilization. N Engl J Med 1997;336: 762–767.
214. Hillis SD, Marchbanks PA, Taylor LR, Peterson HB: Poststerilization regret: Findings from the U.S. Collaborative Review of Sterilization. Obstet Gynecol 1999;93:889–895.
215. Wilcox LS, Chu SY, Eaker ED, et al: Risk factors for regret after tubal sterilization: 5 years of follow-up in a prospective study. Fertil Steril 1991;55:927–933.
216. Wilcox LS, Chu SY, Peterson HB: Characteristics of women who considered or obtained tubal reanastomosis: Results from a prospective study of tubal sterilization. Obstet Gynecol 1990;75:661–665.
217. Rock JA, Guzick DS, Katz E, et al: Tubal anastomosis: Pregnancy success following reversal of Falope ring or monopolar cautery sterilization. Fertil Steril 1987;48:13–17.
218. Westhoff C, Davis A: Tubal sterilization: Focus on the U.S. experience. Fertil Steril 2000;73:913–922.
219. Henderson SR: The reversibility of female sterilization with the use of microsurgery: A report on 102 patients with more than one year of follow-up. Am J Obstet Gynecol 1984;149:57–65.
220. Spivak MM, Librach CL, Rosenthal DM: Microsurgical reversal of sterilization: A six-year study. Am J Obstet Gynecol 1986;154:355–361.
221. DeCherney AH, Mezer HC, Naftolin F: Analysis of failure of microsurgical anastomosis after midsegment non-coagulation tubal ligation. Fertil Steril 1983;39:618–622.
222. Gentile G, Kaufman S, Helbig D: Is there any evidence for a post-tubal ligation syndrome? Fertil Steril 1998;69:179–186.
223. Wilcox LS, Martinez-Schnell B, Peterson HB, et al: Menstrual function after tubal sterilization. Am J Epidemiol 1992;135: 1368–1381.
224. Hillis S, Marchbanks P, Taylor PA, Taylor LR, Peterson HB: Tubal sterilization and long-term risk of hysterectomy: Findings from the United States collaborative review of sterilization. The U.S. Collaborative Review of Sterilization Working Group. Obstet Gynecol 1997;89:609–614.
225. Bhuiyan SN, Begum R: Quinacrine non-surgical female sterilization in Bangladesh. Contraception 2001;64:281–286.
226. Benagiano G: Non-surgical female sterilization with quinacrine: An update. Contraception 2001;63:239–245.
227. Barclay DL, Hawks BL, Frueh DM, et al: Elective cesarean hysterectomy: A 5 year comparison with cesarean section. Am J Obstet Gynecol 1976;124:900–911.
228. Bukovsky I, Schneider DF, Langer R, et al: Elective caesarean hysterectomy. Indications and outcome: A 17-year experience of 140 cases. Aust N Z J Obstet Gynaecol 1989;29:287–290.
229. Levgur M, Duvivier R: Pelvic inflammatory disease after tubal sterilization: A review. Obstet Gynecol Surv 2000;55:41–50.
230. Mosher WD, Pratt WF: Contraceptive use in the United States, 1973–1988. Vital and health statistics, no. 182. Hyattsville, MD, National Center for Health Statistics, 1990.
231. Schwingl PJ, Guess HA: Safety and effectiveness of vasectomy. Fertil Steril 2000;73:923–926.
232. Haldar N, Cranston D, Turner E, et al: How reliable is vasectomy? Long-term follow-up of vasectomized men [letter]. Lancet 2000;356:43–44.
233. Hendry WF: Vasectomy and vasectomy reversal. Br J Urol 1994;73:337–344.
234. Sharlip ID: What is the best pregnancy rate that may be expected from vasectomy reversal?. J Urol 1993;149:1469–1471.
235. Belker AM, Thomas AJ, Jr., Fuchs EF, et al: Results of 1,469 microsurgical vasectomy reversals by the Vasovasostomy Study Group. J Urol 1991;145:505–511.
236. Hewitt G, Logan CJ, Curry RC: Does vasectomy cause testicular cancer? Br J Urol 1993;71:607–608.
237. Moller H, Knudsen LB, Lynge E: Risk of testicular cancer after vasectomy: Cohort study of over 73,000 men. BMJ 1994;309:295–299.
238. Cox B, Sneyd MJ, Paul C, et al: Vasectomy and risk of prostate cancer. JAMA 2002;287:3110–3115.
239. Dennis LK, Dawson DV, Resnick MI: Vasectomy and the risk of prostate cancer: A meta-analysis examining vasectomy status, age at vasectomy, and time since vasectomy. Prostate Cancer Prostatic Dis 2002;5:93–203.
240. Manson JE, Ridker PM, Spelsberg A, et al: Vasectomy and subsequent cardiovascular disease in U.S. physicians. Contraception 1999;59:181–186.
241. Lee CY, Madroazo B, Drukker BH: Ultrasonic evaluation of the postpartum uterus in the management of postpartum bleeding. Obstet Gynecol 1981;58:227.
242. King PA, Duthie, SJ, Dong ZG, et al: Secondary postpartum haemorrhage. Aust N Z Obstet Gynecol 1989;29:394.
243. Smaill F, Hofmeyer G: Cochrane review: Antibiotic prophylactics for caesarean section. Cochrane Database 4, 2000.
244. French LM, Smaill F: Cochrane review: Antibiotic regimens for endometritis after delivery. Cochrane Database 4, 2000.

245. Ridgway LE: Puerperal emergency. Vaginal and vulvar hematomas. Obstet Gynecol Clin North Am 1995;22:275.
246. Benrubi G, Neuman C, Nuss RC, Thompson RJ: Vulvar and vaginal hematomas: A retrospective study of conservative versus operative management. South Med J 1987;80:991.
247. Chin HG, Scott DR, Resnik R, et al: Angiographic embolization of intractable puerperal hematomas. Am J Obstet Gynecol 1989;160:434.
248. Trussel J, et al: Contraceptive Technology, 17th ed. New York, Ardent Media, 1998.

CHAPTER 79

Major Obstetric Hemorrhage and Disseminated Intravascular Coagulation

John Anthony

INTRODUCTION

Maternal death from obstetric hemorrhage remains a global problem. In developing countries it ranks among the leading three causes of maternal death, and industrialized nations continue to report mortality rates in cases in which problems could have been anticipated and prevented.[1,2] In developing countries, postpartum hemorrhage accounts for a higher percentage of deaths due to hemorrhage. The combination of uterine atony with retained products of conception leading to hypovolemic shock and coagulopathy are the most common complications giving rise to death from obstetric hemorrhage.

The U.K. Confidential Enquiries into Maternal Mortality have emphasized the need to recognize the antenatal woman at risk of obstetric hemorrhage and to ensure that a multidisciplinary consultant-led team including hematologists, anesthetists, and obstetricians are available to provide adequate care. The unpredictability of obstetric hemorrhage is also acknowledged in this report and the importance of having protocols to deal with massive hemorrhage is stressed.

MAJOR OBSTETRIC HEMORRHAGE

Definition

"Major obstetric hemorrhage" is an imprecise term, more often applied to the consequences of hemorrhage than arising from any clinical appreciation of excessive blood loss that is notoriously underestimated. This chapter deals with the risks and management of severe or major obstetric hemorrhage in which there is a risk of hypovolemic shock. Inevitably, there will be some overlap with other chapters, which are cross referenced.

Incidence

The incidence is difficult to estimate because the definition includes all severe episodes of antepartum, intrapartum, primary, and secondary postpartum hemorrhage, and these figures are not recorded collectively or statutorily. The incidence is likely to be about 0.5%, with the largest number of cases being due to primary postpartum hemorrhage.

Etiology

Major obstetric hemorrhage is generally caused by the following:

- Placental abruption (see also Chapter 59)
- Placenta previa (see also Chapter 59)
- Causes of primary postpartum hemorrhage (see also Chapter 77)
- Ruptured uterus (see also Chapter 77).

However, underlying disease may contribute to the bleeding, including the following:

- Bleeding disorders (e.g., von Willebrand disease)
- Acquired hemostatic disorders due to liver failure (e.g., fulminant hepatitis, acute fatty liver of pregnancy)
- Severe disseminated intravascular coagulation (discussed in this chapter)
- Platelet dysfunction (e.g., severe preeclampsia, thrombotic thrombocytopenic purpura).

Antepartum hemorrhage accounts for fewer deaths than postpartum hemorrhage in developing countries, although this pattern is reversed in industrialized countries.

Maternal Risks

Death

Deaths due to major antepartum hemorrhage are usually due to placental abruption. Maternal death from placental abruption is attributable to the effects of hypovolemia (see following discussion) combined with the complications that may arise from underlying predisposing conditions such as preeclampsia. The resting uterine tone may be increased (up to 25 mm Hg) and labor may be triggered by placental separation with the sudden onset of frequent contractions.[3,4] Although hypovolemic shock and its sequelae may develop as a result of acute blood loss, hypertension may precede or follow abruptio placentae.[5] The coincident occurrence of hypertension due to preeclampsia together with hypovolemia as a result of abruptio placentae increases the risk of renal failure due to tubular necrosis.[6] Up to one third of pregnancy-related cases of acute renal failure are due to abruptio placentae.[6] Proteinuria is usually found in cases of abruptio placentae and the pattern of glomerular protein loss is similar to that seen in acute ischemic renal failure.[7]

The mother is at risk of severe hypovolemia from placenta previa also, especially as a result of morbidly adherent implantation over a previous cesarean section scar. Placenta previa is also associated with recurrent antepartum hemorrhage and operative delivery.

Severe primary postpartum hemorrhage can lead to hypovolemic shock. Other complications are those associated with the treatment of the underlying condition such as from transfusion-related injury and surgical complications of hysterectomy.

The reported risk of maternal death following uterine rupture varies widely, being very low in industrialized countries but up to 38% in developing countries with limited resources.[8–10] Maternal morbidity rates associated with uterine rupture includes all the complications that may follow severe hypovolemic shock, postoperative complications, and reproductive sequelae that include loss of fertility and the need for future operative delivery.

Hypovolemic Shock

Shock is a clinical condition characterized by inadequate tissue perfusion due to any one of the following:

- Impaired peripheral circulation because of diminished intravascular blood volume (hypovolemic shock)—only this form of shock is covered in this chapter
- Left ventricular failure (cardiogenic shock)
- Disruption of vasoregulatory homeostasis as a result of inappropriate peripheral vasodilation (distributive shock).

Hypovolemia leads to a reduction in peripheral blood flow through the splanchnic and cutaneous circulation as a result of selective vasoconstriction mediated by the central nervous system and a baroreceptor sympathetic response. These differential changes in vascular tone allow selective preservation of blood flow to the brain, heart, and adrenal glands. Venous return to the heart is augmented by a reduction in venous capacitance mediated by catecholamine-induced venoconstriction. This sustains cardiac filling pressures, stroke volume, cardiac output, and critical organ oxygenation. Intravascular volume is also replenished by renal conservation of sodium and water triggered by increased formation of angiotensin. The secretion of antidiuretic hormone further contributes to the renal adaptation.

Sympathetic stimulation and an increase in circulating catecholamines both lead to a rising heart rate and increased myocardial contractility that further increase myocardial oxygen demand. Ongoing hemorrhage and the development of anaerobic metabolism with acidosis may lead to left ventricular failure and the development of irreversible shock.

The immunologic and metabolic response to injury is characterized by the development of the systemic inflammatory response syndrome (SIRS). This process, triggered by hypovolemia and hypoxia, gives rise to diffuse effects as a result of damage to the vascular endothelium.[11] The initial endothelial response to hypoxia includes the expression of adhesion molecules that bind lymphocytes and leukocytes as well as platelets. The activated white blood cells produce and release a range of proinflammatory cytokines and oxygen free radicals.[12] The latter species augment oxidative stress and promote lipid peroxidation once antioxidant mechanisms are saturated. Lipid peroxidation of cell membranes is presumed to result in the loss of vascular integrity with increased vascular permeability. This mechanism is the basis for the development of adult respiratory distress syndrome (ARDS) in the lung and also contributes to the development of multiorgan failure.

Reperfusion injury is also implicated in the development of multiorgan failure. When hypoxic cells can no longer sustain anaerobic metabolism because of glycogen depletion, ATP (adenosine triphosphate) levels fall and homeostatic regulation of ionic flux across the cell membrane fails with rising intracellular sodium and calcium levels. Changes in intracellular calcium concentration adversely affect various enzymes, including xanthine dehydrogenase, converting the enzyme to xanthine oxidase. This switch allows the metabolism of accumulating hypoxanthine (derived from purine catabolism) to superoxide anion and hydrogen peroxide once perfusion and oxygenation are restored.[13] The subsequent release of reactive oxygen species and peroxide augments oxidative stress giving rise to further endothelial damage. Reperfusion injury often arises from delayed restoration of flow through the splanchnic circulation even after adequate resuscitation. The ischemic gut contains xanthine oxidase and is able to generate oxygen free radicals that on reperfusion may overwhelm the hepatic antioxidant defense mechanisms trigerring systemic endothelial damage and contributing to the onset of multiorgan failure. In addition, reduced splanchnic flow alters gut mucosal permeability, allowing the absorption of intestinal bacteria and toxins into the portal circulation.

Disseminated Intravascular Coagulation

Changes in the coagulation system accompany acute blood loss and will vary according to the extent of the blood loss and the underlying pathology associated with bleeding. The acute-phase response elicited by any form of trauma is characterized by increased hepatic synthesis of clotting factors and hyperhomocysteinemia. The resultant hypercoagulability is seldom clinically evident because these effects are usually overwhelmed in women with acute obstetric blood loss by consumptive coagulopathy.

The clotting defect seen in women after obstetric hemorrhage usually develops because of consumption of clotting factors, leading to a bleeding tendency. Disseminated intravascular coagulation (DIC) is frequently also present and develops whenever procoagulant mechanisms promote fibrin formation in the circulation. The hematologic consequences of DIC are often clinically insignificant but are sometimes associated with a profound coagulopathy (typically seen in the anaphylactoid syndrome of pregnancy but also seen in severe sepsis in which liver dysfunction and thrombocytopenia add to the risk of coagulopathy). DIC contributes to the development of organ failure as a result of SIRS, although the management of this complication is the management of the underlying condition rather than the DIC itself. The numerous mechanisms that trigger DIC do so by endothelial or platelet activation and via the release of thromboplastin into the circulation. Hence, procoagulant changes accompany the development of SIRS and are induced by leukocyte activation and endothelial dysfunction.[14] The presence of placental tissue or amniotic fluid in the maternal circulation initiates intravascular coagulation, and thromboplastin release into the circulation is known to occur in cases of abruptio placentae.

Fibrin formation initiates fibrinolysis, leading to the formation of plasmin and the elaboration of fibrin degradation products that are readily measurable in the peripheral circulation (for example, quantitative D-dimer levels). Although these breakdown products of fibrin are used to diagnose intravascular coagulation, the protection of vascular integrity during normal pregnancy includes sufficient intravascular coagulation to increase D-dimer levels with an increase in circulating thrombin-antithrombin complexes. Accelerated formation of fibrin stimulates fibrinolysis. Plasmin may stimulate the complement cascade, which further contributes to the development of increased capillary permeability.

The physiologic adaptations of pregnancy protect the mother from the hemodynamic and hemostatic effects of hemorrhage at the time of delivery. These changes include a 30% increase in blood volume as a result of plasma volume expansion combined with an increase in red blood cell mass. These changes are accompanied by physiologic peripheral vasodilation to accommodate the increased blood volume and cardiac output. The combined effects of these changes allow more extensive hemorrhage prior to the development of shock and the net gain of 1 to 2 L of intravascular volume exceeds the estimated blood loss of 500 to 600 mL at the time of normal delivery. Hemostasis is augmented by increased hepatic production of clotting factors, especially fibrinogen, while the anticlotting mechanism is impeded by a reduction in the level of free protein S. Fibrinolysis also diminishes in response to placental production of plasminogen activator inhibitor II.

Clinical Presentation

The development of hypovolemic shock is recognized by a progressive fall in blood pressure and a rising pulse rate. The severity of the blood loss can be classified on the basis of clinical signs alone (Table 79–1).

Hemodynamic monitoring will confirm low ventricular filling pressures (central venous pressure or pulmonary capillary wedge pressure) and a low cardiac output. In addition, measurement of central venous oxygen saturation will confirm increased rates of oxygen extraction (<65%) as cardiac output and peripheral perfusion diminish. In determining the diagnosis of acute hypovolemia, investigations are of limited utility. This is especially true of hemoglobin concentration estimation because the hematocrit will only fall as transcapillary rehydration from interstitial fluid takes place slowly over several hours.

TABLE 79–1

Clinical Classification of the Severity of Blood Loss

CLINICAL SIGN	BLOOD LOSS <15%	BLOOD LOSS 15–30%	BLOOD LOSS 30–40%	BLOOD LOSS >40%
Pulse rate (beats/min)	<100	>100	>120	>140
Blood pressure	Normal	Normal	Decreased	Decreased
Urinary output (mL/h)	>30	20–30	5–15	<5
Neurologic status	Anxiety	Anxiety	Confusion	Lethargy

From Marino PL: The ICU Book. New York, Williams & Wilkins, 1998, p 209.

Coagulopathy may be very obvious in the woman who presents with bleeding gums and oozing from all venipuncture sites. In many cases of coagulopathy, however, these signs will not be evident and the diagnosis will depend upon measurement of the international normalized ratio (INR), activated partial thromboplastin time (aPTT), and platelet count.

Renal Failure

Acute oliguric renal failure will develop as a consequence of hypovolemic shock. The loss of 15% to 30% of the intravascular blood volume will result in reduced renovascular perfusion and readily reversible changes in urinary output and blood urea and creatinine levels. Ongoing blood loss leads to the development of acute tubular necrosis in which ischemic injury to the tubules results in tubular epithelial cells becoming detached and blocking the tubules. This adds an obstructive component to the renal ischemia that will further reduce glomerular filtration. The development of SIRS may also add an immunologic component to the pathogenesis of renal tubular dysfunction.

Adult Respiratory Distress Syndrome

ARDS develops as part of the systemic inflammatory response syndrome but may also arise as a consequence of multiple blood transfusions. In the latter case, human leukocyte antibodies present in transfused plasma may be responsible for activation of the complement cascade with subsequent pulmonary vascular injury. ARDS is characterized clinically as a form of noncardiogenic pulmonary edema. The underlying pathophysiology is based upon inflammatory changes rather than an accumulation of interstitial edema fluid (usually associated with high pulmonary capillary wedge pressures).

Complications of Blood Transfusion

The immediate complications include incompatible transfusion, hyperkalemia, and citrate intoxication. Hyperkalemia arises because of the leakage of potassium from stored red blood cells and is a potential problem in those who require transfusion despite renal failure. The development of hyperkalemia may be suspected if the electrocardiogram shows peaked T waves with wide PR and QRS intervals. Citrate intoxication develops because calcium ions are chelated, leading to hypocalcemia (manifest as irritability, hypotension, and a prolonged QT interval on the electrocardiogram). Conversely, the U.K. Confidential Enquiries into Maternal Mortality has demonstrated that some maternal deaths from major obstetric hemorrhage have resulted from a failure to give sufficient blood replacement.

Transfusion-related lung injury presents as noncardiogenic pulmonary edema within several hours of transfusion and requires mechanical ventilation for up to 48 hours. Longer-term risks are those related to infection with hepatitis viruses, HIV, and bacterial infection.

Endocrinopathy

During pregnancy the pituitary gland increases in size several-fold. The blood supply to the anterior pituitary gland is dependent on flow through the superior hypophyseal artery and is susceptible to avascular necrosis. The likely clinical presentation includes failure of lactation, amenorrhea, and loss of secondary sexual characteristics, followed by the evolution of hypothyroidism and adrenocortical insufficiency (Sheehan's syndrome). Sheehan's syndrome may evolve over a lengthy period of time after the precipitating event. The diagnosis should be suspected in the woman who fails to lactate, and confirmatory tests of hypothalamic and pituitary function are carried out. Neuroradiologic investigation will usually reveal an abnormal or empty sella turcica.

Anemia

Anemia may be a late complication of massive hemorrhage. Replenishment of the red blood cell mass will require hematopoiesis dependent on adequate iron stores associated with a normal dietary intake of folic acid.

Fetal Risks

Death

Fetal loss in association with placental abruption is due to hypoxia and prematurity with perinatal mortality rates as high as 12%.[15] Placental abruption is the leading cause of perinatal death in many countries.[16,17] Fetomaternal hemorrhage is a common occurrence following abruptio placentae.[18]

Major obstetric hemorrhage due to placenta previa less commonly causes perinatal death, but again, this is due to prematurity or fetal hypoxia.[19–21]

The fetal risks following uterine rupture depend on the nature of the rupture and vary from no adverse effects to severe asphyxia and death.

Cerebral Hypoxia

Antepartum or intrapartum hypoxia may result in an infant in poor condition at delivery, with subsequent development of convulsions, intracerebral edema, and hemorrhage. This may lead to conditions such as periventricular leukomalacia and porencephalic cysts and long-term neurologic handicap. Pulmonary hemorrhage and necrotizing enterocolitis may also occur after an hypoxic episode.

Consequences of Prematurity

These complications account for most of the cases of neonatal death if the infant has survived the initial insult, and include respiratory distress syndrome and persistent fetal circulation with patent ductus arteriosus. Complications associated with prolonged neonatal intensive care such as sepsis and bronchopulmonary dysplasia are relatively common.

Management Options

(See also Chapters 59 and 77)

Prenatal: Identification of "At-Risk" Patients

ANY BLEEDING

Massive blood loss cannot always be anticipated or prevented. Some high risk patients can be identified more easily, such as those with placenta previa. However, the prediction of such an event in the general obstetric population is poor. If a woman is anemic prior to labor, or states that she will refuse blood products on religious grounds, she is at increased risk should she bleed excessively in association with delivery. It is good practice in such cases for delivery to occur in a large unit with appropriate staff and facilities.

Patients who have had a previous hemorrhage in pregnancy are at risk of recurrence and should be counseled about such risk and delivered in larger obstetric units with full resuscitative measures available. They should be aware of the procedures for urgent admission to the unit and the need to attend with any degree of bleeding. Iron prophylaxis is advisable in this group (although the risk of major hemorrhage is not generally seen as an indication for routine iron therapy).

PLACENTA PREVIA

Advancing age and parity are associated with the development of placenta previa, although the relative importance of these two factors is disputed.[22,23] Uterine scars, previous miscarriages, terminations, and dilation and curettage are reported as predisposing factors, possibly due to endometrial damage.[24] Placenta previa is more common in multiple pregnancy, owing to increased placental size. Maternal age is an important factor in recurrent placenta previa, and the risk of recurrence is quoted as between 10% and 15%.[25] There is an association between a previous cesarean section and the subsequent development of placenta previa (3%–10%); the risk increases with the number of previous cesarean sections.[22,26] This group of patients is also at risk of placenta accreta (reported as 10%–67%), again increasing with the number of previous cesarean sections. Any patient with a placenta previa and previous cesarean section should be informed of the possible necessity of a hysterectomy. The repeat cesarean section should be booked in an appropriate unit and performed by a senior obstetrician with blood cross-matched and immediately available.

However, only 15% to 20% of cases of placenta previa have major bleeding episodes.[27,28] It should be stressed to the woman with a placenta previa that she is much more likely not to have a severe hemorrhage than she is to have one, especially as ultrasonographic diagnosis has led to increased detection of asymptomatic placenta previa that may prove to be of uncertain clinical significance.

Although bleeding with a placental previa is assumed to be of maternal origin, it has been suggested that a proportion of the blood loss may be fetal in origin.[23] A denaturation test to detect the presence of fetal cells should be carried out in the presence of hemorrhage if delivery is not planned.[28]

PLACENTAL ABRUPTION

The causative factors are known in only a minority of cases of placental abruption but an association with increasing parity, smoking, low socioeconomic status, intrauterine growth restriction, and preeclampsia is reported.[29–31]

The importance of maternal factors is shown by the recurrence rate of 6% to 16% after one placental abruption and 20% to 25% after two previous placental abruptions.[29] Interventions in women at risk have not been shown unequivocally to reduce the occurrence or consequences of placental abruption. Thus, maintenance of a normal blood pressure and cessation of smoking may reduce the risk, although this has not been proved in controlled trials. Similarly, both folic acid supplementation and low-dose aspirin therapy, though advocated by some, have not been shown to reduce the risk of recurrent abruption.

RISK OF POSTPARTUM HEMORRHAGE

Any woman having a baby is at some risk of postpartum hemorrhage (3%–5% of deliveries) and women contemplating a home delivery should be informed of this, as many cases occur unexpectedly. If there has been a previous postpartum hemorrhage, the risks of recurrence are increased to approximately 8% to 10%. Women with a history of retained placenta and those with multiple pregnancy are also at risk. Active management of the third stage of labor should be advised.[32]

Active Bleeding: General Management

The essential management of major bleeding is the same, whatever the underlying cause of hemorrhage, and involves the following steps:

- Stop the bleeding
- Restore the circulating blood volume and oxygen-carrying capacity
- Correct any coagulation defect
- Maintaining vigilance for and dealing with the consequences of hypovolemia.

MANAGEMENT PROTOCOL

Every obstetric unit should have its own protocol for management of massive hemorrhage available on the delivery unit for all nursing and medical staff. This enables the appropriate clinical and laboratory staff to be summoned early and a clear management strategy to be adopted. An example of a general management protocol for major hemorrhage is given in Table 79–2, and these guidelines should be followed without delay as soon as a major bleeding episode is recognized. This protocol clearly outlines the necessary steps to be taken. Similar guidelines could be drawn up for any obstetric unit customized to local circumstances.

TABLE 79–2

Sample Major Hemorrhage Protocol

Organization

1. Switchboard operator sends urgently for the following:
   a. Obstetric resident if not present
   b. Duty obstetric anesthetist
   c. Obstetric nursing officer to arrange extra staff
   d. Blood bank technician
   e. Porter to maternity unit (for transfer of samples)
2. Consultant hematologist and obstetrician are informed of the clinical situation.
3. One nurse to be solely assigned to record keeping:
   a. Patient vital signs, central venous pressure, and urine output
   b. Amount and type of all fluids the patient receives
   c. Dosage and types of drugs given
4. Prepare for theater as soon as possible—most diagnoses require surgical intervention.

Clinical Management

1. Insert two large-bore (preferably 14-gauge) cannulas. Take 20 mL of blood for complete blood count, baseline clotting studies, and cross-matching and order at least 6 units of blood together with 3 units of fresh frozen plasma.
2. Give oxygen via face mask.
3. Commence fluid replacement quickly. (All fluids and blood should be given through a warming device.)
   a. Initially crystalloid and colloid. Hartmann's solution to a maximum of 1.5–2 L.
   b. Uncrossed blood. Rh-negative, matched with the patient's ABO blood group should be given next if cross-matched blood not ready.
   c. Cross-matched blood given as soon as possible.
   d. Give O-negative blood only if none of the above are available (but it may be lifesaving).
4. Insert central venous line and urinary catheter.
5. Stop the bleeding
   a. If ante partum, deliver the fetus (see text).
   b. If postpartum, deliver the placenta if still in utero, commence bimanual compression of the uterus, and give ergometrine 0.5 mg IV. Commence syntocinon infusion of 40 units in 500 mL of Hartmann's solution to run over 4 hours.
   c. If bleeding because of genital tract trauma or retained products, take the patient to theater promptly to explore the uterine cavity and repair damage.
   d. If bleeding continues, consider coagulation failure. Temporary direct aortic compression may give valuable time.
   e. Other surgical measures:
      Direct intramyometrial injection of prostaglandin E_2 0.5 mg, or prostaglandin F_{2a} 0.25 mg
      Insertion of Lynch suture
      Ligation of uterine arteries on both sides
      Ligation of internal iliac arteries
      Hysterectomy

SITE OF MANAGEMENT

The setting will vary with local resources and established practices. Many units have a high dependency area where such patients can be managed. However, there will be a stage in the management of these patients at which admission to an intensive care unit is indicated. These indications will also vary with local resources and practices but an arbitrary list of possible indicators is given in Table 79–3.

MONITORING

The woman bleeding as a result of obstetric hemorrhage may require increasingly invasive monitoring, depending on the extent of the hemorrhage.

- Clinical monitoring should include measurement of blood pressure, pulse rate, urinary output combined with an estimation of the extent of the blood loss on a half-hourly to hourly basis.
- Hypovolemic patients should all have invasive hemodynamic monitoring to assess intravascular volume and ventricular filling pressures (either a central venous pressure line or, in the case of preeclampsia, a pulmonary artery catheter)—see later discussion.
- The extent of the coagulation defect and the hemoglobin concentration must also be assessed, the frequency of which will be determined by the severity and duration of the hemorrhage.
- Organ function may be compromised by massive blood loss and the sequelae associated with resuscitation and massive transfusion. Hence, organ-specific complications such as renal failure and acute lung injury should be considered and laboratory monitoring of renal function, peripheral oxygenation (Astrup), and chest x-rays may all be required on a daily basis. In high dependency units, peripheral oxygen saturation is commonly monitored continuously during resuscitation.

FLUID, BLOOD, AND BLOOD PRODUCT REPLACEMENT

Restoration of the circulating blood volume and reperfusion of ischemic organs is an essential priority and needs

TABLE 79–3

Indications for Intensive Care

1. All patients requiring mechanical ventilation
2. All patients with ongoing hemorrhage
3. All patients requiring inotropic support
4. All patients with organ failure
   a. Renal failure (urine output <30 mL/h, creatinine >150 mmol/L)
   b. Respiratory distress
5. All patients with underlying complicating disorders
   a. Preeclampsia/eclampsia/HELLP syndrome
   b. Acute fatty liver of pregnancy
   c. Other causes of acute liver failure
   d. Anaphylactoid syndrome
6. All patients with invasive monitoring

to be accomplished within 6 hours of developing hypovolemia if inflammatory sequelae are to be avoided.[33] Intravenous fluids must be infused as rapidly as possible until the pulse rate begins to decline. Thereafter, the volume infused should be titrated against a number of clinical parameters, including blood pressure (mean arterial pressure >60 mm Hg), peripheral capillary filling, urinary output, and central venous pressure. In the intensive care setting, other indices of tissue oxygenation (oxygen delivery and consumption indices) as well as mixed venous oxygen saturation levels may be used to optimize fluid management.[33,34]

The rapid administration of fluids depends upon the viscosity of the fluid chosen and the physical properties of the cannula used to establish the infusion. Acellular fluids (rather than blood or packed red blood cells) can be infused rapidly and should be used to initiate resuscitation. Randomized studies have shown no benefit associated with the use of colloidal solutions; consequently, they should only be used as an adjunct to crystalloids in specific situations in which low oncotic pressure may complicate the presentation (e.g., severe preeclampsia with abruptio placentae). Crystalloids commonly used for resuscitation include lactated Ringer's solution or normal saline. The choice of the cystalloid is probably less important than the volume and the rate at which the solution is given. The rate of fluid infusion is determined by the bore and length of the infusion cannula with short large-bore peripheral cannulas (ideally, two 14-gauge cannulae) being preferable to long central lines. The initial goal of fluid therapy is a fall in pulse rate with a rise in mean blood pressure to above 60 mm Hg. As a rule of thumb, the amount of crystalloid required will be three times the volume of blood lost. Central venous pressure measurement after resuscitation should rise to between 10 and 12 mm Hg and fluid should be administered as a bolus challenge against the CVP until a sustained rise in pressure beyond these values can be demonstrated. If central venous oxygen saturation monitoring is utilized, values of less than 65% are associated with abnormally high rates of oxygen extraction from blood perfusing the peripheral tissues as a result of ongoing hypovolemia and indicate the need for ongoing resuscitation.

Occasionally, severe persistent hypotension despite fluid resuscitation indicates the need for inotropic support to maintain sufficient cardiac output. This can be attained using adrenaline, dopamine, or dobutamine. Vasopressor doses of adrenaline range from 0.01 to 0.1 μg/kg/minute and should be titrated against the blood pressure. Dopamine in a dose of 4 to 7 μg/kg/minute stimulates β-receptors and increases cardiac output. Dobutamine is primarily a β_1-receptor stimulant and is mostly used for treating left ventricular failure in a dose of 5 to 15 μg/kg/minute. Control of hemorrhage and adequate fluid replacement should allow rapid weaning from inotropic support.

Correction of the coagulation defect usually requires the administration of fresh frozen plasma (FFP) in a ratio of 1 unit to every unit of packed red blood cells considered necessary to restore the oxygen-carrying capacity.[35] Each unit of FFP will restore procoagulant activity by about 10% and will also raise the fibrinogen level by 40 mg/dL. Cryoprecipitate contains factor VIII, fibrinogen, and von Willebrand factor and should be given when the fibrinogen levels fall below 100 mg/dL. Each unit of cryoprecipitate will raise the fibrinogen level by 100 mg/dL. The advice of a hematologist should be sought when correcting the coagulation defect that develops after massive hemorrhage. Platelets do not need to be infused to restore hemostasis until the count falls below 50×10^9 cells/L providing the platelets are functionally normal (women with preeclampsia may have qualitative platelet defects as well as thrombocytopenia). Each unit of platelet concentrate will raise the platelet count by 5×10^9/L. Administration of FFP should be continued until the aPTT and INR are measurably normal.

For the patient with uncontrollable hemorrhage where all other measures have failed, evidence is accumulating that recombinant factor VIIa is proving successful.[36–38]

Correction of the red blood cell mass deficit is guided by the rule that each unit of packed cells will restore hemoglobin concentration by 1 g/dL. There is no consensus regarding what would be generally considered a desirable hemoglobin concentration. Hemoglobin concentrations equal to or less than 6 g/dL probably merit transfusion and in obstetric patients with ongoing blood loss a more liberal transfusion policy is necessary. Full cross-match is preferred prior to transfusion, although with massive hemorrhage, type-specific partially cross-matched blood can be used (5 minute cross-match). Most labor units will also have a limited supply of type O negative blood available for obstetric emergencies. Because of the risks associated with transfusion of donated blood, in circumstances in which the need for transfusion may be foreseeable, autologous blood transfusion should be offered and can be accomplished either by predonation or preoperative normovolemic hemodilution.

During resuscitation, supplemental oxygen delivery should be provided by means of a 40% facemask and the patient should be kept warm with space blankets or commercially available pneumatic blanket warming device. Additional intensive care monitoring of blood pressure via a radial artery line is also helpful both to allow continuous monitoring of the systemic pressure and to facilitate repeated hematologic investigation.

Specific Management

PLACENTAL ABRUPTION

In severe abruption, the woman is usually in severe pain and may be in shock due to hypovolemia. The amount of vaginal bleeding will vary. Coagulopathy occurs in about one third of cases when the fetus is dead, but is comparatively rare with a live fetus. Labor occurs spontaneously in approximately 50% of patients.

Maternal resuscitation, as described in the previous section, is the immediate priority. Adequate analgesia should be given if required, usually by intravenous narcotics supplemented by nitrous oxide/oxygen mixtures self-administered by mask. Epidural analgesia is contraindicated in any woman who is actively bleeding because of the peripheral vasodilation associated with lumbar sympathetic blockade.

The only treatment for severe placental abruption is to empty the uterus as soon as feasible. If the fetus is dead, then normal management is to aim for a vaginal delivery, except where there is an obvious obstetric indication for cesarean section such as transverse lie. In rare situations uterine contractions cannot be stimulated or maternal shock is uncorrectable. Cesarean section may have to be undertaken in such cases, although there is a significant maternal risk from blood loss, especially if there is also a coagulopathy. If there is no response to oxytocin, prostaglandins may be administered with appropriate surveillance in an attempt to stimulate uterine contractions. The management of labor in patients with abruptio placentae is uninformed by any randomized evidence, and no clear guidelines are thus available. There is an increased risk of uterine rupture with a large abruption, particularly if there is a Couvelaire uterus.

Determining if the fetus is alive by auscultation may be difficult because of a tender, hypertonic uterus, especially if there is a retroplacental clot and anterior placenta. Accordingly, visualization of the heart using ultrasound is usually the quickest method if a machine is available. If not, it may be necessary to rupture the membranes and attach a fetal ECG electrode providing the patient is known to have been screened for HIV infection. Exclusion of placenta previa may be difficult on clinical grounds if the presenting part cannot be palpated, and the two conditions may coexist. Ideally, location of the placental site is checked by ultrasonography before any vaginal examination.

If the fetus is alive, then consideration should be given to early delivery by cesarean section for fetal reasons. This will depend on the gestation, as it is extremely improbable that a fetus under 26 weeks will survive such an asphyxial episode. The mode of delivery will also depend on the fetal condition as judged by cardiotocography. If the fetal heart rate pattern is totally normal (which is unlikely), induction of labor with continuous monitoring can be considered. An abnormal cardiotocograph tracing is usually an indication for cesarean delivery providing that the fetal heart beat is confirmed to be present immediately prior to the cesarean section.

The clinical diagnosis of abruptio placentae in the woman who has had a previous cesarean delivery must lead to consideration of whether the clinical presentation could be due to uterine rupture. Signs of generalized peritonitis, cessation of labor, hematuria, and malpresentation may all indicate uterine rupture; abdominal paracentesis may also reveal hemoperitoneum. A high index of clinical suspicion necessitates laparotomy to exclude the diagnosis.

PLACENTA PREVIA

Massive hemorrhage from placenta previa follows smaller "warning" bleeds in the majority of cases, and the placental site will often already be known. The fetal heart is usually still present, and additionally, there may be evidence of uterine contractions or premature rupture of membranes in about 20% of cases.

Initial management involves maternal resuscitation as described earlier. A patient with such a severe hemorrhage due to placenta previa will require delivery by cesarean section irrespective of whether the fetus is dead or alive. The cesarcan section may need to be performed as resuscitative efforts are under way if the mother's condition cannot be stabilized. Occasionally, vaginal delivery may be contemplated if the fetus is dead or extremely premature. Where there is any possibility of placenta previa, a digital examination should only occur in theater after the decision has been made to deliver and the diagnosis of placenta previa is in doubt. Cesarean section for placenta previa is often a difficult procedure associated with fetal malpresentation, a poorly developed lower uterine segment, and excessive blood loss that further compromises the condition of the patient. The operation should be performed by a senior obstetrician in association with a senior anesthetist and with extra blood immediately available.

Several aspects of cesarean delivery present additional unresolved dilemmas. These include the choice of anesthesia, the technique by which the amniotic cavity is reached, and the method of delivery of the baby. Regional anesthesia, which is the generally preferred technique of obstetric anesthesia, is associated with peripheral vasodilation that could be deleterious in women who experience massive intraoperative hemorrhage. Reaching the amniotic cavity in women with an anterior placenta previa presents the surgeon with a choice of dissecting the placenta free from the decidua in order to open the amniotic cavity at the edge of the placenta or the alternative choice of transecting the placenta to open the amniotic cavity directly beneath the uterine incision. These techniques have not been subject to randomized comparison and most practice is informed only by prevailing surgical habit. Delivery of the baby may similarly challenge the surgeon to attempt a potentially difficult cephalic delivery compared to internal podalic version and breech extraction.

Placenta previa accreta may be encountered in about 5% of cases with no previous scar in the uterus, and in up to 67% of cases with multiple cesarean sections. Early recourse to hysterectomy may be necessary but conservative management has been attempted, including oxytocics, uterine devascularization procedures, brace sutures, and catheter compression techniques (see later discussion). Postpartum hemorrhage is also more common because of the inability of the lower uterine segment to contract efficiently and should be anticipated and similar prophylactic measures taken (see later discussion).

PRIMARY POSTPARTUM HEMORRHAGE

Initial Management. Most cases of massive postpartum hemorrhage are primary and occur within the first hour after delivery. It is relatively uncommon for secondary hemorrhage to present with blood loss of more than 1000 mL.

The principles of management are as follows:

- Arrest the hemorrhage
- Resuscitation (see earlier discussion)
- Definitive management of the underlying problem.

In the labor ward initial treatment should include rubbing up the fundus to expel clots and to provoke a uterine contraction. Massive hemorrhage in excess of the attainable rate of fluid replacement may lead to rapidly progressive hypovolemia and cardiac arrest. This situation should be recognized when it develops and temporizing measures are necessary to allow resuscitative measures time to restore circulating blood volume. The temporizing measures employed are those of controlling blood loss by direct pressure on the bleeding vessels. In the case of uterine hemorrhage, this is achieved by bimanual compression of the uterine fundus. The fundus of the uterus is sandwiched between the fist of the obstetrician placed in the anterior vaginal fornix and the abdominal hand that compresses the body of the uterus against the vaginal hand. In desperate circumstances, aortic compression should also be considered. This can be executed by placing the palm of the hand on the abdomen above the umbilicus and applying firm pressure to occlude the aorta.

The cause of the bleeding should be identified early in the management. The main causes are uterine atony (including retained placental tissue), trauma, and coagulation defects.

Management of the Underlying Cause. Few of the necessary interventions can be sustained on the basis of randomized studies. However, the role of oxytocic drugs has been reviewed and their utility in active management of the third stage of labor is well established.[39]

More than one etiologic factor may be present. The commonest cause is uterine atony. Pharmacologic intervention must include a range of oxytocic drugs. First-line treatment requires the use of oxytocin and ergometrine. Oxytocin is administered as a bolus of 5 units intravenously followed by an infusion of 20 units in a liter of Ringer's lactate or normal saline. Ergometrine is given, either in combination with oxytocin (syntometrine) or on its own in a dose of 0.5 mg IM or IV. This dose may be repeated. Ergometrine may be of limited utility in developing countries with poor facilities for refrigeration and storage away from light.[40,41] There is some evidence that rectal misoprostol may be an effective agent for controlling severe hemorrhage and should be used in combination with oxytocin and ergometrine.[39,42,43] Other pharmacologic options include the use of methylated prostaglandin $F_{2\alpha}$ preparations (Hemabate), although the side effect profile of the prostaglandin $F_{2\alpha}$ analogues include hypertension, bronchospasm, and diarrhea that limit the utility of these agents even if they are effective in controlling uterine hemorrhage.[44]

Persistent uterine hemorrhage unresponsive to pharmacologic manipulation may need to be dealt with surgically in a series of increasingly radical procedures. The choice of procedure will be influenced by the specific individual circumstances that may include bleeding due to retained products, hemorrhage as a result of persistent uterine atony, bleeding at the time of cesarean section, bleeding from the lower segment following delivery of a placenta previa, and bleeding as a result of trauma. The surgical options include evacuation of the uterus, devascularization of the uterus, compression techniques, and definitive management in the form of hysterectomy.[42,45,46]

Evacuation of the uterine cavity should be preceded by careful examination under anesthesia to exclude uterine rupture. Removal of placental tissue may be achieved by a combination of digital evacuation, the use of Desjardin forceps, and curettage with a large curette (Baum's curette).

Stepwise devascularization of the uterus commences with ligation of the uterine arteries adjacent to the lower segment. This may necessitate opening the leaves of the broad ligament by dividing the round ligaments.[42] The supposition upon which this intervention is based is that a reduction in the perfusing pressures within the uterine circulation may allow the hemostatic mechanism to reassert itself. Failure to control hemorrhage in this way should lead to ligation of the infundibulopelvic vessels, taking care to avoid damage to the fallopian tubes. Devascularization may also be achieved by occluding the internal iliac artery either by ligation or embolization.[42] Ligation of the internal iliac artery requires careful dissection of the retroperitoneal space and identification of the ureter. This technique should not be attempted without adequate surgical experience in pelvic dissection, and the reported success rates vary from a 42% to 65% chance of avoiding hysterectomy.[47]

Various compression techniques are described. The B-Lynch brace is transfixed through the lower segment with two loops of chromic catgut over the fundus, applying pressure to the body of the uterus in the same way that a pair of braces would be worn.[48] Simpler techniques include sutures that traverse both anterior and posterior walls of the uterus in the form of two parallel sutures inserted into the upper uterine segment.[49]

Bleeding from the lower segment of the uterus after delivery of a placenta previa may be difficult to control because the lower segment does not retract to the same extent as the upper segment. Transcervical catheters with a large bulb (Sengstaken-Blakemore tube) may be used to compress these vessels and have even been advocated as an alternative to uterine packing as a way of controlling postpartum hemorrhage.[50] Uterine packing using gauze packs, previously advocated, as a mechanism for controlling blood loss is no longer practiced because of the difficulty of packing the distensible postpartum uterus and because of concerns about infection.

Hysterectomy remains the final resort in controlling intractable uterine bleeding and may be indicated a priori in cases of uterine rupture. Concern about loss of fertility should not deter the surgeon faced with life-threatening hemorrhage from taking this, sometimes unavoidable, step.

SECONDARY POSTPARTUM HEMORRHAGE

Massive blood loss occurring after the first 24 hours following delivery is less common than primary postpartum hemorrhage and is usually due to subinvolution of the uterus caused by retained pieces of placenta or membrane and superimposed infection. About 1% of secondary postpartum hemorrhage patients will require hysterectomy.

Severe hemorrhage will require maternal resuscitation (see earlier discussion). Definitive treatment comprises exclusion of retained products of conception, treatment for possible sepsis, and the exclusion of underlying trophoblastic disease. None of these interventions have been tested in randomized studies.[51] Antibiotic therapy will generally include a combination of penicillin with an aminoglycoside and anaerobic cover using metronidazole. Alternatives may include the use of cephalosporins or quinolones. Uterine evacuation should be performed if there is any question of retained products or trophoblastic disease.

Pelvic hematoma formation from vulval or vaginal trauma is dealt with conservatively in cases of supralevator retroperitoneal hemorrhage, although this remains a life-threatening source of hemorrhage. Ongoing resuscitation may be required until the bleeding tamponades spontaneously. If this fails to occur, either surgery or radiologic embolization of the traumatized vessel(s) should be considered. The surgical approach may necessitate both hysterectomy and internal iliac ligation. Infralevator hematomas are usually evacuated and either packed for 24 hours or repaired with mattress sutures to obliterate the cavity.

RUPTURED UTERUS AND OTHER GENITAL TRACT TRAUMA

The immediate pre- and postoperative management will include all the previously described principles of dealing with acute hypovolemia and coagulopathy. Experienced anesthetic support is essential.

The suspected diagnosis of uterine rupture necessitates a laparotomy at which time the decision to repair or remove the uterus will need to be made. These decisions need to be individualized, and few generalizations are possible.

Scar dehiscence can be dealt with by simple repair, but more catastrophic rupture (especially of the unscarred uterus) will require hysterectomy. If contiguous injury to the bladder is identified, urologic assistance will usually be required.

Significant bleeding from other genital tract trauma will require surgical repair. The important principles of management are as follows:

- Prompt and effective resuscitation (see previous discussion)
- Prompt surgical exploration and repair to identify and repair the injury
- Effective anesthesia
- Input from other specialists (colorectal, urologic) as indicated.

SUMMARY OF MANAGEMENT OPTIONS

Massive Obstetric Hemorrhage

Management Options (See also Chapters 41, 59, and 77)	Quality of Evidence	Strength of Recommendation	References
Prenatal—Identification of the At-Risk Patient			
Criteria for risk (though no evidence of measures to prevent/ameliorate bleeding) are as follows:	–	GPP	–
Anemia			
Refusal of blood products			
Previous antepartum hemorrhage, postpartum hemorrhage (PPH), cesarean section, placenta previa			
Value of prophylactic iron therapy is uncertain.	–	GPP	–
Perform delivery in adequately resourced unit.	–	GPP	–

Continued

SUMMARY OF MANAGEMENT OPTIONS
Massive Obstetric Hemorrhage *(Continued)*

Management Options (See also Chapters 41, 59, and 77)	Quality of Evidence	Strength of Recommendation	References
Provide additional counseling in pregnancy.	–	GPP	–
Preparations/precautions for delivery:			
Senior obstetrician	IV	C	1,2
Cross-match blood	IV	C	1,2
Advise active management of third stage with previous primary PPH	Ia	A	32
General Measures			
Have detailed guideline/protocol for unit to include the following guidance:	IV	C	1,2
Setting/site of management (high dependency area or equivalent)	IV	C	1,2
Give facial oxygen and warm patient	–	GPP	–
Monitoring	IV	C	1,2
Fluid, blood, and blood product replacement on basis of clinical condition and laboratory results	IV	C	35–39
Recombinant factor VIIa if all else fails	III	B	36–38
Liaison with laboratories and hematologic colleagues	IV	C	1,2
Placental Abruption			
General measures (see above)	IV	C	1,2
Adequate analgesia (not epidural)	–	GPP	–
Empty uterus—method depends on	–	GPP	–
Gestation			
Fetal condition (?alive; ?suspected asphyxia)			
Placenta Previa			
General measures (above)	IV	C	1,2
Delivery by cesarean section:	IV	C	1,2
Cross-match several units of blood			
Experienced obstetrician			
Experienced anesthetist			
See measures under primary PPH (below) for persistent bleeding.	–	GPP	–
Primary PPH			
General measures (see above)	IV	C	1,2
Stop bleeding with first aid measures:	–	GPP	–
"Rub up" a contraction			
Bimanual compression			
Aortic compression			
Atony:	Ia	A	39
Syntocinon bolus and infusion	Ia	A	39
Ergometrine	III	B	40,41
Prostaglandins	Ib	A	44
Misoprostol	III	B	42,43
Trauma:	–	GPP	–
Repair trauma			
Evacuate retained placenta			

SUMMARY OF MANAGEMENT OPTIONS

Massive Obstetric Hemorrhage *(Continued)*

Management Options (See also Chapters 41, 59, and 77)	Quality of Evidence	Strength of Recommendation	References
Persistent bleeding despite the foregoing measures in order:	III	B	45,47,48,50
Devascularization of uterus	IV	C	42,46,49
Uterine compression techniques			
Hysterectomy			
Pelvic hematoma (procedure depends on site):	III	B	45,47,48,50
Evacuate and pack	IV	C	42,46,49
Devascularization of uterus			
Hysterectomy			
Secondary PPH			
General measures (see above)	IV	C	1,2
Antibiotics (not tested in RCTs)	–	GPP	–
	Ia	A	51
Evacuate retained products (not tested in RCTs)	–	GPP	–
	Ia	A	51
Uterine Rupture and Other Genital Tract Trauma			
General measures (see above)	IV	C	1,2
Effective anesthesia	–	GPP	–
Surgical repair (hysterectomy in extreme)	–	GPP	–
Other specialist surgical input as indicated (e.g., colorectal or urologic)	–	GPP	–

PPH, postpartum hemorrhage; RCT, randomized controlled trial.

DISSEMINATED INTRAVASCULAR COAGULATION

Definition

Disseminated intravascular coagulation is the widespread activation of intravascular coagulation leading to the deposition of fibrin within the circulation. Consumption of clotting factors usually leads to a bleeding diathesis, although a small percentage of affected individuals may go on to develop widespread thrombosis with peripheral organ ischemia. Some degree of DIC accompanies most forms of obstetric hemorrhage; however, the greater risk of coagulopathy usually arises from consumption of clotting factors and platelets as a result of massive hemorrhage. The combination of massive hemorrhage and coagulation failure is recognized as one of the most serious complications in pregnancy. DIC may arise from a wide variety of clinical situations in obstetrics but is always a secondary phenomenon following a "trigger" of generalized coagulation activity. The clinical manifestations of coagulation failure can vary from mild disorders detected on laboratory tests only, to massive uncontrollable hemorrhage with very low fibrinogen and platelet levels. A failure to anticipate or detect the early stages of DIC is cited as a major deficiency in the care of women who die from obstetric hemorrhage, and despite advances in obstetric care and hematologic services, hemorrhage with associated DIC remains a major cause of maternal death and morbidity.

Mechanisms

DIC is triggered by various mechanisms (summarized in Table 79–4):

- Blood loss itself with transfusion and volume replacement
- Release of thromboplastic agents into the circulation
- Endothelial damage to small vessels
- Procoagulant phospholipids produced in response to intravascular hemolysis.

With obstetric complications associated with coagulation failure, there may be interaction of several mechanisms. Once DIC has occurred, there is a potential for a vicious circle, with further consumption of clotting fac-

TABLE 79–4

Mechanism of Disseminated Intravascular Coagulation Occurring During Pregnancy

A. Injury to vascular endothelium:
   Preeclampsia
   Hypovolemic shock
   Septicemic shock
B. Release of thromboplastic tissue factors:
   Placental abruption
   Amniotic fluid embolism
   Retained dead fetus
   Chorioamnionitis
   Hydatidiform mole
   Placenta accreta
   Hypertonic saline used to induce abortion
   Acute fatty liver
C. Production of procoagulant:
   Fetomaternal hemorrhage
   Phospholipids
   Incompativile blood transfusion
   Septicemia
   Intravascular hemolysis
D. In many obstetric complications, there may be interaction between several mechanisms and more than one trigger factor present.

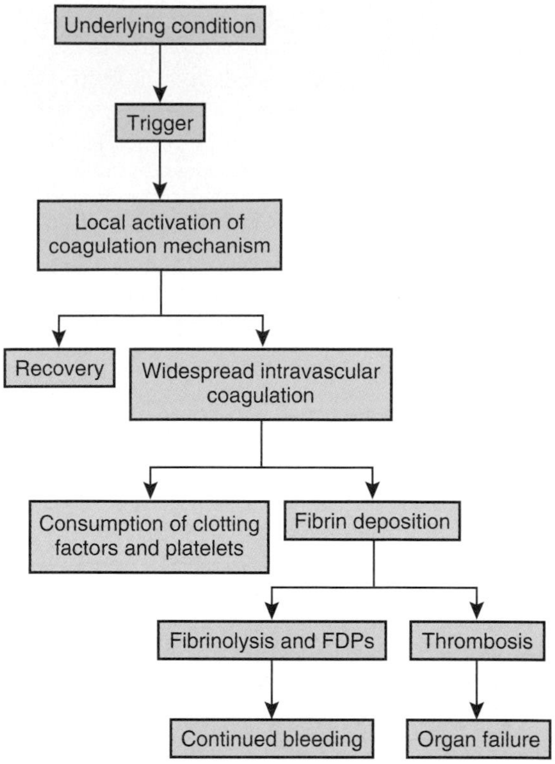

FIGURE 79–1
Once disseminated intravascular coagulation has occurred, there is a potential for a vicious circle, with further consumption of clotting factors and platelets and bleeding until the underlying cause is corrected.

tors and platelets and bleeding until the underlying cause is corrected (Fig. 79–1).

Risks

The risks to both the mother and fetus from coagulation failure in terms of death and morbidity are the same as those discussed earlier under major obstetric hemorrhage. The specific situations in which DIC and coagulation failure may occur and the risks of each underlying condition are considered here.

Placental Abruption

Placental abruption remains the most common cause of coagulation failure in obstetrics and is related to the degree of placental separation and hypovolemic shock. In severe placental abruption with a dead fetus, profound hypofibrinogenemia has been reported in about one third of cases but is much less common if the fetus is alive.[28,52] Earlier stages of DIC are common with mild to moderate abruption but can usually be corrected early if delivery is not delayed.[53] The initial mechanism is due to the release of thromboplastins, but in severe abruption hypovolemic shock, large volume transfusion, and high levels of fibrin degradation products (FDPs) that act as anticoagulants themselves will exacerbate the situation.

Amniotic Fluid Embolism

Amniotic fluid embolism occurs during labor, during cesarean section, or within a short time after delivery. This condition may lead to maternal death as a result of severe pulmonary hypertension following embolization of the pulmonary vessels by fetal squames. If the mother survives this acute event, there may be an anaphylactoid reaction to the presence of the fetal tissues in the maternal circulation associated with cardiovascular collapse, pulmonary edema, seizure activity, and the development of an intractable bleeding diathesis due to severe DIC. The diagnosis is suggested by the detection of fetal squames within the maternal lungs at the time of postmortem, and therefore, the incidence of successfully treated cases is difficult to determine as the diagnosis is only suggestive and cannot be proved. The incidence of death from amniotic fluid embolism between 1970 and 1987 in England and Wales was 7.1 per million maternities. In most cases, the maternal death is unpredictable and unavoidable, and as obstetric care improves, amniotic fluid embolism has been responsible for an increasing proportion of maternal deaths and is now the fifth most common cause of death in the United Kingdom.

Retention of a Dead Fetus

A gradual reduction in clotting factors occurs following intrauterine fetal death, but these changes are not detectable on laboratory testing for 3 to 4 weeks. Approximately 80% of patients with a retained dead fetus will go into spontaneous labor within 3 weeks, but 30% of patients who remain undelivered for more than 4 weeks will develop DIC, usually of a mild degree.[54] Release of thromboplastic substances from the dead fetus into the maternal circulation is thought to be the trigger mechanism.

Preeclampsia

Preeclampsia is associated with endothelial perturbation currently thought to be due to oxidative stress and the release of reactive oxygen species by the ischemic placenta. The changes in endothelial function predispose to multiorgan systems involvement, including the clotting system.[55]

All preeclamptic patients have an increased rate of platelet turnover, and some develop overt thrombocytopenia. Activation of the coagulation cascade leads to a low-grade DIC that only rarely results in a clinically significant hemorrhage in the occasional patient with severe liver necrosis due to the HELLP syndrome.[56] Excessive bleeding, which is often observed at the time of cesarean delivery, is more likely to be due to a qualitative platelet defect in thrombocytopenic individuals than any deficit in clotting factors.

Sepsis

Endotoxic shock can be associated with chorioamnionitis, septic abortion, or postpartum intrauterine infection. Gram-negative organisms are the most common isolated, although *Clostridium welchi* and *Bacteroides* species may be encountered, particularly in septic abortion. The bacterial endotoxin produces severe endothelial damage leading to fibrin deposition and DIC. Secondary intravascular hemolysis, which produces hematuria and oliguria characteristic of the condition, then occurs, and microangiopathic hemolysis can also cause purpuric skin lesions. Hypotension and coagulation failure are poor prognostic features in the presence of sepsis.[57,58]

Other Risk Factors

Other rarer conditions of pregnancy that have been associated with DIC and coagulation failure include induced abortion with hypertonic saline, acute fatty liver of pregnancy, and other hepatic disorders.[59,60] Hydatidiform mole and placenta accreta are associated with DIC because of loss of the intact decidua basalis, and passage of amniotic fluid and other thromboplastic substances into the maternal circulation is more likely.[61,62] Incompatible blood transfusions, large fetomaternal hemorrhage, and other causes of intravascular hemolysis, including drug reactions and the use of other replacement fluids, can also precipitate or exacerbate existing DIC.[63]

Management Options

General

There is a wide spectrum in the manifestation of the process of DIC, but the aims of management are as follows:[64,65]

- To manage the underlying disorder in order to remove the initiating stimulus
- To maintain circulating blood volume
- To replace clotting factors and red blood cells

Management of the underlying disorder will depend upon the specific condition. In the case of placental abruption, delivery will usually lead to rapid recovery once the mother is adequately resuscitated. Amniotic fluid embolism and acute fatty liver of pregnancy will typically result in more resistant coagulopathy that may not be readily corrected despite vigorous attempts at resuscitation.[66]

Laboratory Investigation

If DIC is suspected, blood should be taken and sent for cross-matching and appropriate laboratory tests before commencing definitive treatment (Table 79–5). Blood can be observed for evidence of clotting, but there is little point in performing whole blood clotting tests at the bedside as they are unreliable and time-consuming.[67] Generally, the laboratory assessment of coagulation requires measurement of the aPTT, the INR, the platelet count, and fibrinogen concentrations together with some estimation of FDPs or D-dimers as an index of intravascuular fibrinolysis.

Fluid Replacement in Coagulation Failure

The management of coagulation failure is often subsidiary to management of massive hypovolemia. The urgent necessity in the initial stages is to maintain circulatory volume and tissue perfusion, and resuscitation with

TABLE 79–5

Laboratory Investigations

1. Complete blood count including platelet estimation (2.5 mL in EDTA bottle)
2. Coagulation screen:
   Prothrombin time (extrinsic system)
   Partial thromboplastin time (intrinsic system)
   Thrombin time
   Fibrinogen titer (4.5 mL with 0.5 mL citrate anticoagulant)
3. Fibrin degradation products/D-dimers (2.0 mL in special bottle with antifibrinolytic agent)
4. Cross-matching, at least 6 units (10 mL in plain tube)
   Ideally, 20 mL of blood should be sent, but 10 mL is sufficient for essential tests. The sample should be collected as atraumatically and quickly as possible, and any heparinized IV lines avoided.

crystalloid and colloid solutions should be undertaken as soon as possible, as outlined in the previous section. Dextran solutions should not be used because they interfere with platelet function and can aggravate bleeding and DIC, as well as invalidate the laboratory investigations.[68] Prompt and adequate fluid replacement will also prevent renal failure and help in the clearance of elevated levels of FDPs from the circulation via the liver, aiding the restoration of normal hemostasis.

Replacement of Blood Products

Blood products should be given as soon as available. Fresh frozen plasma (FFP) and stored red blood cells provide all the necessary components in fresh whole blood apart from platelets, and the clotting factors in FFP are well preserved for at least 12 months provided the sample is stored correctly.[35] The use of fresh whole blood should not be encouraged, as it cannot be screened for possible infections. Furthermore, it is not easily obtained in an emergency. It is occasionally necessary to give extra fibrinogen in the form of cryoprecipitate, although sufficient amounts are usually provided in FFP, which also contains factors V, VIII, and antithrombin III in higher concentrations. Platelets are not found in FFP, and their functional activity rapidly deteriorates in stored blood. The platelet count reflects both the degree of DIC and the amount of transfused blood given. If there is persistent bleeding and the platelet count is very low (definitions vary but $<50 \times 10^9$ is often used), the patient may be given concentrated platelets, but these are not usually necessary to gain hemostasis.[67]

Other Treatment Options

Heparin therapy has been used to treat DIC from many different underlying causes, but there is no evidence to suggest that its use confers any benefit over supportive therapy. Heparin is contraindicated if there is hypovolemia and obviously this would include that secondary to placental abruption.[69] Heparin therapy has been suggested in the management of amniotic fluid embolism, but in the face of massive coagulation failure and clinical hemorrhage, it is difficult to justify.[66] It has likewise been suggested in the management of sepsis, although the most recent literature suggests that recombinant protein C may have advantages in terms of preventing fibrin deposition and stimulating the immune response.[69–73] Antifibrinolytic drugs have also been used, but there is the risk that their use would prevent the removal of microvascular thrombi from organs such as kidney or brain as the DIC resolves, leading to long-term sequelae.

SUMMARY OF MANAGEMENT OPTIONS

Disseminated Intravascular Coagulation

Management Options	Quality of Evidence	Strength of Recommendation	References
Remove Insult/"Trigger"			
Empty uterus with major antepartum hemorrhage, retained dead fetus, molar pregnancy	See Major Obstetric Hemorrhage Box (above) and Chapters 4 and 26		
Treat uterine atony/repair trauma with postpartum hemorrhage (PPH)	See Chapter 77		
End pregnancy with preeclampsia	See Preeclampsia, Chapter 36		
Antibiotics with sepsis	–	GPP	–
General			
Involve hematologist and support services (blood transfusion, etc.) early	IV	C	64
Investigations			
See Table 72–5	–	GPP	–
Maintain Circulation			
See Major Obstetric Hemorrhage Box (above)	IV	C	64
Colloids (rather than crystalloid) initially but blood ideally	IV	C	64
Avoid dextran	III	B	68

SUMMARY OF MANAGEMENT OPTIONS

Disseminated Intravascular Coagulation *(Continued)*

Management Options	Quality of Evidence	Strength of Recommendation	References
Replacement of Blood Products			
Hematologic priorities are to replace blood constituents and coagulation factors (fresh frozen plasma and cryoprecipitate first-line rather than platelets)	III	B	35,70
Other Treatment			
Heparin and antithrombolytic therapy have both been used in DIC to break the cycle of consumptive coagulopathy. Neither has been subjected to controlled trials.	IV III	C B	64,66 65
Concentrates of anticoagulant proteins such as antithrombin, protein C, and activated protein C are possibly useful in DIC due to severe sepsis.	III	B	70,71
Recombinant activated protein C is very effective in severe DIC due to sepsis outside pregnancy; limited experience in pregnancy.	III IV	B C	72 73

CONCLUSIONS

- Hemorrhage and its consequences remain an unpredictable and potentially lethal complication of pregnancy.
- A clear understanding is required of the causes as well as the principles of managing obstetric hemorrhage.
- Much of what we practice and teach remains uninformed by high-quality studies, although there is much accumulated experience from which we can learn.
- Although we should continue to strive for better evidence of effective care, indecision in the management of individual patients is not an option when faced with major obstetric hemorrhage.
- The skills required to care for these women include those of the obstetrician, anesthetists, intensivists, hematologists, renal physicians, and radiologists.
- The obstetrician will usually be the physician most involved with the care of these patients and should have regular "fire-drills" in all aspects of resuscitation and the management of major hemorrhage.

REFERENCES

1. A review of maternal deaths in South Africa during 1998. National Committee on Confidential Enquiries into Maternal Deaths. S Afr Med J 2000;90(4):367–373.
2. de Swiet M: Maternal mortality: Confidential enquiries into maternal deaths in the United Kingdom. Am J Obstet Gynecol 2000;182(4):760–766.
3. Odendaal HJ: Uterine contraction patterns in patients with severe abruptio placentae. S Afr Med J 1980;57(22):908–910.
4. Odendaal HJ, Burchell H: Raised uterine resting tone in patients with abruptio placentae. Int J Gynaecol Obstet 1985;23(2):121–124.
5. Abdella TN, Sibai BM, Hays JM Jr, Anderson GD: Relationship of hypertensive disease to abruptio placentae. Obstet Gynecol 1984;63(3):365–370.
6. Drakeley AJ, Le Roux PA, Anthony J, Penny J: Acute renal failure complicating severe preeclampsia requiring admission to an obstetric intensive care unit. Am J Obstet Gynecol 2002;186(2):253–256.
7. Robson JS: Proteinuria and the renal lesion in preeclampsia and abruptio placentae. Perspect Nephrol Hypertens 1976;5:61–73.
8. Ekele BA, Audu LR, Muyibi S: Uterine rupture in Sokoto, Northern Nigeria—Are we winning? Afr J Med Med Sci 2000;29(3–4):191–193.
9. Lynch JC, Pardy JP: Uterine rupture and scar dehiscence. A five-year survey. Anaesth Intensive Care 1996;24(6):699–704.
10. Aboyeji AP, Ijaiya MD, Yahaya UR: Ruptured uterus: A study of 100 consecutive cases in Ilorin, Nigeria. J Obstet Gynaecol Res 2001;27(6):341–348.
11. Galley HF, Webster NR: The immuno-inflammatory cascade. Br J Anaesth 1996;77(1):11–16.
12. Scannell G: Leukocyte responses to hypoxic/ischemic conditions. New Horiz 1996;4(2):179–183.
13. Biffl WL, Moore EE: Splanchnic ischaemia/reperfusion and multiple organ failure. Br J Anaesth 1996;77(1):59–70.

14. Dries DJ: Activation of the clotting system and complement after trauma. New Horiz 1996;4(2):276–288.
15. Ananth CV, Wilcox AJ: Placental abruption and perinatal mortality in the United States. Am J Epidemiol 2001;153(4):332–337.
16. Haddad B, Mercer BM, Livingston JC, Sibai BM: Obstetric antecedents to apparent stillbirth (Apgar score zero at 1 minute only). Obstet Gynecol 2001;97(6):961–964.
17. Fretts RC, Boyd ME, Usher RH, Usher HA: The changing pattern of fetal death, 1961–1988. Obstet Gynecol 1992;79(1):35–39.
18. Cardwell MS: Ultrasound diagnosis of abruptio placentae with fetomaternal hemorrhage. Am J Obstet Gynecol 1987;157(2): 358–359.
19. Spinillo A, Fazzi E, Stronati M, et al: Early morbidity and neurodevelopmental outcome in low-birthweight infants born after third trimester bleeding. Am J Perinatol 1994;11(2):85–90.
20. Vintzileos AM, Ananth CV, Smulian JC, et al: The impact of prenatal care on neonatal deaths in the presence and absence of antenatal high-risk conditions. Am J Obstet Gynecol 2002;186(5):1011–1016.
21. Gruenberger W, Gerstner GJ: The causes of antepartum fetal death: A clinico-pathological study. Clin Exp Obstet Gynecol 1980;7(4):210–214.
22. Clark SL, Koonings PP, Phelan JP: Placenta previa/accreta and prior cesarean section. Obstet Gynecol 1985;66(1):89–92.
23. Naeye RL: Placenta previa. Predisposing factors and effects on the fetus and surviving infants. Obstet Gynecol 1978;52(5): 521–525.
24. Brenner WE, Edelman DA, Hendricks CH: Characteristics of patients with placenta previa and results of "expectant management." Am J Obstet Gynecol 1978;132(2):180–191.
25. Gorodeski IG, Bahari CM, Schachter A, Neri A: Recurrent placenta previa. Eur J Obstet Gynecol Reprod Biol 1981;12(1):7–11.
26. Singh PM, Rodrigues C, Gupta AN: Placenta previa and previous cesarean section. Acta Obstet Gynecol Scand 1981;60(4):367–368.
27. Cotton DB, Read JA, Paul RH, Quilligan EJ: The conservative aggressive management of placenta previa. Am J Obstet Gynecol 1980;137(6):687–695.
28. Green-Thompson RW: Antepartum haemorrhage. Clin Obstet Gynaecol 1982;9(3):479–515.
29. Hibbard BM, Jeffcoate TN: Abruptio placentae. Obstet Gynecol 1966;27(2):155–167.
30. Naeye RL, Harkness WL, Utts J: Abruptio placentae and perinatal death: A prospective study. Am J Obstet Gynecol 1977;128(7):740–746.
31. Naeye RL: Abruptio placentae and placenta previa: Frequency, perinatal mortality, and cigarette smoking. Obstet Gynecol 1980;55(6):701–704.
32. Elbourne DR, Prendville WJ, Carroli G, et al: Active versus expectant management in the third stage of labour. The Cochrane Library, Issue 4. Oxford: Update Software, 2001.
33. Pinsky MR: Targets for resuscitation from shock. Minerva Anestesiol 2003;69(4):237–244.
34. Rivers EP, Ander DS, Powell D: Central venous oxygen saturation monitoring in the critically ill patient. Curr Opin Crit Care 2001;7(3):204–211.
35. Conteras M, Ala FA, Greaves M, et al: Guidelines for the use of fresh frozen plasma. British Committee standards in Haematology, working paper of Blood Transfusion Task Force. Transfusion Medicine 1992;2:57–63.
36. O'Connell NM, Perry DJ, Hodgson AJ, et al: Recombinant factor VIIa in the management of uncontrolled haemorrhage. Transfusion 2003;43:1649–1651.
37. Zupancic SS, Sokolic V, Viskovic T, et al: Successful use of recombinant factor VIIa for massive bleeding after cesaerean section due to HELLP syndrome. Acta Haematol 2002;108: 162–163.
38. Moscardo F, Perez F, de la Rubia J, et al: Successful treatment of severe intraabdominal bleeding associated with disseminated intravascular coagulation using recombinant activated factor VIIa. Br J Haematol 2001;114:174–176.
39. Mousa HA, Alfirevic Z: Treatment for primary postpartum haemorrhage. Cochrane Database Syst Rev 2003;(1):CD003249.
40. Hogerzeil HV, Walker GJ: Instability of (methyl)ergometrine in tropical climates: An overview. Eur J Obstet Gynecol Reprod Biol 1996;69(1):25–29.
41. de Groot AN, Hekster YA, Vree TB, van Dongen PW: Ergometrine and methylergometrine tablets are not stable under simulated tropical conditions. J Clin Pharm Ther 1995;20(2): 109–113.
42. Jouppila P: Postpartum haemorrhage. Curr Opin Obstet Gynecol 1995;7(6):446–450.
43. Bjornerem A, Acharya G, Oian P, Maltau JM: [Postpartum hemorrhage—Prophylaxis and treatment in Norway.] Tidsskr Nor Laegeforen 2002;122(26):2536–2537.
44. Lamont RF, Morgan DJ, Logue M, Gordon H: A prospective randomised trial to compare the efficacy and safety of hemabate and syntometrine for the prevention of primary postpartum haemorrhage. Prostaglandins Other Lipid Mediat 2001;66(3):203–210.
45. Vandelet P, Gillet R, Pease S, et al: [Limits to arterial embolization treatment of severe postpartum hemorrhage.] Ann Fr Anesth Reanim 2001;20(4):317–324.
46. Bonnar J: Massive obstetric haemorrhage. Baillieres Best Pract Res Clin Obstet Gynaecol 2000;14(1):1–18.
47. Clark SL, Phelan JP, Yeh SY, et al: Hypogastric artery ligation for obstetric hemorrhage. Obstet Gynecol 1985;66(3):353–356.
48. Lynch C, Coker A, Lawal AH, et al: The B-Lynch surgical technique for the control of massive postpartum haemorrhage: An alternative to hysterectomy? Five cases reported. BJOG 1997;104(3):372–375.
49. Mousa HA, Walkinshaw S: Major postpartum haemorrhage. Curr Opin Obstet Gynecol 2001;13(6):595–603.
50. Johanson R, Kumar M, Obhrai M, Young P: Management of massive postpartum haemorrhage: Use of a hydrostatic balloon catheter to avoid laparotomy. BJOG 2001;108(4): 420–422.
51. Alexander J, Thomas P, Sanghera J: Treatments for secondary postpartum haemorrhage. Cochrane Database Syst Rev 2002;(1): CD002867.
52. Pritchard JA, Brekken AL: Clinical and laboratory studies on severe abruptio placentae. Am J Obstet Gynecol 1967;97(5): 681–700.
53. Knab DR: Abruptio placentae. An assessment of the time and method of delivery. Obstet Gynecol 1978;52(5):625–629.
54. Pritchard JA: Fetal death in utero. Obstet Gynecol 1959;14: 573–580.
55. Redman CW: Current topic: Pre-eclampsia and the placenta. Placenta 1991;12(4):301–308.
56. Weinstein L: Syndrome of hemolysis, elevated liver enzymes, and low platelet count: A severe consequence of hypertension in pregnancy. Am J Obstet Gynecol 1982;142(2):159–167.
57. Beller FK, Uszynski M: Disseminated intravascular coagulation in pregnancy. Clin Obstet Gynecol 1974;17(4):250–278.
58. Hawkins DF, Sevitt LH, Fairbrother PF, Tothill AU: Management of septic chemical abortion with renal failure. Use of a conservative regimen. N Engl J Med 1975;292(14):722–725.
59. Stander RW, Flessa HC, Glueck HI, Kisker CT: Changes in maternal coagulation factors after intra-amniotic injection of hypertonic saline. Obstet Gynecol 1971;37(5):660–666.
60. Harpey JP, Charpentier C: Acute fatty liver of pregnancy. Lancet 1983;1(8324):586–587.
61. Breen JL, Neubecker R, Gregori CA, Franklin JE Jr: Placenta accreta, increta, and percreta. A survey of 40 cases. Obstet Gynecol 1977;49(1):43–47.

62. Read JA, Cotton DB, Miller FC: Placenta accreta: Changing clinical aspects and outcome. Obstet Gynecol 1980;56(1):31–34.
63. Hewitt PE, Machin SJ: ABC of transfusion. Massive blood transfusion. BMJ 1990;300(6717):107–109.
64. Giles AR: Disseminated intravascular coagulation. In Bloom AL, Forbes CD, Thomas DP, Taddenham EGD (eds): Haemostasis and Thrombosis, 3rd ed. Vol. 2. Edinburgh, Churchill Livingstone, 1994.
65. Levi M, TenClate H: Disseminated intravascular coagulation. N Engl J Med 1999;341:586–592.
66. Chung AF, Merkatz IR: Survival following amniotic fluid embolism with early heparinisation. Obstet Gynecol 1973;42: 809–881.
67. Letsky EA: Disseminated intravascular coagulation. Best Pract Res Clin Obstet Gynaecol 2001;15(4):623–644.
68. Suzuki K, Nishioka J, Hashimoto S: Inhibition of factor VIII–associated platelet aggregation by heparin and dextran sulphate. Biochim Biophys Acta 1979;585:416–426.
69. Levi M, de Jonge E, Van Der PT: New treatment strategies for disseminated intravascular coagulation based on current understanding of the pathophysiology. Ann Med 2004;36(1): 41–49.
70. Maki M, Teraco T, Ikeraire T, et al: Clinical evaluation of antithrombin III concentrate (BI 6.013) for disseminated intravascular coagulation in obstetrics. Well-controlled multicenter trial. Gynecol Obstet Invest 1987;23:230–240.
71. Matthay MD: Severe sepsis–A new treatment with both anticoagulant and anti-inflammatory properties. N Engl J Med 2001;344:759–762.
72. Bernard GR, Vincent J-L, Laterrie PF, et al: Efficancy and safety of recombinant human activated protein C for severe sepsis. N Engl J Med 2001;344:699–709.
73. Kobayashi T, Teraco T, Maktri M, Ikenaire T: Activated protein C is effective for DIC associated with placental abruption (letter). Thromb Haemostasis 1999;82(4):1363.

CHAPTER 80

Critical Care of the Obstetric Patient

John Anthony

INTRODUCTION

Maternal mortality accounts for half a million deaths annually.[1] The risk of obstetric mortality varies according to the socioeconomic development of different countries, and many deaths could be avoided with better access to medical care. Industrialized countries, however, continue to focus on maternal deaths because many are associated with substandard care, some of which could be avoided by greater attention to critical care management.[2]

The admission of obstetric patients to critical care facilities is low (published intensive care unit [ICU] admission rates are 0.29% to 1.5% of deliveries in industrialized countries).[1,3] No standardized criteria define the requirement for critical care among pregnant women. The reasons for ICU admission range from obstetric complications (usually due to preeclampsia, hemorrhage, and sepsis) through medical disorders exacerbated by pregnancy (e.g., cardiac disease and thromboembolism) to conditions incidental to pregnancy (e.g., respiratory disease, complications of HIV infection). Only one dedicated obstetric ICU published its experience several years ago, and the pattern of admissions may be changing in developing countries due to the evolving HIV pandemic, with a far greater burden of sick patients being admitted as a result of infection and postoperative sepsis.[3]

Provision of critical care to the pregnant woman requires knowledge of intensive care principles as well as relevant aspects of maternal and fetal physiology.

RELEVANT PHYSIOLOGY OF PREGNANCY

Cardiovascular Changes

The dominant cardiovascular change in pregnancy is the increase in cardiac output leading to accelerated delivery of oxygenated blood to the peripheral tissues including the uterus and choriodecidual space. Stroke volume and cardiac output rise by 40%, and blood pressure falls due to peripheral vasodilation and because the placental circulation functions as an arteriovenous fistula. These changes precede and exceed the fetal and maternal metabolic requirements of pregnancy to such an extent that the difference in arteriovenous oxygen declines in normal pregnancy.[4] Increased cardiac output is achieved largely by a rise in circulating blood volume due to physiologic hyperreninism that increases aldosterone levels 10-fold.[5] This adaptation leads to water and electrolyte retention and a 50% increase in plasma volume.[6,7] Doppler ultrasound has been used to redefine the cardiac changes that accompany the increase in cardiac output. Both filling phases of the left ventricle show increased filling velocities. The peak mitral flow velocity in early diastole (E wave) and the peak velocity during atrial systole (A wave) both increase. The increase in early wave velocity occurs by the end of the first trimester, whereas the peak A-wave velocity changes occur in the third trimester. The E/A ratio increases in the first trimester but falls again as the A-wave velocity increases and is accompanied by decreasing left ventricular isovolumetric relaxation time.[8,9] Left ventricular mass increases significantly while fractional shortening and velocity of shortening diminish throughout pregnancy.[10] Systolic function is preserved by falling systemic (including uterine artery) resistance.[8,9] Peak left ventricular wall stress, an indicator of afterload, has been demonstrated in early pregnancy and normalizes as ventricular mass increases in the midtrimester.[10] Giva and colleagues report a 45% increase in cardiac output in normal pregnancy accompanied by an increase in left ventricular end-diastolic volume and increased end-systolic wall stress accompanied by transient left ventricular hypertrophy.[11] These authors also report a reversible decline in left ventricular function during the second and third trimesters.

The pulmonary circulation shows increased flow during pregnancy with some reduction in vascular resistance without any significant alteration in blood pressure. These changes are evident by 8 weeks' gestation without any subsequent alteration and return to prepregnancy values by 6 months postpartum.[12] Systemic arterial vascular compliance is thought to diminish because of reduced vascular tone.[13]

Plasma volume expansion is matched by enhanced oxygen-carrying capacity brought about by a 14% to 28% increase in red cell mass.[14] Fetal respiration depends on maternal hyperventilation that creates a partially compensated respiratory alkalosis. The partial pressure of carbon dioxide ($Paco_2$) in a pregnant woman will fall approximately 15% with a reduction in plasma bicarbonate, although arterial pH remains unaltered.[15]

Effective renal plasma flow rises with increasing cardiac output and blood volume, leading to a 50% increase in glomerular filtration.[16] This results in increased fractional excretion of glucose as well as other metabolites and drugs.

Coagulation

The mother is protected against the effects of hemorrhage at the time of delivery by her increased blood volume and also by enhanced coagulation. Coagulation changes include increased estrogen-dependent hepatic synthesis of fibrinogen and factors VII, VIII, X, and XIII.[17] The anticlotting mechanism is physiologically impaired by reduced levels of protein S. Pregnancy is therefore a state of physiologic resistance to the action of activated protein C because free protein S is a necessary cofactor in this reaction. The fibrinolytic system is also impeded by increased levels of both plasminogen activator inhibitor-I (PAI-I, derived from endothelial cells) and PAI-II, derived from the placenta. Expression of procoagulant activity takes place normally during pregnancy and may be detected by measuring levels of circulating thrombin-antithrombin III complexes.[17]

Effect of Delivery

These physiologic changes in pregnancy are progressive during pregnancy and revert to normal at varying rates during the puerperium. Hence, labor stimulates a further increase in cardiac output, peaking out at 10 L/min as a result of autotransfusion of blood from the choriodecidual circulation during the third stage of labor.[18] Blood pressure fluctuates during pregnancy, falling by 10% to 15% in the midtrimester but rises again toward prepregnancy levels by the end of the third trimester, with a further rise occurring in some patients during labor.

Uteroplacental Effects

Blood flow to the choriodecidual space is determined by both the cardiac output and dilation of the spiral arteries prior to the 20th week of pregnancy. These dilated vessels cannot vasoregulate blood flow to the placenta, which remains directly proportional to changes in maternal cardiac output and blood pressure. Vasoconstriction in the uterine circulation can develop in response to catecholamines, while uterine contractions restrict flow through these vessels by compression of the vessel wall. Transplacental gas exchange takes place by simple diffusion, and even at low partial pressures, fetal hemoglobin binds oxygen avidly because the oxyhemoglobin dissociation curve is shifted to the left. Even minor changes in the partial pressure of oxygen (Pao_2) in the maternal circulation may significantly improve fetal hemoglobin saturation operating on the steep part of the oxyhemoglobin dissociation curve. Fetal well-being is therefore critically dependent on maternal cardiac output, uterine blood flow, and maternal Pao_2.

Anatomic Changes

The enlarged uterus compresses the inferior vena cava and aorta. This may lead to supine hypotension as a result of diminished venous return, although the adrenergic response to aortocaval compression tends to maintain or increase blood pressure. Diminished cardiac output can nevertheless critically impair uterine perfusion, especially during labor.

The diaphragm is displaced by the enlarging uterus resulting in a 10% to 20% reduction in residual volume and functional residual capacity. Under the influence of progesterone, the respiratory center increases chest wall movement, leading to an increase in tidal volume. This leads to respiratory alkalosis and hypocapnia.

METHODS OF MONITORING

Oxygen Saturation Monitoring

Spectrophotometry is the detection of specific light frequencies reflected by a range of molecules. Specific molecules reflect specific frequencies, and their reflective properties differ with changes in molecular conformation. Oximetry is the detection of oxygenated and deoxygenated blood. The oxygenated hemoglobin reflects more light at 660 nm, whereas at 940 nm deoxyhemoglobin reflects infrared light more strongly. This allows the simultaneous acquisition of peripheral signals from which the ratio of oxyhemoglobin to deoxyhemoglobin can be calculated and expressed as a percentage of oxyhemoglobin saturation.

Oximetry may be based on transcutaneous measurements or can be derived from mixed venous blood via a probe located in a pulmonary artery catheter. The peripheral pulse oximetry devices rely on detection of pulsed alterations in light transmitted between a transmitter and a photodetector.

Although oximetry is regarded as an effective method of monitoring oxygenation, some limitations are recognized. They include the assumptions that methemoglobin and carboxyhemoglobin are not present in significant concentrations. Invasive mixed venous oxygen saturation monitoring is less frequently used than peripheral oxygen saturation monitoring. It also shows greater spontaneous variation than peripheral monitors but has a clinical role to play in determining the balance between peripheral oxygen delivery and peripheral oxygen consumption. This is a robust measurement that will reflect changes in cardiac output, hemoglobin concentration, and arterial and venous hemoglobin oxygen saturation. This provides useful clinical information in many clinical circumstances.

Hemodynamic Monitoring of Cardiac Output

Hemodynamic monitoring is an integral part of intensive care management and is especially important in cases of severe hemorrhage, severe preeclampsia, and septic shock. An adequate cardiac output is essential in delivering oxygenated blood to the peripheral tissues. Low output will reflect either hypovolemia or ventricular failure. Knowledge of the cardiac output will determine management and will also allow calculation of other derived hemodynamic values, including vascular resistance and oxygen delivery and consumption indices.

Cardiac output was previously most commonly measured using the Fick principle. This principle states that the amount of a substance taken up by the body per unit time equals the difference between the arterial and venous levels multiplied by the blood flow. Hence, oxygen consumption by the body divided by the arteriovenous oxygen difference equals the cardiac output. This principle has been modified to use other markers, including dye dilution techniques and the thermodilution principle of the pulmonary artery catheter. In the latter case, iced water is the marker injected into the right atrium, with a probe measuring the temperature of the blood flowing through the pulmonary artery, thus allowing the derivation of the cardiac output from the area under the curve. This technique, although clinically robust, may produce results confounded by variations in catheter position and variations in injectate temperature and volume, as well as changes in the rate of saline injection. Despite these limitations, this technology remains the gold standard against which newer techniques are assessed. The need to cannulate peripheral and central vessels has been associated with some risk of injury and noninvasive techniques of measuring cardiac output have been sought.

Ultrasound in the form of echocardiography allows estimation of cardiac output by measuring changes in left ventricular dimensions during systole measured in the plane below the level of the mitral valve. By assuming that the ventricle is ellipsoid in shape and that the long axis is double the short axis, stroke volume can be calculated from the cube of the change in left ventricular dimension. This measurement is inaccurate when the assumptions on which it is based are no longer true. Hence, the dilated ventricle and the pregnant woman with an increased volume and end-diastolic dimensions violate these assumptions and may overestimate stroke volume and cardiac output. Doppler ultrasound has now added to the utility of echocardiography by allowing an estimation of blood velocity. The Doppler principle measures the frequency of a reflected ultrasound beam striking moving erythrocytes, where the change in frequency detected is proportional to the velocity of the red cells moving in the axis of the beam. The velocity of a column of red cells multiplied by the period of ejection provides a measure of the distance traveled by a column of blood during systole. The use of ultrasound to measure the diameter of the vessels containing the blood will allow calculation of cross-sectional area with subsequent derivation of stroke volume and cardiac output. The velocity of blood flow can also be related to the pressure gradient down which the blood is moving, providing a way of calculating intracardiac pressure gradients and pulmonary artery pressures.

Doppler probes may be range-gated (pulsed) to allow the measurement of a signal from a given depth of tissue. The pulsed Doppler signal usually allows simultaneous ultrasound imaging and estimation of the angle of insonation between the Doppler probe and the vessel. This latter measurement is important because the calculation of velocity from the reflected Doppler signal requires a knowledge of the angle between the ultrasound beam and the column of blood from which the signal is being reflected. Where the signal is perpendicular to the moving column of blood, no movement will be detected, and the closer the beam moves to being parallel to the vessel, the more completely the reflected vector represents the velocity of the cells in the path of the beam.

The combination of cross-sectional echocardiography and Doppler measurement of flow velocity at specific points in the heart and great vessels allows the determination of volumetric flow. The mitral and aortic valve orifices and the root or arch of the aorta have all been studied using both suprasternal and intraesophageal Doppler probes. Potential for error exists in these techniques, both in the calculation of the insonation angle and the measurement of the cross-sectional area of the vessel. Of the different sites studied, the best correlation between the Doppler technique and thermodilution studies was documented in the aortic valve orifice measurements. Although transthoracic Doppler studies are the most widely accessible tool, transesophageal Doppler allows the posterior structures of the heart to be more clearly imaged with more accurate diagnosis of cardiac pathology and precise alignment to the aortic valve in both the long and short axis as well as providing long axis views of the ascending aorta.[19] The use of multiplanar transesophageal echocardiography allows precise measurements of asymmetrical ventricles that cannot be reliably imaged using a transthoracic probe.[20] The probe has particular utility in the diagnosis of aortic dissection and thromboembolism, although the need for esophageal endoscopy limits the application of this technology to specific situations including intraoperative and postoperative care.[21]

Doppler echocardiography has provided a ready means of studying women at risk of developing hypertensive complications during pregnancy. The most detailed study, to date, by Borghi and associates described detailed cardiac findings among 40 women with mild preeclampsia compared with a control cohort of pregnant women and nonpregnant controls.[22] This study showed a progressive rise in left ventricular mass between nonpregnant women and women with a normal pregnancy, with a further increase in mass among women with preeclampsia. Ejection fraction and fractional shortening decreased in normal pregnancy though this did not reach statistical significance. However, women with preeclampsia had a significant reduction in both these parameters compared with nonpregnant women. In addition, left ventricular end-diastolic volume rose significantly in preeclampsia. Together with a fall in cardiac output in the preeclamptic group, these findings suggest a compensatory increase in ventricular size to maintain cardiac output against an elevated systemic vascular resistance.

The latter study also showed changes in the peak filling velocities of the left ventricle during diastole. The E/A ratio fell significantly during pregnancy, partly reflecting increased preload. In preeclampsia further augmentation of the A-wave peak velocity resulted in further significant reduction in the ratio. Collectively these data support the notion of changes in both cardiac systolic and diastolic function. The authors also measured atrial natriuretic peptide (ANP) levels. In keeping with previous studies, elevated levels of ANP were found in pregnancy, with further increments occurring in preeclampsia. These could not be accounted for by differences in atrial size although a significant correlation was found between left ventricular mass and volume in women with preeclampsia.[22]

Transesophageal Doppler monitoring of hemodynamic data has been carried out in adult ICUs and found to be equivalent to data derived from pulmonary artery catheter measurements.[23] Pregnancy data are few, and only one study has reported the use of transesophageal Doppler monitoring in pregnancy compared with pulmonary artery catheters. That study showed that the Doppler consistently underestimated cardiac output by 40% in women under the age of 35 years.[24] This error may be due to the assumptions implicit in the algorithm used to calculate output. These assumptions include a fixed aortic diameter during systole and a fixed percentage of blood perfusing upper and lower parts of the body. Pregnancy physiologic changes probably invalidate these assumptions. The authors nevertheless conclude that esophageal Doppler may contribute to the estimation of trends over time.

Other techniques of measuring cardiac output include impedance cardiography based on changes in transthoracic electrical resistance associated with the ejection of blood into the pulmonary circulation. This technique has been shown to overestimate low cardiac output, with the opposite error in high cardiac output states.

Invasive Pressure Monitoring

Invasive pressure monitoring includes the insertion of lines used for the measurement of intra-arterial pressure and central venous and pulmonary artery pressure.

Intra-arterial lines allow for continuous assessment of systemic blood pressure and also eliminate the need for repeated venesection, often a prerequisite in the management of the critically ill patient. Various noninvasive blood pressure monitors are also available that measure pressure using an oscillometric principle. These monitors have been shown to be significantly inaccurate when measuring blood pressure from women with preeclampsia, consistently underestimating pressures measured by direct arterial line measurement and auscultation.[25]

Central venous pressure (CVP) monitoring is employed as a measure of right ventricular filling pressure and intravascular blood volume. These lines may be inserted as long lines via the antecubital fossa or can be introduced via the internal jugular or subclavian veins. The long-line technique is preferred in any patient with a bleeding diathesis and also in anyone who cannot tolerate positioning in the Trendelenburg position for internal jugular catheterization (e.g., women with pulmonary edema). CVP in the normovolemic patient should measure between 10 and 12 mm Hg. When managing hypovolemia fluid should be administered as repeated bolus dose infusions until the CVP shows a sustained rise above 10 to 12 mm Hg over a 30-minute period. Central venous lines allow the withdrawal of mixed venous blood in which estimation of the PaO_2 will indicate the extent of peripheral oxygen extraction. In normally oxygenated and perfused individuals, central venous oxygen saturation should remain above 65%. CVP monitoring should not be used to monitor fluid management in severe preeclampsia because left ventricular diastolic dysfunction in this condition results in left-sided changes in pressure that are not reflected by similar changes in right ventricular filling pressures. Hence, a bolus of intravenous fluid may lead to a rapid increase in pulmonary capillary wedge pressure without any change in CVP.

Pulmonary artery catheterization, although controversial, remains a standard intensive care monitoring technique.

Current evidence indicates that pulmonary artery catheters (PAC) do not alter ICU mortality and morbidity, although their utility is recognized in specific patients.[26] In obstetric practice, severe preeclampsia and maternal cardiac disease justify the measurement of left ventricular filling pressures, and measurement of cardiac output allows the calculation of derived hemodynamic parameters such as the systemic vascular resistance and left ventricular stroke work volume. Knowledge of these parameters is a useful guide to appropriate fluid and vasodilator therapy. In preeclampsia, rapid plasma volume expansion has been shown repeatedly to cause a sharp rise in left-sided filling pressures, often without any changes in CVP.[27–29] This occurs despite evidence of normal systolic ventricular function and is a reflection of reduced ventricular compliance during diastole.

PACs, like CVP lines, are inserted either via the internal jugular vein or as a long-line insertion through the antecubital fossa. Catheter placement may lead to a number of complications, especially in inexperienced hands, and should not be undertaken without adequate training and supervision. The incidence of complications may also be lower in pregnant patients than in other ICU populations; the Groote Schuur Obstetric ICU reported no major complications over a 3-year period.[30]

The indications for the insertion of a PAC are similar to those in nonpregnant patients. In addition, severe preeclampsia is recognized to be a condition in which changes in left ventricular diastolic function necessitate monitoring of pulmonary capillary wedge pressure after fluid loading. The Groote Schuur Obstetric ICU audit showed that most catheters were inserted for the management of preeclampsia in patients who also had renal failure (56%), pulmonary edema (32%), or eclampsia (6%).[30]

Although the Pulmonary Artery Catheter Consensus Conference concluded that PAC monitoring did not reduce complications and mortality in patients with preeclampsia, the statement recognized the utility of the catheter in specific circumstances including oliguria unresponsive to fluids, pulmonary edema, and resistant hypertension.[26]

Capnometry

Exhaled gas can be evaluated using an infrared probe and a photodetector set to detect carbon dioxide. This is usually found in the expiratory limb of a ventilator circuit. Expired gas shows a pattern of increasing carbon dioxide concentration related to the sequential expiration of air in the upper airway followed by air from the alveoli. The end-expiratory (or end-tidal) carbon dioxide concentration should approximate the $Pa{CO_2}$ in arterial blood. The development of a gradient between these measurements reflects an increase in anatomic or physiologic dead space. In the latter event, low cardiac output and pulmonary embolism may both affect the measurement. Changes in end-tidal $Pa{CO_2}$ have been correlated to changes in cardiac output and may be used as a means of monitoring the efficacy of resuscitation.

INDICATIONS FOR MONITORING (CAUSES OF CRITICAL ILLNESS IN PREGNANCY)

The main causes of critical illness in pregnancy are listed in Table 80–1.

MANAGEMENT OF CRITICALLY ILL MONITORED PATIENTS

Severe Preeclampsia (See also Chapter 36)

The preeclampsia syndrome can develop into multiorgan failure (including neurologic, renal, liver, hematologic, and cardiorespiratory disease). Preeclampsia affects 2% to 6% of pregnant women and remains among the leading global causes of maternal mortality.[31–33] Eclampsia with or without evidence of intracranial hemorrhage is the single most lethal complication of preeclampsia/eclampsia. Deaths have also been associated with pulmonary edema; hemolysis, elevated liver enzymes, low platelets (HELLP) syndrome; renal failure; and the development of hypovolemia (commonly due to concurrent abruptio placentae).

The pathogenesis involves chronic placental ischemia that predisposes to an accelerated production of lipid peroxides and oxygen free radicals. Systemic endothelial injury and altered vascular reactivity develop subsequently and are assumed to be a consequence of endothelial damage. The onset of clinical disease is marked by the development of hypertension, proteinuria, and intrauterine fetal growth restriction. Impaired prostacyclin

TABLE 80–1

Main Conditions Causing Critical Illness in Pregnancy

Preeclampsia and its variants
Eclampsia*
HELLP
Thrombotic thrombocytopenic purpura
Acute fatty liver
Hemorrhage*
Sepsis*
Thromboembolism*
Cardiac problems*
Arrythmias
Cardiomyopathy
Neurologic problems*
Trauma
Metabolic
Anaphylactoid syndrome of pregnancy*
Others

*Indicates patients who may present with "collapse."
HELLP, hemolysis, elevated liver enzymes, low platelets.

production and increased release of vasoconstrictors (including thromboxane, endothelin, serotonin, and possibly catecholamines) lead to rising peripheral vascular resistance.[34–38] Endothelial damage leads to expression of cell adhesion molecules that interact with activated leukocytes and platelets.[39,40] Platelet turnover accelerates and may end in thrombocytopenia. Activated platelets also release cytokines that trigger intravascular coagulation.[39,41] Endothelial damage leads to interstitial edema, intravascular dehydration, intensified peripheral vasospasm, and diminished cardiac output. Low cardiac output translates into a critically low rate of oxygen delivery to the peripheral tissues, and multiorgan failure in severe preeclampsia can be attributed to multiorgan ischemia, developing because of vasospasm, low cardiac output, and intravascular coagulation.[28,42]

Management of Renal Failure

The presentation of renal impairment is commonly that of oliguria (a urine output of <30 mL/hr over 4 hr) with or without hematuria. Provided that the patient is not already in positive fluid balance, plasma volume expansion should be attempted. If two fluid challenges (300 mL of colloidal solution) fail to improve the urinary output, low-dose dopamine should be commenced at an infusion rate of 1 to 5 μg/kg/minute. Low-dose dopamine is thought to act as a selective renal artery vasodilator, and although of questionable benefit in general critical care, two randomized studies have demonstrated efficacy without adverse effects in the oliguric preeclamptic patient.[43,44] Patients who fail to respond to either of these measures require more intensive monitoring. Pulmonary artery catheters are a useful adjunct in securing optimal left ventricular preload and afterload. The volume-replete vasodilated patient who fails to pass urine over a 4-hour period should be considered to have intrinsic renal pathology, namely acute tubular necrosis. A single large dose of furosemide (0.5–1 g IV) may convert these patients to high-output renal failure. Should this measure also fail, care must be taken to avoid fluid overload by restricting IV fluid administration to output plus 500 mL/24 hours (to allow for insensible loss), and the patient should be prepared for dialysis.

Management of Respiratory Distress

Respiratory distress in the preeclamptic patient can be caused by or associated with

- Upper airway edema
- Pulmonary edema (patients with severe preeclampsia are predisposed to the development of pulmonary edema because of low oncotic pressure, leaky capillaries, and left ventricular dysfunction; diastolic dysfunction cannot be detected without invasive monitoring or access to echocardiography; iatrogenic fluid overload, even with small amounts of fluid, is also a frequent cause of pulmonary edema; cardiomyopathy and valvular heart disease may be indistinguishable from other causes of pulmonary edema without echocardiography or invasive monitoring)
- Aspiration pneumonia (especially if the patient has had a cesarean section under general anesthetic) (see also Chapter 38)
- Postoperative atelectasis (it also occurs in some women with the HELLP syndrome from "splinting" of the right hemidiaphragm because of liver pain) (see also Chapter 38)
- Pulmonary embolism (see following discussion and also Chapter 43)
- Adult respiratory distress syndrome (ARDS) (though not a primary complication of preeclampsia, it may follow aspiration pneumonia or prolonged ventilation) (see also Chapter 38).

Clearly patients who present with respiratory distress are a diagnostic challenge. Where the diagnosis remains in doubt after clinical examination and special investigation, echocardiography or pulmonary artery catheterization are indicated.

Pulmonary edema will need to be managed according to the hemodynamic findings. Elevated pulmonary capillary wedge pressure may result from high systemic vascular resistance, left ventricular failure, or fluid overload. These complications may require vasodilation with agents such as dihydralazine, the use of diuretics, or a combination of both. Drugs that are negatively inotropic are generally avoided. In the absence of iatrogenic fluid overload, afterload reduction by vasodilation may be the most important aspect of management.

The development of localized lung signs and purulent sputum should alert the clinician to the possibility of aspiration pneumonia. Radiographic findings vary from normal lung fields to unilateral shadowing, atelectasis, and collapse. Bronchoscopy may be necessary if aspiration of particulate matter is suspected. Treatment with broad-spectrum (including anaerobic) antibiotics and physiotherapy would be indicated.

Management of other causes of respiratory distress are covered in the relevant chapters.

Management of Resistant Hypertension (See also Chapter 36)

Hypertension that fails to respond to standard vasodilator therapy has been cited as an indication for invasive hemodynamic monitoring.[45] The purpose of this is to distinguish hypertension due to high cardiac output from that arising from elevated systemic vascular resistance. Treatment aimed at reducing a high cardiac output may seem counterintuitive, but life-threatening hypertension due to this cause should be treated with drugs such as labetalol rather than the more traditionally used calcium channel blockers and direct-acting vasodilators such as dihydralazine.

Eclampsia (See also Chapter 36)

Eclampsia is the occurrence of generalized tonic-clonic seizures in a pregnant patient with proteinuric hypertension. Most seizures occur prior to delivery, although 40% occur within 24 hours of delivery. Eclampsia may be preceded by prodromal symptoms of headaches and visual disturbances (blurred vision, photopsia, scotomata, and diplopia).[46] The blood pressure at the time of seizure activity varies from levels that are mildly elevated or even normal, although they more commonly have moderate to severe hypertension.[47] Seizure activity is, however, associated with a sharp increase in blood pressure and decreased peripheral oxygen saturation levels. This is important because severe hypertension has been linked to the risk of cerebrovascular hemorrhage.

The differential diagnosis of seizure activity in pregnancy is extensive and includes epilepsy, systemic lupus erythematosus, thrombotic thrombocytopenic purpura (TTP), amniotic fluid embolus, cerebral venous thrombosis, malaria, and cocaine intoxication.[48–50] Late postpartum eclampsia (seizures first developing between 48 hours and 4 weeks after delivery) requires neuroradiologic investigation to exclude alternative diagnoses.[51–53]

The critical care management of eclampsia is centered on the prevention of recurrent seizures, control of the airway to prevent aspiration pneumonia, control of severe hypertension, management of other organ failure, and termination of the pregnancy.

Seizure Prophylaxis

Magnesium sulfate is the drug of choice for seizure prophylaxis. Randomized evidence clearly demonstrates a significantly lower risk of recurrent seizures with magnesium sulfate than for phenytoin and benzodiazepines.[54,55] Magnesium sulfate is a weak calcium channel blocker that regulates intracellular calcium flux through the *N*-methyl-D-aspartate receptor in neuronal tissue and may inhibit ischemic neuronal damage brought about by anion flux through this receptor.[56] Parenterally administered magnesium results in systemic vasodilation and improved cardiac output as well as cerebral vasodilation distal to the middle cerebral artery. Retinal artery vasospasm has been reversed by magnesium sulfate infusion.[57–59] The myocardial effects of parenteral magnesium include slowing of the cardiac conduction times and in high doses magnesium is significantly negatively inotropic.[60] Intravenous magnesium sulfate reduces serum calcium levels possibly as a result of increased renal magnesium and calcium excretion.[61] Falling serum calcium inhibits acetylcholine release at the motor endplate, the extent of which is directly related to the level of the serum magnesium and inversely proportional to the calcium concentration. This is the origin of magnesium sulfate toxicity leading to neuromuscular blockade and respiratory arrest.[62,63] Dosage regimens vary, but the majority of women in the Collaborative Eclampsia Trial were treated with a 4-g IV loading dose followed by a constant infusion of 1 g/hour. Magnesium sulfate is excreted by the kidney, and impaired renal function may lead to toxicity, manifested as weakness, absent tendon reflexes, and respiratory arrest. Patients with undiagnosed myasthenia gravis may have their disease unmasked by magnesium sulfate, even when the drug only reaches normal therapeutic levels.[64]

Patients who experience recurrent seizures in spite of magnesium sulfate are best treated with intubation and ventilation. Sedation using continuous high-dose benzodiazepine or pentothal infusions will be necessary and will serve to prevent further seizures. Following multiple seizures, these women are likely to have cerebral edema with raised intracranial pressure. Consequently care should be taken to maintain a mean arterial pressure in excess of 100 mm Hg in order to preserve cerebral blood flow.[65]

Control of the Airway

Clearing the airway is an important first-aid measure accomplished by suctioning and positioning the patient head-down on her side. Endotracheal intubation is indicated in women with recurrent seizures, those who are inadequately oxygenated, and when the patient remains persistently obtunded more than 30 minutes after the seizure. Ventilatory care should be maintained for a minimum of 24 hours postpartum, until the patient is fully conscious, and any upper airway edema has dissipated.

Obstetric Management

Vaginal delivery, if foreseeable within a short period may be contemplated in the woman with no complicating features other than a single seizure. Induction of labor should not be protracted, and an arbitrary time limit should be set as a goal for attaining a vaginal delivery.

HELLP Syndrome (See also Chapter 36)

This complication of preeclampsia is due to hepatic ischemia, giving rise to periportal hemorrhage and necrosis along with microangiopathic hemolytic anemia and thrombocytopenia.[66] The mnemonic, HELLP stands for: **h**emolysis, **e**levated **l**iver enzymes and **l**ow **p**latelets. These patients present with epigastric pain and, in severe cases, are usually obviously ill because of associated complications including renal failure (characterized by rising urea and creatinine levels and the passage of small quantities of bloodstained or “Coke”-colored urine) and eclampsia. Many women with HELLP syndrome, however, seem to have unremarkable clinical disease.

Liver failure may arise from conditions that mimic preeclampsia, such as TTP and acute fatty liver of pregnancy.[67,68] Obstetric cholestasis and viral hepatitis may also enter the differential diagnosis in milder cases of

HELLP syndrome. Distinguishing between these conditions may be difficult, but the hallmark of preeclamptic disease is that it resolves after delivery.[69]

Subcapsular liver hematoma is a rare complication of the HELLP syndrome. The surface of the liver is covered in petechial hemorrhages that may coalesce to form one large hematoma. Rupture of this lesion leads to right upper quadrant pain and sudden hypovolemia.

Coagulopathy is uncommon, but thrombocytopenia and impaired platelet function both give rise to impaired coagulation. Prolonged partial thromboplastin times and international normalized ratios (INRs) are more likely to occur in association with acute fatty liver than HELLP syndrome. Hypoglycemia may occur in some cases, but is more characteristic of acute fatty liver of pregnancy.

The management of HELLP syndrome is delivery, whereas the associated complications (renal failure, eclampsia, and respiratory distress) may require critical care on their individual merits. Thrombocytopenia should reach a nadir within 72 hours of delivery, and if it is persistent beyond this point, a search for alternative diagnoses should commence (e.g., sepsis, folate deficiency, thrombotic thrombocytopenic purpura, systemic lupus erythematosus).

Thrombotic Thrombocytopenic Purpura

TTP is one of a spectrum of microangiopathic hemolytic conditions that include preeclampsia, hemolytic uremic syndrome (HUS), acute fatty liver of pregnancy, and autoimmune conditions such as systemic lupus erythematosus. TTP is a condition in which multimers of von Willebrand's factor, derived from the endothelium, accumulate in the circulation. Von Willebrand's factor binds platelets to the endothelium, and high concentrations are associated with peripheral platelet consumption and the formation of platelet microthrombi. Von Willebrand's factor is usually broken down by a specific metalloproteinase, but may accumulate if this enzyme is deficient or if endothelial damage provokes excessive release of von Willebrand's factor. The metalloproteinase enzyme deficiency exists either as a hereditary condition or can be acquired as a consequence of autoimmune disease due to a specific IgG inhibitor of the enzyme. Many factors can precipitate both the congenital and acquired forms of TTP, including drugs, malignancy, bacterial infection, HIV, and other viral infections. Pregnancy is the precipitating factor in 10% to 25% of cases.[70,71]

TTP presents with a clinical pentad of features:

- Microangiopathic hemolytic anemia
- Fever
- Neurologic disturbance
- Renal impairment
- Thrombocytopenia

The neurologic features of the syndrome may be transitory, and mild hypertension and proteinuria may make the condition indistinguishable from HELLP syndrome. TTP does not, however, remit after delivery, whereas HELLP syndrome invariably resolves. Other diagnostic features that may help to distinguish between the two conditions include evidence of marked hemolysis on examination of the peripheral blood smear (this is more characteristic of TTP than HELLP).

Without appropriate management TTP has a high mortality rate. Treatment consists of plasmapheresis, infusion of fresh frozen plasma, and high-dose steroids.[70] Renal failure and the neurologic manifestations may require appropriate intensive care management.

Acute Fatty Liver of Pregnancy (See also Chapter 48)

Developing in the latter half of pregnancy, acute fatty liver of pregnancy (AFLP) is a condition characterized by microvesicular fatty infiltration of the liver. The incidence is approximately 1:12,000 deliveries. Clinical disease severity varies, with some patients having only mild right upper quadrant discomfort associated with prodromal nausea and vomiting. Others develop fulminant liver failure leading to coma. A depressed level of consciousness may arise from either hypoglycemia or the onset of hepatic encephalopathy. Hypoglycemia is a common feature of AFLP and should alert the clinician to the possible diagnosis. More than 50% of affected patients will have mild hypertension and proteinuria, making the distinction from HELLP syndrome difficult. Jaundice is often present at the time of diagnosis. Liver enzymes are increased, and transaminases may rise above 1000 IU/L in severe cases. Liver failure leads to severe coagulopathy and a prolonged partial thromboplastin time and INR. DIC with microangiopathic hemolytic anemia develop together a mild neutrophil leukocytosis.[72,73]

Management principles include delivery of the fetus and treatment of the acute liver failure.[74] Coagulopathy may complicate the delivery and must be corrected beforehand. Management of liver failure also includes maintenance of the blood glucose level, the use of lactulose to limit the effects of intestinal bacteria, and administration of vitamin K to mother and baby. Intubation and ventilation may be necessary in the comatose mother who cannot protect her airway. Associated complications of renal failure and pancreatitis need to be managed individually.

Obstetric Hemorrhage

This occurs as a result of bleeding from the placental site or as a consequence of trauma to the genital tract. These issues, including medical, surgical, and critical care management of shock and coagulopathy are dealt with in Chapter 79.

Severe Sepsis

The systemic inflammatory response syndrome (SIRS) consists of markers of a systemic immune response (Table 80–2).[75] SIRS may develop from any noxious stimulus including preeclampsia and hypovolemia. When infection causes SIRS, the condition is named sepsis. Sepsis leading to multiorgan dysfunction is termed severe sepsis, and severe sepsis plus refractory hypotension is septic shock. Collectively, infection arising during pregnancy or that resulting from underlying HIV infection is by far the single largest cause of maternal mortality in developing countries. In South Africa these two entities account for 40% of the maternal deaths: double the number of the next most prevalent cause of mortality.

The sources of sepsis vary. Pelvic infection after delivery, wound sepsis, respiratory infection, and urosepsis are all common and can all lead to life-threatening illness requiring critical care.

Pelvic Sepsis

Pelvic sepsis usually results from infection with gram-negative organisms, although gram-positive organisms and fungi can be implicated. Tuberculosis can also present with abdominal sepsis. Prolonged rupture of the membranes, obstructed labor, instrumentation of the genital tract, retained products of conception, trauma, and operative delivery, together with immunosuppression all contribute to the pathogenesis of sepsis.

Recognition of pelvic sepsis is based on the presence of SIRS together with localizing signs of pelvic infection, including peritonitis, a tender subinvoluted uterus, and malodorous lochia. Coexisting organ dysfunction, such as impaired renal function, gastrointestinal signs (ileus), hyperbilirubinemia or elevated liver enzymes, DIC, ARDS, neurologic dysfunction, and cardiorespiratory disease including left ventricular failure, will define the syndrome of severe sepsis and will indicate the need for intensive care.

TABLE 80–2

The Systemic Inflammatory Response Syndrome

Any two or more of the following features:
- Temperature >38 or <36°C
- Heart rate >90 bpm
- Respiratory rate >20 breaths/min or $PaCO_2$ <32 mm Hg
  - WBC >12,000 or <4,000/mm^3 or >10% immature (band forms)

WBC, white blood cell count.

Intensive care principles are self-evident. Supportive therapy will be necessary to maintain organ function by ensuring adequate peripheral perfusion, and the source of sepsis will need to be managed by medical and surgical intervention. Supportive therapy consists of fluid replacement measured against the CVP. Women with distributive shock due to peripheral vasodilation may require large amounts of fluid and blood products. Persistent hypotension due to left ventricular failure may require inotropic support using adrenaline, dopamine, or dobutamine. Coagulopathy due to liver dysfunction and DIC will need to be corrected prior to any surgical intervention, and oxygen-carrying capacity of the blood should be optimized by packed cell transfusion in women who are anemic. Appropriate respiratory support may take the form of facemask oxygen or intubation and ventilation in cases of respiratory distress with inadequate peripheral oxygen saturation or respiratory failure.

Managing the sepsis will require broad-spectrum antibiotic cover tailored to the specific infecting organism if bacteriologic surveillance from blood cultures and pus swabs identify a specific pathogen. Surgical intervention may include evacuation of retained products of conception, drainage of pelvic abscesses, and hysterectomy. The last option is often delayed because of understandable concern about future fertility. However, the woman with multiorgan failure precipitated by sepsis who fails to respond to 24 hours of appropriate antibiotic treatment is at risk of developing septic shock that may progress rapidly and is associated with mortality rates of between 20% and 50%.[76] Under these circumstances, hysterectomy to remove the source of sepsis may be a lifesaving procedure.

Respiratory Infection

This may be community acquired (often gram-positive organisms like *Streptococcus pneumoniae*) or nosocomial (usually gram-negatives e.g., *Pseudomonas*, *Acinetobacter*, *Escherichia coli*, and others).

The clinical presentation is that of SIRS together with respiratory symptoms of dyspnea, pleuritic chest pain, cough, sputum production, and clinical signs of pulmonary crepitations or consolidation with bronchial breathing. Radiographic signs may take time to develop, but new pulmonary infiltrates should be identified if the diagnosis of pulmonary infection is correct. Sputum specimens should be routinely examined bacteriologically to identify the infecting organism. Tuberculosis should also be excluded as a diagnosis, especially in areas where there is a high prevalence of HIV infection.

Critical care management must maintain oxygenation while treating the underlying infection. Peripheral oxygen saturation levels will determine the necessary respiratory support, which may include the use of facemask oxygen, the administration of continuous positive airways pressure oxygen (CPAP) or intubation, and ventilation. Generally, respiratory infection has not been regarded as an indication for delivery of the baby, even among ventilated patients. Antibiotic therapy for community-acquired infection is usually a cephalosporin or an aminoglycoside with penicillin, whereas nosocomial infections due to gram-positive organisms will need treatment with vancomycin. A suspicion of mixed aerobic infection or anaerobic infection may lead to the use of imipenem or a combination of clindamycin/metronidazole with an aminoglycoside. Bacteriologic advice should be sought and treatment adapted to organisms identified from blood and sputum culture.

Sepsis in the Immunocompromised Patient

HIV infection predisposes the affected individual to pelvic, respiratory, and neurologic infection. Respiratory infection may be due to atypical organisms (*Mycoplasma* and *Legionella*), tuberculosis, cytomegalovirus, or the protozoan *Pneumocystis jiroveci* [formerly *carinii*] (PCP). The clinical presentation and radiographic signs may not discriminate between these different disorders, and sputum should be obtained (or bronchoscopic lavage used) to arrive at a bacteriologic diagnosis. Radiologically, PCP may present with patchy changes that progress to a diffuse pattern of bilateral pulmonary infiltrates resembling ARDS. Management consists of supportive treatment including ventilation together with high doses of trimethoprim and sulfamethoxazole (dose 20/100 mg/kg/day for 21 days) and corticosteroids. The prognosis for women with PCP who require ventilation is poor, with only one in three surviving ventilatory care that extends for more than 2 weeks.[77] Suspected atypical pneumonia requires treatment with erythromycin.

Pelvic and wound sepsis seems to occur more readily in HIV-infected women. Antibiotic prophylaxis against postoperative sepsis should be extended to 48 hours for elective surgery and for 5 days in those having emergency cesarean delivery. In managing puerperal sepsis, surgical intervention, including hysterectomy, has been practiced more aggressively than in immunocompetent women. These approaches are unsubstantiated by randomized evidence but have developed in units faced with a large burden of HIV-infected women.

Thromboembolism (See also Chapter 43)

Thromboembolism is the leading direct cause of maternal mortality in the United Kingdom. The incidence of venous thromboembolism lies between 0.5 and 1 per 1000 deliveries.[78–81] The predisposing factors giving rise to thromboembolism are pregnancy itself, underlying thrombophilia, age, and circumstantial risk factors such as surgery and immobilization. Pregnancy is a procoagulant condition because of increased hepatic synthesis of clotting factors, decreased protein S activity leading to activated protein C resistance, and inhibition of fibrinolysis by placental production of PAI-II. Underlying hereditary or acquired thrombophilias add to the risk. These conditions include deficiencies in protein C, protein S, and antithrombin. The Leiden and prothrombin gene mutations have been described more recently. Hereditary defects also exist in factor VIII and fibrinogen genes, giving rise to increased concentrations of these clotting factors. Hyperhomocysteinemia is also considered to be a thrombogenic condition, which arises either because of a dietary deficiency in cofactors such as folate, vitamin B_6, and B_{12}, or because of enzyme deficiencies. Common mutations affect the enzyme methylene tetrahydrofolate reductase, which is required to convert folate to tetrahydrofolate. The other rarer enzyme defect is linked to cystathionine β-synthase deficiency. Thrombophilia may also be acquired as part of the antiphospholipid syndrome due to the presence of the lupus anticoagulant that interferes with the protein C mechanism and also promotes platelet activation through the release of platelet-activating factor by endothelial cells. Finally, the sticky platelet syndrome may increase the risk of clot formation.

Ileofemoral vein thrombosis occurs more commonly in pregnancy; the presenting features of venous thromboembolism are those of a swollen, red, and tender leg. These signs are unreliable, and investigation is sometimes also unhelpful. Compression ultrasound is useful in identifying proximal thrombosis, but venography remains the gold standard against which other investigations are assessed. Pulmonary embolism classically presents with sudden-onset pleuritic chest pain, dyspnea, and hemoptysis. Investigations may confirm hypoxemia and right ventricular strain ($S_1Q_3T_3$ ECG pattern). Radiologic investigation may show no lesion or an elevated hemidiaphragm. Ventilation-perfusion scanning identifies mismatched areas of ventilation and perfusion that may be indicative of embolization. More recently, spiral CT is helpful in diagnosing segmental rather than subsegmental emboli.[82,83] It is notable that measurement of D-dimer concentrations during pregnancy is not a useful way of diagnosing excessive fibrinolysis associated with venous thrombosis because D-dimer levels are normally elevated in pregnancy.

Treatment of thromboembolism consists of anticoagulation to arrest clot propagation until the clot resolves followed by prophylactic doses of low-molecular-weight heparin to prevent further clot formation. The detailed description of how heparin and warfarin are used are covered in Chapter 43. In the critical care setting, unfractionated heparin is given intravenously in a dose of 20,000 units in 200 mL of saline beginning at 13 mL/hour, with the dose titrated against the aPTT to maintain values 1.5 to 2 times the control value. Other supportive therapy may be necessary to maintain oxygenation, up to and including intubation and ventilation.

Cardiac Problems

Arrhythmias (See also Chapter 37)

The patient experiencing cardiac arrest should be resuscitated according to standard protocols, including defibrillation, external cardiac massage, and ventilatory support. The pregnant uterus restricts venous return as a result of aortocaval compression, and cesarean delivery will facilitate resuscitation. If this is to be done, it should take place within 5 minutes of the arrest.

Ventilatory support, when required, should aim for slight hyperventilation to mimic pregnancy physiology in which $Pa\text{CO}_2$ falls to allow fetal excretion of carbon dioxide down a concentration gradient. Extreme hypocarbia may affect uterine blood flow adversely, and maternal $Pa\text{CO}_2$ levels must be maintained above 2 kPa. Where pressure considerations permit, tidal volumes of 10 to 15 mL/kg should be used, and the ventilator rate adjusted to achieve an appropriate $Pa\text{CO}_2$. The maximum ventilatory plateau pressure should (ideally) not exceed 35 cm H_2O.[84]

Arrhythmias occur more frequently in pregnancy and occasionally lead to hypotension. In the critical care setting, the drugs most likely to be used to treat arrhythmias are adenosine, short-acting β-blockers, and amiodarone.[85] Adenosine is used to treat supraventricular tachycardia, Wolf-Parkinson-White syndrome, and arrhythmias involving the AV node. Because it can cause bronchospasm, it should be avoided in asthmatics. Lignocaine has been used in pregnancy, but there is limited experience. Although β-adrenergic blocking agents given to the mother have been linked to fetal growth restriction, fetal hypoglycemia, and hyperbilirubinemia, short-acting drugs such as esmolol may be used during pregnancy for specific indications such as the treatment of arrhythmias. Amiodarone is a drug with a long half-life (>50 days) and has been linked to a risk of neonatal hypothyroidism. The use of amiodarone should therefore be restricted to the treatment of life-threatening arrhythmias unresponsive to other treatment.

Other Cardiac Problems

Arrhythmias were discussed in detail in the previous section but can additionally cause sudden hypotension. Acute pulmonary edema can result from peripartum cardiomyopathy or valvular heart disease, especially thrombosis of a prosthetic valve. Myocardial infarction is rare but can result in cardiogenic shock. Aortic dissection and pulmonary hypertension giving rise to acute right ventricular failure also enter the differential diagnosis. The reader is referred to Chapter 37 for detailed discussion of the management of these conditions.

Neurologic Disorders

Cerebral ischemia or hemorrhage will present with neurologic signs. There may also be a sudden onset of neurogenic pulmonary edema.[86,87] Management should be directed to protecting the airway. Urgent neuroradiologic investigation is required to exclude a surgical remedial cause, and the management of these cases must always take place in consultation with a neurologist. The reader is referred to Chapter 49 for detailed discussion of the management of these conditions.

Trauma

Motor vehicle accidents and assault are the most serious causes of trauma in pregnancy. Pregnancy does not increase the risk of maternal death due to trauma, but the fetus is at exaggerated risk of death due to maternal hypovolemia, placental abruption, and direct trauma to the uterus and fetus.[88]

Direct trauma to the abdomen can lead to placental separation and abruptio placentae, the clinical signs of which may be delayed by up to 6 hours after the event. More forceful blunt trauma has the potential to cause uterine rupture, although this is a rare occurrence among pregnant trauma victims. Other obstetric consequences of blunt trauma are those of premature rupture of the membranes and fetomaternal hemorrhage, which can lead to isoimmunization of babies whose blood groups are incompatible with those of the mother.

Penetrating injury to the abdomen and uterus may lead to direct fetal trauma. Conservative management of penetrating injuries below the level of the uterine fundus has been advocated, but in pregnancies in which the fetus is considered to be viable (usually over 28 weeks) many obstetricians would resort to laparotomy and operative delivery in the presence of a penetrating uterine injury.

Resuscitation and critical care should be based on normal trauma guidelines, although monitoring must be extended to include an assessment of the fetal condition. The reader is referred to Chapter 55 for detailed discussion of the management of these conditions.

Metabolic Problems

Hypoglycemia, hyperglycemia, hypocalcemia, and hyponatremia should always be considered in any patient who collapses acutely. Management will be based on the specific cause and diagnosis.

Anaphylactoid Syndrome of Pregnancy

This complication of labor or cesarean delivery gives rise to peripartum collapse as a result of embolization of amniotic fluid and fetal squames into the maternal circulation. The syndrome may be rapidly lethal in women who develop a true embolus of fetal squamae that obstruct the pulmonary circulation, leading to severe pulmonary hypertension and cardiac arrest. However, those who survive for longer periods develop an anaphylactoid type of response to the presence of amniotic fluid in the circulation.[50]

The clinical syndrome is diagnosed in 1 in 8000 to 1 in 80,000 pregnancies. A national registry of cases that has been opened in the United States is currently the most authoritative source of information about this condition.[50] The condition usually presents during labor but may occur at the time of cesarean delivery or immediately after birth. There are no demographic predisposing factors, and obstetric practices such as prior amniotomy and oxytocin administration do not seem to influence the risk of developing amniotic fluid embolus. The onset of the condition is abrupt, and hypotension is universally present. Most patients develop pulmonary edema with cyanosis and a profound coagulopathy, which should immediately give rise to a suspicion of the diagnosis. The single most common initial presenting symptom in antenatal patients is seizure activity, which may be confused with eclampsia. The patients who survive the initial embolus and who develop the anaphylactoid picture have markedly depressed left ventricular function. Cardiac electromechanical dissociation may develop, and there is a high risk of cardiopulmonary arrest. The prognosis is poor; in the U.S. national registry, 61% of the patients died, and only 15% survived neurologically intact.

Diagnosis must be prompt, and continuous vigorous resuscitation will be needed immediately. Intensive care is mandatory and inotropic support necessary from the beginning. Hemorrhage should be anticipated, and hypovolemia is also likely to be a problem as a result of postpartum hemorrhage or bleeding after cesarean section. Continuous transfusion with blood and coagulation factors will be necessary, and obstetric intervention in the form of oxytocic drugs and hysterectomy may be necessary to control bleeding (see also Chapters 77 and 79). Intubation and mechanical ventilation along with pulmonary artery catheterization are likely adjuncts to intensive care management.

Other Causes of Acute Collapse

Several other conditions may result in acute collapse requiring emergency intensive care. The same general principles apply to all these cases: namely secure the airway, maintain respiration and circulation, and then look for and correct the underlying cause.

Respiratory Disorders

Air embolism may develop during delivery as a result of air entering the venous system and becoming trapped in the right ventricle. Paradoxical arterial emboli can develop in any individual with a patent foramen ovale. Presenting features include acute collapse, coronary insufficiency, and cerebral artery occlusion, leading to seizures and a depressed level of consciousness. Specific management is based on the use of hyperbaric oxygen to decrease the volume of the gas.

Other Systemic Disorders

These include thyroid storm, myasthenic crisis, sickle cell crisis, anaphylaxis, and transfusion reactions. The description of these disorders is found in the relevant chapters.

CONCLUSIONS

- This chapter has given an overview rather than an exhaustive discussion of a very broad subject.
- Some would argue that many of the complications reviewed are more appropriately managed exclusively by intensivists, anesthetists, and physicians. However, the pregnant woman presents a unique challenge because of both the physiologic changes that accompany pregnancy and also the need to address the requirements of the fetus in a mother who is critically ill. Thus, obstetricians must remain involved in the care of these women if the mother and her unborn child are to receive optimal care. More importantly, there should be a thorough understanding of those conditions that commonly lead to maternal mortality.
- Substandard care of the critically ill woman arising from ignorance should not be an issue raised by confidential enquiries into maternal mortality.

SUMMARY OF MANAGEMENT OPTIONS
Critical Care of the Obstetric Patient

Management Options	Quality of Evidence	Strength of Recommendation	References
Preeclampsia-Renal Impairment			
See also Chapter 36.	–	–	–
Give two fluid challenges.	–	GPP	–
Pulmonary artery catheterization	III	B	27–29
IV dopamine	Ib	A	43,44
Single dose of furosemide in volume-replete patient who does not respond to IV dopamine		GPP	–
Dialysis if these measures do not work	–	GPP	–
Preeclampsia-Respiratory Distress			
See also Chapter 36.	–	–	–
Diagnosis is critical—management depends on cause	–	GPP	–
Pulmonary edema	–	GPP	–
Options for monitoring			
a. Noninvasive			
b. Invasive			
Diuretics			
Fluid restriction			
Ventilation in extreme			
Pulmonary aspiration/atelectasis	–	GPP	–
Antibiotics			
Physiotherapy			
See relevant chapters for specific management options with other conditions	–	–	–
Preeclampsia-Resistant Hypertension			
See also Chapter 36.	–	–	–
Invasive monitoring to distinguish high output from increased systemic vascular resistance	III	B	46
Labetalol and/or doxazocin better for high-output failure than calcium channel blockers and/or hydralazine	–	GPP	–
Eclampsia			
See also Chapters 36 and 49.	–	–	–
Consider the differential diagnosis especially with late-onset presentation.	–	GPP	–
Seizure control and prophylaxis with magnesium sulfate	Ia	A	54,55
Intubation and ventilation in the extreme	III	B	65
Control of airway	III	B	65
Deliver baby—though not necessarily by cesarean section	–	GPP	–
HELLP			
See also Chapter 36.	–	–	–
Delivery	–	GPP	–
Appropriate supportive therapy for coagulation, liver, and renal function	–	GPP	–
Consider alternative causes for low platelets if they do not start to recover within 72 hr after delivery.	–	GPP	–

SUMMARY OF MANAGEMENT OPTIONS

Critical Care of the Obstetric Patient *(Continued)*

Management Options	Quality of Evidence	Strength of Recommendation	References
TTP			
See also Chapter 42.	–	–	–
Plasmapheresis	III	B	70
FFP transfusion	III	B	70
High-dose steroids	III	B	70
Appropriate supportive therapy for renal failure and neurological features	–	GPP	–
Acute Fatty Liver			
See also Chapter 48.	–	–	–
Delivery	–	GPP	–
Treat liver failure with	IV	C	67
Maintenance of blood glucose			
Lactulose			
Vitamin K			
Intubation and ventilation in the extreme	–	GPP	–
Appropriate supportive therapy for coagulation abnormalities, renal failure, and pancreatitis	–	GPP	–
Obstetric Hemorrhage			
See Chapter 79.	–	–	–
Severe Sepsis			
Appropriate supportive therapy for organ failure (coagulation, renal failure, liver, ARDS, cardiorespiratory, neurologic)	–	GPP	–
Antibiotic therapy determined by blood culture results	–	GPP	–
Surgical options (abscess, removal of retained products, hysterectomy in the extreme)	–	GPP	–
Fluid replacement monitored with CVP	–	GPP	–
Thrombo-Embolism			
See also Chapter 43.	–	–	–
IV unfractionated heparin (maintain APTT at 1.5–2 × control)	–	GPP	–
Oxygen and ventilation according to pulse oximetry	–	GPP	–
Cardiac Arrythmias			
See also Chapter 37.	–	–	–
Standard resuscitation	IV	C	84
External cardiac massage			
Ventilation			
Defibrillation			
Drugs dependent on diagnosis/type	IV	C	86
Adenosine			
Lignocaine			
Short-acting beta-blockers			
Amiodarone			
Deliver fetus if no response to resuscitation after 5 min.	–	GPP	–

SUMMARY OF MANAGEMENT OPTIONS
Critical Care of the Obstetric Patient *(Continued)*

Management Options	Quality of Evidence	Strength of Recommendation	References
Other Cardiac Problems			
See Chapter 37.	–	–	–
Neurologic (CVA)			
See Chapter 49.	–	–	–
Trauma			
See Chapter 55.	–	–	–
Anaphylactoid Syndrome of Pregnancy			
Resuscitation	–	GPP	–
Intensive care setting and ventilatory support as indicated; invasive monitoring (including pulmonary artery catheter)	–	GPP	–
Inotropic support	–	GPP	–
Blood clotting factor support	–	GPP	–
Management if the cause is PPH—see Chapter 77.	–	GPP	–
Other Conditions			
General supportive measures	–	GPP	–
Secure airway			
Support respiration			
Support ventilation			
Find and treat underlying condition.	–	GPP	–

PTT, activated partial thromboplastin time; ARDS, acute respiratory distress syndrome; FFP, A fresh frozen plasma; IV, intravenous; PPH, postpartum hemorrhage.

REFERENCES

1. Royston E, Abouzahr C: Measuring maternal mortality. BJOG 1992;99(7):540–543.
2. de Swiet M: Maternal mortality: Confidential enquiries into maternal deaths in the United Kingdom. Am J Obstet Gynecol 2000;182(4):760–766.
3. Mabie WC, Sibai BM: Treatment in an obstetric intensive care unit. Am J Obstet Gynecol 1990;162(1):1–4.
4. Bader ME, Bader RA: Cardiovascular hemodynamics in pregnancy and labor. Clin Obstet Gynecol 1968;11(4):924–939.
5. Geelhoed GW, Vander AJ: Plasma renin activities during pregnancy and parturition. J Clin Endocrinol Metab 1968;28(3): 412–415.
6. Nolten WE, Ehrlich EN: Sodium and mineralocorticoids in normal pregnancy. Kidney Int 1980;18(2):162–172.
7. Pirani BB, Campbell DM, MacGillivray I: Plasma volume in normal first pregnancy. J Obstet Gynaecol Br Commonw 1973; 80(10):884–887.
8. Valensise H, Novelli GP, Vasapollo B, et al: Maternal cardiac systolic and diastolic function: Relationship with uteroplacental resistances. A Doppler and echocardiographic longitudinal study. Ultrasound Obstet Gynecol 2000;15(6):487–497.
9. Mesa A, Jessurun C, Hernandez A, et al: Left ventricular diastolic function in normal human pregnancy. Circulation 1999;99(4):511–517.
10. Mone SM, Sanders SP, Colan SD: Control mechanisms for physiological hypertrophy of pregnancy. Circulation 1996;94(4): 667–672.
11. Geva T, Mauer MB, Striker L, et al: Effects of physiologic load of pregnancy on left ventricular contractility and remodeling. Am Heart J 1997;133(1):53–59.
12. Robson SC, Hunter S, Boys RJ, Dunlop W: Serial changes in pulmonary haemodynamics during human pregnancy: A non-invasive study using Doppler echocardiography. Clin Sci (Lond) 1991;80(2):113–117.
13. Poppas A, Shroff SG, Korcarz CE, et al: Serial assessment of the cardiovascular system in normal pregnancy. Role of arterial compliance and pulsatile arterial load. Circulation 1997;95(10): 2407–2415.

14. Taylor DJ, Lind T: Red cell mass during and after normal pregnancy. BJOG 1979;86(5):364–370.
15. Eng M, Butler J, Bonica JJ: Respiratory function in pregnant obese women. Am J Obstet Gynecol 1975;123(3):241–245.
16. Dunlop W, Davison JM: Renal haemodynamics and tubular function in human pregnancy. Baillieres Clin Obstet Gynaecol 1987;1(4):769–787.
17. Halligan A, Bonnar J, Sheppard B, et al: Haemostatic, fibrinolytic and endothelial variables in normal pregnancies and pre-eclampsia. BJOG 1994;101(6):488–492.
18. Robson SC, Dunlop W, Boys RJ, Hunter S: Cardiac output during labour. BMJ 1987;295(6607):1169–1172.
19. Flachskampf FA, Hoffmann R, Verlande M, et al: Initial experience with a multiplane transoesophageal echo-transducer: Assessment of diagnostic potential. Eur Heart J 1992;13(9): 1201–1206.
20. Krebs W, Klues HG, Steinert S, et al: Left ventricular volume calculations using a multiplanar transoesophageal echoprobe; in vitro validation and comparison with biplane angiography. Eur Heart J 1996;17(8):1279–1288.
21. Lee LC, Black IW, Hopkins A, Walsh WF: Transoesophageal echocardiography in heart disease—old technologies, new tricks. Aust N Z J Med 1992;22(5 Suppl):527–531.
22. Borghi C, Esposti DD, Immordino V, et al: Relationship of systemic hemodynamics, left ventricular structure and function, and plasma natriuretic peptide concentrations during pregnancy complicated by preeclampsia. Am J Obstet Gynecol 2000;183(1): 140–147.
23. Singer M, Clarke J, Bennett ED: Continuous hemodynamic monitoring by esophageal Doppler. Crit Care Med 1989;17(5):447–452.
24. Penny JA, Anthony J, Shennan AH, et al: A comparison of hemodynamic data derived by pulmonary artery flotation catheter and the esophageal Doppler monitor in preeclampsia. Am J Obstet Gynecol 2000;183(3):658–661.
25. Penny JA, Shennan AH, Halligan AW, et al: Blood pressure measurement in severe pre-eclampsia. Lancet 1997;349(9064): 1518.
26. Pulmonary Artery Catheter Consensus conference: Consensus statement. Crit Care Med 1997;25(6):910–925.
27. Belfort MA, Anthony J, Buccimazza A, Davey DA: Hemodynamic changes associated with intravenous infusion of the calcium antagonist verapamil in the treatment of severe gestational proteinuric hypertension. Obstet Gynecol 1990;75(6): 970–974.
28. Belfort MA, Anthony J, Kirshon B: Respiratory function in severe gestational proteinuric hypertension: The effects of rapid volume expansion and subsequent vasodilatation with verapamil. BJOG 1991;98(10):964–972.
29. Visser W, Wallenburg HC: Central hemodynamic observations in untreated preeclamptic patients. Hypertension 1991;17(6 Pt 2):1072–1077.
30. Gilbert WM, Towner DR, Field NT, Anthony J: The safety and utility of pulmonary artery catheterization in severe preeclampsia and eclampsia. Am J Obstet Gynecol 2000;182(6):1397–1403.
31. Duley L: Maternal mortality associated with hypertensive disorders of pregnancy in Africa, Asia, Latin America and the Caribbean. BJOG 1992;99(7):547–553.
32. Hogberg U, Innala E, Sandstrom A: Maternal mortality in Sweden, 1980–1988. Obstet Gynecol 1994;84(2):240–244.
33. Geographic variation in the incidence of hypertension in pregnancy. World Health Organization International Collaborative Study of Hypertensive Disorders of Pregnancy. Am J Obstet Gynecol 1988;158(1):80–83.
34. Roberts JM, Taylor RN, Musci TJ, et al: Preeclampsia: An endothelial cell disorder. Am J Obstet Gynecol 1989;161(5): 1200–1204.
35. McCarthy AL, Woolfson RG, Raju SK, Poston L: Abnormal endothelial cell function of resistance arteries from women with preeclampsia. Am J Obstet Gynecol 1993;168(4):1323–1330.
36. Nova A, Sibai BM, Barton JR, et al: Maternal plasma level of endothelin is increased in preeclampsia. Am J Obstet Gynecol 1991;165(3):724–727.
37. Clark BA, Halvorson L, Sachs B, Epstein FH: Plasma endothelin levels in preeclampsia: Elevation and correlation with uric acid levels and renal impairment. Am J Obstet Gynecol 1992;166(3):962–968.
38. Walsh SW: Preeclampsia: An imbalance in placental prostacyclin and thromboxane production. Am J Obstet Gynecol 1985;152(3):335–340.
39. Redman CW: Platelets and the beginnings of preeclampsia. N Engl J Med 1990;323(7):478–480.
40. Lyall F, Greer IA, Boswell F, et al: The cell adhesion molecule, VCAM-1, is selectively elevated in serum in pre-eclampsia: Does this indicate the mechanism of leucocyte activation? BJOG 1994; 101(6):485–487.
41. Taylor RN, Casal DC, Jones LA, et al: Selective effects of preeclamptic sera on human endothelial cell procoagulant protein expression. Am J Obstet Gynecol 1991;165(6 Pt 1): 1705–1710.
42. Belfort MA, Anthony J, Saade GR, et al: The oxygen consumption/oxygen delivery curve in severe preeclampsia: Evidence for a fixed oxygen extraction state. Am J Obstet Gynecol 1993;169(6):1448–1455.
43. Mantel GD, Makin JD: Low dose dopamine in postpartum preeclamptic women with oliguria: A double-blind, placebo controlled, randomised trial. BJOG 1997;104(10):1180–1183.
44. Clark SL, Greenspoon JS, Aldahl D, Phelan JP: Severe preeclampsia with persistent oliguria: Management of hemodynamic subsets. Am J Obstet Gynecol 1986;154(3):490–494.
45. Wasserstrum N, Cotton DB: Hemodynamic monitoring in severe pregnancy-induced hypertension. Clin Perinatol 1986;13:781–799.
46. Duncan R, Hadley D, Bone I, et al: Blindness in eclampsia: CT and MR imaging. J Neurol Neurosurg Psychiatry 1989;52(7): 899–902.
47. Lindheimer MD: Pre-eclampsia-eclampsia 1996: Preventable? Have disputes on its treatment been resolved? Curr Opin Nephrol Hypertens 1996;5(5):452–458.
48. Hauser WA, Kurland LT: The epidemiology of epilepsy in Rochester, Minnesota, 1935 through 1967. Epilepsia 1975;16(1):1–66.
49. Towers CV, Pircon RA, Nageotte MP, et al: Cocaine intoxication presenting as preeclampsia and eclampsia. Obstet Gynecol 1993;81(4):545–547.
50. Clark SL, Hankins GD, Dudley DA, et al: Amniotic fluid embolism: Analysis of the national registry. Am J Obstet Gynecol 1995;172(4 Pt 1):1158–1167.
51. Douglas KA, Redman CW: Eclampsia in the United Kingdom. BMJ 1994;309(6966):1395–1400.
52. Lubarsky SL, Barton JR, Friedman SA, et al: Late postpartum eclampsia revisited. Obstet Gynecol 1994;83(4):502–505.
53. Tetzschner T, Felding C: Postpartum eclampsia. Impossible to eradicate? Clin Exp Obstet Gynecol 1994;21(2):74–76.
54. Coetzee EJ, Dommisse J, Anthony J: A randomised controlled trial of intravenous magnesium sulphate versus placebo in the management of women with severe pre-eclampsia. BJOG 1998;105(3):300–303.
55. Anon: Which anticonvulsant for women with eclampsia? Evidence from the Collaborative Eclampsia Trial. Lancet 1995;345(8963): 1455–1463.
56. Altura BT, Altura BM: Interactions of Mg and K on cerebral vessels—Aspects in view of stroke. Review of present status and new findings. Magnesium 1984;3(4–6):195–211.

57. Belfort MA, Saade GR, Moise KJ Jr: The effect of magnesium sulfate on maternal retinal blood flow in preeclampsia: A randomized placebo-controlled study. Am J Obstet Gynecol 1992;167(6):1548–1553.
58. Belfort MA, Moise KJ Jr: Effect of magnesium sulfate on maternal brain blood flow in preeclampsia: A randomized, placebo-controlled study. Am J Obstet Gynecol 1992;167(3):661–666.
59. Belfort MA: The effect of magnesium sulphate on blood flow velocity in the maternal retina in mild pre-eclampsia: A preliminary colour flow Doppler study. BJOG 1992;99(8):641–645.
60. Arsenian MA: Magnesium and cardiovascular disease. Prog Cardiovasc Dis 1993;35(4):271–310.
61. Cruikshank DP, Chan GM, Doerrfeld D: Alterations in vitamin D and calcium metabolism with magnesium sulfate treatment of preeclampsia. Am J Obstet Gynecol 1993;168(4): 1170–1176.
62. Ramanathan J, Sibai BM, Pillai R, Angel JJ: Neuromuscular transmission studies in preeclamptic women receiving magnesium sulfate. Am J Obstet Gynecol 1988;158(1):40–46.
63. Richards A, Stather-Dunn L, Moodley J: Cardiopulmonary arrest after the administration of magnesium sulphate. A case report. S Afr Med J 1985;67(4):145.
64. Bashuk RG, Krendel DA: Myasthenia gravis presenting as weakness after magnesium administration. Muscle Nerve 1990;13(8): 708–712.
65. Richards AM, Moodley J, Graham DI, Bullock MR: Active management of the unconscious eclamptic patient. BJOG 1986;93(6):554–562.
66. Weinstein L: Syndrome of hemolysis, elevated liver enzymes, and low platelet count: A severe consequence of hypertension in pregnancy. Am J Obstet Gynecol 1982;142(2):159–167.
67. Kaplan MM: Acute fatty liver of pregnancy. N Engl J Med 1985;313(6):367–370.
68. Atlas M, Barkai G, Menczer J, et al: Thrombotic thrombocytopenic purpura in pregnancy. BJOG 1982;89(6):476–479.
69. Chandran R, Serra-Serra V, Redman CW: Spontaneous resolution of pre-eclampsia-related thrombocytopenia. BJOG 1992;99(11):887–890.
70. Proia A, Paesano R, Torcia F, et al: Thrombotic thrombocytopenic purpura and pregnancy: A case report and a review of the literature. Ann Hematol 2002;81(4):210–214.
71. Chang JC, Kathula SK: Various clinical manifestations in patients with thrombotic microangiopathy. J Investig Med 2002;50(3):201–206.
72. Strauss AW, Bennett MJ, Rinaldo P, et al: Inherited long-chain 3-hydroxyacyl-CoA dehydrogenase deficiency and a fetal-maternal interaction cause maternal liver disease and other pregnancy complications. Semin Perinatol 1999;23(2):100–112.
73. Rahman TM, Wendon J: Severe hepatic dysfunction in pregnancy. QJM 2002;95(6):343–357.
74. Kaplan MM: Acute fatty liver of pregnancy. N Engl J Med 1985;313:367–370.
75. Afessa B, Green B, Delke I, Koch K: Systemic inflammatory response syndrome, organ failure, and outcome in critically ill obstetric patients treated in an ICU. Chest 2001;120(4): 1271–1277.
76. Vincent JL, de Carvalho FB, De Backer D: Management of septic shock. Ann Med 2002;34(7–8):606–613.
77. Ahmad H, Mehta NJ, Manikal VM, et al: Pneumocystis carinii pneumonia in pregnancy. Chest 2001;120(2):666–671.
78. Zotz RB, Gerhardt A, Scharf RE: Prediction, prevention, and treatment of venous thromboembolic disease in pregnancy. Semin Thromb Hemost 2003;29(2):143–154.
79. Bates SM: Treatment and prophylaxis of venous thromboembolism during pregnancy. Thromb Res 2002;108(2–3):97–106.
80. Soomro RM, Bucur IJ, Noorani S: Cumulative incidence of venous thromboembolism during pregnancy and puerperium: A hospital-based study. Angiology 2002;53(4):429–434.
81. Heit JA: Venous thromboembolism epidemiology: Implications for prevention and management. Semin Thromb Hemost 2002;28(Suppl 2):3–13.
82. Rocha AT, Tapson VF: Venous thromboembolism in intensive care patients. Clin Chest Med 2003;24(1):103–122.
83. Powell T, Muller NL: Imaging of acute pulmonary thromboembolism: Should spiral computed tomography replace the ventilation-perfusion scan? Clin Chest Med 2003;24(1):29–38.
84. James MFM, Anthony J: Critical care management of the pregnant patient. In Birnbach DJ, Gatt SP, Datta S (eds): Textbook of Obstetric Anesthesia. Philadelphia, Churchill Livingstone, 2000, pp 716–732.
85. Gowda RM, Khan IA, Mehta NJ, et al: Cardiac arrhythmias in pregnancy: Clinical and therapeutic considerations. Int J Cardiol 2003;88(2):129–133.
86. Deehan SC, Grant IS: Haemodynamic changes in neurogenic pulmonary oedema: Effect of dobutamine. Intensive Care Med 1996;22(7):672–676.
87. Theodore J, Robin ED: Pathogenesis of neurogenic pulmonary oedema. Lancet 1975;2(7938):749–751.
88. Drost TF, Rosemurgy AS, Sherman HF, et al: Major trauma in pregnant women: Maternal/fetal outcome. J Trauma 1990;30(5):574–578.

CHAPTER 81

Domestic Violence

Loraine Bacchus / Susan Bewley

INTRODUCTION

Over the last decade awareness of the importance of domestic violence has increased. Obstetricians, gynecologists, and midwives have a key role in identifying women who are experiencing domestic violence; documenting the abuse; and ensuring that appropriate advice, support, and interventions are offered.

"Domestic violence" is defined in this chapter as "any behavior within an intimate relationship that causes physical, psychological, or sexual harm to those in the relationship."[1] It can be physical (hitting, slapping, kicking, punching, burning, scalding, choking, hair pulling, throwing objects, and the use of weapons), psychological (verbal threats; intimidation; isolation of the woman from friends and family; constant belittling and humiliation; deprivation of sustenance such as food, money, clothing, transportation, and health care; and restricting access to information and source of support), or sexual (forced sexual contact, rape, being forced to watch or reenact pornographic material, and sexual assault with objects).

Domestic violence is rarely isolated and the abusive behavior often begins insidiously, growing more oppressive and harmful with time.[2] In most cases, violence is directed toward a woman by her male partner.[3] Women are more likely than men to sustain physical injuries, to experience repeated assaults, report fear, emotional distress, and seek medical attention as a result of the violence.[4] This chapter will deal with violence by men against female partners in pregnancy.

PREVALENCE

Surveys in the United Kingdom show that domestic violence is common, affecting one in three to four women at some point in their lives[4,5] and one in nine in the preceding year.[6] Similar rates have been reported in surveys from Canada[7] and the United States.[8] Higher reported rates of domestic violence have been found among women attending health care settings. Two U.K. studies conducted in primary health care settings reported higher lifetime rates of about 40%.[9,10] Domestic violence accounts for a significant number of homicides amongst women. In Australia, Canada, Israel, South Africa, the United States, and England and Wales, between 40% and 70% of female murder victims were killed by their husbands or partners.[1] The corresponding figure for male victims of homicide is 8%.[11] It is often assumed that the violence will end once the woman leaves her abusive partner. However, women assume a greater risk of escalating or even fatal violence when they leave or attempt to leave the relationship.[12]

In most cases of domestic abuse that are identified in pregnancy there is pre-existing violence that continues throughout the pregnancy and following the baby's birth.[13] However, in a minority the first incident of violence takes place during pregnancy.[14] The prevalence of domestic violence in pregnancy is between 2.5%[15] and 33.7%,[16] with the greatest risk occurring during the postpartum period.[17,18] Higher rates of violence during pregnancy have been found among pregnant teenagers.[19,20] Thus domestic violence is commoner than many obstetric complications such as preeclampsia.

Domestic violence was the cause of death in 14 cases in the two most recent Confidential Enquiries into Maternal Deaths in the UK (CEMD).[21,22] In the 1997–1999 enquiry, of the 378 reported deaths, 45 (12%) women had voluntarily disclosed domestic violence to a health professional during their pregnancy. This figure could be an underestimate of the problem since women rarely volunteer information about abuse experiences.[22]

RECOGNITION

Significant associations with domestic violence include:

Demographic and Psychosocial Factors

- Young women who are single, separated, or divorced and have children living at home[5,23]
- Women who have a history of childhood physical or sexual abuse are at increased risk of experiencing violence within their adult relationships.[24]
- Psychiatric illness (depression, suicide, self-harming, post traumatic stress disorder, anxiety, and phobic symptoms.[25-28] The development of a psychological disorder resulting from domestic violence is positively correlated to the frequency and severity of the violence.[29,30]
- Higher prescription rates for tranquillizers, antidepressants, and pain medication and higher admissions rates for psychiatric illness.[31,32]
- Alcohol and substance misuse is associated with both the experience and perpetration of domestic violence.[17,23,33,34] These factors can have a significant influence on the power dynamics of an abusive relationship and isolate the woman from potential sources of support.

Behavioral Factors

- Unwanted pregnancy, sexually transmitted infections, and rapid repeat pregnancy (within 24 months)[35-38]
- Increased parity and younger age at first pregnancy[15,23,39]

Contact with Health Services

- Increased access to emergency and nonemergency health services, requiring treatment for injuries and symptoms resulting from the violence.[40-42] In most cases enquiry about domestic violence is not made.
- Late initiation of antenatal care[15,43]
- Frequent clinic or hospital visits with vague complaints or symptoms.[15]

Interactions with Partner Indicative of a Controlling Relationship

- Partner may accompany the woman to all her antenatal appointments, answer questions directed at her, or appear reluctant to leave the room.
- The woman may present as nervous, avoid eye contact with the health professional, or be afraid to speak openly in front of her partner.
- Noncompliance with treatment regimens, lack of independent transportation or access to finances, and difficulties in communicating by telephone[44]
- Failure to attend clinics with visible injuries
- Where domiciliary care is available, difficulties in gaining access can be experienced by health professionals.[45-47]

Clinical Presentations

- See Table 81–1 for the common presentations.[48,49]
- Delay in seeking treatment for injuries
- Woman's explanation for how an injury occurred seems implausible.
- Forced sex that can lead to infection of perineal sutures and delay the healing process[50]
- Difficulties having pelvic examinations in prenatally or during labor, with the woman becoming distressed, withdrawn, or even hostile.[39] This may be significant when a woman requests a female health professional for such examinations.

Although the presence of these risk factors and indicators may raise a health professional's index of suspicion, no single factor will accurately identify which women are likely to be affected by domestic violence. Abused women

TABLE 81–1

Physical Signs and Injuries Associated with Domestic Violence

Head, neck, or facial injuries	Multiple bruises or lacerations in various stages of healing
Back, chest, or abdominal pain or tenderness	Patterned injuries that show the imprint of the object used
Injuries to the breasts, abdomen, or genitals	Burns from cigarettes, appliances, rope, or friction
Vaginal bleeding, sexually transmitted, infections	Scalding from boiling water
Dizziness, black outs	Strangulation marks
Numbness	Fractures
Injuries to the extremities	Broken bones
Delay in seeking treatment	Knife wounds
Premature removal of and infection of perineal sutures	Dental injuries (e.g., broken or lost teeth)
Distress, aggression, or withdrawn behavior during pelvic examinations, labor, and delivery	Hair loss consistent with hair pulling
Partial loss of hearing or vision	Bite marks or scratches

may present with a range of these symptoms and behaviors or none at all.

RISKS

Maternal Risks

Women who experience domestic violence have significantly poorer health outcomes than nonabused women including

- Chronic pain[51,52] (e.g., headaches, backaches, pelvic pain), hearing or vision problems,[53] sleep disturbance, poor appetite,[54] and gastrointestinal disorders such as irritable bowel syndrome.[55] These effects may be caused directly by recurrent physical or sexual injury or indirectly from underlying stress.[56]
- Gynecologic problems (e.g., urinary tract infections, pelvic inflammatory disease, vaginal bleeding, menstrual irregularities, genital irritation, and pain during intercourse.[57,58] Possible mechanisms include stress and depression, which can affect the immune system, and infection from forced and unprotected sex.[58]
- Psychosocial stress (e.g., stressful life events, financial problems, feeling unhappy about the pregnancy; perceiving her partner or family to be unhappy about the pregnancy; lack of partner or family support, and housing problems)[23,33,59,60]
- Depression,[60] especially in the postpartum period when domestic violence may get worse[17,18,61]

Fetal and Neonatal Risks

These include

- Low-birth-weight babies[62,63]
- Trauma to the abdomen may result in separation of the placenta, premature rupture of membranes, premature labor, miscarriage, and fetal death.[64–66]
- Bruising, fractures, hemorrhaging, and deformity.[67]

MANAGEMENT OPTIONS

General

Women suffering domestic violence are more likely to seek help from health care personnel than from any other statutory organization. However, qualitative studies have reported unhelpful and ineffective responses from health professionals, including a tendency to prescribe antidepressants; not enquiring directly about domestic violence; and failing to offer information about sources of support, document the abuse, and offer follow-up planning.[42,68,69] In recognition of the serious health implications of domestic violence, in the United Kingdom the Royal College of Midwives[44] and the Royal College of Obstetricians and Gynaecologists[70] have published guidelines for the identification and support of women affected by domestic violence. The Department of Health[71] has also produced a domestic violence manual for health care professionals. Similarly, guidelines for health practitioners have been developed in North America.[45,72]

Five key stages to the clinical management of domestic violence are applicable to any stage of the pregnancy and postpartum period:[44]

- Awareness and recognition of domestic violence
- Provision of a safe and quiet environment
- Identification and aiding disclosure
- Documenting the abuse
- Safety assessment, information giving, and ongoing support

Stage 1: Awareness and Recognition of Domestic Violence

All health professionals providing care for pregnant women should be aware of the potential indicators (see earlier discussion) of domestic violence and the maternal and fetal risks. Women may present with a range of physical and emotional indicators or none at all. Although these indicators may increase the index of suspicion, if abuse is suspected, enquiry about domestic violence should be made using stages 2 and 3. Health professionals should also be aware of their personal feelings about the subject and that they too can be affected by domestic violence, either as victims or perpetrators. However, their duty of care and professionalism requires them to provide an informed and nonjudgmental response to women. To this end, maternity services should work toward the development of guidelines and good practice protocols for identifying and supporting women experiencing domestic violence.

Stage 2: Provision of a Safe and Quiet Environment

The woman should be provided with a safe and quiet environment before any enquiry about domestic violence takes place. If a partner, friend, or family member has accompanied the woman, an excuse should be sought to see her alone without raising suspicion.[71] Strategies for creating private consulting time may include: requesting to see the woman alone as a routine procedure, asking the partner to wait outside at the end of the appointment to conduct a physical examination, or taking the woman to another part of the clinic for a urine sample, blood test, or weight check. Issues of safety and confidentiality should be paramount when working with women experiencing domestic violence. Children as young as 2 years may report back to the partner or family members that abuse was discussed. The woman should be reassured that any information she provides will not be shared with her partner, family members, or friends. However, the woman must be advised about the limitations of confidentiality. If the woman does not feel safe discussing the violence in depth with her partner waiting nearby, it may be preferable to make another appointment at a time when the partner is unable to attend. Health professionals working in the community could offer to meet women at the clinic or at the home of a trusted friend or family member. If a woman has hearing difficulties or her first language is not English, arrange for a professional interpreter, preferably female, to be present. Family or friends should never be asked to translate when discussing domestic violence. Health professionals may be confronted with an angry or threatening partner who refuses to leave the room, which may be indicative of a problem within the relationship and makes it difficult to assess for partner violence. Therefore, it is best to offer a confidential time to all women at some point during pregnancy so that it becomes easier with practice. Health professionals have the right to protect themselves and withdraw from any situation where they feel their personal safety is at risk, but must also think sympathetically about the women and children who are also at risk.

Occasionally, a health professional may become aware that a child or other vulnerable person living with the abused woman is also at risk of harm. Child protection procedures should be followed. The other exceptional circumstance in which confidentiality may be breached is when the health professional becomes aware that a victim of domestic violence is at risk of serious harm or death from a violent partner. Any referrals to social services should be discussed with the mother and her consent and cooperation sought.[70,73] Much more is likely to be achieved by working openly with the woman and reassuring her that social services are able to support her in protecting herself and her children. Any information disclosed to a third party without consent should be the minimum necessary to secure the best interests of the woman and her children.[71]

Stage 3: Identification and Aiding Disclosure

Studies conducted in a range of health care settings have shown that the use of direct questions about domestic violence, asked routinely of all patients, increases the rate of detection.[74,75] Evidence shows that the majority of women find routine enquiry for domestic violence during health care appointments acceptable.[9,10]

A woman's willingness to discuss the abuse will partly depend on the approach of the health professional, and disclosure is more likely if a sensitive and nonjudgmental manner is adopted.[76,77] Important principles are to listen and offer validation of the woman's experiences, to acknowledge the seriousness of the situation, to emphasize that domestic violence is very common, that she is not to blame for the violence, and that she does not have to deal with it by herself. An expression of shock or disbelief could dissuade the woman from telling you more, so acknowledge her courage for being able to discuss it. These skills of providing an empathic response are similar to those used in cases of bereavement, for example.

It is recommended that the health professional begin by asking a few open-ended questions before following up with specific questions about abuse. For example:

"How are things at home?"
"Are you getting the support you need?"
"Is there anything you are unhappy about?"

This will help to establish some degree of rapport with the woman.[44,70] Women often talk around the issue of domestic violence, for example, referring to feeling stressed, overwhelmed, not coping, financial worries, or housing problems. When asking directly about domestic violence, the question should be framed in a way that conveys you recognize domestic violence is an important health issue and difficult to talk about. For example:

"Many of the women I see are experiencing some form of emotional or physical abuse from their partner, but find it difficult to bring the subject up themselves. That is why I've started to ask about it routinely."

This can be followed up with one or more direct questions that are appropriate to the situation. For example:

"Do you ever feel afraid of your partner?"

"Do you and your partner argue or fight? Do the arguments get physical?"

"I've noticed a number of bruises/cuts/scratches; has someone at home hurt you?"

"Some women tell me that their partners are cruel, sometimes emotionally and sometimes physically hurting them—is this happening to you?"

"Does your partner ever treat you badly such as shout at you, constantly call you names, push you around, or threaten you?"

If a woman makes a disclosure of abuse, stages 4 and 5 should be followed. If a woman tells you that she has not been abused, it is important to accept her response even if you suspect otherwise as this conveys respect. However, it is important to allow the opportunity for future disclosure, by reminding her that she can talk to you about any concerns or problems at home at any time. It has been demonstrated that repeated enquiry about domestic violence increases the detection rate and it can facilitate detection of violence that begins later in pregnancy.[78]

A study from the United States tested the effectiveness of routine questioning for domestic violence in maternity settings, followed by various interventions such as referral to community resources, a counseling intervention, and counseling plus regular support from an outreach advocacy worker. This has proven to be effective in helping women to initiate seeking help and adopt safety behaviors. It has also reduced the severity of the violence over time.[79–81] A randomized controlled trial of a community-based advocacy intervention for women entering a refuge to escape from domestic violence found that 2 years later, 1 in 4 of the intervention group did not experience further violence compared with 1 in 10 of the control group. Women who received the intervention reported a higher quality of life, increased effectiveness in obtaining their goals, and improved ability to access community resources.[82] A qualitative study of women's experiences of routine questioning during pregnancy demonstrated that simply asking about domestic violence is an important intervention in itself, by reducing the stigma attached to it, creating an environment that encourages disclosure of abuse, and directing women to sources of help.[76] Health professionals have a key role in providing women with information about services and options available to them, assessing current and future risk, and documenting the abuse. Maternity services can raise public awareness of domestic violence as an important health issue and convey the message that violence of any kind is unacceptable. Posters and leaflets about domestic violence and support services should be placed in clinic waiting rooms and areas where women will be able to access the information safely (e.g., the toilets, baby-changing rooms). These should be available in a range of languages that reflect the local community.

Stage 4: Documenting the Abuse

The medical records of treatment for any injuries or symptoms resulting from the violence are important documents. Women experiencing domestic violence are often required to provide evidence of the abuse when seeking help from agencies (e.g., housing, divorce proceedings, obtaining injunctions), and medical evidence can be important to support her statement. Documentation is also important to ensuring the flow of information to other health professionals involved in the woman's care, which will facilitate ongoing support and monitoring. Inform the woman of the benefits of documentation, even if she does not wish to take immediate action.[44,70] To maintain the woman's safety and confidentiality, domestic violence should never be recorded in places accessible to her partner (e.g., in hand-held maternity records) but in a separate record that is kept in the clinic or hospital.[71] Clear and accurate notes are important, including:

- Date and time that the abuse took place
- Where the incident occurred
- Name and relationship of the perpetrator to the woman
- Any new or old injuries sustained including psychological symptoms, information, advice or treatment offered, and whether the woman accepted this
- A body map picture can be used to indicate the location of any injuries sustained.[83]

Injuries consistent with domestic violence that are explained implausibly should also be documented in the confidential records. Records should be signed and dated. The woman's permission to share the information with other relevant health professionals must be obtained, emphasizing that information will only be shared on a "need to know" basis.

Stage 5: Safety Assessment, Information Giving, and Ongoing Support

The immediate safety of the mother and her children should be assessed by asking whether it is safe for her to return home. Inform the woman of her options and of the specialist domestic violence services in and out of her area that can provide emergency help and long-term support.[71] Provide written information about domestic violence organizations and other support services, after confirming that it is safe for her to take the information away with her. Discreet credit-sized cards may be preferable. The woman may prefer to use a telephone in a private room to contact the agencies herself, if she cannot do this at home. It is always best to encourage the woman to talk to the agencies herself so that she is in control of her sources of help and gains confidence in explaining her situation and asking for help. Health professionals can best facilitate the woman's exploration of her options by maintaining a supportive position, but avoiding personal and emotional investment in the choices she makes. Within the context of an abusive relationship, the woman's position is generally one of powerlessness.[28] By exerting medical power and seeking to control events, the health professional may increase the woman's sense of isolation and entrapment. Although it may be frustrating for the health professional when a woman does not act on advice offered, it is important to be aware of the dangers of coercing her into taking action that she is uncomfortable with. Domestic violence tends to escalate in frequency and severity when the woman attempts to leave or has left the abusive relationship, and many women are at increased risk of being murdered by their partners. Each week in the United Kingdom, two women are killed by former or current partners.[84]

Women require time to assess the risks and benefits of pursuing different options available to them. A variety of emotional and situational factors make leaving an abusive relationship difficult, and women often return to their partners several times before terminating the relationship. Isolation from friends and family, lack of self-esteem, guilt, and self-blame are just some of the reasons that women may find it difficult to confide in health professionals and other individuals for assistance. Even when women do attempt to leave, they are often forced to return to their partners because of the difficulties they encounter in trying to remain hidden.[28] For example, inappropriate accommodation, financial hardship, lack of support, loss of social networks, unemployment, loneliness, and living in constant fear of retaliation by the abuser. Other factors that may undermine the woman's capacity to initiate change or increase her dependence on her partner include alcohol and substance misuse, mental health needs, pregnancy, having dependent children, and cultural or religious values that emphasize family and marriage over the woman's well-being.[28]

When providing information about services, health professionals should be mindful of the needs of women who may have additional issues (e.g., women with disabilities or mental health needs, black women and women from ethnic minority, asylum seekers, refugees, travelers, and lesbians). All organizations should ensure that the service they provide is accessible and competent to handle language needs and cultural sensitivity when working with women who face additional problems.

It is suggested that each woman is provided with a mutually agreed basic safety plan that can be modified over time.[71] This may include the following:

- Making a list of important phone numbers, including emergency numbers that can be called at any time of the day or night (e.g., social services, housing, the police, refuges)
- Identifying a trusted friend or family member that the woman can stay with in an emergency
- Leaving a bag packed with clothes, medicines, other essential items with a trusted friend or family member
- Having money for bus, train, cab fares
- Getting an extra set of house and car keys
- Taking original copies or photocopies of any important legal and financial papers (e.g., passport, birth and marriage certificate, bank book, rent book, credit cards)

If the woman agrees to being referred to a specialized domestic violence service, the health professional can offer to speak to someone from the organization to make an introduction, give basic details of the situation, and identify any needs. It is good practice to ensure that, wherever possible, the woman is given the option of seeing the same health professional at subsequent appointments.[71] Reconciliation work with the couple should not be attempted, as this may jeopardize the safety of both the woman and the health professional.

Domestic violence cannot be approached or managed within the traditional medical model. One public health parallel may be smoking; clinicians ask about it routinely and give advice. Even though some women will act on the advice, others may continue to smoke, though over time when the circumstances are right, many will stop. Early identification of domestic violence and support may result in improved outcomes for the mother and her baby in the long term. A woman may not take up referral options immediately, but keep the information and call for help in the future. Therefore, the quality of the health professional's response will influence future help-seeking attempts by the woman. Domestic violence is a complex issue, and health professionals should not work in isolation since many local and national initiatives offer expertise on the subject, and no single agency or professional will meet the varied needs of women and children affected by domestic violence. All statutory and voluntary organizations have a responsibility to work together to provide a high-quality, coordinated response. This requires the individuals within these organizations to have a better understanding of one another and an appreciation of the services they provide. Having a lead practitioner on domestic violence can facilitate and maintain the process of change in health professionals' attitudes and practice. Health professionals should equip themselves with the skills and knowledge necessary to provide an informed response to women affected by violence by requesting and accessing opportunities for training and education.

Finally, health professionals working with abused women should take their concerns about domestic violence to their clinical supervisor, named child protection nurse, and peers for support and supervision, while being mindful of the boundaries of confidentiality. Given the frequency of domestic violence, it is important to recognize that health professionals may themselves have experienced domestic violence, which can affect their ability to work supportively with women.[85] In these circumstances, confidential support and advice may be sought from occupational counseling services, a supervisor, or specialist domestic violence services in the community.

CONCLUSIONS

- Domestic violence is common, affecting one in three women at some point in their lives and may begin during pregnancy or escalate in frequency and severity.
- Domestic violence is an important public health issue that has serious consequences for women's physical and mental well-being. During pregnancy, there are risks to the fetus.
- No woman is immune, but those most at risk are young women, who are single, separated or divorced, and have children living at home. Other risk factors include a history of childhood sexual abuse, depression, suicide attempts, and substance misuse. Not all abused women present in the same way.
- Asking direct questions routinely about domestic violence in health settings increases the detection rate.

CONCLUSIONS (*Continued*)

- The woman should be provided with a private environment, and direct questions about domestic violence should be asked in a sensitive and nonjudgmental manner. Any disclosure of abuse should be followed up with an assessment of the immediate safety of the woman and any children, referral to the appropriate community resources, and clear documentation of the abuse and information offered in the confidential medical record. Ongoing monitoring and support should be provided at follow-up appointments.
- Referral to community resources may result in a reduction in the violence and increased use of community resources. Working in partnership with other health professionals and community organizations will result in a coordinated response to women and children affected by domestic violence.
- Health professionals must accept the limitations of their intervention and should not expect immediate results.

SUMMARY OF MANAGEMENT OPTIONS
Domestic Violence

Management Options (any stage of pregnancy or the postpartum)	Quality of Evidence	Strength of Recommendation	References
Stage 1: Awareness and Recognition			
Increase awareness and recognition of domestic violence and its health effects through training and education.*	IV	C	70,71
Develop guidelines for identifying and supporting women affected by domestic violence, in conjunction with other health professionals and community groups.	IV	C	70
Stage 2: Provision of Safe Environment			
Provide the woman with a safe and private environment away from partners, family, or friends.	IV	C	70,71
Stage 3: Identification and Aiding Disclosure			
When language translation is required, professional interpreters, preferably female, should be arranged.	IV	C	70,71
Ask direct questions about domestic violence, routinely.	IV	C	79,89,90
Adopt a supportive and nonjudgmental response.	III	B	70,71
Stage 4: Documenting the Abuse			
Document the abuse and any interventions offered in the confidential maternity record.	IV	C	70,71,73
Stage 5: Safety Assessment, Information Giving, and Ongoing Support			
Offer referral information about local and national organizations that provide immediate and long-term support to women and children affected by domestic violence.†	IV	C	79–81,89
Assess the immediate safety of the woman and any children.	III	B	71,73
Provide ongoing support and monitoring at subsequent appointments, ensuring continuity of care wherever possible.	IV	C	71
Display and disseminate information about local and national domestic violence organizations and other helpful agencies so that it is accessible to users and providers of maternity services.	IV	C	70,71,73
Work in partnership with local multiagency domestic violence initiatives.	IV	C	70,71,91

*Good evidence from qualitative work about the effectiveness of education and training, in increasing health professionals' knowledge and confidence in supporting abused women.[85–88]

†Little experimental work on interventions, but one randomized controlled trial showing a reduction in violence, decreased difficulty in obtaining community resources and a higher quality of life at 2 years in the intervention group compared with the control group.[82] Good evidence from qualitative work on referral systems, support, and advocacy to services outside the health sector.[92,93]

REFERENCES

1. Krug EG, Dahlberg DL, Mercey JA, et al: World Report on Violence and Health. Geneva, World Health Organisation, 2002, pp 89–121.
2. Fishwick NJ: 1998 Assessment of women for partner abuse. J Obstet Gynecol Neonatal Nurs 1998;27:661–670.
3. Kershaw C, Budd T, Kinshott G, et al: The 2000 British Crime Survey. England and Wales. Home Office Statistical Bulletin 18/00. London, Home Office, 2000, p 36.
4. Mirlees-Black C: Domestic violence: Findings from a new British Crime Survey self-completion questionnaire. Research Study 191. Home Office, London, 1999, p 22.
5. Mooney J: The Hidden Figure: Domestic Violence in North London. Islington Council, London, 1993, p 29.
6. Stanko EA, Crisp D, Hale C, Lucraft H: Counting the Costs: Estimating the Impact of Domestic Violence in the London Borough of Hackney. Crime Concern, Wiltshire, 1998, p 21.
7. Johnson H, Sacco VF: Researching violence against women: Statistics Canada's national survey. Can J Criminol 1995;37: 281–304.
8. McFarlane J, Christoffel K, Bateman L, et al: Assessing for abuse: Self-report versus nurse interview. Public Health Nurse 1991;8:245–250.
9. Bradley F, Smith M, Long J, O'Dowd T: Reported frequency of domestic violence: Cross sectional survey of women attending general practice. BMJ 2002;324:271–274.
10. Richardson J, Coid J, Petruckevitch A, et al: Identifying domestic violence: Cross sectional study in primary care. BMJ 2002;324:274–277.
11. Home Office Research and Statistics Directorate. Criminal Statistics England and Wales 1995. Stationary Office, London, 1996, p 70.
12. Kurz D: Separation, divorce and woman abuse. Violence Against Women 1996;2:63–81.
13. Campbell JC, Oliver C, Bullock L: Why battering during pregnancy? AWHONNS Clin Issues Perinat Womens Health Nurs 1993;4:343–349.
14. Helton A, McFarlane J, Anderson ET: Battered and pregnant: A prevalence study. Am J Pub Health 1987;77:1337–1339.
15. Mezey G, Bacchus L, Bewley S, Haworth A: An exploration of the prevalence, nature and effects of domestic violence in pregnancy. Economic and Social Research Council, Violence Research Programme, 2001. Available at: http://www1.rhul.ac.uk/sociopolitical-science/VRP/Findings/Findings.htm
16. Huth-Bocks AC, Levendosky AA, Bogat GA: The effects of domestic violence during pregnancy on maternal and infant health. Violence Vict 2002;17:169–185.
17. Gielen A, O'Campo PJ, Faden RR, et al: Interpersonal conflict and physical violence during the childbearing year. Soc Sci Med 1994;39:781–787.
18. Hedin-Widding L: Postpartum, also a risk period for domestic violence. Eur J Obstet Gynecol 2000;89:41–45.
19. Curry MA, Perrin N, Wall E: Effects of abuse on maternal complications and birth weight in adult and adolescent women. Obstet Gynecol 1998;92:530–534.
20. Gazmararian JA, Lazorick A, Spitz AM, et al: Prevalence of violence against pregnant women. JAMA 1996;275:1915–1920.
21. Department of Health: Why Mothers Die. Report on Confidential Enquiries into Maternal Deaths in the United Kingdom 1994–1996. Department of Health, London, 1998.
22. National Institute for Clinical Excellence, Scottish Executive Health Department, Department of Health, Social Service and Public Safety Northern Ireland: Why Mothers Die 1997–1999. The Confidential Enquiries into Maternal Deaths in the United Kingdom. RCOG Press, London, 2001.
23. Cokkinides VE, Coker AL: Experiencing physical violence during pregnancy: Prevalence and correlates. Fam Community Health 1998;20:19–37.
24. Coid J, Petruckevitch A, Feder G, et al: Relation between childhood sexual and physical abuse and risk of revictimisation in women: A cross-sectional survey. Lancet 2001;358:450–454.
25. Gleason WJ: Mental disorders in battered women: An empirical study. Violence Vict 1993;8:53–68.
26. Scott-Gliba E, Minnie C, Mezey G: The psychological, behavioural and emotional impact of surviving an abusive relationship. J Forensic Psychiatry 1995;6:343–358.
27. Stark E, Flitcraft A: Killing the beast within: Woman battering and female suicidality. Int J Health Serv 1995;25:43–64.
28. Royal College of Psychiatrists. Domestic Violence. Council Report CR102. RCP, London, 2002, p 11.
29. Mullen RE, Romans-Clarkson SE, Walton VA, Herbison GP: Impact of sexual and physical abuse on women's mental health. Lancet 1988;1:841–845.
30. Kemp A, Rawlings EL, Green BL: Post-traumatic stress disorder (PTSD) in battered women: A shelter sample. J Trauma Stress 1991;4:137–148.
31. Stark E, Flitcraft A, Frazier W: Medicine and patriarchal violence: The social construction of a "private" event. Int J Health Serv 1979;9:461–493.
32. Webster J, Chandler J, Battistutta D: Pregnancy outcomes and health care use: Effects of abuse. Am J Obstet Gynecol 1996;174:760–767.
33. Campbell JC, Poland ML, Waller JB, Ager J: Correlates of battering during pregnancy. Res Nurs Health 1992;15:219–226.
34. Martin SL, English KT, Clark KA, et al: Violence and substance use among North Carolina pregnant women. Am J Pub Health 1996;86:991–998.
35. Gazmararian JA, Adams MM, Saltzman LE, et al: The relationship between pregnancy intendedness and physical violence in mothers of newborns. Obstet Gynecol 1995;85:1031–1038.
36. El-Bassel N, Gilbert L, Krishnan S, et al: Partner violence and sexual HIV-risk behaviours among women in an inner-city emergency department. Violence Vict 1998;13:377–393.
37. Martin SL, Kilgallen B, Tsui AO, et al: Sexual behaviours and reproductive outcomes. Associations with wife abuse in India. JAMA 1999;282:1967–1972.
38. Jacoby M, Gorenflo D, Black E, et al: Rapid repeat pregnancy and experiences of interpersonal violence among low-income adolescents. Am J Prevent Med 1999;16:318–321.
39. Hillard PJ: Physical abuse in pregnancy. Obstet Gynecol 1985;66:185–190.
40. Kernic MA, Wolf ME, Holt VL: Rates and relative risk of hospital admission among women in violent intimate partner relationships. Am J Pub Health 2000;9:1416–1420.
41. Roberts GL, Lawrence JM, O'Toole BI, Raphael B: Domestic violence in the emergency department: I Two case-control studies of victims. Gen Hosp Psychiatry 1997;19:5–11.
42. Dobash RE, Dobash RP, Cavanagh K: The contact between battered women and social and medical agencies. In Pahl J (ed): Private Violence and Public Policy. The Needs of Battered Women and the Response of the Public Services. Routledge and Kegan, London, 1985.
43. Taggart L, Mattson S: Delay in prenatal care as a result of battering in pregnancy: Cross-cultural implications. Health Care Women Int 1995;17:25–34.
44. Royal College of Midwives: Domestic Abuse in Pregnancy: A Position Paper. RCM, London, 1997.
45. American Medical Association: Diagnostic and treatment guidelines on domestic violence. Arch Fam Med 1992;1:39–47.

46. McCoy M: Domestic violence: Clues to victimisation. Ann Emerg Med 1996;27:764–765.
47. Orloff LE: Effective advocacy for domestic violence victims. Role of the nurse-midwife. J Nurse Midwifery 1996;41:473–494.
48. Royal College of Nursing: Domestic Violence. Guidance for Nurses. RCN, London, 2000.
49. Crowley P: Sensitive vaginal examination. In Bewley S, Friend J, Mezey G (eds): Violence Against Women. Royal College of Obstetricians and Gynaecologists Press, London, 1997, pp 262–279.
50. Bohn DK, Parker B: Domestic violence and pregnancy. Health effects and implications for nursing practice. In Campbell JC, Humphreys J (eds): Nursing Care of Survivors of Family Violence. Mosby, London, 1987.
51. Lent B, Morris P, Rechner S: Understanding the effect of domestic violence on pregnancy, labour, and delivery. Can Fam Physician 2000;46:505–507.
52. Walling MK, Reiter RC, O'Hara MW, et al: Abuse history and chronic pain in women: I. Prevalences of sexual abuse and physical abuse. Obstet Gynecol 1994;84:193–199.
53. Ratner PA: Indicators of exposure to wife abuse. Can J Nurs Res 1995;27:31–46.
54. Eby K, Campbell J, Sullivan C, Davidson WS: Health effects of experiences of sexual violence for women with abusive partners. Health Care Women Int 1995;16:563–576.
55. Sutherland C, Bybee D, Sullivan C: The long-term effects of battering on women's health. Women's Health 1998;4:41–70.
56. Drossman DA, Talley NJ, Leserman J, et al: Sexual and physical abuse and gastrointestinal illness. Review and recommendations. Ann Intern Med 1995;123:782–794.
57. Schei B, Bakketeig LS: Gynaecological impact of sexual and physical abuse by spouse. A study of a random sample of Norwegian women. BJOG 1989;94:1379–1383.
58. Campbell JC: Health consequences of intimate partner violence. Lancet 2002;359:1331–1336.
59. Dye TD, Tollivert NJ, Lee RV, Kenney CJ: Violence, pregnancy and birth outcome in Appalachia. Paediatr Perinat Epidemiol 1995;9:35–47.
60. Nayak MB, Al-Yattama M: Assault victim history as a factor in depression during pregnancy. Obstet Gynecol 1999;94:204–208.
61. Stewart DE: Incidence of postpartum abuse in women with a history of abuse during pregnancy. CMAJ 1994;151:1601–1604.
62. Fernandez FM, Krueger PM: Domestic violence: Effect on pregnancy outcome. J Am Osteopath Assoc 1999;99:254–256.
63. Valdez-Santiago R, Sanin-Aguirre LH: Domestic violence during pregnancy and its relation to birth weight. Salud Publica Mex 1996;38:352–362.
64. Jejeebhoy SJ: Associations between wife-beating and fetal and infant death: Impressions from a survey in rural India. Stud Fam Plan 1998;29:300–308.
65. Pak LL, Reece EA, Chan L: Is adverse pregnancy outcome predictable after blunt abdominal trauma? Am J Gynaecol Obstet 1998;179:1140–1144.
66. Shumway J, O'Campo P, Gielen A, et al: Preterm labour, placental abruption and premature rupture of membranes in relation to maternal violence or verbal abuse. J Matern Fetal Med 1999;8:76–80.
67. Robinson J: The battered fetus. Br J Midwifery 1996;4:496–498.
68. Pahl J: The general practitioner and the problems of battered women. J Med Ethics 1979;5:117–123.
69. Kurz D: Interventions with battered women in health care settings. Violence Vict 1990;5:243–256.
70. Bewley S, Friend J, Mezey G (eds): Violence Against Women. Royal College of Obstetricians and Gynaecologists Press, London, 1997.
71. Department of Health: Domestic Violence: A Resource Manual for Health Care Professionals. DOH, London, 2000.
72. American College of Obstetricians and Gynecologists: ACOG Technical Bulletin 209. Domestic Violence. ACOG, Washington DC, 1995.
73. British Medical Association: Domestic Violence: A Health Care Issue? London, British Medical Association Science. Department and the Board of Science and Education, London, 1998, pp 51–52.
74. Norton LB, Peipert JF, Zierler S, et al: Battering in pregnancy: An assessment of two screening methods. Obstet Gynecol 1995;85:321–325.
75. McLeer SV, Anwar R: A study of battered women presenting in an emergency department. Am J Pub Health 1989;79:65–66.
76. Bacchus L, Mezey G, Bewley S: Women's perceptions and experiences of routine screening for domestic violence in a maternity service. BJOG 2002;109:9–16.
77. Rodriguez MA, Szkupinski S, Bauer HM: Breaking the silence. Arch Fam Med 1996;5:153–158.
78. Covington DL, Diehl SJ, Wright BD, Piner M: Assessing for violence during pregnancy using a systematic approach. Matern Child Health J 1997;1:129–133.
79. McFarlane J, Wiist W: Preventing abuse to pregnant women: Implementation of a "mentor mother" advocacy model. J Community Health Nurs 1997;14:237–249.
80. McFarlane J, Parker B, Soeken K, et al: Safety behaviours of abused women after an intervention during pregnancy. J Obstet Gynecol Neonatal Nurs 1998;27:64–69.
81. McFarlane J, Soeken K, Wiist W: An evaluation of interventions to decrease intimate partner violence to pregnant women. Public Health Nurs 2000;17:443–451.
82. Sullivan CM, Bybee DI: Reducing violence using community-based advocacy for women with abusive partners. J Consult Clin Psychol 1999;67:43–53.
83. Sheridan DJ: Forensic documentation of battered pregnant women. J Nurse Midwifery 1996;41:467–472.
84. Home Office and Cabinet Office: Living without fear: An integrated approach to tackling violence against women. Home Office, London, 1999, p 12.
85. Mezey G, Bacchus L, Haworth S, Bewley S: Midwives' perceptions and experiences of routine screening for domestic violence. BJOG 2003;110:774–752.
86. Cant B, Irvine A: A report of a group interview with health professionals about their experience of a pilot project organised by the Domestic Violence Health Care Project in Redbridge and Waltham Forest. Faculty of Health, London, 2001. Available at: http://www.sbu.ac.uk/~regeneva/documents/domesticstaff(4).pdf
87. Green J, Spibey H, Protheroe L: Midwifery Responses Towards Women Who Are Experiencing Violence in Pregnancy. University of Leeds, Mother and Infant Research Unit, London, 2001. Paper in preparation.
88. Taket A: Tackling domestic violence: the role of health professional. Home office, London, 2004.
89. Wiist WH, McFarlane J: The effectiveness of an abuse assessment protocol in public health prenatal clinics. Am J Pub Health 1999;89:17–21.
90. Morrison LJ, Allan R, Grunfield A: Improving the emergency department detection rate of domestic violence using direct questioning. J Emerg Med 2000;19:117–124.
91. Hague G: Interagency work and domestic violence in the UK. Womens Stud Int Forum 1997;21:441–449.
92. Humphreys C, Thiara R: Routes to Safety: Protection Issues Facing Abused Women and Children and the Role of Outreach Services. Women's Aid Federation of England, Bristol, 2002.
93. Humphreys C, Hester M, Hague G, et al: From Good Intentions to Good Practice: Mapping Services Working with Families Where There Is Domestic Violence. Policy Press, Bristol, 2000.

CHAPTER 82

Resuscitation and Immediate Care of the Newborn

Neil Marlow / Philip Baker

INTRODUCTION

> "Every maternity unit, whether or not care of sick babies is undertaken, must have clearly established arrangements for the prompt, safe and effective resuscitation of babies and for the care of babies who require continuing support, either in the maternity unit or by safe transfer elsewhere."
>
> From: Standards for Hospitals Providing Neonatal Intensive and High Dependency Care (2nd Edition) London: BAPM 2001

Few babies need any assistance to establish normal respiration and circulation at birth, and of those who do most require only simple measures. Less than 5% of babies will need more than simple mouth suction, and most of these will require only initial help with lung inflation by mask ventilation. Very few need full resuscitation with intubation, chest compressions, and the use of drugs. All babies need care to maintain their temperature.

Formal resuscitation for about 20% of babies who require it is not predictable from clinical observations in pregnancy and during labor.[1] Prompt resuscitation of babies without apparent signs of life at birth will result in a significant number of healthy survivors.[2] Hence, wherever babies are delivered someone must be present who is trained and experienced to commence neonatal resuscitation, and someone must be available to provide expert back up for the complicated resuscitation. Generally, the local pediatric neonatal service provides the necessary expertise for the anticipated resuscitation problem, but other professionals must be prepared to commence resuscitation when it has not been anticipated. All professionals attending delivery must understand the principles of neonatal resuscitation and be able to institute effective respiration with a suitable mask ventilation system or intubation.[3]

Many centers conduct their own neonatal resuscitation training programs, which all obstetricians and midwives should attend. In addition neonatal life support courses (NLS or NALS) are now widely available. Formal training and certification by an appropriate route is encouraged for all staff.

Therefore the obstetrician must:

- Ensure the adequate provision of facilities and staff for resuscitation
- Understand the principles of resuscitation of the newborn
- Be prepared to institute neonatal resuscitation if pediatric support is unavailable, at least until help arrives

STRUCTURE OF A NEONATAL RESUSCITATION SERVICE

In many settings the service is provided by a neonatal team. However, in some settings where pediatric support is not available the obstetrician (or midwife) must assume this role. The critical elements are described in the British Paediatric Association document, "Neonatal Resuscitation,"[3] and comprise:

- Provision of training in resuscitation for all professionals involved
- Establishment of unit protocols
- Rostering individuals who are to be responsible for neonatal resuscitation and distribution of rotas to appropriate areas, such as labor suite, switchboard, neonatal unit

- Ensuring that equipment is available and working (Table 82–1)—local policy should determine who is responsible for checking this on a daily basis
- A protocol for summoning expert assistance where resuscitation is anticipated
- Ensuring a draught-free delivery room with a temperature of 24°C or greater

PHYSIOLOGY AND PERINATAL ADAPTATION

All professionals should be familiar with the normal respiratory and cardiovascular changes at birth. Acute total hypoxia in animals at delivery results in primary apnea. This is associated with initial tachycardia and rise in blood pressure, followed by bradycardia. Redistribution of blood flow occurs to essential organs (brain and heart) at the expense of others (skin, gut, and kidneys). If hypoxia persists, deep slow gasping occurs every 10 to 20 seconds before a further final period of apnea occurs, called terminal apnea. During this phase, hypotension, progressive bradycardia, and decreased cardiac output result in organ damage and death unless active resuscitation is commenced. A similar sequence of changes seems to occur in the human newborn, but it is not always possible to differentiate primary from terminal apnea: a baby in poor condition should be assumed to be in terminal apnea, and cardiopulmonary resuscitation must be initiated without delay.

ANTICIPATION OF HIGH RISK DELIVERIES

Normal practice should be to call pediatric assistance when resuscitation may be likely (Table 82–2). Few randomized studies have been conducted in this area; evidence from them is summarized at the end of the chapter. One study identified that attending 20% of deliveries resulted in identification of 50% of deliveries with low or medium Apgar scores.[4] Most services, however, now identify three levels of pediatric input at delivery: those where attendance is required, those where pediatric help may be informed that a delivery is taking place, and those where early postnatal review is necessary (see Table 82–2). For these services, where pediatric help is readily and immediately available it may be possible simply to inform the rostered individual of the impending delivery of a fetus that is unlikely to require assistance (elective cesarean delivery at term with regional analge-

TABLE 82–1

Delivery Room Resuscitation Equipment

Equipment	
Warmed towels and plastic bag	
Gloves	
Resuscitation trolley with overhead heater, lighting, and stop-clock	
Oxygen and air supply (with reducing valve, flow meter, pressure blowoff device [set at 30 cm H_2O], pressure measuring device [e.g., manometer], and connecting tubes to supply air or oxygen to a bag and mask and (with a side hole) an endotracheal tube	
Face masks (e.g., Bennett sizes 2 and 3)	
500-mL resuscitation bag with a fitting for a face mask and an endotracheal tube adaptor and blowoff valve (e.g., Ambu, Laerdal)	
Laryngoscopes with preterm- and term-sized straight blades (e.g., Wisconsin, Magill) and spare bulbs and batteries	
Endotracheal tubes (2.5, 3.0, and 3.5 mm) with connectors and fixation devices and an endotracheal tube introducer (nylon or metal)	
Oropharyngeal airways (sizes 00 and 0)	
Nasogastric tubes (sizes 5 and 8)	
Suction device and suction catheters (no. 4, 6, or 8 French)	
Oral mucus extractors	
Stethoscope	
Sterile towel, scissors, and cord clamps	
Antiseptic cleaning solution (e.g., povidone-iodine, chlorhexidine)	
Intravenous cannulaes, three-way taps, and connecting tubing	
Sterile syringes (2, 5, and 10 mL) and needles	
Adhesive tape	
Capillary blood sugar test strips	
Alcohol swabs	
Sterile containers and specimen bottles for blood tests (e.g., complete blood count, packed cell volume, electrolytes, blood sugar, bilirubin, blood typing, and Coomb's test)	
Equipment for umbilical catheterization	
Pneumothorax drains and Heimlich valves	
Drugs and Fluids	
Epinephrine	1:10,000 (10-mL ampule)
Dextrose	10% solution
Sodium chloride	0.9% solution for injection
Water for injection	
Naloxone	400 µg/mL
Volume expanders	Plasma and albumin solutions
Blood	Fresh group O Rh-negative (cytomegalovirus-negative)

TABLE 82–2

Risk Factors That Require Pediatric Staff or Staff Trained in Resuscitation

FACTOR	PRESENT	INFORMED*
Labor and Delivery		
Cesarean section for fetal indications	✓	
Cesarean section for nonfetal reasons, with regional anesthesia		✓†
Breech delivery or other malpresentation	✓	
Forceps or ventouse delivery (not simple "lift-outs")	✓	
Delivery after significant antepartum hemorrhage	✓	
Prolapsed cord	✓	
Maternal		
Maternal medical disorder that may affect the fetus	✓	
Current maternal drug or alcohol abuse		✓
Delivery under heavy sedation or general anesthesia	✓	
Fever		✓
Fetal		
Multiple pregnancy (one pediatrician for each infant)	✓	
Preterm delivery (<37 wk)	✓‡	
Prolonged membrane rupture (>24 hr) or suspected chorionamnionitis		✓
Hydramnios	✓	
Fetal distress	✓	
Known or suspected Fetal abnormality or disease	✓	
Isoimmunization	✓	

*Informed of delivery and freely available to attend within 3 to 4 minutes, if required.
†Elective cesarean section at term if the individual is available to attend, as discussed above.
‡Two individuals are advisable before 31 weeks' gestation or if the anticipated birth weight is <1500 g.

sia,[5–7] deliveries for maternal [nonfetal] reasons, simple "lift-out" forceps deliveries, certain maternal medical problems, prolonged rupture of membranes with no other risk factors). If a pediatrician is not present at delivery, prime responsibility for initiating resuscitation and summoning help, if required, remains with the delivery suite team.

PREPARATION FOR RESUSCITATION

Any individual who expects to initiate neonatal resuscitation should always introduce themselves to the parents and explain what is happening or likely to happen. He or she should obtain as full a history as possible from the mother, midwife, or obstetrician and examine the mother's chart notes to establish:

- Gestational age
- Drugs given to mother
- Evidence of fetal distress (e.g., heart rate abnormality, acidosis, meconium)
- Presence of vaginal bleeding
- Prolonged rupture of membranes
- Maternal health in labor[8]
- Number of fetuses[9]
- Relevant obstetric or medical history

In addition the person performing the resuscitation should check and prepare the necessary equipment

- Ensure the delivery room is warm (>24°C) and free of drafts
- Check that equipment is available and in working order
- Turn on overhead heater
- Ensure that warmed towels are available
- If the mother has recently received a narcotic such as pethidine (meperidine), ensure that antagonist (naloxone [Narcan]) is readily available[10]
- Wash hands, put on gloves, or take other precautions against blood-borne viruses as per hospital policy

TIMING OF BIRTH

The time of the baby's birth should be recorded so that the timing of subsequent interventions can be accurately documented.

ASSESSMENT OF CONDITION AT BIRTH

Apgar Score

Condition at birth is traditionally assessed using the Apgar score (Table 82–3), which was designed as a guide for the need for resuscitation. Measures may be made at 1 and 5 minutes with further recordings at 5-minute intervals if resuscitation continues. Ideally the Apgar score should be assessed and recorded at the time of resuscitation (originally this was done by a second observer)—retrospective assignation is fraught with errors. The Apgar score is a poor prognostic guide for later outcome, except that low Apgar scores that persist beyond 10 minutes suggest significant

TABLE 82-3
Apgar Score

	0	1	2
Heart Rate	Absent	<100 beats min	>100 beats min
Respiratory Effort	Absent	Weak	Good, crying
Muscle Tone	Flaccid	Some flexion of extremities	Well flexed
Reflex Irritability	No response	Grimace	Cough or sneeze
Color	Pale or blue	Body pink with blue extremities	Completely pink

hypoxia.[11] In practice, careful assessment of heart rate and respiration may be preferable as a simpler guide to condition of the newborn (Figs. 82–1, through 82–4).

Cord Blood Acid–Base

For babies born after fetal distress or for those needing resuscitation, the cord blood pH and base excess may indicate the severity of perinatal asphyxia. Blood from both the umbilical artery and vein should be sampled. Some infants, however, may have suffered significant intrapartum asphyxia despite a normal pH. As is true with the Apgar score, extremes of acidosis are most strongly associated with poor outcome. Cord blood acid–base status cannot be used to determine the need for resuscitation.

DIVIDING THE UMBILICAL CORD

Modern obstetric practice usually involves division of the cord while the placenta is still in utero. The time of occlusion of the umbilical cord determines the distribution of blood between the infant and placenta. Optimal distribution has not been clearly defined, but for preterm infants in particular, even a short delay in cord clamping may cause major hemodynamic advantage. The optimum distribution of blood volume and the least hemodynamic

Time of birth

Note time to calculate timings of other events if needed/start clock.

Dry and wrap baby

Even healthy babies have difficulty maintaining body temperature after birth, the risk is increased if the baby is growth impaired, preterm, ill, or sedated.

- *Minimize heat loss* by drying immediately, discarding the wet towels and wrapping the infant in a warm towel. For tiny babies, place baby inside a plastic bag without drying.
- Cover head—up to 85% heat loss may be via the head and therefore a bonnet is used during prolonged resuscitation or for very preterm children.
- *Use a radiant heater*–If resuscitation is required place the baby under a radiant heater–note that silver foil should not be used as it will reflect heat away from the baby.
- *Use an incubator or silver foil wrap (swaddler)* to transfer at risk babies.

Clear airway

Most babies do not require aspiration of the upper airway with a suction device–wipe the lips and nares during drying or with gauze (if suction is required see Figure 82-2)

Assess condition at 1 minute

- *Regular respiration and heart rate about 100 bpm*
  - Wrap infant to prevent heat loss and hand to mother or lay on mother's chest and cover with warm towels
  - Reassure mother that all is well
  - Return to make surface examination of infant when delivery procedure complete
- *No regular respiration or heart rate below 100 bpm*
  - Transfer to resuscitaire/radiant heater
  - Summon pediatric help
  - Commence resuscitation (see below)
  - Start clock to time events
  - Go to Figure 82-2

FIGURE 82–1
Basic neonatal Management after birth (1). If meconium present at birth, see Figure 82–4.

disturbance may be achieved by clamping the cord about 30 seconds after delivery.[12] By this time the infant usually has taken his or her first breath and will have received a partial placental transfusion.

After division, the cord should be firmly occluded about 2 cm from the umbilicus using a suitable umbilical cord clamp.

TREATMENT OF THE NORMAL INFANT AT BIRTH

When early assessment reveals no resuscitative problems or congenital abnormality, the baby should be handed at once to the mother. This may be done even before dividing the umbilical cord, but care should be taken to prevent heat loss (see Fig. 82–1).[13,14] The baby may be wrapped in a warmed towel or nursed skin-to-skin on the mother's chest, covered with a warm towel. If the mother intends to breast-feed, the baby should be put to the breast. This not only improves the success of lactation,[15,16] but also may aid delivery of the placenta, by encouraging the release of endogenous oxytocin. Extra care to avoid cold stress must be taken when a baby is preterm or growth restricted.

MANAGEMENT WHEN RESUSCITATION IS REQUIRED

This is approached differently for the very preterm infant (<30 wks' gestation) (see below).

RESUSCITATION OF THE FULL-TERM AND NEAR-TERM INFANT

Algorithms for management of poor condition at birth are given in Figures 82–2, 82–3, and 82–4.

Airway suction must be performed gently. There is little value in blind probing with the catheter, and pharyngeal suction should never be attempted except under direct vision using a laryngoscope. When suction is required do not use direct mouth suction because of the risk of virus transmission—a double mucus trap system or mechanical suction is preferred. The place of suction in uncomplicated resuscitation is detailed in Figure 82–1 and in the face of meconium stained liquor in Figure 82–4.[17-19]

If obstruction is suspected (cyanosis despite good respiratory effort with no audible breath sounds), direct inspection using a laryngoscope is preferred to blind aspiration;

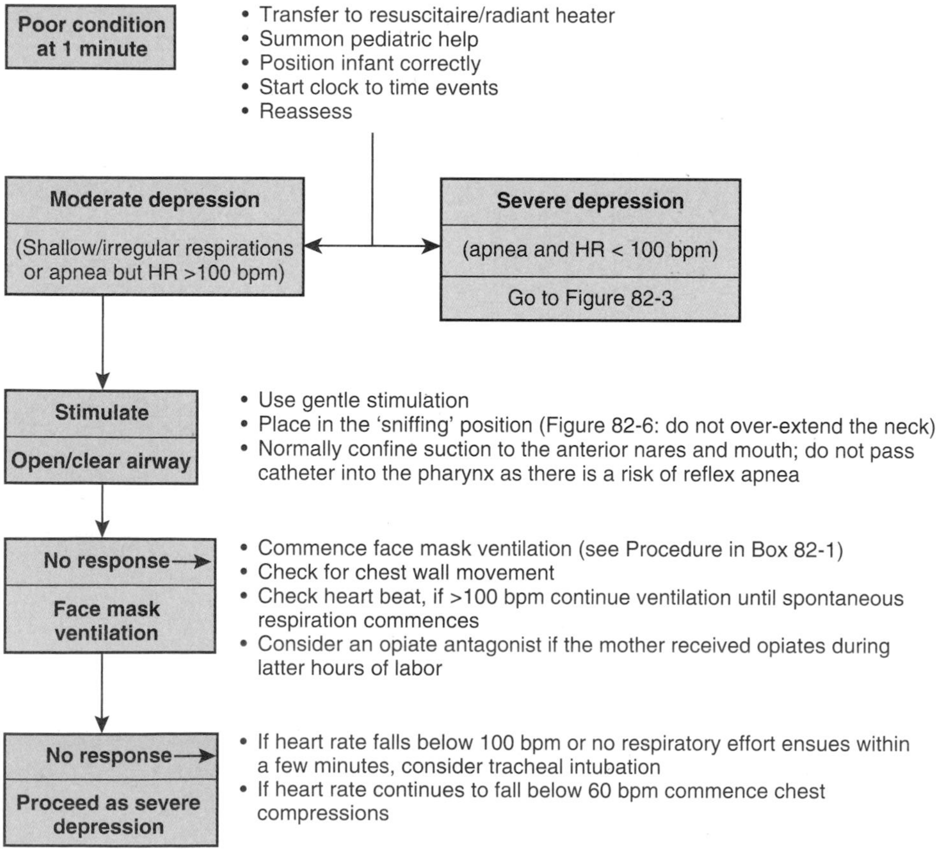

FIGURE 82–2
Management of the moderately depressed newborn (2). If meconium present at birth, see Figure 82–4.

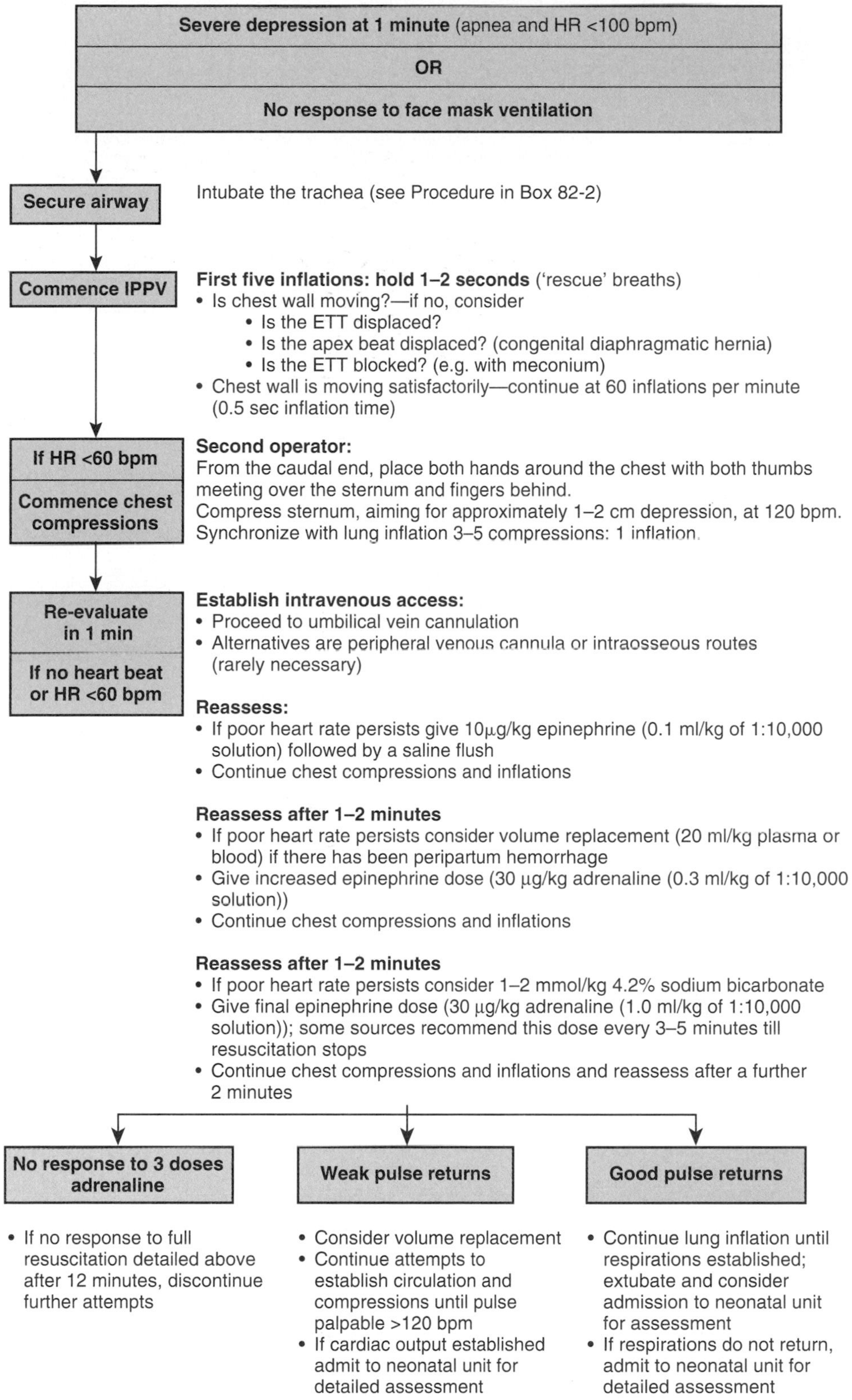

FIGURE 82–3
Management of the severely depressed newborn (3).

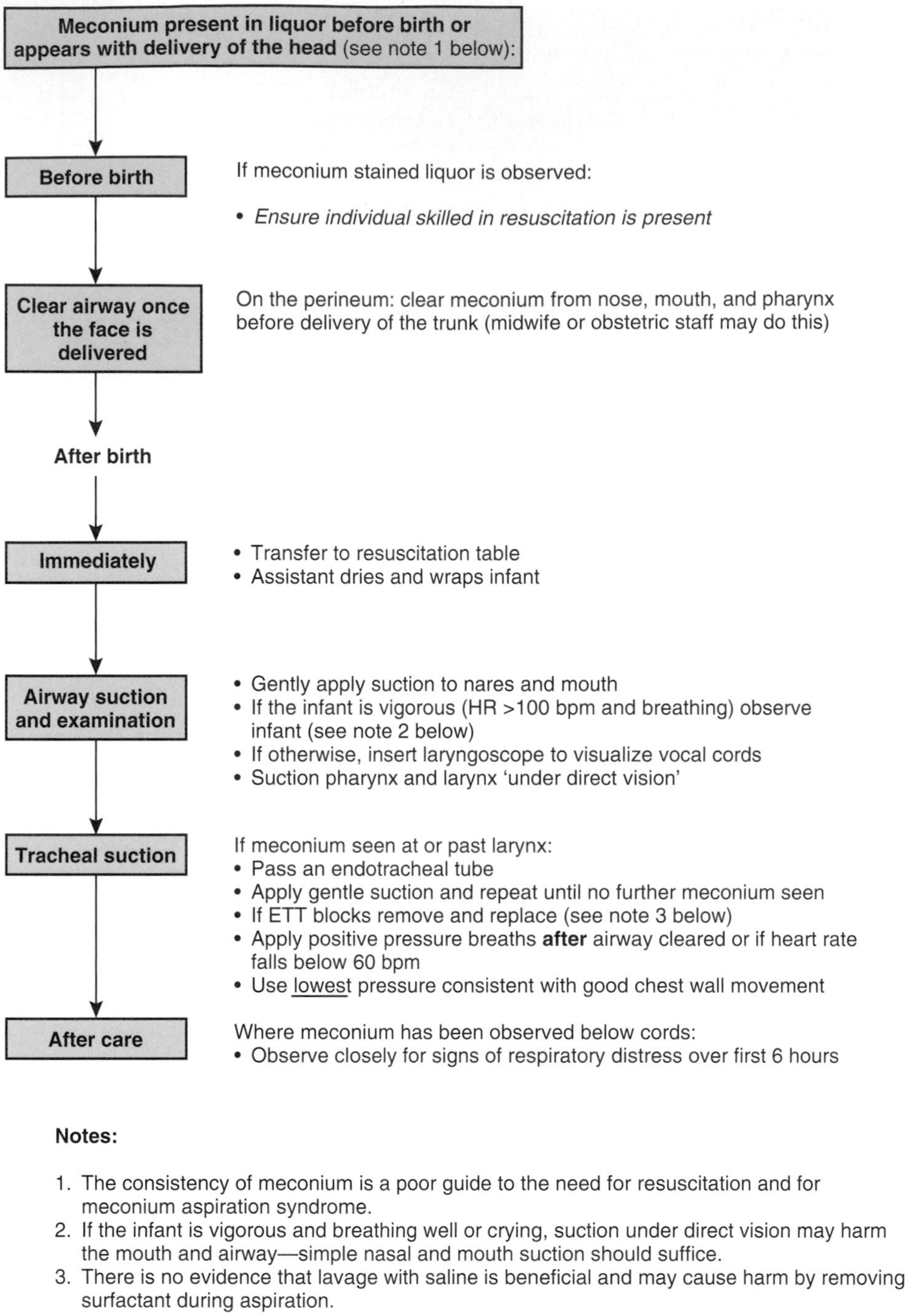
Meconium present in liquor before birth or appears with delivery of the head (see note 1 below):
Before birth
If meconium stained liquor is observed:
• Ensure individual skilled in resuscitation is present
Clear airway once the face is delivered
On the perineum: clear meconium from nose, mouth, and pharynx before delivery of the trunk (midwife or obstetric staff may do this)
After birth
Immediately
• Transfer to resuscitation table
• Assistant dries and wraps infant
Airway suction and examination
• Gently apply suction to nares and mouth
• If the infant is vigorous (HR >100 bpm and breathing) observe infant (see note 2 below)
• If otherwise, insert laryngoscope to visualize vocal cords
• Suction pharynx and larynx 'under direct vision'
Tracheal suction
If meconium seen at or past larynx:
• Pass an endotracheal tube
• Apply gentle suction and repeat until no further meconium seen
• If ETT blocks remove and replace (see note 3 below)
• Apply positive pressure breaths after airway cleared or if heart rate falls below 60 bpm
• Use lowest pressure consistent with good chest wall movement
After care
Where meconium has been observed below cords:
• Observe closely for signs of respiratory distress over first 6 hours
Notes:
1. The consistency of meconium is a poor guide to the need for resuscitation and for meconium aspiration syndrome.
2. If the infant is vigorous and breathing well or crying, suction under direct vision may harm the mouth and airway—simple nasal and mouth suction should suffice.
3. There is no evidence that lavage with saline is beneficial and may cause harm by removing surfactant during aspiration.

FIGURE 82–4
Management after birth when meconium present in liquor (4).

this should be followed by the placement of an oral airway. Obstruction is usually nasal and due to debris or choanal atresia/stenosis:

- Check nasal patency with stethoscope (while obstructing contralateral side).
- Aspirate nose (in choanal atresia a clear gel cast of the nasal cavity may be aspirated).
- Check for small jaw and cleft palate (in Pierre Robin syndrome, the posteriorly placed tongue may obstruct the airway in the cleft).

Face Mask Ventilation

All medical, midwifery, and nursing staff involved in care in labor must know how to instigate face mask ventilation using either a bag and mask or a mask and Y or T piece. This technique provides the initial intervention in neonatal resuscitation.[20] It is usually all that is required and may be preferred when the resuscitator is not experienced in placing an endotracheal tube; in this situation intubation may be more dangerous than continuing well-applied mask ventilation. Regular updating of skills in mask ventilation is mandatory for all staff. Initial resuscitation should include five larger prolonged inflations (or "rescue breaths"), as a way of stimulating Heads', paradoxical reflex (a well described respiratory reflex) and starting respiration.

The relative advantages of mask ventilation using a bag set versus a Y or T piece are poorly defined and depend on local practice.

PROCEDURE

MASK VENTILATION

Apply the correct size of face mask to fit well over the nose and mouth providing a close fit (it should not extend over the eyes or tip of the mandible (Fig. 82–5).

Hold the chin gently forward using a finger under the tip of the mandible or upward from the angle of the jaw.

Using a bag, valve, and mask (blow-off valve set at 30 cm H_2O):

- Squeeze slowly to produce an inflation time of 1 to 2 seconds for the first five ("rescue") breaths.

Using a Y or T piece:

- Check pressure relief valve set at 30 cm H_2O or manometer in line.
- Occlude Y or T-piece for 2-second breaths for five breaths.

Assess chest movement, if satisfactory proceed at 30 to 40 breaths/minute. If not satisfactory check:

- Is the mask application satisfactory?
- Is the airway obstructed? Consider position, oral airway.
- Is higher pressure required?

The Use of Oxygen and Air in Resuscitation

The use of air to resuscitate newborn infants is controversial.[21] For most full-term or near-term infants, it probably does not matter. However in a well-conducted randomized trial, infants of 31 weeks' gestation or more were satisfactorily resuscitated using room air,[22] oxygen concentration being increased if cyanosis persisted. For preterm infants high arterial oxygen concentrations should be avoided (generally this is taken to be above 80 mm Hg or 10 kPa[23]; there is evidence that hyperoxia may lead to cerebral vasoconstriction.[24] Moreover, oxygen-induced retinal vasoconstriction may be crucial to the early pathogenesis of retinopathy of prematurity in preterm infants.

For best practice, a device for varying the inspired oxygen concentration is therefore necessary. Self-inflating (e.g., Laerdal) bags rely on the oxygen (or mixed gas) supply filling a reservoir to provide gas for ventilation. They may be used without reservoirs and with low flow rates of oxygen (4 L/min) to produce low inspired oxygen concentrations (25%–40%); this may provide a useful alternative method of resuscitating with low oxygen concentrations in the absence of a mixing device. If resuscitation is difficult, or the infant remains cyanotic, the

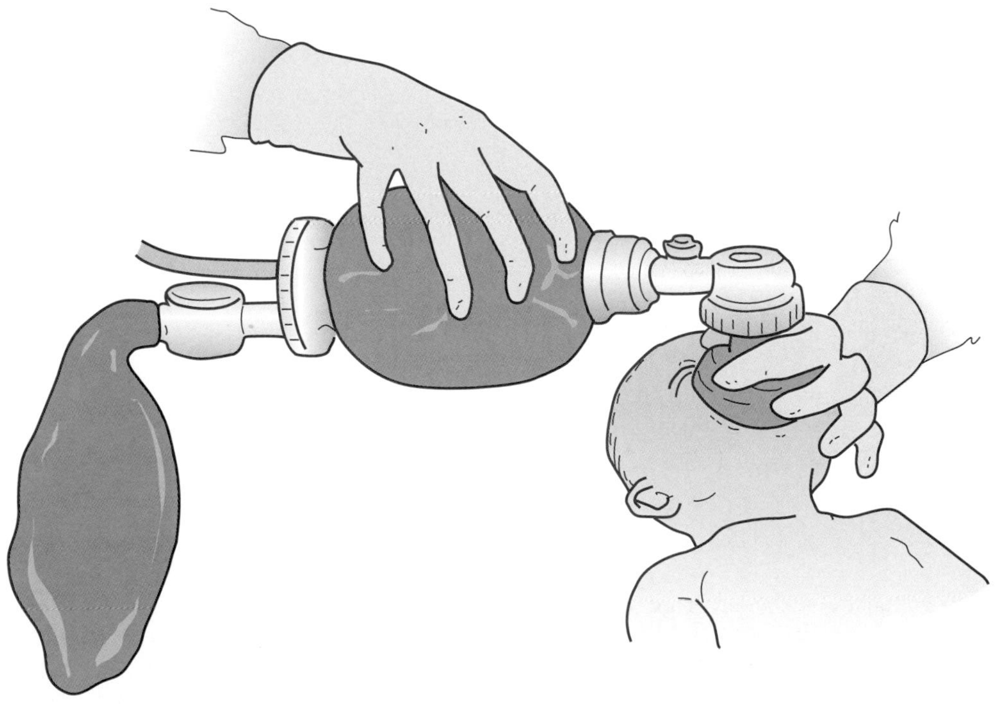

FIGURE 82–5
Using a bag, valve, and mask. (Reproduced with permission from Textbook of Neonatal Resuscitation, The American Heart Association.)

reservoir must be reattached before high concentrations of oxygen can be achieved.

Endotracheal Intubation

This method of ventilation is preferred for infants not responding rapidly to mask ventilation (within 1 min)[20] see Figure 82–7. Training in intubation should be undertaken by those likely to be required to perform intubation reasonably frequently, for example those likely to be called to difficult resuscitations. Formal training using models is useful before attempting it in the clinical situation.

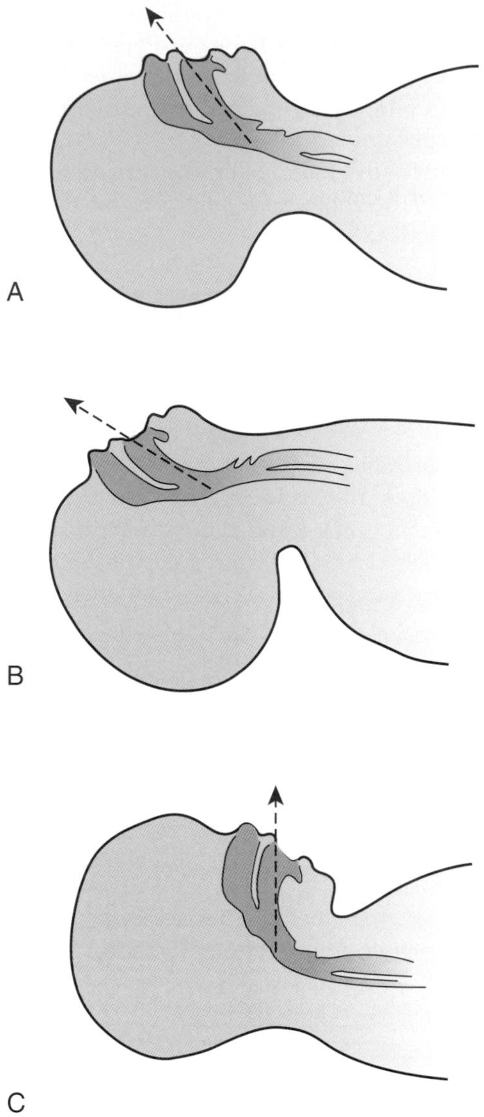

FIGURE 82–6
Positioning the head for resuscitation. a, Correct; b, incorrect; c, incorrect.

PROCEDURE

NEONATAL ENDOTRACHEAL INTUBATION

Endotracheal Tube Sizes

TUBE SIZE (MM)	GESTATIONAL AGE (WK)	ESTIMATED OR ACTUAL WEIGHT (G)
2.5	<29	<1000
3.0	30–34	1000–2000
3.0 or 3.5	34–36	2000–3000
3.5	>36	>3000

Technique

- Ensure head and neck are in line with body and neck, in the "sniffing" position (Fig. 82–6).
- Insert the laryngoscope blade over the tongue to the back of the larynx, the uvula and epiglottis will come into view (Fig. 82–7).
- Lift the epiglottis forward by exerting traction parallel to the handle of the laryngoscope—do not tilt the blade handle.

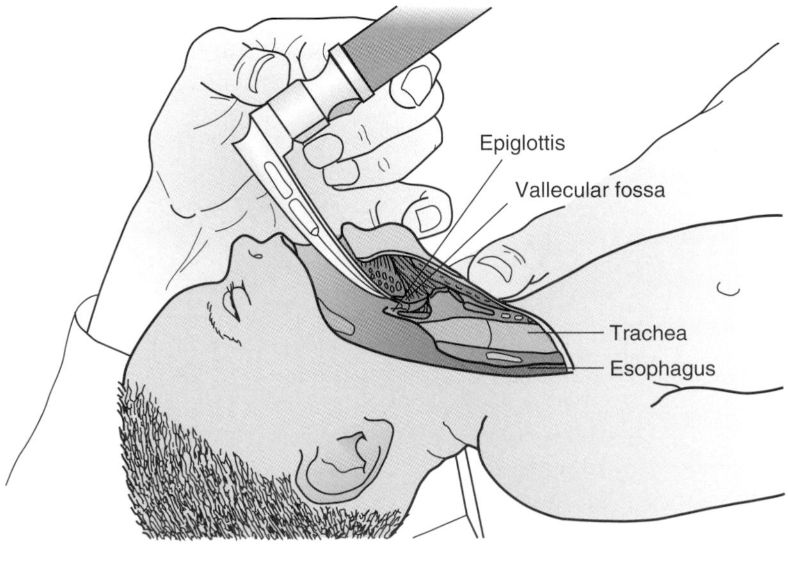

FIGURE 82–7
The technique for endotracheal intubation. (Reproduced with permission from Fleming PJ, Speidel BD, Marlow N, Dunn PM (1991). A Neonatal Vade-Mecum. London, Edward Arnold.)

- The vocal cords should then be visible. Brief suction to clear secretions may be needed. Apply gentle cricoid pressure with the fifth finger of the left hand, or an assistant may help your view.
- Keeping the trachea central, insert the appropriate size endotracheal tube (ETT) through the cords until the shoulder or 2-cm mark is at the vocal cords.
- Firmly fix the position of the ETT with the thumb and forefinger of the right hand while fixing the hand against the side of face and jaw with the other three fingers.
- Carefully remove the laryngoscope from the mouth.
- Ask an assistant to connect ETT to the ventilation device (mask or bagging set).
- Observe chest movement with ventilation, auscultate both sides—unequal air entry usually means the ETT is too far down and should be withdrawn slightly.

After intubation and five long breaths (approximately 1-second inflation time), chest wall movement is usually observed. Careful assessment to determine if the infant has improved after 30 seconds of positive pressure breaths is necessary. Tube displacement, misplacement, blockage, or congenital abnormalities may be responsible for a lack of improvement (Table 82–4). Ventilation at 40 to 60 inflations/minute (approximately 0.5-second inflation time) should continue until the infant has regular spontaneous respirations. Extubation may then be performed after mouth suction.

An ETT should never be disconnected from positive pressure for other than brief periods because of the danger of progressive atelectasis after removal of a positive end-expiratory pressure.

TABLE 82–4

Causes of Difficulty at Resuscitation

Respiratory
Meconium aspiration syndrome
Diaphragmatic hernia
Pneumothorax or pneumomediastinum
Pleural or pericardial effusion
Congenital pneumonia or sepsis
Pulmonary edema or hemorrhage
Pulmonary hypoplasia
Extreme prematurity or severe respiratory distress syndrome
Malformation of the respiratory tract, such as congenital lobar emphysema
Cardiovascular
Congenital heart disease
Persistent fetal circulation
Hypovolemia as a result of blood loss
Neurologic
Cerebrospinal trauma, hypoxia, of malformation
Cerebral depression caused by drugs
Other
Severe metabolic disturbance

Chest Compressions and Cardiac Massage

Chest compressions should be commenced if the heart rate does not respond to ventilation (see Fig. 82–3). Two techniques are described: the two-hand approach has advantage under experimental conditions and is preferred. Chest compressions are performed by an assistant:

- From the caudal end, place both hands around the chest with both thumbs meeting over the sternum and fingers behind the infant's back.
- Compress the sternum using thumbs acting against fingers, aiming for approximately 1 to 2 cm depression, at a rate of about 100 to 120 compressions per minute.
- Compressions should be coordinated with lung inflations (3 compressions:1 inflation; count aloud "1-2-3-breath" until a rhythm is established). The combined rhythm should produce 30 to 40 breaths and 100 to 120 compressions per minute.

(An alternative technique is often used if a sole resuscitator is providing cardiopulmonary support: place two fingers over the sternum at the level of the nipples, depressing the sternum as previously described.)

Compressions should continue until a palpable pulse of >120 beats/minute returns or until resuscitation is discontinued. Overvigorous chest compression may cause rib fractures or liver injury.

Intravenous Drugs

Before progressing to the administration of drugs it is mandatory that the following are secured:

- Airway
- Breathing
- Chest compressions

If the infant fails to respond, intravenous drugs should be administered.

ESTABLISH INTRAVENOUS ACCESS

The umbilical venous route is the most effective for establishing intravenous access. Alternative routes are via peripheral cannulae and intraosseous infusions. Intracardiac administration is rarely necessary and dangerous in the ventilated infant as a pneumothorax could be precipitated. There is a vogue for the intratracheal instillation of epinephrine; this is an unproven route with no evidence-based dosage guidelines. Generally this route should be avoided and umbilical venous access sought.

EPINEPHRINE

Epinephrine is the first-line medication in the face of bradycardia.[25] Recent recommendations[26,27] have concurred that a first dose of 10 μg/kg (0.1 mL/kg of 1:10,000 solution) should be followed by increased doses of 30 μg/kg (0.3 mL/kg of 1:10,000 solution). If intratracheal instillation is desired, doses of 10, 20, 30 or 100 μg/kg have all been recommended. Current practice is to give 20 μg/kg followed by 5mL saline and five long inflation breaths. In between doses of adrenaline, chest compressions per inflations should continue for at least 1 minute before reassessment. Further doses are unnecessary once the heart rate has risen above 60 beats/minute and pulses are palpable.

COLLOID (PLASMA/WHOLE BLOOD)

Hypovolemia should be considered if there is:

- Evidence of bleeding or twin-twin transfusion
- Poor pulse volume after adequate resuscitation
- Poor peripheral circulation despite adequate pulse volume
- Suspicion of hemolysis

A dose of 10 to 20 mL/kg should be administered over 5 to 10 minutes and repeated depending on response.

SODIUM BICARBONATE

Administration of alkali during resuscitation is controversial; sodium bicarbonate is a negative inotrope and correction of extracellular acidosis may worsen intracellular pH. However, one unevaluated justification for its use may be the vasodilation of coronary arteries and improvement of adrenaline delivery to the myocardium. It is not necessary to correct acidosis fully. Many neonatal units do not use sodium bicarbonate, those that do recommend 1 to 2 mmol/kg (2–4 mL 4.2% $NaHCO_3$), which may be given before the *third* dose of adrenaline.

NALOXONE

Naloxone is an opiate antagonist and is not administered as part of resuscitation after hypoxia. It may be of value for infants who have established good cardiac output but in whom respiratory depression persists and the mother has received an opiate in labor. Care should be taken not to give naloxone to infants of opiate-dependent mothers as it may precipitate acute withdrawal. Dosage is 100 mg/kg intramuscularly.[28]

OTHER MEDICATIONS

Calcium is no longer given as part of resuscitation because it may cause coronary artery constriction. Glucose solutions are generally unnecessary except as flush solutions. Hypoglycemia is unusual during the first 30 minutes because of high circulating stress hormone concentrations, but it may occur occasionally. Current recommendations are to give 2.5 mL/kg glucose intravenously if the resuscitation is prolonged (>10 min).

Failure to Respond to Resuscitation

The decision to cease resuscitative efforts should be taken by a senior and experienced doctor. Usually the obstetrician is not faced with this problem as the neonatal team will have arrived. Rarely this does not occur. Generally, if the full resuscitation process has been carried out as detailed earlier, efforts may be stopped if there is no response after 12 minutes. However, in practice, resuscitation is rarely that efficient. It is wise to consider stopping after 20 minutes if there is no response. One senior member of the resuscitation team should discuss this with the parents wherever possible.

RECORDING OF INFORMATION

As much information about the procedures taken should be entered into the clinical notes, including the persons present (and the time of arrival if summoned), procedures undertaken, and medications given with doses and times. The results of telephone discussions should be accurately recorded.

STABILIZATION OF THE VERY PRETERM BABY AFTER BIRTH

Although most conventional teaching suggests that an identical approach is taken to the very preterm infant (babies born at 30 weeks' gestation or less), recent evidence suggests that a different approach may have value. Although this is the province of the neonatal intensive care team, all staff should be aware of the differences if called upon to help. Furthermore the use of surfactant replacement therapy is often best commenced in the delivery room for maximal effect. Many centers use endotracheal intubation less frequently and allow infants longer to establish their own respiratory drive or use continuous positive airways pressure (CPAP) from soon after birth. Where the baby is in poor condition and not responding to simple measures, including intubation, resuscitation should progress in a similar manner to that described earlier. The major areas of difference are as follows.

Prior Discussion with Parents

When possible and well before delivery, members of the neonatal team should meet with women and their partners who are expecting a very preterm baby, and both parents should visit the neonatal intensive care unit. This allows for a planned approach to the stabilization of the infant. The preliminary discussions with parents concerning prognosis should be shared between obstetric and neonatal staff, and agreed prognostic information should be available.

Thermal Care

Allowing a very preterm baby to get cold may significantly worsen the likelihood of death through increasing the severity of the respiratory illness. Current best practice is to:

- Place the infant immediately into a plastic bag (before drying) and bring the bag up to the neck.[29]
- Dry the head and put on a bonnet before continuing with resuscitation. Leave the infant inside the bag until stabilized in an incubator.
- Cover the infant and bag with warm towels before transfer.

Surfactant Replacement Therapy

The smallest babies (i.e., babies of 26 wks' or less gestational age) should be intubated immediately after being placed in the plastic bag, and surfactant should be administered as soon as is practicable afterward.[30] Some doctors prefer to give surfactant before the first breath. For more mature babies, surfactant is given in the neonatal unit.

Inflation Breaths

There is evidence from animal studies that large tidal volumes given after birth may produce lung injury.[31] The use of large inflation breaths should be avoided and positive end-expiratory pressure (PEEP) should be provided during resuscitation with either mask or endotracheal support. The chest excursions should be barely visible during initial inflations.

These variations from standard practice are really the province of the specialist neonatal team and we therefore reemphasize that they should be called early to provide for optimal stabilization.

CONCLUSIONS

- Someone trained in neonatal resuscitation should be immediately available for all deliveries.
- In most hospitals, a pediatrician is available to perform neonatal resuscitation.
- As far as possible deliveries where such skills may be required should be identified in advance and the pediatric staff alerted in well in advance of the delivery.
- Since some deliveries occur for which such specialists are not immediately available, all health professionals responsible for delivery (obstetricians, midwives) should receive training in and be competent to carry out effective neonatal resuscitation using, as a minimum, face mask ventilation.
- Only those who can maintain skills should receive formal training in intubation.

SUMMARY OF MANAGEMENT OPTIONS

Neonatal Resuscitation (Obstetric Perspective)

Management Options	Quality of Evidence	Strength of Recommendation	References
General and Organizational Issues			
Planning			
Wherever babies are delivered, someone capable of initiating expert resuscitation must be present.	IV	C	3, 26
Training			
Obstetricians must be able to institute effective neonatal resuscitation because neonatal staff may not be immediately available at every delivery.	–	GPP	–
Resources			
Service requirements: • Training of all professionals involved in delivery room care • Written protocols and lines of communication • Published list of available individuals who are on call for resuscitation • Resuscitation equipment available and working • Delivery room temperature at least 75°F (24°C) and no drafts	IV	C	3,26,27

Continued

SUMMARY OF MANAGEMENT OPTIONS
Neonatal Resuscitation (Obstetric Perspective) *(Continued)*

Management Options	Quality of Evidence	Strength of Recommendation	References
Need for Staff Experienced in Neonatal Resuscitation (See also Table 82–2)			
Factors Related to Labor and Delivery			
Cesarean section	III	B	4
Breech delivery or other malpresentation	III	B	4
Forceps of ventouse delivery (not "lift-outs")	III	B	4
Delivery after significant antepartum hemorrhage	III	B	4
Prolapsed cord	III	B	4
Maternal Factors			
Maternal medical disorder that may affect the fetus	–	GPP	–
Current maternal drug or alcohol abuse	IIa	B	32
Delivery under heavy sedation or general anesthesia	Ia, III	A, B	5–7
Fever	IIa	B	8
Fetal Factors			
Multiple pregnancy (one pediatrician for each infant)	III	B	9
Preterm delivery (<37 weeks)	IIa	B	33
Prolonged membrane rupture or suspected chorioamnionitis	–	GPP	–
Hydramnios	–	GPP	–
Fetal distress	III	B	4
Known or suspected fetal abnormality	–	GPP	–
Isoimmunization	IV	C	34
Management Options			
Preparation			
Introduce yourself.	–	GPP	–
Obtain a relevant history.	–	GPP	–
Check the equipment and turn on the heater.	–	GPP	–
Management			
Thermal control: Dry and wrap infant (see Fig. 82–1), and then follow ABCD as described later.	III	B	13,14
Airway: Suction as necessary (see Figs. 82–1 and 82–2).	IV	C	17
Meconium-stained liquor: perform tracheal suction when indicated (see Fig. 82–4).	Ib, III, IV	A, B, C	17–19
Breathing: Consider face mask ventilation or endotracheal intubation and ventilation, as appropriate (see Figs. 82–2 and 82–3).	IIb, IV	B, C	17,20
There is no difference in resuscitation between room air and 100% oxygen.	Ib	A	22,35
Maintain adequate levels of humidity.	Ib	A	36
Chest compressions: Consider drugs or other volume replacement if the patient has a poor response (see Fig. 82–3).	IV	C	17
Drugs: Consider epinephrine IV when no effect of ventilation is seen on a heart rate of <60 beats/min for longer than 30 sec (see Fig. 82–3).	IV	C	17
Consider naloxone to reverse the possible opioid effects on respiratory efforts (See Fig. 82–3).	Ib	A	10,28

REFERENCES

1. Palme-Kilander C: Methods of resuscitation in low-Apgar-score newborn infants: A national survey. Acta Paediatr 1992;81:739–744.
2. Casalaz DM, Marlow N, Speidel BD: Outcome of resuscitation following unexpected apparent stillbirth. Arch Dis Child Fetal Neonatal Ed 1998;78:F112–F115.
3. British Paediatric Association: Neonatal resuscitation. London, BPA, 1993.
4. Primhak RA, Herber SM, Whincup G, Milner RD: Which deliveries require paediatricians in attendance? BMJ 1984;289 (6436):16–18.
5. Levine EM, Ghai V, Barton JJ, Strom CM: Pediatrician attendance at cesarean delivery: Necessary or not? Obstet Gynecol 1999;93:338–340.
6. Kolatat T, Somboonnanonda A, Lertakyamanee J, et al: Effects of general and regional anesthesia on the neonate (a prospective, randomized trial). J Med Assoc Thai 1999;82:40–45.
7. Ong BY, Cohen MM, Palahniuk RJ: Anesthesia for cesarean section: Effects on neonates. Anesth Analg 1989;68:270–275.
8. Lieberman E, Eichenwald E, Mathur G, et al: Intrapartum fever and unexplained seizures in term infants. Pediatrics 2000;106: 983–988.
9. Prins RP: The second-born twin: Can we improve outcomes? Am J Obstet Gynecol 1994;170:1649–1656; discussion 1656–1657.
10. Wiener PC, Hogg MI, Rosen M: Effects of naloxone on pethidine-induced neonatal depression: Part I. Intravenous naloxone. BMJ 1977;2(6081):228–229.
11. Nelson KB, Ellenberg JH: Antecedents of cerebral palsy: Multivariate analysis of risk. N Engl J Med 1986;315:81–86.
12. Kinmond S, Aitchison TC, Holland BM, et al: Umbilical cord clamping and preterm infants: A randomised trial. BMJ 1993; 306(6871):172–175.
13. MacDonald HM, Mulligan JC, Allen AC, Taylor PM: Neonatal asphyxia: I. Relationship of obstetric and neonatal complications to neonatal mortality in 38,405 consecutive deliveries. J Pediatr 1980;96:898–902.
14. Blackfan KD, Yaglou CP: The premature infant: A study of the effects of atmospheric conditions on growth and development. Am J Dis Child 1933;46:1175.
15. Taylor PM, Maloni JA, Taylor FH, Campbell SB: Extra early mother-infant contact and duration of breast-feeding. Acta Paediatr Scand (Suppl) 1985;316:15–22.
16. Woolridge MW, Greasley V, Silpisornkosol S: The initiation of lactation: The effect of early versus delayed contact for suckling on milk intake in the first week post-partum. A study in Chiang Mai, Northern Thailand. Early Hum Dev 1985;12: 269–278.
17. Kattwinkel J, Niermeyer S, Nadkarni V, et al: Resuscitation of the newly born infant: An advisory statement from the Pediatric Working Group of the International Liaison Committee on Resuscitation. Resuscitation 1999;40:71–88.
18. Wiswell TE, Gannon CM, Jacob J, et al: Delivery room management of the apparently vigorous meconium-stained neonate: Results of the multicenter, international collaborative trial. Pediatrics 2000;105(1 Pt 1):1–7.
19. Halliday H, Sweet D: Endotracheal intubation at birth for preventing morbidity and mortality in vigorous, meconium-stained infants born at term. Cochrane Library issue 1;2005.
20. Milner AD, Vyas H, Hopkin IE: Efficacy of facemask resuscitation at birth. BMJ 1984;289(6458):1563–1565.
21. Niermeyer S, Van Reempts P, Kattwinkel J, et al: Resuscitation of newborns. Ann Emerg Med 2001;37(4 Suppl):S110–S125.
22. Saugstad OD, Rootwelt T, Aalen O: Resuscitation of asphyxiated newborn infants with room air or oxygen: An international controlled trial. The Resair 2 study. Pediatrics 1988;102:e1.
23. American Academy of Pediatrics and American College of Obstetrics and Gynecology: Guidelines for Prenatal Care, 2nd ed. AAP and ACOG 1988, p 247.
24. Lundstrom KE, Pryds O, Greisen G: Oxygen at birth and prolonged cerebral vasoconstriction in preterm infants. Arch Dis Child Fetal Neonatal Ed 1995;73:F81–F86.
25. Ziino AJ, Davies MW, Davis PG: Epinephrine for the resuscitation of apparently stillborn or extremely bradycardic newborn infants. Cochrane Database Syst Rev 2003:CD003849.
26. Royal College of Pediatrics and Child Health, Royal College of Obstetricians and Gynaecologists: Resuscitation of babies at birth. London, BMJ Publishing 1997.
27. Richmond S (ed): Resuscitation at Birth: The Newborn Life Support Provider Course Manual. London, Resuscitation Council 2001.
28. Wiener PC, Hogg MI, Rosen M: Effects of naloxone on pethidine-induced neonatal depression: Part II. Intramuscular naloxone. BMJ 1977;2(6081):229–231.
29. Vohra S, Frent G, Campbell V, et al: Effect of polyethylene occlusive skin wrapping on heat loss in very low birth weight infants at delivery: A randomized trial. J Pediatr 1999;134:547–551.
30. Soll R, Morley C: Prophylactic versus selective use of surfactant in preventing morbidity and mortality in preterm infants. Cochrane Library issue 1:2005.
31. Bjorklund LJ, Werner O: Should we do lung recruitment maneu vers when giving surfactant? Pediatr Res 2001;50:6–7.
32. Eyler FD, Behnke M, Conlon M, et al: Prenatal cocaine use: A comparison of neonates matched on maternal risk factors. Neurotoxicol Teratol 1994;16:81–87.
33. Rogers JF, Graves WL: Risk factors associated with low Apgar scores in a low-income population. Paediatr Perinat Epidemiol 1993;7:205–216.
34. Bowman J: The management of hemolytic disease in the fetus and newborn. Semin Perinatol 1997;21:39–44.
35. Saugstad OD: Resuscitation of newborn infants with room air or oxygen. Semin Neonatol 2001;6:233–239.
36. Silverman WA, Blanc WA: The effect of humidity on the survival of newly born premature infants. Pediatrics 1957;20:477–487.

APPENDIX

Normal Values

CONTENTS

INTRODUCTION

What Is a "Normal" Value?

"Normal" has different meanings. In the context of physical or laboratory measurements, "normal" may mean "average," "disease-free," or "within a given statistical range." However, it is important to know the characteristics of the population yielding "normal" values before deciding whether these values provide an appropriate reference range with respect to an individual. Many laboratories now print reference ranges on their reports and highlight test values that fall outside these values as "abnormal." When the test subject is a pregnant woman, a fetus, or a newborn, and the reference population is composed predominantly of middle-aged men, then comparisons are patently inappropriate. It is important to understand how the physiologic changes of pregnancy affect the results of various tests and measurements before deciding whether an out-of-range result is actually abnormal.

Changes in Pregnancy

Pregnancy results in profound changes in maternal physiology and metabolism, orchestrated by hormonal changes. Thus, physical and laboratory measurements may be very different in the pregnant state compared with the nonpregnant state and may change as pregnancy advances. Similarly, physical, biochemical, hormonal, and hematologic measurements of the fetus change markedly as the fetus increases in size and maturity. Thanks to ultrasound techniques, the fetus, once hidden within the uterus, is now accessible. Fetal structures can be measured, fetal behavior observed, and blood velocity measured with Doppler ultrasound, and a sampling needle can be used to access blood, liquor, urine, and placental and other tissues.

Statistical Terms

The terms used to define normal values depend on the distribution characteristics of data points. The entire range of values encountered in a healthy population may be quoted as reference points, or distribution may be described by terms that express central tendency and scatter. When data are distributed symmetrically around a central value (i.e., normal distribution), mean, standard deviation (SD), and standard error of the mean (SEM) are the appropriate statistics. From these, ranking values, or percentiles, may be calculated (e.g., 5th and 95th percentiles, which encompass the central 90% of data points, with 5% on either side of them). When the data distribution is skewed, median and percentiles should be used. When the data distribution is exponential, median and multiples of the median (MOM) can be used rather than percentiles. Specialized texts provide a more detailed critical appraisal of the statistical analyses used in these studies (Altman, 1991).

Study Methods Used to Derive Normal Values During Pregnancy

Two basic designs are used for studies addressing changes in physical or laboratory values during pregnancy.

1. Longitudinal studies follow a group of women sequentially through pregnancy and compare measurements of a particular parameter with those obtained well before or at an interval after the pregnancy. Because these studies are very labor-intensive and require committed research subjects, they usually do not involve large numbers of subjects. They are very effective at showing changes with time, either between the nonpregnant and pregnant states or with advancing gestation. The variability of the data is small because the same subjects are studied sequentially. These studies are very helpful in showing how pregnancy affects measurement of a particular parameter. This benefit has particular relevance when prepregnancy values are known and the effect of pregnancy must be differentiated from disease-related changes over time. A limitation of longitudinal studies is that a narrow range of "normal" values is defined from a small number of subjects. This narrow range may not correspond to the wider range of values found in a larger group of healthy subjects studied on a single occasion.
2. Cross-sectional studies involve large numbers of subjects, each contributing one data point to the study. If the number of study subjects is large enough, then the findings provide a good idea of the true scatter of data points. These studies allow accurate characterization of mean values, standard deviations, and percentiles. For pregnancy studies, subjects must be evenly distributed throughout gestation and values must not be extrapolated beyond the gestational range actually included. These studies are essential when the ranking of a particular measurement must be determined (e.g., fetal ultrasonic measurement of abdominal circumference for a known gestational age). Most studies of fetal ultrasonic measurements and Doppler waveform indices are of this design, and their statistical methods have been described in detail (Altman and Chitty, 1994).

Opportunistic studies are also used. For example, fetal blood sampling may be done to identify infection or karyotype in a fetus unaffected by the condition. The portion of the blood sample that is not used for specific tests can be used to measure other substances. Much information available about fetal hematologic, biochemical, and endocrine function has been collected in this way. There are obvious ethical concerns about planning studies in normal fetuses requiring invasive sampling because of the risks of fetal injury and loss. However, the selection of fetuses for study after exclusion of a particular problem means that they are not truly normal or representative of the entire fetal population. Opportunistic studies do not cover the entire range of gestational ages. Nevertheless, they provide information that would not be known otherwise.

The pregnancy studies in the literature are of mixed quality in terms of numbers of subjects included, selection criteria for subjects, sampling and laboratory techniques, and statistical interpretation. The best studies found are reported here. The methods used for each study included are described briefly and presented alongside the results. Comment sections provide interpretation of the data or a discussion of the robustness of the statistical methods, and references to the original papers are given for readers who wish to explore in greater detail. Few studies address the possible effect of maternal age, gravidity, or ethnic differences on the parameters under study. Data on many normal ranges are deficient or limited and are occasionally unreliable.

Use of Normal Ranges in Pregnancy

Some disease states are diagnosed from characteristic symptoms or signs, but others have agreed biochemical definitions. For example, diabetes mellitus is diagnosed with reference to fasting blood glucose measurements and those after a known glucose challenge (see Fig. 24). These values represent the upper limits of the normal ranges found in studies of healthy subjects. Differences in blood glucose values in pregnancy led to the suggestion that diagnostic criteria for diabetes should be adjusted in pregnancy.

Disease or organ dysfunction does not always occur at a given value of a physical or laboratory measurement outside its derived normal range. Elevated liver enzyme levels indicative of liver cell dysfunction may be 2, 10, or 50 times the normal values. However, even minimal deviation of pH from its closely clustered normal values may be biologically important.

Another use of normal values is to calculate odds ratios. Assessment of the risk or likelihood of genetic abnormalities (e.g., Down syndrome) is possible from measurement of serum α-fetoprotein, chorionic gonadotropin, or placental protein A (see Figs. 44–46). Measured values of these hormones are compared with expected values at known gestational age (derived from healthy pregnancies). The degree of difference is expressed in terms of multiples of the median values. Absolute values cannot be used for mathematical calculations because these hormonal concentrations change with gestation. For each hormone, multiple regression analysis has shown the relationships between deviations in values and the risk of Down syndrome. Thus, a woman's age-related risk of aneuploidy may be adjusted after measurement of serum hormones (Wald and associates, 1996).

Units of Measurement

When possible, both SI and traditional units are given for ease of interpretation. It is important to check the units of measurement carefully when comparing a physical or laboratory value with a normal range. In SI units, grams (g) and liters (L) are used, whereas traditional units commonly use milligrams (mg) and deciliters (dL). To avoid errors of interpretation, the prefixes d-, m-, μ-, and n-, signifying 10^{-1}, 10^{-3}, 10^{-6}, and 10^{-9} must be observed and used with care.

The terminology milliequivalents (mEq) has not been used because it has been superseded by millimoles (mmol). For monovalent ions (Na^+, K^+, Cl^-), 1 mmol = 1 mEq. For divalent ions (Mg^{2+}, Ca^{2+}, PO_4^{2+}, SO_4^{2-}), 1 mmol = 2 mEq.

FURTHER READING

Altman DG: Practical Statistics for Medical Research. London, Chapman and Hall, 1991.

Altman DG, Chitty LS: Charts of fetal size: 1. Methodology. BJOG 1994;101:29–34.

Wald NJ, George L, Smith D, et al: Serum screening for Down's syndrome between 8 and 14 weeks of pregnancy. BJOG 1996; 103:407–412.

MATERNAL VALUES

Physiology

Nutrition

WEIGHT GAIN

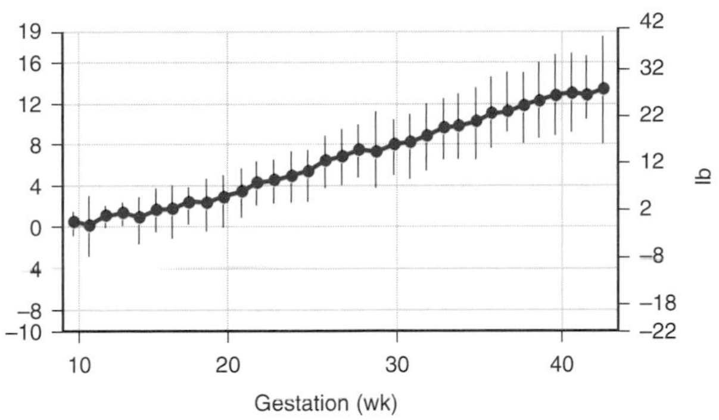

FIGURE 1
Longitudinal study of maternal weight gain (mean ± SD) in 988 normal women who had uneventful pregnancies. All of the study subjects underwent initial evaluation at less than 20 weeks' gestation and were delivered between 37 and 41 weeks. *Data source:* ref. 1, with permission.

Weight-for-height category	Recommended total weight gain	
	kg	lb
Low (BMI <19.8)	12.5–18	28–40
Normal (BMI 19.8–26.0)	11.5–16	25–35
High (BMI 26.0–29.0)	7–11.5	15–25
Obese (BMI >29.0)	7	15
BMI = weight/height^2		

FIGURE 2
Recommended ranges for total weight gain during pregnancy for women with a singleton gestation, classified by prepregnancy body mass index (BMI). *Data source:* ref. 2, with permission.

Comment: Average total weight gain during pregnancy is approximately 10 kg. Low weight gain during pregnancy in nonobese women has been associated with delivery of small-for-gestational-age infants.[3] However, overweight women often deliver large-for-gestational-age infants, regardless of their weight gain during pregnancy.[3]

NUTRITIONAL REQUIREMENTS

Nutritional requirements		
Nutrient (unit)	Pregnant	Lactating
Energy (kcal)	+300	+500
Protein (g)	60	65
Fat-soluable vitamins		
Vitamin A (µg retinol equivalents)	800	1300
Vitamin D (µg as cholecalciferol)	10	10
Vitamin E (mg α-tocopherol equivalents)	10	12
Vitamin K (µg)	65	65
Water-soluable vitamins		
Vitamin C (mg)	70	95
Thiamin (mg)	1.5	1.6
Riboflavin (mg)	1.6	1.8
Niacin (mg niacin equivalent)	17	20
Vitamin B_6 (mg)	2.2	2.1
Folate (µg)	400	280
Vitamin B_{12} (µg)	2.2	2.6
Minerals		
Calcium (mg)	1200	1200
Phosphorous (mg)	1200	1200
Magnesium (mg)	300	355
Iron (mg)	30	15
Zinc (mg)	15	19
Iodine (µg)	175	200
Selenium (µg)	65	75

FIGURE 3
Recommended daily dietary allowance and energy intake for pregnant and lactating women. These should be used as a guide to nutritional requirements when formulating a balanced diet. *Data source:* ref. 4, with permission.

Comment: The increased requirements for vitamins and minerals during pregnancy can usually be met through the diet. Therefore, routine supplementation with multivitamin preparations is not necessary. However, periconceptual supplementation with folic acid for all women is now advocated in an attempt to reduce the incidence of neural tube defects. Vitamin supplementation should be considered in women with inadequate standard diets, heavy smokers, those who abuse drugs or alcohol, and those with multiple pregnancies. Excessive intake (i.e., more than twice the recommended daily allowance) of fat- or water-soluble vitamins may have toxic effects.

Cardiovascular Function

BLOOD PRESSURE

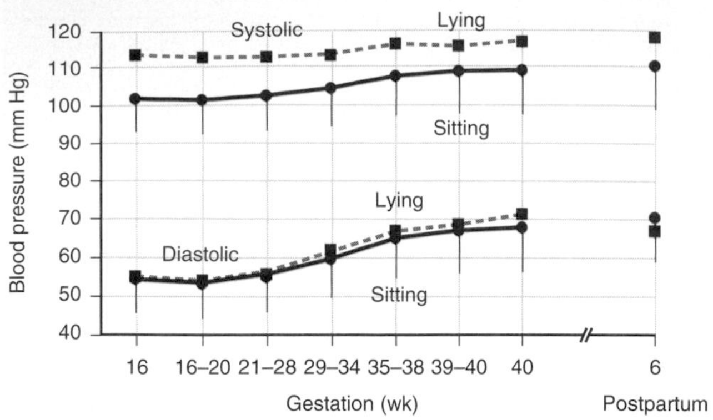

FIGURE 4
Blood pressure measurements (mean and standard deviation) from a longitudinal study of 226 primigravidae whose first attendance at the antenatal clinic was before 20 weeks' gestation. Their mean age was 24.3 years (SD, 4.9). Blood pressure measurements were taken with the London School of Hygiene sphygmomanometer to avoid terminal digit preference and observer bias. Diastolic pressures were recorded at the point of muffling (phase 4). *Data source:* ref. 5, with permission.

> **Comment:** Systolic pressure changes little during pregnancy, but diastolic pressure decreases markedly toward midpregnancy, then rises to near nonpregnant levels by term. Thus, widening of pulse pressure occurs for most of pregnancy.

PULSE RATE

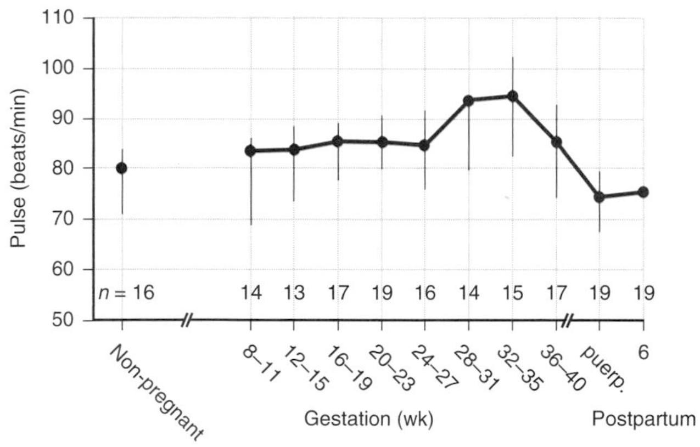

FIGURE 5
Pulse rate (median and interquartile ranges) from a longitudinal study of 20 healthy women recruited in early pregnancy and studied every 2 weeks thereafter. "Nonpregnant" measurements were made 8 to 12 months after delivery. All women finished the study, but not all participated in every visit. *Data source:* ref. 6, with permission.

> **Comment:** The typical increase in heart rate during pregnancy is approximately 15 beats/min, beginning as early as 4 weeks after the last menstrual period.[7]

CARDIAC OUTPUT

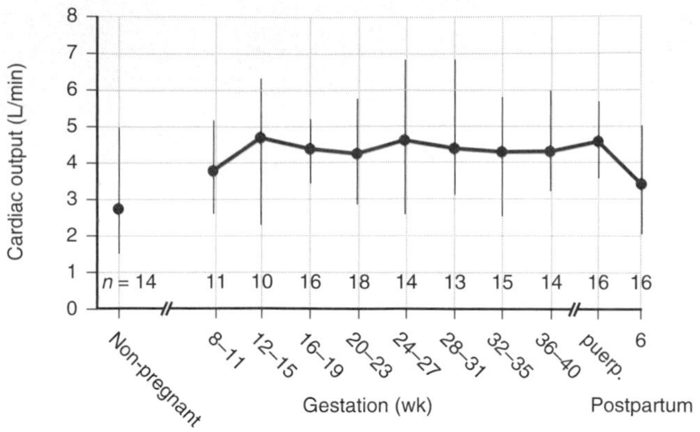

FIGURE 6
Cardiac output (median and interquartile ranges) from a longitudinal study of 20 healthy women recruited in early pregnancy and studied every 2 weeks thereafter. "Nonpregnant" measurements were made 8 to 12 months after delivery. All women finished the study, but not all participated in every visit. Cardiac output was measured by an indirect Fick method. *Data source:* ref. 6, with permission.

> **Comment:** Cardiac output increases significantly during the first trimester and remains elevated until the puerperium. When changes in body weight are considered, it is apparent that cardiac output reaches maximal values at 12 to 15 weeks' gestation and then declines gradually toward term.

INVASIVE MONITORING

Invasive monitoring		
	Non-pregnant	Pregnant
Cardiac output (L/min)	4.3 ± 0.9	6.2 ± 1.0
Heart rate (beats/min)	71 ± 10	83 ± 10
Systemic vascular resistance (dyne/sec/cm^5)	1530 ± 520	1210 ± 266
Pulmonary vascular resistance (dyne/sec/cm^5)	119 ± 47	78 ± 22
Colloid oncotic pressure (mm Hg)	20.8 ± 1.0	18.0 ± 1.5
Colloid oncotic pressure—pulmonary capillary wedge pressure (mm Hg)	14.5 ± 2.5	10.5 ± 2.7
Mean arterial pressure (mm Hg)	86.4 ± 7.5	90.3 ± 5.8
Pulmonary capillary wedge pressure (mm Hg)	6.3 ± 2.1	7.5 ± 1.8
Central venous pressure (mm Hg)	3.7 ± 2.6	3.6 ± 2.5
Left ventricular stroke work index (g–m/beat/m^2)	41 ± 8	48 ± 6

FIGURE 7
Findings of a study involving 10 healthy, primigravid women with a singleton pregnancy who were examined at 36 to 38 weeks' gestation and again 11 to 13 weeks postpartum. All women were younger than 26 years old. They did not smoke and were not anemic. Fetal anatomy and growth and amniotic fluid volume were normal. A pulmonary artery catheter was placed through the subclavian vein, and baseline hemodynamic assessment was made in the left lateral position after 30 minutes' rest. Cardiac output was measured with a thermodilution technique. For each subject, the result represented the mean of five independent measurements, with the highest and lowest values excluded. Central pressures were measured over three consecutive respiratory cycles. Results quoted are mean ± SD. *Data source:* ref. 8, with permission.

Comment: Systemic vascular resistance is 21% lower and pulmonary resistance is 34% lower in the late third trimester than in the nonpregnant state. Both colloid oncotic pressure and the colloid oncotic–pulmonary capillary wedge pressure gradient are lower (by 14% and 28%, respectively). Mean arterial pressure, central venous pressure, pulmonary capillary wedge pressure, and left ventricular stroke work index show no significant changes in the third trimester. These results indicate that the systemic and pulmonary vascular beds accommodate higher vascular volumes at normal pressures during pregnancy. The ventricles are dilated, and cardiac contractility does not change significantly. Because the colloid oncotic pressure–pulmonary capillary wedge pressure gradient is reduced in pregnancy, an increase in cardiac preload or an alteration in pulmonary capillary permeability predisposes the patient to pulmonary edema.

Pulmonary Function and Respiration

ARTERIAL BLOOD GASES

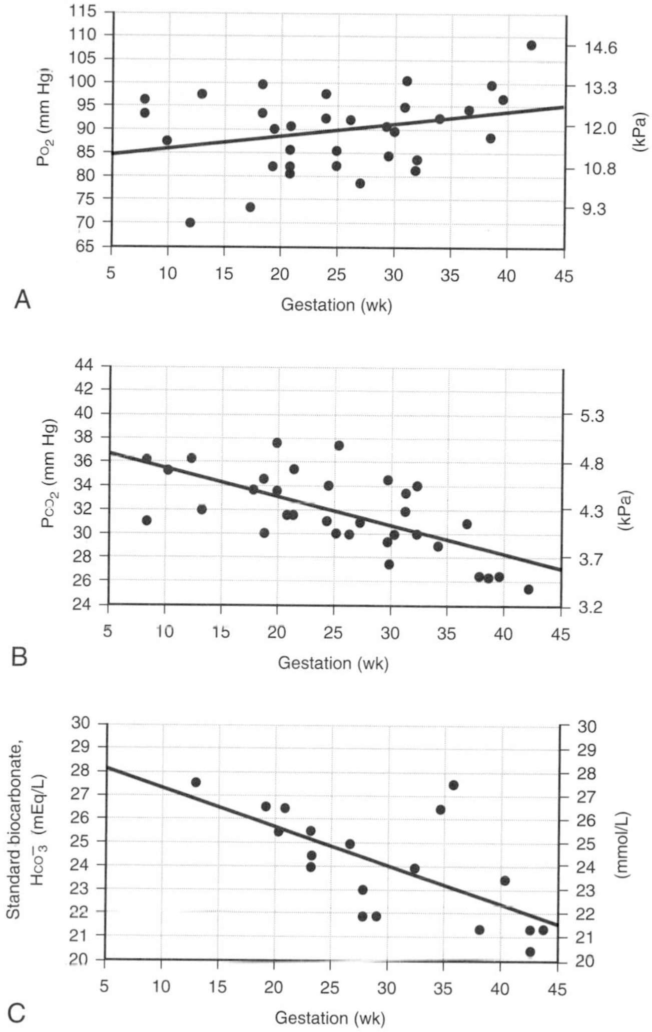

FIGURE 8
Arterial blood gas pressures: *A*, oxygen (Po_2), *B*, carbon dioxide (Pco_2), and *C*, standard bicarbonate (individual values, with regression lines shown) from a cross-sectional study of 37 women at 8 to 42 weeks' gestation. Blood sampling was done from a cannula inserted into the brachial artery under local anesthesia, after 30 minutes' rest in a quiet, darkened room. *Data source:* ref. 9, with permission of Elsevier Science NL, Amsterdam, The Netherlands.

Comment: Arterial pH was constant (7.47) during pregnancy in this study. Pco_2 and standard bicarbonate levels showed a significant decrease with advancing gestation, but Po_2 levels did not change significantly.

TRANSCUTANEOUS GASES

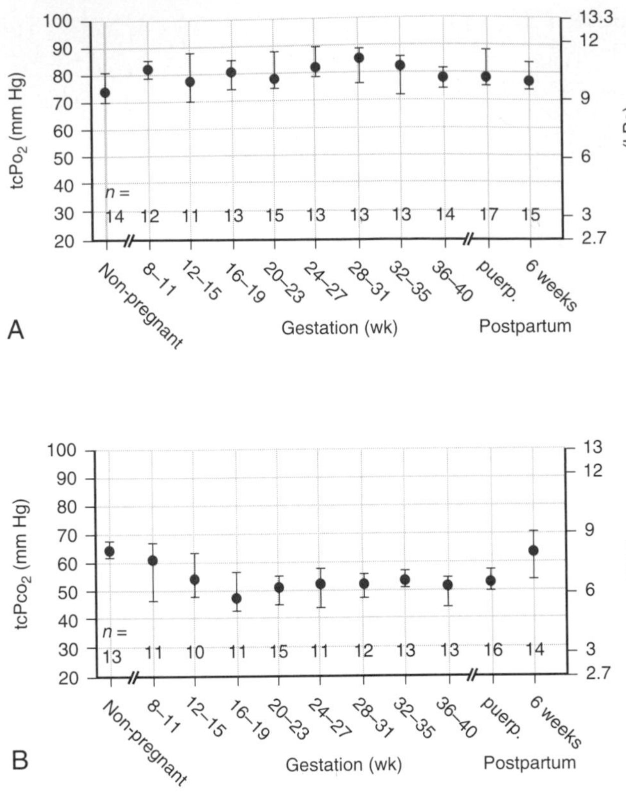

FIGURE 9
A, Transcutaneous oxygen (tcPO_2) and *B*, carbon dioxide (tcPCO_2) pressures (median and interquartile ranges) from a longitudinal study of 20 healthy women recruited in early pregnancy and studied every 2 weeks thereafter. Nonpregnant measurements were made 8 to 12 months after delivery. All women finished the study, but not all participated in every visit. *Data source:* ref. 6, with permission.

> ***Comment:*** Transcutaneous PCO_2 is higher than arterial PCO_2 as a result of temperature differences between the skin surface and blood as well as the addition of CO_2 by skin metabolism (conversion factor, approximately 1.4).[6] Transcutaneous PO_2 values in adults are 10% to 20% lower than arterial PO_2 values. In this study, the increase in tcPO_2 and the decrease in tcPCO_2 during pregnancy were significant.

RESPIRATION RATE

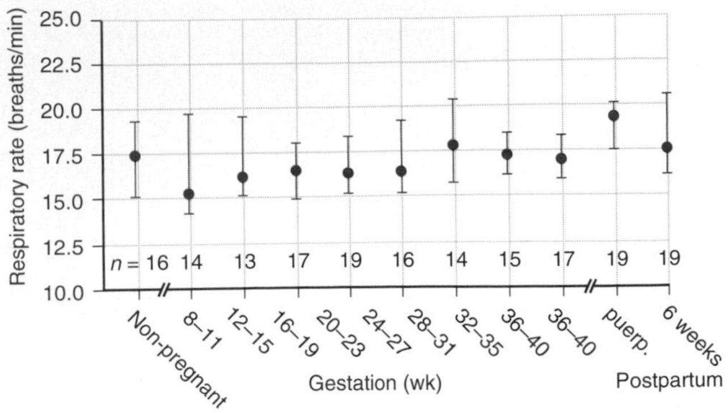

FIGURE 10
Respiration rate (median and interquartile ranges) from a longitudinal study of 20 healthy women recruited in early pregnancy and studied every 2 weeks thereafter; nonpregnant measurements were made 8 to 12 months after delivery. All women finished the study, but not all participated in every visit. *Data source:* ref. 6, with permission.

> ***Comment:*** The respiration rate is similar in pregnant and nonpregnant women.

TIDAL VOLUME

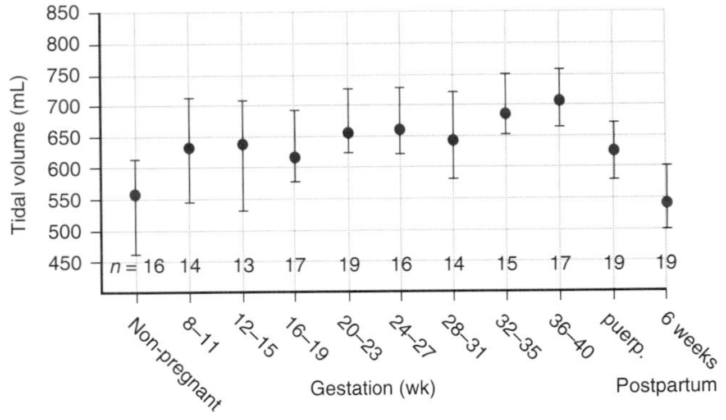

FIGURE 11
Tidal volume (median and interquartile ranges) from a longitudinal study of 20 healthy women recruited in early pregnancy and studied every 2 weeks thereafter. Nonpregnant measurements were made 8 to 12 months after delivery. All women finished the study, but not all participated in every visit. *Data source:* ref. 6, with permission.

> ***Comment:*** Tidal volume increases early in pregnancy and continues to rise until term; overall, a 30% to 40% rise occurs. By 6 to 8 weeks postpartum, tidal volumes return to nonpregnant values. Minute ventilation increases in parallel with tidal volume; typical values are 7.5 L/min in nonpregnant women and 10.5 L/min in late pregnancy.[10]

RESPIRATORY FUNCTION TESTS

Respiratory function tests				
	During pregnancy			After delivery
	10 weeks	24 weeks	36 weeks	10 weeks postpartum
Vital capacity (L)	3.8	3.9	4.1	3.8
Inspiratory capacity (L)	2.6	2.7	2.9	2.5
Expiratory reserve volume (L)	1.2	1.2	1.2	1.3
Residual volume (L)	1.2	1.1	1.0	1.2

FIGURE 12
Respiratory volumes (mean values) from a longitudinal study of eight healthy women 18 to 29 years old who were studied through pregnancy and again 10 weeks postpartum. All tests were done with the patient in the sitting position. *Data source:* ref. 10, with permission.

Comment: In some women, vital capacity increases by 100 to 200 mL during pregnancy, but the converse is seen in obese women.[11] Anatomic changes (flaring of the lower ribs, a rise in the diaphragm, and an increase in the transverse diameter of the chest) are responsible for alterations in lung volume subdivisions.[11] Forced expiratory volume in 1 second (FEV_1) and peak expiratory flow rate (PEFR) are unaffected by normal pregnancy.[10] The gas transfer factor (i.e., pulmonary diffusing capacity with carbon monoxide) decreases in pregnancy.[10] This decrease has been attributed to altered mucopolysaccharides in the alveolar capillary walls as well as lower circulating levels of hemoglobin.

Chromosomal Abnormalities

Maternal age at delivery (years)	Risk of Down's syndrome
15	1 : 1578
20	1 : 1528
25	1 : 1351
30	1 : 909
31	1 : 796
32	1 : 683
33	1 : 574
34	1 : 474
35	1 : 384
36	1 : 307
37	1 : 242
38	1 : 189
39	1 : 146
40	1 : 112
41	1 : 85
42	1 : 65
43	1 : 49
44	1 : 37
45	1 : 28
46	1 : 21
47	1 : 15
48	1 : 11
49	1 : 8
50	1 : 6

FIGURE 13
The risk of having a pregnancy affected by Down syndrome according to maternal age at the time of birth. *Data source:* ref. 12, with permission.

Maternal age	Rate per 1000				
	Trisomy 21	Trisomy 18	Trisomy 13	XXY	All chromosomal anomalies
35	3.9	0.5	0.2	0.5	8.7
36	5.0	0.7	0.3	0.6	10.1
37	6.4	1.0	0.4	0.8	12.2
38	8.1	1.4	0.5	1.1	14.8
39	10.4	2.0	0.8	1.4	18.4
40	13.3	2.8	1.1	1.8	23.0
41	16.9	3.9	1.5	2.4	29.0
42	21.6	5.5	2.1	3.1	37.0
43	27.4	7.6		4.1	45.0
44	34.8			5.4	50.0
45	44.2			7.0	62.0
46	55.9			9.1	77.0
47	70.4			11.9	96.0

FIGURE 14
Chromosomal abnormalities by maternal age at the time of amniocentesis performed at 16 weeks' gestation (expressed as rate per 1000). *Data source:* ref. 13, with permission.

Comment: The incidence of chromosomal disorders increases with maternal age but is not affected by paternal age.[13] Trisomy 21 (Down syndrome) is the most important numerically of these disorders, with an overall population incidence of 1 in 650 live births. Trisomies 13, 18, and 22 are rare in live births. Other autosomal trisomies are nonviable and are common in spontaneous abortions.

Biochemistry

Hepatic Function

TOTAL SERUM PROTEIN AND ALBUMIN

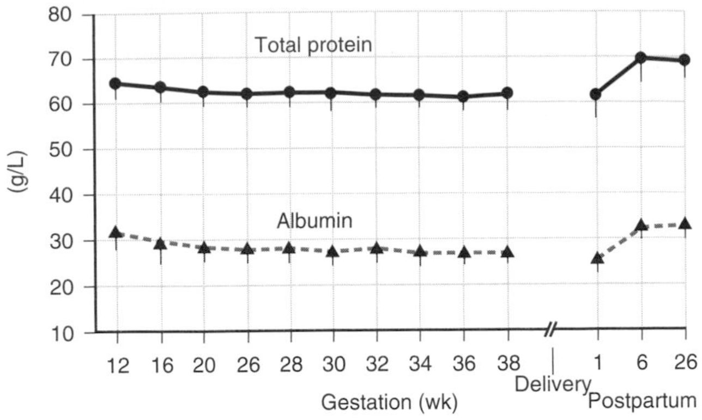

FIGURE 15
Total serum protein and albumin (mean and SD) from a longitudinal study of 83 healthy pregnant women (77 of whom were primigravidae) who were recruited at 12 weeks' gestation. Samples were collected every 4 weeks during pregnancy, 7 days postpartum, and again 6 and 26 weeks postpartum. *Data source:* ref. 14, with permission.

> ***Comment:*** Decreased total serum protein and albumin concentrations in pregnancy are associated with a decrease in colloid osmotic pressure.[14] Serum immunoglobulin levels do not change significantly in pregnancy.[15]

LIVER ENZYMES, SERUM BILE ACIDS, BILIRUBIN, AMYLASE, COPPER, AND ZINC

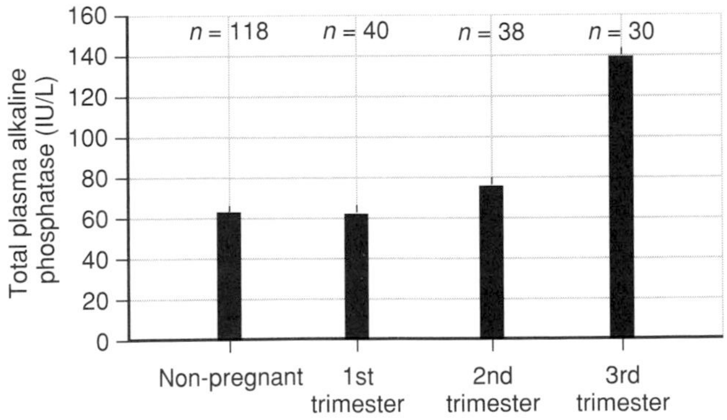

FIGURE 16
Total alkaline phosphatase levels (mean and SEM) from a cross-sectional study of 108 women attending a hospital antenatal clinic in Nigeria. The nonpregnant control subjects of similar age were patients attending the gynecologic clinic. No patients were clinically anemic, and all were normotensive. *Data source:* ref. 16, with permission.

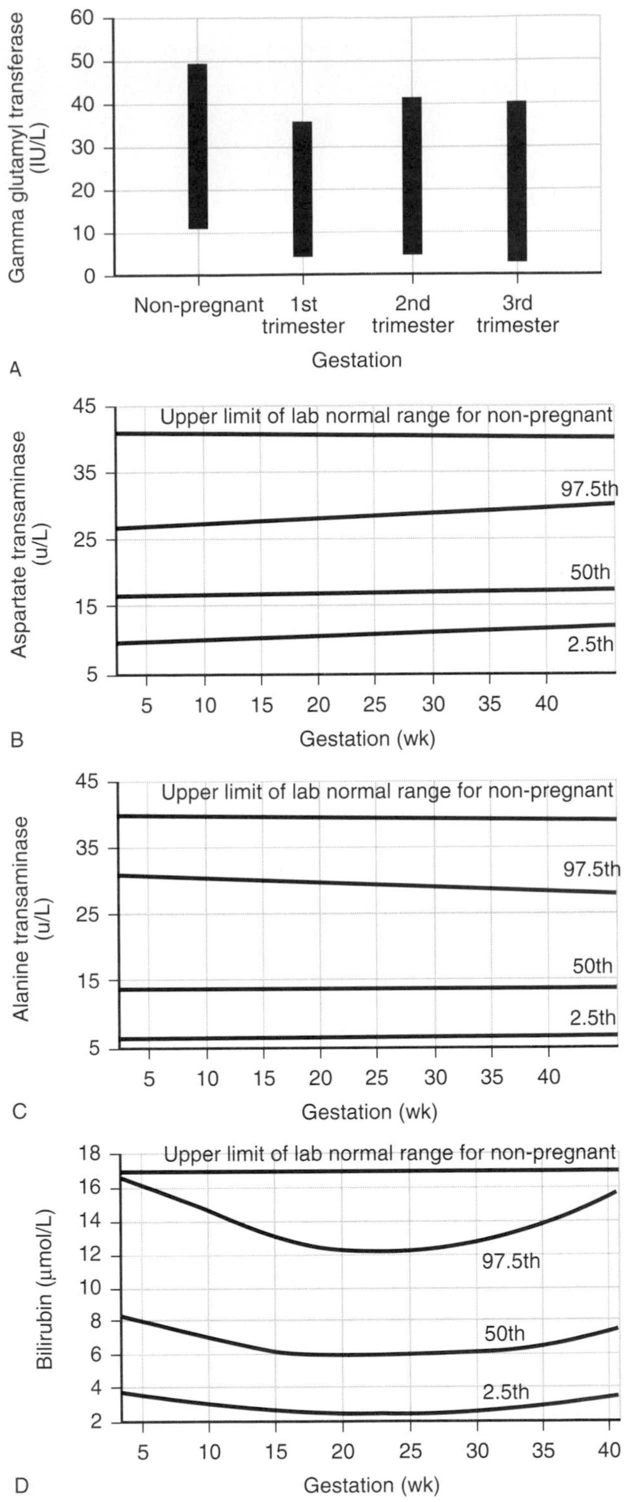

FIGURE 17
A, Serum γ-glutamyl transferase (GGT), *B*, aspartate transaminase (AST), *C*, alanine transaminase (ALT), and *D*, bilirubin (95% reference ranges) from a cross-sectional study of 430 women with uncomplicated singleton pregnancies. No subjects had hypertension or liver disease, were taking drugs associated with liver dysfunction, or were consuming more than 10 units of alcohol weekly. Data for GGT were not normally distributed, and the results presented are calculated from the nonparametric determination of percentiles. Data for AST, ALT, and bilirubin were normally distributed after logarithmic transformation, allowing gestation-specific percentiles to be calculated. *Data source:* ref. 17, with permission.

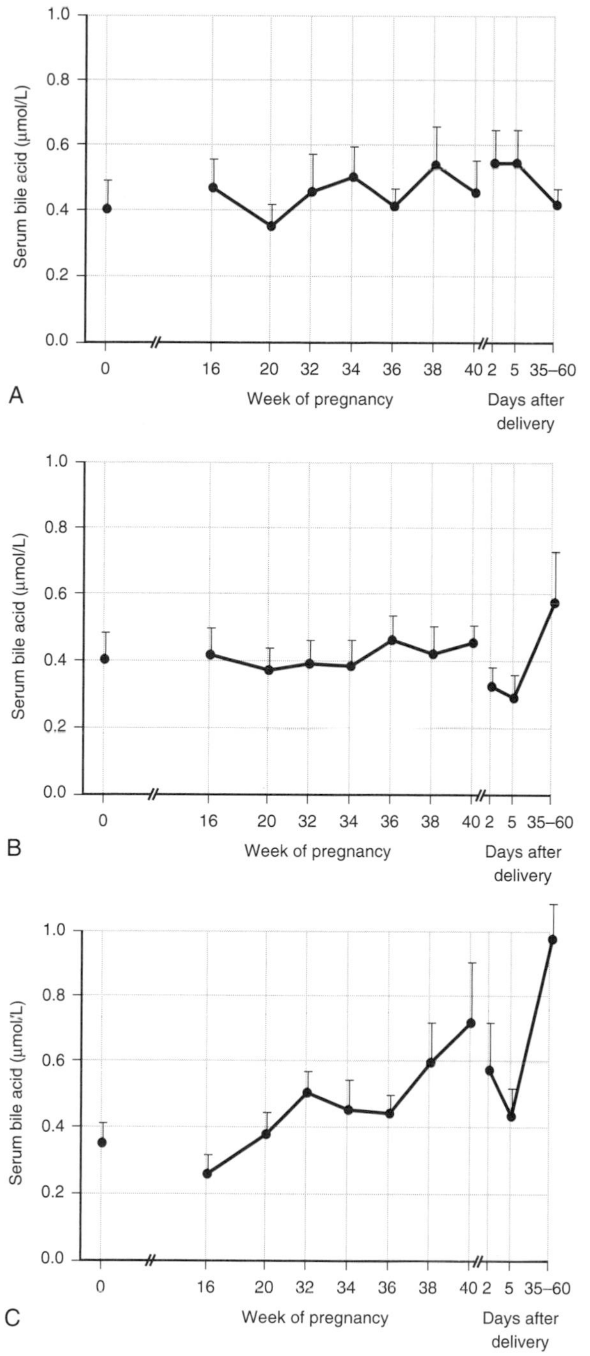

FIGURE 18

A, Serum cholic acid (CA), *B*, deoxycholic acid (DCA), and *C*, chenodeoxycholic acid (CDCA) (mean and SD) from a longitudinal study of 30 healthy pregnant women. The subjects had uncomplicated pregnancies and no history of hepatobiliary disease. Blood samples were taken after an overnight fast. Most women were recruited at 12 to 17 weeks' gestation and gave blood samples at 18 to 22 weeks, every 2 weeks in the third trimester, and on three occasions up to 35 to 60 days after delivery. Bile acids were measured separately by radioimmunoassay, and the results presented are for total concentrations (i.e., free plus conjugated bile acid). *Data source:* ref. 18, with permission.

Comment: Total plasma alkaline phosphatase (AP) levels are approximately doubled by late pregnancy. Almost half of the total plasma AP in pregnancy is placental AP isoenzyme, but bone AP isoenzyme levels are also markedly increased. Liver AP isoenzyme levels do not change significantly in pregnancy.[16] Serum γ-glutamyl transferase (GGT) and transaminase levels overall are lower in pregnancy than in the nonpregnant adult population. There are no significant gestational changes in GGT, AST, or ALT, but all increase after delivery, especially after cesarean section.[19] During pregnancy, bilirubin levels remain within the normal range for adults.[20] Serum concentrations of the primary bile acid, cholic acid (CA), and the secondary bile acid, deoxycholic acid (DCA), do not change during pregnancy, but chenodeoxycholic acid (CDCA) levels increase significantly toward term.[18] These minor changes in serum bile acid levels may be caused by changes in bile acid metabolism and excretion as a result of high circulating levels of estrogen and progesterone, but may show a tendency to cholestasis in normal pregnancy. No data are available on serum amylase in pregnancy, but decreased concentrations may be expected as a dilutional effect. Serum copper levels are increased in pregnancy, but zinc levels are decreased compared with those in nonpregnant women.[21] There are considerable differences between laboratories with regard to liver enzyme assays and resultant variability in "normal ranges" in adults. These differences should be borne in mind when interpreting individual results from pregnant women.

LIPIDS: CHOLESTEROL AND TRIGLYCERIDE

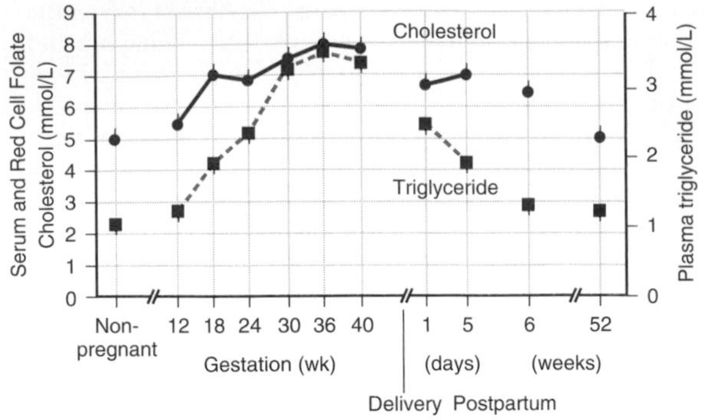

FIGURE 19
Plasma cholesterol and triglyceride levels (mean and SEM) from a longitudinal study of 43 women 20 to 41 years old. Samples were taken after an overnight fast and 10 minutes' supine rest at 4- to 6-week intervals through pregnancy, during labor, and in the puerperium. Samples were also taken 12 months after delivery in 14 of the subjects. The nonpregnant reference samples were obtained from 15 subjects of comparable age. No dietary restrictions were imposed. *Data source:* ref. 22, with permission. *Conversion factors:* cholesterol, mmol/L × 38.5 = mg/dL; triglyceride, mmol/L × 88 = mg/dL.

Comment: During pregnancy, plasma cholesterol doubles and a threefold increase in plasma triglyceride concentration occurs. The lipid content of low-density lipoproteins increases in pregnancy, as does the high-density lipoprotein triglyceride content.[22] Serum lipid levels decrease rapidly after delivery, but cholesterol and triglyceride concentrations remain elevated 6 to 7 weeks postpartum. Lactation does not affect lipid levels.[22]

Renal Function

SERUM URATE

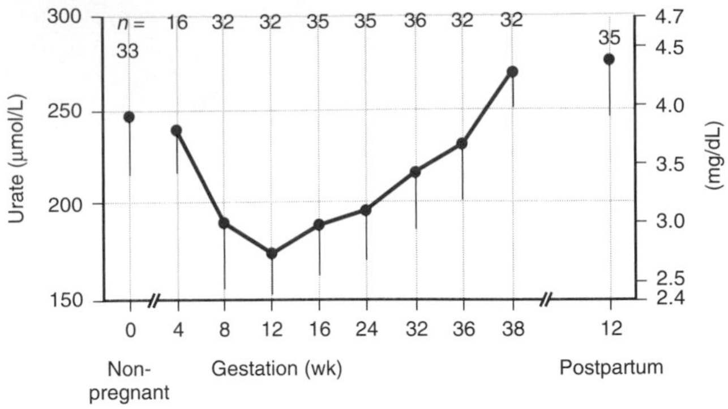

FIGURE 20
Serum urate levels (mean and SD) from a longitudinal study of 31 healthy women 23 to 37 years old, five of whom were studied during two pregnancies. Subjects were studied preconceptually, at least 3 months after discontinuing oral contraceptives (if used), in the luteal phase of their menstrual cycle, monthly during pregnancy, and again 12 weeks postpartum. All samples were taken between 9:00 AM and 9:30 AM, after overnight fasting. *Data source:* ref. 23, with permission.

Comment: Serum urate levels decrease during the first trimester, probably as a result of altered renal handling of uric acid.[23] During late pregnancy, the serum urate level increases to levels higher than nonpregnant values at term. Levels may remain elevated for 12 weeks after delivery.[23]

SERUM OSMOLALITY, ELECTROLYTES, AND UREA

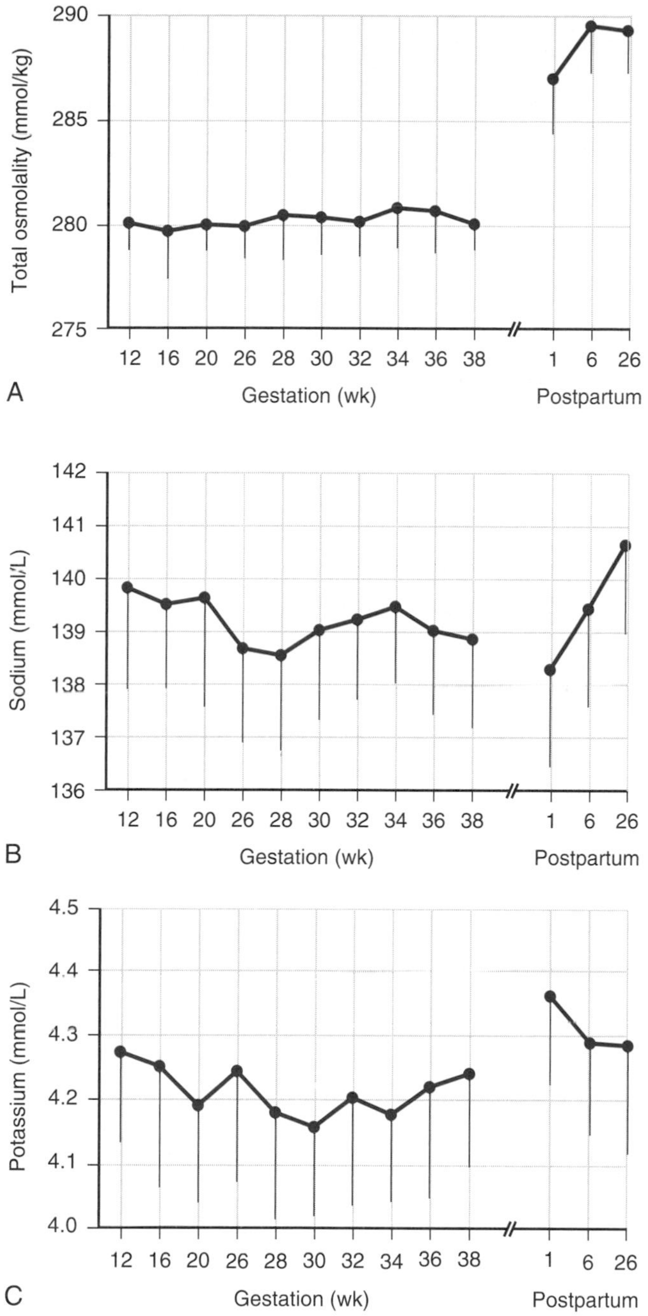

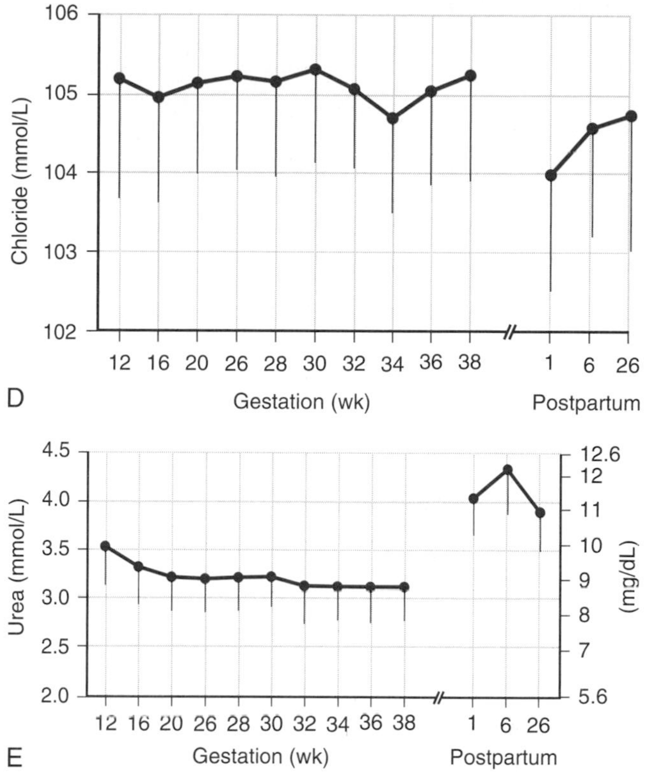

FIGURE 21

Serum osmolality (*A*), electrolytes (*B–D*), and urea (*E*), (mean and SD) from a longitudinal study of 83 healthy pregnant women (77 of whom were primigravidae), recruited at 12 weeks' gestation. Samples were collected every 4 weeks during pregnancy, 7 days postpartum, and then 6 and 26 weeks postpartum. *Data source:* ref. 14, with permission.

Comment: Total osmolality decreases by the end of the first trimester to a nadir 8 to 10 mmol/kg below nonpregnant values. Concentrations of the major serum electrolytes (sodium, potassium, chloride) are almost unchanged during pregnancy. Bicarbonate and phosphate concentrations decrease during pregnancy.[24] Plasma urea and creatinine decrease during pregnancy; typical mean (SD) values for plasma creatinine are 60 (8), 54 (10), and 64 (9) μmol/L in the first, second, and third trimesters, respectively, increasing to 73 (10) μmol/L by 6 weeks postpartum[25,26] (see also Fig. 22b).

CREATININE CLEARANCE AND PLASMA CREATININE

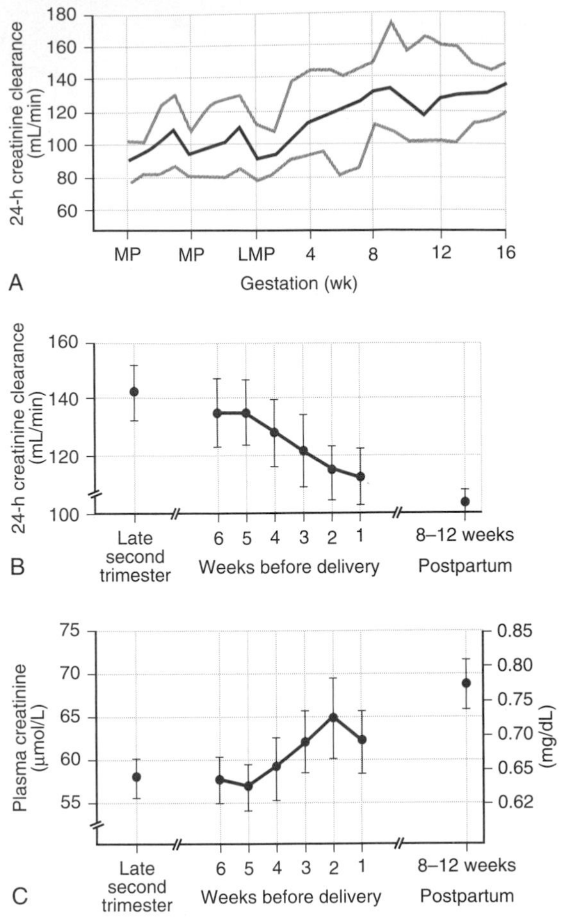

FIGURE 22
A, Creatinine clearance (mean and range) in early pregnancy from a longitudinal study of nine healthy women who were recruited before pregnancy. Measurements of 24-hour creatinine clearance were made weekly, through the different phases of the menstrual cycle, and up to 16 weeks' gestation. No diet, fluid, or exercise restrictions were imposed. *Data source:* ref. 27, with permission. *B*, Creatinine clearance and *C*, plasma creatinine (mean ± SEM) in the second and third trimesters from a longitudinal study of 10 healthy pregnant women. Creatinine clearance was measured once between 25 and 28 weeks' gestation, weekly from 32 weeks until delivery, and once between 8 and 12 weeks postpartum. *Data source:* ref. 28, with permission.

Comment: The glomerular filtration rate (GFR) and effective renal plasma flow increase in early pregnancy to levels approximately 50% above nonpregnant values. In the third trimester, the GFR decreases by approximately 15%.[28] The 24-hour creatinine clearance measurements mirror these changes. During the menstrual cycle, a 20% mean increase in creatinine clearance occurs between the week of menstruation and the late luteal phase.[27]

URINE COMPOSITION: GLUCOSE, AMINO ACIDS, AND PROTEIN

Comment: Glycosuria is common in pregnant women whose plasma glucose concentrations and glucose tolerance test results are normal. It is believed to arise because of increased glomerular filtration plus decreased tubular resorption of glucose.[29] Aminoaciduria is also reported during pregnancy,[30] and urinary albumin excretion is increased.[31]

Carbohydrate Metabolism

FASTING PLASMA GLUCOSE

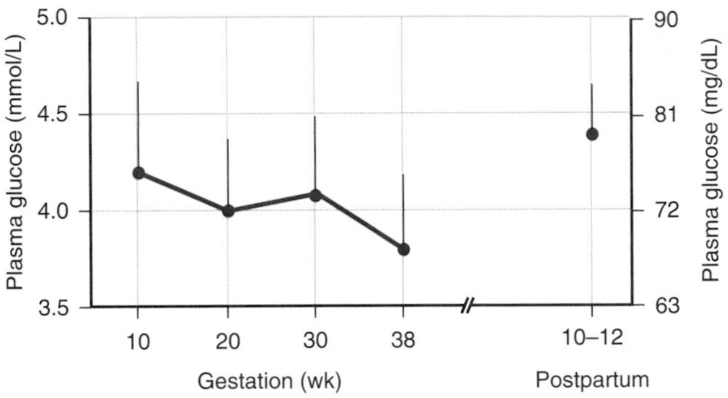

FIGURE 23
Longitudinal study of plasma glucose levels (mean and SD) after an overnight fast of at least 10 hours in 19 healthy women. The subjects were not obese and had no family history of diabetes mellitus. *Data source:* ref. 32, with permission.

Comment: Other studies[33] confirmed these findings that fasting plasma glucose levels decrease in pregnancy. In most women, the decline occurs by the end of the first trimester. Thereafter, most studies show further decreases in the second and third trimesters.[33] Severely obese women (body mass index [BMI] >30.0 kg/m^2) studied throughout pregnancy did not show these changes, but had progressively increasing plasma glucose levels.[33] Plasma insulin levels increase in the third trimester.[32,34] Ethnic differences are seen in insulin production (as measured by C-peptide concentrations) and insulin resistance (as indicated by insulin-to-glucose ratios) during pregnancy.[34]

GLUCOSE TOLERANCE TEST (GTT)

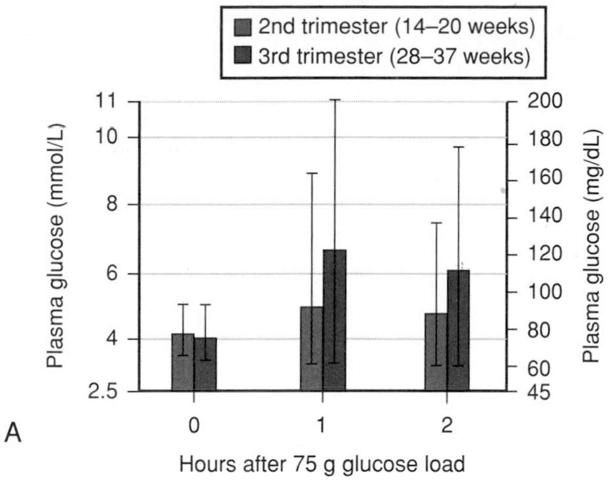

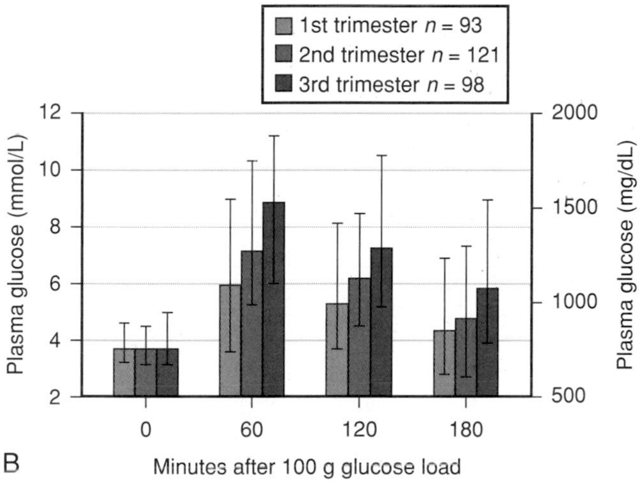

FIGURE 24
A, Plasma glucose values (median, 2.5th, and 97.5th percentiles) after a 75-g oral glucose load. Cross-sectional study of 111 healthy women younger than 35 years old, weighing less than 85 kg, with singleton pregnancies (n = 43 and 168 in the second and third trimesters, respectively). None had a personal or family history of diabetes mellitus. *Data source:* ref. 35, with permission. *B*, Plasma glucose values (median, 5th, and 95th percentiles) after a 100-g oral glucose load. The study involved 93 women in the first trimester, 121 in the second trimester, and 98 in the third trimester. All were healthy, were not obese, had no family history of diabetes, and had no obstetric complications. *Data source:* ref. 36, with permission.

Comment: Women in the third trimester have decreased glucose tolerance, as judged by criteria used to diagnose diabetes outside pregnancy. Gestational diabetes may be diagnosed when two or more of the following plasma glucose levels are found on 100-g GTT: ≥105 mg/dL (fasting), ≥190 mg/dL (1 hour), 165 mg/dL (2 hours), and ≥145 mg/dL (3 hours). These values are 5.8 mmol/L (fasting), 10.6 mmol/L (1 hour), 9.2 mmol/L (2 hours), and 8.1 mmol/L (3 hours).[37]

SERUM FRUCTOSAMINE AND GLYCOSYLATED HEMOGLOBIN

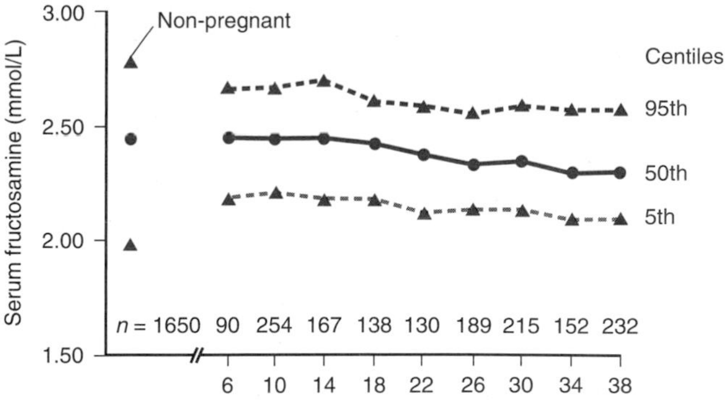

FIGURE 25
Serum fructosamine (median, 5th, and 95th percentiles) from a cross-sectional study of 1200 pregnant women at different gestational ages, compared with 1650 nonpregnant women 15 to 40 years old. Women with known diabetes or previous gestational diabetes were excluded from the study. *Data source:* ref. 38, with permission.

Comment: Serum fructosamine concentrations are significantly lower in the second and third trimesters than in the first trimester or the nonpregnant state. Decreasing total protein and albumin concentrations in pregnancy may contribute to this reduction.[38] In some studies, values for glycosylated hemoglobin (Hb A_1 and Hb A_{1c}) during pregnancy in healthy women were lower in the first and second trimesters,[33,39] but in other studies, they were similar to values in nonpregnant women.[40]

AMNIOTIC FLUID INSULIN, GLUCOSE, AND C-PEPTIDE

Amniotic fluid insulin, glucose, and C-peptide					
		Glucose (nmol/L)	Immunoreactive insulin (pmol/L)	C-peptide (pmol/L)	C-peptide/insulin molar ratio
Early pregnancy	n = 77	3.44 ± 0.22	44.2 ± 2.1	38 ± 2.0	0.97 ± 0.06
Late pregnancy	n = 33	0.72 ± 0.11	45.5 ± 2.6	218 ± 54	4.3 ± 1.2

FIGURE 26
Insulin, glucose, and C-peptide levels in amniotic fluid (mean ± SD) from a cross-sectional study of 110 nondiabetic women who had amniocentesis in pregnancy (mostly for karyotyping). *Data source:* ref. 41, with permission.

Comment: Insulin and C-peptide levels in amniotic fluid can be studied as markers of fetal pancreatic β cell function. C-peptide and insulin are normally secreted in equimolar amounts from β cells. C-peptide may be the more reliable marker because insulin is degraded in the fetal liver and circulating insulin antibodies may be present.[41] In pregnant women with diabetes, concentrations of these substances are greater and third-trimester values are correlated with neonatal complications (macrosomia, hypoglycemia, jaundice, respiratory distress).[42] The midtrimester insulin concentration in amniotic fluid is also greater in women who subsequently had gestational diabetes.[43]

Antioxidants

Comment: In pregnancy, levels of vitamin E (a free radical scavenger that opposes the effects of lipid peroxides) are increased compared with the nonpregnant state.[43] Vitamin E levels increase progressively with gestation, whereas lipid peroxide levels are constant.[44] Ascorbic acid concentrations in maternal serum during the third trimester and in breast milk during lactation are related to dietary consumption of fruit and vegetables.[45]

Hematology

White Blood Cell Count (Total and Differential)

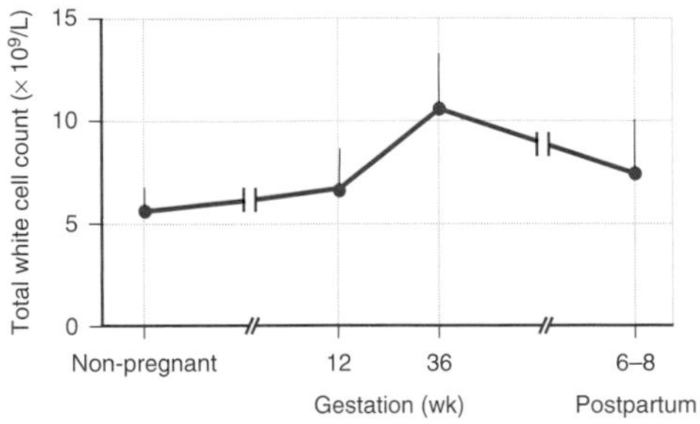

A

	Week 33 (*n* = 151)	Week 36 (*n* = 146)	Week 39 (*n* = 130)	Postpartum (*n* = 91)	Non-pregnant range
Total white cell count (WBC) 10^9/L	9.1 (5.7–14)	8.9 (6.1–15)	9.0 (6.0–16)	16 (9.4–25)	(4.0–9.0)
Neutrophils 10^9/L	6.5 (3.5–11)	6.4 (4.1–11)	6.5 (3.7–13)	14 (6.6–23)	(1.8–6.7)
Lymphocytes 10^9/L	1.7 (0.9–2.8)	1.8 (1.1–2.8)	1.8 (1.1–2.9)	1.1 (0.5–2.4)	(0.8–4.0)
Monocytes 10^9/L	0.50 (0.2–1.0)	0.50 (0.3–1.0)	0.50 (0.28–0.90)	0.53 (0.3–1.2)	(0.10–0.90)
Eosinophils 10^9/L	0.10 (0.0–0.40)	0.10 (0.0–0.30)	0.10 (0.0–0.40)	0.0 (0.0–0.50)	(0.0–0.50)
Basophils 10^9/L	0.0 (0.0–0.10)	0.03 (0.0–0.10)	0.04 (0.0–0.10)	0.08 (0.0–0.20)	(0.0–0.10)

B

FIGURE 27
A, Total white cell count (mean and SD) from a longitudinal study of 24 women who were recruited at 12 weeks and were delivered after 37 weeks. Nonpregnant samples were taken 4 to 6 months after delivery. Samples were analyzed in a Coulter counter. *Data source:* ref. 46, with permission. *B*, Total and differential white cell counts from a semilongitudinal study of 153 healthy pregnant women who were taking iron supplementation. All of the subjects had at least one previous normal pregnancy. Postpartum samples taken from women who were eventually delivered by cesarean section were excluded from analysis. *Data source:* ref. 47, with permission.

Comment: Supplementation with iron and folate does not affect the total white blood cell (WBC) count during or after pregnancy.[46] No studies reported WBC values during labor, but in the early postpartum period, very high values (up to 25 × 10^9/L) may be normal.[47] Pregnancy-related changes in the WBC count are still present 6 to 8 weeks after delivery. Immature granulocytes (myelocytes and metamyelocytes) are often found in peripheral blood smears during pregnancy.[48]

Hemoglobin and Red Blood Cell Indices

Hemoglobin and red blood cell indices				
Parameter	Non-pregnant (SD)	12 weeks (SD)	36 weeks (SD)	Postpartum (SD)
Red blood cell count (× 10^{12}/L)	4.688 (0.309)	4.008 (0.247)	3.880 (0.304)	4.493 (0.338)
Hemoglobin concentration (g/dl)	13.20 (0.77)	12.03 (0.70)	11.07 (0.84)	12.69 (0.92)
Hematocrit (L/L)	0.3936 (0.0233)	0.3515 (0.0226)	0.3311 (0.0232)	0.3787 (0.0289)
Mean cell volume (fL)	83.7 (3.1)	86.2 (3.6)	85.0 (5.3)	84.1 (3.8)
Mean cell hemoglobin (pg)	28.39 (1.06)	30.07 (1.16)	28.65 (2.00)	28.23 (1.45)
Mean cell hemoglobin concentration (g/dl)	33.75 (0.68)	34.23 (1.13)	33.46 (0.82)	33.47 (0.93)

A

Hemoglobin and red blood cell indices				
Parameter	Non-pregnant (SD)	12 weeks (SD)	36 weeks (SD)	Postpartum (SD)
Red blood cell count (× 10^{12}/L)	4.621 (0.238)	4.109 (0.227)	4.119 (0.246)	4.370 (0.169)
Hemoglobin concentration (g/dl)	13.42 (0.66)	12.06 (0.57)	12.66 (0.81)	13.03 (0.45)
Hematocrit (L/L)	0.3971 (0.0190)	0.3539 (0.020)	0.3666 (0.020)	0.3880 (0.0123)
Mean cell volume (fL)	85.7 (2.2)	86.0 (3.3)	88.8 (2.9)	88.4 (3.3)
Mean cell hemoglobin (pg)	29.00 (0.77)	29.43 (1.03)	30.76 (1.24)	29.86 (1.20)
Mean cell hemoglobin concentration (g/dl)	33.63 (0.69)	34.05 (1.08)	34.50 (0.82)	33.59 (0.66)

B

FIGURE 28
A, Hemoglobin and red blood cell indices (mean and SD) from a longitudinal study of women who were recruited at 12 weeks and were delivered after 37 weeks (*n* = 24). No iron or folate supplements were given. Nonpregnant samples were taken 4 to 6 months after delivery. Samples were analyzed in a Coulter counter. *B*, Hemoglobin and red blood cell indices (mean and SD) from a longitudinal study of women who were recruited at 12 weeks and were delivered after 37 weeks (*n* = 21). All were given iron and folate supplements from 12 weeks' gestation. Nonpregnant samples were taken 4 to 6 months after delivery. Samples were analyzed in a Coulter counter. *Data source:* ref. 46, with permission.

Comment: Hemoglobin concentration decreases in the first trimester, regardless of whether iron and folate supplements are given. Pregnancy-induced hematologic changes are still present 6 to 8 weeks postpartum.

Platelet Count and Indices

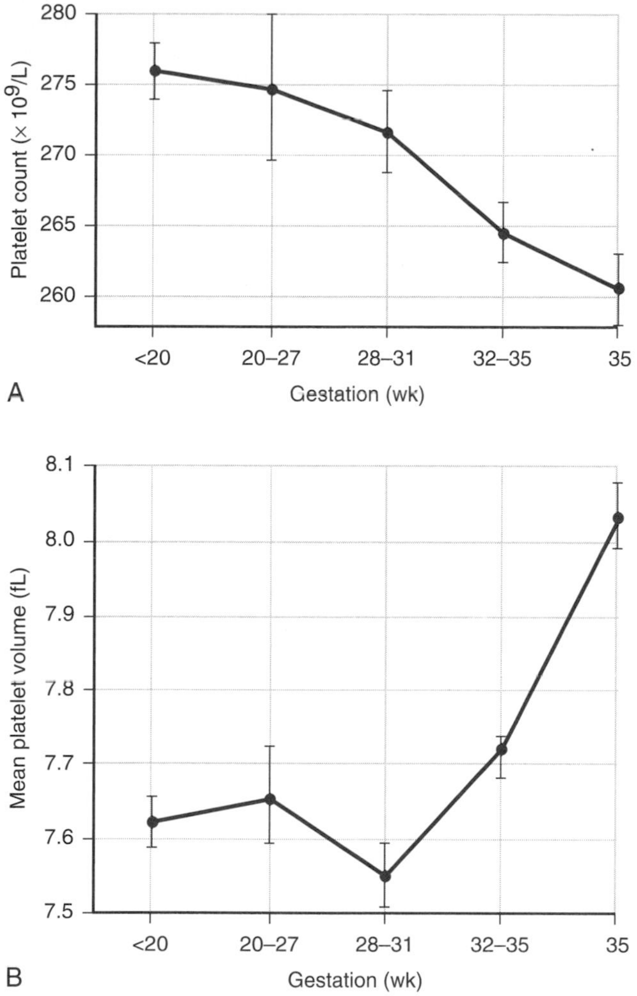

FIGURE 29

A, Platelet count and *B*, mean platelet volume (mean ± SEM) during pregnancy. The study was largely cross-sectional in design (2881 samples from 2114 women). Samples were analyzed in a Coulter counter. At the end of the study, patients who had hypertension were excluded. *Data source:* ref. 49, with permission.

Comment: Hyperdestruction of platelets may occur in pregnancy, with a consequent decrease in platelet life span. Young platelets are larger than old platelets. In a large study of 6770 women in late pregnancy, mean platelet counts were 213×10^9/L and the 2.5th percentile value was 116×10^9/L.[50] Another longitudinal study[51] with much smaller numbers (n = 44) did not find evidence of a significant change in platelet count with gestational age.

Iron Metabolism

Iron metabolism					
Patients	Hb (g/dL)	Serum iron (μmol/L)	Serum iron (mg/dL)	Transferrin/TIBC saturation (%)	Serum ferritin (mg/L)
Non-treated (n = 30)					
First trimester	12.9	23	129	36	96
Term	12.0	14	78	13	13
Given $FeSO_4$ (n = 82)					
First trimester	12.5	22	123	33	67
Term	12.5	25	140	27	41

A

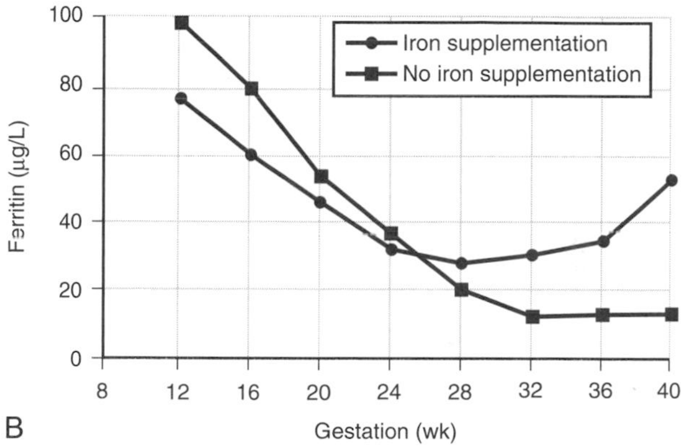

FIGURE 30

A, Mean hemoglobin (Hb) and iron indices from a longitudinal study of women recruited in the first trimester. At the start of the study, 72 were randomized to the no-treatment group, but any whose Hb fell below 11 g/dL were prescribed ferrous sulfate 60 mg three times daily. Only 30 progressed through pregnancy without iron supplements. *B*, In all of the subjects studied, serum ferritin levels rose rapidly postpartum, reaching values similar to those found in early pregnancy by 5 to 8 weeks after delivery. No iron supplements were given after delivery. *Data source:* ref. 52, with permission.

Comment: Iron stores, as indicated by the serum ferritin level, are depleted during pregnancy, regardless of whether iron supplements are given.

Serum and Red Cell Folate

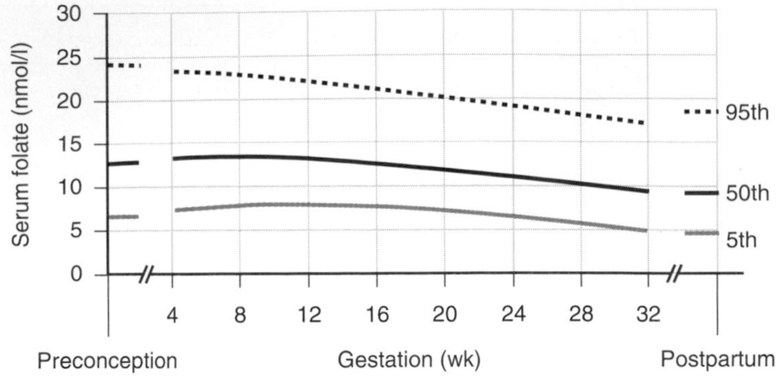

A

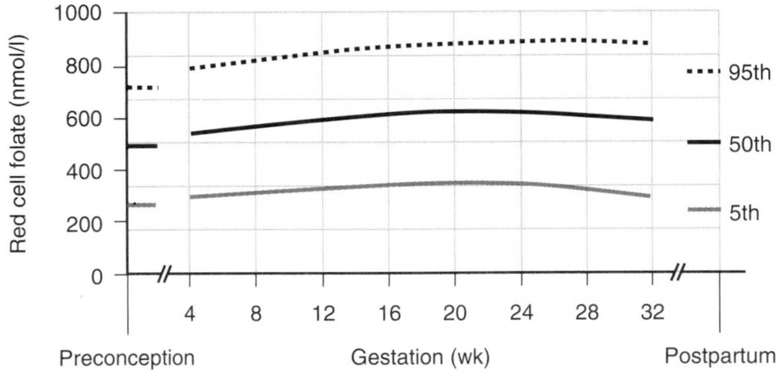

B

FIGURE 31
Longitudinal study of (*A*), serum and (*B*), red cell folate levels (5th, 50th, and 95th percentiles) in healthy nulliparous women during an uneventful singleton pregnancy. None of the study subjects took iron or vitamin supplements (n = 102). Nonfasting blood samples were taken within 3 months of conception, at 6, 10, 20, and 32 weeks' gestation, and again 6 weeks postpartum. All women had spontaneous labor at term and had infants of normal size. *Data source:* ref. 53, with permission. *Conversion factor for folate:* nmol/L × 0.044 = µg/dL.

Comment: In other studies, red cell folate levels showed a slight downward trend with advancing gestation, and patients with low red cell folate levels at the beginning of pregnancy had megaloblastic anemia in the third trimester.[54] These differences may relate to dietary folate intake. In a cross-sectional study of 155 women, red cell folate concentration increased with gestation and was significantly higher in subjects who took supplemental folic acid (1 mg daily) than in those who did not (1056 nmol/L vs. 595 nmol/L, respectively).[55] Serum and red cell folate levels are lower in pregnancy in women who smoke.[56] By 6 weeks after delivery, red cell folate levels return toward preconception values, although serum folate levels remain low. Lactation, which is an added folate stress, may be one reason.[57] Serum folate levels may remain low for up to 6 months after delivery.[53]

Homocysteine

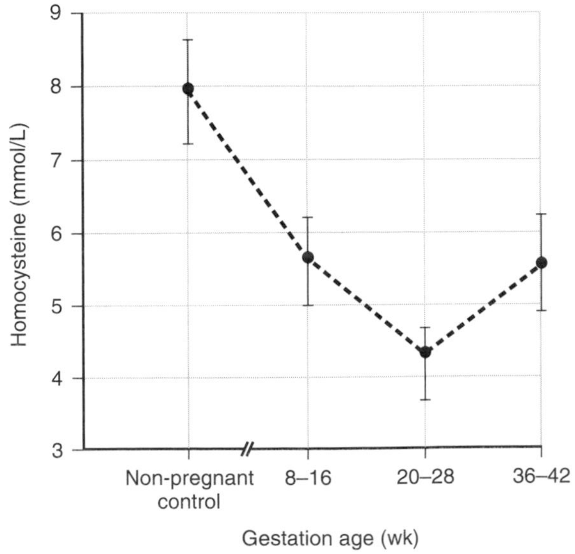

Comment: Plasma homocysteine levels are significantly lower in all trimesters of pregnancy compared with nonpregnant control values. A small longitudinal study confirmed these findings.[53] The lowest levels are found in the second trimester. Homocysteine is 70% to 80% albumin-bound, so these gestational changes mirror those of serum albumin (Fig. 15). Homocysteine is negatively correlated with red cell folate, and lower concentrations are found in women who take folic acid supplements.[55] Hyperhomocysteinemia, which can result from genetic and environmental factors, is associated with deep venous thrombosis, recurrent miscarriage, abruption, stillbirth, and neural tube defects.

FIGURE 32
Plasma homocysteine (mean and 95% confidence interval [CI]) in a cross-sectional study of 155 normal women in the first, second, and third trimesters of pregnancy and in nonpregnant control subjects. Homocysteine concentrations were determined by high-pressure liquid chromatography. *Data source:* ref. 55, with permission.

Vitamin B_{12}

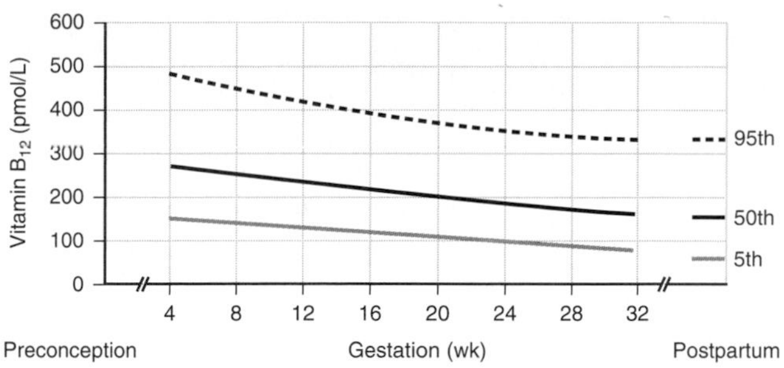

FIGURE 33
Serum vitamin B_{12} levels (5th, 50th, and 95th percentiles) in 102 healthy nulliparous women during an uneventful singleton pregnancy. Subjects were those described in Figure 31. *Data source:* ref. 53, with permission.

Comment: Serum vitamin B_{12} levels are approximately 100 pmol/L lower in pregnancy, but recovery occurs by 6 weeks postpartum.[53] Levels tend to be lower in women who smoke.[56] Muscle and red cell vitamin B_{12} concentrations also fall during pregnancy; however, vitamin B_{12} absorption does not change.[57,58] Saturation of vitamin B_{12}-binding proteins decreases steadily during pregnancy.[58] These changes in vitamin B_{12} status do not represent a deficiency state, however, because they are not associated with evidence of reduced red blood cell count or hemoglobin or homocysteine concentrations, once correction is made for serum ferritin concentrations.[58]

Other Vitamins

Comment: Vitamin concentrations during pregnancy are available from a large longitudinal study performed in the Netherlands on women who were not using iron, folate, or other vitamin supplementation. Vitamins studied included retinol, thiamin, riboflavin, pyridoxal 5′-phosphate, and α-tocopherol.[53]

Coagulation Factors

Coagulation factors									
No. of patients		41	48	47	66	62	48	61	61
Weeks		11–15	16–20	21–25	26–30	31–35	36–40	Post-delivery	Postnatal
Factor VII	Mean range	111 60–206	129 68–244	150 80–280	158 75–332	162 84–312	171 87–336	134 70–255	94 52–171
Fibrinogen (g/L)	Mean range	3.63 2.64–5.00	3.65 2.55–5.22	3.65 2.53–5.26	3.78 2.67–5.35	4.17 2.90–6.00	4.23 2.90–6.15	4.61 2.98–7.14	2.65 1.71–4.11
Factor X	Mean range	103 62–169	111 74–166	115 74–177	126 78–203	123 78–194	127 72–208	117 72–191	90 54–149
Factor V	Mean range	93 46–188	84 46–155	82 36–185	82 34–214	82 34–195	85 39–184	91 36–233	81 42–155
Factor II	Mean range	125 70–224	128 75–218	125 73–214	124 79–193	115 74–179	115 68–194	112 74–170	106 68–165
Factor VIII: C	Mean range	122 53–283	150 53–419	141 44–453	188 67–528	185 69–499	212 79–570	206 74–569	95 46–193
Factor VIII: R Ag	Mean range	133 56–318	156 55–439	167 66–427	203 84–492	262 95–718	376 133–1064	421 169–1042	89 29–272
Factor VIIIR: Ag/VIII: C ratio	Mean range	1.09 0.43–2.74	1.04 0.40–2.72	1.18 0.43–3.27	1.08 0.41–2.81	1.42 0.48–4.21	1.77 0.62–5.09	2.05 0.71–5.92	0.95 0.36–2.52

FIGURE 34
Coagulation factors (mean and 95% ranges) from a longitudinal study of 72 women, 19 to 42 years old (healthy primigravidae or multigravidae whose previous pregnancies were uncomplicated). Postdelivery samples were taken between 6 hours and 4 days after delivery (mean, 52 hours); postnatal samples were taken after 6 weeks. The postnatal samples yielded values similar to those from an age-matched nonpregnant group of women (n = 66). Where no units are stated, values are expressed as percentage of standard. *Data source:* ref. 59, with permission.

Comment: Normal pregnancy is a hypercoagulable state associated with increased levels of factors VII, VIII, and X and a marked increase in fibrinogen levels as a result of increased synthesis. Factor IX levels increase, whereas factor XI levels decrease.[57] Not shown is the first-trimester increase in fibrinopeptide A.

Naturally Occurring Anticoagulants and Fibrinolytic Factors

Naturally occuring anticoagulants and fibrinolytic factors									
No. of patients		41	48	47	66	62	48	61	61
Weeks		11–15	16–20	21–25	26–30	31–35	36–40	Post-delivery	Postnatal
FDPs (μg/mL)	Mean	1.07 –	1.06 –	1.09 –	1.13 –	1.28 –	1.32 –	1.66 –	1.04 –
Fibrinolytic activity (lysis time in hours)	Min Max	7.6 13.25	7.4 13.5	7.3 13.75	5.5 18.25	4.5 22.25	5.6 17.8	6.75 14.8	5.75 17.4
Antithrombin III: C	Mean range	85 49–120	90 46–133	87 42–132	94 47–141	87 42–132	86 40–132	87 48–127	92 38–147
Antithrombin III: Ag	Mean range	93 60–126	94 56–131	93 56–130	97 56–138	96 59–132	93 50–136	95 58–133	100 64–134
α1-Antitrypsin	Mean range	124 66–234	136 86–214	125 53–295	146 85–249	149 89–250	154 91–260	172 84–352	77 44–135
α2-Macroglobulin	Mean range	176 100–309	178 98–323	170 92–312	160 88–294	157 85–292	153 85–277	146 81–265	142 82–245

FIGURE 35
Naturally occurring anticoagulants and fibrinolytic factors (mean and 95% ranges), fibrinolytic activity (full range), and fibrin degradation products (mean values) from a longitudinal study. Where no units are stated, values are expressed as percentage of standard. Patients were those described in Figure 34. *Data source:* ref. 59, with permission.

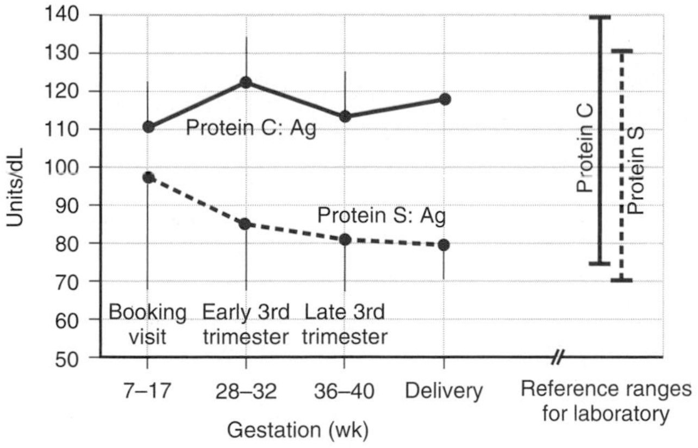

FIGURE 36
Protein S and protein C levels (mean ± SD) from a longitudinal study in 14 healthy women 24 to 38 years old. *Data source:* ref. 60, with permission.

Comment: Free protein S levels fall progressively during pregnancy but remain within the normal reference ranges; protein C levels change little. Antithrombin III levels are stable during pregnancy, decrease in labor, and then increase 1 week postpartum.[57] Fibrinolysis is depressed during pregnancy; fibrinogen and plasminogen levels are elevated, but levels of circulating plasminogen activator are decreased.[61] In late normal pregnancy, D-dimer levels are also elevated.[47]

Immunology

Complement System and Immune Complexes

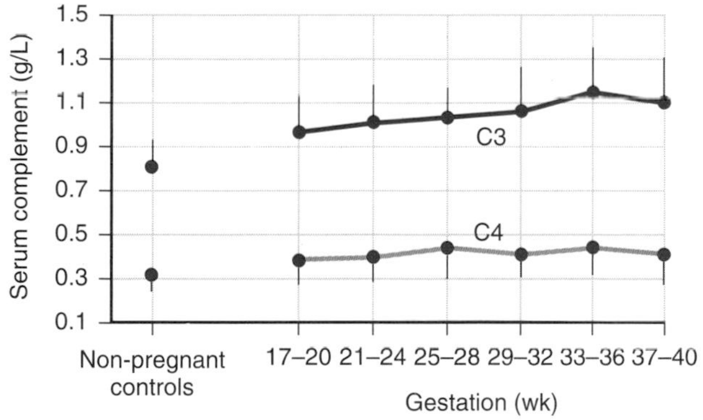

FIGURE 37
Complement factors C3 and C4 (mean and SD) from a longitudinal study of 147 healthy women who were normotensive throughout pregnancy. The control population was 32 normal nonpregnant women 15 to 41 years old, 11 of whom were taking oral contraceptives. *Data source:* ref. 62, with permission.

Comment: Levels of C3 and C4 are significantly elevated during the second and third trimesters. Another cross-sectional study[63] showed elevated levels of C4, but not C3, during the first trimester. Levels of circulating immune complexes are low during pregnancy.[63] There is disagreement as to whether levels of C3 degradation products are elevated[63] or normal[64]; no longitudinal studies have been done.

Markers of Inflammation

ERYTHROCYTE SEDIMENTATION RATE (ESR) AND C-REACTIVE PROTEIN (CRP)

Comment: The erythrocyte sedimentation rate (ESR) is high in pregnancy (typically >30 mm in the first hour) as a result of elevated plasma globulins and fibrinogen.[65] Thus, the ESR cannot be used as a marker for inflammation. Levels of C-reactive protein are the same in healthy pregnant women as in nonpregnant adults[47]; elevations are caused by intercurrent disease.

Endocrinology

Thyroid Function

TOTAL THYROXINE (T_4), TRI-IODOTHYRONINE (T_3), THYROID UPTAKE, AND THYROID-BINDING GLOBULIN (TBG)

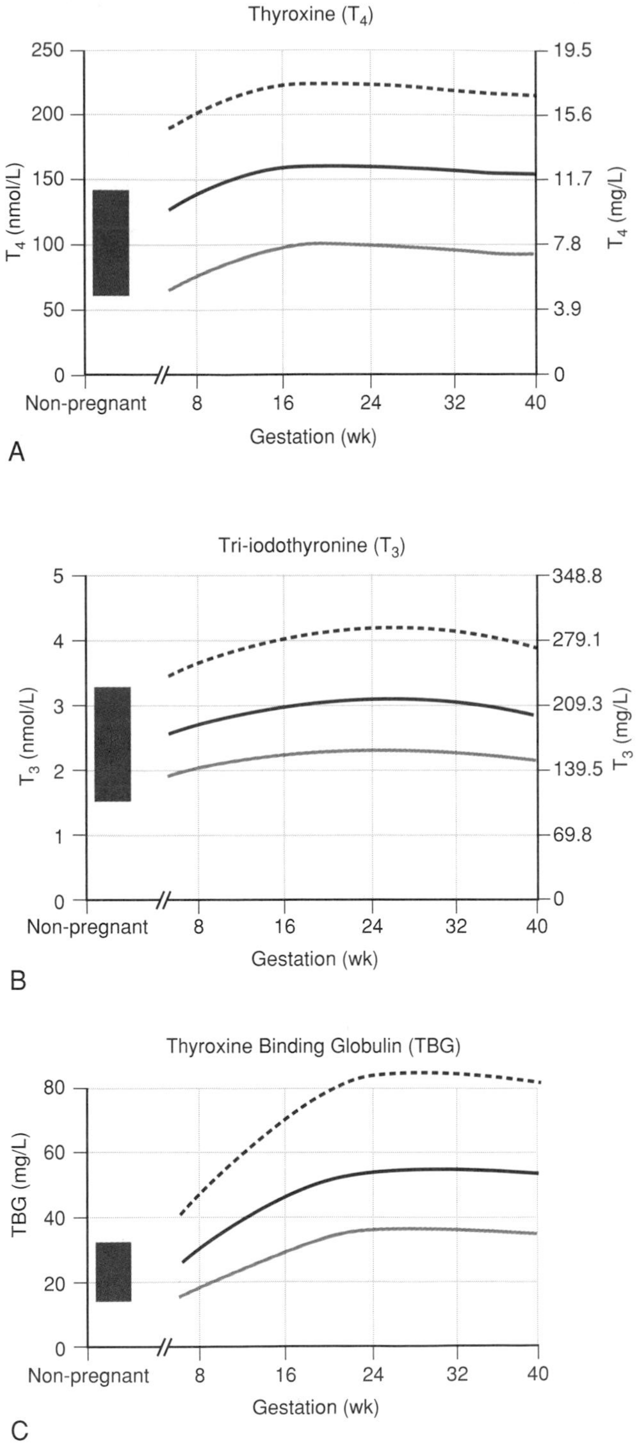

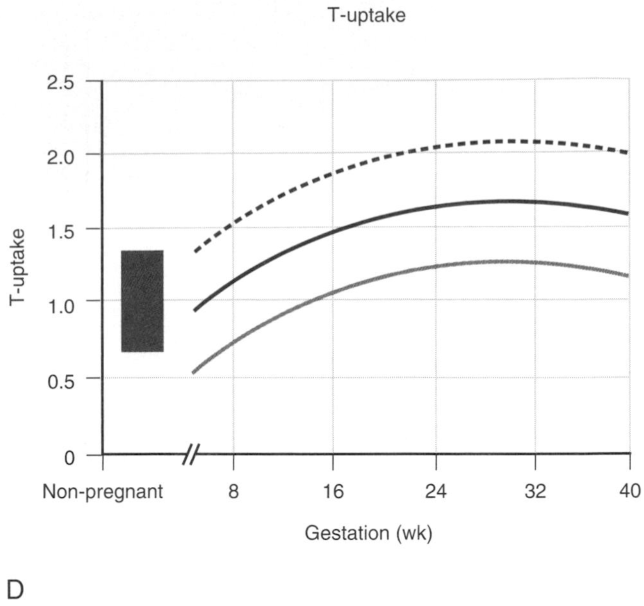

FIGURE 38
A, Total T_4, *B*, total T_3, *C*, thyroid-binding globulin, and *D*, T uptake (2.5th, 50th, and 97.5th percentiles) from a longitudinal study of 60 women who each had blood samples three times during pregnancy, once each trimester. Control values were taken from 30 healthy nonpregnant women. *Data source:* ref. 66, with permission.

Comment: Serum total T_4 and T_3 concentrations are elevated in pregnancy. Thyroid-binding globulin concentrations are doubled by the end of the first trimester, remain elevated throughout pregnancy, and decrease slowly in the 6 weeks after delivery.[67] T_3 uptake is believed to represent total serum thyroxine-binding capacity rather than unoccupied binding site concentration.[66] Other cross-sectional studies found decreased T_3 uptake during pregnancy.[68]

FREE THYROXINE (FREE T_4), FREE THYROXINE INDEX (FTI), THYROID-STIMULATING HORMONE (TSH), AND FREE TRI-IODOTHYRONINE (FREE T_3)

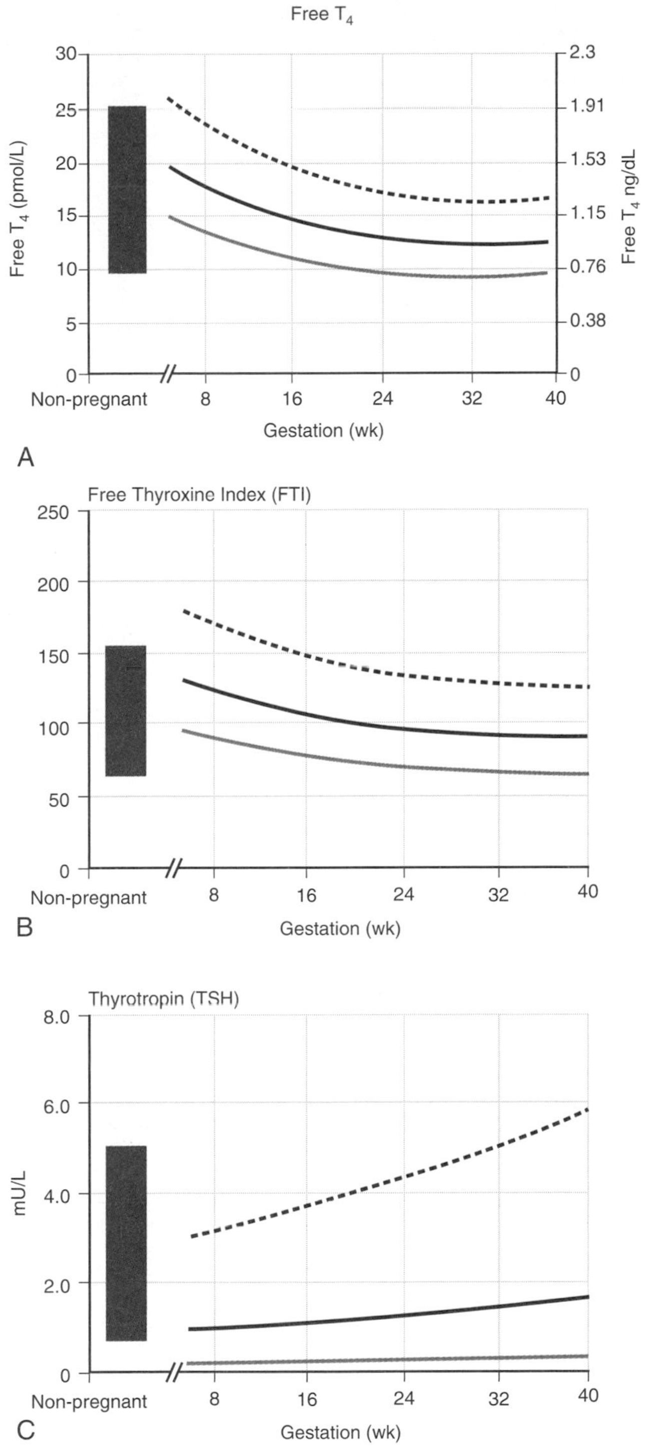

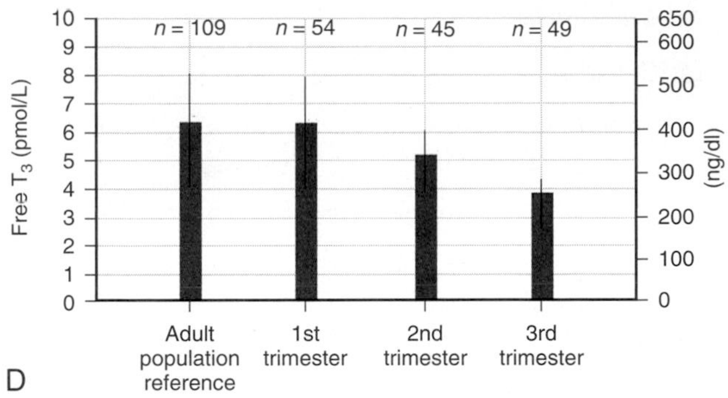

FIGURE 39

A, Free T_4 levels, *B*, free T_4 index, and *C*, thyroid-stimulating hormone (TSH) levels (2.5th, 50th, and 97.5th percentiles) from the same study described in Figure 38. *Data source:* ref. 66, with permission. *D*, Free T_3 concentrations (mean ± 2 SDs) from a cross-sectional study of 159 women attending antenatal clinics; none had metabolic illness. The control samples were obtained from 109 patients (male and female), taken from the routine workload of the laboratory (excluding those with thyroid disease, diabetes, cardiac disease, or carcinoma, and postoperative patients). *Data source:* ref. 69, with permission.

Comment: Free T_4 and free T_3 concentrations, measured directly (rather than derived from resin uptake measurements) decrease during pregnancy but remain within normal nonpregnant ranges.[66,69,70] TSH levels increase with gestation but remain within the reference range for nonpregnant women.[66] Some studies found low TSH levels toward the end of the first trimester in association with the highest circulating concentrations of hCG.[68] The increase in TSH in response to thyrotropin-releasing hormone during early pregnancy is enhanced, similar to responses found in central hypothyroidism.[71]

Adrenal Function

CATECHOLAMINES

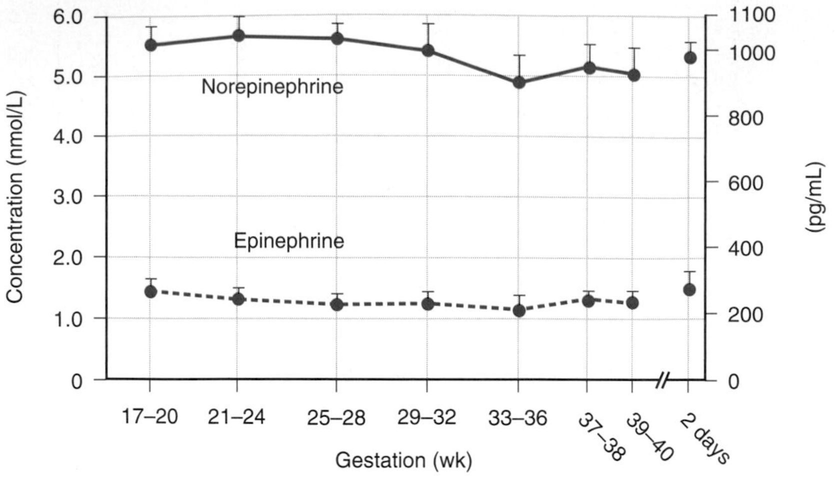

FIGURE 40
Epinephrine and norepinephrine concentrations (mean and SEM) from a longitudinal study of 52 women, mean age 28 years, who were normotensive throughout pregnancy; 39 were primigravidae. Samples were taken by venepuncture after 20 minutes' rest in the left lateral position. A radioenzymic method was used for the assays. *Data source:* ref. 72, with permission.

Comment: This study showed a decrease in plasma levels of both epinephrine and norepinephrine as pregnancy progressed. Other studies (in which blood samples were taken from indwelling intravenous cannulas) showed steady levels throughout pregnancy, with no difference between values during pregnancy and those in the early puerperium.[73] In healthy pregnant women, plasma epinephrine and norepinephrine levels show a diurnal pattern, with the lowest levels reported at night.[74] Urinary vanillylmandelic acid (VMA) excretion has not been studied in healthy pregnancies but is likely to be within the normal adult range.

GLUCOCORTICOIDS

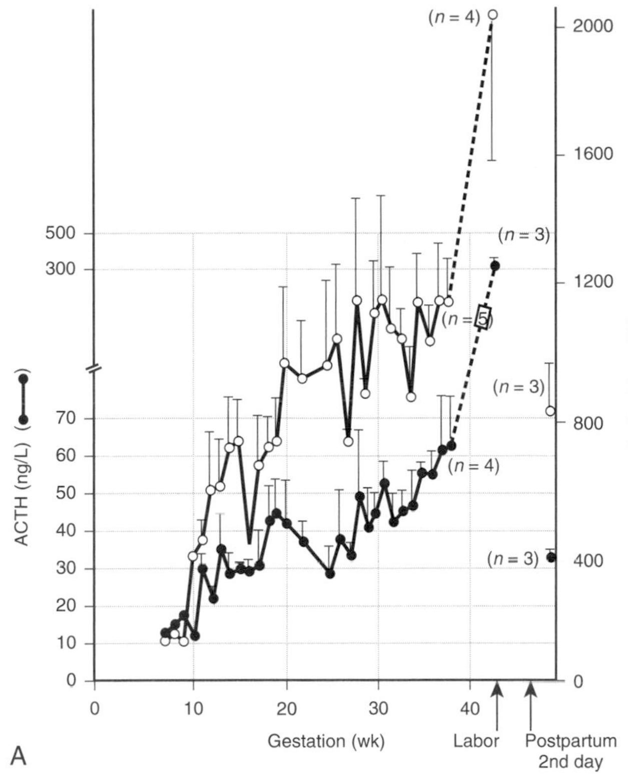

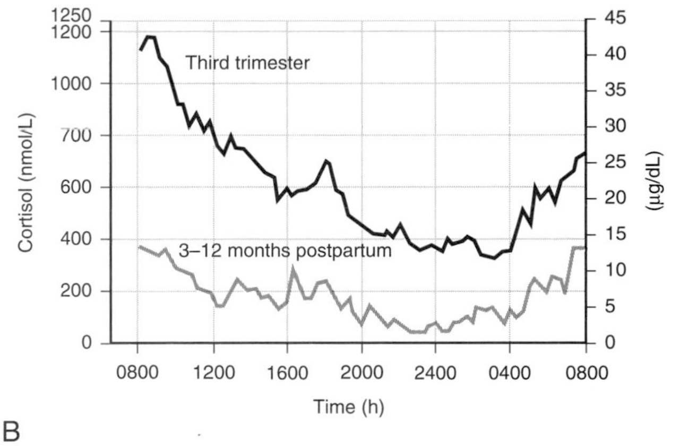

	Plasma cortisol (nmol/L)			Free cortisol index	
	Minimum	Mean (in 24-h period)	Maximum	Minimum	Maximum (in 24-h period)
Pregnant third trimester ($n = 7$)	197 (25)	581 (28)	1206 (94)	2.2 (0.3)	15.7 (1.7)
Non-pregnant ($n = 3$)	22 (6)	175 (25)	450 (3)	0.22 (0.05)	5.7 (0.9)

C

FIGURE 41

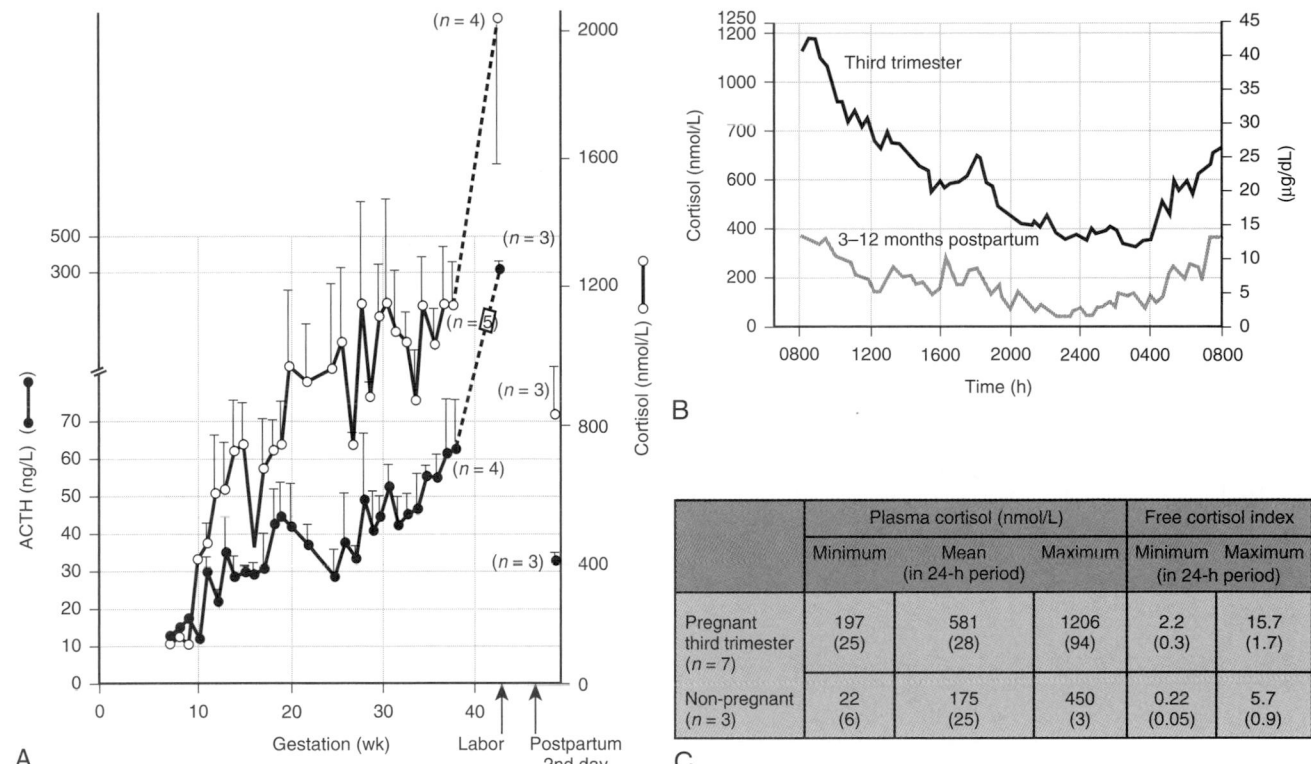

A, Adrenocorticotropic hormone (ACTH) and cortisol concentrations (mean and SEM) from a longitudinal study of five healthy pregnant women 17 to 28 years old. Blood samples were taken weekly, from early pregnancy until delivery. Samples were obtained between 8:00 AM and 9:00 AM after an overnight fast. Samples for ACTH measurement were collected improperly from one woman and had to be discarded. Samples were also taken from three of these subjects during labor and on the second postpartum day. *Data source:* ref. 75, with permission. *B*, Mean plasma cortisol levels throughout a 24-hour period from a study of seven primigravidae in the third trimester and three nonpregnant women, two of whom had been studied during pregnancy. The nonpregnant women were at least 3 months postdelivery and were not breast-feeding or using oral contraceptives. Samples were taken every 20 minutes. *Data source:* ref. 76, with permission. *C*, Plasma cortisol and free cortisol index (mean and SD) from a study of seven primigravidae in the third trimester and three nonpregnant women, two of whom had been studied during pregnancy. Subjects were those described in Figure 41b. *Data source:* ref. 76, with permission.

Comment: The total, bound, and free plasma cortisol levels and the free cortisol index are increased in pregnancy compared with the nonpregnant state.[76,77] ACTH levels during pregnancy are variously reported as remaining within the normal range for non-pregnant subjects, increasing, or decreasing,[75,78] but there is agreement that levels increase with advancing gestation. The rise in ACTH during pregnancy is attributed to placental production of the peptide.[78] Despite overall elevated levels, normal diurnal patterns of cortisol are found during pregnancy (i.e., lowest values at 12:00 AM, highest values at 8:00 AM).[76,77] The biologic half-life of cortisol is increased in pregnancy.[76] Cortisol-binding globulin (CBG) concentrations rise steadily during pregnancy, reaching twice the normal values by midgestation.[77,79] The cortisol production rate during pregnancy has been described as depressed[80] or elevated.[76] Urinary free cortisol more than doubles during pregnancy.[81] After 1 mg dexamethasone given orally at 11:00 PM, plasma cortisol levels measured at 8:00 AM are less than 139 nmol/L or 5 μg/dL (a normal response).[82] However, urinary cortisol levels are not suppressed as much in pregnant subjects as in nonpregnant subjects.[78] The cortisol response to an ACTH challenge (Synacthen test) is unchanged in pregnancy.[83]

Prolactin

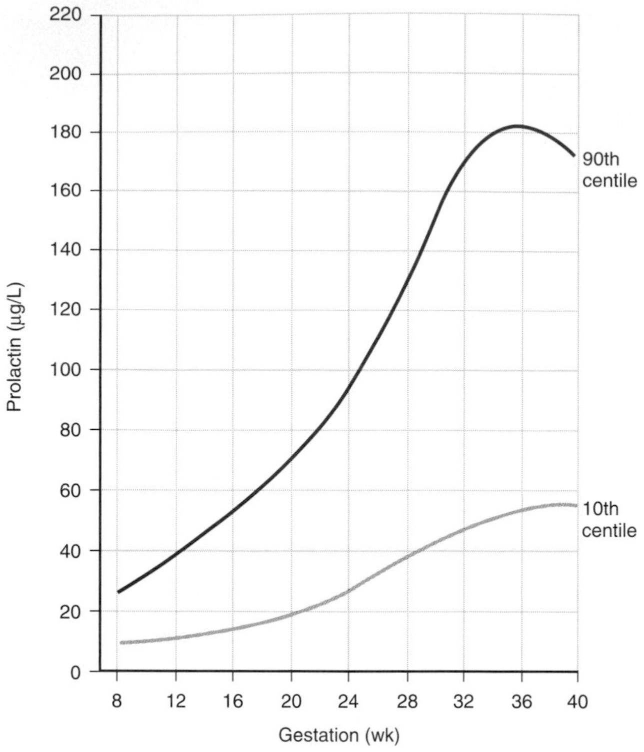

FIGURE 42
Serum prolactin (10th and 90th percentiles) from a mostly cross-sectional study of 839 women with uncomplicated singleton pregnancies at 8 to 40 weeks' gestation; 980 blood samples were taken. All of the samples were collected between 9:00 AM and 11:00 AM. Women who had a pregnancy complication were rejected from the normal series. *Data source:* ref. 84, with permission.

Comment: Prolactin concentrations increase 10- to 20-fold during pregnancy. The concentrations show a normal circadian rhythm, with a nocturnal rise.[85] In labor, levels decrease acutely, followed by a postpartum surge during the first 2 hours after delivery.[86] These changes are not seen in women undergoing elective cesarean delivery. Prolactin levels approach the normal range 2 to 3 weeks after delivery in nonlactating women, but remain elevated in those who breast-feed their infants.[87]

Calcium Metabolism

TOTAL AND IONIZED CALCIUM, MAGNESIUM, ALBUMIN, PARATHYROID HORMONE (PTH), CALCITONIN, AND VITAMIN D

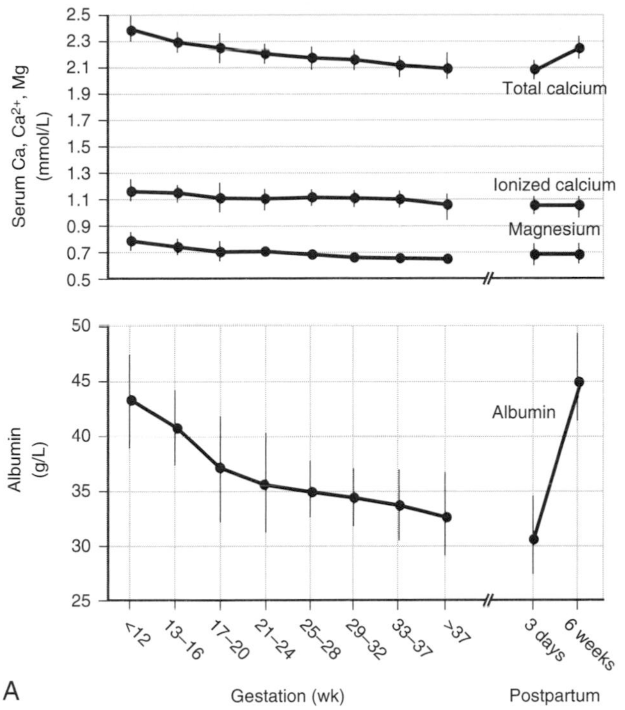

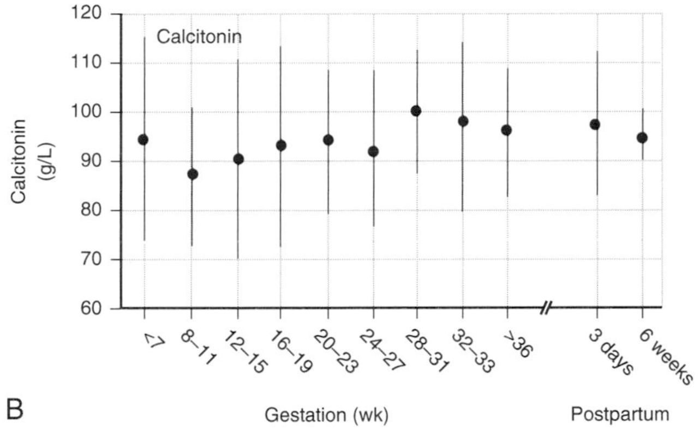

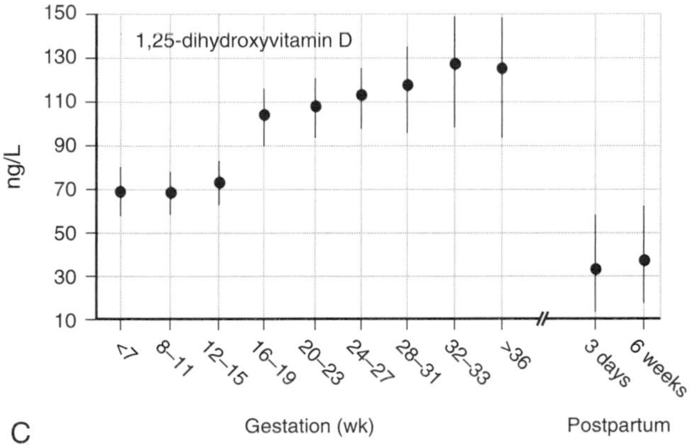

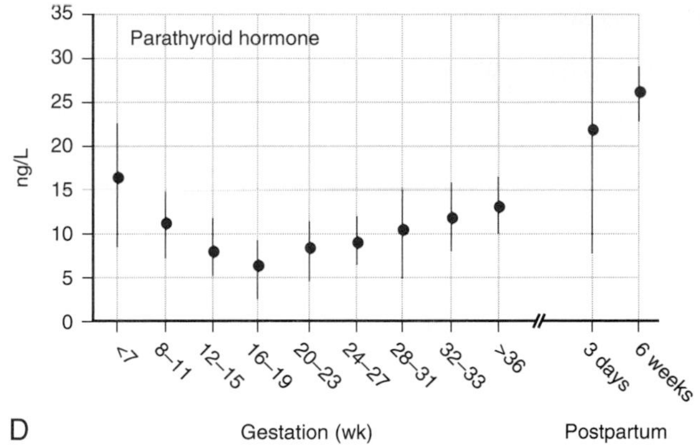

FIGURE 43
A, Total and ionized calcium, magnesium, and albumin (mean ± SD) from a longitudinal study of 30 women who were recruited in the first trimester and studied at 4-week intervals. Samples were taken on the third postpartum day and during the sixth postpartum week. Subjects ranged in age from 19 to 33 years; 20 were primigravidae. Samples were collected by venepuncture after an overnight fast. Calcium, mmol/L × 4 = mg/dL; magnesium, mmol/L × 2.4 = mg/dL. *Data source:* ref. 88, with permission. *B*, Calcitonin, *C*, 1,25-dihydroxyvitamin D, and *D*, parathyroid hormone (PTH) (mean ± SD) from a longitudinal study of 20 women 22 to 34 years old, 12 of whom were nulliparous. All had uncomplicated pregnancies of more than 38 weeks' gestation. The only medication they received was ferrous sulfate. Blood samples were taken in the morning after an overnight fast. Samples were collected at 4-week intervals, with the first taken before 7 weeks' gestation. Samples were also taken on the third postpartum day and during the sixth postpartum week. *Data source:* ref. 89, with permission.

Comment: Total serum calcium decreases during pregnancy, in association with the fall in serum albumin; however, ionized calcium levels remain constant. Serum intact PTH levels are lower in pregnancy than at 6 weeks postpartum; they reach a nadir in midpregnancy. A menstrual cyclicity in PTH has also been noted, with higher values corresponding to times of increased estrogen secretion.[88] Calcitonin levels are not significantly altered in pregnancy. 1,25-Dihydroxyvitamin D levels increase with advancing gestation and are significantly higher than during the puerperium. 1α-Hydroxylation of 25-hydroxyvitamin D in the placenta accounts for this increase and the consequent suppression of PTH.[89]

Placental Biochemistry

PLASMA PROTEIN A (PAPP-A)

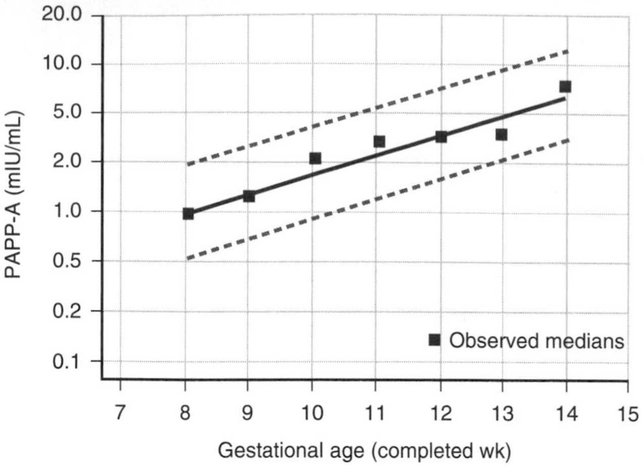

FIGURE 44
Plasma protein A (PAPP-A) levels in maternal serum (median, 0.5 MoM and 2 MoM) from a cross-sectional study of 379 healthy women at 8 to 14 weeks' gestation. These women had been selected to match 77 women whose fetuses had Down syndrome. Their median age was 39 years (10th and 90th percentiles, 34 and 42 years, respectively). *Data source:* ref. 90, with permission.

> **Comment:** PAPP-A and free βhCG are useful markers for discriminating pregnancies affected by Down syndrome from normal pregnancies at 8 to 14 weeks' gestation. PAPP-A levels are lower in affected pregnancies than in normal pregnancies (particularly at 11 weeks' gestation or less).[90,91]

SERUM α-FETOPROTEIN (SAFP)

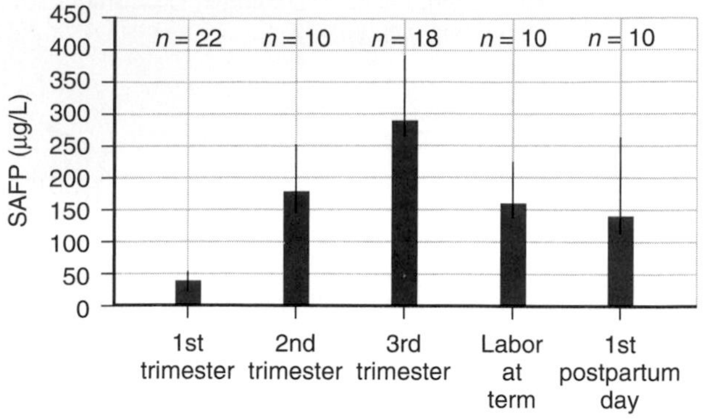

FIGURE 45
Serum α-fetoprotein (SAFP) (median and interquartile ranges) from a cross-sectional study. Samples from women in labor and samples obtained on the first postpartum day were paired. SAFP was measured by radioimmunoassay. *Data source:* ref. 92, with permission.

> **Comment:** In the second trimester, SAFP increases by approximately 15% weekly.[93] Individual screening laboratories establish reference ranges for SAFP in the second trimester for their own populations. These ranges are usually expressed as multiples of the median (MoM) for gestation. In twin pregnancies, SAFP levels are approximately twice as high as those in singleton pregnancies.[93] Maternal weight is inversely related to SAFP levels, probably because of the dilutional effect of a larger vascular compartment.[93]

HUMAN CHORIONIC GONADOTROPIN (HCG)

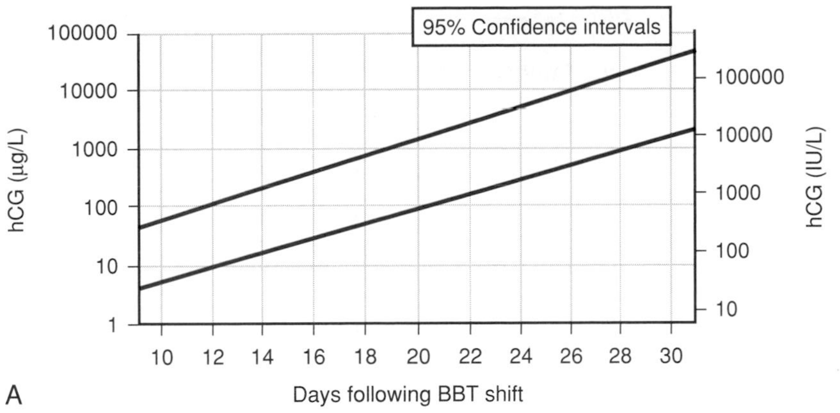

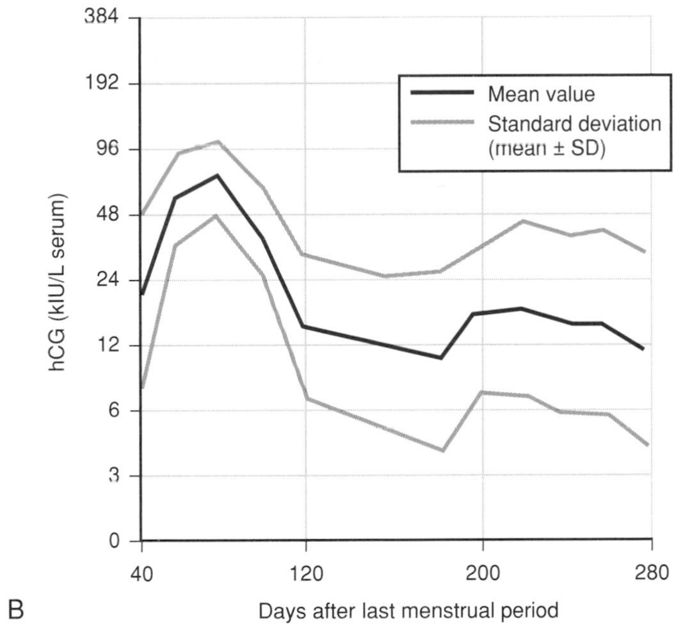

FIGURE 46
A, Serum values of the β subunit of hCG (95% CI) measured in 189 women who subsequently had successful pregnancies (total of 280 samples analyzed). The study subjects were patients in an infertility clinic and were keeping basal body temperature (BBT) charts to indicate the timing of ovulation. Some conceptions were spontaneous; other patients were treated with clomiphene citrate, human menopausal gonadotropin, or hCG (a single injection of 5000 IU to induce ovulation). A radioimmunoassay was used for βhCG. *Data source:* ref. 94, with permission. *B*, Total serum hCG (mean ± SD) from a longitudinal study of 20 healthy women. The first samples were obtained as early in pregnancy as possible, with subsequent samples obtained every 3 to 4 weeks. The last sample was taken during labor. Samples were classified into groups, with a class interval of 30 days. Radioimmunoassay was used to obtain the hCG level; the international hCG standard was used as a reference. *Data source:* ref. 95, with permission.

Comment: The mean doubling time of βhCG is 2.2 days ± 1.0 (2 SDs).[94] Low hCG values that do not double to within this range are associated with ectopic pregnancy or spontaneous abortion.[94] Women with male fetuses have significantly lower hCG levels than those with female fetuses.[95]

HUMAN PLACENTAL LACTOGEN (HPL)

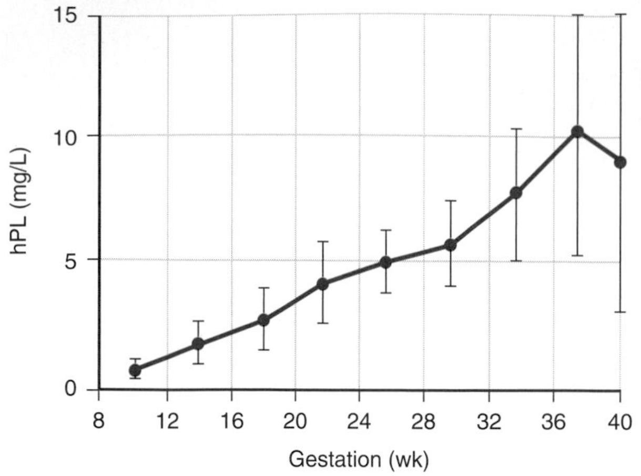

FIGURE 47
Serum human placental lactogen (hPL) values (mean ± SD) from a cross-sectional study of 151 normal women with singleton pregnancies attending a antenatal clinic. Radioimmunoassay was used to measure hPL. *Data source:* ref. 96, with permission.

> ***Comment:*** In women with multiple pregnancies, hPL levels are outside these ranges; however, if values are corrected for predicted placental weight, then they are appropriate for gestational age.[96] Four hours after delivery of the placenta, plasma hPL is virtually undetectable; the half-life of hPL in the plasma is 21 to 23 minutes.[97]

ESTRIOL (E_3)

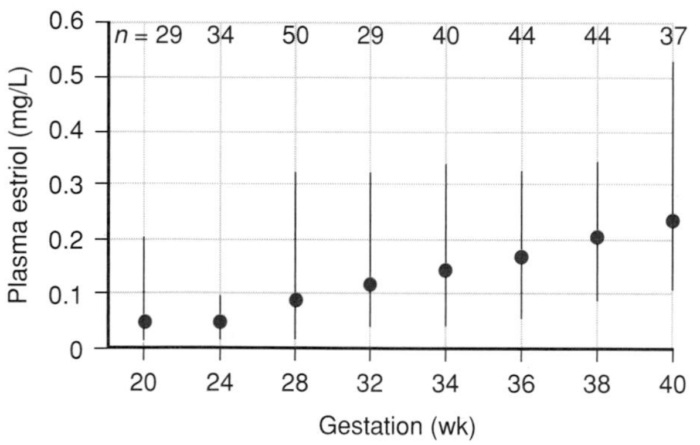

FIGURE 48
Plasma estriol (mean and range) from a cross-sectional study in women with uncomplicated pregnancies. Plasma estriol was measured fluorometrically. *Data source:* ref. 98, with permission.

> ***Comment:*** The normal range of plasma estriol in pregnancy is wide. To assess the significance of values outside this range, trends should be studied over several days.

FETAL VALUES

Physiology

Early Embryonic Structures

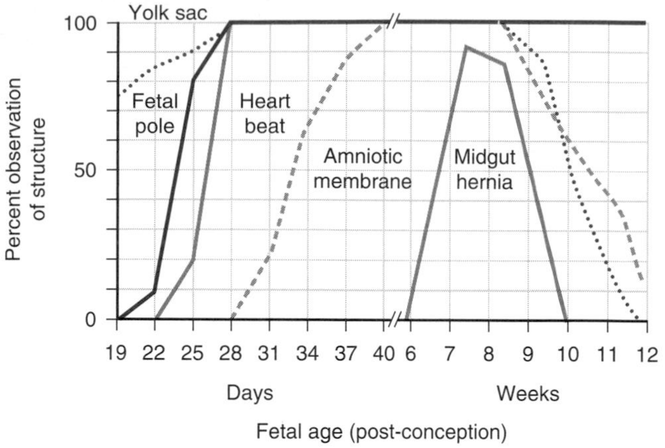

FIGURE 49
Ultrasound visualization of the yolk sac, fetal pole, heartbeat, amniotic membrane, and midgut hernia from a longitudinal study of 39 women with known dates of ovulation; most were patients from an assisted conception unit. Once pregnancy was confirmed, patients were scanned with a vaginal probe weekly, starting as early as 18 days after conception. Five subjects had twin pregnancies. *Data source:* ref. 99, with permission.

> ***Comment:*** Transvaginal ultrasound scanning yields better images in the first trimester than does transabdominal scanning. By 28 days after conception, fetal viability may be confirmed by visualization of a heartbeat. The fetal heart rate increases from 90 beats/min to 145 beats/min by 7 weeks after conception.[99]

Biometry

CROWN–RUMP LENGTH (CRL)

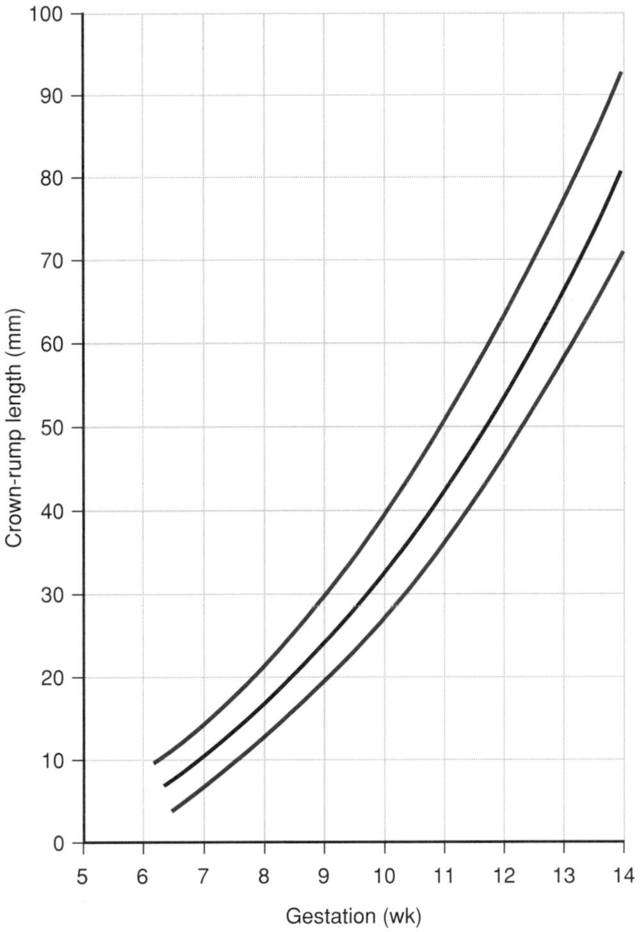

FIGURE 50
Crown–rump length (CRL) (mean ± 2 SDs) from a cross-sectional study of 334 women who were certain of the date of their last menstrual period (LMP) and had normal, regular menstrual cycles. The study covered the period from 6 to 14 weeks after the LMP. A transabdominal ultrasound technique was used, and the longest length of fetal echoes was found and measured. *Data source:* ref. 100, with permission.

Comment: CRL measurements can be used effectively only in the first trimester. Other studies found similar CRL values; measurements are not affected by maternal age, height, or parity.[101] In a smaller longitudinal study, CRL was significantly lower in female than in male fetuses.[101] No differences in CRL measurements have been found between Asian and European patients.[102]

NUCHAL TRANSLUCENCY (NT)

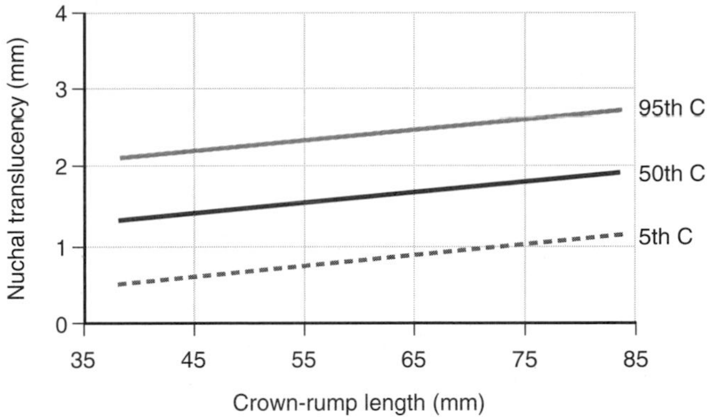

FIGURE 51
Nuchal translucency (NT) measurements (5th, 50th, and 95th percentiles) from a cross-sectional study of 20,217 chromosomally normal fetuses examined at 10 to 14 weeks' gestation. Most examinations were done with transabdominal ultrasound, and all operators were carefully trained in the technique before the study. A saggital section of the fetus was obtained perpendicular to the ultrasound beam, allowing measurement of crown–rump length and the maximum thickness of the subcutaneous translucency between skin and soft tissue overlying the cervical spine.[103] Care was taken to avoid confusion between fetal skin and amnion, both of which appear as thin membranes. *Data source:* ref. 104, with permission.

Comment: Abnormal fluid collections in the cervical region (as shown by increased NT measurements) are strongly associated with chromosomal abnormalities. The upper limit of normal may be set at 2.5 or 3.0 mm when these measurements are used as a screening test.[104,105] However, it is preferable to use the 95th percentile of NT as plotted against CRL, because measurements increase with gestational age.[104]

BIPARIETAL DIAMETER (BPD)

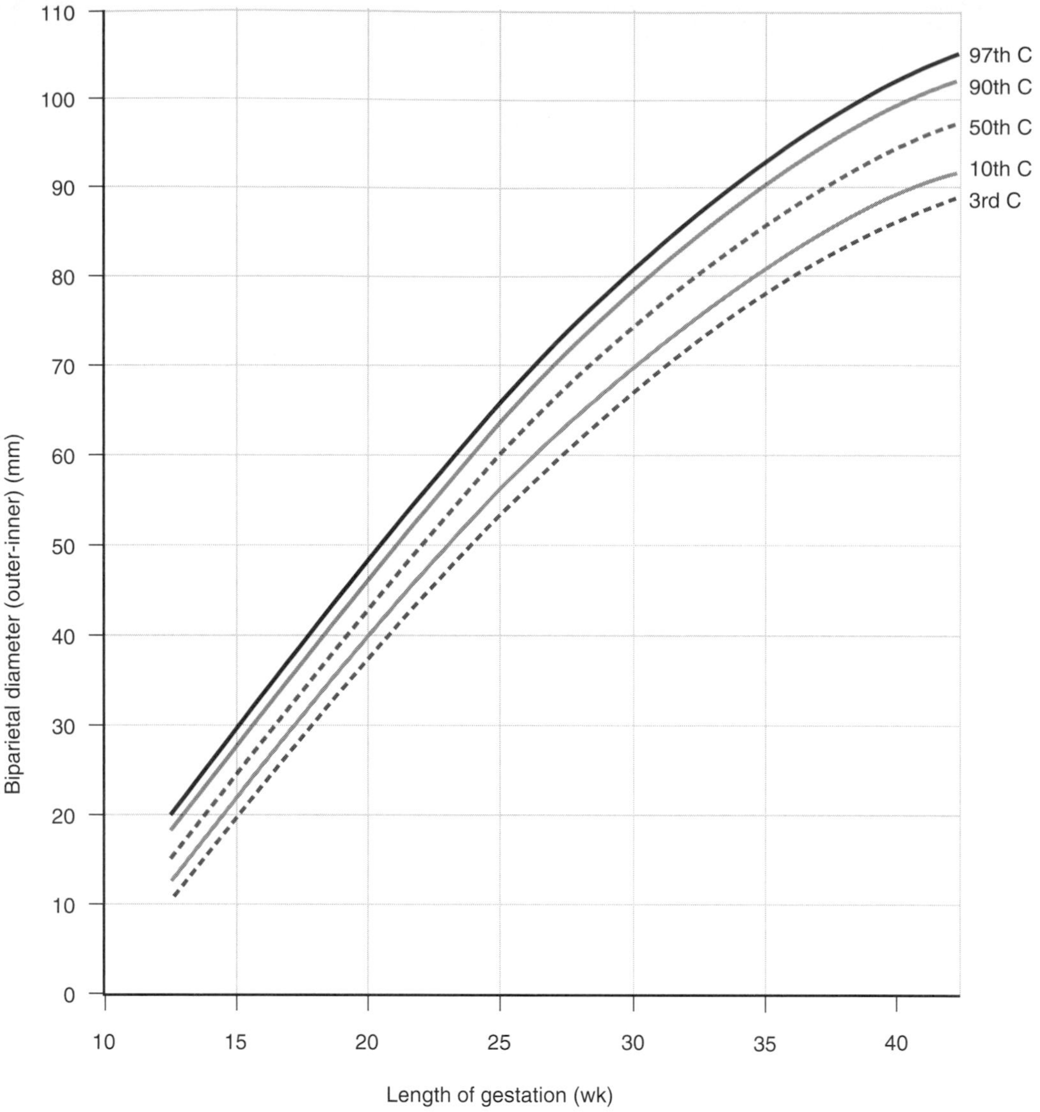

FIGURE 52

Biparietal diameter (BPD) (3rd, 10th, 50th, 90th, and 97th percentiles) of 594 fetuses from a prospective cross-sectional study of 663 women with singleton pregnancies carried out in London. Each fetus was measured only once between 12 and 42 weeks' gestation for the study. All women had certain menstrual dates, and menstrual and ultrasound ages at 18 to 22 weeks did not differ by more than 10 days. The study population consisted of 75% Western European and 25% African Caribbean women. No women had disease or used medication that was likely to affect fetal growth (e.g., diabetes, hypertension, renal disease). Measurements from two fetuses subsequently found to have abnormal karyotypes were excluded from the study. BPD measurements were obtained in the axial plane of the skull at the level where the continuous midline echo is broken by the cavum septum pellucidum in the anterior third. Measurements presented are those from the proximal edge of the skull closest to the transducer to the proximal edge of the deep border (i.e., outer-inner edges of bone). The statistical methods used to derive graphs and tables from the raw data are described in detail. *Data source:* refs. 106 and 107, with permission.

Comment: Other large studies are in close agreement with these measurements.[108,109] Information about growth in BPD is available from a longitudinal study.[110] Charts and graphs are also available for outer-outer BPD measurements,[107] and regression equations are given for both parameters. Racial differences in fetal measurements are likely to be found, so charts or percentile graphs appropriate for the population should be used. A small study found no significant differences between Asian and European women living in the same city.[102]

HEAD CIRCUMFERENCE (HC)

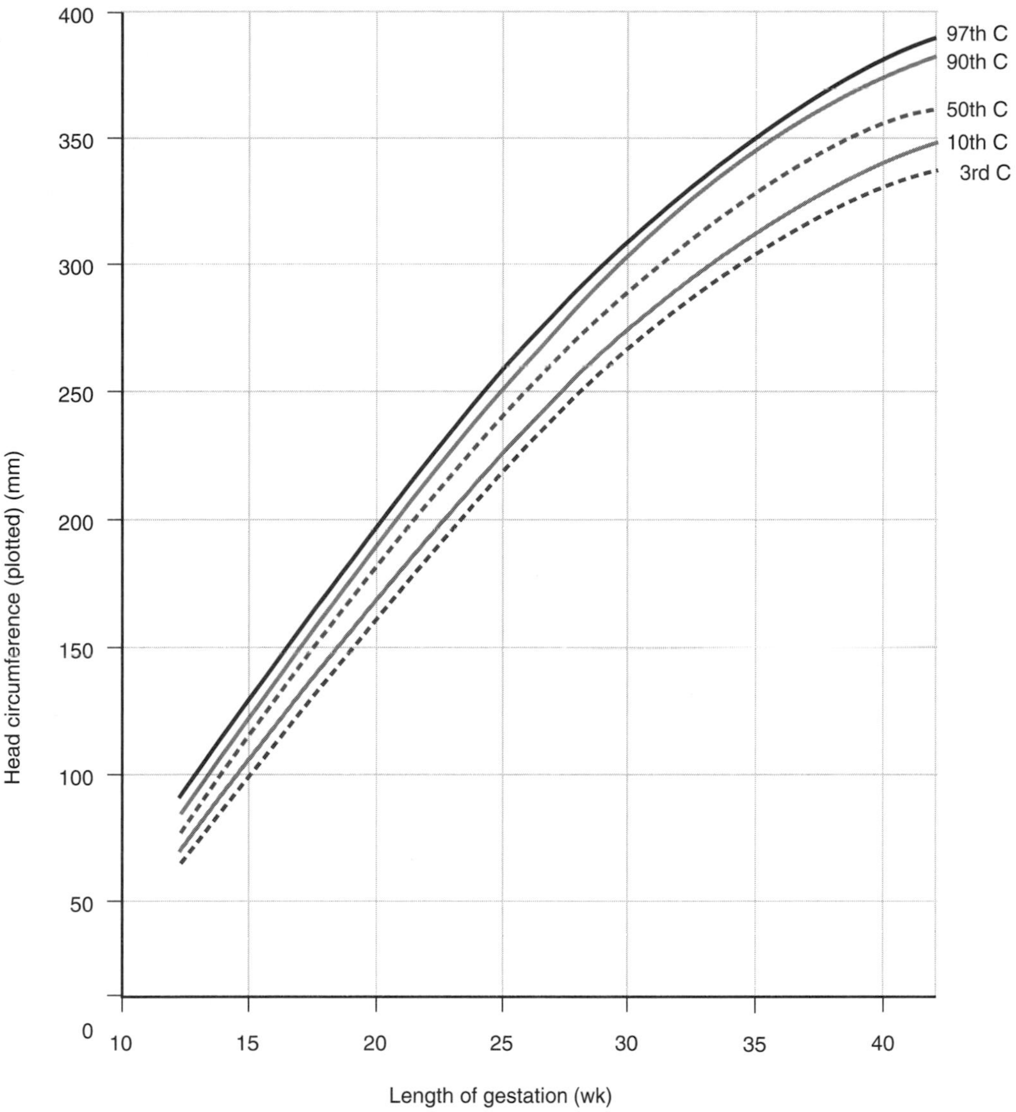

FIGURE 53
Head circumference (HC) (3rd, 10th, 50th, 90th, and 97th percentiles) from a prospective cross-sectional study of 594 fetuses, as described in Figure 52. HC was measured directly by tracing around the perimeter of the skull in the same plane used for biparietal diameter measurements. *Data source:* refs. 106 and 107, with permission.

Comment: HC measurements as derived from the biparietal and occipitofrontal diameters are also available[107,108] as well as regression equations for each parameter. Other studies yielded similar data, with some differences seen in the late third trimester.[108,111] These differences have been attributed to patient recruitment characteristics (whether only women delivering at term were included in the study) and the numbers of ultrasound operators used to collect data. HC measurements are particularly useful in the assessment of gestational age when the fetal head shape is abnormal (e.g., dolichocephaly).

ABDOMINAL CIRCUMFERENCE (AC)

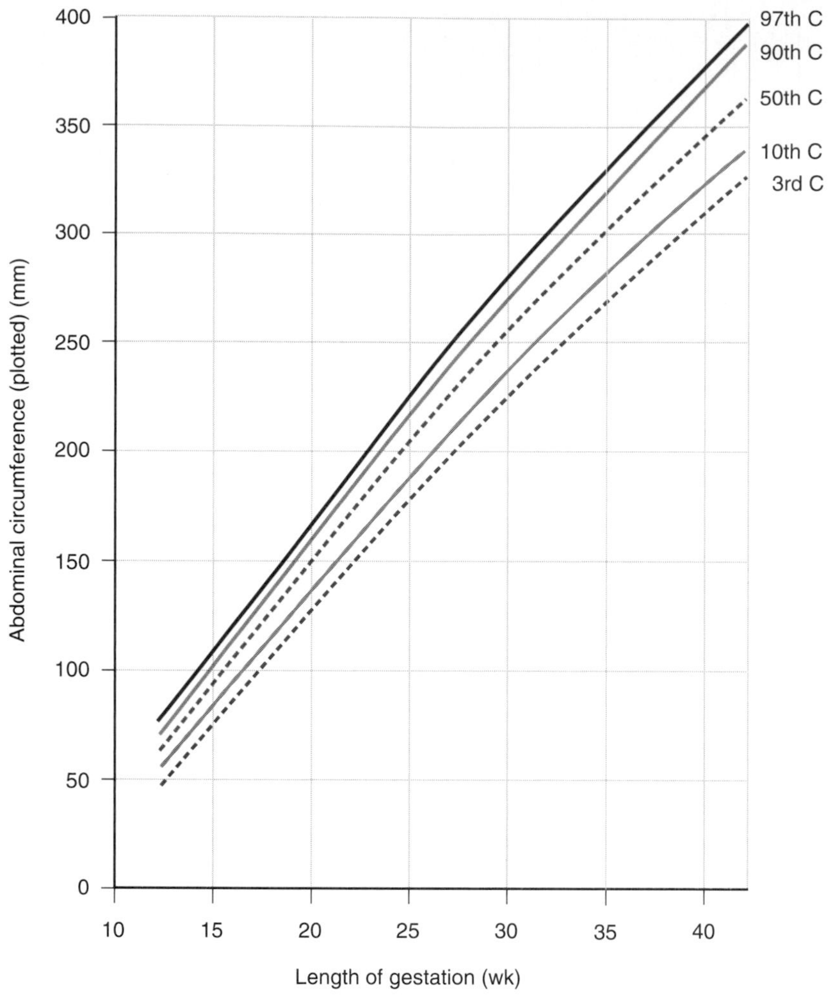

FIGURE 54
Abdominal circumference (AC) (3rd, 10th, 50th, 90th, and 97th percentiles) from 610 fetuses in the prospective cross-sectional study described in Figure 52. The fetal abdomen was measured in a transverse section, with the spine and descending aorta posterior, the umbilical vein in the anterior third, and the stomach bubble in the same plane. Care was taken to ensure that the section was as close as possible to circular, perpendicular to the spine. The circumference was measured by tracing around the perimeter. *Data source:* refs. 106 and 112, with permission.

Comment: Variability in AC increases with gestational age, as shown by widening of the percentiles. Other large studies are in close agreement[109,113,114] with these findings. Studies in which all women delivered at term did not find flattening of the growth velocity curves in late pregnancy.[115,116] Some of the discrepancies are the result of differences in mathematical curve-fitting techniques applied to the experimental data and differences in study design and the numbers of subjects and operators involved. AC is not a good indication of gestational age, but is used to assess fetal size (e.g., in relation to head and limb measurements). A method has been described[113] for assigning Z-scores to measurements, so that deviation from median values can be expressed without graphic presentation of the data. Measurements can also be compared between subjects or between the same subject at different times. Regression equations for AC, both plotted and derived from abdominal diameter measurements, are described.[112,113]

FEMUR LENGTH (FL)

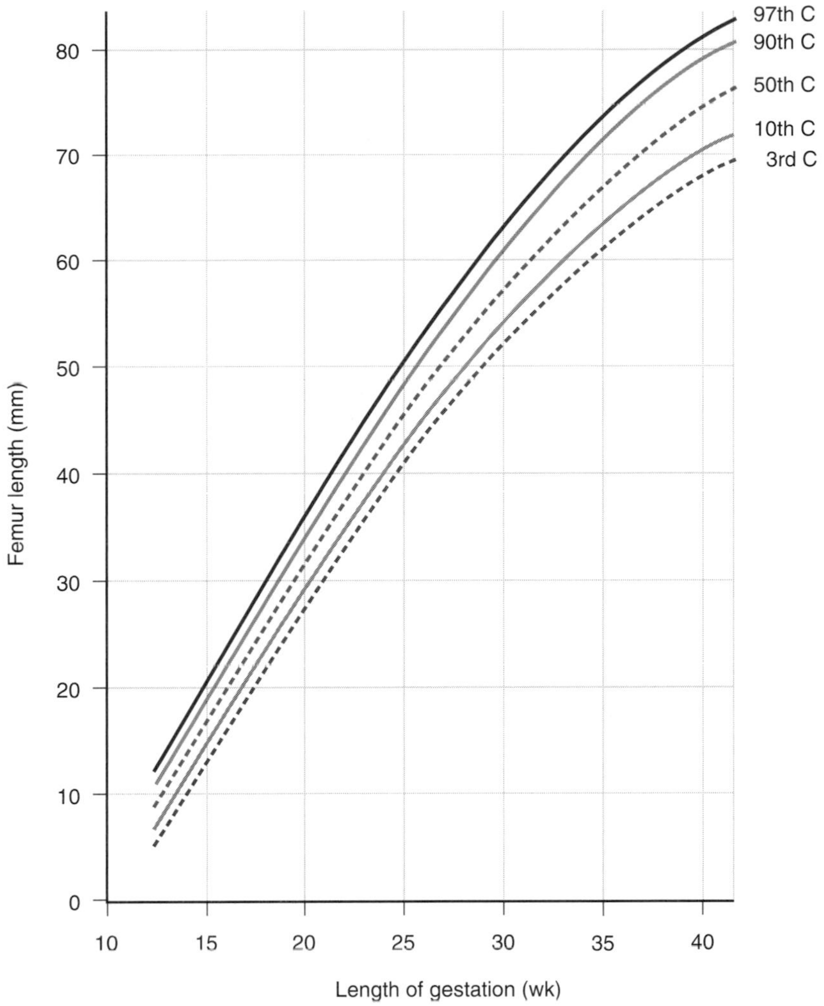

FIGURE 55
Femur length (FL) (3rd, 10th, 50th, 90th, and 97th percentiles) from 649 fetuses in the prospective cross-sectional study described in Figure 52. The femur was identified and the transducer rotated until the full femoral diaphysis was seen in a plane almost at a right angle to the ultrasound beam. The measurement was made from one end of the diaphysis to the other, disregarding curvature and ignoring the distal femoral epiphysis. *Data source:* refs. 106 and 117, with permission.

Comment: Other cross-sectional studies of FL provide similar measurements,[109,113] although one has wider percentiles in late pregnancy.[118] This difference is likely to be related to a difference in the statistical approach to the calculation of percentiles from the regression line. Regression equations are available.[109,113,117]

LIMB BONE LENGTHS

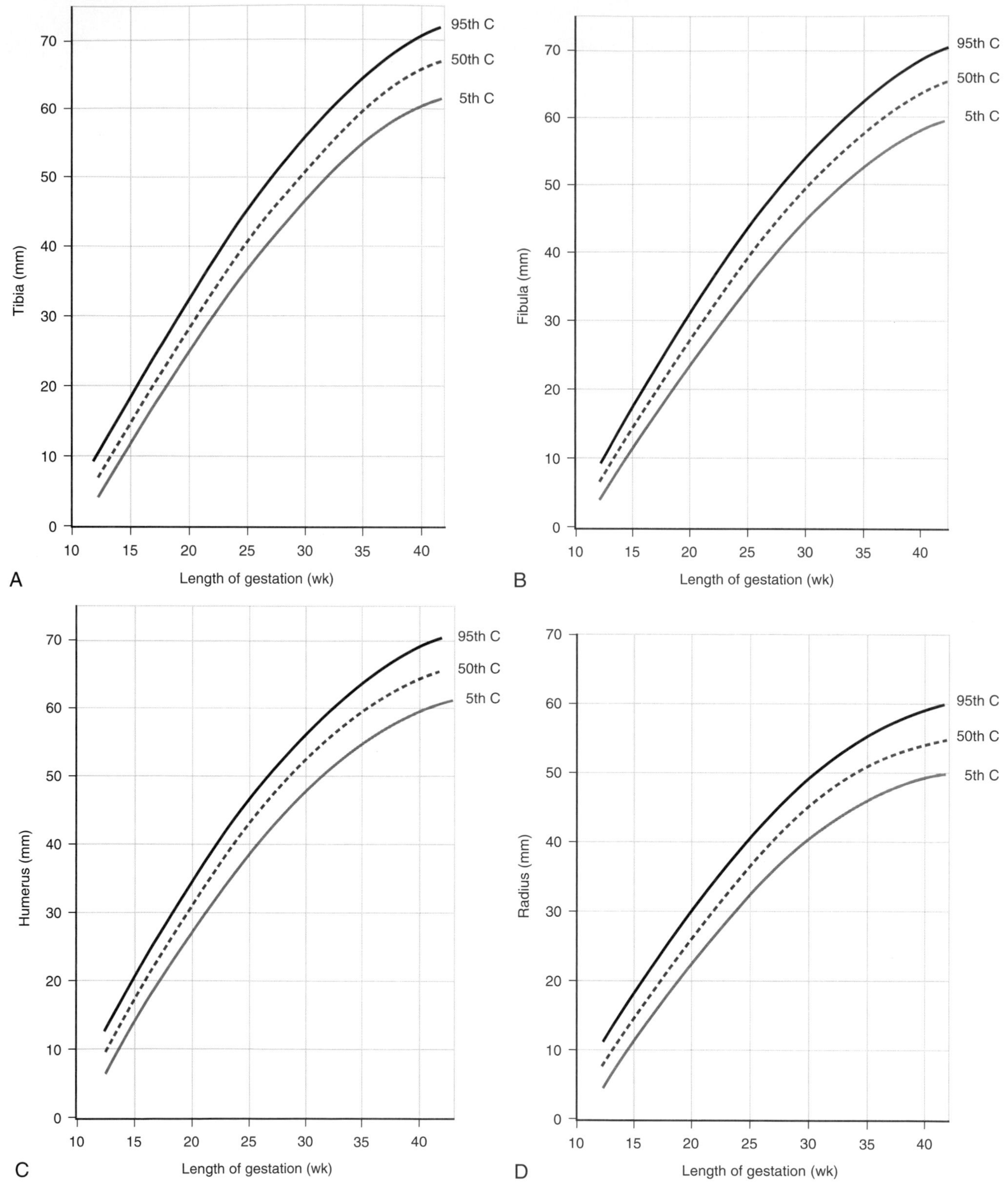

Continued

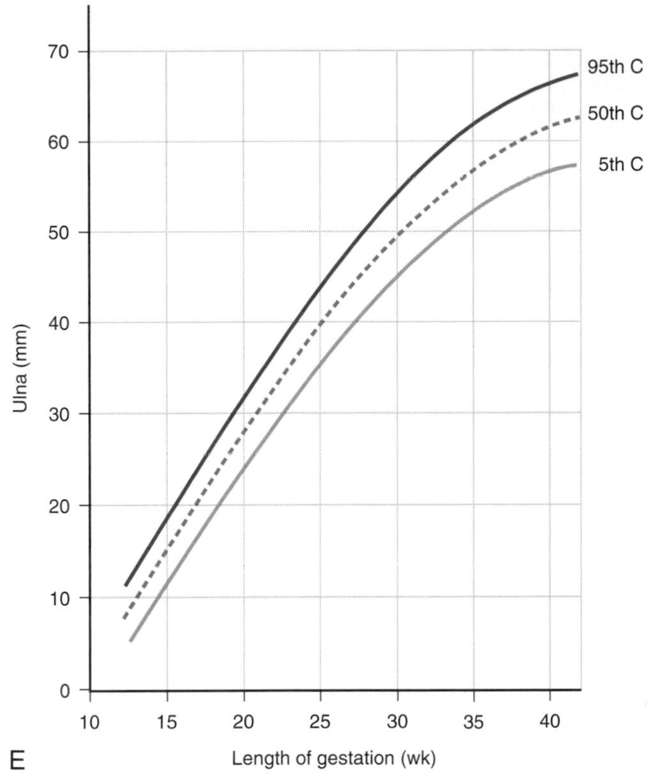

FIGURE 56 cont'd
Lengths of the *A*, tibia, *B*, fibula, *C*, humerus, *D*, radius, and *E*, ulna (5th, 50th, and 95th percentiles) from a cross-sectional study of 669 healthy women with singleton pregnancies. Women who subsequently delivered an infant with an abnormal karyotype, a significant malformation, or any other disease were excluded from the analysis. In all women, menstrual dating was certain and there was agreement between menstrual age and ultrasound dates at the time of the initial scan. Approximately 20 measurements were obtained for each parameter for each week of gestation from 12 to 42 weeks. *Data source:* ref. 119, with permission.

FOOT

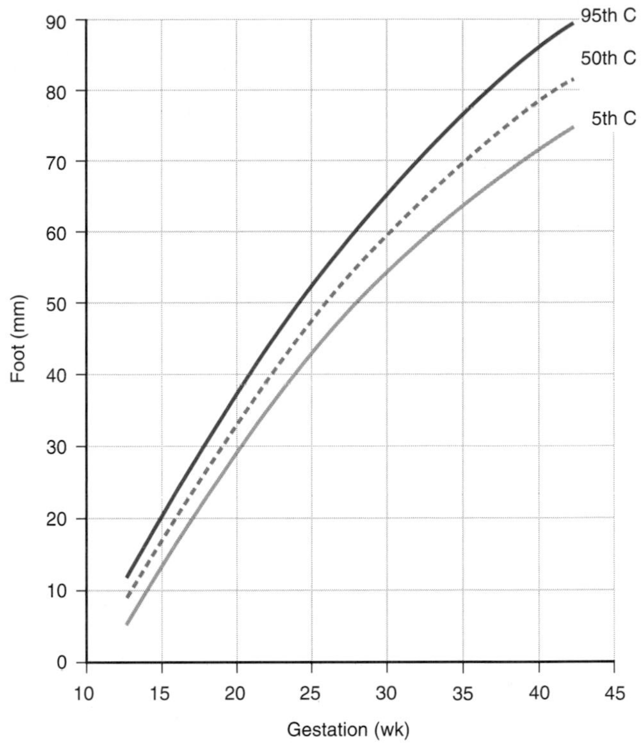

FIGURE 57
Length of the foot (5th, 50th, and 95th percentiles) from the cross-sectional study of 669 healthy women with singleton pregnancies described in Figure 56. Approximately 20 measurements were obtained for each variable for each week of pregnancy at 12 to 42 weeks' gestation. *Data source:* ref. 119, with permission.

Comment: All limb bones show linear growth from 13 to 25 weeks' gestation; thereafter, growth is nonlinear. Other studies confirmed these findings.[120] Good agreement has been found between ultrasound and x-ray measurements of limb bone lengths. Tables are available to allow assessment of gestational age from measurement of limb bone lengths.[121] This use of limb bone measurements should be distinguished from tables or graphs of normal measurements at known gestational age that allow assessment of possible skeletal dysplasia.[119,122]

KIDNEY

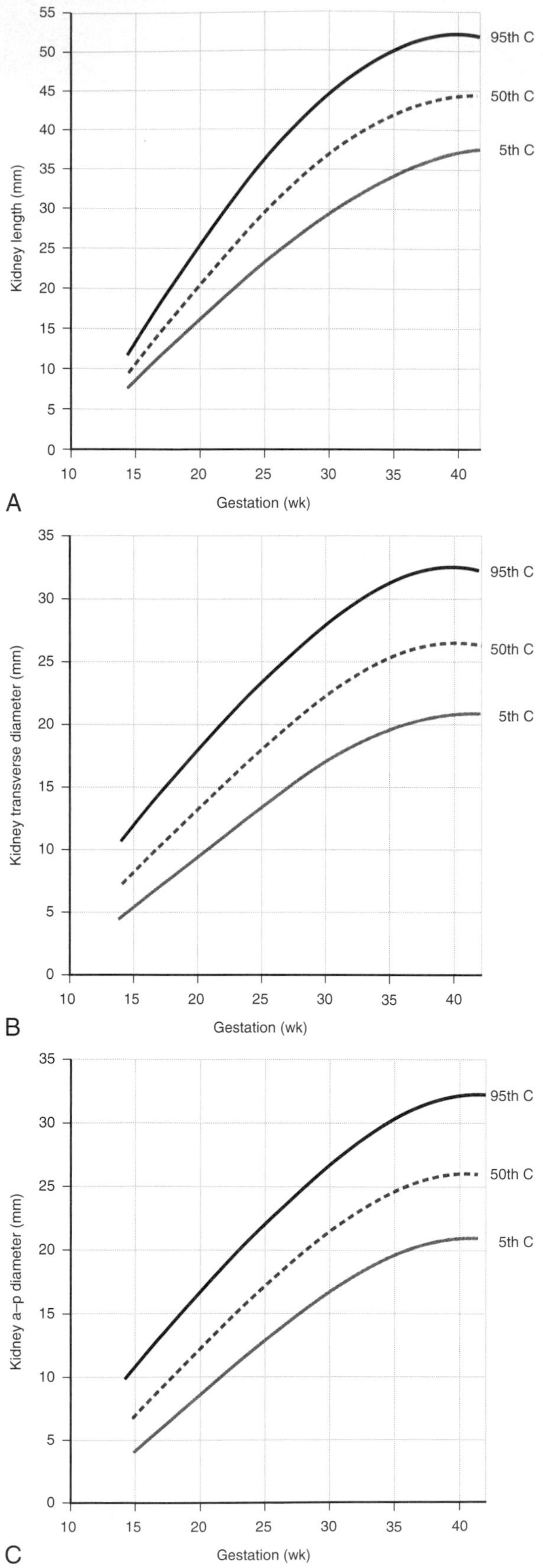

FIGURE 58
Kidney measurements; *A*, length, *B*, transverse diameter, *C*, antero-posterior diameter (5th, 50th, and 95th percentiles) from the cross-sectional study of 669 healthy women with singleton pregnancies described in Figure 56. Approximately 20 measurements were obtained for each variable for each week from 12 to 42 weeks' gestation. *Data source:* ref. 119, with permission.

> ***Comment:*** The ratio of transverse renal circumference to abdominal circumference (in a section at the level of the umbilical vein) is a simple way to assess normal kidney size. This ratio is 0.27 to 0.30 from 17 weeks' gestation until term.[123]

ORBITAL DIAMETERS

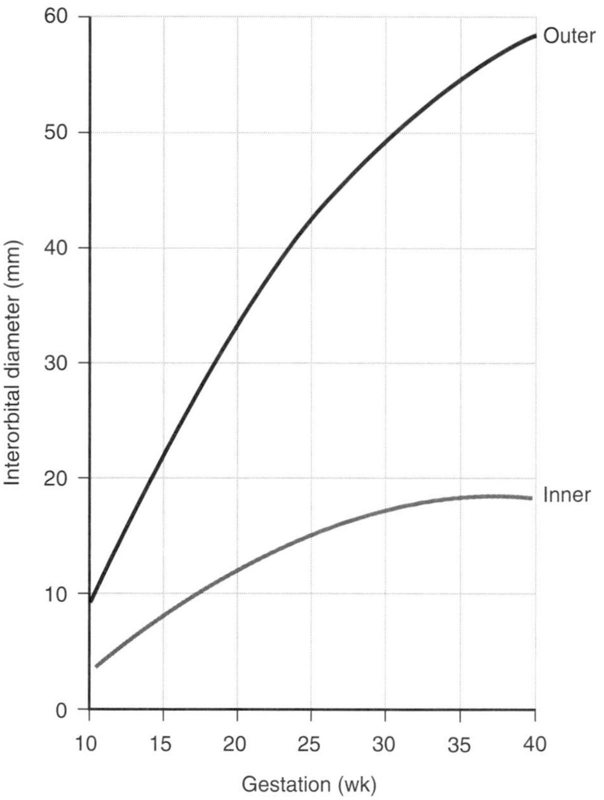

FIGURE 59
Interorbital distance (mean) from a cross-sectional study of 180 healthy women at 22 to 40 weeks' gestation. The scan plane that was used transected the occiput, orbits, and nasal processes. *Data source:* ref. 124, with permission.

> ***Comment:*** Outer-orbital diameter is closely related to biparietal diameter. This measurement is useful when the fetal position precludes accurate measurement of biparietal diameter.

CEREBRAL VENTRICLES

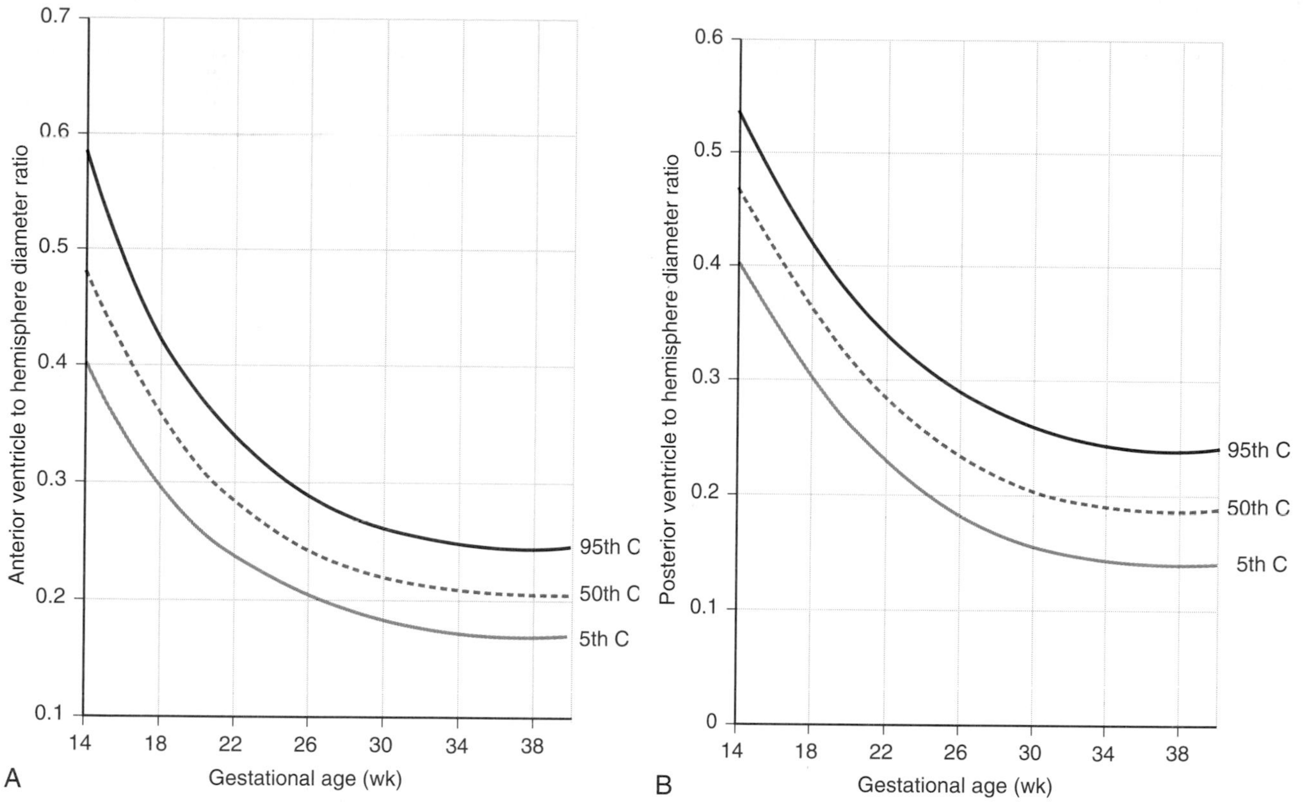

FIGURE 60
Ventriculohemispheric ratios (5th, 50th, and 95th percentiles) from a cross-sectional study of 1040 singleton pregnancies at 14 to 40 weeks' gestation, selected from a large database. All women had known last menstrual period dates, with a cycle length of 26 to 30 days. They had no pregnancy complications. Only data from structurally normal fetuses who were liveborn at 37 weeks' gestation or more and who had birth weights between the 3rd and 97th percentiles for gestation were included. For each week, measurements from 40 fetuses were obtained. Each fetus contributed measurements to the data pool on only one occasion. *A*, Measurement of the anterior horn of the lateral cerebral ventricle was made in a transverse axial plane of the fetal head (as for biparietal diameter or head circumference measurements), from the lateral wall of the anterior horn to the midline. *B*, Posterior horn measurements were made from the medial to the lateral wall of the posterior horn. Hemispheric measurements were made from the midline to the inner border of the skull. *Data source:* ref. 109, with permission.

Comment: The most reliable measurements of the ventricular system are made with the frontal horns of the lateral cerebral ventricles because they are the easiest to identify. In general, ventricular diameter should be less than 10 mm.

CEREBELLUM

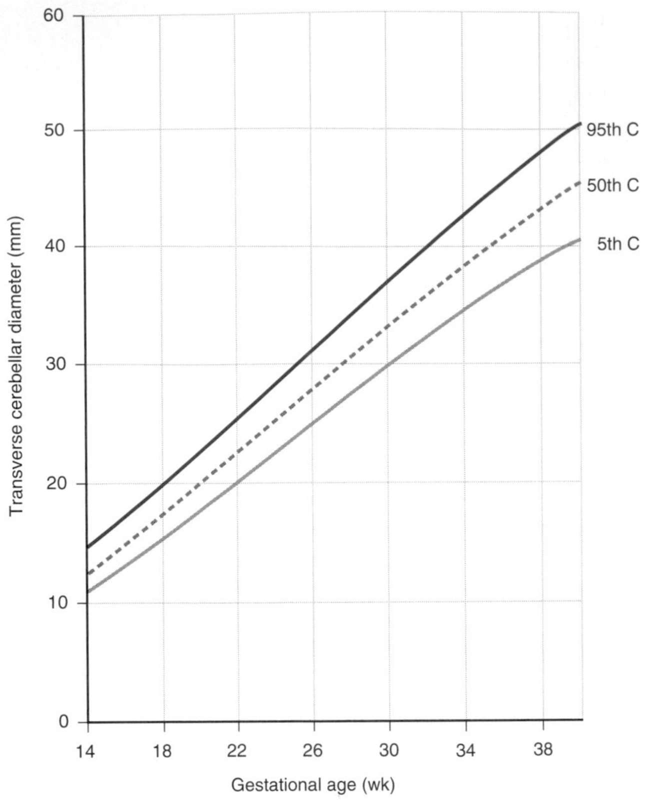

FIGURE 61
Transverse cerebellar diameter (5th, 50th, and 95th percentiles) from the cross-sectional study of 1040 singleton pregnancies described in Figure 60. Measurements were made in the suboccipitobregmatic plane of the fetal head. *Data source:* ref. 109, with permission.

Comment: The cerebellum may be visualized as early as 10 to 11 weeks' gestation. Other studies found similar measurements.[125]

OTHER FETAL MEASUREMENTS

Comment: Normal ranges for many other fetal structures are described in the literature. Each may be useful under certain circumstances. Charts of liver length are useful in the assessment of isoimmunized fetuses, where liver length is inversely correlated with fetal hemoglobin levels.[126] Fetal ear measurements are helpful in the detection of fetuses with abnormal karyotypes.[127,128]

BIOMETRY IN MULTIPLE GESTATIONS

Comment: A study of ultrasound measurements in twin pregnancies after 24 weeks' gestation (involving 884 sets of twins, each of whom contributed only one measurement to the data set) found that the growth pattern for femur length was similar to that of singletons.[129] Abdominal circumference measurements in twins were lower than those in singletons after 32 weeks; biparietal diameter measurements were greater than those in singletons before 32 weeks.[129] A longitudinal study of 35 healthy women with twin pregnancies did not find clinically important differences between measurements of fetal size (head circumference, biparietal diameter, limb bone lengths) in twins compared with singletons.[130,131] Studies in normal triplet pregnancies found delay in growth patterns after midgestation.[132]

BIRTH WEIGHT

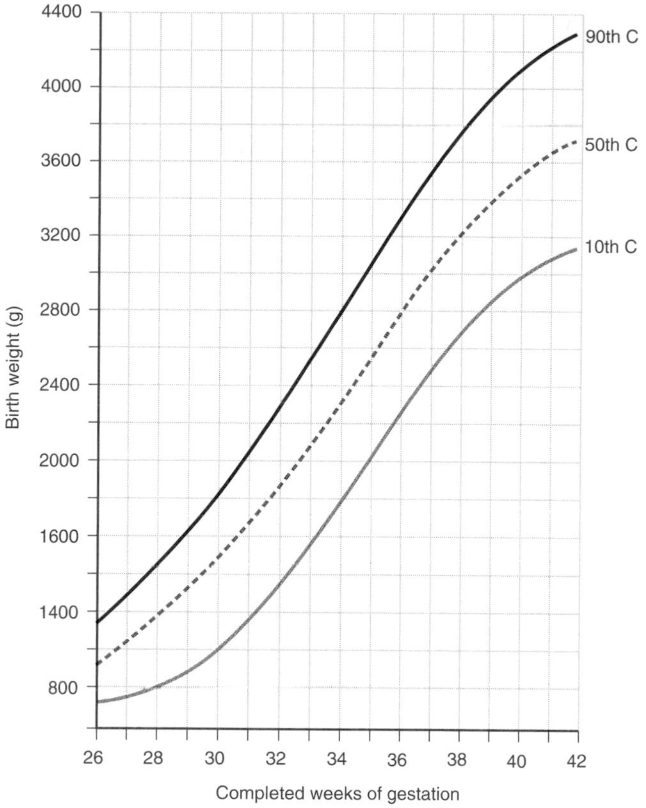

FIGURE 62
Birth weight (10th, 50th, and 90th percentiles) from an analysis of 41,718 singleton births in Nottingham, UK, between 1986 and 1991. All women had dates confirmed by ultrasound measurements (crown–rump length up to 13 weeks and biparietal diameter thereafter) before 24 weeks, and they delivered between 168 and 300 days' gestation. The population was of mixed ethnicity. *Data source:* ref. 133, with permission.

> ***Comment:*** This study differs from previous reports[134,135] (which did not have ultrasound confirmation of gestational age) in that it found a continued increase, rather than flattening, of birth weight curves toward term. Birth weights of preterm infants (≤32 weeks' gestation) were negatively skewed, consistent with the observation that growth-restricted infants may be born earlier than those of appropriate size.[133] Birth weight is also dependent on ethnic origin, altitude, socioeconomic factors, maternal size, birth order, and maternal cigarette smoking.[133,136,137] All of the studies described here are for singletons. Different ranges apply to multiple pregnancies.

WEIGHT ESTIMATED FROM ULTRASOUND MEASUREMENTS

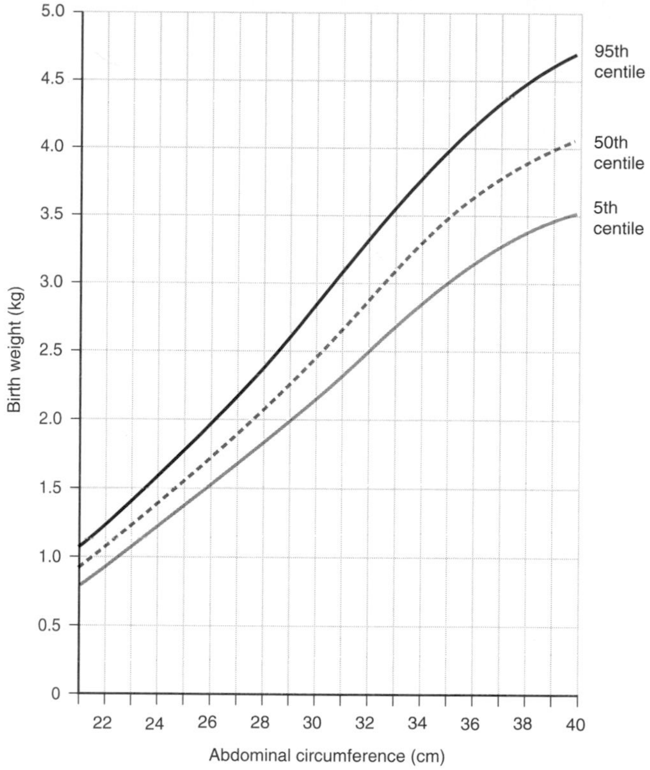

FIGURE 63
Weight estimated from ultrasound measurements (5th, 50th, and 90th percentiles) in a study of 138 women who underwent ultrasound examination within 48 hours of delivery for the measurement of fetal abdominal circumference (AC). Actual birth weights were compared with AC measurements, and a polynomial equation was derived to describe the relationship. *Data source:* ref. 138, with permission.

> ***Comment:*** Equations have been derived for estimating fetal weight from various combinations of ultrasonic measurements (AC, biparietal diameter, head circumference, and femur length).[139,140] These estimates are reported to be more accurate than those based on AC measurements alone.

Amniotic Fluid

TOTAL VOLUME

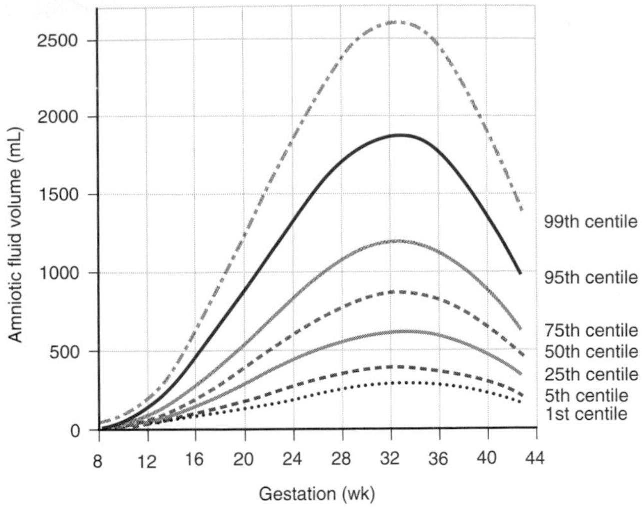

FIGURE 64
Total amniotic fluid volume (1st, 5th, 25th, 50th, 75th, 95th, and 99th percentiles). Composite analysis of 12 published reports of amniotic fluid volume in human pregnancy, totaling 705 measurements. Amniotic fluid volume was measured directly at the time of hysterotomy or indirectly with an indicator dilution technique. Only healthy pregnancies were included; any complicated by fetal death or anomaly or by maternal disease were excluded. *Data source*: ref. 141, with permission.

AMNIOTIC FLUID INDEX (AFI)

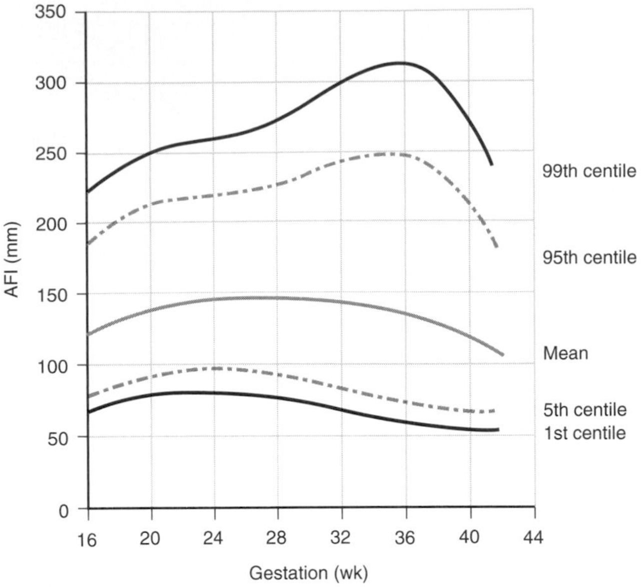

FIGURE 65
Amniotic fluid index (AFI) (1st, 5th, 50th, 95th, and 99th percentiles) from a prospective study of 791 patients. Any who did not have a normal pregnancy outcome (i.e., infant born at term, between the 10th and 90th percentiles for birth weight, with a 5-minute Apgar score >6, and without congenital anomaly) were subsequently excluded. Ultrasound imaging was performed, and the uterus was divided into four quadrants along the sagittal midline and midway up the fundus. The AFI was calculated as the sum of the deepest vertical dimension (in millimeters) of the amniotic fluid pocket in each quadrant of the uterus. *Data source:* ref. 142, with permission.

Comment: The volume of amniotic fluid increases to a plateau of 700 to 850 mL between 22 and 39 weeks' gestation. This volume corresponds to an AFI of 140 to 150 mm. After term, amniotic fluid volume decreases significantly.

PRESSURE

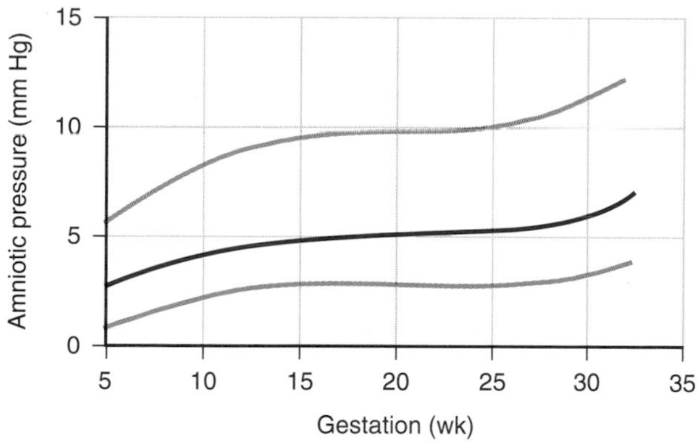

FIGURE 66
Amniotic fluid pressure (mean and 95% CI) from a cross-sectional study of 171 singleton pregnancies subsequently shown to have a normal karyotype. Amniotic fluid volume was subjectively assessed as normal, based on ultrasonic appearance. All patients were scheduled to undergo an invasive diagnostic transamniotic procedure or therapeutic termination of pregnancy. Amniotic fluid pressure was measured with a manometry technique referenced to the top of the maternal abdomen. *Data source:* ref. 143, with permission.

Comment: Amniotic fluid pressure increases with gestation, reaching a midtrimester plateau of 4 to 5 mm Hg. Pressure was not affected by parity or maternal age and was similar in twin and singleton pregnancies.[143]

OSMOLALITY

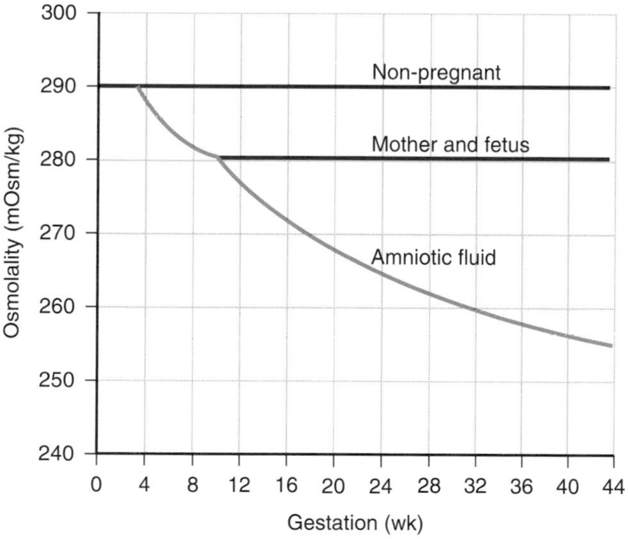

FIGURE 67
Amniotic fluid osmolality (mean) from a composite analysis of six published reports. *Data source:* ref. 144, with permission.

Comment: In early pregnancy, the composition of amniotic fluid is consistent with a transudate of maternal or fetal plasma.[145] The fetal skin becomes keratinized by midpregnancy, and amniotic fluid solute concentrations decrease as fetal urine becomes more dilute.[145] Thus, there is an osmotic gradient between amniotic fluid and both maternal and fetal plasma.

Cardiac Dimensions

CARDIAC CIRCUMFERENCE

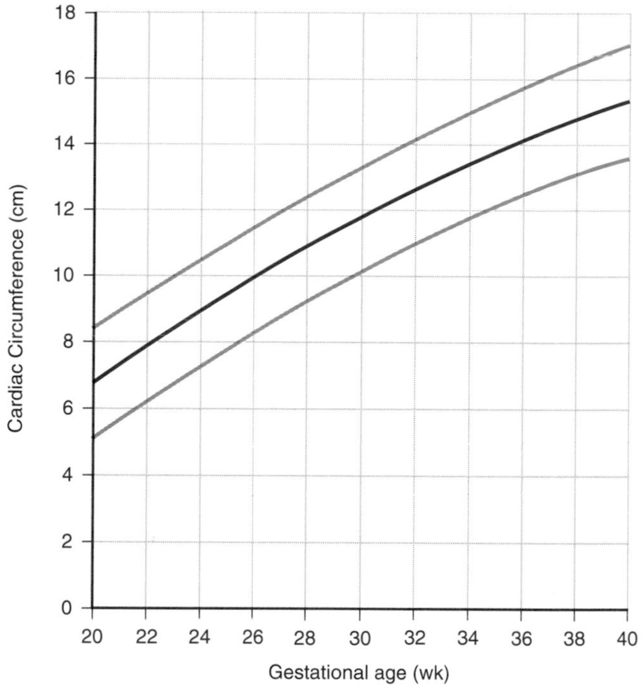

FIGURE 68
Cardiac circumference (mean and 95% CI) from a longitudinal study of 45 healthy women with known menstrual dates that were confirmed by early ultrasound scan. Study subjects were recruited before 20 weeks' gestation and underwent scanning every 4 weeks. Fetal cardiac and thoracic circumference was measured in a transverse plane through the chest, at the level of the four-chamber view of the fetal heart. *Data source:* ref. 146, with permission.

Comment: The cardiac-to-thoracic circumference ratio is normally approximately 0.5 (95% CI at 20 weeks, 0.40–0.58; at 30 weeks, 0.44–0.60; at 40 weeks, 0.46–0.65).[146]

VENTRICULAR DIMENSIONS

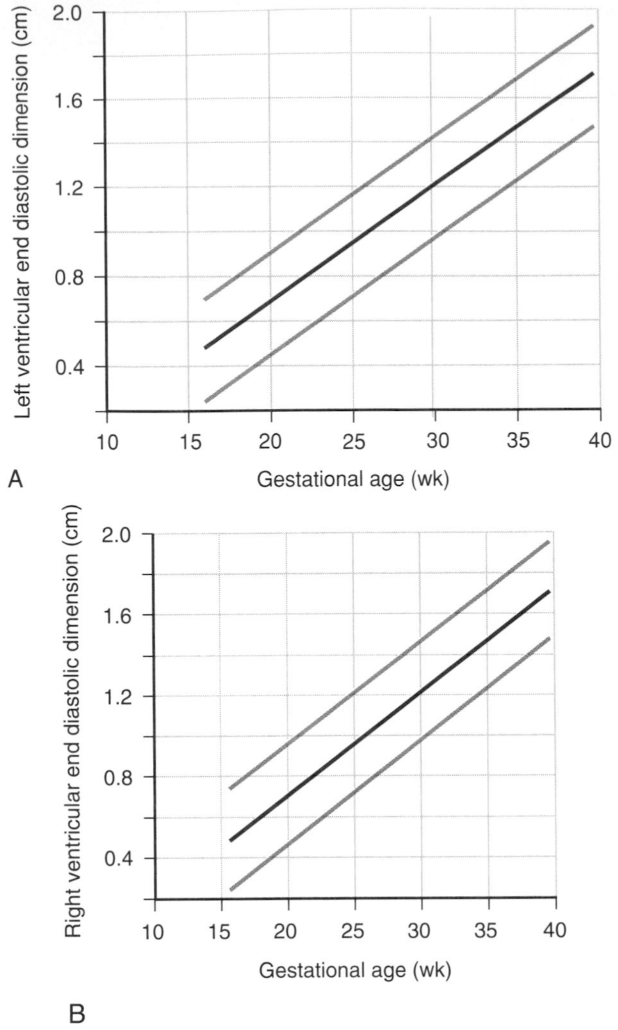

FIGURE 69
End-diastolic dimensions of *A*, the left ventricle and *B*, the right ventricle (regression line and 95% prediction interval) from a cross-sectional study of 117 normal women at 16 to 41 weeks' gestation. All fetuses were anatomically normal, and gestational age was confirmed by first-trimester ultrasound measurements. A four-chamber view of the heart was obtained in a transverse plane through the fetal chest. The transducer was adjusted so that the intraventricular septum was perpendicular to the ultrasound beam. In this view, transverse endocardial–endocardial dimensions of both ventricles were measured just below the valves, at the end of diastole. *Data source:* ref. 147, with permission.

> ***Comment:*** This study found narrower confidence intervals for cardiac measurements than those described in earlier reports.[148] This finding was attributed to improved resolution of newer ultrasound equipment and the use of imaging planes perpendicular to the ultrasound plane (which reduces lateral resolution error). Close correlation was seen between measurements made by two observers in this study.

VENTRICULAR AND SEPTAL WALL THICKNESS

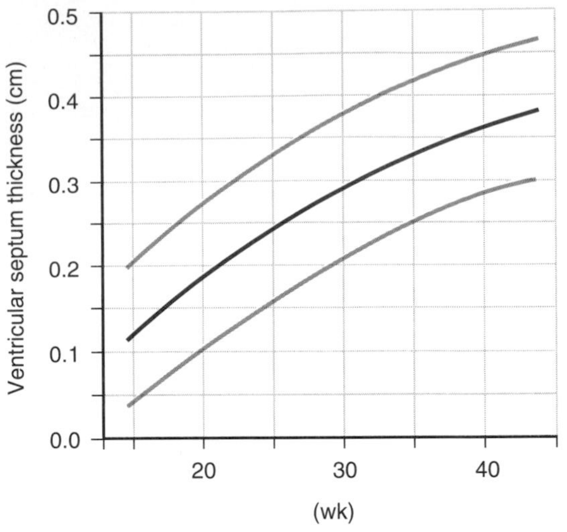

FIGURE 70
Thickness of the interventricular septum (regression line and 95% CI) from a study with cross-sectional and longitudinal data (*n* = 100 observations). Subjects were healthy and had their menstrual dates confirmed by ultrasound measurements; all subsequently were delivered at term. Interventricular septal thickness was measured in the four-chamber view of the fetal heart, just below the atrioventricular valves. *Data source:* ref. 148, with permission.

> ***Comment:*** The thickness of the left or right ventricular wall is similar to that of the interventricular septum.

ASCENDING AORTA AND PULMONARY ARTERY DIAMETER

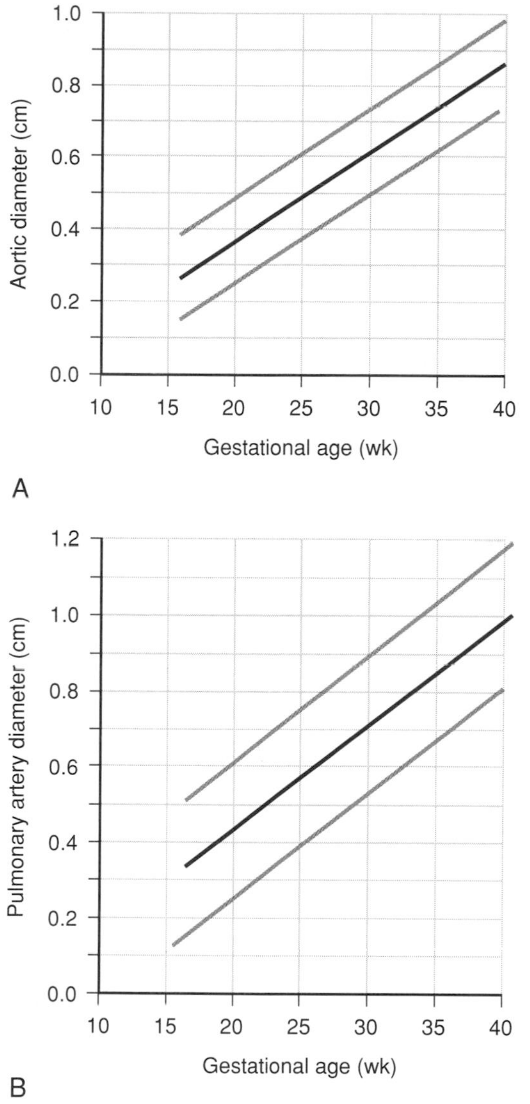

FIGURE 71
Diameter of *A*, the ascending aorta and *B*, the main pulmonary artery (regression line and 95% prediction interval) from a cross-sectional study of 117 fetuses at 16 to 41 weeks' gestation, as described in Figure 69. The aorta was measured in a long axis view of the heart, found by moving cephalad from the four-chamber view. Measurements were made between intimal surfaces when the aorta had been aligned perpendicular to the ultrasound beam, just above the sinuses of Valsalva. The main pulmonary artery was measured in a long axis view, with its vessel walls perpendicular to the ultrasound beam. *Data source:* ref. 147, with permission.

Comment: During intrauterine life, the diameter of the pulmonary artery is slightly larger than that of the aorta. It may not be possible to obtain good views of these vessels in the planes described. However, similar values were reported in other studies in which measurements were made in different scan planes.[148]

Cardiovascular Doppler Indices

DUCTUS VENOSUS

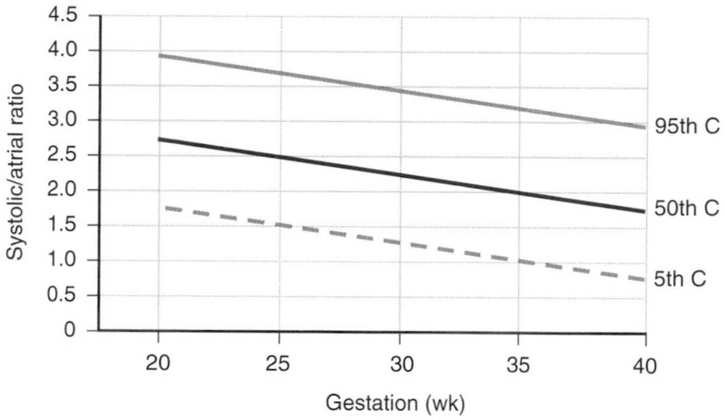

FIGURE 72
Systolic-to-atrial ratio (5th, 50th, and 95th percentiles) from ductus venosus Doppler flow velocity waveforms recorded in a cross-sectional study of 164 fetuses at 16 to 42 weeks' gestation. Fetal size was appropriate for gestational age, and no structural or chromosomal abnormalities were reported. Velocity waveforms were recorded from the ductus venosus at its origin from the umbilical vein, as visualized in a transverse section of the fetal abdomen with color and pulsed Doppler recordings. The angle of insonation of the vessel was kept low; recordings in which this angle exceeded 20 degrees were rejected. Ductus venosus waveforms were recognized by their characteristic biphasic pattern. The ratio between peak systolic velocity and velocity during atrial contraction (nadir of the waveform) was calculated. *Data source:* ref. 149, with permission.

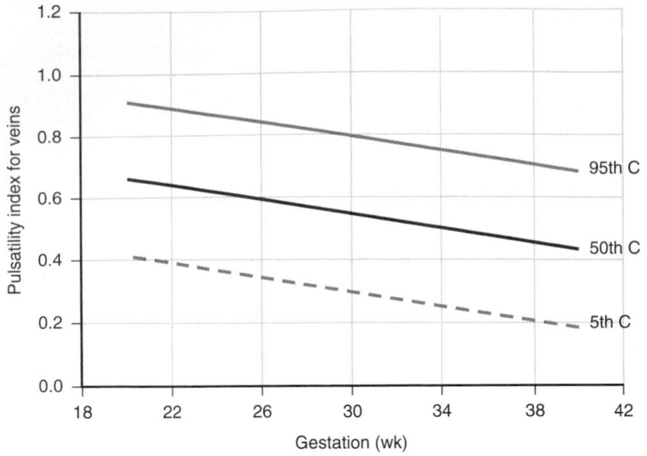

FIGURE 73
Pulsatility index for veins from the ductus venosus (5th, 50th, and 95th percentiles) from a cross-sectional study of 143 women with singleton pregnancies at 20 to 40 weeks' gestation. All fetuses were anatomically normal. Gestational age was calculated from menstrual history and confirmed by fetal measurements made at 20 weeks' amenorrhea. At the time of the study, measurements of fetal head and abdominal circumference were within the 90% CI for gestational age. Movements, amniotic fluid volume, and umbilical artery Doppler pulsatility index were also normal. All measurements were made in the absence of fetal breathing movements. Flow velocity waveforms were recorded from the ductus venosus and visualized in an oblique transverse plane through the upper abdomen or in a midsagittal longitudinal plane. Good signals were obtained from 134 cases. The pulsatility index for veins was calculated as (peak systolic velocity – minimum atrial velocity/time-averaged maximum velocity). *Data source:* ref. 150, with permission.

> ***Comment:*** Color-flow mapping Doppler equipment is necessary for correct identification of the ductus venosus. Waveforms from the intrahepatic portion of the umbilical vein and the inferior vena cava are different. The decreasing systolic-to-atrial ratio is interpreted as indicating a relative increase in blood flow during end diastole (i.e., improved cardiac filling).

INFERIOR VENA CAVA

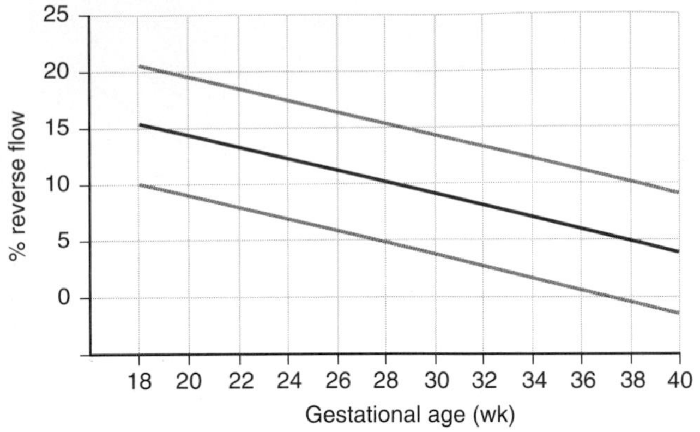

FIGURE 74
Percentage of reverse flow from the inferior vena cava (mean and linear regression of the 95th CI) from a cross-sectional study of 118 appropriate-for-gestational-age fetuses at 18 to 40 weeks' gestation. All pregnancies were singleton and were dated by certain last menstrual period and early second-trimester ultrasonography. All fetuses were structurally normal and of appropriate size for gestation at the time of study. Flow velocity waveforms were recorded with color and pulsed Doppler equipment from the inferior vena cava, which was identified in a saggital view of the fetal trunk between the entrance of the renal vein and the ductus venosus. Measurements were made in the absence of fetal body or breathing movements. Three components of the waveform were identified: systolic peak (S), diastolic wave (D), and reverse flow during atrial contraction (A). The percentage of reverse flow was calculated as the percentage of the time–velocity intervals during the A wave, with respect to the total forward time–velocity intervals (S + D). *Data source:* ref. 151, with permission.

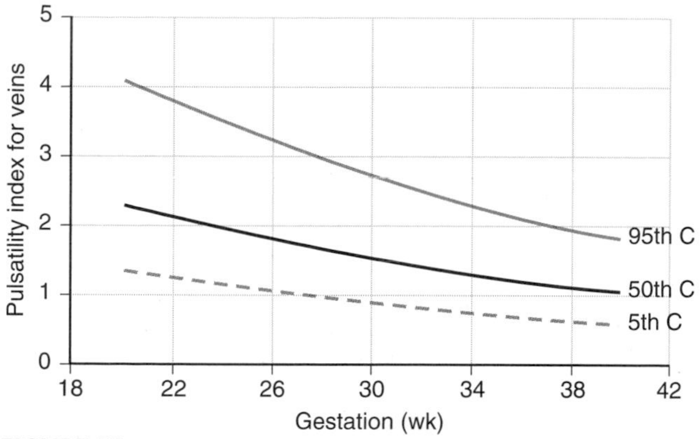

FIGURE 75
Pulsatility index for veins from the inferior vena cava (5th, 50th, and 95th percentiles) from the cross-sectional study of 143 women described in Figure 73. Flow velocity waveforms were recorded from the inferior vena cava in a longitudinal section of the fetal abdomen, with the sample volume placed in the portion between the renal and hepatic veins. Clear signals were obtained from 127 fetuses. The pulsatility index for veins was calculated as (peak systolic velocity – minimum atrial velocity/time-averaged maximum velocity). *Data source:* ref. 150, with permission.

> ***Comment:*** Flow velocity waveforms in the inferior vena cava are characteristically triphasic, with reverse velocities found during atrial contraction. These reverse velocities decrease significantly with advancing gestation. This decrease is attributed to a decrease in the pressure gradient between the right atrium and right ventricle at end diastole as a result of improved ventricular compliance and reduced end-diastolic pressure. Right ventricular afterload declines with decreasing placental resistance, contributing to the reduction in end-diastolic pressure. In studies in which Doppler waveforms were recorded from the inferior vena cava and ductus venosus in growth-restricted fetuses before cordocentesis, fetal hypoxemia, and acidemia were associated with more reverse flow and more pulsatile waveforms.[152,153]

CARDIAC FUNCTION

> ***Comment:*** Normal ranges have been defined for Doppler flow velocity waveform indices derived from across the mitral, tricuspid, aortic, and pulmonary valves.[150,154,155] These have potential use in the assessment of cardiac function in growth-restricted fetuses and fetuses with structural heart defects. Waveforms from the ductus arteriosus show considerable individual variability[156] and do not appear to be useful in the detection of fetal compromise. Waveforms from peripheral pulmonary arteries show decreasing pulsatility with advancing gestation in healthy fetuses.[157]

CARDIAC OUTPUT

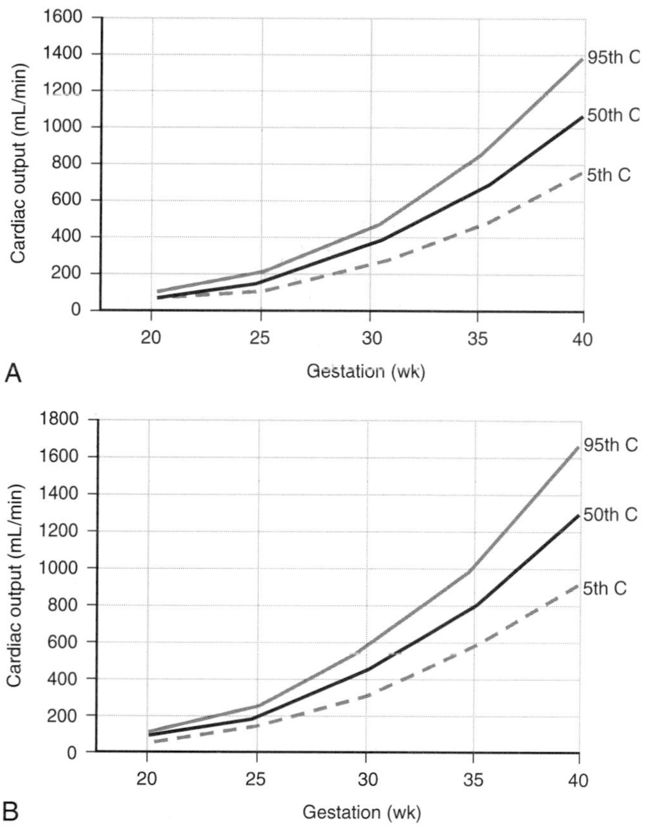

FIGURE 76
A, Left cardiac output (LCO) *B*, right cardiac output (RCO) calculated at the level of the outflow tracts (5th, 50th, and 95th percentiles) from a longitudinal study of 26 healthy singleton fetuses studied at weekly intervals. Velocity waveforms were recorded from the ascending aorta and pulmonary artery with the flow parallel to the Doppler beam. Recordings obtained with a beam angle greater than 20 degrees were rejected. Valve diameter measurements were made from videotape images, and valve areas were calculated by assuming a circular cross-section. *Data source:* ref. 154, with permission.

> ***Comment:*** Cardiac output rises progressively with gestation, with RCO slightly higher than LCO (RCO/LCO ratio, approximately 1.3). Peak flow velocity at both the aortic and pulmonary valves increases with gestation. This increase is attributed to progressive improvement in cardiac contractility, reduction in afterload, and increase in preload.[154] This type of calculation of volume flow is susceptible to high coefficients of variation because an error in the measurement of diameter (e.g., valve ring diameter) is magnified as the cross-sectional area is computed.

MIDDLE CEREBRAL ARTERY

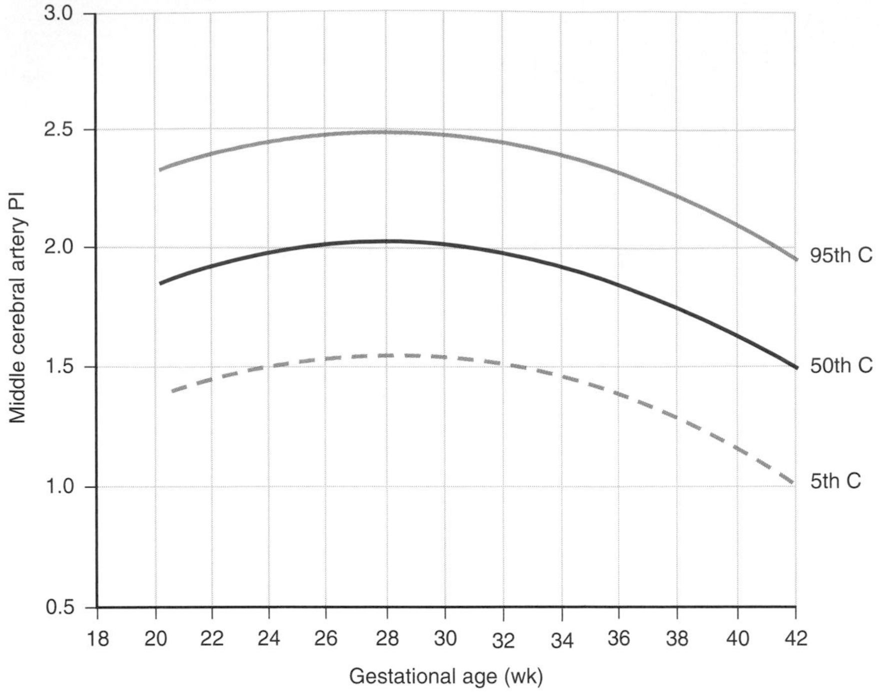

FIGURE 77
Pulsatility index from the middle cerebral artery (5th, 50th, and 95th percentiles) from a cross-sectional study of 1556 fetuses at 20 to 42 weeks' gestation. All fetuses were singletons, and gestational age was confirmed by early ultrasound measurement of crown–rump length. Color flow imaging was used to identify the fetal middle cerebral artery, and waveforms were recorded at a low angle of insonation. Good signals were obtained from 1467 fetuses. Pulsatility index was calculated as (maximum systolic velocity – diastolic velocity/mean velocity). *Data source:* ref. 158, with permission.

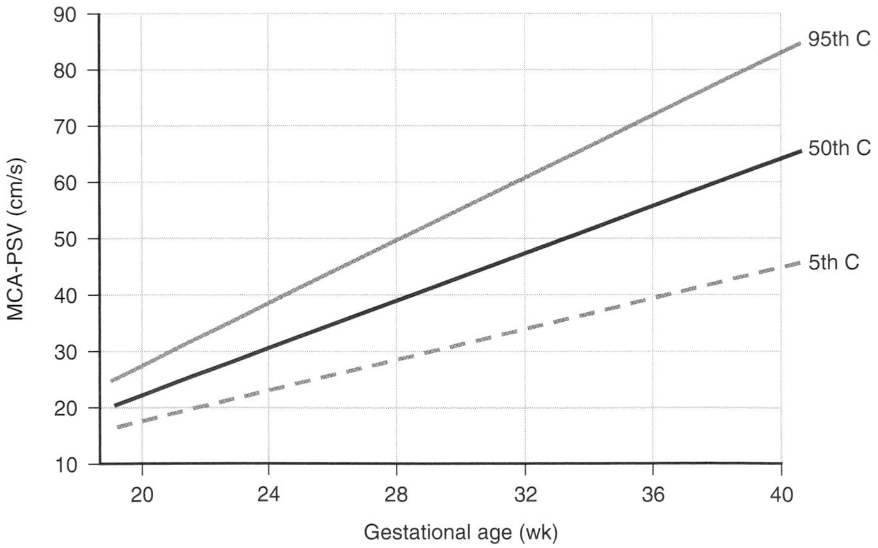

FIGURE 78
Peak systolic velocity from the middle cerebral artery (5th, 50th, and 95th percentiles) from a cross-sectional study of 331 women at 19 to 40 weeks' gestation. All fetuses were singletons, and none of the pregnancies were complicated by blood group antibodies, hypertension, diabetes, or congenital abnormalities. Only one measurement from each fetus was included in the study. The middle cerebral artery was identified in an axial section of the fetal brain and insonated at a low angle. The highest point on the waveform (peak systolic velocity) was measured. *Data source:* ref. 159, with permission.

Comment: A longitudinal study of middle cerebral artery (MCA) Doppler waveforms found that pulsatility index values are higher at 25 to 30 weeks' gestation than those at 15 to 20 weeks, or toward term.[160] Diameter of the fetal MCA increases with gestational age. In one study,[161] calculated volume blood flow in the artery increased from 23 mL/min at 19 weeks' gestation to 133 mL/min at term. Doppler waveforms from the MCA may also be quantitated with a resistance index (maximum systolic velocity – minimum diastolic velocity/systolic velocity).[162] When MCA waveforms are recorded, care must be taken to apply minimal pressure to the maternal abdomen because fetal skull compression may alter MCA flow.[163] Different signals are obtained in the distal portion of the MCA, and most studies have concentrated on the proximal portion, close to the circle of Willis.[164] Changes in MCA Doppler waveforms are noted in growth-restricted fetuses, suggesting that fetal cardiac output may be redistributed to preserve brain blood.[60,163,164] High MCA peak systolic velocities are associated with fetal anemia in pregnancies complicated by maternal alloimmunization.[165,166]

DESCENDING AORTA

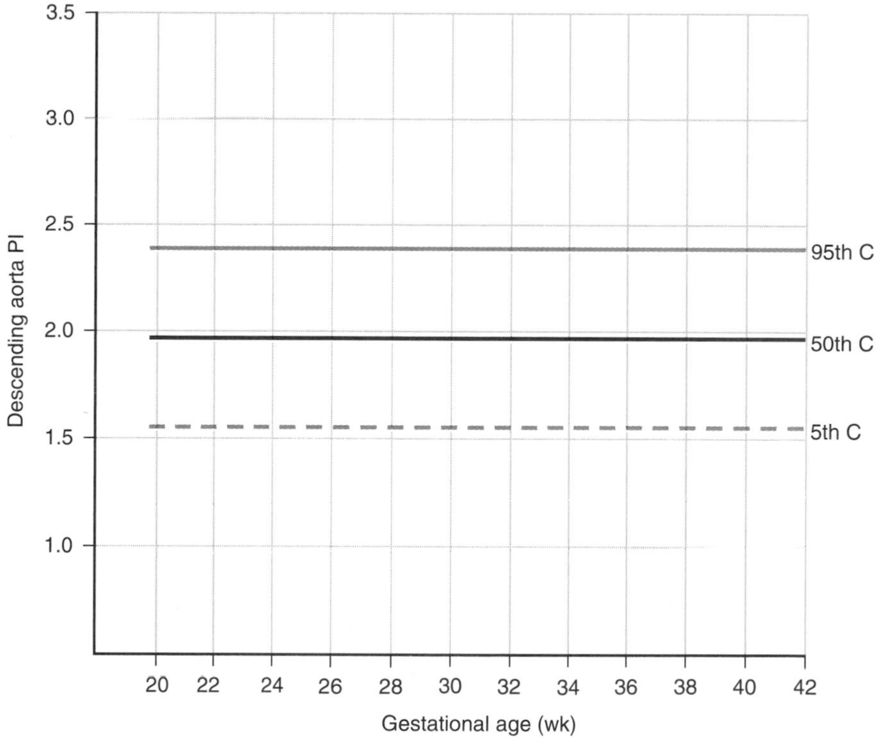

FIGURE 79
Descending aorta pulsatility index (5th, 50th, and 95th percentiles) from a cross-sectional study of 1556 healthy pregnancies at 20 to 42 weeks' gestation. All fetuses were singletons, and gestational age was confirmed by early ultrasound measurement of crown–rump length. Recordings from the thoracic portion of the descending aorta were made in the absence of fetal body or breathing movements. Satisfactory recordings were obtained in 1398 fetuses. The pulsatility index was calculated as (systolic velocity – diastolic velocity/mean velocity). *Data source:* ref. 158, with permission.

Comment: Unlike in other fetal vessels, no significant change with gestation was seen in the aortic pulsatility index.

UMBILICAL ARTERY

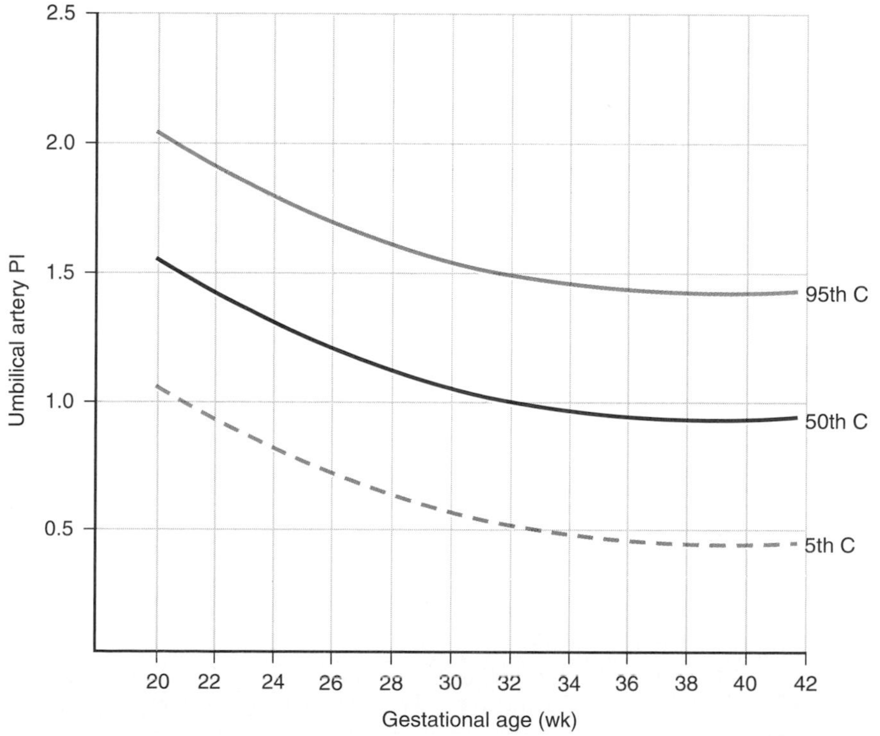

FIGURE 80
Umbilical artery pulsatility index (5th, 50th, and 95th percentiles) from a cross-sectional study of 1556 healthy pregnancies at 20 to 42 weeks' gestation. All fetuses were singletons, and gestational age was confirmed by early ultrasound measurement of crown–rump length. Recordings from the umbilical artery were made in the absence of fetal body or breathing movements. The pulsatility index was calculated as (systolic velocity – diastolic velocity/mean velocity). *Data source:* ref. 158, with permission.

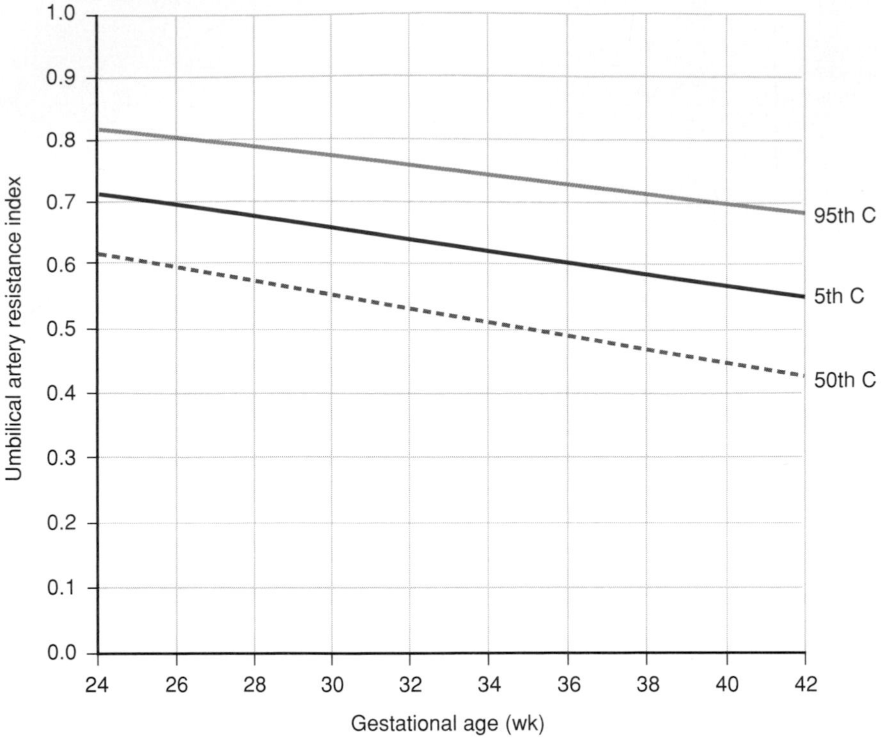

FIGURE 81
Umbilical artery resistance index (5th, 50th, and 95th percentiles) from a cross-sectional study of 1675 pregnancies at 24 to 42 weeks' gestation. Each fetus contributed only one measurement to the study. Signals were recorded from a free-floating loop in the middle of the umbilical cord. Resistance (Pourcelot) index was calculated as (systolic diastolic velocity/systolic velocity). *Data source:* ref. 162, with permission.

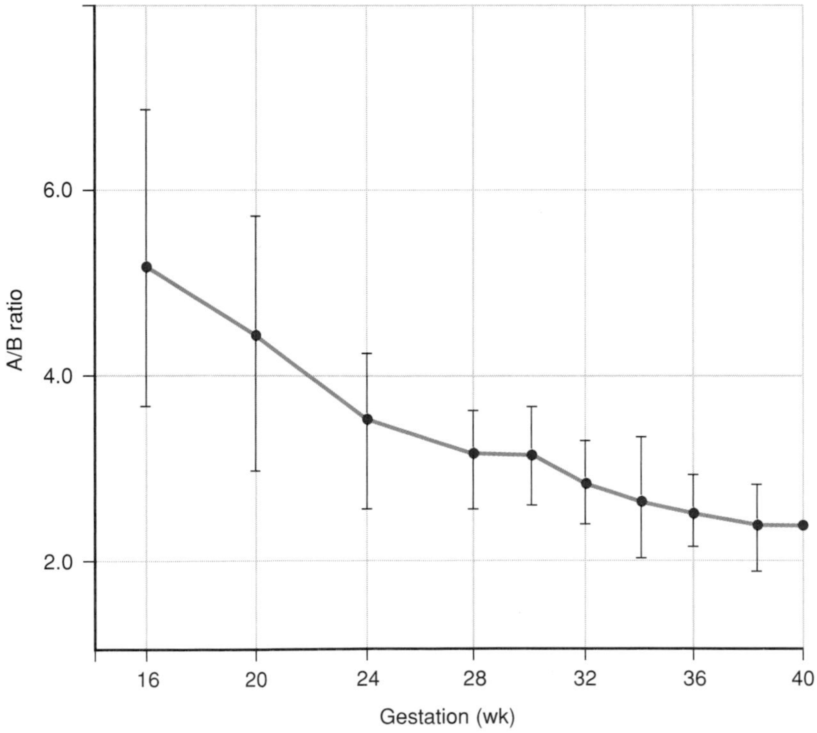

FIGURE 82
Systolic-to-diastolic ratio (A/B ratio) calculated from umbilical artery flow velocity waveforms (mean ± 2 SDs) obtained in a longitudinal study of 15 normal pregnancies. Study subjects were scanned every 2 weeks, from 24 to 28 weeks' gestation until delivery. Eight of the study subjects had been recruited at 16 weeks and were also scanned every 4 weeks throughout the second trimester. In all subjects, gestational age was confirmed by ultrasound scanning at 16 weeks' gestation. A range-gated pulsed Doppler beam was guided from the ultrasound image to insonate the umbilical artery. *Data source:* ref. 167, with kind permission from Elsevier Science Ireland Ltd, Co. Clare, Ireland.

Comment *(Figs. 80–82):* After 16 weeks' gestation, forward flow occurs in umbilical arteries throughout the cardiac cycle, as evidenced by positive Doppler shift frequencies, even at the end of diastole. Decreasing values for the resistance index, pulsatility index, and A/B ratio with gestation are interpreted as indicating decreasing resistance in the placental circulation.

FETAL–PLACENTAL DOPPLER RATIOS

Comment: Various ratios have been suggested to compare fetal cerebral flow velocity waveforms with those from the umbilical artery or aorta. These waveforms may be useful in detecting alterations in fetal cardiac output distribution (e.g., in response to fetal hypoxemia ["brain-sparing" effect]). The placentocerebral ratio[162] describes resistance indices from the umbilical artery and middle cerebral artery. The cerebroplacental ratio[168] describes resistance indices from the middle cerebral artery and umbilical artery. The umbilical artery-to-middle cerebral artery ratio[158] describes pulsatility indices from the umbilical artery and middle cerebral artery. The descending thoracic aorta-to-middle cerebral artery ratio[158] describes pulsatility indices from the descending thoracic aorta and middle cerebral artery.

Cardiovascular and Behavioral Parameters

UMBILICAL VENOUS PRESSURE (UVP)

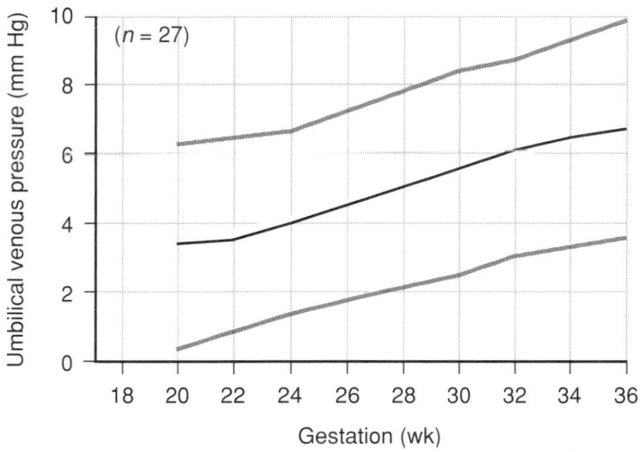

FIGURE 83
Umbilical venous pressure (mean and 95% CI) from 27 fetuses referred for assessment of possible intrauterine infection or hemolysis, but subsequently shown to be unaffected. All of the fetuses underwent cordocentesis; after the necessary blood samples were obtained, the needle was connected to a pressure transducer. The transducer was placed at the level of the fetal heart, and the pressure was read at its nadir. The needle was confirmed to be in the umbilical vein by the nonpulsatile pressure tracing that was obtained and by observing the direction of flow of injected saline. As the needle was withdrawn, pressure in the amniotic cavity was recorded. Umbilical venous pressure was calculated by subtracting the amniotic pressure from the measured umbilical venous pressure. *Data source:* ref. 169, with permission.

Comment: Umbilical venous pressure increases with advancing gestation, but remains within a narrow range. Values above the confidence interval are associated with cardiac failure.[170]

MEAN UMBILICAL ARTERIAL PRESSURE (MAP)

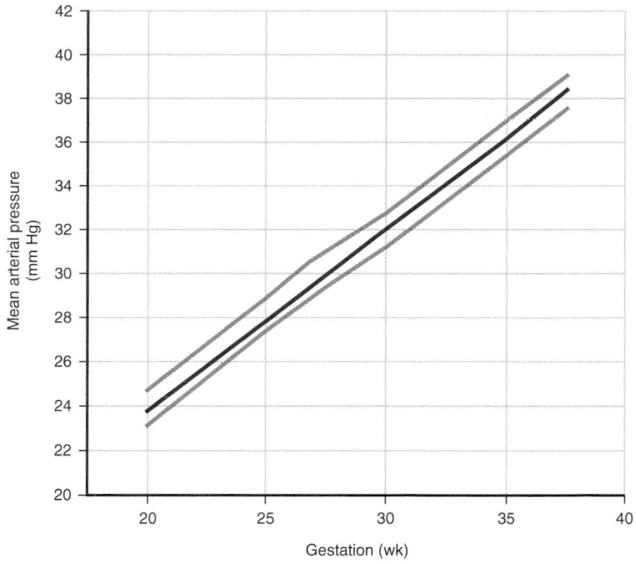

FIGURE 84
Mean umbilical arterial pressure (mean and 95% CI) from 30 normal fetuses referred for assessment of possible infection or hemolysis, but found to be unaffected. The method was identical to that described in Figure 66. It was apparent that the needle tip was in an umbilical artery rather than a vein (because of a pulsatile pressure signal). *Data source:* ref. 171, with permission.

Comment: The normal range of arterial pressure in the fetus is much more narrow than the range of umbilical venous pressure. Arterial pressure increases with gestational age.

FETAL HEART RATE (FHR)

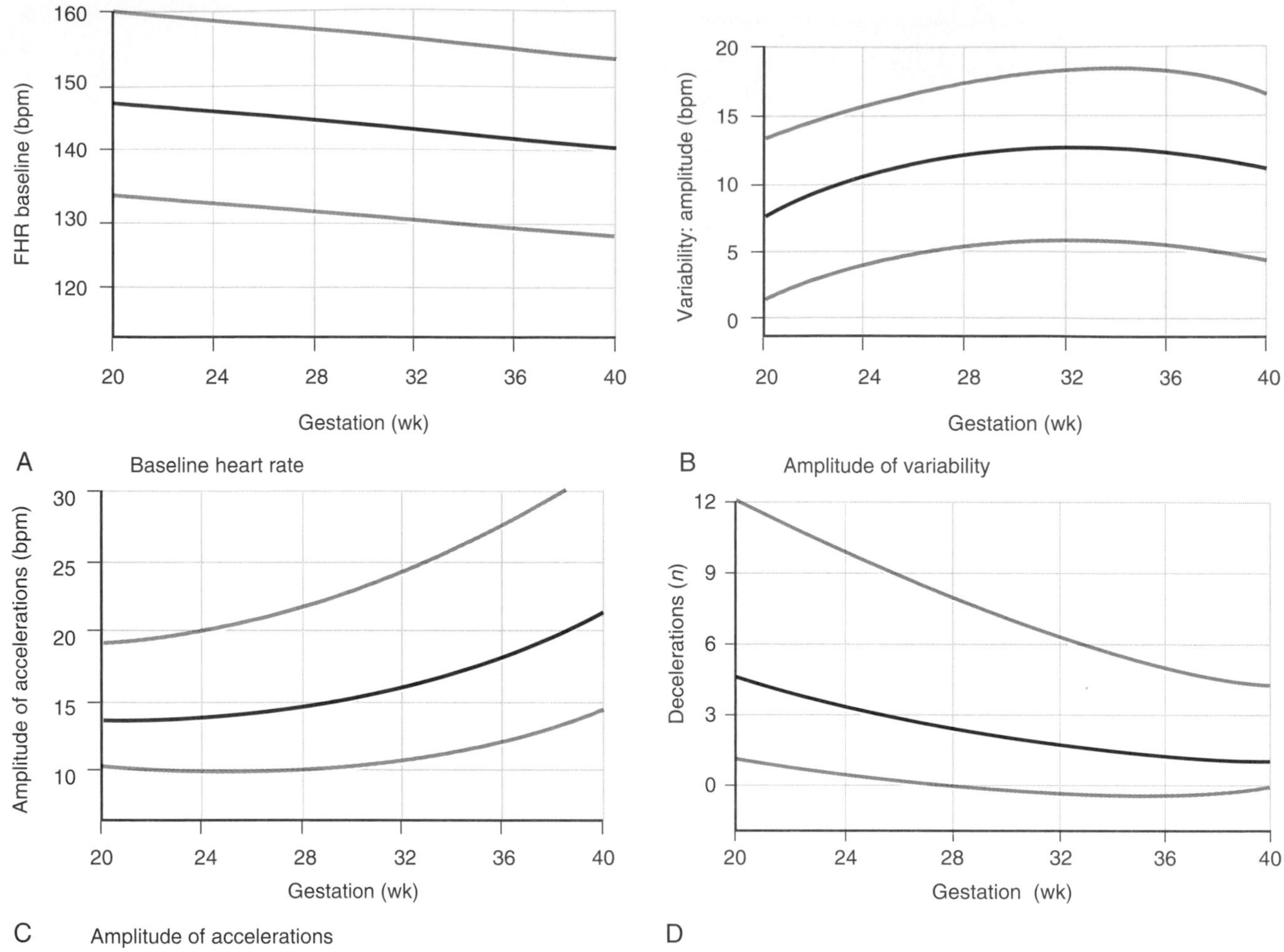

FIGURE 85

Fetal heart rate (FHR) parameters (mean and 95% CI) showing *A*, the baseline heart rate, *B*, the amplitude of variability, Fetal heart rate (FHR) Parameters (mean and 95% CI) showing *C*, the amplitude of accelerations, and *D*, the number of decelerations. Data were obtained from a cross-sectional study of 119 pregnancies at 20 to 39 weeks' gestation. Study subjects were referred for prenatal diagnosis by cordocentesis. In all cases, fetal blood gas values, hemoglobin, and karyotype were subsequently shown to be normal; none of the fetuses had hydrops fetalis or a cardiac defect. FHR monitoring was performed immediately before cordocentesis for 30 minutes, and tracings were examined for baseline heart rate, variability, accelerations, and decelerations. *Data source:* ref. 172, with permission from S Karger AG, Basel.

- At least two accelerations (>15 beats for >15 s) in 20 min, baseline heart rate 110–150 bpm, baseline variability 5–25 bpm, absence deacceleration.
- Sporadic deaccelerations amplitude <40 bpm are acceptable if duration <15 s, or <30 s following an acceleration.
- When there is moderate tachycardia (150–170 bpm) or bradycardia (100–110 bpm) a reactive trace is reassuring of good health.

FIGURE 86

Features of a normal antepartum cardiotocogram (nonstress test). *Data source:* ref. 173, with permission.

Comment: Baseline FHR decreases with gestation, but the variability of the baseline increases. The number and amplitude of accelerations increase with gestation. Spontaneous decelerations are common in the second and early third trimesters, but rarely in healthy fetuses approaching term. Definitions of the features of normal and abnormal cardiotocograms are available.[174] During labor, criteria for the interpretation of FHR tracings are different (see Fig. 104).

BIOPHYSICAL PROFILE SCORE (BPS)

Fetal variable	Normal behavior (score = 2)	Abnormal behavior (score = 0)
Fetal breathing movements	More than one episode of 30 s duration, intermittent within a 30 min overall period. Hiccups count. (Not continuous throughout the observation time)	Repetitive or continuous breathing without cessation. Completely absent breathing or no sustained episodes
Gross body/limb movements	Three or more discrete body/limb movements in a 30 min period. Continuous active movement episodes are considered as a single movement. Also included are fine motor movements, positional adjustments and so on.	Two or fewer body/limb movements in a 30 min observation period
Fetal tone and posture	Demonstration of active extension with rapid return of flexion of fetal limbs, brisk repositioning/trunk rotation. Opening and closing of hand, mouth, kicking, etc.	Only low-velocity movements, incomplete return to flexion, flaccid extremity positions; abnormal fetal posture. Includes score = 0 when FM absent
Fetal heart rate reactivity	Greater than 2 significant accelerations associated with maternally palpated fetal movement during a 20 min cardiotocogram. (Accelerations graded for gestation: 10 beats/min for 10 s before 26 weeks; 15 beats/min for 15 s after 26 weeks; 20 beats/min for 20 s at term)	Fetal movement and accelerations not coupled. Insufficient accelerations, absent accelerations, or decelerative trace. Mean variation <20 on numerical analysis of CTG
Amniotic fluid volume evaluation	One pocket of >3 cm without umbilical cord loops. More than 1 pocket of >2 cm without cord loops. No elements of subjectively reduced amniotic volume.	No cord-free pocket >2 cm, or elements of subjectively reduced amniotic fluid volume definite

FIGURE 87

Scoring system for five fetal biophysical variables (breathing movements, gross body and limb movements, tone and posture, heart rate reactivity, and amniotic fluid volume) developed for the assessment of patients with high risk pregnancies. This scoring system was evaluated in 216 patients who were studied in the week before delivery and whose eventual pregnancy outcome was documented. No perinatal deaths occurred in this study when all five variables were present at the time of examination with ultrasound and cardiotocography. Low scores (≤6 of 10) were associated with an increased incidence of adverse outcomes (i.e., fetal distress in labor, Apgar scores ≤7 at 5 minutes, perinatal death). *Data source:* ref. 175, with permission.

Comment: Various means of monitoring fetal well-being antenatally have been proposed (i.e., cardiotocography, observation of fetal breathing patterns, measurement of amniotic fluid volume). Scoring systems that consider a combination of behavioral parameters are better able to detect a compromised fetus and allow early delivery.[176] The use of these scoring systems led to improved perinatal mortality rates, even in a high risk group of pregnant women.[176] Fetal behavior is periodic and is affected by external factors (e.g., maternal ingestion of stimulant or depressant drugs, maternal hypoglycemia or hyperglycemia) and by structural or genetic abnormalities. Fetal behavior changes abruptly from a quiescent pattern to an active pattern and vice versa; therefore, ultrasound observation may need to be extended for 30 or 40 minutes to confirm the absence of fetal movements or breathing. Most biophysical profile score (BPS) studies are completed in less than 10 minutes.[175] Acute events may occur that invalidate the predictive accuracy of the BPS (e.g., abruptio placentae, diabetic ketoacidosis, eclampsia).

Biochemistry

Proteins

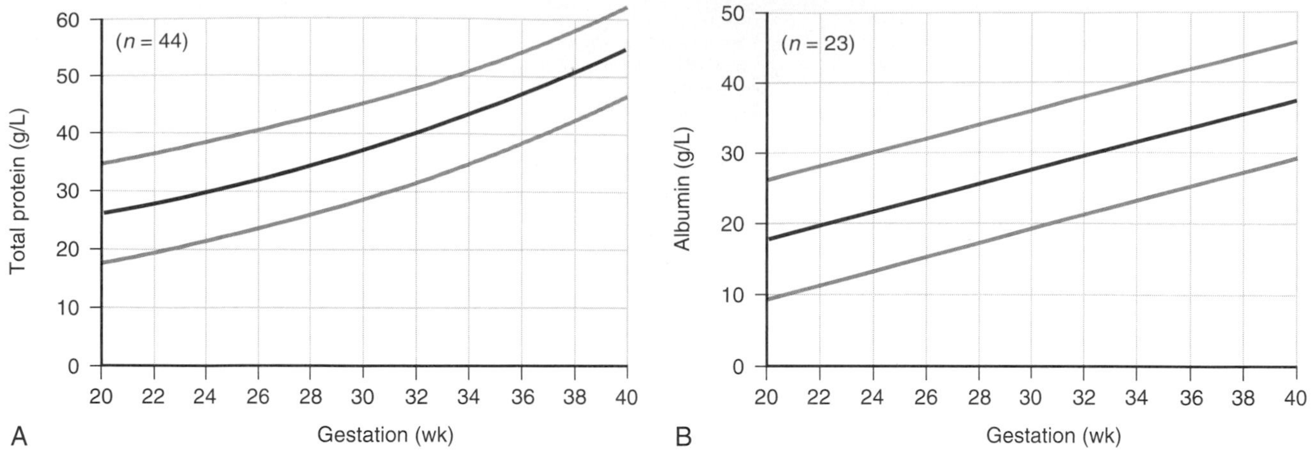

FIGURE 88
A, Total protein and *B*, albumin concentrations (regression curve and 95% CI) from a cross-sectional study of 45 fetuses subsequently shown to be normal at birth. Blood samples were obtained by ultrasound-guided cordocentesis. *Data source:* ref. 177, with permission.

Renal Function Tests, Liver Function Tests, and Glucose

	SI units (mean ± SD)	Traditional units (mean ± SD)
Glucose	4.3 ± 0.6 mmol/L	7.7 ± 1.1 mg/dL
Cholesterol	1.5 ± 0.3 mmol/L	59 ± 11 mg/dL
Uric acid	179 ± 39 mol/L	2.8 ± 0.6 mg/dL
Triglycerides	4.5 ± 1.1 µmol/L	40 ± 10 mg/dL
Total bilirubin	26.3 ± 5.8 µol/L	15 ± 0.3 mg/dL
Alkaline phosphatase	260 ± 65 IU/L	
Gamma glutamyl transferase	60 ± 34 IU/L	
Asparate transaminase	17 ± 6.5 IU/L	
Creatinine	1.8 ± 0.3 mol/L	0.02 ± 0.003 mg/dL
Calcium	2.3 ± 0.2 mmol/L	9.2 ± 0.8 mg/dL

FIGURE 89
Glucose, calcium, liver function, and renal function test results (mean ± SD) from a cross-sectional study of 78 fetuses at 20 to 26 weeks' gestation; all fetuses were subsequently shown to be healthy at birth. Blood samples were obtained by ultrasound-guided cordocentesis. *Data source:* ref. 178, with permission.

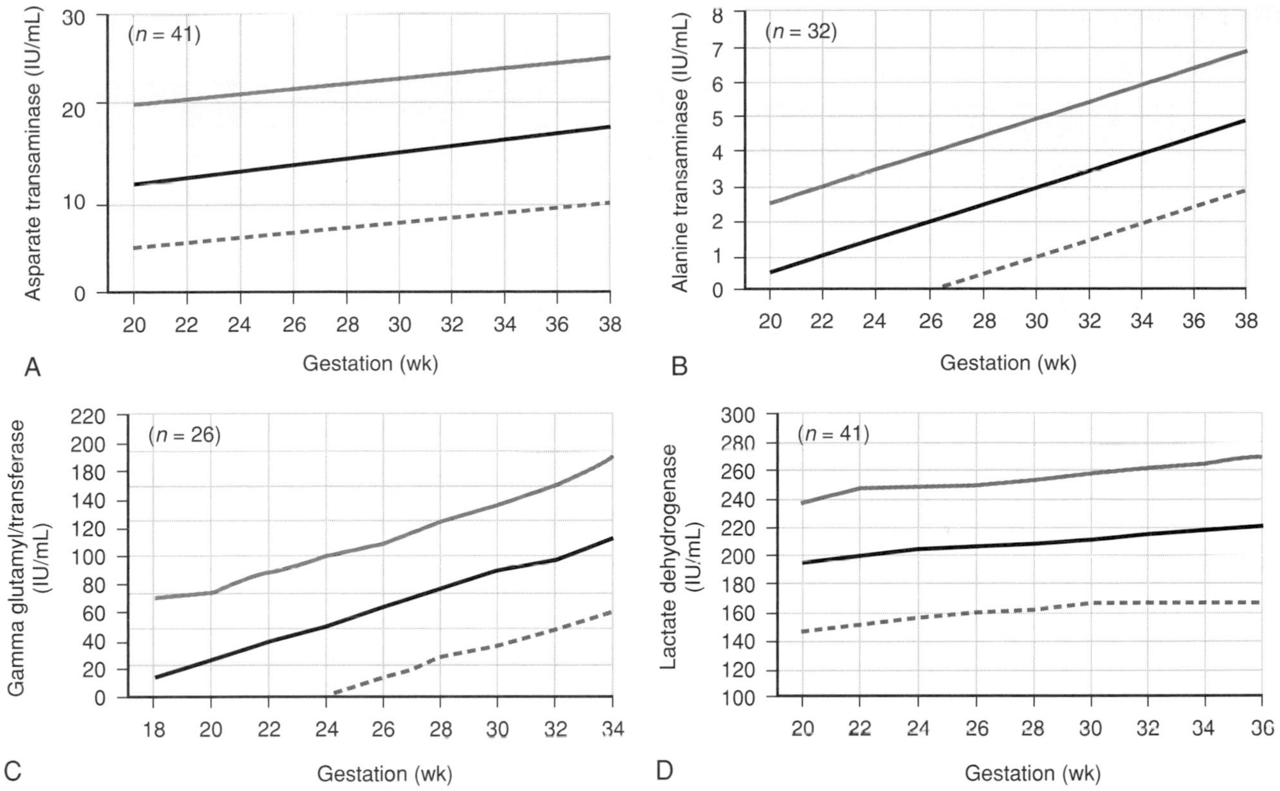

FIGURE 90

A, Aspartate transaminase (AST), *B*, alanine transaminase (ALT), *C*, γ-glutamyl transferase (GGT), and *D*, lactate dehydrogenase (LDH) concentrations (regression line and 95% CI) from a cross-sectional study of 80 fetuses referred for assessment of possible intrauterine infection or hemolysis, but subsequently shown to be unaffected. All study subjects underwent cordocentesis, and blood samples were obtained for liver enzyme assays. Individual graphs show the number of assays performed for each enzyme. *Data source:* ref. 169, with permission.

***Comment** (Figs. 88–90):* Plasma total protein and albumin concentrations increase significantly with gestational age.[177] Little information is available about many other biochemical variables. Triglyceride levels decrease with advancing gestation,[178] bilirubin levels increase,[179] and liver enzyme concentrations (other than LDH) increase.[169] Fetal concentrations of bilirubin are higher and triglyceride and cholesterol concentrations are lower than those in maternal serum.[178] Fetal plasma insulin levels increase with gestation.[180]

Urinary Biochemistry

	16 weeks	33 weeks
Phosphate (mmol/L)	0.91	0.10
Creatinine (µmol/L)	99.9	172.9
(mean values)		

A

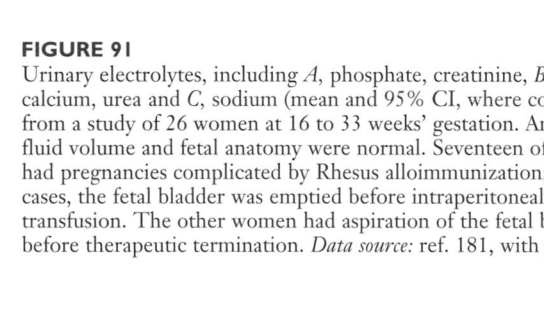

	Mean value	95% confidence intervals (CI)
Potassium (mmol/L)	3.0	0–6.1
Calcium (µmol/L)	0.21	0.04–1.2
Urea (µmol/L)	7.9	2.6–13.1

B

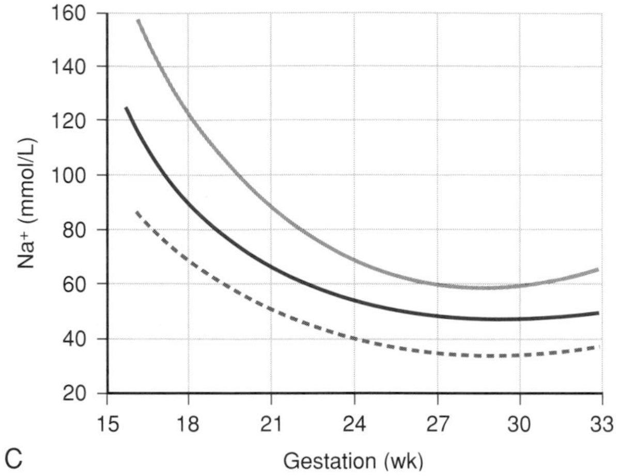

C

FIGURE 91
Urinary electrolytes, including *A*, phosphate, creatinine, *B*, potassium, calcium, urea and *C*, sodium (mean and 95% CI, where computed) from a study of 26 women at 16 to 33 weeks' gestation. Amniotic fluid volume and fetal anatomy were normal. Seventeen of the women had pregnancies complicated by Rhesus alloimmunization; in these cases, the fetal bladder was emptied before intraperitoneal blood transfusion. The other women had aspiration of the fetal bladder before therapeutic termination. *Data source:* ref. 181, with permission.

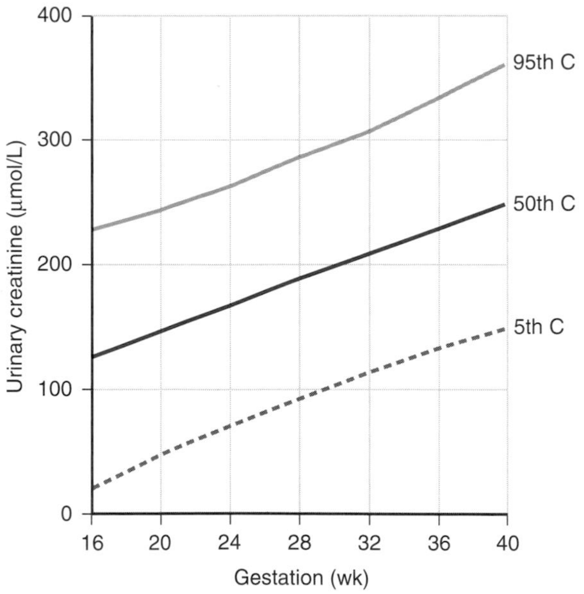

FIGURE 92
Urinary creatinine (5th, 50th, and 95th percentiles) from a study of 20 fetuses with obstructive uropathy and no features of renal dysplasia. All fetuses had normal postnatal renal function. Ultrasound-guided needle aspiration of fetal urine was performed. The fetal bladder was aspirated when it was distended, and both kidneys appeared similar; the renal pelvis was aspirated when unilateral pelvicalyceal dilation was seen. In all cases, the fetal karyotype was normal. *Data source:* ref. 182, with permission.

***Comment** (Figs. 91 and 92):* Previously, fetal urinary biochemistry had been studied only indirectly from examination of the amniotic fluid.[145] These direct studies found that urinary sodium and phosphate levels decreased significantly with gestational age over the period studied (16–33 weeks); creatinine levels increased. Urinary potassium, calcium, and urea did not show gestational changes. The pattern of electrolyte changes suggests parallel maturation of glomerular and tubular function with advancing gestation. Fetuses with obstructive uropathy but normal postnatal renal function[182] had sodium and urea values similar to those shown in Figure 91. However, reference ranges for urinary calcium were calculated as 0.25, 0.95, and 1.65 mmol/L (5th, 50th, and 95th percentiles, respectively).[182] Various groups have suggested urinary electrolyte values that predict an adverse outcome (e.g., sodium level >100 mmol/L, creatinine level >150 µmol/L [1.7 mg/dL], calcium level >2 mmol/L [8 mg/dL], osmolality >200 mOsm/L). However, these values are not universally accepted.[183,184] These data show that sodium concentration of greater than 100 mmol/L may be normal for fetuses at less than 20 weeks' gestation.

Blood Gases

OXYGEN PRESSURE (PO_2), CARBON DIOXIDE PRESSURE (PCO_2), PH, AND BASE DEFICIT

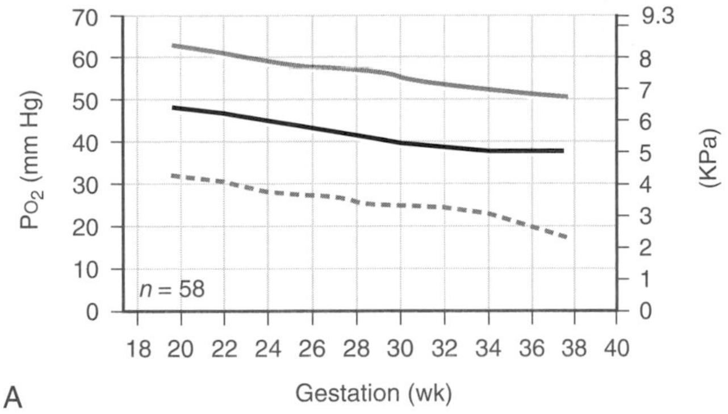

A

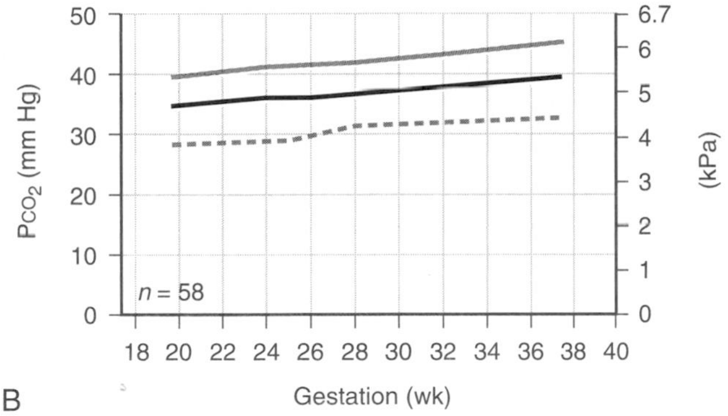

B

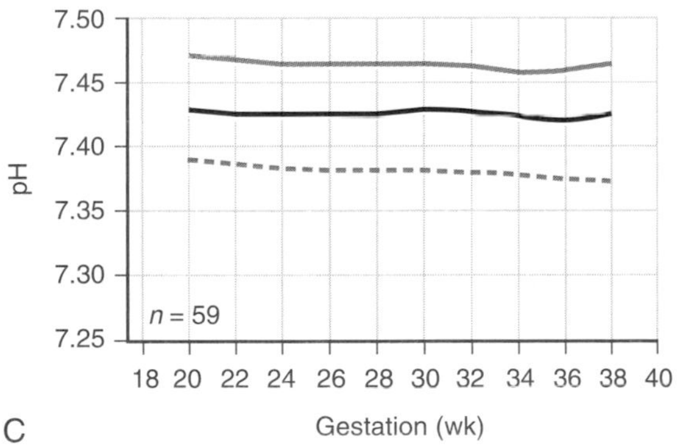

C

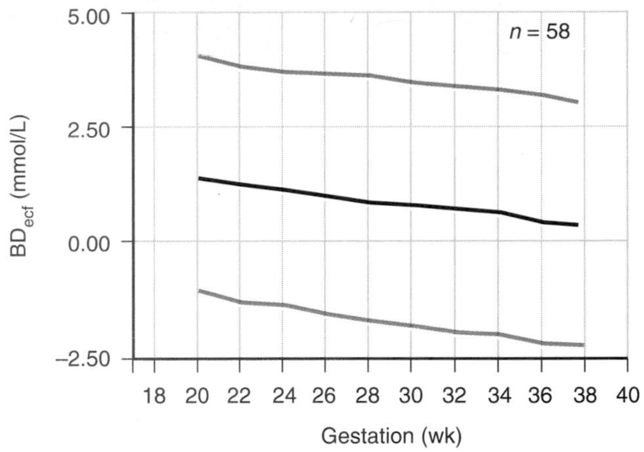

D

FIGURE 93

A, Umbilical venous PO_2, *B*, PCO_2, *C*, pH, and *D*, base deficit of the extracellular fluid (2.5th, 50th, and 97.5th percentiles) from a cross-sectional study of 59 fetuses referred for assessment of possible intrauterine infection or hemolysis, but found to be unaffected. All were healthy at birth and appropriately grown. *Data source:* ref. 185, with permission.

Comment: Umbilical arterial and venous PO_2 and pH decrease, and PCO_2 increases with gestational age.[186] Concentrations of lactate do not change with gestation; mean (SD) values are 0.99 mmol/L (0.32) for the umbilical vein and 0.92 mmol/L (0.21) for the umbilical artery.[186] Intervillous blood has higher PO_2 and lower PCO_2 than umbilical venous blood, but similar pH and lactate concentrations.[187] The decrease in PO_2 in umbilical venous blood that is seen with advancing gestation is offset by the increasing fetal hemoglobin concentration. As a result, the blood oxygen content remains constant; mean umbilical venous oxygen content is 6.7 mmol/L (0.6).[187]

Hematology

Complete Blood Count (CBC)

Gestational age (weeks)	WBC (10^9/L)	PLT (10^9/L)	RBC (10^{12}/L)	Hb (g/dL)	MCV (fL)
18–23 (*n* = 771)	4.41 ± 1.2	241 ± 45	2.87 ± 0.2	11.7 ± 0.8	131.2 ± 7.3
24–29 (*n* = 407)	4.6 ± 1.3	267 ± 49	3.38 ± 0.32	12.8 ± 1.1	119.1 ± 5.6
30–35 (*n* = 55)	5.8 ± 1.6	265 ± 59	3.86 ± 0.43	14.1 ± 1.4	114.3 ± 7

FIGURE 94
White blood cell count (WBC), platelet count (PLT), red blood cell count (RBC), hemoglobin (Hb), and mean cell volume (MCV) from a cross-sectional study of 1233 normal fetuses at 18 to 36 weeks' gestation (mean ± SD). Study subjects were referred for fetal blood sampling for prenatal diagnosis (mostly toxoplasmosis), but the fetuses were normal and subsequently shown to be healthy at birth. Fetal blood samples were taken by ultrasound-guided cordocentesis. *Data source:* ref. 178, with permission.

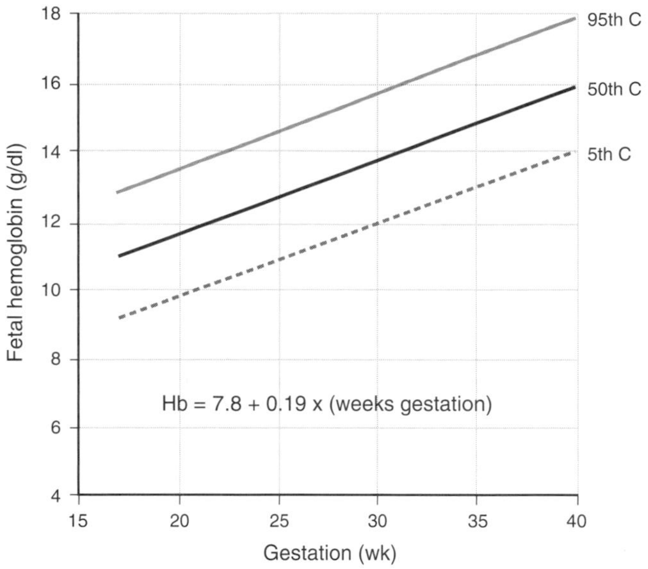

FIGURE 95
Hemoglobin (5th, 50th, and 95th percentiles) from a study of 194 fetuses at 17 to 40 weeks' gestation. The fetuses were undergoing prenatal diagnosis, but were unaffected for the condition tested. *Data source:* ref. 188, with permission.

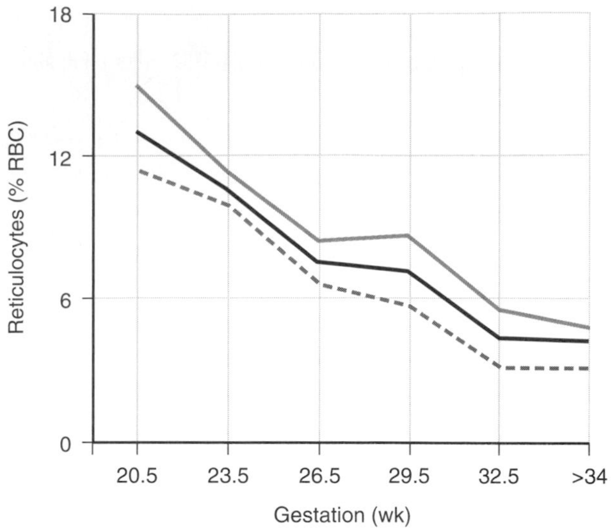

FIGURE 96
Fetal reticulocyte count (mean and 95% CI) from a cross-sectional study of 81 fetuses referred for prenatal diagnosis for a variety of indications, but subsequently shown to be unaffected. Ultrasound-guided cordocentesis was performed to obtain blood samples. *Data source:* ref. 189, with permission.

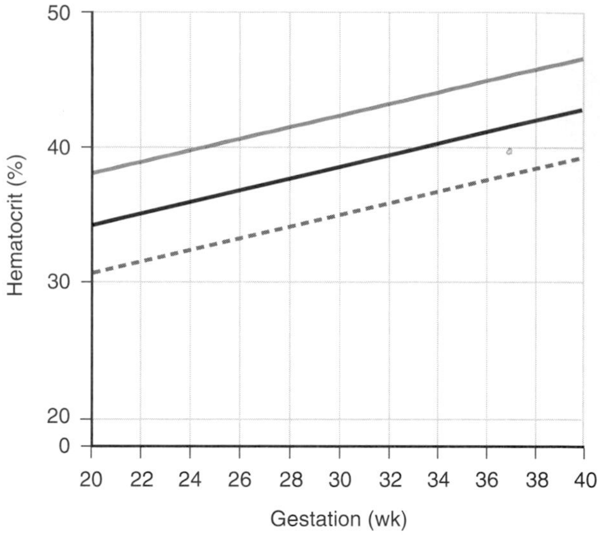

FIGURE 97
Hematocrit (regression line and 95% CI) from a cross-sectional study of 81 fetuses referred for prenatal diagnosis for a variety of indications, but subsequently shown to be unaffected. Ultrasound-guided cordocentesis was performed to obtain blood samples. *Data source:* ref. 189, with permission.

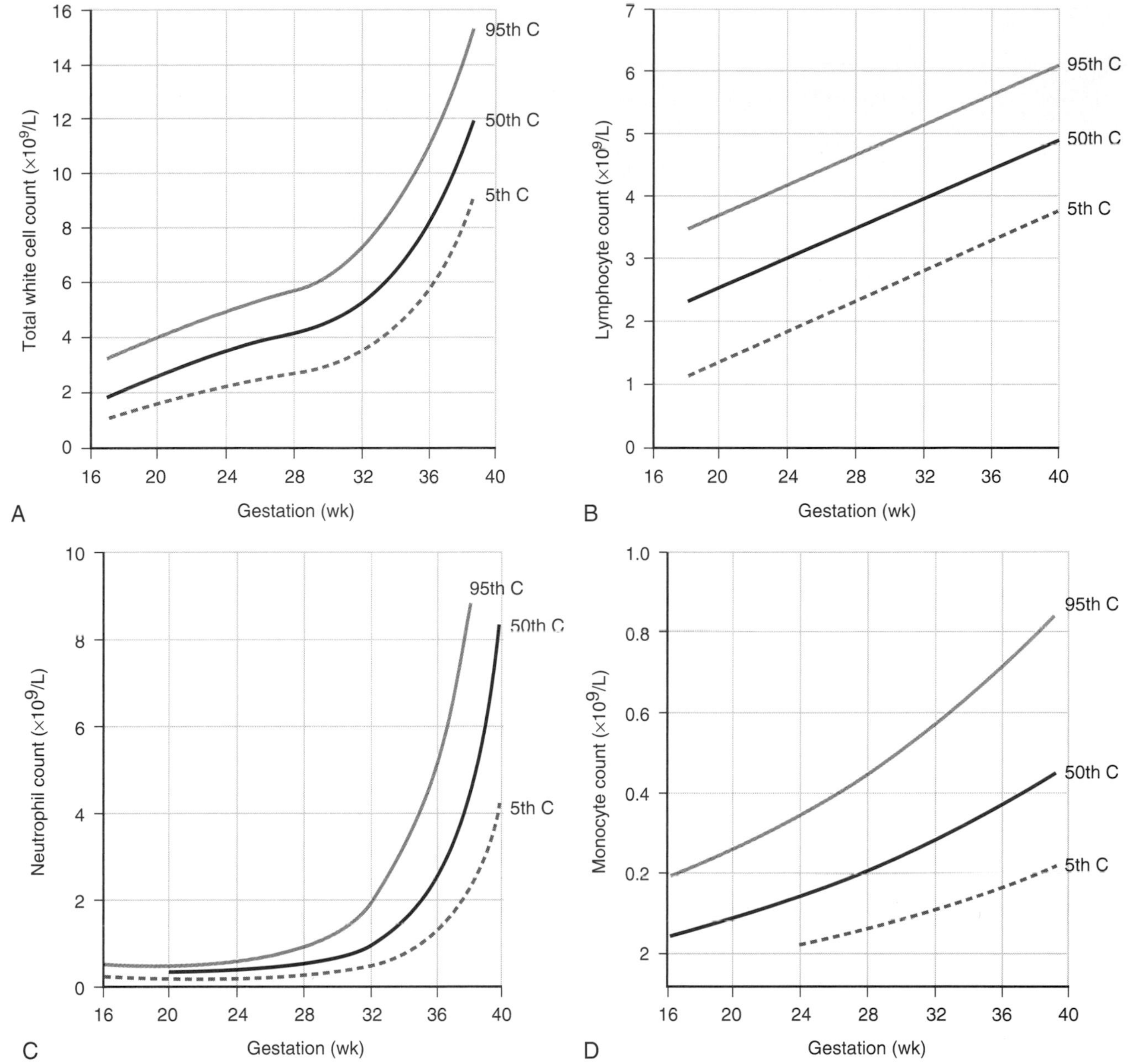

FIGURE 98

A, Total white blood cell, *B*, lymphocyte, *C*, neutrophil, and *D*, monocyte counts (5th, 50th, and 95th percentiles) from umbilical cord blood samples obtained at cordocentesis (n = 316) or elective cesarean delivery (n = 11) from fetuses at 18 to 40 weeks' gestation. Cordocentesis was performed for karyotyping, prenatal diagnosis, evaluation of infection, or blood typing, but all fetuses included in the study were unaffected by the condition being studied. The fetuses studied at the time of elective cesarean delivery were normal and appropriately grown; the indication for cesarean delivery was breech presentation or uterine scar. *Data source:* ref. 190, with permission.

Comment *(Figs. 94–98):* Fetal red blood cell count and total hemoglobin increase linearly, reticulocyte count decreases linearly, and erythroblast count decreases exponentially with gestation.[188–190] Platelet count does not change.[178] Lymphocytes form the main population of white cells in the fetus until 37 to 38 weeks' gestation.[190] From 32 weeks onward, neutrophils become more plentiful, and by term, they form approximately 60% of the total white cell count.[190] Natural killer cells are the main type of circulating white cell in the first trimester.[190,191] Interferon-γ concentrations (5th–95th percentiles) are high in the first trimester (0.4–3.1 U/mL) and decrease to 0.2 to 1.7 U/mL in the third trimester.[191] Fetal hemoglobin decreases with advancing gestation, from more than 80% of total hemoglobin in midpregnancy to approximately 70% by term.[178]

Coagulation Factors

Coagulation factors	%	Inhibitors	%
VIIIC	40 ± 12	Fibronectin	40 ± 10
VIIIRAg	60 ± 13	Protein C	11 ± 3
VII	28 ± 5	α2-Macroglobulin	18 ± 4
IX	9 ± 3	α1-Antitrypsin	40 ± 4
V	47 ± 10	AT III	30 ± 3
II	12 ± 3	α2-Antiplasmin	61 ± 6
XII	22 ± 3		
Prealllikrein	19 ± 2		
Fibrin-stabilizing factor	30 ± 5		
Fibrinogen	40 ± 15		
Plasminogen	24 ± 15		

FIGURE 99

Coagulation factors (percentage of normal adult values; mean ± SD) from a cross-sectional study of 103 fetuses at 19 to 27 weeks' gestation. All fetuses were subsequently shown to be healthy. Blood samples were obtained by ultrasound-guided cordocentesis. *Data source:* ref. 178, with permission.

Comment: No changes in the level or activity of the various coagulation factors and their inhibitors were observed through the 8 weeks of gestation studied.

Iron Metabolism

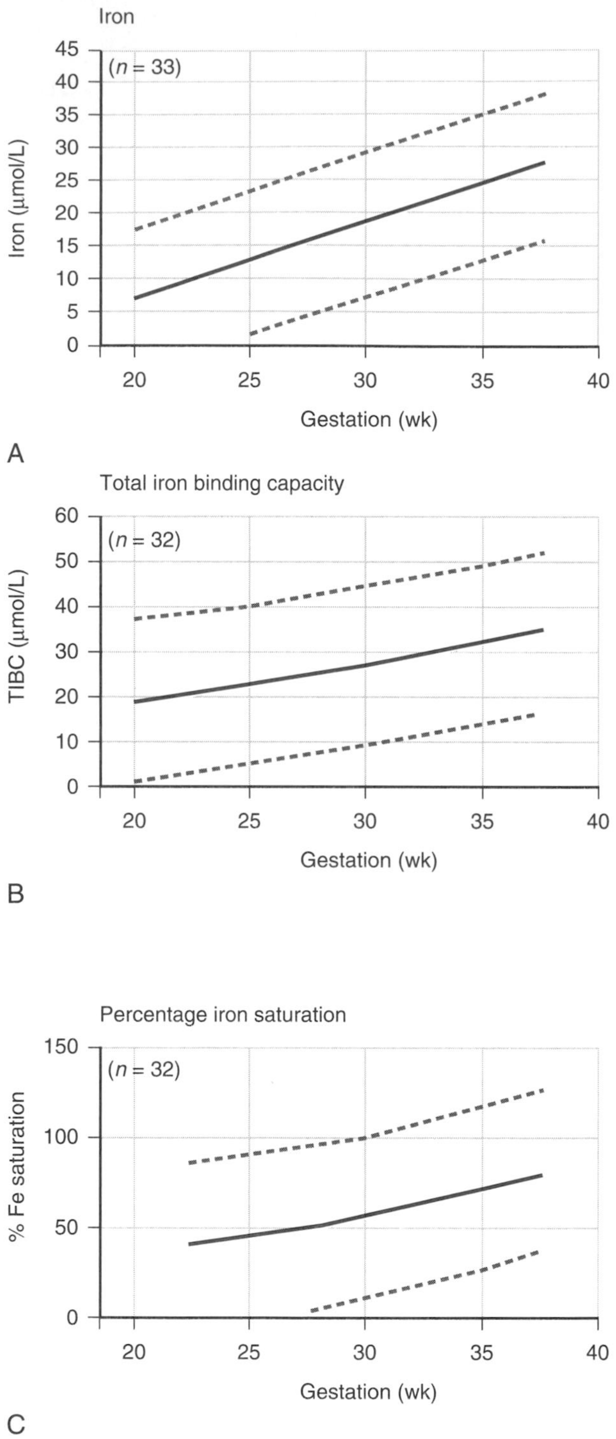

FIGURE 100

A, Fetal iron, *B*, total iron-binding capacity (TIBC), and *C*, percentage of iron saturation from a cross-sectional study of 33 fetuses referred for prenatal diagnosis for a variety of indications, but subsequently found to be unaffected. Blood samples were taken by ultrasound-guided cordocentesis. *Data source:* ref. 192, with permission.

Comment: Fetal iron, TIBC, and percentage of iron saturation increase with advancing gestation.

Amniotic Fluid Bilirubin

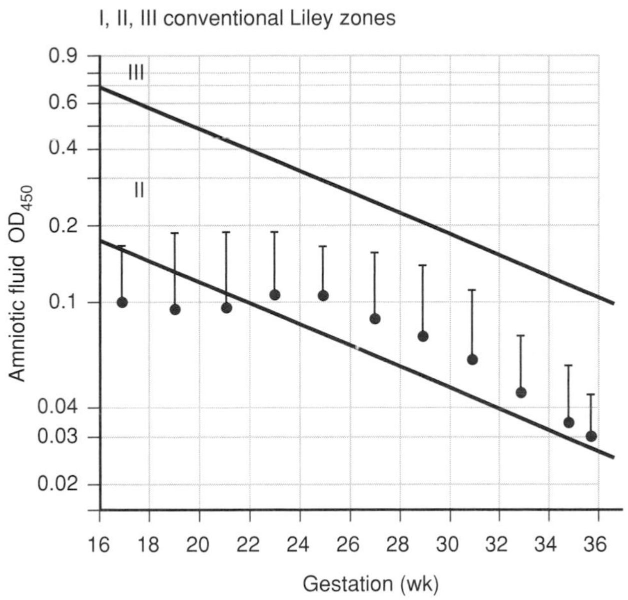

FIGURE 101
Amniotic fluid bilirubin ΔOD_{450} (mean ± 2 SDs) from 475 samples of amniotic fluid obtained from pregnancies at 16 to 36 weeks' gestation. The pregnancies were not complicated by fetal hemolysis. Amniotic fluid samples obtained at fetoscopy or by amniocentesis were placed in darkened containers to protect against photodecomposition and centrifuged to remove vernix and cellular debris. The bilirubin concentration was measured spectrophotometrically by the deviation in optical density of the amniotic fluid at a wavelength of 450 nm. *Data source:* ref. 193, with permission.

Comment: The normal range of liquor ΔOD_{450} does not change between 16 and 25 weeks' gestation, but values decrease during the third trimester and are widely scattered.

Endocrinology

Thyroid Function

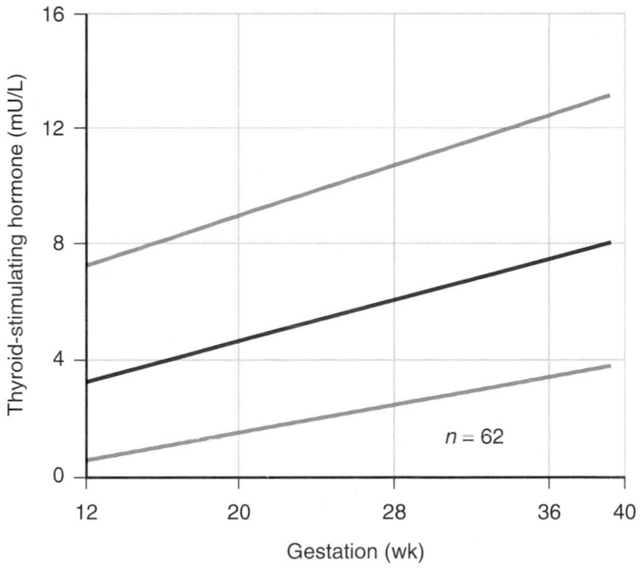

A

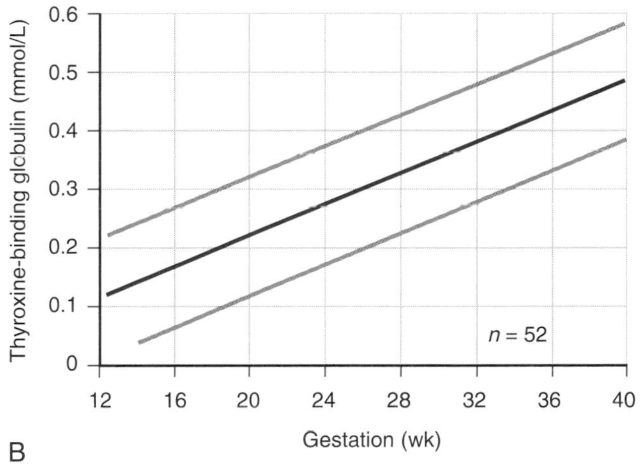

B

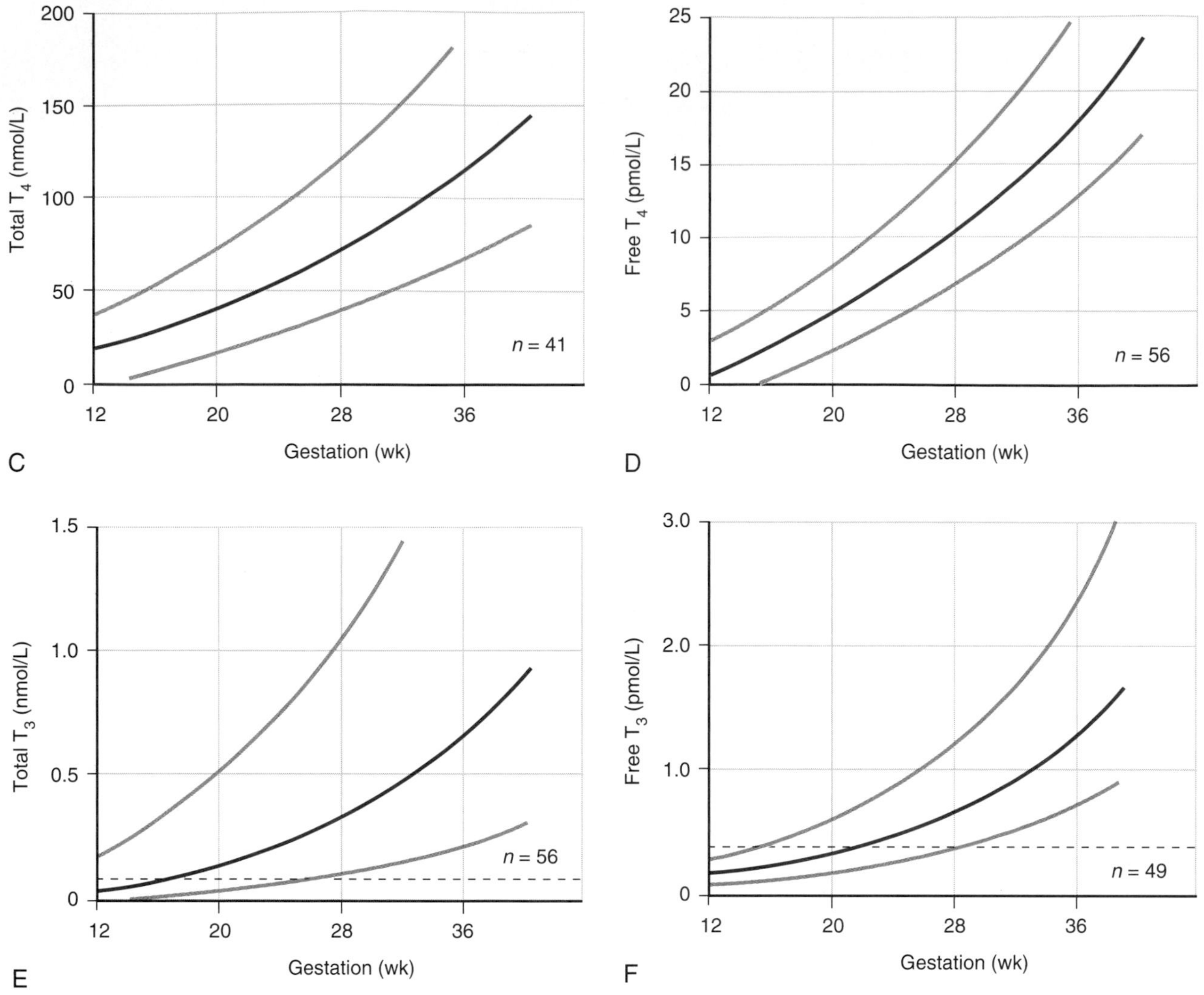

FIGURE 102

A, Thyroid-stimulating hormone (TSH), *B*, thyroid-binding globulin (TBG), *C*, total thyroxine (total T_4), *D*, free thyroxine (free T_4), *E*, total tri-iodothyronine (T_3), and *F*, free tri-iodothyronine (T_3) from a study of 62 women who underwent cordocentesis or cardiocentesis for prenatal diagnosis. Fetuses were subsequently found to be normal (mean, 5th, and 95th percentiles). The cross-hatched area is the lower limit of sensitivity of the assay. *Data source:* ref. 194, with permission.

Comment: No significant associations have been found between fetal and maternal thyroid hormones and TSH concentrations, suggesting that the fetal pituitary-thyroid axis is independent of the maternal axis.[194] Fetal TSH levels are always higher than maternal levels. Fetal free and total T_4 levels and TBG levels increase throughout pregnancy and reach adult levels by 36 weeks' gestation; however, fetal free and total T_3 levels are always substantially lower than adult levels. The increase in fetal levels of TSH, thyroid hormones, and TBG during pregnancy indicates independent and autonomous maturation of the pituitary, thyroid, and liver, respectively.[194] There does not appear to be feedback control of pituitary secretion of TSH by circulating thyroid hormones in utero.

LABOR

Progress of Labor

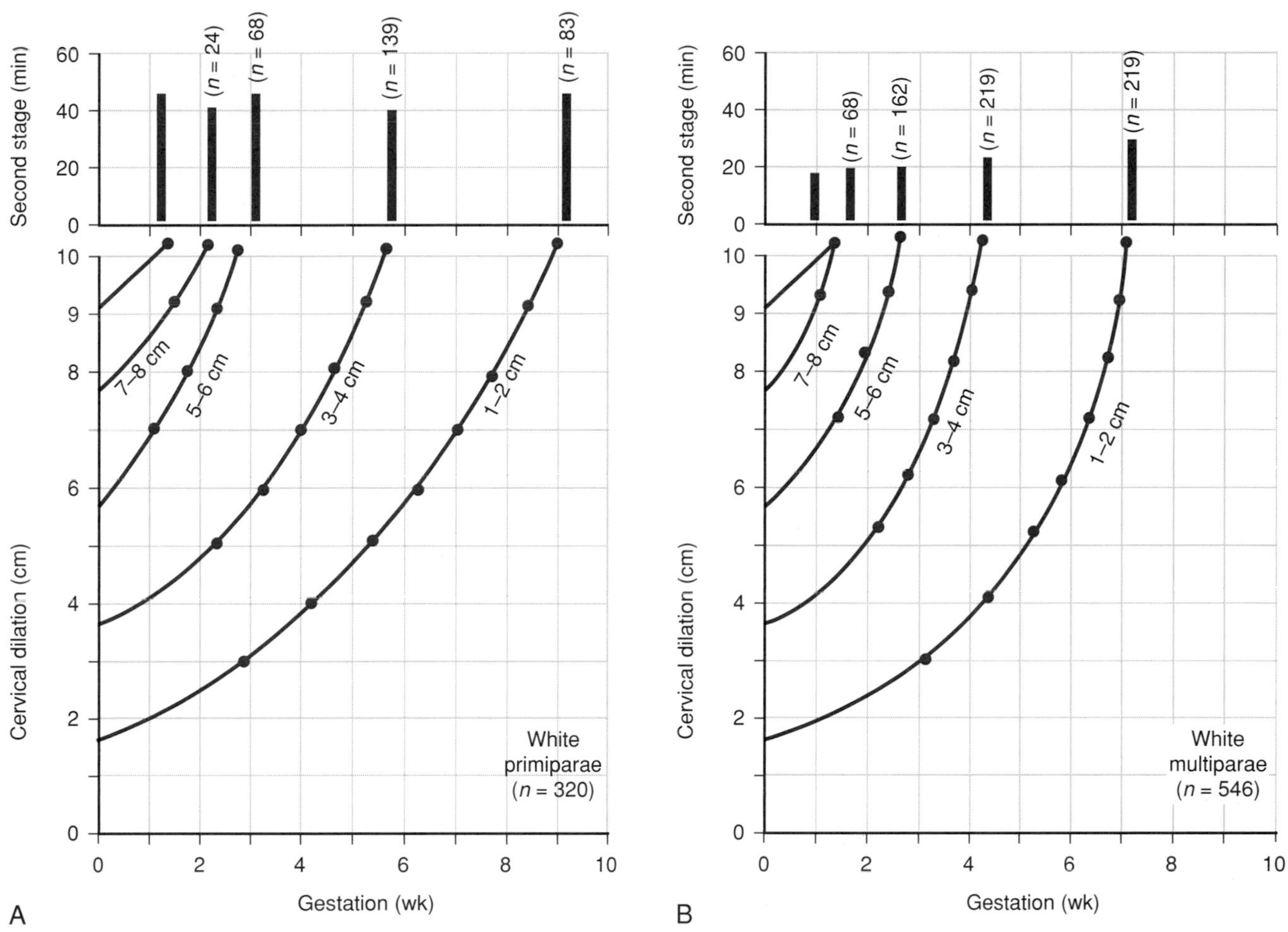

FIGURE 103
Mean cervimetric progress of *A*, white primigravidae and *B*, white multigravidae from a study of 3217 consecutive women in labor, from which a group of 1306 who had normal labor were identified (i.e., women with a cephalically presenting fetus who did not have epidural block, receive oxytocic drugs, or require instrumental delivery). The progress of labor was followed by vaginal examination to establish cervical dilation. The first examination was performed soon after admission to the labor suite. The onset of the second stage was confirmed when full cervical dilation was found on routine examination or when the patient was beginning to bear down. *Data source:* ref. 195, with permission.

Comment: This study found that mean cervimetric progress from 1 to 7 cm was faster in white multiparae than in primiparae, but thereafter, progress in the two groups was similar. No significant differences in the cervimetric progress of labor between women from different racial groups has been found.[195] The mean duration of the second stage of labor is approximately 42 minutes in primiparae and 17 minutes in multiparae,[195] although the precise onset of full cervical dilation is difficult to establish.

Fetal Heart Rate Parameters by Cardiotocography (CTG)

Admission test CTG
- At least two accelerations (>15 beats for >15 s) in 20 minutes.
- Baseline heart rate 110–150 bpm.
- Baseline variability 5–25 bpm.
- Absence of decelerations.
- Moderate tachycardia/bradycardia and accelerations.

First stage intrapartum CTG
- At least two accelerations (>15 beats for >15 s) in 20 minutes.
- Baseline heart rate 110–150 bpm.
- Baseline variability 5–25 bpm.
- Early decelerations (in late first stage of labor).

Second stage intrapartum CTG
- Normal baseline heart rate, normal baseline variability and no decelerations, both periodic and scattered.
- Baseline heart rate 110–150 bpm and baseline variability 5–25 bpm or >25 bpm, with or without early and/or variable decelerations.

FIGURE 104
Features of the normal CTG in labor. *Data source:* ref. 173, with permission.

Comment: Guidelines defining the parameters for normal cardiotocography (CTG) have been established by working groups, but are based on opinion and clinical experience rather than research evidence. The definitions here are taken from the International Federation of Obstetricians and Gynecologists (FIGO). Different interpretations are available from the Royal College of Obstetricians and Gynaecologists in Britain[196] and the American College of Obstetricians and Gynecologists in the United States.[174] There are differences in the range of baseline heart rates accepted as normal (lower limit, 110–120 beats/min; upper limit, 150–160 beats/min) and the definitions of variability. Decelerations that are considered abnormal if identified antepartum (see Fig. 86) often occur intrapartum. Early decelerations (i.e., synchronous with contractions) are common toward the end of the first stage of labor; during the second stage of labor, both early and variable decelerations can be normal findings. Accelerations and normal baseline variability are important features of a normal CTG finding.

Umbilical Cord Blood Sampling

BLOOD GASES

Blood Gases		Umbilical artery	Umbilical vein
pH		7.06–7.36	7.14–7.45
Po_2			
	(kPa)	1.3–5.5	1.7–6.0
	(mmHg)	9.8–41.2	12.3–45.0
Pco_2			
	(kPa)	9.1–3.7	7.5–3.2
	(mm Hg)	68.3–27.8	56.3–24.0
BD ecf	(mmol/L)	15.3–0.5	12.6–0.7

FIGURE 105
Umbilical arterial and venous blood gas values (pH, Po_2, Pco_2, and extracellular base deficit) from a 2-year-long study in a university hospital in the Netherlands, where cord blood samples were taken from all deliveries (95% CI). A piece of umbilical cord was isolated as soon as possible after delivery, and arterial and venous samples were taken into two heparinized syringes. Samples were analyzed within 75 minutes of delivery by an automated blood gas machine. If the difference between pH valu es in the umbilical artery and the vein was not at least 2 pH units, the arterial sample was rejected. Thus, 4667 arterial and 5151 venous pH samples were obtained. Smaller numbers of samples also had Po_2 and Pco_2 values measured. *Data source:* ref. 197, with permission.

Comment: The overall distribution of pH values was negatively skewed. This data set was large enough to allow for subanalysis. Values for pH were lower after cesarean section or breech delivery than after spontaneous vertex delivery. The 10th percentiles for pH in these groups were 7.12, 7.11, and 7.15, respectively. Optimal cases (no problems antenatally or during labor, spontaneous labor, second stage lasting <30 minutes, vertex presentation, and a normally grown infant in good condition at birth) had 10th percentile pH values of 7.17. There were only small differences in pH between samples obtained from premature, mature, and postmature infants. Guidelines are available for optimal collection and analytical techniques.[185]

LACTATE

Comment: Mean umbilical cord lactate values were reported as 1.87 mmol/L (SD, 0.94) in a study of more than 3000 spontaneous vaginal deliveries.[198] Lower values were found after elective cesarean delivery (mean, 1.44 mmol/L; SD, 0.10; $n = 300$).

COMPLETE BLOOD COUNT

Complete blood count			
Analyte	25th centile	50th centile	75th centile
Red cell count ($\times 10^{12}$/L)	4.13	4.40	4.62
Hemoglobin (mmol/L)	9.5	10.0	10.7
(g/dl)	15.3	16.1	17.2
Hematocrit (%)	45.2	47.9	50.9
Mean cell volume (fl)	107.4	109.8	113.3
Mean cell hemoglobin (fmol)	2.2	2.3	2.4
(pg)	35.4	37.1	38.7
Reticulocyte count ($\times 10^9$/L)	145.8	170.0	192.6
Platelet count ($\times 10^9$/L)	237	270	321
Total white cell count ($\times 10^9$/L)	11.1	13.3	16.2
Neutrophil ($\times 10^9$/L)	5.4	7.4	8.8
Lymphocyte ($\times 10^9$/L)	3.3	3.8	5.1
Monocyte ($\times 10^9$/L)	1.2	1.6	2.3
Eosinophil ($\times 10^9$/L)	0.23	0.39	0.54
Basophil ($\times 10^9$/L)	0.04	0.06	0.09

FIGURE 106
Red blood cell count, hemoglobin, hematocrit, mean cell volume, mean cell hemoglobin, reticulocyte count, platelet count, and differential white blood cell count (25th, 50th, and 75th percentiles) from a study of 89 women who had been healthy during pregnancy and were nonsmokers. All were delivered after 34 weeks' gestation, and their infants were of normal birth weight and had umbilical cord pH greater than 7.20. Umbilical venous samples were taken and analyzed within 3 hours. *Data source:* ref. 199, with permission.

Comment: In this study, infants of smokers had lower reticulocyte and neutrophil counts.[199] Reticulocyte counting was done by flow cytometry, which is more precise than manual counting. Full-term cord blood has more immature reticulocyte forms than does adult blood.[200] Another recent study found similar blood counts[201] and recommended that the lower limit for normal hemoglobin be designated as 12.5 g/dL for term newborns.

BIOCHEMISTRY

Analyte	Cord arterial (n = 179)	Cord venous (n = 390)	Adult
Na^+ (mmol/L)	135–143	135–143	136–146
K^+ (mmol/L)	3.7–6.4	3.8–6.8	3.6–4.8
Cl^- (mmol/L)	102–111	102–112	96–110
Glucose (mmol/L)	2.3–6.7	2.9–7.4	4.4–6.1
Urea (mmol/L)	1.8–5.6	1.8–5.4	2.5–8.5
Creatinine (μmol/L)	45–96	51–97	65–125
Urate (μmol/L)	186–480	200–456	150–480
Phosphate (mmol/L)	1.23–2.14	1.31–2.18	0.80–1.60
Ca^{2+}(mmol/L)	2.16–2.94	2.32–2.99	2.10–2.60
Albumin (g/L)	26–40	30–41	35–48
Total protein (g/L)	43–67	46–68	60–80
Cholesterol (mmol/L)	0.8–2.5	0.9–2.5	<5.2
ALP (U/L)	77–285	87–303	36–135 (20–55 years) 37–160 (55–74 years) 50–200 (>75 years)
ALT (U/L)	4–24	4–27	5–40
AST (U/L)	16–63	17–59	10–30
CK (U/L)	71–475	82–528	10–180
LD (U/L)	206–580	201–494	90–230
CO_2 (mmol/L)	13–29	15–28	24–30
GGT (U/L)	20–302	27–339	8–50 (male) 6–50 (female)
Triglyceride (mmol/L)	0.10–1.04	0.13–0.97	0.55–1.7
Mg^{2+} (mmol/L)	0.49–0.80	0.50–0.79	0.6–1.0

ALP, alkaline phosphatase; ALT, alanine aminotransferase; AST, aspartate aminotransferase; LD, lactate dehydrogenase

FIGURE 107
Clinical chemistry analytes (95% CI) from umbilical arterial and venous blood compared with adult blood values. Samples were taken into heparinized tubes from the umbilical cords of 397 infants delivered at 37 to 41 weeks' gestation, before placental expulsion from the uterus. There were 310 vaginal deliveries and 87 cesarean deliveries. All infants included in the study had 5-minute Apgar scores of 8 or greater. Samples were stored at 40°C until analysis. Complete biochemistry profiles were obtained from 390 venous plasma and 179 arterial plasma samples. These were compared with the adult reference ranges from the institution (Ottawa Civic Hospital, Ottawa, Canada). *Data source:* ref. 202, with permission.

Comment: All cord blood chemistry values were significantly different from adult values. No male-to-female differences were identified. Cord creatine kinase concentrations were very high, although they were similar in infants after vaginal or cesarean delivery, suggesting that this change did not relate to physical trauma.

REFERENCES

1. Dawes MG, Grudzinkas JG: Patterns of maternal weight gain in pregnancy. BJOG 1991;98:195–201.
2. National Academy of Sciences: Nutrition During Pregnancy. Washington, DC, National Academy Press, 1990.
3. Rosso P: A new chart to monitor weight gain during pregnancy. Am J Clin Nutr 1985;41:644–652.
4. National Academy of Sciences: Recommended Dietary Allowances, 10th ed. Washington, DC, National Academy Press, 1989.
5. MacGillivray I, Rose GA, Rowe B: Blood pressure survey in pregnancy. Clin Sci 1969;37:395–407.
6. Spatling L, Fallenstein F, Huch A, et al: The variability of cardiopulmonary adaptation to pregnancy at rest and during exercise. BJOG 1992;99(suppl 8):1–40.
7. Clapp JF III: Maternal heart rate in pregnancy. Am J Obstet Gynecol 1985;152:659–660.
8. Clark SL, Cotton DB, Lee W, et al: Central hemodynamic assessment of normal term pregnancy. Am J Obstet Gynecol 1989;161:1439–1442.
9. Lucius H, Gahlenbeck H, Kleine H-O, et al: Respiratory functions, buffer system, and electrolyte concentrations of blood during human pregnancy. Resp Physiol 1970;9:311–317.
10. Gazioglu K, Kaltreider NL, Rosen M, Yu PN: Pulmonary function during pregnancy in normal women and in patients with cardiopulmonary disease. Thorax 1970;25:445–450.
11. De Swiet M: The respiratory system. In Hytten F, Chamberlain G (eds): Clinical Physiology in Obstetrics, 2nd ed. Oxford, Blackwell, 1991, pp 83–100.
12. Cuckle HS, Wald NJ, Thompson SG: Estimating a woman's risk of having a pregnancy associated with Down's syndrome using her age and serum α-fetoprotein level. BJOG 1987;94:387–402.
13. Ferguson-Smith M: Prenatal chromosome analysis and its impact on the birth incidence of chromosome disorders. Br Med Bull 1983;39:355–364.
14. Robertson EG, Cheyne GA: Plasma biochemistry in relation to the oedema of pregnancy. J Obstet Gynaecol Br Commonw 1972;79:769–776.
15. Mendenhall HW: Serum protein concentrations in pregnancy. Am J Obstet Gynecol 1970;106:388–399.
16. Adeniyi FA, Olatunbosun DA: Origins and significance of the increased plasma alkaline phosphatase during normal pregnancy and pre-eclampsia. BJOG 1984;91:857–862.
17. Girling JC, Dow E, Smith JH: Liver function tests in pre-eclampsia: Importance of comparison with a reference range derived for normal pregnancy. BJOG 1997;104:246–250.
18. Heikkinene J, Mäentausta O, Ylöstalo P, Jänne O: Changes in serum bile acid concentrations during normal pregnancy, in patients with intrahepatic cholestasis of pregnancy and in pregnant women with itching. BJOG 1981;88:240–245.
19. David AL, Kotecha M, Girling JC: Factors influencing postnatal liver function tests. BJOG 2000;107:1421–1426.
20. McNair RD, Jaynes RV: Alterations in liver function during normal pregnancy. Am J Obstet Gynecol 1960;80:500–505.
21. Kiilholma P, Gronroos M, Liukko P, et al: Maternal serum copper and zinc concentrations in normal and small-for-date pregnancies. Gynecol Obstet Invest 1984;18:212–216.
22. Potter JM, Nestel PJ: The hyperlipidaemia of pregnancy in normal and complicated pregnancies. Am J Obstet Gynecol 1979;133:165–170.
23. Lind T, Godfrey KA, Otun H: Changes in serum uric acid concentrations during normal pregnancy. BJOG 1984;91:128–132.
24. Newman RL: Serum electrolytes in pregnancy, parturition, and puerperium. Obstet Gynecol 1957;10:51–55.
25. Kuhlback B, Widholm O: Plasma creatinine in normal pregnancy. Scand J Clin Lab Invest 1966;18:654–656.
26. Davison J: Renal disease. In De Swiet M (ed): Medical Disorders in Obstetric Practice, 2nd ed. Oxford, Blackwell, 1989, pp 306–407.
27. Davison JM, Noble MCB: Serial changes in 24 hour creatinine clearance during normal menstrual cycles and the first trimester of pregnancy. BJOG 1981;88:10–17.
28. Davison JM, Dunlop W, Ezimokhai M: 24-hour creatinine clearance during the third trimester of normal pregnancy. BJOG 1980;87:106–109.
29. Davison JM, Dunlop W: Renal haemodynamics and tubular function in normal human pregnancy. Kidney Int 1980; 18:152–161.
30. Hytten FE, Cheyne GA: The aminoaciduria of pregnancy. J Obstet Gynaecol Br Commonw 1972;79:424–432.
31. Lopez-Espinola I, Dhar H, Humphreys S, Redman CWG: Urinary albumin excretion in pregnancy. BJOG 1986;93: 176–181.
32. Lind T, Billewicz WZ, Brown G: A serial study of changes occuring in the oral glucose tolerance test during pregnancy. J Obstet Gynaecol Br Commonw 1973;80:1033–1039.
33. Mills JL, Jovanovic L, Knopp R, et al: Physiological reduction in fasting plasma glucose concentration in the first trimester of normal pregnancy: The diabetes in early pregnancy study. Metabolism 1998;47:1140–1144.
34. Chen X, Scholl TO: Ethnic differences in C-peptide/insulin/glucose dynamics in young pregnant women. J Clin Endocrinol Metab 2002;87:4642–4646.
35. Hatem M, Anthony F, Hogston P, et al: Reference values for 75 g oral glucose tolerance test in pregnancy. Br Med J 1988;296:676–678.
36. Forest J-C, Garrido-Russo M, LeMay A, et al: Reference values for the oral glucose tolerance test at each trimester of pregnancy. Am J Clin Pathol 1983;80:828–831.
37. Dicknson JE, Palmer SM: Gestational diabetes: Pathophysiology and diagnosis. Semin Perinatol 1990;14:2–11.
38. Roberts AB, Baker JR: Serum fructosamine: A screening test for diabetes in pregnancy. Am J Obstet Gynecol 1986;154: 1027–1030.
39. Feige A, Nossner U: Das Verhalten des glykosylierten Haemoglobins (Hb-A1) in normaler und pathologischer Schwangerschaft. Z Geburtshilfe Perinatol 1985;189:13–16.
40. Ylinen K, Hekalir R, Teramo K: Haemoglobin A_{1c} during pregnancy of insulin-dependent diabetic and healthy control. J Obstet Gynaecol 1981;1:223–228.
41. Falluca F, Sciullo E, Napoli A, et al: Amniotic fluid insulin and C-peptide levels in diabetic and nondiabetic women during early pregnancy. J Clin Endocrinol Metab 1995;81:137–139.
42. Falluca F, Gargiulo P, Troili F, et al: Amniotic fluid insulin, C-peptide concentrations, and fetal morbidity in infants of diabetic mothers. Am J Obstet Gynecol 1985;153:534–540.
43. Carpenter MW, Canick JA, Star J, et al: Fetal hyperinsulinism at 14–20 weeks and subsequent gestational diabetes. Obstet Gynecol 1996;87:89–93.
44. Wang Y, Walsh SW, Guo J, Zhang J: Maternal levels of prostacyclin, thromboxane, vitamin E, and lipid peroxides throughout normal pregnancy. Am J Obstet Gynecol 1991;165:1690–1694.
45. Ortega RM, Quintas ME, Andres P, et al: Ascorbic acid levels in maternal milk: Differences with respect to ascorbic acid status during the third trimester of pregnancy. Br J Nutr 1998;79: 431–437.
46. Taylor DJ, Lind T: Red cell mass during and after normal pregnancy. BJOG 1979;86:364–370.
47. Edelstam G, Lowbeer C, Kral G, et al: New reference values for routine blood samples and human neutrophilic lipocalin during

third trimester pregnancy. Scand J Clin Lab Invest 2001;61:583–592.
48. Kuvin SF, Brecher G: Differential neutrophil counts in pregnancy. N Engl J Med 1962;266:877–878.
49. Fay RA, Hughes AO, Farron NT: Platelets in pregnancy: Hyperdestruction in pregnancy. Obstet Gynecol 1983;61: 238–240.
50. Boehlen F, Hohlfeld P, Extermann P, et al: Platelet count at term pregnancy: A reappraisal of the threshold. Obstet Gynecol 2000;95:29–33.
51. Fenton V, Saunders K, Cavill I: The platelet count in pregnancy. J Clin Pathol 1977;30:68–69.
52. Fenton V, Cavill I, Fisher J: Iron stores in pregnancy. Br J Haematol 1977;37:145–149.
53. Cikot R, Steegers-Theunissen R, Thomas C, et al: Longitudinal vitamin and homocysteine levels in normal pregnancy. Br J Nutr 2001;85:49–58.
54. Chanarin I, Rothman D, Ward A, Perry J: Folate status and requirement in pregnancy. Br Med J 1968;2:390–394.
55. Walker MC, Smith GN, Perkins SL, et al: Changes in homocysteine levels during normal pregnancy. Am J Obstet Gynecol 1999;180:660–664.
56. McDonald SD, Perkin SL, Jodouin CA, Walker MA: Folate levels in pregnant women who smoke: An important gene/environment interaction. Am J Obstet Gynecol 2002;187:620–625.
57. Letsky E: The haematological system. In Hytten F, Chamberlain G (eds): Clinical Physiology in Obstetrics, 2nd ed. Oxford, Blackwell, 1991, pp 39–82.
58. Koebnick C, Heins UA, Dagnelie PC, et al: Longitudinal concentrations of vitamin B12-binding proteins during uncomplicated pregnancy. Clin Chem 2002;48:928–933.
59. Stirling Y, Woolf L, North WRS, et al: Haemostasis in normal pregnancy. Thromb Haemost 1984;52:176–182.
60. Warwick R, Hutton RA, Goff L, et al: Changes in protein C and free protein S during pregnancy and following hysterectomy. J R Soc Med 1989;82:591–594.
61. Bonnar J, McNicol GP, Douglas AS: Fibrinolytic enzyme system and pregnancy. Br Med J 1969;3:387–389.
62. Gallery ED, Raftos J, Gyory AZ, Wells JV: A prospective study of serum complement (C3 and C4) levels during normal human pregnancy: Effect of the development of pregnancy-associated hypertension. Aust N Z J Med 1981;11:243–245.
63. Schena FP, Manno C, Selvaggi L, et al: Behaviour of immune complexes and the complement system in normal pregnancy and pre-eclampsia. J Clin Lab Immunol 1982;7:21–26.
64. Jenkins JS, Powell RJ: C3 degradation products (C3d) in normal pregnancy. J Clin Pathol 1987;40:1362–1363.
65. Hytten FE, Lind T: Volume and composition of the blood. In Diagnostic Indices in Pregnancy. Basel, Switzerland, Documenta Geigy, 1973, pp 36–54.
66. O'Leary PC, Boyne P, Atkinson G, et al: Longitudinal study of serum thyroid hormone levels during normal pregnancy. Int J Gynecol Obstet 1992;38:171–179.
67. Man EB, Reid WA, Hellegers AE, Jones WS: Thyroid function in human pregnancy. Am J Obstet Gynecol 1969;103:338–347.
68. Harada A, Hershman JM, Reed AW, et al: Comparison of thyroid stimulators and thyroid hormone concentrations in the sera of pregnant women. J Clin Endocrinol Metab 1979;48:793–797.
69. Parker JH: Amerlex free triiodothyronine and free thyroxine levels in normal pregnancy. BJOG 1985;92:1234–1238.
70. Osathanondh R, Tulchinsky D, Chopra IJ: Total and free thyroxine and triiodothyronine in normal and complicated pregnancy. J Clin Endocrinol Metab 1976;42:98–102.
71. De Leo V, La Marca A, Lanzetta D, Morgante G: Thyroid function in early pregnancy: I. Thyroid-stimulating response to thyrotropin-releasing hormone. Gynecol Endocrinol 1998;12: 191 196.
72. Natrajan PG, McGarrigle HHG, Lawrence DM, Lachelin GCL: Plasma noradrenaline and adrenaline levels in normal pregnancy and in pregnancy-induced hypertension. BJOG 1982; 89:1041–1045.
73. Rubin PC, Butters L, McCabe R, Reid JL: Plasma catecholamines in pregnancy-induced hypertension. Clin Sci 1986;71:111–115.
74. Beilin LJ, Deacon J, Michael CA, et al: Diurnal rhythms of blood pressure, plasma renin activity, angiotensin II and catecholamines in normotensive and hypertensive pregnancies. Clin Exp Hypertens; Hypertens in Pregnancy 1983;B2(2):271–293.
75. Carr BR, Parker CR, Madden JD, et al: Maternal plasma adrenocorticotrophin and cortisol relationships throughout human pregnancy. Am J Obstet Gynecol 1981;139:416–422.
76. Nolten WE, Lindheimer MD, Rueckert PA, et al: Diurnal patterns and regulation of cortisol secretion in pregnancy. J Clin Endocrinol Metab 1980;51:466–472.
77. Demey-Ponsart E, Foidart JM, Sulon J, Sodoyez JC: Serum CBG, free and total cortisol and circadian patterns of adrenal function in normal pregnancy. J Steroid Biochem 1982;16: 165–169.
78. Rees LH, Burke CW, Chard T, et al: Possible placental origin of ACTH in normal human pregnancy. Nature 1975;254:620–622.
79. Doe RP, Fernandez R, Seal US: Measurement of corticosteroid-binding globulin in man. J Clin Endocrinol 1964;24:1029–1039.
80. Migeon CJ, Kenny FM, Taylor FH: Cortisol production rate: VIII. Pregnancy. J Clin Endocrinol 1968;28:661–666.
81. Pearson Murphy BE, Okouneff LM, Klein GP, Ngo SH: Lack of specificity of cortisol determinations in human urine. J Clin Endocrinol Metab 1981;53:91–99.
82. Nolten WE, Lindheimer MD, Oparil S, Ehrlich EN: Desoxycorticosterone in normal pregnancy: I. Sequential studies of the secretory patterns of desoxycorticosterone, aldosterone, and cortisol. Am J Obstet Gynecol 1978;132:414–420.
83. Garner PR: Pituitary and adrenal disorders. In Burrow GN, Ferris TF (eds): Medical Complications during Pregnancy, 4th ed. Philadelphia, WB Saunders, 1995, pp 188–209.
84. Biswas S, Rodek CH: Plasma prolactin levels during pregnancy. BJOG 1976;83:683–687.
85. Boyer RM, Finkelstein JW, Kapen S, Hellman L: Twenty-four hour prolactin (Prl) secretory patterns during pregnancy. J Clin Endocrinol Metab 1975;40:1117–1120.
86. Rigg LA, Yen SSC: Multiphasic prolactin secretion during parturition in human subjects. Am J Obstet Gynecol 1977;128: 215–218.
87. Jacobs HS: The hypothalamus and pituitary gland. In Hytten F, Chamberlain G (eds): Clinical Physiology in Obstetrics, 2nd ed. Oxford, Blackwell, 1991, pp 345–356.
88. Pitkin RM, Reynolds WA, Williams GA, Hargis GK: Calcium metabolism in normal pregnancy: A longitudinal study. Am J Obstet Gynecol 1979;133:781–787.
89. Seki K, Makimura N, Mitsui C, et al: Calcium-regulating hormones and osteocalcin levels during pregnancy: A longitudinal study. Am J Obstet Gynecol 1991;164:1248–1252.
90. Wald NJ, George L, Smith D, et al: Serum screening for Down's syndrome between 8 and 14 weeks of pregnancy. BJOG 1996;103:407–412.
91. Biagiotti R, Brizzi L, Periti E, et al: First trimester screening for Down's syndrome using maternal serum PAPP-A and free β-HCG in combination with fetal nuchal translucency thickness. BJOG 1998;105:917–920.
92. Seppala M, Ruoslahti E: Radioimmunoassay of maternal alpha fetoprotein during pregnancy and delivery. Am J Obstet Gynecol 1972;112:208–212.
93. Haddow JE, Palomaki GE: Maternal protein enzyme analyses. In Reece EA, Hobbins JC, Mahoney MJ, Petrie RH (eds): Medicine of the Fetus and Mother. Philadelphia, JB Lippincott, 1992, pp 653–667.
94. Batzer FR, Schlaff S, Goldfarb AF, Corson SL: Serial β-subunit human chorionic gonadotrophin doubling time as a prognosticator of pregnancy outcome in an infertile population. Fertil Steril 1981;35:307–311.

95. Brody S, Carlstrom G: Human chorionic gonadotrophin pattern in serum and its relation to the sex of the fetus. J Clin Endocrinol 1965;25:792–797.
96. Josimovich JB, Kosor B, Boccella L, et al: Placental lactogen in maternal serum as an index of fetal health. Obstet Gynecol 1970;36:244–250.
97. Beck P, Parker ML, Daughaday WH: Radioimmunologic measurement of human placental lactogen in plasma by a double antibody method during normal and diabetic pregnancies. J Clin Endocrinol 1965;25:1457–1462.
98. Mathur RS, Leaming AB, Williamson HO: A simplified method for estimation of estriol in pregnancy plasma. Am J Obstet Gynecol 1972;113:1120–1129.
99. Mills MS: Ultrasonography of early embryonic growth and fetal development. MD Thesis, University of Bristol, 1992.
100. Robinson HP, Fleming JEE: A critical evaluation of sonar 'crown-rump length' measurements. BJOG 1975;82:702–710.
101. Pedersen JF: Fetal crown-rump length measurement by ultrasound in normal pregnancy. BJOG 1982;89:926–930.
102. Parker AJ, Davies P, Newton JR: Assessment of gestational age of the Asian fetus by the sonar measurement of crown-rump length and biparietal diameter. BJOG 1982;89:836–838.
103. Nicolaides KH, Azar G, Byrne D, et al: Fetal nuchal translucency: Ultrasound screening for chromosomal defects in first trimester of pregnancy. Br Med J 1992;304:867–869.
104. Pandya PP, Snijders RM, Johnson SP, et al: Screening for fetal trisomies by maternal age and fetal nuchal translucency thickness at 10–14 weeks of gestation. BJOG 1995;102:957–962.
105. Nicolaides KH, Brizot ML, Snijders RJM: Fetal nuchal translucency: Ultrasound screening for fetal trisomy in the first trimester of pregnancy. BJOG 1994;101:782–786.
106. Altman DG, Chitty LS: Charts of fetal size: 1. Methodology. BJOG 1994;101:29–34.
107. Chitty LS, Altman DG, Henderson A, Campbell S: Charts of fetal size: 2. Head measurements. BJOG 1994;101:35–43.
108. Kurmanavicius J, Wright EM, Royston P, et al: Fetal ultrasound biometry: 1. Head reference values. BJOG 1999;106: 126–135.
109. Snijders RJM, Nicolaides KH: Fetal biometry at 14–40 weeks' gestation. Ultrasound Obstet Gynecol 1994;4:34–48.
110. Erikson PS, Secher NJ, Weis-Bentzon M: Normal growth of the fetal biparietal diameter and the abdominal diameter in a longitudinal study. Acta Obstet Gynecol Scand 1985;64:65–70.
111. Hadlock FP, Deter RL, Harrist RB, Park SK: Fetal head circumference: Relation to menstrual age. Am J Roentgenol 1982; 138:647–653.
112. Chitty LS, Altman DG, Henderson A, Campbell S: Charts of fetal size: 3. Abdominal measurements. BJOG 1994;101: 125–131.
113. Kurmanavicius J, Wright EM, Royston P, et al: Fetal ultrasound biometry: 2. Abdomen and femur length reference values. BJOG 1999;106:136–143.
114. Hadlock FP, Deter RL, Harrist RB, Park SK: Fetal abdominal circumference as a predictor of menstrual age. Am J Roentgenol 1982;139:367–370.
115. Deter RL, Harrist RB, Hadlock FP, Poindexter AN: Longitudinal studies of fetal growth with the use of dynamic image ultrasonography. Am J Obstet Gynecol 1982;143: 545–554.
116. Tamura RK, Sabbagha RE: Percentile ranks for sonar fetal abdominal circumference measurements. Am J Obstet Gynecol 1980;138:475–479.
117. Chitty LS, Altman DG, Henderson A, Campbell S: Charts of fetal size: 4. Femur length. BJOG 1994;101:132–135.
118. Warda AH, Deter RL, Rossavik IK, et al: Fetal femur length: A critical reevaluation of the relationship to menstrual age. Obstet Gynecol 1985;66:69–75.
119. Chitty LS, Altman DG: Charts of fetal size. In Dewbury K, Meire H, Cosgrove D (eds): Ultrasound in Obstetrics and Gynaecology. Edinburgh, Churchill Livingstone, 1993, pp 513–595.
120. Merz E, Kim-Kern M-S, Pehl S: Ultrasonic mensuration of fetal limb bones in the second and third trimesters. J Clin Ultrasound 1987;15:175–183.
121. Jeanty P: Fetal biometry. In Fleischer AC, Romero R, Manning FA, et al (eds): The Principles and Practice of Ultrasonography in Obstetrics and Gynecology, 4th ed. Norwalk, Conn, Appleton & Lange, 1991, pp 93–108.
122. Romero R, Athanassiadis AP, Sirtori M, Inati M: Fetal skeletal anomalies. In Fleischer AC, Romero R, Manning FA, et al (eds): The Principles and Practice of Ultrasonography in Obstetrics and Gynecology, 4th ed. Norwalk, Conn, Appleton & Lange, 1991, pp 277–306.
123. Grannum P, Bracken M, Silverman R, Hobbins JC: Assessment of fetal kidney size in normal gestation by comparison of ratio of kidney circumference to abdominal circumference. Am J Obstet Gynecol 1980;136:249–254.
124. Mayden KL, Tortora M, Berkowitz RL, et al: Orbital diameters: A new parameter for prenatal diagnosis and dating. Am J Obstet Gynecol 1982;144:289–297.
125. Goldstein I, Reece EA, Pilu G, et al: Cerebellar measurements with ultrasonography in the evaluation of fetal growth and development. Am J Obstet Gynecol 1987;156:1065–1069.
126. Roberts AB, Mitchell JM, Pattison NS: Fetal liver length in normal and isoimmunized pregnancies. Am J Obstet Gynecol 1989;161:42–46.
127. Shimizu T, Salvador L, Allanson J, et al: Ultrasonographic measurements of fetal ear. Obstet Gynecol 1992;80:381–384.
128. Birnholz JC, Farrell E: Fetal ear length. Pediatrics 1988;81:555–558.
129. Ong S, Lim M-N, Fitzmaurice A, et al: The creation of twin centile curves for size. BJOG 2002;109:753–758.
130. Reece EA, Yarkoni S, Abdalla M, et al: A prospective longitudinal study of growth in twin gestations compared with growth in singleton pregnancies: I. The fetal head. J Ultrasound Med 1991;10:439–443.
131. Reece EA, Yarkoni S, Abdalla M, et al: A prospective longitudinal study of growth in twin gestations compared with growth in singleton pregnancies: II. The fetal limbs. J Ultrasound Med 1991;10:445–450.
132. Shushan A, Mordel N, Zajicek G, et al: A comparison of sonographic growth curves of triplet and twin fetuses. Am J Perinatol 1993;10:388–391.
133. Wilcox M, Gardosi J, Mongelli M, et al: Birth weight from pregnancies dated by ultrasonography in a multicultural British population. Br Med J 1993;307:588–591.
134. Yudkin PL, Aboualfa M, Eyre JA, et al: New birthweight and head circumference centiles for gestational ages 24 to 42 weeks. Early Hum Dev 1987;15:45–52.
135. Thompson AM, Billewicz WZ, Hytten FE: The assessment of fetal growth. J Obstet Gynaecol Br Commonw 1968;75:903–916.
136. Wilcox MA, Johnson IR, Maynard PV, et al: The individualised birthweight ratio: A more logical outcome measure of pregnancy than birthweight alone. BJOG 1993;100:342–347.
137. Williams RL, Creasy RK, Cunningham GC, et al: Fetal growth and perinatal viability in California. Obstet Gynecol 1982;59: 624–632.
138. Campbell S, Wilkin D: Ultrasonic measurement of fetal abdomen circumference in the estimation of fetal weight. BJOG 1975;82:689–697.
139. Shepard MJ, Richards VA, Berkowitz RL, et al: An evaluation of two equations for predicting fetal weight by ultrasound. Am J Obstet Gynecol 1982;142:47–54.
140. Hadlock FP, Harrist RB, Carpenter RJ, et al: Sonographic estimation of fetal weight. Radiology 1984;150:535–540.
141. Brace RA, Wolf EJ: Normal amniotic fluid volume changes throughout pregnancy. Am J Obstet Gynecol 1989;161:382–388.
142. Moore TR, Cayle JE: The amniotic fluid index in normal human pregnancy. Am J Obstet Gynecol 1990;162:1168–1173.

143. Fisk NM, Ronderos-Dumit D, Tannirandorn Y, et al: Normal amniotic pressure throughout gestation. BJOG 1992;99:18–22.
144. Gilbert WM, Moore TR, Brace RA: Amniotic fluid volume dynamics. Fetal Med Rev 1991;3:89–104.
145. Lind T, Parkin FM, Cheyne GA: Biochemical and cytological changes in liquor amnii with advancing gestation. J Obstet Gynaecol Br Commonw 1969;76:673–683.
146. Saddiqi TA, Meyer RA, Korfhagen J, et al: A longitudinal study describing confidence limits of normal fetal cardiac, thoracic and pulmonary dimensions from 20 to 40 weeks gestation. J Ultrasound Med 1993;12:731–736.
147. Steed RD, Strickland DM, Swanson MS, et al: Normal fetal cardiac dimensions obtained by perpendicular imaging. Am J Cardiol 1998;81:1059–1061.
148. Tan J, Silverman NH, Hoffman JIE, et al: Cardiac dimensions determined by cross-sectional echocardiography in the normal human fetus from 18 weeks to term. Am J Cardiol 1992;70: 1459–1467.
149. Rizzo G, Capponi A, Arduini D, Romanini C: Ductus venosus velocity waveforms in appropriate and small for gestational age fetuses. Early Hum Dev 1994;39:15–26.
150. Hecher K, Campbell S, Snijders R, Nicolaides K: Reference ranges for fetal venous and atrioventricular blood flow parameters. Ultrasound Obstet Gynecol 1994;4:381–390.
151. Rizzo G, Arduini D, Romanini C: Inferior vena cava flow velocity waveforms in appropriate- and small-for-gestational-age fetuses. Am J Obstet Gynecol 1992;166:1271–1280.
152. Rizzo G, Capponi A, Talone PE, et al: Doppler indices from inferior vena cava and ductus venosus in predicting pH and oxygen tension in umbilical blood at cordocentesis in growth-retarded fetuses. Ultrasound Obstet Gynecol 1996;7:401–410.
153. Hecher K, Snijders R, Campbell S, Nicolaides K: Fetal venous, intracardiac, and arterial blood flow measurements in intrauterine growth retardation: Relationship with fetal blood gases. Am J Obstet Gynecol 1995;173:10–15.
154. Rizzo G, Arduini D: Fetal cardiac function in intrauterine growth retardation. Am J Obstet Gynecol 1991;165:876–882.
155. Van Splunder P, Stijnen T, Wladimiroff JW: Fetal atrioventricular, venous and arterial flow velocity waveforms in the small for gestational age fetus. Pediatr Res 1997;42:765–775.
156. Mari G, Deter RL, Uerpairojkit B: Flow velocity waveforms of the ductus arteriosus in appropriate and small-for-gestational age fetuses. J Clin Ultrasound 1996;24:185–196.
157. Rizzo G, Capponi A, Chaoui R, et al: Blood flow velocity waveforms from peripheral pulmonary arteries in normally grown and growth-retarded fetuses. Ultrasound Obstet Gynecol 1996;8:87–92.
158. Arduini D, Rizzo G: Normal values of pulsatility index from fetal vessels: A cross-sectional study on 1556 healthy fetuses. J Perinat Med 1990;18:165–172.
159. Kurmanavicius J, Streicher A, Wright EM, et al: Reference values of fetal peak systolic blood velocity in the middle cerebral artery at 19–40 weeks of gestation. Ultrasound Obstet Gynecol 2001;17:50–53.
160. Mari G, Deter RL: Middle cerebral artery flow velocity waveforms in normal and small-for-gestational-age fetuses. Am J Obstet Gynecol 1992;166:1262–1270.
161. Veille J-C, Hanson R, Tatum K: Longitudinal quantitation of middle cerebral artery blood flow in normal human fetuses. Am J Obstet Gynecol 1993;169:1393–1398.
162. Kurmanavicius J, Florio I, Wisser J, et al: Reference resistance indices of the umbilical, fetal middle cerebral and uterine arteries at 24–42 weeks of gestation. Ultrasound Obstet Gynecol 1997;10:112–120.
163. Vyas S, Nicolaides KH, Bower S, Campbell S: Middle cerebral artery flow velocity waveforms in fetal hypoxaemia. BJOG 1990;97:797–803.
164. Sherer DM: Prenatal ultrasonographic assessment of the middle cerebral artery: A review. Obstet Gynecol Surv 1997;52:444–455.
165. Mari G, Adrignolo A, Abuhamad AZ, et al: Diagnosis of fetal anemia with Doppler ultrasound in the pregnancy complicated by maternal blood group immunisation. Ultrasound Obstet Gynecol 1995;5:400–405.
166. Mari G: Noninvasive diagnosis by Doppler ultrasonography of fetal anemia due to maternal red-cell alloimmunization. N Engl J Med 2000;342:9–14.
167. Erskine RLA, Ritchie JWK: Umbilical artery blood flow characteristics in normal and growth-retarded fetuses. BJOG 1985;92:605–610.
168. Bahado-Singh RO, Kovanci E, Jeffres A, et al: The Doppler cerebroplacental ratio and perinatal outcome in intrauterine growth restriction. Am J Obstet Gynecol 1999;180:750–756.
169. Weiner CP, Sipes SL, Wenstrom K: The effect of fetal age upon normal fetal laboratory values and venous pressure. Obstet Gynecol 1992;79:713–718.
170. Weiner CP, Heilskov J, Pelzer G, et al: Normal values for human umbilical venous and amniotic fluid pressures and their alteration by fetal disease. Am J Obstet Gynecol 1989;161:714–717.
171. Weiner CP: Intrauterine pressure: Amniotic and fetal circulation. In Ludomirski A, Nicolini U, Bhutani UK (eds): Therapeutic and Diagnostic Interventions in Early Life. New York, Futura, 1995.
172. Sadovsky G, Nicolaides KH: Reference ranges for fetal heart rate patterns in normoxaemic nonanaemic fetuses. Fetal Ther 1989;4:61–68.
173. Arulkumaran S, Ingemarsson I, Montan S, et al: Guidelines for Interpretation of Antepartum and Intrapartum Cardiotocography. Bracknell, Berks, U.K. Hewlett Packard, 1992.
174. NIH Workshop: Electronic fetal heart rate monitoring. Research guidelines for interpretation. Am J Obstet Gynecol 1997;177:1385–1390.
175. Manning FA, Platt LD, Sipos L: Antepartum fetal evaluation: Development of a fetal biophysical profile. Am J Obstet Gynecol 1980;136:787–795.
176. Manning FA, Baskett TF, Morrison I, Lange I: Fetal biophysical profile scoring: A prospective study in 1184 high-risk patients. Am J Obstet Gynecol 1981;140:289–294.
177. Takagi K, Tanaka H, Nishijima S, et al: Fetal blood values by percutaneous umbilical blood sampling. Fetal Ther 1989;4:152–160.
178. Forestier F: Some aspects of fetal biology. Fetal Ther 1987;2:181–187.
179. Weiner CP: Human fetal bilirubin levels and fetal hemolytic disease. Am J Obstet Gynecol 1992;166:1449–1454.
180. Ecomomides DL, Nicolaides KH, Campbell S: Metabolic and endocrine findings in appropriate and small for gestational age fetuses. J Perinat Med 1991;19:97–105.
181. Nicolini U, Fisk NM, Rodeck CH, Beacham J: Fetal urine biochemistry: An index of renal maturation and dysfunction. BJOG 1992;99:46–50.
182. Nicolaides KH, Cheng HH, Snijders RJM, Moniz CF: Fetal urine biochemistry in the assessment of obstructive uropathy. Am J Obstet Gynecol 1992;166:932–937.
183. Evans MI, Sacks AJ, Johnson MP, et al: Sequential invasive assessment of fetal renal function and the intrauterine treatment of fetal obstructive uropathies. Obstet Gynecol 1991;77: 545–550.
184. Wilkins IA, Chitkara U, Lynch L, et al: The nonpredictive value of fetal urinary electrolytes: Preliminary report of outcomes and correlations with pathological diagnosis. Am J Obstet Gynecol 1987;157:694–698.
185. Huch A, Huch R, Rooth G: Guidelines for blood sampling and measurement of pH and blood gas values in obstetrics. Eur J Obstet Gynaecol Reprod Biol 1994;54:165–175.
186. Nicolaides KH, Economides DL, Soothill PW: Blood gases, pH, and lactate in appropriate- and small-for-gestational-age fetuses. Am J Obstet Gynecol 1989;161:996–1001.
187. Soothill PW, Nicolaides KH, Rodeck CH, Campbell S: Effect of gestational age on fetal and intervillous blood gas and acid-base values in human pregnancy. Fetal Ther 1986;1:168–175.

188. Nicolaides KH, Thilaganathan B, Mibashan RS: Cordocentesis in the investigation of fetal erythropoiesis. Am J Obstet Gynecol 1989;161:1197–1200.
189. Weiner CP, Williamson RA, Wenstrom KD, et al: Management of fetal hemolytic disease by cordocentesis: I. Prediction of fetal anemia. Am J Obstet Gynecol 1991;165:546–553.
190. Davies NP, Buggins AGS, Snijders RJM, et al: Blood leucocyte count in the human fetus. Arch Dis Child 1992;67:399–403.
191. Abbas A, Thilaganathan B, Buggins AGS, et al: Fetal plasma interferon gamma concentration in normal pregnancy. Am J Obstet Gynecol 1993;168:1414–1416.
192. Weiner CP: Unpublished data, 1995.
193. Nicolaides KH, Rodeck CH, Mibashan RS, Kemp JR: Have Liley charts outlived their usefulness? Am J Obstet Gynecol 1986;155:90–94.
194. Thorpe-Beeston JG, Nicolaides KH, Felton CV, et al: Maturation of the secretion of thyroid hormone and thyroid stimulating hormone in the fetus. N Engl J Med 1991;324:532–536.
195. Duignan NM, Studd JWW, Hughes AO: Characteristics of normal labour in different racial groups. BJOG 1975;82:593–601.
196. The use of electronic fetal monitoring. Royal College of Obstetricians and Gynaecologists Guideline. London, RCOG Press, 2001.
197. Eskes TKAB, Jongsma HW, Houx PCW: Percentiles for gas values in human umbilical cord blood. Eur J Obstet Gynecol Reprod Biol 1983;14:341–346.
198. Westgren M, Divon M, Horal M, et al: Routine measurements of umbilical artery lactate levels in the prediction of perinatal outcome. Am J Obstet Gynecol 1995;173:1416–1422.
199. Mercelina-Roumans P, Breukers R, Ubachs J, Van Wersch J: Hematological variables in cord blood of neonates of smoking and nonsmoking mothers. J Clin Epidemiol 1996;49:449–454.
200. Paterakis GS, Lykopoulou L, Papassotiriou J, et al: Flow-cytometric analysis of reticulocytes in normal cord blood. Acta Haematol 1993;90:182–185.
201. Walka MM, Sonntag J, Kage A, et al: Complete blood counts from umbilical cords of healthy term newborns by two automated cytometers. Acta Haematol 1998;100:167–173.
202. Perkins SL, Livesey JF, Belcher J: Reference intervals for 21 clinical chemistry analytes in arterial and venous cord blood. Clin Chem 1993;39:1041–1044.

INDEX

Note: Page numbers followed by f indicate figures; those followed by t indicate tables; those followed by b indicate boxed material.

B

C

D

E

F

G

H

I

J

K

L

M

Q

R

S